英汉医学辞典

第3版·新媒体版

AN ENGLISH-CHINESE MEDICAL DICTIONARY

3rd Edition

主　编　陈维益

副主编　李定钧

编　者　孙庆祥　陈雪雷　蔡和兵　凌秋虹

林谋济　陈社胜　赵世澄　殷建国

唐　伟　杨　霞　肖　英　吴德雯

上海科学技术出版社

图书在版编目(CIP)数据

英汉医学辞典/陈维益主编.—3版.—上海:上海科学技术出版社,2009.4(2018.11重印)
ISBN 978－7－5323－9488－3/R·2560

Ⅰ.英...　Ⅱ.陈...　Ⅲ.医学－词典－英、汉
Ⅳ.R－61

中国版本图书馆CIP数据核字(2008)第094996号

英汉医学辞典(第3版·新媒体版)

主编　陈维益　**副主编**　李定钧

上海世纪出版股份有限公司
上海科学技术出版社 出版
(上海钦州南路71号　邮政编码200235)

上海世纪出版股份有限公司发行中心发行
200001　上海福建中路193号　www.ewen.co
苏州望电印刷有限公司印刷
开本　850×1168　1/32　印张39　插页4
字数:3000千字
1984年5月第1版　1997年5月第2版
2009年4月第3版　2018年11月第24次印刷
ISBN 978－7－5323－9488－3/R·2560
定价:88.00元

本书如有缺页、错装或坏损等严重质量问题,
请向工厂联系调换

目录 Contents

序

回顾·思考·期望

我曾供职的母校三易其名，1952年我调入工作时，校名已由上海医学院改为上海第一医学院，后改称上海医科大学，现为复旦大学上海医学院；我曾执教的外文教研室还在，但已并入复旦外文学院大学英语部。当初和我一起编写《英汉医学辞典》的老师们都已相继退休。这些年承蒙在职的中青年教师积极参与，更兼上海科学技术出版社的大力支持，《英汉医学辞典》第3版修订工作终于顺利完成。

《英汉医学辞典》自1984年问世以来，已两次修订，发行数量超过45万册，深受读者欢迎，对我国的医学教育和医学发展做出了一定的贡献。

此时此刻回首往日的点点滴滴，我颇感人生有期，学海无涯。记得1976年我从江西开门办学回沪，随即参加《英汉医学辞典》的编写工作。当时医学院的教务长金问涛教授专门召集一次有各科医学专家参加的编审会，出席的专家有妇产科的王淑贞教授、眼科的郭秉宽教授、外科的陈化东教授和内科的朱无难教授等。在初版前言中，我们仅笼统地表示对专家教授的感谢，而未提及他们的名字；其实他们对辞典原稿的审阅尤为严谨、细致。譬如说王淑贞教授对一些胎位的译名提出不同的看法，如LMA（left mentoanterior），最早按英文的顺序译为“左颏前”，但王教授改译为“颏左前”，后来被《英汉医学词汇》（第二版，人民卫生出版社，2000年）所认同，说明这一学术观点并不是王教授的一家之说。如今这些专家教授有些已离开了人世，但他们所付出的辛勤劳动及认真负责的态度却让我终身难忘。

我一生中最难忘的是医学院的两位教授。一位是原外文教研室主任、哈佛大学博士杨昌毅教授。他一方面举荐我主持《英汉医学辞典》的编写工作，另一方面大力支持我参加卫生部主持的《汉英医学大词典》核查工作，让我有机会广泛接触国内的医学专家，对辞典的编写与修订工作起到了积极的作用。数年前我惊悉杨教授在纽约寓所不幸去世，尤为哀伤。

另一位是已故医学院副院长朱益栋教授。当年为编写医学辞典，我常向他请教新词的译名；他总是能很快解决我的难题，足见他的博学多才。20 世纪 80 年代初卫生部曾委托医学专家编写《汉英医学大词典》，由于稿源来自各方，译名不统一，编委会决定成立核查小组，朱教授推荐我去北京参加核查工作，后来曾一起乘船前往大连参加核查汇报会。在核查、汇报与交流期间，我获益匪浅，由此结识了不少医学专家，有的后来成为挚友，如原武汉同济医科大学张强华教授，就是我在核查小组工作时认识的。1994 年我赴美探亲期间，读到纽约《世界日报》关于细胞适时死亡(apoptosis)的报道，回国后致函张教授，请教如何翻译较为妥当，他说应译成"细胞凋亡"，后来证实他的译名是准确的。

回顾辞典编写初期的艰辛，我无法不提到已故人民卫生出版社资深编辑赵师震医师。我们曾造访他在上海南昌路的寓所，分几次从他那里借阅《英汉医学词汇》清样稿；记得有一次还稿闲谈中，我向赵老问起这些译名是从哪里来的，他笑答："都是从你们学校教科书中来的。"他对香港当时出版一本英汉医学详解辞典颇为感慨，因为当时内地还是空白。可告慰赵老的，现在国内已出版多种此类辞典。而他推崇医学详解辞典的一番话，启迪我在个别词条列出译名外，再加上必要的释义，现在看来是颇受读者欢迎的。

第 3 版辞典的修订主要涉及两大内容，一是增补新词，二是译名进一步规范。

我是根据《*Dorland's Illustrated Medical Dictionary*》(2003 年第 30 版，以下简称 Dorland 本)增补新词及少量词组，共增补 4 000 余条。许多新增单词的规范译名大多可以找到出处。例如，"Cubomedusae(立方水母目)"见于《拉汉无脊椎动物名称》(科学出版社，1978 年)；"abciximab(阿昔单抗)"见于《中国药品通用名称》(卫生部药典委员会编，化学工业出版社，1997 年)。对于新增补的单词，如找不到译名，我不敢擅自妄译，更不敢以音译来搪塞。近年来，音译之风愈演愈烈，如有的辞典竟将"attapolgite(绿坡缕石)"，音译为"阿塔朴尔盖特"，其实此译名早已见之于《英汉药学词汇》(人民卫生出版社，1984 年)。又如 Medicago(苜蓿属)、Malpighia(金虎尾属)、Phillyrea(连翘属)、Phleum(梯牧草属)被音译成"麦迪开格属"、"马尔皮吉属"、"非丽属"、"弗利草属"，真的让人感到不知为何物。

新的药名可以音译，但必须采用卫生部药典委员会编译的《中国药品通用名称》(1997)一书中的规范译名，如"abciximab(阿昔单抗)"、"penciclovir(喷昔洛韦)"。如果有的新药名在该书中未能刊载，可根据世界卫生组织(WHO)编订的"国际通用(非专利)药名(International Nonproprietary

Names for Pharmaceutical Substances, INN)”采用的词干及其中文译名表翻译。例如,免疫系统药“-mab”需译为“单抗”,抗病毒药“-vir”需译成“韦”,均有明确的规定,切不可随意音译。收词丰富的《中国药品通用名称》也许跟不上新药的发展,但作为词典编写者,应根据药典委员会公布的有关药名命名原则试译,即根据英文名称、药品性质和结构等,采用音译、意译或音意合译,以保持药品汉语译名的规范性、统一性和系统性。其次,任何药名音译后必须注明其用途,如果只音译不加必要的释义,就会令读者感到疑惑。如果嫌原文的释义太长,不妨采用《中国药品通用名称》中诸如“抗病毒药”之类的说明。

医药译名的规范化正日益引起医学界的重视,为了避免出现医药名词的混乱局面,全国科学技术名词审定委员会就医药名词在专业性、科学性和准确性三个方面进行严格的审定。我们作为医学辞典的编写者应当积极推进医药译名的规范化,全面采用全国科学技术名词审定委员会公布的名词(以下简称审定本),弥补第2版出版时因审定本未出全,未能全面修订规范译名的遗憾。我们的修订原则是审定本具有一定的权威性与指令性,作为辞典编写者应该最大限度地执行。但是,我们也会重新甄别与校正一些译名。最明显的例子是审定本《人体解剖学》中的“mitral valve”汉译为“左房室瓣”,不用“二尖瓣”,而后出版的审定本在其他学科涉及该病名时,却采用“二尖瓣”,如“mitral stenosis(二尖瓣狭窄)”。这就使我想起上世纪50年代卫生部审定的《医学名词汇编》,用“红细胞”、“白细胞”取代“红血球”、“白血球”一事,半个世纪过去了,但习惯上还是有人采用旧称。这次审定本推荐“心肌梗死”取代“心肌梗塞”,有些人依旧故我,尤其是患者宁愿说“心肌梗塞”,而不愿说“心肌梗死”。又譬如“rheumatoid arthritis(类风湿关节炎)”,不译“类风湿性关节炎”,“amyloidosis(淀粉样变性)”,不译“淀粉样变”,“adrenergic(拟肾上腺素药)”,不译“肾上腺素能药”,“mood disorder(情感障碍)”,不推荐“心境障碍”,都是比较突出的例子。因此,在推进译名规范化的同时,出现几个值得我思考的问题。

1. 译名的统一 尽可能做到统一,这是编者的责任。审定本公布的名词为数甚少,对某一词的同义词和派生词就需要做到译名统一。例如审定本《医学名词1》只审定“acanthocytosis(刺状红细胞增多)”一个词,其同义词“acanthrocytosis”也要做到译名统一,而其源词“acanthocyte”与同义词“acanthrocyte”就应改译为“刺状红细胞”。

2. 译名的甄别 审定本推荐的个别词存有疑问,需要加以鉴别与区分。如"enthesis"一词，审定本《医学名词1》推荐的译名为"肌腱末端病"，Dorland本列有三个词"enthesis, enthesitis, enthesopathy"，按原文释义enthesopathy(disorder of the muscular or tendinous attachment to bone)才是"肌腱末端病"。

3. 译名的准确性 关于译名的准确与否，我的依据只能是Dorland本。审定本《医学名词1》推荐的"Sjögren syndrome"译名为"干燥综合征"，但据Dorland本，此综合征的特点为角膜结膜炎、口腔干燥和结缔组织病三联症，而干燥综合征(sicca syndrome)则不伴有结缔组织病，故此译为"舍格伦综合征"加注方为准确。又如"Hailey-Hailey disease"，据Dorland本释义(benign familial pemphigus)译为"良性家族性天疱疮"，我未采用审定本《医学名词7》的译名"家族性良性天疱疮"，因审定本释义(familial benign pemphigus)不符合Dorland本书写规范。

4. 译名的选择 推荐的两个译名不统一时，把两个译名都列上。例如"mental retardation"，审定本《医学名词4》译为"精神发育迟缓"，而《医学名词3》推荐译名为"智力低下"，不推荐"精神发育迟缓"。其次，推荐的两个译名相互矛盾时，作为编者必须作出选择。如《医学名词1》对"Behşet syndrome"推荐译名为"贝赫切特综合征"，不推荐译"白塞综合征"，而《医学名词5》的说法正好与此相反，如果人名的译名同时并列，岂非误以为两个人。据Dorland本，"Behşet"为土耳其皮肤科医师，"白塞"听上去像是法语的发音，但又查不到他是否法裔，故只能根据Dorland本的音标译"贝赫切特"，不译"白塞"。

英文的规范，似乎不是一个问题，只要按照原文排印即可。殊不知，问题就出在各有各的原版，书写不一，也就谈不上规范了。目前介绍到国内的重要医学辞书有Dorland, Stedman, Butterworth三种，据我所知，有的专家偏爱Stedman，因为它释义简洁，而Dorland收词多，Butterworth则是英式拼写，各有千秋。不过国内的词典译编大多以Dorland本为准。审定本中除少数明显拼写错误外，也有书写不规范的问题。例如，审定本《医学名词1》中的"tubo-eruptive xanthoma(结节丘疹性黄瘤)"，根据审定本推荐的译名，英文应该是"tuberoeruptive xanthoma"，除拼写错误以外，第一个字中间的连字符号，不符合Dorland本的书写。又如审定本对冠名名词一律不加所有格符号's，可能出于某种理由，但也不符合Dorland本的规范。

我原先参考的2000年第29版Dorland本也有问题，特别是新增补的词和词组。例如，在"angioplasty"词项下的词组书写成"transluminal coronary angioplasty",根据 Dorland 本的释义为 PTCA,结果造成漏词,全文应该是"percutaneous transluminal coronary angioplasty",根据审定本《医学名词 4》的译名"经皮腔内冠状动脉成形术",同时考虑 PTCA 手术目前在国内已广泛应用,故我在本辞典中除修正其错误外,还在本书 P 部增补这一条缩写词。2003 年第 30 版 Dorland 本证实了我的判断。

值得一提的是第 30 版 Dorland 本开始引介中医中药,百年来是第一次,实属罕见,如 di huang(地黄),dong guai(当归),feng shui(风水),huang-qi(黄芪)、jing(精),ma huang(麻黄),qi 或 chi(气),qi gong(气功)、sheng(神)、tai chi(太极),tui na(推拿),yang(阳),yin(阴),令人瞩目。本辞典对这些词条仅列其名,不注音标,也不加释义。

辞典的每一次修订,我都期望读者从中获得正确的译名和信息。例如,"abciximab(阿昔单抗)"除了说明此药用作抗血栓药外,还传递此药在 PTCA 手术时使用的信息。有些词如"addressin(地址素)",若不加必要的释义,读者未必明了。至于医学冠名术语,更应加以说明,如"Down syndrome"仅译为"唐氏综合征",我就感到很不踏实,总希望能让读者获得更多的信息,不厌其烦加以释义。本辞书的修订秉承"精益求精"的编写理念,诚惶诚恐,一路求证。例如,"Brueghel's syndrome"是以 16 世纪画家命名的综合征,此人为佛兰德斯画家(Flemish painter),其人名译为(老)勃鲁盖尔,这是约定俗成的(见《英汉大词典》及《辞海》)。至于命名的缘由为老年妇女脸上出现的症状,有些词典的释义显然不准确,因为画家是无法画出卵巢纤维瘤或其他盆腔肿瘤的。

《英汉医学辞典》第 3 版现以崭新的面貌呈现在读者面前,我期望读者能购得一本称心如意的辞典。考虑到在上世纪 70 年代读者很难购得一部普通英汉辞典(尤指《新英汉辞典》),经出版社认可,我们在编写时适当增加一些普通词和词组,以适应当时读者的需要。如今情况不同了,书坊间可见到各类英汉辞典及电子辞典。为使本辞典更加专业化,有必要删去大部分普通词或词组以及词条中非医学专业的译名,仅保留与医学相关的普通词或词组,例如"show"词项下的 bloody show(见红),access 项下的 arteriovenous access(动静脉入口),这样可节省篇幅,增补新词。当然删除的内容还包括药名中的异名和别名,仅用《中国药品通用名称》中的译名;至于各种药品的商品名也在删除之列,其中理由之一是因为早在 20 世纪 90 年代初就有人主张用非专有名(generic names)(美国采用药名),不用商品名(trade name)(*Dorland's Medical Abbreviation*, 1992 及 Neil M. Davis:

Medical Abbreviation, 1993)。

其次,我期望读者尽可能查阅到所需要的医学新词。Dorland 本每次新版增补大量新词和词组,且绝大部分是词组,同时新版中必删去大致相等篇幅的旧词和词组。本辞典对 Dorland 各版(第 25 ~ 30 版)中出现的词条基本全部收录,至于 Dorland 本词条下的大量词组,仅收录一小部分,从这个意义上说,本辞典是一部中型辞典,但基本上可以满足读者的需要。同时,本辞典也增补一些近年来出现的新词,如 SARS。正如上世纪 70 年代末和 80 年代初 AIDS(艾滋病)暴发时,1981 年第 26 版 Dorland 本来不及收录一样,2003 年第 30 版 Dorland 本也未能收录 SARS,但 2004 年第 27 版《*Dorland's Pocket Medical Dictionary*》填补这一空白,读者可在本辞典"syndrome"词项下 severe acute respiratory syndrome(SARS)见到简短的释义。

此外,为了便于读者检索,我们在附录中收录部分拉英汉对照的动脉名、肌名、神经名、骨名和静脉名,标以[TA](解剖学术语)取代[NA](解剖学名词),这样更有利于医学生在攻读解剖学时背诵记忆。在体例排列上,本辞典不拘泥于 Dorland 模式,如人名中的 Mc 和 Mac 读音相同,Mc 按 Mac 排序(Dorland),也可分开各自排序(Webster 大词典)。我们采用后一种排序,以利读者检索。顺便说一下,人名后的 's 及其后的名词可以不计排序(Dorland),也可以参与排序(Webster 大词典),我们采用后一种。

平心而论,我不希望一本辞典有任何差错,哪怕是十万分之一的差错,尤其是译名上的差错,毕竟医药名词术语是医学研究及其学术理论构建的基础,有待于我们不断地对那些经翻译而来的医药名词术语进行勘查、甄别与校正,确保医学研究及相关学术理论建设的精密性与准确性。30 年来,我始终把辞典的编写与修订看作是一项繁琐、艰辛和细致的综合研究工作,需要不断查找资料进行对比研究;我同时也衷心地希望与我一起工作的同事们继续保持这种敬业精神。令我欣慰的是许多中青年教师结合辞书编写开展医学语词的学术研究,矢志不移,日趋成熟,尤其是我十余年前带教过的医学英语研究生李定钧协助我完成本辞典的编写工作,庆幸后继有人,传承有望。是为序。

陈维益

2008 年 3 月于上海寓所

体例说明

(一) 词　　条

一个单词立为一个词条,附有国际音标、词性及释义。有的词条还收有医学词组(以名词为主)、派生词和同义词。

有些词组如药名、化学名、冠名名词(如 Addison's disease)等立为词条,按首词字母编排。

缩写词、字母、符号等立为词条,注明来源及释义。

构词成分、前缀、后缀立为词条,不注音标,但注明释义。

(二) 本　　词

一个词有不同拼法时,若相隔很近,排在同一词条内,用圆括号表明;若相隔较远,则分立词条。

每个单词的音标后注明词性,词性用英语缩写形式注出,如名词(*n*),代词(*pron*),形容词(*a*),数词(*num*),副词(*ad*),及物动词(*vt*),不及物动词(*vi*),助动词(*v aux*),前置词(*prep*),连接词(*conj*),冠词(*art*)。

名词的复数形式,或单数复数同形的,则在方括号内加以注明,如[复]、[单复同]。

列为词条的词组,一般全部注明读音,但部分药名词组(如 benzhydramine hydrochloride),化学名词组(如 salicylic acid),只对第一个词注音,冠名名词的音标,只对其原姓加以注音(如 Addison's disease,只对 Addison 注音)。

本词如源自希腊语、拉丁语、德语、法语、俄语、葡萄牙语、西班牙语、意大利语、日语、梵语、汉语等,则分别注以【希】、【拉】、【德】、【法】、【俄】、【葡】、【西】、【意】、【日】、【梵】、【汉】。

(三) 释　　义

不同释义时,用分号分开;如词义较近的,则用逗号分开。

可省略的字放在方括号内,说明部分放在圆括号内。

部分单词、词组,除释义外,有时也用参见形式。如:

anatoxireaction 类毒素反应(见 Moloney's test)

Oestreicher's reaction 伊斯特赖歇尔反应,黄嘌呤醇反应(xanthydrol reaction,见 reaction 项下相应术语)

(四) 词组与派生词

列在词条内的词组,其本词以代字号(~)表示之。各词组之间均以斜线号(/)分隔。在本词、医学词组、派生词之间以直线号(|)分隔。

以-ly, -ness 结尾的派生词,一般不作释义。

A

A accommodation 调节；adenine 腺嘌呤；adenosine 腺苷；alanine 丙氨酸；ampere 安培；anode 阳极，正极；anterior 前的；alveolar gas 肺泡气（用作下角标）

A. annum【拉】年

A absorbance 吸光度；activity 放射性；admittance 导纳；area 心影区；mass number［原子］质量数

AⅠ first auditory area 第一听区

AⅡ second auditory area 第二听区

A_2 aortic second sound 主动脉瓣第二音

Å angstrom 埃（长度单位 = 10^{-10} m）

a accommodation 调节；atto-阿［托］（10^{-18}）；arterial blood 动脉血（用作下角标）

a. annum【拉】年；aqua【拉】水，水剂；arteria【拉】动脉

a acceleration 加速度；activity（化学物质热力）效能；specific absorptivity 比吸光系数

a-［前缀］【希】不，无，缺（在元音或 h 前则用 an-）；【拉】离

$\bar{a}$ ante【拉】［在］前

α alpha 希腊语的第 1 个字母；本生（Bunsen）系数、IgA 重链，血红蛋白 α 链和第一类错误概率的符号

α- 前缀，表示①邻近主要功能基的碳原子，例如 α-氨基酸类；②旋光物的比旋，例如 α-D-葡萄糖；③环外原子或基团的定向，例如 3α-羟-5α-雄甾烷-17-酮（雄酮）；④蛋白电泳时随 α 带（可再分为 α_1 和 α_2 带）移动的一种血浆蛋白，例如甲胎蛋白；⑤一系列相关化合物中的一种，特指立体异构形、同分异构形、多聚形和同素异形型，例如 α-胡萝卜素；⑥一组相关实体中的一种，例如 α-射线

AA achievement age 智力成就年龄；Alcoholic Anonymous 嗜酒者互诫协会，戒酒者协会；amino acid 氨基酸

$\overline{AA}$，$\overline{aa}$ ana【希】各，各个（处方上用）

aa. arteriae【拉】动脉

AAA American Association of Anatomists 美国解剖学家协会

AAAS American Association for the Advancement of Science 美国科学发展协会

AABB American Association of Blood Banks 美国血库协会

AACP American Academy of Child Psychiatry 美国儿童精神病学会

AAD American Academy of Dermatology 美国皮肤病学会

AADP American Academy of Denture Prosthetics 美国义齿修复学会

AADR American Academy of Dental Radiology 美国牙科放射学会

AADS American Association of Dental Schools 美国牙科学校协会

AAE American Association of Endodontists 美国牙髓病学家协会

AAFP American Academy of Family Physicians 美国家庭医师学会

AAI American Association of Immunologists 美国免疫学家协会

AAID American Academy of Implant Dentistry 美国口腔种植学会

AAIN American Association of Industrial Nurses 美国工业护士协会

AAMA American Association of Medical Assistants 美国助理医师协会

AAMC American Association of Medical Colleges 美国医学院校协会

AAMD American Association of Mental Deficiency 美国心理缺陷协会

AAMT American Association for Medical Transcription 美国医学转录协会

AAN American Academy of Neurology 美国神经病学学会

AANP American Association of Naturopathic Physicians 美国自然医术医师协会

AAO American Academy of Ophthalmology 美国眼科学会；American Association of Orthodontists 美国口腔正畸学家协会；American Academy of Otolaryngology 美国耳鼻喉科学会

AAOP American Academy of Oral Pathology 美国口腔病理学会

AAOS American Academy of Orthopaedic Surgeons 美国矫形外科医师学会

AAP American Academy of Pediatrics 美国儿科学会；American Academy of Pedodontics 美国儿童口腔医学学会；American Academy of Periodontology 美国牙周病学会；American Association of Pathologists 美国病理学家协会

AAPA American Academy of Physician Assistants 美国内科助理医师学会

AAPB American Association of Pathologists and Bacteriologists 美国病理学家及细菌学家协会

AAPMR American Academy of Physical Medicine and Rehabilitation 美国物理医学与康复学会

AARC American Association for Respiratory Care 美国呼吸监护协会

Aaron's sign [ˈɛərən] (Charles D. Aaron) 艾伦征(阑尾炎时压麦克伯尼〈McBurney〉点,在腹上部或心前区有痛觉)

Aarskog-Scott syndrome [ˈɑːskɔg skɔt] (D. C. Aarskog; C. I. Scott, Jr.) 阿-斯综合征(见 Aarskog syndrome)

Aarskog syndrome [ˈɑːskɔg] (D. C. Aarskog) 阿斯柯格综合征(一种 X 连锁综合征,特征为两眼距离过远,鼻孔前倾,上唇宽,特有的阴囊"围巾"包在阴茎上方,手小。亦称面-指〈趾〉-生殖器综合征)

Aase syndrome [eiz] (J. M. Aase) 艾氏综合征(一种家族性综合征,特征为轻度发育迟缓,再生不良性贫血,程度不等的白细胞减少,三指骨拇指,肩狭窄,前囟闭合延迟,有时有唇裂、腭裂、视网膜病及蹼颈)

AATA American Art Therapy Association 美国艺术疗法协会

AAV adeno-associated virus 腺伴随病毒

AB Artium Baccalaureus【拉】文学士

Ab antibody 抗体

ab [æb] *prep*【拉】从

ab- [前缀]【拉】离,从

abacavir sulfate [əˈbækvir] 硫酸阿巴卡韦(一种非核苷反转录酶抑制剂,用作抗反转录病毒药,治疗人免疫缺陷病毒感染,口服给药)

abacteremic [ˌeibæktəˈriːmik] *a* 非菌血症的

abacterial [ˌeibækˈtiəriəl] *a* 非细菌性的;无菌的

Abadie's sign [ɑːbɑːˈdiː] (Charles Abadie) 阿巴迪征(上睑提肌痉挛,突眼性甲状腺肿的一种体征);(Jean Abadie)阿巴迪征(跟腱受压无感觉,见于脊髓痨时)

abaissement [əbeisˈmɔŋ] *n*【法】降下;针拨术,内障摘出术

abaptiston [əbæpˈtistən] ([复] **abaptista** [əbæpˈtistə]) *n* 安全开颅圆锯

abarognosis [ˌeibærəgˈnəusis] *n* 压觉缺失,辨重不能

abarthrosis [ˌæbɑːˈθrəusis] *n* 动关节

abarticular [ˌæbɑːˈtikjulə] *a* 不影响关节的;关节外的

abarticulation [ˌæbɑːˌtikjuˈleiʃən] *n* 关节脱位;滑膜关节,动关节

abasia [əˈbeiziə] *n* 步行不能 | ~ astasia 站立行走不能 / paroxysmal trepidant ~, spastic ~ 阵发性震颤性步行不能,痉挛性步行不能 / trembling ~ 震颤性步行不能 | **abasic** [əˈbeisik], **abatic** [əˈbætik] *a*

abate [əˈbeit] *vt, vi* 减少,减轻(痛或症状) | **~ment** *n*

abaxial [æbˈæksiəl] *a* 远轴的,离轴的,轴外的

abbau [ˈæbau] *n*【德】分解代谢产物

Abbe's condenser [əˈbe] (Ernst K. Abbe) 阿贝聚光镜(放在显微镜载物台下有两个透镜构成的聚光镜结合装置)

Abbe's flap [ˈæbi] (Robert Abbe)阿贝皮瓣(取自下唇正中部的三角形全层瓣,用以填补上唇的缺损) | ~ operation 阿贝手术(用肠线环做肠侧面吻合术;用线割法治食管狭窄)

Abbe-Zeiss counting cell, counting chamber [əˈbe ˈtsais] (E. K. Abbe; Carl Zeiss) 阿-蔡计数池(血细胞计数器)

Abbott-Miller tube [ˈæbət ˈmilə] (William O. Abbott; T. Grier Miller) 艾-米管(见 Miller-Abbott tube)

Abbott-Rawson tube [ˈæbət ˈrɔːsn] (William O. Abbott; Arthur J. Rawson)艾-罗管(一种注入及抽出两用的双筒管,用于洗胃或胃减压)

Abbott's method [ˈæbət] (Edville G. Abbott) 艾博特法(用石膏绷带及石膏短上衣矫治脊柱侧弯)

ABC aspiration biopsy cytology 针吸活检细胞学

ABCD doxorubicin, bleomycin, lomustine, and dacarbazine 多柔比星-博来霉素-洛莫司汀-达卡巴嗪(联合化疗治癌方案)

abciximab [æbˈsiksimæb] *n* 阿昔单抗(抑制血小板凝集的人鼠单克隆抗体 Fab 片段,经皮腔内冠状动脉成形术时用作抗血栓药,静脉输注给药)

Abderhalden's reaction (dialysis, test) [ˈɑːbdəˌhɑːldən] (Emil Abderhalden) 阿布德尔哈尔顿反应(透析法、试验)(根据一个废弃的假说而进行的血清反应,当异种蛋白进入血液时,机体产生一种能分解该蛋白的酶,称为保护性酶或防御酶,该酶对促使其形成的蛋白质有特异性)

abdomen [ˈæbdəmen, æbˈdəumen] *n* 腹 | acute ~, surgical ~ 急腹症 / scaphoid ~, boat-shaped ~, carinate ~, navicular ~ 舟状腹(见于患脑病的儿童) / pendulous ~ 悬垂腹 | **abdominal** [æbˈdɔminl] *a*

abdomino- [构词成分] 腹

abdominocentesis [æbˌdɔminəusenˈtiːsis] *n* 腹腔穿刺术

abdominocystic [æbˌdɔminəuˈsistik] *a* 腹胆囊的

abdominogenital [æbˌdɔminəuˈdʒenitl] *a* 腹生殖器的

abdominohysterectomy [æbˌdɔminəuˌhistəˈrektəmi] *n* 剖腹子宫切除术,腹式子宫切除术

abdominohysterotomy [æbˌdɔminəuˌhistəˈrɔtə-

mi], **abdominouterotomy** [æbˌdɔminəuˌjuː-təˈrɔtəmi] *n* 剖腹子宫切开术,腹式子宫切开术
abdominoscopy [æbˌdɔmiˈnɔskəpi] *n* 腹腔镜检查术
abdominoscrotal [æbˌdɔminəuˈskrəutl] *a* 腹阴囊的
abdominothoracic [æbˌdɔminəuθɔːˈræsik] *a* 腹胸的,腹部胸廓的
abdominovaginal [æbˌdɔminəuˈvædʒinəl] *a* 腹阴道的
abdominovesical [æbˌdɔminəuˈvesikəl] *a* 腹膀胱的
abducent [æbˈdjuːsnt] *a* 外展的,展的(如展神经)
abduct [æbˈdʌkt] *vt* 外展,展 | ~ **ion** [æbˈdʌk-ʃən] *n* | ~ **or** *n* 外展肌
ABE acute bacterial endocarditis 急性细菌性心内膜炎
abed [əˈbed] *ad* 在床上
Abelin's reaction (test) [ˈæbilin] (Isaak Abelin) 阿贝林反应(试验)(检尿中胂凡纳明)
abembryonic [ˌæbembriˈɔnik] *a* 胚外的
abepithymia [ˌæbəpiˈθaimiə] *n* 太阳神经丛麻痹
abequose [ˈæbikwəus] *n* β-脱氧岩藻糖(一种沙门菌菌体多糖抗原)
Abercrombie's degeneration (syndrome) [ˈæbəˌkrʌmbi] (John Abercrombie) 淀粉样变性
Abernethy's fascia [ˌæbəˈneθi] (John Abernethy) 髂筋膜 | ~ sarcoma 艾伯内西肉瘤(主要在躯干上的一种变性的脂肪瘤)
aberrancy [æˈberənsi] *n* 差异传导 | acceleration-dependent ~ 加速依赖性差异传导
aberrant [æˈberənt] *a* 偏离常轨的;迷乱的,迷行的;畸变的;异常的,失常的
aberration [ˌæbəˈreiʃən] *n* 偏离常规;(精神)迷乱;像差;差异传导 | chromatic ~, newtonian ~ 色[像]差,牛顿像差 / chromosome ~ 染色体畸变 / distantial ~ 距离像差 / heterosomal ~ 异源染色体畸变 / mental ~ 精神错乱 / meridional ~ 子午圈像差 / penta-X chromosomal ~ 5-X 染色体畸变 / tetra-X chromosomal ~ 4-X 染色体畸变 / triple-X chromosomal ~ 3-X 染色体畸变
aberrometer [ˌæbəˈrɔmitə] *n* 像差计
abesterase [æˈbestəreis] *n* 脂族酯酶
abetalipoproteinemia [eiˌbeitəˌlipəuˌprəutiːˈniːmiə] *n* 无 β 脂蛋白血症
abfraction [æbˈfrækʃən] *n* 牙结构病理性缺失
ABG arterial blood gases 动脉血气
abhor [əbˈhɔː] *vt* 憎恶,厌恶
abhorrence [əbˈhɔrəns] *n* 憎恶
ABI ankle-brachial index 踝-臂指数
abiatrophy [ˌæbaiˈætrəfi] *n* 生活力缺损
abient [ˈæbiənt] *a* 避开的(指对刺激的反应)
Abies [ˈeibiiz] *n* 冷杉属
abietate [ˈæbiəteit] *n* 松香酸盐
abietic acid [ˌæbiˈetik] 松香酸
abietinic acid [ˌæbiəˈtinik] 松香酸
abiogenesis [ˌeibaiəuˈdʒenisis] *n* 自然发生说,非生源说 | **abiogenetic** [ˌeiˌbaiəudʒiˈnetik], **abiogenous** [ˌeibaiˈɔdʒinəs] *a* 自然发生的 | **abiogenist** [ˌeibaiˈɔdʒinist] *n* 自然发生论者
abiophysiology [ˌeibaiəuˌfiziˈɔlədʒi] *n* 无机生理学
abiosis [ˌeibaiˈəusis] *n* 无生命;生活力缺损 | **abiotic** [ˌeibaiˈɔtik] *a*
abiotrophy [ˌeibaiˈɔtrəfi] *n* 生活力缺损 | retinal ~ 视网膜生活力缺损(如色素性视网膜炎、家族黑矇性白痴) | **abiotrophia** [ˌeibaiəuˈtrəufiə], **abionergy** [ˌeibaiˈɔnədʒi] *n* / **abiotrophic** [ˌeibaiəuˈtrɔfik] *a*
abirritant [æbˈiritənt] *a* 减轻刺激的,缓和的 *n* 缓和药
abirritation [ˌæbiriˈteiʃən] *n* 应激性减弱;张力缺乏,弛缓
abirritative [æbˈiriˌteitiv] *a* 减弱应激性的,和缓的
abiuret [əiˈbaijuəret], **abiuretic** [əˌbaijuəˈretik] *a* 双缩脲反应阴性的,无双缩脲反应的
ablactation [ˌæblækˈteiʃən] *n* 断乳;泌乳停止
ablastemic [eiblæsˈtemik] *a* 非芽生的
ablastin [əbˈlæstin] *n* 抑殖素,抗殖素(防止入侵微生物繁殖的一种抗体)
ablate [æbˈleit] *vt, vi* 切除;摘除 | **ablation** [æbˈleiʃən] *n* 分离,脱离;摘除;部分切除[术];消融[术]
ablatio [æbˈleiʃiəu] *n*【拉】脱离;部分切除术 | ~ placentae 胎盘脱离
ablepharia [ˌeibleˈfɛəriə], **ablepharon** [eiˈblefərɔn], **ablephary** [eiˈblefəri] *n* 无睑[畸形] | **ablepharous** [eiˈblefərəs] *a*
ablepsia [əˈblepsiə], **ablepsy** [əˈblepsi] *n* 视觉缺失,盲
abluent [ˈæbluənt] *a* 清洗的,洗净的 *n* 清洗剂,洗净剂,去污剂
abluminal [æbˈljuminæl] *a* 来自管腔的
ablution [əˈbluːʃən] *n* 擦浴,沐浴;清洗法
ablutomania [æbˌluːtəuˈmeinjə] *n* 清洗癖,沐浴癖
abmortal [æbˈmɔːtl] *a* 来自死亡或损伤部位的(尤指电流)
ABMT autologous bone marrow transplantation 自体骨髓移植
abnegate [ˈæbnigeit] *vt* 放弃;拒绝;克制 | **abnegation** [ˌæbniˈgeiʃən] *n*
abnerval [æbˈnəːvəl] *a* 来自神经的(指电流)

abnormal [æbˈnɔːməl] *a* 反常的,异常的;变态的
abnormality [ˌæbnɔːˈmæləti] *n* 异常 | potential ~ of glucose tolerance (pot AGT) 葡萄糖耐量潜在异常 / previous ~ of glucose tolerance (prev AGT) 葡萄糖耐量既往异常
abnormity [æbˈnɔːməti] *n* 反常,异常;畸形
abolish [əˈbɔliʃ] *vt* 废除,取消 | **abolition** [ˌæbəˈliʃən] *n*
abomasitis [ˌæbəuməˈsaitis] *n* 皱胃炎
abomasopexy [ˌæbəuˈmeisəuˌpeksi] *n* 皱胃固定术
abomasotomy [ˌæbəumeiˈsɔtəmi] *n* 皱胃切开术
abomasum [ˌæbəuˈmeisəm] *n* 皱胃(反刍动物的第四胃)
A-bomb [ˈei bɔm] *n* 大麻和海洛因混制香烟
abominate [əˈbɔmineit] *vt* 厌恶,憎恨 | **abomination** [əˌbɔmiˈneiʃən] *n*
aborad [æˈbɔːræd] *a* 离口的
aboral [æˈbɔːrəl] *a* 离口的,远口的;对口的
aboriginal [ˌæbəˈridʒənl] *a* 土著的 *n* 土著居民;土生动植物
aborigine [ˌæbəˈridʒən] *n* 土著居民;[复] [ˌæbəˈridʒəˌniːz] 土生动植物群
abort [əˈbɔːt] *vi* 流产,小产;(动植物器官)发育不全,退化 *vt* 使流产;顿挫(抑制病的发展)
aborticide [əˈbɔːtisaid] *n* 堕胎;堕胎药
abortifacient [əˌbɔːtiˈfeiʃənt], **abortient** [əˈbɔːʃənt] *a* 堕胎的 *n* 堕胎药
abortin [əˈbɔːtin] *n* 流产菌素(流产杆菌的甘油浸出物,用途与结核菌素同,但用于诊断人的布鲁杆菌病)
abortion [əˈbɔːʃən] *n* 流产,小产;流产儿;发育不全,(病势的)顿挫 | accidental ~ 意外流产 / afebrile ~ 无热性流产 / ampullar ~ 输卵管壶腹部流产 / artificial ~ 人工流产 / cervical ~ 子宫颈流产 / complete ~ 完全流产 / criminal ~ 违法流产,堕胎 / habitual ~, recurrent ~ 习惯性流产 / imminent ~ 紧迫流产 / incomplete ~ 不全流产 / induced ~ 人工流产 / missed ~ 稽留流产 / ~ in progress, inevitable ~ 进行性流产,难免流产 / septic ~ 流产感染 / spontaneous ~ 自然流产 / therapeutic ~, justifiable ~ 治疗性流产,合法流产 / threatened ~ 先兆流产 / tubal ~ 输卵管流产
abortionist [əˈbɔːʃənist] *n* 堕胎者
abortive [əˈbɔːtiv] *a* 发育不全的;流产的;顿挫性(指病程)
abortus [əˈbɔːtəs] *n*【拉】流产儿(体重少于 500 g)
abouchement [əbuːʃˈmɔŋ] *n*【法】注入,汇入(指血管在一个较大的血管内终止)
ab-oukine *n* 阿布奥开病,雅司病(即 yaws,加蓬土名)
aboulia [əˈbjuːliə] *n* 意志缺失
aboulomania [əˌbuːləuˈmeinjə] *n* 意志缺失狂
ABP arterial blood pressure 动脉血压
abrachia [əˈbreikiə], **abrachiatism** [əˈbreikiəˌtizəm] *n* 无臂[畸形]
abrachiocephalia [əˌbreikiəusiˈfeiliə] *n* 无头无臂[畸形]
abrachiocephalus [əˌbreikiəuˈsefələs] *n* 无头无臂畸胎
abrachius [əˈbreikiəs] *n* 无臂畸胎
abradant [əˈbreidənt] *a* 擦除的,擦伤的;磨损的 *n* 摩擦剂
abrade [əˈbreid] *vt* 擦除,擦伤;磨损
Abrahams' sign [ˈeibrəhæm] (Robert Abrahams) 亚伯拉罕(①早期肺尖结核时,叩诊肩峰突可听到浊音和实音之间的音;②膀胱结石时,在脐和第九右肋软骨之间中部施加压力即引起剧痛)
Abrami's disease [əˈbrɑːmi] (Pierre Abrami) 溶血性贫血
Abrams' heart reflex [ˈeibrəmz] (Albert Abrams) 艾布勒姆斯心反射(刺激心前区皮肤引起心肌收缩,心浊音区减少)
abrasio [əˈbreisiəu] *n*【拉】擦伤;磨损 | ~ corneae 角膜上皮擦伤
abrasion [əˈbreiʒən] *n* 擦除,擦伤;磨损[症] | dental ~ 牙质磨损
abrasive [əˈbreisiv] *a* 致擦伤的;致磨损的 *n* 磨擦剂
abrasor [əˈbreizə] *n* 擦除器,刮除器;磨[除]器
abreaction [ˌæbri(ː)ˈækʃən] *n* 疏泄,精神发泄 | motor ~ 运动[表达]性精神疏泄
abreuography [ˌæbruːˈɔgrəfi] *n* 荧光 X 线摄影[术]
Abrikosov's (Abrikosoff's) tumor [ˌæbriˈkɔsɔf] (Aleksei I. Abrikosov) 粒细胞瘤
abrin [ˈeibrin] *n* 相思豆毒素
abrism [ˈeibrizəm] *n* 相思豆中毒
abrosia [əˈbrəuziə] *n* 断食,禁食
abruptio [əˈbrʌpʃiəu] *n*【拉】分离,分开 | ~ placentae 胎盘早剥
abruption [əˈbrʌpʃən] *n* 突然分离;分裂,断裂 | placental ~ 胎盘早剥
Abrus [ˈeibrəs] *n* 相思子属
abs- [前缀] 离,从
abscess [ˈæbsis] *n* 脓肿 | alveolar ~, acute dentoalveolar ~ 牙槽脓肿,急性牙槽脓肿 / arthrifluent ~ 蚀关节性脓肿 / bartholinian ~ 前庭大腺脓肿 / bicameral ~ 双腔脓肿 / bilharziasis ~ 裂体吸虫病脓肿 / bone ~ 骨髓炎;化脓性骨膜炎 / canalicular ~ 乳小管脓肿 / cholangitic ~, bile duct ~ 胆管脓肿 / cold ~, chronic ~ 寒性脓肿,慢性脓肿 / circumscribed ~ 局限性脓肿 /

encysted ~ 包囊性脓肿 / extradural ~, epidural ~ 硬膜外脓肿 / epiploic ~ 网膜脓肿 / frontal ~ 额叶脓肿 / gastric ~ 胃脓肿,蜂窝织炎性胃炎 / glandular ~ 淋巴结脓肿 / gravitation ~, gravity ~ 流注[性]脓肿,引力性脓肿 / ischiorectal ~ 坐骨直肠窝脓肿 / lateral ~, lateral alveolar ~, parietal ~, peridental ~, periodontal ~ [根]侧脓肿,牙周脓肿 / lymphatic ~ 淋巴结脓肿 / milk ~ 哺乳期(乳腺)脓肿 / mother ~ 原[发]脓肿 / mural ~ 腹壁脓肿 / nocardinal ~ 诺卡菌性脓肿 / ossifluent ~ 蚀骨性脓肿 / pelvic ~ 盆腔脓肿 / periapical ~ (急性牙根)尖周脓肿 / peritonsillar ~, circumtonsillar ~ 扁桃体周脓肿 / serous ~ 浆膜脓肿,蛋白性骨膜炎 / shirt-stud ~, collar-button ~ 哑铃形脓肿 / sudoriparous ~ 汗腺脓肿 / tuberculous ~, scrofulous ~, strumous ~ 结核性脓肿 / tympanitic ~, emphysematous ~, gas ~ 气脓肿 / urinary ~ 尿[外渗性]脓肿 / wandering ~, hypostatic ~, migrating ~ 游走性脓肿,坠积性脓肿

abscessus [æbˈsesəs] *n* 【拉】脓肿 | ~ siccus corneae 盘状角膜炎

abscissa [æbˈsisə] *n* 横坐标

abscis(s)in [æbˈsisin] *n* 脱落素

abscission [æbˈsiʒən] *n* 切除 | corneal ~ 角膜切除术

absconsio [æbˈskɔnsiəu] ([复]**absconsiones** [æbskɔnsiˈəuniːz]) *n* 【拉】骨窝

abscopal [æbˈskɔpəl] *a* 伴随远隔的(指对未经照射组织所产生的效应)

absence [ˈæbsəns] *n* 缺失,缺如;失神 | ~ of penis 阴茎缺失 / ~ of radius 桡骨缺如

absent [ˈæbsənt] *a* 缺失的,缺如的;失神的

absentia [æbˈsenʃiə] *n* 【拉】失神 | ~ epileptica 癫痫[小发作]性失神

absent-minded [ˈæbsənt ˈmaindid] *a* 心不在焉的 | **~ness** *n*

abs. feb. absente febre【拉】无[发]热时

Absidia [æbˈsidiə] *n* 犁头霉属

absinth(e) [ˈæbsinθ] *n* 苦艾;苦艾酒

absinthin [æbˈsinθin] *n* 苦艾苷,苦艾素

absinthium [æbˈsinθiəm] *n* 苦艾

absolute [ˈæbsəljuːt] *a* 绝对的;纯粹的;确实的

absorbable [əbˈsɔːbəbl] *a* 可吸收的 | **absorbability** [əbˌsɔːbəˈbiləti] *n*

absorbance [əbˈsɔːbəns], **absorbency** [əbˈsɔːbənsi] *n* 吸光度(放射学中指一种介质吸收放射能力的量度)

absorbefacient [əbˌsɔːbiˈfeiʃənt] *a* 吸收性的,促吸收的 *n* 吸收剂

absorbent [əbˈsɔːbənt] *a* 能吸收的 *n* 吸收体;吸收剂

absorptiometer [əbˌsɔːpʃiˈɔmitə] *n* 液体吸气计;吸收比色计(用作血分光镜)

absorptiometry [əbˌsɔːpʃiˈɔmitri] *n* 吸收测定法 | dual energy X-ray ~ (DEXA) 双能 X 线吸收测定法 / dual photon ~ 双光子吸收测定法

absorption [əbˈsɔːpʃən] *n* 吸收[作用];吸能;全神贯注 | agglutinin ~ 凝集素吸收(从免疫血清中除去抗体,即以与该抗体同种的颗粒性抗原〈一般是细菌〉处理之,然后离心和分离抗原抗体复合物) / cutaneous ~ 皮肤吸收 / internal ~, enteral ~ 内吸收,肠吸收 / external ~ 外吸收 / interstitial ~ 组织间吸收 / intestinal ~ 肠吸收 / parenteral ~ 肠胃外吸收,非肠胃吸收 / pathologic(al) ~, excrementitial ~ 病理吸收,排泄物吸收 | **absorptive** *a* 能吸收的,吸收的

absorptivity [ˌæbsɔːpˈtivəti] *n* 吸光系数,吸光度 | molar ~ 摩尔吸光系数 / specific ~ 比吸光系数

abst., abstr. abstract 摘要,提要

abstemious [æbˈstiːmjəs] *a* 饮食有度的;有节制的

abstention [əbˈstenʃən] *n* 戒除

absterge [əbˈstəːdʒ] *vt* 清洗;使净化 | **~nt** *a* 洗涤的 *n* 洗涤剂

abstinence [ˈæbstinəns] *n* 节制,戒瘾,禁戒(如禁酒,节欲) | alimentary ~ 饮食节制,断食 | **abstinent** *a*

abstract [ˈæbstrækt] *a* 抽象的 *n* 摘要,提要(指书、论文、病史的);提出物,萃取物(化学) [æbˈstrækt] *vt* 提取

abstraction [æbˈstrækʃən] *n* 抽象[化];提取,抽出;拉长

abterminal [æbˈtəːminl] *a* 离末端的,从末端向中心的(指肌肉本体中的电流)

abtorsion [æbˈtɔːʃən] *n* 眼外转

abtropfung [ˈɑːbtrɔpfuŋ] *n* 【德】痣细胞团下移(从表皮到真皮中)

abulia [əˈbjuːliə] *n* 意志缺失 | cyclic ~ 周期性意志缺失 | **abulic** *a*

abulomania [əˌbjuːləuˈmeinjə] *n* 意志缺乏性精神障碍

abundance [əˈbʌndəns] *n* 丰富;丰度

abuse [əˈbjuːz] *vt* 滥用[əˈbjuːs] *n* 滥用;虐待,伤害 | child ~ 虐待儿童(见 syndrome 项下 battered-child syndrome) / drug ~ 药物滥用 / psychoactive substance ~ 精神作用物质滥用(见 dependence 项下相应术语) / substance ~ [精神作用]物质滥用

abusive [əˈbjuːsiv] *a* 滥用的;恶习的

abut [əˈbʌt] *vi*, *vt* 接触,毗连,接界;支托

abutment [əˈbʌtmənt] *n* 桥基

ABVD doxorubicin, bleomycin, vinblastine, and

dacarbazine 多柔比星-博来霉素-长春碱-达卡巴嗪(联合化疗治癌方案,用于治霍奇金〈Hodgkin〉病)

abwehrfermente [ɑːbˈvɛəfəˌmentə] *n*【德】防护[性]酶

AC acromioclavicular 肩[峰]锁[骨]的;air conduction 空气传导;alternating current 交流电;anodal closure 阳极通电;aortic closure 主动脉瓣关闭;axiocervical 轴颈的;doxorubicin and cyclophosphamide 多柔比星-环磷酰胺(联合化疗治癌方案)

Ac actinium 锕

a. c. ante cibum【拉】饭前[服]

ACA American College of Angiology 美国血管学学会;American College of Apothecaries 美国药剂师学会

Acacia [əˈkeiʃə] *n*【拉】阿拉伯胶属,金合欢胶属

acacia [əˈkeiʃə] *n* 阿拉伯胶,金合欢胶

acalcerosis [əˌkælsəˈrəusis] *n* 缺钙

acalcicosis [əˌkælsaiˈkəusis] *n* 缺钙症

acalculia [əkælˈkjuːliə] *n* 计算不能,失算症

acampsia [əˈkæmpsiə] *n* 屈挠不能(指身体某一部位或关节)

acantha [əˈkænθə] *n* 棘;棘突

acanthaceous [ˌækənˈθeiʃəs] *a* 有棘的

acanthamebiasis [əˌkænθəmiˈbaiəsis] *n* 棘阿米巴病

Acanthamoeba [əˌkænθəˈmiːbə] *n* 棘阿米巴属

Acantharea [ˌækənˈθɛəriə] *n* 等幅骨虫纲

acantharian [ˌækənˈθɛəriən] *a* 等幅骨虫的

acanthesthesia [əˌkænθisˈθiːzjə] *n* 针刺感

Acanthia lectularia [əˈkænθiə ˌlektjuˈlɛəriə] 温带臭虫(即 Cimex lectularius)

acanthion [əˈkænθiːən] *n* 鼻前棘点

acantho- [构词成分] 棘

Acanthobdellidea [əˌkænθədeˈlidiə] *n* 棘蛭目

Acanthocephala [əˌkænθəˈsefələ] *n* 棘头门

acanthocephalan [əˌkænθəˈsefələn] *n* 棘头虫

acanthocephaliasis [əˌkænθəˌsefəˈlaiəsis] *n* 棘头虫病

acanthocephalous [əˌkænθəˈsefələs] *a* 棘头虫的

Acanthocephalus [əˌkænθəˈsefələs] *n* 棘头虫属

Acanthocheilonema [əˌkænθəˌkailəˈniːmə] *n* 棘唇线虫属 | ~ perstans 常现棘唇线虫,常现丝虫(即 Mansonella perstans) / ~ streptocerca 链尾棘唇线虫(即 Mansonella streptocerca)

acanthocheilonemiasis [əˌkænθəˌkailəniˈmaiəsis] *n* 棘唇虫病

acanthocyte [əˈkænθəsait] *n* 刺状红细胞

acanthocytosis [əˌkænθəsaiˈtəusis] *n* 刺状红细胞增多;无β脂蛋白血症

acanthoid [əˈkænθɔid] *a* 棘样的

acantholysis [ˌækənˈθɔlisis] *n* 棘层松解 | **acantholytic** [əˌkænθəˈlitik] *a*

acanthoma [ˌækænˈθəumə] ([复] **acanthomas** 或 **acanthomata** [ˌækænˈθəumətə]) *n* 棘皮瘤 | ~ adenoides cysticum 囊性腺样棘皮瘤,多发性毛发上皮瘤

acanthopelvis [əˌkænθəˈpelvis], **acanthopelyx** [əˌkænθəˈpeliks] *n* 棘状骨盆

Acanthophacetus [əˌkænθəufəˈsitəs] *n* 食孑孓鱼属 | ~ reticulatus 网状食孑孓鱼(即 Lebistes reticulatus)

Acanthophis [əˈkænθəfis] *n* 棘蛇属 | ~ antarctica 澳洲蝮

Acanthopodina [əˌkænθəpəuˈdainə] *n* 棘足亚目

Acanthopterygii [əˌkænθətiˈridʒiiː] *n* 棘鳍超目

acanthorrhexis [əˌkænθəˈreksis] *n* 皮肤棘层破裂

acanthosis [ˌækənˈθəusis] *n* 棘层肥厚 | ~ nigricans 黑棘皮病 | **acanthotic** [ˌækənˈθɔtik] *a*

acanthrocyte [əˈkænθrəsait] *n* 刺状红细胞

acanthrocytosis [əˌkænθrəsaiˈtəusis] *n* 刺状红细胞增多

acapnia [əˈkæpniə] *n* 缺碳酸血[症],血液二氧化碳缺乏 | **acapnic** [eiˈkæpnik], **acapnial** [əˈkæpniəl] *a*

Acarapis [əˈkɑːrəpis] *n* 螨属 | ~ woodi 伍[德]氏螨

acarbia [əˈkɑːbiə] *n* 血液碳酸盐缺乏,缺碳酸盐血[症]

acarbose [ˈeikɑːbəus] *n* 阿卡波糖(一种 α-葡糖苷酶抑制剂,用作抗低血糖药,治疗非胰岛素依赖型糖尿病,口服给药)

acardia [eiˈkɑːdiə] *n* 无心[畸形]

acardiac [eiˈkɑːdiæk] *a* 无心的 *n* 无心畸胎

acardius [əˈkɑːdiəs], **acardiacus** [əkɑːˈdaiəkəs] *n* 无心畸胎

acari [ˈækərai] acarus 的复数

acarian [əˈkɛəriən] *a* 螨的,粉螨的

acariasis [ˌækəˈraiəsis] *n* 螨病 | chorioptic ~ 皮螨病 / demodectic ~ 毛囊螨病 / psoroptic ~ 痒螨病 / sarcoptic ~ 疥螨病

acaricide [əˈkærisaid] *a* 杀螨的 *n* 杀螨药

acarid [ˈækərid], **acaridan** [əˈkæridən] *n* 螨,粉螨

Acaridae [əˈkæraidiː] *n* 粉螨科

acaridiasis [əˌkæriˈdaiəsis] *n* 粉螨病

Acarina [ˌækəˈrainə] *n* 螨目,蜱螨目

acarine [ˈækərain] *n* 螨类,蜱螨类

acarinosis [əˌkæriˈnəusis], **acariosis** [əˌkæriˈəusis] *n* 螨病

acar(o)- [构词成分]螨

acarodermatitis [ˌækərəudəːməˈtaitis] *n* 螨皮炎 | ~ urticarioides 荨麻疹样螨皮炎,谷痒病

acaroid [ˈækərɔid] *a* 螨样的
acarology [ˌækəˈrɔlədʒi] *n* 螨类学,蜱螨学 | **acarologist** *n* 螨类学家,蜱螨学家
acarophobia [ˌækərəˈfəubjə] *n* 螨恐怖症,细小物恐怖
acarotoxic [ˌækərəˈtɔksik] *a* 灭螨的,毒螨的
Acarpomyxea [əˌkɑːpəˈmiksiə] *n* 微胶丝纲
Acartomyia [əˌkɑːtəˈmaijə] *n* 茸蚊属(库蚊亚科)
Acarus [ˈækərəs] *n*【拉】粉螨属 | ~ folliculorum 毛囊蠕螨(即 Demodex folliculorum) / ~ gallinae 鸡皮刺螨(即 Dermanyssus gallinae) / ~ hordei 麦螨 / ~ rhyzoglypticus hyacinthi 洋葱螨 / ~ scabiei 疥螨(即 Sarcoptes scabiei) / ~ siro 粗足粉螨
acarus [ˈækərəs] ([复] **acari** [ˈækərai]) *n* 螨
acaryote [əˈkɛəriəut] *a* 无核的 *n* 无核细胞
ACAT acyl CoA: cholesterol acyltransferase 酰基辅酶 A:胆固醇酰基转移酶
acatalasemia [ˌeikætəleiˈsiːmiə] *n* 无过氧化氢酶血症
acatalasia [ˌeikætəˈleiziə] *n* 过氧化氢酶缺乏症
acatalepsia [əˌkætəˈlepsiə] *n* 领悟不能;诊断不明
acatamathesia [eiˌkætəməˈθiːziə] *n* 理解不能(理解言语的能力丧失)
acataphasia [eiˌkætəˈfeiziə] *n* 连贯表意不能(中枢神经系统损害所致)
acatastasia [ˌækətæsˈteiziə] *n* 反常,失规 | **acatastatic** [ˌækətæsˈtætik] *a*
acathexia [ˌækəˈθeksiə] *n* 排泄失禁 | **acathectic** *a*
acathexis [ˌækəˈθeksis] *n* 无贯注,心力贯注缺乏,感情贯注缺乏
acathisia [ˌækəˈθiziə] *n* 静坐不能
acaudate [eiˈkɔːdeit], **acaudal** [eiˈkɔːdl] *a* 无尾的
acaulinosis [eiˌkɔːliˈnəusis] *n* 无茎真菌病
ACC American College of Cardiology 美国心脏病学学会
Acc accommodation 调节(眼);适应
accelerant [əkˈselərənt] *a* 加速的,促进的 *n* 促进剂,催化剂
acceleration [əkˌseləˈreiʃən] *n* 加速[作用];促进;加速度 | negative ~ 负加速度,减速
accelerative [əkˈselərətiv] *a* 加速的,促进的
accelerator [əkˈseləreitə] *n* 加速剂,加速器;加速神经,加速肌 | C3b inactivator ~ C3b 灭活加速剂(即 H 因子) / linear ~ 直线加速器(加速逊原子微粒) / serum prothrombin conversion ~ (SPCA) 血清凝血酶原转变加速因子(因子Ⅶ) / ~ urinae 球海绵体肌
accelerin [əkˈselərin] *n* 加速因子,加速球蛋白(因子Ⅵ)
accelerometer [əkˌseləˈrɔmitə] *n* 加速计
accentuation [ækˌsentjuˈeiʃən] *n* 增强,亢进
acceptor [əkˈseptə] *n* [接]受体,受器;接纳体 | hydrogen ~ 氢受体 / oxygen ~ 氧受体
access [ˈækses] *n* 接近;进入;入口 | arteriovenous ~ 动静脉入口 / vascular ~ 血管入口
accessible [ækˈsesəbl] *a* 能接近的 | **accessibility** [ækˌsesiˈbiləti] *n* 可及性;易接近,可亲
accessiflexor [ækˈsesiˌfleksə] *n* 副屈肌
accession [ækˈseʃən] *n* 增加;增加物;发病,发作
accessorius [ˌækseˈsɔːriəs] *a*【拉】副的
accessory, accessary [ækˈsesəri] *a* 附属的,副的,辅助的 *n* 附件 | **accessorial** [æksəˈsɔːriəl] *a* 附属的
accident [ˈæksidənt] *n* 意外,事故,意外伤害 | cerebrovascular ~ 脑血管意外,[脑]卒中综合征
accidental [ˌæksiˈdentl] *a* 偶然的,意外的
accidentalism [ˌæksiˈdəntəlizəm] *n* 唯症象论(这派医学说,只看病的症状,不顾病因和病理)
accident-prone [ˈæksidənt ˌprəun] *a* (因心理因素)易致事故的
accipiter [ækˈsipitə] *n* 鹰爪带(一种面部绷带)
ACCl anodal closure clonus 阳极通电阵挛
acclimate [əˈklaimit], **acclimatize** [əˈklaimətaiz] *vt, vi* 习服 | **acclimation** [ˌæklaiˈmeiʃən], **acclimatation** [əˌklaiməˈteiʃən], **acclimatization** [əˌklaimətaiˈzeiʃən] *n* 习服
accommodate [əˈkɔmədeit] *vt* 容纳;供应,使适应;调节 *vi* 适应
accommodation [əˌkɔməˈdeiʃən] *n* 适应,顺应;调节(尤指眼对不同距离的调节作用) | absolute ~ 绝对调节,单眼调节 / binocular ~ 双眼调节 / excessive ~ 调节过度 / negative ~ 负调节(视远调节) / nerve ~ 神经适应(直流电持续通电时,阈值的上升) / positive ~ 正调节(视近调节) / subnormal ~ 低常调节
accommodative [əˈkɔməˌdeitiv] *a* 适应的;调节的
accommodometer [əˌkɔməˈdɔmitə] *n* 调节计
accompaniment [əˈkʌmpənimənt] *n* 伴随;伴随物
accompany [əˈkʌmpəni] *vt* 伴随
accomplice [əkɔmˈpliːs] *n*【法】协同菌(混合感染时伴随主要传染物并影响其毒性的一种细菌)
accord [əˈkɔːd] *vt* 使一致 *vi* 符合;一致 *n* 一致;和谐
accordance [əˈkɔːdəns] *n* 一致
accouchement [əkuːʃˈmɔŋ] *n*【法】分娩,生产 | ~ forcé 强促分娩,强迫分娩
accoucheur [ˌækuːˈʃəː] *n*【法】男助产士;男产科医师
accoucheuse [ˌækuːˈʃez] *n* 女助产士;女产科

医师
ACCP American College of Chest Physicians 美国胸内科医师学会
accrementition [ˌækrimenˈtiʃən] *n* 增生
accretio [æˈkriːʃiəu] *n*【拉】粘连 | ~ cordis, ~ pericardii 心包粘连
accretion [æˈkriːʃən] *n* 增积,增加;增积[物];粘连
accumbent [əˈkʌmbənt] *a* 横卧的
accumulate [əˈkuːmjuleit] *vt, vi* 蓄积,累积 | **accumulation** [əˌkuːmjuˈleiʃən] *n* / **accumulator** *n* 蓄电池;累加器,存储器
accumulative [əˈkjuːmjuːlətiv] *a* 积累的,聚集的
accuracy [ˈækjurəsi] *n* 准确[度],精确
ACD acid citrate dextrose [枸橼]酸-枸橼酸盐-葡萄糖(见 solution)
ACE adrenocortical extract 肾上腺皮质浸膏;angiotension converting enzyme 血管紧张素转化酶
acebutolol [ˌæsiˈbjutələul] *n* 醋丁洛尔(心脏选择性 β_1-肾上腺素能受体阻滞药)
acecainide hydrochloride [ˌæsiˈkeinaid] 盐酸乙酰卡尼(抗心律失常性心脏抑制药)
aceclidine [əˈseklidiːn] *n* 醋克利定(合成胆碱能促效药,青光眼时用于降低眼内压)
acedapsone [æsiˈdæpsəun] *n* 醋氨苯砜(抗疟药,抗麻风药)
acedia [əˈsiːdiə] *n* 淡漠性忧郁症
acellular [eiˈseljulə] *a* 无细胞的,非细胞的
acelomate [eiˈsiːləmeit] *n* 无体腔的
acelous [eiˈsiːləs] *a* 无凹[面]的(指某些动物的脊椎)
acenesthesia [əˌsenisˈθiːzjə] *n* 存在感觉缺失;自身感觉不良(见于忧郁症及疑病症)
acenocoumarol [əˌsiːnəuˈkuːmərɔl], **acenocoumarin** [əˌsiːnəuˈkuːmərin] *n* 醋硝香豆素(抗凝药)
acentric [eiˈsentrik] *a* 偏心的,非正中的;无着丝粒的(染色体)
ACEP American College of Emergency Physicians 美国急救医师学会
acephalia [ˌeisiˈfeiliə], **acephalism** [eiˈsefəlizəm] *n* 无头[畸形]
Acephalina [eiˌsefəˈlainə] *n* 无头亚目
acephalobrachia [eiˌsefələuˈbreikiə] *n* 无头无臂[畸形]
acephalobrachius [eiˌsefələuˈbreikiəs] *n* 无头无臂畸胎
acephalocardia [eiˌsefələuˈkɑːdiə] *n* 无头无心[畸形]
acephalocardius [eiˌsefələuˈkɑːdiəs] *n* 无头无心畸胎
acephalochiria [eiˌsefələuˈkaiəriə] *n* 无头无手[畸形]
acephalochirus [eiˌsefələuˈkaiərəs] *n* 无头无手畸胎
acephalocyst [eiˈsefələusist] *n* 无头囊
acephalogaster [eiˌsefələuˈgæstə] *n* 无头胸上腹畸胎
acephalogastria [eiˌsefələuˈgæstriə] *n* 无头胸上腹[畸形]
acephalopodia [eiˌsefələuˈpəudiə] *n* 无头无足[畸形]
acephalopodius [eiˌsefələuˈpəudiəs] *n* 无头无足畸胎
acephalorhachia [eiˌsefələuˈreikiə] *n* 无头无脊柱[畸形]
acephalostomia [eiˌsefələuˈstəumiə] *n* 无头无口[畸形]
acephalostomus [eiˌsefəˈlɔstəməs] *n* 无头无口畸胎
acephalothoracia [eiˌsefələuθɔːˈreisiə] *n* 无头无胸[畸形]
acephalothorus [eiˌsefələuˈθɔːrəs] *n* 无头无胸畸胎
acephalous [eiˈsefələs] *a* 无头的
acephalus [eiˈsefələs] ([复] **acephali** [eiˈsefəlai]) *n* 无头畸胎
acephaly [eiˈsefəli] *n* 无头[畸形]
acepromazine maleate [ˌæsiˈprəuməziːn] 马来酸乙酰丙嗪(安定药,在兽医中用作大动物的止动剂)
Acer [ˈeisə] *n* 槭属
Aceraria [ˌæsəˈrɛəriə] *n* 无角线虫属 | ~ spiralis 螺旋无角线虫
acerbic [əˈsəːbik], **acerb** [əˈsəːb] *a* 酸[味]的,涩的
acerbity [əˈsəːbiti] *n* 酸涩
acerin [ˈæsərin] *n* 槭素(有抗菌作用)
acerola [ˌæsəˈrəulə] *n* 金虎尾(西印度群岛的樱桃果)
acervuline [əˈsəːvjulain] *a* 堆集的,集合的(指腺)
acervulus [əˈsəːvjuləs] ([复] **acervuli** [əˈsəːvjulai]) *n* 分生孢子盘
acescent [əˈsesnt] *a* 变酸的;微酸的 | **acescence** [əˈsesns] *n* 酸度;变酸
acesodyne [əˈsesədain] *n* 止痛药 *a* 止痛的
Acetabularia [ˌæsəˌtæbjuˈlɛəriə] *n* 伞藻属
acetabulectomy [ˌæsəˌtæbjuˈlektəmi] *n* 髋臼切除术
acetabuloplasty [ˌæsəˈtæbjuləuˌplæsti] *n* 髋臼成形术
acetabulum [ˌæsəˈtæbjuləm] ([复] **acetabula** [ˌæsəˈtæbjulə]) *n* 髋臼;腹吸盘 | sunken ~ [髋]关节内陷 | **acetabular** *a*
acetal [ˈæsitæl] *n* 乙缩醛

acetaldehydase [ˌæsiˈtældiːˌhaideis] *n* 乙醛[氧化]酶
acetaldehyde [ˌæsiˈtældihaid] *n* 乙醛
acetaldehyde dehydrogenase [ˌæsiˈtældihaid diː-ˈhaidrədʒəneis] 乙醛脱氢酶,醛脱氢酶(NAD^+)
acetaldehyde reductase [ˌæsiˈtældiːhaid riˈdʌk-teis] 乙醛还原酶,醇脱氢酶(NAD^+)
acetamide [ˌæsiˈtæmaid] *n* 乙酰胺
acetamidine [ˌæsiˈtæmidain] *n* 乙脒
***p*-acetamidobenzene sulfonamide** [ˌæsiˌtæmid-*ə*uˈbenziːn] 对乙酰氨基苯磺酰胺
acetaminophen [ˌæsiˈtæmin*ə*ufen] *n* 对乙酰氨基酚(解热镇痛药)
acetanilid [ˌæsiˈtænilid], **acetanilide** [ˌæsiˈtæ-nilaid] *n* 乙酰苯胺(镇痛、解热药,治神经痛及风湿病)
acetannin [ˌæsiˈtænin] *n* 乙酰丹宁,乙酰鞣酸
acetarsone [ˌæsiˈtɑːsəun], **acetarsol** [ˌæsiˈtɑːs-ɔl] *n* 乙酰胂胺(抗原虫药)
acetas [əˈsiːtəs] *n*【拉】乙酸盐,醋酸盐
acetate [ˈæsiteit] *n* 乙酸盐,醋酸盐
acetate-CoA ligase [ˈæsiteit kəuˈei ˈlaigeis] 乙酸辅酶 A 连接酶(亦称乙酰辅酶 A 合成酶)
acetazolamide [ˌæsitəˈzɔləmaid] *n* 乙酰唑胺(利尿药,为碳酸酐酶抑制药,可使眼内压降低,用于治青光眼)
acetenyl [əˈsiːtənil] *n* 乙炔基
aceteugenol [ˌæsiˈtjuːdʒinɔl] *n* 乙酰丁香酚
acetic [əˈsiːtik, əˈsetik] *a* 醋的,醋酸的 | ~ alde-hyde 乙醛
acetic acid [əˈsiːtik] 醋酸,乙酸 | glacial ~ 冰醋酸
aceticoceptor [əˌsiːtik*ə*uˈseptə] *n* 乙酸受体,乙酸基团
acetify [əˈsetifai] *vt*, *vi* 醋化,醋酸化 | **acetifica-tion** [əˌsetifiˈkeiʃən] *n*
acetimeter [ˌæsiˈtimitə] *n* 醋酸[比重]计
acetin [ˈæsitin] *n* 乙酸甘油酯
Acetivibrio [əˌsiːtiˈvibriəu] *n* 醋酸弧菌属
acet(o)- [前缀]乙酰
acetoacetate [əˌsiːt*ə*uˈæsiteit] *n* 乙酰乙酸盐,乙酰乙酸
acetoacetic acid [əˌsiːtəuəˈsiːtik] 乙酰乙酸
acetoacetyl-CoA [ˌæsət*ə*uˈæsitil, əˈsiːtəæsiˌtil, kəuˈei] 乙酰乙酰辅酶 A
acetoacetyl-CoA reductase [ˌæsət*ə*uˈæsitil kəu-ˈei riˈdʌkteis] 乙酰乙酰辅酶 A 还原酶
acetoacetyl-CoA thiolase [ˌæsət*ə*uˈæsitil, əˈsiː-təæsiˌtil kəuˈei ˈθaiəleis] 乙酰乙酰辅酶 A 硫解酶
acetoacetyl coenzyme A [ˌæsət*ə*uˈæsitil, əˈsiː-təæsiˌtil kəuˈenzaim] 乙酰乙酰辅酶 A
Acetobacter [əˌsiːt*ə*uˈbæktə] *n* 醋酸杆菌属
Acetobacteraceae [əˌsiːt*ə*uˌbæktəˈreisiiː] *n* 醋酸杆菌科
acetoform [əˈsiːtəfɔːm] *n* 乌洛托品(尿路抗菌药)
acetohexamide [ˌæsit*ə*uˈheksəmaid] *n* 醋磺己脲(降血糖药)
acetohydroxamic acid [ˌæsit*ə*uˌhaidrɔkˈsæmik] 醋羟胺酸(尿素酶抑制药,用于防治鸟粪石性肾结石)
acetoin [əˈsetəuin] *n* 3-羟基丁酮
acetokinase [ˌæsit*ə*uˈkaineis] *n* 乙酸激酶
acetolase [əˈsetəleis] *n* 醋酸[生成]酶
acetolysis [ˌæsiˈtɔlisis] *n* 醋酸分解,醋酸酐分解
acetomeroctol [ˌæsit*ə*uməˈrɔktɔl] *n* 醋辛酚汞(消毒防腐药)
acetometer [ˌæsiˈtɔmitə] *n* 醋酸[比重]计
acetomorphine [ˌæsit*ə*uˈmɔːfiːn] *n* 二乙酰吗啡,海洛因
acetonaphthone [ˌæsit*ə*uˈnæfθəun] *n* 萘乙酮
acetonation [ˌæsit*ə*uˈneiʃən] *n* 丙酮化合[作用]
acetone [ˈæsitəun] *n* 丙酮 | ~ diethyl-sulfone 丙酮缩二乙砜,二乙眠砜 | **acetonic** [ˌæsiˈtɔnik] *a*
acetonemia [ˌæsit*ə*uˈniːmiə] *n* 丙酮血[症] | **ac-etonemic** [ˌæsit*ə*uˈniːmik] *a*
acetonglycosuria [ˌæsitəunˌglaik*ə*uˈsjuəriə] *n* 丙酮糖尿(丙酮中毒所致)
acetonitrile [ˌæsit*ə*uˈnaitril, -trail] *n* 乙腈,氰化甲烷
acetonum [ˌæsiˈtəunəm] *n*【拉】丙酮
acetonumerator [ˌæsit*ə*uˈnjuːməˌreitə] *n* 尿丙酮定量器
acetonuria [ˌæsit*ə*uˈnjuəriə] *n* 丙酮尿
aceto-orcein [ˈæsitəˈɔːsiːn] *n* 乙酸地衣红(地衣红溶于乙酸中,用于制作多线染色体压剂标本)
acetophenazine maleate [ˌæsit*ə*uˈfenəziːn] 马来酸醋奋乃静(强安定药)
acetophenetidin [ˌæsit*ə*ufiˈnetidin], **acetphene-tidin** [ˌæsitfiˈnetidin] *n* 非那西丁(解热镇痛药)
acetosal [əˈsiːtəsæl] *n* 乙酰水杨酸(解热镇痛药)
acetosoluble [ˌæsit*ə*uˈsɔljubl] *a* 醋酸溶性的
acetosulfone sodium [ˌæsit*ə*uˈsʌlfəun] 磺胺苯砜钠(抗麻风药)
acetous [ˈæsitəs], **acetose** [ˈæsitəus] *a* 醋的;醋酸的
acetowhite [əˌsiːtə*h*wait] *a* 醋酸增白的
acetowhitening [əˌsiːtəˈ*h*waitəniŋ] *n* 醋酸增白(皮肤或黏膜,尤其是人乳头瘤病毒所致的疣,某些亚临床损害经局部使用醋酸时暂时变白的过程)
acetphenarsine [ˌæsitfeˈnɑːsiːn] *n* 乙酰胂胺(抗

滴虫药)

acetpyrogall [ˌæsitˈpaiərəgəl] *n* 乙酰没食子酚(表面腐蚀剂和角质层分离剂)

acetrizoate [ˌæsitraiˈzəueit] *n* 醋碘苯酸盐(水溶性造影剂,其钠盐用于子宫输卵管造影)

acetrizoic acid [ˌæsitriˈzəuik] 醋碘苯酸

acetum [əˈsiːtəm] ([复]**aceta** [əˈsiːtə]) *n*【拉】醋;醋剂

aceturate [əˈsetjuːreit] *n* *N*-乙酰甘氨酸盐(*N*-acetylglycinate 的 USAN 缩约词)

acetyl [ˈæsitil] *n* 乙酰[基] | ~ chloride 乙酰氯,氯化乙酰 / ~ peroxide 过氧化乙酰 / ~ sulfisoxazole 醋磺胺异噁唑(抗菌药)

acetylaminobenzene [ˌæsitilˌæminəuˈbenziːn] *n* 乙酰苯胺(解热镇痛药)

acetylaminobenzene sulfonate [ˌæsitilˌæminəuˈbenziːn ˈsʌlfəneit] 磺酸乙酰苯胺

acetylaminobenzoic acid [ˌæsitilˌæminəubenˈzəuik] 乙酰氨基苯甲酸

acetylaminofluorene [ˌæsitilˌæminəuˈfluəriːn] *n* 乙酰氨基芴

acetylandromedol [ˌæsitilænˈdrɔmədɔl] *n* 梫木毒素

acetylaniline [ˌæsitilˈæniliːn] *n* 乙酰苯胺(解热镇痛药)

acetylase [əˈsetileis] *n* 乙酰基转移酶,转乙酰基酶

acetylate [əˈsetileit] *vt* 乙酰化 | **acetylation** [əˌsetiˈleiʃən] *n* 乙酰化[作用]

acetylator [əˌsetiˈleitə] *n* 乙酰化者,乙酰化个体(在人类,乙酰化者状态〈快速或慢速〉是由磺胺二甲嘧啶的乙酰化速度决定的)

acetylcholine (ACh) [ˌæsitilˈkəuliːn] *n* 乙酰胆碱(副交感神经阻滞药) | ~ chloride 氯乙酰胆碱(缩瞳药)

acetylcholinesterase (AChE) [ˌæsitilˌkəuliˈnestəreis] *n* 乙酰胆碱酯酶

acetyl-CoA acetyltransferase [ˈæsitil kəuˈei ˌæsitilˈtrænsfəreis] 乙酰辅酶 A 乙酰基转移酶(亦称乙酰乙酰辅酶 A 硫解酶,乙酰乙酰硫解酶)

acetyl-CoA *C*-acetyltransferase [ˈæsitil kəuˈei ˌæsitilˈtrænsfəreis] 乙酰辅酶 A *C*-乙酰转移酶

acetyl-CoA acyltransferase [ˈæsitil kəuˈei ˌæsilˈtrænsfəreis] 乙酰辅酶 A 酰基转移酶

acetyl-CoA *C*-acyltransferase [ˈæsitil kəuˈei ˌæsilˈtrænsfəreis] 乙酰辅酶 A *C*-酰基转移酶(亦称 β-酮硫解酶)

acetyl-CoA carboxylase [ˈæsitil kəuˈei kɑːˈbɔksileis] 乙酰辅酶 A 羧化酶

acetyl-CoA: *α*-glucosaminide-*N*-acetyltransferase [ˈæsitil kəuˈei ˌgluːkəuˈsæminaid ˌæsitilˈtrænsfəreis] 乙酰辅酶 A: α-氨基葡糖苷-*N*-乙酰基转移酶,乙酰肝素-α-氨基葡糖苷乙酰基转移酶

acetyl-CoA: heparan-*α*-D-glucosaminide *N*-acetyltransferase [ˈæsitil kəuˈei ˈhepəræn ˌgluːkəuˈsæminaid ˌæsitilˈtrænsfəreis] 乙酰辅酶 A: 乙酰肝素-α-D-氨基葡糖苷-*N*-乙酰基转移酶(亦称乙酰肝素-α-氨基葡糖苷乙酰基转移酶)

acetyl-CoA synthetase [ˈæsitil kəuˈei ˈsinθiteis] 乙酰辅酶 A 合成酶,乙酰辅酶 A 连接酶

acetylcoenzyme A [ˌæsitilkəuˈenzaim], **acetyl-CoA** 乙酰辅酶 A

acetylcysteine [ˌæsitilˈsistiin] *n* 乙酰半胱氨酸(黏液溶解药)

acetyldigitoxin [ˌæsitilˌdidʒiˈtɔksin] *n* 醋洋地黄毒苷(强心药)

acetyldihydrolipoamide [ˌæsitildaiˌhaidrəulipəuˈæmaid] *n* 乙酰二氢硫辛酰胺

acetylene [əˈsetiliːn] *n* 乙炔

acetylenic acid [əˌsetiˈliːnik] 乙炔酸,炔酸

acetyleugenol [ˌæsitilˈjuːdʒənɔl] *n* 乙酰丁香油酚

***N*-acetylgalactosamine (GalNac)** [ˌæsitilgəlækˈtəusəmiːn] *n* *N*-乙酰半乳糖胺

***N*-acetylgalactosamine-4-sulfatase** [ˌæsitilgəlækˈtəusəmiːn ˈsʌlfəteis] *N*-乙酰半乳糖胺-4-硫酸酯酶(此酶的遗传性缺乏为一种常染色体隐性性状,可致黏多糖贮积症Ⅵ型)

***N*-acetylgalactosamine-6-sulfatase** [ˌæsitilgəlækˈtəusəmiːn ˈsʌlfəteis] *N*-乙酰半乳糖胺-6-硫酸酯酶(此酶缺乏为一种常染色体隐性性状,可致莫基奥尔〈Morquio〉综合征 A 型,即黏多糖贮积症ⅣA 型,亦称软骨素硫酸酯酶)

***N*-acetylgalactosamine-4-sulfatase deficiency** *N*-乙酰半乳糖胺-4-硫酸酯酶缺乏症,马-拉(Maroteaux Lamy)综合征

α-*N*-acetylgalactosaminidase [ˌæsitilgəˌlæktəusəˈminideis] α-*N*-乙酰氨基半乳糖苷酶(亦称 α-D-半乳糖苷酶 B)

β-*N*-acetylgalactosaminidase [ˌæsitilgəˌlæktəusəˈminideis] β-*N*-乙酰氨基半乳糖苷酶(此酶有两种同工酶:A〈$\alpha\beta_2$〉和 B〈β_4〉〈氨基己糖苷酶 A 和 B〉。同工酶 A〈α-链〉的常染色体隐性遗传缺陷可致泰-萨克斯〈Tay-Sachs〉病。同工酶 A 和 B〈β-链〉的遗传缺陷亦为一种常染体隐性性状,可致桑霍夫〈Sandhoff〉病。亦称 *N*-乙酰-β-氨基己糖苷酶 A)

***N*-acetylglucosamine (GlcNac)** [ˌæsitilgluːˈkəusəmiːn] *n* *N*-乙酰氨基葡糖

***N*-acetylglucosamine-6-sulfatase** [ˌæsitilgluːˈkəusəmiːn ˈsʌlfəteis] *N*-乙酰氨基葡糖-6-硫酸酯酶(此酶的缺陷为一种常染色体隐性性状,可致桑菲利波〈Sanfilippo〉综合征 D 型。亦称 *N*-乙酰-

α-D-氨基葡糖苷-6-硫酸酯酶）

α-N-acetylglucosaminidase [ˌæsitilgluːˌkəusəˈm-inideis] α-N-乙酰氨基葡糖苷酶（此酶的遗传性缺陷为一种常染色体隐性性状，可致桑菲利波〈Sanfilippo〉综合征B型）

β-D-acetylglucosaminidase [ˌæsitilgluːˌkəusəˈm-inideis] *n* β-D-乙酰氨基葡糖苷酶

N-acetyl-α-D-glucosaminide-6-sulfatase [ˌæsi-til-, æsiˌtilgluːˈkəusəmiˌnaid ˈsʌfəteis] N-乙酰-α-D-氨基葡糖苷-6-硫酸酯酶，N-乙酰氨基葡糖-6-硫酸酯酶

N⁴-β-N-acetylglucosaminyl-L-asparaginase [ˌæsitilgluːˌkəusəˈminil ˌæspəˈrædʒineis] N⁴-β-N-乙酰氨基葡糖基-L-天冬酰氨酶（aspartylglucosaminidase 的 EC 名称）

β-N-acetylglucosaminylglycopeptide β-1, 4-galactosyltransferase [ˌæsitilgluːkəˌsæminil-ˌgl-aikəuˈpeptaid gəˌlæktəsilˈtrænsfəreis] β-N-乙酰氨基葡糖基糖肽β-1, 4-半乳糖基转移酶（glycoprotein 4-β-galactosyltransferase 的 EC 名称）

N-acetylglucosaminylphosphotransferase [ˌæsi-tilgluːkəˌsæminilˌfɔsfəˈtrænsfəreis] N-乙酰氨基葡糖基磷酸转移酶，尿苷二磷酸-N-乙酰葡糖胺溶酶体酶，N-乙酰葡糖胺磷酸转移酶

N-acetylglutamate [ˌæsitilˈgluːtəmeit] *n* N-乙酰谷氨酸

N-acetylglutamate synthetase [ˌæsitilˈgluːtəm-eit ˈsinθiteis] N-乙酰谷氨酸合成酶，氨基酸N-乙酰转移酶

N-acetylglutamic acid [ˌæsitilgluːˈtæmik] N-乙酰谷氨酸

N-acetylhexosamine [ˌæsitilhekˈsɔsəmiːn] *n* N-乙酰己糖胺

β-N-acetylhexosaminidase [ˌæsitilhekˌsɔsəˈmini-deis] *n* β-N-乙酰氨基己糖苷酶

N-acetyl-β-hexosaminidase A [ˌæsitil-, æsiˌtil-ˌheksəusəˈminideis] N-乙酰-β-氨基己糖苷酶A, β-N-乙酰-D-氨基半乳糖苷酶的同工酶A

acetylization [əˌsetilaiˈzeiʃən] *n* 乙酰化作用

N-acetylmanosamine [ˌæsitilməˈnəusəmin] *n* N-乙酰甘露糖胺

acetylmethadol [ˌæsitilˈmeθədəul] *n* 醋美沙朵（镇痛药）

N-acetylmuramate [ˌæsitilˈmjuərəmeit] *n* N-乙酰胞壁酸盐（酯或阴离子型）

N-acetylmuramic acid [ˌæsitilmjuəˈræmik] N-乙酰胞壁酸

N-acetylneuraminate [ˌæsitilmjuəˈræmineit] *n* N-乙酰神经氨酸盐（酯或阴离子型）

N-acetylneuraminate lyase [ˌæsitil-, æsiˌtilnjuə-ˈræmineit ˈlaieis] N-乙酰神经氨酸裂合酶

N-acetylneuraminic acid [ˌæsitilˌnjuərəˈminik] N-乙酰神经氨酸

acetylphenylhydrazine [ˌæsitilˌfenilhaiˈdreiziːn] *n* 乙酰苯肼（红细胞抑制药，治真性红细胞增多）

acetylphosphatase [ˌæsitilˈfɔsfəteis] *n* 乙酰磷酸酶

acetylpropionic acid [ˌæsitilˌprəupiˈɔnik] 乙酰丙酸，块茎糖酸

acetylsalicylic acid [ˌæsitilsæliˈsilik] 乙酰水杨酸，阿司匹林（解热镇痛药）

acetylstrophanthidin [ˌæsitilstrəˈfænθidin] *n* 醋毒毛花苷元（强心药）

acetylsulfadiazine [ˌæsitilˌsʌlfəˈdaiəziːn] *n* 乙酰磺胺嘧啶

acetylsulfaguanidine [ˌæsitilˌsʌlfəˈgwænidiːn] *n* 乙酰磺胺胍

acetylsulfanilamide [ˌæsitilˌsʌlfəˈniləmaid] *n* 乙酰氨苯磺胺

acetylsulfathiazole [ˌæsitilˌsʌlfəˈθaiəzəul] *n* 乙酰磺胺噻唑

acetyltannic acid [ˌæsitilˈtænik] 乙酰鞣酸

acetyltannin [ˌæsitilˈtænin] *n* 乙酰鞣酸

acetyltransferase [ˌæsitilˈtrænsfəreis] *n* 乙酰基转移酶 | phosphate ~ 磷酸乙酰基转移酶

acetyltributyl citrate [ˌæsitiltraiˈbjuːtil] 枸橼酸乙酰三丁酯（药物制剂时用作增塑剂）

ACG American College of Gastroenterology 美国胃肠学学会；angiocardiography 心血管造影[术]；apexcardiogram 心尖搏动图

AcG accelerator globulin 凝血因子V（促凝血球蛋白）

ACh acetylcholine 乙酰胆碱

ACHA American College of Hospital Administrators 美国医院管理人员学会

achalasia [ˌækəˈleiziə] *n* 弛缓不能，失弛缓症（亦称贲门痉挛） | pelvirectal ~ 直肠弛缓不能，先天性巨结肠 / sphincteral ~ 括约肌弛缓不能

Achard-Castaigne method, test [əˈʃɑː kəsˈtein]（Emile C. Achard; Joseph Castaigne）亚甲蓝试验（检肾渗透性）

Achard-Thiers syndrome [əˈʃɑː ˈtiəz]（Emile C. Achard; Joseph Thiers）阿夏-蒂斯综合征（绝经后妇女糖尿病、多毛症及其他男性化特征的综合征，系由肾上腺皮质雄激素分泌过多所致）

Achatina [ˌækəˈtainə] *n* 玛瑙螺属

Achatinidae [ækˈtinidiː] *n* 玛瑙螺科

AChE acetylcholinesterase 乙酰胆碱酯酶

ache [eik] *vi* 痛 *n* 疼痛

acheilia [əˈkailiə] *n* 无唇[畸形] | **acheilous** *a*

acheiria [əˈkaiəriə] *n* 无手[畸形]；无手感

acheiropodia [əˌkaiərəuˈpəudiə] *n* 无手足[畸形]

acheirus [ə'kaiərəs] *n* 无手畸胎
achievement [ə'tʃiːvmənt] *n* 成就,成绩
Achillea [ˌæki'liə] *n*【拉】蓍属
Achilles [ə'kiliːz] (Achilleus) 阿基里斯(希腊神话中的英雄,其母握其踝将他在冥河水中浸过) | ~ bursa 跟腱囊 / ~ jerk, ~ tendon reflex 跟腱反射,踝反射 / ~ tendon 跟腱
achillobursitis [əˌkiləubəː'saitis] *n* 跟腱滑囊炎
achillodynia [ˌækiləu'diniə] *n* 跟腱痛;跟腱滑囊炎
achillorrhaphy [ˌæki'lɔrəfi] *n* 跟腱缝合术
achillotenotomy [əˌkiləuti'nɔtəmi], **achillotomy** [ˌæki'lɔtəmi] *n* 跟腱切断术 | plastic ~ 成形跟腱切断术
aching ['eikiŋ] *a* 疼痛的
achiria [ə'kairiə] *n* 无手[畸形]
achirus [ə'kairəs] *n* 无手畸胎
achlorhydria [ˌeiklɔː'haidriə] *n* 胃酸缺乏 | **achlorhydric** *a*
achloropsia [ˌeiklɔː'rɔpsiə], **achloroblepsia** [əˌklɔːrə'blepsiə] *n* 绿色盲
Achlya ['ækliə] *n* 绵霉属
Acholeplasma [əˌkəuli'plæzmə] *n* 无胆甾原体属 | ~ granularum 粒[状]无胆甾原体 / ~ laidlawii 莱德劳无胆甾原体
Acholeplasmataceae [əˌkəuliˌplæzmə'teisiiː] *n* 无胆甾原体科
acholia [ə'kəuliə] *n* 无胆汁[症]
acholic [ə'kɔlik] *a* 无胆汁的
acholuria [əkəu'ljuəriə] *n* 无胆色素尿 | **acholuric** *a*
achondrogenesis [əˌkɔndrəu'dʒenisis] *n* 软骨成长不全
achondroplasia [əˌkɔndrəu'pleiziə], **achondroplasty** [ə'kɔndrəuˌplæsti] *n* 软骨发育不全 | **achondroplastic** [əˌkɔndrəu'plæstik] *a*
achordate [ei'kɔːdeit], **achordal** [ei'kɔːdəl] *a* 无脊索的
Achorion [ə'kɔːriən] *n* 毛[癣]菌属,发癣菌属
achrestic [ə'krestik] *a* 失利用性的,利用不能的(如失利用性贫血时,身体不能利用抗贫血素)
achroacytosis [əˌkrəuəsai'təusis] *n* 淋巴细胞增多
achromasia [ˌækrəu'meiziə] *n* 色素缺乏(指皮肤缺乏正常色素的现象);染色性缺乏(指某一组织或细胞对染色不能发生正常的染色反应)
achromat ['ækrəmæt] *n* 消色差物镜;全色盲者
achromate [ə'krəumeit] *n* 全色盲者
Achromatiaceae [ˌækrəu'meiʃi'eisiiː] *n* 无色[杆]菌科
achromatic [ˌækrəu'mætik] *a* 无色的;不易染色的;非染色质的;消色差的;全色盲的
achromatin [ə'krəumətin] *n* 非染色质 | **~ic** [əˌkrəumə'tinik] *a*
achromatism [ə'krəumətizəm] *n* 消色差[性];全色盲
Achromatium [ˌækrəu'meiʃiəm] *n* 无色[杆]菌属
achromatize [ə'krəumətaiz] *vt* 使无色;消…色差
achromatolysis [əˌkrəumə'tɔlisis] *n* 非染[色]质溶解
achromatophil [ˌeikrəu'mætəfil] *a* 不染色的 *n* 不染体
achromatophilia [əˌkrəumətəu'filiə] *n* 不染色性,拒染性
achromatopia [ˌeikrəumə'təupiə], **achromatopsia** [əˌkrəumə'tɔpsiə] *n* 色盲,全色盲 | **achromatopic** [əˌkrəumə'tɔpik] *a*
achromatosis [əˌkrəumə'təusis] *n* 色素缺乏(如皮肤和虹膜内);染色性缺乏
achromatous [ə'krəumətəs] *a* 无色的
achromaturia [əˌkrəumə'tjuəriə] *n* 无色尿
achromia [ə'krəumiə] *n* 色素缺乏,无色性 | congenital ~ 先天性色素缺乏,白化病 / cortical ~ 皮质色素缺乏(大脑皮质的无节细胞区) / ~ parasitica 寄生性色素缺乏,白糠疹 | **achromic** *a*
achromin [ə'krəumin] *n* 非染色质
Achromobacter [əˌkrəumə'bæktə] *n* 无色[杆]菌属
Achromobacteraceae [əˌkrəuməˌbæktə'reisiiː] *n* 无色[杆]菌科
achromocyte [ə'krəuməsait] *n* 无色红细胞,新月形小体
achromophil [ə'krəuməfil] *a* 不染色的 *n* 不染体
achromophilous [ˌækrəu'mɔfiləs] *a* 非嗜色的,不染色的
achromotrichia [eiˌkrəuməu'trikiə] *n* 毛发色素缺乏
achrooamyloid [eiˌkrəuə'æmilɔid] *n* 无色淀粉样蛋白
achroocytosis [əˌkrəuəsai'təusis] *n* 淋巴细胞增多
achroodextrin [əˌkrəuə'dekstrin] *n* 消色糊精,无色糊精(一种低分子量糊精,遇碘不呈色)
Achroonema [ˌækrəuə'niːmə] *n* 无色线菌属
Achucárro's stain [ˌætʃu'kɑːrəu] (Nicolás Achucárro) 阿丘卡罗染剂(银鞣酸染剂,用以浸染结缔组织)
achylia [ə'kailiə] *n* 胃液缺乏
achymia [ə'kaimiə], **achymosis** [ˌækai'məusis] *n* 食糜缺乏
acicular [ə'sikjulə] *a* 针形的
aciculum [ə'sikjuləm] *n* 针毛(鞭毛虫的)
acid ['æsid] *a* 酸的,酸性的 *n* 酸(对个别特殊的酸,见各有关条目) | bile ~s 胆汁酸 / ~ citrate

dextrose (ACD) (枸橼)酸-枸橼酸盐-葡萄糖 / essential amino ~ 必需氨基酸 / essential fatty ~ 必需脂肪酸

acidalbumin [ˌæsidˈælbjumin] *n* 酸清蛋白,酸白蛋白

Acidaminococcus [ˌæsidəˌmiːnəuˈkɔkəs] *n* 氨基酸球菌属

acidaminuria [ˌæsidˌæmiˈnjuəriə] *n* 氨基酸尿

acid-CoA ligase (GDP-forming) [ˈæsis kəuˈei ˈlaigeis] 酸性辅酶 A 连接酶(GDP 形成的)

acidemia [ˌæsiˈdiːmiə] *n* 酸血[症] | argininosuccinic ~ 精氨基琥珀酸血[症] / glutaric ~ 戊二酸血[症] / methylmalonic ~ 甲基丙二酸血[症] / propionic ~ 丙酸血[症]

acid-fast [ˈæsidfɑːst] *a* 耐酸的,抗酸的

acidic [əˈsidik] *a* 酸的,酸性的

acidifier [əˈsidiˌfaiə] *n* 酸化器;酸化剂,致酸剂

acidify [əˈsidifai] *vt*, *vi* 变酸,酸化 | **acidifiable** [əˈsidiˌfaiəbl] *a* 可酸化的 / **acidification** [əˌsidifiˈkeiʃən] *n*

acidimeter [ˌæsiˈdimitə] *n* 酸定量器 | **acidimetric** [əˌsidiˈmetrik] *a* 酸定量的,酸量滴定的 / **acidimetry** *n* 酸定量法,酸量滴定法

acidism [ˈæsidizəm], **acidismus** [ˌæsiˈdizməs] *n* 酸[类]中毒

acidity [əˈsiditi] *n* 酸度,酸性

acid lipase [ˈæsid ˈlaipeis] 酸性脂肪酶(①甾醇酯酶;②酸性 pH 最适的脂肪酶)

acid lipase deficiency 酸性脂[肪]酶缺乏症(①渥尔曼病,见 Wolman's disease;②胆固醇酯贮积症)

acid maltase [ˈæsid ˈmɔːlteis] 酸性麦芽糖酶,葡聚糖 1, 4-α-葡糖苷酶

acid-maltase deficiency [ˈæsidˈmɔlteis] 酸性麦芽糖酶缺乏症,糖原贮积症Ⅱ型

acidogenic [ˌæsidəuˈdʒenik] *a* 生酸的,成酸的(尤指尿酸度)

acidology [ˌæsiˈdɔlədʒi] *n* 外科器械学

acidophil [əˈsidəfil], **acidophile** [əˈsidəfail] *a* 嗜酸的 *n* 嗜酸细胞(尤指垂体前叶);嗜酸菌 | **acidophilic** [əˌsidəˈfilik] *a* 嗜酸的

acidophilism [ˌæsiˈdɔfilizəm] *n* 垂体嗜酸性腺瘤病(导致肢端肥大症)

acidosis [ˌæsiˈdəusis] *n* 酸中毒 | diabetic ~ 糖尿病酸中毒 / hypercapnic ~, respiratory ~ 血碳酸过多性酸中毒,呼吸性酸中毒 / renal hyperchloremia ~, renal tubular ~ 肾性高氯血症酸中毒,肾小管性酸中毒 / uremic ~ 尿毒症酸中毒 | **acidosic, acidotic** [ˌæsiˈdɔtik] *a*

acidosteophyte [ˌæsiˈdɔstiəfait] *n* 针状骨赘

acid phosphatase [ˈæsid ˈfɔsfəteis] 酸性磷酸酶(测定血清酸性磷酸酶为一重要诊断试验,前列腺癌已转移者,此酶显著增高,佩吉特〈Paget〉病、甲状旁腺功能亢进、骨癌和其他病理病变时中度增高。亦称酸性磷酸单酯酶)

acidulate [əˈsidjuleit] *vt* 酸化 | **~d** *a* / **acidulation** [əˌsidjuˈleiʃən] *n*

acidulous [əˈsidjuləs], **acidulent** [əˈsidjulənt] *a* 微酸的,带酸味的

acidum [ˈæsidəm] *n*【拉】酸

aciduria [ˌæsiˈdjuəriə] *n* 酸尿 | acetoacetic ~ 乙酰乙酸尿 / argininosuccinic ~ 精氨基琥珀酸尿,精氨基琥珀酸裂合酶缺乏症 / betaaminoisobutyric ~ β-氨基异丁酸尿 / ethylmalonic-adipic ~ 乙基丙二酸己二酸尿 / glutaric ~ (GA) 戊二酸尿 / methylmalonic ~ 甲基丙二酸尿 / orotic ~ 乳清酸尿 / pyroglutamic ~ 焦谷氨酸尿,5-羟脯氨酸尿

aciduric [ˌæsiˈdjuərik] *a* 耐酸的

acidyl [ˈæsidil] *n* 酸基;酰基

acidylation [əˌsidiˈleiʃən] *n* 酰化[作用]

acinesia [ˌæsiˈniːziə] *n* 运动不能,失运动能 | **acinetic** [ˌæsiˈnetik] *a*

Acinetobacter [ˌæsiˌnetəuˈbæktə] *n* 不动杆菌属 | ~ anitratus 硝酸盐阴性不动杆菌 / ~ calcoaceticus 醋酸钙不动杆菌(亦称阴道赫尔菌 Herellea vaginicola,多形模仿菌 Mima polymorpha) / ~ lwoffi 鲁氏不动杆菌

aciniform [əˈsinifɔːm] *a* 腺泡状的,葡萄状的

acinitis [ˌæsiˈnaitis] *n* 腺泡炎

acinitrazole [ˌæsiˈnaitrəzəul] *n* 醋胺硝唑(抗滴虫药)

acinotubular [ˌæsinəuˈtjuːbjulə] *a* 管状腺泡的

acinus [ˈæsinəs] *n* 腺泡 | **acinar** [ˈæsinə], **acinic** [əˈsinik] *a* 腺泡的 / **acinous** [ˈæsinəs], **acinose** [ˈæsinəus] *a* 腺泡状的,葡萄状的;腺泡的

acipenserin [ˌæsiˈpensərin] *n* 鳣鱼毒素

acitretin [ˌæsiˈtretin] *n* 阿维 A(阿维 A 酯的主要代谢产物,用于治疗重度银屑病,口服给药)

acivicin [ˌæsiˈvaisin] *n* 阿西维辛(谷氨酰胺拮抗剂,用于治疗各种实体瘤,静注给药)

ackee [ˈækiː] *n* 西非荔枝果(见 akee)

acladiosis [ˌæklædiˈəusis] *n* 皮疡真菌病,皮疡霉菌病

Acladium [əˈkleidiəm] *n* 皮疡真菌属

aclasis [ˈækləsis] *n* 续连症,病态连接(如软骨营养不良时) | diaphyseal ~ 骨干性续连症,软骨发育障碍 / tarsoepiphyseal ~ 半肢畸形骨骺发育不良 | **aclasia** [əˈkleiziə] *n* / **aclastic** [eiˈklæstik] *a* 续连症的;不折射的

acleistocardia [əˌklaistəuˈkɑːdiə] *n* [心]卵圆孔未闭

aclusion [əˈkluːʒən] *n* 无殆

acme [ˈækmi] *n* 极期

acmesthesia [ˌækmisˈθiːzjə] *n* [皮肤]尖端触觉感,针刺感

acne [ˈækni] *n* 痤疮 | beatle ~ 皮脂溢性皮炎 / chlorine ~, halowax ~ 氯痤疮 / ~ excoriée des jeunes filles 少女人工痤疮 / ~ keloid 瘢痕疙瘩性痤疮 / ~ neonatorum 新生儿痤疮 / ~ rosacea 红色痤疮,酒渣鼻 / ~ varioliformis, ~ frontalis 痘样痤疮,额面痤疮 / ~ vulgaris, common ~ 寻常痤疮

acnegen [ˈæknidʒən] *n* 致痤疮物质

acnegenic [ˌækniˈdʒenik] *a* 致痤疮的

acneiform [ækˈniːifɔːm], **acneform** [ˈæknifɔːm] *a* 痤疮样的

acnemia [ækˈniːmiə] *n* 腓肠部萎缩

acnitis [ækˈnaitis] *n* 痤疮炎,丘疹坏死性结核疹

acnitrazole [ækˈnaitrəzəul] *n* 醋胺硝唑,胺硝噻唑(抗滴虫药)

ACNM American College of Nurse-Midwives 美国助产护士学会

acoasma [ˌeikəuˈæsmə] *n* 幻听,听幻觉

Acocanthera, Acokanthera [ˌækəukænˈθiərə] *n* 箭毒木属(夹竹桃科)

acocantherin [ˌækəuˈkænθərin] *n* 乌本[箭毒]苷,毒毛旋花苷 G

Acoela [əˈsiːlə] *n* 无腔目

acoelomate [əˈsiːləmeit] *a* 无体腔的 *n* 无体腔动物(如扁蠕虫)

acoenesthesia [əˌsenesˈθiːzjə] *n* 存在感觉缺失

ACOG American College of Obstetricians and Gynecologists 美国妇产科医师学会

acognosia [ˌækɔgˈnəusiə], **acognosy** [əˈkɔgnəsi] *n* 治疗论

acology [əˈkɔlədʒi] *n* 治疗学

acolumellate [ˌeikɔljuˈmeleit] *a* 无囊轴的(指某些原虫和真菌)

aconative [əˈkɔnətiv] *a* 意向缺失的,非意志的,无意念的

Aconchulinida [əˌkɔntʃuˈlinidə] *n* 无壳目

aconine [ˈækənin] *n* 乌头原碱

aconitase [əˈkɔniteis] *n* 顺乌头酸酶

***cis*-aconitate** [əˈkɔniteit] *n* 顺乌头酸

aconitate hydratase [əˈkɔniteit ˈhaidrəteis] 乌头酸水合酶(亦称乌头酸酶)

aconite [ˈækənait] *n* 乌头

aconitine [əˈkɔnitin] *n* 乌头碱

Aconitum [ækəˈnaitəm] *n*【拉】乌头属

aconuresis [ˌækɔnjuəˈriːsis] *n* 小便失禁

acoprosis [ˌækəˈprəusis] *n* 肠内空虚(肠内粪便缺乏) | **acoprous** [əˈkɔprəs] *a*

acor [ˈeikɔː] *n*【拉】酸涩;辛辣

acorea [ˌækəˈriə] *n* 无瞳

acoria [əˈkɔːriə] *n* 贪食,不饱[症]

acorin [ˈækərin] *n* 菖蒲苦苷

acorn [ˈeikɔːn] *n* 槲果,橡子

acortan [eiˈkɔːtən] *n* 促皮质素,促肾上腺皮质激素

Acorus [ˈækərəs] *n*【拉】菖蒲属

ACOS American College of Osteopathic Surgeons 美国整骨疗法外科医师学会

Acosta's disease [əˈkɔstə] (José d'Acosta) 急性高山病

acou- [构词成分] 听,听觉

acouesthesia [əˌkuːesˈθiːzjə] *n* 听觉

acoumeter [əˈkuːmitə], **acouometer** [ˌækuːˈɔmitə] *n* 听力计,听力测验器 | **acoumetry** *n* 听力测验法

acouophone [ˈækuːəfəun] *n* 助听器

acousma [əˈkuːsmə], **acouasm** [əˈkuːæzəm] *n* 幻听,听幻觉

acousmatamnesia [əˌkuːsmætæmˈniːzjə] *n* 听觉性健忘[症]

acoustic(al) [əˈkuːstik(əl)] *a* 听的;声学的

acoustician [ˌækuːsˈtiʃən] *n* 声学家,声学工作者

acousticophobia [əˌkuːstikəuˈfəubjə] *n* 听声恐怖,恐声症

acoustics [əˈkuːstiks] *n* 声学

acoustogram [əˈkuːstəgræm], **acoustigram** [əˈkuːstigræm] *n* 关节音图(一种记录关节运动所发声音的频率曲线图)

acoutometer [ˌækuːˈtɔmitə] *n* 听力计,听力测验器

ACP American College of Pathologists 美国病理学家学会;American College of Physicians 美国内科医师学会

ACPS acrocephalopolysyndactyly 尖头多指并指[畸形],尖头多趾并趾[畸形]

acquiescence [ˌækwiˈesns] *n* 默认

acquired [əˈkwaiəd] *a* 获得的,后天的

acquisition [ˌækwiˈziʃən] *n* 习得,获得

acquisitus [əˈkwisitəs] *a*【拉】获得的,后天的

ACR American College of Radiology 美国放射学会

acragnosis [ˌækrəgˈnəusis] *n* 肢体感觉缺失

acral [ˈækrəl] *a* 肢的,肢端的

acrania [əˈkreiniə] *n* 无颅盖

acranial [əˈkreiniəl] *a* 无颅的

Acraniata [əˌkreiniˈeitə] *n* 无头亚门

acranius [əˈkreiniəs] *n* 无颅畸胎

Acrasia [əˈkreisiə] *n* 混胶丝纲

Acrasida [əˈkreisidə] *n* 混胶丝目

Acrasis [əˈkreisis] *n* 混胶丝虫属

acraturesis [əˌkrætjuəˈriːsis] *n* 排尿无力

Acrel's ganglion [ˈækrəl] (Olof 或 Olaf Acrel) 阿克雷尔腱鞘囊肿(腕伸肌腱鞘囊肿)

Acremoniella [ˌækriməuniˈelə] *n* 小支顶孢属

acremoniosis [ˌækriməuniˈəusis] *n* 支顶孢病

Acremonium [ˌækriˈməuniəm] *n* 支顶孢属
acribometer [ˌækriˈbɔmitə] *n* 精微测量器
acrid [ˈækrid] *a* 辛辣的;腐蚀性的
acridine [ˈækridin] *n* 吖啶,一氮蒽 | ~ orange 吖啶橙
acriflavine [ˌækriˈfleivin] *n* 吖啶黄(消毒防腐药) | ~ hydrochloride 盐酸吖啶黄 / neutral ~ 中性吖啶黄,吖啶黄
acrinyl sulfocyanate [æˈkrainil] 羟苄基硫氰酸酯,硫氰酸对羟基苯甲酯
acrisorcin [əkriˈsɔːsin] *n* 吖啶琐辛(抗感染药,外用治疗花斑癣)
acritical [əˈkritikəl] *a* 无极期的,无危象的(尤指热病消退)
acritochromacy [ˌəkritəuˈkrəuməsi] *n* 色盲
ACRM American Congress of Rehabilitation Medicine 美国康复医学协会
acroagnosis [ˌækrəuægˈnəusis] *n* 肢体感觉缺失
acroanesthesia [ˌækrəuˌænisˈθiːzjə] *n* [四]肢麻木,肢端麻木
acroarthritis [ˌækrəuɑːˈθraitis] *n* 肢关节炎
acroblast [ˈækrəblæst] *n* 原顶体(精细胞的高尔基〈Golgi〉物质,由此长出顶体)
acrobrachycephaly [ˌækrəuˌbrækiˈsefəli] *n* 扁头[畸形]
acrobystiolith [ˌækrəuˈbistiəliθ] *n* 包皮结石
acrobystitis [ˌækrəubisˈtaitis] *n* 包皮炎
acrocentric [ˌækrəˈsentrik] *a* 近端着丝粒的
acrocephalia [ˌækrəusiˈfeiliə] *n* 尖头[畸形] | **acrocephalic** [ˌækrəusiˈfælik], **acrocephalous** [ˌækrəˈsefələs] *a*
acrocephalopolysyndactyly (**ACPS**) [ˌækrəuˌsefələu, pɔlisinˈdæktili] *n* 尖头多指并指[畸形],尖头多趾并趾[畸形]
acrocephalosyndactyly [ˌækrəuˌsefələu sinˈdæktili], **acrocephalosyndactylia** [ˌækrəuˌsefələuˌsindækˈtiliə], **acrocephalosyndactylism** [ˌækrəuˌsefələusinˈdæktilizəm] *n* 尖头并指[畸形],尖头并趾[畸形]
acrocephaly [ˌækrəˈsefəli] *n* 尖头[畸形] | ~ syndactyly 尖头并指[畸形],尖头并趾[畸形]
acrochordon [ˌækrəˈkɔːdən] *n* 软垂疣(一般发生在颈或眼睑的有蒂新生物)
acrocinesis [ˌækrəusaiˈniːsis] *n* 运动过度 | **acrocinetic** [ˌækrəusaiˈnetik] *a*
acrocontracture [ˌækrəukənˈtræktʃə] *n* [四]肢挛缩
acrocyanosis [ˌækrəuˌsaiəˈnəusis] *n* 肢端发绀,手足发绀
acrodermatitis [ˌækrəuˌdəːməˈtaitis] *n* 肢端皮炎
acrodermatosis [ˌækrəuˌdəːməˈtəusis] ([复] **acrodermatoses** [ˌækrəuˌdəːməˈtəusiːz] *n* 肢端皮病
acrodolichomelia [ˌækrəuˌdɔlikəuˈmiliə] *n* 手足过长
acrodont [ˈækrədɔnt] *a* 颌缘牙的,端生牙的
acrodynia [ˌækrəuˈdiniə] *n* 肢痛症(一种婴儿病,特征为指和趾痛、肿及红色,有急躁、不安、怕光、出汗等症状。亦称红皮水肿性多发性神经病)
acrodysplasia [ˌækrəudisˈpleisiə] *n* 尖头并指[畸形],尖头并趾[畸形]
acroesthesia [ˌækrəuesˈθiːzjə] *n* 感觉过敏;肢痛
acrogenous [əˈkrɔdʒənəs] *a* 顶生的(指分生孢子)
acrognosis [ˌækrɔgˈnəusis] *n* 肢体感
acrohypothermy [ˌækrəuˌhaipəuˈθəːmi] *n* 手足温度过低
acrohysterosalpingectomy [ˌækrəuˌhistərəuˌsælpinˈdʒektəmi] *n* 子宫底输卵管切除术
acrokeratosis [ˌækrəuˌkerəˈtəusis] *n* 肢端角化症
acrokinesia [ˌækrəukaiˈniːziə] *n* 运动过度
acrolein [əˈkrəuliːn] *n* 丙烯醛
acromacria [ˌækrəuˈmækriə] *n* 细长指,细长趾,蜘蛛脚样指,蜘蛛脚样趾
acromania [ˌækrəuˈmeinjə] *n* 重躁狂
acromastitis [ˌækrəumæsˈtaitis] *n* 乳头炎
acromegalogigantism [ˌækrəu ˌmegələu ˈdʒaigæntizəm] *n* 肢端肥大性巨大畸形
acromegaloidism [ˌækrəuˈmegəlɔidizəm] *n* 类肢端肥大症
acromegaly [ˌækrəuˈmegəli], **acromegalia** [ˌækrəumiˈgeiliə] *n* 肢端肥大症 | **acromegalic** [ˌækrəumiˈgælik] *a*
acromelalgia [ˌækrəumiˈlældʒiə] *n* 红斑性肢痛病
acromelic [ˌækrəuˈmiːlik] *a* 肢端的
acrometagenesis [ˌækrəuˌmetəˈdʒenisis] *n* 四肢发育过度
acromial [əˈkrəumiəl] *a* 肩峰的
acromicria, acromikria [ˌækrəuˈmikriə] *n* 肢端过小症
acromi(o)- [构词成分] 肩峰
acromioclavicular [əˌkrəumiəukləˈvikjulə] *a* 肩峰锁骨的
acromiocoracoid [əˌkrəumiəuˈkɔːrəkɔid] *a* 肩峰喙突的
acromiohumeral [əˌkrəumiəuˈhjuːmərəl] *a* 肩峰肱骨的
acromion [əˈkrəumiɔn] *n* 肩峰
acromionectomy [əˌkrəumiəuˈnektəmi] *n* 肩峰切除术
acromioscapular [əˌkrəumiəuˈskæpjulə] *a* 肩峰肩胛的
acromiothoracic [əˌkrəumiəuθɔ(ː)ˈræsik] *a* 肩峰

胸廓的
acromphalus [əˈkrɔmfələs] *n* 脐膨出;脐心
acromyotonia [ˌækrəumaiəˈtəuniə], **acromyotonus** [ˌækrəumaiˈɔtənəs] *n* 肢肌强直
acronarcotic [ˌækrəunɑːˈkɔtik] *a* 辛辣麻醉的
acroneurosis [ˌækrəunjuəˈrəusis] *n* 肢体神经[功能]病,肢体神经症
acronine [ˈeikrənin] *n* 阿克罗宁(抗肿瘤药)
acronym [ˈækrənim] *n* 首字母缩略词,头字语(如 laser,由 *l*ight *a*mplication by *s*timulated *e*mission of *r*adiation 中各主要词的第一个字母缩合而成)
acro-osteolysis [ˌækrəuˌɔstiˈɔlisis] *n* 肢端骨质溶解
acropachia [ˌækrəuˈpækiə] *n* 杵变病(指犬)
acropachy [ˈækrəuˌpæki] *n* 杵状指,肥大性肺性骨关节病
acropachyderma [ˌækrəuˌpækiˈdəːmə] *n* 肢端厚皮病
acroparalysis [ˌækrəupəˈrælisis] *n* 肢麻痹,肢瘫痪
acroparesthesia [ˌækrəuˌpærisˈθiːzjə] *n* 肢端感觉异常
acropathology [ˌækrəupəˈθɔlədʒi] *n* [四]肢病理学
acropathy [əˈkrɔpəθi] *n* [四]肢病
acropeptide [ˌækrəuˈpeptaid] *n* 无色肽(蛋白质在非水溶剂中加热至 140 ℃以上所得到的部分)
acropetal [əˈkrɔpitl] *a* 趋向顶端的
acrophobia [ˌækrəˈfəubjə] *n* 高处恐怖,恐高症
acropleurogenous [ˌækrəupluːˈrɔdʒənəs] *a* 顶侧生的(指分生孢子)
acroposthitis [ˌækrəupɔsˈθaitis] *n* 包皮炎
acropurpura [ˌækrəuˈpəːpjurə] *n* 肢端紫癜(尤指指、趾)
acropustulosis [ˌækrəuˌpʌstjuˈləusis] *n* 肢端脓疱病 | infantile ~ 婴儿肢端脓疱病
acrosclerosis [ˌækrəuskliəˈrəusis], **acroscleroderma** [ˌækrəuˌskliərəuˈdəːmə] *n* 肢端硬化病
acrosin [ˈækrəsin] *n* 顶体蛋白,顶体素
acrosome [ˈækrəusəum] *n* 顶体(精子)
acrosphenosyndactylia [ˌækrəuˌsfinəuˌsindækˈtiliə] *n* 尖头并指[畸形],尖头并趾[畸形]
acrospiroma [ˌækrəuspiˈrəumə] *n* 顶端螺旋瘤 | eccrine ~ 小汗腺顶端螺旋瘤,透明细胞汗腺瘤
acrostealgia [æˌkrɔstiˈældʒiə] *n* 肢骨痛
acrosyndactyly [ˌækrəusinˈdæktili] *n* 末端并指,末端并趾
acroteric [ˌækrəuˈterik] *a* 末梢的,周围的
Acrotheca [ˌækrəˈθiːkə] *n* 产色芽生菌属
Acrothecium [ˌækrəˈθiːsiəm] 表皮癣菌属
acrotic [əˈkrɔtik] *a* 无脉的,弱脉的
acrotism [ˈækrətizəm] *n* 无脉,弱脉,脉搏微茫
acrotrophodynia [ˌækrəuˌtrɔfəuˈdiniə] *n* 营养性肢痛症
acrotrophoneurosis [ˌækrəuˌtrɔfəunjuəˈrəusis] *n* 肢端营养神经病
acrylaldehyde [ˌækrilˈældihaid] *n* 丙烯醛
acrylamide [əˈkriləmaid] *n* 丙烯酰胺
acrylate [ˈækrileit] *n* 丙烯酸盐(或酯)
acrylic [əˈkrilik] *a* 丙烯酸的 | ~ acid 丙烯酸
acrylonitrile [ˌækriləuˈnaitril, -trail] *n* 丙烯腈
ACS American Cancer Society 美国癌症学会; American Chemical Society 美国化学学会; American College of Surgeons 美国外科医师学会
ACSM American College of Sports Medicine 美国运动医学会
act [ækt] *n* 行为,动作;法令,条例 *vi* 行动;充任,担任;起作用 | compulsive ~, imperious ~ 强迫动作 / impulsive ~ 冲动性动作 / reflex ~ 反射动作
Actaea [ækˈtiːə] *n* 类叶升麻属
actaplanin [ˌæktəˈpleinin] *n* 阿克他宁,阿克他菌素(抗生素类药)
ACTe anodal closure tetanus 阳极通电强直
ACTH adrenocorticotropic hormone 促肾上腺皮质激素,促皮质素
actin [ˈæktin] *n* 肌动蛋白
Actineliida [ˌæktiniˈlaiidə] *n* 辐射虫目
acting out [ˈæktiŋ aut] 潜意识显露
actinic [ækˈtinik] *a* 光化[性]的 | **~ity** [ˌæktiˈnisəti] *n* 光化力
actiniform [ækˈtinifɔːm] *a* 放射形的,放线状的
α-actinin [ˈæktinin] *n* α-辅肌动蛋白
actinine [ˈæktinin] *n* 海葵素
actinism [ˈæktinizəm] *n* 光化力;射线化学
actinium(Ac) [ækˈtiniəm] *n* 锕(化学元素)
actinobacillosis [ˌæktinəuˌbæsiˈləusis] *n* 放线杆菌病
Actinobacillus [ˌæktinəubəˈsiləs] *n* 放线杆菌属 | ~ actinoides 类放线杆菌 / ~ actinomycetemcomitans 放线共生放线杆菌,伴放线放线杆菌 / ~ lignieresii 利尼耶尔放线杆菌 / ~ mallei 鼻疽放线杆菌
Actinobifida [ˌæktinəuˈbifidə] *n* 双歧放线菌属
actinobolin [ˌæktiˈnɔbəlin] *n* 放线菌光素
Actinocephalus [ˌæktinəuˈsefələs] *n* 辐头属
actinochemistry [ˌæktinəuˈkemistri] *n* 光化学
actinochitin [ˌæktinəuˈkaitin] *n* 放线菌壳多糖
actinocongestin [ˌæktinəukənˈdʒestin] *n* 海葵[毒]素

actinocutitis [ˌæktinəukjuːˈtaitis], **actinodermatitis** [ˌæktinəuˌdəːməˈtaitis] *n* X 线皮炎,射线皮炎
actinodaphnine [ˌæktinəuˈdæfnin] *n* 樟碱,黄肉楠碱
actinodiastase [ˌæktinəuˈdaiəsteis] *n* 腔肠淀粉酶
actinoerythrin [ˌæktinəuˈeriθrin] *n* 赤海葵红素,海葵赤素
actinogen [ækˈtinədʒən] *n* 射线质
actinogenesis [ˌæktinəuˈdʒenisis] *n* 射线发生 | **actinogenic** [ˌæktinəuˈdʒenik] *a*
actinogenics [ˌæktinəuˈdʒeniks] *n* 射线发生学
actinograph [ækˈtinəgrɑːf] *n* 光力计,[日光]光化力测定器,光化线强度记录器
actinohematin [ˌæktinəuˈhemətin] *n* 海葵正铁血红素
actinoid [ˈæktinɔid] *a* 放射线状的
actinolite, actinolyte [ækˈtinəlait] *n* 光化[学产]物;阳起石
actinology [ˌæktiˈnɔlədʒi] *n* 光化学;射线学
Actinomadura [ˌæktinəuˈmædjurə] *n* 马杜拉放线菌属 | ~ madurae 足肿马杜拉放线菌 / ~ pelletierii 白乐杰马杜拉放线菌
actinometer [ˌæktiˈnɔmitə] *n* 感光计;光化线强度计 | **actinometric** [ˌæktinəuˈmetrik] *a* / **actinometry** *n* 感光测定;光化线强度测定
actinomorphous [ˌæktinəuˈmɔfəs] *a* 放射型的,放射状的
actinomycelial [ˌæktinəumaiˈsiːliəl] *a* 放线菌丝体的;放线菌的
Actinomyces [ˌæktinəuˈmaisiːz] *n* 放线菌属 | ~ actinoides 类放线菌 / ~ bovis 牛型放线菌 / ~ israelii 以色列放线菌(不耐酸的厌氧放线菌)
actinomyces [ˌæktinəuˈmaisiːz] ([复] **actinomycetes** [ˌæktinəumaiˈsiːtiːz]) *n* 放线菌 | **actinomycetic** [ˌæktinəumaiˈsetik] *a*
Actinomycetaceae [ˌæktinəuˌmaisiˈteisiiː] *n* 放线菌科
Actinomycetales [ˌæktinəuˌmaisiˈteiliːz] *n* 放线菌目
actinomycete [ˌæktinəuˈmaisiːt] *n* 放线菌 | **actinomycetous** [ˌæktinəumaiˈsiːtəs] *a*
actinomycetin [ˌæktinəumaiˈsiːtin] *n* 白放线菌素
actinomycetoma [ˌæktinəuˌmaisiˈtəumə] *n* 放线菌性足分支菌病
actinomycin [ˌæktinəuˈmaisin] *n* 放线菌素
actinomycoma [ˌæktinəumaiˈkəumə] *n* 放线菌肿
actinomycosis [ˌæktinəumaiˈkəusis] *n* 放线菌病 | **actinomycotic** [ˌæktinəumaiˈkɔtik] *a*
actinomycotin [ˌæktinəuˈmaikətin] *n* 放线菌体素
Actinomyxia [ˌæktinəuˈmiksiə] *n* 放射孢子亚纲
Actinomyxida [ˌæktinəuˈmiksidə] *n* 放射孢子目
actinon [ˈæktinɔn] *n* 锕射气(氡 219)
actinoneuritis [ˌæktinəunjuəˈraitis] *n* 放射性神经炎
actinophage [ækˈtinəfeidʒ] *n* 放线菌噬菌体
Actinophryida [ˌæktinəuˈfriːidə] *n* 太阳虫目
actinophytosis [ˌæktinəufaiˈtəusis] *n* 放线菌病,诺卡菌病
Actinoplanaceae [ˌæktinəupləˈneisiiː] *n* 游动放线菌科
Actinoplanes [ˌæktinəuˈpleiniːz] *n* 游动放线菌属
Actinopoda [ˌæktiˈnɔpədə] *n* 辐足亚纲(原生动物)
actinoquinol sodium [ækˈtinəkwinəul] 阿克汀喹钠(紫外线遮蔽剂)
Actinosporea [ˌæktinəuˈspɔːriə] *n* 放线孢子纲
actinotherapy [ˌæktinəuˈθerəpi], **actinotherapeutics** [ˌæktinəuˌθerəˈpjuːtiks] *n* 射线疗法(用紫外线或光化射线治病)
actinotoxemia [ˌæktinəutɔkˈsiːmiə] *n* 放射性毒血症
actinotoxin [ˌæktinəuˈtɔksin] *n* 海葵触须毒[素]
actinouranium [ˌæktinəujuəˈreinjəm] *n* 锕铀(铀的同位素)
action [ˈækʃən] *n* 行动,行为,活动;功能;作用 | ball-valve ~ 球瓣作用(异物所致的间歇性阻塞) / buffer ~, tampon ~ 缓冲作用 / calorigenic ~ 生热作用 / capillary ~ 毛细[管]吸引 / contact ~ 接触催化[作用] / cumulative ~ 蓄积作用(突然增加强度的作用,如服用某一药物数剂后其生物效应比服用第一剂后为大) / diastasic ~, diastatic ~ 淀粉糖化作用 / opsonic ~ 调理素作用(调理素对细菌和其他细胞所起的作用,使其增加对吞噬作用的易感性) / reflex ~ 反射动作 / specific dynamic ~ 特殊动力作用(食物消化和同化作用促使新陈代谢超过基础代谢率,脂肪和碳水化合物增加 4% ~6%,蛋白质增加 30%) / thermogenic ~ 升温作用,产热作用 / trigger ~ 激发作用(一种释放能量的作用,其性质与其释放能量的过程无关)
activable [ˈæktivəbl] *a* 能被活化的
activate [ˈæktiveit] *vt* 使活动;活化,激活 | **activation** [ˌæktiˈveiʃən] *n*
activator [ˈæktiˌveitə] *n* 活化剂,激活剂;双颌式功能矫正器 | functional ~, monoblock ~ 功能矫正器 / plasminogen ~ 纤溶酶原激活物 / polyclonal ~ 多克隆活化因子 / tissue ~ 纤维蛋白激活酶
active [ˈæktiv] *a* 活动的;积极的;有效的,活性的;自动的,主动的 | optically ~ 有旋光力的
activin [ˈæktivin] *n* 激活素(一种非类固醇调节

素,促卵泡激素分泌,其作用与抑制素〈inhibin〉相反)

activity [æk'tivəti] *n* 活动[度];活性 | displacement ~ 替换活动(生物体内两个相冲突的内驱力,其中过多的一个所产生的无关系活动)/ enzyme ~ 酶活性 / leukemia-associated inhibitory ~ (LIA) 白血病相关抑制活性 / nonsuppressible insulin-like ~ (NSILA) 非抑制性胰岛素样活性 / optical ~ 旋光性,旋光度 / specific ~ 比活性,比放射性

activize, activise ['æktivaiz] *vt* 使活动;活化,激活

actodigin [ˌæktəu'didʒin] *n* 阿托地近(强心药)

actometer [æk'tɔmitə] *n* 活动度测量计(如运动过度时,测量水平面运动所反映出的活动度)

actomyosin [ˌæktəu'maiəsin] *n* 肌动球蛋白

Actonia [æk'təuniə] *n* 假膜形成酵母菌属

actor ['æktə] *n* 行为者;作用物,反应物

ACTP adrenocorticotropic polypeptide 促肾上腺皮质多肽(一种促肾上腺皮质激素的水解产物)

acu- [构词成分] 针,尖锐

Acuaria [ˌækju'ɛəriə] *n* 锐形[线虫]属

acuclosure [ˌækju'kləuʒə] *n* 针止血法

acuesthesia [ˌækjuis'θiːzjə] *n* 听觉

acufilopressure [ˌækju'failəpreʃə] *n* 针线压迫法(针压与结扎并用以止血)

acuity [ə'kju(ː)iti] *n* 敏度(尤指视力) | visual ~ 视敏度,视力

aculeate [ə'kjuːliit] *a* 有刺的,尖的

acumen [ə'kjuːmen] *n* 敏锐,聪明

acumeter [ə'kuːmitə] *n* 听力计,听力测验器

acuminate [ə'kjuːminit] *a* 尖的,尖锐的 [ə'kjuːmineit] *vt* 使尖,使尖锐 | **acumination** [əˌkjuːmi'neiʃən] *n*

acupoint ['ækjupɔint] *n* [针刺]穴位

acupressure ['ækjuˌpreʃə], **acupression** [ˌækju'preʃən] *n* 针压法(插针于相邻组织压迫血管止血)

acupuncture ['ækjupʌŋktʃə] *n* 针刺疗法,针术,针刺 [ˌækju'pʌŋktʃə] *vt* 对…施行针疗 | auricular ~ 耳针[术]

acupuncturist [ˌækju'pʌŋktʃərist] *n* 针灸医师,针疗医师

acus ['eikəs] *n*【拉】针;针状突

acusection ['ækjuˌsekʃən] *n* 电针切开术

acusector ['ækjuˌsektə] *n* 电针刀(分离组织用)

acute [ə'kjuːt] *a* 急性的

acutorsion [ˌækju'tɔːʃən] *n* 针扭转法(控制出血)

acyanoblepsia [əˌsaiənəu'blepsiə], **acyanopsia** [əˌsaiə'nɔpsiə] *n* 蓝色盲

acyanotic [eiˌsaiə'nɔtik] *a* 不发绀的

acyclia [ə'saikliə] *n* 体液循环停止

acyclic [ei'saiklik, ei'si-] *a* 无环族的,开链式的;无周期性的(如月经周期)

acyclovir [ei'saikləvi(r)] *n* 阿昔洛韦(抗病毒药)

acyesis [ˌæsai'iːsis] *n* 不孕,不育;无妊娠

acyl ['æsil] *n* 酰[基]

acylase ['æsileis] *n* 酰基转移酶

acylation [ˌæsi'leiʃən] *n* 酰化作用

acylcholine acylhydrolase [ˌæsil'kəulin ˌæsil'haidrəleis] 酰基胆碱酰基水解酶,胆碱酯酶

acyl-CoA ['æsil kəu'ei] 酰基辅酶 A

acyl-CoA: cholesterol acyltransferase ['æsil kəu'ei kə'lestərɔl ˌæsil'trænsfəreis] 酰基辅酶 A:胆固醇酰基转移酶,固醇 *O*-酰基转移酶

acyl-CoA dehydrogenase ['æsil kəu'ei diː'haidrədʒəneis] 酰基辅酶 A 脱氢酶 | long-chain ~ ~ (LACD) deficiency 长链酰基辅酶 A 脱氢酶缺乏症(临床上类似 MCAD 缺乏症,尿排泄长链二羧酸,可能有骨骼肌软弱无力和心脏扩大)/ medium-chain ~ ~ (MCAD) deficiency 中链酰基辅酶 A 脱氢酶缺乏症(特征为低血糖、呕吐和嗜眠反复发作,伴有尿排泄中链二羧酸、最小酮体生成及血浆和组织肉碱浓度低)/ short-chain ~ ~ (SCAD) deficiency 短链酰基辅酶 A 脱氢酶缺乏症(临床显示不定,但常存在肌病和肉碱累积与排泄异常)

acyl-CoA desaturase ['æsil kəu'ei diː'sætʃəreis] 酰基辅酶 A 去饱和酶(亦称硬脂酰基辅酶 A 去饱和酶)

acyl-CoA synthetase ['æsil kəu'ei 'sinθiteis] 酰基辅酶 A 合成酶

acyl-CoA synthetase (GDP-forming) ['æsil kəu'ei 'sinθiteis] 酰基辅酶 A(GDP 形成的),酸性辅酶 A 连接酶(GDP 形成的)

acyl coenzyme A ['æsil kəu'enzaim] 酰基辅酶 A

acylglycerol [ˌæsil'glisərɔl] *n* 酰基甘油,甘油酯

2-acylglycerol *O*-acyltransferase [ˌæsil'glisərɔl ˌæsil'trænsfəreis] 2-酰基甘油 *O*-酰基转移酶(此反应发生于肠黏膜,亦称酰基甘油棕榈酰转移酶和单酸甘油酯酰基转移酶)

acylglycerol lipase [ˌæsil'glisərɔl 'laipeis] 酰基甘油脂[肪]酶

acylglycerol palmitoyltransferase [ˌæsil'glisərɔl ˌpælmiˌtɔil'trænsfəreis] 酰基甘油棕榈酰转移酶,2-酰基甘油 *O*-酰基转移酶

acylmutase [ˌæsil'mjuteis] *n* 酰基变位酶

***N*-acylneuraminate cytidylyltransferase** [ˌæsilnjuə'ræmineit ˌsaitidilil'trænsfəreis] *N*-酰基神经氨酸胞苷酰[基]转移酶

***N*-acylneuraminic acid** [ˌæsilˌnjuərə'minik] *N*-酰基神经氨酸,唾液酸

acylphosphatase [ˌæsil'fɔsfəteis] *n* 酰基磷酸

酯酶

***N*-acylsphingosine** [æsilˈsfiŋgəsi:n] *N*-酰基[神经]鞘氨醇,神经酰胺

acylsphingosine deacylase [ˌæsil-, ˌeisilˈsfiŋgəu-si(:)n di:ˈæsileis, di:ˈeisileis] 酰基[神经]鞘氨醇脱酰[基]酶(此酶的遗传性缺乏为一种常染色体隐性性状,可致神经酰胺与神经节苷脂的贮积。亦称神经酰胺酶)

acyltransferase [ˌæsilˈtrænsfəreis] *n* 酰基转移酶

acystia [eiˈsistiə] *n* 无膀胱[畸形]

acystinervia [əˌsistiˈnə:viə], **acystineuria** [əˌsi-stiˈnjuəriə] *n* 膀胱神经无力

Acystosporidia [əˌsistəuspəˈridiə] *n* 无囊孢子虫目

AD alcohol dehydrogenase 醇脱氢酶; anodal duration 阳极期间; auris dextra【拉】右耳

ad [æd] *prep*【拉】加,加到,至 | ~ nauseam 至恶心为度 / ~ libitum 任意

ad- [前缀] 至,向,近

-ad [后缀] 向

ADA adenosine deaminase 腺苷脱氨酶; American Dental Association 美国牙科协会; American Diabetes Association 美国糖尿病协会; American Dietetic Association 美国饮食学协会

adactyly [eiˈdæktili], **adactylia** [ədækˈtiliə], **adactylism** [eiˈdæktilizəm] *n* 先天性无指,先天性无趾 | **adactylous** [eiˈdæktiləs] *a*

Adair Dighton's syndrome [əˈdɛəˈdaitən] (Charles Allen Adair Dighton) 成骨不全(Ⅰ型)

adamantine [ˌædəˈmæntin] *a* 釉质的

adamantinoma [ˌædəˌmæntiˈnəumə] *n* 成釉质细胞瘤 | pituitary ~ 颅咽管瘤 | **adamantoblastoma** [ˌædəˌmæntəublæsˈtəumə], **adamantoma** [ˌædəmænˈtəumə] *n*

adamantoblast [ˌædəˈmæntəblæst] *n* 成釉质细胞

ADAMHA Alcohol, Drug Abuse, and Mental Health Administration 乙醇、药物滥用与精神卫生管理局(属美国公共卫生署)

Adami's theory [æˈdæmi] (John G. Adami) 阿达米学说(一种解释遗传的假说,类似埃利希〈Ehrlich〉免疫侧锁学说)

Adamkiewicz's arteries [ədæmˈki:vitʃ] (Albert Adamkiewicz) 椎动脉脊支

adamsite [ˈædəmzait] *n* 亚当毒气,二苯胺氯胂(喷嚏性毒气)

Adams'operation [ˈædəmz] (William Adams) 亚当斯手术(股骨颈皮下囊内切断术,治髋关节强硬;掌腱膜皮下切断术,治掌挛缩病;矫正睑外翻的眼睑边缘楔形切除术) | ~ saw 亚当斯长柄小锯(切骨用)

Adams-Stokes disease (syncope, syndrome) [ˈædəmz ˈstəuks] (Robert Adams; William Stokes) 亚-斯病(晕厥、综合征),心源性脑缺氧综合征(一种心脏传导阻滞引起的病,其特征为突然神志丧失,有或无抽搐)

Adansonia [ˌædənˈsəuniə] (Michel Adanson) *n* 猴饼树属,猴面包属

adansonian [ˌædənˈsəuniən] *a* 亚当森(Michel Adanson)的,数值分类的

adapalene [əˈdæpəli:n] *n* 阿达帕林(一种合成维A酸类似物,局部用于治疗寻常痤疮)

adaptation [ˌædæpˈteiʃən] *n* 适应[作用] | dark ~, scotopic ~ 暗适应(指眼) / genetic ~ 遗传适应(突变种后代的自然选择更能适应新环境) / phenotypic ~ 表型适应(环境改变时,生物体表型起变化,遗传型不起变化) / retinal ~ 视网膜适应

adapter, adaptor [əˈdæptə] *n* 接合器;接合体

adaptometer [ˌædæpˈtəmitə] *n* 适应计(用于检夜盲、维生素A缺乏及色素性视网膜炎)

adaxial [ædˈæksiəl] *a* 近轴的,向轴的

ADC anodal duration contraction 阳极期间收缩; axiodistocervical 轴远中颈的

ADCC antibody-dependent cell-mediated cytotoxicity 抗体依赖性细胞介导的细胞毒作用

add [æd] *vt* 加,加上 *vi* 增加,增进 | **~able, ~ible** *a* 可添加的

add. adde 或 addetur【拉】加,加到,至 adde [ˈædi]【拉】加,加到,至

Ad def. an. ad defectionem animi【拉】至昏厥时

Ad deliq. ad deliquium【拉】至昏厥时

addendum [əˈdendəm] ([复] **addenda** [əˈdendə]) *n* 补遗;附录

adder¹ [ˈædə] *n* 添加者;加法器

adder² [ˈædə] *n* 蝰蛇(一种小毒蛇) | death ~ 致死毒蛇 / puff ~ 吹气蝰

addict [əˈdikt] *vt* 使吸毒成瘾 [ˈædikt] *n* 癖嗜者,成瘾者(尤指吸毒或饮酒成瘾的人)

addiction [əˈdikʃən] *n* 瘾,癖嗜,成瘾性(尤指吸毒成瘾) | drug ~ 药瘾 / polysurgical ~ [寻求]外科治疗癖

Addis count (method, test) [ˈædis] (Thomas Addis) 艾迪斯计数(法、试验)(测红细胞、白细胞、上皮细胞、管型及蛋白含量的数目,诊断和处理肾病)

addisin [ˈædisin] *n* 胃液抗贫血素(胃液中促骨髓形成的物质,如从猪胃液中的浸出物,用于治恶性贫血)

addisonian [ˌædiˈsəuniən] *a* 艾迪生(Thomas Addison)的(如 ~ anemia 恶性贫血, ~ disease 艾迪生病)

addisonism [ˈædisnizəm] (Thomas Addison) 类艾迪生病,艾迪生病型,类青铜色皮病(此病与结核有关,有色素沉着和虚弱等症状,类似艾迪生病的症状)

Addison's anemia [ˈædisn] (Thomas Addison) 恶性贫血,慢性肾上腺皮质功能不全性恶性贫血 | ~ disease 艾迪生病(肾上腺皮质功能减退,慢性肾上腺皮质功能不全) / ~ keloid 局限性皮硬化,硬斑病

Addison's planes [ˈædisn] (Christopher Addison) 艾迪生平面(一系列平面用作胸和腹局部解剖学的界标) | ~ point 艾迪生点(腹上区的中点)

additament [əˈditəmənt] *n* 附加物

additive [ˈæditiv] 加的,添加的,加性的(如加性效应) *n* 添加剂(一物质如调味剂、防腐剂或维生素加在另一物质上以改进它的外形,增加它的营养价值等)

addresin [əˈdresin] *n* 地址素(血管内皮细胞表面上的分子,使特异白细胞尤其是淋巴细胞附着在内皮上,与归巢淋巴细胞受体相结合)

adducent [əˈdjuːsnt] *a* 收的,内收的

adducin [əˈdjuːsin] *n* 内收蛋白(使肌动蛋白和血影蛋白结合的一种蛋白,据认为在红细胞膜血影蛋白-肌动蛋白复合物中起到一定作用)

adduct¹ [əˈdʌkt] *vt* 收,内收

adduct² [ˈædʌkt] *n* 加合物

adduction [əˈdʌkʃən] *n* 内收[作用]

adductor [əˈdʌktə] *n* 收肌

Adelea [əˈdeliə] *n* 匿虫属

Adeleina [ˌædəliˈainə] *n* 匿虫亚目

Adelmann's method [ˈɑːdəlmən] (Georg F. B. Adelmann) 阿德尔曼法(急救时用力弯屈肢体控制动脉出血) | ~ operation 阿德尔曼手术(掌指关节断离术)

adelomorphous [əˌdeləuˈmɔːfəs], **adelomorphic** [əˌdeləuˈmɔːfik] *a* 隐形的,不显形的

-adelphus [构词成分] 寄生胎

adenalgia [ˌædiˈnældʒiə] *n* 腺痛

adenase [ˈædineis] *n* 腺嘌呤[脱氨]酶

adenasthenia [ˌædənæsˈθiːniə] *n* 腺功能衰弱

adendritic [ˌeidənˈdritik], **adendric** [eiˈdendrik] *a* 无树突的

adenectomy [ˌædiˈnektəmi] *n* 腺切除术

adenectopia [ˌædinekˈtəupiə] *n* 腺异位

adenia [əˈdiːniə] *n* 淋巴腺增生病;假白血病

adenic [əˈdiːnik] *a* 腺的;腺样的

adeniform [əˈdenifɔːm] *a* 腺样的

adenine [ˈædəniːn] *n* 腺嘌呤 | ~ arabinoside 阿糖腺苷,腺嘌呤阿糖苷(抗病毒药) / ~ hypoxanthine 腺嘌呤次黄嘌呤 / ~ nucleotide 腺嘌呤核苷酸

adenine deaminase [ˈædəniːn, ˈædiniːn diːˈæmineis] 腺嘌呤脱氨酶

adenine phosphoribosyl transferase [ˈædəniːn ˌfɔsfəuˈraibəsil ˈtrænsfəreis] 腺嘌呤磷酸核糖基转移酶(此酶缺乏为一种常染色体稳性性状,可致婴儿绞痛、血尿及2, 8-二羟腺嘌呤性尿石)

adenine phosphoribosyl transferase deficiency 腺嘌呤磷酸核糖基转移酶缺乏症

adenitis [ˌædiˈnaitis] *n* 腺炎 | cervical ~ 颈腺炎,颈淋巴结炎 / mesenteric ~ 肠系膜淋巴结炎 / phlegmonous ~ 蜂窝织炎性腺炎 / ~ tropicalis 性病性淋巴肉芽肿

Adenium [əˈdiːniəm] *n* 箭毒胶属(夹竹桃科)

adenization [ˌædinaiˈzeiʃən] *n* 腺样变性,腺样化

aden(o)- [构词成分] 腺

adenoacanthoma [ˌædinəuˌækənˈθəumə], **adenocancroid** [ˌædinəuˈkæŋkrɔid] *n* 腺棘皮瘤

adenoameloblastoma [ˌædinəuəˌmeləublæsˈtəumə] *n* 腺性成釉质细胞瘤

adenoblast [ˈædinəuˌblæst] *n* 成腺细胞

adenocarcinoma [ˌædinəuˌkɑːsiˈnəumə] *n* 腺癌 | mucinous ~ 黏蛋白性腺癌 / papillary ~, polypoid ~ 乳头状腺癌,息肉状腺癌

adenocele [ˈædinəˌsiːl] *n* 腺囊肿

adenocellulitis [ˌædinəuˌseljuˈlaitis] *n* 腺蜂窝织炎

adenochondroma [ˌædinəukənˈdrəumə] *n* 腺软骨瘤

adenocystoma [ˌædinəusisˈtəumə], **adenocyst** [ˈædinəsist] *n* 腺囊瘤

adenocyte [ˈædinəsait] *n* 腺细胞

adenodynia [ˌædinəuˈdiniə] *n* 腺痛

adenoepithelioma [ˌædinəuˌepiˌθiːliˈəumə] *n* 腺上皮瘤

adenofibroma [ˌædinəufaiˈbrəumə] *n* 腺纤维瘤 | ~ edematodes 水肿性腺纤维瘤(如鼻息肉)

adenofibrosis [ˌædinəufaiˈbrəusis] *n* 腺纤维变性,腺纤维化

adenogenous [ˌædiˈnɔdʒinəs] *a* 腺源的,腺性的

adenography [ˌædiˈnɔgrəfi] *n* 腺X线摄影[术] | **adenographic** [ˌædinəuˈgræfik] *a*

adenohypophysectomy [ˌædinə u haiˌpɔfiˈsektəmi] *n* 腺垂体切除术

adenohypophysis [ˌædinəuhaiˈpɔfisis] *n* 腺垂体 | **adenohypophyseal, adenohypophysial** [ˌædinəuˌhaipəuˈfiziəl] *a*

adenoid [ˈædinɔid] *a* 腺样的,腺样体的 *n* [复]腺样体(指小儿的咽扁桃体)

adenoidal [ædiˈnɔidl] *a* 腺样的,腺样体的

adenoidectomy [ˌædinɔiˈdektəmi] *n* 腺样体切除术

adenoidism [ˈædinɔidizəm] *n* 腺样体病

adenoiditis [ˌædinɔiˈdaitis] *n* 腺样体炎

adenoleiomyofibroma [ˌædinəuˌlaiəˌmaiəufaiˈbrəumə] *n* 腺平滑肌纤维瘤

adenolipoma [ˌædinəuliˈpəumə] *n* 腺脂瘤

adenolipomatosis [ˌædinəuˌlipəuməˈtəusis] *n* 腺

脂瘤病

adenologaditis [ˌædinəuˌlɔgəˈdaitis] *n* 新生儿眼炎;眼腺结膜炎

adenology [ˌædiˈnɔlədʒi] *n* 腺学

adenolymphitis [ˌædinəulimˈfaitis] *n* 淋巴结炎(旧名淋巴腺炎)

adenolymphocele [ˌædinəuˈlimfəsiːl] *n* 淋巴结囊肿

adenolymphoma [ˌædinəulimˈfəumə] *n* 腺淋巴瘤

adenoma [ˌædiˈnəumə], ([复]**adenomata** [ˌædiˈnəumətə]或 **adenomas**) *n* 腺瘤 | acidophilic ~ 嗜酸性腺瘤(一般见于垂体前叶) / basophil ~, basophilic ~ 嗜碱性腺瘤(垂体前叶) / chromophobe ~, chromophobic ~ 嫌色性腺瘤(垂体前叶) / islet ~, langerhansian ~ 胰岛[腺]瘤 / malignant ~ 恶性腺瘤,腺癌 / racemose ~ 葡萄状腺瘤 / sebaceous ~ 皮脂腺腺瘤 | **~tous** [ˌædiˈnɔmətəs] *a*

adenomalacia [ˌædinəuməˈleiʃiə] *n* 腺软化

adenomatoid [ˌædiˈnəumətɔid] *a* 腺瘤样的

adenomatosis [ˌædinəuməˈtəusis] *n* 腺瘤病

adenomectomy [ˌædinəuˈmektəmi] *n* 腺瘤切除术

adenomegaly [ˌædinəuˈmegəli] *n* 腺[肿]大

adenomere [ˈædinəumiə] *n* 腺节

adenomyoepithelioma [ˌædinəuˌmaiəuˌepiˌθiːliˈəumə] *n* 腺肌上皮瘤

adenomyofibroma [ˌædinəuˌmaiəfaiˈbrəumə] *n* 腺肌纤维瘤

adenomyoma [ˌædinəumaiˈəumə] *n* 腺肌瘤 | ~ psammopapillare 沙粒乳头状腺肌瘤 | **~tous** [ˌædinəuˌmaiˈəumətəs] *a*

adenomyomatosis [ˌædinəuˌmaiəuməˈtəusis] *n* 腺肌瘤病

adenomyometritis [ˌædinəuˌmaiəumiˈtraitis] *n* 子宫腺肌炎

adenomyosarcoma [ˌædinəuˌmaiəusɑːˈkəumə] *n* 腺肌肉瘤 | embryonal ~ 胚性腺肌肉瘤,胚性癌肉瘤

adenomyosis [ˌædinəumaiˈəusis] *n* 子宫内膜异位 | ~ externa 子宫外子宫内膜异位 / stromal ~ 基质性子宫内膜异位

adenoncus [ˌædiˈnɔŋkəs] *n* 腺[肿]大

adenoneural [ˌædinəuˈnjuərəl] *a* 腺与神经的

adenopathy [ˌædiˈnɔpəθi] *n* 腺病(腺肿大,尤指淋巴结肿大)

adenopharyngitis [ˌædinəuˌfærinˈdʒaitis] *n* 咽扁桃体炎

adenophlegmon [ˌædinəuˈflegmən] *n* 蜂窝织炎性腺炎

adenophthalmia [ˌædinɔfˈθælmiə] *n* 睑板腺炎

adenopituicyte [ˌædinəupiˈtjuisait] *n* 腺垂体细胞

adenosarcoma [ˌædinəusɑːˈkəumə] *n* 腺肉瘤 | embryonal ~ 胚性腺肉瘤,胚性癌肉瘤

adenosclerosis [ˌædinəuskliəˈrəusis] *n* 腺硬化

adenosinase [ædiˈnəusineis] *n* 腺苷酶

adenosine [əˈdenəsi(ː)n] *n* 腺[嘌呤核]苷 | cyclic ~ monophosphate (cAMP) 环腺苷酸 / ~ diphosphate (ADP) 腺苷二磷酸 / ~ monophosphate (AMP) 腺苷[一磷]酸 / ~ phosphate 腺苷磷酸 / ~ triphosphate (ATP) 腺苷三磷酸

adenosine deaminase (ADA) [əˈdenəsi(ː)n diˈæmineis] 腺苷脱氨酶(此酶缺乏为一种常染色体隐性性状,已从很多有严重联合免疫缺陷综合征患者中发现)

adenosine kinase [əˈdenəsi(ː)n ˈkaineis] 腺苷激酶(亦称腺苷酸激酶)

adenosinetriphosphatase [əˌdenəsiːntraiˈfɔsfəteis] *n* 腺苷三磷酸酶

adenosis [ˌædiˈnəusis] *n* 腺病 | blunt duct ~ 闭塞性乳腺导管增生症 / ~ vaginae 阴道腺病

adenosyl [əˈdenəˌsil] *n* 腺苷基

adenosylcobalamin (AdoCbl) [əˌdenəsilkəuˈbæləmin] *n* 腺苷钴胺

***S*-adenosylhomocysteine** [əˌdenəsilˌhəuməˈsistiiːn] *n* *S*-腺苷高半胱氨酸

***S*-adenosylmethionine** [əˌdenəsilmeˈθaiəniːn] *n* *S*-腺苷甲硫氨酸

adenotome [ˈædinətəum] *n* 腺样体刀

adenotomy [ˌædiˈnɔtəmi] *n* 腺解剖术,腺切除术;腺样体切除术

adenotonsillectomy [ˌædinəuˌtɔnsiˈlektəmi] *n* 腺样体扁桃体切除术

adenous [ˈædinəs] *a* 腺的

adenoviral [ˌædinəuˈvaiərəl] *a* 腺病毒的

Adenoviridae [ˌædinəuviˈraidiː] *n* 腺病毒科

adenovirus [ˌædinəuˈvaiərəs] *n* 腺病毒

adenyl [ˈædənil] *n* 腺嘌呤[基]

adenylate [əˈdenileit] *n* 腺[嘌呤核]苷酸

adenylate cyclase [əˈdenileit ˈsaikleis] 腺苷酸环化酶

adenylate deaminase [əˈdenileit diːˈæmineis] 腺苷酸脱氨酶

adenylate kinase [əˈdenileit ˈkaineis] 腺苷酸激酶

adenyl cyclase [ˈædənil ˈsaikleis] 腺苷酸环化酶

adenylic acid [ˌædəˈnilik] 腺苷[一磷]酸

adenylic acid deaminase [ˌædəˈnilikˈæsid diːˈæmineis] 腺苷酸脱氨酶

adenylosuccinase [ˌædiniləuˈsʌksineis] *n* 腺苷酸[基]琥珀酸[裂合]酶

adenylosuccinate [ˌædiniləuˈsʌksineit] *n* 腺苷酸[基]琥珀酸 | **~lyase** 腺苷酸[基]琥珀酸裂合酶

adenylosuccinate synthase [ˌædənilə*u*ˈsʌksineit ˈsinθeis] 腺苷酸[基]琥珀酸合酶
adenylpyrophosphatase [ˌædənilˌpaiərə*u*ˈfɔsfəteis] *n* 腺苷酰焦磷酸酶
adenylpyrophosphate [ˌædinilˌpaiərə*u*ˈfɔsfeit] *n* 腺苷三磷酸
adenylyl [ˈædənilil] *n* 腺[嘌呤核]苷酰[基]
adenylyl cyclase [ˈædənilil ˈsaikleis] 腺苷酰环化酶,腺苷酸环化酶
adenylyltransferase [ˌædənililˈtrænsfəreis] *n* 腺苷酰[基]转移酶
adeps [ˈædeps] *n*【拉】豚脂,动物脂(软膏制剂用) | ~ anserinus 鹅脂 / ~ benzoinatus 安息香豚脂,苯甲酸豚脂 / ~ lanae 无水羊毛脂 / ~ lanae hydrosus 含水羊毛脂 / ~ ovillus 羊脂 / ~ porci 豚脂 / ~ renis 肾脂肪囊 / ~ suillus 豚脂
adept [ˈædept] *a* 熟练的,内行的 *n* 专家,能手
adequacy [ˈædikwəsi] *n* 适当;足够,充分 | ~ of perfusion 灌注充分 / velopharyngeal ~ 腭咽关闭良好
adermia [əˈdəːmiə] *n* 无皮[畸形]
adermine [əˈdəːmiːn] *n* 吡哆醇,维生素 B_6
adermogenesis [əˌdəːmə*u*ˈdʒenisis] *n* 皮肤发育不全
Ad grat. acid. ad gratum aciditatem【拉】至适宜酸度
ADH alcohol dehydrogenase 醇脱氢酶; antidiuretic hormone 抗利尿激素,血管升压素
Adhatoda [ædˈhætədə] *n* 鸭嘴花属
adhere [ədˈhiə] *vi* 黏附;粘连;依附
adherence [ədˈhiərəns] *n* 依附;粘连 | immune ~ 免疫粘连(一种补体依赖性现象)
adherent [ədˈhiərənt] *a* 粘连的;附着的
adhesin [ədˈhiːsin] *n* 黏附素
adhesio [ədˈhiːziəu] ([复] **adhesiones** [ədhiːziˈəuniːz]) *n*【拉】连接带,连接体 | ~ interthalamica 丘脑间黏合
adhesiolysis [ædˌhiːsiˈɔlisis] *n* 粘连[物]切离术
adhesion [ədˈhiːʒən] *n* 粘连;黏着物 | primary ~ 原发性粘连(第一期愈合) / secondary ~ 继发性粘连(第二期愈合) / serological ~ 血清学粘连(抗体和补体存在时,非特异性颗粒物质粘连到颗粒性抗原的现象) / traumatic uterine ~s 创伤性子宫粘连
adhesiotomy [ædˌhiːziˈɔtəmi] *n* 粘连[物]切离术
adhesive [ədˈhiːsiv] *a* 黏着的;粘连性的 *n* 黏附剂 | dental ~ 牙科黏胶 / denture ~ 义齿黏附剂
adhesiveness [ədˈhiːsivnis] *n* 粘连性 | platelet ~ 血小板粘连
Adhib. adhibendus【拉】给服药
adhibit [ædˈhibit] *vt* 贴,粘;用(药等)
adiabatic [ˌædaiəˈbætik] *a* 绝热的
adiactinic [əˌdaiækˈtinik] *a* 绝射的(不容光化线透过的)
adiadochokinesia, adiadokokinesia [əˌdaiəˌdəukə*u*kiˈniːsiə], **adiadochocinesia** [əˌdaiəˌdəukə*u*siˈniːsiə], **adiadochocinesis** [əˌdaiəˌdəukə*u*siˈniːsis], **adiadochokinesis, adiadokokinesis** [əˌdaiəˌdəukə*u*kiˈniːsis] *n* 轮替动作不能
Adiantum [ˌædiˈæntəm] *n* 铁线蕨属
adiaphoria [ˌeidaiəˈfɔːriə] *n* 无反应,无活动
adiaspiromycosis [ˌædiəˌspaiərə*u*maiˈkəusis] *n* 不育大孢子菌病
adiaspore [ˈædiəˌspɔː] *n* 不育大孢子
adiasporosis [ˌædiəspɔːˈrəusis] *n* 大孢子菌病
adiathermancy [əˌdaiəˈθəːmənsi], **adiathermance** [əˌdaiəˈθəːməns] *n* 不透热,绝热
adicillin [ˌædiˈsilin] *n* 阿地西林(抗生素类药,治疗伤寒和淋病)
adiemorrhysis [əˌdaiəˈmɔrisis] *n* 血液循环停止
adient [ˈædiənt] *a* 趋近的,趋向的
Adie's pupil [ˈeidi] (William J. Adie) 埃迪瞳孔,紧张性瞳孔 | ~ syndrome 埃迪综合征(病理性瞳孔反应综合征,表现在患侧瞳孔对近距目标的辐辏性收缩反应较对侧瞳孔迟缓,复原时,瞳孔开大也较迟缓)
Adinida [əˈdinidə] *n* 无凹鞭毛虫目
adipectomy [ˌædiˈpektəmi] *n* 脂肪切除术
adiphenine hydrochloride [ˌædiˈfeniːn] 盐酸阿地芬宁(抗胆碱能药,解痉药)
adipic [əˈdipik] *a* 脂肪的 | ~ acid 己二酸
adip(o)-[构词成分]脂
adipocele [ˈædipə*u*ˌsiːl] *n* 脂肪突出
adipocellular [ˌædipə*u*ˈseljulə] *a* 脂肪结缔组织的
adipocellulose [ˌædipə*u*ˈseljuləus] *n* 脂纤维素
adipocere [ˈædipə*u*ˌsiə] *n* 尸蜡 | **adipoceratous** [ˌædipə*u*ˈserətəs] *a* 尸蜡[样]的
adipocyte [ˈædipəˌsait] *n* 脂肪细胞
adipofibroma [ˌædipə*u*faiˈbrəumə] *n* 脂肪纤维瘤
adipogenesis [ˌædipə*u*ˈdʒenisis] *n* 脂肪形成
adipogenic [ˌædipə*u*ˈdʒenik], **adipogenous** [ˌædiˈpɔdʒinəs] *a* 脂肪形成的,生脂的
adipohepatic [ˌædipə*u*hiˈpætik] *a* 肝脂肪变性的
adipoid [ˈædipɔid] *a* 脂样的,类脂的
adipokinesis [ˌædipə*u*kiˈniːsis] *n* 脂肪移动(释出游离脂肪酸至血浆内) | **adipokinetic** [ˌædipə*u*kiˈnetik] *a* 脂肪移动的,促脂肪移动的
adipokinin [ˌædipə*u*ˈkainin] *n* 脂肪动用激素(从垂体前叶分离出来的一种脂肪氧化激素)
adipolysis [ˌædiˈpɔlisis] *n* 脂肪分解[作用] | **adipolytic** [ˌædipə*u*ˈlitik] *a*

adipometer [ˌædiˈpɔmitə] *n* 皮厚度计(测定肥胖)
adiponecrosis [ˌædipəuneˈkrəusis] *n* 脂肪坏死
adipopexis [ˌædipəuˈpeksis], **adipopexia** [ˌædipəuˈpeksiə] *n* 积脂 | **adipopectic** [ˌædipəuˈpektik], **adipopexic** [ˌædipəuˈpeksik] *a*
adiposalgia [ˌædipəuˈsældʒiə] *n* 脂肪痛
adipose [ˈædipəus] *a* 脂肪的,脂的;脂肪多的,肥胖的 *n* (脂肪组织细胞内存在的)脂肪
adiposis [ˌædiˈpəusis] *n* 肥胖症 | ~ cerebralis [大]脑性肥胖症 / ~ dolorosa 痛性肥胖症 / ~ universalis 全身性肥胖症
adipositas [ˌædiˈpɔsitəs] *n*【拉】肥胖[症] | ~ cordis 心脏脂肪症,脂肪心 / ~ ex vacuo 肥胖性萎缩,脂性萎缩
adipositis [ˌædipəuˈsaitis] *n* 脂肪织炎,脂膜炎
adiposity [ˌædiˈpɔsəti] *n* 肥胖[症] | cerebral ~ [大]脑性肥胖症 / pituitary ~ 垂体性肥胖症
adiposuria [ˌædipəuˈsjuəriə] *n* 脂肪尿
adipsa [əˈdipsə] *n* 止渴剂
adipsia [əˈdipsiə], **adipsy** [əˈdipsi] *n* 渴感缺乏,不渴症
adipsous [əˈdipsəs] *a* 止渴的(如某些水果)
adit [ˈædit] *n* 入口,进口
aditus [ˈæditəs] *n*【拉】入口,口
adjacency [əˈdʒeisənsi] *n* 毗邻,接近;[复]邻接物
adjacent [əˈdʒeisənt] *a* 相邻的,毗连的
adjection [əˈdʒekʃən] *n* 附加作用(尤指对体内活的微生物添加许多微生物,并与之结合而构成适当剂量使病人免疫的原理)
adjunct [ˈædʒʌŋkt] *n* 附件,附属品,附属物;辅助物 *a* 附属的;辅助的;附加的
adjunctive [əˈdʒʌŋktiv] *a* 附属的;辅助的
adjustment [əˈdʒʌstmənt] *n* 调整,调节;适应 | occlusal ~ 调称,咬合调整
adjuvant [ˈædʒuvənt] *a* 辅助的 *n* 辅药,佐药;佐剂(在免疫学中指与抗原混合增加抗原性,并产生较大免疫应答的物质) | mycobacterial ~ 分枝杆菌佐剂(弗氏佐剂,见 Freund's adjuvant)
adjuvanticity [ˌædʒuvənˈtisəti] *n* 佐剂性(改变免疫应答的能力)
ADL activities of daily living 日常生活活动
Adler's test [ˈɑːdlə] (Oscar Adler) 联苯胺试验(检血)
Adler's theory [ˈɑːdlə] (Alfred Adler) 阿德勒学说(认为神经症的发病是因社会或身体代偿力低劣而产生)
ad lib. ad libitum【拉】任意,随意
adlumidine [ædˈluːmidiːn] *n* 紫罂粟次碱
adlumine [ædˈluːmin] *n* 紫罂粟碱
admeasure [ædˈmeʒə] *vt* 分配 | ~ment *n* 分配;尺寸,大小
admedial [ædˈmiːdiəl] *a* 近正中[面]的
admedian [ædˈmiːdiən] *a* 向正中[面]的
adminicle [ædˈminikl] *n* 辅助;辅助物 | **adminicular** [ˌædmiˈnikjulə] *a*
adminiculum [ˌædmiˈnikjuləm] ([复] **adminicula** [ˌædmiˈnikjulə]) *n*【拉】支座
administer [ədˈministə] *vt* 管理,支配;执行;给予,用(药等)
administration [ədˌminisˈtreiʃən] *n* 管理;(药的)服法,用法;给予 | continuous ~ of low flow oxygen 持续低流量给氧
administrator [ədˈministreitə] *n* 管理人;行政官员
admissible [ədˈmisəbl] *a* 容许的
admission [ədˈmiʃən] *n* 住院,入院
admit [ədˈmit] *vt* 住院,入院
admittance(A) [ədˈmitəns] *n* 导纳(导纳的单位是西门子〈Siemens〉) | acoustic ~ 声导纳
admix [ədˈmiks] *vt, vi* 掺和
admixture [ədˈmikstʃə] *n* 掺和;加药配液 | venous ~ 静脉血掺和
admov. admove, admoveatur【拉】加,加入
adnerval [ædˈnəːvəl], **adneural** [ædˈnjuərəl] *a* 近神经的;向神经的(指经肌肉通向神经进入点通过的电流)
adnexa [ædˈneksə] *n* 附件,附器 | ~l *a* 附件的(尤指子宫附件)
adnexectomy [ˌædnekˈsektəmi] *n* [子宫]附件切除术
adnexitis [ˌædnekˈsaitis] *n* 子宫附件炎
adnexogenesis [ædˌneksəuˈdʒenisis] *n* 附件发生
adnexorganogenic [ædˌneksɔːgənəuˈdʒenik] *a* 子宫附件原的
ado [əˈduː] *n* 忙乱;烦恼
AdoCbl adenosylcobalamin 腺苷钴胺
adolescence [ˌædəuˈlesns] *n* 青春期,青春(11 ~ 19 岁)
adolescent [ˌædəuˈlesnt] *a* 青春期的 *n* 青少年
adonin [əˈdəunin] *n* 福寿草苷,侧金盏花苷
Adonis [əˈdəunis] *n* 福寿草属,侧金盏花属
adonitol [əˈdɔnitɔl], **adonite** [ˈædənit] *n* 福寿草醇,侧金盏花醇,核糖醇
adoral [ædˈɔːrəl] *a* 向口的;近口的
ADP adenosine diphosphate 腺苷二磷酸; aminohydroxypropylidene diphosphate (pamidronate) 氨基羟基亚丙基二膦酸(帕米膦酸)
ADPKD autosomal dominant polycystic kidney disease 常染色体显性遗传多囊肾病
Ad pond. om. ad pondus omnium【拉】至全部的重量

adrenal [əˈdriːnl] *a* 肾上腺的;肾旁的 *n* 肾上腺
adrenalectomize [əˌdriːnəˈlektəmaiz] *vt* 切除肾上腺
adrenalectomy [əˌdriːnəˈlektəmi] *n* 肾上腺切除术
adrenaline [əˈdrenəlin] *n* 肾上腺素 | ~ acid tartrate 重酒石酸肾上腺素
adrenalinemia [əˌdrenəliˈniːmiə] *n* 肾上腺素血症
adrenalinogenesis [əˌdrenəlinəuˈdʒenisis] *n* 肾上腺素生成
adrenalinuria [əˌdrenəliˈnjuəriə] *n* 肾上腺素尿
adrenalism [əˈdrenəlizəm] *n* 肾上腺功能病
adrenalitis [əˌdrenəˈlaitis] *n* 肾上腺炎
adrenalone [əˈdrenələun] *n* 肾上腺酮(拟肾上腺素药,具有收缩血管作用)
adrenalopathy [əˌdrenəˈlɔpəθi] *n* 肾上腺病
adrenalotropic [əˌdrenələuˈtrɔpik] *a* 促肾上腺的
adrenarche [ˌædrenˈɑːki] *n* 肾上腺功能初现(尤指雄激素增进,大约 8 岁时发生的一种生理变化)
adrenergic [ˌædreˈnəːdʒik] *a* 肾上腺素能的 *n* 拟肾上腺素药(亦称拟交感神经药)
adrenic [əˈdrenik] *a* 肾上腺的
adrenin(e) [əˈdriːnin] *n* 肾上腺素
adrenitis [ˌædriːˈnaitis] *n* 肾上腺炎
adren(o)- [构词成分]肾上腺
adrenoceptive [əˈdriːnəuˈseptiv] *a* 肾上腺素受体的
adrenoceptor [əˈdriːnəuˈseptə] *n* 肾上腺素受体
adrenochrome [əˈdriːnəuˌkrəum] *n* 肾上腺色素,肾上腺素红(用于试验性控制毛细管出血,产生心理效应,并可用以局部止血)
adrenocortical [əˌdriːnəuˈkɔːtikəl] *a* 肾上腺皮质的
adrenocorticohyperplasia [əˌdriːnəuˌkɔːtikəu-ˌhaipəˈpleiziə] *n* 肾上腺皮质增生
adrenocorticoid [əˌdriːnəuˈkɔːtikɔid] *n* 肾上腺类皮质激素
adrenocorticomimetic [æˌdriːnəuˌkɔːtikəumai-ˈmetik] *a* 类肾上腺皮质激素的
adrenocorticotrophic [æˌdriːnəuˌkɔːtikəuˈtrɔfik], **adrenocorticotropic** [æˌdriːnəuˌkɔːtikəuˈtrɔpik] *a* 促肾上腺皮质的
adrenocorticotrophin [æˌdriːnəuˌkɔːtikəuˈtrɔfin], **adrenocorticotropin** [æˌdriːnəuˌkɔːtikəuˈtrɔpin] *n* 促肾上腺皮质激素,促皮质素
adrenodontia [æˌdrenəuˈdɔnʃiə] *n* 肾上腺牙式(犬牙大而尖,釉面变棕色)
adrenodoxin [əˌdriːnəuˈdɔksin] *n* (肾上腺)皮质铁氧还蛋白
adrenogenic [əˌdriːnəuˈdʒenik] *a* 肾上腺原的
adrenogenous [ˌædreˈnɔdʒinəs] *a* 肾上腺原的,肾上腺性的
adrenogram [æˈdrenəgræm] *n* 肾上腺 X 线[照]片
adrenokinetic [æˌdriːnəukaiˈnetik, -kiˈn-] *a* 刺激肾上腺的
adrenoleukodystrophy [əˌdriːnəuˌljuːkəuˈdistrəfi] *n* 肾上腺脑白质营养不良
adrenolutin [əˌdriːnəuˈljuːtin] *n* 肾上腺黄素,1-甲基-3,5,6-茚三醇(肾上腺素的降解产物)
adrenolytic [ˌædrenəuˈlitik] *a* 抗肾上腺素[作用]的,抑肾上腺素[作用]的
adrenomedullary [əˌdriːnəuˈmedələri] *a* 肾上腺髓质的
adrenomedullotropic [əˌdriːnəuˌmedʌləuˈtrɔpik] *a* 促肾上腺髓质的(对肾上腺髓质产生激素影响的)
adrenomegaly [æˌdrenəuˈmegəli] *n* 肾上腺[增]大
adrenomimetic [ˌədriːnəumaiˈmetik] *a* 类肾上腺素能作用的 *n* 拟肾上腺素药
adrenopathy [ˌædreˈnɔpəθi] *n* 肾上腺病
adrenopause [æˈdrenəpɔːz] *n* 肾上腺功能停滞
adrenoprival [æˈdriːnəuˌpraivəl] *a* 肾上腺缺乏的,肾上腺切除的
adrenoreceptor [əˌdriːnəuriˈseptə] *n* 肾上腺素受体
adrenostatic [əˌdriːnəuˈstætik] *a* 抑制肾上腺[作用]的 *n* 肾上腺抑制药
adrenosterone [ˌædriːˈnəustəˌrəun] *n* 肾上腺雄[甾]酮
adrenotoxin [əˌdriːnəuˈtɔksin] *n* 肾上腺毒素
adrenotrophin [əˌdriːnəuˈtrəufin], **adrenotropin** [əˌdriːnəuˈtrəupin] *n* 促肾上腺皮质激素,促皮质素
adrenotropic [əˌdriːnəuˈtrɔpik], **adrenotrophic** [əˌdriːnəuˈtrɔfik] *a* 促肾上腺的,亲肾上腺的
adrenoxidase [ˌædreˈnɔksideis] *n* 肾上腺氧化酶
adromia [əˈdrəumiə] *n* 肌神经传导缺失
adrue [əˈdruːei] *n* 有节莎草(西印度群岛的草样植物,其根有强壮、止吐、驱虫作用)
ADS antidiuretic substance 抗利尿物质
adscititious [ˌædsiˈtiʃəs] *a* 外加的,附加的
Adson's forceps [ˈædsən] (Alfred W. Adson) 艾德生镊(一种小按捏镊) | ~ maneuver(test) 艾德生手法(试验)(检查胸廓出口综合征的一种试验)
Adson-Brown forceps [ˈædsən braun] (A. W. Adson; James B. Brown) 艾-布镊(一种按捏镊;用于夹精细组织)
adsorb [ædˈsɔːb] *vt* 吸附
adsorbate [ædˈsɔːbit] *n* 吸附物

adsorbent [æd'sɔːbənt] *a* 吸附的 *n* 吸附剂
adsorption [æd'sɔːpʃən] *n* 吸附[作用] | agglutinin ~ 凝集素吸附[反应] / immune ~ 免疫吸附
adsternal [æd'stəːnəl] *a* 向胸骨的,近胸骨的
adst. feb. adstante febre【拉】发热时
ADTA American Dance Therapy Association 美国舞蹈疗法协会
ADTe 强直性收缩(tetanic contraction)的符号
adterminal [æd'təːmin] *a* 向[肌肉]末端的(指电流)
adtorsion [æd'tɔːʃən] *n* [眼]内旋
adult ['ædʌlt] *a* 成年人的,成熟的 *n* 成人,成年;成虫 | **~hood** *n* 成年期,成熟期
adulterant [ə'dʌltərənt] *n* 假药,掺杂物 *a* 掺杂用的
adulterate [ə'dʌltəreit] *vt* 掺杂,掺假 *a* 掺假的 | **adulteration** [əˌdʌltə'reiʃən] *n*
adumbration [ˌædʌm'breiʃən] *n* 轮廓;双像形成,阴影产生
Adv. adversum【拉】抗,对
advance [əd'vɑːns, əd'væns] *vt* 推进;促进;做徙前术
advanced [əd'vɑːnst, əd'vænst] *a* 高级的;年老的;先进的;晚期的
advancement [əd'vɑːnsmənt, -'væns-] *n* 改进,促进;徙前术(主要用于斜视手术,有时将子宫圆韧带前移,以纠正子宫后移位) | capsular ~ (眼球)囊徙前术 / tendon ~ 腱徙前术 / urethral ~ 尿道前移术
adventitia [ˌædvən'tiʃiə] *n* [血管]外膜 | **~l** *a*
adventitious [ˌædven'tiʃəs] *a* 外来的;偶生的,偶发的;异位的;附加的
adverse ['ædvəːs] *a* 不利的
Ad 2 vic. ad duas vices【拉】两次,两剂
advice [əd'vais] *n* 劝告;意见(如医嘱)
adynamia [eidai'neimiə] *n* 动力缺失;无力 | ~ episodica hereditaria 遗传性周期性麻痹症,周期性麻痹Ⅱ型 | **adynamic** [eidai'næmik] *a*
adysplasia [ˌeidis'pleiziə] *n* 发育不良 | hereditary renal ~ 遗传性肾发育不良
A-E, AE above elbow 肘上(截肢)
ae- 以 ae-起始的词,同样见以 e-起始的词
Aeby's muscle ['eibi] (Christopher T. Aeby) 降下唇肌,下唇方肌 | ~ plane 埃比平面(即通过鼻根点和颅底点,与颅腔正中平面垂直的平面)
aec- 以 aec-起始的词,同样见以 ec-起始的词
aeciospore ['iːsiəˌspɔː] *n* 锈孢子,夏孢子
aecium ['iːsiəm] ([复] **aecia** ['iːsiə]) *n* 锈子器
AED automatic external defibrillator 自动体外除颤器
Aedes [ei'iːdiːz] *n* 伊蚊属 | ~ aegypti 埃及伊蚊 / ~ africanus 非洲伊蚊 / ~ albopictus 白纹伊蚊 / ~ chemulpoensis 仁川伊蚊 / ~ cinereus 灰色伊蚊 / ~ dorsalis 背点伊蚊 / ~ flavescens 黄色伊蚊 / ~ ingrami 英氏伊蚊 / ~ leucocelaenus 白星伊蚊 / ~ polynesiensis 波利尼西亚伊蚊 / ~ pseudoscutellaris 假鳞斑伊蚊 / ~ scapularis 肩胛伊蚊 / ~ scutellaris 鳞斑伊蚊 / ~ simpsoni 辛[普森]氏伊蚊 / ~ sollicitans 烦扰伊蚊 / ~ spencerii 斯[潘塞]氏伊蚊 / ~ taeniorhynchus 带喙伊蚊 / ~ togoi 海滨伊蚊,东乡伊蚊 / ~ varipalpus 变须伊蚊 / ~ vexans 刺扰伊蚊
Aedini [eii'dainai] *n* 伊蚊族
aedoeocephalus [ˌediə'sefələs] *n* 生殖器状头畸胎(无嘴,鼻似阴茎,单眼眶)
Aeg. aeger, aegra【拉】病人
Aegyptianella [iːˌdʒipʃiə'nelə] *n* 埃及小体属 | ~ pullorum 雏埃及小体
aelurophobia [iːˌluːrəu'fəubjə] *n* 猫恐怖,恐猫症
aeluropsis [ˌiːluː'rɔpsis] *n* 猫眼样细睑裂
Aelurostrongylus [iːˌljurəu'strɔŋdʒiləs] *n* 猫圆线虫属
AEP auditory evoked potential 听(觉)诱发电位
aequator [i'kweitə] *n* 中纬线(即 **equator**)
aequorin [iː'kwɔːrin] *n* 水母发光蛋白(注入活细胞检钙离子存在)
aequum ['iːkwəm] *n*【拉】维持量,平衡量(营养)
aer ['eiə] *n* 气压单位(见 atmos)
aer- [构词成分]见 aero-
aerase ['eiəreis] *n* 需氧菌呼吸酶
aerasthenia [ˌeiəræs'θiːniə] *n* 飞行员精神衰弱,飞行员神经功能病
aerate ['eiəreit] *vt* 使暴露于空气中;通过呼吸供氧给(血液);使充气,充[碳酸]气于 | **~ed** *a* 曝气的;充[二氧化碳]气的;充氧的 / **aeration** [ˌeiə'reiʃən] *n* 换气(肺内血液二氧化碳换氧);充气,曝气 / **aerator** *n* 曝气池;充气器,灌气器
aeremia [ˌeiə'riːmiə] *n* 气泡栓塞,气栓;减压病
aerial ['ɛəriəl] *a* 空气的
aeriferous [ˌɛə'rifərəs] *a* 带空气的,传气的(如支气管)
aeriform ['ɛərifɔːm] *a* 气样的
aerify ['ɛərifai] *vt* 使气体化;充气于 | **aerification** [ˌɛərifi'keiʃən] *n* 气体化;充满气体[状态]
aero-, aer- [构词成分]气,空气
aeroasthenia [ˌeiərəuæs'θiːniə] *n* 飞行员精神衰弱,飞行员神经功能病
Aerobacter [ˌɛərəu'bæktə] *n* 气杆菌属 | ~ aerogenes 产气气杆菌(即产气肠杆菌 Enterobacter aerogenes) / ~ cloacae 阴沟气杆菌(即阴沟肠杆菌 Enterobacter cloacae)
aerobe ['ɛərəub] *n* 需氧菌 | facultative ~s 兼性需氧菌(在需氧或厌氧的情况下均能生长的) /

obligate ~s 专性需氧菌(需氧生长的)
aerobic [ɛəˈrəubik] *a* 有氧的;需氧的
aerobiology [ˌɛərəubaiˈɔlədʒi] *n* 空气生物学 | **aerobiological** [ˌɛərəubaiəˈlɔdʒikəl] *a*
aerobiosis [ˌɛərəubaiˈəusis] *n* 需氧生活 | **aerobiotic** [ˌɛərəubaiˈɔtik] *a*
aerobullosis [ˌɛərəubjuˈləusis] *n* 减压病
aerocele [ˈɛərəusiːl] *n* 气肿(如喉囊肿和气管黏膜疝样突出)
Aerococcus [ˌɛərəuˈkɔkəs] *n* 气球菌属 | ~ viridans 绿色气球菌
aerocolpos [ˌɛərəuˈkɔlpəs] *n* 阴道积气
aerocystography [ˌɛərəusisˈtɔgrəfi] *n* 膀胱充气造影[术]
aerocystoscope [ˌɛərəuˈsistəskəup] *n* 充气膀胱镜
aerocystoscopy [ˌɛərəusisˈtɔskəpi] *n* 充气膀胱镜检查
aerodermectasia [ˌɛərəuˌdəːmekˈteiziə] *n* 皮下气肿
aerodigestive [ˌɛərəudiˈdʒestiv] *a* 呼吸消化道的
aerodontalgia [ˌɛərəudɔnˈtældʒiə] *n* 航空牙痛
aerodontics [ˌɛərəuˈdɔntiks], **aerodontia** [ˌɛərəuˈdɔnʃiə] *n* 航空牙科学
aerodrome [ˈɛərədrəum] *n* 飞机场
aerodynamics [ˌɛərəudaiˈnæmiks] *n* 气体动力学 | **aerodynamic** *a*
aeroembolism [ˌɛərəuˈembəlizəm] *n* 气栓(可能在头、颈和心脏手术、人工流产以及严重减压病时发生)
aeroemphysema [ˌɛərəuˌemfiˈsiːmə] *n* 肺气肿(由于大气迅速减压,肺组织内氮气泡聚集所致的肺气肿和肺水肿)
aerogastria [ˌɛərəuˈgæstriə] *n* 胃积气 | blocked ~ 阻滞性胃积气
aerogel [ˈɛərədʒel] *n* 气凝胶[体]
aerogen [ˈɛərədʒən] *n* 产气菌
aerogenesis [ˌɛərəuˈdʒenisis] *n* 产气
aerogenic [ˌɛərəuˈdʒenik], **aerogenous** [ɛəˈrɔdʒinəs] *a* 产气的(指细菌)
aerogram [ˈɛərəˌgræm] *n* [器官]充气造影[照]片
aeroionotherapy [ˌɛərəuˌaiənəuˈθerəpi] *n* 空气离子化疗法
aeromedicine [ˌɛərəuˈmedsin] *n* 航空医学 | **aeromedical** *a*
aerometer [ɛəˈrɔmitə] *n* 气体比重计,量气计 | **aerometric** [ˌɛərəuˈmetrik] *a* 气体比重计的,量气计的;量气学的 / **aerometry** *n* 量气学
Aeromonas [ˌɛərəuˈməunəs] *n* 气单胞菌属 | ~ hydrophila 嗜水气单胞菌 / ~ punctata 斑点气单胞菌 / ~ salmonicida 杀鲑气单胞菌

aeronautic(al) [ˌɛərəˈnɔːtik(əl)] *a* 航空的;航空学的
aeronautics [ˌɛərəˈnɔːtiks] *n* 航空学;飞行术
aero-odontalgia [ˌɛərəuˌɔdɔnˈtældʒiə], **aero-odontodynia** [ˌɛərəuɔˌdɔntəˈdiniə] *n* 航空牙痛
aero-otitis [ˌɛərəuəuˈtaitis] *n* 气压损伤性中耳炎
aeropathy [ˌɛəˈrɔpəθi] *n* 航空病(大气压所致的疾病,如减压病、晕机病)
aeropause [ˈɛərəupɔːz] *n* 乏气[压]层(同温层和外层空间之间的地区,实际上无大气存在)
aeroperitoneum [ˌɛərəuˌperitəuˈniːəm], **aeroperitonia** [ˌɛərəuˌperiˈtəuniə] *n* 腹膜腔积气,气腹
aerophagia [ˌɛərəuˈfeidʒiə], **aerophagy** [ˌɛəˈrɔfədʒi] *n* 吞气症(功能性胃肠失调时常见之)
aerophil [ˈɛərəuˌfil] *n* 嗜气菌
aerophilic [ˌɛərəuˈfilik], **aerophilous** [ˌɛəˈrɔfiləs] *a* 嗜气的,需气的
aerophobia [ˌɛərəuˈfəubjə] *n* 气流恐怖
aerophyte [ˈɛərəufait] *n* 气生植物(亦指从空气中得到营养的任何微生物或其他植物菌)
aeropiesotherapy [ˌɛərəupaiˌiːsəuˈθerəpi] *n* 压缩气疗法(将空气压缩或使之稀薄以治病)
aeroplankton [ˌɛərəuˈplæŋktɔn] *n* 气中生物,空浮生物(指空气中的生物体,如细菌、花粉等)
aeroplethysmograph [ˌɛərəupləˈθizməgrɑːf, -græf] *n* 呼吸气量描记器
aeroporotomy [ˌɛərəupəˈrɔtəmi] *n* 呼吸道通气术(如用插管法或气管切开术)
aerosialophagy [ˌɛərəuˌsaiəˈlɔfədʒi] *n* 咽气涎癖
aerosinusitis [ˌɛərəuˌsainəˈsaitis] *n* 气压损伤性鼻窦炎,航空性鼻窦炎,飞行员鼻窦炎
aerosis [ɛəˈrəusis] *n* 产气(组织或器官内)
aerosol [ˈɛərəusɔl] *n* 气溶胶;烟雾剂,气雾剂(用于空气消毒或吸入疗法)
aerosolization [ˌɛərəuˌsɔliˈzeiʃən] *n* 烟雾化[作用]
aerosolology [ˌɛərəusɔˈlɔlədʒi] *n* 气溶胶[治疗]学
aerospace [ˈɛərəuspeis] *n* 宇宙航空
aerosphere [ˈɛərəsfiə] *n* 大气
aerostatics [ˌɛərəuˈstætiks] *n* 气体静力学 | **aerostatic** *a*
aerotaxis [ˌɛərəuˈtæksis] *n* 趋氧性(指细菌)
aerotitis [ˌɛərəuˈtaitis] *n* 气压损伤性中耳炎
aerotolerant [ˌɛərəuˈtɔlərənt] *a* 耐氧的
aerotonometer [ˌɛərəutəˈnɔmitə] *n* [血内]气体张力计
aerotropism [ˌɛəˈrɔtrəpizəm] *n* 向氧性
aerotympanal [ˌɛərəuˈtimpənl] *a* [空]气鼓室的
aerourethroscope [ˌɛərəujuəˈriːθrəskəup] *n* 充

气尿道镜,充气膀胱镜

aerourethroscopy [ˌɛərəuˌjuəriˈθrɔskəpi] *n* 充气尿道镜检查

aeruginous [iəˈruːdʒinəs] *a* 蓝绿色的,铜锈色的

aes-, aet- 以 aes-, aet-起始的词,同样见以 es-, et-起始的词

Æsculapius [ˌiːskjuˈleipjəs] *n* 艾斯库累普(希腊罗马神话中的医神) | **aesculapian** *a* 艾斯库累普的;医术的 *n* 医师

aesculin [ˈeskjulin] *n* 见 esculin

Aesculus [ˈeskjuləs] *n* 七叶树属

aesthesi(o)- 以 aesthesi(o)-起始的词,同样见以 esthesi(o)-起始的词

aesthetic [iːsˈθetik] *a* 见 esthetic

aesthetics [iːsˈθetiks] *n* 见 esthetics

aestival [iːsˈtaivəl] *a* 见 estival

aestivation [ˌiːstiˈveiʃən] *n* 见 estivation

aet. aetas【拉】年龄

aether [ˈiːθə] *n* 见 ether

Aethusa [iːˈθuːsə] *n* 犬毒芹属

aethylenum [ˌeθiˈliːnəm] *n*【拉】乙烯;次乙基,乙撑 | ~ pro narcosi 麻醉用乙烯

aetiology [iːtiˈɔlədʒi] *n* 见 etiology

AF albumose-free 脱脲(结核菌素); atrial fibrillation 心房纤颤,心房颤动

AFCR American Federation for Clinical Research 美国临床研究联合会

afebrile [eiˈfiːbrail, eiˈfebril] *a* 无热的

afetal [əˈfiːtl] *a* 无胎的

affect [əˈfekt] *vt* 影响;(疾病)侵袭 [ˈæfekt] *n* 感情,情感 | blunted ~ 情感迟钝 / flat ~ 情感淡漠

affected [əˈfektid] *a* 受(疾病等)侵袭的;受影响的;感染的

affection¹ [əˈfekʃən] *n* 疾患,病,病变;影响 | celiac ~ 粥状泻,乳糜泻,婴儿型非热带口炎性腹泻

affection² [əˈfekʃən] *n* 感情 | **~al** *a*

affective [əˈfektiv] *a* 感情的,情感的 | **affectivity** [ˌæfekˈtivəti] *n* 感触性,易感性,情感性

affectomotor [əˌfektəˈməutə] *a* 情感运动(亢进)的

affektepilepsie [əˌfektˌepiˈlepsi] *n* 情感性痉挛(见于精神衰弱和强迫观念状态)

affenspalte [ˈɑːfənˌspɑːltə] *n*【德】月状沟(大脑枕叶)

afferent [ˈæfərənt] *a* 传入的(如传入神经)

afferentia [ˌæfəˈrenʃiə] *n*【拉】传入管,输入管(血管或淋巴管);淋巴管(统称)

affiliation [əˌfiliˈeiən] *n* 亲近,交往(一种社交动机)

affinin [ˈæfinin] *n* 阿菲宁,假向日葵酰胺(有杀虫和局部麻醉作用)

affinity [əˈfinəti] *n* 姻亲关系;(语言等的)类同,似近;亲合势,亲合力(对特殊元素、器官或结构的一种特殊吸引力,在热力学上是一种推动力) | chemical ~ 化学亲合力(将原子结合成分子);化学亲合势(物质有相互起反应的倾向) / elective ~ 选择性亲合力(指一物质选择另一物质结合,而不与其他物质结合) / residual ~ 剩余亲合力(使分子结合成较大的聚集体)

affluence [ˈæfluəns] *n* 流入;丰富 | **affluent** *a*

afflux [ˈæflʌks], **affluxion** [əˈflʌkʃən] *n* (血液或液体的)流向,流入,汇流

affusion [əˈfjuːʒən] *n* 冲浴,泼水疗法(使发烧减退,此法现在很少用)

AFib atrial fibrillation 心房纤颤,心房颤动

afibrinogenemia [əˌfaibrinədʒəˈniːmiə] *n* 纤维蛋白原缺乏血症 | congenital ~ 先天性纤维蛋白原缺乏血症(一种不常见的出血性凝血疾病,可能由常染色体隐性基因遗传,特征为血液完全不能凝固)

AFl atrial flutter 心房扑动

aflatoxicosis [ˌæfləˌtɔksiˈkəusis] *n* 黄曲霉[毒素]中毒(流传很广的流行病,死亡率高,亦称 X 病)

aflatoxin [ˌæfləˈtɔksin] *n* 黄曲霉毒素

AFO ankle-foot orthosis 踝-足矫形器,踝-足支具

AFP alpha-fetoprotein 甲胎蛋白

africate [ˈæfricət], **africative** [əˈfricətiv] *n* 塞擦音

AFS American Fertility Society 美国生育学会

afteraction [ˈɑːftəˌækʃən] *n* 后作用(可引起反应的刺激停止后所产生的效应)

afterbirth [ˈɑːftəˌbəːθ] 胞衣

afterbrain [ˈɑːftəˌbrein] *n* 后脑

aftercare [ˈɑːftəkɛə] *n* [术]后疗法(恢复期病人,尤指手术后病人的治疗与护理)

aftercurrent [ˌɑːftəˈkʌrənt] *n* 后电流(肌肉和神经在通电停止尚有电流)

afterdepolarization [ˌɑːftədiːˌpəuləraiˈzeiʃən, -riˈz-] *n* 后除极

afterdischarge [ˌɑːftədisˈtʃɑːdʒ] *n* 后发放(刺激物停止后,对感觉神经有兴奋作用的反应部分仍存在)

aftereffect [ˈɑːftəriˌfekt] *n* 后效应,后作用

aftergilding [ˌɑːftəˈgildiŋ] *n* 硬后镀金(在组织学中指神经组织在固定和硬化后,用金盐即氯金酸钠镀于其上)

afterhearing [ˌɑːftəˈhiəriŋ] *n* 余听觉,余音觉(产生听觉的刺激停止后,余音犹在)

afterimage [ˈɑːftəˌimidʒ] *n* 后像(引起原像的刺激停止后,视觉余像仍短暂存在)

afterload [ˈɑːftəˌləud] *n* 后负荷(心脏生理学中指抗心肌收缩之力)

aftermath [ˈæftəmæθ] *n* 再生草

aftermovement [ˌɑːftəˈmuːvmənt] *n* 后继性运动(手臂用力压刚硬物体使之麻木后,由于肌自身收缩,手臂自行上举)

afterpains [ˈɑːftəˌpeinz] [复] *n* 产后宫缩痛(子宫收缩所致)

afterperception [ˌɑːftəpəˈsepʃən] *n* 后知觉(产生知觉的刺激停止后,知觉仍存在)

afterpotential [ˌɑːftəpəuˈtenʃəl] *n* 后电位

aftersensation [ˌɑːftəsenˈseiʃən], **afterimpression** [ˌɑːftərimˈpreʃən] *n* 后感觉(产生感觉的刺激已经消除后,感觉仍存在)

aftersound [ˈɑːftəˌsaund] *n* 余音,余声,后音觉(振动停止后,余音犹在)

aftertaste [ˈɑːftəˌteist] *n* 余味(产生味觉的物质去除后,味觉感仍存在)

aftertreatment [ˌɑːftəˈtriːtmənt] *n* 术后治疗(见 aftercare)

aftervision [ˌɑːftəˈviʒən] *n* 后视觉(产生视觉的刺激停止后,视觉暂留)

aftosa [æfˈtəusə] *n*【西】口蹄疫

afunction [eiˈfʌnkʃən] *n* 功能缺失

AFX atypical fibroxanthoma 非典型纤维黄瘤

AG atrial gallop 心房性奔马律

A/G albumin / globulin (ratio) 白蛋白球蛋白(比率)

Ag antigen 抗原;argentum【拉】银

AGA American Gastroenterological Association 美国胃肠病学协会; American Geriatrics Association 美国老年病学协会

agalactia [ˌeigəˈlækʃiə] *n* 乳泌缺乏,无乳 | contagious ~ 接触传染性无乳(指山羊有时为绵羊的一种接触传染性疾病) | **agalactosis** [eiˌgælækˈtəusis] *n*

agalactosuria [eiˌgælæktəuˈsjuəriə] *n* 无半乳糖尿

agalactous [ˌeigəˈlæktəs] *a* [制]止乳[腺]分泌的;不用母乳的,人工喂养的

agalorrhea [eiˌgæləˈriə] *n* 乳泌停止,无乳

agamete [ˈægəmiːt] *n* 无性生殖体

agametic [ˌeigəˈmetik] *a* 无生殖细胞的,无配子的

agammaglobulinemia [eiˌgæməˌglɔbjuliˈniːmiə] *n* 无丙种球蛋白血症 | acquired ~ 获得性无丙种球蛋白血症 / common variable ~ 常见可变型无丙种球蛋白血症 / congenital ~ 先天性无丙种球蛋白血症 / lymphopenic ~ 淋巴细胞减少性无丙种球蛋白血症(即重度联合免疫缺陷) / Swiss type ~ 瑞士型无丙种球蛋白血症(一种致死的混合免疫缺乏综合征,伴有胸腺发育不全、无淋巴细胞症、迟发性免疫或细胞介导免疫形成能力缺乏等) / X-linked ~, X-linked infantile ~ X 连锁无丙种球蛋白血症,X 连锁婴儿无丙种球蛋白血症

agam(o)- [构词成分]无性的

Agamococcidiida [əˌgæməuˌkɔksiˈdiːidə] *n* 无性球孢子目

Agamodistomum [ˌægəməuˈdistəuməm] *n* 缺母吸虫属 | ~ ophthalmobium 眼缺母吸虫

Agamofilaria [əˌgæməufaiˈlɛəriə] *n* 缺母丝虫属

agamogenesis [ˌægəməuˈdʒenisis] *n* 无性生殖[期],裂殖生殖[期] | **agamogenetic** [ˌægəməudʒəˈnetik] *a* 裂殖生殖的 | **agamocytogeny** [əˌgæməusaiˈtɔdʒini], **agamogony** [ˌægəˈmɔgəni] *n*

Agamomermis culicis [ˌægəməuˈməːmis ˈkjuːlisis] 库蚊缺母线虫

Agamonema [ˌægəməuˈniːmə] *n* 缺母线虫属

Agamonematodum migrans [ˌægəməu ˌniːməˈtəudəm ˈmaigrəns] 游走缺母小线虫

agamont [ˈægəmɔnt] *n* 裂殖体

agamous [ˈægəməs] *a* 无性的;无性器官的;隐花的

aganglionic [eiˌgæŋgliˈɔnik] *a* 无神经节细胞的

aganglionosis [əˌgæŋgliəˈnəusis] *n* 无神经节症(副交感神经节细胞先天性缺乏,如先天性巨结肠)

agar [ˈeigɑː] *n* 琼脂(用作细菌固体培养基中的支持物以及用作免疫扩散和免疫电泳的支持物等)

Agarbacterium [ˌægɑːbækˈtiəriəm] *n* 琼脂菌属

agaric [ˈægərik, əˈgærik] *n* 伞菌,落叶松蕈;火绒(由干蕈类制成的引火物) | fly ~ 毒绳蕈 / larch ~, purging ~, white ~ 落叶松蕈 / surgeons' ~ 外科用落叶松蕈,干落叶松蕈(止血药)

Agaricaceae [əˌgæriˈkeisiiː] *n* 伞菌科

agaric acid [əˈgærik, ˈægərik] 松蕈三酸

Agaricales [əˌgæriˈkeiliːz] *n* 伞菌目

agaricic acid [ˌægəˈrisik] 松蕈三酸,落叶松蕈酸

Agaricus [əˈgærikəs] *n* 伞菌属,落叶松蕈属 | ~ campestris 洋蘑菇 / ~ muscarius 捕蝇蕈

agastria [əˈgæstriə] *n* 无胃[畸形]

agastric [əˈgæstrik] *a* 无胃的;无消化道的

Agave [əˈgeivi] *n*【拉】龙舌兰属

AGCT Army General Classification Test 陆军通用分类测验(美国安置军队人员的一种智力测验)

age [eidʒ] *n* 年龄;时期 *vi*, *vt* (ag⟨e⟩ing) 变老,老化 | achievement ~ 智力成就年龄 / bone ~ 骨龄 / chronological ~ 实足年龄 / emotional ~ 情感发育龄 / gestation ~ 孕龄 / menstrual ~ 月经龄 / mental ~ 智力年龄

ageing [ˈeidʒiŋ] *n* = **aging**
Agelenidae [ˌeidʒiˈlenidiː] *n* 漏斗网蛛科
agency [ˈeidʒənsi] *n* 力量;[能动]作用;代理处;机构
agenesis [eiˈdʒenisis], **agenesia** [ˌeidʒəˈniːziə] *n* 发育不全;无生殖力
agenitalism [eiˈdʒenitəlizəm] *n* 生殖腺功能缺失
agenized [ˈeidʒinaizd] *a* 用三氯化氮处理的(用于漂白)
agenosomia [eiˌdʒenəˈsəumiə] *n* 无生殖器[畸形],生殖器发育不全
agenosomus [eiˌdʒenəˈsəuməs] *n* 无生殖器畸胎
agent [ˈeidʒənt] *n* 剂,物;动因,因素,因子 | adrenergic blocking ~ 肾上腺素能阻滞药 / alkylating ~ 烷化剂;烃化剂 / Bittner ~ 比特纳因子,小鼠乳腺瘤病毒 / blocking ~ 阻滞药 / causative ~ 病原体 / chimpanzee coryza ~ 黑猩猩鼻炎病原因子,呼吸道合胞体病毒 / chelating ~ 螯合剂 / cholinergic blocking ~ 胆碱能阻断剂 / fixing ~s 固定剂;定像剂 / Marcy ~ 马尔西因子(可致人类无热性腹泻的一种病毒) / mouse mammary tumor ~ 小鼠乳腺瘤病毒 / Norwalk ~ 诺沃尔克因子(为急性感染性胃肠炎的病原体,可能是一种病毒) / Agent Orange 橙剂(除莠剂) / Pittsburgh pneumonia ~ 匹兹堡肺炎病原体 / progestational ~s 促孕剂 / reducing ~ 还原剂 / transforming ~ 转化因素 / vacuolating ~ 空泡因子 / virus inactivating ~ 病毒灭活素,病毒灭活因子 / wetting ~s 润湿剂
ageotropic [əˌdʒiːəuˈtrɔpik] *a* 非向地性的(指某些植物的根)
AGEPC acetyl glyceryl ether phosphoryl choline 乙酰甘油醚磷酸胆碱
agerasia [ˌædʒəˈreiziə] *n* 容颜不老,驻颜
ageusia [əˈgjuːziə], **ageustia** [əˈguːstiə] *n* 味觉缺失 | **ageusic** [əˈgjuːsik] *a*
agger [ˈædʒə] ([复] **aggeres** [ˈædʒəriːz]) *n* 【拉】堤,丘
agglomerate [əˈglɔməreit] *vt*, *vi* 凝聚;结块 [əˈglɔmərit] *a* 凝聚的;结块的 [əˈglɔmərit] *n* 大块;聚集;附聚物 | **~d** *a* 团集的,聚结的 / **agglomeration** [əˌglɔməˈreiʃən] *n* 成团;凝聚[反应];附聚[作用]
agglutinable [əˈgluːtinəbl] *a* 可凝集的
agglutinant [əˈgluːtinənt] *a* 黏合的 *n* 黏合剂
agglutinate [əˈgluːtinit] *a* 胶着的;凝集的 [əˈgluːtineit] *vt*, *vi* 黏结;凝集
agglutination [əˈgluːtiˈneiʃən] *n* 凝集[作用](创伤治愈时)愈合[过程];凝集[反应] | acid ~ 酸凝集[反应](细菌在氢离子浓度较低时的非特异性凝集) / bacteriogenic ~ 细菌促成性凝集[反应](由于细菌作用促成细胞凝集) / chief ~ 主[要]凝集[反应] / cold ~ 冷凝集[反应](只在低温时发生) / cross ~ 交叉凝集[反应](颗粒性抗原的凝集反应,在抗体碰到不同的、但相关的抗原而出现) / group ~ 群凝集[反应](如伤寒杆菌的特异性凝集素可以凝集结肠伤寒属中的大肠杆菌等) / H ~ H凝集,鞭毛凝集(抗体存在时游动细菌对不耐热鞭毛抗原的凝集) / intravascular ~ 血管内凝集(颗粒性成分在血管内聚集,常用于表示红细胞聚集) / macroscopic ~ 肉眼凝集[反应](用肉眼可看到反应产物——凝集物) / microscopic ~ 显微镜凝集[反应] / minor ~, part ~ 副凝集[反应] / O ~ O凝集,菌体凝集(抗体存在时,细菌向耐热菌体抗原凝集) / passive ~ 被动凝集[反应](抗血清中颗粒的凝集,颗粒上已吸附着特异性可溶性抗原) / platelet ~ 血小板凝集[反应](有时与凝聚反应交替使用) / spontaneous ~ 自发凝集[反应](细菌或其他细胞在生理盐水溶液中的凝集) / Vi ~ Vi凝集反应(含有Vi抗原的细菌如有特异性凝集素即在其表面上凝集)
agglutinative [əˈgluːtinətiv] *a* 黏结的;凝集的
agglutinator [əˈgluːtiˌneitə] *n* 凝集物,凝集素
agglutinin [əˈgluːtinin] *n* 凝集素 | anti-Rh ~ 抗Rh凝集素(一种正常不存在于人类血浆中的凝集素,但Rh阴性妇女怀有Rh阳性胎儿后或Rh阴性者接受Rh阳性输血后方可产生) / chief ~, haupt ~, major ~ 主[要]凝集素(动物经传染原免疫后,血液中的特异性免疫凝集素,在血清较高稀释度时,仍具有活性) / cold ~ 冷凝集素(只有在相当低的温度〈0 ~ 20 ℃〉时起反应) / complete ~s 完全凝集素(此种凝集素如IgM血凝素,可由简单直接试验说明之) / cross ~ 交叉凝集素(在对颗粒性抗原应答时所产生的凝集素,同时对不同的但有关的抗原同样发生特异性反应) / expected ~s 预期凝集素(针对血型A和〈或〉血型B红细胞抗原的正常人凝集素) / flagellar ~ 鞭毛凝集素 / group ~ 群凝集素(对某些细菌或细胞有特异作用,但同样也凝集其他密切相关的物种) / H ~ H凝集素,鞭毛凝集素(能动型菌株的鞭毛抗原所特有的凝集素) / immune ~ 免疫凝集素(血中特异性凝集素,由于病痊愈或注射了引起疾病的微生物而产生) / incomplete ~ 不完全凝集素(在合适浓度时不能与同种抗原凝集,只有当悬浮于高分子量介质中或用血清抗球蛋白反应方能证实) / leukocyte ~ 白细胞凝集素(针对中性粒细胞和其他白细胞的一种凝集素,见于多种疾病) / MG ~ MG(链球菌)凝集素 / normal ~ 正常凝集素(人或动物血中的特异性凝集素) / O ~ O凝集素,菌体凝集素(微生物菌体抗原特有的凝集素) / partial ~, minor ~,副凝集素(凝集血清中的凝集素,与特异性抗原密切相关

的细菌和细胞起反应,但在较低的稀释度时反应)/ platelet ~ 血小板凝集素(可在若干疾病中见到,或许与已证实的血小板减少症并不总是相关的,它在血小板分类法中很重要)/ somatic ~ 菌体凝集素(微生物体特有的凝集素)/ unexpected ~ 非预期凝集素(针对红细胞抗原,而不是针对血型 A 和血型 B 抗原的正常凝集素或免疫凝集素)/ warm ~ 温[型]凝集素(在 37 ℃反应最强)

agglutinogen [ˌæglu:ˈtinədʒən] *n* 凝集原(指任何引起产生凝集素的抗原,也指做凝集试验用的颗粒性抗原) | **~ic** [əˌglu:tinəˈdʒenic], **agglutogenic** [əˌglu:təˈdʒenik] *a* 产生凝集素的

agglutinophilic [əˌglu:tinəˈfilik] *a* 易凝集的

agglutinoscope [əˈglu:tinəˌskəup] *n* 凝集反应镜

agglutometer [ˌæglu:ˈtɔmitə] *n* 凝集反应器(伤寒凝集试验用,不用显微镜)

aggrandize [əˈgrændaiz] *vt* 增大;提高 | **~ment** [əˈgrændizmənt] *n*

aggravate [ˈægrəveit] *vt* 加重;使恶化 | **aggravation** [ˌægrəˈveiʃən] *n*

aggred. feb. aggrediente febre【拉】热续升时

Aggregata [ˌægriˈgeitə] *n* 丛集球虫属

aggregate [ˈægrigit] *a* 聚集的,集合的;凝聚的;合计的 *n* 聚集,集合;聚集体,凝聚物 | leukocyte ~ 白细胞聚集体 [ˈægrigeit] *vt*, *vi* 聚集;凝聚 | **aggregation** [ˌægriˈgeiʃən] *n* 聚集,集合;集合物;凝聚反应 / **aggregative** [ˈægrigeitiv] *a* 聚集的

aggregen [ˈægrədʒin] *n* [细胞]集合体

aggregometer [ægriˈgɔmitə] *n* 集合度计(检测由血小板〈或微粒〉群引起血浆〈或溶液〉旋光密度的变化)

aggregometry [ˌægriˈgɔmitri] *n* 集合度测定

aggrephore [ˈægrəfɔ:] *n* 集合管

aggressin [əˈgresin] *n* 攻击素(曾认为由病原菌产生的物质,较易侵入宿主组织并在体内扩散传染因子)

aggression [əˈgreʃən] *n* 攻击行为(一种行为型)

aggressive [əˈgresiv] *a* 攻击性的;有进取心的;(行为)过分的

aging [ˈeidʒiŋ] *n* 老龄化,衰老;老化 | successful ~ 健康老龄化

agitate [ˈædʒiteit] *vt* 搅动,振荡;焦急不安,激越,激动 | **~d** *a* 焦虑不安的;激越的 / **agitation** [ˌædʒiˈteiʃən] *n* / **agitator** [ˈædʒiteitə] *n* 搅拌器,振荡器

agitographia [ˌædʒitəuˈgræfiə] *n* 急躁性错写

agitophasia [ˌædʒitəuˈfeiziə], **agitolalia** [ˌædʒitəuˈleiliə] *n* 急躁性错语

Agit. vas. agitato vase【拉】振摇容器

Agkistrodon [ægˈkistrədɔn] *n* 蝮蛇属

aglaucopsia, aglaukopsia [ˌæglɔ:ˈkɔpsiə] *n* 绿色盲

aglomerular [ˌægləuˈmerjulə] *a* 肾小球缺乏的

aglossia [eiˈglɔsiə] *n* 无舌畸形

aglossostomia [ˌeiglɔsəuˈstəumiə] *n* 无舌锁口(畸形)

aglucon [əˈglu:kɔn], **aglucone** [əˈglu:kəun] *n* 配基,糖苷配基

aglutition [eiglu:ˈtiʃən] *n* 吞咽不能

aglycemia [ˌeiglaiˈsi:miə] *n* 血糖缺乏

aglycon [əˈglaikɔn], **aglycone** [əˈglaikəun] *n* 配基,糖苷配基

aglycosuric [eiˌglaikəuˈsjuərik] *a* 无糖尿的

agmatology [ˌægməˈtɔlədʒi] *n* 骨折学

agminated [ˈægmiˌneitid] *a* 簇状的,成簇的;集合的,聚集的

agnail [ˈægneil] *n* 逆剥,甲刺(甲上的逆刺皮)

agnate [ˈægneit] *n* 男方亲属,父系亲属(按苏格兰法律,指判为精神病的一方的父系亲属,并任命为同一方的监护人) *a* 男方的,父系的 | **agnatic** [ægˈnætik] *a* 男方的,父系的

Agnatha [ˈægneiθə] *n* 无颌纲

agnathia [ægˈneiθiə] *n* 无颌畸形 | **agnathous** [ægˈneiθəs] *a*

agnathus [ægˈneiθəs] *n* 无下颌

agnea [ægˈniə] *n* (对物体)认识不能,失认

Agnew's splint [ˈægnju:] (David H. Agnew) 阿格纽夹板(髌骨掌骨骨折用)

agnogenic [ˌægnəuˈdʒenik] *a* 起因不明的,病因不明的

agnosia [ægˈnəuziə] *n* 失认[症] | acoustic ~, auditory ~ 听觉失认[症] / body-image ~ 体像失认[症]

agnosterol [ægˈnɔstərɔl] *n* 羊毛脂甾醇

agnostic [ægˈnɔstik] *n* 不可知论者 *a* 不可知论的 | **agnosticism** *n* 不可知论

agnus castus [ˈægnəs ˈkæstəs]【拉】羊荆,荆子

agofollin [əˈgɔfəlin] *n* 雌二醇

-agogue [构词成分]催,利

agomphiasis [ˌægɔmˈfaiəsis], **agomphosis** [ˌægɔmˈfəusis] *n* 无牙,缺牙;牙动,松动牙 | **agomphious** [əˈgɔmfiəs] *a*

agonad [eiˈgɔnæd] *n* 无生殖腺者 *a* 无生殖腺的

agonadal [eiˈgɔnədl] *a* 无生殖腺的,无性腺的

agonadism [eiˈgəunədizəm] *n* 无性腺症

agonal [ˈægənl] *a* 濒死痛苦的;末期传染的

agoniadin [ˌægəˈnaiədin] *n* 鸡蛋花苷(解热药)

agonist [ˈægənist] *n* 主动肌,主缩肌(与拮抗肌对立);激动药

agony [ˈægəni] *n* 剧痛,极度痛苦;濒死挣扎

agoraphilia [ˌægərəˈfiliə] *n* 嗜广场癖,恋旷野癖

agoraphobia [ˌægərəˈfəubjə] *n* 广场恐怖症

Agostini's test (reaction) [ˌægəsˈtini] (C. Agostini) 阿戈斯蒂尼试验(反应)(检葡萄糖)

agouti [əˈguːti] *n* 刺鼠,南美豚鼠;野鼠色

-agra [构词成分]急性疼痛发作

agraffe [əˈgrɑːf] *n*【法】对合钳(使伤口对合)

agrammatism [eiˈgræmətizəm], **agrammatica** [ˌægrəˈmætikə], **agrammatologia** [eiˌgræmətəuˈləudʒiə] *n* 语法缺失(说话不能合乎语法,由于脑损伤或脑病所致)

agranulocyte [eiˈgrænjuləuˌsait] *n* 无粒白细胞

agranulocytosis [eiˌgrænjuləusaiˈtəusis], **agranulosis** [eiˌgrænjuˈləusis] *n* 粒细胞缺乏 | infantile genetic ~ 婴儿遗传性粒细胞缺乏[症](亦称科斯曼〈Kostmann〉综合征) / infectious feline ~ 猫传染性粒细胞缺乏[症],猫瘟

agranuloplastic [eiˌgrænjuləuˈplæstik] *a* 只形成无粒细胞的,不形成粒细胞的

agraphia [əˈgræfiə] *n* 书写不能,失写[症](大脑皮质损害所致) | literal ~ 字母书写不能 / mental ~, cerebral ~ 精神性书写不能,大脑性书写不能 / optic ~ 视觉性书写不能 | **agraphic** *a*

agria [ˈægriə] *n*【拉】脓疱,疱疹

Agriolimax [ˌægriəˈlaimæks] *n* 野蛞蝓属 | ~ laevis 光润蛞蝓

agrius [ˈeigriəs] *a*【拉】剧烈的(指皮肤发疹)

Agrobacterium [ˌægrəubækˈtiəriəm] *n* 土壤杆菌属 | ~ radiobacter 放射形土壤杆菌

agromania [ˌægrəuˈmeinjə] *n* 隐居癖,野居癖

Agropyron [ˌægrəuˈpaiərɔn] *n* 冰草属

Agropyrum [ˌægrəuˈpaiərəm] *n* 冰草属

Agrostemma [ˌægrəˈstemə] *n* 麦仙翁属

Agrostis [əˈgrɔstis] *n* 禾草属

agrypnia [əˈgripniə] *n* 失眠

agrypnocoma [əˌgripnəuˈkəumə] *n* 醒态昏迷,睁眼昏迷

agrypnotic [ˌægripˈnɔtik], **agrypnode** [əˈgripnəud] *a* 醒态的 *n* 阻睡药

AGS American Geriatrics Society 美国老年医学会

AGT antiglobulin test 抗球蛋白试验

AGTH adrenoglomerulotropin 促醛固酮激素

aguamiel [ˌægwəmiˈel] *n* 龙舌兰汁

ague [ˈeigjuː] *n* 疟[疾],疟状发热;寒战 | brass-founders' ~ 黄铜铸工热病(吸入锌尘所致) / dumb ~ 哑疟(无寒战疟疾) / quartan ~ 三日疟 / quintan ~ 四日疟 / quotidian ~ 日发疟/ shaking ~ 寒战疟 / tertian ~ 间日疟 | **aguish** [ˈeigju(ː)iʃ] *a*

AGV aniline gentian violet 苯胺龙胆紫(染色剂)

agyria [eiˈdʒaiəriə] *n* 无脑回[畸形] | **agyric** *a*

ah 远视散光(hyperopic astigmatism)的符号

AHA American Heart Association 美国心脏协会; American Hospital Association 美国医院协会

ahaptoglobinemia [eiˌhæptəuˌgləubiˈniːmiə] *n* 触珠蛋白缺乏血症

AHCPR Agency for Health Care Policy and Research 卫生保健政策与研究处(属美国公共卫生署)

AHF antihemophilic factor 抗血友病因子(凝血因子Ⅷ)

AHG antihemophilic globulin 抗血友病球蛋白(凝血因子Ⅷ)

ahistidasia [əˌhistiˈdeiziə] *n* 组氨酸酶缺乏

AHP Assistant House Physician 内科助理住院医师

AHS Assistant House Surgeon 外科助理住院医师

Ahumada-del Castillo syndrome [ɑːuːˈmɑːθæ deil kɑːsˈtiːjəu] (Juan C. Ahumada; E. B. del Castillo) 阿-卡综合征(乳溢闭经综合征伴促性腺激素分泌过少)

AI anaphylatoxin inhibitor 过敏毒素抑制剂; aortic incompetence 主动脉瓣关闭不全; aortic insufficiency 主动脉瓣关闭不全; apical impulse 心尖冲动; artificial insemination 人工授精

AIC Association des Infirmières Canadiennes 加拿大医务所协会

Aicardi's syndrome [iˈkɑːdi] (J. Aicardi) 伊卡第综合征(累及女婴的一种综合征,特征为胼胝体发育不全、不连续的大面积脉络膜视网膜病、痉挛与强直发作以及智力迟钝)

AICC anti-inhibitor coagulant complex 抗抑制剂促凝剂复合物

AICD activation-induced cell death 激活诱发细胞死亡; automatic implantable cardioverter-defibrillator 埋藏式自动复律除颤器

aichmophobia [ˌeikməuˈfəubjə] *n* 锋刃恐怖,尖端恐怖

AID artificial insemination by donor 他精人工授精

aid [eid] *n* 帮助;救护;辅助器 | first ~ 急救 / hearing ~ 助听器 / pharmaceutic ~, pharmaceutical ~ 调剂辅佐剂 / prosthetic speech ~ 助语假腭托 / speech ~ 助话器;助话疗法

AIDS acquired immunodeficiency syndrome 获得性免疫缺陷综合征,艾滋病

AIH American Institute of Homeopathy 美国顺势疗法学会; artificial insemination by husband 夫精人工授精

AIHA American Industrial Hygiene Association 美国工业卫生协会; autoimmune hemolytic anemia 自身免疫性溶血性贫血

ail [eil] *vt* 使受病痛,使苦恼 *vi* 有病痛,生病

Ailanthus [eiˈlænθəs], **Ailantus** [eiˈlæntəs] *n* 臭椿属,樗属

ailantic acid [eiˈlæntik] 高樗酸,樗酸

AILD angioimmunoblastic lymphadenopathy with

dysproteinemia 血管免疫母细胞淋巴结病伴异常蛋白血症
ailment ['eilmənt] *n* 疾病,失调(一般指轻微疾病)
ailurophilia [aiˌljuərə'filiə] *n* 嗜猫癖
ailurophobia [aiˌljuərə'fəubjə] *n* 猫恐怖,恐猫症
ainhum ['einhəm] *n* 箍趾病(自发性断趾病,主要见于热带国家)
AIP acute intermittent porphyria 急性间歇性卟啉病
air [ɛə] *n* 气,空气 | alveolar ~ 肺泡气 / factitious ~ 一氧化二氮,氧化亚氮 / liquid ~ 液态空气 / reserve ~ 储气(补呼气) / residual ~ 余气 / tidal ~ 潮[流]气 / venous alveolar ~ 静脉血平衡性肺泡气
airborne ['ɛəbɔːn] *a* 空气传播的
air-condition ['ɛəkənˌdiʃən] *vt* 调节空气
air-cooled ['ɛəkuːld] *a* 空气冷却的
airdent ['ɛədənt] *n* 气磨洞形器(牙科用)
airflow ['ɛəˌfləu] *n* 气流;气流速度
airsacculitis [ˌɛəsækjuː'laitis] *n* 肺泡炎(指鸟类)
airsick ['ɛəˌsik] *a* 晕机的 | **~ness** *n* 空晕病
airstream ['ɛəˌstriːm] *n* 气流
airtight ['ɛətait] *a* 不漏气的,密封的
airway ['ɛəˌwei] *n* 气道;导气管(全身麻醉时保证空气毫无阻碍地进出肺部) | esophageal obturator ~ 食管充填器导气管 / nasopharyngeal ~ 鼻咽导气管 / oropharyngeal ~ 口咽导气管
AIUM American Institute of Ultrasound in Medicine 美国医用超声学会
Ajellomyces [əˌdʒeləu'maisiːz] *n* 阿杰罗菌属,组织胞浆菌属
A-K, AK above knee 膝上(截肢)
ak- 以 ak-起始的词,同样见以 ac-起始的词
akaryocyte [ei'kæriəˌsait], **akaryota** [eiˌkæri'əutə], **akaryote** [ei'kæriəut] *n* 无核细胞(如红细胞)
akaryomastigont [eiˌkæriəu'mæstigɔnt] *n* 无核鞭毛
akatama [ˌækə'tæmə] *n* 慢性周围神经炎(曾见于西非洲)
akatamathesia [əˌkætəmə'θiːziə] *n* [言语]理解不能
akatanoesis [əˌkætə'nəuəsis] *n* 自我理解不能
akathisia [ˌækə'θiːziə] *n* 静坐不能(见于酚噻嗪的毒性反应,亦称静坐恐怖)
akee ['ækiː] *n* 阿开木果实,西非荔枝果(儿童食其生果子会引起致命性中毒)
akembe [ə'kembiː] *n* 阿肯病,血小板减少性紫癜症(非洲病名)
Åkerlund deformity ['ekəlund] (Åke O. Åkerlund) 阿克隆德变形(十二指肠溃疡时,十二指肠冠在X线照片中的变形,除龛影以外还有切迹)
akidogalvanocautery [ˌækaidəˌgælvənəu'kɔːtəri] *n* 电针烙术
akin [ə'kin] *a* 同族的,有亲缘关系的;同类的,相近似的
akinesia [ˌeiki'niːzjə], **akinesis** [ˌeiki'niːsis] *n* 运动不能,无动力
akinesthesia [əˌkinis'θiːzjə] *n* 运动[感]觉缺失
akinetic [ˌeiki'netik] *a* 运动不能的;无丝分裂的
akiyami [ˌɑːki'jɑːmi] *n* 七日热(钩端螺旋体病)
aklomide ['ækləmaid] *n* 阿克洛胺(家禽抑球虫药)
aknephascopia [ˌæknefə'skəupiə] *n* 黄昏盲,雀盲症
Akokanthera [ˌækəkæn'θiərə] *n* 箭毒木属(夹竹桃科)
akoria [ə'kɔriə] *n* 贪食,不饱[症]
Akureyri disease [ə'kjuəreiri] (Akureyri 为冰岛一地名)阿库雷里病,良性肌痛性脑脊髓炎
Al aluminium 铝
-al [后缀]表示醛基,如 choral;同样用于构成形容词,如 arterial 和名词,如 denial
ALA aminolevulinic acid 氨基乙酰丙酸,氨基-γ-酮戊酸
Ala alanine 丙氨酸
ala ['eilə] ([复]**alae** ['eiliː]) *n*【拉】翼,翼膜
alacrima [ei'lækrimə] *n* 无泪
alactasia [əlæk'teiziə] *n* 乳糖酶缺乏
Alagille syndrome [ɑːlɑː'ʒiːl] (Daniel Alagille) 阿拉惹综合征(一种常染色体显性遗传综合征:新生儿黄疸胆汁淤积伴周围肺动脉瓣狭窄,有时为中隔缺损或动脉导管未闭,系由肝内胆管缺少或缺如所致,特征为异常面容和眼、脊椎及神经系统异常)
Alajouanine's syndrome [ˌæləʒuə'niːn] (T. Alajouanine)阿拉让宁综合征(第六、七对脑神经对称性损伤,双侧面瘫及双侧外直肌麻痹,伴双侧畸形足)
alalia [ə'leiliə] *n* 哑;失语[症] | ~ cophica 聋哑症 | **alalic** [ə'lælik] *a*
alamecin [ælə'miːsin] *n* 阿来霉素(抗生素类药)
Åland eye disease ['ɑːlənd] (Åland Islands 为芬兰在波罗的海的群岛,20世纪60年代首次在此发现此病)阿兰群岛眼病(见 Forsius-Eriksson syndrome)
alangine [ə'lændʒin] *n* 八角枫碱
Alangium [ə'lændʒiəm] *n* 八角枫属
alanine (Ala, A) ['æləniːn] *n* 丙氨酸
***β*-alanine** ['æləniːn] *n* β-丙氨酸
alanine aminotransferase ['æləniːn əˌmiːnəu-'trænsfəreis] 丙氨酸转氨酶(亦称谷[氨酸]-丙

[酮酸]转氨酶)

alanine-glyoxylate aminotransferase [ˈæləniːn glaiˈɔksileit əˌminəuˈtrænsfəreis] 丙氨酸乙醛酸转氨酶(见 alanine-glyoxylate transaminase)

alanine-glyoxylate transaminase [ˈæləniːn glai-ˈɔksileit trænsˈæmineis] 丙氨酸乙醛酸转氨酶(肝性过氧物酶体酶缺乏为一种常染色体隐性性状,可致原发性Ⅰ型高草酸尿)

β-alanine-α-ketoglutarate transaminase [ˈæləniːn ˌkiːtəuˈgluːtəreit trænsˈæmineis] β-丙氨酸-α-酮戊二酸转氨酶(此酶活性缺乏可致高β-丙氨酸血症)

β-alaninemia [ˌæləniˈniːmiə] *n* β-丙氨酸血症,高β-丙氨酸血症

β-alanine-pyruvate aminotransferase [ˈæləniːn ˈpaiəruːveit əˌmiːnəuˈtrænsfəreis] β-丙氨酸丙酮酸转氨酶(即 β-alanine-pyruvate transaminase)

β-alanine-pyruvate transaminase [ˈæləniːn ˈpaiəruːveit trænsˈæmineis] β-丙氨酸丙酮酸转氨酶

alanine transaminase (ALT) [ˈæləniːn trænsˈæminesis] 丙氨酸转氨酶

β-alanine transaminase [ˈæləniːn trænsˈæmineis] β-丙氨酸转氨酶

Alanson's amputation [ˈælənsn] (Edward Alanson) 阿兰森切断术(环形切断术,残肢呈空心圆锥状)

alantin [əˈlæntin] *n* 菊粉,土木香粉

alanyl [ˈælənil] *n* 丙氨酰[基]

alanyl-leucine [ˌælənil-ˈljuːsin] *n* 丙氨酰亮氨酸

alar [ˈeilə] *a* 翼的,翅的;腋的

ALARA as low as reasonably achievable (exposure dose of radiation) 达到尽可能低的(放射照射剂量)

Alaria [əˈleiriə] *n* 重翼[吸虫]属

alarm [əˈlɑːm] *n* 警报;惊恐

ALAS 5-aminolevulinate synthase 5 氨基乙酰丙酸合酶

alastrim [əˈlæstrim] *n* 类天花 | **~ic** [ˌæləsˈtrimik], **alastrinic** [ˌæləsˈtrinik] *a*

ALAT alanine aminotransferase 丙氨酸氨基转移酶,丙氨酸转氨酶

alate [ˈeileit] *a* 有翼的

alatrofloxacin mesylate [əˌlætrəuˈflɔksəsin] 甲磺阿拉沙星(抗菌药)

alba [ˈælbə] *a* 【拉】白的(用于解剖学名词,如 substantia ~ 白质;用于某些疾病,如 pityriasis ~ 白糠疹)

Albarrán's disease [ˌælbɑːˈrɑːn] (Joaquin Albarrán y Dominguez) 大肠杆菌尿 | ~ gland 阿尔巴朗腺(膀胱悬雍垂下前列腺中叶部) / ~ test 多尿试验(检肾功能不全) / ~ tubules 前列腺小管

albedo [ælˈbiːdəu] *n* 【拉】白色 | ~ retinae 视网膜水肿

Albee's operation [ˈɔːlbiː] (Fred. H. Albee) 阿尔比手术(股骨头髋臼融合术,治髋关节强硬)

albendazole [ælˈbendəzəul] *n* 阿苯达唑(抗蠕虫药)

Albers-Schönberg disease [ˈɑːlbəz ˈʃiːnbəːg] (Heinrich E. Albers-Schönberg) 骨硬化病

Albertini's treatment [ælbəˈtini] (Ippolito F. Albertini) 阿尔贝蒂尼疗法(主动脉动脉瘤时绝对休息和节制饮食)

Albert's diphtheria stain [ˈælbət] (Henry Albert) 艾伯特白喉杆菌染剂(含有苯甲胺蓝和甲基绿或孔雀绿的染剂)

Albert's operation [ˈælbət] (Eduard Albert) 阿尔贝特手术(膝关节强直术,作为连枷关节的疗法) | ~ suture 阿尔贝特缝合术(一种肠缝合术,第一排缝线穿过肠管全层厚度)

albescent [ælˈbesənt] *a* 正在变白的,微白的

albicans [ˈælbikənz] ([复] **albicantia** [ˌælbiˈkænʃiə]) *a* 【拉】白色的 *n* 白体;乳头状体

albiduria [ˌælbiˈdjuəriə] *n* 白尿;乳糜尿

albidus [ˈælbidəs] *a* 【拉】带白的

albinism [ˈælbinizəm] *n* 白化病(皮肤、毛发、眼睛先天性色素缺乏) | autosomal recessive ocular ~ (AROA) 常染色体隐性遗传眼白化病 / ocular ~ (OA) 眼白化病 / oculocutaneous ~ (OCA) 眼皮肤白化病 / partial ~, localized ~ 局部白化病 / total ~ 全身白化病 / tyrosinase-negative (ty-neg) oculocutaneous ~ 酪氨酸酶阴性眼皮肤白化病 / tyrosinase-positive (ty-pos) oculocutaneous ~ 酪氨酸酶阳性眼皮肤白化病 / X-linked ocular ~ (Nettleship) (XOAN) X 连锁眼白化病(Nettleship 型) | **albinotic** [ˌælbiˈnɔtik] *a*

albinismus [ˌælbiˈnizməs] *n* 【拉】白化病

Albini's nodules [ælˈbini] (Giuseppe Albini) 阿尔比尼小结(灰色小结,谷粒状大小,有时见于幼儿房室瓣游离缘,为胎儿结构的残留)

albino [ælˈbiːnəu] *n* 白化病患者

albinoidism [ælbiˈnɔidizəm] *n* 不完全白化病,类白化病(毛发、皮肤、眼睛内色素缺乏,但还未到白化病所见的程度) | oculocutaneous ~ 眼皮肤类白化病 / punctate oculocutaneous ~ 点状眼皮肤类白化病

albinuria [ˌælbiˈnjuəriə] *n* 白尿;乳糜尿

Albinus muscle [ælˈbiːnəs] (Bernard S. Albinus) 笑肌;中斜角肌

Albrecht's bone [ˈɑːlbreʃt] (Karl MP. Albrecht) 耳底骨

Albright's syndrome [ˈɔːlbrait] (Fuller Albright) 奥尔布赖特综合征(多骨纤维性结构不良症、斑

片状皮肤色素沉着和内分泌功能障碍)

albuginea [ˌælbjuˈdʒiniə] *n*【拉】白膜 | ~ oculi 巩膜

albugineotomy [ˌælbjuˌdʒiniˈɔtəmi] *n* [睾丸]白膜切开术

albugineous [ˌælbjuˈdʒiniəs] *a* 白膜的

albuginitis [ˌælbjudʒiˈnaitis] *n* 白膜炎

albugo [ælˈbjuːgəu] *n*【拉】角膜白斑

albumen [ˈælbjumin] *n*【拉】卵白;白蛋白,清蛋白

albumin [ˈælbjumin] *n* 白蛋白,清蛋白 | ~ A 白蛋白 A(血清的一种成分,癌患者白蛋白 A 数量减少,但在癌细胞中大量聚集) / circulating ~ 体液白蛋白 / derived ~ 衍生白蛋白 / egg ~ 卵白蛋白 / hematin ~ 高铁血红素白蛋白 / iodinated ^{125}Ⅰ serum ~, radioiodinated(^{125}Ⅰ) serum ~ (human) 放射碘(^{125}Ⅰ)人血清白蛋白(诊断用以测定血容量和心排出量) / normal human serum ~ 正常人血清白蛋白(用于防治休克及治疗低蛋白血症) / soap ~ 皂合白蛋白,蛋白脂 / serum ~, blood ~ 血清白蛋白,血液白蛋白(人血清中主要蛋白成分) / ~ tannate 鞣酸蛋白(用于腹泻)

albuminate [ælˈbjuːmineit] *n* 变性蛋白

albuminaturia [ælˌbjuːminəˈtjuəriə] *n* 变性蛋白尿

albuminemia [ælˌbjuːmiˈniːmiə] *n* 白蛋白血症

albuminimeter [ælˌbjuːmiˈnimitə], **albumimeter** [ælˌbjuˈmimitə], **albuminometer** [ælˌbjuːmiˈnɔmitə] *n* 白蛋白定量器 | **albuminimetry** [ælˌbjuːmiˈnimitri] *n* 白蛋白定量法

albuminocholia [ælˌbjuːminəuˈkəuliə] *n* 蛋白胆汁症

albuminocytological [ælˌbjuːminəuˌsaitəˈlɔdʒikəl] *a* 白蛋白细胞学的

albuminoid [ælˈbjuːminɔid] *a* 蛋白样的 *n* 纤维白蛋白;硬蛋白

albuminolysin [ˌælbjumiˈnɔlisin] *n* 白蛋白溶素;过敏素

albuminolysis [ælˌbjuːmiˈnɔlisis] *n* 白蛋白分解

albuminoptysis [ˌælbjumiˈnɔptisis] *n* 白蛋白痰

albuminoreaction [ælˌbjuːminəuri(ː)ˈækʃən] *n* 白蛋白反应(检痰白蛋白试验,痰内有白蛋白〈阳性反应〉是肺炎的指征)

albuminorrhea [ælˌbjuːminəˈriə] *n* 白蛋白溢

albuminous [ælˈbjuːminəs] *a* 白蛋白的

albuminuretic [ælˌbjuːminjuəˈretik] *a* 蛋白尿的,促蛋白尿的 *n* 促蛋白尿剂

albuminuria [ælˌbjuːmiˈnjuəriə] *n* 蛋白尿 | **albuminuric** [ˌælbjumiˈnjuərik] *a*

albuminurophobia [ælˌbjuːmiˌnjuərəˈfəubjə] *n* 蛋白尿恐怖

albumoscope [ælˈbjuːməˌskəup] *n* (尿)白蛋白测定器

albumose [ˈælbjuməus] *n* [蛋白]脲

albuterol [ælˈbjuːtərəul] *n* 沙丁胺醇(亦称 salbutamol,支气管扩张药) | ~ sulfate 硫酸沙丁胺醇

Alcaligenes [ˌælkəˈlidʒiniːz] *n* 产碱[杆]菌属 | ~ dentrificans 反硝化产碱菌 / ~ faecalis 粪产碱菌 / ~ odorans 臭味产碱菌

alcapton [ælˈkæptɔn] *n* 尿黑酸

alcaptonuria [ælˌkæptəuˈnjuəriə] *n* 尿黑酸尿症 | **alcaptonuric** *a*

alchemy [ˈælkimi] *n* 炼丹术

alclofenac [ælˈkləufenæk] *n* 阿氯芬酸(镇痛、解热、抗炎药,用于治疗类风湿关节炎)

alclometasone dipropionate [ˌælkləuˈmetəsəun] 二丙酸阿氯米松(合成皮质类固醇,皮质类固醇反应性皮病时局部用于缓解炎症和瘙痒症)

Alcock's canal [ˈælkɔk] (Benjamin Alcock) 阴部管

alcogel [ˈælkədʒel] *n* 醇凝胶

alcohol [ˈælkəhɔl] *n* 醇,乙醇,酒精 | amyl ~ 戊醇 / anisyl ~ 茴香醇,对甲氧基苄醇,对甲氧基苯甲醇 / batyl ~ 鲨肝醇 / benzyl ~ 苄醇,苯甲醇 / bornyl ~, camphyl ~ 冰片 / butyl ~ 丁醇 / carnaubyl ~ 二十四[烷]醇,巴西棕榈醇 / ceryl ~ 蜡醇,二十六[烷]醇 / cetyl ~ 鲸蜡醇,十六烷醇 / cinnamyl ~ 肉桂醇 / dehydrated ~, absolute ~ 无水醇 / denatured ~ 变性醇 / deodorized ~ 去味乙醇 / dihydric ~ 二羟醇,二元醇 / diluted ~ 稀醇 / ethyl ~ 乙醇 / fatty ~ 脂肪醇 / glyceryl ~, glycyl ~ 甘油/ isoamyl ~ 异戊醇 / isobutyl ~ 异丁醇 / isopropyl ~ 异丙醇 / ketone ~ 酮醇 / methyl ~ 甲醇 / monohydric ~ 一元醇 / palmityl ~ 棕榈醇 / primary ~ 伯醇 / *n*-propyl ~ 正丙醇 / secondary ~ 仲醇 / stearyl ~ 十八[烷]醇 / tertiary ~ 叔醇 / tertiary amyl ~ 叔戊醇,水合戊烯 / tribromoethyl ~ 三溴乙醇 / trihydric ~ 三元醇 / wood ~ 甲醇,木醇

alcoholase [ˈælkəhɔˌleis] *n* 醇酶

alcohol dehydrogenase [ˈælkəhɔl diːˈhaidrədʒəneis] 醇脱氢酶(亦称乙醛还原酶)

alcohol dehydrogenase (NADP$^+$) [ˈælkəhɔl diːˈhaidrədʒəneis] 醇脱氢酶(NADP$^+$)

alcohol dehydrogenase [NAD(P)$^+$] 醇脱氢酶[NAD(P)$^+$]

alcoholemia [ˌælkəhɔˈliːmiə] *n* 醇血症

alcoholic [ˌælkəˈhɔlik] *a* 醇的,乙醇的,酒精的 *n* 酗酒者,嗜酒者

alcoholism [ˈælkəhɔlizəm] *n* 酒精中毒 | acute ~ 急性酒精中毒 / chronic ~ 慢性酒精中毒

alcoholize [ˈælkəhɔlaiz] *vt* 用乙醇处理,用乙醇治疗;使醇化 | **alcoholization** [ˌælkəˌhɔlaiˈzeiʃən] *n* 乙醇疗法;醇化[作用]

alcoholometer [ˌælkəhɔˈlɔmitə] *n* 酒精比重计,醇定量计

alcoholuria [ˌælkəhɔˈljuəriə] *n* 醇尿

alcoholysis [ˌælkəˈhɔlisis] *n* 醇解

alcosol [ˈælkəsɔl] *n* 醇溶胶

alcuronium chloride [ælkjuˈrɔniəm] 阿库氯铵(骨骼肌松弛药)

aldaric acid [ælˈdærik] 醛糖二羧酸

aldehydase [ˌældiˈhaideis] *n* 醛酶

aldehyde [ˈældihaid] *n* 醛 | acetic ~ 乙醛 / acrylic ~ 丙烯醛 / amylic ~ [正]戊醛 / anisic ~ 茴香醛(甲氧基苯甲醛) / benzoic ~ 苯[甲]醛 / cinnamic ~ 肉桂醛,桂皮醛 / cumic ~ 枯醛,对异丙基苯甲醛 / glyceric ~, glycerin ~ 甘油醛/ trichloracetic ~ 三氯乙醛,氯醛 / valeric ~ 戊醛

aldehyde dehydrogenase (NAD⁺) [ˈældihaid diːˈhaidrədʒəneis] 醛脱氢酶(NAD⁺)(亦称乙醛脱氢酶)

aldehyde-lyase [ˈældihaidˈlaieis] *n* 醛裂合酶

aldehyde oxidase [ˈældihaid ˈɔksideis] 醛氧化酶

aldehyde reductase [ˈældihaid riˈdʌkteis] 醛还原酶(半乳糖激酶缺乏所致的半乳糖血症时,晶状体内醛还原酶催化半乳糖还原成半乳糖醇,可致白内障形成。亦称醛糖还原酶)

Alder-Reilly anomaly [ˈɔːldə ˈraili] (Albert von Alder; William A. Reilly) 奥-里异常(见 Alder's anomaly) | ~ bodies 奥-里小体(粗大嗜苯胺蓝颗粒,见于奥-里异常时的白细胞内)

Alder's anomaly, constitutional granulation anomaly [ˈɔːldə] (Albert von Alder) 奥尔德异常,体质性颗粒性异常(一种常染色体遗传病,骨髓细胞系白细胞,有时为全部白细胞均含有粗大嗜苯胺蓝颗粒。这种异常现象通常在临床上是无关紧要的,但有时和胡尔勒〈Hurler〉综合征或其他病理情况有关)

aldesleukin [ˌældəsˈljuːkin] *n* 阿地白介素(一种重组体白细胞介素 2 产物,用作抗肿瘤药及生物反应调节剂,治疗转移性肾细胞癌,静注给药)

aldicarb [ˈældikɑːb] *n* 涕灭威(一种氨基甲酸酯杀虫剂,用作杀虫药,有些国家亦用作杀鼠药)

aldin [ˈældin] *n* 醛碱

alditol [ˈælditɔl] *n* 糖醇

aldobionic acid [ˌældəubaiˈɔnik] 醛糖二糖酸

aldohexose [ˌældəuˈheksəus] *n* 己醛糖

aldolase [ˈældəleis] *n* 醛缩酶

aldonic acid [ælˈdɔnik] 醛糖酸

aldopentose [ˌældəˈpentəus] *n* 戊醛糖

aldose [ˈældəus] *n* 醛糖

aldose 1-epimerase [ˈældəus iˈpiməreis] 醛糖 1-差向异构酶(常称变旋酶)

aldose reductase [ˈældəus riˈdʌkteis] 醛糖还原酶,醛还原酶

aldoside [ˈældəsaid] *n* 醛糖苷

aldosterone [ælˈdɔstərəun] *n* 醛固酮

aldosteronism [ælˈdɔstərəunizəm] *n* 醛固酮症

aldosteronogenesis [ælˌdɔstərəunəuˈdʒenisis] *n* 醛固酮生成

aldosteronoma [ælˌdɔstərəuˈnəumə] *n* 醛固酮瘤

aldosteronopenia [ælˌdɔstərəunəuˈpiːniə] *n* 醛固酮减少症

aldosteronuria [ælˌdɔstərəuˈnjuəriə] *n* 醛固酮尿

aldotetrose [ˌældəuˈtetrəus] *n* 丁醛糖

aldotriose [ˌældəuˈtraiəus] *n* 丙醛糖

aldoxime [ælˈdɔksaim] *n* 醛肟

Aldrich-McClure test [ˈɔːldritʃ meˈkluə] (Charles A Aldrich; William B. McClure) 奥尔德里奇-麦克卢尔试验(见 McClure-Aldrich test)

Aldrich-Mees lines [ˈældritʃ miːz] (C. J. Aldrich; R. A. Mees) 阿-米线(见 Mees' lines)

Aldrich mixture [ˈɔːldritʃ] (Robert H. Aldrich) 奥尔德里奇合剂(1% 甲紫水溶液,治烧伤)

Aldrich syndrome [ˈɔːldritʃ] (Robert A Aldrich) 奥尔德里奇综合征(一种 X 连锁遗传的免疫缺陷综合征,其特征为湿疹、血小板减少以及反复化脓性感染)

aldrin [ˈældrin] *n* 艾氏剂,氯甲桥萘(有机杀虫药)

alecithal [əˈlesiθəl] *a* 无卵黄的

Alectorobius [ˌæliktəˈrəubiəs] *n* 钩缘蜱属 | ~ talaje 臭虫阿蜱,臭虫钩缘蜱,麦虱

alembic [əˈlembik] *n* 蒸馏器,蒸馏瓶

alembroth [əˈlembrɔθ] *n* 氯化汞铵(曾用作防腐敷料)

alemtuzumab [ˌæləmˈtʌzjumæb] *n* 阿妥单抗(一种重组 DNA 衍生的人源化单克隆抗体,旨在抗 CD 抗原 CD52,静脉内给药,用作抗肿瘤药,治疗 B 细胞慢性淋巴细胞白血病)

alendronate sodium [əˈlendrəneit] 阿仑膦酸钠(双膦酸钙调节药,用于抑制骨吸收,治疗畸形性骨炎、绝经后期骨质疏松和恶性肿瘤相关的高钙血症,口服给药)

alepric acid [əˈleprik] 环戊烯壬酸

aleprylic acid [əˈleprilik] 环戊烯庚酸

aletocyte [əˈliːtəsait] *n* 游走细胞

Aletris farinosa L. (Liliaceae) [ˈælitris fɔriˈnəusə] 北美肺筋草,美粉条儿菜(干根用作利尿及子宫收缩药,冷水泡制叶浸剂治急腹痛和胃病)

aleukemia [ˌeiljuːˈkiːmiə] *n* 白细胞缺乏症 | **aleukemic** *a*

aleukia [eiˈljuːkiə] *n* 白细胞缺乏症,白细胞减少

| alimentary toxic ~ (ATA) 饮食中毒性白细胞缺乏症(一种真菌毒素中毒症,与摄食田里过冬的谷物有关)

aleukocytic [eiˌljuːkəˈsitik] *a* 无白细胞的,白细胞缺乏的

aleukocytosis [eiˌljuːkəsaiˈtəusis] *n* 白细胞减少

aleurioconidium [əˌljuəriəukəˈnidiəm] *n* 侧生[厚垣]孢子,粉生孢子

aleuriospore [əˈljuəriəspɔː] *n* 侧生孢子

Aleurisma [ˌæljuəˈrizmə] *n* 糊蕈属

Aleurobius farinae [əljuəˈrəubiəs fəˈrainiː] 粗足粉螨

aleurone [ˈæljuərəun] *n* 麦粉蛋白粒,糊粉 | **aleuronic** [ˌæljuəˈrɔnik] *a*

aleuronoid [əˈljuərənɔid] *n* 麦粉样的

Alexander-Adams operation [ˌæligˈzændə ˈædəmz] (William Alexander; James A. Adams) 亚历山大-亚当斯手术(缩短圆韧带,矫正子宫移位)

Alexander's deafness (hearing loss) [ˌæligˈzændə] (Gustav Alexander) 亚历山大聋(一种耳蜗发育不全的先天性聋,主要累及螺旋器及其相邻的耳蜗底螺旋神经节细胞,出现高频听觉丧失)

Alexander's disease [ˌæligˈzændə] (W. Stewart Alexander)亚历山大病(一种婴儿型脑白质营养不良,组织学特征为脑表面及其血管周围有嗜酸性物质,导致脑膨大)

Alexander's operation [ˌæligˈzændə] (Samuel Alexander)亚历山大手术(前列腺切除术,耻骨上正中及会阴正中做切口);(William Alexander)亚历山大手术(缩短圆韧带,矫正子宫移位)

Alexander technique [ˌæligˈzændə] (Frederick M. Alexander) 亚历山大法(一种身体活动法,利用身心再训练,以改正姿势和运动的功能不良习惯)

alexeteric [əˈleksiˈterik] *a* 解[外]毒的

alexia [əˈleksiə] *n* 失读[症] | cortical ~ 皮质性失读 / musical ~ 读乐谱不能 / optical ~ 视觉性失读,文字盲 / subcortical ~ 皮质下失读

alexic [əˈleksik] *a* 补体性的;失读的

alexidine [əˈleksidiːn] *n* 阿来西定(抗菌药)

alexin [əˈleksin] *n* 防御素,补体(存在于血清中的不耐热物质,有别于感染或免疫作用产生的致敏物质〈抗体〉,在这层意义上,与 complement 同义) | leukocytic ~ 白细胞防御素 | **~ic** [ˌælekˈsinik] *a*

alexipharmac [əˌleksiˈfɑːmæk] *a* 解毒的 *n* 解毒药

alexithymia [əˌleksiˈθaimiə] *n* 情感表达不能

alexocyte [əˈleksəsait] *n* 产补体白细胞

aleydigism [əˈlaidigizəm] *n* 睾丸间质细胞(即 Leydig 细胞)功能缺失

Alezzandrini's syndrome [ˌælizænˈdriːni] (A. S. Alezzandrini) 眼-皮肤-耳综合征(单侧毯层视网膜变性,随后在同侧出现面部白斑及白发,有时伴耳聋)

alfacalcidol [ˌælfəˈkælsidɔl] *n* 阿法骨化醇(一种合成的骨化三醇类似物,用于治疗低钙血症、低磷酸盐血症、佝偻病和骨营养不良)

alfalfa [ælˈfælfə] *n* 苜蓿

alfentanil hydrochloride [ælˈfentənil] 盐酸阿芬太尼(一种得自芬太尼〈fentanyl〉的快速短效麻醉性镇痛药,用作诱导全身麻醉的主要药物,也用作维持全身麻醉的辅助药物,静脉内给药)

alfresco [ælˈfreskəu] *ad*, *a* 在户外(的)

ALG antilymphocyte globulin 抗淋巴细胞球蛋白

alga [ˈælgə] ([复] **algae** [ˈældʒiː]) *n* [常用复]藻 | **~l** [ˈælgəl] *a*

alganesthesia [ælˌgænisˈθiːzjə] *n* 痛觉缺失

algarroba, algaroba [ˌælgəˈrəubə] *n* 角豆树,角豆树果实;牧豆树,牧豆树荚果

alge- 见 algesi(o)-

algebra [ˈældʒibrə] *n* 代数学

algedonic [ˌældʒiˈdɔnik] *a* 欣快痛感的,痛觉快感的,苦乐的

algefacient [ˌældʒiˈfeiʃənt] *a* 清凉的 *n* 清凉剂

algeldrate [ælˈdʒeldreit] *n* 水合氢氧化铝(抗酸药)

algeoscopy [ˌældʒiˈɔskəpi] *n* 压痛测定法(作加压体检,以确定压力是否产生疼痛,常用于神经病学检查及用于确定昏迷的深度)

algesia [ælˈdʒiːziə] *n* 痛觉;感觉过敏

algesic [ælˈdʒiːzik] *a* 疼痛的

algesichronometer [ælˌdʒiːzikrəˈnɔmitə] *n* 痛觉时间计

algesimeter [ˌældʒiˈsimitə], **algesiometer** [ælˌdʒiziˈɔmitə] *n* 痛觉计 | **algesimetry** [ˌældʒiˈsimitri] *n* 痛觉测定法

algesi(o)-, alge-, algi(o)-, alg(o)- [构词成分]痛

algesiogenic [ælˌdʒiziəˈdʒenik] *a* 产生疼痛的

algesthesia [ˌældʒisˈθiːzjə], **algesthesis** [ˌældʒisˈθiːsis] *n* 痛觉

algestone acetophenide [ælˈdʒestəun] 醋苯阿尔孕酮(孕激素)

algetic [ælˈdʒetik] *a* 疼痛的

-algia [构词成分]痛

algicide [ˈældʒisaid] *n* 灭藻剂

algid [ˈældʒid] *a* 寒冷的 | **~ity** [ælˈdʒidəti] *n*

algin [ˈældʒin] *n* 藻胶,藻酸钠

alginate [ˈældʒineit] *n* 藻酸盐

alginic acid [ælˈdʒinik] 藻酸

Alginobacter [ˌældʒinəuˈbæktə] *n* 藻杆菌属
Alginomonas [ˌældʒinəuˈməunəs] *n* 藻单孢菌属
alginuresis [ˌældʒinjuəˈriːsis] *n* 痛性排尿
algi(o)- 见 algesi(o)-
algioglandular [ˌældʒiəuˈglændjulə] *a* 痛性腺活动的
algiometabolic [ˌældʒiəuˌmetəˈbɔlik] *a* 痛性代谢改变的
algiomotor [ˌældʒiəuˈməutə] *a* 痛性运动的(如痉挛或蠕动障碍)
algiomuscular [ˌældʒiəuˈmʌskjulə] *a* 痛性肌活动的
algiovascular [ˌældʒiəuˈvæskjulə] *a* 痛性血管活动的
alglucerase [ælˈgluːsəˌreis] *n* 阿糖脑苷酶(葡糖脑苷脂酶的改良型,从混合人胎盘组织制得,用以置换葡糖脑苷脂酶〈葡糖神经酰胺酶〉,治疗Ⅰ型戈谢〈Gaucher〉病,静脉输注给药)
alg(o)- 见 algesi(o)-
algodystrophy [ˌælgəuˈdistrəfi] *n* 痛性营养障碍
algogenesia [ˌælgəudʒiˈniːziə], **algogenesis** [ˌælgəuˈdʒenisis] *n* 疼痛产生
algogenic [ælgəuˈdʒenik] *a* 产生疼痛的;产生寒冷的
algolagnia [ˌælgəuˈlægniə] *n* 虐淫,痛淫
algology [ælˈgɔlədʒi] *n* 藻类学 | **algological** [ælgəˈlɔdʒikəl] *a* / **algologist** *n* 藻类学家
algometer [ælˈgɔmitə] *n* 痛觉计 | pressure ~ 压痛计 | **algometry** *n* 痛觉测验法
algophobia [ˌælgəuˈfəubjə] *n* 疼痛恐怖,恐痛症
algopsychalia [ˌælgəusaiˈkeiliə] *n* 精神性[头]痛
algorithm [ˈælgəriðəm] *n* 算法,规则系统(解决某些类型数学问题的一种机械操作法);运算法,推导(逐步解决某一问题的方法,如作诊断时即用此法)
algosis [ælˈgəusis] *n* 海藻病,藻害
algospasm [ˈælgəspæzəm] *n* 痛性痉挛
algovascular [ˌælgəuˈvæskjulə] *a* 痛性血管活动的
aliasing [ˈeiliəsiŋ] *n* 假象;伪象;伪影,混叠
Alibert's disease [ɑːliˈbəː] (Jean L. M. Alibert) 蕈样真菌病
alible [ˈælibl] *a* 可食的,有营养的
alices [ˈælisiːz] [复] *n* 天花红斑
alicyclic [ˌæliˈsaiklik] *a* 脂环族的
alienation [ˌeiljəˈneiʃən] *n* 情感疏远,疏隔感
alienia [eilaiˈiːniə] *n* 无脾[畸形]
alienism [ˈeiljənizəm] *n* 精神错乱;精神病学(旧名)
alienist [ˈeiljənist] *n* 精神病学家,精神科医生(旧名);精神科法医
ali-esterase [ˌæliˈestəreis] *n* 脂族酯酶,羧酸酯酶
aliflurane [ˌæliˈfluːrein] *n* 阿列氟烷(吸入麻醉药)
aliform [ˈælifɔːm] *a* 翼状的
alignment [əˈlainmənt] *n* 牙排列
alimentary [ˌæliˈmentəri] *a* 营养的,饮食的;消化器官的
alimentation [ˌælimenˈteiʃən] *n* 营养法,饮食法 | parenteral ~ 胃肠外营养 / total parenteral ~ 全胃肠外营养,全静脉营养(亦称胃肠外高营养,静脉高营养)
alimentology [ˌælimentˈɔlədʒi] *n* 营养学
alimentotherapy [ˌæliˌmentəuˈθerəpi] *n* 营养疗法,饮食疗法
alinasal [ˌæliˈneizəl] *a* 鼻翼的
alinement [əˈlainmənt] *n* 牙排列
alipamide [əˈlipəmaid] *n* 阿利帕胺(利尿、降压药)
aliphatic [ˌæliˈfætik] *a* 脂[肪]族的 | ~ acid 脂肪族酸
alipogenic [eiˌlipəuˈdʒenik] *a* 不生脂肪的
alipoidic [ˌeiliˈpɔidik] *a* 无脂的
alipotropic [ˌælipəuˈtrɔpik] *a* 不亲脂肪的(对脂肪代谢无影响的)
aliquorrhea [əˌlikwɔˈriːə] *n* 脑脊液缺乏,脑脊液不足
aliquot [ˈælikwɔt] *n* 可分量
alismin [əˈlismin] *n* 泽泻浸出物
alisphenoid [æliˈsfiːnɔid] *a* 蝶骨大翼的 *n* 翼蝶骨
alitretinoin [ˌæliˈtretiˌnɔin] *n* 阿利维A酸(一种内源性类维生素A,用作局部抗肿瘤药,治疗艾滋病相关皮肤卡波西〈Kaposi〉肉瘤)
alizarin [əˈlizərin] *n* 茜素 | ~ monosulfonate, ~ red 磺酸茜素,茜素红 / ~ yellow 茜素黄
alizarinopurpurin [ˌæliˌzærinəuˈpəːpjuərin] *n* 紫色素,红紫素,1, 2, 4-三羟蒽醌
alkalemia [ˌælkəˈliːmiə] *n* 碱血[症](血液pH增加或氢离子浓度减少)
alkalescence [ˌælkəˈlesns] *n* 微碱性,弱碱性 | **alkalescent** *a*
alkali [ˈælkəlai] ([复] **alkali〈e〉s**) *n* 碱,强碱 | caustic ~ 苛性碱
alkalify [ˈælkəlifai, ælˈkælifai] *vt, vi* 碱化;加碱
Alkaligenes [ˌælkəˈlidʒiniːz] *n* 产碱杆菌属
alkaligenous [ˌælkəˈlidʒinəs] *a* 产碱的,生碱的
alkalimeter [ˌælkəˈlimitə] *n* 碱定量器,碳酸定量器 | **alkalimetry** *n* 碱定量法
alkaline [ˈælkəlain] *a* 碱的,碱性的 | **alkalinity** [ˌælkəˈlinəti] *n* 碱度,碱性
alkaline phosphatase (ALP) [ˈælkəlain, -lin-ˈfɔsfəteis] 碱性磷酸酶(骨型碱性磷酸酶遗传性缺乏为一种常染色体隐性性状,可致低磷酸酶血症。亦称磷酸单酯酶) | leucocyte ~ ~

(LAP) 白细胞碱性磷酸酶(慢性髓性白血病及其他病变时,此酶的活性降低)

alkalinuria [ˌælkəliˈnjuəriə] *n* 碱尿

alkalitherapy [ˌælkəlaiˈθerəpi] *n* 碱疗法

alkalize [ˈælkəlaiz], **alkalinize** [ˈælkəlinaiz] *vt* 碱化 | **alkalization** [ˌælkəlaiˈzeiʃən], **alkalinization** [ˌælkəˌliniˈzeiʃən] *n* 碱化[作用]

alkalizer [ˌælkəˈlaizə] *n* 碱化剂

alkalogenic [ˌælkələuˈdʒenik] *a* 生碱性的

alkaloid [ˈælkəlɔid] *n* 生物碱 | animal ~ 动物性生物碱(尸碱;蛋白碱) / artificial ~ 人工[合成]生物碱 / vinca ~s 长春花碱

alkalometry [ˌælkəˈlɔmitri] *n* 生物碱剂量规定

alkalosis [ˌælkəˈləusis] *n* 碱中毒 | altitude ~ 高空碱中毒 / compensated ~ 代偿性碱中毒(代偿性机制已使 pH 趋于正常) / metabolic ~ 代谢性碱中毒 / respiratory ~ 呼吸性碱中毒 | **alkalotic** [ˌælkəˈlɔtik] *a*

alkalotherapy [ˌælkələuˈθerəpi] *n* 碱疗法

alkaluria [ˌælkəˈljuəriə] *n* 碱尿

alkamine [ˈælkəmin] *n* 氨基醇

alkane [ˈælkein] *n* 链烷

alkanet [ˈælkənit] *n* 紫朱草[根]

alkannin [ˈælkənin] *n* 紫草素,紫草红

alkapton [ælˈkæptɔn] *n* 尿黑酸

alkaptonuria [ælˌkæptəuˈnjuəriə] *n* 尿黑酸尿 | spontaneous ~ 自发性尿黑酸尿(一种遗传性先天性酪氨酸代谢失常,患者尿内排出尿黑酸) | **alkaptonuric** [ælˌkæptəˈnjuərik] *a* 尿黑酸尿的 *n* 尿黑酸尿患者

alkatriene [ˌælkəˈtraiiːn] *n* 三烯烃

alkavervir [ˌælkəˈvəːvə] *n* 绿藜芦碱(抗高血压药)

alkene [ˈælkiːn] *n* 链烯

alkyl [ˈælkil] *n* 烷基

alkylamine [ˌælkiləˈmiːn] *n* 烷基胺

alkylation [ˌælkiˈleiʃən] *n* 烷基取代,烷基化 | **alkylate** [ˈælkilit] *n* 烷基化物 [ˈælkileit] *vt* 烷基化,用烷化剂处理

alkylogen [ælˈkilədʒən] *n* 烷基卤,卤代烷

alkyne [ˈælkain] *n* 炔

ALL acute lymphoblastic leukemia 急性淋巴细胞白血病

allachesthesia [ˌæləkisˈθiːzjə] *n* 异处感觉 | optical ~ 视觉异位,异处视觉

allanic acid [əˈlænik], **allanturic acid** [ˌælənˈtjuərik] 脲乙醛酸

allantiasis [ˌælənˈtaiəsis] *n* 腊肠中毒

allanto- [构词成分]腊肠;尿囊

allantochorion [əˌlæntəuˈkɔːriɔn] *n* 尿囊绒[毛]膜

allantogenesis [əˌlæntəuˈdʒenisis] *n* 尿囊生成

allantoic [ˌælənˈtəuik] *a* 尿囊的 | ~ acid 尿囊酸

allantoicase [ˌælənˈtəuikeis] *n* 尿囊酸酶

allantoid [əˈlæntɔid] *a* 尿囊样的;腊肠样的

allantoidean [ˌælənˈtɔidiən] *a* 尿囊的 *n* 尿囊动物

allantoidoangiopagus [ˌælənˌtɔidəuændʒiˈɔpəgəs] *n* 脐血管联胎 | **allantoidoangiopagous** *a*

allantoin [əˈlæntəuin] *n* 尿囊素

allantoinase [ˌælənˈtəuineis] *n* 尿囊素酶

allantoinuria [əˌlæntəuinˈjuəriə] *n* 尿囊素尿

allantois [əˈlæntəuis] *n* 尿囊

allantotoxicon [əˌlæntəuˈtɔksikɔn] *n* 尿囊毒

allassotherapy [əˌlæsəuˈθerəpi] *n* 变质疗法(基于促使生物体的一般性生物环境发生变化的一种疗法)

allaxis [əˈlæksis] *n* 【希】变形,变态;变化,转化

allele [əˈliːl] *n* 等位基因(遗传学中指能占据一个特定染色体座位的基因的交替型) | multiple ~s 复等位基因(可能在任何一个位点上的两个以上的等位基因) / silent ~ 不活动等位基因(无法测到任何效应的等位基因) | **allel** [əˈlel], **allelomorph** [əˈliːləmɔːf] *n* **allelic** [əˈliːlik], **allelomorphic** [əˌliːləˈmɔːfik] *a* 等位的,等位基因的

allelism [ˈælilizəm], **allelomorphism** [əˌliːləˈmɔːfizəm] *n* 等位性(指等位基因的存在或指等位基因间的相互关系)

allel(o)- [构词成分]对偶

allelocatalysis [əˌliːləukəˈtælisis] *n* 交互催化(细菌培养物中增加其他同一型的细胞,促使细胞生长) | **allelocatalytic** [əˌliːləukætəˈlitik] *a*

allelochemics [əˌliːləˈkemiks] *n* 种间交互化学

allelotaxis [əˌliːləˈtæksis], **allelotaxy** [əˈliːləˌtæksi] *n* 异源发生(一个器官由数种胚胎的构造发育而成)

Allemann's syndrome [ˈæləmɑːn] (Richard Allemann) 阿尔曼综合征(重复肾和杵状指同时并存,有时伴有面部不对称和各种运动神经变性)

Allen-Doisy test [ˈælənˈdɔisi] (Edgar V. Allen; Edward A Doisy) 艾伦-多伊西试验(检实验动物的雌激素)

Allen's fossa [ˈælən] (Harrison Allen) 艾伦窝(股骨颈窝)

Allen's paradoxic law [ˈælən] (Frederick M. Allen) 艾伦反常定律(对正常人供糖愈多,其利用量也愈多,而糖尿病患者则相反) | ~ treatment 艾伦疗法,禁食疗法(治糖尿病)

Allen's test [ˈælən] (Alfred H Allen) 艾伦试验(检尿葡萄糖、检酚); (Edgar V. Allen) 艾伦试验(检尺动脉或桡动脉闭塞)

allergen [ˈælədʒen] *n* 变应原(能引起变态反应性或过敏性的物质;亦指某种食物、细菌或花粉

的提纯蛋白,用以检查病人对某种物质是否有超敏反应) | pollen ~ 花粉变应原(亦称花粉抗原) | **~ic** [ˌæləˈdʒenik] *a*

allergic [əˈləːdʒik] *a* 变应性的,过敏性的

allergid [ˈælədʒid] *n* 变应疹(一种丘疹或结节性变应性皮肤反应)

allergie [ˈælədʒi] *n* 变应性

allergin [ˈælədʒin] *n* 变应素(可致过敏性的抗体;一种结核菌素无菌标定溶液,1% ~5% 溶液用于眼试验,25% 用于皮肤试验)

allergist [əˈləːdʒist] *n* 变态反应学家

allergization [ˌælədʒiˈzeiʃən] *n* 变应化[作用],致敏作用(自动致敏或将变应原引入体内)

allergize [ˈælədʒaiz] *vt* 变态反应化,致敏

allergoid [ˈæləgɔid] *n* 类变应原

allergology [ˌæləˈgɔlədʒi] *n* 变态反应学 | **allergological** [ˌæləgəuˈlɔdʒikəl] *a* / **allergologist** *n* 变态反应学家

allergosis [ˌæləˈgəusis] ([复] **allergoses** [ˌæləˈgəusiːz]) *n* 变态反应病

allergy [ˈælədʒi] *n* 变[态反]应性;变态反应,过敏反应 | atopic ~, hereditary ~, spontaneous ~ 特应性变态反应,遗传性变态反应,自发性变态反应 / bacterial ~ 细菌性变态反应(对一个特指的细菌抗原,如结核分枝杆菌,有特异的超敏反应) / contact ~ 接触性变态反应 / delayed ~ 迟发型变态反应(使用或吸收变应原后数小时或几天后出现的变应性反应,包括接触性皮炎和细菌性变态反应) / drug ~ 药物变态反应,药物变应性,药物过敏 / immediate ~ 速发型变态反应(使用和吸收变应原后在一个短时期内,即从几分钟到一小时出现的变应性反应) / induced ~, normal ~, physiologic ~ 诱发性变态反应,普通变态反应,生理性变态反应 / latent ~ 潜伏[性]变态反应(不表现症状的变态反应,能通过试验测出) / nonatopic ~ 非特应性变态反应(包括接触性皮炎及某种食物和药物变态反应) / pollen ~ 花粉变态反应,枯草热,花草气喘,花粉病 / polyvalent ~ 多价变态反应(对多种抗原均呈现变态反应)

allescheriasis [ˌæləskəˈraiəsis], **allescheriosis** [ˌæləskiriˈəusis] *n* 霉样真菌病

Allescheria [ˌæləsˈkiəriə] *n* 阿利什利菌属

allescheriasis [ˌæləskəˈraiəsis], **allescheriosis** [ˌæləskiriˈəusis] *n* 阿利什利菌病

allesthesia [ˌælisˈθiːzjə] *n* 异处感觉

allethrin [ˈæliθrin] *n* 丙烯除虫菊酯(杀虫药)

alleviate [əˈliːvieit] *vt* 减轻(痛苦等),缓和 | **alleviation** [əˌliːviˈeiʃən] *n* / **alleviator** *n* 缓和剂 / **alleviative, alleviatory** [əˈliːviətəri] *a*

alliaceous [ˌæliˈeiʃəs] *a* 蒜的,蒜样的

alliance [əˈlaiəns] *n* 同盟;联合,联结 | therapeutic ~ 联合治疗,治疗配合 / working ~ 联合工作

allicin [ˈælisin] *n* 蒜素(具有抗菌活性)

allied [əˈlaid, ˈælaid] *a* 联合的;同类的

alligation [ˌæliˈgeiʃən] *n* 合剂求值

alligator [ˈæligeitə] *n* 短吻鳄 | ~ boy 干皮病儿(患严重鳞癣的孩子)

Allingham's operation[1] [ˈæliŋəm] (Herbert W. Allingham) 阿林厄姆手术(一种腹股沟结肠切开术,在与腹股沟韧带上方 1.4 cm 处平行切开)

Allingham's operation[2] [ˈæliŋəm] (William Allingham) 阿林厄姆手术(一种直肠切除术,绕直肠切入坐骨直肠窝,向后延伸至尾骨)

Allis's inhaler [ˈælis] (Oscar H. Allis) 艾利斯吸入器(用点滴法吸入醚、氯仿等一类麻醉剂) | ~ sign 艾利斯征(股骨颈折断时,髂嵴和大转子之间的筋膜松弛)

alliteration [əˌlitəˈreiʃən] *n* 同音韵错语症,同音韵言语障碍

allithiamine [ˌæliˈθaiəmin] *n* 蒜硫胺,大蒜硫胺素

Allium [ˈæliəm] *n*【拉】葱属

all(o)- [构词成分]别,异常,障碍,倒错,错

alloalbumin [ˌæləuælˈbjuːmin] *n* 异白蛋白

alloantibody [ˌæləuˈæntiˌbɔdi] *n* 异型抗体

alloantigen [ˌæləuˈæntidʒən] *n* 异型抗原

alloantiserum [ˌæləuˌæntiˈsiərəm] *n* [同种]异型抗血清

allobar [ˈæləbɑː] *n* 异组分体,同素异重体(化学元素的一种形式,它具有的原子量不同于天然存在的原子量)

allobarbital [ˌæləuˈbɑːbitæl] *n* 阿洛巴比妥(催眠镇静药)

allobiosis [ˌæləubaiˈəusis] *n* 反应特性改变(指生物体)

allocentric [ˌæləuˈsentrik] *a* 非自我中心的,他人中心的

allochesthesia [ˌæləukisˈθiːzjə] *n* 感觉定位不能

allochiria, allocheiria [ˌæləuˈkaiəriə] *n* 感觉定侧不能 | **allochiral** *a*

allochroism [ˌæləuˈkrəuizəm] *n* 变色,色变化 | **allochroic** [ˌæləuˈkrəuik] *a*

allochromacy [ˌæləuˈkrəuməsi] *n* 异色形成,异染色性

allochromasia [ˌæləukrəuˈmeiziə] *n* 变色(皮肤,毛发)

allochthonous [əˈlɔkθənəs] *a* 引入的,外生的,外来的

allocinesia [ˌæləusaiˈniːziə] *n* 对侧运动,异侧运动

allocolloid [ˌæləuˈkɔlɔid] *n* 同素异形胶体

allocortex [ˌæləuˈkɔːteks] *n* 异形皮质

allocrine [ˈæləkrin] *a* 多种分泌的
allocytophilic [ˌæləusaitəˈfilik] *a* 嗜同种细胞的
Allodermanyssus [ˌæləudəːməˈnisəs] *n* 异刺皮螨属 | ~ sanguineus 血异刺皮螨
allodesmism [ˌæləuˈdesmizəm] *n* 异质同晶异物[现象]
allodiploid [ˌæləuˈdiplɔid] *a* 异源二倍体的 *n* 异源二倍体(指某一个体或细胞具有来自异种来源的两组染色体) | **~y** *n* 异源二倍性
allodynia [ˌæləuˈdiniə] *n* 异常性疼痛(正常皮肤受无害性刺激所致的疼痛)
alloerotic [ˌæləuiˈrɔtik] *a* 异体恋的,异体性欲的
alloeroticism [ˌæləueˈrɔtisizəm], **alloerotism** [ˌæləˈerətizəm] *n* 异体恋
alloesthesia [ˌæləuisˈθiːzjə] 感觉定位不能
allogamy [əˈlɔgəmi] *n* 异体受精,交叉受精 | **allogamous** [əˈlɔgəməs] *a*
allogeneic [ˌæləudʒiˈneiik], **allogenic** [ˌæləuˈdʒenik] *a* 同种[异体]的;同种异基因的
allogotrophia [ˌæləugəˈtrəufiə] *n* 自耗营养
allograft [ˈæləgrɑːft, -græft] *n* [同种]异基因移植物
Allogromiina [ˌæləugrəˈmaiinə] *n* 异网足虫亚目
allogroup [ˈæləuˌgrəup] *n* 同种异群
alloimmune [ˌæləuiˈmjuːn] *a* 同种免疫的
alloimmunization [ˌæləuˌimju(ː)naiˈzeiʃən] *n* 同种异型免疫
alloisomerism [ˌæləuaiˈsɔmərizəm] *n* 立体异构[现象]
allokeratoplasty [ˌæləuˈkerətəuplæsti] *n* 异质角膜成形术
allokinesis [ˌæləukaiˈniːsis, -kiˈn-] *n* 被动运动;反射运动 | **allokinetic** [ˌæləukaiˈnetik, -kiˈn-] *a*
allolactose [ˌæləuˈlæktəus] *n* 异乳糖
allolalia [ˌæləuˈleiliə] *n* 言语障碍
allomerism [əˈlɔmərizəm] *n* 异质同形,异质同晶 | **allomerous** *a*
allometric [ˌæləuˈmetrik] *a* 体形变异的;体形变异测定的
allometron [ˌæləuˈmetrɔn] *n* 体形变异
allometry [əˈlɔmitri] *n* 体形变异测定法
Allomonas [ˌæləuˈməunəs] *n* 异单孢菌属
allomorphism [ˌæləˈmɔːfizəm] *n* 同质异晶[现象]
allongement [əlɔnʒˈmɔŋ] *n* 【法】(尤指子宫瘤的)伸长术
allonomous [əˈlɔnəməs] *a* 受外部(刺激)节制的
allopath [ˈæləpæθ], **allopathist** [əˈlɔpəθist] *n* 对抗疗法派,顺治派
allopathy [əˈlɔpəθi] *n* 对抗疗法 | **allopathic** [ˌæləˈpæθik] *a*
allophanamide [æləˈfænəmaid] *n* 双脲,双缩脲
allophanate [əˈlɔfəneit] *n* 脲基甲酸盐
allophanic acid [ˌæləˈfænik] 脲基甲酸
allophasis [əˈlɔfəsis] *n* 语无伦次,谵妄
allophenic [ˌæləuˈfiːnik] *a* 异表型的;嵌合体的
allophore [ˈæləfɔː] *n* 红色素细胞
allophthalmia [ˌælɔfˈθælmiə] *n* 两眼轴向不等,斜眼;两眼异色
alloplasia [ˌæləuˈpleiziə] *n* 发育异常
alloplasmatic [ˌæləuplæzˈmætik] *a* 异质的(以细胞质的分化而形成的)
alloplast [ˈæləplæst] *n* 异源体(用以移植至组织)
alloplastic [ˌæləˈplæstik] *a* 兴趣外向的,变更环境性适应的;异源体的
alloplasty [ˈæləplæsti] *n* 兴趣外向,变更环境性适应
alloploid [æləˈplɔid] *a* 异源倍体的 *n* 异源倍体(指某一个体或细胞具有来自异种来源的任何数目〈二组或多组〉的染色体) | **~y** *n* 异源倍性
allopolyploid [ˌæləuˈpɔliˌplɔid] *a* 异源多倍的 *n* 异源多倍体(指某一个体或细胞具有来自异种来源的两组以上的染色体) | **~y** *n* 异源多倍性
allopregnandiol [ˌæləupregˈnændiɔl] *n* 别孕二醇
allopregnane [æləuˈpregnein] *n* 别孕烷
allopregnanediol [ˌæləuˌpregneinˈdaiɔl] *n* 别孕二醇
allopregnenolone [ˌæləupregˈnenələun] *n* 别孕烯醇酮
allopsychic [ˌæləuˈsaikik] *a* 对外心理的(指对周围环境的心理过程)
allopsychosis [ˌæləusaiˈkəusis] *n* 外界感知障碍性精神病(有错觉、幻觉,但言语、动作正常)
allopurinol [ˌæləuˈpjuərinɔl] *n* 别嘌醇,别嘌呤醇(抗痛风药)
alloreactive [ˌæləuri(ː)ˈæktiv] *a* 同种异体反应的
allorhythmia [ˌæləuˈriθmiə] *n* 节律异常 | **allorhythmic** [ˌæləˈriθmik] *a*
all or none 全或无(心肌受刺激,将收缩至极限,或不全收缩,亦称全或无定律)
allorphine [ˈæləfiːn] *n* 烯丙吗啡(吗啡拮抗药)
allose [ˈæləus] *n* 阿洛糖
allosensitization [ˌæləuˌsensitaiˈzeiʃən, -tiˈz-] *n* 同种致敏作用(亦称同族致敏作用)
allosome [ˈæləsəum] *n* 异染色体(进入胞浆的异体成分) | paired ~ 双心体 / unpaired ~ 单体
allosteric [ˌæləuˈsterik] *a* 别构的
allosterism [ˈæləˌsterizəm] *n* 立体异构,别构效应
allostery [ˌæləˈstiəri] *n* 别构状态,别构效应
allotetraploid [ˌæləuˈtetrəplɔid] *n* 异源四倍体(指某一个体具有异种来源的两组染色体)
allotherm [ˈæləθəːm] *n* 变温动物;异温动物

allotope [ˈælətəup] *n* 同种异型位(抗体分子恒定区上能被其他抗体结合簇识别的位置)

allotopia [ˌæləˈtəupiə] *n* 异位,错位 | **allotopic** [ˌæləˈtɔpik] *a*

allotoxin [ˌæləuˈtɔksin] *n* 防异毒素(体内组织变化时形成的物质,使毒素的毒性中和,从而对毒素起到防护的作用)

allotransplantation [ˌæləuˌtrænsplɑːnˈteiʃənplæn-] *n* [同种]异基因移植(即将某一个体的组织移植到同一种内但与供体的基因型不同的异体之中)

allotri(o)- [构词成分]异

allotriodontia [əˌlɔtriəˈdɔnʃiə] *n* 牙移植术;异位牙(如生长在皮样瘤中的牙)

allotriogeustia [əˌlɔtriəˈgjuːstiə] *n* 味觉异常,味觉倒错

allotriolith [ˌæləˈtraiəliθ] *n* 异位结石;异质结石

allotriophagy [əˌlɔtriˈɔfədʒi], **allotriophagia** [əˌlɔtriəˈfeidʒiə] *n* 异食癖,异嗜癖,食欲倒错

allotriosmia [ˌæləutraiˈɔsmiə] *n* 嗅觉异常,嗅觉倒错

allotriuria [əˌlɔtriˈjuəriə] *n* 异尿症,尿液异常

allotrope [ˈælətrəup] *n* 同素异形体

allotrophic [ˌæləˈtrɔfik] *a* 营养异常的

allotropic [ˌæləˈtrɔpik] *a* 同素异形的;异向的,外向的(指精神病学中愿受他人意想为主的一种人格型,即非自我中心的)

allotropism [əˈlɔtrəpizəm], **allotropy** [əˈlɔtrəpi] *n* 同素异形

allotrylic [ˌæləˈtrilik] *a* 异物侵入的

allotype [ˈælətaip] *n* [同种]异型 | **allotypic** [ˌæləˈtipik] *a*

allotypy [ˌæləˈtaipi] *n* [同种]异型性

allowance [əˈlauəns] *n* 供给量 | recommended daily ~ 推荐日供给量 / recommended dietary ~ (RDA) 推荐膳食供给量

alloxan [əˈlɔksən] *n* 四氧嘧啶

alloxanic acid [ˌælɔkˈsænik] 阿脲酸

alloxantin [əˈlɔksəntin] *n* 双阿脲,双四氧嘧啶

alloxazine [əˈlɔksəziːn] *n* 咯嗪

alloxuremia [ˌælɔksjuəˈriːmiə] *n* 嘌呤碱血(血内有嘌呤碱即引起中毒)

alloxuria [ˌælɔkˈsjuəriə] *n* 嘌呤碱尿 | **alloxuric** *a*

alloxyproteic acid [əˌlɔksiˈprəutiik] 氧化蛋白酸

alloy [ˈælɔi] *n* 合金 *vt* 合铸 | amalgam ~ 汞合金

alloyage [əˈlɔiidʒ] *n* 合金法

allspice [ˈɔːlspais] *n* 药椒,牙买加胡椒

alluranic acid [ˌæljuəˈrænik] 脲合四氧嘧啶酸

allyl [ˈælil] *n* 烯丙基 | ~ aldehyde 烯丙醛 / ~ isothiocyanate 异硫氰酸烯丙酯 / ~ sulfide 烯丙基化硫,烯丙基硫醚 / ~ sulfocarbamide, ~ thiocarbamide, ~ thiourea 烯丙基硫脲

allylamine [ˌæliˈlæmin] *n* 烯丙胺

allylguaiacol [ˌælilˈgwaiəkɔl] *n* 丁香酚,烯丙愈创木酚

allylnormorphine hydrochloride [ælilnəˈmɔːfiːn] 盐酸烯丙吗啡(吗啡拮抗药)

allysine [eiˈlaisiːn] *n* ε-醛[基]赖氨酸

almadrate sulfate [ˈælmədreit] 铝硫酸镁(抗酸药)

Almeida's disease [ælˈmeidə] (Floriano P. de Almeida) 巴西芽生菌病,类球孢子菌病

Almén's reagent [ælˈmein] (August T. Almén) 阿尔门试剂(240 ml 内含 0.325 g 鞣酸的 50% 乙醇中加 10 ml 25% 的乙酸) | ~ test 阿尔门试验(检尿白蛋白、血或血色素、葡萄糖)

almond [ˈɑːmənd] *n* 杏仁,扁桃,巴旦杏

almoner [ˈælmənə] *n* 救济[品]分发人员 | hospital ~ (英国的)医院社会服务基金分发人员,医院社会服务员

almotriptan malate [ˌæməuˈtriptæn] 马来酸阿莫曲坦(一种选择性 5-羟色胺受体拮抗药,用于治疗急性偏头痛,口服给药)

alochia [əˈləukiə] *n* 无恶露

Alocinma [ˌæləˈsinmə] *n* 涵螺属 | ~ longiocornis 长角涵螺

Aloe [ˈæləwi] *n* 【希】芦荟属

aloe [ˈæləu] *n* 芦荟 | **~tic** [ˌæləuˈetik] *a* 芦荟制的;[含]芦荟的

aloe-emodin [ˈæləu ˈemədin] *n* 芦荟泻素

alogia [əˈləudʒiə] *n* 精神性失语症(中枢损害所致)

aloin [ˈæləuin] *n* 芦荟素,芦荟总苷

alonimid [əˈlɔnimid] *n* 阿洛米酮,(催眠镇静药)

alopecia [ˌæləuˈpiːʃiə] *n* 脱发,秃 | **alopecic** [æləuˈpiːsik] *a*

aloxanthin [ˌælɔkˈsænθin] *n* 芦荟黄质

aloxiprin [æˈlɔksiprin] *n* 阿洛普令(镇痛药)

ALP alkaline phosphatase 碱性磷酸酶

alpenstich [ˈɑːlpənstiʃ] *n* 【德】阿尔卑斯山肺炎

Alpers' disease [ˈælpəz] (Bernard J. Alpers) 阿尔珀斯病(幼儿的一种罕见病,特征为大脑皮质和其他部位的神经元退变,伴进行性精神衰退、运动障碍、癫痫发作和早期死亡。亦称脑灰质营养不良症,进行性脑灰质营养不良症或婴儿灰质营养不良症)

alpertine [ælˈpəːtiːn] *n* 阿尔哌汀(安定药)

alpha-amylose [ˌælfə ˈæmiləus] *n* α-直链淀粉

alpha$_1$-antitrypsin [ˌælfə ˌæntiˈtripsin] *n* α_1-抗胰蛋白酶(此蛋白缺乏与肺气肿的发生有关)

alpha$_2$-antiplasmin [ˌælfə ˌæntiˈplɑːzmin] *n* α_2-抗纤维蛋白溶酶

alpha-dinitrophenol [ˌælfə daiˌnaitrəuˈfiːnɔl] *n* α-二硝基酚,2,4-二硝基苯酚

alphadione [ˌælfəˈdaiəun] *n* 安泰酮(甾类麻醉剂)
alpha-endorphin [ˌælfə enˈdɔːfin] *n* α-内啡肽
alpha-estradiol [ˌælfə ˌestrəˈdaiɔl] *n* α-雌二醇
alpha fetoprotein [ˌælfəˌfiːtəuˈprəutiːn] 甲胎蛋白
alpha-galactosidase [ˌælfə gəˌlæktəˈsaideis] *n* α-半乳糖苷酶
alpha globulin [ˌælfəˈglɔbjulin] α 球蛋白
alpha-1, 4-glucosidase deficiency [ˈælfə gluːˈkəusideis] α-1, 4-葡糖苷酶缺乏症,糖原贮积症Ⅱ型
Alphaherpesvirinae [ˌælfəˌhəːpizviˈrainiː] *n* α-疱疹病毒亚科
alpha-hypophamine [ˌælfə ˈhaiˈpɔfəmin] *n* [垂体后叶]催产素
alpha-lipoprotein [ˌælfə lipəˈprəutiːn] *n* α-脂蛋白,甲脂蛋白,高密度脂蛋白
alpha-lobeline [ˌælfə ˈlɔbilin] *n* α-北美山梗菜碱,洛贝林(呼吸中枢兴奋药)
alphalytic [ˌælfəˈlitik] *a* 抗 α-肾上腺素能的 *n* 抗 α-肾上腺素能药
alpha$_2$-macroglobulin [ˌælfə ˌmækrəuˈglɔbjulin] *n* α_2-巨球蛋白
alphamimetic [ˌælfəmaiˈmetik] *a* 拟 α-肾上腺素能的,类 α-肾上腺素能的 *n* 拟 α-肾上腺素能药
alphanaphthol [ˌælfəˈnæfθɔl] *n* α-萘酚
alphaprodine hydrochloride [ˌælfəˈprəudiːn] 盐酸阿法罗定(麻醉镇痛药)
alpharsonic acid [ˌælfɑːˈsɔnik] α-胂酸
alpha-tocopherol [ˌælfətəˈkɔfərɔl] *n* α-生育酚
alphatoluic acid [ˌælfətəˈluːik] 苯乙酸
alpha-tropeine [ˌælfə ˈtrəupiːin] *n* α-托品因
Alphavirus [ˈælfəˌvaiərəs] *n* α-病毒属
alphavirus [ˈælfəˌvaiərəs] *n* α-病毒
alphitomorphous [ˌælfitəˈmɔːfəs] *a* 麦粉形的(指植物某些真菌寄生物)
alphonsin [ælˈfɔnsin] (Alphonse Ferri) *n* 三爪取弹钳
alphos [ˈælfɔs] *n*【拉;希】牛皮癣
Alport's syndrome [ˈælpɔːt] (Arthur Alport) 奥尔波特综合征(一种遗传性障碍,特征为进行性感音神经性聋、进行性肾盂肾炎或肾小球肾炎以及偶有眼缺损,属常染色体显性遗传或 X 连锁特性遗传)
alprazolam [ælˈpreizələm] *n* 阿普唑仑(安定药)
alprenolol hydrochloride [ælˈprenələl] 盐酸阿普洛尔(β 肾上腺素能阻滞药)
alprostadil [ælˈprɔstədil] *n* 前列地尔(治疗先天性心脏病时,用作动脉导管的暂时性维持药)
alrestatin sodium [ˈælriˌstætin] 阿司他丁钠(醛糖还原酶抑制药)
ALROS American Laryngological, Rhinological, and Otological Society 美国耳鼻咽喉科学会
ALS amyotrophic lateral sclerosis 肌萎缩性侧索硬化; antilymphocyte serum 抗淋巴细胞血清
alseroxylon [ˌælsəˈrɔksilɔn] *n* 阿舍西隆(降压镇静药)
alstonine [ˈɔːlstəniːn] *n* 鸡骨常山碱,解热树碱
Alstroemeria [ælstrəˈmiːriə] *n* 石蒜属
Alström's syndrome [ˈɑːlstrem] (Carl H. Alström)阿尔斯特伦综合征(常染色体隐性遗传综合征,表现为视网膜色素变性伴眼球震颤和中心视力过早丧失、耳聋、肥胖及糖尿病)
ALT alanine transaminase 丙氨酸转氨酶
alt. dieb. alternis diebus【拉】隔日
alteplase [ˈæltəpleis] *n* 阿替普酶(组织纤维蛋白溶酶原激活药,由重组 DNA 技术产生,用于纤维蛋白溶解疗法,治疗急性心肌梗死)
alter [ˈɔːltə] *vi* 改变;阉,阉割(如家畜) *vi* 变样 | **alterable** [ˈɔːltərəbl] *a* 可改变的,可改动的
alteration [ˌɔːltəˈreiʃən] *n* 改变,变更
alteregoism [ˌɔːltəˈriːgəizəm] *n* 同病相怜症
alternans [ɔːlˈtəːnənz]【拉】*a* 交替的 *n* 交替脉 | electrical ~ 心电交替 / ~ of the heart 心脏交替[现象] / pulsus ~ 心音交替(提示左心室衰竭)
Alternaria [ˌɔːltəˈnɛəriə] *n* 链格孢属(可致数种植物病及发现于人类肺病与皮肤感染,也是人类支气管哮喘常见的变应原)
alternariatoxicosis [ˌɔːltəˌnæriətɔksiˈkəusis] *n* 链格孢中毒
alternariosis [ˌɔːltənɛəriˈəusis] *n* 链格孢病
alternate [ɔːlˈtəːnit] *a* 交替的,轮流的;互生的(植物)
alternating [ˌɔːltəneitiŋ] *a* 更迭的;交替的
alternation [ˌɔːltəˈneiʃən] *n* 交替,更迭;互生(植物) | ~ of generations 世代交替 / ~ of the heart 心脏交替
alternative [ɔːlˈtəːnətiv] *a* 可选择的;替代的 *n* (可供选择的)两者之一;选择对象;替代办法
Alteromonas [ˌɔːltərəˈməunəs] *n* 互生单胞菌属 | ~ putrefaciens 腐败互生单胞菌,腐败假单胞菌
Althaea [ælˈθiːə] *n*【拉】蜀葵属
Althausen test [ˈɔːlthauzən] (Theodore L. Althausen) 阿尔陶森试验(口服糖后,间隔时间抽血测定半乳糖浓度以检肠吸收速度)
althea [ælˈθiːə] *n* 药蜀葵[根]
althiazide [ælˈθaiəzaid] *n* 阿尔噻嗪(利尿、降压药)
Alt. hor. alternis horis【拉】每 2 小时,每隔 1 小时
altitude [ˈæltitjuːd] *n* 高,高度 | equivalent ~ 等

效高度

Altmann-Gersh method ['ɑːltmɑːn gəːʃ] (Richard Altmann; Isidore Gersh) 阿尔特曼-格什法(用冰冻干燥法制备组织,供组织学研究用)

Altmann's fluid ['ɑːltmɑːn] (Richard Altmann) 阿尔特曼液(组织固定液,由等量的2%锇酸溶液和5%重铬酸钾溶液组成) | ~ granule 线粒体 / ~ theory 阿尔特曼学说(认为细胞原浆由微细的小粒所组成,这种小粒为生活物质的单位,称为原生粒)

altofrequent [ˌæltəu'friːkwənt] *a* 高频率的

altretamine [æl'retəmiːn] *n* 六甲蜜胺(抗肿瘤药)

altricious [æl'triʃəs] *a* 长期护理的

altronic acid [æl'trɔnik] 阿卓糖酸

altrose ['æltrəus] *n* 阿卓糖

altruism ['æltruizəm] *n* 利他主义

alum ['æləm] *n* 明矾 | exsiccated ~, burnt ~, dried ~ 煅明矾,干燥明矾

alumina [ə'ljuːminə] *n* 矾土;氧化铝 | ~ and magnesia 铝镁片,氧化铝和氧化镁(抗酸药)

aluminate [ə'ljuːmineit] *n* 铝酸盐

aluminated [ə'ljuːmiˌneitid] *a* 含明矾的

aluminosis [əˌljuːmi'nəusis] *n* 铝质沉着病,铝尘肺,肺矾土沉着病,矾土肺

aluminous [ə'ljuːminəs] *a* 铝土的;矾的

aluminum (Al) [ə'ljuːminəm] *n* 铝 | ~ acetate 醋酸铝(收敛、防腐药) / ~ ammonium sulfate 硫酸铝铵;铵矾 / ~ hydroxide 氢氧化铝(外用作干燥粉,内用作抗酸药和吸收药) | **aluminium** [ˌæljuː'minjəm] *n*

alundum [ə'lʌndəm] *n* 钢铝石

Alv. adst. alvo adstricta【拉】便秘

Alv. deject. alvi dejectiones【拉】便通

alvei ['ælviai] alveus 的复数

alveobronchiolitis [ˌælviəubrɔŋkiə'laitis] *n* 支气管肺炎

alveolalgia [ˌælviəu'lældʒiə] *n* (术后)牙槽窝痛

alveolar [æl'viələ] *a* 牙槽的;小泡的

alveolate [æl'viəlit] *a* 蜂窝状的,槽形的 | **alveolation** [ælˌviə'leiʃən] *n*

alveolectomy [ˌælviə'lektəmi] *n* 牙槽骨切除术

alveoli [æl'viəlai] alveolus 的复数

alveolitis [ˌælviə'laitis] *n* 牙槽炎;肺泡炎 | fibrosing ~ 纤维化肺泡炎 / ~ sicca dolorosa 干槽症(牙槽窝骨髓炎)

alveol(o)- [构词成分] 牙槽;小泡

alveolocapillary [ælˌviələu'kæpiləri] *a* 肺泡[与]毛细管的

alveoloclasia [ælˌviələu'kleiziə] *n* 牙槽崩解,牙槽溃坏

alveolodental [ælˌviələu'dentl] *a* 牙槽牙的

alveololabial [ælˌviələu'leibiəl] *a* 牙槽唇的

alveololabialis [ælˌviələuleibi'eilis] *n* 颊肌

alveololingual [ælˌviələu'liŋgwəl] *a* 牙槽舌的

alveolomerotomy [ælˌviələumi'rɔtəmi] *n* 牙槽突部分切除术

alveolonasal [ælˌviələu'neizəl] *a* 牙槽鼻的

alveolopalatal [ælˌviələu'pælətl] *a* 牙槽腭的

alveoloplasty [æl'viələˌplæsti], **alveoplasty** [ælˌviə'plæsti] *n* 牙槽成形术,牙槽骨修整术

alveolotomy [ˌælviəu'lɔtəmi] *n* 牙槽切开术

alveolus [æl'viələs] ([复] **alveoli** [æl'viəlai]) *n* 牙槽;小泡,小窝;肺泡 | dental alveoli 牙槽 / alveoli pulmonis, alveoli pulmonum 肺泡

alverine citrate ['ælvəriːn] 枸橼酸阿尔维林(抗胆碱能药,胃肠道和生殖泌尿道疾病时用作平滑肌松弛药)

alveus ['ælviəs] ([复] **alvei** ['ælviai]) *n*【拉】槽;海马槽,海马白质

alvus ['ælvəs] *n*【拉】腹,腹脏

alymphia [ə'limfiə] *n* 淋巴液缺乏

alymphocytosis [əˌlimfəusai'təusis] *n* 淋巴细胞缺乏(血内)

alymphoplasia [əˌlimfəu'pleiziə] *n* 淋巴[组织]发育不全 | thymic ~ 胸腺淋巴[组织]发育不全(重症联合免疫缺陷)

alymphopotent [əˌlimfəu'pəutənt] *a* 淋巴细胞再生不能的

Alzheimer's cells ['æltshaimə] (Alois Alzheimer) 阿尔茨海默细胞(①巨大星形胶质细胞,见于肝豆状变性与肝昏迷时的脑内;②变性星形胶质细胞) | ~ dementia (disease, sclerosis) 早老性痴呆 / ~ stain 阿尔茨海默染剂(一种亚甲蓝与曙红的多色染剂,染内格里〈Negri〉小体)

AM artium magister【拉】文科硕士

Am americium 镅

am ametropia 屈光不正; meterangle 米角; myopic astigmatism 近视散光

AMA Aerospace Medical Association 航空航天医学协会; American Medical Association 美国医学协会; Australian Medical Association 澳大利亚医学协会

ama ['eimə] ([复] **amae** ['eimiː]) *n* 半规管膨隆(在壶腹对侧)

amaas ['ɑːməs] *n* 乳白痘,类天花

amacratic [ˌæmə'krætik] *a* 焦聚的,聚光的(透镜)

amacrinal [ˌæmə'krainl] *a* 无长突的

amacrine, amakrine ['æməkriːn] *a* 无长突的(神经细胞) *n* 无长突细胞

amadinone acetate [ə'mædinəun] 醋酸阿马地酮(孕激素类药)

Amadori product [ˌɑːmɑː'dɔːri] (Marie Amadori) 阿马多里产物(结合希夫〈Schiff〉碱形成

化学可逆产物)
amadou [ˈæmədu:] *n*【法】火绒(从前用于裹伤和止血)
AMAL Aero-Medical Acceleration Laboratory 航空医学加速实验室
amalgam [əˈmælgəm] *n* 汞合金,汞齐 | dental ~ 银汞合金(一种银、锡和汞的合金,充填牙用)
amalgamable [əˈmælgəməbl] *a* 可合汞的,可成合金的
amalgamate [əˈmælgəmeit] *vt* 调制汞合金,混合 *vi* 汞齐化 | **amalgamation** [əˌmælgəˈmeiʃən] *n* 汞齐化法,汞合金调制;研制[法]/ **amalgamator** [əˈmælgəmeitə] *n* 混汞[合金]器,汞合金调制器;研制器
amandin [ˈæməndin] *n* 苦扁桃仁球蛋白,苦杏仁球蛋白
Amanita [ˌæməˈnaitə] *n* 捕蝇蕈属
Amanitaceae [ˌæmənaiˈteisii:] *n* 捕蝇蕈科
amanitine [əmæˈniti:n] *n* 蝇蕈素,鹅膏蕈碱
amanitotoxin [əˌmænitəuˈtɔksin] *n* 蝇蕈毒素
amantadine hydrochloride [əˈmæntədi:n] 盐酸金刚烷胺(抗病毒药,抗震颤麻痹药)
amaranth [ˈæməræn θ] *n* 苋紫,蓝光酸性红(用作食品、化妆品和药物的着色剂)
Amaranthus [ˌæməˈrænθəs] *n* 苋属
amaril [ˈæməril] *n* 黄热病毒质(一种过去认为致黄热病的假设性毒质) | virus ~ 黄热病 | **~lic** [ˌæməˈrilik] *a*
amarine [ˈæməri:n] *n* 苦杏素,苦木精,苦杏精
amaroid [ˈæmərɔid] *n* 苦味质
amaroidal [æməˈrɔidl] *a* 苦味质的
amarthritis [ˌæmɑ:ˈθraitis] *n* 多[数]关节炎
amasesis [ˌæməˈsi:sis] *n* 咀嚼不能
amass [əˈmæs] *vt* 积聚 | **~ment** *n*
amasthenic [ˌæmæsˈθenik] *a* 焦聚的,聚光的(透镜)
amastia [əˈmæstiə] *n* 无乳房,乳房缺如
amastigote [əˈmæstigəut] *n* 无鞭毛体
amathophobia [əˌmæθəˈfəubjə] *n* 飞尘恐怖,尘埃恐怖
amativeness [ˈæməˌtivnis] *n* 恋爱嗜好,好色
amatol [ˈæmətɔl] *n* 阿马托炸药(由硝酸铵和三硝基甲苯组成)
amatoxin [ˌæməˈtɔksin] *n* 蝇蕈毒素
amaurosis [ˌæmɔ:ˈrəusis] *n* 黑矇 | albuminuric ~ 蛋白尿性黑矇 / central ~ 中枢性黑矇 / cerebral ~ 脑性黑矇 / ~ fugax 一时性黑矇 / saburral ~ 胃炎性黑矇 | **amaurotic** [ˌæmɔ:ˈrɔtik] *a*
amazia [əˈmeiziə] *n* 无乳腺[畸形]
amb- 见 ambi-
Ambard's formula (coefficient, constant, equation) (Leon Ambard) [əmˈbɑ:] 昂巴公式(系数、常数、方程式)(肾病时找出脲指数〈*K*〉,其公式为:$\dfrac{U_r}{\sqrt{D\times\dfrac{70}{P}\times\sqrt{\dfrac{C}{25}}}}=K$,其中 U_r 表示血内脲的比例,*D* 表示 24 h 总脲量〈g〉,*P* 表示患者的体重〈kg〉,*C* 表示尿中脲的比例)
ambenonium chloride [ˌæmbiˈnəuniəm] 安贝氯铵(胆碱酯酶抑制药,用于重症肌无力)
amber [ˈæmbə] *n*, *a* 琥珀(的),琥珀色(的)
ambergris [ˈæmbəgri(:)s] *n* 龙涎香
Amberg's line [ˈæmbə:g] (Emil Amberg) 安伯格线(为乳突前缘和颞线所成之角的中分线,本线最靠近侧窦。亦称侧窦线)
ambi-, amb- [前缀]两,复,双,两侧
ambidexterity [ˌæmbideksˈterəti], **ambidextrality** [ˌæmbideksˈtræləti], **ambidextrism** [ˌæmbiˈdekstrizəm] *n* 双利手,两手同利 | **ambidextrous** [æmbiˈdekstrəs] *a*
ambient [ˈæmbiənt] *a* 周围的,环境的
ambilateral [ˌæmbiˈlætərəl] *a* 两侧的
ambilevosity [ˌæmbiliˈvɔsəti] *n* 两手不利 | **ambilevous** [ˌæmbiˈli:vəs] *a*
ambiopia [ˌæmbiˈəupiə] *n* 复视
ambisexual [ˌæmbiˈseksjuəl] *a* 两性的(指两性共有的性特征,如阴毛)
ambisinister [ˌæmbisiˈnistə] *a* 两手不利的 *n* 两手不利者
ambisinistrous [ˌæmbisiˈnistrəs] *a* 两手不利的
ambivalence [ˌæmbiˈveiləns, æmˈbivələns] *n* 矛盾意向(对同一事物既爱又恨) | **ambivalent** [æmˈbivələnt] *a* 矛盾意向的;矛盾的
ambiversion [ˌæmbiˈvə:ʒən] *n* 中向人格(介于内向和外向人格之间)
ambivert [ˈæmbivə:t] *n* 中向人格者
ambly- [构词成分]钝,弱
amblyacousia [ˌæmbliəˈku:siə], **amblykusis** [ˌæmbliˈkju:sis] *n* 听觉迟钝
amblyaphia [æmbliˈeifiə] *n* 触觉迟钝
amblychromasia [ˌæmblikrəuˈmeiziə] *n* 弱染性
amblychromatic [ˌæmblikrəuˈmætik] *a* 弱染性的
amblygeustia [ˌæmbliˈgju:stiə] *n* 味觉迟钝
Amblyomma [ˌæmbliˈɔmə] *n* 钝眼蜱属 | ~ americanum 美洲钝眼蜱 / ~ cajennense 卡延钝眼蜱 / ~ hebraeum 希伯来钝眼蜱 / ~ maculatum 斑点钝眼蜱 / ~ ovale 卵圆钝眼蜱 / ~ tuberculatum 结节钝眼蜱 / ~ variegatum 彩饰钝眼蜱
amblyope [ˈæmbliəup] *n* 弱视者
amblyopia [ˌæmbliˈəupiə] *n* 弱视 | color ~ 色弱视 / crossed ~ 交叉性弱视 / postmarital ~ 婚后弱视 / quinine ~ 奎宁毒性弱视 | **amblyopic**

[ˌæmbliˈəupik] *a*
amblyopiatrics [ˌæmbliˌəupiˈætriks] *n* 弱视矫正法
amblyoscope [ˈæmbliəˌskəup] *n* 弱视镜
Amblyospora [ˌæmbliˈɔspɔrə] *n* 钝孢子属
Amblystoma [æmˈblistəumə] *n* 美西螈属
ambo [ˈæmbəu] *n* 关节盂缘
ambo- [构词成分]两,复,双,两侧
amboceptor [ˌæmbəuˈseptə] *n* 介体 | bacteriolytic ~ 溶菌介体 / hemolytic ~ 溶血性介体
amboceptorgen [ˌæmbəuˈseptədʒən] *n* 介体原(产生介体的抗原)
ambomalleal [ˌæmbəuˈmæliəl] *a* 砧骨锤骨的
ambomycin [ˌæmbəˈmaisin] *n* 安波霉素,二霉素(抗生素类药)
ambon [ˈæmbɔn] *n* 关节盂缘
ambosexual [ˌæmbəuˈseksjuəl] *a* 两性的(见 ambisexual)
ambrin [ˈæmbrin], **ambrain** [æmˈbreiin], **ambrein** [æmˈbriːin] *n* 龙涎香脂,龙涎精
Ambrosia [æmˈbrəuzjə] *n* 豕草属(一年生草本,产生大量风播花粉,引致枯草热)
ambrosterol [æmˈbrɔstərɔl] *n* 豕草甾醇,豕草固醇
ambruticin [ˌæmbruːˈtaisin] *n* 安布替星(抗真菌药)
ambulance [ˈæmbjuləns] *n* 救护车
ambulant [ˈæmbjulənt], **ambulatory** [ˈæmbjulətəri] *a* 能走动的,不卧床的
ambulate [ˈæmbjuleit] *vi* 行走,移动 | **ambulation** [ˌæmbjuˈleiʃən] *n* 离床活动
ambuphylline [æmˈbjuːfiliːn] *n* 安布茶碱(利尿药,平滑肌松弛药)
ambustion [æmˈbʌstʃən] *n* 灼伤,烫伤
ambutoxate hydrochloride [ˌæmbjuˈtɔkseit] 盐酸氨布卡因(脊髓麻醉药)
Ambystoma [æmˈbistəmə] *n* 美西螈属
amcinafal [æmˈsinəfəl] *n* 安西法尔(抗炎药)
amcinafide [æmˈsinəfaid] *n* 安西非特(抗炎药)
amcinonide [æmˈsinəˌnaid] *n* 安西奈德(合成皮质类固醇)
amdinocillin [æmˈdiːnəˌsilin] *n* 甲亚胺青霉素(用于治疗尿路感染,亦称美西林 mecillinam)
ameba [əˈmiːbə] ([复] **amebae** [əˈmiːbiː] 或 **amebas**) *n* 阿米巴,变形虫 | artificial ~ 人工阿米巴 / coprozoic ~ 粪生阿米巴 | **amebic** [əˈmiːbik] *a*
amebacidal [əˌmiːbəˈsaidl] *a* 杀阿米巴的
amebacide [əˈmiːbəsaid] *a* 杀阿米巴的 *n* 杀阿米巴药
amebadiastase [əˌmiːbəˈdaiəsteis] *n* 阿米巴淀粉酶
amebaism [əˈmiːbəizəm] *n* 阿米巴样运动力
ameban [əˈmiːbən] *n* 卡巴胂(即 carbarsone,抗阿米巴药)
amebevan [əˈmiːbəvən] *n* 卡巴胂(即 carbarsone,抗阿米巴药)
amebiasis [ˌæmiˈbaiəsis] *n* 阿米巴病 | ~ cutis 皮肤阿米巴病 / hepatic ~ 肝阿米巴病,阿米巴[性]肝炎 / intestinal ~ 肠阿米巴病,阿米巴[性]痢疾
amebicidal [əˌmiːbiˈsaidl] *a* 杀阿米巴的
amebicide [əˈmiːbisaid] *a* 杀阿米巴的 *n* 杀阿米巴药
amebiform [əˈmiːbifɔːm] *a* 阿米巴样的,变形虫样的
ameb(i)(o)- [构词成分]阿米巴的(同样见以 amoeb(i)(o)-起始的词)
amebiosis [ˌæmibaiˈəusis] *n* 阿米巴病
amebism [ˈæmibizəm] *n* 阿米巴样运动;阿米巴病
amebocyte [əˈmiːbəsait] *n* 阿米巴样细胞,变形[虫样]细胞
amebodiastase [əˌmiːbəuˈdaiəsteis] *n* 阿米巴淀粉酶
ameboflagellate [əˌmiːbəuˈflædʒəleit] *n* 阿米巴鞭毛虫
ameboid [əˈmiːbɔid] *a* 阿米巴样的,变形虫样的
ameboidism [əˈmiːbɔidizəm] *n* 阿米巴样运动
ameboma [ˌæmiˈbəumə] *n* 阿米巴瘤
amebosis [ˌæmiˈbəusis] *n* 阿米巴病
amebula [əˈmiːbjulə] *n* 变形虫样孢子,假孢子虫
ameburia [ˌæmiˈbjuəriə] *n* 阿米巴尿,变形虫尿
amedalin hydrochloride [əˈmiːdəlin] 盐酸氨甲达林(抗抑郁药)
ameiosis [ˌeimaiˈəusis] *n* 不减数分裂(如单性生殖中所发生的)
AMEL Aero-Medical Equipment Laboratory 航空医学设备实验室
amelanosis [əˌmeləˈnəusis] *n* 无黑素病,黑素缺失症
amelanotic [ˌæmeləˈnɔtik] *a* 无黑素的
amelia [əˈmiːliə] *n* 无肢,先天性无肢
amelification [əˌmelifiˈkeiʃən] *n* 成釉[作用],釉质化
ameloblast [əˈmeləublæst] *n* 成釉[质]细胞
ameloblastoma [əˌmeləublæsˈtəumə] *n* 成釉细胞瘤 | melanotic ~, pigmented ~ 黑素沉着性成釉细胞瘤,色素沉着性成釉细胞瘤;黑素沉着性神经外胚层瘤 / pituitary ~ 垂体性成釉细胞瘤,颅咽管瘤
amelodentinal [ˌæmiləuˈdentinl] *a* 釉牙本质的
amelogenesis [ˌæmiləuˈdʒenisis] *n* 釉质发生 | ~ imperfecta 釉质发生不全

amelogenic [ˌæmiləuˈdʒenik] *a* 釉质发生的,釉原性的

amelogenin [ˌæmiləuˈdʒenin] *n* 牙釉蛋白

amelus [ˈæmiləs] *n* 无肢畸胎

amenia [əˈmiːniə] *n* 闭经

amenorrhea [eiˌmenəˈriə] *n* 闭经 | dysponderal ~ 体重失常性闭经,代谢性闭经/ hypothalamic ~ 下丘脑性闭经 / ovarian ~ 卵巢性闭经 / physiologic ~ 生理闭经,妊娠期闭经 / relative ~ 月经减少 | **~l** [eiˌmenəˈriəl] *a*

amensalism [eiˈmensəlizəm] *n* 偏害共生,偏害共栖(一群体或个体受到损害,而另一群体或个体则不受影响的共生)

ament [ˈeimənt] *n* 白痴,低能者,精神发育不全者

amentia [əˈmenʃiə] *n* 白痴,低能,精神发育不全;精神错乱 | nevoid ~ 痣性低能,痣性精神障碍 / phenylpyruvic ~ 苯丙酮酸性白痴 | **~l** *a*

American Type Culture Collection(ATCC) 美国模式培养物保藏所

americium(Am) [ˌæməˈrisiəm] *n* 镅(化学元素)

amerism [ˈæmərizəm] *n* 不分节 | **ameristic** [ˌæməˈristik] *a*

Ames test [eimz] (Bruce Ames) 埃姆斯试验,细菌回复突变试验

ametabolon [ˌæmeˈtæbəlɔn] *n* 不变态类(指动物)

ametabolous [ˌeimeˈtæbələs] *a* 不变态的

ametachromophil [ˌeimetəˈkrəuməfil], **ametaneutrophil** [ˌeimetəˈnjuːtrəfil] *a* 非偏染的,正染色的

amethocaine [əˈmeθəkein] *n* 丁卡因(局部或表面麻醉药)

amethopterin [əmeˈθɔptərin] *n* 甲氨蝶呤(抗肿瘤药,免疫抑制剂)

ametria [eiˈmiːtriə] *n* 无子宫[畸形]

ametrometer [ˌæmiˈtrɔmitə] *n* 屈光不正测量器

ametropia [ˌæmiˈtrəupiə] *n* 屈光不正 | axial ~ 轴性屈光不正 / curvature ~ 曲率性屈光不正 | **ametropic** [ˌæmiˈtrɔpik] *a*

amfenac sodium [ˈæmfənæk] 氨芬酸钠(抗炎药)

amfonelic acid [ˌæmfəˈniːlik] 安福萘酸(中枢神经系统兴奋药)

Amh mixed astigmatism with myopia predominating 近视为主混合散光

AMI acute myocardial infarction 急性心肌梗死

amianthoid [ˌæmiˈænθɔid] *a* 石棉样的(指肋软骨和喉软骨坏变时所见的某些纤维)

amibiarson [ˌæmibaiˈɑːsəun] *n* 卡巴胂(即 carbarsone,抗阿米巴药)

amichloral [ˌæmiˈklɔːrəl] *n* 阿米氯醛(兽用食物添加剂)

amicine [ˈæmisin] *n* 生长抑制素

Amici's disk(line), striae [əˈmitʃi] (Giovanni B. Amici) 阿米契盘(线)、纹(Z 盘,克劳泽〈Krause〉膜,横纹肌间线)

amicloral [ˌæmiˈklɔːrəl] *n* 阿米氯醛(与吡喃葡萄糖密切相关的一种化合物,作为兽医饲料添加剂给药)

amicrobic [ˌeimaiˈkrəubik] *a* 无菌的,非微生物性的

amicron [eiˈmaikrɔn], **amicrone** [eiˈmaikrəun] *n* 超视粒,绝微子(直径约 10^{-7} cm 的一种胶粒,只有用超显微镜方可看到)

amicroscopic [əˌmaikrəˈskɔpik] *a* 超显微镜的

amiculum [əˈmikjuləm] ([复] **amicula** [əˈmikjulə]) *n* 包膜;橄榄核套

amidapsone [ˌeimiˈdæpsəun] *n* 阿米氨苯砜(家禽抗病毒药)

amidase [ˈæmideis] *n* 酰胺酶

amide [ˈæmaid] *n* 酰胺 | niacin ~, nicotinic acid ~ 烟酰胺,尼克酰胺

amide synthetase [ˈæmaid ˈsinθiteis] 酰胺合成酶

amidin [ˈæmidin] *n* 淀粉溶素

amidine [ˈæmidiːn] *n* 脒 | insoluble ~, tegumentary ~ 支链淀粉

amidine-lyase [ˈæmidiːn-ˈlaieis] *n* 脒裂合酶

amidino [æmiˈdiːnəu] *n* 脒基

amidinohydrolase [æmiˌdiːnəuˈhaidrəleis] *n* 脒基水解酶

amidinotransferase [ˌæmiˌdinəˈtrænsfəreis] *n* 转脒酶,脒基转移酶

amido- [前缀][酰]氨基

amidoazotoluene [ˌæmidəu ˌeizəˈtɔljuiːn, əˌmiːdəu-] *n* 氨基偶氮甲苯

amidobenzene [ˌæmidəuˈbenziːn, əˌmiːdəu-] *n* 苯胺,阿尼林(aniline)

amidogen [əˈmiːdəˌdʒən] *n* 氨基

amidohexose [ˌæmidəuˈheksəus, əˌmiːdəu-] *n* 氨基己糖

amidohydrolase [ˌæmidəuˈhaidrəleis, əˌmiːdəu-] *n* 氨基水解酶

amido-ligase [ˌæmidəuˈlaigeis, əˌmiːdəu-] *n* 酰氨基连接酶

amidophosphoribosyltransferase [əˌmiːdəu ˌfɔsfəˌraibəu silˈtrænsfəreis] *n* 酰胺磷酸核糖基转移酶

amidopyrine [ˌæmidəuˈpaiərin] *n* 氨基比林(解热镇痛药)

Amidostomum [ˌæmiˈdɔstəməm] *n* 裂口线虫属 | ~ anseris 鹅裂口线虫

amidoxime [æmiˈdɔksaim] *n* 氨肟

amidulin [əˈmidjulin] *n* 可溶性淀粉

amifostine [ˌæmiˈfɔstiːn] *n* 氨磷汀(一种化学防

护剂,用于预防顺铂化疗时的肾毒性,静脉输注给药。本品在放疗时,亦用作放射防护剂)

amikacin [ˌæmiˈkeisin] *n* 阿米卡星(抗生素类药)

amilocellulose [ˌæmiləuˈseljuləus] *n* 直链淀粉

amiloride hydrochloride [əˈmiləraid] 盐酸阿米洛利(利尿药)

amiloxate [ˌæmiˈlɔkseit] *n* 阿米洛沙(防晒药)

amimia [əˈmimiə] *n* 表情不能,无表情,拟态缺失,摹仿不能 | amnesic ~ 遗忘性表情不能

aminacrine hydrochloride [æmiˈnækrin] 盐酸氨吖啶(表面抗感染药,主要治感染性创伤)

aminarsone [æmiˈnɑːsəun] *n* 卡巴胂(即 carbarsone,抗阿米巴药)

amination [ˌæmiˈneiʃən] *n* 胺化作用

amine [əˈmiːn, ˈæmiːn] *n* 胺 | catechol ~ 儿茶酚胺

amine-lyase [əˌmiːnˈlaieis] *n* 胺裂合酶

amine oxidase (copper-containing) [əˈmiːn ˈɔksideis] 胺氧化酶(含铜)(亦称二胺氧化酶)

amine oxidase (flavin-containing) [əˈmiːn ˈɔksideis] 胺氧化酶(含黄素)(亦称单胺氧化酶)

aminergic [ˌæmiˈnəːdʒik] *a* 胺能的

aminitrozole [ˌæmiˈnaitrəzəul] *n* 醋胺硝唑(抗滴虫药)

aminoacetic acid [əˌmiːnəuəˈsiːtik] 氨基乙酸,甘氨酸(氨基酸类药)

amino acid (AA) [ˈæminəu, əˈmiːnəu] 氨基酸 | essential ~ ~s 必需氨基酸 / nonessential ~ ~s 非必需氨基酸

amino-acid *N*-acetyltransferase [əˌmiːnəuˈæsid ˌæsitilˈtrænsfəreis] 氨基酸 *N*-乙酰转移酶(此酶缺乏可致高氨血症,而无乳清酸尿,类似氨甲酰基磷酸合成酶缺乏症所见。亦称 *N*-乙酰谷氨酸合成酶)

aminoacidemia [əˌmiːnəuˌæsiˈdiːmiə] *n* 氨基酸血

aminoacidopathy [əˌmiːnəuˌæsiˈdɔpəθi] *n* 氨基酸代谢病

D-amino-acid oxidase [əˈmiːnəu ˈæsid ˈɔksideis] D-氨基酸氧化酶

L-amino-acid oxidase [əˈmiːnəu ˈæsid ˈɔksideis] L-氨基酸氧化酶

aminoaciduria [əˌmiːnəuˌæsiˈdjuəriə] *n* 氨基酸尿

aminoacridine hydrochloride [əˌmiːnəu ˈækridiːn] 盐酸氨吖啶(消毒防腐药)

aminoacyl [əˌmiːnəuˈæsil] *n* 氨酰基 | ~-tRNA 氨酰[基]转移核糖核酸,氨酰[基]-tRNA

aminoacylase [əˌmiːnəuˈæsileis] *n* 酰化氨基酸水解酶

aminoacyl-histidine dipeptidase [əˌmiːnəuˈæsil ˈhistidiːn daiˈpeptideise] 氨酰基组氨酸二肽酶(即 X-His dipeptidase)

aminoacyltransferase [əˌmiːnəuˈæsilˈtrænsfəreis] *n* 氨酰基转移酶

aminoacyl-tRNA synthetase [əˌmiːnəuˈæsil ˈsinθiteis] 氨酰[基]转移核糖核酸合成酶,氨酰[基]-tRNA 合成酶

***α*-aminoadipate** [əˌmiːnəuəˈdipeit] *α*-氨基己二酸(*α*-aminoadipic acid 的阴离子型)

2-aminoadipate transaminase [əˌmiːnəuəˈdipeit trænsˈæmineis] 2-氨基己二酸转氨酶(亦称 2-aminoadipate aminotransferase)

***α*-aminoadipic acid** [əˌminəuəˈdipik] *α*-氨基己二酸(亦可写成 2-aminoadipic acid)

***α*-aminoadipicaciduria** [əˌminəuəˌdipikˌæsiˈdjuəriə] *α*-氨基己二酸尿(尿内排泄 *α*-氨基己二酸)

***α*-aminoadipic semialdehyde synthase** [əˌmiːnəuəˈdipik ˌsemiˈældihaid ˈsinθeis] *α*-氨基己二酸半醛合酶(此酶缺乏,为一种常染色体隐性性状,可致高赖氨酸血症)

***p*-aminoazobenzene** [əˌmiːnəuˌeizəˈbenziːn] *n* 对氨基偶氮苯(一种黄色偶氮染料,致癌)

***o*-aminoazotoluene** [əˌmiːnəu-, ˌæminəu ˌæzəˈtɔljuiːn] *n* *O*-氨基偶氮甲苯(有力的致癌物质)

aminobenzene [əˌmiːnəu-, ˌæminəuˈbenziːn] *n* 氨基苯,苯胺

aminobenzoate [əˌmiːnəuˈbenzəueit] *n* 对氨苯甲酸(盐或酯) | ~ potassium 对氨苯甲酸钾(口服用作抗纤维变性药,治疗以纤维变性或非化脓性炎症为特点的皮肤疾病,与水杨酸钾结合,用于镇痛药制剂) / ~ sodium 对氨苯甲酸钠(与水杨酸钠结合,用于镇痛药制剂)

***p*-aminobenzoic acid (PAB, PABA)** [əˌmiːnəu-benˈzəuik] 对氨苯甲酸(防晒药)

***p*-aminobiphenyl** [əˌmiːnəubaiˈfenil] *n* 对氨基联苯(从前用于制作染料,由于本品具有毒性和致癌性,现主要用于诱发实验动物癌症。本词也可写成 4-aminobiphenyl)

***γ*-aminobutyrate** [əˌmiːnəuˈbjuːtireit] *n* *γ*-氨基丁酸

aminobutyrate aminotransferase [əˌmiːnəu-ˈbjuːtireit əˌmiːnəuˈtrænsfəreis] 氨基丁酸转氨酶(此酶的先天性缺乏为一种常染色体隐性性状,可致高 *β*-丙氨酸血症。亦称 *β*-丙氨酸 *α*-酮戊二酸转氨酶,*β*-丙氨酸转氨酶)

4-aminobutyrate transaminase [əˌminəu ˈbjuːtireit trænsˈæmineis] 4-氨基丁酸转氨酶(此酶缺乏,为一种常染色体隐性性状,可致精神运动性阻抑、张力减低、反射亢进和加速直线性生长,脑脊液中有高浓度 GABA、高肌肽和 *β*-丙氨酸)

***γ*-aminobutyric acid (GABA)** [əˌmiːnəu bjuˈtirik] γ-氨基丁酸(用作脑内主要抑制性神经递质)

ε-aminocaproic acid [əˌmiːnəukə'prəuik] ε-氨基己酸(用于治疗大量纤维蛋白溶解所致的急性出血综合征)

7-aminocephalosporanic acid [əˌmiːnəu ˌsefələu-spɔː'rænik] 7-氨基头孢烷酸

aminodinitrophenol [ˌæminəudaiˌnaitrəu'fiːnɔl] *n* 氨基二硝基酚

***p*-aminodiphenyl** [əˌmiːnəudai'fenil] *n* 对氨基联苯(即 *p*-aminobiphenyl)

2-aminoethanol [ˌæminəu'eθənɔl] *n* 2-氨基乙醇

aminofluorene [ˌæminəu'fluəriːn] *n* 氨基芴

aminoform [ə'minəfɔːm] *n* 乌洛托品,环六亚甲基四胺(尿路消毒药)

aminoglutaric acid [ˌæminəugluː'tærik] 谷氨酸,氨基戊二酸

aminoglutethimide [əˌminəuglu'teθimaid] *n* 氨鲁米特(抗惊厥药,治癫痫)

aminoglycoside [ˌæminəu'glaikəusaid] *n* 氨基糖苷

aminogram ['æminəgræm] *n* 氨基酸谱

aminoheterocyclic [əˌmiːnəuˌhetərəu'siklik] *a* 氨基杂环的

aminohippurate [ˌæminəu'hipjureit] *n* 氨基马尿酸盐

***p*-aminohippurate** [əˌmiːnəu -'hipjureit] *n* 对氨基马尿酸盐 | ~ sodium 对氨基马尿酸钠

***p*-aminohippuric acid (PAH, PAHA)** [əˌmiː-nəu hi'pjuərik] 对氨基马尿酸

aminohydrolase [əˌmiːnəu'haidrəleis] *n* 氨基水解酶

aminohydroxybenzoic acid [əˌmiːnə u haiˌdrɔ-ksiben'zəuik] 氨基羟基苯甲酸(用于治疗抗酸杆菌感染的一组化疗药物)

aminoisobutyrate [əˌmiːnəuˌaisəu'bjuːtireit] *n* 氨基异丁酸(aminoisobutyric acid 的阴离子型)

***β*-aminoisobutyrate-pyruvate transaminase** [ə-ˌmiːnəuˌaisəu'bjuːtireit 'paiəruveit træns'æmineis] β-氨基异丁酸丙酮酸转氨酶(此酶缺乏,为一种常染色体隐性性状,可致 β-氨基异丁酸尿症)

aminoisobutyric acid [əˌmiːnəuˌaisəubjuː'tirik] 氨基异丁酸

***β*-aminoisobutyricaciduria** [əˌmiːnəuˌaisəubjuː-ˌtirikæsi'djuəriə] *n* β-氨基异丁酸尿(亦称高 β-氨基异丁酸尿)

aminolevulinate [əˌmiːnəuˌlevju'lineit] *n* 氨基-γ-酮戊酸,氨基乙酰丙酸

aminolevulinate dehydratase [əˌmiːnəu ˌlevju-'lineit diː'haidrəteis] 氨基-γ-酮戊酸脱水酶,氨基乙酰丙酸脱水酶,胆色素原合酶

5-aminolevulinate synthase [əˌmiːnə u ˌlevju'li-neit 'sinθeis] 5-氨基-γ-酮戊酸合酶,5-氨基乙酰丙酸合酶

aminolevulinic acid (ALA) [əˌmiːnəu ˌlevju'li-nik] 氨基-γ-酮戊酸,氨基乙酰丙酸

aminolipid [əˌmiːnəu -, ˌæminəu'lipid], **aminolipin** [əˌmiːnəu -, ˌæminəu 'laipin] *n* 氨基脂

aminolysis [ˌæmi'nɔlisis] *n* 氨解[作用]

aminomethane [əˌmiːnəu'meθein] *n* 甲胺(即 methylamine)

aminomethyl [əˌmiːnəu'meθil] *n* 氨甲基

(*R*)-3-amino-2-methylpropionate-pyruvate transaminase [əˌmiːnəuˌmeθil'prəupiəneit 'paiə-ruveit træns'æmineis] (*R*)-3-氨基-2-丙酸甲酯丙酮酸转氨酶

aminometradine [əˌmiːnəu -,ˌæminəu'metrədiːn], **aminometramide** [əˌmiːnəu -, ˌæminəu 'metr-əmaid] *n* 氨美啶(利尿药)

aminonitrogen [əˌmiːnəu -, ˌæminəu'naitrədʒən] *n* 氨基氮

aminonitrothiazole [ˌæminəuˌnaitrəu'θaiəzəul] *n* 氨硝噻唑(用于防治火鸡的黑头病,即组织滴虫病)

6-aminopenicillanic acid [əˌmiːnəuˌpenisi'læ-nik] 6-氨基青霉烷酸

aminopentamide sulfate [əˌmiːnəu, ˌæminəu -'pentəmid] 硫酸氨戊酰胺(抗胆碱药,胃肠解痉药)

aminopeptidase [əˌmiːnəu'peptideis] *n* 氨肽酶

aminophenazone [ˌæminəu'fenəzəun] *n* 氨基比林(解热镇痛药)

***p*-aminophenol** [əˌmiːnəu'fiːnɔl] *n* 对氨基酚

aminopherase [ˌæmi'nɔfəreis] *n* 转氨酶,氨基转移酶

aminophylline [ˌæmi'nɔfilin] *n* 氨茶碱(平滑肌松弛药,利尿药)

aminopolypeptidase [əˌmiːnəu, ˌæminəupɔli'pe-ptideis] *n* 氨基多肽酶

2-aminopropionic acid [ˌæminəuprəupi'ɔnik] 2-氨基丙酸

aminopterin [ˌæmi'nɔptərin] *n* 氨蝶呤(抗肿瘤药) | ~ sodium 氨蝶呤钠盐(治儿童急性白血病)

aminopteroylglutamic acid [ˌæminɔpterəuilglu-'tæmik] 氨基叶酸,氨蝶呤(抗肿瘤药)

aminopurine [əˌmiːnəu'pjuərin] *n* 氨基嘌呤

aminopyrine [əˌmiːnəu -, ˌæminəu'paiərin] *n* 氨基比林(解热镇痛药)

aminoquin ['æminəkwin] *n* 氨基喹(扑疟喹啉的一种)

aminoquinoline [əˌmiːnəu'kwinəliːn] *n* 氨基喹啉 | 4- ~s 4-氨基喹啉(一组抗疟化合物,对红细

胞型疟原虫有效,其中包括阿莫地喹、氯喹和羟氯喹) / 8- ~s 8-氨基喹啉(一组抗疟化合物,对红细胞外型疟原虫有效,其中只有伯氨喹〈primaquine〉被广泛使用)

aminorex [ə'minəreks] *n* 阿米雷司(拟交感性食欲抑制药)

aminosaccharide [əˌmiːnəu, ˌæminəu'sækəraid] *n* 氨基糖

aminosalicylate [əˌmiːnəusə'lisileit] *n* 氨基水杨酸盐 | calcium ~ 氨基水杨酸钙(抗菌药,治结核病)

***p*-aminosalicylate** [əˌmiːnəusə'lisəleit] *n* 对氨[基]水杨酸盐

***p*-aminosalicylic acid (PAS, PASA)** [əˌmiːnəuˌsæli'silik] 对氨水杨酸(抗结核药)

5-aminosalicylic acid (5-ASA) [əˌmiːnəusæli'silik] 5-氨基水杨酸(见 mesalamine)

aminosidine sulfate [əˌminəu'saidin] 硫酸氨基杀菌素,硫酸巴龙霉素(即 paromomycin sulfate)(抗阿米巴药)

aminosis [ˌæmi'nəusis] *n* 氨基酸过多[症]

aminostiburea [əˌmiːnəu-, ˌæminəustai'bjuəriə] *n* 脲锑胺苷(治黑热病)

aminosuccinic acid [ˌæminəusək'sinik] 氨基丁二酸

aminosuria [əˌmiːnəu-, ˌæminəu'sjuəriə] *n* 胺尿

aminothiazole [əˌmiːnəu-, ˌæminəu'θaiəzəul] *n* 氨噻唑(抗甲状腺药)

aminotoluene [əˌmiːnəu'tɔljuiːn] *n* 氨基甲苯,甲苯胺

aminotransferase [əˌmiːnəu'trænsfəreis] *n* 氨基转移酶

aminotrate ['æminətreit] *n* 三硝酸三乙醇胺[酯] | ~ phosphate 磷酸三硝乙醇胺

aminotriazole [əˌmiːnəu'traiəzəul] *n* 氨基三唑

3-aminotriazole [əˌmiːnəu'traiəzəul] *n* 3-氨基三唑(见 amitrole)

aminoxyacetic acid [ˌæmiˌnɔksiæ'siːtik] 氨氧醋酸

aminuria [ˌæmi'njuəriə] *n* 胺尿

amiodarone hydrochloride [ə'miːədəˌrəun] 盐酸胺碘酮(心血管扩张药,抗心律失常药)

amiphenazole hydrochloride [ˌæmi'fenəzəul] 盐酸阿米苯唑(中枢兴奋药)

amiquinsin hydrochloride [ˌæmi'kwinsin] 盐酸氨喹新(抗高血压药)

amisometradine [ˌæmisəu'metrədiːn] *n* 阿米美啶(利尿药)

amithiozone [ˌæmi'θaiəzəun] *n* 缩氨硫脲

amitosis [ˌæmi'təusis] *n* 无丝分裂 | **amitotic** [ˌæmi'tɔtik] *a*

amitriptyline hydrochloride [ˌæmi'triptiliːn] 盐酸阿米替林(抗抑郁药)

amitrole ['æmitrəul] *n* 氨基三唑,杀草强(一种除草剂,因是基因外致癌物故限制使用。亦称 3-aminotriazole)

AML acute myelogenous leukemia 急性粒细胞白血病

amlexanox [æm'leksənɔks] *n* 氨来占诺(局部抗溃疡药,用于治疗复发性阿弗他口炎)

amlodipine besylate [æm'ləudiˌpiːn] 苯磺氨氯地平(钙通道阻滞药,用以治疗高血压和慢性稳定性及血管痉挛性心绞痛,口服给药)

ammeter ['æmitə] *n* 安培计

Ammi ['æmi] *n* 阿密属 | ~ visnaga 阿密茴(治尿道痉挛及肾绞痛)

ammoaciduria [ˌæməuˌæsi'djuəriə] *n* 氨氨基酸尿

ammonemia [ˌæmə'niːmiə] *n* 氨血症

ammonia [ə'məuniə] *n* 氨 | ~ hemate 苏木红质氨

ammoniac [ə'məuniæk] *n* 阿摩匿,阿摩尼亚脂,氨草胶(兴奋药和祛痰药)

ammoniacal [ˌæmə'naiəkəl] *a* 氨的,含氨的

ammonia-lyase [ə'məuniə 'laieis] *n* 氨裂解酶,解氨酶

ammoniate [ə'məunieit] *vt* 氨合(与氨化合) *n* 氨合物 | **ammoniation** [əˌməuni'eiʃən] *n* 氨合作用

ammoniemia [əˌməuni'iːmiə] *n* 氨血症

ammonification [əˌməunifi'keiʃən] *n* 氨化作用(细菌作用于蛋白质而形成氨)

ammonirrhea [ˌæməni'riə] *n* 氨排泄

ammonium [ə'məunjəm] *n* 铵 | ~ acetate 醋酸铵(利尿、发汗、解热药,并用作赋形剂) / ~ benzoate 苯甲酸铵(兴奋药和利尿药) / ~ chloride, ~ muriate 氯化铵(用作全身性酸化剂) / ~ ichthyolate 鱼石脂铵 / ~ ichthyosulfonate, ~ sulfoichthyolate 鱼石脂磺酸铵,鱼石脂(局部皮肤消毒防腐药) / ~ mandelate 杏仁酸铵(泌尿系统消毒剂) / ~ oxalate 草酸铵(用作试验溶液) / ~ purpurate 紫尿酸铵 / ~ valerate 戊酸铵,缬草酸铵(镇静药)

ammoniuria [əˌməuni'juəriə] *n* 氨尿症

ammonolysis [ˌæmə'nɔlisis] *n* 氨解[作用]

ammonotelic [əˌməunəu'telik] *a* 排氨的(以氨作为氮代谢的主要排泄产物,如淡水鱼)

Ammon's fissure ['æmən] (Friedrich A. von Ammon)阿蒙裂(胎儿时,巩膜下部的梨状小裂) | ~ operation 阿蒙手术(①睑成形术;②泪囊切开术;③用于内眦赘皮)

Ammon's horn [ˌæmən] 阿蒙角,海马

Ammospermophilus [ˌæməspə'mɔfiləs] *n* 羚松鼠属 | ~ leucurus 白尾羚松鼠

amnalgesia [ˌæmnæl'dʒiːziə] *n* 遗忘止痛[法]

（使用药物或催眠术）

amnesia [æm'niːzjə] *n* 遗忘[症] | anterograde ~ 顺行性遗忘 / auditory ~ 听语遗忘,辨语聋 / immunologic ~ 免疫遗忘(对抗原不发生回忆免疫应答) / lacunar ~, patchy ~ 空隙性遗忘 / olfactory ~ 嗅觉丧失 / retroactive ~, retrograde ~ 逆行性遗忘 / tactile ~ 实体觉缺失 / verbal ~ 遗忘性失语症 / visual ~ 文字盲,视性失语 | **~c** [æm'niːziæk] *a* 遗忘的 *n* 遗忘者 / **amnesic** [æm'niːzik] *a* 遗忘的

amnestic [æm'nestik] *a* 遗忘的;引起遗忘的

amni(o)- [构词成分] 羊膜

amniocele ['æmniəusiːl] *n* 脐突出

amniocentesis [ˌæmniəusen'tiːsis] *n* 羊膜腔穿刺术

amniochorial [ˌæmniəu'kɔːriəl] *a* 羊膜绒[毛]膜的

Amniocolidae [ˌæmniəu'kɔlidiː] *n* 鳚螺科

amniocyte ['æmniəsait] *n* 羊水细胞

amniogenesis [ˌæmniəu'dʒenisis] *n* 羊膜形成

amniography [ˌæmni'ɔgrəfi] *n* 羊膜腔造影术

amnioinfusion [ˌæmniəuin'fjuːʒən] *n* 羊膜输注(输液于羊膜,如人工流产、抵消脐带压迫引起的晚期减速或稀释厚胎粪)

amnion ['æmniən] *n* 羊膜 | ~ nodosum 结节性羊膜(羊膜多灶性损害) | **~ic** [ˌæmni'ɔnik] *a*

amnionitis [ˌæmniəu'naitis] *n* 羊膜炎

amniorrhea [ˌæmniə'riə] *n* 羊水溢

amniorrhexis [ˌæmniə'reksis] *n* 羊膜破裂

amnioscope ['æmniəˌskəup] *n* 羊膜镜 | **amnioscopy** [ˌæmni'ɔskəpi] *n* 羊膜镜检查(经子宫颈直接观察胎儿及羊水的颜色和数量)

Amniota [æmni'əutə] *n* 羊膜动物类

amniote ['æmniəut] *n* 羊膜动物

amniotic [ˌæmni'ɔtik] *a* 羊膜的

amniotome ['æmniəˌtəum] *n* 羊膜穿刺器,羊膜刀

amniotomy [ˌæmni'ɔtəmi] *n* 羊膜穿刺术(引产)

amobarbital [ˌæməu'bɑːbitæl] *n* 异戊巴比妥(镇静催眠药) | ~ sodium 异戊巴比妥钠(镇静催眠药)

amodiaquine [ˌæmə'daiəkwin] *n* 阿莫地喹(抗疟药)

amoeb-, amoebi-, amoebo- [构词成分] 阿米巴的;同样见以 ameb(i)(o)-起始的词

Amoeba [ə'miːbə] *n* 阿米巴属,变形虫属 | ~ buccalis 颊阿米巴,龈内阿米巴(即 Entamoeba gingivalis) / ~ coli 结肠阿米巴(即 Entamoeba coli) / ~ dentalis 牙阿米巴,龈内阿米巴(即 Entamoeba gingivalis) / ~ limax 微小内蜒阿米巴(即 Endolimax nana) / ~ proteus 变形阿米巴 / ~ urinae granulata 尿粒形阿米巴 / ~ verrucosa 疣状核阿米巴

amoeba [ə'miːbə] ([复] **amoebas** 或 **amoebae** [ə'miːbiː]) *n* 阿米巴,变形虫(即 ameba)

Amoebida [ə'miːbidə] *n* 阿米巴目,变形目

Amoebobacter [əˌmiːbəu'bæktə] *n* 阿米巴细菌属

amoebocyte [ə'miːbəsait] *n* = **amebocyte**

Amoebotaenia [əˌmiːbəu'tiːniə] *n* 变形带[绦虫]属

amoebula [ə'miːbjulə] *n* 小阿米巴

amok [ə'mɔk] *n* 杀人狂(抑郁后暴发)

Amomum [ə'məuməm] *n* 【拉】豆蔻属

amopyroquin hydrochloride [ˌæməu'paiərəkwin] 盐酸阿莫吡喹(抗疟药)

amorph [ə'mɔːf] *n* 无效等位基因(一种不表现其效应的突变等位基因)

amorpha [ə'mɔːfə] *n* 无定形病(无一定结构上改变的疾病)

amorphia [ə'mɔːfiə], **amorphism** [ə'mɔːfizəm] *n* 无定形(现象);非晶形[现象]

amorphic [ə'mɔːfik] *a* 无定形的;非晶形的;无效的(遗传学中指几乎完全不活跃的,如无效等位基因)

amorphinism [ə'mɔːfinizəm] *n* 吗啡断瘾状态

Amorphosporangium [əˌmɔːfəspɔ'rændʒiəm] *n* 无定形孢囊菌属

amorphosynthesis [əˌmɔːfə'sinθəsis] *n* 形态错觉

amorphous [ə'mɔːfəs] *a* 无定形的;非晶形的

amorphus [ə'mɔːfəs] *n* 无定形畸胎

amosite ['eiməˌsait] *n* 长纤维石棉,铁石棉,铁直闪石(亦称棕石棉)

Amoss' sign ['eimɔs] (Harold L. Amoss) 阿莫斯征(脊柱痛性弯曲时,患者双手扶在背后床边支撑身体,方能起坐)

amotio [ə'məuʃiəu] *n* 【拉】脱落,剥落 | ~ retinae 视网膜脱离

amoxapine [ə'mɔksəpin] *n* 阿莫沙平(抗抑郁药)

amoxicillin [əˌmɔk'silin] *a* 阿莫西林(抗生素类药)

AMP adenosine monophosphate 腺苷[一磷]酸;3′,5′-AMP, cyclic AMP 环腺苷酸

amp ampere 安培

AMP deaminase [diː'æmineis] AMP 脱氨酶,腺苷酸脱氨酶

ampelotherapy [ˌæmpiləu'θerəpi] *n* 葡萄疗法

amperage ['æmpəridʒ] *n* 安培度

ampere(A) ['æmpɛə] *n* 安培(电流单位)

amphamphoterodiplopia [ˌæmfæmˌfəutərəu di'pləupiə] *n* 两眼复视;单眼复视

ampheclexis [ˌæmfi'kleksis] *n* 两性选择

amphetamine [æm'fetəmiːn] *n* 苯丙胺(中枢兴奋药) | dextro ~ sulfate 硫酸右[旋]苯丙胺 / ~ phosphate 磷酸苯丙胺 / ~ sulfate 硫酸苯丙胺

amph(i)- [前缀] 两,两侧,两端,周围
amphiarkyochrome [ˌæmfiˈɑːkiəkrəum] *n* [双]网染细胞
amphiarthrosis [ˌæmfiɑːˈθrəusis] *n* 微动关节 | **amphiarthrodial** [ˌæmfiɑːˈθrəudiəl] *a*
amphiaster [ˈæmfiˌæstə] *n* 双星[体]
Amphibia [æmˈfibiə] *n* 两栖纲
amphibious [æmˈfibiəs] *a* 两栖的
amphiblastula [ˌæmfiˈblæstjulə] *n* 两极囊胚 | **amphiblastic** *a*
amphiblestritis [ˌæmfiblesˈtraitis] *n* 视网膜炎
amphibolia [ˌæmfiˈbəuliə] *n* 动摇期,不稳定期
amphibolic [ˌæmfiˈbɔlik], **amphibolous** [ˌæmˈfibələs] *a* 模棱两可的;动摇的,不稳定的,预后未定的;两用代谢的(具有分解和合成代谢两种作用)
amphicarcinogenic [ˌæmfiˌkɑːsinəuˈdʒenik] *a* 两向性生癌的(指增加或减少致癌活性)
amphicelous [ˌæmfiˈsiːləs] *a* 两[边]凹的(指某些冷血动物脊椎体)
amphicentric [ˌæmfiˈsentrik] *a* 起止同源的(指在同一血管中起始与终止的)
amphichroic [ˌæmfiˈkrəuik], **amphichromatic** [ˌæmfikrəuˈmætik] *a* 双变色的,两性反应的(对红色和蓝色石蕊试纸均呈反应)
amphicreatine [ˌæmfiˈkriːətin] *n* 两性肌酸
amphicreatinine [ˌæmfikriːˈætinin] *n* 两性肌酸酐
amphicyte [ˈæmfisait] *n* 套细胞
amphicytula [ˌæmfiˈsitjulə] *n* 受精卵,受精端黄卵
amphidiarthrosis [ˌæmfiˌdaiɑːˈθrəusis] *n* 屈戍动关节(如下颌关节既有屈戍动关节,又有摩动关节)
amphidiploid [ˌæmfiˈdiplɔid] *n* 双二倍体(见 allotetraploid)
amphigastrula [ˌæmfiˈgæstrulə] *n* 两极原肠胚
amphigenetic [ˌæmfidʒiˈnetik] *a* 两性生殖的
amphigonadism [ˌæmfiˈgɔnədizəm] *n* 两性[生殖]腺共存(真两性畸形)
amphigony [æmˈfigəni] *n* 有性生殖
amphikaryon [ˌæmfiˈkæriɔn] *n* 倍数核
Amphileptus branchiarum [ˌæmfiˈleptəs brənˈkiərəm] 住腮纤毛虫
amphileukemic [ˌæmfiljuːˈkiːmik] *a* 两向性白血病的(显示白血病的病变,随着器官的病变而轻重有所不同)
Amphimerus [æmˈfimərəs] *n* 对体[吸虫]属
amphimorula [ˌæmfiˈmɔrələ] *n* 两歧桑葚胚
amphinucleus [ˌæmfiˈnjuːkliəs] *n* 双质核,中心核,中央核(原虫核的一般型)
Amphioxus [ˌæmfiˈɔksəs] *n* 文昌鱼,蛞蝓鱼
amphipath [ˈæmfipɑːθ] *n* 两歧性分子(指一个分子中含有不同性质的基,如亲水性和疏水性的基) | **~ic** [ˌæmfiˈpæθik] *a*
amphipyrenin [ˌæmfiˈpairinin] *n* [细胞]核模质
amphiregulin [ˌæmfiˈregjulin] *n* 双向调节蛋白
Amphistoma [æmˈfistəmə], **Amphistomum** [æmˈfistəməm] *n* 端盘[吸虫]属,双口吸虫属 | ~ conicum 圆锥端盘吸虫(即 Paramphistomum cervi) / ~ hominis 人似端盘吸虫(即 Gastrodiscoides hominis) / ~ watsoni 互[生]氏端盘吸虫(即 Watsonius watsoni)
amphistome [æmˈfistəum] *n* 端盘吸虫
amphistomiasis [ˌæmfistəuˈmaiəsis] *n* 端盘吸虫病,双口吸虫病
amphitene [ˈæmfitiːn] *n* 偶线期(见 zygotene)
amphitheater [ˌæmfiˈθiətə] *n* 手术示教室,看台式教室(内有梯形座位,供学生或参观者就座)
amphitrichous [æmˈfitrikəs] *a* 两端有鞭毛的(指菌细胞)
amphitypy [æmˈfitipi] *n* 两型[状态]
ampho- [前缀] 两
amphochromatophil [ˌæmfəukrəuˈmætəfil], **amphochromophil** [ˌæmfəˈkrəuməfil] *n* 两染细胞 *a* 两染性的
amphocyte [ˈæmfəsait] *n* 两染细胞
amphodiplopia [ˌæmfəudiˈpləupiə] *n* 两眼复视
amphogenic [ˌæmfəˈdʒenik] *a* 两性生殖的
ampholyte [ˈæmfəlait] *n* 两性电解质;两性物
amphomycin [ˌæmfəˈmaisin] *n* 安福霉素(抗生素类药)
amphophil [ˈæmfəfil], **amphophile** [ˈæmfəfail] *n* 两染细胞(易染酸性或碱性染剂) *a* 两染性的
amphophilic [æmfəˈfilik] *a* 两染性的 | ~-basophil 嗜碱性两染的 / gram- ~ 革兰两染性的 / ~-oxyphil 嗜酸性两染的 | **amphophilous** [æmˈfɔfiləs] *a*
amphoric [æmˈfɔrik] *a* 空瓮性的 | **~ity** [ˌæmfəˈrisəti] *n* 空瓮性
amphoriloquy [ˌæmfəˈriləkwi] *n* 空瓮性语音
amphorophony [ˌæmfəˈrɔfəni] *n* 空瓮性语音
amphoteric [ˌæmfəˈterik] *a* 两性的,兼性的
amphotericin(B) [ˌæmfəˈterisin] 两性霉素 B(抗真菌抗生素,治隐球菌所致的脑膜炎及全身性真菌感染)
amphoterism [ˌæmˈfəutərizəm], **amphotericity** [ˌæmfətəˈrisəti] *n* 两性,酸碱兼性
amphoterodiplopia [æmˌfɔtərəudiˈpləupiə] *n* 两眼复视
amphoterous [æmˈfɔtərəs] *a* 两性的,酸碱兼性的
amphotony [æmˈfɔtəni] *n* 交感迷走神经过敏;交感神经系紧张
ampicillin [ˌæmpiˈsilin] *n* 氨苄西林(对多种革兰

阴性和革兰阳性菌有效）

AMP kinase [ˈkaineis] AMP 激酶，腺苷酸激酶

amplexation [ˌæmplekˈseiʃən] *n* [锁骨骨折]围合疗术

amplexus [æmˈpleksəs] *n*【拉】(雄雌蛙性交时)抱合

amplification [ˌæmplifiˈkeiʃən] *n* 放大，扩大，扩增 | biological ~ 生物放大效应

amplifier [ˈæmplifaiə] *n* 放大器，扩大器 | microelectrode ~ 微电极放大器

amplify [ˈæmplifai] *vt* 放大，增强

amplitude [ˈæmplitjuːd] *n* 振幅，幅度；范围 | ~ of accommodation 调节幅度 / ~ of convergence 集合幅度

amprenavir [æmˈprenəvir] *n* 安普纳韦(HIV 蛋白酶抑制剂，可致未成熟非感染性病毒颗粒形成，用于治疗人免疫缺陷病毒感染，口服给药)

amprolium [æmˈprəuliəm] *n* 安普罗铵(兽医用于预防和治疗球虫病)

amprotropine phosphate [ˌæmprəˈtrəupiːn] 磷酸安普洛托品(抗胆碱能药)

ampule, ampoule, ampul [ˈæmpuːl] *n* 安瓿(密封的小玻璃筒内含灭菌的溶液，主要供皮下注射)

ampulla [æmˈpulə] ([复] **ampullae** [æm-ˈpuliː]) *n*【拉】壶腹 | ~ chyli 乳糜池 / ~ ductus deferentis 输精管壶腹 / hepatopancreatic ~ 肝胰管壶腹 / ampullae lactiferae 输乳管壶腹，输乳管窦 | **~r**, **~ry** [ˈæmpuləri] *a*

Ampullariella [ˌæmpuˌlɛəriˈelə] *n* 小瓶菌属

ampullate [æmˈpulit] *a* 壶腹状的

ampullitis [ˌæmpuˈlaitis] *n* 壶腹炎(尤指输精管壶腹)

ampullula [æmˈpuljulə] *n*【拉】小壶腹

amputate [ˈæmpjuteit] *vt* 切断；截肢

amputation [ˌæmpjuˈteiʃən] *n* 切断术，截肢术 | aperiosteal ~ 除骨膜性切断术 / chop ~ 无瓣切断术 / cinematic ~, cineplastic ~, kineplastic ~ 运动成形性切断术 / closed ~, flap ~ 瓣状切断术 / coat-sleeve ~ 袖形切断术 / ~ in contiguity 关节切断术，关节断离术 / ~ in continuity 关节外切断术 / diaclastic ~ 穿骨切断术 / eccentric ~ 偏心切断术 / guillotine ~, flapless ~, open ~ 斩断术，无瓣切断术 / galvanocaustic ~ 电烙切断术 / interilioabdominal ~, interinnominoabdominal ~, hindquarter ~ 髂腹间切断术(下肢切断术，包括全部或部分髋骨) / intermediary ~, intermediate ~, intrapyretic ~, mediate ~ 间期切断术，热期内切断术(反应期及化脓前) / interscapulothoracic ~, forequarter ~ 肩胸间切断术，上肢切断术(包括肩胛骨和锁骨) / multiple ~ 多处切断术 / phalangophalangeal ~ 指节间切断术，趾节间切断术 / primary ~ 早期切断术(在休克期后及炎症形成前施行) / quadruple ~ 四肢切断术 / racket ~ 球拍形切断术 / secondary ~ 二期切断术(在肉芽面愈合期间施行) / tertiary ~ 三期切断术(在炎症反应第二阶段消退后施行) / triple ~ 三肢切断术

amputator [ˈæmpjuteitə] *n* 施行切断手术者，施行截肢手术者

amputee [ˌæmpjuˈtiː] *n* 被截肢者

AMRA American Medical Record Association 美国医学档案协会

amrinone [ˈæmrinəun] *n* 氨力农(口服强心药)

AMRL Aerospace Medical Research Laboratories 航空航天医学研究所

AMS American Meteorological Society 美国气象学会

ams amount of a substance 物质量

amsacrine [ˈæmsəkriːn] *n* 安吖啶(抑制 DNA 合成的抗肿瘤药，用于治疗几种白血病，静脉内给药)

Amsler's charts [ˈɑːmzlə] (Marc Amsler) 阿姆斯勒图(用以检测中心视野缺损) | ~ marker 阿姆斯勒标志器(用于戈南〈Gonin〉手术，用以标明应烧烙的部位)

AMTA American Music Therapy Association 美国音乐疗法协会

amu atomic mass unit 原子质量单位

amuck [əˈmʌk] *a*, *n* 杀人狂(的)

amusia [əˈmjuːziə] *n* 失乐感[症] | instrumental ~ 奏乐器不能 / vocal motor ~ 歌唱不能

Amussat's operation [ˌæmuˈsɑː] (Jean Z. Amussat) 阿谬萨手术(作长的横切口以暴露结肠) | ~ probe 阿谬萨探子(用于碎石术)

AMWA American Medical Women's Association 美国女医务人员协会；American Medical Writers' Association 美国医学作家协会

amyasthenia [əˌmaiæsˈθiːniə] *n* 肌无力 | **amyasthenic** [əˌmaiæsˈθenik] *a*

amychophobia [əˌmaikəuˈfəubje] *n* 抓伤恐怖(如怕给猫抓伤)

amyctic [əˈmiktik] *a* 腐蚀性的，刺激性的

amydricaine hydrochloride [əˈmaidrikein] 盐酸戊胺卡因(局部麻醉药，现在罕用)

amyelencephalia [əˌmaiəlensəˈfeiliə] *n* 无脑脊髓[畸形]

amyelencephalus [əˌmaiəlenˈsefələs] *n* 无脑脊髓畸胎

amyelia [ˌæmaiˈiːliə] 无脊髓[畸形]

amyelic [ˌæmaiˈelik] *a* 无脊髓的

amyelinic [əmaiəˈlinik] *a* 无髓鞘的

amyelonic [əˌmaiəˈlɔnik] *a* 无脊髓的；无骨髓的

amyelotrophy [əˌmaiəˈlɔtrəfi] *n* 脊髓萎缩

amyelus [əˈmaiələs] *n* 无脊髓畸胎

amygdala [əˈmigdələ] *n* 苦扁桃，苦巴旦杏；扁桃体；杏仁核 | accessory ~ 舌扁桃体 / ~ amara

苦扁桃[仁],苦巴旦杏 / ~ of cerebellum 小脑扁桃体 / ~ dulcis 甜扁桃[仁],甜巴旦杏仁

amygdalase [əˈmigdəleis] *n* 苦杏仁苷酶

amygdalectomy [əˌmigdəˈlektəmi] *n* 扁桃体切除术

amygdalic acid [əˌmigdəlik] 杏仁酸

amygdalin [əˈmigdəlin] *n* 苦杏仁苷

amygdaline [əˈmigdəliːn] *a* 杏形的,扁桃形的;扁桃体的

amygdalitis [əˌmigdəˈlaitis] *n* 扁桃体炎

amygdal(o)- [构词成分]扁桃,杏

amygdalohippocampectomy [əˌmigdələuˌhipəu-kæmˈpektəmi] *n* 杏仁核海马切除术

amygdaloid [əˈmigdəlɔid], **amygdaloidal** [əˌmigdəˈlɔidl] *a* 扁桃样的,杏仁样的

amygdalolith [əˈmigdələliθ] *n* 扁桃体石

amygdalopathy [əˌmigdəˈlɔpəθi] *n* 扁桃体病

amygdalophenin [əˌmigdəˈlɔfinin] *n* 杏仁酰对乙氧基苯胺

amygdalose [əˈmigdələus] *n* 苦杏仁糖

amygdalothrypsis [əˌmigdələˈθripsis] *n* 扁桃体压碎术

amygdalotome [əˈmigdələtəum] *n* 扁桃体刀

amygdalotomy [əˌmigdəˈlɔtəmi] *n* 杏仁核毁损术;扁桃体切开术,扁桃体部分切除术

amyl [ˈæmil] *n* 戊基 | ~ acetate 醋酸戊酯 / ~ chloride 戊基氯 / ~ nitrite 亚硝酸异戊酯(治心绞痛及解氰化物中毒药)

amylaceous [ˌæmiˈleiʃəs] *a* 淀粉的

amylase [ˈæmileis] *n* 淀粉酶 | α-~ α-淀粉酶(亦称淀粉糖化酶,内淀粉酶,糖原酶,唾液淀粉酶) / β-~ β-淀粉酶(亦称淀粉糖化酶,外淀粉酶) / γ-~ γ-淀粉酶(即葡聚糖 1,4-α-葡糖苷酶) / endo-~ 内淀粉酶 / exo-~ 外淀粉酶 / pancreatic ~ 胰淀粉酶(即胰 α-淀粉酶) / salivary ~ 唾液淀粉酶,涎液素

amylasuria [ˌæmileiˈsjuəriə] *n* 淀粉酶尿(为胰腺炎病征)

amylatic [æmiˈlætik] *a* 水解淀粉的(淀粉转化为糖)

amylemia [ˌæmiˈliːmiə] *n* 淀粉血症

amylene [ˈæmiliːn] *n* 戊烯 | ~ chloral [水合]戊烯氯醛(曾用作安眠药) / ~ hydrate 水合戊烯(用作溶剂、安眠药等)

amylenization [ˌæmilinaiˈzeiʃən] *n* 戊烯麻醉

amylic [əˈmilik] *a* 戊基的

amylin [ˈæmilin] *n* 支链淀粉(亦称淀粉不溶素,淀粉粒纤维素)

amylism [ˈæmilizəm] *n* 戊醇中毒

amyl(o)- [构词成分] 淀粉

amylobarbitone [ˌæmiləuˈbɑːbitəun] *n* 异戊巴比妥(催眠镇静药)

amyloclast [ˈæmiləklæst] *n* 淀粉分解酶 | **~ic** [ˌæmiləˈklæstik] *a* 分解淀粉的,消化淀粉的

amylocoagulase [ˌæmiləukəuˈægjuleis] *n* 淀粉凝固酶

amylodextrin [ˌæmiləuˈdekstrin] *n* 极限糊精

amylodyspepsia [ˌæmiləudisˈpepsiə] *n* 淀粉消化不良

amylogen [əˈmilədʒən] *n* 淀粉溶质

amylogenesis [ˌæmiləuˈdʒenisis] *n* 淀粉生成

amylogenic [ˌæmiləuˈdʒenik] *a* 生成淀粉的

amylo-1, 6-glucosidase [ˌæmiləu gluːˈkəusideis] *n* 淀粉-1,6-葡糖苷酶(此酶的遗传性缺乏为一种常染色体隐性性状,可致糖原贮积症Ⅲ型)

amylo-1, 6-glucosidase deficiency 淀粉-1,6-葡糖苷酶缺乏症,糖原贮积症Ⅲ型

amylohemicellulose [ˌæmiləuˌhemiˈseljuləus] *n* 类直链淀粉

amylohydrolysis [ˌæmiləuhaiˈdrɔlisis] *n* 淀粉水解,淀粉分解

amyloid [ˈæmilɔid] *a* 淀粉样的 *n* 淀粉样蛋白(很可能是一种糖蛋白);[硫酸]胶化纤维素(借硫酸作用于纤维素而成,用碘处理呈蓝色)

amyloidemia [ˌæmilɔiˈdiːmiə] *n* 淀粉样蛋白血症

amyloidoma [ˌæmilɔiˈdəumə] *n* 淀粉样蛋白瘤

amyloidosis [ˌæmilɔiˈdəusis] *n* 淀粉样变性 | cutaneous ~ 皮肤淀粉样变性 / hereditary ~, heredofamilial ~, familial ~ 遗传性淀粉样变性,家族遗传性淀粉样变性,家族性淀粉样变性 / immunocyte-derived ~, AL ~, light-chain-related ~, primary ~ 免疫细胞衍生性淀粉样变性,AL 型淀粉样变性,原发性淀粉样变性 / immunocytic ~ 免疫细胞淀粉样变性 / lichen ~ 苔藓样淀粉样变性,淀粉变性苔藓 / macular ~ 斑疹性淀粉样变性 / nodular ~ 结节性淀粉样变性 / reactive systemic ~, AA ~ 反应性系统性淀粉样变性,AA 型淀粉样变性 / secondary ~ 继发性淀粉样变性 / senile ~, ~ of aging 老年淀粉样变性

amylolysis [ˌæmiˈlɔlisis] *n* 淀粉分解 | **amylolytic** [ˌæmiləˈlitik] *a*

amylopectin [ˌæmiləuˈpektin] *n* 支链淀粉(亦称淀粉不溶素、淀粉粒纤维素)

amylopectinosis [ˌæmiləuˌpektiˈnəusis] *n* 支链淀粉病(糖原贮积症Ⅳ型)

amylophagia [ˌæmiləuˈfeidʒiə] *n* 食淀粉癖

amyloplast [əˈmiləuˌplæst] *n* 淀粉形成体,造粉体

amyloplastic [ˌæmiləuˈplæstik] *a* 造成淀粉的

amylopsin [ˌæmiˈlɔpsin] *n* 胰淀粉酶

amylorrhea [ˌæmiləˈriə] *n* 淀粉溢(粪便中)

amylorrhexis [ˌæmiləˈreksis] *n* 淀粉酶解[作用]

amylose [ˈæmiləus] *n* 直链淀粉 | alpha-~ 支链淀粉

amylosis [ˌæmiˈləusis] *n* 淀粉样变性
amylosuria [ˌæmiləuˈsjuəriə] *n* 淀粉尿
amylosynthesis [ˌæmiləuˈsinθisis] *n* 淀粉合成作用
amylo-1∶4, 1∶6-transglucosidase [ˌæmiləu-ˌtrænsgluːˈkəusideis] 淀粉-1∶4, 1∶6-转葡糖苷酶, 1, 4-α-葡聚糖分支酶
amylo-1∶4, 1∶6-transglucosidase deficiency 淀粉-1∶4, 1∶6-转葡糖苷酶缺乏症,糖原贮积症Ⅳ型
amylum [ˈæmiləm] *n*【拉】淀粉 | ~ iodatum 碘化淀粉
amyluria [ˌæmiˈljuəriə] *n* 淀粉尿
amyoesthesia [eiˌmaiəesˈθiːziə], **amyoesthesis** [eiˌmaiəesˈθiːsis] *n* 肌觉缺失
amyoplasia [eiˌmaiəˈpleiziə] *n* 肌[肉]发育不良
amyostasia [eiˌmaiəˈsteiziə] *n* 肌静止不能,肌震颤(见于运动性共济失调) | **amyostatic** [eiˌmaiəˈstætik] *a*
amyosthenia [eiˌmaiəˈsθiːniə] *n* 肌无力(常见于癔症) | **amyosthenic** [eiˌmaiəˈsθenik] *a*
amyotaxia [əˌmaiəˈtæksiə], **amyotaxy** [əˈmaiə-ˌtæksi] *n* 肌运动失调,肌共济失调
amyotonia [ˌeimaiəˈtəuniə] *n* 肌张力缺失
amyotrophy [ˌeimaiˈɔtrəfi], **amyotrophia** [eiˌmaiəˈtrəufiə] *n* 肌萎缩 | **amyotrophic** [eiˌmaiəˈtrɔfik] *a*
amyous [ˈæmiəs] *a* 无肌的
amyrol [ˈæmirɔl] *n* 白檀油醇
amyxia [əˈmiksiə] *n* 黏液缺乏
amyxorrhea [əˌmiksəˈriə] *n* 黏液分泌缺乏 | ~ gastrica 胃黏液分泌缺乏
An anode 阳极,正极; anodal 阳极的,正极的
an- [前缀]缺乏,无(用于元音或 h 前,见 a-);向上;向后;过度;再(用于元音或 h 前,见 ana-)
ANA American Nurses' Association 美国护士协会 antinuclear antibodies 抗核抗体
ana [ˈænə] *ad*【拉】各(通常写成 $\bar{a}\,\bar{a}$)
ana-, an- [前缀]向上;向后;过度;再
anabasine [əˈnæbəsin] 新烟碱(杀虫药)
anabasis [əˈnæbəsis] ([复] **anabases** [əˈnæbəsiːz]) *n*【希】[疾]病加重期 | **anabatic** [ˌænəˈbætik] *a* 加剧的,加重的;[疾]病加重期的
Anabena, Anabaena [ˌænəˈbinə] *n* 鱼腥藻属(一种蓝绿藻属,使水污臭)
anabiosis [ˌænəbaiˈəusis] *n*【希】复苏,回生 | **anabiotic** [ˌænəbaiˈɔtik] *a*
anabolism [əˈnæbəˌlizəm] *n* 合成代谢 | **anabolic** [ˌænəˈbɔlik], **anabolistic** [əˌnæbəˈlistik] *a*
anabolite [əˈnæbəˌlait], **anabolin** [əˈnæbəlin] *n* 合成代谢产物,同化产物
anacamptic [ˌænəˈkæmptik] *a* 折射的(如声或光)
anacamptometer [ˌænəkæmpˈtɔmitə] *n* 反射计
anacardic acid [ˌænəˈkɑːdik] 漆树酸
Anacardium [ˌænəˈkɑːdiəm] *n* 槚如树属
anacardol [ˌænəˈkɑːdɔl] *n* 槚如酚(3-十五二烯基苯酚)
anacatadidymus [ˌænəˌkætəˈdidiməs] *n* 中腰联胎
anacatesthesia [ˌænəˌkætesˈθiːzjə] *n* 徬徨[不安]感
anachoresis [ˌænəkəˈriːsis] *n* 摄引作用,引菌作用,摄菌作用 | **anachoretic** [ˌænəkəˈretik], **anachoric** [ˌænəˈkɔrik] *a*
anachronobiology [ˌænəˌkrɔnəubaiˈɔlədʒi] *n* 生物成长学
anacidity [ˌænəˈsidəti] *n* 酸缺乏 | gastric ~ 胃酸缺乏
anaclasimeter [ˌænəkləˈsimitə] *n* 屈光检查计
anaclasis [əˈnækləsis] *n* 光折射;反射作用;骨复折法;肢强屈法
anaclitic [ˌænəˈklitik] *a* 斜倚的;情感依附的 | **anaclisis** [ˌænəˈklaisis] *n* 斜卧位;情感依附
anacmesis [æˈnækmisis] *n* 成熟受阻(见 anakmesis)
anacobra [ˌænəˈkəubrə] *n* 灭活眼镜蛇毒(用甲醛及加热法处理后的眼镜蛇毒)
anacousia [ˌænəˈkuːziə], **anacusis** [ˌænəˈkuːsis] *n* 听觉缺失,聋
anacrotic [ˌænəˈkrɔtik] *a* 升线一波[脉]的;升线二波[脉]的
anacrotism [əˈnækrətizəm] *n* 升线一波脉
Anacystis [ˌænəˈsistis] *n* 组囊藻属
anadicrotic [ˌænədaiˈkrɔtik] *a* 升线二波[脉]的
anadidymus [ˌænəˈdidiməs] *n* 双下身联胎,上身联胎
anadipsia [ˌænəˈdipsiə] *n* 剧渴
anadrenalism [ˌænəˈdriːnəlizəm], **anadrenia** [ˌænəˈdriːniə] *n* 肾上腺功能缺失
anaerase [əˈneiəˌreis] *n* 厌氧酶
anaerobe [əˈneiərəub] *n* 厌氧菌 | facultative ~s 兼性厌氧菌 / obligate ~s 专性厌氧菌 / spore-forming ~ 梭状芽胞杆菌
anaerobiase [əˌneiərəuˈbaieis] *n* 厌氧[蛋白分解]酶
anaerobic [əˌneiˈrɔbik] *a* 厌氧的
anaerobiosis [əˌneiərəubaiˈəusis] *n* 厌氧生活
Anaerobiospirillum [ˌeinəˌrəubiəuspaiəˈriləm] *n* 厌氧螺菌属
anaerogenic [əˌneiərəuˈdʒenik] *a* 不产气的
Anaeroplasma [əˌneiərəuˈplæzmə] *n* 厌氧支原体属
anaeroplasty [əˈneiərəˌplæsti] *n* 排气疗法(如用水排出伤口内的空气)

anaerosis [ˌæneiəˈrəusis] *n* 呼吸间断(尤指新生儿)
Anaerovibrio [ˌeinərəuˈvibriəu] *n* 厌氧弧菌属
anagen [ˈænədʒən] *n* 毛发生长初期
Anagnostakis' operation [əˌnægnɔsˈteikis] (Andreas Anagnostakis)阿纳诺斯塔基斯手术(①睑内翻手术;②倒睫手术)
anagocytic [æˌnægəˈsitik] *a* 抑制细胞再生的
anagogy, anagoge [ˌænəˈgəudʒi] *n* 理想精神[内容] | **anagogic(al)** [ˌæneˈgɔdʒik(əl)] *a* 理想精神的;神秘的
anagotoxic [æˌnægəˈtɔksik] *a* 抗毒的
anagrelide hydrochloride [æˈnəgrəlaid] 盐酸阿那格雷(一种用以降低血小板计数升高和减少血栓形成风险的药物,治疗出血性血小板增多,口服给药)
anahormone [ˌænəˈhɔːməun] *n* 类激素
anakatadidymus [ˌænəˌkætəˈdidiməs] *n* 中腰联胎
anakatesthesia [ˌænəˌkætisˈθiːzjə] *n* 徬徨[不安]感
anakhré [ɑːnɑːˈkrei] *n* 鼻骨增生性骨膜炎,根度病(见 goundou)
anakmesis [æˈnækmisis] *n* 成熟受阻(特指骨髓内早期粒细胞〈干细胞〉增多,缺乏进一步成熟,如粒性白细胞缺乏症时骨髓中所见者)
anakusis [ˌænəˈkuːsis] *n* 全聋
anal [ˈeinl] *a* 肛门的
analbuminemia [ˌænælˌbjuːmiˈniːmiə] *n* 白蛋白缺乏血症(血清内白蛋白缺乏)
analeptic [ˌænəˈleptik] *a* 提神的,强身的 *n* 苏醒药(如咖啡因、苯丙胺等)
analgesia [ˌænəlˈdʒiːzjə] *n* 痛觉缺失;镇痛 | ~ algera, ~ dolorosa 痛区感觉缺失 / audio ~ 听音镇痛 / patient controlled ~ 病人控制镇痛
analgesic [ˌænəlˈdʒiːzik], **analgetic** [ˌænəlˈdʒetik] *a* 镇痛的;痛觉缺失的 *n* 镇痛药
analgia [æˈnældʒiə] *n* 痛觉缺失 | **analgic** [æˈnældʒik] *a*
analgin [əˈnældʒin] *n* 安乃近(解热镇痛药)
anality [eiˈnæləti] *n* 肛恋,肛恋色情固结
anallergic [ˌænəˈləːdʒik] *a* 非变应性的,非过敏性的
analog [ˈænəlɔg] *a* 模拟计算机的,模拟数据的 *n* [结构]类似物
analogic(al) [ænəˈlɔdʒik(əl)] *a* 相似的,类似的
analogous [əˈnæləgəs] *a* 类似的,类同的
analogue [ˈænəlɔg] *n* 类似器官;类似物 | base ~ 碱基类似物 / homologous ~ 同系类似物
analogy [əˈnælədʒi] *n* 类似;同功(器官)
analphalipoproteinemia [æˌnælfəˌlipəu ˌprəutiːˈniːmiə] *n* α-脂蛋白缺乏血[症];丹吉尔(Tangier)病
analysand [əˈnælisænd] *n* 精神分析对象
analysis [əˈnæləsis] ([复] **analyses** [əˈnæləsiːz]) *n* 分析,分解;精神分析 | activation ~ 活化分析 / antigenic ~ 抗原分析(测定菌种抗原嵌合体的成分) / bradycinetic ~ 活动照相分析(对运动状态) / character ~ 性格分析/ densimetric ~ 比重分析 / endgroup ~ 末端分析/ organic ~ 有机分析 / qualitative ~, qualitive ~ 定性分析 / quantitative ~, quantitive ~ 定量分析 / ultimate ~ 元素分析 / ~ of variance (ANOVA)方差分析
analysor [ˈænəlaizə] *n* 分析器
analyst [ˈænəlist] *n* 分析者;化验员
analyte [ˈænəlait] *n* 分析物
analytic(al) [ˌænəˈlitik(əl)] *a* 分析的;分解的
analyzer [ˈænəˌlaizə] *n* 分析器;检偏振器,大脑皮质分析器 | amino acid sequence ~ 氨基酸顺序分析器/ voice ~ 语声分析器
Aname [ˈænəmi] *n* 安纳米蜘蛛属
Anamirta [ˌænəˈməːtə] *n* 印防己属 | ~ cocculus 印防己,毒鱼防己
anamirtin [ˌænəˈməːtin] *n* 印防己苷
anamnesis [ˌænæmˈniːsis] *n* 记忆力;既往症,既往病历;回忆性(在免疫学中指免疫回忆的能力) | **anamnestic** [ænəmˈnestik] *a*
Anamniota [ˌænæmniˈəutə] *n* 无羊膜动物类
anamniote [æˈnæmniəut] *n* 无羊膜动物
anamniotic [ˌænæmniˈɔtik] *a* 无羊膜的
anamorph [ˈænəmɔːf] *n* 无性型(真菌的无性〈不完全〉状态)
anamorphosis [ˌænəmɔːˈfəusis] *n* 渐进形态
ananabolic [ˌænænəˈbɔlik] *a* 组成代谢缺乏的
ananaphylaxis [ænˌænəfiˈlæksis] *n* 抗过敏[性],脱过敏
ananastasia [ænˌænəsˈteisiə] *n* 起立不能
anancastic [ˌænənˈkæstik] *a* 强迫观念与行为的
anandia [æˈnændiə] *n* 运动性失语,运动性言语不能
anangioid [æˈnændʒiɔid] *a* 似无血管的
anapepsia [ˌænəˈpepsiə] *n* 胃蛋白酶缺乏
anaphalantiasis [ænˌæfəlænˈtaiəsis] *n* 【希】眉毛脱落
anaphase [ˈænəfeiz] *n* [分裂]后期(细胞分裂的一个时期) | flabby ~ 呆滞后期(在细胞分裂的后期中,由于细胞中毒,干扰了纺锤体的形成,两条子染色体不能分开)
anaphia [æˈneifiə] *n* 触觉缺失
anaphoresis [ˌænəfəˈriːsis] *n* 阴离子电泳
anaphoria [ˌænəˈfəuriə] *n* 上隐斜眼
anaphrodisiac [ˌænəfrəˈdiziæk] *a* 制欲的 *n* 制欲药
anaphylactin [ˌænəfiˈlæktin] *n* 过敏素
anaphylactogen [ˌænəfiˈlæktədʒən] *n* 过敏原

anaphylactogenesis [ˌænəfiˌlæktəuˈdʒenisis] *n* 过敏性发生,过敏反应发生
anaphylactogenic [ˌænəˌfilæktəuˈdʒenik] *a* 发生过敏性的
anaphylactoid [ˌænəfiˈlæktɔid] *a* 过敏性样的
anaphylatoxin [ˌænəˌfailəˈtɔksin], **anaphylactotoxin** [ˌænəfiˌlæktəuˈtɔksin], **anaphylotoxin** [ˌænəˌfailəˈtɔksin] *n* 过敏毒素(补体结合时血清中产生的一种物质)
anaphylaxin [ˌænəfiˈlæksin] *n* 过敏素
anaphylaxis [ˌænəfiˈlæksis] *n* 过敏性,过敏反应 | acquired ~ 获得性过敏性,获得性过敏反应 / active ~ 主动过敏反应(个体注射异免疫原时产生) / active cutaneous ~ 主动皮肤过敏反应(用于花粉变态反应试验) / aggregate ~ 凝聚物过敏反应(药理介质所致) / cytotoxic ~ 细胞毒性过敏反应 / cytotropic ~ 亲细胞性过敏反应 / generalized ~ 全身性过敏反应 / inverse ~ 反转过敏反应(休克剂是抗体〈过敏素〉,而不是抗原〈过敏原〉;过敏性休克由一次静脉注射福斯曼〈Forssman〉抗体于豚鼠体内产生) / local ~ 局部过敏性,局部过敏反应 / passive ~, antiserum ~ 被动过敏反应,抗血清过敏反应 / passive cutaneous ~ (PCA)被动皮肤过敏反应(用于研究引起速发型超敏感性反应的抗体) / reverse ~ 逆转过敏反应(先注射抗血清再注射抗原后发生的过敏反应;同样是由血循环中的抗体与组织细胞所固定的抗原相结合的局部反应) / systemic ~ 全身性过敏反应 | **anaphylactic** [ˌænəfiˈlæktik] *a*
anaphylodiagnosis [ˌænəˌfiləuˌdaiəgˈnəusis] *n* 过敏性诊断法
anaplasia [ˌænəˈpleiziə] *n* 退行发育,间变 | monophasic ~ 单形退行发育 / polyphasic ~ 多形退行发育 | **anaplastia** [ˌænəˈplæstiə] *n*
Anaplasma [ˌænəˈplæzmə] *n* 无形体属
Anaplasmataceae [ˌænəˌplæzməˈteisiiː] *n* 无形体科
anaplasmodastat [ˌænəplæzˈməudəˌstæt] *n* 抗无形体药
anaplasmosis [ˌænəplæzˈməusis] *n* 无形体病
anaplastic [ˌænəˈplæstik] *a* 还原成形术的,整形术的;退行发育的(指细胞)
anaplerosis [ˌænəpliˈrəusis] *n* (组织)补缺术 | **anaplerotic** [ˌænəpliˈrɔtik] *a*
anapnotherapy [ˌænæpnəuˈθerəpi] *n* [气体]吸入疗法(如复苏术时)
anapophysis [ˌænəˈpɔfisis] *n* 副突(尤指胸椎或腰椎的副突)
anaptic [æˈnæptik] *a* 触觉缺失的
anarchic [əˈnɑːkik] *a* 反常的
anaric [əˈnɛərik] *a* 无鼻的
anarithmia [ˌænəˈriθmiə] *n* 计算不能(由于中枢损害)
anarrhexis [ˌænəˈreksis] *n* 骨复折术
anarthria [æˈnɑːθriə] *n* 构音不全
anasarca [ˌænəˈsɑːkə] *n* 全身性水肿 | **anasarcous** [ˌænəˈsɑːkəs] *a*
anascitic [ˌænəˈsitik] *a* 无腹水的
anastalsis [ˌænəˈstælsis] *n* 逆蠕动
anastaltic [ˌænəˈstæltik] *a* 收敛的;止血的 *n* 抗敛药;止血药
anastate [ˈænəˌsteit] *n* 组成代谢产物,同化产物
anastigmatic [ˌænəstigˈmætik] *a* 无散光的;矫正散光的
anastole [əˈnæstəli] *n* 退缩,收缩(如伤口边缘)
anastomose [əˈnæstəməuz] *vt, vi* (使)吻合
anastomosis [əˌnæstəˈməusis] ([复] **anastomoses** [əˌnæstəˈməusiːz]) *n* 吻合;吻合术 | antiperistaltic ~ 逆蠕动吻合[术] / arteriovenous ~ 动静脉吻合;动静脉吻合术 / crucial ~ 十字形吻合(一种动脉吻合) / heterocladic ~ 异支吻合术 / homocladic ~ 同支吻合术 / intestinal ~ 肠吻合术 / isoperistaltic ~ 顺蠕动吻合[术] / postcostal ~ 肋后吻合 / precapillary ~ 前毛细管吻合 / stirrup ~ 镫形吻合 / terminoterminal ~ 端端吻合术 / transureteroureteral ~ 经输尿管两段吻合术 / ureterotubal ~ 输尿管输卵管吻合术 / ureteroureteral ~ 输尿管两段吻合术 | **anastomotic** [əˌnæstəˈmɔtik] *a* 吻合的
anastral [æˈnæstrəl] *a* 无星的,无星状体的(指有丝分裂)
anastrophic [ˌænəˈstrɔfik] *a* 反向的,可钝化又再活化的(指某些蛋白酶)
anastrozole [æˈnæstrəzəul] *a* 阿那司唑(非类固醇芳香酶抑制剂,能使血清雌二醇水平降低,化疗时用以治疗乳腺癌,尤其用于绝经后妇女,口服给药)
anat. anatomical 解剖的,解剖学的; anatomy 解剖学
anatherapeusis [ˌænəˌθerəˈpjuːsis] *n* 增剂疗法
anatomic(al) [ˌænəˈtɔmik(əl)] *a* 解剖的;解剖学的
anatomicomedical [ænəˌtɔmikəuˈmedikəl] *a* 医用解剖学的
anatomicopathological [ˌænəˌtɔmikəuˌpæθəˈlɔdʒikəl] *a* 病理解剖学的
anatomicophysiological [ˌænəˌtɔmikəuˌfiziəˈlɔdʒikəl] *a* 解剖生理学的
anatomicosurgical [ˌænəˌtɔmikəuˈsəːdʒikəl] *a* 解剖学与外科学的,外科解剖学的
anatomist [əˈnætəmist] *n* 解剖学家
anatomize, anatomise [əˈnætəmaiz] *vt, vi* 解剖;剖析 | **anatomization** [əˌnætəmaiˈzeiʃən,

-mi'z-] *n*

anatomopathology [ˌænətəməupə'θɔlədʒi] *n* 病理解剖学

anatomy [ə'nætəmi] *n* 解剖学;解剖 | applied ~ 应用解剖学 / clastic ~ 分层[模型]解剖学 / comparative ~ 比较解剖学 / corrosion ~ 腐蚀解剖 / descriptive ~, systematic ~ 记载解剖学,系统解剖学 / developmental ~ 发育解剖学,胚胎学 / general ~ 解剖学总论 / gross ~, macroscopic ~ 大体解剖学 / histologic ~ 组织解剖学,组织学 / homologic ~ 相关部位解剖学 / medical ~ 医用解剖学 / microscopic ~, minute ~ 显微解剖学,组织学 / morbid ~, pathological ~ 病理解剖学 / physiognomonic ~ 表征解剖学,相法解剖学(尤指面部的) / physiological ~ 功能解剖学 / plastic ~ 模型解剖学 / practical ~ 实地解剖学,解剖学实习 / special ~ 解剖学各论 / topographic ~ 局部解剖学 / transcendental ~ 直观解剖学

anatoxin [ˌænə'tɔksin] *n* 类毒素,变性毒素 | diphtheria ~, ~-Ramon 白喉类毒素 | **anatoxic** [ˌænə'tɔksik] *a*

anatoxireaction [ˌænəˌtɔksiri(ː)'ækʃən] *n* 类毒素反应(见 Moloney's test)

anatricrotic [ˌænətrai'krɔtik] *a* 升线三波[脉]的

anatriptic [ˌænə'triptik] *a* 揉擦的 *n* 揉擦药

anatrophic [ˌænə'trɔfik] *a* 防衰的 *n* 防衰药

anatropia [ˌænə'trəupiə] *n* 上隐斜眼 | **anatropic** [ˌænə'trɔpik] *a*

anavenin [ˌænə'venin] *n* 去活毒液,去毒[动物]毒液(加甲醛后变成无毒的一种动物毒液,但仍保持其抗原特性)

anaxon [æ'næksɔn] *n* 无轴索[神经]细胞

anazolene sodium [æ'næzəliːn] 阿那佐林钠(诊断用药,用以测定血容量和心排血量)

ANCA antineutrophil cytoplasmic autoantibody (or antibody) 抗嗜中性粒细胞胞质自身抗体(或抗体)

Ancalomicrobium [ænˌkeiləumai'krəubiəm] *n* 臂微菌属

anchor ['æŋkə] *n* 锚;抗基 | endosteal implant ~ 骨内膜植入物抗基(种植义齿下部结构的一部分,深植于骨内,牙修复术时作固定之用)

anchorage ['æŋkəridʒ] *n* 支抗 | cervical ~ 颈支抗 / extraoral ~ 口外支抗 / occipital ~ 枕支抗 / stationary ~ 固定支抗

anchyl(o)- [构词成分]弯曲;粘连

ancillary [æn'siləri, 'ænsiˌlɛəri] *a* 辅助的,附属的

ancipital [æn'sipitl] *a* 二头的,二边的

Ancistrodon [æn'sistrədɔn] *n* 蝮蛇属

ancistroid [æn'sistrɔid] *a* 钩样的

anconad ['æŋkənæd] *ad* 向肘,向鹰嘴

anconagra [ˌæŋkɔ'nægrə] *n* 肘痛风症

anconeal [æŋ'kəuniəl], **anconal** ['æŋkənəl] *a* 肘的

anconitis [ˌæŋkə'naitis] *n* 肘关节炎

anconoid ['æŋkənɔid] *a* 肘样的

ANCOVA analysis of covariance 协方差分析

ancrod ['ænkrɔd] *n* 安克洛酶(抗凝药)

ancyl(o)- [构词成分]弯曲;粘连

Ancylostoma [ˌæŋki'lɔstəmə, ˌænsi-] *n* 钩口[线虫]属 | ~ americanum 美洲钩虫(即 Necator americanus) / ~ braziliense, ~ ceylonicum 巴西钩[口线]虫,猫钩虫 / ~ caninum 犬钩口线虫,犬钩虫 / ~ duodenale 十二指肠钩口线虫,十二指肠钩虫 | **Ancylostomum** [ˌæŋkilɔs'təuməm, ˌænsi-] *n*

ancylostomatic [ˌænkiləustəu'mætik, ˌænsi-] *a* 钩虫性的

Ancylostomatidae [ˌæŋkiləustə'mætidiː, ˌænsi-] *n* 钩口[线虫]科

ancylostome [æn'kiləstəum, -'si-] *n* 钩虫,钩口线虫

ancylostomiasis [ˌænkiˌlɔstə'maiəsis] *n* 钩虫病 | ~ braziliensis 巴西钩虫病,游走性幼虫病

Ancylostomidae [ˌæŋkiləu'stəumidiː, ˌænsi-] *n* 钩口[线虫]科

ancyroid ['ænsirɔid] *a* 锚样的,钩样的

Anda ['ændə] *n*【巴西】安达树属

Andernach's ossicles ['ɑːndənɑːh] (Johann W. von Andernach) 缝间骨

Andersch's ganglion ['ændəʃ] (Carolus S. Andersch) 岩神经节 | ~ nerve 鼓室神经

Anders' disease ['ændəz] (James M. Anders) 单纯结节性肥胖症

Andersen's disease ['ændəsn] (Dorothy H. Andersen) 安德森病(糖原贮积症Ⅳ型) | ~ syndrome (triad) 安德森综合征(三征)(支气管扩张、胰腺囊性纤维化、维生素 A 缺乏)

Anderson-Hynes pyeloplasty ['ændəsn hainz] (J. C. Anderson; W. Hynes) 安-海肾盂成形术,断离性肾盂成形术

Anderson splint ['ændəsn] (Roger Anderson) 安德森夹板(内外固定骨折用)

Andira [æn'daiərə] *n* 柯桠树属

andirine [æn'daiərin] *n* 柯桠树碱,甲基酪氨酸

Andrade's indicator [æn'dreid] (Eduardo P. Andrade) 安德雷德指示剂(酸性品红水溶液,可被氢氧化钠溶液脱色成黄色,加到葡糖肉汤培养基内,此肉汤培养的一种产酸菌使培养基变为品红色)

Andrade type familial amyloid polyneuropathy (syndrome) [æn'drɑːdei] (Corino M. Andrade) 安德拉德型家族性淀粉样蛋白多神经病(综合征),葡萄牙型家族性淀粉样蛋白多神经病

Andral's decubitus (sign) [æn'drɑːl] (Gabriel

Andral)昂德拉尔卧位(征)(卧于健侧,为胸膜炎早期卧位)

andreioma [ændriː'əumə], **andreoblastoma** [ˌændriəblæs'təumə] *n* 男性细胞瘤(卵巢)

Andresen appliance ['ændrisən] (V. Andresen) 安德森矫正器,功能矫正器

André Thomas sign [ɑːn'drei təu'mɑːs] (André A. H. Thomas)安德烈·托马斯征(①若在指鼻试验时,令患者将一臂高举过头,然后令其将臂落在头上,患者手臂即出现反跳,见于小脑疾病;②捏斜方肌可在脊髓损害水平上方引起鸡皮疙瘩)

Andrewes' test ['ændruːz] (Christopher H. Andrewes) 安德鲁斯试验(检尿毒症)

Andrews' disease ['ændruːz] (George C. Andrews)脓疱性细菌疹

andrin ['ændrin] *n* 睾丸雄激素(统称,即睾酮、雄甾酮和脱氢雄酮)

andr(o)- [构词成分] 男,雄

androblastoma [ˌændrəublæs'təumə] *n* 塞尔托利(Sertoli)细胞瘤,足细胞瘤(睾丸);男性细胞瘤(卵巢)

androcyte ['ændrəsait] *n* 精子细胞(尤指未成熟期)

androdedotoxin [ˌændrəuˌdiːdə'tɔksin] *n* 杜鹃花毒素

androecium [æn'driːʃiəm, ˌændrəu'iːʃiəm] *n* 雄蕊

androgalactozemia [ˌændrəugəˌlæktə'ziːmiə] *n* 男子泌乳

androgamone [ˌændrəu'gæməun] *n* 雄[性交]配素

androgen ['ændrədʒən] *n* 雄激素 | **~ic** [ˌændrəu'dʒenik] *a* 雄激素的;生男性征的,产生雄性征的

androgenesis [ˌændrəu'dʒenisis] *n* 雄核发育;单雌生殖

androgenicity [ˌændrəudʒi'nisəti] *n* 生男性征性能,产生雄性征性能

androgenization [ˌændrəudʒeni'zeiʃən] *n* 雄激素化[作用](女子产生过多雄激素;男子正常的男性化)

androgenized [æn'drɔdʒinaizd] *a* 雄激素化的(女子产生或存在过多雄激素;男子正常男性化)

androgenous [æn'drɔdʒinəs] *a* 生男性征的,产生雄性征的

androglossia [ˌændrəu'glɔsiə] *n* 女性男声

androgone ['ændrəgəun] *n* 精原细胞,生精细胞

androgyne ['ændrədʒain] *n* 两性体,雌雄同体;女性假两性体

androgyneity [ˌændrəudʒi'niːiti], **androgynism** [æn'drɔdʒinizəm], **androgyny** [æn'drɔdʒini] *n* 女性假两性同体 | **androgynous** [æn'drɔdʒinəs] *a*

androgynoid [æn'drɔdʒinɔid] *n* 假两性体 *a* 女性假两性畸形的

android ['ændrɔid], **androidal** [æn'drɔidəl] *a* 男性样的

andrology [æn'drɔlədʒi] *n* 男科学,男性生殖器病学

androma [æn'drəumə] *n* 男性细胞瘤(卵巢)

Andromeda [æn'drɔmidə] *n* 梫木属(其中数种含麻醉性毒质)

andromedotoxin [ænˌdrɔmidə'tɔksin] *n* 梫木毒素(抑制呼吸中枢及催眠)

andromerogon [ˌændrə'merəgɔn] *n* 雄核卵片 | **andromerogone** [ˌændrə'merəgəun] *n*

andromerogony [ˌændrəumə'rɔgəni] *n* 雄核卵片发育

andromimetic [ˌændrəumi'metik] *a* 男子样的,生男性征的

andromorphous [ˌændrəu'mɔːfəs] *a* 男性形态的,男形的

andropathy [æn'drɔpəθi] *n* 男性病

androphile ['ændrəfail], **androphilous** [æn'drɔfiləs] *a* 嗜人血的(指蚊)

androphobia [ˌændrəu'fəubjə] *n* 男性恐怖,恐男症

Andropogon [ˌændrəu'pəugɔn] *n* 须芒草属

androstane ['ændrəstein] *n* 雄[甾]烷

androstanediol [ˌændrə'steindiɔl] *n* 雄[甾]烷二醇

androstanedione [ˌændrəu'steindiəun] *n* 雄[甾]烷二酮

androstanolone [ˌændrəu'steinələun] *n* 雄诺龙,雄[甾]烷醇酮

androstene ['ændrəstiːn] *n* 雄[甾]烯

androstenediol [ˌændrəu'stiːndiɔl] *n* 雄[甾]烯二醇

androstenedione [ˌændrəu'stiːndiəun] *n* 雄[甾]烯二酮

androsterone [æn'drɔstərəun] *n* 雄酮

-ane [词尾]饱和烃;烷[烃]

anecdotal [ˌænik'dəutəl] *a* 无对照的(不是根据对照临床试验的)

anecdysis [æ'nekdisis] *n* 不蜕皮期,蜕皮间期(指节肢动物)

anechoic [ˌæni'kəuik] *a* 无回声的,无反响的,消声的(指消声室)

anectasin [æ'nektəsin] *n* 缩脉管性菌毒素

anectasis [æ'nektəsis] *n* 先天性扩张不全,原发性肺不张

anejaculation [ˌæniˌdʒækju'leiʃən] *n* 射精不能

anelectrotonus [ˌænilek'trɔtənəs] *n* 阳极电紧张

| **anelectrotonic** [ˌænilektrəuˈtɔnik] *a*

Anel's operation [ɑːˈnel] (Dominique Anel) 阿内尔手术(用探子扩张泪管,然后注射收敛剂) | ~ probe 阿内尔探子(用于泪点及泪管) / ~ syringe 泪道注射器

anemia [əˈniːmiə] *n* 贫血 | achylic ~ 胃液缺乏性贫血 / anhematopoietic ~, anhemopoietic ~ 造血功能不良性贫血 / aplastic ~, aregenerative ~ 再生障碍性贫血 / autoimmune hemolytic ~ (AIHA) 自身免疫性溶血性贫血(获得性溶血性贫血,其血清抗体一般为 IgG 类,与红细胞起反应,血清抗球蛋白试验为阳性) / cameloid ~, elliptocytary ~, elliptocytotic ~ 椭圆形红细胞性贫血 / congenital ~ of newborn 新生儿先天性贫血 / cow's milk ~ 牛乳性贫血,食乳性贫血 / deficiency ~, nutritional ~ 营养[缺乏]性贫血 / drug-induced immune hemolytic ~ 药物诱发免疫性溶血性贫血 / familial megaloblastic ~ 家族性巨成红细胞性贫血 / glucose-6-phosphate dehydrogenase deficiency ~ 葡糖-6-磷酸脱氢酶缺乏性贫血 / ground itch ~ 钩虫性贫血,钩虫病 / hemolytic ~ 溶血性贫血 / hemorrhagic ~ 出血性贫血 / hypochromic ~ 低色指数性贫血 / hypochromic microcytic ~ 低色小红细胞性贫血 / iron deficiency ~ 缺铁性贫血 / leukoerythroblastic ~, myelopathic ~, myelophthisic ~ 成白红细胞性贫血,骨髓病性贫血 / macrocytic ~, megalocytic ~ 大红细胞性贫血,巨红细胞性贫血 / Mediterranean ~ 珠蛋白生成障碍性贫血,地中海贫血 / microcytic ~ 小红细胞性贫血 / miners' ~ 矿工贫血,钩[口线]虫病 / normocytic ~ 正常红细胞性贫血 / pernicious ~ 恶性贫血 / phenylhydrazine ~ 苯肼中毒性贫血 / polar ~ 极地贫血 / primary ~ 原发性贫血 / pure red cell ~ 纯红细胞性贫血 / refractory ~ 顽固性贫血 / refractory sideroblastic ~ 顽固性铁粒幼细胞贫血 / scorbutic ~ 坏血病性贫血 / secondary ~ 继发性贫血 / sickle cell ~ 镰状细胞贫血 / sideroblastic ~, sideroachrestic ~ 铁粒幼细胞贫血,铁失利用性贫血 / slaty ~ 石板样贫血 / splenic ~ 脾性贫血(先天性脾肿大) | **anemic** [əˈniːmik] *a*

anem(o)- [构词成分]风

anemometer [ˌæniˈmɔmətə] *n* 风速计 | **anemometry** *n* 风速测量法

Anemone [əˈneməni] *n* 银莲花属(毛茛科)

anemonin [əˈnemənin] *n* 白头翁素

anemonism [əˈneməniʐəm] *n* 白头翁中毒

anemonol [əˈnemənɔl] *n* 白头翁脑

anemophilous [ˌæniˈmɔfiləs] *n* 风媒的

anemophobia [ˌæniməuˈfəubjə] *n* 通风恐怖,畏风,恐风症

Anemonopsis [əˌneməˈnɔpsis] *n* 蕺菜属

anemotaxis [ˌæniməuˈtæksis] *n* 向风性,趋风性

anemotrophy [ˌæniˈmɔtrəfi] *n* 血液滋养不足

anemotropism [ˌæniˈmɔtrəpizəm] *n* 趋风性,向风性

anencephalus [ˌænenˈsefələs] *n* 无脑儿

anencephaly [ˌænenˈsefəli], **anencephalia** [ˌænensiˈfeiliə] *n* 无脑[畸形] | **anencephalic** [ˌænensiˈfælik], **anencephalous** [ˌænenˈsefələs] *a*

anenterous [æˈnentərəs] *a* 无肠的

anenzymia [ˌænenˈzaimiə] *n* 无酶症 | ~ catalasea 触酶缺乏症,过氧化氢酶缺乏症

anephric [eiˈnefrik] *a* 无肾脏的

anephrogenesis [ˌeinefrəuˈdʒenisis] *n* 肾缺如

anepiploic [æˌnepiˈpləuik] *a* 无网膜的

anepithymia [æˌnepiˈθimiə] *n* 食欲不振,食欲缺乏

anerethisia [æˌneriˈθiziə] *n* 兴奋缺乏

aneretic [ˌæniˈretik] *a* 破坏的(对动物组织)

anergasia [ˌænəˈgeiziə] *n* 活动力缺失(指功能活动缺失,亦指与中枢神经系统结构损害有关的一种精神病)

anergastic [ˌænəˈgæstik] *a* 器质性精神病的

anergy [ˈænədʒi] *n* 无力;无反应性 | absolute ~ 绝对无反应性(对抗原〈或变应原〉的一时性无反应性或完全无反应性) / cachectic ~ 恶病质无反应性(致敏个体由于虚弱,对变应原的反应性一时的减低) / negative ~ 负无反应性(致敏个体由于恶病质,对变应原的反应性一时性的减低) / positive ~ 正无反应性(致敏个体由于疾病〈如结核〉过程中免疫反应的改变,对变应原反应性减低) | **anergia** [æˈnəːdʒiə] *n* / **anergic** [æˈnəːdʒik] *a*

aneroid [ˈænərɔid] *a* 无液的,不湿的

anerythroplasia [ˌæniˌriθrəuˈpleiziə] *n* 红细胞发生不能 | **anerythroplastic** [ˌæniˌriθrəuˈplæstik] *a*

anerythropoiesis [ˌæniˌriθrəupɔiˈiːsis] *n* 红细胞生成不足

anerythropsia [ˌæneriˈθrɔpsiə], **anerythroblepsia** [ˌæniˌriθrəuˈblepsiə] *n* 红色盲

anerythroregenerative [ˌæniˌriθrəuriˈdʒenəreitiv] *a* 红细胞再生不能的

anesthecinesia [æˌnisθiːsiˈniːziə], **anesthekinesia** [æˌnisθiːkiˈniːziə] *n* 感觉[与]运动能力缺失

anesthesia [ˌænisˈθiːzjə] *n* 感觉缺失;麻醉 | acupuncture ~ 针刺麻醉 / angiospastic ~ 血管痉挛性感觉缺失 / balanced ~ 平衡麻醉 / basal ~ 基础麻醉 / block ~ 阻滞麻醉 / bulbar ~ 延髓性感觉缺失 / caudal ~ 脊尾麻醉,骶管麻醉 / central ~ 中枢性感觉缺失 / cerebral ~ 大脑性感觉缺失 / closed ~ 紧闭式麻醉 / colonic ~ 结肠麻醉 / compression ~ 压迫性感觉缺失 / conduction ~ 传导阻滞麻醉 / crossed ~ 交叉性感觉缺失 / dissociated ~, dissociation ~ 分离

麻醉 / doll's head ~ 木偶式感觉缺失(影响头、颈和胸上部) / electric ~ 电麻醉 / epidural ~ 硬[脊]膜外阻滞 / facial ~ 面[神经]麻木 / gauntlet ~, glove ~ 手套式感觉缺失 / general ~ 全身麻醉 / girdle ~ 束带状感觉缺失 / gustatory ~ 味觉丧失 / high pressure ~ 压力麻醉 / hypothermic ~ 低温麻醉 / infiltration ~ 浸润麻醉 / inhalation ~ 吸入麻醉 / insufflation ~ 吹入麻醉 / intracostal ~ 肋间神经阻滞麻醉 / intranasal ~ 鼻内麻醉 / intraoral ~ 口内麻醉 / intraosseous ~ 骨内麻醉 / intravenous ~ 静脉麻醉 / local ~ 局部麻醉 / mental ~ 精神性感觉缺失 / mixed ~ 混合麻醉 / muscular ~ 肌觉缺失 / olfactory ~ 嗅觉丧失 / parasacral ~ 骶旁麻醉 / partial ~ 部分感觉缺失 / peridural ~ 硬脊膜外麻醉 / peripheral ~ 末梢性感觉缺失 / permeation ~ 渗入麻醉 / refrigeration ~ 冷冻麻醉 / regional ~ 区域麻醉 / sacral ~ 骶[管]麻醉 / saddle block ~ 鞍状阻滞麻醉 / segmental ~ 分节性感觉缺失 / semiopen ~ 半开放式麻醉 / sexual ~ 性欲缺失 / spinal ~ 脊椎麻醉;脊髓性感觉缺失 / splanchnic ~ 内脏神经麻醉 / surface ~ 表面麻醉 / surgical ~ 外科麻醉 / thalamic hyperesthetic ~ 丘脑感觉过敏性感觉缺失,丘脑综合征 / thermal ~, thermic ~ 温度觉缺失 / topical ~ 表面麻醉 / total ~ 全[部]感觉缺失 / transsacral ~ 经骶麻醉 / traumatic ~ 外伤性感觉缺失 / twilight ~ 朦胧麻醉,朦胧睡眠,半麻醉 / unilateral ~ 偏身麻木 / vein ~ 静脉麻醉 / visceral ~ 内脏感觉缺失

anesthesimeter [ˌænisθiˈzimitə] *n* 麻醉度计,麻醉剂量调节计;感觉缺失测量器

anesthesiology [ˌænisθiːziˈɔlədʒi] *n* 麻醉学 | **anesthesiologist** *n* 麻醉学家

anesthesiophore [ˌænisˈθiːziəˌfɔː] *a* 有麻醉作用的 *n* 麻醉功能簇

anesthetic [ˌænisˈθetik] *a* 感觉缺失的;麻醉的 *n* 麻醉药,麻醉剂 | general ~ 全身麻醉药 / local ~ 局部麻醉药 / topical ~ 表面麻醉药

anesthetist [æˈniːsθətist, -əˈnes-] *n* 麻醉师

anesthetize [æˈniːsθətaiz, -əˈnes-] *vt* 使麻醉;使麻木 | **anesthetization** [æˌniːsθətaiˈzeiʃən, -tiˈz-] *n* 麻醉法

anesthetometer [æˌniːsθəˈtɔmitə] *n* 麻醉气计量器

anesthetospasm [ˌænisˈθetəspæzəm] *n* 麻醉期痉挛

anestrus [æˈniːstrəs, -əˈnes-], **anestrum** [æˈniːstrəm, əˈnes-] *n* 动情间期

anethene [ˈæniθiːn] *n* 莳萝烃,莳萝烯

anethole [ˈænəθəul] *n* 茴香脑(升白细胞药)

Anethum [əˈniːθəm] *n* 【拉】莳萝属

anetic [əˈnetik] *a* 弛缓的,缓和的

anetiological [æˌniːtiəˈlɔdʒikəl] *a* 非病原学的,病原不明的

anetoderma [ˌænitəˈdəːmə] *n* 皮肤松垂 | perifollicular ~ 毛囊周围皮肤松垂 / postinflammatory ~ 炎症后皮肤松垂

aneugamy [æˈnjuːgəmi] *n* 非整倍配合

aneuploid [ˈænju ˈplɔid] *a* 非整倍的 *n* 非整倍体(指一个体或细胞具有多于或少于正常二倍体数的染色体数) | **~y** *n* 非整倍体性

aneurin(e) [ˈænjuərin] *n* 硫胺,维生素 B_1 | ~ hydrochloride 盐酸硫胺,盐酸维生素 B_1

aneurogenic [ˌeinjuərəuˈdʒenik] *a* 无神经源[性]的

aneurysm [ˈænjuərizəm] *n* 动脉瘤 | abdominal ~ 腹主动脉瘤 / arteriovenous ~ 动静脉瘤 / arteriovenous pulmonary ~ 肺动静脉瘤,动静脉瘘 / berry ~, brain ~, cerebral ~ 颅内小动脉瘤,脑动脉瘤 / dissecting ~ 夹层动脉瘤 / mycotic ~, bacterial ~ 真菌性动脉瘤,细菌性动脉瘤 / venous ~ 静脉瘤 | **aneurysmal** [ˌænjuəˈrizməl], **aneurysmatic** [ˌænjuərizˈmætik] *a*

aneurysmectomy [ˌænjuərizˈmektəmi] *n* 动脉瘤切除术

aneurysmoplasty [ˌænjuəˈrizməˌplæsti] *n* 动脉瘤成形术

aneurysmorrhaphy [ˌænjuərizˈmɔrəfi] *n* 动脉瘤缝闭术

aneurysmotomy [ˌænjuərizˈmɔtəmi] *n* 动脉瘤切开术

ANF antinuclear factor 抗核因子

anfractuosity [ænˌfræktjuˈɔsəti] *n* 纡曲,弯曲;曲折,错综;脑沟

anfractuous [ænˈfræktjuəs] *a* 纡曲的,弯曲的

angei- 见 angi-

Angelica [ænˈdʒelikə] *n* 【拉】当归属(白芷属)

angelica [ænˈdʒelikə] *n* 当归 | Chinese ~ 当归

angelic acid [ænˈdʒelik] 当归酸,欧白芷酸

angeline [ˈændʒəlin] *n* *N*-甲基酪氨酸

Angelman's syndrome [ˈeindʒəlmən] (Harry Angelman)安吉尔曼综合征,快乐木偶综合征(见 syndrome 项下 happy puppet syndrome)

Angelucci's syndrome [ˌændʒiˈlutʃi] (Arnaldo Angelucci)昂杰路契综合征(春季结膜炎综合征:激动、心悸及血管运动障碍)

Anger camera [ˈæŋgə] (Hal O. Anger)安格照相机(用以在病人身上形成一种发射放射性核素 γ 线分布的影像。亦称 γ 照相机,闪烁照相机)

Anghelescu's sign [ɑːndʒəˈleskuː] (Constantin Anghelescu)安杰利斯库征(脊椎结核患者仰卧时只能靠头和足跟移动,脊椎不能前弯)

angi- 见 angio-

angialgia [ˌændʒiˈældʒiə] *n* 血管痛
angiasthenia [ˌændʒiæsˈθiːniə] *n* 血管无力
angiectasis [ˌændʒiˈektəsis] *n* 血管扩张 | **angiectatic** [ˌændʒiekˈtætik] *a*
angiectomy [ˌændʒiˈektəmi] *n* 血管切除术
angiectopia [ˌændʒiekˈtəupiə] *n* 血管异位
angiitis [ˌændʒiˈaitis] ([复] **angiitides** [ˌændʒiˈaitidiːz]) *n* 血管炎,脉管炎 | allergic granulomatous ~ 变应性肉芽肿性血管炎 / leukocytoclastic ~ 白细胞破碎性血管炎,过敏性血管炎 / necrotizing ~ 坏死性血管炎
angina [ænˈdʒainə, ˈændʒinə] *n* 咽峡炎,咽痛;绞痛(现在几乎专指心绞痛) | abdominal ~ 腹绞痛 / agranulocytic ~ 粒细胞缺乏性咽峡炎 / benign croupous ~ 疱疹性咽峡炎 / ~ cordis 心绞痛 / exudative ~ 渗出性咽峡炎,格鲁布(croup) / hippocratic ~ 咽后脓肿 / hysteric ~ 癔症性心绞痛 / intestinal ~ 肠绞痛 / lacunar ~ 扁桃体炎 / malignant ~ 恶性咽峡炎 / neutropenic ~ 粒细胞缺乏性咽峡炎/ ~ pectoris 心绞痛 / ~ phlegmonosa 扁桃体周脓肿 / ~ sine dolore 无痛性心绞痛 / vasomotor ~ 血管舒缩性心绞痛 | **~l** [ænˈdʒainəl, ˈændʒinəl], **anginose** [ˈændʒinəus], **anginous** [ˈændʒinəs] *a*
anginiform [ænˈdʒinifɔːm], **anginoid** [ˈændʒinɔid] *a* 咽峡炎样的;绞痛样的
anginophobia [ˌændʒinəuˈfəubjə] *n* 心绞痛恐怖
anginosis [ˌændʒiˈnəusis] *n* 咽峡炎病,咽痛病;绞痛病
angi(o)- [构词成分]血管
angioaccess [ˌændʒiəuˈækses] *n* 血管入口
angioasthenia [ˌændʒiəuæsˈθiːniə] *n* 血管无力
angioataxia [ˌændʒiəuəˈtæksiə] *n* 血管紧张失调
angioblast [ˈændʒiəuˌblæst] *n* 成血管细胞 | **~ic** [ˌændʒiəuˈblæstik] *a*
angioblastoma [ˌændʒiəublæsˈtəumə] *n* 成血管细胞瘤
angiocardiogram [ˌændʒiəuˈkɑːdiəɡræm] *n* 心血管造影[照]片
angiocardiography [ˌændʒiəuˌkɑːdiˈɔɡrəfi] *n* 心血管造影[术]
angiocardiokinetic [ˌændʒiəuˌkɑːdiəukaiˈnetik] *a* 心血管运动的 *n* 心血管运动药
angiocardiopathy [ˌændʒiəuˌkɑːdiˈɔpəθi] *n* 心血管病
angiocarditis [ˌændʒiəukɑːˈdaitis] *n* 血管心脏炎
angiocavernous [ˌændʒiəuˈkævənəs] *a* 海绵状血管瘤的
angiocentric [ˌændʒiəuˈsentrik] *a* 血管中心的
angioceratoma [ˌændʒiəuˌserəˈtəumə] *n* 血管角质瘤,血管角化瘤
angiocheiloscope [ˌændʒiəuˈkailəˌskəup] *n* 唇血管镜
angiochondroma [ˌændʒiəukənˈdrəumə] *n* 血管软骨瘤
angioclast [ˈændʒiəuˌklæst] *n* 血管压轧钳
Angiococcus [ˌændʒiəuˈkɔkəs] *n* 管球菌属
angiocrine [ˈændʒiəukrain] *a* 内分泌性血管[舒缩]障碍的
angiocrinosis [ˌændʒiəukriˈnəusis] *n* 内分泌性血管[舒缩]障碍
angiocyst [ˈændʒiəuˌsist] *n* 成血管囊
angioderm [ˈændʒiəudəːm] *n* 成血管层(成血管细胞)
angiodermatitis [ˌændʒiəudəːməˈtaitis] *n* 血管皮炎 | disseminated pruritic ~ 播散性瘙痒性血管皮炎,痒性紫癜
angiodiascopy [ˌændʒiəudaiˈæskəpi] *n* 肢血管透视法
angiodiathermy [ˌændʒiəuˈdaiəˌθəːmi] *n* 血管透热凝固术
angiodynia [ˌændʒiəuˈdiniə] *n* 血管痛
angiodysplasia [ˌændʒiəudisˈpleiziə] *n* 血管发育不良
angiodystrophia [ˌændʒiəudisˈtrəufiə], **angiodystrophy** [ˌændʒiəuˈdistrəfi] *n* 血管营养障碍
angioectatic [ˌændʒiəuekˈtætik] *a* 血管扩张的
angioedema [ˌændʒiəuiˈdiːmə] *n* 血管性水肿 | hereditary ~ 遗传性血管性水肿 / vibratory ~ 振动性血管性水肿 | **~tous** *a*
angioelephantiasis [ˌændʒiəuˌelifənˈtaiəsis] *n* 血管象皮病
angioendothelioma [ˌændʒiəuˌendəuˌθiːliˈəumə] *n* 血管内皮瘤
angioendotheliomatosis [ˌændʒiəuˌendəuˈθiːliəuməˈtəusis] *n* 血管内皮瘤病 | systemic proliferating ~ 系统性增生性血管内皮瘤病
angiofibroma [ˌændʒiəufaiˈbrəumə] *n* 血管纤维瘤 | nasopharyngeal ~, juvenile ~ 鼻咽血管纤维瘤,幼年血管纤维瘤
angiofollicular [ˌændʒiəufəˈlikjulə] *a* 血管滤泡的
angiogenesis [ˌændʒiəuˈdʒenisis] *n* 血管发生 | tumor ~ 肿瘤血管发生
angiogenic [ˌændʒiəuˈdʒenik] *a* 血管源[性]的,生成血管的
angioglioma [ˌændʒiəuɡlaiˌəumə] *n* 血管神经胶质瘤
angiogliomatosis [ˌændʒiəuˌɡlaiəməˈtəusis] *n* 血管神经胶质瘤病
angiogram [ˈændʒiəuˌɡræm], **angiograph** [ˈændʒiəuˌɡrɑːf, -ɡræf] *n* 血管造影[照]片
angiogranuloma [ˌændʒiəuˌɡrænjuˈləumə] *n* 血管

肉芽肿
angiography [ˌændʒiˈɔgrəfi] *n* 血管造影术;血管学 | cerebral ~ 脑血管造影[术] / coronary ~ 冠状血管造影[术] / intra-arterial digital subtraction ~ 动脉数字减影血管造影[术] / intravenous digital subtraction ~ 静脉数字减影血管造影[术] / magnetic resonance ~ (MRA)磁共振血管造影[术]
angiohemophilia [ˌændʒiəuˌhiːməˈfiliə] *n* 血管性血友病
angiohyalinosis [ˌændʒiəuˌhaiəliˈnəusis] *n* 血管[肌层]透明变性
angioid [ˈændʒiɔid] *a* 血管样的
angioinvasive [ˌændʒiəuinˈveisiv] *a* 侵入血管(壁)的
angiokeratoma [ˌændʒiəuˌkerəˈtəumə] *n* 血管角化瘤,血管角质瘤(亦称血管角化病,血管扩张性疣) | ~ circumscriptum 局限性血管角化瘤 / corporis diffusum, diffuse ~ 弥漫性躯体性血管角化瘤 / ~ of scrotum 阴囊血管角化瘤 / solitary ~ 孤立性血管角化瘤
angiokeratosis [ˌændʒiəuˌkerəˈtəusis] *n* 血管角化病,血管角质瘤
angiokinesis [ˌændʒiəukiˈniːsis] *n* 血管舒缩 | **angiokinetic** [ˌændʒiəukiˈnetik] *a*
angioleiomyoma [ˌændʒiəuˌlaiəumaiˈəumə] *n* 血管平滑肌瘤
angioleucitis [ˌændʒiəuljuːˈsaitis], **angioleukitis** [ˌændʒiəuljuːˈkaitis] *n* 淋巴管炎
angiolipoleiomyoma [ˌændʒiəuˌlipəulaiəmaiˈəumə] *n* 血管脂肪平滑肌瘤
angiolipoma [ˌændʒiəuliˈpəumə] *n* 血管脂肪瘤
angiology [ˌændʒiˈɔlədʒi], **angiologia** [ˌændʒiəuˈləudʒiə] *n* 血管学,脉管学,血管淋巴管学
angiolupoid [ˌændʒiəuˈljuːpɔid] *n* 毛细管扩张性狼疮疹(主要生在鼻两侧)
angiolymphangioma [ˌændʒiəulimˌfændʒiˈəumə] *n* 血管淋巴管瘤
angiolymphitis [ˌændʒiəulimˈfaitis] *n* 淋巴管炎
angiolysis [ˌændʒiˈɔlisis] *n* 血管破坏(指血管退化或闭塞,例如发生在胚胎发育期间)
angioma [ˌændʒiˈəumə] *n* 血管瘤 | carvernous ~ 海绵状血管瘤 / fissural ~ 胚裂血管瘤 / hypertrophic ~ 肥大性血管瘤 / spider ~ 蜘蛛状血管瘤,蜘蛛痣 / telangiectatic ~ 毛细管扩张性血管瘤 | **~tous** [ˌændʒiˈɔmətəs] *a*
angiomatoid [ˌændʒiˈəumətɔid] *a* 类血管瘤的
angiomatosis [ˌændʒiəuməˈtəusis] *n* 血管瘤病,多发性血管瘤
angiomegaly [ˌændʒiəuˈmegəli] *n* 血管增大(尤指眼睑)
angiometer [ˌændʒiˈɔmitə] *n* 血管口径张力计
angiomyolipoma [ˌændʒiəuˌmaiəuliˈpəumə] *n* 血管肌脂瘤
angiomyoma [ˌændʒiəumaiˈəumə] *n* 血管肌瘤
angiomyoneuroma [ˌændʒiəuˌmaiəunjuəˈrəumə] *n* 血管肌神经瘤,血管球瘤
angiomyosarcoma [ˌændʒiəuˌmaiəusɑːˈkəumə] *n* 血管肌肉瘤
angiomyxoma [ˌændʒiəumikˈsəumə] *n* 血管黏液瘤
angionecrosis [ˌændʒiəuneˈkrəusis] *n* 血管壁坏死
angioneoplasm [ˌændʒiəuˈni(ː)əuplæzəm] *n* 血管瘤
angioneuralgia [ˌændʒiəunjuəˈrældʒiə] *n* 血管神经痛
angioneurectomy [ˌændʒiəunjuəˈrektəmi] *n* 血管神经切除术
angioneuroma [ˌændʒiəunjuəˈrəumə], **angioneuromyoma** [ˌændʒiəuˌnjuərəumaiˈəumə] *n* 血管神经瘤,血管神经肌瘤(亦称血管球瘤)
angioneuropathy [ˌændʒiəunjuəˈrɔpəθi] *n* 血管神经病 | **angioneuropathic** [ˌændʒiəuˌnjuərəˈpæθik] *a*
angioneurotic [ˌændʒiəunjuəˈrɔtik] *a* 血管神经病的
angioneurotomy [ˌændʒiəunjuəˈrɔtəmi] *n* 血管神经切断术
angionoma [ˌændʒiəuˈnəumə] *n* 血管溃疡
angioparalysis [ˌændʒiəupəˈrælisis] *n* 血管麻痹
angioparesis [ˌændʒiəuˈpærisis] *n* 血管不全麻痹,血管轻麻痹
angiopathology [ˌændʒiəupəˈθɔlədʒi] *n* 血管病理学
angiopathy [ændʒiˈɔpəθi] *n* 血管病
angiophakomatosis [ˌændʒiəuˌfækəuməˈtəusis] *n* 囊肿性视网膜血管瘤病(小脑及视网膜内血管瘤样囊肿形成)
angioplasty [ˈændʒiəuˌplæstik] *n* 血管成形术 | percutaneous transluminal ~ 经皮腔内血管成形术 / percutaneous transluminal coronary ~ (PTCA)经皮腔内冠状动脉成形术
angiopoiesis [ˌændʒiəupɔiˈiːsis] *n* 血管形成 | **angiopoietic** [ˌændʒiəupɔiˈetik] *a*
angiopressure [ˈændʒiəuˌpreʃə] *n* 血管压迫法(控制出血)
angiopsathyrosis [ˌændʒiəuˌsæθiˈrəusis] *n* 血管脆弱
angioreticuloendothelioma [ˌændʒiəuriˌtikjuləu-ˌendəuθiliˈəumə] *n* 血管网状内皮瘤
angioreticuloma [ˌændʒiəuriˌtikjuˈləumə] *n* 血管网状细胞瘤
angiorrhaphy [ˌændʒiˈɔrəfi] *n* 血管缝合术 | arte-

riovenous ~ 动静脉缝合术
angiosarcoma [ˌændʒiəusɑːˈkəumə] *n* 血管肉瘤
angiosclerosis [ˌændʒiəuskliəˈrəusis] *n* 血管硬化 | **angiosclerotic** [ˌændʒiəuskliəˈrɔtik] *a*
angioscope [ˈændʒiəuˌskəup] *n* 毛细血管显微镜
angioscopy [ˌændʒiˈɔskəpi] *n* 光导血管镜检查;毛细血管显微镜检查
angioscotoma [ˌændʒiəuskəˈtəumə] *n* 血管暗点(视网膜血管暗影所致)
angioscotometry [ˌændʒiəuskəˈtɔmitri] *n* 血管暗点测量法(特别用于诊断青光眼)
angiospasm [ˌændʒiəuˌspæzəm] *n* 血管痉挛 | **angiospastic** [ˌændʒiəuˈspæstik] *a*
angiosperm [ˈændʒiəuˌspəːm] *n* 被子植物
angiospermin [ˌændʒiəuˈspəːmin] *n* 被子植物素(据说具有类似激素的性质)
angiostenosis [ˌændʒiəustiˈnəusis] *n* 血管狭窄
angiosteosis [ˌændʒiˌɔstiˈəusis] *n* 血管骨化,血管钙化
angiosthenia [ˌændʒiɔsˈθiːniə] *n* 动脉张力,动脉压
angiostomy [ˌændʒiˈɔstəmi] *n* 血管造口术
angiostrongyliasis [ˌændʒiəuˌstrɔndʒiˈlaiəsis] *n* 管圆线虫病
Angiostrongylidae [ˌændʒiəustrɔnˈdʒilidiː] *n* 管圆[线虫]科
angiostrongylosis [ˌændʒiəuˌstrɔndʒiˈləusis] *n* 管圆线虫病
Angiostrongylus [ˌændʒiəuˈstrɔndʒiləs] *n* 管圆[线虫]属 | ~ cantonensis 广州管圆线虫 / ~ vasorum 脉管圆线虫
angiostrophe, angiostrophy [ˌændʒiˈɔstrəfi] *n* 血管扭转术(止血法)
angiotelectasis [ˌændʒiəutiˈlektəsis] *n* 毛细血管扩张
angiotensin [ˌændʒiəuˈtensin] *n* 血管紧张素,血管紧张肽 | ~ amide 血管紧张素胺,增压素(升压药)
angiotensinase [ˌændʒiəˈtensineis] *n* 血管紧张肽酶
angiotensin-converting enzyme [ˌændʒiəu ˈtensin] 血管紧张肽-转化酶,肽基二肽酶 A
angiotensinogen [ˌændʒiəˈtensinədʒən] *n* 血管紧张素原,血管紧张肽原
angiotitis [ˌændʒiəuˈtaitis] *n* 耳血管炎
angiotome [ˌændʒiəuˌtəum] *n* 血管节
angiotomy [ˌændʒiˈɔtəmi] *n* 血管切开(血管或淋巴管切开或切断)
angiotonase [ˌændʒiəuˈtəuneis] *n* 血管紧张肽酶
angiotonia [ˌændʒiəuˈtəuniə] *n* 血管紧张
angiotonic [ˌændʒiəuˈtɔnik] *a* 血管紧张的
angiotonin [ˌændʒiəuˈtəunin] *n* 血管紧张素,血管紧张肽
angiotribe [ˈændʒiəuˌtraib] *n* 血管压轧钳,血管压轧器
angiotripsy [ˈændʒiəuˌtripsi] *n* 血管压轧术
angiotrophic [ˌændʒiəuˈtrɔfik] *a* 血管营养的
angitis [ænˈdʒaitis] *n* 血管炎,脉管炎
angle [ˈæŋgl] *n* 角;角度 | ~ of aberration 像差角,偏向角 / alpha ~ α 角(视线与视轴在节点交叉所形成的角) / beta ~ β 角(枕外粗隆点与囟枕线间的角) / biorbital ~ 眶间角 / cardiohepatic ~ 心肝角 / carrying ~ 臂外偏角 / ~ of convergence 会聚角,集合角 / critical ~, limiting ~ 临界角,极限角 / ~ of declination 偏角,倾斜角 / ~ of deviation 偏向角 / ~ of direction 注视角 / facial ~ 颜面角 / filtration ~ 滤角,虹膜[角膜]角 / gamma ~ γ 角(固定线与视轴在眼旋转中心连接所形成的角) / gonial ~ 下颌角 / ~ of incidence 入射角 / ~ of inclination 倾斜角,骨盆倾斜度 / kappa ~ κ 角,瞳孔轴间角 / lambda ~ λ 角(瞳孔轴与视线间角) / mesial ~s 近中角(牙近中面与其他面形成的角) / metafacial ~ 面后角(颅底与翼突间角) / nu ~ ν 字角(固定半径与蝶枕点及鼻根点连线之间的角) / parietal ~ 顶角(通过两颧间横径两端及最大额横径两端的两线接合所形成的角) / refracting ~, principal ~ 折射棱角,主角 / rolandic ~ 中央沟角(正中平面与中央沟汇合形成) / sigma ~ σ 形角(固定半径与后鼻棘点至蝶枕点线之间的角) / Y ~ Y 形角(固定半径与人字缝尖及枕外隆凸尖连线之间的角)
Angle's classification [ˈæŋgl] (Edward H. Angle)安格尔错殆分类(共分四类,第一类中性殆,第二类远中殆,第三类近中殆,第四类不用) | ~ splint 安格尔夹板(下颌骨骨折用)
Anglesey leg [ˌæŋglsi] 安格尔西假腿(一种有关节的假腿,因 Anglesey 侯爵而得名)
anglicus sudor [ˌæŋglikəs ˈsjuːdə] 英国黑汗热
angophrasia [ˌæŋgəˈfreiziə] *n* 言语涩滞(痴呆时发生)
angor [ˈæŋgɔː] *n*【拉】绞痛;极度痛苦
angry [ˈæŋgri] *a* (患处)肿痛发炎的
angstrom (Å) [ˈæŋstrəm] *n* 埃(长度单位,= 10^{-10} m)
Angström's law [ˈæŋstrəm] (Anders J Angström) 埃[格斯特勒姆]氏定律(物质吸收光的波长与物质发光时释放的波长相同) | ~ unit 埃单位,埃(见 angstrom)
Anguillula [æŋˈgwiljulə] *n* 鳗形线虫属 | ~ aceti 醋鳗形线虫,醋线虫(即 Turbatrix aceti) / ~ intestinalis, ~ stercoralis 粪鳗形线虫,粪类圆线虫(即 Strongyloides stercoralis)
Anguillulina putrefaciens [æŋˌgwiljuˈlainəˌpjutrəˈfeiʃiənz] 腐败小鳗线虫

angular [ˌæŋgjulə] *a* 角的;角形的
angulation [ˌæŋgju'leiʃən] *n* 角度形成(如肠、输尿管内形成的阻塞性尖角);歪曲(如接骨不好,偏离直线)
angulus ['æŋgjuləs]([复] **anguli** ['æŋgjulai]) *n*【拉】角
anhalamine [æn'hæləmin] *n* 老头掌胺
anhalonine [ˌænhə'ləunin] *n* 老头掌碱
Anhalonium lewinii [ˌænhə'ləuniəmlju'winii] 威廉斯仙人球
anhaphia [æn'heifiə] *n* 触觉缺失
anhedonia [ˌænhiː'dəuniə] *n* 快感缺乏
anhidrosis [ˌænhi'drəusis] *n* 无汗症 | thermogenic ~ 生热无汗症,热带性汗闭性衰弱
anhidrotic [ˌænhi'drɔtik] *a* 止汗的,无汗的 *n* 止汗药
anhydrase [æn'haidreis] *n* 脱水酶,去水酶 | carbonic ~ 碳酸酐酶
anhydration [ˌænhai'dreiʃən] *n* 脱水[作用],去水[作用]
anhydremia [ˌænhai'driːmiə] *n* 缺水血[症]
anhydride [æn'haidraid] *n* 酐,脱水物 | arsenous ~ 亚砷酸酐,三氧化二砷 / carbonic ~ 碳酸酐,二氧化碳 / chromic ~ 铬[酸]酐,三氧化铬 / perosmic ~ 锇酐,四氧化锇 / silicic ~ 硅酐,硅石,二氧化硅 / sulfurous ~ 亚硫[酸]酐,二氧化硫
anhydrochloric [ˌænhaidrəu'klɔːrik] *a* 无盐酸的
anhydrohydroxyprogesterone [ænˌhaidrəuhaiˌdrɔksiprəu'dʒestərəun] *n* 脱水羟基孕酮,孕烯炔醇酮,乙炔基睾丸酮
anhydromuscarine [ˌænhaidrəu'mʌskərin] *n* 脱水毒蕈碱(用于实验医学)
anhydrosugar [ˌænhaidrəu'ʃugə] *n* 脱水糖,去水糖
anhydrous [æn'haidrəs] *a* 脱水的,无水的
aniacinamidosis [əˌnaiəsiˌnæmai'dəusis] *n* 烟酰胺缺乏症
aniacinosis [əˌnaiəsi'nəusis] *n* 烟酸缺乏症
anianthinopsy [ˌæni'ænθiˌnɔpsi] *n* 紫色盲
Anichkov's (Anitschkow's) myocyte (cell) [ə'nitʃkɔf](Nikolai N Anichkov)阿尼齐科夫肌细胞(风湿热小体中的肌细胞,核内有锯齿棒状染色质。亦称心肌组织细胞)
anicteric [ˌænik'terik] *n* 无黄疸的
anideus [ə'nidiəs] *n* 无体形畸胎,不成形寄生胎畸胎 | embryonic ~ 无体形畸胚 | **anidean** [ə'nidiən] *a*
anidoxime [ˌæni'dɔksiːm] *n* 阿尼多昔(镇痛药)
anidrosis [æni'drəusis] *n* 无汗[症]
anidrotic [ˌæni'drɔtik] *a* 止汗的,无汗的 *n* 止汗药
anile ['einail] *a* 老妪样的;痴愚的
anileridine [ˌæni'ləːridiːn] *n* 阿尼利定(麻醉性镇痛药)
anilid ['ænilid], **anilide** ['ænilaid] *n* 酰基苯胺
anilinction [ˌeini'liŋkʃən] *n* 舔肛,舐肛色情 | **anilinctus** [ˌeini'liŋktəs] *n*
aniline ['æniliːn] *n* 苯胺,阿尼林 | ~ sulfate 硫酸苯胺
anilingus [ˌeini'liŋgəs] *n* 舔肛者,舐肛色情者
anilinism ['ænilinizəm], **anilism** ['ænilizəm] *n* 苯胺中毒
anilinparasulfonic acid [ˌænilinˌpærəsʌl'fɔnik] 对氨基苯磺酸
anility [ə'niləti] *n* 老妪样状态;衰老
anilopam hydrochloride ['æniləˌpæm] 盐酸阿尼洛泮(镇痛药)
anil-quinoline [ˌænil'kwinəlin] *n* 缩苯胺喹啉
anima ['ænimə] *n*【拉】灵气,灵;精,精华(药品的有效成分);阿妮玛,女性意象(精神分析用词)
animal ['æniməl] *n* 动物 *a* 动物的 | control ~ 对照动物 / decerebrate ~ 去大脑动物 / experimental ~ 实验动物 / nuclein ~核素[注射]动物/ slime ~ 黏液动物
animalcule [ˌæni'mælkjuːl] *n* 微小动物
animalculist [ˌæni'mælkjulist] *n* 精源论者(认为未发育的胚胎已预先形成而存于精子内)
animality [ˌæni'mæləti] *n* 动物性
animation [ˌæni'meiʃən] *n* 生存,生活;生气,活泼 | suspended ~ 生活暂停,假死
animism ['ænimizəm] *n* 泛灵论,万物有灵论
animus ['æniməs] *n* 女性的男性意向
anion ['ænaiən] *n* 阴离子,阳向离子 | **anionic** [ˌænai'ɔnik] *a*
anionotropy [ˌæniə'nɔtrəpi] *n* 阴离子移变[现象]
aniridia [ˌæni'ridiə] *n* 无虹膜
anisakiasis [ˌænisei'kaiəsis] *n* 异尖线虫病
Anisakidae [əˌni'sækidiː] *n* 异尖科
Anisakis [ˌæni'seikis] *n* 异尖属 | ~ marina 海生异尖线虫
anisate ['æniseit] *n* 茴香酸盐
anise ['ænis] *n* 茴香(驱风、祛痰药) | Chinese ~, Indian ~, star ~ 八角茴香,大茴香
aniseikonia [ˌænaisai'kəuniə] *n* 影像不等(指一眼所见物象的大小和形状与另一眼所见不同) | **aniseikonic** [ˌænaisai'kɔnik] *a*
anisic acid [ə'nisik] 茴香酸,对甲氧基苯甲酸
***o*-anisidine** [ə'nisidiːn] *n o*-茴香胺
anisindione [ˌænisin'daiəun] *n* 茴茚二酮(抗凝药)
anisine ['ænisin] *n* 茴香碱
anis(o)- [构词成分]不等,不同,不均,参差
anisoaccommodation [æˌnaisə-əˌkɔmə'deiʃən] *n*

两眼调节参差
anisochromasia [æˌnaisəkrəuˈmeiziə] *n* 色素不均(仅红细胞周围区着色)
anisochromatic [æˌnaisəkrəuˈmætik] *a* 色素不均的(将正常眼和色盲眼均能辨别的两种色素溶液混合,供测色盲用)
anisochromia [ˌænisəˈkrəumiə] *n* 色素不均(由于血红蛋白容量不同所致的红细胞颜色不一)
anisocoria [ˌænisəˈkɔːriə] *n* 瞳孔不等
anisocytosis [æˌnaisəsaiˈtəusis] *n* 红细胞大小不均
anisodactyly [æˌnaisəˈdæ-ktili] *n* 指长短不均,趾长短不均 | **anisodactylous** [æˌnaisəˈdæktiləs] *a*
anisodiametric [æˌnaisədaiəˈmetrik] *a* 不等直径的
anisodont [æˈnaisədɔnt] *n* 牙长短不齐者;大小不等牙
anisogamete [ˌænisəˈgæmiːt] *n* 异形配子 | **anisogametic** [ˌænisəgəˈmetik] *a*
anisogamy [ˌæniˈsɔgəmi] *n* 异配生殖 | **anisogamous** [ˌæniˈsɔgəməs] *a*
anisoic [ˌæniˈsəuik] *a* 茴香的
anisoiconia [æˌnaisəaiˈkəuniə] *n* 物象不等(见 aniseikonia)
anisokaryosis [æˌnaisəˌkæriˈəusis] *n* 核[大小]不均
Anisolobis [ænˌaisəuˈləubis] *n* 肥螋属
anisomastia [æˌnaisəˈmæstiə] *n* 乳房大小不等
anisomelia [æˌnaisəˈmiːliə] *n* 对称肢体大小不等
anisomeric [æˌnaisəˈmerik] *a* 非异物性的,非同质异构的
anisometrope [æˌnaisəˈmetrəup] *n* 屈光参差者
anisometropia [æˌnaisəmiˈtrəupiə] *n* 屈光参差(两眼屈光不等) | **anisometropic** [æˌnaisəmiˈtrɔpik] *a*
Anisomorpha [æˌnaisəˈmɔːfə] *n* 竹节虫属 | ~ buprestoides 二纹竹节虫
anisophoria [ˌænaisəˈfɔːriə] *n* 不等隐斜
anisopia [ˌænaiˈsəupiə] *n* 两眼视力不等
anisopiesis [æˌnaisəpaiˈiːsis] *n* 各部血压不等
anisopoikilocytosis [æˌnaisəˌpɔikiləusaiˈtəusis] *n* [大小]不均性红细胞异形[症]
anisosmotic [ˌænisɔsˈmɔtik] *a* 渗透压不等的
anisospore [æˌnaisəˈspɔː] *n* 有性孢子;异形孢子 | **anisosporous** [æˌnaiˈsɔspərəs] *a*
anisosthenic [æˌnaisəˈsθenik] *a* 力量不等的(指配对肌肉)
anisotonic [æˌnaisəˈtɔnik] *a* 张力不等的;不等渗的
anisotropic [æˌnaisəˈtrɔpik], **anisotropal** [ˌænaiˈsɔtrəpəl] *a* 各向异性的;双折射的 | **anisotropy** [ˈænaiˈsɔtrəpi], **anisotropism** [ˌænaiˈsɔtrəpizəm] *n* 各向异性;双折射性
anisotropine methylbromide [ænˌaisəuˈtrəupiːn] 甲溴辛托品(抗胆碱药,解痉药)
anistreplase [æniˈstrepleis] *n* 阿尼普酶(溶纤维蛋白药)
anisum [æˈnaisəm] *n*【拉】茴香
anisuria [ˌænaiˈsjuəriə] *n* 尿量不等
anisuric acid [ˌæniˈsjuərik] 茴香酰甘氨酸
anitrogenous [ˌænaiˈtrɔdʒinəs] *a* 非氮性的
Anitschkow = Anichkow
Anixiopsis [əˌniksiˈɔpsis] *n* 裸囊菌属
ankle [ˈæŋkl] *n* 踝;踝关节;距骨;后踝 | deck ~s 船员踝肿 / tailors' ~ 裁缝踝(外踝滑囊炎)
ankyl(o)- [构词成分]弯曲;粘连
ankyloblepharon [ˌæŋkiləuˈblefərɔn] *n* 睑缘粘连 | ~ filiforme adnatum 丝状睑缘粘连[畸形] / ~ totale 隐眼[畸形]
ankylocheilia [ˌæŋkiləuˈkailiə] *n* 唇粘连
ankylocolpos [ˌæŋkiləuˈkɔlpəs] *n* 阴道闭锁
ankylodactyly [ˌæŋkiləuˈdæktili] *n* 并指,并趾
ankyloglossia [ˌæŋkiləuˈglɔsiə] *n* 舌系带短缩,舌系带过短
ankylophobia [ˌæŋkiləuˈfəubjə] *n* 关节强硬恐怖
ankylopoietic [ˌæŋkiləupɔiˈetik] *a* 关节强硬的
Ankyloproglypha [ˌæŋkiləuprəuˈglifə] *n* 前牙类,沟牙类
ankylose [ˌæŋkiləuz] *vt*, *vi* (关节)变强直 | **~d** *a* 关节强直的
ankylosis [ˌæŋkiˈləusis] ([复] **ankyloses** [ˌæŋkiˈləusiːz]) *n* 关节强直 | artificial ~ 人工关节强直 / bony ~, true ~ 骨质性关节强直,真性关节强直 / dental ~ 牙与牙槽骨粘连 / extracapsular ~ 关节囊外强直 / fibrous ~, false ~, spurious ~ 纤维性关节强直,假性关节强直 / intracapsular ~ 关节囊内强直 | **ankylotic** [ˌæŋkiˈlɔtik] *a*
Ankylostoma [ˌæŋkiˈlɔstəmə] = Ancylostoma
ankylostomiasis [ˌæŋkiˌlɔstəˈmaiəsis] *n* 钩[口线]虫病
ankylotia [ˌæŋkiˈləuʃiə] *n* 外耳道闭锁
ankylotomy [ˌæŋkiˈlɔtəmi] *n* 舌系带切除术
ankylurethria [ˌæŋkiljuəˈriːθriə] *n* 尿道粘连性狭窄
ankyrin [ˈæŋkirin] *n* 锚蛋白(红细胞和脑的膜蛋白,使血影蛋白固定于阴离子通道处的质膜)
ankyroid [ˈæŋkirɔid] *a* 钩样的
anlage [ˈɑːnlɑːgə, ˈænleidʒ] ([复] **anlagen** [ˈɑːnlɑːgən]或 **anlages**) *n*【德】原基
ANLL acute nonlymphocytic leukemia 急性非淋巴细胞白血病

ANNA-1 type 1 antineuronal antibody 1 型抗神经元抗体
ANNA-2 type 2 antineuronal antibody 2 型抗神经元抗体
Annandale's operation [ˈænəndeil] (Thomas Annandale)安南代尔手术(股骨髁切除术,治膝外翻;膝软骨固定术,用缝线固定膝关节内移位的软骨)
anneal [əˈniːl] *vt* 退火,炼韧(使金属等物控制加热和冷却以使回韧)
annectent [əˈnektənt] *a* 连接的,接合的
annelid [ˈænəlid] *n* 环节动物
Annelida [əˈnelidə] *n* 环节动物门
annexin [əˈneksin] *n* 膜联蛋白(亦称脂皮质蛋白)
Annona [əˈnəunə] *n* 番荔枝属
annotto [əˈnɔtəu] *n* 胭脂树红,果红(用作干酪、乳酪等食品的着色剂)
annoyer [əˈnɔiə] *n* 厌恶物,不快感刺激
annular [ˈænjulə] *a* 环状的,环形的
annulate(d) [ˈænjuleit(id)] *a* 有环的,有环纹的
annulation [ˌænjuˈleiʃən] *n* 环的形成;环;环形物
annulet [ˈænjulit] *n* 小环
annuloaortic [ˌænjuləueiˈɔːtik] *a* 环主动脉的(主动脉与主动脉环的)
annuloid [ˈænjulɔid], **annulose** [ˈænjuləus] *a* 环状的;有环的
annuloplasty [ˌænjuləuˈplæsti] *n* 瓣环成形术
annulorrhaphy [ˌænjuˈlɔrəfi] *n* [疝]环[形]缝合术
annulus [ˈænjuləs] ([复] **annuli** [ˈænjulai]) *n* 【拉】环,终环 | ~ abdominalis 腹股沟管环 / ~ migrans 地图样舌
Anocentor [ˌeinəˈsentə] *n* 暗眼蜱属 | ~ nitans 明暗眼蜱
anochromasia [ˌænəkrəuˈmeisiə] *n* 不染色性(指组织或细胞对普通染色无反应);色素不均(指血红蛋白在红细胞周围集积,而中心呈淡白色)
anociassociation [əˌnəusiəˌsəusiˈeiʃən], **anociation** [əˌnəusiˈeiʃən], **anocithesia** [əˌnəusiˈθiːzjə] *n* 创伤性休克防止法(一种旨在减少外科休克作用的麻醉法)
anociated [əˈnəusiˌeitid] *a* 创伤性休克防止的
anococcygeal [ˌeinəukɔkˈsidʒiəl] *a* 肛尾的
anode [ˈænəud] *n* 阳极,正极 | hooded ~ 有罩阳极 | **anodal** [æˈnəudl], **anodic** [əˈnɔdik] *a*
anoderm [ˈeinədəːm] *n* 肛膜
anodmia [æˈnɔdmiə] *n* 嗅觉丧失,失嗅
anodontia [ˌænəuˈdɔnʃiə], **anodontism** [ˌænəuˈdɔntizəm] *n* 无牙,无牙症
anodyne [ˈænəudain] *a* 止痛的 *n* 止痛药 | **anodynic** [ænəˈdinik] *a*
anodynia [ˌænəuˈdiniə] *n* 无痛,痛觉缺失
anodynin [ˌænəˈdainin] *n* 镇痛素(吗啡样物质)
Anogeissus [ˌænəˈdʒaisəs] *n* 使君子属
anoia [əˈnɔiə] *n* 精神错乱;白痴
***p*-anol** [ˈeinɔl] *n* 对丙烯基苯酚
anomalad [əˈnɔmələd] *n* 形态缺陷
anomalistic(al) [əˈnɔməˈlistik(əl)] *a* 不规则的,异常的
anomal(o)- [构词成分] 不规则,异常,反常
anomalopia [əˌnɔməˈləupiə] *n* 视觉异常
anomaloscope [əˈnɔmələˌskəup] *n* 色盲检查镜
anomalotrophy [əˌnɔməˈlɔtrəfi] *n* 营养异常
anomalous [əˈnɔmələs] *a* 不规则的,异常的,反常的
anomaly [əˈnɔməli] *n* 异常,反常 | chromosomal ~, chromosome ~ 染色体异常 / developmental ~ 发育异常,发育反常
anomer [ˈænəmə] *n* 异头物,端基异构体(糖类的 α 或 β 异构体) | **~ic** [ˌænəˈmerik] *a*
anomia [əˈnəumiə] *n* 称名不能,忘名症
anonacein [ˌænəˈneisiin] *n* 阿诺纳辛,胡椒番荔枝碱
anonychia [ˌænəˈnikiə] *n* 甲缺如
anonymous [əˈnɔniməs] *a* 无名的
anoopsia [ˌænəuˈɔpsiə] *n* 上斜视
anoperineal [ˌeinəuperiˈniːəl] *a* 肛门会阴的
Anopheles [əˈnɔfiliːz] *n* 按蚊属 | ~ aconitus 乌头按蚊 / ~ albimanus 白魔按蚊 / ~ albitarsis 白蹠按蚊 / ~ amictus 具饰按蚊 / ~ annularis 环斑按蚊 / ~ annulipes annulipes 环须按蚊 / ~ aquasalis 咸水按蚊 / ~ atroparvus 黑小按蚊 / ~ bancroftii 斑[克罗夫特]氏按蚊 / ~ barbirostris barbirostris 须喙按蚊 / ~ bellator 挑战按蚊 / ~ claviger 带棒按蚊 / ~ culicifacies 库态按蚊 / ~ darlingi 达[林]氏按蚊 / ~ farauti 法老按蚊 / ~ fluviatilis 溪流按蚊 / ~ funestus 催命按蚊 / ~ gambiae 冈比亚按蚊 / ~ hyrcanus nigerrimus 最黑按蚊,赫坎按蚊最黑亚种 / ~ hyrcanus sinensis 中华按蚊,赫坎按蚊中华亚种 / ~ jeyporiensis candidiensis 日月潭按蚊,杰普按蚊日月潭亚种 / ~ jeyporiensis jeyporiensis 杰普按蚊 / ~ kochi 可赫按蚊,腹簇按蚊 / ~ labranchiae atroparvus 羽斑按蚊黑小亚种 / ~ labranchiae labranchiae 羽斑按蚊唇边亚种 / ~ leucosphyrus leucosphyrus 白踝按蚊 / ~ maculatus maculatus 多斑按蚊 / ~ maculipennis 五斑按蚊 / ~ messeae 麦赛按蚊,米赛按蚊 / ~ minimus 微小按蚊 / ~ minimus flavirostris 微小按蚊黄喙亚种 / ~ moucheti moucheti 毛捷蒂按蚊 / ~ multicolor 多色按蚊 / ~ nili 乌有按蚊 / ~ pattoni 伯[顿]氏按蚊 / ~ pharoensis 法氏按蚊

/ ~ philippinensis 菲律宾按蚊 / ~ pseudopunctipennis pseudopunctipennis 伪点翅按蚊/ ~ punctimacula 点斑按蚊 / ~ punctulatus punctulatus 点体按蚊 / ~ quadrimaculatus 四斑按蚊 / ~ sacharovi 萨[卡洛]氏按蚊,黑背按蚊 / ~ sergentii 萨[京特]氏按蚊 / ~ stephensi stephensi 史[蒂芬斯]氏按蚊,斑须按蚊 / ~ subpictus subpictus 浅色按蚊 / ~ sundaicus 圣代克按蚊 / ~ superpictus 深色按蚊 / ~ umbrosus 荫影按蚊 / ~ varuna 瓦容按蚊,印神按蚊

anophelicide [əˈnɔfilisaid] *a* 杀蚊的 *n* 杀蚊药

anophelifuge [əˈnɔfilifjuːdʒ] *a* 驱蚊的,防蚊的 *n* 驱蚊药,防蚊药

Anophelinae [əˌnɔfiˈlainiː] *n* 按蚊亚科

anopheline [əˈnɔfilain] *a* 按蚊的

Anophelini [əˌnɔfiˈlaini] *n* 按蚊族

anophelism [əˈnɔfilizəm] *n* 蚊害,蚊病

anophoria [ˌænəuˈfɔːriə] *n* 上隐斜视

anophthalmia [ˌænɔfˈθælmiə], **anophthalmos** [ˌænɔfˈθælmɔs] *n* 无眼[畸形]

anophthalmus [ˌænɔfˈθælməs] *n* 无眼畸胎

anopia [æˈnəupiə] *n* 无眼[畸形];废用性弱视;上斜视

anoplasty [ˈeinəuˌplæsti] *n* 肛门成形术

Anoplocephala [ˌænəpləuˈsefələ] *n* 裸头绦虫属

Anoplocephalidae [ˌænəpləusiˈfælidiː] *n* 裸头[绦虫]科

Anoplura [ˌænəˈpluərə] *n* 虱目,吸虱目

anopsia [æˈnɔpsiə] *n* 废用性弱视;上斜视

anorchia [æˈnɔːkiə] *n* 无睾丸,无睾症

anorchid [æˈnɔːkid], **anorchis** [æˈnɔːkis] *n* 无睾者

anorchism [æˈnɔːkizəm], **anorchidism** [æˈnɔːkidizəm] *n* 无睾畸形 | **anorchidic** [ˌænɔːˈkidik] *a* 无睾的

anorectal [ˌeinəuˈrektəl] *a* 肛门直肠的

anorectitis [ˌeinəurekˈtaitis] *n* 肛门直肠炎

anorectocolonic [ˌeinəuˌrektəukəˈlɔnik] *a* 肛门直肠结肠的

anorectoplasty [ˌeinəuˈrektəuˌplæsti] *n* 肛门直肠成形术

anorectum [ˌeinəuˈrektəm] *n* 肛门直肠

anorexia [ˌænəuˈreksiə] *n* 食欲缺乏 | **anorectic** [ˌænəuˈrektik], **anoretic** [ˌænəuˈretik], **anorexic** [ˌænəuˈreksik] *a* 食欲缺乏的 *n* 减食欲物质,减食欲药

anorexigenic [ˌænəureksiˈdʒenik], **anorexiant** [ˌænəuˈreksiənt] *a* 使食欲不振的 *n* 减食欲药

anorganic [ˌænɔːˈgænik] *a* 除(去)有机质的(如骨)

anorgasmy [ˌænɔːˈgæzmi], **anorgasmia** [ˌænɔːˈgæzmiə] *n* 性快感缺失

anorthography [ˌænɔːˈθɔgrəfi] *n* 正规书写不能

anorthopia [ˌænɔːˈθəupiə] *n* 偏视;斜视

anorthoscope [æˈnɔːθəskəup] *n* 弱视镜(将两个分离像连在一起成为一个完整的视像)

anorthosis [ˌænɔːˈθəusis] *n* (阴茎)挺直不能,无勃起功能(一种阳萎型)

anoscope [ˈeinəskəup] *n* 肛门镜 | **anoscopy** [əˈnɔskəpi] *n* 肛门镜检查[术]

anosigmoidoscopy [ˌeinəuˌsigmɔiˈdɔskəpi] *n* 直肠乙状结肠镜检查 | **anosigmoidoscopic** [ˌeinəusigˌmɔidəˈskɔpik] *a*

anosmatic [ˌænɔzˈmætik] *a* 嗅觉缺失的,嗅觉迟钝的

anosmia [æˈnɔzmiə], **anosphresia** [ˌænɔsˈfriːziə] *n* 嗅觉缺失 | **anosmic** [æˈnɔzmik] *a*

anosognosia [æˌnəusəˈnəuziə] *n* 病感失认[症]

anospinal [ˌeinəuˈspainl] *a* 肛门脊髓的

anosteoplasia [æˌnɔstiəuˈpleiziə] *n* 骨成形不全

anostosis [ˌænɔsˈtəusis] *n* 骨发育不全

anotia [æˈnəuʃiə] *n* 无耳畸形

anotropia [ˌænəˈtrəupiə] *n* 上显斜视(上斜视)

anotus [æˈnəutəs] *n* 无耳畸胎

anourethral [ˌeinəujuəˈriːθrəl] *a* 肛门尿道的

ANOVA analysis of variance 方差分析

anovaginal [ˌeinəuˌvædʒinl] *a* 肛门阴道的

anovarism [æˈnəuvərizəm], **anovaria** [ˌænəuˈvɛəriə], **anovarianism** [ˌænəuˈvɛəriənizəm] *n* 无卵巢[畸形]

anovesical [ˌeinəuˈvesikəl] *a* 肛门膀胱的

anovular [æˈnɔvjulə], **anovulatory** [æˈnɔvjuləˌtəri] *a* 不排卵的,无排卵性的

anovulation [ˌænɔvjuˈleiʃən] *n* 不排卵

anovulomenorrhea [æˌnɔvjuləuˌmenəˈriːə] *n* 不排卵性月经,无卵月经

anoxemia [ˌænɔkˈsiːmia] *n* 缺氧血症,血缺氧 | **anoxemic** [ˌænɔkˈsiːmik] *a*

anoxia [æˈnɔksiə] *n* 缺氧[症] | altitude ~ 高空缺氧 / anemic ~ 贫血性缺氧 / anoxic ~ 缺氧性缺氧 / ~ neonatorum 新生儿缺氧 / stagnant ~ 淤滞性缺氧,循环障碍性缺氧 | **anoxic** [æˈnɔksik] *a*

anoxiate [əˈnɔksieit] *vt* 使缺氧

Anoxyphotobacteria [əˌnɔksiˌfəutəubækˈtiəriə] *n* 厌氧发光杆菌纲

ANP atrial natriuretic peptide 心房钠尿肽

ANS anterior nasal spine 鼻前棘; autonomic nervous system 自主神经系统

ansa [ˈænsə] ([复] **ansae** [ˈænsiː]) *n*【拉】襻

ansate [ˈænseit] *a* 有柄的,襻状的

Ansbacher unit [ˈɑːnsbɑːkə] (Stefan Ansbacher) 安施巴克单位(一种维生素 K 剂量单位)

anseriform [ˈænseriˌfɔːm] *a* 雁形目的

Anseriformes [ˌænseriˈfɔːmiːz] *n* 雁形目
anserine [ˈænsərain] *a* 鹅的,鹅状的 [ˈænsəriːn] *n* 鹅肌肽
anserinus [ˌænsəˈrainəs] *a* 鹅的,鹅状的
ansiform [ˈænsifɔːm] *a* 襻状的
Anstie's limit(rule) [ˈænsti] (Francis E. Anstie) 安斯提极限(人寿保险检查规则:成人能饮用纯乙醇而无损害的最大限量为每日 42.5 g) | ~ reagent 安斯提试剂(重铬酸钾 3.33 g,浓硫酸 250 ml,加水配成 500 ml) / ~ test 安斯提试验(检尿醇)
ant [ænt] *n* 蚁 | fire ~ 火蚁
ant- 见 anti
ant. anterior 前的
antacid [æntˈæsid] *a* 抗酸的 *n* 抗酸药
antagonism [ænˈtægənizəm] *n* 拮抗,相反
antagonist [ænˈtægənist] *n* 对抗肌,拮抗肌;拮抗物,拮抗药,拮抗剂;对殆牙 | aldosterone ~ 醛固酮拮抗剂 / associated ~s 协同对抗肌 / competitive ~ 竞争性拮抗物,抗代谢[产]物 / direct ~s 直接对抗肌,直接拮抗肌 / enzyme ~ 酶拮抗物,抗代谢[产]物 / metabolic ~ 抗代谢[产]物 / narcotic ~ 麻醉药拮抗药 / sulfonamide ~ 磺胺对抗药
antagonistic [ænˌtægəˈnistik] *a* 对抗[性]的;有反作用的
antalgesic [æntælˈdʒiːzik], **antalgic** [ænˈtældʒik] *a* 止痛的 *n* 镇痛药
antalkaline [ænˈtælkəˌlain] *a* 解碱的 *n* 解碱药
antaphrodisiac [ˌæntæfrəuˈdiziæk] *a* 抗性欲的,抑制性欲的 *n* 制欲药
antapoplectic [ˌæntæpəˈplektik] *a* 防止中风的 *n* [防止]中风药
antarthritic [ˌæntɑːˈθritik] *a* 抗关节炎的 *n* 抗关节炎药
antasthenic [ˌæntæsˈθenik] *a* 恢复体力的 *n* 恢复体力药
antasthmatic [ˌæntæsˈmætik] *a* 止喘的,镇喘的 *n* 止喘药,镇喘药
antatrophic [ˌæntəˈtrɔfik] *a* 防萎缩的
antazoline [ænˈtæzəliːn] *n* 安他唑啉(抗心律失常药,抗组胺药) | ~ hydrochloride 盐酸安他唑啉 / ~ phosphate 磷酸安他唑啉
ante- [前缀][在]前
antebrachium [ˌæntiˈbreikiəm] *n* 前臂
antecardium [æntiˈkɑːdiəm] *n* 腹上部
antecedent [ˌæntiˈsiːdənt] *n* 前体,先质 | plasma thromboplastin ~ (PTA) 血浆凝血激酶前质(凝血因子Ⅺ)
ante cibum [ˈænti ˈsaibəm]【拉】饭前[服]
antecubital [ˌæntiˈkjubitl] *a* 肘前的
antecurvature [ˌæntiˈkəːvətʃə] *n* 前弯,轻度前屈
antefebrile [ˌæntiˈfiːbrail] *a* 发热前的
anteflect [ˈæntiflekt] *vi* 前屈
anteflexed [ˌæntiˈflekst] *a* 前屈的
anteflexio [ˌæntiˈfleksiəu] *n*【拉】前屈 | ~ uteri 子宫前屈
anteflexion [ˌæntiˈflekʃən] *n* 前屈;子宫前屈
antegrade [ˈæntigreid] *a* 前进的,顺行的
antelocation [ˌæntiləuˈkeiʃən] *n* 前移(指器官)
antemeridian [ˌæntiməˈridiən] *a* 午前的
ante meridiem [ˌænti məˈridiəm]【拉】午前,上午
antemetic [ˌæntiˈmetik] *a* 止吐的 *n* 止吐药,镇吐药
ante mortem [ˈænti ˈmɔːtəm]【拉】死前
antemortem [ˌæntiˈmɔːtəm] *a* 死前的
antenatal [ˌæntiˈneit] *a* 出生前的,产前的
antenna [ænˈtenə] ([复] **antennae** [ænˈteniː] 或 **antennas**) *n* 触角 | **~ry** [ænˈtenəri] *a*
antepartal [ˌæntiˈpɑːtl] *a* 分娩前的,产前的
antepartum [ˌæntiˈpɑːtəm] *a*【拉】分娩前的,产前的
ante partum [ˈænti ˈpɑːtəm]【拉】分娩前,产前
antephase [ˈæntifeiz] *n* (核分裂)前期
antephialtic [ˌæntefiˈæltik] *a* 抗梦魇的,抗夜惊的
anteposition [ˌæntipəˈziʃən] *n* 前位(如子宫)
anteprostate [ˌæntiˈprɔsteit] *n* 尿道球腺
anteprostatitis [ˌæntiprɔstəˈtaitis] *n* 尿道球腺炎
antepyretic [ˌæntipaiˈretik] *a* 发热前的
antergia [ænˈtəːdʒiə], **antergy** [ˈæntədʒi] *n* 对抗作用,拮抗作用
antergic [ænˈtəːdʒik] *a* 对抗的,拮抗的(用于拮抗肌)
anteriad [ænˈtiəriæd] *ad* 向前
anterior [ænˈtiəriə] *a* 前的
antero- [前缀]前
anteroclusion [ˌæntərɔˈkluːʒən] *n* 前咬合,下颌前突样殆(亦称近中殆)
anteroexternal [ˌæntərəueksˈtəːnl] *a* 前外的,前外侧的(最好用 anterolateral)
anterograde [ˈæntərəugreid] *a* 前进的,顺行的
anteroinferior [ˌæntərəuinˈfiəriə] *a* 前下的
anterointernal [ˌæntərəuinˈtəːnl] *a* 前内的,前内侧的(最好用 anteromedial)
anterolateral [ˌæntərəuˈlætərəl] *a* 前外侧的
anteromedial [ˌæntərəuˈmiːdiəl] *a* 前内侧的
anteromedian [ˌæntərəuˈmiːdiən] *a* 前正中的
anteroposterior [ˌæntərəupɔsˈtiəriə] *a* 前后[位]的(X 线学中指光束的方向)
anteroseptal [ˌæntərəuˈseptl] *a* (房室)隔前的
anterosuperior [ˌæntərəusju(ː)ˈpiəriə] *a* 前上的
anterotic [ˌæntiˈrɔtik] *a* 制欲的 *n* 制欲药

anteroventral [ˌæntərəuˈventrəl] *a* 前腹侧的
antetorsion [ˌæntiˈtɔːʃən] *n* 前扭转
antetype [ˈæntitaip] *n* 先型,原型
anteversion [ˌæntiˈvəːʃən] *n* 前倾
antevert [ˈæntivəːt] *vt* 前倾
antexed [ænˈtekst] *a* 前屈的
antexion [ænˈtekʃən] *n* 前屈(如脊柱前凸)
anthelix [ˈænthiːliks] *n* 对耳轮
anthelmintic [ˌænthelˈmintik], **anthelminthic** [ˌænthelˈminθik] *a* 抗蠕虫的 *n* 抗蠕虫药
anthelmycin [ænθelˈmaisin] *n* 安太霉素(抗蠕虫药)
anthelone [æntˈhiːləun] *n* 尿抑胃素;抗溃疡素
anthelotic [ˌænthiːˈlɔtik] *a* 除胼胝的 *n* 除胼胝药,鸡眼药
Anthemis [ˈænθimis] *n* 春黄菊属;罗马甘菊
anthemorrhagic [ˌænthemәˈrædʒik] *a* 止血的 *n* 止血药
anther [ˈænθə] *n* 花粉囊,花药
antheridium [ˌænθəˈridiəm] ([复] **antheridia** [ˌænθəˈridiə]) *n* 雄器
antherozoid [ˈænθərəˌzɔid] *n* 游动精子
antherpetic [ˌænthəːˈpetik] *a* 防治疱疹的
anthiolimine [ˌænθaiˈəulimiːn] *n* 安锑锂明(抗血吸虫药)
anthocyanidin [ˌænθəusaiˈænidin] *n* 花色素
anthocyanin [ˌænθəuˈsaiənin] *n* 花色苷
anthocyaninemia [ˌænθəusaiəniˈniːmiə] *n* 花色苷血症
anthocyaninuria [ˌænθəusaiəniˈnjuəriə] *n* 花色苷尿
Anthomyia [ˌænθəˈmaijə] *n* 花蝇属
Anthomyiidae [ˌænθəumaiˈaiidiː] *n* 花蝇科
anthophobia [ˌænθəˈfəubiə] *n* 花恐怖,恐花症
Anthoxanthum [ˌænθəuˈzænθəm] *n* 禾本属
Anthoxium [ænˈθɔksiəm] *n* 芳香膜菊属
Anthozoa [ˌænθəˈzəuə] *n* 珊瑚动物纲
anthracene [ˈænθrəsiːn] *n* 蒽
anthracenedione [ˌænθrəsiːnˈdaiən] *n* 蒽二酮(任何一类蒽醌衍生物,有些具有抗肿瘤性质)
anthracic [ænˈθræsik] *a* 炭疽的;炭疽样的
anthrac(o)- [构词成分]煤;炭;痈
anthracoid [ˈænθrəkɔid] *a* 炭疽样的;痈样的
anthracometer [ˌænθrəˈkɔmitə] *n* 二氧化碳测量器
anthracomucin [ˌænθrəkəuˈmjuːsin] *n* 炭疽菌黏液素
anthraconecrosis [ˌænθrekəuneˈkrəusis] *n* 黑色干性坏死
anthracosilicosis [ˌænθrəkəusiliˈkəusis] *n* 炭末石末沉着病
anthracosis [ænθrəˈkəusis] *n* 炭末沉着[病] | ~ linguae 黑舌[病] | **anthracotic** [ˌænθrəˈkɔtik] *a*
anthracotherapy [ˌænθrəkəuˈθerəpi] *n* 炭疗法
anthracycline [ˌænθrəˈsaikliːn] *n* 蒽环类抗生素
anthragallol [ˌænθrəˈgælɔl] *n* 三羟基蒽醌
anthralin [ˈænθrəlin] *n* 地蒽酚(外用治疗皮肤真菌病、慢性湿疹及其他皮肤病)
anthramycin [ˌænθrəˈmaisin] *n* 安曲霉素(抗肿瘤抗生素)
anthranilate [ˌænθrəˈnileit] *n* 邻氨基苯甲酸
anthranilic acid [ˌænθrəˈnilik] 邻氨基苯甲酸,氨茴酸
anthraquinone [ˌænθrəˈkwinəun] *n* 蒽醌
anthrarobin [ˌænθrəˈrəubin] *n* 1, 2, 10-蒽三酚(10% ~20% 软膏剂,用于治牛皮癣及各种皮肤病,亦用作杀寄生虫药)
anthrax [ˈænθræks] *n* 炭疽 | cutaneous ~ 皮肤炭疽 / inhalational ~ 吸入性炭疽 / meningeal ~, cerebral ~ 脑膜炭疽,脑炭疽 / pulmonary ~ 肺炭疽 / symptomatic ~ 气肿性炭疽,黑腿病
anthrop(o)- [构词成分]人类,人
anthropobiology [ˌænθrəpəubaiˈɔlədʒi] *n* 人类生物学
anthropocentric [ˌænθrəpəuˈsentrik] *a* 人类中心的
anthropodesoxycholic acid [ˌænθrəpəu diˌzɔksiˈkəulik] 12-脱氧胆酸,鹅脱氧胆酸
anthropogeny [ˌænθrəˈpɔdʒini] *n* 人类发生,人类起源
anthropography [ˌænθrəˈpɔgrəfi] *n* 人类分布学,人种志
anthropoid [ˈænθrəpɔid] *a* 似人的,类人的 *n* 类人猿
Anthropoidea [ˌænθrəˈpɔidiə] *n* 类人猿亚目
anthropokinetics [ˌænθrəpəukiˈnetiks] *n* 人类活动学(从生物和自然科学、心理学以及社会学的特殊领域中,研究整体人类的活动)
anthropology [ˌænθrəˈpɔlədʒi] *n* 人类学 | criminal ~ 人类犯罪学 / cultural ~ 文化人类学 / physical ~ 人类体格学 | **anthropologic(al)** [ˌænθrəpəˈlɔdʒik(əl)] *a* / **anthropologist** *n* 人类学者,人类学家
anthropometer [ˌænθrəˈpɔmitə] *n* 人体测量器
anthropometry [ˌænθrəˈpɔmitri] *n* 人体测量学 | **anthropometric(al)** [ˌænθrəpɔˈmetrik(əl)] *a* / **anthropometrist** *n* 人体测量学家
anthropomorphic [ˌænθrəpəuˈmɔːfik] *a* 有人形的,拟人的
anthropomorphism [ˌænθrəpəuˈmɔːfizəm] *n* 拟人说(用人类的形象或性格来解释非人类的对象,如各种动物、无生物等)
anthropomorphous [ˌænθrəpəuˈmɔːfəs] *a* 有人形的,似人的

anthroponomy [ˌænθrəˈpɔnəmi] *n* 人体进化论,人类进化学
anthroponosis [ˌænθrəpəˈnəusis] *n* 人类传染病 | **anthroponotic** [ˌænθrəpəˈnɔtik] *a*
anthropopathy [ˌænθrəˈpɔpəθi] *n* 情感拟人说(用人类的情感来解释非人类的对象)
anthropophagy [ˌænθrəˈpɔfədʒi] *n* 嗜食人肉;食人肉色情倒错
anthropophilic [ˌænθrəpəuˈfilik] *a* 嗜人类的,嗜人血的(指蚊)
anthropophobia [ˌænθrəpəuˈfəubiə] *n* 人群恐怖
anthroposcopy [ˌænθrəˈpɔskəpi] *n* 人类体型审定(根据目观而不用测量方法)
anthroposophy [ˌænθrəˈpɔsəfi] *n* 人智学
anthropozoonosis [ˌænθrəpəuˌzəuəˈnəusis] ([复] **anthropozoonoses** [ˌænθrəpəuˌzəuəˈnəusiːz]) *n* 人兽病,人与动物病
anthropozoophilic [ˌænθrəpəuˌzəuəˈfilik] *a* 嗜人兽血的(指蚊)
anthysteric [ˌænthisˈterik] *a* 抗癔症的 *n* 抗癔症药
anti-, ant- [前缀]抗,解,抑制,取消
antiabortifacient [ˌæntiəˌbɔːtiˈfeiʃənt] *a* 防流产的,安胎的,促受孕的 *n* 防流产药,安胎药,促受孕药
antiabortionist [ˌæntiəˈbɔːfənist] *n* 反对堕胎者
antiaditis [ˌæntiəˈdaitis] *n* 扁桃体炎
antiadrenergic [ˌæntiədreˈnəːdʒik] *a* 抗肾上腺素能的 *n* 抗肾上腺素药
antiagglutinating [ˌæntiəˈgluːtineitiŋ] *a* 抗凝集[作用]的
antiagglutinin [ˌæntiəˈgluːtinin] *n* 抗凝集素
antiaggressin [ˌæntiəˈgresin] *n* 抗攻击素(重复注射攻击素在体内形成的一种物质,以对抗攻击素的作用)
antialbumin [ˌæntiˈælbjumin] *n* 抗清蛋白
antialexin [ˌæntiəˈleksin] *n* 抗补体 | **antialexic** *a*
antiamboceptor [ˌæntiˈæmbəˌseptə] *n* 抗介体,抗体(对抗介体作用的物质,亦称抗免疫体)
antiamebic [ˌæntiəˈmiːbik] *a* 抗阿米巴的 *n* 抗阿米巴药
antiamylase [ˌæntiˈæmileis] *n* 抗淀粉酶
antianaphylactin [ˌæntiænəfiˈlæktin] *n* 抗过敏素
antianaphylaxis [ˌæntiænəfiˈlæksis] *n* 抗过敏,脱[过]敏
antiandrogen [ˌæntiˈændrədʒən] *n* 抗雄激素[物质]
antianemic [ˌæntiəˈniːmik] *a* 抗贫血的,补血的 *n* 抗贫血药,补血药
antianginal [ˌæntiænˈdʒainəl] *a* 抗心绞痛的 *n* 抗心绞痛药
antianopheline [ˌæntiəˈnɔfiliːn] *a* 抗按蚊的
antiantibody [ˌæntiˈæntiˌbɔdi] *n* 抗抗体(旨在对抗其他抗体〈免疫球蛋白〉分子上的抗原决定簇的一种抗体)
antiantidote [ˌæntiˈæntiˌdəut] *n* 抗解毒药
antiantitoxin [ˌæntiˌæntiˈtɔksin] *n* 抗抗毒素(用抗毒素免疫时所形成的一种抗体,以对抗抗毒素的作用)
antianxiety [ˌæntiæŋˈzaiəti] *a* 抗焦虑的 *n* 抗焦虑药
antiapoplectic [ˌæntiˌæpəˈplektik] *a* 防止中风的
antiapoptotic [ˌæntiˌæpɔpˈtɔtik] *a* 抗[细胞]凋亡的,抑制[细胞]凋亡的
antiarachnolysin [ˌæntiˌærəkˈnɔlisin] *n* 抗蛛毒溶血素
antiarin [ænˈtiərin] *n* 见血封喉苷,弩箭子苷(从前用作心脏抑制药)
Antiaris [ˌæntiˈɛəris] *n* 见血封喉属 | ~ toxicaria 见血封喉(用作箭毒)
antiarrhythmic [ˌæntiəˈriθmik] *a* 抗心律失常的 *n* 抗心律失常药
antiarsenin [ˌæntiˈɑːsinin] *n* 抗砷素(由于亚砷酸免疫剂量而在体内产生的非砷性物质)
antiarthritic [ˌæntiɑːˈθritik] *a* 抗关节炎的 *n* 抗关节炎药
antiasthmatic [ˌæntiæsˈmætik] *a* 止喘的,镇喘的 *n* 止喘药,镇喘药
antiatherogenic [ˌæntiˌæθərəuˈdʒenik] *a* 抗动脉粥样化的
antiautolysin [ˌæntiɔːˈtɔlisin] *n* 抗自[身]溶素
antiauxin [æntiˈɔːksin] *n* 抗促长素,抗植物生长素
antibacterial [ˌæntibækˈtiəriəl] *a* 抗细菌的 *n* 抗菌药,抗菌物
antibechic [ˌæntiˈbekik] *a* 镇咳的 *n* 镇咳药
antibiosis [ˌæntibaiˈəusis] *n* 抗生作用
antibiotic [ˌæntibaiˈɔtik] *a* 抗生的 *n* 抗生素 | bactericidal ~ 杀菌性抗生素 / bacteriostatic ~ 抑菌性抗生素 / broad-spectrum ~ 广谱抗生素 / oral ~ 口服抗生素
antibiotin [ˌæntiˈbaiətin] *n* 抗生物素
antiblastic [ˌæntiˈblæstik] *a* 抑制细菌发育的,制菌的
antiblennorrhagic [ˌæntiblenəˈrædʒik] *a* 抗淋病的,防治淋病的 *n* 抗淋病药,防治淋病药
antibody [ˈæntiˌbɔdi] *n* 抗体 | acetylcholine receptor antibodies 乙酰胆碱受体抗体 / anaphylactic ~ 过敏抗体 / anti-acetylcholine receptor (anti-AChR) antibodies 抗乙酰胆碱受体抗体 / anti-cardiolipin ~ 抗心脂抗体 / anti-centromere ~ 抗着丝点抗体 / anti-D ~ 抗 D 抗体 / anti-DNA ~ 抗 DNA 抗体 / anti-ENA ~ 抗 ENA 抗体 /

anti-glomerular basement membrane (anti-GBM) anti-bodies 抗肾小球基膜抗体 / anti-bodies 抗肾小球基膜抗体/ anti-histone ~ 抗组蛋白抗体 / anti-idiotype ~ 抗独特型抗体 / anti-microsomal antibodies 抗微粒体抗体 / antimitochondrial anti-bodies 抗线粒体抗体(亦称线粒体抗体) / anti-nuclear antibodies(ANA) 抗核抗体 / anti-nucle-olar ~ 抗核仁抗体 / anti-RNA ~ 抗 RNA 抗体 / antireceptor antibodies 抗受体抗体 / antithyro-globulin antibodies 抗甲状腺球蛋白抗体 / anti-thyroid antibodies 抗甲状腺抗体 / auto-anti-idio-typic antibodies 自身抗独特型抗体 / autologous ~自身抗体 / bispecific ~ 双重特异性抗体(亦称杂交抗体) / blocking ~, inhibiting ~ 封闭性抗体,抑制性抗体 / cold ~, cold reactive ~ 冷[型]抗体,冷反应性抗体 / complement-fixing ~ 补体结合性抗体 / complete ~ 完全抗体(一种 Rh 抗体,能在盐水中直接凝集 Rh 阳性红细胞) / cross-reacting ~ 交叉反应[性]抗体 / cy-totropic ~, cytophilic ~ 亲细胞抗体,嗜细胞[性]抗体 / despeciated ~ 去种特异性抗体 / duck virus hepatitis yolk ~ 鸭病毒性肝炎卵黄抗体 / heterocytotropic ~ 亲异种细胞抗体 / heter-ogenetic ~ 异种抗体 / heterophile ~ 嗜异性抗体 / homocytotropic ~ 亲同种细胞抗体 / hybrid ~ 杂交抗体,双重特异性抗体 / incomplete ~ 不完全抗体(指能与抗原结合但不出现可见反应的抗体,亦指单价抗体的一种丙种球蛋白) / lipoidotropic ~ 亲类脂抗体 / maternal ~ 母体抗体(在母体内产生并传至胎循环的抗体,例如 IgG 类抗体) / mitochondrial antibodies 线粒体抗体,抗线粒体抗体 / monoclonal antibodies 单克隆抗体 / natural antibodies 天然抗体 / neutrali-zing ~ 中和抗体 / polyclonal ~ 多克隆抗体 / protective ~ 保护[性]抗体(对传染性因子具有免疫性的抗体,见于被动免疫) / reaginic ~ 反应素 / Rh ~ Rh 抗体(Rh 抗原的对应抗体) / TSH displacing ~ (TDA) 促甲状腺激素置换性抗体,促甲状腺激素结合抑制性免疫球蛋白/ warm ~, warm-reactive ~ 温[型]抗体,温反应性抗体(在 37 ℃时反应较强) / xenocytophilic ~ 嗜异种细胞抗体 / 7S ~ 7S 抗体(具有沉降系数 7S 的抗体,包括所有免疫球蛋白类 IgG 和 IgD 以及某些 IgA 类)

antibrachium [ˌæntiˈbreikiəm] *n* 前臂

antibromic [ˌæntiˈbrəumik] *a* 除臭的,抗臭的 *n* 除臭剂

antibubonic [ˌæntibju(ː)ˈbɔnik] *a* 抗腺鼠疫的

anticachectic [ˌæntikəˈkektik] *a* 抗恶病质的 *n* 抗恶病质药

anticalculous [ˌæntiˈkælkjuləs] *a* 抗石的;防牙垢的

anticancer [ˌæntiˈkænsə] *n* 抗癌 | **anticancerous** [ˌæntiˈkænsərəs] *a* 抗癌的

anticarcinogen [ˌæntikɑːˈsinədʒən] *n* 抗癌药

anticarcinogenic [ˌæntikɑːˌsinəˈdʒenik] *a* 防癌的,抗癌的

anticardium [ˌæntiˈkɑːdiəm] *n* 腹上部

anticariogenic [ˌæntiˌkɛəriəuˈdʒenik], **anticarious** [ˌæntiˈkɛəriəs] *a* 防龋的 *n* 防龋[齿]药

anticatalyst [ˌæntiˈkætəlist], **anticatalyzer** [ˌæntiˈkætəlaizə] *n* 反催化剂,抗催化剂

anticataphylaxis [ˌæntiˌkætəfiˈlæksis] *n* 抗防卫力毁灭 | **anticataphylactic** [ˌæntiˌkætəfiˈlæktik] *a* 抗防卫力毁灭的 *n* 抗防卫力毁灭药

anticathexis [ˌæntikəˈθeksis] *n* 相反贯注,相反注情

anticathode [ˌæntiˈkæθəud] *n* 对阴极(真空管与阴极对面的部分);靶

anticephalalgic [ˌæntisefəˈlældʒik] *a* 抗头痛的

anticheirotonus [ˌæntikaiˈrɔtənəs] *n* 拇指痉曲

antichlorotic [ˌæntikləˈrɔtik] *a* 抗萎黄病的

anticholelithogenic [ˌæntiˌkəuliˌliθəˈdʒenik] *a* 消胆结石的 *n* 消胆结石药

anticholerin [ˌæntiˈkɔlərin] *n* 抗霍乱菌素

anticholesteremic [ˌæntikəˌlestəˈriːmik], **anticholesterolemic** [ˌæntikeˌlestərəuˈliːmik] *a* 抗胆固醇血的 *n* 抗胆固醇血药

anticholinergic [ˌæntiˌkəuliˈnəːdʒik] *a* 抗胆碱能的 *n* 抗胆碱药(亦称副交感神经阻滞药)

anticholinesterase [ˌæntikəuliˈnestəreis] *n* 抗胆碱酯酶

antichymosin [ˌæntiˈkaiməsin] *n* 抗凝乳酶

anticipate [ænˈtisipeit] *vt* 提前出现,先期发生(指病或症状)

anticipation [ænˌtisiˈpeiʃən] *n* 提前出现;早现[遗传](指某种遗传病的发病时间一代比一代早,现在认为是一种赝象,这可能与检查方法有关)

anticlinal [ˌæntiˈklain] *a* 对向倾斜的,倾向对侧的

anticnemion [ˌæntikˈniːmiɔn] *n* 胫

anticoagulant [ˌæntikəuˈægjulənt] *a* 抗凝的 *n* 抗凝血药,抗凝剂

anticoagulation [ˌæntikəuˌægjuˈleiʃən] *n* 抗凝[作用]

anticoagulative [ˌæntikəuˈægjuˌleitiv] *a* 抗凝的

anticoagulin [ˌæntikəuˈægjulin] *n* 抗凝血素

anticoccidial [ˌæntikɔkˈsidiəl] *n* 抗球虫药,球虫抑制药

anticodon [ˌæntiˈkəudən] *n* 反密码子(转移 RNA 上的核苷酸三联体与信使 RNA 内的密码子成互补关系)

anticollagenase [ˌæntikɔˈlædʒineis] *n* 抗胶原酶

anticomplement [ˌæntiˈkɔmplimənt] *n* 抗补体 |

anticomplementary [ˌæntiˌkɔmpliˈmentəri] *a*
anticonceptive [ˌæntikənˈseptiv] *a* 避孕的 *n* 避孕药
anticoncipiens [ˌæntikənˈsipiənz] *n* 避孕药
anticonvulsant [ˌæntikənˈvʌlsənt], **anticonvulsive** [ˌæntikənˈvʌlsiv] *a* 抗惊厥的 *n* 抗惊厥药
anticrotin [ˌæntiˈkrəutin] *n* 抗巴豆毒素
anticurare [ˌæntikjuˈrɑːri] *n* 抗箭毒药(抗箭毒对骨骼肌的作用)
anticus [ænˈtaikəs] *a*【拉】前的
anticutin [æntiˈkjuːtin] *n* 中和结核菌素[皮肤反应]抗体(某些结核病人血内的一种抗体,加入结核菌素使之中和,因此不会产生皮肤反应)
anticyclic acid [ˌæntiˈsaiklik] 抗环酸
anticytolysin [ˌæntisaiˈtɔlisin] *n* 抗溶细胞素
anticytotoxin [ˌæntiˌsaitəuˈtɔksin] *n* 抗细胞毒素
anti-D 抗 D 抗体
antidepressant [ˌæntidiˈpresənt] *a* 抗抑郁的 *n* 抗抑郁药 | tricyclic ~s 三环抗抑郁药
antidiabetic [ˌæntiˌdaiəˈbetik] *a* 抗糖尿病的 *n* 抗糖尿病药
antidiabetogenic [ˌæntidaiəˌbiːtəuˈdʒenik] *a* 抗糖尿病发生的 *n* 抗糖尿病发生药
antidiarrheal [ˌæntiˌdaiəˈriəl], **antidiarrheic** [ˌæntiˌdaiəˈriːik] *a* 止泻的 *n* 止泻药
antidiastase [ˌæntiˈdaiəsteis] *n* 抗淀粉[水解]酶
antidinic [ˌæntiˈdinik] *a* 防止眩晕的
antidipsetic [ˌæntidipˈsetik] *a* 止渴的
antidipticum [ˌæntiˈdiptikəm] *n* 止渴药
antidiuresis [ˌæntiˌdaijuəˈriːsis] *n* 抗利尿
antidiuretic [ˌæntiˌdaijuəˈretik] *a* 抗利尿的 *n* 抗利尿药
antidiuretin [ˌæntidaijuəˈriːtin] *n* 后叶加压素,抗利尿素
antidote [ˈæntidəut] *n* 解毒药;矫正方法 | ~ against arsenic 解砷毒药 / "universal" ~ "万能"解毒药 | **antidotal** [ˌæntiˈdəutl], **antidotic** [ˌæntiˈdɔtik] *a* 解毒的
antidromic [ˌæntiˈdrɔmik] *a* 逆向的,逆行的(指脊髓后根的神经元)
antidysenteric [ˌæntiˌdisənˈterik] *a* 抗痢疾的 *n* 抗痢疾药
antidysentericum [ˌæntiˌdisənˈterikəm] *n* 抗痢疾药
antidyskinetic [ˌæntiˌdiskiˈnetik] *a* 抗运动障碍的 *n* 抗运动障碍药
antieczematic [ˌæntiekziˈmætik] *a* 抗湿疹的 *n* 抗湿疹药 | **antieczematous** [ˌæntiekˈzemətəs] *a*
antiedemic [ˌæntii(ː)ˈdemik] *a* 消水肿的 *n* 消水肿药 | **antiedematous** [ˌæntii(ː)ˈdemətəs] *a*
antiemetic [ˌæntiiˈmetik] *a* 止吐的 *n* 止吐药,镇吐药
antiemulsin [ˌæntiiˈmʌlsin] *n* 抗苦杏仁酶,抗氰糖酶
antiendotoxin [ˌæntiˌendəuˈtɔksin] *n* 抗内毒素 | **antiendotoxic** [ˌæntiˌendəuˈtɔksik] *a*
antienzyme [ˌæntiˈenzaim] *n* 抗酶
antiepileptic [ˌæntiˌepiˈleptik] *a* 抗癫痫的 *n* 镇癫痫药
antiepithelial [ˌæntiˌepiˈθiːliəl] *a* 抗上皮的
antierotica [ˌæntiiˈrɔtikə] *n* 制欲药
antiesterase [ˌæntiˈestəreis] *n* 抗酯酶
antiestrogen [ˌæntiˈestrədʒən] *a* 抗雌激素的 *n* 抗雌激素
antiestrogenic [ˌæntiˌestrəˈdʒenik] *a* 抗雌激素的
antifebrile [ˌæntiˈfiːbrail, -ˈfebril] *a* 退热的 *n* 退热药
antifebrin [ˌæntiˈfebrin] *n* 退热冰,乙酰苯胺
antifertilizin [ˌæntiˈfəːtiˌlaizin] *n* 抗受精素
antifibrillatory [ˌæntiˈfibriləˌtəri] *a* 抗心脏纤颤的 *n* 抗心脏纤颤药
antifibrinolysin [ˌæntiˌfaibriˈnɔlisin] *n* 抗纤维蛋白溶素,抗纤维蛋白溶酶
antifibrinolytic [ˌæntiˌfaibrinəˈlitik] *a* 抗纤维蛋白溶解的
antifibrotic [ˌænifaiˈbrɔtik] *a* 抗纤维化的 *n* 抗纤维化药
antifilarial [ˌæntifiˈlεəriəl] *a* 抗丝虫的 *n* 抗丝虫药
antiflatulent [ˌæntiˈflætjulənt] *a* 抗[肠胃]气胀的 *n* 抗[肠胃]气胀药
antiflux [ˈæntiflʌks] *n* 抗焊媒
antifol [ˈæntifəul] *n* 抗叶酸剂,叶酸拮抗剂
antifolate [ˌæntiˈfəuleit] *n* 抗叶酸剂,叶酸拮抗剂
antifungal [ˌæntiˈfʌŋgəl] *a* 抗真菌的 *n* 抗真菌药
antigalactic [ˌæntigəˈlæktik] *a* 制乳的 *n* 制乳药
antigametocyte [ˌæntigəˈmiːtəsait] *n* 抗配子体
antigen [ˈæntidʒən] *n* 抗原 | acetone-insoluble ~ 丙酮不容性抗原 / allergic ~ 变应性抗原,变应原 / allogeneic ~ 同种异体抗原 / Am ~s Am 抗原 / Au ~, Australia ~ 澳大利亚抗原,乙型肝炎表面抗原 / B ~ B[血型]抗原(K 抗原复合物的抗原成分) / beef heart ~ 牛心抗原 / blood group ~s 血型抗原 / capsular ~ 荚膜抗原 / carbohydrate ~s 糖抗原 / carcinoembryonic ~ (CEA) 癌胚抗原 / chick embryo ~ 鸡胚抗原 / cholesterinized ~ 胆固醇抗原 / class Ⅰ ~s Ⅰ类抗原(主要组织相容性抗原,几乎见于所有细胞,人类红细胞为唯一明显例外) / class Ⅱ ~s Ⅱ类抗原(主要组织相容性抗原,仅见于免疫活性细胞,主要为 B 淋巴细胞和巨噬细胞) / class Ⅲ ~s Ⅲ类抗原(指定位在组织相容性复合物,如补体成分 C2, C4 和 B 因子的非组织相容性抗原) / common ~ 共同抗原(两种或两种以上

不同抗原分子中的抗原决定簇常导致抗原分子之间的交叉反应）/ common acute lymphoblastic leukemia ~（CALLA）急性淋巴细胞白血病共同抗原 / common leukocyte ~s 白细胞共同抗原 / complete ~ 完全抗原（能刺激免疫应答，并能与该应答的产物〈如抗体〉发生反应的抗原）/ conjugated ~ 结合抗原 / cross-reacting ~ 交叉反应（性）抗原 / D ~ D（血型）抗原（Rh 血型系的红细胞抗原）/ delta ~ δ 抗原（包有一层乙型表面抗原的一种 32 ~ 37 nm 的 RNA 颗粒）/ E ~ E（血型）抗原（Rh 血型系的红细胞抗原）/ envelope ~s 包膜抗原（即 K 抗原）/ extratable nuclear ~s（ENA）可提取的核抗原 / F ~ F 抗原（见 Forssman antigen）/ febrile ~s 热病抗原（用于进行凝集反应试验，检肠道传染病）/ fetal ~s 胎儿抗原 / flagellar ~ 鞭毛抗原（即 H 抗原）/ Gm group ~ Gm 组抗原（在人的 γ 重链上 20 多种异型标记之一，一般位于 γ 链的 Fc 或 Fd 片段）/ H ~ H 抗原（有动力细菌的鞭毛抗原，亦称鞭毛抗原；H 物质，见 H substance）/ H-2 ~s H-2 抗原，小鼠组织相容性抗原 2（小鼠的主要组织相容性抗原）/ hepatitis B core ~（HBcAg）乙型肝炎核心抗原 / hepatitis B e ~（HBeAg）乙型肝炎 e 抗原 / hepatitis B surface ~（HBsAg）乙型肝炎表面抗原（原称澳大利亚抗原，因首次在澳大利亚土著居民中发现，故名。以前称肝炎相关抗原，血清肝炎抗原）/ heterogenetic ~，heterologous ~，heterophile ~ 异种抗原，嗜异性抗原 / Hikojima ~ 彦岛抗原（霍乱弧菌三种血清型之一）/ histocompatibility ~s 组织相容性抗原 / HLA ~ HLA 抗原（有核细胞表面的组织相容性抗原）/ homologous ~ 同种抗原 / H-Y ~ H-Y 抗原（由 Y 染色体基因决定的一种组织相容性抗原）/ Ia ~（Ⅰ region-associated）Ⅰ区相关抗原（见于小鼠 B 细胞、巨噬细胞、辅助细胞表面的Ⅱ类组织相容性抗原）/ Inaba ~ 稻叶抗原（霍乱弧菌三种血清型之一）/ Inv group ~ Inv 组抗原（三种同种抗原之一，在人免疫球蛋白 *k* 型轻链的恒定区）/ isogeneic ~ 同基因抗原，同源抗原 / isophile ~ 同种抗原 / K ~ K 抗原（一种细菌荚膜抗原）/ Kveim ~ 克温抗原（用人肉样组织，一般用淋巴结或脾脏制备的一种抗原）/ LD ~s，lymphocyte-defined ~s 淋巴细胞限定抗原 / lens ~s 晶状体抗原（眼晶状体在发育过程中形成的一系列蛋白质）/ lymphogranuloma venereum ~ 性病淋巴肉芽肿抗原 / M ~ M 抗原（一种型特异性抗原）/ major histocompatibility ~s 主要组织相容性抗原 / minor histocompatibility ~s 次要组织相容性抗原 / mouse brain ~ 鼠脑抗原 / Nègre ~ 内格雷抗原，结核杆菌抗原（用于血清试验，检结核病）/ NP ~ NP 抗原（痘病毒的核蛋白抗原）/ O ~，somatic ~ O 抗原，菌体抗原 / Ogawa ~ 小川抗原（霍乱弧菌三种血清型之一）/ oncofetal ~ 癌胚抗原 / organ-specific ~ 器官特异性抗原 / Oz ~ Oz 抗原（人类免疫球蛋白 λ 链上的抗原性标记）/ pancreatic oncofetal ~（POA）胰腺瘤胎抗原 / partial ~ 部分抗原，半抗原 / P-K ~s，Prausnitz-Küstner ~s P-K 抗原，被动转移皮肤反应抗原 / pollen ~ 花粉抗原 / private ~s 稀有抗原（低频率血型抗原，仅在个别宗族的成员中测出，故名）/ public ~s 常见抗原，共同抗原 / R ~ R 抗原（一种型特异性抗原，与 M 抗原相似，但不受胰蛋白酶消化作用）/ residue ~s 残余抗原（经自溶或经制备提纯抗原的方法从抗原复合物中分裂出的天然半抗原）/ S ~ S 抗原（一种耐热的可溶性病毒抗原）/ SD ~s，sero-defined（SD）~s，serologically defined（SD）~s SD 抗原，血清学鉴定抗原 / sequestered ~s 隐蔽抗原 / shock ~ 休克抗原 / species-specific ~s 种特异性抗原 / Stein's ~ 斯坦抗原，回归热螺旋体抗原 / T ~ T 抗原（一种非结构性补体结合病毒抗原）/ Tac ~ Tac 抗原（白细胞介素 2 受体）/ T-dependent ~ T 依赖性抗原 / T-independent ~ 非 T[细胞]依赖性抗原 / tissue-specific ~ 组织特异性抗原，器官特异性抗原 / transplantation ~s 组织相容性抗原 / tumor-associated ~ 肿瘤相关抗原 / tumor-specific ~ 肿瘤特异性抗原 / tumor-specific transplantation ~（TSTA）肿瘤特异性移植抗原 / V ~，Vi ~，virulence ~ 病毒抗原，毒力抗原 / VDRL ~（美国）性病研究所梅毒检查试验抗原（含心脂 0.03%、胆固醇 0.99% 和足量的卵磷酯〈以产生标准反应性〉的一种乙醇溶液）/ W ~ W 抗原（与鼠疫杆菌毒力有关的抗原）/ yolk sac ~ 卵黄囊抗原

antigenemia [ˌæntidʒiˈniːmiə] *n* 抗原血症

antigenemic [ˌæntidʒiˈniːmik] *a* 抗原血症的

antigenic [æntiˈdʒenik] *n* 抗原的 | **~ity** [ˌæntidʒiˈnisəti] *n* 抗原性

antigenotherapy [ˌæntiˌdʒenəuˈθerəpi]，**antigentotherapy** [ˌæntiˌdʒentəuˈθerəpi] *n* 抗原疗法

antigentophil [ˌæntiˈdʒentəfil]，**antigenophil** [ˌæntiˈdʒenəfil] *a* 嗜抗原的

antiglaucoma [ˌæntiˌglɔːˈkəumə] *n* 抗青光眼的，预防青光眼的

antiglobulin [ˌæntiˈglɔbjulin] *n* 抗球蛋白

antiglyoxalase [ˌæntiˌglaiˈɔksəleis] *n* 抗乙二醛酶

antigoitrogenic [ˌæntiˌgɔitrəuˈdʒenik] *a* 抗甲状腺肿发生的

antigonadotropic [ˌæntigɔnədəuˈtrɔpik] *a* 抗促性腺激素的

antigonorrheic [ˌæntiˌgɔnəˈriːik] *a* 抗淋病的

antigravity [ˌæntiˈgrævəti] *n* 抗重力

antigrowth [ˈæntigrəuθ] *a* 抗生长的

anti-HAA antibody hepatitis-associated antigen 抗肝炎相关抗原
antihallucinatory [ˌæntihəˈluːsinəˌtəri] *a* 抗幻觉的
anti-HBc antibody to hepatitis B core antigen (HBcAg) 抗乙型肝炎核心抗原的抗体
anti-HBs antibody to hepatitis B surface antigen (HBsAg) 抗乙型肝炎表面抗原的抗体
antihelix [ˌæntiˈhiːliks] *n* 对耳轮
antihelmintic [ˌætihelˈmintik] *a* 抗蠕虫的 *n* 抗蠕虫药
antihemagglutinin [ˌæntihemәˈgluːtinin] *a* 抗血凝素
antihemolysin [ˌæntihiːˈmɔlisin] *n* 抗溶血素
antihemolytic [ˌæntiˌhiːməˈlitik] *a* 抗溶血[性]的
antihemophilic [ˌæntiˌhiːməˈfilik] *a* 抗血友病的 *n* 抗血友病药
antihemorrhagic [æntiˌheməˈrædʒik] *a* 抗出血的 *n* 抗出血药
antiheterolysin [ˌæntiˌhetəˈrɔlisin] *n* 抗异种溶素
antihidrotic [ˌæntihiˈdrɔtik] *a* 止汗的 *n* 止汗药
antihistamine [ˌæntiˈhistəmi(ː)n] *n* 抗组胺药 | **antihistaminic** [ˌæntihistəˈminik] *a* 抗组胺的 *n* 抗组胺药
antihormone [ˌæntiˈhɔːməun] *n* 抗激素
antihyaluronidase [ˌæntihaiəljuːˈrɔnideis] *n* 抗透明质酸酶
antihydrophobic [ˌæntihaidrəˈfəubik] *a* 抗狂犬病的
antihypercholesterolemic [ˌæntiˌhaipə(ː)kɔˌlestərəˈliːmik] *a* 抗高胆固醇血的 *n* 抗高胆固醇[血]药
antihyperglycemic [ˌæntiˌhaipə(ː)glaiˈsiːmik] *a* 抗高血糖的 *n* 抗高血糖药
antihyperkalemic [ˌæntiˌhaipə(ː)kəˈliːmik] *a* 抗高钾血的 *n* 抗高钾血药
antihyperlipidemic [ˌæntiˌhaipə(ː)ilipidiːmik] *a* 抗高血脂的 *n* 抗高血脂药
antihyperlipoproteinemic [ˌæntiˌhaipə(ː)ˌlipəuprəutiːˈniːmik] *a* 抗高脂蛋白血的 *n* 抗高脂蛋白[血]药
antihypertensive [ˌæntiˌhaipə(ː)ˈtensiv] *a* 抗高血压的 *n* 抗高血压药
antihypnotic [ˌæntihipˈnɔtik] *a* 抗眠的 *n* 抗眠药
antihypoglycemic [ˌæntiˌhaipəuglaiˈsiːmik] *a* 抗低血糖的 *n* 抗低血糖药
antihypotensive [ˌæntiˌhaipəuˈtensiv] *a* 抗低血压的 *n* 抗低血压药
antihysteric [ˌæntihisˈterik] *a* 治癔症的 *n* 抗癔症药
anti-icteric [ˌænti ikˈterik] *a* 治黄疸的
anti-idiotype [ˌænti ˈidiətaip] *n* 抗独特型
anti-immune [ˌænti iˈmjuːn] *a* 抗免疫的
anti-infectious [ˌænti inˈfekʃəs] *a* 抗感染的
anti-infective [ˌænti inˈfektiv] *a* 抗感染的 *n* 抗感染药
anti-inflammatory [ˌænti inˈflæməˌtəri] *a* 抗炎的,消炎的 *n* 消炎药
anti-insulin [ˌænti ˈinsjulin] *n* 抗胰岛素
anti-invasin [ˌænti inˈveisin] *n* 抗侵袭素(能对抗透明质酸酶的一种酶) | ~ Ⅰ 抗侵袭素 Ⅰ(正常血浆中一种对抗透明质酸酶的酶) / ~ Ⅱ 抗侵袭素 Ⅱ(正常血浆中一种对抗透明质酸酶前体的酶)
anti-isolysin [ˌænti aiˈsɔlisin] *n* 抗同种溶素
antikataphylactic [ˌæntiˌkætəfiˈlæktik] *a* 抗[防]卫力毁灭的
antikenotoxin [ˌæntiˌkiːnəˈtɔksin] *n* 抗疲倦毒素
antiketogen [ˌæntiˈkiːtədʒən] *n* 抗生酮物质
antiketogenesis [ˌæntiˌkiːtəuˈdʒenisis] *n* 抗生酮[作用] | **antiketogenic** [ˌæntiˌkiːtəuˈdʒenik], **antiketogenetic** [ˌæntiˌkiːtəudʒiˈnetik], **antiketoplastic** [ˌæntiˌkiːtəuˈplæstik] *a*
antikinase [ˌæntiˈkaineis] *n* 抗激酶
antikinesis [ˌæntikaiˈniːsis] *n* 逆向运行(指生物体)
antilactase [ˌæntiˈlækteis] *n* 抗乳糖酶
antilactoserum [ˌæntiˌlæktəuˈsiərəm] *n* 抗乳血清
antileishmanial [ˌæntileʃˈmeiniəl] *a* 抗利什曼虫的 *n* 抗利什曼虫药
antileprotic [ˌæntileˈprɔtik] *a* 抗麻风的 *n* 抗麻风药
antilethargic [ˌæntileˈθɑːdʒik] *a* 抗嗜眠的 *n* 抗嗜眠药
antileukocidin [ˌæntiˌljuːkəˈsaidin, -ˈkəusai-], **antileukotoxin** [ˌæntiˌljuːkəˈtɔksin] *n* 抗杀白细胞素,抗白细胞毒素
antileukocytic [ˌæntiˌljuːkəˈsitik] *a* 破坏白细胞的,抗白细胞的
antileukoprotease [ˌæntiˌljuːkəˈprəutieis] *n* 抗白细胞蛋白酶
antilewisite [ˌæntiˈlju(ː)isait] *n* 二巯丙醇
antilipase [ˌæntiˈlipeis] *n* 抗脂酶
antilipemic [ˌæntiliˈpiːmik] *a* 抗高血脂的 *n* 抗高血脂药
antilipoid [ˌæntiˈlipɔid] *n* 抗类脂(物质)(有能力能同类脂质起作用的一种抗体)
antilipotropism [ˌæntiliˈpɔtrəpizəm] *n* 抗亲脂性 | **antilipotropic** [ˌæntiˌlipəuˈtrɔpik] *a* 抗亲脂的
antilithic [ˌæntiˈliθik] *a* 防结石的 *n* 防结石药
antiluetic [ˌæntilju(ː)ˈetik] *a* 抗梅毒的 *n* 抗梅毒药

antilysin [ˌænti'laisin] *n* 抗溶[菌]素
antilysis [ˌænti'laisis] *n* 抗溶解作用 | **antilytic** [ˌænti'litik] *a*
antilyssic [ˌænti'lisik] *a* 抗狂犬病的，防治狂犬病的
antimalarial [ˌæntimə'lɛəriəl] *a* 抗疟的 *n* 抗疟[疾]药
antimaniacal [ˌæntimə'naiəkəl] *a* 抗躁狂的 *n* 抗躁狂药
antimephitic [ˌæntimə'fitik] *a* 抗臭的
antimere ['æntimiə] *n* 对称部
antimeristem [ˌæntimi'ristəm] *n* 抗分生霉素(制剂名)
antimesenteric [ˌæntimesən'terik] *a* 系膜小肠对向部的，系膜小肠游离部的
antimetabolite [ˌæntime'tæbəlait] *n* 抗代谢物
antimetastatic [ˌæntiˌmetə'stætik] *a* 抗转移的，抑制转移的
antimethemoglobinemic [ˌæntimetˌhiːməu ˌgləubi'niːmik] *a* 抗高铁血红蛋白血的 *n* 抗高铁血红蛋白血药
antimetropia [ˌæntime'trəupiə] *n* 屈光参差(例如一眼远视，他眼近视)
antimiasmatic [ˌæntiˌmaiəz'mætik] *a* 抗瘴毒的
antimicrobial [ˌæntimai'krəubiəl] *a* 抗微生物的，抗菌的 *n* 抗微生物药
antimineralocorticoid [ˌæntiˌminərələu'kɔːtikɔid] *n* 抗盐皮质激素药，抗矿质皮质素物质
antimitotic [ˌæntimai'tɔtik] *a* 抗有丝分裂的
antimongolism [ˌænti'mɔŋgəlizəm] *n* 反[相]先天愚型，反[相]先天性痴呆症
antimongoloid [ˌænti'mɔŋgəlɔid] *a* 反[相]先天愚型样的
antimonial [ˌænti'məunjəl] *a* 锑的，含锑的
antimonic [ˌænti'mɔnik] *a* 五价锑的 | ~ acid 锑酸
antimonid [ˌænti'məunid] *n* 锑化物
antimonious [ˌænti'məuniəs], **antimonous** [ˌænti'məunəs] *a* 亚锑的，三价锑的；含锑的
antimonium [ˌænti'məuniəm] *n*【拉】锑
antimony ['æntiməni] *n* 锑(化学元素) | ~ lithium thiomalate 硫代苹果酸锑锂(治淋巴肉芽肿、锥虫病、丝虫病和血吸虫病) / ~ pentoxide 五氧化二锑 / ~ potassium tartrate 酒石酸锑钾(治寄生虫感染，如血吸虫病或利什曼病) / ~ sodium tartrate 酒石酸锑钠(治锥虫病及其他热带病) / ~ sodium thioglycollate 巯基乙酸锑钠 / ~ thioglycollamide 巯基乙酰胺锑(治腹股沟肉芽肿、黑热病及丝虫病) / ~ trioxide 三氧化锑(用于吐酒石制剂)
antimonyl [æn'timəˌnil] *n* 锑氧基(一价)
antimorph ['æntimɔːf] *n* 反效等位基因(指一突变基因阻抑相对等位基因的活动，或使之失效) | **~ic** [ˌænti'mɔːfik] *a*
antimuscarinic [ˌænti'mʌskəˌrinik] *a* 抗毒蕈碱的
antimutagen [ˌænti'mjuːtədʒən] *n* 抗变剂，抗变物质(能抑制其他物质致突变作用的一种物质)
antimüllerian [ˌæntimi'liəriən] *a* 抗副中肾管的
antimyasthenic [ˌæntiˌmaiæs'θenik] *a* 抗重症肌无力的 *n* 抗重症肌无力药
antimycobacterial [ˌæntiˌmaikəubæk'tiəriəl] *a* 抗分枝杆菌的
antimycotic [ˌæntimai'kɔtik] *a* 抗真菌的
antinarcotic [ˌæntinɑː'kɔtik] *a* 抗麻醉的
antinatriuresis [ˌæntiˌneitrijuə'riːsis] *n* 抗钠尿排泄，抑制钠尿排泄
antinauseant [ˌænti'nɔːziənt] *a* 止恶心的 *n* 止恶心药，防晕药
antineoplastic [ˌæntiˌni(ː)əu'plæstik] *a* 抗肿瘤的 *n* 抗肿瘤药
antineoplaston [ˌæntiˌniːəu'plæstɔn] *n* 抗癌肽类
antineoplastons [ˌæntiˌniːəu'plæstɔnz] *n* 抗肿瘤药物(一组抗肿瘤肽和氨基酸衍生物，原先从血管和尿中分离而得，可抑制肿瘤细胞生长，用于研究治疗癌症)
antinephritic [ˌæntine'fritik] *a* 抗肾炎的
antineuralgic [ˌæntinjuə'rældʒik] *a* 止神经痛的
antineuritic [ˌæntinjuə'ritik] *a* 抗神经炎的
antineurotoxin [ˌæntiˌnjuərə'tɔksin] *n* 抗神经毒素
antineutrino [ˌæntinjuː'triːnəu] *n* 反中微子
antineutron [ˌænti'njuːtrɔn] *n* 反中子
antiniad [æn'tiniæd] *ad* 向额极，向对枕尖
antinion [æn'tiniɔn] *n* 额极，对枕尖 | **antinial** [æn'tiniəl] *a*
antinociceptive [ˌæntiˌnəusi'septiv] *a* 防感受伤害的(具有镇痛作用的，减少疼痛刺激的感受性)
antinuclear [ˌænti'njuːkliə] *a* 抗(细胞)核的
antiodontalgic [ˌæntiˌɔdɔn'tældʒik] *a* 止牙痛的
antioncogene [ˌænti'ɔŋkədʒin] *n* 抗癌基因，肿瘤抑制基因
antioncotic [ˌæntiɔŋ'kɔtik] *a* 消肿的 *n* 消肿药
antiophidica [ˌæntiɔ'fidikə] *n* 解蛇毒药，治蛇咬药
antiophthalmic [ˌæntiɔf'θælmik] *a* 抗眼炎的
antiopsonin [ˌænti'ɔpsənin] *n* 抗调理素
antiotomy [ˌænti'ɔtəmi] *n* 扁桃体切除术
antiovotransferrin [ˌæntiˌəuvətræns'ferin] *n* 抗卵转铁蛋白
antiovulatory [ˌænti'əuvjuləˌtəri] *a* 抗排卵的，抑制排卵的
antioxidant [ˌænti'ɔksidənt], **antioxygen** [ˌænti'ɔksidʒən] *n* 抗氧剂

antioxidase [ˌæntiˈɔksideis] *n* 抗氧化酶
antioxidation [ˌæntiɔksiˈdeiʃən] *n* 抗氧化[作用],氧化抑制[作用]
antipaludian [ˌæntipəˈljuːdiən] *a* 抗疟的 *n* 抗疟药
antiparallel [ˌæntiˈpærərel] *a* 反[向]平行的,逆平行的
antiparalytic [ˌæntiˌpærəˈlitik] *a* 抗麻痹的 *n* 抗麻痹药
antiparasitic [ˌæntiˌpærəˈsitik] *a* 抗寄生虫的 *n* 抗寄生虫药
antiparastata [ˌæntipəˈræstətə] *n* 尿道球腺
antiparastatitis [ˌæntiˌpærəstəˈtaitis] *n* 尿道球腺炎
antiparasympathomimetic [ˌæntiˌpærəˌsimpəθəu-miˈmetik] *a* 抗拟副交感[神经]的
antiparkinsonian [ˌæntiˌpɑːkinˈsəuniən] *a* 抗帕金森病的,抗震颤麻痹的 *n* 抗震颤麻痹药
antiparticle [æntiˈpɑːtikl] *n* 反粒子
antipathogen [ˌæntiˈpæθədʒin] *n* 抗病原物质
antipathy [ænˈtipəθi] *n* 反感,厌恶;相克疗法 | **antipathic** [ˌæntiˈpæθik] *a* 反感的,厌恶的;相克症状的
antipedicular [ˌæntipiˈdikjulə] *a* 抗虱的,灭虱的 *n* 抗虱药,灭虱药
antipediculotic [ˌæntipiˌdikjuˈlɔtik] *a* 抗虱的,灭虱的 *n* 抗虱药,灭虱药
antipepsin [ˌæntiˈpepsin] *n* 抗胃蛋白酶
antiperiodic [ˌæntiˌpiəriˈɔdik] *a* 抗疟的(如疟疾时防止症状定期复发)
antiperistalsis [ˌæntiˌperiˈstælsis] *n* 逆蠕动 | **antiperistaltic** [ˌæntiˌperiˈstæltik] *a* 逆蠕动的;减少蠕动的 *n* 减少蠕动药
antiperspirant [ˌæntiˈpəːspiˌrənt] *a* 止汗的 *n* 止汗药
antiphagin [ˌæntiˈfeidʒin] *n* 抗吞噬素(一种假想的物质,曾被认为是毒性菌的特异成分,并能使毒性菌对抗吞噬作用)
antiphagocytic [ˌæntifægəˈsitik] *a* 抗吞噬作用的
antiphlogistic [ˌæntifləuˈdʒistik] *a* 抗炎的,消炎的 *n* 消炎药
antiphone [ˈæntifəun] *n* 防声器
antiphrynolysin [ˌæntifriˈnɔlisin] *n* 抗蟾蜍溶血素
antiphthiriac [ˌæntiˈθəːriæk] *a* 灭虱的
antiphthisic [ˌæntiˈtizik] *a* 抗痨的,抗结核的
antiplasmin [ˌæntiˈplæzmin] *n* 抗纤维蛋白溶酶
antiplasmodial [ˌæntiplæzˈməudiəl] *a* 杀疟原虫的
antiplastic [ˌæntiˈplæstik] *a* 妨碍愈合的;抑制细胞成形的;骨髓抑制的
antiplatelet [ˌæntiˈpleitlit] *a* 抗血小板的
antipneumococcal [ˌæntiˌnjuːməuˈkɔkəl], **antipneumococcic** [ˌæntiˌnjuːməˈkɔk(s)ik] *a* 抗肺炎球菌的
antipodagric [ˌæntipəˈdægrik] *a* 治痛风的
antipode [ˈæntipəud] *n* 对映体 | **antipodal** [ænˈtipədl] *a* 对跖的,对掌的
antipolycythemic [ˌæntiˌpɔlisaiˈθiːmik] *a* 抗红细胞增生的 *n* 抗红细胞增生药
antiport [ˈæntipɔːt] *n* 反向转运,逆向转运
antiporter [ˈæntiˌpɔːtə] *n* 反向转运蛋白
antiposia [ˌæntiˈpəusiə] *n* 厌饮
antiprecipitin [ˌæntipriˈsipitin] *n* 抗沉淀素
antiprogestin [ˌæntiprəˈdʒestin] *n* 抗孕激素药(抑制促孕药形成的物质,最常见的例子是米非司酮〈mifepristone〉)
antiprostate [ˌæntiˈprɔsteit] *n* 尿道球腺
antiprostatitis [ˌæntiˌprɔstəˈtaitis] *n* 尿道球腺炎
antiprotease [ˌæntiˈprəutieis] *n* 抗蛋白酶
antiprothrombin [ˌæntiprəˈθrɔmbin] *n* 抗凝血酶原
antiprotozoal [ˌæntiˌprəutəuˈzəuəl], **antiprotozoan** [ˌæntiˌprəutəuˈzəuən] *a* 抗原生动物的 *n* 抗原生动物药
antipruritic [ˌæntipruəˈritik] *a* 止痒的 *n* 止痒药
antipsoriatic [ˌæntiˌsɔriˈætik] *a* 治牛皮癣的 *n* 治牛皮癣药
antipsychomotor [ˌæntiˌsaikəuˈməutə] *a* 抑制精神运动的
antipsychotic [ˌæntisaiˈkɔtik] *a* 抑制精神的,抗精神活动的 *n* 精神抑制药(如安定药)
antiputrefactive [ˌæntiˌpjuːtriˈfæktiv] *a* 防腐的
antipyogenic [ˌæntiˌpaiəˈdʒenik] *a* 防止化脓的
antipyresis [ˌæntipaiˈriːsis] *n* 退热[疗]法
antipyretic [ˌæntipaiˈretik] *a* 退热的,解热的 *n* 解热药
antipyrine [ˌæntiˈpaiəriːn] *n* 安替比林(解热镇痛药) | ~ camphorate 樟脑酸安替比林(曾用于盗汗) / ~ mandelate 杏仁酸安替比林
antipyrotic [ˌæntipaiˈrɔtik] *a* 治灼伤的 *n* 治灼伤剂
antirabic [ˌæntiˈræbik] *a* 防治狂犬病的,防狂犬病的
antirachitic [ˌæntirəˈkitik] *a* 抗佝偻病的
antiradiation [ˌæntiˌreidiˈeiʃən] *a* 抗辐射的,抗辐射性损伤的
antirennin [ˌæntiˈrenin] *n* 抗凝乳酶
antiretroviral [ˌæntiˌretrəuˈvaiərəl] *a* 抗反转录病毒的 *n* 抗反转录病毒药
antirheumatic [ˌæntiru(ː)ˈmætik] *a* 抗风湿[病]的 *n* 抗风湿药
antiricin [ˌæntiˈraisin] *n* 抗蓖麻毒蛋白(动物体内注射蓖麻毒素后产生的抗毒素)

antirickettsial [ˌæntiriˈketsiəl] *a* 抗立克次体的 *n* 抗立克次体药
antirobin [ˌæntiˈrəubin] *n* 抗刺槐毒素
antisaluresis [ˌæntiˌsæljuˈriːsis] *n* 抗钠尿排泄，抑制钠尿排泄
antiscabietic [ˌæntiˌskeibiˈetik]，**antiscabious** [ˌæntiˈskeibjəs] *a* 抗疥的 *n* 抗疥药
antiscarlatinal [ˌæntiskɑːləˈtiːnl] *a* 抗猩红热的
antischistosomal [ˌæntiˌskistəˈsəuməl] *a* 抗血吸虫的 *n* 抗血吸虫药
antiscorbutic [ˌæntiskɔːˈbjuːtik] *a* 抗坏血病的 *n* 抗坏血病药
antiseborrheic [ˌæntiˌsebəˈriːik] *a* 抗皮脂溢的 *n* 抗皮脂溢药
antisecretory [ˌæntisiˈkriːtəri] *a* 抑制分泌的 *n* 抑制分泌药
antisense [ˌæntiˈsens] *a* 反义的(分子遗传学中指双链 DNA 中互补有义链的那一条链)
antisensibilisin [ˌæntisensiˈbilizin] *n* 抗致敏素，抗过敏素
antisensitizer [ˌæntiˈsensitaizə] *n* 抗致敏物质(如抗抗体或抗介体)；抗致敏药
antisepsis [ˈæntiˌsepsis] *n* 防腐；抗菌术 | physiologic ~ 生理性抗菌
antiseptic [ˌæntiˈseptik] *a* 防腐的，抗菌的 *n* 抗菌防腐药
antisepticism [ˌæntiˈseptisizəm] *n* 防腐法，抗菌法
antisepticize [ˌæntiˈseptisaiz] *vt* 防腐，抗菌
antiserum [ˌæntiˈsiərəm] *n* 抗血清 | Erysipelothrix rhusiopathiae ~ 猪红斑丹毒丝菌抗血清，猪丹毒丹毒抗血清 / Reenstierna ~ 里恩施坦纳抗血清，麻风抗血清 / Rh ~ Rh 抗血清(此血清含有部分人和全部恒河猴所共有的与抗原决定簇相对应的抗体)
antisialagogue [ˌæntisaiˈæləgɔg] *a* 止涎的 *n* 止涎药
antisialic [ˌæntisaiˈælik] *a* 止涎的 *n* 止涎药
antisideric [ˌæntisiˈderik] *a* 抗铁的，忌铁的
antisocial [ˌæntiˈsəuʃəl] *a* 反社会的(变态人格)；厌恶社交的
antisocialism [ˌæntiˈsəuʃəlizəm] *n* 反社会性(变态人格)；厌恶社交
antispasmodic [ˌæntispæzˈmɔdik] *a* 镇痉的(一般指缓解平滑肌、随意肌的痉挛) *n* 解痉药 | biliary ~ 胆道解痉药 / bronchial ~ 支气管解痉药
antispastic [ˌæntiˈspæstik] *a* 镇痉的(特指骨骼肌的痉挛) *n* 镇痉药
antispermotoxin [ˌæntiˌspəːməuˈtɔksin] *n* 抗精子毒素
antistaphylococcic [ˌæntiˌstæfiləuˈkɔk(s)ik] *a* 抗葡萄球菌的
antistaphylolysin [ˌæntiˌstæfiˈlɔlisin]，**antistaphylohemolysin** [ˌæntiˌstæfiləuhiːˈmɔlisin] *n* 抗葡萄球菌溶血素
antisteapsin [ˌæntistiˈæpsin] *n* 抗胰脂酶
antisterility [ˌæntisteˈriləti] *a* 抗不育的
antistreptococcic [ˌæntiˌstreptəuˈkɔk(s)ik] *a* 抗链球菌的 *n* 抗链球菌药
antistreptokinase [ˌæntiˌstreptəuˈkaineis] *n* 抗链[球菌]激酶
antistreptolysin [ˌæntistrepˈtɔlisin] *n* 抗链[球菌]溶[血]素
antisubstance [ˌæntiˈsʌbstəns] *n* 抗体
antisudorific [ˌæntiˌsjuːdəˈrifik]，**antisudoral** [ˌæntiˈsjuːdərəl] *a* 止汗的 *n* 止汗药
antisympathetic [ˌæntiˌsimpəˈθetik] *a* 抗交感神经的 *n* 抗交感神经药
antisyphilitic [ˌæntiˌsifiˈlitik] *a* 抗梅毒的 *n* 抗梅毒药
antitemplate [ˌæntiˈtempleit] *n* 抗丝裂质(一种设想的能抑制正常细胞有丝分裂的物质)
antitetanic [ˌæntitiˈtænik] *a* 抗破伤风的
antitetanolysin [ˌæntitetəˈnɔlisin] *n* 抗破伤风溶血[毒]素
antithenar [ˌæntiˈθiːnə] *n* 小鱼际
antithermic [ˌæntiˈθəːmik] *a* 退热的，解热的 *n* 退热药，解热药
antithrombin [ˌæntiˈθrɔmbin] *n* 抗凝血酶
antithromboplastin [ˌæntiˌθrɔmbəuˈplæstin] *n* 抗凝血激酶
antithrombotic [ˌæntiθrɔmˈbɔtik] *a* 抗血栓[形成]的 *n* 抗血栓药
antithyroid [ˌæntiˈθairɔid] *a* 抗甲状腺的
antithyrotoxic [ˌæntiˌθairəuˈtɔksik] *a* 抗甲状腺毒性的
antithyrotropic [ˌæntiˌθairəuˈtrɔpik] *a* 抗促甲状腺[激素]的
antitonic [ˌæntiˈtɔnik] *a* 抗紧张的
antitoxic [ˌæntiˈtɔksik] *a* 抗毒的；抗毒素的
antitoxigen [ˌæntiˈtɔksidʒən]，**antitoxinogen** [ˌæntitɔkˈsinədʒən] *n* 抗毒素原
antitoxin [ˌæntiˈtɔksin] *n* 抗毒素 | botulism ~，botulinum ~，botulinus ~ 肉毒抗毒素(用于被动免疫) / bovine ~ 牛抗毒素(用于对马血清过敏者) / diphtheria ~ 白喉抗毒素(用于被动免疫) / gas gangrene ~ 气性坏疽抗毒素 / normal ~ 标准抗毒素 / scarlet fever streptococcus ~ 猩红热链球菌抗毒素 / tetanus ~ 破伤风抗毒素(用于被动免疫)
antitoxinum [æntitɔkˈsainəm] *n* 【拉】抗毒素
antitragicus [ˌæntiˈtrædʒikəs] *n* 对耳屏肌
antitragus [ˌæntiˈtreigəs] *n* 对耳屏
antitreponemal [ˌæntiˌtrepəˈniːməl] *a* 抗密螺旋

体的 *n* 抗密螺旋体药

antitrichomonal [ˌæntitrikəˈməunəl] *a* 抗滴虫的 *n* 抗滴虫药

antitrismus [ˌæntiˈtrizməs] *n* 张口痉挛（不能合口）

antitrope [ˌæntitrəup] *n* 对称体（指器官）；抗体

antitropic [ˌæntiˈtrɔpik] *a* 相似对称的

antitropin [ˌæntiˈtrəupin] *n* 抗调理素

antitrypanosomal [ˌæntitriˌpænəˈsəuməl] *a* 抗锥体虫的 *n* 抗锥体虫药

α_1-antitrypsin [ˌæntiˈtripsin] *n* α_1-抗胰蛋白酶

antitryptase [ˌæntiˈtripteis] *n* 抗胰蛋白酶

antitryptic [ˌæntiˈtriptik], **antitrypsic** [ˌæntiˈtripsik] *a* 抗胰蛋白酶的

antituberculin [ˌæntitju(ː)ˈbəːkjulin] *n* 抗结核菌素

antituberculotic [ˌæntitju(ː)ˌbəːkjuˈlɔtik] *a* 抗结核的 *n* 抗结核药

antituberculous [ˌæntitju(ː)ˈbəːkjuləs] *a* 抗结核的

antitubulin [ˌæntiˈtjuːbjulin] *n* 抗微管蛋白剂

antitumorigenic [ˌæntiˌtjuːməriˈdʒenik] *a* 抗肿瘤发生的

antitussive [ˌæntiˈtʌsiv] *a* 镇咳的 *n* 镇咳药

antityphoid [ˌæntiˈtaifɔid] *a* 抗伤寒的，防治伤寒的

antityrosinase [ˌæntitaiˈrəusineis] *n* 抗酪氨酸酶

antiulcerative [ˌæntiˈʌlsərətiv] *a* 抗溃疡的 *n* 抗溃疡药

antiuratic [ˌæntijuəˈrætik] *a* 抗尿酸盐的

antiurease [ˌæntiˈjuərieis] *n* 抗尿素酶，抗脲酶

antiurokinase [ˌæntiˌjuərəˈkaineis] *n* 抗尿激酶

antiurolithic [ˌæntiˌjuərəˈliθik] *a* 防尿石形成的 *n* 防尿石形成药

antivaccinationist [ˌæntiˌvæksiˈneiʃənist] *n* 反对种痘者，反对接种者

antivenereal [ˌæntiviˈniəriəl] *a* 抗性病的

antivenin [ˌæntiˈvenin] *n* 抗蛇毒血清 | ～ (Crotalidae) polyvalent, polyvalent crotaline ～ 多价抗响尾蛇抗毒血清 / ～ (*Latrodectus mactan*), black widow spider ～ 黑寡妇蜘蛛毒抗毒血清 / ～ (*Micrurus fluvius*) 抗斑色蛇抗毒血清 | **antivenene** [ˌæntiviˈniːn], **antivenom** [ˌæntiˈvenəm] *n*

antivenomous [ˌæntiˈvenəməs] *a* 抗蛇毒的

antiviral [ˌæntiˈvaiərəl] *a* 抗病毒的 *n* 抗病毒药

antivirotic [ˌæntivaiəˈrɔtik] *a* 抗病毒的 *n* 抗病毒药

antivirulin [ˌæntiˈvirjulin] *n* 抗狂犬病毒质

antivirus [ˌæntiˈvaiərəs] *n* 细菌[培养]滤液

antivitamer [ˌæntiˈvaitəmə] *n* 抗同效维生素

antivitamin [ˌæntiˈvaitəmin] *n* 抗维生素

antivivisection [ˌæntiˌviviˈsekʃən] *n* 反对活体解剖，反对动物实验手术 | **~ist** *n* 反对活体解剖者，反对动物实验手术者

antixenic [ˌæntiˈziːnik] *a* 异物反应的

antixerophthalmic [ˌæntiˌziərɔfˈθælmik] *a* 抗干眼病的

antixerotic [ˌæntiziəˈrɔtik] *a* 抗干燥症的

antizyme [ˌæntizaim] *n* 抗酶蛋白

antizymohexase [ˌæntiˌzaiməuˈhekseis] *n* 抗醛缩酶

antizymotic [ˌæntizaiˈmɔtik] *a* 抗发酵的

antodontalgic [ˌæntɔdɔnˈtældʒik] *a* 止牙痛的

Anton-Babinski syndrome [ˈæntən bəˈbinski] (G. Anton; Jeseph F. F. Babinski) 安东-巴宾斯基综合征（见 Anton's syndrome）

Anton's syndrome (symptom) [ˈæntən] (Gabriel Anton) 安东综合征（症状）（盲症状，患者否认自已失明，平常并不觉得，如见于双侧枕叶梗死所致的皮质性盲）

antophthalmic [ˌæntɔfˈθælmik] *a* 抗眼炎的

antorphine [ænˈtɔːfiːn] *n* 烯丙吗啡（吗啡拮抗药）

antra [ˈæntrə] antrum 的复数

antracele [ˈæntrəsiːl] *n* 上颌窦囊肿

antral [ˈæntrəl] *a* 窦的

antrectomy [ænˈtrektəmi] *n* 胃窦切除术（如胃幽门窦切除术）

Antricola [ænˈtrikələ] *n* 蝠蜱属

antritis [ænˈtraitis] *n* 窦炎（主要指上颌窦炎）

antr(o)- [构词成分] 窦

antroatticotomy [ˌæntrəuˌætiˈkɔtəmi] *n* 鼓窦隐窝切开术，上鼓室鼓窦切开术

antrobuccal [ˈæntrəuˈbʌkəl] *a* 窦颊的（上颌窦与口腔前庭相通的）

antrocele [ˈæntrəsiːl] *n* 上颌窦囊肿

antroduodenal [ˌæntrəuˌdju(ː)əuˈdinəl] *a* 胃窦十二指肠的

antroduodenectomy [ˌæntrəuˌdju(ː)əudiˈnektəmi] *n* 胃窦十二指肠[溃疡]切除术

antrodynia [ˌæntrəuˈdiniə] *n* 上颌窦痛

antronalgia [ˌæntrəuˈnældʒiə] *n* 上颌窦痛

antronasal [ˌæntrəuˈneizəl] *a* 上颌窦鼻的，鼻上颌窦的

antroneurolysis [ˌæntrəunjuəˈrɔlisis] *n* 幽门窦除神经支配[法]

antrophore [ˈæntrəfɔː] *n* 安特罗弗尔（一种可溶性含药栓剂）

antrophose [ˈæntrəfəuz] *n* [眼]中枢性光幻觉

antropyloric [ˌæntrəupaiˈlɔːrik] *a* 窦[与]幽门的

antroscope [ˈæntrəˌskəup] *n* 窦透照器，上颌窦镜 | **antroscopy** [ænˈtrɔskəpi] *n* 上颌窦镜检查[法]

antrostomy [æn'trɔstəmi] *n* 窦造口术,窦开窗术
antrotome ['æntrətəum] *n* 窦刀
antrotomy [æn'trɔtəmi] *n* 窦切开术
antrotympanic [ˌæntrəutim'pænik] *a* 鼓窦鼓室的
antrotympanitis [ˌæntrəuˌtimpə'naitis] *n* 鼓窦鼓室炎
antrum ['æntrəm] ([复] **antrums** 或 **antra** ['æntrə]) *n* 窦,房 | cardiac ~ 贲门窦 / gastric ~, pyloric ~ 幽门窦 / mastoid ~, tympanic ~ 鼓窦,鼓房 / maxillary ~ 上颌窦
ANTU alpha-naphthylthiourea α-萘硫脲(一种强力灭鼠药)
anuclear [ei'nju:kliə] *a* 无核的(指细胞,如失去核的红细胞)
anucleated [ei'nju:klieitid] *a* 除核的,失核的
ANUG acute necrotizing ulcerative gingivitis 急性坏死溃疡性龈炎
anuloplasty [ˌænjuləu'plæsti] *n* 瓣膜成形术
anulus ['ænjuləs] ([复] **anuli** ['ænjulai]) *n* 【拉】环,终环
Anura [ə'nju:rə] *n* 无尾目(两栖动物)
anuran [ə'nju:rən] *n* 无尾动物
anuresis [ˌænjuə'ri:sis] *n* 尿闭;无尿 | **anuretic** [ˌænjuə'retik] *a*
anuria [ə'njuəriə] *n* 无尿 | angioneurotic ~ 血管神经性无尿 / calculous ~ 结石性无尿 / obstructive ~ 阻塞性无尿 / postrenal ~ 肾后性无尿,输尿管闭塞性无尿 / prerenal ~ 肾前性无尿 / renal ~ 肾性无尿 / suppressive ~ 抑制性无尿 | **anuric** [ə'njuərik] *a*
anurous [ə'njuərəs] *a* 无尾的
anus ['einəs] [单复同] *n* 【拉】肛门 | artificial ~ 人工肛门 / imperforate ~, ectopic ~ 肛门闭锁 / preternatural ~ 异位肛门 / vulvovaginal ~, ~ vestibularis 外阴阴道肛门[畸形],前庭肛门[畸形]
anusitis [einə'saitis] *n* 肛门炎
anvil ['ænvil] *n* 砧骨
anxietas [æŋɡ'zaiətəs] *n* 【拉】焦虑,(心神)不宁 | ~ presenilis 更年期焦虑 / ~ tibiarum 腿动不宁性焦虑,下肢不宁综合征
anxiety [æŋɡ'zaiəti] *n* 焦虑 | castration ~ 去势焦虑 / freefloating ~ 游离性焦虑 / situation ~ 境遇性焦虑
anxiolytic [ˌæŋɡzaiə'litik] *a* 抗焦虑的 *n* 抗焦虑药
anydremia [ˌæni'dri:miə] *n* 缺水血[症]
AO anodal opening 阳极断电;opening of the atrioventricular valves 房室瓣开张
AOA American Optometric Association 美国视力测定协会;American Orthopaedic Association 美国矫形外科协会;American Orthopsychiatric Association 美国行为精神病学协会;American Osteopathic Association 美国整骨疗法协会
AOC anodal opening contraction 阳极断电收缩
AOCl anodal opening clonus 阳极断电阵挛
AOMA American Occupational Medical Association 美国职业医学协会
AOO anodal opening odor 阳极断电气味
AOP anodal opening picture 阳极断电图
aorta [ei'ɔ:tə] ([复] **aortae** [ei'ɔ:ti:] 或 **aortas**) *n* 主动脉 | abdominal ~ 腹主动脉 / ascending ~ 升主动脉 / descending ~ 降主动脉 / palpable ~ 易扪主动脉 / primitive ~ 原[始]主动脉 / thoracic ~ 胸主动脉 / ventral ~ 腹侧主动脉(鱼类、两栖动物中以及高等脊椎动物胚胎时,心脏与主动脉弓之间相连的短管) | **aortic** [ei'ɔ:tik], **-l** [ei'ɔ:tl] *a*
aortalgia [ˌeiɔ:'tældʒiə] *n* 主动脉痛
aortectomy [ˌeiɔ:'tektəmi] *n* 主动脉部分切除术
aorticomediastinal [eiˌɔ:tikəumi:diə'stainəl] *a* 主动脉[与]纵隔的
aorticopulmonary [eiˌɔ:tikə'pʌlmənəri] *a* 主动脉[与]肺动脉间的
aorticorenal [eiˌɔ:tikə'ri:nl] *a* 主动脉[与]肾的
aortitis [ˌeiɔ:'taitis] *n* 主动脉炎 | nummular ~ 钱币状主动脉炎 / syphilitic ~, luetic ~ 梅毒性主动脉炎
aortobifemoral [eiˌɔ:təubai'femərəl] *a* 主动脉[与]双股动脉的
aortocaval [eiˌɔ:təu'keivəl] *a* 主动脉[与]腔静脉的
aortocoronary [eiˌɔ:təu'kɔrənəri] *a* 主动脉冠状动脉的
aortoduodenal [eiˌɔ:təuˌdju:əu'di:nəl] *a* 主动脉[与]十二指肠的
aortoenteric [eiˌɔ:təuen'terik] *a* 主动脉[与]胃肠道的
aortoesophageal [eiˌɔ:təui:ˌsɔfə'dʒi:əl] *a* 主动脉[与]食管的
aortofemoral [eiˌɔ:təu'femərəl] *a* 主动脉[与]股动脉的
aortogastric [eiˌɔ:təu'gæstrik] *a* 主动脉[与]胃的
aortogram [ei'ɔ:təgræm] *n* 主动脉造影[照]片
aortography [ˌeiɔ:'tɔgrəfi] *n* 主动脉造影[术] | retrograde ~ 逆行主动脉造影[术] / translumbar ~ 经腰部主动脉造影[术]
aortoiliac [eiˌɔ:təu'iliæk] *a* 主动脉[与]髂动脉的
aortopathy [ˌeiɔ:'tɔpəθi] *n* 主动脉病
aortopexy [ei'ɔ:təuˌpeksi] *n* 主动脉固定术
aortoplasty [ˌeiɔ:təu'plæsti] *n* 主动脉成形术
aortopulmonary [eiˌɔ:təu'pʌlmənəri] *a* 主动脉[与]肺动脉的,主动脉[与]肺动脉间的

aortorenal [ei,ɔːtəu'riːnəl] *a* 主动脉[与]肾动脉的
aortorrhaphy [,eiɔː'tɔrəfi] *n* 主动脉缝合术
aortosclerosis [ei,ɔːtəuskliə'rəusis] *n* 主动脉硬化
aortotomy [,eiɔː'tɔtəmi] *n* 主动脉切开合术
AOS anodal opening sound 阳极断电音
aosmic [ei'ɔzmik] *a* 无气味的
AOTA American Occupational Therapy Association 美国职业疗法协会
AOTe anodal opening tetanus 阳极断电强直
AP action potential 动作电位;angina pectoris 心绞痛;anterior pituitary(gland) 垂体前叶;anteroposterior 前后的;arterial pressure 动脉压
ap- 见 apo-
APA American Pharmaceutical Association 美国药学协会;American Physiotherapy Association 美国理疗协会;American Podiatric Association 美国手足医术协会;American Psychiatric Association 美国精神病学协会;American Psychoanalytic Association 美国精神分析协会;American Psychological Association 美国心理学协会;American Psychopathological Association 美国精神病理学协会
apaconitine [,æpə'kɔnitin] *n* 阿扑乌头碱
apallesthesia [ə,pælis'θiːzjə] *n* 振动觉缺失
apancrea [ə'pæŋkriə] *n* 无胰,胰[腺]缺失
apancreatic [ə,pæŋkri'ætik] *a* 无胰的;非胰性的
Apansporoblastina [,eipæŋ,spɔːrəblæs'tainə] *n* 无膜泛成孢子虫亚目
APAP acetaminophen 对乙酰氨基酚(解热镇痛药)
aparalytic [ə,pærə'litik] *a* 无麻痹的
aparathyrosis [ə,pærəθai'rəusis], **aparathyreosis** [ə,pærəθairi'əusis], **aparathyroidism** [ə,pærə'θairɔidizəm] *n* 甲状旁腺功能缺失
apareunia [eipə'ruːniə] *n* 性交不能
aparthrosis [,æpɑː'θrəusis] *n* 动关节,滑膜关节
apastia [ə'pæstiə] *n* 拒食,绝食 | **apastic** [ə'pæstik] *a*
apathetic [,æpə'θetik] *a* 无情感的,情感淡漠的
apathic [ə'pæθik] *a* 无情感的
apathism ['æpəθizəm] *n* 兴奋迟钝,兴奋性缺失
apathy ['æpəθi] *n* 无欲貌,情感淡漠
apatite ['æpətait] *n* 磷灰石
apazone ['æpəzəun] *n* 炎爽痛(具有抗炎、镇痛、解热、促尿酸排泄作用,用于治疗类风湿关节炎和骨关节炎。亦称阿扎丙宗〈azapropazone〉)
APB atrial premature beat 房性期前收缩,房性早搏
APC atrial premature complex 房性期前复合波
APCA anti-Purkinje cell antibody 抗浦肯野细胞抗体
APD atrial premature depolarization 房性期前除极;pamidronate(aminohydroxypropylidene diphosphonate)帕米膦酸(氨基羟基亚丙基二膦酸)
APE anterior pituitary extract 垂体前叶提取物
ape [eip] *n* 无尾猿,类人猿 | anthropoid ~ 类人猿
apeidosis [,æpai'dəusis] *n* 形态渐失
apellous [ei'peləs] *a* 无皮的;无包皮的
aperient [ə'piəriənt] *a* 轻泻的 *n* 轻泻药
aperiodic [,eipiəri'ɔdik] *a* 不定期的,无定期的,非周期的 | **~ity** [ei,piəriə'disəti] *n* 不定期性,非周期性
aperistalsis [,eiperi'stælsis] *n* 蠕动停止
aperitive [ə'peritiv] *a* 开胃的 *n* 润肠药
Apert-Crouzon disease [ə'pεə kru'zɔn] (Eugène Apert; Octava Crouzon)阿佩尔-克鲁宗病(一种常染色体显性遗传病,包括手足畸形,伴阿佩尔综合征〈尖头并指(趾)畸形〉和克鲁宗病〈颅骨面发育不全〉的面部特征。亦称尖头并指〈趾〉畸形Ⅰ型)
apertognathia [ə,pɑːtɔg'neiθiə] *n* 无殆,开殆
apertometer [,æpə'tɔmitə] *n* 数值口径计,物镜口径计(测显微镜物镜口径的角度)
Apert's disease (syndrome) [ə'pεə] (Eugène Apert)阿佩尔病(综合征),尖头并指[畸形],尖头并趾[畸形]
apertura ['æpə'tjuərə] ([复] **aperturae** [,æpə'tjuəriː]) *n*【拉】口,孔
aperture ['æpətjuə] *n* 口,孔 | angle of ~, angular ~, ~ of lens 角孔径(显微镜) / numerical ~ 数值孔径,数值口径(显微镜) / orbital ~ 眶口 / periform ~ 梨状孔 / spinal ~ 椎孔
apex ['eipeks] ([复] **apexes** 或 **apices** ['eipisiːz]) *n*【拉】顶,顶点;尖,尖端 | darwinian ~ 耳郭尖 / ~ of lung 肺尖 / ~ of tongue 舌尖
apexcardiogram [,eipeks'kɑːdiəgræm] *n* 心尖心动图
apexcardiography [,eipeks,kɑːdi'ɔgrəfi] *n* 心尖心动描记法
apexification [ei,peksifi'keiʃən] *n* 根尖诱导形成术
APF acidulated phosphate fluoride 酸化的磷酸氟化物
Apgar score (scale) ['æpgə] (Virginia Apgar)阿普加评分(评分表)(评定新生儿在产后60s时的心率、呼吸力、肌张力、反射应激性和肤色所获得的得分总数)
APH anterior pituitary hormone 垂体前叶激素
APH antepartum hemorrhage 产前出血
APHA American Protestant Hospital Association 美国耶稣教医院协会;American Public Health Association 美国公共卫生协会
APhA American Pharmaceutical Association 美国药

学协会

aphagia [ə'feidʒiə], **aphagopraxia** [əˌfeigə'præksiə] *n* 吞咽不能

aphakia [ə'feikiə], **aphacia** [ə'feisiə] *n* 无晶状体 | **aphakic** [ə'feikik], **aphacic** [ə'feisik] *a*

aphalangia [eifə'lændʒiə] *n* 无指趾[畸形]

Aphanizomenon [əˌfænizə'menɔn] *n* 束丝藻属

Aphanoascus [əˌfænə'æskəs] *n* 裸囊菌属

Aphanozoa [ˌæfənə'zəuə] *n* 超视生物类(即超显微生物,病毒)

aphasia [ə'feizjə] *n* 失语[症] | ageusic ~ 味觉性失语 / amnemonic ~, amnesic ~, amnestic ~ 遗忘性失语 / anomic ~ 命名性失语 / associative ~ 联络性失语 / ataxic ~, motor ~ 运动失调性失语 / auditory ~, acoustic ~ 听觉性失语,听言不能 / central ~ 中枢性失语 / cortical ~, expressive-receptive ~, global ~ 皮质性失语,感觉表达性失语,完全失语 / gibberish ~ 呓语性失语 / graphomotor ~ 失写性失语 / receptive ~, impressive ~, sensory ~, temporoparietal ~ 感觉性失语,记言不能,颞顶性失语 / semantic ~ 语义性失语 / true ~, intellectual ~ 真性失语 / syntactical ~ 语法性失语 / verbal ~ 词汇性失语 / visual ~ 视觉性失语,文字盲 | **aphasic** [ə'feizik] *a* 失语的 *n* 失语者 / **~c** [ə'feiziæk] *n* 失语者

aphasiology [əˌfeizi'ɔlədʒi] *n* 失语症学(研究失语症及产生失语症的特定的神经病学损害) | **aphasiologist** *n* 失语症学家(如神经病学家或心理学家)

aphasmid [ei'fæzmid] *n* 无尾觉器线虫

Aphasmidia [eifæz'midiə] *n* 无尾觉器亚纲

apheliotropism [əˌfiːli'ɔtrəpizəm] *n* 背日性,远日性,远阳性 | **apheliotropic** [əˌfiːliəu'trɔpik] *a*

aphemesthesia [ˌæfiːmis'θiːzjə] *n* 听读不能

aphemia [ə'fiːmiə] *n* 运动性失语,运动性语言失能症 | **aphomic** [ə'fəmik] *a*

apheresis [eifə'riːsis] *n* 单采血液成分术(从供者抽取血液,一部分〈血浆、白细胞、血小板等〉分离并保留,剩下的再输回给供者的方法。此法包括白细胞去除术〈leukapheresis〉,血小板去除术〈thrombocytapheresis〉等,亦称去除术〈pheresis〉)

apheter ['æfitə] *n* 肌肉收缩质促解物

Aphiochaeta ferruginea [ɑːfiəu'kiːtə feru'giniə] 锈色蚤蝇

aphonia [ei'fəunjə] *n* 失声 | ~ clericorum 过用性失声,慢性咽喉炎性发声困难 / spastic ~ 痉挛性失声 | **aphonic** [ei'fɔnik] *a*

aphonogelia [ˌæfəunə'dʒiːliə] *n* 大笑不能症

aphose [ə'fəuz] *n* 影幻视

aphosphagenic [eiˌfɔsfə'dʒenik] *a* 缺磷的

aphosphorosis [eiˌfɔsfə'rəusis] *n* 缺磷症

aphotesthesia [ˌeifɔtis'θiːzjə] *n* 视网膜光感减退

aphotic [ei'fɔtik] *a* 无光的

aphrasia [ei'freiziə] *n* 组句不能

aphrenia [ə'friːniə] *n* 痴呆

aphrodisia [ˌæfrəu'diziə] *n* 性欲炽盛;交合,交媾

aphrodisiac [ˌæfrəu'diziæk] *a* 催欲的 *n* 催欲药

aphtha ['æfθə] ([复] **aphthae** ['æfθiː]) *n*【拉;希】口疮;阿弗他溃疡 | chronic intermittent recurrent ~e, ~e resistentiae 慢性间歇性复发性口疮 / contagious ~e, epizootic ~e [接]触[传]染性口疮,兽疫性口疮(即牛的口蹄疫) / recurring scarring ~e 复发性疤痕性口疮 | **aphthous** ['æfθəs] *a*

aphthoid ['æfθɔid] *a* 口疮样的 *n* 口疮样疹

aphthongia [æf'θɔndʒiə] *n* 痉挛性失语

aphthosis [æf'θəusis] *n* 口疮病

Aphthovirus [ˌæfθəu'vaiərəs] *n* 口疮病毒,口蹄疫病毒;口疮病毒属(可致口蹄疫)

aphylaxis [ˌeifi'læksis] *n* 无防御力,防御力缺失 | **aphylactic** [ˌeifi'læktik] *a*

Aphyllophorales [əˌfiləfə'reiliːz] *n* 多孔菌目

apical ['æpikəl] *a* 顶的;尖的,尖端的

apicalis [ˌæpi'keilis] *a*【拉】尖的,顶的;位于尖端的

apicectomy [ˌeipi'sektəmi] *n* 岩尖切除术(颞骨岩部顶切除术)

apices ['eipisiːz] apex 的复数

apicitis [ˌeipi'saitis] *n* 根尖炎(如牙尖、肺尖或颞骨岩部顶发炎)

apic(o)- [前缀]尖,顶

apicoectomy [ˌeipikə'ektəmi] *n* 根尖切除术

apicolysis [ˌeipi'kɔlisis] *n* 肺尖萎陷术

Apicomplexa [ˌeipikɔm'pleksə] *n* 顶复[原虫]亚门

apicomplexan [ˌeipikɔm'pleksən] *n*, *a* 顶复虫(的)

apicostomy [ˌeipi'kɔstəmi] *n* 根尖造口术

apicotomy [ˌeipi'kɔtəmi] *a* 岩尖切开术(颞骨岩部顶穿刺术)

apiculate [ə'pikjuleit, -lit] *a* 具细尖的

apiculus [ə'pikjuləs] *n* 细尖

Apidae ['æpidiː] *n* 蜂科

apii fructus ['eipiai 'frʌktəs] 芹[菜]实

APIM Association Professionnelle Internationale des Médecins【法】国际专业医师协会

apinealism [ə'piniəlizəm] *n* 松果体功能缺失

apinoid ['æpinɔid] *a* 清洁的,洁净的

apiotherapy [ˌeipiəu'θerəpi] *n* 蜂毒疗法

apiphobia [ˌeipi'fəubiə] *n* 蜂恐怖

Apis ['eipis] *n* 蜂属

apish ['eipiʃ] *a* 猿一样的

apisination [ˌeipisiˈneiʃən] *n* 蜂螫中毒
apitoxin [ˌeipiˈtɔksin] *n* 蜂毒素
apituitarism [ˌeipiˈtju(ː)itəˌrizəm] *n* 垂体功能缺失;先天性无垂体(如无脑畸形)
Apium [ˈeipiəm] *n*【拉】芹属
aplacental [ˌeipləˈsentl] *a* 无胎盘的
aplanatic [ˌæpləˈnætik] *a* 消球[面]差的,等光程的
aplanatism [əˈplænətizəm] *n* 消球[面]差
aplasia [əˈpleizjə] *n* 不发育,发育不全 | ~ axialis extracorticalis congenita 家族性脑中叶硬化 / ~ cutis congenita 先天性皮肤发育不全 / dental ~ 牙发育不全 / gonadal ~, germinal ~ 性腺发育不全 / hereditary retinal ~ 遗传性视网膜发育不全,先天性黑矇 / nuclear ~ 神经核发育不全 / ~ of ovary 卵巢发育不全 / pure red cell ~ 纯红细胞再生障碍 / retinal ~ 视网膜发育不全 / thymic ~ 胸腺发育不全 / thymic-parathyroid ~ 胸腺-甲状旁腺发育不全
aplasmic [eiˈplæzmik] *a* 无原生质的,无原浆的
aplastic [eiˈplæstik] *a* 发育不全的,成形不全的;再生障碍的
Aplectana [əˈplektənə] *n* 双刺蛲虫属
apleuria [eiˈpluəriə] *n* 无肋
APM Academy of Physical Medicine 物理医学学会,理疗学学会;Academy of Psychosomatic Medicine 心身医学学会
apnea [ˈæpniːə] *n* 呼吸暂停 | deglutition ~ 吞咽[时]呼吸暂停 / ~ neonatorum 新生儿呼吸暂停 / traumatic ~ 创伤性窒息 | **apneic** [ˈæpniːik] *a*
apneumatic [ˌæpnju(ː)ˈmætik] *a* 无气的
apneumatosis [ˌæpnju(ː)məˈtəusis] *n* 肺无气,先天性肺膨胀不全
apneumia [æpˈnjuːmiə] *n* 无肺[畸形]
apneusis [æpˈnjuːsis] *n* 长吸 | **apneustic** [æpˈnjuːstik] *a*
apo-, ap- [前缀]远,离,分离;脱,去
apoatropine [ˌæpəuˈætrəpin] *n* 阿扑阿托品(一种镇痉生物碱)
apocamnosis [ˌæpəukæmˈnəusis] *n* 疲劳症
apocenosis [ˌæpəusiˈnəusis] *n* 排液,排脓
apochromat [ˌæpəˈkrəumæt] *n* 复消色差物镜
apochromatic [ˌæpəkrəuˈmætik] *a* 复消色差的
apocope [əˈpɔkəpi] *n* 切断术
apocoptic [ˌæpəˈkɔptik] *a* 切断的
apocrine [ˈæpəkrin] *a* 顶质分泌的
apocrinitis [ˌæpəkriˈnaitis] *n* 顶[质分]泌腺炎
apocrustic [ˌæpəˈkrʌstik] *a* 收敛的 *n* 收敛剂
apocynin [əˈpɔsinin] *n* 夹竹桃麻素,乙酰香草酮(强心药)
Apocynum [əˈpɔsinəm] *n* 茶叶花属
apodal [əˈpəudəl] *a* 无足的
Apodemus [ˌæpəuˈdiːməs] *n* 姬鼠属 | ~ agarius 黑线姬鼠 / ~ sylvaticus 小林姬鼠
apodia [eiˈpəudiə] *n* 无足[畸形]
apoenzyme [ˌæpəuˈenzaim], **apoferment** [ˌæpəˈfəːmənt] *n* 脱辅[基]酶
apoferritin [ˌæpəˈferitin] *n* 阿扑铁蛋白,脱铁铁蛋白
apogamia [ˌæpəˈgæmiə], **apogamy** [əˈpɔgəmi] *n* 无配[子]生殖
apogee [ˈæpədʒiː] *n* 病危期 | **apogean** [ˌæpəˈdʒiːən], **apogeal** [ˌæpəˈdʒiːl] *a*
apokamnosis [ˌæpəukæmˈnəusis] *n* 疲劳症,病态疲劳
apolar [eiˈpəulə] *a* 无极的,非极的;无突的
apolegamy [ˌæpəˈlegəmi] *n* 性选择,选配 | **apolegamic** [ˌæpəliˈgæmik] *a*
apolepsis [ˌæpəˈlepsis] *n* 分泌停止
apolipoprotein [ˌæpəulipəˈprəutiːn] *n* 载脂蛋白
apolipoprotein C-Ⅱ (apo C-Ⅱ) deficiency, familial [ˌæpəulipəˈprəutiːn] 家族性载脂蛋白 C-Ⅱ缺乏症(即家族性高脂蛋白血症Ⅰ和Ⅴ型,由于缺损的载脂蛋白 C-Ⅱ所致)
apomixia [ˌæpəˈmiksiə], **apomixis** [ˌæpəˈmiksis] *n* 无融合生殖
apomorphine [ˌæpəuˈmɔːfiːn] *n* 阿扑吗啡 | ~ hydrochloride 盐酸阿扑吗啡(催吐药)
aponeurectomy [ˌæpənjuəˈrektəmi] *n* 腱膜切除术
aponeurology [ˌæpənjuəˈrɔlədʒi] *n* 腱膜学
aponeurorrhaphy [ˌæpənjuəˈrɔrəfi] *n* 腱膜缝合术,腱膜修补术
aponeurosis [ˌæpənjuəˈrəusis] ([复] **aponeuroses** [ˌæpənjuəˈrəusiːz]) *n* 腱膜 | abdominal ~ 腹肌腱膜 / bicipital ~ 肱二头肌腱膜 / crural ~ 小腿筋膜 / epicranial ~, ~ of occipitofrontal muscle 帽状腱膜,枕额肌腱膜 / ~ of insertion 止腱,止端腱膜 / perineal ~ 会阴腱膜,尿生殖膈下筋膜 / pharyngeal ~, pharyngobasilar ~ 咽腱膜,咽颅底筋膜 / plantar ~ 跖腱膜 / subscapular ~ 肩胛下肌筋膜 / superficial perineal ~ 会阴浅腱膜,盆膈下筋膜 / superior perineal ~ 会阴上腱膜,盆膈上筋膜 / supraspinous ~ 冈上筋膜 / temporal ~ 颞筋膜 / vertebral ~ 腰背筋膜 | **aponeurotic** [ˌæpənjuəˈrɔtik] *a*
aponeurositis [ˌæpənjuərəˈsaitis] *n* 腱膜炎
aponeurotome [ˌæpəˈnjuərətəum] *n* 腱膜刀
aponeurotomy [ˌæpənjuəˈrɔtəmi] *n* 腱膜切开术
aponic [əˈpəunik] *a* 止痛的;减疲劳的
Aponomma [ˌæpəˈnɔmə] *n* 盲花蜱属
apophlegmatic [ˌæpəuflegˈmætik] *a* 化痰的,祛痰的 *n* 祛痰药

apophylaxis [ˌæpəufiˈlæksis] *n* 防御力减退 | **apophylactic** [ˌæpəufiˈlæktik] *a*
apophyseopathy [ˌæpəfiziˈɔpəθi] *n* 骨突病
apophysis [əˈpɔfisis] ([复] **apophyses** [əˈpɔfisiːz]) *n*【希】骨突 | basilar ~ [枕骨]底部 / cerebral ~ 松果体 / genial ~ 颏棘 / ~ of Ingrassia 蝶骨小翼 / **apophyseal, apophysial** [ˌæpəˈfiziəl], **apophysary** [əˈpɔfizəri], **apophysiary** [ˌæpəˈfiziəri] *a*
apophysitis [əˌpɔfiˈzaitis] *n* 骨突炎
Apophysomyces [ˌæpəuˌfizəuˈmaisiːz] *n* 毛霉菌属
apoplasmatic [ˌæpəuplæzˈmætik] *a* 原地胞质[产生]的(指由细胞产生的物质,此物质是组织的一个组成部分,如结缔组织的纤维,或骨和软骨的基质)
apoplectiform [ˌæpəˈplektifɔːm], **apoplectoid** [æpəˈplektɔid] *a* 卒中样的
apoplexia [ˌæpəˈpleksiə] *n*【拉】[脑]卒中
apoplexy [ˈæpəˌpleksi] *n* [脑]卒中 | abdominal ~ 腹卒中 / cerebral ~ 脑卒中 / heat ~ 中暑,热射病 / renal ~ 肾卒中,肾猝出血 | **apoplectic(al)** [ˌæpəˈplektik(əl)] *a*
apoprotein [ˌæpəuˈprəutiːn] *n* 脱辅蛋白质
apoptosis [ˌæpɔpˈtəusis] *n* [细胞]凋亡(与程序性细胞死亡同义) | **apoptotic** [ˌæpɔpˈtɔtik] *a*
aporepressor [ˌæpəriˈpresə] *n* 阻抑物原,阻遏蛋白(阻抑基因的产物,结构不明,它与低分子量的辅阻抑物结合形成完全的阻抑物质,专门阻抑某一特定结构基因的活动)
aposome [ˈæpəsəum] *n* 胞质小体(由细胞活动而产生的包涵物)
aposorbic acid [ˌæpəˈsɔːbik] 从山梨糖酸
apostasis [əˈpɔstəsis] *n* 脓肿;病情骤变
aposthia [əˈpɔsθiə] *n* 无包皮[畸形]
Apostomatida [ˌæpəstəˈmætidə] *n* 后口目
Apostomatidea [ˌæpəstəməˈtiːdiə] *n* 后口总目
Apostomatina [ˌæpəstəˈmætinə] *n* 后口亚目
apothanasia [ˌæpəuθəˈneiziə] *n* 延命术
apothecary [əˈpɔθikəri] *n* 药剂师;药商 | surgeon ~ 外科医师兼药剂师(英国)
apothecium [ˌæpəˈθiːsiəm] *n* 子囊盘
apothem [ˈæpəθəm], **apotheme** [ˈæpəθiːm] *n* 浸剂沉淀物
apotoxin [ˌæpəˈtɔksin] *n* 过敏毒素(可引起过敏反应的症状)
apotransferrin [ˌæpətrænsˈferin] *n* 脱铁运铁蛋白
apotripsis [ˌæpəˈtripsis] *n* 角膜翳擦除法
apotropaic [ˌæpətrəˈpeiik] *a* 预防的(古希腊医学中指避邪去病之意)
apoxemena [ˌæpɔkˈseminə] *n* 牙周刮出物
apoxesis [ˌæpɔkˈsiːsis] *n* 刮除术(牙周袋腐质刮除)
apozem [ˈæpəzem], **apozema** [əˈpɔzəmə], **apozeme** [ˈæpəziːm] *n* 煎剂
apozymase [ˌæpəˈzaimeis] *n* 发酵酶蛋白
apparatus [ˌæpəˈreitəs] ([复] **apparatus** 或 **apparatuses**) *n* 仪器,器[械];装置;器官 | absorption ~ 吸收器(气体分析用) / auditory ~, acoustic ~ 听器,听感受器 / biliary ~ 胆器[官] / central ~ 中心器 / chromidial ~ 核外染色质 / ciliary ~ 睫状体 / cytopharyngeal ~ [细]胞咽器 / digestive ~ 消化器 / juxtaglomerular ~ [肾小]球旁器 / lacrimal ~ 泪器 / masticatory ~ 咀嚼器 / mental ~ 精神结构(即自我保存,自我,超我) / parabasal ~ 副基器 / pilosebaceous ~ 毛囊皮脂腺器 / respiratory ~ 呼吸器 / sound-conducting ~ 传声器 / sound-perceiving ~ 感声器,觉声器 / spindle ~ 纺锤体 / steadiness ~ 运动失调描记器 / sucker ~ 吸器,吸盘,吸足 / urogenital ~, genitourinary ~ 尿生殖器 / vocal ~ 发声器官
appearance [əˈpiərəns] *n* 出现,呈现;外貌;表象,形,状 | torpid ~ 无欲貌 / urea nitrogen ~ 脲氮出现
appendage [əˈpendidʒ] *n* 附件,附器 | atrial ~, auricular ~ 心耳 / cecal ~ 阑尾 / epiploic ~s 肠脂垂 / ~s of the eye 眼附属器(睑、眉、泪器及结膜) / ~s of the fetus 胎儿附件(脐带、胎盘及胎膜) / ovarian ~ 卵巢冠 / ~s of the skin 皮肤附件(毛、爪、皮脂腺、汗腺及乳腺) / testicular ~, ~ of the testis 睾丸附件 / uterine ~s 子宫附件(子宫韧带、输卵管及卵巢) / vermicular ~ 阑尾
appendagitis [əˌpendəˈdʒaitis] *n* 附件炎(尤指肠脂垂炎) | epiploic ~ 肠脂垂炎
appendectomy [ˌæpənˈdektəmi] *n* 阑尾切除术 | auricular ~ 心耳切除术 | **appendicectomy** [əˌpendiˈsektəmi] *n*
appendiceal [æpənˈdisiəl], **appendical** [əˈpendikəl] *a* 阑尾的
appendices [əˈpendisiːz] appendix 的复数
appendicitis [əˌpendiˈsaitis] *n* 阑尾炎 | acute ~ 急性阑尾炎 / amebic ~ 阿米巴性阑尾炎 / chronic ~ 慢性阑尾炎 / ~ by contiguity 接触性阑尾炎 / foreign-body ~ 异物性阑尾炎 / left-sided ~ 左位阑尾炎 / lumber ~ 腰位阑尾炎 / obstructive ~ 梗阻性阑尾炎 / perforating ~, perforative ~ 穿孔性阑尾炎 / protective ~, ~ obliterans 闭塞性阑尾炎 / recurrent ~, relapsing ~ 复发性阑尾炎 / skip ~ 分隔局限性阑尾炎 / stercoral ~ 粪石性阑尾炎 / subperitoneal ~ 腹膜下阑尾炎 / suppurative ~ 化脓性阑尾炎 / verminous ~, helminthic ~ 肠虫性阑尾炎

appendic(o)- [构词成分]附件(尤指阑尾)
appendicocecostomy [əˌpendikəusiˈkɔstəmi] *n* 阑尾盲肠吻合术
appendicocele [əˈpendikəˌsiːl] *n* 阑尾疝
appendicoenterostomy [əˌpendikəuentəˈrɔstəmi] *n* 阑尾小肠吻合术;阑尾造口术
appendicolithiasis [əˌpendikəuliˈθaiəsis] *n* 阑尾石病
appendicolysis [əˌpendikəuˈlaisis] *n* 阑尾粘连分离术
appendicopathy [əˌpendiˈkɔpəθi], **appendicopathia** [əˌpendikəuˈpæθiə] *n* 阑尾病
appendicostomy [əˌpendiˈkɔstəmi] *n* 阑尾造口术
appendicovesical [əˌpendikəuˈvesikəl] *a* 阑尾膀胱的
appendicovesicostomy [əˌpendikəuˌvesiˈkɔstəmi] *n* 阑尾膀胱造口术
appendicular [ˌæpənˈdikjulə] *a* 阑尾的;附件的
appendix [əˈpendiks] ([复] **appendixes** 或 **appendices** [əˈpendisiːz]) *n* 附件;阑尾 | auricular ~ 心耳 / cecal ~, vermiform ~ 阑尾 / ensiform ~, xiphoid ~ 剑突 / epiploic appendices, omental appendices 肠脂垂 / ~ of ventricle of larynx 喉室附部,喉室
appendolithiasis [əˌpendəuliˈθaiəsis] *n* 阑尾石病
apperception [ˌæpə(ː)ˈsepʃən] *n* 统觉,明觉,感知 | **apperceptive** [ˌæpə(ː)ˈseptiv] *a*
appersonation [ˌæpəːsəˈneiʃən] *n* 自我[人格]变换[妄想],易身妄想
appersonification [ˌæpəˌsɔnifiˈkeiʃən] *n* 自我[人格]变换[妄想]
appestat [ˈæpistæt] *n* 食欲中枢
appetite [ˈæpitait] *n* 食欲 | excessive ~ 贪食,食欲过盛 / perverted ~ 异食癖,食欲倒错 | **appetitive** [əˈpetitiv] *a*
appetition [ˌæpiˈtiʃən] *n* 欲望,渴望
appetizer [ˈæpitaizə] *n* 开胃剂(正餐前的开胃食品或饮料)
appetizing [ˈæpitaiziŋ] *a* 促进食欲的,开胃的
applanation [ˌæpləˈneiʃən] *n* 扁平(如角膜扁平)
applanometer [ˌæpləˈnɔmitə] *n* 眼压计(检青光眼时测眼内压)
apple [ˈæpl] *n* 苹果 | Adam's ~ 喉结 / bitter ~ 药西瓜瓤 / Indian ~, May ~ 鬼臼[根] / thorn ~ 曼陀罗
appliance [əˈplaiəns] *n* 器具,用具;设备;器械;矫正器,装置 | craniofacial ~ 颅面[制动]器 / extraoral ~ 口外[制动]器,口外装置 / fixed ~ [牙]固定器,固定装置 / orthodontic ~ 正牙矫正器 / prosthetic ~ 修复器 / universal ~ 通用[矫正]器
application [ˌæpliˈkeiʃən] *n* 应用,用法;敷贴 | for external ~ (药)供外用
applicator [ˈæpliˌkeitə] *n* 声极;敷料器,涂药器 | sonic ~ 声头(超声治疗用)
appliqué [ˌæpliˈkei] *a* 【法】(见 form)
apposition [ˌæpəˈziʃən] *n* 并置,并列;对合
apprehension [ˌæpriˈhenʃən] *n* 理解,领会;恐惧,忧虑 | irresistible ~ 强迫性恐怖症
approach [əˈprəutʃ] *n* 接近;进路,入门;探讨,方法 | combined craniofacial ~ 颅面联合进路 / far lateral ~ 远外侧入路
appropriate [əˈprəupriit] *a* 适当的 | ~ for gestational age infant 适于胎龄儿
approval [əˈpruːvəl] *n* 认可,批准;同意 | social ~ 社会认可,社会同意
approximal [əˈprɔksiməl] *a* 邻接的
approximate [əˈprɔksimit] *a* 近似的,大约的
approximation [əˌprɔksiˈmeiʃən] *n* 接近,近似;近似值 | successive ~ 逐步渐近,渐次趋近(见 shaping)
apractagnosia [əˌpræktægˈnəuziə] *n* [立体]空间关系失认[症]
apramycin [ˌæprəˈmaisin] *n* 安普霉素(抗菌抗生素)
apraxia [əˈpræksiə] *n* 失用[症] | amnestic ~ 遗忘性失用[症] / cortical ~ 皮质性失用[症] / ideokinetic ~ 意想运动性失用[症] / ideomotor ~ 观念-运动性失用[症] / limb-kinetic ~ 肢体运动性失用[症] / motor ~, innervation ~ 运动性失用[症] | **apraxic** [əˈpræksik], **apractic** [əˈpræktik] *a*
aprindine [əˈprindin] *n* 阿普林定(心脏抑制药,用作抗心律失常药) | ~ hydrochloride 盐酸阿普林定
apriority [ˌei-praiˈɔrəti] *n* 先验法;先验性
aprobarbital [ˌæprəuˈbɑːbitæl] *n* 阿普比妥(催眠镇静药)
aproclonidine hydrochloride [ˌæprəˈklɔnidiːn] 盐酸阿可乐定(α_2-肾上腺素能受体激动药,用以降低眼压,治疗开角型青光眼和高眼压症,局部给药)
Aprocta [əˈprɔktə] *n* 无疣丝虫属
aproctia [əˈprɔkʃiə] *n* 锁肛,无肛
apron [ˈeiprən] *n* 围裙 | Hottentot ~, pudendal ~ 小阴唇展长,阴门帘
aprosody [eiˈprɔsədi], **aprosodia** [ˌeiprəˈsəudiə] *n* 失语韵症
aprosopia [ˌæprəˈsəupiə] *n* 无面[畸形]
aprosopus [əˈprəusəpəs] *n* 无面畸胎
aprotic [eiˈprəutik] *a* 质子惰性的
aprotinin [ˌæprəˈtainin] *n* 抑肽酶,抑胰肽酶(抑制蛋白酶及激肽释放酶,用于治疗胰腺炎)
APS American Pediatric Society 美国儿科学会;

American Physiological Society 美国生理学会；American Proctologic Society 美国直肠病学会；American Psychological Society 美国心理学会；American Psychosomatic Society 美国心身医学会
APTA American Physical Therapy Association 美国物理疗法协会
apterous [ˈæptərəs] *a* 无翅的，无翼的
Apterygiformes [ˌæptəˌridʒiˈfɔːmiːz] *n* 无翼鸟目
aptitude [ˈæptitjuːd] *n* 能力；倾向；资质，才能；敏悟，颖悟
APTT, aPTT activated partial thromboplastin time 活化部分促凝血酶原激酶时间
aptyalia [ˌæptaiˈeiliə], **aptyalism** [æpˈtaiəlizəm] *n* 唾液缺乏
APUD amine precursor uptake (and) decarboxylation 胺与胺前体摄取[和]脱羧(细胞)
apudoma [ˌeipjuːˈdəumə] *n* APUD 瘤，apud 瘤
apulmonism [eiˈpʌlmənizəm] *n* 无肺[畸形]
apurinic acid [əˈpjuəri(ː)nik] 无嘌呤核酸
apus [ˈeipəs] *n* 无足畸胎
apyetous [eiˈpaiitəs] *a* 无脓的，不化脓的
apyknomorphous [əˌpiknəˈmɔːfəs] *a* 非密形的，非固缩状的(指某些神经细胞)
apyogenous [ˌeipaiˈɔdʒinəs] *a* 非化脓性的
apyous [eiˈpaiəs] *a* 无脓的
apyrase [ˈæpireis] *n* 腺苷三磷酸双磷酸酶
apyrene [ˈeipaiəriːn] *a* 无核的
apyretic [ˌeipaiˈretik] *a* 无热的，不发热的
apyrexia [ˌeipaiˈreksiə] *n* 无热；无热期，热歇期 | **~l** *a*
apyrogenic [eiˌpaiərəuˈdʒenik] *a* 不致热的
AQ achievement quotient 成就商数，成绩商数
Aq. aqua【拉】水，水剂 | ~ dest. aqua destillata【拉】蒸馏水 / ~ pur. aqua pura【拉】纯水 / ~ tep. aqua tepida【拉】温水
aqua [ˈækwə, ˈɑːkwə] ([复] **aquae** [ˈækwiː, ˈɑːkwiː]) *n*【拉】水，水剂 | ~ amnii 羊[膜]水 / ~ anisi 洋茴香水 / ~ astricta 冰水 / ~ bulliens 沸水 / ~ communis 普通水，常水 / ~ destillata 蒸馏水 / ~ destillata sterilis 无菌蒸馏水 / ~ fervens 热水 / ~ foeniculi 茴香水 / ~ fortis 硝水 / ~ oculi 前房液 / ~ pericardii 心包液 / ~ pro injection 注射用水 / ~ regia 王水 / ~ rosae 玫瑰水 / ~ sterilisata 无菌水 / ~ tepida 温水 / ~ vitae 白兰地
Aquabirnavirus [ˌɑːkwəˈbəːnəˌvaiərəs] *n* 水双节 RNA 病毒属
aquagenic [ˌækwəˈdʒenik] *a* 水源性的
aquaphobia [ˌækwəˈfəubjə] *n* 溺水恐怖，恐水症
aquapuncture [ˈækwəˌpʌŋktʃə] *n* 皮下注水法
Aquareovirus [ˌækwəˈriːəuˌvaiərəs] *n* 呼肠孤病毒属
Aquaspirillum [ˌækwəspaiəˈriləm] *n* 水螺菌属
aquatic [əˈkwætik] *a* 水生的，水栖的 *n* 水生动植物
aqueduct [ˈækwidʌkt] *n* 水管 | cerebral ~, ventricular ~, ~ of midbrain 大脑水管，脑室水管，中脑水管 / ~ of cochlea 蜗小管 / fallopian ~ 面神经管 / ~ of the vestibule 前庭小管；内淋巴管
aqueductus, aquaeductus [ˌækwiˈdʌktəs] *n*【拉】水管
aqueous [ˈeikwiəs] *a* 水的，用水制备的 *n* 眼房水
aquiparous [æˈkwipərəs] *a* 生水的
aquocapsulitis [ˌeikwəuˌkæpsjuˈlaitis] *n* 浆液性虹膜炎
aquula [ˈækwulə] *n*【拉】耳迷路淋巴液
AR alarm reaction 警戒反应，惊恐反应；aortic regurgitation 主动脉瓣反流；artificial respiration 人工呼吸
Ar argon 氩
ARA American Rheumatism Association 美国风湿病协会
ara-A adenine arabinoside 阿糖腺苷(抗病毒药)
araban [ˈærəbæn] *n* 阿拉伯聚糖
arabanase [əˈræbineis] *n* 阿拉伯聚糖酶
arabate [ˈærəbeit] *n* 阿拉伯酸盐
arabic acid [ˈærəbik] 阿拉伯酸
arabin [ˈærəbin] *n* 阿拉伯胶素(亦称阿拉伯酸)
arabinose [əˈræbinəus] *n* 阿拉伯糖
arabinoside [ˌærəˈbinəusaid] *n* 阿拉伯糖苷
arabinosis [əˌræbiˈnəusis] *n* 阿拉伯糖中毒(可致肾病变)
arabinosuria [əˌræbinəuˈsjuəriə] *n* 阿拉伯糖尿
arabinosylcytosine [əˌræbinəusilˈsaitəsiːn] *n* 阿糖胞苷(抗病毒、抗肿瘤药)
arabinulose [ˌærəˈbinjuləus] *n* 阿[拉伯]酮糖
arabitol [əˈræbitɔl], **arabite** [ˈærəbait] *n* 阿[拉伯]糖醇
arabonic acid [ˌærəˈbɔnik] 阿[拉伯]糖酸
arabopyranose [ˌærəbəuˈpairənəus] *n* 阿[拉伯]吡喃糖
ara-C arabinosylcytosine 阿糖胞苷(抗肿瘤药，抗病毒药)
arachic acid [əˈrækik] 花生酸
arachidate [əˈrækideit] *n* 花生酸盐
arachidic [ˌærəˈkidik] *a* [落]花生的(花生仁所致的，如花生仁吸入性支气管炎) | ~ acid 花生酸
arachidonate [əˌrækiˈdɔneit] *n* 花生四烯酸(盐或酯)
arachidonate 5-lipoxygenase [əˌrækiˈdɔneit liˈpɔksidʒəneis] 花生四烯酸 5-脂[肪]氧合酶(亦称脂[肪]氧合酶)

arachidonate 12-lipoxygenase [əˌræki'dɔneit li-'pɔksidʒəneis] 花生四烯酸 12-脂[肪]氧合酶(亦称脂[肪]氧合酶)

arachidonate 15-lipoxygenase [əˌræki'dɔneit li-'pɔksidʒeneis] 花生四烯酸 15-脂[肪]氧合酶

arachidonic acid [ˌærəki'dɔnik] 花生四烯酸

arachis ['ærəkis] *n* 花生

arachnephobia [əˌrækni'fəubjə] *n* 蜘蛛恐怖,恐蛛症

Arachnia [ə'ræknia] *n* 蛔网菌属 | ~ propionica 丙酸蛛网菌

arachnid [ə'ræknid] *n* 蜘蛛(蛛形纲动物) | **~an** [ə'ræknidən] *a*, *n*

Arachnida [ə'ræknidə] *n* 蛛形纲

arachnidism [ə'ræknidizəm] *n* 蛛毒中毒

arachnitis [ˌæræk'naitis] *n* 蛛网膜炎

arachn(o)- [构词成分]蛛网膜,蜘蛛

arachnodactyly [əˌræknəu'dæktili], **arachnodactylia** [əˌræknəudæk'tiliə] *n* 蜘蛛样指,蜘蛛样趾

arachnogastria [əˌræknəu'gæstriə] *n* 蛛状腹(腹水所致,尤见于肝硬化时)

arachnoid [ə'ræknɔid] *a* 蛛网样的 *n* 蛛网膜 | ~ of brain, cranial ~ 脑蛛网膜 / spinal ~, ~ of spinal cord 脊髓蛛网膜 | **~al** [ˌæræk'nɔidl] *a* 蛛网膜的

arachnoidea [ˌæræk'nɔidiə] ([复] **arachnoideae** [ˌæræk'nɔidiiː]) *n*【拉】蛛网膜

arachnoidea mater [ˌæræk'nɔidiəː'meitə, 'mɑːtə] 蛛网膜

arachnoidism [ə'ræknɔiˌdizəm] *n* 蛛毒中毒

arachnoiditis [əˌræknɔi'daitis] *n* 蛛网膜炎

arachnolysin [ˌæræk'nɔlisin] *n* 蛛毒溶血素

arachnomelia [əˌræknəu'miːliə] *n* 蜘蛛样肢(指小牛和羔羊)

arachnophobia [əˌræknəu'fəubjə] *n* 蜘蛛恐怖,恐蛛症

arachnorhinitis [əˌræknəurai'naitis] *n* 蜘蛛性鼻炎

arack [ə'ræk] *n* 粕酒

Aradidae [ə'rædidiː] *a* 扁蝽科

Aralia [ə'reiliə] *n*【拉】楤木属

aralia [ə'reiliə] *n* 美楤木

aralkyl [ə'rælkil] *n* 芳烷基

Aran-Duchenne muscular atrophy (disease) [ɑː'rɑːn du'ʃen] (François A. Aran; Guillaume B. A. Duchenne) 脊髓性肌萎缩

Araneae [ə'reiniiː], **Araneida** [ˌærə'niidə] *n* 蜘蛛目

araneid [ə'reiniid] *n* 蜘蛛 | **~an** [ˌærə'niidən] *a*

araneism [ə'reiniizəm] *n* 蛛毒中毒

araneous [ə'reiniəs] *a* 蛛网状的

Aran's law [ɑː'rɑːn] (François A. Aran) 阿朗定律(由颅顶受伤所致的颅底骨折〈除反冲伤外〉,其折线沿最短的圆周线作放射状延伸)

Arantius' bodies [ə'rænʃiəs] (Julius C. Arantius 或 Aranzi) 阿朗希乌斯体(主动脉瓣小结,半月瓣结) | ~ canal, ~ duct 静脉导管 / ~ ligament 静脉导管索 / ~ nodules 半月瓣结 / ~ ventricle 阿朗希乌斯室(第四脑室终凹)

Aranzi 见 Arantius

araphia [ə'reifiə] *n* 神经管闭合不全

araroba [ɑːrə'rəubə] *n* 柯桠木;柯桠粉

arbaprostil [ˌɑːbə'prɔstil] *n* 阿巴前列素(胃酸分泌抑制药,终止妊娠药)

arbor ['ɑːbə] ([复] **arbores** [ɑː'bɔːriːz]) *n*【拉】树(树状结构) | ~ vitae 侧柏(其叶的油用作祛痰药、抗风湿药和通经药,外用作抗刺激药及治疗皮肤病) | ~ vitae cerebelli 小脑活树 / ~ vitae uteri 棕榈襞(子宫)

arboreal [ɑː'bɔːriəl] *a* 树的;树状的;树上生活的

arborescent [ˌɑːbə'resnt] *a* 树状的

arborization [ˌɑːberai'zeiʃən, -ri'z-] *n* [树状]分枝

arborize ['ɑːbəraiz] *vt*, *vi* 成树状分枝

arboroid ['ɑːbərɔid] *a* 树样分枝的

arbovirology [ˌɑːbəvai'rɔlədʒi] *n* 虫媒病毒学

arbovirus [ˌɑːbə'vaiərəs], **arborvirus** [ɑːbɔː'v-aiərəs] *n* 虫媒病毒(包括黄热病、病毒性脑炎等的病原体) | **arboviral** [ˌɑːbə'vaiərəl] *a*

arbutamine hydrochloride [ɑː'bjuːtəˌmin] 盐酸阿布他明(一种合成的儿茶酚胺,用作心脏负荷试验诊断辅助用药)

arbutin ['ɑːbjutin] *n* 熊果苷,对苯二酚葡糖苷

Arbutus ['ɑːbjutəs] *n* 树莓属(含熊果苷,一种氢醌糖苷,用作利尿及尿路抗菌) | ~ uva-ursi 熊果(树)

ARC AIDS-related complex 艾滋病相关复征; American Red Cross 美国红十字会; anomalous retinal correspondence 异常视网膜对应

arc [ɑːk] *n* 弧,弓 | auricular ~, binauricular ~ 耳弧(耳道间距) / bregmatolambdoid ~ 冠矢弓,顶弓 / mercury ~ 汞弧(通过汞蒸气的放电) / nasobregmatic ~ 鼻前囟弓 / neural ~, sensorimotor ~ 神经弧,感觉运动弧 / nuclear ~ 晶状体涡 / reflex ~ 反射弧

arcade [ɑː'keid] *n* 弓形组织,连拱 | arterial ~s 动脉连拱

Arcanobacterium [ɑːˌkeinəubæk'tiəriəm] *n* 秘菌属 | ~ haemolyticus 溶血性秘菌

arcanum [ɑː'keinəm] ([复]**arcana** [ɑː'keinə]) *n*【拉】秘密,奥秘;秘方药

arcate ['ɑːkeit] *a* 弓形的

Arcella [ɑː'selə] *a* 表壳虫属

Arcellinida [ˌɑːsiˈlinidə] *n* 表壳虫目
arch [ɑːtʃ] *n* 弓;拱门;弓形;弓形纹 | alveolar ~ 牙槽弓 / anterior ~ of atlas 寰椎前弓 / anterior carpal ~ 腕掌侧网 / aortic ~es 主动脉弓 / branchial ~es, pharyngeal ~es, visceral ~es 鳃弓,咽弓 / costal ~, ~ of ribs 肋弓 / dorsal carpal ~, posterior carpal ~ 腕背侧网 / epiphyseal ~ 脑上体弓 / glossopalatine ~, palatoglossal ~ 舌腭弓 / hemal ~ 椎体椎突肋胸弓 / malar ~, zygomatic ~ 颧弓 / palatal ~, maxillary ~, oral ~, palatomaxillary ~ 腭弓,上颌弓,口弓,腭上颌弓 / paraphyseal ~ [脑上]旁突体弓 / pharyngopalatine ~, palatopharyngeal ~ 咽腭弓 / superficial femoral ~ 股浅弓,腹股沟韧带
arch- 见 archi-
archae(o)- 见 archi-
Archaeobacteria [ˌɑːkiəbækˈtiəriə], **Archaebacteria** [ˌɑːkibækˈtiəriə] *n* 古细菌属
archaeocerebellum [ˌɑːkiəˌseriˈbeləm] *n* 原小脑
archaeocortex [ˌɑːkiəˈkɔːteks] *n* 原皮质
archaic [ɑːˈkeiik] *a* 原始的(早期进化阶段的)
archamphiaster [ɑːˈkæmfiˌæstə] *n* 原双星体
Archangelica [ˌɑːkænˈdʒelikə] *n* 【拉】独活属(植物)
Archangiaceae [ɑːˌkændʒiˈeisiiː] *n* 原囊黏菌科
Archangium [ɑːˈkændʒiəm] *n* 原囊黏菌属
archebiosis [ˌɑːkibaiˈəusis], **archegenesis** [ˌɑːkiˈdʒenisis], **archegony** [ɑːˈkegəni] *n* 生物自生,自然发生
archecentric [ˌɑːkiˈsentrik] *a* 原始中心的
arched [ɑːtʃt] *a* 弓形[结构]的
archegonium [ˌɑːkiˈgəuniəm] *n* 雌器,藏卵器(植物) | **archegonial** [ˌɑːkiˈgəuniəl] *a*
archencephalon [ˌɑːkenˈsefələn] *n* 原脑
archenteron [ɑːˈkentərən] *n* 原肠
arche(o)- [构词成分]第一;初,原始
archeocerebellum [ɑːkiəˌseriˈbeləm] *n* 原小脑
archeocortex [ɑːkiəˈkɔːteks] *n* 原皮质
archeocyte [ˈɑːkiəsait] *n* 原细胞(游走变形细胞)
archeokinetic [ˌɑːkiəkaiˈnetik], **archeocinetic** [ˌɑːkiəsaiˈnetik] *a* 原始运动的(指原始型运动神经机制,如见于外周神经系统与神经节神经系统)
archesporium [ˌɑːkiˈspɔːriəm], **archespore** [ˈɑːkispɔː] *n* 孢原组织,原孢子
archetype [ˈɑːkitaip] *n* 原[始]型 | **archetypal**, **archetypical** [ɑːkiˈtipikəl] *a*
archi- [构词成分]主要;初,原始
archiblast [ˈɑːkiblæst] *n* 卵质,卵浆;主胚层 | **~ic** [ˌɑːkiˈblæstik] *a*
archicarp [ˈɑːkikɑːp] *n* 育胚器(子囊菌的雌性生殖器)
archicenter [ɑːkiˈsentə] *n* 原始中心 | **archicentric** [ɑːkiˈsentrik] *a*
archicerebellum [ˌɑːkiˌseriˈbeləm] *n* 原小脑
archicortex [ˌɑːkiˈkɔːteks] *n* 原皮质(见 archipallium)
archicyte [ˈɑːkisait] *n* 原卵细胞
archicytula [ˌɑːkiˈsitjulə] *n* 原始受精卵
archigaster [ˈɑːkiˌgæstə] *n* 原肠
archigastrula [ˌɑːkiˈgæstrulə] *n* 初原肠胚
archigenesis [ɑːkiˈdʒenisis] *n* 自然发生,生物自生
Archigregarinida [ˌɑːkiˌgregəˈrainidə] *n* 原簇虫目
archikaryon [ˌɑːkiˈkæriən] *n* 原始核,初核
archil [ˈɑːkil] *n* 海石蕊紫
archimorula [ɑːkiˈmɔːrjulə] *n* 原始桑葚体
archinephron [ˌɑːkiˈnefrən] *n* 原肾
archineuron [ˌɑːkiˈnjuərən] *n* 原始神经元
archipallium [ˌɑːkiˈpæliəm] *n* 原皮质(指嗅脑、海马结构等区域皮质) | **archipallial** [ˌɑːkiˈpæliəl] *a*
archispore [ˈɑːkispɔː] *n* 孢原组织,原孢子
Archistomatina [ˌɑːkiˌstəuməˈtainə] *n* 原口纤毛亚目
archistome [ˈɑːkistəum] *n* 胚孔
archistriatum [ˌɑːkistraiˈeitəm] *n* 原纹状体
architectonic [ˌɑːkitekˈtənik] *a* 构造的,构型的 *n* 构造(如脑)
arch(o)- [构词成分]直肠,肛门
archocystosyrinx [ˌɑːkəˌsistəˈsiriŋks] *n* 肛门膀胱瘘
archusia [ɑːˈkjuːsiə] *n* 细胞生长素(一种假想物质)
arciform [ˈɑːsifɔːm] *a* 弓状的,弓形的
arclamp [ˈɑːklæmp], **arclight** [ˈɑːklait] *n* 弧光灯
arc-quadrant [ɑːk ˈkwədrənt] *n* 90°弧弧导系统
arctation [ɑːkˈteiʃən] *n* 孔道狭窄
Arctomys [ˈɑːktəmis] *n* 土拨鼠属
Arctostaphylos uva-ursi [ˌɑːktəˈstæfiləs ˈjuvəˈəːsai] 熊果(其叶可用作收敛剂和利尿茶)
arcual [ˈɑːkjuəl] *a* 弓的
arcualia [ˌɑːkjuˈeiliə] *n* 弧片,弓片
arcuate [ˈɑːkjuit] *a* 弓形的
arcuation [ɑːkjuˈeiʃən] *n* 弯曲
arcus [ˈɑːkəs] *n* 【拉】弓
ARD acute respiratory disease 急性呼吸道疾病; acute respiratory distress 急性呼吸窘迫
ardanesthesia [ˌɑːdænisˈθiːzjə] *n* 温觉缺失
ardeparin sodium [ɑːdiˈpɑːrin] 阿地肝素钠(抗

凝药,抗血栓药)

ardo(u)r [ˈɑːdə] *n* 灼热;热心,热情 | ~ urinae 小便灼痛

ARDS acute respiratory distress syndrome 急性呼吸窘迫综合征; adult respiratory distress syndrome 成人型呼吸窘迫综合征

area [ˈɛəriə] ([复] **areae** [ˈɛəriiː] 或 **areas**) *n* 面积;区域;区 | acoustic ~, auditory ~, vestibular ~ 前庭区,听觉区 / apical ~ [牙]根尖区 / association ~s 联络区(大脑皮质区) / basal seat ~ 基托区,底座区 / B-dependent ~ B 细胞依赖区,胸腺依赖区 / cribriform ~ of renal papilla 肾乳头筛状区 / ~ of critical definition 影像清晰区 / denture-bearing ~, denture foundation ~, denture-supporting ~ 义齿承托区 / dermatomic ~ 皮区 / embryonic ~ 胚区,胚盘 / eye ~ 侦视中枢(在额叶) / genital ~s 性区(月经时鼻部充血之区) / germinal ~ 胚区,胚盘 / glove ~ 手套区(手套可遮盖的部分〈手指、手及腕〉,有时与多神经病病例感觉缺失的分布相符) / impression ~ 印模区(口腔构造表面,可供取模) / mirror ~ 镜面区(裂隙灯透视时,角膜与晶状体的反射面) / motor ~, excitable ~, excitomotor ~, precentral ~, psychomotor ~, rolandic ~ 运动区,兴奋区,兴奋运动区,中央前区,心理运动区,皮质运动分析区 / piriform ~, pyriform ~ 梨状区,梨状叶 / postcentral ~, postrolandic ~ 中央后区 / silent ~ 静区(有病理情况,但不产生症状的大脑区) / stress-bearing ~ 应力承受区 / subcallosal ~ 旁嗅区 / thymus-dependent ~, T-dependent ~ 胸腺依赖区,T 细胞依赖区 / thymus-independent ~, T-independent ~ 非胸腺依赖区,非 T 细胞依赖区 / trigger ~ 引发区,扳机区(刺激此一区域会引起另一区域生理或病理变化) / visuopsychic ~ 视觉心理区 / vocal ~ 声门区 | **~l** *a*

areata [ˌæriˈeitə], **areatus** [ˌæriˈeitəs] *a* 簇状的

Areca [ˈærikə] *n* 【拉;东印度】槟榔属

areca [ˈærikə] *n* 槟榔

arecoline [əˈrekəlin] *n* 槟榔碱 | ~ hydrobromide 氢溴酸槟榔碱

areflexia [ˌeiriˈfleksiə] *n* 无反射,反射消失

aregenerative [ˌeiriˈdʒenərətiv] *a* 再生障碍[性]的

arenaceous [ˌæriˈneiʃəs] *a* 沙状的

Arenaviridae [ˌəriːnəˈviridiː] *n* 沙粒病毒科

Arenavirus [əˈriːnəˌvaiərəs] *n* 沙粒病毒属

arenavirus [ˌærinəˈvaiərəs] *n* 沙粒病毒

arenoid [ˈærinɔid] *a* 沙状的

areola [əˈriələ] ([复] **areolae** [əˈriəliː] 或 **areolas**) *n* 晕;细隙,小区 | ~ of mammary gland, ~ of nipple 乳[房]晕 / second ~ 第二乳晕,妊娠乳[房]晕 / vaccinal ~ 接种红晕 | **~r** *a*

areolitis [ˌæriəˈlaitis] *n* 乳晕炎

areometer [ˌæriˈɔmitə] *n* 液体比重计

areometry [ˌæriˈɔmitri] *n* 液体比重测定法 | **areometric** [ˌæriəˈmetrik] *a*

Arey's rule [ˈɛəri] (Leslie B. Arey) 艾里规律(妊娠前 5 个月胎儿身长度〈以英寸计〉等于妊娠起以前的月数的数字之和,而妊娠后 5 个月的身长等于月数乘以 2 所得之积)

ARF acute renal failure 急性肾[功能]衰竭

Arg arginine 精氨酸

arg. argentum 【拉】银

argamblyopia [ˌɑːgæmbliˈəupiə] *n* 废用性弱视

Argand burner [ɑːˈgɑː] (Aimé Argand) 阿尔甘灯(一种燃油或燃气灯,空气经内管进入以助燃)

Argas [ˈɑːgəs] *n* 锐缘蜱属,隐喙属 | ~ brumpti 布氏锐缘蜱 / ~ persicus, ~ americanus, ~ miniatus 波斯锐缘蜱,美洲锐缘蜱,微小锐缘蜱 / ~ reflexus 鸽锐缘蜱

Argasidae [ɑːˈgæsidiː] *n* 软蜱科,隐喙蜱科

argasid [ˈɑːgəsid] *a*, *n* 锐缘蜱(的)

argatroban [ɑːˈgætrəˌbæn] *n* 阿加曲班(抗凝药,抗血栓药)

argema [ˈɑːdʒimə] *n* 角膜缘溃疡

Argemone [ɑːˈdʒemɔni] *n* 蓟罂粟属

argentaffin [ɑːˈdʒentəfin] *a* 嗜银的,亲银的(指组织)

argentaffinoma [ˌɑːdʒənˌtæfiˈnəumə] *n* 嗜银细胞瘤

argentation [ɑːdʒənˈteiʃən] *n* 银染法,镀银

argentic [ɑːˈdʒentik] *a* 高价银的

argentoproteinum [ɑːˌdʒentəuˌprəutiˈainəm] *n* 蛋白银

argentum [ɑːˈdʒentəm] *n* 【拉】银

argilla [ɑːˈdʒilə] *n* 黏土,陶土

argillaceous [ˌɑːdʒiˈleiʃəs] *a* 黏土的,陶土的

arginase [ˈɑːdʒineis] *n* 精氨酸酶

arginase deficiency [ˈɑːdʒineis] 精氨酸酶缺乏症(亦称精氨酸血症,高精氨酸血症)

arginine [ˈɑːdʒini(ː)n] *n* 精氨酸 | ~ glutamate 谷氨酸精氨酸 / ~ hydrochloride 盐酸精氨酸 / suberyl ~ 辛二酰精氨酸

arginine carboxypeptidase [ˈɑːdʒini(ː)n kɑːˌbɔksiˈpeptideis] 精氨酸羧肽酶

argininemia [ˌɑːdʒiniˈniːmiə] *n* 精氨酸血症,精氨酸酶缺乏症

argininosuccinase [ˌɑːdʒininəuˈsʌksineis] *n* 精氨[基]琥珀酸酶,精氨[基]琥珀酸裂合酶

argininosuccinase deficiency 精氨[基]琥珀酸酶缺乏症,精氨[基]琥珀酸尿

argininosuccinate [ˌɑːdʒininəuˈsʌksineit] *n* 精氨基琥珀酸

argininosuccinate lyase [ˌɑːdʒininəuˈsʌksineit ˈlaieis] 精氨[基]琥珀酸裂合酶(亦称精氨[基]琥珀酸酶)

argininosuccinate synthase [ɑːdʒininəu ˈsʌksineit ˈsinθeis] 精氨[基]琥珀酸合酶(亦可写成 argininosuccinate synthetase)

argininosuccinate synthase deficiency 精氨[基]琥珀酸合酶缺乏症(一种常染色体隐性遗传氨基酸病,特征为瓜氨酸血浆和尿浓度明显升高,伴高氨血症,有时伴继发性乳清酸尿症。新生儿及晚发型均存在,临床所见严重程度各异,其中包括精神发育迟缓和神经系统异常。亦称瓜氨酸血症和瓜氨酸尿症)

argininosuccinate synthetase [ˌɑːdʒininəu ˈsʌksineit ˈsinθiteis] 精氨[基]琥珀酸合成酶(此酶的遗传性缺陷可致瓜氨酸血症)

argininosuccinate (ASA) synthetase (ASAS, ASS) deficiency 精氨[基]琥珀酸合成酶缺乏症(亦称瓜氨酸血症,瓜氨酸尿)

argininosuccinic acid [ˌɑːdʒiˌninəusʌkˈsinik] 精氨[基]琥珀酸

argininosuccinicacidemia [ˌɑːdʒiˌninəusʌkˌsinikˌæsiˈdiːmiə] *n* 精氨[基]琥珀酸血[症]

argininosuccinicaciduria [ˌɑːdʒininəusʌkˌsinikˌæsiˈdjuəriə] *n* 精氨[基]琥珀酸尿[症],精氨[基]琥珀酸裂合酶缺乏症

arginyl [ˈædʒinil] *n* 精氨酰[基]

argipressin [ˌɑːdʒiˈpresin] *n* 精氨加压素

argon (Ar) [ˈɑːgɔn] *n* 氩(化学元素)

Argyll Robertson pupil (sign) [ɑːˈdʒail ˈrɔbətsən] (Douglas M. C. L. Argyll Robertson) 阿·罗瞳孔(征)(瞳孔缩小,对调节尚有反应,对光则无反应)

argyremia [ˌɑːdʒiˈriːmiə] *n* 银血[病]

argyria [ɑːˈdʒiriə], **argyriasis** [ˌɑːdʒiˈraiəsis], **argyrism** [ˈɑːdʒirizəm], **argyrosis** [ˌɑːdʒiˈrəusis] *n* 银沉着病

argyric [ɑːˈdʒirik] *a* 银的

argyrophil [ˈɑːdʒirəufil] *a* 嗜银的(指组织)

arhigosis [ˌeiriˈgəusis] *n* 冷觉缺失

arhinencephalia [ˌeirinˌensiˈfeiliə] *n* 无嗅脑[畸形]

arhinia [əˈriniə] *n* 无鼻[畸形]

arhythmia [əˈriθmiə] *n* 心律不齐

Arias-Stella reaction [ˈæriəs-ˈstelə] (Javier Arias-Stella) 阿-斯反应(子宫内膜上皮细胞中产生的变化,主要包括细胞核深染、增大和奇形怪状,细胞极性消失,细胞质偶有空泡形成。这些变化据认为与子宫内或子宫外存在绒毛膜组织有关,可见于某些异位妊娠病例)

ariboflavinosis [eiˌraibəuˌfleiviˈnəusis] *n* 核黄素缺乏病

aril [ˈæril] *n* 假种皮

arildone [ˈærildəun] *n* 阿立酮(抗病毒药)

arillode [ˈæriləud] *n* 类假种皮

aristin [əˈristin] *n* 马兜铃素

aristogenesis [əˌristəuˈdʒenisis] *n* 优生

aristogenics [əˌristəuˈdʒeniks] *n* 优生学

Aristolochia [əˌristəˈləukiə] *n* 马兜铃属

aristolochic acid [əˌristəˈləukik] 马兜铃酸

aristolochine [ərisˈtɔlətʃiːn] *n* 马兜铃酸

Aristotle's anomaly [ˈæristɔtl] (Aristotle 为古希腊哲学家)亚里士多德异常,双笔错觉(拇示两指交叉握笔时,有两支笔的错觉)

arithmetic [əˈriθmətik] *n* 算术;计算 | **arithmetic(al)** [ˌæriθˈmetik(əl)] *a*

arithmomania [əˌriθməˈmeiniə] *n* 计算狂,计算癖

Arizona [ˌæriˈzəunə] *n* 亚利桑那菌属

arkyochrome [ˈɑːkiəkrəum] *n* 网染细胞

arkyostichochrome [ˌɑːkiəˈstikəkrəum] *n* 网纹染细胞

Arloing-Courmont test [ɑːˈljɑːŋ ˈkuəmɔnt] (Saturnin Arloing) 阿尔里安-库亚蒙特试验,结核凝集试验(结核病的肥达〈Widal〉试验)

Arlt's operation [ɑːlt] (Carl F. R. von Arlt) 阿尔特手术(眼和眼睑手术) | ~ recess 阿尔特隐窝(有时在泪囊下部的小窦) / ~ sinus 阿尔特窦,泪囊隐窝 / ~ trachoma 沙眼,颗粒性结膜炎

ARM artificial rupture of membranes 人工破膜

arm [ɑːm] *n* 臂,支臂 | bird ~ 鸟状臂(肌肉萎缩使前臂细小) / chromosome ~ 染色体臂 / golf ~ 高尔夫臂(高尔夫球手过度运动后的一种神经功能症) / lawn tennis ~ 网球员肘病 / with folded ~s 抱着胳膊

armadillo [ˌɑːməˈdiləu] *n* 犰狳

armament [ˈɑːməmənt] *n* (动植物的)防护器官

armamentarium [ˌɑːməmənˈtɛəriəm], **armarium** [ɑːˈmɛəriəm] *n*【拉】医疗设备

Armanni-Ebstein cells [ɑːˈmiːniˈebstain] (Luciano Armanni; Wilhelm Ebstein) 阿-埃细胞(近端肾直小管含有糖原沉积的空泡上皮细胞) | ~ kidney 阿-埃肾(具有阿-埃损害的肾) / ~ lesion (degeneration) 阿-埃损害(变性)(因糖原沉积,近端肾直小管上皮细胞空泡形成,见于未治疗的糖尿病患者)

armature [ˈɑːmətjuə] *n* 衔铁;甲胄

armed [ɑːmd] *a* (动植物)有防护器官的

Armigeres [ɑːˈmidʒəriːz] *n* 阿蚊属 | ~ obturbans 骚扰阿蚊

Armillifer [ɑːˈmilifə] *n* 蛇舌状虫属,洞头虫属 | ~ armillatus 腕带蛇舌状虫 / ~ moniliformis 串珠蛇舌状虫

Armophorina [ˌɑːməufəˈrainə, ˌɑːmɔfəˈrainə] *n* 甲鞘亚目

Armoracia [ˌɑːməˈreiʃə] *n* 辣根属

armo(u)r [ˈɑːmə] *n* (动植物的)防护器官

armpit [ˈɑːmpit] *n* 腋,腋窝

Arndt's law, Arndt-Schulz law [ɑːnt ʃults] (Rudolf Arndt; Hugo Schulz) 阿恩特定律,阿恩特-舒尔茨定律(弱刺激增强生理活动,强刺激抑制生理活动)

Arneth classification, count, formula, index [ɑːˈneit] (Joseph Arneth) 阿尔内特分类法、计数、公式、指数(不同类型多形核白细胞正常比例的表示法,依核显示的叶数〈1到5〉而定:1叶5%,2叶35%,3叶41%,4叶17%,5叶2%)

Arnica [ˈɑːnikə] *n*【拉】山金车属

arnica [ˈɑːnikə] *n* 山金车花

ARNMD Association for Research in Nervous and Mental Disease 神经病与精神病研究协会

Arnold-Chiari malformation (deformity, syndrome) [ˈɑːnɔld kiˈæri] (Julius Arnold; Hans Chiari)阿诺尔德-基亚里畸形(综合征),小脑扁桃体下疝畸形(一种脑各部先天畸形,小脑及延髓变得细长、扁平,经枕骨大孔突出于脊髓管中,可能有许多其他缺损,其中包括隐性脊柱裂、脊髓脊膜突出)

Arnold's bodies [ˈɑːnɔld] (Julius Arnold) 阿诺尔德体(血中红细胞碎片或红细胞影)

Arnold's canal [ˈɑːnɔld] (Philipp F. Arnold) 阿诺尔德管(颞骨岩骨中的小管,为迷走神经耳支的通道) | ~ ganglion 耳神经节;颈动脉球 / ~ ligament 砧骨上韧带 / ~ nerve 迷走神经耳支 / ~ nerve reflex cough syndrome 阿诺尔德神经反射性咳嗽综合征(由于刺激迷走神经耳支分布区所致,此区是外耳道的后下部及鼓膜的后半部)

Arnold's test [ˈɑːnɔld] (Vincenz Arnold) 阿诺尔德试验(检尿乙酰乙酸;生物碱试验)

arnotto [ɑːˈnɔtəu] *n* 胭脂树红,果红(见 annotto)

Arnott's bed [ˈɑːnɔt] (Neil Arnott) 阿诺特水褥(防止褥疮)

ARO Association for Research in Ophthalmology 眼科学研究协会

AROA autosomal recessive ocular albinism 常染色体隐性遗传眼白化病

aroma [əˈrəumə] *n* 芳香,香味

aromatase [əˈrəuməteis] *n* 芳香酶

aromatherapy [əˈrəuməˌθerəpi] *n* 植物精油香味疗法

aromatic [ˌærəuˈmætik] *a* 芳香的,有香味的;芳族的 *n* 芳香剂 | ~ acid 芳香族酸

aromatic-L-amino-acid decarboxylase [ˌærəu-ˈmætik əˈmiːnəu ˈæsid ˌdiːkɑːˈbɔksileis] 芳香-L-氨基酸脱羧酶

aromatization [əˌrəumətaiˈzeiʃən, -tiˈz-] *n* 芳香化

aromine [əˈrəumin] *n* 尿芳香碱

Aron's test [ˈɑːrɔn] (Hans Aron) 阿龙试验(检癌)

arousal [əˈrauzəl] *n* 唤醒,觉醒(对感觉刺激的反应状态);激发,引发 | drive ~ 欲动唤起 / sexual ~ 性欲唤起

ARPKD autosomal recessive polycystic kidney disease 常染色体隐性遗传多囊肾病

arprinocid [ɑːˈprainəsid] *n* 阿普西特(抗球虫药)

arrachement [ɑːrəʃˈmɔŋ] *n*【法】拔除术(拔除膜性内障)

arrack [ˈærək] *n* 粕酒

arrangement [əˈreindʒmənt] *n* 布置;排列;安排 | gene ~ 基因排列

array [əˈrei] *n* 列,排列;数列,数阵 | ~ of means 平均数数列 / phased ~ 相控阵

arrector [əˈrektə] ([复] **arrectores** [ˌærek-ˈtɔːriːz]) *n*【拉】立肌 | ~ pili, arrectores pilorum 立毛肌

arrest [əˈrest] *n* 停止,停搏 | cardiac ~, heart ~ 心脏停搏 / developmental ~ 发育停止 / sinus ~ 窦性停搏

arrested [əˈrestid] *a* 阻住的;停止的(在产科学中,指胎头在骨盆中阻住而不是阻塞时,胎头内旋转停止)

arrestin [əˈrestin] *n* 抑制蛋白

arrhaphia [əˈreifiə] *n* 神经管闭合不全

Arrhenius' equation [əˈriːniəs] (Svante A. Arrhenius) 阿里纽斯方程式(温度与反应速率常数的依从关系,$k = Ae^{-\Delta E_a} / RT$, k 表示速率常数,e 为自然对数的底,ΔE_a 为活化能,R 为气体常数,T 为绝对温度,A 是名为频率因子的常数) / ~ formula 阿里纽斯公式($\log x = \theta c$, x 是溶液的黏度,c 是悬浮粒子所占容积的百分比,θ 是常数) / ~ theory(doctrine) 阿里纽斯学理论(学说)(电解质离解学说)

arrheno- [构词成分]男,雄

arrhenoblastoma [əˌriːnəublæsˈtəumə], **arrhenoma** [ˌæriˈnəumə] *n* 卵巢男胚瘤

arrhenogenic [ˌærinəuˈdʒenik] *a* 产雄的,生男的

arrhenokaryon [ˌærinəuˈkæriɔn] *n* 雄核生殖体

arrhenoplasm [əˈriːnəplæzəm] *n* 雄质,雄胚浆

arrhenotoky [ˌæriˈnɔtəki], **arrhenotocia** [ˌærinəˈtəusiə] *n* 产雄单性生殖

arrhigosis [ˌæriˈgəusis] *n* 冷觉缺失

arrhinencephalia [ˌærinˌensiˈfeiliə] *n* 无嗅脑[畸形]

arrhinia [əˈriniə] *n* 无鼻[畸形]

arrhythmia [əˈriðmiə] *n* 心律失常,心律不齐,无节律 | continuous ~, perpetual ~ 持续性心律

失常,永久性心律失常, / sinus ~, phasic ~, respiratory ~ 窦性心律不齐,呼吸性心律失常 | **arrhythmic(al)** *a*

arrhythmogenesis [əˌriðməu'dʒenisis] *n* 心律失常形成

arrhythmogenic [əˌriðmə'dʒenik] *a* 致心律不齐的

arrhythmokinesis [əˌriðməukai'niːsis] *n* 节律运动障碍

arrival [ə'raivəl] *n* 到来,到达;到达者 | a new ~ 新生儿

arrow ['ærəu] *n* 箭 | caustic ~ 腐蚀箭(箭状的硝酸银或其他腐蚀剂)

arrowroot ['ærəuruːt] *n* 竹芋,竹芋淀粉(为婴儿饮食、老年病学饮食以及恢复期饮食重要成分)

Arroyo's sign [ə'rɔiəu] (Carlos F. Arroyo) 瞳孔反应迟钝

ARRS American Roentgen Ray Society 美国伦琴射线学会

ARS American Radium Society 美国镭学会

arsambide [ɑː'sæmbaid] *n* 卡巴胂(见 carbarsone)

arsanilic acid [ˌɑːsə'nilik] 氨苯胂酸(抗寄生虫药)

arsenate ['ɑːsinit] *n* 砷酸盐 | ferric ~ 砷酸铁(治贫血) / ferrous ~ 砷酸亚铁(杀虫药)

arseniasis [ˌɑːsi'naiəsis] *n* 慢性砷中毒

arsenic[1] (As) [ɑː'senik] *n* 砷;三氧化二砷 | ~ disulfide 二硫化二砷,雄黄 / ~ trichloride, ~ chloride 三氯化砷 / ~ trioxide, white ~ 三氧化二砷,白砷,砒霜 / ~ trisulfide, ~ yellow 三硫化二砷,雌黄

arsenic[2] [ɑː'senik] *a* 砷的;含砷的(五价的) | ~ acid 砷酸

arsenical [ɑː'senikəl] *a* 砷的 *n* 砷剂

arsenicalism [ɑː'senikəlizəm] *n* 慢性砷中毒

arsenicophagy [ˌɑːsini'kɔfədʒi] *n* 吞砷癖

arsenicum [ɑː'senikəm] *n* 【拉】砷

arsenide ['ɑːsinaid] *n* 砷化物

arsenious [ɑː'siːnjəs, ɑː'senjəs] *a* 亚砷的,三价砷的

arsenism ['ɑːsinizəm] *n* 慢性砷中毒

arsenite ['ɑːsinait] *n* 亚砷酸盐

arsenium [ɑː'siːniəm] *n* 【拉】砷

arsenization [ˌɑːsini'zeiʃən] *n* 砷疗法

arseno- [前缀]砷;偶砷基

arsenoactivation [ˌɑːsinəuˌækti'veiʃən] *n* 砷剂促动作用(砷剂治疗梅毒时,梅毒症状增多)

arsenoautohemotherapy [ˌɑːsinəuˌɔːtəuˌhiːməu'θerəpi] *n* 砷剂自血疗法(治梅毒)

arsenobenzene [ˌɑːsinəu'benziːn] *n* 偶砷苯(治螺旋体病)

arsenoblast [ɑː'senəblæst] *n* 雄胚质,雄性原核

arsenoceptor [ɑː'senəˌseptə] *n* 砷受体,嗜砷体(指细胞)

arsenolysis [ˌɑːsi'nɔlisis] *n* 砷分解

arsenophagy [ˌɑːsi'nɔfədʒi] *n* 吞砷癖

arsenorelapsing [ɑːˌsenəuri'læpsiŋ] *a* 砷疗后复发的(指一些梅毒患者)

arsenoresistant [ɑːˌsenəuri'zistənt] *a* 抗砷的(如抗砷凡纳明,指某些梅毒病例)

arsenotherapy [ˌɑːsinəu'θerəpi] *n* 砷疗法

arsenous ['ɑːsinəs] *a* 亚砷的(低价或三价的) | ~ acid 亚砷酸

arsenoxide [ˌɑːsi'nɔksaid] *n* 盐酸氧芬胂

arsenum [ɑː'siːnəm] *n* 【拉】砷

arsine ['ɑːsin] *n* 胂,三氢化砷

arsinic acid [ɑː'sinik] 次胂酸

arsinosalicylic acid [ˌɑːsinəuˌsæli'silik] 胂基水杨酸

arsonic acid [ɑː'sɔnik] 胂酸

arsonium [ɑː'səuniəm] *n* 砷[基],氢化砷基

arsonvalization [ˌɑːsənvæli'zeiʃən] *n* 高频电疗法

arsphenamine [ɑːs'fenəmin] *n* 胂凡纳明,六〇六(曾用于治梅毒、雅司及其他螺菌感染,先后由盐酸氧芬胂及青霉素所取代。亦称 salvarsan〈德〉,arsenobenzol〈法〉,diarsenol〈加拿大〉,arsaminol〈日〉,606, Ehrlich-Hata 或 Hata's preparation 以及 magic bullet) | ~ sulfoxylate 新胂凡纳明,九一四

arsthinol ['ɑːsθinɔl] *n* 胂噻醇(抗原虫药)

ART Accredited Record Technicians 合格的记录技术员;assisted reproductive technology 辅助生殖技术;automated reagin test 自动反应素试验

artarine ['ɑːtərin] *n* 椒根碱

artefact ['ɑːtifækt] *n* 人为现象,人工产物(见 artifact)

Artemisia [ɑːti'misiə] *n* 蒿属,苦艾属

arteralgia [ˌɑːtə'rældʒiə] *n* 动脉[散射]痛(如头痛,由颞动脉炎散射所致)

arterectomy [ˌɑːtə'rektəmi] *n* 动脉切除术

arterenol [ˌɑːtə'riːnɔl] *n* 去甲肾上腺素(升压药)

arteria [ɑː'tiəriə] ([复] **arteriae** [ɑː'tiərii:]) *n* 【拉,希】动脉(详见附录)

arterial [ɑː'tiəriəl] *a* 动脉的

arterialization [ɑːˌtiəriəlai'zeiʃən, -li'z-] *n* 动脉化(手术改变静脉,使之起到动脉的作用)

arteriectasis [ˌɑːtəri'ektəsis], **arteriectasia** [ˌɑːtəriek'teiziə] *n* 动脉扩张

arteriectomy [ˌɑːtəri'ektəmi] *n* 动脉切除术

arteriectopia [ˌɑːtəriek'təupiə] *n* 动脉异位

arteri(o)- [构词成分]动脉

arteriocapillary [ɑːˌtiəriəu'kæpiləri] *a* 动脉毛细

管的

arteriodilating [ɑːˌtiəriəudaiˈleitiŋ] *a* 动脉扩张的(尤指小动脉)

arteriogenesis [ɑːˌtiəriəuˈdʒenisis] *n* 动脉生成

arteriogram [ɑːˈtiəriəgræm] *n* 动脉造影[照]片

arteriograph [ɑːˈtiəriəgrɑːf, -græf] *n* 动脉造影[照]片 | ~y [ˌɑːtəriˈɔgrəfi] *n* 动脉造影[术]

arteriola [ɑːˌtiəriˈəulə]([复] **arteriolae** [ɑːˌtiəriˈəuliː]) *n* 小动脉,微动脉

arteriole [ɑːˈtiəriəul] *n* 小动脉,微动脉 | afferent glomerular ~ 入球小动脉,入球微动脉 / efferent glomerular ~ 出球小动脉,出球微动脉 / ellipsoid ~s 有鞘动脉 / inferior macular ~ 黄斑下小动脉 / inferior nasal ~ of retina 视网膜鼻侧下小动脉 / inferior temporal ~ of retina 视网膜颞侧下小动脉 / superior macular ~ 黄斑上小动脉 / superior nasal ~ of retina 视网膜鼻侧上小动脉 / superior temporal ~ of retina 视网膜颞侧上小动脉 | **arteriolar** [ɑːˌtiəriˈəulə] *a*

arteriolith [ɑːˈtiəriəˌliθ] *n* 动脉石

arteriolitis [ɑːˌtiəriəuˈlaitis] *n* 小动脉炎

arteriol(o)- [构词成分]小动脉

arteriology [ɑːˌtiəriˈɔlədʒi] *n* 动脉学

arteriolonecrosis [ɑːˌtiəriˌəuləuneˈkrəusis] *n* 小动脉坏死(见于肾硬化)

arteriolopathy [ɑːˌtiəriəˈlɔpəθi] *n* 小动脉病

arteriolosclerosis [ɑːˌtiəriˌəuləuskliəˈrəusis] *n* 小动脉硬化 | **arteriolosclerotic** [ɑːˌtiəriˌəuləu-skliˈrɔtik] *a*

arteriomotor [ɑːˌtiəriəuˈməutə] *a* 动脉运动的,动脉舒缩的

arteriomyomatosis [ɑːˌtiəriəuˌmaiəuməˈtəusis] *n* 动脉肌瘤病

arterionecrosis [ɑːˌtiəriəuneˈkrəusis] *n* 动脉坏死

arteriopathy [ˌɑːtiəriˈɔpəθi] *n* 动脉病 | hypertensive ~ 高血压性动脉病

arterioplasty [ɑːˌtiəriəuˈplæsti] *n* 动脉成形术

arteriopressor [ɑːˌtiəriəuˈpresə] *a* 升动脉血压的 *n* 升动脉血压药

arteriorenal [ɑːˌtiəriəuˈriːnl] *a* 肾动脉的

arteriorrhaphy [ɑːˌtiəriˈɔrəfi] *n* 动脉缝合术

arteriorrhexis [ɑːˌtiəriəuˈreksis] *n* 动脉破裂

arteriosclerosis [ɑːˌtiəriəuskliəˈrəusis] *n* 动脉硬化 | cerebral ~ 脑动脉硬化 / coronary ~ 冠状动脉硬化 / intimal ~ 动脉内膜硬化 / medial ~ 动脉中层硬化 / ~ obliterans 闭塞性动脉硬化 | **arteriosclerotic** [ɑːˌtiəriəuskliəˈrɔtik] *a*

arteriosity [ɑːˌtiəriˈɔsəti] *n* 动脉性

arteriospasm [ɑːˈtiəriəˌspæzəm] *n* 动脉痉挛 | **arteriospastic** [ɑːˌtiəriəˈspæstik] *a*

arteriostenosis [ɑːˌtiəriəstiˈnəusis] *n* 动脉狭窄

arteriosteogenesis [ɑːˌtiəriˌɔstiəuˈdʒenisis] *n* 动脉钙化

arteriostosis [ɑːˌtiəriɔsˈtəusis] *n* 动脉骨化

arteriostrepsis [ɑːˌtiəriəuˈstrepsis], **arteriotrepsis** [ɑːˌtiəriəˈtrepsis] *n* 动脉扭转术(止血)

arteriosympathectomy [ɑːˌtiəriəuˌsimpəˈθektəmi] *n* 动脉交感神经切除术

arteriotomy [ɑːˌtiəriˈɔtəmi] *n* 动脉切开术

arteriotony [ɑːˌtiəriˈɔtəni] *n* 动脉张力,[动脉]血压

arterious [ɑːˈtiəriəs] *a* 动脉的

arterio-venous [ɑːˌtiəriəu ˈviːnəs] *a* 动静脉的

arteritis [ˌɑːtəˈraitis]([复] **arteritides** [ˌɑːtəˈritidiːz]) *n* 动脉炎 | brachiocephalic ~ 无脉病 / coronary ~ 冠状动脉炎 / localized visceral ~ 变应性血管炎 / temporal ~, cranial ~, giant cell ~ 颞动脉炎 / tuberculous ~ 结核性动脉炎

Arteriviridae [ɑːˌtiəriˈviridiː] *n* 动脉炎病毒科

Arterivirus [ɑːˌtiəriˈvaiərəs] *n* 动脉炎病毒属

arterivirus [ɑːˌtiəriˈvaiərəs] *n* 动脉炎病毒

artery [ˈɑːtəri] *n* 动脉(详见附录) | common carotid ~ 颈总动脉 / common iliac ~ 髂总动脉 / conducting arteries 传导动脉 / copperwire arteries 铜线样动脉(见于视网膜动脉硬化) / corkscrew arteries 黄斑螺旋状小动脉 / deep facial ~ 面深动脉,上颌动脉 / end ~ 终动脉 / external maxillary ~ 颌外动脉,面动脉 / external spermatic ~ 精索外动脉,睾提肌动脉 / facial ~ 面动脉;颈外动脉 / fallopian ~ 输卵管动脉,子宫动脉 / frontal ~ 额动脉,滑车上动脉 / funicular ~ 精索动脉,睾丸动脉 / inferior capsular ~ 肾上腺下动脉 / internal auditory ~ 迷路动脉 / middle capsular ~ 肾上腺中动脉 / nasopalatine ~ 鼻腭动脉,蝶腭动脉 / nutrient ~, medullary ~ 滋养动脉,髓动脉 / posterior pelvic ~ 骨盆后动脉,髂内动脉 / ~ of the pulp 髓动脉(脾) / pyloric ~ 幽门动脉,胃右动脉 / quadriceps ~ of femur 股四头肌动脉,旋股外侧动脉降支 / radicular arteries 根动脉(与脊神经及前后根伴行) / ranine ~ 舌深动脉 / revehent ~ 出球小动脉 / right auricular ~ 右冠状动脉 / small iliac ~ 髂腰动脉 / transverse scapular ~ 肩胛横动脉,肩胛上动脉 / sciatic ~ 坐骨神经伴行动脉 / sheathed arteries 鞘动脉 / sylvian ~ 大脑中动脉 / venous arteries 静脉性动脉,肺静脉

arthr- 见 arthro-

Arthracanthida [ˌɑːθrəˈkænθidə] *n* 节棘虫目

arthragra [ɑːˈθrægrə] *n* 关节痛风[发作]

arthral [ˈɑːθrəl] *a* 关节的

arthralgia [ɑːˈθrældʒiə] *n* 关节痛 | ~ saturnina 铅[中]毒性关节痛 | **arthralgic** [ɑːˈθrældʒik] *a*

arthrectomy [ɑːˈθrektəmi] *n* 关节切除术

arthrempyesis [ˌɑːθrempaiˈiːsis] *n* 关节化脓

arthresthesia [ˌɑːθresˈθiːziə] *n* 关节感觉

arthrifuge [ˈɑːθrifjuːdʒ] *n* 治痛风药

arthritide [ˈɑːθritaid] *n* 关节炎[性皮]疹

arthritis [ɑːˈθraitis] ([复] **arthritides** [ɑːˈθritidiːz]) *n* 关节炎 | acute rheumatic ~ 急性风湿性关节炎,风湿[性]热 / chronic inflammatory ~ 慢性炎症性关节炎 / degenerative ~, hypertrophic ~ 变性关节炎,增殖性关节炎(即骨关节炎) / gouty ~, uratic ~ 痛风性关节炎,尿酸性关节炎 / menopausal ~, climactic ~ 绝经期关节炎,更年期关节炎 / proliferative ~ 增生性关节炎 / rheumatoid ~ 类风湿关节炎 | **arthritic** [ɑːˈθritik] *a* 关节炎的 *n* 关节炎患者

arthritism [ˈɑːθritizəm] *n* 关节病体质,痛风素质

arthr(o)- [构词成分]关节

Arthrobacter [ˌɑːθrəuˈbæktə] *n* 节杆菌属

arthrobacterium [ˌɑːθrəubækˈtiəriəm] *n* 节孢子杆菌

Arthrobotrys [ˌɑːθrəˈbəutris] *n* 线虫捕捉菌属

arthrocace [ɑːˈθrɔkəsi] *n* 关节疡

arthrocele [ˈɑːθrəsiːl] *n* 关节肿大

arthrocentesis [ˌɑːθrəusenˈtiːsis] *n* 关节穿刺术

arthrochalasis [ˌɑːθrəuˈkæləsis] *n* 关节松弛 | ~ multiplex congenita 先天性多发性关节松弛

arthrochondritis [ˌɑːθrəukənˈdraitis] *n* 关节软骨炎

arthroclasia [ˌɑːθrəuˈkleiziə] *n* 关节活动术

arthroclisis [ˌɑːθrəuˈklaisis] *n* 关节强直

arthroconidium [ˌɑːθrəukəˈnidiəm] *n* 节分生孢子,节孢子

Arthroderma [ˌɑːθrəuˈdəːmə] *n* 节皮真菌属

arthrodesis [ˌɑːθrəuˈdiːsis], **arthrodesia** [ˌɑːθrəuˈdiːsiə] *n* 关节融合术

arthrodia [ɑːˈθrəudiə] *n* 摩动关节 | **~l** *a*

arthrodynia [ˌɑːθrəuˈdiniə] *n* 关节痛

arthrodysplasia [ˌɑːθrəudisˈpleiziə] *n* 关节发育不良

arthroempyesis [ˌɑːθrəuˌempaiˈiːsis] *n* 关节化脓

arthroendoscopy [ˌɑːθrəuenˈdɔskəpi] *n* 关节内镜检查

arthroereisis [ˌɑːθrəuiˈraisis] *n* 关节制动术

arthrogenous [ɑːˈθrɔdʒinəs] *a* 分节的(如分节孢子);关节[源]性的

arthrogram [ˈɑːθrəgræm] *n* 关节造影[照]片

Arthrographis [ˌɑːθrəˈgræfis] *n* 白癣菌属 | ~ langeroni 爪甲白癣菌

arthrography [ɑːˈθrɔgrəfi] *n* 关节造影[术] | air ~ 关节气造影[术]

arthrogryposis [ˌɑːθrəugriˈpəusis] *n* 关节弯曲 | congenital multiple ~, ~ multiplex congenita 先天性多发性关节弯曲

arthrokatadysis [ˌɑːθrəukəˈtædisis] *n* [髋]关节内陷

arthrokleisis [ˌɑːθrəuˈklaisis] *n* 关节强直

arthrolith [ˈɑːθrəliθ] *n* 关节石

arthrolithiasis [ˌɑːθrəuliˈθaiəsis] *n* 关节石病,痛风

arthrologia [ˌɑːθrəuˈləudʒiə] *n* 关节学(以前称韧带学 syndesmologia)

arthrology [ɑːˈθrɔlədʒi] *n* 关节学

arthrolysis [ɑːˈθrɔlisis] *n* 关节松解术

arthromeningitis [ˌɑːθrəuˌmeninˈdʒaitis] *n* 滑膜炎

arthrometer [ɑːˈθrɔmitə] *n* 关节动度计(测关节活动角度) | **arthrometry** *n* 关节动度测量法

Arthromitaceae [ˌɑːθrəumaiˈteisiiː] *n* 节线菌科

Arthromitus [ɑːˈθrɔmitəs] *n* 节线菌属

arthroncus [ɑːˈθrɔŋkəs] *n* 关节肿大

arthroneuralgia [ˌɑːθrəunjuəˈrældʒiə] *n* 关节神经痛

arthronosos [ˌɑːθrəuˈnəusɔs] *n* 关节病 | ~ deformans 变形性关节病

arthro-onychodysplasia [ˌɑːθrəu ˌɔnikəudisˈpleiziə] *n* 关节指甲发育不良(一种遗传性综合征)

arthro-ophthalmopathy [ˌɑːθrəu ɔfθælˈmɔpəθi] *n* 关节眼病 | hereditary progressive ~ 遗传性进行性关节眼病

arthropathia [ˌɑːθrəuˈpæθiə] *n* 【拉】关节病 | ~ ovaripriva 绝经期关节炎 / ~ psoriatica 银屑病性关节病

arthropathology [ˌɑːθrəupəˈθɔlədʒi] *n* 关节病理学

arthropathy [ɑːˈθrɔpəθi] *n* 关节病 | inflammatory ~ 炎性关节病,关节炎 / neuropathic ~, neurogenic ~ 神经病性关节病,神经源性关节病 / osteopulmonary ~ 肺性骨关节病 / static ~ 平衡不良性关节病 | **arthropathic** [ˌɑːθrəuˈpæθik] *a*

arthrophyma [ˌɑːθrəuˈfaimə] *n* 关节肿大

arthrophyte [ˈɑːθrəfait] *n* 关节赘疣

arthroplasty [ˈɑːθrəuˌplæsti] *n* 关节成形术 | gap ~ 裂隙关节成形术 / interposition ~ 插入关节成形术 / intracapsular temporomandibular joint ~ 囊内颞下颌关节成形术 | **arthroplastic** [ˌɑːθrəuˈplæstik] *a*

arthropneumoradiography [ˌɑːθrəu ˌnjuːməu ˌreidiˈɔgrəfi], **arthropneumography** [ˌɑːθrəunju(ː)ˈmɔgrəfi] *n* 关节充气造影[术]

arthropod [ˈɑːθrəpɔd] *n* 节肢动物 | **~an** [ˈɑːθrəˌpəudən], **~ic** [ˌɑːθrəuˈpəudik], **~ous** [ɑːˈθrɔpədəs] *a*

Arthropoda [ɑːˈθrɔpədə] *n* 节肢动物门
arthropyosis [ˌɑːθrəupaiˈəusis] *n* 关节化脓
arthrorheumatism [ˌɑːθrəuˈruːmətizəm] *n* 关节风湿病
arthrorisis [ˌɑːθrəuˈraisis] *n* 关节制动术
arthroscintigram [ˌɑːθrəuˈsintigræm] *n* 关节闪烁[扫描]图
arthroscintigraphy [ˌɑːθrəusinˈtigrəfi] *n* 关节闪烁[扫描]术
arthrosclerosis [ˌɑːθrəuskliəˈrəusis] *n* 关节硬化
arthroscope [ˈɑːθrəskəup] *n* 关节镜
arthroscopy [ɑːˈθrɔskəpi] *n* 关节镜检查
arthrosis [ɑːˈθrəusis] *n*【希】关节;关节病 | ~ deformans 变形性关节病
arthrospore [ˈɑːθrəspɔː] *n* 节孢子
arthrosteitis [ˌɑːθrɔstiˈaitis] *n* 关节骨炎
arthrostomy [ɑːˈθrɔstəmi] *n* 关节造口术
arthrosynovitis [ˌɑːθrəuˌsinəˈvaitis] *n* 关节滑膜炎
arthrotome [ˈɑːθrətəum] *n* 关节刀
arthrotomy [ɑːˈθrɔtəmi] *n* 关节切开术
arthrotropic [ˌɑːθrəuˈtrɔpik] *a* 亲关节的,向关节的
arthrotyphoid [ˌɑːθrəuˈtaifɔid] *n* 风湿型伤寒
arthroxerosis [ˌɑːθrəuziəˈrəusis] *n* 关节干燥症,慢性骨关节炎
arthroxesis [ɑːˈθrɔksəsis] *n* 关节[面]刮[除]术
Arthus reaction (phenomenon) [ɑːˈtjuːs] (Nicolas-Maurice Arthus) 阿蒂斯反应(现象),局部过敏坏死反应(以水肿、出血和坏死为特征的炎症反应,对已有沉淀抗体的动物皮内注射对应抗原可引起此反应) | ~-type reaction 阿蒂斯型反应,局部过敏坏死型反应
articaine hydrochloride [ˈɑːtiˌkein] 盐酸阿替卡因(局部麻醉药)
artichoke [ˈɑːtiˌtʃəuk] *n* 朝鲜蓟;朝鲜蓟叶制剂(具有利胆汁尿和利尿性质,用于治消化不良和高脂血症)
article [ˈɑːtikl] *n* 关节,节
articular [ɑːˈtikjulə] *a* 关节的
articulare [ɑːˌtikjuˈlɛəri] *n* 关节点
articulate[1] [ɑːˈtikjuleit] *vt* 清晰发音;用发声器发音;以连贯言语表达;关节分开或联结;人造义齿整列
articulate[2] [ɑːˈtikjulit] *a* 分节发音的;善于表达的;发音清晰的;由关节分开或联结的
articulated [ɑːˈtikjuˌleitid] *a* 联接的;关节联接的
articulatio [ɑːˌtikjuˈleiʃiəu] ([复] **articulationes** [ɑːˌtikjuˌleiʃiˈəuniːz]) *n*【拉】关节
articulation [ɑːˌtikjuˈleiʃən] *n* 关节;分节发音;咬合;排牙面 | ambomalleolar ~ 砧槌关节 / atlantooccipital ~, craniovertebral ~, occipital ~, occipitoatiantal ~ 寰枕关节 / ball-and-socket ~ 球窝关节 / brachiocarpal ~ 桡腕关节 / brachioradial ~ 肱桡关节 / capitular ~ 肋头关节 / carpal ~s 腕关节 / composite ~, compound ~ 复关节 / confluent ~ 混合发声 / distal radioulnar ~, inferior radioulnar ~ 桡尺远侧关节 / femoral ~, ~ of hip 髋关节 / ~ of humerus 肩关节 / mandibular ~, temporomandibular ~ 下颌关节 / pisocuneiform ~ 豌豆[骨]关节 / pivot ~ 车轴关节 / talocalcaneonavicular ~ 距跟舟关节 / talocrural ~ 踝关节,距骨小腿关节 / ~ of tubercle of rib 肋横突关节
articulator [ɑːˈtikjuleitə] *n* 联接器;殆架 | adjustable ~ 可调式殆架 / dental ~ 殆架 / hinge ~, plain-line ~ 铰链殆架,平线殆架 / semiadjustable ~ 半调整性殆架,可半调整式殆架
articulatory [ɑːˈtikjulətəri] *a* 发言的,言语的,分节发音的
articulo [ɑːˈtikjuləu] *n*【拉】危急时刻 | ~ mortis 濒死
articulus [ɑːˈtikjuləs] ([复] **articuli** [ɑːˈtikjulai]) *n*【拉】关节
artifact [ˈɑːtifækt] *n* 人为现象,人工产物(在组织学及显微镜检查指切片过程中所产生的任何结构);伪影(见于 X 线片)
artifactitious [ˌɑːtifækˈtiʃəs] *a* 人为现象的,人工产物的;伪影的
artifice [ˈɑːtifis] *n* 技巧 | **~r** [ɑːˈtifisə] *n* 技工;牙技工
artificial [ˌɑːtiˈfiʃəl] *a* 人工的,人造的,假的 | **~ity** [ˌɑːtifiʃiˈæləti] *n* 人造性,人造物
artificialize [ˌɑːtiˈfiʃəlaiz] *vt* 使人工化
artiodactyl [ˌɑːtiəuˈdæktil] *n* 偶蹄动物 | **~ous** [ˌɑːtiəuˈdæktiləs] *a* 偶[蹄]的;偶蹄目的
Artiodactyla [ˌɑːtiəuˈdæktilə] *n* 偶蹄目
Artyfechinostomum [ˌɑːtiˌfekiˈnɔstəmən] *n* 刺口吸虫属 | ~ sufrartyfex 多棘刺口吸虫
Arum [ˈɛərəm] *n* 海芋属
Arvin [ˈɑːvin] *n* 蝮蛇抗栓酶,抗栓酶(马来亚蝮蛇蛇毒的提纯部分,在血栓栓塞性疾病中用作抗凝剂)
ARVO Association for Research in Vision and Ophthalmology 视力与眼科学研究协会
aryepiglottic [ˌæriˌepiˈglɔtik] *a* 杓会厌的
aryepiglotticus [ˌæriˌepiˈglɔtikəs] *n* 杓会厌肌
aryepiglottidean [ˌæriˌepiglɔˈtidiən] *a* 杓会厌的
aryl [ˈæril] *n* 芳[香]基
aryl- [化学前缀]芳[香]基
arylamine [ˌæriləˈmiːn, ˌæriˈlæmin] *n* 芳基胺
arylaminopeptidase [ˌæriləˌmiːnəuˈpeptideis] *n* 芳[香]基氨肽酶,胞液氨肽酶

arylarsonic acid [ˌærilɑːˈsɔnik] 芳[香族]基胂酸
aryldialkylphosphatase [ˌærildaiˌælkilˈfɔsfəteis] *n* 芳[香]基二烷基磷酸酶
arylesterase [ˌærilˈestəreis] *n* 芳[香]基酯酶(亦称芳[香]基-酯水解酶)
aryl-ester hydrolase [ˈæril ˈestə] 芳[香]基-酯水解酶,芳[香]基酯酶
arylformamidase [ˌærilfɔːˈmæmideis] *n* 芳[香]基甲酰胺酶(亦称甲酰犬尿氨酸水解酶)
aryl 4-hydroxylase [ˈæril haiˈdrɔksileis] 芳[香]基4-羟化酶,非特异性单加氧酶
arylsulfatase [ˌærilˈsʌlfəteis] *n* 芳[香]基硫酸酯酶
arylsulfatase A deficiency 芳[香]基硫酸酯酶A缺乏症,异染性脑白质营养不良
arylsulfatase B(ARSB) deficiency 芳[香]基硫酸酯酶B缺乏症
arytenoepiglottic [æˌritinəuˌepiˈglɔtik] *a* 杓会厌的
arytenoideus [ˌæritiˈnɔidiəs] *n*【拉】杓肌
arytenoid [ˌæriˈtiːnɔid] *a* 杓状的
arytenoidectomy [ˌæriˌtiːnɔiˈdektəmi] *n* 杓状软骨切除术
arytenoiditis [æˌritinɔiˈdaitis] *n* 杓状软骨炎;杓肌炎
arytenoidopexy [ˌæritiˈnɔidəˌpeksi] *n* 杓状软骨固定术;杓肌固定术
Arzberger's pear [ˈɑːzbəːgə] (Friedrich Arzberger) 梨形直肠施冷器
AS[1] auris sinistra【拉】左耳
AS[2] aortic stenosis 主动脉瓣狭窄; arteriosclerosis 动脉硬化
As arsenic 砷; astigmatism 散光[眼]
ASA acetylsalicylic acid 乙酰水杨酸; American Society of Anesthesiologists 美国麻醉学家学会; American Standards Association 美国标准协会; American Surgical Association 美国外科协会; antisperm antibody 抗精子抗体; argininosuccinic acid 精氨[基]琥珀酸
5-ASA 5-aminosalicylic acid 5-氨基水杨酸(消炎药)
asacria [əˈseikriə] *n* 无骶[畸形]
asafetida [ˌæsəˈfetidə] *n* 阿魏(用作祛风、祛痰和镇痉药)
asaphia [əˈseifiə] *n* 语声不清
asaron [ˈæsərɔn] *n* 细辛脑
Asarum [ˈæsərəm] *n* 细辛属
ASAS American Society of Abdominal Surgeons 美国腹部外科医师学会
ASAT aspartate aminotransferase 天冬氨酸转氨酶
ASB American Society of Bacteriologists 美国细菌学家学会
asbestiform [æzˈbestifɔːm, æsˈbes-] *a* 石棉状的
asbestos [æzˈbestɔs, æsˈbes-] *n* 石棉
asbestosis [ˌæzbesˈtəusis, ˌæs-] *n* 石棉沉着病
A-scan A型[超声]扫描
ascariasis [ˌæskəˈraiəsis] *n* 蛔虫病
ascaricidal [æsˌkæriˈsaidl] *a* 杀蛔虫的
ascaricide [æsˈkærisaid] *n* 驱蛔虫药
ascarid [ˈæskərid] *n* 蛔虫
Ascarididae [ˌæskəˈrididiː] *n* 蛔虫科
ascarides [æsˈkæridiːz] ascaris 的复数
Ascaridia [ˌæskəˈridiə] *n* 鸡蛔虫属 | ~ galli 鸡蛔虫 / ~ lineata 线形禽蛔虫
ascaridiasis [ˌæskæriˈdaiəsis] *n* 蛔虫病
Ascaridoidea [ˌæskəriˈdɔidiə] *n* 蛔[虫]总科
ascaridole [əsˈkæriˌdəul] *n* 土荆芥油精,驱蛔素
ascaridosis [ˌæskæriˈdəusis] *n* 蛔虫病
Ascaris [ˈæskəris] *n*【拉】蛔虫属 | ~ lumbricoides 人蛔虫,蛔虫
ascaris [ˈæskəris] ([复] **ascarides** [æsˈkæridiːz]) *n* 蛔虫
Ascarops [ˈæskərɔps] *n* 斜环咽线虫属
ascending [əˈsendiŋ] *a* 上行的,升的
ascension [əˈsenʃən] *n* 上升,升高 | **~al** *a*
ascensive [əˈsensiv] *a* 上升的
ascensus [əˈsensəs] *n*【拉】上升 | ~ uteri 子宫高位
ascertainment [ˌæsəˈteinmənt] *n* 查明,确认;系谱调查,查证法(在遗传学研究中,研究者选择或发现带有某一特性或疾病者的方法) | complete ~ 完全查证[法] / incomplete ~ 部分查证[法] / multiple ~ 复式查证[法] / single ~ 单个查证[法] / truncate ~ 分段查证[法]
asceticism [əˈsetisizəm] *n* 禁欲主义
Ascetospora [ˌæskiˈtɔspɔːrə] *n* 囊孢子门
ASCH American Society of Clinical Hypnosis 美国临床催眠术学会
aschelminth [ˈæskelminθ] *n* 袋虫
Aschelminthes [ˌæskelˈminθiːz] *n* 袋虫动物门
Ascher's negative glass-rod phenomenon [ˈæʃə] (Karl W. Ascher) 阿谢尔阴性玻璃棒现象,血液输入现象 | ~ positive glass-rod phenomenon 阿谢尔阳性玻璃棒现象,房水输入现象 / ~ syndrome 阿谢尔综合征(睑皮松垂,同时伴甲状腺肿,上唇黏膜及黏膜下组织过多)
Ascherson's membrane [ˈɑːʃəsɔn] (Ferdinand M. Ascherson) 阿谢尔森乳脂球膜(包裹乳球体的酪蛋白膜) | ~ vesicles 阿谢尔森小泡(油与液状白蛋白一起摇荡而成的小泡,油滴外包有一薄层白蛋白)
Aschheim-Zondek hormone [ˈɑːʃhaim ˈtsɔndek] (Selmar Aschheim; Bernhardt Zondek) 促黄体素 | ~ test 阿希海姆-仓德克试验,小白鼠妊娠试

验(检孕)

aschistodactylia [əˌskistəudækˈtiliə] *n* 并指畸形,并趾畸形

Aschner's reflex(phenomenon) [ˈɑːʃnə] (Bernhard Aschner) 阿施内反射(现象),眼心反射(压迫眼球或压迫颈动脉窦,心律即减慢)

Aschoff's bodies(nodules) [ˈɑːʃɔf] (Karl A. L. Aschoff) 阿孝夫小体(小结)(风湿性心肌炎时心肌间质中的小粟状细胞集团) | ~ cells 阿孝夫细胞(一种巨细胞,见于心肌中风湿小结) / ~ node 阿孝夫结,房室结

Aschoff-Tawara node [ˈɑːʃɔf təˈwɑːrə] (Karl A. L. Aschoff; Sunao Tawara 田源淳)阿孝夫-田原结,房室结

Asch's forceps [æʃ] (Morris J. Asch) 阿希钳(鼻骨骨折复位和固定用) | ~ operation 阿希手术(一种鼻中隔偏曲矫正术) / ~ splint 阿希夹板(鼻骨骨折用)

ASCI American Society for Clinical Investigation 美国临床研究学会

asci [ˈæsai] ascus 的复数

ascia [ˈæsiə] *n* 回反绷带(一种螺旋形绷带)

ascites [əˈsaitiːz] *n* 腹水 | bile ~ 胆汁性腹水,胆汁性腹膜炎 / hemorrhagic ~, bloody ~ 血性腹水 / hydremic ~ 稀血性腹水 / milky ~ 油脂性腹水 | **ascitic** [əˈsitik] *a*

ascitogenous [ˌæsiˈtɔdʒinəs] *a* 产生腹水的

asclepiadin [ˌæskləˈpaiədin] *n* 马利筋苦素

Asclepias [æsˈkliːpiəs] *n*【拉】马利筋属

ASCLT American Society of Clinical Laboratory Technicians 美国临床实验技师学会

ASCO American Society of Clinical Oncology 美国临床肿瘤学会; American Society of Contemporary Ophthalmology 美国当代眼科学会

Ascobolaceae [ˌæskəubəuˈleisiiː] *n* 粪盘菌科

Ascobolus [æsˈkɔbələs] *n* 粪盘菌属

ascocarp [ˈæskəkɑːp] *n* 子囊果

Ascocotyle [ˌæskəˈkəutili] *n* 凹管线虫属 | ~ pithecophagicola 猿鹰凹管线虫

ascogenous [æsˈkɔdʒənəs] *a* 产子囊的(指菌丝)

ascogonium [ˌæskəˈgəuniəm] *n* 产囊体(子囊菌的雌性生殖器)

Ascoli's test [æsˈkəuli] (Alberto Ascoli) 阿斯科利试验,炭疽环状试验(一种热沉淀素试验,用于炭疽的血清学诊断) | ~ treatment 阿斯科利疗法(对疟疾患者注射肾上腺素,使脾收缩,迫使脾内含物包括疟原虫进入循环,以利诊断)

ascoma [æsˈkəumə] *n* 子囊果

ascomycete [ˌæskəumaiˈsiːt, æsˈkəumaisiːt] *n* 子囊菌 | **ascomycetous** [ˌæskəumaiˈsiːtəs] *a*

Ascomycetes [ˌæskəumaiˈsiːtiːz], **Ascomycetae** [ˌæskəuˈmaisitiː] *n* 子囊菌纲

Ascomycota [ˌæskəumaiˈkəutə] *n* 子囊菌门

Ascomycotina [ˌæskəuˌmaikəuˈtainə] *n* 子囊菌亚门

ascorbate [æsˈkɔːbeit] *n* 抗坏血酸盐

ascorbemia [ˌæskɔˈbiːmiə] *n* 抗坏血酸血

ascorbic acid [əsˈkɔːbik] 抗坏血酸,维生素 C

ascorburia [æskɔːˈbjuəriə] *n* 抗坏血酸尿

ascorbyl palmitate [əsˈkɔːbil ˈpælmiteit] 抗坏血酸棕榈酸酯(制药时用作防腐剂)

ascospore [ˈæskəspɔː] *n* 子囊孢子

ASCP American Society of Clinical Pathologists 美国临床病理学家协会

ascus [ˈæskəs] ([复] **asci** [ˈæsai]) *n* 子囊

ASCVD arteriosclerotic cardiovascular disease 动脉硬化性心血管病

-ase [后缀]酶

asecretory [eiˈsiːkrətəri] *a* 无分泌的

Aselli's pancreas(glands) [əˈseli] (Gasparo Aselli) 阿塞利胰腺(肠系膜根部淋巴结集合)

asemantic [eisiˈmæntik] *a* 无信息的(指一种分子,并非由生物体产生,因此也不受生物体内带信息分子的影响)

asemasia [ˌæsiˈmeiziə] *n* 示意不能

asemia [əˈsiːmiə] *n* 说示不能

asepsis [eiˈsepsis] *n* 无菌;无菌术 | integral ~ 完全无菌

Aseptatina [ˌeiseptəˈtainə] *n* 无隔亚目

aseptic [eiˈseptik] *a* 无菌的 | ~ acid 抗菌酸剂 | ~ -antiseptic 无菌防腐的 | **~ally** *ad*

asepticism [eiˈseptisizəm] *n* 无菌外科学说

asetake [ˌæsiˈtæki] *n*【日】汗茸,毒茸

asexual [eiˈseksjuəl] *a* 无性的 | **~ity** [eiˌseksjuˈæləti] *n* 性欲缺乏

asexualization [eiˌseksjuælaiˈzeiʃən] *n* 绝育,阉割(如睾丸或卵巢切除)

ASF 苯胺硫甲醛树脂(一种含有苯胺〈aniline〉、甲醛〈formaldehyde〉和硫〈sulfur〉的合成树脂,用于封固显微镜标本)

ASG American Society for Genetics 美国遗传学会

ASGE American Society for Gastrointestinal Endoscopy 美国胃肠内窥镜检查学会

ASH American Society for Hematology 美国血液学学会; asymmetrical septal hypertrophy 非对称性间隔肥大

As H hypermetropic astigmatism 远视散光

ash¹ [æʃ] *n* 灰,灰分;[复]骨灰

ash² [æʃ] *n* 梣,白蜡树

ASHA American School Health Association 美国学校卫生协会; American Speech and Hearing Association 美国言语与听力协会

ASHD arteriosclerotic heart disease 动脉硬化性心脏病

ashen [ˈæʃn] *a* 灰的,灰白的,苍白的
Asherman's syndrome [ˈæʃəmən] (Joseph G. Asherman) 阿谢曼综合征,子宫腔粘连综合征(由于子宫内粘连和闭锁引起的闭经和继发不孕,通常为子宫刮除术的结果)
Asherson's syndrome [ˈæʃəsn] (N. Asherson) 阿谢逊综合征(咽下困难的一种综合征,因神经肌肉协调不能、环咽括约肌弛缓不能及吞咽第三期环咽肌松弛不足所致,导致液体转向进入气道而促使一阵剧咳。亦称环咽失弛缓症综合征)
Ashhurst's splint [ˈæʃhəːst] (John Ashhurst) 阿希赫斯特夹板(膝关节切除后使用)
ASHI Association for the Study of Human Infertility 人类不育症研究协会
ASHP American Society of Hospital Pharmacists 美国医院药剂师协会
ASI Addiction Severity Index 成瘾严重程度指数
ASIA American Spinal Injury Association 美国脊椎损伤协会
asialia [ˌeisaiˈeiliə] *n* 唾液缺乏
asialo [eiˈsaiələu] *a* 无唾液酸[基]的
asiaticoside [ˌeiʒiˈætikəsaid] *n* 亚细亚皂苷,积雪草苷(用于各种皮肤病,包括创伤或烧伤)
asiderosis [ˌæsidəˈrəusis] *n* 铁缺乏[症]
ASII American Science Information Institute 美国科学情报研究所
ASIM American Society of Internal Medicine 美国内科学会
Asimina [əˈsiminə] *n* 泡泡树属
asiminine [əˈsiminin] *n* 泡泡树碱
-asis [后缀]状态,情况(病的)
asitia [əˈsiʃiə] *n* 厌食
asjike [əsˈdʒaiki] *n* 脚气[病]
Askanazy cells [ˈæskˌnɑːzi] (Max Askanazy) 阿斯克纳齐细胞(大颗粒嗜酸粒细胞,富有线粒体,见于自身免疫性甲状腺炎和许特尔〈Hürthle〉细胞瘤的甲状腺肿)
Askin's tumor [ˈæskin] (Frederic B. Askin) 阿斯金肿瘤(见于儿童胸肺区软组织的恶性小细胞肿瘤,为周围神经外胚层肿瘤之一)
Ask-Upmark kidney [ɑːsk ˈʌpmɑːk] (Erik Ask-Upmark) 阿斯克-厄普马克肾(一种发育不良性肾,小叶比一般少,其表面有裂纹;大多数患者患有严重高血压,有时伴高血压脑病和视网膜病变。本病可能是先天性的,或继发于膀胱输尿管反流合并肾盂肾炎。亦称节段性肾发育不良)
ASL antistreptolysin 抗链球菌溶血素
ASM American Society for Microbiology 美国微生物学会
As M myopic astigmatism 近视散光
ASN American Society of Nephrology 美国肾病学会
Asn asparagine 天冬酰胺
ASO antistreptolysin O 抗链球菌溶血素 O; arteriosclerosis obliterans 闭塞性动脉硬化
asoma [eiˈsəumə]([复] **asomata** [eiˈsəumətə]) *n* 无躯干畸胎
asomatognosia [əˌsəumətɔgˈnəusiə] *n* 身体失认,躯体辨认不能
asomatophyte [eiˈsəumətəˌfait] *n* 无体植物
asonia [əˈsəuniə] *n* 音调聋,音调失认
Asopia [əˈsəupiə] *n* 谷粉蛾属
ASP American Society of Parasitologists 美国寄生虫学家协会
Asp aspartic acid 天冬氨酸
aspalasoma [ˌæspæləˈsəumə] *n* 田鼠体畸胎
asparaginase [ˌæspəˈrædʒineis, əˈspærədʒiˌneis] *n* 天冬酰胺酶;门冬酰胺酶(临床上用于治疗儿童急性淋巴细胞白血病)
asparagine [əˈspærədʒi(ː)n] *n* 天冬酰胺
asparaginyl [əˈspærəˌdʒinil] *n* 天冬酰胺酰[基]
Asparagus [əˈspærəgəs] *n*【拉】天门冬属
aspartame [əˈspɑːteim] *n* 阿司帕坦(营养性甜味药,比蔗糖甜 200 倍)
aspartase [ˈæspɑːteis] *n* 天冬氨酸酶
aspartate [əˈspɑːteit] *n* 天冬氨酸盐;天冬氨酸(解离型)
aspartate aminotransferase [əˈspɑːteit əˌmiːnəu-ˈtrænsfəreis] 天冬氨酸转氨酶
aspartate carbamoyltransferase [əˈspɑːteit kɑː-ˌbæmɔilˈtrænsfəreis] 天冬氨酸氨甲酰[基]转移酶
aspartate transaminase (AST, ASAT) [əˈspɑː-teit trænsˈæmineis] 天冬氨酸转氨酶
aspartate transcarbamoylase [əˈspɑːteit ˌtræn-skɑːˈbæmɔileis] 天冬氨酸转氨甲酰酶
asparthione [əˈspɑːθaiˌəun] *n* 天冬胱甘肽
aspartic acid [əˈspɑːtik] 天冬氨酸;门冬氨酸(氨基酸类药)
aspartic endopeptidase [əˈspɑːtik ˌendəu ˈpept-ideis] 天冬氨酸内肽酶
aspartic proteinase [əˈspɑːtik ˈprəutiːneis] 天冬氨酸蛋白酶
aspartoacylase [əˌspɑːtəuˈæsileis] *n* 天冬氨酸酰基转移酶
aspartocin [əˈspɑːtəsin] *n* 门冬托星(抗生素类药)
aspartokinase [əˌspɑːtəˈkaineis] *n* 天冬氨酸激酶
aspartyl [əˈspɑːtil] *n* 天冬氨酰[基]
β-aspartyl-*N*-acetylglucosaminidase [əˈspɑːtil ˈæsitilgluːˌkɔsəˈminideis] β-天冬氨酰-*N*-乙酰氨基葡糖苷酶(此酶的遗传性缺乏为一种常染色体隐性性状,可致天冬氨酰氨基葡糖尿。亦称

天冬氨酰氨基葡糖苷酶)
aspartylglucosamine [əˌspɑːtilgluːˈkəusəmiːn] *n* 天冬氨酰葡糖胺
aspartylglucosaminuria [əˌspɑːtilˌgluːkəuˌsæmiˈnjuəriə] *n* 天冬氨酰葡糖胺尿
aspartylglycosaminidase [əˈspɑːtilˌglaikəuˈsæmineideis] *n* 天冬氨酰氨基葡糖苷酶,*β*-天冬氨酰-*N*-乙酰氨基葡糖苷酶
aspartylglycosaminuria [əˈspɑːtilˌglaikəu sæmiˈnjuəriə] *n* 天冬氨酰氨基葡糖尿,天冬氨酰葡糖胺尿(一种遗传病,为常染色体隐性遗传的粘脂贮积病,是由*β*-天冬氨酰-*N*-乙酰氨基葡糖苷酶缺乏所致。本病主要在芬兰后裔病人中发现,其特征为异常代谢物排出、智力迟钝及粗陋面容,伴有腹泻和频发感染)
aspecific [ˌeispiˈsifik] *a* 非特异性的,无特异性的
aspect [ˈæspekt] *n* 方面,局面;外观 | dorsal ~ 背面 / ventral ~ 腹面
Asperger's syndrome [ˈæspəːgə] (Hans Asperger) 阿斯珀格综合征(孤独症者其智力或技能过度发育)
aspergillar [ˌæspəˈdʒilə] *a* 曲霉的
aspergilli [ˌæspəˈdʒilai] aspergillus 的复数
aspergillic acid [ˌæspəˈdʒilik] 曲霉酸
aspergillin [ˌæspəˈdʒilin] *n* 曲霉菌素
aspergilloma [ˌæspədʒiˈləumə] *n* 曲霉肿
aspergillosis [ˌæspədʒiˈləusis], **aspergillomycosis** [ˌæspəˌdʒiləumaiˈkəusis] *n* 曲霉病
Aspergillus [ˌæspəˈdʒiləs] *n* 曲霉属(旧名箒状菌属) | ~ auricularis 耳曲霉 / ~ barbae 须曲霉 / ~ clavatus 棒曲霉 / ~ concentricus 同心曲霉 / ~ flavus 黄曲霉 / ~ fumigatus 烟曲霉 / ~ giganteus 巨曲霉 / ~ glaucus 灰绿曲霉 / ~ gliocladium 胶性曲霉 / ~ mucoroides 黏液样曲霉 / ~ nidulans 构巢曲霉 / ~ niger 黑曲霉 / ~ ochraceus 赭曲霉 / ~ parasiticus 寄生曲霉 / ~ pictor 色斑曲霉 / ~ repens 匍匐曲霉 / ~ terreus 土曲霉
aspergillus [ˌæspəˈdʒiləs] ([复] **aspergilli** [ˌæspəˈdʒilai]) *n* 曲霉(旧名箒状菌)
aspergillustoxicosis [ˌæspəˌdʒiləsˌtɔksiˈkəusis], **aspergillotoxicosis** [ˌæspəˌdʒiləuˌtɔksiˈkəusis] *n* 曲霉中毒
asperkinase [əspəˈkaineis] *n* 米曲霉酶
aspermatogenesis [əˌspəːmətəuˈdʒenisis] *n* 无精子发生
aspermia [əˈspəːmiə], **aspermatism** [əˈspəːmətizəm] *n* 无精,精液缺乏
ASPET American Society for Pharmacology and Experimental Therapeutics 美国药理学与实验治疗学会
asphalgesia [ˌæfælˈdʒiːziə] *n* 触物感痛症(催眠状态中出现)
asphyctic [æsˈfiktik], **asphyctous** [æsˈfiktəs] *a* 窒息的,患窒息的
asphygmia [æsˈfigmiə] *n* 脉搏消失,无脉
asphyxia [æsˈfiksiə] *n* 窒息 | ~ livida, blue ~ 青紫窒息 / ~ pallida, white ~ 苍白窒息 / traumatic ~ 创伤性窒息 | **~l** *a* / **~nt** *a* 窒息的 *n* 窒息剂
asphyxiate [æsˈfiksieit] *vt, vi* (使)窒息 | **asphyxiation** [æsˌfiksiˈeiʃən] *n*
Aspidium [æsˈpidiəm] *n* 叉蕨属
aspidium [æsˈpidiəm] *n* 绵马
aspidosperma [ˌæspideˈspəːmə] *n* 白坚木(治哮喘和呼吸困难)
aspidospermine [ˌæspidəˈspəːmiːn] *n* 白坚木碱
aspirate [ˈæspəreit] *vt* 抽吸 *n* 抽出物,吸出物;送气音
aspiration [ˌæspəˈreiʃən] *n* 吸入;抽吸;吸引[术] | fine-needle ~ 细针抽吸 / meconium ~ 胎粪吸入
aspirator [ˈæspəreitə] *n* 吸气器;吸引器,抽吸器
aspirin [ˈæspərin] *n* 阿司匹林(解热镇痛药)
asplenia [eiˈspliːniə] *n* 无脾 | **asplenic** [eiˈsplenik] *a*
asporogenic [ˌæspɔːrəˈdʒenik], **asporogenous** [ˌæspəˈrɔdʒinəs] *a* 不产生孢子的,非孢子性生殖的
asporous [əˈspɔːrəs] *a* 无孢子的,无芽胞的
ASRT American Society of Radiologic Technologists 美国放射技术员学会
ASS anterior superior spine 前上棘
assanation [ˌæsəˈneiʃən] *n* 环境卫生
assay [əˈsei, ˈæsei] *n* 测定,含量测定 | biological ~ 生物学鉴定法 / blastogenesis ~ 胚细胞样转变测定(见 test 项下 lymphocyte proliferation test) / cell-mediated lympholysis(CML) ~ 细胞介导淋巴细胞溶解测定 / CH_{50} ~ CH_{50} 测定,50%补体溶血单位测定(补体总活力的功能性测定。亦称溶血补体测定,补体总量测定,补体全量测定) / E rosette ~ E 玫瑰花结测定,红细胞玫瑰花结测定 / ECA rosette ~ ECA 玫瑰花结测定,红细胞-抗体-补体玫瑰花结测定 / enzyme-linked immunosorbent ~ (ELISA) 酶联免疫吸附测定 / four-point ~ 四点测定[法](根据待检物和标准物各 2 份的混合物进行测定的方法) / hemagglutination inhibition(HI, HAI) ~ 血细胞凝集抑制测定 / hemolytic plaque ~ 溶血空斑测定 / immune ~ 免疫测定法 / immune adherence hemagglutination ~ (IAHA) 免疫粘连血凝测定 / immunoradiometric ~ 免疫放射测定 / lymphocyte proliferation ~ 淋巴细胞增生测定(见 test 项下相应术语) / microbiological ~ 微

生物鉴定 / microcytotoxicity ~ 微量细胞毒性测定 / microhemagglutination ~-*Treponema pallidum* (MHA-TP) 梅毒螺旋体微量血凝测定 / mixed lymphocyte culture(MLC) ~ 混合淋巴细胞培养测定 / radioreceptor ~ 放射性受体测定 / *Treponema pallidum* hemagglutination ~ (TPHA) 梅毒螺旋体血凝测定

assembly [ə'sembli] *n* [病毒]装配

assessment [ə'sesmənt] *n* 评定,评价 | personality ~ 人格鉴定 / ~ of vision 视力评价

Assézat's triangle [əsi'zɑː] (Jules Assézat) 阿希扎三角,面三角(facial triangle,见 triangle 项下相应术语)

assignment [ə'sainmənt] *n* 分配 | gene ~ 基因定位,基因配位

assimilation [əˌsimi'leiʃən] *n* 吸收[作用];同化作用(食物转变为活组织)

assistant [ə'sistənt] *a* 辅助的 *n* 助手;辅助物;助剂 | physician ~ 助理医师

Assmann's focus (tuberculous infiltrate) ['ɑːsmən] (Herbert Assmann) 阿斯曼病灶(结核浸润)(肺结核早期渗出性损害,最常发生在肺尖下部)

association [əˌsəusi'eiʃən] *n* 关联;联络;联合征;联想;协会 | clang ~, klang ~ 音联 / controlled ~s 控制联想 / dream ~s 忆梦联想 / free ~ 自由联想 / rhyme ~ 音联

Association Professionnelle Internationale des Médicins(APIM) 国际专业医师协会(一种从经济观点处理医疗行为的国际团体)

assortment [ə'sɔːtmənt] *n* 分类;组合,分配(在第一次成熟分裂的中期非同源染色体可以随机地分配给配子) | independent ~ 自由组合(不同染色体上的基因在配子中的任意分布)

assurin ['æsjuərin] *n* 二氨基双磷脂

AST aspartate transaminase 天冬氨酸转氨酶

Ast. astigmatism 散光[眼]

astacin ['æstəsin], **astacene** ['æstəsiːn] *n* 虾红素

astasia [æ'steiziə] *n* 起立不能 | ~ -abasia 站立行走不能 | **astatic** [æ'stætik] *a*

astatine(At) ['æstətiːn] *n* 砹(放射元素,治甲状腺功能亢进)

astaxanthin [ˌæstə'zænθin] *n* 虾青素

asteatosis [ˌæstiə'təusis], **asteatodes** [ˌæstiə'təudiːz] *n* 皮脂缺乏[症]

astemizole [əˌstemizəul] *n* 阿司咪唑(一种 H_1 受体拮抗剂,用于治疗慢性荨麻疹和季节性变应性鼻炎〈枯草热〉)

aster ['æstə] *n* 星体 | sperm ~ 精星体,精子星状体

Asteraceae [ˌæstə'reisiiː] *n* 翠菊科

astereognosis [əˌstiəriəg'nəusis], **astereocognosy** [əˌstiəriə'kɔgnəsi] *n* 实体感觉缺失

asterion [æs'tiəriɔn] ([复] **asteria** [æs'tiəriə]) *n*【希】星点(头颅表面上人字缝、顶乳缝和枕乳缝的相交点)

asterixis [ˌæstə'riksis] *n* 扑翼样震颤(见于肝昏迷等)

asternal [ei'stəːnl] *a* 不连胸骨的;无胸骨的

asternia [ei'stəːniə] *n* 无胸骨[畸形]

Asterococcus [ˌæstərəu'kɔkəs] *n* 星球菌属 | ~ canis 犬星球菌 / ~ mycoides 放线样星球菌

asteroid ['æstərɔid] *a* 星样的

asterubin [ˌæstə'rubin] *n* 海星红素

Asth. asthenopia 视疲劳

asthenia [æs'θiːnjə] *n* 无力,虚弱,衰弱 | ~ gravis hypophyseogenea 垂体性恶病质 / myalgic ~ 肌痛性衰弱 / neurocirculatory ~ 神经性循环衰弱(亦称奋力综合征,官能性心血管病) / periodic ~ 周期性衰弱 / tropical anhidrotic ~ 热带无汗性衰弱 | **asthenic** [æs'θenik] *a*

asthen(o)- [构词成分]无力,衰弱

asthenobiosis [æsˌθiːnəubai'əusis] *n* 不活动生活,停滞生活(生物活动能力降低的状态,类似冬眠或夏蛰,与温度和湿度并无直接关系)

asthenocoria [æsˌθiːnəu'kɔːriə] *n* 瞳孔反应迟钝(见于肾上腺功能减退)

asthenometer [ˌæsθi'nɔmitə] *n* 肌无力测量器

asthenope ['æsθənəup] *n* 视疲劳患者

asthenopia [ˌæsθi'nəupiə] *n* 视疲劳 | accommodative ~ 调节性视疲劳 / muscular ~ 肌性视疲劳 / nervous ~ 神经性视疲劳 / retinal ~ 视网膜性视疲劳 / tarsal ~ 睑性视疲劳 | **asthenopic** [ˌæsθi'nɔpik] *a*

asthenospermia [ˌæsθinəu'spəːmiə] *n* 精子活力不足

asthenoteratospermia [ˌæsθinəuˌterətəu'spəːmiə] *n* 精子活力不足并畸形精子[症]

asthenoxia [ˌæsθə'nɔksiə] *n* 氧化力不足

asthma ['æsmə, 'æzmə] *n* 哮喘 | allergic ~, atopic ~ 变应性哮喘,特应性哮喘 / bacterial ~ 细菌性哮喘 / bronchial ~ 支气管哮喘 / cardiac ~ 心源性哮喘 / cotton-dust ~ 棉屑沉着病,棉屑肺 / extrinsic ~ 外源性哮喘 / humid ~ 湿性哮喘,痰喘 / intrinsic ~ 内源性哮喘 / millers' ~ 研磨工哮喘 / miners' ~ 矿工哮喘,炭末沉着病,炭肺 / pollen ~ 花粉性哮喘,枯草热 / potters' ~ 陶工哮喘,肺尘埃沉着病 / stone ~ 支气管结石性哮喘 / **~tic** [æs'mætik, æz-] *a*

asthmatiform [æs'mætifɔːm, æz-] *a* 哮喘样的

asthmogenic [ˌæsmə'dʒenik, ˌæz-] *a* 哮喘原的,致哮喘的 *n* 致喘物质

Asticcacaulis [əˌstikə'kɔːlis] *n* 不粘柄菌属

astigmagraph [əˈstigməgrɑːf, græf] *n* 散光描记器
astigmatism [əˈstigmətizəm] *n* 散光[眼] | acquired ~ 后天性散光 / ~ against the rule, inverse ~ 反规性散光 / hypermetropic ~, hyperopic ~ 远视散光 / lenticular ~ 晶状体性散光 / myopic ~ 近视散光 / oblique ~ 斜轴散光 / ~ with the rule, direct ~ 循规性散光 | **astigmatic(al)** [ˌæstigˈmætik(əl)] *a*
astigmatometer [əˈstigməˈtɔmitə] *n* 散光计
astigmatometry [əˌstigməˈtɔmitri] *n* 散光测量法
astigmatoscope [ˌæstigˈmætəskəup] *n* 散光镜 | **astigmatoscopy** [əˌstigməˈtɔskəpi] *n* 散光镜检查
astigmia [əˈstigmiə] *n* 散光 | **astigmic** *a*
astigmometer [ˌæstigˈmɔmitə] *n* 散光计
astigmometry [ˌæstigˈmɔmitri] *n* 散光测量法
astigmoscope [əˈstigməskəup] *n* 散光镜
astigmoscopy [ˌæstigˈmɔskəpi] *n* 散光镜检查
Astomatida [ˌeistəməˈtaidə] *n* 无口目
astomatous [əˈstɔmətəs] *a* 无口的(如某些纤毛虫)
astomia [əˈstəumiə] *n* 无口
astomus [əˈstəuməs] *n* 无口畸胎
astragalar [æsˈtrægələ] *a* 距骨的
astragalectomy [ˌæstrægəˈlektəmi] *n* 距骨切除术
astragalocalcanean [æsˌtrægələukælˈkeiniən] *a* 距跟的
astragalocrural [æsˌtrægələuˈkruərəl] *a* 距骨小腿的
astragaloscaphoid [æsˌtrægələuˈskæfɔid] *a* 距舟的
astragalotibial [æsˌtrægələuˈtibiəl] *a* 距胫的
Astragalus [əˈstrægələs] *n* 黄芪属
astragalus [əˈstrægələs] *n* 距骨
astral [ˈæstrəl] *a* 星体的
astraphobia [ˌæstrəˈfəubiə], **astrapophobia** [ˌæstrəpəˈfəubiə] *n* 闪电恐怖
astriction [əˈstrikʃən] *n* 收敛[作用];便秘
astringency [əˈstrindʒənsi] *n* 收敛性
astringent [əˈstrindʒənt] *a* 收敛的 *n* 收敛药,收敛剂
astro- [构词成分]星,星形
astroblast [ˈæstrəublæst] *n* 成星形细胞
astroblastoma [ˌæstrəublæsˈtəumə] *n* 成星形细胞瘤
astrocinetic [ˌæstəusaiˈnetik] *a* 星球移动的
astroc(o)ele [ˈæstrəusiːl] *n* 中心体腔
astrocyte [ˈæstrəsait] *n* 星形胶质细胞;星形胶质 | gemistocytic ~ 饲肥星形胶质细胞 | **astrocytic** [ˌæstrəuˈsitik] *a*
astrocytin [ˌæstrəuˈsaitin] *n* 星形胶质细胞膜抗原
astrocytoma [ˌæstrəusaiˈtəumə] *n* 星形胶质细胞瘤 | anaplastic ~ 多形性成胶质细胞瘤 / pilocytic ~ 纤维性星形胶质细胞瘤
astrocytosis [ˌæstrəusaiˈtəusis] *n* 星形胶质细胞增生
astroglia [æsˈtrɔgliə] *n* 星形胶质细胞;星形胶质
astroid [ˈæstrɔid] *a* 星形的
astrokinetic [ˌæstrəukiˈnetik] *a* 星球移动的
astrophorous [æsˈtrɔfərəs] *a* 具星形突的
astroplankton [ˌæstrəuˈplæŋktən] *n* 天体浮游生物
astropyle [ˈæstrəpail] *n* 星口(指原生动物)
astrosphere [ˈæstrəsfiə] *n* 星心球;星体
astrostatic [ˌæstrəuˈstætik] *a* 星球静止的,中心体静止的
Astroviridae [ˌæstrəuˈviridiː] *n* 星形病毒科
Astrovirus [ˈæstrəuˌvaiərəs] *n* 星形病毒属
astrovirus [ˈæstrəuˌvaiərəs] *n* 星形病毒
astyclinic [ˌæstiˈklinik] *n* 市立医院,市立诊所
asuerotherapy [ˌæsuˈɛərəuˌθerəpi] (Fernando Asuero) *n* 阿苏埃罗疗法(蝶腭神经节烙术,与暗示疗法并用)
asulfurosis [eisʌlfəˈrəusis] *n* 硫缺乏症
asyllabia [ˌeisiˈleibiə] *n* 缀字不能,拼音不能
asylum [əˈsailəm] *n* 【拉】收容所,养育院,救济院
asymbolia [əsimˈbəuliə], **asymboly** [əˈsimbəli] *n* 说示不能,失示意能
asymmetry [æˈsimitri] *n* 不对称,偏位 | chromatic ~ 两眼虹膜异色 / encephalic ~ 脑不对称,偏位脑 | **asymmetric(al)** [ˌæsiˈmetrik(əl)] *a*
asymphytous [əˈsimfitəs] *a* 不并的,分离的
asymptomatic [ˌeisimptəˈmætik] *a* 无症状的
asynapsis [eisiˈnæpsis] *n* 不联会(在减数分裂时,同源染色体不进行配对)
asynchronism [eiˈsiŋkrənizəm], **asynchrony** [eiˈsiŋkrəni] *n* 不同时性,异步性;协调障碍 | **asynchronous** [eiˈsiŋkrənəs] *a*
asynclitism [əˈsiŋklitizəm] *n* 头盆倾势不均(产位);红细胞生成障碍
asyndesis [əˈsindisis] *n* 思想连贯不能(见于精神分裂症及器质性脑综合征)
asynechia [ˌeisiˈnekiə] *n* 不连续
asynergy [eiˈsinədʒi] *n* 协同动作不能 | truncal ~ 躯干协同动作不能 | **asynergia** [ˌeisiˈnəːdʒiə] *n* / **asynergic** [ˌeisiˈnəːdʒik] *a*
asynodia [ˌeisiˈnəudiə] *n* 阳萎
asynovia [ˌeisiˈnəuviə] *n* 滑液缺乏,无滑液
asyntaxia [ˌeisinˈtæksiə] *n* 胚胎发育不全 | ~ dorsalis 神经沟未闭
asystole [əˈsistəli], **asystolia** [ˌeisisˈtəuliə] *n* 心

搏停搏,无收缩 | **asystolic** [ˌeisisˈtɔlik] *a*
AT atrial tachycardia 房性心动过速
At astatine 砹
ATA alimentary toxic aleukia 食饵中毒性白细胞缺乏症
atactic [əˈtæktik] *a* 协调不能的;不规则的;共济失调的
atactiform [əˈtæktifɔːm] *a* 共济失调样的
ataractic [ˌætəˈræktik], **ataraxic** [ˌætəˈræksik] *a* 心气和平的,心神安定的 *n* 安定药
ataralgesia [ˌætərælˈdʒiːziə] *n* 镇静止痛法
ataraxia [ˌætəˈræksiə], **ataraxy** [ˌætəˈræksi] *n* 心气和平,心神安定
atavism [ˈætəvizəm] *n* 返祖[现象](几代以后再次出现某些祖先的特征的现象) | **atavistic** [ˌætəˈvistik], **atavic** [ˈætəvik] *a* 返祖性的
ataxaphasia [əˌtæksəˈfeiziə] *n* 组句不能
ataxia [əˈtæksiə] *n* 共济失调 | locomotor ~ 运动性共济失调脊髓痨 / ~-telangiectasia 共济失调-毛细血管扩张症 | **ataxic** [əˈtæksik] *a* / **ataxy** [əˈtæksi] *n*
ataxiagram [əˈtæksiəˌgræm] *n* 共济失调描记图
ataxiagraph [əˈtæksiəˌgrɑːf] *n* 共济失调描记器
ataxiameter [əˌtæksiˈæmitə] *n* 共济失调计
ataxiamnesic [əˌtæksiæmˈniːsik] *a* 共济失调及遗忘[症]的
ataxiaphasia [əˌtæksiəˈfeiziə] *n* 组句不能
ataxophemia [əˌtæksəˈfiːmiə], **ataxiophemia** [əˌtæksiəˈfiːmiə] *n* 言语共济失调
ataxophobia [əˌtæksəˈfəubiə], **ataxiophobia** [əˌtæksiəˈfəubiə] *n* 失调恐怖
ATCC American Type Culture Collection 美国模式培养物保藏所
-ate [后缀]构成名词,表示"产物",如 hemolysate; 在化学中表示"…酸盐",如 glycerate; 构成形容词,表示"具有…特征",如 dentate; 构成动词,表示"成为…",如 decussate
atelectasis [ˌætiˈlektəsis] *n* 肺膨胀不全;肺不张;[中耳]不张 | absorption ~, acquired ~, obstructive ~, resorption ~ 吸收性肺膨胀不全,获得性肺膨胀不全,阻塞性肺膨胀不全 / compression ~ 压迫性肺膨胀不全 / congenital ~ 先天性肺膨胀不全 / lobar ~, segmental ~ 肺叶膨胀不全,节段性肺膨胀不全,肺叶不张 / lobular ~, patchy ~ 小叶性肺不张,片状肺不张 / primary ~, initial ~ 原发性肺膨胀不全,原发性肺不张 / relaxation ~ 松弛性肺膨胀不全 / secondary ~ 继发性肺膨胀不全;吸收性肺膨胀不全 | **atelectatic** [ˌætilekˈtætik] *a*
ateleiosis [ˌətiːliˈəusis], **ateliosis** [əˌtiːliˈəusis] *n* 垂体性幼稚型
atelencephalia [əˌtelensiˈfeiliə] *n* 脑发育不全
atelia [əˈtiːliə] *n* 发育不全 | **ateliotic** [əˌtiːliˈɔtik] *a*
atel(o)- [构词成分]发育不全
atelocardia [ˌætiəuˈkɑːdiə] *n* 心发育不全
atelocephalous [ˌætiləuˈsefələs] *a* 头发育不全的
atelocephaly [ˌætiləuˈsefəli] *n* 头颅发育不全
atelocheilia [ˌætiləuˈkailiə] *n* 唇发育不全
atelocheiria [ˌætiləuˈkaiəriə] *n* 手发育不全
ateloencephalia [ˌætiləuˌensiˈfeiliə] *n* 脑发育不全
ateloglossia [ˌætiləuˈglɔsiə] *n* 舌发育不全
atelognathia [ˌætilɔgˈneiθiə] *n* 颌发育不全
atelomyelia [ˌætiləumaiˈiːliə] *n* 脊髓发育不全
atelopidtoxin [eiteˌlɔpidˈtɔksin] *n* 斑足蟾毒素
atelopodia [ˌætiləuˈpəudiə] *n* 足发育不全
ateloprosopia [ˌætiləupraˈsəupiə] *n* 面发育不全
atelorachidia [ˌætiləurəˈkidiə] *n* 脊柱发育不全
Atelosaccharomyces [ˌætiləuˌsækərəuˈmaisiːz] *n* 不全酵母菌属(隐球菌属 Cryptococcus 的旧称)
atelostomia [ˌætiləuˈstəumiə] *n* 口[腔]发育不全
atenolol [əˈtenəlɔl] *n* 阿替洛尔(β 受体阻滞药)
ATG antithymocyte globulim 抗胸腺细胞球蛋白
Athalamida [ˌeiθəˈlæmidə] *n* 无室目
athalposis [ˌeiθælˈpəusis] *n* 温觉缺失
athelia [əˈθiːliə] *n* 无乳头[畸形]
atherectomy [ˌæθəˈrektəmi] *n* [动脉]粥样硬化斑切除术
athermal [əˈθəːməl] *a* 不热的(指泉水的水温在 15 ℃以下)
athermancy [əˈθəːmənsi] *n* 不透[辐射]热性 | **athermanous** [əˈθəːmənəs] *a*
athermic [əˈθəːmik] *a* 无热的,不发热的;不透热的
athermosystaltic [əˌθəːməusisˈtæltik] *a* 无温度性收缩的(指骨骼肌)
ather(o)- [构词成分]脂肪变性;动脉粥样化;粥样斑
atheroembolism [ˌæθərəuˈembəlizəm] *n* [动脉]粥样硬化栓塞
atheroembolus [ˌæθərəuˈembələs] ([复] **atheroemboli** [ˌæθərəuˈembəlai]) *n* [动脉]粥样硬化栓子
atherogenesis [ˌæθərəuˈdʒenisis] *n* [动脉]粥样化形成
atherogenic [ˌæθərəuˈdʒenik] *a* 致动脉粥样化的
atheroma [ˌæθəˈrəumə] *n* 粥样斑 | **~tous** *a*
atheromatosis [ˌæθəˌrəuməˈtəusis] *n* 动脉粥样斑病
atherosclerosis [ˌæθərəuskliəˈrəusis] *n* 动脉粥样硬化 | ~ obliterans 闭塞性动脉硬化 | **atherosclerotic** [ˌæθərəuskliəˈrɔtik] *a*

atherosis [ˌæθəˈrəusis] *n* 粥样斑
athetoid [ˈæθitɔid] *a* 手足徐动症样的,指痉病样的
athetosis [ˌæθiˈtəusis] *n* 手足徐动症 | double ~, double congenital ~ 先天性两侧手足徐动症 / pupillary ~ 虹膜震颤 | **athetotic** [ˌæθiˈtɔtik], **athetosic** [ˌæθiˈtəusik] *a*
athiaminosis [əˌθaiəmiˈnəusis] *n* 硫胺缺乏病,维生素 B_1 缺乏病
Athiorhodaceae [ˌeiθaiərəuˈdeisiiː] *n* 红色无硫菌科(即红螺菌科 Rhodospirillaceae)
athomin [ˈæθəmin] *n* 辣根素(在印度用作止吐药和治疗霍乱。亦称 GL_{54})
athrepsia [əˈθrepsiə], **athrepsy** [ˈæθrepsi] *n* 重度消瘦型营养不良;营养缺乏[性]免疫(埃利希〈Ehrlich〉术语,用以表示瘤接种所产生的免疫性,认为系由于瘤生长所需的特殊营养物质缺乏所致) | **athreptic** [əˈθreptik] *a* 营养不良的
athrocytosis [ˌæθrəsaiˈtəusis] *n* 细胞摄物作用(肾管细胞自肾小管的腔内吸收巨分子)
athrophagocytosis [ˌæθrəuˈfægəusaiˈtəusis] *n* 非营养性吞噬作用(吞噬惰性无关颗粒,如在碳清除试验中,吞噬细胞清除注射至体内的碳粒)
athymia [əˈθaimiə] *n* 痴愚;无胸腺;人事不省
athymic [eiˈθaimik] *a* 无胸腺的
athymism [əˈθaimizəm], **athymismus** [ˌeiθaiˈmisməs] *n* 无胸腺
athyrea [əˈθairiə] *n* 甲状腺功能缺失;无甲状腺
athyreosis [əˌθairiˈəusis] *n* 甲状腺功能缺失;无甲状腺 | **athyreotic** [əˌθairiˈɔtik] *a*
athyria [əˈθairiə] *n* 无甲状腺;甲状腺功能缺失
athyroidemia [eiˌθairɔiˈdiːmiə] *n* 无甲状腺性血症
athyroidism [eiˈθairɔidizəm], **athyroidation** [eiˌθairɔiˈdeiʃən], **athyroidosis** [eiˌθairɔiˈdəusis] *n* 甲状腺功能缺失;无甲状腺
athyrosis [ˌeiθaiˈrəusis] *n* 甲状腺功能缺失;无甲状腺 | **athyrotic** [ˌeiθaiˈrɔtik] *a*
Athysanus [əˈθisənəs] *n* 北非吸血蝇属
ATL adult T-cell leukemia/lymphoma 成人 T 细胞白血病/淋巴瘤
atlantad [ætˈlæntæd] *ad* 向寰椎
atlantal [ætˈlæntl] *a* 寰椎的
atlant(o)- [构词成分]寰椎
atlantoaxial [ætˌlæntəuˈæksiəl] *a* 寰枢椎的
atlantodidymus [ætˌlæntəuˈdidiməs] *n* 寰椎联胎
atlantomastoid [ætˌlæntəuˈmæstɔid] *a* 寰[椎]乳[突]的
atlanto-odontoid [ætˌlæntəuɔˈdɔntoid] *a* 寰[椎]齿[突]的
atlas [ˈætləs] *n* 寰椎(第一颈椎);图谱,图片集
atloaxoid [ˌætləuˈæksɔid] *a* 寰枢椎的
atlodidymus [ætləuˈdidiməs] *n* 寰椎联胎
atloido-occipital [ætˌlɔidəu ɔkˈsipitl] *a* 寰枕的
atm atmosphere 大气压
atmiatrics [ˌætmiˈætriks], **atmiatry** [ætˈmaiətri] *n* 蒸气吸入疗法
atm(o)- [构词成分]气,蒸气
atmograph [ˈætməgrɑːf,-græf] *n* 呼吸描记器
atmolysis [ætˈmɔlisis] *n* 微孔分气法(借通过多孔板,以分离混合的气体,易扩散的气体先通过);有机组织分解法(利用挥发性液体,如苯、乙醚、乙醇等的气体使有机组织分解)
atmometer [ætˈmɔmitə] *n* 汽化计,蒸发计
atmos [ˈætməs] *n* 大气压(大气压单位,每平方厘米面积上受到一个大气压)
atmosphere [ˈætməsfiə] *n* 大气;大气压(压力的单位,在海平面上地球大气的压力约为 101.3 kPa〈 = 760 mmHg〉,缩写为 atm);气氛,氛围 | group ~ 集体气氛 | **atmospheric (al)** [ˌætməsˈferik(əl)] *a*
atmotherapy [ˌætməuˈθerəpi] *n* 蒸气吸入疗法;缩减呼吸气量疗法(循序减少呼吸疗法)
ATN tyrosinase-negative(ty-neg) oculocutaneoua albinism 酪氨酸酶阴性眼皮肤白化病
at no atomic number 原子序数
atocia [əˈtəusiə] *n* 未经产;女性不育
atolide [ˈætəlaid] *n* 阿托利特(抗惊厥药)
atom [ˈætəm] *n* 原子 | activated ~, excited ~ 激活原子,受激原子 / nuclear ~ 核型原子 / recoil ~, rest ~ 反冲原子 / stripped ~ 被剥原子 / tagged ~ 标记原子,示踪原子
atomic [əˈtɔmik] *a* 原子的
atomicity [ˌætəˈmisəti] *n* 原子价;原子性;原子数
atomism [ˈætəmizəm] *n* 原子论,原子学说 | **atomist** [ˈætəmist] *n* 原子学家
atomistic [ˌætəˈmistik] *a* 原子学的,原子学派的
atomize [ˈætəmaiz] *vt* 使雾化,喷雾 | **atomization** [ˌætəmaiˈzeiʃən, -miˈz-] *n*
atomizer [ˈætəmaizə] *n* 喷雾器,雾化器
atonic [æˈtɔnik] *a* 张力缺乏的,失张力的 | **~ity** [ˌætəˈnisəti] *n* 张力缺失性
atony [ˈætəni], **atonia** [əˈtəuniə] *n* 张力缺失
atopen [ˈætəpən] *n* 特应性变应原
atopic [əˈtɔpik] *a* 异位的;特应性的
atopognosia [əˌtɔpɔgˈnəuziə], **atopognosis** [əˌtɔpɔgˈnəusis] *n* 位置失认[症]
atopy [ˈætəpi] *n* 特应性
atorvastatin calcium [eiˌtɔːvəˈstætin] 阿托伐他汀钙(抗高血脂药,其作用为抑制胆固醇合成,用于治疗原发性高胆固醇血症和异常脂血症,口服给药)
atovaquone [əˈtəuvəˌkwəun] *n* 阿托伐醌(抗疟药)

atoxic [ə'tɔksik] *a* 无毒的,非毒性的
atoxigenic [əˌtɔksi'dʒenik] *n* 不产生毒素的
ATP adenosine triphosphate 腺苷三磷酸
ATPase adenosinetriphosphatase 腺苷三磷酸酶
ATP citrate lyase ['saitreit 'laieis] 腺苷三磷酸枸橼酸裂合酶(亦称枸橼酸裂合酶)
ATP-cobalamin adenosyltransferase [kəu'bæləmin əˌdenəsil'trænsfəreis] 腺苷三磷酸钴胺素腺苷转移酶,钴(1)胺素腺苷基转移酶
ATP synthase ['sinθeis] ATP 合酶,腺苷三磷酸合酶,H^+-转运腺苷三磷酸合酶
atrabiliary [ˌætrə'biljəri] *a* 黑胆质的,忧郁质的
atrabilious [ˌætrə'biljəs], **atrabiliar** [ˌætrə'biljə] *a* 忧郁的
Atractaspis [ətræk'tæspis] *n* 穴蝰属
atracurium besylate [ˌætrə'kjuəriəm] 苯磺阿曲库铵(神经肌肉阻断药)
atransferrinemia [eiˌtrænsfəri'niːmiə] *n* 无转铁蛋白血症
atraumatic [ˌeitrɔː'mætik] *a* 无创伤的
Atrax ['eitræks] *n* 澳毒蜘蛛属
atremia [ə'triːmiə] *n* 无震颤;癔症性步行不能
atrepsy ['ætrepsi] *n* 重度消瘦型营养不良 | **atreptic** [ə'trəptik] *a* 营养不良的
atresia [ə'triːziə] *n* 闭锁 | ~ ani 肛门闭锁 / follicle ~ 卵泡闭锁 / tricuspid ~ 三尖瓣闭锁 | **atretic** [ə'tretik], **atresic** [ə'triːzik] *a*
atret(o)- [构词成分]闭锁
atretoblepharia [əˌtriːtəubli'fɛəriə] *n* 睑球粘连,睑闭锁
atretocephalus [əˌtriːtəu'sefələs] *n* 头部孔窍闭锁畸胎
atretocormus [əˌtriːtəu'kɔːməs] *n* 躯干孔窍闭锁畸胎
atretocystia [əˌtriːtəu'sistiə] *n* 膀胱闭锁
atretogastria [əˌtriːtəu'gæstriə] *n* 胃门闭锁
atretolemia [əˌtriːtəu'liːmiə] *n* 咽门闭锁(喉或食管闭锁)
atretometria [əˌtriːtəu'miːtriə] *n* 子宫闭锁
atretopsia [ˌætriː'tɔpsiə] *n* 瞳孔闭锁
atretorrhinia [əˌtriːtəu'riniə] *n* 鼻孔闭锁
atretostomia [əˌtriːtəu'stəumiə] *n* 口闭锁
atreturethria [əˌtriːtjuə'riːθriə] *n* 尿道闭锁
atria ['eitriə] atrium 的复数
atrial ['eitriəl] *a* 房的,前房的
atrichia [ə'trikiə] *n* 无毛症,秃;无鞭毛 | universal congenital ~ 先天性普秃
atrichosis [ˌætri'kəusis] *n* 无毛症,秃
atrichous [ə'trikəs] *a* 无鞭毛的(指细菌);无毛发的
atri(o)- [构词成分][心]房
atriocommissuropexy [ˌeitriəuˌkɔmi'sjuərəˌpeksi] *n* 二尖瓣固定术
atriohisian [ˌeitriəu'hisiən] *a* 心房希氏束的
atriomegaly [ˌeitriə'megəli] *n* 心房肥大
atrionector [ˌeitriə'nektə] *n* 窦房结
atriopeptigen [ˌeitriəu'peptidʒən] *n* 心房钠尿肽原
atriopeptin [ˌeitriəu'peptin] *n* 心房钠尿肽
atrioseptopexy [ˌeitriəuˌseptə'peksi] *n* 房间隔修补术
atrioseptoplasty [ˌeitriəuˌseptə'plæsti] *n* 房间隔成形术
atriotomy [ˌeitri'ɔtəmi] *n* 心房切开术
atrioventricular [ˌeitriəuven'trikjulə] *a* 房室的
atrioventricularis communis [ˌeitriəuˌventrikju'lɛəris kə'mjunis] 房室共通(一种先天性心脏畸形,亦称房室总管存留)
Atriplex [ə'tripleks] *n* 滨藜属
atriplicism [ə'triplisizəm] *n* 滨藜中毒
atrium ['eitriəm] ([复] **atria** ['eitriə]) *n*【拉】房,前房 | ~ cordis 心房 / ~ dextrum, right ~ 右心房 / ~ of glottis, ~ of larynx 喉前庭 / pulmonary ~ 左心房 / ~ sinistrum, left ~ 左心房 / ~ vaginae 阴道前庭
Atropa ['ætrəpə] *n* 颠茄属
atrophedema [əˌtrɔfi'diːmə] *n* 萎缩性水肿(血管神经性水肿)
atrophia [ə'trəufiə] *n*【拉;希】萎缩
atrophic [æ'trɔfik] *a* 萎缩的
atrophie [ætrə'fi] *n*【法】萎缩 | ~ blanche [blɔŋʃ]【法】白色萎缩 / ~ noire [nwɑː]【法】黑色萎缩
atrophied ['ætrəfid] *a* [已]萎缩的
atroph(o)- [构词成分]萎缩
atrophoderma [ˌætrəfə'dəːmə] *n* 皮萎缩,萎缩性皮肤病
atrophodermatosis [ˌætrɔfədəːmə'təusis] *n* 皮萎缩病
atrophodermia [ˌætrəfə'dəːmiə] *n* 皮肤萎缩,萎缩性皮肤病 | ~ vermiculata 蠕虫样皮萎缩,蠕虫样萎缩性皮肤病
atrophy ['ætrəfi] *n* 萎缩 *vt*, *vi* 萎缩 | acute yellow ~ 急性黄色萎缩(亦称急性实质性肝炎,恶性黄疸) / arthritic ~ 关节周肌萎缩(由于损伤或体质病所致) / blue ~ 蓝色萎缩(一种蓝色色素沉着,常因有药瘾者自行注射药物所致) / brown ~ 褐色萎缩(主要见于老年人心、肝及脾) / ~ of disuse 失用性萎缩(指身体某一部分缺少正常活动所致) / healed yellow ~ 愈合性黄色萎缩,坏死后肝硬变 / infantile ~ 婴儿萎缩[症],消瘦 / lobar ~ 脑叶萎缩 / macular ~ 斑状萎缩,皮肤松垂 / optic ~ 视神经萎缩 / peroneal ~ 腓肌型肌萎缩,进行性神经病性[腓]肌

萎缩 / red ~ 红色萎缩(主要指肝萎缩,由于心脏瓣膜病导致慢性充血所致) / reversionary ~ 退行发育,间变 / white ~ 白色萎缩(一种神经萎缩,仅残存白色结缔组织)

atropine [ˈætrəpiːn] *n* 阿托品(抗胆碱药) | ~ methonitrate, ~ methylnitrate 甲硝阿托品,硝酸甲基阿托品 / ~ sulfate 硫酸阿托品

atropinic [ˌætrəˈpinik] *a* 阿托品的

atropinism [ˈætrəpinizəm], **atropism** [ˈætrəpizəm] *n* 阿托品中毒

atropinization [æˌtrəupinaiˈzeiʃən] *n* 阿托品化,阿托品处理[法]

ATS American Thoracic Society 美国胸科学会; antitetanic serum 抗破伤风血清

ATSDR Agency for Toxic Substances and Diseases Registry 有毒物质和疾病登记处(属美国公共卫生署)

attachment [əˈtætʃmənt] *n* 附着,接合;爱慕,依恋;附着体;固位体 | edgewise ~ 边缘矫正器 / epithelial ~ (of Gottlieb) 上皮附着 / extracoronal ~ 牙冠外固位体 / intracoronal ~, frictional ~, internal ~, key-and-keyway ~, parallel ~, precision ~, slotted ~ 牙冠内固位体,摩擦式固位体,内部固位体,键与键槽式固位体,平行固位体,精密固位体,狭槽式固位体

attack [əˈtæk] *n* 发作 | anxiety ~, panic ~ 焦虑发作,惊恐发作 / transient ischemic ~ (TIA) 短暂性脑缺血发作 / vasovagal ~, vagal ~ 血管迷走神经性发作,迷走神经性发作

attapulgite [ˌætəˈpʌldʒait] (Attapalgus 为美国佐治亚州一城市,在该市附近发现) *n* 绿坡缕石(一种含镁的水合硅酸铝,为漂白土的主要成分) | activated ~ 活化绿坡缕石(经加热处理以增加吸附性,用作辅助剂以吸附细菌和毒素治疗痢疾,口服)

attar [ˈætə] *n* 挥发油,精油 | ~ of roses 玫瑰油

attention [əˈtenʃən] *n* 注意;注意力

attenuant [əˈtenjuənt] *a* 稀释的 *n* 稀释剂

attenuate [əˈtenjueit] *vt, vi* 稀释;减毒,减弱;衰减

attenuation [əˌtenjuˈeiʃən] *n* 稀释;(使病原微生物的毒力)减毒,减弱;衰减 | interaural ~ 耳间衰减

attic [ˈætik] *n* 上鼓室

atticitis [ˌætiˈkaitis] *n* 上鼓室炎

atticoantrotomy [ˌætikəuænˈtrɔtəmi] *n* 上鼓室乳突窦切开术

atticomastoid [ˌætikəuˈmæstɔid] *a* 上鼓室乳突的

atticotomy [ˌætiˈkɔtəmi] *n* 上鼓室切开术 | transmeatal ~ 经耳道上鼓室切开术

attitude [ˈætitjuːd] *n* 姿势;态度,意向 | ~ of combat 格斗姿势(在战场上焚烧至死的尸体呈僵直防守姿势) / crucifixion ~ 十字架姿势(身体强直,手臂外展成直角,见于癔症性癫痫及紧张症) / deflexion ~ 反屈胎势 / discobolus ~ 掷铁饼姿势(半规管受刺激引起) / forced ~ 强迫姿势(见于脑膜炎患者) / illogical ~s 不自然姿势(见于癔症性癫痫患者) / ~ passionnelle, passionate ~ 戏剧性姿势(见于癔症患者) / stereotyped ~ 刻板姿势(见于精神病者)

atto- [构词成分] 阿[托](百亿亿分之一, $=10^{-18}$)

attractant [əˈtræktənt] *n* 诱引剂,吸引剂(诱捕昆虫或害虫用)

attraction [əˈtrækʃən] *n* 吸引,引力;上升(殆平面接近耳平面) | capillary ~ 毛细管吸引,毛细吸引 / chemical ~, ~ of affinity 化学吸引,亲和性吸引

attraxin [əˈtræksin] *n* 趋向素(存在于溶液中的特异物质,当溶液注入组织内时,即对上皮细胞起着趋化性影响)

attrition [əˈtriʃən] *n* 磨损,磨耗

at vol atomic volume 原子体积

At wt atomic weight 原子量

atypia [eiˈtipiə], **atypism** [eiˈtipizəm] *n* 不典型性

atypical [eiˈtipikəl] *a* 不典型的

AU aures unitas 双耳; auris uterque 每耳

Au aurum【拉】金; Australian antigen 澳大利亚抗原

AUA American Urological Association 美国泌尿学会

Au-antigenemia [ˌæntidʒiˈniːmiə] *n* 澳大利亚抗原血症

Aub-Dubois table [ɔːb dju(ː)ˈbɔiz] (Joseph C. Aub; Eugene F. Dubois) 奥-杜表(一种不同年龄均适用的正常基础代谢率表)

Auberger blood group [əubɛəˈʒei] (Auberger 为1961年首次报道法国先证者的姓)奥伯惹血型(含有红细胞抗原 Au^a 的血型,与 Lutheran 血型有关)

Aubert's phenomenon [auˈbɛət] (Hermann Aubert) 奥伯特现象(一种视错觉,即当头向一侧倾斜时,有一垂直线斜向另一侧)

AUC area under the curve 曲线下面积

Auchmeromyia [ˌɔːkmərəˈmaijə] *n* 燥蝇属 | ~ luteola 黄燥蝇

audible [ˈɔːdəbl] *a* 听得到的,可听的 | **audibility** [ɔːdiˈbiləti] *n* 可听度,可听性

audiclave [ˈɔːdikleiv] *n* 助听器

audile [ˈɔːdail] *a* 听力的,听觉的(尤指听的回忆);听觉型的

audimutitas [ˌɔːdiˈmjuːtitəs] *n* 听哑(不伴耳聋的哑症)

audio [ˈɔːdiəu] *a* 听觉的,声音的;声频的
audi(o)- [构词成分]听,听觉
audioanalgesia [ˌɔːdiəuˌænælˈdʒiːzjə] *n* 听性止痛,音乐止痛(通过立体声的耳机听录音音乐以止痛)
audiogenic [ˌɔːdiəuˈdʒenik] *a* 听源性的,音源性的
audiogram [ˈɔːdiəˌgræm] *n* 听力图 | cortical ~ 皮质听力图
audiology [ˌɔːdiˈɔlədʒi] *n* 听力学(尤指对听力损伤不能用药物或手术矫治的研究) | **audiological** [ˌɔːdiəˈlɔdʒikəl] *a* / **audiologist** *n* 听力学家
audiometer [ˌɔːdiˈɔmitə] *n* 听力计 | evoked response ~ 诱发反应听力计 | **audiometry** [ˌɔːdiˈɔmitri] *n* 测听[法] / **audiometric** [ˌɔːdiəuˈmetrik] *a* 测听的 / **audiometrist** [ˌɔːdiˈɔmitrist], **audiometrician** [ˌɔːdiəumiˈtriʃən] *n* 测听专家
audioscope [ˈaudiəskəup] *n* 听力镜(检测听力损害的仪器,由耳镜和听力计组成)
audiosurgery [ˌɔːdiəuˈsəːdʒəri] *n* 听力外科,听力手术
audiovisual [ˌɔːdiəuˈvizjuəl] *a* 视听的,声光感觉的
audiphone [ˈɔːdifəun] *n* 助听器
audition [ɔːˈdiʃən] *n* 听觉 | chromatic ~, ~ colorée 色听觉,闻声觉色 / gustatory ~ 味听觉,闻声觉味
auditive [ˈɔːditiv] *n* 听型学习者(听觉为主要感觉的人)
auditognosis [ˌɔːditəgˈnəusis] *n* 听觉
auditory [ˈɔːditəri] *a* 听的,听觉的
Audouin's microsporon [auduˈæn] (Jean-Victor Audouin) 奥杜安小孢子菌(引起青春前期秃发癣最常见的原因)
Auenbrugger's sign [auenˈbruːgə] (Leopold E. von Auenbrugger) 奥恩布鲁格征(上腹部膨起,由于大量心包渗液所致)
Auerbach's ganglion [ˈauəbɑːh] (Leopold Auerbach) 奥尔巴赫神经节(肠肌丛内的小神经节) | ~ plexus 肠肌丛
Auer's bodies (rods) [ˈauə] (John Auer) 奥尔小体(棒状体)(具有酸性磷酸酶活性,见于成髓细胞、髓细胞、成单核细胞及粒状组织细胞的胞浆内,浆细胞内则罕见,成淋巴细胞或淋巴细胞内也无,实质上可确诊为白血病的病征)
Aufrecht's sign [ˈaufreʃt] (Emanual Aufrecht) 奥夫雷希特征(气管狭窄时,在颈静脉窝可听到微弱的呼吸音)
augmentation [ˌɔːgmenˈteiʃən] *n* 增大 | bladder ~ 膀胱扩大成形术 / breast ~ 乳房增大成形术
augmentor [ɔːgˈmentə] *a* 增进的,增加的(指神经或神经细胞体积的增大与心脏收缩力的增强) *n* 促进素
augnathus [ɔːgˈneiθəs] *n* 双下颌
Aujeszky's disease [ɔːˈjeski] (Aladár Aujeszky) 假狂犬病
AUL acute undifferentiated leukemia 急性未分化白血病
aula [ˈɔːlə] *n* 红晕(在接种损害周围形成的红斑状红晕)
aura [ˈɔːrə] ([复] **aurae** [ˈɔːriː] 或 **auras**) *n* 先兆 | epileptic ~ 癫痫先兆 / intellectual ~, reminiscent ~ 梦样先兆(癫痫发作前) / ~ procursiva 向前奔走性先兆
aural[1] [ˈɔːrəl] *a* 听的,听觉的;耳的
aural[2] [ˈɔːrəl] *a* 先兆的
auramine O [ˈɔːrəmiːn] 金胺 O,碱性槐黄
auranofin [ɔːˈreinəfin] *n* 金诺芬(抗风湿病药)
aurantia [ɔːˈrænʃiə] *n* 金橙黄(用于线粒体染色)
aurantiamarin [ɔːˌræntiˈæmərin] *n* 橙皮苷
aurantiasis [ˌɔːrænˈtaiəsis] *n* 皮肤橙色病,胡萝卜素血症
Aurelia [ɔːˈreliə] *n* 海月水母属
Aureobasidium [ɔːˌriəbəˈsidiəm] *n* 短柄霉属,金担子菌属 | ~ pullulans 出芽短柄霉,出芽金担子菌
aureolin [ɔːˈriəlin] *n* 钴黄(钴亚硝酸钾)
aures [ˈɔːriːz] auris 的复数
auri- [构词成分]耳
auriasis [ɔːˈraiəsis] *n* 金质沉着症
auric [ˈɔːrik] *a* 金的,含金的 | ~ acid 金酸
auricle [ˈɔːrikl] *n* 耳郭;心耳(本词曾用来表示心房) | cervical ~ 颈部耳状附件(偶见于颈侧残存的鳃裂外口处) / left ~ of heart 左心耳 / right ~ of heart 右心耳
auricula [ɔːˈrikjulə, əˈrikjulə] ([复] **auriculae** [ɔːˈrikjuliː] *n*【拉】耳郭;心耳(本词曾用作"心房"的同义词)
auricular [ɔːˈrikjulə] *a* 耳的,耳郭的;心耳的(曾用作"心房的")
auriculare [ɔːˌrikjuˈlɛəri] *n* 耳道点(在外耳道口顶)
auricularis [ˌɔːrikjuˈlɛəris] *a*【拉】耳的;心耳的
auriculate [ɔːˈrikjulit] *a* 耳形的,有耳的
auriculocranial [ɔːˌrikjuləuˈkreinjəl] *a* 耳颅[部]的
auriculotemporal [ɔːˌrikjuləuˈtempərəl] *a* 耳颞[部]的
auriculotherapy [ɔːˌrikjuləuˈθerəpi] *n* 耳疗法
auriculoventricular [ɔːˌrikjuləuvenˈtrikjulə] *a* 房室的
aurid [ˈɔːrid] *n* 金剂疹(由于用金盐而产生的一种皮疹)

auriferous [ɔːˈrifərəs] *a* 含金的;产金的
auriform [ˈɔːrifɔːm] *a* 耳形的,耳状的
aurilave [ˈɔːrileiv] *n* 洗耳器,耳冲洗器
aurin [ˈɔːrin] *n* 蔷薇色酸,玫红酸
aurinarium [ˌɔːriˈnɛəriəm] *n* 耳杆剂,外耳道栓剂(用以插入外耳道)
aurinasal [ˌɔːriˈneizəl] *a* 耳鼻的
auriphone [ˈɔːrifəun] *n* 助听喇叭,助听筒
auripigment [ˌɔːriˈpigmənt] *n* 雌黄,三硫化二砷
auripuncture [ˈɔːriˌpʌŋktʃə] *n* 鼓膜穿刺术
auris [ˈɔːris] ([复] **aures** [ˈɔːriːz]) *n*【拉】耳
auriscalpium [ˌɔːriˈskælpiəm] *n* 耳匙(用以刮除耳内异物)
auriscope [ˈɔːriskəup] *n* 耳镜
aurist [ˈɔːrist] *n* 耳科医生,耳科学家
auristics [ɔːˈristiks] *n* 耳科学,治耳术
auristilla [ˌɔːrisˈtilə] ([复] **auristillae** [ˌɔːrisˈtiliː]) *n*【拉】滴耳药
aurochromoderma [ˌɔːrəˌkrəuməˈdəːmə] *n* 金剂性皮肤变色
aurogauge [ˈɔːrəgeidʒ] *n* 听力计检定器,助听效应鉴定器
aurometer [ɔːˈrɔmitə] *n* 听力计
aurotherapy [ˌɔːrəuˈθerəpi] *n* 金疗法
aurothioglucose [ˌɔːrəuˌθaiəˈgluːkəus] *n* 金硫葡糖(消炎镇痛药,治疗类风湿关节炎)
aurothioglycanide [ˌɔːrəuˌθaiəˈglaikənaid], **aurothioglycolanilide** [ˌɔːrəuˌθaiəˌglaikəˈlænilaid] *n* 金硫醋苯胺(消炎镇痛药,治疗类风湿关节炎)
aurothiomalate disodium [ˌɔːrəuˌθaiəˈmeileit] 金硫丁二钠(消炎镇痛药)
aurum [ˈɔːrəm] *n*【拉】金
auscultate [ˈɔːskəlteit], **auscult** [ɔːsˈkʌlt] *vt, vi* 听诊 | **auscultator** [ˌɔːskəlˈteitə] *n* 听诊者;听诊器 / **auscultatory** [ɔːsˈkʌltətəri] *a* 听诊的
auscultation [ˌɔːskəlˈteiʃən] *n* 听诊[法] | direct ~, immediate ~ 直接听诊 / mediate ~ 间接听诊 / obstetric ~ 产科听诊
auscultoplectrum [ɔːsˌkʌltəuˈplektrəm] *n* 叩听诊器
auscultoscope [ɔːsˈkʌltəskəup] *n* 扩音听诊器
Auspitz sign [ˈauspitz] (Heinrich Auspitz)奥斯皮茨征(银屑病的一种征象,刮去鳞屑后出现点状出血)
Austin Flint murmur [ˈɔstin flint] (Austin Flint) 奥斯汀·弗林特杂音(主动脉瓣反流时心尖部的收缩期前杂音) | ~ respiration 空洞呼吸音
Austin Moore arthroplasty [ˈɔstinmuə] (Austin T. Moore) 奥斯丁·穆尔关节成形术(使用奥斯丁·穆尔人工髋关节,施行髋关节重建手术) | ~ prosthesis 奥斯丁·穆尔人工髋关节(一种金属植入物,用于髋关节成形术)
Australorbis [ˌɔːstrəˈlɔːbis] *n* 澳卷螺属(即 Biomphalaria)
aut- 见 auto-
autacoid [ˈɔːtəkɔid] *n* 自身活性物质(即局部激素,指各种具有生理活性的内源性物质,如组胺、血清素、血管紧张素、前列素等的总称)
autarcesiology [ˌɔːtɑːˌsiːsiˈɔlədʒi] *n* 天然免疫学
autarcesis [ɔːˈtɑːsisis] *n* 天然免疫性(有别于抗体型的免疫性) | **autarcetic** [ɔːtɑːˈsetik] *a*
autechoscope [ɔːˈtekəskəup] *n* 自检听诊器
autecic [ɔːˈtiːsik], **autecious** [ɔːˈtiːʃəs] *a* 同种寄生的,终生寄生的
autecology [ˌɔːtiˈkɔlədʒi] *n* 个体生态学
autemesia [ˌɔːtiˈmiːziə] *n* 功能性呕吐,自[发性呕]吐
autism [ˈɔːtizəm] *n* 自闭症,孤独症;孤独性,内向性,自我中心 | akinetic ~ 睁眼昏迷 / infantile ~ 婴儿孤独症
autistic [ɔːˈtistik] *a* 孤独的,内向的,我向的
aut(o)- [前缀]自己,自体,自动,自发
autoactivation [ˌɔːtəuˌæktiˈveiʃən] *n* 自体活化(腺体分泌)
autoagglutination [ˌɔːtəuəˌgluːtiˈneiʃən] *n* 自身凝集
autoagglutinin [ˌɔːtəuəˈgluːtinin] *n* 自体凝集素,自身凝集素
autoallergy [ˌɔːtəuˈælədʒi] *n* 自体变应性,自体变态反应,自身变态反应 | **autoallergic** [ˌɔːtəuəˈləːdʒik] *a*
autoamputation [ɔːtəuˌæmpjuˈteiʃən] *n* 自[行]断离(如息肉)
autoanalysis [ˌɔːtəuəˈnæləsis] *n* 自我分析
autoanamnesis [ˌɔːtəuˌænæmˈniːsis] *n* 自诉病史
autoantibody [ˌɔːtəuˈæntiˌbɔdi] *n* 自身抗体
autoanticomplement [ˌɔːtəuˌæntiˈkɔmplimənt] *n* 自身抗补体
autoantigen [ˌɔːtəuˈæntidʒən] *n* 自身抗原
autoantisepsis [ˌɔːtəuˌæntiˈsepsis] *n* 自体灭菌,生理性抗菌
autoantitoxin [ˌɔːtəuˌæntiˈtɔksin] *n* 自体抗毒素,自身抗毒素
autoaudible [ˌɔːtəuˈɔːdəbl] *a* 可自听的(指心音)
autobacteriophage [ˌɔːtəubækˈtiəriəfeidʒ] *n* 自体噬菌体
autobiography [ˌɔːtəubaiˈɔgrəfi] *n* 自传
autobiotic [ˌɔːtəubaiˈɔtik] *n* 自生素,自生质(指由细胞产生并控制产生细胞行为的物质)
autoblast [ˈɔːtəblæst] *n* 原生子,微生物
autobody [ˈɔːtəuˌbɔdi] *n* 自体(抗体的一种)
autocatalysis [ˌɔːtəukəˈtælisis] *n* 自动催化,自身

催化 | **autocatalytic** [ˌɔːtəukætəˈlitik] *a*

autocatalyst [ˌɔːtəuˈkætəlist] *n* 自动催化剂,自身催化剂

autocatharsis [ˌɔːtəukəˈθɑːsis] *n* 自我疏泄(精神病疗法,鼓励患者写出自己的病情,从而消除他的精神情绪)

autocatheterism [ˌɔːtəuˈkæθitərizəm] *n* 自插导管[法]

autocerebrospinal [ˌɔːtəuˌseribrəuˈspain] *a* 自体脑脊液的(用于治疗流行性脑膜炎)

autocholecystectomy [ˌɔːtəuˌkəulisisˈtektəmi] *n* 胆囊自切除(胆囊套叠入肠道内,最后分离而排出)

autochthon [ɔːˈtɔkθən] ([复] **autochthons** 或 **autochthones** [ɔːˈtɔkθəniːz] *n* 土著;土生土长的动植物 | **~ous**, **~al** *a* 土著的;(动植物)土生的;本处发生的(未转移到新部位的);自身的(指移至同一个体新部位的组织移植物)

autocinesis [ˌɔːtəusaiˈniːsis] *n* 自体动作,随意运动

autoclasia [ˌɔːtəuˈkleiziə] *n* 自体破坏,自身破坏

autoclasis [ɔːˈtɔkləsis] *n* 自破,自裂

autoclave [ˈɔːtəkleiv] *n* 高压灭菌器

autocoid [ˈɔːtəkɔid] *n* 自体有效物质,局部激素(见 autacoid)

autoconduction [ˌɔːtəukənˈdʌkʃən] *n* 自体导电法

autocrine [ˈɔːtəukrin] *n* 自分泌

autocystoplasty [ˌɔːtəuˈsistəˌplæsti] *n* 自体移植膀胱成形术

autocytolysin [ˌɔːtəusaiˈtɔlisin] *n* 自身细胞溶素,自溶素

autocytolysis [ˌɔːtəusaiˈtɔlisis] *n* 自体溶解,自溶 | **autocytolytic** [ˌɔːtəuˌsaitəuˈlitik] *a*

autocytotoxin [ɔːtəuˌsaitəuˈtɔksin] *n* 自体细胞毒素,自身细胞毒素

autodermic [ˌɔːtəuˈdəːmik] *a* 自皮的,自体皮肤的(指皮移植)

autodestruction [ˌɔːtəudisˈtrʌkʃən] *n* 自体破坏[作用],自身破坏[作用](尤指某些酶在溶液中所起的变化)

autodigestion [ˌɔːtəudiˈdʒestʃən, -dai-] *n* 自体消化,自身消化,自身溶解(尤指死后胃壁及附近组织的被消化)

autodiploid [ˌɔːtəuˈdiplɔid] *a* 同源二倍体的 *n* 同源二倍体(指一个体或细胞具有两套染色体) | **~y** *n* 同源二倍性

autodrainage [ˌɔːtəuˈdreinidʒ] *n* 自体导液法

autodyne [ˈɔːtədain] *n* 甘油苯醚(有镇痛作用)

autoecholalia [ˌɔːtəuˌekəˈleiliə] *n* 重复自语,自我重复言语

autoecic [ɔːˈtiːsik], **autoecious** [əˈtiːʃəs] *a* 同种寄生的,终生寄生的

autoeczematization [ˌɔːtəuekˌzemətaiˈzeiʃən, -tiˈz-] *n* 自体湿疹化

autoeroticism [ˌɔːtəueˈrɔtisizəm], **autoerotism** [ˌɔːtəuˈerətizəm] *n* 自体性欲 | **autoerotic** [ˌɔːtəuiˈrɔtik] *a*

autoerythrophagocytosis [ˌɔːtəuiˌriθrəuˌfægəsaiˈtəusis] *n* 自体红细胞吞噬[作用]

autofluorescence [ˌɔːtəufluəˈresns] *n* 自身荧光,自发荧光(指组织内的荧光)

autofluoroscope [ˌɔːtəuˈfluərəskəup] *n* 自身荧光镜(一种闪烁照相机,其探测器内装有碘化钠晶体,尤其适用于研究大器官的小肿瘤)

autofundoscope [ˌɔːtəuˈfʌndəskəup] *n* 自检眼底镜 | **autofundoscopy** [ˌɔːtəufʌnˈdɔskəpi] *n* 自检眼底镜检查

autogamy [ɔːˈtɔgəmi] *n* 自体受精 | **autogamous** [ɔːˈtɔgəməs] *a*

autogenesis [ˌɔːtəuˈdʒenisis] *n* 自然发生 | **autogenetic** [ˌɔːtəudʒiˈnetik] *a*

autogenous [ɔːˈtɔːdʒinəs], **autogeneic** [ˌɔːtəudʒiˈneiik] *a* 自体的,自身的

autognostic [ˌɔːtɔgˈnɔstik] *a* 自[己]诊[断]的(用于精神分析方法)

autograft [ˈɔːtəgrɑːft, -græft] *n* 自体移植物,自身移植物 *vt*, *vi* 自体移植

autografting [ˈɔːtəgrɑːftiŋ, -græf-] *n* 自体移植术,自身移植术

autogram [ˈɔːtəgræm] *n* 压印(用钝器压迫皮肤形成的痕迹)

autohemagglutination [ˌɔːtəuˌhiːməˌgluːtiˈneiʃən] *n* 自体血细胞凝集作用,自身血凝反应

autohemagglutinin [ˌɔːtəuhiːməˈgluːtinin] *n* 自体血细胞凝集素,自身血凝素

autohemic [ˌɔːtəuˈhiːmik] *a* 自体血液的,自身血液的

autohemolysin [ˌɔːtəuˌhiːməˈlaisin, -hiːˈmɔli-] *n* 自体溶血素,自溶血素

autohemolysis [ˌɔːtəuhiːˈmɔləsis] *n* 自血溶解,自身溶血 | **autohemolytic** [ˌɔːtəuˌhiːməˈlitik] *a*

autohemopsonin [ˌɔːtəuˌhemɔpˈsəunin] *n* 自体血细胞调理素,自身血细胞调理素

autohemotherapy [ˌɔːtəuˌhiːməuˈθerəpi] *n* 自血疗法,自体血液疗法

autohemotransfusion [ˌɔːtəuˌhiːməutrænsˈfjuːʒən] *n* 自体输血

autohistoradiograph [ˌɔːtəuˌhistəˈreidiəugrɑːf, -græf] *n* 自体[组织]放射[照]片,放射自显影[照]片

autohormonoclasis [ˌɔːtəuˌhɔːməuˈnɔkləsis] *n* 自体激素破坏

autohypnosis [ˌɔːtəuhipˈnəusis] *n* 自我催眠 | **autohypnotic** [ˌɔːtəuhipˈnɔtik] *a*

autoimmune [ˌɔːtəuiˈmjuːn] *a* 自身免疫的 | **autoimmunity** [ˌɔːtəuiˈmjuːnəti] *n*

autoimmunization [ˌɔːtəuˌimju(ː)naiˈzeiʃən, niˈz-] *n* 自身免疫作用(亦称自身致敏)

autoinfection [ˌɔːtəuinˈfekʃən] *n* 自体感染,自身感染

autoinfusion [ˌɔːtəuinˈfjuːʒən] *n* 自体聚血,自血输注

autoinoculable [ˌɔːtəuiˈnɔkjuləbl] *a* 能自体接种的

autoinoculation [ˌɔːtəuiˌnɔkjuˈleiʃən] *n* 自身接种

autointerference [ˌɔːtəuˌintəˈfiərəns] *n* 自体干扰,自身干扰(用完整的、减毒的或灭活的病毒对同种病毒的复制进行干扰)

autointoxicant [ˌɔːtəuinˈtɔksikənt] *n* 自体毒物

autointoxication [ˌɔːtəuinˌtɔksiˈkeiʃən] *n* 自体中毒,自身中毒 | intestinal ~ 肠性自体中毒,食物性毒血症

autoisolysin [ˌɔːtəuaiˈsɔlisin] *n* 自体同种溶素,自身同族溶素

autokeratoplasty [ˌɔːtəuˈkerətəuˌplæsti] *n* 自体角膜移植术

autokinesis [ˌɔːtəukaiˈniːsis, -kiˈn-] *n* 自体动作,随意运动 | visible light ~ 可视光自体动作 | **autokinetic** [ˌɔːtəukaiˈnetik, -kiˈn-] *a*

autolaryngoscopy [ˌɔːtəuˌlærinˈgɔskəpi] *n* 自检喉镜检查

autolavage [ˌɔːtəuləˈvɑːʒ] *n* 自[己]灌洗胃

autolesion [ˈɔːtəˌliːʒən] *n* 自伤

autoleukoagglutinin [ˌɔːtəuˌljuːkəuəˈgluːtinin] *n* 自体白细胞凝集素

autoleukocytotherapy [ˌɔːtəuˌljuːkəˌsaitəuˈθerəpi] *n* 自体白细胞疗法

autologous [ɔːˈtɔləgəs] *a* 自体固有的,正型结构的;自体的,自身的

autology [ɔːˈtɔlədʒi] *n* 自体论,自身论

autolysate [ɔːˈtɔliseit] *n* 自溶产物(癌组织的自溶产物用于皮下注射以治癌)

autolysin [ɔːˈtɔlisin] *n* 自溶素

autolysis [ɔːˈtɔlisis] *n* 自溶[作用] | postmortem ~ 死后自溶 | **autolytic** [ˌɔːtəˈlitik] *a* 自溶的

autolysosome [ˌɔːtəˈlaisəsəum] *n* 自体溶酶体(细胞溶酶体系统的一种空泡成分,溶酶体融合时水解酶加入其中)

autolyze [ˈɔːtəlaiz] *vt* 使自溶

automatic [ˌɔːtəˈmætik] *a* 自动的;自行运动的,自行调节的

automaticity [ˌɔːtəməˈtisəti] *n* 自动性,自动作用 | triggered ~ 触发自动作用

automatin [ɔːˈtɔmətin] *n* 心自动素(一种牛心肌浸出物,以前用于治疗循环失调)

automation [ˌɔːtəˈmeiʃən] *n* 自动,自动化

automatism [ɔːˈtɔmətizəm] *n* 自动症;自动性,自动[作用] | ambulatory ~ 觉醒游行症,漫游性自动症 / command ~ 从命自动症(催眠后暗示性自动症)

automatograph [ˌɔːtəuˈmætəgrɑːf, -græf] *n* 自动性运动描记器(描记不随意运动)

automaton [ɔːˈtɔmətən] ([复] **automata** [ɔːˈtɔmətə]或 **automatons**) *n* 自动装置;自动开关;自动症患者

Automeris [ɔːˈtɔməris] *n* 蛾属 | ~io 巨斑刺蛾

automixis [ˌɔːtəˈmiksis] *n* 自体融合

automnesia [ˌɔːtəmˈniːziə] *n* 自发回忆(回忆过去自己的生活情况)

automysophobia [ˌɔːtəuˌmaisəˈfəubiə] *n* 自体不洁恐怖,自秽恐怖

autonarcosis [ˌɔːtəunɑːˈkəusis] *n* 自我麻醉,自我催眠

autonephrectomy [ˌɔːtəuneˈfrektəmi] *n* 自截肾

autonephrotoxin [ˌɔːtəuˌnefrəuˈtɔksin] *n* 自体肾毒素

autonomic [ɔːtəuˈnɔmik] *a* 自主的,自律的 *n* 自主神经系统药

autonomotropic [ˌɔːtəunɔməˈtrɔpik] *a* 亲自主神经系统的

autonomy [ɔːˈtɔnəmi] *n* 自主性,自律性 | **autonomous** [ɔːˈtɔnəməs] *a* 自主的,自律的

auto-ophthalmoscope [ˌɔːtəu ɔfˈθælməskəup] *n* 自检眼镜 | **auto-ophthalmoscopy** [ˌɔːtəu ɔfθælˈmɔskəpi] *n* 自检眼镜检查

auto-oxidation [ˌɔːtəu ˌɔksiˈdeiʃən] *n* 自动氧化[作用]

autooxidizable [ˌɔːtəuˌɔksiˈdaizəbl] *a* 能自身氧化的

autopath [ˈɔːtəpəθ] *n* 自发病者,过敏患者(由于自主神经系统过敏而有变应性症状的人)

autopathography [ˌɔːtəpəˈθɔgrəfi] *n* 自病记录

autopathy [ɔːˈtɔpəθi] *n* 自发病

autophagia [ˌɔːtəuˈfeidʒiə] *n* 自食己肉;自体消瘦;自[吞]噬

autophagolysosome [ˌɔːtəuˌfægəuˈlaisəsəum] *n* 自噬溶酶体

autophagosome [ˌɔːtəuˈfægəsəum] *n* 自[吞]噬体

autophagy [ɔːˈtɔfədʒi] *n* 自[吞]噬;自食己肉

autopharmacologic [ˌɔːtəuˌfɑːməkəˈlɔdʒik] *a* 自体药理学的

autopharmacology [ˌɔːtəuˌfɑːməˈkɔlədʒi] *n* 自体药理学(利用身体组织的天然成分对身体功能作化学性的调节)

autophil [ˈɔːtəfil] *n* 自主神经过敏者
autophilia [ˌɔːtəuˈfiliə] *n* 利己狂,自尊癖;自恋
autophobia [ˌɔːtəuˈfəubiə] *n* 孤独恐怖,恐独症
autophonometry [ˌɔːtəufəuˈnɔmitri] *n* 音叉振动自感测验法
autophony [ɔːˈtɔfəni] *n* 自听增强
autophthalmoscope [ˌɔːtɔfˈθælməskəup] *n* 自检眼镜
autophyte [ˈɔːtəfait] *n* 自养植物
autoplasmotherapy [ˌɔːtəuˌplæzməuˈθerəpi] *n* 自体血浆疗法
autoplast [ˈɔːtəplæst] *n* 自体移植物,自身移植物
autoplasty [ˈɔːtəˌplæsti] *n* 自体移植术,自体成形术;自我变更性适应(精神分析名词) | peritoneal ~ 腹膜自体成形术,腹膜被覆术 | **autoplastic** [ˌɔːtəˈplæstik] *a*
autoploid [ˈɔːtəplɔid] *a* 同源体的 *n* 同源体(见 autopolyploid) | **~y** *n* 同源性
autopodium [ˌɔːtəuˈpəudiəm] *n* 端骨(胚胎期的手和足)
autopoisonous [ˌɔːtəuˈpɔiznəs] *a* 自体中毒性的
autopolymer [ˌɔːtəuˈpɔlimə] *n* 自动聚合物,自聚物
autopolymerization [ˌɔːtəuˌpɔliˌməraiˈzeiʃən, -riˈz-] *n* 自动聚合[作用]
autopolyploid [ˌɔːtəuˈpɔliplɔid] *a* 同源多倍体的 *n* 同源多倍体(指一个体或细胞具有两套以上的染色体,由于单倍体倍加而形成) | ~y *n* 同源多倍性
autoprecipitin [ˌɔːtəupriˈsipitin] *n* 自体沉淀素,自身沉淀素(具有沉淀素特点的自身抗体)
autoprotection [ˌɔːtəuprəˈtekʃən] *n* 自体防御[作用],自身保护(例如由于自身抗毒素形成,保护身体不易致病)
autoproteolysis [ˌɔːtəuˌprəutiˈɔlisis] *n* 自体溶解,自身溶解,自溶
autoprothrombin [ˌɔːtəuprəˈθrɔmbin] *n* 自体凝血酶原 | ~Ⅰ,自体凝血酶原Ⅰ,因子Ⅶ / ~Ⅱ 自体凝血酶原Ⅱ,因子Ⅸ / ~ C 自体凝血酶原 C,因子Ⅹ
autoprotolysis [ˌɔːtəuprəˈtɔlisis] *n* 质子自递[作用]
autopsy [ˈɔːtəpsi], **autopsia** [ɔːˈtɔpsiə] *n* 尸体解剖,尸[体剖]检
autopsychic [ˌɔːtəuˈsaikik] *a* 自我意识的,自觉的
autopsychorhythmia [ˌɔːtəusaikəuˈriθmiə] *n* 脑律动(脑的病理性节律性活动)
autopsychotherapy [ˌɔːtəuˌsaikəuˈθerəpi] *n* 自我精神治疗,自我心理治疗
autoradiograph [ˌɔːtəuˈreidiəugrɑːf, -græf], **autoradiogram** [ˌɔːtəuˈreidiəugræm] *n* 放射自显影[照]片 | **autoradiographic** [ˌɔːtəuˌreidiəuˈgræfik] *a* 放射自显影的 / **autoradiography** [ˌɔːtəuˌreidiˈɔgrəfi] *n* 放射自显影[术](已广泛应用于研究以氚标记的前体〈如胸腺嘧啶〉在细胞中 DNA 的合成和定位)
autoreactive [ˌɔːtəuri(ː)ˈæktiv] *a* 自身反应的,自体反应的
autoregulate [ˌɔːtəuˈregjuleit] *vt* 自动调节,自身调节 | **autoregulation** [ˌɔːtəuˌregjuˈleiʃən] *n*
autoreinfusion [ˌɔːtəuˌriːinˈfjuːʒən] *n* 自体输血,自体再注入
autosensitization [ˌɔːtəuˌsensitaiˈzeiʃən, -tiˈz-] 自身致敏 | erythrocyte ~ 红细胞自身致敏[作用]
autosensitized [ˌɔːtəuˈsensitaizd] *a* 自身致敏的
autosepticemia [ˌɔːtəuˌseptiˈsiːmiə] *n* 自体败血病
autoserodiagnosis [ˌɔːtəuˌsiərədaiəgˈnəusis] *n* 自体血清诊断[法]
autoserosalvarsan [ˌɔːtəusiərəˈsælvɑːsən] *n* 自体血清胂凡纳明(治疗)
autoserum [ˌɔːtəuˈsiərəm] *n* 自体血清,自身血清 | **autoserous** [ˌɔːtəuˈsiərəs] *a*
autosexing [ˌɔːtəuˈseksiŋ] *n* 性别自体鉴别,性别自动鉴定(鸟类遗传学中,有意识地培育早期出现的伴性表型以鉴别小鸡的性别)
autosite [ˌɔːtəsait] *n* 联胎自养体 | **autositic** [ˌɔːtəuˈsitik] *a*
autosmia [ɔːˈtɔsmiə] *n* 自嗅,自辨体臭
autosomatognosis [ˌɔːtəuˌsəumətɔgˈnəusis] *n* 断肢存在幻觉 | **autosomatognostic** [ˌɔːtəuˌsəumətɔgˈnɔstik] *a*
autosome [ˈɔːtəusəum] *n* 常染色体;自[吞]噬体 | **autosomal** [ˌɔːtəuˈsəuməl] *a*
autospermotoxin [ˌɔːtəuˌspəːməˈtɔksin] *n* 自体精子毒素,自身精子毒素(能使动物自身精子凝集的物质)
autosplenectomy [ˌɔːtəuspliˈnektəmi] *n* 脾[脏]自切除(由于进行性纤维化和皱缩而使脾脏几乎完全消失,如见于镰状细胞性贫血)
autospray [ˈɔːtəsprei] *n* 自用喷雾器,自身喷雾器(患者自用)
autosterilization [ˌɔːtəuˌsterilaiˈzeiʃən, liˈz-] *n* 自体灭菌(设想某些病毒,例如脊髓灰质炎病毒,短时间后有从组织内消失的倾向,已发现这种想法是错误的)
autostimulation [ˌɔːtəuˌstimjuˈleiʃən] *n* 自体刺激,自身刺激(动物自身组织产生的抗原性物质所起的刺激)
autosuggestibility [ˌɔːtəusəˌdʒestiˈbiləti] *n* 自我暗示性
autosuggestion [ˌɔːtəusəˈdʒestʃən] *n* 自我暗示
autosynthesis [ˌɔːtəuˈsinθisis] *n* 自己生殖

autotemnous [ˌɔːtəuˈtemnəs] *a* 自切的,自分的
autotherapy [ˌɔːtəuˈθerəpi] *n* 自愈;自疗;自体液疗法
autothromboagglutinin [ˌɔːtəuˌθrɔmbəuəˈgluːtinin] *n* 血小板自[身]凝[集]素(一种血小板自身凝集素)
autotomography [ˌɔːtəutəˈmɔgrəfi] *n* 体动X线体层摄影[术],X线自家体层摄影[术](病人身体移动,X线管不动) | **autotomographic** [ˌɔːtəuˌtɔməˈgræfik] *a*
autotomy [ɔːˈtɔtəmi] *n* 自身分裂;自断,自切(如有些无脊椎动物的附器自行脱落) | **autotomic** [ɔːtəuˈtɔmik] *a*
autotopagnosia [ˌɔːtəuˌtɔpægˈnəusiə] *n* 自身部位失认[症]
autotoxicosis [ˌɔːtəuˌtɔksiˈkəusis], **autotoxemia** [ˌɔːtəutɔkˈsiːmiə], **autotoxis** [ˌɔːtəuˈtɔksis] *n* 自体中毒 | **autotoxic** [ˌɔːtəuˈtɔksik] *a*
autotoxin [ˌɔːtəuˈtɔksin] *n* 自体毒素,自身毒素
autotransfusion [ˌɔːtəutrænsˈfuːʒən] *n* 自身输血 | intraoperative ~ 术中自身输血 / postoperative ~ 术后自身输血
autotransplant [ˌɔːtəutrænsˈplɑːnt, -ˈplænt] *n* 自体移植物 *vt* 自体移植
autotransplantation [ˌɔːtəuˌtrænsplɑːnˈteiʃən, -plæn-] *n* 自体移植
autotrepanation [ˌɔːtəuˌtrepəˈneiʃən] *n* 颅侵蚀(脑瘤所致)
autotroph [ˈɔːtətrɔf, -trəuf] *n* 自养生物 | facultative ~ 兼性自养菌 / obligate ~ 专性自养菌 | **~ic** [ˌɔːtəuˈtrɔfik] *a* 自养的 / **~y** [ɔːˈtɔtrəfi] *n* 自养
autotuberculin [ˌɔːtəutju(ː)ˈbəːkjulin] *n* 自体结核菌素,自身结核菌素
autotuberculinization [ˌɔːtəutju(ː)ˌbəːkjulinaiˈzeiʃən, niˈz-] *n* 自体结核菌素反应,自身结核菌素化过程(患者从自身病灶吸收结核菌素或类似产物)
autovaccination [ˌɔːtəuˌvæksiˈneiʃən], **autovaccinotherapy** [ˌɔːtəuˌvæksinəuˈθerəpi] *n* 自体疫苗接种疗法;自体接种
autovaccine [ˌɔːtəuˈvæksiːn] *n* 自身疫苗
autovaccinia [ˌɔːtəuvækˈsiniə] *n* 自体种痘(在种痘最初部位以外的地方出现的一种痘苗反应,系因搔抓致使痘苗病毒转移之故)
autoxemia [ˌɔːtɔkˈsiːmiə] *n* 自体中毒
autoxidation [ˌɔːtɔksiˈdeiʃən] *n* 自动氧化[作用]
autoxidizable [ɔːˌtɔksiˈdaizəbl] *a* 可自动氧化的
autozygous [ˌɔːtəuˈzaigəs] *a* 自系纯合的
auxanogram [ɔːkˈsænəgræm] *n* 生长谱(生长谱法中的平板培养物)
auxanography [ˌɔːksæˈnɔgrəfi] *n* 生长谱法,生长谱测定[法](微生物营养要求的一种快速测定方法) | **auxanographic** [ˌɔːksænəuˈgræfik] *a* 生长谱的
auxesis [ɔːkˈsiːsis] *n* 增大,发育;细胞增大性生长(细胞体积增大,但细胞数量并未增加) | **auxetic** [ɔːkˈsetik] *a* 增大的,发育的 *n* 发育剂,促生长剂
auxiliary [ɔːgˈziljəri, ˌɔːkˈsiliəri] *a* 辅助的 *n* 辅助物 | torquing ~ 扭转辅助线(正牙治疗用的一种辅助弓镍)
auxiliomotor [ɔːkˌsiliəuˈməutə] *a* 辅助运动的,促进运动的
auxilytic [ɔːksiˈlitik] *a* 促溶解的
auximone [ˈɔːksiməun] *n* 苗长激素(一种假想的物质,类似维生素,促植物生长)
auxin [ˈɔːksin] *n* 苗长素 | ~ B 苗长素B,吲哚乙酸 | **~ic** [ɔːkˈsinik] *a*
auxiometer [ˌɔːksiˈɔmitə] *n* 透镜放大率计;测力计
aux(o)- [构词成分]发育;促进,增加,加速
auxoaction [ˌɔːksəuˈækʃən] *n* 促进作用
auxoamylase [ˌɔːksəuˈæmileis] *n* 促淀粉酶
auxochrome [ˈɔːksəkrəum] *n* 助色团(一种化学团,如引入一个色原,将使后者变成染料) | **auxochromous** [ˌɔːksəˈkrəuməs] *a* 助色的
auxocyte [ˈɔːksəsait] *n* 性母细胞(发育初期的卵母细胞、精母细胞或孢子母细胞)
auxodrome [ˈɔːksədrəum] *n* 生长曲线
auxoflore [ˈɔːksəflɔː], **auxoflur** [ˈɔːksəflə] *n* 助荧光物
auxogluc [ˈɔːksəgluk] *n* 致甜基,助甜团(一种无味原子,生甜团与之结合形成有甜味的化合物)
auxohormone [ˌɔːksəuˈhɔːməun] *n* 生长激素(一种维生素)
auxometer [ɔːkˈsɔmitə] *n* 透镜放大率计
auxometry [ɔːkˈsɔmitri] *n* 生长率测量[法] | **auxometric** [ˌɔːksəˈmetrik] *a*
auxoneurotropic [ˌɔːksəuˌnjuərəuˈtrɔpik] *n* 促进向神经性的
auxospireme [ˌɔːksəuˈspaiəriːm] *n* 联会染色丝纽(生长周期中性母细胞的染色质纽)
auxotherapy [ˌɔːksəuˈθerəpi] *n* 代替疗法,置换疗法(如用激素疗法或脏器置换)
auxotonic [ˌɔːksəuˈtɔnik] *a* 增加紧张的
auxotox [ˈɔːksətɔks] *n* 成毒基
auxotroph [ˈɔːksətrɔf] *n* 营养缺陷体,营养缺陷型 | **~ic** [ˌɔːksəˈtrɔfik] *a* 营养缺陷的
auxotype [ˈɔːksətaip] *n* 生长型,营养型
AV, A-V atrioventricular 房室的;arteriovenous 动静脉的
av avoirdupois 常衡

availability [əˌveiləˈbiləti] *n* 有效度,利用度
avalvular [eiˈvælvjulə] *a* 无瓣的
avantin [ˈævəntin] *n* 异丙醇
avariosis [əˌværiˈəusis] *n* 梅毒
avascular [eiˈvæskjulə] *a* 无血管的
avascularization [eiˌvæskjuləraiˈzeiʃən, riˈz-] *n* 驱血法(缚带驱血法)
AVC atrioventricular canal 房室管
Aveling's repositor [ˈeivliŋ] (James H. Aveling) 艾夫林复位器,子宫复位器
Avellis' syndrome (paralysis) [əˈveliːz] (Georg Avellis) 阿韦利斯综合征(麻痹)(同侧声带和软腭麻痹,对侧腿、躯干、臂、颈以及头皮的痛觉和温觉缺失。亦称疑核脊髓丘脑性麻痹)
Avena [əˈviːnə] *n* 燕麦属
avenin [əˈviːnin] *n* 燕麦蛋白
avenolith [əˈviːnəliθ] *n* 燕麦性肠结石
average [ˈævəridʒ] *n* 平均;平均数 *a* 平均的 *vt* 从…得出平均数;平均为 | pure tone ~ 纯音听阈均值
averaging [ˈævəridʒiŋ] *n* 平均技术,叠加技术 | signal ~ 信号平均技术(使噪声干扰周期性信号减少到最低程度的方法)
avermectin [ˌævəːˈmektin] *n* 除虫菌素(用于抗家畜寄生虫药)
aversion [əˈvəːʃən] *n* 厌恶,反感
aversive [əˈvəːsiv] *a* 厌恶的
Aviadenovirus [ˌeiviˌædenəuˈvaiərəs] *n* 禽腺病毒属
avian [ˈeiviən] *a* 鸟的,禽的
Avibirnavirus [ˌeiviˈbəːnəˌvaiərəs] *n* 禽双节RNA病毒属
avidin [ˈævidin] *n* 抗生物素蛋白(卵白蛋白内一种特殊蛋白,与生物素相互作用时,使生物素无法为动物利用,从而产生生物素缺乏综合征)
avidity [əˈvidəti] *n* 亲和力,抗体亲抗原性;贪婪癖
avifauna [ˌeiviˈfɔːnə] *n* (某一地区的)鸟类
Avihepadnavirus [ˌeivihepˈædnəˌvaiərəs] *n* 禽肝DNA病毒属
Avipoxvirus [ˈeiviˌpɔksvaiərəs] *n* 禽痘病毒属
avipoxvirus [ˈeiviˌpɔksvaiərəs] *n* 禽痘病毒
avirulence [eiˈvirjuləns] *n* 无毒力,毒力缺乏,致病力缺乏(不产生病理效应) | **avirulent** *a*
avitaminosis [eiˌvaitəmiˈnəusis] *n* 维生素缺乏,营养缺乏[症] | **avitaminotic** [eiˌvaitəmiˈnɔtik] *a*
avivement [ɑːviːvˈmɔŋ] *n* 【法】再新术(用手术使伤口边缘复新)
AVMA American Veterinary Medical Association 美国兽医协会
AVN atrioventricular node 房室结
avobenzone [ˌævəˈbenzəun] *n* 阿伏苯宗(防晒药)
Avogadro's law [ævəˈgædrəu] (Amadeo Avogadro) 阿伏伽德罗定律(等体积的一切气体,在同温同压下,含有同数的分子) | ~ number (constant) 阿伏伽德罗数(常数)(数值为 $6.022\,46 \times 10^{23}$)
avogram [ˈævəgræm] *n* 皮皮克(10^{-24}g,即picopicogram)
avoidance [əˈvɔidəns] *n* 避免,回避;无效;回避反应
avoidant [əˈvɔidənt] *a* 回避反应的
avoirdupois [ˌævədəˈpɔiz] *n* 常衡(英国常衡制,以16盎司为1磅)
avoparcin [ævəˈpɑːsin] *n* 阿伏帕星(抗菌药)
AVP arginine vasopressin 精氨酸加压素,精氨酸升压素
AVRT atrioventricular reciprocating tachycardia 房室折返性心动过速
avulsion [əˈvʌlʃən] *n* 撕脱术,抽出术;撕脱伤 | phrenic ~ 膈神经撕脱术
awaken [əˈweikən] *vt* 唤醒
awareness [əˈwεənis] *n* 意识,觉知 | ~ of defecation 便意
awu atomic weight unit 原子量单位
ax. axis 轴
axanthopsia [ˌæksənˈθɔpsiə] *n* 黄色盲
Axenfeld's anomaly, syndrome [ˈæksənfelt] (Theodor Axenfeld) 阿克森费尔德异常综合征(一种明显的遗传性综合征,包括后青年角膜弓,伴虹膜底粘连于后弹性层环、角形结构和蝶小梁区发育缺陷及常伴有青光眼)
Axenfeld's test [ˈæksənfelt] (David Axenfeld) 阿克森费尔德试验(检尿白蛋白)
axenic [eiˈzenik] *a* 无外来污染的,无菌的,未被污染的(指微生物纯净培养或无菌动物)
axes [ˈæksiːz] axis 的复数
axial [ˈæksiəl] *a* 轴的,中轴的
axiation [ˌæksiˈeiʃən] *n* 轴[心]化
axifugal [ækˈsifjuːgəl] *a* 远心的,离心的
axilemma [ˌæksaiˈlemə] *n* 轴索膜
axilla [ækˈsilə] ([复] **axillae** [ækˈsiliː] 或 **axillas**) *n* 【拉】腋,腋窝 | **~ry** [ˈæksiləri] *a*
axillobifemoral [ækˌsiləubaiˈfemərəl] *a* 腋双股动脉的
axillofemoral [ækˌsiləuˈfemərəl] *a* 腋股动脉的
axillopopliteal [ækˌsiləupɔpˈlitiəl] *a* 腋腘动脉的
axi(o)- [构词成分] 轴
axiobuccal [ˌæksiəuˈbʌkəl] *a* 轴颊的
axiobuccocervical [ˌæksiəuˌbʌkəuˈsəːvikəl] *a* 轴颊颈的

axiobuccogingival [ˌæksiəuˌbʌkəu'dʒindʒivəl] *a* 轴颊龈的

axiobuccolingual [ˌæksiəuˌbʌkəu'liŋgwəl] *a* 轴颈舌的

axiocervical [ˌæksiəu'səːvikəl] *a* 轴颈的

axiodistal [ˌæksiəu'distl] *a* 轴远中的

axiodistocervical [ˌæksiəuˌdistəu'səːvikəl] *a* 轴远中颈的

axiodistogingival [ˌæksiəuˌdistəu'dʒindʒivəl] *a* 轴远[中]龈的

axiodistoincisal [ˌæksiəuˌdistəuin'saizəl] *a* 轴远[中]切缘的

axiodisto-occlusal [ˌæksiəuˌdistəu ɔ'kluːzəl] *a* 轴远中殆的

axiogingival [ˌæksiəu'dʒindʒivəl] *a* 轴龈的

axioincisal [ˌæksiəuin'saizəl] *a* 轴切的

axiolabial [ˌæksiəu'leibjəl] *a* 轴唇的

axiolabiogingival [ˌæksiəuˌleibiəu'dʒindʒivəl] *a* 轴唇龈的

axiolabiolingual [ˌæksiəuˌleibiəu'liŋgwəl] *a* 轴唇舌的

axiolingual [ˌæksiəu'liŋgwəl] *a* 轴舌的

axiolinguocervical [ˌæksiəuˌliŋgwəu'səːvikəl] *a* 轴舌颈的

axiolinguogingival [ˌæksiəuˌliŋgwəu'dʒindʒivəl] *a* 轴舌龈的

axiolinguo-occlusal [ˌæksiəuˌliŋgwəuɔ'kluːzəl] *a* 轴舌殆的

axiomesial [ˌæksiəu'miːziəl] *a* 轴近中的

axiomesiocervical [ˌæksiəuˌmiːziəu'səːvikəl] *a* 轴近中颈的

axiomesiodistal [ˌæksiəuˌmiːziəu'distl] *a* 轴近中远侧的

axiomesiogingival [ˌæksiəuˌmiːziəu'dʒindʒivəl] *a* 轴近中龈的

axiomesioincisal [ˌæksiəuˌmiːziəuin'saizəl] *a* 轴近中切的

axiomesio-occlusal [ˌæksiəuˌmiːziəu ɔ'kluːzəl] *a* 轴近中殆的

axio-occlusal [ˌæksiəu ɔ'kluːzəl] *a* 轴殆的

axiopodium [ˌæksiəu'pəudiəm] *n* 轴伪足

axiopulpal [ˌæksiəu'pʌlpl] *a* 轴髓的

axipetal [æk'sipitl] *a* 求心的,向心的(向轴索或轴的)

axis ['æksis] ([复] **axes** ['æksiːz]) *n*【拉】轴;枢椎(第二颈椎) | basibregmatic ~ 基底冠矢轴(从颅底点到前囟的垂直线,颅最高点) / basifacial ~, facial ~ 面基轴(连接下颌角点和鼻下点的线) / celiac ~ 腹腔干,腹腔动脉 / cephalocaudal ~ 头尾轴(身体长轴) / costocervical arterial ~ 肋颈干 / hinge ~, condylar ~, mandibular ~ 铰链轴,下颌轴,髁轴 / optic ~ 视轴;光轴 / optical ~, principal ~ 光轴,主轴

axis-cylinder [ˌæksis 'silində] *n* 轴突

ax(o)- [构词成分] 轴;体轴,轴突

axoaxonic [ˌæksəæk'sɔnik] *a* 轴-轴[突触]的

axodendritic [ˌæksəden'dritik] *a* 轴-树[突触]的

axofugal [æk'sɔfjuːgəl] *a* 远心的,离心的(指离轴索或轴)

axograph ['æksəgrɑːf, -græf] *n* 图轴描记器(记纹鼓)

axoid ['æksɔid], **axoidean** [æk'sɔidiən] *a* 枢椎的,第二颈椎的

axolemma [æksə'lemə] *n* 轴膜

axolotl ['æksəlɔtl] *n* 美西螈(实验用动物)

axolysis [æk'sɔlisis] *n* 神经轴分解

axometer [æk'sɔmitə] *n* 轴测器(尤用于调节眼镜)

axon ['æksɔn] *n* 体轴(脊柱);轴突,轴索(指神经细胞) | naked ~, unmyelinated ~ 裸轴索,无鞘轴索 | ~e ['æksəun] *n* / ~al ['æksənəl] *a*

axonapraxia [ˌæksɔnə'præksiə] *n* 神经失用症,功能性麻痹

axoneme ['æksəniːm] *n* 轴纤丝(染色体的轴丝);轴丝(纤毛或鞭毛的中央轴)

axonometer [ˌæksə'nɔmitə] *n* 镜轴计(快速测透镜的圆柱轴)

axonopathy [ˌæksə'nɔpəθi] *n* 轴突病 | distal ~ 远侧轴突病 / proximal ~ 近侧轴突病

axonotmesis [ˌæksɔnɔt'miːsis] *n* 轴突断伤

axopetal [æk'sɔpitl] *a* 求心的,向心的(指向轴索或轴)

axophage ['æksəfeidʒ] *n* 噬髓鞘细胞

axoplasm ['æksəplæzəm] *n* 轴浆,轴质 | ~ic [ˌæksə'plæsmik] *a*

axopodium [ˌæksə'pəudiəm] ([复] **axopodia** [ˌæksə'pəudiə]) *n* 轴伪足

axosomatic [ˌæksəsəu'mætik] *a* 轴-体[突触]的

axospongium [ˌæksə'spʌndʒiəm] *n* 轴索海绵质

axostyle ['æksəstail] *n* 轴柱,伪足轴

axotomy [æk'sɔtəmi] *n* 轴突切开术

Ayala's quotient (equation, index) [ə'jɑːlə] (A. G. Ayala) 阿亚拉系数(方程式,指数)(检查脑脊液压的一种系数,即10 ml 脑脊液排除前的压力除以排除后的压力,并乘以10)

ayapana [ˌɑːjə'pɑːnə] *n* 三脉佩兰叶(热带国家生长的植物,用作芳香、健胃、发汗和兴奋药)

Ayer's test ['eiə, ɛə] (James B. Ayer) 艾尔试验(检椎管阻滞)

Ayer-Tobey test ['eiə 'təubi] (J. B. Ayer; George L. Tobey, Jr.) 艾尔-托比试验(见 Tobey-Ayer test)

Ayerza's disease [ɑː'jeisɑː] (Abel Ayerza) 阿耶萨病(红细胞增多症的一种,主要特征为慢性发

绀、慢性呼吸困难、慢性支气管炎、支气管扩张、骨髓增殖和肺动脉硬化) | ~ syndrome 阿耶萨综合征(原发性肺动脉高压,伴有肺动脉扩张,与肺病有关,以前认为是梅毒所致)

ayurveda [ˌaiˈjuːvedə, ˌaijəːˈveidə] *n*【梵】生命科学 | **ayurvedic** [ˌaijəːˈeidik] *a*

ayurvedism [ˌɑːjəːˈveidizəm] *n* 印度药草治疗法

Az azote【法】氮

azabon [ˈeizəbɔn] *n* 阿扎苯胺(中枢神经系统兴奋药)

azacitidine [ˌeizəˈsaitidiːn] *n* 阿扎胞苷(抗肿瘤药)

azaclorzine hydrochloride [ˌeizəˈklɔːziːn] 盐酸氮氯嗪(冠状动脉扩张药)

azacosterol hydrochloride [ˌæzəˈkɔstərəul] 盐酸阿扎胆醇(降胆固醇药和鸟类化学不育剂)

azacyclonol [ˌeizəˈsaiklənɔl] *n* 阿扎环醇(其盐酸盐用作安定药,治疗精神分裂症)

5-azacytidine [ˌeizəˈsaitidiːn] *n* 阿扎胞苷(抗肿瘤药,用于治疗急性粒细胞白血病)

Azadirachta [ˌæzədiˈræktə] *n* 印度苦楝属

azaguanine [ˌæzəˈgwænin] *n* 氮鸟嘌呤

Azalea [əˈzeiliə] *n* 杜鹃属

azalide [ˈæzəlaid] *n* 阿扎内酯(大环内酯抗生素的子类,抗菌药阿奇霉素〈azithromycin〉即属于此)

azamethonium bromide [ˌeizəmiˈθəuniəm] 阿扎溴铵(神经节阻断药,抗高血压药)

azanator maleate [ˈeizəˌneitə] 马来酸阿扎那托(支气管扩张药)

azanidazole [ˌeizəˈnidəzəul] *n* 阿扎硝唑(抗滴虫药)

azaperone [ˌeizəˈperəun] *n* 阿扎哌隆(安定药,兽医用)

azapetine phosphate [ˌeizəˈpetiːn] 磷酸阿扎培汀(α 肾上腺素能阻滞药,周围血管扩张药)

azapropazone [ˌæzəˈprəupəzəun] *n* 阿扎丙宗(消炎药)

azaribine [ˌeizəˈraibiːn] *n* 阿扎立平(治疗银屑病、蕈样肉芽肿及真性红细胞增多症)

azaserine [ˌeizəˈseriːn] *n* 偶氮丝氨酸(抗真菌抗生素)

azastene [ˈeizəstiːn] *n* 阿扎斯丁(避孕药)

azatadine maleate [əˈzætədiːn] 马来酸阿扎他定(抗组胺药,用于治疗常年性、季节性变应性鼻炎和慢性荨麻疹)

azathioprine [ˌeizəˈθaiəpriːn] *n* 硫唑嘌呤(免疫抑制药)

6-azauridine [ˌeizəˈjuəridiːn] *n* 氮尿苷,6-氮尿苷(抗肿瘤药,用于治疗急性白血病)

azedarach [əˈzedəræk] *n* 苦楝皮

azelaic acid [ˌæzəˈleiik] 壬二酸

azelastine hydrochloride [əˈzeləstiː] 盐酸氮草斯汀(抗组胺药)

azeotrope [ˈeiziəˌtrəup] *n* 共沸[混合]物 | **azeotropic** [ˌeiziəˈtrɔpik] *a* 共沸的

azeotropy [ˌeiziˈɔtrəpi] *n* 共沸性

azepindole [ˌeiziˈpindəul] *n* 氮草吲哚(抗抑郁药)

azerin [ˈæzərin] *n* 捕虫草酶

azid [ˈæzid], **azide** [ˈæzaid] *n* 叠氮化[合]物

3'-azido-3'-deoxythymidine [ˌæziˌdəu diˌɔksiˈθaimidiːn] 3'-叠氮-3'-去氧胸苷(即齐多夫定〈zidovudine〉,抗病毒药)

azidothymidine [ˌæzidəˈθaimidiːn] *n* 叠氮胸苷(能抑制引起获得性免疫缺陷综合征〈即艾滋病〉的人免疫缺陷病毒)

azimuth [ˈæziməθ] *n* 方位,方位角 | **~al** [ˌæziˈmʌθəl] *a* 方位的,方位角的;水平的

azipramine [əˈziprəmiːn] *n* 阿齐帕明(抗抑郁药)

aziridine [əˈziəridiːn] *n* 氮丙啶,氮杂环丙烷

azithromycin [æˌziθrəˈmaisin] *n* 阿奇霉素(抗生素类药)

azlocillin [ˌæzləuˈsilin] *n* 阿洛西林(抗生素类药)

azo- [前缀] 偶氮基

azoamyly [eizəuˈæmili] *n* 糖原缺乏(肝细胞无贮存正常数量糖原的能力)

azobenzene [ˌæzəuˈbenziːn] *n* 偶氮苯

azobilirubin [ˌæzəuˌbiliˈruːbin] *n* 偶氮胆红素

azocarmine [ˌæzəuˈkɑːmin] *n* 偶氮卡红,偶氮胭脂红

azoic [əˈzəuik] *a* 无生物的 *n* 叠氮酸

azoimide [ˌæzəuˈimaid] *n* 偶氮亚胺

azole [ˈæzəul] *n* 氮二烯五环;吡咯

azolimine [əˈzəulimiːn] *n* 阿佐利明(利尿药)

azolitmin [ˌæzəuˈlitmin] *n* 石蕊精,石蕊素(用作 pH 指示剂,pH4.5 时呈红色,pH 8.3 时呈蓝色)

Azomonas [ˌæzəuˈməunəs] *n* 氮单胞菌属

azomycin [ˌæzəuˈmaisin] *n* 氮霉素,2-硝基咪唑

azoospermia [eiˌzəuəuˈspəːmiə], **azoospermatism** [eiˌzəuəuˈspəːmətizəm] *n* 无精子症

azopigment [ˌeizəuˈpigmənt] *n* 偶氮色素

azoprotein [ˌæzəuˈprəutiːn] *n* 偶氮蛋白

Azorean disease [əˈzəuriən] (Azores 亚速尔群岛)亚速尔群岛病(中枢神经系统一种进行性变性疾病)

Azospirillum [ˌeizəuspaiəˈriləm] *n* 固氮螺菌属

azosulfamide [ˌæzəuˈsʌlfəmaid] *n* 偶氮磺酰胺,新百浪多息

azote [ˈæzəut] *n* 氮

azotemia [ˌæzəuˈtiːmiə] *n* 氮质血症 | extrarenal ~ 肾外性氮质血症 / postrenal ~ 肾后性氮质血症 / prerenal ~ 肾前性氮质血症 / renal ~ 肾性

氮质血症 | **azotemic** *a*
azotenesis [ˌæzəutəˈniːsis] *n* 氮质过多症
azothermia [ˌæzəuˈθəːmiə] *n* 氮血热
azotification [æˌzəutifiˈkeiʃən] *n* 定氮[作用],固氮[作用]
azotize [ˈæzətaiz] *vt* 与氮化合,氮化
Azotobacter [əˌzəutəˈbæktə] *n* 固氮菌属
Azotobacteraceae [əˌzəutəˌbæktəˈreisiiː] *n* 固氮菌科
azotometer [ˌæzəˈtɔmitə] *n* 氮定量器,定氮仪 | **azotometry** *n* 氮量分析法
Azotomonas [əˌzəutəˈməunəs] *n* 固氮单胞菌属(即固氮菌属 Azotobacter)
azotomycin [əˌzəutəˈmaisin] *n* 阿佐霉素(抗生素类药)
azotorrhea [ˌæzəutəˈriːə] *n* 氮溢(粪中氮失去过多)
azoturia [ˌæzəˈtjuəriə] *n* 氮尿症 | **azoturic** [ˌæzəˈtjuərik] *a*
azoxybenzene [ˌæzɔksibenˈziːn] *n* 氧化偶氮苯
azoxy [æˈzɔksi] *n* 氧化偶氮基
AZQ diaziquone 地吖醌(抗肿瘤药)
AZT zidovudine 齐多夫定(抗病毒药)
Aztec idiocy, type [ˈæztek] 头小性白痴(Aztec 为土著墨西哥人部落)
aztreonam [ˈæztriəˌnæm] *n* 氨曲南(抗生素类药)
azul [ˈæzul] *n* 阿祖耳,品他病(即 pinta)
azulene [ˈæʒuliːn] *n* 薁,苷菊环烃
azure [ˈæʒə] *n* 天蓝,天青
azuresin [ˈæʒuˈresin] *n* 天青树脂(诊断用药)
azurophil [æˈʒuərəfil] *n* 嗜天青体,嗜天青细胞
azurophile [ˈæʒurəufail] *n* 嗜体,嗜天青细胞 *a* 嗜天青的
azurophilia [ˌæʒurəuˈfiliə] *n* 嗜天青性 | **azurophilic** [ˌæʒurəuˈfilik] *a*
azyg(o)- [构词成分] 不成对的,奇的;奇静脉
azygoesophageal [ˌæzigəuiːˌsɔfəˈdʒiːəl] *a* 奇静脉[与]食管的
azygogram [ˈæzigəgræm] *n* 奇静脉造影[照]片
azygography [ˌæziˈgɔgrəfi] *n* 奇静脉造影[术]
azygomediastinal [ˌæzigəuˌmiːdiəˈstainəl] *a* 奇静脉[与]纵隔的
azygos [ˈæzigɔs] *a* 不成对的;奇数的;单的 *n* 奇,单
azygospore [əˈzaigəˌspɔː], **azygosperm** [əˈzaigəˌspəːm] 拟接合孢子
azygous [ˈæzigəs] *a* 不成对的;奇数的,单的;无配偶的
azymia [əˈzimiə] *n* 酶缺乏

B

B bel 贝[尔];boron 硼
B magnetic flux density 磁通密度
b barn 靶[恩];base 碱基
β beta 希腊语的第2个字母;血红蛋白β链和第二类错误概率的符号
β- 前缀,表示①紧接主要功能基起始的链第2个碳原子,例如β-羟丁酸(见α-);②旋光物的比旋,例如β-D-葡萄糖;③环外原子或基团的定向,例如胆甾-5-烯-3-β-醇(胆固醇);④蛋白电泳时随β带(可再分为β_1和β_2带)移动的一种血浆蛋白;⑤一系列相关化合物中的一种,特指一系列立体异构形、同分异构形、多聚形和同素异形形;例如β-胡萝卜素;⑥一组相关实体中的一种,例如β射线
BA Bachelor of Arts 文学士
Ba barium 钡
Baastrup's disease (syndrome) [ˈbɑːstrup] (Christian I. Baastrup) 巴斯特罗普病(综合征),吻状棘突,接触棘突
Babbit metal [ˈbæbit] (Isaac Babbit) 巴比特合金(锡铜锑合金,用于牙科)
Babcock's operation [ˈbæbkɔk] (William W. Babcock) 巴布科克手术(静脉瘤治疗术)
Babès-Ernst granules (bodies) [ˈbɑːbeiz əːnst] (Victor Babès; Paul Ernst) 巴-恩颗粒(小体),异染颗粒
Babesia [bəˈbiːziə] *n* 巴贝虫属 | ~ argentina 阿根廷巴贝虫 / ~ bigemina 二联巴贝虫 / ~ bovi 牛巴贝虫 / ~ canis 犬巴贝虫 / ~ divergens 分歧巴贝虫 / ~ equi 马巴贝虫 / ~ hominis 人巴贝虫 / ~ major 主巴贝虫 / ~ microti 田鼠巴贝虫 / ~ ovi 绵羊巴贝虫
babesiasis [bəbiˈsaiəsis] *n* 巴贝虫病(见 babesiosis)
Babesiella [bəˌbiːziˈelə] *n* 巴贝虫属(见 Babesia)
Babesiidae [ˌbəbiˈziːidiː] *n* 巴贝虫科
babesiosis [bəˌbiːziˈəusis] *n* 巴贝虫病 | bovine ~ 牛巴贝虫病 / canine ~ 犬巴贝虫病 / equine ~ 马巴贝虫病 / feline ~ 猫巴贝虫病 / ovine ~ 绵羊巴贝虫病 / swine ~, porcine ~ 猪巴贝虫病
Babès' nodules (node, tubercle) [ˈbɑːbeiz] (Victor Babès) 巴贝斯小结(结,结节)(中枢神经系统内神经元周围小胶质细胞集结,见于狂犬病及其他类型病毒性脑炎)
Babès' treatment [ˈbɑːbeiz] (Victor Babès) 巴贝斯疗法(治狂犬病) | ~ tubercles 巴贝斯结节,狂犬病结节
Babinski-Fröhlich syndrome [bəˈbinski ˈfreiliʃ] (J. F. F. Babinski; Alfred Fröhlich) 肥胖性生殖器退化
Babinski-Nageotte syndrome [bəˈbinski nɑːʒˈjɔt] (J. F. F. Babinski; Jean Nageotte) 巴宾斯基-纳若特综合征(小脑动脉血栓所致的延髓被盖综合征)
Babinski's law [bəˈbinski] (Joseph F. F. Babinski) 巴宾斯基定律,电压眩晕定律(正常受检者倾向于阳极一侧,有迷路病者则不能,如迷路损坏,则无反应) | ~ phenomenon 巴宾斯基现象(皮质脊髓束损害时,刺激足底,不是所有趾向跖侧屈曲,而是踇趾背屈,其余趾伸展) / ~ reflex 巴宾斯基反射,划跖反射(锥体束损害时,刺激足底,踇指即背屈,为器质性瘫痪之征,而非癔症性瘫痪) / ~ sign 巴宾斯基征(①坐骨神经痛时跟腱反射缺失或减少,有别于癔病性坐骨神经痛;②巴宾斯基反射;③偏瘫时,健侧颈阔肌收缩比患侧有力,如张口、吹口哨、吹气时所见;④患者仰卧地板上,两臂交叉胸前,令其用力坐起,瘫痪侧大腿向骨盆屈曲,足跟从地面举起,而健侧肢体未动,见于器质性瘫痪而非癔症性瘫痪;⑤当瘫痪前臂置于旋后位时,即转到旋前位,见于器质性瘫痪患者,亦称旋前征) / ~ syndrome 巴宾斯基综合征(各型晚期神经梅毒合并心血管病)
Babinski-Vaquez syndrome [bəˈbinski væˈkei] (J. F. F. Babinski; Louis H. Vaquez) 巴-瓦综合征(各型晚期神经梅毒合并心血管病)
baby [ˈbeibi] *n* 婴儿 | blue ~ 青紫婴儿,发绀婴儿(因先天性心脏损害或先天性肺膨胀不全所致) / "cloud ~" 雾婴(指排出含葡萄球菌传染雾的婴儿,是婴儿室重要传染源之一) / collodion ~ 火棉胶[样]婴儿(出生时完全被一层火棉胶样或羊皮纸样膜包裹的婴儿) | **~hood** *n* 婴儿期
bacampicillin hydrochloride [bəˌkæmpiˈsilin] 盐酸巴氨西林(抗生素类药)
bacca [ˈbækə] ([复] **baccae** [ˈbækiː]) *n*【拉】浆果
baccate [ˈbækeit] *a* 浆果状的
Baccelli's sign [bækˈtʃeli] (Guido Baccelli) 巴切

利征(低音胸语音)

bacciform [ˈbæksifɔːm] *a* 浆果形的

bachelor [ˈbætʃələ] *n* 学士 | Bachelor of Arts (Science, Medicine) 文科(理科、医)学士

Bachman test (reaction) [ˈbɑːkmən] (George W. Bachman) 巴克曼试验(反应)(检旋毛虫病的皮内试验)

Bachmann's bundle [ˈbɑːkmən] (Jean G. Bachmann) 巴克曼束(结间前束的一组纤维,穿过房间隔,在左心房分开,并连接心房)

Bach remedies (flower remedies) [bɑːk] (Edward Bach) 巴克药(花药)(用于治疗心理和情绪疾患,对身体症状无直接影响)

Bacillaceae [ˌbæsiˈleisiiː] *n* 芽胞杆菌科

bacillary [bəˈsiləri, ˈbæsi-] *a* 杆菌的,杆菌性的;杆状的

bacille [bɑːˈsiːl] *n* 【法】杆菌 | ~ Calmette-Guérin (BCG) 卡介菌

bacillemia [ˌbæsiˈliːmiə] *n* 杆菌血症

bacilli [bəˈsilai] bacillus 的复数

bacilli- [构词成分]杆菌

bacilliculture [bəˈsiliˌkʌltʃə] *n* 杆菌培养

bacilliferous [ˌbæsiˈlifərəs] *a* 带杆菌的

bacilliform [bəˈsilifɔːm] *a* 杆状的;杆菌状的

bacilligenic [bəˌsiliˈdʒenik], **bacillogenic** [bəˌsiləuˈdʒenik] *a* 杆菌性的,杆菌所致的;产生杆菌的

bacillin [bəˈsilin] *n* 杆菌素(自枯草杆菌分离出的抗菌物质)

bacilliparous [ˌbæsiˈlipərəs] *a* 产生杆菌的

bacill(o)- 见 bacilli-

bacillogenous [ˌbæsiˈlɔdʒinəs] *a* 杆菌性的,杆菌所致的

bacillosis [ˌbæsiˈləusis] *n* 杆菌病(杆菌感染)

bacillotherapy [bəˌsiləuˌθerəpi] *n* 细菌疗法

bacilluria [ˌbæsiˈljuəriə] *n* 杆菌尿

Bacillus [bəˈsiləs] *n* 【拉】杆菌属,芽胞杆菌属 | ~ aerogenes capsulatus 产气荚膜芽胞杆菌 / ~ anthracis 炭疽芽胞杆菌 / ~ botulinus 肉毒[芽胞]杆菌 / ~ bronchisepticus 支气管败血性杆菌 / ~ cereus 蜡样芽胞杆菌 / ~ coli 大肠杆菌 / ~ dysenteriae 痢疾杆菌 / ~ enteritidis 肠炎杆菌 / ~ faecalis alcaligenes 粪产碱杆菌 / ~ fragilis 脆弱[微小]杆菌 / ~ fusiformis 梭状杆菌 / ~ larvae 幼虫芽胞杆菌 / ~ leprae 麻风杆菌 / ~ mallei 鼻疽杆菌 / ~ megatherium 巨大芽胞杆菌 / ~ necrophorus 坏死杆菌 / ~ oedematiens, ~ oedematis maligni No. Ⅱ 水肿杆菌,恶性水肿杆菌二号 / ~ pneumoniae 肺炎杆菌,肺炎克雷白杆菌 / ~ polymyxa 多黏芽胞杆菌 / ~ pyocyaneus 铜绿假单胞菌 / ~ subtilis 枯草杆菌 / ~ tetani 破伤风杆菌 / ~ typhi, ~ typhosus 伤寒杆菌 / ~ welchii 魏氏芽胞杆菌,产气荚膜杆菌 / ~ whitmori 惠氏杆菌,假鼻疽杆菌

bacillus [bəˈsiləs] ([复] **bacilli** [bəˈsilai]) *n* 杆菌 | Calmette-Guérin ~ 卡介菌 / diphtheria ~ 白喉杆菌,白喉棒状杆菌 / hay ~ 枯草杆菌 / tubercle ~ 结核杆菌

bacilysin [ˌbæsiˈlaisin] *n* 枯草杆菌溶素

bacitracin [ˌbæsiˈtreisin] *n* 杆菌肽

back [bæk] *n* 背 | flat ~ 板样背 / functional ~ 功能性腰背痛 / hollow ~, saddle ~ 脊柱前凸 / hump ~, hunch ~ 脊柱后凸,驼背 / poker ~ 类风湿脊椎炎

backache [ˈbækeik] *n* 背痛

backalgia [bækˈældʒiə] *n* 损伤性背痛

backbone [ˈbækbəun] *n* 脊柱

back-breaking [ˈbæk ˌbreikiŋ] *a* 劳累至极的

back-calculation [bæk ˌkælkjuˈleiʃən] *n* 倒算法(一种统计法,即使用某一疾病目前发生率和潜伏时间,估计该病累计发生率并设计未来发生的病例数)

backcross [ˈbækkrɔs] *vt, vi; n* 回交(在实验遗传学中,杂合子与纯合子之间的交配) | double ~ 双回交(双杂合子与纯合子之间的交配)

backfiltration [ˌbækfilˈtreiʃən] *n* 反向过滤

backflow [ˈbækfləu] *n* 反流 | pyelovenous ~ 肾盂静脉反流

background [ˈbækgraund] *n* 背景;本底

backing [ˈbækiŋ] *n* 背板 | alloy ~ 前牙桥体金属背

backknee [ˈbækniː] *n* 膝反屈

back-raking [bæk ˈreikiŋ] *n* 肛掏粪(由动物的直肠掏出压紧的粪便)

backscatter [ˈbækskætə] *n* 反向散射

Backteriaceae [ˌbæktiriˈeisiiː] *n* 杆菌科

baclofen [ˈbækləfn] *n* 巴氯芬(肌肉松弛药)

BACON bleomycin, doxorubicin, CCNU, vincristine and nitrogen mustard 博来霉素-多柔比星-环己亚硝脲-长春新碱-氮芥(联合化疗治癌方案)

BACOP bleomycin, doxorubicin, cyclophosphamide, vincristine and prednisone 博来霉素-多柔比星-环磷酰胺-长春新碱-泼尼松(联合化疗治癌方案)

Bact. Bacterium [无芽胞]杆菌属

-bacter [构词成分]细菌

bacterascites [ˌækərəˈsaitiːz] *n* 细菌性腹水感染 | monomicrobial non-neutrocytic ~ 单微生物性非中性粒细胞性细菌性腹水感染 / polymicrobial ~ 多种微生物性细菌性腹水感染

bacteremia [ˌbæktəˈriːmiə] *n* 菌血症 | **bacteremic** *a*

Bacteria [bækˈtiəriə] *n* 细菌纲

bacteria [bækˈtiəriə] bacterium 的复数 | **~l** *a* 细

菌的

bacteria-carrier [bækˌtiəriə ˈkæriə] *n* 带菌者

bacteria-free [bækˌtiəriə ˈfriː] *a* 无菌的

bactericide [bækˈtiərisaid] *n* 杀菌剂 | specific ~ 溶菌素 | **bactericidal** [bækˌtiəriˈsaidl] *a* 杀菌的

bactericidin [ˌbæktəriˈsaidin] *n* 杀[细]菌素

bacterid [ˈbæktərid] *n* 细菌疹 | pustular ~ 脓疱性细菌疹

bacteriemia [bækˌtiəriˈiːmiə] *n* 菌血症

bacteriform [bækˈtiərifɔːm] *a* 细菌状的

bacterin [ˈbæktərin] *n* 菌苗 | *Bordetella bronchiseptica* ~ 支气管败血性博德特菌菌苗(用于预防该菌所致的猪萎缩性鼻炎) / *Clostridium chauvoei-septicum* ~ 肖氏梭菌-败血梭菌菌苗(见 bacterin-toxoid 项下相应术语) / *Clostridium haemolyticum* ~ 溶血梭菌菌苗(用于预防牛、绵羊、山羊中的杆菌性血红蛋白尿,即红尿病) / *Erysipelothrix rhusiopathiae* ~ 猪红斑丹毒丝菌菌苗(用于猪的免疫接种,预防丹毒) / *Hemophilus paragallinarum* ~ 副鸡嗜血菌菌苗(用于鸡的免疫接种,预防传染性鼻卡他) / *Leptospira canicola-grippotyphosa-hardjo-icterohaemorrhagiae-pomona* ~ 五联钩端螺旋体菌菌苗,犬钩端螺旋体-流感伤寒钩端螺旋体-哈德焦钩端螺旋体-黄疸出血钩端螺旋体-波摩那钩端螺旋体菌苗(用于牛的免疫接种,预防钩端螺旋体病) / *Pasturella multocide* ~ 多杀巴斯德菌菌苗(①用以预防猪、绵羊、山羊、牛的巴斯德菌病;②用以预防鸡和火鸡的鸡霍乱) / *Pasturella haemolytica-multocida* ~ 二联巴斯德菌菌苗,溶血巴斯德菌-多杀巴斯德菌菌苗(用以预防牛和绵羊的巴斯德菌病) / *Salmonella dublin-typhimurium* ~ 二联沙门菌菌苗,都伯林沙门菌-鼠伤寒沙门菌菌苗(用以预防牛的沙门菌病) / *Staphylococcus aureus* ~ 金黄色葡萄球菌菌苗(用以预防牛的金黄色葡萄球菌感染) / *Streptococcus equi* ~ 马链球菌菌苗(用以预防马的传染性卡他) / *Vibrio fetus* ~ 胎儿弧菌菌苗(用以小母牛和母羊的免疫接种,预防胎儿弯曲杆菌感染所致的不育和流产)

bacterination [ˌbæktəriˈneiʃən] *n* 菌苗接种;菌苗治疗

bacterinia [bæktəˈriniə] *n* 菌苗病,菌苗反应(菌苗接种后有时引起的全身性反应)

bacterin-toxoid [ˈbæktərin ˈtɔksɔid] *n* 菌苗类毒素 | *Clostridium botulium* type C ~ C 型肉毒梭菌菌苗类毒素(用以预防貂的 C 型肉毒中毒) / *Clostridium chauvoei-septicum* ~ 肖氏梭菌-败血梭菌菌苗类毒素(用以预防牛、马、绵羊以及山羊的黑腿病和恶性水肿) / *Clostridium novyi-sordelli* ~ 诺氏梭菌-索氏梭菌菌苗类毒素(用于牛和绵羊的免疫接种,预防这些梭菌引起的疾病,如黑病,大头病) / *Clostridium perfringes* ~ 产气荚膜梭菌菌苗类毒素(用以预防绵羊和牛的肠毒素血症)

bacteri(o)- [构词成分]细菌,菌

bacterioagglutinin [bækˌtiəriəuəˈgluːtinin] *n* 细菌凝集素,凝菌素

bacteriochlorophyll [bækˌtiəriəˈklɔ(ː)rəfil] *n* 细菌叶绿素

bacteriocidin [bækˌtiəriəˈsaidin] *n* 杀菌素

bacteriocin [bækˈtiəriəsin] *n* 细菌素(如大肠埃希杆菌素等)

bacteriocinogen [bækˌtiəriəˈsinədʒən] *n* 细菌素原(控制细菌素合成的一种细菌的质粒)

bacteriocinogenic [bækˌtiəriəˌsinəuˈdʒenik] *a* 产细菌素的

bacterioclasis [bækˌtiəriˈɔkləsis] *n* 裂菌作用,溶菌作用

bacterioerythrin [bækˌtiəriəuˈeriθrin] *n* 菌红素

bacteriofluorescein [bækˌtiəriəufluəˈresiin] *n* 细菌荧光素

bacteriogenic [bækˌtiəriəˈdʒenik], **bacteriogenous** [bækˌtiəriˈɔdʒinəs] *a* 细菌性的

bacteriohemagglutinin [bækˌtiəriəuˌheməˈgluːtinin] *n* 细菌血凝素

bacteriohemolysin [bækˌtiəriəuhiːməˈlaisin] *n* 细菌溶血素

bacterioid [bækˈtiəriɔid] *a* 细菌样的 *n* 类细菌

bacteriology [bækˌtiəriˈɔlədʒi] *n* 细菌学 | **bacteriologic(al)** [bækˌtiəriəˈlɔdʒik(əl)] *a* / **bacteriologist** *n* 细菌学家

bacteriolysant [bækˌtiəriˈɔlisənt] *n* 溶菌剂

bacteriolysin [bækˌtiəriˈɔlisin] *n* 溶菌素

bacteriolysis [bækˌtiəriˈɔlisis] *n* 溶菌[作用] | **bacteriolytic** [bækˌtiəriəˈlitik] *a*

bacteriolyze [bækˈtiəriəlaiz] *vt* 溶菌

Bacterionema [bækˌtiəriəuˈniːmə] *n* 丝杆菌属 | ~ matruchotii 马氏丝杆菌

bacterio-opsonin [bækˌtiəriəu ˈɔpsənin] *n* 细菌调理素

bacteriopexy [bækˌtiəriəuˈpeksi], **bacteriopexia** [bækˌtiəriəuˈpeksiə] *n* 定菌[作用](由组织细胞或其他吞噬细胞使细菌固定)

bacteriophage [bækˈtiəriəˌfeidʒ] *n* 噬菌体 | temperate ~ 温和噬菌体

bacteriophagia [bækˌtiəriəuˈfeidʒiə], **bacteriophagy** [bækˌtiəriˈɔfədʒi] *n* 噬菌现象 | **bacteriophagic** [bækˌtiəriəuˈfædʒik] *a* 噬菌的

bacteriophagology [bækˌtiəriəufəˈgɔlədʒi] *n* 噬菌体学

bacteriophytoma [bækˌtiəriəufaiˈtəumə] *n* 细菌性瘤(细菌所致的瘤样反应性损害)

bacterioplasmin [bækˌtiəriəuˈplæzmin] *n* 细菌胞

浆素

bacterioprecipitin [bæk,tiəriəupri'sipitin] *n* 细菌沉淀素

bacterioprotein [bæk,tiəriəu'prəuti:n] *n* 细菌蛋白

bacteriopsonin [bæk,tiəri'ɔpsənin] *n* 细菌调理素 | **bacteriopsonic** [bæk,tiəriɔp'sɔnik] *a* 调理细菌[作用]的

bacteriopurpurin [bæk,tiəriəu'pə:pjurin] *n* 菌紫素

bacteriorhodopsin [bæk,tiəriərəu'dɔpsin] *n* 菌视紫质

bacterioscopy [bæk,tiəri'ɔskəpi] *n* 细菌[显微]镜检[查]

bacteriosis [bæk,tiəri'əusis] *n* 细菌性疾病

bacteriospermia [bæk,tiəriəu'spə:miə] *n* 含菌精液,菌精症(精液中存在细菌)

bacteriostasis [bæk,tiəriə'steisis] *n* 抑菌作用,制菌作用 | **bacteriostat** [bæk'tiəriəu,stæt] *n* 抑菌剂 / **bacteriostatic** [bæk,tiəriəu'stætik] *a* 抑菌的,制菌的 *n* 抑菌剂

bacteriotherapy [bæk,tiəriəu'θerəpi] *n* 细菌疗法

bacteriotoxemia [bæk,tiəriəutɔk'si:miə] *n* 细菌毒血症

bacteriotoxic [bæk,tiəriəu'tɔksik] *a* 毒害细菌的

bacteriotoxin [bæk,tiəriəu'tɔksin] *n* 细菌毒素

bacteriotropic [bæk,tiəriəu'trɔpik] *a* 亲菌的

bacteriotropin [bæk,tiəri'ɔtrəpin] *n* 亲菌素

bacteriotrypsin [bæk,tiəriəu'tripsin] *n* 细菌胰蛋白酶

bacteritic [,bæktə'ritik] *a* 细菌性的

Bacterium [bæk'tiəriəm] *n*【拉】[无芽胞]杆菌属 | ~ aerogenes 产气杆菌 / ~ aeruginosum 铜绿假单胞菌,绿脓杆菌 / ~ cholerae suis 猪霍乱杆菌 / ~ cloacae 阴沟气杆菌 / ~ coli, ~ coli commune 大肠埃希菌,大肠杆菌 / ~ dysenteriae 痢疾杆菌 / ~ faecalis alcaligenes 粪产碱杆菌 / ~ pestis 鼠疫杆菌 / ~ sonnei 宋内志贺菌 / ~ tularense 土拉热杆菌,土拉热弗朗西丝菌 / ~ typhosum 伤寒杆菌,伤寒沙门菌

bacterium [bæk'tiəriəm] ([复] **bacteria** [bæk'tiəriə]) *n*【拉】细菌;[无芽胞]杆菌 | acid-fast ~ 耐酸菌 / autotrophic ~ 自营菌,自养菌 / beaded ~ 异染菌 / chemoautotrophic ~ 化学自营菌,化学自养菌 / chemoheterotrophic ~ 化学异营菌,化学异养菌 / chromo ~, chromogenic ~ 产色菌 / coliform bacteria 大肠埃希菌群 / corneform bacteria 棒状杆菌 / denitrifying ~ 反硝化菌 / gram-negative ~ 革兰阴性细菌,G^-细菌 / gram-positive ~ 革兰阳性细菌,G^+细菌 / heterotrophic ~ 异营菌,异养菌 / higher bacteria 高等菌 / mantle ~ 衣原体 / pathogenic ~ 病原菌,致病菌 / pyogenic ~ 化脓菌

bacteriuria [bæk,tiəri'juəriə] *n* 菌尿

bacteriuric [bæk,tiəri'juərik] *a* 菌尿的

bacteroid ['bæktərɔid] *a* 似杆菌的 *n* 类菌体

Bacteroidaceae [,bæktərɔi'deisii:] *n* 拟杆菌科,类杆菌科

Bacteroideae [,bæktə'rɔidii:] *n* 拟杆菌族,类杆菌族

Bacteroides [,bæktə'rɔidi:z] *n* 拟杆菌属,类杆菌属 | ~ fragilis 脆弱拟杆菌 / ~ funduliformis 香肠形拟杆菌 / ~ fusiformis 梭状拟杆菌 / ~ melaninogenicus 产黑素拟杆菌 / ~ pneumosintes 侵肺拟杆菌 / ~ ramosus 分枝拟杆菌

bacteroides [,bæktə'rɔidi:z] *n* 多形杆状菌;类杆菌

bacteroidosis [,bæktərɔi'dəusis] *n* 拟杆菌病,类杆菌病

bacteruria [,bæktiə'rjuəriə] *n* 菌尿

Baculoviridae [,bækjuləu'vaiəridi:] *n* 杆状病毒科

baculovirus [,bækjuləu'vaiərəs] *n* 杆状病毒

baculum ['bækjuləm] *n* 阴茎骨(人类以外的某些哺乳动物均有)

Badal's operation [bə'dɑ:l] (Antoine J. Badal)巴达尔手术(将滑车下神经挫碎,治青光眼)

badge [bædʒ] *n* 放射剂量测定软片 | film ~ (防护衣上的)照射剂量测定软片

Baehr-Löhlein lesion [bεə 'lə:lain] (George Baehr; Max H. F. Löhlein)贝-勒损害(见 Löhlein-Baehr lesion)

Baelz's disease ['beilts] (Erwin von Baelz)贝尔茨病,腺性唇炎

BAEP brainstem auditory evoked potential 脑干听觉诱发电位

Baerensporung's erythrasma ['beirənspru:n] (Friedrich W. F. von Baerensprung)贝伦斯普龙红癣(股红癣)

Baer's (Ber's) cavity ['beiə] (Karl E. von Baer ⟨Ber⟩)贝尔腔,囊胚腔 | ~ law 贝尔定律(在胚胎发育中的动物种群所共有的一般特征,比特殊特征出现为早,而特殊特征能区别不同的动物种群。本概念是重演学说的前身)

Baer's method ['beiə] (William S. Baer)贝尔法(用无菌油注入已强硬的关节内,预防再发生粘连)

Baeyer's test ['beijə] (Adolf von Baeyer)贝耶尔试验(检葡萄糖、吲哚)

Bäfverstedt's syndrome ['beifəʃtet] (Bo Erik Bäfverstedt)贝氏综合征,皮肤淋巴细菌瘤

bag [bæg] *n* 袋;囊 | colostomy ~ 结肠造瘘袋 / ice ~ 冰袋 / micturition ~ 排尿袋 / nuclear ~ 核袋(肌梭内肌纤维中央段的中心部分) / testicular ~ 阴囊 / ~ of waters 羊膜囊，羊水囊

bagasse [bəˈgæs] *n* 蔗渣

bagassosis [ˌbægəsˈəusis], **bagasscosis** [ˌbægəsˈkəusis] *n* 蔗尘肺

Baillarger's external band (line, stria, stripe) [baijɑːˈʒei] (Jules G. F. Baillarger) 贝亚尔惹外带(线，纹)，内[颗]粒层纹 / ~ inner band (line, stria, stripe), internal band (line, stria, stripe) 贝亚尔惹内带(线，纹)，内锥体[细胞]层纹 / ~ outer band (line, stria, stripe) 贝亚尔惹外带(线，纹)，内[颗]粒层纹 / ~ sign 贝亚尔惹征(麻痹性痴呆时瞳孔左右不等)

Bainbridge reflex [ˈbeinbridʒ] (Francis A. Bainbridge) 班布里奇反射(大的体静脉或右心房的压力或膨胀度随着心搏加速而增加)

Baker's cyst [ˈbeikə] (William M. Baker) 腘窝囊肿

Baker's velum [ˈbeikə] (Henry Baker) 贝克帆(腭裂充填器)

bakkola [ˈbækəulə] *n* 治癌桦蕈

BAL dimercaprol 二巯丙醇(砷、汞等中毒解毒药)

balance [ˈbæləns] *n* 天平，秤；平衡 | acid-base ~ 酸碱平衡 / analytical ~ 分析天平 / fluid ~, water ~ 液体平衡，水平衡 / genic ~ 基因平衡 / microchemical ~ 微量化学天平 / nitrogen ~ 氮平衡 / occlusal ~ 㕮平衡 / semimicro ~ 半微量天平 / torsion ~ 扭转天平，扭秤

Balamuthia [ˌbæləˈmuːθiə] *n* 细胶丝目阿米巴属

balanic [bəˈlænik] *a* 阴茎头的，龟头的；阴蒂头的

balanitis [ˌbæləˈnaitis] *n* 阴茎头炎 | gangrenous ~, phagedenic ~ 坏疽性阴茎头炎

balan(o)- [构词成分] 阴茎头，龟头

balanoblennorrhea [ˌbælənəuˌblenəˈriːə] *n* 淋病性阴茎头炎

balanocele [ˈbælənəˌsiːl] *n* 阴茎头膨出(自包皮裂口膨出)

balanoplasty [ˈbælənəˌplæsti] *n* 阴茎头成形术

balanoposthitis [ˌbælənəupɔsˈθaitis] *n* 阴茎头包皮炎

balanoposthomycosis [ˌbælənəuˌpɔsθəmaiˈkəusis] *n* 坏疽性阴茎头炎

balanopreputial [ˌbælənəupriˈpjuːʃəl] *a* 阴茎头包皮的

balanorrhagia [ˌbælənəuˈreidʒiə] *n* 阴茎头脓溢

Balanosporida [ˌbælənəuˈspɔːridə] *n* 孔盖孢子目

balantidiasis [ˌbæləntiˈdaiəsis], **balantidiosis** [ˌbæləntidiˈəusis], **balantidosis** [ˌbæləntiˈdəusis] *n* 小袋纤毛虫病

balantidicidal [bəˌlæntidiˈsaidl] *a* 杀小袋[纤毛]虫的

Balantidium [ˌbælənˈtidiəm] *n* 小袋[纤毛]虫属 | ~ coli 结肠小袋[纤毛]虫 / ~ suis 猪小袋[纤毛]虫

balanus [ˈbælənəs] *n* 阴茎头，龟头

balata [ˈbælətə] *n* 巴拉塔树胶，猿脸树胶

Balbiani's nucleus (body) [bɑːlbiˈɑːni] (Edouard G. Balbiani) 卵黄核

baldness [ˈbɔːldnis] *n* 秃头，秃发 | common male ~ 普通男性秃发

Baldwin's operation [ˈbɔːldwin] (James F. Baldwin) 鲍德温手术(人工阴道形成术，即在膀胱与直肠间移植一段回肠)

Baldy's operation [ˈbɔːldi] (John M. Baldy), **Baldy-Webster operation** [ˈbɔːldi ˈwebstə] (John M. Baldy; John C. Webster) 鲍尔迪手术，鲍尔迪-韦伯斯特手术(见 Webster's operation)

baleri [bəˈliəri] *n* 贝娄病(锥虫病的一种)

Balint syndrome [bɑːˈlint] (Rezsoe Balint) 巴林特综合征(表现为注视皮质性麻痹、视性共济失调及视注意力障碍，但自发的和反射性眼运动尚存。双侧顶-枕区损伤可见，常发生在心脏病起始之后)

Balkan frame, splint [ˈbɔːlkən] 巴尔干式架，夹板(用于骨折及脱骱，作伸展之用)

ball [bɔːl] *n* 球，团块；眼球；丸剂 | chondrin ~ 软骨胶球 / fatty ~ of Bichat 吸垫，颊脂体 / food ~ 植物粪石 / fungus ~ 曲霉肿 / hair ~ 毛团，毛粪石(胃肠内) / ~ of the thumb 鱼际 / pleural fibrin ~s 胸膜纤维素球 / wool ~ 羊毛团

Ballance's sign [ˈbæləns] (Charles A. Ballance) 巴兰斯征(患者左侧卧时右胁腹有叩响，提示脾破裂)

Baller-Gerold syndrome [ˈbælə ˈdʒerəld] (F. Baller; M. Gerold) 巴-杰综合征(一种常染色体隐性遗传综合征，特征为颅骨早闭和桡骨发育不良。亦称颅骨早闭-桡骨发育不良综合征)

Ballet's sign [bæˈlei] (Gilbert Ballet) 巴累征(眼外肌麻痹，所有眼球随意运动消失，瞳孔运动及眼反射性运动仍存在，见于突眼性甲状腺肿及癔症患者)

Ballingall's disease [ˈbæliŋgɔːl] (George Ballingall) 足分枝菌病

ballismus [bəˈlizməs], **ballism** [ˈbælizəm] *n* 颤搐；投掷症

ballistic [bəˈlistik] *a* 弹道[学]的；颤搐的；投掷样的

ballistics [bəˈlistiks] *n* 弹道学 | wound ~ 创伤弹道学(研究发射物的射向及速度对其所产生的创伤的关系)

ballistocardiogram [bəˌlistəuˈkɑːdiəgræm] *n* 心冲击描记图

ballistocardiograph [bəˌlistəuˈkɑːdiəgrɑːf] *n* 心冲击描记器 | **~y** [bəˌlistəuˌkɑːdiˈɔgrəfi] *n* 心冲击描记术

ballistospore [bəˈlistəspɔː] *n* 掷孢子

balloon [bəˈluːn] *n* 气囊;球形玻璃容器 *vi* 加气膨胀 | sinus ~ 窦囊(用以支持上颌窦壁凹陷骨折)

ballooning [bəˈluːniŋ] *n* 气胀术(体腔充气,治疗用)

ballotable [bəˈlɔtəbl] *a* 可冲击触诊的

ballottement [bəˈlɔtmənt] *n* 冲击触诊[法] | abdominal ~ . indirect ~ 腹部冲击触诊[法],间接冲击触诊[法] / renal ~ 肾脏冲击触诊[法]

Ball's valve [bɔːl] (Charles B. Ball)肛瓣,直肠瓣

balm [bɑːm] *n* 香膏;香蜂草,密里萨;香脂,香胶 | blue ~, lemon ~, sweet ~ 香蜂叶,密里萨香叶 / ~ of Gilead 几来香脂,麦加香脂

Balme's cough [bɑːlm] (Paul J. Balme) 巴尔姆咳(躺下时咳嗽,见于鼻咽堵塞)

balmony [ˈbælməni] *n* 窄叶蛇头草

balmy [ˈbɑːmi] *a* 有香气的;止痛的

balneology [ˌbælniˈɔlədʒi] *n* 浴疗学

balneotherapy [ˌbælniəuˈθerəpi], **balneotherapeutics** [ˌbælniəuθerəˈpjuːtiks] *n* 浴疗法

balneum [ˈbælniəm]([复] **balnea** [ˈbælniə] *n*【拉】浴,沐浴 | ~ arenae 沙浴 / ~ pneumaticum 空气浴

Baló's disease (concentric sclerosis) [bɑːˈləu] (Jozsef M. Baló) 巴洛病(同心性硬化),同心性轴周性脑炎

balsalazide disodium [bælˈsæləzaid] 巴柳氮二钠(抗溃疡性结肠炎药)

balsam [ˈbɔːlsəm] *n* 香树脂,香脂,香胶 | Canada ~ 加拿大香脂,加拿大松脂 / friars' ~ 复方安息香酊 / gurjun ~ 古云香脂 / Holland ~, silver ~ 荷兰香胶,银香胶,杜松焦油 / Mecca ~, ~ of Gilead 麦加香脂,几来香脂 / peruvian ~ 秘鲁香脂 / tolu ~ 妥鲁香脂,妥鲁香胶 | **~ic** [bɔːlˈsæmik] *a*

balsamo [ˈbælsəməu] *n*【西】香脂,香胶 | ~ de tolu 妥鲁香脂,妥鲁香胶 / ~ del Peru 秘鲁香脂

Balsamodendron [ˌbælsəməuˈdendrɔn] *n*【拉,希】没药属

balsamum [ˈbælsəməm] *n*【拉】香脂,香胶 | ~ peruvianum 秘鲁香脂

Balser's fatty necrosis [ˈbɑːlzə] (Wilhelm A. Balser) 巴尔泽脂肪性坏死(坏疽性胰腺炎,伴网膜黏液囊炎及脂肪组织的散发性片状坏死;胰腺炎伴脂肪坏死)

balteum [ˈbæltiəm] *n*【拉】托带,腰带,束带 | ~ venereum 性病腰带,汞剂膏药

Bamberger-Marie disease [ˈbɑːmbəgə məˈriː] (Eugen Bamberger; Pierre Marie) 肥大性肺性骨关节病

Bamberger's hematogenic albuminuria [ˈbɑːmbəgəː] (Heinrich von Bamberger) 班伯格血原性蛋白尿(发生在严重贫血后期) | ~ disease 班伯格病(①跳跃性痉挛或下肢抽搐;②进行性恶性多发性浆膜炎) / ~ sign 班伯格征(①异侧感觉;②肩胛骨角部呈现实变体征,身体前倾则消失,为心包积液的体征)

bambermycins [ˌbæmbəˈmaisinz] [复] *n* 班贝霉素(一种抗菌抗生素复合物,主要含默诺霉素〈moenomycin〉A和C,用作饲料添加剂和兽用补品)

bamboo brier [bæmˈbuː ˈbraiə] 菝葜(印第安人用作食物)

bamnidazole [bæmˈnidəzəul] *n* 班硝唑(抗毛滴虫有效的抗原虫药)

BAN British Approved Name 英国通用药名(英国药典委员会批准的非专利药品名称)

banana [bəˈnɑːnə] *n* 芭蕉属植物;香蕉

bancroftian [bæŋˈkrɔftiən] *a* 班[克罗夫特]氏的

Bancroft's filariasis [ˈbæŋkrɔft] (Joseph Bancroft), **bancroftosis** [ˌbæŋkrɔfˈtəusis] *n* 班[克罗夫特]氏丝虫病

band [bænd] *n* 带,束,索;带环 | A ~ A带(肌原纤维节染成黑色之区,亦称A盘,Q盘,横盘,暗板) / absorption ~s 吸收光带 / amniotic ~ 羊膜索 / anchor ~ 抗基圈(牙) / atrioventricular ~, auriculoventricular ~ 房室束 / axis ~ 原条(胚) / clamp ~ 夹圈 / coronary ~ 冠状带,冠状垫 / dentate ~ 牙用带环 / free ~ of colon 结肠独立带 / H ~ H带(横纹肌盘,有时见于穿过横纹肌原纤维A带中央的淡色区) / I ~ I带(在横纹肌原纤维内,光显微镜下出现明区,偏振光下出现暗区,亦称J盘,明板) / M ~ M带(肌原纤维节H带中央的狭窄暗带) / Q ~ Q盘,横盘,暗板 / Z ~ Z带(一种薄膜,用以分隔横纹肌的肌原纤维节)

bandage [ˈbændidʒ] *n* 绷带 | figure-of-8 ~ 8字形绷带 / many-tailed ~ 多头绷带 / spica ~ 人字形绷带 / spiral reverse ~ 螺旋反折绷带

bandaletta [ˌbændəˈletə] *n* 绷带;小带 | ~ diagonalis (Broca) 布罗卡斜角小带,布罗卡斜纹

bandelette [ˌbændəˈlet] *n* 小带

bandicoot [ˈbændikuːt] *n* 袋狸(印度硕鼠,鼠咬热病原体小螺菌的贮主)

banding [ˈbændiŋ] *n* 绑扎;显带(染色体染色的各种技术,由此一种特征图式的横暗带和亮带明显可见) | C ~, C-~, centromeric ~ 着丝粒显带(显示染色体带的染色体鉴别染色) / chromosome ~ 染色体显带(使用各种不同的物理的和细胞化学的制片进行的鉴别染色技术) / G ~, G-~, Giemsa ~ 吉姆萨显带(显示染色体带〈B带〉的染色体鉴别染色) / high-resolution ~, prophase ~ 高分辨率显带技术,前期显带技术(一种显带技术) / pulmonary artery (PA) ~

肺动脉环束术(对患某些先天性心脏病的儿童所做的手术,以控制肺动脉血流) / Q ~, Q-~, quinacrine ~ 喹吖因[荧光]显带(显示染色体带〈Q 带〉的染色体鉴别染色) / R ~, R-~, reverse ~ 反带(显示染色体带〈R 带〉的染色体鉴别染色)

Bandl's ring [ˈbændl] (Ludwig Bandl) 班德尔环(病理性收缩环)

bandpass [ˈbændpɑːs, -pæs] *n* 带通(滤波器)

bandwidth [ˈbænwidθ] *n* 带宽

bandy [ˈbændi] *a* 膝向外曲的 | ~-legged *a* 两腿向外弯曲的

bane [bein] *n* 毒,毒物,毒药 | leopard's ~, wolf's ~ 山金车(花、根)

banewort [ˈbeinwəːt] *n* 颠茄叶

bang [bæŋ] *n* = bhang

Bang's bacillus [bæŋ] (Bernhard L. F. Bang) 班氏杆菌,流产布氏菌 | ~ disease 班氏病,(牛)传染性流产 / ~ test 班氏试验(检牛布氏菌病的凝集试验)

Bang's method [bæŋ] (Ivar C. Bang) 班氏法(微量血生化检查;检尿糖)

banian [ˈbænjən] *n* 孟加拉榕树(籽和皮可以健身、退热、利尿)

Banisteria [ˌbæniˈstiriə] *n* 扶栏树属

banisterine [bæˈnistərin] *n* 南美卡皮根碱,骆驼蓬碱,扶栏树碱

bank [bæŋk] *n* 库(如血库、骨库、眼库等) | blood ~ 血库 / eye ~ 眼库

Bannayan-Zonana syndrome [ˈbænəjən zəuˈneinə] (George A. Bannayan; Jonathan Zonana) 巴-佐综合征(一种罕见的常染色体显性遗传综合征,特征为躯干血管瘤、皮肤脂肪瘤、巨头和腹肿胀伴血管瘤)

Bannister's disease [ˈbænistə] (Henry M. Bannister) 班尼斯特病,血管[神经]性水肿

Bannwarth's syndrome [bɑːnˈvɑːrt] (Alfred Bannwarth) 班伐尔特综合征(脑膜多神经炎〈meningopolyneuritis〉的欧洲名称,可能出现在莱姆〈Lyme〉病中)

Banting's treatment (cure, diet) [ˈbæntiŋ] (William Banting), **bantingism** [ˈbæntiŋizəm] *n* 班廷疗法,忌食减瘦疗法(以高蛋白质低碳水化合物饮食治肥胖症)

Banti's disease, syndrome [ˈbænti] (Guido Banti) 班替病、综合征(原来被描述为脾脏的一种原发病,伴有脾肿大和各类血细胞减少,但以后认为是继发于门静脉高血压。亦称充血性脾大和脾性贫血)

Baptisia [bæpˈtiziə] *n* 【拉】灰叶属,野靛属 | ~ tinctoria 靛灰叶,野靛草

baptisin [ˈbæptizin] *n* 灰叶苦苷,野靛苦苷

baptitoxine [bæptiˈtɔksin] *n* 灰叶毒碱,野靛毒碱,金雀花碱

bar¹ [bɑː] *n* 杆,连接杆;跗骨联合;马牙龈上部;马蹄壁 | arch ~ 弓形连接杆(牙) / ~ of bladder 输尿管间嵴,输尿管间襞(膀胱) / hyoid ~s 舌骨板(第二鳃弓,舌骨弓) / lingual ~ 舌连接杆 / median ~ 正中嵴(前列腺) / palatal ~ 腭连接杆 / sternal ~ 胸骨板(胚胎期) / terminal ~s 上皮栏

bar² [bɑː] *n* 巴(压力单位, $=10^6$ dyn / cm^2)

baragnosis [ˌbæræɡˈnəusis] *n* 重量失认[症]

Bárány's symptom (sign, test) [ˈbɑːrəni] (Robert Bárány) 巴拉尼症状(征、试验)(①耳前庭器官障碍时,身体倾倒的方向与头的位置改变有关;②冷热水试验。亦称[迷路]变温试验) | ~ pointing test 巴拉尼指向试验(检脑损害)

barba [ˈbɑːbə] *n* 【拉】胡须

barba amarilla [ˈbɑːbɑː ɑːmɑːˈrijɑː] 黄须蛇,大具窍蝮蛇

barbaloin [ˈbɑːbəlɔin] *n* 芦荟苷

barban [ˈbɑːbæn] *n* 燕麦灵(除草剂)

barbaralalia [ˌbɑːbɑːrəˈleiliə] *n* 异国语言涩滞

barbasco [bɑːˈbæskəu] *n* 巴巴可鱼毒草

barberry [ˈbɑːbəri] *n* 刺檗[实]

Barber's psoriasis [ˈbɑːbə] (Harold W. Barber) 巴伯银屑病,局限性脓疱性银屑病

barbital [ˈbɑːbitæl], **barbitone** [ˈbɑːbitəun] *n* 巴比妥(催眠镇静药)

barbiturate [bɑːˈbitjurit] *n* 巴比土酸盐(催眠镇静药)

barbituric acid [ˌbɑːbiˈtjuərik] 巴比土酸

barbotage [ˌbɑːbəuˈtɑːʒ] *n* 抽液加药注射法(多用于脊髓麻醉时,分次小量抽出脑脊液,将空针内药液稀释,再行注射,直到注射完毕)

barbula [ˈbɑːbjulə] *n* 【拉】稀须,须少

Barcoo disease (rot) [bɑːˈkjuː] (Barcoo 为南澳大利亚州河名) 巴尔库病(坏疽),沙漠疮 | ~ vomit 巴尔库呕吐(表现为呕吐和恶心,伴食欲过盛,发生于南澳大利亚)

Barcroft's apparatus [ˈbɑːkrɔft] (Joseph Barcroft) 巴克罗夫特仪器(一种测压差计,用以研究血液或其他组织标本)

Bardach's test [ˈbɑːdəh] (Bruno Bardach) 巴尔达赫试验(检蛋白)

Bardenheuer's extension [ˈbɑːdənhɔiə] (Bernhard Bardenheuer) 巴登霍伊厄牵伸术(肢骨折牵伸术)

Bardet-Biedl syndrome [bɑːˈdei ˈbiːdl] (Georges Bardet; Arthur Biedl) 巴-比综合征(见 Laurence-Biedl syndrome)

Bard-Pic syndrome [bɑːd pik] (Louis Bard; Adrien Pic) 巴-皮综合征(慢性进行性黄疸)

Bard's sign [bɑːd] (Louis Bard) 巴尔征,眼球震颤征(器质性眼球震颤时,患者眼球随手指左右移动方向震颤增强,先天性眼球震颤时则无此现象)

baresthesia [ˌbærisˈθiːzjə] *n* 压觉,重觉

baresthesiometer [ˌbærisˌθiːziˈɔmitə] *n* 压觉计,压力计

Barėty's method [ˌbæreiˈti] (Jean P. Baréty) 巴雷蒂法(一种治髋病及股骨骨折的牵伸法)

Barfoed's reagent, test [ˈbɑːfed] (Christen T. Barfoed) 巴费德试剂、试验(检单糖)

Bargen's serum [ˈbɑːgən] (J. A. Bargen) 巴根血清,抗溃疡性结肠炎血清(用慢性溃疡性结肠炎病灶中分离的病原菌制备的血清) | ~ streptococcus 巴根链球菌,牛链球菌,抗链球菌血清

bariatrics [ˌbæriˈætriks] *n* 超体重学,肥胖病学(研究体重过度或肥胖的原因、预防和治疗)

baric [ˈbærik] *a* 气压的;钡的

barite [ˈbɛərait] *n* 重晶石

baritosis [bæriˈtəusis] *n* 钡尘沉着病,钡尘肺

barium (Ba) [ˈbɛəriəm] *n* 钡 | ~ cyanoplatinate, ~ platinocyanide 氯亚铂酸钡,四氰铬亚铂酸钡(用于荧光屏面的涂料) / ~ sulfate 硫酸钡(消化道 X 线造影剂)

barium-filled [ˈbɛəriəm ˌfild] *a* 充盈钡剂的

bark [bɑːk] *n* 皮,树皮 | bearberry ~, chittem ~, Persian ~ 波希鼠李皮 / calisaya ~, cinchona ~ 金鸡纳皮 / casca ~ 非洲围涎树皮 / cramp ~ 雪球荚蒾树皮 / Peruvian ~ 秘鲁皮,金鸡纳皮

Barkan's operation [ˈbɑːkən] (Otto Barkan) 巴尔坎手术,前房角切开术

barker [ˈbɑːkə] *n* (患新生期适应不良综合征的)驹子

barley [ˈbɑːli] *n* 大麦 | pearl ~ 去皮大麦粒,大麦米

Barlow's disease [ˈbɑːləu] (Thomas Barlow) 巴洛病,婴儿坏血病

Barlow syndrome [ˈbɑːləu] (John B. Barlow) 巴洛综合征(二尖瓣脱垂综合征)

barn [bɑːn] *n* 靶[恩](核截面单位, $=10^{-24}/cm^2$)

Barnes' bag (dilator) [ˈbɑːnz] (Robert Barnes) 巴恩斯袋(扩张袋),子宫颈扩张袋 | ~ curve 巴恩斯曲线(以骶岬为中心的曲线,其凹面朝向背侧)

bar(o)- [构词成分]重量,压力

baroagnosis [ˌbærəuægˈnəusis] *n* 重量失认[症]

baroceptor [ˌbærəuˈseptə] *n* 压力感受器

barodontalgia [ˌbærəudɔnˈtældʒiə] *n* 气压牙痛,航空牙痛

baroelectroesthesiometer [ˌbærəu iˌlektrəu isˌθiːziˈɔmitə] *n* 压觉电测计

barognosis [ˌbærɔgˈnəusis] *n* 压觉,辨重能

barogram [ˈbærəugræm] *n* 气压图

barograph [ˈbærəugrɑːf] *n* 气压描记器,气压自记器

baromacrometer [ˌbærəuməˈkrɔmitə] *n* (新生儿)体重身长测量器

barometer [bəˈrɔmitə] *n* 气压计,气压表;晴雨计;(反映变化的)标记 | **barometric (al)** [ˌbærəuˈmetrik(əl)] *a* 气压[计]的,测定气压的 / **barometry** *n* 气压测定法

baro-otitis [ˌbærəu əuˈtaitis] *n* 气压损伤性中耳炎 | ~ media 气压中耳炎,航空性中耳炎

baropacer [ˌbærəuˈpeisə] *n* 血压调节器(一种电子装置埋藏入犬颈,用以不断刺激颈动脉窦)

barophilic [ˌbærəuˈfilik] *a* 嗜压的(指菌细胞)

baroreceptor [ˌbærəuriˈseptə] *n* 压力感受器

baroreflex [ˌbærəuˈriːfleks] *n* 压力感受器反射

baroscope [ˈbærəuskəup] *n* 验压器;脲定量器 | **baroscopic** [ˌbærəˈskɔpik] *a*

barosinusitis [ˌbærəuˌsainəˈsaitis] *n* 气压性鼻窦炎,航空性鼻窦炎

barospirator [ˌbærəuˈspaiəreitə] *n* 变压呼吸器(一种人工呼吸器)

barotaxis [ˌbærəuˈtæksis] *n* 趋压性(生物对压力变化的反应)

barothermograph [ˌbærəuˈθəːməgrɑːf] *n* 气压温度计,气压温度记录器

barotitis [ˌbærəuˈtaitis] *n* 气压损伤性中耳炎 | ~ media 气压中耳炎,航空性中耳炎

barotrauma [ˌbærəuˈtrɔːmə] *n* 气压性损伤(耳鼓及咽鼓管) | odontalgia ~ 航空性牙痛 / otitic ~ 航空性中耳炎 / sinus ~ 鼻窦气压损伤,航空性鼻窦炎

barotropism [bəˈrɔtrəpizəm] *n* 向压性(生物对于压力刺激所引起的一种相对固定的反应,经常为一种运动)

Barraquer's disease [bɑːrəˈkəː] (Roviralta J. A. Barraquer) 进行性脂肪营养不良

Barraquer-Simons syndrome [bɑːrɑːˈkei ˈsimənz] (J. A. R. Barraquer; Arthur Simons) 巴-西综合征,部分脂肪营养不良,进行性脂肪营养不良

Barraquer's method, operation [bɑːrəˈkəː] (Ignacio Barraquer) 晶状体吸出法(治内障眼)

Barr body [bɑː] (Murray L. Barr) X 染色质,性染色质

Barré-Guillain syndrome [bɑːˈrei giˈjæn] (Jean A. Barré; Georges Guillain) 急性热病性多神经炎

barrel [ˈbærəl] *n* 桶;一桶(一种容量单位);管;筒;牙管[金属]环

Barré-Lieou syndrome [bɑːˈrei ljuː] (J. A.

Barré; Y. C. Lieou) 巴-吕综合征(后颈交感神经综合征)
Barré's sign [bɑːˈrei] (Jean A. Barré) 巴雷征(智力障碍患者虹膜收缩迟钝)
Barrett's epithelium [ˈbærət] (N. R. Barrett) 巴雷特上皮(食管组织转化的柱状上皮,见于巴雷特综合征时) | ~ syndrome (esophagus) 巴雷特综合征(食管)(食管下段消化性溃疡,常伴有狭窄) / ~ ulcer 巴雷特溃疡(食管慢性消化性溃疡)
barrier [ˈbæriə] *n* 屏障,障壁;屏蔽 | blood-air ~, blood-gas ~ 血-气屏障 / blood-brain ~, blood-cerebral ~ 血-脑屏障 / blood-thymus ~ 血-胸腺屏障 / filtration ~ 滤过屏障 / gastric mucosal ~ 胃黏膜屏障 / placental ~ 胎盘屏障 / primary protective ~s 初级防护屏蔽 / protective ~, radiation ~ 防护屏蔽,辐射屏蔽 / secondary protective ~s 次级防护屏蔽
barrow [ˈbærəu] *n* 手推车;担架
barsati [bɑːsæˈtiː] *n* 马皮疽(即皮肤丽线虫蚴疮,夏疮 cutaneous habronemiasis)
Bar's incision [bɑː] (Paul Bar) 巴尔切口(剖宫产)
Barthélemy's disease [bɑːˈteilimi] (P. T. Barthélemy) 丘疹坏死性皮结核
Barthel index [bɑːˈtel] (D. W. Barthel) 巴特尔指数(一种常用的功能评价方法,即使用标准化分类以测定诸如日常生活活动和活动度的能力)
bartholinian [ˌbɑːtəuˈliniən] *a* 巴托林管的(舌下腺大管的);巴托林腺的(前庭大腺的)
bartholinitis [ˌbɑːtəuliˈnaitis] *n* 前庭大腺炎
Bartholin's abscess [ˈbɑːtəulin] (Caspar T. Bartholin) 巴托林脓肿(前庭大腺分泌管脓肿) | ~ adenitis 前庭大腺炎 / ~ cyst 前庭大腺囊肿 / ~ duct 舌下腺大管 / ~ gland 前庭大腺
Bartholin's anus [ˈbɑːtəulin] (Thomas Bartholin) 中脑水管口
Barth's hernia [bɑːt] (Jean B. P. Barth) 巴尔特疝(位于腹壁与残存的卵黄管之间)
Barton bandage [ˈbɑːtn] (John R. Barton) 巴尔通绷带(下颌双8字形绷带) | ~ fracture 巴尔通骨折(桡骨下端骨折) / ~ operation 巴尔通手术(关节强硬手术)
Bartonella [ˌbɑːtəˈnelə] (A. L. Barton) *n* 巴尔通体属 | ~ bacilliformis 杆菌状巴尔通体
Bartonellaceae [ˌbɑːtəneˈleisiiː] *n* 巴尔通体科
bartonellemia [ˌbɑːtənəˈliːmiə] *n* 巴尔通菌血[症]
bartonelliasis [ˌbɑːtəneˈlaiəsis], **bartonellosis** [ˌbɑːtəneˈləusis] *n* 巴尔通体病
Bart's syndrome [bɑːt] (B. J. Bart) 巴特综合征(营养不良性大疱性表皮松解的一型,为常染色体显性遗传,特征为先天性局限性皮肤缺陷,伴大疱形成,系由机械性外伤和指甲营养不良所致)
Bartter's syndrome [ˈbɑːtə] (Frederic Crosby Bartter) 巴特综合征([肾小]球旁细胞肥大和增生,造成低血钾性碱中毒和醛固酮过多症,其特征为血浆肾素浓度明显增加,但不出现高血压,对血管紧张素的增压作用也不敏感。儿童常患此征,可能是遗传性的,可伴发其他异常,如智力迟钝和身材矮小。亦称[肾小]球旁细胞增生)
Baruch's law [ˈbɑːruk] (Simon Baruch) 巴鲁克定律(水疗时,当水温高于或低于皮肤温度,则起兴奋作用;当水温与皮肤温度相同时,则起镇静作用) | ~ sign 巴鲁克征(患者进行 15 min, 24 ℃水浴后,肛表测得的温度不变,提示伤寒)
baruria [bəˈrjuəriə] *n* 高比重尿
Barwell's operation [ˈbɑːwel] (Richard Barwell) 巴韦尔手术(矫正膝外翻的切骨术)
bary- [构词成分]笨重,困难,迟钝
barye [ˈbæri] *n* 巴列,微巴(压力单位)
baryencephalia [ˌbæriensiˈfeiliə] *n* 智力迟钝
baryesthesia [ˌbærisˈθiːzjə] *n* 压觉,重觉
baryglossia [ˌbæriˈglɔsiə] *n* 言语拙笨(言语重浊迟钝)
barylalia [ˌbæriˈleiliə] *n* 言语不清(由于发音缺陷,形成说话重浊不清)
baryon [ˈbæriɔn] *n* 重子
baryphonia [ˌbæriˈfəuniə] *n* 语音粗重
baryta [bəˈraitə] *n* 氧化钡;硫酸钡
Baryte [ˈbɑːrait] *n* 氧化钡;硫酸钡
barytosis [ˌbæriˈtəusis] *n* 钡尘沉着病,钡尘肺
barytron [ˈbæritrɔn] *n* 介子(亦称重电子)
basad [ˈbeisæd] *ad* 向基底
basal [ˈbeisl] *a* 基底的;基础的
basalis [beiˈseilis] *a*【拉】基底的
basaloid [ˈbeisəlɔid] *a* 基底细胞样的
basaloma [ˌbeisəˈləumə] *n* 基底细胞癌
base [beis] *n* 基底;基质;碱;基托,基板;碱基(核苷酸) | animal ~ 动物碱(一种尸碱) / ~ of heart 心脏基底 / hexone ~s, histone ~s 组蛋白碱,二氨基酸 / ~ of lung 肺底 / purine ~s, xanthine ~s 嘌呤碱,黄嘌呤碱 / record ~, temporary ~, trial ~ 记录基板,临时基板,试基板(即基板 baseplate)
basedoid [ˈbæzədɔid] *n* 类巴塞多病(类突眼性甲状腺肿,但无毒性症状)
basedowian [ˌbæzəˈdəuiən] *n* 巴塞多病者(突眼性甲状腺肿患者)
basedowiform [ˌbæzəˈdəuifɔːm] *a* 类巴塞多病的(类突眼性甲状腺肿的)

Basedow's disease [ˈbɑːzədəu] (Carl A. von Basedow) 巴塞多病(突眼性甲状腺肿) | ~ triad 巴塞多三征(甲状腺肿、突眼、心动过速) / ~ syndrome 巴塞多综合征(甲状腺功能亢进、甲状腺毒症、突眼性甲状腺肿、中毒性甲状腺肿综合征)

baseline [ˈbeislain] *n* 基线;基准

basement [ˈbeismənt] *n* 基,底

baseplate [ˈbeispleit] *n* 基板(亦称记录基板,临时基板,试基板)

bases [ˈbeisiːz] basis 的复数

bas-fond [bɑː ˈfɔːn] *n*【法】底部(尤指膀胱底)

Basham's mixture [ˈbæʃəm] (William R. Basham) 巴沙姆合剂(醋酸铁铵溶液)

basi-, basio- [构词成分]底,基底

basial [ˈbeisiəl] *a* 颅底点的

basialis [ˌbeisiˈeilis] *a*【拉】底的,基底的,颅底点的

basialveolar [ˌbeisiælˈviələ] *a* 颅底牙槽的(即颅底点到牙槽点)

basiarachnitis [ˌbeisiˌærəkˈnaitis], **basiarachnoiditis** [ˌbeisiəˌræknɔiˈdaitis] *n* 颅底蛛网膜炎

basic [ˈbeisik] *a* 基础的;基本的;碱的,盐基的

basicaryoplastin [ˌbeisiˌkæriə*u*ˈplæstin] *n* 嗜碱胞核副网素

basichromatin [ˌbeisiˈkrəumətin] *n* 嗜碱染色质

basichromiole [ˌbeisiˈkrəumiəul] *n* 嗜碱染色微粒

basicity [bəˈsisəti] *n* 碱性;碱度

basicranial [ˌbeisiˈkreinjəl] *a* 颅底的

basicytoparaplastin [ˌbeisiˌsaitə*u*pærəˈplæstin] *n* 嗜碱胞质副网素

basidia [bəˈsidiə] basidium 的复数

Basidiobolaceae [bəˌsidiə*u*bəˈleisiiː] *n* 蛙粪霉科

basidiobolomycosis [bəˌsidiˌɔbələ*u*maiˈkəusis] *n* 蛙粪虫霉病

Basidiobolus [bəˌsidiˈɔbələs] *n* 蛙粪霉属 | ~ haptosporus, ~ meristosporus 固孢蛙粪霉,裂孢蛙粪霉

basidiocarp [bəˈsidiə*u*ˌkɑːp] *n* 担子果

basidiomycete [bəˌsidiə*u*ˈmaisiːt] *n* 担子菌

Basidiomycetes [bəˌsidiə*u*maiˈsiːtiːz] *n* 担子菌纲

basidiomycetous [bəˌsidiə*u*maiˈsiːtəs] *a* 担子菌的

Basidiomycota [bəˌsidiə*u*maiˈkəutə] *n* 担子菌门

Basidiomycotina [bəˌsidiə*u*ˌmaikə*u*ˈtainə] *n* 担子菌亚门

basidiospore [bəˈsidiəspɔː] *n* 担孢子 | **basidiosporous** [bəˌsidiəˈspɔːrəs] *a*

basidium [bəˈsidjəm] ([复] **basidia** [bəˈsidiə]) *n* 担子

basifacial [beisiˈfeiʃəl] *a* 面基的,面下部的

basification [ˌbeisifiˈkeiʃən] *n* 碱化

basify [ˈbeisifai] *vt* 碱化

basigenous [bəˈsidʒinəs] *a* 成碱的,生盐基的

basihyoid [ˌbeisiˈhaiɔid], **basihyal** [ˌbeisiˈhaiəl] *n* 舌骨体

basil [ˈbæzl] *n* 罗勒,矮糠

basilad [ˈbeisilæd] *ad* 向基底;向底面

basilar [ˈbæsilə] *a* 基础的;基底的

basilaris [ˌbæsiˈlɛəris] *a*【拉】基底的

basilateral [ˌbeisiˈlætərəl] *a* 基侧的

basilemma [ˌbeisiˈlemə] *n* 基膜

basilic [bəˈsilik] *a* 贵要的(静脉)

basiliximab [ˌbæsiˈliksimæb] *n* 巴昔单抗(由重组技术产生的一种嵌合鼠/人单克隆抗体;它是一种白细胞介素-2 受体拮抗药,并用作免疫抑制药,预防肾移植后急性器官排斥反应,作为治疗方案的一部分,其中亦包括环孢素和皮质类固醇,静脉注射给药)

basiloma [bæsiˈləumə] *n* 基底细胞癌

basin [ˈbeisn] *n* 盆;骨盆 | eye bath ~ 洗眼受水器

basinasial [ˌbeisiˈneiziəl] *a* 颅底鼻根的(指颅骨测量线:示颅底长度,即枕骨大孔前缘点到鼻根点的距离)

basi(o)- [构词成分]基底;颅底;碱基

basioccipital [ˌbeisiɔkˈsipitl] *a* 枕骨底部的

basioglossus [ˌbeisiə*u*ˈglɔsəs] *n* 舌骨舌肌舌骨部

basion [ˈbeisiɔn] *n* 颅底点(枕骨大孔前缘中点)

basiotic [ˌbeisiˈɔtik] *n* 耳底骨

basiparachromatin [ˌbeisiˌpærəˈkrəumətin] *n* 嗜碱副染色质

basiparaplastin [ˌbeisiˌpærəˈplæstin] *n* 嗜碱副网素

basipetal [beiˈsipətl] *a* 向基的(如孢子)

basiphilic [ˌbeisiˈfilik] *a* 嗜碱的

basirhinal [ˌbeisiˈrainl] *a* 脑底鼻的

basis [ˈbeisis] ([复] **bases** [ˈbeisiːz] *n* 基底,底

basisphenoid [ˌbeisiˈsfiːnɔid] *n* 蝶底骨

basitemporal [ˌbeisiˈtempərəl] *a* 颞骨底部的

basivertebral [ˌbeisiˈvəːtibrəl] *a* 椎骨体的

basket [ˈbɑːskit] *n* 篮;篮状结构;篮状细胞 | cytopharyngeal ~ 胞咽篮(见 cyrtos) / fiber ~s 纤维篮(视网膜)

Basle Nomina Anatomica [ˈbɑːzl ˈnɔminə ænəˈtɔmikə] 巴塞尔解剖学名词{1895 年在瑞士巴塞尔会议决定的,现已为 Terminologia Anatomica [TA](1998)所取代}

bas(o)- 见 basi(o)-

basocatenulate [ˌbeisəukəˈtenjulit, -leit] *a* 基底成链形的,基底串珠状的

basocyte [ˈbeisə*u*sait] *n* 嗜碱粒细胞

basocytopenia [ˌbeisəuˌsaitəuˈpiːniə] *n* 嗜碱粒细胞减少[症]

basocytosis [ˌbeisəusaiˈtəusis] *n* 嗜碱粒细胞增多[症]

basoerythrocyte [ˌbeisəuiˈriθrəsait] *n* 含嗜碱点彩红细胞

basoerythrocytosis [ˌbeisəuiˌriθrəsaiˈtəusis] *n* 含嗜碱点彩红细胞增多[症]

basograph [ˈbeisəugrɑːf, græf] *n* 异常步态描记器

basolateral [ˌbeisəuˈlætərəl] *a* [基]底外侧的

basometachromophil [ˌbeisəuˌmetəˈkrəuməfil] *a* 嗜碱性异染性的

Basommatophora [beiˌsɔməˈtɔfɔrə] *n* 基眼亚目

basopenia [ˌbeisəuˈpiːniə] *n* 嗜碱粒细胞减少

basophil [ˈbeisəufil] *a* 嗜碱的 *n* 嗜碱性粒细胞

basophilia [ˌbeisəuˈfiliə] *n* 嗜碱性;嗜碱粒细胞增多

basophilic [beisəuˈfilik], **basophile** [ˈbeisəufail], **basophilous** [beiˈsɔfiləs] *a* 嗜碱的

basophilism [beiˈsɔfilizəm] *n* 嗜碱粒细胞增多

basophilopenia [ˌbeisəuˌfiləuˈpiːniə] *n* 嗜碱粒细胞减少

basoplasm [ˈbeisəuˌplæzəm] *n* 嗜碱胞质

Bassen-Kornzweig syndrome [ˈbæsən ˈkɔːnzwaig] (Frank A. Bassen; Abraham L. Kornzweig) 巴-康综合征,无β脂蛋白血症

Basset's operation [bəˈsei] (Antoine Basset) 巴塞手术(腹股沟淋巴结清除术,治女外阴癌)

Bassini's operation [bəˈsini] (Edoardo Bassini) 巴西尼手术(腹股沟疝根治手术)

bassorin [ˈbæsərin] *n* 巴索林,黄蓍胶素(用作佐药)

basswood [ˈbæswud] *n* 美椴木(美民间药材,治胆、肝疾病)

bast [bæst] *n* 韧皮,内皮

bastard [ˈbæstəd] *n* 私生子 *a* 私生的;假的

bastardize [ˈbæstədaiz] *vt* 证明…为假(或谬误)的

Bastedo's rule [bæsˈtiːdəu] (Walter A. Bastedo) 巴斯特多规则(将成人剂量乘以儿童年龄再加3,然后除以30,即为小儿用量)

Bastian-Bruns law (sign) [ˈbæstʃən brunz] (Henry C. Bastian; Ludwig Bruns) 巴斯钦-布伦斯定律(征)(如从头部到腰膨大部的脊髓有完全横截损害,下肢腱反射就消失)

basylous [ˈbæsiləs] *a* 碱性的,碱式的

bat [bæt] *n* 蝙蝠 | vampire ~ 吸血蝠,魑蝠

batch [bætʃ] *n* 批,分批;程序组

bate [beit] *vt* 抑制 | with ~d breath 屏息

Bateman's disease [ˈbeitmən] (Thomas Bateman) 贝特曼病,触染性软疣

bath [bɑːθ] ([复]**baths**) *n* 浴;浴剂;浴器 *vt*, *vi* 洗澡 | cold ~ 冷水浴(19 ℃以下) / contrast ~ 冷热交替浴 / douche ~ 冲浴 / earth ~ 沙土浴 / graduated ~ 温度递变浴 / hot ~ 热水浴(37 ~ 40 ℃) / hot-air ~ 热气浴,热汽浴(38 ~ 55 ℃) / hyperthermal ~ 高温浴(40 ℃以上) / immersion ~ 浸浴 / lukewarm ~ 温水浴(34 ~ 36 ℃) / medicated ~ 药浴 / sheet ~ 湿单浴 / shower ~ 淋浴;淋浴装置;淋浴室 / sitz ~ 坐浴 / sponge ~ 擦浴 / sweat ~ 发汗浴 / tepid ~ 微温浴(24 ~ 33 ℃) / warm ~ 温浴(33 ~ 36 ℃)

bathesthesia [ˌbæθesˈθiːzjə] *n* 深部感觉

bathmotropic [ˌbæθməuˈtrɔpik] *a* 变阈性的 | negatively ~ 负变阈性的 / positively ~ 正变阈性的

bathmotropism [bæθˈmɔtrəpizəm] *n* 变阈性,变阈作用

bath(o)- 见 bathy-

bathochrome [ˈbæθəkrəum] *n* 向红团(一原子或基团,它导入一个化合物时会将化合物的吸收峰移向一个较长的波长)

bathochromy [ˌbæθəuˈkrəumi] *n* 向红团作用,向红

bathoflore [ˈbæθəflɔː] *n* 减荧光物

bathometer [bəˈθɔmitə] *n* 水深测量器

bathomorphic [ˌbæθəuˈmɔːfik] *a* 凹眼的;近视眼的

bathorhodopsin [ˌbæθəurəuˈdɔpsin] *n* 红光视紫红质

bathrocephaly [ˌbæθrəˈsefəli] *n* 梯[形]头(颅骨后部梯状突出的发育异常)

bathy- [构词成分]深,底

bathyanesthesia [ˌbæθiˌænisˈθiːzjə] *n* 深部感觉缺失

bathycardia [ˌbæθiˈkɑːdiə] *n* 低位心(由于解剖原因而并非由疾病引起)

bathyesthesia [ˌbæθisˈθiːzjə] *n* 深部感觉

bathyhyperesthesia [ˌbæθiˌhaipərəsˈθiːzjə] *n* 深部感觉过敏

bathyhypesthesia [ˌbæθiˌhipəsˈθiːzjə] *n* 深部感觉迟钝

bathypnea [ˌbæθiˈpniːə] *n* 深呼吸

BATO a boronic acid adduct of technetium complexed to 8-hydroxyquinoline (oxime) 锝络合8-羟基喹啉(肟)的硼酸加合物

batonet [beitəˈnet] *n* 假染色体

batrachoplasty [ˈbætrəkəuˌplæsti] *n* 舌下囊肿修治术

batrachotoxin [ˌbætrəkəuˈtɔksin] *n* 南美蟾毒(一种极其强烈的类固醇毒液,自南美的一种蛙皮中提炼而得)

Batson's plexus [ˈbætsn] (Oscar V. Batson) 巴森丛,脊椎丛

battarism [ˈbætərizəm], **battarismus** [ˈbætərizməs] *n* 口吃,结舌

Batten disease [ˈbætən] (Frederick E. Batten) 巴腾病(①见 Vogt-Spielmeyer disease; ②较普遍的看法,系指构成神经元蜡样脂褐素沉积症的任何一组或全部疾患)

batter¹ [ˈbætə] *vt* 用旧;磨损

batter² [ˈbætə] *vt*, *vi* 内倾;上倾 *n* 内倾度;上倾度

Battern-Mayou disease [ˈbætən meiˈjuː] (F. E. Batten; Marmaduke S. Mayou) 巴-梅病(见 Batten disease)

battery [ˈbætəri] *n* 电池(组);一套(试验) | solar ~ 太阳电池

Battey bacilli [ˈbæti] 巴蒂杆菌(一种未分类的分枝杆菌,使人产生类似结核的疾病)

batteyin [ˈbætiin] *n* 巴蒂杆菌素,细胞内分枝杆菌素(一种巴蒂杆菌产物,类似结核菌素,用作皮肤过敏性试验)

Battle-Jalaguier-Kammerer incision [ˈbætl ʒɑːlɑːgiˈei ˈkæmərə] (W. H. Battle; Adolphe Jalaguier; Frederic Kammerer) 巴-雅-卡切口(见 Kammerer-Battle incision)

Battle's incision [ˈbætl] (William Henry Battle) 巴特尔切口(见 Kammerer-Battle incision) | ~ operation 巴特尔手术(使腹直肌暂时移位的一种阑尾切除术) / ~ sign 巴特尔征(耳后淤血斑)

Battley's sedative [ˈbætli] (Richard Battley) 巴特利镇静剂(由阿片浸膏、沸水、乙醇及凉水制成的一种液剂)

Baudelocque's diameter (line) [bəudˈlɔk] (Jean L. Baudelocque) 鲍德洛克径(线)(骨盆外直径)

Bauhin's gland [ˈbəuæn] (Gaspard 〈Caspard〉 Bauhin) 舌尖腺 | ~ valve 回盲瓣,结肠瓣

Baumès' law [bɔˈme] (Pieere P. F. Baumès) 博梅定律(见 Colles' law)

Baumé's scale [bɔˈmei] (Antoine Baumé) 波美比重标(测液体的密度)

Baumès' symptom [bɔˈme] (Jean B. T. Baumès) 博梅症状(心绞痛征)

bauxite [ˈbɔːksait] *n* 铝土矿,矾土

bay [bei] *n* 湖,湾;凹入处;隐窝 | lacrimal ~ 泪湖 / sick ~ 军舰卫生所,船上诊所

bayberry [ˈbeibəri] *n* 月桂[树]果;蜡果杨梅;玉桂[果]

Bayer 205 [ˈbeiə] 拜耳二〇五,舒拉明钠(治锥虫病与丝虫病药)

Bayes theorem [beiz] (Thomas Bayes) 贝叶斯定理{用以互换条件参数的定理:$P(B \mid A) = \frac{P(A \mid B)P(B)}{P(A \mid B)P(B) + P(A 非 B)P(非 B)}$)式中 P(A)和 P(B)是两项事件的概率,A 和 B 以及 P(A | B)和 P(B | A)是 A 已知 B 和 B 已知 A 的条件概率。举例说,如 A 表示阳性化验结果,B 表示受试病人实际存在的疾病,那么 P(A | B)即为该试验的"诊断敏感性"(真实阳性率),P(B)则为该病的患病率[P(A)为阳性试验的结果]。P(B | A)为阳性试验的预测值,即出现阳性反应的患者实际患有该病的概率}

bayesian statistics [ˈbeiziən] (T. Bayes) 贝叶斯统计(一种统计方法学)

Bayle's disease [beil] (Antoine L. J. Bayle) 贝尔病,麻痹性痴呆

Bayle's granulations [beil] (Gaspard L. Bayle) 贝尔肉芽(肺内已有纤维样变性的灰色结核性结节)

Bayliss effect [ˈbeilis] (Sir William M. Bayliss) 贝利斯效应(灌注压增高及随后的血管平滑肌伸展,可使肌肉收缩和阻抗增加,但灌注压虽高,仍可使血流恢复正常)

Baynton's bandage [ˈbeintn] (Thomas Baynton) 贝恩顿绷带(用绊创膏敷于腿部治疗无痛性溃疡)

Bazex's syndrome [bɑːˈzeks] (J. Bazex) 巴泽克斯综合征(上呼吸道或消化道癌症患者,在耳、鼻、颊、手、足和膝部出现湿疹性和银屑病样损害。亦称类肿瘤性肢端角化症)

Bazillenemulsion [bəˌziləniˈmʌlʃən] *n*【德】杆菌性乳剂

Bazin's disease [bɑːzæn] (Antoine P. E. Bazin) 巴赞病,硬结性红斑,硬红斑

BBB blood-brain barrier 血-脑屏障; bundle branch block 束支传导阻滞

BBBB bilateral bundle branch block 双侧束支传导阻滞

BBT basal body temperature 基础体温

BC bone conduction 骨导

β1C 补体因子 C3 的旧称

BCAA branched chain amino acid 支链氨基酸

B-CAVe bleomycin, lomustine, doxorubicin and vinblastine 博来霉素-洛莫司汀-多柔比星-长春碱(联合化疗治癌方案)

BCDF B cell differentiation factors B 细胞分化因子

BCF basophil chemotactic factor 嗜碱粒细胞趋化因子

BCG bacille Calmette Guérin 卡介菌; ballistocardiogram 心冲击[描记]图; bicolor guaiac test 双色愈创木脂试验(检脑脊液)

BCGF B cell growth factors B[淋巴]细胞生长因子

BCNU carmustine 卡莫司汀(抗肿瘤药)
b. d. bis die【拉】每日 2 次
BDA British Dental Association 英国牙科协会
Bdella [ˈdelə] *n*【希】吸螨属
bdellepithecium [ˌdelipiˈθiːsiəm] *n* 人工吸血管
bdellium [ˈdeliəm] *n* 伪没药,非洲香胶
bdellometer [deˈlɔmitə] *n* 吸血器
bdellotomy [deˈlɔtəmi] *n* 切蛭吸血法
Bdellovibrio [ˌdeləuˈvibriəu] *n* 蛭弧菌属
bdellovibrio [ˌdeləuˈvibriəu] *n* 蛭弧菌
B-DNA B-脱氧核糖核酸
BDS Bachelor of Dental Surgery 牙外科学士
BDSc Bachelor of Dental Science 牙科学士
Be beryllium 铍
β1E 补体因子 C4 的旧称
bead [biːd] *n* 珠;水珠 *vt* 使形成珠状,使形成串珠状 | rachitic ~s 佝偻病性串珠
beaded [ˈbiːdid] *a* 连珠状的,串珠状的
beading [ˈbiːdiŋ] *n* 串珠型(血管局部交替收缩和扩张,因此在血管造影片上类似一串念珠)
beak [biːk] *n* 喙;喙状物
beaker [ˈbiːkə] *n* 烧杯
Beale's ganglion cells [biːl] (Lionel S. Beale) 比尔神经节细胞(双极细胞)
Beals' syndrome [biːlz] (Rodney K. Beals) 比尔斯综合征,先天性挛缩性细长指,先天性挛缩性细长趾
beam [biːm] *n* 梁;道,束,柱(光学用);梁架(牙);射束,射线 *vi* 发光;发热 *vt* 发射;探测 | cantilever ~ 悬臂梁 / continuous ~ 连续架 / simple ~ 简单支架 / useful ~ 有用光束
beamtherapy [biːmˈθerəpi] *n* 光束疗法(光谱疗法;远距镭疗法)
bean [biːn] *n* 豆;豆形果实 | soya ~ 大豆
bearberry [ˈbεəbəri] *n* 熊果
Beard's disease [biəd] (George M. Beard) 比尔德病,神经衰弱
bearing [ˈbεəriŋ] *n* 支承面,支承点 | ~ down 下坠感(盆腔内);分娩时屏气 / central ~ 中心支承(颌间)
Bearn-Kunkel syndrome, Bearn-Kunkel-Slater syndrome [bəːn ˈkuŋkel ˈsleitə] (Alexander Gordon Bearn; Henry George Kunkel; Robert James Slater) 狼疮样肝炎
bearwood [ˈbεəwud] *n* 波希鼠李皮(轻泻药)
beat [biːt] *n* 搏动 | apex ~ 心尖搏动 / dropped ~ 脱漏搏动;脉搏短绌,间隙脉 / ectopic ~ 异位搏动 / escape ~ 逸搏 / premature ~ 期前收缩
beating [ˈbiːtiŋ] *n* 搏动
Beau's disease [bəu] (Joseph H. S. Beau) 博氏病,心功能不全 | ~ lines 博氏线(指甲在全身病时所显横线或横沟,但也由外伤、冠状动脉闭塞、血钙过多、皮肤病等所致) / ~ syndrome 博氏综合征,心脏停搏
Beauveria [bəuˈviəriə] *n* 白僵菌属 | ~ bassiana 巴西安白僵菌 / ~ tenella 纤细白僵菌
bebeerine [biˈbiriːn] *n* 比比林,甘蜜树皮碱(疟疾时用的补药)
bebeeru [biˈbiru] *n* 比比路,甘蜜树皮(疟疾时用的补药)
becanthone hydrochloride [biˈkænθəun] 盐酸贝恩酮(抗血吸虫药)
becaplermin [bəˈkæpləːmin] *n* 贝卡勒明(由重组 DNA 技术产生的人血小板衍生生长因子,其作用类似内源性血小板衍生生长因子,并局部用于治疗下肢已深入或超越皮下组织的神经病性糖尿病性溃疡)
Beccari process [beˈkɑːri] (Giuseppe Beccari) 贝卡里垃圾处理法(利用封闭池内通过细菌发酵处理垃圾)
bechic [ˈbekik] *a* 咳嗽的 *n* 镇咳药
Bechterew [bekˈtəːjev] 见 Bekhterev
Becker's muscular dystrophy, Becker type muscular dystrophy [ˈbekə] (Peter E. Becker) 贝克尔肌萎缩,贝克尔型肌萎缩(十分类似迪谢内〈Duchenne〉肌萎缩的一型,但起病晚,病程进行缓慢,为 X 连锁特性遗传)
Becker's nevus [ˈbekə] (Samuel William Becker) 贝克痣(此痣多见于 20 ~ 30 岁男子,含有表皮黑变病,呈现节段性、均匀、浅色色素沉着,数年后从患部长出黑色长毛。亦称迟发性斑痣、色素性多毛性表皮痣)
Becker's phenomenon (sign) [ˈbekə] (Otto H. E. Becker) 贝克尔现象(征)(突眼性甲状腺肿时视网膜动脉搏动增加) | ~ test 贝克尔试验(检散光)
Beckmann's apparatus [ˈbekmən] (Ernst O. Beckmann) 贝克曼仪器(借溶液的冰点的下降,或沸点的上升,以测定分子量)
Beck's (Bek's) disease [bek] (E. V. Beck〈或 Bek〉) 贝克病(即 Kashin-Bek disease)
Beck's gastrostomy [bek] (Carl Beck) 贝克胃造口术(从胃大弯到腹壁表面构成管道造胃瘘)
Beck's triad [bek] (Claude S. Beck) 贝克三体征(静脉压上升、动脉压下降、心脏小而收缩减弱,为心脏压塞三特征)
Beckwith's syndrome, Beckwith-Wiedemann syndrome [ˈbekwiθ ˈviːdəmɑːn] (John Bruce Beckwitn; Hans Rudolf Wiedemann) 贝克威恩综合征,贝-维综合征(表现程度不等的先天性常染色体显性遗传综合征,特征为脐疝、巨舌和巨大发育,常伴有内脏肥大、肾上腺皮质细胞肥大和肾髓发育不良。亦称脐疝-巨舌-巨大发育综合征)
Béclard's amputation [beiˈklɑː] (Pierre A.

Béclard）贝克拉尔切断术（髋关节处截断时先切割后皮瓣）| ~ hernia 贝克拉尔疝（穿过大隐静脉孔的股疝）/ ~ triangle 贝克拉尔三角（介于舌骨舌肌后缘、二腹肌后腹与舌骨大角之间）

beclomethasone dipropionate [ˌbekləˈmeθəsəun] 二丙酸倍氯米松（糖皮质激素）

becquerel（Bq）[bekəˈrel] *n* 贝克[勒尔]（放射性强度单位）

Becquerel's rays [bekˈrel]（Antoine H. Becquerel）铀射线

bed [bed] *n* 床；褥；底座；床位 | air ~ 气褥 / air fluidized ~ 气垫床 / capillary ~ 毛细血管床 / hydrostatic ~, water ~ 水褥（防止褥疮用）/ metabolic ~ 代谢测定床 / nail ~ 甲床

bedbug [ˈbedbʌg] *n* 臭虫

bedclothes [ˈbedkləuðz] *n* 床上用品（指被、褥等）

bedfast [ˈbedfəst] *a*（因病）卧床不起的

bedlam [ˈbedləm] *n* 精神病院；病狂状态；精神病

bedlamism [ˈbedləmizəm] *n* 疯狂状态，精神病

bedlamite [ˈbedləmait] *n* 精神病患者；疯子

bed-lift [ˈbedlift] *n* 床靠（使伤病员能坐起的病床活动装置）

Bednar's aphtha [ˈbednɑː]（Alois Bednar）贝德纳尔口疮，硬腭口疮（婴儿硬腭后部感染性创伤性溃疡）

bedpan [ˈbedpæn] *n*（尤指病人在床上用的）便盆

bedrid [ˈbedrid], **bedridden**[ˈbedˌridn] *a*（因病或衰老等而长期）卧床不起的

bedside [ˈbedsaid] *n*（尤指病人的）床侧 | ~ teaching 临床教学 / ~ manner 医生对病人的态度

Bedsonia [bedˈsəuniə] *n* 衣原体属

bedsore [ˈbedˌsɔː] *n* 褥疮

bedtime [ˈbedtaim] *n* 就寝时间

bed-wetting [ˈbedˌwetiŋ] *n* 溺褥，遗尿

bee [biː] *n* 蜜蜂

beef [biːf]（[复]**beeves** 或 **beefs**）*n* 牛肉 | ~, iron, and wine 牛肉铁酒（以牛肉膏、枸橼酸铁铵和雪利酒制成，以前用作补血药）

Beer-Lambert law [biə ˈlæmbət]（August Beer; J. H. Lambert）比尔-朗伯定律（见 Beer's law）

Beer's collyrium [biə]（Georg J. Beer）比尔洗眼液（含醋酸铅、玫瑰水、迷迭香酯）| ~ knife 比尔刀（内障刀）/ ~ operation 比尔手术（带结膜瓣的白内障摘出术）

Beer's law [biə]（August Beer）比尔定律（一个溶液的吸光度〈A〉与光路的长度〈b〉和浓度〈c〉成正比；正比常数为摩尔吸光系数〈ε〉，因此 $A = \varepsilon bc$）

beerwort [ˈbiəwəːt] *n* 麦芽汁（啤酒原料）

beeswax [ˈbiːzwæks] *n* 蜂蜡 | bleached ~ 白[蜂]蜡 / unbleached ~ 黄[蜂]蜡

beet [biːt] *n* 甜菜；甜菜根

beetle [ˈbiːtl] *n* 甲虫 | blister ~ 斑蝥 / rove ~ 隐翅虫

Beevor's sign [ˈbiːvə]（Charles E. Beevor）比弗征（①功能性麻痹时，患者不能抑制对抗肌；②患者抬头时脐向上偏移，为下腹肌无力之征）

Begbie's disease [ˈbegbi]（James Begbie）贝格比病（见 Graves' disease）

Beggiatoa [ˌbedʒiəˈtəuə]（F. S. Beggiato）*n* 贝氏硫菌属

Beggiatoaceae [ˌbedʒiətəuˈeisiiː] *n* 贝氏硫菌科

Beggiatoales [ˌbedʒiətəuˈeiliːz] *n* 贝氏硫菌目

Begg's appliance [beg]（Peter R. Begg）贝格矫治器 | ~ technique 贝格正牙术

Béguez César disease [ˈbeigeis ˈseisɑː]（Antonio Béguez César）贝盖斯·赛萨病（即 Chédiak-Higashi syndrome）

behavio(u)r [biˈheivjə] *n* 行为；举止，态度 | automatic ~ 自动症，自动行为 / invariable ~ 固定性活动 / operant ~ 操作性行为 / respondent ~ 应答行为 / variable ~ 可变性活动 | **~al** [biˈheivjərəl] *a* 关于行为的

behavio(u)rism [biˈheivjərizəm] *n* 行为主义 | **behavio(u)rist** *n* 行为主义者

Behçet's syndrome [beihˈtʃet]（Hulusi Behçet）贝赫切特综合征，眼、口、生殖器三联综合征（眼葡萄膜炎、视网膜脉管炎、视神经萎缩、口疮和生殖器溃疡）

behenate [biˈheneit] *n* 山萮酸盐（或酯）；山萮酸（阴离子型）

behenic acid [biˈhenik] 山萮酸

Béhier-Hardy sign（syndrome）[ˈbeihiə ˈhɑːdi]（Louis J. Béhier; Louis P. A. Hardy）贝希厄-哈迪征（综合征）（早期肺坏疽的失声症）

Behla's bodies [ˈbeilə]（Robert F. Behla）贝拉体（见 Plimmer's bodies）

Behring's law [ˈbeiriŋ]（Emil A. von Behring）贝林定律，免疫转移定律（免疫者的血或血清转输给另一个体时能使后者获得免疫）| ~ tuberculin 贝林结核菌素（结核菌浸剂；结核菌蜡）

Behr's disease [bɛə]（Carl Behr）贝尔病（成人视网膜黄斑变性）| ~ pupil 贝尔瞳孔（视束病变时对侧瞳孔散大）

BEI butanol-extractable iodine 丁醇提取碘

Beigel's disease [ˈbaigəl]（Hermann Beigel）拜格尔病，毛孢子菌病

beikost [ˈbaikəust] *n*【德】固体和半固体婴儿食物

bejel [ˈbedʒəl] *n* 地方性梅毒

Békésy audiometry [ˈbeikeʃi]（Georg von Békésy）贝凯西测听法（患者按一信号按钮，描记他的单耳低音音阈，音强在揿按钮时减少，

放开时则增强,连续低音和中断钝音两者均可测听)

Bekhterev's (Bechterew's) spondylitis [bek'tə:jev] (Vladimir M. Bekhterev) 别赫捷列夫脊椎炎,类风湿脊柱炎 | ~ layer 别赫捷列夫层(大脑皮质外粒层的纤维层) / ~ nucleus 前庭神经上核 / ~ reaction 别赫捷列夫反应(肌强直时,引起肌肉收缩所需电流最小量,在电流每次中断或密度变化时,应加以减少,以防止强直性收缩) / ~ reflex 别赫捷列夫反射(深层反射;下腹部反射;倒错性瞳孔反射;鼻反射) / ~ sign 别赫捷列夫征(别赫捷列夫反射;自动运动面肌麻痹) / ~ test 别赫捷列夫试验(检坐骨神经痛)

Bekhterev-Mendel reflex [bek'tə:jev 'mendəl] (V. M. Bekhterev; Kurt Mendel) 别赫捷列夫-孟德尔反射(见 Mendel-Bekhterev reflex)

bel (B) [bel] *n* 贝[尔](电平单位或声的响度单位)

Belascaris [bə'læskəris] *n* 弓蛔虫属

belch [beltʃ] *vt, vi* 嗳气;呕吐 *n* 嗳气;呕吐物

belching ['beltʃiŋ] *n* 嗳气

belemnoid [bi'lemnɔid] *a* 刺状的 *n* (尺骨或颞骨的)茎突

Belfield's operation ['belfi:ld] (William T. Belfield) 输精管切断术

belladonna [ˌbelə'dɔnə] *n* 颠茄;颠茄叶

belladonnine [ˌbelə'dɔni:n] *n* 颠茄碱

bellaradine [be'lɑ:rədin] *n* 红古豆碱

bell-crowned [bel'kraund] *a* 钟形冠的(牙科)

Bellini's ducts (tubules) [be'li:ni] (Lorenzo Bellini) 肾直小管 | ~ ligament 髂转子韧带

Bell-Magendie law ['bel məʒɑ:n'di:, mə'dʒendi] (Charles Bell; François Magendie) 贝-马定律(见 Bell's law)

Bellocq's cannula (sound, tube) [be'lɔk] (Jean J. Bellocq) 贝洛克套管(塞后鼻孔套管,控制鼻出血)

Bell's law [bel] (Charles Bell) 贝尔定律(脊髓神经前根为运动根,后根为感觉根) | ~ nerve 胸长神经 / ~ palsy (paralysis) 贝尔麻痹(面神经麻痹) / ~ phenomenon 贝尔现象(面瘫患者闭眼时,患侧眼珠向外、上方转动)

Bell's mania (disease) [bel] (Luther V. Bell) 急性谵妄

Bell's muscle [bel] (John Bell) 贝尔肌(输尿管口和膀胱悬雍垂之间的肌性索带,形成膀胱三角区的周界)

Bell's treatment [bel] (William B. Bell) 贝尔疗法(注射胶态铅制剂,治癌用)

belly ['beli] *n* 腹;肌腹 | drum ~ 气臌,臌胀 / swollen ~ 膨胀腹(动物的膨胀) / wooden ~ 板样腹

bellyache ['belieik] *n* 腹痛

belly-bound ['beli baund] *a* 便秘的

bellybutton ['beliˌbʌtn] *n* 脐

bellyful ['beliful] *n* 饱,过饱

belonephobia [ˌbelәni'fәubiә] *n* 尖物恐怖,恐锐症

belonoid ['belәnɔid] *a* 针形的;柱状的

belonoskiascopy [ˌbelәnәuskai'æskәpi] *n* 针形检影法(一种他觉视网膜镜检法)

beloxamide [bi'lɔksәmaid] *n* 贝洛酰胺(抗胆固醇血症药)

Belsey Mark IV operation (fundoplication) ['belsi] (Ronald H. R. Belsey) 贝尔西标志 IV 手术(胃底折叠术) | ~ hiatal hernia repair 贝尔西食管裂孔疝修补

bemegride ['bemigraid] *n* 贝美格(中枢兴奋药,用于治疗巴比土酸盐中毒)

bemidone ['bemidәun] *n* 羟基哌替啶,羟基度冷丁(曾用作麻醉药和镇痛药)

bemoan [bi'mәun] *vt* 悲叹;哀泣

bemuse [bi'mju:z] *vt* 使麻木;使出神

benactyzine hydrochloride [be'næktizi:n] 盐酸贝那替秦(抗胆碱能药,用作安定药)

benapryzine hydrochloride [benә'praizi:n] 盐酸贝那利秦(抗胆碱能药,抗震颤麻痹药)

benazepril hydrochloride [be'neizәpril] 盐酸贝那普利(血管紧张素转化酶抑制剂,口服治疗高血压)

Bence Jones albumosuria [benzdʒәunz] (Henry Bence Jones) 本周脲尿(多发性骨髓瘤) | ~ cylinders 本周圆柱体(精囊内圆柱形胶状物) | ~ protein 本周蛋白(多发性骨髓瘤患者尿中含轻链二聚体蛋白,在 45 ~ 55 ℃凝聚,沸点时部分或全部溶解) | ~ proteinuria 本周蛋白尿(尿中出现本周蛋白) | ~ reaction 本周反应(检蛋白)

bend [bend] *n* 弯,曲;弯曲处 | first order ~s 第一步弯曲(水平面曲) / second order ~s 第二步弯曲(垂直曲面) / third order ~s 第三步弯曲(维持或扭转牙的弓) / V ~s V 形弯曲 | the ~s 潜函病;高空病(亦称减压病,因空气栓塞所致的四肢关节、肌肉和腹腔的剧痛)

bendazac ['bendәzæk] *n* 苄达酸(抗炎药)

Bender Visual-Motor Gestalt test ['bendә] (Lauretta Bender) 本德尔视觉-运动完形测验(一种心理学测验,用于评估知觉-运动协调,评定人格动力学〈如器质性脑损伤试验〉以及检测神经系统发育程度。令受试者徒手照画分见于卡片上的 9 个简单的几何图形,或有时令其凭记忆复绘)

bendroflumethiazide [ˌbendrәuˌflumi'θaiәzaid], **bendrofluazide** [ˌbendrәu'fluәzaid] *n* 苄氟噻嗪

(利尿降压药)

bene [ˈbenei]【拉】佳适,无恙

beneceptor [ˈbeniseptə] *n* 良性感受器

Beneckea [biˈnekiə] *n* 贝内克菌属

Benedict's solution [ˈbenidikt] (Stanley R. Benedict) 本内迪克特溶液(用于尿液分析) | ~ test 本内迪克特试验(检尿内葡萄糖;检尿素)

Benedikt's syndrome [ˈbenidikt] (Moritz Benedikt) 贝内迪克特综合征(一侧动眼神经麻痹,对侧运动过度,对侧肢体震颤和轻瘫,一侧运动失调)

benign [biˈnain] *a* 良性的;不复发的;可复原的

benignant [biˈnignənt] *a* 良性的 | **benignancy** *n*

Béniqué's sound [beiniˈkei] (Pierre J. Béniqué) 贝尼凯探子(扩尿道)

benjamin [ˈbendʒəmin] *n* 安息香

Bennet's corpuscles [ˈbenit] (James H. Bennet) 贝内特体(大体,即卵巢囊内经历高度脂肪变性的上皮细胞;小体,即卵巢囊液中所见的透明微小细胞)

Bennett's disease [ˈbenit] (John H. Bennett) 贝内特病,白血病

Bennett's fracture [ˈbenit] (Edward H. Bennett) 贝内特骨折(第一掌骨基底部骨折进入腕关节内及并发半脱位) | ~ operation 贝内特手术(精索静脉曲张手术)

benny [ˈbeni] *n* 安非他明药片(一种兴奋药)

benorterone [biˈnɔːtərəun] *n* 贝诺睾酮(雄激素拮抗药)

benoxaprofen [beˌnɔksəˈprəufən] *n* 苯噁洛芬(消炎镇痛药)

benoxinate hydrochloride [beˈnɔksineit] 盐酸奥布卡因(局部麻醉药)

benserazide [benˈsiərəzaid] *n* 苄丝肼(脱羧酶抑制药)

Benson's disease [ˈbensn] (Alfred H. Benson) 星形玻璃[状]体炎

bentazepam [benˈtæzipæm] *n* 苯他西泮(安定药)

benthos [ˈbenθɔs] *n* 海底生物 | **benthic** [ˈbenθik], **benthonic** [benˈθɔnik] *a* 海底的;海底生物的

bentiromide [benˈtirəmaid] *n* 苯替酪胺(用于对胰外分泌功能不全的非介入性筛选试验及对胰腺替代疗法的监护)

bentonite [ˈbentənait] *n* 皂土(用作充量轻泻剂及皮肤制剂的基质)

bentoquatam [ˈbentəuˌkweitæm] *n* 苯托喹坦(外用护肤药)

benzaldehyde [benˈzældihaid] *n* 苯甲醛(用作口服药的调味剂)

benzalin [ˈbenzəlin] *n* 苯胺黑

benzalkonium chloride [ˌbenzəlˈkəuniəm] 苯扎氯铵(局部防腐杀菌药)

benzamidase [benˈzæmideis] *n* 苯甲酰胺酶

benzamine [ˈbenzəmiːn] *n* 苯沙明(局部麻醉药)

benzanthracene [benˈzænθrəsiːn] *n* 苯并蒽(碳氢化合物之一,其中一些具有致癌性)

benzazoline hydrochloride [benˈzæzəliːn] 盐酸苄唑啉,盐酸妥拉唑啉(见 tolazoline hydrochloride)

benzbromarone [benzˈbrəumərəun] *n* 苯溴马隆(促尿酸排泄药,用于治疗痛风患者的高尿酸血症)

benzcurine iodide [ˈbenzkjuəriːn] 三碘季铵酚,戈拉碘铵(即 gallamine triethiodide)

benzene [ˈbenziːn] *n* 苯 | ~ hexachloride 六氯化苯(杀虫药) / methyl ~ 甲苯

1, 2-benzenedicarboxylic acid [ˌbenziːndaiˌkɑːbɔkˈsilik] 1, 2-苯二羧酸

benzenemethanol [ˌbenziːnˈmeθənɔl] *n* 苄醇,苯甲醇

benzenesulfonic acid [ˌbenziːnsʌlˈfɔnik] 苯磺酸

benzenoid [ˈbenzinɔid] *a* 苯环型的

benzestrofol [benˈzestrəfɔl] *n* 苯甲酸雌二醇

benzestrol [benˈzestrɔl] *n* 苯雌酚

benzethonium chloride [ˌbenzəˈθəuniəm] 苄索氯铵(局部防腐杀菌药)

benzhexol hydrochloride [benzˈheksɔl] 盐酸苯海索(抗胆碱能药,口服治疗震颤麻痹)

benzhydramine hydrochloride [benzˈhaidrəmiːn] 盐酸苯海拉明(抗组胺药)

benzidine [ˈbenzidiːn] *n* 联苯胺(用于检血)

benzilonium bromide [ˌbenziˈləuniəm] 苯咯溴铵(抗胆碱药,用于治疗消化性溃疡和功能性胃肠紊乱)

benzimidazole [ˌbenziˈmidəzɔl] *n* 苯并咪唑

benzin [ˈbenzin], **benzine** [ˈbenziːn] *n* 石油精,苯精 | petroleum ~, purified ~ 石油精,纯石油精

benzoate [ˈbenzəeit] *n* 苯甲酸盐(或酯) | **~d** *a* 含苯甲酸的

benzocaine [ˈbenzəukein] *n* 苯佐卡因(局部麻醉药)

benzodepa [ˌbenzəuˈdepə] *n* 苯佐替派(抗肿瘤药)

benzodiazepine [ˌbenzəudaiˈæzipiːn] *n* 苯[并]二氮䓬类(任何一类弱安定药,其中包括氯氮䓬〈chlordiazepoxide〉,地西泮〈diazepam〉,氟西泮〈flurazepam〉,奥沙西泮〈oxazepam〉,均具有共同的分子结构和相似的药理作用,如抗忧虑、肌肉松弛、镇静和安眠作用)

benzodioxan [ˌbenzəudaiˈɔksən] *n* 苯并二噁烷(α 受体阻滞药)

benzofuran [ˌbenzəuˈfjurən] *n* 苯并呋喃,氧茚,香豆酮

benzogynestryl [ˌbenzəugaiˈnestril] *n* 苯甲酸雌二醇

benzoic [benˈzəuik] *a* 苯甲酸的,安息香的 | ~ acid 苯甲酸,安息香酸

benzoic aldehyde [benˈzəuik] 苯甲醛

benzoin [ˈbenzɔin] *n* 安息香;苯甲酰苯基甲醇

benzol [ˈbenzɔl] *n* 苯

benzoline [ˈbenzəliːn] *n* 汽油

benzolism [ˈbenzəlizəm] *n* 苯中毒

benzonatate [benˈzəunəteit], **benzononatine** [benˌzəunəˈneitiːn] *n* 苯佐那酯(镇咳药)

benzopurpurine [ˌbenzəuˈpəːpjuərin] *n* 苯并红紫 | ~ 4B 苯并红紫 4B(pH 指示剂)

1, 2-benzopyran [ˌbenzəuˈpirən] *n* 1, 2-苯并吡喃

benzo[a]pyrene [ˌbenzəuˈpairiːn] *n* 苯并吡

benzopyrronium bromide [ˌbenzəupiˈrəuniəm] 溴苯吡洛宁(抗胆碱能药)

benzoquinone [ˌbenzəuˈkwinəun] *n* 苯醌

benzosulfimide [ˌbenzəuˈsʌlfimaid] *n* 糖精,邻磺酰苯酰亚胺

benzotherapy [ˌbenzəuˈθerəpi] *n* 苯疗法(用苯甲酸盐类药物治疗,尤指静脉注射苯甲酸钠以治疗肺脓肿)

benzothiadiazide [ˌbenzəuˌθaiəˈdaiəzaid], **benzothiadiazine**[ˌbenzəuˌθaiəˈdaiəziːn] *n* 苯[并]噻二嗪

benzoxiquine [benˈzɔksikwin] *n* 苯甲酰喹(消毒防腐药)

benzoyl [ˈbenzəuil] *n* 苯甲酰[基] | hydrous ~ peroxide, ~ peroxide 过氧苯甲酰(治痤疮药,消毒防腐药)

benzoylaminoacetic acid [ˈbenzəuiˌlæminə *u* əˈsiːtik] 马尿酸

benzoylecgonine [ˌbenzəuilˈekgəniːn] *n* 苯甲酰爱康宁,苯酰芽子碱

benzoylglucuronic acid [ˌbenzəuilˌglukjuəˈrɔnik] 苯甲酰葡糖醛酸

benzoylglycine [ˌbenzəuilˈglaisin] *n* 苯甲酰甘氨酸,马尿酸

benzoylpas calcium [ˌbenzəuˈilpæz] 苯沙酸钙(抗菌药,口服抗结核药)

benzoylphenylcarbinol [ˌbenzəuilˌfenilˈkɑːbinɔl] *n* 苯甲酰苯基甲醇

benzphetamine hydrochloride [benzˈfetəmiːn] 盐酸苄非他明(口服食欲抑制药)

benzpiperylone [ˌbenzpiˈperiləun] *n* 苄哌立隆(消炎药)

3, 4-benzpyrene [benzˈpaiəriːn] *n* 3, 4-苯并吡

benzpyrinium bromide [ˌbenzpaiəˈrinjəm] 苄吡溴铵(胆碱能药,有抗胆碱酯酶作用)

benzpyrrole [benzˈpirɔl] *n* 吲哚

benzquinamide hydrochloride [benzˈkwinəmaid] 盐酸苯喹胺(镇吐药)

benzthiazide [benzˈθaiəzaid] *n* 苄噻嗪(口服利尿、降压药)

benztropine mesylate [ˈbenztrəpiːn] 甲磺苯扎托品(具有抗胆碱、抗组胺和局部麻醉作用,抗震颤麻痹药)

benzurestat [benˈzjuəristæt] *n* 4-氯-*N*-[2-(羟氨基)-2-氧乙基]苯酰胺(尿素酶抑制剂)

benzydamine [benˈzidəmiːn] *n* 苄达明(消炎镇痛药)

benzydroflumethiazide [benˌzidrəflumiˈθaiəzaid] *n* 苄氟噻嗪(利尿降压药)

benzyl [ˈbenzil] *n* 苄基,苯甲基 | ~ benzoate 苯甲酸苄酯(灭疥、灭虱药) / ~ bromide 溴化苄(一种军用毒气) / ~ carbinol 苄甲醇,苯乙醇(具有麻醉作用) / ~ succinate 琥珀酸苄酯(解痉药)

benzylidene [benˈzilidiːn] *n* 苄叉,苯亚甲基

***p*-benzyloxyphenol** [ˌbenziˌlɔksiˈfiːnɔl] *n* 对苄氧酚

benzylpenicillin [ˌbenzilpeniˈsilin] *n* 青霉素(抗生素类药) | ~ potassium 青霉素钾 / ~ procaine 普鲁卡因青霉素

benzylpenicilloyl polylysine [ˌbenzilˌpeniˈsilɔilˌpɔliˈlaisiːn] 青霉噻唑酰聚赖氨酸(一种皮肤试验抗原,用于通过抓痕试验和皮内试验评定青霉素过敏反应)

bephenium [biˈfeniəm] *n* 苄芬宁(抗蠕虫药)

bephenium hydroxynaphthoate [bəˈfiːniəm haiˌdrɔksiˈnæfθəeit] 羟萘苄芬宁(抗蠕虫药)

bepridil hydrochloride [ˈbepridil] 盐酸苄普地尔(钙拮抗药,用于治疗慢性心绞痛,口服给药)

beractant [bəˈræktənt] *n* 含磷脂牛肺浸膏(防治新生儿呼吸窘迫综合征,气管内滴注给药)

Béraneck's tuberculin [beirəˈnek] (Edmund Béraneck) 巴兰内克结核菌素,正磷酸提取结核菌素(结核杆菌在无蛋白胨的、5% 甘油肉汤培养后,过滤,然后将细菌用 1% 正磷酸长期连续振荡法提取,此提取物与等量滤液混合后备用)

Berardinelli-Seip syndrome [bəˌrɑːdiˈneli saip] (Waldemar Berardinelli; Martin F. Seip) 全身性脂肪营养不良

Bérard's aneurysm [beiˈrɑː] (Anguste Bérard) 贝拉动脉瘤(静脉损伤后发生的动静脉瘤) | ~ ligament 贝拉韧带(心包的悬韧带,延伸至第三、第四胸椎)

Béraud's valve [beiˈrəu] (Bruno J. J. Béraud) 贝罗瓣(泪囊襞)

Berberidaceae [ˌbəːbəriˈdeisiiː] *n* 小檗科

berberine [ˈbəːbəriːn] *n* 小檗碱,黄连素

Berberis [ˈbəːbəris] *n*【拉】小檗属

Berdon syndrome [ˈbəːdən] (Walter E. Berdon) 伯顿综合征,巨膀胱-小结肠-肠蠕动迟缓综合征

bereavement [biˈriːvmənt] *n* 居丧,配偶丧亡

Bereitschaftspotential [bəˌreitʃɑːftspəˈtenʃəl] *n*【德】准备电位

bergamot [ˈbəːgəmɔt] *n* 佛手柑,香柑;香柠檬油,薄荷

Bergenhem's operation [ˈbəːgənhem] (Bengt Bergenhem) 伯根海姆手术(将输尿管移植于直肠)

Bergeron's chorea (disease) [ˈbəːʒrɔn] (Étienne J. Bergeron) 贝尔热隆舞蹈症(病)(电击样舞蹈症,其特征为激烈而有规律的痉挛,但为良性病程)

Berger rhythm [ˈbəːgə] (Hans Berger) α-节律(正常脑电图)

Berger's disease [beˈʒei] (Jean Berger) 贝惹病,IgA 肾病

Berger's method [bɛəˈʒei] (Paul Berger) 贝尔惹法(骶骨横骨折缝法) | ~ operation 贝尔惹手术(肩胸间切断术)

Berger's paresthesia [ˈbəːgə] (Oskar Berger) 贝格尔感觉异常(青少年的一侧或两侧下肢感觉异常、无力,但无他觉症状)

Berger's sign (symptom) [ˈbəːgə] (Emile Berger) 贝格尔征(症状)(不规则或椭圆形瞳孔,见于早期脊髓痨、麻痹性痴呆等)

Bergey's classification [ˈbəːgi] (David H. Bergy) 伯吉分类法(一种细菌分类法)

Bergmann's cells [ˈbəːgmən] (Gottlieb H. Bergmann) 贝格曼细胞(小脑皮质分子层内的特殊神经胶质细胞,其树突通过该层向外延伸) | ~ cords 第四脑室髓纹,听髓纹 / ~ fibers 贝格曼纤维(从小脑分子层放射并进入软脑膜的突)

Bergmann's incision [ˈbəːgmən] (Ernst von Bergmann) 贝格曼切口(暴露肾脏的切口)

Bergman's sign [ˈbəːgmən] (Harry Bergman) 贝格曼征(脊髓痨早期、麻痹性痴呆和某些瘫痪患者的瞳孔呈不规则形或椭圆形)

Bergonié treatment (method) [bɛəgɔˈnjei] (Jean A. Bergonié) 贝果尼埃疗法,感应电减肥疗法

Bergonié-Tribondeau law [bɛəgɔˈnjei tribɔnˈdəu] (J. A. Bergonié; Louis Tribondeau) 贝果尼埃-特立邦多定律(细胞对放射线的敏感性与细胞的繁殖力成正比,与细胞分化程度成反比)

beriberi [ˌberiˈberi] *n* 脚气病 | cerebral ~ 大脑性脚气病(见 Wernicke-Korsakoff syndrome) / dry ~, atrophic ~, paralytic ~ 干性脚气病,萎缩性脚气病,麻痹性脚气病 / ship ~ 航行脚气病 / wet ~ 湿性脚气病 | **~c** *a*

Berkefeld filter [ˈbəːkifeld] (Wilhelm Berkefeld) 贝克费尔德滤菌器

berkelium (Bk) [ˈbəːkliəm] *n* 锫(化学元素)

Berke operation [bəːk] (Raynold N. Berke) 伯克手术(一种用于上睑下垂的手术)

Berlin's disease, edema [ˈbəːlin] (Rudolf Berlin) 视网膜震荡

berlock, berloque [bəˈlɔk] *n* 伯洛克皮炎,香料皮炎

Bernard-Horner syndrome [bəˈnɑː ˈhɔːnə] (Claude Bernard; Johann F. Horner) 伯纳-霍纳综合征(见 Horner's syndrome)

Bernard's canal (duct) [bəˈnɑː] (Claude Bernard) 伯纳管,胰副管 | ~ glandular layer 胰腺腺泡层 / ~ puncture 伯纳穿刺术(实验医学时,在第四脑室特定点穿刺引起糖尿。亦称糖尿穿刺) / ~ syndrome 伯纳综合征(见 Horner's syndrome)

Bernard-Soulier disease (syndrome) [bəːˈnɑː suːliˈei] (Jeam Bernard; Jean-Pierre Soulier) 伯-苏病(综合征)(一种常染色体隐性遗传病,其特征为血小板的大小与形态的范围很大。血小板膜缺乏糖蛋白 Ib,而糖蛋白 Ib 可能是血浆冯·维勒布兰德因子 von Willebrand Factor 〈vWF〉的受体;这种缺乏使血小板不能结合 vWF,因而不能黏附血管内皮下面。临床征象包括黏膜皮肤和内脏出血、紫癜和出血时间延长。亦称巨血小板病或巨血小板综合征)

Bernays' sponge [ˈbəːneiz] (Augustus C. Bernays) 伯奈斯海绵(止鼻衄吸收绵)

Bernhardt's disease, paresthesia, Bernhardt-Rot disease, syndrome [ˈbəːnhɑːt rɔt] (Martin Bernhard; Vladimir K. Rot) 感觉异常性股痛

Bernheimer's fibers [ˈbəːnhaimə] (Stefan Bernheimer) 伯恩海默纤维(自视神经束至柳氏〈Luy〉体的一种脑神经纤维束)

Bernheim's syndrome [ˈbəːnhaim] (P. Bernheim) 伯恩海姆综合征(右心力衰竭,系左心室肥大,室间间隔凸入右心室所致,阻塞血流由右心房进入右心室,改变心室充盈和容量)

Bernoulli distribution [bəˈnuːli, bənuːˈiː] (Jakob Bernoulli) 伯努利分布(二项分布) | ~ theorem 伯努利定理(在涉及概率的实验中,试验数愈大,所观察的事件概率接近其理论概率则愈近) / ~ trial 伯努利试验(统计学中,一系列独立试验里,每一试验只有两种互相排斥的结果,常称之为"成功"和"失败",因此如果成功的概率是 p,失败的概率是 q,那么 $p + q = 1$,而成功的概率在整个试验中都是相同的)

berry [ˈberi] *n* 浆果 | bear ~ 熊果[叶] / buckthorn ~ 泻鼠李[果] / elder ~ 接骨木果 / fish ~, Indian ~ 印防己[实] / horse nettle ~ 美洲野茄果 / juniper ~ 杜松[实] / saw palmetto ~

蓝棕果,锯叶棕果 / spice ~ 美槐木(白松糖浆成分之一) | **berried** *a* 结浆果的

Berry's ligament [ˈberi] (James Berry) 甲状腺外侧韧带

Berthelot reaction [bɛətəˈləu] (Pierre E. M. Berthelot) 伯特洛反应(氨与伯特洛试剂的反应,形成一种稳定的深蓝色产物酚-靛酚,用于检氨与尿素的比色法) | ~ reagent 伯特洛试剂(酚和次氯酸盐的碱性溶液,用于伯洛特反应)

Bertiella [ˌbəːtiˈelə] *n* 伯特绦虫属

bertielliasis [ˌbəːtieˈlaiəsis] *n* 伯特绦虫病

Bertin's bones (ossicles) [bɛəˈtæn] (Exupère J. Bertin) 贝坦骨(小骨),蝶骨甲 | ~ column 肾柱 / ~ ligament 髂股韧带

Bertolotti's syndrome [bɛətəˈlɔti] (Mario Bertolotti) 贝托洛蒂综合征(第5腰椎骶化伴坐骨神经痛和脊柱侧弯)

Bertrand's method, test [bɛəˈtrɑːn] (Gabriel Bertrand) 贝特朗法、试验(检葡萄糖) | ~ reagent 贝特朗试剂(硅钨酸试剂)

berylliosis [ˌberiliˈəusis] *n* 铍中毒(尤指铍尘肺)

beryllium (Be) [bəˈriljəm] *n* 铍(化学元素)

berythromycin [bəˌriθrəuˈmaisin] *n* 红霉素B(抗阿米巴、抗菌药)

Berzelius' test [bɛəˈzeiliəs] (Jöns J. Berzelius) 贝泽利乌斯试验(检尿中白蛋白)

besiclometer [ˌbesiˈklɔmitə] *n* 眼镜架宽度计

besmear [biˈsmiə] *vt* 涂抹

Besnier-Boeck disease [beˈniə ˈbek] (Ernest Besnier; Caesar P. M. Boeck) 结节病,肉样瘤病

Besnier's prurigo [bəˈniə] (Ernest Besnier) 贝尼埃痒疹(一种皮炎,儿科医师对婴儿和幼儿得此痒疹称为婴儿湿疹,皮肤科医师对婴儿、青少年和成人得此痒疹称为特应性皮炎)

Besnoitia [besˈnɔitiə] *n* 贝西诺原虫属(以前亦称球虫属 Globidium)

besnoitiosis [besˌnɔitiˈəusis] *n* 贝西诺原虫病(以前称球虫病 globidiosis)

Besredka's antivirus [besˈredkə] (Alexandre Besredka) 贝斯雷德卡细菌滤液(肉汤中细菌经过加热过滤的培养物,用以产生局部免疫性) | ~ reaction 贝斯雷特卡反应(一种对结核病补体转向反应)

bestial [ˈbestjəl] *a* 兽性的

bestiality [ˌbestiˈæləti] *n* 兽奸

Best's disease [best] (Franz Best) 贝斯特病(先天性黄斑变性)

besylate [ˈbesileit] *n* 苯磺酸盐(或酯)(benzenesulfonate 的 USAN 缩约词)

Beta [ˈbiːtə] *n*【拉】菾菜属,甜菜属 | ~ vulgaris L. 菾菜,甜菜

beta [ˈbiːtə, ˈbeitə] *n* 希腊语的第二个字母(B, *β*);乙种;第二位的东西 *a* 第二位的,*β* 位的(用以区分两个或两个以上的异构体之一,或表示取代某些化合物中原子或基团的位置)

beta-adrenergic [ˈbeitə-, ˈbiːtəˌædrənəːdʒik] *a* *β* 肾上腺素能的

beta-aminobutyric acid [ˈbiːtə ˌæminəubjutirik] *β*-氨基丁酸

Betabacterium [ˌbiːtəbækˈtiəriəm] *n* 异型乳杆菌亚属

beta-blocker [ˌbiːtə ˈblɔkə] *n* β 受体阻滞药

beta-blocking [ˌbiːtə ˈblɔkiŋ] *a* 阻滞 β 受体的

betacarotene [ˌbeitəˈkærətiːn] *n* *β*-胡萝卜素;倍他胡萝卜素(防晒药)

beta-cholestanol [ˌbeitə kəˈlestənɔl] *n* *β*-胆甾烷醇,二氢胆固醇

betacism [ˈbeitəsizəm] *n* (说话中)b 音过多

betacyanin [ˌbiːtəˈsaiənin] *n* *β*-花青苷

betacytotropic [ˌbeitəˌsaitəuˈtrɔpik] *a* 亲 *β* 细胞的

betadex [ˈbeitədeks] *n* *β*-环糊精

beta-endorphin [ˌbiːtəˌenˈdɔːfin] *n* *β*-内啡肽

beta-estradiol [ˌbeitəˌestrəˈdaiɔl] *n* *β*-雌二醇

beta globulin [ˌbeitəˈglɔbjulin] *β*-球蛋白 | pregnancy-specific ~ 妊娠特异性 *β*-球蛋白(由胎盘分泌,其功能不明)

betahemolytic [ˌbeitəˌhiməˈlitik] *a* 乙种溶血的

Betaherpesvirinae [ˌbeitəˌhəːpiːzviˈrainiː] *n* *β*-疱疹病毒亚科

betahistine hydrochloride [ˌbeitəˈhistiːn] 盐酸倍他司丁(口服用作血管扩张药,以减少某些梅尼埃病〈耳性眩晕病〉患者眩晕发作的次数)

beta-hydroxybutyric acid [ˌbiːtə haiˌdrɔksibjuˈtirik] *β*-羟丁酸

beta-hypophamine [ˌbeitə haiˈpɔfəmiːn] *n* [后叶]加压素(亦称抗利尿激素)

betaine [ˈbiːtəiːn, ˈbei-] *n* 甜菜碱(利胆药) | ~ hydrochloride 盐酸甜菜碱

beta-ketobutyric acid [ˌbiːtəˌkiːtəubjuˈtirik] *β*-丁酮酸,乙酰乙酸

beta-ketopalmitic acid [ˌbiːtəˌkiːtəupælˈmitik] *β*-酮软脂酸

beta-lactose [ˌbeitə ˈlæktəus] *n* *β*-乳糖

beta-lipoprotein [ˌbeitə ˌlipəˈprəutiːn] *n* *β*-脂蛋白,低密度脂蛋白

betalipotropin [ˌbiːtəˌlipəˈtrəupin] *n* *β*-脂肪酸释放激素

betalysin [beiˈtælisin] *n* *β*-溶[菌]素,乙型溶[菌]素

betamethasone [ˌbeitəˈmeθəsəun] *n* 倍他米松(糖皮质激素) | ~ acetate 醋酸倍他米松 / ~ benzoate 苯甲酸倍他米松 / ~ dipropionate 二丙酸倍他米松 / ~ sodium phosphate 倍他米松磷

酸酯钠 / ~ valerate 戊酸倍他米松
betamicin sulfate [ˌbeitəˈmaisin] 硫酸倍他米星(抗生素类药)
$beta_2$-microglobulin [ˌbeitə ˌmaikrəuˈglɔbjulin] *n* β_2-微球蛋白
betanaphthol [ˌbeitəˈnæfθɔl] *n* β-萘酚(抗菌药) | ~ benzylamine 苯甲胺萘酚 / ~ bismuth β-萘酚铋(肠内收敛药)
betanaphtholsulfonic acid [ˌbeitəˌnæfθəlsʌlˈfɔnik] β-萘酚磺酸
betanaphthyl [ˌbeitəˈnæfθil] *n* β-萘基 | ~ benzoate 苯甲酸β-萘酯
betanin [ˌbiːtənin] *n* 甜菜苷
betaoxidation [ˌbiːtəˌɔksiˈdeiʃən] *n* β-氧化作用
beta-oxybutyria [ˌbeitə ˌɔksibjuˈtiriə] *n* β-羟酪酸尿
beta-oxybutyric acid [ˌbiːtə ˌɔksibjuˈtirik] β-羟丁酸
beta-phenylpropionic acid [ˌbeitə ˌfenilˌprəupiˈɔnik] β-苯丙酸
betapropiolactone [ˌbeitəˌprəupiəˈlæktəun] *n* β-丙内酯,丙内酯
betaquinine [ˌbeitəˈkwinin] *n* β-奎宁(即奎尼丁)
beta-receptor [ˌbeitə riˈseptə] *n* β[肾上腺素]受体
betatron [ˈbeitətrɔn] *n* 电子回旋加速器
betaxolol hydrochloride [beiˈtæksəlɔl] 盐酸倍他洛尔(β受体阻滞药)
betazole hydrochloride [ˈbeitəzəul] 盐酸倍他唑(促胃液分泌药,胃功能试验用)
betel [ˈbiːtəl] *n* 蒌叶(用蒌叶卷一些槟榔子碎片及石灰作为咀嚼剂,有收敛、强壮及兴奋作用) | ~ leaf 蒌叶 / ~ nut 槟榔子
bête rouge [betˈruːʒ]【法】红恙螨
bethanechol chloride [biˈθeinikɔl] 氯贝胆碱(拟胆碱药)
bethanidine sulfate [biˈθænidiːn] 硫酸倍他尼定(肾上腺素能神经元阻滞药,用以治疗原发性高血压,尤其在恶性期)
Bethea's sign(method) [biˈθeiə] (Oscar W. Bethea)比塞征(法)(当检查者站在患者背后,将指尖置于两侧腋窝上部的肋骨上缘时,患侧肋骨呼吸运动减弱则表示一侧胸廓吸气扩张受损)
Bethesda System [bəˈθezdə] (Bethesda 为美国马里兰州国立癌症研究所所在地)比塞大系统(一种宫颈和阴道细胞学分类,对宫颈和阴道疾病细胞病理学诊断提供标准化命名法。该系统包括3个要素:标本的适当性评价、标本的一般分类和描述性诊断)
Bettendorff's test [ˈbeitəndɔːf] (Anton J. H. M. Bettendorff)贝顿道夫试验(检砷)
Betula [ˈbetjulə] *n* 桦木属
betweenbrain [biˈtwiːnbrein] *n* 间脑
betweenness [biˈtwiːnnis] *n* 中间性
Betz's cells [ˈbets] (Vladimir A. Betz)贝茨细胞(巨锥体细胞) | ~ cell area 贝茨细胞区,心理运动区,运动区
BeV billion electron volts 10亿电子伏,千兆电子伏,10^9 电子伏(现用 giga electron volt, GeV)
Bevan Lewis cells [ˈbevən ˈlju(ː)is] (William Bevan Lewis)贝文·刘易斯细胞(大脑皮质运动区中的某种锥体细胞)
Bevan's incision [ˈbevən] (Arthur D. Bevan)贝文切口(右侧腹直肌外缘纵行切口,以暴露胆囊) | ~ operation 贝文手术(纠正未降睾丸术,使之回到阴囊)
bevel [ˈbevəl] *n* 洞斜面 *vt* 使成洞斜面
beverage [ˈbevəridʒ] *n* 饮料
bexarotene [bekˈsærətiːn] *n* 贝沙罗汀(抗肿瘤药)
bezoar [ˈbiːzɔː] *n*【波斯】胃[肠]石(发生在人或其他动物的胃肠内);牛黄(中药)
Bezold's abscess [ˈbeizɔlt] (Friedrich Bezold)贝佐尔德脓肿(颞骨骨膜下脓肿) | ~ perforation 贝佐尔德穿孔(颞骨乳突内面穿孔) / ~ sign 贝佐尔德征(乳突尖下部炎性肿胀,为乳突炎之征) / ~ triad 贝佐尔德三征(骨传导延长、低音听力减退、林尼〈Rinne〉音叉试验阴性,三者为耳硬化之征)
Bezold's ganglion [ˈbeizɔlt] (Albert von Bezold)贝佐尔德神经节(房中隔一群神经节细胞)
BF blastogenic factor 母细胞生成因子,生殖因子
β1F 补体因子 C5 的旧称
BFP biologic false positive 生物学假阳性(反应)
BFU-E burst-forming unit erythroid 红细胞爆裂型集落生成单位
β1H 补体因子 H 的旧称
BHA butylated hydroxyanisole 丁羟茴醚
bhang [bæŋ] *n*【印度】大麻
BHC benzene hexachloride 六氯化苯(杀虫药)
BHCDA Bureau of Health Care Delivery and Assistance 卫生保健设施与辅助设备处(属美国卫生资源与卫生事业管理局)
BHPR Bureau of Health Professions 卫生专业处(属美国卫生资源与卫生事业管理局)
BHRD Bureau of Health Resources Development 卫生资源开发处(属美国卫生资源与卫生事业管理局)
BHT butylated hydroxytoluene 丁羟甲苯
Bi bismuth 铋
bi- [前缀]二,二倍,双(元音字母前用 bin-)
biacromial [baiəˈkrəumiəl] *a* 双肩峰间的
bialamicol hydrochloride [baiəˈlæmikɔl] 盐酸比拉米可(抗阿米巴药)

biallylamicol [bai|ælil'æmikɔl] *n* 盐酸比拉米可(bialamicol hydrochloride)的旧称

Bial's reagent ['biːəl] (Manfred Bial) 比阿尔试剂(1.5 g 5-苔黑酚、500 g 发烟盐酸、20~30 滴 10%氯化铁制成的试剂) | ~ test 比阿尔试验(检尿戊糖)

Bianchi's nodules [bi'æŋki] (Giovanni B. Bianchi) 比昂基小结,主动脉瓣小结,半月瓣小结 | ~ valve 比昂基瓣(鼻泪管襞)

Bianchi's syndrome [bi'æŋki] (Leonardo Bianchi) 比昂基综合征(为感觉性失语症,伴失用症及失读症,见于左顶叶损伤)

biangular [bai'æŋgjulə] *a* 有两角的

biarticular [|baiɑː'tikjulə] *a* 两关节的

biarticulate [|baiɑː'tikjulit] *a* 有两关节的

bias ['baiəs] *n* 系统误差;偏倚(统计) | selection ~ 选择偏倚

biasteric [|baiəs'terik] *a* 双星体的

biatrial [|bai'eitriəl] *a* 两心房的

biauricular [|baiɔː'rikjulə] *a* 两耳的,双耳的

Bib. bibe【拉】饮

bib [bib] *n* 红细胞碎片(恶性疟原虫新月状配子体在生长中出现)

bibasic [bai'beisik] *a* 二元的;二碱的

bibeveled [bai'bevəld] *a* 双斜面的

bibliomania [|bibliəu'meinjə] *n* 集书癖,藏书癖 | **~c** *a*, *n* 有藏书癖的(人)

bibliotherapy [|bibliəu'θerəpi] *n* 读书疗法,阅读疗法(治疗精神障碍或促进心理卫生)

Bibron's antidote ['bibrɔn] (Gabriel Bibron) 比布隆解毒剂(解蛇毒药,含碘化钾 0.24,二氯化汞 0.12,溴 20)

bibulous ['bibjuləs] *a* 吸水的;吸潮的

bicalutamide [|baikə'ljuːtəmaid] *n* 比卡鲁胺(雄激素拮抗药,用作治疗辅助剂,与黄体素释放素类似物结合使用治疗前列腺癌,口服给药)

bicameral [bai'kæmərəl] *a* 二室的,两室的

bicapsular [bai'kæpsjulə] *a* 二囊的,两囊的

bicarbonate [bai'kɑːbənit] *n* 碳酸氢盐,重碳酸盐 | blood ~, plasma ~ 血液重碳酸盐,血浆重碳酸盐 / ~ of soda 碳酸氢钠,重碳酸钠,小苏打

bicarbonatemia [bai|kɑːbənei'tiːmiə] *n* 重碳酸盐血

bicarbonaturia [bai|kɑːbənei'tjuəriə] *n* 重碳酸盐尿(如见于近端肾小管性酸中毒)

bicaudal [bai'kɔːdl], **bicaudate** [bai'kɔːdeit] *a* 双尾的

bicellular [bai'seljulə] *a* 两细胞的

bicephalus [bai'sefələs] *n* 双头畸胎

biceps ['baiseps] *n* 二头肌 | ~ brachii, ~ femoris 肱二头肌,股二头肌

Bichat's canal [biː'ʃɑː] (Marie F. X. Bichat) 比夏管,蛛网膜管,大脑大静脉池 | ~ fissure 大脑横裂 / ~ foramen 蛛网膜孔 / ~ ligament 骶髂后韧带下束 / ~ membrane 窗膜,内弹性膜 / ~ tunic 血管内膜

bichloroacetic acid [|baiklɔːrə'sitik] 二氯乙酸

bichloride [bai'klɔːraid] *n* 二氯化物,升汞

bichromate [bai'krəumit] *n* 重铬酸盐

bichrome ['baikrəum] *a* 两色的

bicipital [bai'sipitəl] *a* 二头的;二头肌的

biciromab [bai'sirəmæb] *n* 比西单抗(抗纤维蛋白的鼠抗人单克隆抗体,以放射性形式〈与 ^{99m}Tc络合〉诊断深静脉血栓形成)

bicisate [bai'siseit] *n* ECD,乙基半胱氨酸二聚物(一种亲脂胺,具有跨越血-脑屏障和脑内定位的能力,与^{99m}Tc 络合用于脑血管系统成像,使局部脑血流呈现静止影像)

Bickerstaff's migraine ['bikəstæf] (Edwin R. Bickerstaff) 比克斯塔夫偏头痛,基底[动脉]偏头痛

bicollis [bai'kɔlis] *a*【拉】双颈的

bicoronal [baikə'rəunəl] *a* 双放射冠的;双冠状缝的

bicolor ['baikʌlə], **bicolored** ['baikʌləd] *a* 双色的

bicomponent [|baikəm'pəunənt] *n*, *a* 双组分(的)

biconcave [bai'kɔnkeiv] *a* 双凹的

biconvex [bai'kɔnveks] *a* 双凸的

bicornuate [bai'kɔːnjueit], **bicornate** [bai'kɔːneit] *a* 双角的

bicoronial [|baikə'rəuniəl] *a* 双冠的

bicorporate [bai'kɔːpəreit] *a* 双体的,双身的

bicuculline [bai'kjuːkə|liːn] *n* 荷包牡丹碱

bicuspid [bai'kʌspid] *a* 二尖的;左房室瓣的,二尖瓣的 *n* 前磨牙

bicuspidal [bai'kʌspidl] *a* 前磨牙的;二尖的

bicuspidate [bai'kʌspideit] *a* 二尖的

bicuspoid [bai'kʌspɔid] *n* 双尖型

b. i. d. bis in die【拉】每日 2 次

Bidder's ganglia ['bidə] (Heinrich F. Bidder) 比德神经节(心神经的神经节,位于房间隔的下端) | ~ organ 比德器(雄性蟾蜍性腺的前部,其性质似卵巢)

bidental [bai'dentl], **bidentate** [bai'denteit] *a* 双牙的

bidermoma [|baidə'məumə] *n* 双胚叶畸胎瘤(由两个胚层的细胞和组织所组成的一种畸胎瘤)

biduotertian [|baidju(ː)əu'təːʃən] *n* 持续型间日疟

biduous ['bidjuəs] *a* 持续两天的(如发热)

Biederman's sign ['biːdəmən] (Joseph B. Biederman)比德曼征(喉前壁呈暗红色〈而非正常的淡红色〉,见于梅毒患者)

Biedert's cream mixture [ˈbiːdət] (Philipp Biedert)比德特奶油合剂(由奶油、温水及乳糖混成的婴儿食品)

Biedl's disease, syndrome [ˈbiːdl] (Artur Biedl)比德尔病、综合征(肥胖、生殖功能减退、色素性视网膜炎、智能缺陷等综合征)

Bielschowsky-Jansky disease [ˌbiːlˈʃɔvskiˈjænski] (Max Bielschowsky; Jan Jansky)比-杨病(晚发婴儿型神经元蜡样脂褐素沉积症)

Bielschowsky's head tilting test [ˌbiːlˈʃɔvski] (Alfred Bielschowsky)比尔肖夫斯基头倾斜试验(令患者头倾斜至右肩和左肩,注视远方固定物,有可能区别上直肌轻瘫与对侧上斜肌轻瘫)

Bielschowsky's method [ˌbiːlˈʃɔvski] (Max Bielschowsky)比尔肖夫斯基法(一种论证神经轴突及网状纤维的氨银染法)

Biemond syndrome Ⅱ [biːˈmɔːn] (A. Biemond)比蒙综合征Ⅱ型(一种常染色体隐性遗传病,特征为虹膜缺损、肥胖、精神发育迟缓、性腺功能减退和轴后多指〈趾〉畸形)

biennial [baiˈeniəl] *a* 两年生的 *n* 两年生植物

bier [biə] *n* 棺材架;尸体架

Biermer's anemia (disease) [ˈbiəmə] (Anton Biemer)恶性贫血 | ~ sign 比尔默征(水气胸时的金属性叩响,其音调随患者体位的变换而改变,见于气胸)

Biernacki's sign [bjiəˈnɑːtski] (Edmund Biernacki)别尔纳茨基征(脊髓痨及麻痹性痴呆时的尺神经痛觉缺失)

Bier's amputation (operation) [biə] (August K. G. Bier)比尔切断术(手术)(腿骨成形性切断术) | ~ block(anesthesia)比尔阻滞(麻醉法)(静脉局部麻醉法) / ~ passive hyperemia, ~ treatment 比尔被动性充血疗法,收窄性充血法(用薄橡皮带导致静脉充血治关节病)

Biesiadecki's fossa [bjeisiəˈdetski] (Alfred von Biesiadecki)髂筋膜下窝

Biette's collarette [biˈet] (Laurnet T. Biette)比埃特项圈(一种丘疹样梅毒疹,其中心丘疹周围为一圈鳞屑)

biferiens [baiˈfiəriənz] *a* 【拉】重搏的,两次搏动的

biferious [baiˈfiəriəs] *a* 重搏的,两次搏动的

bifid [ˈbaifid] *a* 对裂的,两叉的 | **~ity** *n* / **~ly** *ad*

Bifidobacterium [ˌbaifidəubækˈtiəriəm] *n* 双歧杆菌属 | ~ adolescentis 青春双歧杆菌 / ~ bifidum 两歧双歧杆菌 / ~ cornutum 角状双歧杆菌 / ~ eriksonii 埃氏双歧杆菌 / ~ infantis 婴儿双歧杆菌

bifidobacterium [ˌbaifidəubækˈtiəriəm] ([复] **bifidobacteria** [ˌbaifidəubækˈtiəriə]) *n* 双歧杆菌

bifidus [ˈbifidəs] *a* 【拉】对裂的,两叉的

bifilar [baiˈfailə] *a* 双丝的

biflagellate [baiˈflædʒeleit] *a* 有两个鞭毛的,双鞭毛的

bifocal [baiˈfəukəl] *a* 双焦点的;双焦点镜的 *n* [复]双光眼镜;双焦点眼镜

biforate [baiˈfɔːreit] *a* 双孔的

biform [ˈbaifɔːm] *a* 有两形的;两体的;两形结合的

biformyl [baiˈfɔːmil] *n* 二乙醛

bifunctional [baiːˈfʌŋkʃənəl] *a* 双功能的

bifurcate [ˈbaifəːkeit, baiˈf-] *a* 叉状的;分叉的

bifurcatio [ˌbaifəːˈkeiʃiəu] ([复] **bifurcationes** [ˌbaifəːkeiʃiˈəunis]) *n* 【拉】杈

bifurcation [ˌbaifəːˈkeiʃən] *n* 分叉;杈 | ~ of trachea 气管杈 / ~ of urination 尿流分叉

Bigelow's ligament [ˈbigiləu] (Henry J. Bigelow)髂股韧带 | ~ operation 碎石洗出术,迅速碎石术 / ~ septum 比吉洛隔(股骨颈的一层硬骨组织)

bigemina [baiˈdʒeminə] *n* bigeminum 的复数;二联脉

bigeminum [baiˈdʒeminəm] ([复] **bigemina** [baiˈdʒeminə]) *n* 【拉】二迭体(指胎儿或鸟类的二迭体中的一个)

bigeminy [baiˈdʒemini] *n* 二联律 | nodal ~ (房室)结性二联律 | **bigeminal** *a* 二联的,成对的

bigerminal [baiˈdʒəːminl] *a* 双胚的,双卵的

bighead [ˈbighed] *n* 大头病(动物头颅骨膨胀,由于骨质软化病所致;幼小公羊急性传染病;白面绵羊光敏感症;水貂脑积水;营养性继发性甲状旁腺功能亢进症)

bigjaw [ˈbiˈdʒɔː] *n* 大颌病(牛放线菌病)

bigleg [ˈbigleg] *n* 巨腿病(马腿部淋巴管炎)

bigonial [baiˈgəuniəl] *a* 联颌角的(连结两下颌角点的)

biguanaid [baiˈgwaːnaid] *n* 双缩胍(口服抗高血脂药)

bilabe [ˈbaileib] *n* 尿道异物钳

bilaminar [baiˈlæminə] *a* 二层的,两板的

bilateral [baiˈlætərəl] *a* 两侧的,双边的;对向的,双向的

bilateralism [baiˈlætərəlizəm] *n* 两侧对称

bilayer [ˈbaileiə] *n* 双分子层;双层

bilberry [ˈbilberi] *n* 越橘

bile [bail] *n* 胆汁 | A ~ 总胆管胆汁 / B ~ 胆囊胆汁 / C ~ 肝胆汁 / cystic ~, gallbladder ~ 胆囊胆汁 / limy ~, milk of calcium ~ 钙乳胆汁

bile acid [bail] 胆汁酸

bilestone [ˈbailstəun] *n* 胆石
Bilharzia [bilˈhɑːziə] *n* 裂体吸虫属,血吸虫属
bilharzial [bilˈhɑːziəl], **bilharzic** [bilˈhɑːzik] *a* 裂体吸虫的,血吸虫的
bilharziasis [ˌbilhɑːˈzaiesis], **bilharziosis** [bilˌhɑːziˈəusis] *n* 裂体吸虫病,血吸虫病
bilharzioma [bilˌhɑːziˈəumə] *n* 裂体吸虫瘤,血吸虫瘤
bil(i)- [构词成分]胆汁
biliary [ˈbiljəri] *a* 胆汁的,胆的;胆管的;胆囊的
biliation [ˌbiliˈeiʃən] *n* 胆汁分泌
bilicyanin [ˌbiliˈsaiənin] *n* 胆青素,胆蓝素
bilidigestive [ˌbilidiˈdʒestiv] *a* 胆囊消化道的
biliflavin [ˌbiliˈfleivin] *n* 胆黄素
bilifulvin [ˌbiliˈfʌlvin] *n* 胆黄褐素
bilifuscin [ˌbiliˈfʌsin] *n* 胆褐素
biligenesis [ˌbiliˈdʒenisis] *n* 胆汁生成 | **biligenetic** [ˌbilidʒiˈnetik] *a* 胆汁生成的;生胆汁的
biligenic [ˌbiliˈdʒenik] *a* 生胆汁的
biligrafin [ˌbiliˈgræfin] *n* 胆影葡胺(胆道造影剂)
biligulate [baiˈligjuleit] *a* 双舌状的
bilihumin [ˌbiliˈhjuːmin] *n* 胆土素(胆石中的一种不溶性成分)
bilin [ˈbailin] *n* 胆汁三烯
bilious [ˈbiljəs] *a* 胆汁的,胆汁质的 | **~ness** *n* 胆汁质,胆汁病
biliprasin [ˌbiliˈpreisin] *n* 胆翠素
biliprotein [ˌbiliˈprəutiːn] *n* 胆蛋白质
bilipurpurin [ˌbiliˈpəːpjuərin] *n* 胆紫素
bilirachia, bilirhachia [ˌbiliˈreikiə] *n* 胆汁脊液
bilirubin [ˌbiliˈruːbin] *n* 胆红素 | direct ~, conjugated ~ 直接胆红素,结合胆红素 / indirect ~, unconjugated ~ 间接胆红素,非结合胆红素
bilirubinate [ˌbiliˈruːbineit] *n* 胆红素盐
bilirubinemia [ˌbiliruːbiˈniːmiə] *n* 胆红素血[症]
bilirubinic [ˌbiliruːˈbinik] *a* 胆红素的 | ~ acid 胆红酸,胆红素
bilirubin UDP glucuronyltransferase [ˌbiliˈruːbin gluːˌkjuərənilˈtrænsfəreis] 胆红素 UDP 葡糖醛酸基转移酶,胆红素尿苷二磷酸葡糖醛酸基转移酶,葡糖苷酸[基]转移酶
bilirubinuria [ˌbiliruːbiˈnjuəriə] *n* 胆红素尿
bilis [ˈbailis] *n*【拉】胆汁 | ~ bovina, ~ bubata 牛胆汁
biliuria [ˌbiliˈjuəriə] *n* 胆汁尿
biliverdin [ˌbiliˈvəːdin] *n* 胆绿素
biliverdinate [ˌbiliˈvəːdineit] *n* 胆绿素盐
biliverdin reductase [ˌbiliˈvəːdin riˈdʌkteis] 胆绿素还原酶
bilixanthin [ˌbiliˈzænθin], **bilixanthine** [ˌbiliˈzænθiːn] *n* 胆黄素
bill [bil] *n* 单子;证明书 | ~ of health (车、船、飞机等的)检疫证书,健康证书 / clean ~ of health (船只经检疫后的)无疫证书
Billroth's cords [ˈbilrɔt] (Christian A. T. Billroth)红髓索(脾) | ~ disease 比尔罗特病(假性脑〈脊〉膜突出;淋巴瘤) / ~ operation 比尔罗特手术(胃部分切除术;舌切除术) / ~ strands 脾小梁
bilobate [baiˈləubeit], **bilobated** [baiˈləubeitid], **bilobed** [ˈbailəubd] *a* 二叶的
bilobular [baiˈlɔbjulə], **bilobulate** [baiˈlɔbjuleit] *a* 二小叶的
bilocular [ˈbaiˈlɔkjulə], **biloculate** [baiˈlɔkjuleit] *a* 双房的,二格的
biloma [ˈbailəmə] *n* 胆汁瘤(腹腔包裹性积胆)
Bilophia [baiˈlɔfilə] *n* 嗜胆汁菌属 | ~ wadsworthia 华兹沃斯嗜胆汁菌
bilophodont [baiˈlɔfədɔnt] *a* 两脊形牙的(如袋鼠)
Bimana [ˈbimənə] *n* 二手目(动物)
bimanous [ˈbimənəs, baiˈmeinəs] *a* [有]双手的
bimanual [baiˈmænjuəl] *a* 双手的,用两手的
bimastoid [baiˈmæstɔid] *a* 两乳突的
bimatoprost [biˈmætəuprɔst] *n* 比马前列(一种合成的前列腺素类似物,用作低眼压药,局部用于结膜,治疗开角型青光眼和高眼压症)
bimaxillary [baiˈmæksiləri] *a* 两颌的,双颌的
bimestrial [baiˈmestriəl] *a* 持续两月的;两月一次的
bimeter [ˈbaimitə] *n* 双侧,双度(指双侧颌力计,见 gnathodynamometer)
bimethoxycaine lactate [ˌbaimeˈθɔksikein] 乳酸二甲氧卡因(局部麻醉药)
Bimler's appliance [ˈbimlə] (H. P. Bimler) 比姆勒矫正器(一种可摘正牙矫正器)
bimodal [baiˈməudl] *a* 双峰的(指图示的曲线) | **~ity** [ˌbaiməuˈdæləti] *n*
bimolecular [ˌbaiməuˈlekjulə] *a* 双分子的
bin [bin] *n* 贮藏器,精神病收容所,疯人院
bin- 见 bi-
binal [ˈbainl] *a* 两倍的
binangle [ˈbainæŋgl] *a* 双角的 *n* 双角器(牙科用)
binary [ˈbainəri] *a* 二元的;二进制的 | ~ acid 二元素酸
binate [ˈbaineit] *a* 成对的
binaural [baiˈnɔːrəl] *a* 两耳的
binauricular [ˌbainɔːˈrikjule] *a* 两耳郭的;两心耳的
bind [baind] *vt* 捆;约束;束缚;(用绷带)包扎(伤口);结合;使便秘 *n* 捆绑物;困境 | double ~ 矛盾性支配,对立性牵制 / nail ~ 钉刺痛(指马)
binder [ˈbaində] *n* 黏合剂;结合剂;腹带

binegative [bai'negətiv] *a* 二阴电荷的

Binet's test, Binet-Simon test [bi'nei 'saimən] (Alfred Binet; Théodore Simon) 比奈测验、比奈-西蒙测验(测儿童和青年智力,询问一连串问题,由被测人答复,按其所答而评定其智力年龄)

binge [bindʒ] *n*, *vi* 狂食,狂饮

bingeing ['bindʒiŋ] *n* 狂食,狂饮(尤指狂食)

Bing-Neel syndrome [biŋ neil] (Jens Bing; Axel V. Neel) 宾-内综合征(瓦尔登斯特伦〈Waldenström〉巨球蛋白血症的中枢神经系统表现,症状中包括脑病、出血、卒中、惊厥、谵妄和昏迷)

Bing's test [biŋ] (Albert Bing) 宾氏试验(置振动的音叉于乳突,交替堵塞和开启听道:正常耳和感音神经性聋可感知响度的变化〈宾氏阳性〉,而传导性聋则无甚区别〈宾氏阴性〉)

biniramycin [bi͵niərə'maisin] *n* 比尼霉素(获自比基尼链霉菌 Streptomyces bikiniensis 的一种抗菌物质)

binocular [bi'nɔkjulə, bai'nɔkjulə] *a* 双目的;双目镜的

binoculus [bi'nɔkjuləs] *n* 双眼(看作一个器官)

binomial [bai'nəumjəl] *a* 双名的;二项式的

binophthalmoscope [͵binɔf'θælməskəup] *n* 双目检眼镜(同时可检查患者的两侧眼底)

binoscope ['binəskəup] *n* 双目单视镜

binotic [bi'nɔtik] *a* 两耳的

binovular [bi'nɔvjulə] *a* 双卵性的

Binswanger's disease (dementia, encephalitis) ['binsvɑːŋə] (Otto Binswanger) 宾斯旺格病(痴呆、脑炎)(早老性痴呆的一型,由大脑皮质下白质脱髓鞘作用所致。亦称慢性皮质下脑炎)

binucleate [bai'njuːkliit], **binuclear** [bai'njuːkliə] *a* 双核的

binucleation [͵bainjuːkli'eiʃən] *n* 双核形成

binucleolate [bainjuː'kliːəleit] *a* 双核仁的

Binz's test ['bints] (Karl Binz) 宾茨试验(检尿中奎宁)

bio- [构词成分]生,生命,生物

bioaccumulation [͵baiəuə͵kjuːmju'leifən] *n* 生物累积(生物体内累积有毒化学物质)

bioacoustics [͵baiəuə'kuːstiks] *n* 生物声学

bioactive [͵baiə'æktiv] *a* 生物活性的

bioactivity [͵baiəuæk'tivəti] *a* 生物活性,生物活度

bioaeration [͵baiəu͵eiə'reiʃən] *n* 生物曝气法,生物通气

bioamine [͵baiəu'æmiːn] *n* 生物胺

bioaminergic [͵baiəu͵æmi'nəːdʒik] *a* 生物胺能的

bioartificial [͵baiəu͵ɑːti'fiʃəl] *a* 生物人工制品的

bioassay [͵baiəuə'sei, -'æsei] *n* 生物学鉴定法,生物检定,生物测定

bioastronautics [͵baiəu͵æstrə'nɔːtiks] *n* 生物宇宙航行学(研究宇宙航行对生物体的影响)

bioautograph [͵baiəu'ɔːtəgrɑːf] *n* 生物自显影[照]片 | **~ic** [͵baiəu͵ɔːtə'græfik] *a* 生物自显影的 / **~y** [͵baiəuɔː'tɔgrəfi] *n* 生物自显影

bioavailability [͵baiəuə͵veilə'biləti] *n* 生物利用度(药物或其他物质使用后对靶组织有效的程度)

bioblast ['baiəublæst] *n* 线粒体;原生粒

biocatalyst [͵baiəu'kætəlist] *n* 生物催化剂

biocenosis [͵baiəusi'nəusis] *n* 生物群落 | **biocenotic** [͵baiəusi'nɔtik] *a*

biochemical [͵baiəu'kemikəl] *a* 生物化学的

biochemistry [͵baiəu'kemistri] *n* 生物化学 | **biochemist** *n* 生物化学家

biochemorphology [͵baiəukimɔː'fɔlədʒi] *n* 形态生物化学(研究化学结构及生物活动之间的关系) | **biochemorphic** [͵baiəuki'mɔːfik] *a*

biochore ['baiəutʃɔː] *n* 生态域,生命圈区域界线

biociation [͵baiəusi'eiʃən] *n* 亚生物群落

biocide ['baiəsaid] *n* 杀虫剂 | **biocidal** [͵baiəu'saidl] *a* 杀生物的

bioclean ['baiəukliːn] *a* 无菌的,无病原体的

bioclimatograph [͵baiəuklai'mætəgrɑːf] *n* 生物气候图

bioclimatology [͵baiəu͵klaimə'tɔlədʒi], **bioclimatics** [͵baiəuklai'mætiks] *n* 生物气象学 | **bioclimatologist** *n* 生物气象学家 / **bioclimatic** *a*

biocoenosis [͵baiəusi'nəusis] *n* 生物群落

biocolloid [͵baiəu'kɔlɔid] *n* 生物胶体

biocompatible [͵baiəukəm'pætəbl] *a* 生物相容的 | **biocompatibility** [͵baiəukəm͵pætə'biləti] *n* 生物相容性

bioconversion [͵baiəukən'vəːʃən] *n* 生物转化

biocybernetics [͵baiəu͵saibəː'netiks] *n* 生物控制论

biocycle [͵baiəu'saikl] *n* 生活周期(生物体循环现象)

biocytin [͵baiəu'saitin] *n* 生物胞素

biocytinase [͵baiəu'saitineis] *n* 生物胞素酶

biodegradation [͵baiəu͵degrə'deiʃən] *n* 生物递解,生物降解 | **biodegradable** [͵baiəu di'greidəbl] *a* 生物可降解的

biodetritus [͵baiəudi'traitəs] *n* 生物碎屑,生物腐质

biodynamics [͵baiəudai'næmiks] *n* 生物动力学

bioecology [͵baiəui(ː)'kɔlədʒi] *n* 生物生态学

bioelectricity [͵baiəu͵ilek'trisəti] *n* 生物电

bioelectrogenesis ['baiəui͵lektrəu'dʒenisis] *n* 生

物电发生
bioelectronics [ˌbaiəuˌilekˈtrɔniks] *n* 生物电子学
bioelement [ˌbaiəuˈelimənt] *n* 生物元素(活组织成分中的化学元素)
bioenergetics [ˌbaiəuˌenəˈdʒetiks] *n* 生物能学,生物能量学(研究生物体内能量的转换)
bioengineering (**biomedical engineering**) [ˌbaiəuˌendʒiˈniəriŋ] *n* 生物工程学(生物医学工程学)(工程技术原理在生物学及医学上的应用)
bioenvironment [ˌbaiəuinˈvaiərənˌmənt] *n* 生物环境
bioenvironmental [ˌbaiəuinˌvaiərənˈmentəl] *a* 与生物环境有关的
bioequivalence [ˌbaiəuiˈkwivələns] *n* 生物等效性
bioequivalent [ˌbaiəuiˈkwivələnt] *a* 生物等效的
bioethics [ˌbaiəuˈeθiks] *n* 生物伦理学(研究器官移植等医学活动所涉及的人伦道德问题)
biofeedback [ˌbaiəuˈfiːdbæk] *n* 生物反馈 | alpha ~ α 生物反馈(亦称 α 反馈)
biofilm [ˈbaiəufilm] *n* 生物膜
bioflavonoid [ˌbaiəuˈfleivənɔid] *n* 生物黄酮素
biogen [ˈbaiədʒən] *n* 生源体
biogenesis [ˌbaiəuˈdʒenisis] *n* 生源说(认为一切生物均自生物发生);重演(即 recapitulation,见 theory 项下相应术语) | **biogenetic** [ˌbaiəudʒiˈnetik] *a* 生源的,生物发生的
biogenic [ˌbaiəuˈdʒenik] *a* 生物起源的(如生物胺 biogenic amine)
biogenous [baiˈɔdʒinəs] *a* 生命产生的,产生生命的
biogeochemistry [ˌbaiəuˌdʒi(ː)əuˈkemistri] *n* 生物地理化学
biogeocoenology [ˌbaiəuˌdʒiːəusiˈnɔlədʒi] *n* 生物地理群落学
biogeography [ˌbaiəudʒiˈɔgrəfi] *n* 生物地理学
bioglass [ˈbaiəuglɑːs] *n* 生物玻璃
biograph [ˈbaiəugrɑːf, -græf] *n* 生物运动描记器(用作诊断某些神经病);呼吸描记器
biography [baiˈɔgrəfi] *n* 生物运动摄影术
biohazard [ˈbaiəuˌhæzəd] *n* 生物危害
biohydraulic [ˌbaiəuhaiˈdrɔːlik] *a* 生物水力学的
bioimplant [ˌbaiəuˈimplænt] *n* 生物植入物,生物植入片
bioincompatible [ˌbaiəuˌinkəmˈpætəbl] *a* 生物不相容的(对生物功能具有毒性或损害作用的)
bioinformatics [ˌbaiəuˌinfəˈmætiks] *n* 生物信息学
bioinstrumentation [ˌbaiəuˌinstrumenˈteiʃən] *n* 生物测试设备
biokinetics [ˌbaiəukaiˈnetiks, -kiˈn-] *n* 生物运动学
biologic(al) [ˌbaiəˈlɔdʒik(əl)] *a* 生物学的 | **biologically** *ad*
biologicals [ˌbaiəˈlɔdʒikəlz] [复] *n* 生物制品(包括血清、菌苗、抗原、抗毒素等)
biologos [baiˈɔləgəs] *n* 生物智力
biology [baiˈɔlədʒi] *n* 生物学 | molecular ~ 分子生物学 / radiation ~ 放射生物学 | **biologist** *n* 生物学家
bioluminescence [ˌbaiəuˌljuːmiˈnesns] *n* 生物发光 | **bioluminescent** *a*
biolysis [baiˈɔlisis] *n* 生物分解 | **biolytic** [ˌbaiəuˈlitik] *a* 生物分解的;破坏生命的
biomacromolecule [ˌbaiəuˌmækrəuˈmɔlikjuːl] *n* 生物大分子
biomarker [ˈbaiəuˌmɑːkə] *n* 生物标记;肿瘤标记
biomass [ˈbaiəumæs] *n* 菌体量,生物量,生物质
biomaterial [ˌbaiəuməˈtiəriəl] *n* 生物材料(修复活组织用)
biomathematics [ˌbaiəuˌmæθiˈmætiks] *n* 生物数学(把数学应用于生物学和医学)
biome [ˈbaiəum] *n* 生物群落区
biomechanics [ˌbaiəumiˈkæniks] *n* 生物力学 | **biomechanical** *a*
biomedicine [ˌbaiəuˈmedsin] *n* 生物医学(自然科学如生物学、生物化学及生物物理学在临床医学上的应用) | **biomedical** *a*
biomembrane [ˌbaiəuˈmembrein] *n* 生物膜(如细胞膜) | **biomembranous** [ˌbaiəuˈmembreinəs] *a*
biometeorology [ˌbaiəuˌmiːtjəˈrɔlədʒi] *n* 生物气象学 | **biometeorologist** *n* 生物气象学家
biometer [baiˈɔmitə] *n* 生物计(一种活组织微量二氧化碳测定仪)
biometrician [ˌbaiəumiˈtriʃən] *n* 生物统计学家
biometrics [ˌbaiəuˈmetriks] *n* 生物统计学
biometry [baiˈɔmitri] *n* 生物统计学;寿命预测(人寿保险)
biomicroscope [ˌbaiəuˈmaikrəskəup] *n* 活组织显微镜 | slit-lamp ~ 裂隙灯活组织显微镜(见 Gullstrand's slit lamp)
biomicroscopy [ˌbaiəumaiˈkrɔskəpi] *n* 活组织显微镜检查(亦指用裂隙灯和角膜显微镜作角膜或晶体检查)
biomodulation [ˌbaiəuˌmɔdjuˈleiʃən] *n* 生物调节
biomodulator [ˌbaiəuˈmɔdjuˌleitə] *n* 生物调节剂
biomolecule [ˌbaiəuˈmɔlikjuːl] *n* 生物分子(由活细胞产生的分子,如蛋白质、糖类或脂类)
biomotor [ˌbaiəuˈməutə] *n* 人工呼吸器
Biomphalaria [baiˌɔmfəˈlɛəriə] *n* 扁卷螺属(亦称澳卷螺属 Australorbis)
bion [ˈbaiɔn] *n* 生物个体

bionecrosis [ˌbaiəuneˈkrəusis] *n* 渐进性坏死
bionergy [baiˈɔnədʒi] *n* 生命力
bionic acid [baiˈɔnik] 生物酸
bionics [baiˈɔniks] *n* 仿生学
bionomics [ˌbaiəuˈnɔmiks] *n* 生态学
bionomy [baiˈɔnəmi] *n* 生命规律学
bionosis [baiəuˈnəusis] *n* 生物病,生物性疾病
bionucleonics [ˌbaiəuˌnjuːkliˈɔniks] *n* 生物核子学(研究放射性及稀有稳定同位素在生物学上的应用)
bio-osmotic [ˌbai əuɔzˈmɔtik] *a* 生物渗透的
bioparent [ˌbaiəuˈpɛərənt] *n* 生身父,生身母
biophagism [baiˈɔfədʒizəm], **biophagy** [baiˈɔfədʒi] *n* 食生物作用
biophagous [baiˈɔfəgəs] *a* 食生物的
biopharmaceutical [ˌbaiəuˌfɑːməˈsjutikəl] *a* 生物药剂学的
biopharmaceutics [ˌbaiəuˌfɑːməˈsjutiks] *n* 生物药剂学
biophore [ˈbaiəfɔː] *n* 生源体 | **biophoric** [ˌbaiəuˈfɔrik] *a*
biophotometer [ˌbaiəufəuˈtɔmitə] *n* 光度适应计(用以测眼睛的暗光适应力,检查维生素 A 缺乏的指征)
biophysics [ˌbaiəuˈfiziks] *n* 生物物理学 | dental ~ 牙科生物物理学 | **biophysical** *a* / **biophysicist** *n* 生物物理学家
biophysiography [ˌbaiəufiziˈɔgrəfi] *n* 记载生物学
biophysiology [ˌbaiəufiziˈɔlədʒi] *n* 生物生理学
bioplasia [baiəuˈpleiziə] *n* 储能生长(以生长的形式储存食物能量)
bioplasm [ˈbaiəuplæzəm] *n* 原生质,活质;主浆质 | **~ic** [ˌbaiəuˈplæzmik] *a*
bioplast [ˈbaiəuplæst] *n* 原生质体;细胞(一种阿米巴样细胞)
biopoiesis [ˌbaiəupɔiˈiːsis] *n* 生命自生(生命起源于无机物)
biopolymer [ˌbaiəuˈpɔlimə] *n* 生物聚合体,生物高分子
bioprosthesis [ˌbaiəuprɔsˈθiːsis] *n* 生物假体(由生物材料制成的假体) | **bioprosthetic** [ˌbaiəuprɔsˈθetik] *a*
biopsy [ˈbaiɔpsi] *n*, *vt* 活组织检查,活检 | aspiration ~, needle ~ 针吸活组织检查 / brush ~ 刷拭活检 / cone ~ 锥形活检 / cytological ~ 细胞学活检 / endoscopic ~ 内镜活检 / punch ~ 钻取活组织检查 / sternal ~ 胸骨活组织检查 / surgical ~ 手术活组织检查 / total ~ 完整活组织检查(整个肿瘤活组织检查,此法具有治疗和诊断价值) | **bioptic** [baiˈɔptik] *a*
biopsychic(al) [ˌbaiəuˈsaikik(əl)] *a* 生物心理的
biopsychology [ˌbaiəusaiˈkɔlədʒi] *n* 生物心理学;精神生物学
biopterin [baiˈɔptərin] *n* 生物蝶呤
bioptome [ˈbaiɔpˌtəum] *n* 活组织检查刀
biopyoculture [ˌbaiəuˌpaiəˈkʌltʃə] *n* 脓细胞培养
bioradiography [ˌbaiəuˌreidiˈɔgrəfi] *n* 生物 X 线摄影[术]
biorational [ˌbaiəuˈræʃənl] *a* 生物合理的(通过天然方法产生效果的,指以病毒、细菌、原生动物、真菌或天然存在的生化物质之类的杀虫剂)
biorbital [baiˈɔːbitl] *a* 二眶的
bioresearch [ˌbaiəuriˈsəːtʃ] *n* 生物学研究
bioreversible [ˌbaiəuriˈvəːsəbl] *a* 生物可逆[性]的(指药物)
biorgan [ˈbaiɔːgən] *n* 生理器官(指与形态器官不同而言)
biorheology [ˌbaiəuriˈɔlədʒi] *n* 生物流变学
biorhythm [ˈbaiəuriðəm] *n* 生物节律
bioroentgenography [ˌbaiəurɔntgeˈnɔgrəfi] *n* 生物 X 线摄影[术]
bios [ˈbaiɔs] *n* 生物活素(促单细胞生物如酵母生长的因素) | ~ Ⅰ 肌醇,环己六醇 / ~ Ⅱ 生物素
biosatellite [ˌbaiəuˈsætəlait] *n* 生物卫星(一种宇宙飞船研究宇宙辐射、失重等对地球生物的生理影响)
bioscience [ˌbaiəuˈsaiəns] *n* 生物科学(用一切能应用的科学,如物理学、化学等研究生物学)
bioscopy [baiˈɔskəpi] *n* 生死检定法
biose [ˈbaiəus] *n* 二碳糖;二糖
biosis [baiˈəusis] *n* 生活力;生命现象
biosmosis [ˌbaiɔzˈməusis] *n* 生物渗透
biospectrometry [ˌbaiəuspekˈtrɔmitri] *n* 活组织分光度测量术
biospectroscopy [ˌbaiəuspekˈtrɔskəpi] *n* 活组织分光镜检查
biosphere [ˈbaiəsfiə] *n* 生物圈
biostatics [ˌbaiəuˈstætiks] *n* 生物静力学,生物功能结构学
biostatistics [ˌbaiəustəˈtistiks] *n* 生物统计学;生命统计 | **biostatistical** *a* / **biostatistician** *n* 生物统计学家
biostereometrics [ˌbaiəustiəriəˈmetriks] *n* 生物立体测量技术
biosynthesis [ˌbaiəuˈsinθisis] *n* 生物合成 | **biosynthetic** [ˌbaiəusinˈθetik] *a* / **biosynthetically** *ad*
biota [baiˈəutə] *n* 生物区[系]
biotaxis [ˌbaiəuˈtæksis] *n* 活细胞趋性(活细胞选择和排列的能力)
biotaxy [ˌbaiəuˈtæksi] *n* 活细胞趋性;生物分类学
biotelemetry [ˌbaiəutiˈlemitri] *n* 生物遥测术(远

距离记载和测定生物体某些生命现象)
biotherapy [ˌbaiəuˈθerəpi] *n* 生物制剂疗法
biothesiometer [ˌbaiəuˌθiːziˈɔmitə] *n* 生物震感阈测量器
biotic [baiˈɔtik] *a* 生命的;生物的;生物区系的 | ~ acid 生物酸
biotics [baiˈɔtiks] *n* 生命学(研究生物体特有的功能和性质)
biotin [ˈbaiətin] *n* 生物素(维生素 H,辅酶 R)
biotinidase [ˌbaiəˈtinideis] *n* 生物素酶(此酶缺乏,为一种常染色体隐性性状,可致多羧化酶缺乏症)
biotinyl [ˌbaiəˈtinil] *n* 生物素[酰]基
biotinylation [ˌbaiəˌtiniˈleiʃən] *n* 生物素[酰]基化
biotomy [baiˈɔtəmi] *n* 生物解剖学;活体解剖法
biotoxication [ˌbaiəuˌtɔksiˈkeiʃən] *n* 生物毒中毒
biotoxicology [ˌbaiəuˌtɔksiˈkɔlədʒi] *n* 生物毒理学
biotoxin [ˌbaiəuˈtɔksin] *n* 生物毒
biotransformation [ˌbaiəuˌtrænsfəˈmeiʃən] *n* 生物转化(化合物如药物在生物体内由于酶的作用所发生的一系列化学转化)
biotrepy [baiˈɔtrəpi] *n* 生体化学反应学
biotron [ˈbaiətrɔn] *n* 生物气候室
Biot's respiration (breathing, sign) [biˈɔː] (Camille Biot) 比奥呼吸(征)(其特征为无规律的呼吸暂停期,与四至五次相等深度呼吸交替出现,见于颅内压增高的患者)
biotype [ˈbaiətaip] *n* 同型小种生物属型;生物型 | **biotypic** [baiəuˈtipik] *a*
biotypology [ˌbaiəutaiˈpɔlədʒi] *n* 生物属型学
biovular [baiˈɔvjulə] *a* 双卵性的
biparasitic [ˌbaipærəˈsitik] *a* 重寄生的(在寄生物上寄生的)
biparental [ˌbaipəˈrentl] *a* 来自双亲的
biparietal [ˌbaipəˈraiitl] *a* 二顶骨的,双顶的
biparous [ˈbipərəs] *a* 双胎的,两胎的(经产两次的)
bipartite [baiˈpaːtait] *a* 两部分的;两分的(如哺乳动物的双子宫);双枝的
bipartition [ˌbaipaːˈtiʃən] *n* 分成两部分;两分,对分
biped [ˈbaiped] *a* 两足的 *n* 两足动物
bipedal [ˈbaiˌpedl] *a* 两足的
bipenniform [baiˈpenifɔːm] *a* 二回羽状的;有双翅的
biperforate [baiˈpəːfəreit] *a* 二[穿]孔的
biperiden [baiˈperidin] *n* 比哌立登(抗胆碱能药,抗震颤麻痹药)
biphenamine hydrochloride [baiˈfenəmiːn] 盐酸珍尼柳酯(抗菌、抗真菌、局部麻醉药)
biphenyl [baiˈfiːnil] *n* 联苯 | polybrominated ~s (PBB_s) 多溴化联苯 / polychlorinated ~s (PCB_s) 多氯化联苯
***p*-biphenylamine** [baiˌfiːnilˈæmiːn] *n* 对苯基苯胺,对氨基联苯
bipolar [baiˈpəulə] *a* 有两极的;双极的,两极的(指双极神经元、双极细菌染色法,以及既有躁狂又有抑郁发作的双极情感性精神病) | **bipolarity** [ˌbaipəuˈlærəti] *n* 双极性,两极性
Bipolarina [ˌbaipəuləˈrainə] *n* 双极虫亚目
Bipolaris [baipəˈleiris] *n* 离蠕孢霉属
bipositive [baiˈpɔzətiv] *a* 二正价的(带有两个正电荷的)
bipotential [ˌbaipəuˈtenʃəl] *a* 双潜能的
bipotentiality [ˌbaipəuˌtenʃiˈæləti] *n* 双潜能 | ~ of the gonad 生殖腺两性潜能(可发育成卵巢或睾丸)
bipus [ˈbaipəs] *a* 两足的
biramous [baiˈreiməs] *a* 二支的
birch [bəːtʃ] *n* 桦
bird-arm [ˈbəːd ɑːm] *n* 鸟状臂(前臂肌萎缩所致)
bird-face [ˈbəːdfeis] *n* 鸟状脸(颅骨小而面骨大)
bird-leg [ˈbəːdleg] *n* 鸟状腿(下肢肌萎缩所致)
bird-lime [ˈbəːdlaim] *n* 粘鸟胶(捕小鸟用;旧时敷伤口及溃疡用)
Bird's formula [bəːd] (Golding Bird) 伯德公式(尿比重最后两个数目相近于每英两所含固体的格令〈grain〉数) | ~ treatment 伯德疗法(应用小量直流电治疗褥疮)
Bird's sign [bəːd] (Samuel D. Bird) 伯德征(肺棘球蚴病时呼吸音消失而呈现局限性浊音区)
birefractive [ˌbairiˈfræktiv] *a* 双折射的
birefringence [ˌbairiˈfrindʒəns] *n* 双折射 | crystalline ~, intrinsic ~ 晶体双折射,特性双折射 / flow ~, streaming ~ 流动双折射 / form ~ 形状双折射 / strain ~ 应变双折射 | **birefringent** *a*
birhinia [baiˈrainiə] *n* 双鼻
Birkett's hernia [ˈbəːket] (John Birkett) 伯基特疝,滑膜突出
Birkhaug's test [ˈbəːkhɔːg] (Konrad E. Birkhaug) 伯克豪格试验(风湿病皮肤试验)
Birnaviridae [ˈbəːnəˌviridiː] *n* 双段双链 RNA 病毒科
Birnavirus [ˈbəːnəˌvaiərəs] *n* 双段双链 RNA 病毒属
birnavirus [ˈbəːnəˌvaiərəs] *n* 双节段双链 RNA 病毒
Birnberg bow [ˈbəːnbəːg] (Charles H. Birnberg) 伯恩伯格弓(一种宫内节育器)
birth [bəːθ] *n* 生产,分娩 | complete ~ 完全产 / cross ~ 横产 / dead ~ 死产 / head ~ 头位产 /

multiple ~ 多胎产 / post-term ~ 过期产 / premature ~ 早产 / still ~ 死产

birthmark [ˈbəːθmɑːk] *n* 胎记 | physiologic ~ 生理胎记

birthrate [ˈbəːθreit] *n* 出生率

bis- [前缀]二,两个,双;两次

bisacodyl [bisˈækədil, ˌbisəˈkəudil] *n* 比沙可啶(泻药) | ~ tannex 鞣酸比沙可啶(泻药)

bisacromial [ˌbisəˈkrəumiəl] *n* 二肩峰的

bisalbuminemia [ˌbisælˌbjuːmiˈniːmiə] *n* 双白蛋白血[症]

bisaxillary [biˈsæksiləri] *a* 两腋的

bis(chloromethyl)ether [bisˌklɔːrəuˈmeθilˈiːθə] *n* 二(氯甲基)醚(一种烷化剂,在工业上用作化学中间体,对眼睛与黏膜具有刺激性,并致癌。亦称对称二氯甲基醚)

Bischoff's crown (corona) [ˈbiʃɔf] (Theodor L. W. von Bischoff) 比绍夫冠(卵巢周围粒层细胞的放射冠)

Bischoff's myelotomy [ˈbiʃɔf] (W. Bischoff) 比绍夫脊髓切开术(通过腰区纵向手术切开脊髓,以缓解痉挛状态)

Bischoff's test [ˈbiʃɔf] (Carl A. Bischoff) 比绍夫试验(检胆汁酸)

biscuit [ˈbiskit] *n* 瓷饼,瓷面(牙科) | hard ~ 硬烤瓷饼,硬瓷面 / medium ~ 适中瓷饼,适中瓷面 / soft ~ 软烤瓷饼,软瓷面

biscuiting [ˈbiskitiŋ] *n* 瓷饼形成,瓷面形成

bisect [baiˈsekt] *vt* 把…分为二,把…二等分;对切 | **~ion** [baiˈsekʃən] *n* 二等分;对切,平分;平分的两部分之一 / **~ional** [baiˈsekʃənəl] *a* 对切的,平分的

bisector [baiˈsektə] *n* 二等分物;平分线

bisegmentectomy [ˌbaisegmenˈtektəmi] *n* 双段切除术,肝叶切除术

biseptate [baiˈsepteit] *a* 二分隔的,分隔为二的

biserial [baiˈsiəriəl] *a* 二列的

bisexual [baiˈseksjuəl] *a* 两性的 *n* 两性体

bisexuality [baiˌseksjuˈæləti] *n* 两性现象(两性具有;雌雄同体)

bisferiens [bisˈfiəriənz] *a* 【拉】重搏的,两次重搏的

bisferious [bisˈfiəriəs] *a* 重搏的,两次搏动的

BIS-GMA dimethacrylate 二异丁烯酸

Bishop's sphygmoscope [ˈbiʃəp] (Louis F. Bishop) 毕晓普脉搏检视器(测血压,尤指舒张压)

bishydroxycoumarin [ˌbishaiˌdrɔksiˈkuːmərin] *n* 双香豆素(抗凝药)

bisiliac [baiˈsiliæk] *a* 二髂嵴的

bis in die [bis in ˈdiːei] 【拉】每日 2 次(缩写为 b. d. 或 b. i. d.)

bismuth(Bi) [ˈbizməθ] *n* 铋 | ~ albuminate 白蛋白铋(用于治疗胃肠痉挛) / ~ and ammonium citrate 枸橼酸铋铵(肠收敛剂) / ~ magma 铋乳 / ~ subcarbonate 碱式碳酸铋,次碳酸铋(止泻药) / ~ subnitrate, ~ white 次硝酸铋,铋白(解酸药) / ~ tannate 鞣酸铋 | **~al** *a* 含铋的

bismuthia [bizˈmʌθiə] *n* 铋线,铋剂性变色(由于服用铋剂皮肤和黏膜呈蓝变色)

bismuthic acid [ˈbizməθik] 铋酸

bismuthosis [ˌbizməˈθəusis], **bismuthism** [ˈbizməθizəm] *n* 铋中毒

bisobrin lactate [ˈbisəbrin] 乳酸比索布啉(纤维蛋白溶解药)

bisoprolol fumarate [ˌbisəˈprəulɔl] 延胡索酸比索洛尔(合成 β 受体阻滞药,用于治疗高血压,口服给药)

1, 3-bisphosphoglycerate [ˌbisfɔsfəuˈglisəreit] *n* 1, 3-二磷酸甘油酸

2, 3-bisphosphoglycerate [bisˌfɔsfəuˈglisəreit] *n* 2, 3-二磷酸甘油酸

bisphosphoglycerate mutase [bisˌfɔsfəu ˈglisəreit ˈmjuːteis] 二磷酸甘油酸变位酶(此酶缺乏为一种常染色体隐性性状,可致溶血性贫血)

bisphosphoglycerate phosphatase [bisˌfɔsfəu-ˈglisəreit ˈfɔsfəteis] 二磷酸甘油酸磷酸酶

bisphosphoglyceric acid [ˌbisfɔsfəuˈglisərik] 二磷酸甘油酸

bisphosphoglyceromutase [bisˌfɔsfəu ˌglisərəˈmjuːteis] *n* 二磷酸甘油酸变位酶

bisphosphonate [bisˈfɔsfəneit] *n* 二膦酸;二膦酸盐(或酯)

bispore [ˈbaispɔː] *n* 双孢子

bisque [bisk] *n* 【法】瓷饼,瓷面 | hard ~ 硬烤瓷饼,硬瓷面 / medium ~ 适中瓷饼,适中瓷面 / soft ~ 软烤瓷饼,软瓷面

bistephanic [ˌbaistiˈfænik] *a* 二冠状点的

Biston betularia [ˈbistn bitjuˈlɛəriə] 桦尺蛾(用在研究工业黑化现象)

bistort [ˈbistɔːt] *n* 拳参(其根含有鞣酸,具有收敛和强壮作用)

bistoury [ˈbisturi] *n* 细长小刀(用以切开脓肿及扩大窦道、瘘管等)

bistratal [baiˈstreitl] *a* 双层的

bisulfate, bisulphate [baiˈsʌlfeit] *n* 硫酸氢盐

bisulfide, bisulphide [baiˈsʌlfaid] *n* 二硫化物

bisulfite, bisulphite [baiˈsʌlfait] *n* 亚硫酸氢盐

bit [bit] *n* 二进制位,二进制数字(即 binary digit);比特(二进制信息单位)

bitartrate [baiˈtɑːtreit] *n* 酒石酸氢盐

bite [bait] *n* 殆,咬合;咬力;殆印模;咬面;咬伤;一口食物 | balanced ~ 平衡咬合,平衡殆 / check ~ 正殆法,殆校正法 / cross ~ 反殆,错殆

/ edge-to-edge ~, end-to-end ~ 对切殆,对刃殆 / open ~ 开殆,无殆 / over ~ 覆殆 / stork ~s 毛细血管扩张斑;焰色痣 / underhung ~ 下超殆 / wax ~ 蜡殆法 / X- ~ 反殆

bite-block [ˈbait blɔk] *n* 殆堤,殆缘

bitegage [ˈbaitgeidʒ] *n* 殆尺,咬合计

bitelock [ˈbaitlɔk] *n* 殆锁,咬合锁

bitemporal [baiˈtempərəl] *a* 双颞的

biteplane [ˈbaitplein] *n* 殆平面

biteplate [ˈbaitpleit] *n* 殆板

biterminal [baiˈtəːminl] *a* 双端钮的

bite-wing [ˈbaitwiŋ] *n* 殆翼片(牙科用的一种 X 线片)

bithionol [baiˈθaiənɔl] *n* 硫氯酚(消毒防腐药)

bithionolate sodium [baiˈθaiənəleit] 硫氯酚钠

Bithynia [biˈθiniə] *n* 豆螺属 | ~ longicornus 长角豆螺

biting [ˈbaitiŋ] *a* 刺痛的;辛辣的,腐蚀性的

Bitis [ˈbaitis] *n* 蝰属(一种毒蛇属)

bitolterol mesylate [baiˈtəultərəul] 甲磺比托特罗(β 肾上腺素能支气管扩张药)

Bitot's spots (patches) [biˈtəu] (Pierre A. Bitot) 比奥斑,结膜干燥斑(营养不良维生素 A 缺乏时,结膜上的斑点)

bitrochanteric [ˌbaitrəukənˈterik] *a* 二转子的

bitter [ˈbitə] *a* 苦的 *n* [复]苦味药

bitterling [ˈbitəliŋ] *n* 苦鳑鲏,苦鱼(检孕试验用)

bitters [ˈbitəz] *n* 苦味药酒 | aromatic ~ 芳香苦味药 / styptic ~ 收敛性苦味药 / Swedish ~ 瑞典苦味药,复方芦荟酊

bitterwood [ˈbitəwuːd] *n* 苦木,牙买加苦树

Bittner virus [ˈbitnə] (John J. Bittner) 比特纳病毒,小鼠乳腺瘤病毒

Bittorf's reaction [ˈbitɔf] (Alexander Bittorf) 比托夫反应(肾绞痛发作时,压卵巢或睾丸引起的疼痛放射至肾脏)

bitumen [ˈbitjumin, biˈtjuː-] *n*【拉】沥青 | sulfonated ~ 磺化沥青,鱼石脂

bituminize [biˈtjuːminaiz] *vt* 使成沥青;与沥青混合 | **bituminization** [biˌtjuːminaiˈzeiʃən, -niˈz-] *n*

bituminosis [ˌbitjumiˈnəusis] *n* 沥青末沉着病,沥青末肺

bituminous [biˈtjuːminəs] *n* 沥青的,含沥青的

Bitunicatae [baiˌtjuːniˈkeitiː] *n* 双囊壁子囊亚门

biurate [ˈbaijuəreit] *n* 酸性尿酸盐,重尿酸盐

biuret [ˈbaijuəret] *n* 双缩脲

bivalence [baiˈveiləns, ˈbivə-] *n* 二价

bivalent [baiˈveilənt, ˈbivə-] *a* 二价的;双价的 *n* 二价体

bivalirudin [baiˈvæliruːdin] *n* 比伐柔定(抗凝药)

bivalve [ˈbaivælv] *a* 双瓣的,两片的;双壳的 *n* 双壳类;牡蛎

Bivalvia [baiˈvælviə] *n* 双壳纲(即斧足类 Pelecypoda)

Bivalvulida [ˌbaivælˈvjuːlidə] *n* 双壳目

biventer [baiˈventə] *n* 二腹肌

biventral [baiˈventrəl] *a* 二腹的 *n* 二腹肌

biventricular [ˌbaivenˈtrikjulə] *a* 两心室的

bivitelline [ˌbaivaiˈtelin] *a* 双卵黄的

bixin [ˈbiksin] *n* 红木素,胭脂树橙

bizarre [biˈzɑː] *a* 奇异的,奇特的

bizygomatic [ˌbaizaigəˈmætik] *a* 两颧的

Bizzozero's cells, corpuscles, platelets [biˈtsɔtserəu] (Giulio Bizzozero) 比佐泽罗细胞、小体、小板(血小板)

Bjerrum's scotoma (sign) [ˈbjerum] (Jannik P. Bjerrum) 布耶鲁姆暗点(征)(早期青光眼盲点,镰刀状暗点的进一步发展)

Bjerrum's screen [ˈbjerum] (J. Bjerrum) 布耶鲁姆屏(正切暗点计屏,正面视野计屏)

Björnstad's syndrome [biˈɔnstæd] (R. Björnstad) 比翁施塔德综合征(一种常染色体隐性遗传性疾病,特征为先天性感音神经性聋和扭发)

Bk berkelium 锫

B-K, BK below-knee 膝下(截肢)

BKV BK virus BK 病毒(一种人多瘤病毒)

black [blæk] *a* 黑的;黑色的;黑人的 *n* 黑色;黑斑;黑人 | animal ~, bone- ~, ivory ~, Paris ~ 动物炭,骨炭,象牙炭,巴黎骨炭 / indulin ~ 苯胺黑 / lamp ~ 油烟,煤烟;灯黑

Blackberg and Wanger's test [ˈblækbəːg, ˈwæŋgə] (Solon N. Blackberg; J. O. Wanger) 布莱克伯格和旺格试验(检尿中黑素)

blackberry [ˈblækbəri] *n* 黑刺莓;黑刺莓浆果

blackdamp [ˈblækdæmp] *n* 乌烟,窒息性气体(主要为一氧化碳,矿内空气缺氧)

Blackfan-Diamond anemia (syndrome) [ˈblækfæn ˈdaimənd] (Kenneth D. Blackfan; Louis K. Diamond) 布-戴贫血(综合征),先天性再生不良性贫血

black haw [blæk hɔː] 樱叶荚蒾,(北美)荚蒾

blackhead [ˈblækhed] *n* 黑头粉刺,开放性粉刺;(火鸡)黑冠病,组织滴虫病

blackleg [ˈblækleg], **blackquarter** [blækˈkwɔːtə] *n* 黑腿病,气肿性炭疽

blackout [ˈblækaut] *n* 一时性黑矇

Black's classification [blæk] (Greene V. Black) 布莱克分类(一种龋分类法,根据治疗的相似性,将龋牙分成 5 类)

Black's formula [blæk] (J. A. Black) 布莱克公式($F = \langle W + C \rangle - H$,W 表示体重磅数,C 为深吸气胸围英寸数,H 为身高英寸数,当 F 大于 120,此人为非常强壮,110 ~ 120 时为强壮,100 ~ 110 时为良好,90 ~ 100 时为尚可,80 ~ 90 时为衰弱,

80 以下时为非常衰弱)

blacksnake [ˈblæksneik] *n* 黑蛇;黑脊游蛇,响导黑锦蛇

Black's test [blæk] (Otis F. Black)布莱克试验(检尿中β-羟丁酸)

blacktongue [blækˈtʌŋ] *n* 黑舌病(犬糙皮病)

bladder [ˈblædə] *n* 囊;膀胱 | allantoic ~ 尿囊 / atonic ~ 弛缓性膀胱,无张力性膀胱 / autonomous ~, autonomic ~ 自主性膀胱 / brain ~ 脑泡 / chyle ~ 乳糜池 / gall ~ 胆囊 / irritable ~ 膀胱过敏,刺激性膀胱 / urinary ~ 膀胱

bladdery [ˈblædəri] *a* 囊状的;有囊的

blade [bleid] *n* 扁骨 | shoulder ~ 肩胛骨

blain [blein] *n* 水疱,脓疱;炭疽;肉刺

Blainville's ear [blænˈviːl] (Henri M. D. de Blainville)布兰维尔耳(两耳不对称)

Blake's disks [bleik] (Clarence J. Blake)布莱克盘(修补鼓膜纸片,黏贴鼓膜穿孔用)

Blalock-Hanlon operation [ˈbleilɔk ˈhænlən] (Alfred Blalock; C. Rollins Hanlon)布-汉手术(造成房间隔缺损的大血管转位姑息性手术)

Blalock-Taussig operation (shunt) [ˈbleilɔk ˈtɔːsig] (Alfred Blalock; Helen B. Taussig)布莱洛克-陶西格手术(分流术)(锁骨下动脉肺动脉吻合术)

blanc [blɔŋ] *a*【法】白[色]的 | ~ fixé 硫酸钡(造影剂)

Blanchard's method, treatment [ˈblæntʃɑːd] (Wallace Blanchard)布兰查德法、疗法(用白蜡、矿脂混合物填入结核骨腔中)

Blandin and Nuhn's glands [blənˈdæn nuːn] (P. F. Blandin; Anton Nuhn)布-努腺,舌尖腺

Blandin's ganglion [blənˈdæn] (Philippe F. Blandin)下颌下神经节 | ~ glands 舌尖腺

blanket [ˈblæŋkit] *n* 毯,毡 | electric ~ 电[热]毯

blankophore [ˈblæŋkəfɔː] *n* 荧光增白剂

Blasius' duct [ˈblɑːsiuz] (Gerhard Blasius)腮腺管

blast [blɑːst] *n* 爆炸;冲击波,气浪;胚细胞,原始细胞,未成熟细胞;分裂球丝(分裂球间的丝状纺锤体) | ~ form of red cells 有核红细胞 / immersion ~ 水下爆炸性震伤(深水炸弹爆炸造成水下工作人员的内伤)

blastation [blæsˈteiʃən] *n* 种质变异

blastema [blæsˈtiːmə] *n* 原生质;胚基,芽基 | **blastemic** [blæsˈtemik] *a*

blastic [ˈblæstik] *a* 芽殖[产孢]的,芽生的

blastid [ˈblæstid], **blastide** [ˈblæstaid] *n* 胚痕

blastin [ˈblæstin] *n* 胚素,促细胞增生素

blast(o)- [构词成分]胚,芽

Blastobacter [ˌblæstəuˈbæktə] *n* 芽生杆菌属

blastocatenate [ˌblæstəuˈkætəneit] *a* 顶链形的,顶串珠状的

Blastocaulis [blæstəuˈkɔːlis] *n* 芽柄菌属

blastochyle [ˈblæstəukail] *n* 囊胚腔液

blastoc(o)ele [ˈblæstəusiːl] *n* 囊胚腔 | **blastoc(o)elic** [ˌblæstəuˈsiːlik] *a*

blastoconidium [ˌblæstəukəˈnidiəm] *n* 芽分生孢子

Blastocrithidia [ˌblæstəukriˈθidiə] *n* 芽生短膜虫属

blastocyst [ˈblæstəusist] *n* 胚泡

Blastocystis [ˌblæstəuˈsistis] *n* 酵母菌属 | ~ hominis 人酵母菌

blastocyte [ˈblæstəusait] *n* 胚细胞

blastocytoma [ˌblastəusaiˈtəumə] *n* 胚细胞瘤

blastodendriosis [ˌblæstəuˌdendriˈəusis] *n* 芽枝酵母病

blastoderm [ˈblæstəudəːm] *n* 胚盘,胚层 | bilaminar ~ 二层胚盘 / embryonic ~ 胎部胚盘 / extraembryonic ~ 膜部胚盘 / trilaminar ~ 三层胚盘 | **~al** [ˌblæstəuˈdəːməl], **~ic** [ˌblæstəuˈdəːmik] *a*

blastodisc [ˈblæstəudisk] *n* 胚盘

blastogenesis [ˌblæstəuˈdʒenisis] *n* 芽生;种质遗传(通过生殖细胞将遗传性状传给后代);胚细胞样转变,母细胞化(小淋巴细胞接触植物血凝素后或接触用于免疫宿主的抗原后,变为较大的、相似于胚细胞样的过程) | **blastogenic** [ˌblæstəuˈdʒenik], **blastogenetic** [ˌblæstəudʒiˈnetik] *a*

blastogeny [blæsˈtɔdʒini] *n* 种质演变

Blastogregarinina [ˌblæstəuˌgregəˈrainìnə] *n* 芽生簇虫亚目

blastokinin [ˌblæstəuˈkainin] *n* 胚泡激肽(亦称子宫球蛋白)

blastolysis [ˌblæsˈtɔlisis] *n* 种质破坏 | **blastolytic** [ˌblæstəuˈlitik] *a*

blastoma [blæsˈtəumə] ([复] **blastomas** 或 **blastomata** [blæsˈtəumətə]) *n* 母细胞瘤 | pleuricentric ~ 多中心母细胞瘤 / unicentric ~ 单中心母细胞瘤 | **~tous** *a*

blastomatoid [blæsˈtəumətɔid] *a* 母细胞瘤样的

blastomatosis [ˌblæstəuməˈtəusis] *n* 母细胞瘤形成

blastomere [ˈblæstəumiə] *n* 卵裂球

blastomerotomy [ˌblæstəumiəˈrɔtəmi] *n* 卵裂球分离

blastomogenic [ˌblæstəuməuˈdʒenik], **blastomogenous** [ˌblæstəˈmɔdʒinəs] *a* 生肿瘤的

Blastomyces [ˌblæstəuˈmaisiːz] *n* 芽生菌属 | ~ brasiliensis 巴西芽生菌 / ~ coccidioides 粗球类

芽生菌(粗球孢子菌〈Coccidioides immitis〉的旧称) / ~ dermatitidis 皮炎芽生菌 / ~ farciminosus 马淋巴管炎芽生菌(马淋巴管炎组织胞浆菌〈Histoplasma farciminosus〉的旧称)

blastomyces [ˌblæstəu'maisiːz] ([复] **blastomycetes** [ˌblæstəumai'siːtiːz]) *n* 芽生菌

blastomycete [ˌblæstəu'maisiːt] *n* 芽生菌;酵母样微生物

blastomycin [ˌblæstəu'maisin] *n* 芽生菌素

Blastomycoides immitis [ˌblæstəumai'kɔidiːz i'maitis] 粗球类芽生菌(粗球孢子菌〈Coccidioides immitis〉的旧称)

blastomycosis [ˌblæstəumai'kəusis] *n* 芽生菌病 | Brazilian ~, South American ~ 巴西芽生菌病,南美芽生菌病,类球孢子菌病 / European ~ 欧洲芽生菌病 / keloidal ~ 瘢痕疙瘩性芽生菌病 / North American ~, systemic ~ 北美芽生菌病,全身性芽生菌病

blastoneuropore [ˌblæstəu'njuərəpɔː] *n* 胚神经孔

blastophthoria [ˌblæstəf'θɔːriə] *n* 胚细胞变性 | **blastophthoric** *a*

blastophyllum [ˌblæstəu'filəm] *n* 胚层

blastophyly [blæs'tɔfili] *n* (生物体)种族史

blastopore ['blæstəupɔː] *n* 胚孔

Blastoschizomyces [ˌblæstəuˌskizəu'maisiːz] *n* 芽生裂殖菌属,芽裂菌属

blastosphere ['blæstəusfiə] *n* 囊胚

blastospore ['blæstəuspɔː] *n* 芽生孢子

blastostroma [ˌblæstəu'strəumə] *n* 囊胚基质

blastotomy [blæs'tɔtəmi] *n* 卵裂球分离

blastozooid [ˌblæstəu'zəuɔid] *n* 芽生体

blastula ['blæstjulə] ([复] **blastulae** ['blæstjuliː]) *n* 【拉】囊胚 | **~r** *a*

blastulation [ˌblæstju'leiʃən] *n* 囊胚形成

Blatin's sign, syndrome [blɑː'tæn] (Marc Blatin)布拉坦征、综合征(棘球蚴震颤)

Blatta ['blætə] *n* 【拉】蠊属 | ~ (Blattela) germanica 德国[小]蠊 / ~ orientalis 东方蠊,蟑螂

Blattabacterium [ˌblætəbæk'tiəriəm] *n* 蟑螂杆状体属

Blattaria [blæ'tɛəriə] *n* [蜚]蠊目

Blattella [blæ'telə] *n* 小蠊属

blattic acid ['blætik] 蟑螂酸

Blattidae ['blætidiː] *n* [蜚]蠊科

Blaud's pills [blu] (Pierre Blaud)布洛丸(碳酸亚铁丸,补血药)

blaze [bleiz] *n* 头发白纹

bleaching ['bliːtʃiŋ] *n*, *a* 漂白(的) | coronal ~ 牙冠漂白

blear-eye ['bliərai] *n* 睑缘炎

bleb [bleb] *n* 疱疹,大疱(直径至少 1 cm);气泡 | pleural ~ 胸膜下疱 / subpleural ~ 胸膜下肺小泡

bleeder ['bliːdə] *n* 易出血者;手术时切开的大血管;放血者,静脉切开者

bleeding ['bliːdiŋ] *n* 出血;放血,静脉切开术 | functional ~ 功能性出血(子宫) / implantation ~ 卵植入期出血 / occult ~ 潜出血 / placentation ~ 胎盘形成期出血 / summer ~ 夏季出血,寄生性皮出血

blend [blend] *n* 混合;混合物 | **~er** *n* 搅拌器(搅拌或液化食物的电器)

blennadenitis [ˌblenædi'naitis] *n* 黏液腺炎

blennaphrosin [ble'næfrəsin] *n* 椒钾盐制剂(曾用于治疗淋病和膀胱炎)

blennemesis [blen'emisis] *n* 黏液呕吐

blenn(o)- [构词成分]黏液

blennogenic [ˌblenəu'dʒenik], **blennogenous** [ble'nɔdʒinəs] *a* 生黏液的

blennoid ['blenɔid] *a* 黏液样的

blennorrhagia [ˌblenə'reidʒiə] *n* 黏液溢出,脓溢;淋病(gonorrhea 的旧称) | **blennorrhagic** [ˌblenə'rædʒik] *a*

blennorrhea [ˌblenə'riːə] *n* 脓性卡他,脓溢;淋病(gonorrhea 的旧称) | ~ adultorum 成人淋病性眼炎 / inclusion ~ 包涵体脓溢,包涵体结膜炎 / ~ neonatorum 新生儿眼炎 | **~l** *a*

blennostasis [ble'nɔstəsis] *n* 黏液制止法 | **blennostatic** [ˌblenəu'stætik] *a* 黏液制止的

blennothorax [ˌblenəu'θɔːræks] *n* 黏液胸

blennuria [ble'njuəriə] *n* 黏液尿

bleomycin [bliə'maisin] *n* 博来霉素,争光霉素(抗生素类药) | ~ sulfate 硫酸博来霉素(抗肿瘤药)

blepharadenitis [ˌblefəˌrædi'naitis] *n* 睑板腺炎

blepharal ['blefərəl] *a* 眼睑的

blepharectomy [ˌblefə'rektəmi] *n* 睑切除术

blepharelosis [ˌblefərə'ləusis] *n* 睑内翻

blepharism ['blefərizəm] *n* 睑痉挛;连续瞬目

blepharitis [ˌblefə'raitis] *n* 睑缘炎 | ~ angularis 睑角炎 / ~ ciliaris, ~ marginalis 睑缘炎 / nonulcerative ~, seborrheic ~, squamous seborrheic ~ 非溃疡性睑缘炎,脂溢性睑缘炎,鳞屑脂溢性睑缘炎 / ~ squamosa 鳞屑性睑缘炎 / ~ ulcerosa 溃疡性睑缘炎

blephar(o)- [构词成分]眼睑,睫

blepharoadenitis [ˌblefərəuˌædi'naitis] *n* 睑板腺炎

blepharoadenoma [ˌblefərəuˌædi'nəumə] *n* 眼睑腺瘤

blepharoatheroma [ˌblefərəuˌæθə'rəumə] *n* 眼睑粉瘤

blepharochalasis [ˌblefərəu'kæləsis] *n* 眼睑皮肤

松垂症,眼睑皮肤松弛症
blepharochromidrosis [ˌblefərəukrəumiˈdrəusis] *n* 睑色汗症(常带浅蓝色)
blepharoclonus [ˌblefəˈrɔklənəs] *n* 睑阵挛
blepharoconjunctivitis [ˌblefərəukənˌdʒʌŋktiˈvaitis] *n* 睑缘结膜炎
Blepharocorynthina [ˌblefərəuˌkəurinˈθainə] *n* 毛篮亚目
blepharodiastasis [ˌblefərəudaiˈæstəsis] *n* 睑裂扩大
blepharoncus [ˌblefəˈrɔŋkəs] *n* 睑瘤
blepharopachynsis [ˌblefərəupæˈkinsis] *n* 睑肥厚
blepharophimosis [ˌblefərəufiˈməusis] *n* 睑裂狭小
blepharoplast [ˈblefərəuˌplæst] *n* 生毛体,毛基体
blepharoplasty [ˈblefərəuˌplæsti] *n* 眼睑成形术
blepharoplegia [ˌblefərəuˈpliːdʒiə] *n* 睑瘫痪,睑[肌]麻痹
blepharoptosis [ˌblefərɔpˈtəusis] *n* [上]睑下垂
blepharopyorrhea [ˌblefərəupaiəˈriːə] *n* 睑脓溢,化脓性眼炎
blepharorrhaphy [ˌblefəˈrɔrəfi] *n* 睑缝合术
blepharospasm [ˈblefərəuˌspæzəm] *n* [眼]睑痉挛 | essential ~ 自发性睑痉挛 / symptomatic ~ 症状性睑痉挛
blepharosphincterectomy [ˌblefərəuˌsfiŋktəˈrektəmi] *n* 睑轮匝肌切除术(以缓解睑痉挛时眼睑对角膜的压力)
blepharostat [ˈblefərəuˌstæt] *n* 开睑器;睑牵开器
blepharostenosis [ˌblefərəustiˈnəusis] *n* 睑裂狭窄
blepharosynechia [ˌblefərəusiˈniːkiə] *n* 睑粘连
blepharotomy [ˌblefəˈrɔtəmi] *n* 睑切开术,睑板切开术
blepharoxysis [ˌblefərəuˈzaisis] *n* 睑摩擦法(治沙眼)
Blessig's cysts (spaces, lacunae) [ˈblesig] (Robert Blessig)布勒西格囊肿(间隙、陷窝)(常见于近锯齿缘视网膜外周的囊性间隙,不影响视觉。亦称囊样变性) | ~ groove 布勒西格沟(胚胎发育时眼内的痕迹,与将来的视网膜锯齿缘部位相当)
Blighia [ˈblaijə] *n* 无患子属
blight [blait] *n* 枯萎病(植物)
blind [blaind] *a* 盲的,失明的;盲的,隐蔽的(指临床试验,如单盲试验、双盲试验和三盲试验)
blindgut [ˈblaindgət] *n* 盲肠
blindness [ˈblaindnis] *n* 盲 | color ~ 色盲 / day ~ 昼盲[症](夜视) / flight ~ 飞行盲 / green ~ 绿色盲,第二型色盲 / letter ~ 字盲 / night ~ 夜盲[症](昼视) / snow ~ 雪盲 / taste ~ 味觉丧失 / twilight ~ 黄昏盲,雀盲症 / word ~, text ~ 文字盲,视觉性失读
blister [ˈblistə] *n* 水疱;疱;发疱药 *vt* 发疱,起疱 | blood ~ 血疱 / fever ~ 发热性疱疹,单纯疱疹 / water ~ 水疱
bloat [bləut] *n* 胃气胀(反刍动物);幼兔气胀病(幼兔肠炎伴腹部气胀)
Bloch's scalc [blɔh] (Marcel Bloch)布洛赫标(测蛋白混浊度)
Bloch-Sulzberger syndrome [blɔh sulzˈbəːgə] (Bruno Bloch; Marion B. Sulzberger)布洛克-苏兹贝格综合征,色素失禁
block [blɔk] *n* 阻滞,阻塞;封闭,阻断;传导阻滞;区域麻醉 *vt* 阻塞,阻滞 | adrenergic ~ 肾上腺素能阻滞 / arborization ~ 树状分支性传导阻滞 / bundlebranch ~ 束支传导阻滞 / caudal ~ 骶管阻滞 / comparator ~ 比色架 / dynamic ~ 脊髓蛛网膜下[腔]阻滞 / ear ~, tubal ~ 咽鼓管阻塞 / field ~ 区域阻滞 / heart ~ 心传导阻滞 / nerve ~ 神经传导阻滞 / parasacral ~ 骶旁阻滞 / sinoatrial ~, sinoauricular ~ 窦房传导阻滞 / sympathetic ~ 交感神经阻滞术
blockade [blɔˈkeid] *n* 阻塞,阻滞,阻断;区域麻醉 | adrenergic ~ 肾上腺素能阻滞 / adrenergic neuron ~ 肾上腺素能神经元阻滞 / alpha-adrenergic ~, alpha-~ α 肾上腺素能阻滞 / betaadrenergic ~, beta-~ β 肾上腺素能阻滞 / cholinergic ~ 胆碱能阻滞 / narcotic ~ 麻醉药阻滞 / renal ~ 肾阻塞(肾性无尿) / virus ~ 病毒干扰
blockage [ˈblɔkidʒ] *n* 阻滞,阻塞,阻断;封锁 | tendon ~ 腱固定[术]
blocker [ˈblɔkə] *n* 阻滞药 | α-~ α 受体阻滞药 / β-~ β 受体阻滞药 / calcium channel ~ 钙通道阻滞药
blocking [ˈblɔkiŋ] *n* 阻滞,阻断;传道阻滞;思维中断;标本封块 *a* 阻滞的 | adrenergic ~ 肾上腺能阻滞 / ~ of thought 思维中断
blockout [ˈblɔkaut] *n*, *vt* [倒凹]勾画修整(消除主模型中不合意的倒凹区)
Blocq's disease [blɔk] (Paul O. Blocq)布劳克病,站立行走不能
Blom-Singer puncture [blɔm ˈsiŋə] (Eric D. Blom; Mark I. Singer)布-辛穿刺,气管食管穿刺
Blondlot rays [blɔndˈlɔ] (Prosper R. Blondlot)布朗德罗射线,n 射线(见 n rays)
blood [blʌd] *n* 血,血液 | cord ~ 脐带血 / defibrinated ~ 去纤维蛋白血 / laky ~ 已溶血 / occult ~ 隐血 / oxalated ~ 草酸盐血 / sludged ~ 凝血块 / venous ~ 静脉血 / whole ~ 全血
blood flow [blʌd fləu] 血流量
Bloodgood's disease [ˈblʌdgud] (Joseph C.

Bloodgood)布拉德古德病,乳腺囊性病

blood group [ˈblʌd gruːp] 血型 | ABO ~ ~ ABO 血型(人类主要血型系) / high frequency ~ ~ 高频率血型(99% 以上个体中发现的红细胞抗原,故亦称常见抗原) / I ~ ~ I 血型(包括最冷反应血凝素的受血者) / low frequency ~ ~ 低频率血型(1% 以下个体中发现的红细胞抗原,亦称稀有抗原) / MNSs ~ ~ MNSs 血型(一种复杂的血型系,主要包括两对抗原,并为紧密的连锁基因决定的) / P ~ ~ P 血型(一种血型系,原来只包括 P〈现为 P1〉,但发现包括一种高频率抗原 P2〈Pj^a〉及一种低频率抗原 P3〈P^K〉, P1 在黑人中最常见〈90%〉,白人次之〈75%〉,东方人最少见〈30%〉) / Rh ~ ~ Rh 血型(人类血型系中最为复杂,主要抗原 Rh1〈Rh_0 D〉具有高度免疫性,在被动免疫预防形成之前,是新生儿严重溶血病的原因)

bloodless [ˈblʌdlis] *a* 失血的,贫血的,无血的;无失血的(操作时几乎或完全不失血的)

bloodroot [ˈblʌdruːt] *n* 血根

blood serum [blʌd ˈsiərəm] 血清 | glycerin ~ ~ 甘油血清

bloodstream [ˈblʌdstriːm] *n* 血流

bloom [bluːm] *n* 菌绒;水华

Bloom's syndrome [bluːm] (David Bloom)布卢姆综合征,蝴蝶状红斑综合征(为常染色体隐性遗传综合征,在婴儿期开始形成,包括面部红斑和毛细血管扩张呈蝴蝶状分布、对光敏感及出生前发生的侏儒症。染色体结构〈姊妹染色单体交换〉及免疫球蛋白有异常,而且恶性肿瘤发生率高,尤其是白血病。约有一半病人为犹太人血统)

Bloor's method [blɔː] (Walter R. Bloor)布卢尔法(检磷脂;检胆固醇) | ~ test 布卢尔试验(检脂肪及血中胆固醇)

blot [blɔt] *n* 印迹

blotch [blɔtʃ] *n* 污斑,污点

blotting [ˈblɔtiŋ] *n* 印迹,印迹法

Blount's brace [blʌnt] (W. P. Blount)布朗特支具(脊柱矫形器) | ~ disease 布朗特病(胫骨内翻)

blowfly [ˈbləuflai] *n* 丽蝇

blowpipe [ˈbləupaip] *n* 吹管

BLROA British Laryngological, Rhinological, and Otological Association 英国耳鼻喉科协会

blue [bluː] *a* 蓝色的 *n* 蓝色;蓝,蓝染料 | alcian ~ 阿尔新蓝 / alizarin ~, anthracene ~ 茜素蓝,蒽蓝 / alkali ~, isamine ~ 碱性蓝,衣胺蓝 / aniline ~, China ~, marine ~, soluble ~ (3M. or 2R.), water ~ 苯胺蓝,中国蓝,海军蓝,可溶性蓝(3M. 或 2R.) / brilliant cresyl ~, C. brilliant ~ 煌焦油蓝,煌蓝 / bromchlorphenol ~ 溴氯酚蓝 / bromophenol ~ 溴酚蓝 / bromothymol ~ 麝香草酚蓝 / Coomassie ~ 库马西蓝(商品名,测血容量的指示剂) / Evans ~ 伊文思蓝,偶氮蓝(静脉注射测血容量) / indigo ~ 靛蓝 / methyl ~ 甲基蓝 / methylene ~ 亚甲蓝,美蓝(用于染料及指示剂等) / Nile ~ sulfate 尼罗蓝(染脂肪酸) / trypan ~ 锥虫蓝,台盼蓝(用作活体染色和杀原虫剂) / ~ vitriol 蓝矾,硫酸铜

bluegrass [ˈbluːgræs] *n* 六月禾

blu(e)ing [ˈblu(ː)iŋ] *n* 上蓝剂

bluenose [ˈbluːnəus] *n* 青鼻(马的感光过敏作用)

bluensomycin [ˌbluənsəuˈmaisin] *n* 布鲁霉素(抗生素类药)

bluestone [ˈbluːstəun] *n* 胆矾,硫酸铜

bluetongue [ˈbluːtʌŋ] *n* 蓝舌病(绵羊、牛、山羊等的一种病毒性疾病)

Blumberg's sign [ˈblumbəːg] (Jacob M. Blumberg)布卢姆伯格征,反跳痛(腹膜炎时,手压迫腹壁突然放手则有剧痛)

Blumenau's nucleus [ˈblumənau] (Leonid W. Blumenau)布路门奥核(楔核外侧部)

Blumenbach's clivus [ˈblumənbɑːh] (Johann F. Blumenbach)布卢门巴赫斜坡(与枕骨底突相连的蝶骨斜坡) | ~ plane 布卢门巴赫平面(除去下颌的颅底平面) / ~ process 筛骨钩突

Blumenthal's disease [ˈbluməntɑːl] (Ferdinand Blumenthal)红白血病

Blum's reagent, test [blum] (Léon Blum)布卢姆试剂、试验(检尿白蛋白)

Blum's syndrome [blum] (Paul Blum)缺氯性氮血[症]

blunthook [ˈblʌnthuk] *n* 钝钩(主要用于碎胎术)

blur [bləː] *vt, vi* 涂片(检验);弄模糊;变模糊 *n* 模糊 | ~ring of vision 视力模糊

Blyth's test [blaiθ] (Alexander W. Blyth)布莱思试验(检饮水中铅)

BM balneum maris【拉】海水浴;Bachelor of Medicine 医学士;bowel movement 通便,排便

BMA British Medical Association 英国医学会

BMI body mass index 体重指数

BMR basal metabolic rate 基础代谢率

BMS Bachelor of Medical Science 医学士

BMT behavioral marital therapy 行为婚姻疗法;bone marrow transplantation 骨髓移植

BNA Basle Nomina Anatomica 巴塞尔解剖学名词

BNP brain natriuretic peptide 脑钠尿肽

BOA British Orthopaedic Association 英国矫形外科协会

board [bɔːd] *n* 板;部门;委员会 | angle ~ 投射角板

Boari flap [bəuˈɑːri] (Achille Boari)博厄里瓣(用于输卵管膀胱吻合术时)

Boas' algesimeter [ˈbɔːəz] (Ismar I. Boas) 博亚斯痛觉计(测腹上部敏感性) | ~ point 博亚斯点(胃溃疡病人第12胸椎左侧的一个压痛点) / ~ test 博亚斯试验(检胃盐酸,亦称间苯二酚试验;检胃游离盐酸;检胃乳酸;叶绿素试验)

Boas-Oppler bacillus (lactobacillus) [ˈbɔːəz ˈɔplə] (Ismar I. Boas; Bruno Oppler) 博亚斯-奥普勒杆菌(乳杆菌)(首先在胃癌患者胃液内发现的一种细菌,与保加利亚乳杆菌即使不相同也很相似)

Bobath method [ˌbəubaːt] (Berta and Karel Bobath) 博巴特法(一种医疗体操法,此法的设计是为了通过改变姿势抑制痉挛状态,并有助于新反射反应及平衡反应的发展,从而在婴儿神经系统发育的基础上从简单的运动到复杂的运动循序渐进)

bobbing [ˈbɔbiŋ] *n* 上下快速摆动 | ocular ~ 眼球浮动(眼球快速向下偏斜,然后缓慢回到中间位置,见于昏迷患者,据认为系脑桥损伤所致)

Bobroff's operation [ˈbɔbrəf] (V. F. Bobroff) 鲍布罗夫手术(脊柱裂成形术)

Bochdalek's duct [ˈbɔhdəlek] (Vincent A. Bochdalek) 甲状舌管 |~ foramen (gap, sinus) 胸腹膜裂孔 / ~ ganglion (pseudoganglion) 上牙丛 / ~ hernia 胸腹膜裂孔疝 / ~ valve 博赫达勒克瓣(泪点襞)

Bockhart's impetigo [ˈbɔkhaːt] (Max Bockhart) 博克哈特脓疱病(一种浅表毛囊炎,一般为金黄色酿脓葡萄球菌所致,在毛囊皮脂腺口形成脓性小脓疱,尤其患及头皮和四肢。亦称浅脓疱性毛囊周炎)

Bock's ganglion [bɔk] (August C. Bock) 颈动脉神经节 | ~ nerve 迷走神经咽支

BOD biochemical oxygen demand 生化需氧量

Bodansky unit [bɔˈdænski] (Aaron Bodansky) 博丹斯基单位(一种磷酸酶效能单位)

bodenplatte [ˌbɔːdənˈplaːtə] *n*【德】神经管底板

Bodo [ˈbəudəu] *n* 波陀虫属,胞滴虫属

Bodonina [ˌbəudə*u*ˈnainə] *n* 波陀虫亚目

body [ˈbɔdi] *n* 体;物体;尸体;躯体 | adrenal ~ 肾上腺 / alkapton bodies 黑尿酸类 / anaphylactic reaction ~ 过敏素 / anococcygeal ~ 肛尾韧带 / anti-immune ~, antiintermediary ~ 抗免疫体,抗中间体(抗抗体) / apical ~ 顶体(精子) / asteroid ~ 星状小体 / basal ~ 基体 / brassy ~ 黄铜色小体(一种皱缩红细胞,见于疟疾) / carotid ~, intercarotid ~ 颈动脉球 / coccoid x bodies 鹦鹉热小体(血中) / crescent ~, demilune ~ 新月形小体,半月体(无色细胞) / elementary ~ 血小板;原[生小]体(包涵体) / end ~ 末体(补体末段) / epithelial ~ 甲状旁腺 / falciform ~ 镰刀状体,子孢子 / filling bodies 胀大小体(神经胶质细胞退化) / flagellated ~ 疟原虫配子体 / foreign ~ 异物 / glass ~ 半月体(无色细胞) / glomus bodies 球腺 / habenular ~ 缰核 / hyaloid ~ 玻璃体 / immune ~ 抗体;免疫体 / inclusion bodies 包涵体 / infundibular ~ 漏斗体,垂体后叶 / metachromatic ~ 异染小体,异染粒 / onion bodies, pearly bodies 上皮珠 / paranuclear ~ 中心体 / parolivary bodies 副橄榄核 / pheochrome ~ 嗜铬体,副神经节 / pituitary ~ (大脑)垂体 / residual ~ 溶酶后体;残体 / selenoid ~ 无色细胞 / suprarenal ~ 肾上腺 / thermostabile ~ 耐热小体 / thyroid ~ 甲状腺 / vitelline ~ 卵黄体(卵黄核) / zebra ~ 斑马体

body rocking [ˈbɔdi ˈrɔkiŋ] 身体[前后]摇摆(在坐位时)

body snatching [ˈbɔdi ˈsnætʃiŋ] 盗尸

bodywork [ˈbɔdiwəːk] *n* 健身法(身体治疗法的通称,其中包括按摩、各种触、揉、放松法等)

Boeck's disease, sarcoid [bek] (Caesar P. M. Boeck) 结节病

Boedeker's test [ˈbeidəkə] (Carl H. D. Boedeker) 伯德克尔试验(检白蛋白)

Boerhaave's glands [buəˈhaːvi] (Hermann Boerhaave) 汗腺 | ~ syndrome 伯尔哈维综合征,自发性食管破裂症

Boettcher 见 Böttcher

Boettger 见 Böttger

Bogomolets' serum [bəgəˈmɔlets] (Aleksandr A. Bogomolets) 抗网状细胞毒性血清

Bogros' space [bɔgˈrɔː] (Annet J. Bogros) 博格罗间隙(此部位上界为腹膜,下界为横筋膜,在此区域内不需切开腹膜即可发现髂外动脉的下部。亦称腹股沟后间隙)

Böhler splint [ˈbeilə] (Lorenz Böhler) 伯勒尔夹板(上肢外展夹,一种木夹板,上端为圆形以适合腋部用)

Bohr effect [bɔːr] (Christian Bohr) 波尔效应(二氧化碳分压或 pH 值改变导致氧合血蛋白解离曲线的偏移)

Bohun upas [ˈbəuhən ˈjuːpəs] 见血封喉(爪哇一种毒树的毒汁,用作箭毒)

boil [bɔil] *n* 疖 | blind ~ 盲疖,无头疖 / gum ~ 龈脓肿,龈疖 / oriental ~, tropical ~ 东方疖,热带疮(皮肤利什曼病) / shoe ~ 肘水囊瘤,帽状肘

Bol. bolus【拉】丸剂

bolasterone [bəuˈlæstərəun] *n* 勃拉睾酮(雄激素类药)

boldenone undecylenate [ˈbəuldənəun] 十一烯酸勃地酮(同化激素类药)

boldine [bɔlˈdiːn] *n* 波耳丁(从波耳多树叶取得的一种生物碱,有利尿作用)

boldo [ˈbɔldəu], **boldoa** [ˈbɔldəuə] *n* 波耳多叶(利胆、利尿、健胃、镇静、驱肠虫药)

boldoin [ˈbɔldəuin] 波耳多因(波耳多叶中含有的一种糖苷)

bolenol [ˈbəulənɔl] *n* 勃来诺(同化激素类药)

Boletus [bəuˈliːtəs] *n*【拉】牛肝菌属(真菌,有些可食,有些含毒) | ~ satanus 魔牛肝菌(引起胃肠蕈中毒)

Bolk's retardation theory [bɔlk] (Louis Bolk) 博尔克发育停滞学说(认为人类发育阶段仍处于高等灵长类动物的胎儿阶段)

Bollinger's bodies [ˈbɔliŋə] (Otto von Bollinger) 博林格尔体(鸡痘包涵体) | ~ granules 博林格尔粒(葡萄状菌病肉芽组织中所见的桑葚状黄白色小粒,内含球菌)

bolograph [ˈbəuləgrɑːf] *n* 测辐射热器 | **~ic** [ˌbəuləˈgræfik] *a*

bolometer [bəuˈlɔmitə] *n* 心搏力计;放射热测定计,辐射热计

boloscope [ˈbəuləskəup] *n* 金属异物探测器

Boltz test(reaction) [bɔlts] (Oswald H. Boltz) 博尔茨试验(反应)(诊断精神分裂症)

Boltzmann's constant [ˈbəultsmɑːm] (Ludwig E. Boltzmann) 玻尔茨曼常数(用阿伏加得罗〈Avogadro〉数去除气体常数;$1.380\,66 \times 10^{-23}$ 焦耳/开尔文。符号为 *k*)

bolus [ˈbəuləs] *n* 团,块(如大药丸、食团);造影剂团(静脉注射造影剂或放射性同位素形成的浓缩药团,作诊断用);填充物(放疗用) | ~ alba 白陶土,高岭土 / alimentary ~ 食团

bomb [bɔm] *n* 弹,炮(含有大量镭或放射性元素的容器,用于体外照射) | cobalt ~ 钴炮 / radium ~ 镭[放射]炮

bombard [bɔmˈbɑːd] *vt* 轰击(射线)

Bombay phenotype [bɔmˈbei] 孟买表型(见 phenotype 项下相应术语)

bombesin [ˈbɔmbəsin] *n* 铃蟾肽

bombicesterol [bɔmbiˈsestərɔl] *n* 蚕甾醇

Bombina [bɔmˈbaɪnə] *n* 蟾蜍属

Bombinator [ˈbɔmbiˈneitə] *n* 蛉蟾属

Bombus [ˈbɔmbus] *n* 蜂属

bombykol [ˈbɔmbikɔl] *n* 蚕蛾醇

Bombyx mori [ˈbɔmbiks ˈmɔrai] 家蚕(用于实验遗传学)

bond [bɔnd] *n* 结合力;联结;黏结剂;键 *vt* 使结合 *vi* 结合 | energy-rich ~, high-energy ~ 高能键 / high-energy phosphate ~ 高能磷酸键 / hydrogen ~ 氢键 / ionic ~ 离子键,电价键 / pair ~ 配偶关系(在个体生态学中,指雌雄之间便于交配和抚育后代的相对永久关系) / peptide ~ 肽键

bonding [ˈbɔndiŋ] *n* 黏合,结合 | tooth ~ 牙黏合术

Bond's splint [bɔnd] (Thomas Bond) 邦德夹板(桡骨下端骨折用)

Bondy's mastoidectomy [ˈbɔndi] (G. Bondy) 邦迪乳突切除术(乳突改良根治术)

bone [bəun] *n* 骨 *vt* 剔骨 | alar ~ 蝶骨 / alveolar ~ 牙槽骨 / ankle ~ 距骨 / back ~ 脊柱 / basihyal ~ 基舌骨,舌骨体 / basilar ~, basioccipital ~ 基骨,基枕骨 / basiotic ~ 耳底骨 / breast ~ 胸骨 / brittle ~ 脆骨,成骨不全 / calf ~ 腓骨 / cancellated ~ 骨松质 / capitate ~ 头状骨 / cartilage ~, endochondral ~, replacement ~, substitution ~ 软骨[内]成骨 / chalky ~s 白垩状骨,骨硬化病 / cheek ~ 颧骨 / collar ~ 锁骨 / compact ~ 骨密质 / ear ~s 听小骨 / ethmoid ~ 筛骨 / frontal ~ 额骨 / hamate ~, unciform ~, uncinate ~ 钩骨 / heel ~ 跟骨 / hip ~, innominate ~, pelvic ~ 髋骨 / hyoid ~ 舌骨 / incarial ~, interparietal ~ 顶间骨 / ivory ~s, marble ~s 象牙样骨,大理石样骨,骨硬化病,骨[质]石化病 / maxillary ~ 上颌骨 / occipital ~ 枕骨 / palate ~, palatine ~ 腭骨 / parietal ~ 顶骨 / petrosal ~, petrous ~ 颞骨岩部 / pneumatic ~ 含气骨 / resurrection ~, sacral ~ 骶骨 / scaphoid ~ 舟骨 / sesamoid ~s 籽骨 / shin ~ 胫骨 / sphenoid ~ 蝶骨 / spongy ~ 骨松质 / squamous ~ 颞骨鳞部 / tarsal ~s 跗骨 / temporal ~ 颞骨 / thigh ~ 股骨 / triquetral ~ 三角骨 / tympanic ~ 颞骨鼓部 / ulnal ~ 尺骨 / whettle ~s 胸椎 / xiphoid ~ 剑突骨

boneless [ˈbəunlis] *a* 无骨的

bonelet [ˈbəunlit] *n* 小骨

bone-setter [ˈbəunˌsetə] *n* 正骨者

bonesetting [ˈbəunˌsetiŋ] *n* 正骨法

Bonhoeffer's symptom [ˈbɔnhefə] (Karl Bonhoeffer) 博恩霍弗尔症状(舞蹈症时正常肌张力减退)

Bonnet's capsule [bɔˈnei] (Amédée Bonnet) 眼球鞘,眼球囊 | ~ sign 邦内征(大腿内收时疼痛,见于坐骨神经痛)

Bonnier's syndrome [bɔniˈɛə] (Pierre Bonnier) 邦尼埃综合征,前庭外侧核综合征(前庭神经外侧核损害或与之有关的前庭束损害所致的一组症状,包括眩晕、苍白及不同的听觉和视觉障碍)

Bonwill crown [ˈbɔnwil] (William G. A. Bonwill) 邦威尔冠,桩冠(一种人造瓷冠) | ~ triangle 邦威尔三角(由下颌骨颗状突中心连线、各中心与下颌内切牙近中接触区的连线所组成的等边三角,每边约长 10.2 cm)

book-lung [ˈbuklʌŋ] *n* 书肺(见 lung 项下相应术语)

Böök's syndrome [beik] (Jan Arvid Böök) 培克综合征(即 PHC syndrome,见 syndrome 项下相应术语)

boomslang [ˈbumslæŋ] *n* 南非树蛇(一种毒蛇)
Boophilus [bəuˈɔfiləs] *n* 牛蜱属,方头蜱属 | ~ annulatus, ~ bovis 具环牛蜱 / ~ decoloratus 消色牛蜱 / ~ microplus 微小牛蜱
BOOP bronchiolitis obliterans with organizing pneumonia 闭塞性细支气管炎伴机化性肺炎
Booponus [bəuˈɔpənəs] *n* 牛螯蝇属
booster [ˈbuːstə] *n* 升压机,升压器;增压泵;加强剂量
boot [buːt] *n* 靴;脚鞘护套
bootstrap [ˈbuːtstræp] *n* 自助法,靴襻法(在统计学上,指根据从观察的数据随机重新抽样以计算值的分布的一种方法)
boracic [bəˈræsik] *a* 硼的;含硼的 | ~ acid 硼酸
borate [ˈbɔːreit] *n* 硼酸盐 *vt* 使与硼砂(或硼酸)混合 | **~d** *a* 含硼砂(或硼酸)的
borax [ˈbɔːræks] *n* 硼砂(消毒防腐药)
borborygmus [ˌbɔːbəˈrigməs] ([复] **borborygmi** [ˌbɔːbəˈrigmai]) *n*【拉】腹鸣
Borchardt's test [ˈbɔːʃɑːt] (Leo Borchardt) 博尔夏特试验(检尿内果糖)
border [ˈbɔːdə] *n* 边缘 *vi* 接界 | brush ~, striated ~ 刷状缘,纹状缘(上皮细胞)
borderline [ˈbɔːdəlain] *n* 边缘,临界
Bordetella [ˌbɔːdəˈtelə] (Jules J. B. V. Bordet) 博代杆菌属 | ~ bronchiseptica 支气管败血性博代杆菌 / ~ parapertussis 副百日咳博代杆菌 / ~ pertussis 百日咳博代杆菌,百日咳杆菌
Bordet-Gengou agar (culture media) [bɔːˈdei ʒɑːnˈguː] (Jules J. B. V. Bordet; Octave Gengou) 博代-让古琼脂(培养基)(分离百日咳杆菌和结核分枝杆菌用) | ~ bacillus 百日咳杆菌 / ~ phenomenon(reaction) 补体结合
Bordet's phenomenon, test [bɔːˈdei] (Jules J. B. V. Bordet) 博代现象、试验,血清试验
Borago [bəˈreigəu] *n*【拉】琉璃苣属,紫草科植物属
boric [ˈbɔːrik] *a* 硼的;含硼的 | ~ acid 硼酸(消毒防腐药)
boride [ˈbɔːraid] *n* 硼化物
borism [ˈbɔːrizəm] *n* 硼中毒(硼酸或硼砂中毒)
Börjeson-Forssman-Lehmann syndrome [ˈbɔriəsun ˈfɔːsmɑːn ˈleimɑːn] (M. G. Borjeson; Hans A. Forssman; Orla Lehmann) 博-福-莱综合征(见 Börjeson's syndrome)
Börjeson's syndrome [ˈbɔːriəsun] (Mats G. Börjeson) 博力逊综合征(一种 X 连锁综合征,特征为严重智力迟钝、癫痫、性腺功能减退、代谢减退、显著肥胖、面部皮下组织肿胀以及耳大)
borjom [ˈbɔːdʒɔm] *n* 博焦姆矿水(高加索的一种矿水)
Borna disease [ˈbɔːnə] (Borna 为德国萨克森州一地区,该地区曾流行此病) 博纳病(马、牛、羊的致命性地方性脑炎,由病毒所致。亦称地方性马脑炎和马脑炎)
Bornaviridae [ˌbɔːnəˈviridiː] *n* 博纳病毒科
Bornavirus [ˌbɔːnəˈvaiərəs] *n* 博纳病毒属
borneol [ˈbɔːniɔl] *n* 冰片,龙脑,莰醇 | ~ acetate 乙酸冰片酯
Bornholm disease [ˈbɔːnhəum] (Bornholm 为丹麦一岛名) 博恩霍尔姆病,流行性肌痛,流行性胸膜痛
bornyl [ˈbɔːnil] *n* 冰片基,龙脑基 | ~ acetate 乙酸冰片基,乙酸龙脑基 / ~ alcohol 冰片,龙脑,莰醇 / ~ chloride 氯化冰片,氯化龙脑(防腐剂)
borocitric acid [ˌbɔːrəuˈsitrik] 硼酸枸橼酸
boroglycerin [ˌbɔːrəuˈglisərin] *n* 硼酸甘油 | ~ glycerite 硼酸甘油,甘油剂(以前用作抗菌药) | **boroglyceride** [ˌbɔːrəuˈglisəraid], **boroglycerol** [ˌbɔːrəuˈglisərɔl] *n*
boron (B) [ˈbɔːrɔn] *n* 硼 | ~ carbide 碳化硼(核反应堆中用作中子吸收料,工业和牙科用作研磨料)
borophenylic acid [ˌbɔːrəufeˈnilik] 硼酸苯酯
borosalicylic acid [ˌbɔːrəusæliˈsilik] 硼水杨酸
Borrel bodies [bɔˈrel] (Amédée Borrel) 包柔包涵体(组成博林格尔〈Bollinger〉体的含细小病毒颗粒)
Borrelia [bəˈreliə] *n* 包柔螺旋体属,疏螺旋体属 | ~ berbera 北美洲回归热螺旋体 / ~ buccalis 口腔螺旋体 / ~ carteri 卡氏疏螺旋体,印度回归热螺旋体 / ~ caucasica 高加索疏螺旋体 / ~ duttonii 达氏疏螺旋体,中非洲回归热螺旋体 / ~ novyi 诺氏疏螺旋体,北美洲回归热螺旋体 / ~ persica 波斯疏螺旋体 / ~ recurrentis 回归热螺旋体 / ~ venezuelensis 委内瑞拉疏螺旋体
borreliosis [bəˌreliˈəusis] *n* 包柔螺旋体病,疏螺旋体病
Borrmann's classification [ˈbɔːmɑːn] (R. Borrmann) 博尔曼分类(胃癌分类法,即分为息肉样、溃疡型、溃疡浸润型或浸润型)
Borsieri's sign (line) [ˌbɔːsiˈeri] (Giovanni B. Borsieri) 博西埃里征(线)(猩红热早期皮肤白色划痕,迅即变红)
Borthen's operation [ˈbɔːtən] (Johan Borthen) 虹膜展开术
Bose's hooks [ˈbɔːsə] (Heinrich Bose) 博塞钩(气管造口术时用) | ~ operation 博塞手术(气管造口术的一种方法)
Bosker implant [ˈbɔskə] (Hans Bosker) 博斯卡植入物(经下颌骨植入物的普通型)
boss [bɔs] *n* 圆凸,隆起 | parietal ~es 顶骨隆起,顶骨结节
bosselated [ˈbɔsəleitid] *a* 有圆凸的

bosselation [ˌbɔsəˈleiʃən] *n* 小圆凸,圆凸形成

Bossi's dilator [ˈbɔsi] (Luigi M. Bossi)博西扩张器(一种子宫颈扩张器)

Bostock's catarrh (disease) [ˈbɔstɔk] (John Bostock)花粉症

Boston's sign [ˈbɔstən] (L. N. Boston)博斯顿征(突眼性甲状腺肿时,患者眼球下转,眼睑下降受阻并发生痉挛)

bot [bɔt] *n* 肤蝇[类]蛆(寄生于动物胃内,有时亦寄生于人胃中) | sheep nose ~ 羊鼻狂蝇蛆

Botallo's duct [bəuˈtɑːləu] (Leonardo Botallo)动脉导管 | ~ foramen 卵圆孔(胎儿心房) / ~ ligament 动脉导管索,动脉韧带

botanic [bəˈtænik] *a* 植物[学]的

botanical [bəˈtænikəl] *a* 植物[学]的 *n* 植物性药材

botanist [ˈbɔtənist] *n* 植物学家

botany [ˈbɔtəni] *n* 植物学;植物生态 | medical ~ 医学植物学

Botelho's test [bəˈteljəu] 波特尔约[血清]试验(检癌)

botfly [ˈbɔtflai] *n* 肤蝇[类]

bothridium [bɔˈθridjəm] *n* 吸叶(绦虫)

bothriocephaliasis [ˌbɔθriəuˌsefəˈlaiəsis] *n* 裂头绦虫病

Bothriocephalus [ˌbɔθriəuˈsefələs] *n* 裂头[绦虫]属

bothrium [ˈbɔθriəm] *n* 吸沟,吸槽(见于绦虫头部两侧)

bothropic [bəˈθrɔpik] *a* 具窍蝮蛇的

Bothrops [ˈbɔːθrɔps] *n* 具窍蝮蛇属

botogenin [bɔtəˈdʒenin] *n* 薯吉宁,薯苷配基(得自墨西哥薯蓣,可用以部分合成甾类激素)

botryoid [ˈbɔtriɔid] *a* 葡萄簇状的

botryomycoma [ˌbɔtriəumaiˈkəumə] *n* 葡萄状菌肿

botryomycosis [ˌbɔtriəumaiˈkəusis] *n* 葡萄状菌病 | ~ hominis 脓性肉芽肿 | **botryomycotic** [ˌbɔtriəumaiˈkɔtik] *a*

botryotherapy [ˌbɔtriəuˈθerəpi] *n* 葡萄疗法

botrytimycosis [bəuˌtraitimaiˈkəusis] *n* 葡萄孢霉菌病

Botrytis [bəuˈtraitis] *n* 葡萄孢属 | ~ bassiana 蚕白僵病葡萄孢 / ~ tenella 柔弱葡萄孢

bots [bɔts] [复] *n* [用作单]肤蝇[类]蛆病(马及其他动物)

Böttcher's cells [ˈbetʃə] (Arthur Böttcher)伯特歇尔细胞(耳蜗) | ~ crystals 伯特歇尔结晶(前列腺液中加入磷酸铵液时出现的显微结晶) / ~ space 伯特歇尔间隙,内淋巴囊

Böttger's test [ˈbetgə] (Rudolf Böttger)伯特格尔试验(检一氧化碳);(Wilhelm C. Böttger)伯特格尔试验(检尿内葡萄糖)

Bottini's operation [bəuˈtiːni] (Enrico Bottini)博蒂尼手术(前列腺电灼术,治前列腺增生)

bottle [ˈbɔtl] *n* 瓶 | hot-water ~ 热水袋 / nursing ~ 奶瓶 / wash ~ 洗瓶(洗化学物质或气体)

botuliform [bɔˈtjuːlifɔːm] *a* 腊肠状的

botulin [ˈbɔtjulin] *n* 肉毒杆菌毒素

botulinal [ˌbɔtjuˈlainəl] *a* 肉毒[杆菌]的;肉毒杆菌毒素的

botulinic acid [ˌbɔtjuˈlinik] 尿囊毒酸

botulinogenic [ˌbɔtjuˌlinəuˈdʒenik] *a* 产生肉毒杆菌毒素的

botulism [ˈbɔtjulizəm] *n* 肉毒中毒

botulismotoxin [ˌbɔtjuˌlizməˈtɔksin] *n* 肉毒[杆菌]毒素

bouba [ˈbubə] *n* 雅司病(即 yaws) | ~ braziliana 黏膜皮肤利什曼病

Bouchardat's test [buʃɑːˈdɑː] (Apollinaire Bouchardat)布夏达试验(检生物碱) | ~ treatment 布夏达疗法(饮食中排除含富有糖类的物质,以治疗糖尿病)

Bouchard's coefficient [buˈʃɑː] (Charles J. Bouchard)布夏尔系数(尿中液体与固体的比率);尿毒系数 | ~ disease 布夏尔病(由于胃功能不足造成的胃扩张) / ~ nodes (nodules)布夏尔结节(近端指关节的结节形成,为关节变性的症状) / ~ sign 布夏尔征(检脓性尿:加数滴费林〈Fehling〉溶液于尿中,振荡后,如脓来自肾,则将形成小泡,而把因加热形成的凝块浮向表面)

bouche [buːʃ] *n* 【法】嘴,口 | ~ de tapir 貘嘴,突唇口,撅嘴

Bouchut's respiration [buˈʃu] (Jean A. E. Bouchut)布舒呼吸(小儿患支气管肺炎时吸气较呼气短) | ~ tubes 布舒管(喉插管时用)

Boudin's law [buˈdæn] (Jean C. M. J. Boudin)布丹定律(认为疟疾与结核病之间有拮抗作用)

boufée délirante [buːˈfei deiliˈrɑːnt] 【法】谵妄型暴发

bougie [buˈʒiː] *n* 【法】探条;栓剂,杆剂 | ~ à boule 球头探条 / caustic ~ 烧灼探条 / dilating ~ 扩张探条(常用作扩张尿道狭窄部) / medicated ~ 含药杆剂,含药笔剂

bougienage, bouginage [buːʒiˈnɑːʒ] *n* 探条扩张[术]

Bouillaud's disease [buiˈju] (Jean B. Bouillaud)风湿性心内膜炎 | ~ sign 布优征(心前区胸廓永久性下陷,为心包粘连之征) / ~ syndrome 布优综合征(急性关节风湿病并发心包炎及心内膜炎)

bouillon [ˈbuːjɔːŋ] *n* 【法】肉汤(牛肉或鸡肉等清汤,用作细菌培养基)

Bouin's fluid (solution) [bwæn] (Paul Bouin)

布安液(一种组织学固定液)
boulimia [bu'limiə] *n* 贪食,食欲过盛
bound [baund] *a* 受限的,束缚的
boundary ['baundəri] *n* 分界线,边界;界限,限界
bouquet [bu'kei] *n*【法】花束;香味,酒香;丛(花束状结构,如血管、神经、纤维等)
Bourgery's ligament ['buədʒəri] (Marc J. Bourgery)腘斜韧带
Bourget's test [buə'ʒei] (Louis Bourget)布尔惹试验(检尿及唾液碘化物)
Bourneville-Pringle syndrome [buən'vi:l 'priŋgəl] (V. M. Bourneville; John J. Pringle)结节性硬化
Bourneville's disease ['buənivi:] (Désiré-Magloire Bourneville)节结性硬化
bout [baut] *n* (疾病等)发作
bouton [bu'tɔŋ] *n*【法】疖,小结(哑铃状脓肿) | ~s terminaux 终结,突触结
boutonneuse [bu:tə'nu:z] *n* 南欧斑疹热(见 fever)
boutonnière [ˌbu:tə'njεə] *n*【法】钮孔状切开(尿道)
Bouveret's disease (syndrome) [bu:və'rei] (Léon Bouveret) 阵发性室上性心动过速 | ~ ulcer 布佛雷溃疡(伤寒患者咽扁桃体溃疡)
Boveri's test ['bəuveiri:] (Piero Boveri) 博韦里试验(检脑脊液球蛋白)
Bovimyces pleuropneumoniae [ˌbəuvi'maisi:z ˌpluərəunju(:)'məunii:] 胸膜肺炎牛丝菌,蕈状支原体
bovine ['bəuvain] *a* 牛的
bovovaccination [ˌbəuvəuˌvæksi'neiʃən] *n* 牛结核菌苗接种
bovovaccine [ˌbəuvəu'væksi:n] *n* 牛结核菌苗
bow [bəu] *n* 弓,弓形物;弯曲,弧形物 *a* 弯曲的;弓形的
Bowen technique ['bəuən] (Thomas A. Bowen) 鲍恩法(一种身体治疗法,软组织动员是通过拇指和手指轻压完成的;主要用于治疗肌骨骼疾病和应激相关障碍,并用于慢性病症状缓解)
Bowditch's law ['bauditʃ] (Henry P. Bowditch) 鲍迪奇定律(见 all or none) | ~ staircase phenomenon 鲍迪奇阶梯现象(见 treppe)
bowel ['bauəl] *n* [常用复]肠
bowenoid ['bəuənɔid] *a* 退行发育的,间变的
Bowen's disease (precancerous dermatosis) ['bəuən] (John T. Bowen)鲍恩病(癌前皮炎)(表皮内鳞状细胞癌)
bowl [bəul] *n* 碗;碗状物
bowleg ['bəuleg] *n* 弓形腿,膝内翻 | nonrachitic ~ 非佝偻病性弓形腿,胫骨畸形骨软骨病 | ~ged *a*
Bowman's capsule ['bəumən] (William Bowman) 肾小囊 | ~ membrane [角膜]前界层 / ~ muscle 睫状肌 / ~ probe 鲍曼探子(鼻泪管用) / ~ theory 鲍曼学说(关于泌尿的学说,即肾小球分泌水分和无机盐,肾曲管的上皮细胞则分泌尿素和有关代谢物质) / ~ tube 角膜板层管
box [bɔks] *n* 箱,盒,框 | anatomical snuff ~ 鼻烟窝 / CAT ~ CAT 框(遗传学中,指基因转录起点上方约 80 个碱基对的一段保留的未编码"启动子"顺序) | fracture ~ 骨折箱 / Hogness ~, TATA ~ 霍格内斯框,TATA 框(遗传学中,指基因转录起点上方约 30 个碱基对的一段保留的未编码"启动子"顺序) / viewing ~ 看片灯,读片灯(看 X 线片)
boxing ['bɔksiŋ] *n* 围模(牙科)
box-note ['bɔksnəut] *n* 空匣音(叩诊肺气肿患者的胸部时所听到的空洞音)
Boyce's sign ['bɔisə] (Frederick F. Boyce) 波依斯征(患食管憩室时,手压颈侧可听到一种气过水声)
Boyer's bursa [bwɑ:'jεə] (Alexis Boyer) 布瓦耶黏液囊,舌骨下囊 | ~ cyst 舌骨下囊肿
Boyle's law [bɔil] (Robert Boyle) 波义耳定律(在恒温下,理想气体的体积与压力成反比,而压力又与体积成反比)
Bozeman-Fritsch catheter ['bəuzmən fritʃ] (Nathan Bozeman; Heinrich Fritsch) 博-弗导管,双流子宫导管
Bozeman's catheter ['bəuzmən] (Nathan Bozeman) 博兹曼导管,双流子宫导管 | ~ operation 博兹曼手术,子宫膀胱缝术 / ~ position 膝肘卧位 / ~ speculum 博兹曼窥器(一种双瓣阴道窥器)
Bozzolo's sign ['bɔtsəuləu] (Camillo Bozzolo) 博佐洛征(鼻孔内动脉的搏动表明胸主动脉瘤)
BP blood pressure 血压;British Pharmacopoeia 英国药典
bp base pair 碱基对;boiling point 沸点
BPA British Paediatric Association 英国儿科协会
B Ph British Pharmacopoeia 英国药典
BPI bactericidal permeability increasing protein 杀菌性通透性增强蛋白
BPIG bacterial polysaccharide immune globulin 细菌性多糖免疫球蛋白
Bq becqurel 贝克[勒尔](放射性强度单位)
Br bromine 溴
Braasch bulb catheter [bræʃ] (William Braasch) 布拉什小球导管(顶端有一小球的输尿管导管,用于扩张和测量输尿管内径)
brace [breis] *n* 支架;(用以支架病体的)支具;[复](正牙)固定器,矫正器 | bow leg ~ 弓形腿支具
bracelet ['breislit] *n* 手镯;腕带;腕纹

brachia [ˈbreikjə] brachium 的复数
brachial [ˈbreikjəl] *a* 臂的,肱的
brachialgia [ˌbreikiˈældʒiə] *n* 臂痛
brachiation [ˌbreikiˈeiʃən] *n* 臂力摆荡
brachi(o)- [构词成分]臂
brachiocephalic [ˌbrækiəuseˈfælik] *a* 头臂的
brachiocrural [ˌbrækiəuˈkruərəl] *a* 臂腿的
brachiocubital [ˌbrækiəuˈkjuːbitl] *a* 臂肘的,臂前臂的
brachiocyrtosis [ˌbrækiəusəˈtəusis], **brachiocyllosis** [ˌbrækiəusiˈləusis] *n* 臂弯曲
brachiofaciolingual [ˌbrækiəuˌfeiʃiəuˈliŋgwəl] *a* 臂面舌的
brachio-thoraco-omphalo-ischiopagus [ˌbreikiəu ˌθɔrəkəu ˌɔmfeləu ˌiskiˈɔpagəs] *n* 臂-胸-脐-坐骨联胎 | ~ bipus 双足性臂-胸-脐-坐骨联胎
brachium [ˈbreikiəm] ([复]**brachia** [ˈbreikjə]) *n*【拉】臂
Brachmann-de Lange's syndrome [ˈbrækmɑːn dei ˈlɑːŋgə] (W. Brachmann; Cornelia de Lange) 布-德综合征(见 de Lange's syndrome)
Bracht's maneuver [brækt] (Erich F. Bracht) 布拉赫特手法(用于臀先露)
Bracht-Wächter lesion [brækt ˈvektə] (Erich F. E. Bracht; Hermann J. G. Wächter) 布-韦损害(淋巴细胞和单核细胞在心肌层呈灶状集聚)
brachy- [构词成分]短
Brachyarcus [ˌbrækiˈɑːkəs] *n* 短弓菌属
brachybasia [ˌbrækiˈbeiziə] *n* (曳行)小步,短步(见于两侧瘫)
brachycardia [ˌbrækiˈkɑːdiə] *n* 心动过缓
brachycephaly [ˌbrækiˈsefəli], **brachycephalia** [ˌbrækisiˈfeiliə], **brachycephalism** [ˌbrækiˈsefəlizəm], *n* 短头[畸形](颅指数为 81.0～85.4) | **brachycephalic** [ˌbrækiseˈfælik] **brachycephalous** [ˌbrækiˈsefələs] *a*
brachycheilia [ˌbrækiˈkailiə], **brachychily** [bræˈkikili] *n* 短唇
brachychronic [ˌbrækiˈkrɔnik] *a* 急性的,急促的
brachycnemic [ˌbrækiˈniːmik] *a* 短小腿的,短胫的
brachycranial [ˌbrækiˈkreiniəl] *a* 短颅的
brachycranic [ˌbrækiˈkreinik] *a* 短颅的(颅指数为 80.0～84.9)
brachydactyly [ˌbrækiˈdæktili] *n* 短指,短趾 | **brachydactylous** [ˌbrækiˈdæktiləs] *a*
brachyesophagus [ˌbrækii(ː)ˈsɔfəgəs] *n* 食管过短
brachyfacial [ˌbrækiˈfeiʃəl] *a* 短面的(面指数为 90 或小于 90)
brachygnathia [brækigˈneiθiə] *n* 短颌(下颌过短) | **brachygnathous** [brəˈkignəθəs] *a*
brachykerkic [brækiˈkəːkik] *a* 短前臂的,短腕的(桡肱指数小于 75)
brachyknemic [ˌbrækiˈniːmik] *a* 短小腿的,短胫的(胫股指数为 82 或小于 82)
brachymetacarpia [ˌbrækiˌmetəˈkɑːpiə], **brachymetacarpalism** [ˈbrækiˌmetəˈkɑːpəlizəm] *n* 掌骨过短
brachymetapody [ˌbrækimeˈtæpədi] *n* 掌骨过短,跖骨过短
brachymetatarsia [ˌbrækiˌmetəˈtɑːsiə] *n* 跖骨过短
brachymetropia [ˌbrækimeˈtrəupiə] *n* 近视 | **brachymetropic** [ˌbrækimeˈtrɔpik] *a*
brachymorphic [ˌbrækiˈmɔːfik] *a* 短形的,矮型的
brachyphalangia [ˌbrækifəˈlændʒiə] *n* 指骨过短,趾骨过短
brachyskelous [ˌbrækiˈskiːləs] *a* 短腿的
brachystaphyline [ˌbrækiˈstæfiliːn] *a* 短腭的(腭指数为 85.0 或大于 85.0)
brachystasis [brəˈkistəsis] *n* 肌肉短滞
brachytherapy [ˌbrækiˈθerəpi] *n* 近距[放射]治疗
brachytypical [ˌbrækiˈtipikəl] *a* 短形的,矮型的
brachyuranic [ˌbrækijuəˈrænik] *a* 短上颌的,短牙槽的(颌牙槽指数为 115.0 或大于 115.0)
bracing [ˈbreisiŋ] *n* 支撑;支柱;嚼力支柱(对咀嚼力水平部分的耐力)
bracken [ˈbrækən] *n* 羊齿,欧洲蕨(一种有毒的蕨类植物)
bracket [ˈbrækit] *n* 托架;托槽
bract [brækt] *n* 苞,苞片;托叶
Bradbury-Eggleston syndrome [ˈbrædbəri ˈegəlstən] (Samuel Bradbury; Cary Eggleston) 布-埃综合征(一种直立性低血压综合征,无心动过速,但有视力障碍、少汗、阳痿、基础代谢率降低、眩晕、晕厥以脉搏迟缓无变化。主要见于老年男性,在夏天清晨发生,系因周围血管收缩受损所致,通常病程是进行性的)
Bradford frame [ˈbrædfəd] (Edward H. Bradford) 布莱德福架(用作病人必须保持固定的床架)
Bradley's disease [ˈbrædli] (W. H. Bradley) 布拉德利病,流行性恶心呕吐
bradshot [ˈbrædʃɔt], **bradsot** [ˈbrædsɔt] *n* 羊快疫,羊炭疽
brady- [构词成分] 徐缓,缓慢;迟钝
bradyacusia [ˌbrædiəˈkuːsiə] *n* 听觉迟钝
bradyarrhythmia [ˌbrædiəˈriθmiə] *n* 心动过缓性心律失常
bradyarthria [ˌbrædiˈɑːθriə] *n* 言语过慢(脑损害所致)
bradyauxesis [ˌbrædiɔːkˈsiːsis] *n* 部分发育缓慢

Bradybaena [ˌbrædi'biːnə] *n* 巴蜗牛属

bradycardia [ˌbrædi'kɑːdiə] *n* 心动过缓 | sinus ~ 窦性心动过缓

bradycardiac [ˌbrædi'kɑːdiæk], **bradycardic** [ˌbrædi'kɑːdik] *a* 心动过缓的 *n* 减缓心率药

bradycinesia [ˌbrædisi'niːziə] *n* 运动徐缓

bradycrotic [ˌbrædi'krɔtik] *a* 脉搏过缓的

bradydiastole [ˌbrædidai'æstəli] *n* 舒张期延长

bradydysrhythmia [ˌbrædidis'riθmiə] *n* 心动过缓性心律失常

bradyecoia [ˌbrædii'kɔiə] *n* 重听,部分聋

bradyesthesia [ˌbrædiis'θiːzjə] *n* 感觉过慢;感觉迟钝

bradygenesis [brædi'dʒenisis] *a* 发育过慢

bradyglossia [ˌbrædi'glɔsiə] *n* 言语过慢

bradykinesia [ˌbrædiki'niːziə] *n* 运动徐缓

bradykinetic [ˌbrædiki'netik] *a* 运动过慢的;慢动的(影片放映)

bradykinin [ˌbrædi'kainin] *n* 缓激肽(血管舒张药)

bradylalia [ˌbrædi'leiliə] *n* 言语徐缓(脑损害所致)

bradylexia [ˌbrædi'leksiə] *n* 阅读过慢

bradylogia [ˌbrædi'ləudʒiə] *n*【希】[精神性]言语过慢

bradymenorrhea [ˌbrædiˌmenə'riːə] *n* 经期延长

bradypepsia [ˌbrædi'pepsiə] *n* 消化徐缓

bradyphagia [ˌbrædi'feidʒiə] *n* 慢食癖

bradyphasia [ˌbrædi'feiziə] *n* 言语过慢(脑损害所致)

bradyphemia [ˌbrædi'fiːmiə] *n* 言语过慢

bradyphrasia [ˌbrædi'freiziə] *n* [精神性]迟语症

bradyphrenia [ˌbrædi'friːniə] *n* 智力迟钝(流行性脑炎所致)

bradypnea [ˌbrædi'ni(ː)ə, brædip-] *n* 呼吸缓慢,呼吸过慢

bradypragia [ˌbrædi'preidʒiə] *n* 动作过慢

Bradyrhizobium [ˌbreidirai'zəubiəm] *n* 短根瘤菌属

bradyrhythmia [ˌbrædi'riθmiə] *n* 心动过缓,心搏徐缓

bradyspermatism [ˌbrædi'spəːmətizəm] *n* 射精过慢

bradysphygmia [ˌbrædi'sfigmiə] *n* 脉搏过缓,心搏徐缓

bradystalsis [ˌbrædi'stælsis] *n* 蠕动过慢

bradytachycardia [ˌbrædiˌtæki'kɑːdiə] *n* 心搏快慢交替

bradyteleokinesis [ˌbrædiˌteliəuki'niːsis], **bradyteleocinesia** [ˌbrædiˌteliəusai'niːziə] *n* 运动终末过慢

bradytocia [ˌbrædi'təusiə] *n* 分娩延缓,滞产

bradytrophia [ˌbrædi'trəufiə] *n* 营养作用过慢 | **bradytrophic** [ˌbrædi'trɔfik] *a*

bradyuria [ˌbrædi'juəriə] *n* 排尿过慢

bradyzoite [ˌbrædi'zəuit] *n* 缓殖子,缓殖体

Bragard's sign [brɑː'gɑːd] (Karl Bragard) 布拉加德征(膝挺直,下肢向臀部屈曲直至感到疼痛为止,然后足背屈,如疼痛加重提示神经根疾患)

braidism ['breidizəm] (得名于 James Braid) *n* 催眠术,催眠状态

Braid's strabismus [breid] (James Braid) 布雷德斜视(诱导催眠时)

Brailey's operation ['breili] (William A. Brailey) 布雷利手术(滑车上神经伸展术,以缓解青光眼疼痛)

braille [breil] *n* 盲人点字法(法国盲文教师布莱叶〈Louis Braille〉所创制)

brain [brein] *n* 脑;[复]脑髓;[常用复]脑力;智能 | new ~ 新脑(大脑皮质及其所属)/ old ~ 旧脑,原脑 / olfactory ~, smell ~ 嗅脑 / 'tween ~ 间脑 / water ~ 蹒跚病 / wet ~ 脑水肿

Brain airway [brein] (A. I. Brain) 布雷恩导气管(喉面罩导气管)

Brain's reflex [brein] (Walter R. Brain) 布雷恩反射(当病人采取四足动物位时,偏瘫的曲臂伸直。亦称四足伸直反射)

brainstem ['breinstem] *n* 脑干

brainstorm ['breinstɔːm] *n* 脑猝变,脑猝病

brainwashing ['breinwɔːʃiŋ] *n* 洗脑(强制性改变思想)

brake [breik] *n* 制动器;制动机制 *vt, vi* 制动 | duodenal ~ 十二指肠制动机制

bran [bræn] *n* 麸,糠

branch [brɑːntʃ, bræntʃ] *n* 分支,支,分科,部门 | bundle ~ 希氏束支,房室束支 / left bundle ~ 左束支 / right bundle ~ 右束支

branched-chain-amino-acid transaminase [bræntʃt tʃein ə'miːnəu 'æsid træns'æmineis] 支链氨基酸转氨酶

branched-chain α-keto acid decarboxylase 支链 α-酮酸脱羧酶,支链 α-酮酸脱氢酶

branched-chain α-keto acid dehydrogenase 支链 α-酮酸脱氢酶(缺乏此复合体中某一成分可致枫糖尿病)

brancher enzyme, branching enzyme 分支酶,1, 4-α-葡聚糖分支酶

brancher enzyme deficiency 分支酶缺乏[症],糖原贮积症Ⅳ型

branchia ['bræŋkiə] ([复] **branchiae** ['bræŋkiiː]) *n*【希】鳃 ~l *a*

branchiogenic [ˌbræŋkiəu'dʒenik], **branchiogenous** [ˌbræŋki'ɔdʒinəs] *a* 鳃源[性]的

branchioma [ˌbræŋkiˈəumə] *n* 鳃瘤

branchiomere [ˈbræŋkiəˌmiə] *n* 鳃节 | **branchiomeric** [ˌbræŋkiəuˈmerik] *a*

branchiomerism [ˌbræŋkiˈɔmərizəm] *n* 鳃分节

Branchiostoma [ˌbræŋkiəˈstəumə] *n* 文昌鱼属(即 Amphioxus)

Brand bath [brɑːnt] (Ernst Brand) 布兰特浴(冷水按摩浴)

Brande's test [brænd] (William T. Brande) 布兰德试验(检奎宁)

Brandt-Andrews maneuver [brɑːnt ˈændruːz] (Thure Brandt; Henry R. Andrews) 布-安手法(于第三产程从子宫逼出胎盘的方法:左手持脐带,右手置于产妇腹部,手指放在子宫前面,在右手轻轻地向后稍向上压时,左手轻轻牵引脐带)

Brânemark implant [ˈbrænəmɑːk] (Per-Ingmar Brânemark) 布兰内马克植入物(一种骨内整合性植入物)

Branhamella [ˌbrænhəˈmelə] (Sara Elizabeth Branham) *n* 布兰汉球菌属 | ~ catarrhalis 卡他布兰汉球菌

Branham's sign (bradycardia) [ˈbrænhæm] (H. H. Branham) 布兰汉姆征(心动过缓)(用手指紧压动静脉瘘近侧的动脉引起的心动过缓)

branny [ˈbræni] *a* 糠[麸]状的

brash [bræʃ] *n* 胃灼热 | water ~ 胃灼热,吞酸嘈杂 / weaning ~ 断奶腹泻

brass [brɑːs] *n* 黄铜　*a* 黄铜制的

Brassica [ˈbræsikə] *n*【拉】芥属,芸苔属

brassic acid [ˈbræsik], **brassidic acid** [bræˈsidik] 顺芜酸,顺二十二碳烯-12-酸

brassiere [ˈbræsiə] *n* 奶罩

brassilic acid [bræˈsilik] 十三碳二酸

Braun-Husler test (reaction) [brɔːn ˈhuslə] (Ludwig Braun) 布劳恩-胡斯勒试验(反应)(检脑脊液中过量球蛋白)

Braune's muscle [ˈbraunə] (Christian W. Braune) 布劳内肌,耻骨直肠肌

Braun's anastomosis [brɔːn] (Heinrich Braun) 布劳吻合[术](胃肠吻合术时,为防止胃和十二指肠内含物恶性循环,而在输出和输入肠襻间即在胃肠造口的远端施行手术)

Braun's canal [brɔːn] (Carl von Braun) 神经肠管

Braun's hook [brɔːn] (Gustav Braun) 布劳恩钩(胎儿断头术用)

Braun's test [brɔːn] (Christopher H. Braun) 布劳恩试验(检尿葡萄糖)

Braunwald's sign [ˈbraunwɑːld] (Eugene Braunwald) 布劳恩怀尔德征(心室期前收缩后立即出现弱脉,而不是强脉)

Bravais-jacksonian epilepsy [brɑːˈvei dʒækˈsəuniə] 布-杰癫痫,杰克逊癫痫(见 jacksonian epilepsy)

Braxton Hicks' contraction (sign) [ˈbrækstən hiks] (J. Braxton Hicks) 布拉克斯顿·希克斯收缩(征)(妊娠 3 个月后子宫的间歇性收缩) | ~ version 布拉克斯顿·希克斯转胎位术(内足转胎位术,用于已不能存活的胎儿)

braxy [ˈbræksi] *n* 羊快疫,羊炭疽

brayera [brəˈjerə] *n* 苦苏花(驱虫药、杀绦虫药)

braze [breiz] *vt* 焊接(牙科)

brazilin [brəˈzilin] *n* 巴西木素(主要用作染料,亦可作指示剂)

breadth [bredθ] *n* 宽度 | ~ of accommodations 调视范围,调视限度 / ~ of oral fissure 口裂宽

break [breik] *n* 断路;断裂

breakage [ˈbreikidʒ] *n* (染色体)断裂

breakdown [ˈbreikdaun] *n* (身体、精神等方面的)衰竭,崩溃 | nervous ~ 精神崩溃

breaker [ˈbreikə] *n* 碎裂机;断路器,开关;缓冲衬层

breakfast [ˈbrekfəst] *n* 早餐 | early light ~ 清淡的早早餐

breast [brest] *n* 前胸;乳房 | caked ~ 乳汁潴留性乳腺炎 / funnel ~ 漏斗[状]胸 / hysterical ~ 癔症性乳房(癔症性乳房肿痛) / irritable ~ 乳腺过敏 / pigeon ~, chicken ~ 鸡胸(由于婴儿呼吸阻塞或佝偻病所致) / proemial ~ 先兆乳腺病(女性乳房先兆性病变) / shoe-makers' ~ 鞋工胸(胸骨下部及剑突因受制鞋工具压迫,致使制鞋工人的胸骨凹陷) / shotty ~ 弹丸状乳腺(增生性乳腺炎,亦称纤维性囊肿病) / thrush ~ 鸫鸟胸状心肌

breastbone [ˈbrestbəun] *n* 胸骨

breast-fed [ˈbrest ˌfed] *a* 母乳喂养的

breast-feed [ˈbrest ˌfiːd] *vt* 母乳喂养

breast-feeding [ˈbrest ˈfiːdiŋ] *n* 母乳喂养

breath [breθ] *n* 呼吸 | foul ~ 口臭 / lead ~ 铅中毒口臭 / liver ~ 肝病口臭 / vesicular ~ 肺泡呼吸

breathe [briːð] *vi*, *vt* 呼吸

breathing [ˈbriːðiŋ] *n* 呼吸;一次呼吸;呼吸音 | bronchial ~ 支气管呼吸音 / frog ~, glossopharyngeal ~ 蛙式呼吸,舌咽式呼吸 / intermittent positive pressure ~ 间歇性正压呼吸 / periodic ~ 周期性呼吸

Breda's disease [ˈbreidə] (Achille Breda) 雅司病(即 yaws)

bredouillement [breidwiˈmɔŋ] *n*【法】语词缺落(由于发音过速造成单词未能完整读出)

breech [briːtʃ] *n* 臀 | frank ~ 伸腿臀位

bregma [ˈbregmə] *n*【拉;希】前囟点 | **~tic**

[breg'mætik] *a*

bregmatodymia [ˌbregmətəu'dimiə] *n* 前囟联胎畸形

Brehmer's treatment (method) ['breimə] (Hermann Brehmer) 布雷默疗法(肺结核的膳食及物理疗法)

brei [brai] *n*【德】糊,浆

Breisky's disease ['braiski] (August Breisky) 外阴干皱

Bremer's test ['bremə] (Ludwig Bremer) 布雷默试验(检糖尿病者血液)

bremsstrahlung ['bremˌʃtrɑːluŋ] *n*【德】韧致辐射

Brennemann's syndrome ['brenimən] (Joseph Brennemann) 布伦尼曼综合征(肠系膜淋巴结炎及腹膜后淋巴结炎,为咽喉感染的后遗症)

Brenner operation ['brenə] (Alexander Brenner) 布伦纳手术(巴西尼〈Bassini〉术的改良法,将腹肌缝在睾提肌上)

Brenner's formula (test) ['brenə] (Rudolf Brenner) 布伦纳公式(试验)(用电流刺激听神经,检听觉)

Brenner tumor ['brenə] (Fritz Brenner) 卵巢纤维上皮瘤

brenz- [前缀]【德】焦,焦性(同样见 pyro-起始的词)

brenz-catechin sulfuric acid [brents 'kætikin] 邻羟苯硫酸酯

brephic ['brefik] *a* 胚胎期的,发育初期的

brepho- [构词成分]胚胎;胎儿,新生儿

brephoplastic [ˌbrefəu'plæstik] *a* 胚胎期形成的

brephotrophic [ˌbrefəu'trɔfik] *a* 婴儿营养的

Breschet's canals [brə'ʃei] (Gilbert Breschet) 板障管 | ~ hiatus 蜗孔 / ~ sinus 蝶顶窦 / ~ veins 板障静脉

Brescia-Cimino fistula ['breʃiə si'miːnəu] (Michael J. Brescia; James E. Cimino) 布-西瘘(血液透析用的一种动静脉瘘,包括头静脉和桡动脉的端-端吻合术)

Bretonneau's angina, disease [bretə'nəu] (Pierre F. Bretonneau) 布雷托诺咽峡炎、病(咽白喉)

bretylium tosylate [bri'tiljəm] 托西溴苄铵(抗心律失常药)

Breus mole [brɔis] (Carl Breus) 布罗伊斯胎块(流产时胎盘的病理性改变,突向绒毛膜间隙的大量绒毛间血肿积聚。亦称血肿性胎块)

brevi- [构词成分]短

Brevibacteriaceae [ˌbrevibækˌtiəri'eisiiː] *n* 短杆菌科,短颈细菌科

Brevibacterium [ˌbrevibæk'tiəriəm] *n* 短杆菌属,短颈细菌属

brevicollis [ˌbrevi'kɔlis] *n* 短颈

breviductor [ˌbrevi'dʌktə] *n* 短收肌

breviflexor [ˌbrevi'fleksə] *n* 短屈肌

brevilineal [ˌbrevi'liniəl] *a* 短形的;矮短[体]型的

breviradiate [ˌbrevi'reidieit] *a* 短突的(本词亦适用于某一类神经胶质细胞)

Brewer's infarcts ['bru(ː)ə] (George E. Brewer) 布鲁尔梗死(肾盂肾炎时肾切片上所见类似梗死的暗红色楔形病灶) | ~ point 布鲁尔点(肾脏感染时肋椎角压痛点)

Bricker's technique (operation) ['brikə] (Eugene M. Bricker) 布里克技术(手术),回肠膀胱术(手术造一个回肠通道,形成扁平瘘口以收集尿,将回肠黏膜缝到皮肤上形成此扁平外形)

Brickner's sign ['briknə] (Richard M. Brickner) 布里克纳征(面神经功能损伤时,眼耳的协调活动减弱)

brickpox ['brikpɔks] *n* 猪丹毒

BrIDA mebrofenin 甲溴菲宁(诊断用药)

bridge [bridʒ] *n* 桥;齿桥;跗骨结合;胞间桥 | arteriolovenular ~ 小动静脉桥 / cantilever ~ 悬臂,单端固定桥(牙) / cell ~s, intercellular ~s 胞间桥 / cytoplasmic ~ 胞质桥,胞浆桥;胞间桥 / ~ of the nose 鼻梁

bridgework ['bridʒwəːk] *n* 桥托,局部义齿 | removable ~ 可摘桥托,可摘局部义齿

bridle ['braidl] *n* 系带;约束丝

bridou [bri'duː] *n* 口角炎,念珠菌性口角炎

Brieger's cachexia reaction ['briːgə] (Ludwig Brieger) 布里格恶病质反应(血清中抗胰蛋白酶的增加,见于恶性病及以恶病质为特征的其他疾病) | ~ test 布里格试验(检尿中焦儿茶酚及士的宁)

bright [brait] *a* 亮的 | ~**ness** *n* 亮度

brightic ['braitik] *a* 患肾小球肾炎的 *n* 肾小球肾炎患者

brightism ['braitizəm] *n* 肾炎(急性或慢性)

Bright's disease [brait] (Richard Bright) 布赖特肾病(一般指肾小球肾炎) | ~ eye 布赖特眼(慢性肾病眼)

Brill's disease, Brill-Zinsser disease [bril 'zinsə] (Nathan E. Brill; Hans Zinsser) 布里尔病,布里尔-津泽病,复发性斑疹伤寒

Brill-Symmers disease [bril 'siməz] (Nathan E. Brill; Douglas Symmers) 结节状淋巴瘤

brim [brim] *n* 边,缘;骨盆上口

brimonidine tartrate [bri'məunədiːn] 酒石酸溴莫尼定(α 受体激动药)

Brinell hardness number [bri'nel] (Johann A. Brinell) 布氏硬度数(表示某物质相对硬度的数值)

brinolase [ˈbrainəleis] *n* 米曲纤溶酶
Brinton's disease [ˈbrintən] (William Brinton) 皮革状胃,硬变性胃炎
brinzolamide [brinˈzəuləmaid] *n* 布林佐胺(碳酸酐酶抑制药)
Brion-Kayser disease [briˈɔn ˈkaizə] (Albert Brion; Heinrich Kayser) 副伤寒
Briquet's ataxia [briˈkei] (Paul Briquet) 布里凯共济失调(癔症患者皮肤及腿肌麻木) | ~ syndrome 布里凯综合征(癔症性膈麻痹所致的气促及失声)
brisement [briːzˈmɔŋ] *n* 【法】裂断;折断 | ~ forcé 强力裂断法(强力折断骨质性关节强硬)
brise-pierre [briːs piˈɛə] *n* 【法】碎石器,碎石钳
brisket [ˈbriskət] *n* 胸肉(反刍动物)
Brissaud-Marie syndrome [briˈsu məˈriː] (Edouard Brissaud; Pierre Marie) 布-马综合征,癔症性半侧舌唇痉挛
Brissaud's dwarf [briˈsu] (Edouard Brissaud) 布里索侏儒(伴有黏液性水肿的侏儒) ~ infantilism 布里索幼稚型(婴儿黏液性水肿) / ~ reflex 布里索反射(轻搔足底引起阔筋膜张肌收缩) / ~ scoliosis 坐骨神经痛性脊柱侧凸
Brissaud-Sicard syndrome [briˈsu siˈkɑː] (Edouard Brissaud; Jean A. Sicard) 布里索-西卡综合征(由脑桥病灶引起的痉挛性偏瘫)
bristle [ˈbrisl] *n* 鬃,刚毛 | bacterial ~ 细菌刚毛
Bristowe's syndrome [ˈbristəu] (John S. Bristowe) 布里斯托综合征(胼胝体瘤引起的一系列症状,其中包括偏瘫和运用不能)
BRM biologic response modifier 生物反应调节剂
broach [brəutʃ] *n* 髓针(牙科用) | barbed ~ 倒钩拔髓针 / root-canal ~, pathfinder ~ 根管针 / smooth ~ 平滑髓针
Broadbent's sign [ˈbrɔːdbent] (William H. Broadbent) 布罗德本特征(与心包粘连有关的在背部左侧靠近第十一、第十二肋骨处可见到凹陷)
broad-spectrum [ˈbrɔːd ˈspektrəm] *a* 广谱的
Broca's amnesia [ˈbrɔkə] (Pierre P. Broca) 语言遗忘 | ~ aphasia 运动性失语[症] / ~ area 布罗卡皮层区 / ~ ataxia 癔症性共济失调 / ~ band 布罗卡带(胚胎嗅脑的一部) / ~ center 言语中枢 / ~ convolution (gyrus, region) 左额下回 / ~ diagonal band 布罗卡斜角带(斜纹) / ~ fissure 布罗卡裂(围绕布罗卡回之裂) / ~ motor speech area 布罗卡运动语言区 / ~ parolfactory area 布罗卡旁嗅区(胼胝下区) / ~ plane 视平面 / ~ point 耳穴 / ~ pouch 女阴囊(大阴唇内梨状囊)
Brockenbrough's sign [ˈbrɔkənbrəu] (Edwin C. Brockenbrough) 布劳肯布罗征(心室期前收缩后立即出现弱脉,而不是强脉,提示特发性肥厚性主动脉瓣下狭窄)
Brock's infundibulectomy [brɔk] (Sir Russell Claude Brock) 布洛克动脉圆锥切除术(切除右心室肥厚的流出道的内部,有助于缓解法洛〈Fallot〉四联症时的肺动脉瓣狭窄) / ~ operation 布洛克手术,经室封闭式瓣膜切开术 / ~ syndrome 布洛克综合征,中叶综合征(右肺中叶膨胀不全,兼有慢性肺炎)
Brödel's bloodless line, white line [ˈbrəːdel] (Max Brödel) 布勒德尔无血线、白线(肾脏表面靠近凸面缘处的纵行浅色带,据认为比其他区血管形成少,因为这是动脉分布两个区之间的边缘)
Broders' index (classification) [ˈbrəudəz] (Albert C. Broders) 布罗德斯指数(分级)(以原始细胞或未分化细胞的多少表示肿瘤的恶性程度,第 1 级含 1/4 未分化细胞,第 2 级含 1/2 未分化细胞,第 3 级含 3/4 未分化细胞,第 4 级则全部细胞未分化)
Brodie's abscess [ˈbrəudi] (Benjamin C. Brodie) 骨骺端脓肿 | ~ disease 布罗迪病(①慢性滑膜炎,尤指膝部,患部有髓样退化;②癔症性脊柱假骨折) / ~ knee 布罗迪膝(慢性膝关节滑膜炎) / ~ sign 布罗迪征(龟头上呈现一黑斑,为尿液外渗至海绵体的体征)
Brodie's ligament [ˈbrəudi] (J. G. Brodie) 肱骨横韧带
brodifacoum [ˈbrəudifəkuːm] *n* 溴法库姆(灭鼠药)
Brodmann's areas [ˈbrɔdmən] (Korbinian Brodmann) 布劳德曼区(大脑皮质细胞结构区分图,按 6 个细胞层的排列不同而分区并给每个区以编号)
Broesike's fossa [ˈbriːzikə] (Gustav Broesike) 空肠旁隐窝
brofoxine [brəuˈfɔksiːn] *n* 溴苯噁嗪酮(安定药)
broken wind [ˈbrəukən wind] 马气喘病
bromate [ˈbrəumeit] *n* 溴酸盐 *vt* 用溴处理;使与溴化合
bromated [ˈbrəumeitid] *a* 含溴的,溴化的
bromatology [ˌbrəuməˈtɔlədʒi] *n* 饮食学,食品学
bromatotherapy [ˌbrəumətəuˈθerəpi], **bromatherapy** [ˌbrəuməˈθerəpi] *n* 饮食疗法
bromatotoxin [ˌbrəumətəuˈtɔksin] *n* 食物毒素(由于发酵作用等形成的食物毒素)
bromatoxism [ˌbrəuməˈtɔksizəm], **bromatotoxismus** [ˌbrəumətəutɔkˈsisməs] *n* 食物中毒,食品中毒
bromauric acid [brɔˈmɔːrik] 溴金酸
bromazepam [brəuˈmæzipæm] *n* 溴西泮(抗焦虑药)
bromelain [ˈbrəuməlein], **bromelin** [ˈbrəuməlin, brəˈmelin] *n* 菠萝蛋白酶

bromelains [ˈbrəuməleinz] *n* 菠萝蛋白酶(用于减少炎症和水肿,并加速组织修复)
bromethol [brɔˈmeθɔl] *n* 三溴乙醇溶液
bromhexine hydrochloride [brɔmˈheksiːn] 盐酸溴己新(祛痰药)
bromhidrosis, bromidrosis [ˌbrəumiˈdrəusis] *n* 臭汗症
bromic [ˈbrəumik] *a* 溴的;含溴的;五价溴的 | ~ acid 溴酸
bromide [ˈbrəumaid] *n* 溴化物
brominated [ˈbrəumiˌneitid] *a* 溴化的,加溴的;含溴的
bromindione [brəuminˈdaiəun] *n* 溴茚二酮(抗凝药)
bromine (Br) [ˈbrəumiːn] *n* 溴(化学元素)
brominism [ˈbrəuminizəm], **bromism** [ˈbrəumizəm] *n* 溴中毒
brominized [ˈbrəuminaizd] *a* 用溴处理;含溴的;溴化的,加溴的
bromisovalum [ˌbrəumisəˈvæləm] *n* 溴米索伐(催眠镇静药)
bromization [ˌbrəumaiˈzeiʃən] *n* 溴化作用;大剂量溴化物使用
bromized [ˈbrəumaizd] *a* 溴化的
brom(o)- [构词成分] 臭;溴
bromobenzene [ˌbrəuməuˈbenziːn] *n* 溴苯
bromochlorotrifluoroethane [ˌbrəuməuˌklɔːrəu-traiˌfluərəuˈeθein] *n* 溴氯三氟乙烷,氟烷(吸入麻醉药)
bromocriptine mesylate [ˌbrəuməuˈkriptiːn] 甲磺溴隐亭(催乳激素抑制药,多巴胺拮抗药)
5-bromodeoxyuridine [ˌbrəuməudiɔksiˈjuəridin] *n* 5-溴脱氧尿苷
bromoderma [ˌbrəuməuˈdəːmə] *n* 溴疹
bromodiphenhydramine hydrochloride [ˌbrəuməuˌdaifenˈhaidrəmin] 盐酸溴马秦(抗组胺药)
bromoform [ˈbrəuməufɔːm] *n* 溴仿,三溴甲烷(镇静、镇咳药)
bromoiodism [ˌbrəuməuˈaiədizəm] *n* 溴碘中毒
bromomania [ˌbrəuməuˈmeinjə] *n* 嗜溴剂癖(因溴化物使用不当所致的精神病)
bromomenorrhea [ˌbrəuməumenəˈriːə] *n* 臭[性月]经
bromopnea [brəˈmɔpniə, ˌbrəuməˈni(ː)ə] *n* 口臭
5-bromouracil [ˌbrəuməuˈjuərəsil] *n* 5-溴尿嘧啶(一种具有致突变作用的嘧啶类似物)
bromoxanide [brəuˈmɔksənaid] *n* 溴沙尼特(抗蠕虫药)
bromperidol [brɔmˈperidəul] *n* 溴哌利多(安定药)
brompheniramine [ˌbrəumfeˈnirəmiːn] *n* 溴苯那敏(抗组胺药)
bromphenol [brəumˈfiːnɔl] *n* 溴[代苯]酚
bromphenylacetylcysteine [brəumˌfenilˌæsitilˌsistiin] *n* 嗅苯乙酰半胱氨酸,溴苯硫醇尿酸
bromphenylmercapturic acid [brɔmˌfenilˌməːkæpˈtjuərik] 溴苯硫醇尿酸
bromsalans [ˈbrɔmsəlænz] *n* 溴沙仑类(一组消毒防腐药,见 dibromsalan, metabromsalan 和 tribromsalan)
bromosaligenin [ˌbrəumsæliˈdʒenin] *n* 溴水杨醇(曾用以治关节炎及抗痉挛药)
bromurated [ˈbrəumjuˌreitid] *a* 含溴或溴盐的;溴化的,加溴的
bromuret [ˈbrəumjurit] *n* 溴化物
bronchadenitis [ˌbrɔŋkædiˈnaitis] *n* 支气管淋巴结炎
bronchi [ˈbrɔŋkai] bronchus 的复数
bronchia [ˈbrɔŋkiə] bronchium 的复数
bronchial [ˈbrɔŋkjəl] *a* 支气管的
bronchiarctia [ˌbrɔŋkiˈɑːkʃiə] *n* 支气管狭窄
bronchiectasis [ˌbrɔŋkiˈektəsis] *n* 支气管扩张 | capillary ~ 细支气管扩张 / dry ~ 干性支气管扩张 | **bronchiectasia** [ˌbrɔŋkiekˈteiziə] *n* / **bronchiectatic** [ˌbrɔŋkietˈtætik], **bronchiectasic** [ˌbrɔŋkiekˈteizik] *a*
bronchiloquy [brɔŋˈkiləkwi] *n* 支气管语音
bronchi(o)- [构词成分]支气管
bronchiocele [ˈbrɔŋkiəusiː] *n* 细支气管扩大
bronchiocrisis [ˌbrɔŋkiəuˈkraisis] *n* 支气管危象(脊髓痨病程中呼吸困难的突然发作)
bronchiogenic [ˌbrɔŋkiəuˈdʒenik] *a* 支气管源的
bronchiole [ˈbrɔŋkiəul] *n* 细支气管 | respiratory ~, alveolar ~ 呼吸细支气管 / terminal ~, lobular ~ 终末细支气管
bronchiolectasis [ˌbrɔŋkiəuˈlektəsis] *n* 细支气管扩张
bronchioli [brɔŋˈkaiəlain] bronchiolus 的所有格和复数
bronchiolitis [ˌbrɔŋkiəuˈlaitis] *n* 细支气管炎 | acute obliterating ~ 急性闭塞性细支气管炎 / ~ exudativa 渗出性细支气管炎 / ~ fibrosa obliterans 纤维闭塞性细支气管炎 / vesicular ~ 肺泡性细支气管炎,支气管肺炎
bronchiolus [brɔŋˈkaiələs] ([复] **bronchioli** [brɔŋˈkaiəlai]) *n* 【拉】细支气管 | bronchioli respiratorii 呼吸细支气管
bronchiospasm [ˈbrɔŋkiəuˌspæzəm], **bronchismus** [brɔŋˈkisməs] *n* 支气管痉挛(痉挛性支气管收缩)
bronchiostenosis [ˌbrɔŋkiəustiˈnəusis] *n* 支气管狭窄
bronchisepticin [ˌbrɔŋkiˈseptisin] *n* 支气管败血菌素(由支气管败血性布鲁菌制备的抗原,用于

犬瘟热的皮肤试验）

bronchitis [brɔŋˈkaitis] *n* 支气管炎 | acute ~ 急性支气管炎 / acute laryngotracheal ~ 急性喉气管支气管炎 / arachidic ~ 花生仁吸入性支气管炎 / capillary ~ 细支气管炎，毛细支气管炎 / catarrhal ~ 卡他性支气管炎 / chronic ~ 慢性支气管炎 / croupous ~, exudative ~, fibrinous ~, membranous ~, plastic ~, pseudomembranous ~ 格鲁布性支气管炎，渗出性支气管炎，纤维蛋白性支气管炎，假膜性支气管炎 / dry ~ 干性支气管炎 / epidemic ~ 流行性感冒 / ether ~ 乙醚性支气管炎 / hemorrhagic ~ 支气管螺旋体病 / infectious asthmatic ~ 传染性哮喘性支气管炎 / infectious avian ~ 传染性家禽支气管炎 / mechanic ~ 机械性支气管炎 / ~ obliterans 闭塞性支气管炎 / parasitic ~ 寄生虫性支气管炎，蠕虫性支气管炎 / phthinoid ~ 结核性支气管炎 / productive ~ 增生性支气管炎 / putrid ~ 腐败性支气管炎 / secondary ~ 继发性支气管炎 / staphylococcus ~ 葡萄球菌性支气管炎 / streptococcal ~ 链球菌性支气管炎 / suffocative ~ 窒息性支气管炎 / vesiculary ~ 肺泡性支气管炎 | **bronchitic** [brɔŋˈkitik] *a*

bronchium [ˈbrɔŋkiəm]（[复] **bronchia** [ˈbrɔŋkiə]）*n*【拉】小支气管（支气管分支，小于支气管，大于细支气管）

bronch(o)- [构词成分]支气管

bronchoadenitis [ˌbrɔŋkəuˌædiˈnaitis] *n* 支气管淋巴结炎

bronchoalveolar [ˌbrɔŋkəuælˈviələ] *a* 支气管肺泡的

bronchoalveolitis [ˌbrɔŋkəuˌælviəuˈlaitis] *n* 支气管肺炎

bronchoaspergillosis [ˌbrɔŋkəuˌæspədʒiˈləusis] *n* 支气管曲霉病

bronchoblastomycosis [ˌbrɔŋkəuˌblæstəumaiˈkəusis] *n* 支气管芽生菌病，肺芽生菌病

bronchoblennorrhea [ˌbrɔŋkəuˌblenəˈriːə] *n* 支气管脓溢

bronchocandidiasis [ˌbrɔŋkəuˌkændiˈdaiəsis] *n* 支气管念珠菌病

bronchocavernous [ˌbrɔŋkəuˈkævənəs] *a* 支气管空洞的

bronchocavitary [ˌbrɔŋkəuˈkævitəri] *a* 支气管腔的

bronchocele [ˈbrɔŋkəusiːl] *n* 支气管囊肿（支气管局部扩张）

bronchocephalitis [ˌbrɔŋkəuˌsefəˈlaitis] *n* 百日咳

bronchoconstriction [ˌbrɔŋkəukənˈstrikʃən] *n* 支气管收缩

bronchoconstrictor [ˌbrɔŋkəukənˈstriktə] *a* 支气管收缩的 *n* 支气管收缩药

bronchodilatation [ˌbrɔŋkəudailəˈteiʃən], **bronchodilation** [ˌbrɔŋkəudaiˈleiʃən] *n* 支气管扩张，支气管舒张

bronchodilator [ˌbrɔŋkəudaiˈleitə] *n* 支气管扩张器；支气管扩张药

bronchoegophony [ˌbrɔŋkəuiˈgɔfəni] *n* 支气管羊音

bronchoesophageal [ˌbrɔŋkəui(ː)ˌsɔfəˈdʒi(ː)əl] *a* 支气管食管的

bronchoesophagology [ˌbrɔŋkəu i(ː)sɔfəˈgɔlədʒi] *n* 支气管食管病学

bronchoesophagoscopy [ˌbrɔŋkəu i(ː)sɔfəˈgɔskəpi] *n* 支气管食管镜检查

bronchofiberscope [ˌbrɔŋkəuˈfaibəskəup] *n* [光导]纤维支气管镜

bronchofiberscopy [ˌbrɔŋkəuˈfaibəskəpi], **bronchofibroscopy** [ˌbrɔŋkəufaiˈbrɔskəpi] *n* [光导]纤维支气管镜检查

bronchogenic [brɔŋkəuˈdʒenik] *a* 支气管源性的

bronchogram [ˈbrɔŋkəugræm] *n* 支气管造影摄[照]片 | air ~ 支气管气像，含气支气管像

bronchography [brɔŋˈkɔgrəfi] *n* 支气管造影[术] | **bronchographic** [ˌbrɔŋkəuˈgræfik] *a*

broncholith [ˈbrɔŋkəuliθ] *n* 支气管[结]石，肺石

broncholithiasis [ˌbrɔŋkəuliˈθaiəsis] *n* 支气管结石症

bronchology [brɔŋˈkɔlədʒi] *n* 支气管病学 | **bronchologic** [ˌbrɔŋkəuˈlɔdʒik] *a*

bronchomalacia [ˌbrɔŋkəuməˈleiʃiə] *n* 支气管软化

bronchomoniliasis [ˌbrɔŋkəuməuniˈlaiəsis] *n* 支气管念珠菌病

bronchomotor [ˌbrɔŋkəuˈməutə] *a* 支气管舒缩的

bronchomucotropic [ˌbrɔŋkəuˌmjuːkəuˈtrɔpik] *a* 促支气管分泌的

bronchomycosis [ˌbrɔŋkəumaiˈkəusis] *n* 支气管真菌病，支气管霉菌病

bronchonocardiosis [ˌbrɔŋkəunəuˌkɑːdiˈəusis] *n* 支气管诺卡放线菌病

broncho-oidiosis [ˌbrɔŋkəu əuˌidiˈəusis] *n* 支气管念珠菌病

bronchopancreatic [ˌbrɔŋkəuˌpæŋkriˈætik] *a* 支气管胰腺的

bronchopathy [brɔŋˈkɔpəθi] *n* 支气管病

bronchophony [brɔŋˈkɔfəni] *n* 支气管音 | pectoriloquous ~ 胸语性支气管音 / sniffling ~ 鼻塞支气管音 / whispered ~ 耳语支气管音

bronchoplasty [ˈbrɔŋkəuˌplæsti] *n* 支气管成形术

bronchoplegia [ˌbrɔŋkəuˈpliːdʒiə] *n* 支气管麻痹

bronchopleural [ˌbrɔŋkəuˈpluərəl] *a* 支气管胸膜的

bronchopleuropneumonia [ˌbrɔŋkəuˌpluərəunju(ː)ˈməunjə] *n* 支气管胸膜肺炎

bronchopneumonia [ˌbrɔŋkəunju(ː)ˈməunjə] *n* 支气管肺炎 | postoperative ~ 术后支气管肺炎 / subacute ~ 亚急性支气管肺炎 / virus ~ 病毒性支气管肺炎 | **bronchopneumonic** [ˌbrɔŋkəunju(ː)ˈmɔnik] *a*

bronchopneumonitis [ˌbrɔŋkəuˌnjuːməˈnaitis] *n* 支气管肺炎

bronchopneumopathy [ˈbrɔŋkəunju(ː)ˈmɔpəθi] *n* 支气管肺病

bronchoprovocation [ˌbrɔŋkəuˌprɔvəˈkeiʃən] *n* 支气管激发

bronchopulmonary [ˌbrɔŋkəuˈpʌlmənəri] *a* 支气管肺的

bronchoradiography [ˌbrɔŋkəureidiˈɔgrəfi] *n* 支气管 X 线造影[术]

bronchorrhagia [ˌbrɔŋkəuˈreidʒiə] *n* 支气管出血

bronchorrhaphy [brɔŋˈkɔrəfi] *n* 支气管缝合术

bronchorrhea [brɔŋkəuˈriːə] *n* 支气管黏液溢

bronchoscope [ˈbrɔŋkəskəup] *n* 支气管镜 | fiberoptic ~ 纤维[光导]支气管镜

bronchoscopic [ˌbrɔŋkəuˈskɔpik] *a* 支气管镜检查的;支气管镜的

bronchoscopically [ˌbrɔŋkəuˈskɔpikəli] *ad* 用支气管镜检查

bronchoscopy [brɔŋˈkɔskəpi] *n* 支气管镜检查[法] | fiberoptic ~ 纤维[光导]支气管镜检查[术]

bronchosinusitis [ˌbrɔŋkəusainəˈsaitis] *n* 支气管鼻窦炎

bronchospasm [ˈbrɔŋkəˌspæzəm] *n* 支气管痉挛

bronchospirochetosis [ˌbrɔŋkəuˌspaiərəukiˈtəusis] *n* 支气管螺旋体病

bronchospirography [ˌbrɔŋkəuspaiəˈrɔgrəfi] *n* 支气管肺量描记法(测定一侧肺的肺活量、摄氧量、二氧化碳排出量的记录)

bronchospirometer [ˌbrɔŋkəuspaiəˈrɔmitə] *n* 支气管肺量计

bronchospirometry [ˌbrɔŋkəuspaiəˈrɔmitri] *n* 支气管肺量测定法(测定一侧肺的肺活量、摄氧量、二氧化碳排出量) | differential ~ 对比支气管肺活量测定法

bronchostaxis [ˌbrɔŋkəuˈstæksis] *n* 支气管出血

bronchostenosis [ˌbrɔŋkəustiˈnəusis] *n* 支气管狭窄

bronchostomy [brɔŋˈkɔstəmi] *n* 支气管造口术

bronchotome [ˈbrɔŋkətəum] *n* 支气管刀

bronchotomy [brɔŋˈkɔtəmi] *n* 支气管切开术

bronchotracheal [ˌbrɔŋkəutrəˈkiːəl, -ˈtreiki-] *a* 支气管气管的,气管支气管的

bronchotyphoid [ˌbrɔŋkəuˈtaifɔid] *n* 支气管炎型伤寒

bronchotyphus [ˌbrɔŋkəuˈtaifəs] *n* 支气管炎型斑疹伤寒

bronchovesicular [ˌbrɔŋkəuviˈsikjulə] *a* 支气管肺泡的

bronchus [ˈbrɔŋkəs] ([复] **bronchi** [ˈbrɔŋkai]) *n* 【拉】支气管 | apical ~, segmental ~ 肺尖[段]支气管 / cardiac ~ 肺底心段支气管 / eparterial ~ 动脉上支气管 / hyparterial bronchi 动脉下支气管 / primary ~ 主支气管,初级支气管(由气管分出的左和右支气管) / secondary ~ 次[级]支气管(主支气管的分支,包括肺叶支气管和肺段支气管) / stem ~ 支气管干/ tracheal ~ 气管[延续性]支气管(一种异位或额外支气管,从气管直接延伸到右肺上叶尖段,对某些动物来说是正常的,在人类则为先天性异常)

brontophobia [ˌbrɔntəˈfəubiə] *n* 雷电恐怖

bronze [brɔnz] *n* 青铜 *a* 青铜的 *vt* 镀青铜于,上青铜色于 *vi* 变成青铜色 | **~d** *a* 青铜色的

brood [bruːd] *n* 同窝,同巢,一窝 *vi* 孵,育

Brooke's disease [bruk] (Henry A. G. Brooke) 布鲁克病(触染性毛囊角化病;多发性乳头状毛发上皮瘤) | ~ tumor 布鲁克瘤(囊状腺样上皮瘤,多发性乳头状毛发上皮瘤)

broom [bruːm] *n* 金雀花 | **~y** *a* 金雀花的

Brophy's operation [ˈbrəufi] (Truman W. Brophy) 布罗菲手术(一种腭裂手术)

brosse [brɔs] *n* 花粉刷(见于某些原虫的刷状纤毛细胞器)

broth [brɔ(ː)θ] *n* 肉汤,肉汁;液体培养基

Broviac catheter [ˈbrəuviæk] (J. W. Broviac) 布路维阿克导管(一种中央静脉导管)

brow [brau] *n* 眉;额 | olympian ~, olympic ~ [先天梅毒性]凸额

brown [braun] *a* 棕色的 *n* 棕色,褐色 *vt*, *vi* 变褐,变成棕色 | aniline ~, Bismarck ~, Manchester ~, phenylene ~ 苯胺棕,俾斯麦棕,曼彻斯特棕,亚苯基棕 | **~ish**, **~y** *a* 带棕色的

Brown-Adson forceps [braun ˈædsən] (James B. Brown; Alfred W. Adson) 布-艾镊(见 Adson-Brown forceps)

brownian movement [ˈbrauniən] (Robert Brown) 布朗运动(由于溶剂分子的碰撞引起悬浮微粒的跳跃运动)

Browning's vein [ˈbrauniŋ] (William Browning) 布朗宁静脉(下吻合静脉的上部)

Brown-Roberts-Wells apparatus [braun ˈrɔːbəts welz] (R. A. Brown; T. S. Roberts; T. H. Wells) 布-罗-韦立体定向仪(用于立体定向手术的布-罗-韦技术) | ~ technique 布-罗-韦技术(一种立体定向技术,用一环套头固位,一环使计算机体层摄影影像定向,并使用一个弧导

系统）

Brown-Séquard's injection [ˈbraun seiˈkɑː] (Charles E. Brown-Séquard) 布朗-塞卡尔注射剂（睾丸浸出液注射剂）| ~ paralysis 布朗-塞卡尔麻痹（布朗-塞卡尔综合征；一种弛缓性麻痹，见于尿路疾患）/ ~ syndrome (disease, sign) 布朗-塞卡尔综合征（病、征）（脊髓偏侧损害时，身体同侧有运动麻痹，对侧有感觉缺失）/ ~ treatment 器官疗法，内脏制剂疗法

Brown's test (reaction) [braun] (Thomas K. Brown) 布朗试验（反应）（检孕；检尿氨定量）

Brown-Symmers disease [braun ˈsiməz] (Charles L. Brown; Douglas Symmers) 布-西病，儿童致死性急性浆液性脑炎

Brown-Vialetto-van Laere syndrome [braun viɑːˈleetəu vɑːnˈliː] (C. H. Brown; E. Vialetto; J. van Laere) 布-维-范综合征（一种常染色体隐性遗传综合征，包括进行性延髓性麻痹，伴若干重度障碍中的任何一种，其中有神经性聋、构音困难和吞咽困难）

Browne operation [braun] (Sir Denis J. Browne) 布朗手术（为尿道下裂修补的一种尿道成形术）

BRS British Roentgen Society 英国伦琴学会

Brucea [ˈbruːsiə] *n* 鸦胆子属

Brucella [bruːˈselə] (David Bruce) *n* 布氏菌属 | ~ abortus 流产布氏菌，流产杆菌 / ~ bronchiseptica 支气管败血性布氏菌 / ~ melitensis 马耳他布氏菌 / ~ suis 猪布氏菌 / ~ tularensis 野兔热布氏菌

brucella [bruːˈselə] *n* 布氏菌

Brucellaceae [ˌbruːseˈleisiiː] *n* 布氏菌科

brucellar [bruːˈselə] *a* 布氏菌属的

brucellin [bruːˈselin] *n* 布氏菌素（用于诊断布氏菌病）

brucellosis [ˌbruːseˈləusis], **brucelliasis** [ˌbruːseˈlaiəsis] *n* 布氏菌病

Bruce's septicemia [bruːs] (David Bruce) 布氏败血病，布氏菌病

Bruce's tract [bruːs] (Alexander Bruce) 隔缘束

Bruch's glands [bruh] (Karl W. L. Bruch) 布鲁赫腺（下睑结膜内淋巴滤泡）| ~ membrane (layer)（脉胳膜）玻璃膜

brucine [ˈbruːsi(ː)n] *n* 番木鳖碱，二甲氧基马钱子碱

Brücke's line [ˈbriːkə] (Ernst W. von Brücke) 布吕克线（横纹肌肌原纤维中与 Z 带交替的宽带）| ~ muscle 布吕克肌（睫状肌纵行纤维）/ ~ reagent 布吕克试剂（改良的麦耶〈Meyer〉试剂，50 g 碘化钾，120 g 碘化汞，加水至 1 000 ml / ~ test 布吕克试验（检尿内胆色素、蛋白质、脲）/ ~ tunic 布吕克膜（视网膜大脑层，不包括杆层和圆锥层及其纤维与核）

Bruck's disease [bruk] (Alfred Bruck) 布鲁克病（主征为骨畸形、多发性骨折、关节强硬及肌萎缩）

Bruck's reaction [bruk] (Carl Bruck) 布鲁克（硝酸）反应（检梅毒）

Brudzinski's sign (reflex) [bruːdˈzinski] (Józef Brudzinski) 布鲁金斯基征（反射）（①脑膜炎时，颈部前屈，可致髋、膝屈曲亦称颈征；②脑膜炎时，令一侧下肢被动地屈曲，则对侧下肢可见到同样的运动。亦称对侧征）

Brueghel's syndrome [ˈbrɔigəl] (Pieter Brueghel, the Elder 为佛兰德斯画家，其画 *De Gaper* 显示此综合征）（老）勃鲁盖尔综合征（面肌和口下颌肌张力障碍伴眼睑痉挛，歪嘴运动，舌前突，常发生于老年妇女。同样见 Meige's syndrome②解）

Brugia [ˈbrʌdʒiə] *n* 布［鲁格］氏丝虫属 | ~ malayi 马来丝虫 / ~ pahangi 彭亨丝虫

brugian [ˈbruːdʒiən] *a* 布［鲁格］氏的

Brug's filaria [bruːg] (S. L. Brug) 布［鲁格］氏丝虫，马来丝虫

bruise [bruːz] *n* 青肿；挫伤；捣碎 | stone ~ 石伤

bruit [bruːt] *n*【法】杂音 | ~ d'airain 金属音 / ~ de craquement 爆裂音 / ~ de diable 静脉哼鸣 / ~ de galop 奔马心音，奔马律 / ~ de pot fêlé 破壶音 / ~ de soufflet 风箱音

Brunati's sign [bruːˈnɑːti] (M. Brunati) 布鲁纳蒂征（肺炎或伤寒时出现角膜混浊）

Brunner's glands [ˈbrunə] (Johann C. Brunner) 十二指肠腺

Brünninghausen's method [ˈbriniŋˌhausən] (Herrmann J. Brünninghausen) 布林宁豪森法（扩张子宫颈导引早产）

Brunn's membrane [brun] (Albertvon Brunn) 布龙膜（鼻嗅区上皮）| ~ epithelial nests 布龙上皮细胞巢（健康输尿管内实性的或分支的细胞集落）

Brunschwig's operation [ˈbrunʃviʃ] (Alexzander Brunschwig) 胰十二指肠切除术

Bruns' disease [brʌnz] (John D. Bruns) 肺型疟疾，疟性肺尖硬变

Bruns' syndrome (sign) [brunz] (Ludwig Bruns) 布伦斯综合征（征）（头部突然转动时，可发生间歇性头痛、眩晕、呕吐及视力障碍，为第四脑室囊尾蚴感染等特有症状）

Brunsting's syndrome [ˈbruːnstiŋ] (Louis A. Brunsting) 布鲁斯汀综合征（一种多发性发疹性综合征，通常累及中年男子，在头颈部发生成簇的水疱性病损，并导致瘢痕形成）

Brunnstrom method [ˈbrʌnstrəm] (Signe Brunnstrom) 布伦斯特伦姆法（通过协同运动的感觉刺激来抑制痉挛的一套医疗体操）

brush [brʌʃ] *n* 刷 | stomach ~ 胃刷

Brushfield's spots [ˈbrʌʃfiːld] (Thomas Brushfield）布拉什菲尔德斑（虹膜周围的小白斑，通常呈月牙形，凹面向外，常见于患唐氏〈Down〉综合征的儿童，但并非特有）

Brushfield-Wyatt Syndrome [ˈbrʌʃfiːld ˈwaiət]（Thomas Brushfield; W. Wyatt）布-怀综合征（为一种先天性综合征，包括广泛性单侧鲜红斑痣、影响两眼右或左半侧视野的偏盲、对侧偏瘫、大脑血管瘤及智力迟钝；本征可能与斯-韦〈Sturge-Weber〉综合征有关）

brushite [ˈbrʌʃait] *n* 透碱磷石

Bruton's agammaglobulinemia, disease [ˈbrutən]（Ogden C. Bruton）布鲁顿无丙种球蛋白血症，布鲁顿病（X 连锁无丙种球蛋白血症）

brux [brʌks] *vi* 磨牙

bruxism [ˈbrʌksizəm] *n* 夜磨牙症（睡着时磨牙）| centric ~ 正中磨牙症

bruxomania [ˌbrʌksəuˈmeinjə], **brychomania** [ˌbraikəuˈmeinjə] *n* 磨牙癖（醒着时磨牙）

Bryant's line [ˈbraiənt]（Thomas Bryant）布赖恩特线（①髂股三角的垂直边；②一种试验线，测股骨短缩）| ~ traction 布赖恩牵引（股骨干骨折时作过头的垂直牵引）

Bryce's test [ˈbraisi]（James Bryce）布赖斯试验（测定天花预防接种免疫程度的试验，在过几天后重复接种，如第一次接种成功，则第二次反应很快就赶上第一次的反应）

Bryce-Teacher ovum [ˈbrais ˈtiːtʃə]（Thomas H. Bryce; John H. Teacher）布赖斯-蒂切卵（一种人卵，在 1908 年时期的研究中认为是已知最年幼的卵，现已知是一种病理标本）

Bryobia [braiˈəubiə] *n* 苔螨属 | ~ praetiosa 苜蓿苔螨

Bryonia [braiˈəuniə] *n* 泻根属

bryonia [braiˈəuniə] *n* 泻根

bryonidin [braiˈəunidinə] *n* 泻根素

bryonin [ˈbraiənin] *n* 泻根苦苷，拜俄尼苦苷

Bryson's sign [ˈbraisn]（Alexander Bryson）布赖森征（胸部扩张力减弱，有时见于突眼性甲状腺肿）

BS Bachelor of Science 理学士；Bachelor of Surgery 外科学士；breath sounds 呼吸音；blood sugar 血糖

BSA body surface area 体表面积

B-scan B 型[超声]扫描

BSF B lymphocyte stimulatory factor B 淋巴细胞刺激因子

BSP bromsulphalein 磺溴酞钠（测肝功能）

B'sp bronchospasm 支气管痉挛

BSS Bernard-Soulier syndrome 巨血小板综合征

BThU, BTU British thermal unit 英国热量单位

buba [ˈbubə] *n* 布巴病（皮肤黏膜利什曼病，南美各国的土名）

bubo [ˈbjuːbən] *n*【拉】腹股沟淋巴结炎（俗名横痃，由于鼠疫、梅毒、淋病、结核等所致）| bullet ~ 初期梅毒性腹股沟淋巴结炎 / chancroidal ~, virulent ~ 软下疳性腹股沟淋巴结炎，毒性腹股沟淋巴结炎 / climatic ~ 性病性淋巴肉芽肿，腹股沟淋巴肉芽肿 / malignant ~ 恶性腹股沟淋巴结炎 / primary ~ 原发性腹股沟淋巴结炎 / syphilitic ~ 梅毒性腹股沟淋巴结炎 | **bubonic** [bju(ː)ˈbɔnik] *a*

bubon [bjuˈbɔn] *n*【法】腹股沟淋巴结炎，横痃

bubonalgia [ˌbju(ː)bəuˈnældʒiə] *n* 腹股沟痛

bubonocele [bju(ː)ˈbɔnəsiːl] *n* 腹股沟突出（指在腹股沟部形成隆起的腹股沟疝或股疝）

bubonulus [bju(ː)ˈbɔnjuləs] *n*【拉】阴茎背小结

bucainide maleate [bjuˈkeinaid] 马来酸布卡尼（具有抗心律失常作用的心脏抑制药）

bucardia [bjuˈkɑːdiə] *n* 巨心，牛心症

bucca [ˈbʌkə] *n*【拉】颊

buccal [ˈbʌkəl] *a* 颊的 | **~ly** *ad* 向颊

buccinator [ˈbʌksiˌneitə] *n* 颊肌

bucc(o)- [构词成分] 颊

buccoaxial [ˌbʌkəuˈæksiəl] *a* 颊轴的

buccoaxiogingival [ˌbʌkəuˌæksiəuˈdʒindʒivəl], **buccoaxiocervical** [ˌbʌkəuˌæksiəˈsəːvikəl] *a* 颊轴龈的，颊轴颈的

buccocervical [ˌbʌkəuˈsəːvikəl] *a* 颊颈的；后牙颈颊面的；颊龈的

buccoclusion [ˌbʌkəuˈkluːʒən] *n* 颊殆，颊咬合 | **buccoclusal** [ˌbʌkəuˈkluːsəl] *a*

buccodistal [ˌbʌkəuˈdistl] *a* 颊[侧]远中的

buccogingival [ˌbʌkəuˈdʒindʒivəl] *a* 颊龈的

buccoglossopharyngitis [ˌbʌkəuˈglɔsəuˌfærinˈdʒaitis] *n* 颊舌咽炎 | ~ sicca 干性颊舌咽炎

buccolabial [ˌbʌkəuˈleibjəl] *a* 颊唇的

buccolingual [ˌbʌkəuˈliŋgwəl] *a* 颊舌的 | **~ly** *ad* 自颊向舌地

buccomaxillary [ˌbʌkəuˈmæksiləri] *a* 颊上颌的

buccomesial [ˌbʌkəuˈmiːziəl] *a* 颊[侧]近中的

bucco-occlusal [ˌbʌkəu ɔˈkluːzəl] *a* 颊殆的，颊咬合的

buccopharyngeal [ˌbʌkəufəˈrindʒi(ː)əl] *a* 颊咽的

buccoplacement [ˌbʌkəuˈpleismənt] *n* 颊向移位，颊侧移位

buccopulpal [ˌbʌkəuˈpʌlpl] *a* 颊髓的

buccostomy [bʌˈkɔstəmi] *n* 颊造口术

buccoversion [ˌbʌkəuˈvəːʃən] *n* 颊向错位

Bucephalus [bjuˈsefələs] *n* 牛头[吸虫]属 | ~ papillosus 乳头牛头吸虫

Buchner's bodies [ˈbuhnə]（Hans Buchner）布赫纳体，防御性蛋白（defensive protein，见 protein 项下相应术语）

buchu [ˈbjuːkjuː] *n* 布枯（芸香科植物，用作祛

风、利尿及尿路消毒防腐剂）

buckeye [ˈbʌkai] *n* 七叶树；七叶树的果实（有毒）

Buckley's syndrome [ˈbʌkli]（Rebecca H. Buckley）巴克利综合征，高免疫球蛋白E血症（即 hyperimmunoglobulinemia E syndrome，见 syndrome 项下相应术语）

buckling [ˈbʌkliŋ] *n* 扣带 | scleral ~ 巩膜扣带术

Buck's extension [buk]（Gurdon Buck）布克牵伸法（利用滑车及重量，使用于骨折的一肢牵伸）| ~ fascia 阴茎筋膜（会阴浅筋膜的延续）/ ~ operation 布克手术（髌骨和胫腓骨端楔形切除）

buckwheat [bʌkˈhwiːt] *n* 荞麦

Bucky diaphragm [ˈbʌki]（Gustav P. Bucky）布凯活动[X线]滤线栅（X线台的组成部分，以防次级射线达到胶片上，从而增强对比度和清晰度）| ~ rays 布凯射线，跨界射线（grenz rays，见 ray 项下相应术语）

buclizine [ˈbjukliziːn] *n* 布克力嗪（抗组胺药）| ~ hydrochloride 盐酸布克力嗪（抗组胺药，主要用作止恶心药，以治疗晕动病）

bucnemia [bʌkˈniːmiə] *n* 腿肿大，牛腿症

bucrylate [ˈbjuːkrileit] *n* 丁氰酯（组织粘合剂）

bud [bʌd] *n* 芽 / bronchial ~ 支气管芽 / end ~ 终蕾 / limb ~ 肢芽 / liver ~ 肝芽 / lung ~ 肺芽 / taste ~，gustatory ~ 味蕾 / tooth ~ 牙蕾 / ureteric ~，metanephric ~ 输尿管芽，后肾芽 / vascular ~ 血管芽

Budd-Chiari syndrome (disease) [bʌdʃiˈɑːri]（George Budd；Hans Chiari）巴德-基亚里综合征（肝静脉症状性闭塞，一般原因不明，或许由于各种情况造成，其中包括赘生物、狭窄、肝病、外伤、全身性感染以及血液病等。亦称闭塞性肝静脉内膜炎）

budding [ˈbʌdiŋ] *n* 出芽，芽生

budesonide [bjuˈdesənaid] *n* 布地萘德（一种抗炎糖皮质素，用于治疗鼻炎和哮喘，粉状口服或鼻内喷雾吸入）

budgerigar [ˈbʌdʒərigɑ]，**budgie** [ˈbʌdʒi] *n* 澳洲长尾小鹦鹉（用于鹦鹉病实验）

Budge's center [ˈbudgə]（Julius L. Budge）布格中枢①睫脊中枢，脊髓散瞳中枢；②脊髓生殖中枢）

Budin's joint [buˈdæn]（Pierre-Constant Budin）布丹关节（出生时枕骨鳞部与两个髁部之间的软骨带）| ~ rule 布丹[喂养]规则（每日喂牛奶量不得超过婴儿体重的1/10）

BUDR 5-bromodeoxyuridine 5-溴脱氧尿苷

Buerger's disease [ˈbəːgə]（Leo Buerger）血栓闭塞性脉管炎 | ~ symptom 伯格症状（血栓闭塞性脉管炎患者躺下时，只有将受累腿悬于床边才能减少疼痛）

Buergi's theory [ˈbjugi]（Emil Buergi）布吉学说（引起相同治疗表现的两种不同物质，如具有相同的药物学作用点，在合并使用时，其疗效增加）

buffer [ˈbʌfə] *n* 缓冲器；缓冲液，缓冲剂；缓冲[系] | bicarbonate ~ 碳酸氢盐缓冲系（一种缓冲系统，在体内对决定血液的pH是一个重要的因素）/ cacodylate ~ 二甲胂酸盐缓冲液（用以配制电子显微镜检查用的固定液）/ phosphate ~ 磷酸盐缓冲系（一种缓冲系统，在体内调节肾小管液的pH是重要的）/ TRIS ~ 三羟甲基氨基甲烷缓冲液 / veronal ~ 佛罗那缓冲液（一种巴比妥缓冲液，常用作配制电子显微镜检查用的固定液）

buffering [ˈbʌfəriŋ] *n* 缓冲作用

bufilcon A [bjuˈfilkɔn] 布费尔康A（一种疏水性接触镜材料）

bufin [ˈbjuːfin] *n* 蟾腮腺素

Bufo [ˈbjuːfəu] *n*【拉】蟾蜍属

buformin [bjuˈfɔːmin] *n* 丁福明（口服降血糖药）

bufotalin [ˌbjuːfəˈtælin] *n* 蟾毒配基B[乙酸]酯

bufotenin [bjuːˈfəutənin]，**bufotenine** [ˌbjuːfəˈteniːn] *n* 蟾毒色胺

bufotherapy [ˌbjuːfəuˈθerəpi] *n* 蟾蜍疗法（用蟾毒素治疗疾病）

bufotoxin [ˌbjuːfəˈtɔksin] *n* 蟾毒素

bug [bʌg] *n* 昆虫，虫；臭虫；病菌 *vi*（眼球）暴突 | assassin ~，kissing ~ 猎蝽 / barley ~ 麦螨 / blister ~ 斑蝥 / blue ~，miana ~，Mianeh ~ 波斯锐缘蜱 / cone-nose ~ 锥蝽 / croton ~ 德国小蠊 / harvest ~，red ~ 沙螨（沙虱、恙虫、恙螨、秋蜱）/ hematophagous ~ 吸血昆虫 / Malay ~ 莱末蝽 / wheat ~ 袋腹蒲螨（虱状恙虫、谷螨、虱螨）

Buhl-Dittrich law [buːl ˈditriʃ]（Ludwig von Buhl；Franz Dittrich）布尔-迪特里希定律（一种假定的学说，认为急性粟粒性结核时，体内至少存在着一个干酪性坏死的旧病灶）

Buhl's disease [buːl]（Ludwig von Buhl）布尔病（新生儿败血症，表现为皮肤、黏膜、肠及脐出血兼发绀与黄疸）| ~ desquamative pneumonia 布尔脱屑性肺炎，干酪样肺炎

buiatrics [ˌbjuːiˈætriks] *n* 牛病疗法

Buist's method [bjust]（Robert C. Buist）布伊斯特法（一种人工呼吸法，用于新生儿窒息，即交替压婴儿胃部与背部）

bulb [bʌlb] *n* 球；延髓；壶腹 | ~ of aorta 主动脉球 / auditory ~ 听球（膜迷路及耳蜗）/ ~ of corpus cavernosum，~ of penis，~ of urethra 尿道球 / duodenal ~ 十二指肠冠，十二指肠[上]部 / end ~ 终球 / gustatory ~，taste ~ 味蕾 /

~ of hair 毛球 / ~ of heart 心球,动脉球 / vaginal ~ 阴道芽;阴道前庭球
bulbar [ˈbʌlbə] *a* 球的;延髓的
bulbi [ˈbʌlbai] bulbus 的复数
bulbiform [ˈbʌlbifɔːm] *a* 球状的
bulbitis [bʌlˈbaitis] *n* 尿道球炎
bulboatrial [ˌbʌlbəuˈeitriəl] *a* 心球[与]心房的
bulbocapnine [ˌbʌlbəuˈkæpnin] *n* 褐鳞碱(旧名紫堇碱,治肌震颤及前庭性眼球震颤)
bulbocavernosus [ˌbʌlbəuˈkævəˈnəusəs], **bulbospongiosus** [ˌbʌlbəuˌspɔndʒiˈəusəs] *n* 球海绵体肌
bulbogastrone [ˈbʌlbəuˈgæstrəun] *n* [十二指肠]球抑胃素(抑制犬胃酸分泌)
bulboid [ˈbʌlbɔid] *a* 球状的
bulbopontine [ˌbʌlbəuˈpɔntain] *a* 延髓脑桥的
bulbospiral [ˌbʌlbəuˈspairəl] *a* 球螺旋的(指某些心肌纤维束)
bulbourethral [ˌbʌlbəujuəˈriːθrəl] *a* 尿道球部的
bulbous [ˈbʌlbəs] *a* 球状的,球的
bulbus [ˈbʌlbəs] ([复] **bulbi** [ˈbʌlbai]) *n*【拉】球;延髓 | ~ oculi 眼球 / ~ olfactorius 嗅球 / ~ penis 尿道球 / ~ pili 毛球
bulesis [bjuˈliːsis] *n*【希】意志,意志活动
bulge [bʌldʒ] *n* 肿胀,膨出,隆起物
bulimia [bjuːˈlimiə] *n* 贪食症,食欲过盛 | ~ nervosa 神经性贪食 | **~c** [bjuːˈlimiæk], **bulimic** *a*
Bulimidae [bjuːˈlimiːdiː] *n* 拟锥螺科
Buliminae [bjuːˈliminiː] *n* 拟锥螺亚科
Bulimus [bjuːˈlaiməs] *n* 螺属 | ~ fuchsianus 莲馨螺(华支睾吸虫和后睾吸虫的中间宿主)
Bulinus [bjuːˈlainəs] *n* 泡螺属(埃及血吸虫和后睾吸虫的中间宿主)
bulk [bʌlk] *n* 大体积纤维性物质(不为肠所吸收,但可促进肠蠕动)
bulkage [ˈbʌlkidʒ] *n* 膨胀性食品(增加肠内容,从而促进蠕动)
Bull. bulliat【拉】使煮沸
bulla [ˈbulə, ˈbʌlə] ([复] **bullae** [ˈbuliː]) *n*【拉】大疱;大泡 | ~ ossea 耳骨泡(外耳道骨泡样肥大部)
bullate [ˈbʌleit] *a* 有大疱的;吹张的
bullation [bʌˈleiʃən] *n* 大疱形成;吹张
bullectomy [bəˈlektəmi] *n* 大疱切除术(切除大疱,尤其切除见于大疱性肺气肿的巨大大疱之一,以改进肺功能)
Buller's shield (bandage) [ˈbʌlə] (Frank Buller) 布勒罩(绷带)(一种预防感染的护眼罩)
bullet [ˈbulit] *n* 弹,子弹 | magic ~ 胂凡纳明(见 arsphenamine)
bullneck [ˈbulnek] *n* 公牛颈
bullnose [ˈbulnəuz] *n* 公牛鼻,坏死性鼻炎
bullosis [bʌˈləusis] *n* 大疱生成 | diabetic ~ 糖尿病性大疱生成,糖尿病性大疱病
bullous [ˈbʌləs] *a* 大疱的,大泡的
bumblefoot [ˈbʌmblfut] *n* 禽掌炎
bumetanide [bjuːˈmetənaid] *n* 布美他尼(利尿药)
Bumke's pupil [ˈbuːmkə] (Oswald C. E. Bumke) 布姆克瞳孔(精神刺激后瞳孔散大)
bump [bʌmp] *vt* 撞伤;撞击 *vi* 冲撞 *n* 撞击;肿块;(头盖骨上的)隆起部分;[复]结节性红斑(有时见于原发性球孢子虫病)
BUN blood urea nitrogen 血尿素氮
bunamidine hydrochloride [bjuːˈnæmidiːn] 盐酸丁萘脒(抗蠕虫药)
bunamiodyl [ˌbjuːnəˈmaiədil] *n* 丁碘桂酸(不透 X 线造影剂,用于胆道 X 线摄影)
bunchbacked [ˈbʌntʃbækt] *a* 驼背的
bundle [ˈbʌndl] *n* 束 | aberrant ~ 迷行束 / atrioventricular ~, a-v ~ 房室束 / basis ~, fundamental ~, ground ~ 固有束 / ~ of His 希氏束,房室束 / longitudinal medial ~ 内侧纵束 / sinoatrial ~ 窦房结
bundle branch [ˈbʌndl bræntʃ] 束支
bungarotoxin [ˌbʌŋgərəuˈtɔksin] *n* 银环蛇毒素 | α- ~ α-银环蛇毒素(与乙酰胆碱受体结合产生神经肌肉阻滞)
Bungarus [ˈbʌŋgərəs] *n* 金环蛇属
Bunge's amputation [ˈbuŋgə] (Richard Bunge) 除骨膜性切断术
Bunge's law [ˈbuŋgə] (Gustav von Bunge) 崩格定律(犬、猫、兔等乳腺的分泌细胞自血浆中摄取各种矿物盐类的比例,恰与其所哺养后代发育所需的比例相符)
Bunge's spoon [ˈbuŋgə] (Paul Bunge) 崩格匙(取眼球匙)
bungeye [ˈbʌŋai] *n* 眼蝇蛆病(马)
Büngner's bands (cell cordons) [ˈbiŋnə] (Otto von Büngner) 宾格内带(细胞层)(周围神经再生时鞘细胞融合而形成细胞带)
bungpagga [bʌŋˈpægə] *n* 热带性脓性肌炎
buninoid [ˈbuninɔid] *a* 丘状的;圆形的(指肿瘤)
buniodyl [bjuːˈnaiədil] *n* 丁碘桂酸
bunion [ˈbʌnjən] *n* 踇滑囊肿 | tailor's ~ 小趾囊肿
bunionectomy [bʌnjəˈnektəmi] *n* 踇滑囊肿切除术
bunionette [bʌnjəˈnet] *n* 小趾囊肿
Bunnell suture [bəˈnel] (Sterling Bunnell) 邦内尔缝合(肌腱修补用的 8 字形缝合)
bunodont [ˈbjuːnədɔnt] *n* 丘牙型
bunolol hydrochloride [ˈbjuːnələul] *n* 盐酸布诺

洛尔(β 受体阻滞药)

bunolophodont [ˌbjuːnəˈlɔfədɔnt] *n* 丘嵴牙型

bunoselenodont [ˌbjuːnəusiˈliːnədɔnt] *n* 丘月牙型

Bunostomum [ˌbjuːnəˈstəumәm] *n* 仰口[线虫]属

bunostomiasis [ˌbjuːnəustəˈmaiəsis] *n* 仰口线虫病

Bunsen burner [ˈbunsn] (Robert W. E. von Bunsen) 本生灯(一种实验室用的煤气灯) | ~ coefficient 本生吸收系数(表示一气体在温度0 ℃和压力在100 kPa时被一单位体积的液体所吸收之量)

Bunyaviridae [ˌbʌnjəˈviridiː] *n* 本雅病毒科

Bunyavirus [ˌbʌnjəˈvaiərəs] *n* 本雅病毒属

bunyavirus [ˌbʌnjəˈvaiərəs] *n* 本雅病毒

buphthalmos [bjuːfˈθælmɔs], **buphthalmia** [bjuːfˈθælmiə], **buphthalmus** [bjuːfˈθælməs] *n* 先天性青光眼(亦称巨眼,牛眼)

bupicomide [bjuːˈpikəmaid] *n* 丁吡考胺(抗高血压药)

bupivacaine hydrochloride [bjuˈpivəkein] 盐酸布比卡因(局部麻醉药)

buprenorphine hydrochloride [ˌbjuːpriˈnɔːfiːn] 盐酸丁丙诺啡(镇痛药)

bupropion hydrochloride [bjuːˈprəupiən] 盐酸安非他酮(抗抑郁药)

bur[1], **burr** [bəː] *n* 多刺果;黏附物

bur[2] [bəː] *n* 牙钻 | carbide ~ 碳化钨钻

burbulence [ˈbəːbjuˌləns] *n* 肠气(一组肠源性症状,其中包括饱满感,胃气胀或膨胀、腹鸣及气胀)

Burch procedure (colposuspension) [bəːtʃ] (John C. Burch) 布奇手术(膀胱颈悬吊术)

Burdach's cuneate fasciculus (bundle, columns, fibers, tract) [ˈbuədʌh] (Karl F. Burdach) 布尔达赫楔束,脊髓楔束 | ~ fasciculus 布尔达赫束(大脑上纵束;胼胝体辐射颞部;脊髓楔束) / ~ fissure 布尔达赫裂(脑岛外侧面和岛盖内面间裂) / ~ nucleus 布尔达赫核;楔束核

buret, burette [bjuəˈret] *n* 滴定管,量管

Bürger-Grütz syndrome [ˈbirgə griːts] (Max Bürger; Otto Grütz) 比-格综合征,家族性高脂蛋白血症 I 型

Burghart's symptom (sign) [ˈbuəghɑːt] (Hans G. Burghart) 布格哈特症状(征)(肺前下缘有细啰音,为肺结核的早期体征)

burial [ˈberiəl] *n* 埋葬;埋藏

burimamide [bjuːˈriməmaid] *n* 布立马胺(组胺 H_2 受体阻滞药)

Burkholderia [ˌbəːkhəlˈderiə] *n* 假单胞菌属

Burkitt's lymphoma [ˈbəːkit] (Penis P. Burkitt) 伯基特淋巴瘤(小而未分裂细胞的淋巴瘤,通常见于中非,但其他地区也有报道,最常表现为颌骨有一个大的溶骨性损害,或为一个腹部肿块。一种疱疹病毒EB病毒,即从伯基特淋巴瘤分离出来,并作为致病因子。亦称伯基特瘤和非洲淋巴瘤)

burn [bəːn] *n* 烧伤;[复]烧伤学 | cement ~, concrete ~ 水泥烧伤 / brush ~, friction ~ 擦伤 / first degree ~ 一度烧伤 / flash ~ 闪光烧伤 / full-thickness ~ 三度烧伤 / second degree ~ 二度烧伤 / X-ray ~ X线灼伤

Burnam's test [ˈbəːnəm] (Curtis F. Burnam) 伯纳姆试验(检尿甲醛)

burner [ˈbəːnə] *n* 灯,煤气灯;燃烧器,燃烧炉

Burnett's disinfecting fluid (solution) [bə(ː)ˈnet] (William Burnett) 伯内特消毒液(一种浓氯化锌水溶液)

Burnett's syndrome [bəˈnet] (Charles H. Burnett) 乳-碱综合征(即 milk-alkali syndrome,见 syndrome 项下相应术语)

burning [ˈbəːniŋ] *a* 燃烧的;高热的 *n* 灼热,烧灼感 | rectal ~ 直肠烧灼

burnish [ˈbəːniʃ] *vt, vi* 磨光 | ~er *n* 磨光器(牙科)

burnishing [ˈbəːniʃiŋ] *n* 磨光,磨平(牙科)

Burns' amaurosis [bəːnz] (John Burns) 婚后弱视

Burns' ligament [bəːnz] (Allan Burns) 伯恩斯韧带,隐静脉裂孔镰状缘 | ~ space 颈静脉窝

Burow's operation [ˈbuːrɔv] (Karl A. Burow) 布罗夫手术(切除肿瘤后的成形术) | ~ solution 醋酸铝溶液 / ~ vein 布罗夫静脉(由两支腹壁下静脉和来自膀胱分支所形成的连于门静脉的血管)

burquism [ˈbəːkizəm] (V. B. Burq) 伯克疗法(一种金属疗法,贴用数种金属于患部,治疗癔病及其他精神病)

burr [bəː], **burr-drill** [ˈbəːdril] *n* = **bur**[2]

burrow [ˈbʌrəu] *n* 穴,窦,地洞;寄生虫(如螨)造成的皮下通道

bursa [ˈbəːsə] ([复] **bursae** [ˈbəːsiː]或 **bursas**) *n* 囊,黏液囊 | acromial ~, subdeltoid ~ 三角肌下囊 / adventitious ~, supernumerary ~ 偶发性黏液囊,附加囊,摩擦囊 / calcaneal ~ 跟腱囊 / coracobrachial ~ 喙肱肌囊 / deltoid ~ 肩峰下囊 / gastrocnemiosemimembranous ~, retrocondyloid ~ 腓肠半膜肌囊,髁后囊(半膜肌囊) / gluteal ~ 臀大肌囊 / humeral ~ 肱骨囊(肩峰下囊;腓肠肌外侧腱下囊) / hyoid ~, subhyoid ~ 舌骨囊,舌骨下囊(喉结皮下囊) / ischiadic ~, tuberoischiadic ~ 坐骨囊,坐骨结节囊(闭孔内肌坐骨囊) / pyriform ~

梨状肌囊 / semitendinous ~ 半腱肌囊(股二头肌上囊) / subachilleal ~ 跟腱下囊,跟腱囊 | **~l** *a*

bursa-equivalent [ˈbəːsə iˈkwivələnt] *n* 腔上囊类同器官

bursalogy [bəːˈsælədʒi] *n* 黏液囊论,黏液囊学

Bursata [bəːˈseitə] *n* 交尾囊类(线虫纲)

bursatti [bəːˈsæti], **bursautee** [bəːˈsɔːti] *n* 腐霉病;皮肤丽线虫蚴疮,夏疮(马)

bursectomy [bəːˈsektəmi] *n* 黏液囊切除术

bursic acid [ˈbəːsik], **bursinic acid** [bəːˈsinik] 荠菜酸

bursicon [ˈbəːsikɔn] *n* [角皮]鞣化激素(在蜕皮后的昆虫血液中出现的一种激素,它能促使新的表皮变色和硬化)

bursitis [bəːˈsaitis] *n* 滑囊炎,黏液囊炎 | olecranon ~ 鹰嘴滑囊炎,矿工肘 / radiohumeral ~ 桡肱骨滑囊炎,网球员肘 / retrocalcaneal ~ 跟后滑囊炎,跟腱痛

bursolith [ˈbəːsəliθ] *n* 黏液囊石

bursopathy [bəːˈsɔpəθi] *n* 黏液囊病

bursotomy [bəˈsɔtəmi] *n* 黏液囊切开术

burst [bəːst] *n* 突然发作;爆发,爆裂;阵发快速 | respiratory ~, metabolic ~ 突发性呼吸,突发性代谢(白细胞吞噬时氧耗量明显增加,超氧物和氧化物形成)

bursula [ˈbəːsjulə] *n*【拉】小囊,小黏液囊

Burton's line (sign) [ˈbəːtn] (Henry Burton) 伯顿线(征)(慢性铅中毒时,龈缘呈蓝线)

Buruli ulcer [ˈbuːrəli] (Buruli 为乌干达一地区) 布路里溃疡(由溃疡分枝杆菌引起的一种皮肤感染,表现为小而坚硬、无痛但可移动的皮下小结,可扩大有波动感,进而形成溃疡,留下一条潜行性边缘)

Bury's disease [ˈbjuəri, ˈberi] (Judson S. Bury) 持久隆起红斑

Buscaino's test (reaction) [busˈkainəu] (Vito M. Buscaino) 布斯卡伊诺试验(反应)(脑病时的尿沉淀反应)

Buschke-Löwenstein's tumor [ˈbuʃke ˈleivenstain] (Abraham Buschke; Ludwig W. Löwenstein) 巨大尖锐湿疣

Buschke-Ollendorff syndrome [ˈbuʃke ˈəulendɔːf] (Abraham Buschke; Helene Ollendorff) 播散性豆状皮肤纤维瘤病

Buschke's disease [ˈbuʃkə] (Abraham Buschke) 隐球菌病 | ~ scleredema 布施克硬肿病(慢性扩散性皮肤和皮下组织发硬)

Buselmeier shunt [ˈbuːsəlˌmiə] (T. J. Buselmeier) 布塞密尔分流(昆-斯〈Quinton-Scribner〉分流的一种改良:将硅橡胶管植入皮下,两个通道突出皮肤)

buserelin acetate [ˌbjuːsəˈrelin] 醋酸布舍瑞林(一种合成的促黄体素释放激素类似物,用于晚期前列腺癌的姑息疗法,鼻内给药)

bushmaster [ˈbuʃmɑːstə] *n* 巨蝮,丛林王(南美热带大毒蛇)

buspirone hydrochloride [bjuˈspairəun] 盐酸丁螺环酮(安定药)

Busquet's disease [busˈkei] (P. Busquet) 布斯凯病(跖骨的骨膜炎所致的足背外生骨疣)

Buss disease [bʌs] (Buss 为一农场主的名字,他的牲畜首次被观察到患有此病)巴斯病(侵犯美国和日本牛的一种病毒性脑脊髓炎伴胸膜炎。亦称散发性牛脑脊髓炎)

Busse-Buschke disease [ˈbusə ˈbuʃkə] (Otto Busse; Abraham Buschke) 隐球菌病

busulfan [bjuˈsʌlfən] *n* 白消安(抗肿瘤药,主要用于治疗慢性粒细胞白血病)

But. butyrum【拉】酪,奶油,乳脂

butabarbital sodium [bjutəˈbɑːbitæl] 仲丁比妥钠(催眠镇静药)

butacaine sulfate [ˈbjuːtəkein] 硫酸布他卡因(局部麻醉药)

butaclamol hydrochloride [ˌbjuːtəˈkleimɔl] 盐酸布他拉莫(安定药)

butadiazamide [ˌbjuːtədaiˈæzəmaid] *n* 布他酰胺(降血糖药)

butadiene [ˌbjuːtəˈdaiiːn] *n* 丁二烯

butalbital [bjuˈtælbitæl] *n* 布他比妥(催眠镇静药)

butallylonal [ˌbjuːtəˈiilənəl] *n* 丁溴比妥(催眠镇静药)

butamben [bjuˈtæmbən] *n* 氨苯丁酯(局部麻醉药,用以缓解疼痛和瘙痒症) | ~ picrate 苦味酸氨苯丁酯(局部麻醉药,用以暂时缓解轻度烧伤所致的疼痛)

butamirate citrate [ˌbjuːtəˈmaireit] 枸橼酸布他米酯(镇咳药)

butamisole hydrochloride [bjuˈtæmisəul] 盐酸布他米唑(抗蠕虫药)

butamoxane hydrochloride [ˌbjuːtəˈmɔksein] 盐酸布他莫生(安定药)

butane [ˈbjuːtein] *n* 丁烷 | normal ~ 正丁烷

butanoic acid [ˌbjuːtəˈnəuik] 丁酸

butaperazine [ˌbjuːtəˈperəziːn] *n* 布他哌嗪(抗精神病药) | ~ maleate 马来酸布他哌嗪

butcher's broom [ˈbutʃə] 假叶树;假叶树根茎制剂(用于痔和静脉供血不足的症状疗法)

Butcher's saw [ˈbutʃə] (Richard G. H. Butcher) 布彻锯(锯片可安置在各种不同角度上的切断锯)

BUTE phenylbutazone 保泰松(消炎镇痛药)

butenafine hydrochloride [bjuˈtenəfiːn] 盐酸布

替萘芬(抗真菌药)

butethal [ˈbjuːtəθəl] *n* 正丁巴比妥(镇静药)

butethamine hydrochloride [bjuˈteθəmiːn] 盐酸丁胺卡因(牙科用局部麻醉药)

Buthus [ˈbjuːθəs] *n* 钳蝎属 | ~ carolinianus 卡罗来纳钳蝎 / ~ quinquestriatus 五纹钳蝎

butirosin sulfate [bjuˈtiərəsin] 硫酸布替罗星(抗生素类药)

Butler-Albright syndrome [ˈbʌtlə ˈɔːlbrait] (Alan M. Butler; Fuller Albright) 巴-奥综合征(一型远端肾小管性酸中毒,婴儿期后发生,为常染色体显性遗传)

butoconazole nitrate [ˌbjuːtəˈkɔnəzəul] 硝酸布康唑(抗真菌药,阴道内用药,治疗外阴阴道念珠菌病)

butonate [ˈbjuːtəneit] *n* 布托酯(杀虫药,抗蠕虫药)

butoprozine hydrochloride [ˌbjuːtəˈprəuziːn] 盐酸布托丙茚(心脏抑制药,抗心绞痛药)

butopyronoxyl [ˌbjuːtəˌpaiərəˈnɔksil] *n* 避蚊酮(驱昆虫药)

butorphanol [bjuˈtɔːfənəul] *n* 布托啡诺(镇痛药,镇咳药) | ~ tartrate 酒石酸布托啡诺(镇痛药)

butoxamine hydrochloride [bjuˈtɔksəmiːn] 盐酸布他沙明(β-肾上腺素能阻滞药)

butriptyline hydrochloride [bjuˈtriptiliːn] 盐酸布替林(抗抑郁药)

Bütschlia [ˈbitʃliə] *n* 贝氏纤毛虫属

Bütschli's nuclear spindle [ˈbitʃliː] (Otto Bütschli) 贝奇利核纺锤体(细胞分裂)

butter [ˈbʌtə] *n* 酪,奶油,乳脂 | ~ of antimony 三氯化锑 / ~ of arsenic 三氯化砷 / cacao ~, cocoa ~ 可可脂,可可豆油 / ~ of tin 氯化锡;四氯化锡/ ~ of zinc 氯化锌

butterfat [ˈbʌtəˈfæt] *n* 乳脂

butterfly [ˈbʌtəflai] *n* 蝴蝶;蝶形胶黏带;蝶状皮疹;纸蝶(麻醉时将一纸片置于患者口及鼻孔处,以测知呼吸) *a* 蝶形的

Buttiauxella [ˌbʌtiɔːkˈselə] *n* 布替肠杆菌属

buttock [ˈbʌtək] *n* 半边臀部,[复]臀部

button [ˈbʌtn] *n* 钮(钮状突出或结构,或手术用的肠吻合钮) | bromide ~ 溴疖,溴疣 | dog ~, quaker ~ 马钱子,番木鳖 / iodide ~ 碘疖,碘疣 / mescal ~ 威廉斯仙人球[花] / oriental ~ 东方疖,皮肤利什曼病 / peritoneal ~ 腹膜钮 / terminal ~s 终钮

buttonhole [ˈbʌtnhəul] *n* 钮孔(体腔或器官的短直切口,或指一种结构口径的异常缩窄) | mitral ~ 二尖瓣口钮孔状缩窄

butyl [ˈbjuːtil] *n* 丁基 | ~ acetate 醋酸丁酯 / ~ aminobenzoate 氨苯丁酯(局部麻醉药) / ~ hydride 丁烷(其蒸气为一种不安全的麻醉药)

butylated hydroxyanisole (BHA) [ˈbjuːtileitid haiˌdrɔksiˈænisəul] 丁羟茴醚(食品等抗氧化药)

butylated hydroxytoluene (BHT) [ˈbjuːtileitid haiˌdrɔksiˈtɔljuiːn] 丁羟甲苯(食品等抗氧化药)

butylcarboxylic acid [ˌbjuːtilˌkɑːbɔkˈsilik] 戊酸,缬草酸

butylene [ˈbjuːtiliːn] *n* 丁烯

butylethylbarbituric acid [ˌbjuːtileθilˌbɑːbiˈtjuərik] 丁基乙基巴比土酸,丁巴比妥

butylmercaptan [ˌbjuːtilməˈkæptən] *n* 丁硫醇

butylparaben [bju(ː)tilˈpærəbən] *n* 羟苯丁酯(防腐药)

butyraceous [ˌbjuːtiˈreiʃiəs] *a* 酪状的,含酪的

butyrate [ˈbjuːtireit] *n* 丁酸盐

butyrate-CoA ligase [ˈbjuːtireit kəuˈei ˈlaigeis] 丁酸辅酶 A 连接酶

Butyribacterium [bjuˌtiribækˈtiəriəm] *n* 丁酸杆菌属

butyric [bju(ː)ˈtirik] *a* 丁酸的 | ~ acid 丁酸

butyrin [ˈbjuːtirin] *n* 丁酸甘油酯

butyrinase [bjuˈtirineis], **butyrase** [ˈbjuːtireis] *n* 丁酸甘油酯酶

butyrine [ˈbjuːtiriːn] *n* α-氨基丁酸

Butyrivibrio [bjuˌtiriˈviːbriəu] *n* 丁酸弧菌属

butyr(o)- [构词成分]酪,奶油,乳脂

butyroid [ˈbjuːtirɔid] *a* 酪状的

butyromel [bjuˈtirəmel] *n* 酪蜜

butyrometer [ˌbjuːtiˈrɔmitə] *n* 乳脂计

butyrophenone [ˌbjuːtirəˈfiːnəun] *n* 丁酰苯

butyroscope [bjuˈtairəskəup] *n* 乳脂计,乳脂测定器

butyrous [ˈbjuːtirəs] *a* 酪样的

butyryl [ˈbjuːtiril] *n* 丁酰

butyryl CoA synthetase [ˈbjuːtiril kəuˈei ˈsinθiteis] 丁酰辅酶 A 合成酶,丁酰辅酶 A 连接酶

BVAD biventricular assist device 两心室辅助装置

bypass [ˈbaipɑːs] *n* 分路,旁路;旁路术,分流术(外科) | aortocoronary ~ 主动脉冠状动脉旁路术 / aortoiliac ~ 主动脉髂动脉旁路术 / cardiopulmonary ~ 心肺转流术(体外循环) / femoropopliteal ~ 股动脉腘动脉旁路术 / gastric ~ 胃旁路术 / jejunoileal ~ 空肠回肠旁路术 / left heart ~ 左心转流术

by-product [ˈbaiˌprɔdʌkt] *n* 副产物

byssaceous [biˈseiʃiəs] *a* 麻丝的

byssinosis [ˌbisiˈnəusis] *n* 棉尘肺,棉屑沉着病

byssinotic [ˌbisiˈnɔtik] *a* 棉尘肺的 *n* 棉尘肺患者

byssocausis [ˌbisəuˈkɔːsis] *n* [艾]灸术

byssoid [ˈbisɔid] *a* 伞丝状的

byssus [ˈbisəs] ([复] **byssuses** 或 **byssi** [ˈbisai]) *n* 亚麻布,棉花;足丝(软体动物)

bystander [ˈbaistændə] *n* 旁观者(指只是偶尔卷入某一过程者) | innocent ~ 无辜受殃者(指药物诱发的溶血性贫血或血小板减少)

Bythnia [ˈbiθniə] *n* 小沼螺属,豆螺属(即 Bithynia)

Bythnya [ˈbiθniə] *n* 小沼螺属

Bywaters' syndrome [baiˈwɔːtəz] (Eric G. L. Bywaters) 拜沃特斯综合征,挤压综合征(即 crush syndrome,见 syndrome 项下相应术语)

C

C canine tooth 尖牙;carbon 碳;large calorie 大卡;cathod 阴极;Celsius 摄氏(温标);cervical vertebrae 颈椎;clonus 阵挛;closure 关闭,闭合;color sense 色觉;complement 补体;contraction 收缩;coulomb 库伦;cylinder 圆柱体;cylindrical lens 柱镜片;cytidine 胞苷;cytosine 胞嘧啶

C capacitance 电容;compliance 顺应性(C_L lung compliance 肺顺应性,C_T thoracic compliance 胸顺应性,C_{LT} total lung-thoracic compliance 肺胸总顺应性);clearance 清除率(C_{in} inulin clearance 菊粉清除率,C_{cr} creatinine clearance 肌酐清除率);heat capacity 热容

C. congius【拉】加仑

C_H constant region of an immunoglobulin heavy chain 免疫球蛋白重链恒定区

C_L constant region of an immunoglobulin light chain 免疫球蛋白轻链恒定区

℃ degree Celsius 摄氏度(百分度)

c small calorie 小卡;centi- 厘,百分之一

c. cibus【拉】食物,餐;cum【拉】和,与

c molar concentration 摩尔浓度;specific heat capacity 比热容;velocity of light in a vacuum 真空中光速

c̄ cum【拉】和,与

χ chi 希腊语的第 22 个字母

χ^2 chi-squared χ^2 的,卡方的

CA cardiac arrest 心脏停搏;chronological age 实足年龄;coronary artery 冠状动脉;croup-associated (virus) 哮吼相关(病毒),致哮吼(病毒)

CA_2 a colloid antigen lacking iodine 缺碘的胶体抗原(在甲状腺胶体中第 2 常见的抗原〈最常见的抗原为甲状腺球蛋白〉,血清中存在抗 CA_2 是自身免疫性疾病,如桥本〈Hashimoto〉病的体征)

CA 125 cancer antigen 125 癌抗原 125

Ca calcium 钙;cancer 癌

ca circa【拉】大约

Ca^{2+}-ATpase [eitiː'peis] 钙腺苷三磷酸酶(在 EC 命名法中亦称钙转运腺苷三磷酸酶)

cabbage ['kæbidʒ] *n* 甘蓝,卷心菜,洋白菜

cabergoline [kə'bəːgəuliːn] *n* 卡麦角胺(多巴胺受体激动药,用以治疗以高催乳素血症为特征的疾病,口服给药)

CABG coronary artery bypass graft 冠状动脉旁路移植物

cabin ['kæbin] *n* 小室;舱,座舱 | hyperbaric ~ 高压舱

cabinet ['kæbinit] *n* 小室;柜

Cabot's ring bodies ['kæbət] (Richard C. Cabot) 卡伯特环状体(环状或 8 字形线条,见于严重贫血时染色的红细胞内)

Cabot's splint ['kæbət] (Arthur T Cabot) 卡伯特夹板(一种置于腿后的铁夹板)

cabufocon [ˌkæbjuː'fəukən] *n* 醋酸丁酸纤维素(两种疏水性接触透镜材料之一,定名为 A 或 B)

cacaerometer [ˌkækεə'rɔmitə] *n* 空气纯度测定器

cacanthrax [kæ'kænθræks] *n* 恶性炭疽

cacao [kə'kɑːəu] *n* 可可;可可树;可可豆

cacation [kæ'keiʃən] *n* 排粪

cacatory ['kækətəri] *a* 严重腹泻的

Cacchi-Ricci disease ['kɑːki 'riːtʃi] (Roberto Cacchi; Vincenzo Ricci) 卡-里病,海绵肾

cacesthesia [ˌkækis'θiːzjə] *n* 感觉异常 | **cacesthenic** [ˌkækis'θenik] *a*

cachectin [kə'kektin] *n* 恶病质素

cachet [kæ'ʃei] *n*【法】扁[形胶]囊剂

cachexia [kə'keksiə] *n* 恶病质 | cancerous ~ 癌性恶病质,癌血症 / fluoric ~ 氟中毒恶病质 / lymphatic ~ 假白血病 / pachydermic ~ 黏液性水肿 / saturnine ~ 铅毒恶病质(见于慢性铅中毒) / thyroid ~ 甲状腺性恶病质,突眼性甲状腺肿 / uremic ~ 尿毒症性恶病质 | **cachexy** *n* / **cachectic** [kə'kektik], **cachexic** [kə'keksik] *a*

cachinnation [ˌkæki'neiʃən] *n* 癔症性狂笑

cac(o)- [构词成分]恶,有病

cacodemonomania [ˌkækəˌdiːmənəu'meinjə] *n* 魔附妄想,凭魔妄想狂

cacodyl ['kækəudail] *n* 卡可基 | ~ cyanide 卡可基氰 / ~ hydride 卡可基氢

cacodylate [ˌkækəu'dailit] *n* 卡可基酸盐

cacodylic acid [ˌkækə'dilik] 卡可基酸

cacoethic [ˌkækəu'iːθik] *a* 恶性的,不良的

cacogenesis [ˌkækə'dʒenisis] *n* 构造异常;畸形,劣生(指发育上的缺陷)

cacogenic [ˌkækə'dʒenik] *a* 种族退化的(由于性选择不适当所致);劣生的

cacogenics [ˌkækə'dʒeniks] *n* 种族退化学,劣生学

cacogeusia [ˌkækəˈgjuːsiə] *n* 劣味,恶味
cacomelia [ˌkækəˈmiːliə] *n* 肢畸形
cacomorphosis [ˌkækəmɔːˈfəusis] *n* 畸形
cacoplastic [ˌkækəˈplæstik] *a* 成形不良的
cacorhythmic [ˌkækəˈriθmik] *a* 节律不齐的
cacosmia [ˌkəˈkɔzmiə] *n* 恶臭;恶臭幻觉
cacothenics [ˌkækəˈθeniks] *n* 种族退化学,劣生学(由于环境有害影响所致) | **cacothenic** [ˌkækəˈθenik] *a* 种族退化的
cacothymia [ˌkækəˈθaimiə] *n* 胸腺功能障碍
cacotrophy [kəˈkɔtrəfi] *n* 营养不良
cactinomycin [ˌkæktinəˈmaisin] *n* 放线菌素C(抗生素类药,以前用作抗肿瘤药)
cacuminal [kæˈkjuːminəl] *a* 尖端的
CAD coronary artery disease 冠状动脉病
cadaver [kəˈdeivə] *n* 尸体(尤指解剖用的人尸) | **~ic** [kəˈdævərik] *a*
cadaverine [kəˈdævərin] *n* 尸胺
cadaverous [kəˈdævərəs] *a* 尸体样的,似尸体的,惨白的(指皮色苍白)
caddis [ˈkædis] *n* 毛翅蝇
cadherin [kædˈhiərin] *n* 钙粘连蛋白,钙粘着蛋白(依钙的细胞粘着分子一族中的任何一种)
cadmiferous [kædˈmifərəs] *a* 含镉的
cadmiosis [ˌkædmiˈəusis] *n* 镉尘肺
cadmium(Cd) [ˈkædmiəm] *n* 镉(化学元素) | ~ sulfide 硫化镉(治头皮的皮脂溢性皮炎)
caduca [kəˈdjuːkə] *n* 蜕膜
caduceus [kəˈdjusiəs] *n* 医神杖(希腊神话中众神信使 Hermes 或 Mercury 的杖,杖上盘绕二蛇,杖顶有双翼,作为医学的标志和美陆军卫生队的队徽)
caducity [kəˈdjuːsəti] *n* 衰退
caducous [kəˈdjuːkəs] *a* 脱落的
cae- 以 cae-起始的词,同样见以 ce-起始的词
caecitas [ˈsesitəs] *n*【拉】视觉丧失,盲
caec(o)- 以 caec(o)-起始的词,同样见以 cec(o)-起始的词
caecum [ˈsiːkəm] *n* 盲肠;盲端 | **caecal** *a* 盲的;盲肠的
caecus [ˈsiːkəs] *n*【拉】盲囊
Caedibacter [ˌsiːdiˈbæktə] *n* 脱节菌属
caen(o)- [构词成分]新
caeruleus [siˈrjuːljəs] *a* 蓝色的,蔚蓝色的
caerulin [siˈrjuːlin] *n* 雨蛙肽
caesarean [si(ː)ˈzeəriən] *a* 剖宫产术的
caesium [ˈsiːziəm] *n* 铯
cafard [kəˈfɑː] *n*【法】精神沮丧
caffea [ˈkæfiə] *n*【法】咖啡
caffeic acid [kəˈfiːik] 咖啡酸,二羟[基]肉桂酸
caffeine [ˈkæfiːn] *n* 咖啡因(利尿药,中枢兴奋药) | ~ and sodium benzoate 苯甲酸钠咖啡因(利尿药,中枢兴奋药)
caffeinism [ˈkæfiːnizəm] *n* 咖啡因中毒
caffetannic acid [ˌkæfiˈtænik] 咖啡鞣酸
Caffey's disease [ˈkæfi] (John Caffey) 卡菲病,婴儿骨外层肥厚病
caffuric acid [kəˈfjuərik] 咖啡尿酸(咖啡因氧化后的产物)
cage [keidʒ] *n* 笼;骨架构造;护架,支架 | population ~ 群体饲育箱(供果蝇群体遗传学研究用,可以将果蝇进行连续若干代的饲养) / thoracic ~ 胸廓
Cagot ear [kɑːˈgəu] (Cagot 为比利牛斯山一地区)卡戈族人耳,无耳垂耳
CAH congenital adrenal hyperplasia 先天性肾上腺增生
cain(o)- 见 cen(o)-(第一解)
caisson [kəˈsuːn, ˈkeisən] *n* 潜涵,沉箱
Cajal's cells [kəˈhɑːl] (Santiago Ramón y Cajal) 卡哈尔细胞(星形胶质细胞;神经胶质细胞之一,横列于大脑皮质分子层内) | ~ interstitial nucleus 卡哈尔间质核 / ~ method 卡哈尔染色法(氯化金与氯化汞的化合物使星形胶质细胞着色) / ~ double method 卡哈尔双重染色法(显示神经节细胞) / ~ stain 卡哈尔染剂(见卡哈尔染色法)
cajeput, cajuput [ˈkædʒəpət] *n* 白千层,玉树
cajeputol [ˈkædʒipətɔl] *n* 白千层脑,玉树油精,桉油精,桉树脑
Cal large calorie 大卡,千卡
cal calorie [小]卡
Calabar bean [ˈkæləbɑː] (Calabar 为尼日利亚东南一河流和地区)卡拉巴豆(毒扁豆) | ~ edema(swelling) 卡拉巴水肿(丝虫肿)(丝虫引起的水肿)
calage [kəˈlɑːʒ] *n*【法】垫身防晕船法
calamine [ˈkæləmain] *n* 炉甘石(弱收敛剂和保护剂,皮肤病局部用药)
calamus [ˈkæləməs] *n* 羽根,翮;菖蒲(其根茎为祛风、驱虫药)
calcaneal [kælˈkeiniəl], **calcanean** [kælˈkeiniən] *a* 跟骨的
calcaneitis [kælˌkeiniˈaitis] *n* 跟骨炎
calcane(o)- [构词成分]跟骨
calcaneoapophysitis [kælˌkeiniəuæpɔfiˈzaitis] *n* 跟骨突炎
calcaneoastragaloid [kælˌkeiniəuəˈstrægəlɔid] *a* 跟距的
calcaneocavus [kælˌkeiniəuˈkeivəs] *n* 仰趾弓形足
calcaneocuboid [kælˌkeiniəuˈkjuːbɔid] *a* 跟骰的
calcaneodynia [kælˌkeiniəuˈdiniə] *n* 跟痛

calcaneofibular [kælˌkeiniəuˈfibjulə] *a* 跟腓的
calcaneonavicular [kælˌkeiniəunəˈvikjulə], **calcaneoscaphoid** [kælˌkeiniəuˈskæfɔid] *a* 跟舟的
calcaneoplantar [kælˌkeiniəuˈplæntə] *a* 跟跖的
calcaneotibial [kælˌkeiniəuˈtibiəl] *a* 跟胫的
calcaneovalgocavus [kælˌkeiniəuˌvælgəuˈkeivəs] *n* 仰趾外翻足
calcaneum [kælˈkeiniəm] ([复] **calcanea** [kælˈkeiniə]) *n*【拉】跟骨
calcaneus [kælˈkeiniəs] ([复] **calcanei** [kælˈkeinai]) *n*【拉】跟骨;仰趾足
calcanodynia [ˌkælkənəuˈdiniə] *n* 跟[部]痛
calcar [ˈkælkɑː] *n*【拉】距 | ~ avis 禽距
calcarea [kælˈkɛəriə] *n*【拉】石灰,氧化钙 | ~ chlorata 含氯石灰,漂白粉 / ~ hydrica 石灰水,氢氧化钙溶液 / ~ phosphorica 磷化石灰 / ~ usta 生石灰,氧化钙
calcareous, calcarious [kælˈkɛəriəs] *a* 石灰质的,钙质的;含钙的
calcariferous [ˌkælkəˈrifərəs] *a* 有距的
calcarine [ˈkælkərin] *a* 距状的;距的
calcariuria [kælˌkɛəriˈjuəriə] *n* 石灰盐尿,钙盐尿
calcaroid [ˈkælkərɔid] *a* 钙样的(指脑组织某些沉积物,似钙化,但不呈钙的特异性反应)
calcemia [kælˈsiːmiə] *n* 钙血症,高钙血症
calc(i)- [构词成分]钙,钙盐
calcibilia [ˌkælsiˈbiliə] *n* 钙胆汁
calcic [ˈkælsik] *a* 石灰的,钙的
calcicosilicosis [ˌkælsikəuˌsiliˈkəusis] *n* 钙硅沉着病,钙硅尘肺
calcicosis [ˌkælsiˈkəusis] *n* 灰石沉着病,灰石肺
calcidiol [ˌkælsiˈdaiəul] *n* 25-羟胆钙化[固]醇,25-羟维生素 D_3
calcifames [kælˈsifəmiːz] *n* 钙饥饿,缺钙症
calcifediol [ˌkælsifiˈdaiəul] *n* 骨化二醇(钙代谢调节药);25-羟胆钙化[固]醇,25-羟维生素 D_3
calciferol [kælˈsifərɔl] *n* 维生素 D_2,麦角钙化[固]醇
calciferous [kælˈsifərəs] *a* 含钙的
calcific [kælˈsifik] *a* 钙化的,石灰化的
calcification [ˌkælsifiˈkeiʃən] *n* 钙化 | dystrophic ~ 营养不良性钙化 / metastatic ~ 转移性钙化
calcify [ˈkælsifai] *vt, vi* 钙化,骨化
calcigerous [kælˈsidʒərəs] *a* 含钙的
calcimeter [kælˈsimitə] *n* 钙定量器
calcine [ˈkælsain] *vt, vi* 煅烧,灰化 | **calcination** [ˌkælsiˈneiʃən] *n*
calcineurin [ˌkæliˈnjuərin] *n* 钙调神经磷酸酶
calcinosis [ˌkælsiˈnəusis] *n* 钙质沉着[症](亦称渗出钙化性筋膜炎、钙质性痛风) | ~ circumscripta 局限性钙质沉着 / ~ cutis 皮肤钙质沉着 / ~ interstitialis 间质性钙质沉着 / ~ intervertebralis 椎间盘钙质沉着 / tumoral ~ 肿瘤性钙质沉着 / ~ universalis 全身性钙质沉着,普遍性钙质沉着
calciokinesis [ˌkælsiəukaiˈniːsis] *n* 钙动用 | **calciokinetic** [ˌkælsiəukaiˈnetik] *a* 激钙的
calciorrhachia [ˌkælsiəˈreikiə] *n* 含钙脊液
calciotropism [ˌkælsiˈɔtrəpizəm] *n* 向钙性(指细胞对摄入钙的反应增加)
calcipenia [ˌkælsiˈpiːniə] *n* 钙缺乏,钙质减少(体内) | **calcipenic** [ˌkælsiˈpiːnik] *a*
calcipexy [ˈkælsiˌpeksi], **calcipexis** [ˌkælsiˈpeksis] *n* 钙固定 | **calcipectic** [ˌkælsiˈpektik], **calcipexic** [ˌkælsiˈpeksik] *a* 固定钙的
calciphilia [ˌkælsiˈfiliə] *n* 嗜钙性
calciphylaxis [ˌkælsifiˈlæksis] *n* 钙化防御 | systemic ~ 全身性钙化防御 / topical ~ 局部性钙化防御 | **calciphylactic** [ˌkælsifiˈlæktik] *a*
calcipotriene [ˌkælsipəˈtraiiːn] *n* 卡泊三烯(维生素 D_3 合成衍生物,局部用作抗银屑病药)
calciprivia [ˌkælsiˈpriviə] *n* 钙缺失 | **calciprivic** [ˌkælsiˈprivik] *a* 缺钙的
calcipyelitis [ˌkælsipaiiˈlaitis] *n* 结石性肾盂炎
calcitonin [ˌkælsiˈtəunin] *n* 降钙素(钙代谢调节药,用以治疗重度高钙血症和佩吉特〈Paget〉骨病。亦称甲状腺降钙素)
calcitriol [ˌkælsiˈtraiɔl] *n* 骨化三醇,1, 25-二羟胆钙化[固]醇,1, 25-二羟维生素 D_3
calcium(Ca) [ˈkælsiəm] *n* 钙(化学元素) | ~ benzamidosalicylate 苯沙酸钙(抗结核药) / ~ bromide 溴化钙(以前用作镇静药和抗惊厥药) / ~ caseinate 酪蛋白钙 / ~ chloride 氯化钙(矿物质补充药) / ~ cyanamide 氰氨化钙(杀灭血吸虫卵药) / ~ disodium edetate, ~ edetate disodium 依地酸钙钠(用于诊断和治疗铅中毒) / ~ gluconate 葡萄糖酸钙(矿物质补充药) / ~ lactate 乳酸钙(矿物质补充药) / ~ levulinate 戊酮酸钙(矿物质补充药) / ~ pantothenate 泛酸钙(维生素类药) / precipitated ~ carbonate 沉淀碳酸钙(抗酸药) / racemic ~ pantothenate 消旋泛酸钙 / ~ trisodium pentetate 喷替酸钙钠(解毒药)
calciumedetate sodium [ˌkælsiəˈmediteit] 依地酸钙钠(用于诊断和治疗铅中毒)
calciuria [ˌkælsiˈjuəriə] *n* 钙尿
calc(o)- 见 calci-
calcoglobule [ˌkælkəuˈglɔbjuːl] *n* 钙小球
calcoglobulin [ˌkælkəuˈglɔbjulin] *n* 钙球蛋白
calcospherite [ˌkælkəuˈsfiərait] *n* 钙球
calculary [ˈkælkjuləri] *a* 结石的
calculi [ˈkælkjulaii] calculus 的复数
calculifragous [ˌkælkjuˈlifrəges] *a* 碎石的(尤指

击碎膀胱结石)
calculogenesis [ˌkælkjuləuˈdʒenisis] *n* 结石形成,生石
calculosis [ˌkælkjuˈləusis] *n* 结石病
calculous [ˈkælkjuləs] *a* 结石的
calculus [ˈkælkjuləs]([复] **calculuses** 或 **calculi** [ˈkælkjulai]) *n* 结石,石 | alternating ~, combination ~ 分层石,混合结石(一种泌尿道结石,各层组成的化学成分各不相同)/ articular ~, joint ~ 关节结石 / biliary calculi 胆石 / decubitus ~ 久卧结石 / dental ~ 牙垢,牙[积]石 / encysted ~, pocketed ~ 箝闭结合,被囊性结石 / hemp seed ~ 大麻子样结石(草酸钙石)/ indigo ~ 尿靛石 / mammary ~, lacteal ~ 乳石(乳腺管石)/ salivary ~ 涎石;龈上结石 / vesical ~ 膀胱结石
Caldani's ligament [kəlˈdɑːni](Leopoldo M. Caldani)卡尔达尼韧带(起自喙突内缘,达于锁骨下缘、第一肋骨及锁骨下肌腱。亦称喙锁韧带)
caldesmon [kælˈdezmən] *n* 钙调[蛋白]结合蛋白
Caldwell-Luc operation [ˈkɔːldwəl luk](George W. Caldwell; Henry Luc)考-吕手术,上颌窦根治术(经由前磨牙对侧上牙窝处切开,开口进入上颌窦的手术)
Caldwell-Moloy classification [ˈkɔːldwəl ˈmɔlɔi](William E. Caldwell; Howard C. Moloy)考德威尔-莫洛伊分类(对女子骨盆的分类:女子型骨盆、男子型骨盆、人猿型骨盆和扁骨盆)
Caldwell's position [ˈkɔːldwel](Eugene W. Caldwell)考德威尔位(以前额和鼻部靠着 X 线[硬]片的一种 X 线投照位置)| ~ projection 考德威尔投照(头颅后前位投照,用以观察额窦和前筛窦)
Calef. calefactus, calefac【拉】温,加温
calefacient [ˌkæliˈfeiʃənt] *a* 使暖的,发暖的 *n* 发暖剂
calefaction [ˌkæliˈfækʃən] *n* 发暖[作用];热污染
calefactory [ˌkæliˈfæktəri] *a* 温暖的;生热的
Calendula [kəˈlendjulə] *n*【拉】金盏花属
calentura [kələnˈturə] *n*【西】中暑;热病
calenture [ˈkæləntjuə] *n* 中暑;热病
calf [kɑːf] *n* 腓肠(俗名小腿肚);小牛
calfactant [kælˈfæktənt] *n* 小牛肺表面活性药(来自小牛肺的肺表面活性药,内含磷脂、中性脂和若干表面活性剂相关蛋白质,用于防治新生儿呼吸窘迫综合征,滴入气管内导管以便气管内给药)
caliber, calibre [ˈkælibə] *n* 管径,口径
calibrate [ˈkælibreit] *vt* 校正;管径测量 | **calibration** [ˌkæliˈbreiʃən] *n* / **calibrator** [ˈkælibreitə] *n* 管径扩张器;管径测量器
caliceal [ˌkæliˈsiəl] *a* 盏的
calicectasis [ˌkæliˈsektəsis] *n* 肾盏扩张
calicectomy [ˌkæliˈsektəmi] *n* 肾盏切除术
calices [ˈkælisiːz] calix 的复数
calicine [ˈkælisiːn] *a* 盏的;盏状的,杯状的
caliciviral [kəˌlisiˈvaiərəl] *a* 杯状病毒的
Caliciviridae [kəˌlisiˈviridiː] *n* 杯状病毒科
Calicivirus [kəˈlisiˌvaiərəs] *n* 杯状病毒属
calicivirus [ˌkælisiˈvaiərəs] *n* 杯状病毒,嵌杯样病毒(RNA 级病毒的亚型,包括小疱疹病毒)
calicle [ˈkælik] *n* 杯状小体
Calicophoron [ˌkæliˈkɔfərən] *n* 杯殖[吸虫]属
calicular [kəˈlikjulə] *a* 杯状的;杯状小体的
caliculus [kəˈlikjuləs]([复] **caliculi** [kəˈlikjulai]) *n*【拉】小杯;杯状器官;副萼 | ~ gustatorius 味蕾 / ~ ophthalmicus 视杯
caliectasis [ˌkeiliˈektəsis] *n* 肾盏扩张
caliectomy [ˌkeiliˈektəmi] *n* 肾盏切除术
Call-Exner bodies [kɑːl ˈeksnə](Friedrich von Call; Siegmund Exner)卡-埃小体(见于卵巢粒层细胞内)
californium (Cf) [ˌkæliˈfɔːniəm] *n* 锎(化学元素)
caligo [kəˈlaigəu], **caligation** [ˌkæliˈgeiʃən] *n* 视力不清,眼朦
calipers [ˈkælipəz] [复] *n* 测径器;两脚规 | skinfold ~ 皮褶测径器(用于研究营养状况和体质)
calisthenics [ˌkælisˈθeniks] *n* [复]健美操练法 | **calisthenic(al)** [kælisˈθenik(ə)l] *a*
calix [ˈkeiliks]([复] **calices** [ˈkælisiːz]) *n* 盏 | renal calices 肾盏
CALLA common acute lymphoblastic leukemia antigen 急性淋巴细胞白血病共同抗原
Callander's amputation [ˈkæləndə](C. L. Callander)卡兰德切断术(膝韧带成形切断术)
Callaway's test [ˈkæləwei](Thomas Callaway)卡拉韦试验(检肱骨脱位,患侧肩部从肩峰经腋测得的周径较无病侧大)
Calleja's islets (islands) [kəˈljeihə](C. Callejay Sanchez)卡耶哈岛(海马回嗅觉小岛)
callicrein [ˌkæliˈkriːn] *n* = **kallikrein**
Callimastix [ˌkæliˈmæstiks] *n* 丽鞭毛虫属
Calliphora [kəˈlifərə] *n* 丽蝇属 | ~ vomitoria 反吐丽蝇
calliphorid [kəˈlifərid] *n* 丽蝇
Calliphoridae [ˌkæliˈfɔridiː] *n* 丽蝇科
Callison's fluid [ˌkælisn](James S. Callison)卡利森液(红细胞计数时用作稀释液)
Callista [kəˈlistə] *n* 仙女蛤属
Callitroga [ˌkæliˈtrəugə] *n* 锥蝇属(即 Cochliomyia)

callomania [ˌkæləu'meinjə] *n* 美貌狂,美貌妄想
callosal [kə'ləusəl] *a* 胼胝体的
callositas [kə'lɔsitəs] *n*【拉】胼胝
callosity [kə'lɔsəti] *n* 胼胝
callosomarginal [kəˌləusəu'mɑːdʒinəl] *a* 胼胝体额上回的,扣带缘上回的
callosotomy [ˌkælə'sɔtəmi] *n* 胼胝体切开术
callosum [kə'ləusəm] *n* 胼胝体
callous ['kæləs] *a* 硬的;胼胝状的
callus ['kæləs] *n* 胼胝;骨痂;愈伤组织 | central ~, inner ~, medullary ~, myelogenous ~ 中央骨痂,内骨痂,骨髓骨痂,骨髓原性骨痂 / definitive ~, intermediate ~ 中间骨痂 / permanent ~ 永久骨痂 / ensheathing ~ 鞘样骨痂,暂时骨痂
calmative ['kælmətiv] *a* 镇静的 *n* 镇静药
Calmette-Guérin bacillus [kɑːl'met gei'rei] (A. L. C. Calmette; Camille Guérin) 卡介菌(现已转意为卡介苗)
Calmette's reaction (ophthalmoreaction, test) [kəl'met] (Albert L. C. Calmette) 卡尔梅特反应(眼反应、试验) (ophthalmic reaction, 见 reaction 项下相应术语) | ~ serum 抗蛇毒血清 / ~ tuberculin 卡尔梅特结核菌素(一种精制结核菌素,滴入结核或伤寒患者结膜上能引起严重局部反应,亦称沉淀结核菌素)/ ~ vaccine 卡介苗(结核菌苗)
calmodulin [kæl'mɔdjulin] *n* 钙调蛋白
Calobata [kə'ləubətə] *n* 躁蝇属
calomel ['kæləmel] *n* 甘汞 | vegetable ~ 鬼臼[根]
calor ['keikə] *n*【拉】热,灼热
caloradiance [ˌkælə'reidiəns] *n* 热辐射[线](介于 250 和 55 000 μm 之间的辐射或射线)
calorescence [ˌkælə'resns] *n* 发光热线,热光(从不发光转化为发光的热射线)
calori- [构词成分]热
caloric [kə'lɔrik] *n* 热[量] *a* 热[量]的,卡的
caloricity [ˌkælə'risəti] *n* 生热力
calorie ['kæləri] *n* 卡[路里](旧热量单位) | gram ~, small ~, standard ~ 克卡,小卡,标准卡 / IT ~, International Table ~ 国际表卡(旧热量单位, =4.186 8 J〈焦耳〉) / large ~ 大卡,千卡 / mean ~ 平均卡(使 1 g 水的温度从 0 ℃ 到 100 ℃升高所需热量的百分之一) / thermochemical ~ 热化学卡(热量单位,相当于 4.184 J〈焦耳〉)
calorifacient [kəˌlɔri'feiʃənt] *a* 生热的,产热的
calorific [ˌkælə'rifik] *a* 生热的,产热的
calorigenic [kəˌlɔri'dʒenik], **calorigenetic** [kəˌlɔridʒi'netik] *a* 发生热量[或能量]的;增加热量[或能量产生]的;增加氧耗量的
calorimeter [ˌkælə'rimitə] *n* 测热计,热量计 | bomb ~ 弹式测热计 / compensating ~ 抵偿式测热计 / respiration ~ 呼吸热量计
calorimetry [ˌkælə'rimitri] *n* 测热法 | direct ~ 直接测热法 / indirect ~ 间接测热法 | **calorimetric(al)** [kəˌlɔri'metrik(əl)] *a* 测热的,测热法的
caloripuncture [ˌkæləri'pʌŋktʃə] *n* 火针术
Calori's bursa [kə'lɔri] (Luigi Calori) 卡洛里囊(位于气管与主动脉弓之间)
caloriscope [kə'lɔriskəup] *n* 热量器(用以显示育婴食物的热值)
caloritropic [kəˌlɔri'trɔpik] *a* 向热的
calory ['kæləri] ([复] **calories** ['kæləriz]) 卡[路里](旧热量单位)
Calot's operation [kə'lɔː] (Jean-François Calot) 卡洛手术(在麻醉下用牵伸法对脊柱后凸施行强迫性复位术) / ~ treatment 卡洛疗法(用石膏背夹治疗脊椎结核) / ~ triangle 卡洛三角(胆囊动脉在上,胆囊管在下,肝管在中间所形成的三角)
calotte [kə'lɔt] *n*【法】小帽,纤毛帽;眼球帽样切块(病理组织检查用)
calpain ['kælpein] *n* [需]钙蛋白酶
calreticulin [ˌkælrə'tikjulin] *n* [肌]钙网蛋白
calsequestrin [ˌkælsi'kwestrin] *n* 贮钙素,贮钙蛋白,收钙蛋白(一种结合蛋白,其作用为螯合和贮存钙离子)
calumbic acid [kə'lʌmbik] 非洲防己酸
calusterone [kə'ljuːstərəun] *n* 卡鲁睾酮, 7β, 17α-二甲睾酮(抗肿瘤药)
calutron ['kæljutrɔn] *n* 卡留管(一种铀同位素分离器)
calvacin ['kælvəsin] *n* 马勃素(一种抗肿瘤物质)
calvaria [kæl'vɛəriə], **calvarium** [kæl'vɛəriəm] *n*【拉】颅盖 | **calvarial** *a*
Calvatia [kæl'veiʃiə] *n* 马勃属 | ~ gigantea 大马勃
Calvé-Perthes disease [kəl'vei pə'teis] (Jacques Calvé; Georg C. Perthes) 卡凡-佩特斯病(股骨小头骺端骨软骨病)
calves [kɑːvz] calf 的复数
Calvin cycle ['kælvin] (Melvin Calvin) 卡尔文循环(植物光合作用时发生的一种暗反应,在此反应中二氧化碳附着于五碳糖分子,继而还原而形成其他糖)
calvities [kæl'viʃiiːz] *n*【拉】秃[发],脱发
calx [kælks] *n*【拉】白垩;跟(亦称跟区,足跟);煅余物;石灰,氧化钙 | ~ chlorata, ~ chlorinata 氯化石灰,漂白粉 / ~ sulfurata 硫化石灰
calyceal [ˌkæli'siəl] *a* 盏的,杯状体的;[花]萼的
calycectasis [ˌkæli'sektəsis] *n* 肾盏扩张

calycectomy [ˌkæliˈsektəmi] *n* 肾盏切除术
calycine [ˈkælisin] *a* 盏的,盏状的,杯状的;萼的,萼状的
calycle [ˈkælikl] *n* 杯状器官;副萼
calyculus [kəˈlikjuləs] ([复] **calyculi** [kəˈlikjulai]) *n*【拉】小杯;杯状器官;副萼 | ~ gustatorius 味蕾 / ~ ophthalmicus 视杯
calymma [kəˈlimə] *n* 胶泡
Calymmatobacterium [kəˌlimətəubækˈtiəriəm] *n* 鞘杆菌属 | ~ granulomatis 肉芽肿鞘杆菌
calyx [ˈkeiliks, ˈkæ-] ([复] **calyces** [ˈkeilisiːz, ˈkæ-]或 **calyxes**) *n* 盏;[花]萼
CAM cell adhesion molecules 细胞黏附分子;complementary and alternative medicine 补充和选择性医学
Camallanus [kæməˈleinəs] *n* 驼形丝虫属(寄生于鱼、爬虫类、两栖动物的肠内)
Cambaroides [ˌkæmbəˈrɔidiːz] *n* 蝲蛄属(体内有并殖吸虫属的后囊蚴)
cambendazole [kæmˈbendəzəul] *n* 坎苯达唑(抗蠕虫药)
cambium [ˈkæmbiəm] *n* 新生层,新生组织;形成层(植)
cambogia [kæmˈbəudʒiə] *n*【拉】藤黄
cambric [ˈkeimbrik] *n* 细薄布;麻纱;细夏布
Camellia [kəˈmeliə] *n* 山茶属
cameloid [ˈkæməlɔid] *a* 骆驼状的
camelpox [ˈkæməlpɔks] *n* 骆驼痘
camera [ˈkæmərə] ([复] **cameras** 或 **camerae** [ˈkæməriː]) *n* 照相机;暗室;电视摄像机;房,室 | ~ anterior bulbi 眼前房 / ~ lucida 投影描绘器 / ~ obscura 暗箱 / ~ pulpi 髓腔 / recording ~ 记录照相机,光转筒记录器 / scintillation ~ 闪烁照相机
Camerer's law [ˈkæmərə] (Johann F. W. Camerer)凯麦勒定律(体重相同的儿童,不拘年龄,所需食物量相同)
Camey neobladder [kɑːˈmei] (M. Camey)卡梅新膀胱(以前广泛使用的一型回肠新膀胱,从回肠U形切片制得)
camisole [ˈkæmisəul] *n*【法】约束衣,保护衣
Cammann's stethoscope [ˈkæmən] (George P. Cammann)卡曼听诊器,双耳听诊器
Cammidge reaction (test) [ˈkæmidʒ] (Percy J. Cammidge)坎米奇反应(试验),胰反应(确定胰腺炎或胰脏恶性病的存在)
camouflage [ˈkæmuflɑːʒ] *n* 伪装 | neurotic ~ 神经症性伪装
CAMP cyclophosphamide, doxcrubicin, methotrexate, and procarbazine 环磷酰胺-多柔比星-甲氨蝶呤-丙卡巴肼(联合化疗治癌方案)
cAMP adenosine 3′, 5′-cyclic phosphate 腺苷3′, 5′-环磷酸,环腺苷酸;cyclic AMP 环腺苷酸
campanula [kəmˈpænjulə] *n* 钟形物
Campbell's ligament [ˈkæmbl] (William F. Campbell)坎贝尔韧带(腋悬韧带)
cAMP-dependent protein kinase [diˈpendənt ˈprəutiːn ˈkaineis] 环腺苷酸依赖性蛋白激酶
campe(a)chy [kæmˈpiːtʃi] *n* 苏木精,苏木紫
Camper's facial angle [ˈkæmpə] (Pieter Camper)坎珀尔颜面角(前鼻棘底所形成之角) | ~ fascia 坎珀尔筋膜(腹壁浅筋膜浅层) / ~ ligament 坎珀尔韧带(会阴深筋膜,尿生殖膈) / ~ line 坎珀尔线(由鼻翼下缘至耳屏上缘的假想线)
campesterol [kæmˈpestərɔl] *n* 菜油甾醇,菜油固醇
camphechlor [ˈkæmfəklɔː] *n* 毒杀芬(即 toxaphene,杀虫药)
camphene [ˈkæmfiːn] *n* 莰烯
camphoglycuronic acid [ˌkæmfəuˌglaikjuəˈrɔnik] 樟脑葡萄糖醛酸
camphol [ˈkæmfɔl] *n* 龙脑,冰片,莰醇
campholic acid [ˈkæmfəlik] 四甲基环戊烷羧酸,龙脑酸
camphor [ˈkæmfə] *n* 樟脑,莰酮 | artificial ~ 人造樟脑(氯化蒎烯) / blumea ~ 艾纳香脑,艾片 / Borneo ~ 龙脑,冰片 / carbolated ~ 酚樟脑(用作创伤防腐敷料) / chloral ~ 氯醛樟脑(外用镇静药) / mace ~ 肉豆蔻衣脑 / mentholated ~ 薄荷脑樟脑(局部抗刺激药及喷雾药) / monobromated ~ 一溴樟脑(镇静药) / naphthol ~ β-萘酚樟脑(外用防腐剂) / peppermint ~ 薄荷脑,薄荷醇 / phenol ~ 酚樟脑(杀菌及止牙痛药) / resorcinated ~ 间苯二酚樟脑(治虱病及瘙痒) / ~ salicylate 水杨酸樟脑(外用软膏治各种皮肤病,内服治腹泻) / salol ~ 萨罗樟脑(局部防腐剂) / thyme ~ 麝香草脑(抗菌药) / turpentine ~ 松节油脑,松油二醇
camphora [kæmˈfɔrə] *n*【拉】樟脑
camphoraceous [ˌkæmfəˈreiʃəs] *a* 樟脑样的,似樟脑的
camphorate [ˈkæmfəreit] *vt* 使与樟脑化合;加樟脑在…中 | **~d** *a* 含樟脑的;樟脑酊的
camphoric acid [kæmˈfɔrik] 樟脑酸
camphorism [ˈkæmfərizəm] *n* 樟脑中毒(症状为惊厥、昏迷和胃炎)
camphoronic acid [ˌkæmfəˈrɔnik] 分解樟脑酸,樟脑三酸
campimeter [kæmˈpimitə] *n* 平面视野计 | **campimetry** *n* 平面视野计检查法
campotomy [kæmˈpɔtəmi] *n* 区切开术(指在丘脑下方福雷尔〈Forel〉区造成损害的一种立体定向

性外科手术，以治疗帕金森（Parkinson）病的震颤）

camptocormia [ˌkæmptəuˈkɔːmiə], **camptocormy** [ˌkæmptəuˈkɔːmi], **campospasm** [ˈkæmpəspæzəm], **camptospasm** [ˈkæmptəspæzəm] *n* 躯干前屈症

camptodactyly [ˌkæmptəuˈdæktili], **camptodactylia** [ˌkæmptəudækˈtiliə], **camptodactylism** [ˌkæmptəuˈdæktilizəm] *n* 先天性指屈曲

camptomelia [ˌkæmptəuˈmiːliə] *n* 肢弯曲，弯肢 | **camptomelic** [ˌkæmptəuˈmiːlik] *a*

Campylobacter [ˌkæmpiləuˈbæktə] *n* 弯曲菌属 | ~ fecalis 粪弯曲菌 / ~ fetus 胎儿弯曲菌（亦称胎儿弧菌）/ ~ fetus subsp. fetus 胎儿弯曲菌胎儿亚种 / ~ fetus subsp. intestinalis 胎儿弯曲菌肠亚种 / ~ fetus subsp. jejuni 胎儿弯曲菌空肠亚种 / ~ fetus subsp. venerealis 胎儿弯曲菌性病亚种 / ~ sputorum 痰液弯曲菌 / ~ sputorum subsp. bubulus 痰液弯曲菌牛亚种 / ~ sputorum subsp. mucosalis 痰液弯曲菌黏膜亚种 / ~ sputorum subsp. sputorum 痰液弯曲菌痰液亚种

campylobacter [ˌkæmpiləuˈbæktə] *n* 弯曲菌

campylobacteriosis [ˌkæmpiləubækˌtiəriˈəusis] *n* 弯曲菌病 | bovine genital ~, ovine genital ~ 牛生殖道弯曲菌病，绵羊生殖道弯曲菌病

campylognathia [ˌkæmpiləuˈneiθiə] *n* 颌弯曲畸形；唇裂

camsylate [ˈkæmsileit] *n* 樟脑磺酸盐（camphorsulfonate的 USAN 缩约词）

Camurati-Engelmann disease [kɑːmuːˈrɑːti ˈeŋgəlmɑːn]（Mario Camurati; Guido Engelmann）卡-恩病，骨干发育异常

can [kæn] 容器（如罐、壶、桶等）| douche ~ 冲洗罐

Canada-Cronkhite syndrome [ˈkænədə ˈkrɔŋkait]（Wilma J. Canada; Leonard W. Cronkhite, Jr.）卡纳达-克朗凯特综合征（家族性胃肠息肉病，伴外胚层缺陷，如甲萎缩、脱发以及皮肤色素沉着等，见 Cronkhite-Canada syndrome）

Canadian repair [kəˈneidjən] 加拿大修复术（见 Shouldice repair）

canal [kəˈnæl] *n* 管，道 | abdominal ~ 腹股沟管 / alimentary ~, digestive ~ 消化道 / anterior ethmoid ~ 前筛管，眶颅管 / arterial ~ 动脉导管 / basipharyngeal ~ 颅底咽管 / birth ~, obstetric ~, parturient ~ 产道 / bony ~s of ear 骨性半规管 / bullular ~s, ruffed ~ 小带间隙，皱纹管 / ciliary ~s 睫状管，虹膜角膜角间隙 / crural ~ 股管 / diploic ~s 板障管 / eustachian ~ 咽鼓管 / external auditory ~ 外耳道 / facial ~, fallopian ~, spiroid ~ 面神经管 / flexor ~ 腕管 / ganglionic ~（内耳）螺旋神经节管，蜗轴螺旋管 / genital ~ 生殖管 / gynecophoral ~, gynecophorous ~ 抱雌沟（指血吸虫）/ hemal ~ 脉弧管（胚）/ iliac ~ 髂肌管，肌腔隙 / inguinal ~ 腹股沟管 / internal auditory ~ 内耳道 / lacrimal ~ 鼻泪管 / medullary ~ 椎管；骨髓腔 / musculotubal ~ 肌咽鼓管 / nasal ~, nasolacrimal ~ 鼻泪管 / neural ~, spinal ~, vertebral ~ 神经管，脊椎管，椎管 / omphalomesenteric ~ 脐肠系膜管，卵黄管，卵黄蒂 / optic ~ 视神经管 / osseous eustachian ~ 骨性咽鼓管，肌咽鼓管 / pelvic ~ 小骨盆腔 / perivascular ~ 血管周隙（血管周围的淋巴隙）/ pleural ~s 胸管 / posterior ethmoid ~ 筛后管，筛后孔，眶筛管 / pterygoid ~, recurrent ~, vidian ~ 翼管 / pterygopalatine ~ 腭大管；腭鞘管 / root ~ 牙根管 / sacculocochlear ~ 连合管（耳蜗）/ serous ~ 浆液管（微淋巴隙）/ sheathing ~ 鞘管，腹膜鞘突 / spermatic ~ 精索管（男性的腹股沟管）/ subsartorial ~ 收肌管 / tarsal ~ 跗骨管，跗骨窦 / tubal ~ 咽鼓管半管 / urogenital ~s 尿生殖窦 / uterine ~ 子宫管，子宫腔 / utriculosaccular ~ 椭圆球囊管 / vaginal ~, vulvouterine ~ 阴道腔 / ventricular ~ 胃道，胃管 / vestibular ~ 前庭阶 / vulvar ~ 阴道前庭。

canales [kəˈneiliːz] canalis 的复数

canalicular [ˌkænəˈlikjulə] *a* 小管的，小管样的

canaliculitis [ˌkænəˌlikjuˈlaitis] *n* 泪小管炎

canaliculization [ˌkænəˌlikjulaiˈzeiʃən, -liˈz-] *n* 小管形成，成小管

canaliculodacryocystostomy [ˌkænəˌlikjuləuˌdækriəsisˈtɔstəmi] *n* 泪小管泪囊吻合术

canaliculorhinostomy [ˌkænəˌlikjuləu ˌraiˈnɔstəmi] *n* 泪小管鼻腔吻合术

canaliculus [ˌkænəˈlikjuləs]（[复] **canaliculi** [ˌkænəˈlikjulai]）*n*【拉】小管

canalis [kəˈneilis]（[复] **canales** [kəˈneiliːz]）*n*【拉】管，道

canalith [ˈkænəˌliθ] *n* 管石（半规管内淋巴内一种自由浮动颗粒，管石的存在可致良性阵发性体位性眩晕）

canalization [ˌkænəlaiˈzeiʃən, -liˈz-] *n* 管道形成，成管；造管术；穿通，血管再通；沟通，新径路形成（在心理学上，指在中枢神经系统中由神经冲动反复的通过而形成新的径路）

canaloplasty [kəˈnæləˌplæsti] *n* 管道整复术，管道成形术（如外耳道）

canalplasty [kəˈnælplæsti] *n* 管道成形术

canarypox [kəˈnɛəripɔks] *n* 金丝雀痘

Canavalia [ˌkænəˌvæliə] *n* 刀豆属

canavalin [ˌkænəˈvælin] *n* 刀豆素，刀豆抗菌素

canavanase [kəˈnævəneis] *n* 刀豆氨酸酶

canavanine [kəˈnævənin] *n* 刀豆氨酸
Canavan's disease [ˈkænəvæn] (Myrtelle M. Canavan)卡纳范病,中枢神经系统海绵状变性
Canavan-van Bogaert-Bertrand disease [ˈkænəvæn vɑːn ˈbɔgət bɛəˈtrein] (M. M. Canavan; Ludo van Bogaert; Ivan G. Bertrand)卡-鲍-贝病,中枢神经系统海绵状变性
cancellated [ˈkænsəleitid] *a* 网状的,网状结构的
cancellous [ˈkænsələs] *a* 网眼状的;海绵状的;网状骨质的
cancellus [kænˈseləs] ([复] **cancelli** [kænˈselai]) *n*【拉】网状骨质
cancer [ˈkænsə] *n* 癌,恶性肿瘤;癌症;弊端 | acinar ~, acinous ~ 腺泡癌 / adenoid ~ 腺样癌 / ~ à deux 配偶癌(共同生活的两人同时或先后患癌) / alveolar ~ 蜂窝状癌 / aniline ~ 苯胺癌 / betel ~, buyo cheek ~ 槟榔癌,萎叶性颊癌 / black ~, melanotic ~ 恶性黑色素瘤,黑色素癌 / boring ~ 穿通性癌(面部) / claypipe ~ 烟管癌(唇) / dendritic ~ 乳头[状]癌 / duct ~ 管癌(乳腺) / dyeworkers' ~ 染工[膀胱]癌 / ~ encuirasse, corset ~, jacket ~ 铠甲状癌(在胸部皮肤周围) / ~ in situ 原位癌 / kang ~, kangri ~ 热炕癌,火炉癌(大腿或腹部的上皮癌) / latent ~ 潜在癌,隐匿癌肿(指无临床表现,但组织切片检查发现的一种前列腺癌) / occult ~ 隐性癌(探察前临床明显转移的一种小前列腺癌) / rodent ~ 侵蚀性溃疡 / roentgenologist's ~ 放射线工作者癌(手部) / tubular ~ 管癌(一种排列成管状的腺癌) / villous duct ~ 绒毛管癌
canceremia [ˌkænsəˈriːmiə] *n* 癌细胞血症
cancericidal [ˌkænsəriˈsaidl], **cancerocidal** [ˌkænsərəuˈsaidl] *a* 灭癌的
cancerigenic [ˌkænsəriˈdʒenik], **cancerogenic** [ˌkænsərəuˈdʒenik] *a* 致癌的
cancerin [ˈkænsərin] *n* 尿癌素
cancerism [ˈkænsərizəm] *n* 癌体质
cancerous [ˈkænsərəs] *a* 癌性的,癌的
cancerphobia [ˌkænsəˈfəubjə], **cancerophobia** [ˌkænsərəuˈfəubjə] *n* 癌病恐怖,恐癌症
cancer-ulcer [ˈkænsə ˈʌlsə] *n* 癌性溃疡
cancriform [ˈkæŋkrifɔːm] *a* 癌样的,似癌的
cancroid [ˈkæŋkrɔid] *a* 癌样的 *n* 角化癌
cancrum [ˈkæŋkrəm] *n*【拉】(坏疽性)溃疡 | ~ nasi 鼻坏疽 / ~ oris 走马疳,坏疽性口炎 / ~ pudendi 外阴溃疡
candela(cd) [kænˈdiːlə] *n* 堪[德拉],[新]烛光(旧发光强度单位,缩写为 cd,现用 lx 勒〈克斯〉)
candelilla [ˌkændəˈlilə] *n* 蜡大戟
candicidin [ˌkændiˈsaidin] *n* 克念菌素(抗生素类药)
Candida [ˈkændidə] *n* 念珠菌属 | ~ albicans 白念珠菌 / ~ mesenterica 管道念珠菌 / ~ parapsilosis 近平滑念珠菌 / ~ tropicalis 热带念珠菌 / ~ vini 酸酒念珠菌
candidal [ˈkændidəl] *a* 念珠菌的
candidemia [ˌkændiˈdiːmiə] *n* 念珠菌血[症]
candidiasis [ˌkændiˈdaiəsis] *n* 念珠菌病 | cutaneous ~ 皮肤念珠菌病 / endocardial ~ 心内膜念珠菌病 | **candidosis** [ˌkændiˈdəusis] *n*
candidid [ˈkændidid] *n* 念珠菌疹
candidin [ˈkændidin] *n* 制念珠菌素
candiduria [ˌkændiˈdjuəriə] *n* 念珠菌尿
candiru [kændiˈruː] *n* 亚马逊小鲶(据说会进入在该河中沐浴的男子的尿道或妇女的阴道中)
candle [ˈkændl] *n* 烛;滤柱;烛光 | foot ~ 呎(英尺)烛光(旧照度单位) / international ~ 国际烛光(旧发光强度单位) / meter ~ 米烛光(=1 lx)
candlefish [ˈkændlfiʃ] *n* 烛鱼(产生一种固定油,其作用类似鱼肝油)
candol [ˈkændɔl] *n* 干麦芽浸膏
cane [kein] *n* 手杖 | adjustable ~ 可调节手杖 / English ~ 英式手杖(医疗用) / quadripod ~ 四脚手杖 / tripod ~ 三脚手杖
canescent [kəˈnesənt] *a* 变得灰白的;带灰色的;有灰白毛的
canine [ˈkeinain] *a* 犬的 *n* 尖牙
caniniform [keiˈnainifɔːm] *a* 犬牙样的
caninus [keiˈnainəs] *n* 尖牙肌(口角提肌)
canister [ˈkænistə] *n* 罐;滤毒罐
canities [kəˈniʃiiːz] *n*【拉】白发,头发灰白,灰发[症]
canker [ˈkæŋkə] *n* (坏疽性)溃疡;马蹄疮;(犬、猫的)外耳道炎 | **~ous** [ˈkæŋkərəs] *a* 溃疡的,似溃疡的;引起溃疡的,患溃疡的
canna [ˈkænə] *n*【拉】小腿骨 | ~ major 胫骨 / ~ minor 腓骨
cannabidiol [ˌkænəbiˈdaiəul] *n* 大麻二酚
cannabin [ˈkænəbin] *n* 大麻苷;大麻碱
cannabinoid [kəˈnæbinɔid, ˈkænəbinɔid] *n* 大麻素(可指任何一种大麻的化学成分,如大麻醇、四氢大麻醇等)
cannabinol [kəˈnæbinɔl, ˈkænəbinɔl] *n* 大麻酚
Cannabis [ˈkænəbis] *n* 大麻属
cannabis [ˈkænəbis] *n* 大麻
cannibalism [ˈkænibəlizəm] *n* 同种相残,同类相食(指恶性细胞互相吞噬作用)
Cannizzaro's reaction [ˌkæniˈzɑːrəu] (Stanislao Cannizzaro)康尼扎罗反应(指醛在碱中的反应,当醛与动物组织接触时,醛的一个分子还原为相应的醇,另一个分子同时被氧化为相应的酸)
Cannon-Bard theory [ˈkænən bɑːd] (W. B. Cannon; Philip Bard)坎-巴学说,应急学说(即emer-

gency theory,见 theory 项下相应术语)

Cannon's ring (point) ['kænən] (Walter B. Cannon)坎农环(点)(钡剂造影时右半侧结肠的紧张性收缩环)

cannula ['kænjulə] ([复] **cannulae** ['kænjuliː] 或 **cannulas**) *n* 套管,插管 | perfusion ~ 灌流套管 / washout ~ 冲洗套管

cannulate ['kænjuleit] *vt* 插套管

cannulation [ˌkænju'leiʃən], **cannulization** [ˌkænjulai'zeiʃən, -li'z-] *n* 插管[术],套管插入术

canon ['kænən] *n* 规范

canonical [kə'nɔnikəl] *a* 规范的,典范的

canrenoate potassium [kæn'renəeit] 坎利酸钾(醛固酮拮抗药)

canrenone [kæn'renəun] *n* 坎利酮(醛固酮拮抗药)

cant [kænt] *n* 斜面 | ~ of mandible 下颌骨斜面

canthal ['kænθəl] *a* 眦的,眼角的

canthariasis [ˌkænθə'raiəsis] *n* 斑蝥虫病

cantharidal [kæn'θæridl] *a* 含斑蝥的,斑蝥制的,含芫青的

cantharidate [kæn'θærideit] *n* 斑蝥酸盐

cantharidés [kæn'θæridiːz] *n*【拉】斑蝥,芫青

cantharidic acid [kænθə'ridik] 斑蝥酸

cantharidin [kæn'θæridin] *n* 斑蝥素,芫青素(抗肿瘤药)

cantharidism [kæn'θæridizəm] *n* 斑蝥中毒

Cantharis ['kænθəris] *n* 斑蝥属,芫青属 | ~ vesicatoria 斑蝥,西班牙绿芫青

canthectomy [kæn'θektəmi] *n* 眦切除术

canthi ['kænθai] canthus 的复数

canthitis [kæn'θaitis] *n* 眦炎

canth(o)- [构词成分]眦,眼角

cantholysis [kæn'θɔlisis] *n* 眦切开术(指眦或眦韧带离断术)

canthoplasty ['kænθəˌplæsti] *n* 眦成形术 | provisional ~ 暂时性眦切开术

canthorrhaphy [kæn'θɔrəfi] *n* 眦缝合术

canthotomy [kæn'θɔtəmi] *n* 眦切开术(指外眦切开)

canthus ['kænθəs] ([复] **canthi** ['kænθai]) *n* 眦,眼角

Cantor tube ['kæntə] (Meyer O. Cantor)坎特尔管(一端装有汞的管,作肠插管用)

Cantrell's pentalogy [kæn'trel] (James R. Cantrell)坎特雷尔五联症(胸骨下部裂,伴中线腹缺损,如脐突出、缺损性心包和心包腔与腹膜腔之间沟通膈缺损以及心脏异常,如室间隔缺损或不常见的房间隔缺损、法洛〈Fallot〉四联症或左心室憩室)

cantus galli ['kæntəs 'gæli]【拉】喘鸣性喉痉挛

canula ['kænjulə] *n* 套管,插管

caoutchouc ['kautʃuk] *n*【法】橡皮,弹性树胶,生橡胶

CAP College of American Pathologists 美国病理学家学会

Cap. capiat【拉】取服

cap [kæp] *n* 盖,帽,罩,套;菌盖;髓盖,人造冠;避孕帽;海洛因丸,致幻毒品胶囊 | anterior head ~ 顶体(精子) / bishop's ~, duodenal ~, pyloric ~ 十二指肠冠 / cradle ~ 乳痂 / dutch ~ 阴道隔(避孕用) / enamel ~ 釉帽 / knee ~ 髌,膝盖骨 / metanephric ~s 后肾帽 / phrygian ~ 弗里及亚帽,倒圆锥形帽(显示胆囊体和胆囊底之间的扭结) / postnuclear ~, posterior head ~ 后帽,核后盖 / skull ~ 颅盖

capability [ˌkeipə'biləti] *n* 能力 | civil ~ 民事行为能力

capacitance(*C*) [kə'pæsitəns] *n* 电容 | membrane ~ 膜电容(指细胞膜的电容)

capacitate [kə'pæsiteit] *vt* 使(精子)获能

capacitation [kəˌpæsi'teiʃən] *n* 获能(精子到达输卵管壶腹部后能使卵受精的过程)

capacitor [kə'pæsitə] *n* 电容器

capacity [kə'pæsəti] *n* 容量;能量;能力;电容 | cranial ~ 颅容积,颅容量 / diffusing ~, diffusion ~ 弥散量 / functional residual ~ 功能残气量 / inspiratory ~ 吸气量 / maximal breathing ~ 最大通气量 / maximal tubular excretory ~ 肾小管最大排泄量 / molar heat ~ 摩尔热容 / respiratory ~ 呼吸容量 / specific heat ~ 比热容 / thermal ~, heat ~ 热容量 / total lung ~ 肺总量 / virus neutralizing ~ 病毒中和能量 / vital ~ 肺活量

CAPD continuous ambulatory peritoneal dialysis 持续不卧床腹膜透析

capecitabine [kæpə'saitəbiːn] *n* 卡西他滨(抗肿瘤药,在活体内转化成氟尿嘧啶,用以治疗转移性乳腺癌和结肠直肠癌,口服给药)

capelet ['kæpəlit] *n* 马踝肿,马肘肿

capeline ['kæpəlin] *n*【法】帽式绷带,裹颅双头带

Capgras syndrome ['kæpgrɑː] (Jean M. J. Capgras)卡普格拉斯综合征,替身综合征(一种妄想,患者对面前的其他人,认为不是真的本人,而是替身)

capillarectasia [ˌkæpiˌlærek'teiziə] *n* 毛细管扩张

Capillaria [ˌkæpi'lɛəriə] *n* 毛细线虫属 | ~ contorta 扭转毛细线虫 / ~ hepatica 肝毛细线虫 / ~ philippinensis 菲律宾毛细线虫

capillariasis [ˌkæpilə'raiəsis] *n* 毛细线虫病

capillariomotor [ˌkæpiˌlæriəu'məutə] *a* 毛细管运动的

capillaritis [ˌkæpiləˈraitis] *n* 毛细管炎
capillarity [ˌkæpiˈlæriti] *n* 毛细作用,毛细现象
capillaropathy [ˌkæpiləˈrɔpəθi] *n* 毛细管病
capillaroscopy [ˌkæpiləˈrɔskəpi], **capillarioscopy** [ˌkæpiˌlæriˈɔskəpi] *n* 毛细管显微镜检查
capillary [kəˈpiləri, ˈkæpi-] *a* 毛样的;毛细的 *n* 毛细管 | bile capillaries 胆小管;毛细胆管 / erythrocytic capillaries 红细胞毛细管 / lymph ~, lymphatic ~ 毛细淋巴管
capillitium [ˌkæpiˈliʃiəm] *n* 孢丝
capillomotor [kəˈpiləuˈməutə] *a* 毛细管运动的
capillus [kəˈpiləs] ([复] **capilli** [kəˈpilai]) *n* 【拉】头发
capistration [ˌkæpisˈtreiʃən] *n* 包茎
capita [ˈkæpitə] caput 的复数
capital [ˈkæpitl] *a* 重要的,首要的;股骨头的
capitate [ˈkæpiteit] *a* 头状的
capitation [ˌkæpiˈteiʃən] *n* 按人计算,按人收费(每一个参加保健规划者付给医生的年费)
capitatum [ˌkæpiˈteitəm] *n* 【拉】头状骨
capitellocondylar [ˌkæpiˌteləuˈkɔndilə] *a* 肱骨小头与踝的(如指肘假肢)
capitellum [ˌkæpiˈteləm] *n* 肱骨小头
capitonnage [ˌkæpitəˈnɑːʒ] *n* 【法】囊腔闭合术
capitopedal [ˌkæpitəˈpedl] *a* 头足的
capitulum [kəˈpitjuləm] ([复] **capitula** [kəˈpitjulə]) *n* 小头 | **capitular** *a*
Caplan's syndrome [ˈkæplən] (Anthony Caplan) 卡布兰综合征(尘肺伴类风湿关节炎,X线摄影显示边缘界线清晰的多个球形结节性损害遍及两肺。亦称类风湿尘肺)
capneic [ˈkæpniik] *a* 适二氧化碳的
capn(o)- [构词成分]烟的,煤烟状的;二氧化碳
Capnocytophaga [ˌkæpnəusaiˈtɔfəgə] *n* 嗜二氧化碳细胞菌属 | ~ canimorsus 犬咬嗜二氧化碳细胞菌(以前称 DF2 杆菌)
capnogram [ˈkæpnəgræm] *n* 二氧化碳分析,二氧化碳描记图
capnograph [ˈkæpnəˌgrɑːf] *n* 二氧化碳分析仪
capnography [kæpˈnɔgrəfi] *n* 二氧化碳分析法
capnohepatography [ˌkæpnəuˌhepəˈtɔgrəfi] *n* 肝二氧化碳充气摄影[术]
capnometer [kæpˈnɔmitə] *n* 二氧化碳监测仪
capnometry [kæpˈnɔmitri] *n* 二氧化碳测定[法]
capnophilic [kæpnəuˈfilik] *a* 嗜二氧化碳的(指细菌)
capobenate sodium [ˌkæpəuˈbeneit] 卡泊酸钠(抗心律失常药)
capobenic acid [ˌkæpəuˈbenik] 卡泊酸(血管扩张药,用以防治心肌梗死)
capon [ˈkeipən] *n* 阉鸡 | **~ize** [ˈkeipənaiz] *vt* 阉(鸡),(鸡)去势
capotement [kəpɔtˈmɔŋ] *n* 【法】胃振水声(胃膨胀时听到的一种声音)
capped [kæpt] *a* 帽状的(指关节,尤指马腿或牛腿关节肿大)
cappie [ˈkæpi] *n* (幼绵羊)薄颅骨病
capping [ˈkæpiŋ] *n* 盖帽;帽化,成帽(由于抗原与特异性抗体交叉连接而使细胞表面抗原向细胞表面的一小区移动);髓盖,盖髓术;顶裂 | pulp ~ 盖髓术
caprate [ˈkæpreit] *n* 癸酸盐,癸酸酯;癸酸
capreolate [ˈkæpriəleit], **capreolary** [ˈkæpriələri] *a* 卷曲的
capreomycin [ˌkæpriəuˈmaisin] *n* 卷曲霉素(抗生素类药)
capric acid [ˈkæprik] 癸酸
caprillic [kəˈprilik] *a* 山羊样的(叫声)
capriloquism [kəˈpriləkwizəm] *n* 羊音
caprin [ˈkæprin] *n* 癸酸甘油酯
caprine [ˈkæprain] *a* 羊的 *n* 正亮氨酸
Capripoxvirus [ˈkæpriˌpɔksvaiərəs] *n* 山羊痘病毒属
caprizant [ˈkæprizənt] *a* 羊跳式的(指脉搏)
caproate [ˈkæprəueit] *n* 己酸盐(同样是 hexanoate 的 USAN 缩约词)
caproic acid [kəˈprəuik] 己酸
caproin [kəˈprəuin] *n* 己酸甘油酯
caproleic acid [ˌkæprəˈliːik] 癸烯酸
caprone [ˈkæprəun] *n* 卡普隆,聚己内酰胺纤维
caproyl [kəˈprəuil] *n* 己酰基
caproylamine [ˌkæprəuiˈlæmin] *n* 己胺
capryl [ˈkæpril] *n* 癸酰基;辛基,辛酰基
caprylate [ˈkæprileit] *n* 辛酸盐
caprylic acid [kəˈprilik] 辛酸
caprylin [ˈkæprilin] *n* 辛酸甘油酯
capsaicin [kæpˈseiisin] *n* 辣椒素,辣椒辣素
capsic acid [ˈkæpsik] 辣椒酸
Capsicum [ˈkæpsikəm] *n* 【拉】辣椒属
capsicum [ˈkæpsikəm] *n* 辣椒
capsid [ˈkæpsid] *n* [病毒]壳体
capsitis [kæpˈsaitis] *n* 晶状体囊炎
capsomer [ˈkæpsəmə], **capsomere** [ˈkæpsəmiə] *n* [病毒]壳粒
capsotomy [kæpˈsɔtəmi] *n* 关节囊切开术;晶状体囊切开术
Capsul. capsula【拉】囊,被膜
capsula [ˈkæpsjulə] ([复] **capsulae** [ˈkæpsjuliː]) *n* 【拉】囊,被膜
capsulation [ˌkæpsjuˈleiʃən] *n* 装胶囊
capsule [ˈkæpsjuːl] *n* 囊,被膜;胶囊[剂];荚膜 | adherent ~ 黏着囊 / adrenal ~ 肾上腺 / articular ~, joint ~, synovial ~ 关节囊 / auditory ~ 耳被囊,听囊(胚) / bacterial ~ 细菌荚膜 / ~s

of the brain 脑被,脑囊(大脑白质层) / brood ~s 育囊,雏囊 / cartilage ~ 软骨囊 / dental ~ 牙周组织,牙槽骨膜 / external ~ 外囊 / ~ of heart 心包 / hepatobiliary ~ 肝胆管囊,血管周纤维囊 / internal ~ 内囊 / malpighian ~, müllerian ~ 肾小球囊 / ocular ~ 眼球囊 / optic ~ 眼被囊(胚) / otic ~ 耳囊(胚) / pelvioprostatic ~ 前列腺囊,前列腺筋膜 / periodic 耳周囊(胚) / telemetering ~, radiotelemetering ~ 遥测囊,无线电遥测囊(一种小型无线电发送装置,装在一个大小像通常装药胶囊的囊内,吞入或用其他方法插入体内,可提供器官内有关压力、温度、pH 等信息) / triasyn B ~s 三种维生素 B 胶囊(内含维生素 B_1、维生素 B_2 和烟酰胺)

capsulectomy [ˌkæpsjuˈlektəmi] *n* 关节囊切除术;晶状体囊切除术 | renal ~ 肾被膜剥除术

capsulitis [ˌkæpsjuˈlaitis] *n* 囊炎 | adhesive ~ 粘连性囊炎 / hepatic ~ 肝周炎

capsulize [ˈkæpsjulaiz] *vt* 把…装入胶囊

capsulolenticular [ˌkæpsjuləulenˈtikjulə] *a* 晶状体基质及晶状体囊的

capsuloma [ˌkæpsjuˈləumə] *n* (肾)被膜瘤

capsuloplasty [ˈkæpsjuləˌplæsti] *n* 关节囊成形术

capsulorrhaphy [ˌkæpsjuˈlɔrəfi] *n* 关节囊缝合术

capsulorrhexis [ˌkæpsələuˈreksis] *n* 撕囊术

capsulotome [kæpˈsjuːlətəum] *n* 晶状体囊刀

capsulotomy [ˌkæpsjuˈlɔtəmi] *n* 关节囊切开术;晶状体囊切开术 | renal ~ 肾被膜切开术

captamine hydrochloride [ˈkæptəmiːn] 盐酸卡普他明(脱色素药)

captan [ˈkæptæn] *n* 克菌丹(杀菌药)

captodiame hydrochloride [ˌkæptəuˈdaiəm] 盐酸卡普托胺(安定药,肌肉松弛药)

captodiamine hydrochloride [ˌkæptəuˈdaiəmiːn] 盐酸卡普托胺(安定药,肌肉松弛药)

captopril [ˈkæptəupril] *n* 卡托普利(抗高血压药)

capture [ˈkæptʃə] *n*, *vt* 俘获,夺获 | atrial ~ 心房夺获 / electron ~ 电子俘获

capuride [ˈkæpjuəraid] *n* 卡普脲(催眠镇静药)

caput [ˈkeipət, ˈkæp-] ([复] **capita** [ˈkæpitə]) *n* 【拉】头

CAR Canadian Association of Radiologists 加拿大放射学家协会

caraate [ˌkɑːrəˈɑːti] *n* 品他病(即 pinta)

Carabelli cusp (sign, tubercle) [kɑːrəˈbeli] (George C. Carabelli)卡腊贝利尖(征、结节)(磨牙舌侧副尖)

caramel [ˈkærəmel] *n* 焦糖(用作制药着色剂)

caramiphen [kəˈræmifən] *n* 卡拉美芬(镇咳药) | ~ edisylate, ~ ethanedisulfonate 二乙磺酸卡拉美芬(镇咳药) / ~ hydrochloride 盐酸卡拉美芬(主要用于治疗帕金森〈Parkinson〉病和帕金森综合征)

Carassini's spool [kærəˈsini] 肠端吻合轴

carat [ˈkærət] *n* 开(金属纯度单位,24 开为纯金);克拉(珠宝的重量单位,=205.5 mg)

caraway [ˈkærəwei] *n* 葛缕子,贳蒿(药物调味剂)

carbacephem [ˌkɑːbəˈsefəm] *n* 卡巴头孢菌素(抗生素类药)

carbachol [ˈkɑːbəkɔl] *n* 卡巴胆碱(拟胆碱药,局部使用于结膜,以使瞳孔收缩)

carbadox [ˈkɑːbədɔks] *n* 卡巴多司(兽用抗菌药)

carbamate [ˈkɑːbəmeit] *n* 氨基甲酸酯 | ethyl ~ 氨基甲酸乙酯

carbamazepine [ˌkɑːbəˈmæzəpiːn] *n* 卡马西平(用作抗惊厥和镇痛药)

carbamic acid [kɑːˈbæmik] 氨基甲酸

carbamide [ˈkɑːbəmaid] *n* 脲,尿素

carbaminohemoglobin [kɑːˌbæminəuˌhiːməuˈgləubin] *n* 氨[基]甲酰血红蛋白

carbamoyl [ˈkɑːbəmɔil] *n* 氨甲酰基

carbamoylaspartate [kɑːˌbæməiləˈspɑːteit] *n* 氨甲酰天冬氨酸

carbamoylation [kɑːˌbæməiˈleiʃən] *n* 氨甲酰化

carbamoyl-phosphate synthase (ammonia) [kɑːˈbæməil ˈfɔsfeit ˈsinθeis] 氨甲酰-磷酸合酶(氨)(此酶缺乏为一种常染色体隐性性状,可致高氨血症Ⅱ型)

carbamoyl-phosphate synthetase (glutamine-hydrolyzing) [ˈgluːtəmiːnˈhaidrəlaiziŋ] 氨甲酰-磷酸合成酶(谷氨酰胺水解的)

carbamoyl phosphate synthetase (CPS) [kɑːˈbæməii ˈfɔsfeit ˈsinθiteis] 氨甲酰磷酸合成酶(①氨甲酰磷酸合酶〈氨〉,亦可写成 carbamoyl phoaphate synthetase Ⅰ〈CPS Ⅰ〉;②氨甲酰磷酸合酶〈谷氨酰胺水解的〉,亦可写成 carbamoyl phosphate synthetase Ⅱ〈CPS Ⅱ〉)

carbamoyl phosphate synthetase deficiency [ˈkɑːbəmɔil ˈfɔsfeit ˈsinθiteis] 氨甲酰磷酸合成酶缺乏症(亦称先天性高氨血症Ⅰ型)

carbamoyltransferase [kɑːˌbæməilˈtrænsfəreis] *n* 氨甲酰基转移酶(亦称转氨甲酰酶)

carbamyl [ˈkɑːbəmil] *n* 氨甲酰基

carbamylation [kɑːˌbæmiˈleiʃən] *n* 氨甲酰化

carbamylcholine chloride [ˌkɑːbəmil ˈkəuliːn] 氯化氨甲酰胆碱,卡巴胆碱(即 carbachol)

carbantel lauryl sulfate [ˈkɑːbəntəl] 十二烷基硫酸卡班太尔(抗蠕虫药)

carbaril [ˈkɑːbəril] *n* 卡巴立(杀虫药) | **carbaryl** *n*

carbarsone [ˈkɑːbəsəun] *n* 卡巴胂(抗阿米巴药)

carbaspirin calcium [kɑːˈbæspərin] 卡巴匹林钙

（解热镇痛药）
carbazide [ˈkɑːbəzaid] *n* 卡巴氮，二肼羰
carbazochrome salicylate [kəˈbæzəkrəum] 卡络柳钠（毛细管止血药）
carbazocine [kɑːˈbɑːzəsiːn] *n* 卡巴佐辛（镇痛药）
carbazole [ˈkɑːbəzəul] *n* 咔唑
carbazotate [kɑːˈbæzəteit] *n* 苦味酸盐
carbenicillin [ˌkɑːbeniˈsilin] *n* 羧苄西林 | ~ disodium 羧苄西林二钠 / ~ indanyl sodium 卡茚西林钠 / ~ phenyl sodium 卡非西林钠 / ~ potassium 羧苄西林钾 / ~ sodium 羧苄西林钠
carbenoxolone sodium [ˌkɑːbəˈnɔksələun] 甘珀酸钠（抗溃疡病药）
carbetapentane [kɑːˌbeitəˈpentein] *n* 喷托维林（镇咳药）
carbethyl salicylate [kɑːˈbeθil] 柳碳乙酯（镇痛药，抗关节炎药）
carbhemoglobin [ˌkɑːbhiːməuˈgləubin] *n* 碳酸血红蛋白
carbide [ˈkɑːbaid] *n* 碳化物
carbidopa [kɑːbiˈdəupə] *n* 卡比多巴（脱羧酶抑制药）
carbimazol [kɑːˈbaiməzəul] *n* 卡比马唑（抗甲状腺药）
carbinol [ˈkɑːbinɔl] *n* 甲醇；原醇 | acetylmethyl ~ 乙酰甲基原醇 / dimethyl ~ 二甲基原醇，异丙醇
carbinoxamine maleate [ˌkɑːbiˈnɔksəmiːn] 马来酸卡比沙明（抗组胺药）
carbo [ˈkɑːbəu] *n*【拉】碳，木炭
carbocholine [ˌkɑːbəuˈkəuliːn] *n* 氯化氨甲酰胆碱，卡巴胆碱（即 carbachol）
carbocloral [ˌkɑːbəuˈklɔrəl] *n* 卡波氯醛（催眠药）
carbocromen hydrochloride [ˌkɑːbəuˈkrəumiːn] 盐酸卡波罗孟（抗心绞痛药）
carbocyclic [ˌkɑːbəuˈsaiklik, -ˈsik-] *a* 碳环型的
carbocysteine [ˌkɑːbəusisˈtiːin] *n* 羧甲司坦，羧甲半胱氨酸（祛痰药）
carbodiimide [ˌkɑːbəudaiˈimaid] *n* 碳化二亚胺
carbogaseous [ˌkɑːbəuˈgæsjəs] *a* 含二氧化碳气的
carbogen [ˈkɑːbədʒən] *n* 卡波金（含 5% 二氧化碳的氧）
carbohemia [ˌkɑːbəuˈhiːmiə] *n* 碳酸血症，二氧化碳血症
carbohemoglobin [ˌkɑːbəuhiːməuˈgləubin] *n* 碳酸血红蛋白
carbohydrase [ˌkɑːbəuˈhaidreis] *n* 糖酶
carbohydrate [ˌkɑːbəuˈhaidreit] *n* 糖类 | reserve ~s 贮存糖类
carbohydraturia [ˌkɑːbəuhaidrəˈtjuəriə] *n* 糖类尿，糖尿
carbohydrogenic [ˌkɑːbəuˌhaidrəˈdʒenik] *a* 生糖的
carbolate [ˈkɑːbəleit] *n* 石炭酸盐，酚盐 *vt* 加石炭酸，加酚
carbol-fuchsin [ˌkɑːbəl ˈfuːksin] *n* 石炭酸品红
carbolic acid [kɑːˈbɔlik] 石炭酸
carboligase [ˌkɑːbəˈlaigeis] *n* 醛连接酶
carbolism [ˈkɑːbəlizəm] *n* 石炭酸中毒，酚中毒
carbolize [ˈkɑːbəlaiz] *vt* 加石炭酸，加酚；用石炭酸处理，用酚处理
carboluria [ˌkɑːbəuˈljuəriə] *n* 石炭酸尿，酚尿
carbolxylene [ˌkɑːbɔlˈzailiːn] *n* 石炭酸二甲苯混合液（清洁显微镜切片用）
carbomer [ˈkɑːbəmə] *n* 卡波姆（制药时用作乳化剂和悬浮剂）
carbomycin [ˌkɑːbəuˈmaisin] *n* 卡波霉素（抗生素类药）
carbon(C) [ˈkɑːbən] *n* 碳 | ^{13}C（碳的天然同位素）/ ^{14}C（碳的放射性同位素）/ ~ dioxide 二氧化碳 / ~ disulfide 二硫化碳 / ~ monoxide 一氧化碳 / ~ oxysulfide 氧硫化碳 / radioactive ~ 放射性碳 / ~ tetrachloride 四氯化碳 / ~ trichloride 六氯乙烷
carbonaceous [ˌkɑːbəˈneiʃəs] *a* 碳质的；碳色的
carbonate [ˈkɑːbənit] *n* 碳酸盐 | ferrous ~ 碳酸亚铁（用于治缺铁性贫血）
carbonate dehydratase [ˈkɑːbəneit diːˈhaidrəteis] 碳酸脱水酶
carbonemia [ˌkɑːbəuˈniːmiə] *n* 碳酸血症，二氧化碳血症
carbonic [kɑːˈbɔnik] *a* 碳的 | ~ acid 碳酸
carbonic anhydrase [kɑːˈbɔnik ænˈhaidreis] 碳酸酐酶（亦称碳酸脱水酶）
carbonize [ˈkɑːbənaiz] *vt* 使碳化 | **carbonization** [kɑːbənaiˈzeiʃən, -niˈz-] *n* 碳化［作用］
carbonuria [ˌkɑːbəˈnjuəriə] *n* 碳酸尿［症］| dysoxidative ~ 氧化不足性碳酸尿［症］
carbonyl [ˈkɑːbənil] *n* 碳酰，羰基 | ~ chloride 碳酰氯，光气 | **~ic** [kɑːbəˈnilik] *a*
carbophilic [kɑːbəuˈfilik] *a* 嗜碳酸气的（指细菌）
carboplatin [ˈkɑːbəuˌplætin] *n* 卡铂（抗肿瘤药）
carboprost [ˈkɑːbəuprɔst] *n* 卡前列素（催产药）| ~ methyl 卡前列素甲酯（催产药）/ ~ tromethamine 卡前列素氨丁三醇（催产药）
carboxydismutase [kɑːˌbɔksiˈdismjuteis] *n* 羧基歧化酶，核酮糖二磷酸羧化酶
Carboxydomonas [kɑːˌbɔksidəˈməunəs] *n* 碳氧单胞菌属
γ-carboxyglutamate [kɑːˌbɔksiˈgluːtəmeit] *n* γ-

羧基谷氨酸

γ-carboxyglutamic acid [kɑːˌbɔksigluːˈtæmik] γ-羧基谷氨酸

carboxyhemoglobin [kɑːˌbɔksiˌhiːməuˈgləubin] *n* 碳氧血红蛋白

carboxyhemoglobinemia [kɑːˌbɔksiˌhiːməuˌgləubiˈniːmiə] *n* 碳氧血红蛋白血[症]

carboxyl [kɑːˈbɔksil] *n* 羧基

carboxylase [kɑːˈbɔksileis] *n* 羧化酶 | multiple ~ deficiency(MCD) 多发性羧化酶缺乏症(临床征象包括发育迟缓、弥漫性红疹、脱发和酮酸中毒症,亦称全羧化酶合成酶缺乏症)

carboxylate [kɑːˈbɔksileit] *n* 羧化物;羧酸盐(或酯) | **carboxylation** [kɑːˌbɔksiˈleiʃən] *n* 羧化[作用]

carboxylesterase [kɑːˌbɔksiˈlestəreis] *n* 羧酸酯酶

carboxylic [kɑːbɔkˈsilik] *a* (含)羧基的 | ~ acid 羧酸

carboxylic ester hydrolase [kɑːbɔkˈsilik ˈestə ˈhaidrəleis] 羧酸酯水解酶,羧酸酯酶

carboxyl (acid) proteinase [kɑːˈbɔksilˈprəutiːˌneis] 羧基[酸]蛋白酶,天冬氨酸蛋白酶

carboxyltransferase [kɑːˌbɔksilˈtrænsfəreis] *n* 羧基转移酶

carboxy-lyase [kɑːˈbɔksi ˈlaieis] *n* 羧基裂合酶

carboxymethylcellulose [kɑːˌbɔksiˌmeθilˈseljuləus] *n* 羧甲纤维素(药物制剂时用作悬浮剂、片剂赋形剂和黏度增加剂)

carboxymyoglobin [kɑːˌbɔksiˌmaiəuˈgləubin] *n* 碳氧肌红蛋白

carboxypeptidase [kɑːˌbɔksiˈpeptideis] *n* 羧肽酶 | metallo ~ 金属羧肽酶 / serine ~ 丝氨酸羧肽酶

carboxypeptidase A [kɑːˌbɔksiˈpeptideis] *n* 羧肽酶 A

carboxypeptidase B [kɑːˌbɔksiˈpeptideis] *n* 羧肽酶 B

carboxypeptidase N [kɑːˌbɔksiˈpeptideis] *n* 羧肽酶 N,精氨酸羧肽酶

carboxypolypeptidase [kɑːˌbɔksiˌpɔliˈpeptideis] *n* 羧基多肽酶

carbromal [kɑːˈbrəumæl] *n* 卡溴脲(催眠镇静药)

carbuncle [ˈkɑːbʌŋkl] *n* 痈 | malignant ~ 恶性痈(人类炭疽) | **carbuncular** [kɑːˈbʌŋkjulə] *a*

carbunculoid [kɑːˈbʌŋkjulɔid] *a* 似痈的

carbunculosis [kɑːˌbʌŋkjuˈləusis] *n* 痈病

carbutamide [kɑːˈbjutəmaid] *n* 氨磺丁脲(降血糖药)

carbuterol hydrochloride [kɑːˈbjuːtərəul] 盐酸卡布特罗(拟肾上腺素药,支气管扩张药)

carcass, carcase [ˈkɑːkəs] *n* 屠体,动物尸体

Carcassonne's ligament [kɑːkəˈsɔn] (Bernard G. Carcassonne) 耻骨前列腺韧带 | ~ perineal ligament 骨盆横韧带

carceag, carciag [ˈkɑːsiəg] *n* 羊巴贝虫病,绵羊梨浆虫病

carcinectomy [ˌkɑːsiˈnektəmi] *n* 癌切除术

carcinemia [ˌkɑːsiˈniːmiə] *n* 癌血症,癌性恶病质

carcin(o)- [构词成分]癌

carcinocythemia [ˌkɑːsinəusaiˈθiːmiə] *n* 癌细胞血[症]

carcinoembryonic [ˌkɑːsinəuembriˈɔnik] *a* 癌胚的(抗原)

carcinogen [kɑːˈsinədʒən] *n* 致癌剂,致癌物,致癌原

carcinogenesis [ˌkɑːsinəuˈdʒenisis] *n* 致癌作用,癌发生

carcinogenic [ˌkɑːsinəuˈdʒenik] *a* 致癌的

carcinogenicity [ˌkɑːsinəudʒiˈnisəti] *n* 致癌性

carcinoid [ˈkɑːsinɔid] *n* 类癌

carcinolysin [ˌkɑːsiˈnɔlisin] *n* 溶癌素

carcinolysis [ˌkɑːsiˈnɔlisis] *n* 癌细胞溶解 | **carcinolytic** [ˌkɑːsinəuˈlitik] *a* 溶癌的

carcinoma [kɑːsiˈnəumə] ([复] **carcinomas** 或 **carcinomata** [ˌkɑːsiˈnəumətə]) *n* 癌 | acinar ~, acinous ~ 腺泡癌 / adenoid cystic ~, adenocystic ~ 腺样囊性癌,腺囊性癌 / ~ of adrenal cortex 肾上腺皮质癌 / alveolar ~ 蜂窝状癌 / alveolar cell ~ 肺泡细胞癌 / basal cell ~, hair-matrix ~ 基底细胞癌 / basaloid ~ 类基底细胞癌 / basosquamous cell ~ 基底鳞状细胞癌 / breast ~ 乳腺癌 / bronchioalveolar ~, bronchiolar ~ 细支气管肺泡癌,细支气管癌 / bronchogenic ~ 支气管癌 / cerebriform ~ 髓样癌 / cholangiocellular ~ 胆管细胞癌 / corpus ~ 宫体癌 / cribriform ~ 筛状癌 / cylindrical(cell) ~ 柱状细胞癌 / duct ~ 管癌(乳腺) / ~ en cuirasse 铠甲状癌 / exophytic ~ 外生性癌 / giant cell ~ 巨细胞癌 / granulosa cell ~ 粒层细胞癌 / hepatocellular ~ 肝细胞癌 / hypernephroid ~ 肾上腺样癌 / infantile embryonal ~ 幼稚型胚胎性癌 / ~ in situ, preinvasive ~ 原位癌 / intraepidermal ~ 表皮内癌 / intraepithelial ~ 上皮内癌 / large-cell ~ 大细胞癌 / lymphoepithelial ~ 淋巴上皮癌 / medullary ~, ~ molle 髓样癌,软癌 / mucinous ~, mucous ~, colloid ~, gelatinous ~ 黏液癌,胶样癌 / mucoepidermoid ~ 黏液表皮样癌 / nasopharyngeal ~ 鼻咽癌 / oat cell ~, reserve cell ~ 燕麦细胞癌,储备细胞癌 / signet-ring cell ~ 印戒细胞癌 / spindle cell ~ 梭形细胞癌 / squamous(cell) ~, prickle cell ~ 鳞状细胞癌,棘细胞癌 / string ~ 绳捆癌(大肠〈最常见为升结肠或横结肠〉

的一种癌,形似绳捆) / transitional cell ~ 移形细胞癌,过渡型细胞癌 / tuberous ~ 结节性皮癌 | **~tous** [kɑːsiˈnəumətəs] *a*

carcinomatoid [ˌkɑːsiˈnɔmətɔid] *a* 癌样的

carcinomatophobia [ˌkɑːsiˌnəumətəuˈfəubjə], **carcinophobia** [ˌkɑːsinəuˈfəubjə] *n* 癌症恐怖,恐癌症

carcinomatosis [ˌkɑːsinəuməˈtəusis] *n* 癌病

carcinomectomy [ˌkɑːsinəuˈmektəmi] *n* 癌切除术

carcinophilia [ˌkɑːsinəuˈfiliə] *n* 嗜癌性 | **carcinophilic** *a*

carcinosarcoma [ˌkɑːsinəusɑːˈkəumə] *n* 癌肉瘤 | embryonal ~ 胚胎性癌肉瘤

carcinosis [ˌkɑːsiˈnəusis] *n* 癌病 | miliary ~ 粟粒性癌病 / ~ pleurae 胸膜癌病 / pulmonary ~ 肺癌病,肺泡细胞癌

carcinostatic [ˌkɑːsinəuˈstætik] *a* 制癌的

carcinous [ˈkɑːsinəs] *a* 癌[性]的

card [kɑːd] *n* 卡,卡片 | test ~ 视力卡

cardamom [ˈkɑːdəməm] *n* 豆蔻,小豆蔻

Cardarelli's sign (symptom) [kɑːdɑːˈreli] (Antonio Cardarelli)卡达雷利征(症状)(动脉瘤和主动脉弓扩张时喉气管的侧方搏动)

cardelmycin [kɑːdəlˈmaisin] *n* 新生霉素

Carden's amputation [ˈkɑːdn] (Henry D. Carden)卡登切断术(单瓣切断术,紧邻膝关节上方切断股骨)

cardia [ˈkɑːdiə] *n* 贲门;胃贲门部 | ~ of stomach 贲门

cardiac [ˈkɑːdiæk] *a* 心[脏]的;贲门的 *n* 强心药;心脏病患者

cardialgia [ˌkɑːdiˈældʒiə] *n* 心痛

cardiant [ˈkɑːdiənt] *n* 心兴奋药

cardiasthenia [ˌkɑːdiæsˈθiːniə] *n* 心神经衰弱

cardiasthma [kɑːdiˈæsmə] *n* 心病性哮喘

cardiectasis [ˌkɑːdiˈektəsis] *n* 心扩张

cardiectomized [ˌkɑːdiˈektəmaizd] *a* 心部分切除的(动物实验中)

cardiectomy [ˌkɑːdiˈektəmi] *n* 贲门切除术

cardinal [ˈkɑːdinl] *a* 主要的

cardi(o)- [构词成分]心脏;胃贲门部

cardioaccelerator [ˌkɑːdiəuækˈselereitə] *a* 心动加速的 *n* 心动加速药

cardioactive [ˌkɑːdiəuˈæktiv] *a* 作用于心脏的

cardioangiography [ˌkɑːdiəuˌændʒiˈɔgrəfi] *n* 心血管造影[术]

cardioangiology [ˌkɑːdiəuˌændʒiˈɔlədʒi] *n* 心血管学

cardioaortic [ˌkɑːdiəueiˈɔːtik] *a* 心主动脉的

cardioarterial [ˌkɑːdiəuɑːˈtiəriəl] *a* 心动脉的

Cardiobacterium [ˌkɑːdiəubækˈtiəriəm] *n* 心杆菌属 | ~ hominis 人心杆菌

cardiocairograph [ˌkɑːdiəuˈkaiərəgrɑːf, -græf] *n* 心选择性显影机

cardiocele [ˈkɑːdiəˌsiːl] *n* 心突出

cardiocentesis [ˌkɑːdiəusenˈtiːsis] *n* 心穿刺术

cardiochalasia [ˌkɑːdiəukəˈleiziə] *n* 贲门松弛

cardiocinetic [ˌkɑːdiəusiˈnetik] *a* 促心动的 *n* 强心药

cardiocirculatory [ˌkɑːdiəuˈsəːkjulətəri] *a* 心循环的

cardiocirrhosis [ˌkɑːdiəusiˈrəusis] *n* 心源性肝硬化

cardiocyte [ˈkɑːdiəuˌsait] *n* 心肌细胞,肌细胞

cardiodiaphragmatic [ˌkɑːdiəuˌdaiəfrægˈmætik] *a* 心膈的

cardiodilatin [ˌkɑːdiəuˈdailətin] *n* 心扩张素

cardiodilator [ˌkɑːdiəudaiˈleitə] *n* 贲门扩张器

cardiodiosis [ˌkɑːdiəudaiˈəusis] *n* 贲门扩张术

cardiodynamics [ˌkɑːdiəudaiˈnæmiks] *n* 心[脏]动力学

cardiodynia [ˌkɑːdiəuˈdiniə] *n* 心痛

cardioesophageal [ˌkɑːdiəui(ː)ˌsɔfəˈdʒi(ː)əl] *a* 贲门食管的

cardiogenesis [ˌkɑːdiəuˈdʒenisis] *n* 心脏发生(胚胎) | **cardiogenic** *a* 心源性的;心脏发生的

cardiogram [ˈkɑːdiəgræm] *n* 心动图,心动描记曲线 | apex ~ 心尖搏动图 / esophageal ~ 食管心动图 / negative ~ 负性心动图 / precordial ~ 心振动图 / vector ~ 心电向量图

cardiograph [ˈkɑːdiəgrɑːf, -græf] *n* 心动描记器

cardiography [kɑːdiˈɔgrəfi] *n* 心动描记术 | apex ~ 心尖搏动描记术 / ultrasonic ~ 超声心动描记术 / vector ~ 心电向量描记术 | **cardiographic** [ˌkɑːdiəuˈgræfik] *a* 心动描记的

cardiohepatic [ˌkɑːdiəuhiˈpætik] *a* 心肝的

cardiohepatomegaly [ˌkɑːdiəuˌhepətəuˈmegəli] *n* 心肝肿大

cardioid [ˈkɑːdiɔid] *a* 心脏形的

cardioinhibitor [ˌkɑːdiəuinˈhibitə] *n* 心动抑制药

cardioinhibitory [ˌkɑːdiəuinˈhibitəri] *a* 心动抑制的

cardiokinetic [ˌkɑːdiəukaiˈnetik] *a* 促心动的 *n* 强心药

cardiokymography [ˌkɑːdiəukaiˈmɔgrəfi] *n* 心动描记术 | **cardiokymographic** [ˌkɑːdiəuˌkaiməuˈgræfik] *a*

cardiolipin [ˌkɑːdiəuˈlipin] *n* 心磷脂(由新鲜牛心提取的一种物质,与卵磷脂和胆固醇结合时,形成一种抗原,用于絮状反应试验和沉淀试验以检梅毒)

cardiology [ˌkɑːdiˈɔlədʒi] *n* 心脏病学 | **cardiologist** *n* 心脏病学家

cardiolysin [ˌkɑːdiˈɔlisin] *n* 溶心肌素
cardiolysis [ˌkɑːdiˈɔlisis] *n* 心松解术(松解心包与纵隔粘连的手术,即切除心包前的肋骨和胸骨)
cardiomalacia [ˌkɑːdiəumәˈleiʃiә] *n* 心肌软化
cardiomegalia [ˌkɑːdiəumiˈgeiliә] *n* 心肥大 | ~ glycogenica circumscripta 糖原储积性心肥大 / ~ glycogenica diffusa 糖原贮积症Ⅱ型
cardiomegaly [ˌkɑːdiəuˈmegәli] *n* 心肥大 | glycogenic ~ 糖原储积性心肥大
cardiomelanosis [ˌkɑːdiəuˌmelәˈnәusis] *n* 心[脏]黑变(心肌黑色素沉着)
cardiometer [ˌkɑːdiˈɔmitә] *n* 心力测量器,心力计 | **cardiometry** *n* 心力测量法
cardiomotility [ˌkɑːdiəumәuˈtilәti] *n* 心脏活动,心脏移动
cardiomyoliposis [ˌkɑːdiəuˌmaiəuliˈpәusis] *n* 心肌脂变
cardiomyopathy [ˌkɑːdiəumaiˈɔpәθi] *n* 心肌病(常指原因不明的原发性心肌病) | alcoholic ~ 酒精中毒性心肌病 / congestive ~ 充血性心肌病 / infiltrative ~ 浸润性心肌病 / peripartum ~ 围生期心肌病 / postpartum ~ 产后心肌病 / primary ~ 原发性心肌病 / restrictive ~ 限制型心肌病 / secondary ~ 继发性心肌病
cardiomyopexy [ˌkɑːdiәˈmaiәˌpeksi] *n* 心肌固定术
cardiomyotomy [ˌkɑːdiəumaiˈɔtәmi] *n* 贲门肌切开术
cardionatrin [ˌkɑːdiəuˈneitrin] *n* 心钠素(亦称心房促钠尿排泄因子)
cardionecrosis [ˌkɑːdiəuneˈkrәusis] *n* 心坏死
cardionector [ˌkɑːdiəuˈnektә] *n* 心传导系统
cardionephric [ˌkɑːdiəuˈnefrik] *a* 心肾的
cardioneural [ˌkɑːdiəuˈnjuәrәl] *a* 心神经的
cardioneurosis [ˌkɑːdiəunjuәˈrәusis] *n* 心[脏]神经症,神经性循环衰弱
cardio-omentopexy [ˌkɑːdiəuәuˈmentәˌpeksi] *n* 心网膜固定术
cardiopaludism [ˌkɑːdiəuˈpæljudizәm] *n* 疟疾性心脏病
cardiopath [ˈkɑːdiәpæθ] *n* 心脏病患者
cardiopathy [ˌkɑːdiˈɔpәθi] *n* 心脏病 | infarctoid ~ 类梗死性心脏病 | **cardiopathia** [ˌkɑːdiәˈpæθiә] *n* / **cardiopathic** [ˌkɑːdiәˈpæθik] *a*
cardiopericardiopexy [ˌkɑːdiəuˌperiˈkɑːdiәˌpeksi] *n* 心心包固定术
cardiopericarditis [ˌkɑːdiəuˌperikɑːˈdaitis] *n* 心心包炎
cardiophobia [ˌkɑːdiəuˈfәubjә] *n* 心脏病恐怖
cardiophrenia [ˌkɑːdiəuˈfriːniә] *n* 心血管神经衰弱
cardioplasty [ˈkɑːdiәˌplæsti] *n* 贲门成形术
cardioplegia [ˌkɑːdiəuˈpliːdʒiә] *n* 心脏停搏[法] | **cardioplegic** [ˌkɑːdiəuˈpledʒik] *a*
cardiopneumatic [ˌkɑːdiəunju(ː)ˈmætik] *a* 心肺的
cardiopneumograph [ˌkɑːdiəuˈnjuːmәgrɑːf, -græf] *n* 心肺运动描记器
cardiopneumonopexy [ˌkɑːdiəunju(ː)ˈmɔnәˌpeksi] *n* 心肺叶固定术
cardioprotectant [ˌkɑːdiəuprәˈtektәnt], **cardioprotective** [ˌkɑːdiəuprәˈtektiv] *a* 保护心脏的; *n* 保心药
cardioptosis [ˌkɑːdiˈɔptәsis], **cardioptosia** [ˌkɑːdiɔpˈtәusiә] *n* 心脏下垂
cardiopulmonary [ˌkɑːdiəuˈpʌlmәnәri] *a* 心肺的
cardiopuncture [ˌkɑːdiəuˈpʌŋktʃә] *n* 心穿刺术
cardiopyloric [ˌkɑːdiəupaiˈlɔːrik] *a* 贲门幽门的
cardiorenal [ˌkɑːdiəuˈriːnәl] *a* 心肾的
cardiorespiratory [ˌkɑːdiəuˈrespirәtәri] *a* 心呼吸的,心肺的
cardiorrhaphy [ˌkɑːdiˈɔrәfi] *n* 心肌缝合术
cardiorrhexis [ˌkɑːdiəuˈreksis] *n* 心破裂
cardiosclerosis [ˌkɑːdiəuskliәˈrәusis] *n* 心硬化
cardioscope [ˈkɑːdiәskәup] *n* 心脏检查器,心脏镜
cardioselective [ˌkɑːdiəusiˈlektiv] *a* 心选择性的(对心脏组织比对其他组织具有更大的活性)
cardiospasm [ˈkɑːdiәspæzәm] *n* 贲门痉挛 | tropical ~ 热带性贲门痉挛,热带性咽下困难
cardiosphygmogram [ˌkɑːdiəuˈsfigmәgræm] *n* 心动脉搏图
cardiosphygmograph [ˌkɑːdiəuˈsfigmәgrɑːf, -græf] *n* 心动脉搏描记器
cardiosplenopexy [ˌkɑːdiəuˈsplenәˌpeksi] *n* 心脾固定术
cardiotachometer [ˌkɑːdiəutәˈkɔmitә] *n* 心动计数计,心率计 | **cardiotachometry** *n* 心动计数法,心率测量法
cardiotherapy [ˌkɑːdiəuˈθerәpi] *n* 心脏病疗法
cardiothyrotoxicosis [ˌkɑːdiəuˌθairәuˌtɔksiˈkәusis] *n* 心[脏]甲状腺中毒病(甲状腺功能亢进性心脏并发症)
cardiotocograph [ˌkɑːdiəuˈtәukәgrɑːf, -græf] *n* 心分娩力描记器
cardiotocography, cardiotokography [ˌkɑːdiəutәˈkɔgrәfi] *n* 心分娩力描记法
cardiotomy [ˌkɑːdiˈɔtәmi] *n* 心切开术;贲门切开术
cardiotonic [ˌkɑːdiəuˈtɔnik] *a* 强心的 *n* 强心药
cardiotopometry [ˌkɑːdiəutәˈpɔmitri] *n* 心浊音区测定法

cardiotoxic [ˌkɑːdiəu'tɔksik] *a* 心脏[中]毒的
cardiotoxicity [ˌkɑːdiəutɔk'sisəti] *n* 心脏[中]毒性
cardiovalvular [ˌkɑːdiəu'vælvjulə] *a* 心瓣的
cardiovalvulitis [ˌkɑːdiəˌvælvju'laitis] *n* 心瓣炎
cardiovalvulotome [ˌkɑːdiəu'vælvjulətəum] *n* 心瓣刀
cardiovalvulotomy [ˌkɑːdiəuˌvælvju'lɔtəmi] *n* 心瓣切开术,心瓣膜分离术
cardiovascular [ˌkɑːdiəu'væskjulə] *a* 心血管的
cardiovascular-renal [ˌkɑːdiəu'væskjulə 'riːnl] *a* 心血管肾的
cardiovasology [ˌkɑːdiəuvæ'sɔlədʒi] *n* 心血管学
cardioversion ['kɑːdiəˌvəːʃən] *n* 心脏复律(用电休克使窦性节律复位)
cardioverter ['kɑːdiəˌvəːtə] *n* 心脏复律器(放出直流电震使心脏恢复正常节律)
Cardiovirus ['kɑːdiəuˌvaiərəs] *n* 心脏病毒属
cardiovirus ['kɑːdiəuˌvaiərəs] *n* 心脏病毒
carditis [kɑː'daitis] *n* 心炎 | rheumatic ~ 风湿性[全]心炎 / verrucous ~ 疣性心炎
care [kεə] *n* 关怀;照料;监护,护理;保健 | antenatal ~ 产前保健 / coronary ~ 冠心病监护 / critical ~, intensive ~ 危重症监护,重症监护 / medical ~ 医疗保健 / terminal ~ 临终照料
carfecillin sodium [ˌkɑːfi'silin] 卡非西林钠(抗生素类药)
carfentanil citrate [kɑː'fentənil] 枸橼酸卡芬太尼(镇痛药和麻醉药)
Carica ['kærikə] *n* 番木瓜属
caricous ['kærikəs] *a* 无花果状的
caries ['kεəriiːz] [单复同] *n* 【拉】龋;骨疡,骨疽 | backward ~, internal ~ 逆行性龋,内向性龋 / central ~ 中心性骨疽 / dental ~ 龋(牙) / dry ~ 干性骨疽 / lateral ~ 侧延龋 / spinal ~ 脊柱骨疽
carina [kə'rainə] ([复] **carinae** [kə'rainiː]) *n* 【拉】隆凸 | ~ of trachea 气管杈隆凸 / urethral ~ of vagina 阴道尿道隆凸 | **~l** *a*
carinate ['kærineit], **carinated** ['kærineitid] *a* 有隆凸的,船骨状的
carination [ˌkæri'neiʃən] *n* 嵴状,船骨状
carindacillin sodium [ˌkɑːrində'silin] 卡茚西林钠(抗生素类药)
cariogenesis [ˌkεəriəu'dʒenisis] *n* 龋发生
cariogenic [ˌkεəriəu'dʒenik] *a* 生龋的
cariogenicity [ˌkεəriəudʒe'nisəti] *n* 生龋性
cariology [ˌkæri'ɔlədʒi] *n* 龋病学
cariostatic [ˌkæriəu'stætik] *a* 止龋的
carious ['kεəriəs] *a* 龋的 | **cariosity** [ˌkεəri'ɔsəti] *n* 龋蚀性
carisoprodol [ˌkærai'səuprədɔl] *n* 卡立普多(骨骼肌松弛药)
Carlens' tube ['kɑːlənz] (Eric Carlens)卡伦士管(一种支气管导管,左肺通气用)
Carleton's spots ['kɑːltən] (Bukk G. Carleton)卡尔顿斑(淋病患者骨中的硬化斑)
carmalum [kɑː'mæləm] *n* 卡红明矾染液
Carman-Kirklin sign (meniscus sign) ['kɑːmən 'kəːklin] (R. D. Carman; Byrl R. Kirklin)卡-柯征(半月征)(即 meniscus sign,见 sign 项下相应术语)
Carman's sign ['kɑːmən] (Russell D. Carman)卡曼征,半月征(即 meniscus sign,见 sign 项下相应术语)
carmantadine [kɑː'mæntədiːn] *n* 卡金刚酸(抗震颤麻痹药)
Carmichael's crown ['kɑːmaikl] (J. P. Carmichael)克麦克尔冠(部分罩冠)
carminative ['kɑːminətiv] *a* 祛风的,排气的(减轻胃肠气胀) *n* 祛风药
carmine ['kɑːmain, 'kɑːmin] *n* 卡红,胭脂红 | alizarin ~ 茜素卡红,茜红 / indigo ~ 靛卡红,靛胭脂,靛蓝二磺酸钠 / lithium ~ 锂卡红(用于巨噬细胞的活体染料) | **carminum** [kɑː'mainəm] *n*
carminic acid [kɑː'minik] 胭脂红酸,卡红酸
carminophil [kɑː'minəfil] *a* 嗜卡红的 *n* 嗜卡红细胞;嗜卡红体
carmustine [kɑː'mʌstiːn] *n* 卡莫司汀(抗肿瘤药)
carnassial [kɑː'næsiəl] *a* 裂齿的 *n* 裂齿
carnauba [kɑː'naubə] *n* 巴西棕榈
carnaubic acid [kɑː'nɔːbik] 巴西棕榈酸
Carnegie stages ['kɑːnəgi] (华盛顿市卡内基研究所于 1913 ~ 1920 年间研究发展此分期)卡内基分期(根据解剖学特征如发育中肢体的出现所定义的 23 个编码的分期)
carneous ['kɑːniəs] *a* 肉的,肉性的
Carnett's sign [kɑː'net] (J. B. Carnett)卡奈特征(显示腹壁触痛或腹内病损的试验)
Carney's complex (syndrome, triad) ['kɑːni] (J. A. Carney)卡内复征(综合征、三联征)(一种常染色体显性症状复征,包括软组织黏液瘤,多斑点皮肤色素沉着,肾上腺、垂体和睾丸瘤以及周围神经神经鞘瘤)
carnidazole [kɑː'nidəzəul] *n* 卡硝唑(抗原虫药)
carnification [ˌkɑːnifi'keiʃən] *n* 肉质变
carnitine ['kɑːnitin] *n* 肉碱
carnitine acyltransferase ['kɑːnitiːn ˌæsil'trænsfəreis] 肉碱酰基转移酶,肉碱 *O*-棕榈酰基转移酶
carnitine *O*-palmitoyltransferase ['kɑːnitin ˌpælmiˌtəuil'trænsfəreis] 肉碱 *O*-棕榈酰基转移酶(此酶缺乏可致脂肪酸氧化作用缺损)

carnitine palmityltransferase deficiency [ˈkɑː-niːtiːn ˌpælmitilˈtrænsfəreis] 肉碱棕榈酰基转移酶缺乏症(一种脂质代谢病,已改变的酶经受异常调节,导致肌肉疼痛、容易疲劳和肌红蛋白尿,但经过长期锻炼,尤其是在冷天或禁食之后无脂质积贮。本症为一种常染色体隐性性状,妇女外显率减少)

Carnivora [kɑːˈnivərə] *n* 食肉目

carnivore [ˈkɑːnivɔː] *n* 食肉生物

carnivorous [kɑːˈnivərəs] *a* 食肉的

carnosinase [ˈkɑːnəsineis] *n* 肌肽酶,氨酰基组氨酸二肽酶(即 X-His dipeptidase) | serum ~ deficiency 血清肌肽酶缺乏症(一种常染色体隐性遗传性肌肽代谢氨基酸病,可致肌阵挛发作,严重精神发育迟缓和强直状态。亦称肌肽血症,高β-肌肽血症)

carnosine [ˈkɑːnəsin] *n* 肌肽

carnosinemia [ˌkɑːnəusiˈniːmiə] *n* 肌肽血

carnosinuria [ˌkɑːnəusiˈnjuəriə] *n* 肌肽尿

carnosity [kɑːˈnɔsəti] *n* 赘肉

Carnot's test [kɑːˈnɔː] (Paul Carnot) 卡诺试验(检胃弛张)

carnutine [kɑːˈnjuːtin] *n* 卡纽丁,α-羟基-γ-三甲基丁基甜菜碱(肌组织中的尸碱)

caro [ˈkɛərəu] ([复] **carnes** [ˈkɑːniːz]) *n*【拉】肌,肉

carob [ˈkærəb] *n* 角豆树

carolic acid [kəˈrɔlik] 肉霉酸

Caroli's disease [ˈkɑːrəli] (Jacques Caroli) 卡罗利病(先天性肝内胆管扩张)

carota [kəˈrəutə] ([复] **carotae** [kəˈrəutiː]) *n*【拉】胡萝卜

carotenase [kəˈrɔtineis] *n* 胡萝卜素酶

carotene [ˈkærətiːn] *n* 胡萝卜素

β-carotene 15, 15′-dioxygenase [ˈkærətiːn daiˈɔk-sidʒiˌneis] β-胡萝卜素 15,15′-双加氧酶

carotenemia [ˌkærətiˈniːmiə] *n* 胡萝卜素血[症]

carotenoderma [kəˈrɔtinəˌdəːmə], **carotenodermia** [kəˌrɔtinəˈdəːmiə] *n* 胡萝卜素性黄皮病

carotenoid [kəˈrɔtinɔid] *n* 类胡萝卜素 *a* 黄色的

carotenosis [ˌkærətiˈnəusis] *n* 胡萝卜素性黄皮病

carotic [kəˈrɔtik] *a* 迷睡的

caroticotympanic [kəˌrɔtikəutimˈpænik] *a* 颈鼓的,颈[动脉]鼓室的

caroticovertebral [kəˌrɔtikəuˈvəːtəbrəl] *a* 颈动脉椎动脉的

carotid [kəˈrɔtid] *a* 颈动脉的 *n* 颈动脉

carotidynia [kəˌrɔtiˈdiniə] *n* 颈动脉痛

carotin [ˈkærətin] *n* 胡萝卜素

carotinase [ˈkærətineis] *n* 胡萝卜素酶

carotinemia [ˌkærətiˈniːmiə] *n* 胡萝卜素血[症]

carotinosis [ˌkærətiˈnəusis] *n* 胡萝卜素沉着,皮橙色病,胡萝卜素血[症]

carotodynia [kəˌrɔtəˈdiniə] *n* 颈动脉痛

caroxazone [kəˈrɔksəzəun] *n* 卡罗沙酮(抗抑郁药)

carp [kɑːp] *n* 子实体(真菌)

carpal [ˈkɑːpl] *a* 腕的

carpale [kɑːˈpeil] *n* 腕骨

carpectomy [kɑːˈpektəmi] *n* 腕骨切除术

carpel [ˈkɑːpel] *n* 心皮;果爿(植物)

Carpenter's syndrome [ˈkɑːpentə] (George Carpenter) 卡彭特综合征,尖头多指并指[畸形] Ⅱ型,尖头多趾并趾[畸形] Ⅱ型

carphenazine maleate [kɑːˈfenəziːn] 马来酸卡奋乃静(抗精神病药)

carphology [kɑːˈfɔlədʒi], **carphologia** [ˌkɑːfəˈləudʒiə] *n* 摸空,捉空摸床(见于严重发热和极度衰竭)

carpitis [kɑːˈpaitis] *n* 腕关节炎(家畜)

carpocarpal [ˌkɑːpəuˈkɑːpl] *a* 腕腕的

Carpoglyphus [ˌkɑːpəˈglaifəs] *n* 果螨属 | ~ passularum 干果虫

carpogonium [ˌkɑːpəˈgəuniəm] *n* 育胚器(子囊菌的雌性生殖器)

carpometacarpal [ˌkɑːpəuˌmetəˈkɑːpl] *a* 腕掌的

carpopedal [ˌkɑːpəˈpedl] *a* 腕足的

carpophalangeal [ˌkɑːpəufəˈlændʒiəl] *a* 腕指的

carpoptosis [ˌkɑːpɔpˈtəusis] *n* 腕下垂

carpospore [ˈkɑːpəspɔː] *n* 果孢子

carprofen [kɑːˈprəufən] *n* 卡洛芬(抗炎药)

Carpue's operation, rhinoplasty [ˈkɑːpjuː] (Joseph C. Carpue) 卡普手术,卡普鼻成形术(印度式鼻成形术,额部皮瓣鼻成形术)

carpus [ˈkɑːpəs] ([复] **carpi** [ˈkɑːpai]) *n*【拉】腕;腕骨 | ~ curvas 曲腕畸形

carrageenan [ˌkærəˈgiːnən], **carragheenin** [ˌkærəˈgiːnin] *n* 角叉菜胶,爱兰苔胶(润药)

carrag(h)een [ˈkærəgiːn] *n* 角叉菜,爱兰苔

carrefour [ˌkærəˈfuə] *n*【法】十字路,交叉

Carrel-Dakin fluid [kəˈrel ˈdeikin] (Alexis Carrel; Henry D. Dakin) 卡莱尔-达金液(稀氯酸钠溶液) | ~ treatment 卡莱尔-达金疗法(清创法,见 Carrel's treatment)

Carrel's method [kəˈrel] (Alexis Carrel) 卡莱尔法(①血管对端吻合法;②清创法,见卡莱尔疗法;③创口第二期愈合时间测定法,即自伤口取标本涂于玻片上,染色及计算细菌的数目) | ~ treatment 卡莱尔疗法(清创法,即彻底打开创口,除去异物及死组织等,仔细清洗并用稀次氯酸钠反复冲洗) / ~ tube 卡莱尔管(卡莱尔疗法所用的有小孔的细橡皮管)

carrier [ˈkæriə] *n* 带菌者,带[病]毒者;载体;输

送器;携带者(指只带一个隐性基因的杂合型个体) | amalgam ~ 汞合金输送器(牙科用) / female ~ 女性携带者,女性带基因者(X染色体上某一隐性基因呈杂合状态的女性) / foil ~ 持箔器(牙科用) / gametocyte ~ 带配子体者(疟疾传染源) / hemophilia ~ 血友病传递者 / lentulo paste ~, paste ~ 根管糊剂螺旋形输送器

carrier-free [ˈkæriə friː] *a* 无载体的,不含载体的(放射性同位素)

Carrión's disease [kæriˈɔn] (Daniel A. Carrión) 卡里翁病(巴尔通体病,秘鲁疣)

carrot [ˈkærət] *n* 胡萝卜

carrotene [ˈkærətiːn] *n* 胡萝卜素

Carr-Price test [ˈkɑː ˈprais] (Francis H. Carr; E. A. Price) 卡尔-普赖斯试验(检油中维生素A的定量比色试验)

cart [kɑːt] *n* 手推车 | dressing ~ 敷料车 / resuscitation ~, crash ~ 抢救车,救生车

cartazolate [kɑːˈtæzəleit] *n* 卡它唑酯(抗抑郁药)

carteolol hydrochloride [ˈkɑːtiələul] 盐酸卡替洛尔(抗肾上腺素能药,β受体阻滞药)

Carter's operation [ˈkɑːtə] (William W. Carter) 卡特手术(鼻梁重建术,即自肋骨移植一骨片形成一人工鼻梁) | ~ intranasal splint 卡特鼻内夹(用于凹陷鼻梁的鼻梁夹板手术)

carthamic acid [kɑːˈθæmik] 红花酸

Carthamus [kɑːˈθeiməs] *n* 红花属

cartilage [ˈkɑːtilidʒ] *n* 软骨 | articular ~, arthrodial ~, investing ~, obducent ~ 关节软骨 / circumferential ~ 关节盂唇,盂缘 / conchal ~ 耳郭软骨 / costal ~, sternal ~ 肋软骨 / cricoid ~, innominate ~ 环状软骨 / epactal ~s, minor ~s, accessory nasal ~s, sesamoid ~s of nose 鼻副软骨,鼻籽软骨 / eustachian ~, tubal ~ 咽鼓管软骨 / falciform ~s 镰状软骨 / intervertebral ~s 椎间盘(椎间纤维软骨) / ossifying ~, temporary ~, precursory ~ 骨化软骨,暂时性软骨 / palpebral ~s, tarsal ~s 睑板 / sigmoid ~ 关节半月板 / slipping rib ~ 肋软骨松动变形 / stratified ~ 纤维软骨 / subvomerine ~s, vomeronasal ~ 犁鼻软骨 / supra-arytenoid ~ 小角状软骨 / xiphoid ~ 胸骨剑突 / Y ~ Y形软骨(髋臼)

cartilagin [ˈkɑːtiˌlædʒin] *n* 软骨素原

cartilaginification [ˌkɑːtiləˌdʒinifiˈkeiʃən] *n* 软骨化

cartilaginiform [ˌkɑːtiləˈdʒinifɔːm], **cartilaginoid** [ˌkɑːtiˈlædʒinɔid] *a* 软骨样的

cartilaginous [ˌkɑːtiˈlædʒinəs] *a* 软骨的

cartilago [kɑːtiˈleigəu] ([复] **cartilagines** [ˌkɑːtiˈlædʒiniːz]) *n* 【拉】软骨

cartilagotropic [ˌkɑːtilægəuˈtrɔpik] *a* 亲软骨的

Cartwright blood group [ˈkɑːtrait] (从1956年首次观察到的先证者得名) Yt血型

carubicin hydrochloride [kəˈruːbisin] 盐酸卡柔比星(一种蒽环类抗生素,具有抗肿瘤效用,试验性用于治疗急性白血病和实体瘤)

Carukia [kəˈruːkiə] *n* 水母属

Carum [ˈkɑːrəm] *n* 页蒿属

caruncle [ˈkærəŋk] *n* 小阜,肉阜 | hymenal ~s, myrtiform ~s 处女膜痕 / lacrimal ~ 泪阜 / major ~ of Santorini 十二指肠乳头 / morgagnian ~ 中叶(前列腺) / sublingual ~ 舌下阜 | **caruncular** [kəˈrʌŋkjulə], **caruncuIous** [kəˈrʌŋkjuləs], **carunculate** [kəˈrʌŋkjulit] *a*

caruncula [kəˈrʌŋkjulə] ([复] **carunculae** [kəˈrʌŋkjuliː]) *n* 【拉】小阜,肉阜

Carus curve (circle) [ˈkɑːrus] (Karl G. Carus) 卡鲁斯环(骨盆轴曲线)

Carvallo sign [kɑˈvɑːjəu] (J. M. Rivero-Carvallo) 卡氏征(三尖瓣反流时,吸气可使全收缩期杂音增加)

carvedilol [ˈkɑːvəˌdilɔl] *n* 卡维地洛(β受体阻滞药,用以治疗原发性高血压,并用作辅助药治疗轻度或中度充血性心力衰竭,口服给药)

carver [ˈkɑːvə] *n* 雕刻器(牙科用)

carvone [ˈkɑːvəun] *n* 页蒿[萜]酮,香芹酮

cary(o)- [构词成分]核(见 karyo-)

caryochrome [ˈkæriəkrəum] *n* 核染[色]细胞

Caryococcus [ˌkæriəuˈkɔkəs] *n* 核球菌属

Caryophanaceae [ˌkæriəufəˈneisiiː] *n* 显核菌科

Caryophanales [ˌkæriəufəˈneiliːz] *n* 显核菌目

Caryophanon [ˌkæriˈɔfənɔn] *n* 显核菌属

caryophil [ˈkæriəfil] *a* 嗜噻嗪铵(染料)的

caryophyllic acid [ˌkæriəuˈfilik] 丁香酸

Carysomyia [ˌkærisəˈmaijə] *n* 金蝇属(即 Chrysomyia)

carzenide [ˈkɑːzinaid] *n* 卡西尼特(碳酸酐酶抑制剂)

CASA computer-aided (or assisted) semen analysis 计算机辅助精液分析; computer-assisted sperm analysis 计算机辅助精子分析

Casal's necklace (collar) [kəˈsæl] (Gaspar Casal) 颈蜀黍红疹

casanthranol [kəˈsænθrənəul] *n* 鼠李蒽酚

cascade [kæsˈkeid] *n* 串联,级联

cascara [kæsˈkɑːrə] *n* 【西】波希鼠李皮 | ~ amarga 苦皮 / ~ sagrada 波希鼠李皮

case[1] [keis] *n* 病例,病案,患者;修复体 | basket ~ 全肢断离者 / borderline ~ 疑似病例 / custodial ~ 管制病案,监护病例 / index ~ 索引病例,先证者(指一个家系中最先发现某种遗传病患者)

case² [keis] *n* 箱,盒 | trial ~ 试镜箱(测验视力)
casease [ˈkeisieis] *n* 酪蛋白酶
caseation [ˌkeisiˈeiʃən] *n* 干酪性坏死;干酪化
casebook [ˈkeisbuk] *n* 病案簿
caseidin [keiˈsiːidin] *n* 酪蛋白免疫素
casein [ˈkeisiin, keiˈsiːn] *n* 酪蛋白 | ~-calcium 酪蛋白钙 / gluten ~ 谷胶酪蛋白 / serum ~ 血清酪蛋白,副球蛋白 / ~ sodium 酪蛋白钠 / vegetable ~ 植物酪蛋白
caseinate [ˈkeisiəneit, keiˈsiːneit] *n* 酪蛋白酸盐;酪蛋白合金(酪蛋白与金属的结合)
caseinogen [ˌkeisiˈinədʒən, keiˈsiːn-] *n* 酪蛋白原
caseinogenate [ˌkeisiˈinədʒineit, ˌkeisiˈnɔ-] *n* 酪蛋白原酸盐
caseogenous [ˌkeisiˈɔdʒinəs] *a* 引起干酪化的
caseoserum [ˌkeisiəuˈsiərəm] *n* 酪蛋白血清
caseous [ˈkeisiəs] *a* 干酪样的
caseum [ˈkeisiəm] *n*【拉】酪状碎屑(指细胞)
caseworm [ˈkeiswəːm] *n* 棘球绦虫
casing [ˈkeisiŋ] *n* 包装;套管
Casoni's intradermal test (reaction) [kəˈsəuni] (Tommaso Casoni) 卡索尼皮内试验(反应)(检棘球蚴病:将棘球蚴囊泡液作皮内注射,接着速发或迟发产生风团潮红反应,即显示棘球蚴病)
caspofungin acetate [ˌkæspəuˈfʌndʒin] 醋酸卡泊芬净(抗真菌药)
cassava [kəˈsɑːvə] *n* 木薯
Casselberry's position [ˈkæsəlbəri] (William E. Casselberry) 卡斯尔伯里位置(施行插管术后,患者采取俯卧位,以防止饮水进入插管)
casserian [kəˈsiəriən] *a* 卡塞(Giulio Casserio)的(如 ~ fontanelle 乳突囟)
Casser's (Casserio's, Casserius') fontanelle [ˈkɑːsə] (Giulio Casserio) 卡塞囟门(乳突囟) | ~ ligament 锤骨外侧韧带 / ~ muscle 锤骨前韧带
cassette [kəˈset] *n* 贮片盒,暗盒,片匣(放X线片用);胶卷盒,磁带盒
Cassia [ˈkæsiə] *n* 山扁豆属
cast [kɑːst] *n* 管型,圆柱;铸模,模型;斜视 | bacterial ~ [细]菌管型 / blood ~ 血细胞管型 / coma ~ 昏迷管型(见于糖尿病性昏迷) / decidual ~ 蜕膜管型(宫外妊娠破裂时) / diagnostic ~, preextraction ~, preoperative ~, study ~ 诊断模型,拔牙前模型,术前模型,研究模型 / false ~ 假管型 / hair ~ 毛团,毛粪石(胃肠内) / hemoglobin ~ 血红蛋白管型 / investment ~, refractory ~ 包埋材模型,耐高温模型 / leucocyte ~ 白细胞管型 / master ~ 主模型 / plaster ~ 管形石膏 / urinary ~, renal ~, tube ~ 尿管型,尿圆柱,肾小管管型 / waxy ~ 蜡样管型 / white cell ~ 白细胞管型
Castanea [kæsˈteiniə] *n* 栗属
Castellanella [ˌkæsteləˈnelə] *n* 卡[斯太拉尼]氏锥虫属 | ~ castellani 罗得西亚锥虫 / ~ gambiense 冈比亚锥虫
Castellani-Low symptom [kæsteˈlɑːniˈlɔː] (Aldo Castellani; George C. Low) 卡斯太拉尼-洛症状(昏睡病时舌细震颤)
Castellani's bronchitis (disease) [kæsteˈlɑːni] (Aldo Castellani) 支气管螺旋体病 | ~ mixture 卡斯太拉尼合剂(一种治雅司病合剂,含吐酒石、水杨酸钠、碘化钾、碳酸氢钠和水) / ~ paint 碳酸品红液 / ~ test 卡斯太拉尼试验(①检蛋白尿;②测数种微生物混合感染的凝集试验)
casting [ˈkɑːstiŋ] *n* 铸件;铸造 | vacuum ~ 真空铸造
Castleman's disease [ˈkæsəlmən] (Benjamin Castleman) 卡斯尔曼病,巨淋巴结增生
Castle's intrinsic factor [ˈkɑːsl] (William B. Castle) 卡斯尔内因子(胃液内的黏蛋白为吸收氰钴胺即维生素 B_{12}〈外因子〉所必需)
castrate [kæsˈtreit] *vt* 阉,阉割(切除睾丸或卵巢) *n* 去生殖腺者,阉者,去势者
castration [kæsˈtreiʃən] *n* 阉,阉割,去势(睾丸或卵巢切除术) | female ~ 女性阉,卵巢切除术 / parasitic ~ 寄生物性阉
castroid [ˈkæstrɔid] *n* 类阉者,类无睾者
casual [ˈkæʒjuəl] *a* 意外的,偶然的 *n* 急救入院者
casualty [ˈkæʒjuəlti] *n* 事故,伤亡;(事故中)受害者,伤亡人员;(意外伤害者)抢救室;失踪者
casuistics [ˌkæʒjuˈistiks] *n* 病案讨论
CAT computerized axial tomography 计算机轴向体层摄影[术]
cat [kæt] *n* 猫 | calico ~, tortoiseshell ~ 玳瑁猫,龟甲纹毛猫,三色猫(毛色为黑、白、橙黄,大部分是雌猫,受患雄猫不育,具有额外 X 染色体,如 XXY, XXXY 等)
cata- [前缀]下,向下,在下;依,照;对抗(见 kata-)
catabasial [kætəˈbeiziəl] *a* 颅底点低的
catabasis [kəˈtæbəsis] *n* 缓解期(指病) | **catabatic** [kætəˈbætik] *a* 缓解的,减退的
catabiosis [ˌkætəbaiˈəusis] *n* 细胞衰老变性,老化现象 | **catabiotic** [ˌkætəbaiˈɔtik] *a* 细胞衰老变性的;异化消耗的
catabolergy [ˌkætəˈbɔlədʒi] *n* 异化能量消耗
catabolism [kəˈtæbəlizəm] *n* 分解代谢 | antibody ~ 抗体分解代谢(体内异丙球蛋白迅速降解,即缩短了的半衰期) | **catabolic** [ˌkætəˈbɔlik] *a*
catabolite [kəˈtæbəlait], **catabolin** [kəˈtæbəlin] *n* 分解代谢
catabolize [kəˈtæbəlaiz] *vi*, *vt* 发生分解代谢
catachronobiology [ˌkætəˌkrɔnəubaiˈɔlədʒi] *n* 生

物衰老学

catacrotism [kə'tækrətizəm] *n* 降线一波脉[现象] | **catacrotic** [ˌkætə'krɔtik] *a*

catadicrotism [ˌkætə'daikrətizəm] *n* 降线二波脉[现象] | **catadicrotic** [ˌkætədai'krɔtik] *a*

catadidymus [ˌkætə'didiməs] *n* 下身联胎,双上身联胎

catadioptric [ˌkætədai'ɔptrik] *a* 反[射]折射的

catagen ['kætədʒən] *n* 毛发生长中期

catagenesis [ˌkætə'dʒenisis] *n* 退化 | **catagenetic** [ˌkætədʒi'netik] *a*

catagmatic [ˌkætəg'mætik] *a* 促骨折愈合的

catalase ['kætəleis] *n* 过氧化氢酶 | **catalatic** [ˌkætə'lætik] *a*

catalepsy ['kætəlepsi] *n* 僵住(见于器质性疾病和心理失调以及在催眠状态下发生) | **cataleptic** [ˌkætə'leptik] *a* 僵住的 *n* 僵住患者

cataleptiform [ˌkætə'leptifɔːm], **cataleptoid** [ˌkætə'leptɔid] *a* 僵住[症]样的

catalogia [ˌkætə'ləudʒiə] *n* 言语重复

Catalpa [kə'tælpə] *n* 梓属

catalysis [kə'tælisis] *n* 催化[作用] | contact ~, heterogeneous ~ 接触催化[作用],多相催化[作用] / surface ~ 表面催化[作用]

catalyst ['kætəlist] *n* 催化剂 | negative ~ 负催化剂,缓化剂

catalytic [ˌkætə'litik] *a* 催化的 *n* 催化剂

catalyze ['kætəlaiz] *vt* 催化 | **catalyzator** [ˌkætəli'zeitə], **~r** ['kætəlaizə] *n* 催化剂

catamenia [ˌkætə'miːniə] *n* 月经 | **~l** *a*

catamenogenic [ˌkætəmenə'dʒenik] *a* 促月经的

catamite ['kætəmait] *n* 受鸡奸男童,娈童

catamnesis [ˌkætəm'niːsis] *n* 随访病历;诊后病历 | **catamnestic** [ˌkætəm'nestik] *a*

catapasm ['kætəpæzəm] *n* 扑粉(用于表面伤口)

cataphasia [ˌkætə'feiziə] *n* 言语重复

cataphora [kə'tæfərə] *n* 嗜睡样昏迷(可暂醒的昏迷)

cataphoresis [ˌkætəfə'riːsis] *n* 阳离子电泳 | **cataphoretic** [ˌkætəfə'retik] *a*

cataphoria [ˌkætə'fəuriə] *n* 下隐斜

cataphoric [ˌkætə'fɔrik] *a* 阳离子电泳的;下隐斜的

cataphrenia [ˌkætə'friːniə] *n* 可逆性痴呆

cataplasia [ˌkætə'pleisiə], **cataplasis** [kə'tæpləsis] *n* [组织]退化,返祖性组织变态 | **cataplastic** [ˌkætə'plæstik] *a*

cataplasm ['kætəplæzəm] *n* 泥罨剂,泥敷剂 | kaolin ~ 白陶土泥罨剂,白陶土敷剂

cataplasma [ˌkætə'plæzmə] *n* 【拉】泥罨剂,泥敷剂

cataplectic [ˌkætə'plektik] *a* 猝倒的;暴发的

cataplexie ['kætəˌpleksi] *n* 【法】猝倒 | ~ du réveil 觉醒猝倒(猝倒时,神志觉醒在身体恢复之前)

cataplexy ['kætəpleksi], **cataplexis** ['kætəˌpleksis] *n* 猝倒[症]

catapophysis [ˌkætə'pɔfisis] *n* 骨突;脑髓突起

cataract ['kætərækt] *n* 白内障 | after-~ 后发性白内障 / blue ~, blue dot ~, cerulean ~ 蔚蓝色白内障 / bony ~ 骨化白内障 / capsulolenticular ~ 囊性皮质性白内障 / floriform ~ 花状白内障 / fluid ~, lacteal ~, milky ~ 液化白内障,乳液状白内障 / general ~, mixed ~ 混合白内障 / glassblowers' ~, bottlemakers' ~ 玻璃工人白内障 / glaucomatous ~ 青光眼性白内障 / heat-ray ~ 热辐射白内障 / hypermature ~, overripe ~ 过熟白内障 / lightning ~ 电击性白内障 / morgagnian ~ 莫尔加尼白内障 / naphthalinic ~ 萘性白内障 / nuclear ~, axial ~ 核性白内障,轴性白内障 / puddler's ~ 铁匠白内障 / punctate ~ 点状白内障 / siliculose ~, siliquose ~, dryshelled ~, aridosiliculose ~, aridosiliquate ~ 干荚状白内障 / snowflake ~, snowstorm ~ 雪花状白内障(常见于青年糖尿病患者) / sunflower ~ 葵花状白内障 / total ~ 全白内障 / zonular ~ 板层白内障

cataracta [ˌkætə'ræktə] *n* 【拉】内障,白内障

cataractogenic [ˌkætəˌræktəu'dʒenik] *a* 致白内障的

cataractous [ˌkætə'ræktəs] *a* 白内障性的

cataria [kə'teəriə] *n* 【拉"catnip"】假荆芥,樟脑草(用作祛风剂和温和的神经刺激剂,其香气吸引猫)

catarrh [kə'tɑː] *n* 卡他,黏膜炎 | atrophic ~ 萎缩性鼻卡他 / autumnal ~ 枯草热 / epidemic ~ 流行性感冒,流感 / hypertrophic ~ (黏膜)肥大性卡他 / postnasal ~ 慢性鼻咽炎 / Russian ~ 流行性感冒 / suffocative ~ 气喘,哮喘 / vernal ~, spring ~ 春季结膜炎 | **~al**, **~ous** *a* 卡他性的

Catarrhina [ˌkætə'rainə] *n* 狭鼻类

catarrhine ['kætərain] *a* 狭鼻的(指动物,亦指具有鼻孔紧贴而朝下特征的)

catastaltic [ˌkætə'stæltik] *a* 抑制的 *n* 抑制剂

catastate ['kætəsteit] *n* 分解代谢产物 | **catastatic** [ˌkætə'stætik] *a*

catatasis [kə'tætəsis] *n* 牵伸术(用于脱臼或骨折复位术)

catathermometer [ˌkætəθə'mɔmitə] *n* 干湿球温度计

catathymia [ˌkætə'θaimiə] *n* 激情 | **catathymic** *a*

catatonia [ˌkætə'təuniə], **catatony** [kə'tætəni] *n*

紧张症(紧张性精神分裂症) | **catatoniac** [ˌkætəˈtəuniæk], **catatonic** [ˌkætəˈtɔnik] *a* 紧张性的;紧张症的 *n* 紧张症患者

catatricrotism [ˌkætəˈtraikrətizəm] *n* 降线三波脉[现象] | **catatricrotic** [ˌkætətraiˈkrɔtik] *a*

catatropia [ˌkætəˈtrəupiə] *n* 下隐斜视

catechin [ˈkætikin] *n* 儿茶素,儿茶酸

catechol [ˈkætitʃəul, ˈkætəkəul] *n* 儿茶酚;邻苯二酚

catecholamine [ˌkætiˈkəuləmiːn] *n* 儿茶酚胺(有拟交感神经作用,此类化合物包括多巴胺、去甲肾上腺素和肾上腺素)

catecholaminergic [ˌkætikəˌlæmiˈnəːdʒik] *a* 儿茶酚胺能的

catechol *O*-methyltransferase [ˈkætikɔl ˌmeθilˈtrænsfəreis] 儿茶酚 *O*-甲基转移酶

catechol oxidase [ˈkætəkəul ˈɔksideis] 儿茶酚氧化酶

catechu [ˈkætitʃuː, ˈkætəkjuː] *n* 儿茶(亦称 black catechu);黑儿茶,棕儿茶(即 gambir) | pale ~ 黑儿茶,棕儿茶(即 gambir)

catechuic acid [ˌkætəˈtʃuːik -ˈkjuː-] 儿茶酸,儿茶素

catechutannic acid [ˌkætətʃuːˈtænik] 儿茶鞣酸

catelectrotonus [ˌkætilekˈtrɔtənəs] *n* 阴极电紧张

catena [kəˈtiːnə] ([复] **catenas** 或 **catenae** [kəˈtiːniː]) *n* 连锁;链条

Catenabacterium [ˌkætinəbækˈtiəriəm] *n* 链状细菌属

catenarian [ˌkætiˈnεəriən], **catenary** [kəˈtiːnəri] *n*, *a* 悬链线(的);链状(的)

catenate [ˈkætineit] *vt* 链接 | **catenation** [ˌkætiˈneiʃən] *n*

catenating [ˈkætineitiŋ] *a* 链接的

catenoid [ˈkætinɔid], **catenulate** [kəˈtenjulit] *a* 链状的

caterpillar [ˈkætəˌpilə] *n* 毛虫,蠋

catgut [ˈkætgʌt] *n* 肠线 | chromic ~, chromicized ~ 铬肠线 / formaldehyde ~ 甲醛肠线 / I. K. I. ~, iodine ~ 碘碘化钾肠线,碘肠线 / iodochromic ~ 碘铬肠线 / silverized ~ 银肠线

Cath. catharticus【拉】泻药,泻剂

Catha [ˈkɑːθə] *n* 卡他属 | ~ edulis 阿拉伯茶树

cathaeresis [kəˈθiərisis] *n* 虚弱(用药后引起);轻作用

catharmos [kəˈθɑːmɔs] *n* 驱病咒语

catharometer [ˌkæθəˈrɔmitə] *n* 导热析气计

catharsis [kəˈθɑːsis] *n* 导泻,泻法;(精神或心理)发泄,宣泄

cathartic [kəˈθɑːtik] *a* 导泻的;导泄的 *n* 泻药 | bulk ~ 增量泻药 / lubricant ~ 润滑泻药 / saline ~ 盐水泻药 / stimulant ~ 刺激性泻药

cathartic acid, cathartinic acid [kəθɑːˈtinik] 泻酸

cathectic [kəˈθektik] *a* 精神集中发泄的,聚精会神的

cathemoglobin [ˌkæθeməuˈgləubin] *n* 变性高铁血红蛋白

cathepsin [kəˈθepsin] *n* 组织蛋白酶

catheresis [kəˈθiərisis] *n* 虚弱(用药后引起);轻作用

catheretic [ˌkæθəˈretik] *a* 轻腐蚀性的;虚弱的

catheter [ˈkæθitə] *n* 导管 | bicoudate ~, ~ bicoudé 双弯导管 / cardiac ~ 心导管 / ~ coudé, elbowed ~ 单弯导管,弯头导管 / ~ à demeure, indwelling ~ 留置导尿管 / double-current ~, two-way ~ 双腔导管 / eustachian ~ 咽鼓管导管 / faucial ~ 咽导管 / female ~ 女导尿管 / flexible ~ 软导管 / lobster-tail ~ 虾尾状导管 / prostatic ~ 前列腺导尿管 / railway ~ 槽式导管 / self-retaining ~ 自留导尿管,潴留导尿管 / tracheal ~ 气管导管 / vertebrated ~ 分节导管(由许多小节配合而成的导管,以便能弯曲) / whistle-tip ~ 笛口样导管 / winged ~ 翼状导管

catheterization [ˌkæθitəraiˈzeiʃən, -riˈz-] *n* 插管术;导尿术 | cardiac ~ 心导管插入术,心导管检查 / hepatic vein ~ 肝静脉导管插入术 / retrourethral ~ 逆行导尿管插入术 / umbilical ~ 脐插管

catheterize [ˈkæθitəraiz] *vt* 插入导管

catheterostat [kæˈθiːtərəstæt] *n* 导管保持器(放置及消毒导管用)

cathetometer [ˌkæθiˈtɔmitə] *n* 高差计

cathexis [kəˈθeksis] *n* 精神集中发泄,聚精会神,贯注

cathisophobia [ˌkæθisəuˈfəubjə] *n* 静坐恐怖,恐坐症;静坐不能

cathode [ˈkæθəud] *n* 阴极,负极 | **cathodal** [ˈkæθədl], **cathodic** [kəˈθɔdik] *a*

catholicon [kəˈθɔlikən] *n* 万灵药

catholyte [ˈkæθəlait] *n* 阴极电解质

cation [ˈkætaiən] *n* 阳离子,阴向离子 | **~ic** [ˌkætiˈɔnik, -taiˈɔ-] *a*

cationogen [ˌkætiˈɔnədʒən] *n* 阳离子发生物

cativi [kəˈtivi] *n* 品他病(即 pinta)

catlin [ˈkætlin], **catling** [ˈkætliŋ] *n* 两刃切断刀(截肢用)

catnip [ˈkætnip], **catnep** [ˈkætnep] *n* 假荆芥,樟脑草(见 cataria)

catoptrics [kəˈtɔptriks] *n* 反射光学 | **catoptric(al)** [kəˈtɔptrik(əl)] *a* 反射[光]的

catoptroscope [kəˈtɔptrəskəup] *n* 反光检查器,

反光镜

catotropia [ˌkætəˈtrəupiə] *n* 下隐斜视

Ca^{2+}-transporting ATPase [trænsˈpɔːtiŋ eitiːpiːˈeis] 钙转运腺苷三磷酸酶(Ca^{2+}-ATPase 的 EC 命名法)

Cattani's serum [kəˈtɑːni] (Giuseppina Cattani) 卡塔尼血清(一种氯化钠、碳酸钠及煮沸过的蒸馏水混合剂,传染病注射用)

cauda [ˈkɔːdə] ([复] **caudae** [ˈkɔːdiː]) *n*【拉】尾

caudad [ˈkɔːdæd] *ad* 向尾[侧]的

caudal [ˈkɔːdl] *a* 尾的;尾侧的

caudalis [kɔːˈdeilis] *a*【拉】尾的;尾侧的

caudalward [ˈkɔːdlwɔːd] *ad* 向尾侧

caudamoeba sinensis [ˌkɔːdəˈmiːbə siˈnensis] 中华尾形阿米巴(见 Entamoeba histolytica)

Caudata [kauˈdeitə] *n* 有尾目

caudate [ˈkɔːdeit], **caudated** [ˈkɔːdeitid] *a* 有尾的

caudatolenticular [kɔːˌdeitəulenˈtikjulə] *a* 尾状核与豆状核的

caudatum [kɔːˈdeitəm] *n*【拉】尾状核

caudectomy [kɔːˈdektəmi] *n* 尾切除术(如切除狗的尾巴)

caudocephalad [kɔːdəuˈsefəlæd] *ad* 从尾向头侧;向头及向尾侧

caul [kɔːl] *n* 胎头羊膜;网膜(通常指大网膜)

cauliflower [ˈkɔliflauə] *n* 花椰菜(菜花)

Caulk's punch [kɔːlk] (John R. Caulk) 考克钻孔器(用于前列腺正中嵴肥大切除)

Caulobacter [ˌkɔːləuˈbæktə] *n* 柄杆菌属

Caulobacteraceae [ˌkɔːləubæktəˈreisiiː] *n* 柄杆菌族

Caulobacteriineae [ˌkɔːləubæktiəriˈiniiː] *n* 柄杆菌亚目

Caulococcus [ˌkɔːləuˈkɔkəs] *n* 柄球菌属

Caulophyllum [ˌkauləuˈfiləm] *n* 葳严仙属

caumesthesia [ˌkɔːmisˈθiːzjə] *n* 触冷感热,(遇冷)灼热感

causalgia [kɔːˈzældʒiə] *n* 灼性神经痛(由于周围神经损伤所致)

causality [kɔːˈzæləti] *n* 诱发性;因果关系,因果律

causation [kɔːˈzeiʃən] *n* 引起,导致;因果关系

causative [ˈkɔːzətiv] *a* 原因的,成因的

cause [kɔːz] *n* 原因;病因 *vt* 引起;促使 | constitutional ~ 全身性原因,体质性原因 / exciting ~ 激发原因,直接原因 / immediate ~, precipitating ~ 直接原因,诱因 / local ~ 局部原因 / predisposing ~ 易感因素 / primary ~ 原发性原因,主因 / proximate ~ 近因 / remote ~ 远因,诱因 / secondary ~ 继发性原因,辅因 / ultimate ~ 远因

caustic [ˈkɔːstik] *a* 腐蚀[性]的,苛性的 *n* 腐蚀剂 | lunar ~ 银丹,硝酸银 / mitigated ~ 弱银丹,弱硝酸银 / Vienna ~ 维也纳腐蚀剂,钾石灰 / zink ~ 锌腐蚀剂(一份氯化锌和三份面粉的混合物) | **~ity** [kɔːsˈtisəti] *n* 苛性[度],腐蚀性

causticize [ˈkɔːstisaiz] *vt* 苛化,腐蚀,致腐蚀 | **causticization** [ˌkɔːstisaiˈzeiʃən, -siˈz-] *n*

cauterant [ˈkɔːtərənt] *a* 腐蚀的 *n* 腐蚀剂

cauterize [ˈkɔːtəraiz] *vt* 烙,烧灼 | **cauterization** [ˌkɔːtəraiˈzeiʃən, -liˈz-] *n* 烙术,烧灼术

cautery [ˈkɔːtəri] *n* 烙术,烧灼术;烙器 | actual ~ 火烙术;烙铁 / button ~ 钮式烙器 / chemical ~ 化学烙术 / cold ~ 冻烙术,碳酸霜烙术 / electric ~, galvanic ~ 电烙器 / gas ~ 喷气烙术 / potential ~, virtual ~ 腐蚀剂烙术 / solar ~, sun ~ 日光烙术

cava [ˈkeivə] *n* cavum 的复数;腔静脉

caval [ˈkeivəl] *a* 腔静脉的

cavascope [ˈkævəskəup] *n* 窥腔镜,映腔镜

CAVB complete atrioventricular block 完全性房室传导阻滞

cave [keiv] *n* 小腔

cave-in [ˈkeivin] *n* 塌方(矿井、地道等的坍陷)

caveola [keiviˈəulə] ([复] **caveolae** [keiviˈəuliː]) *n*【拉】小凹、小腔

cavern [ˈkævən] *n* 腔,[空]洞 | ~s of corpus spongiosum(阴茎)海绵体腔

caverna [keiˈvəːnə] ([复] **cavernae**, [keiˈvəːniː]) *n*【拉】腔,[空]洞,盂

caverniloquy [ˌkævəˈniləkwi] *n* 空洞语音(有肺结核空洞时)

cavernitis [ˌkævəˈnaitis], **cavernositis** [ˌkævənəˈsaitis] *n* (阴茎)海绵体炎

cavernoma [ˌkævəˈnəumə] ([复] **cavernomas** 或 **cavernomata** [ˌkævəˈnəumətə]) *n* 海绵状血管瘤

cavernosal [ˌkævəˈnəusəl] *a* 海绵体的;空洞的

cavernoscope [ˈkævənəˌskəup] *n* 空腔镜 | **cavernoscopy** [ˌkævəˈnɔskəpi] *n* 空腔镜检查

cavernosography [ˌkævənəuˈsɔgrəfi] *n* (阴茎)海绵体造影[术]

cavernosometry [ˌkævənəuˈsɔmətri] *n* 海绵体血管压测量法

cavernostomy [ˌkævəˈnɔstəmi] *n* 空腔造口术 | renal ~ 肾病灶清除术

cavernous [ˈkævənəs] *a* 空洞的

Cavia [ˈkeiviə] *n* 豚鼠属 | ~ cobaya 豚鼠

cavilla [kəˈvilə] *n* 蝶骨

cavitary [ˈkævitəri] *a* 腔的,空洞的 *n* 腔肠虫

cavitas [ˈkævitəs] ([复] **cavitates** [kæviˈte-

itiːz]) *n*【拉】腔,[空]洞,盂
cavitation [ˌkæviˈteiʃən] *n* 空腔形成;空洞化
Cavite fever [kəˈviːtə] 卡维太热,类登革热(卡维太为菲律宾一地名)
cavitis [keiˈvaitis] *n* 腔静脉炎
cavity [ˈkæviti] *n* 腔,[空]洞,盂;窝洞 | alveolar cavities 牙槽腔 / body ~ 体腔(指内脏腔) / buccal ~ 颊面[龋]洞;口腔前庭 / cotyloid ~ 髋臼 / fissure ~ 裂龋洞 / gastrovascular ~ 消化腔(腔肠动物的体腔,亦称 coelenteron) / glenoid ~ 关节盂(肩胛骨) / hemal ~ 血腔 / labial ~ 唇面[龋]洞 / lingual ~ 舌面龋洞 / occlusal ~ 𬌗面[龋]洞 / orbital ~ 眶腔 / pelvic ~ 骨盆腔 / pericardial ~ 心包腔 / peritoneal ~, greater peritoneal ~ 腹膜腔,大腹膜腔 / pharyngolaryngeal ~ 咽喉腔 / popliteal ~ 腘窝 / prepared ~ 备填洞,制备洞 / proximal ~ 邻面[龋]洞 / pulp ~, nerve ~ 牙髓腔 / rectoischiadic ~ 坐骨直肠窝 / serous ~ 浆膜腔 / sigmoid ~ of radius 尺骨切迹(桡骨) / somatic ~ 体腔 / somite ~ 肌节腔 / subarachnoid ~ 蛛网膜下腔 / subdural ~ 硬膜下腔 / thoracic ~, pectoral ~ 胸腔 / tympanic ~ 鼓室 / uterine ~ 子宫腔 / visceral ~, splanchnic ~ 内脏腔
cavography [keiˈvɔgrəfi] *n* 腔静脉造影[术]
cavosurface [ˈkeivəuˌsəːfis] *n* 洞面(牙)
cavovalgus [ˌkeivəuˈvælgəs] *n* 空凹外翻足
cavum [ˈkeivəm] ([复] **cava** [ˈkeivə]) *n*【拉】腔,[空]洞
cavus [ˈkævəs] *n* 弓形足
cavy [ˈkeivi] *n* 豚鼠
cayenne [keiˈjen, kai-] *n* 辣椒,红辣椒
Cazenave's disease [kɑːzˈnɑːv] (Pierre L. A. Cazenave) 卡泽纳夫病,落叶性天疱疮 / ~ vitiligo 斑形脱发,斑秃
CB Chirurgiae Baccalaureus【拉】外科学士
Cb columbium 钶(现称铌 niobium)
cbc complete blood count 全血细胞计数
CBF cerebral blood flow 脑血流量
CBG corticosteroid-binding globulin 皮质类固醇结合球蛋白
C3b INA C3b inactivator C3b 灭活因子(补体因子Ⅰ的旧称)
Cbl cobalamin 钴胺素,维生素 B_{12}
CBS chronic brain syndrome 慢性脑综合征
CC chief complaint 主诉
cc cubic centimeter 立方厘米
CC 914 对脲苯基双(羧甲基硫醇)胂(治肠阿米巴病)
CC 1037 对脲苯基双(2-羧基苯硫醇)胂(治肠阿米巴病)
CCA chimpanzee coryza agent 猩猩鼻炎因子(呼吸道合胞体病毒);congenital contractural arachnodactyly 先天性挛缩性细长指,先天性挛缩性细长趾
CCAT conglutinating complement absorption test 胶固补体吸收试验
CCC cathodal closure contraction 阴极通电收缩
CCCl cathodal closure clonus 阴极通电阵挛
CCF crystal-induced chemotactic factor 晶体诱导趋化因子
CCK cholecystokinin 缩胆囊素,缩胆囊肽
CCK-179 双氢麦角毒碱的三种生物碱(dihydroergocornine, dihydroergocristine, dihydroergocryptine)的合剂(降压药和血管扩张药,用于治疗外周血管病)
ccm cubic centimeter 立方厘米
CCNU lomustine 洛莫司汀(抗肿瘤药); methyl CCNU semustine 司莫司汀(抗肿瘤药)
CCP complement control protein 补体控制蛋白
CCPD continuous cycling peritoneal dialysis 持续循环腹膜透析
CCTe cathodal closure tetanus 阴极通电强直
CCU coronary care unit 冠心病监护治疗病房,冠心病监护室;critical care unit 危重症监护室
CD cadaveric donor 尸体供者;cluster designation 细胞表面标记分类法;conjugata diagonalis【拉】对角径;curative dose 治愈量
CD_{50} median curative dose 半数治愈量(使 50% 受试者症状消失的剂量)
Cd cadmium 镉;caudal 尾的;coccygeal 尾骨的
cd candela 堪[德拉],[新]烛光
CDC Centers for Disease Control and Prevention 疾病控制与预防中心
CDC/AIDS Centers for Disease Control and Prevention for the diagnosis of AIDS 疾病控制与预防中心/艾滋病诊断
CDDP cisplatin (*cis*-diaminedichloroplatinum) 顺铂(抗肿瘤药)
cdf cumulative distribution function 累积分布函数
CDH congenital dislocation of the hip 先天性髋关节脱臼,先天性髋脱位
cDNA complementary DNA 互补 DNA; copy DNA 复制 DNA
CDP cytidine diphosphate 胞苷二磷酸
CDP diacylglycerol [daiˌæsilˈglisərɔl] 胞苷二磷酸二酰甘油
CDP diacylglycerol-inositol 3-phosphatidyltransferase [daiˌæsilˈglisərɔl iˈnəusitɔl ˌfɔsfəˌtidilˈtrænsfəreis] 胞苷二磷酸二酰甘油-肌醇 3-磷脂酰转移酶
Ce cerium 铈
CEA carcinoembryonic antigen 癌胚抗原
ceasmic [siˈæsmik] *a* 裂开的(指胚胎期的裂隙生后仍旧存在)
cebocephalus [ˌsiːbəuˈsefələs] *n* 猴头畸胎

cebocephaly [ˌsiːbəuˈsefəli] *n* 猴头畸形
ceca [ˈsiːkə] cecum 的复数
cecal [ˈsiːkəl] *a* 盲端的；盲肠的；盲斑的
cecectomy [siˈsektəmi] *n* 盲肠切除术
Cecil's operation (urethroplasty) [ˈsesil] (Arthur B. Cecil) 塞西尔手术(尿道成形术)(①一种二期尿道成形术，以修补尿道下裂，即作一段新的尿道，并埋入阴囊，然后将新尿道与阴囊分离；②一种三期尿道成形术，以修补尿道狭窄，即通过阴茎的腹面切口切除狭窄区，然后用上述手术步骤修补尿道下裂)
cecitis [siˈsaitis] *n* 盲肠炎
cec(o)- [构词成分] 盲肠
cecocele [ˈsiːkəsiːl] *n* 盲肠疝
cecocentral [ˌsikəuˈsentrəl] *a* 中心盲点的
cecocolic [ˌsiːkəuˈkɔlik] *a* 盲[肠]结肠的
cecocolon [ˌsiːkəuˈkəulən] *n* 盲[肠]结肠
cecocolopexy [ˌsiːkəuˈkəuləˌpeksi] *n* 盲肠升结肠固定术
cecocolostomy [ˌsiːkəukəˈlɔstəmi] *n* 盲肠结肠吻合术
cecocystoplasty [ˌsiːkəuˈsistəuˌplæsti] *n* 盲肠膀胱扩大术
cecoileostomy [ˌsiːkəuˌiliˈɔstəmi] *n* 回肠盲肠吻合术
cecopexy [ˈsiːkəˌpeksi], **cecofixation** [ˌsiːkəu-fikˈseiʃən] *n* 盲肠固定术
cecoplication [ˌsiːkəuplaiˈkeiʃən] *n* 盲肠折叠术
cecorrhaphy [siˈkɔrəfi] *n* 盲肠缝合术
cecosigmoidostomy [ˌsiːkəuˌsigmɔiˈdɔstəmi] *n* 盲肠乙状结肠吻合术
cecostomy [siˈkɔstəmi] *n* 盲肠造口术
cecotomy [siˈkɔtəmi] *n* 盲肠切开术
cecum [ˈsiːkəm] ([复] **ceca** [ˈsiːkə]) *n* 盲肠；盲端 | cupular ~ of cochlear duct 顶盲端(蜗管) / hepatic ~ 肝盲管(胚) / high ~ 高位盲肠
cedar [ˈsiːdə] *n* 雪松；柏 | red ~ 红刺柏，铅笔柏 / western red ~ 大侧柏 / white ~ 白扁柏，金钟柏
Cedecea [ˈsiːdiːsiː] (以 Centers for Disease Control 命名) *n* 肠杆菌属
Cediopsylla [ˌsiːdiəuˈsilə] *n* 蚤属
cefaclor [ˈsefəklɔː] *n* 头孢克洛(抗生素类药)
cefadroxil [ˌsefəˈdrɔksil] *n* 头孢羟氨苄(抗生素类药)
cefamandole [ˌsefəˈmændəul] *n* 头孢孟多(抗生素类药) | ~ nafate 头孢孟多酯钠(抗生素类药)
cefaparole [ˈsefəpərəul] *n* 头孢帕罗(抗生素类药)
cefatrizine [ˌsefəˈtraiziːn] *n* 头孢曲秦(抗生素类药)
cefazaflur sodium [siˈfæzəfləː] 头孢氮氟钠(抗生素类药)
cefazolin [siˈfæzəlin] *n* 头孢唑林(抗生素类药) | ~ sodium 头孢唑林钠(抗生素类药)
cefdinir [ˈsefdini] *n* 头孢地尼(抗生素类药)
cefepime [ˈsefəpiːm] *n* 头孢吡肟(抗生素类药)
cefixime [səˈfiksiːm] *n* 头孢克肟(抗生素类药)
cefmenoxime hydrochloride [ˌsefmeˈnɔksiːm] 盐酸头孢甲肟(抗生素类药)
cefmetazole [sefˈmetəzəul] *n* 头孢美唑(抗生素类药)
cefonicid sodium [səˈfɔnisid] 头孢尼西钠(抗生素类药)
cefoperazone sodium [ˌsefəˈperəzəun] 头孢哌酮钠(抗生素类药)
ceforanide [siˈfɔːrənaid] *n* 头孢雷特(抗生素类药)
cefotaxime [ˌsefəˈtæksiːm] *n* 头孢噻肟(抗生素类药) | ~ sodium 头孢噻肟钠(抗菌药)
cefotetan [ˈsefəˌtiːtən] *n* 头孢替坦(抗生素类药) | ~ disodium 头孢替坦二钠
cefotian hydrochloride [ˌsefəˈtaiəm] 盐酸头孢替安(抗生素类药)
cefoxitin [siˈfɔksitin] *n* 头孢西丁(抗生素类药)
cefpiramide [sefˈpirəmaid] *n* 头孢匹胺(抗生素类药)
cefpodoxime proxetil [ˌsefpəˈdɔksiːm ˈprɔksətil] 头孢泊肟酯(抗生素类药)
cefprozil [sefˈprəuzil] *n* 头孢丙烯(抗生素类药)
ceftazidime [ˈsefteiziˌdiːm] *n* 头孢他啶(抗生素类药)
ceftibuten [sefˈtaibjutən] *n* 头孢布烯(抗生素类药)
ceftiofur sodium [sefˈtaiəfju] 头孢噻呋钠(半合成头孢菌素，用于家畜)
ceftizoxime sodium [ˌseftiˈzɔksiːm] 头孢唑肟钠(抗菌药)
ceftriaxone sodium [ˌseftraiˈæksəun] 头孢曲松钠(抗生素类药)
cefuroxime [ˌsefjuˈrɔksiːm] *n* 头孢呋辛(抗生素类药) | ~ sodium 头孢呋辛钠
Cegka's sign [ˈtʃegkɑː] (Josephus J. Cegka) 切卡征(呼吸不同时期心浊音不变，为粘连性心包的体征)
Cel Celsius 摄氏的(温标)
cel [sel-] *n* 厘米/秒(cm/s，速度单位)
cel- 见 celo-
celarium [siˈlɛəriəm] *n* 体腔膜
-cele [构词成分] 腔；瘤；膨出，突出，疝，肿大
celecoxib [ˌseləˈkɔksib] *n* 塞勒考昔(COX-2 抑制药类中的一种非甾体消炎药，用作骨关节炎和类风湿关节炎的症状治疗，口服给药)

celectome [siˈlektəum] *n* 取瘤质刀,瘤组织剪钳
celenteron [siˈlentərɔn] *n* 原肠;腔肠
celiac [ˈsiːliæk] *a* 腹的,腹腔的
celiectomy [ˌsiːliˈektəmi] *n* 内脏切除术;迷走神经腹支切除术(以缓解原发性高血压)
celi(o)- [构词成分]腹,腔,腹腔;以 celi(o)-起始的词,同样见以 cel(o)-和 coel(o)-起始的词
celiocentesis [ˌsiːliəusenˈtiːsis] *n* 腹腔穿刺术
celiocolpotomy [ˌsiːliəukɔlˈpɔtəmi] *n* 腹式阴道切开术
celioenterotomy [ˌsiːliəuˌentəˈrɔtəmi] *n* 剖腹肠切开术
celiogastrotomy [ˌsiːliəugæsˈtrɔtəmi] *n* 剖腹胃切开术
celiohysterectomy [ˌsiːliəuˌhistəˈrektəmi] *n* 腹式子宫切除术;剖腹产子宫切除术
celioma [siːliˈəumə] *n* 腹瘤(尤指腹膜间皮瘤)
celiomyomectomy [ˌsiːliəuˌmaiəuˈmektəmi] *n* 剖腹肌瘤切除术
celiomyomotomy [ˌsiːliəuˌmaiəuˈmɔtəmi] *n* 剖腹肌瘤切开术
celiomyositis [ˌsiːliəuˌmaiəˈsaitis] *n* 腹肌炎
celioparacentesis [ˌsiːliəuˌpærəsenˈtiːsis] *n* 腹腔穿刺术
celiopathy [ˌsiːliˈɔpəθi] *n* 腹病
celiorrhaphy [ˌsiːliˈɔrəfi] *n* 腹壁缝合术
celiosalpingectomy [ˌsiːliəuˌsælpinˈdʒektəmi] *n* 腹式输卵管切除术
celiosalpingotomy [ˌsiːliəuˌsælpiŋˈgɔtəmi] *n* 腹式输卵管切开术
celioscope [ˈsiːliəskəup] *n* 腹腔镜 | **celioscopy** [ˌsiːliˈɔskəpi] *n* 腹腔镜检查
celiotomy [ˌsiːliˈɔtəmi] *n* 剖腹术 | vaginal ~ 阴道式剖腹术 / ventral ~ 腹式剖腹术
celitis [siˈlaitis] *n* 腹内器官炎,内脏炎
cell [sel] *n* 细胞;室,小房;电池 | A ~, alpha ~s 辅助细胞,α 细胞(胰岛或垂体前叶内) / acid ~s 壁细胞,泌酸细胞 / acidophilic ~ [垂体]嗜酸性细胞 / acoustic hair ~ 听毛细胞,听细胞 / adventitial ~s 外膜细胞,周皮细胞 / air ~ 气泡(肺) / alveolar ~ 肺泡细胞,肺细胞 / alveolar ~s, type Ⅰ Ⅰ型肺泡细胞 / alveolar ~s, type Ⅱ Ⅱ型肺泡细胞(亦称颗粒性肺细胞,大肺泡细胞) / amine precursor uptake and decarboxylation ~s, APUD ~s 胺与胺前体摄取与脱羧细胞 / antigen-presenting ~s 抗原呈递细胞 / antigen-reactive ~s 抗原反应细胞 / antigen-sensitive ~s 抗原敏感细胞 / apotrophic ~s 顶端滋养细胞 / argentaffin ~s, 嗜银细胞 / auditory ~s 听细胞 / B ~s, beta ~s 腔上囊依赖淋巴细胞;β 细胞(胰岛或垂体前叶内) / balloon ~s 气球样细胞(带状疱疹水疱变性细胞) / band ~ 杆状核细胞 / basal ~ 基细胞 / basket ~ 篮细胞 / basophilic ~ [垂体]嗜碱性细胞 / battery ~ 电池 / beaker ~ 杯状细胞 / berry ~ 浆果样细胞 / bipolar ~ (视网膜)双极细胞 / bladder ~s 泡状细胞 / blast ~ 胚细胞 / bloated ~ 肿胀细胞 / border ~s 边缘细胞 / breviradiate ~s 短突神经胶质细胞 / bristle ~s 毛细胞(耳蜗) / bronchic ~ 肺泡 / brood ~ 母细胞 / burr ~ 钝锯齿状红细胞,棘红细胞(见于氮血症、胃癌、出血性消化性溃疡) / C ~s C 细胞(胰岛) / caliciform ~ 杯状细胞 / capsule ~ 被膜细胞 / castration ~s 阉割细胞(性功能不足时垂体前叶中的一种细胞) / caudate ~s 尾状细胞,彗星细胞 / centroacinar ~ 泡心细胞 / chalice ~ 杯状细胞 / chief ~s 主细胞 / clear ~s 明细胞 / collenchyma ~s 厚角细胞 / cometal ~s 彗星细胞,尾状细胞 / contractile fiber ~s 平滑肌纤维细胞,可收缩纤维细胞 / contrasuppresor ~ 抗抑制细胞 / counting ~ 计数池 / cover ~ 盖细胞 / cytotoxic T ~s 细胞毒性 T 细胞 / D ~s D 细胞(胰岛) / daughter ~ 子细胞 / dome ~s 圆顶细胞(构成胎儿皮上层的大细胞) / dust ~ 尘细胞 / encasing ~ 盖细胞 / enterochromaffin ~s 肠嗜铬细胞 / epithelial ~s 上皮细胞 / epithelioid ~s 上皮样细胞 / fat-storing ~s of liver 肝贮脂细胞 / floor ~s 底细胞(耳蜗) / foam ~s 泡沫细胞(细胞内充满类脂体,常见于黄瘤内,亦称黄瘤细胞;米库利奇细胞,见 Mikulicz's cells) / foot ~s 基底细胞;足细胞(见 Sertoli's cells) / formative ~ 胚性细胞 / fusiform ~ 梭形细胞 / G ~s G 细胞,胃泌素细胞(胃幽门部黏膜中的颗粒性肠嗜铬细胞,是胃泌素的来源) / gametoid ~ 配子样细胞 / germ ~s 生殖细胞 / germinal ~ 生发细胞 / ghost ~ 血影细胞 / giant ~s 巨细胞 / gitter ~s 格子细胞,小神经胶质(细胞) / glia ~ 神经胶质细胞 / glomus ~s 球细胞 / goblet ~ 杯形细胞 / grape ~ 葡萄状细胞 / heckel ~ 棘细胞 / HeLa ~s 人宫颈癌传代细胞 / helper ~ 辅助性细胞(能协助 B 细胞形成抗体的 T 细胞) / homozygous typing ~s (HTC) 纯合子分型细胞 / horn ~s 角质细胞;角细胞(脊髓角的节细胞) / I- ~ I 细胞(见于 I 细胞病) / immunologically competent ~ 免疫活性细胞 / incasing ~s 被盖细胞(味蕾内) / indifferent ~ 平凡细胞 / inflammatory ~ 炎症细胞 / initial ~s 胚细胞,生殖细胞 / intercalary ~s 闰细胞 / interdigitating ~s 交错突细胞 / interstitial ~s 间质细胞 / islet ~s 胰岛细胞 / juvenile ~ 幼稚细胞 / juxtaglomerular ~s [肾小]球旁细胞 / K ~s 杀伤细胞(即 killer cells);K 细胞(主要位于十二指肠和空肠黏膜中层的细胞,合成抑胃多肽) / killer T ~s T 杀伤细胞,细胞毒性 T 淋巴细胞 / L ~s L 细胞(①经过多年组织培养而成长的一株〈C3H〉小鼠成纤

维细胞中的细胞;②上段肠黏膜中有大胞质颗粒的嗜银基底粒细胞,亦称大颗粒细胞)/ large granule ~s 大颗粒细胞(见 L ~s ②)/ L. E. ~ 红斑狼疮细胞 / lepra ~ 麻风细胞 / littoral ~s 衬细胞(衬于淋巴窦或血窦壁内面的扁平细胞)/ malpighian ~ 角质形成细胞 / mast ~ 肥大细胞 / mastoid ~s 乳突小房 / megaspore mother ~ 大孢子母细胞 / memory ~s 记忆细胞(介导免疫学记忆的 T 和 B 淋巴细胞)/ mesangial ~s 系膜细胞,球内系膜细胞(肾小球)/ messenchymal ~s 间充质细胞 / metallophil ~s 嗜金属细胞 / mossy ~ 苔藓细胞(原浆性星形细胞;少突神经胶质或小神经胶质细胞)/ mother ~ 母细胞 / mouth ~ 口[咽]细胞 / mucoalbuminous ~s, mucoserous ~s 黏浆液细胞 / mucous neck ~s 颈黏液细胞 / myoepithelial ~s 肌上皮细胞 / myoid ~s 类肌细胞 / myointimal ~ 肌内膜细胞 / neutrophilic ~ 中性细胞 / nevus ~s 痣细胞 / niche ~ 中隔细胞,肺细胞 / NK ~s 自然杀伤细胞(即 natural killer cells)/ noble ~s 分化细胞 / null ~s 无标记细胞,裸细胞 / nurse ~s, nursing ~s [胸腺]抚育细胞 / osteoprogenitor ~s 骨原细胞 / owl's eye ~s 枭眼细胞,肾脱屑上皮细胞 / oxyntic ~s 壁细胞 / packed human blood ~s, packed red blood ~s (human) 浓缩人红细胞(用于输血疗法)/ parent ~ 母细胞 / parietal ~s 壁细胞(亦称酸细胞,边缘细胞,泌酸细胞)/ pavement ~s 扁平细胞 / pediculated ~ 有足(神经胶质)细胞 / peg ~s 闰细胞 / pericapillary ~s 毛细血管周细胞 / perithelial ~ 周皮细胞,外膜细胞 / pessary ~ 子宫托形红细胞 / photoautotrophic ~s 光合自养细胞 / photoreceptor ~s 感光细胞 / plasma ~ 浆细胞 / pneumatic ~s 气小房 / PNH ~s PNH 细胞,阵发性睡眠性血红蛋白尿(paroxysmal nocturnal hemoglobinuria)细胞 / polar ~s 极体 / PP ~ PP 细胞(胰岛和外分泌胰腺内分泌胰多肽〈pancreatic polypeptide〉的细胞之一)/ pre-B ~s 前 B[淋巴]细胞 / prefollicle ~s, primitive granulosa ~s 前卵泡细胞,原始粒层细胞 / pre-T ~ 前 T 细胞 / prickle ~ 棘细胞 / primary ~ 原电池 / prokaryotic ~ 原核细胞 / prolactin ~ 促乳素细胞,催乳素细胞 / prop ~s 浦肯野(Purkinje)细胞 / psychic ~s 精神细胞(大脑皮质细胞)/ RA ~ RA 细胞(即类风湿细胞 ragocyte)/ red ~, red blood ~ 红细胞 / reserve ~s 补充细胞,储备细胞 / residential ~ 居留细胞(非游走细胞)/ resting ~ 休止细胞 / resting wandering ~ 休止游走细胞,破折细胞 / reticular ~s 网状细胞 / reticuloendothelial ~ 网状内皮细胞 / rhagiocrine ~ 巨噬细胞 / rod ~s 视杆细胞 / scavenger ~ 清除细胞(吸收和清除有刺激的物质)/ sclerenchyma ~s 厚壁组织细胞 / segmented ~ 分节核细胞 / seminal ~s 精小管上皮细胞 / seminoma ~ 精原细胞瘤细胞 / sentinal ~s 血管球旁细胞,[肾小]球旁细胞 / septal ~ 隔细胞 / shadow ~ 血影细胞 / sickle ~ 镰状细胞 / signetring ~ 印戒细胞 / silver ~s 嗜银细胞 / smudge ~s 破碎细胞 / sperm ~ 精子 / spermatogonial ~ 精原细胞 / sphenoid ~s 蝶窦 / spindle ~ 梭形细胞 / squamous ~ 扁平细胞,鳞状上皮细胞 / stab ~, staff ~ 杆状核细胞 / star ~ 星状空泡细胞 / stellate ~ 星形细胞 / stem ~ 干细胞 / stipple ~ 点彩红细胞 / supporting ~s [味蕾]支持细胞 / suppresor ~s 抑制细胞(抑制抗体合成或细胞介导免疫的分化的 T 淋巴细胞)/ target ~ 靶细胞 / tart ~ 果馅饼样细胞 / T_{DTH} ~s T_{DTH} 细胞(产生淋巴因子介导迟发型超敏反应〈delayed-type hypersensitivity〉的激活 T 细胞)/ $T\gamma$ ~s $T\gamma$ 细胞(带有可与 IgG 结合的 Fc 受体的淋巴细胞,显示抑制细胞的功能)/ $T\mu$ ~s $T\mu$ 细胞(带有可与 IgM 结合的 Fc 受体的淋巴细胞,显示辅助细胞的功能)/ totipotential ~ 全[潜]能细胞 / touch ~ 触细胞,触觉小体 / trophochrome ~s 拒染细胞,黏浆液细胞 / tubal air ~s 咽鼓管气房 / type Ⅰ ~s Ⅰ型肺泡细胞(即 alveolar ~s, type Ⅰ)/ type Ⅱ ~s Ⅱ型肺泡细胞(即 aleveolar ~s, type Ⅱ)/ veil ~s, veiled ~s 褶皱细胞,面纱细胞(输入淋巴管和淋巴窦内具有无数表面皱褶或面纱样突起的抗原呈递细胞)/ ventricular ~ 室细胞 / veto ~ 否决细胞(抑制细胞的一个亚类)/ voltaic ~ 伏打电池 / water-clear ~ 明细胞(甲状旁腺中大而透明的细胞)/ white ~, white blood ~ 白细胞

cella [ˈselə] ([复] **cellae** [ˈseliː]) *n*【拉】小房,小室

cellaburate [ˌseləˈbjuəreit] *n* 纤维醋丁酯

cellacefate [seˈlæsəfeit] *n* 纤维醋法酯(药用辅料)

Cellfalcicula [ˌselfælˈsikjulə] *n* 镰状纤维菌属

Cellia [ˈseliə] (Angelo Celli) 塞蚊亚属(即按蚊属 Anopheles)

cellicolous [seˈlikələs] *a* 居留细胞内的

celliferous [seˈlifərəs] *a* 生细胞的,含细胞的

celliform [ˈselifɔːm] *a* 细胞样的

cellifugal [seˈlifjugəl] *a* 离细胞的

cellipetal [seˈlipitl] *a* 向细胞的

cellobiase [ˌseləuˈbaieis] *n* 纤维二糖酶

cellobiose [ˌseləuˈbaiəus] *n* 纤维二糖

cellobiuronic acid [ˌseləuˈbaijuəˈrɔnik] 纤维二糖醛酸

cellohexose [ˌseləuˈheksəus] *n* 纤维己糖

celloidin [seˈlɔidin] *n* 火棉;火棉液,火棉胶(用于显微镜检查,作为埋置标本或切片之用)

cellon [ˈselɔn] *n* 四氯乙烷

cellophane [ˈseləfein] *n* 赛璐玢,玻璃纸,透明纸

cellose [ˈseləus] *n* 纤维二糖
cellotetrose [ˌseləuˈtetrəus] *n* 纤维四糖
cellotriose [ˌseləuˈtraiəus] *n* 纤维三糖
cellula [ˈseljulə]（[复] **cellulae** [ˈseljuliː]）*n*【拉】细胞；小房
cellular [ˈseljulə] *a* 细胞的 | **~ity** [ˌseljuˈlærəti] *n* 细胞构成
cellulase [ˈseljuleis] *n* 纤维素酶（助消化药）
cellule [ˈseljuːl] *n* 小细胞；小房 | ~ claire 明细胞 / ethmoidal ~s 筛小房
cellulicidal [ˌseljuliˈsaidl] *a* 杀细胞的
celluliferous [ˌseljuˈlifərəs] *a* 生成细胞的，含细胞的
cellulifugal [ˌseljuˈlifjugəl] *a* 离细胞的
cellulipetal [ˌseljuˈlipitl] *a* 向细胞的
cellulitis [ˌseljuˈlaitis] *n* 蜂窝[组]织炎 | dissecting ~ of scalp 头皮切割性蜂窝织炎，头部脓肿性穿凿性毛囊周围炎 / finger ~ 瘭疽，指头脓炎 / orbital ~ 眼眶蜂窝织炎 / pelvic ~ 盆腔蜂窝织炎，子宫旁[组织]炎 / phlegmonous ~ 蜂窝织炎/ streptococcus ~ 链球菌性蜂窝织炎（常表现为丹毒）
cellulofibrous [ˌseljuləuˈfaibrəs] *a* 细胞与纤维的
celluloid [ˈseljulɔid] *n* 赛璐珞，假象牙
Cellulomonas [ˌseljuləuˈməunəs] *n* 纤维单胞菌属
celluloneuritis [ˌseljuləunjuəˈraitis] *n* 神经细胞炎 | acute anterior ~ 急性前角神经细胞炎
cellulose [ˈseljuləus] *n* 纤维素 | microcrystalline ~ 微晶纤维素（赋形剂）/ oxidized ~, absorbable ~ 氧化纤维素，可吸收[性]纤维素（局部止血药）/ starch ~ 淀粉粒纤维素，支链淀粉
cellulosic acid [ˌseljuˈləusik] 纤维素酸，氧化纤维素（局部止血药）
cellulosity [ˌseljuˈlɔsəti] *n* 细胞构成
cellulotoxic [ˌseljuləuˈtɔksik] *a* 细胞毒的
cellulous [ˈseljuləs] *a* 细胞性的
Cellvibrio [selˈvibriəu] *n* 纤维弧菌属
cel(o)- [构词成分]瘤，肿胀；腔，见 coel(o)-；腹，腹腔，见 celi(o)-
celology [siˈlɔlədʒi] *n* 疝学，赫尼亚论
celom [ˈsiːlɔm] *n* 体腔 | **~ic** [siˈlɔmik] *a*
celophlebitis [ˌsiːləufliˈbaitis] *n* 腔静脉炎
celoschisis [siˈlɔskisis] *n* 腹裂
celoscope [ˈseləskəup] *n* 体腔镜（尤指腹腔镜）| **celoscopy** [siˈlɔskəpi] *n* 体腔镜检查（尤指腹腔镜检查）
celosomia [ˌsiləuˈsəumiə] *n* 露脏畸形
celosomus [ˌsiːləuˈsəuməs] *n* 露脏畸胎
celothel [ˈsiːləθəl]，**celothelium** [ˌsiːləuˈθiːljəm] *n* 间皮
celothelioma [ˌsiːləuθiːliˈəumə] *n* 间皮瘤
celotomy [siˈlɔtəmi] *n* 疝切开术
celovirus [ˌseləuˈvaiərəs] *n* 鸡胚致死孤病毒
celozoic [ˌsiːləuˈzəuik] *a* 体腔寄生的
Celsius scale [ˈselsjəs]（Anders Celsius）摄氏温标 | ~ thermometer 摄氏温度计
Celsus quadrilateral [ˈselsəs]（Aurelius Cornelius）塞尔萨斯四症候（炎症的四个主要症候：红、肿、热、痛）
CEM contagious equine metritis 马[接]触[传]染性子宫炎
cement [siˈment] *n* 黏固剂；牙骨质 | intercellular ~ 细胞间胶质 / interprismatic ~ 釉柱间质 / muscle ~ 肌胶质 / nerve ~ 神经胶质 / resin ~ 树脂黏固剂 / root canal ~ 根管黏固剂 / silicate ~ 硅酸盐黏固剂 / zinc eugenol ~ 锌-丁香油酚黏固剂 / zinc phosphate ~ 磷酸锌黏固剂
cementation [ˌsiːmenˈteiʃən] *n* 黏固
cementicle [siˈmentikl] *a* 牙骨质小体 | adherent ~, attached ~ 连结性牙骨质小体 / free ~, interstitial ~ 游离性牙骨质小体
cementification [siˌmentifiˈkeiʃən] *n* 牙骨质形成
cementin [siˈmentin] *n* 黏合质
cementitis [ˌsiːmenˈtaitis] *n* 牙骨质炎
cement(o)-[构词成分]牙骨质
cementoblast [siˈmentəblæst] *n* 成牙骨质细胞
cementoblastoma [siˌmentəublæsˈtəumə] *n* 成牙骨质细胞瘤
cementoclasia [siˌmentəuˈkleiziə] *n* 牙骨质破坏
cementoclast [siˈmentəˌklæst] *n* 破牙骨质细胞
cementocyte [siˈmentəsait] *n* 牙骨质细胞
cemento-exostosis [siˌmentəuˌeksɔsˈtəusis] *n* 牙骨质疣，牙骨小体
cementogenesis [siˌmentəuˈdʒenisis] *n* 牙骨质发生
cementoid [siˈmentɔid] *n* 类牙骨质
cementoma [ˌsiːmenˈtəumə] *n* 牙骨质瘤
cementopathia [siˌmentəuˈpæθiə] *n* 牙骨质病变，牙周病变
cementoperiostitis [siˌmentəuˌperiɔsˈtaitis] *n* 牙周炎，牙骨质膜炎
cementosis [ˌsiːmenˈtəusis] *n* 牙骨质增生
cementum [siˈmentəm] *n*【拉】牙骨质
cenadelphus [ˌsiːnəˈdelfəs] *n* 完全对称性双畸胎
cenencephalocele [ˌsiːnenˈsefələsiːl] *n* 脑膨出
cenesthesia [ˌsiːnisˈθiːzjə]，**cenesthesis** [ˌsiːnisˈθiːsis] *n* 普通感觉，存在感觉，器官功能正常感觉 | **cenesthesic** [ˌsiːnisˈθiːsik]，**cenesthetic** [ˌsiːnisˈθetik] *a*
cenesthesiopathy [ˌsiːnisˌθiːziˈɔpəθi] *n* 体觉违和，全身违和
cenesthopathy [ˌsiːnisˈθɔpəθi] *n* 体觉违和，全身违和

ceno- [构词成分]新;共同特性或特征
cenobium [si'nəubiəm] *n* 菌团
cenocyte ['si:nəsait] *n* 多核细胞
cenogenesis [ˌsi:nə'dʒenisis] *n* 新性发生(指对外界环境的适应性反应)
cenopsychic [ˌsi:nə'saikik] *a* 精神发展最新表现的
cenosis [si'nəusis] *n* (病理)排泄 | **cenotic** [si'nɔtik] *a*
cenosite ['si:nəsait] *n* 半自由寄生物
cenotoxin [ˌsi:nə'tɔksin] *n* 疲倦毒素
cenotype ['si:nətaip] *n* 共通型,初型
censor ['sensə] *n* 监察员;检查员;潜意识稽查 | freudian ~, psychic ~ 潜意识稽查 | **~ial** [sen'sɔ:riəl] *a* / **~ship** *n* 督察;检查;潜意识压抑力
census ['sensəs] *n* 人口调查,人口普查
Centaurea [sen'tɔ:riə] *n* 矢车菊属
centenarian [senti'nɛəriən] *n* 百岁
center ['sentə] *n* 中心,中央;中枢; | accelerating ~, cardioaccelerating ~ 加速中枢,心加速中枢 / apneustic ~ 长吸中枢 / auditopsychic ~ 认音中枢 / auditory ~, acoustic ~ 听[觉]中枢 / ciliospinal ~ 脊髓散瞳中枢,睫脊中枢 / community mental health ~ (CMHC) 社区心理卫生中心 / Centers for Disease Control and Prevention (CDC) 疾病控制与预防中心(以前称 Communicable Disease Center〈1946〉, Center for Disease Control〈1970〉和 Centers for Diseaes Control〈1980〉) / cortical ~ [大脑]皮质中枢 / dentary ~ 下颌骨化中心 / epiotic ~ 乳突骨化中心 / genital ~, genitospinal ~ 脊髓生殖中枢 / germinal ~, reaction ~ 生发中心,反应中心 / health ~ 卫生院;医学中心(包括医学校以及各种有关的卫生职业学校) / heat-regulating ~s 热调节中枢 / inhibitory ~ 抑制中枢 / kinetic ~ 受精卵中心球 / motor ~ 运动中枢 / nerve ~ 神经中枢 /ossification ~ 骨化中心 / optic ~ 光心 / phrenic ~, tendinous ~ 中心腱[膈] / polypneic ~, panting ~ 呼吸加速中枢 / rectovesical ~ 直肠膀胱反射中枢 / rotation ~ 旋转中枢 / semioval ~ 半卵圆中心 / sensory ~ 感觉中枢 / sex-behavior ~ 性行为中枢(下丘脑内侧核) / somatic ~ [大脑]垂体 / sphenotic ~ 蝶骨骨化中心 / splenial ~ 下颌内板骨化中心 / vesical ~, vesicospinal ~ 膀胱中枢,排尿中枢 / vomiting ~ 呕吐中枢 / visual word ~ 视词中枢
centesimal [sen'tesiməl] *a* 百分之一的,分成百份的,百进位的
centesis [sen'ti:sis] *n* 穿刺术
-centesis [构词成分]穿刺术
centi- [构词成分]厘,百分;一百
centibar ['sentibɑ:] *n* 厘巴(旧气压单位,现用 Pa 帕[斯卡],1 厘巴 = 10^3 Pa)
centigrade ['sentigreid] *a* 百分度的 *n* 百分度
centigram ['sentigræm] *n* 厘克(=10^{-2} g)
centigray (cGy) ['sentigrei] *n* 厘戈瑞(=10^{-2} Gy)(吸收剂量单位,百分之一戈瑞)
centilitre, centiliter (cL) ['sentiˌli:tə] *n* 厘升(=10^{-2} L)
centimetre, centimeter (cm) ['sentiˌmi:tə] *n* 厘米(=10^{-2} m)
centimorgan ['sentimɔ:gən] *n* 厘摩(连锁基因间的图距单位,百分之一摩。亦称图单位)
centinormal [ˌsenti'nɔ:məl] *a* 厘规的,百分之一当量浓度的
centipede ['sentipi:d] *n* 蜈蚣
centipoise ['sentipɔiz] *n* 厘泊(旧物黏度单位,1 cP = 1 mPa · s,百分之一泊)
centistoke ['sentistəuk] *n* 厘沲(旧运动黏度单位,1 cSt = 10^{-6} m^2/s,百分之一沲)
centiunit [ˌsenti'ju:nit] *n* 百分单位
centra ['sentrə] centrum 的复数
centrad ['sentræd] *ad* 向中心 *n* 厘弧度(偏向角的度量单位, = 0.57°)
centrage ['sentreidʒ] *n* (折射)中心线(眼球各折射面的中心点均在同一条直线上)
central ['sentrəl] *a* 中央的,中心的;中枢的
centralis [sen'treilis] *n*【拉】中心结构
centralism ['sentrəlizəm] *n* 中枢功能论
centrality [sen'træləti] *n* 中心性
centraphose ['sentrəfəuz] *n* 中枢性暗觉
centration [sen'treiʃən] *n* 定心作用(不能每次注意一个以上的显著特点,这是人类发育的正常阶段)
centraxonial [ˌsentræk'səuniəl] *a* 中轴的
centre ['sentə] *n* = **center**
centrencephalic [ˌsentrensi'fælik] *a* 脑中心的
centri- [构词成分]中心,中央;中枢
centric ['sentrik] *a* 中央的,中心的;中枢的 *n* 中心
centriciput [sen'trisipət] *n* 头中部
centrifugal [sen'trifjugəl] *a* 离心的,离中的;传出的
centrifugalize [sen'trifju:gəlaiz] *vt* 离心[法],离心分离 | **centrifugalization** [senˌtrifjugəlai'zeiʃən, -li'z-] *n*
centrifugate [sen'trifjugeit] *n* 离心分离物
centrifugation [senˌtrifju'geiʃən] *n* 离心[法],离心分离 | density gradient ~ 密度梯度离心 / differential ~ 差示离心,鉴别离心 / isopyknic ~ 等密度离心
centrifuge ['sentrifju:dʒ] *n* 离心机 *vt* 离心(分离) | microscope ~ 显微镜离心机

centrilobular [ˌsentriˈlɔbjulə] *a* 小叶中心的
centriole [ˈsentriəu] *n* 中心粒 | distal ~, posterior ~ 远侧中心粒,后中心粒 / proximal ~, anterior ~ 近侧中心粒,前中心粒
centripetal [senˈtripitl] *a* 向心的,向中的;传入的
centr(o)- [构词成分] 中心,中央;中枢(见 centri-)
centroblast [ˈsentrəuˌblæst] *n* 中心母细胞
centrocecal [ˌsentrəuˈsiːkəl] *a* 中心盲点的
Centrocestus [ˌsentrəuˈsestəs] *n* 棘带[吸虫]属 | ~ cuspidatus 尖端棘带吸虫
centrocyte [ˈsentrəuˌsait] *n* 中心细胞
centrodesmus [ˌsentrəuˈdesməs], **centrodesmose** [ˌsentrəuˈdesməus] *n* 中心体连丝(某些原虫在细胞分裂期核内中心粒之间的连结)
Centrohelida [ˌsentrəuˈhiːlidə] *n* 中阳目
centrokinesia [ˌsentrəukaiˈniːziə], **centrocinesia** [ˌsentrəusaiˈniːziə] *n* 中枢性运动 | **centrokinetic** [ˌsentrəukaiˈnetik], **centrocinetic** [ˌsentrəusaiˈnetik] *a*
centrolecithal [ˌsentrəuˈlesiθəl] *a* 卵黄居中的,中黄的
centrolobular [ˌsentrəuˈlɔbjulə] *a* 小叶中心的
centromere [ˈsentrəmiə] *n* 着丝粒(指染色体明显的缩窄部分) | **centromeric** [ˌsentrəuˈmerik] *a*
centron [ˈsentrɔn] *n* 中心基质(在淋巴结皮质内)
centronucleus [ˌsentrəuˈnjuːkliəs] *n* 中心核,中央核,双质核
centro-osteosclerosis [ˌsentrəuˌɔsti-əuskliəˈrəusis] *n* 骨髓腔骨化
centrophenoxine [ˌsentrəufiˈnɔksiːn] *n* 甲氯芬酯(精神振奋药)
centrophose [ˈsentrəfəuz] *n* 中枢性光幻觉
centroplasm [ˈsentrəplæzəm] *n* 中心质
centroplast [ˈsentrəplæst] *n* 中心质体
centrosclerosis [ˌsentrəuskliəˈrəusis] *n* 骨髓腔骨化
centrosome [ˈsentrəsəum] *n* 中心体
centrosphere [ˈsentrəsfiə] *n* 中心球;中心体
centrostaltic [ˌsentrəuˈstæltik] *a* 运动中心的
centrotherapy [ˌsentrəuˈθerəpi] *n* [趋]中枢疗法(从体外作用于神经中枢的疗法)
centrum [ˈsentrəm] ([复] **centra** [ˈsentrə] 或 **centrums**) *n*【拉】中心;中枢;椎体;壳心
Centruroides [ˌsentruːˈrɔidiːz] *n* 刺尾蝎属
Cenurus [seˈnjuərəs] *n* 多头[绦虫]蚴属(即 Coenurus) | ~ cerebralis 脑多头(绦虫)蚴(即 Coenurus cerebralis)
CEP congenital erythropoietic porphyria 先天性红细胞生成性卟啉病
cephacetrile sodium [ˈsefəsitrail] 头孢乙腈钠(抗生素类药)
Cephaelis [ˌsefeiˈiːlis] *n* 吐根属
cephal- 见 cephalo-
cephalad [ˈsefəlæd] *ad* 向头侧
cephalalgia [ˌsefəˈlældʒiə] *n* 头痛 | histamine ~ 组胺性头痛 / pharyngotympanic ~ 咽鼓室炎性头痛 / quadrantal ~ 象限性头痛 | **cephalgia** [siˈfældʒiə] *n*
cephaledema [ˌsefəliˈdiːmə] *n* 头水肿
cephalematocele [ˌsefəliˈmætəsiːl] *n* 头血囊肿
cephalematoma [ˌsefəˌleməˈtəumə] *n* 头颅血肿
cephalexin [ˌsefəˈleksin] *n* 头孢氨苄(抗生素类药)
cephalhematocele [ˌsefəlhiːˈmætəsiːl] *n* 头血囊肿
cephalhematoma [ˌsefəlˌhiːməˈtəumə] *n* 头颅血肿 | ~ deformans 畸形性头颅血肿
cephalhydrocele [ˌsefəlˈhaidrəsiːl] *n* 头水囊肿 | ~ traumatica 创伤性头水囊肿
cephalic [siˈfælik] *a* 头的;头侧的;向着头部的
cephalin [ˈsefəlin] *a* 脑磷脂
Cephalina [ˌsefəˈlainə] *n* 隔簇虫亚目(即 Septatina)
cephalitis [ˌsefəˈlaitis] *n* 脑炎
cephalization [ˌsefəlaiˈzeiʃən, -liˈz-] *n* 头部优势发育(胚胎的生长趋势集中或开始于头端)
cephal(o)- [构词成分]头
cephalocathartic [ˌsefələukəˈθɑːtik] *a* 清脑的 *n* 清脑药
cephalocaudad [ˌsefələuˈkɔːdæd] *ad* 从头至尾;向头尾端
cephalocaudal [ˌsefələuˈkɔːdl] *a* 从头至尾的
cephalocele [siˈfæləsiːl] *n* 脑膨出
cephalocentesis [ˌsefələusenˈtiːsis] *n* 头颅穿刺术
cephalochord [ˈsefələkɔːd] *n* 头索(胚胎脊索的颅内部分)
Cephalochordata [ˌsefələukɔːˈdeitə] *n* 头索亚门,无头亚门
cephalochordate [ˌsefələuˈkɔːdeit] *n* 头索动物
cephalocyst [ˈsefələˌsist] *n* 头囊
cephalodactyly [ˌsefələuˈdæktili] *n* 头指畸形,头趾畸形
cephalodiprosopus [ˌsefələudaiˈprɔsəpəs] *n* 头部寄生胎
cephalodymia [ˌsefələuˈdimiə] *n* 头部联胎畸形
cephalodymus [ˌsefəˈlɔdiməs] *n* 头部联胎
cephalodynia [ˌsefələuˈdiniə] *n* 头痛
cephalogaster [ˌsefələuˈgæstə] *n* 头肠(胚胎肠管的前端)
cephalogenesis [ˌsefələuˈdʒenisis] *n* 头部形成

cephaloglycin [ˌsefələuˈglaisin] *n* 头孢来星(抗生素类药)
cephalogram [ˈsefələgræm] *n* 测颅X线[照]片
cephalography [ˌsefəˈlɔgrəfi] *n* 测颅术
cephalogyric [ˌsefələuˈdʒaiərik] *a* 头回旋的
cephalohematocele [ˌsefələuhiːˈmætesiːl] *n* 头血囊肿
cephalohematoma [ˌsefələuˈhiːməˈtəumə] *n* 头颅血肿
cephalomelus [ˌsefəˈlɔmiləs] *n* 头部寄生肢畸胎
cephalomenia [ˌsefələuˈmiːniə] *n* 头部倒经(如行经时鼻出血)
cephalometer [ˌsefəˈlɔmitə] *n* 头颅定位器
cephalometrics [ˌsefələuˈmetriks] *n* 头影测量学
cephalometry [ˌsefəˈlɔmitri] *n* 头影测量学,头影测量[法] | fetal ~ 胎头影测量法
cephalomotor [ˌsefələuˈməutə] *a* 头运动的
Cephalomyia [ˌsefələuˈmaijə] *n* 狂蝇属(即 Oestrus)
cephalonia [ˌsefəˈləuniə] *n* 巨头症
cephalont [ˈsefəlɔnt] *n* 头胞体(簇虫发育的一个时期)
cephalopagus [ˌsefəˈlɔpəgəs] *n* 头联双胎
cephalopathy [ˌsefəˈlɔpəθi] *n* 头[部]病
cephalopelvic [ˌsefələuˈpelvik] *a* 胎头骨盆的
cephalopelvimetry [ˌsefələupelˈvimitri] *n* 胎头骨盆测量法
cephalopharyngeus [ˌsefələufəˈrindʒiəs] *n* 咽上缩肌
cephaloplegia [ˌsefələuˈpliːdʒiə] *n* 头[面]肌麻痹,头[面]肌瘫痪
Cephalopoda [ˌsefəˈlɔpəde] *n* 头足纲
cephalorhachidian [ˌsefələurəˈkidiən] *a* 头与脊柱的
cephaloridine [ˌsefəˈlɔridiːn] *n* 头孢噻啶(抗生素类药)
cephalosporin [ˌsefələuˈspɔːrin] *n* 头孢菌素 | ~ C 头孢菌素 C / ~ N 头孢菌素 N, 氨羧丁青霉素,阿地西林 (adicillin) / ~ P 头孢菌素 P
cephalosporinase [ˌsefələuˈspɔːrineis] *n* 头孢菌素酶,*β*-内酰胺酶
cephalosporiosis [ˌsefələuˌspɔːriˈəusis] *n* 头孢子菌病
Cephalosporium [ˌsefələuˈspɔːriəm] *n* 头孢子菌属 | ~ falciforme 镰状头孢子菌 / ~ granulomatis 肉芽肿头孢子菌(可引起人体树胶肿样损害)
cephalostat [ˈsefələstæt] *n* 头固定器(用于牙放射学)
cephalostyle [ˈsefələˌstail] *n* 脊索颅端
cephalotetanus [ˌsefələuˈtetənəs] *n* 头部破伤风
cephalothin [ˈsefələθin] *n* 头孢噻吩(抗生素类药) | ~ sodium 头孢噻吩钠
cephalothoracic [ˌsefələuθɔːˈræsik] *a* 头[与]胸廓的
cephalothoracopagus [ˌsefələuˌθɔːrəˈkɔpəgəs] *n* 头胸联双胎
cephalotome [ˈsefələtəum] *n* 胎头刀
cephalotomy [ˌsefəˈlɔtəmi] *n* 胎头切开术,穿颅术;胎头解剖
cephalotropic [ˌsefələuˈtrɔpik] *a* 向脑的
cephalotrypesis [ˌsefələutraiˈpiːsis] *n* 颅骨环锯术
cephalous [ˈsefələs] *a* 有头的
-cephalus [构词成分]头
-cephaly [构词成分]头
cephamycin [ˌsefəˈmaisin] *n* 头霉素
cephapirin [sefəˈpaiərin] *n* 头孢匹林(抗生素类药) | ~ sodium 头孢匹林钠(抗生素类药)
cepharanthine [ˌsefəˈrænθin] *n* 千金藤碱(抗矽肺药)
cephradine [ˈsefrədiːn] *n* 头孢拉定(抗生素类药)
-ceptor [构词成分]感受器
ceptor [ˈseptə] *n* 受体;感受器 | nerve ~ 感受器
cera [ˈsiərə] *n*【拉】蜂蜡,蜡
ceraceous [siˈreiʃəs] *a* 蜡状的
ceramic [siˈræmik] *a* 陶瓷的 *n* 陶瓷;金属氧化物
ceramics [siˈræmiks] *n* 制陶术;陶瓷学;陶器 | dental ~ 牙科陶瓷学
ceramidase [seˈræmideis] *n* 神经酰胺酶
ceramidase deficiency 神经酰胺酶缺乏症,法伯(Farber)病
ceramide [ˈserəmaid] *n* 神经酰胺 | ~ aminoethyl phosphate 神经酰胺氨乙基磷酸 | galactosyl ~ 半乳糖[基]神经酰胺,脑苷脂 / ~ lactoside 神经酰胺乳糖苷 / ~ trihexoside 神经酰胺三己糖苷
ceramide cholinephosphotransferase [ˈserəmaid ˌkəuliːnˌfɔsfəˈtrænsfəreis] 神经酰胺转磷酸胆碱酶
ceramide trihexosidase [ˈserəmaid ˌtraihekˈsəusideis] 神经酰胺三己糖苷酶,α-半乳糖苷酶 A
ceramide trihexosidase deficiency 神经酰胺三己糖苷酶缺乏症,法布莱(Fabry)病
ceramidosis [seˌræmiˈdəusis] *n* 神经酰胺病 | lactosyl ~ 乳糖基神经酰氨病
ceramodontics [siˌræməˈdɔntiks] *n* 牙科陶瓷学
cerasin [ˈserəsin] *n* 樱胶素;角苷脂
cerasine [ˈserəsain] *n* 黄光油溶红
Cerastes [siˈræstiːz] *n* 蝰属
cerasus [ˈserəsəs] *n*【拉】樱桃树
cerate [ˈsiərit] *n* 蜡膏,蜡剂 | simple ~ 单蜡膏(安息香豚脂与白蜂蜡熔合而成)

ceratectomy [ˌserəˈtektəmi] *n* 角膜切除术
ceratin [ˈserətin] *n* 角蛋白
Ceratiomyxa [siˌreiʃiəuˈmiksə] *n* 鹅绒黏菌属
ceratitis [ˌserəˈtaitis] *n* 角膜炎
Ceratium [siˈreiʃiəm] *n* 角藻属,角甲藻虫属
cerat(o)- [构词成分]角质;角膜(见 kerato-)
ceratocricoid [ˌserətəuˈkraikɔid] *a* 下角环状软骨的,环甲关节的
ceratocricoideus [ˌserətəukraiˈkɔidiəs] 角环肌
ceratohyal [ˌserətəuˈhaiəl] *a* 舌骨小角的
Ceratomyxa [siˌreitəuˈmiksə] *n* 角形虫属
Ceratonia [ˌsirəˈtəuniə] *n* 长角豆属
ceratonosus [ˌserəˈtɔnəsəs] *n* 角膜病
Ceratophyllus [ˌserəˈtɔfiləs] *n* 角叶蚤属 | ~ acutus 山角叶蚤,山穿手蚤 / ~ fasciatus 具带角叶蚤,具带病蚤 / ~ gallinae 鸡[角叶]蚤 / ~ idahoensis 爱达荷角叶蚤,爱达荷山蚤 / ~ punjabensis 旁遮普角叶蚤 / ~ silantiewi 谢[兰季耶夫]氏角叶蚤,谢[兰季耶夫]氏山蚤 / ~ tesquorum 黄鼠角叶蚤
Ceratopogonidae [ˌserətəupəuˈgɔnidiː] *n* 蠓科
ceratum [siˈreitəm] *n*【拉】蜡剂,蜡膏
cerberin, cerberine [ˈsəːbərin] *n* 海杧果苷(强心药)
cercaria [səːˈkɛəriə] ([复] **cercariae** [səːˈkɛəriiː]) *n* 尾蚴
cercaricidal [səːˌkɛəriˈsaidl] *a* 杀尾蚴的
cercarienhullenreaktion [səːˌkɛərienˌhʌlənri(ː)ˈækʃən] *n* 尾蚴膜反应(检曼氏裂体吸虫试验)
cerci [ˈsəːsai] cercus 的复数
cerclage [sɛəˈklɑːʒ] *n*【法】环扎法(以环或线圈将某一部分作环形裹扎,如对宫颈松弛的环扎,或以金属环或金属线圈将折骨端束紧)
cerc(o)- [构词成分]尾
cercocystis [ˌsəːkəuˈsistis] *n* 小似囊尾蚴
cercoid [ˈsəːkɔid] *n* 似尾蚴
cercomonad [səˈkɔmənəd] *n* 单鞭滴虫
Cercomonas [səˈkɔmənəs] *n* 单鞭滴虫属 | ~ hominis 人单鞭滴虫 / ~ longicauda 长尾单鞭滴虫
Cercopithecidae [ˌsəːkəupiˈθesidiː] *n* 猕猴科
cercopithecoid [ˌsəːkəuˈpiθikɔid] *n* 猕猴
Cercopithecoidea [ˌsəːkəuˌpiθiˈkɔidiə] *n* 猕猴总科
Cercosphaera addisoni [səːkəuˈsfiərə ædiˈsəuni] 艾迪生小孢子菌(见 Microsporum audouini)
Cercospora [ˌsəːkəuˈspɔːrə] *n* 尾孢[霉]属 | ~ apii 尖尾孢霉(引起人的尾孢霉病)
Cercosporalla vexans [ˌsəːkəuspəˈræləˈveksəns] [皮肤]鞭毛孢子菌
cercosporamycosis [ˌsəːkəuˌspɔːrəmaiˈkəusis] *n* 尾孢霉病
cercus [ˈsəːkəs] ([复] **cerci** [ˈsəːsai]) *n* 尾突,尾须
cerea flexibilitas [ˈsiəriə ˌfleksiˈbilitæs]【拉】蜡样屈曲(见于紧张型精神分裂症,保持所施于的任何身体位置。亦称僵住症)
cerealin [siˈriəlin] *n* 谷淀粉酶
cerealose [ˈsiəriələus] *n* 饴糖
cerebella [ˌseriˈbelə] cerebellum 的复数
cerebellar [ˌseriˈbelə] *a* 小脑的
cerebellifugal [ˌseribeˈlifjuqəl] *a* 离小脑的,小脑传出的
cerebellipetal [ˌseribeˈlipitl] *a* 向小脑的,传入小脑的
cerebellitis [ˌseribeˈlaitis] *n* 小脑炎
cerebell(o)- [构词成分]小脑
cerebellofugal [ˌseribeˈlɔfjugəl] *a* 离小脑的,小脑传出的
cerebello-olivary [ˌseriˌbeləuɔlivəri] *a* 小脑橄榄体的
cerebellopontile [ˌseribeləuˈpɔntail], **cerebellopontine** [ˌseribeləuˈpɔntiːn] *a* 小脑脑桥的,桥小脑的
cerebellorubral [ˌseriˌbeləuˈruːbrəl] *a* 小脑红核的
cerebellorubrospinal [ˌseriˌbeləuˌruːbrəuˈspainl] *a* 小脑红核脊髓的
cerebellospinal [ˌseriˌbeləuˈspainl] *a* 小脑脊髓的
cerebellum [ˌseriˈbeləm] ([复] **cerebellums** 或 **cerebella** [ˌseriˈbelə]) *n* 小脑
cerebra [ˈseribrə] cerebrum 的复数
cerebral [ˈseribrəl] *a* 大脑的
cerebrate [ˈseribreit] *vi* 用脑,思考
cerebration [ˌseriˈbreiʃən] *n* 思考;大脑功能活动,精神活动 | unconscious ~ 无意识的精神(或心理)活动
cerebriform [siˈrebrifɔːm] *a* 脑形的,脑质样的
cerebrifugal [ˌseriˈbrifjugəl] *a* 离大脑的,大脑传出的
cerebripetal [ˌseriˈbripitl] *a* 向大脑的,传入大脑的
cerebritis [ˌseriˈbraitis] *n* 大脑炎,脑炎 | saturnine ~ 铅中毒性脑炎
cerebr(o)- [构词成分]大脑
cerebrocardiac [ˌseribrəuˈkɑːdiæk] *a* 大脑心脏的
cerebrocentric [ˌseribrəuˈsentrik] *a* 大脑中枢的(指人格控制中心在大脑的学说)
cerebrocerebellar [ˌseribrəuˌseriˈbelə] *a* 大脑小脑的
cerebrocuprein [ˌseribrəuˈkjuːpriːn] *n* 脑铜蛋白,超氧化物歧化酶
cerebrogalactose [ˌseribrəugəˈlæktəus] *n* 脑半乳糖,脑糖

cerebrogalactoside [ˌseribrəugəˈlæktəsaid] *n* 脑半乳糖苷,脑苷脂
cerebrohyphoid [ˌseribrəuˈhaifɔid] *a* 脑组织样的
cerebroid [ˈseribrɔid] *a* 脑[质]样的
cerebrology [ˌseriˈbrɔlədʒi] *n* 脑学
cerebroma [ˌseriˈbrəumə] *n* 脑瘤
cerebromacular [ˌseribrəuˈmækjulə] *a* 脑黄斑的
cerebromalacia [ˌseribrəuməˈleiʃiə] *n* 脑软化
cerebromedullary [ˌseribrəumeˈdʌləri, -ˈmedə-] *a* 脑脊髓的
cerebromeningeal [ˌseribrəumiˈnindʒiəl] *a* 脑脑膜的
cerebromeningitis [ˌseribrəuˌmeninˈdʒaitis] *n* 脑脑膜炎
cerebron [ˈseribrɔn] *n* 羟脑苷脂
cerebronic acid [ˌseriˈbrɔnik] 脑羟脂酸
cerebro-ocular [ˌseribrəuˈɔkjulə] *a* 脑[与]眼的
cerebropathia [ˌseribrəuˈpæθiə] *n*【拉】脑病 | ~ psychica toxemica 精神中毒性脑病
cerebropathy [ˌseriˈbrɔpəθi] *n* 脑病
cerebrophysiology [ˌseribrəuˌfiziˈɔlədʒi] *n* 大脑生理学
cerebropontile [ˌseribrəuˈpɔntail] *a* 大脑脑桥的
cerebrorachidian [ˌseribrəurəˈkidiən] *a* 脑脊髓的
cerebrosclerosis [ˌseribrəuskliəˈrəusis] *n* 脑硬化
cerebrose [ˈseribrəus] *n* 脑半乳糖,脑糖
cerebroside [ˈseribrəsaid] *n* 脑苷脂
cerebroside *β*-galactosidase [ˈseribrəsaid gəˌlæktəuˈsaideis] 脑苷脂*β*-半乳糖苷酶,半乳糖[基]神经酰胺酶
cerebroside *β*-glucosidase [ˈseribrəsaid gluːˈkəusideis] 脑苷脂*β*-葡糖苷酶
cerebroside sulfatase [ˈseribrəsaid ˈsʌlfəteis] 脑苷脂硫酸酯酶(此酶缺乏为一种常染色体隐性性状,是异染性脑白质营养不良的原因之一)
cerebrosidosis [ˌseribrəusaiˈdəusis] *n* 脑苷脂贮积病
cerebrosis [ˌseriˈbrəusis] *n* 脑病
cerebrospinal [ˌseribrəuˈspainl] *a* 脑脊髓的
cerebrospinant [ˌseribrəuˈspainənt] *n* 脑脊髓药
cerebrospinase [ˌseribrəuˈspaineis] *n* 脑脊液氧化酶
cerebrostomy [ˌseriˈbrɔstəmi] *n* 脑切开[造口]术
cerebrotendinous [ˌseribrəuˈtendinəs] *a* 脑腱的
cerebrotomy [ˌseriˈbrɔtəmi] *n* 脑切开术
cerebrovascular [ˌseribrəuˈvæskjulə] *a* 脑血管的
cerebrum [ˈseribrəm] ([复] **cerebra** [ˈseribrə] 或 **cerebrums**) *n*【拉】大脑
cerecloth [ˈsiəklɔθ] *n* 蜡布
cerement [ˈsiəmənt] *n* 蜡布;[复]寿衣
Cerenkov radiation [ˈkeirenkɔv] (P. A. Cerenkov) 切伦科夫辐射(电子快速通过液体,其速率大于该液体中的光速时所产生的能量)
cereolus [siˈriələs] ([复] **cereoli** [siˈriəlai]) *n*【拉】药制杆剂,烛剂
ceretopharyngeus [ˌserətəufəˈrindʒiəs] *n* 大角咽肌
cerevisia [ˌseriˈviziə] ([复] **cerevisiae** [ˌseriˈviziiː]) *n*【拉】啤酒,麦酒
Cerithidia [ˌseriˈθidiə] *n* 拟蟹守螺属 | ~ cingulata 珠带拟蟹守螺
cerium(Ce) [ˈsiəriəm] *n*【拉】铈(化学元素) | ~ oxalate 草酸铈(治妊娠呕吐、反射性咳等)
cerivastatin sodium [səˈrivəˌstætin] 西伐他汀钠(降血脂药,美国不发售,因其与横纹肌溶解风险增加有关)
cermet [ˈsəːmet] *n* 金属陶瓷,合金陶瓷(牙黏固粉及耐热固体物质的成分)
ceroid [ˈsiərɔid] *n* 蜡样质(肝、神经系统、肌肉内一种不溶性脂质色素)
cerolipoid [ˌsiərəuˈlipɔid] *n* 植物类脂,蜡脂质(植物中含有的蜡样物质)
cerolysin [siˈrɔlisin] *n* 溶蜡素
ceroma [siˈrəumə] *n* 蜡[样变]瘤
ceroplastic [ˌsiərəuˈplæstik] *a* 成蜡型的
ceroplasty [ˈsiərəuˌplæsti] *n* 蜡成型术
cerotic acid [siˈrɔtik], **cerotinicacid** [ˌsiərəuˈtinik] 蜡酸
cerotin [ˈsiərətin] *n* 蜡醇
certifiable [ˈsəːtifaiəbl] *a* 可证明的;法定的(指传染病,根据法律,传染病病例须向卫生当局报告)
certificate [səˈtifikit] *n* 证[明]书,证,合格证件,许可证
cerulean [siˈruːljən] *a* 天蓝色的,蔚蓝色的
cerulein [siˈruːliːn] *n* 蛙皮缩胆囊肽
ceruleus [siˈruːliəs] *a* 天蓝色的,蔚蓝色的
ceruloplasmin [siˌruːləuˈplæzmin] *n* 血浆铜蓝蛋白
cerumen [siˈruːmen] *n* 耵聍 | impacted ~ 耵聍栓塞 / inspissated ~ 干耵聍 | **ceruminal** [siˈruːminl], **ceruminous** [siˈruːminəs] *a* **ceruminolysis** [siˌruːmiˈnɔlisis] *n* 耵聍溶解 | **ceruminolytic** [siˌruːminəˈlitik] *a* 溶耵聍的 *n* 溶耵聍药
ceruminoma [siˌruːmiˈnəumə] *n* 耵聍腺瘤
ceruminosis [siˌruːmiˈnəusis] *n* 耵聍分泌过多
ceruse [ˈsiəruːs] *n* 铅白,碳酸铅白,碱性碳酸铅
cervical [ˈsəːvikəl] *a* 颈的(如宫颈的)
cervicalis [səːviˈkeilis] *a*【拉】颈的(如宫颈的)
cervicectomy [ˌsəːviˈsektəmi] *n* 宫颈切除术

cervices [ˈsəːvisiːzˌsəːˈvaisiːz] cervix 的复数
cervicitis [ˌsəːviˈsaitis] *n* 宫颈炎 | granulomatous ~ 肉芽肿性宫颈炎 / traumatic ~ 创伤性宫颈炎
cervicoaxillary [ˌsəːvikəuækˈsiləri, -ˈæksi-] *a* 颈腋的
cervicobrachial [ˌsəːvikəuˈbreikiəl] *a* 颈臂的
cervicobrachialgia [ˌsəːvikəuˌbrækiˈældʒiə] *n* 颈臂痛
cervicobuccal [ˌsəːvikəuˈbʌkəl] *a* 颈颊的
cervicocolpitis [ˌsəːvikəukɔlˈpaitis] *n* 宫颈阴道炎 | ~ emphysematosa 气肿性宫颈阴道炎
cervicodorsal [ˌsəːvikəuˈdɔːsəl] *a* 颈背的
cervicodynia [ˌsəːvikəuˈdiniə] *n* 颈痛
cervicofacial [ˌsəːvikəuˈfeiʃiəl] *a* 颈颜面的
cervicolabial [ˌsəːvikəuˈleibiəl] *a* 颈唇的
cervicolingual [ˌsəːvikəuˈlingwəl] *a* 颈舌的
cervico-occipital [ˌsəːvikəuɔkˈsipitl] *a* 颈枕的
cervicopexy [ˈsəːvikəuˌpeksi] *n* 宫颈固定术
cervicoplasty [ˌsəːvikəuˈplæsti] *n* 颈成形术
cervicoscapular [ˌsəːvikəuˈskæpjulə] *a* 颈肩胛的
cervicothoracic [ˌsəːvikəuθɔ(ː)ˈræsik] *a* 颈胸[廓]的
cervicotomy [ˌsəːviˈkɔtəmi] *n* 颈切开术;宫颈切开术
cervicovaginitis [ˌsəːvikəuˌvædʒiˈnaitis] *n* 宫颈阴道炎
cervicovesical [ˌsəːvikəuˈvesikəl] *a* 宫颈膀胱的
cervimeter [səːˈvimitə] *n* 宫颈测量器
cervix [ˈsəːviks] ([复] **cervices** [ˈsəːvisiːz, səːˈvaisiːz] 或 **cervixes**) *n*【拉】颈;宫颈 | ~ of axon 轴索颈 / ~ glandis 阴茎颈 / incompetent ~ 宫颈功能不全 / tapiroid ~ 长唇宫颈 / ~ uteri 宫颈 / ~ vesicae 膀胱颈
ceryl [ˈsiəril] *n* 蜡基
ces central excitatory state 中枢兴奋状态
cesarean [si(ː)ˈzɛəriən] *n* 剖宫产术
Cesaris Demel bodies [ˈtʃeisɑːrisˈdemel] (Antonio C. Demel) 切萨里斯·德麦尔体(严重贫血后白细胞的退行性变所形成的小体)
CESD cholesteryl ester storage disease 胆固醇酯贮积病
cesium(Cs) [ˈsiːzjəm] *n* 铯(化学元素)
Cestan-Chenais syndrome [sesˈtɑːŋ ʃeˈnei] (Raymond Cestan; Louis J. Chenais) 塞斯丹-舍奈综合征(锥体、小脑下脚、疑核、瞳孔中枢的病变)
Cestan-Raymond syndrome [sesˈtɑːŋ reiˈmɔŋ] (Etienne J. M. R. Cestan; Fulgence Raymond) 塞斯丹-雷蒙综合征(见 Raymond-Cestan syndrome)
Cestan's syndrome [sesˈtɑːŋ] (Raymond J. Cestan) 塞斯丹综合征(见 Cestan-Chenais syndrome)
cesticidal [ˌsestiˈsaidəl] *a* 杀绦虫的
Cestoda [sesˈtəudə] *n* 多节绦虫亚纲
Cestodaria [sestəuˈdɛəriə] *n* 单节亚纲
cestode [ˈsestəud] *n* 绦虫 *a* 似绦虫的
cestodiasis [ˌsestəuˈdaiəsis] *n* 绦虫病
cestodology [ˌsestəuˈdɔlədʒi] *n* 绦虫学
cestoid [ˈsestɔid] *a* 似绦虫的
Cestoidea [sesˈtɔidiə] *n* 绦虫纲
Cestrum [ˈsestrəm] *n* 茄科热带植物属
cestus [ˈsestəs] *n*【拉】后脑带
cetaben sodium [ˈsiːtəbən] 西他苯钠(降血脂药)
cetaceum [siˈteisiəm] *n* 鲸蜡
cetalkonium chloride [ˌsetælˈkəuniəm] 西他氯铵(局部抗感染药和消毒药)
cetanol [ˈsiːtənɔl] *n* 鲸蜡醇
cetiedil citrate [siˈtaiidil] 枸橼酸西替地尔(周围血管扩张药,用于治疗动脉炎、雷诺〈Raynaud〉病和手足发绀)
cetirizine hydrochloride [səˈtiriziːn] 盐酸西替利嗪(抗过敏药)
cetocycline hydrochloride [ˌsiːtəuˈsaikliːn] 盐酸西托环素(抗菌药)
cetohexazine [ˌsiːtəuˈheksəziːn] *n* 西托沙嗪(即 ketohexazine,催眠镇静药)
Cetraria [siˈtrɛəriə] *n* 冰岛衣属
cetrimide [ˈsiːtrimaid] *n* 西曲溴铵(消毒防腐药)
cetrimonium bromide [ˌsetriˈməuniəm] 西曲溴铵(消毒防腐药)
cetrorelix acetate [ˌsetrəuˈreliks] 醋酸西曲瑞克(抗肿瘤药)
cetyl [ˈsiːtil] *n* 鲸蜡基
cetylpyridinium chloride [ˌsiːtilˌpiriˈdiniəm] 西吡氯铵(消毒防腐药,局部抗感染药)
cetyltrimethylammonium bromide [ˌsiːtilˌmeθiləˈməuniəm] 西曲溴铵(即 cetrimonium bromide)
cevimeline hydrochloride [səˈviməliːn] 盐酸西维美林(胆碱能激动药)
cevitamic acid [ˌsiːvaiˈtæmik] 维生素 C,抗坏血酸
Ceylancyclostoma [ˌsiːlænsaiˈklɔstəumə] *n* 锡兰钩口线虫属,锡兰钩虫属(即巴西钩虫 Ancylostoma braziliense)
ceyssatite [ˈsiːsətait] *n* 赛萨白土(Ceyssat 赛萨为法国一村名,所产白土可作湿疹与多汗症的吸附药粉,亦用以调制油膏与糊剂)
CF carbolfuchsin 石炭酸品红; cardiac failure 心力衰竭; Christmas factor 克里斯马斯因子(凝血因子Ⅸ); citrovorum factor 橙菌因子,亚叶酸
Cf californium 锎

cf confer【拉】比较,参阅
CFC chlorofluorocarbon 含氯氟烃
cff critical fusion frequency 临界融合频率
CFT complement-fixation test 补体结合试验
CFTR cystic fibrosis transmembrane conductance regulator 囊性纤维化跨膜传导调节蛋白
CFU colony-forming unit 集落生成单位,菌落形成单位
CFU-C colony-forming unit-culture 培养集落生成单位
CFU-E colony-forming unit-erythroid 红细胞集落生成单位
CFU-GM colony-forming unit-granulocyte-macrophage 粒细胞巨噬细胞集落生成单位
CFU-S colony-forming unit-spleen 脾集落生成单位
CGD chronic granulomatous disease 慢性肉芽肿病
cGMP cyclic guanosine monophosphate 环鸟苷酸
CGS, cgs centimeter-gram-second 厘米-克-秒(制)
cGy centigray 厘戈瑞(=10^{-2}Gy,吸收剂量单位)
CH crown-heel 顶踵长(指胎长)
Ch[1] Christchurch chromosome 克里斯丘奇染色体(指短臂缺失的 G 组染色体)
CH50, CH_{50} 50% 补体溶血单位
Chabertia [ʃɑːˈbəːtiə] 夏氏线虫属 | ~ ovina 绵羊夏氏线虫
chabertiasis [ʃaibəˈtaiəsis] *n* 夏氏丝虫病
Chabert's disease [ʃɑːˈbɛə] (Philebert Chabert) 症状性炭疽,气肿性炭疽,黑腿病
Chaddock's reflex (sign) [ˈtʃædɔk] (Charles G. Chaddock) 查多克反射(征)(锥体束损害时,刺激足外踝下部即引起踇趾伸直)
Chadwick's sign [ˈtʃædwik] (James R. Chadwick) 查德威克征(阴道黏膜出现紫色斑点,为妊娠之征)
Chaetomium [kiˈtəumiəm] *n* 毛壳[菌]属
Chagas' disease, Chagas-Cruz disease [ˈtʃɑːgəs kruz] (Carlos Chagas; Oswald Cruz) 恰加斯病,恰加斯-克鲁兹病,美洲锥虫病(分布于中美洲、南美洲的一种锥虫病,儿童呈急性型,成人呈慢性型。亦称南美洲锥虫病)
Chagasia [tʃəˈgæsiə] *n* 恰氏蚊亚属
chagasic [tʃəˈgæsik] *a* 恰加斯(Chagas)病的,南美洲锥虫病的
chagoma [tʃəˈgəumə] *n* 恰加斯病结节,美洲锥虫肿
Chagres fever [ˈtʃægris] *n* 恰格尔斯热,巴拿马热(巴拿马恰格尔斯河流域的一种恶性疟疾)
Chailletia [keiiˈliːʃiə] *n* 毒鼠子属
chain [tʃein] *n* 链 | branched ~ 支链 / closed ~ 闭链 /food ~ 食物链 / H ~, heavy ~ 重链 / J ~ J 链,连接链 / kappa ~ κ 链 / lambda ~ λ 链 / light ~ 轻链 / nuclear ~ 核链 / open ~ 开链 / side ~, lateral ~ 侧链 / sympathetic ~ 交感[神经]干
Chakra [ˈtʃʌkrə, ˈʃaikrə] *n*【梵】人体精神心灵力量中心(瑜珈哲学)
Chalara [kəˈlærə] *n* 横节霉菌属
chalasia [kəˈleiziə] *n* 松弛,弛缓(如贲门括约肌松弛,为婴儿呕吐的原因)
chalastodermia [kəˌlæstəuˈdəːmiə], **chalazodermia** [kəˌlæzəuˈdəːmiə] *n* 皮肤松垂
chalaza [kəˈleizə] *n*【希】合点(植物);卵带 | ~ l *a*
chalazion [kəˈleiziən] ([复] **chalazia** [kəˈleiziə]或 **chalazions**) *n* 睑板腺囊肿
chalcitis [kælˈsaitis] *n* 黄铜屑眼炎
chalcone [ˈkælkəun] *n* 查耳酮,苯基苯乙烯酮
chalcosis [kælˈkəusis] *n* 铜屑肺,铜屑沉着病
chalicosis [kæliˈkəusis] *n* 石末肺,石末沉着病
chalinoplasty [ˈkælinəuˌplæsti] *n* 口角成形术
chalk [tʃɔːk] *n* 白垩 | French ~ 滑石 / prepared ~ 精制白垩,沉淀碳酸钙
chalkitis [kælˈkaitis] *n* 黄铜屑眼炎
chalkstone [ˈtʃɔːkstəun] *n* 痛风石
chalky [ˈtʃɔːki] *a* 白垩的;像白垩的
challenge [ˈtʃælindʒ] *n* 激发(在免疫学中指注入抗原以激发免疫应答) *vt* 激发 | bronchial ~ 支气管激发 / food ~ 食物激发 / inhalational ~ 吸入性激发
chalone [ˈkæləun] *n* 抑素,细胞分裂抑制素(一种具有组织特异性,但没有种属特异性的水溶性物质,据说能抑制细胞增殖) | **chalonic** [kəˈlɔnik] *a*
chaluni [tʃæˈluːni] *n* 跖沟状角皮病
chalybeate [kəˈlibiit] *a* 含铁的 *n* 铁剂,含铁物
cham(a)ecephaly [ˌkæmiˈsefəli] *n* 扁头 | **cham(a)ecephalic** [ˌkæmisiˈfælik] *a*
Chamaemelum [ˌkæmiˈmiːləm] *n* 地瓜属
cham(a)eprosopy [ˌkæmiˈprɔsəpi] *n* 扁脸 | **cham(a)eprosopic** [ˌkæmiprəˈsɔpik] *a*
chamber [ˈtʃeimbə] *n* 腔,房,室 | air-equivalent ionization ~ 空气等效电离室 / aqueous ~ 眼房 / cloud ~ 雾室 / counting ~ 计数池 / detonating ~ 起爆箱,爆发室 / diffusion ~ 扩散盒 / ~s of the eye 眼房 / free -air ionization ~ 自由空气电离室 / ~s of the heart 心腔 / hyperbaric ~ 高压舱 / ionization ~ 电离室 / lethal ~ 致死室 / pulp ~ 髓室 / relief ~ 缓冲腔 / thimble ~ 针箍状电离室 / tissue-equivalent ionization ~ 组织等效电离室 / vitreous ~ 玻璃体腔
Chamberland filter [ʃɑːmbəˈlɑːŋ] (Charles E. Chamberland) 尚伯郎细菌滤器(素陶瓷滤器)
Chamberlen forceps [ˈtʃeimbələn] (Peter 〈Pierre〉 Chamberlen) 钱伯伦产钳

chamfer [ˈʃæmfə] *n* 凹线

chamomile [ˈkæməmiːl] *n* 春黄菊

Champetier de Ribes' bag [ʃɑːmptiˈɛədəˈriːb] (Camille L. A. Champetier de Ribes) 尚普提埃·德里伯(宫颈锥形)扩张袋(一种装水的圆锥形丝袋或橡皮袋,扩张宫颈用)

Chance fracture [tʃæns] (G. Q. Chance) 尚斯骨折(神经弓和椎骨体水平分裂,通常在腰区,系由屈曲-骨质分离力所致。亦称座椅安全带骨折)

chancre [ˈʃæŋkə] *n* 下疳 | fungating ~ 蕈样下疳(软下疳) / hard ~, hunterian ~ 硬下疳 / mixed ~ 混合性下疳(亦称混合性溃疡) / monorecidive ~, ~ redux 再发性下疳,复发性下疳 / soft ~ 软下疳 / sporotrichotic ~ 孢子丝菌性下疳 / true ~ 硬下疳 / tuberculous ~ 结核性初疮 | **chancrous** [ˈʃæŋkrəs] *a*

chancriform [ˈʃæŋkrifɔːm] *a* 下疳样的

chancroid [ˈʃæŋkrɔid] *n* 软下疳 | phagedenic ~ 崩蚀性软下疳 / serpiginous ~ 匐行性软下疳 | **~al** [ʃæŋˈkrɔidl] *a*

change [tʃeindʒ] *vt* 改变; *vi* 变化; *n* 改变;变化 | harlequin color ~ 小丑样颜色改变(身体一半纵向地一过性变红,另一半同时变白,为一种新生儿暂时性血管舒缩障碍)

Ch'ang Shan 常山(对疟疾有杀虫及退热功效)

channel [ˈtʃænl] *n* 通道;管,沟 | blood ~s 血管道(见于新鲜肉芽组织) / central ~ 中心管 / false ~ 假通道 / lymph ~s 淋巴隙 / perineural ~ 神经周淋巴隙 / thoroughfare ~ 末端小动静脉间通路

Ch'an su 蟾酥(中国各种蟾蜍的干毒素)

Chantemesse' reaction [ʃɑːntˈmes] (André Chantemesse) 尚特梅斯反应(检伤寒的眼反应)

Chaoborus [ˌkeiəˈbɔrəs] *n* 幽蚊属 | ~ lacustris 湖幽蚊

Chaos chaos [ˈkeiɔs ˈkeiɔs] 大变形虫(即卡罗林多核变形虫 Pelomyxa carolinensis)

Chaoul therapy [ʃaul] (Henri Chaoul) 沙乌尔[X线]疗法(短距低压X线疗法) | ~ tube 沙乌尔管(用于低压X线治疗)

chaperone [ˈʃæpərəun] *n* 陪伴分子,侣伴蛋白 | molecular ~ 分子陪伴,分子侣伴

chaperonine [ˌʃæpəˈrəunin] *n* 陪伴蛋白

chappa [ˈtʃæpə] *n* 查帕病(非洲西部的地方病,类似梅毒或雅司病)

Chaput's method [ʃɑːˈpuː] (Henri Chaput) 夏浦法(治骨髓炎的刮削术)

character [ˈkæriktə] *n* 特征,特性;性格;性状 *vt* 使具有特性 | acquired ~ 获得性状 / dominant ~ 显性性状 / imvic ~s 大肠菌分类特征(指吲哚、甲基红、V-P〈Voges-Proskauer〉反应、枸橼酸盐) / mendelian ~s 孟德尔式性状(符合于孟德尔遗传定律的性状,见 Mendel's law) / primary sex ~s 第一性征 / recessive ~ 隐性性状 / secondary sex ~s 第二性征,副性征 / sex-conditioned ~, sex-influenced ~ 从性性状 / sex -limited ~ 限性性状/ sex-linked ~ 性连锁性状

characteristic [ˌkæriktəˈristik] *a* 特异的;特有的;表示特性的 *n* 特性,特征 | demand ~s 需求特征(关于研究目的或预期行为的线索,期望实验对象察觉并作出反应)

characterization [ˌkæriktəraiˈzeiʃən, -liˈz-] *n* 特性,特征 | denture ~ 义齿特征化

characterize, characterise [ˈkæriktəraiz] *vt* 表示…的特性,成为…的特性

characterology [ˌkæriktəˈrɔlədʒi] *n* 性格论,性格学

charas [ˈtʃɑːrəs] *n* 大麻树脂

charbon [ʃɑːˈbɔŋ] *n*【法】炭疽 | ~ symptomatique 症状性炭疽,气肿性炭疽,黑腿病

charcoal [ˈtʃɑːkəul] *n* 炭,木炭 | activated ~ 活性炭 / animal ~ 动物炭,骨炭 / purified animal ~ 精制动物炭

Charcot-Bouchard aneurysm [ʃɑːˈkəu buˈʃɑː] (J. M. Charcot; Charles J. Bouchard) 夏-布动脉瘤(一型粟粒动脉瘤,见于小血管内,受高血压影响,据认为并非出血所致)

Charcot-Leyden crystals [ʃɑːˈkəu ˈlaidən] (J. M. Charcot; Ernst V. von Leyden) 夏科-莱登晶体(嗜酸粒细胞碎裂时呈现的晶体,亦称气喘晶体,白细胞晶体)

Charcot-Marie atrophy (type), Charcot-Marie-Tooth atrophy (disease, type) [ʃɑːˈkəu məˈriːtuːθ] (J. M. Charcot; Pierre Marie; Howard H. Tooth) 进行性神经性腓骨肌萎缩症

Charcot-Neumann crystals [ʃɑːˈkəu ˈnɔimən] 夏科-诺伊曼晶体(精液和各种动物组织中的磷酸精胺结晶)

Charcot's arthritis (arthropathy, arthrosis, disease, joint) [ʃɑːˈkəu] (Jean M. Charcot) 神经病性关节病 | ~ cirrhosis 原发性胆汁性肝硬化 / ~ fever 肝病性间歇热 / ~ foot 夏科足(脊髓痨性关节病患者的畸形足) / ~ gait 家族性共济失调步态 / ~ syndrome 夏科综合征(①肌萎缩性〈脊髓〉侧索硬化;②间歇性跛行;③肝病性间歇热) / ~ triad 夏科三联征(①眼球震颤、意向性震颤、断音言语,以前认为是多发性硬化症的体征;②胆绞痛、黄疸、发冷发热为间歇性胆管炎的特征)

Charcot-Vigouroux sigh [ʃɑːˈkəu viguːˈruː] (J. M. Charcot; Romain Vigouroux) 夏科-维古鲁征(见 Vigouroux sign)

Charcot-Weiss-Baker syndrome [ʃɑːˈkəu wais ˈbeikə] (J. M. Charcot; Soma Weiss; James P.

Baker)夏-魏-贝综合征,颈动脉窦综合征(即 carotid sinus syndrome,见 syndrome 项下相应术语)
charge(*Q*, *q*) [tʃɑːdʒ] *n* 电荷 | energy ~ 能荷
charlatan [ˈʃɑːlətən] *n*【法】庸医,江湖医 | ~ism, ~ry *n* 江湖医术
Charles' law [ʃɑːlz] (Jacques A. C. Charles) 查理定律(一定质量的理想气体,其容积在恒压下与绝对温度成正比)
charley horse [ˈtʃɑːlihɔːs] 四头肌僵痛(过劳所致)
Charlin's syndrome [ˈtʃɑːlin] (Carlos Charlin) 查林综合征(眼眶疼痛、虹膜炎、角膜炎和鼻部疼痛,为鼻睫神经神经痛的结果。亦称鼻睫部神经痛)
Charlouis's disease [ˌʃɑːluˈiːz] (M. Charlouis) 雅司病(即 yaws)
Charnley's hip arthroplasty [ˈtʃɑːnli] (John Charnley) 查利髋关节成形术(一种髋关节置换手术,包括插入查利髋关节假肢以形成低摩擦关节) | ~ prosthesis 查利髋关节假肢(一种髋关节成形术用的植入物,包括髋臼杯和比较小的股骨头组成部分,形成低摩擦关节)
Charrière scale[ˌʃɑːriˈɛə] (Joseph F. B. Charrière) 夏利艾尺度制(标明尿道探子和尿道导管的大小型号)
charring [ˈtʃɑːriŋ] *n* 烧焦,炭化[作用]
Charrin's disease [ʃɑːˈræn] (Albert Charrin) 绿脓杆菌感染
Chart. charta【拉】纸剂;药纸
chart [tʃɑːt] *n* 图,图表 *vt* 用图表表示 | alignment ~ 列线图,计算图 / reading ~ 近视力表 / test ~ 视力表
charta [ˈkɑːtə] ([复] **chartae** [ˈkɑːtiː]) *n*【拉】纸剂;药纸
chartaceous [kɑːˈteiʃəs] *a* 纸状的
chartreuse [ʃɑːˈtrəːz] *n* 滋补药酒
chartula [ˈkɑːtjulə] ([复] **chartulae** [ˈkɑːtjuliː]) *n*【拉】分包散剂,纸剂
chasma [ˈkæzmə], **chasmus** [ˈkæzməs] *n*【拉;希】呵欠
chasmatoplasson [kæzˈmætəˌplæsɔn] *n* 无核胞质膨胀
Chassaignac's tubercle [ˌʃɑːseiˈnjɑːk] (Charles M. E. Chassaignac) 夏桑亚克结节(第6颈椎横突的颈动脉结节)
chaste tree [ˈtrestˌtriː] 淡紫花牡荆;淡紫花牡荆果实和根皮制备的浸膏(用于经前期综合征和经绝期的症状疗法;亦用于顺势疗法)
chaude-pisse [ʃəudˈpiːs] *n*【法】尿灼热
chauffage [ʃəuˈfɑːʒ] *n* 烘烙[疗]法
Chauffard's syndrome, Chauffard Still syndrome [ʃəuˈfɑːˈstil] (Anatole M. E. Chauffard; George F. Still) 肖法综合征,肖法-斯蒂尔综合征(感染非人型结核后发生多关节炎,并伴有发热、脾大和淋巴结肿大)
chaulmoogric acid [tʃɔlˈmuːgrik] 大风子油酸
Chaunacanthida [ˌtʃɔnəˈkænθidə] *n* 松棘目
Chaussier's areola [ˌʃəusiˈɛə] (Francois Chaussier) 肖西埃晕(皮肤炭疽硬结晕) | ~ line 肖西埃线(胼胝体正中缝)
Chauveau's bacillus (bacterium) [ʃəuˈvəu] (Auguste Chauveau) 肖氏梭菌
ChB Chirurgiae Baccalaureus【拉】外科学士
CHD congenital heart disease 先天性心脏病; coronary heart disease 冠状动脉性心脏病(冠心病)
ChD Chirurgiae Doctor【拉】外科博士
ChE cholinesterase 胆碱酯酶
Cheadle's disease [ˈtʃiːdl] (Walter B. Cheadle) 婴儿坏血病
check-bite [ˈtʃek bait] *n* 正殆法,殆校正法
checker board [ˈtʃekəbɔːd] *n* 棋盘,方格图案(一种有边缘的网格,在边缘内表示每个亲代的配子,方格内表示其可能的后代,亦称庞纳特方格 Punnett square)
checkup [ˈtʃekʌp] *n* 检查;查对;体格检查
Chédiak-Higashi syndrome [ʃeiˈdjɑːk hiˈgɑːʃi] (Alejandro Chédiak; Otakata Higashi) 白细胞异常色素减退综合征(一种致命的常染色体隐性全身性疾病,伴眼皮肤白化病、大量白细胞包涵体〈巨大溶酶体〉、身体多种器官组织细胞浸润、各类血细胞减少的形成,以及可能患恶性淋巴瘤)
Chédiak-Steinbrinck-Higashi anomaly [ˈtʃeidiɑːk ˈʃtainbriŋk hiˈgɑːʃi] (M. Ché diak; W. Steinck; O. Higashi) 谢-施-东异常(见 Chédiak-Higashi syndrome)
Chédiak test (reaction) [ʃeiˈdjɑːk] (Alejandro Chédiak) 谢迪亚克试验(反应)(检梅毒)
cheek [tʃiːk] *n* 颊 | cleft ~ 颊裂[畸形]
cheekbone [ˈtʃiːkˌbəun] *n* 颧骨
cheese [tʃiːz] *n* 干酪
cheesy [ˈtʃiːzi] *a* 干酪样的
cheil- 见 cheilo-
cheilectomy [kaiˈlektəmi] *n* 唇切除术;凿骨术(凿除关节腔中妨碍运动的不规则骨缘)
cheilectropion [ˌkailekˈtrəupiɔn] *n* 唇外翻
cheilitis [kaiˈlaitis] *n* 唇炎 | apostematous ~ 脓肿性唇炎,脓肿性腺性唇炎 / commissural ~ 口角炎 / ~ exfoliativa 剥脱性唇炎 / ~ glandularis 腺性唇炎 / migrating ~ 传染性口角炎
Cheillanthes [kaiˈlænθiːz] *n* 碎米蕨属
cheil(o)- [构词成分]唇
cheiloangioscopy [ˌkailəuˌændʒiˈɔskəpi] *n* 唇血

管镜检查
cheilocarcinoma [ˌkailəuˌkɑːsiˈnəumə] *n* 唇癌
cheilognathopalatoschisis [ˌkailəuˌneiθəuˌpæləˈtɔskisis] *n* 唇颌腭裂[畸形]
cheilognathoprosoposchisis [ˌkailəuˌneiθəuˌprɔsəˈpɔskisis] *n* 唇颌面裂[畸形]
cheilognathoschisis [ˌkailəuneiˈθɔskisis] *n* 唇颌裂[畸形]
cheilognathouranoschisis [ˌkailəuˌneiθəujuərəˈnɔskisis] *n* 唇颌腭裂[畸形]
cheilophagia [ˌkailəuˈfeidʒiə] *n* 啮唇癖
cheiloplasty [ˈkailəˌplæsti] *n* 唇成形术
cheilorrhaphy [kaiˈlɔrəfi] *n* 唇裂修复术
cheiloschisis [kaiˈlɔskisis] *n* 唇裂[畸形]
cheiloscopy [kaiˈlɔskəpi] *n* 唇检术,唇镜检查
cheilosis [kaiˈləusis] *n* 唇干裂(缺乏核黄素) | angular ~ 口角干裂
cheilostomatoplasty [ˌkailəustəuˈmætəˌplæsti] *n* 唇口成形术
cheilotomy [kaiˈlɔtəmi] *n* 骨唇切开术;部分唇切除术
cheir- 见 cheiro-
Cheiracanthium [ˌkaiərəˈkænθiəm] *n* 红螯蛛属(即 Chiracanthium)
Cheiracanthus [ˌkairəˈkænθəs] *n* 颚口[线虫]属(即 Gnathostoma)
cheiragra [kaiˈrægrə] *n* 手痛风
cheiralgia [kaiˈrældʒiə] *n* 手痛
cheirarthritis [ˌkairɑːˈθraitis] *n* 手关节炎
cheir(O)- [构词成分]手
cheirobrachialgia [ˌkairəuˌbreikiˈældʒiə] *n* 手臂痛
cheirognomy [kaiˈrɔgnəmi] *n* 手相术
cheirognostic [ˌkairəgˈnɔstik] *a* 能辨别左右的
cheirokinesthesia [ˌkairəuˌkinisˈθiːzjə], **cheirocinesthesia** [ˌkairəuˌsinisˈθiːzjə] *n* 手运动觉(尤指书写时) | **cheirokinesthetic** [ˌkairəu-ˌkinisˈθetik] *a*
cheirology [kaiˈrɔlədʒi] *n* 手[势]语
cheiromegaly [kairəuˈmegəli] *n* 巨手
cheiroplasty [ˈkairəˌplæsti] *n* 手成形术
cheiropodalgia [ˌkairəupəˈdældʒiə] *n* 手足痛
cheiropompholyx [ˌkairəˈpɔmfəliks] *n* [掌跖]汗疱
cheiroscope [ˈkairəskəup] *n* 手导镜,斜视手矫器,手实体镜
cheirospasm [ˈkairəspæzəm] *n* 手[肌]痉挛
chelate [ˈkiːleit] *a* 螯合的 *n* 螯合物 *vt* 与…结合成螯合物 *vi* 生成螯合物 | **chelation** [kiːˈleiʃən] *n* 螯合作用
chelen [ˈkiːlen] *n* 氯乙烷
chelicera [kiˈlisərə] *n* 螯肢
cheloid [ˈkiːlɔid], **cheloma** [kiˈləumə] *n* 瘢痕疙瘩,疤痕疙瘩
chelonian [kiˈləuniən] *a* 蠵龟科的;海龟的
chemabrasion [kiːməˈbreiʃən], **chemexfoliation** [ˌkiːmeksˌfəuliˈeiʃən] *n* 化学脱皮法,化学整平法(如用苯酚、三氯乙酸等化学药品蚀平皮肤)
chemamnesia [ˌkiːmæmˈniːziə] *n* 药物[性]健忘
chemasthenia [ˌkemæsˈθiːniə] *n* (身体)化学过程减弱
chemi- 见 chem(o)-
chemiatry [ˈkemiətri] *n* 化学医学派 | **chemiatric** [ˌkemiˈætrik] *a*
chemical [ˈkemikəl] *a* 化学的 *n* 化学药品,化学制剂
chemic(o)- 见 chem(o)-
chemicobiological [ˌkemikəuˌbaiəˈlɔdʒikəl] *a* 化学生物学的,生物化学的
chemicocautery [ˌkemikəuˈkɔːtəri] *n* 化学烙术
chemicogenesis [ˌkemikəuˈˌdʒenisis] *n* 化学发生(利用化学作用促使卵发育)
chemicophysical [ˌkemikəuˈfizikəl] *a* 化学物理的
chemicophysiologic [ˌkemikəuˌfiziəˈlɔdʒik] *a* 化学生理学的
chemiluminescence [ˌkemiljuːmiˈnesns] *n* 化学发光
cheminosis [ˌkemiˈnəusis] *n* 化学因素病,化学物质病
chemiosmosis [ˌkemiɔsˈməusis] *n* 化学渗透[作用]
chemiosmotic [ˌkemiɔsˈmɔtik] *a* 化学渗透的
chemiotaxis [ˌkemiəuˈtæksis] *n* 趋化性
chemiotherapy [ˌkemiəuˈθerəpi] *n* 化学疗法,化学治疗
chemism [ˈkemizəm] *n* 化学[反应]历程,化学机制,化学作用
chemisorb [ˈkemisɔːb] *vt* 化学吸附,化学吸着 | **chemisorption** [ˌkemiˈsɔːpʃən] *n*
chemist [ˈkemist] *n* 化学家,化学师;药剂师
chemistry [ˈkemistri] *n* 化学 | applied ~, industrial ~ 应用化学,工业化学 / biological ~, metabolic ~, physiologic ~ 生物化学,代谢化学,生理化学 / forensic ~ 法[医]化学 / inorganic ~, mineral ~ 无机化学,矿质化学 / organic ~ 有机化学 / pharmaceutical ~ 药物化学 / synthetic ~ 合成化学
chemo- [构词成分]化学
chemoattractant [ˌkiːməuəˈtræk tənt] *n* 化学吸引剂,化学引诱物
chemoautotroph [ˌkiːməuˈɔːtətrɔf, ˌkem-] *n* 化学自养菌 | **~ic** [ˌkiːməuˌɔːtəˈtrɔfik, ˌkem-] *a*

化学自养的

chemobiotic [ˌkiːməubaiˈɔtik, ˌkem-] *n* 化学抗生素

chemocautery [ˌkiːməuˈkɔːtəri, ˌkem-] *n* 化学烙术

chemocephaly [ˌkiːməuˈsəfəli, ˌkem-], **chemocephalia** [ˌkiːməusiˈfeiliə, ˌkem-] *n* 扁头

chemoceptor [ˈkiːməuseptə, ˈkem-] *n* 化学感受器;化学受体

chemocoagulation [ˌkiːməukəuˌægjuˈleiʃən, ˌkem-] *n* 化学凝固[法]

chemodectoma [ˌliːməudekˈtəumə, ˌkem-] *n* 化学感受器瘤(非嗜铬性副神经节瘤)

chemodifferentiation [ˌkiːməuˌdifərenʃiˈeiʃən, ˌkem-] *n* 化学分化

chemodynesis [ˌkiːməuˈdainisis, ˌkem-] *n* 药物致原生质流动

chemoembolization [ˌkiːməuˌembəliˈzeiʃən, ˌkem-] *n* 化学栓塞术

chemoendocrine [ˌkiːməuˈendəukrin, ˌkem-] *a* 化学内分泌的,化学激素的

chemoheterotroph [ˌkiːməuˈhetərətrɔf, ˌkem-] *n* 化学异养菌 | **~ic** [ˌkiːməuˌhetərəˈtrɔfik, ˌkem-] *a* 化学异养的(细菌)

chemohormonal [ˌkiːməuhɔːˈməunl, ˌkem-] *a* 化学激素的

chemoimmunology [ˌkiːməuimjuˈnɔlədʒi, ˌkem-] *n* 化学免疫学

chemokine [ˈkiːməkain] *n* 趋化因子

chemokinesis [ˌkiːməukaiˈniːsis, ˌkem-] *n* 化学增活现象,化学激动作用 | **chemokinetic** [ˌkiːməukaiˈnetik, ˌkem-] *a*

chemolithotroph [ˌkiːməuˈliθɔtrəuf, ˌkem-] *n* 化能无机营养菌 | **~ic** [ˌkiːməuˌliθɔˈtrɔfik, ˌkem-] *a* 化能无机营养的

chemoluminescence [ˌkiːməuˌljuːmiˈnesns, ˌkem-] *n* 化学发光

chemolysis [kiˈmɔlisis] *n* 化学分解

chemomorphosis [ˌkiːməumɔːˈfəusis, ˌkem-] *n* 化学性变态,化学诱变

chemonucleolysis [ˌkiːməuˌnjuːkliˈɔlisis, ˌkem-] *n* 髓核化学溶解法(如注射木瓜凝乳蛋白酶溶解椎间盘髓核,以治椎间盘突出)

chemoorganotroph [ˌkiːməuˈɔːgənəuˌtrəuf, ˌkem-] *n* 化能有机营养菌 | **~ic** [ˌkiːməu ˌɔːgənəuˈtrɔfik, ˌkem-] *a* 化能有机营养的

chemopallidectomy [ˌkiːməu pæliˈdektəmi, ˌkem-] *n* 苍白球化学破坏术

chemopallidothalamectomy [ˌkiːməuˌpælidəu-ˌθæləˈmektəmi, ˌkem-] *n* 苍白球丘脑化学破坏术

chemopharmacodynamic [ˌkiːməuˌfɑːməkəudaiˈnæmik, ˌkem-] *a* 药理化学的

chemophysiology [ˌkiːməufiziˈɔlədʒi, ˌkem-] *n* 生理化学

chemoprevention [ˌkiːməupriˈvenʃən, ˌkem-] *n* 化学预防,药物预防

chemoprotectant [ˌkiːməuprəˈtektənt, ˌkem-] *a* 化疗药保护的 *n* 化疗药保护剂

chemoprophylaxis [ˌkiːməuˌprɔfiˈlæksis, ˌkem-] *n* 化学预防,药物预防 | primary ~ 初级化学预防 / secondary ~ 次级化学预防 | **chemoprophylactic** [ˌkiːməuˌprɔfiˈlæktik, ˌkem-] *a*

chemopsychiatry [ˌkiːməusaiˈkaiətri] *n* 精神病化学治疗学,精神药理学

chemoradiotherapy [ˌkeməuˌreidiəuˈθerəpi, ˌkiːməu-] *n* 化学放射疗法

chemoreception [ˌkiːməuriˈsepʃən, ˌkem-] *n* 化学感受[作用]

chemoreceptor [ˌkiːməuriˈseptə, ˌkem-] *n* 化学感受器;化学受体 | **chemoreceptive** [ˌkiːməuriˈseptiv, ˌkem-] *a*

chemoresistance [ˌkiːməuriˈzistəns, ˌkem-] *n* 化学抗性,药物抗性

chemosensitive [ˌkiːməuˈsensitiv, ˌkem-] *a* 化学敏感的

chemosensory [ˌkiːməuˈsensəri, ˌkem-] *a* 化学感觉的

chemoserotherapy [ˌkiːməuˌsiərəuˈθerəpi, ˌkem-] *n* 化学血清疗法

chemosis [kiˈməusis] *n* 结膜水肿

chemosmosis [ˌkiːmɔzˈməusis, ˌkem-] ([复] **chemosmoses** [ˌkiːmɔzˈməusiːz, ˌkem-]) *n* 化学渗透[作用]

chemosmotic [ˌkiːmɔsˈmɔtik, ˌkem-] *a* 化学渗透的

chemosorption [ˌkiːməuˈsɔːpʃən, ˌkem-] *n* 化学吸附,化学吸着

chemosphere [ˈkiːməsfiə, ˈkem-] *n* 光化层,臭氧层(大气的一个区层,30 ~ 80 km)

chemostat [ˈkiːməstæt, ˈkem-] *n* 恒化器

chemosterilant [ˌkiːməuˈsterilent, ˌkem-] *n* 化学绝育剂(用于控制昆虫和害虫)

chemosterilization [ˌkiːməuˌsteriliˈzeiʃən, ˌkem-] *n* 化学不育

chemosurgery [ˌkiːməuˈsəːdʒəri, ˌkem-] *n* 化学外科

chemosynthesis [ˌkiːməuˈsinθisis, ˌkem-] *n* 化学合成 | **chemosynthetic** [ˌkiːməusinˈθetik, ˌkem-] *a*

chemotaxin [ˌkiːməuˈtæksin, ˌkem-] *n* 化学吸引素(即趋化因子 chemotactic factor)

chemotaxis [ˌkiːməuˈtæksis, ˌkem-] *n* 趋化作用,趋化性 | leukocyte ~ 白细胞趋化性 | **chemo-**

tactic [ˌkiːməuˈtæktik] *a*

chemothalamectomy [ˌkiːməuθæləˈmektəmi, ˌkem-] *n* 丘脑化学破坏术

chemotherapy [ˌkiːməuˈθerəpi, ˌkem-] **chemotherapeutics** [ˌkiːməuθerəˈpjuːtiks, ˌkem-] *n* 化学疗法,化学治疗学 | **chemotherapeutic** [ˌkiːməuθerəˈpjuːtik, ˌkem-] *a*

chemotic [kiˈmɔtik] *a* 结膜水肿的 *n* 促结膜淋巴生成剂

chemotrophic [ˌkiːməuˈtrɔfik, ˌkem-] *a* 化能营养的(指细菌)

chemotropism [kiˈmɔtrəpizəm] *n* 向化性 | **chemotropic** [ˌkiːməuˈtrɔpik, ˌkem-] *a*

chemurgy [ˈkeməːdʒi] *n* 农艺化学 | **chemurgic** [keˈməːdʒik] *a*

chenodeoxycholate [ˌkiːnəudiːɔksiˈkəuleit] *n* 鹅脱氧胆酸盐

chenodeoxycholic acid [ˌkiːnəudiːɔksiˈkəulik] 鹅[脱氧]胆酸

chenodeoxycholylglycine [ˌkiːnəudiːˌɔksiˌkəulilˈglaisiːn] *n* 鹅脱氧胆酰甘氨酸(亦称甘氨鹅脱氧胆酸)

chenodeoxycholyltaurine [ˌkiːnəudiːˌɔksiˌkəulilˈtɔːri(ː)n] *n* 鹅脱氧胆酰牛磺酸(亦称牛磺鹅脱氧胆酸)

chenodiol [ˌkenəuˈdaiəul] *n* 鹅二醇(即鹅脱氧胆酸)

Chenopodium [ˌkiːnəuˈpəudiəm] *n* 藜属

chenotaurocholic acid [ˌkiːnəuˌtɔːrəˈkəulik] 鹅牛磺胆酸

chenotherapy [ˌkenəuˈθerəpi] *n* 鹅[脱氧]胆酸疗法(以溶解胆石)

cheoplasty [ˈkiːəˌplæsti] *n* 低溶(金属)铸型 | **cheoplastic** [ˌkiːəˈplæstik] *a*

Cherchevski's (Cherchewski's) disease [ʃəˈʃevski] (Mikhail Cherchevski) 谢尔舍夫斯基病(神经性肠梗阻)

cherry [ˈtʃeri] *n* 樱桃;樱桃色 *a* 樱桃[色]的 | choke ~ 野桃樱 / ~ laurel 月桂樱 / rum ~ (黑)野樱(树) / wild ~ (黑)野樱(树);野黑樱皮

cherubism [ˈtʃerəbizəm] *n* (家族性)巨颌症

Chervin's treatment (method) [ʃəˈvæn] (Claudius Chervin) 舍万疗法(矫治口吃的一种方法)

chest [tʃest] *n* 胸,胸廓 | barrel ~ 桶状胸 / blast ~ 爆炸性肺震荡 / cobbler's ~ 鞋匠胸 / flat ~, alar ~, phthinoid ~, pterygoid ~ 扁平胸,翼状胸,痨型胸 / funnel ~, foveated ~ 漏斗胸 / pigeon ~, keeled ~ 鸡胸 / tetrahedron ~ 菱形胸(鸡胸)

chestnut [ˈtʃesnʌt] *n* 栗

chew [tʃuː] *vt*, *vi*, *n* [咀]嚼

Cheyletiella [ˌkailətiˈelə] *n* 姬螯螨属 | ~ blakei 布氏姬螯螨 / ~ parasitovorax 寄食姬螯螨 / ~ yasguri 牙氏姬螯螨

Cheyletiellidae [ˌkailətiˈelidiː] *n* 姬螯螨科

cheyletiellosis [ˌkailəˌtiːeˈləusis] *n* 姬螯螨病

Cheyne's nystagmus [tʃein] (John Cheyne) 切恩眼球震颤(见 Cheyne-Stokes nystagmus)

Cheyne-Stokes asthma [ˈtʃein stəuks] (John Cheyne; William Stokes) 心源性哮喘 | ~ nystagmus 切-斯眼球震颤(一种特异的、节律性眼球运动,其节律与切-斯呼吸相似) / ~ psychosis 切-斯精神病(类似心源性哮喘,偶见于慢性心脏病) / ~ respiration (sign) 切-斯呼吸(征),潮式呼吸

CHF congestive heart failure 充血性心力衰竭; chronic heart failure 慢性心力衰竭

chi¹ [kai] 希腊语的第 22 个字母(Χ, χ)

chi², ch'i 气

Chiari-Arnold syndrome [kiˈɑːri ˈɑːnɔld] (Hans von Chiari, Julius Arnold) 基亚里-阿诺尔德综合征(见 Arnold-Chiari deformity)

Chiari-Frommel diseaes (syndrome) [kiˈɑːri ˈfrɔməl] (Johann B. Chiari; Richard Frommel) 基亚里-弗罗梅尔病(综合征)(见 Frommel's disease)

Chiari's network (reticulum) [kiˈɑːri] (Hans von Chiari) 基亚里网(从冠状窦瓣和下腔静脉瓣穿过右心房内部延伸至界嵴的纤维网) | ~ syndrome (disease) 基亚里综合征(病)(闭塞性肝静脉内膜炎的综合征)

chiasm [ˈkaiæzəm] *n* 交叉 | ~ of digits of hand 指腱交叉 | **~atic** [kaiəzˈmætik], **~al** [kaiˈæzməl], **~ic** [kaiˈæzmik] *a*

chiasma [kaiˈæzmə] ([复] **chiasmata** [kaiˈæzmətə] 或 **chiasmas**) *n*【拉;希】交叉(在遗传学上指染色体交叉)

chiasmatypy [kaiˈæzməˌtaipi] *n* 互换,交换(染色体间遗传物质的交换)

chiastometer [ˌkaiæzˈtɔmitə], **chiasmometer** [ˌkaiæzˈmɔmitə] *n* 视轴偏斜测量器

Chiba needle [ˈtʃiːbə] [日本千叶(Chiba)大学] 千叶针(日本千叶大学创用的抽吸细针,用于经皮经肝胆管造影。即细针 fine needle)

chichism [ˈtʃiːtʃizəm] *n* 糙皮病(南美洲北部使用的名称)

chickenpest [ˈtʃikinpest] *n* 家禽疫,鸡瘟;纽卡斯尔病(见 Newcastle disease)

chickenpox [ˈtʃikinpɔks] *n* 水痘

chick-pea [ˈtʃik piː] *n* 鹰嘴豆(产于南欧一种植物,其种子可供食用,但可能引起中毒)

Chido-Rodgers blood group [tʃiːdəu ˈrɔdʒəs]

(从20世纪60年代首次观察到的先征者得名)奇多-罗杰士血型

Chiene's operation [ʃiːn] (John Chiene) 希恩手术(大腿内髁楔形切除以矫正膝外翻)

Chievitz's layer [ˈtʃiːwits] (Johan H. Chievitz)契维茨层(分隔视杯内外成神经细胞层的纤维层) | ~ organ 契维茨器官(指腮腺后的胚胎赘疣)

chigger [ˈtʃigə] *n* 沙螨,沙虱,恙螨,恙虫

chigo(e) [ˈtʃigəu] *n* 沙蚤

chikungunya [ˌtʃikuŋˈgunjə] (东非斯瓦希里语意为屈曲)*n* 奇昆古尼亚病(一种甲病毒引起的热病,类似登革热,但无头痛,奇昆古尼亚为坦桑尼亚地名)

Chilaiditi's sign [ˌkiːləˈθiːti] (Demetrios Chilaiditi)奇氏征(结肠定位,见 hepatoptosis 第二解) / ~ syndrome 奇氏综合征(①膈肌下结肠嵌入:肝与膈之间置有结肠,本病征在成人一般无症状,但儿童则症状明显,包括呕吐、腹痛、食欲缺乏、便秘和吞气症,体征包括腹膨胀及肝部浊音消失;②结肠定位,见 hepatoptosis 第二解)

chilblain [ˈtʃilblein] *n* 冻疮 | necrotized ~ 坏死性冻疮,肉样瘤病 | **~ed** *a* 生冻疮的

child [tʃaild]([复]**children** [ˈtʃildrən] *n* 儿童 | preschool ~ 学龄前儿童(2~6岁) / school ~ 学龄儿童(6~10岁或12岁) | **~less** [ˈtʃaildlis] *a* 无子女的

child-bearing [ˈtʃaild ˌbɛəriŋ] *n* 分娩,生产

childbed [ˈtʃaildbed] *n* 产褥,产褥期

childbirth [ˈtʃaildbəːθ] *n* 分娩,生产

childhood [ˈtʃaildhud] *n* 儿童期(从出生到青春期)

chilitis [kaiˈlaitis] *n* 唇炎

chill [tʃil] *n* 寒冷,受寒;寒战 | brass ~, brazier's ~ 铸工热 / congestive ~ 充血性寒战(恶性疟疾,寒战后有胃肠道充血及腹泻) / creeping ~ 寒冷感 / shaking ~ 恶寒战栗 / spelter ~s, zinc ~ 锌中毒性寒战 / urethral ~ (导管)排尿寒战

chil(o)- 见 cheilo-

Chilodon [ˈkailədɔn] *n* 唇纤毛虫属

Chilodonella [ˌkailədəˈnelə] *n* 斜管虫属

Chilognatha [kaiˈlɔgnəθə] *n* 唇颚目

chilomastigiasis [ˌkailəuˌmæstiˈgaiəsis], **chilomastixiasis** [ˌkailəuˌmæstikˈsaiəsis] *n* 唇鞭毛虫病

Chilomastix [ˌkailəuˈmæstiks] *n* 唇鞭毛虫属 | ~ mesnili 迈氏唇鞭毛虫

chilopod [ˈkailəpɔd] *n* 蜈蚣

Chilopoda [kaiˈlɔpəde] *n* 唇足纲

chimaera [kaiˈmiərə] *n* [异源]嵌合体

chimera [kaiˈmiərə] *n* [异源]嵌合体(指体内含有不同合子的同种或不同种的细胞群) | heterologous ~ 异种嵌合体 / homologous ~ 同种嵌合体(但基因型不同) / isologous ~ 异源嵌合体 / radiation ~ 放射性嵌合体

chimerism [kaiˈmiərizəm] *n* 嵌合性(在遗传学上指个体中出现异源细胞的情形,如来自双卵双生的血细胞)

chimpanzee [ˌtʃimpænˈziː, tʃimˈpænzi] *n* 黑猩猩

chin [tʃin] *n* 颏 | galoche ~ 凸颏

chinaberry [ˈtʃainəˌberi] *n* 楝

chinacrine [ˈkinəkriːn] *n* 米帕林(即 mepacrine,抗疟药)

chincap [ˈtʃinkæp] *n* 颏兜

chiniofon [ˈkiniəfɔn] *n* 喹碘方(抗阿米巴药)

chionablepsia [ˌkaiənəˈblepsiə] *n* 雪盲

chip [tʃip] *n* 片屑,碎片;芯片(集成电路块) | bone ~s 碎骨片

chip-blower [tʃip ˈbləuə] *n* 气枪,牙孔[洞]吹洁器,吹器

Chiracanthium [ˌkaiərəˈkænθiəm] *n* 红螯蛛属

chiral [ˈkaiərəl] *a* 手[征]性的 | **~ity** [kaiˈræləti] *n* 手性(在镜像上不能重叠的手性;一个不对称分子的手性)

chir(o)- [构词成分]手

chirobrachialgia [ˌkaiərəuˌbreikiˈældʒiə] *n* (感觉异常性)手臂痛

chirognostic [ˌkaiərɔgˈnɔstik] *a* 能辨别左右的

chiromegaly [ˌkaiərəuˈmegəli] *n* 巨手

Chironex [ˈkairəneks] *n* 立方水母属

Chironomidae [ˌkaiərəˈnɔmidiː] *n* 摇蚊科

Chironomus [kaiˈrɔnəməs] *n* 摇蚊属

chiroplasty [ˈkaiərəˌplæsti] *n* 手成形术

chiropodalgia [ˌkaiərəupəuˈdældʒiə] *n* 手足痛

chiropody [kiˈrɔpədi, kaiəˈrɔpədi] *n* 手足医术 | **chiropodical** [ˌkaiərəˈpɔdikəl] *a* / **chiropodist** [kiˈrɔpədist, kaiəˈrɔpədist] *n* 手足医

chiropractic [ˌka-iərəuˈpræktik], **chiropraxis** [ˌkaiərəuˈpræksis] *n* 脊柱推拿疗法 | **chiropractor** [ˌkaiərəˈpræktə] *n* 脊柱推拿疗法师

Chiropsalmus [ˌkairəˈsɑːlməs] *n* 立方水母属

chiroscope [ˈkaiərəskəup] *n* 手导镜,斜视手矫器,手实体镜

chirospasm [ˈkaiərəspæzəm] *n* 手[肌]痉挛

chi-squared [ˈkai skwɛəd] *a* 卡方的,χ^2 的

chitin [ˈkaitin] *n* 壳多糖,甲壳质 | **~ous** *a*

chitinase [ˈkaitineis] *n* 壳多糖酶

chitobiose [ˌkaitəuˈbaiəus] *n* 壳二糖

chitoneure [ˈkaitənjuə] *n* 神经膜鞘

chitonic acid [kaiˈtɔnik] 缩水甘露糖酸

chitosan [ˈkaitəsæn] *n* 脱乙酰壳多糖

chitose [ˈkaitəus] *n* 壳糖

chitotriose [ˌkaitəuˈtraiəus] *n* 壳三糖

chiufa [tʃi'uːfə] *n* 坏疽性直肠结肠炎(见于南美、南非山区)
CHL crown-heel length 顶踵长
chlamydemia [klæmi'diːmiə] *n* 衣原体血症
Chlamydia [klə'midiə] *n* 衣原体属 | ~ psittaci 鹦鹉热衣原体 / ~ trachomatis 沙眼衣原体
chlamydia [klə'midiə] ([复] **chlamydiae** [klə'midiiː]) *n* 衣原体 | **~l** *a*
Chlamydiaceae [kləˌmidi'eisiiː] *n* 衣原体科
Chlamydiales [klə'midiəliːz] *n* 衣原体目
chlamydiosis [kləˌmidi'əusis] *n* 衣原体病
Chlamydobacteriaceae [ˌklæmidəu bækˌtiəri'ei-siiː] *n* 衣菌科
Chlamydobacteriales [ˌklæmidəubækˌtiəri'eiliːz] *n* 衣菌目
chlamydoconidium [ˌklæmidəukə'nidiəm] *n* 厚膜孢子
Chlamydodontina [kləˌmidəudɔn'tainə] *n* 戎装虫亚目
Chlamydomonas [kləˌmidəu'məunəs] *n* 衣滴虫目
Chlamydophrys [klə'midəfris] *n* 足衣虫属 | ~ anchelys, ~ stercorea 粪池足衣虫
chlamydospore ['klæmidəspɔː] *n* 厚壁孢子
Chlamydozoaceae [ˌklæmidəuzə'eisiiː] *n* 衣原体科
Chlamydozoon [ˌklæmidəu'zəuɔn] *n* 衣原体属
chloasma [kləu'æzmə] *n* 褐黄斑 | ~ hepaticum 肝性褐黄斑,肝斑
chlophedianol hydrochloride [ˌkləufi'daiənɔl] 盐酸氯苯达诺(镇咳药)
chloracetic acid [ˌklɔːrə'siːtik] 氯乙酸
chloracetization [klɔːˌræsiti'zeiʃən] *n* 氯仿冰醋酸局部麻醉法(此法不再使用)
chloracne [klɔː'rækni] *n* 氯痤疮
chloral ['klɔːrəl] *n* 氯醛,三氯乙醛;水合氯醛 | ~ betaine 氯醛甜菜碱(催眠镇静药) / butyl ~ 丁基氯醛 / ~ carmine 氯醛卡红 / ~ hydrate 水合氯醛(催眠药)
chloralism ['klɔːrəlizəm] *n* 氯醛瘾
chloralization [ˌklɔːrəli'zeiʃən] *n* 氯醛瘾;氯醛麻醉
chloralose ['klɔːrələus] *n* 氯醛糖(催眠药,亦称 α-氯醛糖)
chlorambucil [klɔː'ræmbjusil] *n* 苯丁酸氮芥(抗肿瘤药)
chloramine-T ['klɔːrəmiːn] *n* 氯胺 T(消毒防腐药)
chloramphenicol [ˌklɔːræm'fenikɔl] *n* 氯霉素(抗菌、抗立克次体药) | ~ palmitate 氯霉素棕榈酸酯,无味氯霉素(抗菌、抗立克次体药) / ~ sodium succinate 氯霉素琥珀酯钠,氯霉素丁二酸酯钠(抗菌、抗立克次体药)
chloranilic acid [klɔːrə'nilik] 氯醌酸
chlorate ['klɔːrit] *n* 氯酸盐
chlorauric acid [klɔː'rɔːrik] 氯金酸
chlorazanil hydrochloride [klə'rɑːzənil] 盐酸氯拉扎尼(利尿药)
chlorbutol [klɔː'bjuːtɔl] *n* 三氯叔丁醇(局部麻醉药,催眠镇静药)
chlorcyclizine hydrochloride [klɔː'saikliziːn] 盐酸氯环利嗪(抗组胺药)
chlordan ['klɔːdæn], **chlordane** ['klɔːdein] *n* 氯丹(杀虫药)
chlordantoin [klɔː'dæntəin] *n* 氯登妥因(抗真菌药)
chlordecone ['klɔːdəˌkəun] *n* 十氯酮(杀虫、杀真菌药)
chlordiazepoxide [klɔːdaiˌæzə'pɔksaid] *n* 氯氮䓬(安定药)
chlordimorine hydrochloride [klɔː'dimәriːn] 盐酸氯地吗啉(抗真菌药)
Chlorella [klɔː'relə] *n* 小球藻属
chlorellin [klɔː'relin] *n* 绿藻素,小球藻素
chloremia [klɔː'riːmiə] *n* 氯血症,高氯血
chlorenchyma [klə'reŋkimə] *n* 绿色组织
chloretic [klə'retik] *n* 利胆药
chlorguanide [klɔː'gwænaid] *n* 氯胍,白乐君(抗疟药)
chlorhexidine [ˌklɔː'heksidiːn] *n* 氯己定(消毒防腐药) | ~ acetate 醋酸氯己定(抗菌药) / ~ gluconate 葡萄糖酸氯己定 / ~ hydrochloride 盐酸氯己定
chlorhistechia [ˌklɔːhis'tekiə] *n* 组织内氯[化物]过多
chlorhydria [klɔː'haidriə] *n* (胃内)盐酸过多,胃酸过多症
chlorhydric acid [klɔː'haidrik] 盐酸,氢氯酸
chloric ['klɔːrik] *a* 氯的
chloric acid ['klɔːrik] 氯酸
chloride ['klɔːraid] *n* 氯化物 | acid ~ 酰基氯,氯化酰基 / ferric ~ 氯化铁 / mercuric ~ 氯化汞,升汞 / mercurous ~ 氯化亚汞,甘汞 / stannous ~ 氯化亚锡,二氯化锡(药物辅料)
chloridimeter [ˌklɔːri'dimitə], **chloridometer** [ˌklɔːri'dɔmitə] *n* 氯化物定量器 | **chloridimetry** *n* 氯化物定量法
chloridion [ˌklɔːri'daiɔn] *n* 氯离子
chloridorrhea [ˌklɔːri'dɔriə] *n* 高氯性腹泻
chloriduria [ˌklɔːri'djuəriə] *n* 氯尿[症]
chlorinate ['klɔːrineit] *vt* 使氯化 | **~d** *a* 含氯的,氯化了的,加氯的 | **chlorination** [ˌklɔːri'neiʃən] *n* 氯化[作用],加氯(消毒)法
chlorindanol [klɔː'rindənɔl] *n* 氯茚酚(杀精子药)

chlorine (Cl) [ˈklɔːriːn] *n* 氯 | ~ dioxide 二氧化氯(氧化剂,消毒药)
chloriodized [klɔːˈraiədaizd] *a* 含氯碘的
chlorisondamine chloride [ˌklɔːraiˈsɔndəmiːn] 松达氯铵(抗高血压药)
chlorite [ˈklɔːrait] *n* 亚氯酸盐
chlormadinone [klɔːˈmædinəun] 氯地孕酮(曾用作口服避孕药)
chlormerodrin [klɔːˈmerədrin] *n* 氯汞君(利尿药) | ~ [^{197}Hg]氯汞[^{197}Hg]君(诊断用药)/ ~ [^{203}Hg]氯汞[^{203}Hg]君(诊断用药)
chlormethyl [klɔːˈmeθil] *n* 氯甲烷
chlormezanone [klɔːˈmezənəun], **chlormethazanone** [ˌklɔːmeˈθæzənəun] *n* 氯美扎酮(肌肉松弛药,安定药)
chlor(o)- [构词成分]绿;氯
chloroacetaldehyde [ˌklɔːrəuˌæsəˈtældəhaid] *n* 氯乙醛
chloroacetic acid [ˌklɔːrəuəˈsiːtik] 氯醋酸,一氯醋酸
chloroacetophenone (CN) [ˌkləurəuˌæsətəu-ˈfiːnəun] *n* 氯乙酰苯(常用催泪毒气)
chloroazodin [klɔːrəuˈæzədin] *n* 氯脒佐定(消毒防腐药)
Chlorobacteriaceae [ˌklɔːrəubækˌtiəriˈeisiiː] *n* 绿杆菌科
Chlorobacterium [ˌklɔːrəubækˈtiəriəm] *n* 绿杆菌属
***o*-chlorobenzylidenemalonitrile (CS)** [ˌkləu-rəubenˌzilidiːnˌmæləˈnaitrail] *n* 邻-氯亚苄基丙二腈(常用催泪毒气)
Chlorobiaceae [ˌklɔːrəubiːˈeisiiː] *n* 绿杆菌科
Chlorobium [kləˈrəubiəm] *n* 绿杆菌属
chlorobrightism [ˌklɔːrəuˈbraitizəm] *n* 萎黄病[性]肾炎(萎黄病伴蛋白尿)
chlorobutanol [ˌklɔːrəuˈbjuːtənɔl] *n* 三氯叔丁醇(局部麻醉药,催眠镇静药)
Chlorochromatium [ˌklɔːrəkrəuˈmeitiəm] *n* 染绿菌属
chlorocruorin [ˌklɔːrəuˈkruərin] *n* 血绿蛋白
2-chlorodeoxyadenosine [ˌklɔːrəudiˌɔksiəˈdenə-siːn] *n* 2-氯脱氧腺苷,克拉屈滨(即 cladribine,抗肿瘤药)
chloroerythroblastoma [ˌklɔːrəuiˌriθrəublæsˈtəu-mə] *n* 绿色成红细胞瘤
chloroethane [klɔːrəuˈeθein] *n* 氯乙烷
chloroethylene [ˌkləurəuˈeθiliːn] *n* 氯乙烯
chlorofluorocarbon (CFC) [ˌkləurəuˈfluərəu-ˌkɑːbən] *n* 含氯氟烃
chloroform [ˈklɔːrəfɔːm] *n* 氯仿 *vt* 用氯仿处理,用氯仿麻醉,用氯仿杀死 | acetone ~ 三氯叔丁醇,氯丁醇 / alcoholized ~ 含醇氯仿,氯仿醇
chloroformism [ˈklɔːrəˌfɔːmizəm] *n* 氯仿[慢性]中毒;氯仿麻醉
chloroformization [ˌklɔːrəˌfɔːmaiˈzeiʃən] *n* 氯仿麻醉
chlorogenic acid [ˌklɔːrəuˈdʒenik] 绿原酸,氯原酸
chloroguanide hydrochloride [ˌklɔːrəuˈɡwænaid] 盐酸氯胍(抗疟药)
chlorolabe [ˈklɔːrəleib] *n* 绿敏素,感绿色素
chloroleukemia [ˌklɔːrəuljuːˈkiːmiə] *n* 绿色白血病,绿色瘤
chlorolymphosarcoma [ˌklɔːrəuˌlimfəsɑːˈkəumə] *n* 绿色淋巴肉瘤,淋巴肉瘤性绿色瘤
chloroma [kləˈrəumə] *n* 绿色瘤
***p*-chloromercuribenzoate** [ˌklɔːrəuˌməːkjuriˈben-zəueit] *n* 对氯汞基苯甲酸盐
chloromethapyriline citrate [ˌklɔːrəuˌmeθəˈpai-riliːn] 枸橼酸氯吡林(抗组胺药)
chlorometry [klɔːˈrɔmitri] *n* 氯定量法
chloromonad [ˌklɔːrəuˈməunæd] *n* 绿滴虫
Chloromonadida [ˌklɔːrəuməˈnædidə] *n* 绿滴虫目
chloromyeloma [ˌklɔːrəumaiəˈləumə] *n* 绿色骨髓瘤
chloronaphthalene [ˌklɔːrəuˈnæfθəliːn] *n* 氯萘
chloropexia [ˌklɔːrəuˈpeksiə] *n* 氯结合
chlorophane [ˈklɔːrəfein] *n* 视网膜绿色素
***p*-chlorophenol** [ˌklɔːrəuˈfiːnɔl] *n* 对氯酚,对氯苯酚(消毒药)
chlorophenothane [ˌklɔːrəuˈfiːnəθein] *n* 滴滴涕(杀虫药)
chlorophylase [ˈklɔːrəfileis] *n* 叶绿素酶
chlorophyll [ˈklɔːrefil] *n* 叶绿素 | **chlorophyllous** [ˌklɔːreˈfiləs] *a*
chlorophyllin [ˈklɔːrəfilin] *n* 叶绿酸
Chlorophyllum [kləˈrɔfiləm] *n* 叶绿蕈属
chloropia [klɔːˈrəupiə] *n* 绿视症
Chloropidae [klɔːˈrɔpidiː] *n* 黄潜蝇科
chloroplast [ˈklɔːrəplæst], **chloroplastid** [ˌklɔː-rəˈplæstid] *n* 叶绿体
chloroplatinic acid [ˌklɔːrəupləˈtinik] 氯铂酸
chloroprene [ˈklɔːrəpriːn] *n* 氯丁二烯
chloroprivic [ˌklɔːrəˈpraivik] *a* 氯化物缺失的,缺氯的
chloroprocaine hydrochloride [ˌklɔːrəˈprəuke-in] 盐酸氯普鲁卡因(局部麻醉药)
chloroprocaine penicillin [ˌklɔːrəˈprəukein] 氯普鲁卡因青霉素(抗生素类药)
chloropropylene oxide [ˌklɔːrəuˈprəupiliːn] 氯环氧丙胺,表氯醇(见 epichlorohydrin)

Chloropseudomonas [ˌklɔːrəusjuːdəu'məunəs] *n* 绿假单胞菌属
chloropsia [klɔː'rɔpsiə] *n* 绿视症
chloroquine ['klɔːrəkwin] *n* 氯喹(抗疟药,抗阿米巴药) | ~ phosphate 磷酸氯喹(抗疟药,抗阿米巴药,红斑狼疮抑制药)
chlorosis [klə'rəusis] *n* 缺绿症,萎黄病,绿色贫血
Chlorostigma [ˌklɔːrə'stigmə] *n* 萝藦属
chlorostigmine [ˌklɔːrəu'stigmiːn] *n* 绿蕊萝藦碱,塔西草碱(催乳药)
chlorosulfonic acid [ˌklɔːrəusʌl'fɔnik] 氯磺酸
chlorothen citrate ['klɔːrəθen], **chlorothenium citrate** [ˌklɔːrə'θeniəm] 枸橼酸氯吡林(抗组胺药)
chlorothiazide [ˌklɔːrəu'θaiəzaid] *n* 氯噻嗪(利尿降压药)
chlorothymol [ˌklɔːrəu'θaimɔl] *n* 氯麝酚(抗菌药)
chlorotic [klə'rɔtik] *a* 萎黄病的
chlorotrianisene [ˌklɔːrəutrai'ænisiːn] *n* 氯烯雌醚(合成的雌激素,尤用于缓解经绝期的症状)
chlorous [ˌklɔːrəs] *a* 亚氯的 | ~ acid 亚氯酸
chlorovinyldichloroarsine [ˌklɔːrəuˌvinildaiˌklɔːrəu'ɑːsin] *n* 氯乙烯基二氯胂,路易士毒气
chloroxine [klə'rɔksin] *n* 氯喔星,二氯羟喹(抗菌药,抗皮脂溢药)
chloroxylenol [ˌklɔːrə'zailənɔl] *n* 氯二甲酚(抗菌药,主要用于皮肤消毒)
chlorphenesin [klɔ'fenəsin] *n* 氯苯甘醚(抗菌药,抗真菌药,抗滴虫药) | ~ carbamate 氯苯甘油氨酯(骨骼肌松弛药)
chlorpheniramine [ˌklɔːfe'nirəmiːn] *n* 氯苯那敏(抗组胺药) | ~ maleate 马来酸氯苯那敏(抗组胺药)
chlorphenoxamine hydrochloride [ˌklɔːfe'nɔksəmiːn] 盐酸氯苯沙明(抗胆碱药,用作骨骼肌松弛药,治疗帕金森〈Parkinson〉病,口服)
chlorphentermine hydrochloride [klɔː'fentəmiːn] 盐酸对氯苯丁胺(食欲抑制药,口服)
chlorpromazine [klɔː'prəuməziːn] *n* 氯丙嗪(止吐药,安定药) | ~ hydrochloride 盐酸氯丙嗪(强安定药)
chlorpropamide [klɔː'prəupəmaid] *n* 氯磺丙脲(口服降血糖药)
chlorprophenpyridamine [ˌklɔːprəufenpai'ridəmiːn] *n* 氯苯那敏(抗组胺药)
chlorprothixene [klɔːprəu'θiksiːn] *n* 氯普噻吨(抗精神病药)
chlorquinaldol [klɔː'kwinəldɔl] *n* 氯喹那多(杀菌药,杀真菌药)
chlortetracycline [ˌklɔːtetrə'saiklain] *n* 金霉素(广谱抗生素) | ~ hydrochloride 盐酸金霉素(抗菌药,抗原虫药)
chlorthalidone [klɔː'θælidəun] *n* 氯噻酮(利尿药)
chlorum ['klɔːrəm] *n*【拉】氯
chloruresis [ˌklɔːjuə'riːsis] *n* 尿氯排泄 | **chloruretic** [ˌklɔːjuə'retik] *a* [促]尿氯排泄的 *n* 促尿氯排泄药
chloruria [klɔː'rjuəriə] *n* 氯尿[症]
chlorzoxazone [klɔː'zɔksəzəun] *n* 氯唑沙宗(骨骼肌松弛药)
Chlumsky's button ['klʌmskiː] (Vitezslav Chlumsky) 克路姆斯基钮(肠缝合钮)
ChM Chirurgiae Magister 外科硕士
CHO Chinese hamster ovary 中国仓鼠卵巢
choana ['kəuənə] ([复] **choanae** ['kəuəniː]) *n*【拉】漏斗;[复]鼻后孔 | primary ~ 初鼻后孔 / secondary ~ 次鼻后孔 | **~l** *a*
choano- [构词成分]漏斗
choanocyte ['kəuəˌnəusait] *n* 领细胞,襟细胞(海绵动物等)
choanoflagellate [ˌkəuənəu'flædʒileit] *n* 领鞭毛虫
Choanoflagellida [ˌkəuənəu'flædʒiˌlaidə] *n* 领鞭毛目
choanoid ['kəuənɔid] *a* 漏斗状的
choanomastigote [ˌkəuənəu'mæstigəut] *n* 领鞭毛体
Choanotaenia [kəuˌeinəu'tiːniə] *n* 领绦虫属 | ~ infundibulum 漏斗领绦虫
choc [ʃɔk] *n*【法】休克;震荡
chocolate ['tʃɔkəlit] *n* 巧克力 *a* 巧克力制的;含有巧克力的
choice [tʃɔis] *n* 选择,选用 | ~ of drug 药物选用
choke [tʃəuk] *vt* 阻塞;噎塞;抑制;阻止 *vi* 窒息;塞住 *n* 窒息;噎;气哽,气阻,气窒 | ophthalmovascular ~ 视网膜血管扼阻 / thoracic ~ 食管(胸段)梗阻 / water ~ 吸水性气哽
cholagogic [ˌkəulə'gɔdʒik] *a* 利胆的 *n* 利胆药
cholagogue ['kəuləgɔg] *n* 利胆药
cholaic acid [kəu'leiik] 牛磺胆酸
cholane ['kəulein] *n* 胆[甾]烷
cholaneresis [ˌkəulə'nerisis] *n* 胆酸类物质排出增多
cholangeitis [ˌkəulændʒi'aitis] *n* 胆管炎
cholangiectasis [kəuˌlændʒi'ektəsis] *n* 胆管扩张
cholangi(o)- [构词成分]胆管
cholangioadenoma [kəuˌlændʒiəuˌædi'nəumə] *n* 胆管腺瘤
cholangiocarcinoma [kəuˌlændʒiəuˌkɑːsi'nəumə] *n* 胆管癌
cholangiocholecystocholedochectomy [kəuˌlæn-

dʒiəu,kəuli,sistəu,kəulidə'kektəmi] *n* 肝胆道切除术(肝管胆总管胆囊切除术)

cholangioenterostomy [kəu,lændʒiəu,entə'rɔstəmi] *n* 胆管小肠吻合术

cholangiogastrostomy [kəu,lændʒiəugæs'trɔstəmi] *n* 胆管胃吻合术

cholangiogram [kəu'lændʒiə,græm] *n* 胆管造影[照]片

cholangiography [kəu,lændʒi'ɔgrəfi] *n* 胆管造影[术] | fine needle transhepatic ~ (FNTC) 细针经肝[穿刺]胆管造影[术] / transhepatic ~ 经肝胆管造影[术] / transjugular ~ 经颈静脉胆管造影[术]

cholangiohepatitis [kəu,lændʒiəu,hepə'taitis] *n* 胆管肝炎

cholangiohepatoma [kəu,lændʒiəu,hepə'təumə] *n* 胆管肝细胞瘤

cholangiojejunostomy [kəu,lændʒiəudʒidʒu'nɔstəmi] *n* 胆管空肠吻合术 | intrahepatic ~ 肝内胆管空肠吻合术

cholangiole [kəu'lændʒiəul] *n* 胆小管 | **cholangiolar** [,kəulæn'dʒiələ] *a*

cholangiolitis [kəu,lændʒiəu'laitis] *n* 胆小管炎

cholangioma [kəu,lændʒi'əumə] *n* 胆管瘤

cholangiopancreatography [kəu,lændʒiəu,pæŋkriə'tɔgrəfi] *n* 胰胆管造影[术] | endoscopic retrograde ~ (ERCP) 内镜逆行胰胆管造影[术]

cholangiosarcoma [kəu,lændʒiəu'sɑːkəumə] *n* 胆管肉瘤 | hilar ~ 肝门胆管肉瘤(亦称克拉斯金〈Klatskin〉瘤) / peripheral ~ 肝周胆管肉瘤

cholangiostomy [,kəulændʒi'ɔstəmi] *n* 胆管造口术

cholangiotomy [,kəulændʒi'ɔtəmi] *n* 胆管切开术

cholangitis [,kəulæn'dʒaitis] *n* 胆管炎 | catarrhal ~ 卡他性胆管炎,传染性肝炎 / chronic nonsuppurative destructive ~ 慢性非化脓性破坏性胆管炎,原发性胆汁性肝硬变 / ~ lenta 慢性感染性胆管炎 / primary sclerosing ~ 原发性硬化性胆管炎 / progressive nonsuppurative ~ 进行性非化脓性胆管炎,原发性胆汁性肝硬变

cholanic acid [kəu'lænik] 胆[甾]烷酸

cholanopoiesis [,kəulənəupɔi'iːsis] *n* 胆盐酸生成 | **cholanopoietic** [,kəulənəu,pɔi'etik] *a* 促胆酸盐生成的 *n* 促胆酸盐生成药

cholanthrene [kəu'lænθriːn] *n* 胆蒽(具有高度致癌性)

cholate ['kəuleit] *n* 胆酸盐(或酯)

chole- 见 chol(o)-

cholebilirubin [,kəuli,bili'ruːbin] *n* 直(接反)应胆红素

cholecalciferol [,kəulikæl'sifərɔl] *n* 胆钙化[甾]醇,维生素 D_3

cholechromopoiesis [,kəuli,krəuməupɔi'iːsis] *n* 胆色素生成

cholecyanin [,kəuli'saiənin] *n* 胆青素

cholecyst ['kəulisist] *n* 胆囊

cholecystagogic [,kəuli,sistə'gɔdʒik] *a* 促胆囊排空的,排胆的,促胆囊收缩的

cholecystagogue [,kəuli'sistəgɔg] *n* 利胆药

cholecystalgia [,kəulisis'tældʒiə] *n* 胆绞痛;胆囊痛

cholecystatony [,kəulisis'tætəni] *n* 胆囊弛缓

cholecystectasia [,kəuli,sistek'teiziə] *n* 胆囊扩张

cholecystectomy [,kəulisis'tektəmi] *n* 胆囊切除术

cholecystenteric [,kəuli,sisten'terik] *a* 胆囊小肠的

cholecystenterorrhaphy [,kəulisis,tentə'rɔrəfi] *n* 胆囊小肠缝合术

cholecystenterostomy [,kəulisis,tentə'rɔstəmi], **cholecystenteroanastomosis** [,kəulisis,tentərəu-ə,næstə'məusis] *n* 胆囊小肠吻合术

cholecystgastrostomy [,kəulisistgæs'trɔstəmi] *n* 胆囊胃吻合术

cholecystic [,kəuli'sistik] *a* 胆囊的

cholecystis [,kəuli'sistis] *n* 胆囊

cholecystitis [,kəulisis'taitis] *n* 胆囊炎 | acute ~ 急性胆囊炎 / chronic ~ 慢性胆囊炎 / emphysematous ~, ~ emphysematosa, gaseous ~ 气肿性胆囊炎 / follicular ~ 滤泡性胆囊炎 / ~ gradularis proliferans 腺样增生性胆囊炎

cholecystnephrostomy [,kəuli,sistni'frɔstəmi] *n* 胆囊肾盂吻合术

cholecystocholangiogram [,kəuli,sistəukəu'lændʒiəgræm] *n* 胆囊胆管造影[照]片

cholecystocolonic [,kəuli,sistəukə'lɔnik] *a* 胆囊结肠的

cholecystocolostomy [,kəuli,sistəukə'lɔstəmi] *n* 胆囊结肠吻合术

cholecystocolotomy [,kəuli,sistəukə'lɔtəmi] *n* 胆囊结肠切开术

cholecystoduodenostomy [,kəuli,sistəu,dju(ː)-əudi'nɔstəmi] *n* 胆囊十二指肠吻合术

cholecystoenterostomy [,kəulisistəu,entə'rɔstəmi] *n* 胆囊小肠吻合术

cholecystogastric [,kəuli,sistəu'gæstrik] *a* 胆囊胃的

cholecystogastrostomy [,kəuli,sistəugæs'trɔstəmi] *n* 胆囊胃吻合术

cholecystogogic [,kəuli,sistəu'gɔdʒik] *a* 促胆囊收缩的

cholecystogram [,kəuli'sistəgræm] *n* 胆囊造影[照]片

cholecystography [ˌkəulisisˈtɔgrəfi] *n* 胆囊造影术
cholecystoileostomy [ˌkəuliˌsistəuˌiliˈɔstəmi] *n* 胆囊回肠吻合术
cholecystointestinal [ˌkəuliˌsistəuinˈtestinl] *a* 胆囊小肠的
cholecystojejunostomy [ˌkəuliˌsistəudʒidʒjuˈnɔstəmi] *n* 胆囊空肠吻合术
cholecystokinase [ˌkəuliˌsistəuˈkaineis] *n* 缩胆囊素酶
cholecystokinetic [ˌkəuliˌsistəukaiˈnetik] *a* 促胆囊收缩的
cholecystokinin(CCK) [ˌkəuliˌsistəuˈkainin] *n* 缩胆囊素,缩胆囊肽,胆囊收缩素
cholecystolithiasis [ˌkəuliˌsistəuliˈθaiəsis] *n* 胆囊结石病
cholecystolithotomy [ˌkəuliˌsistəuliˈθɔtəmi] *n* 胆囊切开取石术
cholecystolithotripsy [ˌkəuliˌsistəˈliθəˌtripsi] *n* 胆囊碎石术
cholecystonephrostomy [ˌkəuliˌsistəuniˈfrɔstəmi] *n* 胆囊肾盂吻合术
cholecystopathy [ˌkəulisisˈtɔpəθi] *n* 胆囊病
cholecystopexy [ˌkəuliˈsistəˌpeksi] *n* 胆囊固定术
cholecystoptosis [ˌkəuliˌsistəpˈtəusis] *n* 胆囊下垂
cholecystopyelostomy [ˌkəuliˌsistəuˌpaiəˈlɔstəmi] *n* 胆囊肾盂吻合术
cholecystorrhaphy [ˌkəulisisˈtɔrəfi] *n* 胆囊缝合术
cholecystosis [ˌkəulisisˈtəusis] *n* 胆囊病 | hyperplastic ~ 增生性胆囊病
cholecystostomy [ˌkəulisisˈtɔstəmi] *n* 胆囊造口术
cholecystotomy [ˌkəulisisˈtɔtəmi] *n* 胆囊切开术
cholecystotyphoid [ˌkəuliˌsistəuˈtaifɔid] *n* 胆囊型伤寒
choledochal [ˌkɔliˈdɔkəl] *a* 胆总管的
choledochectomy [ˌkɔlidəuˈkektəmi] *n* 胆总管部分切除术
choledochendysis [ˌkɔlidəuˈkendisis] *n* 胆总管切开术
choledochitis [ˌkɔlidəuˈkaitis] *n* 胆总管炎
choledoch(o)- [构词成分] 胆总管
choledochocele [kəˈledəkəsiːl] *n* 胆总管囊肿
choledochocholedochostomy [kəˌledəkəuˌkɔlidəˈkɔstəmi] *n* 胆总管端端吻合术
choledochoduodenostomy [kəˌledəkəuˌdju(ː)əudiˈnɔstəmi] *n* 胆总管十二指肠吻合术
choledochoenterostomy [kəˌledəkəuˌentəˈrɔstəmi] *n* 胆总管小肠吻合术
choledochogastrostomy [kəˌledəkəugæsˈtrɔstəmi] *n* 胆总管胃吻合术
choledochogram [kəˈledəkəˌgræm] *n* 胆总管造影[照]片
choledochography [kəˌledəˈkɔgrəfi] *n* 胆总管造影[术]
choledochohepatostomy [kəˌledəkəuˌhepəˈtɔstəmi] *n* 胆总管肝管吻合术
choledochoileostomy [kəˌledəkəuiliˈɔstəmi] *n* 胆总管回肠吻合术
choledochojejunostomy [kəˌledəkəudʒidʒjuˈnɔstəmi] *n* 胆总管空肠吻合术
choledocholith [kəˈledəkəˌliθ] *n* 胆总管结石
choledocholithiasis [kəˌledəkəuliˈθaiəsis] *n* 胆总管结石病
choledocholithotomy [kəˌledəkəuliˈθɔtəmi] *n* 胆总管石切除术
choledocholithotripsy [kəˌledəkəuˈliθəˌtripsi] *n* 胆总管碎石术
choledochoplasty [kəˌledəkəuˈplæsti] *n* 胆总管成形术
choledochorrhaphy [kəˌledəˈkɔrəfi] *n* 胆总管缝合术
choledochoscope [kəˈledəkəskəup] *n* 胆总管镜
choledochostomy [kəˌledəuˈkɔstəmi] *n* 胆总管造口术
choledochotomy [kəˌledəuˈkɔtəmi] *n* 胆总管切开术
choledochus [kəˈledəkəs] *n* 胆总管
choleglobin [ˌkəuliˈgləubin] *n* 胆珠蛋白,胆绿蛋白
cholehematin [ˌkəuliˈhemətin] *n* 胆紫素
choleic [kəˈliːik] *a* 胆的 | ~ acid 胆酸
cholelith [ˈkəuliliθ] *n* 胆石
cholelithiasis [ˌkəuliliˈθaiəsis] *n* 胆石症
cholelithic [ˌkəuliˈliθik] *a* 胆石的
cholelithotomy [ˌkəuliliˈθɔtəmi] *n* 胆石切除术
cholelithotripsy [ˌkəuliˈliθətripsi], **cholelithotrity** [ˌkəuliliˈθɔtriti] *n* 碎胆石术
cholemesis [kəˈlemisis] *n* 呕胆
cholemia [kəˈliːmiə] *n* 胆血症 | familial ~ 家族性胆血症(见 Gilbert syndrome) | **cholemic** *a*
cholemimetry [ˌkəuliˈmimitri] *n* 胆色素定量法
choleophosphatase [ˌkəuliəˈfɔsfəteis] *n* 胆碱磷酸酶
cholepathia [ˌkəuliˈpæθiə] *n* 胆管病
choleperitoneum [ˌkəuliˌperitəuˈniːəm], **choleperitonitis** [ˌkəuliˌperitəuˈnaitis] *n* 胆汁性腹膜炎
cholepoiesis [ˌkəulipɔiˈiːsis] *n* 胆汁生成 | **cholepoietic** [ˌkəulipɔiˈetik] *a*
choleprasin [ˌkəuliˈpreisin] *n* 胆翠质
cholera [ˈkɔlərə] *n* 霍乱 | Asiatic ~ 亚洲霍乱/

automatic ~ 自动症性霍乱 / bilious ~, European ~, ~ nostrus 胆汁性霍乱,欧洲霍乱,假霍乱 / chicken ~ 鸡霍乱 / fowl ~, ~ gallinarium 禽霍乱 / ~ infantum 婴儿吐泻病,婴儿假霍乱 / ~ morbus, summer ~ 假霍乱,夏季吐泻 / pancreatic ~ 胰性霍乱 / ~ sicca, dry ~ 干性霍乱 | **~ic** [ˌkɔləˈreiik] *a*

choleragen [ˈkɔlərədʒən] *n* 霍乱原,霍乱肠菌素

choleraphage [ˈkɔlərəfeidʒ] *n* 霍乱(弧菌)嗜菌体

choleresis [kəˈlerisis] *n* 胆汁分泌 | **choleretic** [ˌkəuləˈretik] *a* 促胆汁分泌的 *n* 利胆药

choleric [ˈkɔlərik] *a* 急躁的,易怒的

choleriform [kəˈlerifɔːm] *a* 霍乱样的

cholerigenic [ˌkɔləriˈdʒenik], **cholerigenous** [ˌkɔləˈridʒinəs] *a* 引起霍乱的

cholerine [ˈkɔlərin] *n* 轻霍乱

cholerization [ˌkɔləraiˈzeiʃən, -riˈz-] *n* 霍乱预防接种

choleroid [ˈkɔlərɔid] *a* 霍乱样的

choleromania [ˌkɔlərəˈmeinjə] *n* 霍乱躁狂[症]

cholescintigram [ˌkəuliˈsintigræm] *n* 胆道闪烁图

cholescintigraphy [kəuliˈsintigrəfi] *n* 胆道闪烁显像[术]

cholestane [ˈkɔlestein] *n* 胆甾烷

5β-cholestane-3α, 7α, 12α, 25-tetraol 24S-hydroxylase [kɔˈlestein ˈtetrəˈɔl haiˈdrɔksileis] 5β-胆甾烷-3α, 7α, 12α, 25-四醇 24S 羟化酶(此酶缺乏为一种常染色体隐性性状,可致脑腱黄瘤病。亦称 24-羟化酶)

cholestanetriol [kəˌlesteinˈtraiɔl] *n* 胆甾烷三醇

cholestanetriol 26-monooxygenase [kəˌlesteinˈtraiɔl ˌmɔnəuˈɔksidʒineis] 胆甾烷三醇 26-单加氧酶(此酶缺乏为一种常染色体隐性性状,可致脑腱黄瘤病。亦称 26-羟化酶)

cholestanol [kəˈlestənɔl] *n* 胆甾烷醇

cholestasis [ˌkəuliˈsteisis], **cholestasia** [ˌkəuliˈsteiziə] *n* 胆汁淤积 | **cholestatic** [ˌkəuliˈstætik] *a*

cholesteatoma [ˌkəuliˌstiəˈtəumə] *n* 胆脂瘤 | congenital ~ 先天性胆脂瘤,表皮样瘤 | **~tous** *a*

cholesteatosis [ˌkəuliˌstiəˈtəusis] *n* 胆固醇沉着性变性

cholestene [ˈkɔlestiːn] *n* 胆甾烯

cholesteremia [kəˌlestəˈriːmiə], **cholesterinemia** [kəˌlestəriˈniːmiə] *n* 胆固醇血

cholesterin [kəˈlestərin] *n* 胆固醇,胆甾醇

cholesterinosis [kəˌlestəriˈnəusis] *n* 胆固醇沉着[病]

cholesterinuria [kəˌlestəriˈnjuəriə] *n* 胆固醇尿

cholesterogenesis [kəˌlestərəuˈdʒenisis] *n* 胆固醇产生

cholesterohistechia [kəˌlestərəuhisˈtekiə] *n* 组织胆固醇沉着

cholesterohydrothorax [kəˌlestərəuˌhaidrəuˈθɔːræks] *n* 胆固醇性水胸

cholesterol [kəˈlestərɔl] *n* 胆固醇

cholesterol acyltransferase [kəˈlestərɔl ˌæsilˈtrænsfəreis] 胆固醇酰基转移酶,固醇*O*-酰基转移酶

cholesterol desmolase [kəˈlestərɔl ˈdezməleis] 胆固醇碳链[裂解]酶,胆固醇单加氧酶(裂解侧链的)

cholesterol desmolase deficiency 胆甾醇碳链[裂解]酶缺乏症,脂质肾上腺增生

cholesterolemia [kəˌlestərɔˈliːmiə] *n* 胆固醇血

cholesteroleresis [kəˌlestərɔˈlerisis] *n* 胆汁内胆固醇增多

cholesterol esterase [kəˌlestərɔl ˈestəreis] 胆固醇酯酶,固醇酯酶

cholesterolestersturz [kəˌlestərɔˈlestəʃtuəts] *n* 【德】血内胆固醇酯[部分]减少

cholesterol monooxygenase (sidechain cleaving) (P_{450} SCC) [kəˈlestərɔl ˌmɔnəuˈɔksidʒəneis] 胆固醇单加氧酶(裂解侧链的)(此酶缺乏,为一种带染色体隐性性状,可致类脂肾上腺增生〈先天性肾上腺增生症 I 型〉。亦称胆固醇碳链〈裂解〉酶)

cholesterolopoiesis [kəˌlestəˌrɔləpɔiˈiːsis] *n* 胆固醇生成

cholesterolosis [kəˌlestərɔˈləusis] *n* 胆固醇贮积病

cholesterol sulfatase [kəˈlestərɔlˈsʌlfəteis] 胆固醇硫酸酯酶,类固醇硫酸酯酶

cholesterosis [kəˌlestəˈrəusis] *n* 胆固醇贮积病 | ~ cutis 皮肤胆固醇贮积病,黄瘤病 / extracellular ~ 细胞外胆固醇贮积病

cholesteryl [kəˈlestəˌril] *n* 胆固醇基

cholestyramine [ˌkəulisˈtaiərəmiːn] *n* 考来烯胺(降血脂药)

cholestyramine [ˌkəuləˈstairəmiːn] *n* 考来烯胺(降血脂药)

choletelin [kəˈletilin] *n* 胆黄素

choletherapy [ˌkəuliˈθerəpi] *n* 胆汁疗法

choleuria [ˌkəuliˈjuəriə] *n* 胆汁尿

choleverdin [ˌkəuliˈvəːdin] *n* 胆绿素

cholic acid [ˈkəulik] 胆酸

choline [ˈkəuliːn] *n* 胆碱 | acetyl glyceryl ether phosphoryl ~ 乙酰甘油醚磷酰胆碱(血小板活化因子) / ~ magnesium trisalicylate 三水杨酸胆碱镁 / phosphatidyl ~ 磷脂酰胆碱,卵磷脂 / ~ salicylate 水杨酸胆碱(镇痛、解热、抗风湿药) / ~ theophyllinate 胆茶碱(支气管扩张药,平滑肌松弛药)

choline acetylase [ˈkəulin əˈsetileis] 胆碱乙酰化酶,胆碱乙酰基转移酶

choline *O*-acetyltransferase [ˈkəuliːn ˌæsitilˈtrænsfəreis] 胆碱*O*-乙酰转移酶(亦称胆碱乙酰化酶)

choline esterase Ⅰ [ˈkəulin ˈestəreis] 胆碱酯酶Ⅰ,乙酰胆碱酯酶

choline esterase Ⅱ (unspecific) 胆碱酯酶Ⅱ(非特异性的),胆碱酯酶

cholinergic [ˌkəuliˈnəːdʒik] *a* 胆碱能的 *n* 胆碱能药,拟副交感神经药

cholinesterase (CHS) [ˌkəuliˈnestəreis] *n* 胆碱酯酶(亦称胆碱酯酶Ⅱ〈非特异性的〉,血清胆碱酯酶,假胆碱酯酶) | serum ~ (SChE) 血清胆碱酯酶,假胆碱酯酶 / true ~ 乙酰胆碱酯酶

cholinoceptive [ˌkəulinəuˈseptiv] *a* 胆碱受体的

cholinoceptor [ˌkəulinəuˈseptə] *n* 胆碱受体

cholinolytic [ˌkəulinəuˈlitik] *a* 抗胆碱[作用]的,胆碱阻滞的 *n* 抗胆碱药,胆碱阻滞药

cholinomimetic [ˌkəulinəumiˈmetik, -maiˈm-] *a* 拟胆碱[作用]的 *n* 拟胆碱药

chol(o)-, chole- [构词成分]胆汁

cholochrome [ˈkɔləkrəum] *n* 胆色素

cholocyanin [ˌkɔləuˈsaiənin] *n* 胆青素

chologenetic [ˌkɔləudʒiˈnetik] *a* 生胆汁的

cholohematin [ˌkɔləuˈhemətin] *n* 胆紫素

cholohemothorax [ˌkəuləuˌhiːməˈθɔːræks] *n* 胆血胸

choloidanic acid [kəulɔiˈdænik] 胆丹酸,破-AC-四羧胆酸

chololith [ˈkɔləliθ] *n* 胆石

chololithiasis [ˌkɔləuliˈθaiəsis] *n* 胆石病

chololithic [ˌkɔləuˈliθik] *a* 胆石的

cholopoiesis [ˌkɔləupɔiˈiːsis] *n* 胆汁生成

cholothorax [ˌkəuləuˈθɔːræks] *n* 胆汁胸

choluria [kəˈljuəriə] *n* 胆汁尿 | **choluric** *a*

cholylglycine [ˌkəulilˈglaisin] *n* 胆酰甘氨酸(亦称甘胆酸,甘氨胆酸)

cholyltaurine [ˌkəulilˈtɔːri(ː)n] *n* 胆酰牛磺酸(亦称牛磺胆酸,胆酸)

chondodendrine [ˌkɔndəˈdendriːn] *n* 甘密树皮碱,比比林

Chondodendron [ˌkɔndəˈdendrɔn] *n* 南美防己属 | ~ tomentosum Ruiz et Pavon 南美防己(外科用作骨骼肌松弛药及重症肌无力的诊断用药)

chondral [ˈkɔndrəl] *a* 软骨的

chondralgia [kɔnˈdrældʒiə] *n* 软骨痛

chondralloplasia [ˌkɔndrələuˈpleiziə] *n* 软骨发育异常,软骨发育不良

chondrectomy [kɔnˈdrektəmi] *n* 软骨切除术

chondric [ˈkɔndrik] *a* 软骨的

Chondrichthyes [kɔnˈdrikθiiːz] *n* 软骨鱼纲

chondrification [ˌkɔndrifiˈkeiʃən] *n* 软骨化,软骨形成

chondrigen [ˈkɔndridʒən] *n* 软骨素原

chondrin [ˈkɔndrin] *n* 软骨胶

Chondrina [kɔnˈdrainə] *n* 软蛹螺属

chondri(o)- [构词成分]粒,颗粒;软骨

chondriome [ˈkɔndriəum] *n* 线粒体系

chondriosome [ˈkɔndriəsəum] *n* 线粒体

chondritis [kɔnˈdraitis] *n* 软骨炎 | costal ~ 肋软骨炎 / ~ intervertebralis calcanea 椎间盘钙质沉着

chondr(o)- [构词成分]软骨

chondroadenoma [ˌkɔndrəuˌædiˈnəumə] *n* 软骨腺瘤

chondroangioma [ˌkɔndrəuˌændʒiˈəumə] *n* 软骨血管瘤

chondroblast [ˈkɔndrəublæst] *n* 成软骨细胞

chondroblastoma [ˌkɔndrəublæsˈtəumə] *n* 软骨母细胞瘤 | benign ~ 良性软骨母细胞瘤

chondrocalcinosis [ˌkɔndrəuˌkælsiˈnəusis] *n* 软骨钙沉着症(如伴有痛风样症状发作时,称为假痛风)

chondrocarcinoma [ˌkɔndrəuˌkɑːsiˈnəumə] *n* 软骨癌

chondroclast [ˌkɔndrəuklæst] *n* 破软骨细胞

Chondrococcus [ˌkɔndrəuˈkɔkəs] *n* 粒球黏细菌属

chondroconia [ˌkɔndrəuˈkəuniə] *n* 软骨微粒

chondrocostal [ˌkɔndrəuˈkɔstl] *a* 肋与肋软骨的

chondrocranium [ˌkɔndrəuˈkreinjəm] ([复] **chondrocrania** [ˌkɔndrəuˈkreinjə]) *n* 软骨颅

chondrocyte [ˈkɔndrəusait] *n* 软骨细胞 | isogenous ~s 同源软骨细胞

chondrodermatitis [ˌkɔndrə u ˌdəːməˈtaitis] *n* 软骨皮炎 | ~ nodularis chronica helicis 慢性结节性耳轮软骨皮炎

chondrodynia [ˌkɔndrəuˈdiniə] *n* 软骨痛

chondrodysplasia [ˌkɔndrəudisˈpleiziə] *n* 软骨发育不良,软骨发育不全 | hereditary deforming ~ 遗传畸形性软骨发育不良 / ~ punctata 斑点状软骨发育不良

chondrodystrophia [ˌkɔndrəudisˈtrəufiə] *n* 软骨营养障碍,软骨营养不良 | ~ calcificans congenita, ~ congenita punctata, ~ fetalis calcificans 先天性钙化软骨营养不良,先天性斑点状软骨营养不良,胎儿钙化软骨营养不良(即斑点状软骨发育不良)

chondrodystrophy [ˌkɔndrəuˈdistrəfi] *n* 软骨营养障碍,软骨营养不良 | hereditary deforming ~, familial ~ 遗传畸形性软骨营养障碍,软骨发育异常 / hyperplastic ~ 增生性软骨营养障碍

/ hypoplastic ~ 发育不全性软骨营养障碍 / hypoplastic fetal ~ 胎儿发育不全性软骨营养障碍（即点状软骨发育不全）/ ~ malacia 软化性软骨营养障碍

chondroendothelioma [ˌkɔndrəuˌendəuˌθiːliˈəumə] *n* 软骨内皮瘤

chondroepiphyseal [ˌkɔndrəuˌepiˈfiziəl] *a* 软骨骺的

chondroepiphysitis [ˌkɔndrəuˌepifiˈzaitis] *n* 软骨骺炎

chondrofibroma [ˌkɔndrəufaiˈbrəumə] *n* 软骨纤维瘤

chondrogen [ˈkɔndrəudʒən] *n* 软骨素原

chondrogenesis [ˌkɔndrəuˈdʒenisis] *n* 软骨发生 | **chondrogenic** [ˌkɔndrəuˈdʒenik] *a*

chondroglossus [ˌkɔndrəuˈglɔsəs] 小角舌肌（见附录〈二〉肌名对照表）

chondroglucose [ˌkɔndrəuˈgluːkəus] *n* 软骨葡萄糖

chondrography [kɔnˈdrɔgrəfi] *n* 软骨论

chondroid [ˈkɔndrɔid] *a* 软骨样的

chondroitic [ˌkɔndrəuˈitik] *a* 软骨的;软骨样的 | ~ acid 软骨酸

chondroitin [kɔnˈdrəuitin] *n* 软骨素

chondroitin sulfatase [kɔnˈdrəuitinˈsʌlfəteis] 软骨素硫酸酯酶,*N*-乙酰[基]半乳糖胺-6-硫酸酯酶

chondroitin sulfate [kɔnˈdrəuitin ˈsʌlfeit] 硫酸软骨素

chondroitin-sulfuric acid [kɔnˈdrəuitin sʌlˈfjuərik] 硫酸软骨素

chondroitinuria [kɔnˌdrəuitiˈnjuəriə] *n* 软骨素尿

chondrolipoma [ˌkɔndrəuliˈpəumə] *n* 软骨脂瘤

chondrology [kɔnˈdrɔlədʒi] *n* 软骨学

chondrolysis [kɔnˈdrɔlisis] *n* 软骨溶解

chondroma [kɔnˈdrəumə]（[复] **chondromas** 或 **chondromata** [kɔnˈdrəumətə]）*n* 软骨瘤 | true ~ 真性软骨瘤,内生软骨瘤

chondromalacia [ˌkɔndrəuməˈleiʃiə] *n* 软骨软化

chondromatosis [ˌkɔndrəuməˈtəusis] *n* 软骨瘤病

chondromatous [kɔnˈdrɔmətəs] *a* 软骨瘤的

chondromere [ˈkɔndrəmiə] *n* 软骨节

chondrometaplasia [ˌkɔndrəuˌmetəˈpleiziə] *n* 软骨化生,软骨组织变形

chondromitome [ˌkɔndrəuˈmaitəum] *n* 副核

chondromucin [ˌkɔndrəuˈmjuːsin], **chondromucoid** [ˌkɔndrəuˈmjuːkɔid] *n* 软骨黏蛋白

chondromucoprotein [ˌkɔndrəuˌmjuːkəuˈprəutiːn] *n* 软骨黏蛋白质

Chondromyces [ˌkɔndrəuˈmaisiːz] *n* 软骨[霉]菌属

chondromyoma [ˌkɔndrəumaiˈəumə] *n* 软骨肌瘤

chondromyxoma [ˌkɔndrəumikˈsəumə] *n* 软骨黏液瘤

chondromyxosarcoma [ˌkɔndrəuˌmiksəu sɑːˈkəumə] *n* 软骨黏液肉瘤

chondronecrosis [ˌkɔndrəuneˈkrəusis] *n* 软骨坏死

chondro-osseous [ˌkɔndrəuˈɔsiəs] *a* 软骨与骨的

chondro-osteodystrophy [ˌkɔndrəuˌɔstiəˈdistrəfi] *n* 骨软骨营养不良

chondropathia [ˌkɔndrəuˈpæθiə] *n* 软骨病 | ~ tuberosa 结节状软骨病

chondropathology [ˌkɔndrəupəˈθɔlədʒi] *n* 软骨病理学

chondropathy [kɔnˈdrɔpəθi] *n* 软骨病

chondrophyte [ˈkɔndrəufait] *n* 软骨疣

chondroplasia [ˌkɔndrəuˈpleiziə] *n* 软骨生成 | ~ punctata 点状骨骺发育不良

chondroplast [ˈkɔndrəuplæst] *n* 成软骨细胞

chondroplasty [ˈkɔndrəuˌplæsti] *n* 软骨成形术 | **chondroplastic** [ˌkɔndrəuˈplæstik] *a*

chondroporosis [ˌkɔndrəupəˈrəusis] *n* 软骨疏松

chondroprotein [ˌkɔndrəuˈprəutiːn], **chondroproteid** [ˌkɔndrəuˈprəutiːd] *n* 软骨蛋白

chondrosamine [kɔnˈdrəusəmin] *n* 软骨糖胺,半乳糖胺,2-氨基半乳糖

chondrosaminic acid [ˌkɔndrəusəˈminik] 软骨氨酸,氨基半乳糖酸

chondrosarcoma [ˌkɔndrəusɑːˈkəumə] *n* 软骨肉瘤 | ~tous *a*

chondrosarcomatosis [ˌkɔndrəusɑːˌkəuməˈtəusis] *n* 软骨肉瘤病

chondroseptum [ˌkɔndrəuˈseptəm] *n* 鼻中隔软骨部

chondrosin [ˈkɔndrəsin] *n* 软骨胶素（软骨素水解产物）

chondrosis [kɔnˈdrəusis] *n* 软骨形成

chondroskeleton [ˌkɔndrəuˈskelitn] *n* 软骨骼

chondrosome [ˈkɔndrəsəum] *n* 线粒体

chondrosteoma [kɔnˌdrɔstiˈəumə] *n* 软骨骨瘤

chondrosternal [ˌkɔndrəuˈstəːnl] *a* 肋软骨胸骨的

chondrosternoplasty [ˌkɔndrəuˈstəːnəˌplæsti] *n* 漏斗胸矫正术,肋软骨胸骨成形术

chondrotome [ˈkɔndrətəum] *n* 软骨刀

chondrotomy [kɔnˈdrɔtəmi] *n* 软骨切开术

chondrotrophic [ˌkɔndrəuˈtrɔfik] *a* 软骨营养的

chondroxiphoid [ˌkɔndrəuˈzaifɔid] *a* 剑突的

Chondrus [ˈkɔndrəs] *n* 角叉菜属

chondrus [ˈkɔndrəs] *n* 角叉菜,爱兰苔

chonechondrosternon [ˌkəuniˌkɔndrəuˈstəːnən] *n* 漏斗[状]胸

CHOP cyclophosphamide, doxorubicin, vincristine, and prednisone 环磷酰胺-多柔比星-长春新碱-泼尼松(联合化疗治癌方案)

Chopart's amputation (**operation**) [ʃəu'pɑː] (François Chopart) 肖帕尔切断术(手术)(跗中切断术) | ~ articulation (joint) 跗横关节

CHOP-BLEO bleomycin, doxorubicin, cyclophosphamide, vincristine, and prednisone 博来霉素-多柔比星-环磷酰胺-长春新碱-泼尼松(联合化疗治癌方案)

chorangioma [kɔːˌrændʒi'əumə] *n* 绒[毛]膜血管瘤

chord [kɔːd] *n* 索,带

chorda ['kɔːdə] ([复] **chordae** ['kɔːdiː]) *n* 【拉】索,带 | ~ spinalis 脊髓 / ~ umbilicalis 脐带 | **~l** *a*

chorda-mesoderm [ˌkɔːdə 'mezədəːm] *n* 脊索中胚层

Chordata [kɔː'deitə] *n* 脊索门,脊索动物门

chordate ['kɔːdeit] *n* 脊索动物 *a* 有脊索的

chordectomy [kɔː'dektəmi] *n* 声带切除术

chordee ['kɔːdiː, 'kɔːdei] *n* 【法】阴茎下弯畸形 | ~ of penis 阴茎下弯

chorditis [kɔː'daitis] *n* 声带炎;精索炎

chordo- [构词成分]索,带

chordoblastoma [ˌkɔːdəublæs'təumə] *n* 成脊索细胞瘤

chordocarcinoma [ˌkɔːdəukɑːsi'nəumə] *n* 脊索癌,脊索瘤

chordoepithelioma [ˌkɔːdəuˌepiθiːli'əumə] *n* 脊索上皮瘤,脊索瘤

chordoid ['kɔːdɔid] *a* 脊索状的

chordoma [kɔː'dəumə] *n* 脊索瘤

chordopexy ['kɔːdəˌpeksi] *n* 声带固定

Chordopoxvirinae [ˌkɔːdəˌpɔksvi'rainiː] *n* 脊髓动物痘病毒亚科

chordosarcoma [ˌkɔːdəusɑː'kəumə] *n* 脊索肉瘤,脊索瘤

chordoskeleton [ˌkɔːdəu'skelitn] *n* 脊索骨骼(脊索四周的骨骼)

chordotomy [kɔː'dɔtəmi] *n* 脊髓前外侧束切断术

chorea [kɔ'riə] *n* 舞蹈症 | automatic ~ 自动性舞蹈症 / button-makers' ~ 纽扣工抽动症 / diaphragmatic ~, laryngeal ~ 膈痉挛,喉舞蹈症(无痛性抽搐者发出一种特别的喊叫) / electric ~ 电击样舞蹈症 / epidemic ~ 流行性舞蹈症,舞蹈狂 / fibrillary ~ 肌纤维性肌阵挛 / hemilateral ~, onesided ~ 单侧舞蹈症,偏身舞蹈症 / hyoscine ~ 莨菪碱中毒性舞蹈症 / hysterical ~, ~ major 癔症性舞蹈症,大舞蹈症 / limp ~, ~ mollis 麻痹性舞蹈症,瘫痪性舞蹈症 / local ~ 局部舞蹈症,局部性抽动,职业性神经功能病 / malleatory ~ 拳击样舞蹈症 / posthemiplegic ~ 偏瘫后舞蹈症,手足徐动症,指痉病 / saltatory ~, dancing ~ 跳跃性舞蹈症 / simple ~, ~ minor 舞蹈症,小舞蹈症 | **~l** ['kɔːriəl], **~tic** [ˌkɔːri'ætik], **choreic** [kɔ'riːik] *a*

choreiform [kɔː'riifɔːm], **choreoid** ['kɔːriɔid] *a* 舞蹈症样的

choreoacanthocytosis [ˌkɔriəueiˌkænθəusai'təusis] *n* 舞蹈样运动刺状红细胞增多(为常染色体隐性遗传综合征,特征为抽搐、舞蹈症和人格改变,血内有刺状红细胞。亦称神经刺状红细胞增多)

choreoathetosis [ˌkɔːriəuæθi'təusis] *n* 舞蹈徐动症 | **choreoathetoid** [ˌkɔːriəu'æθitɔid] *a* 舞蹈徐动症的,舞蹈徐动症样的

choreomania [ˌkɔːriəu'meinje] *n* 舞蹈狂,流行性舞蹈症

choreophrasia [keˌriəu'freiziə] *n* 片语重复症

chorial ['kɔːriəl] *a* 绒[毛]膜的

chori(o)- [构词成分]绒毛膜

chorioadenoma [ˌkɔːriəuædi'nəumə] *n* 绒[毛]膜腺瘤,恶性葡萄胎 | ~ destruens 恶性葡萄胎

chorioallantois [ˌkɔːriəuə'læntəuis] *n* 绒[毛]膜尿囊 | **chorioallantoic** [ˌkɔːriəuˌælən'təuik] *a*

chorioamnionitis [ˌkɔːriəuˌæmniə'naitis] *n* 绒[毛]膜羊膜炎

chorioangiofibroma [ˌkɔːriəuˌændʒiəufai'brəumə] *n* 绒[毛]膜血管纤维瘤

chorioangioma [ˌkɔːriəuˌændʒi'əumə] *n* 绒[毛]膜血管瘤

chorioblastoma [ˌkɔːriəublæs'təumə] *n* 成绒[毛]膜细胞瘤,成绒[毛]膜瘤,绒[毛]膜癌

chorioblastosis [ˌkɔːriəublæs'təusis] *n* 绒[毛]膜增殖

choriocapillaris [ˌkɔːriəuˌkæpi'lɛəris] *n* 脉络膜血管层

choriocarcinoma [ˌkɔːriəuˌkɑːsi'nəumə] *n* 绒毛膜癌

choriocele ['kɔːriəsiːl] *n* 脉络膜膨出

chorioepithelioma [ˌkɔːriəuˌepiˌθiːli'əumə] *n* 绒[毛]膜上皮癌,绒[毛]膜上皮瘤,绒[毛]膜癌 | ~ malignum 恶性绒[毛]膜上皮癌,恶性合胞体瘤

choriogenesis [ˌkɔːriəu'dʒenisis] *n* 绒[毛]膜发生

choriogonadotropin [ˌkəuriəu'gɔnədəˌtrəupin] *n* 绒[毛]膜促性腺激素

chorioidea [ˌkɔːri'ɔidiə], **chorioid** ['kɔriɔid] *n* 脉络膜

chorioid(o)- 见 choroid(o)-

chorioma [ˌkɔːri'əumə] *n* 绒[毛]膜瘤

choriomammotropin [ˌkɔːriəuˌmæməu'trəupin] *n*

绒毛膜催乳激素，人胎盘催乳素

choriomeningitis [ˌkɔːriəuˌmeninˈdʒaitis] *n* 脉络丛脑膜炎 | lymphocytic ~ 淋巴细胞[性]脉络丛脑膜炎(一种病毒性脑膜炎)

chorion [ˈkɔːriɔn] *n*【希】绒毛膜；子宫内膜基质；卵壳 | ~ frondosum, shaggy ~ 叶状绒毛膜 / ~ leave 平滑绒毛膜 / primitive ~ 原绒毛膜 | **~ic** [ˌkɔːriˈɔnik] *a*

chorionepithelioma [ˌkɔːriɔnˌepiˌθiliˈəumə] *n* 绒[毛]膜上皮癌，绒[毛]膜癌

chorioplacental [ˌkɔːriəupləˈsentl] *a* 绒[毛]膜胎盘的

Chorioptes [ˌkɔːriˈɔptiːz] *n* 皮螨属

chorioptic [ˌkɔːriˈɔptik] *a* 皮螨[属]的

chorioretinal [ˌkɔːriəuˈretinəl] *a* 脉络膜视网膜的

chorioretinitis [ˌkɔːriəuˌretiˈnaitis] *n* 脉络膜视网膜炎 | toxoplasmic ~ 弓形虫性脉络膜视网膜炎

chorioretinopathy [ˌkɔːriəuˌretiˈnɔpəθi] *n* 脉络膜视网膜病变

chorista [kəˈristə] *n* 原基异位性发育异常

choristoma [ˌkɔːrisˈtəumə], **choristoblastoma** [kəˌristəublæsˈtəumə] *n* 迷芽瘤，成迷芽细胞瘤

choroid [ˈkɔːrɔid] *n* 脉络膜 *a* 绒毛膜样的 | **~al** [kəˈrɔidl] *a* 脉络膜的

choroidea [kəˈrɔidiə] *n* 脉络膜

choroidectomy [ˌkɔːrɔiˈdektəmi] *n* 脉络膜切除术

choroideremia [ˌkɔːrɔidəˈriːmiə] *n* 无脉络膜

choroiditis [ˌkɔːrɔiˈdaitis] *n* 脉络膜炎 | acute diffuse serous ~ 急性弥漫性浆液性脉络膜炎 / areolar ~, areolar central ~ 晕轮状脉络膜炎，晕轮状中心性脉络膜炎(由黄斑区或其附近开始至外周) / central ~ 中心性脉络膜炎(黄斑区) / diffuse ~ 弥漫性脉络膜炎 / disseminated ~ 播散性脉络膜炎 / exudative ~ 渗出性脉络膜炎 / focal ~ 局灶性脉络膜炎(一种局限性脉络膜炎) / ~ guttata senilis 老年性点状脉络膜炎 / senile macular exudative ~ 老年性黄斑渗出性脉络膜炎 / ~ serosa 青光眼，绿内障 / suppurative ~ 化脓性脉络膜炎

choroidocyclitis [kəˌrɔidəusikˈlaitis] *n* 脉络膜睫状体炎

choroidoiritis [kəˌrɔidəuaiˈraitis] *n* 脉络膜虹膜炎

choroidopathy [ˌkɔːrɔiˈdɔpəθi] *n* 脉络膜病变

choroidoretinitis [kəˌrɔidəuˌretiˈnaitis] *n* 脉络膜视网膜炎

chorology [kɔːˈrɔlədʒi] *n* 分布学，生物分布学；生物地理学

choromania [ˌkɔːrəuˈmeinjə] *n* 舞蹈狂

chortosterol [kɔːˈtɔstərɔl] *n* 草甾醇，草固醇

chosen [ˈtʃəuzn] choose 的过去分词 *a* 挑选出来的，精选的

Chotzen's syndrome [ˈkɔtzən] (F. Chotzen) 科曾综合征(为常染色体显性遗传病，特征为尖头并指〈趾〉畸形，其中并指〈趾〉畸形为轻度的，器官距离过远，睑下垂，有时智力迟钝。亦称尖头并指〈趾〉畸形Ⅲ型)

Chr Chromobacterium 色杆菌属

Christchurch chromosome [ˈkristtʃəːtʃ] 克里斯丘奇染色体(指短臂缺失的 G 组染色体，最早是在患有慢性淋巴细胞白血病病人中发现)

Christensen-Krabbe disease [ˈkristənsən ˈkrɑːbə] (Erna Christensen; Knud H. Krabbe) 克-克病(见 Alpers' disease)

Christian's disease (syndrome) [ˈkristjən] (Henry A. Christian) 克里斯琴病(综合征)(见 Hand-Schüller-Christian disease)

Christian-Weber diseaes [ˈkristjən ˈwebə] (H. A. Christian; Frederick P. Weber) 克-韦病，复发性发热性结节性非化脓性脂膜炎

Christison's formula [ˈkristisn] (Robert Christison) 克里斯提森公式(见 Trapp's formula)

Christmas disease [ˈkristməs] 克里斯马斯病，凝血因子Ⅸ缺乏，B 型血友病(Christmas 为第一个患者的名字) | ~ factor 克里斯马斯因子，抗血友病因子 B

Christ-Siemens-Touraine syndrome [krist ˈsiːmənz tuːˈrein] (J. Christ; Hermann Werner Siemens; Henri Touraine) 克-西-图综合征，无汗性外胚层发育不良

chromaffin [krəuˈmæfin] *a* 嗜铬的

chromaffinity [ˌkrəuməˈfinəti] *n* 嗜铬性

chromaffinoma [ˌkrəumæfiˈnəumə] *n* 嗜铬细胞瘤，副神经节瘤 | medullary ~ 嗜铬细胞瘤，副神经节瘤

chromaffinopathy [ˌkrəumæfiˈnɔpəθi] *n* 嗜铬器官病

chromaphil [ˈkrəuməfil] *a* 嗜铬的

chromargentaffin [ˌkrəumɑːˈdʒentəfin] *a* 嗜铬及嗜银的

chromate [ˈkrəumit] *n* 铬酸盐 [ˈkrəumeit] *vt* 铬酸盐处理

chromatelopsia [ˌkrəumætəˈlɔpsiə] *n* 色盲，色觉不全

Chromatiaceae [ˌkrəuməti'eisiiː] *n* 着色菌科

chromatic [krəuˈmætik] *a* 色的，可染色的；染色质的

chromatid [ˈkrəumətid] *n* 染色单体 | nonsister ~s 非姐妹染色单体 / sister ~s 姐妹染色单体

chromatin [ˈkrəumətin] *n* 染色质 | nucleolar-associated ~, nucleolus-associated ~ 核仁结合性染色质 / sex ~ 性染色质 | **~ic** [ˌkrəuməˈtinik] *a*

chromatin-negative [ˈkrəumətin ˈnegətiv] *a* 染色质阴性的(正常雄性个体的细胞核中缺乏性染色质)
chromatinolysis [ˌkrəuməti'nɔlisis] *n* 染色质溶解
chromatinorrhexis [ˌkrəumətinə'reksis] *n* 染色质碎裂
chromatin-positive ['krəumətin'pɔzətiv] *a* 染色质阳性的(正常雌性个体的细胞核中具有性染色质)
chromatism ['krəumətizəm] *n* 异常色素沉着
Chromatium [krə*u*'meitiəm] *n* 色素菌属
chromatize ['krəumətaiz] *vt* 加铬,铬处理
chromatoblast [krəu'mætəblæst] *n* 成色素细胞
chromatocinesis [ˌkrəumətə*u*sai'niːsis] *n* 染色质移动
chromatodysopia [ˌkrəumətə*u*dis'əupiə] *n* 色盲,色觉不全
chromatogenous [ˌkrəumə'tɔdʒinəs] *a* 产色的
chromatogram ['krəumətəgræm, krəu'mæt-] *n* 色谱图,层析谱
chromatograph ['krəumətəgrɑːf, -græf, krəu-'mæt-] *n* 色谱仪,层析仪 *vt* 色谱法分析,层析分析
chromatography [ˌkrəumə'tɔgrəfi] *n* 色谱法,层析 | adsorption ~ 吸附色谱法,吸附层析 / gas ~ (GC) 气相色谱法 / gas-liquid ~ (GLC) 气液色谱法 / gas-solid ~ (GSC) 气固色谱法 / gel-filtration ~, gel permeation ~ 凝胶过滤色谱法,凝胶渗透色谱法 / high-performance liquid ~, high-pressure liquid ~ (HPLC) 高效液相色谱法,高压液相层析 / liquid-liquid ~ 液-液色谱法 / molecular exclusion ~ 分子排阻色谱法 / molecular sieve ~ 分子筛色谱法 / paper ~ 纸色谱法 / partition ~ 分配色谱法 / thin-layer ~ (TLC) 薄层色谱法 | **chromatographic** [ˌkrəumətə*u*'græfik] *a*
chromatoid ['krəumətɔid] *a* 浓染的 *n* 拟染色体
chromatokinesis [ˌkrəumətə*u*kai'niːsis] *n* 染色质移动
chromatology [ˌkrəumə'tɔlədʒi] *n* 色彩学
chromatolysis [ˌkrəumə'tɔlisis], **chromatolysm** [krə*u*'mætəlizəm] *n* (神经元)染质溶解,尼氏(Nissl)体溶解 | **chromatolytic** [ˌkrəum-ətə*u*'litik] *a*
chromatometer [ˌkrəumə'tɔmitə] *n* 色觉计
chromatopexis [ˌkrəumətə*u*'peksis] *n* 色素固定 | **chromatopectic** [ˌkrəumətə*u*'pektik] *a*
chromatophagus [ˌkrəumə'tɔfəgəs] *a* 破坏色素的,噬色素的
chromatophil ['krəumətəˌfil] *n* 嗜染细胞,易染细胞
chromatophile ['krəumətəˌfail] *n* 嗜染细胞,易染细胞 *a* 嗜染的,易染的
chromatophilia [ˌkrəumətəu'filiə] *n* 嗜染性,易染性
chromatophilic [ˌkrəumətə*u*'filik], **chromatophilous** [ˌkrəumə'tɔfiləs] *a* 嗜染的,易染的
chromatophore ['krəumətəˌfɔː] *n* 载色素细胞;载色体
chromatophorotropic [ˌkrəumətə*u*ˌfɔrə'trɔpik] *a* 向色素细胞的
chromatoplasm ['krəumətəplæzəm] *n* 色素质
chromatopseudopsis [ˌkrəumətə*psj*uː'dɔpsis] *n* 色幻视,色觉异常
chromatopsia [ˌkrəumə'tɔpsiə] *n* 色视症;部分色盲,色觉异常
chromatoptometer [ˌkrəumətɔp'tɔmitə] *n* 色觉计 | **chromatoptometry** *n* 色觉检查
chromatoscope ['krəumətəskəup, krəu'mæt-] *n* 彩光折射率计
chromatoscopy [ˌkrəumə'tɔskəpi] *n* 色觉检查法,尿色检查法 | gastric ~ 胃内容物颜色检查法(检胃液缺乏)
chromatoskiameter [ˌkrəumətə*u*skai'æmitə] *n* 色觉测量计
chromatosome [krəu'mætəsəum] *n* 染色小体
chromatotaxis [ˌkrəumətə*u*'tæksis] *n* 趋核染质性
chromatotropism [ˌkrəumə'tɔtrəpizəm] *n* 趋色性,亲色性
chromaturia [ˌkrəumə'tjuəriə] *n* 色素尿
chrome [krəum] *n* 铬
-chrome [后缀]色
1, 2-chromene ['krəumiːn] *n* 1, 2-色稀,1, 2-苯并吡喃
chromesthesia [ˌkrəumis'θiːzjə] *n* 色联觉,连带色觉,假色觉
chromhidrosis [ˌkrəumi'drəusis] *n* 色汗症
chromic ['krəumik] *a* 铬的 | ~ acid 铬酸
chromicize ['krəumisaiz] *vt* 加铬,铬处理
chromidien [krə'midien] *n* 【德】非生殖性核外染色粒
chromidiosis [ˌkrəumidi'əusis], **chromidiation** [ˌkrəumidi'eiʃən] *n* 核染质溢出
chromidium [krəu'midiəm] ([复] **chromidia** [krə*u*'midiə]) *n* 核外染色粒 | **chromidial** [krə*u*-'midiəl] *a*
chromidrosis [ˌkrəumi'drəusis] *n* 色汗症
chromiole ['krəumiəul] *n* 染色微粒
chromium (**Cr**) ['krəumjəm] *n* 铬(化学元素) | ~ trioxide 三氧化铬,铬酸(腐蚀收敛剂)
chrom(o)- [构词成分]色
Chromobacterium [ˌkrəumə*u*bæk'tiəriəm] *n* 色

杆菌属 | ~ violaceum 紫色色杆菌
chromoblast [ˈkrəuməblæst] *n* 成色素细胞
chromoblastomycosis [ˌkrəuməuˌblæstəumaiˈkəusis] *n* 着色芽生菌病
chromocenter [ˈkrəuməˌsentə] *n* 染色质核仁,核粒;染色中心
chromocholoscopy [ˌkrəuməukəˈlɔskəpi] *n* 排色[素]检胆[功能]法
chromoclastogenic [ˌkrəuməuˌklæstəuˈdʒenik] *a* 染色体诱裂的
chromocrinia [ˌkrəuməuˈkriniə] *n* 泌色作用
chromocystoscopy [ˌkrəuməusisˈtɔskəpi] *n* [尿]染色膀胱镜检查(亦称染色输尿管镜检查)
chromocyte [ˈkrəuməsait] *n* 色素细胞
chromodacryorrhea [ˌkrəuməuˌdækriəˈriːə] *n* 血泪症
chromodiagnosis [ˌkrəuməuˌdaiəgˈnəusis] *n* 色泽诊断[法];色素[排泄]诊断[法]
chromoflavine [ˌkrəuməuˈfleivin] *n* 吖啶黄
chromogen [ˈkrəumədʒən] *n* 色原
chromogene [ˈkrəumədʒiːn] *n* 染色体基因
chromogenesis [ˌkrəuməuˈdʒenisis] *n* 色素形成 | **chromogenic** [ˌkrəuməuˈdʒenik] *a* 产色的,产色素的
chromogranin [ˌkrəuməuˈgrænin] *n* 嗜铬粒蛋白
chromoisomerism [ˌkrəuməuaiˈsɔmərizəm] *n* 异色异构(现象)
chromolipoid [ˌkrəuməuˈlipɔid] *n* 脂色素
chromolysis [krəˈmɔlisis] *n* 染色质溶解
chromomere [ˈkrəuməmiə] *n* 染色粒;(血小板)颗粒区 | **chromomeric** [ˌkrəuməuˈmerik] *a* 染色粒的
chromometer [krəuˈmɔmitə] *n* 色觉计;比色计 | **chromometry** *n* 比色法;色觉检查
chromomycosis [ˌkrəuməumaiˈkəusis] *n* 着色芽生菌病,着色酿母菌病,着色真菌病
chromonar hydrochloride [ˈkrəumənɑː] 盐酸卡波罗孟(冠状动脉扩张药)
chromone [ˈkrəuməun] *n* 色酮
chromonema [ˌkrəuməuˈniːmə] ([复] **chromonemata** [ˌkrəuməuˈniːmətə]) *n* 染色线 | **~l** *a* / **chromoneme** [ˈkrəuməniːm] *n*
chromonucleic acid [ˌkrəuməunjuːˈkliːik] 染色质核酸,脱氧核糖核酸
chromoparic [ˌkrəuməuˈpærik] *a* 产色的
chromopathy [krəuˈmɔpəθi] *n* 皮肤着色症
chromopexy [ˈkrəuməˌpeksi] *n* 色素固定 | **chromopectic** [ˌkrəuməuˈpektik], **chromopexic** [ˌkrəuməuˈpeksik] *a*
chromophage [ˈkrəuməfeidʒ] *n* 噬色细胞
chromophane [ˈkrəuməfein] *n* 视色质
chromophil [ˈkrəuməfil] *n* 嗜染细胞,易染细胞
chromophile [ˈkrəuməfail] *n* 嗜染细胞,易染细胞 *a* 嗜染的,易染的
chromophilic [ˌkrəuməuˈfilik], **chromophilous** [krəuˈmɔfiləs] *a* 嗜染的,易染的
chromophobe [ˈkrəuməfəub] *n* 嫌色细胞,难染细胞 *a* 嫌色的,难染的
chromophobia [ˌkrəuməuˈfəubjə] *n* 嫌色性,难染性
chromophore [ˈkrəuməfɔː] *n* 发色团,生色团(亦称色基) | **chromophoric** [ˌkrəuməuˈfɔːrik], **chromophorous** [krəuˈmɔfərəs] *a* 发色团的,生色团的;发色的
chromophose [ˈkrəuməfəus] *n* 色幻视
chromophototherapy [ˌkrəuməuˌfəutəuˈθerapi] *n* 色光疗法,光谱疗法
chromoplasm [ˈkrəuməplæzəm] *n* 易染浆,染色浆(即染色质)
chromoplastid [ˌkrəuməuˈplæstid], **chromoplast** [ˈkrəuməplæst] *n* 有色粒,有色体
chromoprotein [ˌkrəuməuˈprəutiːn] *n* 色蛋白
chromopsia [krəuˈmɔpsiə] *n* 色视症;部分色盲
chromoptometer [ˌkrəumɔpˈtɔmitə] *n* 色觉计
chromoradiometer [ˌkrəuməuˌreidiˈɔmitə] *n* X线量感色计
chromoretinography [ˌkrəuməuˌretiˈnɔgrəfi] *n* 视网膜彩色摄影术
chromorhinorrhea [ˌkrəuməuˌrainəˈriːə] *n* 有色鼻液溢
chromosantonin [ˌkrəuməuˈsæntənin] *n* 黄色山道年,有色山道年
chromoscope [ˈkrəuməskəup] *n* 色觉检查器
chromoscopy [krəuˈmɔskəpi] *n* 色觉检查;染色检查(肾功能) | gastric ~ 染色胃液检查(检胃液缺乏症)
chromosome [ˈkrəuməsəum] *n* 染色体 | accessory ~s 副染色体,性染色体 / acentric ~ 无着丝粒染色体 / B ~ B 染色体(即超数染色体) / bivalent ~ 二价染色体 / daughter ~s 子染色体 / dicentric ~ 双着丝粒染色体 / gametic ~ 配子染色体 / giant ~s 巨染色体(多线染色体;刷形染色体) / homologous ~s 对应染色体,同源染色体,同等染色体 / lampbrush ~s 刷形染色体,灯刷染色体(低等动物卵母细胞的巨大染色体) / metacentric ~ 中央着丝粒染色体,等臂染色体 / mitochondrial ~, m- ~ 线粒体染色体 / nucleolar ~s 核仁染色体 / odd ~s 奇染色体,性染色体 / Ph^1 ~, Philadelphia ~ Ph^1 染色体,费城染色体(多数慢性白血病患者巨核细胞粒细胞和红细胞中发现有一个异常的最小近端染色体,其特点为长臂异常短小) / polytene ~s 多线染色体 / ring ~ 环形染色体 / sex ~s 性染色体

(与性别的决定有关的染色体) / somatic ~ 体细胞染色体 / submetacentric ~ 近中央着丝粒染色体 / supernumerary ~ 超数染色体 / telocentric ~ 具端着丝粒染色体 / W ~s, Z ~s W 染色体,Z 染色体(某些昆虫、鸟类、鱼类的性染色体,雌性为异型配子,即有一个 W 染色体和一个 Z 染色体,雄性则为同型配子,只有 Z 染色体) / X ~ X 染色体(雌性性染色体) / Y ~ Y 染色体(雄性性染色体) | **chromosomal** [ˌkrəuməu'səuməl] *a*

chromospermism [ˌkrəuməu'spəːmizəm] *n* 精子着色

chromotherapy [ˌkrəuməu'θerəpi] *n* 色光疗法,光谱疗法(亦称光束疗法)

chromotoxic [ˌkrəuməu'tɔksik] *a* 破坏血红蛋白的

chromotrichia [ˌkrəuməu'trikiə] *n* 毛[发]着色 | **~l** *a*

chromotropic [ˌkrəuməu'trɔpik] *a* 向色的,亲色的

chromoureteroscopy [ˌkrəuməujuəˌriːtə'rɔskəpi] *n* 染色输尿管镜检查

chromourinography [ˌkrəuməuˌjuəri'nɔgrəfi] *n* 染色检尿法

chronaximeter [ˌkrɔnæk'simitə] *n* 时值计 | **chronaximetry** [ˌkrɔnæk'simitri] *n* 时值测量[法] / **chronaximetric** [ˌkrɔnæksi'metrik] *a* 时值计的;时值测量法的

chronaxy ['krəunæksi], **chronaxia** [krə'næksiə], **chronaxie** ['krəunæksi] *n* 时值(电流必须在电压大于基强度一倍时以引起肌肉收缩的最短时间)

chronic ['krɔnik] *a* 慢性的 | **~ally** ['krɔnikəli] *ad* / **~ity** [krə'nisəti] *n* 慢性;长期性

chrono- [构词成分]时

chronobiology [ˌkrɔnəbai'ɔlədʒi] *n* 时间生物学 | **chronobiologic(al)** [ˌkrɔnəbaiə'lɔdʒik(əl)] *a* 时间生物学的,生物钟学的 / **chronobiologist** [ˌkrɔnəbai'ɔlədʒist] *n* 时间生物学家,生物钟学家

chronognosis [ˌkrɔnɔg'nəusis] *n* 时觉

chronograph ['krɔnəgrɑːf, -græf] *n* 微时计

chronometry [krə'nɔmitri] *n* 记时法 | mental ~ 精神记时法

chronomyometer [ˌkrɔnəumai'ɔmitə] *n* 时值计,时值测定器

chronon ['krəunɔn] *n* 定时因子,定时转录子(遗传信息持久性单位)

chronophobia [ˌkrɔnəu'fəubiə] *n* 时间恐怖(见于长期拘禁的囚犯)

chronophotograph [ˌkrɔnəu'fəutəgrɑːf, -græf] *n* 连续摄影[照]片

chronoscope ['krɔnəskəup] *n* 微时测定器,瞬时计

chronosphygmograph [ˌkrɔnəu'sfigməgrɑːf, -græf] *n* 记时脉搏描记器

chronotaraxis [ˌkrɔnəutə'ræksis] *n* 定时不能(丘脑或额叶损害后一时性症状)

chronotherapy ['krəunəuˌθerəpi] *n* 择时治疗[法]

chronotropic [ˌkrɔnəu'trɔpik] *a* 变时性的(如影响心脏收缩的速率)

chronotropism [krə'nɔtrəpizəm] *n* 变时现象(对周期性运动规律性如心搏的干扰)

chrotoplast ['krəutəplæst] *n* [表]皮细胞

chrysalis ['krisəlis] ([复] **chrysalides** [kri'sælidiːz] 或 **chrysalises** ['krisəlisiz]) *n* 【拉】蛹,蝶蛹

Chrysanthemum [kri'sænθəməm] *n* 菊属

chrysarobin [ˌkrisə'rəubin] *n* 柯桠素(局部用于治疗牛皮癣及其他慢性皮肤病)

chrysazin ['krisəzin] *n* 1, 8-二羟蒽醌,丹蒽醌(即 danthron, 导泻药)

chrysene ['kraisiːn] *n* 䓛(一种致癌四环烃)

chrysenic acid [krai'senik] 䓛酸,苯萘甲酸

chrysiasis [kri'saiəsis] *n* 金质沉着症,金沉着性皮病

chrys(o)- [构词成分] 金

chrysoderma [ˌkrisəu'dəːmə] *n* 金沉着性皮病(亦称金质沉着症)

chrysomonad [ˌkrisəu'məunæd] *n* 金滴虫

Chrysomonadida [ˌkrisəumə'nædidə] *n* 金滴虫目

Chrysomyia [ˌkrisəu'maijə] *n* 金蝇属 | ~ albiceps 白头金绳 / ~ bezziana 倍[赞]氏金蝇 / ~ macellaria 腐败金蝇,腐败锥蝇 / ~ megacephala 大头金蝇

chrysophanic acid, medicinal [ˌkraisəu'fænik] 药用大黄酚酸(chrysarobin 的不正确名)

chrysophoresis [ˌkrisəufə'riːsis] *n* 金渗散(金剂治疗后,由于巨噬细胞及多形核白细胞的作用,使金微粒渗散在身体各器官内)

Chrysops ['krisɔps] *n* 斑虻属 | ~ cecutiens 黑尾斑虻 | ~ dimidiata 分斑虻 / ~ discalis 中室斑虻 / ~ silacea 静斑虻

chrysosis [kri'səusis] *n* 金质沉着症

Chrysosporium [ˌkrisəu'spɔːriəm] *n* 金孢子菌属

chrysotherapy [ˌkrisəu'θerəpi] *n* 金疗法(现只用于治类风湿关节炎,使用的制剂为硫代苹果酸金钠)

chrysotile ['krisəutail] *n* 纤蛇纹石,温石棉(吸入其粉尘可致石棉肺,间皮瘤和其他肺癌型则少见)

Chrysozona [ˌkrisəu'zəunə] *n* 麻[翅]虻属

CHS cholinesterase 胆碱酯酶

chthonophagia [ˌθɔnəˈfeidʒiə], **chthonophagy** [θɔˈnɔfədʒi] *n* 食土癖
chunk [tʃʌŋk] *n* 组块,记忆单位(指在学习学说中的一种信息单位,在开始学习包括该单位在内的新材料之前,该信息单位已经储存在记忆之中)
Churg-Strauss syndrome (vasculitis) [tʃəːg straus] (Jacob Churg; Lotte Strauss) 丘—施综合征(血管炎),变应性肉芽肿性血管炎
churn [tʃəːn] *n* 搅乳器 *vt*, *vi* 搅拌
churus [ˈtʃʌrəs] *n* 大麻树脂
Chvostek's anemia [ˈvɔstek] (Franz Chvostek) 沃斯特克贫血(胰腺性贫血) | ~ sign 低钙击面征(轻叩腮腺区的面神经时可引起面肌痉挛,见于手足搐搦)
Chvostek-Weiss sign [ˈvɔstek vais] (Franz Chvostek; Nathan Weiss) 沃-魏征(见 Chvostek's sign)
chylangioma [ˌkailændʒiˈəumə] *n* 乳糜管瘤
chylaqueous [kaiˈleikwiəs] *a* 乳糜水样的
chyle [kail] *n* 乳糜 | **chylaceous** [kaiˈleiʃəs] *a*
chylectasia [ˌkailekˈteisiə] *n* 乳糜管扩张
chylemia [kaiˈliːmiə] *n* 乳糜血[症]
chylifaction [ˌkailiˈfækʃən], **chylification** [ˌkailifiˈkeiʃən] *n* 乳糜形成 | **chylifacient** [ˌkailiˈfeiʃənt], **chylifactive** [ˌkailiˈfæktiv] *a* 形成乳糜的
chyliferous [kaiˈlifərəs] *a* 形成乳糜的;输送乳糜的
chyliform [ˈkailifɔːm] *a* 乳糜样的
chylocele [ˈkailəsiːl] *n* 睾丸鞘膜乳糜囊肿,阴囊乳糜囊肿 | parasitic ~ 寄生虫性阴囊乳糜囊肿,阴囊象皮病
chylocyst [ˈkailəsist] *n* 乳糜池
chyloderma [ˌkailəuˈdəːmə] *n* 阴囊象皮病,丝虫性象皮病
chyloid [ˈkailɔid] *a* 乳糜样的
chylology [kaiˈlɔlədʒi] *n* 乳糜学
chylomediastinum [ˌkailəuˌmiːdiæsˈtainəm] *n* 纵隔乳糜症
chylomicrograph [ˌkailəuˈmaikrəgrɑːf, -græf] *n* 乳糜微粒图
chylomicron [ˌkailəuˈmaikrɔn] ([复] **chylonmicrons, chylomicra** [ˌkailəuˈmaikrə]) *n* 乳糜微粒(血尘)
chylomicronemia [ˌkailəuˌmaikrəuˈniːmiə] *n* 乳糜微粒血[症],高乳糜微粒血症
chylopericarditis [ˌkailəuˌperikɑːˈdaitis] *n* 乳糜性心包炎
chylopericardium [ˌkailəuˌperiˈkɑːdiəm] *n* 乳糜心包,乳糜性心包积液
chyloperitoneum [ˌkailəuˌperitəuˈniːəm] *n* 乳糜性水腹
chylophoric [ˌkailəuˈfɔrik] *a* 带乳糜的
chylopneumothorax [ˌkailəuˌnjuːməuˈθɔːræks] *n* 乳糜气胸
chylopoiesis [ˌkailəupɔiˈiːsis] *n* 乳糜形成,乳糜生成 | **chylopoietic** [ˌkailəupɔiˈetik] *a*
chylorrhea [ˌkailəˈriːə] *n* 乳糜溢
chylosis [kaiˈləusis] *n* 乳糜化[作用]
chylothorax [ˌkailəuˈθɔːræks], **chylopleura** [ˌkailəuˈpluərə] *n* 乳糜胸
chylous [ˈkailəs] *a* 乳糜的
chyluria [kaiˈljuəriə] *n* 乳糜尿
chylus [ˈkailəs] *n* 【拉】乳糜
chymase [ˈkaimeis] *n* 类糜蛋白酶,胃促胰酶
chyme [kaim] *n* 食糜
chymification [ˌkaimifiˈkeiʃən] *n* 食糜生成
chymodenin [ˌkaiməuˈdenin] *n* 促凝乳蛋白酶原释放素,糜蛋白酶素
chymopapain [ˌkaiməupəˈpeiin] *n* 木瓜凝乳蛋白酶
chymorrhea [ˌkaiməˈriːə] *n* 食糜溢
chymosin [kaiˈməusin] *n* 凝乳酶
chymosinogen [ˌkaiməˈsinədʒən] *n* 凝乳酶原
chymotrypsin [ˌkaiməˈtripsin] *n* 胰凝乳蛋白酶,糜蛋白酶
chymotrypsinogen [ˌkaimətripˈsinədʒən] *n* 胰凝乳蛋白酶原,糜蛋白酶原
chymous [ˈkaiməs] *a* 食糜的
chymus [ˈkaiməs] *n* 食糜
Chytridiales [kaiˌtridiˈeiliːz] *n* 壶菌目
Chytridiomycetes [kaiˌtridiəumaiˈsiːtiːz] *n* 壶菌亚纲
Chytridium [kaiˈtridiəm] *n* 壶菌属
CI color index 血色指数; Colour Index 染料索引
Ci 居里(curie)的符号(旧放射性强度单位,现用 Bq〈贝克勒尔〉, 1Ci = 37GBq〈3.7×10^{10} Bq〉)
Ciaccio's glands [ˈtʃɑːtʃəu] (Giuseppe V. Ciaccio) 副泪腺
Ciaccio's method [ˈtʃɑːtʃəu] (Carmelo Ciaccio) 恰乔法(细胞内脂质固定染色法,即处理组织使能见到细胞内的脂质,用酸性酪酸盐溶液固定,再以苏丹Ⅲ染色) | ~ stain 恰乔染剂(显示脂质的染剂)
cib. cibus 【拉】食物,餐
cibarian [siˈbɛəriən] *a* 食物的
cibisotome [siˈbisətəum] *n* 截囊刀
cicatrectomy [ˌsikəˈtrektəmi] *n* 瘢痕切除术
cicatricotomy [ˌsikətraiˈkɔtəmi] *n* 瘢痕切开术
cicatrix [siˈkeitriks, ˈsikətriks] ([复] cicatrices [siˈkeitrisiːz, ˌsikəˈtraisiːz]) *n* 【拉】瘢痕 | filtering ~ 过滤性瘢痕,漏液瘢痕 / manometric ~ 压动性瘢痕(鼓膜) / vicious ~ 不良瘢痕,恶性

瘢痕 | **cicatricial** [ˌsikəˈtriʃəl] *a*
cicatrizant [siˈkætrizənt] *n* 结瘢剂
cicatrize [ˈsikətraiz] *vt*, *vi* 结瘢 | **cicatrization** [ˌsikətriˈzeiʃən, -triˈz-] *n* 瘢痕形成
Cicer [ˈsaisə] *n* 豆科植物属
ciclafrine hydrochloride [ˈsikləfriːn] 盐酸环拉福林(升压药)
ciclopirox olamine [ˌsaikləuˈpiərɔks] 环吡酮胺(抗真菌药)
cicloprofen [ˌsaikləuˈprəufən] *n* 环洛芬(抗炎药)
Cicuta [ˈsikjutə] *n* 毒芹属 | ~ maculata 毒[水]芹 / ~ virosa 毒芹
cicutoxin [ˌsikjuˈtɔksin] *n* 毒芹素
-cide [后缀]杀者,杀灭剂,杀
cidofovir [siˈdɔfəvir] *n* 西多福韦(一种抗病毒核苷类似物,用以治疗获得性免疫缺陷综合征患者巨细胞病毒性视网膜炎,静脉输注给药)
CIE counterimmunoelectrophoresis 对流免疫电泳[法]
CIF clonal inhibitory factor 克隆抑制因子
ciguatera [ˌsiːgwəˈterə] *n*【西】鱼肉毒
ciguatoxin [ˌsiːgwəˈtɔksin] *n* 鱼肉毒素
CIH Certificate in Industrial Health 工业卫生证书
Ci-hr curie-hour 居里小时(旧放射性强度单位)
cilastatin sodium [ˌsailəˈstætin] 西司他丁钠(一种肾性二肽酶抑制药,阻断亚胺培南〈imipenem〉代谢,与亚胺培南结合使用,以增加亚胺培南的尿水平)
cilia [ˈsiliə] cilium 的复数
ciliaris [ˌsiliˈeiris] *n* 睫状肌
ciliariscope [ˌsiliˈæriskəup] *n* 睫区镜
ciliarotomy [ˌsiliəˈrɔtəmi] *n* 睫状体切开术(治青光眼)
ciliary [ˈsiliəri] *a* 睫的,睫状的
Ciliata [ˌsiliˈeitə] *n* 纤毛纲
ciliate [ˈsiliit] *a* 纤毛的 *n* 纤毛虫 | **~d** [ˈsilieitid] *a* 有纤毛的
ciliectomy [ˌsiliˈektəmi] *n* 睑缘切除术;睫状体切除术
cili(o)- [构词成分]睫毛,纤毛;睫状结构
ciliogenesis [ˌsiliəˈdʒenisis] *n* 纤毛形成,纤毛发生
Ciliophora [ˌsiliˈɔfərə] *n* 纤毛门
ciliophoran [ˌsiliˈɔfərən] *n* 纤毛虫 *a* 纤毛虫的
cilioretinal [ˌsiliəuˈretinəl] *a* 睫状体视网膜的
cilioscleral [ˌsiliəuˈskliərəl] *a* 睫状体巩膜的
ciliospinal [ˌsiliəuˈspainl] *a* 睫状体脊髓的
cilostazol [siˈləustəzɔl] *n* 西洛他唑(抗凝药)
ciliotomy [ˌsiliˈɔtəmi] *n* 睫状神经切断术
cilium [ˈsiliəm]([复] cilia [ˈsiliə]) *n* 睫;[复]睫毛;纤毛 | olfactory cilia 嗅毛
Cillobacterium [ˌsiləubækˈtiəriəm] *n* 运动杆菌属
cillosis [siˈləusis], **cillo** [ˈsiləu] *n* 痉挛性睑抽动
cimbia [ˈsimbiə] *n*【拉】大脑脚横束
cimetidine [saiˈmetidiːn] *n* 西咪替丁(组胺 H_2 受体拮抗药,治疗消化性溃疡尤为有效)
Cimex [ˈsaimeks] *n*【拉】臭虫属 | ~ boueti 卜[埃特]氏臭虫 / ~ hemipterus, ~ rotundatus 热带臭虫 / ~ lectularius 温带臭虫 / ~ pilosellus 蝠臭虫 / ~ pipistrella 小蝠臭虫
cimex [ˈsaimeks]([复] **cimices** [ˈsimisiːz]) *n*【拉】臭虫
cimicid [ˈsaimisid] *a* 臭虫的
Cimicidae [saiˈmisidiː] *n* 臭虫科
Cimicifuga [ˌsimiˈsifjugə] *n* 升麻属
cimicosis [ˌsimiˈkəusis] *n* 臭虫痒症
CIN cervical intraepithelial neoplasia 宫颈上皮内瘤病
cinanserin hydrochloride [siˈnænsərin] 盐酸辛那色林(5-羟色胺拮抗药)
cinching [ˈsintʃiŋ] *n* 眼肌折叠术
cinchocaine [ˈsinkəuˌkein] 辛可卡因(局部麻醉药)
cinchomeronic acid [ˌsiŋkəməˈrɔnik] 3, 4-吡啶二羧酸
Cinchona [siŋˈkəunə] *n* 金鸡纳树属
cinchona [siŋˈkəunə] *n* 金鸡纳[树]皮
cinchonic acid [siŋˈkɔnik] 喹啉甲酸,金鸡纳酸
cinchonidine [siŋˈkɔnidiːn] *n* 辛可尼丁(抗疟药)
cinchonine [ˈsiŋkəniːn] *n* 辛可宁(抗疟药)
cinchoninic acid [ˌsiŋkəˈninik] 辛可宁酸
cinchonism [ˈsiŋkənizəm] *n* 金鸡纳反应
cinchophen [ˈsiŋkəfen] *n* 辛可芬(消炎镇痛药)
cinclisis [ˈsiŋklisis] *n* 急速眨眼;呼吸促迫
cincture [ˈsiŋktʃə] *n* 围绕;束带,腰带 *vt* 用带子绕
cine- [构词成分]运动,活动
cineangiocardiography [ˌsiniˌændʒiəuˌkɑːdiˈɔgrəfi] *n* 电影心血管造影[术]
cineangiogram [ˌsiniˈændʒiəgræm] *n* 电影血管造影[照]片
cineangiograph [ˌsiniˈændʒiəgrɑːf] *n* 血管造影用电影摄影机
cineangiography [ˌsiniˌændʒiˈɔgrəfi] *n* 电影血管造影[术] | radionuclide ~ 放射核素电影血管造影[术]
cinedensigraphy [ˌsinidenˈsigrəfi] *n* 运动密度测定法,内部结构活动摄影[术]
cinefluorography [ˌsiniˌfluəˈrɔgrəfi] *n* 电影荧光摄影[术],X 线活动间接摄影[术]
cinemascopia [ˌsiniməsˈkəupiə], **cinemascopy** [ˌsiniˈmæskəpi] *n* 人体运动电影摄影[术]
cinematics [ˌsiniˈmætiks] *n* 运动学

cinematization [ˌsinimætiˈzeiʃən, -tiˈz-] *n* 运动成形切断术
cinematography [ˌsiniməˈtɔgrəfi] *n* 电影摄影[术]
cinematoradiography [ˌsinimətəˌreidiˈɔgrəfi] *n* 电影 X 线摄影[术]
cinemicrography [ˌsinimaiˈkrɔgrəfi] *n* 显微镜电影摄影[术] | time-lapse ~ 定时显微镜电影摄影[术](定时慢转速拍摄显微镜下微小物体的活动情况,再以普通转速放映)
cineol [ˈsiniɔl] *n* 桉油醇,桉树脑(祛痰、局部麻醉、驱虫药)
cinepazet maleate [ˌsiniˈpæzit] 马来酸桂哌酯(冠状动脉扩张药)
cinephlebography [ˌsinifliˈbɔgrəfi] *n* 电影静脉造影[术]
cineplastics [ˌsiniˈplæstiks] *n* 运动成形切断术
cineplasty [ˈsiniˌplæsti] *n* 运动成形切断术
cineradiofluorography [ˌsinəˌreidiəuˌfluəˈrɔgrəfi] *n* 电影 X 线摄影[术]
cineradiography [ˌsiniˌreidiˈɔgrəfi] *n* 电影 X 线摄影[术]
cinerary [ˈsinərəri] *a* 灰的;骨灰的
cineration [ˌsinəˈreiʃən] *n* 灰化;煅灰法
cinerator [ˈsinireitə] *n* (尸体或垃圾的)焚化炉
cinerea [siˈniəriə] *n* 灰质(神经系统) | **~l** [siˈniəriəl] *a*
cinereous [siˈniəriəs], **cineritious** [ˌsinəˈriʃəs] *a* 灰色的,似灰的,烬灰色的
cineroentgenofluorography [ˌsiniˌrɔntgənəuˌfluəˈrɔgrəfi] *n* 电影 X 线荧光摄影[术]
cineroentgenography [ˌsiniˌrɔntgəˈnɔgrəfi] *n* 电影 X 线摄影[术]
cinesalgia [ˌsiniˈsældʒiə] *n* 动作性[肌]痛,肌动痛
cinesi- 以 cinesi-起始的词,同样见以 kinesi-起始的词
cinet(o)- 以 cinet(o)-起始的词,同样见以 kinet(o)-起始的词
cineurography [ˌsinijuəˈrɔgrəfi] *n* 电影尿路造影[术]
cingestol [sinˈdʒestəul] *n* 烯孕醇(孕激素类药)
cingulate [ˈsiŋgjuleit] *a* 扣带的
cingule [ˈsiŋgjuːl] *n* 带;扣带
cingulectomy [ˌsiŋgjuˈlektəmi] *n* 扣带回切除术
cingulotomy [ˌsiŋgjuˈlɔtəmi] *n* 扣带回切开术
cingulum [ˈsiŋgjuləm] ([复] **cingula** [ˈsiŋgjulə]) *n*【拉】带;扣带;舌面隆凸;基嵴
cingulumotomy [ˌsiŋgjuləˈmɔtəmi] *n* 扣带回切开术
C 1 INH C 1 inhibitor C 1 抑制因子
cinnabar [ˈsinəbɑː] *n* 朱砂,一硫化汞
cinnamaldehyde [sinəˈmældihaid] *n* 桂皮醛,肉桂醛
cinnamene [ˈsinəmiːn], **cinnamol** [ˈsinəmɔl] *n* 桂皮烯,苯乙烯
cinnamic [siˈnæmik] *a* 桂皮的,肉桂的 | ~ acid 肉桂酸,桂皮酸
Cinnamomum [ˌsinəˈməuməm] *n* 樟属
cinnamon [ˈsinəmən] *n* 桂皮,肉桂
cinnarizine [siˈnɑːriziːn] *n* 桂利嗪(抗组胺药)
cinnopentazone [ˌsinəuˈpentəzəun] *n* 辛喷他宗(抗炎药)
cinology [siˈnɔlədʒi] *n* 运动学
cinometer [siˈnɔmitə] *n* 运动测量器;皮肤感觉计
cinoplasm [ˈsinəplæzəm] *n* 动质,动浆
cinoxacin [siˈnɔksəsin] *n* 西诺沙星(抗菌药)
cinoxate [siˈnɔkseit] *n* 西诺沙酯(防晒药)
cinromide [ˈsinrəmaid] *n* 桂溴胺(抗惊厥药)
cintazone [ˈsintəzəun] *n* 辛喷他宗(抗炎药)
cionectomy [ˌsaiəˈnektəmi] *n* 悬雍垂切除术
Cionella [ˌsaiəˈnelə] *n* 槲果螺属
Cionellidae [ˌsaiəˈnelidiː] *n* 槲果螺科
cionitis [ˌsaiəˈnaitis] *n* 悬雍垂炎
cionoptosis [ˌsaiənɔpˈtəusis] *n* 悬雍垂过长
cionorrhaphy [ˌsaiəˈnɔrəfi] *n* 悬雍垂缝合术
cionotome [saiˈɔnətəum] *n* 悬雍垂刀
cionotomy [ˌsaiəˈnɔtəmi] *n* 悬雍垂部分切除术
ciprocinonide [ˌsiprəuˈsainənaid] *n* 环丙奈德(肾上腺皮质激素类药)
ciprofibrate [ˌsaiprəuˈfaibreit] *n* 环丙贝特(降血脂药)
ciprofloxacin [ˌsiprəuˈflɔksəsin] *n* 环丙沙星(抗菌药) | ~ hydrochloride 盐酸环丙沙星(抗菌药)
circa [ˈsəːkə] *prep* 大约
circadian [səːˈkeidjən] *a* 昼夜节律的,(24 小时)生理节奏的
circannual [səːˈkænjuəl] *a* 年节律的,以一年为周期的
circellus [səˈseləs] *n* 小环
circinate [ˈsəːsineit] *a* 环状的
circle [ˈsəːkl] *n* 环,圈 | ~ of confusion 模糊圈(显示透镜理论上某一点影像的圆盘) / defensive ~ 防御环(相互对抗或抑制的两种病理情况的共存,如痛风和结核病) / diffusion ~ 弥散圈(视网膜上的朦胧圈) / ~ of dispersion, ~ of dissipation 分散圈(视网膜) / greater ~ of iris 虹膜大环 / lesser ~ of iris 虹膜小环 / sensory ~ 感觉点环 / vicious ~ 恶性循环
circlet [ˈsəːklit] *n* 小圈,小环
circling [ˈsəːkliŋ] *n* 环状运动(如患李斯特菌病〈listeriosis〉的动物所表现的)
circuit [ˈsəːkit] *n* 回路;电路 | gate ~ 门电路 / neural ~ 神经回路 / open ~ 断路,切断电路 / reflex ~ 反射路 / short ~ 捷径,短路

circular [ˈsəːkjulə] *a* 圆形的,环状的;循环的
circulate [ˈsəːkjuleit] *vi* 循环;传播,流传 *vt* 使循环;传播 | **circulative** [ˈsəːkjuleitiv], **circulatory** [ˈsəːkjulətəri] *a* 循环的;促进循环的 / **circulator** [ˈsəːkjuleitə] *n* 传播者;循环器
circulation [ˌsəːkjuˈleiʃən] *n* 循环 | allantoic ~, umbilical ~ 尿囊循环,脐循环 / collateral ~, compensatory ~ 侧支循环 / cross ~ 交叉循环 / derivative ~ 动静脉吻合(动静脉血不经过毛细管而进入静脉) / enterohepatic ~ 肝肠循环/ hypophyseoportal ~ 垂体门脉循环 / portal ~ 门脉循环 / primitive ~, first ~ 原始循环 / pulmonary ~, lesser ~ 肺循环,小循环 / sinusoidal ~ 血窦循环 / systemic ~, greater ~ 体循环 / thebesian ~ 心最小静脉循环 / vitelline ~, omphalomesenteric ~ 卵黄区循环
circulus [ˈsəːkjuləs] ([复] circulli [ˈsəːkjuːlai]) *n* 【拉】环
circum- [前缀] 周[围],环
circumambient [ˌsəːkəmˈæmbiənt] *a* 围绕的,周围的 | **circumambience** [ˌsəːkəmˈæmbiəns], **circumambiency** [ˌsəːkəmˈæmbiənsi] *n*
circumanal [səːkəmˈeinl] *a* 肛门周[围]的
circumarticular [ˌsəːkəmɑːˈtikjulə] *a* 关节周[围]的
circumaxillary [ˌsəːkəmækˈsiləri, -ˈmæksi-] *a* 腋周[围]的
circumbulbar [ˌsəːkəmˈbʌlbə] *a* 眼球周[围]的
circumcallosal [ˌsəːkəmkəˈləusəl] *a* 胼胝体周[围]的
circumcise [ˈsəːkəmsaiz] *vt* (施行包皮)环切[术]
circumcision [ˌsəːkəmˈsiʒən] *n* 包皮环切[术] | female ~ 阴蒂切开术 / pharaonic ~ 锁阴术
circumclusion [ˌsəːkəmˈkluːʒən] *n* 环压止血法
circumcorneal [ˌseːkəmˈkɔːniəl] *a* 角膜周[围]的
circumcrescent [ˌsəːkəmˈkresnt] *a* 环形生长的
circumduction [ˌsəːkəmˈdʌkʃən] *n* 环行[运动](指肢或眼的主动或被动环行运动)
circumference [səˈkʌmfərəns] *n* 圆周,周围;周缘,环状面 | articular ~ 环状关节面 | **circumferential** [səˌkʌmfəˈrenʃəl] *a*
circumferentia [səˌkʌmfəˈrenʃiə] *n* 【拉】周缘,环状面
circumflex [ˈsəːkəmfleks] *a* 弯曲的,卷曲的,旋绕的
circumflexus [ˌsəːkəmˈfleksəs] *a*【拉】弯曲的,卷曲的,旋绕的
circumgemmal [ˌsəːkəmˈdʒeməl] *a* 芽周的
circuminsular [ˌsəːkəmˈinsjulə] *a* 脑岛周[围]的
circumintestinal [ˌsəːkəminˈtestinl] *a* 肠周[围]的
circumlental [ˌsəːkəmˈlentl] *a* 晶状体周[围]的
circumnuclear [ˌsəːkəmˈnjuːkliə] *a* 核周[围]的
circumocular [ˌsəːkəmˈɔkjulə] *a* 眼周的
circumoral [ˌsəːkəmˈɔːrəl] *a* 口周的
circumorbital [ˌsəːkəmˈɔːbitl] *a* [眼]眶周的
circumpolarization [ˌsəːkəmˌpəuləraiˈzeiʃən, -ri-ˈz-] *n* 圆偏振[光]
circumrenal [ˌsəːkəmˈriːnl] *a* 肾周[围]的
circumscribe [ˈsəːkəmskraib] *vt* 限制;使外接,使外切 | **~d** *a* 局限的
circumscription [ˌsəːkəmˈskripʃən] *n* 界限,限制;区域,范围;外接
circumscriptus [ˌsəːkəmˈskriptəs] *a*【拉】局限的
circumstantiality [ˌsəːkəmˌstænʃiˈæləti] *n* 病理性赘述(一种精神症状)
circumtractor [ˈsəːkəmˌtræktə] *n* 环形拉钩,环形牵引器
circumvallate [ˌsəːkəmˈvæleit] *vt* 围绕 *a* 轮廓状的
circumvascular [ˌsəːkəmˈvæskjulə] *a* 血管周[围]的
circumventricular [ˌsəːkəmvenˈtrikjulə] *a* 脑室周[围]的
circumvolute [ˌsəːkəmˈvəuljuːt] *a* 搓合的,缠绕的
circumvolutio [ˌsəːkəmvəˈljuːʃiəu] *n* 包绕;回,脑回
cirolemycin [ˌsirəuliˈmaisin] *n* 西罗霉素(抗肿瘤和抗菌物质)
cirrhogenous [siˈrɔdʒinəs] *a* 致硬变的
cirrhonosus [siˈrɔnəsəs] *n* 胸腹膜黄变病(胎儿)
cirrhosis [siˈrəusis] *n* 硬变,肝硬化 | alcoholic ~ 酒精性肝硬化 / biliary ~ 胆汁性肝硬化 / ~ of liver 肝硬化(亦称慢性间质性肝炎) / ~ of lung, pulmonary ~ 肺硬变,间质性肺炎 / pipe stem ~ 门脉周性肝硬化 / postnecrotic ~, multilobar ~, periportal ~, toxic ~ 坏死后肝硬化,多小叶性肝硬化,门脉周肝硬化,中毒性肝硬化 / primary biliary ~, hypertrophic ~, unilobular ~, 原发性胆汁性肝硬化,肥大性肝硬化,单小叶性肝硬化 / ~ of stomach 胃硬变,皮革状胃,硬变性胃炎 | **cirrhotic** [siˈrɔtik] *a*
cirrus [ˈsirəs] ([复] **cirri** [ˈsirai]) *n* 交接刺(蠕虫);孢子角
cirsectomy [səˈsektəmi] *n* 曲张静脉切除术
cirsenchysis [səˈsenkisis] *n* 曲张静脉注射[疗]法
cirs(o)- [构词成分] 静脉曲张,曲张静脉
cirsocele [ˈsəːsəsiːl] *n* 精索静脉曲张
cirsodesis [səˈsɔdisis] *n* 曲张静脉结扎术
cirsoid [ˈsəːsɔid] *a* 曲张样的
cirsomphalos [səˈsɔmfəlɔs] *n* 脐周静脉曲张

cirsophthalmia [ˌsəːsɔfˈθælmiə] *n* 结膜静脉曲张
cirsotome [ˈsəːsətəum] *n* 曲张静脉刀
cirsotomy [səˈsɔtəmi] *n* 曲张静脉切开术
cis [sis] [前缀] 在一边,在同侧,在近侧;顺式(在有机化学中,指某些原子或基在分子的同侧;在遗传学中,指拟等位基因的两个突变基因在同一的染色体上)
cis- [前缀] 在一边,在同侧,在近侧
cisapride [ˈsisəpraid] *n* 西沙必利(肠肌丛乙酰胆碱释放药,用以促进胃排空,治疗胃食管反流疾病和胃麻痹,口服给药)
cisatracurium besylate [ˌsisætrəˈkjuəriəm] 苯磺西沙库铵(非极化神经肌肉阻断药,静脉给药,作为全身麻醉的佐药,以利气管内插管,手术时诱发骨骼肌松弛和促使机械通气)
cisclomiphene [sisˈkləumifiːn] *n* 恩氯米芬(即 enclomiphene,抗不育症药)
cismatan [ˈsismətən] *n* 埃及决明子
cisplatin [ˈsisplətin] *n* 顺铂(抗肿瘤药)
cis-platinum [sis ˈplætinəm] *n* 顺铂(即 cisplatin,抗肿瘤药)
11-*cis* retinal [sisˈretinəl] 11-顺视黄醛
cissa [ˈsisə] *n* 异食癖
Cissampelos [siˈsæmpilɔs] *n* 锡生藤属(防己科)
cistern [ˈsistən] *n* 池 | cerebellomedullary ~, great ~, posterior ~ 小脑延髓池 / ~ of fossa of Sylvius, ~ of lateral fossa of cerebrum, ~ of Sylvius 大脑外侧窝池 / interpenduncular ~, basal ~ [脑]脚间池 | **~al** [sisˈtəːnl] *a* 池的(尤指小脑延髓池)
cisterna [sisˈtəːnə] ([复] **cisternae** [sisˈtəːniː]) *n*【拉】池
cisternography [ˌsistəːˈnɔgrəfi] *n* 脑池造影[术] | **cisternographic** [ˌsistəːnəuˈgræfik] *a*
cistron [ˈsistrɔn] *n* 顺反子(遗传物质的最小单位,它决定一个多肽链的氨基酸顺序,通过顺反测验所测定,现在常用作基因的同义词)
citalopram hydrobromide [saiˈtæləpræm] 氢溴酸西酞普兰(抗抑郁药)
Citelli's syndrome [tʃiˈteli] (Salvatore Citelli) 契太利综合征(精神减退、注意力不易集中、瞌睡或失眠,见于腺样体炎或鼻窦炎患者)
Citellus [saiˈteləs] *n* 黄鼠属
citraconic acid [ˌsitrəˈkɔnik] 柠康酸,顺甲基丁烯二酸
citral [ˈsitrəl] *n* 枸橼醛,橙花醛
citrate [ˈsitreit] *n* 枸橼酸,柠檬酸;枸橼酸盐,柠檬酸盐 | cupric ~ 枸橼酸铜(防腐剂,收敛药) / ferric ~ 枸橼酸铁(用作试剂) / ~ phosphate dextrose (CPD) 枸橼酸盐磷酸盐葡萄糖(亦称抗凝血枸橼酸盐磷酸盐葡萄糖溶液,抗凝药) / ~ phosphate dextrose adenine (CPDA-1) 枸橼酸盐磷酸盐葡萄糖腺嘌呤(抗凝溶液)
citrate condensing enzyme [ˈsitreit kənˈdensiŋ ˈenzaim] 枸橼酸缩合酶,ATP 枸橼酸裂酶
citrated [ˈsitreitid] *a* 含枸橼酸盐的
citrate (*si*)-synthase [ˈsitreit ˈsinθeis] 枸橼酸合酶
citreoviridin [ˌsitriəˈviridin] *n* 黄绿青霉素
citric acid [ˈsitrik] 枸橼酸,柠檬酸
citrinin [ˈsitrinin] *n* 桔霉素
Citrobacter [ˌsitrəˈbæktə] *n* 枸橼酸杆菌属 | ~ freundii 弗[罗因德]氏枸橼酸杆菌 / ~ intermedius 中间型枸橼酸杆菌
Citromyces [ˌsitrəuˈmaisiːz] *n* 枸橼酸霉菌属
citron [ˈsitrən] *n* 枸橼 *a* 枸橼状的
citronella [ˌsitrəˈnelə] *n* 香茅,雄刈萱(用于香料和驱虫)
citrophosphate [ˌsitrəˈfɔsfeit] *n* 枸橼磷酸盐
citrulline [siˈtrʌliːn] *n* 瓜氨酸,氨基甲酰鸟氨酸
citrullinemia [siˌtrʌliˈniːmiə] *n* 瓜氨酸血症,精氨基琥珀酸合成酶缺乏症
citrullinuria [siˌtrʌliˈnjuəriə] *n* 瓜氨酸尿
Citrullus [siˈtrʌləs] *n* 西瓜属
Citrus [ˈsitrəs] *n*【拉】柑橘属
citta [ˈsitə], **cittosis** [siˈtəusis] *n* 异食癖
Civatte's poikiloderma [siˈvɑːt] (Achille Civatte) 西瓦特皮肤异色病(脸、颈、胸上部红棕色网状色素沉着,常对称发生,由于日晒或搽化妆品中的化学物品所致)
Civiale's operation [ˌsiviˈɑːl] (Jean Civiale) 西维亚勒手术(正中偏侧膀胱切开取石术)
Civinini's ligament [ˌtʃiːviˈniːni] (Filippo Civinini) 翼棘韧带 | ~ process (spine) 翼棘突
CK creatine kinase 肌酸激酶
Cl chlorine 氯
cl centiliter 厘升
cladiosis [ˌklædiˈəusis] *n* 屠宰工人帚霉病(亦称树胶肿样淋巴管炎)
cladistics [kləˈdistiks] *n* 分支系统学
Cladonia [kləˈdəuniə] *n* 石蕊属
Cladorchis watsoni [kleiˈdɔːkis wætˈsəunai] 瓦[生]氏瓦生吸虫(即 Watsonius watsoni)
Cladorchis watsoni [kləˈdɔːkis wɔtˈsəuni] 互[生]氏互生吸虫(即 Watsonius watsoni)
Clado's anastomosis [ˈklɑːdəu] (Spiro Clado) 克拉多吻合术(阑尾动脉和卵巢动脉之间的吻合术) | ~ band 卵巢悬韧带 / ~ ligament 阑尾卵巢韧带
cladosporiosis [ˌklædəuˌspɔːriˈəusis] *n* 分枝孢子菌病
Cladosporium [ˌklædəˈspɔːriəm] *n* 分枝孢子菌属
cladothricosis [ˌklædəuθriˈkəusis] *n* 分枝丝菌病
Cladothrix [ˈklædəθriks] *n* 分枝丝菌属

cladribine [ˈkleidribiːn] *n* 克拉屈滨(一种嘌呤抗代谢物,用作抗肿瘤药,治疗毛细胞白血病,静脉给药。亦称2-氯脱氧腺苷)

clairaudience [klɛərˈɔːdjəns] *n* 神听,超人的听力

clairsentience [klɛəˈsenʃiəns] *n* 神视,超人的视力

clairvoyance [klɛəˈvɔiəns] *n*【法】神视,超人的视力

clamoxyquin hydrochloride [kləˈmɔksikwin] 盐酸氯胺羟喹(抗阿米巴药)

clamp [klæmp] *n* 夹;夹具 | bulldog ~ 动脉夹 / cotton roll rubber dam ~ 棉卷橡皮障夹 / gingival ~ 龈夹 / pedicle ~ 蒂夹 / rubber dam ~ 橡皮障夹

clamping [ˈklæmpiŋ] *n* 血糖钳夹术(测胰岛素分泌和作用时,输注葡萄糖液的速率要经常调节到足以维持预先测定的血糖浓度)

clang [klæŋ] *n* 音质,音响

clanging [ˈklæŋiŋ] *n* 声音代词语(见于精神分裂症及躁狂症)

clap [klæp] *n* 淋病

clapotement [klæpɔːtˈmɔŋ], **clapotage** [klæpəˈtɑːʒ] *n*【法】振荡音

claquement [klækˈmɔŋ] *n*【法】掌拍(按摩)法;毕剥声(心瓣膜闭时的) | ~ d'ouverture 开瓣锐声

Clara cell [ˈklɑːrɑː] (Max Clara) 克拉拉细胞(细支气管细胞)

clarificant [klæˈrifikənt] *n* 澄清剂

clarithromycin [kləˌriθrəˈmaisin] *n* 克拉霉素(抗生素类药)

clarity [ˈklærəti] *n* 澄清度

Clark Ⅱ [klɑːk] *n* 二苯氰化胂(即 diphenylcyanoarsine,一种刺激性毒气)

Clark-Collip method [klɑːk ˈkɔlip] (Earl P. Clark; James B. Collip) 克拉克-科利晋法(检血清钙及检血中)

Clarke-Hadfield syndrome [klɑːk ˈhædfiːld] (Cecil Clarke; Geoffrey Hadfield) 克-哈综合征(幼稚型先天性胰腺病,患儿有肝大,大量脂粪,胰腺广泛萎缩,身材矮小和体重不足)

Clarke's cells [klɑːk] (Jacob A. L. Clarke) 克拉克细胞(脊髓胸核中的色素细胞) | ~ nucleus, ~ column of spinal cord, nucleus of ~ column 胸核

clasmatocyte [klæzˈmætəsait] *n* 破折细胞

clasmatocytosis [klæzˌmætəsaiˈtəusis] *n* 破折细胞增多

clasmatodendrosis [klæzˌmætədenˈdrəusis] *n* 星形细胞突破折

clasmatosis [ˌklæzməˈtəusis] *n* 细胞破碎

clasmocytoma [ˌklæzməusaiˈtəumə] *n* 网状细胞肉瘤

clasp [klɑːspˌklæsp] *n* 卡环(保持和固定托牙用,亦称直接固位体) | arrow ~, arrowhead ~ 箭头卡环 / bar ~ 杆形卡环 / circumferential ~ 环形卡环 / continuous ~, continuous lingual ~ 连续卡环,连续舌侧卡环

class [klɑːsˌklæs] *n* 纲(生物分类);级,组 *vt* 把…分类

classic [ˈklæsik] *a* 古典的;典型的

classical [ˈklæsikəl] *a* 经典的;典型的

classification [ˌklæsifiˈkeiʃən] *n* 分类[法] | adansonian ~ 数值分类法 / Chicago ~ 芝加哥分类法(人类染色体分类法,于1966年在芝加哥为遗传学家所采纳,以鉴定染色体带和区及染色体结构异常定位) / Denver ~ 丹佛分类法(人类染色体根据大小及着丝粒位置的分类法,于1960年在丹佛为遗传学家所采纳,23对染色体按长度减少的顺序排列为A到G7组) / New York Heart Association(NYHA) ~ 纽约心脏协会分类法(第一类病人活动不受限制,平常活动不出现症状;第二类病人活动稍加限制,休息或轻度劳力时无不适感;第三类病人活动明显限制,只有休息时才无不适感;第四类病人应完全休息,卧床或静坐,任何体力活动均会产生不适感) / numerical ~ 数值分类法 / Paris ~ 巴黎分类法(1971年在巴黎对芝加哥人类染色体分类法所作的修正,并提供更详细的遗传信息)

-clast [构词成分]破碎,破裂

clastic [ˈklæstik] *a* 分裂的

clastogen [ˈklæstədʒən] *n* 诱裂剂(致染色体畸变物质)

clastogenic [ˌklæstəuˈdʒenik] *a* 诱裂的(指对染色体) | **~ity** [ˌklæstəudʒeˈnisəti] *n* 诱裂性

clastothrix [ˈklæstəθriks] *n* 结节性脆发症

clathrate [ˈklæθreit] *n* 笼形[化合]物 *a* 格子状的;笼形[化合]物的

clathrin [ˈklæθrin] *n* 网格蛋白

Clathrochloris [ˌklæθrəˈklɔːris] *n* 绿硫菌属

Clauberg's culture medium [ˈklaubəːg] (Karl Wm. Clauberg) 克劳伯格培养基(含有牛、羊血清与甘油和亚碲酸钾凝结的培养基) | ~ test 克劳伯格试验,黄体激素试验(测定黄体制剂或黄体酮标准的生物鉴定法) / ~ unit 克劳伯格单位(一种孕激素单位)

Claude's hyperkinesis sign [klɔːd] (Henri Claude) 克洛德运动增强征(疼痛刺激时瘫痪肌肉的反射性动作) | ~ syndrome 克洛德综合征(一侧第三脑神经〈动眼神经〉麻痹,对侧协同不能,伴有构音障碍)

claudicant [ˈklɔːdikənt] *a* 跛行的 *n* (间歇性)跛行者

claudication [ˌklɔːdiˈkeiʃən] *n* 跛行 | intermittent ~ 间歇性跛行(如见于闭塞性血管性动脉炎) / venous ~ 静脉性跛行(静脉停滞所致) | **claudicatory** [ˈklɔːdikətəri] *a*
Claudius' cells [ˈklaudiəs] (Friedrich M. Claudius) 克劳狄乌斯细胞(螺旋柱弓两侧大而有核细胞)
claustrophilia [ˌklɔːstrəˈfiliə] *n* 幽居癖
claustrophobia [ˌklɔːstrəˈfəubjə] *n* 幽闭恐怖 | **claustrophobic** [ˌklɔːstrəˈfəubik] *a*
claustrum [ˈklɔːstrəm] ([复] **claustra** [ˈklɔːstrə]) *n*【拉】屏状核 | **claustral** [ˈklɔːstrəl] *a*
clausura [klɔːˈsjuərə] *n*【拉】闭锁[畸形],无孔,不通
clava [ˈkleivə] *n*【拉】棒状体,薄束核结节 | **~l** [ˈkleivəl] *a* 棒状体的 / **~te** [ˈkleiveit] *a* 棒状体的;棒状的
clavacin [ˈkleivəsin] *n* 棒曲霉素
clavelization [ˌklævəlaiˈzeiʃən, -liˈz-] *n* 羊痘接种
Claviceps [ˈklæviseps] *n* 麦角菌属
Clavicipitaceae [ˌklæviˌsipiˈteisiiː] *n* 麦角[菌]科
Clavicipitales [ˌklæviˌsipiˈteiliːz] *n* 麦角[菌]目
clavicle [ˈklævikl] *n* 锁骨 | **clavicular** [kləˈvikjulə] *a*
clavicotomy [ˌklæviˈkɔtəmi] *n* 锁骨切断术
clavicula [kləˈvikjulə] *n*【拉】锁骨
claviculus [kləˈvikjuləs] ([复] **claviculi** [kləˈvikjulai]) *n*【拉】钉合纤维
claviform [ˈklævifɔːm] *a* 棍棒状的
claviformin [ˌklæviˈfɔːmin] *n* 棒曲霉素
clavipectoral [ˌklæviˈpektərəl] *a* 锁骨胸部的
Clavispora [kləˈvispərə] *n* 酵母目真菌属
clavulanate potassium [ˈklævjuləneit] 克拉维酸钾(β-内酰胺酶抑制药)
clavus [ˈkleivəs] ([复] **clavi** [ˈkleivai]) *n*【拉】鸡眼 | ~ durus 硬鸡眼 / ~ hystericus 癔症性钉脑痛 / ~ mollis 软鸡眼 / ~ secalinus 麦角
claw [klɔː] *n* 爪;牙钳爪
clawfoot [ˈklɔːˈfut] *n* 爪形足
clawhand [ˈklɔːˈhænd] *n* 爪形手
clay [klei] *n* 土,黏土 | China ~ 白陶土,高岭土
clazolam [ˈkleizəlæm] *n* 克拉唑仑(弱安定药)
clazolimine [kleiˈzəulimiːn] *n* 氯苯唑胺(利尿药)
clazuril [ˈklæzjuril] *n* 克拉珠利(抗球虫药,用于鸟类)
cleaner [ˈkliːnə] *n* 洗洁器;除垢剂
cleanse [klenz] *vt* 使清洁;净化 | **~r** *n* 清洁剂
clear [kliə] *a* 清晰的,透明的,澄明的
clearance [ˈkliərəns] *n* 清除,清理;清除率;间隙 | *p*-aminohippurate ~ 对氨基马尿酸清除率 / blood-urea ~, urea ~ 血脲清除率,脲清除率 / creatinine ~ 肌酸酐清除率 / free water ~ 自由水清除率 / immune ~ 免疫清除,免疫排除 / interocclusal ~ 休止𬌗间隙 / inulin ~ 菊粉清除率 / occlusal ~ 𬌗间隙,咬合间隙 / osmolar ~ 渗透清除率 / plasma ~ 血浆清除率 / plasma iron ~ 血浆铁清除率
clearer [ˈkliərə] *n* 清洗剂
cleavage [ˈkliːvidʒ] *n* 裂,分裂;卵裂 | accessory ~ 副裂 / adequal ~ 近等裂 / determinate ~ 定裂 / discoidal ~ 盘[状卵]裂 / equatorial ~ 中纬[卵]裂 / holoblastic ~, complete ~, total ~ 全裂 / latitudinal ~ 纬线裂 / meridional ~ 经线裂 / meroblastic ~, incomplete ~, partial ~ 部分分裂,不全[卵]裂 / superficial ~ 表[面卵]裂
cleft [kleft] *n* 裂,裂口 | anal ~, clunial ~ 肛裂,臀裂 / branchial ~, visceral ~ 鳃裂 / facial ~ 面裂 / genital ~ 生殖裂 / hyobranchial ~ 舌鳃裂 / hyomandibular ~, hyoid ~ 舌颌裂 / intergluteal ~, natal ~ 臀沟 / transverse facial ~ 面横裂,巨口,颊横裂 / vulval ~ 外阴裂
clegs [klegz] *n* 虻类
cleidagra [klaiˈdægrə] *n* 锁骨痛风
cleidal [ˈklaidl] *a* 锁骨的
cleidarthritis [ˌklaidɑːˈθraitis] *n* 锁骨痛风
cleid(o)- [构词成分]锁骨
cleidocostal [ˌklaidəuˈkɔstl] *a* 锁骨肋骨的
cleidocranial [ˌklaidəuˈkreinjəl] *a* 锁骨头颅的
cleidoic [klaiˈdəuik] *a* 闭锁的
cleidomastoid [ˌklaidəuˈmæstɔid] *a* 锁骨乳突的
cleidorrhexis [ˌklaidəˈreksis] *n* 锁骨折术
cleidotomy [klaiˈdɔtəmi] *n* 锁骨切断术
cleidotripsy [ˈklaidəˌtripsi] *n* 锁骨压碎术
cleisagra [klaiˈsægrə] *n* 锁骨痛风
cleistothecium [ˌklaistəˈθiːsiəm] *n* 闭囊壳
clemastine [ˈklemæstiːn] *n* 氯马斯汀(抗组胺药) | ~ fumarate 延胡索酸氯马斯汀(抗组胺药,用于治疗变应性鼻炎和变应性皮肤病)
Clematis [ˈklemətis] *n* 铁线莲属
clemizole [ˈklemizəul] *n* 克立咪唑(抗组胺药) | ~ hydrochloride 盐酸克立咪唑(抗组胺药,用于治疗皮肤变态反应、食品和化妆品过敏以及血清病) / ~ penicillin 克咪西林(抗生素类药)
clenbuterol [klenˈbjuːtərɔl] *n* 克仑特罗(长效 β_2 受体激动药,用于治疗马支气管痉挛)
clenching [ˈklentʃiŋ] *n* 磨牙癖
cleoid [ˈkliːɔid] *n* 爪状挖匙(牙)
cleptomania [ˌkleptəuˈmeinjə] *n* 偷窃狂
cleptophobia [ˌkleptəuˈfəubiə] *n* 偷窃恐怖
Clérambault 见 de Clérambault
Clérambault-Kandinsky complex (syndrome) [ˌkleirəˈbəu kænˈdinski] (Gatian de Clérambault;

Viktor Kandinsky）克雷朗波-坎迪斯基复征（综合征）（一种精神状态，病人认为其精神受外界影响或受他人控制）
clerk [klɑːk, kləːk] *n* 见习医学生，见习生
clerkship [ˈklɑːkʃip, ˈkləːkʃip] *n* 见习医学生期；见习医学生制
Clethrionomys [ˌkleθriˈɔnəmis] *n* 岸鼯属
Clevelandellina [kləˌvelænˈdelinə] *n* 克利夫兰纤毛虫亚目
click [klik] *n* 喀喇音 | ejection ~s 喷射喀喇音 / systolic ~s 收缩期喀喇音
clicking [ˈklikiŋ] *n* 弹响；碎裂声
clidinium bromide [kliˈdiniəm] 克利溴铵（季铵类抗胆碱药，用作治疗消化性溃疡和其他胃肠道疾病的辅助疗法）
clid(o)- 以 clid(o)-起始的词，见 cleid(o)-起始的词
client [ˈklaiənt] *n*（私人医生的）病人，病家 | **~al** *a*
climacteric [klaiˈmæktərik, ˌklaimækˈterik] *n*, *a* 更年期（的）
climacterium [ˌklaimækˈtiəriəm] *n* 更年期 | ~ praecox 早发更年期，早期绝经
climactic [klaiˈmæktik] *a* 顶点的，极点的
climate [ˈklaimit] *n* 气候 | **climatic** [klaiˈmætik] *a*
climatology [ˌklaiməˈtɔlədʒi] *n* 气候学，风土学 | medical ~ 医用气候学
climatotherapy [ˌklaimətəuˈθerəpi], **climatotherapeutics** [ˌklaimətəuˌθerəˈpjuːtiks] *n* 气候疗法
climax [ˈklaimæks] *n* 顶点；极期；性欲高潮
climograph [ˈklaiməgrɑːfˌ-græf] *n* 气候（对人体）影响图
clinarthrosis [ˌklinɑːˈθrəusis] *n* 关节骨偏斜
clindamycin [ˌklindəˈmaisin] *n* 克林霉素（抗生素类药）| ~ hydrochloride 盐酸克林霉素 / ~ palmitate hydrochloride 盐酸克林霉素棕榈酸酯 / ~ phosphate 克林霉素磷酸酯
cline [klain] *n* 梯度变异
clinic [ˈklinik] *n* 诊所，门诊部；临床讲解；临床［学］科 | ambulant ~ 门诊部 / dry ~ 无病例临床讲解
clinical [ˈklinikəl] *a* 临床的，临证的
clinician [kliˈniʃən] *n* 临床医师；临床教师 | nurse ~ 临床护士
clinicogenetic [ˌklinikəudʒiˈnetik] *a* 临床遗传的
clinicopathologic [ˌklinikəuˌpæθəˈlɔdʒik] *a* 临床病理［学］的
clinocephaly [ˌklainəuˈsefəli], **clinocephalism** [ˌklainəuˈsefəlizəm] *n* 鞍形头
clinodactyly [ˌklainəuˈdæktili], **clinodactylism** [ˌklainəuˈdæktilizəm] *n* 先天性指侧弯，先天性趾侧弯
clinography [kliˈnɔgrəfi] *n* 临床记录
clinoid [ˈklinɔid] *a* 床形的
clinology [klaiˈnɔlədʒi] *n* 动物退化学
clinoscope [ˈklainəskəup], **clinometer** [klaiˈnɔmitə] *n* 旋斜视计（检眼肌麻痹）
clinostatic [ˌklinəuˈstætik] *a* 卧位的
clinostatism [ˈklainəˌstætizəm] *n* 卧位
clinotherapy [ˌklinəuˈθerəpi] *n* 卧床疗养
clioquinol [ˌklaiəuˈkwinɔl] *n* 氯碘羟喹（即 indochlorhydroxyquin，抗阿米巴药，局部抗菌药）
clioxanide [klaiˈɔksənaid] *n* 氯碘沙尼（抗蠕虫药）
CLIP corticotropin-like intermediate lobe peptide 中间叶促皮质样肽
clip [klip] *n* ［小］夹，钳
cliprofen [kliˈprəufən] *n* 克利洛芬（抗炎药）
cliseometer [ˌklisiˈɔmitə] *n* 骨盆斜度计
clitellum [klaiˈteləm] *n* 环带，生殖带
clithridium [kliˈθridiəm] *n* 钥孔状菌，8 字形菌
clition [ˈklitiɔn] *n* 斜坡前中点
Clitocybe [klaiˈtɔsibi] *n* 杯伞属
clitocybine [ˌklitəuˈsaibin] *n* 杯伞素
clitoral [ˈklitərəl, ˈklai-, kliˈtɔr-] *a* 阴蒂的
clitorectomy [ˌklitəuˈrektəmi, ˌklai-] *n* 阴蒂切除术
clitoridauxe [ˈklitəriˌdɔːksi] *n* 阴蒂肥大
clitoridean [ˌklitəˈridiən, ˌklai-] *a* 阴蒂的
clitoridectomy [ˌklitəriˈdektəmi, ˌklai-, kliˌtɔr-] *n* 阴蒂切除术
clitoriditis [ˌklitəriˈdaitis, ˌklai-, kliˌtɔr-], **clitoritis** [ˌklitəˈraitis, ˌklai-] *n* 阴蒂炎
clitoridotomy [ˌklitəriˈdɔtəmi, ˌklai-, kliˌtɔr-], **clitorotomy** [ˌklitəˈrɔtəmi, ˌklai-] *n* 阴蒂切开术
clitorimegaly [ˌklitəriˈmegəli, ˌklai-], **clitoromegaly** [ˌklitərəuˈmegəli, ˌklai-] *n* 阴蒂增大
clitoris [ˈklitəris, ˈklai-, kliˈtɔr-] *n* 阴蒂 | **clitoric** [kliˈtɔrik, klai-] *a*
clitorism [ˈklitərizəm, ˈklai-] *n* 阴蒂肥大；阴蒂异常勃起
clitoroplasty [ˈklitərəuˌplæsti, ˌklai-] *n* 阴蒂成形术
clivography [klaiˈvɔgrəfi] *n* 斜坡造影术（颅后窝 X 线摄影显示）
clivus [ˈklaivəs] *n*【拉】斜坡 | basilar ~ 枕骨斜坡 | **clival** [ˈklaivəl] *a*
clo [kləu] *n* 克漏（测量人体普通日常衣着绝热的单位）
cloaca [kləuˈeikə]（［复］**cloacae** [kləuˈeikiː]）*n*【拉】泄殖腔；骨瘘 | ectodermal ~ 外胚层性泄

殖腔 / entodermal ~ 内胚层性泄殖腔 / persistent ~, congenital ~ 泄殖腔存留,先天性泄殖腔 | ~l *a*

cloacitis [ˌkləuə'saitis] *n* 泄殖腔炎

cloacogenic [ˌkləuəkəu'dʒenik] *a* 泄殖腔原的

clobazam ['kləubəzæm] *n* 氯巴占(弱安定药)

clobetasol propionate [klə'beitəsɔl] 丙酸氯倍他索(肾上腺皮质激素类药)

clobetasone butyrate [kləu'beitəsəun] 丁酸氯倍他松(肾上腺皮质激素类药)

clock [klɔk] *n* [时]钟 | biological ~ 生物钟(生物生命活动的内在节奏性) / inner ~ 体内时钟,生物钟

clocortolone pivalate [klə'kɔːtələun] 特戊酸氯可托龙(糖皮质激素)

clodanolene [klə'dænəliːn] *n* 氯达诺林(骨骼肌松弛药)

clodazon hydrochloride ['kləudəzəun] 盐酸氯达酮(抗抑郁药)

clodronate disodium [klə'drəuneit] 氯膦酸二钠(钙调节药,抑制骨吸收,用于治疗畸形性骨炎和与恶性肿瘤相关的高血钙,口服或静脉给药)

clodronic acid [klə'drɔnik] 氯膦酸(骨钙调节药)

clofazimine [klə'fæzimiːn] *n* 氯法齐明(抗菌药,具有抑制结核菌及麻风菌作用)

clofedanol [klə'fedənɔl] *n* 氯苯达诺(镇咳药)

clofenamic acid [ˌkləufə'næmik] 氯芬那酸(镇痛、抗炎药)

clofibrate [klə'faibreit] *n* 氯贝丁酯(降血脂药)

clogestone acetate [klə'dʒestəun] 醋酸氯孕酮(孕激素类药)

cloison [klwɑː'zɔŋ] *n*【法】肾柱(贝尔坦〈Bertin〉为肾柱使用的原名)

clomacran phosphate ['kləuməkræn] 磷酸氯马克仑(安定药)

clomiphene citrate ['kləumifiːn] 枸橼酸氯米芬(抗不育症药)

clomipramine hydrochloride [klə'miprəmiːn] 盐酸氯米帕明(抗抑郁药)

clonality [klə'næləti] *n* 克隆形成能力

clonazepam [klə'næzipæm] *n* 氯硝西泮(抗惊厥药)

clone [kləun] *n* 克隆 | forbidden ~ 禁忌克隆 | **clonal** *a*

clonic ['klɔnik] *a* 阵挛性的 | **~ity** [klə'nisəti] *n* 阵挛性

clonicotonic [ˌklɔnikəu'tɔnik] *a* 阵挛紧张的

clonidine hydrochloride ['kləunidiːn] *n* 盐酸可乐定(拟肾上腺素药,降压药)

cloning ['kləuniŋ] *n* 克隆[化] | DNA ~ DNA 克隆[化]

clonism ['klɔnizəm], **clonismus** [klə'nizməs] *n* 连续阵挛

clonitrate [klə'naitreit] *n* 氯硝甘油(冠状动脉扩张药)

clonixeril [klə'niksəril] *n* 氯尼塞利(镇痛药)

clonixin [klə'niksin] *n* 氯尼辛(镇痛药)

clonogenic [ˌkləunəu'dʒenik] *a* 促克隆形成的

clonograph ['klɔnəgrɑːf, -græf] *n* 阵挛描记器

clonorchiasis [ˌkləunɔː'kaiəsis], **clonorchiosis** [kləuˌnɔːki'əusis] *n* 支睾吸虫病

Clonorchis [kləu'nɔːkis] *n* 支睾[吸虫]属

clonospasm ['klɔnəspæzəm] *n* 阵发痉挛

Clonothrix ['kləunəθriks] *n* 细枝发菌属 | ~ fusca 褐色细枝发菌

clonotype ['kləunətaip] *n* 克隆型

clonus ['kləunəs] *n* 阵挛 | ankle ~, foot ~ 踝阵挛,足阵挛 / anodal closure ~ (ACCl) 阳极通电阵挛 / anodal opening ~ (AOCl) 阳极断电阵挛 / cathodal closure ~ (CCCl) 阴极通电阵挛 / cathodal opening ~ (COCl) 阴极断电阵挛 / patellar ~ 髌阵挛

clopamide [klə'pæmaid] *n* 氯帕胺(利尿药)

clopenthixol [ˌkləupen'θiksəul] *n* 氯哌噻吨(安定药,治疗精神分裂症)

clopidogrel bisulfate [klə'pidəgrel] 硫酸氢氯吡格雷(血小板凝集抑制药,用作抗血栓药,预防动脉粥样硬化患者心肌梗死、卒中和血管死亡,口服给药)

clopidol ['kləupidəul] *n* 氯吡多(家禽抗球虫药)

clopimozide [klə'piməzaid] *n* 氯哌莫齐(安定药)

clopirac ['kləupiræk] *n* 氯吡酸(抗炎药)

cloprednol [klə'prednəul] *n* 氯泼尼醇(糖皮质激素)

cloprostenol sodium [klə'prɔstinəul] 氯前列醇钠(前列腺素类药)

Cloquet's canal [kləu'kei] (Jules G. Cloquet) 玻璃体管 | ~ fascia, ~ septum 股环隔 / ~ hernia 耻骨下股疝 / ~ ligament 鞘突遗迹 / ~ needle sign 克洛凯针征(将清洁的针刺入二头肌中,如生命一息尚存,该针于20~60分钟内即生锈)

Cloquet's ganglion (pseudoganglion) [kləu'kei] (Hippolyte Cloquet)鼻腭神经节

clorazepate [klə'ræzəpeit] *n* 氯氮䓬(安定药) | ~ dipotassium 氯氮䓬二钾(弱安定药) / ~ monopotassium 氯氮䓬一钾(弱安定药)

clorazepic acid [ˌklɔːrə'zepik] 氯氮䓬酸

clorexolone [klə'reksələun] *n* 氯索隆(利尿药)

cloroperone hydrochloride [ˌkləurə'piərəun] 盐酸氯哌隆(安定药)

clorophene ['kləurəfiːn] *n* 氯苄酚(消毒药)

clorprenaline hydrochloride [klɔː'prenəliːn] 盐

酸氯丙那林(拟肾上腺素药,支气管扩张药)

clorsulon [ˈklɔːsjulɔn] *n* 氯舒隆(抗蠕虫药)

clortermine hydrochloride [klɔːˈtəːmiːn] 盐酸氯特胺(拟肾上腺素药,口服用作食欲抑制药,短期治疗外源性肥胖症)

closantel [ˈkləusəntəl] *n* 氯生太尔(抗蠕虫药)

closiramine aceturate [kləˈsiərəmiːn] 乙酰甘氨酸氯西拉敏(抗组胺药)

clostridiopeptidase [clɔˌstridiəuˈpeptideis] *n* 梭状[芽胞]杆菌肽酶

clostridiosis [klɔˈstridiˈəusis] *n* 梭状芽胞杆菌病

Clostridium [klɔˈstridiəm] *n* 梭菌属,梭状芽胞杆菌属 | ~ acetobutylicum 丙酮丁醇梭菌 / ~ agni 魏氏 B 型梭菌,B 型产气荚膜梭菌 / ~ bifermentans 双酶梭菌,双酶梭状芽胞杆菌 / ~ botulinum 肉毒梭菌,肉毒杆菌 / ~ butyricum 丁酸梭菌,酪酸梭菌 / ~ cadaveris 尸毒梭菌 / ~ chauvoei 肖[韦]氏梭菌 / ~ clostridiiforme 梭菌样梭菌/ ~ difficile 艰难梭菌 / ~ feseri 费[斯尔]氏梭菌 / ~ haemolyticum 溶血梭菌 / ~ histolyticum 溶组织梭菌 / ~ innocum 无害梭菌 / ~ kluyveri 克[鲁佛]氏梭菌 / ~ limosum 泥渣梭菌 / ~ novyi, ~ oedematiens 诺[维]氏梭菌,水肿梭菌 / ~ ovitoxicus 绵羊毒梭菌 / ~ paludis 魏氏 C 型梭菌 / ~ parabotulinum 副肉毒梭菌 / ~ parabotulinum equi 马副肉毒梭菌,D 型肉毒梭菌 / ~ pasteurianum, ~ pastorianum 巴[斯德]氏[固氮]梭菌 / ~ perfringens 产气荚膜梭菌 / ~ septicum 败血梭菌 / ~ ramosum 多枝梭菌 / ~ sordellii 污泥梭菌 / ~ sphenoides 楔形梭菌 / ~ sporogenes 产孢梭菌 / ~ subterminale 近端梭菌 / ~ tertium 第三梭菌 / ~ tetani 破伤风梭菌 / ~ welchii 魏氏梭菌

clostridium [klɔˈstridiəm] ([复] **clostridia** [klɔˈstridiə]) *n* 梭状芽胞杆菌 | **clostridial** [klɔˈstridiəl] *a*

closure [ˈkləuʒə] *n* 关闭,闭合;通电 | aortic valve ~ 主动脉瓣关闭

closylate [ˈkləusileit] *n* 对氯苯磺酸盐(*p*-chlorobenzesulfonate 的 USAN 缩约词)

clot [klɔt] *n* 凝块;血块 | agonal ~, agony ~ 濒死期心脏内血块 / antemortem ~ 死前血块(心脏或大血管内) / blood ~ 血块 / chicken fat ~ 鸡脂状血块 / currant jelly ~ 果酱状血块 / distal ~ 远侧血块 / external ~ 血管外血块 / internal ~ 血管内血块,血栓 / laminated ~, stratified ~ 层状血块,层状血栓 / marantic ~ 消耗性血块,衰弱性血栓 / muscle ~ 肌浆凝块 / passive ~ 被动性血块(血液通过动脉瘤囊时停止循环而形成的血块) / plastic ~ 成形性血块 / postmortem ~ 死后血块(心脏或大血管内) / proximal ~ 近侧血块 / washed ~, white ~ 冲积性血块,白色血块,白色血栓(纤维蛋白和血小板组成)

clothiapine [kləˈθaiəpiːn] *n* 氯噻平(安定药)

clotrimazole [kləuˈtriməzɔl] *n* 克霉唑(抗真菌药)

clotting [ˈklɔtiŋ] *n* 凝固

cloud [klaud] *n* 云雾 | infectious ~ 传染雾

clouding [ˈklaudiŋ] *n* 混浊,模糊 | ~ of consciousness 意识混浊

Cloudman's melanoma S91 [ˈklaudmən] (Arthur M. Claudman) 克劳德曼黑素瘤 S91(坚硬的黑色皮下瘤)

Clough-Richter syndrome [kləu ˈriktər] (Mildred C. Clough; Ina M. Richter) 克-里综合征(红细胞显示严重自体凝集的贫血)

Clouston's syndrome [ˈklaustən] (H. R. Clouston) 出汗性外胚层发育不良

clove [kləuv] *n* 丁香

cloven [ˈkləuvn] *a* 裂开的,分趾的

clover [ˈkləuvə] *n* 三叶草,苜蓿属植物

clownism [ˈklaunizəm] *n* 丑态(歇斯底里性怪异动作)

cloxacillin [klɔksəˈsilin] *n* 氯唑西林(抗生素类药) | ~ sodium 氯唑西林钠(抗生素类药)

cloxyquin [ˈklɔksikwin] *n* 氯羟喹(抗菌药)

clozapine [ˈkləuzəpiːn] *n* 氯氮平(镇静药)

cloze [kləuz] *a* (对阅读理解能力的)填充测验法的

club [klʌb] *n* 棒节(蚤触角)

clubbed [klʌbd] *a* 棍棒状的;杵状的

clubbing [ˈklʌbiŋ] *n* 杵状肥大(指,趾)

clubfoot [ˈklʌbfut] ([复] **clubfeet** [ˈklʌbfiːt]) *n* 畸形足 | ~**ed** [ˈklʌbfutid] *a*

clubhand [ˈklʌbhænd] *n* 畸形手

clubroot [ˈklʌbruːt] *n* 指趾病(即 finger and toe disease, 甘蓝根肿病)

clump [klʌmp] *n* 凝块(细菌) *vt, vi* 结块

clumping [ˈklʌmpiŋ] *n* 凝集

clunis [ˈkluːnis] ([复] **clunes** [ˈkluːniːz]) *n* 【拉】臀 | **cluneal, clunial** [ˈkluːniəl] *a*

clupanodonic acid [ˌkluːpænəˈdɔnik] 鲦鱼酸

clupeine [ˈkluːpiin] *n* 鲱精蛋白

cluster [ˈklʌstə] *n* 聚簇

clusterin [ˈklʌstərin] *n* 蔟连蛋白

cluttering [ˈklʌtəriŋ] *n* 语言急促

Clutton's joint [ˈklʌtn] (Henry H. Clutton) 克拉顿关节(无痛性对称性关节积水,尤指膝关节,见于先天梅毒)

clyers [ˈklaiəz] *n* 放线菌病(牛)

clysis [ˈklaisis] *n* 灌洗,冲洗;补液,补液法;补液剂

clyster [ˈklistə], **clysma** [ˈklizmə] ([复] **clysmata** [ˈklizmətə]) *n* 灌肠[法];灌肠剂

clysterize [ˈklistəraiz] *vt* 施行灌肠
clytocybine [ˌklaitəˈsaibiːn] *n* 杯伞菌素
CM Chirurgiae Magister【拉】外科硕士
Cm curium 锔
cM centimorgan 厘摩
cm centimeter 厘米
cm² square centimeter 平方厘米
cm³ cubic centimeter 立方厘米
CMA Canadian Medical Association 加拿大医学会；Certified Medical Assistant 持证助理医师
CMAP compound muscle action potential 复合肌肉动作电位
CMD cerebromacular degeneration 大脑黄斑变性
CMF cyclophosphamide, methotrexate, and 5-fluorouracil 环磷酰胺-甲氨蝶呤-氟尿嘧啶(联合化疗治癌方案)
CMHC community mental health center 社区精神卫生中心
cmH₂O centimeter of water 厘米水柱(旧压力单位,现用 Pa 帕〈斯卡〉)
CMI cell-mediated immunity 细胞介导免疫,细胞免疫
CML cell-mediated lympholysis 细胞介导淋巴细胞溶解
c mm cubic millimeter 立方毫米
C-MOPP cyclophosphamide, mechlorethamine, vincristine, procarbazine, and prednisone 环磷酰胺-氮芥-长春新碱-丙卡巴肼-泼尼松(联合化疗治癌方案)
CMP cytidine monophosphate 胞苷[一磷]酸
CMR cerebral metabolic rate 大脑代谢率
c. m. s. cras mane sumendus【拉】明晨服用
CMT California Mastitis test 加利福尼亚乳腺炎试验; Certified Medical Transcriptinist 持证医学资料译录员
CMV cytomegalovirus 巨细胞病毒
c. n. cras nocte【拉】明晚
CNA Canadian Nurses' Association 加拿大护士协会
CN-Cbl cyanocobalamin 氰钴胺,维生素 B_{12}
C3 NeF C3 nephritic factor C3 致肾炎因子
cnemiall [ˈniːmiəl] *a* 胫的
Cnemidocoptes [ˌniːmidəˈkɔptiːz] *n* 脚螨属(即 Knemidokoptes)
cnemis [ˈniːmis] *n* 胫骨;胫,小腿
cnemitis [niːˈmaitis] *n* 胫骨炎
cnemoscoliosis [ˌniməuskəuliˈəusis] *n* 腿侧弯
cnicin [ˈnaisin] *n* 蓟[苦]素
Cnidaria [naiˈdεəriə] *n* 刺胞动物门
cnidarian [naiˈdεəriən] *a*, *n* 刺胞动物(的)
Cnidian [ˈnaidiən] *a* 尼达斯(Cnidos)(学派)的(尼达斯为古希腊小亚细亚西南沿海一城市,尼达斯学派强调对疾病作全面彻底的诊断和分类〈尤其是病理〉,达到无视病人的程度)
cnid(o)- [构词成分]荨麻
cnidoblast [ˈnaidəblæst] *n* 刺细胞(腔肠动物)
cnidocil [ˈnaidəsil] *n* 刺毛,刺针(腔肠动物)
cnidosis [naiˈdəusis] *n* 荨麻疹
Cnidospora [ˌnaidəˈspɔːrə] *n* 丝孢子虫亚门(即微孢子门 Microspora)
Cnidosporidia [ˌnaidəspɔːˈridiə] *n* 丝孢子虫亚纲(即微孢子目 Microsporida)
CNM Certified Nurse-Midwife 持证助产护士
CNS central nervous system 中枢神经系统
c. n. s. cras nocte sumendus【拉】明晚服用
CNV contingent negative variation 关联性负变,伴随负电位
CO cardiac output 心排血量,心输出量
Co cobalt 钴;coccygeal 尾骨的
co- [前缀]一同,并合(见 con-)
COA Canadian Orthopaedic Association 加拿大矫形外科协会
CoA coenzyme A 辅酶 A
coacervate [kəuˈæsəveit] *n* 凝聚层;团聚体
coacervation [kəuˌæsəˈveiʃən] *n* 凝聚;团聚
coaction¹ [kəuˈækʃən] *n* 强制力,强迫 | **coactive** *a*
coaction² [kəuˈækʃən] *n* 共同行动;种间相互作用
coadaptation [ˌkəuædæpˈteiʃən] *n* 共适应
coadunate [ˌkəuˈædʒunit] *a* 接合的;联合的;合生的 | **coadunation** [ˌkəuædʒuˈneiʃən], **coadunition** [ˌkəuædʒuˈniʃən] *n*
coagglutination [ˌkəuəˌgluːtiˈneiʃən] *n* 协同凝集[反应]
coagglutinin [ˌkəuəˈgluːtinin] *n* 副凝集素,部分凝集素
coagula [kəuˈægjulə] coagulum 的复数
coagulable [kəuˈægjuləbl] *a* 可凝固的 | **coagulability** [kəuˌægjuləˈbiləti] *n* 凝固性
coagulant [kəuˈægjulənt] *a* 促凝的 *n* 促凝剂,凝血药
coagulase [kəuˈægjuleis] *n* 凝固酶
coagulate [kəuˈægjuleit] *vt*, *vi* 凝结,凝固 | **coagulative** [kəuˈægjuleitiv] *a* 可凝固的,促凝固的 / **coagulator** [kəuˌægjuˈleitə] *n* 凝固器;凝固剂
coagulation [kəuˌægjuˈleiʃən] *n* 凝结,凝固 | blood ~ 血液凝固,凝血 / diffuse intravascular ~, disseminated intravascular ~ (DIC)弥散性血管内凝血 / electric ~ 电凝术 / massive ~ 脑脊液凝固
coagulogram [kəuˈægjuləˌgræm] *n* 凝血时间图[表]
coagulopathy [kəuˌægjuˈlɔpəθi] *n* 凝血病 | consumption ~ 消耗性凝血病

coagulum [kəu'ægjuləm] ([复] **coagula** [kəu'ægjulə]) *n*【拉】凝块,血块 | closing ~ 闭性凝块(子宫内)

coamilozide [ˌkəuə'miləzaid] *n* 盐酸阿米洛利-氢氯噻嗪(利尿药)

coamoxiclav [ˌkəuə'mɔksiklæv] *n* 阿莫西林-克拉维酸钠(抗生素和β-内酰胺酶抑制药,对β-内酰胺酶产生的细菌所致感染有效)

COAP cyclophosphamide, vincristine, ara-C, and prednisone 环磷酰胺-长春新碱-阿糖胞苷-泼尼松(联合化疗治癌方案)

coapt [kəu'æpt] *vt* 接合 | **coaptation** [kəuæp'teiʃən] *n* 接合;接骨术

coarctate [kəu'ɑːkteit] *vt* 紧压,收缩,使缩小 *a* 紧压的,缩小的

coarctation [ˌkəuɑːk'teiʃən] *n* 缩窄 | ~ of the aorta 主动脉缩窄 / ~ of aorta, adult type 成人型主动脉缩窄 / ~ of aorta, infantile 婴儿型主动脉缩窄 / reversed ~ 反向[主动脉]缩窄,无脉病

coarse [kɔːs] *a* 粗的

coarticulation [ˌkəuɑːˌtikju'leiʃən] *n* 不动关节

CoA-SH coenzyme A 辅酶 A

coat [kəut] *n* 外衣;外壳;衣,膜,层;涂层 | adventitial ~ 外膜 / adventitious ~ of uterine tube, subserous ~ 输卵管外膜,浆膜下组织 / albugineous ~ 白膜 / buffy ~ 血沉棕黄层 / cremasteric ~ of testis 睾提肌 / dartos ~ 肉膜 / enteric ~ 肠溶衣 / fibrous ~ of ovary 卵泡膜 / fibrous ~ of testis, proper ~ of testis 睾丸白膜 / mucous ~ 黏膜 / muscular ~ 肌层 / pharyngobasilar ~ 咽腱膜,咽颅底筋膜,咽颅底板 / proper ~ 固有膜,固有层

coating ['kəutiŋ] *n* 包被;包衣;外衣;涂层

CoA-transferase ['kəuei'trænsfəreis] 辅酶 A 转移酶

Coats's disease, retinitis [kəuts] (George Coats) 外层渗出性视网膜病变

coaxial [kəu'æksiəl] *a* 并轴的,合轴的

cobalamin [kəu'bæləmin] *n* 钴胺素,钴胺,维生素 B_{12} | ~ concentrate 浓缩钴胺素(用作维生素 B_{12}的补充)

cob(1)alamin adenosyltransferase [kəu'bæləmin əˌdenəsil'trænsfəreis] 钴(1)胺素腺苷转移酶(此酶缺乏,为一种常染色体隐性性状,可致甲基丙二酸单酰-CoA 变位酶的缺乏,并导致甲基丙二酸血症,形成钴胺素 B)

cobalamin reductase [kəu'bæləmin ri'dʌkteis] 钴胺素还原酶

cobalophilin [kəubə'lɔfilin] *n* 嗜钴素,R 蛋白

cobalt(Co) ['kəubɔːlt] *n* 钴(化学元素) | ~ salipyrine 撒利比林钴(水杨酸钴和安替比林,形成淡红色粉末) / ~ 60 ^{60}Co(钴的放射性同位素,工业放射摄影时用作放射源) | **~ic** [kəu'bɔːltik] *n*

cobaltosis [ˌkəubəl'təusis] *n* 钴尘肺

cobaltous [kəu'bɔːltəs] *a* [正]钴的;二价钴的

cobamide ['kəubəmaid] *n* 钴胺酰胺

COBMAM cyclophosphamide, vincristin, bleomycin, methotrexate, doxorubicin, and semustine 环磷酰胺-长春新碱-博来霉素-甲氨蝶呤-多柔比星-司莫司汀(联合化疗治癌方案)

cobra ['kəubrə] *n* 眼镜蛇 | blacknecked ~, spitting ~ 黑颈眼镜蛇 / Indian ~ 印度眼镜蛇 / king ~ 扁颈眼镜蛇

cobraism ['kəubrəizəm] *n* 眼镜蛇毒中毒

cobralysin [kəu'brælisin] *n* 眼镜蛇毒溶血素

COBS cesarean-obtained barrier-sustained 剖腹取出并隔离培育的(实验动物)

cobucafAPAP [ˌkəubju'kæfəpæp] *n* 布他比妥-咖啡因-对乙酰氨基酚(镇痛药)

cobweb ['kɔbweb] *n* 蜘蛛网(有时用作止血药,用于灸料,也用作家用退热药和解痉药)

COC cathodal opening contraction 阴极断电收缩

coca ['kəukə] *n* 古柯(曾用于中枢神经系统兴奋药,在南美地区广泛用作引起欣快的咀嚼剂)

cocaine [kə'kein, 'kəukein] *n* 可卡因(局部麻醉药) | ~ hydrochloride 盐酸可卡因(麻醉药)

cocainism [kə'keinizəm, 'kəukən-] *n* 可卡因瘾,可卡因慢性中毒

cocainist [kə'keinist] *n* 可卡因瘾者

cocainize [kə'keinaiz, 'kəukən-] *vt* 可卡因化;用可卡因麻醉 | **cocainization** [kəˌkeinai'zeiʃən, -ni'z-; ˌkəukəni'z-] *n* 可卡因麻醉法

cocarboxylase [ˌkəukɑː'bɔksileis] *n* 辅羧酶,脱羧辅酶,焦磷酸硫胺

cocarcinogen [kəu'kɑːsinədʒən] *n* 辅致癌物,助癌剂 | **~ic** [kəuˌkɑːsinə'dʒenik] *a*

cocarcinogenesis [kəuˌkɑːsinə'dʒenisis] *n* 辅致癌作用,助致癌作用

cocardiform [kəu'kɑːdifɔːm] *a* 花结形的

cocareldopa [ˌkəukærəl'dəupə] *n* 卡比多巴-左旋多巴(抗震颤麻痹药)

cocatannic acid [ˌkəukə'tænik] 柯卡丹宁酸

coccal ['kəukəl] *a* 球菌的

coccerin ['kɔksərin] *n* 胭脂虫蜡

cocci ['kɔkai, 'kɔksai] coccus 的复数

Coccidae ['kɔksidiː] *n* 介壳虫科

Coccidia [kɔk'sidiə] *n* 球虫亚纲

coccidia [kɔk'sidiə] coccidium 的复数 | **~l** *a* 球虫的

coccidian [kɔk'sidiən] *a*, *n* 球虫(的)

coccidioidal [kɔkˌsidi'ɔidl] *a* 球孢子菌的

Coccidioides [kɔkˌsidi'ɔidiːz] *n* 球孢子菌属

coccidioidin [ˌkɔksidiˈɔidin] *n* 球孢子菌素
coccidioidoma [kɔkˌsidiɔiˈdəumə] *n* 球孢子菌瘤
coccidioidomycosis [kɔkˌsidiˌɔidəumaiˈkəusis] *n* 球孢子菌病 | primary extrapulmonary ~ 原发性肺外球孢子菌病,下疳样综合征 | **coccidioidosis** [kɔkˌsidiɔiˈdəusis] *n*
coccidiosis [ˌkɔksidiˈəusis] *n* 球虫病
coccidiostat [kɔkˈsidiəstæt] *n* 抗球虫药,球虫抑制药 | **~ic** [kɔkˌsidiəˈstætik] *a* 抑制球虫生长的 *n* 抑制球虫生长药
Coccidium [kɔkˈsidiəm] *n* 球虫属 | ~ bigeminum 双孢子球虫,二联等孢子球虫(即 Isospora bigemina) / ~ cuniculi 兔艾美球虫,啮齿艾美球虫(即 Eimeria stiedae) / ~ oviforme 卵形球虫,啮齿艾美球虫(即 Eimeria stiedae) / ~ tenellum 禽艾美球虫(即 Eimeria tenella)
coccidium [kɔkˈsidiəm] ([复] **coccidia** [kɔkˈsidiə]) *n* 球虫
coccigenic [ˌkɔksiˈdʒenik] *a* 球菌原的,球菌引起的
coccillana [ˌkɔksiˈjɑːnə] *n* 南美祛痰楝皮,柯西拉那楝皮(曾用作催吐、祛痰和泻药)
coccinella [ˌkɔksiˈnelə] *n* 胭脂虫
coccinellin [ˌkɔksiˈnelin] *n* 卡红,胭脂红
cocco- [构词成分] 浆果;球菌
coccobacillary [ˌkɔkəubəˈsiləri, -ˈbæs-] *a* 球杆菌的;球杆菌样的
Coccobacillus [ˌkɔkəubəˈsiləs] *n* 球杆菌属,星球菌属
coccobacillus [ˌkɔkəubəˈsiləs] ([复]) **coccobacilli** [ˌkɔkəubəˈsilai]) *n* 球杆菌
coccobacteria [ˌkɔkəubækˈtiəriə] *n* 球菌
coccode [ˈkɔkəud] *n* 球状小粒
coccogenic [ˌkɔkəuˈdʒenik], **coccogenous** [kɔˈkɔdʒinəs] *a* 球菌原的
coccoid [ˈkɔkɔid] *a* 球菌样的;球形的
coccolith [ˈkɔkəliθ] *n* 球石粒(某些海洋原生动物形成的钙板外骨骼)
Coccolithus [ˌkɔkəˈliθəs] *n* 钙板金藻属
cocculin [ˈkɔkjulin] *n* 印防己毒素
cocculus [ˈkɔkjuləs] *n* 印防己[实] | ~ indicus 印防己[实]
Coccus [ˈkɔkəs] *n* 胭脂虫属
coccus [ˈkɔkəs] ([复] **cocci** [ˈkɔksai]) *n*【拉】球菌
coccyalgia [ˌkɔksiˈældʒiə], **coccydynia** [ˌkɔksiˈdiniə], **coccygalgia** [ˌkɔksiˈgældʒiə] *n* 尾骨痛
coccycephalus [ˌkɔksiˈsefələs] *n* 喙形头畸胎
coccygeal [kɔkˈsidʒiəl] *a* 尾骨的
coccygectomy [ˌkɔksiˈdʒektəmi] *n* 尾骨切除术
coccygerector [ˌkɔksidʒiˈrektə] *n* 尾伸肌,尾立肌
coccygeus [kɔkˈsidʒiəs] *a*【拉】尾骨的 *n* 尾骨肌
coccygodynia [ˌkɔksigəuˈdiniə], **coccyodynia** [ˌkɔksiəuˈdiniə] *n* 尾骨痛
coccygotomy [ˌkɔksiˈgɔtəmi] *n* 尾骨切开术
coccyx [ˈkɔksiks] ([复]) **coccyxes** 或 **coccyges** [kɔkˈsaidʒiːz] *n* 尾骨 **cochineal** [ˈkɔtʃiniːl] *n* 胭脂虫
cochl. cochleare【拉】匙,一匙量;cochl. amp. 见 cochleare amplum; cochl. mag. 见 cochleare magnum; cochl. med. 见 cochleare medium; cochl. parv. 见 cochleare parvum
cochlea [ˈkɔkliə] ([复] **cochleae** [ˈkɔkliiː] 或 **cochleas**) *n*【拉】蜗,耳蜗 | membranous ~ 蜗管(耳) | **~r** [ˈkɔkliə] *a*
cochleare [ˈkɔkliˈɛəri] *n*【拉】匙,一匙量 | ~ amplum 一满匙量 / ~ magnum 一大匙量,一汤匙量 / ~ medium 一中匙量 / ~ parvum 一茶匙量
Cochlearia [ˌkɔkliˈɛəriə] *n*【拉】辣根属(十字花科) | ~ officinalis 辣根菜(曾用作抗坏血病药)
cochleariform [ˌkɔkliˈærifɔːm] *a* 匙形的
cochleitis [ˌkɔkliˈaitis] *n* 耳蜗炎
cochleosacculotomy [ˌkɔkliəuˌsækjuˈlɔtəmi] *n* 耳蜗球囊切开术
cochleotopic [ˌkɔkliəuˈtɔpik] *a* 耳蜗分布的
cochleotoxicity [ˌkɔkliəutɔkˈsisəti] *n* 耳蜗毒性
cochleovestibular [ˌkɔkliəuvesˈtibjulə] *a* 耳蜗前庭的
Cochliobolus [ˌkɔkliˈɔbələs] *n* 旋孢菌属
Cochliomyia [ˌkɔkliəuˈmaijə] *n* 锥蝇属 | ~ bezziana 倍氏锥虫(即 Chrysomia bezziana) / ~ hominivorax, ~ americana 嗜人锥蝇,美洲锥蝇
cochlitis [kɔkˈlaitis] *n* 耳蜗炎
cocillana [ˌkəusiˈjɑːnə] *n* 南美祛痰楝皮,柯西拉那楝皮(曾用作催吐、祛痰和泻药)
cockade [kɔˈkeid] *n* 花结(一种皮肤病灶的表现,见于多形红斑、复发性结核样麻风)
Cockayne's syndrome (disease) [kɔˈkein] (E. A. Cockayne) 科凯恩综合征(病)(一种遗传性综合征,作为常染色体隐性性状遗传,包括视网膜萎缩、侏儒、耳聋,伴有早衰、精神发育迟缓及光敏感性)
cockleburr [ˈkɔklbər] *n* 苍耳
cockroach [ˈkɔkrəutʃ] *n* 蟑螂
Cock's operation [kɔk] (Edward Cock) 科克手术(沿会阴中线行尿道切开术)
cocktail [ˈkɔkteil] *n* 鸡尾酒(一种各种成分混合的饮料);混合剂,合剂 | frostbite ~ 冻疮混合剂(一种含乙醇、普鲁卡因和肝素的 5% 葡萄糖溶液,曾推荐治疗冻疮) / lytic ~ 抗自主神经合剂,冬眠合剂,(精神)安定性鸡尾酒剂
COCl cathodal opening clonus 阴极断电阵挛
coclimasone [kəuˈklaiməsəun] *n* 克霉唑-二丙酸倍他米松(局部抗真菌药)

coco [ˈkəukəu] *n* 椰子;椰子树

cocoa [ˈkəukəu] *n* 可可

cocodAPAP [kəuˈkəudəpæp] *n* 磷酸可待因-阿司匹林(镇痛药)

coconscious [kəuˈkɔnʃəs] *a* 并[存]意识的 | **~ness** *n*

cocontraction [ˌkəukənˈtrækʃən] *n* 协同收缩

coconut [ˈkəukənʌt] *n* 椰子

cocoon [kəˈkuːn] *n* 茧

Cocos [ˈkəukəus] *n* 棕榈属

Coct. coctio【拉】煮沸

coction [ˈkɔkʃən] *n* 煮沸;消化

coctoantigen [ˌkɔktəuˈæntidʒən] *n* 加热抗原

cocto-immunogen [ˌkɔktəu iˈmjuːnədʒən] *n* 加热免疫原

coctolabile [ˌkɔktəuˈleibail] *a* 不耐热的(加热至沸点时被破坏或改变的)

coctoprecipitin [ˌkɔktəupriˈsipitin] *n* 加热沉淀素(用加热抗原免疫接种所产生的沉淀素)

coctoprotein [ˌkɔktəuˈprəutiːn] *n* 加热蛋白

coctostabile [ˌkɔktəuˈsteibail], **coctostable** [ˌkɔktəuˈsteibl] *a* 耐热的(加热至沸水温度时而不改变的)

coculine [ˈkɔkjuliːn] *n* 汉防己碱,青藤碱

cocultivation [ˈkəukʌltiˈveiʃən] *n* 协同培养(如正常未感染的人细胞与感染的或潜在感染的同种细胞一起培养)

cod [kɔd] *n* 鳕鱼

code [kəud] *n* 法典,法规 | degeneracy of ~ 密码简并 / genetic ~ 遗传密码(指核苷酸内四种含氮碱基的不同排列组合) / triplet ~ 三联体密码(DNA 分子中三个碱基顺序〈核苷酸〉决定某一氨基酸)

codehydrogenase Ⅰ [ˌkəudiːˈhaidrədʒəˌneis] *n* 辅脱氢酶 Ⅰ,烟酰胺腺嘌呤二核苷酸 | ~Ⅱ 辅脱氢酶 Ⅱ,烟酰胺腺嘌呤二苷酸磷酸

codeine [ˈkəudiːn] *n* 可待因(镇咳、麻醉止痛药) | ~ phosphate 磷酸可待因(镇咳、麻醉止痛药) / ~ sulfate 硫酸可待因(麻醉止痛药)

codeposition [ˌkəuˌdepəˈziʃən] *n* 共积作用

codex [ˈkəudeks] ([复] **codices** [ˈkəudisiːz]) *n*【拉】药方集;药典(特指法国药典 Codex medicamentarium)

Codivilla's extension [ˌkəudiˈvilə] (Alessandro Codivilla) 科迪维拉牵伸术(肢骨折牵伸术,用钉穿过骨的下端以牵引骨折肢体) | ~ operation 科迪维拉手术(一种假关节的手术,用取自胫骨内面的薄骨骨膜板围绕假关节)

Codman's sign [ˈkɔdmən] (Ernest A. Codman) 科德曼征(三角)(冈上肌腱断裂时,手臂可无痛地被动外展,但当手臂失去支持时,则三角肌突然收缩,疼痛又出现) | ~ triangle 科特曼三角(骨膜被骨肿瘤顶起时,X 片可见与正常骨皮质形成一个三角区)

codocyte [ˈkəudəsait] *n* 靶细胞

codominance [kəuˈdɔminəns] *n* 共显性(杂合型合子中两等位基因都能表现为显性,如血型为 AB 型者) | **codominant** [kəuˈdɔminənt] *a*, *n*

codon [ˈkəudɔn] *n* 密码子(DNA 或 RNA 分子的多核苷酸链中决定一个特定的氨基酸的三个相邻的碱基联结,亦称三联体) | chain-initiation ~s 链起始密码子 / chain-termination ~s, nonsense ~s 链终止密码子,无义密码子

coe- 以 coe-起始的词,同样见以 ce-起始的词

coefficient [ˌkəuiˈfiʃənt] *n* 系数 | confidence ~ 置信系数(置信区间含总体参数真值的概率) / cryoscopic ~ 冰点降低系数 / ~ of demineralization 矿盐滤除率(系数) / ~ of extinction(抗体作用)消退系数 / homogeneity ~ 均匀系数(在放射学中指半价层与第二半价层之比) / isometric ~ of lactic acid 乳酸等溶系数 / linear absorption ~ 线性吸收系数 / linear attenuation ~ 线性衰减系数 / mass absorption ~ 质量吸收系数 / mass attenuation ~ 质量衰减系数 / ~ of partage 醚溶酸系数(酸在水醚系统中分配系数) / product-moment ~ 积距系数(两个随机变量的协方差除以其标准差的积。符号为 *r*。亦称皮尔逊相关系数 Pearson's correlation coefficient) / ~ of relationship 亲缘系数(两个个体从共同的祖先承袭某一确定基因的概率,或他们从共同祖先获得所有基因的比例) / sedimentation ~ [离心]沉降系数 / selection ~ 选择系数(一定基因型生存值的不利条件与群体标准基因型不利条件相比较的一种定量尺度) / ~ of thermal conductivity 热传导系数 / ~ of thermal expansion 热膨胀系数 / ~ of variability 可变性系数 / velocity ~ 速率系数 / ~ of viscosity 黏滞系数 / volume ~ 容积系数

coel- [构词成分] 腔,穴,孔

coelarium [siˈlɛəriəm] *n* 体腔膜,间皮,体腔上皮

-coele [后缀] 腔,穴,孔(有时拼写成-cele 和 -coel)

Coelenterata [siˌlentəˈreitə] *n* 腔肠动物门

coelenterate [siˈlentəreit] *a*, *n* 腔肠动物(的)

coelenteron [siˈlentərɔn] ([复] **coelentera** [siˈlentərə]) *n* 原肠(即 archenteron);体肠腔(即 gastrovascular cavity)

coeliac [ˈsiːliæk] *a* 腹的,腹腔的

coel(o)- [构词成分] 腹,腔,腹腔(有时拼写成 cel〈o〉-)

coeloblastula [ˌsiːləˈblæstjulə] *n* 有腔囊胚

coelom [ˈsiːləm] *n* 体腔 | extraembryonic ~ 胚外体腔 | **~ic** [siˈlɔmik] *a*

coeloma [siˈləumə] *n* 体腔

coelomate [ˈsiːləmeit] *a* 有体腔的 *n* 体腔动物

coelomyarian [ˌsiːləumaiˈɛəriən] *n* 体腔肌(指线虫的一种肌肉系统)
Coelomycetes [ˌsiːləumaiˈsiːtiːz] *n* 腔孢纲
coelosomy [ˌsiːləuˈsəumi] *n* 露脏畸形
coelothel [ˈsiːləθel] *n* 体腔上皮,间皮
coen(o)-见 cen(o)-第三解
coenocyte [ˈsiːnəsait] *n* 多核细胞,多核体 | **coenocytic** [ˌsiːnəˈsitik] *a*
coenuriasis [ˌsiːnjuəˈraiəsis] *n* 多头[绦虫]蚴病
coenurosis [ˌsiːnjuəˈrəusis] *n* 多头蚴病
Coenurus [siˈnjuərəs] *n* 多头[绦虫]蚴属 | ~ cerebralis 脑多头[绦虫]蚴
coenurus [siˈnjuərəs] *n* 多头蚴
coenzyme [kəuˈenzaim] *n* 辅酶 | ~ A 辅酶 A,泛酸 / ~ Ⅰ 辅酶Ⅰ,烟酰胺腺嘌呤二核苷酸(即 NAD) / ~ Ⅱ 辅酶Ⅱ,烟酰胺腺嘌呤二核苷酸磷酸(即 NADP) / ~ Q 辅酶 Q,泛醌(类似维生素 K) / ~ R 辅酶 R,维生素 H,生物素
coenzymometer [ˌkəuenzaiˈmɔmitə] *n* 辅酶测定器
COEPS cortically originating extrapyramidal system 皮质源性锥体外系统
coerce [kəuˈəːs] *vt* 强制;迫使 | **coercible** [kəuˈəːsibl] *a* 可强迫的;(气体)可压凝的;可凝结的
coercive [kəuˈəːsiv] *a* 强制的 | **~ly** *ad*
coeruleus [siˈruːljəs] *a* 青的,蓝色的
coerynsulfisox [ˌkəuerinˈsʌlfəzɔks] *n* 琥乙红霉素-磺胺乙酰异噁唑(抗菌药)
coetaneous [ˌkəuiˈteiniəs], **coeval** [kəuˈiːvəl] *a* 同年龄的
coeur [kəː] *n*【法】心【脏】 | ~ en sabot 靴状心(见于法乐〈Fallot〉四联症)
coexcitation [kəuiksaiˈteiʃən] *n* 同时兴奋
coexistence [kəuigˈzistəns] *n* 共存 | ~ of transmitters 递质共存
cofactor [kəuˈfæktə] *n* 辅因子 | platelet ~ Ⅰ 血小板辅因子Ⅰ,凝血因子Ⅷ / platelet ~ Ⅱ 血小板辅因子Ⅱ,凝血因子Ⅸ
co-ferment [kəu ˈfəːmənt] *n* 辅酶
Coffea [ˈkɔfiə] *n* 咖啡属
coffee [ˈkɔfi] *n* 咖啡,咖啡豆
coffeurin [kɔfiˈjuərin] *n* 咖啡尿质
Coffey-Humber treatment [ˈkɔfi ˈhʌmbə] (Walter B. Coffey; John D. Humber) 科菲-亨伯疗法(注射绵羊肾上腺皮质浸膏,治癌用)
Coffin-Lowry syndrome [ˈkɔfin ˈləuri] (George S. Coffin; R. B. Lowry) 科-洛综合征(生后时期起始的病征,特征为不能言语,严重智力缺陷以及肌肉、韧带和骨骼异常,本征为 X 连锁中间性遗传的)
Coffin-Siris syndrome [ˈkɔfin ˈsiris] (G. S. Coffin; Evelyn Siris) 科-西综合征(第 5 指和趾甲发育不全或缺如,伴生长和智力缺陷,粗糙面容,轻度小头畸形,张力减低,关节松弛,轻度多毛,有时为心脏、椎骨或胃肠道异常)
Cogan's oculomotor apraxia [ˈkɔgən] (David G. Cogan) 科根动眼失用[症],先天性动眼失用[症](亦称科根综合征) | ~ syndrome 科根综合征(①非梅毒性角膜炎,伴前庭听觉症状;②科根动眼失用[症])
cogener [ˈkəudʒinə] *n* 协同肌
cognition [kɔgˈniʃən] *n* 认识,识别;认知 | **~al**, **cognitive** [ˈkɔgnitiv] *a*
coherence [kəuˈhiərəns], **coherency** [kəuˈhiərənsi] *n* 黏着;黏合性;黏结;连接,连贯;内聚性,内聚力
coherent [kəuˈhiərənt] *a* 黏着的,黏结的,黏附的;连贯的
cohesion [kəuˈhiːʒən] *n* 内聚性,内聚力;黏着,结合,黏结力
cohesive [kəuˈhisiv] *a* 黏着的,内聚[性]的
Cohnheim's areas (fields) [ˈkəunhaim] (Julius F. Cohnheim) 孔海姆区(肌原纤维的深色多边形区,在肌纤维的横切面上可见) | ~ theory 孔海姆学说(认为肿瘤是由胚胎剩余组织发生的,这些剩余组织并不参与正常外周组织的形成)
Cohn's solution [kəun] (Ferdinand J. Cohn) 科恩溶液(培养酵母和霉的合成培养基,含有磷酸一钾酸、磷酸钙、硫酸镁和酒石酸铵,溶于水中)
Cohn's test [kəun] (Hermann L. Cohn) 科恩试验(检色觉)
cohoba [kəˈhəubə] *n* 帕立卡(见 parica)
cohobation [ˌkəuhəˈbeiʃən] *n* 回流蒸馏,再蒸馏
cohort [ˈkəuhɔːt] *n* 队列,群组(在流行病学中指有共同点的一组人,如同年出生的人,为出生队列或出生群组 birth cohort);股(生物分类,相当于部〈division〉、目〈order〉或亚目〈suborder〉) | age ~ 同龄人
cohosh [kəˈhɔʃ] *n* 升麻类药草(指多种毛茛科植物)
cohycodAPAP [ˌkəuhaiˈkəudəpæp] *n* 重酒石酸氢可酮-对乙酰氨基酚(镇痛药)
cohydrogenase [ˌkəuhaiˈdrɔdʒineis] *n* 辅酶
Co Ⅰ coenzyme Ⅰ 辅酶Ⅰ(烟酰胺腺嘌呤二核苷酸)
Co Ⅱ coenzyme Ⅱ 辅酶Ⅱ(烟酰胺腺嘌呤二核苷酸磷酸)
coil [kɔil] *n* 圈,线圈;蟠管,旋管;螺旋 | random ~ 无规线圈,无规卷曲(指蛋白质没有规则的反复的二级结构,如 α-螺旋或 β-层)
coinfection [ˌkəuinˈfekʃən] *n* 同时感染
coin(o)-见 cen(o)-第二解
coinosite [ˈkɔinəsait] *n* 半自由寄生物

coisogeneic [kəuˌaisəudʒiˈneiik] *a* 同类系的(指生物品系)
coisogenic [kəuˌaisəuˈdʒenik] *a* 同类系的
coition [kəuˈiʃən] *n* 性交,交媾
coitophobia [ˌkəuitəˈfəubjə] *n* 性交恐怖
coitus [ˈkəuitəs] *n* 性交 | ~ incompletus, ~ interruptus 不完全性交,中断性交 / ~ reservatus 含蓄性交 | **coital** [ˈkəuitl] *a*
Coix [ˈkəuiks] *n* 薏苡属
coke [kəuk] *n* 焦炭
Cokeromyces [ˌkəukərəuˈmaisiːz] *n* 枝霉菌属
Col. cola【拉】漉过,滤过
col [kɔl] *n* 龈谷(为牙间组织的一个小凹)
col- 见 con-
cola [ˈkəulə] colon 的复数
colamine [ˈkəuləmin] *n* 胆胺,乙醇胺
colander [ˈkʌləndə,ˈkɔləndə] *n* 滤器,滤锅
colaspase [kəˈlæspeis] *n* 门冬酰胺酶(asparaginase 的 BAN 名)
Colat. colatus【拉】漉过的,滤过的
colation [kəˈleiʃən] 漉过,滤过;漉液,滤液
colatorium [ˌkɔləˈtɔːriəm]([复] **colatoria** [ˌkɔləˈtɔːriə]) *n*【拉】漉药器,滤器;筛网
colature [ˈkəulətʃə] *n* 漉液,滤液
colchicine [ˈkɔltʃisiːn] *n* 秋水仙素,秋水仙碱(用于治疗痛风性关节炎)
colchicinic acid [ˌkɔltʃiˈsinik] 秋水仙酸
Colchicum [ˈkɔltʃikəm] *n* 秋水仙属
cold [kəuld] *a* 冷的 *n* 感冒,伤风 | allergic ~, June ~ 枯草热 / common ~ 感冒 / head ~ 头伤风,鼻伤风 / rose ~ 玫瑰花粉热
COLD chronic obstructive lung disease 慢性阻塞性肺疾病
cold-blooded [ˈkəuldˈblʌdid] *a* 冷血的
coldsore [ˈkəuldsɔː] *n* 单纯性疱疹,唇疱疹
colectomy [kəˈlektəmi] *n* 结肠切除术
Coleman-Shaffer diet [ˈkəulmən ˈʃæfə](Warren Coleman; Philip A. Shaffer) 科尔曼-谢弗饮食(高糖、高蛋白质饮食,宜少量多餐,曾为伤寒病饮食)
cole(o)- [构词成分] 阴道;鞘
Coleomitus [ˌkəuliəuˈmaitəs] *n* 鞘丝菌属
Coleoptera [ˌkɔliˈɔptərə] *n* 鞘翅目
coles [ˈkəuliːz] *n* 阴茎 | ~ femininus 阴蒂
colesevelam hydrochloride [ˌkəuləˈsevəlæm] 盐酸考来西仑(作为降低原发性高胆固醇血症患者 LDL 胆固醇水平增高的辅助治疗,口服给药)
Colesiota [kəuˌliːsiˈəutə](J. D. W. A. Coles) *n* 科尔斯小体属
Cole's sign [kəul](Lewis G. Cole) 科尔征(X 线片所见的十二指肠轮廓变形,为十二指肠溃疡之征)
Cole's test [kəul](Sidney W. Cole) 科尔试验(检葡萄糖、乳糖、尿酸)
colestipol hydrochloride [kəˈlestipəul] 盐酸考来替泊(降血脂药)
Colet. coletur【拉】(使被)滤过,漉过
Colettsia [kəˈletsiə](J. D. W. A. Coles) *n* 科尔次体属
Coley's fluid (mixture), toxin [ˈkəuli](William B. Coley) 科利液(混合物)、毒素(某些细胞培养物的未过滤过的混合物,曾用于治不能进行手术的恶性肿瘤)
colfosceril palmitate [kɔlˈfɔsəril] 棕榈胆磷(合成肺表面治性药,与鲸蜡醇和泰洛沙泊结合使用,防治新生儿呼吸窘迫综合征,滴注气管内导管,以便气管内给药)
coli- 大肠杆菌的,大肠埃希杆菌的
colibacillemia [ˌkəulibæsiˈliːmiə] *n* 大肠杆菌菌血症
colibacillosis [ˌkəulibæsiˈləusis] *n* 大肠杆菌病 | ~ gravidarum 妊娠期大肠杆菌病
colibacilluria [ˌkəuliˌbæsiˈljuəriə] *n* 大肠杆菌尿
colibacillus [ˌkəulibəˈsiləs] *n* 大肠杆菌,大肠埃希杆菌
colic [ˈkɔlik] *a* 结肠的 *n* 绞痛,急腹痛 | biliary ~, gallstone ~, hepatic ~ 胆绞痛,胆石绞痛,肝绞痛 / bilious ~ 吐胆性绞痛 / copper ~ 铜绞痛(铜中毒所致) / endemic ~ 地方性绞痛 / flatulent ~ 气绞痛,气鼓,鼓胀 / infantile ~ 婴儿腹痛 / lead ~, painter's ~, saturnine ~ 铅绞痛 / menstrual ~ 痛经,经期绞痛 / ovarian ~ 卵巢绞痛 / renal ~, nephric ~ 肾绞痛 / stercoral ~ 便秘绞痛 / tubal ~ 输卵管绞痛 / ureteral ~ 输尿管绞痛 / uterine ~ 子宫绞痛 / vermicular ~, appendicular ~ 阑尾绞痛 / verminous ~, worm ~ 蠕虫性绞痛 / wind ~ 气绞痛 / zinc ~ 锌绞痛(慢性锌中毒所致)
colica [ˈkɔlikə] *n*【拉】绞痛,急腹痛 | ~ pictonum 铅绞痛
colicin [ˈkɔlisin] *n* 大肠[杆]菌素
colicinogen [ˌkɔliˈsinədʒən] *n* 大肠杆菌素原(亦称产杆菌素因子)
colicinogeny [ˌkɔlisiˈnɔdʒini] *n* 产大肠杆菌素性,大肠杆菌素产生 | **colicinogenic** [ˌkɔliˌsinəˈdʒenik] *a* 产大肠杆菌素的
colicky [ˈkɔliki] *a* 绞痛的,腹痛的,急腹痛的
colicoplegia [ˌkɔlikəuˈpliːdʒiə] *n* 绞痛麻痹(指铅绞痛和铅毒性麻痹同时存在)
colicystitis [ˌkəulisisˈtaitis] *n* 大肠杆菌性膀胱炎
colicystopyelitis [ˌkəuliˌsistəuˌpaiiˈlaitis] *n* 大肠杆菌性膀胱肾盂炎
coliform [ˈkəulifɔːm] *n* 大肠菌类;大肠菌 *a* 大肠杆菌状的

colinearity [ˌkəulini'æləti] *n* 共线性
colinephritis [ˌkəuline'fraitis] *n* 大肠杆菌性肾炎
colipase [kəu'laipeis] *n* 辅脂肪酶,共脂肪酶
coliphage ['kɔlifeidʒ] *n* 大肠杆菌噬菌体
coliplication [ˌkəuliplai'keiʃən] *n* 结肠折术
colipuncture ['kəuliˌpʌŋktʃə] *n* 结肠穿刺术
colisepsis [ˌkəuli'sepsis] *n* 大肠杆菌性脓毒病
colistatin [ˌkəuli'steitin] *n* 制大肠杆菌素
colistimethate sodium [kəˌlisti'meθeit] 多黏菌素 E 甲磺酸钠(抗生素类药)
colistin [kə'listin] *n* 多黏菌素 E(抗生素类药) | ~ sulfate 硫酸多黏菌素 E
colitis [kɔ'laitis] ([复] **colitides** [kɔ'litidiːz]) *n* 结肠炎 | amebic ~ 阿米巴性结肠炎,阿米巴痢疾 / antibiotic-associated ~ 抗生素性结肠炎 / balantidial ~ 毛囊虫性结肠炎,袋虫性结肠炎 / ischemic ~ 缺血性结肠炎 / mucous ~, myxomembranous ~ 黏液性结肠炎,黏液膜性结肠炎 / regional ~, segmental ~ 局限性结肠炎,节段性结肠炎 / transmural ~ 透壁性结肠炎 / ulcerative ~, ~ gravis 溃疡性结肠炎
colitose ['kɔlitəus] *n* 大肠杆菌糖
colitoxemia [ˌkəulitɔk'siːmiə] *n* 大肠杆菌毒血症
colitoxicosis [ˌkəuliˌtɔksi'kəusis] *n* 大肠杆菌毒素中毒
colitoxin [ˌkəuli'tɔksin] *n* 大肠杆菌毒素
coliuria [ˌkəuli'juəriə] *n* 大肠杆菌尿
colla ['kɔlə] collum 的复数
collacin ['kɔləsin] *n* 胶质素
collagen ['kɔlədʒən] *n* 胶原 | fibrous long-spacing (FLS) ~ 长间距纤维胶原 / segment long-spacing(SLS) ~ 长间距节段胶原
collagenase [kə'lædʒineis] *n* 胶原酶 | Clostridium histolyticum ~ 溶组织梭菌胶原酶(亦称梭菌肽酶 A) / vertebrate ~ 脊椎动物胶原酶
collagenation [kɔ'lædʒi'neiʃən] *n* 胶原生成
collagenic [ˌkɔlə'dʒenik] *a* 胶原的,产生胶原的
collagenitis [kəˌlædʒi'naitis] *n* 胶原炎
collagenoblast [kɔ'lædʒinəblæst] *n* 成胶原细胞
collagenocyte [kɔ'lædʒinəˌsait] *n* 胶原细胞
collagenogenic [ˌkɔlədʒenəu'dʒenik] *a* 产生胶原的,胶原生成的;形成胶原的,形成胶原纤维的
collagenolysis [ˌkɔlədʒe'nɔlisis] *n* 胶原溶解 | **collagenolytic** [kɔˌlædʒinə'litik] *a* 溶胶原的
collagenosis [kɔˌlædʒi'nəusis] *n* 胶原性疾病
collagenous [kɔ'lædʒinəs] *a* 胶原的;产生胶原的,形成胶原的
collapse [kə'læps] *n* 虚脱;萎陷 | circulatory ~ 循环性虚脱 / ~ of the lung 肺萎陷 / massive ~ (肺)大块萎陷
collar ['kɔlə] *n* 颈圈;假牙颈;(噬菌体)颈部 | ~ of pearls, venereal ~, ~ of Venus 颈部梅毒白斑病 / periosteal bone ~ 骨领 / Spanish ~ 箝顿包茎
collarbone ['kɔləbəun] *n* 锁骨
collarette [ˌkɔlə'ret] *n* 蜀黍红疹颈圈;角线;囊领
collastin [kə'læstin] *n* 胶质素
collateral [kɔ'lætərəl] *a* 并行的;附属的;伴随的;侧的,副的 *n* 侧突(轴索);侧支
collect [kə'lekt] *vt* 收集
collection [kə'lekʃən] *n* 收集,采集;收集品,标本收藏
collective [kə'lektiv] *a* 集合的,共同的;集体的
collector [kə'lektə] *n* 收集者;收集器
college ['kɔlidʒ] *n* 学院 | medical ~ 医学院
Colles-Baumès law ['kɔliːz bɔ'mei] (Abraham Colles; Pierre P. F. Baumès) 柯莱斯-博梅定律(见 Colles'law)
Colles' fascia ['kɔliːz] (Abraham Colles) 尿生殖膈下筋膜 | ~ fracture 柯莱斯骨折(桡骨下端骨折,下部碎片向后移位,如其下部碎片向前移位,则称史密斯〈Smith〉骨折) / ~ law 柯莱斯定律(患先天梅毒的儿童,其母无症状,也不传染其母) / ~ ligament 腹股沟翻转韧带 / ~ space 会阴筋膜下隙
Colletotrichum [ˌkɔlətəu'trikəm] *n* 刺盘孢属
Collet's syndrome, Collet-Sicard syndrome [kɔ'lei si'kɑː] (Frédéric J. Collet; Jean A. Sicard) 科莱综合征,科莱-西卡尔综合征(第 9、10、11、13 脑神经完全损伤所致的舌喉肩胛咽偏瘫)
colliculectomy [kɔˌlikju'lektəmi] *n* 精阜切除术
colliculitis [kɔˌlikju'laitis] *n* 精阜炎
colliculus [kɔ'likjuləs] ([复] **colliculi** [kɔ'likjulai]) *n*【拉】小丘 | facial ~ 面神经丘 / inferior ~ 下丘(四叠体) / seminal ~ 精阜 / superior ~ 上丘(四叠体)
colligative ['kɔliˌgeitiv] *a* 依数[性]的(在物理化学中指依赖于存在一定空间的分子数,而并不依赖于分子的大小、分子量或化学结构)
collimate ['kɔlimeit] *vt* 校准,使准直,使(光线)平行 | **collimation** [ˌkɔli'meiʃən] *n* 准直 / **collimator** [ˌkɔli'meitə] *n* 准直仪,平行光管
Collinsonia [ˌkɔlin'səuniə] (Peter Collinson) *n* 二蕊紫苏属 | ~ canadensis 二蕊紫苏(利尿、强壮药)
Collin's osteoclast ['kɔlin] (Anatole Collin) 柯林碎骨器,柯林折骨器(用以折断任何一点上的骨)
Collip unit ['kɔlip] (James B. Collip) 科利普单位(一种甲状旁腺浸膏的剂量单位)
colliquation [ˌkɔli'kweiʃən] *n* 溶化,液化,液化变性(组织) | ballooning ~ (细胞原生质)肿大性液化 / reticulating ~ (细胞原生质)网状液化

colliquative [kəˈlikwətiv] *a* 过多排液的;液化的,溶化的

collision [kəˈliʒən] *n* 碰撞

collocate [ˈkɔləukeit] *vt* 把…并置排列,配置 | **collocation** [ˌkɔləuˈkeiʃən] *n* 并置,排列,配置

collochemistry [ˌkɔləuˈkemistri] *n* 胶体化学

collodiaphyseal [ˌkɔləuˌdaiəˈfiziəl] *a* 颈及骨干的(尤指股骨)

collodion [kəˈləudjən] *n* 火棉胶[剂] | flexible ~, ~ elastique 弹性火棉胶(表面保护剂) / salicylic acid ~ 水杨酸火棉胶(角质分离剂)

colloid [ˈkɔlɔid] *a* 胶体的,胶态的 *n* 胶体,胶质;胶态 | amyl ~, anodyne ~ 戊基胶体,止痛胶 / antimony trisulfide ~ 三硫化二锑胶体(制药辅剂) / association ~ 联合胶体 / bovine ~ 胶固素,黏合素 / emulsion ~, hydrophilic ~, lyophilic ~, lyotropic ~ 乳胶体,亲液胶体 / suspension ~, hydrophobic ~, lyophobic ~ 悬胶体,疏液胶体 / stannous sulfur ~ 亚锡硫胶体(骨、肝和脾成像的诊断辅剂)

colloidal [kəˈlɔidl] *a* 胶体的,胶质的;胶态的

colloidin [kəˈlɔidin] *n* 胶[体]变[性]质,胶体素

colloidoclasia [kəˌlɔidəuˈkleisiə], **colloidoclasis** [kəˌlɔidəuˈkleisis] *n* 胶体性猝衰(产生过敏性休克)

colloidophagy [ˌkɔlɔiˈdɔfədʒi] *n* 胶体吞噬(在促甲状腺激素影响下胶体为巨噬细胞所吸收)

colloxylin [kəˈlɔksilin] *n* 火棉,低氮硝化纤维素

collum [ˈkɔləm] ([复] **colla** [ˈkɔlə]) *n*【拉】颈

collunarium [ˌkɔljuˈnɛəriəm] ([复] **collunaria** [ˌkɔljuˈnɛəriə]) *n*【拉】洗鼻剂

Collut. collutorium【拉】漱口剂

collutorium [ˌkɔljuˈtɔːriəm] ([复] **collutoria** [ˌkɔljuˈtɔːriə]) *n*【拉】漱口剂

collutory [ˈkɔljutəri] *n* 漱口剂

Collyr. collyrium【拉】洗眼剂

Collyriculum [ˌkɔliˈrikjuləm] *n* 瘤吸虫属 | ~ faba 鸟瘤吸虫

collyrium [kəˈliriəm] ([复] **collyria** [kəˈliriə]) *n* 洗眼剂,洗眼液

colo- [构词成分]结肠

coloboma [ˌkɔləˈbəumə] ([复] **colobomas** 或 **colobomata** [ˌkɔləˈbəumətə]) *n* 缺损(指眼组织) | bridge ~ 桥形缺损(指虹膜) / ~ of choroid 脉络膜缺损 / ~ of iris 虹膜缺损 / ~ of retina 视网膜缺损 / retinochoroidal ~, ~ of fundus 视网膜脉络膜缺损,眼底缺损 / ~ of vitreous 玻璃状体缺损

colocecostomy [ˌkəuləusiˈkɔstəmi] *n* 结肠盲肠吻合术

colocentesis [ˌkəuləusenˈtiːsis] *n* 结肠穿刺术

colocholecystostomy [ˌkəuləuˌkɔlisisˈtɔstəmi] *n* 结肠胆囊吻合术,胆囊结肠吻合术

coloclysis [ˌkəuləuˈklaisis], **coloclyster** [ˌkəuləuˈklistə] *n* 结肠灌洗,灌肠

colocolostomy [ˌkəuləukəˈlɔstəmi] *n* 结肠结肠吻合术

colocutaneous [ˌkəuləukjuˈteinjəs] *a* 结肠[与]皮肤的

colocynth [ˈkɔləsinθ], **colocynthis** [ˌkɔləˈsinθis] *n* 药西瓜瓤(可作泻药)

colocynthidism [ˌkɔləˈsinθidizəm] *n* 药西瓜中毒

colocynthin [ˌkɔləˈsinθin] *n* 药西瓜苦

colodyspepsia [ˌkəuləudisˈpepsiə] *n* 结肠性消化不良

coloenteritis [ˌkəuləuˌentəˈraitis] *n* 小肠结肠炎,大小肠炎

colofixation [ˌkəuləufikˈseiʃən] *n* 结肠固定术

colography [kəˈlɔgrəfi] *n* 结肠造影术

colohepatopexy [ˌkəuləuˈhepətəˌpeksi] *n* 结肠肝固定术

coloileal [ˌkəuləuˈiliəl] *a* 结肠回肠的

colOlysis [kəˈlɔlisis] *n* 结肠松解术

colometrometer [ˌkəuləumiˈtrɔmitə] *n* 结肠活动测定器

colon [ˌkəulən] ([复] **cola** [ˈkəulə] 或 **colons**) *n* 结肠 | ascending ~ 升结肠 / descending ~ 降结肠 / giant ~ 巨结肠 / irritable ~ 过敏性结肠,结肠过敏,激惹性结肠 / lead-pipe ~ 结肠强直 / sigmoid ~ 乙状结肠 / transverse ~ 横结肠 | **~ic** [kəˈlɔnik] *a*

colonalgia [ˌkəuləˈnældʒiə] *n* 结肠痛

colonial [kəˈləunjəl] *a* 集群的,群体的;菌落的

colonitis [ˌkɔləˈnaitis] *n* 结肠炎

colonize [ˈkɔlənaiz] *vt* 移生,移地发育;集中护理(精神病人);建群,定居 | **colonization** [ˌkɔlənaiˈzeiʃən,-niˈz-] *n*

Colonna's operation [kəˈləunə] (Paul Colonna) 科隆纳手术(①股骨颈囊内骨折修复术;②髋部囊关节成形术)

colonography [ˌkəuləˈnɔgrəfi] *n* 结肠造影术

colonopathy [ˌkəuləˈnɔpəθi] *n* 结肠病

colonorrhagia [ˌkəulənəˈreidʒiə] *n* 结肠出血

colonorrhea [ˌkəulənəˈriːə] *n* 结肠黏液溢,黏液性结肠炎

colonoscope [kəˈlɔnəskəup] *n* 结肠镜

colonoscopy [ˌkəuləˈnɔskəpi] *n* 结肠镜检查[术]

colony [ˈkɔləni] *n* 菌落,集落;集群;群体 | bitten ~, nibbled ~ 缺蚀菌落 / butyrous ~ 奶油样菌落 / checker ~ 棋盘菌落 / daisy-head ~ 雏菊花头菌落 / daughter ~ 子菌落 / disgonic ~ 微弱菌落 / dwarf ~, D ~ 侏儒型菌落 / effuse ~ 弥散菌落 / H ~ H 菌落(能动型菌落) / matte ~ 无光泽菌落 / motile ~ 运动菌落 / mucoid

~, M ~ 黏稠菌落 / O ~ O 菌落(不动型菌落) / rough ~, R ~ 粗糙型菌落 / satellite ~ 卫星菌落,卫星菌,陪菌(如在葡萄球菌菌落附近的流感嗜血杆菌) / smooth ~, S ~ 光滑型菌落
colopathy [kəˈlɔpəθi] *n* 结肠病
colopexotomy [ˈkəuləupekˈsɔtəmi] *n* 结肠固定切开术
colopexy [ˈkəuləˌpeksi], **colopexia** [ˌkəuləˈpeksiə] *n* 结肠固定术
colophony [kəˈlɔfəni] *n* 松香(rosin 的旧名)
coloplication [ˌkəuləuplaiˈkeiʃən] *n* 结肠折术
coloproctectomy [ˌkəuləuprɔkˈtektəmi] *n* 结肠直肠切除术
coloproctitis [ˌkəuləuprɔkˈtaitis] *n* 结肠直肠炎
coloproctostomy [ˌkəuləuprɔkˈtɔstəmi] *n* 结肠直肠吻合术
coloptosis [ˌkəulɔpˈtəusis] *n* 结肠下垂
colopuncture [ˈkəuləˌpʌŋktʃə] *n* 结肠穿刺术
Color. coloretur【拉】需着色
color [ˈkʌlə] *n* 色,色泽 *vt* 着色 *vi* 变色 | complementary ~s 补色 / confusion ~s 混淆色 / contrast ~ 反衬色 / incidental ~ 后遗色[觉] / primary ~s 原色 / pseudoisochromatic ~s 假同色 / pure ~ 纯色 / saturation ~ 饱和色
colorable [ˈkʌlərəbl] *a* 可着色的
coloration [ˌkʌləˈreiʃən] *n* 着色,显色 | protective ~ 保护色 / warning ~ 警戒色
color-blind [ˈkʌlə blaind] *a* 色盲的 | **~ness** *n*
colorectal [kɔləˈrektl] *a* 结肠直肠的
colorectitis [ˌkəulərekˈtaitis] *n* 结肠直肠炎
colorectostomy [ˌkəulərekˈtɔstəmi] *n* 结肠直肠吻合术
colorectum [ˌkɔləˈrektəm] *n* 结肠直肠
colorimeter [ˌkʌləˈrimitə] *n* 比色计 | titration ~ 滴定比色计 | **colorimetry** *n* 比色法 / **colorimetric** [ˌkʌləriˈmetrik] *a* 比色[法]的
coloring [ˈkʌləriŋ] *n* 着色[法];面色;特质
colorrhaphy [kəˈlɔrəfi] *n* 结肠缝合术
colorrhea [ˌkəuləˈriːə] *n* 结肠黏液溢,黏液性结肠炎
coloscope [ˈkɔləskəup] *n* 结肠镜
coloscopy [kəˈlɔskəpi] *n* 结肠镜检查
colosigmoidostomy [ˌkəuləˌsigmɔiˈdɔstəmi] *n* 结肠乙状结肠吻合术
colostomy [kəˈlɔstəmi] *n* 结肠造口术 | dry ~ 干性结肠造口术 / ileotransverse ~ 横结肠造口术 / wet ~ 湿性结肠造口术
colostrorrhea [kəˌlɔstrəˈriːə] *n* 初乳溢
colostrous [kəˈlɔstrəs] *a* 初乳的
colostrum [kəˈlɔstrəm] *n*【拉】初乳 | ~ gravidarum 妊娠初乳 / ~ puerperarum 产褥初乳 | **colostric** [kəˈlɔstrik] *a*
colotomy [kəˈlɔtəmi] *n* 结肠切开术
colotyphoid [ˌkəuləuˈtaifɔid] *n* 结肠型伤寒
colour [ˈkʌlə] *n*, *vt*, *vi* =color
colovaginal [ˌkəuləuvəˈdʒainəl,-ˈvædʒi-] *a* 结肠阴道的
colovesical [ˌkəuləu ˈvesikəl] 结肠膀胱的
colp- 见 colpo-
colpalgia [kɔlˈpældʒiə] *n* 阴道痛
colpatresia [ˌkɔlpəˈtriːziə] *n* 阴道闭锁
colpectasia [ˌkɔlpekˈteiziə], **colpectasis** [kɔlˈpektəsis] *n* 阴道扩张
colpectomy [kɔlˈpektəmi] *n* 阴道切除术
colpeurynter [ˈkɔlpjuˌrintə] *n* 阴道扩张袋(即宫颈扩张袋)
colpeurysis [kɔlˈpjuərisis] *n* 阴道扩张术
colpismus [kɔlˈpizməs] *n* 阴道痉挛
colpitis [kɔlˈpaitis] *n* 阴道炎 | ~ emphysematosa, emphysematous ~ 气肿性阴道炎 / ~ mycotica 真菌性阴道炎,霉菌性阴道炎(即阴道霉菌病) | **colpitic** [kɔlˈpitik] *a*
colp(o)-[构词成分]阴道
colpocele [ˈkɔlpəsiːl] *n* 阴道疝;阴道脱垂
colpoceliocentesis [ˌkɔlpəuˌsiːliəusenˈtiːsis] *n* 经阴道腹腔穿刺术,阴道式腹腔穿刺术
colpoceliotomy [ˌkɔlpəuˌsiːliˈɔtəmi] *n* 经阴道剖腹术,阴道式剖腹术
colpocephaly [ˌkɔlpəuˈsefəli] *n* 侧脑室枕角增大
colpocleisis [ˌkɔlpəuˈklaisis] *n* 阴道闭合术
colpocystitis [ˌkɔlpəusisˈtaitis] *n* 阴道膀胱炎
colpocystocele [ˌkɔlpəuˈsistəsiːl] *n* 阴道内膀胱膨出
colpocystoplasty [ˌkɔlpəuˈsistəˌplæsti] *n* 阴道膀胱成形术
colpocystotomy [ˌkɔlpəusisˈtɔtəmi] *n* 阴道膀胱切开术
colpocystoureterocystotomy [ˌkɔlpəuˌsistəujuəˌriːtərəusisˈtɔtəmi] *n* 阴道膀胱壁切开输尿管露出术
colpocytogram [ˌkɔlpəuˈsaitəgræm] *n* 阴道细胞涂片谱
colpocytology [ˌkɔlpəusaiˈtɔlədʒi] *n* 阴道细胞学
Colpodida [kɔlˈpəudidə] *n* 肾形[纤虫]目
colpodynia [ˌkɔlpəuˈdiniə] *n* 阴道痛
colpohyperplasia [ˌkɔlpəuhaipəˈpleiziə] *n* 阴道黏膜增生 | ~ cystica 囊肿性阴道黏膜增生 / ~ emphysematosa 气肿性阴道黏膜增生
colpomicroscope [ˌkɔlpəuˈmaikrəskəup] *n* 阴道显微镜 | **colpomicroscopy** [ˌkɔlpəumaiˈkrɔskəpi] *n* 阴道显微镜检查 / **colpomicroscopic** [ˌkɔlpəumaikrəsˈkɔpik] *a* 阴道显微镜的;阴道显微镜

检查的

colpomyomectomy [ˌkɔlpəuˌmaiəuˈmektəmi] *n* 阴道[式]子宫肌瘤切除术

colpoperineoplasty [ˌkɔlpəuˌperiˈniːəuˌplæsti] *n* 阴道会阴成形术

colpoperineorrhaphy [ˌkɔlpəuˌperiniːˈɔrəfi] *n* 阴道会阴缝合术

colpopexy [ˈkɔlpəˌpeksi] *n* 阴道固定术

colpoplasty [ˈkɔlpəˌplæsti] *n* 阴道成形术

colpopoiesis [ˌkɔlpəupɔiˈiːsis] *n* 阴道成形术

colpoptosis [ˌkɔlpəˈptəusis] *n* 阴道下垂

colporectopexy [ˌkɔlpəˈrektəˌpeksi] *n* 阴道直肠固定术

colporrhagia [ˌkɔlpəˈreidʒiə] *n* 阴道出血

colporrhaphy [kɔlˈpɔrəfi] *n* 阴道缝合术；阴道缩窄术

colporrhexis [ˌkɔlpəˈreksis] *n* 阴道破裂

colposcope [ˈkɔlpəskəup] *n* 阴道镜 | **colposcopy** [kɔlˈpɔskəpi] *n* 阴道镜检查 / **colposcopic** [ˌkɔlpəˈskɔpik] *a* 阴道镜的；阴道镜检查的

colpospasm [ˈkɔlpəspæzəm] *n* 阴道痉挛

colpostat [ˈkɔlpəstæt] *n* 阴道镭置器

colpostenosis [ˌkɔlpəustiˈneusis] *n* 阴道狭窄

colpostenotomy [ˌkɔlpəustiˈnɔtəmi] *n* 阴道狭窄切开术

colposuspension [ˌkɔlpəusəsˈpenʃən] *n* 膀胱颈悬吊术

colpotherm [ˈkɔlpəθəːm] *n* 阴道电热器

colpotomy [kɔlˈpɔtəmi] *n* 阴道切开术 | posterior ~ 阴道后穹窿切开术，子宫直肠陷凹切开术

colpoureterocystotomy [ˌkɔlpəujuəˌriːtərəusisˈtɔtəmi] *n* 阴道膀胱输尿管切开术

colpoureterotomy [ˌkɔlpəujuəˌriːtəˈrɔtəmi] *n* 阴道输尿管切开术

colpoxerosis [ˌkɔlpəuziəˈrəusis] *n* 阴道干燥

colterol mesylate [ˈkəultərɔl] 甲磺酸可尔特罗（支气管扩张药）

Coltivirus [ˈkɔltiˌvaiərəs] *n* 科罗拉多蜱传热病毒属

Colton blood group [ˈkəultən]（从 1965 年首次报道的挪威先证者得名）柯尔顿血型

Coluber [ˈkɔljubə] *n* 游蛇属

colubrid [ˈkɔljubrid] *n* 游蛇 *a* 游蛇科的

Colubridae [kɔˈljuːbridiː] *n* 游蛇科

columbium [kəˈlʌmbiəm] *n* 钶（元素铌〈niobium〉的旧名）

columella [ˌkɔljuˈmelə]（[复] **columellae** [ˌkɔljuˈmeliː]）*n*【拉】小柱；囊轴 | ~ cochleae 蜗轴 / ~ nasi 鼻小柱

columellate [ˌkɔljuˈmeleit] *a* 小柱的；具囊轴的

column [ˈkɔləm] *n* 柱 | ~s of abdominal ring 腹股沟管皮下环脚 / anal ~s 肛柱，直肠柱 / fat ~s 皮下脂肪柱 / fractionating ~ 分馏柱 / fundamental ~ 固有束 / muscle ~ 肌柱，肌原纤维 / ~ of nose 鼻中隔 / rectal ~s 肛柱，直肠柱 / ~s of rugae of vagina, ~s of vagina 阴道柱，阴道嵴柱 / vertebral ~, dorsal ~, spinal ~ 脊柱 | **~ar** [kəˈlʌmnə], **~ed** [ˈkɔləmd] *a*

columna [kəˈlʌmnə]（[复] **columnae** [kəˈlʌmniː]）*n*【拉】柱

columnella [ˌkɔləmˈnelə] *n*【拉】小柱

columnization [ˌkɔləmnaiˈzeiʃən, -niˈz-], **columning** [ˈkɔləmniŋ] *n* 棉塞支托法（用于子宫脱垂）

colypeptic [ˌkəuliˈpeptik] *a* 抑制消化的，调整消化的

coma [ˈkəumə] *n* 昏迷；斜射球面象差 | alcoholic ~ 酒精中毒昏迷 / alpha ~ α 昏迷（脑电波显示明显的 α 波活动）/ apoplectic ~ 中风昏迷，卒中昏迷 / diabetic ~ 糖尿病昏迷 / hepatic ~, ~ hepaticum 肝[性]昏迷 / hyperosmolar nonketotic ~ 高渗性非酮症性昏迷 / irreversible ~ 不可逆性昏迷，脑死亡 / metabolic ~ 代谢性昏迷/ ~ somnolentium 嗜睡样昏迷 / trance ~ 催眠性昏睡 / uremic ~ 尿毒症昏迷 / ~ vigil, agrypnodal ~ 睁眼昏迷，醒状昏迷 | **~tose** [ˈkəumətəus] *a*

comanic acid [kəuˈmænik] 哌啶甲酸

COMB cyclophosphamide, vincristine, semustine, and bleomycin 环磷酰胺-长春新碱-司莫司汀-博来霉素（联合化疗治癌方案）

combination [ˌkɔmbiˈneiʃən] *n* 联合，结合；化合；复合

combinative [ˈkɔmbinətiv] *a* 结合的

combing [ˈkəumiŋ] *n* 神经纤维松解法

combining [kəmˈbainiŋ] *a* 结合性的；化合的

combustible [kəmˈbʌstəbl] *a* 易燃的，可燃的 *n* 易燃物，可燃物

combustion [kəmˈbʌstʃən] *n* 燃烧 | **combustive** [kəmˈbʌstiv] *a*

comedo [ˈkɔmidəu]（[复] **comedos** 或 **comedones** [ˌkɔmiˈdəuniːz]）*n* 粉刺

comedocarcinoma [kɔˌmidəukɑːsiˈnəumə] *n* 粉刺性癌

comedogenic [ˌkɔmidəuˈdʒenik] *a* 产生粉刺的，引起粉刺的

comedomastitis [kəˌmidəumæsˈtaitis] *n* 粉刺状乳腺炎，乳腺管扩张

comenic acid [kəuˈmenik] 可孟酸，羟基吡喃羰酸

comes [ˈkəumiːz]（[复] **comites** [ˈkəumitiːz]）*n*【拉】伴行血管，并行血管（伴同神经的动脉或静脉，如坐骨神经伴行动脉）

comfimeter [kʌmˈfimitə] *n* 空气冷却力计（用于室内保持舒适）

comfortization [ˌkʌmfətai'zeiʃən] *n* 使舒适(应用生理学原理力求在潜在紧张的处境中达到舒适,如用于飞机设计)

comfrey ['kʌmfri] *n* 聚合草

comites ['kəumitiːz] comes 的复数

commasculation [kəˌmæskju'leiʃən] *n* 男性互恋,男子同性恋

commensal [kə'mensəl] *a* 共生的,共栖的 *n* 共生体,共栖体 | **~ism** *n* 偏利共栖(两种生物共同生活在一起,一方从另一方获取营养,而后者既无得益,亦不受损)

commentary ['kɔməntəri] *n* 评论;注解 | medical ~ 病案附注

Commiphora [kɔ'mifərə] *n* 没药属

commissura [ˌkɔmi'sjuərə] ([复] **commissurae** [ˌkɔmi'sjuəriː]) *n* 【拉】连合

commissure ['kɔmisjuə] *n* 连合,接缝处 | anterior ~ of cerebrum 大脑前连合 / anterior ~ of labia 阴唇前连合 / ~ of fornix, hippocampal ~ 穹窿连合,海马连合 / interthalamic ~ , middle ~ of cerebrum 中间块,大脑中连合(即丘脑间黏合) / ~ of lips of mouth 唇连合,口角 / medial ~ of eyelids 睑内侧连合,内眦 / posterior ~ (大脑)后连合 / supraoptic ~s 视上连合 | **commissural** [ˌkɔmi'sjuərəl] *a*

commissurorrhaphy [ˌkɔmisjuə'rɔrəfi] *n* 连合部缝合术

commissurotomy [ˌkɔmisjuə'rɔtəmi] *n* 连合部切开术

commotio [kə'məuʃiəu] *n* 【拉】震荡(震荡性休克) | ~ cerebri 脑震荡,脑震伤 / ~ retinae 视网膜震荡 / ~ spinalis 脊椎震荡

communicable [kə'mjuːnikəbl] *a* 传染的,传播的 | **communicability** [kəˌmjuːnikə'biləti] *n* 传染性 / **communicably** *ad*

communicans [kə'mjuːnikənz] *a* 【拉】交通的(如神经)

communis [kə'mjuːnis] *a* 【拉】普通的

community [kə'mjuːnəti] *n* 社会;社区;群落 | biotic ~ 生物群落 / climax ~ 顶极群落 / seral ~ 演替系列群落 / therapeutic ~ 治疗中心(专门组织安排好的精神病院或病房,运用集体疗法和环境疗法鼓励病人在社会规范内活动)

Comolli's sign [kɔ'mɔli] (Antonio Comolli) 科莫利征(肩胛骨骨折后很快在肩胛区出现重现肩胛骨形状的三角形肿胀)

Comp. compositus【拉】复方的,复合的

compact [kəm'pækt] *a* 紧密的,致密的

compacta [kəm'pæktə] *n* 致密层(蜕膜)

compaction [kəm'pækʃən] *n* 双胎紧贴

compages [kəm'peidʒiz] [单复同] *n* 【拉】综合结构;骨架 | ~ thoracis 胸廓

companion [kəm'pænjən] *n* 同伴;[复]伴生种

comparascope [kəm'pærəskəup] *n* 双片对比显微镜

comparative [kəm'pærətiv] *a* 比较的 *n* 比拟物

comparator ['kɔmpəreitə] *n* 比较器,比值器,比色器

compartimentum [kəmˌpɑːti'mentəm] *n* 隔室,隔间;间隙

compartment [kəm'pɑːtmənt] *n* 区室;隔室,隔间 | muscular ~ 肌腔隙 / vascular ~ 血管腔隙

compartmentalization [ˌkɔmpɑːtˌmentəlai'zeiʃən, -li'z-], **compartmentation** [kəmˌpɑːtmen'teiʃən] *n* 区室化,区室作用(选择性渗透膜在细胞内造成天然分隔,并围住每一个分隔的部分〈线粒体、溶酶体、高尔基复合体等〉,而使每一个部分得以调节各自的内含物)

compatibility [kəmˌpætə'biləti] *n* 相容性;可配伍性 | ~ of drugs 药物配伍

compensation [ˌkɔmpen'seiʃən] *n* 代偿(功能),补偿[作用] | broken ~ 代偿功能不全 / dosage ~ 剂量补偿(遗传学中指使正常女性两个 X 染色体的效应与正常男性一个 X 染色体的效应相等的机制) | **~al** *a*

compensator ['kɔmpenˌseitə] *n* 补偿器,伸缩器

competence ['kɔmpitəns] *n* 能力;胜任性;活性;感受态 | embryonic ~ 胚反应能力 / immunologic ~ 免疫活性 | **competency** ['kɔmpitənsi] *n*

competent ['kɔmpitənt] *a* 有能力的,能胜任的;活性的;感受态的

competition [kɔmpi'tiʃən] *n* 竞争(两种结构相似的分子"竞争"第三种分子上的一个结合部位) | antigenic ~ 抗原竞争(同时或短时内给予两种免疫原所引起的对免疫原应答的改变,对第一种免疫原应答正常,而对第二种免疫原的应答则抑制或减弱)

compimeter [kəm'pimitə] *n* 视野计

complain [kəm'plein] *vi* 陈诉,主诉

complaint [kəm'pleint] *n* 陈诉,主诉;病 | chief ~ 主诉 / summer ~ 假霍乱,欧洲霍乱

complement ['kɔmplimənt] *n* 补体 | dominant ~ 显性补体(各种补体中显示特异性作用者) / endocellular ~ (红细胞)内补体

complementary [ˌkɔmpli'mentəri], **complemental** [ˌkɔmpli'mentl] *a* 补偿的;补充的;互补的

complementation [ˌkɔmplimen'teiʃən] *n* 互补 | intercistronic ~ , intergenic ~ 顺反子间互补,基因间互补 / intracistronic ~ , intragenic ~ , interallelic ~ 顺反子内互补,基因内互补

complemented ['kɔmpliˌmentid] *a* 补体致活的

complementoid [ˌkɔmpli'mentɔid] *n* 类补体(在早期免疫学说中,指补体已失去活性,但不影响

它与介体的结合力，类补体由补体加热后产生，注射时能产生抗补体）

complementophil [ˌkɔmpliˈmentəfil] *a* 嗜补体的（在早期免疫学说中指介体对补体有亲和力）

complex [ˈkɔmpleks, kəmˈpleks] *a* 复杂的；综合的；络合的；复合的 [ˈkɔmpleks] *n* 复(合)体；络合物；复征，综合征；情结；复合波（心电图）| adrenochrome monosemicarbazone sodium salicylate ~ 肾上腺色素缩氨脲水杨酸钠复合物 / AIDS-related ~ (ARC) 艾滋病相关复征（代表人免疫缺陷病毒感染一型的复合体征和症状，其病情较典型的获得性免疫缺陷综合征为轻，特征为慢性全身性淋巴结病伴发热、体重减轻、长期腹泻、轻微条件致病菌感染、血细胞减少以及与艾滋病有关的T细胞异常）/ amygdaloid ~ 杏仁体 / amyotrophic lateral sclerosis-parkinsonism-de-mentia ~ 肌萎缩性侧索硬化-帕金森神经功能障碍-痴呆复征（一种常染色体显性遗传疾病）/ anomalous ~ 异常复合波 / antigen-antibody ~ 抗原抗体复合物（抗原和抗体以非共价结合而形成的复合物，亦称免疫复合物 immune complex，但此术语特别在讨论疾病时使用）/ atrial ~ 心房复合波（心电图的P波）/ avian leukosis ~ 家禽造白细胞组织增生综合征 / basal ~ of choroid 脉络膜基底层 / Cain ~ 兄弟情结 / calcarine ~ 禽距 / castration ~ 阉割情结 / EAHF ~ 湿症、哮喘、枯草热复征 / Electra ~，father ~ 恋父情结 / factor Ⅸ ~ 因子Ⅸ复合物（一种无菌干冻粉末，含有从健康人供血者静脉血浆中提取的部分纯化的因子Ⅸ成分以及浓缩的因子Ⅱ，Ⅶ和Ⅹ成分）/ H-2 ~ H-2复合体（鼠的主要组织相容性复合体）/ hapten-carrier ~ 半抗原-载体复合物（半抗原与载体蛋白结合而成的抗原）/ HLA ~ HLA复合体（人类主要组织相容性复合体）/ immune ~ 免疫复合物（即 antigen-antibody ~）/ inclusion ~es 包涵体复合物 / inferiority ~ 自卑情结，自卑感 / jumped process ~ 脊椎关节突脱位 / junctional ~ 连接复合体（相邻的柱状上皮细胞之间的细胞排列，含有密闭小带，黏着小带和桥粒）/ α-ketoglutarate dehydrogenase ~ α-酮戊二酸脱氢酶复合体 / α-ketoisovalerate dehydrogenase ~ α-酮异戊酸脱氢酶复合体 / major histocompatibility ~ (MHC) 主要组织相容性复合体（人类为HLA复合体，鼠为H-2复合体）/ membrane attack ~ (MAC) 膜攻击复合体 / Oedipus ~，mother ~ 恋母情结 / perihypoglossal ~，perihypoglossal nuclear ~ 舌下周复合体，舌下周核复合体（亦称舌下周灰质）/ pore ~ 核孔复合体 / primary ~ 原发复合征（指实质性肺损害和相应的淋巴结病灶的复征，常见于儿童原发性结核）/ primary inoculation ~，primary tuberculosis ~ 原发性接种性复征，原发性结核性复征（即原发性接种性结核）/ sex ~ 性复[合]体 / superiority ~ 自尊情结，优越感 / symptom ~ 综合征 / synaptonemal ~ 联会丝复合体 / ureterotrigonal ~ 输尿管膀胱三角复合体（即输尿管膀胱连接）/ urobilin ~ 尿胆囊络合物 / ventricular ~es 心室复合波 / zymase ~ 酿酶复体

complexion [kəmˈplekʃən] *n* 面色，面容；肤色 | **~al** *a*

complexus [kəmˈpleksəs] *n*【拉】复[合]体 | ~ basalis choroideae 脉络膜基底层

compliance [kəmˈplaiəns] *n* 顺应性 | dynamic ~ 动态顺应性 / lung ~ 肺顺应性 / specific ~ 比顺应性 / static ~ 静态顺应性

complicate [ˈkɔmplikeit] *vt*, *vi* 并发

complicated [ˈkɔmplikeitid] *a* 并发的

complication [ˌkɔmpliˈkeiʃən] *n* 并发症，并发病

complon [ˈkɔmplɔn] *n* 互补单位，顺反子（见 cistron）

compomer [ˈkɔmpəmə] *n* 树脂基质复合填料

component [kəmˈpəunənt] *a* 组成的，合成的 *n* 组分，成分；组元（神经组元）| anterior ~ 殆向前动力 / complement ~s，~s of complement 补体成分 / group-specific ~ 组特异成分（维生素D结合蛋白）/ M ~ M成分（任何一类同种免疫球蛋白在电泳上出现一个非常窄的带，见于多发性骨髓瘤、原发性巨球蛋白血症、重链病及黏液水肿性苔藓）/ plasma thromboplastin ~ (PTC) 血浆凝血激酶组分，凝血因子Ⅸ / secretory ~ (SC) 分泌成分（分泌型IgA中的一种分子量为70 000的糖蛋白。亦称分泌片）/ somatic motor ~ 躯体运动组元 / somatic sensory ~ 躯体感觉组元 / splanchnic motor ~ 内脏运动组元 / splanchnic sensory ~ 内脏感觉组元

compos mentis [ˈkɔmpɔs ˈmentis]【拉】精神健全

composure [kəmˈpəuʒə] *n* 镇静，沉着

compound [kəmˈpaund] *vt* 使合成，使化合 [ˈkɔmpaund] *a* 复合的，复方的 *n* 化合物，复合物 | ~ A 化合物A，11-脱氢皮质[甾]酮 / acyclic ~ 无环化合物，开链化合物 / addition ~ 加成化合物 / aliphatic ~ 脂肪族化合物 / APC ~ 复方APC制剂 / ~ B 化合物B，皮质[甾]酮 / clathrate ~s 笼形化合物 / closed-chain ~ 闭链化合物 / condensation ~ 缩合物 / diazo ~ 偶氮化合物 / ~ E 可的松 / ~ F 氢化可的松 / high-energy ~s，energy-rich ~s 高能化合物 / inorganic ~ 无机化合物 / isocyclic ~ 碳环化合物，纯环化合物；等(原子数)环化合物 / low-energy ~s 低能化合物 / nonpolar ~s 非极性化合物 / open-chain ~ 开链化合物 / organic ~ 有机化合物 / paraffin ~ 烷属化合物 / quaternary ~ 四元化合物 / quaternary ammonium ~ 季铵化合物 / substitution ~ 取代化合物 / ternary ~，tertiary ~ 三元化合物

compress [kəm'pres] *vt* 压缩;浓缩 ['kɔmpres] *n* 敷布,压布 | cribriform ~ 筛形敷布 / fenestrated ~ 开孔敷布 / graduated ~ 梯形敷布,分级敷布 | **compressibility** [kəm,presi'biləti] *n* 可压性,压缩性;压缩系数

compression [kəm'preʃən] *n* 压迫;加压;压缩;发育期缩短 | ~ of the brain 脑受压 / digital ~ 指压法(止血) / instrumental ~ 器械压迫法(止血) / spinal ~ 脊髓受压

compressive [kəm'presiv] *a* 有压力的,压缩的

compressor [kəm'presə] *n*【拉】压迫器;压肌 | shot ~ 缝线珠镊

compressorium [,kɔmpre'sɔːriəm] ([复] **compressoria** [,kɔmpre'sɔːriə]) *n*【拉】压迫装置(显微镜检查)

compromised ['kɔmprəmaizd] *a* 妥协的(指由于某一疗程如照射等或某一疾病如白血病等的影响,对感染缺乏充分的抵抗力或免疫反应的能力)

Compton effect ['kʌmptən] (Arthur H. Compton)康普顿效应(指 X 射线和 γ 射线波长的变化) | ~ scattering 康普顿散射

compulsion [kəm'pʌlʃən] *n* 强迫,强制;强迫行为

compulsive [kəm'pʌlsiv] *a* 强迫的,强迫症的

computer [kəm'pjuːtə] *n* 计算机,电子计算机;计算员

computerize [kəm'pjuːtəraiz] *vt* 用计算机操作;使计算机化 *vi* 计算机化 | **~d** *a* 计算机(操作、辅助、处理)的;计算机化的

con- [前缀] 合,同(co-用在元音或 h 前;col-用在另一个字母 l 前;com-用在 b, m, p 前;cor-用在另一个字母 r 前)

ConA concanavalin A 伴刀豆球蛋白 A

conal ['kəunəl] *a* 圆锥的,锥体的

conalbumin [,kɔnæl'bjuːmin] *n* 伴清蛋白

conarium [kəu'nɛəriəm] *n* 松果体 | **conarial** *a*

conation [kəu'neiʃən] *n* 意动,意图 | **~al** *a*

conative ['kəunətiv] *a* 意动的

conavanine [kɔnə'vænin] *n* 豆氨酸

c-*onc* [cellular *onc*ogene] 细胞癌基因

concanavalin A (ConA) [,kɔnkə'nævəlin] 伴刀豆球蛋白 A

concassation [,kɔnkə'seiʃən] *n* 捣碎,摇碎(使根的有效成分更易提取)

concatenate [kɔn'kætineit] *a* 链状结合的,连结的 *vt* 连结;链状结合,连环 | **concatenation** [kɔn,kæti'neiʃən] *n* 链状结合,连结

Concato's disease [kɔn'kɑːtəu] (Luigi M. Concato)孔卡托病(进行性恶性多浆膜炎,伴大量渗出液渗入心包、胸膜和腹膜腔)

concave ['kɔnkeiv] *a* 凹的,凹面的 *n* 凹面

concavity [kɔn'kævəti] *n* 凹,凹面;成凹形;凹性

concavoconcave [kɔn'keivəu'kɔnkeiv] *a* 对凹的,双凹的

concavoconvex [kɔn,keivəu'kɔnveks] *a* 凹凸的

concentrate ['kɔnsentreit] *vt*, *vi* 集中;浓缩 *n* 浓缩物,浓缩剂 | liver ~ 浓缩肝(从哺乳动物肝中提取,用作补血药) / plant protease ~ 植物蛋白酶浓缩剂(用于消炎、消肿和加速组织修复) / vitamin ~ 浓缩维生素

concentration [,kɔnsen'treiʃən] *n* 集中;浓缩;浓度 | hydrogen ion ~ 氢离子浓度 / ionic ~ 离子浓度 / limiting isorrheic ~ (LIC)最大[水]平衡浓度 / mass ~ 质量浓度 / maximum urinary ~ (MUC) 最高尿浓度 / minimal bactericidal ~ (MBC) 最小杀菌浓度 / minimal inhibitory ~ (MIC) 最低抑制浓度 / minimal isorrheic ~ (MIC) 最低[水]平衡浓度 / minimal lethal ~ (MLC) 最小致死浓度 / molar ~ 摩尔浓度

concentric [kɔn'sentrik] *a* 同心的,共心的

concept ['kɔnsept] *n* 概念 | second messenger ~ 第二信使概念(认为激素〈第一信使〉在其靶组织的表面膜上激活腺苷酸环化酶,增加充当"第二信使"的环腺苷酸的胞间水平,并在靶细胞内执行该激素的工作)

conception [kən'sepʃən] *n* 受孕

conceptive [kən'septiv] *a* 能受孕的;能使受精的

conceptus [kən'septəs] *n*【拉】孕体

concha ['kɔŋkə] ([复] **conchae** ['kɔŋkiː]) *n*【拉】甲;蚌壳 | ~ of auricle 耳甲 / ~ of cranium 颅盖 / ~ of eye 眼眶 / inferior nasal ~, inferior turbinate ~ 下鼻甲 / middle nasal ~, inferior ethmoidal ~ 中鼻甲 / nasoturbinal ~ 鼻堤 / sphenoidal ~ 蝶骨甲;蝶骨小翼 / superior nasal ~, superior ethmoidal ~ 上鼻甲 / supreme ethmoidal ~ 最上鼻甲

conchiform ['kɔŋkifɔːm] *a* 甲壳形的

conchiolin [kɔŋ'kaiəlin] *n* 贝壳素,贝壳硬蛋白

conchiolinosteomyelitis [kɔŋ,kaiəlin,ɔstiə,maiə'laitis] *n* 珍珠工骨髓炎

conchitis [kɔŋ'kaitis] *n* 鼻甲炎

conchoidal [kɔŋ'kɔidl] *a* 甲状的,甲介形的

conchoscope ['kɔŋkəskəup] *n* 鼻[腔]镜

conchotome ['kɔŋkətəum] *n* 鼻甲刀

conchotomy [kɔŋ'kɔtəmi] *n* 鼻甲切开术,鼻甲切除术

Concis. concisus【拉】割,切

conclination [,kɔnkli'neiʃən] *n* 两眼内旋

concoct [kən'kɔkt] *vt* 调制,混合 | **~ion** [kən'kɔkʃən] *n* 加热合剂(药物);消化过程

concomitant [kən'kɔmitənt] *a* 伴随的,伴发的,副的 *n* 相伴物,伴随物

conconscious [kən'kɔnʃəs] *a* 并存意识的

concordance [kən'kɔːdəns] *n* 一致性(在遗传学中指一对孪生个体同样出现某一遗传性状,就称为一致性或和谐性)

concrement ['kɔnkrimənt] *n* 凝结物,凝结体,结石

concrescence [kɔn'kresns] *n* 结合,共同生长,合生;增殖;结合牙

concretio [kən'kriːʃiəu] *n*【拉】凝结物,结石;粘连;凝结[作用] | ~ cordis, ~ pericardii 心包腔粘连

concretion [kən'kriːʃən] *n* 凝结物,结石;粘连;凝结[作用] | alvine ~ 粪石,胃肠结石 / calculous ~ 关节结石,痛风石 / preputial ~ 包皮垢结石 / prostatic ~s 前列腺凝结体 / tophic ~ 痛风石

concupiscence [kən'kjuːpisəns] *n* 性欲,色欲

concurrent [kən'kʌrənt] *a* 同时发生的,并发的,共存的

concuss [kən'kʌs] *vt* 震荡,震动

concussion [kən'kʌʃən] *n* 震荡,震伤 | air ~ 空气振荡 / ~ of the brain 脑震荡 / hydraulic abdominal ~ 潜水性腹震荡 / ~ of the labyrinth 迷路震荡 / pulmonary ~ 肺震伤 / ~ of he retina 视网膜震荡 / ~ of the spinal cord 脊髓震荡 | **concussive** [kən'kʌsiv] *a*

condensation [ˌkɔnden'seiʃən] *n* 冷凝;凝缩;缩合;凝聚

condense [kən'dens] *vt*, *vi* 冷凝;缩合;浓缩 | **condensability** [kənˌdensə'biləti] *n* 凝缩性;冷凝性

condenser [kən'densə] *n* 冷凝器;聚光器;电容器;充填器(用以填塞塑料补牙材料的充填器) | back-action ~ , reverse ~ 回力充填器,反向充填器 / cardioid ~ 心形聚光器 / darkfield ~ 暗视野聚光器 / foot ~ 足形充填器 / gold ~ 金充填器 / mechanical ~ , automatic ~ 机械充填器,自动充填器 / paraboloid ~ 抛物面聚光器

condition [kən'diʃən] *n* 情况,状态;条件;健康状况,病

conditioner [kən'diʃənə] *n* 调节器;调节剂;空气调节器,空调设备

conditioning [kən'diʃəniŋ] *n* 条件反射;健身训练 | aversive ~ 反向条件作用,厌恶性条件[反射]作用 / classical ~ , respondent ~ 经典性条件反射,反应性条件反射 / instrumental ~ , operant ~ 工具性条件反射,操作性条件反射

condom ['kɔndəm] *n* 阴茎套,避孕套

conductance(*C*) [kən'dʌktəns] *n* 传导率 | airway ~ 气道传导率

conductible [kən'dʌktəbl] *a* 能(被)传导的 | **conductibility** [kənˌdʌkti'biləti] *n* 传导性

conduction [kən'dʌkʃən] *n* 传导 | aerial ~ [空]气传导 / aerotympanal ~ 气鼓传导 / antidromic ~ 逆向传导 / avalanche ~ 雪崩状传导 / bone ~ , cranial ~ , osteotympanic ~ , tissue ~ 骨导,颅骨传导,骨鼓传导,组织传导 / delayed ~ [心]传导迟延 / synaptic ~ 突触传导

conductive [kən'dʌktiv] *a* 传导性的

conductivity [ˌkɔndʌk'tivəti] *n* 传导率;传导性

conductor [kən'dʌktə] *n* 指导者;导体;导管(外科用有槽导子)

conduit ['kɔndit, 'kɔndjuit] *n* 导管;管道 | ileal ~ 回肠膀胱术

conduplicate [kɔn'djuːplikit] *a* 折合状的,纵叠的

conduplicatio [kənˌdjuːpli'keiʃiəu] *n* 折合,重叠 | ~ coporis 胎体屈叠

conduplicato corpore [kənˌdjuːpli'keitəu'kɔːpəri]【拉】自然旋出

condurangin [ˌkɔndju'ræŋgin] *n* 康德郎皮苷,南美牛奶菜皮苷

condurango [ˌkɔndju'ræŋgəu] *n* 康德郎皮,南美牛奶菜皮

condylarthrosis [ˌkɔndilɑː'θrəusis] *n* 髁状关节(椭圆关节)

condyle ['kɔndil] *n* 髁 | external ~ 外侧髁 / internal ~ 内侧髁 | **condylar** ['kɔndilə], **condylicus** [kən'dilikəs] *a*

condylectomy [ˌkɔndi'lektəmi] *n* 髁切除术

condyli ['kɔndilai] condylus 的复数

condylion [kən'diliɔn] *n* 髁状突外点(下颌骨)

condyloid ['kɔndilɔid] *a* 髁状的

condyloma [ˌkɔndi'ləumə] ([复] **condylomata** [ˌkɔndi'ləumətə]), *n*【希】湿疣 | ~ acuminatum, pointed ~ 尖锐湿疣 / ~ latum, flat ~ 扁平湿疣,梅毒湿疣

condylomatoid [ˌkɔndi'ləumətɔid] *a* 湿疣样的

condylomatosis [ˌkɔndiˌləumə'təusis] *n* 湿疣病

condylomatous [ˌkɔndi'ləumətəs] *a* 湿疣的,湿疣性的

condylotomy [ˌkɔndi'lɔtəmi] *n* 髁切断术,髁切开术

condylus ['kɔndiləs]([复] **condyli** ['kɔndilai]) *n*【拉】髁

Condy's fluid ['kɔndi] (Henry B. Condy)康迪液(高锰酸钾钠消毒溶液)

cone ['kəun] *n* 锥,圆锥;锥体;遮光筒,放射筒 | adjusting ~s 调节锥(测量眼轴距离) / arterial ~ 动脉圆锥 / bifurcation ~ 分歧锥 / cerebellar pressure ~ 小脑压迫圆锥 / ectoplacental ~ 绒[毛]膜锥 / fertilization ~ , attraction ~ 受精锥 / implantation ~ 轴索丘 / medullary ~ , terminal ~ of spinal cord 脊髓圆锥 / theca interna ~ 内膜锥 / twin ~s (视网膜)双锥[体] / visual ~

视锥;视网膜锥[体]

cone-nose [ˈkəun nəuz] *n* 猎蝽

conexus [kəˈneksəs] [单复同] *n*【拉】结合,结合体 | ~ intertendineus 腱间结合 / interthalamicus 丘脑间黏合

coney [ˈkəuni] *n* 蹄兔

confabulation [kənˌfæbjuˈleiʃən] *n* 虚构

confectio [kənˈfekʃiəu] *n*【拉】糖膏[剂]

confection [kənˈfekʃən] *n* 糖膏[剂] | ~ of senna 番泻叶糖膏

confertus [kənˈfəːtəs] *a*【拉】融合的,汇合的

confidentiality [ˌkɔnfiˌdenʃiˈæləti] *n* 机密性(医学伦理学的原则,即病人向医生透露的内情纯属私人性质的,以什么方式和什么时候向第三方公开都有一定的限度,通常医生必须得到病人的许可方能作出如此的公开)

configuration [kənˌfigjuˈreiʃən] *n* 构型 | cis ~ 顺式构型(拟等位基因的两个突变基因在同一染色体上,两个野生型基因在同源染色体上) / trans ~ 反式构型(两个同源染色体,各含有拟等位基因的一个突变基因和一个野生型基因)

confine [kənˈfain] *vt* 使闭门不出 | be ~d 分娩,生产 / **~ment** [kənˈfainmənt] *n* 分娩,生产

conflict [ˈkɔnflikt] *n* 冲突,矛盾 | approach-approach ~ 趋向-趋向冲突,接近-接近冲突(指两种可以达到的、欲得而又不相容的目标所引起的心理冲突) / approach-avoidance ~ 趋向-回避冲突,接近-回避冲突(指一种目标,既欲求取又欲回避所引起的心理冲突) / avoidance-avoidance ~ 回避-回避冲突(指希望回避两个都不称心的抉择所引起的心理冲突) / extrapsychic ~ 心理外冲突 / intrapsychic ~ , intrapersonal ~ 心理内冲突

confluence [ˈkɔnfluəns] *n* 汇合,融合,合流点,汇合处 | ~ of sinuses 窦汇 | **conflux** [ˈkɔnflʌks] *n*

confluens [ˈkɔnfluəns] *n*【拉】汇合,融合 | ~ sinuum 窦汇

confluent [ˈkɔnfluənt] *n* 汇合的,融合的

conformation [ˌkɔnfɔːˈmeiʃən] *n* 符合,一致;构象(一个分子中原子在单键周围旋转所产生的空间排列)

conformer [kənˈfɔːmə] *n* 构象异构体(一个分子中在单键周围旋转所产生的任何一组结构)

confounder [kənˈfaundə] *n* 混淆变量(间接歪曲其他两个变量之间关系的第三变量)

confounding [kənˈfaundiŋ] *n* 混淆(受第三变量的干预,以至歪曲两个其他变量之间正在研究中的关联) *a* 致混淆的

confrication [ˌkɔnfriˈkeiʃən] *n* 磨碎,捣细(指将药物磨碎成粉末)

confront [kənˈfrʌnt] *vt* 比较,对照 | **~ation** [ˌkɔnfrʌnˈteiʃən] *n* 对抗;对诊法(一种治疗心理病症的方法,即使患者直接注意矛盾的说法或行动)

confusion [kənˈfjuːʒən] *n* 混乱;混淆;慌乱;意识错乱

cong. congius【拉】加仑

congeal [kənˈdʒiːl] *vt*, *vi* 冻结,凝结

congelation [ˌkɔndʒiˈleiʃən] *n* 冻[结]伤

congeneic [ˌkɔndʒiˈneiik] *a* 同基因异系的,异系同基因的

congener [ˈkɔndʒinə] *n* 同源物;协同肌 | **congeneric** [ˌkɔndʒiˈnerik], **congenerous** [kənˈdʒenərəs] *a* 同源的;协同的

congenial [kənˈdʒiːniəl] *a* 同属的,同类的

congenic [kənˈdʒenik] *a* 同类系的

congenital [kənˈdʒenitl] *a* 先天的,天生的

congest [kənˈdʒest] *vt*, *vi* 充血 | **~ed** *a* / **~ive** *a* 充血的

congestin [kənˈdʒestin] *n* 海葵毒[素]

congestion [kənˈdʒestʃən] *n* 充血,淤血 | active ~ 自动充血 / hypostatic ~ 沉下性充血,沉积性充血 / passive ~ ,venous ~ 被动性充血,淤血,静脉性充血

congius [ˈkɔndʒiəs] *n*【拉】加仑

conglobate [ˈkɔngləubeit] *vt*, *vi* 成球形;成团,成块 *a* 成球形的;成团的,成块的 | **conglobation** [ˌkɔngləuˈbeiʃən] *n*

conglomerate [kənˈglɔməreit] *vt*, *vi* 成球形;堆积[kənˈglɔmərit] *a* 聚成球形的;堆积的 | **conglomeration** [kənˌglɔməˈreiʃən] *n*

conglutin [kənˈgluːtin] *n* 羽扇豆球蛋白

conglutinant [kənˈgluːtinənt] *a* 黏合的,促创口愈合的

conglutinate [kənˈgluːtineit] *vt*, *vi* 胶固;黏附,黏合 | **conglutination** [kənˌgluːtiˈneiʃən] *n* 胶固反应(红细胞依赖于补体和抗体的凝集反应);胶着,黏合(指组织)

conglutinatio [kənˌgluːtiˈneiʃiəu] *n*【拉】胶着,黏合

conglutinin [kənˈgluːtinin] *n* 胶固素

conglutinogen [kənˈgluːtinədʒən] *n* 胶固素原

congophilic [ˌkɔngəuˈfilik] *a* 嗜刚果红的

congregate [ˈkɔŋgrigeit] *vt*, *vi* 集合 *a* 集合的;集体的

congressus [kənˈgresəs] *n* 性交,交媾

coni [ˈkəunai] conus 的复数

conic [ˈkɔnik] *a* 圆锥形的 *n* 圆锥曲线,二次曲线 | **~al** *a*

Conidae [ˈkɔnidiː] *n* 芋螺科

Conidiobolus [kəuˌnidiˈɔbələs] *n* 耳霉属

conidiogenesis [kəˌnidiəuˈdʒenəsis] *n* 分生孢子形成

conidiogenous [kəˌnidiˈɔdʒənəs] *a* 产孢的,产分生孢子的

conidioma [kəˌnidiˈəumə] ([复] **conidiomata** [kəˌnidiˈəumətə]) *n* 分生孢子瘤

conidiophore [kə*u*ˈnidiəfɔː] *n* 分生孢子梗

Conidiosporales [kəuˌnidiəuspəˈreiliːz] *n* 分生孢子菌目(念珠菌目 Moniliales 的旧称)

conidium [kə*u*ˈnidiəm] ([复] **conidia** [kə*u*ˈnidiə]), **conidiospore** [kə*u*ˈnidiəspɔː] *n* 分生孢子 | **conidial** [kə*u*ˈnidiəl] *a*

coniform [ˈkəunifɔːm] *a* 圆锥形的

coniine [ˈkəunii(ː)n] *n* [欧]毒芹碱

coni(o)- [构词成分]尘,尘埃

coniofibrosis [ˌkəuniə*u*faiˈbrəusis] *n* 肺尘性纤维变性,纤维性肺尘病

coniology [ˌkəuniˈɔlədʒi] *n* 尘埃学

coniolymphstasis [ˌkəuniə*u*ˈlimfstəsis] *n* 淋巴阻塞性尘肺

coniometer [ˌkəuniˈɔmitə] *n* 尘埃计算器

coniophage [ˈkəuniəfeidʒ] *n* 噬尘细胞

coniosis [ˌkəuniˈəusis] *n* 粉尘病,尘埃沉着病

Coniosporium [ˌkəuniə*u*ˈspɔːriəm] *n* 梨孢霉属 | ~ corticale 皮质梨孢霉(可致梨孢霉病)

coniosporosis [ˌkəuniə*u*spəˈrəusis] *n* 梨孢霉病

coniotomy [ˌkəuniˈɔtəmi] *n* 喉弹性圆锥切开术,环甲膜切开术

coniotoxicosis [ˌkəuniə*u*ˌtɔksiˈkəusis] *n* 肺尘中毒症

Conium [kə*u*ˈnaiəm] *n* 欧毒芹属,毒茴属 | ~ maculatum L. 欧毒芹,斑毒茴

conization [ˌkɔniˈzeiʃən] *n* 锥形切除术(如宫颈部分切除时) | ~ of cervix 宫颈锥切术 / cold ~ 冷冻锥形切除术

conjoined [kənˈdʒɔind] *a* 联体的(如 conjoined twins〈联体儿〉)

conjugant [ˈkɔndʒugənt] *n* 接合体

conjugata [ˌkɔndʒuˈgeitə] *n* 结合径,(骨盆)直径;正中直径(真直径) | ~ anatomica 解剖学直径,真直径 / ~ diagonalis 对角径 / ~ vera 真结合径,真直径 / ~ vera obstetrica 产科结合径,产科直径

conjugate [ˈkɔndʒugit] *n* 结合径,(骨盆)直径;轭合物,结合物 [ˈkɔndʒugeit] *vt* 结合,连接;使成对 *vi* 成婚;配合;成对 | anatomic ~ 解剖学直径,真直径(骨盆入口) / diagonal ~ 对角径 / external ~ 骶耻外径 / obstetric ~ 产科结合径(骨盆入口最小的前后径)

conjugation [ˌkɔndʒuˈgeiʃən] *n* 结合;接合[作用];共轭

conjugon [ˈkɔndʒugɔn] *n* 接合子,促接合因子(促使结合的一种附加体)

conjunct [kənˈdʒʌŋkt] *a* 结合的,联合的;连接的

conjunctiva [ˌkɔndʒʌŋ*k*ˈtaivə] ([复] **conjunctivae** [ˌkɔndʒʌŋ*k*ˈtaiviː]) *n* 【拉】结膜 | ~l *a*

conjunctive [kənˈdʒʌŋ*k*tiv] *a* 连接的,联合的

conjunctiviplasty [kənˈdʒʌŋktiviˌplæsti] *n* 结膜成形术

conjunctivitis [kənˌdʒʌŋ*k*tiˈvaitis] *n* 结膜炎 | actinic ~ 光化性结膜炎 / acute contagious ~, acute epidemic ~, epidemic ~ 急性触染性结膜炎,急性流行性结膜炎,流行性结膜炎 / allergic ~, anaphylactic ~ 变应性结膜炎,过敏性结膜炎,枯草热 / angular ~ 眦结膜炎 / arc-flash ~ 电光性结膜炎 / atopic ~ 特应性结膜炎 / croupous ~ 格鲁布性结膜炎,假膜性结膜炎 / Egyptian ~ 埃及结膜炎,沙眼 / granular ~ 颗粒性结膜炎,沙眼 / inclusion ~, swimming pool ~ 包涵体结膜炎,游泳池结膜炎 / infantile purulent ~ 婴儿脓性结膜炎,新生儿眼炎 / larval ~ 结膜蛆病 / membranous ~ 膜性结膜炎 / nodular ~ 结节性眼炎 / phlyctenular ~, eczematous ~, scrofular ~ 小疱性结膜炎,湿疹性结膜炎,瘰疬性结膜炎 / prairie ~ 白点状慢性结膜炎 / pseudomembranous ~ 假膜性结膜炎 / shipyard ~ 船坞结膜炎,流行性角膜结膜炎 / tularemic ~, squirrel plague ~ 土拉热杆菌性结膜炎 / uratic ~ 尿酸盐沉着性结膜炎 / vernal ~, spring ~ 春季[卡他性]结膜炎 / welder's ~ 电焊工结膜炎(电光性眼炎)

conjunctivodacryocystostomy [ˌkɔndʒʌŋ*k*ˌtaivə*u*ˌdækriə*u*sisˈtɔstəmi] *n* 结膜泪囊吻合术

conjunctivoma [kənˌdʒʌŋ*k*tiˈvəumə] *n* 结膜瘤

conjunctivoplasty [ˌkɔndʒʌŋ*k*ˈtaivəˌplæsti] *n* 结膜成形术

conjunctivorhinostomy [ˌkɔndʒʌŋ*k*ˌtaivə*u*raiˈnɔstəmi] *n* 结膜鼻腔吻合术

connatal [kəˈneitl], **connate** [ˈkɔneit] *a* 同生的,同源的;出生时的(在生产时发生的)

connectin [kəˈnektin] *n* 肌联蛋白

connection [kəˈnekʃən] *n* 接合,连接 | clamp ~ 锁状连合 / intertendinous ~ 腱结合 / total cavopulmonary ~ 全腔静脉-肺动脉连接术

connective [kəˈnektiv] *a* 连接的,结合的,结缔的 *n* 连接物

connectology [kənekˈtɔlədʒi] *n* 连接学(本词指用于连接体外透析器与腹内导管的设备和方法)

connector [kəˈnektə] *n* 联合突;连接体 | major ~, saddle ~ 大连接体,鞍状连接杆 / minor ~ 小连接体(亦称连接杆)

Connell's suture [ˈkɔnəl] (Frank G. Connell)康内尔缝合,连续全层内翻缝合(U 形连续缝合,用于肠吻合术)

connexin [kəˈneksin] *n* 连结蛋白

connexin 26 [kəˈneksin] *n* 连接蛋白 26(间隙连

接处连接子的初级蛋白质组分,其基因中的突变是听力丧失的常见原因)

connexon [kə'neksɔn] *n* 连接子

connexus [kə'neksəs] [单复同] *n* 结合质(亦可拼写成 conexus) | ~ intertendineus 腱结合

connivent [kə'naivənt] *a* 会接的,靠合的;聚合的

Conn's syndrome [kɔn] (Jerome W. Conn) 原发性醛固酮症

cono- [构词成分]圆锥

conoid ['kəunɔid] *a* 锥形的 *n* 类锥体 | **~al** [kəu'nɔidəl] *a* 圆锥状的

Conolly's system ['kɔnəli] (John Conolly) 康诺利制,(精神病患者)废除约束制(一种不约束疗法制,治精神病)

conomyoidin [ˌkəunəumai'ɔidin] *n* 视网膜锥体原生质

conophthalmus [ˌkəunɔf'θælməs] *n* 角膜葡萄肿

Conopodina [ˌkəunəpəu'dainə] *n* 锥足亚目

Conorhinus [ˌkəunə'rainəs] *n* 锥蝽属

conquinine [kən'kwinin] *n* 康奎宁(抗心律失常药)

Conradi-Hünermann syndrome [kən'rɑːdi 'hjuːnəmɑːn] (E. Conradi; Carl Hünermann) 康-休综合征(为常染色体显性遗传型点状软骨发育不良,特征为肢体不对称性缩短和脊柱侧凸,智力与预期寿命正常,本征也与孕妇在妊娠期使用华法林钠〈warfarin sodium〉有关)

Conradi's disease (syndrome) [kən'rɑːdi] (Erich Conradi) 康拉迪病(综合征),点状软骨发育不良

Conradi's line [kən'rɑːdi] (Andreas C. Conradi) 康拉迪线(从剑突底部到心尖跳动点的连线,示左叶肝叩诊浊音的上界)

Cons. conserva【拉】保存

consanguineous [ˌkɔnsæŋ'gwiniəs] *a* 同宗的;同血缘的,血亲的

consanguinity [ˌkɔnsæŋ'gwinəti] *n* 近亲

conscience ['kɔnʃəns] *n* 良心,道德,意识

consciousness ['kɔnʃəsnis] *n* 意识 | collective ~ 集体意识 / colon ~ 结肠意识(慢性便秘时,患者意识到结肠的活动) / double ~ 双重意识(患者似过两种生活的一种异常状况) / noetic ~ 理智意识

conscious-sedation ['kɔnʃəs si'deiʃən] *n* 清醒性镇静[作用](牙科麻醉)

consenescence [ˌkɔnsi'nesns] *n* 衰老,老朽

consensual [kən'senʃuəl] *a* 同感的,交感的(反射刺激引起,尤指刺激于一瞳孔时,两瞳孔的相似反应) | **~ly** *ad*

consensus [kən'sensəs] *n* 一致;同感,交感

consent [kən'sent] *vi*, *n* 同意,赞同 | informed ~ 知情同意(病人或监护人得知治疗的目的、方法、步骤、效果和风险后表示的同意)

conservative [kən'səːvətiv] *a* 保存的,防腐的;保守的 *n* 防腐剂

conserve ['kɔnsəːv] *n* 糖剂,糖膏剂

consistency [kən'sistənsi] *n* 一致性 | ~ of an estimator 估计量一致性

consolidant [kən'sɔlidənt] *a* 促创口愈合的,收创的 *n* 愈合剂

consolidation [kənˌsɔli'deiʃən] *n* 实变(如肺炎时的一肺)

consonation [ˌkɔnsə'neiʃən] *n* 谐和(啰音)

conspecific [ˌkɔnspi'sifik] *a* 同种的 *n* 同种生物

constancy ['kɔnstənsi] *n* 恒有度,恒定性;常性 | cell ~ 细胞常数 | object ~ 对象常性

constant ['kɔnstənt] *n* 常数 | absorption ~ 吸收常数 / association ~, binding ~ 结合常数 / decay ~, disintegration ~, radioactive ~ 蜕变常数,衰变常数,放射性常数 / dielectric ~ 介电常数,电容率 / dissociation ~ 离解常数,电离常数 / equilibrium ~ 平衡常数 / quantum ~ 量子常数 / sedimentation ~ 沉降常数,沉降系数

constipate ['kɔnstipeit] *vt*, *vi* 便秘 | **~d** ['kɔnstipeitid] *a* 便秘的

constipation [ˌkɔnsti'peiʃən] *n* 便秘 | atonic ~ 无力性便秘 / gastrojejunal ~ 胃空肠性便秘 / proctogenous ~ 直肠性便秘 / spastic ~ 痉挛性便秘

constituent [kən'stitjuənt] *a* 形成的;组成的 *n* 成分 | effective ~有效成分

constitution [ˌkɔnsti'tjuːʃən] *n* 体质,素质 | lymphatic ~ 淋巴体质 / neuropathic ~ 神经病体质 / vasoneurotic ~ 血管神经病体质

constitutional [ˌkɔnsti'tjuːʃənl] *a* 全身的;体质的,素质的

constitutive ['kɔnstitjuːtiv] *a* 组成的,基本的,要素的

constriction [kən'strikʃən] *n* 狭窄,缩窄;紧窄感;缢痕(中期染色体上的凹缢的区域) | duodenopyloric ~ 十二指肠幽门狭窄 / primary ~ 主缢痕,初级缢痕 / secondary ~ 副缢痕,次级缢痕,二级缢痕

constrictive [kən'striktiv] *a* 狭窄的,缩窄的

constrictor [kən'striktə] *n* 缩窄器;缩肌

constringent [kən'strindʒənt] *a* 引起收缩的,收缩性的

constructive [kən'strʌktiv] *a* 构成的;合成代谢的(生理学)

consult [kən'sʌlt] *vi* 会诊 *vt* 找(医生)看病 | **~ing** *a* 咨询的,顾问的;会诊的,诊疗的

consultant [kən'sʌltənt] *n* 顾问医师,会诊医师;顾问,咨询者

consultation [ˌkɔnsəl'teiʃən] *n* 会诊

consumption [kən'sʌmpʃən] *n* 消耗,消费;痨病,结核 | luxus ~ 过量消耗(指摄食过量蛋白质) / oxygen ~ 氧耗量,氧消耗

consumptive [kən'sʌmptiv] *a* 消耗性的;[患]肺结核的 *n* 痨病患者,肺结核患者

Cont. contusus【拉】挫伤的;捣碎的

contact ['kɔntækt] *n* 接触,联系;(曾与传染病)接触者;接触物;触点[kən'tækt] *vt, vi* 接触 | complete ~ 全邻面接触(牙) / deflective occlusal ~ 偏侧咬合接触 / direct ~, immediate ~ 直接接触 / indirect ~, mediate ~ 间接接触 / interceptive occlusal ~ 阻隔性咬合接触 / premature occlusal ~ 早咬合接触 / working ~ 工能性接触

contactant [kən'tæktənt] *n* 接触物(一种变应原,接触一两次后能引起动物或人的表皮迟发性接触型过敏反应)

contactology [ˌkɔntæk'tɔlədʒi] *n* 接触镜学 | **contactologist** *n* 接触镜技师

contagion [kən'teidʒən] *n* [接]触[传]染;[接触性]传染病;[接]触[传]染物 | direct ~, immediate ~ 直接触染 / mediate ~ 间接触染 / psychic ~ 心理感染,精神感染

contagiosity [kənˌteidʒi'ɔsəti] *n* [接]触[传]染性

contagious [kən'teidʒəs] *a* [接]触[传]染的

container [kən'teinə] *n* 容器

contaminant [kən'tæminənt] *n* 污染物

contaminate [kən'tæmineit] *vt* 污染 | **contaminative** *a* / **contaminator** *n* 污染物

contamination [kənˌtæmi'neiʃən] *n* 污染

content ['kɔntent] *n* 含量,内容 | carbon dioxide ~ 二氧化碳含量 / latent ~ 潜隐内容(梦或思想) / manifest ~ (梦的)显示内容 / oxygen ~ 氧含量

Contin. continuetur【拉】继续

continence ['kɔntinəns] *n* 节制;节欲 | fecal ~ 排便节制 / urinary ~ 排尿节制

continent ['kɔntinənt] *a* 节制的,节欲的

contingency [kən'tindʒənsi] *n* 偶然[性];可能[性]

contingent [kən'tindʒənt] *a* 可能发生的;偶然的;应急的;伴随的

continued [kən'tinju(ː)d] *a* 连续的

continuity [ˌkɔnti'nju(ː)əti] *n* 连续[性],持续[性]

continuous [kən'tinjuəs] *a* 连续的;持续的

contology [kən'tɔlədʒi] *n* 接触镜学 | **contologist** *n* 接触镜技师

contour ['kɔntuə] *n* 外形,轮廓 *vt* 勾划…的轮廓;成形,塑形 | height of ~ 外形凸度 / ~ of nasal tip 鼻尖形态

contoured ['kɔntuəd] *a* 波状外形的,波状轮廓的(细菌菌落)

contouring [kən'tuəriŋ] *n* 外形修整,外形修复 | occlusal ~ 殆外形修复

contra- [前缀] 反,抗,逆,对

contra-angle [ˌkɔntrə 'æŋgl] *n* 反角

contra-aperture [ˌkɔntrə'æpətjuə] *n* 对口(脓肿处作第二开口,以利排脓)

contraception [ˌkɔntrə'sepʃən] *n* 避孕 | intrauterine ~ 子宫内避孕

contraceptive [ˌkɔntrə'septiv] *a* 避孕的 *n* 避孕药;避孕器 | intrauterine ~ 子宫内避孕器 / oral ~ 口服避孕药

contract [kən'trækt] *vt* 得(病),感染;收缩 | **~ibility** [kənˌtræktə'biləti] *n* 收缩性 | **~ible** [kən'træktəbl] *a* 会缩的,可缩的

contractile [kən'træktail] *a* 收缩的,有收缩力的

contractility [ˌkɔntræk'tiləti] *n* 收缩性 | cardiac ~ 心肌收缩性 / galvanic ~ 电流收缩性 / idiomuscular ~ 肌自身收缩性 / neuromuscular ~ 神经肌肉收缩性(正常收缩性,以区别肌自身收缩性)

contraction [kən'trækʃən] *n* 收缩;挛缩;缩约词;感染;牙弓内缩 | anodal closure ~ (ACC)阳极通电收缩 / anodal opening ~ (AOC)阳极断电收缩 / cathodal closure ~ (CCC)阴极通电收缩 / cathodal opening ~ (COC)阴极断电收缩 / clonic ~ 阵挛性收缩 / closing ~ 通电收缩 / escaped ventricular ~, automatic ventricular ~ 心室自动收缩 / galvanotonic ~ 电紧张性收缩 / hourglass ~ 葫芦状收缩(胃或子宫) / idiomuscular ~ 肌自身收缩 / isometric ~ 等长收缩 / isotonic ~ 等张收缩 / myotatic ~ 肌伸张性收缩 / opening ~ 断路收缩,断电收缩 / paradoxical ~ 反常收缩 / premature ~ 过早收缩,期前收缩 / rheumatic ~ 手足搐搦 / tetanic ~, tonic ~ 强直性收缩,紧张性收缩 / uterine ~ 子宫收缩 / wound ~, cicatricial ~ 伤口收缩,瘢痕收缩

contractive [kən'træktiv] *a* 收缩的

contracture [kən'træktʃə] *n* 挛缩 | ischemic ~ 缺血性挛缩 / organic ~ 器质性挛缩 / postpoliomyelitic ~ 脊髓灰质炎后挛缩 / veratrin ~ 藜芦碱挛缩

contraextension [ˌkɔntrəiks'tenʃən] *n* 对抗牵伸术

contrafissure [kɔntrə'fiʃə], **contrafissura** [kəntrəfi'sjuərə] *n* 对裂

contraincision [ˌkɔntrəin'siʒən] *n* 对口切开

contraindicant [ˌkɔntrə'indikənt] *a* 禁忌的

contraindicate [ˌkɔntrə'indikeit] *vt* 禁忌 | **contraindication** [ˌkɔntrəˌindi'keiʃən] *n* 禁忌证

（尤指不宜使用某种疗法的任何病情）/ **contraindicative** [ˌkɔntrəinˈdikətiv] *a*
contrainsular [ˌkɔntrəˈinsjulə] *a* 抑胰岛素分泌的
contralateral [ˌkɔntrəˈlætərəl] *a* 对侧的
contraparetic [ˌkɔntrəpəˈretik] *a* 抗麻痹性痴呆的 *n* 抗麻痹性痴呆药
contrasexual [ˌkɔntrəˈseksjuəl] *a* 异性的，异性特征的
contrast [kənˈtræst] *vt* 使对比，使对照 *vi* 形成对照 [ˈkɔntræst] *n* 对比，对照 | long-scale ~, low ~ 长阶对比，低对比（影像）/ short-scale ~, high ~ 短阶对比，高对比（影像）/ subject ~ 自身对比，组织对比（组织中对不同部位X线的吸收差异）
contrastimulant [ˌkɔntrəˈstimjulənt] *a* 抗兴奋的 *n* 抗兴奋药
contrastimulism [ˌkɔntrəˈstimjulizəm] *n* 抗刺激法，抗兴奋疗法
contrastimulus [ˌkɔntrəˈstimjuləs] *n* 抗兴奋药
contrecoup [kɔntrəˈkuː] *n*【法】对侧[外]伤
contrectation [ˌkɔntrekˈteiʃən] *n* 接触异性欲
Cont. rem. continuetur remedium【拉】继续使用此药
control [kənˈtrəul] *n* 控制，调节，节制；监督，管理；对照 | associative automatic ~ 联合性自动控制（起于纹状体的神经冲动，作用于最后的总神经束，因而达于各肌）/ aversive ~ 厌恶控制（在行为疗法中使用令人不愉快的刺激以改变不良行为）/ birth ~ 节育，避孕 / feedback ~ 反馈控制 / idiodynamic ~ 肌营养神经控制 / reflex ~ [肌]反射控制 / sex ~ 性别控制（人工控制后代性别）/ stimulus ~ 刺激控制 / synergic ~（活动）协调控制（来自小脑）/ tonic ~ 肌张力控制 / vestibuloequilibratory ~ 前庭平衡控制 / volitional ~, voluntary ~ 意志控制，随意控制
Controlled Substances Act 药物控制条例（1970年颁布的美国联邦法令）
controller [kənˈtrəulə] *n* 控制器；管理员
contund [kənˈtʌnd] *vt* 研碎，捣碎；挫伤
contuse [kənˌtjuːz] *vt* 挫伤
contusion [kɔnˈtjuːʒən] *n* 挫伤 | brain ~ 脑挫伤 / contrecoup ~ 对侧挫伤 / ~ of spinal cord 脊髓挫伤
contusive [kənˈtjuːsiv] *a* 挫伤的
conular [ˈkɔnjulə] *a* 圆锥形的
Conus [ˈkəunəs] *n* 芋螺属
conus [ˈkəunəs]（[复] **coni** [ˈkəunai]）*n* 圆锥，锥体；弧形斑 | distraction ~ 视神经乳头颞侧弧形斑 / myopic ~ 近视性圆锥，眼后葡萄肿 / supertraction ~ 视神经乳头鼻侧弧形斑
convalesce [ˌkɔnvəˈles] *vi* 恢复健康，渐愈
convalescence [ˌkɔnvəˈlesns] *n* 恢复[期]，康复[期]
convalescent [ˌkɔnvəˈlesnt] *a* 恢复[期]的 *n* 恢复期病人
convection [kənˈvekʃən] *n*（热的）对流 | **convective** *a*
convergence [kənˈvəːdʒəns] *n* 趋同；会聚；集合；收敛 | accommodative ~ 调节性集合 / amplitude of ~ 集合幅度 / far point of ~ 集合远点 / fusional ~ 融合集合 / near point of ~ 集合近点 / negative ~ 负集合（视轴向外偏斜）/ positive ~ 正集合（视轴向内偏斜）| **convergency** [kənˈvəːdʒənsi] *n* / **convergent** [kənˈvəːdʒənt] *a* 会聚的，集合的
convergiometer [kənˌvəːdʒiˈɔmitə] *n* 隐斜[眼]计
Converse method [ˈkɔnvəːs]（John Marquis Converse）康氏法（重建耳垂法）
conversion [kənˈvəːʃən] *n* 转化，转变；转换（指情绪转换为躯体症状的过程）；（胎儿）倒转术；基因转变
convert [kənˈvəːt] *vt* 转变，变换；转化；倒转
convertase [kənˈvəːteis] *n* 转化酶 | C3 ~ C3 转化酶 / C3 proactivator ~（C3PAase）C3 活化因子前体转化酶 / C5 ~ C5 转化酶
converter, convertor [kənˈvəːtə] *n* 转化器，变流器；变频器
convertible [kənˈvəːtəbl] *a* 可改变的，可变换的 | **convertibility** [kənˈvəːtəˈbiləti] *n*
convertin [kənˈvəːtin] *n* 转变加速因子（凝血因子Ⅶ）
convex [kɔnˈveks, ˈkɔn-] *a* 凸的，凸面的 *n* 凸面；凸状 | low ~ 低凸面的 | **~ity** [kɔnˈveksəti] *n* 凸，凸面 / **~ly** *ad*
convexobasia [kɔnˌveksəuˈbeisiə] *n* 颅骨隆凸畸形
convexoconcave [kɔnˌveksəuˈkɔnkeiv] *a* 凸凹的
convexoconvex [kɔnˌveksəuˈkɔnveks] *a* 对凸的，双凸的
convolute [ˈkɔnvəluːt] *a* 卷曲的，回旋的 *vt, vi* 卷曲 | **~d** *a* 卷曲的，回旋的
convolution [ˌkɔnvəˈluːʃən] *n* 卷曲，回旋；回，脑回 | ~s of cerebrum 大脑回 / occipitotemporal ~ 枕颞回，梭状回 | **~al**, **~ary** *a*
convolve [kənˈvɔlv] *vt, vi* 卷，缠绕
Convolvulaceae [kənˌvɔlvjuˈleisiiː] *n* 旋花科
Convolvulus [kənˈvɔlvjuləs] *n* 旋花属
convulsant [kənˈvʌlsənt] *a* 引起惊厥的 *n* 惊厥药
convulse [kənˈvʌls] *vt* 使剧烈震动；使痉挛，使抽搐
convulsibility [kənˌvʌlsiˈbiləti] *n* 惊厥性

convulsion [kən'vʌlʃən] *n* 惊厥,抽搐 | central ~ essential ~, spontaneous ~, 中枢性惊厥,自发性惊厥 / clonic ~ 阵挛性惊厥 / coordinate ~ 协调性惊厥 / crowing ~ 喘鸣性喉痉挛 / epileptiform ~ 癫痫样惊厥 / febrile ~s 热性惊厥 / hysterical ~ 癔症性惊厥 / hysteroid ~ 癔症样惊厥 / mimetic ~, mimic ~ 面肌痉挛,面肌抽搐 / puerperal ~ 产惊,子痫 / salaam ~ 点头状痉挛 / tonic ~, tetanic ~ 强直性惊厥 / uremic ~ 尿毒症性惊厥 | **convulsive** [kən'vʌlsiv] *a*

convulsivant [kən'vʌlsivənt] *n* 惊厥药

Cooke's formula (count, criterion, index) [kuk] (William E. Cooke)库克公式(分类计数、标准、指数)(阿尔内特〈Arneth〉公式的一种简化法,如果核材料有核带,除连接白细胞核不同部分的染色质丝状体之外,那么这样的核是不可分的)

cooler ['kuːlə] *n* 冷却器

Cooley's anemia (disease) ['kuːliː] (Thomas B. Cooley)库利贫血(病),重型珠蛋白生成障碍性贫血

Coolidge tube ['kuːlidʒ] (William D. Coolidge)库利奇管(热阴极 X 线管)

cooling ['kuːliŋ] *n* 冷却,降温 | peritoneal ~ 腹腔降温 / pleural ~ 胸膜腔降温 / surface ~ 体表降温

Coombs' test [kuːmz] (R. R. A. Coombs) 库姆斯试验,抗球蛋白试验(使用各种抗血清,一般用于检红细胞表面的蛋白〈通常是抗体〉的存在,如用于胎儿成红细胞增多病试验)

cooperativity [kəuˌɔpərə'tivəti] *n* 协同性 | negative ~ 负协同性(每一个连续的配体结合的解离常数高于前一个,因此其结合亲和力连续减低) / positive ~ 正协同性(每一个连续的配体结合的解离常数低于前一个,因此其结合亲和力连续增加)

Cooperia [ku'piəriə] *n* 古珀线虫属 | ~ oncophora, ~ pectinata, ~ punctata 肿孔古珀线虫,篦形古珀线虫,点状古珀线虫

cooperiasis [ˌkuːpə'raiəsis] *n* 古珀线虫病

cooperid ['kuːpərid] *n* 古珀线虫

Coopernail's sign ['kuːpəneil] (George P. Coopernail) 库珀内尔征(会阴和阴囊或阴唇上出现的小瘀血斑,为骨盆骨折之征)

Cooper's fascia ['kuːpə] (Astley P. Cooper) 库珀筋膜(提睾筋膜;脚间纤维) | ~ hernia 库珀疝(股疝并有附加束进入阴囊,或走向大阴唇或闭孔) / ~ irritable breast 库珀乳腺过敏,乳腺神经痛 / ~ ligament 耻骨梳韧带 / ~ suspensory ligaments 乳房悬韧带

coordinate [kəu'ɔːdinət] *n* 坐标; [kəu'ɔːdineit] *vt*, *vi* 协调 | **coordinator** [kəu'ɔːdineitə] *n* 协调器,共济器;坐标测定器

coordination [kəuˌɔːdi'neiʃən] *n* 协调,协同作用,共济

coossify [kəu'ɔsifai] *vi* 共同骨化 | **coossification** [kəuˌɔsifi'keiʃən] *n* 共同骨化[作用]

cooxycodAPAP [ˌkəuɔksi'kəudəpæp] *n* 盐酸羟考酮-对乙酰氨基酚(镇痛药)

COP cyclophosphamide, vincristine, and prednisone 环磷酰胺-长春新碱-泼尼松(联合化疗治癌方案)

copaiba [kəu'paibə] *n* 玷玔香脂,玷玔香胶

copal [kəu'pæl] *n* 玷玔脂,岩树脂

coparaffinate [kəu'pɑːrəˌfineit] *n* 液体石蜡合剂(一种不溶于水的异链烷烃酸与异辛基羟苄基二烃基胺部分中和的合剂,用作皮肤抗感染药)

COP-BLAM cyclophosphamide, vincristine, prednisone, bleomycin, doxorubicin, and proearbazine 环磷酰胺-长春新碱-泼尼松-博来霉素-多柔比星-丙卡巴肼(联合化疗治癌方案)

COPD chronic obstructive pulmonary disease 慢性阻塞性肺病

cope [kəup] *n* 根端盖;顶盖

copepod ['kəupipɔd] *n* 挠足虫

Copepoda [kəu'pepədə] *n* 挠足亚纲

Copernicia [ˌkəupəː'niʃiə] *n* 杯形花属

Cope's sign [kəup] (Vincent Cope) 科普征,腰大肌征(常见于阑尾炎)

coping ['kəupiŋ] *n* 顶盖 | transfer ~ 转移盖(用于牙印膜中的代型定位)

copiopia [kɔpi'əupiə] *n* 眼疲劳

copolymer [kəu'pɔlimə] *n* 共聚物 | **~ic** [kəuˌpɔli'merik] *a*

Copolymer 1 [kə'pɔlimə] 共聚物 1(一种合成多肽的商品名,含有丙氨酸、谷氨酸、赖氨酸和酪氨酸;本品模拟髓磷脂碱性蛋白,试验性用于治疗复发性和间歇性多发性硬化症)

copolymerization [kəuˌpɔlimərai'zeiʃən, -ri'z-] *n* 共聚,作用 | **copolymerize** [kəu'pɔliməraiz] *vt*, *vi* 共聚

COPP cyclophosphamide, vincristine, procarbazine, and prednisone 环磷酰胺-长春新碱-丙卡巴肼-泼尼松(联合化疗治癌方案)

copper(co) ['kɔpə] *n* 铜 | ~ abietinate 松香酸铜(兽用抗蠕虫药和驱虫药) / ~ citrate 枸橼酸铜 / ~ iodide 碘化亚铜 / ~ oxyphosphate 氧磷酸铜 / ~ phenolsulfonate 酚磺酸铜 / ~ sulfate 硫酸铜 | **~y** *a* 含铜的,似铜的

copperas ['kɔpərəs] *n* 绿矾,硫酸亚铁(消毒剂和除臭剂)

copper-colo(u)red ['kɔpə ˌkʌləd] *a* 古铜色的,紫铜色的

copperhead ['kɔpəhed] *n* 铜头蛇

copracrasia [ˌkɔprə'kreisiə] *n* 大便失禁,肛门失禁

copragogue [ˈkɔprəgɔg] *n* 泻药
coprecipitin [ˌkəupriˈsipitin] *n* 共沉淀素(在同一血清中与一种或多种其他沉淀素共同存在的沉淀素)
copremesis [kɔpˈremisis] *n* 呕粪,吐粪
Coprinaceae [ˌkəupriˈneisiiː] *n* 鬼伞科
coprine [ˈkəupriːn] *n* 鬼伞
Coprinus [kəuˈprainəs] *n* 鬼伞属
copro- [构词成分] 粪
coproantibody [ˌkɔprəˈæntibɔdi] *n* 粪抗体(存在于肠道内的一种抗体,主要是分泌型 IgA)
Coprococcus [ˌkɔprəˈkɔkəs] *n* 粪球菌属
coprod(a)eum [ˌkɔprəˈdiːəm] *n* 粪道,排粪道
coprolagnia [ˌkɔprəˈlægniə] *n* 弄粪色情,恋粪色情
coprolalia [ˌkɔprəˈleiliə], **coprolalomania** [ˌkɔprəˌlæləuˈmeinjə] *n* 秽语[症]
coprolith [ˈkɔprəliθ] *n* 粪石
coprology [kɔˈprɔlədʒi] *n* 粪便学
coproma [kɔˈprəumə] *n* 粪结,粪瘤(肠内结粪)
Copromastix [ˌkɔprəˈmæstiks] *n* 粪鞭毛虫属 | ~ prowazeki 普[鲁瓦策克]氏粪鞭毛虫
Copromonas [kɔˈprɔmənəs] *n* 粪滴虫属 | ~ subtilis 枯草粪滴虫
coprophagia [ˌkɔprəˈfeidʒiə], **coprophagy** [kɔˈprɔfədʒi] *n* 食粪症,食粪癖
coprophagous [kɔˈprɔfəgəs] *a* 食粪的
coprophil [ˈkɔprəfil] *n* 嗜污菌
coprophile [ˈkɔprəfail] *n* 嗜污菌 *a* 嗜污的
coprophilia [ˌkɔprəˈfiliə] *n* 嗜粪癖
coprophiliac [ˌkɔprəˈfiliæk] *n* 嗜粪癖者(精神病)
coprophilic [ˌkɔprəˈfilik], **coprophilous** [kɔˈprɔfiləs] *a* 嗜粪癖的;嗜粪的(指某些细菌和原虫)
coprophobia [ˌkɔprəˈfəubjə] *n* 粪便恐怖,排便恐怖,恐粪症
coprophrasia [ˌkɔprəˈfreiziə] *n* 秽语,秽亵言语
coproporphyria [ˌkɔprəpɔːˈfiriə] *n* 粪卟啉症 | erythropoietic ~ 红细胞生成性粪卟啉症 / hereditary ~ 遗传性粪卟啉症
coproporphyrin [ˌkɔprəˈpɔːfirin] *n* 粪卟啉
coproporphyrinogen [ˌkɔprəˌpɔːfiˈrinədʒən] *n* 粪卟啉原
coproporphyrinogen oxidase [ˌkɔprəˌpɔːfiˈrinədʒən ˈɔksideis] 粪卟啉原氧化酶(此酶缺乏为一种常染色体显性性状,可致遗传性粪卟啉症)
coproporphyrinuria [ˌkɔprəˌpɔːfiriˈnjuəriə] *n* 粪卟啉尿
coprostanol [ˌkɔprəˈsteinɔl], **coprosterin** [ˌkɔprəˈstiərin], **coprosterol** [ˌkɔprəˈstiərɔl] *n* 粪[甾]醇
coprostasis [kɔˈprɔstəsis] *n* 便结,粪积
coproxAPAP [kəuˈprɔksəpæp] *n* 萘磺酸丙氧芬-对乙酰氨基酚(镇痛药)
coprozoa [ˌkɔprəˈzəuə] *n* 粪内寄生动物,粪生动物
coprozoic [ˌkɔprəˈzəuik] *a* 粪内寄生的,粪生的
Coptis [ˈkɔptis] *n*【拉】黄连属
copula [ˈkɔpjulə] *n* 联合突;(舌)联体 | **~r** *a*
copulate [ˈkɔpjuleit] *vi* 交合,交媾;接合 | **copulation** [ˌkɔpjuˈleiʃən] *n* **copulative** [ˈkɔpjulətiv] *a* 连接的;交合的,交媾的;结合的
Coq. coque【拉】煮沸
Coq. in s. a. coque in sufficiente aqua【拉】用足量水煮沸
Coq. s. a. coque secundum artem【拉】适当煮沸,按常法煮沸
coquille [kəuˈkwiːl] *n* 有色眼镜罩
Coquillettidia [kəuˌkwiləˈtidiə] *n* 科蚊属 | ~ perturbans 骚扰科蚊 | ~ venezuelensis 委内瑞拉科蚊
cor- 见 con-
cor [kɔː] *n*【拉】心
coracidium [ˌkɔrəˈsidiəm] ([复]**coracidia** [ˌkɔrəˈsidiə]) *n* 钩球蚴,纤毛蚴
coracoacromial [ˌkɔrəkəuəˈkrəumiəl] *a* 喙肩的,喙突肩峰的
coracoclavicular [ˌkɔrəkəukləˈvikjulə] *a* 喙锁的,喙突锁骨的
coracohumeral [ˌkɔrəkəuˈhjuːmərəl] *a* 喙肱的,喙突肱骨的
coracoid [ˈkɔrəkɔid] *a* 喙状的 *n* 喙突
coracoiditis [ˌkɔrəkɔiˈdaitis] *n* 喙突炎
coracoradialis [ˌkɔrəkəuˌreidiˈeilis] *n* 肱二头肌短头
coracoulnaris [ˌkɔrəkəuʌlˈnɛəris] *n* 肱二头肌腱膜
coral [ˈkɔrəl] *a*, *n* 珊瑚(的)
coralliform [kəˈrælifɔːm], **coralloid** [ˈkɔrəlɔid] *a* 珊瑚状的
corallin [ˈkɔrəlin] *n* 珊瑚精;玫红酸 | yellow ~ 黄玫红酸
corasthma [kɔˈræsmə] *n* 花粉症
Corbus' disease [ˈkɔːbəs] (Budd C. Corbus) 坏疽性阴茎头炎
cord [kɔːd] *n* 索,带;[复]束 | dental ~ 牙索 / enamel ~ 釉索 / false vocal ~ 假声带,室襞 / ganglionated ~ 交感[神经]干 / genital ~ 生殖索 / gubernacular ~ 睾丸引带 / hepatic ~s 肝索 / lumbosacral ~ 腰骶干 / medullary ~s 髓索 / nephrogenic ~ 生肾索 / nerve ~ 神经干 / ovigerous ~s 生卵索 / psalterial ~ 血管纹 / red pulp ~s, splenic ~s 红髓索,脾索 / rete ~s 网索

/ sex ~s 网索,性索 / sexual ~s 生殖索 / spermatic ~ 精索 / spinal ~脊髓 / true vocal ~ 声带,声襞 / umbilical ~ 脐带 | **~al** *a* 索的,带的(尤指声带或声襞的)
cordate [ˈkɔːdeit] *a* 心形的
cordectomy [kɔːˈdektəmi] *n* 声带切除术,索带切除术
cordial [ˈkɔːdjəl] *a* 强心的 *n* 香酒
cordiale [kɔːdiˈeili] *n*【拉】香酒
cordiform [ˈkɔːdifɔːm] *a* 心形的
cording-up [ˌkɔːdiŋ ˈʌp] *n* 氮尿症(马)
corditis [kɔːˈdaitis] *n* 精索炎
cordocentesis [ˌkɔːdəusenˈtiːsis] *n* 脐穿刺(亦称经皮脐血取样)
cordon [ˈkɔːdən] *n* 封锁线 | sanitary ~ 防疫线,(国境)交通检疫封锁线
cordopexy [ˈkɔːdəˌpeksi] *n* 声带固定术
cordotomy [kɔːˈdɔtəmi] *n* 声带切开术;脊髓前外侧束切断术
Cordyceps [ˈkɔːdiseps] *n* 冬虫夏草属 | ~ sinensis 冬虫夏草
Cordylobia [ˌkɔːdiˈləubiə] *n* 瘤蝇属 | ~ anthropophaga 嗜人瘤蝇
core [kɔː] *n* 核,核心;(感应圈或电磁铁的)铁芯;病毒体核心;铸模核;片心;(噬菌体)髓部 | cast ~ 铸模核
core-, cor(o)- [构词成分] 瞳孔;同样见以 irid(o)-起始的词
coreclisis [ˌkɔːriˈklaisis] *n* 瞳孔闭合,虹膜箝顿术
corectasis [kɔːˈrektəsis] *n* 瞳孔开大,瞳孔散大,瞳孔扩大
corectome [kɔːˈrektəum] *n* 虹膜刀
corectomedialysis [kɔˌrektəuˌmiːdiˈælisis] *n* 人造瞳孔术,假瞳术
corectomy [kɔˈrektəmi] *n* 虹膜切除术
corectopia [kɔːrekˈtəupiə] *n* 瞳孔异位
coredialysis [ˌkɔːridaiˈælisis] *n* 虹膜根部分离术
corediastasis [ˌkɔːridaiˈæstəsis] *n* 瞳孔扩大
coregonin [kəˈregənin] *n* 白鲑精蛋白
corelysis [kɔˈrelisis] *n* 虹膜后粘连分离术
coremium [kəˈriːmiəm] *n* 菌丝束
coremorphosis [ˌkɔːrimɔːˈfəusis] *n* 瞳孔形成
corenclisis [ˌkɔːrenˈklaisis] *n* 虹膜箝顿术
coreometer [ˌkɔːriˈɔmitə] *n* 瞳孔计 | **coreometry** *n* 瞳孔测量法
coreoplasty [ˈkɔːriəˌplæsti] *n* 瞳孔成形术,造瞳术
corepressor [ˌkəuriˈpresə] *n* 辅阻遏物(与阻遏物蛋白结合形成控制酶合成的小分子物质)
corestenoma [ˌkɔːristiˈnəumə] *n* 瞳孔狭窄 | ~ congenitum 先天性瞳孔部分狭窄
Corethra [kəˈriːθrə] *n* 短嘴蚊属(即 Chaoborus)
coretomedialysis [ˌkɔːritəmidiˈælisis] *n* 假瞳术,造瞳术
coretomy [kɔˈretəmi] *n* 虹膜切开术
coriaceous [ˌkɔriˈeiʃəs] *a* 革样的,粗糙的(指细菌培养物)
coriamyrtin [ˌkɔːriəˈməːtin] *n* 马桑苷,马桑内酯,马桑毒内酯
coriander [ˌkɔriˈændə] *n* 芫荽,胡荽(曾用作驱风剂及芳香剂,现用作调味品)
Coriandrum [ˌkəuriˈændrəm] *n* 芫荽属
Coriaria [kɔriˈɛəriə] *n* 马桑属
Cori cycle [ˈkɔːri] (Carl F. Cori; Gerty T. Cori) 科里循环,葡萄糖乳酸循环 | ~ disease 糖原贮积症Ⅲ型 / ~ ester 科里酯,葡糖-1-磷酸
coriin [ˈkɔːriin] *n* 柯里因(用碱处理纤维结缔组织所形成的物质)
corrinoid [ˈkɔːrinɔid] *n* 类咕啉
corium [ˈkɔːriəm] ([复]**coria** [ˈkɔːriə]) *n*【拉】真皮
cork [kɔːk] *n* 木栓
corm [kɔːm] *n* 球茎
cormethasone acetate [kɔːˈmeθəsəun] 醋酸可米松(局部抗炎药)
corn[1] [kɔːn] *n* 玉米;谷物
corn[2] [kɔːn] *n* 鸡眼;钉胼 | hard ~ 硬鸡眼 / soft ~ 软鸡眼
corn cockle [kɔːnˈkɔkəl] 麦仙翁,毒莠草
cornea [ˈkɔːniə] *n* 角膜 | conical ~ 圆锥形角膜 / ~ farinata 角膜粉样变性 / ~ globosa 球形角膜 / ~ guttata 角膜点状变性 / ~ opaca 巩膜 / ~ plana 扁平角膜 | **~l** *a*
corneitis [ˌkɔːniˈaitis] *n* 角膜炎
Cornelia de Lange [kəːˈneiliə deiˈlɑːŋə] 见 de Lange
corneoblepharon [ˌkɔːniəuˈblefərɔn] *n* 角膜睑粘连
corneocyte [ˈkɔːniəˌsait] *n* 角膜细胞
corneoiritis [ˌkɔːniəuaiəˈraitis] *n* 角膜虹膜炎
corneosclera [ˌkɔːniəuˈskliərə] *n* 角巩膜
corneoscleral [ˌkɔːniəuˈskliərəl] *a* 角膜巩膜的
corneous [ˈkɔːniəs] *a* 角样的;角质的
corner [ˈkɔːnə] *n* 角齿,侧门牙(马)
Corner-Allen test [ˈkɔːnə ˈælin] (George W. Corner; Willard M. Allen) 康纳-艾伦试验(生物鉴定法,测黄体酮或黄体制剂) | ~ unit 康纳-艾伦单位(一种黄体激素的剂量单位)
Corner's tampon [ˈkɔːnə] (Edred M. Corner) 康纳塞子(网膜塞,插入胃或肠伤口用)
Cornet's forceps [ˈkɔːnit] (George Cornet) 科内特钳(用以夹住盖玻片的钳)
corneum [ˈkɔːniəm] *n*【拉】角质层
corniculate [kɔːˈnikjulit] *a* 小角状的

corniculum [kɔːˈnikjuləm] *n*【拉】小角软骨

cornification [ˌkɔːnifiˈkeiʃən] *n* 角化;复层鳞状上皮化

cornified [ˈkɔːnifaid] *a* 角[质]化的

Corning's anesthesia (method) [ˈkɔːniŋ] (James L. Corning) 脊髓麻醉 | ~ puncture 腰椎穿刺

cornoid [ˈkɔːnɔid] *a* 角样的

cornstarch [ˈkɔnstɑːtʃ] *n* 玉米淀粉

cornu [ˈkɔːnju] ([复] **cornua** [ˈkɔːnjuə]) *n*【拉】角 | coccygeal ~ 尾骨角 / ethmoid ~ 中鼻甲 / sacral ~ 骶骨角 / ~ a of spinal cord 脊髓角 | **~al**, **~ate** [ˈkɔːnjuit] *a*

cornucommissural [ˌkɔːnjukəˈmisjurəl] *a* 角的;角连合的

cornucopia [ˌkɔːnjuˈkəupjə] *n* 外侧隐窝(第四脑室)

Cornus [ˈkɔːnəs] *n*【拉】梾木属(山茱萸科) | ~ florida 北美山茱萸(其干根皮用作收敛性苦味药)

cor(o)- 见 core-

corodiastasis [ˌkɔrəudaiˈæstəsis] *n* 瞳孔扩大

corolla [kəˈrɔlə] *n* 卵冠;花冠

corometer [kɔˈrɔmitə] *n* 瞳孔计

corona [kəˈrəunə] ([复] **coronas** 或 **coronae** [kəˈrəuniː]) *n*【拉】冠 | dental ~ 牙冠,齿冠 / ~ of glandis penis 阴茎头冠 / ~ veneris 额(发缘)梅毒疹

coronad [ˈkɔrənæd] *ad* 向冠;向头顶

coronal [kəˈrəunəl, ˈkɔrənl] *n* 冠;花冠 *a* 冠的;冠状的;头冠状缝的

coronale [kɔrəˈneili] *n* 冠状缝(额径端点);额骨

coronalis [kɔrəˈneilis] *a*【拉】冠的(指位于冠状缝方向的)

coronaritis [ˌkɔrənəˈraitis] *n* 冠状动脉炎

coronarography [kəˈrəunəˈrɔgrəfi] *n* 冠状动脉造影[术]

coronary [ˈkɔrənəri] *a* 冠状的

Coronaviridae [kəˌrəunəˈviridiː] *n* 冠状病毒科

Coronavirus [kəˈrəunəˌvaiərəs] *n* 冠状病毒属

coronavirus [kəˈrəunəˌvaiərəs] *n* 冠状病毒,日冕形病毒(一组形态相似、醚致敏的病毒,或许是RNA,引起鸟传染性支气管炎、鼠肝炎、猪胃肠炎、人呼吸道感染,由于在电子显微镜下酷似冠,故名)

corone [kəˈrəuni] *n* 下颌冠状突

coroner [ˈkɔrənə] *n* 验尸官

coronet [ˈkɔrənit] *n* 马蹄冠

coronion [kəˈrəuniɔn] *n* 冠状突尖(下颌)

coronitis [ˌkɔrəˈnaitis] *n* 冠状垫炎(马)

coronoid [ˈkɔrənɔid] *a* 喙状的;冠状的

coronoidectomy [ˌkɔrənɔiˈdektəmi] *n* (下颌骨)冠突切除术

coronoidotomy [ˌkɔːrənɔiˈdɔtəmi] *n* (下颌骨)冠突切除术

coroparelcysis [ˌkɔrəpəˈrelsisis] *n* 瞳孔旁移术

coroplasty [ˈkɔrəˌplæsti] *n* 瞳孔成形术,造瞳术

coroscopy [kəˈrɔskəpi] *n* 瞳孔检影法

corotomy [kəˈrɔtəmi] *n* 虹膜切开术

corpora [ˈkɔːpərə] corpus 的复数

corporeal [kɔːˈpɔːriəl], **corporal** [ˈkɔːpərəl] *a* 体的

corporic [kɔːˈpɔːrik] *a* 体的(器官)

corps [kɔː] ([复] **corps** [kɔːz]) *n* 队,团;体,物体 | medical ~ 医疗队(陆、海军外科军医官等组成) / ~ ronds 圆体,圆体细胞(见于毛囊角化症)

corpse [kɔːps] *n* 尸体

corpulence [ˈkɔːpjuləns], **corpulency** [ˈkɔːpjulənsi] *n* 肥胖

corpulent [ˈkɔːpjulənt] *a* 肥胖的

corpus [ˈkɔːpəs] ([复] **corpora** [ˈkɔːpərə]) *n*【拉】体 | ~ albicans, ~ fibrosum 白体,纤维体 / ~ alienum 异物,外物 / ~ luteum 黄体

corpuscallosotomy, corpus callosotomy [ˈkɔːpəs kæləˈsɔtəmi] 胼胝体切开术(亦称 callosotomy)

corpuscle [ˈkɔːpʌsl] *n* 小体,细胞;微粒,粒子 | amylaceous ~s, amyloid ~s 淀粉样体 / articular ~s 关节内(触觉)小体 / axile ~, axis ~ 轴小体(触觉小体的中心部分) / blood ~s 血细胞 / bone ~ 骨小体,骨细胞 / cement ~ 牙骨质细胞 / chyle ~ 乳糜小体 / colloid ~s 胶状小体,淀粉样体 / colostrum ~s 初乳小体,初乳细胞 / concentric ~s, thymus ~s 胸腺小体 / dust ~s 血尘 / marginal ~ 边缘小体(红细胞内) / meconium ~ 胎粪小体 / milk ~ 乳脂微粒 / nerve ~s 神经细胞,神经元;神经膜细胞 / pessary ~ 子宫托形红细胞 / phantom ~, ghost ~, shadow ~ 红细胞影 / red blood ~s 红细胞 / splenic ~s 脾小结,脾淋巴滤泡 / tactile ~s, touch ~s 触觉小体 / taste ~s 味细胞 / white blood ~s 白细胞 | **corpuscular** [kɔːˈpʌskjulə] *a*

corpusculum [kɔːˈpʌskjuləm] ([复] **corpuscula** [kɔːˈpʌskjulə]) *n*【拉】小体,细胞

correction [kəˈrekʃən] *n* 矫正;校正;校正数

corrective [kəˈrektiv] *a* 矫正的 *n* 矫味药

corrector [kəˈrektə] *n* 矫正器 | function ~ 功能矫正器(畸牙矫正用,亦称弗伦克尔矫正器 Fränkel appliance)

correlation [ˌkɔriˈleiʃən] *n* 相关[性]

correspondence [ˌkɔrisˈpɔndəns] *n* 对应,相对 | anomalous retinal ~ 异常视网膜对应 / normal retinal ~ 正常视网膜对应 / retinal ~ 视网膜对应

Corridor disease [ˈkɔridɔː] (The Corridor 为南

非一地区,首次在此报道此病)科立多病(一种蜱传性原虫病,对牛有高度致病性,水牛为其贮存宿主)
Corrigan's cautery [ˈkɔrigən] (Dominic J. Corrigan)科里根烙器(钮式烙器) | ~ disease 主动脉瓣反流 / ~ line 科里根线(铜中毒时,牙龈上所见的紫线) / ~ pulse 科里根脉(水冲状脉,主动脉瓣反流时发生) / ~ respiration 科里根呼吸(低热时浅而频繁的吹气样呼吸) / ~ sign 科里根征(①慢性铜中毒时龈缘有紫色线;②腹主动脉瘤时搏动特别扩张;③低热时浅而频繁的吹气样呼吸)
corrigent [ˈkɔridʒənt] *a* 矫正的 *n* 矫味药
corrin [ˈkɔːrin] *n* 咕啉
corroborant [kəˈrɔbərənt] *a* 滋补的
corrode [kəˈrəud] *vt* 腐蚀 *vi* 起腐蚀作用
corroid [ˈkɔːrɔid] *n* 咕啉类(含一个咕啉环系统的化合物,如钴胺)
corrosion [kəˈrəuʒən] *n* 腐蚀[作用]
corrosive [kəˈrəusiv] *a* 腐蚀的 *n* 腐蚀剂
corrugator [ˈkɔruˌgeitə] *n* 皱眉;皱眉肌
corsair [ˈkɔːsɑː] *n* 猎蝽
corset [ˈkɔːsit] *n* 围腰,胸衣(如脊髓损伤或畸形者所穿)
Cort. cortex【拉】(树)皮;皮质,皮层
cortex [ˈkɔːteks] ([复] **cortices** [ˈkɔːtisiːz] 或 **cortexes**) *n* [树]皮;皮质,皮层 | adrenal ~ 肾上腺皮质 / cerebellar ~, ~ of cerebellum 小脑皮质,小脑皮层 / cerebral ~, ~ of cerebrum 大脑皮质,大脑皮层 / nonolfactory ~ 新[大脑]皮质,新皮层 / olfactory ~ 原始外表(嗅脑),旧皮质,旧皮层 / provisional ~ 临时皮质(肾上腺) / renal ~, ~ of kidney 肾皮质 | **cortical** [ˈkɔːtikəl] *a*
cortexone [kɔːˈteksəun] *n* Ⅱ-脱氧皮质[甾]酮
cortiadrenal [ˌkɔːtiəˈdriːnl] *a* 肾上腺皮质的
corticalosteotomy [ˌkɔːtikɔləstiˈɔtəmi] *n* 经皮质切骨术
corticate(d) [ˈkɔːtikeit(id)] *a* 有皮质的;有(树)皮的
corticectomy [ˌkɔːtiˈsektəmi] *n* [脑]皮质切除术(治病灶性癫痫)
cortices [ˈkɔːtisiːz] cortex 的复数
corticifugal [ˌkɔːtiˈsifjugəl] *a* 离皮质的,离皮层的
corticipetal [ˌkɔːtiˈsipitl] *a* 向皮质的,向皮层的
cortic(o)- [构词成分]皮质,皮层
corticoadrenal [ˌkɔːtikəuəˈdriːnl] *a* 肾上腺皮质的
corticoafferent [ˌkɔːtikəuˈæfərənt] *a* [向]皮质传入的,[向]皮层传入的
corticoautonomic [ˌkɔːtikəuˌɔːtəuˈnɔmik] *a* 皮质自主的,皮层自主的
corticobulbar [ˌkɔːtikəuˈbʌlbə] *a* 皮质延髓的
corticocancellous [ˌkɔːtikəuˈkænsələs] *a* 皮质网状体的
corticocerebral [ˌkɔːtikəuˈseribrəl] *a* 大脑皮质的,大脑皮层的
corticodiencephalic [ˌkɔːtikəuˌdaiensiˈfælik] *a* 皮质间脑的,皮层间脑的
corticoefferent [ˌkɔːtikəuˈefərənt] *a* [从]皮质传出的,[从]皮层传出的
corticofugal [ˌkɔːtiˈkɔfjugəl] *a* 离皮质的,离皮层的
corticoid [ˈkɔːtikɔid] *n* 肾上腺皮质激素
corticoliberin [ˌkɔːtikəuˈlibərin] *n* 促肾上腺皮质素释放素
corticolipotrope [ˌkɔːtikəuˈlipəuˌtrəup] *n* 促皮质激素细胞
corticomedullary [ˌkɔːtikəuˈmedjuləri] *a* 皮质髓质的
corticomesencephalic [ˌkɔːtikə u ˌmesensiˈfælik] *a* 皮质中脑的,皮层中脑的
corticopeduncular [ˌkɔːtikəupiˈdʌŋkjulə] *a* 皮质大脑脚的,皮层大脑脚的
corticopetal [ˌkɔːtiˈkɔpitl] *a* 向皮质的,向皮层的
corticopleuritis [ˌkɔːtikəupluəˈraitis] *n* 胸膜壁层炎
corticopontine [ˌkɔːtikəuˈpɔntain] *a* 皮质脑桥的
corticorelin ovine triflutate [ˌkɔːtikəuˈrelin] 羊三氟醋酸可的瑞林(诊断辅助药)
corticospinal [ˌkɔːtikəuˈspainl] *a* 皮质脊髓的
corticosteroid [ˌkɔːtikəuˈstiərɔid] *n* 皮质类固醇
corticosterone [ˌkɔːtiˈkɔstərəun] *n* 皮质酮
corticosterone methyl oxidase [ˌkɔːtiˈkɔstərəun ˈmeθil ˈɔksideis] 皮质酮甲基氧化酶,皮质酮 18-单加氧酶
corticosterone methyl oxidase deficiency 皮质酮甲基氧化酶缺乏症(一种类固醇生成疾病,皮质酮 18-单加氧酶缺乏有损于醛甾酮生物合成并导致盐消耗。亦称 18-羟化酶缺乏症)
corticosterone 18-monooxygenase [ˌkɔːtiˈkɔstərəun ˌmɔnəuˈɔksidʒəneis] 皮质酮 18-单加氧酶
corticotensin [ˌkɔːtikəuˈtensin] *n* 皮质加压素
corticothalamic [ˌkɔːtikəuθəˈlæmik] *a* 皮质丘脑的,皮层丘脑的
corticotrope [ˈkɔːtikətrəup] *n* 促肾上腺皮质激素细胞
corticotroph [ˈkɔːtikətrəuf] *n* 促肾上腺皮质激素细胞
corticotroph-lipotroph [ˈkɔːtikətrəuf ˈlipətrəuf] *n* 促肾上腺皮质-促脂细胞(即促肾上腺皮质激素细胞 corticotroph)
corticotropic [ˌkɔːtikəuˈtrɔpik], **corticotrophic**

[ˌkɔːtikəuˈtrɔfik] *a* 促肾上腺皮质的

corticotropin [ˌkɔːtikəuˈtrəupin], **corticotrophin** [ˌkɔːtikəuˈtrəufin] *n* 促皮质素；（垂体前叶激素类药）；促肾上腺皮质激素

corticotropinoma [ˌkɔːtikəuˌtrəupiˈnəumə] *n* 促肾上腺皮质[激]素瘤，促肾上腺皮质[激]素腺瘤

cortilymph [ˈkɔːtiˌlimf] *n* 科尔蒂淋巴，第三淋巴（充满科尔蒂器细胞间隙的液体）

cortin [ˈkɔːtin] *n* 皮质素（旧名，即肾上腺皮质浸膏）

Cortinariaceae [ˌkɔːtiˌnεəriˈeisiiː] *n* 丝膜蕈属

Corti's arch [ˈkɔːti] (Alfonso Corti)科尔蒂弓（螺旋柱弓）| ~ canal 科尔蒂管（内隧道）/ ~ cell 科尔蒂细胞（听毛细胞）/ ~ fiber 科尔蒂纤维（柱细胞）/ ~ ganglion 科尔蒂神经节（蜗神经节）/ ~ membrane 科尔蒂膜（蜗管覆膜）/ ~ organ 科尔蒂器（螺旋器）/ ~ pillar 科尔蒂柱（柱细胞）/ ~ rods 科尔蒂杆（柱细胞）/ ~ tunnel 科尔蒂小管（内隧道）

cortisol [ˈkɔːtisɔl] *n* 皮质醇

cortisone [ˈkɔːtisəun] *n* 可的松（天然糖皮质激素）| ~ acetate 醋酸可的松（抗炎药）

cortivazol [kɔːˈtivəzəul] *n* 可的伐唑（合成糖皮质激素）

corundum [kəˈrʌndəm] *n* 刚玉，金刚砂（牙科中用作磨料）

coruscation [ˌkɔrəsˈkeiʃən] *n* 闪光感

Corvisart's disease [ˌkɔːviˈsɑː] (Jean N. Corvisart)科维萨尔病（①以前称慢性肥大性心肌炎；②法洛〈Fallot〉四联症伴右主动脉弓）

corybantism [ˌkɔːriˈbæntizəm], **corybantiasm** [ˌkɔːriˈbæntiæzəm] *n* 精神狂乱

corydaline [kəˈridəliːn] *n* 紫堇碱，延胡索碱（利尿强壮药）

corydalis [kəˈridəlis] *n* 紫堇

corymb [ˈkɔrim*b*] *n* 伞房花序 | **~iform** [kəˈrimbifɔːm], **~ose** [ˈkɔrimbəus], **~ous** [kəˈrimbəs] *a* 伞房花形的

Corynebacteriaceae [kəˌrainibækˌtiəriˈeisiiː] *n* 棒状杆菌科

Corynebacterium [kəˌrainibækˈtiəriəm] *n* 棒状杆菌属 | ~ acnes 粉刺棒状杆菌，痤疮棒状杆菌 / ~ diphtheriae 白喉棒状杆菌，白喉杆菌 / ~ diphtheroides 类白喉棒状杆菌，白喉杆菌 / ~ equi 马棒状杆菌 / ~ genitalium 生殖器棒状杆菌 / ~ granulosum 粒状棒状杆菌 / ~ haemolyticum 溶血棒状杆菌 / ~ infantisepticum 婴儿败血症棒状杆菌 / ~ kutscheri 库[彻]氏棒状杆菌 / ~ minutissimum 微小棒状杆菌，红癣菌 / ~ murisepticum 鼠败血棒状杆菌 / ~ necrophorum 坏疽热棒状杆菌，犊白喉杆菌 / ~ parvulum 产单核细胞李斯特菌（即 Listeria monocytogenes）/ ~ parvum 短小棒状杆菌 / ~ pseudodiphtheriticum, ~ hofmannii 假白喉棒状杆菌，霍夫曼棒状杆菌 / ~ pseudotuberculosis, ~ ovis 假结核棒状杆菌，绵羊棒状杆菌 / ~ pyogenes 化脓棒状杆菌 / ~ renale 肾棒状杆菌 / ~ tenuis 纤细棒状杆菌，腋毛癣菌 / ~ ulcerans 溃疡棒状杆菌 / ~ vesiculare 泡囊棒状杆菌 / ~ xerosis 干燥棒状杆菌

corynebacterium [kəˌrainibækˈtiəriəm] ([复] **corynebacteria** [kəˌrainibækˈtiəriə]) *n* 棒状[杆]菌 | group JK ~ JK 型棒状杆菌 / group 3 ~ 3 型棒状杆菌，迟缓真杆菌（即 Eubacterium lentum）

Coryneform [kəˈrainifɔːm] *n* 棒状杆菌群

coryneform [kəˈrainifɔːm] *a* 棒状杆菌的

Corynespora [ˌkɔːriˈnespɔːrə] *n* 棒状孢菌属

corytuberine [ˌkɔriˈtjuːbəriːn] *n* 紫堇块茎碱

coryza [kəˈraizə] *n*【拉】鼻卡他，鼻炎，感冒（俗名伤风）| allergic ~ 变应性鼻炎，枯草热 / ~ foetida 恶臭性鼻炎，臭鼻症 / infectious avian ~ 传染性禽鼻炎 / ~ oedematosa 水肿性鼻卡他

coryzavirus [kəˌraizəˈvaiərəs] *n* 感冒病毒，鼻炎病毒（现称鼻病毒 rhinovirus）

COS Canadian Ophthalmological Society 加拿大眼科学会

Coschwitz' duct [ˈkɔʃwits] (Georgius D. Coschwitz)科施维茨管（一条假定的涎管，在舌背侧形成弓状，由 von Haller 证明实为一条静脉）

cosensitize [kəuˈsensitaiz] *vt* 共同敏感，多敏感

cosmesis [kɔzˈmiːsis] *n* 美容术

cosmetic [kɔzˈmetik] *a* 美容的 *n* 化妆品，美容剂

cosmetology [ˌkɔzməˈtɔlədʒi] *n* 美容学 | **cosmetologist** *n* 美容专家

cosmid [ˈkɔzmid] *n* 黏粒

cospironozide [ˌkəuspiˈrɔnəzaid] *n* 螺内酯-氢氯噻嗪（利尿药）

costa [ˈkɔstə] ([复] **costae** [ˈkɔstiː]) *n*【拉】肋骨 | **~l** *a*

costalgia [kɔsˈtældʒiə] *n* 肋痛；肋肌痛

costalis [kɔsˈteilis] *a*【拉】肋的

costate [ˈkɔsteit] *a* 有肋骨的；肋骨状的

costectomy [kɔsˈtektəmi], **costatectomy** [ˌkɔstəˈtektəmi] *n* 肋骨切除术

Costen's syndrome [ˈkɔstən] (James B. Costen) 科斯滕综合征，颞下颌关节功能障碍综合征（即 temporomandibular dysfunction syndrome，见 syndrome 项下相应术语）

costicartilage [ˌkɔstiˈkɑːtilidʒ] *n* 肋软骨

costicervical [ˌkɔstiˈsəːvikəl] *a* 肋颈的

costiferous [kɔsˈtifərəs] *a* 有肋的

costiform [ˈkɔstifɔːm] *a* 肋状的

costispinal [kɔsti'spainl] *a* 肋椎的
costive ['kɔstiv] *a* 便秘的 *n* 肠蠕动抑制药 | ~ **ness** *n* 便秘
cost(o)- [构词成分]肋骨,肋
costocentral [ˌkɔstəu'sentrəl] *a* 肋骨[与]椎体的
costocervicalis [ˌkɔstəusəːvi'keilis] *n* 颈髂肋肌
costochondral [ˌkɔstəu'kɔndrəl] *a* 肋骨(肋)软骨的
costoclavicular [ˌkɔstəuklə'vikjulə] *a* 肋锁的
costocoracoid [ˌkɔstəu'kɔrəkɔid] *a* 肋[骨]喙突的
costogenic [ˌkɔstəu'dʒenik] *a* 肋骨性的(由肋骨产生的,尤指由肋骨髓缺陷产生的)
costoinferior [ˌkɔstəuin'fiəriə] *a* 下肋的
costophrenic [ˌkɔstəu'frenik] *a* 肋膈的(胸膜)
costopleural [ˌkɔstəu'pluərəl] *a* 肋胸膜的
costopneumopexy [ˌkɔstəu'njuːməˌpeksi] *n* 肋骨肺固定术
costoscapular [ˌkɔstəu'skæpjulə] *a* 肋骨肩胛的
costoscapularis [ˌkɔstəuˌskæpju'lɛəris] *n* 前锯肌
costosternal [ˌkɔstəu'stəːnəl] *a* 肋胸[骨]的
costosternoplasty [ˌkɔstəu'stəːnəˌplæsti] *n* 肋骨胸骨成形术(漏斗胸成形术)
costosuperior [ˌkɔstəusju(ː)'piəriə] *a* 上肋的
costotome ['kɔstətəum] *n* 肋骨刀,断肋器
costotomy [kɔs'tɔtəmi] *n* 肋骨切开术
costotransverse [ˌkɔstətræns'vəːs] *a* 肋(椎骨)横突的
costotransversectomy [ˌkɔstəuˌtrænsvəː'sektəmi] *n* 肋骨横突切除术
costovertebral [ˌkɔstəu'vəːtibrəl] *a* 肋椎的
costoxiphoid [ˌkɔstəu'zifɔid] *a* 肋剑突的
cosyntropin [kəusin'trəupin] *n* 替可克肽,二十四肽促皮质素,α^{1-24}促皮质素(一种合成的促皮质素,用于检诊肾上腺功能不全)
cot¹ [kɔt] *n* 吊床;儿童摇床;儿童病床
cot² [kɔt] *n* 指套,趾套
Cotard's syndrome [kɔ'tɑː] (Jules Cotard)科塔尔综合征(妄想狂的一型,伴有虚无妄想、自杀倾向等)
cotarnine chloride [kəu'tɑːniːn] 氯化可他宁(曾用作止血药)
COTe cathodal opening tetanus 阴极断电强直
cotenidone [kəu'tenidəun] *n* 阿替洛尔-氯噻酮(β受体阻滞药,噻嗪类利尿药)
cothromboplastin [kəuˌθrɔmbəu'plæstin] *n* 辅促凝血酶原激酶(凝血因子Ⅶ)
cotinine ['kəutiniːn] *n* 可替宁(精神振奋药) | ~ fumarate 延胡索酸可替宁(抗抑郁药)
cotransfection [ˌkəutræns'fekʃən] *n* 共转染(指两个分离的互不相关的核酸分子同时转染)
cotransport [kəu'trænspɔːt] *n* 协同转运(指两个物质跨越膜朝同一方向同时转运)
Cotrel-Dubousset instrumentation [kəu'trel djubus'sei] (Y. Cotrel; J. Dubousset)科-杜器械用法(一套杆、钩和螺钉用于脊柱融合术治疗胸腰区脊柱侧凸) | ~ rod 科-杜杆(一种坚硬的波状外形杆,用于科-杜器械用法)
cotriamterzide [ˌkəutrai'æmtəzaid] *n* 氨苯蝶啶-氢氯噻嗪(利尿药)
co-trimoxazole [ˌkəutrai'mɔksəzəul] *n* 增效磺胺甲噁唑,复方磺胺甲噁唑,甲氧苄啶-磺胺甲噁唑复合剂
Cotte's operation [kɔt] (Gaston Cotte)科特手术(骶前神经切除术)
Cotting's operation ['kɔtiŋ] (Benjamin E. Cotting)科廷手术(嵌甲手术)
cotton ['kɔtn] *n* 棉,棉花 | absorbent ~ 脱脂棉,吸水棉,药棉 / collodion ~, gun ~, soluble gun ~ 火棉胶,硝酸纤维素 / purified ~ 精制棉 / salicylated ~ 水杨酸棉 / styptic ~ 止血棉
cottonmouth ['kɔːtnmauθ] *n* 棉口蛇,水生噬鱼蝮蛇
cottonpox ['kɔtnpɔks] *n* 乳白痘,类天花
cottonseed ['kɔtənsiːd] *n* 棉籽
cotton-wool ['kɔtn'wul] *n* 原棉;脱脂棉,药棉
Cotugno's disease [kəu'tuːnjɔ] (Domenico Cotugno)坐骨神经痛
Cotunnius' aqueduct, canal [kəu'tuniəs] (Domenico Cotugno)科图尼约水管(前庭小管;蜗小管) | ~ nerve 鼻腭神经 / ~ space 科图尼约间隙(膜迷路间隙)
coturnism [kə'təːnizəm] *n* 鹑肉中毒症
co-twin ['kəu twin] *n* 双胎
cotyledon [ˌkɔti'liːdən] *n* 子叶(植物);绒毛叶(盘状胎盘母体面的分叶)
Cotyledon [ˌkɔti'liːdən] *n* 子叶属
cotyledontoxin [ˌkɔtiˌliːdən'tɔksin] *n* 瓦松毒素
Cotylogonimus [ˌkɔtilou'gɔnimɔs] *n* 异形吸虫属(即 Heterophyes)
cotyloid ['kɔtilɔid] *a* 杯状的,臼状的;髋臼的
Cotylophoron [ˌkɔti'lɔfərɔn] *n* 殖盘[吸虫]属
cotylopubic [ˌkɔtiləu'pjuːbik] *a* 髋臼耻骨的
cotylosacral [ˌkɔtiləu'seikrəl] *a* 髋臼骶骨的
cotype ['kəutaip] *n* 全模标本
couch [kautʃ] *n* 诊察台;休息处 *vt* (用压下术)除去(白内障)
couch grass ['kautʃ grɑːs] 匍匐冰草,茅草,偃麦草(其长根为利尿剂,曾用于治膀胱炎,且有润滑和镇咳作用)
couching ['kautʃiŋ] *n* 内障压下术
cough [kɔf] *vi* 咳嗽 *vt* 咳出 *n* 咳,咳嗽 | aneurysmal ~ 动脉瘤性咳(有时伴声带麻痹) / barking ~ 犬吠样咳嗽 / compression ~, dog ~ 压迫性

咳,犬吠样咳 / dry ~ 干咳(无痰) / hacking ~ 频咳 / minute gun ~ 密接阵发性咳(百日咳) / privet ~ 水蜡树花粉过敏咳 / productive ~ 排痰性咳 / wet ~ 湿咳(有痰) / whooping ~ 百日咳 / winter ~ 冬季咳(冬季发生的慢性支气管炎)

coulomb(C) [ˈkuːlɔm] *n* 库仑(电量单位)

Coulter counter [ˈkəultə] (Wallace H. Coulter) 库尔特计数器(一种自动血细胞计数器,根据细胞导电性小于生理盐水的原理,进行血细胞计数)

coumaric acid [kuˈmærik] 香豆酸

coumarin [ˈkumərin] *n* 香豆素

coumermycin [kuməˈmaisin], **coumamycin** [kuməˈmaisin] *n* 库马霉素(抗菌药)

Councilmania [ˌkaunsilˈmeiniə] (William Thomas Councilman) *n* 康西尔曼变形虫属,内变形虫属 | ~ dissimilis 异形变形虫,结肠内变形虫 / ~ lafleuri 拉夫勒尔变形虫,结肠内变形虫

Councilman's bodies (lesions) [ˈkaunsilmən] (William T. Councilman)康西尔曼体(损害)(肝细胞内嗜酸性圆体,见于病毒性肝炎、黄热病及其他肝病)

counsel [ˈkaunsəl] *n* 咨询 *vt*, *vi* 咨询,指导 | genetic ~ing 遗传咨询

count [kaunt] *n* 计数 | blood ~ 血细胞计数 / complete blood ~ 全血细胞计数 / differential ~ 白细胞分类计数 / direct platelet ~ 血小板直接计数 / filament-nonfilament ~ 白细胞分核计数 / indirect platelet ~ 血小板间接计数 / neutrophil lobe ~ 中性粒细胞分叶计数

counter [ˈkauntə] *n* 计数器;柜台 | proportional ~ 正比计数器 / scintillation ~ 闪烁计数器

counteract [ˌkauntəˈrækt] *vt* 对抗,中和 | **~ion** [ˌkauntəˈrækʃən] *n* 对抗作用,反作用,中和 / **~ive** *a* 对抗的,中和性的 *n* 反作用剂,中和力

counterbalance [ˈkauntəˌbæləns] *n* 等衡,抗衡 [ˌkauntəˈbæləns] *vt* 使平衡,抵消 | renal ~ 肾脏相互平衡(一侧正常肾或部分肾呈代偿性肥大,其对侧患侧肾或部分肾处于相对萎缩状态)

countercathexis [ˌkauntəkəˈθeksis] *n* 相反贯注,相反注情

countercurrent [ˈkauntəˌkʌrənt] *n* 逆流,反流;反向电流 *a* 逆流的

counterdie [ˈkauntədai] *n* 反代型(一般由较软的低熔金属制成)

counterelectrophoresis [ˌkauntəiˌlektrəufəˈriːsis] *n* 对流免疫电泳

counterextension [ˌkauntəriksˈtenʃən] *n* 对抗牵伸术

counterimmunoelectrophoresis [ˌkauntəiˌmjunəuiˌlektrəufəˈriːsis] *n* 对流免疫电泳

counterincision [ˌkauntərinˈsiʒən] *n* 对口切开

counterinvestment [ˌkauntərinˈvestmənt] *n* 相反贯注,相反注情

counterirritant [ˌkauntərˈiritənt] *a* 抗刺激的 *n* 抗刺激剂

counterirritation [ˌkauntərˌiriˈteiʃən] *n* 对抗刺激[作用]

counteropening [ˌkauntərˈəupəniŋ] *n* 对口切开

counterphobia [ˌkauntəˈfəubjə] *n* 反恐怖症 | **counterphobic** [ˌkauntəˈfəubik] *a* 反恐怖的

counterpoise [ˈkauntəpɔiz] *n* 平衡,平衡力;衡重[体],配衡[体] *vt* 使平衡

counterpoison [ˈkauntəˌpɔizn] *n* 抗毒剂

counterpulsation [ˌkauntəpʌlˈseiʃən] *n* 对抗搏动法,反搏术 | intra-aortic balloon (IAB) ~ 主动脉内球囊反搏

counterpuncture [ˌkauntəˈpʌŋktʃə] *n* 对口穿刺术

countershock [ˈkauntəʃɔk] *n* 对抗电震,对抗休克(治心房纤维性颤动的一种疗法)

counterstain [ˈkauntəstein] *n* 复染剂

counterstroke [ˈkauntəˌstrəuk] *n* 反击;对侧外伤

countersuggestion [ˌkauntəsəˈdʒestʃən] *n* 反暗示

countertraction [ˌkauntəˈtrækʃən] *n* 对抗牵引

countertransference [ˌkauntətrænsˈfəːrəns] *n* 反转移法,反移情作用

countertransport [ˌkauntəˈtrænspɔːt] *n* 反向转运(指两个物质跨越膜朝相反方向同时转运)

counting [ˈkauntiŋ] *n* 计数 | liquid scintillation ~ 液体闪烁计数

coup [kuː] ([复] **coups** [kuːz, kuː]) *n*【法】发作;中,击 | ~ de fouet 足骤伤,跖肌破裂 / en ~ de sabre 军刀状头面伤 / ~ de sang 中风 / ~ de soleil 日射病,中暑 / ~ sur coup 小剂量短间隔服药

couple [ˈkʌpl] *n* 力偶,电偶

coupler [ˈkʌplə] *n* 联结器,偶联器;联结剂

couplet [ˈkʌplət] *n* 连搏(在心脏学中指两个连续期前收缩)

coupling [ˈkʌpliŋ] *n* 联结,连接,偶联;相偶,相引(遗传学上指两个突变型等位基因的双杂合子在同一染色体上);联律(心脏病学上指一次正常心搏后紧接着出现一次期前收缩) | excitation-contraction ~ 兴奋-收缩耦联 / fixed ~ 固定间距联律

courap [kuˈræp] *n* 库腊普病(印度的一种皮肤病,腋窝、腹股沟、乳房及面部有疹和瘙痒)

courbature [ˈkuəbətʃə] *n*【法】肌肉痛;减压病

court [kɔːt] *n* 庭院,场所;法庭,法院 | infection ~ 传染部位

Courvoisier's law (sign) [kuəˌvwɑːziˈjei] (Ludwig G. Courvoisier)库瓦西耶定律(征)(胆石堵塞胆总管时,很少引起胆囊扩张,如出于其他原因使胆管受阻时,则胆囊扩张是常见的)

Courvoisier-Terrier syndrome [kuəˌvwɑːziˈjei təˈjei](L. G. Courvoisier; Louis F. Terrier)库瓦西耶-泰耶综合征(胆囊扩张、潴留性黄疸和粪便变色,为法特〈Vater〉壶腹瘤梗死征)

Coutard's method [kuˈtɑː](Henri Coutard)库塔法(一种 X 线照射法)

couvade [kuːˈvɑːd] *n* 拟娩(原始部落的风俗,在妻子生产和产褥期,丈夫也卧床模仿分娩)

Couvelaire uterus [ˌkuvəˈlɛə](Alexandre Couvelaire)库弗莱尔子宫,子宫胎盘卒中(胎盘剥离性子宫猝出血)

couvercle [ˈkuːvəkl] *n*【法】血管外凝血块

covalence [kəuˈveiləns] *n* 共价 | **covalent** *a*

covariance [kəuˈvɛəriəns] *n* 协方差(两个随机变量数值与其均数之差的乘积的期望值)

covariate [kəuˈvɛəriət] *n* 共变量

coverglass [ˈkʌvəglɑːs], **coverslip** [ˈkʌvəslip] *n* 盖[玻]片

covering [ˈkʌvəriŋ] *n* 覆盖(物);套,罩 | hernial ~ 疝被盖

cowage [ˈkauidʒ] *n* 黎豆;黎豆荚毛

Cowden disease (syndrome) [ˈkaudən](Cowden 为首次报道病例的姓)考登病(综合征)(一种常染色体显性遗传疾病,构成一组外胚层、中胚层和内胚层异常,表现为形成广泛多发性错构瘤性损害,尤见于皮肤、口腔黏膜、乳房、甲状腺、结肠和小肠,受累器官癌变率高,亦称多发性错构瘤综合征)

Cowdria [ˈkaudriə](Edmund V. Cowdry) *n* 考德里体属,考德里立克次体属 | ~ ruminantium 反刍动物考德里体(牛羊水胸病的病原体,对人无致病性)

cowdriosis [ˌkaudriˈəusis] *n* 考德里立克次体病,牛羊水心胸病

Cowen's sign [ˈkauən](J. P. Cowen)考恩征(光线进入一侧瞳孔时,对侧瞳孔痉挛性收缩,为突眼性甲状腺肿的体征)

cowl [kaul] *n* 帽,罩;胎头羊膜

cowperian [kauˈpiəriən](William Cowper) *a* 考珀的

cowperitis [ˌkaupəˈraitis] *n* 尿道球腺炎

Cowper's gland [ˈkaupə](William Cowper)库珀腺(尿道球腺) | ~ ligament 耻骨筋膜

cowpox [ˈkaupɔks] *n* 牛痘

coxa [ˈkɔksə]([复] **coxae** [ˈkɔksiː]) *n*【拉】髋;髋关节 | ~ valga 髋外翻 / ~ vara 髋内翻

coxalgia [kɔkˈsældʒiə] *n* 髋关节病;髋痛

coxarthria [kɔksˈɑːθriə], **coxarthritis** [ˌkɔksɑːˈθraitis] *n* 髋关节炎

coxarthrocace [ˌkɔksɑːˈθrɔkəsi] *n* 髋关节真菌病

coxarthropathy [ˌkɔksɑːˈθrɔpəθi] *n* 髋关节病

coxarthrosis [kɔksɑːˈθrəusis] *n* 髋关节变性病,髋关节骨关节炎

coxib [ˈkɔksib] *n* 考昔(任何一类非甾体消炎药,其作用为抑制环加氧酶的作用,如塞勒考昔〈celecoxib〉和罗非考昔〈rofecoxib〉)

Coxiella [ˌkɔksiˈelə](Herald R. Cox) *n* 柯克斯体属,柯克斯立克次体属 | ~ burnetii 伯纳特柯克斯体,伯纳特立克次体(Q 热的病原体)

coxitis [kɔkˈsaitis] *n* 髋关节炎 | ~ fugax 暂时性良性髋关节炎 / senile ~ 老年性髋关节炎(髋关节变性关节炎)

coxodynia [ˌkɔksəˈdiniə] *n* 髋痛

coxofemoral [ˌkɔksəˈfemərəl] *a* 髋股的

coxotomy [kɔkˈsɔtəmi] *n* 髋关节切开术

coxotuberculosis [ˌkɔksəutju(ː)ˌbəːkjuˈləusis] *n* 髋关节结核

Cox proportional hazards model [kɔks](David R. Cox)科克斯比例危险模式(分析多种因素〈变量〉的一种方法,这些因素影响保险计算出来的表示一定的负结果如疾病的发生或死亡的危险曲线。对每一个单独的变量〈如有多少病人并在什么时候受到该因素的影响而罹患负结果〉计算出危险率,对实际情况中已存在的这些变量的组合计算出累积的危险率)

coxsackievirus [kɔkˈsækiˌvaiərəs] *n* 柯萨奇病毒(肠道病毒的一种,柯萨奇是美国地名)

coyotillo [kɔiəˈtiːjəu] *n* 山枸矮毒木,洪堡鼠李

cozymase [kəuˈzaimeis] *n* 辅酶 I,烟酰胺腺嘌呤二核苷酸

CP chemically pure 化学纯;candle power 烛光

C'p chickenpox 水痘

cP centipoise 厘泊

C3PA C3 proactivator C3 活化因子前体

C3PAase C3 proactivator convertase C3 活化因子前体转化酶

CPAP continuous positive airway pressure 连续气道正压通气

CPC clinicopathological conference 临床病理讨论会

CPD citrate phosphate dextrose 枸橼酸-磷酸-葡萄糖

CPDA-1 citrate phosphate dextrose adenine 枸橼酸-磷酸-葡萄糖-腺嘌呤

CPDD calcium pyrophosphate deposition disease 焦磷酸钙沉积症

C Ped Certified Pedorthist 持证矫形鞋制造者

CPH Certificate in Public Health 公共卫生学证书

CPI California Personality Inventory 加利福尼亚人格调查表;congenital palatopharyngeal incompetence 先天性腭咽功能不全

CPK creatine phosphokinase 肌酸磷酸激酶

cpm counts per minute 计数/分钟(每分钟计数,表示给予放射性物质如^{131}I后发射的粒子)
CPP cerebral perfusion pressure 大脑灌注压
CPPD calcium pyrophosphate dihydrate 双水焦磷酸钙
CPR cardiac pulmonary reserve 心肺储备; cardiopulmonary resuscitation 心肺复苏
CPS carbam(o)yl phosphate synthetase 氨甲酰基磷酸合成酶
cps cycles per second 每秒周数
CPS Ⅰ carbamoyl phosphate synthetase Ⅰ 氨甲酰磷酸合成酶Ⅰ
CPS Ⅱ carbamoyl phosphate synthetase Ⅱ 氨甲酰磷酸合成酶Ⅱ
Cr complement receptor 补体受体; conditioned response 条件反应; crown-rump 顶臀长度(指胚胎学中的胎儿测量轴); dibenz(b, f)-1, 4-oxazepine 二苯(b, f)-1, 4-氧氮䓬(常用催泪毒气)
CR3 complement receptor type 3 补体受体3型
Cr chromium 铬
crab [kræb] *n* 蟹;阴虱(俗名)
crack [kræk] *n* 破裂声;裂缝,裂,裂开;沙裂,马蹄裂 | quarter ~ (马的)蹄侧裂 / sand ~ 沙裂,马蹄裂;(在热沙上行走引起的)足裂 / toe ~ (马的)蹄裂病,蹄趾裂
crackle ['krækl] *n* 湿啰音
cradle ['kreidl] *n* 婴儿期支架;摇床 | electric ~, heat ~ 光电温床,加热温床 / ice ~ 冰床罩(降低病人体温用)
Crafts' test [krɑːfts] (Leo M. Crafts) 克拉夫茨试验(检锥体束病)
Craigia ['kreigiə] (Charles F. Craig) *n* 克雷格鞭毛虫属,副变形虫属
Cramer's splint ['krɑːmə] (Friedrich Cramer) 克拉默夹板,钢丝夹板
cramp¹ [kræmp] *n* 痛性痉挛 | accessory ~ 副神经性[痉挛性]斜颈 / heat ~ 热痉挛 / intermittent ~ 间歇性痉挛 / recumbency ~s 躺卧性痉挛 / writers' ~ 书写痉挛
cramp² [kræmp] *n* 夹,钳
Crampton's muscle ['kræmptən] (Philip Crampton) 克兰顿肌(鸟类睫状肌的前部)
Crampton's test ['kræmptən] (Charles W. Crampton) 克兰顿试验(根据斜卧和站立时脉搏与血压之间的差异测身体抗力状况,若相差70或70以上表明良好,相差65或65以下则不良)
crania ['kreinjə] cranium 的复数
craniad ['kreiniæd] *ad* 向颅
cranial ['kreinjəl] *a* 颅的,颅侧的
cranialis [ˌkreini'eilis] *a*【拉】颅的,颅侧的
craniamphitomy [ˌkreiniæm'fitəmi] *n* 颅周切开术
Craniata [ˌkreini'eitə] *n* 头盖亚门
craniectomy [ˌkreini'ektəmi] *n* 颅骨切除术 | linear ~ 线状颅骨切除术
cranii ['kreiniai] cranium 的所有格
crani(o)- [构词成分]颅,颅骨
cranioacromial [ˌkreiniəuə'krəumiəl] *a* 颅肩峰的
cranioaural [ˌkreiniə'ɔːrəl] *a* 颅耳的
craniobuccal [ˌkreiniəu'bʌkəl] *a* 颅颊的
craniocele ['kreiniəˌsiːl] *n* 脑膨出
craniocerebral [ˌkreiniəu'seribrəl] *a* 颅[与]脑的
craniocervical [ˌkreiniəu'səːvikəl] *a* 颅颈的
cranioclasis [ˌkreini'ɔkləsis], **cranioclasty** ['kreiniəˌklæsti] *n* 碎颅术
cranioclast ['kreiniəklæst] *n* 碎颅钳
craniocleidodysostosis [ˌkreiniəuˌklaidəuˌdisɔs'təusis] *n* 锁骨颅骨发育不全
craniodidymus [ˌkreiniəu'didiməs] *n* 双头畸胎
craniofacial [ˌkreiniəu'feiʃəl] *a* 颅面的
craniofenestria [ˌkreiniəufi'nestriə] *n* 颅顶骨多孔[畸形]
craniognomy [kreini'ɔgnəmi] *n* 颅形学;相颅术
craniograph ['kreiniəgrɑːf, -græf] *n* 颅形描记器
craniography [ˌkreini'ɔgrəfi] *n* 颅形论(用照片、图表等研究头颅)
craniolacunia [ˌkreiniəulə'kjuːniə] *n* 颅顶骨内面凹陷
craniology [ˌkreini'ɔlədʒi] *n* 颅骨学
craniomalacia [ˌkreiniəumə'leiʃiə] *n* 颅骨软化
craniomeningocele [ˌkreiniəumə'niŋgəsiːl] *n* 颅部脑膜膨出
craniometer [ˌkreini'ɔmitə] *n* 颅测量器 | **craniometry** *n* 颅测量法 / **craniometric** [ˌkreiniəu'metrik] *a* 颅测量的,测颅的
craniopagus [ˌkreini'ɔpəgəs] *n* 颅联体,头联双胎
craniopathy [ˌkreini'ɔpəθi] *n* 颅病 | metabolic ~ 代谢性颅病
craniopharyngeal [ˌkreiniəufə'rindʒiəl] *a* 颅咽的
craniopharyngioma [ˌkreiniəufəˌrindʒi'əumə] *n* 颅咽管瘤
craniophore ['kreiniəfɔː] *n* 颅位保持器
cranioplasty ['kreiniəˌplæsti] *n* 颅[骨]成形术
craniopuncture ['kreiniəˌpʌŋktʃə] *n* 颅穿刺术
craniorachischisis [ˌkreiniəurə'kiskisis] *n* 颅脊柱裂[畸形]
craniosacral [ˌkreiniəu'seikrəl] *a* 颅骶的;副交感神经的
cranioschisis [ˌkreini'ɔskisis] *n* 颅裂
craniosclerosis [ˌkreiniəuskliə'rəusis] *n* 颅骨硬化
cranioscopy [ˌkreini'ɔskəpi] *n* 颅检查术
craniospinal [ˌkreiniəu'spainl] *a* 颅脊柱的
craniostenosis [ˌkreiniəusti'nəusis] *n* 颅狭[窄]

症,狭颅症
craniostosis [ˌkreiniɔs'təusis] *n* 颅缝早闭
craniosynostosis [ˌkreiniəuˌsinɔs'təusis] *n* 颅缝早闭
craniotabes [ˌkreiniəu'teibiːz] *n* 颅骨软化
craniotome ['kreiniəˌtəum] *n* 开颅器
craniotomy [ˌkreini'ɔtəmi] *n* 开颅术
craniotonoscopy [ˌkreiniəutə'nɔskəpi] *n* 颅叩听诊法
craniotopography [ˌkreiniəutə'pɔgrəfi] *n* 颅脑局部解剖学
craniotrypesis [ˌkreiniəutri'piːsis] *n* 颅骨环锯术
craniotympanic [ˌkreiniəutim'pænik] *a* 颅鼓[室]的
cranitis [krei'naitis] *n* 颅骨炎
cranium ['kreinjəm] ([复] **craniums** 或 **crania** ['kreinjə]) *n*【拉】颅 | cerebral ~ 脑颅 / visceral ~ [骨性]面颅,面骨
crapulence ['kræpjuləns] *n* 暴饮暴食;酗酒 | **crapulent**, **crapulous** *a*
craquelé [kræk'lei] *a*【法】有裂隙的,裂开的(如裂隙性湿疹 eczema craquelé)
-crasia [构词成分]混合
crasis ['kreisis] ([复] **crases** ['kreisiːz]) *n*【拉】体质
crassamentum [ˌkræsə'mentəm] *n*【拉】凝块;血块
Crast. crastinus【拉】明日
Crataegus [krə'tiːgəs] *n* 山楂属
crater ['kreitə] *n* 火山口;壁龛(急性消化性溃疡的外形,见于X线检查)
crateriform [krei'terifɔːm] *a* 杯状的,火山口状的;漏斗状的(指菌落)
craterization [ˌkreitərai'zeiʃən, -ri'z-] *n* 火山口状切除术(指切除火山口状的骨)
craunology [krɔː'nɔlədʒi] *n* 矿泉疗养学
craunotherapy [ˌkrɔːnəu'θerəpi] *n* 矿泉疗法
cravat [krə'væt] *n* 三角布绷带
craw [krɔː] *n* 嗉囊
craw-craw ['krɔːkrɔː] *n* 科罗病,盘尾丝虫病
crayfish ['kreifiʃ] *n* 蝲蛄,小龙虾(并殖吸虫的中间宿主)
crazing ['kreiziŋ] *n* 裂纹(如瓷牙的)
cream [kriːm] *n* 乳油,乳皮;乳膏,霜 | cold ~ 冷膏,冷霜,玫瑰水软膏 / leukocytic ~ 白细胞层 / ~ of tartar 酒石,酒石酸氢钾
creamometer [kri'mɔmitə] *n* 乳脂测定器
crease [kriːs] *n* 褶痕,皱褶 | ear lobe ~ 耳垂褶 / palmar ~, flexion ~ 掌屈褶痕,屈褶痕 / simian ~ 猿褶,猿线
creasote ['kri(ː)əsəut] *n* 木溜油,杂酚油
creatinase [kri'ætineis] *n* 肌酸酶
creatine ['kriːətin] *n* 肌酸 | ~ phosphate 磷酸肌酸
creatine kinase (CK) ['kriːətin 'kaineis] 肌酸激酶
creatinemia [ˌkriːəti'niːmiə] *n* 肌酸血
creatine phosphokinase ['kriːətin ˌfɔsfəu'kaineis] 肌酸磷酸激酶(亦称肌酸激酶)
creatine phosphotransferase ['kriːətin ˌfɔsfəu'trænsfəreis] 肌酸磷酸转移酶(亦称肌酸激酶)
creatininase [ˌkriːə'tinineis] *n* 肌酸酐酶
creatinine [kri'ætinin] *n* 肌酸酐
creatinuria [kriˌæti'njuəriə] *n* 肌酸尿
creatorrhea [ˌkriːətə'riə] *n* 肉质下泄,肉质溢出(粪便中有未消化的肌肉纤维)
creatotoxism [ˌkriːətə'tɔksizəm] *n* 肉中毒
creatoxicon [ˌkriːə'tɔksikɔn] *n* 肉毒质
creatoxin [ˌkriːə'tɔksin] *n* 肉毒素,尸碱
crèche [kreiʃ] *n*【法】托儿所
Credé's method (maneuver) [krei'dei] (Karl S. F. Credé) 克勒德法(①腹外用手压出胎盘法;②用同法挤压膀胱排尿,尤其在麻痹性膀胱时;③新生儿硝酸银滴眼法,以防止新生儿眼炎)
Credé's ointment [krei'dei] (Benno C. Credé) 克勒德软膏(含胶体银软膏,擦用治败血病、脓毒症、疖等)
creep [kriːp] *n* 蠕变
CREG cross-reactive group 交叉反应组(HAL抗原)
cremaster [kri'mæstə] *n*【拉】提睾肌 | **cremasteric** [ˌkrimæs'terik] *a*
cremate [kri'meit] *vt* 火葬 | **cremation** [kri'meiʃən] *n*
crematory ['kremətəri], **crematorium** [kremə'tɔriəm] ([复] **crematoriums** 或 **crematoria** [ˌkremə'tɔːriə]) *n* 火葬场
cremnocele ['kremnəsiːl] *n* 阴唇疝
cremor ['kriːmə] *n*【拉】乳油,乳皮;乳膏,霜 | ~ tartari 酒石,酒石酸氢钾
crena ['kriːnə] ([复] **crenae** ['kriːniː]) *n*【拉】裂,裂隙
crenate(d) ['kriːneit(id)] *a* 钝锯齿形的
crenation [kri'neiʃən] *n* 钝锯齿形;皱缩(红细胞)
crenilabrin [kreni'leibrin] *n* 青鲈精蛋白,锯隆头鱼精蛋白
crenocyte ['kriːnəsait] *n* 皱缩红细胞
crenocytosis [ˌkriːnəsai'təusis] *n* 皱缩红细胞症
crenology [kri'nɔlədʒi] *n* 矿泉疗养学
Crenosoma [ˌkriːnə'səumə] *n* 环体[线虫]属
Crenosomatidae [ˌkriːnəsə'mætidiː] *n* 环体[线虫]科
crenotherapy [ˌkrenəu'θerəpi] *n* 矿泉疗法
Crenothrix ['kriːnəθriks] *n* 铁细菌属

Crenotrichaceae [ˌkriːnətriˈkeisiiː] *n* 铁细菌科
crenulation [ˌkrenjuˈleiʃən] *n* (红细胞)皱缩
creophagism [kriˈɔfədʒizəm], **creophagy** [kriˈɔfədʒi] *n* 肉食癖
creosol [ˈkriəsɔl] *n* 甲氧甲酚,2-甲氧基-4-甲基苯酚,木溜油酚
creosote [ˈkriəsəut] *n* 木溜油,杂酚油(外用作防腐药,内服用作祛痰药,治慢性支气管炎) | ~ carbonate 碳酸木溜油(用作祛痰、防腐药)
creotoxin [ˌkriəˈtɔksin] *n* 肉毒素
creotoxism [ˌkriəˈtɔksizəm] *n* 肉中毒
crepe, crêpe [kreip] *n* 皱布,皱纱
crepitate [ˈkrepiteit] *vi* 发碎裂声,发咿轧音 | **crepitant** *a* 咿轧咿轧地响爆裂声的,捻发音的 / **crepitation** [ˌkrepiˈteiʃən] *n* 捻发音;骨擦音
crepitus [ˈkrepitəs] *n*【拉】肠排气,屁;捻发音;咿轧音 | bony ~ 骨咿轧音,骨摩擦音 / ~ indux (肺炎)渐重期咿轧音,(肺炎)渐重期捻发音 / joint ~, articular ~, false ~ 关节咿轧音,假咿轧音 / ~ redux (肺炎)消退期咿轧音,(肺炎)消退期捻发音 / silken ~ 丝绸样咿轧音
crepuscular [kriˈpʌskjulə] *a* 黄昏的,朦胧的
crescendo [kriˈʃendəu] *n* 逐渐增强
crescent [ˈkresnt] *n* 新月,半月体 *a* 新月形的 | articular ~ 关节半月板 / epithelial ~ 上皮新月 / gray ~ 灰质新月(脊髓) / malarial ~s 疟原虫半月体 / myopic ~ 眼后葡萄肿,近视性圆锥 / sublingual ~ 舌下新月形区 | **~ic** [kriˈsentik] *a* 新月形的
cresol [ˈkriːsɔl] *n* 甲酚(消毒防腐药)
cresolphthalein [ˌkrisəlˈθæliin] *n* 甲酚酞
cresorcin [kriˈsɔːsin], **cresorcinol** [kriˈsɔːsinɔl] *n* 荧光黄
cresotic acid [kriˈsɔtik], **cresotinic acid** [ˌkresəˈtinik] 甲基水杨酸
cresoxydiol [kreˌsɔksiˈdaiɔl], **cresoxypropanediol** [kreˌsɔksiprəˈpeindaiɔl] *n* 甲酚甘油醚,甲苯丙醇,美芬新(即 mephenesin)
crest [krest] *n* 嵴 | acoustic ~ 听嵴,壶腹嵴 / acusticofacial ~ 听面神经嵴(胚) / cross ~ 横嵴 / deltoid ~ 三角肌粗隆(肱骨) / fimbriated ~ 伞襞 / inguinal ~ 腹股沟嵴(胚) / neural ~ 神经脊(胚) / orbital ~ 眶上缘 / ~ of ridge 嵴顶
crestomycin sulfate [ˌkrestəuˈmaisin] 硫酸巴龙霉素(即 paromomycin sulfate,抗生素类药)
cresylic acid [kriˈsilik] 甲酚
cretin [ˈkretin, ˈkriːtin] *n*【法】呆小病者
cretinism [ˈkretinizəm] *n* 呆小病 | athyreotic ~, sporadic nongoitrous ~ 甲状腺功能缺失性呆小病,散发性非甲状腺肿呆小病 / goitrous ~ 甲状腺肿呆小病 / spontaneous ~, sporadic ~ 自发性呆小病,散发性呆小病 | **cretinistic** [ˌkretiˈnistik], **cretinous** [ˈkretinəs] *a*
cretinoid [ˈkretinɔid] *a* 呆小病样的
Creutzfeldt-Jakob disease [ˈkrɔitsfelt ˈjækɔb] (Hans G. Creutzfeldt; Alfons M. Jakob)克罗伊茨费尔特-雅各布病,克-雅病(一种罕见的、致命的、可传染的海绵状病毒性脑病,发生在中年,锥体和锥体外系统部分变性,伴进行性痴呆,有时肌肉消瘦、震颤、指痉病以及阵挛性口吃。亦称痉挛性假麻痹) | new variant Creutzfedt-Jakob disease(nvCJD) 新变异型克-雅病(亚急性海绵状脑病)
crevice [ˈkrevis] *n* 缝,裂隙 | gingival ~ 龈缝,龈沟,龈下隙 | **crevicular** [kriˈvikjulə] *a*
CRF chronic renal failure 慢性肾衰竭
CRH corticotropin-releasing hormone 促肾上腺皮质[激]素释放[激]素
crib [krib] *n* 槽;栏床;正牙器 | clinical ~ 病院栏床(观察小儿用)
crib-biting [ˈkribbaitiŋ] *n* 咬槽咽气癖(马)
cribrate [ˈkribreit] *a* 筛状的,多孔的
cribration [kriˈbreiʃən] *n* 过筛;多孔性
cribriform [ˈkribrifɔːm] *a* 筛状的,多孔的
cribrum [ˈkribrəm] ([复] **cribra** [ˈkribrə]) *n* 筛板 | **cribral** [ˈkribrəl] *a* 筛板的;筛的,筛状的
Cricetulus [kraiˈsiːtjuləs] *n* 仓鼠属 | ~ griseus 灰仓鼠
Cricetus [kraiˈsiːtəs] *n* 仓鼠属
Crichton-Browne's sign [ˈkraitn braun] (James Crichton-Browne)克赖顿·布朗征(早期麻痹性痴呆的外眦及唇连合震颤)
crick [krik] *n* (颈或背的)痛性痉挛,痛痉 *vt* 引起(颈、背等)痛性痉挛
cricoarytenoid [ˌkraikəuˌæriˈtiːnɔid] *a* 环杓软骨的
cricoid [ˈkraikɔid] *a* 环状的 *n* 环状软骨
cricoidectomy [ˌkraikɔiˈdektəmi] *n* 环状软骨切除术
cricoidynia [ˌkraikɔiˈdiniə] *n* 环状软骨痛
cricopharyngeal [ˌkraikəufəˈrindʒiəl] *a* 环咽的
cricothyreotomy [ˌkraikəuˌθairiˈɔtəmi] *n* 环甲软骨切开术
cricothyroid [kraikəuˈθairɔid] *a* 环甲软骨的
cricothyrotomy [ˌkraikəuθaiˈrɔtəmi], **cricothyroidotomy** [ˌkraikəuθairɔiˈdɔtəmi] *n* 环甲膜切开术
cricotomy [kraiˈkɔtəmi] *n* 环状软骨切开术
cricotracheotomy [ˌkraikəuˌtreikiˈɔtəmi] *n* 环状软骨气管切开术
cri du chat [kri dju ʃɑː]【法】猫叫(见 syndrome 项下相应术语)
Crigler-Najjar syndrome [ˈkriglə ˈneidʒə] (John F. Crigler; Victor A. Najjar)克里格勒-纳贾尔综

合征(一种常染色体隐性遗传型非溶血性黄疸,由于肝脏酶的葡糖苷酰基转移酶缺乏所致,特征为血内存在大量非结合胆红素,伴有核黄疸及中枢神经系统严重紊乱,亦称先天性高胆红素血[症],先天性非溶血性黄疸)

Crile-Matas operation [krail ˈmætəs] (George W. Crile; Rudolph Matas) 克-马手术(神经内浸润区域麻醉法)

criminology [ˌkrimiˈnɔlədʒi] *n* 犯罪学

crinin [ˈkrinin] *n* 激泌素

crinis [ˈkrainis] ([复] **crines** [ˈkrainiːz]) *n*【拉】毛,发

crinogenic [ˌkrainəˈdʒenik] *a* 促分泌的

crinology [kraiˈnɔlədʒi] *n* 分泌学

crinophagy [kriˈnɔfədʒi] *n* 分泌自噬

Crinum [ˈkrainəm] *n* 文殊兰属

cripple [ˈkripl] *n* 跛者;残缺 *vt* 使跛;使丧失活动能力 | immunologic ~ 免疫残缺(先天性的或人工造成的免疫无活性状态)

crisantaspase [ˌkrisənˈtæspeis] *n* 门冬酰胺酶(asparaginase 的 BAN 名)

crisis [ˈkraisis] ([复] **crises** [ˈkraisiːz]) *n* 危机,危象;骤退,临界,极期 | addisonian ~ 艾迪生病危象,肾上腺皮质危象 / aplastic ~ 再生障碍性危象 / asthmatic ~ 气喘危象,气喘状态 / bronchial ~ 支气管危象(脊髓痨时) / cardiac ~ 心危象(脊髓痨时) / cholinergic ~ 胆碱能危象(因治疗重症肌无力使用过量的胆碱酯酶药所致去极化阻滞而引起的肌软弱) / clitoris ~ 阴蒂危象(女性脊髓痨患者发作性性欲亢进) / colloidoclastic ~ 胶体性猝衰 / false ~ 假(热度)骤退 / gastric ~, intestinal ~ 胃危象,肠危象(脊髓痨时) / glaucomatocyclitic ~ 青光眼睫状体炎危象(一种罕见的复发性单侧型继发性开角青光眼) / identity ~ 性格认同危机,(个人)同一性危机(个人的心理社会发展的一个时期,通常发生在青春期,一般表现为缺乏个人性格的同一性和历史连贯性的认识,或者不能接受社会期望他应扮演的角色) / myasthenic ~ 肌无力危象(重症肌无力时) / nefast ~ 实验性钩端螺旋体病危象 / nitritoid ~ 亚硝酸盐样危象(注射胂凡纳明后有时会发生一组症状,包括面部发红、呼吸困难、痛苦感觉、咳嗽以及心前区疼痛,由于此病类似亚硝酸戊酯中毒,故名) / salt-losing ~, salt-depletion ~ 失盐危象,缺盐危象,缺盐综合征(见 syndrome 项下相应术语) / thoracic ~ 胸危象(脊髓痨时)

Crismer's test [ˈkrismə] (Leon Crismer) 克里斯默试验(检葡萄糖)

crispation [krisˈpeiʃən] *n* 卷缩,短缩(指肌肉挛缩)

crisscross [ˈkriskrɔs] *n* 十字形 *a* 十字形的,交叉的

crista [ˈkristə] ([复] **cristae** [ˈkristiː]) *n*【拉】嵴

cristal [ˈkristl] *a* 嵴的

Cristispira [ˌkristiˈspaiərə] *n* 脊膜螺旋体属,鸡冠波体属

cristobalite [krisˈtəubəlait] *n* 方英石(用于铸造包埋材模)

Critchett's operation [ˈkritʃet] (George Critchett) 克里切特手术(前半眼球切除)

criterion [kraiˈtiəriən] ([复] **criteria** [kraiˈtiəriə]或 **criterions**) *n* 标准,准则

crith [kriθ] *n* 克瑞(气体重量的单位,相当于 1 L 氢气在标准状况下的重量,合 0.089 6 g)

Crithidia [kriˈθidiə] *n* 短膜[鞭毛]虫属

crithidia [kriˈθidiə] *n* 短膜[鞭毛]虫;短膜虫型(血锥虫类发育的一个阶段)

crithidial [kriˈθidiəl] *a* 短膜[鞭毛]虫的;短膜虫型的

critical [ˈkritikəl] *a* 危急的;危象的;临界的,极期的

CRL crown-rump length 顶臀长度(胎长)

CRM cross-reacting material 交叉反应物质

CRNA Certified Registered Nurse Anesthetist 持证注册护士麻醉师

cRNA complementary RNA 互补 RNA

crocein [ˈkrəusiːn] *n* 藏花精

crocidismus [ˌkrəusiˈdizməs] *n* 摸索,摸空,捉空摸床

crocidolite [krəuˈsidəlait] *n* 青石棉(亦称 blue asbestos)

croconic acid [krəˈkɔnik] 克铜酸,邻二羟环戊烯三酮

Crocq's disease [krɔk] (Jean B. Crocq) 手足发绀

crofilicon A [krəˈfilkɔn] 聚酰胺光学纤维 A

Crohn's disease [krəun] (Burrill B. Crohn) 克罗恩病,局限性肠炎

cromoglycate [ˌkrəuməˈglaikeit] *n* 色甘酸盐(用于治支气管哮喘)

cromoglycic acid [ˌkrəuməuˈglaisik] 色甘酸

cromolyn [ˈkrəumәlin] *n* 色甘酸 | ~ sodium 色甘酸钠,色甘酸二钠

Cronin Lowe test (reaction) [ˈkrəunin ləu] (E. Cronin Lowe) 克罗宁・洛试验(反应)(一种诊断癌症的沉淀试验)

Cronin method [ˈkrəunin] (Thomas Dillon Cronin) 克朗宁法(用一短柱将鼻孔底两侧皮瓣抬起,以校正扁平的鼻尖)

Cronkhite-Canada syndrome [ˈkrɔŋkait ˈkænədə] (Leonard W. Cronkhite, Jr.; Wilma Jeanne Canada) 克朗凯特-卡纳达综合征,变应性肉芽肿性血管炎(亦称 Canada-Cronkhite syndrome)

Crooke's changes [kruk] (Arthur C. Crooke) 克鲁克变化(垂体前叶嗜碱性细胞胞质的透明变性)
Crookes' space [kruks] (William Crookes) 克鲁克斯暗区(在近乎衰竭的 X 线管阴极附近有一个暗区,电流经此通过,亦称阴极暗区) | ~ tube 克鲁克斯管(早期 X 线真空管)
crop [krɔp] *n* 嗉囊
cropropamide [krə'prəupəmaid] *n* 克罗丙胺(镇痛药)
cross [krɔs] *n* 十字,十字形;异种交配,杂交 *a* 交叉的;杂交的 | clavicular ~ 锁骨十字形绷带 / phage ~ 噬菌体杂交 / silver ~ 银十字(神经纤维) / two-factor ~ 二因子杂交(涉及两对遗传标记的遗传重组) / yellow ~ 黄十字,二氯二乙硫醚,芥子气(毒气)
crossbite ['krɔsbait] *n* 反(牙合),反咬合 | anterior ~ 前反(牙合) / buccal ~ 颊反(牙合) / lingual ~ 舌反(牙合) / posterior ~ 后反(牙合) / scissors-bite ~, telescoping ~ 套叠式反(牙合)
crossbreeding ['krɔsbriːdiŋ] *n* 杂交育种,杂交繁育
cross-bridges [krɔs 'bridʒiz] *n* 横桥,交叉桥(肌原纤维)
cross-dressing ['krɔs dresiŋ] *n* 异性装扮[癖]
crossed [krɔst] *a* 十字形的,交叉的
cross-eye ['krɔs ai] *n* 内斜视 | **~d** *a*
crossfertilize [ˌkrɔs'fəːtilaiz] *vt*, *vi* 异体受精;异花受精 | **crossfertilization** [ˌkrɔsfəːtilai'zeiʃən, -li'z-] *n*
crossfoot ['krɔsfut] *n* 内翻足
crossing ['krɔsiŋ] *n* 杂交,交叉 | ~ over 交换(在第一次成熟分裂时期,同源染色体间遗传物质的交换,导致基因新的组合)
cross-link ['krɔs ˌlink] *n* 交联
cross-linking ['krɔs ˌlinkiŋ] *n* 交联
crossmatch ['krɔsmætʃ] *n* 交叉配血;(器官)移植前交叉配血,HLA 配型
crossmatching [krɔs'mætʃiŋ] *n* 交叉配血
Cross-McKusick-Breen syndrome [krɔs mə'kjusik briːn] (H. E. Cross; Victor A. McKusick; William Breen) 克罗斯-麦库西克-布林综合征(见 Cross syndrome)
crossover [krɔs'əuvə] *n* 交换(染色体间遗传物质相互交换的结果);交换型 *a* 交换的;交换型的
cross-reactivation [ˌkrɔs ri(ː)ækti'veiʃən] *n* 交叉复活
cross-reactivity [ˌkrɔs ˌriːæk'tivəti] *n* 交叉反应性
cross-reference [krɔs 'refərəns] *n*, *vt* 相互参照
cross-resistance [krɔs ri'zistəns] *n* 交叉抗药性
cross-sensitization [krɔs ˌsensitai'zeiʃən, -ti'z-] *n* 交叉致敏[作用],交叉敏化[作用]
Cross syndrome [krɔs] (Harold E. Cross) 克罗斯综合征(一种常染色体隐性遗传综合征,特点为眼皮肤白化病,小眼,角膜小而不透明,伴痉挛状态的智力发育不全,硬腭高拱,龈肥大及脊柱侧弯。亦称眼大脑色素减退综合征)
crosstalk ['krɔstɔːk] *n* 串扰(在心脏病学中指通过心室传感机制对心房刺激检测不当,通常植有双心腔起搏器者可见之)
cross-tolerance ['krɔs tɔlərəns] *n* 交叉耐受[性]
crossway ['krɔswei] *n* 交叉路;交叉
Crotalaria [krəutə'lɛəriə] *n* 猪屎豆腐,野百合属
crotalid ['krəutəlid] *n* 响尾蛇 *a* 响尾蛇科的
Crotalidae [krəu'tælidiː] *n* 响尾蛇科(蝮蛇科)
crotalin ['krəutəlin] *n* 响尾蛇素(曾用以治癫痫)
Crotalinae [krəu'tæliniː] *n* 响尾蛇亚科
crotaline ['krəutəlin] *n* 响尾蛇 *a* 响尾蛇的
crotalotoxin [ˌkrəutələu'tɔksin] *n* 响尾蛇毒素
Crotalus ['krəutələs] *n* 响尾蛇属
crotamine ['krəutəmiːn] *n* 响尾蛇胺
crotamiton [ˌkrəutə'maitɔn] *n* 克罗米通(抗疥螨药)
crotaphion [krəu'tæfiɔn] *n* 蝶骨大翼尖点
crotch [krɔtʃ] *n* 叉状物;人体两腿分叉处,胯部
crotethamide [krə'teθəmaid] *n* 克罗乙胺(镇痛药)
crotin ['krəutin] *n* 巴豆毒蛋白
Croton ['krəutən] *n*【拉】巴豆属
crotonic acid [krəu'tɔnik] 巴豆酸
crotonism ['krəutənizəm] *n* 巴豆中毒
crotoxin [krəu'tɔksin] *n* 响尾蛇毒素
crounotherapy [ˌkruːnəu'θerəpi] *n* 矿泉疗法
croup [kruːp] *n* 格鲁布,哮吼 | catarrhal ~ 卡他性格鲁布,痉挛性支气管炎 / diphtheritic ~ 白喉性哮吼,喉白喉 / false ~, spasmodic ~ 假性格鲁布,痉挛性格鲁布,喘鸣性喉痉挛 / membranous ~, pseudomembranous ~ 膜炎喉炎,假膜性格鲁布(亦称喉白喉) | **~ous**, **~y** *a* 格鲁布性的,哮吼性的
Crouzon's disease [kru'zɔn] (Octave Crouzon) 颅面骨发育不全
crowding ['kraudiŋ] *n* 牙列拥挤
Crowe's sign [krəu] (Frank W. Crowe) 克劳征(腋下雀斑,见于神经纤维瘤病)
Crow-Fukase syndrome [krəu fuː'kɑːsi] (R. S. Crow; Masaichi Fukase) 克罗-深濑综合征,POEMS 综合征(即 POEMS syndrome,见 syndrome 项下相应术语)
crown [kraun] *n* 冠;人造冠 | anatomical ~ 解剖冠 / artificial ~ 人造冠 / cap ~, shell ~ 帽冠,壳冠 / ciliary ~ 睫状冠,睫状区 / clinical ~, extraalveolar ~ 临床冠,牙槽外冠 / collar ~ 颈

圈冠 / jacket ~ 甲冠 / post ~ 桩冠 / veneered ~, window ~ 罩冠,开面冠
crowning [ˈkrauniŋ] *n* 胎头着冠(分娩);造冠术(牙)
crozat [ˈkrəuzæt] (G. B. Crozat) *n* 克罗扎矫治器
Crozat appliance [ˈkrəuzæt] (George B. Crozat) 克罗扎矫治器(一种可摘正畸矫治器) | ~ clasp 克罗扎卡环(一种可摘矫治器的金属固位体,适用于楔状隙)
CRP C-reactive protein C 反应蛋白
CRRT continuous renal replacement therapy 持续肾置换治疗
CRS Chinese restaurant syndrome 中国餐馆综合征(见 syndrome 项下相应术语)
cruces [ˈkruːsiːz] crux 的复数
crucial [ˈkruːʃəl, ˈkruːʃjəl] *a* 决定性的;十字形的
cruciate [ˈkruːʃiit] *a* 十字形的
crucible [ˈkruːsibl] *n* 坩埚
cruciform [ˈkruːsifɔːm] *a* 十字形的
crude [kruːd] *a* 生的;粗制的
cruentation [ˌkruenˈteiʃən] *n* 受害尸体出血
crufomate [ˈkruːfəmeit] *n* 克芦磷酯(兽用抗蠕虫药)
cruor [ˈkruːɔː] ([复] **cruores** [kruˈɔːrəs]) *n*【拉】血块
crural [ˈkruərəl] *a* 脚的,股的
crureus [kruˈriəs] *n* 股间肌
crus [krʌs] ([复] **crura** [ˈkruərə]) *n*【拉】小腿;脚
crust [krʌst] *n* 痂;壳 | buffy ~ 血沉棕黄层 / milk ~ 乳痂(乳婴头皮脂溢)
crusta [ˈkrʌstə] ([复] **crustae** [ˈkrʌstiː]) *n*【拉】痂;壳;(大脑)脚底 | ~ lactea 乳痂
Crustacea [krʌsˈteiʃjə] *n* 甲壳纲
crustaceorubin [krʌsˌteisiəˈruːbin] *n* 甲壳红素,动物红素,四红素
crustosus [krʌsˈtəusəs] *a*【拉】结痂的
crutch [krʌtʃ] *n* 腋杖,拐杖,支器;会阴区(尤指动物) | Canadian ~ 加拿大式拐杖
Crutchfield tongs [ˈkrʌtʃfiːld] (William G. Crutchfield) 克拉奇费尔德钳,颅骨牵引钳
Cruveilhier-Baumgarten syndrome (cirrhosis) [kruveiˈjei ˈbɔːmgɑːtn] (Jean Cruveilhier; Paul C. von Baumgarten) 克吕韦耶-鲍姆加滕综合征(肝硬变和门静脉高血压,伴脐静脉或附脐静脉先天性未闭)
Cruveilhier's atrophy (paralysis) [kruːveiˈjei] (Jean Cruveilhier) 脊髓性肌萎缩 | ~ disease 脊髓性肌萎缩;单纯性胃溃疡 / ~ joint 寰枕关节
crux [krʌks] ([复] **cruxes** 或 **cruces** [ˈkruːsiːz]) *n*【拉】十字,十字形 | ~ of heart 心十字,房室交叉
Cruz's trypanosomiasis, Cruz-Chagas disease [krʌz ˈtʃɑːgəs] (Oswaldo Cruz; Carlos Chagas) 克鲁斯锥虫病,克鲁斯-恰加斯病(见 Chagas' disease)
cry [krai] *vi* 叫,喊;哭 *n* 喊叫,呼号 | epileptic ~ 癫痫性喊叫 / hydrocephalic ~ 脑积水喊叫 / night ~, arthritic ~, articular ~, joint ~ (关节病)夜叫
cryalgesia [ˌkraiælˈdʒiːziə] *n* 冷痛觉
cryanaesthesia [ˌkraiænisˈθiːzjə] *n* 冷觉缺失
Cryer's elevator [ˈkraiə] (Matthew H. Cryer) 克里厄牙挺(三角牙根挺)
cryesthesia [ˌkraiisˈθiːzjə] *n* 冷觉过敏
crym(o)- [构词成分]寒冷,冷
crymoanesthesia [ˌkraiməuænisˈθiːzjə] *n* 冷冻麻醉
crymodynia [ˌkraiməuˈdiniə] *n* 冷痛
crymophilic [ˌkraiməuˈfilik] *a* 嗜冷的(细菌)
crymophylactic [ˌkraiməufiˈlæktik] *a* 抗冷的,耐冷的(细菌)
crymotherapeutics [ˌkraiməuˌθerəˈpjuːtiks], **crymotherapy** [ˌkraiməˈθerəpi] *n* 冷冻疗法,冷凝疗法
cry(o)- [构词成分]冷
cryoablation [ˌkraiəuæbˈleiʃən] *n* 冷冻消融[术]
cryoanalgesia [ˌkraiəuˌænəlˈdʒiːzjə] *n* 冷止痛法
cryoanesthesia [ˌkraiəuˌænisˈθiːziə] *n* 冷冻麻醉
cryobank [ˈkraiəuˌbæŋk] *n* 冷库(低温冷冻和保存精液)
cryobiology [ˌkraiəubaiˈɔlədʒi] *n* 低温生物学 | **cryobiologist** *n* 低温生物学家
cryocardioplegia [ˌkraiəuˌkɑːdiəuˈpliːdʒiə] *n* 低温心搏停止法
cryocautery [ˌkraiəuˈkɔːtəri] *n* 冻烙术,碳酸霜烙术
cryocrit [ˈkraiəkrit] *n* 冷沉[淀]比容
cryodamage [ˈkraiəuˌdæmidʒ] *n* 冷冻损伤
cryoextraction [ˌkraiəuiksˈtrækʃən] *n* 冷冻[内障]摘出术
cryoextractor [ˌkraiəuiksˈtræktə] *n* 冷冻[内障]摘出器
cryofibrinogen [ˌkraiəufaiˈbrinədʒən] *n* 冷沉[淀]纤维蛋白原
cryofibrinogenemia [ˌkraiəufaiˌbrinədʒəˈniːmiə] *n* 冷沉[淀]纤维蛋白原血[症]
cryogammaglobulin [ˌkraiəugæməˈglɔbjulin] *n* 冷丙球蛋白,冷球蛋白,冷沉[淀]γ-球蛋白
cryogen [ˈkraiədʒən] *n* 冷冻剂
cryogenic [ˌkraiəˈdʒenik] *a* 致冷的,降温的,产低温的
cryoglobulin [ˌkraiəuˈglɔbjulin] *n* 冷球蛋白

cryoglobulinemia [ˌkraiəuˌglɔbjuliˈniːmiə] *n* 冷球蛋白血症
cryohydrate [ˌkraiəuˈhaidreit] *n* 冰盐,低共溶冰盐结晶
cryohypophysectomy [ˌkraiəuˌhaipəufizˈektəmi] *n* 垂体冷凝破坏法
cryolesion [ˈkraiəuˌliʒən] *n* 冷冻损害
cryolite [ˈkraiəlait] *n* 冰晶石
cryometer [kraiˈɔmitə] *n* 低温计,低温温度表
cryopathy [kraiˈɔpəθi] *n* 寒冷病
cryophile [ˈkraiəuˌfail] *n* 嗜冷微生物
cryophilic [ˌkraiəuˈfilik] *a* 嗜冷的(细菌)
cryophylactic [ˌkraiəufiˈlæktik] *a* 抗冷的,耐冷的(细菌)
cryoprecipitability [ˌkraiəupriˌsipitəˈbiləti] *n* 冷沉[淀]性
cryoprecipitate [ˌkraiəupriˈsipiteit] *n* 冷沉淀物
cryoprecipitation [ˌkraiəupriˌsipiˈteiʃən] *n* 冷沉淀[作用],冷沉淀反应
cryopreservation [ˌkraiəuprezəːˈveiʃən] *n* 深低温保藏[法],冷冻保存(贮存切除的组织或器官)
cryoprobe [ˈkraiəprəub] *n* 冷冻探子,冷冻器,冷刀
cryoprotective [ˌkraiəuprəˈtektiv] *a* 低温防护的,冷冻防护的(如甘油保护冷冻的红细胞)
cryoprotein [ˌkraiəuˈprəutiːn] *n* 冷沉[淀]蛋白
cryoscope [ˈkraiəskəup] *n* 冰点测定器 | **cryoscopy** [kraiˈɔskəpi] *n* (溶液)冰点测定法,冰点降低测定法 / **cryoscopic(al)** [ˌkraiəˈskɔpik(əl)] *a* 冰点测定的
cryospray [ˈkraiəusprei] *n* 冷冻喷雾(冷冻手术时使用液氮喷雾)
cryostat [ˈkraiəstæt] *n* 低温控制器,恒冷箱;恒冷切片机
cryosurgery [ˌkraiəuˈsəːdʒəri] *n* 冷冻术,冷冻破坏法 | **cryosurgical** *a*
cryothalamectomy [ˌkraiəuˌθæləˈmektəmi] *n* 丘脑冷冻破坏法
cryothalamotomy [ˌkraiəuˌθæləˈmɔtəmi] *n* 丘脑冷冻破坏法
cryotherapy [ˌkraiəuˈθerəpi] *n* 冷冻疗法
cryotolerant [ˌkraiəuˈtɔlərənt] *a* 耐冷的
crypt [kript] *n* 隐窝;滤泡,腺管 | anal ~s 肛门陷凹,肛窦 / dental ~ 牙囊 / mucous ~s of duodenum 十二指肠腺 / odoriferous ~s of prepuce 包皮腺 / synovial ~ 滑膜憩室 / ~s of tongue 舌滤泡陷凹 | **~al** *a*
crypta [ˈkriptə] ([复] **cryptae** [ˈkriptiː]) *n*【拉】隐窝;滤泡,腺管
cryptanamnesia [ˌkriptænæmˈniːziə] *n* 潜隐记忆,潜忆
cryptectomy [kripˈtektəmi] *n* 隐窝切除术
cryptenamine [kripˈtenəmain] *n* 绿藜安(抗高血压药) | ~ acetates 醋酸绿藜安(治子痫和高血压性脑病) / ~ tannates 鞣酸绿藜安(口服可控制中度至重度高血压)
cryptesthesia [ˌkriptisˈθiːzjə] *n* 潜在感觉,潜觉
cryptic(al) [ˈkriptik(əl)] *a* 隐蔽的,潜在的
cryptitis [kripˈtaitis] *n* 隐窝炎 | anal ~ 肛窦炎
crypt(o)- [构词成分]隐,隐窝
Cryptobia [kripˈtəubiə] *n* 隐鞭虫属(亦称锥浆虫属 Trypanoplasma)
Cryptobiidae [ˌkriptəuˈbaiidiː] *n* 隐鞭虫科
cryptocephalus [ˌkriptəuˈsefələs] *n* 隐头畸胎
Cryptococales [ˌkriptəukɔˈkeiliːz] *n* 隐球菌目
Cryptococcaceae [ˌkriptəukɔˈkeisiiː] *n* 隐球菌科
cryptococcoma [ˌkriptəukɔˈkəumə] *n* 隐球菌肿块
cryptococcosis [ˌkriptəukɔˈkəusis] *n* 隐球菌病
Cryptococcus [ˌkriptəuˈkɔkəs] *n* 隐球菌属 | ~ capsulatus 荚膜隐球菌 / ~ gilchristi 吉[尔克里斯特]氏隐球菌 / ~ neoformans, ~ histolyticus, ~ hominis, ~ meningitidis 新型隐球菌,溶组织隐球菌,人类隐球菌,脑膜炎隐球菌
cryptocrystalline [ˌkriptəuˈkristəlain] *a* 隐晶体的
Cryptocystis trichodectis [ˌkriptəuˈsistis ˌtrikəuˈdektis] 犬似囊尾蚴
cryptodeterminant [ˌkriptəudiˈtəːminənt] *n* 隐蔽决定簇(即 hidden determinant)
cryptodidymus [ˌkriptəuˈdidiməs] *n* 胎内胎
cryptoempyema [ˌkriptəuˌempaiˈiːmə] *n* 隐性积脓,隐性脓胸
cryptogam [ˈkriptəgæm] *n* 隐花植物
cryptogamic [ˌkriptəˈgæmik], **cryptogamous** [ˌkripˈtɔgəməs] *a* 隐花植物的
cryptogenic [ˌkriptəˈdʒenik], **cryptogenetic** [ˌkriptəudʒiˈnetik] *a* 隐源性的,原因不明的
cryptoglandular [ˌkriptəuˈglændjulə] *a* 肛腺与肛窦的
cryptoglioma [ˌkriptəuglaiˈəumə] *n* 隐神经胶质瘤(视网膜)
cryptoleukemia [ˌkriptəuljuːˈkiːmiə] *n* 隐白血病
cryptolith [ˈkriptəliθ] *n* 隐窝结石
cryptomenorrhea [ˌkriptəuˌmenəˈriːə] *n* 隐性月经
cryptomere [ˈkriptəmiə] *n* 隐窝状,囊状
cryptomerorachischisis [ˌkriptəuˌmiərəurəˈkiskisis] *n* 隐性脊柱裂
cryptomnesia [ˌkriptɔmˈniːziə] *n* 潜隐记忆,潜忆 | **cryptomnesic** [ˌkriptɔmˈniːsik] *a*
cryptomonad [ˌkriptəuˈmɔnæd] *n* 隐滴虫
Cryptomonadida [ˌkriptəuməˈnædidə] *n* 隐滴

虫目
Cryptomonas [ˌkriptəuˈməunəs] *n* 隐滴虫属
cryptoneurous [ˌkriptəuˈnjuərəs] *a* 无明显神经系统的,隐性神经系统的
cryptophanic acid [ˌkriptəˈfænik] 隐尿酸
cryptophthalmos [ˌkriptɔfˈθælməs], **cryptophthalmia** [ˌkriptɔfˈθælmiə], **cryptophthalmus** [ˌkriptɔfˈθælməs] *n* 隐眼[畸形]
Cryptophyceae [ˌkriptəˈfisiiː] *n* 隐藻目
cryptopine [ˈkriptəpin] *n* 克利多平(阿片中的一种生物碱)
cryptoplasmic [ˌkriptəuˈplæzmik] *a* 隐伏的(感染)
cryptopodia [ˌkriptəuˈpəudiə] *n* 隐足病,足肿病
cryptopsychic [ˌkriptəuˈsaikik] *a* 潜隐精神的,潜隐心理的
cryptopsychism [ˌkriptəuˈsaikizəm] *n* 心灵学,心灵心理学
cryptopyic [ˌkriptəuˈpaiik] *a* 隐脓的
cryptoradiometer [ˌkriptəuˌreidiˈɔmitə] *n* X 线透度计
cryptorchid [kripˈtɔːkid] *a* 隐睾病的 *n* 隐睾者
cryptorchidectomy [ˌkriptɔːkiˈdektəmi] *n* 隐睾切除术
cryptorchidia [kriptɔːˈkiːdiə] *n* 隐睾病 | **cryptorchic** [kripˈtɔːkik], **cryptorchidic** [kripˈtɔːˈkidik] *a*
cryptorchidism [kripˈtɔːkidizəm], **cryptorchidy** [kripˈtɔːkidi], **cryptorchism** [kripˈtɔːkizəm] *n* 隐睾[症](睾丸未降)
cryptorchidopexy [kripˌtɔːkidəuˈpeksi] *n* 隐睾固定术
cryptorrhea [ˌkriptəˈriːə] *n* 内分泌异常 | **cryptorrhetic** [ˌkriptəˈretik], **cryptorrheic** [ˌkriptəˈriːik] *a* 内分泌的;内分泌异常的
cryptoscope [ˈkriptəskəup] *n* 荧光镜,荧光屏 | **cryptoscopy** [kripˈtɔskəpi] *n* 荧光镜透视检查,X 线透视检查
cryptosporidiosis [ˌkriptəuspɔːˌridiˈəusis] *n* 隐孢子虫病
Cryptosporidium [ˌkriptəuspɔːˈridiəm] *n* 隐孢子虫属
cryptosterol [kripˈtɔstərɔl] *n* 酵母甾醇,隐花植物甾醇
Cryptostroma [ˌkriptəuˈstrəumə] *n* 隐子座菌属 | ~ corticale 皮质隐子座菌(即皮质梨孢霉 Coniosporium corticale)
cryptotia [kripˈtəuʃiə] *n* 隐耳
cryptotoxic [ˌkriptəuˈtɔksik] *a* 隐毒的
cryptoxanthin [ˌkriptəuˈzænθin] *n* 隐黄素,玉米黄质(能在体内变成维生素 A)
cryptozoite [ˌkriptəuˈzəuait] *n* 潜隐体
cryptozygous [kripˈtɔzigəs] *a* 隐颧的(宽颅窄面的)
Crys. crystal 晶体,结晶
crystal [ˈkristl] *n* 晶体,结晶 | asthma ~s, leukocytic ~s 气喘晶体,白细胞晶体(嗜酸粒细胞破碎后晶体) / blood ~s 血晶(血内胆红素结晶) / coffin lid ~s, knife rest ~s 棺盖状晶体,刀架状晶体 / dumbbell ~s 哑铃形晶体 / ear ~ 位觉砂,耳石 / hedgehog ~s 尿酸铵结晶 / liquid ~s 液晶 / rock ~ 水晶,石英(二氧化硅) / sperm ~s, spermin ~s 精液结晶 / thorn-apple ~s 尿酸铵结晶 / whetstone ~s 砥石结晶,磨石结晶
crystalbumin [ˌkristəlˈbjuːmin] *n* (血清)晶白蛋白
crystalli [krisˈtæli] *n* 水痘
crystallin [krisˈtælin] *n* 晶体蛋白
crystalline [ˈkristəlain] *a* 结晶的,晶状的
crystallitis [kristəˈlaitis] *n* 晶状体炎
crystallize [ˈkristəlaiz] *vt*, *vi* 结晶 | **crystallization** [ˌkristəlaiˈzeiʃən, -liˈz-] *n* 结晶[作用]
crystallography [ˌkristəˈlɔgrəfi] *n* 结晶学,晶体学 | X-ray ~ X 线衍射晶体分析法,X 射线晶体学
crystalloid [ˈkristəlɔid] *a* 晶体样的,类晶体的 *n* 拟晶体,类晶体
crystalloiditis [ˌkristəlɔiˈdaitis] *n* 晶状体炎
crystalluria [kristəˈljuəriə] *n* 结晶尿
CS cesarean section 剖宫产术; conditioned stimulus 条件刺激; coronary sinus 冠状窦; *o*-chlorobenzylidenemalonitrile 邻-氯亚苄基丙二腈(常用催泪毒气)
Cs cesium 铯
CSAA Child Study Association of America 美国儿童研究协会
CSC coup sur coup 小剂量短间隔服药
CSF cerebrospinal fluid 脑脊液; colony-stimulating factor 集落刺激因子
CSGBI Cardiac Society of Great Britain and Ireland 大不列颠及爱尔兰心脏学会
CSII continuous subcutaneous insulin infusion 胰岛素皮下持续输注
CSM cerebrospinal meningitis 脑脊膜炎
CST convulsive shock therapy 惊厥休克疗法; contraction stress test 宫缩应激试验
CT computed tomography 计算机体层摄影[术]
CTA Canadian Tuberculosis Association 加拿大结核病协会
CTBA cetrimonium bromide 西曲溴铵
cteinophyte [ˈtainəfait] *n* 有害寄生菌
cteno- [构词成分]栉
Ctenocephalides [ˌtiːnəusiˈfælidiːz] *n* 栉头蚤属 | ~ canis 犬栉头蚤 / ~ felis 猫栉头蚤
Ctenophora [teˈnɔfərə] *n* 栉水母门

ctenophore [ˈtenəfɔː] *n*, *a* 栉水母(的)
Ctenophthalmus [ˌtiːnɔfˈθælməs] *n* 栉眼蚤属 | ~ agrytes 欧洲鼠栉眼蚤
Ctenus [ˈtiːnəs] *n* 栉蜘蛛属
C-terminal [ˈtəːminl] *n* C 端,羧基端(肽链的一端,带有最后一个氨基酸的游离 α 羧基者,习惯写在右侧)
ctetology [tiˈtɔlədʒi] *n* 获得性生物学(研究获得性状的生物学分支)
ctetosome [ˈtetəsəum] *n* 额外染色体(性染色体)
CTL cytotoxic lymphocytes 细胞毒性淋巴细胞; cytotoxic T lymphocytes 细胞毒性 T[淋巴]细胞
CTP cytidine triphosphate 胞苷三磷酸
CTP synthase [ˈsinθeis] CTP 合酶,胞苷三磷酸合酶
Cu cuprum 铜
cuajani [kwəˈhɑːni] *n* 夸哈尼(成药,祛痰药)
cubeb [ˈkjuːbeb] *n* 荜澄茄(曾用作利尿药和尿路消毒药)
cubebic acid [kjuˈbebik] 荜澄茄酸
cubebin [kjuˈbiːbin] *n* 荜澄茄素(曾用作尿路消毒药)
cubebism [ˈkjuːbebizəm] *n* 荜澄茄中毒
cubic [ˈkjuːbik] *a* 立方体的,立方形的,立方的
cubical [ˈkjuːbikəl] *a* 立方体的;立方的
cubicle [ˈkjuːbikl] *n* (宿舍或病室中的)小隔间
cubiform [ˈkjuːbifɔːm] *a* 立方形的
cubilose [ˈkjuːbiləus] *n* 燕窝膏
cubit [ˈkjuːbit] *n* 肘尺(测量单位,从肘到中指尖的长度,在 46 ~ 53 cm 之间)
cubital [ˈkjuːbitl] *a* 肘的;尺骨的,前臂的
cubitalis [kjuːbiˈteilis] *a*【拉】肘的;尺骨的,前臂的
cubitocarpal [ˌkjuːbitəuˈkɑːpl] *a* 尺腕的
cubitoradial [ˌkjuːbitəuˈreidjəl] *a* 尺桡的
cubitus [ˈkjuːbitəs] *n*【拉】肘;前臂;尺骨 | ~ valgus 肘外翻 / ~ varus 肘内翻
cuboid [ˈkjuːbɔid] *a* 骰状的 *n* 骰骨 | **~al** [kju(ː)ˈbɔidəl] *a*
Cubomedusae [ˌkjuːbəuməˈdjuːsiː] *n* 立方水母目
cubomedusan [ˌkjuːbəuməˈdjuːsən] *a* 立方水母目的 *n* 立方水母目
cu cm cubic centimeter 立方厘米
cucoline [ˈkjuːkəliːn] *n* 汉防己碱,青藤碱
cucullaris [kjukəˈlɛəris] *n* 斜方肌
cucumber [ˈkjuːkəmbə] *n* 黄瓜 | bitter ~ 药西瓜瓤
Cucumis [ˈkjuːkəmis] *n* 黄瓜属
cucurbit [kju(ː)ˈkəːbit] *n* 南瓜;葫芦
Cucurbita [kjuˈkəːbitə] *n* 南瓜属
cucurbitol [kjuˈkəːbitɔl] *n* 西瓜子甾醇,西瓜子固醇
cucurbitula [ˌkjukəˈbitjulə] *n*【拉】吸[疗]杯,吸罐 | ~ cruenta 湿吸杯 / ~ sicca 干吸杯
cucurbocitrin [ˌkjuːkəbəˈsitrin] *n* 西瓜子素(用以降低血压)
cud [kʌd] *n* (反刍时的)食团
cudbear [ˈkʌdbɛə] *n* 地衣紫
cudding [ˈkʌdiŋ] *n* 吐草症(见 quidding)
cuff [kʌf] *n* 袖口(状构造);套囊 | musculotendinous ~, rotator ~ 肌腱套,旋转套(肩关节囊的) / vaginal ~ 阴道断端
cuffing [ˈkʌfiŋ] *n* 成套(如见于某些病毒病,血管周围白细胞聚集如套状)
Cuignet's method [kuiːnˈjei] (Ferdinand L. J. Cuignet)视网膜镜检查,视网膜检影法
cuirass [kwiˈræs] *n* 护胸甲(皮革制) | tabetic ~ 骨髓痨性护胸甲状麻木
Cuj. cujus【拉】其中,那一个的,那一些的
cul-de-sac [ˌkul də ˈsæk] ([复] **cul-de-sacs** 或 **culs-de-sac**) *n*【法】盲管,陷凹 | conjunctival ~ 结膜穹窿 / dural ~ 硬膜腔终部
culdocentesis [ˌkʌldəusenˈtiːsis] *n* 后穹窿穿刺术
culdoscope [ˈkʌldəskəup] *n* 后陷凹镜,后穹窿镜 | **culdoscopy** [kʌlˈdɔskəpi] *n* 后陷凹镜检查,后穹窿镜检查
culdotomy [kʌlˈdɔtəmi] *n* 子宫直肠陷凹切开术
Culex [ˈkjuːleks] *n*【拉】库蚊属 | ~ fatigans, ~ quinquefasciatus 致倦库蚊,致乏库蚊 / ~ pipiens 尖音库蚊 / ~ tarsalis 跗斑库蚊 / ~ tritaeniorhyncus 三带喙库蚊
Culicidae [kjuˈlisidiː] *n* 蚊科
culicidal [kjuliˈsaidl] *a* 杀蚊的,灭蚊的
culicide [ˈkjulisaid], **culicicide** [kjuˈlisisaid] *n* 杀蚊剂
culicifuge [kjuˈlisifjuːdʒ] *n* 驱蚊剂
Culicinae [ˌkjuliˈsainiː] *n* 库蚊亚科
culicine [ˈkjuːlisin, ˈkjuːlisain] *n* 库蚊 *a* 库蚊的
Culicini [kjuliˈsainai] *n* 库蚊族
Culicoides [kjuliˈkɔidiːz] *n* 库蠓属 | ~ austeni 奥[斯汀]氏库蠓 / ~ furens 毛库蠓 / ~ grahami 格[雷厄姆]氏库蠓
Culiseta [ˌkjuːliˈsiːtə] *n* 脉毛蚊属(以前称赛保蚊属 Theobaldia) | ~ melanura 黑尾赛蚊,黑尾脉毛蚊(东、西方马脑炎病毒的传播媒介)
Cullen's sign [ˈkʌlən] (Thomas S. Cullen)卡伦征(脐周皮肤颜色变蓝,有时伴腹膜内出血,尤发生于宫外孕时输卵管破裂之后,同样见于急性出血性胰腺炎)
culling [ˈkʌliŋ] *n* 剔除,拣除(指脾脏从血液中除去不正常红细胞等)
culmen [ˈkʌlmən] ([复] **culmina** [ˈkʌlminə]) *n*

【拉】山顶;小脑山顶 | **culminal** [ˈkʌlminəl] *a*

Culp-De Weerd ureteropelvioplasty [kʌlp diː-ˈwiəd] (Ormond S. Culp; James H. De Weerd) 克-迪输尿管肾盂成形术(将螺旋形肾盂皮瓣翻下,使之合并于邻近的输尿管上)

culprit [ˈkʌlprit] *n* 元凶;事故的原因

cult [kʌlt] *n* 巫术

cultivate [ˈkʌltiveit] *vt* 培养 | **cultivation** [ˌkʌl-tiˈveiʃən] *n*

culturable [ˈkʌltʃərəbl] *a* 可培养的

cultural [ˈkʌltʃərəl] *a* 培养的

culture [ˈkʌltʃə] *n* 培养;培养物 *vt* 培养 | asynchronous ~ 不同步培养 / attenuated ~ 减毒培养物,减弱培养物,弱化培养物 / cell ~ 细胞培养 / chorioallantoic ~ (鸡胚)绒毛膜尿囊培养[物] / continuous flow ~ 连续流动培养 / enrichment ~ 增菌培养 / flask ~ 玻瓶培养 / fractional ~ 分级培养法 / hanging-block ~ 悬块培养[物] / hanging-drop ~ 悬滴培养[物] / mixed lymphocyte ~ (MLC) 混合淋巴细胞培养(亦称混合淋巴细胞反应) / plate ~ 平板培养物 / pure ~ 纯培养物 / radioisotopic ~ 放射性同位素培养[物] / secondary ~ 继代培养物 / selective ~ 选择性培养[物] / sensitized ~ 致敏培养 / shake ~ 振荡培养 / slope ~ 斜面培养 / spinner ~ 搅拌培养 / stab ~, needle ~, thrust ~ 穿刺培养物 / stock ~ 原培养物 / subculture ~ 传代培养物培养 / suspended cell ~ 悬浮细胞培养 / suspension ~ 悬浮培养 / tissue ~ 组织培养 / tube ~ 试管培养 / type ~ 模式培养物

culture medium [ˈkʌltʃə ˈmiːdjəm] 培养基 | agar ~ ~ 琼脂培养基 / beer wort ~ ~ 麦芽汁培养基 / bile ~ ~, bile salt ~ ~ 胆汁培养基,胆盐培养基 / dextrose ~ ~ 右旋糖培养基(琼脂) / eosin-methylene blue (EMB) ~ ~ 曙红亚甲蓝培养基(琼脂,儿用于分离志贺菌) / fuchsin ~ ~, fuchsin sulfite ~ ~ 品红培养基(琼脂) / glycerin ~ ~ 甘油培养基(肉汤) / indicator ~ ~ 指示培养基 / iron ~ ~ 含铁培养基(肉汤) / lead ~ ~ 含铅培养基,醋酸铅肉汤 / milk ~ ~ 牛奶培养基(脱脂) / milk-rice ~ ~ 乳米糊培养基(培养产色细菌) / N. N. N. ~ ~ N. N. N. 培养基(含琼脂、盐、兔血,用以培养黑热病病原体) / selective ~ ~ 选择培养基 / serum ~ ~ 血清培养基(马血清和营养肉汤) / silicate jelly ~ ~ 硅酸胶质培养基(培养固氮细菌) / sugar ~ ~ 糖培养基,含糖肉汤(检细菌发酵特性) / tellurite ~ ~ 亚碲酸盐培养基(白喉杆菌初级培养) / wheat ~ ~ 小麦培养基(肉汤)

cum [kʌm]【拉】*prep* 和,与;附有

cumic acid [ˈkjuːmik], **cuminic acid** [kjuː-ˈminik] 枯茗酸,异丙苯甲酸,枯酸

cumidine [ˈkjuːmidin] *n* 对异丙基苯胺,枯胺

cuminuric acid [ˌkjuːmiˈnjuərik] 枯茗尿酸,异丙马尿酸

cu mm cubic millimeter 立方毫米

cumulative [ˈkjuːmjulətiv] *a* 累积的

cumulus [ˈkjuːmjuləs] ([复] **cumuli** [ˈkjuːmjulai]) *n*【拉】丘 | ovarian ~ 卵丘

cuneate [ˈkjuːniit], **cuneiform** [ˈkjuːniifɔːm] *a* 楔状的

cuneocuboid [ˌkjuniəˈkjuːbɔid] *a* 楔骰的

cuneonavicular [ˌkjuniənəˈvikjulə] *a* 楔舟的

cuneoscaphoid [ˌkjuniəˈskæfɔid] *a* 楔舟的

cuneus [ˈkjuːniəs] ([复] **cunei** [ˈkjuːniai]) *n*【拉】楔叶(大脑)

Cuniculus [kjuˈnikjuləs] *n* 穴鼠属

cuniculus [kjuˈnikjuləs] ([复] **cuniculi** [kju-ˈnikjulai]) *n*【拉】(疥虫)隧道

Cunila [kjuˈnailə] *n* 白藓属(唇形科)

cunnilinctus [ˌkʌniˈlinktəs] *n* 舔阴

cunnilinguism [ˌkʌniˈliŋgwizəm] *n* 舔阴欲

cunnilingus [ˌkʌniˈliŋgəs] *n* 舔阴

Cunninghamella [ˌkʌniŋhæˈmelə] *n* 小克银汉霉属

Cunninghamellacae [ˌkʌniŋhæməˈleisiiː] *n* 小克银汉霉科

cunnus [ˈkʌnəs] *n* 女阴,外阴

cuorin [ˈkjuːərin] *n* 心磷脂

cup [kʌp] *n* 杯;杯状物;火罐 | dry ~ 干吸杯,火罐 / glaucomatous ~ 青光眼杯(青光眼性视神经乳头陷凹) / ocular ~, ophthalmic ~ 视杯 / optic ~ 生理凹;视杯 / physiologic ~ 生理凹(视神经乳头陷凹) / wet ~ 湿吸杯

cupola [ˈkjuːpələ] *n* 顶

cupped [kʌpt] *a* 杯状的,凹陷的

cupping [ˈkʌpiŋ] *n* 杯吸法,拔火罐;杯状陷凹形成 | pathologic 病理凹(疾病引起的视神经乳头陷凹)

cuprammonia [ˌkjuːprəˈməuniə] *n* 铜氨液,氢氧化铜氨溶液

cupreine [ˈkjupriiːn] *n* 铜色树碱(具有抗疟性质)

cupremia [kjuˈpriːmiə] *n* 铜血

cupreous [ˈkjuːpriəs] *a* 含铜的;铜色的

cupric [ˈkjuːprik] *a* 含铜的,铜的;高铜的,二价铜的 | ~ sulfate 硫酸铜

cupriferous [kju(ː)ˈprifərəs] *a* 含铜的

cuprimyxin [ˌkʌpriˈmiksin] *n* 铜迈星(兽用抗菌药和抗真菌药)

cupriuria [ˌkjuːpriˈjuəriə] *n* 铜尿

cuprophane [ˈkjuːprəfein] *n* 铜铵薄膜,铜纺(用于血液透析器)

cuprous [ˈkjuːprəs] *a* 亚铜的,一价铜的

cupruresis [ˌkjuːpruˈriːsis] *n* 铜尿排泄 | **cupruretic** [ˌkjuːpruˈretik] *a* [促]铜尿排泄的

cupula [ˈkjuːpjuːlə] ([复] **cupulae** [ˈkjuːpjuːliː]) *n*【拉】顶 | ~ of ampullary crest 壶腹嵴顶 / ~ of cochlea 蜗顶 / ~ of pleura 胸膜顶

cupulogram [ˈkjuːpjuləˌgræm] *n* 嵴帽敏度图,嵴帽图

cupulolithiasis [ˌkjuːpjuːləuliˈθaiəsis] *n* 嵴帽沉石病

cupulometry [ˌkjuːpjuˈlɔmitri] *n* 嵴帽[敏度]测量[法]

curable [ˈkjuərəbl] *a* 可治愈的 | **curability** [ˌkjuərəˈbiləti] *n*

curage [kjuˈrɑːʒ] *n*【法】刮除术(尤指使用手指刮除)

curandera [kuːrɔnˈdeirɑː] *n*【西】女治疗师

curanderismo [kuːˌrɔndiˈrizməu] *n* 墨西哥印第安人传统治疗法

curandero [kuːrɔnˈdeirəu] *n*【西】男治疗师

curare, curari [kjuˈrɑːri] *n* 箭毒

curaremimetic, curarimimetic [kjuˌrɑːrimaiˈmetik] *n* 箭毒样[神经]阻断剂 *a* 箭毒样作用的

curariform [kjuˈrɑːrifɔːm] *a* 箭毒样的

curarine [ˈkjuərəriːn] *n* 箭毒碱

curarize [ˈkjuərəraiz] *vt* 用箭毒于,用箭毒处理 | **curarization** [ˌkjuərəraiˈzeiʃən, -riˈz-] *n* 箭毒化(使用箭毒,直至产生其生理作用)

curative [ˈkjuərətiv] *a* 治疗的,有疗效的;治愈的 *n* 治疗物;药品

curb [kəːb] *n* 节制,控制;(马后腿上可引起跛足的)飞节肿大

Curcuma [ˈkəːkjumə] *n* 姜黄属 | ~ longa 姜黄

curcuma [ˈkəːkjumə] *n* 姜黄

curcumin [ˈkəːkjumin] *n* 姜黄色素

curd [kəːd] *n* 凝乳 | alum ~ 明矾乳

curdy [ˈkəːdi] *a* 多凝乳的,凝乳状的

cure [kjuə] *n* 疗程;治愈;疗法,治疗;良药;加工处理 *vt* 治愈 *vi* 起治疗作用;受治疗 | diet ~ 饮食疗法 / economic ~ 经济疗法 / faith ~ 信仰疗法 / grape ~ 葡萄饮食疗法 / hunger ~ 饥饿疗法 / liman ~ 咸水浴疗法 / milk ~ 乳疗法 / mind ~ 精神疗法,心理疗法 / potato ~ 马铃薯疗法(消化道异物的治疗法) / starvation ~ 禁食疗法 / thirst ~ 节饮疗法 / whey ~ 乳清疗法

curet [kjuəˈret] *n* 刮器,刮匙 *vt* (用刮器)刮除

curettage [ˌkjuriˈtɑːʒ, ˌkjuəˈretidʒ] *n*【法】刮除术 | medical ~ 药物刮宫法 / periapical ~, apical ~ 牙根周刮除术 / subgingival ~ 龈下刮除术 / surgical ~ 外科刮除术(牙科) / ultrasonic ~ 超声刮除术(牙科) / vacuum ~, suction ~ 真空吸刮术,(子宫)吸刮术

curette [kjuˈret] *n*【法】刮匙

curettement [kjuˈretmənt] *n* 刮术 | physiologic ~ 生理性刮除,酶清创术

curie(Ci) [ˈkjuəri] (Marie S. Curie; Pierre Curie) *n* 居里(旧放射性强度单位,现用 Bq〈贝克勒尔〉,1 Ci = 37 GBq〈3.7 × 10^{10} Bq〉)

curiegram [ˈkjuərigræm] *n* 氡[射]线照片

curie-hour [ˈkjuəri ˌauə] *n* 居里小时(旧放射剂量单位,相当于放射性物质在每秒分裂蜕变 3.7 × 10^{10} 原子下暴露一小时所获得的剂量,现用 Bq〈贝克勒尔〉)

Curie's law [ˈkjuəri] (Pierre Curie)居里定律(任何物质均可受到镭射气影响而具放射性,如将此物质被封在不能透过射气的材料中,则其放射性可维持较久) | ~ therapy 居里疗法,镭疗法

curietherapy [ˌkjuəriˈθerəpi] *n* 放射疗法(原指镭疗法或氡疗法,现指用任何放射源的射气疗法)

curing [ˈkjuəriŋ] *n* 食物加工法(用腌、熏等方法);加工法 | denture ~ 义齿加工法(义齿基质聚合或变硬的过程)

curioscopy [ˌkjuːriˈɔskəpi] *n* 核辐射检查法,放射核素显像

curium(Cm) [ˈkjuəriəm] *n* 锔(化学元素)

Curling's ulcer [ˈkəːliŋ] (Thomas B. Curling)柯林溃疡(体表严重烧伤后胃或十二指肠急性溃疡)

Currarino-Silverman syndrome [ˌkuːrəˈriːnəu ˈsilvəmən] (Guido Currarino; Frederic N. Silverman)库-西综合征(胸缝及骨连接过早消失,胸骨柄突出,导致鸡胸;其他异常也可能存在,如肋骨骨肥厚或前膈营养不足。亦称西尔弗曼〈Silverman〉综合征)

Currarino's triad [ˌkuːrəˈriːnəu] (Guido Currarino)库拉里诺三联症(肛尾区严重先天性畸形,包括短弯刀状骶骨;骶骨前前方脑[脊]膜膨出、畸胎瘤或囊肿;直肠畸形如狭窄、异位性闭锁)

current [ˈkʌrənt] *n* 流;电流 | abnerval ~ 离神经电流 / action ~, nerve-action ~ 动作电流,神经动作电流(在神经或肌肉细胞膜内产生) / alternating ~ 交流电 / axial ~ 轴流(血流中部的有色部分) / centrifugal ~, descending ~ 离心电流,下行电流(在体内,神经中枢附近为正极,周围为负极) / centripetal ~, ascending ~ 向心电流,上行电流(通过身体的电流,在神经或周围为正极,神经中枢附近为负极) / demarcation ~, ~ of injury 损伤电流 / direct ~ 直流电 / electric ~ 电流 / electrotonic ~ 紧张电流 / faradic ~ 感应电流,法拉第电流 / surgical ~ 外科用高频电流

curriculum [kəˈrikjuləm] ([复] **curriculums** 或 **curricula** [kəˈrikjulə]) *n*【拉】课程,学程

Curschmann-Batten-Steinert syndrome [ˈkuːʃmɑːn ˈbætən ˈʃtainert] (Hans Curschmann; Frederick E. Batten; Hans Steinert)库-巴-斯综合征,肌强直性营养不良

Curschmann's disease [ˈkuːʃmen] (Heinrich Curschmann)慢性增生性肝周炎,糖衣肝 | ~ mask 库施曼吸药罩(曾用以吸入松节油蒸气) / ~ spirals 库施曼螺旋物(黏蛋白状的原纤维,有时见于支气管性哮喘患者的痰内)

Curtius' syndrome [ˈkuətius] (Friedrich Curtius)库齐乌斯综合征(全身一侧肥大或偏身肥大,如面偏侧肥大)

curvatura [ˌkəːvəˈtjuərə] ([复] **curvaturae** [ˌkəːvəˈtjuəriː]) *n*【拉】弯,曲

curvature [ˈkəːvətʃə] *n* 弯,曲;曲率 | gingival ~ 龈曲 / greater ~ of stomach 胃大弯 / lesser ~ of stomach 胃小弯 / occlusal ~ 殆曲 / spinal ~ 脊柱弯曲

curve [kəːv] *n* 曲线,曲线图表;弯曲,弯曲部分 | alignment ~ 排列曲线,整列曲线(指牙列曲线) / dose-effect ~, dose-response ~ 剂量效应曲线,剂量反应曲线(表示放射剂量与所产生的特殊生物效应程度之间的相互关系) / frequency ~, probability ~ 频率曲线,概率曲线 / growth ~ 生长曲线(指儿童或细菌的) / isodose ~s 等剂量曲线(放射治疗时用) / muscle ~ 肌肉收缩曲线,肌动[描记]图 / ~ of occlusion, dental ~ 殆曲线,牙列曲线 / oxygen dissociation ~, oxygen-hemoglobin dissociation ~, oxyhemoglobin dissociation ~ 氧解离曲线(表示与血红蛋白结合的氧量正常变化曲线) / pulse ~ 脉搏描记图,脉搏曲线 / visibility ~ 可见度曲线

curvea [kəːviə] *n* 曲线 | ~ occlusalis 殆曲线

Curvularia [kəːvjuˈlɛəriə] *n* 弯孢[霉]属 | ~ lunata 月状弯孢霉

cuscamidine [kʌsˈkæmidin] *n* 古柯米定(一种金鸡纳属生物碱)

cuscamine [kʌsˈkæmin] *n* 古柯明(一种金鸡纳属生物碱)

cuscohygrine [kʌskəˈhaigrin] *n* 红古豆碱(抗胆碱药)

cushingoid [ˈkuʃiŋgɔid] *a* 类库欣综合征的(指体征和症状)

Cushing-Rokitansky ulcers [ˈkuʃiŋ rɔːkiˈtʌnski] (Harvey W. Cushing; Karl F. von Rokitanski)库-罗溃疡(见 Rokitansky-Cushing ulcers)

Cushing's disease [ˈkuʃiŋ] (Harvey W. Cushing)库欣病(为库欣综合征,其肾上腺功能亢进继发于垂体前叶过度分泌促肾上腺皮质激素,伴或不伴垂体腺瘤) | ~ law 库欣定律(颅内张力增高引起血压增高) / ~ operation 库欣手术(一种输尿管缝合法) / ~ phenomenon 库欣现象(颅内压增高所致的全身性血压增高) / ~ syndrome 库欣综合征(①肾上腺皮质功能亢进,症状为肥胖、多毛、阳痿等,当继发于垂体过度分泌促肾上腺皮质激素时,则称库欣病,亦称垂体嗜碱细胞增殖;②小脑脑桥角及听神经生瘤时,引起耳鸣、重听及同侧第6、7脑神经功能损害及颅内压升高)

Cushing's suture [ˈkuʃiŋ] (Hayward W. Cushing)库欣缝合,连续浆肌层内翻缝合(一种连续缝术,用于胃肠道手术)

cushion [ˈkuʃən] *n* 垫;减震器,缓冲器 | coronary ~ 冠状垫 / endocardial ~s 心内膜垫 / ~ of epiglottis 会厌垫(会厌软骨柄;会厌结节) / eustachian ~, ~ of eustachian orifice 咽鼓管圆枕 / intimal ~s 内膜垫 / sucking ~ 颊脂体,吸垫,颊脂垫

cuskohygrine [ˌkʌskəˈhaigrin] *n* 红古豆碱

cusp [kʌsp] *n* 尖 | aortic ~ 主动脉瓣前尖 | semilunar ~ 半月形尖 / dental ~ 牙尖

cuspid [ˈkʌspid] *a* 尖[端]的 *n* 尖牙

cuspidate(d) [ˈkʌspideit(id)] *a* 有尖的

cuspis [ˈkʌspis] ([复] **cuspides** [ˈkʌspidiːz]) *n*【拉】尖

custodian [kʌsˈtəudjən] *n* 监护人

cut [kʌt] *vt, vi* 切,割,剪,砍,削 *n* 切伤;刀伤;切面;切磨(牙);切口

cutaneous [kju(ː)ˈteinjəs] *a* 皮[肤]的

cutdown [ˈkʌtdaun] *n* 切开(切一小口,以利静脉切开术)

Cuterebra [ˌkjuːtəˈriːbrə] *n* 黄蝇属

Cuterebridae [ˌkjuːtəˈrebridiː] *n* 黄蝇科

cuticle [ˈkjuːtikl] *n* 小皮;甲上皮;角质层 | dental ~, enamel ~ 牙小皮,釉小皮 / keratose ~ 角化小皮(眼的色素细胞外表面层) / primary ~ 原发性釉小皮,釉小皮 / ~ of root sheath 毛根鞘小皮 / secondary ~ 继发性釉小皮,牙小皮 | **cutlcular** [kju(ː)ˈtikjulə] *a*

cuticula [kjuˈtikjulə] ([复] **cuticulae** [kjuˈtikjuliː]) *n*【拉】小皮;角质层 | ~ dentis 牙小皮

cuticularization [kjuˌtikjuləraiˈzeiʃən, -riˈz-] *n* 小皮形成;角质层形成

cuticulin [kjuˈtikjulin] *n* 壳脂蛋白

cuticulum [kjuˈtikjuləm] *n* 表皮;护膜

cutidure [ˈkjuːtidjuə], **cutiduris** [ˌkjuːtiˈdjuəris] *n* 冠状垫

cutin [ˈkjuːtin] *n* 角质(植物);角质素

cutinization [ˌkjuːtinaiˈzeiʃən, -niˈz-] *n* 表皮埋植术

cutireaction [ˌkjuːtiri(ː)ˈækʃən] *n* 皮肤反应(在某些传染病中,以该病病原制剂注射或应用于皮肤时,皮肤发生的炎症或刺激性反应) | differential ~ 鉴别皮肤反应(一次同时接种旧结核

菌素〈人型结核菌素滤液〉及牛型结核菌素滤液,以决定患者是否感染结核,若已感染,则鉴别属人型还是属牛型)

cutis [ˈkjuːtis]([复] **cutes** [ˈkjuːtiːz]或 **cutises**) *n*【拉】皮肤 | ~ anserina 鸡皮(亦称鸡皮疙瘩)/ ~ elastica 弹力性皮肤 / ~ hyperelastica 皮肤弹性过度,弹力过度性皮肤 / ~ laxa 皮肤松弛症,皮肤松垂 / ~ marmorata 大理石样皮肤 / ~ rhomboidalis nuchae 颈部菱形

cuttlebone [ˈkʌtəlbəun] *n* 乌贼骨,海螵蛸,墨鱼骨

cuvette [kjuˈvet] *n* 杯,吸收池

Cuvier's canal, duct(sinus) [ˈkuviei](Georges L. C. F. Dagobert)静脉导管

CV cardiovascular 心血管的;closing volume 闭合容积,闭合气量;coefficient of variation 变异系数

C. V. cras vespere【拉】明晚;conjugata vera【拉】真结合径

CVA cardiovascular accident 心血管意外;cerebrovascular accident 脑血管意外 costovertebral angle 肋椎角

CVB cyclophosphamide, etoposide, and carmustine 环磷酰胺-依托泊苷-卡莫司汀(高剂量移植方案);lomustine, vinblastine, and bleomycin 洛莫司汀-长春碱-博来霉素(联合化疗治癌方案)

CVID common variable immunodeficiency 普通可变型免疫缺陷

CVP central venous pressure 中心静脉压;cyclophosphamide, vincristine, and prednisone 环磷酰胺-长春新碱-泼尼松(联合化疗治癌方案)

CVS cardiovascular system 心血管系统;chorionic villus sampling 绒膜绒毛取样

Cx cervix 颈;convex 凸的,凸面的

Cy cyanogen 氰

Cyamopsis [ˌsaiəˈmɔpsis] *n* 豆科植物属

cyanalcohol [ˌsaiənˈælkəhɔl] *n* 氰醇

cyanamide [saiˈænəmaid] *n* 氰酰胺;氰氨化钙

cyanate [ˈsaiəneit] *n* 氰酸盐

cyanemia [ˌsaiəˈniːmiə] *n* 青血症,绀血症

cyanhematin [ˌsaiənˈhiːmətin] *n* 氰[化]高铁血红素

cyanhemoglobin [ˌsaiənˌhiːməuˈgləubin] *n* 氰血红蛋白

cyanhydric acid [ˌsaiənˈhaidrik] 氢氰酸

cyanic acid [saiˈænik] 氰酸

cyanide [ˈsaiənaid] *n* 氰化物 *vt* 用氰化物处理 | mercuric ~ 氰化汞

cyanin [ˈsaiənin] *n* 花青苷,矢车菊苷(用作pH7 ~ 8 的指示剂)

cyanmethemoglobin [ˌsaiənˌmethiːməuˈgləubin] *n* 氰化高铁血红蛋白(此色素广泛用于临床血红蛋白测定法)

cyanmetmyoglobin [ˌsaiənmetˌmaiəuˈgləubin] *n* 氰化高铁肌球蛋白

cyan(o)- [构词成分]青紫,绀,蓝;氰

cyanoacrylate [ˌsaiənəuˈækrileit] *n* 氰基丙烯酸酯

cyanoalcohol [ˌsaiənəuˈælkəhɔl] *n* 氰醇

Cyanobacteria [ˌsaiənəubækˈtiəriə] *n* 蓝藻目

cyanobacterium [ˌsaiənəubækˈtiəriəm]([复] **cyanobacteria** [ˌsaiənəubækˈtiəriə]) *n* 蓝细菌

cyanocobalamin [ˌsaiənəukəˈbæləmin] *n* 氰钴铵,维生素 B_{12}(防治恶性贫血及大红细胞性贫血) | radioactive ~ 放射性氰钴铵(诊断恶性贫血)

cyanocrystallin [ˌsaiənəuˈkristəlin] *n* 蓝晶质(由虾、蟹等十足类动物外壳所得的一种蓝色物质)

cyanoform [saiˈænəfɔːm] *n* 氰仿

cyanogen [saiˈænədʒin] *n* 氰 | ~ bromide 溴化氢 / ~ chloride 氯化氰

cyanogenesis [ˌsaiənəuˈdʒenisis] *n* 生氰作用

cyanogenetic [ˌsaiənəudʒiˈnetik], **cyanogenic** [ˌsaiənəuˈdʒenik] *a* 生氰的

cyanohydrin [ˌsaiənəuˈhaidrin] *n* 氰醇

cyanolabe [ˈsaiənəˌleib] *n* 蓝敏素,感蓝色素

cyanophil [saiˈænəfil] *a* 嗜蓝的,嗜青的 *n* 嗜蓝细胞,嗜青细胞

cyanophilous [ˌsaiəˈnɔfiləs] *a* 嗜蓝的,嗜青的

cyanophoric [ˌsaiənəuˈfɔːrik] *a* 氰基的

cyanophose [ˈsaiənəfəuz] *n* 蓝光幻视

Cyanophyceae [ˌsaiənəuˈfaisiiː] *n* 蓝藻纲

cyanopsia [ˌsaiəˈnɔpsiə], **cyanopia** [ˌsaiəˈnəupiə] *n* 蓝视症

cyanose [ˈsaiəˌnəus] *n*【法】发绀,青紫 | ~ tardive 迟发性发绀

cyanosed [ˈsaiənəuzd] *a* 发绀的,青紫的

cyanosis [ˌsaiəˈnəusis] *n* 发绀,青紫 | central ~ 中央性发绀 / enterogenous ~, autotoxic ~ 肠源性发绀,自身中毒性发绀(肠吸收亚硝酸盐和硫化物所引起的综合征)/ false ~ 假性发绀 / hereditary methemoglobinemic ~ 遗传性正铁血红蛋白血性发绀 / ~ lienis 脾性发绀,淤血脾 / peripheral ~ 外周性发绀 / pulmonary ~ 肺性发绀 / ~ retinae 视网膜发绀 / shunt ~ 短路性发绀 / tardive ~ 迟发性发绀(先天性心脏病) | **cyanotic** [ˌsaiəˈnɔtik] *a*

cyanuria [ˌsaiəˈnjuəriə] *n* 蓝色尿,青色尿

cyanuric acid [saiəˈnjuərik] 氰尿酸,三聚氰酸,三羟均三嗪

cyanurin [ˌsaiəˈnjuərin] *n* 尿靛蓝

Cyath. cyathus【拉】一杯

Cyathostoma [ˌsaiəˈθɔstəmə] *n* 比翼线虫属

cyathostomiasis [ˌsaiəθɔstəuˈmaiəsis] *n* 圆线虫病

Cyathostomum [ˌsaiəθɔˈstəuməm] *n* 圆线虫属

Cycas [ˈsaikəs] *n* 苏铁属
cybernetics [ˌsaibəˈnetiks] *n* 控制论
CYC cyclophosphamide 环磷酰胺
cycad [ˈsaikæd] *n* 苏铁科植物
cycasin [ˈsaikəsin] *n* 苏铁苷
cyclacillin [saikləˈsilin] *n* 环青霉素,氨环己青霉素(抗菌药)
cyclamate [ˈsaikləmeit] *n* 环拉酸盐
Cyclamen [ˈsikləmən] *n* 仙客来属
cyclamic acid [saiˈklæmik] 环拉酸(甜味药)
cyclamin [ˈsikləmin] *n* 仙客来苷(有催泻和催吐作用)
cyclandelate [saiˈklændileit] *n* 环扁桃酯(解痉药,周围血管扩张药)
cyclarthrosis [ˌsiklɑːˈθrəusis] ([复] **cyclarthroses** [ˌsiklɑːˈθrəusiːz]) *n* 车轴关节,屈戌关节,回旋关节 | **cyclarthrodial** *a*
cyclase [ˈsaikleis] *n* 环化酶 | adenyl ~, adenylate ~ 腺苷酸环化酶
cyclazocine [ˌsaikləˈzəusin] *n* 环佐辛(麻醉拮抗药,镇痛药)
cycle [ˈsaikl] *n* 周期;环,循环;周波数 *vi* 循环 | aberrant ~ 迷行循环 / anovulatory ~ 无排卵周期 / asexual ~ 无性生殖周期 / biliary ~ 胆汁循环(胆酸盐循环) / carbon ~ 碳循环 / cardiac ~ 心动周期 / cell ~ 细胞周期 / citrate-pyruvate ~ 枸橼酸-丙酮酸循环 / citric acid ~ 枸橼酸循环 / cytoplasmic ~ 胞质[内生活]环(寄生物) / estrous ~ 动情周期 / exogenous ~ 外生环,外生期(原生动物) / forced ~ 强迫周期(一种心搏周期) / futile ~ 无效周期 / gastric ~ 胃周期(蠕动) / genesial ~ 生殖周期 / glucose-lactate ~ 葡萄糖乳酸盐循环 / glyoxylate ~ 乙醛酸循环,乙醛酸支路 / gonotrophic ~ 生殖成熟周期(昆虫) / hair ~ 毛发周期 / intranuclear ~ 细胞核内[生长]环 / life ~ 生活史,生活环,生活周期 / masticating ~, masticatory ~, chewing ~ 咀嚼周期 / menstrual ~ 月经周期 / mosquito ~ 蚊体内生环 / nitrogen ~ 氮循环 / ornithine ~ 鸟氨酸循环 / ovarian ~, oogenetic ~ 卵巢周期,卵发生周期 / pregnancy ~ 妊娠周期 / reproductive ~ 生殖周期 / restored ~ 复原周期(心搏) / returning ~ 恢复周期(由期外收缩开始的心搏周期) / schizogenic ~, schizogenous ~ 裂殖周期 / sex ~, sexual ~ 性周期 / sporogenic ~, sporogenous ~ 孢子生殖周期 / tricarboxylic acid ~ 三羧酸循环 / uterine ~ 子宫周期 / vaginal ~ 阴道周期
cyclectomy [sikˈlektəmi] *n* 睫状体切除术;睑缘切除术
cyclencephalus [ˌsiklenˈsefələs] *n* (大脑)两半球并合畸胎,并脑畸胎
cyclic [ˈsiklik, ˈsaiklik] *a* 周期的;循环的,环[状]的
cyclic AMP cyclic adenosine monophosphate 环腺苷酸
cyclic-AMP-dependent protein kinase [ˈsaiklik diˈpendənt ˈprəutiːn ˈkaineis] 环腺苷酸依赖性蛋白激酶
cyclic GMP cyclic guanosine monophosphate 环鸟苷酸
3′, 5′-cyclic GMP phosphodiesterase [ˈsaiklik ˌfɔsfəudaiˈestəreis] 3′, 5′-环鸟苷酸磷酸二酯酶
cyclicotomy [ˌsikliˈkɔtəmi] *n* 睫状肌切开术
cyclin [ˈsiklin] *n* 细胞周期蛋白
cyclindole [saiˈklindəul] *n* 胺氢咔唑(抗抑郁药)
cyclitis [sikˈlaitis] *n* 睫状体炎
cyclization [ˌsaiklaiˈzeiʃən, -liˈz-] *n* 环化[作用];成环作用
cyclizine [ˈsaikliziːn] *n* 赛克利嗪(抗组胺药) | ~ hydrochloride 盐酸赛克利嗪 / ~ lactate 乳酸赛克利嗪(止吐、止恶心药,尤用于预防和缓解晕动病)
cycl(o)- [构词成分]环,圆形;睫状体
cycloanemization [ˌsaikləuˌænimaiˈzeiʃən] *n* 睫状体贫血术(在青光眼手术治疗时将睫状长动脉阻塞)
cyclobarbital [ˌsaikləuˈbɑːbitæl] *n* 环己巴比妥(口服安眠药) | ~ calcium 环己巴比妥钙
cyclobendazole [ˌsaikləuˈbendəzəul] *n* 环苯达唑(抗蠕虫药)
cyclobenzaprine hydrochloride [ˌsaiklə*u* ˈbenzəpriːn] 盐酸环苯扎林(肌肉松弛药)
cyclocephalus [ˌsaikləuˈsefələs] *n* [大脑]两半球并合独眼畸胎,并脑独眼畸胎
cycloceratitis [ˌsaikləuˌserəˈtaitis] *n* 睫状体角膜炎
cyclochoroiditis [ˌsaikləuˌkɔːrɔiˈdaitis] *n* 睫状体脉络膜炎
cyclocryotherapy [ˌsaikləuˌkraiəuˈθerəpi] *n* 睫状体冷冻疗法(治青光眼)
cyclocumarol [ˌsaikləuˈkuməraul] *n* 环香豆素(抗凝血药)
cyclodamia [ˌsaikləuˈdeimiə] *n* 调节受抑(指眼)
cyclodextrin [ˌsaikləuˈdekstrin] *n* 环[化]糊精
cyclodialysis [ˌsaikləudaiˈælisis] *n* 睫状体分离术
cyclodiathermy [ˌsaikləuˈdaiəˌθəːmi] *n* 睫状体透热术
cycloduction [ˌsaikləuˈdʌkʃən] *n* 眼球旋转
cycloelectrolysis [ˌsaikləuˌilekˈtrɔlisis] *n* 睫状体电解术
cyclogeny [saiˈklɔdʒini] *n* (细菌)周期发育,生活周期
cyclogram [ˈsaikləgræm] *n* 视野图;排卵周期图,内分泌周期图

cycloguanide embonate [ˌsaiklə'gwænaid] 恩波环氯胍,双羟萘酸环氯胍(抗疟药)
cycloguanil pamoate [saikləu'gwænil] 双羟萘酸环氯胍(抗疟药,亦称恩波环氯胍)
cyclohexane [ˌsaikləu'heksein] *n* 环己烷
cyclohexanehexol [ˌsaikləuˌheksein'heksɔl] *n* 环己六醇,肌醇
cyclohexanesulfamic acid [ˌsaiklə u ˌheksinsʌl-'fæmik] 环拉酸(即 cyclamic acid)
cyclohexanol [ˌsaikləu'heksənɔl] *n* 环己醇,环糖
cycloheximide [ˌsaikləu'heksimaid] *n* 放线酮(抗真菌药)
cycloid ['saiklɔid] *a* 环状的;循环性情感的,躁郁性气质的 *n* 循环性情感气质者,躁郁性气质者
cycloisomerase [ˌsaikləuai'sɔməreis] *n* 环异构酶
cyclokeratitis [ˌsaikləukerə'taitis] *n* 睫状体角膜炎
cyclo-ligase [ˌsaikləu 'laigeis] *n* 环连接酶
cyclomastopathy [ˌsaikləumæs'tɔpəθi] *n* 乳腺(结缔组织及上皮)增生症
cyclomethycaine sulfate [ˌsaikləu'meθikein] 硫酸环美卡因(局部麻醉药)
cyclooxygenase [ˌsaikləu'ɔksidʒineis] *n* 环氧合酶,环加氧酶
cyclooxygenation [ˌsaikləuˌɔksidʒi'neiʃən] *n* 环氧合作用,环加氧作用
cyclopentamine hydrochloride [ˌsaikləu'pen-təmiːn] 盐酸环喷他明(拟肾上腺素药)
cyclopentane [ˌsaikləu'pentein] *n* 环戊烷
cyclopentanoperhydrophenanthrene [ˌsaikləu-ˌpentənəupəːˌhaidrəufə'nænθriːn] *n* 环戊烷多氢菲
cyclopentenophenanthrene [ˌsaikləupenˌtiːnəfi-'nænθriːn] *n* 环戊烯菲
cyclopenthiazide [ˌsaikləupen'θaiəzaid] *n* 环戊噻嗪(利尿降压药)
cyclopentolate hydrochloride [ˌsaiklə u 'pen-təleit] 盐酸环喷托酯(抗胆碱药,散瞳药)
cyclophenazine hydrochloride [ˌsaiklə u 'fenə-ziːn] 盐酸环丙奋乃静(安定药)
cyclophoria [ˌsaikləu'fəuriə] *n* 旋转隐斜 | accommodative ~ 调节性旋转隐斜(斜轴散光所致) / minus ~, negative ~ 内旋转隐斜 / plus ~, positive ~ 外旋转隐斜
cyclophorometer [ˌsaikləufə'rɔmitə] *n* 旋转隐斜计
cyclophosphamide (CYC) [ˌsaikləu'fɔsfəmaid] *n* 环磷酰胺(免疫抑制药及抗肿瘤药)
Cyclophyllidea [ˌsaikləufi'lidiə] *n* 圆叶目
cyclopia [sai'kləupiə] *n* 独眼
cyclopin ['saikləpin] *n* 圆弧素(圆弧青霉 Penicillium cyclopium 的蛋白成分,已证明能抑制虫媒病毒 A 组和 B 组的代表性病毒的繁殖)
cycloplegia [ˌsaikləu'pliːdʒiə] *n* 睫状肌麻痹 | **cycloplegic** [ˌsaikləu'pliːdʒik] *a* 睫状肌麻痹的 *n* 睫状肌麻痹剂
cyclopropane [ˌsaikləu'prəupein] *n* 环丙烷(吸入麻醉药,因其能燃烧,现很少使用)
cyclopropanone hydrate [ˌsaikləu'prəupənəun 'haidreit] 环丙酮水合物
Cyclops ['saiklɔps] *n* 剑水蚤属
cyclops ['saiklɔps] *n* 独眼畸胎 | ~ hypognathus 下颌不全独眼畸胎
cyclopterin [sai'klɔptərin] *n* 环蝶呤
cyclorotary [ˌsaikləu'rəutəri] *a* 睫状体旋转的
cyclorotation [ˌsaikləurəu'teiʃən] *n* 睫状体旋转
cycloscope ['saikləskəup] *n* 视野镜
cyclose ['saikləuz] *n* 环糖
cycloserine [ˌsaikləu'seriːn] *n* 环丝氨酸(抗结核药,有时用于治疗尿路感染)
cyclosis [sai'kləusis] *n* 胞质环流
cyclospasm ['saikləspæzəm] *n* 调节痉挛(指眼)
Cyclospora [sai'klɔspərə] *n* 圆孢子球虫属
cyclosporiasis [ˌsaikləuspə'raiəsis] *n* 圆孢子球虫病
cyclosporin A [ˌsaikləu'spɔːrin] *n* 环孢菌素 A
cyclosporine [ˌsaikləu'spɔːrin] *n* 环孢菌素(具有免疫抑制和抗真菌作用,用于防止器官移植的排斥)
cyclostat ['saikləstæt] *n* [实验]动物旋转瓶
cyclotate ['saikləteit] *n* 双环辛烯酸盐,4-甲基双环[2.2.2]环辛-2-烯-1-羧酸盐(4-methylbicyclo-[2.2.2] oct-2-ene-1-carboxylate 的 USAN 缩约词)
cyclotherapy [ˌsaikləu'θerəpi] *n* 自行车疗法
cyclothiazide [ˌsaikləu'θaiəzaid] *n* 环噻嗪(利尿降压药)
cyclothyme ['saiklə'θaim] *n* [躁郁]环性气质者
cyclothymia [ˌsaikləu'θaimiə] *n* [躁郁]环性气质 | **cyclothymic** *a* / **~c** [ˌsaikləu'θimiæk] *n* [躁郁]环性气质者
cyclotol ['saiklətɔl] *n* 多羟环己烷
cyclotome ['saiklətəum] *n* 睫状肌刀
cyclotomy [sai'klɔtəmi] *n* 睫状肌切开术
cyclotron ['saiklətrɔn] *n* 回旋加速器
cyclotropia [ˌsaikləu'trəupiə] *n* 旋转斜视 | minus ~, negative ~ 内旋转斜视 / plus ~, positive ~ 外旋转斜视
cycrimine hydrochloride ['saikrimiːn] 盐酸赛克立明(抗胆碱药,治帕金森神经功能障碍)
cyema [sai'iːmə] *n* 胚胎
cyemology [ˌsaii'mɔlədʒi] *n* 胚胎学
cyesis [sai'iːsis] *n* 妊娠
cyestein [sai'estiːn], **cyesthein** [sai'esθiːn] *n* 孕

尿翳(孕妇尿表面有膜样形成)
cyl cylinder 圆柱体;cylindrical lens 柱镜片
cylicotomy [ˌsiliˈkɔtəmi] *n* 睫状肌切开术
cylinder [ˈsilində] *n* 圆柱;圆柱体(尤指圆柱管型或柱镜片) | crossed ~s 正交圆柱[透]镜 / terminal ~s 终柱 / urinary ~ 尿圆柱,尿管型
cylindrarthrosis [ˌsilindrɑːˈθrəusis] *n* 柱状关节
cylindraxile [ˌsilinˈdræksil] *n* 轴索,轴突,神经轴
cylindric(al) [siˈlindrik(ə)l] *a* 圆柱的,圆柱状的
cylindriform [siˈlindrifɔːm] *a* 圆柱状的
Cylindrocarpon [siˌlindrəuˈkɑːpɔn] *n* 柱盘孢属
cylindrocellular [ˌsilindrəuˈseljulə] *a* 柱状细胞的
cylindrodendrite [ˌsilindrəuˈdendrait] *n* 轴索侧支,旁轴索
cylindroid [ˈsilindrɔid] *a* 圆柱状的 *n* 圆柱状体
cylindroma [ˌsilinˈdrəumə] *n* 圆柱瘤;腺样囊性癌 | **~tous** [ˌsilinˈdrɔmətəs] *a*
Cylindrothorax [siˌlindrəuˈθɔːræks] *n* 斑蝥属 | ~ melanocephala 黑头斑蝥
cylindruria [ˌsilinˈdrjuəriə] *n* 管型尿,圆柱尿
cylite [ˈsailait] *n* 溴化苄
cyllosis [siˈləusis] *n* 畸形足
cyllosoma [ˌsiləˈsəumə], **cyllosomus** [ˌsiləˈsəuməs] *n* 下侧腹露脏下肢不全畸胎
cymarose [ˈsaimərəus] *n* 磁麻糖
cymba [ˈsimbə] ([复] **cymbae** [ˈsimbiː]) *n*【拉】艇,舟状物
cymbiform [ˈsimbifɔːm] *a* 舟形的,舟状的
cymb(o)- [构词成分]凹,舟形
cymbocephaly [ˌsimbəuˈsefəli], **cymbocephalia** [ˌsimbəusiˈfeiliə] *n* 舟状头[畸形] | **cymbocephalic** [ˌsimbəuseˈfælik], **cymbocephalous** [ˌsimbəuˈsefələs] *a*
Cymbopogon [ˌsimbəˈpəugɔn] *n* 香茅属
cyme [saim] *n* 聚伞花序
cymograph [ˈsaiməgrɑːf, -græf] *n* 记波[纹]器
cynanche [siˈnænki] *n* 锁喉,咽峡炎 | ~ maligna 坏疽性咽峡炎 / ~ tonsillaris 扁桃体周脓肿
cynanthropy [siˈnænθrəpi] *n* 变犬妄想
cynarase [ˈsainəreis] *n* 洋蓟酶
cynic [ˈsinik] *a* 犬的,似犬的
cyn(o)- [构词成分]犬,狗
cynocephalic [ˌsainəuseˈfælik] *a* 狗[状]头的
Cynodon [ˈsainədɔn] *n* 狗牙根属
cynodont [ˈsainədɔnt] *n* 尖牙
cynomolgus [ˌsinəuˈmɔlgəs] *n* 猕猴,食蟹猴
Cynomyia [ˌsainəuˈmaijə] *n* 蓝蝇属
Cynomys [ˈsainəmis] *n* 草原犬属(有传播瘟疫的蚤寄生)
cynophobia [ˌsainəuˈfəubjə] *n* 犬恐怖
cynorexia [ˌsainəˈreksiə] *n* 贪食,食欲过盛,犬样善饥
cyogenic [ˌsaiəuˈdʒenik] *a* 引起妊娠的,致孕的
cyonin [ˈsaiənin] *n* 胎盘促性腺激素
Cyon's experiment [ˈsiːɔn] (Elie de Cyon)齐翁实验(刺激完整的脊神经前根所引起的肌肉收缩,较同样刺激一根切断的神经根远侧端所引起的肌肉收缩为强) | ~ nerve 齐翁神经(一种减压神经,为兔迷走神经的分支,一经刺激,即导致血压下降)
cyophoria [ˌsaiəˈfɔriə] *n* 妊娠 | **cyophoric** [ˌsaiəˈfɔrik] *a*
cyopin [ˈsaiəpin] *n* 绿脓色素
cyotrophy [saiˈɔtrəfi] *n* 胎儿营养
Cyperus [saiˈpiːrəs] *n*【拉】莎草属
cyph(o)- 以 cyph(o)-起始的词,同样见以 kyph(o)-起始的词
cypionate [ˈsipiəuneit] *n* 环戊丙酸盐(或酯)(cyclopentanepropionate 的 USAN 缩约词)
cypothrin [ˈsaipəθrin] *n* 螺茚扁腈酯(兽用抗螨虫药)
cyprazepam [saiˈpræzəpæm] *n* 环丙西泮(安定药)
cypridology [ˌsipriˈdɔlədʒi] *n* 性病学
cypridopathy [ˌsipriˈdɔpəθi] *n* 性病
cyprinin [ˈsiprinin] *n* 鲤精蛋白甲
cyproheptadine hydrochloride [ˌsaiprəuˈheptədiːn] 盐酸赛庚啶(抗组胺药,止痒药)
cyproquinate [ˌsaiprəuˈkwineit] *n* 环丙喹酯(家禽抗球虫药)
cyproterone acetate [saiˈprəutərəun] 醋酸环丙孕酮(雄激素拮抗药)
Cyriax's syndrome [ˈsiriæks] (Edward F. Cyriax)西里阿克斯综合征(滑动的肋软骨压迫软骨间关节神经,导致软骨区疼痛,并辐射至肩和臂,或类似心绞痛样疼痛)
cyrto- [构词成分]弯曲
cyrtograph [ˈsəːtəgrɑːf, -græf] *n* 胸动描记器
cyrtometer [səːˈtɔmitə] *n* 曲面测量计,曲度计
Cyrtophorida [ˌsəːtəuˈfɔridə] *n* 管口目
cyrtos [ˈsəːtəs] *n* 弯咽管(一种经常弯曲的管状胞咽器,其壁由线带支持,亦称胞咽篮)
cyrtosis [səːˈtəusis] *n* 驼背,脊柱后凸;骨弯曲
Cys cysteine 半胱氨酸
Cys-Cys cystine 胱氨酸
cyst [sist] *n* 囊;囊肿;孢囊,包囊 | adventitious ~, false ~ 异物周[围]囊肿,假囊肿 / apopletic ~ 中风性囊肿(一部分由于血液外渗所形成) / blood ~ 血囊肿 / blue dome ~ 蓝顶囊肿(乳腺) / branchial ~, branchialcleft ~, branchiogenetic ~, branchiogenous ~ 鳃裂囊肿 / bronchogenic ~, bronchial ~ 支气管源性囊肿,支气管

囊肿 / butter ~ 黄油样囊肿；乳腺潴留囊肿 / cervical ~ 颈部先天性囊肿 / chocolate ~ 巧克力样囊肿(常见于乳房切除术后或卵巢子宫内膜异位时的卵巢内) / compound ~ 多房性囊肿 / daughter ~ 子囊 / epidermal ~ 表皮囊肿 / epidermal inclusion ~ 表皮包涵囊肿 / eruption ~ 萌出期囊肿 / gas ~ 含气囊肿 / hydatid ~, echinococcus ~ 棘球囊,棘球蚴 / lacteal ~ 乳腺囊肿 / mother ~, parent ~ 母囊 / multilocular ~ 多房性囊肿 / neural ~ 神经系[统]囊肿 / neurenteric ~ 神经管原肠囊肿 / pilar ~ 藏毛囊肿 / piliferous ~, pilonidal ~ 藏毛囊肿 / placental ~ 胎盘囊肿 / radicular ~, radiculodental ~, root ~ [牙]根端囊肿,牙根囊肿 / secondary ~ 次生囊,子囊 / urachal ~, allantoic ~ 脐尿管囊肿 / urinary ~ 尿[液]囊肿 / vitellointestinal ~ 卵黄管囊肿,脐囊肿

cystadenocarcinoma [sisˌtædinəuˌkɑːsiˈnəumə] *n* 囊腺癌

cystadenoma [ˌsistædiˈnəumə] *n* 囊腺瘤 | ~ adamantinum 釉质[上皮]瘤,成釉细胞瘤 / papillary ~ 乳头状囊腺瘤 / papillary ~ lymphomatosum 乳头状淋巴性囊腺瘤 / pseudomucinous ~, mucinous ~ 假黏液性囊腺瘤,黏液性囊腺瘤 / serous ~ 浆液性囊腺瘤

cystalgia [sisˈtældʒiə] *n* 膀胱痛

γ-cystathionase [ˌsistəˈθaiəneis] *n* γ-胱硫醚酶(见 cystathionine γ-lyase)

cystathionine [ˌsistəˈθaiəniːn] *n* 胱硫醚

cystathionine γ-lyase [ˌsistəˈθaiəniːn ˈgæmə ˈlaieis] 胱硫醚 γ-裂合酶(此酶缺乏为一种常染色体隐性性状,可致胱硫醚尿症。亦称胱硫醚酶)

cystathionine β-synthase [ˌsistəˈθaiəniːn ˈbeitə ˈsinθeis] 胱硫醚 β-合酶(此酶缺乏为一种常染色体隐性性状,可致高胱氨酸尿症)

cystathionine β-synthase deficiency 胱硫醚 β-合酶缺乏症(为一种常染色体隐性遗传氨基酸病,特征为高胱氨酸尿伴高蛋氨酸血症。临床异常主要发生在眼和骨骼、神经与血管系统;晶状体异位、骨质疏松、智力迟钝和血栓形成是最常见的表现。在旧文献中,本征有时称为高胱氨酸尿)

cystathioninuria [ˌsistəˌθaiəniˈnjuəriə] *n* 胱硫醚尿

cystatrophia [ˌsistəˈtrəufiə] *n* 膀胱萎缩

cystauchenitis [ˌsistɔːkiˈnaitis] *n* 膀胱颈炎

cystauchenotomy [ˌsistɔːkiˈnɔtəmi] *n* 膀胱颈切开术

cystauxe [ˈsistɔːksi] *n* 膀胱增大

cysteamine [ˈsistiəˌmiːn] *n* 半胱胺,β-巯基乙胺

cystectasia [ˌsistekˈteizjə], **cystectasy** [sisˈtektəsi] *n* 膀胱扩张术

cystectomy [sisˈtektəmi] *n* 囊切除术;膀胱切除术

cysteic acid [sisˈtiːik] 磺基丙氨酸

cysteine [sisˈtiːin] *n* 半胱氨酸 | ~ hydrochloride 盐酸半胱氨酸(治皮肤溃疡)

cysteine endopeptidase [sisˈtiːin ˌendəuˈpeptideis] 半胱氨酸内肽酶(亦称硫醇内肽酶)

cysteine-type carboxypeptidase [ˈsistiiːnˌtaip kɑːˌbɔksiˈpeptideis] 半胱氨酸型羧肽酶

cysteinyl [ˈsistiːnil, sisˈtiːinil] *n* 半胱氨酰

cystelcosis [ˌsistelˈkəusis] *n* 膀胱溃疡

cystencephalus [ˌsistenˈsefələs] *n* 囊状脑畸胎

cystendesis [ˌsistenˈdiːsis] *n* 胆囊缝术;膀胱缝术

cysterethism [sisˈteriθizəm] *n* 膀胱过敏

cysthypersarcosis [sistˌhaipə(ː)sɑːˈkəusis] *n* 膀胱肌肥厚

cysti- 见 cyst(o)-

cystic [ˈsistik] *a* 囊的;膀胱的;胆囊的

cysticercoid [sistiˈsəːkɔid] *n* 似囊尾蚴

cysticercosis [ˌsistisəˈkəusis] *n* 猪囊尾蚴病(俗名囊虫病)

Cysticercus [ˌsistiˈsəːkəs] *n* 囊尾蚴属 | ~ bovis 牛囊尾蚴 / ~ cellulosae 猪囊尾蚴 / ~ ovis 羊囊尾蚴 / ~ tenuicollis 细颈囊尾蚴

cysticercus [ˌsistiˈsəːkəs] ([复] **cysticerci** [ˌsistiˈsəːsai]) *n* 囊尾蚴

cysticolithectomy [ˌsistiˌkəuliˈθektəmi] *n* 胆囊管石切除术

cysticolithotripsy [ˌsistikəuˈliθətripsi] *n* 胆囊管碎石术

cysticorrhaphy [sistiˈkɔrəfi] *n* 胆囊管缝合术

cysticotomy [ˌsistiˈkɔtəmi] *n* 胆囊管切开术

cystides [ˈsistidiːz] cystis 的复数

cystid(o)- 见 cyst(o)-

cystidolaparotomy [ˌsistidəuˌlæpəˈrɔtəmi], **cystidoceliotomy** [ˌsistidəuˌsiliˈɔtəmi] *n* 剖腹膀胱切开术

cystidotrachelotomy [ˌsistidəutreikiˈlɔtəmi] *n* 膀胱颈切开术

cystifellotomy [ˌsistifeˈlɔtəmi] *n* 胆囊切开术

cystiferous [sisˈtifərəs] *a* 含囊的

cystiform [ˈsistifɔːm] *a* 囊样的,囊状的

cystigerous [sisˈtidʒərəs] *a* 含囊的

cystine [ˈsisti(ː)n] *n* 胱氨酸

cystinemia [ˌsistiˈniːmiə] *n* 胱氨酸血[症]

cystinosis [ˌsistiˈnəusis] *n* 胱氨酸贮积症

cystinuria [ˌsistiˈnjuəriə] *n* 胱氨酸尿症 | **cystinuric** *a*

cystirrhagia [ˌsistiˈreidʒiə] *n* 膀胱出血

cystirrhea [ˌsistiˈriːə] *n* 膀胱黏液溢,膀胱卡他

cystis [ˈsistis] ([复] **cystides** [ˈsistidiːz]) *n* 囊;

囊肿 | ~ fellea 胆囊
cystistaxis [ˌsistiˈstæksis] *n* 膀胱渗血
cystitis [sisˈtaitis] *n* 膀胱炎 | allergic ~ 变应性膀胱炎 / bacterial ~ 细菌性膀胱炎 / chronic interstitial ~, panmural ~ 慢性间质性膀胱炎 / cystic ~ 囊性膀胱炎 / diphtheritic ~, croupous ~ 白喉性膀胱炎 / eosinophilic ~ 嗜酸细胞性膀胱炎 / incrusted ~ 结痂性膀胱炎
cystitome [ˈsistitəum] *n* 截囊刀
cystitomy [sisˈtitəmi] *n* 囊切开术;晶状体囊切开术
cyst(o)- [构词成分]囊;囊肿;膀胱
cystoadenoma [ˌsistəuædiˈnəumə] *n* 囊腺瘤
Cystobacter [ˌsistəuˈbæktə] *n* 囊孢杆菌属
Cystobacteraceae [ˌsistəuˌbæktiəˈreisiiː] *n* 囊孢杆菌科
cystoblast [ˈsistəblæst] *n* 囊层,羊膜腔细胞层
cystocarcinoma [ˌsistəukɑːsiˈnəumə] *n* 囊性癌
Cystocaulus [ˌsistəuˈkɔːləs] *n* 原圆线虫属
cystocele [ˈsistəsiːl] *n* 膀胱膨出(经由阴道壁膨出)
cystochrome [ˈsistəkrəum] *n* 尿着色合剂(靛卡红和乌洛托品的合剂,作肌肉或静脉注射,用于检测肾功能的靛卡红试验)
cystochromoscopy [ˌsistəukrəuˈmɔskəpi] *n* [尿]染色膀胱镜检查(肾功能)
cystocolostomy [ˌsistəukəˈlɔstəmi] *n* 膀胱结肠造口吻合术
cystodiaphanoscopy [ˌsistəuˌdaiəfəˈnɔskəpi] *n* 膀胱透照检查
cystoduodenostomy [ˌsistəuˌdju(ː)əudiˈnɔstəmi] *n* 囊肿十二指肠吻合[引流]术
cystodynia [ˌsistəuˈdiniə] *n* 膀胱痛
cystoelytroplasty [ˌsistəuiˈlitrəˌplæsti] *n* 阴道膀胱成形术
cystoenterocele [ˌsistəuˈentərəsiːl] *n* 膀胱肠疝
cystoepiplocele [ˌsistəuiˈpipləsiːl] *n* 膀胱网膜疝
cystoepithelioma [ˌsistəuˌepiˌθiːliˈəumə] *n* 囊性上皮瘤
cystofibroma [ˌsistəufaiˈbrəumə] *n* 囊性纤维瘤
cystogastrostomy [ˌsistəugæsˈtrɔstəmi] *n* 囊肿胃吻合[引流]术
cystogenesis [ˌsistəuˈdʒenisis] *n* 囊形成
cystogram [ˈsistəgræm] *n* 膀胱[照]片,膀胱造影[照]片
cystography [sisˈtɔgrəfi] *n* 膀胱造影[术] | delayed ~ 延迟膀胱造影[术] / voiding ~ 排尿式膀胱造影[术]
cystoid [ˈsistɔid] *a* 囊样的 *n* 类囊肿
Cystoisospora [ˌsistəuaiˈsɔspərə] *n* 囊等孢子球虫属
cystojejunostomy [ˌsistəudʒidʒuːˈnɔstəmi] *n* 囊肿空肠吻合[引流]术
cystolith [ˈsistəliθ] *n* 膀胱结石 | **~ic** [ˌsistəˈliθik] *a*
cystolithectomy [ˌsistəuliˈθektəmi] *n* 膀胱切开取石术
cystolithiasis [ˌsistəuliˈθaiəsis] *n* 膀胱结石病
cystolithotomy [ˌsistəuliˈθɔtəmi] *n* 膀胱切开取石术
cystolutein [ˌsistəuˈljuːtiːn] *n* 囊肿黄素(卵巢)
cystoma [sisˈtəumə] *n* 囊瘤 | **~tous** *a*
cystomatitis [ˌsistəuməˈtaitis] *n* 囊瘤炎
cystometer [sisˈtɔmitə] *n* 膀胱测压器
cystometrogram [ˌsistəuˈmetrəgræm] *n* 膀胱内压[测量]图
cystometrography [ˌsistəumiˈtrɔgrəfi] *n* 膀胱内压描记法
cystometry [sisˈtɔmitri] *n* 膀胱测压 | filling ~ 充盈性膀胱测压
Cystomonas [sisˈtɔmənəs] *n* 胞滴虫属(即波陀虫属 Bodo)
cystomorphous [ˌsistəuˈmɔːfəs] *a* 囊形的
cystonephrosis [ˌsistəuneˈfrəusis] *n* 肾囊状肿大
cystoneuralgia [ˌsistəunjuəˈrældʒə] *n* 膀胱神经痛
cystoparalysis [ˌsistəupəˈrælisis] *n* 膀胱麻痹
cystoparesis [ˌsistəupəˈriːsis] *n* 膀胱麻痹
cystopexy [ˈsistəˌpeksi] *n* 膀胱固定术
cystophorous [sisˈtɔfərəs] *a* 含囊的
cystophotography [ˌsistəufəˈtɔgrəfi] *n* 膀胱内照相术
cystophthisis [sisˈtɔfθisis] *n* 膀胱结核
cystoplasty [ˈsistəˌplæsti] *n* 膀胱成形术 | cecal ~ 盲肠膀胱扩大术
cystoplegia [ˌsistəuˈpliːdʒə] *n* 膀胱麻痹
cystoproctostomy [ˌsistəuprɔkˈtɔstəmi] *n* 膀胱直肠造口吻合术
cystoprostatectomy [ˌsistəuprɔstəˈtektəmi] *n* 膀胱前列腺切除术
cystoptosis [ˌsistɔpˈtəusis] *n* 膀胱下垂
cystopyelitis [ˌsistəuˌpaiiˈlaitis] *n* 膀胱肾盂炎
cystopyelography [ˌsistəuˌpaiiˈlɔgrəfi] *n* 膀胱肾盂 X 线造影[术]
cystopyelonephritis [ˌsistəuˌpaiiləuneˈfraitis] *n* 膀胱肾盂肾炎
cystoradiography [ˌsistəuˌreidiˈɔgrəfi] *n* 膀胱 X 线造影[术]
cystorectostomy [ˌsistəurekˈtɔstəmi] *n* 膀胱直肠造口吻合术
cystorrhagia [ˌsistəuˈreidʒiə] *n* 膀胱出血
cystorrhaphy [sisˈtɔrəfi] *n* 膀胱缝合术
cystorrhea [ˌsistəuˈriːə] *n* 膀胱黏液溢,膀胱卡他
cystosarcoma [ˌsistəusɑːˈkəumə] *n* 囊性肉瘤

cystoschisis [sis'tɔskisis] *n* 膀胱裂
cystosclerosis [ˌsistəuskliə'rəusis] *n* 囊肿硬化
cystoscope ['sistəˌskəup] *n* 膀胱镜
cystoscopy [sis'tɔskəpi] *n* 膀胱镜检查[术] | air ~ 充气膀胱镜检查 / water ~ 充水膀胱镜检查 | **cystoscopic** [ˌsistə'skɔpik] *a*
cystose ['sistəus] *a* 囊的;含囊的
cystospasm ['sistəspæzəm] *n* 膀胱痉挛
cystospermitis [ˌsistəuspəː'maitis] *n* 精囊炎
cystosphincterometry [ˌsistəuˌsfiŋktə'rɔmətri] *n* 膀胱括约肌测压
cystostaxis [ˌsistəu'stæksis] *n* 膀胱渗血
cystostomy [sis'tɔstəmi] *n* 膀胱造口术
cystotome ['sistətəum] *n* 膀胱刀;截囊刀
cystotomy [sis'tɔtəmi] *n* 膀胱切开术 | suprapubic ~ 耻骨上膀胱切开术
cystotrachelotomy [ˌsistəuˌtreiki'lɔtəmi] *n* 膀胱颈切开术
cystoureteritis [ˌsistəujuˌriːtə'raitis] *n* 膀胱输尿管炎
cystoureterogram [ˌsistəujuə'riːtərəgræm] *n* 膀胱输尿管[照]片,膀胱输尿管造影[照]片
cystoureteropyelonephritis [ˌsistəujuəˌriːtərəuˌpaiiləune'fraitis], **cystoureteropyelitis** [ˌsistəujuəˌriːtərəuˌpaii'laitis] *n* 膀胱输尿管肾盂肾炎
cystourethritis [ˌsistəuˌjuəri'θraitis] *n* 膀胱尿道炎
cystourethrocele [ˌsistəujuə'riːθrəsiːl] *n* 膀胱尿道膨出(女性尿道及膀胱脱垂)
cystourethrogram [ˌsistəujuə'riːθrəgræm] *n* 膀胱尿道[照]片,膀胱尿道造影[照]片
cystourethrography [ˌsistəujuəri'θrɔgrəfi] *n* 膀胱尿道造影[术] | chain ~ 链标膀胱尿道造影[术] / voiding ~ 排尿式膀胱尿道造影[术]
cystourethroscope [ˌsistəujuə'riːθrəskəup] *n* 膀胱尿道镜
cystourethroscopy [ˌsistəuˌjuərə'θrɔskəpi] *n* 膀胱尿道镜检查术
cystous ['sistəs] *a* 囊的;含囊的
cystyl ['sistil] *n* 胱氨酰[基]
cytapheresis [ˌsaitəfə'riːsis] *n* 细胞单采法,细胞去除术
cytarabine(ara-c) [sai'tɛərəbiːn] *n* 阿糖胞苷(抗病毒、抗肿瘤药) | ~ hydrochloride 盐酸阿糖胞苷(抗病毒药)
cytarme [si'tɑːmi] *n* 分裂球变扁
cytase ['saiteis] *n* 细胞溶[解]酶,溶胞酶
cytaster ['saitæstə] *n* [细胞]星体
Cytauxzoon [ˌsaitɔːk'zəuɔn] *n* 胞质虫属
cytauxzoonosis [ˌsaitɔːkˌzəuə'nəusis] *n* 胞质虫病
-cyte [后缀]细胞
cythemolysis [ˌsaiθi'mɔlisis] *n* 血细胞溶解
cytheromania [ˌsiθərəu'meinjə] *n* 慕男狂,女子色情狂
cytidine ['saitidiːn] *n* 胞苷 | ~ diphosphate (CDP) 胞苷二磷酸 / ~ monophosphate(CMP) 胞苷[一磷]酸 / ~ triphosphate(CTP) 胞苷三磷酸
cytidine deaminase ['saitidiːn diː'æmineis] 胞苷脱氨酶
cytidylate [saiti'dileit] *n* 胞[嘧啶核]苷酸
cytidylate kinase [ˌsaiti'dileit 'kaineis] 胞[嘧啶核]苷酸激酶
cytidylic acid [ˌsaiti'dilik] 胞苷[一磷]酸
cytidylyl [ˌsaiti'dilil] *n* 胞苷酰
cytisine ['sitisin] *n* 金雀花碱,野靛碱(中枢兴奋药)
cytisism ['sitisizəm] *n* 金雀花中毒
Cytisus ['sitisəs] *n* 金雀花属
cyt(o)- [构词成分]细胞
cytoanalyzer [ˌsaitəu'ænəˌlaizə] *n* 细胞分析器(一种电子光学仪器,检测恶性细胞)
cytoarchitecture [ˌsaitəu'ɑːkiˌtektʃə], **cytoarchitectonics** [ˌsaitəuˌɑːkitek'tɔniks] *n* 细胞结构(尤指大脑皮质内的细胞结构) | **cytoarchitectural** [ˌsaitəuˌɑːki'tektʃərəl], **cytoarchitectonic** [ˌsaitəuˌɑːkitek'tɔnik] *a*
cytobiology [ˌsaitəubai'ɔlədʒi] *n* 细胞生物学
cytobiotaxis [ˌsaitəubaiəu'tæksis] *n* 细胞互应性
cytoblast ['saitəblæst] *n* 细胞形成核,细胞核
cytoblastema [ˌsaitəublæs'tiːmə] *n* 细胞胚基,细胞形成质
cytocentrum [ˌsaitəu'sentrəm] *n* 中心体
cytocerastic [ˌsaitəusi'ræstik] *a* 细胞发育的
cytochalasin [ˌsaitəu'kæləsin] *n* 松胞菌素 | ~ B 松胞菌素 B
cytochemism [ˌsaitəu'kemizəm] *n* 细胞化学作用
cytochemistry [ˌsaitəu'kemistri] *n* 细胞化学
cytochrome ['saitəkrəum] *n* 细胞色素
cytochrome oxidase ['saitəkrəum 'ɔksideis] 细胞色素氧化酶
cytochrome-c oxidase ['saitəkrəum 'ɔksideis] 细胞色素 c 氧化酶
cytochrome-*c* oxidase deficiency 细胞色素 *c* 氧化酶缺乏症
cytochrome-b_5 reductase ['saitəkrəum ri'dʌkteis] 细胞色素 b_5 还原酶
cytochrome P-450 reductase ['saitəkrəum ri'dʌkteis] 细胞色素 P-450 还原酶
cytochylema [ˌsaitəukai'liːmə] *n* 细胞液
cytocidal [ˌsaitəu'saidl] *a* 杀细胞的
cytocide ['saitəsaid] *n* 杀细胞药
cytocinesis [ˌsaitəusai'niːsis, -si'n-] *n* 胞质分裂
cytoclasis [sai'tɔkləsis] *n* 细胞解体,细胞破碎 |

cytoclastic [ˌsaitəuˈklæstik] *a*
cytoclesis [ˌsaitəuˈkiːsis] *n* 细胞互应性 | **cytocletic** [ˌsaitəuˈkletik] *a*
cytoctony [saiˈtɔktəni] *n* 细胞杀害[作用]
cytocuprein [ˌsaitəuˈkjuːprin] *n* 超氧[化]物歧化酶
cytocyst [ˈsaitəsist] *n* 胞囊
cytode [ˈsaitəud] *n* 无核细胞
cytodendrite [ˌsaitəuˈdendrait] *n* [胞体]树突
cytodesma [ˌsaitəuˈdezmə] *n* 细胞[间]桥
cytodiagnosis [ˌsaitəuˌdaiəgˈnəusis] *n* 细胞诊断 | exfoliative ~ 脱落细胞诊断(检癌) | **cytodiagnostic** [ˌsaitəuˌdaiəgˈnɔstik] *a*
cytodieresis [ˌsaitəudaiˈiərisis] *n* 胞体分裂
cytodifferentiation [ˌsaitəuˌdifəˌrenʃiˈeiʃən] *n* 细胞分化
cytodistal [ˌsaitəuˈdistl] *a* 远离细胞的(轴索远端)
Cytoecetes [ˌsaitəuəˈsiːtiz] *n* 细胞立克次体属
cytoflav [ˈsaitəflæv] *n* 细胞黄(核黄素的一种磷酸酯,见于肝与心脏内)
cytoflavin [ˌsaitəuˈfleivin] *n* 细胞黄素,核黄素磷酸酯
cytogene [ˈsaitədʒiːn] *n* 细胞质基因
cytogenesis [ˌsaitəuˈdʒenisis] *n* 细胞发生
cytogenetics [ˌsaitəudʒiˈnetiks] *n* 细胞遗传学 | **cytogenetic(al)** *a* / **cytogeneticist** [ˌsaitəudʒiˈnetisist] *n* 细胞遗传学家
cytogenic [ˌsaitəuˈdʒenik] *a* 细胞发生的;细胞形成的,细胞产生的
cytogenous [saiˈtɔdʒinəs] *a* 细胞发生的
cytogeny [saiˈtɔdʒini] *n* 细胞发生;细胞谱系
cytoglomerator [ˌsaitəuˌglɔməˈreitə] *n* 血细胞团集器
cytoglycopenia [ˌsaitəuˌglaikəuˈpiːniə], **cytoglucopenia** [ˌsaitəuˌgluːkəuˈpiːniə] *n* 血细胞糖分过少
cytogony [saiˈtɔgəni] *n* 细胞性繁殖,细胞性生殖
cytohistogenesis [ˌsaitəuˌhistəuˈdʒenisis] *n* 细胞[组织]发生
cytohistology [ˌsaitəuhisˈtɔlədʒi] *n* 细胞组织学 | **cytohistologic** [ˌsaitəuˌhistəˈlɔdʒik] *a*
cytohormone [ˌsaitəuˈhɔːməun] *n* 细胞激素
cytohyaloplasm [ˌsaitəuˈhaiələˌplæzəm] *n* 细胞透明质
cytohydrolist [ˌsaitəuˈhaidrəlist] *n* 细胞膜水解酶
cytoid [ˈsaitɔid] *a* 细胞状的
cyto-inhibition [ˌsaitəu ˌinhiˈbiʃən] *n* 细胞抑制
cytokalipenia [ˌsaitəuˌkæliˈpiːniə] *n* 细胞钾缺乏,细胞钾过少
cytokerastic [ˌsaitəukəˈræstik] *a* 细胞发育的
cytokeratin [ˌsaitəuˈkerətin] *n* 细胞角蛋白
cytokine [ˌsaitəuˈkain] *n* 细胞因子,细胞活素
cytokinesis [ˌsaitəukaiˈniːsis, -kiˈn-] *n* 胞质分裂 | **cytokinetic** [ˌsaitəukaiˈnetik, -kiˈn-] *a*
cytokinin [ˌsaitəuˈkainin] *n* 细胞分裂素,细胞激肽
cytolipin H [saiˈtɔlipin] *n* 细胞糖苷脂 H,神经酰胺乳糖苷
cytolist [ˈsaitəlist] *n* 溶细胞素
cytology [saiˈtɔlədʒi] *n* 细胞学 | aspiration biopsy ~ (ABC) 针吸活组织检查细胞学 / exfoliative ~ 脱落细胞学 | **cytologic(al)** [ˌsaitəuˈlɔdʒik(əl)] *a* **cytologist** *n* 细胞学家
cytolymph [ˈsaitəlimf] *n* 细胞液
cytolysate [saiˈtɔliseit] *n* 细胞溶解液 | blood ~ 血细胞溶解液
cytolysin [saiˈtɔlisin] *n* 溶细胞素,细胞溶素
cytolysis [saiˈtɔlisis] *n* 细胞溶解 | **cytolytic** [ˌsaitəuˈlitik] *a* 细胞溶解的,溶细胞的
cytolysosome [ˌsaitəuˈlaisəsəum] *n* 细胞溶酶体
cytoma [saiˈtəumə] *n* 细胞瘤
cytomachia [ˌsaitəuˈmækiə] *n* 细胞抗争(身体的防御细胞与细菌之间的斗争)
cytomegalic [ˌsaitəuməˈgælik] *a* 巨细胞的
cytomegaloviruria [ˌsaitəuˌmegələuvaiˈruəriə] *n* 巨细胞病毒尿
Cytomegalovirus [ˌsaitəuˈmegələuˌvaiərəs] *n* 巨细胞病毒属
cytomegalovirus (CMV) [ˌsaitəuˌmegələuˈvaiərəs] *n* 巨细胞病毒(亦称涎腺病毒)
cytomegaly [ˌsaitəuˈmegəli] *n* 巨细胞,细胞肥大
cytomere [ˈsaitəmiə] *n* 裂殖子胚;精子胞浆部,胞质区
cytometaplasia [ˌsaitəuˌmetəˈpleiziə] *n* 细胞变异
cytometer [saiˈtɔmitə] *n* 血细胞计数器 | **cytometry** *n* 血细胞计数
cytomitome [ˌsaitəuˈmaitəum] *n* 胞质网丝
cytomorphology [ˌsaitəumɔːˈfɔlədʒi] *n* 细胞形态学
cytomorphosis [ˌsaitəumɔːˈfəusis] *n* 细胞形成;细胞变形
cytomycosis [ˌsaitəumaiˈkəusis] *n* 细胞真菌病
cyton [ˈsaitɔn] *n* (神经元)细胞体
cytonecrosis [ˌsaitəuneˈkrəusis] *n* 细胞坏死
cytopathic [ˌsaitəuˈpæθik] *a* 细胞病变的
cytopathogenesis [ˌsaitəuˌpæθəˈdʒenisis] *n* 细胞病变发生 | **cytopathogenetic** [ˌsaitəuˌpæθədʒiˈnetik] *a*
cytopathogenic [ˌsaitəuˌpæθəˈdʒenik] *a* 致细胞病变的 | **~ity** [ˌsaitəuˌpæθədʒiˈnisəti] *n* 致细胞病变性

cytopathologist [ˌsaitəupəˈθɔlədʒist] *n* 细胞病理学家
cytopathology [ˌsaitəupəˈθɔlədʒi] *n* 细胞病理学 | **cytopathologic(al)** [ˌsaitəuˌpæθəˈlɔdʒik(əl)] *a*
cytopenia [ˌsaitəuˈpiːniə] *n* 血细胞减少[症]
Cytophaga [saiˈtɔfəgə] *n* 噬纤维菌属
Cytophagaceae [ˌsaitəufəˈgeisiiː] *n* 噬纤维菌科
Cytophagales [ˌsaitəufəˈgeiliːz] *n* 噬纤维菌目
cytophagous [saiˈtɔfəgəs] *a* 吞噬细胞的
cytophagy [saiˈtɔfədʒi], **cytophagocytosis** [ˌsaitəuˌfægəsaiˈtəusis] *n* 细胞吞噬作用(吞噬细胞吞噬其他细胞的作用)
cytopharynx [ˌsaitəuˈfæriŋks] *n* 胞咽
cytopherometric [ˌsaitəuˌferəˈmetrik] *a* 细胞移动测定的(试验)
cytophil [ˈsaitəfil] *n* 亲细胞体,嗜细胞体
cytophilic [saitəuˈfilik] *a* 亲细胞的,嗜细胞的(如嗜细胞抗体)
cytophotometer [ˌsaitəufəuˈtɔmitə] *n* 细胞光度计 | **cytophotometry** [ˌsaitəufəuˈtɔmitri] *n* 细胞光度测定法,细胞分光光度法 / **cytophotometric** [ˌsaitəuˌfəutəˈmetrik] *a* 细胞光度测定的
cytophylaxis [ˌsaitəufiˈlæksis] *n* 细胞防御;细胞活性增强 | **cytophylactic** [ˌsaitəufiˈlæktik] *a*
cytophyletic [ˌsaitəufaiˈletik] *a* 细胞谱系的
cytophysics [ˌsaitəuˈfiziks] *n* 细胞物理学
cytophysiology [ˌsaitəufiziˈɔlədʒi] *n* 细胞生理学
cytopigment [ˌsaitəˈpigmənt] *n* 细胞色素
cytopipette [ˌsaitəupaiˈpet] *n* 细胞吸管
cytoplasm [ˈsaitəˌplæzəm] *n* 细胞质 | **~ic** [ˌsaitəuˈplæzmik] *a*
cytoplast [ˈsaitəuplæst] *n* 胞质体
cytopreparation [ˌsaitəuˌprepəˈreiʃən] *n* 细胞制备 | **cytopreparatory** [ˌsaitəuˈprepərətəri] *a*
cytoproct [ˈsaitəuprɔkt], **cytopyge** [ˈsaitəupaidʒ] *n* 胞肛(原生动物)
cytoprotectant [ˌsaitəuprəˈtektənt] *n* 细胞保护药
cytoprotection [ˌsaitəuprəˈtekʃən] *n* 细胞保护作用
cytoprotective [ˌsaitəuprəˈtektiv] *a* 细胞保护的 *n* 细胞保护药
cytoproximal [ˌsaitəuˈprɔksiməl] *a* 近细胞的
cytoreduction [ˌsaitəuriˈdʌkʃən] *n* 细胞减数;缩小体积手术,细胞减数外科(见 debulking)
cytoreductive [ˌsaitəuriˈdʌktiv] *a* 细胞减数的
cytoreticulum [ˈsaitəuriˈtikjuləm] *n* 细胞网
cytorrhyctes [ˌsaitəuˈriktiːz] *n* 细胞包涵体
cytoscopy [saiˈtɔskəpi] *n* 细胞检查
cytosiderin [ˌsaitəuˈsidərin] *n* 胞铁[色]素
cytosine [ˈsaitəsin] *n* 胞嘧啶 | ~ arabinoside 阿糖胞苷 / 5-hydroxymethyl ~ 5-羟甲基胞嘧啶
cytosine deaminase [ˈsaitəsiːn diːˈæmineis] 胞嘧啶脱氨[基]酶
cytoskeleton [ˌsaitəuˈskelitn] *n* 细胞骨架 | **cytoskeletal** [ˌsaitəuˈskelitl] *a*
cytosol [ˈsaitəsɔl] *n* 细胞溶胶 | **~ic** [ˌsaitəˈsɔlik] *a*
cytosol aminopeptidase [ˈsaitəsɔl ˌæminəuˈpeptideis] 细胞溶胶氨肽酶(亦称亮氨酰氨基肽酶)
cytosome [ˈsaitəsəum] *n* [细]胞质体
cytospongium [ˌsaitəuˈspɔndʒiəm] *n* (细胞)海绵质
cytost [ˈsaitɔst] *n* 细胞损伤毒素
cytostasis [saiˈtɔstəsis] *n* 白细胞郁滞(炎症初期)
cytostatic [ˌsaitəuˈstætik] *a* 抑制细胞的 *n* 细胞[增殖]抑制药
cytostome [ˈsaitəstəum] *n* [细]胞口(原生动物)
cytostromatic [ˌsaitəustrəˈmætik] *a* 细胞基质的
cytotaxigen [ˌsaitəuˈtæksidʒən] *n* 细胞趋化素原
cytotaxin [ˌsaitəuˈtæksin] *n* 细胞趋化素
cytotaxis [saitəuˈtæksis] *n* 细胞趋性 | **cytotactic** *a*
cytotherapy [ˌsaitəuˈθerəpi] *n* 细胞疗法(应用动物细胞进行治疗;应用溶细胞血清或细胞毒血清进行治疗)
cytothesis [saiˈtɔθisis] *n* 细胞修复,细胞再生
cytotoxic [ˌsaitəuˈtɔksik] *a* 细胞毒素的;细胞[中]毒的
cytotoxicity [ˌsaitəutɔkˈsisəti] *n* 细胞毒性(能对特殊器官的细胞产生特异性毒性作用的能力) | antibody-dependent cell-mediate ~, antibody-dependent cellular ~ (ADCC) 抗体依赖性细胞介导的细胞毒性
cytotoxicosis [ˌsaitəuˌtɔksiˈkəusis] *n* 细胞毒素中毒
cytotoxin [ˌsaitəuˈtɔksin] *n* 细胞毒素
cytotrochin [ˌsaitəuˈtrəukin] *n* [毒素]亲胞体簇
cytotrophoblast [ˌsaitəuˈtrɔfəblæst] *n* 细胞滋养层 | **~ic** [ˌsaitəuˌtrɔfəˈblæstik] *a*
cytotropic [ˌsaitəuˈtrɔpik] *a* 向细胞的,亲细胞的(尤指抗体)
cytotropism [saiˈtɔtrəpizəm] *n* 细胞向性;向细胞性,亲细胞性(指病毒、细菌、药物等)
cytozoic [ˌsaitəuˈzəuik] *a* 细胞[内]寄生的
cytozyme [ˈsaitəzaim] *n* 凝血[酶]致活酶,凝血激酶
cyttarrhagia [ˌsitəˈreidʒiə] *n* 牙槽出血
cytula [ˈsitjulə] *n* 受精卵
cytuloplasm [ˈsitjuləˌplæzəm] *n* 受精卵胞质
cyturia [siˈtjuəriə] *n* 细胞尿[症]

CyVADIC cyclophosphamide, vincristine, doxorubicin, and imidazole carboxamide 环磷酰胺-长春新碱-多柔比星-咪唑羧胺(联合化疗治癌方案)

Czapek-Dox agar (solution) [ˈtʃɑːpek dɔks] (Friedrich J. F. Czapek; Arthur W. Dox)查-多琼脂(溶液)(一种琼脂培养基,含蔗糖、硝酸钠、硫酸镁、氯化钾、硫酸亚铁和钾缓冲液,用于培养诺卡菌属、链霉菌属和真菌)

Czermak's spaces (lines) [ˈtʃɛəmɑːk] (Johann N. Czermak)球间隙(在牙质的外表面)

Czerny-Lembert suture [ˈtʃɛəni ləˈbɛə] (Vincenz Czerny; Antoine Lembert)策-郎缝术(肠环形缝术)

Czerny's anemia [ˈtʃɛəni] (Adalbert Czerny)策尔尼贫血(婴儿营养性贫血)

Czerny's suture [ˈtʃɛəni] (Vincenz Czerny)策尔尼缝术(①仅穿过肠黏膜的肠管缝术;②筋膜末端修补缝术)

D

D dalton 道尔顿；deciduous（teeth）乳牙；decimal reduction time 拾一存活时间；density 密度；deuterium 氘；died 已故；diffusing capacity 弥散量；diopter 屈光度；distal 远侧的；dorsal vertebrae 胸椎；dose 剂量；duration 持续时间；dwarf（colony）侏儒型（菌落）

2，4-D 2，4-dichlorophenoxyacetic acid 二四滴，2，4-二氯苯氧乙酸（植物生长刺激素）

D. da【拉】给予；detur【拉】须给予；dexter【拉】右的；dosis【拉】剂量

D_L diffusing capacity of the lung 肺弥散量

D_{37} D_{37} 剂量（使细胞存活部分减至 e^{-1} 或 0.37 所需的剂量）

D-［前缀］D［构］型的

d 天（day），十分之一（deci-）和脱氧核糖（deoxyribose）的符号

d. da【拉】给予；detur【拉】须给予；dexter【拉】右的；dosis【拉】剂量

d 密度（density）和直径（diameter）的符号

d-［diː］右旋的

Δ 希腊语字母 delta 的大写；增量的符号（如 ΔG）；change 变化（如温度）

δ 希腊语的第 4 个字母；IgD 重链和血红蛋白 δ 链的符号

dA deoxyadenosine 脱氧腺苷

DA developmental age 发育年龄；diphenylchlorarsine 二苯氯胂

da- 十（10^1）（米制前缀 deka-的罕用符号）

Daae's disease［ˈdɑːə］（Anders Daae）流行性胸痛

Dabney's grip［ˈdæbni］（William C. Dabney）流行性胸痛

Daboia［dəˈbɔiə］*n* 大蒲蛇属｜～ russelli 鲁氏大蒲蛇

DAC decitabine 地西他滨

dacarbazine（DTIC）［dəˈkɑːbəˌziːn］*n* 达卡巴嗪（抗肿瘤药）

d'Acosta 见 Acosta

Da Costa's disease［dəˈkɔstə］（Jacob M. DaCosta）达科斯塔病（①异位性痛风；②神经性循环衰弱）｜～ syndrome 达科斯塔综合征（神经性循环衰弱）

dacry- 见 dacryo-

dacryadenalgia［ˌdækriædiˈnældʒiə］*n* 泪腺痛

dacryadenitis［ˌdækriˌædiˈnaitis］*n* 泪腺炎

dacryagogatresia［ˌdækriəˌgɔgəˈtriːziə］*n* 泪管闭锁

dacryagogic［ˌdækriəˈgɔdʒik］*a* 催泪的；排泪的

dacryagogue［ˈdækriəˌgɔg］*n* 催泪剂；排泪管

dacrycystalgia［ˌdækrisisˈtældʒiə］*n* 泪囊痛

dacrycystitis［ˌdækrisisˈtaitis］*n* 泪囊炎

dacryelcosis［ˌdækrielˈkəusis］*n* 泪器溃疡（泪囊或泪管溃疡）

dacry(o)-［构词成分］泪

dacryoadenalgia［ˌdækriəuædiˈnældʒiə］*n* 泪腺痛

dacryoadenectomy［ˌdækriəuˌædiˈnektəmi］*n* 泪腺切除术

dacryoadenitis［ˌdækriəuˌædiˈnaitis］*n* 泪腺炎

dacryoblennorrhea［ˌdækriəuˌblenəˈriə］*n* 泪管黏液溢

dacryocanaliculitis［ˌdækriəuˌkænəˌlikjuˈlaitis］*n* 泪小管炎

dacryocele［ˈdækriəsiːl］*n* 泪囊突出

dacryocyst［ˈdækriəˌsist］*n* 泪囊

dacryocystalgia［ˌdækriəusisˈtældʒiə］*n* 泪囊痛

dacryocystectasia［ˌdækriəuˌsistekˈteiziə］*n* 泪囊扩张

dacryocystectomy［ˌdækriəusisˈtektəmi］*n* 泪囊切除术

dacryocystis［ˌdækriəuˈsistis］*n* 泪囊

dacryocystitis［ˌdækriəusisˈtaitis］*n* 泪囊炎

dacryocystitome［ˌdækriəuˈsistitəum］*n* 泪管刀

dacryocyte［ˈdækriəusait］*n* 泪滴状红细胞（亦称泪滴状细胞）

dacryocystoblennorrhea［ˌdækriəusistəuˌblenəˈriə］*n* 泪囊黏液溢

dacryocystocele［ˌdækriəuˈsistəsiːl］*n* 泪囊突出

dacryocystoptosis［ˌdækriəuˌsistɔpˈtəusis］*n* 泪囊脱垂

dacryocystorhinostenosis［ˌdækriəuˌsistəuˌrainəustiˈnəusis］*n* 鼻泪管狭窄

dacryocystorhinostomy［ˌdækriəuˌsistəuraiˈnɔstəmi］*n* 泪囊鼻腔吻合术

dacryocystorhinotomy［ˌdækriəuˌsistəuraiˈnɔtəmi］*n* 泪囊鼻腔造孔术

dacryocystostenosis［ˌdækriəuˌsistəustiˈnəusis］*n* 泪囊狭窄

dacryocystostomy［ˌdækriəusisˈtɔstəmi］*n* 泪囊造口术

dacryocystosyringotomy [ˌdækriəuˌsistəusiriŋ-ˈgɔtəmi] *n* 泪囊泪管切开术

dacryocystotome [ˌdækriəuˈsistətəum] *n* 泪囊刀

dacryocystotomy [ˌdækriəusisˈtɔtəmi] *n* 泪囊切开术

dacryogenic [ˌdækriəuˈdʒenik] *a* 催泪的

dacryohelcosis [ˌdækriəuhelˈkəusis] *n* 泪器溃疡(泪囊或泪管溃疡)

dacryohemorrhea [ˌdækriəuˌheməˈriːə] *n* 血泪溢

dacryolith [ˈdækriəˌliθ] *n* 泪(囊或泪管结)石

dacryolithiasis [ˌdækriəuliˈθaiəsis] *n* 泪(囊或泪管结)石病

dacryoma [ˌdækriˈəumə] *n* 泪管肿大

dacryon [ˈdækriən] *n* 泪点(泪骨及额骨与上颌骨的会合点)

dacryops [ˈdækriɔps] *n* 泪眼;泪管积液

dacryopyorrhea [ˌdækriəuˌpaiəˈriːə] *n* 脓泪溢

dacryopyosis [ˌdækriəupaiˈəusis] *n* 泪器化脓(泪囊泪管化脓)

dacryorhinocystotomy [ˌdækriə u ˌrainə u sisˈtɔtəmi] *n* 泪囊鼻腔造孔术

dacryorrhea [ˌdækriəuˈriːə] *n* 流泪,泪溢

dacryoscintigraphy [ˌdækriəuˈsintigrəfi] *n* 泪囊闪烁显像[术]

dacryosinusitis [ˌdækriəuˌsainəˈsaitis] *n* 筛窦泪管炎

dacryosolenitis [ˌdækriəusəuliˈnaitis] *n* 泪管炎

dacryostenosis [ˌdækriəustiˈnəusis] *n* 泪管狭窄

dacryosyrinx [ˌdækriəuˈsiriŋks] *n* 泪小管;泪管瘘;泪管注射器

DACT dactinomycin 放线菌素 D

dactinomycin (DACT) [ˌdæktinəuˈmaisin] *n* 放线菌素 D(抗肿瘤抗生素)

dactyl [ˈdæktil] *n* 指,趾

dactyl- 见 dactylo-

Dactylaria [ˌdæktiˈlɛriə] *n* 指孢菌属

dactylate [ˈdæktileit] *a* 有指状的

dactyledema [ˈdæktiliˈdiːmə] *n* 指水肿,趾水肿

dactylion [dækˈtiliɔn] *n* 并指,并趾

dactylitis [ˈdæktiˈlaitis] *n* 指炎,趾炎

dactyl(o)- [构词成分]指,趾

dactylocampsodynia [ˌdæktiləuˌkæmpsəuˈdiniə] *n* 指曲痛

dactylogram [dækˈtiləgræm] *n* 指纹,指印

dactylography [ˌdæktiˈlɔgrəfi] *n* 指纹学

dactylogryposis [ˌdæktiləugriˈpəusis] *n* 弯指

Dactylogyrus [ˌdæktiləuˈdʒairəs] *n* 枝环[吸虫]属

dactylology [ˌdæktiˈlɔlədʒi], **dactylophasia** [ˌdæktiləuˈfeiziə] *n* 手指语,手语

dactylolysis [ˌdæktiˈlɔlisis] *n* 指脱落,趾脱落;截指,截趾 | ~ spontanea 自发性指脱落,自发性趾脱落(如发生于自发性断趾病及麻风)

dactylomegaly [ˌdæktiləuˈmegəli] *n* 巨指,巨趾

dactyloscopy [ˌdæktiˈlɔskəpi] *n* 指纹鉴定法

Dactylosoma [ˌdæktiləuˈsəumə] *n* 指状虫属

dactylospasm [ˈdæktiləspæzəm] *n* 指痉挛,趾痉挛

Dactylosporangium [ˈdæktiləuspəˈrændʒiəm] *n* 指孢囊菌属

dactylus [ˈdæktiləs] *n* 指,趾

DAD delayed after depolarization 延迟后除极

DADDS diacetyl diaminodiphenylsulfone 二乙酰氨苯砜(抗麻风药)

dADP deoxyadenosine diphosphate 脱氧腺苷二磷酸

DAEC diffusely adherent *Escherichia coli* 弥散黏附性大肠埃希杆菌

DAF decay accelerating factor 衰变加速因子

daffodil [ˈdæfədil] *n* 水仙,水仙花

dahlia [ˈdeiljə] *n* 大丽花;大丽紫 | ~ B 龙胆紫

dahlin [ˈdælin] *n* 菊粉

dahllite [ˈdɑːlait] *n* 磷碳酸钙

Dakin-Carrel method [ˈdeikin kəˈrel] (Henry D. Dakin; Alexis Carrel) 达金-卡莱尔法(清创法)

Dakin's fluid (antiseptic solution) [ˈdeikin] (Henry D. Dakin) 达金液,次氯酸钠稀溶液

dakryon [ˈdækriən] *n* 泪点(泪骨及额骨与上颌骨的会合点)

daledalin tosylate [dəˈledəlin] 托西酸达来达林(抗抑郁药)

Dale's reaction (phenomenon) [deil] (Henry H. Dale) 戴尔反应(现象),豚鼠子宫角体外过敏反应(现象)(一种体外试验,检豚鼠过敏反应,用少量抗原加到浸有致敏豚鼠子宫角的组织液中,能引起致敏的子宫肌收缩)

dalfopristin [dælˈfəupristin] *n* 达福普汀(抗菌药)

Dalrymple's disease [ˈdælrimpl] (John Dalrymple) 睫状体角膜炎 | ~ sign 达尔林普尔征(突眼性甲状腺肿时睑孔增大)

dalteparin sodium [dælˈtepərin] 达肝素钠(抗凝药)

dalton (D, Da) [ˈdɔːltən] (John Dalton) 道尔顿(质量单位,为氧原子质量的十六分之一,约 1.657×10^{-24} g)

Dalton-Henry law [ˈdɔːltən ˈhenri] (John Dalton; Joseph Henry) 道尔顿-亨利定律(液体吸收一混合气体时,其对任一气体的吸收量与各气体单独存在时所吸收之量相同)

daltonism [ˈdɔːltənizm] *n* 道尔顿症(红-绿色盲)

Dalton's law [ˈdɔːltən] (John Dalton) 道尔顿定律(气体混合物的总压力等于各气体的分压之和)

dam [dæm] *n* 水坝;屏障,障碍物;(牙科用的)橡皮障 | rubber ~ 橡皮障
damage ['dæmidʒ] *n* 损伤,损害
Damalinia [ˌdæmə'liniə] *n* 啮虱属 | ~ caprae 山羊啮虱 / ~ equi 马啮虱 / ~ hermsi 赫姆斯啮虱 / ~ pilosus 马啮虱
D'Amato's sign [dɑː'mɑːtəu] (Luigi D'Amato) 达马托征(胸膜腔积液患者由坐位改为健侧卧位时,浊音由脊柱区移向心脏区)
damiana [dæmi'einə] *n* 达米阿那,特纳草叶(据说有强状、回苏、利尿、催欲等作用)
dammar ['dæmə] *n* 达玛脂(显微镜检查用作封固剂以及制作动植物标本时用以防腐)
dämmerschlaf ['deməʃlɑːf] *n*【德】朦胧麻醉(皮下注射吗啡及东莨菪碱引起的半麻醉状态)
Damoiseau's curve (sign) [dæmwɑː'zəu] (Louis H. C. Damoiseau) 达莫瓦索曲线(征)(胸膜积液时胸部呈 S 形线)
dAMP deoxyadenosine monophosphate 脱氧腺苷酸
damp [dæmp] *n* 矿内毒气;潮湿,湿气 *a* 有湿气的,潮湿的 *vt* 使潮湿;抑止;阻尼;使衰减 *vi* 变潮湿;减幅,衰减 | after- ~ [矿]爆炸后毒气(含氮、二氧化碳,通常亦含一氧化碳) / black ~, choke ~ 乌烟,窒息毒气(矿内煤长期吸收氧而排出二氧化碳所致) / cold ~ 冷毒气(含二氧化碳的雾样蒸气) / fire ~ 引火毒气(气态烃,主要是沼气) / white ~ 白色毒气,一氧化碳
dampen ['dæmpən] *vt* 使潮湿,使衰减 *vi* 变潮湿
damper ['dæmpə] *n* 抑制因素;阻尼器,减震器
damping ['dæmpiŋ] *n* 阻尼,减幅,衰减(指电或声波)
danaparoid sodium [də'næpərɔid] 达那帕罗钠(抗血栓药)
danazol ['dænəzɔl] *n* 达那唑(垂体前叶抑制药)
Danbolt-Closs syndrome [dɑːn'bəult klɔs] (Niels C. Danbolt; Karl Closs) 丹-克综合征,肠病性肢端皮炎
dance [dɑːns, dæns] *n* 舞蹈 | brachial ~ 肱动脉扭曲(见于老年动脉硬化患者) / hilar ~ 肺门血管搏动过度 / St. Anthony's ~, St. Guy's ~, St. John's ~, St. Vitus' ~ 舞蹈症,小舞蹈症(即 Sydenham's chorea) / St. Vitus' ~ of the voice 口吃
Dancel's treatment [dæn'sel] (Jean François Dancel) 丹塞尔疗法(尽量减少饮食中的含水量,治疗肥胖病)
D and C dilatation and curettage 刮宫术
dandelion ['dændilaiən] *n* 蒲公英
dander ['dændə] *n* 毛皮垢屑
dandruff ['dændrəf] *n* 头皮屑;头皮脂溢性皮炎
Dandy's operation ['dændi] (Walter E. Dandy) 丹迪手术(使用经颅后窝的切口施行三叉神经脊神经根切断术)
Dandy-Walker syndrome (deformity) ['dændi 'wɔːkə] (Walter E. Dandy; Arthur E. Walker) 丹迪-沃克综合征(畸形)(先天性脑积水,由于第四脑室正中孔及第四脑室外侧孔阻塞所致)
Dane particle [dein] (D. S. Dane) 丹氏粒(乙型肝炎病毒完整的颗粒)
daniell ['dænjəl] (John F. Daniell) *n* 丹聂尔(旧电动势单位, =1.124 V)
Danlos' syndrome (disease) ['dænlɔs] (Henri A. Danlos) 当洛斯综合征(见 Ehlers-Danlos syndrome)
DANS 5-dimethylamino-1-naphthelenesulphonic acid 5-二甲氨基-1-萘磺酸
dansyl chloride ['dænsil] 丹酰氯
danthron ['dænθrɔn] *n* 丹蒽醌(导泻药)
dantrolene sodium ['dæntrəliːn] 丹曲林钠(骨骼肌松弛药)
Danysz's phenomenon (effect) ['dæniːz] (Jan Danysz) 丹尼什现象(效应),毒素抗毒素分批中和现象(毒素分批加入时,抗毒素中和影响减少)
Daphne ['dæfni] *n* 瑞香属
daphnetin [dæf'niːtin] *n* 瑞香素
Daphnia ['dæfniə] *n* 溞属,水蚤属
daphnin ['dæfnin] *n* 瑞香苷
daphnism ['dæfnizəm] *n* 瑞香中毒
dapiprazole hydrochloride [də'piprəzəul] 盐酸达哌唑(α 受体阻滞药,局部用于结膜)
dapsone (DDS) ['dæpsəun] *n* 氨苯砜(抗菌药) | diacetyl ~ 二乙酰氨苯砜
Dare's method [dɛə] (Arthur Dare) 戴尔法(检血红蛋白)
Dar es Salaam bacterium [dɑːr es sə'lɑːm] 达累斯萨拉姆细菌(证实是一种沙门菌血清型,即萨拉姆沙门菌〈salmonella salamae〉)
Darier-Roussy sarcoid [dɑːri'ei ruː'si] (F. J. Darier; Gustave Roussy) 达-罗肉样瘤(肉样瘤病的一型,其特征为结节较大,且常位于皮下)
Darier's disease [dɑːri'ei] (Ferdinand J. Darier) 毛囊角化病 | ~ sign 达里埃征(摩擦色素性荨麻疹可出现荨麻疹和瘙痒)
Darier-White disease [dɑːri'ei hwait] (F. J. Darier; James Clarke White) 达-怀病,毛囊角化病
dark [dɑːk] *a* 黑暗的;黑色的,深色的 *n* 黑暗;暗色
darkroom ['dɑːkruːm] *n* 暗室
Darkshevich's fibers [dɑːk'ʃeivitʃi] (Liverij O. Darkshevich) 达克谢维奇纤维(自视神经索至缰神经节的大脑神经纤维) | ~ nucleus (ganglion) 达克谢维奇核(神经节)(在中脑水管和第

三脑室交界处）

Darling's disease [ˈdɑːliŋ] (Samuel T. Darling) 组织胞浆菌病

darmous [ˈdɑːmus] *n* 氟中毒（北非俗名）

darnel [ˈdɑːnel] *n* 黑麦草，毒麦

d'Arsonval current [dɑːsənˈvɑːl] (Jacques A. d'Arsonval) 达松伐电流（高频低压电流）

dartos [ˈdɑːtɔs] *n*【希】肉膜 | **dartoic** [dɑːˈtəuik], **dartoid** [ˈdɑːtɔid] *a* 肉膜状的

dartre [dɑːtr] *n*【法】皮肤病（尤指疱疹）

dartrous [ˈdɑːtrəs] *a* 肉膜的，肉膜状的；疱疹的

Darwin's ear [ˈdɑːwin] (Charles R. Darwin) 达尔文耳（耳轮边上有隆起的耳） | ~ tubercle 耳郭结节

darwinian [dɑːˈwiniən] *a* 达尔文（C. R. Darwin）的

darwinism [ˈdɑːwinizəm] (Charles R. Darwin) 达尔文学说，进化论

dassie [ˈdæsi] *n* 蹄兔

dasymeter [dæˈsimitə] *n* 气体密度计

Dasyprocta [ˌdæsiˈprɔktə] *n* 刺豚鼠属

data [ˈdeitə] datum 的复数

date [deit] *n* 日期 | expected ~ of confinement 预产期 / expiry ~ 失效期，有效期

dATP deoxyadenosine triphosphate 脱氧腺苷三磷酸

datum [ˈdeitəm] ([复] **data** [ˈdeitə]) *n* 数据

Datura [dəˈtjuərə] *n* 曼陀罗属 | ~ metel 白曼陀罗（东莨菪碱的来源，抗胆碱药）

dauernarkose [ˈdauənɑːkəus], **dauerschlaf** [ˈdauəslɑːf] *n*【德】持续麻醉法，持续睡眠法

daughter [ˈdɔːtə] *n* 子体（衰变产物） *a* 子代的（细胞分裂形成的，如子细胞）

daunomycin [dɔːnəˈmaisin] *n* 道诺霉素，柔红霉素（抗肿瘤药）

daunorubicin [dɔːnəˈrubisin] *n* 柔红霉素（抗肿瘤药） | ~ hydrochloride 盐酸柔红霉素

daunosamine [dɔːˈnəusəmiːn] *n* 六碳氨糖（见于蒽环类抗生素）

Davainea [deiˈveiniə] *n* 代凡绦虫属，斧钩绦虫属 | ~ proglottina 节代凡绦虫，舌形斧钩绦虫

Davaineidae [ˌdeiveiˈniːidiː] *n* 代凡（绦虫）科

Davidoff's (Davidov's) cells [ˈdɑːvidɔf] (M. von Davidoff) 达维多夫细胞（见 Paneth's cells）

David's disease [dɑːˈviːd] (Jean P. David) 脊椎结核病

Davidsohn differential absorption test [ˈdeividsən] (lsrael Davidsohn) 戴维森鉴别吸收试验（见 Paul-Bunnell-Davidsohn test）

Davidsohn's sign [ˈdɑːvidsɔn] (Hermann Davidsohn) 达维逊征（用电灯置于口腔内透照时，瞳孔光度减弱，作为上颌窦积液或肿瘤生长的体征）

Daviel's operation [dɑːviˈel] (Jacques Daviel) 达维尔手术（在不切除虹膜情况下，经由角膜切口取出白内障手术） | ~ spoon 达维尔匙（用以清除残余晶状体皮质）

Davis graft [ˈdeivis] (John S. Davis) 戴维斯移植皮片（小移植皮片，一块直径约 1 cm 的皮肤）

Davy's test [ˈdeivi] (Edmund W. Davy) 戴维试验（检酚）

Dawbarn's sign [ˈdɔːbɑːn] (Robert H. M. Dawbarn) 道巴恩征（急性肩峰下滑囊炎时，臂下垂，触诊此滑液囊即引起疼痛，但当臂外展时，痛即消失）

day-care [ˈdei kεə] *a* 日托的

DAy Doctor of Ayurvedic Medicine 印度草药医学博士

day-mare [ˈdeiˌmεə] *n* 昼魇，昼惊

Day's test [dei] (Richard H. Day) 戴伊试验（检血）

daytime [ˈdeitaim] *n* 白天，日间

dazadrol maleate [ˈdeizədrɔl] 马来酸苯唑吡醇（抗抑郁药）

dB, db decibel 分贝（响度单位）

DBA dibenzanthracene 二苯蒽

DBS deep brain stimulation 深部脑刺激

DC direct current 直流电；Doctor of Chiropractic 按摩疗法博士

D & C dilation and curettage 刮宫术

dC deoxycytidine 脱氧胞苷

DCA desoxycorticosterone acetate 醋酸去氧皮质酮

DCc double concave 双凹的

dCDP deoxycytidine diphosphate 脱氧胞苷二磷酸

DCF direct centrifugal flotation 直接离心浮集法

DCH Diploma in Child Health 儿童保健学文凭

DCI dichloroisoproterenol 二氯异丙肾上腺素

DCIS ductal carcinoma in situ 原位导管癌

dCMP deoxycytidine monophosphate 脱氧胞苷酸

dCMP deaminase [diːˈæmineis] 脱氧胞苷酸脱氨[基]酶

DCOG Diploma of the College of Obstetricians and Gynaecologists 妇产科医师学会证书（英国）

dCTP deoxycytidine triphosphate 脱氧胞苷三磷酸

DCx double convex 双凸的

d. d. detur ad【拉】给予

ddC dideoxycytidine 双去氧胞苷（见 zalcitabine）

DDD dichlorodiphenyldichloroethane 二氯二苯二氯乙烷（杀虫药）

DDH developmental dysplasia of the hip 发育性髋关节发育不良

ddI dideoxyinosine 双去氧肌苷（见 didanosine）

o, p'-DDD mitotane 米托坦

DDP, *cis*-DDP cisplatin 顺铂

DDS diaminodiphenylsulfone 二氨二苯砜，氨苯砜；

Doctor of Dental Surgery 牙外科学博士

DDSc Doctor of Dental Science 牙科学博士

DDT dichlorodiphenyltrichloroethane 滴滴涕,二氯二苯三氯乙烷(杀虫药,以前广泛使用,因其造成生态破坏,现在美国禁用)

de- [前缀]脱,去,除,离,解除

deacetyllanatoside C [ˌdiːˌæsitilə'nætəsaid] 去乙酰毛花苷(强心药)

deacidification [ˌdiːəˌsidifi'keiʃən] *n* 脱酸[作用],去酸[作用]

deactivate [diː'æktiveit] *vt* 使不活动;使减活,使失活;使无效 | **deactivation** [diːˌækti'veiʃən] *n* 灭活;失活,活动性消失

deacylase [diː'æsileis] *n* 脱酰[基]酶

dead [ded] *a* 死亡的 | ~ on arrival 到院死亡

deaf [def] *a* 聋的

deaf-aid ['defeid] *n* 助听器

deafen ['defn] *vt* 使聋

deafferentate [diː'æfərənteit] *vt* 传入神经阻滞 | **deafferentation** [diːˌæfərən'teiʃən] *n* 去传入

deaf-mute ['def 'mjuːt] *n* 聋哑人 *a* 聋哑的

deaf-mutism ['def 'mjuːtizəm] *n* 聋哑

deafness ['defnis] *n* 耳聋 | apoplectiform ~ 中风样聋,梅尼埃(Ménière)征 / bass ~ 低音聋 / ceruminous ~ 耵聍性聋 / paradoxic ~ 威利斯(Willis)误听 / postlingual ~ 学语后聋 / prelingual ~ 学语前聋 / sensorineural ~ 感音神经性聋 / tone ~ 音乐聋,感觉性学歌不能 / word ~ 辨语聋

dealbation [ˌdiːæl'beiʃən] *n* 漂白

dealcoholization [diːˌælkəhɔlai'zeiʃən, -li'z-] *n* 脱醇[作用]

deallergization [diːˌælədʒai'zeiʃən] *n* 脱敏[作用]

deamidase [diː'æmideiz] *n* [脱]酰胺酶

deamidization [diːˌæmidai'zeiʃən, -di'z-], **deamidation** [diːˌæmi'deiʃən] *n* 脱酰胺[作用]

deaminase [diː'æmineis] *n* 脱氨酶

deaminate [diː'æmineit], **deaminize** [diː'æminaiz] *vt* 使脱去氨基 | **deamination** [diːˌæmi'neiʃən], **deaminization** [diːˌæminai'zeiʃən, -ni'z-] *n* 脱氨基[作用]

deanol acetamidobenzoate ['diːənɔl ˌæsitˌæmidəu'benzəeit] 醋氨苯酸地阿诺(大脑兴奋剂,具有拟副交感神经活性,在治疗儿童某些行为和学习障碍时用作抗抑郁药)

deaquation [ˌdiːə'kweiʃən] *n* 脱水[作用]

dearterialization [diːɑːˌtiəriəlai'zeiʃən, -li'z-] *n* 供血中断

dearticulation [ˌdiːɑːˌtikju'leiʃən] *n* 脱位,关节脱臼

death [deθ] *n* 死亡 | black ~ 黑死病(腺鼠疫的旧名) / brain ~ 脑死亡 / cot ~, crib ~ 卧床死亡,婴儿猝死综合征(典型发生在身体健康的1~6个月的婴儿突然死亡,尸体解剖研究也无法说明原因) / early fetal ~ 早期死胎(妊娠20周内) / genetic ~ 遗传死亡 / intermediate fetal ~ 中期死胎(妊娠21~28周) / late fetal ~ 晚期死胎(妊娠28周后) / liver ~ 肝性死亡 / local ~ 局部死亡 / programmed cell ~ 程序性细胞死亡(亦称细胞凋亡) / somatic ~ 整体死亡

deathbed ['deθbed] *n* 临终床;临终 *a* 临终时作的

Deaver's incision ['diːvə] (John B. Deaver) 迪弗切口(阑尾手术时切开右侧腹直肌前鞘,然后将该肌推之向内)

DeBakey forceps [də'beiki] (Michael E. DeBakey) 德贝凯镊(无创伤组织镊,攫精细组织用)

debanding [diː'bændiŋ] *n* 去带环(正牙法)

Debaryomyces [ˌdiːbæriə'maisiːz] *n* 德巴利酵母菌属 | ~ hensenii 汉森德巴利酵母菌 / ~ hominis, ~ neoformans 人德巴利酵母菌,新型德巴利酵母菌(新型隐球菌的旧称)

debilitate [di'biliteit] *vt* 使衰弱 | **debilitation** [diˌbili'teiʃən] *n* 虚弱

debility [di'biləti] *n* 虚弱

débouchement [deibuʃ'mɔŋ] *n*【法】开口

Débove's disease ['debɔv] (Georges M. Débove) 脾肿大 | ~ membrane 德博夫膜(气管、支气管、肠黏膜的上皮与固有膜之间的一层薄膜 / ~ treatment 德博夫疗法(强迫给予特殊饮食治结核病)

debrancher enzyme [di'bræntʃə'enzaim] 脱支酶

debrancher enzyme deficiency 脱支酶缺乏症,糖原贮积症Ⅲ型

debranching enzyme [di'brɑːntʃiŋ, di'bræntʃiŋ] 脱支酶,(淀粉-1, 6-葡糖苷酶;异淀粉酶)

Debré-Sémélaigne syndrome [də'brei seimei'leniə] (Robert Debré; Georges Sémélaigne) 德-塞综合征(为常染色体隐性遗传的甲状腺功能缺失性呆小病,伴肌强直及假性肌肥大)

Debré's phenomenon [də'brei] (Robert Debré) 德布雷现象(注射恢复期麻疹血清的部位不发疹,但该血清未能防止全身出疹)

débride [dei'briːd] *vt* 清创

débridement [deibriːd'mɔŋ] *n*【法】清创术 | enzymatic ~ 酶溶痂术 / surgical ~ 外科清创术

debris ['deibriː də'briː] *n* 碎屑,碎片 | word ~ 碎语(失语症患者发出的无意义声调)

debrisoquin sulfate [de'brisəkwin] 硫酸异喹胍(抗高血压药)

debrisoquine [de'brisəkwin] *n* 异喹胍(抗高血压药)

Deb. spis. debita spissitudine【拉】按适当稠度
debt [det] *n* 债 | oxygen ~ 氧债
debulking [diːˈbʌlkiŋ] *n* 减体治疗(切除组成大部分损害的物质,如切除大部分肿瘤,以便为以后的治疗〈如化疗或放疗〉有较少的肿瘤负荷。亦称细胞减数外科)
debye [deˈbai] *n* 德拜(电偶极矩单位,符号为D)
Dec. decanta【拉】倾泻,倾析
deca- [构词成分]十,癸
decacurie [ˌdekəˈkjuəri] *n* 10 居里(旧放射能单位)
decade [ˈdekeid] *n* 十;十倍程
decagram [ˈdekəgræm] *n* 十克,10 g
decalcify [diːˈkælsifai] *vt* 使脱钙 | **decalcification** [ˌdiːkælsifiˈkeiʃən] *n* 脱钙[作用];除石灰质[作用]
decaliter, decalitre [ˈdekəˌliːtə] *n* 十升,10 L
decameter, decametre [ˈdekəˌmiːtə] *n* 十米,10 m
decamethonium [ˌdekəmiˈθəuniəm] *n* 十烃季铵 | ~ bromide 十烃溴铵(骨骼肌松弛药) / ~ iodide 十烃碘铵(骨骼肌松弛药)
decane [ˈdekein] *n* 癸烷
decannulation [diˌkænjuˈleiʃən] *n* 除套管术(尤指气管造口术套管)
decanoate [ˌdekəˈnəueit] *n* 癸酸盐,癸酸酯;癸酸
decanoic acid [ˌdekəˈnəuik] 癸酸
decanormal [ˌdekəˈnɔːməl] *a* 十当量的(指溶液)
decant [diˈkænt] *vt* 滗析,倾析(从沉淀物中泻去上面的清液层);移注,倾注 | **decantation** [ˌdiːkænˈteiʃən] *n*
decanter [diˈkæntə] *n* 滗析器,倾析器;(有玻璃塞的)细颈盛水瓶
decapacitation [ˈdiːkəˌpæsiˈteiʃən] *n* (精子在女性生殖道内的)去[获]能
decapeptide [ˌdekəˈpeptaid] *n* 十肽
decapitate [diˈkæpiteit] *vt* 将…断头 | **decapitation** [diˌkæpiˈteiʃən] *n* 断头[术] | **decapitator** [diˈkæpiˌteitə] *n* 断[胎]头器
decapod [ˈdekəpɔd] *a* 十足的 *n* 十足目动物
Decapoda [dikəˈpəudə] *n* 十足目
decapsulation [diːˌkæpsjuˈleiʃən] *n* 被膜剥除术
decarbonate [diːˈkɑːbəneit] *vt* 除去二氧化碳 | **decarbonation** [ˌdiːˌkɑːbəˈneiʃən] *n*
decarbonize [diːˈkɑːbənaiz] *vt* (使)脱碳 | **decarbonization** [diːˌkɑːbənaiˈzeiʃən, -niˈz-] *n*
decarboxylase [ˌdiːkɑːˈbɔksileis] *n* 脱羧酶
decarboxylation [ˌdiːkɑːˌbɔksiˈleiʃən] *n* 脱羧[作用]
decavitamin [ˌdekəˈvaitəmin] *n* 十维他,复合维生素
decay [diˈkei] *vi*, *n* 腐烂,腐蚀;衰退,衰变 | beta ~ β 衰变 / radioactive ~ 放射衰变 / tone ~ [阈]音衰减
decease [diˈsiːs] *n*, *vi* 死亡,亡故
deceased [diˈsiːst] *a* 已死的
decedent [dəˈsiːdənt] *n* 死者(刚去世者)
deceit [diˈsiːt] *n* 欺骗 | facial ~ 假表情
decelerate [diːˈseləreit] *vt*, *vi* (使)减速
deceleration [diːˌseləˈreiʃən] *n* 减速 | early ~ 早期减速 / late ~ 晚期减速 / variable ~ 变异减速
decenter [diːˈsentə] *vt* 偏心
decentered [diːˈsentəd] *a* 偏心的
decentration [ˌdiːsenˈtreiʃən] *n* 偏心
deception [diˈsepʃən] *n* 诈骗,迷惑;装病,诈病
deceration [ˌdiːsiəˈreiʃən] *n* 除蜡法
decerebellation [diːˌseribeˈleiʃən] *n* 去小脑,小脑切除[法]
decerebrate [diˈseribreit] *vt* 去脑,切除大脑(经脑干作横切消除大脑功能) *n* 去脑动物;去脑样患者
decerebration [ˌdiːseriˈbreiʃən] *n* 去脑[法],大脑切除[法]
decerebrize [diˈseribraiz] *vt* 去脑,去大脑(消除大脑功能)
dechloridation [diːˌklɔːriˈdeiʃən], **dechlorination** [diːˌklɔːriˈneiʃən] *n* 脱氯,除氯;除盐
dechlorurant [diːˈklɔːrjuərənt] *n* 减尿氯药
dechloruration [diːˌklɔːrjuəˈreiʃən] *n* 减尿氯[作用]
decholesterinization [ˌdiːkɔˌlestərinaiˈzeiʃən, -niˈz-], **decholesterolization** [ˌdiːkɔˌlestərəlaiˈzeiʃən, -liˈz-] *n* 除胆固醇[作用]
deci- [构词成分]分,十分之一
decibel [ˈdesibel] *n* 分贝(响度单位,符号为db)
decidua [diˈsidjuə] *n* 蜕膜 | basal ~ 基蜕膜 / capsular ~, reflex ~ 包蜕膜 / menstrual ~ 经期蜕膜/ parietal ~, true ~ 壁蜕膜,真蜕膜 | ~l [diˈsidjuəl] *a*
deciduate [diˈsidjuit] *a* 有蜕膜的
deciduation [diˈsidjuˈeiʃən] *a* 蜕膜脱落
deciduitis [diˌsidjuˈaitis] *n* 蜕膜炎
deciduoma [diˌsidjuˈəumə] *n* 蜕膜瘤 | ~ malignum 恶性蜕膜瘤,绒毛膜癌
deciduomatosis [diˌsidjuəuməˈtəusis] *n* 蜕膜异常形成(在非孕期)
deciduosis [diˌsidjuˈəusis] *n* 蜕膜病(子宫以外的局部出现异位的子宫蜕膜或类妊娠期的子宫内膜组织)
deciduous [diˈsidjuəs] *a* (在成熟期)脱落的(如乳牙)
decigram(me) [ˈdesigræm] *n* 分克(dg,十分之一克)
decile [ˈdesil, ˈdesail] *n*, *a* 十分位数(的)

deciliter (dL) [ˈdesiˌliːtə] *n* 分升(十分之一升)

decimal [ˈdesiməl] *a* 十进的;小数的 *n* 小数,十进分数

decinormal [ˌdesiˈnɔːməl] *a* 分当量的(十分之一当量的,现用 mol/L 摩[尔]/升)

decipara [deˈsipərə] *n* 十产妇

decitabine (DAC) [diˈsaitəˌbiːn] *n* 地西他滨(抗肿瘤药,用于治疗急性白血病,静脉输液给药)

deckplatte [ˈdekplətə] *n*【德】顶板

declawing [diːˈklɔːiŋ] *n* 甲切除术

de Clérambault syndrome [dəˌkleirɑːmˈbəu] (Gaetan G. de Clérambault) 色情狂

declination [ˌdekliˈneiʃən] *n* 偏斜;偏角,偏差;偏转(眼球)

declinator [ˈdeklineitə] *n* (脑膜)牵开器

decline [diˈklain] *vi*, *vt* 下降,下垂;偏斜;衰退 *n* 减退期(指疾病或发作);衰退期(指体力或精力逐渐衰退或消耗)

declive [diˈklaiv] *n* 山坡(小脑山坡)

declivis [diˈklaivis] *n*【拉】山坡

decoagulant [ˌdiːkəuˈægjulənt] *a* 脱凝血质的 *n* 抗凝剂

Decoct. decoctum【拉】煎[剂]

decoct [diˈkɔkt] *vt* 煎[药]

decoction [diˈkɔkʃən] *n* 煎法;煎剂,汤药

decoctum [diˈkɔktəm] *n*【拉】煎[剂]

decoic acid [diˈkəuik] 癸酸

decollate [diˈkɔleit] *vt* 断头 | **decollation** [ˌdiːkəˈleiʃən] *n* 断头术(主要用于难产时的胎儿)

decoloration [diːˌkʌləˈreiʃən] *n* 脱色[作用];漂白;色消失,失色

decolorize [diːˈkʌləraiz] *vt* 脱色;漂白 | **decolorization** [diːˌkʌləraiˈzeiʃən, -riˈz-] *n*

decompensation [diːˌkɔmpenˈseiʃən] *n* 代偿失调

decomplementize [diːˈkɔmpliˌmentaiz] *vt* 脱补体 | **decomplementation** [ˌdiːˌkɔmplimənˈteiʃən] *n* 脱补体作用

decompose [diːkəmˈpəuz] *vt*, *vi* 分解;解体;腐解,腐败 | **decomposable** [ˌdiːkəmˈpəuzəbl] *a* 可分解的

decomposition [ˌdiːkɔmpəˈziʃən] *n* 分解;解体;腐解,腐败 | anaerobic ~ 无氧分解 / ~ of movement 动作分解(指运动失调)

decompress [ˌdiːkəmˈpres] *vt* 减压

decompression [ˌdiːkəmˈpreʃən] *n* 减压 | cardiac ~ 心减压术 / cerebral ~ 脑减压术

deconditioning [ˌdiːkənˈdiʃəniŋ] *n* 去适应[作用](指长期失重后心血管功能的一种改变)

decongestant [ˌdiːkənˈdʒestənt] *a* 减轻充血的 *n* 减充血剂

decongestive [ˌdiːkənˈdʒestiv] *a* 减轻充血的

decontaminate [ˌdiːkənˈtæmineit] *vt* 清除污垢;去除(毒气、放射性等)污染 | **decontamination** [ˌdiːkəntæmiˈneiʃən] *n* 去污染[法]

decoquinate [dikəˈkwineit] *n* 地考喹酯(抗球虫药,用于家禽)

decorticate [diˈkɔːtikeit] *vt* 剥除皮质,去皮质;剥外皮,去皮

decortication [diːˌkɔːtiˈkeiʃən] *n* (树、果等)剥外皮法;(脑、肾、肺等)皮质剥除术 | arterial ~ 动脉外层剥除术,动脉周交感神经切除术 / chemical ~, enzymatic ~ 化学去皮质法,酶去皮质法 / ~ of lung 胸膜外纤维层剥除术 / renal ~ 肾被膜剥除术

decrease [ˈdiːkriːs] *n* 减小;减少[量] [di(ː)ˈkriːs] *vi*, *vt* 减小,减少

decrement [ˈdekrimənt] *n* 减少;减量;减退期(疾病)

decrepit [diˈkrepit] *a* 老弱的;衰老的

decrepitate [diˈkrepiteit] *vt*, *vi* 烧爆 | **decrepitation** [diˌkrepiˈteiʃən] *n* 烧爆作用;烧爆声(指某些物质如盐、晶体受热时的爆裂声)

decrudescence [ˌdiːkruˈdesns] *n* (症状)减退

decrustation [ˌdiːkrʌsˈteiʃən] *n* 痂皮脱落,脱痂

dectaflur [ˈdektəfluː] *n* 氢氟酸十八烯胺(牙龋预防剂)

Decub. decubitus【拉】卧,卧位

decubation [ˌdiːkjuˈbeiʃən] *n* 恢复期(传染病)

decubital [diˈkjuːbitl] *a* 褥疮的

decubitus [diˈkjuːbitəs] *n* 卧,卧位;褥疮 | dorsal ~ 仰卧位 / lateral ~ 侧卧位 / ventral ~ 腹卧位;伏卧位

decumbin [diˈkʌmbin] *n* 蓝菌素,斜卧菌素(一种毒性物质,获自斜卧青霉菌,引起呼吸窘迫和出血,鼠口服 50% 致死量约 275 mg/kg)

decurrent [diˈkʌrənt] *a* 向下的

decussate [diˈkʌseit] *vt*, *vi* 交叉 *a* 交叉的

decussatio [ˌdekʌˈseiʃiəu] ([复] **decussationes** [ˌdekʌseiʃiˈəuniːz]) *n*【拉】交叉

decussation [ˌdekʌˈseiʃən] *n* 交叉 | ~, of fillet, ~ of lemniscus 丘系交叉 / motor ~, pyramidal ~, ~ of pyramids 锥体交叉 / ~ of superior cerebellar peduncles 小脑上脚交叉 / tegmental ~s, ~s of tegmentum 被盖交叉

decussorium [ˌdiːkʌˈsɔːriəm] *n* 硬脑膜压下器

dedentition [ˌdiːdenˈtiʃən] *n* 脱牙

dedifferentiation [diːˌdifərenʃiˈeiʃən] *n* 去分化,脱分化(分化的消退,即一种组织的逆向分化、退行发育)

de d. in d. de die in diem【拉】天天

dedolation [ˌdedəˈleiʃən] *n* 伤肢感;斜切开(取皮)

deduction [diˈdʌkʃən] *n* 推论;演绎[法]

deemanate [diːˈemәneit] *vt* 去射气
Deen's test [diːn] (Izaac A. van Deen) 迪恩试验(检胃液血)
de-epicardialization [ˌdiːepiˌkɑːdiәlaiˈzeiʃәn] *n* 除心外膜[法](以往用于缓解顽固性心绞痛,即用石炭酸处置或用其他腐蚀剂破坏心外膜组织,以促进侧支循环发展)
deet [diːt] *n* 二乙甲苯酰胺(即 diethyltoluamide)
Deetjen's bodies [ˈdeitjәn] (Hermann Deetjen) 血小板
DEF decayed, extracted, and filled 乳牙龋数(率)(D=需补牙数,e=需拔牙数,F=已补牙数)
defatigation [diːˌfætiˈgeiʃәn] *n* (肌肉或神经)疲劳过度
defatted [diːˈfætid] *a* 脱脂的(饮食)
defaunate [diːˈfɔːneit] *vt* 灭虫,除虫
defaunation [diːfɔːˈneiʃәn] *n* 除[原虫]动物区系[作用]
defeat [diˈfiːt] *vt*, *n* 战胜
defecate [ˈdefikeit] *vt* 澄清,净化 *vi* 排粪
defecation [ˌdefiˈkeiʃәn] *n* 澄清,净化;排粪 | fragmentary ~ 断续性多次排粪
defecography [ˌdefәˈkɔgrәfi] *n* 排粪造影(用以评估大便失禁)
defect [diˈfekt] *n* 缺损,缺陷 | acquired ~ 后天缺损 | aortic septal ~, aorticopulmonary septal ~ 主动脉间隔缺损,主动脉肺动脉间隔缺损 / atrial septal ~s, atrioseptal ~s 房间隔缺损 / congenital ~, birth ~ 先天缺损,出生缺陷 / endocardial cushion ~s 心内膜垫缺损 / filling ~ 充盈缺损(钡灌肠 X 线造影) / neural-tube ~ 神经管缺损 / ostium primum ~ 原发孔型房间隔缺损 / ostium secundum ~ 继发孔型房间隔缺损 / retention ~ 记忆缺损 / salt-losing ~ 失盐缺陷 / subperiosteal cortical ~ 骨膜下皮质缺陷 / ventricular septal ~ 室间隔缺损
defective [diˈfektiv] *a* 有缺陷的 *n* 身心缺陷者
defeminization [diːˌfeminaiˈzeiʃәn, -niˈz-] *n* 失女性态,女态缺失(女性特征缺失)
defend [diˈfend] *vt* 防御;保护(from, against) | ~**er** *n* 防御者;保护人
defense, defence [diˈfens] *n* 防御,防护 | character ~ 性格防御(可以用作防御机制的任何性格特征,如作态、姿势或矫饰) / insanity ~ 精神障碍防御(如果一个人在犯罪时由于精神障碍而缺乏犯罪责任能力,那就不能宣判该人有罪的一种法律概念) / muscular ~ 肌性防御(局限性炎症时) / ur ~ 原始信念,基本信念
defensin [diˈfensin] *n* 防卫素(嗜中性粒细胞和巨噬细胞内发生的抗菌肽)
defensive [diˈfensiv] *a* 防御的
deferens [ˈdefәrәnz] *a*【拉】输送的
deferent [ˈdefәrәnt] *a* 输送的,输出的
deferentectomy [ˌdefәrәnˈtektәmi] *n* 输精管切除术
deferential [defәˈrenʃәl] *a* 输精管的
deferentitis [ˌdefәrәnˈtaitis] *n* 输精管炎
deferoxamine [difәˈrɔksәmiːn] *n* 去铁胺(螯合剂) | ~ hydrochloride 盐酸去铁胺 / ~ mesylate 甲磺酸去铁胺,去铁敏(用作铁中毒的解毒药)
defervescence [ˌdiːfәˈvesәns] *n* 退热期
defervescent [ˌdiːfәˈvesәnt] *a* 退热的 *n* 退热药
defibrillate [diːˈfaibriˌleit] *vt* 除颤 | **defibrillation** [diːˌfaibriˈleiʃәn] *n* 心脏除颤(电休克使心房或心室纤颤停止);组织纤维分离[法] / **defibrillator** [diːˌfaibriˈleitә] *n* 除颤器
defibrinated [diːˈfaibriˌneitid] *a* 去纤维蛋白的
defibrination [diːˌfaibriˈneiʃәn] *n* 去纤维蛋白法
defibrinogenation [ˌdiːfaiˌbrinәdʒәˈneiʃәn] *n* 致去纤维蛋白法(如在血栓溶解疗法中用蛇毒蛋白酶〈ancrod〉所引起的去纤维蛋白法)
deficiency [diˈfiʃәnsi] *n* 缺乏,不足;缺陷,缺损 | congenital sucrase-isomaltase ~ 先天性蔗糖酶-异麦芽糖酶缺乏 / debrancher ~ 脱支酶缺乏 / 17-hydroxylase ~ 17-羟化酶缺乏(见 syndrome 项下相应术语) / immune ~ 免疫缺陷 / intestinal sucrase-α-dextrinase ~ 肠蔗糖酶-α-糊精酶缺乏 / isolated IgA ~, selective IgA ~ 孤立性 IgA 缺乏,选择性 IgA 缺乏(最常见的免疫缺陷病:IgA 缺乏,其他免疫球蛋白种类水平正常及细胞免疫正常。特点为复发性肺窦感染以及变态反应、胃肠道疾病〈乳糜泻、溃疡性结肠炎、局限性回肠炎〉和自身免疫病〈类风湿关节炎、系统性红斑狼疮〉的发病率增加。许多患者有抗 IgA 抗体,可引起严重的输血反应) / kapa-chain ~ κ 链缺乏(带 κ 轻链的免疫球蛋白分子缺乏) / leukocyte G6PD ~ 白细胞葡糖-6-磷酸脱氢酶缺乏(一种 X 连锁遗传病,临床上类似慢性肉芽肿病) / oxygen ~ 缺氧 / thymus-dependent ~ 非胸腺依赖性缺陷(由于胸腺发育不全所引起的细胞介导免疫缺陷病,但体液免疫比较完整) / thymus-independent ~ 不依赖胸腺的缺陷(B 淋巴细胞增生时的缺陷病,其中包括丙球蛋白缺乏血症和丙球蛋白异常血症) / vitamin ~ 维生素缺乏
deficient [diˈfiʃәnt] *a* 缺乏的,不足的
deficit [ˈdefisit] *n* 缺乏,短缺;缺陷,缺损 | oxygen ~ 缺氧 / pulse ~ 脉搏短绌 / saturation ~ 饱和不足
definitive [diˈfinitiv] *a* 确定的,决定的;发育完全的,最后的,终局的(宿主)
defloration [ˌdiːflɔːˈreiʃәn] *n* 处女膜破裂
deflorescence [ˌdeflɔːˈresns] *n* 皮疹消退
defluvium [diːˈfluviәm] *n*【拉】脱落;流下 | postpartum ~ 产后脱发 / ~ unguium 脱甲

defluxio [di'flʌkʃiəu] *n*【拉】脱落;流下

defluxion [di'flʌkʃən] *n* 突然消失;(分泌物)溢出,流出;(毛发)脱落

defoam [diː'fəum] *vt* 去泡沫 | **~er** *n* 消泡剂,消沫剂

deformability [diˌfɔːmə'biləti] *n* 变形性(如红细胞通过微血管时的变形能力)

deformation [ˌdiːfɔː'meiʃən] *n* 畸形;变形(过程)(指红细胞通过毛细血管时的变形)

deforming [di'fɔːmiŋ] *a* 致畸形的,使变形的

deformity [di'fɔːməti] *n* 变形,畸形 | boutonnière ~ 钮孔状变形(一种手指变形,特征为近侧指间关节屈曲及远侧关节过度伸展) / buttonhole ~ 钮孔状畸形(见 boutonnière ~);钮孔状二尖瓣狭窄(见 stenosis 项下 buttonhole mitral stenosis) / gun stock ~ 枪托状变形,肘内翻 / lobster claw ~ 虾螯状畸形(手指) / reduction ~ 短缺畸形(尤指肢体缺如) / rocker-bottom ~ 摇椅底变形,凸底变形(见 foot 项下相应术语) / rolled edge ~ 卷边变形(梅毒所致的主动脉瓣尖十分典型的变形) / seal-fin ~ 海豹鳍状畸形(手指) / silver fork ~ 银叉样变形(见于柯莱斯〈Colles〉骨折) / thumb-in-palm ~ 拇指内收畸形

defundation ['diːfʌn'deiʃən], **defundectomy** [ˌdiːfʌn'dektəmi] *n* 子宫底切除术

Deg. degeneration 变性;退化,变质;degree 度;程度

degassing [diː'gæsiŋ] *n* 除气,排气;解[除]毒气[法]

degeneracy [di'dʒenərəsi] *n* 退化,变质;精神变质,堕落;简并[性],简并密码 | ~ of code, code ~ 简并密码(在遗传密码中存在一个以上的密码子,可决定一个氨基酸,并将其插入一条增长中的肽链)

degenerate [di'dʒenərit] *a* 退化的,变质的;变性的;(密码等)简并的 *n* 精神变质者 [di'dʒenəreit] *vi* 退化;变质,变性

degeneratio [diˌdʒenə'reiʃiəu] *n*【拉】退化,变质;变性

degeneration [diˌdʒenə'reiʃən] *n* 退化;变质;变性 | adiposogenital ~ 肥胖性生殖器退化 / albuminoid ~, albuminous ~ 蛋白样变性,浊肿 / amyloid ~, bacony ~, cellulose ~, chitinous ~, hyaloid ~, lardaceous ~, waxy ~ 淀粉样变性 / anemic ~ 贫血性变性,(红细胞)多染性 / angiolithic ~ 血管石变性,血管壁钙化 / atrophic pulp ~ 萎缩性芽髓变性,牙髓萎缩 / black ~ of brain 大脑黑变病(一种真菌病) / calcareous ~, earthy ~ 石灰变性 / cerebromacular ~ (CMD), cerebroretinal ~ 大脑黄斑变性,大脑视网膜变性 / comma ~ (脊髓)束间束变性 / corticostriatal-spinal ~ 皮质纹状体-脊髓变性症,克-雅(Creutzfeldt-Jakob)综合征 / disciform macular ~ 盘状黄斑变性 / dystrophic ~ 营养不良性变性/ elastoid ~ (动脉)弹力组织变性 / endoglobular ~ [血]细胞内变性(见于巨红细胞) / fatty ~, adipose ~ 脂肪变性 / glistening ~ 闪光性变性(见于神经胶质组织) / hepatolenticular ~, lenticular ~, progressive lenticular ~ 肝豆状核变性 / hyaline ~, vitreous ~ 透明变性,玻璃样变性 / macular ~ 黄斑变性(视网膜) / olivopontocerebellar ~ 橄榄体脑桥小脑变性 / parenchymatous ~ 实质[性]变性,浊肿 / red ~ 红色变性(妊娠时子宫平滑肌瘤的红色软化) / retrograde ~ 逆向变性,轴索反应 / senile exudative macular ~ 老年渗出性黄斑变性 / spongy ~ of central nervous system, spongy ~ of white matter 中枢神经系统海绵状变性,白质海绵状变性(一种罕见的常染色体隐性遗传型脑白质营养不良,特征为发病早,脑白质广泛性去髓鞘及空泡形成,因而外形呈海绵状,有严重精神发育迟缓,巨头,颈肌无力,臂与腿强直,一般在年龄 18 个月左右死亡。亦称卡纳万〈Canavan〉病) / trabecular ~ 小梁状变性(支气管) / uratic ~ 尿酸盐性变性 / vacuolar ~ 空泡变性 | **degenerative** [di'dʒenərətiv] *a*

degenitalize [di'dʒenitəlaiz] *vt* 去性(精神分析,指对性的情感转移到其他方面)

degerm [diː'dʒəːm] *vt* 消毒;灭菌

deglycerolize [diː'glisərəlaiz] *vt*, *vi* 去甘油化(从冷冻红细胞中除去深低温保藏的甘油培养基,代之以等渗溶液,以便输注)

degloving [di'glʌviŋ] *n* 下颌骨颏部口腔内显露法

Deglut. deglutiatur【拉】吞服

deglutible [diː'gluːtəbl] *a* 可吞咽的

deglutition [ˌdiːgluː'tiʃən] *n* 吞服 | **deglutitive** [diː'gluːtitiv], **deglutitory** [diː'glutitəri] *a*

Degos' disease, syndrome [də'gəuz] (Robert Degos) 恶性萎缩性丘疹病

degradation [ˌdegrə'deiʃən] *n* 降解[作用];退化,劣化

degranulation [diːˌgrænju'leiʃən] *n* 脱粒,去粒,失粒(指某些粒细胞)

degree [di'griː] *n* 度;程度;学位 | ~s of freedom 自由度(样本组成中可独立变化的项数) / prism ~ 棱镜度

degrowth ['diːgrəuθ] *n* 生长度减退

degustation [ˌdiːgʌs'teiʃən] *n* 尝味

dehab ['diːhəb] *n* 苏拉病(surra),伊[凡士]氏锥虫病(家畜的一种恶性贫血病)

dehematize [diː'hemətaiz] *vt* 去血,除血

dehemoglobinize [ˌdiːhiːməu'gləubinaiz] *vt* 去血红蛋白

dehepatized [di'hepətaizd] *a* 去肝的

Dehio's test [ˈdeihiəu] (Karl K. Dehio) 杰希奥试验(注射阿托品,若心动过缓情况减轻,则与迷走神经紧张有关,否则与心肌病有关)
dehiscence [diˈhisns] *n* 裂开 | wound ~ 伤口裂开
dehumanization [diːˌhjuːmənaiˈzeiʃən, -niˈz-] *n* 人性丧失(指某些严重的患精神病状态)
dehumidifier [ˌdiːhjuˈmidifaiə] *n* 除湿器
dehydrant [diːˈhaidrənt] *a* 脱水的 *n* 脱水剂
dehydratase [diːˈhaidrəteis] *n* 脱水酶
dehydrate [diːˈhaidreit] *vt* 脱水 | **dehydration** [ˌdiːhaiˈdreiʃən] *n* 脱水[作用];失水(病理)/ **dehydrator** [diːˈhaidreitə] *n* 脱水器
dehydro- [构词成分]脱氢
dehydroandrosterone [diːˌhaidrəuænˈdrɔstərəun] *n* 脱氢雄(甾)酮
dehydroascorbic acid [diːˌhaidrəuæsˈkɔːbik] 脱氢抗坏血酸
dehydrobilirubin [diːˌhaidrəubiliˈruːbin] *n* 脱氢胆红素,胆绿素
dehydrochlorinase [diːˌhaidrəˈklɔrineis] *n* 脱氯化氢酶
dehydrocholaneresis [diːˌhaidrəuˌkəuləˈnəːrisis] *n* 脱氢胆酸排出增多(胆汁中)
dehydrocholate [diːˌhaidrəuˈkəuleit] *n* 脱氢胆酸盐
7-dehydrocholesterol [diːˌhaidrəukəˈlestərɔl] *n* 7-脱氢胆固醇(皮肤内的一种固醇) | activated 7-~ 活化7-脱氢胆固醇,胆钙化[甾]醇,维生素 D_3
dehydrocholic acid [diːˌhaidrəuˈkəulik] 脱氢胆酸
11-dehydrocorticosterone [diːˌhaidrəukɔːtiˈkɔstərəun] *n* 11-脱氢皮质[甾]酮
dehydrocorydaline [diːˌhaidrəukəˈridəlin] *n* 脱氢紫堇碱
dehydroemetine [diːˌhaidrəuˈemətiːn] *n* 去氢依米丁(抗原虫药)
dehydroepiandrosterone (DHEA) [diːˌhaidrəu-ˌepiænˈdrɔstərəun], **dehydroisoandrosterone** [diːˌhaidrəuˌaisəuænˈdrɔstərəun] *n* 脱氢表雄酮,脱氢异雄酮
dehydrogenase [diˈhaidrədʒəneis] *n* 脱氢酶 | acetaldehyde ~ 乙醛脱氢酶 / alcohol ~ [乙]醇脱氢酶 / anaerobic ~ 不需氧脱氢酶 / glutamate ~ 谷氨酸脱氢酶 / lactate ~ 乳酸脱氢酶
dehydrogenate [diːˈhaidrədʒəneit] *vi* 脱氢 | **dehydrogenation** [diːˌhaidrədʒəˈneiʃən] *n*
dehydromorphine [diːˌhaidrəuˈmɔːfiːn] *n* 脱氢吗啡,假吗啡
dehydropeptidase [diːˌhaidrəuˈpeptideis] *n* 脱氢肽酶
dehydropeptidase Ⅱ [diːˌhaidrəuˈpeptideis] 脱氢肽[水解]酶Ⅱ,酰化氨基酸水解酶
dehydroretinal [diːˌhaidrəuˈretinəl] *n* 脱氢维生素A醛,脱氢视黄醛
dehydroretinol [diːˌhaidrəuˈretinɔl] *n* 脱氢维生素A醇,脱氢视黄醇,维生素 A_2
dehydrotestosterone [diːˌhaidrəuteˈstɔstərəun] *n* 去氢睾酮
dehypnotize [diːˈhipnətaiz] *vt* 解除催眠状态
deiodination [diːˌaiədiˈneiʃən] *n* 脱碘作用
deionization [diːˌaiɔnaiˈzeiʃən, -niˈz-] *n* 除离子[作用],消电离[作用]
deiteral [ˈdaitərəl] *a* 前庭神经外侧核的
Deiters' cell [ˈdaitəz] (Otto F. C. Deiters) 外指细胞 | ~ nucleus 前庭外侧核 / ~ phalanges 戴特斯指节(听器外指细胞的末端) / ~ process 轴突,轴索 / ~ terminal frame 戴特斯终末装置(连接代特斯指节与亨森〈Hensen〉细胞的网状板) / ~ tract 前庭脊髓束
déjà entendu [deiˈʒɑː ɑːŋtɑːŋˈdjuː]【法】似曾听闻症
déjà éprouvé [deiˈʒɑː ˌeipruːˈvei]【法】似曾实践症
déjà fait [deiˈʒɑː fei]【法】似曾从事症
déjà pensé [deiˈʒɑː pɔŋˈsei]【法】似曾思及症
déjà raconté [deiˈʒɑː ˌrækɔnˈtei]【法】似曾讲述症
déjà vécu [deiˈʒɑː veiˈkjuː]【法】似曾经历症
déjà voulu [deiˈʒɑː vəuˈljuː]【法】似曾要求症
déjà vu [deiˈʒɑː ˈvjuː]【法】似曾相识症
Dejean's syndrome [dəˈʒɑːn] (M. C. Dejean) 眶底综合征(即 orbital floor syndrome,见 syndrome 项下相应术语)
dejecta [diˈdʒektə] *n* 排泄物,粪便
dejection [diˈdʒekʃən] *n* 排泄物,粪便;排粪
Dejerine-Klumpke paralysis [ˌdeʒəˈriːn ˈklʌmpki] (Augusta Dejerine-Klumpke) 德热里纳-克隆普克麻痹(见 Klumpke's paralysis)
Dejerine-Landouzy dystrophy (type) [ˌdeʒəˈriːn lɑːnduˈzi] (J. J. Dejerine; Louis T. J. Landouzy) 德热里纳-朗杜齐营养不良(型)(见 Landouzy-Dejerine dystrophy)
Dejerine-Lichtheim phenomenon [ˌdeʒəˈriːn ˈliʃtaim] (J. J. Dejerine; Ludwig Lichtheim) 德热里纳-利希特海姆现象(见 Lichtheim sign)
Dejerine-Roussy syndrome [ˌdeʒəˈriːn ruˈsi] (J. J. Dejerine; Gustav Roussy) 丘脑综合征(thalamic syndrome,见 syndrome 项下相应术语)
Dejerine's disease [ˌdeʒəˈriːn] (Joseph J. Dejerine) 进行性肥大性间质性神经病 | ~ sign 德热里纳征(咳嗽、喷嚏及用力大便时神经根炎症状加重) / ~ syndrome 德热里纳综合征 ① 神经

根炎症状；② 延髓综合征；③ 类似脊髓痨的多神经病

Dejerine-Sottas disease (atrophy) [ˌdeʒəˈriːn ˈsɔtəz] (J. J. Dejerine; Jules Sottas) 德热里纳-索塔斯病(萎缩)，进行性肥大性间质性神经病

Dejerine-Thomas syndrome [ˌdeʒəˈriːn tɔˈmɑːs] (J. J. Dejerine; André A. H. Thomas) 德-托综合征，橄榄体脑桥小脑萎缩

deka- [构词成分] 十，癸(见 deca-)

delacrimation [diˌlækriˈmeiʃən] *n* 泪液过多，多泪

delactation [ˈdiːlækˈteiʃən] *n* 断乳；停乳，泌乳停止

Delafield's fluid [ˈdeləfiːld] (Francis Delafield) 德拉菲尔德液(一种固定液，为精细的组织学组织用，含有锇酸、铬酸、醋酸和乙醇) | ~ hematoxylin 德拉菲尔德苏木精染剂(染核用)

delamination [ˌdiːlæmiˈneiʃən] *n* 分层，离层

de Lange's syndrome [dei ˈlɑːŋə] (Cornelia de Lange) 德朗热综合征(一种先天性综合征：严重智力迟钝，伴有多种畸形，其中包括身材矮小〈阿姆斯特丹侏儒〉，短头，低位耳，蹼颈，鲤鱼嘴，鼻梁凹陷伴鼻尖上翘与鼻孔朝前，浓眉且与中线相连，前额与颈部长有低位不整齐的粗发，扁平铲样手伴短而逐渐变细的手指)

delavirdine mesylate [ˌdeləˈvirdiːn] 甲磺地拉维啶(一种非核苷反转录酶抑制药，与其他抗反转录病毒药结合使用，治疗人免疫缺陷病毒 I 型〈HIV-1〉感染，口服给药)

delay [diˈlei] *n* 延误 | atrio-ventricular ~ 房-室延搁 / ~ in case-finding 病例发现延误

delayed-release [diˈleid riˈliːs] 延迟释放，缓释(释放药物的时间比立即服药后的时间稍晚)

Delbet's sign [delˈbei] (Pierre Delbet) 德尔贝征(肢体主要血管发生动脉瘤时，如肢体远端营养保持良好，虽无脉搏，侧支循环仍充分形成)

del Castillo's syndrome [del kɑːsˈtiːjəu] (E. B. del Castillo) 戴尔·卡斯蒂育综合征(见 Sertoli-cell-only syndrome)

de-lead [di ˈled] *vt* (从组织中)除铅(排除铅中毒)

DeLee catheter [diˈliː] (Joseph B. DeLee) 德李导管(用以从新生儿鼻咽和口咽部抽吸胎便和羊膜碎屑) | ~ forceps 德李产钳(一种改良的辛普森〈Simpson〉产钳)

DeLee-Hillis obstetric stethoscope [diˈliː ˈhilis] (J. B. DeLee; David S. Hillis) 德李-希利斯产科听诊器(一种戴在检查者头上用以听胎儿心音的听诊器)

deleterious [ˌdeliˈtiəriəs] *a* 有害的

deletion [diˈliːʃən] *n* 缺失(在遗传学中指染色体遗传物质部分丧失) | antigenic ~ 抗原性部分消失(子细胞中的抗原决定簇丧失或掩蔽) / clonal ~ 克隆排除

delimit [diːˈlimit], **delimitate** [di(ː)ˈlimiteit] *vt* 定…的界限 | **delimitation** [di(ː)ˌlimiˈteiʃən] *n* 定界，定限

delinquency [diˈliŋkwənsi] *n* 失职；过失；少年犯罪；违法，反社会行为

delinquent [diˈliŋkwənt] *a* 失职的；有过失的；违法的 *n* 失职者；违法者(尤指少年犯罪者) | juvenile ~ 少年罪犯

deliquesce [ˌdeliˈkwes] *vi* 溶化；潮解(使物质从大气中吸收水分而逐渐液化) | **deliquescence** [ˌdeliˈkwesns] *n* / **deliquescent** [ˌdeliˈkwesnt] *a*

deliriant [diˈliriənt] *a* 致谵妄的 *n* 致谵妄药；谵妄者

delirifacient [diˌliriˈfeiʃiənt] *a* 致谵妄的 *n* 致谵妄药

delirious [diˈliriəs] *a* 谵妄的

delirium [diˈliriəm] ([复] **deliriums** 或 **deliria** [diˈliriə]) *n* 谵妄 | acute ~ 急性谵妄 / ~ alcoholicum 酒精中毒性谵妄，震颤性谵妄 / alcohol withdrawal ~ 酒精脱瘾性谵妄，震颤性谵妄 / febrile ~ 热病谵妄，发热谵妄 / low ~ [意识]模糊性精神迟钝 / senile ~ 老年性谵妄 / toxic ~ 中毒性谵妄 / traumatic ~ 外伤性谵妄 / ~ tremens 震颤性谵妄(亦称酒精脱瘾性综合征)

delitescent [ˌdeliˈtesənt] *a* 潜伏[期]的 | **delitescence** [ˌdeliˈtesns] *n* 骤退，突然消退；(毒物或致病因子的)潜伏期

deliver [diˈlivə] *vt* 分娩；传递，传送；除去，摘除

delivery [diˈlivəri] *n* 交付；传递，传送；分娩，生产；除去，摘除(如眼睛晶状体) | abdominal ~ 剖宫产 / breech ~ 臀位分娩 / high forceps ~ 高位产钳术 / low forceps ~ 低位产钳术 / midforceps ~ 中位产钳术 / postmature ~ 逾期分娩 / postmortem ~ 死后分娩 / premature ~ 早产

dell [del] *n* 小凹，浅窝

delle [ˈdele] *n* 小凹(染色红细胞的中央透明区)

dellen [ˈdelən] *n* 角膜浅凹

delling [ˈdeliŋ] *n* 小凹形成

delmadinone [delˈmædinəun] *n* 地马孕酮(孕激素类药)

delmadinone acetate [delˈmædinəun] 醋酸地马孕酮(孕激素类药，具有抗雄激素和抗雌激素作用，用于兽医)

Delmege's sign [delˈmeʒə] (Jean A. Delmege) 戴尔梅惹征(三角肌变平，据认为是结核病的早期体征)

delomorphous [delə'mɔːfəs], **delomorphic** [delə'mɔːfik] *a* 显形的(如细胞或组织)
Delore's method [dei'lɔː](Xavier Delore) 德劳尔法(膝外翻矫正手法)
delouse [diː'laus] *vt* 灭虱 | **~r** *n* 灭虱器
delousing [di'lausiŋ] *n* 灭虱[法]
Delpech's abscess [del'peʃ] (Jacques M. Delpech) 德尔北希脓肿(脓肿形成迅速,使人极度衰竭,但很少发热)
Delphian node ['delfiən](Delphi 为古希腊城市)特尔斐结(包埋在中线筋膜内的一个淋巴结,正好位于甲状腺峡部的前面,其得名系由于手术时首先暴露出来,如此结有病时,提示甲状腺有疾病,但并非特殊疾病的过程)
delphinine ['delfiniːn], **delphine** ['delfiːn] *n* 翠雀碱,翠雀宁
Delphinium [del'finiəm] *n* 翠雀,飞燕草
delphinoidine ['delfi'nɔidiːn] *n* 翠雀次碱
delphisine ['delfisiːn] *n* 异翠雀碱
delta ['deltə] *n* 希腊语的第4个字母(Δ, δ);丁种;三角,三角形区 | ~ mesoscapulae 肩胛冈三角
deltacortisone [ˌdeltə'kɔːtisəun] *n* 泼尼松(合成糖皮质激素)
deltamethrin [ˌdeltə'meθrin] *n* 溴氰菊酯(杀虫药,局部用于牛、猪)
Deltavirus ['deltəˌvaiərəs] *n* 丁型肝炎病毒属
deltoid ['deltɔid] *a* 三角形的 *n* 三角肌
delusion [di'ljuːʒən] *n* 妄想 | ~ of being controlled, ~ of control 受控妄想(认为自己的思想、情感和行动不属于自己的,而是由别人或某种外力所强加的) / bizarre ~ 奇异妄想(如受控妄想或思想被广播) / encapsulated ~ 包藏妄想(对行为没有很大影响的妄想) / expansive ~ 夸大妄想 / fragmentary ~s 不连贯妄想 / ~ of grandeur 夸大妄想 / mood-congruent ~ 心境协调妄想(心境混乱表现的妄想) / mood-in-congruent ~ 心境不协调妄想(精神病表现的妄想) / ~ of negation 虚无妄想(认为身体某部缺失或世界已不复存在) / nihilistic ~ 虚无妄想(否认某事物或一切事物存在) / ~ of persecution 被害妄想 / poverty ~ 贫穷妄想(认为失去或即将失去物质财富的妄想) / ~ of reference 关系妄想,牵连妄想 / somatic ~ 器官变异妄想,躯体(疾患)妄想(认为身体的器官及其功能有些变异) | **~al** *a*
demand [di'mɑːnd] *vt* 要求,需要;查问 *vi* 要求;查问 *n* 需要,需求[量]
Demansia [di'mænsiə] *n* 褐眼镜蛇属
demarcation [ˌdiːmɑː'keiʃən] *n* 分界,划界 | surface ~ 表面分界(划分坏死与存活组织)
Demarquay's sign [demɑː'kei](Jean N. Demarquay) 德马凯征(发声和吞咽时,喉部固定或下移,为气管梅毒的一种体征)
demasculinization [diːˌmæskjulinai'zeiʃən, -ni'z-] *n* 男性征丧失(伴睾丸萎缩及前列腺退化)
dematerialize [diːmə'tiəriəlaiz] *vi, vt* 非物质化
Dematiaceae [diˌmæti'eisiiː] *n* 暗色孢科
dematiacious [diˌmæti'eiʃəs] *a* 暗色孢科真菌的
Dematium [di'meiʃiəm] *n* 暗色孢属
deme [diːm] *n* 繁殖群,同类群,混交群体
demecarium [ˌdemi'kɛəriəm] *n* 癸二胺苯酯(抗胆碱酯酶药)
demecarium bromide [ˌdemi'kɛəriəm] 地美溴铵(胆碱酯酶抑制药)
democlocycline [ˌdemikləu'saikliːn] *n* 地美环素 | ~ hydrochloride 盐酸地美环素(抗生素类药)
demecycline [demi'saikliːn] *n* 去甲环素(抗生素类药)
dement [di'ment] *n* 痴呆者
demented [di'mentid] *a* 痴呆的
dementia [di'menʃiə] *n* 痴呆 | dialysis ~ 透析性痴呆(一种进行性脑病,特征为伴有举名性失语症的构音障碍、痴呆、肌阵挛性反射、癫痫大发作及精神病,发生在长期做血液透析的患者,可能由于透析液中使用的水含有高浓度的铝所致) / epileptic ~ 癫痫性痴呆 / multi-infarct ~ 多发性脑梗死性痴呆(伴逐步退化过程〈一系列小发作〉和脑血管病所致的神经缺损"斑片"状分布〈影响一些功能,但不影响其他功能〉的痴呆) / paralytic ~, paretic ~ 麻痹性痴呆 / presenile ~ 早老性痴呆 / primary degeneration ~ 原发性退变性痴呆(属阿尔茨海默〈Alzheimer〉型,此病开始是隐袭性的,以后病程逐步发展,几乎所有病例都发生于50岁以后。按65岁以前或以后发病可分为早老性或老年性的。大多数病例有阿尔茨海默病的组织病理学特点,匹克〈Pick〉病的特点则为罕见) / senile ~ 老年性痴呆,老年前期痴呆
demethylation [ˌdiːmeθi'leiʃən] *n* 脱甲基[作用]
demethylchlortetracycline [diːˌmeθilˌklɔːtetrə'saikliːn] *n* 地美环素(抗生素类药)
demi- [前缀]半
Demianoff's sign [ˌdemiə'nɔf](G.S.Demianoff) 德米阿诺夫征(检腰痛:令患者仰卧,腿伸直抬高到10°以上即剧痛,为腰区骶棘肌损害之征)
demibain ['demibein] *n*【法】坐浴
demifacet [ˌdemi'fæsit] *n* 半面(关节) | inferior ~ for head of rib 下肋凹 / superior ~ for head of rib 上肋凹
demigauntlet [demi'gɔːntlit] *n* 半手套状绷带
demilune ['demiljuːn] *n* 半月体,新月(细胞) *a* 新月形的

demimonstrosity [ˌdemimɔn'strɔsəti] *n* 半畸形(不影响功能的畸形)
demineralization [diːˌminərəlai'zeiʃən, -li'z-] *n* 失矿质[作用],脱矿质[作用],去矿质[作用](矿质或无机盐排泄过多,见于肺结核、癌、骨软化患者)
demipenniform [ˌdemi'penifɔːm] *a* 半羽形的(指某些肌肉)
demodectic [demə'dektik] *a* 蠕螨的
Demodex ['demədeks] *n* 蠕螨属 | ~ aurati 金鼠蠕螨 / ~ brevis 皮脂蠕螨 / ~ canis 犬蠕螨 / ~ equi 马蠕螨 / ~ folliculorum 毛囊蠕螨 / ~ myotis 鼠耳蝠蠕螨
Demodicidae [ˌdemə'disidiː] *n* 蠕螨科
demodicidosis [ˌdemə'disi'dəusis] *n* 蠕形螨病
demodicosis [ˌdemədi'kəusis] *n* 犬毛囊蠕螨病;蠕形螨病
demogram ['diːməgræm] *n* 人口统计图
demography [diː'mɔgrəfi] *n* 人口学,人口统计学 | dynamic ~ 动态人口学(社区集体性的生理学,对出生、结婚、死亡等的统计)/ static ~ 静态人口学(社区集体性的解剖学及其环境的研究) | **demographic** [ˌdiːmə'græfik] *a* 人口统计的
demoniac [di'məuniæk] *a* 魔凭的,疯狂的 *n* 疯病者,魔凭精神错乱者
demonopathy [ˌdiˌmə'nɔpəθi], **demonomania** [ˌdiːmənəu'meinjə] *n* 魔附妄想,魔凭妄想
demonophobia [ˌdiːmənəu'fəubjə] *n* 魔鬼恐怖,恐魔症
demonstration [ˌdemənsˈtreiʃən] *n* 示教,实物教学
demonstrator ['demənstreitə] *n* 示教者
De Morgan's spots [də'mɔːgən] (Campbell de Morgan) 樱桃色血管瘤
demorphinization [diːˌmɔːfinai'zeiʃən, -ni'z-] *n* 吗啡脱瘾法
de Morsier's syndrome [dəmɔːsi'ei] (Georges de Morsier) 德摩西埃综合征,[透明]隔-视发育不良
Demours' membrane [dei'muəz] (Pierre Demours) 角膜后界膜,角膜后弹性膜
demoxepam [di'mɔksipæm] *n* 地莫西泮(安定药)
demucosation [ˌdiːmjukə'seiʃən] *n* 黏膜剥离术
demulcent [di'mʌlsnt] *a* 缓和的,润的 *n* 缓和药,润药
de Musset 见 Musset
de Mussy's point (sign) [dəmi'siː] (Noel François Odon Gueneau de Mussy) 德米西点(征)(胸骨左缘线第十肋末端水平上剧痛的压痛点,为膈胸膜炎的一个症状)
demustardization [diːˌmʌstədai'zeiʃən, -di'z-] *n* 除芥子气[作用];解芥子毒气法
demutization [ˌdiːmjuːtai'zeiʃən] *n* 聋哑教练法(教练唇读或手语)
demyelinate [diː'maiəlineit] *vt* 脱髓鞘 | **demyelination** [diːˌmaiəli'neiʃən], **demyelinization** [diːˌmaiəlinai'zeiʃən, -ni'z-] *n* 脱髓鞘[作用]
denarcotize [diː'nɑːkətaiz] *vt* 脱麻醉药(解除麻醉药瘾)
denasality [ˌdinei'zæləti] *n* 去鼻音,鼻音过少
denatality [ˌdiːnei'tæləti] *n* 出生率降低
denatonium benzoate [ˌdiːnə'təuniəm] 苯甲酸地那铵(乙醇变性剂,用作药用辅料)
denature [diː'neitʃə] *vt* 使失去自然属性;变性 | **denaturant** [diː'neitʃərənt] *n* 变性剂 / **denaturation** [diːˌneitʃə'reiʃən] *n* 变性[作用]
denatured [diː'neitʃəd] *a* 变性的
dendraxon [den'dræksɔn] *n* 短轴索细胞
dendriceptor ['dendriˌseptə] *n* (神经元的)树突受体
dendriform ['dendrifɔːm] *a* 树状的
dendrite ['dendrait] *n* (神经元的)树突 | **dendric** ['dendrik], **dendritic** [den'dritik] *a* 树突的,树状的
dendr(o)- [构词成分]树
dendroarcheology [ˌdendrəuˌɑːki'ɔlədʒi], **dendrochronology** [ˌdendrəukrə'nɔlədʒi] *n* 树木年代学
Dendroaspis [ˌdendrəu'æspis] *n* 树眼镜蛇属
dendrodendritic [ˌdendrəuden'dritik] *a* 树状树突的
dendrodochiotoxicosis [denˌdrəudəkiːəˌtɔksi'kəusis] *n* 半知菌中毒
Dendrodochium [den'drɔdəkiːəm] *n* 半知菌属
Dendrohyrax [ˌdendrəu'hairæks] *n* 树蹄兔属
dendroid ['dendrɔid] *a* 树状的
dendron ['dendrən] *n*【希】树突
dendrophagocytosis [ˌdendrəuˌfægəsai'təusis] *n* 噬胞突作用(变性的星形细胞的破损部分被小神经胶质细胞所吸收)
denervate [diː'nəːveit] *vt* 去神经 | **denervation** [ˌdiːnəː'veiʃən] *n* 去神经,失神经支配
dengue ['deŋgi] *n*【西】登革热(一种出疹发热性传染病,由病毒引起,藉埃及伊蚊、白纹伊蚊等传播) | hemorrhagic ~ 出血性登革热
denial [di'naiəl] *n* 否定,否认
denicotinize [diː'nikətinaiz] *vt* 除烟碱 | **denicotinization** [diːˌnikətinai'zeiʃən, -ni'z-] *n*
denicotinized [diː'nikətinaizd] *a* 除烟碱的
denidation [ˌdeni'deiʃən] *n* 卵床脱落,落床(经期的子宫黏膜脱落)
Denigès' test [deni'ʒeiz] (Georges Denigès) 代尼惹试验(检尿酸、尿丙酮、吗啡)

denileukin diftitox [ˌdeniˈljuːkinˈdiftitɔks] 地尼白介素地弗托司(抗肿瘤药,治疗皮肤 T 细胞淋巴瘤,静脉内给药)

Denis Browne splint [ˈdenis braun] (Denis J. Browne) 丹尼斯·布朗夹板(由一对足夹板和十字形杆连接而成,用以矫正马蹄内翻足)

Denis' method [ˈdenis] (Wiley G. Denis) 丹尼斯法(检血清镁)

Denisonia [deniˈsəuniə] *n* 铜头蛇属

Dennie's sign [ˈdeni] (Charles C. Dennie) 丹尼征(异位性皮炎时,下睑继发性皮皱)

denitrifier [diːˈnaitriˌfaiə] *n* 脱氮菌

denitrify [diːˈnaitrifai] *vt* 反硝化脱氮 | **denitrification** [diːˌnaitrifiˈkeiʃən] *n*

denitrogenation [diːˌnaitrədʒiˈneiʃən] *n* 除氮法(除去体内溶解的氮,预防潜水员病、气栓等)

Denman's spontaneous evolution (version, method) [ˈdenmən] (Thomas Denman) 登曼式自然旋出(横产倒转术,肩产式时偶或可见的自然转向)

Dennie-Marfan syndrome [ˈdeni mɑːˈfɑːŋ] (C. C. Dennie; Antoine B. J. Marfan) 丹–马综合征(痉挛性麻痹和智力迟钝,伴先天性梅毒)

Denny-Brown's sensory neuropathy (sensory radicular neuropathy), syndrome [ˈdeni braun] (Derek E. Denny-Brown) 丹尼·布朗感觉神经病变(感觉根性神经病变)、综合征,遗传性感觉根性神经病变

denofungin [ˌdiːnəˈfʌŋdʒin] *n* 地奴真菌素(抗真菌抗生素)

Denonvilliers' fascia (aponeurosis) [denɔnviːˈjeiz] (Charles P. Denonvillers) 直肠前列腺筋膜 | ~ operation 鼻成形术

denote [diˈnəut] *vt* 表示

dens [dens] ([复] **dentes** [ˈdentiːz]) *n*【拉】牙,齿;齿突;齿状结构

densimeter [ˌdenˈsimitə] *n* 密度计(测液体密度)

densitometer [densiˈtɔmitə] *n* 密度计(测液体密度);光密度计;暗度计(测显像或 X 线片的深浅度) | gas ~ 气体密度计 | **densitometry** *n* 密度测定法

density [ˈdensəti] *n* 密度 | arciform ~ 弓形致密 / background ~ 背景密度(在 X 线摄影中冲洗过的胶片密度) / inherent ~ 固有密度 / ionization ~ 电离密度 / optical ~ (OD) 光密度,吸光度

densography [denˈsɔgrəfi] *n* X 线底片密度检定法

dent-, denta- 见 dento-

dentagra [denˈtægrə, ˈdentəgrə] *n* 拔牙钳;牙痛

dental [ˈdentl] *a* 牙的,齿的 *n* 齿音字母;齿音

dentalgia [denˈtældʒiə] *n* 牙痛

dentaphone [ˈdentəfəun] *n* 牙助听器(使声波通过牙齿令聋者闻及)

dentata [denˈteitə] *n* 枢椎

dentate [ˈdenteit] *a* 有齿的;齿状的

dentatothalamic [denˌteitəuθəˈlæmik] *a* 齿状核丘脑的

dentatum [denˈteitəm] *n*【拉】齿状核

Dent disease [dent] (Charles E. Dent) 丹特病(近端肾小管的肾小管病变,伴低分子量蛋白尿、高钙血症、肾钙沉着症、佝偻病和进行性肾[功能]衰竭)

dentes [ˈdentiːz] dens 的复数

denti- 见 dent(o)-

dentia [ˈdenʃiə] *n*【拉】出牙 | ~ praecox 早出牙,乳牙早出 / ~ tarda 迟出牙

dentibuccal [ˌdentiˈbʌkəl] *a* 牙颊的

denticle [ˈdentikl] *n* 小牙;髓石 | adherent ~, attached ~ 附着髓石 / embedded ~, interstitial ~ 包藏性髓石,组织间隙小牙 / false ~ 假髓石 / free ~ 游离髓石 / true ~ 真髓石

denticulate [denˈtikjulit], **denticulated** [denˈtikjuleitid] *a* 有小牙的

dentification [ˌdentifiˈkeiʃən] *n* 牙本质形成

dentiform [ˈdentifɔːm] *a* 牙形的

dentifrice [ˈdentifris] *n* 洁牙剂,牙粉

dentigerous [denˈtidʒərəs] *a* 含牙的

dentilabial [ˌdentiˈleibjəl] *a* 牙唇的

dentilingual [ˌdentiˈliŋgwəl] *a* 牙舌的

dentimeter [denˈtimitə] *n* 牙测量器

dentin [ˈdentin] *n* 牙[本]质 | adventitious ~, irregular ~, secondary ~ 继发性牙本质/ circumpulpar ~ 髓周牙本质 / cover ~ 罩牙本质/ hereditary opalescent ~ 遗传性乳光牙本质 / primary ~ 原发性牙本质 / reparative ~ 修复性牙本质 / transparent ~, sclerotic ~ 透明牙本质,硬化牙本质 | **dentine** [ˈdentiːn] *n* / **~al** *a*

dentinalgia [ˌdentiˈnældʒiə] *n* 牙本质痛

dentinification [denˌtinifiˈkeiʃən] *n* 牙本质形成

dentinoblast [ˈdentinəblæst] *n* 成牙本质细胞

dentinoblastoma [ˌdentinəublæsˈtəumə] *n* 成牙本质细胞瘤

dentinogenesis [ˌdentinəuˈdʒenisis] *n* 牙本质发生 | ~ imperfecta 牙本质发生不全

dentinogenic [ˌdentinəuˈdʒenik] *a* 牙本质生成的

dentinoid [ˈdentinɔid] *a* 似牙本质的 *n* 前期牙本质

dentinoma [ˌdentiˈnəumə] *n* 牙本质瘤

dentinosteoid [ˌdentiˈnɔstiɔid] *n* 牙本质骨质瘤

dentinum [denˈtainəm] *n* 牙[本]质

dentiparous [denˈtipərəs] *a* 成牙的

dentist [ˈdentist] *n* 口腔科医师

dentistry [ˈdentistri] *n* 口腔医学 | cosmetic ~, esthetic ~ 口腔美容学 / forensic ~ 口腔法医学

/ geriatric ~ 老年口腔医学 / operative ~ 牙体外科学 / pediatric ~ 儿童口腔医学 / preventive ~ 预防口腔医学 / prosthetic ~ 口腔修复学 / psychosomatic ~ 身心口腔医学

dentition [den'tiʃən] *n* 出牙;牙列 | artificial ~ 人工牙列,托牙 / deciduous ~, primary ~ 乳牙列 / mixed ~, transitional ~ 混合牙列 / permanent ~, secondary ~ 恒牙列 / precocious ~ 出牙过早 / predeciduous ~ 乳牙前出牙 / retarded ~, delayed ~ 出牙迟延

dent(o)- [构词成分]牙,齿

dentoalveolar [ˌdentəuæl'viələ] *a* 牙槽的

dentoalveolitis [ˌdentəuælviə'laitis] *n* 牙槽炎(牙周病)

dentofacial [ˌdentəu'feiʃəl] *a* 牙面的

dentography [den'tɔgrəfi] *n* 牙符记法

dentoid ['dentɔid] *a* 牙形的;似牙的

dentoidin [den'tɔidin] *n* 牙(有机或蛋白)基质

dentolegal [ˌdentəu'liːgəl] *a* 口腔法医学的

dentoma [den'təumə] *n* 牙本质瘤

dentomechanical [ˌdentəumi'kænikəl] *a* 口腔机械学的,牙科机械学的

dentonomy [den'tɔnəmi] *n* 口腔医学名词,牙科学名词,牙科命名法

dentosurgical [ˌdentəu'səːdʒikəl] *a* 口腔外科的,牙外科的

dentotropic [ˌdentəu'trɔpik] *a* 亲牙的,向牙的

dentulous ['dentjuləs] *a* 有天然牙的

denture ['dentʃə] *n* 义齿;牙列 | complete ~, full ~ 全口义齿 / conditioning ~ 调试义齿 / distal extension partial ~ 远中延伸性部分义齿 / fixed partial ~ 固定性部分义齿 / immediate ~, immediate-insertion ~ 即刻义齿 / implant ~ 种植义齿 / interim ~, provisional ~ 暂时性义齿 / overlay ~, telescopic ~ 覆盖义齿 / partial ~ 部分义齿 / removable partial ~ 可摘局部义齿 / transional ~ 过渡义齿 / trial ~ 试用义齿 / unilateral partial ~ 单侧部分义齿

denturist ['dentʃrist] *n* 义齿制作技师(为患者镶制修理义齿的牙科技师,但无牙科医师证书) | **denturism** *n* 义齿业

Denucé's ligament [dənju'sei] (Jean H. M. Denucé) 德努塞韧带(在腕关节中连结桡骨与尺骨的宽带)

denucleated [diː'njuːkliˌeitid] *a* 除核的,失核的

denudate ['diːniu(ː)deit], **denude** [di'njuːd] *vt* 剥露,剥脱 | **denudation** [ˌdiːnju'deiʃən] *n* 剥露,剥脱(由于手术、创伤或病理变化致使表皮覆盖从皮肤表面除去)

denutrition [ˌdiːnjuː'triʃən] *n* 营养缺乏

Denys' tuberculin [de'niːs] (Joseph Denys) 结核菌素肉汤滤液

deodorant [diː'əudərənt] *a* 除臭的 *n* 除臭剂,解臭剂

deodorize, deodorise [diː'əudəraiz] *vt* 除臭,解臭 | **deodorization** [diːˌəudərai'zeiʃən, -ri'z-] *n* 除臭作用 / **deodorizer** *n* 除臭剂,解臭剂

deontology [ˌdiːɔn'tɔlədʒi] *n* (医生)职责学,义务学,(医务界)成规学(伦理学的一门)

deoppilant [diː'ɔpilənt] *a* 疏通的

deoppilation [diːˌɔpi'leiʃən] *n* 疏通,去阻塞

deorsumduction [diˌɔːsəm'dʌkʃən] *n* 下转(眼)

deorsumvergence [diˌɔːsəm'vəːdʒəns] *n* 下转(尤指眼)

deorsumversion [diˌɔːsəm'vəːʒən] *n* 下转(尤指两眼同时下转)

deossification [diːˌɔsifi'keiʃən] *n* 除骨质,骨质丧失

deoxidize [diː'ɔksidaiz] *vt* 使脱氧 | **deoxidation** [diːˌɔksi'deiʃən] *n* 脱氧[作用] / ~**r** *n* 去氧剂

deoxy- [前缀]脱氧,去氧(见 desoxy-)

deoxyadenosine [diːˌɔksiə'denəsi(ː)n] *n* 脱氧腺苷 | ~ diphosphate (dADP) 脱氧腺苷二磷酸 / ~ monophosphate (dAMP) 脱氧腺苷一磷酸,脱氧腺苷酸 / ~ triphosphate (dATP) 脱氧腺苷三磷酸

deoxyadenosyl [diːˌɔksiə'denəsil] *n* 脱氧腺苷基

deoxyadenosylcobalamin [diːˌɔksiəˌdenəusilkəu'bæləmin] *n* 脱氧腺苷钴胺素,腺苷钴胺素

5′-deoxyadenosyl transferase [diːˌɔksiə'denəsil] 5-脱氧腺苷转移酶,钴(1)胺素腺苷[基]转移酶

deoxyadenylate [diːˌɔksiə'denileit] *n* 脱氧腺苷酸

deoxyadenylic acid [diːˌɔksiˌædi'nilik] 脱氧腺苷酸

deoxyadenylyl [diːˌɔksiædi'nilil] *n* 脱氧腺苷酰

deoxycholaneresis [diːˌɔksi'kəulə'nəːrisis] *n* 脱氧胆酸排出增多(胆汁中)

deoxycholate [diːˌɔksi'kəuleit] *n* 脱氧胆酸(盐、酯或阴离子型)

deoxycholeic acid [diːˌɔksikəu'liːk] 脱氧络胆酸

deoxycholic acid [diːˌɔksi'kɔlik] 脱氧胆酸;去氧胆酸(利胆药)

deoxycholylglycine [diːˌɔksiˌkəulil'glaisiːn] *n* 脱氧胆酰甘氨酸

deoxycholyltaurine [diːˌɔksiˌkəulil'tɔːri(ː)n] *n* 脱氧胆酰牛磺酸

11-deoxycorticosterone (DOC) [diːˌɔksiˌkɔːti'kɔstərəun, -ˌkɔːtikə'stiərəun] *n* 11-脱氧皮质[甾]酮

11-deoxycortisol [diːˌɔksi'kɔːtisɔl] *n* 11-脱氧皮质[甾]醇

deoxycortone [di'ɔksi'kɔːtəun] *n* 脱氧皮质

[甾]酮
deoxycytidine [diːˌɔksiˈsaitidiːn] *n* 脱氧胞苷 | ~ diphosphate (dCDP) 脱氧胞苷二磷酸 / ~ monophosphate (dCMP) 脱氧胞苷一磷酸,脱氧胞苷酸 / ~ triphosphate (dCTP) 脱氧胞苷三磷酸
deoxycytidylate [diːˌɔksiˌsaitiˈdileit] *n* 脱氧胞苷酸(解离型)
deoxycytidylic acid [diːˌɔksisaitiˈdilik] 脱氧胞苷酸
deoxycytidylyl [diːˌɔksisaitiˈdilil] *n* 脱氧胞苷酰
deoxygenate [diːˈɔksidʒineit] *vt* 去氧,脱氧 | **deoxygenation** [diːˌɔksidʒiˈneiʃən] *n* 排氧,脱氧合[作用]
deoxygenated [diːˈɔksidʒineitid] *a* (血液)血红蛋白还原的
2-deoxy-D-glucose [diːˌɔksi ˈgluːkəus] *n* 2-脱氧-D-葡萄糖(抗病毒药)
deoxyguanosine [diːˌɔksiˈgwɑːnəsin] *n* 脱氧鸟苷 | ~ diphosphate (dGDP) 脱氧鸟苷二磷酸 / ~ monophosphate (dGMP) 脱氧鸟苷一磷酸,脱氧鸟苷酸 / ~ triphosphate (dGTP) 脱氧鸟苷三磷酸
deoxyguanylate [diːˌɔksiˈgwɑːnileit] *n* 脱氧鸟苷酸(解离型)
deoxyguanylic acid [diːˌɔksigwæˈnilik] *n* 脱氧鸟苷酸
deoxyguanylyl [diːˌɔksigwɑːˈnilil] *n* 脱氧鸟苷酰
deoxyhemoglobin [diːˌɔksiˌhiːməuˈgləubin] *n* 脱氧血红蛋白,去氧血红蛋白
deoxyhexose [diːˌɔksiˈheksəus] *n* 脱氧己糖
deoxynivalenol [diːˌɔksiniˈvælənɔl] *n* 脱氧瓜蒌镰菌醇
deoxynucleotidyl transferase (terminal) [diːˌɔksiˌnjuːkliəuˈtaidil] 脱氧核苷酸转移酶(末端),DNA 核苷酸基外转移酶
deoxypentose [diːˌɔksiˈpentəus] *n* 脱氧戊糖
deoxypentosenucleic acid [diːˌɔksiˌpentəusnjuːˈkliːik] 脱氧戊糖核酸
deoxyribonuclease (DNase) [diːˌɔksiˌraibəu ˈnjuːklieis] *n* 脱氧核糖核酸酶
deoxyribonucleic acid (DNA) [diːˌɔksiˌraibəu-njuːˈkliːik] 脱氧核糖核酸 | complementary DNA, copy DNA (cDNA) 互补脱氧核糖核酸,复制脱氧核糖核酸
deoxyribonucleoprotein [diːˌɔksiraibəuˌnjuːkliəuˈprəutiːn] *n* 脱氧核糖核蛋白
deoxyribonucleoside [diːˌɔksiˌraibəuˈnjuːkliəsaid] *n* 脱氧核[糖核]苷
deoxyribonucleotide [diːˌɔksiˌraibəuˈnjukliətaid] *n* 脱氧核[糖核]苷酸
deoxyribose [diːˌɔksiˈraibəus] *n* 脱氧核糖
deoxyribovirus [diːˌɔksiˈraibəuˌvaiərəs] *n* DNA 病毒,脱氧核糖核酸病毒
deoxythymidine [diːˌɔksiˈθaimidiːn] *n* 脱氧胸苷 | ~ diphosphate (dTDP) 脱氧胸苷二磷酸 / ~ monophosphate (dTMP) 脱氧胸苷一磷酸,脱氧胸苷酸 / ~ triphosphate (dTTP) 脱氧胸苷三磷酸
deoxythymidylate [diːˌɔksiˈθaimiˈdileit] *n* 脱氧胸苷酸(解离型)
deoxythymidylic acid [diːɔksiˈθaimiˈdilik] 脱氧胸苷酸
deoxythymidylyl [diːˌɔksiˈθaimidilil] *n* 脱氧胸苷酰
deoxyuridine [diːˌɔksiˈjuəridiːn] *n* 脱氧尿苷 | ~ monophosphate (dUMP) 脱氧尿苷一磷酸,脱氧尿苷酸 / ~ triphosphate (dUTP) 脱氧尿苷三磷酸
deoxyuridylate [diːˌɔksiˌjuəriˈdileit] *n* 脱氧尿苷酸(解离型)
deoxyuridylic acid [diːˌɔksiˌjuəriˈdilik] 脱氧尿苷酸
Dep. depuratus【拉】精制的,纯化的
depancreatize [diːˈpæŋkriətaiz] *vt* 除胰腺
dependence [diˈpendəns] *n* 依靠,相依性;依赖(如药物依赖,即瘾或癖) | psychoactive substance ~ 精神作用物质依赖(即精神作用物质滥用,在此期间耐受性与脱瘾症状并存。DSM Ⅲ-R《美国精神病统计手册》中包括产生特殊物质依赖症的有乙醇、苯丙胺或类似作用的拟交感神经药、大麻、可卡因、致幻剂、吸入剂、烟碱、类阿片、苯环利定或类似作用的芳基环己胺、镇静药、安眠药和抗焦虑药) / substance ~ 物质依赖(见 psychoactive substance ~)
dependency [diˈpendənsi] *n* 依赖性
dependency-prone [diˈpendənsi prəun] *a* (对毒品)有依赖心理倾向的,易产生依赖心理的
dependent [diˈpendənt] *a* 依靠的,依赖的;下垂的,悬垂的
Dependovirus [dəˈpendəuˌvaiərəs] *n* 依赖病毒属
depepsinized [diːˈpepsinaizd] *a* 除胃蛋白酶[作用]的;胃液中胃蛋白酶失活的
depersonalization [diːˌpəːsnəlaiˈzeiʃən, -liˈz-] *n* 人格解体(一种综合征,对自己、身体或环境有不真实和疏远的感觉)
de Pezzer catheter [dəpəˈzei] (Oscar M. B. de Pezzer) 德·佩赞导管(一端呈球形的留存导尿管)
dephosphorylate [ˌdiˈfɔsfərileit] *vt* 脱去磷酸 | **dephosphorylation** [diːˌfɔsfəraiˈleiʃən, -riˈl-] *n* 脱磷酸(作用)
depigmentation [ˌdiːpigmenˈteiʃən] *n* 色素脱失

depilate [ˈdepileit] *vt* 拔毛[发],脱毛[发] | **depilation** [depiˈleiʃən] *n* 脱毛术

depilatory [diˈpilətəri] *a* 脱毛[发]的 *n* 脱毛[发]剂

deplasmolysis [diːˈplæzˈmɔlisis] *n* 质壁分离复原

deplasmolyze [diːˈplæzməlaiz] *vt* 使质壁分离复原

deplete [diˈpliːt] *vt* 排空,排除;减液(如放血);耗尽精力 | **depletive** [diˈpliːtiv] *a*

depletion [diˈpliːʃən] *n* 排空,排除;减液(如放血);衰竭状态(过分失血所致) | plasma ~ 血浆去除法

depolarize [diːˈpəuləraiz] *vt* 除极,去极化;消偏振 | **depolarization** [diːˌpəuləˌraiˈzeiʃən, -riˈz-] *n* / **depolarizer** *n* 去极化剂;消偏振镜;肌松弛药(改变肌受体的电状态,使横纹肌产生麻痹,从而阻滞肌肉对神经冲动的反应)

depollute [ˌdipəˈluːt] *vt* 清除…污染

depollution [ˌdiːpəˈluːʃən] *n* 清除污染

depolymerize [diːˈpɔlimərаiz] *vt* 解聚 | **depolymerization** [diːˌpɔliməraiˈzeiʃən, -riˈz-] *n*

depopulate [diːˈpɔpjuleit] *vt* (战争、疫病等)使人口减少;减少粒子数 | **depopulation** [diːˌpɔpjuˈleiʃən] *n*

deposit [diˈpɔzit] *vt, vi* 沉积,沉淀 *n* 沉淀,沉积物(牙科中指牙垢) | tooth ~ 牙垢

deposition [depəˈziʃən] *n* 沉淀,沉积 | granulocyte ~ 粒细胞沉积

depot [ˈdepəu] *n* 仓库;储存,积存 | fat ~ 脂肪储存

deprave [diˈpreiv] *vt* 恶化,变坏 | **depravation** [ˌdeprəˈveiʃən] *n* / **~d** *a*

L-deprenyl [ˈdeprənəl] *n* 司来吉兰(即 selegiline)

depress [diˈpres] *vt* 降低,抑制

depressant [diˈpresənt] *a* 抑制的,生活力减低的 *n* 抑制药 | cardiac ~ 心抑制药

depressed [diˈprest] *a* 抑郁的;压低的;凹陷的;扁平的

depression [diˈpreʃən] *n* 抑制,压抑;凹陷;凹,窝;抑郁[症] | agitated ~ 激越性抑郁[症] / anaclitic ~ 情感依附性抑郁[症](婴儿突然长期地脱离生母或养母后引起的精神状态) / ~ of cataract 内障摘出术,针拨术 / congenital chondrosternal ~ 先天性肋软骨胸骨凹陷 / endogenous ~ 内因性抑郁症 / freezing point ~ 冰点降低 / involutional ~ 更年期忧郁[症] / major ~ 重性抑郁[症] / neurotic ~ 官能性抑郁症,神经症性抑郁症 / otic ~ 听凹 / pacchionian ~s 颗粒小凹 / postdormital ~ 醒后抑郁[症] / precordial ~ 心窝,胸口 / psychotic ~ 精神病性抑郁症,重性抑郁症 / pterygoid ~ 翼凹 / radial ~ 桡骨窝(肱骨) / reactive ~, situational ~ 反应性抑郁[症] / retarded ~ 运动阻抑性抑郁[症] / tooth ~ 牙内突 / ventricular ~ 心室凹

depressive [diˈpresiv] *a* 抑郁的;阻抑的,压低的;内凹的

depressomotor [diˌpresəˈməutə] *a* 运动抑制的 *n* 运动抑制剂

depressor [diˈpresə] *n* 降肌;抑制剂,阻化剂;压器,压板;减压神经 | tongue ~ 压舌板

deprimens oculi [ˈdeprimənz ˈɔkjuli]【拉】眼下直肌

deprivation [ˌdepriˈveiʃən] *n* 剥夺;丧失,缺乏 | emotional ~ 情感剥夺 / maternal ~ 母爱剥夺,失母爱(见 maternal deprivation syndrome 项下相应术语) / sensory ~ 感觉剥夺 / thought ~ 思维剥夺,思维中断

deprostil [diˈprɔstil] *n* 地前列素(抑制胃液分泌的前列腺素)

deproteinate [diːˈprəutineit] *vt* 除去…中的蛋白质

deproteinization [diːˌprəutinaiˈzeiʃən, -niˈz-] *n* 去蛋白作用

depside [ˈdepsaid] *n* 缩酚酸类

depth [depθ] *n* 深度 | focal ~ 焦点深度,焦深

depula [ˈdepjulə] *n* 初原肠胚

depurant [ˈdepjuərənt] *a* 纯化的,净化的 *n* 净化剂;净化器

depurate [ˈdepjuəreit] *vt* 净化,提纯 | **depuration** [ˌdepjuəˈreiʃən] *n* / **depurative** [diˈpjuərətiv] *a* / **depurator** [ˈdepjuəˌreitə] *n* 净化剂;净化器

de Quervain's disease [dəkɛəˈvæn] (Fritz de Quervain) 德奎尔万病,桡骨茎突狭窄性腱鞘炎(疼痛性腱鞘炎,由于拇长展肌和拇短展肌共同腱鞘的相对狭窄性所致) | ~ fracture 德奎尔万骨折(舟骨骨折伴月骨向掌侧脱位) / ~ thyroiditis 德奎尔万甲状腺炎(亚急性肉芽肿性甲状腺炎)

der- [构词成分]颈

deradelphus [ˌderəˈdelfəs] *n* 并头联胎

deradenitis [ˌderædiˈnaitis] *n* 颈部腺炎

deradenoncus [ˌderædiˈnɔŋkəs] *n* 颈部腺肿大

derailment [diːˈreilmənt] *n* 脱轨,偏向(思维或言语障碍,有时与联系松散同义)

deranencephalia [deˌrænensiˈfeiliə] *n* 无脑有颈畸形(脑及脊髓上端缺损)

derange [diˈreindʒ] *vt* 打乱,使…紊乱 | **derangement** [diˈreindʒmənt] *n* (精神)错乱;紊乱

Dercum's disease [ˈdəːkʌm] (Francis X. Dercum) 痛性脂肪病

derealization [diˌriəlaiˈzeiʃən, -liˈz-] *n* 现实解

体,现实感丧失,非真实感(一种精神状态,对外部世界产生不真实感觉)

dereism [ˈdiːriizəm], **derism** [ˈdiːrizəm] *n* 空想癖 | **dereistic** [ˌdiːriˈistik] *a*

derencephalocele [ˌderensiˈfæləsiːl] *n* 颈椎脑突出

derencephalus [ˌderenˈsefələs] *n* 颈脑畸胎

derepression [ˌdiːriˈpreʃən] *n* 去抑制,脱抑制,消阻遏(据遗传学说,调节基因产生的阻抑物质受抑制,结果操纵基因就可以自由进入多肽合成的过程) | gene ~ 基因消阻遏作用

dericin [ˈderisin] *n* 德里辛(得自蓖麻油的一种浅色油,用作薄荷脑的赋形剂)

derivation [ˌderiˈveiʃən] *n* 衍化;诱导 | **derivant** [ˈderivənt] *a* 衍化的;诱导的 *n* 衍化物;诱导剂

derivative [diˈrivətiv] *a* 衍生的 *n* 衍生物 | hematoporphyrin ~ 血卟啉衍生物(用于光动力疗法)

-derm [构词成分]皮肤,胚层

derma [ˈdəːmə] *n*【希】皮(尤指真皮)

derma- 见 dermat(o)-

dermabrader [dəːməˈbreidə] *n* 擦皮器

dermabrasion [dəːməˈbreiʒən] *n* 皮肤磨削术(用擦皮器磨平皮肤)

Dermacentor [ˈdəːməˈsentə] *n* 革蜱属 | ~ albipictus 棕色蜱 / ~ andersoni 安[德逊]氏革蜱 / ~ halli 黄棕色蜱 / ~ hunteri 棕色蜱 / ~ marginatus 边缘革蜱 / ~ nitens 明暗眼蜱 / ~ occidentalis 西方革蜱 / ~ parumapertus 红棕色蜱 / ~ reticulatus 网纹革蜱 / ~ sylvarum 森林革蜱 / ~ variabilis 变异革蜱 / ~ venustus 安[德逊]氏革蜱

Dermacentroxenus [ˌdəːməˌsentrɔkˈsiːnəs] *n* 革蜱立克次体属 / ~ rickettsi 立氏立克次体 / ~ typhi 地方性斑疹伤寒立克次体

dermad [ˈdəːmæd] *ad* 向皮肤

dermal [ˈdəːməl] *a* 皮[肤]的

dermamyiasis [ˌdəːməmaiˈaiəsis] *n* 皮肤蝇蛆病

Dermanyssidae [ˌdəːməˈnisidiː] *n* 皮刺螨科

Dermanyssus [ˌdəːməˈnisəs] *n* 皮刺螨属 | ~ gallinae 鸡皮刺螨

dermaskeleton [ˌdəːməˈskelitn] *n* 外骨骼

dermat- 见 dermato-

dermatan sulfate [ˈdəːmətæn] 硫酸皮肤素

dermatergosis [ˌdəːmætəˈgəusis] *n* 职业性皮肤病

dermatic [dəːˈmætik] *a* 皮[肤]的

dermatitis [ˌdəːməˈtaitis] ([复] **dermatitides** [ˌdəːməˈtitidiːz]) *n* 皮炎 | actinic ~ 光线性皮炎 / allergic contact ~ 变应性接触性皮炎 / ammonia ~ 氨皮炎(一种尿布皮炎) / ashy ~ 灰色皮炎,持久性变色红斑 / atopic ~, allergic ~ 特应性皮炎,变应性皮炎(亦称婴儿湿疹、变应性湿疹、特应性湿疹、播散性神经性皮炎) / berlock ~, berloque ~, perfume ~ 伯洛克皮炎,香料皮炎 / bhiwanol ~, dhobie mark ~ 朵比癣,洗衣员癣 / brown-tail moth ~ 褐尾蠹皮炎 / ~ bullosa striata pratensis, grass ~ 草地线状大疱性皮炎,青草皮炎 / caterpillar ~ 毛虫皮炎 / contact ~ 接触性皮炎(一种接触各种物质引起的急性变应性皮炎,严重时为中毒性皮炎,另一种为原发性刺激性〈非变应性〉皮炎) / diaper ~, napkinarea ~ 尿布皮炎 / exfoliative ~ 剥脱性皮炎 / halowax ~ 氯萘性皮炎 / industrial ~, occupational ~ 工业性皮炎,职业性皮炎 / io-moth ~ 巨斑刺蛾幼虫皮炎 / irritant ~ 刺激性皮炎 / marine ~ 海水皮炎,海水浴疹 / moth ~ 蛾皮炎 / nummular eczematous ~ 钱币状湿疹性皮炎 / periocular ~ 眼周皮炎 / perioral ~ 口周皮炎 / photocontact ~, photoallergic contact ~ 光接触性皮炎,光变应性接触性皮炎 / phytophototoxic ~ 植物性光毒性皮炎 / poison ivy ~, poison oak ~, poison sumac ~ 野葛皮炎,毒漆树皮炎 / primary irritant ~ 原发性刺激性皮炎 / radiation ~ 放射性皮炎 / sabra ~ 仙人掌皮炎 / ~ striata pratensis bullosa 草地线状大疱性皮炎 / swimmer's ~, schistosome ~ 血吸虫皮炎 / uncinarial ~ 钩虫皮炎,钩虫痒病,着地痒 / ~ venenata 中毒性皮炎(见 contact ~) / weeping ~ 湿疹 / x-ray ~, roentgen-ray ~ X线皮炎

dermat(o)-, derma-, derm(o)- [构词成分]皮,皮肤

dermatoarthritis [ˌdəːmətəuɑːˈθraitis] *n* 皮肤关节炎 | lipid ~, lipoid ~ 脂质皮肤关节炎,多中心性网状组织细胞增生病

dermatoautoplasty [ˌdəːmətəuˈɔːtəuˌplæsti] *n* 自皮移植术

Dermatobia [ˌdəːməˈtəubiə] *n* 皮蝇属 | ~ hominis 人皮蝇

dermatobiasis [ˌdəːmətəuˈbaiəsis] *n* 皮蝇[蛆]病

dermatocandidiasis [ˌdəːmətəuˌkændiˈdaiəsis] *n* 皮肤念珠菌病

dermatocele [ˈdəːmətəsiːl], **dermatochalasis** [ˌdəːmətəuˈkæləsis], **dermatochalazia** [ˌdəːmətəukəˈleiziə] *n* 皮肤松弛

dermatoconjunctivitis [ˌdəːmətəukənˌdʒʌŋktiˈvaitis] *n* 结膜皮肤炎

dermatodysplazia [ˌdəːmətəudisˈpleiziə] *n* 皮肤发育不良

dermatofibroma [ˌdəːmətəuˌfaiˈbrəumə] *n* 皮肤纤维瘤 | ~ protuberans 隆突性皮肤纤维瘤

dermatofibrosarcoma [ˌdəːmətəuˌfaibrəusɑːˈkəumə] *n* 皮肤纤维肉瘤 | ~ protuberans 隆凸性皮肤纤维肉瘤

dermatofibrosis [ˌdəːmətəufaiˈbrəusis] *n* 皮肤纤

维变性,皮肤纤维化 | ~ lenticularis disseminata 播散性豆状皮肤纤维瘤病

dermatogen [dəːˈmætədʒən] *n* 皮肤抗原

dermatoglyphics [ˌdəːmətəuˈglifiks] *n* 肤纹学(对指、趾、手掌、脚掌的皮肤纹理的研究与鉴定)

dermatographia [ˌdəːmətəuˈgræfiə] *n* 皮肤划痕症

dermatographism [ˌdəːməˈtɔgrəfizəm] *n* 皮肤划痕症(物理性变态反应所致的荨麻疹,用钝器在皮肤上划痕,出现白色条痕,两侧红肿) | black ~ 黑色皮肤划痕症 / white ~ 白色皮肤划痕症

dermatoheteroplasty [ˌdəːmətəuˈhetərəˌplæsti] *n* 异种皮肤移植

dermatology [ˌdəːməˈtɔlədʒi] *n* 皮肤病学 | **dermatologic(al)** [ˌdəːmətəˈlɔdʒik(əl)] *a* / **dermatologist** *n* 皮肤病学家,皮肤科医师

dermatolysis [ˌdəːməˈtɔlisis] *n* 皮肤松垂 | ~ palpebrarum 睑皮松垂

dermatome [ˈdəːmətəum] *n* 取皮机,植皮刀,皮刀;皮区(指某一脊神经后根感觉纤维的皮肤分布区);皮板,生皮节(中胚层体节的外侧部) | **dermatomic** [ˌdeːməˈtɔmik] *a*

dermatomegaly [ˌdəːmətəuˈmegəli] *n* 巨皮症,皮肤松弛

dermatomere [ˈdəːmətəˌmiə] *n* 皮[肤]节(胚体节表层)

dermatomyces [ˌdəːmətəuˈmaisiːz] *n* 皮真菌,皮霉菌

dermatomycin [ˌdəːmətəuˈmaisin] *n* 皮真菌素,皮霉菌素(用于诊断、预防和治疗皮肤真菌病)

dermatomycosis [ˌdəːmətəumaiˈkəusis] *n* 皮肤真菌病

dermatomyiasis [ˌdəmətəumaiˈaiəsis] *n* 皮肤蝇蛆病

dermatomyoma [ˌdəːmətəumaiˈəumə] *n* 皮肤[平滑]肌瘤

dermatomyositis [ˌdəːmətəuˌmaiəˈsaitis] *n* 皮肌炎

dermatomeurology [ˌdəːmətəuniuəˈrɔlədʒi] *n* 皮肤神经学

dermato-ophthalmitis [ˌdəːmətəuˌɔfθælˈmaitis] *n* 皮肤眼炎(包括结膜、角膜等)

dermatopathology [ˌdəːmətəupəˈθɔlədʒi] *n* 皮肤(微观解剖)病理学

dermatopathy [ˌdəːməˈtɔpəθi] *n* 皮肤病 | **dermatopathic** [ˌdəːmətəˈpæθik] *a*

Dermatophagoides [ˌdəːməˌtɔfəˈgɔidiːs] *n* 尘螨属,表皮螨属 | ~ pteronyssinus 屋尘螨,欧洲尘螨 / ~ scheremetewskyi 舍雷梅托斯基尘螨

dermatopharmacology [ˌdəːmətə u ˌfɑːməˈkɔlədʒi] *n* 皮肤药理学

Dermatophilaceae [ˌdəːmətəufiˈleisiiː] *n* 嗜皮菌科

dermatophiliasis [ˌdəːmətəufiˈlaiəsis], **dermatophilosis** [ˌdəːmətəufaiˈləusis] *n* 潜蚤病

Dermatophilus [ˌdəːməˈtɔfiləs] *n* 嗜皮菌属;潜蚤属(见 Tunga) | ~ congolensis 刚果嗜皮菌 / ~ penetrans 穿皮潜蚤,沙蚤

dermatophylaxis [ˌdəːmətəufiˈlæksis] *n* 皮肤病预防

dermatophyte [ˌdəːmətəfait] *n* 皮真菌,皮霉菌

dermatophytid [ˌdəːməˈtɔfitid] *n* 皮癣菌疹

dermatophytosis [ˌdəːmətəufaiˌtəusis] *n* 皮肤癣菌病

dermatoplasty [ˌdəːmətəˌplæsti] *n* 皮成形术,植皮术 | **dermatoplastic** [ˌdəːmətəˈplæstik] *a* 皮成形的,植皮的

dermatopolyneuritis [ˌdəːmətəuˌpɔlinjuəˈraitis] *n* 皮肤多神经炎,肢痛症,红皮水肿性多神经病

dermatorrhagia [ˌdəːmətəuˈreidʒiə] *n* 皮肤出血

dermatorrhexis [ˌdəːmətəuˈreksis] *n* 皮肤毛细管破裂

dermatosclerosis [ˌdəːmətəuskliəˈrəusis] *n* 硬皮病

dermatosis [ˌdəːməˈtəusis] ([复] **dermatoses** [ˌdəːməˈtəusiːz]) *n* 皮肤病 | acute febrile neutrophilic ~ 急性发热性嗜中性[细胞]皮肤病,斯威特(Sweet)综合征 / dermatolytic bullous ~ 营养不良性大疱性表皮松解 / industrial ~ 工业皮肤病,职业性皮炎 / stasis ~ (血液)淤积性皮肤病 / transient acantholytic ~ 暂时性棘层松解性皮肤病

dermatosome [ˈdəːmətəusəum] *n* 中纬板小体(有丝分裂时纺锤体纤维在中央区增厚部分)

dermatosparaxis [ˌdəːmətəuspəˈræksis] *n* 皮肤脆裂症(指牛、羊)

dermatotherapy [ˌdəːmətəuˈθerəpi] *n* 皮肤病疗法

dermatotome [ˈdəːmətətəum] *n* 植皮刀,皮刀;皮板,生皮节(中胚层体节的外侧部)

dermatotropic [ˌdəːmətəuˈtrɔpik] *a* 亲皮的,向皮的,嗜皮肤的(指某些微生物)

dermatozoon [ˌdəːmətəuˈzəuɔn] *n* 皮肤寄生虫

dermatozoonosis [ˌdəːmətəuˌzəuəuˈnəusis], **dermatozoiasis** [ˌdəːmətəuzəuˈaiəsis] *n* 皮肤寄生虫病

dermenchysis [dəːˈmenkisis] *n* 皮下投药法

dermic [ˈdəːmik] *a* 皮[肤]的

dermis [ˈdəːmis] *n* 真皮

derm(o)- 见 dermato-

dermoanergy [ˌdəːməˈænədʒi] *n* 皮肤无反应性(皮肤对抗原没有超敏感性反应;皮肤缺乏免疫反应性)

dermoblast [ˈdəːməblæst] *n* 成皮细胞
dermocyma [ˌdəːməˈsaimə], **dermocymus** [ˌdəːməˈsaiməs] *n* 皮下寄生胎(含另一胎畸胎)
dermoglyphics [ˌdəːməˈglifiks] *n* 肤纹学
dermographia [ˌdəːməˈgræfiə], **dermographism** [ˌdəːˈmɔgrəfizəm] *n* 皮肤划痕症 | **dermographic** [ˌdəːməˈgræfik] *a*
dermohygrometer [ˌdəːməhaiˈgrɔmitə] *n* 皮肤湿度计(测定皮肤电阻)
dermoid [ˈdəːmɔid] *a* 皮样的 *n* 皮样囊肿 | implantation ~ 植入性皮样囊肿 / inclusion ~ 包涵性皮样囊肿 / thyroid ~ 甲状腺管皮样囊肿 / tubal ~ 输卵管皮样囊肿
dermoidectomy [ˌdəːmɔiˈdektəmi] *n* 皮样囊肿切除术
dermolipectomy [ˌdəːməˌliˈpektəmi] *n* 皮肤脂肪切除术
dermolipoma [ˌdəːməliˈpəumə] *n* 皮脂瘤(球结膜下先天性黄色脂瘤)
dermolysin [dəːˈmɔlisin] *n* 溶皮素
dermometer [dəːˈmɔmitə] *n* 皮肤电阻计 | **dermometry** *n* 皮肤电阻测量法
dermomycosis [ˌdəːməmaiˈkəusis] *n* 皮真菌病，皮霉菌病
dermomyotome [ˌdəːməˈmaiətəum] *n* 生皮肌节
dermoneurotropic [ˌdəːməˌnjuərəˈtrɔpik] *a* 亲皮肤神经的,向皮肤神经的
dermopathy [dəːˈmɔpəθi] *n* 皮肤病 | diabetic ~ 糖尿病皮肤病变,色素性胫前斑 / infiltrative ~ 胫前黏液性水肿 | **dermopathic** [ˌdəːməˈpæθik] *a*
dermophylaxis [ˌdəːməfiˈlæksis] *n* 皮肤病预防
dermophyte [ˈdəːməfait] *n* 皮真菌,皮霉菌
dermoplasty [ˈdəːməˌplæsti] *n* 皮成形术,植皮术
dermoreaction [ˌdəːməri(ː)ˈækʃən] *n* 皮肤反应
dermoskeleton [ˌdəːməˈskelitn] *n* 外骨骼
dermosynovitis [ˌdəːməsinəˈvaitis] *n* 皮肤黏液囊炎
dermotoxin [ˌdəːməˈtɔksin] *n* 皮肤坏死毒素(一种葡萄球菌毒素,注入皮肤能产生坏死)
dermotropic [ˌdəːməˈtrɔpik] *a* 亲皮的,向皮的,嗜皮肤的(指某些微生物)
dermovaccine [ˌdəːməˈvæksin], **dermovirus** [ˈdəːməˌvaiərəs] *n* 皮肤疫苗(痘苗病毒经皮肤接种得以维持,然后从皮肤损害处刮取配制而成的疫苗,亦称皮肤病毒)
dermovascular [ˌdəːməˈvæskjulə] *a* 皮肤血管的
der(o)- [构词成分]颈
derodidymus [ˌderəˈdidiməs] *n* 双头畸胎
derrengadera [ˌderengəˈdeirə] *n*【西】马锥虫病
derriengue [deriˈeŋge] *n*【西】疯牛病
Derrien's test [ˌdεəriˈæn] (Eugène Derrien) 德廉试验(检尿 α-二硝基酚)
derris [ˈderis] *n* 鱼藤属
Derxia [ˈdeksiə] (H. G. Derx) *n* 戴克斯菌属
DES diethylstilbestrol 己烯雌酚
desalination [ˌdiːseiliˈneiʃən], **desalinization** [diːˌseilinaiˈzeiʃən] *n* 脱盐[作用],去盐[作用]
desalivation [ˌdiːsæliˈveiʃən] *n* 除涎,除唾液
desalt [diːˈsɔːlt] *vt* 脱盐,去盐
desamido-NAD⁺ [desəˈmidəu] 脱氨基-NAD⁺ (即 deaminated-NAD⁺)
De Sanctis-Cacchione syndrome [də ˈsæŋktis ˌkækiˈəuni] (Carlo De Sanctis; Aldo Cacchione) 德·桑蒂斯-卡基奥尼综合征(一种遗传性综合征,为常染色体隐性性状遗传,包括着色性干皮病,伴智力迟钝,性腺发育不全,有时伴神经系统方面的并发症及对光敏感。亦称干皮病性白痴)
desaturate [diːˈsætʃəreit] *vt*, *vi* 去饱和 | **desaturation** [diːˌsætʃəˈreiʃən] *n* 去饱和[作用]
Desault's bandage (apparatus) [deˈsəu] (Pierre J. Desault) 戴佐绷带(锁骨骨折时用以固定上臂) | ~ sign 戴佐征(见于股骨囊内骨折)
Descartes' law [deiˈkɑːt] (René Descartes) 笛卡尔定律(先进入两个已知介质时,其入射角的正弦与折射角的正弦呈恒定关系)
descemetitis [ˌdesimiˈtaitis] *n* 后弹力层炎
descemetocele [ˌdesiˈmetəsiːl] *n* 后弹力层突出
Descemet's membrane [desiˈmei] (Jean Descemet) [角膜]后界层
descend [diˈsend] *vi* 下降;下行;传下,遗传
descended [diˈsendid] *a* (睾丸等)下降的
descendens [diˈsendenz] *a*【拉】下行的,降的 | ~ cervicis 舌下神经降支
descending [diˈsendiŋ] *a* 下降的;下行的
descensus [diˈsensəs] [单复同] *n*【拉】下垂,下降 | ~ testis 睾丸下降 / ~ uteri 子宫脱垂 / ~ ventriculi 胃下垂
descent [diˈsent] *n* 下降,下行;世代,血统 | ~ of man 人类由来
Deschamps' compressor [deiˈʃɔŋ] (Joseph F. L. Deschamps) 德尚压迫器(压动脉器) | ~ needle 德尚针(长柄钩针,用于结扎深部动脉)
desensitization [diːˌsensitaiˈzeiʃən, -tiˈz-] *n* 脱敏 | systematic ~ 系统[精神]脱敏疗法
desensitize, desensitise [diːˈsensitaiz] *vt* 脱敏[感] | **desensitizer** *n* 脱敏剂
deserpidine [diːˈsəːpidiːn] *n* 地舍平(抗高血压药、安定药)
desex [diːˈseks], **desexualize** [diːˈseksjuəlaiz] *vt* 除性征,使无性欲
desferrioxamine [desˌferiˈɔksəmiːn] *n* 去铁胺(解毒药)
desflurane [desˈfluːrein] *n* 地氟醚,地氟烷(吸入

麻醉药）

deshydremia [ˌdeshaiˈdriːmiə] *n* 浓缩血（血液水分减少）

desiccant [ˈdesikənt] *a* 干燥的 *n* 干燥剂

desiccate [ˈdesikeit] *vt* 使干燥 *vi* 变成干燥 | **desiccative** [ˈdesikeitiv] *a* 干燥的

desiccation [ˌdesiˈkeiʃən] *n* 干燥法 | electric ~ 电干燥法（治肿瘤等病）

desiccator [ˈdesikeitə] *n* 干燥器

design [diˈzain] *n* 设计 | factorial ~ 析因设计，因子设计

desipramine [deˈsiprəmiːn] *n* 地昔帕明（抗抑郁药） | ~ hydrochloride 盐酸地昔帕明（抗抑郁药）

desirable [diˈzaiərəbl] *a* 值得的，可取的

desire [diˈzaiə] *vt*, *n* 想望，欲望；要求 | micturition ~ 尿意

-desis [构词成分]固定，固定术

Desjardins' point [ˌdeiʒɑːˈdænz] (Abel Desjardins) 代雅丹点，胰腺头点（在脐至右腋连线上，距脐 5 ~ 7 cm 处）

deslanoside [desˈlænəsaid] *n* 去乙酰毛花苷（强心药）

desloratadine [ˌdesləˈrætədiːn] *n* 地洛拉定（抗组胺药）

desm- 见 desmo-

desmalgia [desˈmældʒiə] *n* 韧带痛

Desmanthos [desˈmænθɔs] *n* 花丛菌属

desmectasis [desˈmektəsis] *n* 韧带伸展

desmepithelium [ˌdesmepiˈθiːljəm] *n* 中胚叶上皮层

desmid [ˈdesmid] *n* 鼓藻

desmin [ˈdezmin] *n* 肌纤丝蛋白，结蛋白

desmiognathus [ˌdesmiəˈnæθəs] *n* 下颌[颈]部寄生畸胎，双头寄头畸胎

desmitis [desˈmaitis] *n* 韧带炎

desm(o)- [构词成分]带，韧带，纤维

Desmobacteriaceae [ˌdezməbækˌtiəriˈeisiiː] *n* 丝状细菌科

desmocranium [ˌdezməuˈkreinjəm] *n* 膜颅（中胚层的）

desmocyte [ˈdezməsait] *n* 成纤维细胞

desmocytoma [ˌdezməsaiˈtəumə] *n* 成纤维细胞瘤，纤维瘤

desmodontium [ˌdesməˈdɔnʃiəm] *n* 牙周纤维

Desmodus [dezˈməudəs] *n* 吸血蝠属

desmodynia [ˌdezməˈdiniə] *n* 韧带痛

desmogenous [dezˈmɔdʒinəs] *a* 韧带[原]性的

desmography [dezˈmɔgrəfi] *n* 韧带学

desmohemoblast [ˌdezməˈhiːməblæst, -ˈhe-] *n* 间[充]质

desmoid [ˈdezmɔid] *a* 纤维性的，纤维样的 *n* 硬纤维瘤

desmolase [ˈdezməleis] *n* 碳链[裂解]酶 | 17, 20- ~ 17α-羟黄体酮醛缩酶 / 20, 22- ~ 胆固醇单加氧酶（裂解侧链的）

desmology [dezˈmɔlədʒi] *n* 韧带学；绷带学

desmolysis [dezˈmɔlisis] ([复] **desmolyses** [dezˈmɔlisiːz]) *n* 解碳链作用 | **desmolytic** [ˌdesməˈlitik] *a*

desmoma [dezˈməumə] *n* 硬纤维瘤

desmon [ˈdezmɔn] *n* 介体

desmoneoplasm [ˌdezməˈni(ː)əuplæzəm] *n* 结缔组织肿瘤

desmopathy [dezˈmɔpəθi] *n* 韧带病

desmoplasia [ˌdezməˈpleiziə] *n* 结缔组织生成

desmoplastic [ˌdezməˈplæstik] *a* 促结缔组织生成的（引起粘连的）

desmopressin acetate [ˌdesməuˈpresin] 醋酸去氨加压素（一种强合成加压素类似物，垂体性尿崩症时用作抗利尿药，鼻内、肌内或静脉内使用，静脉内给药对血友病患者及冯·维勒布兰特〈von Willebrand〉病患者在术前可增加因子Ⅷ活性）

desmopyknosis [ˌdezməpikˈnəusis] *n* 圆韧带缩短术

desmorrhexis [ˌdezməˈreksis] *n* 韧带破裂

desmose [ˈdesməus] *n* 连接纤丝

desmosine [ˈdesməsin, ˈdezməsain] *n* 锁链素

desmosis [dezˈməusis] *n* 结缔组织病

desmosome [ˈdezməsəum] *n* 桥粒

desmosterol [dezˈmɔstərɔl] *n* 链甾醇，24-脱氢胆固醇

Desmothoracida [ˌdesməθɔˈræsidə] *n* 链胸目

desmotomy [dezˈmɔtəmi] *n* 韧带切开术

desmotropism [dezˈmɔtrəpizəm] *n* 稳变异构[现象]

desogestrel [ˌdezəˈdʒestrəl] *n* 去氧孕烯（孕激素类药）

desoleolecithin [desˌəuliəuˈlesiθin] *n* 脱油酸卵磷脂

desomorphine [ˌdesəˈmɔːfin] *n* 地索吗啡（麻醉止痛药）

desonide [ˈdesənaid] *n* 地奈德（抗炎药，治类固醇敏感的皮肤病）

desorb [diːˈsɔb] *vt* 使解除吸附 | **desorption** [diːˈsɔːpʃən] *n* 解吸附作用

desoximetasone [deˌsɔksiˈmetəsəun] *n* 去羟米松（皮质类固醇，具有抗炎、止痒和血管收缩作用）

desoxy- [前缀]脱氧（见 deoxy-）

desoxycorticosterone [dezɔksiˌkɔːtiˈkɔstərəun] *n* 去氧皮质酮 | ~ acetate 醋酸去氧皮质酮 / ~ pivalate，~ trimethylacetate 特戊酸去氧皮质酮

desoxycortone [ˌdezɔksiˈkɔːtəun] *n* 去氧皮质酮

| ~ acetate 醋酸去氧皮质酮
desoxyephedrine [ˌdezɔksieˈfedrin] *n* 去氧麻黄碱
desoxymorphine [ˌdezɔksiˈmɔːfin] *n* 去氧吗啡
desoxyphenobarbital [deˌzɔksiˌfiːnəˈbɑːbitæl] *n* 去氧苯比妥(抗癫痫药)
desoxyribonuclease [deˌzɔksiˌraibəuˈnjuːklieis] *n* 脱氧核糖核酸酶
desoxyribonucleic acid (DNA) [deˌzɔksiˌraibəunjuːˈkliːik], **desoxyribose nucleic acid** [deˌzɔksiˈraibəusnjuːˈkliːik] 脱氧核糖核酸
desoxyribose [ˌdeˌzɔksiˈraibəus] *n* 脱氧核糖
desoxy-sugar [deˌzɔksiˈʃugə] *n* 脱氧糖
despair [disˈpɛə] *n* 绝望
despeciate [diˈspiːʃieit] *vt* 种特性丧失
despeciation [diˌspiːʃiˈeiʃən] *n* 种特性丧失
despecification [diˌspesifiˈkeiʃən] *n* 去种特异性作用
d'Espine's sign [deˈspiːn] (Jean H. A. d'Espine) 德斯平征(正常成人在脊柱听诊棘突附近时,胸语音在气管分支处停止,正常小儿则在第七颈椎的高度消失,如出现在此高度以下,则显示支气管淋巴结肿大)
desquamate [ˈdeskwəmeit] *vi* 脱屑,脱皮
desquamation [ˌdeskwəˈmeiʃən] *n* 脱屑,脱皮 | furfuraceous ~ 糠样脱屑 / lamellar ~ of the newborn 新生儿层板状脱屑
desquamative [ˈdeskwæmətiv], **desquamatory** [ˈdeskwæmətəri] *a* 脱屑的,脱皮的
dest. destilla【拉】蒸馏;destillatus【拉】蒸馏的
destain [diːˈstein] *vt* 使(标本)脱色 | **~er** *n* 脱色液
desthiobiotin [ˌdesθaiəuˈbaiətin] *n* 脱硫生物素
destil. destilla【拉】蒸馏
desulfhydrase [ˌdiːsʌlfˈhaidreis] *n* 脱巯基酶
Desulfobacter [diːˌsʌlfəuˈbæktə] *n* 脱硫杆菌属
Desulfobulbus [diːˌsʌlfəuˈbʌlbəs] *n* 脱硫球茎菌属
Desulfococcus [diːˌsʌlfəuˈkɔkəs] *n* 脱硫球菌属
Desulfomonas [diːˌsʌlfəuˈməunəs] *n* 脱硫单胞菌属
Desulfosarcina [diːˌsʌlfəuˈsɑːsinə] *n* 脱硫叠球菌属
Desulfotomaculum [diːˌsʌlfətəuˈmækjuləm] *n* 脱硫肠状菌属
Desulfovibrio [diːˌsʌlfəuˈvibriəu] *n* 脱磺弧菌属
desulfurase [diːˈsʌlfəreis] *n* 脱硫酶
desulfurize [diːˈsʌlfəraiz] *vt* 使脱硫
Desulfuromonas [diːˌsʌlfjuərəuˈməunəs] *n* 脱硫单胞菌属
desynchronization [diːˌsiŋkrənaiˈzeiʃən, -niˈz-] *n* 去同步化
desynchrony [diːˈsiŋkrəni] *n* 失同步症(飞行时差反应即为一例)
DET diethyltryptamine 二乙色胺(致幻药)
Det. detur【拉】给予
detachment [diˈtætʃmənt] *n* 分离,脱离 | ~ retina, retinal ~ 视网膜脱离
detection [diˈtekʃən] *n* 检测,探测
detective [diˈtektiv] *a* 探测的
detector [diˈtektə] *n* 探测器,检验器,指示器 | lie ~ 多种波动描记器,测谎器 / radiation ~ 辐射探测器
detention [diˈtenʃən] *n* 隔离,拘留;滞留,停滞
deterenol hydrochloride [diˈtiərinəul] 盐酸地特诺(眼科用拟肾上腺素药)
deterge [diˈtəːdʒ] *vt* 洗净(伤口等)
detergent [diˈtəːdʒənt] *a* 去污的 *n* 去污剂,去垢剂;洗涤剂
deteriorate [diˈtiəriəreit] *vt, vi* 恶化;变质;衰退,退化 | **deterioration** [diˌtiəriəˈreiʃən] *n* / **deteriorative** *a*
determinable [diˈtəːminəbl] *a* 可决定的,可确定的,可限定的
determinant [diˈtəːminənt] *n* 决定子;决定因素;决定簇 | antigenic ~ 抗原决定簇 / germ cell ~ 生殖细胞决定体,卵小体 / hidden ~ 隐蔽决定簇(位于分子隐蔽区的抗原决定簇) / immunogenic ~ 免疫原决定簇 / sequential ~ 顺序决定簇
determination [diˌtəːmiˈneiʃən] *n* 决定,确定,测定 | embryonic ~ 胚胎决定 / sex ~ 性别决定
determiner [diˈtəːminə] *n* 决定因素,决定簇
determinism [diˈtəːminizəm] *n* 宿命论,决定论 | psychic ~ 精神决定论 | **deterministic** [diˌtəːmiˈnistik] *a*
detersive [diˈtəːsiv] *a* 去污的 *n* 去污剂
dethyroidism [diˈθairɔidizəm] *n* 甲状腺功能缺失[症]
dethyroidize [diˈθairɔidaiz] *vt* 除甲状腺功能
Det. in dup., Det. in 2 plo. detur in duplo【拉】加倍给予
detonation [ˌdetəuˈneiʃən] *n* 爆燃,爆炸;失调发声,爆鸣
de Toni-Fanconi syndrome [deiˈtəni fənˈkəuni] (Giovanni de Toni; Guido Fanconi) 德-范综合征(见 Fanconi's syndrome 第②解)
detomidine [diˈtəumidiːn] *n* 地托咪啶(镇痛安定药,用于马)
detorsion [diˈtɔːʃən] *n* 扭转矫正法(如睾丸捩转复位);扭转不全
detoxicate [diːˈtɔksikeit] *vt* 解毒
detoxification [diːˌtɔksifiˈkeiʃən] *n* 解毒;解毒疗法 | metabolic ~ 代谢性解毒 | **detoxication**

[ˌdiːˌtɔksiˈkeiʃən] *n*
detoxify [diːˈtɔksifai] *vt* 解毒
Detre's reaction [ˈdetə] (László Detre) 德特反应(鉴别人或牛型结核病的皮肤反应)
detriment [ˈdetrimənt] *n* 损害,伤害
detrimental [ˌdetriˈmentl] *a* 有害的
detrition [diˈtriʃən] *n* 磨耗(如牙齿)
detritivorous [ˌdiːtriˈtivərəs] *a* 食腐质的(生物)
detritus [diˈtraitəs] *n* 腐质,碎屑
detruncate [diːˈtrʌŋkeit] *vt* 截短,削去…的一部分
detruncation [ˌdiːtrʌŋˈkeiʃən] *n* 断头术(主要指胎儿)
detrusor [diˈtruːsə] *n* 逼肌;压出器 | ~ urinae 逼尿肌,耻骨膀胱肌
D. et s. detur et signetur【拉】给予并标记
detubation [ˌdiːtjuˈbeiʃən] *n* 除管法
detumescence [ˌdiːtju(ː)ˈmesns] *n* 退肿,消肿
deutan [ˈdjuːtən] *a* 绿色觉异常的,绿色盲的 *n* 绿色觉异常者,绿色盲患者
deutencephalon [ˌdjuːtenˈsefələn] *n* 间脑
deuteranomal [ˌdjuːtərəˈnɔməl] *n* 绿色弱视者
deuteranomalopia [ˌdjuːtərənɔməˈləupiə], **deuteranomalopsia** [ˌdjuːtərəˌnɔməˈlɔpsiə], **deuteranomaly** [ˌdjuːtərəˈnɔməli] *n* 绿色弱视 | **deuteranomalous** [ˌdjuːtərəˈnɔmələs] *a*
deuteranope [ˈdjuːtərənəup] *n* 绿色盲者,色觉异常者
deuteranopia [ˌdjuːtərəˈnəupiə], **deuteranopsia** [ˌdjuːtərəˈnɔpsiə] *n* 绿色盲,第二型色盲 | **deuteranopic** [ˌdjuːtərəˈnɔpik] *a*
deuterate [ˈdjuːtəreit] *vt* 氘化
deuterion [dju(ː)ˈtiəriɔn] *n* 氘核
deuterium (**D**, ^{2}**H**) [dju(ː)ˈtiəriəm] *n* 氘,重氢 | ~ oxide 氧化氘,重水
deuter(o)-, **deut(o)-** [构词成分]第二,次,亚
deuteroconidium [ˌdjuːtərəukəˈnidiəm] *n* 半[知]分生孢子
deuterofat [ˈdjuːtərəfæt] *n* 氘[化]脂
deuterohemin [ˌdjuːtərəuˈhemin] *n* 次氯血红素
deuterohemophilia [ˌdjuːtərəuˌhiːməˈfiliə] *n* 亚血友病(由于凝血因子缺乏或某些抗凝血剂的作用所致)
Deuteromyces [ˌdjuːtərəuˈmaisiːz], **Deuteromycetae** [ˌdjuːtərəumaiˈsiːtiː] *n* 半知菌纲,不[完]全菌纲
deuteromycete [ˌdjuːtərəuˈmaisiːt] *n* 半知菌,不[完]全菌
Deuteromycetes [ˌdjuːtərəumaiˈsiːtiːz] *n* 半知菌纲,不[完]全菌纲
Deuteromycota [ˌdjuːtərəumaiˈkəutə] *n* 半知菌门,不[完]全菌门
Deuteromycotina [ˌdjuːtərəuˌmaikəuˈtainə] *n* 半知菌亚门,不[完]全菌亚门
deuteron [ˈdjuːtərɔn] *n* 氘核,重氢核
deuteropathy [ˌdjuːtəˈrɔpəθi] *n* 继发病 | **deuteropathic** [ˌdjuːtərəˈpæθik] *a*
deuteropine [ˌdjuːtəˈrəupin] *n* 阿片次碱(一种阿片生物碱)
deuteroplasm [ˈdjuːtərəˌplæzəm] *n* 滋养质,副质(如卵黄)
deuteroporphyrin [ˌdjuːtərəuˈpɔːfirin] *n* 次卟啉
deuterosome [ˈdjuːtərəsəum] *n* 次胞质体(纤毛上皮细胞内)
deuterostome [ˈdjuːtərəuˌstəum] *n* 后口动物
Deuterostomia [ˌdjuːtərəuˈstəumiə] *n* 后口动物
deuterotocia [ˌdjuːtərəuˈtəusiə], **deuterotoky** [ˌdjuːtəˈrɔtəki] *n* 两性单性生殖
deuthyalosome [ˌdjuːθaiˈæləsəum] *n* 成熟卵核
deut(o)- 见 deuter(o)-
deutomerite [ˌdjuˈtɔmmərait] *n* 后节,簇虫后胞
deuton [ˈdjuːtɔn] *n* 氘核,重氢核
deutonephron [ˌdjuːtəuˈnefrɔn] *n* 中肾
deutoplasm [ˈdjuːtəplæzəm] *n* 滋养质,副质(如卵黄)
deutoplasmolysis [ˌdjuːtəplæzˈmɔlisis] *n* 滋养质溶解
Deutschländer's disease [ˌdɔitʃləndə] (Karl E. W. Deutschländer) 多伊奇兰德病(①跖骨瘤;②行军足病〈骨折〉)
DEV duck embryo rabies vaccine 鸭胚狂犬病疫苗
devaluation [diːˌvæljuˈeiʃən] *n* 降低(指心理防御机制)
devascularization [diːˌvæskjuləraiˈzeiʃən, -riˈz-] *n* 血供应阻断,血行阻断
developer [diˈveləpə] *n* 显影液,显影剂;显色剂
development [diˈveləpmənt] *n* 发展;发育;显影,显像;显层(色谱法) | arrested ~ 发育停顿 / cognitive ~ 识知发展(婴儿期开始的智力、意识思维和解决问题能力的发展) / mosaic ~ 镶嵌式发育 / postnatal ~ 产后发育 / prenatal ~ 产前发育 / psychosexual ~ 性心理发育 / regulative ~ 规律性发育 | **~al** [diˌveləpˈmentl] *a* 发育的
deviant [ˈdiːviənt] *a* 不正常的,偏离标准的 *n* 不正常者,偏离标准者 | color ~ 色觉异常者(对红绿色、蓝黄色分辨不清) / sexual ~ 性欲不正常者
deviation [ˌdiːviˈeiʃən] *n* 偏差;(个体发育的变异中的)离差;偏斜,偏向 | animal ~ 动物诱离法(用动物诱使蚊子离开人) / axis ~ 轴偏心(心电图中平均 QRS 复合波的方向) / complement ~ 补体转向,补体偏移(当抗体〈溶血素〉过剩时,补体诱发的免疫溶血作用受到抑制) / con-

jugate ~ 同向偏斜 / immune ~ 免疫偏差,免疫偏向 / latent ~ 隐斜视 / manifest ~ 斜视,斜眼 / minimum ~ 最小偏向 / primary ~ 原偏斜(眼) / sample standard ~ 样本标准差(符号为 *s*) / secondary ~ 副偏斜(眼) / sexual ~ 性欲倒错 / skew ~ 反向偏斜(脑病灶同侧眼球向下向内转,对侧眼球向上向外偏斜) / squint ~ 斜视角 / standard ~ 标准差 / strabismic ~ 斜视偏向 / ~ to the left 偏左 / ~ to the right 偏右

device [di'vais] *n* 器械,装置 | central-bearing ~ 中支器(牙科) / central-bearing tracing ~ 中支描记器(牙科) / contraceptive ~ 避孕器 / intra-uterine ~ (IUD) 宫内节育器

Devic's disease [də'viːk] (Eugène Devic) 视神经脊髓炎

deviometer [ˌdiːvi'ɔmitə] *n* 斜视计,偏向计

devisceration [diːˌvisə'reiʃən] *n* 去脏术,脏器切除术

devitalization [diːˌvaitəlai'zeiʃən] *n* 失活,去生机 | pulp ~ 牙髓失活

devitalize, devitalise [diː'vaitəlaiz] *vt* 失活,去生机

devitrification [diːˌvitrifi'keiʃən] *n* 透明消失

devolution [ˌdiːvə'ljuːʃən, ˌdevə'ljuːʃən] *n* 退行进化,退化;异化 | **devolutive** ['diːvəljuːtiv, 'devəljutiv] *a*

De Vries' theory [də'vriːz] (Hugo de Vries) 德符里学说(突变学说,见 theory of mutations)

dewater [diː'wɔːtə] *vt* 脱水;浓缩 | **~er** *n* 脱水器 / **~ed** *a* 脱水的(指用干燥法或压挤法使淤泥脱水)

dewclaw ['djuːklɔː] *n* 悬蹄(动物的无用残趾或爪)

dewlap ['djuːlæp] *n* (动物颈部)垂肉

deworming [diː'wəːmiŋ] *n* 灭除蠕虫,驱蠕虫

Dew's sign [djuː] (Harold R. Dew) 迪尤征(膈右顶下棘球蚴囊脓肿时,叩响区可因患者取肘膝位而下移)

DEXA dual energy X-ray absorptiometry 双能 X 线吸收测量法

dexamethasone [ˌdeksə'meθəsəun] *n* 地塞米松(合成糖皮质激素) | ~ acetate 醋酸地塞米松 / ~ sodium phosphate 磷酸钠地塞米松

dexamisole [dek'sæmisəul] *n* 右旋咪唑(抗抑郁药)

dexbrompheniramine [ˌdeksbrəmfə'niərəmiːn] *n* 右溴苯那敏(抗组胺药) | ~ maleate 马来酸右溴苯那敏

dexchlorpheniramine [ˌdeksklɔːfə'niərəmiːn] *n* 右氯苯那敏(抗组胺药) | ~ maleate 马来酸右氯苯那敏

dexclamol hydrochloride ['deksklәməul] 盐酸环庚吡喹醇(镇静药)

dexetimide [dek'setimaid] *n* 右苄替米特(抗胆碱药,抗帕金森病药)

dexfenfluramine hydrochloride [ˌdeksfen'fluːrəmiːn] 盐酸右芬氟拉明(拟肾上腺素药,用作食欲抑制药,短期治疗外源性肥胖症,口服给药)

deximafen [dek'siməfən] *n* 苯双咪唑(抗抑郁药)

dexiocardia [ˌdeksiəu'kɑːdiə] *n* 右位心

dexiotropic [ˌdeksiəu'trɔpik] *a* (由左向)右旋的

dexivacaine [dek'sivəkein] *n* 地昔卡因(局部麻醉药)

dexmedetomidine hydrochloride [ˌdeksmedə'təumidiːn] 盐酸右美托咪定(安定药)

dexpanthenol [deks'pænθənɔl] *n* 右[旋]泛醇(胆碱能药)

dexpropranolol [ˌdeksprə'prænəlɔl] *n* 右普萘洛尔 | ~ hydrochloride 盐酸右普萘洛尔(抗心律失常的心脏抑制药)

dexter ['dekstə] *a*【拉】右的

dextrad ['dekstræd] *ad* 向右[侧]

dextral ['dekstrəl] *a* 右[侧]的;右利的,善用右侧器官的 *n* 右利手者 | **~ity** [deks'træləti] *n* 右利,善用右侧器官(如右眼、右手或右足)

dextran ['dekstrən] *n* 葡聚糖(血浆代用品,原名右旋糖酐)

dextranomer [deks'trænəumə] *n* 聚糖酐(用于渗液性创伤的清创术)

dextransucrase [ˌdekstrən'sukreis] *n* 葡聚糖蔗糖酶,蔗糖-6-葡糖基转移酶

dextrates ['dekstreits] *n* 葡萄糖结合剂(一种制片剂用的结合剂兼稀释剂)

dextraural [deks'trɔːrəl] *a* 右利耳的,善用右耳的

dextriferron [ˌdekstri'ferɔn] *n* 糊精铁(治缺铁性贫血)

dextrin ['dekstrin] *n* 糊精

dextrinase ['dekstrineis] *n* 糊精酶

α-dextrinase ['dekstrineis] *n* α-糊精酶

dextrinate ['dekstrineit], **dextrinize** ['dekstrinaiz] *vi* 糊精化

dextrin-1, 6-glucosidase [ˌdekstringluː'kəusideis] *n* 糊精-1, 6-葡萄糖酶,脱支链酶

dextrinose ['dekstrinəus] *n* 糊精糖,异麦芽糖

dextrinosis [ˌdekstri'nəusis] *n* 糖原贮积症,糖原病 | limit ~ 糖原贮积症Ⅲ型

dextrinuria [ˌdekstri'njuəriə] *n* 糊精尿

dextr(o)- [构词成分]右,右旋

dextroamphetamine [ˌdekstrəuæm'fetəmiːn] *n* 右[旋]苯丙胺 | ~ phosphate 磷酸右[旋]苯丙胺(中枢神经兴奋药) / ~ sulfate 硫酸右[旋]

苯丙胺(中枢神经兴奋药)
dextrocardia [ˌdekstrəuˈkɑːdiə] *n* 右位心 | mirror-image ~ 镜影右位心(心脏位于右侧胸腔)/ secondary ~ 继发性右位心
dextrocardiogram [ˌdekstrəuˈkɑːdiəgræm] *n* 右心电图
dextrocerebral [ˌdekstrəuˈseribrəl] *a* 右脑的,右脑优势的
dextroclination [ˌdekstrəukliˈneiʃən], **dextrocycloduction** [ˌdekstrəuˌsaikləuˈdʌkʃən] *n* 右旋(眼)
dextrocompound [ˌdekstrəuˈkɔmpaund] *n* 右旋物
dextrocular [deksˈtrɔkjulə] *a* 右利眼的,善用右眼的 | **~ity** [ˌdekstrɔkjuˈlærəti] *n*
dextroduction [ˌdekstrəuˈdʌkʃən] *n* 右转(眼)
dextrogastria [ˌdekstrəuˈgæstriə] *n* 右位胃
dextroglucose [ˌdekstrəuˈgluːkəus] *n* 葡萄糖,右旋糖
dextrogram [ˈdekstrəgræm] *n* 轴右偏心电图(轴右偏表明右心室肥大)
dextrogyral [ˌdekstrəuˈdʒaiərəl] *n* 右旋的
dextrogyration [ˌdekstrəudʒaiəˈreiʃən] *n* 右旋(指眼的活动及偏振面)
dextromanual [ˌdekstrəuˈmænjuəl] *a* 右利手的,善用右手的
dextromenthol [ˌdekstrəuˈmenθɔl] *n* 右旋薄荷脑
dextromethorphan hydrobromide [ˌdekstrəuˈmeθəfən] 氢溴酸右美沙芬(镇咳药)
dextropedal [deksˈtrɔpedəl] *a* 右利足的,善用右足的
dextroposition [ˌdekstrəupəˈziʃən] *n* 右移位
dextropropoxyphene [ˌdekstrəuprəˈpɔksifiːn] *n* 右[旋]丙氧吩,丙氧吩(镇痛药)
dextrorotary [ˌdekstrəuˈrəutəri] *a* 右旋的
dextrorotation [ˌdekstrəurəuˈteiʃən] *n* 右旋[作用]
dextrorotatory [ˌdekstrəuˈrəuteitəri] *a* 右旋的(指偏振面或光线)
dextrosazone [deksˈtrəusəzəun] *n* 葡糖脎
dextrose [ˈdekstrəus] *n* 葡萄糖
dextrosinistral [ˌdekstrəuˈsinistrəl] *a* 自右至左的 *n* 左利手者(本词亦指对生来善用左手的人,可在某些动作方面加以训练使用右手)
dextrosozone [ˌdekstrəuˈsəuzəun] *n* 葡糖脎
dextrosuria [ˌdekstrəuˈsjuəriə] *n* 葡萄糖尿,右旋糖尿
dextrotartaric acid [ˌdekstrəutɑːˈtærik] 右旋酒石酸
dextrothyroxine sodium [ˌdekstrəuθaiˈrɔksi(ː)n] *n* 右[旋]甲状腺素钠(口服降血脂药)
dextrotorsion [ˌdekstrəuˈtɔːʃən] *n* 右旋(眼)
dextrotropic [ˌdekstrəuˈtrɔpik] *a* 右转的
dextroversion [ˌdekstrəuˈvəːʒən] *n* 右转(尤指眼);右旋(心脏位于右单侧胸廓,左心室仍在左方但位于右心室的前方)
dextroverted [ˌdekstrəuˈvəːtid] *a* 右转的
dezocine [ˈdezəsiːn] *n* 地佐辛,氨甲苯环癸醇(镇痛药)
DF-2 DF-2 杆菌(见 Capnocytophaga canimorsus)
DFDT difluoro-diphenyl-trichloroethane 二氟二苯三氯乙烷(杀虫药)
DFP diisopropyl fluorophosphate 氟磷酸二异丙酯,异氟磷(乙酰胆碱酯酶抑制药)
dG deoxyguanosine 脱氧鸟苷
dg decigram 分克
dGDP deoxyguanosine diphosphate 脱氧鸟苷二磷酸
dGMP deoxyguanosine monophosphate 脱氧鸟苷酸
dGTP deoxyguanosine triphosphate 脱氧鸟苷三磷酸
DH delayed hypersensitivity 迟发型超敏反应
DHA 2, 8-dihydroxyadenine 2, 8-二羟腺嘌呤; docosahexaenoic acid 二十二碳六烯酸
dhava [ˈdɑːvə] *n* 阔叶使君子
diacetoxyscirpenol [daiˌæsiˌtɔksiˈsəːpənɔl] *n* 蛇形菌素
DHEA dehydroepiandrosterone 脱氢表雄[甾]酮,脱氢异雄[甾]酮
d'Herelle phenomenon [dəˈrel] (Félix H. d'Herelle) 代列尔现象(见 Twort-d'Herelle phenomenon)
DHF dihydrofolate or dihydrofolic acid 二氢叶酸
DHFR dihydrofolate reductase 二氢叶酸还原酶
DHg, DHy Doctor of Hygiene 卫生学博士
DHom Doctor of Homeopathic Medicine 顺势疗法医学博士
DHPG 3, 4-dihydroxyphenylglycol 3, 4-二羟[基]苯乙二醇
DHT dihydrotestosterone 双氢睾酮
dhurrin [ˈdjurin] *n* 蜀黍氰苷
di- [前缀]二,两,双
dia- [前缀]通过,透过,横过,分离,间
diabetes [ˌdaiəˈbiːtiːz] *n* 糖尿病;多尿症 | adult-onset ~ 成年型糖尿病(即 non-insulin-dependent ~)/ ~ albuminurinicus 蛋白尿性多尿症 / alloxan ~ 四氧嘧啶糖尿病 / artificial ~, experimental ~ 人为性糖尿病,实验性糖尿病 / bronze ~, bronzed ~ 血色素沉着[症] / growth-onset ~ 生长期糖尿病(即 insulin-dependent ~) / ~ insipidus 尿崩症 / insulin-dependent ~ (IDD) 胰岛素依赖型糖尿病(Ⅰ型糖尿病,特征为症状突然发作、胰岛素减少、依赖外源性胰岛素维持生命,有发生酮酸中毒的倾向) / juvenile ~, juvenile-onset ~ 幼年型糖尿病(即 insulin-depend-

ent ~) / ketosis-prone ~ 趋酮症性糖尿病 / ketosis-resistant ~ 抗酮症性糖尿病 / latent ~ 隐性糖尿病 / masked ~ 隐蔽性糖尿病 / maturity-onset ~ 成年型糖尿病(即 non-insulin-dependent) / maturity-onset ~ youth (MODY) 青年成年型糖尿病(非胰岛素依赖型糖尿病的亚型,特征为常染色体显性遗传,青春晚期或成年早期发病) / ~ mellitus (DM) 糖尿病 / non-insulin-dependent ~ (NIDD) 非胰岛素依赖型糖尿病(Ⅱ型糖尿病,其特征通常为发病缓慢,有轻微或无代谢障碍〈糖尿及其后果〉的症状,不需要外源性胰岛素以预防酮尿和酮酸中毒;控制饮食,加或不加口服降血糖药通常即有效) / overflow ~ 溢出性糖尿病 / pancreatic ~ 胰腺性糖尿病 / preclinical ~ 临床前糖尿病(见 tolerance 项下 impaired glucose tolerance) / puncture ~, piqûre ~ 穿刺性糖尿病 / subclinical ~ 亚临床型糖尿病(葡萄糖耐量降低或以前有葡萄糖耐量异常。见 tolerance 项下 impaired glucose tolerance) / thiazide ~ 噻嗪性糖尿病(噻嗪类利尿药引起的葡萄糖耐量降低或显著的高血糖症,可能通过噻嗪诱发低钾血症抑制胰岛素的分泌)

diabetic [ˌdaiəˈbetik] *a* 糖尿病的 *n* 糖尿病患者

diabetid [ˌdaiəˈbiːtid] *n* 糖尿病疹,糖尿病性皮肤病

diabetogenic [ˌdaiəˌbetəuˈdʒenik] *a* 致糖尿病的

diabetogenous [ˌdaiəbiˈtɔdʒinəs] *a* 糖尿病[源]性的

diabetograph [ˌdaiəˈbiːtəgrɑːf, -græf] *n* 尿糖计

diabetometer [ˌdaiəbiˈtɔmitə] *n* 旋光尿糖计

diabrosis [ˌdaiəˈbrəusis] *n* 溃破,腐蚀(腐蚀性穿孔,穿孔性溃疡)

diabrotic [ˌdaiəˈbrɔtik] *a* 溃破的,腐蚀的 *n* 腐蚀剂

diacele [ˈdaiəsiːl] *n* 第三脑室

diacetate [daiˈæsiteit] *n* 乙酰乙酸盐

diacetemia [ˌdaiæsiˈtiːmiə] *n* 乙酰乙酸血

diacetic acid [ˌdaiəˈsiːtik] 乙酰乙酸

diaceturia [ˌdaiæsiˈtjuəriə], **diaceticaciduria** [ˌdaiəˌsetikˌæsiˈdjuəriə], **diacetonuria** [daiˌæsitəuˈnjuəriə] *n* 乙酰乙酸尿

diacetyl [daiˈæsitil] *n* 二乙酰,双乙酰,丁二酮 | ~ peroxide 二乙酰化过氧,过氧化二乙酰(防腐剂)

diacetylmorphine [ˌdaiəˌsiːtilˈmɔːfiːn] *n* 二乙酰吗啡,海洛因 | ~ hydrochloride 盐酸二乙酰吗啡

diacetyltannic acid [ˌdaiˌæsitilˈtænik] 乙酰鞣酸

Diachlorus [daiəˈklɔrəs] *n* 细虻属

diachorema [ˌdaiəkəˈriːmə] *n*【希】排泄物,粪便

diachoresis [ˌdaiəkəˈriːsis] *n* 排粪

diachylon [daiˈækilɔn], **diachylum** [daiˈækiləm] *n* (油酸)铅硬膏

diacid [daiˈæsid] *n* 二酸

diaclasis [daiˈækləsis] *n* 折骨术

diaclast [ˈdaiəklæst] *n* 穿颅器

diacrinous [daiˈækrinəs] *a* 单纯分泌的,透泌的

diacrisis [daiˈækrisis] *n* 诊断;分泌异常;窘迫排泄

diacritic [ˌdaiəˈkritik] *a* 诊断的,辨别的

diactinic [ˌdaiækˈtinik] *a* 透[过]光化线的

diactinism [daiˈæktinizəm] *n* 光化线透性

diacylglycerol [daiˌæsilˈglisərɔl] *n* 二酰甘油

diacylglycerol *O*-acyltransferase [daiˌæsilˈglisərɔl ˌæsilˈtrænsfəreis] 二酰甘油 *O*-酰基转移酶(亦称甘油二酯酰基转移酶)

diacylglycerol kinase [daiˌæsilˈglisərɔl ˈkaineis] 二酰甘油激酶(亦称甘油二酯激酶)

diad [ˈdaiæd] *n* 二价基;二分体,二联体(见 dyad)

Diadema [ˈdaiədemə] *n* 海胆属

diaderm [ˈdaiədəːm] *n* 二胚层胚,间胚盘 | ~**ic** [ˌdaiəˈdəːmik] *a* 二胚层胚的,间胚盘的;经皮的,透皮的

diadochokinesia [daiˌædəkəukaiˈniːziə], **diadochocinesia** [daiˌædəkəusaiˈniːziə], **diadochokinesis** [daiˌædəkəukaiˈniːsis] *n* 轮替动作(停止某一运动冲动,代之以完全相反的运动冲动) | **diadochokinetic** [daiˌædəkəukaiˈnetik], **diadochocinetic** [daiˌædəkəusaiˈnetik] *a*

diagnose [ˈdaiəgnəuz], **diagnosticate** [ˌdaiəgˈnɔstikeit] *vt, vi* 诊断

diagnosis [ˌdaiəgˈnəusis] ([复] **diagnoses** [ˌdaiəgˈnəusiːz]) *n* 诊断 | biological ~ 生物学诊断 / clinical ~ 临床诊断 / cytologic ~, cytohistologic ~ 细胞学诊断,细胞组织学诊断 / differential ~ 鉴别诊断 / ~ by exclusion 除外诊断 / niveau ~ 定位诊断,平准诊断(如对椎间瘤) / physical ~ 物理诊断 / provocative ~ 激发诊断 / roentgen ~ X[射]线诊断 / serum ~ 血清诊断(免疫诊断)

diagnostic [ˌdaiəgˈnɔstik] *a* 诊断的

diagnostician [ˌdaiəgnɔsˈtiʃən] *n* 诊断医师,诊断学家

diagnostics [ˌdaiəgˈnɔstiks] *n* 诊断学

diagnosticum [ˌdaiəgˈnɔstikəm] *n* 诊断剂,诊断液(用于实验诊断的制剂)

diagonal [daiˈægənl] *a* 对角线的,对顶的;斜的,斜纹的

diagram [ˈdaiəgræm] *n* 图解;图表;线图 | ladder ~ 梯形图(图解表示心脏收缩途径,如由心电图记录测定之,用于诊断心律失常) / scatter ~ 散点图 / vector ~ 矢量图 | ~**matic(al)** [ˌdaiəgrəˈmætik(əl)] *a*

diagraph [ˈdaiəgrɑːf, -græf] *n* 描界器(用于颅测量术等)

diakinesis [ˌdaiəkaiˈniːsis] *n* 终变期(第一次减数分裂前期中的一个阶段)

dial [ˈdaiəl] *n* 盘表,刻度盘 | astigmatic ~ 散光盘表

Dialister [ˌdaiəˈlistə] *n* 小杆菌属(嗜血杆菌族)

diallyl [daiˈælil] *n* 联丙烯;二丙烯基

diallylbarbituric acid [daiˌælilbɑːbiˈtjuərik] 二丙烯巴比土酸

diallylbisnortoxiferin dichloride [daiˌælilbisnɔːˈtɔksifərin] 阿库氯铵(即 alcuronium chloride,横纹肌松弛药)

dialurate [daiˈæljuəreit] *n* 5-羟[基]巴比土酸盐

dialuric acid [ˌdaiəˈljuərik] 5-羟[基]巴比土酸

dialysance [ˌdaiəˈlaisəns] *n* 透析率

dialysate [daiˈæliseit] *n* 透析液

dialysis [daiˈælisis] ([复] **dialyses** [daiˈælisiːz]) *n* 透析 | cross ~ 交叉透析(即渗透性联体生活) / equilibrium ~ 平衡透析(用以测定抗体-半抗原亲和力的一种技术) / lymph ~ 淋巴透析 / peritoneal ~ 腹膜透析 / ~ retinae (在锯齿缘)视网膜断离 | **dialytic** [ˌdaiəˈlitik] *a*

dialyzable [ˌdaiəˈlaizəbl] *a* 可透析的

dialyze [ˈdaiəlaiz] *vt, vi* 透析

dialyzed [ˈdaiəlaizd] *a* 透析了的

dialyzer [ˈdaiəˌlaizə] *n* 透析器

Diamanus [ˌdaiəˈmeinəs] *n* 穿手蚤属 | ~ montanus 山穿手蚤

diameter [daiˈæmitə] *n* 直径,径;(透镜的)放大倍数 | anterotransverse ~ 前横径,颞间径 / biischial ~ 坐骨棘间径(骨盆) / biparietal ~ 顶骨径 / bispinous ~ 坐骨棘间径(骨盆) / cervicobregmatic ~ 颈前囟径 / conjugate ~ (骨盆)直径 / diagonal conjugate ~ 对角径 / inferior longitudinal ~ 下纵径(从盲孔到枕内隆凸) / parietal ~, posterotransverse ~ 顶骨间径,后横径 / sagittal ~ 矢状径(眉间至枕外隆凸) / suboccipitobregmatic ~ 枕下前囟径

diamide [daiˈæmaid] *n* 二酰胺

diamidine [daiˈæmidiːn] *n* 联脒;二脒

diamido- [前缀]二氨基

diamine [ˈdaiəmiːn] *n* 二胺

diamine oxidase [ˈdaiəmiːn ˈɔksideis] 二胺氧化酶

diaminoacetic acid [daiˌæminəuəˈsiːtik] 二氨基乙酸

diamino acid [daiˈæminəu] 二氨基酸

diaminoacridine [daiæminəuˈækridin] *n* 二氨基吖啶,原黄素

α, γ-diaminobutyric acid [daiˌæminəubju(ː)ˈtirik] α, γ-二氨基丁酸

α, ε-diaminocaproic acid [daiˌæminəuˌkəˈprəuik] 二氨己酸,赖氨酸

***p*-diaminodiphenyl** [daiəˌminəudaiˈfenil] *n* 对二氨[基]二苯,联苯胺

diaminodiphenylsulfone (DDS) [daiˌæminəu-daiˌfenilˈsʌlfəun] *n* 氨苯砜,二氨二苯砜(抗麻风药) | diacetyl ~ 双乙酰氨苯砜(抗麻风药)

diaminodiphosphatide [daiˌæminə u daiˈfɔsfətaid] *n* 二氨[基]二磷脂

diaminomonophosphatide [daiˌæminə u ˌmɔnəˈfɔsfətaid] *n* 二氨[基]磷脂

α, ε-diaminopimelic acid [daiˌæminəupiˈmelik] α, ε-二氨基庚二酸

α, δ-diaminovaleric acid [daiˌæminəuvəˈlerik] α, δ-二氨基戊酸,鸟氨酸

diaminuria [daiˌæmiˈnjuəriə] *n* 二胺尿

diamniotic [ˌdaiæmniˈɔtik] *a* 双羊膜囊的

diamocaine cyclamate [daiˈæməkein] 环己氨磺酸二胺卡因(局部麻醉药)

diamond [ˈdaiəmənd] *n* 金刚钻;菱形

Diamond-Blackfan syndrome (anemia) [ˈdaiəmənd ˈblækfæn] (Louis Klein Diamond; Kenneth D. Blackfan) 戴-布综合征(贫血),先天性再生障碍性贫血

diamonds [ˈdaiəmənds] [复] *n* [用作单或复]荨麻疹样丹毒(一种荨麻疹样猪丹毒)

diamorphine [ˌdaiəˈmɔːfiːn] *n* 二醋吗啡(镇痛药,镇咳药)

diamthazole dihydrochloride [daiˈæmθəzəul] 盐酸地马唑(抗真菌药)

diamylene [daiˈæmiliːn] *n* 二戊烯

diandry [daiˈændri] *n* 双雄受精

dianhydroantiarigenin [ˌdaiænˌhaidrə u ˌæntiˈɑːriˌdʒenin] *n* 双脱水弩箭子苷配基

dianoetic [daiəˈniːtik] *a* 智力的,推理的

diantebrachia [ˌdaiæntiˈbreikiə] *n* 双前臂畸形

diapamide [daiˈæpəmaid] *n* 硫米齐特(即 tiamizide,利尿、降压药)

diapason [ˌdaiəˈpeisn] *n* 音叉(检听觉用);音域

diapause [ˈdaiəpɔːz] *n* 滞育(卵细胞、昆虫蛹、种子的发育暂停)

diapedesis [ˌdaiəpəˈdiːsis] ([复] **diapedeses** [ˌdaiəpəˈdiːsiːz]) *n* 血细胞渗出 | **diapedetic** [ˌdaiəpəˈdetik] *a*

diaphane [ˈdaiəfein] *n* 透照灯(用于透射照明)

diaphaneity [ˌdaiəfəˈniːiəti] *n* 透明性,透明[度]

diaphanography [daiˌæfəˈnɔgrəfi] *n* 透照摄影术

diaphanometer [daiˌæfəˈnɔmitə] *n* 透明度计(检乳、小便及其他液体) | **diaphanometry** *n* 透明度测定法

diaphanoscope [daiˈæfənəskəup] *n* [电光]透照镜(供照体腔用) | **diaphanoscopy** [daiˌæf-

əˈnɔskəpi] *n* (电光)透照检查
diaphemetric [ˌdaiəfəˈmetrik] *a* 测量触觉的
diaphorase [daiˈæfəreis] *n* 黄递酶,心肌黄酶;硫辛酰胺脱氢酶
diaphoresis [ˌdaiəfəˈriːsis] *n* 出汗,发汗(尤指大量出汗)
diaphoretic [ˌdaiəfəˈretik] *a* 发汗的 *n* 发汗药
diaphragm [ˈdaiəfræm] 膈;隔膜;光阑 | accessory ~ 尿生殖膈 / contraceptive ~ 阴道隔膜,子宫帽(避孕用具) / ~ of mouth, oral ~ 下颌舌骨肌 / pelvic ~, ~ of pelvis 盆膈 / secondary ~, urogenital ~ 泌尿生殖膈 / ~ of sella turcica 鞍膈 | **~atic** [ˌdaiəfrægˈmætik] *a*
diaphragma [ˌdaiəˈfrægmə] ([复] **diaphragmata** [ˌdaiəˈfrægmətə] *n*【希】膈
diaphragmalgia [ˌdaiəfrægˈmældʒiə], **diaphragmodynia** [ˌdaiəˌfrægməuˈdiniə] *n* 膈痛
diaphragmatitis [ˌdaiəˈfrægməˈtaitis], **diaphragmitis** [ˌdiaəfrægˈmaitis] *n* 膈炎
diaphragmatocele [ˌdaiəfrægˈmætəsiːl] *n* 膈疝
diaphysectomy [ˌdaiəfiˈzektəmi] *n* 骨干[部分]切除术
diaphysis [daiˈæfisis] ([复] **diaphyses** [daiˈæfisiːz]) *n*【希】骨干 | **diaphysary** [daiˈæfisəri], **diaphyseal**, **diaphysial** [ˌdaiəˈfiziəl] *a*
diaphysitis [ˌdaiəfiˈzaitis] *n* 骨干炎 | tuberculous ~ 结核性骨干炎
diapiresis [ˌdaiəpaiˈriːsis] *n* 血细胞渗出
diaplacental [ˌdaiəpləˈsentl] *a* 经胎盘的
diaplasis [daiˈæpləsis] *n*【希】复位术(骨折或脱位) | **diaplastic** [ˌdaiəˈplæstik] *a*
diapophysis [ˌdaiəˈpɔfisis] *n* (椎骨)横突关节面
Diaptomus [daiˈæptəməs] *n* 镖水蚤属
diapyesis [ˌdaiəpaiˈiːsis] *n* 化脓 | **diapyetic** [ˌdaiəpaiˈetik] *a*
diarrheogenic [ˌdaiəˌriəˈdʒenik] *a* 致腹泻的
diarrh(o)ea [ˌdaiəˈriə] *n* 腹泻 | paradoxical ~, stercoral ~ 积粪性腹泻 / serous ~, watery ~ 浆液性腹泻,水泻 | **~l**, **diarrheic** [ˌdaiəˈriik] *a*
diarthric [daiˈɑːθrik], **diarticular** [ˌdaiɑːˈtikjulə] *a* 两关节的
diarthrosis [ˌdaiɑːˈθrəusis] ([复] **diarthroses** [daiɑːˈθrəusiːz]) *n* 动关节 | **diarthrodial** [ˌdaiɑːˈθrəudiəl] *a*
diaschisis [daiˈæskisis] *n* 神经功能联系不能
diascope [ˈdaiəskəup] *n* 透皮玻片,透照片 | **diascopy** [daiˈæskəpi] *n* 玻片压诊法;透照法
diasostic [ˌdaiəˈsɔstik] *a* 保健的,卫生的
diaspironecrobiosis [daiˌæspaiərəuˌnekrəubaiˈəusis] *n* 播散性渐进性(细胞)坏死
diaspironecrosis [daiˌæspaiərəuneˈkrəusis] *n* 播散性坏死
diastase [ˈdaiəsteis] *n* 淀粉酶 | pancreatic ~ 胰淀粉酶 / ~ vera 胰酶 | **diastasic** [ˌdaiəˈsteisik] *a*
diastasemia [ˌdaiəstəˈsiːmiə] *n* 红细胞分解
diastasimetry [ˌdaiəstəˈsimitri] *n* 淀粉酶测定法
diastasis [daiˈæstəsis] *n*【希】脱离,分离;舒张末期 | ~ cordis 心舒张末期 / iris ~ 虹膜[根部]脱离
diastasuria [ˌdaiəsteiˈsjuəriə] *n* 淀粉酶尿
diastatic [ˌdaiəˈstætik] *a* 淀粉酶的;脱离的,分离的;舒张末期的
diastema [ˌdaiəsˈtiːmə] ([复] **diastemata** [ˌdaiəˈstemətə]), **diastem** [ˈdaiəstem] *n* 间隙,裂;牙间隙;胞质分裂面
diastematocrania [ˌdaiəˌstemətəuˈkreinjə] *n* 颅纵裂
diastematomyelia [ˌdaiəˌstemətəumaiˈiːliə] *n* 脊髓纵裂
diastematopyelia [ˌdaiəˌstemətəupaiˈiːliə] *n* 骨盆纵裂
diaster [daiˈæstə] *n* 双星[体]
diastereoisomer [ˌdaiəˌsteriəuˈaisəumə] *n* 非对映[立体]异构物
diastereoisomerism [ˌdaiəˌsteriəuaiˈsɔmərizəm] *n* 非对映[立体]异构[现象] | **diastereoisomeric** [ˌdaiəˌsteriəuˌaisəuˈmerik] *a* 非对映异构的
diastole [daiˈæstəli] *n* 心舒 | **diastolic** [ˌdaiəˈstɔlik] *a* 舒张的
diastomyelia [daiˌæstəmaiˈiːliə] *n* 脊髓纵裂
diastrophic [ˌdaiəˈstrɔfik] *a* 弯曲变形的,畸形的(如骨骼)
diataxia [ˌdaiəˈtæksiə] *n* 两侧共济失调 | cerebral ~ 脑性两侧共济失调
diathermy [ˈdaiəˌθəːmi] *n* 透热疗法 | short wave ~ 短波透热[疗]法 / ultrashort wave ~ 超短波透热[疗]法 | **diathermal** [ˌdaiəˈθəːməl], **diathermic** [ˌdaiəˈθəːmik] *a* 透热的
diathesis [daiˈæθisis] ([复] **diatheses** [daiˈæθisiːz]) *n* 素质 | aneurysmal ~ 动脉瘤素质 / bilious ~ 胆汁素质 / contractural ~ 挛缩素质 / cystic ~ 囊肿素质 / fibroplastic ~ 纤维形成性素质 / gouty ~ 痛风素质 / hemorrhagic ~ 出血素质 / inopectic ~ 血栓素质 / spasmodic ~, spasmophilic ~ 痉挛素质 / uric acid ~ 尿酸素质 | **diathetic** [ˌdaiəˈθetik] *a*
diatom [ˈdaiətəm] *n* 硅藻
diatomaceous [ˌdaiətəuˈmeiʃəs] *a* 硅藻的
diatomic [ˌdaiəˈtɔmik] *a* 二原子的;二元的;二价的;硅藻的
diatomite [daiˈætəmait] *n* 硅藻土
diatrizoate [ˌdaiətraiˈzəueit] *n* 泛影酸盐(心血管造影术及尿路造影术时用作造影剂) | ~

meglumine 泛影葡胺(造影剂) / ~ sodium 泛影酸钠(造影剂)
diatrizoic acid [ˌdaiətraiˈzəuik] 泛影酸
diauchenos [daiˈɔːkinɔs] *n* 双颈双头畸胎
diauxie [daiˈɔːksi] *n* 两阶段生长,双峰生长 | **diauxic** [daiˈɔːksik] *a*
diaveridine [ˌdaiəˈveridiːn] *n* 二氨黎芦啶(抗原虫药和抗菌药)
diaxon [daiˈæksɔn], **diaxone** [daiˈæksəun] *n* 二轴突细胞,双极细胞
diazepam [ˌdaiˈæzəpæm] *n* 地西泮(安定药)
diazine [daiˈæzin] *n* 二嗪,二氮[杂]苯
diaziquone (AZQ) [daiˈeiziˌkwəun] *n* 地吖醌(抗肿瘤药)
diazo-[前缀]重氮基
diazobenzene [daiˌæzəuˈbenziːn] *n* 重氮苯
diazobenzenesulfonic acid [daiˌæzəuˌbenziːnsʌlˈfɔnik] 重氮苯磺酸
diazoma [ˌdaiəˈzəumə] *n* 膈;隔膜
diazomethane [daiˌæzəuˈmeθein] *n* 重氮甲烷
diazonal [ˌdaiəˈzəunəl] *a* 横过两区的;暗带的
diazone [ˈdaiəzəun] *n* 暗带(牙釉质的横断层)
diazosulfobenzol [daiˌæzəuˌsʌlfəuˈbenzɔl] *n* 重氮磺苯(对尿内某些成分起作用,形成苯胺色)
diazotize [daiˈæzətaiz] *vt* 使重氮化 | **diazotization** [daiˌæzətaiˈzeiʃən, -tiˈz-] *n* 重氮化[作用]
5-diazouracil [daiˌæzəuˈjuərəsil] *n* 5-重氮尿嘧啶(癌研究用药)
diazoxide [ˌdaiəˈzɔksaid] *n* 二氮嗪(抗高血压药)
dibasic [daiˈbeisik] *a* 二元的,二碱价的
dibenz(b, f)-1, 4-oxazepine [daiˌbenzɔksˈæzəpiːn] *n* 二苯(b, f)-1, 4-氧氮䓬(常用催泪毒气)
dibenzanthracene [ˌdaibenˈzænθrəsin] *n* 二苯蒽
dibenzazepine [daibenˈzæzəpin] *n* 二苯扎西平(任何一组结构上相关的包括三环抑郁药氯米帕明〈clomipramine〉、地昔帕明〈desipramine〉、米帕明〈imipramine〉和曲米帕明〈trimipramine〉的药物)
dibenz-dibutyl anthraquinol [daiˌbenzdaiˈbjuːtil ˌænθrəˈkwinɔl] 二苯二丁对蒽二酚(一种致癌和产生雌激素的物质)
dibenzepin hydrochloride [daiˈbenzəpin] 盐酸二苯西平(抗抑郁药)
dibenzocycloheptadiene [daiˌbenzəuˌsaikləuˌheptəˈdaiiːn] *n* 二苯环庚二烯(任何一类结构上相关的包括三环抗抑郁药阿米替林〈amitriptyline〉、去甲替林〈nortriptyline〉和普罗替林〈protriptyline〉的药物)
dibenzodiazepine [daiˌbenzəudaiˈæzəpiːn] *n* 二苯二氮䓬(抗精神病药)
dibenzothiazine [daiˌbenzəˈθaiəziːn] *n* 吩噻嗪
dibenzoxazepine [daiˌbenzɔkˈsæzəpiːn] *n* 二苯并氧氮䓬(任何一类结构上相关的杂环药物,其中包括抗精神病药洛沙平〈loxapine〉和抗抑郁药阿莫沙平〈amoxapine〉)
dibenzoxepine [daibenˈzɔksəpiːn], **dibenzoxepin** [daibenˈzɔksəpin] *n* 二苯多塞平(任何一类结构上相关的包括三环抗抑郁药多塞平〈doxepin〉的药物)
dibenzylchlorethamine [ˌdaibenzilkləˈreθəmiːn] *n* 苄氯乙胺(α 受体阻滞药,治周围血管疾病及诊断嗜铬细胞瘤)
diblastula [daiˈblæstjulə] *n* 二叶性囊胚
dibothriocephaliasis [daiˌbɔθriəuˌsefəˈlaiəsis] *n* 裂头绦虫病
Dibothriocephalus [daiˌbɔθriəuˈsefələs] *n* 裂头[绦虫]属(即 Diphyllobothrium)
dibrachia [daiˈbreikiə] *n* 复臂[畸形]
dibrachius [daiˈbreikiəs] *n* 二臂联胎
dibromide [daiˈbrəumaid] *n* 二溴化物
dibromochloropropane [daiˌbrəuməuˌklɔːrəuˈprəupein] *n* 二溴氯丙烷(曾用作杀虫药、土壤熏蒸剂和杀线虫药,因其致癌性现限制使用)
dibromodulcitol [daiˌbrəuməuˈdʌlsitɔl] *n* 二溴卫矛醇(抗肿瘤药)
1, 2-dibromoethane [daiˌbrəuməuˈeθein] *n* 1, 2-二溴乙烷
dibromoketone [daiˌbrəuməˈkiːtəun] *n* 二溴丁酮(战用毒气)
dibromsalan [daiˈbrɔmsəlæn] *n* 二溴沙仑(具有抗菌和抗真菌作用的消毒剂,主要用于药皂)
dibucaine [ˈdaibjukein] *n* 地布卡因(局部麻醉药) | ~ hydrochloride 盐酸地布卡因
dibutoline sulfate [daiˈbjuːtəliːn] 地硫酸地布托林(抗胆碱能药)
dibutyl [daiˈbjuːtil] *n* 二丁基
DIC diffuse or disseminated intravascular coagulation 弥散性血管内凝血
dicacodyl [daiˈkækədail] *n* 双二甲胂,四甲二胂
dicalcic [daiˈkælsik] *a* 二钙的
dicalcium phosphate [daiˈkælsiəm] 磷酸二钙,磷酸氢钙
dicamphendion [ˌdaikæmˈfendiən] *n* 二樟脑萜二酮,二缩莰烯二酮
dicamphor [daiˈkæmfə] *n* 二缩莰酮
dicarbonate [daiˈkɑːbənit] *n* 碳酸氢盐
dicarboxylic acid [daikɑːbɔkˈsilik] 二羧酸
dicarboxylicaciduria [ˌdaikɑːbɔkˌsilikˌæsiˈdjuəriə] *n* 二羧酸尿[症]
dicelous [daiˈsiːləs] *a* 双凹的;有两腔的
Dicentra [daiˈsentrə] *n* 荷包牡丹属
dicentric [daiˈsentrik] *a* 具双着丝粒的

dicephalous [dai'sefələs] *a* 双头[畸形]的
dicephalus [dai'sefələs] *n* 双头畸胎,并体联胎
dicephaly [dai'sefəli] *n* 双头[畸形]
Dichapetalum [ˌdaikə'petələm] *n* 南非树属
dicheilia [dai'kailiə] *n* 复唇[畸形]
dicheiria [dai'kaiəriə] *n* 复手[畸形]
dicheirus [dai'kaiərəs] *n* 复手[畸形]者
Dichelobacter [dai'kiːləuˌbæktə] *n* 偶蹄菌属 | ~ nodosus 节瘤偶蹄菌
dichloracetic acid [daiˌklɔːrə'siːtik] 二氯乙酸
dichloralphenazone [ˌdaiklɔrəl'fenəzəun] *n* 氯醛比林(用作轻度镇静药和弛缓药,与半乳糖二酸异美汀和对乙酰氨基酚结合用于治疗偏头痛和紧张性头痛)
dichlordioxydiamidoarsenobenzol [daiˌklɔːdaiˌɔksidaiˌæmidəuˌɑːsinəu'benzɔl] *n* 二氯二氧二氨联胂苯,胂凡纳明
dichlorhydrin [ˌdaiklɔː'haidrin] *n* 二氯丙醇
dichloride [dai'klɔːraid] *n* 二氯化物
dichlorisone [dai'klɔːrisəun] *n* 二氯松(糖皮质激素,用于治疗对类固醇敏感的瘙痒性炎症和变应性炎症)
***o*-dichlorobenzene** [daiˌklɔːrəu'benziːn] *n* 邻二氯苯(一种溶剂、熏剂和杀虫剂,有时用作喷雾剂,如摄入或吸入,则中毒)
3, 3-dichlorobenzidine [daiˌklɔrəu'benzidiːn] *n* 3, 3-二氯联苯胺(用于制造染料和塑料,具有致癌性)
dichlorodiethyl sulfide [daiˌklɔːrəudai'eθil] 二氯二乙硫醚,芥子气(糜烂性毒气)
dichlorodifluoromethane [daiˌklɔːrəudaiˌfluərə'meθein] *n* 二氯二氟甲烷(用作气溶胶抛射剂及致冷剂)
1, 1-dichloroethane [daiˌklɔːrəu'eθein] *n* 1, 1-二氯乙烷,亚乙基二氯
1, 2-dichloroethane [daiˌklɔːrəu'eθein] *n* 1, 2-二氯乙烷,二氯化乙烯
dichloroformoxime [daiˌklɔːrəufə'mɔksim] *n* 二氯甲醛肟(窒息性毒气)
dichloroisoproterenol [daiˌklɔːrəuˌaisəuprə'terinɔl] *n* 二氯异丙去甲肾上腺素(一种 *β* 受体阻滞药,治各种心脏病)
dichlorophen [dai'klɔːrəfən] *n* 双氯酚(抗蠕虫药)
2, 4-dichlorophenoxyacetic acid [daiˌklɔːrəufiˌnɔksiə'siːtik] 2, 4-D, 二四滴,2, 4-二氯苯氧乙酸(植物生长刺激素)
dichlorotetrafluoroethane [daiˌklɔːrəuˌtetrəˌfluərə'eθein] *n* 克立氟烷,二氯四氟乙烷(用作气溶胶抛射剂)
dichlorphenamide [ˌdaiklɔː'fenəmaid] *n* 双氯非那胺(碳酸酐酶抑制药,治青光眼药)
dichlorvos [dai'klɔːvɔs] *n* 敌敌畏(有机磷杀虫药,抗蠕虫药)
dichogeny [dai'kɔdʒəni] *n* 两向发育(指组织随着影响其条件的变化而向不同的方向发育)
dichorionic [ˌdaikɔːri'ɔnik], **dichorial** [ˌdai'kɔːriəl] *a* 双绒[毛]膜的
dichotomize [dai'kɔtəmaiz] *vt*, *vi* 分成两部分,分成两类 | **dichotomization** [daiˌkɔtəmai'zeiʃən] *n* 二分(一分为二);二[分]叉,二歧
dichotomy [dai'kɔtəmi] *n* 二分法,两分法(一分为二);二[分]叉,二歧,二叉分枝 | **dichotomous** *a*
Dichroa [dai'krəuə] *n* 常山属 | ~ febrifuga 黄常山
dichroic [dai'krəuik], **dichroitic** [ˌdaikrəu'itik] *a* 二向色[性]的,二色性的
dichroine [dai'krəuiːn] *n* 黄常山碱
dichroism ['daikrəuizəm] *n* 二向色性,二色性
dichromasy [dai'krəuməsi] *n* 二色性;二色视,二色性色盲
dichromat ['daikrəumæt] *n* 二色视者
dichromate [dai'krəumit] *n* 重铬酸盐
dichromatism [dai'krəumətizəm] *n* 二色性;二色视,二色性色盲 | **dichromatic** [ˌdaikrəu'mætik] *a*
dichromatopsia [ˌdaikrəumə'tɔpsiə] *n* 二色视,二色性色盲(只能辨识两色,一般为蓝和黄)
dichromic [dai'krəumik] *a* 二色性的
dichromophil [dai'krəuməfil] *a* 两染性的 *n* 两染细胞
dichromophilism [ˌdaikrəu'mɔfilizəm] *n* 两染性(能染酸性和碱性色素)
dichuchwa [di'tʃuːtʃwɑː] *n* 非性病性梅毒
dick [dik] *n* 二氯乙胂(毒气)
Dick serum [dik] (George F. Dick) 狄克血清(含猩红热病原菌链球菌红疹毒素抗体的免疫血清) | ~ test (reaction) 狄克试验(反应),猩红热毒素试验(测定人体对猩红热有无免疫力的皮肤试验) / ~ toxin 红疹毒素(检猩红热)
diclidostosis [ˌdiklidɔs'təusis] *n* 静脉瓣骨化
diclofenac [dai'kləufənæk] *n* 双氯芬酸钠(非甾体消炎药)
dicloralurea [ˌdaiklɔːˌræljuː'riːə] *n* 双氯醛脲(动物饲料添加剂)
dicloxacillin sodium [daiˌklɔksə'silin] 双氯西林钠(半合成抗青霉素酶青霉素)
dicoelous [dai'siːləs] *a* 双凹的;有两腔的
dicophane ['daikəfein] *n* 滴滴涕,二氯二苯三氯乙烷(杀虫药)
dicoria [dai'kɔːriə] *n* 重瞳
dicotyledon [daiˌkɔti'liːdən] *n* 双子叶植物

dicoumarin [daiˈkuːmərin] *n* 双香豆素(抗凝药)
dicroceliasis [ˌdikrəusiˈlaiəsis] *n* 双腔吸虫病
Dicrocoelium [ˌdikrəuˈsiːliəm] *n* 双腔[吸虫]属 | ~ dendriticum, ~ lanceolatum 支双腔吸虫,矛形双腔吸虫 / ~ hospes 牛双腔吸虫 / ~ macrostomum 巨口双腔吸虫
dicrotic [daiˈkrɔtik] *a* 二波[脉]的,重搏[脉]的 | **dicrotism** [ˈdaikrətizəm] *n* 二波脉[现象],重波脉[现象]
dictionary [ˈdikʃənəri] *n* 字典 | genetic code ~ 遗传密码字典
dicty(o)-[构词成分]网,网状结构
dictyocaulus [ˌdiktiəuˈkɔːləs] *n* 网尾[线虫]属 | ~ filaria 丝状网尾线虫(亦称丝圆线虫) / ~ viviparus 胎生网尾线虫(亦称小圆线虫)
Dictyocha [ˌdiktiˈəukə] *n* 硅鞭藻属
dictyokinesis [ˌdiktiəukaiˈniːsis] *n* 网体分裂,高尔基(Golgi)体分裂(有丝分裂时高尔基体移居分布到子细胞中)
dictyoma [ˌdiktiˈəumə] *n* 视网膜胚瘤
dictyosome [ˈdiktiəsəum] *n* [分散]高尔基(Golgi)体,网体
Dictyosteliia [ˌdiktiəustiˈlaiiə] *n* 网柱原虫亚纲
Dictyosteliida [ˌdiktiəustiˈlaiidə] *n* 网柱原虫目
dictyotene [ˈdiktiətiːn] *n* 核网期
dicumarol [daiˈkumərɔl] *n* 双香豆素(抗凝药)
dicyclic [daiˈsaiklik] *a* 二周期的;双环的
dicyclomine hydrochloride [daiˈsaikləmiːn] 盐酸双环胺(抗胆碱药,胃肠道疾病时用作解痉药)
dicysteine [ˌdaisisˈtiːn] *n* 胱氨酸
dicytosis [ˌdaisaiˈtəusis] *n* 两种细胞情况(指血内单核白细胞及多核白细胞)
didactic [daiˈdæktik] *a* 释理的,理论的,教导的
didactylism [daiˈdæktilizəm] *n* 两指畸形,两趾畸形 | **didactylous** [daiˈdæktiləs] *a*
didanosine [daiˈdænəsiːn] *n* 去羟肌苷(抗反转录病毒药,用于治疗晚期感染人免疫缺陷病毒-1和获得性免疫缺陷综合征,口服给药。以前称双去氧肌苷〈ddI〉)
didelphia [daiˈdelfiə] *n* 双子宫 | **didelphic** *a*
Didelphis [daiˈdelfis] *n* 负鼠属
2′, 3′-dideoxyadenosine [ˌdaidiˌɔksiəˈdenəsiːn] *n* 2′, 3′-双去氧腺苷(抗反转录病毒药,用于治疗获得性免疫缺陷综合征)
dideoxycytidine [ˌdaidiˌɔksiˈsaitidiːn] *n* 双去氧胞苷(zalcitabine 的旧称)
dideoxyinosine (ddI) [ˌdaidiˌɔksiˈinəsiːn] *n* 双去氧肌苷(即 didanosine)
dideoxynucleoside [ˌdaidiˌɔksiˈnjuːkliəˌsaid] *n* 双去氧核苷(具有抗反转录病毒效用)
didermoma [daidəˈməumə] *n* 双胚叶[畸胎]瘤
Didiée's projection [diːdiːˈei] (J. Didiée) 迪迪耶投照(一种罕见型 X 线投照,以评估不稳定的或反复脱位的肩部可能有诸如希-萨〈Hill-Sachs〉损害的隐匿病变。令患者俯卧,中心射线从侧斜位方向进入肩部)
didymalgia [ˌdidiˈmældʒiə], **didymodynia** [ˌdidiməuˈdiniə] *n* 睾丸痛
didymitis [ˌdidiˈmaitis] *n* 睾丸炎
didymospore [ˈdidimɔspɔː] *n* 双胞孢子
didymous [ˈdidiməs] *a* 双的,双生的
-didymus[构词成分]睾丸
didymus [ˈdidiməs] *n* 睾丸
die [dai] *n* 模圈;代型 | amalgam ~ 汞合金代型(一种牙型)
Dieb. alt. diebus alternis【拉】隔日
Dieb. tert. diebus tertiis【拉】每三日
diechoscope [daiˈekəskəup] *n* 两音听诊器
diecious [daiˈiːʃəs] *a* 雌雄异体的
Dieffenbach's amputation (operation) [ˈdiːfənbʌh] (Johann F. Dieffenbach) 迪芬巴赫切断术(手术)(①髋关节环状切除术;②三角状缺损修补法)
Diego blood group [diːˈeigəu] (Diego 为委内瑞拉家族的名字,1955 年首次报道他血液中的抗原)狄哥血型(血型抗原 Di^a 和 Di^b,系由等位基因决定。Di^a 在南美洲印第安人、日本人和中国人中最常见)
dieldrin [ˈdiːldrin, daiˈeldrin] *n* 狄氏剂,氧桥氯甲桥萘(杀虫药)
dielectric [ˌdaiiˈlektrik] *n* 电介质;电介体 *a* 介电的
dielectrolysis [ˌdaiilekˈtrɔlisis] *n* 电解渗入法
diembryony [daiˈembriˌɔni] *n* 双胎生成
diencephalohypophysial [ˌdaienˌsefələuˌhaipəuˈfiziəl] *a* 间脑垂体的
diencephalon [ˌdaienˈsefəlɔn] *n* 间脑 | **diencephalic** [ˌdaienseˈfælik] *a*
-diene[后缀]二烯
diener [ˈdiːnə] *n*【德】实验室勤杂员
dienestrol [ˌdaiiˈniːstrɔl] *n* 己二烯雌酚(雌激素类药,治绝经期症状和萎缩性阴道炎以及抑制泌乳)
Dientamoeba [ˌdaientəˈmiːbə] *n* 双核阿米巴属 | ~ fragilis 脆弱双核阿米巴
dieresis [daiˈiərisis, daiˈerisis] *n* 分开,分离;(刀切、电烙、烧灼)切开
diesophagus [daii(ː)ˈsɔfəges] *n* 双食管
diester [daiˈestə] *n* 二酯
diestrum [daiˈiːstrəm, -ˈes-] *n* 动情间期
diestrus [daiˈiːstrəs, -ˈes-] *n* 动情间期 | gestational ~ 妊娠间情期 / lactational ~ 授乳间情期
diet [ˈdaiət] *n* 饮食,膳食 | absolute ~ 禁食,绝食

/ acid-ash ~ 酸化饮食 / bland ~ 清淡饮食 / diabetic ~ 糖尿病饮食 / elimination ~ 剔除饮食(饮食中剔除不致过敏的食物) / light ~ 清淡饮食,易消化饮食 / low ~ 素淡饮食 / low caloric ~ 低热量饮食 / low residue ~ 少渣饮食 / low salt ~ 低盐饮食 / provocative ~ 激发性饮食(包括最常见的变应原食物,然后一个个加以去除,作为决定食物变态反应触犯物的方法) / salt-free ~ 无盐饮食 / smooth ~ 细食

dietary [ˈdaiətəri] *n* 规定食物,食谱 *a* 规定食物的,饮食的

dietetic [ˌdaiəˈtetik] *a* 饮食的,营养的 | **~al** *a*

dietetics [ˌdaiəˈtetiks] *n* 饮食学,营养学

diethanolamine [ˌdaieθəˈnɔləmiːn] *n* 二乙醇胺(用作药用辅料〈碱化剂〉)

diethazine hydrochloride [daiˈeθəziːn] 盐酸二乙嗪(抗胆碱药,用作抗震颤麻痹药)

diethyl [daiˈeθil] *a* 二乙基的 | ~ ether, ~ oxide 乙醚

diethylamine [ˌdaieθiˈlæmiːn] *n* 二乙胺

diethylbarbituric acid [daiˌeθilbɑːbiˈtjuərik] 二乙巴比土酸,巴比妥

diethylcarbamazine [daiˌeθilkɑːˈbæməziːn] *n* 乙胺嗪(抗丝虫药,以枸橼酸乙胺嗪使用)

diethylene diamine [daiˌeθiliːn ˈdaiəmiːn] *n* 二乙烯二胺,哌嗪,胡椒嗪

1, 4-diethylene dioxide [daiˈeθiliːn daiˈɔksaid] 二噁烷(即 dioxane)

diethylene glycol [daiˈeθiliːn ˈglaikɔl] 二甘醇

diethylenetriamine pentaacetic acid (DTPA) [daiˌeθiliːnˈtraiəmiːn ˌpentəəˈsiːtik] 二亚乙基三胺五乙酸,喷替酸(解毒药)

diethylpropion hydrochloride [daiˌeθilˈprəupiən] 盐酸安非拉酮(拟肾上腺素药,用作口服食欲抑制药)

diethylstilbestrol (DES) [daiˌeθilstilˈbæstrɔl] *n* 己烯雌酚(治绝经期症状、阴道炎和抑制泌乳) | ~ dipropionate 丙酸己烯雌酚

diethyltoluamide [daiˌeθiltɔˈljuəmaid] *n* 二乙甲苯酰胺(驱避药)

diethyltryptamine (DET) [daiˌeθilˈtriptəmiːn] *n* 二乙色胺(致幻药)

dietitian, dietician [ˌdaiəˈtiʃən] *n* 饮食学家;营养医师

Dietl's crisis [ˈdiːtl] (Józef Dietl) 迪特尔危象(突然性肾痛,伴胃痛、恶心、呕吐及全身性虚脱等症状,据说是由肾脏蒂部部分扭转所致)

dietotherapy [ˌdaiətəuˈθerəpi] *n* 食治

dietotoxicity [ˌdaiətəutɔkˈsisəti] *n* 食物毒性(出现于饮食不均衡时) | **dietotoxic** [ˌdaiətəu ˈtɔksik] *a*

Dieudonné's medium (agar, culture) [djuːdɔˈnei] (Adolf Dieudonné) 迪厄多内培养基(用于分离霍乱弧菌的碱性血液琼脂)

Dieulafoy's aspirator [djuːləˈfwɑː] (Georges Dieulafoy) 迪厄拉富瓦吸引器(双管吸引器) | ~ theory 迪厄拉富瓦学说,阑尾阻塞学说(阑尾炎总是由于阑尾闭锁腔洞引起) / ~ triad 迪厄拉富瓦三征(阑尾炎时的皮肤过敏性、反射性肌收缩和麦克伯尼〈McBurney〉点压痛)

difenoxamide hydrochloride [ˌdaifəˈnɔksəmaid] 盐酸氰苯哌酰胺(抗肠蠕动药)

difenoxin [ˌdaifəˈnɔksin] *n* 地芬诺辛(抗肠蠕动药)

difference [ˈdifrəns] *n* 差,差异,差别 | arteriovenous (AV) oxygen ~ 动静脉血氧差

differential [difəˈrenʃəl] *a* 差别的,差异的 *n* 差异;差异因子

differentiate [difəˈrenʃieit] *vt* 鉴别;分化

differentiation [ˌdifərenʃiˈeiʃən] *n* 鉴别;分化[作用] | correlative ~, dependent ~ 相关分化(组织本身以外的因素所引起的分化) / functional ~ 功能分化 / invisible ~ 难见分化 / regional ~ 局部分化 / self ~ 自身分化(完全在组织内的因素所产生的分化)

difficulty [ˈdifikəlti] *n* 困难 | ~ urination 排尿困难

diffluence [ˈdifluəns] *n* 溶化,液化

diffluent [ˈdifluənt] *a* 易溶化的,液化的

Difflugia [diˈfluːdʒiə] *n* 沙壳虫属

diffraction [diˈfrækʃən] *n* 绕射,衍射 | ~ grating 衍射光栅(分光镜用) / X-ray ~ X 线衍射(研究细胞用,尤用于研究无机和有机晶体)

diffusate [diˈfjuːzit] *n* 渗出液;扩散物,弥散物

diffuse [diˈfuːs] *a* 扩散的,弥散的,弥漫的 [diˈfuːz] *vt, vi* 扩散,散布;弥散;弥漫

diffusible [diˈfjuːzəbl] *a* 可扩散的,弥漫性的 | **diffusibility** [diˌfjuːzəˈbiləti] *n* 扩散性,扩散率

diffusiometer [diˌfjuːziˈɔmitə] *n* 扩散率测定器,弥散率测定器

diffusion [diˈfjuːʒən] *n* 扩散,弥散 | double ~ 双[向]扩散(一种免疫扩散试验,试验时抗原和抗体扩散到一个共同区,若抗原和抗体在相互作用,则它们即结合而形成沉淀带) / gel ~ 凝胶扩散(抗原和抗体通过凝胶介质彼此向对方扩散而形成沉淀的一种试验) / single ~ 单向扩散 / single radial ~ 单向放射扩散(亦称放射免疫扩散)

diffusive [diˈfjuːsiv] *a* 扩散开的,弥散的

diflorasone diacetate [daiˈflɔːrəsəun] 双醋二氟拉松(局部用皮质类固醇,治疗某些皮肤病)

difluanine hydrochloride [daiˈfluːəniːn] 盐酸二氟嗪(中枢神经系统兴奋药)

diflucortolone [ˌdaifluːˈkɔːtələun] *n* 二氟可龙

（糖皮质激素）| ~ valerate 戊酸二氟可龙（糖皮质激素）
diflumidone sodium [daiˈfluːmidəun] 二氟米酮钠（抗炎药）
diflunisal [daiˈfluːnisæl] *n* 二氟尼柳（抗炎药）
difluprednate [ˌdaifluːˈpredneit] *n* 二氟泼尼酯（抗炎药）
diftalone [ˈdiftələun] *n* 地弗他酮（抗炎药）
Dig. digeratur【拉】蒸煮
digallic acid [daiˈgælik] 双没食子酸，鞣酸
digametic [ˌdaigəˈmetik] *a* 雌雄两性配子的；异型配子的
digastric [daiˈgæstrik] *a* 二腹的 *n* 二腹肌
digenesis [daiˈdʒenisis] *n* 世代交替
digenetic [ˌdaidʒiˈnetik] *a* 复殖的，两性（生殖）的（指吸虫和其他寄生虫）
DiGeorge's syndrome [diˈdʒɔːdʒ]（Angelo M. DiGeorge）德乔治综合征（一种先天性病，第三和第四咽囊发育缺陷导致胸腺和甲状旁腺发育不全，常伴先天性心脏缺损、大血管异常、食管闭锁和面部结构异常。亦称胸腺发育不全，咽囊综合征）
digest [diˈdʒest, dai-] *vt* 消化；蒸煮 *vi* 消化 [ˈdaidʒest] *n* 消化液；水解液
digestant [diˈdʒestənt, dai-] *a* 助消化的 *n* 助消化药
digester [diˈdʒestə, daiˈdʒestə] *n* 蒸煮器
digestible [diˈdʒestəbl, dai-] *a* 可消化的，易消化的 | **digestibility** [diˌdʒestəˈbiləti, dai-] *n* 可消化性
digestion [diˈdʒestʃən, dai-] *n* 消化[作用]，消化力；蒸煮[作用]，煮解 | gastric ~，peptic ~ 胃消化 / gastrointestinal ~ 胃肠消化 / parenteral ~ 胃肠外消化 / primary ~ 第一度消化，胃肠消化 / salivary ~ 唾液消化 / sludge ~ 污泥消化法
digestive [diˈdʒestiv, dai-] *a* 消化的 *n* 消化药
digit [ˈdidʒit] *n* 指，趾
digital [ˈdidʒitl] *a* 指的，趾的；指纹样的；数字的
digitalin [ˌdidʒiˈtælin] *n* 毛地黄苷
Digitalis [ˌdidʒiˈteilis] *n* 毛地黄属，洋地黄属
digitalis [ˌdidʒiˈteilis] *n* 毛地黄，洋地黄 | ~ leaf 毛地黄叶 / powdered ~，prepared ~ 毛地黄粉
digitalization [ˌdidʒitəlaiˈzeiʃən, -liˈz-] *n* 毛地黄化，洋地黄化
digitaloid [ˈdidʒitəlɔid] *a* 毛地黄样的，洋地黄样的
digitalose [ˈdidʒitələus] *n* 毛地黄糖，洋地黄糖
digitate [ˈdidʒiteit] *a* 指状[突]的
digitatio [ˌdidʒiˈteiʃiəu]（[复] **digitationes** [ˌdidʒiteiʃiˈəunez]）*n*【拉】指状突
digitation [ˌdidʒiˈteiʃən] *n* 指状突；指叉形切断术，指[畸形]成形术
digiti [ˈdidʒitai] *n* digitus 的复数
digitiform [ˈdidʒitifɔːm] *a* 指状的
digitigrade [ˈdidʒitiˌgreid] *n* 趾行
digitogenin [ˌdidʒiˈtɔdʒinin] *n* 毛地黄皂苷元，洋地黄皂苷元
digitonin [ˌdidʒiˈtəunin] *n* 毛地黄皂苷，洋地黄皂苷
digitoplantar [ˌdidʒitəuˈplæntə] *a* 趾跖的
digitoxigenin [ˌdidʒiˌtɔksiˈdʒenin, -ˈdʒiː-] *n* 洋地黄毒苷元，毛地黄毒苷配基
digitoxin [ˌdidʒiˈtɔksin] *n* 洋地黄毒苷（强心药）
digitoxose [ˌdidʒiˈtɔksəus] *n* 毛地黄毒糖，洋地黄毒糖
digitus [ˈdidʒitəs]（[复] **digiti** [ˈdidʒitai]）*n*【拉】指，趾
diglossia [daiˈglɔsiə] *n* 双舌[畸形]，舌裂[畸形]
diglutathione [daiˌgluːtəˈθaiəun] *n* 二谷胱甘肽
diglyceride [daiˈglisəraid] *n* 甘油二酯
diglyceride acyltransferase [daiˈglisəraid ˌæsilˈtrænsfəreis] 甘油二酯酰基转移酶
diglyceride kinase [daiˈglisəraid ˈkaineis] 甘油二酯激酶，二酰基甘油激酶
diglycoldisalicylic acid [daiˌglaikɔldaiˌsæliˈsilik] 双缩甲醇酰二水杨酸
dignathus [digˈneiθəs] *n* 双[下]颌畸胎
digoxigenin [didʒˌɔksiˈdʒenin, -ˈdʒiː-] *n* 异羟洋地黄毒苷元，毛地黄毒苷
digoxin [didʒˈɔksin] *n* 地高辛（强心药）
Digramma brauni [daiˈgræmə ˈbrɔːnai] *n* 双线绦虫
Di Guglielmo's disease (syndrome) [diː guːgˈliəlməu]（Giovanni Di Guglielmo）迪·古利莫病（综合征）（①巨红细胞性骨髓增殖；②红白血病）
digyny [ˈdaidʒini] *n* 双雌受精
diheterozygote [daiˌhetərəuˈzaigəut] *n* 双因子杂种，双因子杂合子
dihexyverine hydrochloride [ˌdaiheksiˈveəriːn] 盐酸双己维林（抗胆碱药，解痉药）
dihomocinchonine [daiˌhəuməˈsinkəniːn] *n* 二高辛可宁（制自金鸡纳皮的一种生物碱）
di huang【汉】地黄
dihybrid [daiˈhaibrid] *n* 双因子杂种，双因子杂合子
dihydrate [daiˈhaidreit] *n* 二水合物；二羧化物
dihydrated [daiˈhaidreitid] *a* 二水合的
dihydric [daiˈhaidrik] *a* 二氢的
dihydrobiopterin [daiˌhaidrəubaiˈɔptərin] *n* 二氢生物蝶呤
dihydrobiopterin synthetase deficiency [daiˌhaidrəubaiˈɔptərin ˈsinθiteis] 二氢生物蝶呤合

成酶缺乏症,高苯丙氨酸血症Ⅴ型

dihydrocholesterol [daiˌhaidrəukəˈlestərɔl] *n* 二氢胆固醇

dihydrocodeine [daiˌhaidrəuˈkəudiːn] *n* 双氢可待因(麻醉性镇痛药和镇咳药)

dihydrocodeinone [daiˌhaidrəuˈkəudiːnəun] *n* 二氢可待因酮 | ~ bitartrate, ~ tartrate 重酒石酸二氢可待因酮

dihydrocoenzyme Ⅰ [daiˌhaidrəukəuˈenzaim] *n* 二氢辅酶Ⅰ(还原型烟酰胺腺嘌呤二核苷酸)

dihydrocollidine [daiˌhaidrəuˈkɔlidin] *n* 二氢三甲吡啶,二氢可力丁(一种尸碱)

dihydrodiethylstilbestrol [daiˌhaidrəudaiˌeθilsˈtilˈbestrɔl] *n* 己[烷]雌酚,人造雌酚

dihydroergocornine [daiˌhaidrəuˌəːgəˈkɔːnin] *n* 二氢麦角柯宁碱(具有交感神经阻滞和抗肾上腺素作用)

dihydroergocristine [daiˌhaidrəuəːgəˈkristin] *n* 双氢麦角汀(具有交感神经阻滞和抗肾上腺素作用)

dihydroergocryptine [daiˌhaidrəuˌəːgəˈkriptin] *n* 二氢麦角隐亭(具有交感神经阻滞和抗肾上腺素作用)

dihydroergotamine [daiˌhaidrəuəːˈgɔtəmiːn] *n* 双氢麦角胺(抗偏头痛药)

dihydroergotamine mesylate [daiˌhaidrəuəːˈgɔtəmiːn] 甲磺双氢麦角胺(抗肾上腺素能药,用作血管收缩药治疗偏头痛)

dihydrofolate [daiˌhaidrəuˈfəuleit] *n* 二氢叶酸

dihydrofolate reductase [daiˌhaidrəuˈfəuleit riˈdʌkteis] 二氢叶酸还原酶

dihydrofolate reductase (DHFR) deficiency 二氢叶酸还原酶缺乏症

dihydrofolic acid [daiˌhaidrəuˈfəulik] 二氢叶酸

dihydrofolliculin [daiˌhaidrəufəˈlikjulin] *n* 雌二醇

dihydroindolone [daiˌhaidrəuˈindələun] *n* 二氢吲哚酮

dihydrol [daiˈhaidrɔl] *n* 二聚水

dihydrolipoamide [daiˌhaidrəuˌlipəuˈæmaid] *n* 二氢硫辛酰胺

dihydrolipoamide *S*-acetyltransferase [daiˌhaidrəuˌlipəuˈæmaid ˌæsitilˈtrænsfəreis] 二氢硫辛酰胺 *S*-乙酰[基]转移酶

dihydrolipoamide acyltransferase [daiˌhaidrəuˌlipəuˈæmaid ˌæsilˈtrænsfəreis] 二氢硫辛酰胺酰基转移酶

dihydrolipoamide dehydrogenase [daiˌhaidrəuˌlipəuˈæmaid diːˈhaidrədʒəneis] 二氢硫辛酰胺脱氢酶

dihydrolipoamide *S*-succinyltransferase [daiˌhaidrəulipəuˈæmaidˌsʌksinilˈtrænsfəreis] 二氢硫辛酰胺 *S*-琥珀酰[基]转移酶

dihydrolipoyl [daiˌhaidrəuˈlipəuil] *n* 二氢硫辛酰胺酰基

dihydrolipoyltransacetylase [daiˌhaidrəuˌlipəuiltrænsˈæsitileis] 二氢硫辛酰胺转乙酰酶

dihydrolutidine [daiˌhaidrəuˈluːtidin] *n* 二氢路提丁

dihydromorphinone [daiˌhaidrəuˈmɔːfinəun] *n* 二氢吗啡酮

dihydroorotase [daiˌhaidrəuˈɔːrəteis] *n* 二氢乳清酸酶

dihydroorotate [daiˌhaidrəuˈɔːrəteit] *n* 二氢乳清酸盐

dihydroporphyrin [daiˌhaidrəuˈpɔːfirin] *n* 二氢卟啉

dihydropteridine reductase [daiˌhaidrəuˈteridiːn riˈdʌkteis] 二氢蝶啶还原酶(此酶缺乏为一种常染色体隐性性状,可致恶性高苯丙氨酸血症)

dihydropteridine reductase (DHPR) deficiency 二氢蝶啶还原酶缺乏症,高苯丙氨酸血症Ⅳ型

dihydropyrimidine dehydrogenase (NADP) [daiˌhaidrəupəˈrimidiːn diːˈhaidrədʒəneis] 二氢嘧啶脱氢酶(NADP)(此酶缺乏为一种常染色体隐性遗传病,可导致血浆、尿和脑脊液内嘧啶水平增高;临床表现儿童为大脑功能障碍,成人为对药物氟尿嘧啶过敏反应)

dihydrostreptomycin [daiˌhaidrəustreptəuˈmaisin] *n* 双氢链霉素 | ~ sulfate 硫酸双氢链霉素(抗生素类药,由于它对人有毒性,现仅用于兽医)

dihydrotachysterol [daiˌhaidrəutæˈkistərɔl] *n* 双氢速甾醇(治低钙血症药)

dihydrotestosterone [daiˌhaidrəutesˈtɔstərəun] *n* 双氢睾酮(强效雄激素)

dihydrotheelin [daiˌhaidrəuˈθiːlin] *n* 雌二醇

dihydrouracil dehydrogenase ($NADP^+$) [daiˌhaidrəuˈjuərəsil diːˈhaidrədʒəneis] 二氢尿嘧啶脱氢酶($NADP^+$),二氢嘧啶脱氢酶(NADP)

dihydroxy [ˌdaihaiˈdrɔksi] *n* 二羟[基]

3,4-dihydroxyphenylglycol (DHPG) [ˌdaihaiˌdrɔksiˌfenilˈglaikɔl] 3,4-二羟[基]苯乙二醇(去甲肾上腺素的代谢物,嗜铬细胞瘤时水平可能增高)

dihydroxyacetone [ˌdaihaiˌdrɔksiˈæsitəun] *n* 二羟丙酮 | ~ phosphate 磷酸二羟丙酮

2,8-dihydroxyadenine (DHA) [ˌdaihaiˌdrɔksiˈædəniːn] *n* 2,8-二羟腺嘌呤(此嘌呤蓄积可致晶尿症和肾石病)

dihydroxyaluminum [ˌdaihaiˌdrɔksiəˈljuːminəm] *n* 二羟铝 | ~ aminoacetate 甘羟铝(抗酸药)

3, 6-dihydroxycholanic acid [ˌdaihaiˌdrɔksikəu-ˈlænik] 3, 6-二羟基胆烷酸,猪脱氧胆酸
1, 25-dihydroxycholecalciferol [ˌdaihaiˌdrɔksi-ˌkəulikælˈsifərɔl] *n* 1, 25-二羟胆钙化醇,1, 25-二羟维生素 D_3
dihydroxyestrin [ˌdaihaiˌdrɔksiˈiːstrin, -ˈes-] *n* 雌二醇
dihydroxyfluorane [ˌdaihaiˌdrɔksiˈfluərein] *n* 二羟基荧烷,荧光素
2, 5-dihydroxyphenylacetic acid [ˌdaihaiˌdrɔk-siˌfeniləˈsiːtik] 2, 5-二羟苯乙酸,尿黑酸
3, 4-dihydroxyphenylalanine [ˌdaihaiˌdrɔksiˌfe-niˈlæləniːn] *n* 3, 4-二羟苯丙氨酸,多巴(即 dopa)
4, 8-dihydroxyquinaldic acid [ˌdaihaiˌdrɔksikw-iˈnældik] 4, 8-二羟基喹啉甲酸,黄尿酸
dihydroxystearic acid [ˌdaihaiˌdrɔksistiˈærik] 二羟硬脂酸
1, 25-dihydroxyvitamin D [ˌdaihaiˌdrɔksiˈvaitə-min] 1, 25-二羟维生素 D
dihydroxyvitamin D_3 [ˌdaihaiˌdrɔksiˈvaitəmin] 二羟维生素 D_3 | 1, 25- ~ 1, 25-二羟维生素 D_3, 1, 25-羟胆钙化醇
dihypercytosis [daiˌhaipəsaiˈtəusis] *n* 中性粒细胞过多性白细胞增多
dihysteria [ˌdaihisˈtiəriə] *n* 双子宫
diiodide [daiˈaiəudaid] *n* 二碘化物
diiodocarbazol [daiˌaiədəuˈkɑːbəzɔl] *n* 二碘咔唑(防腐剂)
diiodofluorescein [ˌdaiaiˌɔdəuˌfluəˈresin] *n* 二碘荧光素(用作吸收指示剂)
diiodoform [ˌdaiaiˈɔdəfɔːm] *n* 二碘仿(强力结瘢剂)
diiodohydroxyquin [ˌdaiaiˌɔdəuhaiˈdrɔksikwin] *n* 双碘喹啉(抗阿米巴药)
diiodosalicylic acid [daiˌaiədəuˌsæliˈsilik] 二碘水杨酸
3, 5-diiodothyronine [ˌdaiaiˌɔdəuˈθairəniːn] *n* 3, 5-二碘甲状腺氨酸(用于制造甲状腺素)
diiodotyrosine [ˌdaiaiˌɔdəuˈtairəsiːn] *n* 双碘酪氨酸(甲状腺激素类)
diisocyanate [daiˌaisəuˈsaiəneit] *n* 二异氰酸
diisopropyl fluorophosphate (**DFP**) [daiˌai-səuˈprɔpil ˌfluərəuˈfɔsfeit] 氟磷酸二异丙酯,异氟磷(乙酰胆碱酯酶抑制药)
Dikaryomycota [daiˌkæriəumaiˈkəutə] *n* 双核真菌门
dikaryon [daiˈkæriɔn] *n* 双核体
dikaryote [daiˌkæriəut] *n* 双核细胞
dikaryotic [ˌdaikæriˈɔtik] *a* 双核的;双核细胞的
diketone [daiˈkiːtəun] *n* 二酮
diketopiperazine [daiˌkiːtəupaiˈperəzin] *n* 二酮哌嗪,环缩二氨酸
diktyoma [ˌdiktiˈəumə] *n* 视网膜胚瘤
dikwakwadi [ˌdikwækˈwædi] *n* 头皮白痂病(黄癣)
dil. dilue【拉】稀释
dilaceration [daiˌlæsəˈreiʃən] *n* 撕裂,撕除(白内障);弯曲(牙);裂痕(牙)
dilatant [daiˈleitənt] *a* 膨胀的,扩张的 | **dilatancy** *a* 膨胀性,扩张性
dilatation [ˌdailəˈteiʃən] *n* 扩大;扩张;扩张术 | ~ and curettage 刮宫术 / ~ of cervix 宫口扩张 / ~ of the cervix 宫颈扩张术 / digital ~ 指扩张术 / ~ of the heart 心脏扩大 / prognathic ~, prognathion ~ 幽门端扩张 / ~ of the stomach, gastric ~ 胃扩张 | **~al** *a*
dilatator [ˌdailəˈteitə] *n* 扩张器,开大肌
dilate [daiˈleit] *vt, vi* 扩大;扩张
dilation [daiˈleiʃən] *n* 扩大;扩张术 | digital ~ 指扩张术
dilator [daiˈleitə] *n* 开大肌;扩张器 | anal ~ 肛门扩张器 / laryngeal ~ 喉扩张器
dilecanus [dailiˈkeinəs] *n* 双臀畸胎
Dilepididae [ˌdiləˈpididiː] *n* 囊宫[绦虫]科
dill [dil] *n* 莳萝,小茴香
diltiazem hydrochloride [dilˈtaiəzəm] 盐酸地尔硫䓬(冠状动脉扩张药)
Diluc. diluculo【拉】拂晓时,天明时
diluent [ˈdiljuənt] *a* 稀释的 *n* 稀释剂
dilut. dilutus【拉】稀释的
dilute [daiˈljuːt] *vt* 稀释 *a* 稀释的
dilution [daiˈljuːʃən] *n* 稀释;稀释法 | doubling ~ 二倍稀释 / nitrogen ~ 氮稀释 / serial ~ 连续稀释,系列稀释
dim. dimidius【拉】半的,二分之一的
dimargarin [daiˈmɑːgərin] *n* 二珠脂酸甘油酯
Dimastigamoeba [daiˌmæstigəˈmiːbə] *n* 双鞭阿米巴属,双鞭变形虫属(即耐格里原虫属 Naegleria)
dimefadane [daiˈmefədein] *n* 二甲法登(镇痛药)
dimefilcon A [ˌdaiməˈfilkɔn] 地美费康 A(一种亲水性接触镜材料)
dimefline [daiˈmefliːn] *n* 二甲弗林(中枢兴奋药) | ~ hydrochloride 盐酸二甲弗林(呼吸兴奋药)
dimeglumine [daiˌmegluˈmiːn] *n* 双葡[甲]胺盐
dimelia [daiˈmiːliə] *n* 复肢[畸形]
dimelus [daiˈmiːləs] *n* 复肢畸胎
dimenhydrinate [ˌdaimənˈhaidrineit] *n* 茶苯海明(抗晕动病药)
dimension [diˈmenʃən] *n* 尺度;量纲,因次;维,度 | vertical ~ 垂直尺度;垂直距离(牙) | **~al** *a*
dimensionless [diˈmenʃənlis, daiˈmenʃənlis] *a* 无

维的,无因次的

dimer [ˈdaimə] *n* 二[聚]体,二聚物;二壳粒 | thymine ~ 胸腺嘧啶二聚体 | **~ic** [daiˈmerik] *a*

dimercaprol [ˌdaiməˈkæprɔl] *n* 二巯丙醇(解砷及金属中毒药)

dimerous [ˈdimərəs] *a* 由两部分组成的

dimetallic [ˌdaimiˈtælik] *a* 二[原子]金属的

dimethacrylate [ˌdaiməˈθækrileit] *n* 二异丁烯酸

dimethadione [daiˌmeθəˈdaiəun] *n* 二甲双酮(抗惊厥药)

dimethicone [daiˈmeθikəun] *n* 二甲硅油(消泡药)

dimethindene maleate [ˌdaiməˈθindiːn] 马来酸二甲茚定(抗组胺药)

dimethisoquin hydrochloride [ˌdaimeˈθaisəkwin] 盐酸二甲异喹,盐酸奎尼卡因(局部麻醉药)

dimethisterone [ˌdaimeˈθistərəun] *n* 地美炔酮(孕激素类药)

dimethoxanate [daimeˈθɔksəneit] *n* 地美索酯(镇咳药) | ~ hydrochloride 盐酸地美索酯(镇咳药)

2, 5-dimethoxy-4-methylamphetamine (DOM) [ˌdaimeˌθɔksiˌmeθilæmˈfetəmiːn] *n* 2, 5-二甲氧基-4-甲基苯丙胺(致幻药)

3, 4-dimethoxyphenylethylamine (DMPE) [daimeˌθɔksiˌfeniˌleθiˈlæmin] *n* 3, 4-二甲氧基苯乙胺

dimethylacetal [ˌdaimeθiˈlæsitæl] *n* 二甲缩醛

dimethylamine [daiˌmeθiˈlæmin] *n* 二甲胺

***p*-dimethylaminoazobenzene** [daiˌmeθiˌlæminəuˌæzəuˈbenziːn] *n* 二甲氨基偶氮苯,甲基黄

dimethylaminopropionitrile (DMAPN) [daiˌmeθiləˌmiːnəuˌprəupiəuˈnaitril] *n* 二甲氨基丙腈(一种无色水溶性液体,用以制造聚氨酯泡沫,工人过多接触易患泌尿系疾患和神经障碍)

dimethylarsine [daiˌmeθiˈlɑːsin] *n* 二甲胂

dimethylarsinic acid [daiˌmeθilɑːˈsinik] *n* 二甲胂酸

7, 12-dimethylbenz[a]anthracene [daiˌmeθilbenˈzænθrəsiːn] 7, 12-二甲[基]苯并蒽

dimethylbenzene [daiˌmeθilˈbenziːn] *n* 二甲苯

5, 6-dimethylbenzimidazole [ˌdaimeθilˌbenziˈmidəzəul] 5, 6-二甲[基]苯并咪唑

dimethylcarbamyl chloride [daiˌmeθilˈkɑːbəmil] 二甲基氨基甲酰氯(一种无色液体,用作化学中间体,制造药物制品、染料和杀虫剂,具有催泪并致癌性质)

dimethyl carbate [daiˈmeθil ˈkɑːbeit] 驱蚊灵

dimethylcarbinol [daiˌmeθilˈkɑːbinɔl] *n* 异丙醇

dimethylcolchicinic acid [daiˌmeθilˌkɔltʃiˈsinik] 二甲秋水仙酸

dimethylethylpyrrole [daiˌmeθiˌleθilˈpirɔl] *n* 二甲基乙基吡咯

dimethylformamide (DMF) [daiˌmeθilˈfɔːməmaid] *n* 二甲基甲酰胺

***N, N*-dimethylglycine** [daiˌmeθilˈglaisiːn] *n* *N, N*-二甲基甘氨酸

dimethylglycine dehydrogenase [daiˌmeθilˈglaisiːn diːˈhaidrədʒəneis] 二甲基甘氨酸脱氢酶

dimethylguanidine [daiˌmeθilˈguænidin] *n* 二甲胍

dimethylketone [daiˌmeθilˈkiːtəun] *n* 二甲酮,丙酮

dimethylnitrosamine [daiˌmeθilnaiˈtrəusəmiːn] 二甲基亚硝胺,*N*-亚硝基二甲胺

dimethylphenanthrene [daiˌmeθilfiˈnænθriːn] *n* 二甲菲

dimethyl-*p*-phenylenediamine [daiˌmeθilˌfeniliːnˈdaiəmiːn] *n* 二甲[基]-*p*-苯二胺

dimethylphosphine [daiˌmeθilˈfɔsfiːn] *n* 二甲膦

dimethyl phthalate [daiˈmeθil ˈθæleit] 酞酸二甲酯(驱虫药)

dimethyl sulfate [daiˈmeθil ˈsʌlfeit] 硫酸二甲酯(工业毒物及军用毒气)

dimethyl sulfoxide (DMSO) [daiˈmeθil sʌlˈfɔksaid] 二甲亚砜(消炎止痛药)

dimethyltryptamine (DMT) [daiˌmeθilˈtriptəmiːn] *n* 二甲色胺(致幻药)

dimetria [daiˈmiːtriə] *n* 双子宫[畸形]

dimetridazole [ˌdaiməˈtraidəzəul] *n* 地美硝唑(抗原虫药,用于抗火鸡组织滴虫病)

diminazene aceturate [daiˈminəziːn] 乙酰甘氨酸二脒那秦(抗原虫药,用于抗巴贝虫属和锥虫属)

diminish [diˈminiʃ] *vt* 减小,缩减 *vi* 变小,缩小

diminution [dimiˈnjuːʃən] *n* 减少,减小,缩减

diminutive [diˈminjutiv] *a* 小的,小型的

Dimmer's keratitis [ˈdimə] (Friedrich Dimmer) 钱币状角膜炎

dimorphism [daiˈmɔːfizəm] *n* 二形性,二态性,双态现象 | physical ~ 物理二态 / sexual ~ 两性异型

dimorphobiotic [daiˌmɔːfəbaiˈɔtik] *a* 二形生活的,二态生活的

dimorphous [daiˈmɔːfəs], **dimorphic** [daiˈmɔːfik] *a* 二形的,二态的

dimoxamine hydrochloride [daiˈmɔksəmiːn] 盐酸地莫沙明(记忆佐药)

dimoxyline phosphate [daiˈmɔksiliːn] 磷酸地莫昔林(血管扩张药,解痉药)

dimple [ˈdimpl] *n* 小凹,浅凹;颊窝,笑靥 | postanal ~ 尾小凹

dimpling [ˈdimpliŋ] *n* 小凹形成

dineric [daiˈnerik] *a* 二媒液的

dineuric [dai'njuərik] *a* 二轴突的(指神经细)
dinical ['dinikl] *a* 眩晕的
dinitrate [dai'naitreit] *n* 二硝酸盐
dinitrated [dai'naitreitid] *a* 二硝化的
dinitroaminophenol [dai,naitrəu,æminəu'fi:nɔl] *n* 二硝基氨基酚
dinitrobenzene [dai,naitrəu'benzi:n] *n* 二硝基苯
dinitrocellulose [dai,naitrəu'seljuləus] *n* 硝基纤维素,火棉
dinitrochlorobenzene [dai,naitrə u ,klɔ(:)rə'benzi:n] *n* 二硝基氯苯(将致敏剂量用于测生物体对形成迟发接触性变应性反应的能力)
dinitrocresol [dai,naitrəu'kri:sɔl] *n* 二硝基甲酚(杀虫药)
dinitrofluorobenzene [dai,naitrəu,fluərəu'benzi:n] *n* 二硝基氟苯
dinitrogen [dai'naitrədʒən] *a* 二氮 | ~ monoxide 一氧化二氮,氧化亚氮
dinitrophenol [dai,naitrəu'fi:nɔl] *n* 二硝基苯酚(曾建议用以治黏液性水肿及肥胖,据报告为粒细胞缺乏症及内障的原因,现仅用作试剂及指示剂,还常用作半抗原)
dinitroresorcinol [dai,naitrəuri'sɔ:sinɔl] *n* 二硝基间苯二酚(研究神经组织用)
dinitrotoluene [dai,naitrəu'tɔljui:n] *n* 二硝基[甲]苯(一种极毒晶体化合物,用以制造染料和炸药,容易渗入皮肤,为一种潜在致癌物)
Dinobdella [,dainɔb'delə] *n* 恐蛭属
Dinoflagellata [,dainəuflædʒe'leitə] *n* 腰鞭毛目
dinoflagellate [,dainəu'flædʒəleit] *a* 腰鞭毛目的 *n* 腰鞭毛虫
Dinoflagellida [,dainəuflæ'dʒəlidə] *n* 腰鞭毛目
dinogunellin [,dainəu'gʌnəlin] *n* 鳚毒蛋白
dinoprost ['dainəprɔst] *n* 地诺前列素,前列腺素 F_{2a}(堕胎药) | ~ tromethamine, ~ trometanol 前列腺素 F_{2a} 缓血酸胺盐(催产药,堕胎药)
dinoprostone [,dainə'prɔstəun] *n* 地诺前列酮,前列腺素 E_2(PGE_2)(催产药)
dinormocytosis [dai,nɔ:məusai'təusis] *n* 等比例白细胞正常
D. in p. aeq. divide in partes aequales【拉】分成等分
dinsed ['dinsid] *n* 定磺胺(家禽抗球虫药)
dinucleotide [dai'nju:kliətaid] *n* 二核苷酸
Dioctophyme [dai,ɔktə'faim] *n* 膨结线虫属 | ~ renale 肾膨结线虫
Dioctophymidae [dai,ɔktəu'faimidi:] *n* 膨结[线虫]科
Dioctophymoidea [dai,ɔktəu,fai'mɔidiə] *n* 膨结(线虫)总科
dioctyl calcium sulfosuccinate [dai'ɔktil] 多库酯钙(即 docusate calcium)
dioctyl sodium sulfosuccinate [dai'ɔktil] 多库酯钠(即 docusate sodium)
Diodon ['daiədɔn] *n* 刺鲀属
dioecious [dai'i:ʃəs] *a* 雌雄异体的
diogenism [dai'ɔdʒinizəm] *n* (源自公元前5世纪古希腊哲学家 Diogenes)迪奥杰尼斯主义(主张废除文化,返回原始)
diolamine [dai'ɔləmi:n] *n* 二乙醇胺(diethanolamine 的 USAN 缩约词)
diopsimeter [,daiɔp'simitə] *n* 视野计
diopter, dioptre [dai'ɔptə] *n* 屈光度
dioptometer [,daiɔp'tɔmitə], **dioptrometer** [,daiɔp'trɔmitə] *n* 屈光计
dioptometry [,daiɔp'tɔmitri], **dioptrometry** [,daiɔp'trɔmitri] *n* 屈光测量
dioptoscopy [,daiɔp'tɔskəpi], **dioptroscopy** [,daiɔp'trɔskəpi] *n* 屈光测量法
dioptric(al) [dai'ɔptrik(əl)] *a* 屈光(学)的,折射的
dioptrics [dai'ɔptriks] *n* 屈光学
dioptry ['daiəptri] *n* 屈光度
dioscin [dai'ɔskin] *n* 薯蓣皂苷
Dioscorea [,daiɔs'kɔ:riə] *n* 薯蓣属 | ~ mexicana 墨西哥薯蓣
diose ['daiəus] *n* 二糖
diosgenin [dai'ɔsdʒənin] *n* 薯蓣皂苷元薯蓣皂苷配基
diospyrobezoar [,daiɔs,paiərəu'bi:zɔ:] *n* 柿石
diovulatory [dai'əuvjulətəri] *a* 排二卵的
dioxane [dai'ɔksein] *n* 二噁烷
dioxide [dai'ɔksaid] *n* 二氧化物
dioxin [dai'ɔksin] *n* 二噁英,二氧[杂]芑(据认为具有致癌和致畸形性质)
dioxybenzone [dai,ɔksi'benzəun] *n* 二羟苯宗(防晒药)
dioxygen [dai'ɔksidʒən] *n* 分子氧(O_2)
dioxygenase [dai'ɔksidʒəneis] *n* 二氧化酶
dioxyline phosphate [dai'ɔksili:n] *n* 磷酸二氧林(冠状血管及外周血管扩张药)
dipentene [dai'penti:n] *n* 二戊烯
dipeptidase [dai'peptideis] *n* 二肽酶
dipeptide [dai'peptaid] *n* 二肽
dipeptidyl carboxypeptidase I [dai'peptidil kɑ:,bɔksi'peptideis] 二肽酰羧肽酶 I,肽基二肽酶 A
dipeptidyl-peptidase [dai,peptidil'peptideis] 二肽酰肽酶
dipeptidyl-peptidase I [dai'peptidil 'peptideis] 二肽酰肽酶 I(亦称组蛋白酶 C)
diperodon [dai'perədɔn] *n* 地哌冬(局部麻醉药) | ~ hydrochloride 盐酸地哌冬(局部麻醉药)
Dipetalonema [dai,petələ'ni:mə] *n* 棘唇[线虫]

属 | ~ perstans 常现棘唇线虫 / ~ recondium 隐现棘唇线虫 / ~ streptocerca 链尾棘唇线虫

dipetalonemiasis [daiˌpetələniˈmaiəsis] *n* 棘唇线虫病

diphacenone [daiˈfeisənəun] *n* 二苯茚酮(抗凝药)

diphallia [daiˈfæliə] *n* 双阴茎[畸形]

diphallus [ˈdaifæləs] *n* 双阴茎畸胎

diphase [ˈdaifeiz], **diphasic** [daiˈfeizik] *a* 二相性的,双相的

diphebuzol [daiˈfebjuzɔl] *n* 保泰松(治痛风及镇痛药)

diphemanil methylsulfate [daiˈfiːmənil] 甲硫酸二苯马尼(抗胆碱药,用于治疗消化性溃疡、胃酸过多、胃炎和幽门痉挛时的蠕动过强,以及用于治疗多汗症)

diphenadione [daiˌfenəˈdaiəun] *n* 二苯茚酮(抗凝药)

diphenhydramine hydrochloride [ˌdaifenˈhaidrəmiːn] 盐酸苯海拉明(抗组胺药)

diphenicillin [ˌdaifeniˈsilin] *n* 联苯青霉素

diphenidol [daiˈfenidəul] *n* 地芬尼多(镇吐药) | ~ hydrochloride 盐酸地芬尼多 / ~ pamoate 双羟萘酸地芬尼多

diphenol oxidase [daiˈfiːnɔl ˈɔksideis] 二酚氧化酶,儿茶酚氧化酶

diphenoxylate hydrochloride [ˌdaifəˈnɔksileit] 盐酸地芬诺酯(止泻药)

diphenyl [daiˈfiːnil] *n* 二苯基;联[二]苯

diphenylamine [daiˌfeniˈlæmiːn] *n* 二苯胺

diphenylaminearsine chloride [daiˌfeniˌlæmiːnˈɑːsin] 氯化二苯胺胂(喷嚏性毒气)

diphenylamine chlorarsine [daiˈfeniləˌmiːn ˌklɔːˈrɑːsiːn] 二苯胺氯胂

diphenylamino-azo-benzene [daiˌfeniˌlæminəu-ˌæzəuˈbenziːn] *n* 二苯胺[基]偶氮苯(一种指示剂 pH 1.2 ~2.1)

diphenylbutylpiperidine [daiˌfenilˌbjuːtilpiˈperidiːn] *n* 二苯丁基哌啶(任何一类结构上有关的抗精神病药,包括五氟利多 penfluridol 和匹莫齐特 pimozide)

diphenylchlorarsine [daiˌfenilklɔˈrɑːsin] *n* 二苯氯[化]胂(一种刺激呼吸道黏膜的毒气)

diphenylcyanarsine [daiˌfenilˌsaiəˈnɑːsin] *n* 二苯氰[化]胂(一种致死性毒气)

diphenyldiimide [daiˌfenilˈdaiimaid] *n* 二苯基偶氮,偶氮苯

diphenylhydantoin [daiˌfenilhaiˈdæntəuin] *n* 二苯乙内酰脲,苯妥英(抗癫痫药)

diphenylnitrosamine [daiˌfenilnaiˈtrəusəmiːn] *n* 二苯亚硝胺,*N*-亚硝基二苯胺

diphenylpyraline hydrochloride [daiˌfenilˈpiərəliːn] 盐酸二苯拉林(抗组胺药,用于缓解变态反应的症状,口服)

diphonia [daiˌfəuniə] *n* 复音,双音

diphosgene [daiˈfɔsdʒiːn] *n* 双光气,氯甲酸三氯甲酯(一种毒气,对肺有强烈刺激性,可产生肺水肿)

diphosphatidylglycerol [ˌdaifɔsfəˌtaidilˈglisərɔl] *n* 双磷脂酰甘油(1, 3-diphosphatidylglycerol 为心磷脂〈cardiolipin〉)

2,3-diphosphoglycerate [daiˌfɔsfəuˈglisəreit] *n* 2,3-二磷酸甘油酸

diphosphoglycerate mutase [daiˌfɔsfəuˈglisəreit ˈmjuːteis] 二磷酸甘油酸变位酶

diphosphoglycerate phosphatase [daiˌfɔsfəu-ˈglisəreit ˈfɔsfəteis] 二磷酸甘油酸磷酸酶

diphosphonate [daiˈfɔsfəneit] *n* 二膦酸,二膦酸盐(或酯) | methylene ~ (MDP) 亚甲基二膦酸(用于骨扫描)

diphosphonic acid [ˌdaifɔsˈfɔnik] 二膦酸

diphosphopyridine nucleotide (DPN) [daiˌfɔsfəuˈpiridiːn] 二磷酸吡啶核苷酸(烟酰胺腺嘌呤二核苷酸 nicotinamide adenine dinucleotide 〈NAD〉的旧称)

diphosphothiamin [daiˌfɔsfəˈθaiəmin] *n* 焦磷酸硫胺素,辅羧酶

diphosphotransferase [ˌdaifɔsfəuˈtrænsfəreis] *n* 二磷酸转移酶(亦称焦磷酸转移酶)

diphtheria [difˈθiəriə] *n* 白喉 | avian ~, fowl ~ 家禽白喉 / calf ~ 牛白喉 / cutaneous ~ 皮肤白喉 / false ~ 假白喉 / faucial ~ 咽白喉 / laryngeal ~ 喉白喉,膜性喉炎 / malignant ~, ~ gravis 恶性白喉 / pharyngeal ~ 咽白喉 / surgical ~, wound ~ 外科白喉,创伤白喉 | **~l** *a*

diphtheric [difˈθerik], **diphtheritic** [ˌdifθiˈritik] *a* 白喉的

diphtherin [ˈdifθirin] *n* 白喉菌素(多价白喉抗原,用于过敏性皮肤试验)

diphtheritis [ˌdifθiˈraitis] *n* 白喉

diphtheroid [ˈdifθərɔid] *a* 类白喉的,白喉样的 *n* 假白喉;非白喉棒状杆菌;丙酸杆菌

diphtherotoxin [ˌdifθərəuˈtɔksin] *n* 白喉毒素

diphthongia [difˈθɔndʒiə] *n* 复音,双音

Diphylla [daiˈfilə] *n* 吸血蝠属,魑蝠属

diphyllobothriasis [diˌfiləubɔˈθraiəsis] *n* 裂头绦虫病

Diphyllobothriidae [daiˌfiləubɔˈθriidiː] *n* 裂头[绦虫]科

Diphylobothrium [daiˌfiləuˈbɔθriəm] *n* 裂头[绦虫]属 | ~ cordatum 心形裂头绦虫 / ~ erinacei, ~ mansoni 猬裂头绦虫,曼[森]氏裂头绦虫 / ~ latum, ~ taenioides 阔节裂头绦虫 / ~ mansonoides 类曼[森]氏裂头绦虫 / ~ parvum

小裂头绦虫

diphyodont [ˈdifiəˌdɔnt] *a* 双套牙[列]的(有乳牙恒牙的)

dipipanone hydrochloride [daiˈpipənəun] 盐酸地匹哌酮(镇痛药)

dipivefrin [diˈpivəfrin] *n* 地匹福林(眼科用拟肾上腺素药,抗青光眼药)

diplacusis [ˌdipləˈkuːsis] *n* 复听 | binaural ~ 双耳复听 / disharmonic ~ [双耳]不协调性复听 / echo ~ [双耳]回声性复听 / monaural ~ 单耳复听 | **diplacusia** [ˌdipləˈkuːziə] *n*

diplasmatic [ˌdaiplæzˈmætik] *a* 含二要质的(细胞)

diplegia [daiˈpliːdʒiə] *n* 双侧瘫痪,双瘫 | atonic-astatic ~ 弛缓性双瘫 / facial ~ 两侧面瘫 / infantile ~ 婴儿双瘫,产伤瘫痪 / masticatory ~ 两侧嚼肌瘫 / spastic ~ 痉挛性双瘫 | **diplegic** *a*

dipl(o)-[构词成分]双,两

diploalbuminuria [ˌdipləuælˌbjuːmiˈnjuəriə] *n* (生理性及病理性)双蛋白尿

diplobacillus [ˌdipləubəˈsiləs] ([复] **diplobacilli** [ˌdipləubəˈsilai]), **diplobacterium** [ˌdipləubækˈtiəriəm] ([复] **diplobacteria** [ˌdipləubækˈtiəriə]) *n* 双杆菌

diploblastic [ˌdipləuˈblæstik] *n* 二胚层的

diplocardia [ˌdipləuˈkɑːdiə] *n* 心裂[畸形]

diplocephalus [ˌdipləuˈsefələs] *n* 双头畸胎

diplocephaly [ˌdipləuˈsefəli] *n* 双头[畸形]

diplococcoid [ˌdipləuˈkɔkɔid] *a* 双球菌样的 *n* 类双球菌

Diplococcus [ˌdipləuˈkɔkəs] *n* 双球菌属 | ~ constellatus 星形双球菌 / ~ intracellularis 脑膜炎双球菌 / ~ magnus 大双球菌 / ~ morbillorum 麻疹双球菌 / ~ mucosus 黏液双球菌 / ~ paleopneumoniae 厌氧肺炎双球菌 / ~ plagarumbelli 战伤双球菌 / ~ pneumoniae 肺炎双球菌

diplococcus [ˌdipləuˈkɔkəs] ([复] **diplococci** [ˌdipləuˈkɔkai, ˌdipləuˈkɔksai]) *n* 双球菌 | **diplococcal** *a*

diplocoria [ˌdipləuˈkɔːriə] *n* 重瞳[畸形]

Diplodia [diˈpləudiə] *n* 色二孢属

diplodiosis [ˌdipləudiˈəusis], **diplodiatoxicosis** [ˌdipləudaiəˌtɔksiˈkəusis] *n* 色二孢霉菌中毒症

Diplodinium [ˌdipləuˈdiniəm] *n* 倍环纤虫属

diploë [ˈdipləiː] *n* 【希】板障(颅骨间松疏骨质) | **diploetic** [ˌdipləˈetik] *a*

Diplogaster [ˈdipləuˌgæstə] *n* 双胃属

diplogenesis [ˌdipləuˈdʒenisis] *n* 联胎成长,联胎产生

Diplogonoporus [ˌdipləugəˈnɒpərəs] *n* 复殖孔属 | ~ grandis 大复殖孔[绦]虫

diplogram [ˈdipləgræm] *n* 重复 X 线[照]片

diploic [dipˈləuik] *a* 两倍的,双的;板障的

diploid [ˈdiplɔid] *a* 二倍的;二倍体的 *n* 二倍体(含有二组同源染色体的个体或细胞) | **~y** *n* 二倍性

diplokaryon [ˌdipləuˈkæriɔn] *n* 二倍核(染色体)

diplomonad [ˌdipləuˈməunæd] *n*, *a* 双滴虫(的)

Diplomonadida [ˌdipləuməˈnædidə] *n* 双滴虫目

Diplomonadina [ˌdipləuˌmɔnəˈdainə] *n* 双滴虫亚目

diplomyelia [ˌdipləumaiˈiːliə] *n* 双干脊髓

diplon [ˈdiplɔn] *n* 氘核

diplonema [ˌdipləuˈniːmə] *n* 双线(双线期的双染色体)

diplont [ˈdiplɔnt] *n* 二倍性生物(个体由二倍体细胞所构成的生物)

diplopagus [dipˈlɔpəgəs] *n* 对称性联胎

diplophase [ˈdipləufeiz] *n* 二倍期(某些生物体的生活史其核为二倍体的阶段)

diplophonia [ˌdipləuˈfəuniə] *n* 复音,双音

diplopia [diˈpləupiə] *n* 复视 | crossed ~, heteronymous ~, paradoxical ~ 交叉性复视 / direct ~, homonymous ~ 同侧性复视 | **diplopic** *a*

diplopiometer [diˌpləupiˈɔmitə] *n* 复视计

Diplopoda [daiˈplɔpədə] *n* 倍足亚纲

Diplopylidium [ˌdipləupaiˈlidiəm] *n* 复孔[绦虫]属

diploscope [ˈdipləskəup] *n* 两眼视力检器,两眼视力计

diplosomatia [ˌdipləusəuˈmeiʃiə], **diplosomia** [ˌdipləuˈsəumiə] *n* 双躯[畸形]

diplosome [ˈdipləsəum] *n* 双点体(哺乳类动物细胞的两个中心粒)

diplotene [ˈdipləti:n] *n* 双线期(减数分裂过程前期中的一个阶段)

diploteratology [ˌdipləuˌterəˈtɔlədʒi] *n* 联胎畸形学

Dipluridae [dipˈljuəridiː] *n* 长尾蛛科

dipodia [daiˈpəudiə] *n* 复足[畸形];复足并腿[畸形]

dipodial [daiˈpəudiəl] *a* 复足并腿[畸形]的

dipole [ˈdaipəul] *n* 偶极,二极;偶极子 | **dipolar** [daiˈpəulə] *a*

dipotassium phosphate [ˌdaipəˈtæsjəm] 磷酸氢二钾

dipping [ˈdipiŋ] *n* 急压触诊(检肝);浸渍

dippoldism [ˈdipɔldizəm] *n* 鞭挞,鞭打,体罚主义(Dippold 为德国一教师)

diprosopus [daiˈprɔsəpəs] *n* 双面畸胎 | ~ tetrophthalmus 四眼双面畸胎

diprotrizoate [daiprəˈtraizəeit] *n* 尿影酸盐(尿路造影剂)

dipsesis [dip'si:sis] *n* 善渴,烦渴 | **dipsetic** [dip'setik] *a* 善渴的,致渴的
dipsia ['dipsiə] *n* 口渴
dipsogen ['dipsədʒən] *n* 致渴剂,致渴物
dipsogenic [dipsəu'dʒenik] *a* 致渴的
dipsomania [ˌdipsəu'meinjə] *n* 酒狂,嗜酒狂,间发性酒狂
dipsophobia [ˌdipsəu'fəubjə] *n* 饮酒恐怖
dipsosis [dip'səusis] *n* 善渴,烦渴
dipsotherapy [ˌdipsəu'θerəpi] *n* 节饮疗法,限饮疗法
dipstick ['dipstik] *n* 浸渍片,测验片(浸过的纤维素片,测尿中蛋白质、葡萄糖等)
Diptera ['diptərə] *n* 双翅目
Dipterocarpus [ˌdiptərəu'kɑ:pəs] *n* 古云香属,羯布罗香属
dipterous ['diptərəs] *a* 双翅的;双翅目的
Dipteryx ['diptəriks] *n* 香豆属
dipus ['daipəs] *n* 双足联胎
dipygus [dai'paigəs] *n* 双臀畸胎 | ~ parasiticus 不对称性双臀畸胎
dipylidiasis [ˌdipili'daiəsis] *n* 复孔绦虫病
Dipylidiidae [ˌdipili:'daiidi:] *n* 复孔[绦虫]科
Dipylidium [ˌdipi'lidiəm] *n* 复孔[绦虫]属 | ~ caninum 犬复孔绦虫
dipyridamole [ˌdaipi'ridəməul] *n* 双嘧达莫(冠状动脉扩张药)
dipyrithione [ˌdaipiəri'θaiəun] *n* 双硫氧吡啶(抗菌、抗真菌药)
dipyrone ['daipaiərəun] *n* 安乃近(解热镇痛药)
director [di'rektə, dai-] *n* 导子;控制器,引向器 | grooved ~ 有槽导子(导引手术切口的方向和深度)
directoscope [di'rektəskəup, dai-] *n* 直接检喉镜
dirhinic [dai'rainik] *a* 双鼻腔的
dirigomotor [ˌdirigəu'məutə] *a* 控制肌活动的
dirithromycin [daiˌriθrəu'maisin] *n* 地红霉素(抗生素类药)
Dirofilaria [ˌdaiərəufi'lɛəriə] *n* 恶丝虫属 | ~ immitis 犬恶丝虫 / ~ magalhaesi 麦[加尔黑斯]氏恶丝虫 / ~ repens 匐行恶丝虫
dirofilariasis [ˌdaiərəuˌfilə'raiəsis] *n* 恶丝虫病
Dir. prop. directione propria【拉】适当用法
dis- [前缀]分,离;二,两,双
disability [disə'biləti] *n* 失能,无力;伤残,残疾,劳动能力丧失 | developmental ~ 发育性残疾(18岁以前发病,并将无限期延续下去,由于精神发育迟缓、孤独症、大脑性麻痹、癫痫或其他神经病所致)
disaccharidase [dai'sækəriˌdeis] *n* 二糖酶 | intestinal ~ deficiency 肠二糖酶缺乏 / small-intestinal ~s 小肠二糖酶
disaccharide [dai'sækəraid] *n* 二糖 | reducing ~s 还原性二糖
disacchariduria [daiˌsækərai'djuəriə] *n* 二糖尿
disaccharose [dai'sækərəus] *n* 二糖
disacidify [ˌdisə'sidifai] *vt* 除酸,脱酸
disadvantage [ˌdisəd'vɑ:ntidʒ] *n* 不利[条件]
disadvantageous [disˌædvɑ:n'teidʒəs] *a* 不利的
disaggregation [ˌdisˌægri'geiʃən] *n* 感觉综合不能;解聚作用
disarticulate [ˌdisɑ:'tikjuleit] *vt, vi* 关节断离 | **disarticulation** [ˌdisɑ:ˌtikju'leiʃən] *n* 关节断离术,关节切断术
disassemble [ˌdisə'sembl] *vt* 拆卸,分解 | **disassembly** [ˌdisə'sembli] *n*
disassimilate [ˌdisə'simileit] *vt* (使)异化 | **disassimilation** [ˌdisəˌsimi'leiʃən] *n*
disaster [di'zɑ:stə] *n* 灾难 | burn ~ 烧伤灾难
disastrous [di'zɑ:strəs] *a* 灾难性的
disazo- 见 diazo-
disc [disk] *n* 盘,板,[圆]片
disc- 见 disco-
discectomy [dis'kektəmi] *n* 椎间盘切除术
discharge [dis'tʃɑ:dʒ] *vt* 排出;放电(疗法);释放,使出(医院等) *vi* 排出,流出 *n* 排出,流出;分泌物;放电;释放 | brush ~ 刷形放电,电刷疗法 / disruptive ~ 迅烈放电,电容放电疗法 / epileptic ~ 癫痫放电(癫痫引起的病理生理活动) / nervous, neural ~ 神经[冲动]发放 / systolic ~ 收缩期射血
dischronation [ˌdiskrə'neiʃən] *n* 时间觉障碍
disci ['disai] discus 的复数
disciform ['disifɔ:m] *a* 盘状的
discinesia [disai'ni:ziə] *n* 运动障碍
discission [di'siʒən] *n* 刺开,切开 | ~ of cataract 内障刺开术 / ~ of cervix uteri 宫颈切开 / posterior ~ 后路刺囊术(指内障)
discitis [dɪs'kaɪtɪs] *n* 关节盘炎
disclination [ˌdiskli'neiʃən] *n* 眼外转
disc(o)- [构词成分]盘,盘形,盘状
discoblastic [ˌdiskəu'blæstik] *a* 盘状囊胚的;盘形卵裂的
discoblastula [ˌdiskəu'blæstjulə] *n* 盘状囊胚
discocyte ['diskəsait] *n* [正常]盘形红细胞
discogastrula [ˌdiskəu'gæstrulə] *n* 盘形原肠胚
discogenic [ˌdiskəu'dʒenik], **discogenetic** [ˌdiskəudʒi'netik] *a* 椎间盘性的
discogram ['diskəgræm] *n* 椎间盘造影[照]片
discography [dis'kɔgrəfi] *n* 椎间盘造影[术]
discoid ['diskɔid] *a* 盘状的 *n* 盘形药丸;盘形挖器(牙)
discoidectomy [ˌdiskɔi'dektəmi] *n* 椎间盘切除术
discolo(u)r [dis'kʌlə] *vt, vi* (使)变色 | **~ation**

[disˌkʌləˈreiʃən] *n* 变色

Discomyces [ˌdiskəuˈmaisiːz] *n* 盘状菌属

Discomycetes [ˌdiskəumaiˈsiːtiːz] *n* 盘菌纲

discontinue [ˌdiskənˈtinjuː] *vt*, *vi* 中止,中断,停止

discontinuous [ˌdiskənˈtinjuəs] *a* 间断的,不连续的 | **discontinuity** [ˈdisˌkɔntiˈnjuːəti] *n* 间断性,不连续性

discopathy [disˈkɔpəθi] *n* 椎间盘病变

discophorous [disˈkɔfərəs] *a* 有盘的

discoplacenta [ˌdiskəupləˈsentə] *n* 盘状胎盘

discoplasm [ˈdiskəplæzəm] *n* 红细胞浆质

discord [ˈdiskɔːd] *n* 不一致,不调和;音混杂,音不谐和

discordant [disˈkɔːdənt] *a* 不一致的 | **discordance** [disˈkɔːdənz] *n* 不一致性(遗传学中指一对双生子中只有一人出现某种遗传性状)

discoria [disˈkɔːriə] *n* 瞳孔变形

discospondylitis [ˌdiskəuˌspɔndiˈlaitis] *n* (动物)椎间盘脊椎炎

discrepancy [disˈkrepənsi] *n* 差异,不一致 | leg length ~ 下肢不等长 / tooth size ~ 牙形不一致

discrete [disˈkriːt] *a* 分离的,分散的,稀疏的

discrimination [disˌkrimiˈneiʃən] *n* 辨别;歧视 | color ~ 色辨别

discriminator [disˈkrimiˌneitə] *n* 鉴别器,甄别器

discus [ˈdiskəs] ([复] **disci** [ˈdisai]) *n*【拉】盘,板,[圆]片

discutient [disˈkjuːʃiənt], **discussive** [disˈkʌsiv] *a* 消散的 *n* 消散剂

disdiaclast [disˈdaiəklæst] *n* 双折射物质(肌肉)

disdiadochokinesia [disdaiˌædəkəukaiˈniːsiə, -kiˈn-] *n* 轮替性运动障碍

DIS Diagnostic Interview Schedule 诊断性访问调查表

disease [diˈziːz] *n* [疾]病 | accumulation ~ 贮积病,沉积症 / acute demyelinating ~ 急性脱髓鞘病,传染病后脑炎 / adult celiac ~ 成人乳糜泻(非热带性口炎性腹泻) / akamushi ~ 恙虫病 / Aleutian mink ~ 阿留申貂病(阿留申群岛的一种貂的慢性病毒性疾病) / alkali ~ (家畜)硒中毒 / allogeneic ~ 同种[异基因]病(免疫抑制动物接受同种异体淋巴细胞注射后引起的移植物抗宿主反应) / alpha chain ~ α 链病(为最常见的重链病,主要发生于地中海地区的青年,特征为小肠固有层浆细胞浸润导致吸收不良,伴有腹泻、腹痛和体重减轻,十分罕见的特征为肺受累。其胃肠型亦称免疫增生性小肠病) / altitude ~ 高山病,高空病 / alveolar hydatid ~ 泡状棘球蚴病 / anti-glomerular basement membrane (anti-GBM) antibody ~ 抗肾小球基膜抗体病 / arc-welder's ~ 铁质沉着病,铁尘肺 / atopic ~ 异位性疾病,特应性疾病 / attic ~ 隐窝(耳鼓)病 / Australian X ~ 澳洲 X 脑炎 / autoimmune ~ 自身免疫病 / aviators' ~ 航空病,飞行员病 / bleeder's ~ 血友病 / blinding filarial ~ 旋盘尾丝虫病 / brancher glycogen storage ~ 支链淀粉病(糖原贮积症Ⅳ型) / bridegrooms' ~ 新郎病(性行为过度所致的蔓状静脉丛血栓形成) / broad-beta ~ 宽 β 脂蛋白病(家族性高脂蛋白血症Ⅲ型,因电泳时脂蛋白显示有一条 β 脂蛋白宽带,故名) / bronzed ~ 青铜色皮病,艾迪生病(肾上腺皮质功能减退症) / caisson ~ 潜水员病,减压病 / caloric ~ 高温病 / canine parvovirus ~ 犬细小病毒病 / celiac ~ 乳糜泻(一种吸收不良的综合征) / central core ~ 中央轴空病(常染色体显性型肌病,表现为缺少细胞器的肌原纤维中央部有稠密非晶形透明病变。婴儿期起病,尤其引起下肢运动发育延迟) / Chicago ~ 北美芽生菌病 / cholesteryl ester storage ~ (CESD) 胆固醇酯贮积病 / Christmas ~ 克里斯马斯病,凝血因子Ⅸ缺乏(克里斯马斯是第一个病人的姓) / chronic granulomatous ~ (CGD) 慢性肉芽肿性疾病 / chronic obstructive pulmonary ~ (COPD) 慢性阻塞性肺疾病 / chronic respiratory ~ of poultry 家禽慢性呼吸系疾病 / climatic ~ 气候病 / cold agglutinin ~ 冷凝集素病(见 syndrome 项下相应术语) / collagen ~ 胶原性疾病(一组结缔组织疾病的总称,这些疾病包括红斑狼疮、皮肤肌炎、硬皮病、结节性多动脉炎等) / combined immunodeficiency ~ 联合免疫缺陷病(指体液免疫和细胞免疫都有缺陷) / combined system ~ 联合系统病(恶性贫血病的脊髓亚急性联合变性) / communicable ~ 传染病 / complicating ~ 并发病 / compressed-air ~ 减压病 / contagious ~ 接触传染病 / corridor ~ 科立多病(一种蜱传原虫病,首次在南非科立多地区报道,对牛有高度致死性,水牛为传染贮主) / cystic ~ of breast 乳腺囊性病 / cystic ~ of lung 肺囊性病(本词有时用于囊肿性肺气肿。亦称肺假囊肿) / dancing ~ 舞蹈狂(见 tarantism) / debrancher glycogen storage ~ 脱支链糖原贮积症(糖原贮积症Ⅱ型) / deer fly ~ 兔热病 / deficiency ~, deprivation ~ 营养缺乏病 / demyelinating ~ 脱髓鞘病 / dense deposit ~ 致密沉积物病(Ⅱ型膜性增生性肾小球肾炎) / dermopathic herpesvirus ~ 皮肤病性疱疹病毒病(牛的一种疱疹病毒疾病) / elevator ~ 谷仓工人尘肺 / English ~ 英国病(佝偻病) / English sweating ~ 英国黑汗病(英国黑汗热) / eosinophilic endomyocardial ~ 嗜酸性心内膜心肌病,吕弗勒(Löffler) 心内膜炎 / extensor process ~ 锥突部骨炎 / fatigue ~ 职业性神经官能症 / fifth ~ 第五病,传染性红斑 / fifth venereal ~ 第五性病,性病性淋巴肉芽肿 / finger and toe ~

指趾病，根肿病（甘蓝根肿菌所致的一种植物病）/ flint ～ 石末沉着病，石末肺 / floating ～ 宽β脂蛋白病（即 broad-beta ～）/ fourth venereal ～ 第四性病（①特异性坏疽溃疡性龟头包皮炎；②腹股沟肉芽肿）/ functional cardiovascular ～ 功能性心血管病 / gannister ～（肺）硅石末沉着病 / garapata ～ 回归热 / genetotrophic ～ 遗传性营养失调病 / giant platelet ～ 巨血小板病 / glucose-6-phosphate dehydrogenase（G6PD）～ 葡糖-6-磷酸脱氢酶病（为最常见的先天性代谢病）/ glycogen storage ～，glycogen ～ 糖原贮积症，糖原病 / grinder's ～ 磨工病，硅肺 / heart ～ 心脏病 / heavy chain ～s 重链病（一组早见的淋巴浆细胞恶性肿瘤）/ hemoglobin C-thalassemia ～ 血红蛋白 C 型珠蛋白生成障碍性贫血 / hemolytic ～ of newborn 新生儿溶血症，胎儿成红血细胞增多症 / hepatorenal glycogen storage ～ 肝肾型糖原贮积症（糖原贮积症 I 型）/ hereditary ～ 遗传性[疾]病 / hock ～ 骨短粗病 / holoendemic ～ 全地方性疾病（在一个群体的大多数儿童中流行的疾病，而在同一群体中的成人很少患此病）/ hunger ～，hungry ～ 饥饿病，胰岛素分泌过多症 / hyaline membrane ～ 透明膜病（新生儿呼吸道病变引起肺不张）/ hydatid ～ 棘球蚴病（通常为肝感染，其特征为发生膨大的囊肿）/ hyperendemic ～ 高度地方性疾病（在一个群体的所有年龄组都流行的疾病）/ hypopigmentation-immunodeficiency ～ 色素减退-免疫缺陷病 / Iceland ～，Icelandic ～ 冰岛病，流行性神经肌无力症 / I-cell ～ I-细胞病，黏脂病第二型 / immune-complex ～ 免疫复合物病（由抗原抗体复合物引起的疾病）/ immunoproliferative small intestine ～ 免疫增生性小肠病（亦称α-链病，见 alpha chain ～）/ inborn lysosomal ～s 先天性溶酶体病，溶酶体贮积病 / infantile celiac ～ 婴儿乳糜泻（非热带性口炎性腹泻）/ infectious ～ 感染性疾病，传染病 / infectious bursal ～ 传染性黏液囊病（一种高度接触传染性家禽急性病）/ inherited ～ 遗传病 / insect-borne ～s 昆虫传染病 / iron storage ～ 铁贮积病，血色素沉着[症] / island ～ 丛林型斑疹伤寒 / kissing ～ 传染性单核细胞增多[症]（俗称接吻病）/ Kyasanur Forest ～ 夸赛纳森林病（最初在印度夸赛纳森林中流行的一种严重的出血热）/ laughing ～ 笑病（见 kuru，新几内亚震颤病）/ leaf-curl ～ 缩叶病，卷叶病（植物的一种病毒病）/ legionnaires' ～ 军团病（一种致死率高的疾病，由革兰阴性杆菌〈嗜肺性军团杆菌〉引起，人际间接触并不蔓延，特征为高热、胃肠痛、头痛及肺炎，也可累及肾、肝和神经系统。病原菌是在 1976 年夏在费城美国退伍军人大会期间发生的暴发性流行后鉴定的）/ lipid storage ～ 脂质贮积病 / lung fluke ～ 肺吸虫病，寄生虫性咯血 / Lyme ～ 莱姆病（一种复发性多系统疾病，首次在美国康涅狄克州的 Old Lyme 作过报道，此病开始为游走性慢性红斑损害，继以大关节炎、肌痛、不适以及神经系统和心脏症状。病原体为博氏疏螺旋体，媒介为鹿扁虱。亦称莱姆关节炎）/ lysosomal storage ～ 溶酶体贮积症 / maple bark ～ 枫树皮病（吸入枫树皮下一种霉〈皮质梨孢霉〉的孢子而引起的肉芽肿性间质性肺炎）/ maple syrup urine ～（MSUD）枫糖尿病（一种遗传性氨基酸病，由于支链氨基酸〈BACC〉分解代谢第二步某种酶缺乏所致，BACC 及其同类物蓄积在血液及尿内，可致出生后很快就发生的严重酮酸中毒，约半数新生儿的死亡、抽搐、昏迷、身心发育迟缓以及在尿内和体内有特征性的枫糖浆和咖喱气味。亦称酮酸脱羧酶缺乏症、支链酮酸尿症或酮氨基酸血症）/ Marburg ～，Marburg virus ～ 马尔堡病，马尔堡病毒病（一种严重的、常致命的急性病毒性出血热，表现为发热、虚脱、出血、胰腺炎和肝炎，最初原发性病例在德国的马尔堡和法兰克福作过报道）/ mast cell ～ 肥大细胞病，着色性荨麻疹 / Mediterranean ～ 地中海病，珠蛋白生成障碍性贫血 / medullary cystic ～ 髓质囊肿病 / miasmatic ～ 瘴气病 / microdrepanocytic ～ 小镰状细胞病，镰状红细胞珠蛋白生成障碍性贫血[病] / Minamata ～ 水俣病（日本水俣地方所发生的汞中毒）/ mish ～ 密施病（叙利亚的一种痢疾，因食杏子致病）/ mixed connective tissue ～ 混合型结缔组织病（兼有硬皮病、肌炎、系统性红斑狼疮及类风湿关节炎特征，在血清学上表现为有作用于可提取的核抗原的抗体）/ moyamoya ～ [日语 moyamoya 意为烟雾，血管造影时出现]烟雾病（由于脑底异常血管网破裂所致阻塞及小出血而引起的大脑缺血，导致进行性神经系统失能；此病主要发生于日本人）/ mu chain ～ μ 链病（最罕见的重链病，见于慢性淋巴细胞性白血病患者，有肝脾肿大症状）/ mule spinner's ～ 纺纱工病（由锭子油引起的皮肤尤其是阴囊上的疣或溃疡，易癌变）/ organic ～ 器质性病 / pelvic inflammatory ～ 盆腔炎（累及宫颈以上女性生殖管道的任何一种盆腔上行感染）/ phytanic acid storage ～ 植烷酸贮积病 / pink ～ 肢痛症 / polyendocrine autoimmune ～ 多内分泌腺自身免疫病（内分泌腺和非内分泌腺自身免疫病的结合。Ⅰ型发生于婴儿和儿童，伴有念珠菌病、甲状腺功能减退和肾上腺功能不足，也可发生恶性贫血、白斑、性腺功能衰竭、脱发、胰岛素依赖型糖尿病和甲状腺自身免疫病。亦称自身免疫性多内分泌腺-念珠菌病综合征；Ⅱ型称施密特综合征〈Schmidt's syndrome〉）/ rat-bite 鼠咬热 / rice ～ 脚气病 / runt ～ 侏儒病（实验产生的一种综合征，注射免疫活性细胞于异体宿主，而宿主对这些细胞不

能排斥,结果宿主发育迟缓,最后常死亡。亦称移植物抗宿主反应) / sandworm ~ 幼虫移行症 / secondary ~ 二次病,继发病 / self-limited ~ 自限性疾病 / severe combined immunodeficiency ~ (SCID) 重症联合免疫缺陷病 / sexually transmitted ~ 性传播疾病 / shimamushi ~ 丛林型斑疹伤寒 / shipyard ~ 船坞病、流行性角膜结膜炎 / sickle cell-hemoglobin C ~ 镰状细胞血红蛋白 C 病(一种遗传性贫血,红细胞含有血红蛋白 S 和血红蛋白 C) / sickle cell-hemoglobin D ~ 镰状细胞血红蛋白 D 病(一种遗传性贫血,红细胞含有血红蛋白 S 和血红蛋白 D) / sickle cell-thalassemia ~, thalassemia-sickle cell ~ 镰状细胞珠蛋白生成障碍性贫血,小镰状细胞病,血红蛋白 S 珠蛋白生成障碍性贫血 / silo-filler's ~ 地窖装填工病(吸入地窖内青贮饲料产生的氮氧化物等气体所引起的肺炎,常伴有急性肺水肿) / sixth ~ 第六病,猝发疹 / sixth venereal ~ 第六性病,性病性淋巴肉芽肿 / sleeping ~ 发作性睡眠[病],昏睡病 / sod ~ 水疱皮炎 / sterility ~ 不育症(实验动物饮食中缺乏维生素 E 所致) / storsge pool ~ 贮存池病(一种血液凝固障碍,由于血小板不能释放 ADP 对凝聚物质〈胶原、肾上腺素、外源性 ADP、凝血酶等〉反应所致。本病特征为轻度出血,出血时间延长,对胶原或凝血酶的凝聚反应减低) / structural ~ 器质性病 / sweet clover ~ 香草木樨中毒 / tarabagan ~ 土拨鼠[流行]病 / tsetse-fly ~ 非洲锥虫病 / tsusugamushi ~ 恙虫病 / tunnel ~ 隧道病,减压病 / vagabonds' ~, vagrants' ~ 寄生性黑皮病 / vibration ~ 振荡损伤(手臂连续使用振动工具所引起手指变白,屈曲减少,冷、热、痛感丧失及骨关节炎病变) / white-spot ~ 白点病(①硬化性萎缩性苔藓;②点滴状硬斑病;③小瓜虫病) / woolsorters' ~ 拣毛工病(吸入性炭疽病) / X ~ X 病(①角化过度;②黄曲霉中毒) / X-linked lymphoproliferative ~ X-连锁淋巴[细胞]增生症(见 syndrome 项下相应术语) | ~d *a* 害了病的;不健全的

disengage [ˌdisinˈgeidʒ] *vt* 解脱

disengagement [ˌdisinˈgeidʒmənt] *n* 解脱(分娩)

disequilibrium [disˌiːkwiˈlibriəm] *n* 失去平衡,平衡不稳 | linkage ~ 连锁不平衡

disesthesia [ˌdisisˈθiːzjə] *n* 感觉迟钝;触物感痛

disgerminoma [disˌdʒəːmiˈnəumə] *n* 无性细胞瘤

disgorge [disˈgɔːdʒ] *vt, vi* 吐出,呕吐

dish [diʃ] *n* 皿,碟 | culture ~ 培养皿 / evaporating ~ 蒸发皿

disharmony [disˈhɑːməni] *n* 不和谐,失谐,失调 | occlusal ~ 殆失调,咬合失调 | **disharmonious** [ˌdishɑːˈməunjəs] *a*

DISIDA disofenin (diisopropyl iminodiacetic acid) 地索苯宁(二异丙基亚氨基二乙酸)

disimmune [ˌdisiˈmjuːn] *a* 免疫性消失的

disimmunity [ˌdisiˈmjuːnəti] *n* 免疫性消失

disimmunize [disˈimjuːnaiz] *vt* 脱免疫

disimpaction [disimˈpækʃən] *n* 排除胎粪嵌塞(常用手指或灌肠法)

disinfect [ˌdisinˈfekt] *vt* 消毒

disinfectant [ˌdisinˈfektənt] *a* 消毒的 *n* 消毒药,消毒剂 | coal-tar ~ 煤焦油消毒剂,杂酚油,木溜油

disinfection [ˌdisinˈfekʃən] *n* 消毒 | concomitant ~, concurrent ~ 随时消毒,即时消毒 / terminal ~ 终末消毒,终结消毒

disinfest [ˌdisinˈfest] *vt* 灭除害虫 | **disinfestation** [ˌdisinfesˈteiʃən] *n* 灭病媒[法],灭[昆]虫[法]

disinhibition [ˌdisinhiˈbiʃən] *n* 去抑制

disinomenine [ˌdaisiˈnɔmənin] *n* 双青藤碱

disinsected [ˌdisinˈsektid] *a* 灭昆虫的

disinsectization [ˌdisinˌsektaiˈzeiʃən, -tiˈz-], **disinsection** [ˌdisinˈsekʃən] *n* 灭[昆]虫法

disinsector [ˌdisinˈsektə] *n* 灭虫器

disinsertion [ˌdisinˈsəːʃən] *n* 腱断裂;视网膜剥离

disintegrant [disˈintigrənt] *n* 崩解剂(制造片剂用);解磨机,碎磨机

disintegration [ˌdisintiˈgreiʃən] *n* 分裂,分解;解体;衰变 | radioactive ~ 放射性衰变

disintegrin [disˈintəgrin] *n* 分解蛋白,解整连蛋白(极低浓度时亦能抑制血小板聚集)

disjoint [disˈdʒɔint] *vt, vi* 脱位,关节分离

disjunct [disˈdʒʌnkt] *a* 断离的,不接连的

disjunction [disˈdʒʌnkʃən] *n* 分离(在遗传学中指在第一次减数分裂后期同源染色体配对后分别向两极移动);析取 | craniofacial ~ 颅面分离

disk [disk] *n* 盘,板,[圆]片 | A ~, Q ~, anisotropic ~, anisotropous ~ A 盘,Q 盘,双折光盘(横纹肌纤维的暗带) / articular ~, interarticular ~ 关节盘 / blood ~ 血小板 / carborundum ~ 金刚砂磨片 / choked ~ 视神经乳头水肿 / ciliary ~ 睫状环 / cloth ~ 布质磨片 / cupped ~ 视乳头盘凹(视乳头杯状凹陷) / cutting ~ 磨片,磨盘 / dental ~ 牙科切盘 / embryonic ~, germinal ~ 胚盘 / I ~, isotropic ~, J ~ I 盘,单折光盘,J 盘(横纹肌纤维的亮带) / M ~ M 板(亨森〈Hensen〉盘中间的薄带) / optic ~ 视乳头盘,视神经乳头 / proligerous ~ [载]卵丘 / sandpaper ~ 砂纸片 / stenopeic ~ 裂隙盘(检散光) / stroboscopic ~ 动态镜盘(用于眼睛检查,能使目标变形) / tactile ~ 触小板 / Z ~, thin ~ Z 盘,克劳泽(Krause)膜(横纹肌间线)

disk- 见 disko-

diskectomy [disˈkektəmi] *n* 椎间盘切除术

diskiform [ˈdiskifɔːm] *a* 盘状的
diskitis [disˈkaitis] *n* 关节盘炎
disk(o)-[构词成分]盘
diskogram [ˈdiskəgræm] *n* 椎间盘X线[照]片
diskography [disˈkɔgrəfi] *n* 椎间盘X线造影[术]
dislocate [ˈdisləukeit] *vt* 使关节脱位
dislocatio [ˌdisləuˈkeiʃiəu] *n*【拉】脱位 | ~ erecta 竖直脱位(肩关节)
dislocation [ˌdisləuˈkeiʃən] *n* 脱位 | closed ~ 无创脱位 / complete ~ 完全脱位 / complicated ~ 并发脱位 / compound ~, open ~ 哆开脱位 / consecutive ~ 接连性脱位 / divergent ~ 分开性脱位(尺骨与桡骨分开) / fracture ~ 骨折脱位 / habitual ~ 习惯性脱位 / incomplete ~, partial ~ 不全脱位 / primitive ~ 初期脱位,原脱位 / recent ~ 新脱位(无并发炎症)
dismember [disˈmembə] *vt* 肢解 | **~ment** *n* 截肢,肢体(部分)切断
dismutation [ˌdismjuˈteiʃən] *n* 歧化(作用)
disocclude [ˌdisɔˈkluːd] *vt* 使无殆
disodium [daiˈsəudjəm] *n* 二钠
disofenin (DISIDA) [ˌdaisəuˈfenin] *n* 地索苯宁(二异丙基取代的亚氨基二乙酸〈IDA〉类似物,与锝 Tc99m 络合用于肝胆成像)
disome [ˈdaisəum] *n* 二体(双染色体)
disomus [daiˈsəuməs] *n* 双躯干畸胎
disomy [ˈdaisəmi] *n* 二体性 | uniparental ~ 单亲二体
disopyramide [ˌdaisəuˈpiərəmaid] *n* 丙吡胺(抗心律失常药) | ~ phosphate 磷酸丙吡胺(抗心律失常药)
disorder [disˈɔːdə] *n* 障碍,紊乱,疾病 | adjustment ~ 适应性障碍 / amnestic ~ 遗忘症 / anxiety ~s 焦虑症 / anxiety ~s of childhood or adolescence 青少年焦虑症 / attention-deficit hyperactivity ~ 注意缺陷障碍[伴多动](一种有争议的儿童期精神障碍,7岁前发病,特征为坐立不安,静坐困难,容易分心,无耐心等待,问题未提完前迫不及待抢答,不能服从指导,以及其他破坏性行为。亦称脑功能轻微失调) / avoidant ~ of childhood or adolescence 青少年怯生症 / behavior ~, conduct ~ 行为障碍,行为异常 / bipolar ~ 双相性精神障碍(亦称躁郁症,躁郁性精神病) / body dysmorphic ~ 身体变形性精神障碍 / character ~ 性格障碍,人格障碍 / collagen ~ 胶原障碍(先天性代谢病,包括胶原结构或代谢异常) / conversion ~ 转换性障碍(以转换症状〈提示躯体疾病的生理功能的缺失或改变〉为特征的一种精神障碍) / cyclothymic ~ 循环情感性[精神]障碍 / delusional (paranoid) ~ 妄想(类偏执狂)性[精神]障碍 / depersonalization ~ 人格解体性[精神]障碍 / dissociative ~s 分离性障碍 / dysthymic ~ 心境恶劣障碍 / emotional ~ 情绪障碍 / factitious ~ 造作性[精神]障碍(以反复故意模拟躯体和心理症状,除求得治疗外并无明显目的为特征的一种精神障碍) / functional ~ 功能性障碍,功能紊乱 / generalized anxiety ~ 广泛性焦虑症 / genetic ~ 遗传障碍 / identity ~ 同一性障碍 / induced psychotic ~ 感应性精神障碍 / intermittent explosive ~ 间歇性暴发性[精神]障碍 / isolated explosive ~ 孤立性暴发性[精神]障碍 / LDL-receptor ~ 低密度脂蛋白受体病 / major mood ~s 重性心境障碍(双相性精神障碍和重性抑郁症) / manicdepressive ~ 躁郁症 / mendelian ~, monogenic ~ 孟德尔病,单基因[遗传]病 / mental ~ 精神障碍 / multifactorial ~ 多因素障碍,多因素病(由遗传因素和也许是非遗传的环境因素相互作用引起的一种障碍,如某些类型的先天性缺陷和糖尿病) / multiple personality ~ 多重人格障碍 / organic mental ~s 器质性精神障碍 / over anxious ~ 过度焦虑症 / panic ~ 惊恐性障碍,急性焦虑症 / paranoid ~s 偏执性精神障碍 / personality ~ 人格障碍 / post-traumatic stress ~ 创伤后精神紧张性[精神]障碍 / psychoactive substance-induced organic mental ~s 精神作用物质引起的器质性精神障碍 / psychoactive substance use ~s 应用精神作用物质所致精神障碍(见 dependence 项下 psychoactive substance dependence) / psychogenic pain ~ 心因性疼痛症 / psychosomatic ~s, psychophysiologic ~ 心身障碍,心理生理性障碍 / schizoaffective ~ 分裂情感性精神障碍 / schizophreniform ~ 精神分裂症样精神障碍 / seasonal mood ~ 季节性心境障碍 / separation anxiety ~ 分离焦虑症 / shared paranoid ~ 分担类偏执狂(即感应性精神障碍) / single-gene ~ 单基因[遗传]病(孟德尔病) / sleep terror ~ 夜惊症 / sleep-walking ~ 梦游症 / somatization ~ 躯体症状化障碍(为典型的癔病,患者主诉可能包括全身不适或具体的转换症状〈假性神经症状〉、胃肠症状、女性生殖系统症状、性心理症状、心肺症状或疼痛) / somatoform ~s 躯体病样精神障碍 / somatoform pain ~ 躯体病样疼痛症 / substance use ~s 应用精神作用物质所致精神障碍(即 psychactive substance use ~s) / unipolar ~s 单相性精神障碍(重性抑郁症和精神抑郁症)
disorganize [disˈɔːgənaiz] *vt* 结构破坏 | **disorganization** [disˌɔːgənaiˈzeiʃən, -niˈz-] *n*
disorientation [disˌɔːrienˈteiʃən] *n* 定向障碍 | spatial ~ 空间定向障碍(亦称飞行员眩晕)
disoxidation [ˌdisɔksiˈdeiʃən] *n* 脱氧(作用)
dispar [ˈdispɑː] *a*【拉】不等的,不相称的
disparasitized [disˈpærəsitaizd, -si-] *a* 无寄生物的

disparate [ˈdispəreit] *a* 不等的,不相称的;异种[类]的
disparity [disˈpæriti] *n* (双眼像)差异
dispensary [disˈpensəri] *n* 医务所;药房
dispensation [ˌdispenˈseiʃən] *n* 配方
dispensatory [disˈpensətəri] *n* 处方集 | Dispensatory of the United States of America 美国处方集
dispense [disˈpens] *vt* 调剂,配药
dispenser [disˈpensə] *n* 调剂员,配药者
dispermine [daiˈspəːmin] *n* 胡椒嗪,哌嗪,驱蛔灵
dispermy [ˈdaispəːmi] *n* 双精入卵,双精受精
dispersate [ˈdispəseit] *n* 分散质
disperse [disˈpəːs] *vt*, *vi* 分散,弥散 | **dispersible** [disˈpəːsəbl] *a* 可分散的,可弥散的
dispersion [disˈpəːʃən] *n* 分散[作用],弥散[现象];分散体;胶体溶液 | colloid ~ 胶体分散,胶体溶液 / molecular ~ 分子分散
dispersity [disˈpəːsəti] *n* 分散度,分散性
dispersive [disˈpəːsiv] *a* 分散的,弥散的
dispersoid [disˈpəːsɔid] *n* 分散胶体
dispersonalization [disˌpəːsənəlaiˈzeiʃən, -liˈz-] *n* 人格解体
dispert [ˈdispəːt] *n* 干浸出制剂
Dispholidus [disˈfɔlidəs] *n* 多鳞蛇属
dispireme [daiˈspaiəriːm], **dispira** [daiˈspaiərə] *n* 双纽[期](双星体后的细胞分裂期)
displace [disˈpleis] *vt* 取代,置换;移位
displaceability [disˌpleisəˈbiləti] *n* [可]移位性
displacement [disˈpleismənt] *n* 错位;取代,置换;移位;渗漉 | character ~ 性状替位(能使一物种进化并将另一物种从某生态小境中排除的适应特性或性状) / fetal ~ 胎移位 / fish-hook ~ 鱼钩状移位(胃) / gallbladder ~ 游动胆囊 / tissue ~ 组织移位
dispore [ˈdaispɔː] *n* 双孢担孢子(双孢担子上的孢子)
disporous [ˈdaispərəs] *a* 双孢子的
disposable [disˈpəuzəbl] *a* 可处理的;一次性[使用]的
disposition [ˌdispəˈziʃən] *n* 处理;倾向,素质;秉性,性情;素因(躯体或精神对某些疾病的倾向)
disproportion [ˌdisprəˈpɔːʃən] *n* 不相称 | cephalopelvic ~ 头盆不称
disproportionate [ˌdisprəˈpɔːʃənit] *a* 不相称的
disrupt [disˈrʌpt] *vt*, *vi* 破裂 | **~ion** [disˈrʌpʃən] *n*
disruptive [disˈrʌptiv] *a* 破裂的
dissector [diˈsektə] *n* 解剖者;解剖器;解剖[指导]书
disseminate [diˈsemineit] *vt*, *vi* 弥散,播散 | **dissemination** [diˌsemiˈneiʃən] *n* / **~d** *a* 弥散性的,播散性的
Disse's spaces [ˈdisə] (Joseph Disse) 窦周间隙
dissever [disˈsevə] *vt*, *vi* 分裂,分割
dissimilate [diˈsimileit] *vi*, *vt* 异化
dissimilation [ˌdisimiˈleiʃən] *n* 异化作用
dissipation [ˌdisiˈpeiʃən] *n* 逸散[作用]
dissociable [diˈsəuʃjəbl] *a* 可离解的,易离解的
dissociant [diˈsəuʃiənt] *n* 变异菌株
dissociation [diˌsəusiˈeiʃən] *n* 分离;离解;分裂,联想散漫;变异(细菌) | albuminocytologic ~ (脑脊液)蛋白细胞分离 / atrioventricular ~, auriculoventricular ~ 房室分离 / bacterial ~, microbic ~ 细菌变异 / interference ~, ~ by interference 干扰性分离 / peripheral ~ 感觉分离(肢端浅感觉减退,见于多神经炎) / syringomyelic ~ 脊髓空洞症性感觉分离 / tabetic ~ 脊髓痨性感觉分离 | **dissociative** [diˈsəuʃiətiv] *a*
dissogeny [diˈsɔdʒini] *n* 两度性熟(幼虫期及成虫期都有性成熟)
dissoluble [diˈsɔljubl] *a* 可溶解的;可分解的 | **dissolubility** [diˌsɔljuˈbiləti] *n* 溶[解]度;溶[解]性;[可]溶性
dissolution [disəˈljuːʃən] *n* 溶解;分解;液化;松解[法]死亡
dissolve [diˈzɔlv] *vt*, *vi* 分解;溶解 | **dissolvable** [diˈzɔlvəbl] *a* 可溶的,能溶[解]的
dissolvent [diˈzɔlvənt] *n* 溶剂,溶媒;溶化药 *a* 溶解的
dissonance [ˈdisənəns] *n* 不和谐 | cognitive ~ 认知失调(人们的思想、信仰、态度和经历缺乏一致的看法时产生的一种不愉快感觉)
Dist. distilla【拉】蒸馏
distad [ˈdistæd] *ad* 向远侧
distal (**D**) [ˈdistl] *a* 远侧的;末梢的;远中的(牙) | **~ly** *ad* 向远侧
distalis [disˈteilis] *a* 远侧的;末梢的
distance [ˈdistəns] *n* 距离 | focal ~ 焦[点]距[离] / object-film ~ 物-片距离(被照物体与胶片间距离) / targetskin ~ 靶-皮[肤]距离(从X线阳极至体表皮肤的距离) / working ~ 资用距离,焦点距离
distantia [disˈtænʃə] *n* 距离 | ~ intercristalis 髂嵴间距(亦称髂嵴间径) / ~ interspinosa 髂棘间距(亦称髂棘间径)
distemper [disˈtempə] *n* 瘟热(动物传染病,尤指犬瘟热) | canine ~ 犬瘟热 / cat ~ 猫瘟热,猫传染性粒细胞缺乏症
distemperoid [disˈtempərɔid] *n* 犬瘟热减弱病毒
distend [disˈtend] *vt*, *vi* (使)膨胀
distensibility [disˌtensiˈbiləti] *n* 膨胀性;弹性
distention [disˈtenʃən] *n* 膨胀 | gaseous ~ 气胀
distichiasis [ˌdistiˈkaiəsis], **distichia** [disˈtikiə] *n*

双行睫
distil(l) [dis'til] (-ll-) *vt*, *vi* 蒸馏
distillate ['distilit, 'distileit] *n* 馏出物,蒸馏物
distillation [ˌdisti'leiʃən] *n* 蒸馏 | destructive ~, dry ~ 分解蒸馏,干馏 / fractional ~ 分馏
distinct [dis'tiŋkt] *a* 独特的;明显的
distoaxiogingival [ˌdistəuˌæksiəudʒin'dʒaivəl, -'dʒindʒi-] *a* 远中轴龈的
distoaxioincisal [ˌdistəuˌæksiəuin'saizəl] *a* 远中轴切的
distoaxio-occlusal [ˌdistəuˌæksiəuɔ'klu:zəl] *a* 远中轴殆的
distobuccal [ˌdistə'bʌkəl] *a* 远中颊的
distobucco-occlusal [ˌdistəuˌbʌkəuɔ'klu:zəl] *a* 远中颊殆的
distobuccopulpal [ˌdistəuˌbʌkə'pʌlpl] *a* 远中颊髓的
distocervical [ˌdistəu'sə:vikəl] *a* 远中颈的;远中龈的
distoclination [ˌdistəuklai'neiʃən, -ki:'n-] *n* 远中偏斜
distoclusal [ˌdistəu'klu:zəl] *a* 远中殆的
distoclusion [ˌdistəu'klu:ʒən] *n* 远中殆
distogingival [ˌdistəudʒin'dʒaivəl, -'dʒindʒi-] *a* 远中龈的
distolabial [ˌdistəu'leibjəl] *a* 远中唇的
distolabioincisal [ˌdistəuˌleibiəuin'saizəl] *a* 远中唇切的
distolingual [ˌdistəu'liŋgwəl] *a* 远中舌的
distolinguoincisal [ˌdistəuˌliŋgwəuin'saizəl] *a* 远中舌切的
distolinguo-occlusal [ˌdistəuˌliŋgwəuɔ'klu:zəl] *a* 远中舌殆的
distolinguopulpal [ˌdistəuˌliŋgwəu'pʌlpl] *a* 远中舌髓的
Distoma ['distəmə] *n* 双盘吸虫属 | ~ buski 布氏姜片吸虫(即 Fasciolopsis buski) / ~ felineum 猫后睾吸虫(即 Opisthorchis felineus) / ~ haematobium 埃及血吸虫(即 Schistosoma haematobium) / ~ hepaticum 肝片吸虫(即 Fasciola hepatica) / ~ heterophyes 异形异形吸虫(即 Heterophyes heterophyes) / ~ sinensis 华支睾吸虫(即 Clonorchis sinensis) / ~ westermani, ~ ringeri 卫氏并殖吸虫,肺吸虫(即 Paragonimus westermani) | **Distomum** *n*
distomia [dai'stəumiə] *n* 双口[畸形]
distomiasis [ˌdistəu'maiəsis] *n* 双盘吸虫病 | hemic ~ 血吸虫病 / hepatic ~ 肝吸虫病 / intestinal ~ 肠吸虫病,姜片虫病 / pulmonary ~ 肺吸虫病,寄生性咯血
distomolar [ˌdistəu'məulə] *n* 远中磨牙
distomus [dai'stəuməs] *n* 双口畸胎
disto-occlusal [ˌdistəu ɔ'klu:zəl] *a* 远中殆的
disto-occlusion [ˌdistəu ɔ'klu:ʒən] *n* 远中殆
distoplacement [ˌdistəu'pleismənt] *n* 远中移位
distopulpal [ˌdistəu'pʌlpl] *a* 远中髓的
distopulpolabial [ˌdistəuˌpʌlpəu'leibjəl] *a* 远中髓唇的
distopulpolingual [ˌdistəu'pʌlpəu'liŋgwəl] *a* 远中髓舌的
distortion [dis'tɔ:ʃən] *n* 失真;扭转,变形;乖僻 | parataxic ~ 认人失真 / ~ of penis 阴茎扭转
distortor [dis'tɔ:tə] *n* 【拉】扭转者 | ~ oris 口角提肌,颧小肌
distoversion [ˌdistəu'və:ʃən] *n* 远中错位
distract [dis'trækt] *vt* (注意力)分散;迷惑
distractibility [ˌdistrækti'biləti] *n* 随境转移
distraction [dis'trækʃən] *n* 注意力分散;内脱位;骨折分离;撑开牵引[术];牙弓过宽
distress [dis'tres] *vt*, *n* 痛苦,困苦 | idiopathic respiratory ~ of newborn 新生儿特发性呼吸窘迫
distribution [ˌdistri'bju:ʃən] *n* 分配;分布 | chi-squared ~ χ^2(卡方)分布 / density ~ 密度分布 / dose ~ 剂量分布 / frequency ~ 频数分布 / normal ~ 正态分布
distributive [dis'tribjutiv] *a* 分配的;分布的
districhiasis [ˌdistri'kaiəsis] *n* 双毛[症]
disturbance [dis'tə:bəns] *n* 障碍,失调,紊乱 | sexual orientation ~ 性定向障碍 / transient situational ~ 暂时性境遇反应障碍,急性应激反应
disubstituted [dai'sʌbstitju:tid] *a* 二取代的
disulfate [dai'sʌlfeit] *n* 焦硫酸盐
disulfide [dai'sʌlfaid] *n* 二硫化物
disulfiram [dai'sʌlfaiəræm] *n* 双硫仑(治慢性醇中毒药)
disunion [dis'ju:njən] *n* 分离;分裂;不愈合;不连接
dithiazanine iodide [ˌdaiθai'æzəni:n] 碘二噻宁(抗蠕虫药)
dithio [dai'θaiəu] *n* 二硫代,联硫基($-S_2-$)
dithiol [dai'θaiɔl] *n* 二巯基化物
dithranol ['diθrənəl] *n* 地蒽酚(消毒防腐药)
dithymol diiodide [dai'θaimɔl] 麝酚碘,麝香草酚碘(抗真菌药,抗感染药)
Ditropenotus aureoviridis [ˌdaitrəpə'nəutəsˌɔ:riəu'viridis] 袋形虱螨
Dittel's operation ['ditəl] (Leopold R. von Dittel)迪特尔手术(经由外切口摘除肥大前列腺侧叶)
Dittrich's plugs ['ditriʃ] (Franz Dittrich) 迪特里希塞(腐败性支气管炎及支气管扩张时痰中的淡黄色或灰色的干酪样碎屑)
Ditylenchus [diti'leŋkəs] *n* 茎线虫属
diurea [dai'juəriə] *n* 双脲,环二脲

diureide [daiˈjuəriaid] *n* 二酰脲
diurese [ˌdaijuəˈriːs] *n* 利尿
diuresis [ˌdaijuəˈriːsis] ([复] **diureses** [ˌdaijuəˈriːsiːz]) *n* 利尿,多尿 | tubular ~ 肾小管性多尿 / water ~ 水利尿
diuretic [ˌdaijuəˈretik] *a* 利尿的 *n* 利尿药 | cardiac ~ 强心利尿药 / hemopiesic ~ 升压利尿药 / high-ceiling ~s, loop ~s 强效利尿药,襻性利尿药 / hydragogue ~ 排水性利尿药 / mercurial ~s 汞利尿药 / osmotic ~ 渗压性利尿药 / potassium-sparing ~s 保钾利尿药 / thiazide ~ 噻嗪类利尿药
diuria [daiˈjuəriə] *n* 昼间尿频
diurnal [daiˈəːnl] *a* 白天的,昼间的;昼现的(丝虫)
diurnule [daiˈəːnjul] *n* 一日剂量
Div. divide【拉】划分
divagation [ˌdaivəˈgeiʃən] *n* 言语散乱,语无伦次
divalent [ˈdaiˌveilənt, daiˈveilənt] *a* 二价的
divalproex sodium [daiˈvælprəueks] 地伐罗克钠(丙戊酸钠与丙戊酸以 1∶1 摩尔关系的配合物,用于治疗躁狂发作伴双相型障碍和癫痫发作,特别是失神发作以及预防偏头痛,口服给药)
divarication [daiˌværiˈkeiʃən] *n* 分离,脱离
divergence [daiˈvəːdʒəns] *n* 分散,散开;趋异;偏离,偏斜 | negative vertical ~ (–V. D.)负垂直偏斜 / positive vertical ~ (+V. D.)正垂直偏斜
divergent [daiˈvəːdʒənt] *a* 散开的;趋异的;偏斜的
diversine [daiˈvəːsin] *n* 无定形青藤碱
diversion [daiˈvəːʃən] *n* 转向,转移,转换 | antigenic ~ 抗原性转换 / ileal conduit ~ 回肠膀胱尿流改道术 / urinary ~ 尿流改道术
diversity [daiˈvəːsəti] *n* 多样性
divert [daiˈvəːt] *vt* 使转移,使转向
diverticular [ˌdaivəˈtikjulə] *a* 憩室的
diverticularization [ˌdaivəˌtikjuləraiˈzeiʃən, -riˈz-] *n* 憩室形成
diverticulectomy [ˌdaivəˌtikjuˈlektəmi] *n* 憩室切除术
diverticuleve [ˌdaivəˈtikjuliːv] *n* 膀胱憩室起子
diverticulitis [ˌdaivətikjuˈlaitis] *n* 憩室炎
diverticulogram [ˌdaivəˈtikjuləgræm] *n* 憩室造影[照]片
diverticulopexy [ˌdaivəˌtikjuləˈpeksi] *n* 憩室固定术
diverticulosis [ˌdaivəˌtikjuˈləusis] *n* 憩室病(尤指肠憩室)
diverticulum [ˌdaivəˈtikjuləm] ([复] **diverticula** [ˌdaivəˈtikjulə]) *n* 憩室 | acquired ~ 后天性憩室 / allantoic ~ 尿囊憩室(胎生期) / ganglion ~ 腱鞘滑膜憩室 / pressure ~, pulsion ~ 内压性憩室 / thyroid ~ 甲状腺憩室 / vesical ~ 膀胱憩室
divicine [daiˈvaisin] *n* 香豌豆嘧啶
divi-divi [ˌdiviˈdivi] *n* 南美云实荚
divinyl [daiˈvaini] *n* 二乙烯 | ~ oxide 二乙烯醚
divinylbenzene [daiˌvainilˈbenziːn] *n* 二乙烯基苯
divisio [diˈviziəu] ([复] **divisiones** [diˌviziˈəuniːz]) *n*【拉】分开,分裂;分支
division [diˈviʒən] *n* 分裂;部分,门;切断 | cell ~细胞分裂 / maturation ~ 成熟分裂 / reduction ~ 减数分裂 | **~al** *a*
divulse [daiˈvʌls] *vt* 扯裂;扯离 | **divulsion** [daiˈvʌlʃən] *n* 扯裂[术]
divulsor [daiˈvʌlsə] *n* 尿道扩张器
Dixon Mann 见 Mann
dizygotic [ˌdaizaiˈgɔtik], **dizygous** [daiˈzaigəs] *a* 两合子的
dizzy [ˈdizi] *a* 眩晕的 | **dizziness** *n* 眩晕
djenkolic acid [dʒenˈkɔlik] 黎豆氨酸, S-亚甲胱氨酸
djenkolism [dʒenˈkɔlizəm] *n* 黎豆中毒
dk deca- 十,癸
DL doxorubicin and lomustine 多柔比星-洛莫司汀(联合化疗治癌方案)
DL-[化学前缀][外]消旋的
dL deciliter 分升
dl-[化学前缀][外]消旋的
DLE discoid lupus erythematosis 盘状红斑狼疮
DM diabetes mellitus 糖尿病; dermatomyositis 皮肌炎; diphenylamine chlorarsine 二苯胺氯胂
DMAPN dimethylaminopropionitrile 二甲氨基丙腈
DMARD disease-modifying antirheumatic drug 缓解疾病的抗风湿药
DMBA 7, 12-dimethylbenz[a]anthracene 7, 12-二甲基苯并蒽
DMD Doctor of Dental Medicine 口腔牙医学博士
dmelcos [ˈdmelkɔs] *n* 杜克雷(Ducrey)菌苗(曾用于检软下疳及用于轻瘫患者以产生高温)
DMF decayed, missing, filled 龋失补(见 rate 项下相应术语); dimethylformamide 二甲基甲酰胺
DMFO eflornithine 依氟鸟氨酸
DMPE 3, 4-dimethoxyphenylethylamine 3, 4-二甲氧基苯基乙胺
DMRD Diploma in Medical Radio Diagnosis 医疗放射诊断学文凭(英国)
DMRT Diploma in Medical Radio Therapy 医疗放射治疗学文凭(英国)
DMSA succimer 二巯丁二酸(解毒药)
DMSO dimethyl sulfoxide 二甲亚砜
DMT dimethyltryptamine 二甲色胺

DN dibucaine number 地布卡因值

Dn. dekanem 十能母(营养价值单位,相当于 10 g 母乳营养)

dn. decinem 分能母,十分之一能母(相当于 1/10 g 母乳营养)

DNA deoxyribonucleic acid 脱氧核糖核酸 | DNA library DNA 文库 / recombinant DNA 重组 DNA

DNA-directed DNA polymerase DNA 指导的 DNA 聚合酶(亦称 DNA 核苷酸基转移酶,DNA 聚合酶)

DNA-directed RNA polymerase DNA 指导的 RNA 聚合酶(亦称 RNA 聚合酶)

DNA gyrase [ˈdʒaireis] DNA 回旋酶,DNA 拓扑异构酶(ATP-水解的)

DNA ligase(ATP) [ˈlaigeis] DNA 连接酶(ATP)(亦称多脱氧核糖核苷酸合酶〈ATP〉)

DNA nucleotidylexotransferase [ˌnjuːkliə*u*-ˌtaidilˌeksə*u*ˈtrænsfəreis] DNA 核苷酸基外转移酶(临床上测定此酶用以诊断白血病)

DNA nucleotidyltransferase [ˌnjuːkliə*u* ˌtaidil-ˈtrænsfəreis] DNA 核苷酸基转移酶(DNA 聚合酶的旧称)

DNA polymerase [pəˈliməreis] DNA 聚合酶,DNA 指导的 DNA 聚合酶

DNase deoxyribonuclease 脱氧核糖核酸酶

DNA topoisomerase [ˌtɔpəaiˈsɔməreis] DNA 拓扑异构酶(亦称 Ⅰ 型拓扑异构酶)

DNA topoisomerase (ATP-hydrolyzing) [ˌtɔpəai-ˈsɔməreis ˈhaidrəlaiziŋ] DNA 拓扑异构酶(ATP-水解的)(亦称 Ⅱ 型拓扑异构酶,DNA 回旋酶)

DNB dinitrobenzene 二硝基苯; Diplomate of the National Board(of Medical Examiners) 全国(医学主考人)委员会资格证书持有者

DNCB dinitrochlorobenzene 二硝基氯苯

DNFB dinitrofluorobenzene 二硝基氟苯

DNR do not resuscitate 未复苏

DO Doctor of Osteopathy 整骨疗法博士

DOA dead on arrival 到院死亡

Dobell's solution [dəˈbel] (Horace B. Dobell) 复方硼砂溶液

Dobie's globule [ˈdəubiː] (William M. Dobie) 窦比小体(存于肌纤维透明盘的中心,染色后方可见到) | ~ layer(line) 窦比层(线)(横纹肌间线)

Dobrin syndrome [ˈdəubrin] (Robert S. Dobrin) TINU 综合征(见 syndrome 项下相应术语)

dobutamine [dəuˈbjuːtəmiːn] *n* 多巴酚丁胺(强心药) | ~ hydrochloride 盐酸多巴酚丁胺

DOC 11-deoxycorticosterone 11-脱氧皮质[甾]酮

doc [dɔk] *n* 医生

docere [dəuˈsiərə] *vt*【拉】教(医生作为教师是自然医术医学的一个原则,论述病人卫生保健教育的重要性,并强调把病人作为个体予以诊治)

docetaxel [ˌdəusəˈtæksəl] *n* 多西他索(抗肿瘤药,用于化疗,治疗乳腺癌,静脉输注给药)

Dochmius duodenalis [ˈdɔkmiəsˌdju(ː)ə*u*di-ˈneilis] 十二指肠钩虫

docimasia [ˌdəusiˈmeiziə] *n* 检查,检验(一种法定检验) | auricular ~ 耳检验(见 Wreden's sign) / hepatic ~ 肝脏检查(肝脏中糖的检查) / pulmonary ~ 肺[浮沉]检验(将死婴之肺置于水中,视其浮沉以鉴定其是否死产) | **docimastic** [ˌdəusiˈmæstik] *a*

dock [dɔk] *vt* 剪短(动物尾巴),除尾

doconazole [dəuˈkəunəzəul] *n* 多康唑(抗真菌药)

docosahexaenoic acid [ˌdɔkə*u*səˌheksəiːˈnəuik] 二十二碳六烯酸

docosanol [dəuˈkəusənɔl] *n* 二十二[烷]醇(具有抗病毒活性,局部用于治疗复发性唇疱疹)

doctor [ˈdɔktə] *n* 医生,医师;博士

docusate [ˈdɔkjuseit] *n* 多库酯 | ~ calcium 多库酯钙(阴离子表面活性剂,用于软化大便) / ~ potassium 多库酯钾(阴离子表面活性剂,用于软化大便) / ~ sodium 多库酯钠(阴离子表面活性剂,用于软化大便)

dodecadactylitis [ˌdəudekəˌdæktiˈlaitis] *n* 十二指肠炎

dodecadactylon [ˌdəudekəˈdæktilɔn] *n* 十二指肠

dodecenoyl-CoA Δ-isomerase [ˌdəudəsəˈnəuil kəuˈei aiˈsɔməreis] 十二碳烯酰辅酶 A Δ-异构酶(亦称烯酰辅酶 A 异构酶)

Döderlein's bacillus [ˈdedəlain] (Albert S. G. Döderlein) 杜德莱因杆菌(一种大的革兰阳性细菌,常见于阴道内,据说与嗜酸乳杆菌相同)

dofetilide [dəuˈfetəlaid] *n* 多非利特(抗心律失常药)

dogbane [ˈdɔgbein] *n* 夹竹桃麻根

Dogiel's corpuscles [dəuʒlˈel] (Jeanvon Dogiel) 多纪尔小体(眼、鼻、口、生殖器黏膜内的感觉神经终器)

dogma [ˈdɔgmə] *n* 教条,信条

dogmatism [ˈdɔgmətizəm] *n* 教条主义 | **dogmatist** *n* 教条主义者

Dogmatist [ˈdɔgmətist] *n* 公式主义学派,教条主义学派(古希腊希波克拉底〈Hippocrates〉学派以后的第一个重要医派)

Döhle-Heller aortitis [ˈdeləˈhelə] (K. G. P. Döhle; Arnold L. G. Heller) 梅毒性主动脉炎

Döhle's disease [ˈdelə] (Paul Döhle) 梅毒性主动脉炎 | ~ inclusion bodies 窦勒包涵体(见于猩红热等病患者血内多形核白细胞球状小体。亦称白细胞包涵体)

doigt [dwɑː] *n*【法】指,趾

dol [dəul] *n* 多尔(痛强度单位)

dolabrate [dəuˈlæbreit], **dolabriform** [dəuˈlæbrifɔːm] *a* 斧形的

dolasetron mesylate [duˈlæsətrɔn] 甲磺多拉司琼(5-羟色胺受体阻滞药)

Dold's test(reaction) [dɔlt] (Herman Dold) 多尔德试验(反应),梅毒絮状试验(诊断梅毒的一种絮状沉淀反应)

Doléris' operation [dɔleiˈriːz] (Jacques A. Doléris) 多累里手术(用于子宫后倾,先缩短圆韧带,然后通过髂棘上方开口,使圆韧带固定在腹直肌的两端)

dolich(o)- [构词成分]长

dolichocephalic [ˌdɔlikəusəˈfælik], **dolichocephalous** [ˌdɔlikəuˈsefələs] *a* 长头的(头颅指数为75.9或以下的) | **dolichocephaly** [ˌdɔlikəuˈsefəli], **dolichocephalia** [ˌdɔlikəusəˈfeiliə], **dolichocephalism** [ˌdɔlikəuˈsefəlizəm] *n*

dolichocolon [ˌdɔlikəuˈkəulən] *n* 长结肠[畸形]

dolichocranial [ˌdɔlikəuˈkreinjəl], **dolichocranic** [ˌdɔlikəuˈkreinik] *a* 长头的(头颅指数为74.9或以下的)

dolichoderus [ˌdɔlikəuˈdiərəs] *n* 长颈者

dolichofacial [ˌdɔlikəuˈfeiʃəl] *a* 长面的

dolichohieric [ˌdɔlikəuhaiˈəːrik] *a* 长骶骨的(骶骨指数为100以下的)

dolichokerkic [ˌdɔlikəuˈkəːkik] *a* 长前臂的(桡肱指数为80以上的)

dolichoknemic [ˌdɔlikəuˈniːmik] *a* 长腿的(胫股指数为83或以上的)

dolichomorphic [ˌdɔlikəuˈmɔːfik] *a* 长形的

dolichopellic [ˌdɔlikəuˈpelik], **dolichopelvic** [ˌdɔlikəuˈpelvik] *a* 长骨盆的(骨盆指数为95或以上的)

dolichoprosopic [ˌdɔlikəuprəˈsɔpik] *a* 长面的

dolichostenomelia [ˌdɔlikəuˌstiːnəuˈmiːliə] *n* 细长指,细长趾,蜘蛛脚样指,蜘蛛脚样趾

dolichuranic [ˌdɔlikjuəˈrænik] *a* 长腭的(颌牙槽指数为109.9或以下的)

Dölinger's tendinous ring [ˈdeliŋə] (Johann I. J. Dollinger) 窦林格腱环(后弹性层增厚,在角膜缘周围形成一个弹性环)

dolor [ˈdəulə] ([复] **dolores** [dəˈlɔːriːz]) *n* 【拉】疼痛

dolorific [ˌdəuləˈrifik], **dolorogenic** [dəuˌlɔːrəuˈdʒenik] *a* 致痛的

dolorimeter [ˌdəuləˈrimitə] *n* 测痛计 | **dolorimetry** *n* 疼痛测量法

DOM 2,5-dimethoxy-4-methylamphetamine 2,5-二甲氧-4-甲苯丙胺

domain [dəuˈmein] *n* 域,区 | immunoglobulin ~s 免疫球蛋白辖区

domaria [dəˈmæriə] *n* 雅司病(即 yaws)

domazoline fumarate [ˌdəuməˈzəulin] 富马酸多马唑啉(抗胆碱能药)

Dombrock blood group [ˈdɔmbrɔk] (Dombrock 为患者的名字,1965年首次报道他的抗原)道姆布洛克血型(一种红细胞抗原,在白人中最常见〈65%〉,其他人种也并不少见)

domicile [ˈdɔmisail] *n* 住处 | **domiciliary** [ˌdɔmiˈsiljəri] *a* 住所的;家庭的,家用的

dominance [ˈdɔminəns] *n* 优势;显性 | cerebral ~ [单侧]大脑优势 / incomplete ~, partial ~ 不完全显性(对于某一种基因来讲,杂合子表现中间性状的现象) / lateral ~, one-sided ~ 单侧性优势 / ocular ~ 眼优势

dominant [ˈdɔminənt] *a* 优势的;显性的 *n* 显性;显性等位基因;显性性状

domiphen bromide [ˈdəumifən] 度米芬(消毒防腐药)

domoic acid [ˈdɔməik] 软骨藻酸

domperidone [dɔmˈperidəun] *n* 多潘立酮(镇吐药)

Donath-Landsteiner antibody [ˈdəunət ˈlɑːndstainə] (Julius Donath; Karl Landsteiner) 多-兰抗体(一种抗P血型抗原的IgG抗体,首次见于梅毒患者,低温时与红细胞结合,复温时诱发补体介导溶解,为阵发性血红蛋白尿溶血现象的诱因) | ~ test 多-兰试验(检阵发性寒冷性血红蛋白尿)

Donath's phenomenon(test) [ˈdəunət] (Julius Donath) 多纳特现象(试验)(阵发性血红蛋白尿患者血液在体外冷至5℃,然后加热至体温时发生溶血现象)

donaxine [dəuˈnæksiːn] *n* 芦竹碱

Donders' glaucoma [ˈdɔndəz] (Franciscus C. Donders) 单纯性青光眼 | ~ law 东德定律(眼球视物旋转定律,即眼睛在视线周围转动并非随意的,当注视远距离目标时,其转动的程度完全决定于目标正中面及水平面间的角距)

Donec alv. sol. fuerit donec alvus soluta fuerit 【拉】至通便为止

donee [dəuˈniː] *n* 受体;受[血]者

donepenzil hydrochloride [dəuˈnepəzil] 盐酸多奈潘齐(一种可逆性胆碱酯酶抑制药,用于治疗轻度到中度阿尔茨海默〈Alzheimer〉型痴呆症状,口服给药)

dong quai 【汉】当归

Don Juan [dɔn hwɑːn] (源自唐璜,西班牙传奇中的一个贵族和风流浪荡子)男子性乱交者

Don Juanism [dɔnˈhwɑːnizəm] 男子性欲亢进

Donnan's equilibrium [ˈdɔnən] (Frederick G. Donnan) 道南平衡(两种不同的溶液为一膜所分隔,经有些离子〈但不是全部离子〉渗透后所

呈的一种平衡状况,两个溶液之间的离子分布不一致,膜的两边之间产生电位,此两溶液的渗透压也不相同)

Donné's corpuscles (bodies) [dɔ'nei] (Alfred Donné)初乳小体,初乳细胞 | ~ test 多内试验(检尿脓)

Donohue's syndrome ['dɔnəhjuː] (William L. Donohue) 唐纳休综合征,矮妖精貌综合征(即 leprechaunism)

donor ['dəunə] *n* 供者,供血者;供体 | general ~, universal ~ 普适供血者,万能供血者(指具有O型血的人,其血液有时在紧急输血时使用)/ hydrogen ~ 氢供体 / living ~ 活体供者

Donovan bodies ['dɔnəvæn] (Charles Donovan) 杜[诺凡]氏体(肉芽肿杜诺凡菌;利什曼-杜诺凡小体,见 Leishman-Donovan bodies)

Donovania [dɔnə'veiniə] *n* 杜诺凡菌属 | ~ granulomatis 肉芽肿杜诺凡菌

donovanosis [ˌdɔnəvə'nəusis] *n* 杜诺凡菌病,腹股沟肉芽肿

dopa ['dəupə] *n* 多巴,3, 4-二羟苯丙氨酸(治震颤麻痹和锰中毒)

dopamantine [ˌdəupə'mæntiːn] *n* 多巴金刚(抗震颤麻痹药)

dopamine ['dəupəmiːn] *n* 多巴胺(升压药) | ~ hydrochloride 盐酸多巴胺

dopamine β-hydroxylase ['dəupəmiːn hai'drɔksileis] 多巴胺β-羟化酶,多巴胺β-单加氧酶

dopamine β-monoxygenase ['dəupəmiːn ˌmɔnəu'ɔksidʒəneis] 多巴胺β-单加氧酶(亦称多巴胺β-羟化酶)

dopaminergic [ˌdəupəmiː'nəːdʒik] *a* 多巴胺能的

dopant ['dəupənt] *n* 搀杂剂(如对激光晶体或半导体搀杂)

dopa-oxidase [ˌdəupə'ɔksideis] *n* 多巴氧化酶,单酚单加氧酶

dopaquinone [ˌdəupə'kwinəun] *n* 多巴醌(多巴的氧化产物,从酪氨酸合成黑色素的中间产物)

dopase ['dəupeis] *n* 多巴氧化酶,单酚单加氧酶

doped ['dəupt] *a* (搀杂剂)搀杂的

doping ['dəupiŋ] *n* (搀杂剂的)搀杂;服药(如服用增强行为表现的药物) | blood ~ 血搀(给运动员输入血液、红细胞或相关的血液制品以增强表现,经常在此事之前先抽血,以便在失血状态下继续训练)

doppellender ['dɔpəˌlendə] *n* 肌纤维增生

Doppler ['dɔplə] *n* 多普勒超声检查[术] | color ~ 彩色多普勒血流显像

Doppler effect (phenomenon, principle) ['dɔplə] (Christian J. Doppler) 多普勒效应(现象、原理)(运动体所发出的波型辐射〈光波或声波〉随着趋近观测者或远离观测者而分别在波长上增大或减少)

Doppler's operation ['dɔplə] (Karl Doppler) 多普勒手术(性腺交感神经对切或注射石碳酸于其周围组织内,其目的使激素产生增加及产生性的返老还童,亦称生殖腺交感神经毁损术)

Dopter's serum [dɔp'təː] (Charles H. A. Dopter) 多普特血清,副脑膜炎球菌血清(含副脑膜炎球菌抗体的免疫血清)

dorastine hydrochloride ['dɔːrəstiːn] 盐酸哚拉斯汀(抗组胺药)

Dorello's canal [dəu'reləu] (Primo Dorello) 多勒洛管(颞骨外层神经管)

Dorendorf's sign ['dɔrəndɔːf] (Hans Dorendorf) 多伦道夫征(主动脉弓动脉瘤时,患侧的锁骨上沟隆起)

dormancy ['dɔːmənsi] *n* 休眠;不活动,蛰伏

dormant ['dɔːmənt] *a* 休眠的,不活动的,蛰伏的

dormifacient [ˌdɔːmi'feiʃənt] *a* 促睡眠的

dornase ['dɔːneis] *n* 脱氧核糖核酸酶,去氧核糖核酸酶(亦用作构词,如 streptodornase) | pancreatic ~ (胰)去氧核糖核酸酶(用作气雾剂,以减少肺分泌物的黏性)

dornase alfa ['dɔːneis ælfə] 阿法链道酶(重组人脱氧核糖核酸Ⅰ〈Dnase Ⅰ〉,通过把长的细胞外DNA分子水解成较短的片断,减少囊性纤维化患者痰的黏度,吸入给药)

Dorno's rays ['dɔːnəu] (Carl W. Dorno) 多尔诺射线(小于2 890 Å〈埃〉单位紫外线)

Dorn-Sugarman test [dɔːn 'ʃugəmən] (John H. Dorn; Edward J. Sugarman) 多恩-休格曼试验(观察孕妇尿对家兔睾丸的作用,以检测胎儿的性别)

dorsa ['dɔːsə] dorsum 的复数

dorsad ['dɔːsæd] *ad* 向背侧,向背面

dorsal ['dɔːsəl] *a* 背的,背侧的 | **~ly** *ad*

dorsalgia [dɔː'sældʒiə] *n* 背痛

dorsalis [dɔː'seilis] *a*【拉】背的,背侧的

dorsi- 见 dors(o)-

dorsiduct ['dɔːsidʌkt] *vi* 引向背侧

dorsiflexion [ˌdɔːsi'flekʃən] *n* 背[侧]屈(如手或足向后弯曲)

dorsimesad [dɔːsi'mesæd] *ad* 向背中线

dorsimesal [ˌdɔːsi'mesəl] *a* 背中线的

dorsispinal [ˌdɔːsi'spainəl] *a* 脊柱背侧的

dors(o)- [构词成分]背,背侧

dorsoanterior [ˌdɔːsəuæn'tiəriə] *a* 背向前的(胎位)

dorsocephalad [ˌdɔːsəu'sefəlæd] *ad* 向头后,向枕部

dorsodynia [ˌdɔːsəu'diniə] *n* 背痛

dorsointercostal [ˌdɔːsəuˌintə'kɔstl] *a* 背肋间的

dorsolateral [ˌdɔːsəu'lætərəl] *a* 背外侧的

dorsolumbar [ˌdɔːsəu'lʌmbə] *a* 背腰的
dorsomedian [ˌdɔːsəu'miːdjən] *n* 背中线
dorsomesial [ˌdɔːsəu'misiəl] *a* 背中线的
dorsonasal [ˌdɔːsəu'neizəl] *a* 鼻梁的,鼻背的
dorsonuchal [ˌdɔːsəu'njuːkəl] *a* 颈背部的,项背的
dorsoposterior [ˌdɔːsəupɔs'tiəriə] *a* 背向后的(胎位)
dorsoradial [ˌdɔːsəu'reidjəl] *a* 手背桡侧的
dorsoscapular [ˌdɔːsəu'skæpjulə] *a* 肩胛背侧的
dorsoventrad [ˌdɔːsəu'ventræd] *ad* 由背向腹
dorsoventral [ˌdɔːsəu'ventrəl] *a* 背腹的;由背向腹的,后前位的
dorsum ['dɔːsəm] ([复] **dorsa** ['dɔːsə]) *n* 背 | ~ of foot 足背 / ~ of hand 手背 / ~ of penis 阴茎背 / ~ of tongue 舌背
dosage ['dəusidʒ] *n* 剂量
dose [dəus] *n* 量,[一次]剂量,一剂 *vt* 给…服药 *vi* 服药 | absorbed ~ 吸收量 / air ~ 空气量(X线或γ线) / average ~ 平均量 / booster ~ 加强剂量 / challenging ~ 攻击量(见 reacting ~) / cumulative ~, cumulative radiation ~ 累积剂量,累积辐射剂量 / daily ~ 一日量 / depth ~ 深度(剂)量 / divided ~ 均分[剂]量 / effective ~ 有效量,效应量 / emergency ~ 应急剂量 / epilating ~ 脱毛剂量 / erythema ~ 红斑量,红疹量 / exit ~ 出口量 / exposure ~ 照射剂量 / integral ~, integral absorbed ~, volume ~ 总吸收量 / L_+ ~ 致死限量 / lethal ~, fatal ~ 致死量 / Lf ~ 絮状反应限量,絮状沉淀限量 / limes nul ~, L_0 ~ 无毒限量 / Lr ~ 皮肤反应限量,皮肤反应界量 / maximum permissible ~ 最大容许量 / median curative ~ 半数有效量(使50%受试者症状消失的剂量) / median effective ~ 半数有效量,半数效应量 / median infective 半数感染量 / median lethal ~ 半数致死量 / median-tissue culture infective ~ 半数组织培养感染量 / minimum lethal ~ (MLD) 最小致死量 / optimal ~, optimum ~ 最适量 / organ tolerance ~ 器官耐受量 / priming ~ 初次剂量,准备剂量 / reacting ~ 反应量(对一动物第二次给予致敏性抗原能引起速发型超敏的反应量) / sensitizing ~ 致敏剂量 / threshold erythema ~ 红斑阈量 / tolerance ~ [可]耐受量
dorzolamide hydrochloride [dɔː'zəuləmaid] 盐酸多佐胺(抗青光眼药)
dosimeter [dəu'simitə] *n* [放射]剂量计 | **dosimetric** [ˌdəusi'metrik] *a* 剂量测定法的 / **dosimetrist** [dəu'simətrist] *n* [放射]剂量测定者 / **dosimetry** *n* [放射]剂量测定法
dosis ['dəusis] *n*【拉;希】量,[一次]剂量;一剂
dossier ['dɔsiei] *n*【法】病历表册,病历夹
dot [dɔt] *n* 小点,斑点
dotage ['dəutidʒ] *n* 老年性记忆衰退,衰老,老年性精神病
dotard ['dəutəd] *n* 衰老者
dothiepin hydrochloride [dəu'θaiəpin] 盐酸度硫平(抗抑郁药)
dotty ['dɔti] *a* 有点的
double ['dʌbl] *a* 双的
double blind ['dʌblblaind] 双盲(指在药物临床评价时不让病人和医务人员知道所试药物究属何种)
double mask [dʌbl mɑːsk, mæsk] 双盲(即double blind)
doublet ['dʌblit] *n* 成对物;双合透镜;(光谱的)双重线;电子偶;偶极子
doubt [daut] *n* 怀疑 | obsessive ~s 强迫性怀疑
douche [duːʃ] *n*【法】冲洗 | air ~ 空气冲洗 / fan ~ 扇形冲洗 / jet ~ 喷射冲性 / transition ~, alternating ~, Scotch ~ 冷热交替冲洗,交替冲洗
Douglas abscess ['dʌgləs] (James Douglas) 道格拉斯脓肿(直肠子宫陷窝脓肿) | ~ cul-de sac (punch, space) 道格拉斯陷凹(陷窝,间隙)(直肠子宫陷凹) / ~ fold 道格拉斯襞(①直肠子宫襞;②腹直肌鞘弓状线) / ~ ligament 道格拉斯韧带(直肠子宫襞) / ~ line 道格拉斯线(腹直肌鞘弓状线) / ~ septum 道格拉斯隔(胎儿的直肠隔)
Douglas bag ['dʌgləs] (Claude Gordon Douglas) 道格拉斯袋(测劳动代谢的集气袋)
douglascele ['dʌgləsiːl] *n* 阴道后壁膨出
douglasitis [ˌdʌglə'saitis] *n* 直肠子宫陷凹炎
dourine [duː'riːn] *n* [法]马类性病,马类锥虫病
Dover's powder ['dəuvə] (Thomas Dover) 杜佛散,复方吐根散(阿片吐根散)
dowel ['dauəl] *n* 桩,接合钉(以人造冠接于天然牙根所用的钉)
down [daun] *n* 胎毛
downgrowth ['daungrəuθ] *n* 向下生长;向下生长物 | epithelial ~ 上皮向下生长
down-regulation [daun ˌregju'leiʃən] *n* 减量调节,向下调节(某一化学制品或药物在一定区域内细胞表面上的受体数减少,通常由于长期接触该药剂所致)
downstream ['daunˌstriːm] *a* 下游的 *n* 下游区(在分子生物学中,本词用以表示位于基因的3′位的DNA或RNA区,或感兴趣区)
Down syndrome (disease) [daun] (John L. H. Down)唐氏综合征(病)(特征为头型小而前后扁平,鼻梁低平,指〈趾〉骨短,手足第一与第二指〈趾〉间的空隙大,精神发育迟缓,染色体异常,亦称蒙古痴呆症及21-三体综合征)

doxacurium chloride [ˌdɔksəˈkjuəriəm] 多沙氯铵(一种长效非去极化神经肌肉阻断剂,用以在手术时使骨骼肌松弛,并便于气管内插管,静脉内注射给药)
doxapram hydrochloride [ˈdɔksəpræm] 盐酸多沙普仑(呼吸兴奋药)
doxaprost [ˈdɔksəprɔst] *n* 多沙前列素(支气管扩张药)
doxazosin mesylate [dɔkˈsæzəsin] 甲磺多沙唑嗪(抗高血压药)
doxepin hydrochloride [ˈdɔksəpin] 盐酸多塞平(抗焦虑、抗抑郁药,兽用止痒药)
doxercalciferol [ˌdɔksəkælˈsifərɔl] *n* 多塞麦角钙化固醇(一种合成的维生素 D_2 类似物,用以减低循环甲状旁腺菌素水平,治疗继发性甲状旁腺功能亢进症,伴慢性肾[功能]衰竭,口服或静脉内给药)
doxogenic [ˌdɔksəˈdʒenik] *a* 自身概念(所致)的
doxorubicin [ˌdɔksəˈruːbisin] *n* 多柔比星(抗肿瘤抗生素) | ~ hydrochloride 盐酸多柔比星
doxycycline [ˌdɔksiˈsaikliːn] *n* 多西环素(抗生素类药) | ~ calcium 多西环素钙 / ~ hyclate, ~ hydrochloride 盐酸多西环素
doxylamine succinate [dɔkˈsiləmiːn] 琥珀酸多西拉敏(抗组胺药)
Doyen's clamp [dwɑːˈjɑːŋ] (Eugene L. Doyen) 杜瓦扬夹(胃肠道手术时用以止血) | ~ operation 杜瓦扬手术(阴囊鞘膜积水手术)
Doyère's eminence(hillock) [dwɑːˈjɛə] (Louis M. F. Doyère) 杜瓦叶尔隆凸(神经末梢穿入肌纤维所形成乳头状隆凸)
Doyne's familial honeycombed choroiditis [dɔin] (Robert W. Doyne) 多英家族性蜂窝状脉络膜炎(一种遗传性退化性眼异常,特征为在视乳头盘及黄斑附近显浅色斑点)
DP directione propria【拉】按适当用法; Doctor of Pharmacy 药学博士; Doctor of Podiatry 足医术博士
DPH Diploma in Public Health 公共卫生文凭
DPM Diploma in Psychological Medicine 心理医学文凭; Doctor of Podiatric Medicine 足医学博士
DPN diphosphopyridine nucleotide 二磷酸吡啶核苷酸(现称 nicotinamide adenine dinucleotide 〈NAD〉烟酰胺腺嘌呤二核苷酸)
DPN kinase [ˈkaineis] DPN 激酶, NAD^+ 激酶
DPT diphtheria-pertussis-tetanus(vaccine) 白喉-百日咳-破伤风(菌苗)
DR reaction of degeneration 变性反应
Dr Doctor 博士
dr dram 打兰,英钱
drachm [dræm] *n* 打兰,英钱(见 dram)
draconic acid [drəˈkɔnik] 茴香酸,对甲氧基苯甲酸
dracuncular [drəˈkʌŋkjulə] *a* 龙线虫的
dracunculiasis [drəˌkʌŋkjuˈlaiəsis], **dracontiasis** [ˌdrækənˈtaiəsis], **dracunculosis** [drəˌkʌŋkjuˈləusis] *n* 龙线虫病,麦地那丝虫病
Dracunculidae [drəkʌŋˈkjulidiː] *n* 龙线科
Dracunculoidea [drəˌkʌŋkjuˈlɔidiə] *n* 龙线总科
Dracunculus [drəˈkʌŋkjuləs] *n* 龙线[虫]属 | ~ medinensis 麦地那龙线虫
draft [drɑːft, dræft] *n* 顿服(剂) | black ~ 黑色顿服剂,复方番泻叶浸剂 / effervescing ~ 泡腾顿服剂 / mustard ~ 芥子硬膏,芥子泥罨
drag [dræg] *n* 型盒下部(牙模盘)
dragée [drəˈʒei] *n*【法】糖衣丸,糖锭剂
Dragendorff's test [ˈdrægəndɔːf] (Georg J. N. Dragendorff) 德腊根道夫试验(检有无胆色素)
drain [drein] *vt* 引流,导液 *n* 导管,引流管;引流,导液;引流物 | cigarette ~ 烟卷式引流 / controlled ~ 控制式引流管 / quarantine ~ 隔离引流管 / stab wound ~ 刺创引流管
drainage [ˈdreinidʒ] *n* 排水[设备];引流[法],导液[法] | basal ~ 脑底引流法(脑底蛛网膜下腔脑脊液引流法) / button ~ 钮式引流法 / closed ~ 闭合引流[术] / open ~ 开放引流[术];明沟 / postural ~ 体位引流 / through ~ 贯穿引流法 / tidal ~ 潮式引流法
dram [dræm] *n* 打兰,英钱(衡量单位) | fluid ~ 液量打兰(在药衡制中 1 液量打兰为 60 量滴,合 3.697 ml)
dramatism [ˈdræmətizəm] *n* 戏剧样行为(精神病时表现自大及戏剧性言行)
dramatization [ˌdræmətaiˈzeiʃən, -tiˈz-] *n* 戏剧化;梦中剧情
drape [dreip] *n* 布单,被单 | surgical ~ 手术[大]单(覆盖病人全身,只露手术区的布单)
Drash syndrome [dræʃ] (Allan L. Drash) 德拉舒综合征(一种遗传方式不明的家族性综合征,包括维尔姆斯〈Wilms〉瘤,伴肾小球病和男性假两性体)
drastic [ˈdræstik] *a* 剧烈的 *n* 剧泻药,峻泻药
draught [drɑːft] *n* =**draft**
dream [driːm] *n* 梦 *vi*, *vt* 做梦 | clairvoyant ~ 启示性梦 / day ~ 白日梦,幻想 / wet ~ 梦遗[精]
Drechsel's test [ˈdreksel] (Edmund Drechsel) 德雷克塞尔试验(检胆汁或黄嘌呤)
dreg [dreg] *n* [常用复]残渣,废物
drench [drentʃ] *vt* (给牲口)灌药 *n* 兽用顿服药
Drepanidotaenia [ˌdrepənidəuˈtiːniə] *n* 镰带绦虫属(寄生于禽类)
drepanocyte [ˈdrepənəuˌsait] *n* 镰状细胞 | **drepanocytic** [ˌdrepənəuˈsaitik] *a*
drepanocytemia [ˌdrepənəusaiˈtiːmiə] *n* 镰状细

胞血症,镰状细胞性贫血

drepanocytosis [ˌdrepənəusaiˈtəusis] *n* 镰状细胞病

Drepanospira [ˌdrəpənəuˈspaiərə] *n* 镰旋体属

Dresbach's syndrome [ˈdresbɑːh] (Melvin Dresbach) 德雷斯巴赫综合征(椭圆形红细胞增多症)

dresser [ˈdresə] *n* 敷裹员

dressing [ˈdresiŋ] *n* 敷料;敷裹,包扎 | antiseptic ~ 抗菌敷料 / cocoon ~ 茧式敷料 / cross ~ 易装癖 / dry ~ 干敷料 / fixed ~ 固定敷裹 / occlusive ~ 包扎疗法 / paraffin ~ 石蜡敷裹 / protective ~ 保护敷料

Dressler's syndrome [ˈdreslə] (William Dressler) 心肌梗死后综合征

Dreyer and Bennett hypothesis [ˈdraijəˈbenit] 德-贝假说(见 theory 项下 recombinational germline theory)

DRG diagnosis-related group 诊断相关组

drier [ˈdraiə] *n* 干燥器;催干剂

drift [drift] *n* 漂移,漂流;[遗传]漂变(如基因各代的随机变异);连续变异,漂离 | antigenic ~ 抗原性漂移(指某一病毒株的抗原结构的变异) / genetic ~, random genetic ~ 遗传漂变,随机遗传漂变(由于样本机误造成基因频率的随机波动,漂变在所有群体中都能出现,而在很小的群体中效应更为明显) / physiologic ~ 生理性牙移行 / ulnar ~ 尺侧偏移

drill [dril] *n* 锥,钻 | bur ~, dental ~ 牙钻 / cannulated ~ 管状锥

drilling [ˈdriliŋ] *n* 钻孔

drinidene [ˈdrainidiːn] *n* 氨甲茚酮(镇痛药)

drink [driŋk] *vt*, *vi* 饮 *n* 饮料;酒 | sham ~ 假饮(如经食管造口术的狗,其所饮之水不能进入胃内,或不能保存于胃内)

Drinker respirator [ˈdriŋkə] (Philip Drinker) 德林克人工呼吸器(一种金属箱,患者卧于其中,头露在外,用正负压力交替地产生人工呼吸,俗称铁肺)

drip [drip] *n* 流滴;滴注[法] | intravenous ~ 静脉滴注 / nasal ~ 鼻滴法,鼻饲法 / postnasal ~ 后鼻滴涕

drip-feed [ˈdrip ˈfiːd] *vt* 用鼻饲法喂(病人)

drive [draiv] *vt* 驱使;传动;推进 *n* [内]驱力,欲望动力;本能,冲动,传动,推进 | aggressive ~ 攻击冲动,死亡本能(death instinct) / sexual ~ 性驱力,生存本能(life instinct)

drivel [ˈdrivl] *vi* 流涎,垂涎

drivenness [ˈdrivənnəs] *n* 活动过强 | organic ~ 器质性活动过强(见于脑损伤者)

driving [ˈdraiviŋ] *n* 激发作用(脑电图上所见的一种效应,其间某些反复感觉刺激可引起脑电波振幅的变化) | photic ~ 光激发作用(当眼暴露于有节律的闪光时,来自枕部皮质的 α 节律受到改变)

drobuline [ˈdrəubjuːliːn] *n* 羟布林(抗心律失常药)

drocarbil [drəuˈkɑːbil] *n* 槟榔胂胺(兽用抗蠕虫药)

drocinonide [drəuˈsinənaid] *n* 羟西萘德(抗炎药)

drocode [ˈdrəukəud] *n* 双氢可待因(镇痛药,镇咳药)

drom(o)- [构词成分]传导;走,行;加速

dromograph [ˈdrɔməgrɑːf, -græf] *n* 血流速度描记器

dromostanolone propionate [ˌdrəuməuˈstænələun] 丙酸屈他雄酮(雄激素类药,用作抗肿瘤药)

dromotropic [ˌdrɔməˈtrɔpik] *a* 影响神经传导的,变[传]导的

dromotropism [drəˈmɔtrəpizəm] *n* 传导受影响,变导性 | negative ~ 负变导性,传导性减弱 / positive ~ 正变导性,传导性增强

dronabinol [drəˈnæbinɔl] *n* 屈大麻酚(镇吐药)

drool [druːl] *vi* 流口水,流涎 *n* 口水

drop [drɔp] *n* 滴;量滴;[复]滴剂;下垂;降落 | ear ~s 滴耳剂 / enamel ~ 釉质瘤,釉珠 / eye ~s 滴眼剂,眼药水 / foot ~ 足下垂 / nose ~s 滴鼻剂 / wrist ~ 腕下垂

dropacism [ˈdrɔpəsizəm] *n* 硬膏脱毛[发]法

droperidol [drəuˈperidɔl] *n* 氟哌利多(抗精神病药,有抗焦虑、镇静及抗呕吐作用)

droplet [ˈdrɔplit] *n* 飞沫,小滴

dropper [ˈdrɔpə] *n* 滴管

dropping [ˈdrɔpiŋ] *n* 滴下;滴下物;跛行步态(马)

dropsy [ˈdrɔpsi] *n* 积水,水肿 | abdominal ~, ~ of belly, peritoneal ~ 腹水 / ~ of amnion 羊水过多 / articular ~ 关节积水 / ~ of brain, ~ of head 脑积水 / cardiac ~ 心病性水肿 / ~ of chest 水胸,胸膜[腔]积水 / cutaneous ~ 皮下水肿,水肿 / epidemic ~, acute anemic ~ 流行性水肿,急性贫血性水肿 / hepatic ~ 肝性水肿 / nutritional ~, famine ~, war ~ 营养不良性水肿 / renal ~ 肾病性水肿 / salpingian ~ 输卵管积水,输卵管积液 / wet ~ 脚气[病] | **dropsical** [ˈdrɔpsikəl], **dropsied** [ˈdrɔpsid] *a*

dropwort [ˈdrɔpwəːt] *n* 水芹

Drosophila [drəuˈsɔfilə] *n* 果蝇属 | ~ melanogaster 黑腹果蝇(用于遗传学实验)

drosopterin [drəuˈsɔptərin] *n* 果蝇蝶呤

drostanolone propionate [drəˈstænələun] 丙酸屈他雄酮(dromostanolone propionate 的 INN 和 BAN 名)

drought [draut] *n* 旱灾
drowning [ˈdrauniŋ] *n* 溺水 | near ~ 近似溺水(溺水后一息尚存,并暂时窒息,但有时以继发性溺水而告终) / secondary ~ 继发性溺水(迟发性溺水,由于肺泡炎症之类的并发症所致)
droxacin sodium [ˈdrɔksəsin] 屈克沙星钠(抗菌药)
droxifilcon A [ˌdrɔksiˈfilkɔn] 屈若费康 A(一种亲水性接触镜材料)
DrPH Doctor of Public Health 公共卫生学博士
drug [drʌg] *n* 药,药品,药物;麻醉剂;成瘾性毒品 *vt* 给药 *vi* 常用麻醉药;吸毒成癖 | antagonistic ~ 拮抗药 / crude ~ 生药 / habit-forming ~ 成瘾药
druggist [ˈdrʌgist] *n* 药商;药剂师,调剂员
drug-resistant [ˈdrʌgriˌzistənt], **drug-fast** [ˈdrʌgfɑːst] *a* 抗药的,耐药的
drum [drʌm] *n* 鼓膜
drumhead [ˈdrʌmhed] *n* 鼓膜
Drummond's sign [ˈdrʌmənd] (David Drummond) 德拉蒙德征(在主动脉瘤患者呼吸张口时听到的喷气声)
drumstick [ˈdrʌmstik] *n* 鼓槌体(在正常女性个体的多核白细胞中发现约有 3% ~5% 的核有鼓槌状的突起,正常男性则无此现象)
drunkard [ˈdrʌŋked] *n* 嗜酒者
drunken [ˈdrʌŋkən] *a* 酒醉的,酒醉引起的 | ~ness *n* 醉酒,酩酊
drunkometer [drʌŋˈkɔmitə] *n* 酩酊测定器
drupe [druːp] *n* 核果
drusen [ˈdrusən] *n*【德】玻璃疣,脉络膜小疣;放线菌块,硫黄色颗粒
dryer [ˈdraiə] *n* 干燥器
Dryopteris [draiˈɔptəris] *n* 鳞毛蕨属
Drysdale's corpuscles [ˈdraizdeil] (Thomas M. Drysdale) 德赖斯代尔小体(卵巢囊肿液内的透明细胞)
DSC Doctor of Surgical Chiropody 外科手足医术博士
dsDNA double-stranded DNA 双链 DNA
dsRNA double-stranded RNA 双链 RNA
DT diphtheria and tetanus toxoids 白喉破伤风类毒素(儿科用)
Dt duration tetany 通电期间强直
dT deoxythymidine 脱氧胸苷
DTaP diphtheria and tetanus toxoids and acellular pertussis vaccine 白喉破伤风类毒素-无细胞百日咳菌苗
D. T. D. datur talis dosis【拉】给此剂量,给予同剂量
dTDP deoxythymidine diphosphate 脱氧胸苷二磷酸
DTH delayed-type hypersensitivity 迟发型超敏反应
DTIC, Dtic decarbazine 达卡巴嗪(抗肿瘤药)
dTMP deoxythymidine monophosphate 脱氧胸苷酸
dTMP kinase [ˈkaineis] 脱氧胸苷酸激酶
DTP diphtheria and tetanus toxoids and pertussis vaccine 白喉-破伤风类毒素-百日咳菌苗,白百破三联制剂
DTPA pentetic acid 喷替酸(二乙撑三胺五乙酸)
dTTP deoxythymidine triphosphate 脱氧胸苷三磷酸
dU deoxyuridine 脱氧尿苷
dual [ˈdju(ː)əl] *a* 二重的;二元的
dualism [ˈdju(ː)əlizəm] *n* 两重性;二元论(①认为血细胞的形成源于两个不同的干细胞:一个是淋巴细胞,另一个为髓细胞;②认为人类是由两个独立的系统组成,即精神与肉体,并认为心理与生理的现象基本上是独立的,性质上亦不相同)
dualist [ˈdju(ː)əlist] *n* 二元论者
dualistic [ˌdju(ː)əˈlistik] *a* 两重的;二元论的
Duane's syndrome [djuˈein] (Alexander Duane) 杜安综合征(一种遗传性先天性综合征,患眼显示外展的局限或缺失、内收受限制、内收时眼球退缩、内收时睑裂变窄而外展时变宽以及会聚缺乏,这是由常染色体显性性状遗传) | ~ test 杜安试验(使用烛焰及棱镜检隐斜视)
durable [ˈdjuərəbl] *a* 耐久的,持久的 | **durability** [ˌdjuərəˈbiləti] *n*
duazomycin [djuˌæzəuˈmaisin] *n* 达佐霉素(抗生素类药) | ~ A 达佐霉素 / ~ B 阿佐霉素(azotomycin) / ~ C 安波霉素(ambomycin)
dubi [ˈduːbi] *n* 雅司病(非洲加纳称法,即 yaws)
Dubini's chorea (disease) [djuˈbiːni] (Angelo Dubini) 杜比尼舞蹈症(病)(由中枢神经系统急性感染所致的一种电击样舞蹈症)
Dubin-Johnson syndrome [ˈduːbin ˈdʒɔnsən] (Isidore N. Dubin; Frank B. Johnson) 杜宾-约翰逊综合征(一种家族性慢性型非溶血性黄疸,据认为由于肝脏不能排泄结合胆红素和某些其他有机阴离子〈如磺溴酞〉所致,特点为肝细胞内存在棕色粗颗粒色素,为本征的特殊病征)
Dubin-Sprinz syndrome [ˈduːbin ʃprints] (I. N. Dubin; Helmuth Sprinz) 杜-施综合征(见 Dubin-Johnson syndrome)
Duboisia [dju(ː)ˈbɔisiə] *n* 澳洲毒茄属(茄科)
DuBois-Reymond's law [dju(ː)ˌbwɑː raiˈmɔŋ] (Emil H. DuBois-Reymon) 杜布瓦 · 雷蒙定律(对于肌肉及运动神经的刺激是由电流密度的变化所引起,与电流密度的绝对值无关)
Dubois's abscess [dju(ː)ˈbwɑː] (Paul Dubois) 杜布瓦脓肿(先天性梅毒时的胸腺脓肿),亦称胸腺脓肿 | ~ disease 杜布瓦病(先天性梅毒时胸腺内产生多发性脓肿)
Dubois's method (treatment) [dju(ː)ˈbwɑː] (Paul C. Dubois) 杜布瓦精神疗法(向病人说明病情并获得他的配合)

Duboscq colorimeter [dju'bɔsk] (Louis J. Duboscq) 杜博斯克比色计(与标准有色溶液作比较,测定有色溶液的强度)

Dubos enzyme(crude crystals, lysin) [du'bɔs] (René J. Dubos) 短杆菌素 | ~ medium 迪博斯培养基(白蛋白肉汤)

Dubreuil-Chambardel's syndrome [djubruː'iː ʃɑːmbɑː'del] (Louis Dubreuil-Chambardel) 杜布鲁依·尚巴达尔综合征(切牙龋,大多数情况仅为上切牙,通常发生在青春期,几年内损坏牙齿无法修复。有些权威人士认为此综合征不是真正的疾病)

Duchenne-Aran muscular atrophy (disease, type) [dju'ʃen ɑː 'rɑːn] (G. B. A. Duchenne; F. A. Aran) 脊髓性肌萎缩

Duchenne-Erb paralysis [dju'ʃenεəb] (G. B. A. Duchenne; Wilhelm H. Erb) 迪谢内-埃尔布麻痹(见 Erb-Duchenne paralysis)

Duchenne-Griesinger disease [dju'ʃən'griːsingə] (G. B. Duchenne; Wilhelm Griesinger) 迪-格病,迪谢内肌营养不良(假性肥大性肌营养不良)

Duchenne-Landouzy dystrophy (type) [dju'ʃen lɑːn'du'ziː] (G. B. A. Duchenne; L. T. J. Landouzy) 面肩肱型肌营养不良

Duchenne's disease [dju'ʃen] (Guillaume B. A. Duchenne) 迪谢内病(①脊髓病性肌萎缩;②延髓性麻痹;③脊髓痨;④迪谢内肌营养不良) | ~ (type) muscular dystrophy 迪谢内(型)肌营养不良,假性肥大性肌营养不良 / ~ paralysis 延髓性麻痹;埃尔布-迪谢内麻痹(见 Erb-Duchenne paralysis) / ~ sign 迪谢内征(膈麻痹或某些心包积水患者,吸气时上腹部下陷)

Duckworth's phenomenon (sign) ['dʌkwəːθ] (Dyce Duckworth) 达克沃思现象(征)(某些致命性脑病时,在心脏停止跳动前呼吸先行停止)

Ducrey's bacillus [du'krei] (Augosto Ducrey) 杜克雷嗜血杆菌

duct [dʌkt] *n* 管,导管 | aberrant ~ 迷管 / acoustic ~ 外耳道 / allantoic ~ 尿囊柄 / alveolar ~ 肺泡管 / biliary ~s, biliferous ~s, gall ~s 胆管 / canalicular ~s 输乳管 / cloacal ~ 泄殖腔管 / cochlear ~ 蜗管 / common bile ~ 胆总管 / common hepatic ~ 肝总管 / cowperian ~ 库珀腺管(尿道球腺管) / cystic ~ 胆囊管 / deferent ~ 输精管 / efferent ~ 输出小管 / ejaculatory ~ 射精管 / ~ of epoophoron 卵巢冠纵管 / gasserian ~ 加塞管(副中肾管) / guttural ~ 咽鼓管 / hepaticopancreatic ~ 肝胰管 / hepatocystic ~ 胆总管 / hypophyseal ~, craniopharyngeal ~ 垂体管,颅咽管 / incisive ~, incisor ~ 切牙管 / intercalated ~ 闰管 / lymphatic ~s 淋巴导管 / metanephric ~ 后肾管,输尿管 / milk ~s 输乳管 / omphalomesenteric ~, umbilical ~, vitelline ~, vitello intestinal ~ 卵黄管,卵黄柄 / ovarian ~ 输卵管 / papillary ~s 乳头管 / paramesonephric ~, primordial ~ 副中肾管 / pronephric ~ 前肾管,原肾管(胚) / renal ~ 输尿管 / sacculoutricular ~, utriculosaccular ~ 椭圆球囊管 / semicircular ~s 膜半规管 / seminal ~s 精管(包括输精管、精囊、排泄管、射精管) / testicular ~ 输精管 / thoracic ~, alimentary ~, chyliferous ~, left lymphatic ~ 胸导管 / thyroglossal ~, thyrolingual ~ 甲状舌管 | **~less** *a* 无管的

ductal ['dʌktl] *a* 管的,导管的

ductile ['dʌktail] *a* 延[伸]性的

ductility [dʌk'tiləti] *n* 延性;韧性;黏性;可塑性

duction ['dʌkʃən] *n* 转向(眼转动方向)

ductopenia ['dʌktəu'piːniə] *n* 胆管缺乏症

ductule ['dʌktjuːl] *n* 小管 | aberrant ~s 迷管(附睾) / alveolar ~s 肺泡小管 / bile ~s, biliary ~s 胆小管 / transverse ~s of epoophoron 卵巢冠横管

ductulus ['dʌktjuləs] ([复] **ductuli** ['dʌktjulai]) *n*【拉】小管

ductus ['dʌktəs] [单复词] *n*【拉】管,导管 | patent ~ arteriosus 动脉导管未闭

Duddell's membrane ['dʌdel] (Benedict Duddell) 角膜后弹性层,角膜后界层

Duffy blood group ['dʌfi] (从 1954 年首次观察到的先证者得名) 达菲血型(主要由红细胞抗原 Fy^a 和 Fy^b 组成的一种血型,由等位基因所决定。无效等位基因在非洲裔个体中是常见的)

Dugas' test(sign) ['dugəs] (Louis A. Dugas) 杜加斯试验(征)(检肩关节脱位:将患侧手置于对侧肩上,患侧肘部移至胸侧,如此动作不能完成〈杜加斯征〉,即有肩关节脱位)

Duhamel operation [djuɑː'mel] (Bernard G. Duhamel) 杜阿梅尔手术(治疗先天性巨结肠,拖出术的一种改良,在结肠近端神经节段和直肠之间作纵的吻合,使直肠保持原位) | ~ procedure 直肠后拖出吻合巨结肠根治术

Duhot's line [dju'hɔː] (Robert Duhot) 杜霍线(髂前上棘至骶骨尖间线)

Duhring's disease ['djuriŋ] (Louis A. Duhring) 疱疹样皮炎

Dührssen's incisions ['djuəsən] (Alfred Dührssen) 迪尔森切开(在宫颈上做切口,以利导产,即宫颈切开术) | ~ operation 迪尔森手术(阴道式子宫固定术)

Dujarier's clasp [djuʒəri'εə] 杜贾里爱夹(跟骨钩,跟骨骨折用)

Dukes' classification [djuːks] (Cuthbert Esquire Dukes) 杜克斯分类法(根据肿瘤侵害程度,结肠直肠癌可分成 A 到 C 的一种三级分期系统:A 为穿入但未穿透肠壁;B 为穿透肠壁;C 已累及

淋巴结,不论其对肠壁侵害程度如何。对此分类法已有很多改良) | ~ classification for colon cancer 结肠癌杜克斯分类法

Dukes' disease [dju:ks] (Clement Dukes) 杜克斯病,猝发疹,幻儿急疹(一种儿童轻型发热病)

Duke's test (method) [dju:k] (William W. Duke) 杜克试验(法)(测出血时间,即以标准穿刺刺伤耳垂后引起出血持续时间)

dulcite [ˈdʌlsait], **dulcitol** [ˈdʌlsitɔl], **dulcose** [ˈdʌlkəus] *n* 卫矛醇,半乳糖醇

dull [dʌl] *a* 浊音的;迟钝的

dullness, dulness [ˈdʌlnis] *n* 迟钝;浊音 | shifting ~ 移动性浊音 / tympanitic ~ 鼓性浊音

dulse [dʌls] *n* 掌状红皮藻(苏格兰及北欧国家居民食用)

dumas [ˈdju:məs] *n* 足雅司病(斯里兰卡对 tubba 的用语)

dumb [dʌm] *a* 哑的 | **~ness** 哑[症]

Dumdum fever [ˈdʌmdʌm] (Dum Dum 为印度加尔各管的一个区,20 世纪初期首次观察到此病)内脏利什曼病,黑热病

dummy [dʌmi] *n* 哑巴;橡皮奶头;修复体,桥体(托牙上的假牙);安慰剂,无效(对照)剂

Dumontpallier's test [ˌdju:mɔŋpælˈjɛə] (Victor A. A. Dumontpallier) 杜蒙伯利埃试验(检胆色素)

dUMP deoxyuridine monophosphate 脱氧尿苷酸

dumping [ˈdʌmpiŋ] *n* 倾倒(见 syndrome 项下的相应术语);填埋(处理垃圾的一种方法)

Dunbar's serum [ˈdʌnbɑ:] (William P. Dunbar) 邓巴血清,抗花粉血清(含豕草、黄花、黑麦等花粉的一种抗毒素,用于治疗花粉症)

Duncan disease, syndrome [ˈdʌŋkən] (本病最早在 Duncan 家族中发现)邓肯病,综合征(见 syndrome 项下 X-linked lymphoproliferative syndrome)

Duncan's fold [ˈdʌŋkən] (James M. Duncan) 邓肯襞(子宫腹膜襞,即产后立刻覆盖于子宫上的疏松腹膜襞) | ~ mechanism 邓肯机制(母体面娩出式) ~ position 邓肯位置(胎盘排出时,边缘先露于子宫口) / ~ ventricle 邓肯室,透明隔腔,第五脑室

Duncan's method [ˈdʌŋkən] (Charles H. Duncan) 自体疗法

Dunfermline scale [dʌnˈfə:mlin] 登弗姆林营养指标(按儿童营养情况进行分类:1. 优良,2. 一般,3. 需照料,4. 需治疗)

dung [dʌŋ] *n* 粪,粪肥

Dunham's fans (cones, triangles) [ˈdʌnəm] (Henry K. Dunham) 登纳姆扇影(锥面,三角)(见于硅肺患者的肺 X 线片结构,由细线连接的小结组成,呈锥形排列)

dunsiekte [dʌnˈsi:ktə] *n* (南非马)野百合中毒

duodenal [ˌdju(:)əuˈdi:nl] *a* 十二指肠的

duodenectomy [ˌdju(:)əudiˈnektəmi] *n* 十二指肠切除术

duodenitis [ˌdju(:)əudiˈnaitis] *n* 十二指肠炎

duoden(o)- [构词成分] 十二指肠

duodenocholangeitis [ˌdju(:)əuˌdi:nəukəuˌlændʒiˈaitis] *n* 十二指肠胆[总]管炎

duodenocholecystostomy [ˌdju(:)əuˌdi:nəuˌkəulisisˈtɔstəmi] *n* 十二指肠胆囊造口吻合术

duodenocholedochotomy [ˌdju(:)əuˌdi:nəuˌkəuledəˈkɔtəmi] *n* 十二指肠胆总管切开术

duodenocolic [ˌdju(:)əuˌdi:nəuˈkɔlik] *a* 十二指肠结肠的

duodenocystostomy [ˌdju(:)əuˌdi:nəusisˈtɔstəmi] *n* 十二指肠胆囊造口吻合术

duodenoduodenostomy [ˌdju(:)əuˌdi:nəuˌdjuəu-diˈnɔstəmi] *n* 十二指肠十二指肠吻合术

duodenoenterostomy [ˌdju(:)əuˌdi:nəuˌentəˈrɔstəmi] *n* 十二指肠小肠造口吻合术

duodenogram [dju(:)əudi:nəugræm] *n* 十二指肠 X 线[造影]照片

duodenohepatic [dju(:)əuˌdinəuhiˈpætik] *a* 十二指肠肝的

duodenoileostomy [ˌdju(:)əuˌdi:nəuˌiliˈɔstəmi] *n* 十二指肠回肠造口吻合术

duodenojejunostomy [ˌdju(:)əuˌdi:nəudʒidʒuˈnɔstəmi] *n* 十二指肠空肠造口吻合术

duodenolysis [ˌdju(:)əudiˈnɔlisis] *n* 十二指肠松解术

duodenopancreatectomy [ˌdju(:)əuˌdi:nəuˌpænkriəˈtektəmi] *n* 胰十二指肠切除术

duodenorrhaphy [ˌdju(:)əudiˈnɔrəfi] *n* 十二指肠缝合术

duodenoscope [ˌdju(:)əuˈdi:nəskəup] *n* 十二指肠镜 | **duodenoscopy** [ˌdju(:)əudiˈnɔskəpi] *n* 十二指肠镜检查[术]

duodenostomy [ˌdju(:)əudiˈnɔstəmi] *n* 十二指肠造口术

duodenotomy [ˌdju(:)əudiˈnɔtəmi] *n* 十二指肠切开术

duodenum [ˌdju(:)əuˈdi:nəm] ([复] **duodenums** 或 **duodena** [ˈdju(:)əuˈdi:nə]) *n* 十二指肠

duoparental [ˌdju(:)əupəˈrəntl] *a* 双亲的,源于两种生殖细胞的

Duplay's bursitis (disease) [duˈplei] (Simon E. Duplay) 杜普累黏液囊炎(肩峰下或三角肌下黏液囊炎) | ~ operation 杜普累手术(用于先天性阴茎畸形〈尿道上裂和尿道下裂〉的几种成形手术)

duplex [ˈdju:pleks] *a* 双的 *n* 二显性组合;双链

体;双螺旋

duplicate [ˌdjuːplikit] *a* 重复的;复制的;二倍的 *n* 复制品;副本 [ˈdjuːplikeit] *vt* 复制;使重复

duplication [ˌdjuːpliˈkeiʃən] *n* 重叠,双折;重复(染色体上增加某一片段的畸变) | incomplete ~ of spinal cord 脊髓纵裂 / renal ~ 重复肾

duplicitas [djuːˈplisitəs] *n*【拉】双畸胎,联胎 | ~ anterior 双上身联胎 / ~ posterior 双下身联胎

duplitized [ˈdjuːplitaizd] *a* 双面有感光药膜的(指 X 线片)

dupp [dup] *n* 杜普(表示听诊时第二心音)

Dupré's disease (syndrome) [djuˈprei] (Ernest P. Dupré) 假性脑膜炎

Dupuy-Dutemps' operation [djupjuˈiː djuˈtɔŋ] (Louis Dupuy-Dutemps) 杜普伊·杜当手术(下睑成形术)

Dupuytren's contracture [djupwiˈtrɑːn] (Baron G. Dupuytren) 迪皮特朗挛缩(掌腱膜挛缩) | ~ amputation 迪皮特朗切断术(肩关节切断术) / ~ enterotome 迪皮特朗肠刀(做人工肛门用) / ~ fracture 迪皮特朗骨折(见 Pott's fracture 及〈前臂〉Galeazzi's fracture) / ~ hydrocele 迪皮特朗鞘膜积液(二房性睾丸鞘膜积液) / ~ sign 迪皮特朗征(①压迫骨肉瘤时有一种咔嗒感;②先天性股骨头移位时股骨头可上下自由活动) / ~ splint 迪皮特朗夹板(防止腓骨下端骨折外翻) / ~ suture 连续浆肌层缝合

dura [ˈdjuərə] *n* 硬膜 | ~ mater 硬膜 / ~ mater of brain, ~ mater encephali 硬脑膜 / ~ mater of spinal

dural [ˈdjuərəl] *a* 硬膜的

Durand-Nicolas-Favre disease [djuˈrɑːn nikəˈlɑːˈfɑːvr] (J.Durand; Joseph Nicolas; M. Favre) 性病性淋巴肉芽肿

Durand's disease [djuˈræn] (Paul Durand) 杜朗病(一种病毒性疾病,伴有头痛以及上呼吸道、脑膜和胃肠道的症状)

Duran-Reynals' permeability factor [djuˈræn ˈreinlz] (Francisco Duran Reynals) 透明质酸酶

Durante's disease [djuˈrɑːnt] (Gustave Durante) 杜兰特病(成骨不全)

durapatite [djuˈræpəteit] *n* 羟磷灰石(即 hydroxylapatite,用作假体辅料)

duraplasty [ˈdjuərəˌplæsti] *n* 硬脑(脊)膜成形术

duration [djuəˈreiʃən] *n* 期间;持续时间 | expiratory ~ 呼气时间

Dürck's nodes [diək] (Hermann Dürck) 迪尔克结(锥体虫病时大脑皮质肉芽肿性血管周围浸润)

Dur. dolor. durante dolore【拉】疼痛持续时间

Duret's hemorrhages [djuˈrei] (Henri Duret) 迪雷出血(脑干和上脑桥中线线形小出血,由于脑干创伤性向下移位所致)

Durham rule [ˈdʌrəm] (Durham 为美国重罪犯的姓,1954 年被判为犯罪的精神病患者)德拉姆通例(美国联邦法院 1954 年德拉姆 vs. 美国诉讼案中关于犯罪责任的界定,认为"被告如由于精神病或精神缺陷造成不法行为时可不对其行为负责")

Durham's tube [ˈdʌrəm] (Arthur E. Durham) 德拉姆管(一种有接头的气管导管);(Herbert E. Durham) 德拉姆管(一种倒置的小试管,用以测定细菌气体总产量)

duroarachnitis [ˌdjuərəˌærəkˈnaitis] *n* 硬膜蛛网膜炎

Durozier's disease [djuˌrɔziˈe] (Paul L. Durozier) 先天性二尖瓣狭窄 | ~ murmur (sign) 杜罗济埃杂音(征)(主动脉瓣关闭不全时股动脉或其周围动脉双重杂音)

dust [dʌst] *n* 灰尘,尘埃,尘屑,粉尘 | blood ~ (of Müller) 血尘 / chromatin ~ 核染质屑(红色小粒,比豪厄尔〈Howell〉体小,常见于染色的红细胞边缘部) / ear ~ 耳沙,耳石

dust-borne [ˈdʌstbɔːn] *a* 尘埃传播的

Dutcher body [ˈdʌtʃə] (Thomas F. Dutcher) 达切小体(含免疫球蛋白胞质的一种核内内陷,见于肿瘤性浆细胞样淋巴细胞和浆细胞)

dUTP deoxyuridine triphosphate 脱氧尿苷三磷酸

dUTP pyrophosphatase [ˌpaiərəuˈfɔsfəteis] 脱氧尿苷三磷酸焦磷酸酶

Duttonella [dʌtəˈnelə] (J. E. Dutton) *n* 达顿锥虫属

Dutton's disease [ˈdʌtn] (Joseph E. Dutton) 锥虫病 | ~ relapsing fever 达顿回归热(中非洲蜱传回归热) / ~ spirochete 达顿包柔螺旋体(中非洲回归热螺旋体)

Duval's nucleus [djuˈvæl] (Mathias M. Duval) 杜瓦尔核(为一群多极神经节细胞,位于延髓内舌下神经核的腹外侧)

Duverney's foramen [djuvəˈnei] (Joseph G. Duverney) 网膜孔 | ~ gland 前庭大腺

dv double vibrations 双振动(声波频率的测定单位)

DVA Department of Veterans Affairs (formerly the Veterans Administration) 退伍军人事务部(以前为退伍军人管理局)

DVM Doctor of Veterinary Medicine 兽医学博士

DVT deep venous thrombosis 深静脉血栓形成

dwale [dweil] *n* 颠茄叶

dwarf [dwɔːf] *n* 矮小[畸形],侏儒 *a* 矮小的 | achondroplastic ~ 软骨发育不全性侏儒 / asexual ~ 性功能缺乏性侏儒 / ateliotic ~ 发育不全性侏儒 / cretin ~, hypothyroid ~ 愚侏病性侏儒,甲状腺功能减退性侏儒 / hypophysial ~, pituitary ~ 垂体性侏儒 / infantile ~ 幼稚型侏儒

/ micromelic ~ 肢端纤细性侏儒 / normal ~, physiologic ~, pure ~, true ~ 正常侏儒
dwarfish [ˈdwɔːfiʃ] *a* 矮小的,侏儒的,侏儒样的
dwarfism [ˈdwɔːfizəm] *n* 矮小,侏儒症 | deprivation ~ 剥夺性侏儒(即失母爱综合征,见 syndrome 项下 maternal deprivation syndrome)
Dwyer instrumentation [ˈdwiər] (Allen F. Dwyer)杜韦尔器械用法(使用杆、螺钉和U形钉矫正脊柱侧凸以便在腰区施行脊柱融合术的方法)
Dy dysprosium 镝
dyad [ˈdaiæd] *n* 二联体,二分体(由四分体离开而形成一个双染色体) | **dyadic** [daiˈædik] *a*
dyaster [ˈdaiæstə] *n* 双星[体]
dyclonine hydrochloride [ˈdaikləuniːn] 盐酸达克罗宁(局部麻醉药)
dydrogesterone [ˌdaidrəˈdʒestərəun] *n* 地屈孕酮(孕激素类药)
dye [dai] *n* 染色;染料,染剂 *vt* 染 *vi* [染]上色 | acid ~, acidic ~, anioic ~ 酸性染剂 / basic ~, cationic ~ 碱性染剂 / metachromatic ~ 异染染料,多色染料 / orthochromatic ~ 正染染料(只使组织染上一种颜色的染料) / vital ~ 活体染剂
dying [ˈdaiiŋ] *a* 临终的
dying-back [ˈdaiiŋbæk] *n* 变性(指轴突开始从远侧逐渐进展到近侧区的变性)
dyke [daik] *n* 女性同性恋
dynamic [daiˈnæmik] *a* 动力的,动态的;动力学的 | **~al** *a*
dynamics [daiˈnæmiks] *n* 动力学
dynam(o)- [构词成分]力,动力
dynamogenesis [ˌdainəməuˈdʒenisis], **dynamogeny** [ˌdainəˈmɔdʒini] *n* 动力发生,力生成 | **dynamogenic** [ˌdainəməuˈdʒenik] *a*
dynamograph [daiˈnæməgrɑːf, -græf] *n* 肌力描记器
dynamometer [ˌdainəˈmɔmitə] *n* 肌力计,量力器 | squeeze ~ 握力测量计
dynamoneure [daiˈnæmənjuə] *n* 脊髓[运动]神经元
dynamopathic [daiˌnæməˈpæθik] *a* 影响功能的;功能性的
dynamophore [daiˈnæməfɔː] *n* 供能[食]物
dynamoscope [daiˈnæməskəup] *n* 动力测验器,功能测验器 | **dynamoscopy** [ˌdainəˈmɔskəpi] *n* 动力测验法,功能测验法(如用尿道插管法观察肌肉活动或肾功能的情况)
dyn dtne 达因(力的单位)
dyne(dyn) [dain] *n* 达因(旧力的单位),现用N牛[顿], 1dyn = 10^{-5} N)
dynein [ˈdainin] *n* 动力蛋白
dynein ATPase [ˈdainiːn] 动力蛋白腺苷三磷酸酶(ATP-hydrolyzing activity of dynein 的 EC 命名法)
dynorphin [daiˈnɔːfin] *n* 强啡肽
dyphylline [daiˈfilin] *n* 双羟丙茶碱
dys- [构词成分]不良;困难,障碍
dysacusis [ˌdisəˈkuːsis], **dysacousia** [ˌdisəˈkuːziə], **dysacousis** [ˌdisəˈkuːsis], **dysacousma** [ˌdisəˈkuːsmə] *n* 听力减退;听音不适
dysadrenalism [ˌdisəˈdriːnəlizəm], **dysadrenia** [ˌdisəˈdriːniə] *n* 肾上腺功能障碍
dysallilognathia [disˌæliləˈneiθiə] *n* 上下颌不[相]称
dysanagnosia [ˌdisænægˈnəuziə] *n* (词失认性)诵读障碍
dysantigraphia [ˌdisæntiˈgræfiə] *n* 抄写不能,抄写障碍
dysaphia [disˈeifiə] *n* 触觉障碍,触觉迟钝
dysaptation [ˌdisæpˈteiʃən], **dysadaptation** [ˌdisædæpˈteiʃən] *n* 眼调节障碍,眼调节不良
dysarteriotony [ˌdisɑːtiəriˈɔtəni] *n* 血压异常
dysarthria [disˈɑːθriə] *n* 构音困难,(由于损害中枢神经系统所致) | **dysarthric** *a*
dysarthrosis [ˌdisɑːˈθrəusis] *n* 关节变形
dysaudia [disˈɔːdiə] *n* 听力障碍
dysautonomia [ˌdisɔːtəuˈnəumiə] *n* 自主神经功能异常
dysbarism [ˈdisbərizəm] *n* 气压病(统称)
dysbasia [disˈbeiziə] *n* 步行困难,步行障碍(尤指神经性) | ~ lordotica progressiva 进行性脊柱前凸性步行障碍,变形性肌张力不全
dysbetalipoproteinemia [ˌdisˌbeitəˌlipəuˌprəutiːˈniːmiə] *n* 异常β脂蛋白血症,家族性高脂蛋白血症Ⅲ型 | familial ~ 家族性异常β脂蛋白血症,家族性高脂蛋白血症Ⅲ型
dysbolism [ˈdisbəlizəm] *n* [新陈]代谢障碍
dysb(o)ulia [disˈbuːliə] *n* 意志障碍 | **dysb(o)ulic** [disˈbuːlik] *a*
dyscalculia [ˌdiskælˈkjuːliə] *n* 计算困难,计算障碍(脑伤或疾病所致)
dyscephaly [disˈsefəli] *n* 头面骨畸形 | mandibulo-oculofacial ~ 下颌眼面骨畸形,眼下颌面综合征
dyschezia, dyschesia [disˈkiːziə] *n* 大便困难
dyschiasia [diskaiˈeiziə] *n* 定位觉障碍,感觉定位障碍
dyschiria [disˈkaiəriə] *n* 左右感觉障碍(试验触觉时,难于分辨左右)
dyscholia [disˈkəuliə] *n* 胆汁障碍
dyschondroplasia [ˌdiskɔndrəuˈpleiziə] *n* 软骨发育不良
dyschondrosteosis [ˌdiskɔnˌdrɔstiˈəusis] *n* 软骨

骨生成障碍

dyschromatopsia [disˌkrəumə'tɔpsiə], **dyschromasia** [ˌdiskrəu'meiziə] *n* 色觉障碍

dyschromia [dis'krəumiə] *n* 皮肤变色

dyschronism [dis'krəunizəm] *n* 定时障碍(不合时,时间关系紊乱)

dyschylia [dis'kailiə] *n* 乳糜形成障碍

dyscinesia [disi'niːziə] *n* 运动障碍

dyscoimesis [ˌdiskɔi'miːsis] *n* 睡眠困难

dyscontrol [ˌdiskɔn'trəul] *n* (行为)控制不良 | episodic ~ 发作性(行为)控制不良,(行为)控制不良综合征(即 dyscontrol syndrome,见 syndrome 项下相应术语)

dyscoria [dis'kɔːriə] *n* 瞳孔变形(瞳孔反应异常)

dyscorticism [dis'kɔːtisizəm] *n* 肾上腺皮质功能障碍

dyscrasia [dis'kreizjə] *n* 体液不调,恶液质 | blood ~ 血质不调,血恶液质 / lymphatic ~ 淋巴恶液质;淋巴肉芽肿 | **dyscratic**, **dyscrasic** *a*

dyscrinic [dis'krinik] *a* 内分泌失调的

dysdiadochokinesia [ˌdisdaiˌædəkəukai'niːziə, -ki'n-], **dysdiadochocinesia** [ˌdisdaiˌædəkəu-sai'niːziə, -si'n-] *n* 轮替动作困难 | **dysdiadochokinetic** [ˌdisdaiˌædəkəukai'netik, -ki'n-] **dysdiadochocinetic** [ˌdisdaiˌædəkəusai'netik, -si'n-] *a*

dysdipsia [dis'dipsiə] *n* 饮水困难

dysecdysis [dis'ekdisis] *n* 蜕皮不良(指爬形动物)

dysecoia [ˌdisi'kɔiə] *n* 听力减退;听音不适

dysembryoma [disˌembri'əumə] *n* 畸胎瘤

dysembryoplasia [disˌembriəu'pleiziə] *n* 胚胎期发育不良

dysencephalia splanchocystica [disˌensi'feiliə ˌsplæŋknəu'sistikə] 头颅异常和内脏囊肿,梅克尔综合征(见 Meckel's syndrome)

dysenteriform [ˌdisən'terifɔːm] *a* 痢疾样的

dysentery ['disəntri] *n* 痢疾 | amebic ~ 阿米巴[性]痢疾 / asylum ~ 群居性痢疾 / bacillary ~, Japanese ~ 菌痢,杆菌[性]痢疾 / balantidial ~ 小袋虫[性]痢疾 / bilharzial ~ 裂体吸虫[性]痢疾,血吸虫[性]痢疾 / catarrhal ~ 卡他性痢疾,脂肪痢,口炎性腹泻 / ciliary ~, ciliate ~ 纤毛虫[性]痢疾 / epidemic ~ 流行性痢疾 / flagellate ~ 鞭毛虫[性]痢疾 / fulminant ~ 暴发型痢疾 / institutional ~ 团体[性]痢疾(尤在精神病院) / malarial ~ 疟性痢疾 / protozoal ~ 原虫[性]痢疾 / spirillar ~ 螺[旋]菌性痢疾 | **dysenteric** [ˌdisən'terik] *a*

dysequilibrium [ˌdisˌiːkwi'libriəm] *n* 平衡失调

dyserethesia [ˌdiseri'θiːziə], **dyserethism** [dis-'eriθizəm] *n* 应激性不良

dysergasia [ˌdisəː'geiziə] *n* 脑控制[功能]不良,整体反应障碍 | **dysergastic** [ˌdisəː'gæstik] *a*

dysergia [dis'əːdʒiə] *n* 传出性共济失调

dyserythropoiesis [disiˌriθrəupɔi'iːsis] *n* 红细胞生成不良

dysesthesia [ˌdisis'θiːzjə] *n* 感觉迟钝;触物感痛 | auditory ~ 听力减退;听音不适 | **dysesthetic** [ˌdisis'θetik] *a*

dysfibrinogenemia [ˌdisfaibrinəudʒe'niːmiə] *n* 异常纤维蛋白原血症

dysfluency [dis'flu(ː)ənsi] *n* 表达困难

dysfluent [dis'flu(ː)ənt] *a* 表达困难的

dysfunction [dis'fʌŋkʃən] *n* 功能障碍,功能不良(或异常) | constitutional hepatic ~, constitutional ~ of liver 体质性肝功能不良 / minimal brain ~ 脑功能轻微失调(即注意缺陷障碍[伴多动] attention-deficit hyperactivity disorder,见 disorder 项下相关术语) / myofascial pain ~ 肌筋膜疼痛功能障碍(颞颌关节综合征) / ~ uterus 子宫无力 | **~al** *a*

dysgalactia [ˌdisgə'læktiə] *n* 泌乳障碍

dysgammaglobulinemia [disˌgæməˌglɔbjuli'niː-miə] *n* 异常 γ 球蛋白血症(一类或几类 Ig〈不是全部〉缺陷状态,对体液免疫有关的传染病特别易感)

dysgenesia [ˌdisdʒi'niːziə] *n* 生殖力障碍,不孕

dysgenesis [dis'dʒenisis] *n* 发育不全,发育障碍 | seminiferous tubule ~ 细精管发育障碍症,克兰费尔特(Klinefelter)综合征

dysgenic [dis'dʒenik] *a* 种族退化的,非优生学的,劣生的 | **~s** *n* 种族退化学,劣生学

dysgenitalism [dis'dʒenitəlizəm] *n* 生殖器发育障碍

dysgenopathy [ˌdisdʒi'nɔpəθi] *n* 发育障碍病

dysgerminoma [ˌdisdʒəmi'nəumə] *n* 无性细胞瘤

dysgeusia [dis'gjuːziə] *n* 味觉障碍

dysglandular [dis'glændjulə] *a* 腺[功能]障碍的

dysglobulinemia [disˌglɔbjuli'niːmiə] *n* 异常球蛋白血症

dysglycemia [ˌdisglai'siːmiə] *n* 血糖代谢障碍

dysgnathia [dis'neiθiə] *n* 两颌发育异常 | **dysgnathic** [dis'næθik] *a*

dysgnosia [dis'nəuziə] *n* 智力障碍

dysgonesis [ˌdisgə'niːsis] *n* 生殖器功能障碍

dysgonic [dis'gɔnik] *a* 生长不良的(指细菌培养)

dysgrammatism [dis'græmətizəm] *n* 语法错乱,部分语法缺失(由于脑损伤或脑病所致)

dysgraphia [dis'græfiə] *n* 书写困难(由于顶叶障碍或运动系统障碍所致)

dyshematopoiesis [disˌhemətəupɔi'iːsis], **dyshemopoiesis** [disˌhiːməupɔi'iːsis] *n* 造血[功能]不全 | **dyshematopoietic** [disˌhemətəupɔi-

ˈetik], **dyshemopoietic** [disːhiːməupɔiˈetik] *a*

dyshepatia [dishiˈpeiʃiə] *n* 肝功能障碍

dyshesion [disˈhiːʒən] *n* 细胞黏着障碍,细胞间内聚力丧失

dyshidrosis, dyshydrosis [dishiˈdrəusis], **dysidrosis** [disiˈdrəusis] *n* [掌跖]汗疱;出汗障碍

dyshormonal [disˈhɔːməunl], **dyshormonic** [dishɔːˈmɔnik] *a* 内分泌障碍的

dyshormonism [disˈhɔːməunizəm] *n* 内分泌障碍

dysimmunity [disiˈmjuːnəti] *n* 免疫异常(免疫性疾病或异常免疫应答)

dysjunction [disˈdʒʌkʃən] *n* 分离

dyskaryosis [disˌkæriˈəusis] *n* 核异常(如见于孕妇宫颈的上皮细胞内) | **dyskaryotic** [ˌdiskæriˈɔtik] *a*

dyskeratoma [ˌdiskerəˈtəumə] *n* 角化不良瘤 | warty ~ 疣状角化不良瘤(亦称孤立性毛囊角化不良)

dyskeratosis [ˌdiskerəˈtəusis] *n* 角化不良症 | ~ congenita, congenital ~ 先天性角化不良 / hereditary benign intraepithelial ~ 遗传性良性上皮内角化不良 / isolated ~ follicularis 孤立性毛囊角化不良,疣状角化不良 | **dyskeratotic** [ˌdiskerəˈtɔtik] *a*

dyskinesia [ˌdiskaiˈniːziə, -kiˈn-] *n* 运动障碍 | biliary ~ 胆道运动障碍 / ~ intermittens 间歇性运动障碍 / occupational ~ 职业性运动障碍,职业性神经功能病 / tardive ~ 迟发性运动障碍 | **dyskinetic** [ˌdiskaiˈnetik, -kiˈn-] *a*

dyskoimesis [ˌdiskɔiˈmiːsis] *n* 睡眠困难

dyslalia [disˈleiliə] *n* 言语困难

dyslexia [disˈleksiə] *n* 诵读困难(由于中枢损害所致) | **dyslexic** *a*

dyslipidemia [disˌlipiˈdiːmiə] *n* 异常脂血症

dyslipidosis [ˌdislipiˈdəusis] ([复] **dyslipidoses** [ˌdislipiˈdəusiːz]), **dyslipoidosis** [disˌlipɔiˈdəusis] ([复] **dyslipoidoses** [disˌlipɔiˈdəusiːz]) *n* 脂质代谢障碍

dyslipoproteinemia [disˌlipəuˌprəutiːˈniːmiə] *n* 异常脂蛋白血症

dyslochia [disˈləukiə] *n* 恶露障碍

dyslogia [disˈləudʒiə] *n* 推理障碍,逻辑障碍;言语[思想]不连贯

dysmature [disməˈtʃuə] *a* 成熟不良的(指患有成熟障碍综合征的婴儿)

dysmaturity [disməˈtjuərəti] *n* 成熟障碍;成熟障碍综合征(即 dysmaturity syndrome,见 syndrome 项下相应术语) | pulmonary ~ 肺成熟障碍(见 Wilson-Mikity syndrome)

dysmegalopsia [ˌdismegəˈlɔpsiə] *n* 视物显大症

dysmelia [disˈmiːliə] *n* 肢体畸形,肢体发育异常

dysmenorrhea [ˌdismenəˈriːə] *n* 痛经 | congestive ~ 充血性痛经 / essential ~, primary ~ 自发性痛经,原发性痛经 / membranous ~ 膜性痛经 / obstructive ~ 梗阻性痛经 / psychogenic ~ 心因性痛经 / secondary ~, acquired ~ 继发性痛经 / spasmodic ~ 痉挛性痛经 / tubal ~ 输卵管性痛经 / uterine ~ 宫性痛经

dysmetabolism [ˌdismeˈtæbəlizəm] *n* 代谢障碍

dysmetria [disˈmiːtriə] *n* 辨距不良,辨距困难

dysmetropsia [ˌdismiˈtrɔpsiə] *n* 视物[大小]不称症

dysmimia [disˈmimiə] *n* 表情障碍

dysmnesia [disˈniːziə] *n* 记忆障碍 | **dysmnesic** [disˈniːzik] *a*

dysmorphic [disˈmɔːfik] *a* 畸形学的;畸形的

dysmorphism [disˈmɔːfizəm] *n* 同质异晶[现象];异形;畸形

dysmorphology [ˌdismɔːˈfɔlədʒi] *n* 畸形学 | **dysmorphologist** *n* 畸形学家

dysmorphopsia [ˌdismɔːˈfɔpsiə] *n* (眼)曲影症,视物变形症

dysmorphosis [ˌdismɔːˈfəusis] *n* 畸形,变形

dysmotility [disməuˈtiləti] *n* 能动性障碍(如胃肠道内)

dysmyelination [ˌdismaiəliˈneiʃən] *n* 髓鞘形成分解,髓鞘形成缺陷

dysmyelopoiesis [disˌmaiələupɔiˈiːsis] *n* 脊髓发育不良

dysmyotonia [ˌdismaiəuˈtəuniə] *n* 肌张力障碍

dysnomia [disˈnəumiə] *n* 举名困难,部分举名性失语

dysodontiasis [ˌdisədɔnˈtaiəsis] *n* 出牙困难,出牙不良,晚出牙

dysoemia [disˈiːmiə] *n* 死因不明(法医学名词,可归因于慢性无机物中毒)

dysontogenesis [ˌdisɔntəuˈdʒenisis] *n* 胚胎发育不良,个体发育不良 | **dysontogenetic** [ˌdisɔntəudʒiˈnetik] *a*

dysopia [disˈəupiə] *n* 视觉障碍,视觉缺陷 | ~ algera 痛性视觉障碍 | **dysopsia** [diˈsɔpsiə] *n*

dysorexia [ˌdisəˈreksiə] *n* 食欲障碍

dysorganoplasia [disˌɔːgənəuˈpleiziə] *n* 器官发育障碍

dysoria [diˈsɔriə] *n* 脉管渗透异常 | **dysoric** [diˈsɔrik] *a*

dysosmia [diˈsɔzmiə] *n* 嗅觉障碍

dysostosis [ˌdisɔsˈtəusis] *n* 骨发育障碍,骨发育不全,成骨不全 | cleidocranial ~ 颅骨锁骨发育不良 / craniofacial ~ 颅骨面骨发育不全 / mandibulofacial ~ 下颌面骨发育不全 / mandibulofacial ~ with epibulbar dermoids 下颌面骨发育不全伴眼球上皮样囊肿,眼耳脊椎发育不良 / metaphyseal ~ 干骺端成骨不全(亦称干

骺端软骨发育不良) / ~ multiplex 脂肪软骨营养不良 / orodigitofacial ~ 口指(趾)面骨发育不全,口面指(趾)综合征 | **dysosteogenesis** [dis,ɔstiəu'dʒenisis] *n*

dysoxidative [dis'ɔksi,deitiv] *a* 氧化障碍的,氧化不足的

dysoxidizable [dis'ɔksi,dizəbl] *a* 不易氧化的,难氧化的

dyspancreatism [dis'pæŋkriətizəm] *n* 胰腺功能障碍

dyspareunia [,dispə'runiə] *n* 交媾困难,性交疼痛[症]

dyspepsia [dis'pepsiə] *n* 消化不良 | acid ~ 酸性消化不良 / catarrhal ~ 卡他性消化不良 / chichiko ~ 米粉性消化不良(婴儿) / flatulent ~ 胃积气性消化不良 / gastric ~ 胃消化不良 | **dyspeptic** [dis'peptik] *a* 消化不良的 *n* 患消化不良症者

dysperistalsis [,disperi'stælsis] *n* 蠕动障碍

dysphagia [dis'feidʒiə] *n* 吞咽困难 | contractile ring ~ 收缩环性吞咽困难 / ~ inflammatoria (食管)炎性吞咽困难 / ~ lusoria(食管)受压性吞咽困难 / ~ nervosa 神经性吞咽困难,食管痉挛 / ~ paralytica 麻痹性吞咽困难,瘫痪性吞咽困难 / sideropenic ~ 缺铁性吞咽困难 / vallecular ~ 食物存积性吞咽困难 / ~ valsalviana 舌骨大角脱位性吞咽困难 | **dysphagic** [dis'feidʒik] *a* | **dysphagy** [,disfədʒi] *n*

dysphasia [dis'feizjə] *n* 言语困难 | **dysphasic** *a* 言语困难的 *n* 言语困难者

dysphemia [dis'fiːmiə] *n* 口吃,讷吃

dysphonia [dis'fəuniə] *n* 发声困难 | **dysphonic** [dis'fɔnik] *a*

dysphoretic [,disfə'retik] *a* 烦躁不安的,不适的 *n* 致烦躁剂,致烦躁物

dysphoria [dis'fɔːriə] *n* 病理性心境恶劣 | **dysphoric** [dis'fɔːrik] *a*

dysphoriant [dis'fɔːriənt] *a* 使烦躁不安的 *n* 致烦躁剂,致烦躁物

dysphrasia [dis'freiziə] *n* 言语困难,难语症(由于中枢神经或大脑缺陷所致)

dysphrenia [dis'friːniə] *n* 精神障碍,继发性精神障碍

dysphylaxia [,disfi'læksiə] *n* 早醒性失眠

dyspigmentation [,dispigmen'teiʃən] *n* (皮肤或毛发)色素沉着异常

dyspituitarism [,dispi'tjuːitərizəm] *n* 垂体功能障碍

dysplasia [dis'pleiziə] *n* 发育异常,发育不良 | anhidrotic ectodermal ~ 无汗性外胚层发育不良,先天性外胚层缺陷 / anteroposterior facial ~ 前后[颜]面发育异常 / chondroectodermal ~ 软骨外胚层发育不良 / cretinoid ~ 愚侏病样发育不良 / dental ~ 出牙不良,出牙困难 / dentinal ~ 牙本质发育异常,无根牙 / ectodermal ~ 外胚层发育不良症 / encephalo-ophthalmic ~ 脑性眼球发育不全 / epiphyseal ~ 骨骺发育不良 / ~ epiphysealis hemimelica 半肢畸形骨骺发育不良 / ~ epiphysealis multiplex 多发性骨骺发育不良 / ~ epiphysealis punctata 点状骨骺发育不良 / familial white folded mucosal ~ 家族性白色皱襞性黏膜发育不良,白色海绵状痣 / fibrous ~ (of bone) (骨)纤维性结构不良 / fibrous ~ of jaw 颌骨纤维性结构不良,颌骨增大症 / hidrotic ectodermal ~ 出汗性外胚层发育不良 / oculoauricular ~, oculoauriculovertebral (OAV) ~ 眼耳发育不良,眼耳脊椎发育不良(亦称 OAV 综合征) / oculodentodigital (ODD) ~, oculodento-osseous ~ (ODOD) 眼牙指(趾)发育不良,眼牙骨发育不良(亦称 ODD 综合征) / ophthalmomandibulomelic ~ 眼下颌肢发育不全 / thymic ~ 胸腺发育不全(一组遗传性疾病,有些是常染色体隐性遗传,有些是 X 连锁隐性遗传) | **displastic** [dis'plæstik] *a*

dyspnea [dis'pni(ː)ə] *n* 呼吸困难 | expiratory ~ 呼气困难 / inspiratory ~ 吸气困难 / nonexpansional ~ 胸廓扩张不能性呼吸困难 / sighing ~ 叹息式呼吸困难 | **dyspneic** [disp'niːk] *a*

dyspoiesis [,dispɔi'iːsis] *n* 生成障碍(如血细胞)

dysponderal [dis'pɔndərəl] *a* 体重异常的

dysponesis [,dispəu'niːsis] *n* 皮质运动区活动障碍

dyspragia [dis'preidʒiə] *n* 动时感痛,功能性疼痛

dyspraxia [dis'præksiə] *n* 运用障碍

dysprosium (Dy) [dis'prəusiəm] *n* 镝(化学元素)

dysprosody [dis'prɔsədi] *n* 言语声律障碍

dysproteinemia [dis,prəutiː'niːmiə] *n* 蛋白异常血症

dysraphia [dis'reifiə], **dysraphism** [,disrəfizəm] *n* 神经管闭合不全

dysreflexia [,disri'fleksiə] *n* 反射异常 | autonomic ~ 自主(神经)性反射异常

dysrhaphia [dis'reifiə], **dysrhaphism** ['disrəfizəm] *n* [神经管]闭合不全

dysrythmia [dis'riθmiə] *n* 节律障碍 | cerebral ~, electroencephalographic ~ 脑节律障碍,脑电波节律障碍 / esophageal ~ 食管节律障碍,弥漫性食管痉挛

dyssebacia, dyssebacea [,disi'beiʃiə] *n* 皮脂障碍症

dyssomnia [di'sɔmniə] *n* 睡眠障碍

dysspermia [di'spəːmiə] *n* 精液异常;精子异常

dysstasia [di'steiziə] *n* 起立困难 | **dysstatic**

[diˈstætik] *a*

dyssymbolia [ˌdisimˈbəuliə], **dyssymboly** [diˈsimbəli] *n* 构思障碍

dyssymmetry [diˈsimitri] *n* 不对称,偏位

dyssynergia [ˌdisiˈnəːdʒiə] *n* 协同失调,协同动作障碍 | biliary ~ 胆道协同动作障碍

dystasia [disˈteiʃiə] *n* 起立困难 | hereditary ataxic ~ 遗传性共济失调性起立困难

dystaxia [disˈtæksiə] *n* 共济失调

dystectia [disˈtekʃiə] *n* 神经管闭合不全

dysteleology [ˌdistiliˈɔlədʒi] *n* 无用器官学,残存器官学;无目的论

Dysteriina [ˌdistəˈraiinə] *n* 旋毛亚目

dysthymia [disˈθaimiə] *n* 心境恶劣,心境恶劣障碍 | **~c** [disˈθaimiæk] *n* 心境恶劣障碍者

dysthymic [disˈθaimik] *a* 心境恶劣的

dysthyroid [disˈθairɔid], **dysthyroidal** [ˌdisθaiˈrɔidəl] *a* 甲状腺功能障碍的

dysthyroidism [disˈθairɔidizəm], **dysthyreosis** [ˌdisθairiˈəusis], **dysthyroidea** [ˌdisθaiˈrɔidiə] *n* 甲状腺功能障碍

dystimbria [disˈtimbriə] *n* 音色不良

dystithia [disˈtiθiə] *n* 哺乳困难

dystocia [disˈtəuʃiə] *n* 难产 | constriction ring ~, contraction ring ~ 子宫痉挛性狭窄环难产,收缩环性难产 / fetal ~ 胎原性难产 / maternal ~ 母原性难产 / placental ~ 胎盘难产

dystonia [disˈtəuniə] *n* 张力障碍 | torsion ~ 扭转性肌张力障碍 | **dystonic** [disˈtɔnik] *a*

dystopia [disˈtəupiə], **dystopy** [ˈdistəpi] *n* 异位,错位 | **dystopic** [disˈtɔpik] *a*

dystrophia [disˈtrəufiə] *n*【拉】营养障碍,营养不良

dystrophin [distrəfin] *n* 抗肌萎缩蛋白,肌营养不良蛋白

dystrophodextrin [ˌdistrɔfəuˈdekstrin] *n* 血糊精

dystrophoneurosis [disˌtrɔfənjuəˈrəusis] *n* 营养不良性神经病;神经性营养障碍

dystrophy [ˈdistrəfi] *n* 营养不良 | adiposogenital ~ 肥胖性生殖器退化,脑性肥胖症 / asphyxiating thoracic ~ (ATD) 窒息性胸廓营养不良 / craniocarpotarsal ~ 颅腕跗骨营养不良 / hypophyseal ~ 垂体功能减退性营养不良 / tapetochoroidal ~ 无脉络膜(眼) / wound ~ 创伤后营养不良

dystropy [ˈdistrəpi] *n* 行为异常 | **dystropic** [disˈtrəupik] *a*

dystrypsia [disˈtripsiə] *n* 胰蛋白酶(分泌)障碍

dysuria [disˈjuəriə], **dysuresia** [ˌdisjuəˈriːziə] *n* 排尿困难 | **dysuric** [disˈjuərik] *a* / **dysuriac** [disˈjuəriæk] *n* 排尿困难者

dysvascular [disˈvæskjulə] *a* 血供不足的

dysvitaminosis [ˌdisvaitəmiˈnəusis] *n* 维生素失调症

dyszoospermia [diszəuəuˈspəːmiə] *n* 精子形成障碍

E

E emmetropia 正视眼;enzyme 酶;exa- 艾[可萨]

E elastance 弹性; electric intensity 电[场]强度; electromotive force 电动势;energy 能量;expectancy 预期;illumination 照度;redox potential 氧化还原电位

E- 一种用以说明具有双键化合物绝对构型的立体描记器

E_1 estrone 雌酮

E_2 estradiol 雌二醇

E_3 estriol 雌三醇

E_4 estetrol 雌四醇

E_h redox potential 氧化还原电位

$E°$ standard reduction potential 标准还原电位

e electron 电子

e- [前缀]离;外

e 电荷(electric charge)基本单位的符号;自然对数的底(base of natural logarithmus)的符号(约2.718 281 828 5)

e^+ positron 正电子,阳电子

e^- electron 负电子,阴电子

ε epsilon 希腊语的第5个字母;摩尔吸光系数(molar absorptivity)、IgE 的重链(heavy chain of IgE)、血红蛋白的 ε 链(ε chain of hemoglobin)的符号

η 希腊语的第7个字母;绝对黏度(absolute viscosity)的符号

EAC 红细胞(erythrocyte)、抗体(antibody)和补体(complement)的符号,有时用来表示补体复合物,如 $EAC14b2_a$

EACA epsilon-aminocaproic acid ε-氨基己酸,6-氨基己酸(止血药)

EAD early afterdepolarization 早期后除极

ead. eadem【拉】*ad* 同样

EAE experimental allergic encephalomyelitis 实验性变应性脑脊髓炎

EAEC enteroadherent *Escherichia coli* 肠黏附性大肠杆菌

EAggEC enteroaggregative *Escherichia coli* 肠聚集性大肠杆菌

Eagle test [ˈiːgl] (Harry Eagle) 伊格尔试验(检梅毒)

Eagle-Barrett syndrome [iːgəlˈbærət] (J. F. Eagle, Jr.; Norman R. Barrett) 伊-巴综合征(干杏梅状腹综合征)

EAHF *e*czema, *a*sthma, *h*ay *f*ever 湿疹、哮喘、花粉症

Eales's disease [iːlz] (Henry Eales) 伊尔斯病,视网膜静脉周围炎(青年复发性视网膜出血)

EAP epiallopregnanolone 表异孕烷醇酮

Ea. R. Entartungs-Reaktion【德】变性反应

ear [iə] *n* 耳 | acute ~ 急性中耳炎,急性卡他性中耳炎 / aviator's ~ 航空性中耳炎 / beach ~ 海水浴耳病 / cat's ~ 猫耳(耳郭褶叠) / cauliflower ~, prizefighter ~ 菜花状耳,拳击耳 / diabetic ~ 糖尿病性乳突炎 / Hong Kong ~, Singapore ~ 耳真菌病,真菌性耳炎 / hot weather ~ 湿热耳 / lop ~, bat ~ 垂耳,招风耳 / satyr ~ 尖耳轮耳 / scroll ~ 卷耳 / tank ~ 游泳池耳病

earache [ˈiəreik] *n* 耳痛

eardrops [ˈiədrɔps] *n* 耳药水(滴耳剂)

eardrum [ˈiədrʌm] *n* 中耳;鼓膜,鼓室

eared [iəd] *a* 有耳的

earlobe [ˈiələub] *n* 耳垂

early [ˈəːli] *a* 早期的

ear-minded [iəˈmaindid] *a* 听性记忆的

earphone [ˈiəfəun] *n* 耳机

earth [əːθ] *n* 土,土地 | alkaline ~ 碱土 / fuller's ~ 漂白土 / infusorial ~, diatomaceous ~, silicious ~ 硅藻土

earth-nut [ˈəːθnʌt] *n* 落花生

earthquake [ˈəːθkweik] *n* 地震

earwax [ˈiəwæks] *n* 耵聍,耳垢

eating [ˈiːtiŋ] *n* 进食 | binge ~ 狂食

Eaton-Lambert syndrome [ˈiːtənˈlæmbət] (L. M. Eaton; Edward H. Lambert) 伊顿-兰伯特综合征(一种肌无力样综合征,肢体通常软弱无力,而眼肌和眼球肌则幸免,刺激肢体神经时肌肉的动作电位降低,但若反复刺激则动作电位增高。本征常合并肺燕麦细胞癌,亦称肌无力综合征)

EAV electroacupuncture after Voll 福尔电针[刺]术

EB elementary body 血小板,原生小体

Ebbinghaus test [ˈebiŋhaus] (Hermann Ebbinghaus) 埃宾豪斯试验(检精神疾病:检查者给予患者一些已省略几个字的句子,然后由患者完成这些句子)

EBCT electron beam computed tomography 电子束计算体层摄影[术]

Eberthella [ˌiːbəˈθelə] (Karl Joseph Eberth) *n* 埃[伯特]氏杆菌属

Eberth's lines [ˈeibət] (Karl J. Eberth) 埃伯特线（显微镜下心肌细胞交接处的断裂或梯纹状线）

EBL enzootic bovine leukosis 地方流行性牛白血病

Ebner's fibrils [ˈebnə] (Victor Ebner von Rofenstein) 埃伯内原纤维（牙质内）| ~ glands 舌腺，味腺 / ~ reticulum 埃伯内网（细精管内）

Ebola virus, virus disease (hemorrhagic fever) [ˈeibəulə] (Ebola 为刚果北方一条河流名，1976 年首次观察到此病) 埃博拉病毒、病毒病（出血热）（见 virus 项下相应术语）

ebonation [ˌiːbəˈneiʃən] *n* （损伤后）碎骨片清除术

ébranlement [eibrɑːnləˈmɔŋ] *n*【法】息肉扭摘术

ebriety [iˈbraiəti] *n* 沉醉，醉酒；酒癖

Ebstein's angle [ˈebstain] (Wilhelm Ebstein) 心肝角 | ~ anomaly 埃布斯坦异常（右房室瓣畸形，常伴房间隔缺损）/ ~ disease 埃布斯坦病（①肾小管上皮细胞透明变性及坏死，见于糖尿病；②右房室瓣畸形，常伴房间隔缺损）

ebullient [iˈbʌljənt] *a* 沸腾的 | **ebullience, ebulliency** *n*

ebullition [ebəˈliʃən] *n* 沸，沸腾

ebur [ˈiːbə] *n*【拉】象牙 | ~ dentis 牙本质

eburnation [ˌiːbəˈneiʃən] *n* 骨质象牙化；牙本质象牙化 | ~ of dentin 牙本质象牙化

eburneous [iˈbəːniəs] *a* 象牙样的

eburnitis [iːbəˈnaitis] *n* 牙釉质密固

EBV Epstein-Barr virus EB 病毒，非洲淋巴细胞瘤病毒

EC Enzyme Commission 酶学委员会

écarteur [eikɑːˈtəː] *n*【法】牵开器

ecaudate [iˈkɔːdeit] *a* 无尾的

ecbolic [ekˈbɔlik] *a* 催产的 *n* 催产药

ecbovirus [ekbəuˈvaiərəs] (*e*nteric *c*ytopathic *b*ovine *o*rphan virus) *n* ECBO 病毒，牛肠道细胞病变孤儿病毒

eccentric [ikˈsentrik] *a* 偏心的，离心的；怪僻的

eccentricity [ˌeksenˈtrisiəti] *n* 怪僻，偏僻性；偏心度，离心率

eccentro-osteochondrodysplasia [ekˌsentrəu ˌɔstiəuˌkɔndrəudisˈpleiziə], **eccentrochondroplasia** [ekˌsentrəuˌkɔndrəuˈpleiziə] *n* 离心性（骨）软骨发育不良（即 Morquio's syndrome）

eccephalosis [ˌeksefəˈləusis] *n* 穿颅术

ecchondroma [ˌekɔnˈdrəumə], **ecchondrosis** [ˌekɔnˈdrəusis] *n* 外生软骨瘤

ecchondrotome [eˈkɔndrətəum] *n* 软骨刀

ecchordosis physaliphora [ˌekəˈdəusis ˌfisəˈlifərə] 颅内脊索瘤

ecchymoma [ekiˈməumə] *n* 瘀血肿，皮下血肿

ecchymosed [ˈekiməuzd] *a* 有瘀斑的，成瘀斑的

ecchymosis [ˌekiˈməusis] ([复] **ecchymoses** [ˌekiˈməusiːz]) *n* 出血斑，瘀斑 | cadaveric ecchymoses 尸斑 | **ecchymotic** [ekiˈmɔtik] *a*

eccoprotic [ˌekəˈprɔtik] *a* 导泻的 *n* 导泻药

eccrine [ˈekrin] *n* 外分泌物（特指一般的汗腺）*a* 外分泌的

eccrinology [ˌekriˈnɔlədʒi], **eccrisiology** [eˌkrisiˈɔlədʒi] *n* （外）分泌学

eccrisis [ˈekrisis] *n* 排泄

eccritic [eˈkritik] *a* 促排泄的 *n* 排泄剂

eccyesis [ˌeksaiˈiːsis] *n* 异位妊娠，宫外孕

ECD ethyl cysteinate dimer 乙基半胱氨酸二聚物

ecdemic [ekˈdemik] *a* 非地方性的，外地的，外来的（指疾病）

ecdovirus [ˌekdəuˈvaiərəs] (*e*nteric *c*ytopathic *d*og *o*rphan + virus) *n* ECDO 病毒，犬肠道细胞病变孤儿病毒

ecdysiasm [ekˈdaisiəzəm] *n* 脱衣癖

ecdysis [ˈekdisis] *n* 蜕皮；换羽

ecdysone [ekˈdaisɔn] *n* 蜕皮激素

ecdysterone [ˌekdiˈstiərəun] *n* 脱皮【甾】酮

ECF extracellular fluid 细胞外液；eosinophil chemotactic factor 嗜酸性粒细胞趋化因子

ECF-A eosinophil chemotactic factor of anaphylaxis 过敏反应嗜酸性粒细胞趋化因子

ECG electrocardiogram 心电图

ecgonine [ˈekgənin] *n* 爱康宁，芽子碱（局部麻醉药）

echeosis [ˌekiˈəusis] *n* 噪音性神经功能病

echidnase [iˈkidneis] *n* 蛇毒致炎酶

echidnin [iˈkidnin] *n* 蝰[蛇]毒素

Echidnophaga [ˌekidˈnɔfəgə] *n* 冠蚤属 | ~ gallinacea 禽冠蚤

echidnotoxin [iˌkidnəuˈtɔksin] *n* 蝰[蛇]毒素

echidnovaccine [iˌkidnəuˈvæksin] *n* 抗蛇毒疫苗

Echinacea [ˌekiˈneisiə] *n* 紫锥花属

echinate [ˈekineit] *a* 猬棘状的，小棘状的

echinenone [iˈkinənəun] *n* 海胆酮，β-胡萝卜素-4-酮，海胆紫酮

echin(o)- [构词成分] 棘，刺

Echinochasmus [iːˌkainəuˈkæzməs] *n* 棘隙吸虫属 | ~ perfoliatus 抱茎棘隙吸虫，叶形棘隙吸虫

echinochrome [iˈkainəkrəum] *n* 海胆色素

echinococcosis [iˌkainəukɔˈkəusis], **echinococciasis** [iˌkainəukɔˈkaiəsis] *n* 棘球蚴病

echinococcotomy [iˌkainəukɔˈkɔtəmi] *n* 棘球囊切开术

echinococcus [iˌkainəuˈkɔkəs] ([复] **echinococci** [iˌkainəuˈkɔk(s)ai]) *n* 棘球蚴，棘球绦虫

Echinococcus [iˌkainəuˈkɔkəs] *n* 棘球绦虫属 | ~ granulosus 细粒棘球绦虫 / ~ multilocularis,

~ alveolaris 多房棘球绦虫

echinocyte [iˈkainəsait] *n* 棘状红细胞,钝锯齿状红细胞

echinocytosis [iˌkainəsaiˈtəusis] *n* 棘状红细胞增多

echinoderm [iˈkainədəːm] *n* 棘皮动物

Echinodermata [iˌkainəuˈdəːmətə] *n* 棘皮动物门

Echinoidea [ikiˈnɔidiə] *n* 棘皮纲,海胆纲

Echinolaelaps [iˌkainəuˈliːlæps] *n* 棘厉螨属 | ~ echidninus 毒棘厉螨

echinophthalmia [iˌkinɔfˈθælmiə] *n* 倒睫性眼睑炎

Echinorhynchus [iˌkainəuˈriŋkəs] *n* 巨吻棘头虫属

echinosis [ˌekiˈnəusis] *n* 红细胞皱缩

Echinosteliida [iːˌkainəustiˈlaiidə] *n* 棘柱目

Echinostoma [ˌekiˈnɔstəumə] *n* 棘口吸虫属 | ~ ilocanum 伊族棘口吸虫

Echinostomatidae [ˌekinəustəuˈmætidiː] *n* 棘口[吸虫]属

echinostomiasis [iˌkinəustəuˈmaiəsis] *n* 棘口吸虫病

Echinothrix [iˈkainəuθriks] *n* 刺棘海胆属

echinulate [iˈkinjulit] *a* 猬棘状的,小棘状的

Echis [ˈiːkis] *n* 小蝰属(产于印度至北非一带的小形毒蛇)

echo [ˈekəu] *n* 回声,回波;重复,模仿 | amphoric ~ 空瓮性回声(胸部听诊时) / metallic ~ 金属性回声(心包积气和气胸患者的心音)

echoacousia [ˌekəuəˈkuːziə] *n* 回声感觉

echocardiogram [ˌekəuˈkɑːdiəgræm] *n* 超声心动图

echocardiography [ˌekəuˌkɑːdiˈɔgrəfi] *n* 超声心动描记术

echoencephalogram [ˌekəuenˈsefələgræm] *n* 脑回波图,脑声像图

echoencephalograph [ˌekəuenˈsefələgrɑːf, -græf] *n* 脑回波描记器 | **~y** [ˌekəuenˌsefəˈlɔgrəfi] *n* 脑回波检查[法],脑声像图检查

echogenic [ˌekəuˈdʒenik] *a* 回波发生的,产生回声的

echogenicity [ˌekəudʒeˈnisəti] *n* 产生回波[性],产生回声[性]

echogram [ˈekəgræm] *n* 回波[描记]图,声像图

echographia [ekəuˈgræfiə] *n* 模仿书写

echography [iˈkɔgrəfi] *n* 回波描记术,声像图检查

echokinesis [ˌekəukaiˈniːsis] *n* 模仿运动,模仿动作

echolalia [ˌekəuˈleiliə] *n* 模仿言语

echolalus [ekəuˈleiləs] ([复] **echolali** [ˌekəuˈleilai]) *n*【拉】模仿言语者

echolucent [ˌekəuˈljuːsənt] *a* 无回波的(可使超声波通过,该区即透声区,声像图上显示黑色)

echomatism [eˈkəumətizəm] *n* 模仿行动

echomimia [ˌekəuˈmimiə] *n* 模仿表情

echomotism [ˌekəuˈməutizəm] *n* 模仿动作

echopathy [eˈkɔpəθi] *n* 病态模仿,模仿症

echophonocardiography [ˌekəuˌfəunəuˌkɑːdiˈɔgrəfi] *n* 超声心音检查法

echophony [eˈkɔfəni] *n* 胸内回声(胸听诊时)

echophotony [ˌekəˈfɔtəni] *n* 声色联觉(因音响而呈现某种色觉)

echophrasia [ˌekəuˈfreisiə] *n* 模仿言语

echopraxia [ˌekəuˈpræksiə], **echopraxis** [ˌekəuˈpræksis] *n* 模仿动作

echo-ranging [ˌekəuˈreindʒiŋ] *n* 回波测距,回波定位

echothiophate iodide [ˌekəuˈθaiəfeit] 碘依可酯(抗胆碱酯酶药,缩瞳药)

echovirus [ˌekəuˈvaiərəs] (*e*nteric *c*ytopathic *h*uman *o*rphan + virus) *n* 艾柯病毒,ECHO 病毒,人肠道细胞病变孤儿病毒

ECI electrocerebral inactivity 脑电静止

Ecker's fissure [ˈekə] (Alexander Ecker) 枕横沟

Ecker's fluid [ˈekə] (Enrique E. Ecker) 埃克液(见 Rees and Ecker diluting fluid)

Eck's fistula [ek] (Nicolai V. Eck) 埃克瘘(在门静脉与腔静脉间的人造通道) | ~ fistula in reverse 埃克逆瘘(引导身体后部〈下部〉血液经由门静脉和肝脏的人造通道)

eclabium [ekˈleibiəm] *n* 唇外翻

eclampsia [iˈklæmpsiə] *n* 惊厥,子痫 | puerperal ~ 产惊,子痫 / uremic ~ 尿毒性惊厥 | **eclamptic** *a*

eclampsism [iˈklæmpsizəm] *n* 虚性子痫,子痫前期

eclamptism [iˈklæmptizəm] *n* 产惊

eclamptogenic [iˌklæmptəuˈdʒenik] *a* 致惊厥的

eclectic [ekˈlektik] *a* 折衷[主义]的(采用医学各派中最好的)

eclecticism [eˈklektisizəm] *n* 折衷主义;折衷[主义]医学(古时用单一药物治病,而不顾及疾病分类学)

eclipse [iːˈklips] *n* 隐蔽期(指病毒学中的传染期,此时受染的菌细胞不含有传染性噬菌体)

eclysis [ˈeklisis] *n* 轻晕厥

ECM extracellular matrix 细胞外基质

ecmnesia [ekˈniːziə] *n* 近事遗忘

ECMO extracorporeal membrane oxygenation 体外膜式氧合

ecmovirus [ˌekməuˈvaiərəs] (*e*nteric *c*ytopathic *m*onkey *o*rphan + virus) *n* ECMO 病毒,猴肠道

细胞病变孤儿病毒
ECochG electrocochleogram 耳蜗电图
ecochleation [iˌkɔkliˈeiʃən] *n* 耳蜗切除术；剜出术
ecogenetics [ˌekəudʒəˈnetiks] *n* 生态遗传学
E. coli 见 Escherichia coli
ecologic(al) [ˌekəˈlɔdʒik(əl)] *a* 生态的；生态学的
ecology [i(ː)kɔlədʒi] *n* 生态学 | human ~ 人类生态学 | **ecologist** *n* 生态学家
ecomone [ˈekəuməun] *n* 生态激素
econazole nitrate [iˈkɔnəzəul] 硝酸益康唑(抗真菌药)
Economo's disease (encephalitis) [eiˈkɔnəməu] (Constantin von Economo) 昏睡性脑炎
economy [i(ː)ˈkɔnəmi] *n* 经济；节约；系统；整体 | **animal** ~ 机体整体 / token ~ 标记奖酬法，奖券奖酬法(行为疗法用语，从事适当的个人和社会行为的患者可以得到奖券，奖券可调换食品、衣服等，或得到特殊优惠，如看电视，离开医院等)
ecoparasite [ˌiːkəuˈpærəsait], **ecosite** [ˈiːkəsait] *n* 定居寄生物
écorché [ˌeikɔːˈʃei] *n*【法】肌肉部位图
ecostate [iˈkɔsteit] *a* 无肋骨的
ecosystem [ˌiːkəˈsistəm] *n* 生态系[统]
ecotaxis [ˈiːkəuˌtæksis, ˈekəuˌtæksis] *n* 生态趋向性
ecotone [ˈiːkətəun, ˈekətəun] *n* 群落交错区
ecotropic [ˌiːkəuˈtrɔpik] *a* 嗜环境的，亲嗜性的，同向性(指病毒)
écouvillon [eiˌkuviˈjɔŋ] *n*【法】擦洗刷
écouvillonage [eiˌkuvijɔˈnɑːʒ] *n*【法】擦洗术
ecphoria [ekˈfɔriə], **ecphory** [ˈekfəri] *n* 印迹激活，记忆遗迹活动
ecphorize [ˈekfəraiz] *vt* 记忆复起，印迹激活
ecphyaditis [ˌekfaiəˈdaitis] *n* 阑尾炎
ecphylaxis [ˌekfiˈlæksis] *n* 无防卫力(血内抗体无力) | **ecphylactic** [ˌekfiˈlæktik] *a*
écrasement [eikrəzˈmɔŋ] *n*【法】绞勒
écraseur [eikrəˈzəː] *n*【法】绞勒器
ECS electrocerebral silence 脑电静止
ecsomatics [ˌeksəuˈmætiks] *n* 体液检验学
ecsovirus [ˌeksəuˈvaiərəs] (*e*nteric *c*ytopathic *s*wine *o*rphan virus) *n* ECSO 病毒，猪肠道细胞病变孤儿病毒
Ecstasy [ˈekstəsi] *n* 迷魂药(3, 4-甲撑二氧甲基丙醇的俗称)
ecstrophy [ˈekstrəfi] *n* 外翻
ECT electroconvulsive therapy 电休克治疗
ectacolia [ˌektəˈkəuliə] *n* 结肠部分扩张
ectad [ˈektæd] *ad* 向外
ectal [ˈektəl] *a* 外的，外表的
ectasia [ekˈteiziə] *n* 扩张，膨胀 | alveolar ~ 肺泡扩张，肺泡气肿 / diffuse arterial ~ 蜿蜒状动脉瘤 / hypostatic ~ 坠积性(血管)扩张 / papillary ~ 局限性毛细管扩张(皮肤呈红点) | **ectasis** [ˈektəsis], **ectasy** [ˈektəsi] *n* / **ectatic** [ekˈtætik] *a*
ectental [ekˈtentəl] *a* 外[与]内胚层的
ecterograph [ˈektərəgrɑːf] *n* 肠运动描记器
ectethmoid [ekˈteθmɔid] *n* 筛骨侧块，筛骨外侧部
ecthyma [ekˈθaimə] *n* 深脓疱，臁疮
ecthymiform [ekˈθaimifɔːm] *a* 深脓疱样的
ecthyreosis [ekˌθairiˈəusis] *n* 甲状腺缺失；甲状腺功能缺失
ect(o)- [前缀]外
ectoantigen [ˌektəuˈæntidʒən] *n* 菌表抗原，体外抗原(松弛地附着在菌体外的一种抗原，因此将细菌置于生理盐水中摇动很容易将其洗去；亦指在细菌外胞质中形成的一种抗原)
ectobiology [ˌektəubaiˈɔlədʒi] *n* 细胞表面生物学(研究细胞表面及表面上特异酶的性质和生化构造)
ectoblast [ˈektəblæst] *n* 外胚层；外膜 | **~ic** [ˌektəˈblæstik] *a*
ectocardia [ektəuˈkɑːdiə] *n* 异位心
ectocervix [ˌektəuˈsəːviks] *n* 外[子]宫颈，子宫颈阴道部 | **ectocervical** *a*
ectocolon [ˌektəuˈkəulən] *n* 结肠扩张
ectocommensal [ˌektəukəˈmensəl] *n* 外共生体，外共栖体
ectocondyle [ˌektəuˈkɔndail] *n* 外侧髁
ectocuneiform [ˌektəukjuˈniːifɔːm] *n* 外侧楔骨，第三楔骨
ectocytic [ˌektəuˈsaitik] *a* 细胞外的
ectoderm [ˈektədəːm] *n* 外胚层 | blastodermic ~, primitive ~ 胚盘外胚层，原始外胚层 / chorionic ~ 滋养层 | **~al** [ektəuˈdəːməl], **~ic** [ˌektəuˈdəːmik] *a*
ectodermoidal [ˌektəudəːˈmɔidəl] *a* 外胚层的，外胚层样的
ectodermosis [ˌektəudəːˈməusis] *n* 外胚层形成异常，外胚层增殖，外胚层病 | ~ erosiva pluriorificialis 多腔性糜烂性外胚层病 | **ectodermatosis** [ˌektəuˌdəːməˈtəusis] *n*
ectoentad [ˌektəuˈentæd] *ad* 自外向内
ectoenzyme [ˌektəuˈenzaim] *n* [胞]外酶
ectogenous [ekˈtɔdʒinəs], **ectogenic** [ˌektəuˈdʒenik] *a* 外源性的
ectoglia [ekˈtɔgliə] *n* 外[神经]胶质
ectogony [ekˈtɔgəni] *n* 孕势(胎发育对母体的影响)

ectohormone [ˌektəuˈhɔːməun] *n* 外激素（排至体外的激素，如信息激素）
ectolecithal [ˌektəuˈlesiθəl] *n* 外黄的
ectolysis [ekˈtɔlisis] *n* 外[胞]质溶解
ectomere [ˈektəmiə] *n* 成外胚层裂球 | **ectomeric** [ˌektəuˈmerik] *a*
ectomesenchyme [ˌektəuˈmeseŋkaim] *n* 外胚层间质
ectomesoblast [ˌektəuˈmesəblæst] *n* 外(胚层原)中胚层
-ectomize [构词成分]切除
ectomorph [ˈektəmɔːf] *n* 外胚层体型者 | **~ic** [ˌektəuˈmɔːfik] *a* 外胚层体型的 / **~y** *n* 外胚层体型
ectomy [ˈektəmi] *n* 切除术
-ectomy [构词成分]切除术
ectonuclear [ˌektəuˈnjuːkliə] *a* 核外的
ectopagus [ekˈtɔpəgəs] *n* 胸侧联胎畸胎
ectoparasite [ˌektəuˈpærəsait] *n* 外寄生物 | **ectoparasitic** [ˌektəupærəˈsitik] *a*
ectoparasiticide [ˌektəuˌpærəˈsitisaid] *n* 杀外寄生虫药
ectopectoralis [ˌektəuˌpektəˈreilis] *n* 胸大肌
ectoperitoneal [ˌektəuˌperitəuˈniːəl] *a* 腹膜外[面]的
ectoperitonitis [ˌektəuperitəuˈnaitis] *n* 腹膜外层炎
ectophyte [ˈektəfait] *n* 外皮寄生植物；外寄生菌
ectopia [ekˈtəupiə] *n* 异位 | **ectopic** [ekˈtɔpik] *a*
ectoplacenta [ektəupləˈsentə] *n* 外胎盘
ectoplasm [ˈektəplæzəm] *n* 外质 | **~ic** [ˌektəuˈplæzmik], **~atic** [ˌektəuplæzˈmætik] *a*
ectoplast [ˈektəuplæst] *n* 外质体
ectoplastic [ˌektəuˈplæstik] *n* 外形成性的
ectopotomy [ˌektəuˈpɔtəmi] *n* 异位胎切除术
ectopterygoid [ˌektəuˈterigɔid] *n* 翼外肌
ectopy [ˈektəpi] *n* 异位
ectosarc [ˈektəsɑːk] *n* 外质，外膜；外囊(卵)
ectoscopy [ekˈtɔskəpi] *n* 外表检视法
ectoskeleton [ˌektəuˈskelitn] *n* 外骨骼
ectosphere [ˈektəsfiə] *n* 外球，中心球外层
ectosteal [ekˈtɔstiəl] *a* 骨外的
ectostosis [ˌektəuˈstəusis] *n* 软骨膜下软骨骨化，骨膜下骨化
ectosuggestion [ˌektəusəˈdʒestʃən] *n* 外暗示
ectosymbiont [ˌektəuˈsimbiɔnt] *n* 外共生生物
ectotherm [ˈektəθəːm] *n* 外温动物，冷血动物，变温动物
ectothermic [ˌektəˈθəːmik] *a* 变温的
ectothermy [ˌektəˈθəːmi] *n* 变温性
Ectothiorhodospira [ˌektəˌθaiərəuˈdɔspirə] *n* 外红硫螺菌属
ectothrix [ˈektəθriks] *n* 毛外癣菌
Ectotrichophyton [ˌektətraiˈkɔfitɔn] *n* 发外发癣菌属
ectozoon [ˌektəuˈzəuɔn] ([复] **ectozoa** [ˌektəuˈzəuə]) *n*【希】体表寄生虫 | **ectozoal** *a*
ectr(o)- [构词成分]先天性缺损
ectrodactyly [ˌektrəuˈdæktili], **ectrodactylia** [ˌektrəudækˈtiliə], **ectrodactylism** [ˌektrəuˈdæktilizəm] *n* 缺指畸形，缺趾畸形
ectrogeny [ekˈtrɔdʒini] *n* 先天性缺损 | **ectrogenic** [ˌektrəuˈdʒenik] *a*
ectromelia [ˌektrəuˈmiːliə] *n* (先天性)缺肢畸形 | infectious ~ 传染性缺肢畸形，鼠痘 | **ectromelic** [ˌektrəuˈmelik] *a*
ectromelus [ekˈtrɔmiləs] *n* 缺肢畸胎，四肢不全畸胎
ectrometacarpia [ˌektrəuˌmetəˈkɑːpiə] *n* 缺掌骨[畸形]，先天性掌骨缺如畸形
ectrometatarsia [ˌektrəuˌmetəˈtɑːsiə] *n* 缺跖骨[畸形]，先天性跖骨缺如畸形
ectrophalangia [ˌektrəufəˈlændʒiə] *n* 缺指骨[畸形]，缺趾骨[畸形]，先天性指骨缺如畸形，先天性趾骨缺如畸形
ectropion [ekˈtrəupiɔn] *n* 外翻 | flaccid ~ 弛缓性下睑外翻 / paralytic ~ 麻痹性睑外翻 / senile ~ 老年性睑外翻 / spastic ~ 痉挛性[睑]外翻 | **ectropium** *n*
ectropionize [ekˈtrəupiəˌnaiz] *vt* 使外翻
ectrosis [ekˈtrəusis] *n* 流产；顿挫疗法
ectrosyndactyly [ˌektrəusinˈdæktili], **ectrosyndactylia** [ˌektrəusindækˈtiliə] *n* 并指缺指畸形，并趾缺趾畸形
ectrotic [ekˈtrɔtik] *a* 流产的；顿挫的
ectylurea [ˌektiˈljuəriə] *n* 依克替脲，乙巴酰脲（镇静药）
ectype [ˈektaip] *n* 异常型(体质)
ectypia [ekˈtaipiə] *n* 体质型异常
eczema [ˈeksimə, ˈekzimə] *n* 湿疹 | contact ~ 接触性湿疹 / flexural ~ 屈侧性湿疹，异位性皮炎 / impetiginous ~ 传染性湿疹样皮炎 / nummular, orbicular ~ 钱币状湿疹(一种神经性皮炎) / ~ vaccinatum 牛痘性湿疹
eczematid(e) [ekˈzemətid] *n* 湿疹样疹
eczematization [ekˌzemətaiˈzeiʃən, -tiˈz-] *n* 湿疹化
eczematogenic [ekˌzemətəuˈdʒenik] *a* 引起湿疹的
eczematoid [ekˈzemətɔid] *a* 湿疹样的
eczematous [ekˈzemətəs] *a* 湿疹的，湿疹性的
ED effective dose 有效量；erythema dose 红斑量

ED_{50} median effective dose 半数有效量

edathamil [iˈdæθəmil] *n* 依地酸,乙二胺四乙酸 | calcium disodium ~ 依地酸钙钠(解毒药) / ~ disodium 依地酸二钠(解毒药)

EDC expected date of confinement 预产期

Eddowes' syndrome (disease) [ˈedəuz] (Alfred Eddowes) 埃多斯综合征(病),成骨不全(Ⅰ型)

Edebohls' operation [ˈedibəulz] (George M. Edebohls) 埃德博尔手术(为布赖特〈Bright〉病所施行的一种肾被膜剥脱术) | ~ position 埃德博尔卧位(曲膝外展,腿贴近腹部,臀部抬高的一种背卧位)

Edelmann's cell [ˈedəlmən] (Adolf Edelmann) [活]动细胞

edema [i(ː)ˈdiːmə] ([复] **edemas** 或 **edemata** [iːˈdiːmətə]) *n* 水肿 | angioneurotic ~, acute circumscribed ~, giant ~, migratory ~, periodic ~, wandering ~ 血管神经性水肿 / blue ~, hysterical ~ 蓝色水肿,癔症性水肿(见于癔症性瘫痪的一肢) / hereditary angioneurotic ~ (HANE) 遗传性血管神经性水肿 / local intracutaneous ~ 荨麻疹 / neuropathic ~ 神经病性水肿,假脂瘤 / nonpitting ~ 非指压性水肿,非压凹性水肿 / nutritional ~, alimentary ~, famine ~, war ~, hunger ~ 营养不良性水肿 / periretinal ~ 浆液性中心性视网膜炎 / pitting ~ 压凹性水肿 / pulmonary ~ 肺水肿 / solid ~ 实性水肿 / terminal ~ 临终时水肿,末期水肿 / vernal ~ of lung 春季肺水肿,变应性肺水肿

edemagen [iˈdiːmədʒən] *n* 致水肿原(一种促发水肿的刺激物)

edematization [iˌdemətaiˈzeiʃən] *n* 水肿形成

edematogenic [iˌdemətəuˈdʒenik], **edematigenous** [iˌdeməˈtidʒinəs] *a* 致水肿的

edematous [iˈdemətəs] *a* 水肿的

Edentata [ˌiːdenˈteitə] *n* 贫齿目

edentia [iːˈdenʃiə] *n* 无牙,无齿

edentulism [iːˈdentjulizəm] *n* 无牙,无齿

edentulous [iːˈdentjuləs], **edentate** [iːˈdenteit], **edentulate** [iːˈdentjulit] *a* 无牙的

edetate [ˈediteit] *n* 依地酸盐 | ~ calcium disodium, calcium disodium ~ 依地酸钙[二]钠,解铅乐(铅中毒诊断治疗用) / ~ disodium, disodium ~ 依地酸二钠(用于治疗铅和其他重金属中毒) / ~ sodium 依地酸钠(螯合剂) / ~ trisodium 依地酸三钠(其作用有时类似依地酸二钠)

edetic acid [iˈdiːtik] 依地酸,乙二胺四乙酸

edge [edʒ] *n* 边缘,缘 | cutting ~ 刀刃,刀口;切缘(牙) / incisal ~ 边缘

edge-strength [ˈedʒ streŋθ] *n* 边缘韧力

edible [ˈedibl] *a* 可食的,食用的 *n* [复]食品 | **edibility** [ˌediˈbiləti] *n* 可食用性

Edinger's law [ˈediŋgə] (Ludwig Edinger) 埃丁格尔定律(一神经元,如逐渐使其活动增加,能促进其生长,若活动增加不规则与过度,则导致萎缩与退化) | ~ nucleus 动眼神经副核

Edinger-Westphal nucleus [ˈediŋgə ˈvestfəl] (L. Edinger; Carl F. O. Westphal) 动眼神经副核

edipism [ˈedipizəm] *n* 眼自伤,自毁伤目

edisylate [iˈdisileit] *n* 乙二磺酸盐(1, 2-ethanedisulfonate 的 USAN 缩约词)

Edlefsen's reagent [ˈedlefsən] (Gustav J. J. F. Edlefsen) 埃德勒弗森试剂(碱性高锰酸盐溶液试验尿糖用) | ~ test 埃德勒弗森试验(检右旋糖)

EDR effective direct radiation 有效直接辐射;electrodermal response 皮肤电反应

EDRF endothelium-derived relaxing factor 内皮细胞舒血管因子

edrophonium chloride [ˌedrəˈfəuniəm] 依酚氯铵(抗胆碱酯酶药,用于诊断重症肌无力,并用作箭毒拮抗药)

Edsall's disease [ˈedsl] (David L. Edsall) 中暑性痉挛

EDTA ethylenediaminetetraacetic acid 依地酸,乙二胺四乙酸;European Dialysis and Transplant Association 欧洲透析与移植协会

educable [ˈedjukəbl] *a* 可教育的(轻度精神发育迟缓者,智商 50~70)

education [ˌedju(ː)ˈkeiʃən] *n* 教育;训练,培养 | health ~ 卫生教育

educt [ˈiːdʌkt] *n* 离析物,浸提物

edulcorant [iˈdʌlkərənt] *n* 加甜剂

edulcorate [iˈdʌlkəreit] *vt* 使甜

EDV end-diastolic volume 舒张期末容积

Edwardsiella [edˌwɔːsiˈelə] *n* 爱德华菌属 | ~ tarda 迟钝爱德华菌

Edwardsielleae [edˌwɔːsiːˈeliiː] *n* 爱德华菌族

Edwards' syndrome [ˈedwədz] (J. H. Edwards) 爱德华兹综合征,18 三体综合征(即 trisomy 18 syndrome,见 syndrome 项下相应术语)

EEE eastern equine encephalomyelitis 东方马脑脊髓炎

EEG electroencephalogram 脑电图

EEJ electroejaculation 电射精

eelworm [ˈiːlwəːm] *n* 线虫

EENT eye-ear-nose-throat 眼耳鼻喉

EERP extended endocardial resection procedure 扩大心内膜切除术

EFA essential fatty acids 必需脂肪酸

efavirenz [ˈefəˌvairenz] *n* 依法维仑(一种非核苷反转录酶抑制药,与其他抗反转录病毒药结合使用,治疗人免疫缺陷病毒Ⅰ型〈HIV-1〉感染,口服给药)

effacement [iˈfeismənt] *n* 擦掉,抹去;消失(指分娩时宫颈管消失) | ~ of cervix 颈管消失

effect [iˈfekt] *n* 结果;效应;作用,影响 | additive ~ 相加作用(药效) / clasp-knife ~ 折刀式效应(肢伸长反应时突然屈曲) / contrary ~ 反效应(用小剂量化疗药物后传染病病情反而加重) / experimenter ~s 实验者效应(见 characteristic 项下 demand characteristics) / heel ~ 倾斜效应(由于X线管阳极不同角度出现X线差异衰减,使有用光束通过截面时造成强度差异,阴极侧强度较大) / isomorphic ~ 同形反应(同形现象) / position ~ 位置效应(染色体上各种基因相对位置因改变而产生的效应)

effective [iˈfektiv] *a* 有效的

effectiveness [iˈfektivnis] *n* 效力,效率 | relative biological ~ 相对生物效率

effector [iˈfektə] *n* 效应器(神经);效应物,效应基因 | allosteric ~ 别构效应物

effemination [iˌfemiˈneiʃən] *n* [男子]女性化

efferent [ˈefərənt], **efferential** [ˌefəˈrenʃəl] *a* 输出的,传出的,离心的

effervescent [ˌefəˈvesnt] *a* 发泡的,泡腾的

efficacy [ˈefikəsi] *n* 功效,效能,有效性

efficiency [iˈfiʃənsi] *n* 效率,功效 | visual ~ 视觉效率

efficient [iˈfiʃənt] *a* 有效的,高效的

effleurage [efluːˈrɑːʒ] *n*【法】轻擦按摩法

efflorescence [ˌeflɔːˈresns] *n* 风化,粉化;皮疹 | **efflorescent** *a* 风化的

effluence [ˈefluəns] *n* 射出[物];流出[物]

effluent [ˈefluənt] *a* 发出的,流出的 *n* 流出物,坑水

effluve [eˈfluːv] *n* 介流(通过介质的高压放电)

effluvium [eˈfluːvjəm] ([复] **effluvia** [eˈfluːvjə]) *n*【拉】脱落,脱发;散发,放出(指有毒气体);排出物,臭气 | anagen ~ 再生期脱发 / telluric ~ 地气(大地蒸发物,如瘴气) / telogen ~ 静止期脱发 | **effluvial** *a* 恶臭的

efflux [ˈeflʌks], **effluxion** [eˈflʌkʃən] *n* 流出,散发;流出物;消逝;满期外向通量

effraction [eˈfrækʃən] *n* 破裂;衰弱

effuse [eˈfjuːs] *a* 渗散的(指细菌) [eˈfjuːz] *vt, vi* 弥散,流出

effusion [iˈfjuːʒən] *n* 流出,渗出;渗漏液,渗出液 | hemorrhagic ~ 血性渗漏液 / pleural ~ 胸腔积液

effusive [iˈfjuːsiv] *a* 流出的,溢出的

eflornithine hydrochloride [efˈlɔːniˌθiːn] 盐酸依氟鸟氨酸(用以治疗非洲锥虫病,亦用作抗肿瘤药。亦称 DMFO)

egagropilus [ˌiːgəˈgrɔpiləs] *n* 毛团,毛块

EGD esophagogastroduodenoscopy 食管胃十二指肠镜检查

egersimeter [ˌiːgəˈsimitə] *n* 电激相应计(试验神经与肌肉的电兴奋性及其时值的测定器)

egersis [iˈgəːsis] *n*【希】异常觉醒,失眠

egest [iːˈdʒest] *vt* 排泄,排出 | **egestion** [iːˈdʒestʃən] *n* / **egestive** [iːˈdʒestiv] *a*

egesta [iːˈdʒestə] *n* 排泄物

EGF epidermal growth factor 表皮生长因子,上皮生长因子

egg-bound [ˈeg baund] *a* 难产的,不能产卵的 *n* 不能产卵性

Eggers' plate [ˈegəz] (George W. N. Eggers) 爱格士板(用以维持骨折端对位的骨板)

Eggleston's method [ˈeglstən] (Cary Eggleston) 埃格斯顿法(洋地黄定效测定法)

egilops [ˈiːdʒilɔps] *n* 内眦脓肿穿破

eglandulous [iːˈglændjuləs] *a* 无腺的

ego [ˈiːgəu, ˈe-] *n* 自我,自己

ego-alien [ˌiːgəu ˈeiljən, ˌeg-] *a* 自我所排斥的,与自我失谐的

egobronchophony [ˌiːgəubrɔŋˈkɔfəni, ˌeg-] *n* 支气管羊音

egocentric [ˌiːgəuˈsentrik, ˌeg-] *a* 自我中心的,利己的 | **~ity** [ˌiːgəusenˈtrisəti, ˌeg-] *n* 自我中心,自私自利

ego-dystonic [ˌiːgəu disˈtɔnik, ˌeg-] *a* 自我所排斥的,与自我失谐的

ego-ideal [ˌiːgəu aiˈdiəl] *n* 自我理想

egoism [ˈiːgəuizəm, ˈeg-] *n* 自我中心,利己主义 | **egoist** *n* 利己主义者

egomania [ˌiːgəuˈmeinjə, ˌeg-] *n* 极端利己主义;利己狂

egophony [iˈgɔfəni] *n* 支气管羊音

ego-syntonic [ˌiːgəu sinˈtɔnik, eg-] *a* 与自我融洽的,与自我和谐的

egotism [ˈiːgəutizəm, ˈeg-] *n* 利己主义,唯我主义

egotist [ˈiːgəutist, ˈeg-] *n* 利己主义者 | **egotistic(al)** [-ˈtistik(ə)l] *a* 自我中心的,利己主义的

egotropic [ˌiːgəuˈtrɔpik, ˌeg-] *a* 自我中心的,利己的

EGTA egtazic acid 依他酸

egtazik acid [əgˈteizik] 依他酸(药用辅料)

EHBF estimated hepatic blood flow 估计肝血流量

EHDP etidronate (ethane-1-hydroxy-1, 1-diphosphonate) 依替膦酸(乙烷-1-羟基-1, 1-二膦酸)

EHEC enterohemorrhagic *Escherichia coli* 肠出血性大肠杆菌

Ehlers-Danlos syndrome (disease) [ˈeiləz dɑːnˈlɔː] (Edvard Ehlers; Henri A. Danlos) 埃勒斯-当洛综合征(病)(①一种先天性遗传性综合征,

特征为皮肤和关节过度伸展,组织脆性增加,容易损伤出血,伤口难以愈合,皮下有钙化的球状体和假瘤;②皮肤脆裂症)

Ehrenritter's ganglion [ˈerənˌritə] (Johann Ehrenritter) 舌咽神经上节

Ehrlich-Hata preparation, remedy, treatment [ˈɛəliʃ ˈhɑːtə] (Paul Ehrlich; Sahachiro Hata) 胂凡纳明,六〇六

Ehrlich-Heinz granules [ˈɛəliʃ ˈhaints] (Paul Ehrlich; Robert Heinz) 埃利希-海因茨粒(见 Ehrlich's granules)

Ehrlichia [ɛəˈlikiə] (Paul Ehrlich) *n* 埃利希体属 | ~ canis 犬埃利希体

ehrlichia [ɛəˈlikiə] *n* 埃利希体

ehrlichial [ɛəˈlikiəl] *a* 埃利希体属的

Ehrlichieae [ɛəliˈkaiiː] *n* 埃利希体族

ehrlichiosis [ɛəˌlikiˈəusis] *n* 埃利希菌病 | canine ~ 犬埃利希菌病

Ehrlich's acid hematoxylin [ˈɛəliʃ] *n* (Paul Ehrlich) 埃利希酸性苏木素(核染剂) | ~ biochemical theory 埃利希生物化学理论(特殊化学亲和力存在于特殊生活细胞物质与特殊化学物质内) / ~ diazo reaction 埃利希重氮反应(患某些病而在尿中含某种芳香性物质时,可因重氮苯磺酸与氨的作用而产生粉红色或红色反应,此反应对伤寒与麻疹有诊断价值,对结核病有判定预后的价值) / ~ granules 埃利希粒(可用埃利希三酸染剂染色的细胞粒) / ~ hemoglobinemic bodies 埃利希血红蛋白血症小体(在变性红细胞中心的深色小体) / ~ neutral stain 埃利希中性染剂(亚甲蓝与酸性品红的混合液,用以染红细胞) / ~ side-chain theory 埃利希侧链学说(关于免疫与细胞溶解现象的学说,根据这一学说,体细胞的原生质含有高度复合有机分子,内含一稳定的中央簇,与原子或原子簇欠稳定的侧链相接,原生质内通常的化学转变靠这些侧链〈或受体〉进行,分子的稳定中心仍未受影响,侧链含有的原子簇〈结合簇〉能与类似簇的毒素、细菌细胞及体外细胞相结合) / ~ test 埃利希试验(见埃利希重氮反应;苯甲醛试验,检尿胆素原) / ~ triacid stain 埃利希三酸染剂(含酸性品红、橙 G 和甲基绿,用以显示血液中各种有形成分)

EI erythema infectiosum 传染性红斑

EIA electroimmunoassay 电免疫测定;enzyme immunoassay 酶免疫测定

Eichhorst's atrophy (type) [ˈikhɔːst] (Hermann L. Eichhorst) 艾克霍斯特萎缩(型)(股胫型进行性肌萎缩伴趾挛缩) | ~ corpuscles 艾克霍斯特小体(恶性贫血时一种特殊的小红细胞)

Eichstedt's disease [ˈikstet] (Karl F. Eichstedt) 花斑癣

Eicken's method [ˈaikən] (Carl Otto von Eicken) 艾肯法(将环状软骨拉向前,检咽下部)

eiconometer [ˌaikəˈnɔmitə] *n* 影像计,物像计

eicosanoate [aiˌkəusəˈnəueit] *n* 二十[烷]酸盐

eicosanoic acid [ˌaikəusəˈnəuik] 二十[烷]酸,花生酸

eicosanoid [aiˈkəusənɔid] *n* 类二十[烷]酸,类花生酸

eicosapentaenoic acid [aiˌkəusəˌpentəiːˈnəuik] 二十碳五烯酸

eidetic [aiˈdetik] *a* 遗觉的 *n* 具遗觉能力者

eidogen [ˈaidədʒən] *n* (器官)变形质

eidoptometry [ˌaidɔpˈtɔmitri] *n* 形觉测定法

EIEC enteroinvasive *Escherichia coli* 肠侵袭性大肠杆菌

Eijkman's test [ˈaikmən] (Christiaan Eijkman) 艾克曼试验(检酚)

Eikenella [aikəˈnelə] (M. Eiken) *n* 埃肯菌族

eikonometer [ˌaikəˈnɔmitə] *n* 影像计,物像计

eiloid [ˈailɔid] *a* 蟠管状的,线圈形的

Eimeria [aiˈmiəriə] *n* 艾美球虫属 | ~ caviae 豚鼠艾美球虫 / ~ clupearum 鱼艾美球虫 / ~ falciformis 镰形艾美球虫 / ~ meleagridis 吐绶鸡艾美球虫 / ~ mieschulzi 密氏艾美球虫 / ~ necatrix 扁嘴艾美球虫 / ~ perforans 穿孔艾美球虫,兔肠球孢子虫 / ~ sardinae 鳁艾美球虫 / ~ stiedae 啮齿艾美球虫,兔艾美球虫 / ~ tenellum, ~ avium 禽艾美球虫 / ~ zurni 祖[尔尼]氏艾美球虫,牛艾美球虫

Eimeriina [ˌaimiəˈraiinə] *n* 艾美球虫亚目

Einhorn's saccharimeter [ˈainhɔːn] (Max Einhorn) 艾因霍恩糖定量器(测糖发酵管)

einsteinium (Es) [ainˈstainiəm] *n* 锿(化学元素)

Einthoven's formula [ˈaintəuvn] (Willem Einthoven) 艾因托文公式($e^1 + e^3 \times e^2$,见艾因托文三角) | ~ galvanometer 艾因托文电流计,弦(线)电流计 / ~ triangle 艾因托文三角(一种等边三角形,用作标准心电图肢体导联的数学模型,使心脏额平面瞬时向量可投射到三角形的三边,从而证明心电图导联Ⅰ和Ⅲ记录的电位差的代数和,等于导联Ⅱ记录的电位差)

eisanthema [aiˈsænθimə] *n* 黏膜疹

Eisenia [aiˈsiːniə] *n* 爱胜蚓属 | ~ foetida 赤子爱胜蚓

Eisenmenger's complex, syndrome [ˈaisənˌmeŋgə] (Victor Eisenmenger) 艾森门格复合征、综合征(心室间隔缺损,伴有重度肺动脉高血压、右心室肥大和隐性或显性发绀)

eisodic [aiˈsɔdik] *a* 输入的,传入的;向心的

EIT erythrocyte iron turnover 红细胞铁转换

Eitelberg's test [ˈaitəlbəːg] (Abraham Eitelberg) 艾特尔伯格试验(用一大音叉持近耳朵,20 ~ 30

分钟,如此数次,如耳正常,则振荡感觉逐次增加,如传导器官有损害,则感觉减低)
eiweissmilch [ˈaivaismilʃ] *n*【德】白蛋白乳
ejaculate [iˈdʒækjuleit] *vt*, *vi* 射出(液体);射精, *n* (一次射出的)精液
ejaculatio [iˌdʒækjuˈleiʃiəu] *n*【拉】射精
ejaculation [iˈdʒækjuˈleiʃən] *n* 射出,射精 | premature ~ 早泄 | **ejaculatory** [iˈdʒækjulətəri] *a*
ejaculator [iˈdʒækjuleitə] *n* 射出者;喷射器
ejaculum [iˈdʒækjuləm] *n* (一次射出的)精液
eject [i(ː)ˈdʒekt] *vt*, *n* 逐出;喷射,吐出
ejecta [i(ː)ˈdʒektə] *n* 喷出物;排出物
ejection [i(ː)ˈdʒekʃən] *n* 排出;喷射;排出物 | **ejective** *a* 喷出的,射出的
ejector [i(ː)ˈdʒektə] *n* 喷射器;剔出器,排除器 | saliva ~ 排涎器
Ejusd. ejusdem【拉】同样
eka- [前缀]准(元素);第一
eka-iodine [ˈiːkəˈaiədiːn] *n* 准碘(砹的旧称)
Ekbom syndrome [ˈekbɔm] (Karl A. Ekbom) 埃克鲍姆综合征,多动腿综合征(即 restless legs syndrome,见 syndrome 项下相应术语)
EKG electrocardiogram 心电图
ekiri [iˈkiːri] *n* 疫痢(日本幼儿患志贺菌痢疾时发生的一种急性脑和心血管疾病)
Ekman-Lobstein syndrome [ˈekmɑːn ˈləubstain] (O. J. Ekman; Johann F. G. C. Lobstein) 埃-劳综合征,成骨不全(Ⅰ型)
Ekman's syndrome [ˈekmɑːn] (Olof J. Ekman) 埃克曼综合征,成骨不全(Ⅰ型)
ekphorize [ˈekfəraiz] *vt* 记忆复起,印迹激活
EKY electrokymogram 电记波[照]片,心电记波图
elaborate [iˈlæbərit] *a* 精心制作的,[iˈlæbəreit] *vt* 精心制作;从简单成分合成
elaboration [iˌlæbəˈreiʃən] *n* 精心制作
elaborative [iˈlæbərətiv] *a* 精心制作的
elacin [ˈeləsin] *n* 变性弹力蛋白
elae(o)- 见 ele(o)-
Elaeophora [ˌeliːˈɔfərə] *n* 盘尾丝虫属
elaeophoriasis [ˌeliːˌɔfəˈraiəsis], **elaeophorosis** [ˌeliːˌɔfəˈrəusis] *n* 盘尾丝虫病,丝虫性皮炎
elaidate [ˌeləˈideit] *n* 反油酸(盐、酯或阴离子型)
elaidic acid [ˌeləˈidik] 反油酸
elaioma [iliˈəumə] *n* 油肿(见 eleoma)
elaiometer [ˌiːleiˈɔmitə] *n* 油度计,油比重计
elaiopathy [ˌiːleiˈɔpəθi] *n* 脂肪性[水]肿病,脂质浮肿病 | pathomimic ~ 拟脂质浮肿病(皮下注射液状石蜡所致) | **eleopathia** [ˌiːleiəˈpæθiə] *n*
elaioplast [iˈleiəplæst] *n* 脂质体,造油体
elantrine [ˈelæntriːn] *n* 依兰群(抗胆碱能药,用于治疗药物引起的锥体束外综合征)
Elaut's triangle [eiˈləu] (Léon J. S. Elant) 埃劳三角(一个三角区,其底为骶骨岬,其边为左和右髋总动脉)
elapid [ˈeləpid] *n*, *a* 眼镜蛇(的)
Elapidae [iˈlæpidiː] *n* 眼镜蛇科
Elaps [iːˈlæps] *n* 珊瑚毒蛇属
elasmobranch [iːˈlæzməbræŋk] ([复] **elasmobranchs**) *n* 板鳃类鱼 *a* 板鳃类的
elastance [iˈlæstəns] *n* 弹回性,弹回率;弹性 | ~ of lung 肺弹性
elastase [iˈlæsteis] *n* 弹性蛋白酶
elastic [iˈlæstik, iˈlɑːstik] *a* 弹性的 *n* 橡皮带,松紧带,弹性带
elastica [iˈlæstikə] *n*【拉】橡皮,弹性树胶;弹性组织;弹性层
elasticity [ˌelæsˈtisəti] *n* 弹性,弹力
elastin [iˈlæstin], **elasticin** [iˈlæstisin] *n* 弹性蛋白
elastinase [iˈlæstineis] *n* 弹性蛋白酶
elast(o)- [构词成分]弹性;弹性蛋白;弹性组织
elastofibroma [iˌlæstəufaiˈbrəumə] *n* 弹力纤维瘤 | ~ dorsi 背部弹力纤维瘤
elastogel [iˈlæstədʒel] *n* 弹性凝胶
elastoid [iˈlæstɔid] *n* 弹性样物质(见于分娩后子宫血管内)
elastoidosis [iˌlæstɔiˈdəusis] *n* 类弹力纤维病 | nodular ~ 结节性类弹力纤维病
elastolysis [ˌiːlæsˈtɔlisis] *n* 弹力纤维松解 | generized ~ 泛发性弹力纤维松解,皮肤松弛 / perifollicular ~ 毛囊周围弹力纤维松解 / postinflammatory ~ 炎症后弹力纤维松解
elastolytic [iˌlæstəuˈlitik] *a* 促弹性组织离解的
elastoma [ˌiːlæsˈtəumə] *n* 弹性[组织]瘤 | juvenile ~ 少年期弹性组织增生
elastomer [iˈlæstəmə] *n* 弹性体;合成橡胶 | **~ic** [ˌilæstəˈmerik] *a*
elastometer [ˌiːlæsˈtɔmitə] *n* 组织弹性测定器(测水肿程度) | **elastometry** *n* 弹性测定法
elastomucin [iˌlæstəuˈmjuːsin] *n* 弹性[组织]黏蛋白
elastopathy [ˌiːlæsˈtɔpəθi] *n* 弹性组织[缺乏]病
elastorrhexis [iˌlæstəˈreksis] *n* 弹性组织(纤维)破裂
elastose [iˈlæstəus] *n* 弹性蛋百胨
elastosis [ˌiːlæsˈtəusis] *n* 弹性组织变性 | actinic ~ 光线性弹性组织变性 / ~ perforans serpiginosa, perforating ~ 匐行性穿通性弹性组织变性 / solar ~ 日光性弹性组织变性 | **elastotic** [ˌiːlæsˈtɔtik] *a*
elater [elətə] *n* 弹丝
elation [iˈleiʃən] *n* 情感高涨
elbow [ˈelbəu] *n* 肘;肘状物 | baseball pitchers' ~ 垒球投手肘 / miners' ~ 矿工肘,矿工鹰嘴黏液

囊炎/ pulled ~, nursemaids' ~ 牵引肘,乳母肘,桡骨头半脱位 / tennis ~ 网球肘

elcosis [el'kəusis] *n* 溃疡形成

elderberry ['eldəberi] *n* 接骨木(其花含有一种挥发油,用于包裹创伤、烧伤、溃疡等)

elder ['eldə] *a* 年长的 *n* 老年人(不足 70 岁者)

eldrin ['eldrin] *n* 芸香苷,芦丁

elective [i'lektiv] *a* 选择的;有择的 *n* 选修课程

Electra complex [i'lektrə] (Electra 为希腊传说中的人物,她怂恿兄弟杀死她的母亲和继父,为被谋杀的父亲报仇)伊莱克特拉情结,(女)恋父情结(与子恋母情结〈Oedipus complex〉相反,指女性的恋父、妒忌或怨恨母亲,但由于 Oedipus complex 适用于两性,故本术语现已罕用)

electric [i'lektrik] *a* 电的,电动的 *n* 带电体

electrical [i'lektrikəl] *a* 电的

electrician [ilek'triʃən] *n* 电工,电学家

electricity [ilek'trisəti] *n* 电,电学

electro- [构词成分]电

electroacupuncture [iːˌlektrəuˌækju'pʌŋktʃə, -'ækju-] *n* 电针[刺]术

electroaffinity [iˌlektrəuə'finəti] *n* 电亲合性

electroanalgesia [iːˌlektrəuˌænæl'dʒiːzjə] *n* 电止痛法

electroanalysis [iˌlektrəuə'næləsis] *n* 电分析 | **electroanalytic(al)** [iˌlektrəuˌænə'litik(əl)] *a*

electroanesthesia [iˌlektrəuˌænis'θiːzjə] *n* 电麻醉

electroappendectomy [iˌlektrəuˌæpən'dektəmi] *n* 电刀阑尾切除术

electroaugmentation [iˌlektrəuˌɔːgmen'teiʃən] *n* 电起搏法(心)

electrocauterization [iˌlektrəuˌkɔːtərai'zeiʃən, -ri'z-] *n* 电灼术

electrobasograph [iˌlektrəu'beisəgrɑːf, -græf] *n* 步态电图描记器

electrobiology [iˌlektrəubai'ɔlədʒi] *n* 电生物学,生物电学

electrobioscopy [iˌlektrəubai'ɔskəpi] *n* 电鉴定生死法

electroblot [i'lektrəuˌblɔt] *n* 电印迹(通常为蛋白质印迹〈western blot〉,溶质从凝胶转移到膜或其他底物是通过电泳而不是通过毛细管作用来实现的)

electrocardiogram [iˌlektrəu'kɑːdiəgræm] *n* 心电图 | ambulatory ~ 动态心电图 / scalar ~ 无向量心电图

electrocardiograph [iˌlektrəu'kɑːdiəgrɑːf, -græf] *n* 心电图机 | **~ic** [iˌlektrəuˌkɑːdiə'græfik] *a* / **~y** [iˌlektrəuˌkɑːdi'ɔgrəfi] *n* 心电图学

electrocatalysis [iˌlektrəukə'tæləsis] *n* 电催化[作用]

electrocautery [iˌlektrəu'kɔːtəri] *n* 电灼术;电烙器

electrochemistry [iˌlektrəu'kemistri] *n* 电化学 | **electrochemical** *a*

electrocholecystectomy [iˌlektrəuˌkəulisis'tektəmi] *n* 电刀胆囊切除术

electrocholecystocausis [iˌlektrəuˌkəulisistə'kɔːsis] *n* 胆囊电烙

electrochromatography [iˌlektrəuˌkrəumə'tɔgrəfi] *n* 电色谱法,电层析法,电泳

electrocision [iˌlektrəu'siʒən] *n* 电切术

electrocoagulation [iˌlektrəukəuˌægju'leiʃən] *n* 电凝[术],电凝[固]术

electrocochleogram [iˌlektrəu'kɔkliəgræm] *n* 耳蜗电图

electrocochleograph [iˌlektrəu'kɔkliəgrɑːf, -græf] *n* 耳蜗电图仪 | **~ic** [iˌlektrəuˌkɔkliə'græfik] *a* 耳蜗电图检查的 / **~y** [iˌlektrəuˌkɔkli'ɔgrəfi] *n* 耳蜗电图检查

electrocontractility [iˌlektrəukəntræk'tiləti] *n* 电(刺激)收缩性

electroconvulsive [iˌlektrəukən'vʌlsiv] *a* 电惊厥的

electrocorticogram [iˌlektrəu'kɔːtikəˌgræm] *n* 脑皮质电图

electrocorticography [iˌlektrəuˌkɔːti'kɔgrəfi] *n* 脑皮质电图学

electrocortin [iˌlektrəu'kɔːtin] *n* 醛甾酮,醛固酮

electrocryptectomy [iˌlektrəukrip'tektəmi] *n* 扁桃体隐窝电烙术

electrocute [i'lektrəkjuːt] *vt* 使触电而死;以电刑处死(罪犯) | **electrocution** [iˌlektrə'kjuːʃən] *n* [触]电死,电[死]刑

electrocystography [iˌlektrəusis'tɔgrəfi] *n* 膀胱电位描记[法]

electrocystoscope [iˌlektrəu'sistəskəup] *n* 电光膀胱镜

electrode [i'lektrəud] *n* 电极 | active ~, exciting ~, localizing ~, therapeutic ~ 探查电极,作用电极,刺激电极,定位电极,疗用电极 / indifferent ~, dispersing ~, silent ~ 无关电极,弥散电极,无效电极 / point ~ 尖端电极

electrodeposit [iˌlektrəudi'pɔzit] *n* 电淀积物 *vt* 电淀积 | **electrodeposition** [iˌlektrəuˌdepə'ziʃən] *n* 电淀积

electrodermal [iˌlektrəu'dəːməl] *a* 皮肤电的

electrodermatome [iˌlektrəu'dəːmətəum] *n* 电[植]皮刀

electrodesiccation [iˌlektrəuˌdesi'keiʃən] *n* 电干燥法

electrodiagnosis [iˌlektrəuˌdaiəg'nəusis] *n* 电诊断法

electrodiagnostics [iˌlektrəuˌdaiəgˈnɔstiks] *n* 电诊断医学
electrodialysis [iˌlektrə*u*daiˈæləsis] *n* 电渗析
electrodialyzer [iˌlektrə*u*ˌdaiəˈlaizə] *n* 电渗析器，电透析器
electrodiaphake [iˌlektrə*u*daiˈæfəki] *n* 晶状体透热摘出器
electrodiaphane [iˌlektrə*u*ˈdaiəfein], **electrodiaphanoscope** [iˌlektrə*u*daiˈæfənəskəup] *n* 电透照镜
electrodiaphanoscopy [iˌlektrə*u*daiˌæfəˈnɔskəpi] *n* 电透照检查
electrodiaphany [iˌlektrə*u*daiˈæfəni] *n* 电透照
electroejaculation (EEJ) [iˌlektrə*u*iˌdʒækjuˈleiʃən] *n* 电射精
electroencephalogram (EEG) [iˌlektrə*u* enˈsefələˌgræm] *n* 脑电图 | flat ~, isoelectric ~ 平坦脑电图，等电位脑电图
electroencephalograph [iˌlektrə*u*enˈsefələgrɑːf, -græf] *n* 脑电图机 | **~ic** [iˌlektrə*u* enˌsefələˈgræfik] *a* / **~y** [iˌlektrə*u*enˌsefəˈlɔgrəfi] *n* 脑电图学
electroencephaloscope [iˌlektrə*u*enˈsefələskəup] *n* 脑电镜，脑电显示器
electroendosmosis [iˌlektrə*u*ˌendɔsˈməusis] *n* 电渗，内电渗
electroenterostomy [iˌlektrə*u*ˌentəˈrɔstəmi] *n* 电肠造口术
electroexcision [iˌlektrə*u*ekˈsiʒən] *n* 电切除
electrofocusing [iˌlektrə*u*ˈfəukəsiŋ] *n* 电聚焦
electrogastroenterostomy [iˌlektrə*u*ˌgæstrə*u*entəˈrɔstəmi] *n* 胃肠电吻合术
electrogastrogram [iˌlektrə*u*ˈgæstrəgræm] *n* 胃电图
electrogastrograph [iˌlektrə*u*ˈgæstrəgrɑːf, -græf] *n* 胃电描记器 | **~y** [iˌlektrə*u*gæsˈtrɔgrəfi] *n* 胃电描记法
electrogenic [iˌlektrə*u*ˈdʒenik] *a* 生电的
electroglottography [iˌlektrə*u*ˈglɔtəgrəfi] *n* 电声门描记[法]
electrogoniometer [iˌlektrə*u*ˌgəuniˈɔmitə] *n* 电测角计，电角度计
electrogram [iˈlektrəgræm] *n* 电描记图 | His bundle ~ (HBE) 希氏束电图
electrograph [iˈlektrəgrɑːf, -græf] *n* 电描记图 | **~y** [ˌilekˈtrɔgrəfi] *n* 电描记术
electrogustometry [iˌlektrə*u*gʌsˈtɔmitri] *n* 电味觉测定[法]
electrohemostasis [iˌlektrə*u*hiˈmɔstəsis] *n* 电止血[法]
electrohysterography [iˌlektrə*u*ˌhistəˈrɔgrəfi] *n* 子宫电描记[法]
electrohysterogram [iˌlektrə*u*ˈhistərəgræm] *n* 子宫电图
electroimmunoassay [iˌlektrə*u*imjunə*u*ˈæsei] *n* 电免疫测定
electroimmunodiffusion [iˌlektrə*u*ˌimjunə*u*diˈfjuːʒən] *n* 电免疫扩散
electrokinetic [iˌlektrə*u*kaiˈnetik] *a* 动电的，电动的
electrokymogram [iˌlektrə*u*ˈkaiməgræm] *n* 电记波[照]片，心电记波图
electrokymograph [iˌlektrə*u*ˈkaiməgrɑːf, -græf] *n* 电记波器 | **~y** [iˌlektrə*u*kaiˈmɔgrəfi] *n* 电记波摄影[术]
electrolaryngography [iˌlektrə*u*ˈlæriŋgə*u*grəfi] *n* 喉电描记[法]
electrolarynx [iˌlektrə*u*ˈlæriŋks] *n* 人工喉
electrolepsy [iˈlektrəˌlepsi] *n* 电击样舞蹈症
electrolithotrity [iˌlektrə*u*liˈθɔtriti] *n* 电碎石术
electrolysis [ilekˈtrɔlisis] *n* 电解
electrolyte [iˈlektrə*u*lait] *n* 电解质 | amphoteric ~ 两性电解质（能分解成氢离子〈H^+〉和氢氧离子〈OH^-〉的一种物质）/ colloidal ~ 胶体电解质
electrolytic [iˌlektrə*u*ˈlitik] *a* 电解的
electrolyzable [iˌlektrə*u*ˈlaizəbl] *a* 可电解的
electromagnet [iˌlektrə*u*ˈmægnit] *n* 电磁铁；电磁体
electromagnetic [iˌlektrə*u*mægˈnetik] *a* 电磁的
electromagnetism [iˌlektrə*u*ˈmægnitizəm] *n* 电磁；电磁学
electromanometer [iˌlektrə*u*məˈnɔmitə] *n* 电测压计
electrometer [ˌilekˈtrɔmitə] *n* 静电计，静电测量器
electrometrogram [iˌlektrə*u*ˈmetrəgræm] *n* 子宫肌电图，子宫收缩电[描记]图
electromigratory [iˌlektrə*u*ˈmaigrətəri] *a* 电迁移的
electromotive [iˌlektrə*u*ˈməutiv] *a* 电动的
electromyogram [iˌlektrə*u*ˈmaiəgræm] *n* 肌电图
electromyograph [iˌlektrə*u*ˈmaiəgrɑːf] *n* 肌电图描记器 | **~y** [iˌlektrə*u*maiˈɔgrəfi] *n* 肌电图学
electron [iˈlektrɔn] *n* 电子 | emission ~ 发射电子 / free ~ 自由电子 / valence ~ 价电子
electronarcosis [iˌlektrə*u*nɑːˈkəusis] *n* 电[流]麻醉，电麻醉疗法
electron-dense [iˈlektrɔnˌ dens] *a* 电子致密的（电子显微镜检查法中指一种使电子难以透过的密度）
electronegative [iˌlektrə*u*ˈnegətiv] *a* 阴电性的，负电性的 | **electronegativity** [iˌlektrə*u*ˌnegəˈtivəti] *n* 阴电性，电负性

electroneurography [iˌlektrəunjuəˈrɔgrəfi] *n* 神经电图学
electroneurolysis [iˌlektrəunjuəˈrɔlisis] *n* 电针神经松解术
electroneuromyography [iˌlektrə*u*ˌnjuərə*u*maiˈɔgrəfi] *n* 神经肌电描记术
electronic [ˌilekˈtrɔnik] *a* 电子的;带电子的
electronics [ˌilekˈtrɔniks] *n* 电子学
electron-microscopic(al) [iˈlektrɔnˌmaikrəˈskɔpik(əl)] *a* 电镜可见的
electronograph [ˌilekˈtrɔnəgrɑːf, -græf] *n* 电子显微照片
electron transfer flavoprotein: ubiquinone oxidoreductase [iˈlektrɔnˈtrænsfəː ˌfleivə*u*ˈprəutiːn juːˈbikwinəun ˌɔksidə*u*riˈdʌkteis] 电子转移黄素蛋白:泛醌氧化还原酶(该氧化还原酶缺乏为一种常染色体隐性性状,可致戊二酸尿Ⅱ型)
electronystagmogram [iˌlektrə*u*nisˈtægməgræm] *n* 眼震电图
electronystagmograph [iˌlektrə*u*nisˈtægməgrɑːf] *n* 眼震电图描记器 | **~y** [iˌlektrə*u*ˌnistægˈmɔgrəfi] *n* 眼震电图描记[法]
electro-oculogram [iˌlektrə*u*ˈɔkjuləgræm] *n* 眼动电图
electro-oculography [iˌlektrə*u*ˌɔkjuˈlɔgrəfi] *n* 眼动电图描记[法]
electro-olfactogram [iˌlektrə*u*ɔlˈfæktəgræm] *n* 嗅电图
electro-osmosis [iˌlektrə*u*ɔzˈməusis] *n* 电渗
electroparacentesis [iˌlektrə*u*ˌpærəsenˈtiːsis] *n* (眼前房)电穿刺术
electropathology [iˌlektrə*u*pəˈθɔlədʒi] *n* 电病理学
electrophile [iˈlektrəfail] *n* 亲电子试剂
electrophilic [iˌlektrə*u*ˈfilik] *a* 亲电子的
electrophonoide [iˌlektrə*u*ˈfəunɔid] *n* 电助听训练器(用于治疗慢性聋)
electrophoresis [iˌlektrə*u*fəˈriːsis] *n* 电泳 | counter ~ 对流电泳 / disc ~ 圆盘电泳 / lipoprotein ~ 脂蛋白电泳 / protein ~ 蛋白电泳 / pulsed field gradient ~ 脉冲场梯度电泳 | **electrophoretic** [iˌlektrə*u*fəˈretik] *a*
electrophoretogram [iˌlektrə*u*fəˈretəgræm], **electropherogram** [iˌlektrə*u*ˈferəgræm], **electrophoregram** [iˌlektrə*u*ˈfɔrigræm] *n* 电泳图[谱]
electrophorus [ilekˈtrɔfərəs] *n* 起电盘
electrophotometer [iˌlektrə*u*fəˈtɔmitə] *n* 光电比色计
electrophrenic [iˌlektrə*u*ˈfrenik] *a* 膈神经电刺激的
electrophysiology [iˌlektrə*u*fiziˈɔlədʒi] *n* 电生理学 | **electrophysiologic(al)** [iˌlektrə*u*ˌfiziəˈlɔdʒik(əl)] *a* / **electrophysiologist** *n* 电生理学家
electroplating [iˈlektrə*u*ˌpleitiŋ, iˌlektrə*u*ˈpleitiŋ] *n* 电镀[术]
electroplax [iˈlektrə*u*plæks] *n* 电板
electroplexy [iˈlektrə*u*ˌpleksi] *n* 电休克,电休克疗法
electropneumatotherapy [iˌlektrə*u*ˌnjuːmətə*u*ˈθerəpi] *n* 喉感应电疗法
electroporation [iˌlektrə*u*pəˈreiʃən] *n* 电穿孔(应用电场在细胞质膜内引起可逆性穿孔,核酸即可由此引入)
electropositive [iˌlektrə*u*ˈpɔzətiv] *a* 阳电[性]的,正电[性]的
electropuncture [iˈlektrə*u*ˌpʌŋktʃə] *n* 电针术
electroradiometer [iˌlektrə*u*reidiˈɔmitə] *n* 放射测量计
electroresection [iˌlektrə*u*riˈsekʃən] *n* 电切除术
electroretinogram [iˌlektrə*u*ˈretinəgræm] *n* 视网膜电图
electroretinograph [iˌlektrə*u*ˈretinəgrɑːf, -græf] *n* 视网膜电描记器 | **~y** [iˌlektrə*u*ˌretiˈnɔgrəfi] *n* 视网膜电描记[法]
electrosalivogram [iˌlektrə*u*səˈlaivəgræm] *n* 涎腺电图
electroscission [iˌlektrə*u*ˈsiʒən] *n* 电切术
electroscope [iˈlektrəskəup] *n* 验电器 | **electroscopic** [iˌlektrəˈskɔpik] *a*
electrosection [iˌlektrə*u*ˈsekʃən] *n* 电切除术
electroselenium [iˌlektrə*u*siˈliːnjəm] *n* 胶体硒
electroshock [iˈlektrə*u*ʃɔk] *n* 电休克
electrosleep [iˈlektrə*u*sliːp] *n* 电睡眠,电疗睡眠
electrosol [iˈlektrə*u*sɔl] *n* 电溶胶,金属电胶液
electrospectrogram [iˌlektrə*u*ˈspektrəgræm] *n* 电光谱图
electrospectrography [iˌlektrə*u*spekˈtrɔgrəfi] *n* 电光谱描记术
electrospinogram [iˌlektrə*u*ˈspainəgræm] *n* 脊髓电图
electrostatic [iˌlektrə*u*ˈstætik] *a* 静电的;静电学的 | **~s** *n* 静电学
electrostenolysis [iˌlektrə*u*stiˈnɔlisis] *n* 膜孔电析
electrostimulation [iˌlektrə*u*ˌstimjuˈleiʃən] *n* 电刺激术(治疗和实验用)
electrostriatogram [iˌlektrə*u*straiˈeitəgræm] *n* 纹状体电图
electrosurgery [iˌlektrə*u*ˈsəːdʒəri] *n* 电外科
electrosyneresis [iˌlektrə*u*siniˈriːsis] *n* 免疫过滤
electrosynthesis [iˌlektrə*u*ˈsinθisis] *n* 电合成[法]
electrotaxis [iˌlektrə*u*ˈtæksis] *n* 趋电性

electrothanasia [iˌlektrəuθəˈneiziə] *n* [触]电死,电[死]刑

electrotherapeutics [iˌlektrəuθerəˈpjuːtiks] *n* 电疗学,电疗法 | **electrotherapeutist** [iˌlektrəuθerəˈpjuːtist] *n* 电疗学家,电疗医生

electrotherapy [iˌlektrəuˈθerəpi] *n* 电疗学,电疗法 | cerebral ~ (CET) 脑电疗法 | **electrotherapist** [iˌlektrəuˈθerəpist] *n* 电疗学家

electrotherm [iˈlektrəuθəːm] *n* 电热器

electrothermal [iˈlektrəuˈθəːməl] *a* 电热的

electrotome [iˈlektrətəum] *n* 电刀

electrotomy [ilekˈtrɔtəmi] *n* 电切术

electrotonus [ilekˈtrɔtənəs] *n* 电紧张 | **electrotonic** [iˌlektrəuˈtɔnik] *a*

electrotrephine [eˌlektrəuˈtriːfin] *n* 电圆锯

electrotropism [ˌilekˈtrɔtrəpizəm] *n* 向电性;应电性 | negative ~ 阴性向电性 / positive ~ 阳性向电性

electrotubogram [ˌilektrəuˈtjuːbəugræm] *n* 咽鼓管电图

electroultrafiltration [iˌlektrəuˌʌltrəfilˈtreiʃən] *n* 电超滤[作用]

electroureterogram [iˌlektrəujuəˈriːtərəgræm] *n* 输尿管电图

electroureterography [iˌlektrəujuəˌriːtəˈrɔgrəfi] *n* 输尿管电描记术

electrovagogram [iˌlektrəuˈveigəgræm] *n* 迷走神经电图

electrovalence [iˌlektrəuˈveiləns] *n* 电价

electrovalent [iˌlektrəuˈveilənt] *a* 电价的;电价键的

electrovert [iˌlektrəvəːt] *vt* 电复律(以制止心律紊乱) | **electroversion** [iˌlektrəuˈvəːʃən, -ʒən] *n*

electuary [iˈlektjuəri] *n* [干]药糖剂 | ~ of senna 番泻叶糖剂

eledoisin [ˌeləˈdɔisin] *n* 章鱼唾腺精

eleidin [eˈliːidin] *n* 角母蛋白

element [ˈelimənt] *n* 要素,成分;(化学)元素 | appendicular ~s 附件成分(接于胚胎软骨性头颅骨的一组软骨杆,由此而发育成耳骨、舌骨和茎突) / formed ~s (of the blood) (血液)有形成分 / morphological ~, anatomic ~, tissue ~ 形态成分,解剖成分,组织成分 / radioactive ~ 放射性元素 / rare earth ~s 稀土元素 / sarcous ~ 肌成分 / trace ~s 微量元素,痕量元素 / tracer ~s 示踪元素 / transcalifornium ~s 锎后元素,超锎元素 / transuranic ~s, transuranium ~s 铀后元素,超铀元素

elementary [ˌeliˈmentəri] *a* 初级的,基本的;元素的

elemi [ˈelimi] *n* 榄香脂(一种橄榄属树脂)

ele(o)- [构词成分]油

eleoma [ˌeliˈəumə] *n* 油肿(油注射于组织所致的瘤或肿胀)

eleometer [ˌeliˈɔmitə] *n* 油度计,油比重计

eleopathy [ˌeliˈɔpəθi] *n* 脂肪性[水]肿病,脂质浮肿病

eleoplast [eˈliːəplæst] *n* 成油体,含油体(含油滴的原浆球体)

eleopten [ˌeliːˈɔptən] *n* 油萜,挥发油精

eleosaccharum [ˌeliəuˈsækərəm] *n* 油糖剂

eleotherapy [ˌeliəuˈθerəpi] *n* 油疗法

elephantiasis [ˌelifənˈtaiəsis] *n* 象皮病,象皮肿 | ~ arabicum 阿拉伯象皮病 / ~ filariensis 丝虫性象皮病 / lymphangiectatic ~ 淋巴管扩张性象皮病 / nevoid ~ 痣样象皮病 | **elephantiasic** [ˌeliˌfæntiˈæsik] *a*

elephantoid [ˌeliˈfæntɔid] *a* 象皮病样的

Elettaria cardamomum (L.) Maton (Zingiberaceae) [eliˈtɛəriə ˌkɑːdəˈməuməm] 小豆蔻

eleuthero [iˈljuːθərəu] (Eleutherococcus 的缩写) *n* 西伯利亚人参

Eleutherococcus [iˈljuːθərəuˌkɔkəs] *n* 五加属 | ~ senticosus 刺五加(西伯利亚人参,其根作药用)

eleutheromania [iˌljuːθərəuˈmeinjə] *n* 自由狂(追求自由狂热)

elevation [ˌeliˈveiʃən] *n* 提高,上升;隆肿,隆凸 | boiling point ~ 沸点上升 / tactile ~s 触觉隆凸,触觉小珠

elevator [ˈeliveitə] *n* 牙挺;起子 | periosteum ~ 骨膜起子,骨膜分离器 / screw ~ 螺旋牙根挺;螺旋起子

elfazepam [elˈfæzəpæm] *n* 依法西泮(兽用食欲刺激药)

eliminant [iˈliminənt] *a* 排泄的,排除的 *n* 排除剂

eliminate [iˈlimineit] *vt* 排除,消除,消灭

elimination [iˌlimiˈneiʃən] *n* 排除,消除,消灭 | immune ~ 免疫排除,免疫清除

elinguation [ˌiːliŋˈgweiʃən] *n* 去舌术

elinin [ˈelinin] *n* 红细胞脂蛋白(含有 Rh、A、B 因子的红细胞的脂蛋白部分)

ELISA [iˈlaisə] (*E*nzyme *L*inked *I*mmuno *S*orbent *A*ssay) 酶联免疫吸附测定

elixir [iˈliksə] *n* 酏剂

elkosis [ˈelkəsis] *n* 溃疡形成

Ellermann-Erlandsen test (method) [ˈeləmən ˈɛələndsən] (Vilhelm Ellermann; Alfred W. E. Erlandsen) 埃勒曼-厄兰森试验(法)(结核菌素效价试验 tuberculin titer test, 见 test 项下相应术语)

Elliot's operation [ˈeljət] (R. H. Elliot) 埃利奥特手术(巩膜角膜环钻术,用以减轻青光眼时的

眼压升高）
Elliot's position [ˈeljət]（John W. Elliot）埃利奥特卧位（下胸部垫高，用于胆囊手术）
Elliot's sign [ˈeljət]（George T. Elliot）埃利奥特征（①梅毒性皮肤溃疡边缘坚硬；②盲点扩大）
ellipsin [iˈlipsin] *n* 细胞不溶质
ellipsis [iˈlipsis] *n* 脱漏，省略（患者在精神分析中单词或观念的省略）
ellipsoid [iˈlipsɔid] *n* 椭圆体（尤指脾和视网膜杆）
elliptic(al) [iˈliptik(əl)] *a* 椭圆的，椭圆形的
elliptocyte [iˈliptəsait] *n* 椭圆形红细胞 | **elliptocytary** [iˌliptəuˈsaitəri] *a*
elliptocytosis [iˌliptəusaiˈtəusis] *n* 椭圆形红细胞增多症（一种遗传性疾患，大部分红细胞为椭圆形，其特征为不同程度红细胞破坏增加和贫血） | **elliptocytotic** [iˌliptəusaiˈtɔtik] *a*
Ellis-Garland line [ˈelis ˈɡɑːlənd]（Calvin Ellis；George M. Garland）埃利斯-加兰线（见 Ellis's line）
Ellis's line (curve) [ˈelis]（Calvin Ellis）埃利斯线（曲线）（胸部 S 形线，指示胸膜渗出液的上界） | ~ sign 埃利斯征（胸膜渗出液吸收时浊音曲线）
Ellis-van Creveld syndrome [ˈelisvɑːn ˈkriːveld]（Richard W. B. Ellis；Simon van Creveld）埃-范综合征；软骨外胚层发育不良
elm [elm] *n* 榆，榆木
Eloesser flap [eˈlesə]（Leo Eloesser）埃莱塞皮瓣（为慢性脓胸开放引流而在肋上所做的皮瓣）
elongate [ˈiːlɔŋɡeit] *vt*, *vi* 拉长，延长 *a* 拉长的，延伸的，细长的 | **elongation** [ˌiːlɔŋˈɡeiʃən] *n* 拉长，伸长；移动（牙向殆和切方向的病理性移动）；[射野]拉长
Elsberg's test [ˈelsbəːɡ]（Charles A. Elsberg）埃尔斯伯格试验（检嗅觉以测定脑瘤）
Elschnig's bodies (pearls) [ˈelʃniʃ]（Anton P. Elschnig）埃尔斯尼希体（珠）（内障摘出术后上皮细胞增生形成葡萄状串）
Elsner's asthma [ˈelsnə]（Christoph F. Elsner）心绞痛
El Tor vibrio [eltɔː]（El Tor 为埃及西奈半岛的检疫站，1960 年首次在此隔离）埃尔托弧菌，霍乱弧菌埃尔托型
eluate [ˈeljuit] *n* 洗出液；洗出物，洗脱物
elucaine [iˈljuːkein] *n* 依鲁卡因（抗胆碱能药）
eluent [iˈljuːənt] *n* 洗脱液
elute [iˈljuːt] *vt* 洗提，洗脱
elution [iˈljuːʃən] *n* 洗脱 | membrane ~ 膜洗脱
elutriate [iˈljuːtrieit] *vt* 淘析，淘洗 | **elutriation** [iˌljuːtriˈeiʃən] *n* 淘析法
Ely's operation [ˈiːli]（Edward T. Ely）伊利手术（慢性化脓性中耳炎肉芽面植皮术）
Ely's test (sign) [ˈiːli]（Leonard W. Ely）伊利试验（征）（检股侧筋膜挛缩）
elytr(o)- [构词成分] 阴道（见 colpo-）
Elzholz's bodies [ˈeltshɔlts]（Adolf Elzholz）埃尔兹霍兹体（有髓神经纤维变性小体） | ~ mixture 埃尔兹霍兹合剂（计算白细胞用的伊红甘油水溶液）
EM effective masking 有效掩蔽
Em emmetropia 正视眼
emaciate [iˈmeiʃieit] *vt*, *vi* 消瘦 | **emaciation** [iˌmeisiˈeiʃən] *n*
emailloblast [iˈmeiləblæst] *n* 成釉细胞
eman [ˈemən] *n* 唉曼（镭射气在溶液中的浓度单位，$=10^{-10}$ 居里，现用 Bq〈贝可勒尔〉，1Ci〈居里〉$=37$ GBq〈3.7×10^{10} Bq〉）
emanate [ˈeməneit] *vi* 发散，放射
emanation [ˌeməˈneiʃən] *n* 发散，放射；射气 | actinium ~ 锕射气 / radium ~ 氡，镭射气 / thorium ~ 钍射气
emanator [ˈeməˌneitə] *n* 射气投置器
emanatorium [ˌemənəˈtɔːriəm] *n* 射气治疗院
emancipate [iˈmænsipeit] *vt* 解放，使不受束缚 | **emancipation** [iˌmænsiˈpeiʃən] *n* 解放（在发育中胎儿在有限范围内成立局部自主状态）
emasculate [iˈmæskjuleit] *vt* 阉割 [iˈmæskjulit] *a* 阉割了的 | **emasculation** [iˌmæskjuˈleiʃən] *n* 阴茎切除；去睾术，阉割，去势，去雄
Embadomonas [ˌembəˈdɔmənəs] *n* 内滴虫属（即 Retortamonas）
embalm [imˈbɑːm] *vt* 涂香油（或药料等）于尸体防腐 | **~er** *n* 尸体防腐者 / **~ment** *n* 尸体防腐法
embalming [imˈbɑːmiŋ] *n* 尸体防腐
embarrass [imˈbærəs] *vt* 窘迫；妨碍，阻碍 | **~ment** *n*
Embden ester [ˈembdən]（Gustav G. Embden）恩伯登酯（75% ~ 80% 葡糖-6-磷酸和 20% ~ 25% 果糖-6-磷酸的平衡混合液）
Embden-Meyerhof pathway [ˈembdən ˈmaiəhɔf]（G. G. Embden；Oto F. Meyerhof）恩-迈[糖代谢]途径（为葡萄糖无氧转变为乳酸的一系列酶反应，结果以腺苷三磷酸〈ATP〉形式形成能量）
Embden-Meyerhof-Parnas pathway [ˈembdən ˈmaiərhɔf ˈpɑːnɑːs]（G. G. Embden；O. F. Meyerhof；Jakub K. Parnas）恩-迈-帕途径，糖酵解途径（见 Embden-Meyerhof pathway）
embed [imˈbed] *vt* 包埋；植入 | **~ment** *n*
embedding [imˈbediŋ] *n* 包埋；植入

Embelia [emˈbiːliə] *n* 信筒子属 | ~ ribes, ~ robusta 信筒子(其果实用于抗蠕虫和泻药的成分)
embelin [ˈembilin] *n* 信筒子素(曾用作杀绦虫药)
emboitement [ɔŋbwɑːtˈmɔŋ] *n*【法】套装(认为前一代生殖细胞内即装有一个微型个体,此说以后发展为先成说 preformation)
embolalia [ˌembəˈleiliə] *n* 插语症
embole [ˈembəli], **embolia** [emˈbəuliə] *n* 关节复位;(囊胚)套入
embolectomy [ˌembəˈlektəmi] *n* 栓子切除术
emboli [ˈembəlai] embolus 的复数
embolic [emˈbɔlik] *a* 栓子的;栓塞的
emboliform [emˈbɔlifɔːm] *a* 楔形的;栓子状的
embolism [ˈembəlizəm] *n* 栓塞 | air ~ 空气栓塞 / amniotic fluid ~ 羊水栓塞 / bacillary ~ 杆菌栓塞 / bland ~ 非脓毒性栓塞 / cerebral ~ 脑栓塞 / coronary ~ 冠状动脉栓塞 / direct ~ 顺行栓塞 / fat ~, oil ~ 脂[肪]栓塞 / lymph ~, lymphogenous ~ 淋巴管栓塞 / paradoxical ~, crossed ~ 反常栓塞,交叉性栓塞 / plasmodium ~ 疟原虫性栓塞 / pulmonary ~ 肺栓塞 / saddle ~, pantaloon ~ 鞍栓塞(主动脉分叉口栓塞) / spinal ~ 脊髓[动脉]栓塞 / tumor ~ 肿瘤栓塞
embolization [ˌembəlaiˈzeiʃən, -liˈz-] *n* 栓塞,栓子形成 | poppet ~ 笼球阀栓塞(用作心脏瓣膜修复物的笼球阀瓣引起的栓塞)
embolize [ˈembəlaiz] *vt* 栓塞 *vi* 成为栓子
embololalia [ˌembələuˈleiliə], **embolophrasia** [ˌembələuˈfreiziə] *n* 插语症
embolomycotic [ˌembələumaiˈkɔtik] *a* 感染性栓子的
embolotherapy [ˌembələuˈθerəpi] *n* 栓塞疗法
embolus [ˈembələs] ([复] **emboli** [ˈembəlai]) *n* 栓子 | air ~ 气栓,空气栓子 / cancer ~ 癌细胞栓子 / foam ~ 泡沫栓子(气体和血混合形成) / obturating ~ 阻塞性栓子 / riding ~, saddle ~, stradding ~ 血管分叉口栓子,鞍栓
emboly [ˈembəli] *n* (囊胚)套入
embouchment [ɔŋbuʃˈmɔŋ] *n*【法】血管汇入
embrasure [imˈbreiʒə] *n* 楔状隙 | occlusal ~ 殆侧楔状隙
embrocate [ˈembrəukeit] *vt* (用洗液等)涂擦 | **embrocation** [ˌembrəuˈkeiʃən] *n* 擦法;擦剂
embryectomy [ˌembriˈektəmi] *n* 胎切除术(宫外孕时)
embryo [ˈembriəu] *n* 胚[胎] *a* 胚胎的 | hexacanth ~ 六钩蚴,钩球蚴 / previllous ~ 绒毛前胚 / somite ~ 体节胚
embryoblast [ˈembriəˌblæst] *n* 成胚细胞,内细胞团
embryocardia [ˌembriəuˈkɑːdiə] *n* 胎样心音(第一心音与第二心音的性质无甚差异)
embryoctony [ˌembriˈɔktəni] *n* 碎胎术
embryogeny [ˌembriˈɔdʒini], **embryogenesis** [ˌembriəuˈdʒenisis] *n* 胚胎发生 | **embryogenetic** [ˌembriəudʒiˈnetik], **embryogenic** [ˌembriəuˈdʒenik] *a*
embryograph [ˈembriəgrɑːf, -græf] *n* 胚胎描记器 | **~y** [ˌembriˈɔgrəfi] *n* 胚胎描记[法]
embryoid [ˈembriɔid] *a* 胚胎样的
embryoism [ˈembriəizəm] *n* 胚胎状态
embryolethality [ˌembriəuliˈθæləti] *n* 胎仔致死作用
embryology [ˈembriˈɔlədʒi] *n* 胚胎学 | comparative ~ 比较胚胎学 / descriptive ~ 描述胚胎学 / experimental ~, causal ~ 实验胚胎学 | **embryologic(al)** [ˌembriəˈlɔdʒik(əl)] *a* / **embryologist** *n* 胚胎学家
embryoma [ˌembriˈəumə] *n* 胚胎瘤 | ~ of kidney 肾胚胎瘤,维尔姆斯(Wilms)瘤
embryomorphous [ˌembriəuˈmɔːfəs] *a* 胚胎形的(指某些异常组织,被认为是孕体的遗迹)
embryonate [ˈembriəneit] *a* 胚胎的;含胚的;受孕的
embryonic [ˌembriˈɔnik], **embryonal** [ˈembriənəl] *a* 胚胎的
embryoniform [ˌembriˈɔnifɔːm], **embryonoid** [ˈembriənɔid] *a* 胚胎样的
embryonism [ˈembriənizəm] *n* 胚胎状态
embryonization [ˌembriəunaiˈzeiʃən] *n* 胚胎化
embryony [ˈembriəni] *n* 胚形成
embryopathia [ˌembriəuˈpæθiə] *n* 胚胎病 | ~ rubeolaris 风疹性胚胎畸形
embryopathology [ˌembriəupəˈθɔlədʒi] *n* 胚胎病理学
embryopathy [ˌembriˈɔpəθi] *n* 胚胎病 | rubella ~ 风湿性胚胎畸形
embryophore [ˈembriəfɔː] *n* 胚膜(卵);胚托
embryoplastic [ˌembriəuˈplæstik] *a* 胚胎形成的
embryoscope [ˈembriəskəup] *n* 胚胎发育观察器,胚胎镜
embryotocia [ˌembriəuˈtəusiə] *n* 流产
embryotome [ˈembriətəum] *n* 碎胎刀
embryotomy [ˌembriˈɔtəmi] *n* 碎胎术
embryotoxicity [ˌembriəultɔkˈsisəti] *n* 胚胎毒性
embryotoxon [ˌembriəuˈtɔksən] *n* (角膜)胚胎环 | anterior ~ (角膜)前胚胎环(即角膜弓 arcus corneae) / posterior ~ (角膜)后胚胎环,阿克森费尔德(Axenfeld)异常
embryotroph [ˈembriəˌtrəuf] *n* 胎体营养物 | **~y** [ˌembriˈɔtrəfi] *n* 胎体营养

embryulcia [ˌembriˈʌlsiə] *n* 钳胎术
embryulcus [ˌembriˈʌlkəs] *n* 牵胎钩
EMC encephalomyocarditis (virus) 脑心肌炎(病毒)
emedastine difumarate [ˌeməˈdæstiːn] 延胡索酸依美斯汀(抗组胺药〈H_1 受体拮抗药〉,局部用于结膜,治疗变应性结膜炎)
emedullate [iˈmedjuleit] *vt* 去髓
emelocytosis [iːˌmiəusaiˈtəusis] *n* 细胞分泌
emergence [iˈməːdʒəns] *n* 苏醒(从以前的状态中出来的过程,如麻醉后患者恢复到正常的生理状态)
emergency [iˈməːdʒənsi] *n* 紧急,意外;急症
emergent [iˈməːdʒənt] *a* 紧急的,意外的;突生的(如突生进化)
Emericella [ˌeməriˈselə] *n* 翘孢霉属
emery [ˈeməri] *n* 刚砂,金刚砂
Emery-Dreifuss muscular dystrophy [ˈeməri ˈdraifəs] (Alan E. H. Emery; F. E. Dreifuss) 埃-德肌营养不良(一种罕见的 X 连锁型肌营养不良,幼年开始发病,上臂及骨盆带肌缓慢地渐渐变得软弱无力,伴有心肌病及肘屈曲挛缩,肌肉并不肥大。亦称肩腓型肌营养不良)
emesis [ˈeməsis] *n* 呕吐 | ~ gravidarum 孕吐 | **emesia** [iˈmiːziə] *n*
-emesis [构词成分]呕吐
emetatrophia [ˌemitəˈtrəufiə] *n* 吐瘦(由于持续性呕吐所引起的萎缩或消瘦)
emetic [iˈmetik] *a* 催吐的 *n* 催吐药 | direct ~, mechanical ~ 直接催吐药 / indirect ~, central ~, systemic ~ 间接催吐药 / tartar ~ 吐酒石,酒石酸锑钾
emeticology [iˌmetiˈkɔlədʒi], **emetology** [ˌemiˈtɔlədʒi] *n* 催吐学,催吐药物学
emetine [ˈemətiːn] *n* 依米丁,吐根碱(抗阿米巴药) | ~ and bismuth iodide 碘化铋吐根碱(抗阿米巴药,治阿米巴痢疾) / ~ hydrochloride 盐酸依米丁(抗阿米巴药)
emetocathartic [ˌemətəukəˈθɑːtik] *a* 催吐导泻的 *n* 吐泻药
emetogenic [ˌemətəuˈdʒenik] *a* 催吐的
EMF electromotive force 电动势
EMG electromyogram 肌电图
-emia [构词成分]血[液]
emigration [ˌemiˈgreiʃən] *n* (白细胞)游出
emilium tosylate [iˈmiliəm] 托西依米铵(抗心律失常药)
eminectomy [ˌemiˈnektəmi] *n* 结节切除术(颞骨关节隆起切除)
eminence [ˈeminəns] *n* 隆起,隆凸 | articular ~ 关节结节 / bicipital ~ 二头肌结节,桡骨粗隆 / capitate ~ 肱骨小头 / ~ of cartilage of Santorini 小角结节 / caudate ~ of liver 肝尾状突 / coccygeal ~ 骶骨角 / cuneiform ~ of head of rib 肋骨头小嵴 / deltoid ~ 三角肌粗隆(肱骨) / facial ~ of eminentia teres 面神经丘 / frontal ~ 额结节 / genital ~ 生殖隆起,生殖结节(胚) / gluteal ~ of femur 股骨臀肌粗隆 / ~ of humerus 肱骨小头 / hypobranchial ~ 舌联桁 / hypothenar ~, antithenar ~ 小鱼际 / intercondylar ~, intercondyloid ~, intermediate ~ 髁间隆起 / jugular ~ 颈静脉结节(枕骨) / mamillary ~ 乳头体 / nasal ~ 鼻隆起 / oblique ~ of cuboid bone 骰骨粗隆 / occipital ~ 枕隆起(胚) / olivary ~ of sphenoid bone 蝶骨鞍结节 / postchiasmatic ~, postfundibular ~ 视交叉后隆起(第三脑室底) / terete ~ 菱形窝内侧隆起 / thenar ~ 鱼际 / thyroid ~ 喉结 / triangular ~, ~ of triangular fossa of auricle 耳三角窝隆起 / trochlear ~ 肱骨滑车 / ulnar ~ of wrist 腕尺侧隆起 / vagal ~ 迷走神经三角,灰翼
eminentia [ˌemiˈnenʃiə] ([复] **eminentiae** [ˌemiˈnenʃiiː]) *n*【拉】隆起,隆凸
emiocytosis [ˌimiəusaiˈtəusis] *n* 细胞分泌,细胞物质排出(如排出胰岛素)
emissarium [ˌemiˈsɛəriəm] ([复] **emissaria** [ˌemiˈsɛəriə]) *n*【拉】导血管(导静脉)
emissary [ˈemisəri] *n* 导血管
emission [iˈmiʃən] *n* 发射,放射;遗精 | nocturnal ~ 梦遗,遗精 / thermionic ~ 热离子发射
emissive [iˈmisiv] *a* 发出的;发射的
emissivity [ˌeməˈsivəti] *n* 发射率,放射率(辐射能)
EMIT [iˈmit] (*E*nzyme-*M*ultiplied *I*mmunoassay *T*echnique) 酶倍增免疫测定法
emmenagogic [iˌmenəˈgɔdʒik] *a* 通经的
emmenagogue [iˈmenəgɔg] *n* 通经药
emmenia [iˈmiːniə] *n* 月经 | **emmenic** [iˈmenik] *a*
emmeniopathy [iˌmiːniˈɔpəθi] *n* 月经病
emmenology [ˌemiˈnɔlədʒi] *n* 月经学
Emmert-Gellhorn pessary [ˈemət ˈgelhɔːn] (Frederick V. Emmert; George Gellhorn) 埃默特-盖尔霍恩子宫托(空杆子宫托)
emmetrope [ˈemətrəup] *n* 正视者
emmetropia [ˌeməˈtrəupiə] *n* 正视眼 | **emmetropic** [ˌeməˈtrɔpik] *a*
Emmet's operation [ˈemit] (Thomas A. Emmet) 埃米特手术(①修补会阴撕裂术;②子宫颈缝术或宫颈裂缝术;③膀胱阴道瘘造口术,使膀胱炎时的膀胱得以引流)
Emmonsia [əˈmɔnsiə] *n* 金孢子菌属 | ~ crescens 新月金孢子菌 / ~ parva 小金孢子菌
emodin [ˈemədin] *n* 泻素,大黄素
emollient [iˈmɔliənt] *a* 软化的,润滑的 *n* 润肤

剂,润滑药

emotiometabolic [iˌməuʃiəuˌmetəˈbɔlik] *a* 情绪性代谢的

emotiomotor [iˌməuʃiəuˈməutə] *a* 情绪性动作的

emotiomuscular [iˌməuʃiəuˈmʌskjulə] *a* 情绪性肌肉活动的

emotion [iˈməuʃən] *n* 情绪 | **~al** *a*

emotiovascular [iˌməuʃiəuˈvæskjulə] *a* 情绪性血管变化的

emotive [iˈməutiv] *a* 情绪的;动感情的 | **emotivity** [iˌməuˈtivəti] *n* 感触性,易感性

Emp. emplastrum【拉】硬膏剂,贴膏剂

empacho [emˈpɑːkəu] *n* 恩帕寇(墨西哥儿童慢性消化不良,伴腹泻)

empasma [emˈpæzmə] *n* 撒布散剂(外用药粉)

empathize [ˈempəθaiz] *vi* 移情,神入

empathy [ˈempəθi] *n* 移情,神入 | **empathic** [emˈpæθik], **empathetic** [ˌempəˈθetik] *a*

emperipolesis [emˌperipəuˈliːsis] *n* 伸入运动(淋巴细胞在另一个细胞内伸入和活动)

emphraxis [emˈfræksis] *n*【希】闭塞,阻塞

emphysatherapy [ˌemfizəˈθerəpi] *n* 注气疗法

emphysema [ˌemfiˈsiːmə] *n* 气肿;肺气肿 | alveolar ~ 肺泡性气肿 / atrophic ~, small-lunged ~ 萎缩性肺气肿 / ectatic ~ 扩张性肺气肿 / glass blower's ~ 吹玻璃工肺气肿 / pulmonary ~, ~ of lungs 肺气肿 | **~tous** [ˌemfiˈsemətəs] *a*

Empiric [emˈpirik] *n* 经验医学派(古希腊希波克拉底〈Hippocrates〉学派以后的一个医派)

empiric [emˈpirik] *a* 经验主义的 *n* 经验主义者;江湖医

empirical [emˈpirikəl] *a* 经验主义的

empiricism [emˈpirisizəm] *n* 经验主义;经验[主义]医学;江湖医术 | **empiricist** *n* 经验主义者;庸医

emplastic [emˈplæstik] *a* 黏的,黏质的 *n* 便秘药

emplastrum [emˈplæstrəm] *n* 硬膏剂,贴膏剂

emporiatrics [emˌpɔːriˈætriks] *n* 旅行[者]医学

emprosthotonos, emprosthotonus [ˌemprɔsˈθɔtənəs] *n* 前弓反张

empty [ˈempti] *a* 空的 *vt* 排空 *vi* 排空;流入 | gastric ~ing 胃排空

emptysis [ˈemptisis] *n*【希】咯血

Empusa [emˈpjuːsə] *n* 虫霉属,蝇疫霉属

empyema [ˌempaiˈiːmə] *n* 积脓;脓胸 | ~ of gallbladder 胆囊积脓 / interlobar ~ (肺)叶间脓胸 / latent ~ 潜伏性脓胸 / loculated ~ 分房[性]脓胸 / mastoid ~ 乳突积脓 / metapneumonic ~ 肺炎后脓胸 / ~ of pericardium 脓性心包炎,心包积脓 / pneumococcal ~ 肺炎球菌性脓胸 / pulsating ~ 搏动性脓胸 / thoracic ~ 脓性胸膜炎,脓胸 / tuberculous ~ 结核性脓胸 | **~tous**, **empyemic** *a*

empyesis [ˌempaiˈiːsis] *n*【希】眼前房积脓;脓疱

empyocele [emˈpaiəsiːl] *n* 脐脓肿

empyreuma [ˌempaiˈruːmə] *n* (动植物在密封容器中焚烧后)焦臭 | **~tic** [ˌempairuːˈmætik] *a* 焦臭的(有机物质分解蒸馏所产生的气味)

EMS Emergency Medical Service 急诊部(英国)

emul. emulsum【拉】乳剂

emulgent [iˈmʌldʒənt] *a* 泄出的 *n* 泄出血管(肾动脉或肾静脉);利泄药(利胆、利尿药)

emulsify [iˈmʌlsifai] *vt*, *vi* 乳化 | **emulsification** [iˌmʌlsifiˈkeiʃən] *n* 乳化作用 / **emulsifier** [iˈmʌlsifaiə] *n* 乳化剂

emulsin [iˈmʌlsin] *n* 苦杏仁酶

emulsion [iˈmʌlʃən] *n* 乳胶,乳浊液;乳剂 | bacillary ~ 杆菌性乳剂,细菌性乳剂 / chylomicron ~ (血中)乳糜微粒 / kerosene ~ 煤油乳剂 / photographic ~ 照相乳剂 | **emulsive** *a* 乳剂性的;乳化的

emulsoid [iˈmʌlsɔid] *n* 乳胶体

emulsum [iˈmʌlsəm] ([复] **emulsa** [iˈmʌlsə]) *n*【拉】乳剂

emunctory [iˈmʌŋktəri] *a* 排泄的 *n* 排泄器,排泄管

emylcamate [iˈmilkəmeit] *n* 依米氨酯(安定药)

en [ɔŋ] *prep*【法】在…中;在;用 | ~ bloc 整块,整块地;全体,整个 / ~ masse 一起,全体;全部地,整个地 / ~ plaque 平板状

ENA extractable nuclear antigen 可提取的核抗原

enalapril [iˈnæləpril] *n* 依那普利(抗高血压药)

enalaprilat [əˈnæləˌprilət] *n* 依那普利拉(一种依那普利〈enalapril〉活性代谢物的静脉内制剂,治疗高血压危象时使用)

enamel [iˈnæməl] *n* 釉质 | curled ~ 曲形釉质 / dwarfed ~, nanoid ~ 薄釉质 / gnarled ~ 螺状釉质 / hereditary brown ~ 釉质生长不全 / hypoplastic ~ 釉质发育不全 / mottled ~ 斑釉

enameloblast [iˈnæmələblæst] *n* 成釉细胞

enameloblastoma [iˌnæmeləublæsˈtəumə] *n* 成釉细胞瘤

enameloma [iˌnæməˈləumə] *n* 釉质瘤

enameloplasty [iˌnæmələuˈplæsti] *n* 釉质成形术

enamelum [iˈnæmələm] *n* 釉质

enanthate [əˈnænθeit] *n* 庚酸盐(heptanoate 的 USAN 缩约词,庚酸的阴离子型)

enanthema [ˌenænˈθiːmə] ([复] **enanthemas** 或 **enanthemata** [ˌenænˈθiːmətə]), **enanthem** [eˈnænθəm] *n* 黏膜疹 | **enanthematous** [ˌenænˈθemətəs] *a*

enanthic acid [iˈnænθik], **enanthylic acid** [ˌiːnænˈθilik] 庚酸

enanthrope [eˈnænθrəup] *n* 体内病因,疾病内因

enantiobiosis [enˌæntiəubaiˈəusis] *n* 拮抗共生
enantiomerism [eˌnæntiˈɔmərizəm] *n* 对映形态
enantiomorph [enˈæntiəumɔːf], **enantiomer** [enˈæntiəumə] *n* 对映[异构]体 | **enantiomorphic** [enˌæntiəuˈmɔːfik] *a*
enantiomorphism [enˌæntiəuˈmɔːfizəm] *n* 对映形态
enantiopathia [enˌæntiəuˈpæθiə], **enantiopathy** [enˌæntiˈɔpəθi] *n* 对抗病;拮抗疗法
enantiopathic [enˌæntiəuˈpæθik] *a* 引起反感的;拮抗疗法的
Enantiothamnus [enˌæntiəuˈθæmnəs] *n* 结节中央化脓性真菌属
enarkyochrome [eˈnɑːkiəˌkrəum] *n* 单网色细胞
enarthritis [ˌenɑːˈθraitis] *n* 杵臼关节炎
enarthrosis [ˌenɑːˈθrəusis] *n* 杵臼关节 | **enarthrodial** *a*
encainide hydrochloride [enˈkeinaid] 盐酸恩卡尼(抗心律失常药)
encanthis [enˈkænθis] *n* 内眦瘤
encapsulate [inˈkæpsjuleit], **encapsule** [inˈkæpsjul] *vt* 用胶囊包 | **encapsulated** [inˈkæpsjuleitid], **encapsuled** [inˈkæpsjuld] *a* 有[胶]囊包着的,包在荚膜内的,[被]包围的 / **encapsulation** [inˌkæpsjuˈleiʃən] *n* 包围,包囊
encarditis [ˌenkɑːˈdaitis] *n* 心内膜炎
encatarrhaphy [ˌenkæˈtɑːrəfi] *n* 埋藏缝合术
enceinte [ɔŋˈsæŋt] *a* 【法】妊娠的
encelialgia [ˌensiːliˈældʒiə] *n* [腹]内脏痛
enceliitis [enˌsiliˈaitis], **encelitis** [ˌensiˈlaitis] *n* 内脏炎,腹内器官炎
encephalalgia [enˌsefəˈlældʒiə] *n* 头痛
encephalatrophy [enˌsefəˈlætrəfi] *n* 脑萎缩
encephalauxe [ˌensefəˈlɔːksi] *n* 脑肥大
encephalemia [enˌsefəˈliːmiə] *n* 脑充血
encephalic [ˌensəˈfælik] *a* 脑的;颅内的
encephalitis [enˌsefəˈlaitis] ([复] **encephalitides** [enˌsefəˈlitidiːz]) *n* 脑炎,大脑炎 | acute necrotizing ~ 急性坏死性脑炎 / Australian X ~ 澳大利亚 X 脑炎 / benign myalgic ~ 良性肌痛性脑炎(即流行性神经肌无力症) / California ~ 加利福尼亚脑炎(一种由虫媒病毒所致的急性病毒性脑炎,主要为儿童的一种疾病) / eastern equine ~ 东方马脑炎 / epidemic ~ 流行性脑炎 / hemorrhagic arsphenamine ~ 出血性胂凡纳明脑炎 / herpes ~, herpes simplex ~, herpetic ~ 疱疹脑炎,单纯疱疹性脑炎,疱疹性脑炎(由疱疹病毒所致的一种疾病,类似马脑脊髓炎) / influenzal ~ 流感脑炎 / Japanese B ~, ~ B, Russian autumnal ~ 乙型脑炎 / lethargic ~, ~ A. Vienna ~ 昏睡性脑炎,甲型脑炎,维也纳脑炎 / postinfectious ~, acute disseminated ~ 感染后脑炎,急性播散性脑炎 / postvaccinal ~, vaccinal ~ 疫苗接种后脑炎 / Russian forest-spring ~ 俄罗斯森林春季脑炎 / Russian spring-summer ~ 俄罗斯春夏型脑炎 / Russian tick-borne ~, woodcutter's ~ 俄罗斯蜱传脑炎,伐木者脑炎 / Russian vernal ~ 俄罗斯春季脑炎 / St. Louis ~, ~ C 圣路易脑炎,丙型脑炎 / Venezuelan equine ~ 委内瑞拉马脑炎 | **encephalitic** [ˌensefəˈlitik] *a*
encephalitogen [enˌsefəˈlitədʒən] *n* 致脑炎因子
encephalitogenic [enˌsefəlitəuˈdʒenik] *a* 致脑炎的
Encephalitozoon [ˌenseˌfælitəuˈzəuɔn] *n* 脑胞内原虫属(亦称微粒子虫属 Nosema) | ~ cuniculi 家兔脑胞内原虫 / ~ rabiei 内格里(Negri)小体,狂犬病包涵体
encephalitozoonosis [enˌsefəˌlitəzəuˈɔnəsis] *n* 脑胞内原虫病
encephalization [enˌsefəlaiˈzeiʃən, -liˈz-] *n* 大脑化
encephal(o)- [构词成分]脑
encephalo-arteriography [enˌsefələu ɑːˌtiəriˈɔgrəfi] *n* 脑动脉造影[术]
encephalocele [enˈsefələˌsiːl] *n* 脑突出,脑膨出
encephaloclastic [enˌsefələuˈklæstik] *a* 破坏脑的,脑损害[性]的
encephalocoele [enˌsəfələuˈsiːli] *n* 颅腔;脑室,脑腔
encephalocystocele [enˌsəfələuˈsistəsiːl] *n* 积水性脑突出
encephalodialysis [enˌsefələudaiˈælisis] *n* 脑软化,脑松软
encephaloduroarteriosynangiosis [enˌsefələu-ˌdjuːrəuɑːˌtiəriəusinændʒiˈəusis] *n* 脑硬脑膜动脉联合血管病
encephalodysplasia [enˌsefələudisˈpleiziə] *n* 脑发育异常
encephalogram [enˈsefələgræm] *n* 脑 X 线[照]片,脑造影[照]片
encephalography [enˌsefəˈlɔgrəfi] *n* 脑造影[术]
encephaloid [enˈsefəlɔid] *a* 脑样的 *n* 髓样癌
encephalolith [enˈsefələliθ] *n* 脑石
encephalology [ˌensefəˈlɔlədʒi] *n* 脑学
encephaloma [enˌsefəˈləumə] *n* 脑瘤;髓样癌
encephalomalacia [enˌsefələuməˈleiʃiə] *n* 脑软化
encephalomeningitis [enˌsefələuˌmeninˈdʒaitis] *n* 脑脑膜炎
encephalomeningocele [enˌsefələumiˈniŋgəsiːl] *n* 脑脑膜膨出
encephalomeningopathy [enˌsefələuˌmeniŋˈgɔ-

pəθi] *n* 脑脑膜病

encephalomere [en'sefələmiə] *n* 脑节

encephalometer [en͵sefə'lɔmitə] *n* 脑域测定器

encephalomyelitis [en͵sefələu͵maiə'laitis] *n* 脑脊髓炎 | acute disseminated ~ 急性播散性脑脊髓炎,感染后脑炎 / avian ~ 禽脑脊髓炎(鸡的一种病毒性疾病,亦称鸟狂病,流行性震颤) / benign myalgic ~ 良性肌痛性脑脊髓炎 / eastern equine ~ 东方马脑脊髓炎 / experimental allergic ~ (EAE) ~ 实验性变应性脑脊髓炎 / granulomatous ~ 肉芽肿性脑脊髓炎 / infectious porcine ~ 传染性猪脑脊髓炎 / Mengo ~ 门戈脑脊髓炎(其病毒首次在乌干达门戈地区分离而得) / mouse ~, murine ~ 鼠脑脊髓炎 / porcine ~ 猪脑脊髓炎 / postinfectious ~, postvaccinal ~ 感染后脑脊髓炎,疫苗接种后脑脊髓炎 / toxoplasmic ~ 弓形虫脑脊髓炎 / Venezuelan equine ~ 委内瑞拉马脑脊髓炎 / western equine ~ 西方马脑脊髓炎

encephalomyelocele [en͵sefələumai'eləsiːl] *n* 脑脊髓膨出

encephalomyeloneuropathy [en͵sefələu'maiələu-njuə'rɔpəθi] *n* 脑脊髓神经病

encephalomyelopathy [en͵sefələu͵maiə'lɔpəθi] *n* 脑脊髓病 | postinfection ~ 感染后脑脊髓病 / postvaccinal ~ 疫苗接种后脑脊髓病 / subacute necrotizing ~ 亚急性坏死性脑脊髓病(亦称亚急性坏死性脑病,利〈Leigh〉氏病或综合征)

encephalomyeloradiculitis [en͵sefələu͵maiələu-rə͵dikju'laitis] *n* 脑脊髓脊神经根炎

encephalomyeloradiculoneuritis [en͵sefələu͵m-aiələurə͵dikjuləunjuə'raitis] *n* 脑脊髓脊神经根神经炎,急性热病性多神经炎

encephalomyeloradiculopathy [en͵sefələu͵maiə-ləurə͵dikju'lɔpəθi] *n* 脑脊髓脊神经根病

encephalomyocarditis [en͵sefələu͵maiəukɑː'dai-tis] *n* 脑心肌炎(病毒性)

encephalomyopathy [en͵sefələumai'ɔpəθi] *n* 脑肌病 | mitochondrial ~ 线粒体脑肌病

encephalon [en͵sefəlɔn] ([复] **encephala** [en-͵sefələ]) *n* 脑

encephalonarcosis [en͵sefələunɑː'kəusis] *n* 脑病性木僵

encephalopathia [en͵sefələu'pæθiə] *n* 脑病 | ~ alcoholica 酒精中毒性脑病,出血性脑上部灰质炎

encephalopathy [en͵sefə'lɔpəθi] *n* 脑病 | biliary ~, bilirubin ~ 胆汁性脑病,胆红素脑病,核黄疸 / demyelinating ~ 脱髓鞘性脑病 / dialysis ~, progressive dialysis ~ 透析性脑病,进行性透析性脑病(长期应用血液透析而伴发的一种脑变性病) / hepatic ~, portal-systemic ~, portasystemic ~ 肝性脑病,门体脑病 / hypernatremic ~ 高血钠脑病(由渗透压过高伴高血钠和失水所致的严重出血性脑病) / hypoglycemic ~ 低血糖脑病 / lead ~, saturnine ~ 铅毒性脑病 / mink ~ 水貂脑病(水貂中枢神经系统的一种进行性病毒性疾病) / myoclonic ~ of childhood 儿童肌阵挛性脑病 / progressive subcortical ~ 进行性皮质下脑病,席尔德(Schilder)病 / spongiform ~ 海绵状脑病 / subacute necrotizing ~ 亚急性坏死性脑病 / subcortical arteriosclerotic ~ 皮质下动脉硬化性脑病,宾斯万格(Binswanger)痴呆 / transmissible spongiform ~, transmissible spongiform virus ~, subacute spongiform ~ 传染性海绵状脑病,传染性海绵状病毒性脑病,亚急性海绵状脑病 / traumatic ~ 外伤性脑病 | **encephalopathic** [en͵sefələu'pæθik] *a*

encephalopsy [en͵sefə͵lɔpsi] *n* 色联觉,伴生色觉

encephalopuncture [en͵sefələu'pʌŋktʃə] *n* 脑穿刺术

encephalopyosis [en͵sefələupai'əusis] *n* 脑脓肿,脑脓疡

encephalorachidian [en͵sefələurə'kidiən] *a* 脑脊髓的

encephaloradiculitis [en͵sefələurə͵dikju'laitis] *n* 脑脊神经根炎

encephalorrhagia [en͵sefələu'reidʒiə] *n* 脑出血,脑溢血

encephalosclerosis [en͵sefələuskliə'rəusis] *n* 脑硬化

encephaloscope [en͵sefələskəup] *n* 窥脑器,窥脑镜 | **encephaloscopy** [en͵sefə'lɔskəpi] *n* 脑检视法,窥脑术

encephalosepsis [en͵sefələu'sepsis] *n* 脑坏疽

encephalosis [en͵sefə'ləusis] *n* 器质性脑病;退行性脑病

encephalospinal [en͵sefələu'spainl] *a* 脑脊髓的

encephalothlipsis [en͵sefələu'θlipsis] *n* 脑受压

encephalotome [en͵sefələtəum] *n* 脑刀

encephalotomy [en͵sefə'lɔtəmi] *n* 脑切开术

encheiresis [͵enkai'riːsis] *n* 插管术

enchondral [en'kɔndrəl] *a* 软骨内的

enchondroma [͵enkɔn'drəumə] ([复] **enchondromas** 或 **enchondromata** [͵enkɔn'drəu-mətə]) *n* 内生软骨瘤 | multiple congenital ~ 多发性先天性内生软骨瘤,内生软骨瘤病 | **~tous** *a*

enchondromatosis [en͵kɔndrəumə'təusis] *n* 内生软骨瘤病 | multiple ~, skeletal ~ 多发性内生软骨瘤病,骨性内生软骨瘤病

enchondrosarcoma [en͵kɔndrəusɑː'kəumə] *n* 内生软骨肉瘤

enchondrosis [ˌenkɔnˈdrəusis] *n* 软骨疣;内生软骨瘤
enchylema [ˌenkaiˈliːmə] *n* 透明质
enchyma [ˈenkimə] *n* 组织形成液
enclave [ˈenkleiv, ɔŋˈklɑːv] *n*【法】被包围物(指脱离正常联系并被包围在另一个器官或组织内的物质)
enclitic [enˈklitik] *a* 头盆倾势不均的
enclomiphene [enˈkləumifiːn] *n* 恩氯米芬(抗不育症药,亦称 csclomiphene)
encode [inˈkəud] *vt* 编码
encolpism [enˈkɔlpizəm] *n* 阴道投药法
encopresis [enkəˈpriːsis] *n* 大便失禁(并非由于器官缺损或疾病所致)
encranius [enˈkreiniəs] *n* 颅内联胎畸胎
encyesis [ˌensaiˈiːsis] *n* 妊娠(正常的宫孕)
encyopyelitis [enˌsaiəˌpaiiˈlaitis] *n* 妊娠性肾盂炎
encyst [enˈsist] *vt, vi* 包在囊内 | **~ment** *n* 包囊形成 / **~ation** [ˌensisˈteiʃən] *n* 被囊作用,成囊 / **~ed** *a* 包绕的,被囊的
end- 见 endo-
endadelphos [ˌendəˈdelfɔs] *n* 体内联胎畸胎,胎内胎,隐联胎
Endamoeba [ˌendəˈmiːbə] *n* 内阿米巴属,内变形虫属 | ~ blattae 蠊内阿米巴
endangiitis [ˌendændʒiˈaitis] *n* 血管内膜炎
endangium [enˈdændʒiəm] *n* 血管内膜
endaortic [ˌendeiˈɔːtik] *a* 主动脉内的
endaortitis [ˌendeiɔːˈtaitis] *n* 主动脉内膜炎 | bacterial ~ 细菌性主动脉内膜炎
endarterectomize [ˌendɑːtəˈrektəmaiz] *vt* 切除动脉内膜
endarterectomy [ˌendɑːtəˈrektəmi] *n* 动脉内膜切除术 | gas ~ 气体动脉内膜切除术(利用高压二氧化碳以除去冠状血管的斑块沉着物,以治疗动脉粥样硬化)
endarterial [ˌendɑːˈtiəriəl] *a* 动脉内的
endarteritis [ˌendɑːtəˈraitis] *n* 动脉内膜炎 | ~ obliterans 闭塞性动脉内膜炎 / ~ proliferans 增生性动脉内膜炎
endarterium [ˌendɑːˈtiəriəm] *n* 动脉内膜
endarteropathy [ˌendɑːtəˈrɔpəθi] *n* 动脉内膜病 | digital ~ 指动脉内膜病,趾动脉内膜病
end-artery [ˈend ɑːtəri] *n* 终动脉
endaural [endˈɔːrəl] *a* 耳内的
end-body [ˈend bɔdi] *n* 末体,补体末段(见 end-piece)
endbrain [ˈendbrein] *n* 端脑,终脑
end-brush [ˈend brʌʃ] *n* 终树突
end-bud [ˈend bʌd] *n* 终球;终蕾
end-bulb [ˈend bʌlb] *n* 终球
endchondral [endˈkɔndrəl] *a* 软骨内的
endeictic [enˈdaiktik] *a* 症状的
endemia [enˈdiːmiə], **endemy** [ˈendimi] *n* 地方病
endemic [enˈdemik] *a* 地方性的;地方病的 *n* 地方性流行病 | **~al** *a* / **~ity** [ˌendiˈmisəti] *n* 地方性;地方流行性 / **endemial** [enˈdiːmiəl] *a*
endemiology [enˌdiːmiˈɔlədʒi] *n* 地方病学
endemoepidemic [ˌendeməuepiˈdemik] *a* 地方性流行的
endepidermis [ˌendəpiˈdəːmis] *n* 上皮,内表皮
endergic [enˈdəːdʒik] *a* 吸能的(指化学反应)
endergonic [ˌendəˈgɔnik] *a* 吸收能量的,吸能的
enderon [ˈendərɔn] *n* 外皮深层(皮肤深层或黏膜深层) | **~ic** [ˌendəˈrɔnik] *a*
end-flake [ˈendfleik] *n* 终板
end-foot [ˈendfut] *n* 终结,突触结
ending [ˈendiŋ] *n* 末梢 | annulospiral ~s 环螺末梢 / encapsulated nerve ~s 有被囊神经末梢 / epilemmal ~s 梢膜性神经末梢 / flower-spray ~s 花枝状末梢 / free nerve ~s 游离神经末梢 / grape ~s 葡萄状神经末梢 / nerve ~s 神经末梢
end-nucleus [end ˈnjuːkliəs] *n* 终核
end(o)- [前缀]内
endoabdominal [ˌendəuæbˈdɔminl] *a* 腹内的
endo-amylase [ˌendəuˈæmileis] *n* 内淀粉酶,α-淀粉酶
endoaneurysmorrhaphy [ˌendəuˈænjuərizˈmɔrəfi] *n* 动脉瘤内缝合术
endoangiitis [ˌendəuændʒiˈaitis] *n* 血管内膜炎
endoaortitis [ˌendəuˌeiɔːˈtaitis] *n* 主动脉内膜炎
endoappendicitis [ˌendəuəˌpendiˈsaitis] *n* 阑尾黏膜炎
endoarteritis [ˌendəuˌɑːtəˈraitis] *n* 动脉内膜炎
endoauscultation [ˌendəuˌɔːskʌlˈteiʃən] *n* 内听诊法(用管子通入胃内,对胃和胸部器官进行听诊)
endobacillary [ˌendəubəˈsiləri] *a* 杆菌内的
endobiotic [ˌendəubaiˈɔtik] *a* 组织内寄生的
endoblast [ˈendəublæst] *n* 内胚层 | **~ic** [ˌendəuˈblæstik] *a*
endobronchitis [ˌendəubrɔŋˈkaitis] *n* 支气管黏膜炎
endocardial [ˌendəuˈkɑːdiəl] *a* 心内的;心内膜的
endocardiopathy [ˌendəuˌkɑːdiˈɔpəθi] *n* (非炎性)心内膜病
endocardiosis [ˌendəuˌkɑːdiˈəusis] *n* 心内膜病(狗的房室瓣一般为二尖瓣慢性纤维变性,可导致充血性心力衰竭)
endocarditis [ˌendəukɑːˈdaitis] *n* 心内膜炎 | bacterial ~ 细菌性心内膜炎 / constrictive ~ 缩窄性心内膜炎 / malignant ~, septic ~, ulcerative ~ 恶性心内膜炎,脓毒性心内膜炎,溃疡性

心内膜炎 / mycotic ~ 真菌性心内膜炎 / non-bacterial verrucous ~ 非细菌性赘疣状心内膜炎 / pulmonic ~ 肺动脉瓣性心内膜炎 / valvular ~ 瓣性心内膜炎 / verrucous ~, vegetative ~ 赘疣状心内膜炎,增殖性心内膜炎 / viridans ~, subacute bacterial ~ 草绿色链球菌心内膜炎,亚急性细菌性心内膜炎 | **endocarditic** [ˌendəukɑːˈditik] *a*

endocardium [ˌendəuˈkɑːdiəm] *n* 心内膜

endoceliac [ˌendəuˈsiːliæk] *a* 体腔内的

endocellular [ˌendəuˈseljulə] *a* 细胞内的

endocervical [ˌendəuˈsəːvikəl] *a* 宫颈内的

endocervicitis [ˌendəuˌsəːviˈsaitis] *n* 宫颈内膜炎

endocervix [ˌendəuˈsəːviks] *n* 宫颈内膜

endochondral [ˌendəuˈkɔndrəl] *a* 软骨内的

endochorion [ˌendəuˈkɔːriɔn] *n* 绒[毛]膜内层

endochrome [ˈendəkrəum] *n* [细]胞内染色质

endocochlear [ˌendəuˈkɔkliə] *a* [耳]蜗内的

endocolitis [ˌendəukɔˈlaitis] *n* 结肠黏膜炎

endocommensal [ˌendəukəˈmensəl] *a* 内共生体,内共栖体

endoconidiotoxicosis [ˌendəukəuˌnidiəˌtɔksiˈkəusis] *n* 内分生孢菌中毒症

Endoconidium [ˌendəukəˈnidiəm] *n* 内分生孢子属

endocorpuscular [ˌendəukɔːˈpʌskjulə] *a* 小体内的

endocranial [ˌendəuˈkreinjəl] *a* 颅内的

endocraniosis [ˌendəuˌkreiniˈəusis] *n* 颅内骨肥大

endocranitis [ˌendəukreiˈnaitis] *n* 硬脑膜炎

endocranium [ˌendəuˈkreinjəm] *n* 硬脑膜

endocrinasthenia [ˌendəuˌkrinæsˈθiːniə] *n* 内分泌[功能]衰弱,内分泌衰竭 | **endocrinasthenic** [ˌendəuˌkrinæsˈθenik] *a*

endocrine [ˈendəukrain, ˈendəukrin] *n* 内分泌 *a* 内分泌的,激素的

endocrinic [ˌendəuˈkrinik] *a* 内分泌的;内分泌腺的

endocrinism [enˈdɔkrinisəm] *n* 内分泌病

endocrinium [ˌendəuˈkrinjəm] *n* 内分泌系统

endocrinology [ˌendəukriˈnɔlədʒi] *n* 内分泌学 | **endocrinological** [ˌendəukrinəˈlɔdʒikəl] *a* / **endocrinologist** *n* 内分泌学家

endocrinopath [ˌendəuˈkrinəpæθ] *n* 内分泌病患者

endocrinopathy [ˌendəukriˈnɔpəθi] *n* 内分泌病 | **endocrinopathic** [ˌendəuˌkrinəˈpæθik] *a*

endocrinosis [ˌendəukriˈnəusis] *n* 内分泌病(内分泌系统功能失调)

endocrinosity [ˌendəukriˈnɔsiti] *n* 内分泌[状态]

endocrinotherapy [ˌendəuˌkrinəuˈθerəpi] *n* 内分泌疗法,激素疗法

endocrinotropic [ˌendəuˌkrinəuˈtrɔpik] *a* 促内分泌的

endocrinous [enˈdɔkrinəs] *a* 内分泌的;内分泌腺的

endocritic [ˌendəuˈkritik] *a* 内分泌的;激素的 *n* 内分泌

endocuticle [ˌendəuˈkjutikl] *n* 内表皮(指甲壳动物和节肢动物,几乎完全由蛋白质和甲壳质组成)

endocyclic [ˌendəuˈsiklik] *a* 内环的,桥环的(指桥环化合物)

endocyst [ˈendəsist] *n* 内囊(棘球蚴)

endocystitis [ˌendəusisˈtaitis] *n* 膀胱黏膜炎

endocyte [ˈendəusait] *n* 细胞内含物

endocytic [endəˈsitik] *a* [细胞]内吞的,胞吞的

endocytosis [ˌendəusaiˈtəusis] *n* 胞吞作用(细胞的吞噬作用和吞饮作用)

endodeoxyribonuclease [ˌendəudiːˌɔksiˌraibəuˈnjuːklieis] *n* 内切脱氧核糖核酸酶

endoderm [ˈendəudəːm] *n* 内胚层 | **~al** [ˌendəuˈdəːməl] *a*

Endodermophyton [ˌendəudəːˈmɔfitɔn] *n* 皮内癣菌属(现称发癣菌属 Trichophyton)

endodermoreaction [ˌendəuˌdəːməuri(ː)ˈækʃən] *n* 皮内反应(见 Trambusti's reaction)

endodiascope [ˌendəuˈdaiəskəup] *n* 体腔 X 线管 | **endodiascopy** [ˌendəudaiˈæskəpi] *n* 体腔 X 线管检查

endodontics [ˌendəuˈdɔntiks] *n* 牙髓病学 | **endodontic** [ˌendəuˈdɔntik] *a* / **endodontist** [ˌendəuˈdɔntist] *n* 牙髓病学家

endodontitis [ˌendəudɔnˈtaitis] *n* 牙髓炎

endodontium [ˌendəuˈdɔnʃiəm] *n* 牙髓

endodontology [ˌendəudɔnˈtɔlədʒi] *n* 牙髓病学 | **endodontologist** [ˌendəudɔnˈtɔlədʒist] *n* 牙髓病学家

endodyogeny [ˌendəudaiˈɔdʒini] *n* 内芽生增殖(两个子细胞在母细胞壁内形成〈内芽生〉而增殖,其后代由母细胞破裂释出,如弓形体)

endoectothrix [ˌendəuˈektəθriks] *n* 发内外癣菌

endoenteritis [ˌendəuˌentəˈraitis] *n* 肠黏膜炎

endoenzyme [ˌendəuˈenzaim] *n* [胞]内酶

endoepidermal [ˌendəuˌepiˈdəːməl] *n* 表皮内的

endoepithelial [ˌendəuˌepiˈθiːliəl] *a* 上皮内的

endoergic [ˌendəuˈəːdʒik] *a* 吸能的(指化学反应)

endoerythrocytic [ˌendəuiˌriθrəˈsitik] *a* 红细胞内的

endoesophagitis [ˌendəui(ː)ˌsɔfəˈdʒaitis] *n* 食管黏膜炎

endoexoteric [ˌendəuˌeksəuˈterik] *a* 内外因的

endofaradism [ˌendəuˈfærədizəm] *n* 内部感应电

疗法,体腔感应电疗法(如将感应电使用于胃)

endogalvanism [ˌendəuˈgælvənizəm] *n* 内部直流电疗法,体腔[直]流电疗法(如将直流电使用于胃)

endogamy [enˈdɔgəmi] *n* 同族结婚;同系交配 | **endogamous** [enˈdɔgəməs], **endogamic** [ˌendəuˈgæmik] *a*

endogastric [ˌendəuˈgæstrik] *a* 胃内的

endogastritis [ˌendəugæsˈtraitis] *n* 胃黏膜炎

Endogenina [ˌendəudʒiˈnainə] *n* 内生亚目

endogenote [ˌendəuˈdʒiːnəut] *n* 内基因子(在细菌遗传学中指受体细胞遗传信息的自身补体)

endogenous [enˈdɔdʒənəs], **endogenetic** [ˌendəudʒiˈnetik], **endogenic** [ˌendəˈdʒenik] *a* 内生的,内源的

endoglobular [ˌendəuˈglɔbjulə], **endoglobar** [ˌendəuˈgləubə] *a* 血细胞内的

endognathion [ˌendəuˈneiθiən] *n* 内颌骨(切牙骨内部)

endogonidium [ˌendəugəˈnidiəm] *n* 细胞内分生孢子

endoherniorrhaphy [ˌendəuˌhəːniˈɔrəfi] *n* 疝内修补术

endointoxication [ˌendəuinˌtɔksiˈkeiʃən] *n* 内源性中毒,自体中毒

endolabyrinthitis [ˌendəuˌlæbirinˈθaitis] *n* 迷路内膜炎,膜迷路炎

endolaryngeal [ˌendəulərˈindʒiəl] *a* 喉内的

endolarynx [ˌendəuˈlæriŋks] *n* 喉腔

Endolimax [ˌendəuˈlaimæks] *n* 内蜓属 | ~ nana 小内蜓,微小内蜓

endolymph [ˈendəlimf], **endolympha** [ˌendəˈlimfə] *n* 内淋巴(内耳膜迷路内的液体) | **endolymphatic** [ˌendəulimˈfætik] *a*

endolysin [enˈdɔlisin] *n* 内溶菌素

endolysis [enˈdɔlisis] *n* 胞质溶解作用

endomastoiditis [ˌendəuˌmæstɔiˈdaitis] *n* 乳突内[膜]炎

endomesoderm [ˌendəuˈmesədəːm] *n* 内中胚层

endometrectomy [ˌendəuməˈtrektəmi] *n* 子宫内膜切除术

endometria [ˌendəuˈmiːtriə] endometrium 的复数

endometrial [ˌendəuˈmiːtriəl] *a* 子宫内膜的

endometrioid [ˌendəuˈmiːtriɔid] *a* 子宫内膜样的

endometrioma [ˌendəuˌmiːtriˈəumə] *n* 子宫内膜瘤,子宫腺肌瘤

endometriosis [ˌendəuˌmiːtriˈəusis] *n* 子宫内膜异位症 | ~ externa 宫外子宫内膜异位 / ~ interna 宫内子宫内膜异位 / ovarian ~, ~ ovarii 卵巢子宫内膜异位 / stromal ~ 基质性子宫内膜异位 / ~ uterina 子宫内膜异位 / ~ vesicae 膀胱子宫内膜异位 | **endometriotic** [ˌendəuˌmiːtriˈɔtik] *a*

endometritis [ˌendəuməˈtraitis] *n* 子宫内膜炎 | bacteriotoxic ~ 细菌毒性子宫内膜炎 / decidual ~ 蜕膜性子宫内膜炎 / exfoliative ~ 剥脱性子宫内膜炎 / membranous ~ 膜性子宫内膜炎 / puerperal ~ 产后子宫内膜炎 / syncytial ~ 合胞体细胞子宫内膜炎(亦称合胞体细胞瘤) / tuberculous ~ 结核性子宫内膜炎 / ~ tuberosa papulosa 丘疹结节状子宫内膜炎

endometrium [ˌendəuˈmiːtriəm] ([复] **endometria** [ˌendəuˈmiːtriə]) *n* 子宫内膜 | Swiss-cheese ~ 瑞士干酪样子宫内膜

endometry [enˈdɔmitri] *n* 内腔容积测定法

endomitosis [ˌendəumaiˈtəusis] *n* 核内有丝分裂(在分裂过程中未见到染色体向两极移动和细胞质的分裂) | **endomitotic** [ˌendəumaiˈtɔtik] *a*

endomixis [ˌendəˈmiksis] *n* 内融合 | **endomictic** [ˌendəˈmiktik] *a*

endomorph [ˈendəmɔːf] *n* 内胚层体型者 | **~ic** [ˌendəˈmɔːfik] *a* 内胚层体型的 / **~y** [ˈendəˌmɔːfiː] *n* 内胚层体型

Endomyces [ˌendəˈmaisiːz] *n* 内孢霉属,内真菌属 | ~ albicans 白色内孢霉(现名白色念珠菌 Candida albicans) / ~ capsulatus, ~ epidermatidis 荚膜内孢霉,表皮炎内孢霉(现名皮炎芽生菌 Blastomyces dermatitidis)

Endomycetales [ˌendəuˌmaisiˈteiliːz] *n* 内孢霉目

endomyocardial [ˌendəuˌmaiəuˈkɑːdiəl] *a* 心内膜心肌的

endomyocarditis [ˌendəuˌmaiəukɑːˈdaitis] *n* 心肌心内膜炎

endomysium [ˌendəˈmiziəm, -ˈmis-] *n* 肌内膜 | endomysial *a*

endonasal [ˌendəuˈneizəl] *a* 鼻内的

endoneural [ˌendəuˈnjuərəl] *a* 神经内的

endoneurial [ˌendəuˈnjuəriəl] *a* 神经内膜的

endoneuritis [ˌendəunjuəˈraitis] *n* 神经内膜炎

endoneurium [ˌendəuˈnjuəriəm] *n* 神经内膜

endoneurolysis [ˌendəunjuəˈrɔlisis] *n* 神经内松解术,神经纤维松解法

endonuclear [ˌendəuˈnjuːkliə] *a* 细胞核内的

endonuclease [ˌendəuˈnjuːklieis] *n* 内切核酸酶 | restriction ~ 限制性内切核酸酶

endonucleolus [ˌendəunjuːˈkliːələs] *n* 核仁内小体

endo-oxidase [ˌendəu ˈɔksideis] *n* [细]胞内氧化酶

endoparasite [ˌendəuˈpærəsait] *n* 内寄生物,体内寄生物,体内寄生虫

endopelvic [ˌendəuˈpelvik] *a* 骨盆内的

endopeptidase [ˌendəuˈpeptideis] *n* 内肽酶

endopericardial [ˌendəuˌperiˈkɑːdiəl] *a* 心内膜心包的
endopericarditis [ˌendəuˌperikɑːˈdaitis] *n* 心内膜心包炎
endoperimyocarditis [ˌendə*u* ˌperiˌmaiə*u* kɑː-ˈdaitis] *n* 心内膜心包心肌炎，全心炎
endoperineuritis [ˌendəuˌperinjuəˈraitis] *n* 神经束膜内膜炎
endoperitoneal [ˌendəuˌperitəuˈniːəl] *a* 腹膜内的
endoperitonitis [ˌendəuˌperitəuˈnaitis] *n* 腹膜内层炎，腹膜浆层炎
endoperoxide [ˌendə*u*pəˈrɔksaid] *n* 内过氧化物
endoperoxide-D-isomerase [ˌendə*u*pəˈrɔksaid aiˈsɔməreis] 内过氧化物-D-异构酶，前列腺素-D合酶
endoperoxide-E-isomerase [ˌendə*u*pəˈrɔksaid aiˈsɔməreis] 内过氧化物-E-异构酶，前列腺素-E合酶
endoperoxide reductase [ˌendə*u*pəˈrɔksaid ri-ˈdʌkteis] 内过氧化物还原酶
endophasia [ˌendəˈfeiziə] *n* 无声唇语
endophlebitis [ˌendə*u*fliˈbaitis] *n* 静脉内膜炎 | proliferative ~ 增生性静脉内膜炎，静脉硬化
endophotocoagulation [ˌendə*u* ˌfəutə*u* kəuˌæg-juˈleiʃən] *n* 眼内光凝术
endophthalmitis [ˌendɔfθælˈmaitis] *n* 眼内炎 | phacoanaphylactic ~ 晶状体蛋白过敏性眼内炎，晶状体抗原性色素层炎
endophylaxination [ˌendə*u*faiˌlæksiˈneiʃən] *n* 内防御力
endophyte [ˈendə*u*fait] *n* 内寄生菌，植物内寄生菌 | **endophytic** [ˌendə*u*ˈfitik] *a* 内寄生菌的；内部生长的（如肿瘤）
endoplasm [ˈendəplæzəm] *n* 内质 | **~ic** [ˌendəˈplæzmik] *a*
endoplast [ˈendə*u*plæst] *n* 内质体（围绕细胞核的那部分细胞质）
endoplastic [ˌendə*u*ˈplæstik] *a* 内形成性的
endopolyploid [ˌendə*u*ˈpɔliplɔid] *n* 内多倍体 | **~y** *n* 核内有丝分裂；核内多倍性；同源多倍性
endopredator [ˌendə*u*ˈpredətə] *n* 内捕食者
endoprosthesis [ˌendə*u*prɔsˈθiːsis] *n* 内镜置管[术]（一个空心的塑料支架〈stent〉插入胆管，超越梗阻部位施行胆管引流）
endopyelotomy [ˌendə*u*ˌpaiəˈlɔtəmi] *n* 内镜肾盂切开术
endoradiography [ˌendə*u*ˌreidiˈɔgrəfi] *n* 体腔X线摄影[术]，体腔造影[术]
endoradiosonde [ˌendə*u*ˌreidiə*u*ˈsɔnd] *n* 体腔内无线电测压器（如测肠腔内压）
endoreduplication [ˌendə*u*riˌdjuːpliˈkeiʃən] *n* 核内复制
end-organ [end ˈɔːgən] *n* 终器，终末器官
endorhinitis [ˌendə*u*raiˈnaitis] *n* 鼻黏膜炎
endoribonuclease [ˌendə*u*ˌraibə*u*ˈnjuːklieis] *n* 内切核糖核酸酶
endorphin [enˈdɔːfin, ˈendɔːfin] *n* 内啡肽
endosalpingitis [ˌendə*u*ˌsælpinˈdʒaitis] *n* 输卵管内膜炎
endosalpingoma [ˌendə*u*ˌsælpiŋˈgəumə] *n* 输卵管内膜瘤
endosalpingosis [ˌendə*u*ˌsælpiŋˈgəusis] *n* 输卵管子宫内膜异位；卵巢子宫内膜异位
endosalpinx [ˌendə*u*ˈsælpiŋks] *n* 输卵管内膜
endosarc [ˈendəˌsɑːk] *n* 内质
endoscope [ˈendəskəup] *n* 内镜 | **endoscopic** [ˌendəˈskɔpik] *a* 内镜的；内镜检查的 / **endoscopy** [enˈdɔskəpi] *n* 内镜检查术
endosecretory [endə*u*ˈsiːkritəri] *a* 内分泌的
endosepsis [ˌendə*u*ˈsepsis] *n* 内因败血病
endoskeleton [ˌendə*u*ˈskelitn] *n* 内骨骼 | **endoskeletal** *a*
endosmometer [ˌendɔsˈmɔmitə] *n* 内渗压测定器
endosmosis [ˌendɔsˈməusis] *n* 内渗 | **endosmotic** [ˌendɔsˈmɔtik] *a*
endosoma [ˌendə*u*ˈsəumə] *n* 红细胞浆质
endosome [ˈendəsəum] *n* 内体，核内体
endosonography [ˌendə*u*səˈnɔgrəfi] *n* 内镜超声检查
endosperm [ˈendə*u*spəːm] *n* 胚乳 | **~ic** [ˌendə*u* ˈspəːmik]，**~ous** [ˌendə*u*ˈspəːməs] *a*
endospore [ˈendə*u*spɔː] *n* 内生孢子；孢子内壁 | **endosporic** [ˌendə*u*ˈspɔːrik] *a*
endosporium [ˌendə*u*ˈspɔːriəm] *n* 内孢子膜
endosteal [enˈdɔstiəl] *a* 骨内膜的；骨内[生]的
endosteitis [enˌdɔstiˈaitis]，**endostitis** [ˌendɔˈs-taitis] *n* 骨内膜炎
endosteoma [enˌdɔstiˈəumə]，**endostoma** [ˌen-dɔˈstəumə] *n* 骨髓腔肿瘤，内生骨瘤
endostethoscope [ˌendə*u*ˈsteθəskəup] *n* 食管内听心器
endosteum [enˈdɔstiəm] *n* 骨内膜
endosulfan [ˌendə*u*ˈsʌlfən] *n* 硫丹（杀虫剂）
endosymbiont [ˌendə*u*ˈsimbiɔnt] *n* 内共生体（指细胞内共生生物）
endosymbiosis [ˌendə*u*ˌsimbaiˈəusis] *n* 内共生[现象]（指病毒及其宿主细胞间达到的一种状态，细胞分裂受抑制，细胞并未立即受到破坏）
endotendineum [ˌendə*u*tenˈdiniəm]，**endotenon** [ˌendə*u*ˈtenən] *n* 腱内膜
endothelia [ˌendə*u*ˈθiːliə] endothelium 的复数
endothelial [ˌendə*u*ˈθiːliəl] *a* 内皮的

endothelialization [ˌendəuˌθiːliəli'zeiʃən] *n* 内皮愈合
endotheliitis [ˌendəuθili'aitis] *n* 内皮炎
endothelioblastoma [ˌendəuˌθiːliəublæs'təumə] *n* 成内皮细胞瘤
endotheliochorial [ˌendəuˌθiːliəu'kɔːriəl] *a* 内皮[细胞]绒[毛]膜的
endotheliocyte [ˌendəu'θiːliəˌsait] *n* 内皮细胞
endotheliocytosis [endəuˌθiːliəsai'təusis] *n* 内皮细胞增多
endothelioid [ˌendəu'θiːliɔid] *n* 内皮样的
endotheliolysin [ˌendəuˌθiːli'ɔlisin] *n* 内皮溶素
endotheliolytic [ˌendəuˌθiːliə'litik] *a* 溶[解]内皮的，内皮[细胞]分解的
endothelioma [ˌendəuˌθiːli'əumə] *n* 内皮瘤 | dural ~ 硬脑[脊]膜内皮瘤，脑膜瘤
endotheliomatosis [ˌendəuˌθiːliəumə'təusis] *n* 内皮瘤病
endotheliosarcoma [ˌendəuˌθiːliəusɑː'kəumə] *n* 内皮肉瘤
endotheliosis [ˌendəuˌθiːli'əusis] *n* 内皮增生
endotheliotoxin [ˌendəuˌθiːliə'tɔksin] *n* 内皮毒素
endothelium [ˌendəu'θiːliəm] ([复] **endothelia** [ˌendəu'θiːliə]) *n*【拉】内皮
endotherm ['endəθəːm] *n* 温血动物，内温动物 *a* 温血的
endothermic [ˌendəu'θəːmik], **endothermal** [ˌendəu'θəːməl] *a* 吸热的，收热的(指化学反应)
endothermy ['endəˌθəːmi] *n* 透热法，高频电透热法
endothoracic [ˌendəuθɔ(ː)'ræsik] *a* 胸内的
endothrix ['endəθriks] *n* 发内癣菌，毛内癣菌
endothyropexy [endəu'θairəpeksi], **endothyroidopexy** [ˌendəuθai'rɔidəˌpeksi] *n* 甲状腺内固定术
endotoscope [en'dəutəskəup] *n* 耳[内]镜
endotoxemia [ˌendəutɔk'siːmiə] *n* 内毒素血症
endotoxin [ˌendəu'tɔksin] *n* 内毒素 **endotoxic** [ˌendəu'tɔksik] *a*
endotoxoid [ˌendəu'tɔksɔid] *n* 类内毒素
endotracheal [ˌendəutrə'kiːəl, -'treikiəl] *a* 气管内的
endotracheitis [ˌendəutreiki'aitis] *n* 气管内膜炎，气管黏膜炎
endotrachelitis [ˌendəutreikə'laitis] *n* 宫颈内膜炎
endotrypsin [ˌendəu'tripsin] *n* 酵母内胰蛋白酶
endoureteral [ˌendəujuə'riːtərəl], **endoureteric** [ˌendəuˌjuəri'terik] *a* 输尿管内的
endoureterotomy [ˌendəujuə'riːtə'rɔtəmi] *n* 输尿管内切开术
endourethral [ˌendəujuə'riːθrəl] *a* 尿道内的
endourology [ˌendəujuə'rɔlədʒi] *n* 腔道泌尿外科学
endouterine [ˌendəu'juːtərain] *a* 子宫内的
endovaccination [ˌendəuˌvæksi'neiʃən] *n* 内服疫苗法
endovascular [ˌendəu'væskjulə] *a* 血管内的
endovasculitis [ˌendəuˌvæskju'laitis] *n* 血管内膜炎
endovenitis [ˌendəuvi'naitis] *n* 静脉内膜炎
endovenous [ˌendə'viːnəs] *a* 静脉内的
endozoite [ˌendəu'zəuait] *n* 内殖体(即速殖子)
end-piece ['end piːs] *n* 补体末段(在早期免疫学说中指豚鼠血清的拟球蛋白部分，相当于补体的 C2 成分)
end plate, end-plate ['endpleit] *n* 终板 | motor ~ 运动终板
end-pleasure ['end pleʒə] *n* 终期性乐
end point ['endpɔint] 终点(在滴定中，与一定容量的另一物质起反应的某物质的最高稀释度)
end product [end'prɔdʌkt] 终产物
endrin ['endrin] *n* 异狄氏剂(杀虫剂)
endrysone ['endrisəun] *n* 恩甲羟松(眼用抗炎药)
end-tidal [end 'taidəl] *a* 终末潮的(正常潮气量的呼气终末时发生的)
endyma ['endimə] *n* 室管膜
-ene [后缀]烯
enema ['enimə] ([复] **enemas** 或 **enemata** [i'nemətə]) *n*【希】灌肠剂；灌肠法 | analeptic ~, thirst ~ 强壮灌肠剂，解渴灌肠剂 / barium ~, contrast ~ 钡灌肠，对比灌肠 / blind ~ 肛管排气法，导肠气法 / double contrast ~ 双对比灌肠 / flatus ~ 驱气灌肠剂 / nutrient ~, nutritive ~ 营养灌肠剂 / pancreatic ~ 胰酶灌肠剂 / soapsuds ~ 肥皂水灌肠 / turpentine ~ 松节油灌肠
enemator ['enimeitə] *n* 灌肠器
energetics [ˌenə'dʒetiks] *n* 能量学，能力学
energid ['enədʒid] *n* 活质体
energize ['enədʒaiz] *vt* 供以能量，赋能；通电 | **~r** *n* 兴奋药
energometer [ˌenə'gɔmitə] *n* 脉能测量器
energy ['enədʒi] *n* 能，能量 | atomic ~ 原子能 / binding ~ 结合能 / biologic ~, biotic ~ 生物能，生命能 / chemical ~ 化学能 / free ~ 自由能 / kinetic ~ 动能 / nuclear ~ [原子]核能 / ~ of position, potential ~ 势能，位能 / radiant ~ 辐射能
enervate ['enəːveit] *vt* 使衰弱 [i'nəːvit] *a* 无力的，衰弱的 | **enervation** [ˌenəː'veiʃən] *n* 神经

无力;神经切除
enflagellation [ˌenflædʒəˈlaiʃən] *n* 鞭毛形成
enflurane [ˈenflurein] *n* 安氟醚,恩氟烷(吸入麻醉药)
ENG electronystagmogram 眼震[颤]电图; electronystagmography 眼震[颤]电图描记[法]
engagement [inˈgeidʒmənt] *n* 衔接(指胎头或先露部进入骨盆入口开始通过真骨盆腔下降) | ~ of head 胎头入盆
engastrius [enˈgæstriəs] *n* 腹内附胎
Engelmann's disease [ˈeŋgəlmən] (Guido Engelmann) 骨干发育异常
Engelmann's disk [ˈeŋgəlmən] (Theodor W. Engelmann) 恩格尔曼盘(横纹肌盘)
Engel-Recklinghausen disease [ˈeŋgəl ˈrekliŋ ˈhauzən] (Gerhard Engel; Friedrich D. von Recklinghausen) 恩-雷病,囊状纤维性骨炎
Engel's alkalimetry [ˈeŋgəl] (Rodolphe C. Engel) 恩格尔血碱定量法(以正酒石酸溶液滴定稀释的血液标本,直至石蕊纸变红以测定碱度的一种方法,酒石酸溶液的量须能产生指示血液碱度的结果)
Engen orthosis [ˈeŋgen] (Thorkild J. Engen) 恩根支具(用于牵伸膝或肘挛缩的一种支具)
engine [ˈendʒin] *n* 引擎,发动机;工具,器械 | dental ~ 钻牙机 / surgical ~ 手术机
engineering [endʒiˈniəriŋ] *n* 工程[学] | genetic ~ 遗传工程
englobe [inˈgləub] *vt* 摄入,吞噬
Engman's disease [ˈeŋgmən] (Martin F. Engman) 传染性湿疹样皮炎
engorgement [inˈgɔːdʒmənt] *n* 充血;肿胀 | venous ~ 静脉怒张
engraftment [inˈgrɑːftmənt, -ˈgræft-] *n* 植活,移入
engram [ˈengræm] *n* 兴奋痕迹,记忆印迹 | **~ic** [enˈgræmik] *a*
engraphia [enˈgræfiə] *n* 兴奋留迹
engulf [inˈgʌlf] *vt* 吞没,吞食
enhance [inˈhɑːns, enˈhæns] *vt* 增强 | **~ment** *n* 增强[作用],促进[作用](在免疫学中表示肿瘤同种异体移植物在宿主内的有效建立和长期存活,或表示各种特异的和非特异的方法以增加免疫应答量) / **~r** *n* 强化因子;促进剂;增强子
enhemospore [inˈheməspɔː] *n* 血细胞内孢子,裂殖子,裂体性孢子
enhexymal [enˈheksiməl] *n* 环己巴比妥,海索比妥(催眠镇静药)
Enhydrina [ˌenhaiˈdrainə] *n* 海蛇属
eniotypy [ˌeniəˈtaipi] *n* 同种异型[性](一个巨分子基因产物存在于同种的而非其他种的一些个体之中)
enkatarrhaphy [ˌenkəˈtɑːrəfi] *n* 埋藏缝合术
enkephalin [enˈkefəlin] *n* 脑啡肽
enkephalinergic [enˌkefəliˈnəːdʒik] *a* 脑啡肽能的
enlargement [inˈlɑːdʒmənt] *n* 增大,肥大,肿大,膨大 | cardiac ~, ~ of heart 心脏增大 / cervical ~ 颈[部]膨大 / gingival ~ 龈增厚
enniatin [eniˈeitin] *n* 恩镰孢菌素
enol [ˈiːnɔl] *n* 烯醇 | **~ic** [iːˈnɔlik] *a* / **~ization** [ˌenəlaiˈzeiʃən, -liˈz-] *n* 烯醇化(作用)
enolase [ˈiːnəleis] *n* 烯醇化酶
enology [iːˈnɔlədʒi] *n* 酿酒学
enophthalmos [ˌenɔfˈθælmɔs], **enophthalmus** [ˌenɔfˈθælməs] *n* 眼球内陷
enorganic [enɔːˈgænik] *a* 机体固有的
enostosis [ˌenɔsˈtəusis] *n* 内生骨疣
enoxaparin sodium [iˌnɔksəˈpærin] 依诺肝素钠(抗凝药)
enoxidase [iˈnɔksideis] *n* 酒氧化酶
enoximone [iˈnɔksiməun] *n* 依诺昔酮(强心药)
enoyl CoA [ˈiːnəil kəuˈei] 烯酰 CoA,烯酰辅酶 A
enoyl-CoA hydratase [ˈiːnəil kəuˈei ˈhaidrəteis] 烯酰-CoA 水合酶
enoyl CoA isomerase [ˈiːnəil kəuˈei aiˈsɔməreis] 烯酰 CoA 异构酶,十二碳烯酰辅酶 AΔ-异构酶
enoyl coenzyme A [ˈiːnəil kəuˈenzaim] 烯酰辅酶 A
en plaque [ɔŋˈplɑːk]【法】斑块状,平板状
enpromate [ˈenprəmeit] *n* 恩普氨酯(抗肿瘤药)
enrichment [enˈritʃmənt] *n* 强化(食品);富集,增菌法
enrofloxacin [ˌenrəˈflɔksəsin] *n* 恩氟沙星(兽用抗生素,其作用和用途与人体使用的环丙沙星〈ciprofloxacin〉相同)
Enroth's sign [ˈenrɔt] (Emil E. Enroth) 恩罗特征(突眼性甲状腺肿时眼睑异常肿胀)
ens [enz] *n*【拉】本态 | ~ morbi [疾]病本态
ensanguine [inˈsæŋgwin] *vt* 血染,血污;使成血红色
ensiform [ˈensifɔːm] *a* 剑形的
ensisternum [ˌensisˈtəːnəm] *n* 剑突
ensomphalus [enˈsɔmfələs] *n* 双脐畸胎
enstrophe [ˈenstrəfi] *n* 内翻(尤指睑内翻)
ENT ear, nose, and throat 耳鼻喉
ent- 见 ento-
entacapone [enˈtækəpəun] *n* 恩他卡朋(抗震颤麻痹药)
entacoustic [ˌentəˈkuːstik] *a* 听器的,听觉器的
entad [ˈentæd] *ad* 向内,向心
ental [ˈentəl] *a* 内侧的;中央的
entalação [ˌentələˈsɑːjəu] *n* 热带性咽下困难,热带性贲门痉挛(恰加斯〈Chagas〉病的并发症)

entamebiasis [ˌentəmiˈbaiəsis] *n* 内阿米巴病，内变形虫病

Entamoeba [ˌentəˈmiːbə] *n* 内阿米巴属，内变形虫属 | ～ buetschlii 见 Iodamoeba buetschlii / ～ coli 结肠内阿米巴，结肠内变形虫 / ～ gingivalis，～ buccalis 龈内阿米巴，颊内阿米巴 / ～ hartmanni 哈氏内阿米巴 / ～ histolytica 溶组织内阿米巴，痢疾阿米巴 / ～ invadens 侵袭性阿米巴 / ～ nana 微小内蜒阿米巴（即 Endolimax nana）/ ～ polecki 波氏内阿米巴

entanglement [inˈtæŋglmənt] *n* 纠缠；牵连；精神错乱 | cord ～ 脐带缠绕

entasia [enˈteiziə]，**entasis** [ˈentəsis] *n*【希】紧张性痉挛

entelechy [enˈteləki] *n* 完成（行动）；生机，生命力

entepicondyle [enˌtepiˈkɔndail] *n* 内上髁

enteque [enˈteikei] *n* 慢性出血性败血病（指牛、羊）

enter- 见 entero-

enteraden [enˈterædən] *n* 肠腺

enteradenitis [ˌentəˌrædiˈnaitis] *n* 肠腺炎

enteral [ˈentərəl] *a* [小]肠的；肠内的；经肠的

enteralgia [ˌentəˈrældʒiə] *n* 肠痛

enteramine [ˌentəˈræmin] *n* 肠胺，5-羟色胺

enterectasis [ˌentəˈrektəsis] *n* 肠扩张

enterectomy [ˌentəˈrektəmi] *n* 肠切除术

enterepiplocele [ˌentəriˈpipləsiːl] *n* 肠网膜疝，肠网膜突出

enteric [enˈterik] *a* [小]肠的

enteric-coated [enˌterikˈkəutid] *a* 肠溶的（指片剂或胶囊剂）

entericoid [enˈterikɔid] *a* 伤寒样的

enteritis [ˌentəˈraitis] *n* 肠类，小肠类 | cicatrizing ～，chronic cicatrizing ～ 瘢痕性肠炎，局限性肠炎 / diphtheritic ～ 假膜性肠炎，假膜溃疡性肠炎 / membranous ～，mucomembranous ～，mucous ～，myxomembranous ～，pellicular ～ 膜性肠炎，黏液性肠炎，黏液膜性肠炎 / regional ～，segmental ～，terminal ～ 局限性肠炎，节段性肠炎

enter(o)- [构词成分]肠

enteroadherent [ˌentərəuædˈhiərənt] *a* 肠黏附的

enteroaggregative [ˌentərəuˈægrəˌgeitiv] *a* 肠聚集的

enteroanastomosis [ˌentərəuəˌnæstəˈməusis] *n* 肠吻合术

enteroanthelone [ˌentərəuæntˈhiːləun] *n* 肠抑胃素（胃分泌抑制药）

enteroantigen [ˌentərəuˈæntidʒən] *n* 肠抗原

enteroapokleisis [ˌentərəuˌæpəˈklaisis] *n* 肠旷置术

enteroarthric [ˌentərəuˈɑːθrik] *a* 壁节的（指体殖-节生分生孢子发生）

Enterobacter [ˌentərəuˈbæktə] *n* 肠杆菌属 | ～ aerogenes 产气肠杆菌 / ～ agglomerans 聚团肠杆菌 / ～ amnigenus 栖水肠杆菌 / ～ cloacae 阴沟肠杆菌 / ～ hafnia 哈夫尼亚肠杆菌 / ～ intermedium 中间肠杆菌

Enterobacteriaceae [ˌentəˌrəubækˌtiəriˈeisiiː] *n* 肠杆菌科

enterobacteriotherapy [ˌentərəubækˌtiəriəuˈθerəpi] *n* 肠菌疫苗疗法，肠道细菌疗法

enterobactin [ˌentərəuˈbæktin] *n* 肠菌素

enterobiasis [ˌentərəuˈbaiəsis] *n* 蛲虫病

enterobiliary [ˌentərəuˈbiljəri] *a* 肠胆管的

Enterobius [ˌentəˈrəubiəs] *n* 蛲虫属 | ～ vermicularis 蛲虫

enteroblastic [ˌentərəuˈblæstik] *a* 成壁的（指芽殖分生孢子发生）

enterocele [ˈentərəuˌsiːl] *n* 肠疝；阴道后疝

enterocentesis [ˌentərəusenˈtiːsis] *n* 肠穿刺

enterochirurgia [ˌentərəukaiˈrəːdʒiə] *n* 肠外科

enterocholecystostomy [ˌentərəuˌkɔlisisˈtɔstəmi] *n* 小肠胆囊吻合术

enterocholecystotomy [ˌentərəuˌkɔlisisˈtɔtəmi] *n* 肠胆囊切开术

enterochromaffin [ˌentərəuˈkrəuməfin] *a* 肠嗜铬的

enterocinesia [ˌentərəusaiˈniːziə] *n* [肠]蠕动，肠动 | **enterocinetic** [ˌentərəusaiˈnetik] *a* 蠕动的，促蠕动的

enterocleisis [ˌentərəuˈklaisis] *n* 肠缝合；肠闭塞 | omental ～ 肠穿孔网膜覆盖术

enteroclysis [ˌentəˈrɔklisis] *n* 灌肠[法]（将营养素或药用液体注入肠内）；灌肠剂（用于小肠 X 线摄影检查，亦称小肠灌肠剂）

enteroclysm [ˈentərəuklizəm] *n* 灌肠[法]

enterococcemia [ˌentərəukɔkˈsiːmiə] *n* 肠球菌血症

Enterococcus [ˌentərəuˈkɔkəs] *n* 肠道球菌属 | ～ avium 禽肠道球菌 / ～ faecalis，～ faecium 粪肠道球菌

enterococcus [ˌentərəuˈkɔkəs] *n*（[复] **enterococci** [ˌentərəuˈkɔksai]）*n*【希】肠球菌 | **enterococcal** *a*

enterocoel [ˌentərəuˈsiːl]，**enterocoele** [ˌentərəuˈsiːli]，**enterocoelom** [ˌentərəuˈsiːləm] *n* 肠体腔

enterocoelomate [ˌentərəuˈsiːləmeit] *a* 有肠体腔的 *n* 肠体腔动物

enterocolectomy [ˌentərəukəˈlektəmi] *n* 小肠结肠切除术

enterocolitis [ˌentərəukəˈlaitis] *n* 小肠结肠炎 | antibiotic-associated ～ 抗生素性小肠结肠炎（亦

称抗生素性结肠炎) / hemorrhagic ~ 出血性小肠结肠炎 / pseudomembranous ~, necrotizing ~ 假膜性小肠结肠炎,坏死性小肠结肠炎 / regional ~ 局限性小肠结肠炎

enterocolostomy [ˌentərəukəˈlɔstəmi] *n* 小肠结肠吻合术

enterocrinin [ˌentəˈrɔkrinin] *n* 促肠液素

enterocutaneous [ˌentərəukju(ː)ˈteiniəs] *a* 肠皮肤的

enterocyst [ˈentərəuˌsist] *n* 肠囊肿

enterocystocele [ˌentərəuˈsistəsiːl] *n* 肠膀胱疝

enterocystoma [ˌentərəusisˈtəumə] *n* 肠囊瘤

enterocystoplasty [ˌentərəuˈsistəuˌplæsti] *n* 肠膀胱扩大术

enterocyte [ˈentərəuˌsait] *n* 肠细胞,肠上皮细胞

Enterocytozoon [ˌentərəuˌsaitəuˈzəuən] *n* 肠细胞原虫属

enterodynia [ˌentərəuˈdiniə] *n* 肠痛

enteroenterostomy [ˌentərəuˌentəˈrɔstəmi] *n* 肠肠吻合术

enteroepiplocele [ˌentərəuiˈpipləsiːl] *n* 肠网膜疝,肠网膜突出

enterogastric [ˌentərəuˈgæstrik] *a* 肠胃的

enterogastritis [ˌentərəugæsˈtraitis] *n* 肠胃炎

enterogastrone [ˌentərəuˈgæstrəun] *n* 肠抑胃素

enterogenous [ˌentəˈrɔdʒinəs] *a* 肠生的

enteroglucagon [ˌentərəuˈgluːkəgɔn] *n* 肠高血糖素

enterogram [ˈentərəugræm] *n* 肠动[描记]图

enterograph [ˈentərəugrɑːf, -græf] *n* 肠动描记图 | **~y** [ˌentəˈrɔgrəfi] *n* 肠动描记法

enterohemorrhagic [ˌentərəuˌheməˈrædʒik] *a* 肠出血的

enterohepatitis [ˌentərəuhepəˈtaitis] *n* 肠肝炎

enterohepatocele [ˌentərəuˈhepətəˌsiːl] *n* 肠肝脐疝

enterohepatopexy [ˌentərəuˌhepətəˈpeksi] *n* 肠肝固定术

enterohydrocele [ˌentərəuˈhaidrəsiːl] *n* 阴囊积水疝

enteroidea [ˌentəˈrɔidiə] *n* 肠热病[类](肠细菌所致的热病,包括伤寒、副伤寒等)

enterointestinal [ˌentərəuinˈtestinl] *a* 肠肠的(肠不同部分的)

enteroinvasive [ˌentərəuinˈveisiv] *a* 肠侵袭的

enterokinase [ˌentərəuˈkaineis] *n* 肠激酶

enterokinesia [ˌentərəuˌkaiˈniːziə] *n* (肠)蠕动,肠动 | **enterokinetic** [ˌentərəukaiˈnetik] *a* 蠕动的,促蠕动的

enterokinin [ˌentərəuˈkainin] *n* 肠激肽

enterolith [ˈentərəuˌliθ] *n* 肠石

enterolithiasis [ˌentərəuliˈθaiəsis] *n* 肠石病

enterology [ˌentəˈrɔlədʒi] *n* 肠病学

enterolysis [ˌentəˈrɔlisis] *n* 肠粘连松解术

enteromegaly [ˌentərəuˈmegəli], **enteromegalia** [ˌentərəumiˈgeiliə] *n* 巨肠

enteromere [ˈentərəumiə] *n* 肠节

enteromerocele [ˌentərəuˈmiərəsiːl] *n* 股疝

Enteromonadina [ˌentərəuˌməunəˈdainə] *n* 肠滴虫亚目

Enteromonas [ˌentərəuˈməunəs] *n* 肠滴虫属 | ~ hominis 人肠滴虫

enteromycodermitis [ˌentərəuˌmaikəudəːˈmaitis] *n* 肠黏膜炎

enteromycosis [ˌentərəumaiˈkəusis] *n* 肠[真]菌病 | ~ bacteriacea 细菌性肠菌病

enteromyiasis [ˌentərəumaiˈaiəsis] *n* 肠蛆病

enteron [ˈentərɔn] *n* 【希】肠,消化道

enteroneuritis [ˌentərəunjuəˈraitis] *n* 肠神经炎

enteronitis [ˌentərəuˈnaitis] *n* 肠炎

entero-oxyntin [ˌentərəuˈɔksitin] *n* 肠泌酸素

enteroparesis [ˌentərəuˈpærisis] *n* 肠弛缓,肠轻瘫(导致肠扩大)

enteropathogen [ˌentərəuˈpæθədʒən] *n* 肠病原体

enteropathogenesis [ˌentərəuˌpæθəˈdʒenisis] *n* 肠病发生

enteropathogenic [ˌentərəuˌpæθəˈdʒenik] *a* 肠病发生的;肠致病的

enteropathy [ˌentəˈrɔpəθi] *n* 肠病 | gluten ~ 非热带性口炎性腹泻 / protein-losing ~ 蛋白丢失性肠病

enteropeptidase [ˌentərəuˈpeptideis] *n* 肠肽酶,肠激酶

enteropexy [ˈentərəuˌpeksi] *n* 肠固定术

enteroplasty [ˈentərəuˌplæsti] *n* 肠成形术

enteroplegia [ˌentərəuˈpliːdʒiə] *n* 肠麻痹,肠瘫,无力性肠梗阻

enteroproctia [ˌentərəuˈprɔkʃiə] *n* 人工肛门

enteroptosis [ˌentərɔˈptəusis], **enteroptosia** [ˌentərɔˈptəusiə] *n* 肠下垂 | **enteroptotic** [ˌentərəˈptɔtik] *a*

enteroptychia [ˌentərəuˈtaikiə], **enteroptychy** [ˌentərəuˈtaiki] *n* 肠折术

enterorenal [ˌentərəuˈriːnl] *a* 肠肾的

enterorrhagia [ˌentərəuˈreidʒiə] *a* 肠出血

enterorrhaphy [ˌentəˈrɔrəfi] *n* 肠缝合术 | circular ~ 肠环形缝合术

enterorrhea [ˌentərəuˈriə] *n* 腹泻

enterorrhexis [ˌentərəuˈreksis] *n* 肠破裂

enteroscope [ˈentərəskəup] *n* 肠镜

enterosepsis [ˌentərəuˈsepsis] *n* 肠脓毒病

enterosorption [ˌentərəuˈsɔːpʃən] *n* 肠积蓄(外

吸渗超过内吸渗所致)
enterospasm [ˈentərəˌspæzəm] *n* 肠痉挛
enterostasis [ˌentrəuˈsteisis] *n* 肠淤滞
enterostaxis [ˌentərəuˈstæksis] *n* 肠渗血
enterostenosis [ˌentərəustiˈnəusis] *n* 肠狭窄
enterostomy [ˌentəˈrɔstəmi] *n* 肠造口术 | gun-barrel ~ 双管形肠造口术 | **enterostomal** [ˌentərəuˈstəuməl] *a*
enterotome [ˈentərəˌtəum] *n* 肠刀
enterotomy [ˌentəˈrɔtəmi] *n* 肠切开术
enterotoxemia [ˌentərəutɔkˈsiːmiə] *n* 肠[源]性毒血症,肠毒素血症 | hemorrhagic ~ 出血性肠[源]性毒血症,羊肠毒血病 / infectious ~ of sheep 绵羊传染性肠[源]性毒血症
enterotoxication [ˌentərəuˌtɔksiˈkeiʃən] *n* 肠[源]性中毒
enterotoxigenic [ˌentərəutɔksiˈdʒenik] *a* 肠产毒性的,产肠毒素的
enterotoxin [ˌentərəuˈtɔksin] *n* 肠毒素 | cholera ~ 霍乱肠毒素,霍乱源
enterotoxism [ˌentərəuˈtɔksizəm] *n* 肠[源]性中毒
enterotropic [ˌentərəuˈtrɔpik] *a* 向肠的
enterotyphus [ˌentərəuˈtaifəs] *n* 伤寒
enterovaginal [ˌentərəuvəˈdʒainəl, -ˈvædʒi-] *a* 肠阴道的
enterovesical [ˌentərəuˈvesikəl] *a* 肠膀胱的
enteroviral [ˌentərəuˈvaiərəl] *a* 肠病毒的
Enterovirus [ˈentərəuˌvaiərəs] *n* 肠道病毒属
enterovirus [ˈentərəuˌvaiərəs] *n* 肠道病毒
enterozoon [ˌentərəˈzəuɔn] ([复] **enterozoa** [ˌentərəˈzəuə]) *n* 肠寄生虫 | **enterozoic** [ˌentərəˈzəuik] *a*
enteruria [ˌentəˈrjuəriə] *n* 粪尿症
enthalpy [ˈenθælpi] *n* 焓,热函(物理体系中的热含量)
enthesis [enˈθiːsis] *n*【希】填补法(用人造物质以修补身体缺损或畸形);肌腱末端(肌肉或韧带在骨上的附着部位)
enthesitis [enθiˈsaitis] *n* 肌腱末端炎(肌肉或肌腱在骨上附着处的炎症)
enthesopathy [ˌenθiˈsɔpəθi] *n* 肌腱末端病(肌肉或肌腱在骨上附着部位的病变)
enthetic [enˈθetik] *a* 填补的;外来的
enthetobiosis [enˌθetəbaiˈəusis] *n* 体内生命支持法(如靠体内植入起搏器维持生命)
enthlasis [ˈenθləsis] *n* 颅骨骨折内陷
entire [inˈtaiə] *a* 光边的(指菌落)
entiris [enˈtaiəris] *n* 虹膜后色素层
entity [ˈentəti] *n* 实体,实在;本质;病种
ent(o)- [前缀]内,在内
entoblast [ˈentəblæst] *n* 内胚层,内胚叶;细胞核仁
entocele [ˈentəsiːl] *n* 内疝
entochondrostosis [ˌentəuˌkɔndrɔsˈtəusis] *n* 软骨内成骨
entochoroidea [ˌentəukɔːˈrɔidiə] *n* 脉络膜内层
entocnemial [ˌentɔkˈniːmiəl] *a* 胫骨内侧的
entocone [ˈentəkəun] *n* 上内尖(上磨牙的内后尖)
entoconid [ˌentəˈkəunid] *n* 下内尖(下磨牙的内后尖)
entocornea [ˌentəuˈkɔːniə] *n* 角膜后弹性层,角膜后界层
entocranial [ˌentəuˈkreinjəl] *a* 颅内的
entocuneiform [ˌentəuˈkjuːniifɔːm] *n* 内侧楔骨
entocyte [ˈentəsait] *n* 细胞内含物
entoderm [ˈentədəːm] *n* 内胚层 | **~al** [ˌentəˈdəːməl], **~ic** [ˌentəˈdəːmik] *a*
Entodiniomorphida [ˌentəuˌdainiəuˈmɔːfidə] *n* 内毛目
entoectad [ˌentəuˈektæd] *a* 由内向外
entome [ˈentəum] *n* 尿道刀
entomere [ˈentəmiə] *n* 内胚层裂球
entomesoderm [ˌentəuˈmesədəːm] *n* 内中胚层
entomion [enˈtəumiɔn] *n* 乳突凸
entom(o)- [构词成分]昆虫
Entomobrya [ˌentəməuˈbraiə] *n* 跳虫属
entomogenous [ˌentəˈmɔdʒinəs] *a* 昆虫源的;昆虫体内生长的
entomology [ˌentəˈmɔlədʒi] *n* 昆虫学 | medical ~ 医学昆虫学 | **entomologic(al)** [ˌentəməˈlɔdʒik(əl)] *a* / **entomologist** *n* 昆虫学家
entomophagous [ˌentəˈmɔfəgəs] *a* 食虫的
entomophilous [ˌentəˈmɔfiləs] *a* 虫媒的
Entomophthora [ˌentəˈmɔfθərə] *n* 虫霉属 | ~ coronata 冠虫霉 / ~ muscae 蝇虫霉
Entomophthoraceae [ˌentəˌmɔfθəˈreisiiː] *n* 虫霉科
Entomophthorales [ˌentəˌmɔfθəˈreiliːz] *n* 虫霉目
entomophthoromycosis [ˌentəˌmɔfθərəmaiˈkəusis] *n* 虫霉病(如鼻藻菌病,皮下藻菌病)
Entomospira [ˌentəməuˈspaiərə] *n* 疏螺旋体属(现属 Borrelia)
entophthalmia [ˌentɔfˈθælmiə] *n* 眼内炎
entophyte [ˈentəfait] *n* 内寄生菌,植物内寄生菌 | **entophytic** [ˌentəˈfitik] *a*
entopic [enˈtɔpik] *a* 正[常]位[置]的
entoplasm [ˈentəplæzəm] *n* 内质
entoplastic [ˌentəˈplæstik] *a* 内形成性的
entoptic [enˈtɔptik] *a* 内视的
entoptoscope [enˈtɔptəskəup] *n* 眼内媒质镜 |

entoptoscopy [ˌentɔp'tɔskəpi] *n* 眼内媒质镜检查
entoretina [ˌentə'retinə] *n* 视网膜内层(神经层)
entorganism [ent'ɔːgənizəm] *n* 内寄生物
entorhinal [ˌent*əu*'rainəl] *a* 内嗅区的(嗅脑沟的内部)
entosarc ['entəsɑːk] *n* 内质
entosthoblast [en'tɔsθəblæst] *n* 核仁小体
entostosis [ˌentɔs'təusis] *n* 内生骨疣
entotic [en'tɔtik] *a* 耳内的
entotympanic [ˌent*əu*tim'pænik] *n* 鼓室内的
entozoon [ˌentə'zəuɔn] ([复] **entozoa** [ˌentə'zəuə]) *n* 内寄生虫 | **entozoal** [ˌentə'zəuəl], **entozoic** [ˌentə'zəuik] *a*
entrails ['entreilz] *n* [复]内脏,脏腑;(物体的)内部
entrain [in'trein] *vt* 带走(蒸馏或蒸发时蒸汽将雾沫状液体夹带走);诱导,引时(心律) | ~**ment** *n* 导引,复律
entrance ['entrəns] *n* 进入;入口 | ~ of wound tract 伤道入口
entrapment [in'træpmənt] *n* 陷夹(神经或血管受到邻近组织如纤维性或纤维骨性管壁、肌肉、腱或其他组织的压迫)
entripsis [en'tripsis] *n* 敷擦法
entropion [en'trəupjən], **entropium** [en'trəupjəm] *n* 睑内翻
entropionize [en'trəupiənaiz] *vt* 使[睑]内翻
entropy ['entrəpi] *n* 熵(在热力学中,指一个体系中的不能用来做功的这一部分能量);衰退(如衰老)
entsulfon sodium ['entsʌlfɔn] 辛苯氧磺钠(去污剂)
entwicklungsmechanik [ˌentvikˌluŋsmə'kɑːnik] *a* 实验胚胎学
entypy ['entaipi] *n* 反向(原肠胚形成的一种方式,即内胚层位于羊膜外胚层的外部)
enucleate [i'njuːklieit] *vt* 摘出,摘除(瘤、眼球);去核 [i'njuːkliit] *a* 摘出的,摘除的;无核的,去核的 | **~d** [i'njuːkliˌeitid] *a* / **enucleation** [iˌnjuːkli'eiʃən] *n* 摘出[术],摘除术;去核
enuresis [ˌenju'riːsis] *n* 遗尿[症] | **enuretic** [ˌenju'retik] *a*
envelope ['envələup] *n* 包膜;膜,被膜 | cell ~ 细胞被膜 / egg ~ 卵膜 / nuclear ~ 核膜
envenom [in'venəm] *vt* 加毒于;毒化
envenomation [inˌvenə'meiʃən] *n* 螫刺毒作用,蛇咬毒作用
environment [in'vaiərənmənt] *n* 环境,周围 | ~**al** [inˌvaiərən'mentl] *a*
envy ['envi] *n* 羡慕,妒忌 | penis ~ 阴茎妒忌(弗洛伊德〈Freud〉概念,指小女孩对男孩拥有阴茎的妒忌心理;同样亦指女性对男性的一种广泛妒忌心理)
enzootic [ˌenzəu'ɔtik] *a* 地方性兽病的 *n* 地方性兽病
enzygotic [ˌenzai'gɔtik] *a* 同卵性的
enzyme ['enzaim] *n* 酶 | activating ~ 活化酶 / adding ~ 加成酶 / allosteric ~ 别构酶 / angiotensin converting ~ 血管紧张肽转化酶,二肽[基]羧肽酶 I / brancher ~, branching ~ 分支酶,分支因子 / catheptic ~ 组织蛋白酶 / clotting ~, coagulating ~ 凝固酶 / constitutive ~ 组成酶,原有酶 / cryptic ~ 隐蔽酶 / debrancher ~, debranching ~ 脱支酶,淀粉-1, 6-葡萄苷酶 / induced ~, inducible ~, adaptive ~ 诱导酶,适应酶 / milk-curdling ~ 凝乳酶 / old yellow ~ 老黄酶,NADPH 脱氢酶 / proteolytic ~ 蛋白水解酶 / Q ~ Q 酶,1, 4-α-葡聚糖分支酶 / receptor-destroying ~ 受体破坏酶 / redox ~ 氧化还原酶 / repressible ~ 阻遏酶 / restriction ~ 限制酶,限制性内切核酸酶 / transferring ~ 转移酶 | **enzymatic** [ˌenzai'mætik], **enzymic** [en'zimik] *a*
Enzyme Commission (EC) 酶学委员会(国际生物化学联合会于 1956 年成立一个对酶的分类和命名进行规范化工作的国际酶学委员会)
enzymoimmunoelectrophoresis [ˌenzaimə*u*ˌimjunəuiˌlektrəufə'riːsis] *n* 酶免疫电泳(检查和鉴定具有酶活性的蛋白质的免疫电泳)
enzymology [ˌenzai'mɔlədʒi] *n* 酶学 | **enzymologist** [ˌenzai'mɔlədʒist] *n* 酶学家
enzymolysis [ˌenzai'mɔlisis] *n* 酶解作用
enzymopathy [ˌenzai'mɔpəθi] *n* 酶病 | lysosomal ~ 溶酶体酶病,溶酶体贮积病
enzymopenic [ˌenzaim*əu*'penik] *a* (血内)缺酶的
enzymuria [ˌenzai'mjuəriə] *n* 酶尿
EOG electro-olfactogram 嗅电图
EOM extraocular movement 眼外[肌]运动
eonism ['iːənizəm] *n* 男扮女装癖,异性模仿欲(指男性)
eopsia [i'ɔpsiə] *n* 暮视[症]
eosin ['iːəsin] *n* 伊红 | **~ic** [ˌiːə'sinik] *a*
eosinopenia [ˌiːəsinə'piːniə] *n* 嗜酸粒细胞减少
eosinophil [ˌiːə'sinəfil], **eosinocyte** [ˌiːə'sinəsait] *n* 嗜酸粒细胞 | **eosinophilic** [ˌiːəˌsinə'filik], **eosinophilous** [ˌiːəsi'nɔfiləs] *a* 嗜酸性的
eosinophile [ˌiːə'sinəfail] *n* 嗜酸细胞 *a* 嗜酸性的
eosinophilia [ˌiːəˌsinə'filiə] *n* 嗜酸粒细胞增多 | tropical ~, tropical pulmonary ~ 热带嗜酸粒细胞增多症
eosinophilopoietin [ˌiːəˌsin*əu*ˌfil*əu*'pɔiətin] *n* 嗜酸细胞生成素
eosinophilosis [ˌiːəˌsinəfi'ləusis] *n* 嗜酸粒细胞增

多 | pulmonary ~, tropical ~ 肺嗜酸粒细胞增多,热带嗜酸粒细胞增多
eosinophiluria [ˌiːəˌsinəufiˈljuəriə] *n* 嗜酸细胞尿
eosinotactic [ˌiːəˌsinəˈtæktik], **eosinophilotactic** [ˌiːəˌsinəˌfiləˈtæktik] *a* 嗜酸细胞趋化的
eosolate [iˈəusəleit] *n* 木溜磺酸盐
eosolic acid [ˌiːəˈsɔlik] 木溜磺酸
EP evoked potential 诱发电位
ep- 见 epi-
EPA eicosapentaenoic acid 二十碳五烯酸;Environmental Protection Agency 环境保护局
epacme [eˈpækmi] *n* 增进期,增长期,繁盛期(指进化) | **epacmastic** [ˌepækˈmæstik] *a*
epactal [iˈpæktl] *a* 额外的,多余的 *n* 缝间骨
epallobiosis [eˌpæləbaiˈəusis] *n* 体外生命支持法(如靠心肺机或血液透析仪维持生命)
eparsalgia [ˌepɑːˈsældʒiə] *n* 过劳病,伤力病(身体某一部分过度紧张引起的痛性障碍,包括心脏扩张、疝、肠下垂、咳嗽等)
eparterial [ˌepɑːˈtiəriəl] *a* 动脉上的
epaxial [eˈpæksiəl] *a* 轴上的
EPEC enteropathogenic *Escherichia coli* 肠致病性大肠杆菌
epencephalon [ˌepenˈsefəlɔn], **epencephal** [ˌepenˈsefəl] *n* 小脑;后脑 | **epencephalic** [ˌepensiˈfælik] *a*
ependopathy [ˌepenˈdɔpəθi] *n* 室管膜病
ependyma [eˈpendimə] *n* 室管膜 | **~l** [eˈpendiməl] *a*
ependymitis [eˌpendiˈmaitis] *n* 室管膜炎
ependymoblast [eˈpendiməublæst] *n* 室管膜母细胞
ependymoblastoma [eˌpendiməublæsˈtəumə] *n* 室管膜母细胞瘤
ependymocyte [eˈpendiməusait] *n* 室管膜细胞
ependymoma [eˌpendiˈməumə], **ependymocytoma** [eˌpendiməusaiˈtəumə] *n* 室管膜[细胞]瘤
ependymopathy [eˌpendiˈmɔpəθi] *n* 室管膜病
Eperythrozoon [ˌepiˌriθrəˈzəuɔn] *n* 附红细胞体属
eperythrozoonosis [ˌepiriθrəˌzəuəˈnəusis] *n* 附红细胞体病
ephapse [iˈfæps] *n* 神经元间接触 | **ephaptic** [iˈfæptik] *a*
epharmony [epˈhɑːməni] *n* [环境]协调发育
ephebiatrics [iˌfiːbiˈætriks] *n* 青年医学,青春期医学
ephebic [iˈfiːbik] *a* 青春的,青春期的
ephebogenesis [ˌefibəˈdʒenisis] *n* 发身,青春期身体变化 | **ephebogenic** [ˌefibəˈdʒenik] *a*
ephebology [ˌefiˈbɔlədʒi] *n* 青春期学
Ephedra [iˈfedrə, ˈefədrə] *n* 麻黄属 | ~ sinica 麻黄,草麻黄
ephedrine [iˈfedrin, ˈefedrin] *n* 麻黄碱(平喘药,血管收缩药) | ~ hydrochloride 盐酸麻黄碱 / ~ sulfate 硫酸麻黄碱
ephelis [iˈfiːlis] ([复] **ephelides** [iˈfelidiːz]) *n* 【希】雀斑
ephemera [iˈfemərə] ([复] **ephemeras** 或 **ephemerae** [iˈfeməriː]) *n* 暂时状态,暂时事物
ephemeral [iˈfemərəl] *a* 短命的;短暂的,暂时的
Ephemerida [ˌiːfəˈmeridə] *n* 蜉蝣科
Ephemeroptera [iˌfeməˈrɔptərə] *n* 蜉蝣目
Ephemerovirus [iˈfemərəˌvaiərəs] *n* 弹状病毒属
epi-, ep- [前缀]上,在上;在外
epiallopregnanolone [ˌepiˌæləpregˈnænələun] *n* 表异孕烷醇酮
epiandrosterone [ˈepiænˈdrɔstərəun] *n* 表雄[甾]酮
epiblast [ˈepiblæst] *n* 上胚层;外胚层 | **~ic** [ˌepiˈblæstik] *a* 上胚层的
epiblepharon [ˌepiˈblefərɔn] *n* 睑赘皮
epiboly, epibole [iˈpibəli] *n* 外包
epibulbar [ˌepiˈbʌlbə] *a* 眼球上的
epicanthus [ˌepiˈkænθəs] *n* 内眦赘皮 | **epicanthal** [ˌepiˈkænθəl], **epicanthic** [ˌepiˈkænθik], **epicanthine** [ˌepiˈkænθain] *a* 内眦赘皮的;眦上的
epicarcinogen [ˌepikɑːˈsinədʒən] *n* 致癌物(致癌物质的增强因子)
epicardia [ˌepiˈkɑːdiə] *n* 贲门上部
epicardial [ˌepiˈkɑːdiəl] *a* 心外膜的;贲门上部的
epicardiectomy [ˌepiˌkɑːdiˈektəmi] *n* 心外膜切除术
epicardiolysis [ˌepikɑːdiˈɔlisis] *n* 心外膜松解术
epicardium [ˌepiˈkɑːdiəm] *n* 脏层,心外膜,浆膜心包脏层
epicauma [ˌepiˈkɔːmə] *n* 角膜斑
Epicauta [ˌepiˈkautə] *n* 芫菁属
epicentral [ˌepiˈsentrəl] *a* 椎[骨]体上的
epichitosamine [ˌepikiˈtəusəmin] *n* 氨基甘露糖
epichlorohydrin [ˌepiˌklɔːrəˈhaidrin] *n* 表氯醇(树脂、油彩、清漆及其他有机化合物的溶剂,对皮肤有强刺激性,并致癌)
epichordal [ˌepiˈkɔːdəl] *a* 脊索上的
epichorion [ˌepiˈkɔːriɔn] *n* 包蜕膜
epicillin [epiˈsilin] *n* 依匹西林(抗菌药)
epicoeloma [ˌepisiːˈləumə] *n* 上体腔
epicomus [iˈpikəməs] *n* 头顶寄生畸胎
epicondylalgia [ˌepikɔndiˈlældʒiə] *n* 上髁痛
epicondyle [ˌepiˈkɔndil] *n* 上髁 | **epicondylian** [ˌepikɔnˈdailiən], **epicondylic** [ˌepikɔnˈdilik] *a*

epicondylitis [ˌepiˌkɔndiˈlaitis] *n* 上髁炎 | external humeral ~, radiohumeral ~ 肱骨外上髁炎,桡肱骨黏液囊炎,网球员肘

epicondylus [ˌepiˈkɔndiləs] ([复] **epicondyli** [ˌepiˈkɔndilai]) *n*【拉】上髁

epicoracoid [ˌepiˈkɔrəkɔid] *a* 喙突上的

epicorneascleritis [ˌepiˌkɔːniəskliəˈraitis] *n* 角巩膜表层炎(慢性角巩膜炎)

epicostal [ˌepiˈkɔst] *a* 肌[骨]上的

epicotyl [ˌepiˈkɔtil] *n* 上胚轴

epicranium [ˌepiˈkreinjəm] *n* 头被,头皮(头外部皮肤、腱膜、肌肉) | **epicranial** *a*

epicranius [ˌepiˈkreiniəs] *n*【拉】颅顶肌

epicrisis [ˌepiˈkraisis] *n* 第二次骤退,再骤退;病案讨论

epicritic [ˌepiˈkritik] *a* [精]细觉的(指皮肤神经纤维)

epicutaneous [ˌepikju(ː)ˈteinjəs] *a* 皮上的,皮表面的

epicuticle [ˌepiˈkjuːtikl] *n* 上表皮(节肢动物)

epicystitis [ˌepisisˈtaitis] *n* 膀胱上组织炎

epicystotomy [ˌepisisˈtɔtəmi] *n* 耻骨上膀胱切开术

epicyte [ˈepisait] *n* 细胞膜;上皮细胞

epidemic [ˌepiˈdemik] *a* 流行性的 *n* 流行病;(流行病)流行 | **~al** *a*

epidemicity [ˌepidəˈmisəti] *n* 流行性

epidemiogenesis [ˌepiˌdiːmiəˈdʒenisis] *n* 流行病发生

epidemiography [ˌepiˌdiːmiˈɔgrəfi] *n* 流行病纪述,流行病志

epidemiology [ˌepiˌdiːmiˈɔlədʒi] *n* 流行病学 | **epidemiologic(al)** [ˌepiˌdiːmiəˈlɔdʒik(əl)] *a* / **epidemiologist** *n* 流行病学家

epiderm [ˈepidəːm] *n* 表皮

epidermal [ˌepiˈdəːməl] *a* 表皮的;表皮样的

epidermatitis [ˌepidəːməˈtaitis] *n* 表皮炎

epidermatoplasty [ˌepidəːˈmætəˌplæsti] *n* 表皮成形术

epidermic [ˌepiˈdəːmik] *a* 表皮的

epidermicula [ˌepidəːˈmikjulə] *n* 表小皮

epidermidalization [ˌepiˌdəːmidəlaiˈzeiʃən, -liˈz-] *n* 表皮化

epidermis [ˌepiˈdəːmis] ([复] **epidermides** [ˌepiˈdəːmidiːz]) *n*【希】表皮

epidermitis [ˌepidəːˈmaitis] *n* 表皮炎

epidermization [ˌepiˌdəːmaiˈzeiʃən] *n* 表皮形成;皮移植法

epidermodysplasia [ˌepiˌdəːməudisˈpleiziə] *n* 表皮发育不良 | ~ verruciformis 疣状表皮发育不良

epidermoid [ˌepiˈdəːmɔid] *a* 表皮样的 *n* 表皮样瘤 | **~al** [ˌepidəːˈmɔidl] *a* 表皮样的

epidermoidoma [ˌepiˌdəːmɔiˈdəumə] *n* 表皮样瘤

epidermolysin [ˌepiˌdəːˈmɔlisin] *n* 脱叶菌素(即 exfoliatin)

epidermolysis [ˌepidəːˈmɔlisis] *n* 表皮松解(症) | acquired ~ bullosa, ~ bullosa acquisita 获得性大疱性表皮松解[症] / albopapuloid ~ bullosa dystrophica 白色丘疹样大疱性表皮松解[症] / dominant ~ bullosa dystrophica 显性遗传营养不良型大疱性表皮松解[症] / dysplastic ~ bullosa dystrophica 发育不良性营养不良型大疱性表皮松解[症] / hyperplastic ~ bullosa dystrophica 增生性营养不良型大疱性表皮松解[症] / junctional ~ bullosa 交界型大疱性表皮松解[症] / recessive ~ bullosa dystrophica 隐性遗传营养不良型大疱性表皮松解[症] / toxic bullosa ~ 中毒性大疱性表皮松解[症],中毒性表皮坏死松解[症] | **epidermolytic** [ˌepidəːməˈlitik] *a*

epidermomycosis [ˌepiˌdəːməumaiˈkəusis] *n* 表皮霉菌病

epidermophytid [ˌepidəːˈmɔfitid] *n* 表皮癣菌疹

epidermophytin [ˌepidəːˈmɔfitin] *n* 表皮癣菌素

Epidermophyton [ˌepidəːˈmɔfitɔn] *n* 表皮癣菌属 | ~ floccosum 絮状表皮癣菌

epidermophytosis [ˌepiˌdəːməufaiˈtəusis] *n* 表皮癣菌病,表皮真菌病

epidermopoiesis [ˌepiˌdəːməupɔiˈiːsis] *n* 表皮生成(如胚胎期或伤愈时)

epidermotropic [ˌepidəːməuˈtrɔpik] *a* 嗜表皮的,向表皮的

epididymectomy [ˌepiˌdidiˈmektəmi] *n* 附睾切除术

epididymis [ˌepiˈdidimis] ([复] **epididymides** [ˌepidiˈdimidiːz]) *n* 附睾 | **epididymal** *a*

epididymitis [ˌepiˌdidiˈmaitis] *n* 附睾炎 | spermatogenic ~ 精[子]性附睾炎

epididymodeferentectomy [ˌepiˌdidiməuˌdefərənˈtektəmi] *n* 附睾输精管切除术

epididymodeferential [ˌepiˌdidiməuˌdefəˈrenʃəl] *a* 附睾输精管的

epididymo-orchidectomy [ˌepiˌdidiməu ɔːkiˈdektəmi], **epididymo-orchiectomy** [ˌepiˌdidiməu -ɔːkiˈektəmi] *n* 附睾睾丸切除术

epididymo-orchitis [ˌepiˌdidiməuɔːˈkaitis] *n* 附睾睾丸炎

epididymotomy [ˌepiˌdidiˈmɔtəmi] *n* 附睾切开术

epididymovasectomy [ˌepiˌdidiməuvæˈzektəmi] *n* 附睾输精管切除术

epididymovasostomy [ˌepiˌdidiməuvæˈzɔstəmi] *n* 输精管附睾吻合术

epidural [ˌepiˈdjuərəl] *a* 硬膜外的

epidurography [ˌepidjuəˈrɔgrəfi] *n* 硬膜外造影

［术］
epiestriol ［ˌepiˈiːstriɔl, -ˈes-］ *n* 表雌三醇
epifascial ［ˌepiˈfæʃiəl］ *a* 筋膜上的
epigamous ［iˈpigəməs］ *a* ［卵］受精后发生的
epigaster ［ˌepiˈgæstə］ *n* 后肠
epigastralgia ［ˌepigæsˈtrældʒiə］ *n* 上腹部痛
epigastrium ［ˌepiˈgæstriəm］（［复］**epigastria** ［ˌepiˈgæstriə］）*n* 腹上区 | **epigastric** *a* 上腹部的
epigastrius ［ˌepiˈgæstriəs］ *n* 上腹部寄生畸胎
epigastrocele ［ˌepiˈgæstrəusiːl］ *n* 上腹疝
epigenesis ［ˌepiˈdʒenisis］ *n* 渐成论，后生说，后成论（认为个体的发育是在各器官和各部分发育过程中逐渐形成的，而不是预先存在于受精卵中，与错误的先成说相对） | **epigenetic** ［ˌepidʒiˈnetik］ *a* 渐成的，后生的
epigenetics ［ˌepidʒiˈnetiks］ *n* 实验胚胎学
epiglottidectomy ［ˌepiˌglɔtiˈdektəmi］，**epiglottectomy** ［ˌepiglɔˈtektəmi］ *n* 会厌切除［术］
epiglottiditis ［ˌepiˌglɔtiˈdaitis］，**epiglottitis** ［ˌepiˈglɔˈtaitis］ *n* 会厌炎
epiglottis ［ˌepiˈglɔtis］ *n* 会厌 | **epiglottal** ［ˌepiˈglɔt］，**epiglottic** ［ˌepiˈglɔtik］，**epiglottidean** ［ˌepigləˈtidiən］ *a*
epiglottoplasty ［ˌepiˈglɔtəˌplæsti］ *n* 会厌成形术
epignathus ［iˈpignəθəs］ *n* 上颌寄生胎 | **epignathous** *a*
epigonal ［iˈpigənəl］ *a* 性腺上的
epiguanine ［ˌepiˈgwænin］ *n* 7-甲基鸟［便］嘌呤
epihydrinaldehyde ［ˌepiˌhaidrinˈældihaid］ *n* 1,2-内醚丙醛
epihyoid ［ˌepiˈhaiɔid］ *a* 舌骨上的
epikeratophakia ［ˌepiˌkerətəuˈfeikiə］ *n* 表层角膜镜片术
epilamellar ［ˌepiləˈmelə］ *a* 基膜上的
epilate ［ˈepileit］ *vt* 脱毛［发］，拔毛［发］ | **epilation** ［ˌepiˈleiʃən］ *n* 脱毛术
epilemma ［ˌepiˈlemə］ *n* 神经梢膜 | **~l** *a*
epilepsia ［ˌepiˈlepsiə］ *n*【拉；希】癫痫（俗称羊痫疯）
epilepsy ［ˈepilepsi］ *n* 癫痫（俗称羊痫疯） | acquired ～ 后天性癫痫 / activated ～ 诱发性癫痫 / automatic ～ 自发性癫痫，自动症性癫痫 / grand mal ～，major ～ 癫痫大发作 / idiopathic ～ 特发性癫痫 / larval ～，latent ～ 隐性癫痫 / laryngeal ～ 喉性癫痫，阵咳性昏厥 / organic ～ 器质性癫痫 / petit mal ～ 癫痫小发作 / procursive ～ 前奔性癫痫，狂奔发作 / psychomotor ～，temporal lobe ～ 精神运动型癫痫，颞叶癫痫 / rolandic ～ 运动性癫痫 / sleep ～ 发作性睡眠 | **epileptic** ［ˌepiˈleptik］ *a* 癫痫的 *n* 癫痫患者
epileptiform ［ˌepiˈleptifɔːm］，**epileptoid** ［ˌepiˈleptɔid］ *a* 癫痫样的；严重发作的，突然发作的
epileptogenesis ［ˌepiˌleptəuˈdʒenəsis］ *n* 癫痫产生，癫痫发生
epileptogenic ［ˌepileptəuˈdʒenik］，**epileptogenous** ［ˌepilepˈtɔdʒinəs］ *a* 引起癫痫的，致癫痫的
epileptology ［ˌepilepˈtɔlədʒi］ *n* 癫痫学 | **epileptologist** *n* 癫痫学家
epilesional ［ˌepiˈliːʒənəl］ *a* 损伤面上的
epiloia ［ˌepiˈlɔiə］ *n* 结节性硬化［症］
epimandibular ［ˌepimænˈdibjulə］ *a* 下颌上的
epimastigote ［ˌepiˈmæstigəut］ *n* 表鞭毛体，表鞭毛型
epimenorrhagia ［ˌepiˌmenəˈreidʒiə］ *n* 月经过频过多
epimenorrhea ［ˌepimenəˈriə］ *n* 月经过频
epimer ［ˈepimə］ *n* 差向异构体
epimerase ［iˈpiməreis］ *n* 差向异构酶
epimere ［ˈepimiə］ *n* ［中胚层］背段
epimerite ［ˌepiˈmerait］ *n* 中胚层节
epimerization ［iˌpiməraiˈzeiʃən］ *n* 差向异构化
epimestrol ［ˌepiˈmestrəul］ *n* 表美雌醇（垂体前叶激活剂）
epimorphosis ［ˌepimɔːˈfəusis］ *n* 割处再生 | **epimorphic** ［ˌepiˈmɔːfik］ *a*
Epimys ［ˈepimis］ *n* 鼠属（即 Rattus）
epimysiotomy ［ˌepiˌmisiˈɔtəmi］ *n* 肌外膜切开术
epimysium ［ˌepiˈmisiəm］（［复］**epimysia** ［ˌepiˈmisiə］）*n* 肌外膜
epinephrectomy ［ˌepineˈfrektəmi］ *n* 肾上腺切除术
epinephrine ［ˌepiˈnefrin］ *n* 肾上腺素 | ～ bitartrate 重酒石酸肾上腺素
epinephrinemia ［ˌepiˌnefriˈniːmiə］ *n* 肾上腺素血［症］
epinephritis ［ˌepineˈfraitis］ *n* 肾上腺炎
epinephros ［ˌepiˈnefrɔs］ *n* 肾上腺
epinephryl borate ［epiˈnefril］ 环硼肾上腺素（眼科用肾上腺素能药）
epineural ［ˌepiˈnjuərəl］ *a* 神经弓上的
epineurium ［ˌepiˈnjuəriəm］ *n* 神经外膜 | **epineurial** *a*
epinosic ［ˌepiˈnəusik］ *a* ［因病］继发有利的
epinosis ［ˌepiˈnəusis］ *n* 续发性精神病态
eponychium ［ˌepiɔˈnikiəm］ *n* ［指］甲上皮
epiorchium ［ˌepiˈɔːkiəm］ *n* 睾丸外膜，睾丸鞘膜脏层
epiotic ［ˌepiˈɔtik］ *a* 耳上的
epipastic ［ˌepiˈpæstik］ *a* 撒布的 *n* 撒布粉
epipharyngitis ［ˌepiˌfærinˈdʒaitis］ *n* 咽上部炎，鼻咽炎

epipharynx [ˌepiˈfæriŋks] *n* 咽上部，鼻咽 | **epipharyngeal** [ˌepifærinˈdʒiːəl, -fəˈrindʒiəl] *a*
epiphenomenon [ˌepifiˈnɔminən]（[复]**epiphenomena** [ˌepifiˈnɔminə]）*n* 副现象（指疾病过程中的例外现象或偶发现象）| **epiphenomenal** *a*
epiphora [iˈpifərə] *n* 溢泪
epiphyseal, epiphysial [ˌepiˈfiziəl] *a* 骺的
epiphysiodesis, epiphyseodesis [ˌepifiziˈɔdisis] *n* 骺骨干固定术，骨骺过早融合
epiphysioid [ˌepiˈfiziɔid] *a* 骺样的
epiphysiolysis [ˌepifiziˈɔlisis] *n* 骺脱离
epiphysiometer [ˌepiˌfiziˈɔmitə] *n* [骨]骺测量器（用以诊断佝偻病）
epiphysiopathy [ˌepiˌfiziˈɔpəθi] *n* 松果体病；骺病
epiphysis [iˈpifisis]（[复]**epiphyses** [iˈpifisiːz]）*n* 松果体；骺 | slipped ~ 骨骺滑脱，髋内翻 / stippled epiphyses 斑点骺，点状软骨发育不全
epiphysitis [iˌpifiˈsaitis] *n* 骺炎 | vertebral ~ 椎骨骺炎（椎骨骨软骨病）
epiphyte [ˈepifait] *n* 附生植物；体表寄生菌 | **epiphytic** [ˌepiˈfitik] *a*
epipia [ˌepiˈpaiə] *n* 软膜
epipial [ˌepiˈpaiəl] *a* 软膜上的
epipleural [ˌepiˈpluərəl] *a* 胸膜上的
epipl(o)- [构词成分]网膜
epiplocele [iˈpipləusiːl] *n* 网膜疝
epiploectomy [ˌepipləuˈektəmi] *n* 网膜切除术
epiploenterocele [iˌpipləuˈentərəusiːl] *n* 网膜肠疝
epiploic [ˌepiˈpləuik] *a* 网膜的
epiploitis [iˌpipləuˈaitis] *n* 网膜炎
epiplomerocele [iˌpipləuˈmiərəsiːl] *n* 网膜股疝
epiplomphalocele [ˌepiplɔmˈfæləsiːl] *n* 网膜脐疝
epiploon [iˈpipləɔn] *n*【希】网膜 | great ~ 大网膜 / lesser ~ 小网膜
epiplopexy [iˈpipləuˌpeksi] *n* 网膜固定术
epiploplasty [iˈpipləuˌplæsti] *n* 网膜成形术
epiplorrhaphy [ˌiːpipˈlɔrəfi] *n* 网膜缝合术
epiplosarcomphalocele [iˌpipləuˌsɑːkɔmˈfæləsiːl] *n* 网膜肉芽脐疝
epiploscheocele [ˌiːpipˈlɔskiəˌsiːl] *n* 网膜阴囊疝
epipodophyllotoxin [ˌepiˌpɔdəuˌfiləuˈtɔksin] *n* 表鬼臼毒素（鬼臼毒素的化学衍生物，抗肿瘤药依托泊苷〈etoposide〉和替尼泊苷〈teniposide〉由此衍生）
epipropidine [ˌepiˈprəupidiːn] *n* 依匹哌啶（抗肿瘤药）
epipygus [ˌepiˈpaigəs] *n* 臀肢畸胎，臀部寄生肢畸胎
epipyramis [ˌepiˈpirəmis] *n* 上椎骨，上三角骨（额外腕骨）
epiretinal [ˌepiˈretinəl] *a* 视网膜上的
epirizole [iˈpiərizəul] *n* 依匹唑（消炎镇痛药）
epirotulian [ˌepirɔˈtjuːliən] *a* 髌上的
epirubicin [ˌepiˈruːbisin] *n* 表柔比星（抗生素类药）
episarkin [ˌepiˈsɑːkin] *n* 表次黄嘌呤（存在于正常尿及白血病时的尿中）
episclera [ˌepiˈskliərə] *n* 巩膜外层 | **~l** *a* 巩膜上的；巩膜外层的
episcleritis [ˌepiskliəˈraitis], **episclerotitis** [ˌepiskliərəˈtaitis] *n* 巩膜外层炎
episi(o)- [构词成分]阴部，外阴
episioperineoplasty [iˌpiziəuˌperiˈniːəˌplæsti] *n* 外阴会阴成形术
episioperineorrhaphy [iˌpiziəuˌperiniˈɔrəfi] *n* 外阴会阴缝合术
episioplasty [iˈpiziəˌplæsti] *n* 外阴成形术
episiorrhaphy [iˌpiziˈɔrəfi] *n* 外阴缝合术（大阴唇缝合术，会阴撕裂缝合）
episiostenosis [iˌpiziəustiˈnəusis] *n* 外阴狭窄
episiotomy [iˌpiziˈɔtəmi] *n* 外阴切开术
episode [ˈepisəud] *n* 插话；插曲；发作 | psycholeptic ~ 致病性精神创伤 | **episodic(al)** [epiˈsɔdik(əl)] *a*
episome [ˈepisəum] *n* 附加体（在细胞遗传学中，染色体外能复制的辅助性遗传成分，可以游离于细胞质中，也可以与染色体结合在一起，如F因子、大肠杆菌素因子、接合子、抗药性转移因子）
epispadias [ˌepiˈspeidiəs], **epispadia** [ˌepiˈspeidiə] *n* 尿道上裂 | **epispadiac** [ˌepiˈspeidiæk] *a* 尿道上裂的 *n* 尿道上裂者 / **epispadial** *a*
epispinal [ˌepiˈspainl] *a* 脊柱上的，脊髓上的
episplenitis [ˌepispliˈnaitis] *n* 脾被膜炎
epistasis [iˈpistəsis], **epistasy** [iˈpistəsi] *n* 排泄制止（如血、月经或恶露）；尿浮膜；上位性（指在不同位点的基因之间的相互作用，结果一个遗传性状由于另一个遗传性状在其上面的叠合而未显示出来或掩蔽起来了）| **epistatic** [ˌepiˈstætik] *a* 上位的
epistaxis [ˌepiˈstæksis] *n*【希】鼻出血
epistemology [iˌpistəˈmɔlədʒi] *n* 认识论 | **epistemological** [iˌpistəməˈlɔdʒikəl] *a*
episternum [ˌepiˈstəːnəm]（[复]**episterna** [ˌepiˈstəːnə]）*n* 上胸骨（指爬行动物和单孔目动物）| **episternal** [ˌepisˈtəːnl] *a* 胸骨上的；上胸骨的
episthotonos [ˌiːpisˈθɔtənəs] *n* 前弓反张
epistropheus [ˌepiˈstrəufiəs] *n*【希】枢椎（第二

颈椎)

epitarsus [ˌepi'tɑːsəs] *n* 结膜前垂(睑结膜皱褶,亦称先天翼状胬肉)

epitaxy [ˌepi'tæksi] *n* [晶体]取向附生,外延附生

epitela [ˌepi'tiːlə] *n* 前髓帆组织

epitendineum [ˌepiten'diniəm] *n* 腱纤维鞘,腱鞘

epitenon [ˌepi'tiːnɔn] *n* 腱鞘

epithalamus [ˌepi'θæləməs] *n* 上丘脑 | **epithalamic** [ˌepiθə'læmik] *a* 上丘脑的;丘脑上部的

epithalaxia [ˌepiθə'læksiə] *n* 上皮脱屑(尤指肠黏膜)

epithelia [ˌepi'θiːljə] epithelium 的复数

epithelial [ˌepi'θiːliəl] *a* 上皮的

epithelialize [ˌepi'θiːliəlaiz] *vt* 上皮形成,上皮化 | **epithelialization** [ˌepiˌθiːliəlai'zeiʃən, -li'z-] *n*

epitheliitis [ˌepiˌθiːli'aitis] *n* 上皮炎

epitheli(o)- [构词成分]上皮

epithelioceptor [ˌepiˌθiːliəu'septə] *n* 腺细胞感受体

epitheliochorial [ˌepiˌθiːliəu'kɔːriəl] *a* 上皮绒[毛]膜的(胎盘)

epitheliofibril [ˌepi'θiːliəuˌfaibril] *n* 上皮原纤维

epitheliogenesis [ˌepiˌθiːliəu'dʒenəsis] *n* 上皮发生

epitheliogenetic [ˌepiˌθiːliəudʒi'netik] *a* 上皮增殖的

epitheliogenic [ˌepiˌθiːliəu'dʒenik] *a* 生成上皮的,上皮形成的

epithelioglandular [ˌepiˌθiːliəu'glændjulə] *a* 腺上皮[细胞]的

epithelioid [ˌepi'θiːliɔid] *a* 上皮样的

epitheliolysin [ˌepiθiːli'ɔlisin] *n* 溶上皮素

epitheliolysis [ˌepiˌθiːli'ɔlisis] *n* 上皮溶解 | **epitheliolytic** [ˌepiˌθiːliəu'litik] *a* 溶上皮的

epithelioma [ˌepiˌθiːli'əumə] ([复] **epitheliomas** 或 **epitheliomata** [ˌepiˌθiːli'əumətə]) *n* 上皮瘤,上皮癌 | basal cell ~ 基底细胞癌 / benign calcifying ~, calcified ~, calcifying ~ 良性钙化上皮瘤,钙化上皮瘤 / chorionic ~ 绒[毛]膜癌 / columnar ~, cylindrical ~ 柱状上皮瘤 / diffuse ~ 浸润性癌 / glandular ~ 腺性上皮瘤 / multiple benign cystic ~ 多发性良性囊性上皮瘤 / multiple self-heating ~ 多发性自愈性上皮瘤 | **~tous** *a*

epitheliomatosis [ˌepiˌθiːliəumə'təusis] *n* 上皮瘤病

epitheliomuscular [ˌepiˌθiːliəu'mʌskjulə] *a* 上皮肌的

epitheliosis [ˌepiˌθiːli'əusis] *n* 上皮增殖

epitheliotoxin [ˌepiˌθiːliəu'tɔksin] *n* 杀上皮[细胞]毒素

epitheliotropic [ˌepiˌθiːliəu'trɔpik] *a* 亲上皮细胞的

epithelite [ˌepi'θiːlait] *n* 上皮瘢痕(放射线治疗后所致,上皮为纤维性渗出物所取代)

epithelium [ˌepi'θiːljəm] ([复] **epithelia** [ˌepi'θiːljə]) *n* 上皮,上皮组织 | anterior ~ of cornea, corneal ~ 角膜前上皮,角膜上皮 / ciliated ~ 纤毛上皮 / columnar ~ 柱状上皮 / cubical ~, cuboidal ~ 立方上皮 / ~ of lens 晶状体上皮 / mesenchymal ~ 间[充]质上皮 / pavement ~ 扁平上皮,单层鳞状上皮 / simple ~ 单层上皮 / stratified ~, laminated ~ 复层上皮 / tessellated ~ 单层鳞状上皮 / transitional ~ 变移上皮

epithelize [ˌepi'θiːlaiz] *vt* 上皮形成 | **epithelization** [ˌepiˌθiːlai'zeiʃən, -li'z-] *n*

epithermal [ˌepi'θəːməl] *a* 超热的

epithesis [i'piθəsis] *n*【希】(四肢畸形)矫正术;夹板

epithiazide [ˌepi'θaiəzaid] *n* 依匹噻嗪(降压、利尿药)

epitonic [ˌepi'tɔnik] *a* 异常紧张的

epitope ['epitəup] *n* 表位(即抗原决定簇)

epitrichium [ˌepi'trikiəm] *n* 皮上层(胚)

epitriquetrum [ˌepitrai'kwiːtrəm] *n* 上三角骨,上锥骨(额外腕骨)

epitrochlea [ˌepi'trɔkliə] *n* 肱骨内上髁

epitrochlear [ˌepi'trɔkliə] *a* 肱骨内上髁的;滑车上的(如肱骨滑车)

epituberculosis [ˌepitju(ː)ˌbəːkju'ləusis] *n* 浸润型[上部]肺结核

epiturbinate [ˌepi'təːbineit] *n* 鼻甲软组织,鼻甲外组织

epitympanitis [ˌepitimpə'naitis] *n* 上鼓室炎

epitympanum [ˌepi'timpənəm] *n* 鼓室上隐窝 | **epitympanic** [ˌepitim'pænik] *a* 上鼓室的;鼓室上隐窝的

epitype ['epitaip] *n* 表位型(一类或一族相关的抗原决定簇)

epityphlitis [ˌepitif'laitis] *n* 阑尾炎;盲肠旁炎

epityphlon [ˌepi'taiflɔn] *n* 阑尾

epivaginitis [ˌepiˌvædʒi'naitis] *n* 外阴道炎(牛的性病)

epizoicide [ˌepi'zəuisaid] *n* 杀体表寄生虫剂

epizoon [ˌepi'zəuɔn] ([复] **epizoa** [ˌepi'zəuə]) *n*【希】体表寄生虫 | **epizoic** [ˌepi'zəuik] *a* 体表寄生的;体表寄生虫的

epizootic [ˌepizəu'ɔtik] *a* 兽疫流行的 *n* 兽疫

epizootiology [ˌepizəuˌəuti'ɔlədʒi], **epizoology** [ˌepizəu'ɔlədʒi] *n* 兽疫学

épluchage [ˌeiplu'ʃɑːʒ] *n*【法】扩创术,清创术

epivag [epivæg] *n* 附睾阴道炎(牛)

epoetin [i'pəuətin] *n* 红细胞生成素(为重组人红

细胞生成素,用作抗贫血药。有两型:α 型红细胞生成素〈epoetin alfa〉和 β 型红细胞生成素〈epoetin beta〉)

epontic [iˈpɔntik] *a* 表面生长的(植物、动物或矿物)

eponychium [ˌepəˈnikiəm] *n* 甲上皮

epoophorectomy [ˌepəuˌɔfəˈrektəmi] *n* 卵巢冠切除术

epoöphoron [ˌepəuˈɔfərɔn] *n* 卵巢冠

epoprostenol [ˌepəuˈprəustənɔl] *n* 依前列醇(前列素类药)

epornithology [eˌpɔːniˈθɔlədʒi] *n* 鸟类流行病学,禽疫学

epornitic [ˌepɔːˈnitik] *n* 禽疫

epoxide [eˈpɔksaid] *n* 环氧化物

epoxy [iˈpɔksi] *a* 环氧的,环氧化物的 *n* 环氧树脂

epoxytropine tropate [iˌpɔksiˈtrəupiːn ˈtrəupeit] 托品酸环氧托品(副交感神经阻滞药)

EPP equal pressure point 等压点;erythrohepatic or erythropoietic protoporphyria 红细胞肝性原卟啉病,红细胞生成性原卟啉病

EPR electrophrenic respiration 膈神经电刺激呼吸

eprosartan mesylate [ˌeprəuˈsɑːtæn] 甲磺依普沙坦(抗高血压药)

EPS exophthalmos-producing substance 致突眼物质

epsilon [epˈsailən, ˈepsilən] *n* 希腊语的第 5 个字母(Ε, ε)

EPSP excitatory postsynaptic potential 兴奋性突触后电位

Epstein-Barr virus [ˈepstain ˈbɑː] (Michael A. Epstein; Y. M. Barr) EB 病毒,非洲淋巴细胞瘤病毒

Epstein's disease [ˈepstain] (Alois Epstein) 假白喉 | ~ pearls 爱泼斯坦小结(新生儿硬腭缝两侧的黄白小块)

Epstein's nephrosis [ˈepstain] (Albert A. Epstein)爱泼斯坦肾变病(由全身性代谢障碍引起的一种慢性肾小管肾炎,常伴甲状腺功能减退和内分泌功能紊乱) | ~ syndrome 肾病综合征(即 nephrotic syndrome)

eptatretin [ˌeptəˈtriːtin] *n* 黏盲鳗素(一种有效力的心脏兴奋剂)

eptifibatide [ˌeptəˈfibətaid] *n* 依非他特(血小板聚集抑制药)

epulis [eˈpjuːlis] ([复]**epulides** [eˈpjuːlidiːz]) *n* 【希】[牙]龈瘤;末梢骨化性纤维瘤

epuloerectile [ˌepjuləuiˈrektail] *a* 龈瘤样勃起的,龈瘤样竖立的

epulofibroma [ˌepjuləufaiˈbrəumə] *n* 龈纤维瘤

epuloid [ˈepjulɔid] *a* 龈瘤样的

epulosis [ˌepjuˈləusis] *n* 瘢痕成形,结瘢 | **epulotic** [ˌepjuˈlɔtik] *a* 结瘢的,促进瘢痕形成的

equate [i(ː)ˈkweit] *vt* 使相等 [ˈiːkweit] *n* 色融合力(在色觉中使两种不同颜色配成第三种颜色的生理能力,如混合红与绿形成均匀的黄色)

equation [iˈkweiʃən] *n* 等式;方程式 | chemical ~ 化学反应方程式 / personal ~ 人差方程式(某一事物的结果,常因观察者个人而异,遂产生或多或少的差别) | **~al** *a*

equator [iˈkweitə] *n* 赤道,中纬线 | ~ of cell 细胞中纬线 / ~ of crystalline lens, ~ of lens 晶状体赤道 / ~ of eyeball 眼球中纬线 | **~ial** [ˌekwəˈtɔːriəl] *a*

equianalgesic [ˌiːkwiˌænəlˈdʒiːsik] *a* 同等镇痛作用的

equiaxial [ˌiːkwiˈæksiəl] *a* 等长轴的

equicaloric [ˌiːkwikəˈlɔrik] *a* 等卡(热)的

Equidae [ˈekwidiː] *n* 马科

equilateral [ˌiːkwiˈlætərəl] *a* 等边的

equilibrate [ˌiːkwiˈlaibreit] *vt, vi* 平衡,有均势 | **equilibration** [ˌiːkwilaiˈbreiʃən] *n* 平衡,均势 / **equilibrator** [ˌiːkwilaiˈbreitə] *n* 平衡器

equilibrium [ˌiːkwiˈlibriəm] 平衡 | acid-base ~ 酸碱平衡 / fluid ~, water ~ 水平衡 / genetic ~ 遗传平衡(在连续世代中一个群体的基因库在不发生选择或突变的情况下仍保持不变,即群体中每个等位基因频率在连续世代中是保持不变的) / nitrogen ~, nitrogenous ~, protein ~ 氮平衡,蛋白质平衡 / physiologic ~, neutritive ~ 生理平衡,营养平衡 / radioactive ~ 放射平衡

equilin [ˈekwilin] *n* 马烯雌酮(雌激素)

equimolar [ˌiːkwiˈməulə] *a* 等摩尔的

equimolecular [ˌiːkwiməuˈlekjulə] *a* 等分子的

equimultiple [ˌiːkwiˈmʌltipl] *n* 等倍数,等倍量

equination [ˌiːkwiˈneiʃən] *n* 马痘接种

equine [ˈiːkwain] *a* 马的

equinophobia [iˌkwainəˈfəubiə] *n* 马恐怖,恐马症

equinovalgus [iˌkwainəˈvælgəs] *n* 马蹄外翻足

equinovarus [iˌkwainəˈvɛərəs] *n* 马蹄内翻足

equinus [iˈkwainəs] *n* 马蹄足

equipotential [ˌiːkwipəuˈtenʃəl] *a, n* 等势(的),等位(的)

equipotentiality [ˌiːkwipəuˌtenʃiˈæləti] *n* 等势性,等位性

equisetosis [ˌekwisəˈtəusis] *n* 木贼中毒(马)

Equisetum [ˌekwiˈsiːtəm] *n* 木贼属

equivalence [iˈkwivələns], **equivalency** [iˈkwivələnsi] *n* 等值,等量;等价(在免疫学中指抗原与抗体浓度之比,以此比例产生最大量抗原抗体结合,同时产生沉淀或凝聚)

equivalent [iˈkwivələnt] *a* 相等的;等价的,同等

的,等值的 *n* 等同物;当量;等位症,等位发作 | chemical ~, gram ~ 化学当量,克当量 / concrete ~ 混凝土当量 / dose ~ 剂量当量 / endosmotic ~ 内渗当量 / epileptic ~ 癫痫等位发作 / isodynamic ~ 等热当量 / lethal ~ 致死当量(如一组杂合情况中的两个基因,其中每个基因在纯合情况下会导致 50% 携带者死亡) / neutralization ~ 中和当量 / protein ~ 蛋白当量 / psychic ~ 精神性等位发作,精神性癫痫 / starch ~ 淀粉当量 / toxic ~ 毒性当量 / ventilation ~ 通气当量 / water ~ 水当量

equulosis [ˌekwuˈləusis] *n* 马驹病(主要侵袭幼驹的一种化脓性关节炎、滑膜炎和肠炎)

Equus [ˈekwəs] *n* 马属(包括马、驴和斑马)

ER emergency room 急诊室;endoplasmic reticulum 内质网;estrogen receptor 雌激素受体

Er erbium 铒

ERA electric response audiometry 电反应测听[法],电反应测听术

erabutoxin [əˌræbjuˈtɔksin] *n* 埃拉布毒素

eradicate [iˈrædikeit] *vt* 根除;消灭,扑灭 | **eradication** [iˌrædiˈkeiʃən] *n*

erasion [iˈreiʒən] *n* 刮除;刮术 | ~ of a joint 关节刮术

Eratyrus [ˌerəˈtaiərəs] *n* 尔太锥蝽属

Erb-Charcot disease [ˈɛəb ʃɑːˈkəu] (W. H. Erb; Jean M. Charcot) 埃尔布-夏科病(见 Erb's spastic paraplegia)

Erb-Duchenne paralysis [ˈɛəb djuːˈʃen] (Willhelm H. Erb; Guillaume B. A. Duchenne) 埃尔布-迪谢内麻痹(产伤所致的上臂麻痹)

Erben's phenomenon [ˈɛəbən] (Siegmund Erben) 埃尔本现象(某些神经衰弱患者在弯腰或坐下时出现的脉搏暂时变慢) | ~ reflex (sign) 埃尔本反射(征)(低头和躯干过度前倾时脉搏变慢,表示迷走神经时应激性)

ERBF effective renal blood flow 有效肾血流量

Erb-Goldflam disease [ˈɛəb ˈgɔltfləm] (W. H. Erb; Samuel V. Goldflam) 重症肌无力

erbium (Er) [ˈəːbiəm] *n* 铒(化学元素)

Erb's atrophy [ɛəb] (Wilhelm H. Erb) 假肥大性肌营养不良 | ~ disease 进行性肌营养不良 / ~ paralysis 埃尔布麻痹(①见 Erb-Duchenne paralysis;②埃尔布痉挛性截瘫;③假肥大性肌营养不良) / ~ point 埃尔布点(位于锁骨上 2 或 3 cm 胸锁乳突肌后缘之后,第六颈椎横突水平处的一点,如刺激此处可引起手臂各肌收缩) / ~ sclerosis 原发性脊髓侧索硬化 / ~ sign 埃尔布征(①强直性痉挛时运动神经的应电性增强;②肢端肥大症时胸骨柄部叩诊呈浊音) / ~ spastic paraplegia, ~ syphilitic spastic paraplegia 埃尔布痉挛性截瘫,埃尔布梅毒性痉挛性截瘫(一种脑膜血管梅毒) / ~ syndrome 埃尔布综合征(重症肌无力全部体征)

ERCP endoscopic retrograde cholangiopancreatography 内镜逆行胰胆管造影[术]

Erdheim's disease (cystic medial necrosis) [ˈəːdhaim] (Jakob Erdheim) 埃尔德海姆病(囊性中膜坏死)

Erdmann's reagent [ˈɛədmən] (Hugo Erdmann) 埃德曼试剂(硝酸与硫酸的混合液,用以检生物碱)

erect [iˈrekt] *a* 勃起的 *vt* 使勃起 *vi* 勃起 | **~ion** [iˈrekʃən] *n* 勃起

erectile [iˈrektail] *a* 能勃起的

erector [iˈrektə] *n* 勃起肌,立肌

eredosome [iˈredəsəum] *n* 非晶性血红蛋白

eremacausis [ˌeriməˈkɔːsis] *n* 缓慢氧化;缓燃;(有机物的)腐烂

eremophobia [ˌeriməˈfəubiə] *n* 孤独恐怖

erepsin [iˈrepsin] *n* 肠肽酶

erethism [ˈeriθizəm] *n* 兴奋增盛,兴奋增强 | **erethistic** [ˌeriˈθistik], **erethismic** [ˌeriˈθizmik] *a*

erethisophrenia [ˌeriˌθizəˈfriːniə] *n* 精神兴奋过度

erethitic [ˌeriˈθitik] *a* 兴奋的

Erethmapodites [əˌreθməˈpɔditiːs] *n* 埃雷托曼蚊属

ereuth(o)- 见 eryth-

ERG electroretinogram 视网膜电图

erg [əːg] *n* 尔格(旧功或能量的单位,1 erg〈尔格〉= 10^{-7} J〈焦耳〉,或 0.624 × 10^{12} eV〈电子伏〉)

ergasia [əːˈgeiziə] *n*【希】精神活动;(精神)整体功能

ergasiatrics [əːˌgeiziˈætriks], **ergasiatry** [ˌəːgəˈsaiətri] *n* 精神病学

ergasiology [əːˌgeisiˈɔlədʒi] *n* 客观精神生物学

ergastic [əːˈgæstik] *a* 有潜能的,储能的(指被动物质形成或贮存于细胞内,如淀粉、脂肪、纤维素);[精神]整体功能的

ergastoplasm [əːˈgæstəplæzəm] *n* 动质;载粒内质网,粗糙内质网

erg(o)- [构词成分]工作,力,动力

ergobasine [ˌəːgəuˈbeisin] *n* 麦角新碱(即 ergonovine)

ergocalciferol [əːgəukælˈsifərɔl] *n* 麦角钙化[固]醇,维生素 D_2(抗佝偻病维生素)

ergocardiogram [ˌəːgəuˈkɑːdiəgræm] *n* 心电动力图

ergocardiography [ˌəːgəuˌkɑːdiˈɔgrəfi] *n* 心电动力描记术

ergocornine [ˌəːgəuˈkɔːniːn] *n* 麦角柯宁碱

ergocristine [ˌəːgəuˈkristiːn] *n* 麦角克碱,麦角嵴亭

ergocryptine [ˌəːgəuˈkriptiːn] *n* 麦角隐亭,麦角环肽

ergodynamograph [ˌəːgəudaiˈnæməgrɑːf, -græf] *n* 肌动力描记器

ergoesthesiograph [ˌəːgəuesˈθiːsiəgrɑːf, -græf] *n* 肌动感觉描记器

ergogenic [ˌəːgəuˈdʒenik] *a* 生力的,功能亢进的

ergogram [ˈəːgəgræm] *n* 测力图

ergograph [ˈəːgəgrɑːf, -græf] *n* 测力器,肌[动]力描记器 | **~ic** [ˌəːgəˈgræfik] *a*

ergoloid mesylates [ˈəːgəlɔid] 麦角生物碱甲磺酸盐类(含有等比例重量的三种氢化麦角生物碱〈二氢麦角汀碱、二氢麦角柯宁碱和二氢麦角隐亭〉的甲磺酸盐类的混合物,用于治疗老年人心理功能特发性衰退,口服)

ergomaniac [ˌəːgəuˈmeiniæk] *n* 工作狂者

ergometer [əːˈgɔmitə] *n* 测力计 | bicycle ~ 自行车测力计

ergometrine [ˌəːgəuˈmetrin] *n* 麦角新碱(即 ergonovine)

ergon [ˈəːgɔn] *n* 尔冈(基因稳定性的单位;作用量单位)

ergonomics [ˌəːgəˈnɔmiks] *n* 人类工程学,人体功率学(基于解剖、生理、心理以及机械的原理研究人类能量有效应用的科学) | **ergonomical** *a* / **ergonomist** *n* 人类工程学家,人体功率学家

ergonovine [ˌəːgəˈnəuvin] *n* 麦角新碱(用作催产剂及缓解偏头痛) | ~ maleate 马来酸麦角新碱(催产剂)

ergophore [ˌəːgəˈfɔː] *n* 作用簇(在埃利希〈Ehrlich〉侧链学说中,指一个分子中的原子团,在该分子与结合簇已经适当地结合之后,即发挥诸如毒素、凝集素等物质的效能)

ergoplasm [ˈəːgəplæzəm] *n* 颗粒内质网

ergosome [ˈəːgəsəum] *n* 多核糖体

ergostat [ˈəːgəstæt] *n* 练肌器

ergosterol [əːˈgɔstərɔl] *n* 麦角固醇 | activated ~, irradiated ~ 活化麦角固醇,照射麦角固醇(即麦角钙化[固]醇 ergocalciferol)

ergostetrine [ˌəːgəuˈstetrin] *n* 麦角新碱(即 ergonovine)

ergot [ˈəːgət] *n* 麦角 | **~ic** [əːˈgɔtik] *a*

ergotamine [əːˈgɔtəmin] *n* 麦角胺(治偏头痛药) | ~ tartrate 酒石酸麦角胺(治偏头痛药)

ergotaminine [ˌəːgəuˈtæminin] *n* 麦角异胺

ergotherapy [ˌəːgəuˈθerəpi] *n* 运动疗法

ergothioneine [ˌəːgəuˌθaiəˈniːin] *n* 麦角硫因,巯组氨酸三甲[基]内盐

ergotinic acid [ˌəːgəuˈtinik] 麦角碱酸

ergotism [ˈəːgətizəm] *n* 麦角中毒

ergotized [ˈəːgətaizd] *a* 麦角中毒的

ergotocine [ˌəːgəuˈtəusiːn] *n* 麦角新碱(即 ergonovine)

ergotoxicosis [ˌəːgəuˌtɔksiˈkəusis] *n* 麦角菌中毒

ergotoxine [ˌəːgəuˈtɔksiːn] *n* 麦角毒碱

ergusia [əːˈdʒuːsiə] *n* 细胞迁移素(一种假想的类脂质,从细胞中放出,减低表面张力,从而促使细胞迁移)

Erichsen's sign (test) [ˈeriksən] (John E. Erichsen) 埃里克森征(试验)(用力将髂骨相互挤压时,骶髂疾病患者感痛,而髋部患者则无痛感)

Eriodictyon [ˌeriəuˈdiktiɔn] *n* 圣草属,散塔草属

eriodictyon [ˌeriəuˈdiktiɔn] *n* 北美圣草,散塔草

eriometer [ˌeriˈɔmitə] *n* 微粒直径测定器(检红细胞直径) | **eriometry** [ˌeriˈɔmitri] *n* 微粒直径测定法

erionite [ˈeriənait] *n* 毛沸石

erisiphake [eˈrisifeik] *n* 晶状体吸盘(白内障时用)

Eristalis [eˈristəlis] *n* 蜂蝇属 | ~ tenax [绒]蜂蝇

Erlanger's sphygmomanometer [ˈəːlæŋə] (Joseph Erlanger) 厄兰格血压计

Erlenmeyer flask [ˈɛələnˌmaiə] (Emil R. A. C. Erlenmeyer) 埃伦美厄烧瓶(锥形瓶)

Erni's sign [ˈəːni] (H. Erni) 埃尔尼征(一种肺空洞叩征)

erntefieber [ˈəːntiˌfiːbə] *n*【德】秋收热,沼地热(类似钩端螺旋体性黄疸)

erode [iˈrəud] *vt* 腐蚀,侵蚀 *vi* 受腐蚀,遭侵蚀

erodent [iˈrəudənt] *a* 侵蚀的,腐蚀的 *n* 腐蚀药

erogenous [iˈrɔdʒinəs] *a* 催情的,性感的,性欲发生的

erose [iˈrəus] *a* 不整齐的;啮蚀状的,蛀蚀状的

erosio [iˈrəusiəu] *n*【拉】腐蚀,侵蚀;糜烂 | ~ interdigitalis blastomycetica 芽生菌性指间糜烂,芽生菌性趾间糜烂

erosion [iˈrəuʒən] *n* 腐蚀,侵蚀;糜烂 | cervical ~ 宫颈糜烂 / dental ~ 牙侵蚀症

erosive [iˈrəusiv] *a* 腐蚀性的,侵蚀性的 *n* 腐蚀药

erotic(al) [iˈrɔtik(əl)] *a* 性欲的,色情的

eroticism [iˈrɔtisizəm] *n* 性欲,性爱;色情,好色

eroticize [iˈrɔtisaiz] *vt* 使产生性欲,性欲化,力必多化

eroticomania [iˌrɔtikəuˈmeinjə] *n* 色情狂

erotism [ˈerətizəm] *n* 性欲,性爱;色情,好色 | anal ~ 肛欲(性欲),肛欲(色情) / oral ~ 口欲(性欲),口欲(色情)

erotize [ˈerətaiz] *vt* 使产生性欲,性欲化,力必多化

erot(o)- [构词成分]性欲,色情

erotogenesis [iˌrəutəuˈdʒenisis] *n* 性欲发生 | **erotogenic** [iˌrəutəuˈdʒenik] *a*

erotology [ˌerəˈtɔlədʒi] *n* 性爱学

erotomania [iˌrəutəuˈmeinjə] *n* 色情狂
erotomaniac [iˌrəutəuˈmeiniæk] *n* 色情狂者
erotophobia [iˌrəutəuˈfəubjə] *n* 性欲恐怖
erotosexual [iˌrəutəuˈseksjuəl] *a* 性欲的,性爱的
ERP endocardial resection procedure 心内膜切除法
ERPF effective renal plasma flow 有效肾血浆流量
erratic [iˈrætik] *a* 游走的,移动的;乖僻的
errhine [ˈerain] *a* 促鼻液的 *n* 促鼻液剂
error [ˈerə] *n* 谬误,错误;缺陷,误差 | inborn ~ of metabolism 先天性代谢缺陷,先天性代谢病 / random ~ 随机误差 / systemic ~ 系统误差 / Type Ⅰ ~ 第一类误差(在假设检验中对真实的无效假设的摒弃,第一类误差的概率〈显著性水平〉以 α 表示) / Type Ⅱ ~ 第二类误差(在假设检验中,接受不真实的无效假设,第二类误差的概率以 β 表示)
erucic acid [iˈrusik] 芥[子]酸
eruct [iˈrʌkt], **eructate** [iˈrʌkteit] *vi* 嗳气,打嗝 *vt* 嗝出
eructatio [ˌiːrʌkˈteiʃiəu] *n*【拉】嗳气
eructation [ˌiːrʌkˈteiʃən] *n* 嗳气 | nervous ~ 神经性嗳气
eruption [iˈrʌpʃən] *n* 长出,出牙;疹,发疹 | bullous ~ 大疱疹 / continuous ~ 继续长出 / creeping ~ 匐行疹 / delayed ~ 迟萌 / drug ~ 药疹,药物皮炎 / fixed ~ 固定疹(在同一部位数月或若干年后复发的一种局限性炎性皮肤损害) / fixed drug ~ 固定性药疹(在同一部位复发) / passive ~ 被动萌出 / petechial ~ 瘀点疹 / seabather's ~ 海水浴疹 / serum ~ 血清疹 / surgical ~ 经手术牙长出 | **eruptive** *a*
ERV expiratory reserve volume 补呼气量
Erwinia [əːˈwiniə] (Erwin F. Smith) *n* 欧文菌属
Erwinieae [ˌəːwiˈnaiiiː] *n* 欧文菌族
erysipelas [ˌeriˈsipiləs] *n* 丹毒 | coast ~ 蟠尾丝虫结节 | **erysipelatous** [ˌerisiˈpelətəs] *a*
erysipeloid [ˌeriˈsipilɔid] *n* 类丹毒
Erysipelothrix [ˌeriˈsipiləuˌθriks] *n* 丹毒丝菌属 | ~ insidiosa, ~ rhusiopathiae 诡谲丹毒丝菌,猪红斑丹毒丝菌
erysipelotoxin [ˌerisipiləuˈtɔksin] *n* 丹毒毒素
Erysiphaceae [eˌrisiˈfeisiiː] *n* 白粉菌科
erysiphake [eˈrisifeik] *n* 晶状体吸盘
Erysiphales [eˌrisiˈfeiliːz] *n* 白粉菌目
Erysiphe [eˈrisifi] *n* 白粉菌属
erythema [ˌeriˈθiːmə] *n*【希】红斑 | acrodynic ~ 肢痛性红斑 / diaper ~, napkin ~ 尿布红斑 / ~ dyschromicum perstans 持久性色素异常性红斑 / epidemic ~ 肢痛症,红皮水肿性多发性神经病 / ~ induratum 硬结性红斑,硬红斑 / ~ marginatum rheumaticum 风湿性边缘性红斑 / ~ multiforme major 重症多形[性]红斑,斯蒂文斯-约翰逊(Stevens-Johnson)综合征 / ~ multiforme minor 轻症多形红斑,黑布拉(Hebra)病 / necrolytic migratory ~ 坏死松解性游走性红斑 / nine-day ~, ninth-day ~ 九日红斑(注射六〇六等 7 ~ 9 日后出现的红斑) / ~ nodosa 结节性红斑 / ~ nodosum leprosum 麻风性结节性红斑 / ~ nodosum migrans 游走性结节性红斑 / ~ toxicum neonatorum 新生儿中毒性红斑 | **erythemic** [ˌeriˈθiːmik], **~tous** [ˌeriˈθemətəs] *a*
erythematoedematous [ˌeriˌθiːmətəuiˈdemətəs] *a* 红斑水肿的
erythematopultaceous [ˌeriˌθiːmətəupʌlˈteiʃəs] *a* 红斑髓样的(毛细管充血引起)
erythemogenic [ˌeriˌθiːməuˈdʒenik] *a* 引起红斑的
erythermalgia [ˌeriθəˈmældʒiə] *n* 红斑性肢痛病
Erythraea [ˌeriˈθriːə] *n* 百金花属
erythralgia [ˌeriˈθrældʒiə] *n* (皮肤)红痛
erythrasma [ˌeriˈθræzmə] *n* 红癣
erythredema polyneuropathy [iˌriθriˈdiːməˌpɔlinjuəˈrɔpəθi] 红皮水肿性多发性神经病,肢痛病
erythremia [ˌeriˈθriːmiə] *n* 红细胞增多[症],真性红细胞增多
erythremoid [ˌeriˈθriːmɔid] *n* 红细胞增多症样的
erythremomelalgia [eˌriθriməumeˈlældʒiə] *n* 红斑性肢痛病
erythrin [ˈeriθrin] *n* 赤地衣素,地衣红质
Erythrina [ˌeriˈθrainə] *n* 刺桐属
erythrism [iˈriθrizəm] *n* 红须发 | **~al** [ˌeriˈθrizməl], **erythristic** [ˌeriˈθristik] *a*
erythritol [iˈriθritɔl] *n* 赤藓醇
erythrityl [iˈriθritil] *n* 赤藓醇基 | ~ tetranitrate 丁四硝酯(血管扩张药,抗心绞痛药)
erythr(o)- [构词成分]红
Erythrobacillus [iˌriθrəubəˈsiləs] *n* 红杆菌属
erythroblast [iˈriθrəublæst] *n* 幼红细胞,有核红细胞 | basophilic ~, early ~ 嗜碱性幼红细胞,早幼红细胞 / definitive ~s 次级幼红细胞 / orthochromatic ~, eosinophilic ~, acidophilic ~, oxyphilic ~, late ~ 正染性幼红细胞,嗜酸性幼红细胞,晚幼红细胞 / polychromatic ~, intermediate ~ 多染性幼红细胞,中幼红细胞 / primitive ~s 原始幼红细胞 | **~ic** [iˌriθrəuˈblæstik]
erythroblastemia [iˌriθrəublæsˈtiːmiə] *n* 幼红细胞血症
erythroblastoma [iˌriθrəublæsˈtəumə] *n* 幼红细胞瘤
erythroblastomatosis [iˌriθrəuˌblæstəuməˈtəusis] *n* 幼红细胞瘤病
erythroblastopenia [iˌriθrəuˌblæstəˈpiːniə] *n* 幼红细胞减少

erythroblastosis [iˌriθrə*u*blæsˈtəusis] *n* 幼红细胞增多症;红白血病(一种禽类疾病) | ~ fetalis, ~ neonatorum 胎儿幼红细胞增多症,新生儿幼红细胞增多症(亦称新生儿溶血病) | **erythroblastotic** [iˌriθrə*u*blæsˈtɔtik] *a* 幼红细胞增多的
erythrocatalysis [iˌriθrə*u*kəˈtælisis] *n* 红细胞溶解
erythrochloropia [iˌriθrə*u*kləˈrəupiə], **erythrochloropsia** [iˌriθrə*u*kləˈrɔpsiə] *n* 红绿视症,青黄色盲
erythrochromia [iˌriθrə*u*ˈkrəumiə] *n* 脊[髓]液血色症
erythroclasis [ˌeriˈθrɔkləsis] *n* 红细胞破碎 | **erythroclastic** [iˌriθrə*u*ˈklæstik] *a*
erythroclast [iˈriθrəklæst] *n* 破碎红细胞,血影细胞
erythroconte [iˈriθrə*u*kəunt] *n* 红细胞杆状小体(见于恶性贫血)
erythrocruorin [iˌriθrə*u*ˈkruərin] *n* 无脊椎动物血红蛋白
erythrocuprein [iˌriθrə*u*ˈkuːprin] *n* 红细胞铜蛋白
erythrocyanosis [iˌriθrə*u*ˌsaiəˈnəusis] *n* 红绀病
erythrocytapheresis [iˌriθrə*u*ˌsaitəfəˈriːsis] *n* 红细胞去除术
erythrocyte [iˈriθrə*u*sait] *n* 红细胞 | achromic ~ 无色红细胞,红细胞影 / burr ~ 锯齿形红细胞(即 burr cell) / crenated ~ 皱缩红细胞 / hypochromic ~ 低色素红细胞 / "Mexican hat" ~, target ~ 靶红细胞 / nucleated ~ 有核红细胞 / orthochromatic ~ 正染性红细胞 / polychromatic ~, polychromatophilic ~ 多染性红细胞 | **erythrocytic** [iˌriθrə*u*ˈsitik] *a*
erythrocythemia [iˌriθrə*u*saiˈθiːmiə] *n* 红细胞增多[症]
erythrocytin [iˌriθrə*u*ˈsaitin] *n* 红细胞素
erythrocytoblast [iˌriθrə*u*ˈsaitəblæst] *n* 成红细胞,有核红细胞
erythrocytolysin [iˌriθrə*u*saiˈtɔlisin] *n* 红细胞溶解素,溶血素
erythrocytolysis [iˌriθrə*u*saiˈtɔlisis] *n* 红细胞溶解
erythrocytometer [iˌriθrə*u*saiˈtɔmitə] *n* 红细胞计数器 | **erythrocytometry** *n* 红细胞计数法
erythrocyto-opsonin [iˌriθrə*u*ˌsaitə*u*ɔpˈsəunin] *n* 红细胞调理素(血调理素)
erythrocytopenia [iˌriθrə*u*ˌsaitə*u*ˈpiːniə] *n* 红细胞减少
erythrocytophagy [iˌriθrə*u*saiˈtɔfədʒi] *n* 噬红细胞作用 | **erythrocytophagous** [iˌriθrə*u* saiˈtɔfəgəs] *a* 噬红细胞的
erythrocytopoiesis [iˌriθrə*u*ˌsaitə*u*pɔiˈiːsis] *n* 红细胞发生
erythrocytorrhexis [iˌriθrə*u*ˌsaitə*u*ˈreksis] *n* 红细胞破裂
erythrocytoschisis [iˌriθrə*u*saiˈtɔskisis] *n* 红细胞分裂
erythrocytosis [iˌriθrə*u*saiˈtəusis] *n* 红细胞增多症 | leukemic ~, ~ megalosplenica 白血病性红细胞增多症,巨脾性红细胞增多症,真性红细胞增多症 / stress ~ 应激性红细胞增多症
erythrocytotropic [iˌriθrə*u*ˌsaitə*u*ˈtrɔpik] *a* 向红细胞的
erythrocyturia [iˌriθrə*u*saiˈtjuəriə] *n* 红细胞尿,血尿
erythrodegenerative [iˌriθrə*u*diˈdʒenərətiv] *a* 红细胞变性的
erythroderma [iˌriθrə*u*ˈdəːmə] *n* 红皮病;剥脱性皮炎 | bullous congenital ichthyosiform ~ 先天性大疱性鱼鳞病样红皮病,表皮松解性角化过度 / ~ desquamativum 脱屑性红皮病 / nonbullous congenital ichthyosiform ~ 先天性非大疱性鱼鳞病样红皮病(现名层板状鱼鳞病)
erythrodermia [iˌriθrə*u*ˈdəːmiə] *n* 红皮病
erythrodextrin [iˌriθrə*u*ˈdekstrin] *n* 红糊精
erythrodontia [iˌriθrə*u*ˈdɔnʃiə] *n* 红牙
erythrogen [iˈriθrədʒən] *n* 胆血色质
erythrogenesis [iˌriθrə*u*ˈdʒenisis] *n* 红细胞发生 | ~ imperfecta 不全性红细胞发生(先天性再生障碍性贫血)
erythrogenic [iˌriθrə*u*ˈdʒenik] *n* 红细胞发生的;产生红色感觉的;产生或引起红疹的
erythrogenin [iˈriθrədʒinin] *n* 红细胞生成素
erythrogone [iˈriθrə*u*gəun], **erythrogonium** [iˌriθrə*u*ˈgəuniəm] *n* 原巨幼红细胞,原巨红细胞
erythrogranulose [iˌriθrə*u*ˈgrænjuləus] *n* 红淀粉糊精
erythroid [ˈeriθrɔid] *a* 红色的;红细胞系的
β-erythroidine [iˈriθrɔidin] *n* β-刺桐碱(具有箭毒样作用)
erythrokatalysis [iˌriθrə*u*kəˈtælisis] *n* 红细胞溶解
erythrokeratodermia [iˌriθrə*u*ˌkerətə*u*ˈdəːmiə] *n* 红斑角皮病 | ~ variabilis 可变性红斑角皮病
erythrokinetics [iˌriθrə*u*kaiˈnetiks] *n* 红细胞动态学
erythrol [ˈeriθrɔl] *n* 赤藓醇 | ~ tetranitrate 丁四硝酯(抗心绞痛药,血管扩张药)
erythrolabe [iˈriθrəleib] *n* 红敏素,感红色素
erythrolein [ˌeriˈθrəuliːn] *n* 石蕊红素
erythroleukemia [iˌriθrə*u*l*j*uːˈkiːmiə] *n* 红白血病
erythroleukoblastosis [iˌriθrə*u*l*j*uːkəblæsˈtəusis] *n*

幼红白细胞增多症,新生儿重度黄疸
erythroleukosis [iˌriθrəuljuːˈkəusis] *n* 红细胞黄铜色变(疟疾时);幼红细胞增多病(见于禽类)
erythroleukothrombocythemia [iˌriθrəuˌljuːkəuˌθrɔmbəusaiˈθiːmiə] *n* 全血初细胞增生(成红白细胞血小板增生)
erythrolitmin [iˌriθrəuˈlitmin] *n* 结晶性石蕊红素
erythrolysin [ˌeriˈθrɔlisin] *n* 红细胞溶解素,溶血素
erythrolysis [ˌeriˈθrɔlisis] *n* 红细胞溶解
erythromania [iˌriθrəuˈmeinjə] *n* 赧颜症
erythromelalgia [iˌriθrəuməˈlældʒiə] *n* 红斑性肢痛症 | ~ of the head 红斑性头痛(由于组胺引起的血管扩张所致,也可用组胺治愈)
erythrometer [ˌeriˈθrɔmitə] *n* 红度计;红细胞计数器 | **erythrometry** *n* 红度测量[法];红细胞计数法
erythromycin [iˌriθrəuˈmaisin] *n* 红霉素 | ~ B 红霉素 B, 12-脱氧红霉素 / ~ estolate 依托红霉素 / ~ ethylcarbonate 红霉素碳酸乙酯 / ~ ethylsuccinate 琥乙红霉素 / ~ gluceptate 葡庚糖酸红霉素 / ~ lactobionate 乳糖酸红霉素 / ~ propionate 丙酸红霉素 / ~ stearate 硬脂酸红霉素
erythromyeloblastosis [iˌriθrəuˌmaiələublæsˈtəusis] *n* 成红[细胞]成髓细胞增多症(鸡的肿瘤病,由禽肿瘤病毒引起)
erythron [ˈeriθrɔn] *n* 红细胞系(循环中的红细胞及其前身以及与其生成有关的全身一切成分)
erythroneocytosis [iˌriθrəuˌni(ː)əusaiˈtəusis] *n* 幼稚红细胞血症
erythronoclastic [iˌriθrɔnəuˈklæstik] *a* 溶红细胞系的
erythroparasite [iˌriθrəuˈpærəsait] *n* 红细胞寄生物
erythropathy [ˌeriˈθrɔpəθi] *n* 红细胞病
erythropenia [iˌriθrəuˈpiːniə] *n* 红细胞减少
erythrophage [iˈriθrəufeidʒ] *n* 噬红[细胞]细胞
erythrophagia [iˌriθrəuˈfeidʒiə] *n* 噬红细胞现象(噬红细胞作用)
erythrophagocytic [iˌriθrəuˌfægəuˈsitik] *a* 噬红细胞的
erythrophagocytosis [iˌriθrəuˌfægəusaiˈtəusis] *n* 噬红细胞作用 | **erythrophagous** [ˌeriˈθrɔfəgəs] *a* 噬红细胞的
erythropheresis [iˌriθrəufəˈriːsis] *n* 红细胞去除术
erythrophil [iˈriθrəfil] *n* 红染细胞 *a* 嗜红色的
erythrophilous [ˌeriˈθrɔfiləs] *a* 嗜红色的
Erythrophloeum [iˌriθrəˈfliːəm] *n* 围涎树属
erythrophobia [iˌriθrəuˈfəubjə] *n* 赧颜恐怖;红色恐怖
erythrophobic [iˌriθrəuˈfəubik] *a* 疏红性的(指对红染料〈酸性品红〉)
erythrophore [iˈriθrəfɔː] *n* 红色素细胞
erythrophose [iˈriθrəfəuz] *n* 红色幻视
erythrophthisis [iˌriθrəuˈθaisis] *n* 红细胞消耗症,红细胞痨
erythrophthoric [iˌriθrəuˈθɔrik] *a* 红细胞破坏的
erythrophyll [iˈriθrəfil] *n* 叶红素(在植物内)
erythropia [ˌeriˈθrəupiə] *n* 红视症
erythroplakia [iˌriθrəuˈpleikiə] *n* 黏膜红斑 | speckled ~ 斑点状黏膜红斑
erythroplasia [iˌriθrəuˈpleiziə] *n* 增生性红斑
erythroplastid [iˌriθrəuˈplæstid] *n* 无核红细胞(哺乳类动物)
erythropoiesis [iˌriθrəupɔiˈiːsis] *n* 红细胞生成 | **erythropoietic** [iˌriθrəupɔiˈetik] *a*
erythropoietin [iˌriθrəuˈpɔiitin] *n* 红细胞生成素
erythropoietinogen [iˌriθrəuˈpɔiətinədʒən] *n* 红细胞生成素原
erythroprecipitin [iˌriθrəupriˈsipitin] *n* 红细胞沉淀素
erythroprosopalgia [iˌriθrəuˌprɔsəˈpældʒiə] *n* 红斑性面痛
erythropsia [ˌeriˈθrɔpsiə] *n* 红视症
erythropsin [ˌeriˈθrɔpsin], **erythropsine** [ˌeriˈθrɔpsiːn] *n* 视红质
erythropyknosis [iˌriθrəupikˈnəusis] *n* 红细胞固缩
erythrorrhexis [iˌriθrəuˈreksis] *n* 红细胞破裂
erythrose [iˈriθrəus] *n* 赤藓糖
érythrose [eiriˈθrəuz] *n* 【法】皮肤红变 | ~ péribuccale pigmentaire of Brocq 布劳克色素性口周红斑
erythrosedimentation [iˌriθrəuˌsedimenˈteiʃən] *n* 红细胞沉降
erythrosin [iˈriθrəsin] *n* 藻红(组织染剂)
erythrosine sodium [iˈriθrəsiːn] 四碘荧光素钠(着色剂,用于揭示牙菌斑)
erythrosis [ˌeriˈθrəusis] *n* 皮肤红变;造红细胞组织增生 | ~ pigmentata faciei 色素性面部红斑
erythrostasis [iˌriθrəuˈsteisis] *n* 红细胞停滞(在毛细血管内,如镰状细胞性贫血时)
erythrothioneine [iˌriθrəuˌθaiəˈniːin] *n* 麦角硫因,巯组氨酸三甲[基]内盐
erythrotoxin [iˌriθrəuˈtɔksin] *n* 红细胞毒素
Erythrovirus [iˈriθrəuˌvaiərəs] *n* 红病毒属
Erythroxylon [ˌeriˈθrɔksilɔn] *n* 古柯属
erythrulose [iˈriθruləus] *n* 赤藓酮糖
erythruria [ˌeriˈθrjuəriə] *n* 红尿症
Es einsteinium 锿

es [es] *n* 低于模糊意识(低于下意识)
Esbach's method (reagent, test) [ˈesbɑːh] (Georges H. Esbach) 埃斯巴赫法(试剂、试验)(检尿内白蛋白)
escape [isˈkeip] *n* 逃避;脱逸 | aldosterone ~ 醛固酮脱逸 / nodal ~ (房室)结性逸搏 / vagal ~ 迷走[神经]脱逸 / ventricular ~ 室性逸搏
eschar [ˈeskɑː] *n* 焦痂
escharotic [ˌeskəˈrɔtik] *a* 苛性的,腐蚀性的 *n* 苛性剂,腐蚀剂
escharotomy [ˌeskəˈrɔtəmi] *n* 焦痂切开术
Escherich's bacillus [ˈeʃəriʃ] (Theodor Escherich) 埃[舍利]希杆菌,大肠杆菌 | ~ sign (reflex) 埃舍利希征(反射)(手足搐搦时叩击唇或舌内表面,即引起唇、舌和咬肌收缩) / ~ test 埃舍利希试验,结核菌素试验(将结核菌素注射至皮下的一种皮肤试验)
Escherichia [ˌeʃəˈrikiə] *n* 埃[舍利]希杆菌属 | ~ aurescens 金色埃希杆菌 / ~ blattae 蠊埃希杆菌 / ~ coli 大肠埃希杆菌,大肠杆菌 / ~ fergusonii 福氏埃希杆菌 / ~ freundii 弗[罗因德]氏埃希杆菌 / ~ hermanii 黑氏埃希杆菌 / ~ intermedia 中间型埃希杆菌
Escherichieae [ˌeʃəˈrikiiː] *n* 埃[舍利]希杆菌族
eschrolalia [ˌeskrəˈleiliə] *n* 秽亵言语
Eschscholtzia [isˈkɔltʃə, əˈʃɔltsiə] *n* 花菱草属
escin [ˈeskin] *n* 七叶皂苷
escitalopram oxalate [ˌesiˈtæləupræm] 草酸艾他洛普仑(抗抑郁药)
Escobar syndrome [eskəˈbɑː] (Victor Escobar) 埃斯柯巴综合征,多发性翼状赘蹼综合征(即 multiple pterygium syndrome,见 syndrome 项下相应术语)
escorcin [esˈkɔːsin] *n* 七叶酚(用于检测角膜和巩膜损害)
Escudero's test [eskuˈdeirəu] (Pedro Escudero) 埃斯库德罗试验(检痛风的嘌呤餐试验)
esculapian [ˌeskjuˈleipiən] *a*, *n* = **aesculapian**
esculent [ˈeskjulənt] *a* 可食的,食用的
esculin [ˈeskjulin] *n* 七叶苷(有退热作用)
escutcheon [esˈkʌtʃən] *n* 盾式分布(阴毛分布型)
eseptate [iːˈsepteit] *a* 无[中]隔的
eserine [ˈesərin] *n* 依色林,毒扁豆碱(即 physostigmine)
ESF erythropoietic stimulating factor 促红细胞生成因子
-esis [后缀]表示(病的)状态、情况
esmarch [ˈesmɑːh] *n* 埃斯马赫驱血绷带
Esmarch's bandage [ˈesmɑːh] (Johann F. A. von Esmarch) 驱血绷带 | ~ tourniquet 驱血止血带 / ~ tube 埃斯马赫管(用于细菌培养)
ESMO Europian Society for Medical Oncology 欧洲医学肿瘤学学会
esmolol hydrochloride [ˈesmələl] 盐酸艾司洛尔(β受体阻滞药)
eso- [构词成分]在内
esocataphoria [ˌesəukætəˈfəuriə] *n* 内下隐斜
esocine [ˈesəsiːn] *n* 鲩精蛋白
esodeviation [ˌesəuˌdiːviˈeiʃən] *n* 内转,内偏;内隐斜;内斜视
esodic [iˈsɔdik] *a* 传入的(如传入神经)
esoethmoiditis [ˌesəuˌeθmɔiˈdaitis] *n* 筛窦炎
esogastritis [ˌesəugæsˈtraitis] *n* 胃黏膜炎
esomeprazole magnesium [ˌesəuˈmeprəzəul] 艾美哌唑镁(胃酸分泌抑制药)
esophagalgia [i(ː)ˌsɔfəˈgældʒiə] *n* 食管痛
esophageal [i(ː)ˌsɔfəˈdʒi(ː)əl, i(ː)səuˈfeidʒiəl] *a* 食管的
esophagectasia [i(ː)ˌsɔfədʒekˈteiziə], **esophagectasis** [i(ː)ˌsɔfəˈdʒektəsis] *n* 食管扩张
esophagectomy [i(ː)ˌsɔfəˈdʒektəmi] *n* 食管切除术
esophagism [i(ː)ˈsɔfədʒizəm] *n* 食管痉挛 | hiatal ~ 贲门痉挛 | **~us** [i(ː)ˌsɔfəˈdʒizməs] *n*
esophagitis [i(ː)ˌsɔfəˈdʒaitis] *n* 食管炎 | ~ dissecans superficialis 表层脱落性食管炎 / reflux ~, chronic peptic ~ 反流性食管炎,慢性消化性食管炎
esophagobronchial [i(ː)ˌsɔfəgəuˈbrɔŋkiəl] *a* 食管支气管的
esophagocardiomyotomy [i(ː)ˌsɔfəgəuˌkɑːdiəu-maiˈɔtəmi] *n* 食管贲门肌切开术,贲门肌切开术
esophagocele [i(ː)ˈsɔfəgəˌsiːl] *n* 食管膨出,食管疝
esophagocologastrostomy [i(ː)ˌsɔfəgəuˌkəuləu-gæsˈtrɔstəmi] *n* 食管结肠胃吻合术
esophagocoloplasty [i(ː)ˌsɔfəgəuˈkəuləˌplæsti] *n* 食管结肠成形术
esophagoduodenostomy [i(ː)ˌsɔfəgəuˌdju(ː)-əudiːˈnɔstəmi] *n* 食管十二指肠吻合术
esophagodynia [i(ː)ˌsɔfəgəuˈdiniə] *n* 食管痛
esophagoenterostomy [i(ː)ˌsɔfəgəuˌentəˈrɔstəmi] *n* 食管肠吻合术
esophagoesophagostomy [i(ː)ˌsɔfəgəui(ː)-ˌsɔfəˈgɔstəmi] *n* 食管食管吻合术
esophagofundopexy [i(ː)ˌsɔfəgəuˌfʌndəˈpeksi] *n* 食管胃底固定术
esophagogastrectomy [i(ː)ˌsɔfəgəugæsˈtrektəmi] *n* 食管胃切除术
esophagogastric [i(ː)ˌsɔfəgəuˈgæstrik] *a* 食管胃的
esophagogastroanastomosis [i(ː)ˌsɔfəgəuˌgæstrəuəˌnæstəˈməusis] *n* 食管胃吻合术
esophagogastroduodenal [i(ː)ˌsɔfəgəuˌgæs-

trəuˌdju(ː)əu'diːnəl] *a* 食管胃十二指肠的
esophagogastroduodenoscopy (EGD) [i(ː)-ˌsɔfəgəuˌgæstrəuˌdju(ː)əudi'nɔskəpi] *n* 食管胃十二指肠镜检查
esophagogastromyotomy [i(ː)ˌsɔfəgəuˌgæstrəu-mai'ɔtəmi] *n* 食管胃肌切开术,食管贲门肌切开术
esophagogastroplasty [i(ː)ˌsɔfəgəu'gæstrəˌplæs-ti] *n* 食管胃成形术;贲门成形术
esophagogastroscopy [i(ː)ˌsɔfəgəu gæs'trɔskə-pi] *n* 食管胃镜检查
esophagogastrostomy [i(ː)ˌsɔfəgəu gæs'trɔstə-mi] *n* 食管胃吻合术
esophagogram [i(ː)'sɔfəgəgræm] *n* 食管X线[照]片,食管X线造影[照]片
esophagography [i(ː)sɔfə'gɔgrəfi] *n* 食管X线摄影[术],食管X线造影[术]
esophagojejunogastrostomosis [i(ː)ˌsɔfəgəu-dʒiˌdʒuːnəuˌgæstrɔstə'məusis], **esophagojejunogastrostomy** [i(ː)ˌsɔfəgəudʒiˌdʒuːnəugæs-'trɔstəmi] *n* 食管空肠胃吻合术
esophagojejunoplasty [i(ː)ˌsɔfəgəudʒi'dʒuːnə-ˌplæsti] *n* 食管空肠成形术
esophagojejunostomy [i(ː)ˌsɔfəgəudʒidʒuː'nɔs-təmi] *n* 食管空肠吻合术
esophagolaryngectomy [i(ː)ˌsɔfəgəuˌlærin'dʒe-ktəmi] *n* 食管喉切除术
esophagology [i(ː)ˌsɔfə'gɔlədʒi] *n* 食管病学
esophagomalacia [i(ː)ˌsɔfəgəumə'leiʃiə] *n* 食管软化[症]
esophagometer [i(ː)ˌsɔfə'gɔmitə] *n* 食管[长度]测量计
esophagomycosis [i(ː)ˌsɔfəgəumai'kəusis] *n* 食管真菌病,食管霉菌病
esophagomyotomy [i(ː)ˌsɔfəgəumai'ɔtəmi] *n* 食管肌切开术
esophagopharynx [i(ː)ˌsɔfəgəu'færiŋks] *n* 咽下部,下咽[部]
esophagoplasty [i(ː)'sɔfəgəˌplæsti] *n* 食管成形术
esophagoplication [i(ː)ˌsɔfəgəuplai'keiʃən] *n* 食管襞折术
esophagoptosis [i(ː)ˌsɔfəgəp'təusis] *n* 食管下垂,食管脱垂
esophagorespiratory [i(ː)ˌsɔfəgəuris'paiərətəri, -'respir-] *a* 食管呼吸道的
esophagosalivation [i(ː)ˌsɔfəgəuˌsæli'veiʃən] *n* 食管性多涎,食管癌性多涎症
esophagoscope [i(ː)'sɔfəgəskəup] *n* 食管镜 | **esophagoscopy** [i(ː)ˌsɔfə'gɔskəpi] *n* 食管镜检查[术]
esophagospasm [i(ː)'sɔfəgəˌspæzəm] *n* 食管痉挛
esophagostenosis [i(ː)ˌsɔfəgəusti'nəusis] *n* 食管狭窄
esophagostoma [ˌiːsɔfə'gɔstəmə] *n* 食管瘘口
esophagostomiasis [i(ː)ˌsɔfəgəustəu'maiəsis] *n* 结节线虫病
esophagostomy [i(ː)ˌsɔfə'gɔstəmi] *n* 食管造口术
esophagotome [ˌiːsəu'fægətəum] *n* 食管刀
esophagotomy [i(ː)ˌsɔfə'gɔtəmi] *n* 食管切开术
esophagotracheal [i(ː)ˌsɔfəgəutrə'ki(ː)əl, -'treiki-] *a* 食管气管的
esophagram [i(ː)'sɔfəgræm] *n* 食管X线[照]片,食管X线造影[照]片
esophagus [i(ː)'sɔfəgəs] *n* 食管 | nutcracker ~ 胡桃夹样食管(一种能动性障碍,由远侧食管引起,表现为高振幅蠕动收缩,持续时间长)
esophoria [ˌesəu'fəuriə] *n* 内隐斜 | **esophoric** [ˌesəu'fɔrik] *a*
esosphenoiditis [ˌesəuˌsfiːnɔi'daitis] *n* 蝶骨骨髓炎
esotropia [ˌesəu'trəupiə] *n* 内斜视 | **esotropic** [ˌesəu'trɔpik] *a*
ESP extrasensory perception 超感官知觉
espial [is'paiəl] *n* 窥见;观察;发现
espnoic [es'pnəuik] *a* 气注疗法的
esponja [es'pɔŋə] *n* 皮肤丽线虫蚴疮,夏疮(马)
esproquin hydrochloride ['esprəkwin] 盐酸艾司丙喹(拟肾上腺素药)
espundia [es'pundiə] *n* 黏膜皮肤利什曼病,美洲利什曼病
esquillectomy [ˌeskwi'lektəmi] *n* 碎骨片清除术
ESR electron spin resonance 电子自旋共振;erythrocyte sedimentation rate 红细胞沉降率
ESRD end-stage renal disease 终末期肾病
essence ['esns] *n* 要素;露,香精剂(挥发油醇溶液) | ~ of peppermint 欧薄荷酯
essentia [i'senʃiə] *n* 【拉】要素;露,香精剂
essential [i'senʃəl] *a* 基本的;必需的;自发的,特发的
Esser's graft ['esə] (Johannes F. S. Esser) 埃塞移植物(口腔外科用) | ~ operation 埃塞手术(上皮内置法)
essiac ['esiæk] (essiac 为推广此药的加拿大护士 Rene M. Caisse 〈1887 ~ 1978〉姓的反拼法) 艾西阿克(一种草药制剂,当茶用于治癌)
EST electric shock therapy 电休克治疗;electroshock therapy 电休克治疗
estazolam [es'tæzəulæm] *n* 艾司唑仑(催眠镇痛药)
ester ['estə] *n* 酯 | acetoacetic ~ 乙酰乙酸乙酯 / hexosephosphoric ~s 磷酸己糖酯

esterapenia [ˌestərəˈpiːniə] *n* 血胆碱酯酶缺乏
esterase [ˈestəreis] *n* 酯酶
esterify [esˈterifai] *vt*, *vi* 酯化 | **esterification** [esˌterifiˈkeiʃən] *n* 酯化[作用]
esterize [ˈestəraiz] *vt* 使酯化
esterolysis [ˌestəˈrɔləsis] *n* 酯水解[作用] | **esterolytic** [ˌestərəˈlitik] *a*
Estes' operation [ˈestiːz] (William L. Estes, Jr.) 埃斯蒂斯手术(移植卵巢于子宫角内,为了解除输卵管缺如所致的不孕症)
estetrol [ˈestətrɔl] *n* 雌四醇
esthematology [ˌesθeməˈtɔlədʒi] *n* 感觉学,感官学
esthesia [iːsˈθiːzjə, es-] *n* 感觉 | **esthesic** [iːsˈθiːsik, es-] *a*
esthesio- [构词成分]感觉
esthesioblast [esˈθiːziəˌblæst] *n* 成神经节细胞
esthesiodic [esˌθiːziˈɔdik] *a* 感觉传导的
esthesiogen [esˈθiːziədʒən] *n* 激奋质,引奋质
esthesiogenic [esˌθiːziəuˈdʒenik] *a* 发生感觉的
esthesiology [esˌθiːziˈɔlədʒi] *n* 感觉学,感官学
esthesiomene [esˌθiːziˈɔməni] *n* 女阴蚀疮,腹股沟淋巴肉芽肿性女阴象皮病
esthesiometer [esˌθiːziˈɔmitə] *n* 触觉测量器 | **esthesiometry** *n* 触觉测量法
esthesioneure [esˈθiːziənjuə] *n* 感觉神经元
esthesioneuroblastoma [esˌθiːziəuˌnjuərəublæsˈtəumə] *n* 成感觉神经细胞瘤,鼻腔神经胶质瘤
esthesioneurosis [esˌθiːziəunjuəˈrəusis], **esthesionosus** [esˌθiːziˈɔnəsəs] *n* 感觉性神经病
esthesiophysiology [esˌθiːziəuˌfiziˈɔlədʒi] *n* 感觉[器官]生理学
esthesodic [ˌesθiˈzɔdik] *a* 感觉传导的
esthetic(al) [esˈθetik(əl)] *a* 感觉的;美的
esthetics [iːsˈθetiks, es-] *n* 美学
esthiomene [ˌesθiˈɔməni] *n* 女阴蚀疮,腹股沟淋巴肉芽肿性女阴象皮病
estimate [ˈestimeit] *vt*, *vi* 估计,评价 [ˈestimit] *n* 估计;评价;估计量(亦称 estimator) | biased ~ 有偏估计(不是无偏的一种点估计) / consistent ~ 相容估计,一致估计(随着样本大小的增加可使待估参数趋于同样结果的一种统计) / interval ~ 区间估计(一种统计学估计,以特定量信度表明参数在特定区间内) / point ~ 点估计(一种统计学估计,为参数定出一个值) / product-limit ~ 乘积极限估计,卡普兰-迈耶(Kaplan-Meier) 生存曲线 / unbiased ~ 无偏估计(样本分布的均值等于待估参数的一种点估计)
estimation [ˌestiˈmeiʃən] *n* 估计;评价;测定 | ~ of biological potency 生物效价测定
estimator [ˈestimeitə] *n* 估计量,估计值(用以表示总体参数的值的一种统计量)
estival [iːˈstaivəl, ˈesti-] *a* 夏令的,夏季的
estivation [ˌiːstiˈveiʃən, ˌes-] *n* 夏眠,夏蛰
estivoautumnal [ˌestivəuɔːˈtʌmnəl] *a* 夏秋的
Estlander's operation [ˈestlɑːdə] (Jacob A. Estlander) 埃斯特兰德手术(①脓胸时切除一根或数根肋骨,使胸壁萎陷,并关闭腹腔;②从下唇一侧旋转三角瓣,充填外侧上唇缺损)
estolate [ˈestəleit] *n* 丙酸酯十二烷基硫酸盐(propionate lauryl sulfate 的 USAN 缩约词)
eston [ˈestɔn] *n* 醋酸铝
estradiol [ˌestrəˈdaiɔl, esˈtreidiɔl] *n* 雌二醇(雌激素类药) | ~ benzoate 苯甲酸雌二醇 / ~ cypionate 环戊丙酸雌二醇 / ~ dipropionate 二丙酸雌二醇 / ~ enanthate 庚酸雌二醇 / ethinyl ~ 炔雌醇 / ~ undecylate 十一酸雌二醇 / ~ valerate 戊酸雌二醇
estradiol 6*β*-hydroxylase [ˌestrəˈdaiɔl haiˈdrɔksileis] 雌二醇 6*β*-羟化酶,雌二醇 6*β*-单加氧酶
estradiol 6*β*-monooxygenase [ˌestrəˈdaiɔl ˌmɔnəuˈɔksidʒəneis] 雌二醇 6*β*-单加氧酶
estramustine [ˌestrəˈmʌstiːn] *n* 雌莫司汀(抗肿瘤药)
estramustine phosphate [ˌestrəˈmʌstiːn] 磷酸雌莫司汀(抗肿瘤药)
estrane [ˈestrein] *n* 雌[甾]烷
estrapentaene [ˌestrəˈpentəiːn] *n* 五烯甲雌醇核
estratetraene [ˌestrəˈtetrəiːn] *n* 四烯甲雌醇核
estratriene [ˌestrəˈtraiiːn] *n* 三烯甲雌醇核
estrazinol hydrobromide [esˈtræzinɔl] 氢溴酸雌嗪醇(雌激素类药)
estrenol [ˈestrinɔl] *n* 雌烯三醇
estriasis [esˈtraiəsis] *n* 狂蝇蛆病
Estridae [ˈestridiː] *n* 狂蝇科(即 Oestridae)
estrin [ˈestrin] *n* 雌激素
estrinization [ˌestriniˈzeiʃən] *n* 动情期[变]化(使阴道上皮细胞具动情期特征的细胞变化)
estriol [ˈestriɔl] *n* 雌三醇
estrofurate [ˌestrəˈfjuəreit] *n* 雌呋酯(雌激素类药)
estrogen [ˈestrədʒən] *n* 雌激素 | conjugated ~s 结合雌激素 / esterified ~s 酯化雌激素
estrogenic [ˌestrəˈdʒenik], **estrogenous** [esˈtrɔdʒinəs] *a* 动情的,动情期的;雌激素的
estrogenicity [ˌestrədʒiˈnisəti] *n* 动情性,动情力
estrone [ˈestrəun, ˈiːs-] *n* 雌酮
estrophilin [ˌestrəˈfilin] *n* 亲雌[激]素蛋白(雌素受体细胞蛋白)
estropipate [ˈestrəpipeit] *n* 哌嗪雌酮硫酸酯(用作雌酮)
estrostilben [ˌestrəˈstilbən] *n* 己烯雌酚,乙底酚
estrous [ˈestrəs, ˈiːs-], **estrual** [ˈestruəl] *a* 动情

期的
estruation [ˌestruˈeiʃən] *n* 动情期
estrus [ˈestrəs, ˈiːs-], **estrum** [ˈestrəm] *n* 动情期
estuarium [ˌestjuˈɛəriəm] *n*【拉】蒸汽浴
esu electrostatic unit 静电单位
ESV end-systolic volume 收缩期末容积
esylate [ˈesileit] *n* 乙磺酸盐(ethanesulfonate 的 USAN 缩约词)
Et ethyl 乙基
et [et] *conj*【拉】和,以及
eta [ˈiːtə, ˈeitə] *n* 希腊语的第 7 个字母(H, η)
etafedrine hydrochloride [ˌetəˈfedriːn] 盐酸乙非君(肾上腺素能药,口服治疗支气管哮喘)
etafilcon A [ˌeitəˈfilkɔn] 艾塔费康 A(一种亲水性接触镜材料)
et al. et alibi【拉】以及其他地方;et alii【拉】以及其他等等
etanercept [iˈtænəsept] *n* 依地萘塞(一种可溶性肿瘤坏死因子受体,可使肿瘤坏死因子失活,用于治疗类风湿关节炎和幼年型类风湿关节炎,皮下给药)
état [eiˈtɑː] *n*【法】状况,状态 | ~ criblé 筛孔状态(伤寒病时小肠黏膜集合淋巴结坏死而形成不规则小穿孔状态);筛状脑(脑内血管周淋巴隙扩张所致) / ~ lacunaire (脑)陷凹状态 / ~ mammelonné 乳头状态(慢性胃炎时胃黏膜增生所致) / ~ marbré 大理石状态(脑纹状体的一种病变) / ~ vermoulu 虫蚀状态(严重脑动脉硬化时有时在脑表面见有不规则溃疡状态)
etazolate hydrochloride [iˈtæzəleit] 盐酸依他唑酯(安定药)
etc. et cetera [itˈsetrə]【拉】等等;以及其他等等
etch [etʃ] *vt* 蚀刻;浸蚀
etching [ˈetʃiŋ] *n* 蚀刻,蚀刻法
ETEC enterotoxigenic *Escherichia coli* 产肠毒素大肠杆菌,肠产毒性大肠杆菌
Eternod's sinus [eitəˈnəu] (Auguste F. C. Eternod) 埃特诺窦(一种血管襻连接绒毛膜血管以及卵囊下面的血管)
eterobarb [iˈterəbɑːb] *n* 依特比妥(抗惊厥药)
ETF electron transfer flavoprotein 电子传递黄素蛋白
ethacrynate [eθəˈkrineit] *n* 依他尼酸盐 | ~ sodium 依他尼酸钠(利尿药)
ethacrynic acid [ˌeθəˈkrinik] 依他尼酸(利尿药)
ethal [ˈeθəl] *n* 十六醇
ethambutol hydrochloride [iˈθæmbjutɔl] 盐酸乙胺丁醇(抗菌药,治疗肺结核)
ethamivan [eˈθæmiˌvæn] *n* 香草二乙胺(中枢兴奋药)
ethamsylate [iˈθæmsileit] *n* 酚磺乙胺(止血药)
ethanal [ˈeθənəl] *n* 乙醛
ethane [ˈeθein] *n* 乙烷
ethanedial [eθeinˈdaiəl] *n* 乙二醛
ethanedinitrile [ˌeθeindaiˈnaitril] *n* 乙二腈
ethanoic acid [ˌeθəˈnəuik] 醋酸,乙酸
ethanol [ˈeθənɔl] *n* 乙醇
ethanolamine [ˌeθəˈnɔləmiːn] *n* 乙醇胺,氨基乙醇,胆胺(其油酸盐用于治静脉曲张)
ethanolism [ˈeθəˈnɔlizəm] *n* 乙醇中毒(乙醇性低血糖)
ethaverine hydrochloride [ˌeθəˈveriːn] 盐酸依沙维林(解痉药,平滑肌松弛药)
ethchlorvynol [eθˈklɔːvinɔl] *n* 乙氯维诺(催眠镇静药)
ethene [ˈeθiːn] *n* 乙烯;次乙基;乙撑
ethenoid [ˈeθinɔid] *a* 乙烯型的
etheogenesis [ˌiːθiəuˈdʒenisis] *n* 孤雄生殖,雄体单性生殖(指原虫)
ether [ˈiːθə] *n* 醚;乙醚(麻醉药) | anesthetic ~ 麻醉醚,二乙醚 / petroleum ~ 石油醚 / thio ~ 硫醚
ethereal, etherial [i(ː)ˈθiəriəl] *a* 乙醚的;醚制的;挥发性的
etherify [iːˈθerifai] *vt* 醚化 | **etherification** [ˌiːθərifiˈkeiʃən] *n* 醚化[作用]
etherize [ˈiːθəraiz] *vt* 醚麻醉 | **etherization** [ˌiːθəraiˈzeiʃən, -riˈz-] *n* 醚麻醉法
etheromania [ˌiːθərəuˈmeinjə], **etherism** [ˈiːθərizəm] *n* 乙醚瘾,乙醚癖
etherometer [ˌiːθəˈrɔmitə] *n* 乙醚滴定器
ethic [ˈeθik] *a* 伦理的,道德的
ethical [ˈeθikəl] *a* 伦理的,道德的;(药品)合乎规格的,凭处方出售的
ethics [ˈeθiks] *n* 伦理学 | medical ~ 医学伦理学,医德
ethidene [ˈeθidiːn] *n* 亚乙基 | ~ chloride 氯乙烷(溶剂) / ~ diamine 乙二胺
ethidium [iˈθidiəm] *n* 乙啡啶
ethinamate [iˈθinəmeit] *n* 炔己蚁胺(短效镇静药)
ethinyl [ˈeθinil] *n* 乙炔基 | ~ estradiol 炔雌醇(雌激素类药) / ~ trichloride 三氯乙烯(吸入麻醉药)
ethionamide [iˌθaiəˈnæmaid] *n* 乙硫异烟胺(抗结核药)
ethionine [iˈθaiənin] *n* 乙硫氨酸
ethisterone [iˈθistərəun] *n* 炔孕酮(孕激素类药)
ethmocarditis [ˌeθməukɑːˈdaitis] *n* 心结缔织炎
ethmocephalus [eθməuˈsefələs] *n* 头发育不全畸胎
ethmofrontal [ˌeθməuˈfrʌntl] *a* 筛额[骨]的

ethmoid [ˈeθmɔid] *a* 筛状的;筛骨的 *n* 筛骨 | **~al** [eθˈmɔidl] *a* 筛骨的
ethmoidectomy [ˌeθmɔiˈdektəmi] *n* 筛窦切除术,筛房切除术
ethmoiditis [ˌeθmɔiˈdaitis] *n* 筛窦炎
ethmoidotomy [ˌeθmɔiˈdɔtəmi] *n* 筛窦切开术
ethmolacrimal [ˌeθməuˈlækriməl] *a* 筛泪[骨]的
ethmomaxillary [ˌeθməumækˈsiləri, -ˈmæksi-] *a* 筛上颌[骨]的
ethmonasal [ˌeθməuˈneizəl] *a* 筛鼻[骨]的
ethmopalatal [ˌeθməuˈpælətl] *a* 筛腭[骨]的
ethmosphenoid [ˌeθməuˈsfiːnɔid] *a* 筛蝶[骨]的
ethmoturbinal [ˌeθməuˈtəːbinl] *a* 上中鼻甲[骨]的,筛鼻甲[骨]的
ethmovomerine [ˌeθməuˈvəuməriːn] *a* 筛犁[骨]的
ethmyphitis [ˌeθmiˈfaitis] *n* 蜂窝织炎
ethnic [ˈeθnik] *a* 人种的;人种学的 | **~s** *n* 人种学 / **~al** *a*
ethnobiology [ˌeθnəubaiˈɔlədʒi] *n* 人种生物学
ethnobotany [ˌeθnəuˈbɔtəni] *n* 民族植物学
ethnography [eθˈnɔgrəfi] *n* 人种志,人种论 | **ethnographic(al)** [ˌeθnəuˈgræfik(əl)] *a*
ethnology [eθˈnɔlədʒi] *n* 人种学 | **ethnologic(al)** [ˌeθnəuˈlɔdʒik(əl)] *a* / **ethnologist** *n* 人种学者
ethnomedicine [ˌeθnəuˈmedisin] *n* 民族医学 | **ethnomedical** [ˌeθnəuˈmedikəl] *a*
ethnopharmacology [ˌeθnəuˌfɑːməˈkɔlədʒi] *n* 民族药理学
ethobrom [ˈeθəbrəum] *n* 三溴乙醇(吸入麻醉药)
ethocaine [ˈeθəkein] *n* 盐酸普鲁卡因(局部麻醉药)
ethoglucid [ˌeθəuˈgluːsid] *n* 依托格鲁(抗肿瘤药)
ethoheptazine [ˌeθəˈheptəziːn] *n* 依索庚嗪(镇痛药) | ~ citrate 枸橼酸依索庚嗪(镇痛药)
ethohexadiol [ˌeθəuˌheksəˈdaiɔl] *n* 乙基己二醇,驱蚊醇(驱虫药)
ethology [i(ː)ˈθɔlədʒi] *n* 行为学(研究动物的行为,特别是在自然条件下的行为的学科) | **ethologic(al)** [ˌiːθəuˈlɔdʒik(əl)] *a* 行为的 / **ethologist** *n* 行为学家
ethomoxane hydrochloride [ˌeθəuˈmɔksein] 盐酸乙氧莫生(安定药)
ethonam nitrate [ˈeθənəm] 硝酸依托南(抗真菌药)
ethopabate [ˌeθəˈpæbeit] *n* 4-乙酰氨基-2-乙氧基苯甲酸甲酯
ethopropazine hydrochloride [ˌeθəˈprəupəziːn] 盐酸普罗吩胺(抗震颤麻痹药)
ethosuximide [ˌeθəˈsʌksimaid] *n* 乙琥胺(抗惊厥药,用于治疗癫痫小发作)
ethotoin [iˈθəutəin] *n* 乙苯妥英(抗惊厥药,用于治疗癫痫大发作和精神运动性癫痫发作)
ethoxazene hydrochloride [əˈθɔksəziːn] 盐酸依托沙秦(局部镇痛药,用于缓解泌尿道感染疼痛)
ethoxzolamide [ˌeθɔksˈzɔləmaid] *n* 依索唑胺(碳酸酐酶抑制药,用于治疗青光眼和水肿)
ethybenztropine [ˌeθibenzˈtrəupiːn] *n* 乙苄托品(抗胆碱药)
ethyl [ˈeθil, ˈiːθail] *n* 乙基;乙烷基 | ~ acetate 乙酸乙酯 / ~ aminobenzoate 氨基苯甲酸乙酯,苯佐卡因 / ~ bromide 溴乙烷,乙基溴(吸入麻醉药) / ~ carbamate 氨基甲酸乙酯,尿烷 / ~ chaulmoograte 大风子酸乙酯(抗麻风药) / ~ chloride 氯乙烷(局部麻醉药) / ~ cyanide 乙基氰,丙腈 / ~ ether 乙醚 / ~ iodide 乙基碘,碘乙烷(试剂) / ~ mercaptan 乙硫醇 / ~ nitrite 亚硝酸乙酯 / ~ orange 乙橙(指示剂) / ~ oxide 氧化乙烷(极似乙醚,用作制药溶剂)
ethylaldehyde [ˌeθiˈlældihaid] *n* 乙醛
ethylamine [ˌeθiˈlæmin] *n* 乙胺
ethylate [ˈeθileit] *vt* 乙基化 [ˈeθilit] *n* 乙醇盐 | **ethylation** [ˌeθiˈleiʃən] *n* 乙基化[作用]
ethylcellulose [ˌeθilˈseljuləus] *n* 乙基纤维素
ethylene [ˈeθiliːn] *n* 乙烯 | ~ dichloride 二氯乙烷,二氯化乙烯
ethylenediamine [ˌeθiliːnˈdaiəmiːn] *n* 乙二胺
ethylenediaminetetraacetate [ˌeθiliːnˌdaiəmiːnteˈtræsiteit] *n* 依地酸盐,乙二胺四乙酸盐
ethylenediaminetetraacetic acid (EDTA) [ˌeθiliːnˌdaiəmiːnˌtetrəəˈsiːtik] 依地酸,乙二胺四乙酸(螯合剂)
ethyleneimine [ˌeθiˈliːnimiːn], **ethylenimine** [ˌeθiˈlenimiːn] *n* 乙烯亚胺,氮丙啶(一种毒性致癌化合物,其衍生物包括烷化剂用作抗肿瘤药)
ethylestrenol [ˌeθilˈestrinɔl] *n* 乙雌烯醇(雄激素,促蛋白合成类固醇)
ethylic [iˈθilik] *a* 乙基的
ethylidene [eˈθilidiːn] *n* 乙叉,亚乙基
ethylism [ˈeθilizəm] *n* 乙醇中毒,酒精中毒
ethylmalonicadipicaciduria [ˌeθilməˌlɔnikəˌdipikæsiˈdjuəriə] *n* 乙基丙二酸己二酸尿,Ⅱ型戊二酸尿
ethylmorphine hydrochloride [ˌeθilˈmɔːfiːn] 盐酸乙基吗啡
ethylnoradrenaline [ˌeθilnɔːrəˈdrenəlin] *n* 乙诺那林,乙基去甲肾上腺素(拟肾上腺素药,支气管扩张药)
ethylnorepinephrine hydrochloride [ˌeθilnɔːrepiˈnefrin] *n* 盐酸乙基去甲肾上腺素(合成拟肾上腺素药,支气管哮喘时用于缓解支气管痉挛,肌内或皮下给药)
ethylnorsuprarenin [ˌeθilnɔːsjuːprəˈrenin] *n* 乙

基去甲肾上腺素(拟肾上腺素药,支气管扩张药)
ethylparaben [ˌeθil'pærəbin] *n* 羟苯乙酯(抗真菌药,药物制剂时用作防腐药)
ethylphenylhydantoin [ˌeθilˌfenilhai'dæntəin] *n* 乙苯妥英(即 ethotoin)
ethylstibamine [ˌeθil'stibəmiːn] *n* 乙胺胺,新胺生(抗原虫药)
ethylsulfonic acid [ˌeθilsʌl'fɔnik] 乙基磺酸
ethynodiol diacetate [iˌθainə'daiəul] 双醋炔诺醇(孕激素,与雌激素合用为口服避孕药)
ethynyl [e'θainil] *n* 乙炔基
etidocaine hydrochloride [i'tiːdəkein] 盐酸依替卡因(局部麻醉药)
etidronate (EHDP) [iti'drɔneit] *n* 依替膦酸 | ~ disodium 依替膦酸二钠(用于治疗畸形性骨炎和恶性高钙血症,口服或静脉内给药)
etidronic acid [itai'drɔnik] 依替膦酸(骨钙调节药)
etiocholanolone [ˌiːtiəukəu'lænələun] *n* 本胆烷醇酮(还原尿睾酮)
etiogenic [ˌiːtiəu'dʒenik] *a* 成因的,原因的
etiolate ['iːtiəuleit] *vt* 使苍白;使衰弱;黄化,萎黄(指植物和皮肤未受日光所致 | **etiolation** [ˌiːtiəu'leiʃən] *n* 黄化
etiology [ˌiːti'ɔlədʒi] *n* 病原学,病因学 | **etiologic** [ˌiːtiə'lɔdʒik], **etiological** [ˌiːtiə'lɔdʒikəl] *a*
etiopathology [ˌiːtiəupə'θɔlədʒi] *n* 疾病发生学,发病机制(即 pathogenesis)
etioporphyrin [ˌiːtiəu'pɔːfirin] *n* 本卟啉
etiotropic [ˌiːtiəu'trɔpik] *a* 针对病因的
etiquette [ˌeti'ket] *n* (同业间的)成规 | madical ~ 医界成规
ET-NANB enterically transmitted non-A, non-B hepatitis 肠道传播非甲非乙型肝炎
etodolac [itəu'dəulæk] *n* 依托度酸(非甾体消炎药,用于镇痛和抗感染,尤用于治疗关节炎,口服给药)
etodolic acid [itəu'dəulik] 依托度酸(即 etodolac)
etofenamate [itəu'fenəmeit] *n* 依托芬那酯(消炎镇痛药)
etoformin hydrochloride [ˌetə'fɔːmin] 盐酸依托福明(抗糖尿病药)
etomidate [i'tɔmideit] *n* 依托咪酯(镇静催眠药)
etoposide [itəu'pəusaid] *n* 依托泊苷(抗肿瘤药)
etoprine ['etəpriːn] *n* 氯苯乙嘧胺(抗肿瘤药)
etorphine [i'tɔːfiːn] *n* 埃托啡(镇痛药)
etoxadrol hydrochloride [i'tɔksədrəul] 盐酸乙苯噁啶(麻醉药)
etozolin [ˌetə'zəulin] *n* 依托唑啉(利尿药)
etretinate [i'tretineit] *n* 阿维 A 酯(抗银屑病药)
etrotomy [i'trɔtəmi] *n* 下腹切开术(耻骨弓上切开)
etryptamine acetate [i'triptəmin] 醋酸乙色胺(曾用作中枢兴奋药,因有严重毒性反应现不再发售)
Eu europium 铕
eu- [构词成分]好,佳,优,正常,真
euadrenocorticism [ˌjuːəˌdrinəu'kɔːtisizəm] *n* 肾上腺皮质功能正常
euallele [juə'liːl] *n* 优等位基因(两个同源染色体中个别作用子的同一密码子发生突变) | **euallelic** [juə'liːlik] *a*
euangiotic [ˌjuːændʒi'ɔtik] *a* 血管丰富的
Euascomycetidae [juːˌæskəumai'siːtidiː] *n* 真子囊菌亚纲
eubacteria [ˌjuːbæk'tiəriə] *n* 真细菌
Eubacteriales [ˌjuːbæktiəri'eiliːz] *n* 真细菌目
Eubacterium [ˌjuːbæk'tiəriəm] *n* 真细菌属 | ~ alactolyticum 不解乳真细菌 / ~ lentum 迟缓真细菌
eubacterium [ˌjuːbæk'tiəriəm] *n* 真细菌
eubiotics [ˌjuːbai'ɔtiks] *n* 摄生学
eucaine ['juːkein] *n* 优卡因(作用类似可卡因)
eucalyptol [ˌjuːkə'liptɔl] *n* 桉油醇,桉树脑(祛痰、局部麻醉、驱虫药)
Eucalyptus [ˌjuːkə'liptəs] *n* 桉树属
eucapnia [juː'kæpniə] *n* 血碳酸正常 | **eucapnic** [juː'kæpnik] *a*
eucaryon [juː'kæriɔn] *n* 真核,真核生物
eucaryosis [ˌjuːkæri'əusis] *n* 真核形成
Eucaryotae [juːˌkæri'əutiː] *n* 真核生物界
eucaryote [juː'kæriəut] *n* 真核生物
eucaryotic [ˌjuːkæri'ɔtik] *a* 真核的;真核生物的
eucatropine hydrochloride [juː'kætrəpiːn] *n* 盐酸尤卡托品(散瞳药)
Eucestoda [juːses'təudə] *n* 多节亚纲,真绦虫类(即 Cestoda)
euchlorhydria [ˌjuːklɔː'haidriə] *n* 胃液[游离]盐酸正常
eucholia [juː'kəuliə] *n* 胆汁正常
euchromatin [juː'krəumətin] *n* 常染色质 | **euchromatic** [juːkrəu'mætik] *a*
euchromatopsy [juː'krəuməˌtɔpsi] *n* 色觉正常
euchromosome [juː'krəuməsəum] *n* 常染色体
euchylia [juː'kiliə] *n* 乳糜正常
Euciliatia [juːˌsili'eiʃiə] *n* 真纤毛亚纲
Eucoccidia [ˌjuːkɔk'sidiə] *n* 真球虫目
eucoelom [juː'siːləm] *n* 体腔
Eucoelomata [ˌjuːsiːlə'meitə] *n* 体腔动物门
eucoelomate [juː'siːləmeit] *n* 体腔动物
eucolloid [juː'kɔlɔid] *n* 真胶体,大粒胶体
eucrasia [juː'kreisiə] *n* 体质健全,体质正常
eudiemorrhysis [ˌjuːdaiə'mɔrisis] *n* 毛细管血行

正常

eudiometer [ˌjuːdiˈɔmitə] *n* 空气纯度测定仪 | **eudiometric(al)** [ˌjuːdiəˈmetrik(əl)] *a* 空气纯度测定仪的;空气纯度测定[法]的 / **eudiometry** *n* 空气纯度测定法

eudipsia [juːˈdipsiə] *n* 渴感正常

euergasia [ˌjuːəˈgeiziə] *n* 精神整体反应正常,精神健康

euesthesia [ˌjuːisˈθiːzjə] *n* 感觉正常

Euflagellata [juːˌflædʒeˈleitə] *n* 真鞭毛虫目(即 Mastigophora)

euflavine [juːˈfleivin] *n* 吖啶黄(消毒防腐药)

eugamy [ˈjuːgəmi] *n* 整倍配合

Eugenia [juːˈdʒiːniə] *n* 丁子香属,番樱桃属

eugenic [juːˈdʒenik] *a* 优生的

eugenic acid [juːˈdʒenik] 丁子香酚,丁香酸

eugenicist [juːˈdʒenisist], **eugenist** [ˈjuːdʒenist, -ˈdʒe-] *n* 优生学家

eugenics [juːˈdʒeniks] *n* 优生学 | negative ~ 消极优生学(防止具有低劣或不良的遗传性状者生育) / positive ~ 积极优生学(鼓励具有优良或所需的遗传性状者优质生育)

eugenism [ˈjuːdʒənizəm] *n* 优生论

eugenol [ˈjuːdʒənɔl] *n* 丁香酚(牙镇痛药)

eugenothenics [juːˌdʒiːnəˈθeniks] *n* 优生优境学(调整遗传和环境的因素以改良种族素质)

Euglena [juːˈgliːnə] *n* 眼虫属

Euglenamorpha [juːˌglenəˈmɔːfə] *n* 眼形虫属

Euglenamorphina [juːˌgliːnəmɔːˈfainə] *n* 眼形虫亚目

euglenid [juːˈglinid] *n* 眼虫

Euglenida [juːˈgliːnidə] *n* 眼虫目

Euglenina [ˌjuːgliˈnainə] *n* 眼虫亚目

euglenoid [juːˈglinɔid] *a* 眼虫的,眼虫目的 *n* 眼虫

Euglenoidina [juːˌglinɔiˈdainə] *n* 眼虫目

euglobulin [juːˈglɔbjulin] *n* 优球蛋白(其特征为不溶于水而溶于盐溶液)

euglycemia [ˌjuːglaiˈsiːmiə] *n* 血糖正常 | **euglycemic** *a*

Euglypha [juːˈglifə] *n* 鳞壳虫属

eugnathia [juːˈneiθiə] *n* 上下颌正常 | **eugnathic** [juːˈnæθik] *a*

eugnosia [juːˈnəusiə] *n* 感觉正常,知觉正常 | **eugnostic** [juˈnɔstik] *a*

eugonadotropic [juːˌgɔnədəuˈtrɔpik] *a* 正常促性[腺]激素的

eugonic [juːˈgɔnik] *a* 生长旺盛的(指细菌培养)

Eugregarinida [ˌjuːgregəˈrainidə] *n* 真簇虫目

euhydration [juːhaiˈdreiʃən] *n* 水合正常,水分正常

eukaryon [juːˈkæriɔn] *n* 真核;真核生物

eukaryosis [ˌjuːkæriˈəusis] *n* 真核形成

Eukaryotae [juːˌkæriˈəutiː] *n* 真核生物界

eukaryote [juːˈkæriəut] *n* 真核生物

eukaryotic [ˌjuːkæriˈɔtik] *a* 真核的;真核生物的

eukeratin [juːˈkerətin] *n* 优角蛋白

eukinesia [ˌjuːkaiˈniːsiə, -kiˈn-], **eukinesis** [ˌjuːkaiˈniːsis, -kiˈn-] *n* 运动正常,动作正常 | **eukinetic** [ˌjuːkaiˈnetik, -kiˈn-] *a*

eulachon [ˈjuːləkɔn] *n* 香烛鱼(其油的应用和鱼肝油相似)

eulaminate [juːˈlæmineit] *a* 层数正常的(如大脑皮质某几个区)

Eulenburg's disease [ˈɔilənbəːg] (Albert Eulenburg) 先天性肌强直

eumelanin [juːˈmelənin] *n* [真]黑色素

eumenorrhea [ˌjuːmenəˈriə] *n* 月经正常

Eumetazoa [juːˌmetəˈzəuə] *n* 真后生动物

eumetria [juːˈmiːtriə] *n*【希】神经冲动正常

eumorphism [juːˈmɔːfizəm] *n* 形态正常(细胞)

Eumycetes [ˌjuːmaiˈsiːtiːz] *n* 真菌纲

eumycetoma [ˌjuːmaisiˈtəumə] *n* 真足菌肿,真菌性足分支菌病

Eumycetozoea [ˌjuːmaiˌsiːtəuˈzəuiə] *n* 真胶丝菌纲

eumycin [juːˈmaisin] *n* 优霉素

Eumycophyta [juːˌmaikəuˈfaitə] *n* 真菌纲

Eumycota [ˌjuːmaiˈkəutə] *n* 真菌门

eunuch [ˈjuːnək] *n* 去睾者,无睾者,阉人,去势者(青春期前去除睾丸)

eunuchism [ˈjuːnəkizəm] *n* 去势状态,阉病,无睾症,去睾症 | pituitary ~ 垂体性无睾症

eunuchoid [ˈjuːnəkɔid] *a* 类无睾者的 *n* 类无睾者,类无睾

eunuchoidism [ˈjuːnəˌkɔidizəm] *n* 类无睾症 | female ~ 女性类无睾症 / hypergonadotropic ~ 促性腺激素亢进性类无睾症 / hypogonadotropic ~ 促性腺激素不足性类无睾症

euosmia [juːˈɔsmiə] *n* 嗅觉正常;愉快气味

eupancreatism [juːˈpæŋkriəˌtizəm] *n* 胰腺功能正常

eupatorin [ˌjuːpəˈtɔːrin] *n* 佩兰素

Eupatorium [ˌjuːpəˈtɔːriəm] *n* 佩兰属

eupepsia [juːˈpepsiə], **eupepsy** [juːˈpepsi] *n* 消化[力]正常 | **eupeptic** *a*

euperistalsis [juːˌperiˈstælsis] *n* 蠕动正常,蠕动良好

euphenics [juːˈfeniks] *n* 优型学(通过化学的或外科的方法而改变遗传病患者的表型)

Euphorbia [juːˈfɔːbiə] *n* 大戟属

euphoretic [ˌjuːfəˈretik], **euphoriant** [juːˈfɔriənt] *a* 欣快的 *n* 欣快剂

euphoria [juːˈfɔːriə] *n* 欣快 | **euphoric** *a*

euphorigenic [juːˌfɔːriˈdʒenik], **euphoristic** [ˌjuː-fəˈristik] *a* 致欣快的

euphoropsia [ˌjuːfɔːˈrɔpsiə] *n* 视觉舒适

euplastic [juːˈplæstik] *a* 容易机化的,适于组织形成的(如胚胎发育和伤口愈合时)

euploid [ˈjuːplɔid] *a* 整倍体的 *n* 整倍体(指个体或细胞含有整组染色组) | **~y** [juːˈplɔidi] *n* 整倍性

eupnea [juːpˈniːə] *n* 平静呼吸 | **eupneic** [juːp-ˈniːik] *a*

eupraxia [juːˈpræksiə] *n* 【希】协同动作正常 | **eupractic** [juːˈpræktik] *a* 协同动作正常的,促协同动作正常的

eupraxic [juːˈpræksik] *a* 功能正常的;协同动作正常的

euprocin hydrochloride [ˈjuːprəsin] 盐酸尤普罗辛(局部麻醉药)

Euproctis [juːˈprɔktis] *n* 蠹属 | ~ chrysorrhoea (phaeorrhoea) 褐尾蠹

eupyrene [juːˈpaiəriːn], **eupyrous** [juːˈpaiərəs] *a* 有正常核的

eupyrexia [ˌjuːpaiəˈreksiə] *n* 微热

eurhythmia [juəˈriθmiə] *n* 发育均匀;脉搏正常

europium(Eu) [juəˈrəupiəm] *n* 铕(化学元素)

Eurotiaceae [juəˌrəuʃiˈeisiiː] *n* 曲霉菌科

Eurotiales [juəˌrəuʃiˈeiliːz] *n* 曲霉菌目

Eurotium [juəˈrəuʃiəm] *n* 曲霉菌属 | ~ malignum 恶性曲霉菌 / ~ repens 熟物曲霉菌

Eurotransplant [ˌjuərəˈtrænsplɑːnt] *n* 欧洲国家器官储存运输组织

eury- [构词成分]阔

eurycephalic [ˌjuərisəˈfælik], **eurycephalous** [ˌjuəriˈsefələs], **eurycranial** [ˌjuəriˈkreinjəl] *a* 阔头的

eurygnathism [juəˈrignəθizəm] *n* 阔颌[状态] | **eurygnathic** [ˌjuərigˈnæθik] *a* 阔颌的

euryon [ˈjuəriən] *n* 颅阔点

euryopia [ˌjuəriˈəupiə] *n* 阔眼裂

Eurypelma [ˌjuəriˈpelmə] *n* 毒[蜘]蛛属 | ~ hentzii 美洲毒[蜘]蛛

euryphotic [ˌjuəriˈfəutik] *a* 广光性的,宽光域的

eurysomatic [ˌjuərisəuˈmætik] *a* 阔体的

Eurysporina [ˌjuərispɔːˈrainə] *n* 阔孢亚目

eurytherm [ˈjuəriθəːm] *n* 广温生物 | **~al** [ˌjuəriˈθəːməl], **~ous** [ˌjuəriˈθəːməs], **~ic(al)** [ˌjuəriˈθəːmik(əl)] *a* 广温的

eurytopic [ˌjuəriˈtɔpik] *a* 广适性的 | **~ity** [ˌjuəritəuˈpisəti] *n*

Eurytrema [juːriˈtriːmə] *n* 阔盘[吸虫]属

Euscorpius [juːˈskɔːpiəs] *n* 真蝎属 | ~ italicus 意大利真蝎

Eusimulium [ˌjuːsiˈmjuːliəm] *n* 真蚋属

eusitia [juːˈsitiə] *n* 食欲正常

euspermic [juːˈspəːmik] *a* 精子正常的

eusplanchnia [juːˈsplæŋkniə] *n* 内脏正常

eusplenia [juːˈspliːniə] *n* 脾功能正常

eustachian [juːsˈteiʃjən, juːsˈteikiən] (Bartolommeo Eustachio) *a* 欧氏的,咽鼓管的 | ~ canal, ~ tube 咽鼓管 / ~ cartilage 咽鼓管软骨 / ~ catheterization 咽鼓管导管吹张术 / ~ valve 下腔静脉瓣

eustachitis [ˌjuːsteiˈkaitis] *n* 咽鼓管炎

eustachium [juːsˈteikjəm] *n* 咽鼓管

eusthenia [juːˈsθeniə] *n* 体力正常,强壮

eusthenuria [ˌjuːsθeˈnjuəriə] *n* 正渗尿,尿浓缩正常

Eustrongylus [juːˈstrɔndʒiləs] *n* 真圆虫属 | ~ gigas 肾膨结线虫(即 Dioctophyma renale)

eusystole [juːˈsistəli] *n* 心收缩正常 | **eusystolic** [ˌjuːsisˈtɔlik] *a*

Eutamias [juːˈtæmiəs] *n* 金花鼠

eutectic [juːˈtektik] *a* 易熔的,低共熔的(指低熔混合物)

eutelegenesis [juːˌteliˈdʒenisis] *n* 育种人工授精法,优种授精

eutelolecithal [juːˌteləˈlesiθəl] *a* 端黄卵的

euthanasia [ˌjuːθəˈneizjə] *n* 安乐死,安死术(为不治之症患者施行的一种无痛苦死亡术)

euthenic [juːˈθenik] *a* 优境的 | **~s** *n* 优境学

eutherapeutic [juːˌθerəˈpjuːtik] *a* 良效的,疗效好的

Eutheria [juːˈθiəriə] *n* 真兽亚纲

eutherian [juːˈθiəriən] *a* 真兽亚纲的

euthermic [juːˈθəːmik] *a* 增温的

euthymia [juːˈaimiə] *n* 心境愉快,情感正常

euthymism [juːˈθaimizəm] *n* 胸腺功能正常

Euthyneura [juːθiˈnjuərə] *n* 真神经亚纲

euthyphoria [ˌjuːθiˈfəuriə] *n* 直视(视轴正常)

euthyroidism [juːˈθairɔidizəm] *n* 甲状腺功能正常 | **euthyroid** *a*

eutocia [juːˈtəusiə] *n* 顺产,正常分娩

eutopic [juːˈtɔpik] *a* 位置正常的,正位的

Eutreptiina [juːˌtreptiˈainə] *n* 二毛眼虫亚目

Eutriatoma [ˌjuːtriˈætəmə] *n* 真锥蝽属

Eutrombicula [ˌjuːtrɔmˈbikjulə] *n* 真恙螨亚属 | ~ alfreddugèsi 阿氏真恙螨,致痒恙螨 / ~ splendens 华丽真恙螨

eutrophia [juːˈtrəufiə] *n* 营养佳良

eutrophic [juːˈtrɔfik] *a* 营养佳良的;(湖泊等)富营养的

eutrophication [ˌjuːtrəufiˈkeiʃən] *n* (水体的)富营养化[作用]
euvolia [juːˈvəuliə] *n* 正常水含量,液量正常
euxanthon [juːˈzænθɔn] *n* 优咕吨酮,二羟[基]夹氧杂蒽酮
eV, ev electron volt 电子伏[特]
evacuant [iˈvækjuənt] *a* 排泄的,排除的 *n* 排空药(如泻药、吐药或利尿药)
evacuate [iˈvækjueit] *vt* 排泄,排除,排空 *vi* 排粪,排便 | **evacuative** *a* / **evacuator** *n* 排出器 / **evacuation** [iˌvækjuˈeiʃən] *n*
evaginate [iˈvædʒineit] *vt* 外翻;外突,凸出
evagination [iˌvædʒiˈneiʃən] *n* 外翻;外突,凸出 | optic ~ 视外突,眼泡
Evaginogenina [iˌvædʒinəudʒiˈnainə] *n* 外凸亚目
evaluation [iˌvæljuˈeiʃən] *n* 评估 | preanesthetic ~ 麻醉前病情评估
evanescent [ˌiːvəˈnesnt, ˌevə-] *a* 易消散的;短暂的,瞬息的 | **evanescence** *n* 消失,消散
Evans' syndrome [ˈevənz] (Robert S. Evans) 埃文斯综合征(获得性溶血性贫血和血小板减少)
evaporable [iˈvæpərəbl] *a* 可蒸发的;挥发的
evaporate [iˈvæpəreit] *vt* 蒸发;脱水;发射(电子) *vi* 蒸发,发散 | **evaporation** [iˌvæpəˈreiʃən] *n* / **evaporative** *a* 蒸发的 / **evaporator** *n* 蒸发器
evasion [iˈveiʒən] *n* 逃避,回避;借口
eventration [ˌiːvenˈtreiʃən] *n* 腹脏突出;腹脏除去法 | diaphragmatic ~ 膈膨生 / umbilical ~ 脐突出
Eversbusch's operation [ˈeivɛəzbuʃ] (Oskar Eversbusch) 上睑下垂矫正术
eversible [iˈvəːsəbl] *a* 可外翻的,可翻转的
eversion [iˈvəːʃən] *n* 外翻
evert [iˈvəːt] *vt* 外翻,翻转
evertor [iˈvəːtə] *n* 外翻肌
Eve's method [iːv] (Frank C. Eve) 伊夫人工呼吸法(将患者脸向下躺在担架上,用毛毯裹住,腕与踝绑在把手上,然后举起加以摇动,先作头向下倾斜 50°,以产生满意的呼气,然后脚向下倾斜 50°,以产生满意的吸气,这样每次以 50°角摇动,每分钟摇 12 次)
évidement [eiviːdˈmɔŋ] *n*【法】挖除法
évideur [eiviˈdəː] *n*【法】挖除器
evil [ˈiːvl] [疾]病 | quarter ~ 气肿性炭疽,黑腿病 / St. John's ~ 圣约翰病,癫痫 / St. Main's ~ 圣梅因病,疥疮 / St. Martin's ~ 圣马丁病,醇中毒,乙醇中毒
evirate [ˈiːvireit] *vt* 阉割 | **eviration** [ˌiːviˈreiʃən] *n* 阉,阉割;去势,女性化;变女妄想
eviscerate [iˈvisəreit] *vt* 切除内脏;切除(或剜出)器官内容物 *vi* (手术后患部切口处)凸出(如内脏) | **evisceration** [iˌvisəˈreiʃən] *n* 除脏术;脏器除去术;眼内容摘除术(巩膜仍完好)
evocation [ˌevəuˈkeiʃən] *n* 诱发,启发,唤起(经由与组织原接触而唤起形态建成的潜势力)
evocator [ˈevəukeitə] *n* 唤起物,诱发物(由胚胎组织原区产生的化学物质,如与接触,能使胚胎组织诱发特异性形态反应)
evoke [iˈvəuk] *vt* 唤醒;引起
evolution [ˌiːvəˈljuːʃən, ˌevə-] *n* 进化,演化;(气体、热等)放出;旋出(胎儿);先成说,预成说(见 preformation) | bathmic ~, orthogenic ~ 直向进化 / convergent ~ 趋同进化 / determinate ~ 直向进化,定向进化 / emergent ~ 突然进化 / organic ~ 生物进化 / saltatory ~ 飞跃进化 / spontaneous ~ 自然旋出(指横卧胎儿) | **~al, ~ary** *a*
evolutionist [ˌiːvəˈljuːʃənist, ˌevə-] *n* 进化论者 *a* 进化的;进化论的;进化论者的 | **evolutionism** *n* 进化论 / **~ic** [ˌiːvəˌljuːʃəˈnistik] *a*
evolve [iˈvɔlv] *vt* 发展;(气体、热等)放出;进化 *vi* 进展;进化;发育 | **~ment** *n*
evulsio [iˈvʌlsiəu] *n*【拉】撕去
evulsion [iˈvʌlʃən] *n* 撕去 | ~ of eyeball 眼球撕脱
Ewart's sign [ˈjuːət] (William Ewart) 尤尔特征(心包积液征:第一肋骨胸骨端过分隆凸;叩诊左肩胛下角可听到支气管呼吸音和浊音)
evulsion [iˈvʌlʃən] *n* 撕脱
Ewart's sign [ˈjuːət] (William Ewart) 尤尔特征(心包积液征:第一肋骨胸骨端过分隆凸;叩诊左肩胛下角可听到支气管呼吸音和浊音)
Ewingella [ˌjuːiŋˈelə] *n* 尤因杆菌属
Ewing's tumor (sarcoma) [ˈjuːiŋ] (James Ewing) 尤因瘤(肉瘤)(内皮细胞性骨髓瘤)
ex- [前缀]出,离;从;除
exa- [构词成分]艾[可萨] = (10^{18},符号为 E)
exacerbate [ekˈsæsə(ː)beit, igˈz-] *vt* 使(疾病或症状)加重,转剧,恶化 | **exacerbation** [ekˌsæsə(ː)ˈbeiʃən, igˌz-] *n*
exairesis [ekˈserisis] *n*【希】切除术
exalt [igˈzɔːlt] *vt* 使喜悦 *vi* 使人兴奋 | **~ation** [ˌegzɔːlˈteiʃən] *n* 升高;提拔;[异常]兴奋,激越;情感高涨
exametazime [ˌeksəˈmetəziːm] *n* 依沙美肟(即 HMPAO 六甲丙烯胺肟,与 ^{99m}Tc 络合用于大脑局部血流成像,以检测卒中时已改变的局部灌注、鉴别阿尔茨海默〈Alzheimer〉病,评价癫痫以及诊断脑死亡)
examination [igˌzæmiˈneiʃən] *n* 检查;诊察 | double-contrast ~ 双对比检查 / physical ~ 体格检查

exania [ek'seiniə] *n* 脱肛
exanimate [ig'zænimit] *a* 已死的,无生命的;意气消沉的
exanimation [igˌzæni'meiʃən, eg-] *n* 晕厥,昏迷
exanthem [ig'zænθəm, eg-] *n* 疹病;疹 | Boston ~ 波士顿疹(伴人肠道细胞病变孤儿病毒16,但无淋巴结病) | **~atous** [ˌegzæn'θemətəs] *a* 疹的;发疹的
exanthema [ˌegzæn'θiːmə, ˌeks-] ([复] **exanthemas** 或 **exanthemata** [ˌegzæn'θemətə]) *n* 【希】疹病;疹 | ~ subitum 婴儿玫瑰疹,幼儿急疹
exanthrope ['ekzænθrəup] *n* 疾病外因,体外病因 | **exanthropic** [ˌekzæn'θrɔpik] *a*
exarticulation [ˌeksɑːtikju'leiʃən] *n* 关节切断术,关节断离术
exasperate [ig'zɑːspəreit] *vt* 激怒;使(疾病、痛苦等)加剧,使恶化 [ig'zɑːspərit] *a* 具硬突起的,[表面]粗糙的 | **exasperation** [igˌzɑːspə'reiʃən] *n* 激怒;加剧,恶化
excalation [ˌekskə'leiʃən] *n* 部分缺失(正常连续部分的缺失,如脊椎)
excarnation [ˌekskɑː'neiʃən] *n* 修切标本
excavate ['ekskəveit] *vt* 挖,凿 *vi* 凿;挖掘;使变成空洞
excavatio [ˌekskə'veiʃiəu] ([复] **excavationes** [ˌekskəveiʃi'əuniːz]) *n* 【拉】陷凹
excavation [ˌekskə'veiʃən] *n* 挖除;陷凹 | atrophic ~ 萎缩性(视神经盘)陷凹 / dental ~ 龋质挖除 / glaucomatous ~ 青光眼性陷凹 / ischiorectal ~, rectoischiadic ~ 坐骨直肠窝 / ~ of optic disk, physiologic ~ 视[神经]盘陷凹,生理性陷凹
excavator ['ekskəˌveitə] *n* 挖治器
excelsin [ek'selsin] *n* 巴西果蛋白
excementosis [ekˌsiːmən'təusis] *n* 牙骨质增生
excerebration [ˌekseri'breiʃən] *n* 去脑术,大脑切除[法](主要用于碎胎术)
excernent [ek'səːnənt] *a* 促排泄的
excess [ik'ses, 'eks-] *n* 过量,过剩;超过;过度 *a* 过量的;额外的;过度的 | antibody ~ 抗体过剩 / antigen ~ 抗原过剩 | **~ive** *a* 过多的;极度的
exchange [iks'tʃeindʒ] *n* 交换 | plasma ~ 血浆交换 / sister chromatid ~ 姐妹染色单体交换
exchanger [iks'tʃeindʒə] *n* 交换器 | heat ~ 热交换器(体外循环时用)
excipient [ik'sipiənt] *n* 赋形剂
excise [ek'saiz] *vt* 切除;删去 | **excision** [ek'siʒən] *n* 切除[术]
excitable [ik'saitəbl] *a* 应激的,[可]兴奋的 | **excitability** [ikˌsaitə'biləti] *n* 兴奋性

excitant ['eksitənt, ik'saitənt] *a* 刺激性的,使兴奋的 *n* 兴奋剂,刺激物
excitation [ˌeksi'teiʃən, -sai-] *n* 刺激,兴奋;激发 | anomalous atrioventricular ~ 异常房室兴奋,预激综合征 / direct ~ 直接刺激(电极放置肌肉上) / indirect ~ 间接刺激(电极放置神经上)
excitative [ek'saitətiv] *a* 刺激性的;兴奋性的;激发的
excitatory [ek'saitətəri] *a* 刺激性的,兴奋性的;起异化作用的
excitement [ik'saitmənt] *n* 兴奋 | psychomotor ~ 精神运动性兴奋
excitoanabolic [ekˌsaitəuˌænə'bɔlik] *a* 促合成代谢的
excitocatabolic [ekˌsaitəuˌkætə'bɔlik] *a* 促分解代谢的
excitoglandular [ekˌsaitəu'glændjulə] *a* 兴奋腺体的
excitometabolic [ekˌsaitəuˌmetə'bɔlik] *a* 促代谢的
excitomotor [ekˌsaitəu'məutə], **excitomotory** [ekˌsaitəu'məutəri] *a* 兴奋运动的 *n* 激动剂
excitomuscular [əkˌsaitəu'mʌskjulə] *a* 兴奋肌肉的
excitonutrient [əkˌsaitəu'njuːtriənt] *a* 兴奋营养的
excitor [ik'saitə, ek's-] *n* 刺激神经
excitosecretory [ekˌsaitəusi'kriːtəri] *a* 兴奋分泌的
excitotoxic [ek'saitəuˌtɔksik] *a* 兴奋毒的 | **~ity** [ekˌsaitəutɔk'sisəti] *n* 兴奋毒性;兴奋毒力
excitotoxin [ekˌsaitəu'tɔksin] *n* 兴奋毒素(任何一类致神经毒性物质,存在于某些植物中或合成制得,类似谷氨酸并模仿它对中枢神经系统的神经元产生兴奋作用,并在核周体上造成损害)
excitovascular [ekˌsaitəu'væskjulə] *a* 兴奋血管的
exclave ['ekskleiv] *n* 内脏游离部(如胰腺或其他腺)
exclusion [ik'skluːʒən, ek's-] *n* 排斥;排除,除外;分离术(仅使器官的一部分与原器官分离而并不切除) | allelic ~ 等位性排斥 / competitive ~ 竞争性排斥
exclusive [ik'skluːsiv] *a* 排外的;专有的;唯一的;全部的
excochleation [eksˌkɔkli'eiʃən] *n* 刮除术
exconjugant [eks'kɔndʒuːgənt] *n* 接合后体(原虫)
excoriate [ek'skɔːrieit] *vt* 擦伤…的皮肤;剥皮
excoriation [ekˌskɔːri'eiʃən] *n* 抓痕,表皮脱落 | neurotic ~ 神经官能症性表皮剥脱

excrement [ˈekskrimənt] *n* 粪便 | **~al** [ˌekskriˈmentl], **~itious** [ˌekskrimenˈtiʃəs] *a*
excrescence [ikˈskresns] *n* 赘生物,赘疣 | fungating ~, fungous ~ 蕈样赘生物,脐肉芽肿 | **excrescent** *a*
excreta [ekˈskriːtə] [复] *n* 排泄物 | **~l** *a*
excrete [ekˈskriːt] *vt* 排泄,分泌
excretin [ˈekskriːtin] *n* [人]粪素;促胰外泌素
excretion [ekˈskriːʃən] *n* 排泄 | fractional ~ of sodium 钠排泄分数 / pseudouridine ~ 假尿[嘧啶核]苷排泄
excretory [ekˈskriːtəri, ˈekskrə-] *a* 排泄的;促排泄的
excruciate [ikˈskruːʃieit] *vt* 折磨;使苦恼 | **excruciation** [ikˌskruːʃiˈeiʃən] *n* 剧痛;苦恼
excruciating [ikˈskruːʃieitiŋ] *a* 非常痛苦的;剧痛的;极度的,剧烈的
excurrent [ekˈskʌrənt] *a* 排泄的;传出的
excursion [ikˈskəːʃən, ekˈs-] *n* 离题;移动 | lateral ~ 侧移动(颌) / protrusive ~ 前移动(颌) / retrusive ~ 后移动(颌)
excursive [ekˈskəːsiv] *a* 离题的;移动性的
excyclophoria [ˌeksaikləuˈfəuriə] *n* 外旋转隐斜
excyclotropia [ˌeksaikləuˈtrəupiə] *n* 外旋转斜视
excystation [ˌeksisˈteiʃən] *n* 脱囊
exelcin [ekˈselsin] *n* 埃克塞辛(巴西果浸出物)
exelcymosis [ˌekselsaiˈməusis] *n* 拔除(如拔牙)
exemestane [ˌeksəˈmestein] *n* 依西美坦(抗肿瘤药)
exemia [ekˈsiːmiə] *n* 浓缩血[症]
exencephalus [ˌeksenˈsefələs], **exencephalon** [ˌeksenˈsefələn] *n* 露脑畸胎
exencephaly [ˌeksenˈsefəli], **exencephalia** [ˌeksensiˈfeiliə] *n* 露脑 | **exencephalous** [ˌeksenˈsefələs] *a*
exenterate [ekˈsentəreit] *vt* 去除(眼眶、盆腔的)内容物 | **exenteration** [ekˌsentəˈreiʃən] *n* 去脏术,脏器除去术(通常指盆腔廓清术,眼科中为眶内容摘除术) / **exenterative** *a* 去脏术的,挖出术的
exenteritis [ekˌsentəˈraitis] *n* 肠腹膜炎,肠浆膜炎
exercise [ˈeksəsaiz] *n* 锻炼,体操,操练,运动 | active ~ 主动运动(肌肉) / active resistive ~ 主动抗阻运动 / corrective ~, therapeutic ~ 矫形体操,医疗体操 / free ~ 自由操练,主动运动(不借外力协助) / muscle-setting ~, static ~ 肌静态操练,原位运动 / passive ~ 被动运动 / underwater ~ 水中运动
exercitation [egˌzəːsiˈteiʃən] *n* 实习,训练
exeresis [ekˈsəːrisis] *n* 切除术
exergic [ekˈsəːdʒik] *a* 放能的(指化学反应)
exergonic [ˌeksəˈgɔnik] *a* 能量释放的,放能的
exertion [igˈzəːʃən] *n* 用力,劳力,劳累;运用
exertional [igˈzəːʃənl] *a* 劳累性的
exesion [egˈziːʒən] *n* 腐蚀
exfetation [ˌeksfiːˈteiʃən] *n* 宫外孕
exflagellation [ˌeksflædʒeˈleiʃən] *n* 鞭毛突出,小配子形成
exfoliate [eksˈfəulieit] *vt*, *vi* 表皮脱落,鳞片样脱皮,表皮剥脱
exfoliatin [eksˌfəuliˈeitin] *n* 脱叶霉素,脱叶菌素,[表皮]剥脱素
exfoliatio [ˌeksfəuliˈeiʃiəu] *n*【拉】表皮脱落,鳞片样脱皮,表皮剥脱 | ~ areata linguae 良性迁移性舌炎,地图样舌
exfoliation [ˌeksfəuliˈeiʃən] *n* 表皮剥脱 | lamellar ~ of the newborn 新生儿层板状脱落 / **exfoliative** [eksˈfəuliˌeitiv] *a*
exhalant [eksˈheilənt, egˈzeilənt] *a* 呼出的;蒸发[性]的;发散[性]的 *n* 发散管,蒸发管
exhale [eksˈheil, egˈzeil] *vi* 呼气;蒸发,发散 *vt* 呼出;发散出 | **exhalation** [eks*h*əˈleiʃən, egzəˈleiʃən] *n* 蒸发;发散物(如气体、气味);呼出,呼气
exhaust [igˈzɔːst] *vt* 抽空,汲干;用完,耗尽;疲竭 *vi* 排出(气体等) *n* 排出;排气(或水等);排气装置 | **exhaustible** [igˈzɔːstəbl] *a* 可耗尽的,会枯竭的
exhaustion [igˈzɔːstʃən] *n* 耗尽;抽空;排除,排尽;衰竭,虚脱 | heat ~ 热衰竭 / nervous ~ 神经衰弱,脑力衰竭
Exhib. exhibeatur【拉】须给予
exhibit [igˈzibit] *vt* 展览,陈列;显示;投(药),给(药) *vi* 展出
exhibition [ˌeksiˈbiʃən] *n* 显示;投药
exhibitionism [ˌeksiˈbiʃənizəm] *n* 露阴癖 | **exhibitionist** *n* 露阴癖者 / **exhibitionistic** [ˌeksiˌbiʃəˈnistik] *a*
exhibitive [igˈzibitiv] *a* 起显示作用的,表示的
exhibitory [igˈzibitəri] *a* 显示的,表示的
exhilarant [igˈzilərənt] *a* 使欢乐的,提神的 *n* 欢乐剂,提神剂
exhume [eksˈhjuːm] *vt* 掘出,发掘(尸体) | **exhumation** [ˌekshjuːˈmeiʃən] *n* 尸体发掘
exiguous [egˈzigjuəs] *a* 稀少的,微小的 | **exiguity** [ˌeksiˈgjuːəti] *n*
exist [igˈzist] *vi* 存在;生存
existence [igˈzistəns] *n* 存在;生存 | struggle for ~ 生存,竞争
existent [igˈzistənt] *a* 存在的,现存的;目前的 *n* 生存者
existing [igˈzistiŋ] *a* 存在的,现存的;目前的
exit [ˈeksit, ˈegzit] *n* 出口,太平门 | ~ of wound

tract 伤道出口
exitus [ˈeksitəs] [单复同] *n*【拉】死亡;出口 | ~ pelvis 骨盆下口
Exner's plexus [ˈeksnə] (Siegmund Exner) *n* 埃克斯内神经丛,分子丛(接近大脑皮质表面的一层神经纤维)
exo- [前缀]外,在外
exo-amylase [ˌeksəuˈæmileis] *n* 外淀粉酶,β-淀粉酶(即 β-amylase)
exoantigen [ˌeksəuˈæntidʒən] *n* 外抗原(见 ectoantigen)
exoatmosphere [ˌeksəuˈætməsfiə] *n* 外大气层 | **exoatmospheric** [ˌeksəuætməsˈferik] *a*
exobiology [ˌeksəubaiˈɔlədʒi] *n* 宇宙生物学,外[层]空[间]生物学 | **exobiological** [ˌeksəuˌbaiəˈlɔdʒikəl] *a* / **exobiologist** *n* 宇宙生物学者,外[层]空[间]生物学者
exocardia [ˌeksəuˈkɑːdiə] *n* 异位心
exocardial [ˌeksəuˈkɑːdiəl] *a* 心外的
exocarp [ˈeksəukɑːp] *n* 外果皮
exocataphoria [ˌeksəuˌkætəˈfəuriə] *n* 外下隐斜
exocele [ˈeksəusiːl] *n* 外腔,胚外体腔
exocellular [ˌeksəuˈseljulə] *a* 胞外的(细胞膜外的)
exocervix [ˌeksəuˈsəːviks] *n* 外宫颈(宫颈阴道部)
exochorion [ˌeksəuˈkɔːriɔn] *n* 绒[毛]膜外层
exocoelom [ˌeksəuˈsiːləm], **exocoeloma** [ˌeksəusiˈləumə] *n* [胚]外体腔
exocolitis [ˌeksəukɔˈlaitis] *n* 结肠腹膜炎
exocrine [ˈeksəkrain] *a* 外分泌的 *n* 外分泌;外分泌物
exocrinology [ˌeksəukriˈnɔlədʒi] *n* 外分泌学
exocrinosity [ˌeksəukriˈnɔsəti] *n* 外分泌[性]
exocuticle [ˌeksəuˈkjutikl] *n* 外角皮(节肢动物);外表皮(昆虫)
exocyclic [ˌeksəuˈsaiklik] *a* 环外的,不在环上的(指环化合物)
exocytosis [ˌeksəusaiˈtəusis] *n* 胞吐作用(由细胞排出因太大而不能通过细胞壁扩散的颗粒);炎细胞外渗,白细胞凝聚(游走的白细胞向表皮凝聚的过程,作为炎症反应的一个部分)
exodeoxyribonuclease [ˌeksəudiːˌɔksiˌraibəuˈnjuːklieis] *n* 外切脱氧核糖核酸酶
exodeviation [ˌeksəuˌdiːviˈeiʃən] *n* 外转;外斜视
exodic [ekˈsɔdik] *a* 离心的;传出的,输出的
exodontia [ˌeksəuˈdɔnʃiə], **exodontics** [ˌeksəuˈdɔntiks] *n* 拔牙学 | **exodontist** *n* 拔牙学家
exoenzyme [ˌeksəuˈenzaim] *n* 胞外酶,外酶
exoergic [ˌeksəuˈəːdʒik] *a* 放能的(指化学反应)
exoerythrocytic [ˌeksəuiˌriθrəuˈsitik] *a* 红细胞外的
exogamy [ekˈsɔgəmi] *n* 异系配合,异系交配;异族结婚 | **exogamous** [ekˈsɔgəməs], **exogamic** [ˌeksəuˈgæmik] *a*
exogastric [ˌeksəuˈgæstrik] *a* 胃外膜的
exogastritis [ˌeksəugæsˈtraitis] *n* 胃外膜炎
exogastrula [ˌeksəuˈgæstrulə] *n* 外凸原肠胚
exogastrulation [ˌeksəuˌgæstruːˈleiʃən] *n* 原肠胚外凸
Exogenina [ˌeksəudʒiˈnainə] *n* 外生亚目
exogenote [ekˈsɔdʒinəut] *n* 外基因子
exogenous [ekˈsɔdʒinəs], **exogenetic** [ˌeksəudʒiˈnetik], **exogenic** [ˌeksəuˈdʒenik] *a* 外源的,外生的
exognathia [ˌeksɔgˈneiθiə] *n* 凸颌
exognathion [ˌeksɔgˈneiθiɔn] *n* 上颌骨齿槽突;上颌骨
exohemophylaxis [ˌeksəuˌhiːməufiˈlæksis] *n* 抽血注射预防[反应]法
exolever [ˌeksəuˈliːvə] *n* [牙]根挺
exometer [ekˈsɔmitə] *n* 荧光计
exomphalos [ekˈsɔmfələs] *n* 脐凸出;先天性脐疝
exomysium [ˌeksəuˈmisiəm] *n* 肌束膜
exon [ˈeksɔn] *n* 外显子
exonuclease [ˌeksəuˈnjuːklieis] *n* 外切核酸酶
exopathy [ekˈsɔpəθi] *n* 外因病 | **exopathic** [ˌeksəuˈpæθik] *a*
exopeptidase [ˌeksəuˈpeptideis] *n* 外肽酶
Exophiala [ˌeksəˈfaiələ] *n* 外瓶霉属 | ~ werneckii 韦内斯基外瓶霉
exophoria [ˌeksəuˈfəuriə] *n* 外隐斜 | **exophoric** [eksəuˈfɔːrik] *a*
exophthalmic [ˌeksɔfˈθælmik] *a* 眼球突出的,突眼的
exophthalmogenic [ˌeksɔfˌθælməuˈdʒenik] *a* 致突眼的,造成眼球突出的
exophthalmometer [ˌeksɔfθælˈmɔmitə] *n* 突眼计,眼球突出计 | **exophthalmometric** [ˌeksɔfˌθælməuˈmetrik] *a* 眼球突出测量[法]的 / **exophthalmometry** *n* 眼球突出测量[法]
exophthalmos [ˌeksɔfˈθælmɔs] *n* 突眼,眼球突出 | endocrine ~ 内分泌性突眼,内分泌性眼球突出 / malignant ~ 恶性突眼 / thyrotoxic ~ 甲状腺毒性眼球突出 / thyrotropic ~ 促甲状腺激素性眼球突出 | **exophthalmus** [ˌeksɔfˈθælməs] *n*
exophytic [ˌeksəuˈfitik] *a* 外部生长的;外寄生菌的
exoplasm [ˈeksəuplæzəm] *n* 外质
exorbitism [ˈekˈsɔːbitizəm] *n* 眼球突出,突眼
exoribonuclease [ˌeksəuˌraibəuˈnjuːklieis] *n* 外切核糖核酸酶
exosepsis [ˌeksəuˈsepsis] *n* 体外性脓毒症

exoserosis [ˌeksəusiˈrəusis] *n* 血清渗出
exo-α-sialidase [ˌeksəusai ˈælideis] 外-α-唾液酸酶(EC 命名法中称唾液酸酶,见 sialidase)
exoskeleton [ˌeksəuˈskelitn] *n* 外骨骼(如甲壳纲动物的甲壳,在脊椎动物指毛、甲、蹄、牙等) | **exoskeletal** [ˌeksəuˈskelitl] *a*
exosmose [ˈeksɔzməus, -sos-] *vi* 外渗
exosmosis [ˌeksɔzˈməusis, -sos-] *n* 外渗 | **exosmotic** [ˌeksɔzˈmɔtik, -sos-] *a*
exosplenopexy [ˌeksəuˈspliːnəˌpeksi] *n* 脾外固定术
exospore [ˈeksəuspɔː] *n* 外生孢子
exosporium [ˌeksəuˈspɔːriəm] *n* [孢子]外壁
exostosectomy [ekˌsɔstəuˈsektəmi] *n* 外生骨疣切除术
exostosis [ˌeksɔsˈtəusis] ([复] **exostoses** [eksɔsˈtəusiːz]) *n* 外生骨疣 | ivory ~ 象牙质样外生骨疣 / multiple exostoses, hereditary multiple exostoses, multiple cartilaginous exostoses 多发性外生骨疣(亦称骨干性续连症) / osteocartilaginous ~ 骨软骨外生骨疣,骨软骨瘤 | **exostotic** [ˌeksɔsˈtɔtik] *a*
exoteric [ˌeksəuˈterik] *a* 体外的;外源的,外生的 | **~ally** *ad*
exothelioma [ˌeksəuθiːliˈəumə] *n* 脑膜瘤
exothermic [ˌeksəuˈθəːmik], **exothermal** [ˌeksəuˈθəːməl] *a* 放热的
exothymopexy [ˌeksəuˈθaiməˌpeksi] *n* 胸腺外固定术
exothyropexy [ˌeksəuˈθairəpeksi], **exothyroidopexy** [ˌeksəuθaiˈrɔidəuˌpeksi], **exothyropexia** [ˌeksəuˌθairəuˈpeksiə] *n* 甲状腺外固定术
exotic [egˈzɔtik] *a* 外来的 *n* 外来物
exotoxin [ˌeksəuˈtɔksin] *n* 外毒素 | **exotoxic** *a*
exotropia [ˌeksəuˈtrəupiə] *n* 外斜视,散开性斜视 | **exotropic** *a*
expand [ikˈspænd] *vt, vi* 张开,伸展;扩大;膨胀
expander [ikˈspændə, ekˈs-] *n* 膨胀器;膨胀剂,增容剂 | plasma volume ~ 血浆扩容剂
expanse [ikˈspæns] *n* 膨胀;扩张
expansible [ikˈspænsəbl] *a* [可]扩张的;[可]膨胀的 | **expansibility** [ikˌspænsəˈbiləti] *n* 可扩张性;可膨胀性
expansion [ikˈspænʃən, ekˈs-] *n* 伸展;膨胀;扩张,扩大 | ~ of the arch 牙弓扩张 / clonal ~ 克隆扩增(一种免疫学反应,受抗原刺激的淋巴细胞使有关细胞的群体增生和扩大) / cubical ~ 体积膨胀 / hygroscopic ~ 吸湿性膨胀 / setting ~ 凝固性膨胀 / thermal ~ 热膨胀 / wax ~ 蜡型膨胀
expansionary [ikˈspænʃənəri] *a* 扩张性的;发展性的
expansive [ikˈspænsiv] *a* 扩张的;膨胀的;自大狂的,夸张性的 | **~ness** *n*
expect [ikˈspekt] *vt* 期望,期待;预期
expectancy [ikˈspektənsi], **expectance** [ikˈspektəns] 期望,期待;预期 | life ~ (根据概率统计求得的)预期寿命
expectant [ikˈspektənt] *a* 期望的,预期的
expectation [ˌekspekˈteiʃən] *n* 期望;预期 | ~ of life (根据概率统计求得的)估计寿命,预期寿命
expectorant [ekˈspektərənt] *a* 祛痰的 *n* 祛痰药 | liquefying ~ 液化祛痰药
expectorate [ekˈspektəreit] *vt, vi* 咳出(痰等);吐(唾液、血等) | **expectoration** [ekˌspektəˈreiʃən] *n* 咳痰;咳出物,痰
expel [ikˈspel] (-ll-) *vt* 排除,迫出
expellant, expellent [ikˈspelənt] *a* 排除的;排毒的 *n* 排毒剂
expend [ikˈspend] *vt* 花费,耗尽
expendable [ikˈspendəbl] *a* 可消费的;值得消耗的 *n* 消耗物
expenditure [ikˈspenditʃə] *n* 消费,消耗 | rest energy ~ 静息能量消耗
experience [ikˈspiəriəns] *n* 经验;经历;体验 *vt* 感受;体验 | passive ~ 被动体验
experienced [ikˈspiəriənst] *a* 有经验的;熟练的
experiment [ikˈsperimənt, ekˈs-] *n* 实验,试验 [ikˈsperiment] *vi* 进行实验(或试验) | control ~ 对照实验 / crucial ~, check ~ 决定性实验,定局实验 / defect ~ 缺损实验(观察胚胎某一区域或某一部分被破坏后对其生长发育所受的影响) | **~er** [ikˈsperimentə] *n* 实验者,试验者
experimental [ikˌsperiˈmentl, ekˌs-] *a* 实验[性]的,试验[性]的
experimentation [ikˌsperimenˈteiʃən, ekˌs-] *n* 实验[法],试验[法]
expertise [ˌekspəːˈtiːz] *n* 专家评定(或鉴定) | forensic psychiatrics ~ 司法精神病学鉴定
expirate [ˈekspireit] *n* 呼气
expiration [ˌekspaiəˈreiʃən] *n* 呼出,呼气;断气,死亡;期满,终止
expiratory [ikˈspaiərətəri, ekˈs-] *a* 呼气的
expire [ikˈspaiə] *vi* 呼气;断气,死亡;满期;终止 *vt* 呼出
expiry [ikˈspaiəri] *n* 满期,终止
explant [eksˈplɑːnt] *vt* 移动,移植 [ˌeksplɑːnt] *n* 移出物,外植体 | **~ation** [ˌeksplɑːnˈteiʃən] *n*
explode [ikˈspləud, ekˈs-] *vt* (使)爆炸 *vi* 爆炸;爆发,突发(如流行病)
explore [ikˈsplɔː] *vt* 探索,探查,探察,勘探 | **exploration** [ˌeksplәˈreiʃən] *n* / **exploratory** [ikˈsplɔːrətəri], **explorative** [ikˈsplɔrətiv] *a* |

~r [ik'splɔːrə] *n* 探索者,探查者;探针;探察器(尤其用于探察异物)
explosion [ik'spləuʒən, ek's-] *n* 爆炸;爆发,突发;激增
explosive [ik'spləusiv, ek's-] *a* 爆炸[性]的;爆发[性]的
exponent [ik'spəunənt, ek's-] *n* 指数,幂
exponential [ˌekspəu'nenʃəl] *a* 指数的,幂的 *n* 指数
expose [ik'spəuz] *vt* 暴露,露置;曝露,露光
exposure [ik'spəuʒə, ek's-] *n* 暴露;曝光;辐照;照射 | acute ~ 急性照射(短时间射线照射)/ air ~ 空气照射量 / chronic ~ 慢性照射(长期射线照射)
express [ik'spres] *vt* 表示,表达;压出,压榨
expressate [iks'preseit, eks-] *n* 压出物,压榨物
expression [ik'spreʃən] *n* 表达;(面部)表情;词句;式;压出[法],压榨[法](用于产科等);表现 | early ~ 早期(胎盘)压出术 / gene ~ 基因表达
expressivity [ˌekspre'sivəti] *n* 表现度(指带有主要基因的个体所显示的遗传特性的程度)
expulsion [ik'spʌlʃən] *n* 娩出,逼出 | placental ~ 胎盘娩出 | **expulsive** *a*
exsanguinate [eks'sæŋgwineit] *vt* 放血,使无血 *a* 无血的,贫血的 | **exsanguination** [eksˌsæŋgwi'neiʃən] *n* 放血,驱血法
exsanguine [eks'sæŋgwin] *a* 无血的,贫血的
exsanguinotransfusion [eksˌsæŋgwinəutræns'fjuːʒən] *n* 交换输血法
exscind [ek'sind] *vt* 割开,切去,除去
exsect [ek'sekt] *vt* 切除 | **~ion** [ek'sekʃən] *n* 切除术 / **~or** *n* 切除刀
Exserohilum [ˌeksərə'hailəm] *n* 丝状菌属
exsiccant [ek'sikənt] *a* 干燥的 *n* 干燥剂
exsiccate ['eksikeit] *vt* 使干燥 | **exsiccation** [ˌeksi'keiʃən] *n* 干燥[法];结晶脱水
exsmoker [eks'sməukə] *n* 戒了烟的人
exsomatize [ek'səumətaiz] *vt* 使离体
exsorption [ek'sɔːpʃən] *n* 外吸渗
exstrophia [eks'trəufiə] *n* 外翻
exstrophy ['ekstrəfi] *n* 外翻 | ~ of the bladder 膀胱外翻
exsufflation [ˌeksʌ'fleiʃən] *n* 排气(尤指使用排气器对肺作人工排气)
exsufflator [ˌeksʌ'fleitə] *n* 排气器
ext. extract 提取物
extend [ik'stend] *vt, vi* 伸,伸展;延长,扩大;扩散,蔓延(指病变)
extended-release [ik'stendid ri'liːs] 延时释放(指用药次数比常规剂量减少2倍或更多一些)
extender [ek'stendə] *n* 膨胀器;膨胀剂,增容剂 | artificial plasma ~ 人造血浆膨胀剂,人造血浆增容剂
extendible [ik'stendəbl], **extensible** [ik'stensəbl] *a* 可伸展的;可延长的;可扩张的 | **extensibility** [ikˌstensə'biləti] *n* 伸展性;可延展性;可扩张性
extension [ik'stenʃən, ek's-] *n* 伸展,仰伸;扩散,蔓延(指病变);牵伸术 | nail ~ 导钉牵伸术(以钉或针钉入折骨远侧断片,然后施以牵伸术)/ ~ percontiguitatem 邻接性蔓延 / ~ percontinuitatem 连续性蔓延 / ~ per saltam 转移,迁徙 / ridge ~ 牙槽嵴加高
extensive [ik'stensiv] *a* 广大的;广阔的;广泛的;广延的
extensometer [ˌeksten'sɔmitə] *n* 伸长计;伸展计
extensor [ik'stensə, ek's-] *n*【拉】伸肌
extent [ik'stent] *n* 广度;宽度;长度;程度;范围
extenuate [ik'stenjueit] *vt* 减轻,减量 | **extenuation** [ikˌstenju'eiʃən] *n*
exterior [ik'stiəriə] *a* 外的 *n* 外部,外表
exteriorize [ik'stiəriəraiz, ek's-] *vt* 使外表化,使具体化;外向化;外置(取内脏于体外) | **exteriorization** [ikˌstiəriərai'zeiʃən, -ri'z-] *n* (注意、兴趣)外向;外置术
exterminate [ik'stəːmineit] *vt* 根除,灭绝,消灭 | **extermination** [ikˌstəːmi'neiʃən] *n*
exterminatory [ik'stəːminətəri], **exterminative** [ik'stəːminətiv] *a* 根除的,扑灭的,消灭的
external [ik'stəːnl, ek's-] *a* 外的,外部的;外用的 *n* 外部;外面 | for ~ use only 只供外用(指药物)
externalia [ˌekstəː'neiliə] *n* 外生殖器
extern(e) ['ekstəːn] *n* (不住院的)实习医学生
externus [eks'təːnəs] *a* 外的,外部的,外界的(指远离器官或体腔中心的结构)
exteroceptive [ˌekstərəu'septiv] *a* 外感受性的
exteroceptor [ˌekstərəu'septə] *n* 外感受器
exterofection [ˌekstərəu'fekʃən] *n* 对外反应作用(身体通过脑脊髓神经系统对外界环境的变化所起的反应) | **exterofective** *a*
exterogestate [ˌekstərəu'dʒesteit] *a* 宫外发育的; *n* 宫外孕胎
extima ['ekstimə] *n*【拉】外膜
extinct [ik'stiŋkt] *a* 已熄灭了的;灭绝的,绝种的
extinction [ik'stiŋkʃən] *n* 熄灭;灭绝,绝种;消退;消光;消失(在心理学上指条件反应消失)
extirpate ['ekstəːpeit] *vt* 根除,消灭;破除;摘除
extirpation [ˌekstəː'peiʃən] *n* 根除,消灭;破除;摘除 | dental pulp ~ 牙髓摘除
extirpator ['ekstəpeitə] *n* 根除者;摘除器
extorsion [ik'stɔːʃən, ek's-] *n* 外旋
extortor [ik'stɔːtə] *n* 外旋肌

extra- [前缀]外,在外,额外
extra-abdominal [ˌekstrə æbˈdɔminl] *a* 腹外的
extra-adrenal [ˌekstrəəˈdriːnl] *a* 肾上腺外的
extraanatomic [ˌekstrəˌænəˈtɔmik] *a* 解剖外的(不遵循正常解剖途径的,指某些动脉分流术)
extra-anthropic [ˌekstrəænˈθrɔpik] *a* 疾病外因的,体外病因的
extra-articular [ˌekstrəɑːˈtikjulə] *a* 关节外的
extrabronchial [ˌekstrəˈbrɔŋkiəl] *a* 支气管外的
extrabuccal [ˌekstrəˈbʌkəl] *a* 口腔外的
extrabulbar [ˌekstrəˈbʌlbə] *a* 球外的(如尿道球外的,延髓外的)
extracapsular [ˌekstrəˈkæpsjulə] *a* (关节)囊外的
extracardial [ˌekstrəˈkɑːdiəl] *a* 心外的
extracarpal [ˌekstrəˈkɑːpl] *a* 腕外侧的
extracellular [ˌekstrəˈseljulə] *a* 细胞外的
extracerebral [ˌekstrəˈseribrəl] *a* 脑外的
extracorporeal [ˌekstrəkɔːˈpɔːriəl], **extracorporal** [ˌekstrəˈkɔːpərəl] *a* 体外的
extracorpuscular [ˌekstrəkɔːˈpʌskjulə] *a* 小体外的,细胞外的
extracorticospinal [ˌekstrəˌkɔːtikəuˈspainəl] *a* 皮质脊髓束外的
extracranial [ˌekstrəˈkreinjəl] *a* 颅外的
extract [ikˈstrækt] *vt* (用力)取出,拔出;提取;摘录 [ˈekstrækt] *n* 摘录;浸膏,浸出物;提取物 | allergenic ~ 变应原浸出物(用于诊断和脱敏治疗超敏反应) / animal ~ 动物性浸膏 / compound ~ 复方浸膏 / fluid ~ 流浸膏 / poisonivy ~ 野葛浸出物(用于野葛皮炎的脱敏治疗) / pollen ~ 花粉浸液,花粉浸出物
extraction [ikˈstrækʃən, ekˈs-] *n* 摘出术,牵引术,拔出,取出;浸出,提取 | breech ~ 胎臀牵引术 / ~ of a cataract 白内障摘出术 / flap ~ [白内障]瓣状摘出术 / tooth ~ 拔牙
extractive [ikˈstræktiv, ekˈs-] *a* [可]抽出的;[可]提取的 *n* 提取物,浸出物
extractor [ikˈstræktə] *n* 拔出器;提取器
extractum [ekˈstræktəm] ([复] **extracta** [ekˈstræktə]) *n*【拉】浸膏,浸出物
extracystic [ˌekstrəˈsistik] *a* 囊外的;膀胱外的
extradural [ˌekstrəˈdjuərəl] *a* 硬膜外的
extraembryonic [ˌekstrəˌembriˈɔnik] *a* 胚外的
extraepiphyseal [ˌekstrəˌepiˈfiziəl] *a* 骺外的,不连骺的
extrafusal [ˌekstrəˈfjuːzəl] *a* 梭外的
extragenic [ˌekstrəˈdʒenik] *a* 基因外的,非基因的
extragenital [ˌekstrəˈdʒenitl] *a* 生殖器外的,性器官外的
extraglomerular [ˌekstrəgləuˈmerjulə] *a* [肾小]球外的
extrahepatic [ˌekstrəhiˈpætik] *a* 肝外的
extraimmunization [ˌekstrəˌimju(ː)niˈzeiʃən] *n* 额外免疫(使用至少一次剂量疫苗超出推荐数的免疫)
extraligamentous [ˌekstrəˌligəˈmentəs] *a* 韧带外的
extraluminal [ˌekstrəˈljuːminl] *a* 腔外的
extralymphatic [ˌekstrəlimˈfætik] *a* 淋巴系统外的
extramalleolus [ˌekstrəməˈliːələs] *n* 外踝
extramarginal [ˌekstrəˈmɑːdʒinəl] *a* (意识)边缘外的,(意识)域外的
extramastoiditis [ˌekstrəˌmæstɔiˈdaitis] *n* 乳突周炎
extramedullary [ˌekstrəmeˈdʌləri, -ˈmedə-] *a* 髓外的,延髓外的
extrameningeal [ˌekstrəmiˈnindʒiəl] *a* 脑[脊]膜外的
extramural [ˌekstrəˈmjuərəl] *a* 城市(学校、医院等)外的;(器官)壁外的
extraneous [ekˈstreinjəs] *a* 体外的;外部的
extranuclear [ˌekstrəˈnjuːkliə] *a* (细胞)核外的
extraocular [ˌekstrəˈɔkjulə] *a* 眼外的
extraoculogram [ˌekstrəˈɔkjuləgræm] *n* 外眼电图
extraosseous [ˌekstrəˈɔsiəs] *a* 骨外的
extrapancreatic [ˌekstrəˌpænkriˈætik] *a* 胰腺外的
extraparenchymal [ˌekstrəpəˈrenkiməl] *a* 实质外的
extrapelvic [ˌekstrəˈpelvik] *a* 盆外的;盂外的
extrapericardial [ˌekstrəˌperiˈkɑːdiəl] *a* 心包外的
extraperineal [ˌektrəˌperiˈniːəl] *a* 会阴外的
extraperiosteal [ˌekstrəˌperiˈɔstiəl] *a* 骨膜外的
extraperitoneal [ˌekstrəˌperitəuˈniːəl] *a* 腹膜外的
extraplacental [ˌekstrəpləˈsentl] *a* 胎盘外的
extraplantar [ˌekstrəˈplɑːntə, ˈplæn-] *a* 足底外的,跖外的
extrapleural [ˌekstrəˈpluərəl] *a* 胸膜外的
extrapolate [ekˈstræpəleit] *vt, vi* 推断,推知;外推 | **extrapolation** [ekˌstræpəˈleiʃən] *n* 推断,推知;外推法
extraprostatic [ˌekstrəprɔsˈtætik] *a* 前列腺外的
extraprostatitis [ˌekstrəˌprɔstəˈtaitis] *n* 前列腺周炎
extrapsychic [ˌekstrəˈsaikik] *a* 精神外的,心理外的
extrapulmonary [ˌekstrəˈpʌlməˌnəri] *a* 肺外的
extrapyramidal [ˌekstrəpiˈræmidl] *a* 锥体[束]

外的
extrarectus [ˌekstrəˈrektəs] *n* 眼外直肌
extrasensory [ˌekstrəˈsensəri] *a* 超感官的,超感觉的,超感知的
extraserous [ˌekstrəˈsiərəs] *a* 浆膜腔外的
extrasomatic [ˌekstrəsəuˈmætik] *a* 体外的
extrastimulus [ˌekstrəˈstimjuləs] *n* 额外刺激
extrasuprarenal [ˌekstrəˌsjuːprəˈriːnl] *a* 肾上腺外的
extrasystole [ˌekstrəˈsistəli] *n* 期前收缩 | atrioventricular ~, nodal ~ [房室]结性期前收缩 / interpolated ~ 插入[性]期前收缩 / retrograde ~ 逆行性期前收缩 / ventricular ~, infranodal ~ 室性期前收缩,结下性期前收缩
extraterrestrial [ˌekstrətiˈrestriəl] *a* 地球外的,宇宙的
extrathoracic [ˌekstrəθɔːˈræsik] *a* 胸腔外的
extratracheal [ˌekstrətrəˈki(ː)əl, -ˈtreiki-] *a* 气管外的
extratubal [ˌekstrəˈtjuːbl] *a* 管外的
extratympanic [ˌekstrətimˈpænik] *a* 鼓室外的
extrauterine [ˌekstrəˈjuːtərain] *a* 子宫外的
extravaginal [ˌekstrəvəˈdʒainəl, -ˈvædʒi-] *a* 阴道外的;鞘外的
extravasate [ikˈstrævəseit, ekˈs-] *vt, vi* (血液等)外渗
extravasation [ikˌstrævəˈseiʃən, ekˌs-] *n* 外渗;外渗物(如血液) | punctiform ~ 点状外渗
extravascular [ˌekstrəˈvæskjulə] *a* 血管外的
extraventricular [ˌekstrəvenˈtrikjulə] *a* 室外的
extraversion [ˌekstrəˈvəːʃən] *n* 外倾,外向(指个人兴趣、感情、精神趋向的外向);牙弓过宽 | **extravert** [ˈekstrəvəːt] *n* 外倾(性格)者
extreme [ikˈstriːm] *a* 末端的;最远的;极度的;极端的
extremital [ekˈstremitl] *a* 肢的;末端的,远侧的
extremitas [ekˈstremitəs] ([复] **extremitates** [ekˌstremiˈteitiːz]) *n* 【拉】骨端;肢
extremity [ikˈstreməti, ekˈs-] *n* 骨端;四肢 | cartilaginous ~ of rib 肋软骨 / external ~ of clavicle, scapular ~ of clavicle 锁骨外侧端,锁骨肩峰端 / fimbriated ~ of fallopian tube 输卵管伞端,卵巢伞 / internal ~ of clavicle 锁骨内侧端,锁骨胸骨端 / lower ~ 下肢 / upper ~ 上肢 / uterine ~ of ovary, pelvic ~ of ovary 卵巢子宫端
extrinsic [ekˈstrinsik] *a* 外部的;体外的;外源[性]的
extro- [前缀]外
extrogastrulation [ˌekstrəuˌgæstruːˈleiʃən] *n* 肠胚外翻畸形
extrophia [eksˈtrəufiə] *n* 外翻
extrospection [ˌekstrəuˈspekʃən] *n* 自窥癖(时常检视自己皮肤,伴有不洁恐怖)
extroversion [ˌekstrəuˈvəːʃən] *n* 外翻;外倾,外向
extrovert [ˈekstrəvəːt] *n* 外倾[性格]者
extrude [ekˈstruːd] *vt* 挤出;使突出 *vi* 伸出,突出,凸出,凸生芽 | **extrusion** [ekˈstruːʒən] *n* 挤压;伸出;突出,凸出,凸生牙
extrudoclusion [ekˌstruːdəuˈkluːʒən] *n* 上超殆,上超咬合
extubate [eksˈtjuːbeit] *vt* 拔管 | **extubation** [ˌekstjuːˈbeiʃən] *n* 拔管法
exuberance [igˈzjuːbərəns] *n* 繁茂;充溢
exuberant [igˈzjuːbərənt] *a* 繁茂的;充溢的;生成过多的,高度增生的
exudate [ˈeksjudeit] *n* 渗出物,渗出液 | cotton-wool ~s 棉絮状渗出物
exudation [ˌeksjuːˈdeiʃən] *n* 渗出
exudative [igˈzjuːdətiv] *a* 渗出性的
exude [igˈzjuːd] *vt, vi* 渗出,流出;发散
exulcerans [eksˈʌlsərənz] *a* 【拉】形成溃疡的
exulceratio [eksˌʌlsəˈreiʃiəu] *n* 【拉】溃疡
exumbilication [ˌeksʌmbiliˈkeiʃən] *n* 脐凸出;脐疝
exuviate [igˈzjuːvieit] *vt, vi* 蜕皮,脱壳;上皮脱落;(乳牙)脱落 | **exuviation** [igˌzjuːviˈeiʃən, eg-] *n* 上皮脱落;乳牙脱落
ex vivo [ˌeksˈviːvəu] 【拉】在活体外,离体
eye [ai] *n* 眼 | blear ~ 边缘性眼睑炎,睑缘炎 / compound ~ 复眼 / crossed ~s 内斜眼 / cystic ~ 囊状眼 / dark-adapted ~ 暗适应眼 / deviating ~, following ~ 偏斜眼,伴随眼 / epiphyseal ~, pineal ~ 松果眼,顶眼 / exciting ~, primary ~ 激发眼,原发眼(引起交感性眼炎的受伤眼) / fixating ~ 注视眼 / light-adapted ~ 光适应眼 / monochromatic ~ 单色觉眼 / naked ~ 肉眼 / pink ~ 急性结膜炎,红眼 / reduced ~, schematic ~ 简化眼,模型眼 / shipyard ~ 船坞眼,流行性角膜结膜炎 / squinting ~ 斜视眼 / sympathizing ~, secondary ~ 交感眼,继发眼 / wall ~ 角膜白斑;外斜视
eyeball [ˈaibɔːl] *n* 眼球
eyebrow [ˈaibrau] *n* 眉,眉毛
eyecup [ˈaikʌp] *n* 洗眼杯;视杯;生理陷凹(视神经乳头陷凹)
eyeglass [ˈaiglɑːs] *n* 镜片;[复]眼镜;[接]目镜;洗眼杯
eyeground [ˈaigraund] *n* 眼底
eyelash [ˈailæʃ] *n* 睫毛
eyelet [ˈailit] *n* 眼孔(正牙科中用)
eyelid [ˈailid] *n* 眼睑 | third ~ 第三眼睑,瞬膜
eye-minded [ai ˈmaindid] *a* 视觉记忆的

eyepiece [ˈaipiːs] *n* 目镜,接目镜 | comparison ~ 比较目镜 / compensating ~ 补偿目镜 / demonstration ~ 示教目镜 / high-eyepoint ~ 高出射点目镜(出射点比一般要高,供戴眼镜观察者使用) / huygenian ~ 惠更斯(Huygens)目镜(由两个平凸透镜组成,凸面正对物镜) / negative ~ 负目镜 / positive ~ 正目镜 / widefield ~ 宽视野目镜

eyepoint [ˈaipɔint] *n* 出射点

eyespot [ˈaispɔt] *n* 眼点(某些无脊椎动物的感光有色点)

eyestrain [ˈaistrein] *n* 眼疲劳

eyetooth [ˈaituːθ] ([复]**eyeteeth** [ˈaitiːθ]) *n* 上尖牙,上犬牙

eyewash [ˈaiwɔʃ] *n* 洗眼药水(洗眼剂)

eyeworm [ˈaiwəːm] *n* 眼丝虫,罗阿丝虫

F

F Fahrenheit 华氏温标；farad 法拉；fertility 致育力（见 plasmid 项下 F plasmid）；visual field 视野；fluorine 氟；formular 公式；French 法制标度（见 scale 项下）

F. fiat【拉】作成，制成

F Faraday 法拉第；force 力；gilbert 吉伯

F_1 first filial generation 第一子代，子 1 代

F_2 second filial generation 第二子代，子 2 代

℉ degree Fahrenheit 华氏温度

f femto- 飞［母托］；focal length 焦距

f frequency 频率

FA fatty acid 脂肪酸；fluorescent antibody 荧光素标记抗体

FAB French-American-British 法美英分类法（用于鉴别某些白血病）

Fab（*f*ragment，*a*ntigen-*b*inding）Fab 片段，抗原结合片段（IgG 分子经木瓜蛋白酶处理抗体分子后所得到的两个片段之一，它们仍能与抗原结合）

$F(ab')_2$ $F(ab')_2$ 片段（IgG 分子经胃蛋白酶裂解后获得的片段，包含两个 Fab 区及经由键间的二硫键连接这两个区的铰链区）

fabella［fə'belə］（［复］**fabellae**［fə'beliː］）*n*【拉】腓肠豆（腓肠肌内籽状纤维软骨，在膝关节后 X 线可见的小骨影）

Faber's syndrome［'fɑːbə］（Knud H. Faber）低色［指数］性贫血

fabism［'feibizəm］*n* 蚕豆病（见 favism）

fabrication［ˌfæbri'keiʃən］*n* 虚谈症，虚构症

Fabricius' bursa［fə'brisiəs］（Geronimo〈Hieronymus〉Fabrizio）法氏囊，腔上囊（鸡肚泄殖腔的上皮赘生物，长成类似哺乳动物的胸腺形状，到 5 或 6 个月后即萎缩，在性成熟的鸟类中变为纤维性残留物。它含有淋巴样滤泡，退化前是淋巴细胞生成的部位，与体液免疫密切相关）

Fabry's disease（syndrome）［'fɑːbri］（Johannes Fabry）法布里病（综合征）（一种糖鞘脂分解的 X 连锁溶酶体贮积症，是由于 α 半乳糖苷酶 A 缺乏所致，可使神经酰胺三己糖苷蓄积于肾和心血管系统。患者通常死于肾衰竭、心脏或脑血管疾病。亦称弥漫性躯体血管角化瘤、α-半乳糖苷酶 A 缺乏症和神经酰胺三己糖苷酶缺乏症）

fabulation［ˌfæbju'leiʃən］*n* 虚谈症、虚构症

Facb *f*ragment *a*ntigen and *c*omplement *b*inding 抗原和补体结合片段

FACD Fellow of the American College of Dentists 美国口腔科医师学会会员

face［feis］*n* 面；面容 ǀ adenoid ~ 增殖体面容 / bovine ~，cow ~ 牛面（两眼距离过远）/ cleft ~ 巨口，颊横裂 / frog ~ 蛙面（由于鼻内疾病所致的颜面扁平）/ hippocratic ~ 死相，希波克拉底面容 / moon ~，moonshaped ~ 满月脸，月样圆面容（见于多种病情，如库欣〈Cushing〉综合征或使用肾上腺皮质激素类后）

face-bow［'feisbəu］*n* 面弓（在牙科中用以记录上颌弓与颞下颌关节位置关系的一种仪器）ǀ adjustable axis ~，kinematic ~ 可调节轴式面弓，运动式面弓

face-lift［'feisˌlift］*n*（为除去皱纹的）整容术

faceometer［feis'ɔmitə］*n* 面直径测量器

facet［'fæsit］*n* 小平面，小面

facetectomy［ˌfæsi'tektəmi］*n* 椎骨关节面切除术

facette［fə'set］*n*【法】小平面，小面

facial［'feiʃəl］*a* 面［部］的

-facient［构词成分］生，成

facies［'feiʃiiːz］［单复同］*n*【拉】面；面容 ǀ adenoid ~ 增殖体面容 / mitral ~，mitrotricuspid ~ 二尖瓣病面容，二尖瓣三尖瓣病面容 / moon ~ 满月脸，月样圆面容（见 face 项下相应术语）/ myasthenic ~ 肌无力面容 / myopathic ~ 肌病性面容 / typhoid ~，~ typhosa 伤寒病面容，淡漠面容

facilitation［fəˌsili'teiʃən］*n* 推进，促进；易化；接通［作用］ǀ **facilitative**［fə'silitətiv］*a* 促进的

facilitory［fə'silitəri］*a* 容易化的；接通的

facing［'feisiŋ］*n* 牙面

faci(o)-［构词成分］面

faciobrachial［ˌfeiʃiəu'breikiə］*a* 面臂的

faciocephalalgia［ˌfeiʃiəuˌsefə'lældʒiə］*n* 面颈神经痛

faciocervical［ˌfeiʃiəu'səːvikəl］*a* 面颈的

faciolingual［ˌfeiʃiəu'liŋgwəl］*a* 面舌的

facioplasty［ˌfeiʃiəu'plæsti］*n* 面成形术

facioplegia［ˌfeiʃiəu'pliːdʒiə］*n* 面神经麻痹，面瘫

facioscapulohumeral［ˌfeiʃiəuˌskæpjuləu'hjuməral］*a* 面肩胛臂的

faciostenosis［ˌfeiʃiəusti'nəusis］*n* 面狭窄

FACOG Fellow of the American College of Obstetricians and Gynecologists 美国妇产科医师学会

会员

FACP Fellow of the American College of Physicians 美国内科医师学会会员

FACR Fellow of the American College of Radiology 美国放射学会会员

FACS fluorescence-activated cell sorter 荧光激活细胞分类器;Fellow of the American College of Surgeons 美国外科医师学会会员

FACSM Fellow of the American College of Sports Medicine 美国运动医学学会会员

F-actin [ef ˈæktin] *n* F-肌动蛋白,纤维状肌动蛋白

factitial [fækˈtiʃəl] *a* 人造的,人工的,人为的

factitious [fækˈtiʃəs] *a* 人工的,人造的,非自然的

factor [ˈfæktə] *n* 因子,因素,要素(在遗传学上指遗传因子,即基因) | accelerator ~ 前加速因子,[凝血]因子V / accessory ~, accessory food ~ 附属要素,食物附加要素(一种维生素) / activation ~ 致活因子,[凝血]因子Ⅻ / adrenocorticotropic releasing ~ (ACTH-RF) 促肾上腺皮质激素释放因子 / aldosterone stimulating ~ 醛固酮刺激因子 / anabolism-promoting ~ (APF) 促合成代谢因子 / angiogenesis ~ 血管生成因子 / animal protein ~ 动物蛋白因子(维生素 B_{12}) / antiachromotrichia ~ 抗白发因子,泛酸 / antiacrodynia ~ 抗肢痛因子,吡哆醇 / antialopecia ~ 抗脱发因子,肌醇 / antianemia ~ 抗贫血因子,氰钴胺 / antiblack tongue ~ 抗黑舌病因子,烟酸 / anticanities ~, antidermatitis ~ of chicks 抗白发因子,抗鸡皮炎因子,泛酸 / antidermatitis ~ of rats 抗鼠皮炎因子,吡哆醇 / antiegg white ~ 抗卵白因子,生物素 / antigen-specific T-cell helper ~ 抗原特异性 T 细胞辅助因子 / antigen-specific T-cell suppressor ~ 抗原特异性 T 细胞抑制因子 / anti-gray hair ~ 抗白发因子,泛酸 / antihemophilic ~, antihemophilic ~ A 抗血友病因子,抗血友病因子 A,[凝血]因子Ⅷ / antihemophilic ~ B 抗血友病因子 B,[凝血]因子Ⅸ / antihemophilic ~ C 抗血友病因子 C,[凝血]因子Ⅺ / antihemorrhagic ~ 抗出血因子,维生素 K / antineuritic ~ 抗神经炎因子,硫胺,维生素 B_1 / antinuclear ~ (ANF) 抗核因子(一种抗细胞核成分的自身抗体,可用免疫荧光法检出之,存在于系统性红斑狼疮患者的血清中,偶尔见于类风湿关节炎及其他胶原性疾病) / antipellagra ~ 抗糙皮病因子,烟酸 / anti-pernicious anemia ~ 抗恶性贫血因子,氰钴胺,维生素 B_{12} / antirachitic ~ 抗佝偻病因子,维生素 D / antiscorbutic ~ 抗坏血病因子,抗坏血酸,维生素 C / antisterility ~ 抗不育因子,维生素 E / antixerophthalmia ~, antixerotic ~ 抗干眼因子,维生素 A / basophil chemotactic ~ (BCF) 嗜碱细胞趋化因子 / B cell differentication ~s (BCDF) B 细胞分化因子 / blastogenic ~ (BF) 母细胞生成因子,生殖因子 / B-lymphocyte stimulatory ~s (BSF) B 淋巴细胞刺激因子 / bone ~ 骨因子(牙周溃坏的基本因素) / Bx ~ Bx 因子,对氨基苯甲酸 / C3 nephritic ~ (C3NeF) C3 致肾炎因子(某些低补体血症、膜增生性肾小球肾炎患者血浆中的一种非 Ig 的丙球蛋白) / CAMP ~ CAMP 因子(为 Christie Atkins 和 Munch-Petersen 所发现,故取其首字母命名) / chemotactic ~ 趋化因子 / chick antidermatitis ~ 鸡抗皮炎因子,泛酸 / chick antipellagra ~ 鸡抗糙皮病因子,泛酸 / chick growth ~ S 鸡生长因子 S,蛋白促生长肽 / Christmas ~ 克里斯马斯因子,[凝血]因子Ⅸ / chromotrichial ~ 对氨基苯甲酸 / citrovorum ~ 柠胶因子,甲酰四氢叶酸 / clonal inhibitory ~, cloning inhibitory ~, clone-inhibitory ~ (CIF) 克隆抑制因子 / coagulation ~s 凝血因子 / coenzyme ~ 辅酶因子,黄递酶 / colony-stimulating ~s (CSF) 集落刺激因子 / contact ~ 接触因子,[凝血]因子Ⅻ / corticotropin releasing ~ (CRF) 促肾上腺皮质[激]素释放因子 / cryoprecipitated antihemophilic ~ 冷沉淀抗血友病因子 / crystal-induced chemotactic ~ (CCF) 晶体诱发趋化因子 / decay-activating ~ (DAF) 腐蚀激活因子 / diabetogenic ~ 致糖尿病因子 / diffusion ~ 扩散因子,透明质酸酶 / elongation ~ 延长因子(指蛋白质) / eluate ~ 洗脱物因子,吡哆醇 / eosinophil chemotactic ~ (ECF) 嗜酸细胞趋化因子 / eosinophil chemotactic ~ of anaphylaxis (ECF-A) 过敏反应嗜酸细胞趋化因子 / epidermal growth ~ 表皮生长因子 / erythropoietic stimulating ~ (ESF) 促红细胞生成因子 / extrinsic ~ 外因子,维生素 B_{12} (氰钴胺) / F ~, fertility ~ F 因子,致育因子 / fermentation Lactobacillus casei ~ 干酪乳杆菌发酵因子,叶酸 / fibrin stabilizing ~ 纤维蛋白稳定因子,[凝血]因子ⅩⅢ / filtrate ~, filtrate ~ Ⅱ 滤液因子,滤液因子Ⅱ型,泛酸 / follicle stimulating hormone releasing ~ (FRF, FSH-RF) 促卵泡激素释放因子 / galactopoietic ~ 催乳因子,催乳激素 / gastric anti-pernicious anemia ~, gastric intrinsic ~ 胃抗恶性贫血因子,胃内因子 / glass ~ 玻璃因子,[凝血]因子Ⅻ / glucose tolerance ~ 葡萄糖耐受因子 / gonadotropin releasing ~ (GnRF)促性腺激素释放因子 / growth hormone releasing (GRF, GH-RF) 生长激素释放因子 / ~H H 因子(一种与 C3b〈补体第三成分 b 片段〉结合的糖蛋白) / high-molecular-weight neutrophil chemotactic ~ (HMW-NCF) 高分子量中性粒细胞趋化因子,中性粒细胞趋化因子 / histamine releasing ~ 组胺释放因子 / HL-A ~s 人组织相容性抗原因子 / human antihemophilic ~ 人抗血友病因子 / hydrazine-sensitive ~ (HSF)

肼敏感因子 / hyperglycemic-glycogenolytic ~ 高血糖性糖原分解因子(胰高血糖素) / ~ Ⅰ [凝血]因子Ⅰ,纤维蛋白原 / ~ Ⅱ [凝血]因子Ⅱ,凝血酶原;泛酸 / ~ Ⅲ [凝血]因子Ⅲ,组织凝血[酶]致活酶(亦称组织因子) / immunoglobulin-binding ~(IBF) 免疫球蛋白结合因子 / initiation ~ 起动因子,起始因子 / insulin-like growth ~s (IGF) 胰岛素样生长因子 / intermediate lobe inhibiting ~ (垂体)中间叶抑制因子,促黑素细胞激素抑制因子 / intrinsic ~ 内因子 / ~ Ⅳ [凝血]因子Ⅳ,钙离子 / ~ Ⅸ [凝血]因子Ⅸ,血浆促凝血酶原成分(亦称克里斯马斯〈Christmas〉因子,抗血友病因子 B) / Lactobacillus casei ~ 干酪乳杆菌发酵因子,叶酸 / Lactobacillus lactis Dorner ~, LLD ~ 多讷乳酸乳杆菌因子,维生素 B_{12}(氰钴胺) / lactogenic ~ 生乳因子,催乳激素 / LE ~LE 因子,红斑狼疮因子 / lethal ~s 致死因子(由于遗传物质的缺陷引起个体〈包括胚胎期〉死亡的因子) / leukocyte in hibitory ~(LIF) 白细胞抑制因子 / leukocyte mitogenic ~(LMF) 白细胞致有丝分裂因子 / leukocytosis-promoting ~ 促白细胞增多因子 / liver filtrate ~ 肝滤液因子,泛酸 / liver Lactobacillus casei ~ 肝干酪乳杆菌发酵因子,叶酸 / luteinizing hormone releasing ~(LRF, LH-RF) 促黄体激素释放因子,黄体生成素释放因子 / lymphocyte activating ~ 淋巴细胞激活因子 / lymphocyte blastogenic ~(LBF) 淋巴细胞母细胞生成因子 / lymphocyte mitogenic ~ (LMF) 淋巴细胞致有丝分裂因子 / lymphocyte transforming ~(LTF) 淋巴细胞转化因子 / lysogenic ~ 噬菌体 / macrophage-activating ~ (MAF) 巨噬细胞激活因子 / macrophage chemotactic ~(MCF) 巨噬细胞趋化因子 / macrophage-derived growth ~ 巨噬细胞衍生生长因子 / macrophage growth ~(MGF) 巨噬细胞生长因子 / macrophage-inhibitory ~(MIF) 巨噬细胞抑制因子 / mauve ~ 紫红色因子(尿内的一种物质,在纸色谱法上产生紫红色) / melanocyte stimulating hormone inhibiting ~(MIF) 促黑[素细胞]激素抑制因子 / melanocyte stimulating hormone releasing ~(MRF, MSHRF) 促黑[素细胞]激素释放因子 / migration inhibiting ~(MIF) 游走抑制因子 / milk ~ 小鼠乳腺瘤病毒 / mitogenic ~ 促有丝分裂因子 / modifying ~s 修饰因子,修饰基因(影响另一基因表现程度的多基因或多因子) / mouse antialopecia ~ 小鼠抗秃因子,肌醇 / mouse mammary tumor ~ 小鼠乳腺瘤因子 / MSH inhibiting ~ MSH 抑制因子(即促黑素细胞激素抑制因子 melanocyte stimulating hormone inhibiting ~) / müllerian regression ~, müllerian duct inhibitory ~ 副中肾管组织退化因子,副中肾管抑制因子 / multiple ~s 多因子(在遗传学上指两个或两个以上遗传基因合作或混合或累积而产生某一种性状) / myocardial depressant ~(MDF) 心肌抑制因子 / neutrophil chemotactic ~(NCF) 中性粒细胞趋化因子 / osteoclast activating ~(OAF) 破骨细胞激活因子 / pellagra-preventive ~, P.-P. ~ 抗糙皮病因子,P.-P. 因子,烟酸 / platelet activating ~(PAF) 血小板激活因子 / platelet-derived growth ~ 血小板源性生长因子 / prolactin inhibiting ~(PIF) 催乳素抑制因子 / prolactin releasing ~(PRF) 催乳素释放因子 / proliferation inhibitory ~(PIF) 增生抑制因子 / R ~ R 质粒(即 R plasmid,亦称抗性质粒) / rat acrodynia ~ 鼠肢痛症因子,吡哆醇 / recruitment ~ 募集因子,淋巴细胞致有丝分裂因子 / releasing ~ 释放因子(指两个可溶性蛋白质之一,在蛋白合成时,如与终链密码子相遇,可从核糖体中释放出完整的多肽链) / releasing ~s 释放因子,释放激素 / resistance-inducing ~ 抗性诱导因子(见 Rubin's test②解) / resistance transfer ~(RTF) 抗性转移因子(菌细胞内 R 质粒的部分,含有结合和复制基因) / Rh ~, Rhesus ~ Rh [血型] 因子,猕因子 / rheumatoid ~(RF) 类风湿因子 / risk ~ 危险因素 / ~S S 因子,生物素 / separation ~ 分离因子(两种同位素处理前后的相对浓度之比) / sex ~ 性因子,F 质粒 / somatotropin-releasing ~(SRF) 生长激素释放因子 / specific macrophage arming ~(SMAF) 特异性巨噬细胞武装因子 / spreading ~ 扩散因子,透明质酸酶 / stable ~ 稳定因子,[凝血]因子Ⅶ / T-cell growth ~ T 细胞生长因子,白细胞介素 2/ thyrotropin releasing ~(TRF) 促甲状腺激素释放因子 / transfer ~(TF) 转移因子 / tumor-angiogenesis ~ 肿瘤-血管生成因子 / tumor necrosis ~(TNF) 肿瘤坏死因子 / V ~ V[生长]因子(嗜血杆菌属某些菌种生长所必需的一种辅助物质) / ~ V[凝血]因子V,前加速因子(亦称促凝血球蛋白,不稳定因子) / ~ Ⅵ [凝血]因子Ⅵ,促凝血球蛋白 / ~ Ⅶ [凝血]因子Ⅶ,前转化因子(亦称稳定因子) / ~ Ⅷ [凝血]因子Ⅷ,抗血友病因子(亦称抗血友病因子 A) / ~W W 因子,生物素 / ~X [凝血]因子X,斯图尔特(Stuart)因子(亦称自凝血酶原 C,凝血酶原激酶) / X ~ X 因子(嗜血杆菌属某些菌种需氧生长时所必需的一种辅助物质) / ~ Ⅺ [凝血]因子Ⅺ,血浆促凝血酶原激酶因子(亦称抗血友病因子 C) / ~ Ⅻ [凝血]因子Ⅻ,哈格曼(Hageman)因子(亦称玻璃因子,接触因子,致活因子) / ~ ⅩⅢ [凝血]因子ⅩⅢ,纤维蛋白稳定因子(亦称血纤维形成酶,血纤维交链酶) / yeast eluate ~ 酵母洗脱物因子,吡哆醇 / yeast filtrate ~ 酵母滤液因子,泛酸

facultative [ˈfækəltətiv] *a* 任意的;兼性的

faculty [ˈfækəlti] *n* 能力;(大学)院系 | fusion ~ 融合能力(指两眼所见的两个物像融合为一的能力)

FAD flavin adenine dinucleotide 黄素腺嘌呤二核苷酸

$FADH_2$ the reduced form of flavin adenine dinucleotide 黄素腺嘌呤二核苷酸的还原型

fading [ˈfeidiŋ] *n* 幼犬进行性衰竭症

fae- 以 fae-起始的词,同样见以 fe-起始的词

fag [fæg] *n* 疲劳;衰竭,虚脱

Faget's law(sign) [fəˈʒei] (Jean C. Faget) 法盖定律(征)(黄热病时,与正常关系相反,脉搏降低,体温不变,或脉搏不变,体温则上升)

fagopyrism [fəˈgɔpirizəm] *n* 荞麦中毒

Fagopyrum [ˌfægəˈpairəm] *n* 荞麦属

Fahraeus phenomenon, reaction, test [fəˈriːəs] (Robin Fahraeus) 红细胞沉降率

Fahrenheit scale [ˈfærənhait] (Gabriel D. Fahrenheit) 华氏温标 | ~ thermometer 华氏温度计

Fahr-Volhard disease [fɑː ˈfəulhɑːt] (Karl T. Fahr; Franz Volhard) 恶性肾硬化

failure [ˈfeiljə] *n* 衰竭 | heart ~ 心力衰竭 / renal ~, kidney ~ 肾[功能]衰竭

faint [feint] *n* 晕厥

Fajersztajn's crossed sciatic sign [fɑːʒɛəˈstain] (Jean Fajersztajn) 法捷尔斯坦坐骨神经痛交叉征(坐骨神经痛时,小腿屈曲,髋部也能屈曲,但小腿伸直时,髋部则不能伸直;屈曲健侧大腿而小腿伸直,则可引起患侧疼痛)

falcadina [ˌfælkəˈdiːnə] 法耳卡德纳(亚得里亚海伊斯的利亚半岛的地方病,其特征为乳头状瘤形成)

falces [ˈfælsiːz] falx 的复数

falcial [ˈfælʃəl] *a* 镰的

falciform [ˈfælsifɔːm], **falcate** [ˈfælkeit], **falcular** [ˈfælkjulə] *a* 镰形的,镰状的

falling-out [ˈfɔːliŋ aut] *n* 失落症(一种文化特异性综合征,主要发生在南美洲和加勒比海群体,特征为突然虚脱发生,有时无事先警告即伴有言语、视物或行走不能)

fallopian aqueduct [fəˈləupiən] (Gabriele Fallopio) 面神经管 | ~ artery 子宫动脉 / ~ ligament 腹股沟韧带 / ~ tube 输卵管

falloposcopy [fələuˈpɔskəpi] *n* 输卵管镜检查

Fallot's tetralogy (tetrad) [fəˈlɔː] (Etienne-Louis A. Fallot) 法洛四联症(先天性心脏缺损,包括肺动脉瓣狭窄、室间隔缺损、主动脉右位、右心室肥大) | ~ pentalogy 法洛五联症(法洛四联症同时伴有卵圆孔未闭或房间隔缺损) / ~ trilogy 法洛三联症(肺动脉瓣狭窄、房间隔缺损、右心室肥大)

fallout [ˈfɔːlaut] *n* (核)沉降灰,(放射性)尘埃

false-negative [ˈfɔːls ˈnegətiv] *a* 假阴性的 *n* 假阴性

false-positive [ˈfɔːls ˈpɔzətiv] *a* 假阳性的 *n* 假阳性 | biologic ~ (BFP) 生物学假阳性(梅毒不存在时梅毒血清学试验呈阳性)

falsification [ˌfɔːlsifiˈkeiʃən] *n* 错构,曲解;伪造 | retrospective ~ 回溯性错构症,往事错构症

falsifying [ˌfɔːlsiˈfaiiŋ] *n* (表情的)伪装

Falta's coefficient [ˈfʌltə] (Wilhelm Falta) 法尔塔系数(排出体外糖与口服糖量的百分比) | ~ triad 法尔塔三征(糖尿病的发生与胰腺、肝脏、甲状腺三个脏器有关)

falx [fælks] ([复] **falces** [ˈfælsiːz]) *n* 【拉】镰 | inguinal ~, aponeurotic ~ 腹股沟镰 / ligamentous ~ 骶结节韧带镰突

famciclovir [fæmˈsaiklɔvir] *n* 泛昔洛韦(抗病毒药)

fames [ˈfeimiːz] *n* 【拉】饥饿

familial [fəˈmiljəl] *a* 家族的;家庭的;全家的

family [ˈfæmili] *n* 家庭;家属;家族;科(分类) | systematic ~ 科(分类)

famine [ˈfæmin] *n* 饥荒

famotidine [fæˈməutidiːn] *n* 法莫替丁(组胺 H_2 拮抗剂,用于治疗十二指肠溃疡)

famotine hydrochloride [ˈfæmətiːn] 盐酸法莫汀(抗病毒药)

fan [fæn] *n* 扇,风扇;通风机;扇形物

Fanconi's syndrome (anemia, pancytopenia) [fɑːŋˈkəuni] (Guido Fanconi) 范科尼综合征(贫血、全血细胞减少)(①一种罕见的遗传性疾病,由隐性方式遗传,并有不良预后,特征为全血细胞减少、骨髓发育不全以及皮肤斑状棕色变色等。亦称先天性再生障碍性贫血,先天性全血细胞减少;②以近端肾小管功能障碍为特征的一组疾病的总称,表现为全身高氨基酸尿、肾性糖尿、高磷酸盐尿及重碳酸盐和水的丢失,最常见的病因是胱氨酸病,当不伴有胱氨酸病时,本病亦称 de Toni-Fanconi syndrome)

F and R force and rhythm (of pulse) 力与节律(脉搏)

fang [fæŋ] *n* 牙根;尖牙,蛇类毒牙 | **~ed** *a* 有尖牙的,有毒牙的

fango [ˈfæŋgəu] *n* 温泉泥,矿泥

fangotherapy [ˌfæŋgəuˈθerəpi] *n* 温泉泥疗法

Fannia [ˈfæniə] *n* 厕蝇属 | ~ canicularis 黄腹厕蝇 | ~ scalaris 灰腹厕蝇

fantascope [ˈfæntəskəup] *n* 幻视器

fantasy [ˈfæntəsi] *n* 幻想

fantridone hydrochloride [ˈfæntridəun] 盐酸泛曲酮(抗抑郁药)

Fantus' antidote [ˈfæntəs] (Bernard Fantus) 范特斯解毒剂(曾用作解汞中毒药,含硫化钙溶

液,静脉内注射用)

FAPHA Fellow of the American Public Health Association 美国公共卫生协会会员

Farabeuf's amputation [ˌfɑːrəˈbjuf] (Louis H. Farabeuf) 法腊布夫切断术(小腿的大外瓣状切断术) | ~ triangle 法腊布夫三角(在颈上部,其边为颈内静脉和面静脉,底边为舌下神经)

farad(*F*) [ˈfærəd] (Michael Faraday) *n* 法拉(电容单位)

faraday(*F*) [ˈfærədi, ˈfærədei] *n* 法拉第(电量单位,约等于 96 510 C〈库仑〉)

Faraday's constant [ˈfærədi] (Michael Faraday) 法拉第常数(一摩尔电子或一当量的离子所运载的电量:96 493. 5 C/mol〈库伦/摩尔〉) | ~ law 法拉第定律(电解时,任一时间内所沉析的离子的量与通过的电流强度成比例) / ~ dark space 法拉第暗区(分隔克鲁克斯〈Crookes〉管内阴电辉与阳极区的暗区)

faradimeter [ˌfærəˈdimitə] *n* 感应电流计

faradism [ˈfærədizəm] *n* 感应电;感应电疗法 | surging ~ 浪涌式感应电疗法 | **faradic** [fəˈrædik] *a* 感应电的

faradize [ˈfærədaiz] *vt* 用感应电流刺激;用感应电流治疗 | **faradization** [ˌfærədaiˈzeiʃən, -diˈz-] *n* 感应电疗法

faradocontractility [ˌfærədəuˌkɔntrækˈtiləti] *n* 感应电收缩性

faradomuscular [ˌfærədəuˈmʌskjulə] *a* 感应电肌肉的

faradopalpation [ˌfærədəupælˈpeiʃən] *n* 感应电触诊法

far-advanced [ˈfɑːrədˈvɑːnst] *a* 严重晚期的

Farber's disease (lipogranulomatosis, syndrome) [ˈfɑːbə] (Sidney Farber) 法伯病(脂肪肉芽肿病(综合征),由神经酰胺酶缺乏所致的一种神经酰胺代谢溶酶体贮积病,表现为患儿约3月龄起开始出现声音嘶哑、失音和淡褐色脱屑性皮炎,继之为骨和关节有泡沫细胞浸润,导致畸形。淋巴结、心、肺和肾内有肉芽肿性反应及精神运动性阻滞。亦称神经酰胺酶缺乏症)

Farber-Uzman syndrome [ˈfɑːbə ˈuːzmən] (S. Farber; Lahut Uzman) 法-乌综合征,法伯病(见 Farber's disease)

farcy [ˈfɑːsi] *n* 马皮疽,慢性鼻疽 | button ~ 结节性马皮疽 / cryptococcus ~ 隐性菌马皮疽,兽疫性淋巴管炎 / Japanese ~, Neapolitan ~ 日本马皮疽,那不勒斯马皮疽,兽疫性淋巴管炎 / ~ pipes 淋巴管马皮疽

fardel-bound [ˈfɑːdəl baund] *n* 食阻(指牛、羊)

farina [fəˈriːnə] *n* 谷粉,面粉;淀粉 | ~ avena 燕麦片 / ~ tritici 小麦粉

farinaceous [ˌfæriˈneiʃəs] *a* 谷粉的;含淀粉的

farinometer [ˌfæriˈnɔmitə] *n* 面粉谷胶测定器

farinose [ˈfærinəus] *a* 产粉的,含粉的;粉质的

farnoguinone [fɑːnəˈkwinəun] *n* 金合欢醌,维生素 K_2

Farre's tubercles [fɑː] (John R. Farre) 法尔结节(肝囊下方的块,在某些肝癌病例中触诊可摸到)

Farre's white line [fɑː] (Arthur Farre) 法尔白线(卵巢系膜附着卵巢门的线)

Farr's law [fɑː] (William Farr) 法尔定律(传染病流行时发病数逐渐减少)

farsighted [ˈfɑːˈsaitid] *a* 远视的 | **~ness** *n*

fasc. fasciculus *n*【拉】束

fascia [ˈfeiʃə, ˈfæʃiə] ([复] **fasciae** [ˈfæʃiiː]) *n*【拉】筋膜 | anal ~ 盆膈下筋膜 / anoscrotal ~ 会阴浅筋膜 / antebrachial ~, (deep) ~ of forearm 前臂筋膜 / aponeurotic ~, deep ~ 深筋膜 / clavipectoral ~, coracoclavicular ~ 锁胸筋膜,喙锁筋膜 / cribriform ~ 筛状板;股环隔 / crural ~ 小腿筋膜 / fibroareolar ~ 浅筋膜 / hypogastric ~, pelvic ~ 盆筋膜 / iliac ~ 髂筋膜;髂耻弓 / infundibuliform ~, internal spermatic ~ 漏斗状筋膜,精索内筋膜 / intercolumnar ~ 睾提筋膜;脚间纤维 / ischioprostatic ~ 尿生殖膈下筋膜 / ischiorectal ~ 盆膈下筋膜 / palpebral ~ 睑筋膜,眶隔 / prevertebral ~ 椎前筋膜,椎前层 / rectal ~, rectovesical ~ 盆膈上筋膜 / rectoabdominal ~ 腹直肌鞘 / scalene ~ 胸膜上膜 / subperitoneal ~ 腹膜下筋膜;腹膜浆膜下组织 / superficial perineal ~ 会阴浅筋膜 / thoracolumbar ~, lumbodorsal ~ 胸腰筋膜,腰背筋膜 / triangular ~ of abdomen 腹股沟反转韧带 | **~l** *a*

fasciagram [ˈfæʃiəgræm] *n* 筋膜造影[照]片

fasciagraphy [ˌfæʃiˈægrəfi] *n* 筋膜造影[术]

fasciaplasty [ˈfæʃiəˌplæsti] *n* 筋膜成形术

fascicle [ˈfæsikl] *n* 束 | **~d** *a* 成束的;簇生的

fascicular [fəˈsikjulə] *a* 束的;束状的,成束的;簇生的

fasciculate [fəˈsikjulit], **fasciculated** [fəˈsikjuleitid] *a* 束状的,成束的;簇生的

fasciculation [fəˌsikjuˈleiʃən] *n* 成束;(肌纤维)自发性收缩

fasciculus [fəˈsikjuləs] ([复] **fasciculi** [fəˈsikjulai]) *n*【拉】束 | cerebellospinal ~ 脊髓小脑后束 / dorsolateral ~ 背外侧束 / extrapyramidal motor ~ 红核脊髓束

fasciectomy [ˌfæsiˈektəmi] *n* 筋膜切除术

fasciitis [ˌfæsiˈaitis] *n* 筋膜炎 | exudative calcifying ~ 渗出钙化性筋膜炎,钙质沉着

fasciodesis [ˌfæsiˈɔdisis] *n* 筋膜固定术

Fasciola [fəˈsaiələ, fəˈsiələ] *n* 片吸虫属 | ~ cervi 鹿片吸虫(即鹿同盘吸虫 Paramphistomum cervi) / ~ gigantica 大片吸虫 / ~ hepatica 肝片吸虫 / ~ heterophyes 异形片吸虫(即异形异形吸虫 Heterophyes heterophyes)

fasciola [fəˈsaiələ] ([复] **fasciolae** [fəˈsaiəliː]) *n* 【拉】小片,小束;小绷带 | ~ cinerea, ~ cinerea cinguli 束状回 | **~r** [fəˈsaiələ] *a*

Fascioletta [ˌfæsiəuˈletə] *n* 棘口线虫属(即 Echinostoma) | ~ ilocana 伊族棘口吸虫(即 Echinostoma ilocanum)

fascioliasis [ˌfæsiəuˈlaiəsis] *n* 片形吸虫病

fasciolicide [ˌfæsiˈəulisaid] *n* 杀片吸虫药

Fasciolidae [ˌfæsiˈəulidiː] *n* 拟片吸虫科

Fascioloides [ˌfæsiəuˈlɔidiːz] *n* 拟片吸虫属 | ~ magna 巨大拟片吸虫

fasciolopsiasis [ˌfæsiəulɔpˈsaiəsis] *n* 姜片虫病

Fasciolopsis [ˌfæsiəuˈlɔpsis] *n* 姜片虫属 | ~ buski 布氏姜片虫

fascioplasty [ˈfæʃiəˌplæsti] *n* 筋膜成形术

fasciorrhaphy [ˌfæʃiˈɔrəfi] *n* 筋膜缝合术

fasciotomy [ˌfæʃiˈɔtəmi] *n* 筋膜切开术

fascitis [fəˈsaitis] *n* 筋膜炎

fast[1] [fɑːst] *a* 紧的,牢的;不褪色的;快[速]的;抗拒的(指对某种特效药物的作用、染色或退染剂具有抗力)

fast[2] [fɑːst] *vi*, *n* 禁食,节制饮食

fastidious [fæsˈtidiəs] *a* 难养的(指需要复杂营养和培养条件的微生物)

fastidium [fæsˈtidiəm] *n* 【拉】厌食症 | ~ cibi 厌食症 / ~ potus 厌饮症

fastigatum [ˌfæstiˈgeitəm] *a* 【拉】尖的

fastigium [fæsˈtidʒiəm] *n* 【拉】顶,尖顶(第四脑室顶的最高点);极度,顶点(如发热) | **fastigial** [fæsˈtidʒiə] *a*

fasting [ˈfɑːstiŋ] *n* 禁食,绝食 *a* 禁食的,空腹的

fastness [ˈfɑːstnis] *n* 抗拒性(细菌)

fat [fæt] *a* 肥胖的,肥大的,多脂肪的 *n* 脂肪 | brown ~, moruloid ~, mulberry 褐色脂肪 / chyle ~ 乳糜脂,乳化脂肪 / corpse ~, grave ~ 尸脂,尸蜡 / fetal ~ 胎儿性脂肪(此术语在病理学上有时用于指褐脂组织) / hydrous wool ~ 含水羊毛脂 / masked ~, bound ~ 隐性脂肪,结合脂肪 / milk ~ 乳[内]脂 / molecular ~ 分子脂肪 / wool ~ 羊毛脂

fatal [ˈfeitl] *a* 致命的,致死的

fatality [fəˈtæləti] *n* 致命性

fate [feit] *n* 命运;结局 | prospective ~ 预期命运

fat-free [ˈfætfriː] *a* 不含脂肪的

fatigability [ˌfætigəˈbiləti] *n* 易疲[劳]性

fatigue [fəˈtiːg] *n* 疲劳 | combat ~ 战斗疲劳症 / pseudocombat ~ 假性战斗疲劳症 / stimulation ~ 刺激性疲劳

fatty [ˈfæti] *a* 脂肪的

fatty acid [ˈfæti] 脂肪酸 | free ~ ~s(FFA) 游离脂肪酸 / nonesterified ~ ~s(NEFA) 非酯化脂肪酸 / polyunsaturated ~ ~s 多不饱和脂肪酸

fatty acid synthase 脂肪酸合酶

fatty acid thiokinase [ˈfæti ˈæsid ˌθaiəuˈkaineis] 脂肪酸硫激酶

fatuity [fəˈtju(ː)əti] *n* 愚鲁;痴呆

fatuous [ˈfætjuəs] *a* 愚蠢的

fauces [ˈfɔːsiːz] [复] *n* 【拉】咽门 | **faucial** [ˈfɔːʃəl] *a*

Fauchard's disease [fəuˈʃɑː] (Pierre Fauchard) 边缘性牙周炎

faucitis [fɔːˈsaitis] *n* 咽门炎

Faught's sphygmomanometer [fɔːt] (Francis A. Faught) 福特血压计

fauna [ˈfɔːnə] ([复] **faunae** [ˈfɔːniː] 或 **faunas**) *n* 动物志;动物区系 | **~l** *a*

Fauvel's granules [fəuˈvel] (Sulpice A. Fauvel) 支气管周脓肿

fava [ˈfeivə] *n* 蚕豆

faveolate [feiˈviːəlit] *a* 蜂窝状的

faveolus [feiˈviːələs] ([复] **faveoli** [feiˈviːəlai]) *n* 【拉】(小)凹 | **faveolar** *a*

favid [ˈfeivid] *n* 黄癣疹

favism [ˈfeivizəm] *n* 蚕豆病(食用蚕豆或吸入该植物的花粉后所引起的一种急性溶血性贫血)

Favre-Durand-Nicolas disease [ˈfɑːvr djuˈræn nikəˈlɑː] (Maurice J. Favre; J. Durand; Joseph Nicolas) 法-杜-尼病,性病性淋巴肉芽肿

Favre-Racouchot nodular elastosis (syndrome) [ˈfɑːvre rɑːkuːˈʃəu] (Maurice J. Favre; Jean Racouchot) 法-拉结节性弹力纤维病(综合征)(光化性弹力纤维病,主要发生于老年男性,眶周区可见巨大粉刺、毛皮脂腺囊肿及浅黄色多皱皮肤的大褶。亦称结节性类弹力纤维病)

favus [ˈfeivəs] *n* 黄癣

Fay method [fei] (T. Fay) 费伊方法(为消除痉挛的系统医疗体操)

Fazio-Londe atrophy, disease [ˈfɑːziəu ləund] (E. Fazio; P. E. L. Londe) 法齐奥-隆德萎缩、病,儿童期进行性延髓性麻痹

Fc (fragment, crystallizable) Fc 片段(即免疫球蛋白经木瓜蛋白酶水解后的结晶片段)

Fc' Fc' 片段(即免疫球蛋白经胃蛋白酶水解后的结晶片段)

5-FC flucytosine 氟胞嘧啶,5-氟胞嘧啶

fCi femtocurie 飞[母托]居里

Fd Fd 片段(即免疫球蛋白经木瓜蛋白酶水解后的抗原结合片段的重链部分)

Fd' Fd' 片段(即免疫球蛋白经胃蛋白酶水解后的抗原结合片段的重链部分)

FDA fronto-dextra anterior 额右前(胎位);Food

and Drug Administration 食品和药物管理局
FDI Fédération Dentaire Internationale【法】国际牙科联合会
FDP fibrin degradation products 纤维蛋白降解产物; fibrinogen degradation products 纤维蛋白原降解产物; fronto-dextra posterior 额右后(胎位)
FDT fronto-dextra transversa 额右横(胎位)
F-duction [ef-ˈdʌkʃən] F 因子传导(细菌遗传学中的一个过程,一部分细菌染色体附着于自主性 F 因子〈致育因子〉上,因而极其频繁地从供体〈雄性〉细菌转移到受体〈雌性〉细菌。亦称性导)
F-dUMP 5-fluorodeoxyuridine monophosphate 5-氟尿苷一磷酸
FE_{Na} fractional excretion of sodium 钠排泄分数
FE_{Na} excreted fraction of filtered sodium 滤过钠排泄分数(见 test 项下相应术语)
Fe iron 铁(由拉丁名 ferrum 而来)
fear [fiə] *n* 恐惧,畏惧
feasible [ˈfiːzəbl] *a* 可行的;可用的,适宜的 | **feasibility** [ˌfiːzəˈbiləti] *n* 可行性,可能性
feature [ˈfiːtʃə] *n* 容貌;特征,特点
febantel [ˈfebəntəl] *n* 非班太尔(兽用抗蠕虫药)
Feb. dur. febre durante【拉】发热期间
febricant [ˈfebrikənt] *a* 致热的
febricide [ˈfebrisaid] *n* 退热药
febricity [fiˈbrisəti] *n* 发热
febricula [fiˈbrikjulə] *n*【拉】轻热
febrifacient [ˌfebriˈfeiʃənt], **febrific** [fiˈbrifik] *a* 发热性的,致热的
febrifugal [fiˈbrifjugəl, ˌfebriˈfjuːgəl] *a* 退热的,解热的
febrifuge [ˈfebrifjuːdʒ] *n* 退热药,解热药
febrifugine [feˈbrifjudʒin] *n* 退热碱,常山碱
febrile [ˈfiːbrail, ˈfebril] *a* 热性的,发热的
febris [ˈfiːbris] *n*【拉】发热,热
fecal [ˈfiːkəl] *a* 粪便的
fecalith [ˈfiːkəliθ] *n* 粪石
fecaloid [ˈfiːkəlɔid] *a* 粪样的
fecaloma [ˌfiːkəˈləumə] *n* 粪结,粪瘤(肠内积粪)
fecaluria [ˌfiːkəˈljuəriə] *n* 粪尿
feces [ˈfiːsiːz] [复] *n* 粪便
Fechner's law [ˈfeʃnə, ˈfek-] (Gustav T. Fechner) 费希纳定律(不同刺激所产生的感觉的强度与该刺激强度的对数成正比)
fecula [ˈfekjulə] *n* 渣滓;淀粉
feculent [ˈfekjulənt] *n* 有渣滓的;粪便的
fecund [ˈfiːkənd, ˈfekənd] *a* 生殖力旺盛的
fecundability [fəˌkʌndəˈbiliti] *n* 能生育率
fecundate [ˈfiːkəndeit] *vt* 使受孕,使受精
fecundatio [ˈfiːkʌnˈdeiʃiəu] *n*【拉】受孕,受精 | ~ ab extra 体外受精
fecundation [ˌfiːkənˈdeiʃən] *n* 受孕,受精 | artificial ~ 人工受孕,人工受精
fecundity [fiˈkʌndəti] *n* 生殖能,生殖力;产卵力
Federici's sign [fidiˈriːtʃi] (Cesare Federici) 费德里契征(肠穿孔时腹腔充气,听诊腹部可听到心音)
Fede's disease [ˈfeidei] (Francesco Fede) 费代病(见 Riga-Fede disease)
feeblemindedness [ˌfiːblˈmaindidnis] *n* 低能
feedback [ˈfiːdbæk] *n* 反馈 | alpha ~ α-反馈 / negative ~ 负反馈 / positive ~ 正反馈
feeder [ˈfiːdə] *n* 饲养员;奶瓶;喂食器;进料器
feedforward [fiːdˈfɔːwəd] *n* 前馈
feeding [ˈfiːdiŋ] *n* 喂养,饲,哺;加液(组织培养) | artificial ~ 人工喂养 / breast ~ 母乳喂养 / extrabuccal ~ 口外喂养 / forced ~, forcible ~ 强制喂养 / sham ~ 假饲
feeling [ˈfiːliŋ] *n* 触觉;知觉;感觉;情感;感情 | ~ of being controlled 被控制感
Feer's disease [ˈfeiə] (Emil Feer) 肢痛症
fee-splitting [fiːˈsplitiŋ] *n* 收费分成(指专科医师如外科医师所分得的收入与转托患者给他的内科医师之间的分成)
feet [fiːt] foot 的复数
FEF forced expiratory flow 用力呼气流量
Fehleisen's streptococcus [ˈfeilaisən] (Friedrich Fehleisen) 化脓链球菌
Fehling's solution [ˈfeiliŋ] (Hermann C. von Fehling) 费林溶液(检尿糖用) | ~ test 费林试验(检尿葡萄糖)
fel [fel] *n*【拉】胆汁 | ~ bovis 牛胆汁 / ~ bovis purificatum, ~ tauri purificatum 精制牛胆汁
felbamate [ˈfelbəˌmeit] *n* 非尔氨酯(抗惊厥药)
Feldenkrais method [ˈfeldenkrais] (Moshe Feldenkrais) 费尔登克赖斯法(利用探查性技术使患者重新学习功能障碍运动型的专用法)
Felderstruktur [ˌfeldəˈʃtruktur] *n*【德】肌丝结构
Feleky's instrument [feiˈleiki] (Hugó von Feleky) 费累基器(前列腺按摩器)
Felicola [feliˈkəulə] *n* 猫羽虱属
feline [ˈfiːlain] *a* 猫的 *n* 猫;猫科动物
Felix-Weil reaction [ˈfeiliks-vai] (Arthur Felix; Edmund Weil)斐-外反应(见 Weil-Felix reaction)
fellatio [fiˈleiʃiəu] *n* 含阳,舐阳(吮吸阴茎)
felo-de-se [ˌfeiləu dei ˈsei] *n*【西】自杀者
felodipine [fəˈləudipiːn] *n* 非洛地平(抗高血压药)
felon [ˈfelən] *n* 瘭疽,指头脓炎 | bone ~ 骨瘭疽 / deep ~ 深瘭疽 / subcuticular ~, subepithelial ~, superficial ~ 表皮下瘭疽,浅瘭疽 / thecal ~ 滑膜鞘瘭疽
Felton's phenomenon [ˈfeltən] (Lloyd D. Fel-

ton) 费尔顿现象(在小鼠体内注射大剂量抗原引起对肺炎球菌多糖的免疫无反应性或免疫耐受性) | ~ serum 费尔顿血清(浓缩抗肺炎球菌马血清) / ~ unit 费尔顿单位(抗肺炎球菌血清的小鼠保护单位)

feltwork [ˈfeltwəːk] *n* 神经纤维网

Felty's syndrome [ˈfelti] (Augustus R. Felty) 费尔蒂综合征(慢性、类风湿关节炎、脾大、白细胞减少、下肢皮肤色素斑及脾功能亢进等的其他表现,即贫血和血小板减少)

felypressin [feliˈpresin] *n* 苯赖加压素(血管收缩药,升压药)

female [ˈfiːmeil] *a* 女性的,雌性的 *n* 女性,女子;雌性生物

feminine [ˈfeminin] *a* 女性的,雌性的

femininity [ˌfemiˈninəti] *n* 女子本性,女性;女子气

feminism [ˈfeminizəm] *n* 男子女[性]征 | mammary ~ 男子乳房发育,男子女性型乳房

feminization [ˌfeminaiˈzeiʃən, -niˈz-] *n* 女性化(指男子);雌性化 | testicular ~ 睾丸女性化,睾丸雌化(患者表征像女性,但缺少核性染色质,为 XY 染色体性别)

feminize, feminise [ˈfeminaiz] *vt, vi* (使)女性化(指男子);(用卵巢植入术等)使雌性化

feminizing [ˈfemiˌnaiziŋ] *a* 女性化的

feminonucleus [ˌfeminəuˈnjuːkliːəs] *n* 雌性原核

Fem. intern. femoribus internus【拉】股内侧

femme [fem, fɑːm] *n*【法】妇女 | sage ~ 助产士

femor(o)- [构词成分]股骨

femora [ˈfemərə] femur 的复数

femoral [ˈfemərəl] *a* 股骨的;股的

femorocele [ˈfemərəusiːl] *n* 股疝

femorofemoral [ˌfemərəuˈfemərəl] *a* 股股的(左和右股动脉的)

femorofemoropopliteal [ˌfemərəuˌfemərəupɔpˈlitiəl] *a* 股股腘的(左右股动脉和腘动脉的)

femoroiliac [ˌfemərəuˈiliæk] *a* 股髂的

femoropopliteal [ˌfemərəupɔpˈlitiəl] *a* 股腘的(股动脉和腘动脉的)

femorotibial [ˌfemərəuˈtibiəl] *a* 股胫的

femto- [构词成分]飞[母托](10^{-15})

femtocurie(fCi) [ˌfemtəuˈkjuəri] *n* 飞[母托]居里(10^{-15} 居里,1 Ci〈居里〉= 37 GBq〈贝可勒尔〉)

femur [ˈfiːmə] ([复] **femurs** 或 **femora** [ˈfemərə]) *n*【拉】股骨;股

fenalamide [fəˈnæləmaid] *n* 非那拉胺(平滑肌松弛药)

fenamate [ˈfenəmeit] *n* 芬那酸(镇痛消炎药)

fenbendazole [fənˈbendəzəul] *n* 芬苯达唑(抗蠕虫药)

fenbufen [fənˈbjuːfən] *n* 芬布芬(抗炎药)

fenclofenac [fənˈkləufənæk] *n* 芬氯酸(抗炎药)

fenclonine [ˈfenkləniːn] *n* 芬克洛宁(5-羟色胺抑制药)

fenclorac [fənˈklɔːræk] *n* 苯克洛酸(抗炎药)

fendosal [ˈfendəsəl] *n* 芬度柳(抗炎药)

fenestra [fiˈnestrə] ([复]**fenestrae** [fiˈnestriː]) *n*【拉】窗 | ~ of cochlea, ~ cochleae, ~ rotunda 蜗窗,正圆窗 / ~ non-ovalis 人造前庭窗 / ~ vestibuli, ~ ovalis 前庭窗,卵圆窗 | **~l** *a*

fenestrate [ˈfenestreit] *vt, vi* 凿孔,开窗

fenestrated [fiˈnestreitid] *a* 有孔的,有窗的

fenestration [ˌfenisˈtreiʃən] *n* 穿通,穿孔;开窗术(治耳硬化症) | aortopulmonary ~ 主动脉肺动脉穿通(主动脉中隔缺损) / apical ~, alveolar plate ~ 根尖穿孔,牙槽板穿孔

fenestrel [fəˈnestrəl] *n* 芬雌酸(雌激素类药)

fenethylline hydrochloride [fəˈneθiliːn] 盐酸芬乙茶碱(中枢神经系统兴奋药)

fenfluramine hydrochloride [fənˈfluːrəmiːn] 盐酸芬氟拉明(拟肾上腺素药,用作食欲抑制药,短期治疗外源性肥胖症,口服)

feng shui【汉】风水

fenimide [ˈfenimaid] *n* 非尼米特(安定药)

fenisorex [fəˈnaisəreks] *n* 非尼雷司,(食欲抑制药)

fenmetozole hydrochloride [fənˈmetəzəul] 盐酸氯苯氧甲唑(抗抑郁药,麻醉药拮抗药)

fenmetramide [fənˈmetrəmaid] *n* 苯甲吗酮(抗抑郁药)

fennel [ˈfenl] *n* 茴香

fenobam [ˈfenəbæm] *n* 非诺班(安定药)

fenofibrate [ˌfenəuˈfaibreit] *n* 非诺贝特(降血脂药)

fenoldopam mesylate [fiˈnɔldəupæm] 甲磺非诺多泮(血管扩张药)

fenoprofen [ˌfenəˈprəufən] *n* 非诺洛芬(消炎镇痛药)

fenoprofen calcium [ˌfenəuˈprəufən] 非诺洛芬钙(抗炎药,用于治疗类风湿关节炎和骨关节炎)

fenoterol [ˌfenəˈterəul] *n* 非诺特罗(支气管扩张药)

fenpipalone [fənˈpipələun] *n* 苯吡噁二酮(抗炎药)

fenspiride hydrochloride [fənˈspiəraid] 盐酸芬司匹利(支气管扩张药)

fentanyl citrate [ˈfentənil] 枸橼酸芬太尼(麻醉性镇痛药)

fenticlor [ˈfentiklə] *n* 芬替克洛(局部抗感染药,抗真菌药)

fenugreek [ˈfenjugriːk] *n* 胡芦巴(种子)

Fenwick's disease [ˈfenwik] (Samuel Fenwick)

芬威克病(特发性萎缩性胃炎)

FEP free erythrocyte protoporphyrin 游离红细胞原卟啉

fer-de-lance [ˌfɛə də ˈlɑːŋs] *n*【法】枪蝰,矛头蛇,大具窍蝮蛇(南美及中美等地的大毒蛇)

Ferguson Smith epithelioma [ˈfəːgəsən smiθ] (John Ferguson Smith) 弗格森·史密斯上皮瘤,自愈性鳞状上皮瘤

Fergusson's incision (operation) [ˈfəːgəsn] (William Fergusson) 弗格森切口(手术)(上颌骨切除的皮肤切开法) | ~ speculum 弗格森窥器(镀银玻管制的圆柱形阴道窥器)

ferment [ˈfəːment] *n* 酶,酵素;发酵 [fə(ː)ˈment] *vt*, *vi* 发酵

fermentation [ˌfəːmenˈteiʃən] *n* 发酵 | heterolactic ~ 杂乳酸发酵 / homolactic ~ 纯乳酸发酵 / mixed acid ~ 混合酸发酵 / stormy ~ 汹涌发酵 | **fermentative** [fəːˈmentətiv] *a*

fermentemia [ˌfəːmenˈtiːmiə] *n* 酶血症

fermentogen [fəːˈmentedʒən] *n* 酶原

fermentoid [fəːˈmentɔid] *n* 类酶(已失活性的变性酶)

fermentum [fəːˈmentəm] *n*【拉】酵母[菌],酿母[菌]

fermium(Fm) [ˈfɛəmiəm] *n* 镄(化学元素)

fern [fəːn] *n* 蕨,蕨类植物,羊齿植物 | **~y** *a* 蕨的;像蕨的;多蕨的

ferning [ˈfəːniŋ] *n* 蕨样变[现象](子宫颈黏膜的干标本,表明有雌激素存在)

-ferous [构词成分]产生

ferpentetate [fəˈpentəteit] *n* 铁喷替酸(铁和抗坏血酸与喷替酸的一种螯合物,^{99m}Tc 络合用于肾扫描)

ferr(o)- [构词成分]铁

Ferrata's cells [fəˈrɑːtə] (Adolfo Ferrata) 成血细胞

ferrate [ˈfereit] *n* 高铁酸盐

ferrated [ˈfereitid] *a* 含铁的

ferredoxin [ˌferiˈdɔksin] *n* 铁氧还蛋白

Ferrein's canal [ˈferæn] (Antoine Ferrein) 费蓝管,泪河(闭合的眼睑边缘所形成的隙,睡眠时可将眼泪导至泪点) | ~ cords 费蓝带(下或真正声带,声襞) ~ foramen 面神经管裂孔 / ~ ligament 费蓝韧带,颞颌韧带(颞颌关节囊外侧肥厚部) / ~ pyramid 肾皮质小叶辐射部 / ~ tubes 肾曲小管 / ~ tubule 费蓝小管(形成肾皮质小叶辐射部的肾小管部分)

ferreous [ˈferiəs] *a* 铁的,含铁的

ferri [ˈferi] (【拉】ferrum 的所有格) *n* 铁

ferri-albuminic [ˌferi ælbjuˈminik] *a* 含铁[与]白蛋白的

Ferribacterium [ˌferibækˈtiəriəm] *n* 铁杆菌属

ferric [ˈferik] *a* 高铁[基]的,[正]铁的,三价铁的 | ~ fructose 果糖铁(抗贫血药,治疗缺铁) / red ~ oxide 红氧化铁,赤色氧化铁 / yellow ~ oxide 黄色氧化铁

ferricyanic acid [ˌferisaiˈænik] 氰铁酸

ferricytochrome [ˌferiˈsaitəkrəum] *n* 高铁细胞色素

ferriheme [ˈferihiːm] *n* 高铁血红素,高铁原卟啉

ferrihemochrome [ˌferiˈhiːməkrəum] *n* 高铁血色素

ferritin [ˈferitin] *n* 铁蛋白

Ferrobacillus [ˌferəubəˈsiləs] *n* 亚铁[芽胞]杆菌属

ferrochelatase [ˌferəuˈkiːləteis] *n* 亚铁螯合酶(缺乏此酶为一种常染色体显性性状,可致原卟啉病)

ferrocholinate [ˌferəuˈkəulineit] *n* 铁胆盐(亦称枸橼酸铁胆碱,抗贫血药,用于治疗缺铁性贫血)

ferrocyanic acid [ˌferəusaiˈænik] 氰亚铁酸,亚铁氰酸

ferroflavoprotein [ˌferəuˌfleivəuˈprəutiːn] *n* 亚铁黄素蛋白

ferroflocculation [ˌferəuflɔkjuˈleiʃən] *n* 铁絮状反应(用细铁粒抗原对疟疾作絮状试验)

ferroheme [ˈferəuhiːm] *n* [亚铁]血红素

ferrohemochrome [ˌferəuˈhiːməkrəum] *n* 低铁血色素

ferrokinetics [ˌferəukiˈnetiks, -kaiˈn-] *n* 铁动力学(铁在机体内的吸收、利用、代谢等) | **ferrokinetic** *a*

ferroprotein [ˌferəuˈprəutiːn] *n* 铁蛋白

ferroprotoporphyrin [ˌferəuˌprəutəuˈpɔːfirin] *n* 亚铁原卟啉

ferrosilicon [ˌferəuˈsilikɔn] *n* 硅铁(合金)(钢脱氧用)

ferrosoferric [ˌferəusɔˈferik] *a* 亚铁高铁的

ferrotherapy [ˌferəuˈθerəpi] *n* 铁剂疗法

ferrous [ˈferəs] *a* 亚铁的,二价铁的 | ~ fumarate 富马酸亚铁(抗贫血药,用于治疗缺铁) / ~ gluconate 葡萄糖酸亚铁(抗贫血药) / ~ lactate 乳酸亚铁(以前用作补血药) / ~ sulfate 硫酸亚铁(抗贫血药)

ferroxidase [feˈrɔksideis] *n* 亚铁氧化酶

ferruginous [feˈruːdʒinəs] *a* 含铁的;铁锈色的

ferrule [ˈferuːl] *n* 牙环,金属加固环(用于牙根或牙冠)

ferrum [ˈferəm] *n*【拉】铁

Ferry-Porter law [ˈferi ˈpɔːtə] (Ervin S. Ferry; T. C. Porter) 费里-波特定律(临界融合频率与光强度的对数成正比)

fertile [ˈfəːtail, -til] *a* 能生育的

fertility [fəːˈtiləti] *n* 生育力,受精[能]力;生育

率,人口出生率
fertilization [ˌfəːtilaiˈzeiʃən, -liˈz-] *n* 受精,授精 | cross ~ 异体受精 / external ~ 体外受精 / internal ~ 体内受精 / in vitro ~ 体外受精
fertilize, fertilise [ˈfəːtilaiz] *vt* 使受精
fertilizer [ˈfəːtilaizə] *n* 肥料;受精媒介物
fertilizin [ˈfəːtilaizin, ˌfəːtiˈlai-] *n* 受精素
Ferv. fervens【拉】煮沸的,沸腾的
fervescence [fəːˈvesns] *n* 发热,体温升高
FES functional electrical stimulation 功能性电刺激;functional endoscopic sinus surgery 功能性内镜窦外科
fescue [ˈfeskjuː] *n* 羊茅草,酥油草(用作牧草);羊茅病,羊茅足(牛、羊)
fester [ˈfestə] *n* 浅溃疡;脓疱 *vi, vt* 溃烂,化脓(浅表化脓)
festinant [ˈfestinənt] *a* 加速的,慌张的
festination [ˌfestiˈneiʃən] *n* 慌张步态(见于震颤麻痹及其他神经性疾病)
festoon [fesˈtuːn] *n* 缘饰;突彩,龈缘弯肿
Festuca [fesˈtuːkə] *n* 羊茅属
fetal [ˈfiːtl] *a* 胎的,胎儿的
fetalism [ˈfiːtəlizəm], **fetalization** [ˌfiːtəlaiˈzeiʃən, -liˈz-] *n* 胎型(出生后仍有某些胎象存留)
fetation [fiːˈteiʃən] *n* 成胎;胎儿发育;妊娠,[受]孕
feticide [ˈfiːtisaid] *n* 杀胎,堕胎 | **feticidal** [ˌfiːtiˈsaidl] *a*
fetid [ˈfetid] *a* 恶臭的,腐臭的
fetish [ˈfetiʃ, ˈfiːtiʃ] *n* 拜物(原始人认为有神赋力之物);恋物(能引起性满足之物)
fetishism [ˈfetiʃizəm, ˈfiː-] *n* 恋物癖 | transvestic ~ 易装癖
fetishist [ˈfetiʃist, ˈfiː-] *n* 恋物癖者
fetlock [ˈfetlɔk] *n* 距毛;球节(马)
fetoglobulin [ˌfiːtəuˈglɔbjulin] *n* 胎蛋白
fetography [fiːˈtɔgrəfi] *n* 胎儿造影术
fetometry [fiːˈtɔmitri] *n* 胎儿测量法 | roentgen ~ 胎头 X 线测量法
fetopathy [fiːˈtɔpəθi] *n* 胎儿病
fetoplacental [ˌfiːtəupləˈsentl] *a* 胎儿胎盘的
fetoprotein [ˌfiːtəuˈprəutiːn] *n* 胎蛋白
α-fetoprotein [ˌfiːtəuˈprəutiːn] *n* 甲胎蛋白
fetor [ˈfiːtə] *n*【拉】臭气,恶臭 | ~ exore, ~ oris 口臭 / ~ hepaticus 肝病性口臭
fetoscope [ˈfiːtəskəup] *n* 胎儿镜;胎心听诊器
fetoscopy [fiːˈtɔskəpi] *n* 胎儿镜检查 | **fetoscopic** [ˌfiːtəˈskɔpik] *a*
fetoxylate hydrochloride [fiˈtɔksileit] 盐酸非托西酯(平滑肌松弛药)
fetuin [ˈfiːtjuin] *n* 胎球蛋白
fetus [ˈfiːtəs] *n* 胎【儿】 | ~ acardiacus 无心畸胎 / ~ amorphus 不成形寄生胎,不成形无心寄生胎 / calcified ~ 胎儿石化,石胎 / harlequin ~, ichthyosis ~ 斑色胎,先天性鱼鳞癣胎儿 / ~ in fetu 胎中胎 / mummified ~ 木乃伊化胎儿,干瘪胎儿 / paperdoll ~, papyraceous ~ 纸样胎 / ~ papyraceus, ~ compressus 纸样胎,压扁胎 / parasitic ~ 寄生胎 / sireniform ~ 并腿畸胎
Feuerstein-Mims syndrome [ˈfɔiərstain mimz] (Richard C. Feuerstein; Leroy C. Mims) 福-密综合征,雅达逊皮脂腺痣(即 nevus sebaceus of Jadassohn)
Feulgen test(reaction) [ˈfɔilgən] (Robert Feulgen) 福尔根试验(反应)(检动物性核酸及脱氧核糖核酸)
FEV forced expiratory volume 用力呼气量
fever [ˈfiːvə] *n* 发热,热 | African tick ~ 非洲蜱传热,非洲回归热 / algid pernicious ~ 寒冷型恶性疟,恶性疟 / aphthous ~ 口疮热,口蹄疫 / Argentine hemorrhagic ~ 阿根廷出血热(由呼宁〈Junin〉病毒所致的一种出血热,亦称呼宁热 Junin ~) / Assam ~ 阿萨姆热,黑热病 / asthenic ~, adynamic ~ 虚热,无力性发热,衰弱性发热 / autumn ~ 秋季热,七日热(钩端螺旋体病) / biduotertian ~ 持续[发热]型间日疟 / black ~ 落基山斑点热;黑热病(经典型内脏利什曼病) / blackwater ~ 黑尿热 / blue ~ 落基山斑点热 / Bolivian hemorrhagic ~ 玻利维亚出血热(由马丘波〈Machupo〉病毒所致的一种出血热) / boutonneuse ~ 南欧斑疹热 / brain ~ 脑热病,脑膜炎 / brassfounder's ~ 黄铜铸工热 / Brazilian purpuric ~ 巴西紫癜热(儿童的一种急性病,特征为腹痛、呕吐、瘀点、紫癜和近期结膜炎史) / Bullis ~ 布利斯军营热(1942 年得克萨斯州布利斯军营士兵发生的热病,为一种立克次体热) / Bwamba ~ 布汪巴热(乌干达的一种病毒热) / cachectic ~, cachexial ~ 恶病质热,黑热病(经典型内脏利什曼病) / camp ~ 流行性斑疹伤寒 / canicola ~ 犬钩端螺旋体病 / cat-scratch ~ 猫抓热 / central ~ 中枢性热(下丘脑体温调节中枢损害所致的持续性发热) / cerebrospinal ~ 流行性脑脊膜炎 / Chagres ~ 恰格尔斯热(巴拿马恰格尔斯河一带发生的疟疾) / childbed ~ 产褥热 / Choix ~ 北墨西哥斑疹热(与落基山斑点热同) / Colombian tick ~ 哥伦比亚蜱传斑疹热 / Colorado tick ~ 科洛拉多蜱传热(美国西部一种病毒病) / Congolian red ~ 刚果红色热,鼠型斑疹伤寒 / continued ~ 稽留热 / cotton-mill ~ 棉纺热,棉屑沉着病 / Cyprus ~ 波状热,布鲁[杆]菌病 / deer fly ~ 兔热病,土拉菌病 / dengue ~, dandy ~ 登革热 / dehydration ~ 新生儿脱水热;脱水热 / desert ~ 沙漠热(球孢子菌病初期) / double continued ~ 双峰稽留热(类似伤寒,发生在中国) / double

quartan ~ 复三日疟 / Dumdum ~ 黑热病(经典型内脏利什曼病, Dumdum 为印度一地名) / dust ~ 波状热,布鲁[杆]菌病 / East Coast ~, African Coast ~ 罗得西亚热,牛二联巴贝虫病 / enteric ~ 伤寒 / ephemeral ~ 短暂热 / epidemic catarrhal ~ 流行性感冒 / essential ~ 特发性热 / familial Mediterranean ~ 家族性地中海热 / famine ~ 饥饿热(回归热;斑疹伤寒) / flood ~ 洪水热,恙虫病 / glandular ~ 腺热,传染性单核白细胞增多[症] / Gibraltar ~ 直布罗陀热,波状热,布鲁[杆]菌病 / hay ~ 花粉症,枯草热 / hospital ~ 医院热,斑疹伤寒 / inanition ~ (新生儿)脱水热 / intermittent ~ 间歇热 / inundation ~ 洪水热,恙虫病 / island ~ 岛热,恙虫病 / Japanese flood ~, Japanese river ~ 洪水热,恙虫病 / jungle ~ 丛林热(东印度群岛恶性疟) / Junin ~ 呼宁热,阿根廷出血热 / Katayama ~ 片山热(急性全身性血吸虫病,此病首先在日本片山河流域报道) / Kedani ~ 恙虫病 / Kenya ~ 肯尼亚斑疹热 / Kew Gardens spotted ~ 立克次体痘 / Korin ~ 流行性出血热 / Lassa ~ 拉沙热(流行于西非的一种由沙粒病毒所致的高度致死的急性传染病) / Lone Star ~ 布利斯军营热(即 Bullis ~) / lung ~ 肺炎 / malarial ~ 疟疾 / Malta ~, Maltese ~ 马耳他热,波状热,布鲁[杆]菌病 / marsh ~ 沼泽热(钩端螺旋体性黄疸;疟疾) / Mediterranean ~ 地中海热(波状热,布鲁[杆]菌病;南欧斑疹热) / Mediterranean Coast ~ 地中海沿岸热,热带泰累尔梨浆虫病 / milk ~ 生乳热;地方性热(使用不洁牛乳所致);轻性产褥热 / Mossmam ~ 澳洲钩端螺旋体病 / mud ~ 沼地热,泥土热,钩端螺旋体性黄疸 / nanukayami ~ 七日热,钩端螺旋体病 / O'nyong-nyong ~ 翁尼翁-尼翁热(见 O'nyong-nyong) / Oroya ~ 奥罗亚热(巴尔通体病) / paratyphoid ~ 副伤寒 / parenteric ~ 类伤寒 / petechial ~ 瘀点热,脑脊膜炎 / Philippine hemorrhagic ~ 菲律宾出血热,出血性登革热 / phlebotomus ~, pappataci ~ 白蛉热 / Pontiac ~ 庞蒂亚克热(一种自限性疾病,1968 年在美国密执安庞蒂亚克一次暴发中首次发现,特征为发热、咳嗽、肌痛、寒战、胸痛、意识模糊和胸膜炎,现知由一株嗜肺性军团杆菌所致) / protein ~ 蛋白反应热 / puerperal ~ 产褥热 / pulmonary ~, pneumonic ~ 肺炎 / pythogenic ~ 腐败热,伤寒 / Q ~, Australian Q ~, nine-mile ~ Q 热(Q 表示疑问〈query〉,为一种发热性立克次体感染,常侵犯呼吸道) / quartan ~ 三日热,三日疟,四日两头疟 / quintan ~, quintana ~ 五日热 / quotidian ~ 每日热,日发热 / rabbit ~ 兔热病 / rat-bite ~ 鼠咬热 / relapsing ~, recurrent ~ 回归热 / remittent ~ 弛张热 / rheumatic ~ 风湿热,急性关节风湿病 / rice-field ~ 稻田热(一种钩端螺旋体病) / rock ~ 岩石热,波状热,布鲁[杆]菌病 / Rocky Mountain spotted ~ 落基山斑点热 / Roman ~ 罗马热(一种毒型疟疾) / sandfly ~ 白蛉热 / San Joaquin ~ (美国)圣华金河热(球孢子菌病初期) / scarlet ~ 猩红热 / seven-day ~ 七日热(类登革热;钩端螺旋体病) / ship ~ 船热,斑疹伤寒 / slime ~ 钩端螺旋体性黄疸 / sthenic ~ 实热,强壮性发热 / stiffneck ~ 僵颈热,流行性脑脊膜炎 / swamp ~ 沼地热(钩端螺旋体性黄疸;疟疾) / tertian ~ 间日疟 / tetanoid ~ 破伤风样热,脑脊膜炎 / Texas tick ~ 得克萨斯蜱热(见 Bullis ~) / thermic ~ 中暑性热,日射病,中暑 / three-day ~ 三日热,白蛉热 / Tobia ~ 落基山斑点热 / trench ~, five-day ~, shin bone ~ 战壕热,五日热,胫骨热 / trypanosome ~ 锥体虫热,锥虫病 / tsutsugamushi ~ 恙虫病 / typhoid ~ 伤寒 / typhomalarial ~ 伤寒型疟疾 / typhus ~ 斑疹伤寒 / undulant ~ 波状热,布鲁[杆]菌病 / valley ~ 溪谷热(球孢子菌病初期) / viral hemorrhagic ~ 病毒性出血热 / war ~ 流行性斑疹伤寒 / Yangtze Valley ~ 扬子江流域热,日本血吸虫病 / yellow ~ 黄热病(由黄病毒引起的急性传染病)

fever blister [ˈfiːvə ˈblistə] 发热性疱疹,单纯疱疹

feverfew [ˈfiːvəfjuː] *n* 白菊,野甘菊(用于治疗偏头痛、关节炎、风湿性疾病以及变态反应)

feverish [ˈfiːvəriʃ] *a* 发热的,引起热病的

Fèvre-Languepin syndrome [ˈfevrə ˈlæŋgəpen] (Marcel Fèvre; Anne Languepin) 费-兰综合征(腘蹼合并唇与腭裂、下唇瘘、并指〈趾〉畸形、甲发育不良及马蹄内翻足。亦称腘窝翼状赘蹼综合征)

fexofenadine hydrochloride [ˌfeksəˈfenədiːn] 盐酸非索芬定(H_1 受体拮抗药,用作抗组胺药,治疗季节性变应性鼻炎,口服给药)

FFA free fatty acids 游离脂肪酸

FFT flicker fusion threshold 闪光融合阈

F. h. fiat haustus【拉】制成顿服剂

FIA fluorescence immunoassay 荧光免疫测定;fluorescent immunoassay 荧光免疫测定;fluoroimmunoassay 荧光免疫测定

FIAC Fellow of International Academy of Cytology 国际细胞学会会员

fiat [ˈfaiət], **fiant** [ˈfaiənt]【拉】制成,作成

fiber [ˈfaibə] *n* 纤维 | A ~s A 类纤维(神经) / accelerating ~s, accelerator ~s, augmentor ~s, cardiac accelerator ~s [心]加速纤维 / accessory ~s, auxiliary ~s 副纤维 / B ~s B 类纤维(神经) / basilar ~s 基底纤维 / C ~s C 类纤维(神经) / chief ~s, principal ~s, main ~s 主纤维 / chromatic ~ 染色质线 / cilioequatorial ~s 睫状中纬线纤维 / collagenous ~, white ~s 胶原纤

维，白纤维 / continuous ~s 连续丝 / corticobulbar ~s, corticonuclear ~s 皮质核纤维 / elastic ~s, yellow ~s 弹性纤维，黄纤维 / half-spindle ~s 半纺锤丝 / muscle ~ 肌纤维 / reticular ~s, lattice ~s 网状纤维 / spindle ~s 纺锤丝 / sustentacular ~s 支柱纤维 / traction ~s, chromosomal ~s 牵引丝，染色体牵丝 / transilient ~s 逾回神经纤维 / varicose ~s 念珠状[神经]纤维

fibercolonoscope [ˌfaibəkəˈlɔnəskəup] *n* 结肠纤维镜

fibergastroscope [ˌfaibəˈgæstrəskəup] *n* 胃纤维镜

fiber-illuminated [ˈfaibə iˈljuːmiˌneitid] *a* 纤维照明的

fiberoptics [ˌfaibəˈrɔptiks] *n* 纤维光学 | **fiber-optic** *a* 纤维光学的，光学纤维的，光导纤维的，光纤的

fiberscope, fibrescope [ˈfaibəskəup] *n* 纤维镜

fibra [ˈfaibrə]（[复] **fibrae** [ˈfaibriː]）*n*【拉】纤维

fibrates [ˈfaibreits] *n* 纤维酸

fibre [ˈfaibə] *n* 纤维

fibric acid [ˈfaibrik] 纤维酸

fibril [ˈfaibril] *n* 原纤维，纤丝 | ~ acid 神经纤维酸 / border ~s 肌胶质 / collagen ~s 胶原纤维 / fibroglia ~s 纤维胶质原纤维 | **~lar**, **~lary** *a*

fibrilla [faiˈbrilə]（[复] **fibrillae** [faiˈbriliː]）*n*【拉】原纤维，纤丝

fibrillate [ˈfaibrileit] *a* 有原纤维的，有纤维组织的 *vt*, *vi* 形成原纤维

fibrillated [ˈfaibriˌleitid] *a* 原纤维的，原纤维组成的

fibrillation [ˌfaibriˈleiʃən] *n* 肌纤维震颤；原纤维形成 | atrial ~, auricular ~ 心房纤颤，心房颤动 / ventricular ~ 心室纤颤，心室颤动

Fibrillenstruktur [fiˌbrilenˈʃtruktur] *n*【德】[肌]原纤维结构

fibrillin [faiˈbrilin] *n* 微纤维蛋白

fibrilloblast [faiˈbriləblæst] *n* 成牙质细胞

fibrillogenesis [ˌfaibriləuˈdʒenisis] *n* 原纤维形成

fibrillolysis [ˌfaibriˈlɔlisis] *n* 原纤维溶解 | **fibrillolytic** [ˌfaibriləuˈlitik] *a* 溶解原纤维的

fibrin [ˈfaibrin] *n* 纤维蛋白，血纤蛋白 | gluten ~, vegetable ~ 麸纤维蛋白，植物纤维蛋白 / myosin ~ 肌浆（球蛋白）纤维蛋白 / stroma ~ 基质纤维蛋白

fibrinase [ˈfaibrineis] *n* [凝血]因子 XIII，纤维蛋白稳定因子，[血]纤维形成酶，[血]纤维交链酶

fibrinocellular [ˌfaibrinəuˈseljulə] *a* 纤维蛋白细胞的

fibrinogen [faiˈbrinədʒən] *n* 纤维蛋白原，血纤蛋白原

fibrinogenase [ˌfaibriˈnɔdʒineis] *n* [血]纤维蛋白原酶

fibrinogenemia [faiˌbrinədʒiˈniːmiə] *n* 纤维蛋白原血症

fibrinogenesis [ˌfaibrinəuˈdʒenisis] *n* 纤维蛋白形成

fibrinogenic [ˌfaibrinəuˈdʒenik], **fibrinogenous** [ˌfaibriˈnɔdʒinəs] *a* 纤维蛋白原的，产生纤维蛋白的

fibrinogenolysis [ˌfaibrinəudʒiˈnɔlisis] *n* 纤维蛋白原溶解[作用] | **fibrinogenolytic** [ˌfaibrinəuˌdʒenəˈlitik] *a* 溶解纤维蛋白原的

fibrinogenopenia [faiˌbrinəuˌdʒenəˈpiːniə] *n* [血]纤维蛋白原减少 | **fibrinogenopenic** [ˌfaibrinəuˌdʒenəˈpiːnik] *a*

fibrinoid [ˈfaibrinɔid] *a* 纤维蛋白样的 *n* 类纤维蛋白

fibrinokinase [ˌfaibrinəuˈkaineis] *n* 血纤（纤维蛋白溶酶原）激活酶，纤维蛋白激酶，纤维蛋白致活酶

fibrinolysin [ˌfaibriˈnɔlisin] *n* 纤维蛋白溶酶

fibrinolysis [ˌfaibriˈnɔlisis] *n* 纤维蛋白溶解 | **fibrinolytic** [ˌfaibrinəuˈlitik] *a* 溶纤维蛋白的 *n* 溶纤维蛋白药

fibrinopenia [ˌfaibrinəuˈpiːniə] *n* [血]纤维蛋白减少

fibrinopeptide [ˌfaibrinəuˈpeptaid] *n* 纤维蛋白肽，血纤肽

fibrinoplastin [ˌfaibrinəuˈplæstin] *n* 副球蛋白 | **fibrinoplastic** [ˌfaibrinəuˈplæstik] *a* 副球蛋白的，变性球蛋白的

fibrinoplatelet [ˌfaibrinəuˈpleitlit] *a* 血小板纤维蛋白的

fibrinopurulent [ˌfaibrinəuˈpjuərulənt] *a* 脓性纤维蛋白的

fibrinorrhea [ˌfaibrinəuˈriːə] *n* 纤维蛋白溢出

fibrinoscopy [ˌfaibriˈnɔskəpi] *n* 纤维质消化检查

fibrinose [ˈfaibrinəus] *n* 纤维蛋白脲

fibrinous [ˈfaibrinəs] *a* 纤维蛋白的

fibrinuria [ˌfaibriˈnjuəriə] *n* 纤维蛋白尿

fibr(o)- [构词成分] 纤维

fibroadenia [ˌfaibrəuəˈdiːniə] *n* 腺纤维化（尤指班替〈Banti〉病内淋巴细胞减少与肾小体基质增加）

fibroadenoma [ˌfaibrəuædiˈnəumə] *n* 纤维腺瘤 | giant ~ of the breast 乳腺巨大纤维腺瘤

fibroadenosis [ˌfaibrəuˌædiˈnəusis] *n* 纤维囊性乳腺病

fibroadipose [ˌfaibrəuˈædipəus] *a* 纤维脂肪性的

fibroangioma [ˌfaibrəuˌændʒiˈəumə] *n* 纤维血管瘤 | nasopharyngeal ~ 鼻咽纤维血管瘤

fibroareolar [ˌfaibrəuəˈriələ] *a* 纤维蜂窝性的，纤

维蜂窝组织的

fibroatrophy [ˌfaibrəuˈætrəfi] *n* 萎缩纤维化

fibroblast [ˈfaibrəblæst] *n* 成纤维细胞 | pericryptal ~ 腺周成纤维细胞 | **~ic** [ˌfaibrəuˈblæstik] *a*

fibroblastoma [ˌfaibrəublæsˈtəumə] *n* 成纤维细胞瘤 | perineural ~ 神经周成纤维细胞瘤

fibrobronchitis [ˌfibrəubrɔŋˈkaitis] *n* 纤维蛋白性支气管炎，格鲁布性支气管炎

fibrocalcific [ˌfaibrəukælˈsifik] *a* 纤维钙化的

fibrocarcinoma [ˌfaibrəukɑːsiˈnəumə] *n* 纤维癌，硬癌

fibrocartilage [ˌfaibrəuˈkɑːtilidʒ] *n* 纤维软骨 | basal ~ 基底纤维软骨 / basilar ~ 蝶枕软骨结合 / circumferential ~ 关节盂缘，盂缘 / connecting ~，spongy ~ 骨间纤维软骨 / cotyloid ~ 髋关节盂缘，髋臼缘 / elastic ~ 弹性纤维软骨，纤维弹力软骨 / interarticular ~ 关节盘 / intervertebral ~s 椎间盘 / semilunar ~s 关节半月板 | **fibrocartilaginous** [ˌfaibrəuˌkɑːtiˈlædʒinəs] *a*

fibrocartilago [ˌfaibrəukɑːtiˈleigəu] ([复] **fibrocartilagines** [ˌfaibrəuˌkɑːtiˈlædʒiniːz]) *n*【拉】纤维软骨

fibrocaseous [ˌfaibrəuˈkeisiəs] *a* 纤维干酪性的

fibrocellular [ˌfaibrəuˈseljulə] *a* 纤维[与]细胞的

fibrochondritis [ˌfaibrəukɔnˈdraitis] *n* 纤维软骨炎

fibrochondroma [ˌfaibrəukɔnˈdrəumə] *n* 纤维软骨瘤

fibrocollagenous [ˌfaibrəukɔˈlædʒinəs] *a* 纤维胶原的

fibrocyst [ˈfaibrəusist] *n* 囊变性纤维瘤

fibrocystic [ˌfaibrəuˈsistik] *a* 纤维囊性的

fibrocystoma [ˌfaibrəusisˈtəumə] *n* 纤维囊瘤

fibrocyte [ˈfaibrəsait] *n* 纤维细胞，成纤维细胞

fibrocytogenesis [ˌfaibrəuˌsaitəuˈdʒenisis] *n* 结缔组织纤维发生

fibrodysplasia [ˌfaibrəudisˈpleisiə] *n* 纤维发育不良

fibroelastic [ˌfaibrəuiˈlæstik] *a* 纤维[组织与]弹性组织的

fibroelastoma [ˌfaibrəuilæsˈtəumə] *n* 弹力纤维瘤 | papillary ~ 乳头状弹力纤维瘤

fibroelastosis [ˌfaibrəuˌiːlæsˈtəusis] *n* 弹力纤维增生 | endocardial ~ 心内膜弹力纤维增生症

fibroenchondroma [ˌfaibrəuˌenkɔnˈdrəumə] *n* 纤维[内生]软骨瘤

fibroepithelioma [ˌfaibrəuˌepiˌθiːliˈəumə] *n* 纤维上皮瘤 | premalignant ~ 恶变前纤维上皮瘤，恶变前上皮瘤

fibrofascitis [ˌfaibrəufəˈsaitis] *n* 纤维织炎

fibrofatty [ˌfaibrəuˈfæti] *a* 纤维脂肪性的

fibrofibrous [ˌfaibrəuˈfaibrəs] *a* 连结纤维的

fibrofolliculoma [ˌfaibrəufəˌlikjuˈləumə] *n* 纤维毛囊瘤

fibrogenesis [ˌfaibrəuˈdʒenisis] *n* 纤维发生 | ~ imperfecta ossium 骨不完全性纤维发生 | **fibrogenic** *a*

fibroglia [faiˈbrɔgliə] *n* 纤维胶质

fibroglioma [ˌfaibrəuglaiˈəumə] *n* 纤维胶质瘤

fibrohemorrhagic [ˌfaibrəuˌheməˈrædʒik] *a* 纤维蛋白性出血性的

fibrohistiocytic [ˌfaibrəuˌhistiəˈsitik] *a* 纤维组织细胞的

fibroid [ˈfaibrɔid] *a* 纤维性的，纤维样的 *n* 纤维瘤；平滑肌瘤（在临床口语中 fibroids 一词指子宫平滑肌瘤）

fibroidectomy [ˌfaibrɔiˈdektəmi] *n* 子宫纤维瘤切除术

fibroin [ˈfaibrəuin, faiˈbrəuin] *n* 丝心蛋白

fibrolamellar [ˌfaibrəuləˈmelə] *a* 纤维层的

fibrolipoma [ˌfaibrəuliˈpəumə] *n* 纤维脂瘤 | **~tous** *a*

fibrolymphoangioblastoma [ˌfaibrəuˌlimfəuˌændʒiəublæsˈtəumə] *n* 纤维成淋巴管细胞瘤

fibroma [faiˈbrəumə] ([复] **fibromas** 或 **fibromata** [faiˈbrəumətə]) *n* 纤维瘤 | ameloblastic ~ 成釉细胞纤维瘤 / cementifying ~ 成牙骨质细胞瘤 / concentric ~ 同心性[子宫]纤维瘤 / cystic ~ 囊变性纤维瘤，囊性纤维瘤 / hard ~，~ durum 硬纤维瘤 / intracanalicular ~ 小管内纤维瘤（乳腺纤维腺瘤） / juvenile nasopharyngeal ~ 青少年鼻咽纤维瘤（即鼻咽血管纤维瘤 nasopharyngeal angiofibroma） / nonosteogenic ~ 非成骨细胞瘤 / odontogenic ~ 牙原纤维瘤 / ossifying ~，ossifying ~ of bone 骨化性纤维瘤 / osteogenic ~ 成骨细胞瘤 / peripheral ossifying ~ 末梢骨化纤维瘤（即 epulis） / rabbit ~ 兔纤维瘤 / recurrent digital ~ of childhood 复发性指纤维瘤，儿童复发性趾纤维瘤 / soft ~，~ molle 软性纤维瘤 / telangiectatic ~ 血管纤维瘤 | **~tous** [faiˈbrəumətəs] *a*

fibromatogenic [faiˌbrəumətəuˈdʒenik] *a* 产生纤维瘤的

fibromatoid [faiˈbrəumətɔid] *a* 纤维瘤样的

fibromatosis [ˌfaibrəuməˈtəusis] *n* 纤维瘤病 | ~ colli 颈部纤维瘤病 / congenital generalized ~ 先天性泛发性纤维瘤病 / digital ~，infantile digital ~（婴儿）指[部]纤维瘤病 / ~ gingivae，gingival ~ 龈纤维瘤病 / palmar ~ 掌腱膜纤维瘤病 / plantar ~ 跖腱膜纤维瘤病 / subcutaneous pseudosarcomatous ~ 皮下假肉瘤样纤维瘤病，增生性筋膜炎 / ~ ventriculi 胃纤维瘤病，皮革状胃

fibromectomy [ˌfaibrəuˈmektəmi] *n* 纤维瘤切除术

fibromembranous [ˌfaibrəuˈmembrənəs] *a* 纤维膜性的

fibromuscular [ˌfaibrəuˈmʌskjulə] *a* 纤维肌性的

fibromyitis [ˌfaibrəumaiˈaitis] *n* 纤维性肌炎

fibromyoma [ˌfaibrəumaiˈəumə] *n* 纤维肌瘤 | ~ uteri 子宫纤维肌瘤,子宫平滑肌瘤

fibromyomectomy [ˌfaibrəuˌmaiəuˈmektəmi] *n* 纤维肌瘤切除术

fibromyositis [ˌfaibrəuˌmaiəuˈsaitis] *n* 纤维肌炎 | nodular ~ 结节性纤维肌炎

fibromyotomy [ˌfaibrəumaiˈɔtəmi] *n* 纤维肌瘤切除术

fibromyxoma [ˌfaibrəumikˈsəumə] *n* 纤维黏液瘤

fibromyxosarcoma [ˌfaibrəuˈmiksəusɑːˈkəumə] *n* 纤维黏液肉瘤

fibronectin [ˌfaibrəuˈnektin] *n* 纤维连接蛋白,纤连蛋白

fibroneuroma [ˌfaibrəunjuəˈrəumə] *n* 纤维神经瘤,神经纤维瘤

fibronuclear [ˌfaibrəuˈnjuːkliə] *a* 纤维[与]核的

fibroodontoma [ˌfaibrəuˌəudɔnˈtəumə] *n* 纤维牙瘤 | ameloblastic ~ 釉质母细胞纤维牙瘤

fibroosseous [ˌfaibrəuˈɔsiəs] *a* 纤维骨[组织]的

fibro-osteoma [ˌfaibrəuˌɔstiˈəumə] *n* 纤维骨瘤,骨纤维瘤

fibropapilloma [ˌfaibrəuˌpæpiˈləumə] *n* 纤维乳头瘤

fibropituicyte [ˌfaibrəupiˈtju(ː)isait] *n* 纤维垂体后叶细胞

fibroplasia [ˌfaibrəuˈpleiʃə] *n* 纤维增生症 | retrolental ~ (RLF) 晶体后纤维增生症

fibroplastic [ˌfaibrəuˈplæstik] *a* 纤维形成的

fibroplastin [ˌfaibrəuˈplæstin] *n* 副球蛋白

fibroplate [ˈfaibrəpleit] *n* 关节间纤维软骨

fibropolypus [ˌfaibrəuˈpɔlipəs] *n* 纤维息肉

fibropurulent [ˌfaibrəuˈpjuərulənt] *a* 纤维脓性的

fibroreticulate [ˌfaibrəurəˈtikjuleit] *a* 纤维网的

fibrosarcoma [ˌfaibrəusɑːˈkəumə] *n* 纤维肉瘤 | odontogenic ~ 牙原纤维肉瘤

fibrosclerosis [ˌfaibrəuskliəˈrəusis] *a* 纤维硬化

fibrose [ˈfaibrəus] *vt* 使纤维组织形成 *a* 纤维性的

fibroserous [ˌfaibrəuˈsiərəs] *a* 纤维浆液性的

fibrosis [faiˈbrəusis] *n* 纤维变性,纤维化 | diffuse interstitial pulmonary ~ 弥漫性肺间质纤维化,特发性肺纤维化(见 idiopathic pulmonary ~) / idiopathic pulmonary ~ 特发性肺纤维化(肺泡壁的慢性炎症和纤维化,伴有进行性呼吸困难,最后导致因缺氧或右心衰竭而死。亦称弥漫性肺间质纤维化,其急性迅速致死型常称黑-里〈Hamman-Rich〉综合征) / nodular subepidermal ~ 结节性表皮下纤维化 / panmural ~ of the bladder 全膀胱壁纤维化,慢性间质性膀胱炎 / proliferative ~, neoplastic ~ 增生性纤维化 / pulmonary ~ 肺纤维化(见 idiopathic pulmonary ~) / replacement ~ 替代性纤维化 / ~ uteri 子宫纤维化 | **fibrotic** [faiˈbrɔtik] *a*

fibrositis [ˌfaibrəuˈsaitis] *n* 纤维织炎,肌风湿病

fibrothorax [ˌfaibrəuˈθɔːræks] *n* 纤维胸

fibrotuberculosis [ˌfaibrəutju(ː)bəːkjuˈləusis] *n* 纤维性结核

fibrous [ˈfaibrəs] *a* 纤维性的

fibrovascular [ˌfaibrəuˈvæskjulə] *a* 纤维血管的

fibroxanthoma [ˌfaibrəuzænˈθəumə] *n* 纤维黄瘤 | atypical ~ (AFX) 非典型纤维黄瘤

fibroxanthosarcoma [ˌfaibrəuˌzænθəusɑːˈkəumə] *n* 纤维黄肉瘤

fibula [ˈfibjulə] ([复] **fibulas** 或 **fibulae** [ˈfibjuliː]) *n*【拉】腓骨 | **~r** *a*

fibularis [ˌfibjuˈlɛəris] *a*【拉】腓骨的,腓侧的

fibulocalcaneal [ˌfibjuləukælˈkeiniəl] *a* 腓跟的

ficain [ˈfaikein] *n* 无花果蛋白酶

FICD Fellow of the International College of Dentists 国际牙医师学会会员

ficin [ˈfaisin] *n* 无花果蛋白酶

Ficker's diagnosticum [ˈfikə] (Philipp M. Ficker) 菲克尔诊断液(检伤寒)

Fick principle (formula, method) [fik] (Adolph E. Fick) 菲克原理(公式、法)[重述质量守恒定律,例如用于间接测心输出量,即心输出量〈L/min〉= 氧吸收〈ml/min〉÷ 动脉氧-混合静脉氧〈ml/L〉)]

Fick's bacillus [fik] (Rudolph A. Fick) 普通变形杆菌

FICS Fellow of the International College of Surgeons 国际外科医师学会会员

Ficus [ˈfaikəs] *n* 无花果属

fidicinales [faiˌdisiˈneiliːz] [复] *n* 蚓状肌

fieber [ˈfiːbə] *n*【德】发热,热 | gelb ~ 黄热病 / rückfall ~ 回归热

Fiedler's disease [ˈfiːdlə] (Carl L. A. Fiedler) 钩端螺旋体黄疸 | ~ myocarditis 急性孤立性心肌炎

field [fiːld] *n* 区,域,场;领域,范围;视野;生成区(胚胎学) | absolute ~ 绝对区(大脑皮质损伤后常引起麻痹或痉挛的区域) / auditory ~ 听野 / ~ of consciousness 意识域 / cribriform ~ of vision 筛形视野 / dark- ~ 暗视野 / deaf ~ 聋域,聋点 / ~ of fixation 固定视野 / gamma ~ γ 辐射图 / H ~ H 区(见 Forel's field) / high-power ~ 高倍视野 / individuation ~ 个体形成区 / lowpower ~ 低倍视野 / magnetic ~ 磁场 / ~ of a microscope 显微镜视野 / morphogenetic ~ 形态生成区 / myelinogenetic ~ 髓鞘生成区 / overshot ~ of vision 上射视野 / penumbra ~ 半影区 / primary nail ~ 原甲区(胚胎) / relative ~ 相关[皮质]区 / surplus ~ 剩余视野 / ~ of vision 视野 / visual ~ 视野

Fielding's membrane [ˈfiːldiŋ] (George H. Fielding) 菲尔丁膜,毯(脉络膜毯)

Fiessinger-Leroy-Reiter syndrome [ˈfiːsiŋgə ləˈrɔi ˈraitə] (Noël A. Fiessinger; Emile Leroy; Hans C. Reiter) 费-莱-赖综合征(见 Reiter's syndrome)

fièvre [fiˈevrə] *n*【法】发热,热 | ~ boutonneuse, ~ exanthematique de Marseille 南欧斑疹热 / ~ caprine 波状热,布鲁[杆]菌病 / ~ jaune 黄热病 / ~ récurrente 回归热

fig [fig] *n* 无花果

fig. figure(s) 图,图像;数字

FIGLU formiminoglutamic acid 亚胺甲基谷氨酸

FIGO Fédération Internationale de Gynécologie et d'Obstétrique 国际妇产科联合会

figuration [ˌfigjuˈreiʃən] *n* 成形;外形,轮廓

figuratum [ˌfigjuˈreitəm] *a*【拉】带花纹的,有图案的

figure [ˈfigə] *n* 图,图像;图表;数字;(字母、数字)符号 | fortification ~s (偏头痛)闪烁幻象 / mitotic ~s 有丝分裂像

fila [ˈfailə] filum 的复数

filaceous [faiˈleiʃəs] *a* 丝状的,丝性的

filament [ˈfiləmənt] *n* 丝,丝体 | linin ~ 核丝 / spermatic ~ 精子丝 / terminal ~ 终丝,末丝 | **~ary** [ˌfiləˈmentəri], **~ous** [ˌfiləˈmentəs] *a* 丝[状]的,丝性的

filamentum [ˌfiləˈmentəm] ([复] **filamenta** [ˌfiləˈmentə]) *n*【拉】丝,丝体

filamin [ˈfiləmin] *n* [肌动蛋白]细丝蛋白

filar [ˈfailə] *a* 丝状的,丝性的

Filaria [fiˈlɛəriə] *n* 丝虫属 | ~ bancrofti 班[克曼夫特]氏丝虫(即 Wuchereria bancrofti) / ~ conjunctivae, ~ palpebralis 结膜丝虫,结膜吸吮线虫 / ~ demarquayi, ~ juncea, ~ ozzardi 奥[扎尔德]氏曼森线虫(即 Mansonella ozzardi) / ~ diurna 昼现幼

fimbria [ˈfimbriə] ([复] **fimbriae** [ˈfimbriiː]) *n*【拉】伞;菌毛,伞毛,纤毛 | ovarian ~ 卵巢伞 / ~e of tongue 伞襞 / ~e of uterine tube 输卵管伞

Fimbriaria [ˌfimbriˈɛəriə] *n* 绉缘绦虫属 | ~ fasciolaris 片形绉缘绦虫

fimbriate [ˈfimbriit], **fimbriated** [ˈfimbrieitid] *a* 伞状的 | **fimbriation** [ˌfimbriˈeiʃən] *n* 伞形成,有伞

fimbriatum [ˌfimbriˈeitəm] *a*【拉】伞状的

fimbriocele [ˈfimbriəˌsiːl] *n* 输卵管伞突出

filariasis [filəˈraiəsis] *n* 丝虫病 | ~ malayi 马来丝虫病

filaricidal [fiˌlɛəriˈsaidl] *a* 杀丝虫的

filaricide [fiˈlɛərisaid] *n* 杀丝虫药

filariform [fiˈlɛərifɔːm] *a* 丝状的,丝虫状的

Filarioidea [fiˌlɛəriˈɔidiə] *n* 丝虫总科,丝虫目

Filaroides [ˌfiləˈrɔidiːz] *n* 丝虫属

Filaroididae [ˌfiləˈrɔididiː] *n* 丝虫科

Filatov-Dukes disease [fiˈlætɔf djuːks] (N. F. Filatov; Clement Dukes) 费拉托夫-杜克病(见 Dukes' disease)

Filatov's (Filatow's) disease [fiˈlætɔf] (Nils F. Filatov) 传染性单核细胞增多[症]

Fildes enrichment agar [fildz] (Paul G. Fildes) 菲尔兹增菌琼脂(用于培养和分离流感嗜血杆菌和难养链球菌)

file [fail] *n* 锉 | endodontic ~ 牙髓锉 / root canal ~ 根管锉(亦称牙髓锉)

filgrastim [filˈgræstim] *n* 非格司亭(人粒细胞集落刺激因子,由重组 DNA 技术制成,用于刺激中性粒细胞产生,使中性粒细胞减少症的病期缩短,使接受骨髓抑制化学疗法以治疗非骨髓样恶性肿瘤的患者减少感染发生率,皮下或静脉内给药)

filial [ˈfiljəl] *a* 子代的

filicic acid [fiˈlisik], **filicinic acid** [ˌfiliˈsinik] 绵马酸

filicin [ˈfilisin] *n* 绵马酸

filicitannic acid [ˌfilisiˈtænik] 绵马鞣酸

filiform [ˈfilifɔːm] *a* 线形的 *n* 线形探条 | urethral ~ 尿道丝状探子

filioparental [ˌfiliəupəˈrentl] *a* 嗣亲的(子女与双亲间的)

filipin [ˈfilipin] *n* 非律平(抗真菌抗生素)

Filipovitch's (Filipowicz's) sign [fiˈliːpəvitʃ] (Casimir Filipovitch) 费利波维奇征(伤寒病时,掌跖黄色变色,亦称掌跖征)

filix [ˈfailiks] ([复] **filices** [ˈfilisiːz]) *n*【拉】绵马,蕨 | ~ mas 绵马

filixic acid [fiˈliksik] 绵马酸

fillet [ˈfilit] *n* 襻;丘系

filling [ˈfiliŋ] *n* 充填;[充]填料;灌注(安瓿) | complex ~ 多面洞充填 / composite ~ 复合填料 / compound ~ 复[面]洞充填 / permanent ~ 永久充填 / root canal ~ 根管充填 / ventricular ~ 心室充盈

film [film] *n* 薄膜,膜;软片,胶片 | absorbable gelatin ~ 吸水明胶片 / bite-wing ~ 殆翼片 /

fixed blood ~ 固定血膜 / occlusal ~ 殆片 / sulfa ~ 磺胺薄膜 / X-ray ~ X 线胶片,X 线片
film badge [film bædʒ] 照射剂量测定软片
filmy [ˈfilmi] *a* 薄膜似的
Filobasidiella [ˌfailəubəˌsidiˈelə], **Filobasidium** [ˌfailəubəˈsidiəm] *n* 线黑粉菌属
filopodium [ˌfailəˈpəudiəm, ˌfi-] ([复] **filopodia** [ˌfailəˈpɔdiə]), **filopod** [ˈfiləpɔd] *n* 丝足
filopressure [ˈfiləˌpreʃə] *n* 线压法
filose [ˈfailəus] *a* 丝(或线)状的;有线状突起的
Filosea [faiˈləusiə] *n* 丝足纲
filovaricosis [ˈfailəuˌværiˈkəusis] *n* 神经轴索静脉曲张
Filoviridae [ˌfailəuˈviridiː] *n* 纤丝病毒科
Filovirus [ˈfailəuˌvaiərəs] *n* 纤丝病毒(马尔堡〈Marburg〉病毒和埃博拉〈Ebola〉病毒);纤丝病毒属(可致出血性热〈马尔堡病毒病,埃博拉病毒病〉)
filter [ˈfiltə] *n* 滤器;滤纸;滤光片 *vt* 过滤 *vi* 滤过 | intermittent sand ~ 间歇沙滤池 / mechanical ~ 机械过滤池 / roughing ~, scrubbing ~ 粗滤池 / sintered glass ~ 多孔玻璃滤器 / slow sand ~ 慢沙滤池 / sprinkling ~ 喷滤池 / trickling ~, percolating ~ 滴滤池
filterable [ˈfiltərəbl], **filtrable** [ˈfiltrəbl] *a* 可滤过的 | **filterability** [ˌfiltərəˈbiləti] *n* 可滤性;滤过率
filtrate [ˈfiltreit] *vt*, *vi* 过滤 [ˈfiltrit] *n* 滤液 | glomerular ~ 肾小球滤液
filtration [filˈtreiʃən] *n* 过滤,滤清;滤光[作用] | gel ~ 凝胶过滤
filtrum ventriculi [ˈfiltrəm venˈtrikjulai]【拉】喉室沟
filum [ˈfailəm] ([复] **fila** [ˈfailə]) *n*【拉】丝
fimbria [ˈfimbriə] ([复] **fimbriae** [ˈfimbriiː]) *n*【拉】伞;菌毛,伞毛,纤毛 | ovarian ~ 卵巢伞 / ~e of tongue 伞襞 / ~e of uterine tube 输卵管伞
Fimbriaria [ˌfimbriˈɛəriə] *n* 绉缘绦虫属 | ~ fasciolaris 片形绉缘绦虫
fimbriate [ˈfimbriit], **fimbriated** [ˈfimbrieitid] *a* 伞状的 | **fimbriation** [ˌfimbriˈeiʃən] *n* 伞形成,有伞
fimbriatum [ˌfimbriˈeitəm] *a*【拉】伞状的
fimbriocele [ˈfimbriəˌsiːl] *n* 输卵管伞突出
fimbrin [ˈfimbrin] *n* 丝束蛋白
fimbrioplasty [ˈfimbriəuˌplæsti] *n* 输卵管伞成形术
finasteride [fiˈnæstəraid] *n* 非那雄胺(5α-还原酶抑制药,用于治疗良性前列腺增生,口服给药)
Finckh test [fink] (Johann Finckh) 芬克试验(检精神病,令患者解释格言的意义)
finder [ˈfaində] *n* 寻觅器,探示器
finding [ˈfaindiŋ] *n* 发现物;[常用复]调查(或研究)的结果,所见,发现
finger [ˈfiŋgə] *n* 手指 | baseball ~, drop ~, hammer ~, mallet ~ 垒球指,槌状指 / bolster ~s 枕垫指(糖业工人手指为念珠菌感染而发生的肿胀) / clubbed ~, drumstick ~, hippocratic ~s 杵状指 / dead ~, waxy ~, white ~ 死指,蜡指,苍白指 / first ~ 拇指 / giant ~ 巨指 / index ~ 示指 / insane ~ 精神病者瘭疽(慢性指炎) / lock ~ 固定指,指活动障碍 / Madonna ~s 纤细指(见于肢端过小症) / ring ~ 环指,无名指 / spider ~ 蜘蛛状指,细长指 / spring ~ 弹跳指(指伸屈活动障碍) / trigger ~, snapping ~ 扳机指,弹响指 / tulip ~s 山慈姑指(山慈姑皮炎) / washerwoman's ~s 洗衣员[手]指(霍乱脱水的表现) / webbed ~s 蹼指,并指
fingeragnosia [ˌfiŋgəræɡˈnəusiə] *n* 手指失辨觉能,手指认识不能
finger and toe 指趾病,根肿病(甘蓝根菌所致的一种植物病)
fingered [ˈfiŋgəd] *a* 有指的;指状的
fingernail [ˈfiŋgəneil] *n* 指甲
fingerprint [ˈfiŋgəprint] *n* 指印,指纹;指纹图谱,酶解图谱
fingerprinting [ˌfiŋgəˈprintiŋ] *n* 指纹法,酶解图谱法(一种把电泳和色谱法相结合的分析方法,用以分析和分离蛋白质水解后的肽段)
fingerstall [ˈfiŋgəstɔːl] *n* (皮或橡皮制的)护指套
finger-sucking [ˈfiŋgə ˈsʌkiŋ] *n* 吮指癖
fingertip [ˈfiŋgəˌtip] *n* 指尖
Finikoff's treatment [ˈfinikɔf] (Aleksandr P. Finikoff) 菲尼科夫疗法(骨结核疗法,每 5 ~ 8 日肌内注射碘化花生油,每周 3 次静脉注射 10% 钙溶液)
finish [ˈfiniʃ] *n* 完成 | ~ of a denture 义齿的完成
Finkelstein's albumin milk [ˈfinkəlstain] (Heinrich Finkelstein) 芬克尔斯坦白蛋白乳(特殊配制,乳糖和盐类含量低,酪蛋白和脂肪丰富,用于糖尿病及需要高蛋白质饮食的病,如肾病、营养不良性水肿) | ~ feeding 芬克尔斯坦减乳糖哺法(按减少食物中的乳糖以哺养婴儿)
Finkler-Prior spirillium [ˈfinklə ˈpraiə] (Dittmar Finkler; J. Prior) 芬-普螺菌,麦奇尼科夫弧菌(即 Vibrio metschnikovii)
Finney's pyloroplasty(operation) [ˈfini] (John M. T. Finney) 芬尼幽门成形术(手术)(经幽门及邻近胃十二指肠壁作纵切开,使幽门管扩大,然后作倒 U 形胃十二指肠吻合术)
Finochietto's stirrup [fiˌnəukiˈetəu] (Enrique Finochietto) 菲诺切托牵引镫(作骨骼牵引用)

Finsen bath [ˈfinsən] (Niels R. Finsen) 芬森浴(以紫外线照射患者全身) | ~ lamp(apparatus) 芬森弧光灯(50 V 及 50 A 的炭弧灯) / ~ light (rays) 芬森光(芬森弧光灯发出的光,主要为紫射线及紫外线组成,用以治狼疮及类似疾病)

fire [ˈfaiə] *n* 火;发热;炎症 | St. Anthony's ~ 圣安东尼热(麦角中毒的旧称;丹毒的旧称)

firedamp [ˈfaiədæmp] *n* 沼气

fireproof [ˈfaiəpruːf] *a* 防火的;耐火的

firing [ˈfaiəriŋ] *n* (陶瓷的)焙烧,加热;发放

Firmacutes [fəːˈmækjutiːz, ˌfəːməˈkjuːtiːz] *n* 硬壁菌门(即 Firmicutes)

Firmibacteria [ˌfəːmibækˈtiəriə] *n* 硬壁菌纲

Firmicutes [fəːˈmikjutiːz, ˌfəːmiˈkjuːtiːz] *n* 硬壁菌门

firpene [ˈfəːpiːn] *n* 松油萜,松油烃,蒎烯

first aid [ˈfəːsteid] 急救

Fischer's sign [ˈfiʃə] (Louis Fischer) 费希尔征(①支气管淋巴结结核患者头部后仰,则在胸骨柄上的听诊有时可听到由于淋巴结压迫无名静脉所引起的一种杂音;②心包粘连时的收缩期前杂音)

Fischer's test [ˈfiʃə] (Emil Fischer) 费希尔试验(检尿葡萄糖)

Fishberg concentration test [ˈfiʃbəːg] (Arthur M. Fishberg) 菲什伯格浓缩试验(检肾功能)

Fisher exact test [ˈfiʃə] (Sir Ronald A. Fisher) 费希尔精确性检验(根据观察频率的精确样本分布,2×2 列联表中行、列的无关性的统计假说检验,当其中任何期望值很小时,则有用)

Fisher syndrome [ˈfiʃə] (C. Miller Fisher) 费希尔综合征(①急性特发性多神经炎的变异型,特征为反射消失、共济失调和眼肌麻痹;亦称 Miller Fisher syndrome;②一个半综合征,即 one-and-a-half syndrome,见 syndrome 项下相应术语)

fishing [ˈfiʃiŋ] *n* 钓菌法,钓取菌落

fishpox [ˈfiʃpɔks] *n* 鱼痘

fissile [ˈfisail] *a* 可裂变的,可分裂的 | **fissility** [fiˈsiləti] *n* 可裂变性

fission [ˈfiʃən] *n* 分裂;裂殖[法];(原子)核裂变 *vt*, *vi* 裂变 | binary ~ 二分裂 / cellular ~ 细胞分裂 / nuclear ~ (原子)核裂变 | **~able** *a* 可分裂的,可裂变的

fissiparous [fiˈsipərəs] *a* 裂殖的

fissula [ˈfisjulə] *n*【拉】小裂

fissura [fiˈsjuərə] ([复] **fissurae** [fiˈsjuəriː]) *n*【拉】裂,裂隙,裂纹

fissure [ˈfiʃə] *n* 裂,裂隙,裂纹 *vt*, *vi* 裂开 | abdominal ~ 腹壁裂[畸形] / amygdaline ~ 杏仁裂(大脑近颞叶端的裂) / angular ~ 蝶岩裂 / basilar ~ 蝶枕裂 / calcarine ~ 距状沟,距状裂 / callosal ~ 胼胝体沟 / callosomarginal ~ 扣带沟 / central ~ 中央沟(大脑) / cerebral ~s, ~s of cerebrum 大脑沟 / dentate ~ 海马裂 / enamel ~ 牙釉质裂纹 / ethmoid ~ 上鼻道 / inferofrontal ~, subfrontal ~ 额下沟(脑) / intercerebral ~ 半球间裂 / interparietal ~ 顶间沟 / intratonsillar ~ 扁桃体上窝 / portal ~ 肝门 / postcentral ~ 中央后沟(小脑) / precentral ~ 中央前沟 / presylvian ~ 前水平支(大脑侧裂) / pudendal ~ 外阴裂 / sphenoidal ~ 眶上裂 / supertemporal ~ 颞上沟 / ~ of the venous ligament 静脉导管窝,静脉导管索部 / zygal ~ 轭合裂 | **fissural** *a* 裂的

fissurella [ˌfisəˈrelə] *n* 钥孔蝛

fistula [ˈfistjulə] ([复] **fistulas** 或 **fistulae** [ˈfistjuliː]) *n* 瘘,瘘管 | abdominal ~ 腹[壁]瘘 / amphibolic ~ 胆囊[实验]瘘 / blind ~ 单口瘘 / cervical ~ (颈部)鳃瘘;子宫颈瘘 / complete ~ 完全性瘘,双口瘘 / craniosinus ~ 鼻脑脊液瘘 / horseshoe ~ 马蹄形[肛门]瘘 / incomplete ~ 不全性瘘,单口瘘 / thoracic ~ 胸壁瘘

fistulatome [ˈfistjuləˌtəum] *n* 瘘管刀

fistulectomy [ˌfistjuˈlektəmi] *n* 瘘管切除术

fistulization [ˌfistjulaiˈzeiʃən] *n* 瘘管形成

fistuloenterostomy [ˌfistjuləuˌentəˈrɔstəmi] *n* 胆瘘小肠造口术

fistulotomy [ˌfistjuˈlɔtəmi] *n* 瘘管切开术

fistulous [ˈfistjuləs] *a* 瘘的,瘘管的

fit [fit] *n* 突发,阵发,发作;适合 | running ~ 奔驰性发作(犬惊病,犬癔病;奔驰性癫痫)

FITC fluorescein isothiocyanate 异硫氰酸荧光素

fitful [ˈfitful] *a* 间歇的

fitness [ˈfitnis] *n* 适合;合格;健康;适合度(在遗传学中指某一基因与群体平均概率相比时,传给下一代并使其基因存活和传给下一代的概率) | physical ~ 体能

fitting [ˈfitiŋ] *a* 适合的,相称的 *n* 装配,装置

Fitz Gerald method treatment [fitsˈdʒerəld] (William H. H. Fitz Gerald) 体区疗法(zone therapy,见 therapy 项下相应术语)

Fitz-Hugh-Curtis syndrome [ˈfitz hjuː ˈkəːtis] (Thomas Fitz-Hugh, Jr.; Arthur H. Curtis) 菲-科综合征(患淋病妇女并发肝周炎,特点为发热,右上腹疼痛,腹壁紧张与痉挛,肝区有时闻及摩擦音)

Fitz's syndrome [ˈfits] (Reginald H. Fitz) 菲茨综合征(急性胰腺炎一组症状:上腹部痛、呕吐、虚脱,继之以 24 h 上腹部局限性肿胀或气鼓)

fix [fiks] *vt* 使固定;安装;凝视 *vi* 固定;注视 | **~able** *a* 可固定的

fixate [ˈfikseit] *vt*, *vi* (使)固定;注视

fixateur [fiksəˈtəː] *n*【法】抗体,介体

fixation [fikˈseiʃən] *n* 结合,固定;固定法,固定术;固结,固恋;定型;凝视;定影 | alexin ~ 防御

素结合(见 complement ~) / binocular ~ 双目注视 / complement ~, ~ of the complement 补体结合(当抗原与其特异性抗体结合时,如有补体,则补体参与结合而变成不活动或固定,补体的游离或被结合可通过加入致敏红细胞来检查,如有游离补体,则发生溶血,如无游离补体,则不溶血,此反应是诊断许多传染病的血清学试验的基础) / father ~ 父亲固恋,恋父固结 / freudian ~ 精神发育固定 / mother ~ 母亲固恋,恋母固结 / nitrogen ~ 氮固定,定氮作用

fixative [ˈfiksətiv] *a* 固定的 *n* 固定剂;介体

fixator [fikˈseitə] *n* 抗体,介体;固定肌

fixed [fikst] *a* 固定的

fixing [ˈfiksiŋ] *n* 固定;安装;定影

fixity [ˈfiksəti] *n* 固定;入盆(指胎儿头)

fixture [ˈfikstʃə] *n* 固定;固定物;[常用复]固定装置

Fl. fluid 液体,液

FLA fronto-laeva anterior 额左前(胎位)

F. l. a. fiat lege artis【拉】按常规做

flabby [ˈflæbi] *a* (肌肉等)不结实的,松弛的 | **flabbily** *ad* / **flabbiness** *n*

flabellate [fləˈbelit], **flabelliform** [fləˈbelifɔːm] *a* 扇形的

Flabellina [ˌflæbiˈlainə] *n* 扇子介亚目

flaccid [ˈflæksid] *a* (肌肉等)不结实的,柔软的,弛缓的 | **~ity** [flækˈsidəti] *n*

flacherie [flæʃəˈriː] *n*【法】蚕软化病

Flack's node [flæk] (Martin W. Flack) 窦房结 | ~ test 弗拉克体力测验(尽量吸气后,再以5.33 kPa〈=40 mmHg〉之力尽可能久地向水银测压计吹气,以测体力)

flag[1] [flæg] *n* 旗 | sick ~ (检疫站或船的)传染病信号旗,(黄色)疫旗

flag[2] [flæg] *n* 菖蒲

flagella [fləˈdʒelə] flagellum 的复数

flagellantism [ˈflædʒiləntizəm] *n* 鞭挞[色情]狂(包括施鞭或受鞭者)

flagellar [fləˈdʒelə] *a* 鞭毛的

Flagellata [ˌflædʒeˈleitə] *n* 鞭毛虫纲

flagellate [ˈflædʒeleit] *vt* 鞭击 *a* 有鞭毛的;鞭毛状的 *n* 鞭毛虫;鞭毛藻 | animal-like ~ 类动物鞭毛虫 / plant-like ~ 类植物鞭毛虫

flagellated [ˈflædʒeleitid] *a* 有鞭毛的;鞭毛状的

flagellation [ˌflædʒeˈleiʃən] *n* 轻叩法(一种按摩法);鞭击,鞭挞[色情]狂;鞭毛突出

flagelliform [fləˈdʒelifɔːm] *a* 鞭毛状的

flagellin [ˈflædʒəlin] *n* 鞭毛蛋白

flagellosis [ˌflædʒəˈləusis] *n* 鞭毛虫病

flagellospore [fləˈdʒeləspɔː], **flagellula** [fləˈdʒeljulə] *n* 鞭毛芽胞,鞭毛孢子

flagellum [fləˈdʒeləm] ([复] **flagellums** 或 **flagella** [fləˈdʒelə]) *n*【拉】鞭毛

flail [fleil] *n* 连枷(如连枷关节)

Flajani's disease [fləˈdʒæni] (Giuseppe Flajani) 突眼性甲状腺肿

flake [fleik] *n* 薄片;絮片,鳞片

flame [fleim] *n* 火焰 | capillary ~s 毛细血管扩张斑(有时见于新生儿的脸上) / manometric ~ 感压火焰

flange [flændʒ] *n* 翼缘 | buccal ~ 颊侧翼缘 / denture ~ 义齿翼缘 / labial ~ 唇侧翼缘 / lingual ~ 舌侧翼缘

flank [flæŋk] *n* 胁;胁腹

flap [flæp] *n* 皮片,皮瓣;往返翻动(不能控制的),扑动 | island skin ~ 岛状皮瓣 / jump ~ 迁移瓣 / liver ~ 姿势保持不能,扑翼样震颤(见于肝昏迷等) / pedicle ~, gauntlet ~ 蒂状瓣 / skin ~ 皮瓣 / sliding ~, advancement ~, French ~ 滑动瓣,前徙瓣,法式瓣 | **~s** *n* 唇肿胀(马)

flare [flɛə] *n* 闪耀,闪光 | aqueous ~ 房水闪光

flare-up [ˈflɛər ʌp] *n* 突然起燃;(怒气、疾病等的)发作

flaring [ˈflɛəriŋ] *n* 张开 | ~ of alae nasi 鼻翼扇动

flash [flæʃ] *n* 闪光;闪耀;铸模溢出物

flashlamp [ˈflæʃlæmp] *n* 闪光灯

flashlight [ˈflæʃlait] *n* 手电筒;闪光灯

flask [flɑːsk] *n* 瓶,烧瓶;型盒(牙) *vt* 装型盒(牙) | crown ~ 牙冠型盒 / culture ~ 培养瓶 / denture ~ 义齿型盒 / refractory ~, casting ~ 耐火型盒,铸造型盒 / volumetric ~ [容]量瓶

flasket [ˈflɑːskit] *n* 小瓶

flasking [ˈflɑːskiŋ] *n* 装盒(牙)

flat [flæt] *a* 平的;平坦的;扁平的;实音的,低音的 *n* 平面;平坦部分;扁平物 | optical ~ 光学玻璃板

Flatau-Schilder disease [fləˈtau ˈʃildə] (E. Flatau; Paul F. Schilder) 弗-希病(见 Schilder disease)

Flatau's law [fləˈtau] (Edward Flatau) 弗拉托定律(脊髓纤维长度愈长,则愈接近外周)

flatfoot [ˈflætfut] ([复] **flatfeet** [ˈflætfiːt]) *n* 扁平足,平足 | rocker-bottom ~ 摇摆椅足(见 foot 项下相应术语)

flat-footed [ˈflæt ˌfutid] *a* 平脚的

flatness [ˈflætnis] *n* 实音(叩诊)

flattening [ˈflætəniŋ] *n* 平淡,低沉 | ~ affect 情感淡漠,情感低沉

flatulent [ˈflætjulənt] *a* (肠胃)气胀的 | **flatulence** [ˈflætjuləns], **flatulency** [ˈflætjulənsi] *n*

flatus [ˈfleitəs] *n*【拉】肠胃气;屁 | ~ vaginalis 阴道气响

flatworm [ˈflætwəːm] *n* 扁虫
flavanoid [ˈfleivənɔid] *n* 黄烷类
flavanone [ˈfleivənəun] *n* 黄烷酮
flavanonol [ˈfleivənɔnəl] *n* 黄烷酮醇
flavaspidic acid [ˌfleivəˈspidik] 黄绵马酸
flavectomy [fleiˈvektəmi] *n* 黄韧带切除术
flavescent [fləˈvesnt] *a* 淡黄色的,浅黄色的
flavianic acid [ˌfleiviˈænik] 黄萘酸
flavin [ˈfleivin] *n* 黄素 | ~-adenine dinucleotide (FAD) 黄素腺嘌呤二核苷酸 / ~ mononucleotide(FMN) 黄素单核苷酸
flavine [ˈfleivain] *n* 吖啶黄(消毒防腐药)
flavin monooxygenase [ˈfleivin ˌmɔnəu ˈɔksidʒəneis] 黄素单加氧酶,非特异性单加氧酶
Flaviviridae [ˌfleiviˈviridiː] *n* 黄病毒科
Flavivirus [ˈfleiviˌvaiərəs] *n* 黄病毒属
flavivirus [ˈfleiviˌvaiərəs] *n* 黄病毒
flav(o)- [构词成分]黄
Flavobacterium [ˌfleivəubækˈtiəriəm] *n* 黄杆菌属 | ~ breve 短黄杆菌 / ~ meningosepticum 脑膜脓毒性黄杆菌 / ~ odoratum 芳香黄杆菌
flavodoxin [ˌfleivəuˈdɔksin] *n* 黄素氧还蛋白
flavoenzyme [ˌfleivəuˈenzaim] *n* 黄素酶
flavomycin [ˌfleivəuˈmaisin] *n* 黄霉素
flavone [ˈfleivəun] *n* 黄酮
flavonoid [ˈfleivənɔid] *n* 黄酮类
flavonol [ˈfleivənɔl] *n* 黄酮醇
flavoprotein [ˌfleivəuˈprəutiːn] *n* 黄素蛋白
flavorful [ˈfleivəful], **flavorsome** [ˈfleivəsəm], **flavorous** [ˈfleivərəs], **flavory** [ˈfleivəri] *a* 味浓的;有香味的
flavo(u)r [ˈfleivə] *n* 味;风味;香味;调味香料 | **~less** *a* 无味的;乏味的
flavo(u)ring [ˈfleivəriŋ] *n* 调味品
flavoxanthin [ˌfleivəuˈzænθin] *n* 黄黄质
flavoxate hydrochloride [fleiˈvɔkseit] 盐酸黄酮哌酯(平滑肌松弛药,用作泌尿系统解痉药)
falx [flæks] *n* 亚麻
flaxseed [ˈflæksiːd] *n* 亚麻籽,亚麻仁
flazalone [ˈfleizələun] *n* 夫拉扎酮(抗炎药)
fld fluid 液体;液
fl dr fluid dram 液量英钱
flea [fliː] *n* 蚤 | Asiatic rat ~ 亚洲鼠蚤(即 Xenopsylla cheopis) / burrowing ~ 穿皮潜蚤(即 Tunga penetrans) / cat ~ 猫蚤(即 Ctenocephalides felis) / chigoe ~ 沙蚤(即 Tunga penetrans) / common ~ 普通蚤(即 Pulex irritans) / common rat ~ 鼠蚤(即 Nosopsyllus fasciatus) / dog ~ 犬蚤(即 Ctenocephalides canis) / European mouse ~ 欧洲鼠蚤(即 Ctenophthalmus agrytes) / European rat ~ 欧洲鼠蚤(即 Nosopsyllus fasciatus) / human ~ 人蚤(即 Pulex irritans) / Indian rat ~ 印度鼠蚤(即 Xenopsylla astia) / jigger ~ 恙螨(即 Tunga penetrans) / mouse ~ 鼷蚤(即 Leptopsylla segnis) / sand ~ 沙蚤(即 Tunga penetrans) / squirrel ~ 松鼠蚤(即 Hoplopsyllus anomalus) / sticktight ~ 吸着蚤(即 Echidnophaga gallinacea) / suslik ~ 地松鼠蚤 / tropical rat ~ 热带鼠蚤(即 Xenopsylla cheopis)
flecainide acetate [fliˈkeinaid] 醋酸氟卡尼(抗心律失常药)
Flechsig's areas [ˈfleksis] (Paul E. Flechsig) 弗莱西格区(延髓每半边的前、侧、后三个区,有迷走神经及舌下神经纤维可见) | ~ cuticulum 弗莱西格表皮(神经胶质外面的一层扁平细胞) / ~ fasciculus 前固有束;外侧固有束 / ~ field 髓鞘生成区 / ~ myelogenetic law 弗莱西格髓鞘发生定律,髓鞘发生定律(发育中的脑神经纤维,其髓鞘的形成有一定的次序,属于特定功能系统的神经纤维亦同时成熟)
fleck [flek] *n* 斑点;微粒 | tobacco ~s 含铁结节,香烟色斑点(在某些脾肿大患者的脾内可见到的棕色或黄色色素的小结)
fleckfieber [flekˈfiːbə] *n*【德】流行性斑疹伤寒
fleckmilz [ˈflekmilts] *n*【德】斑点脾
flection [ˈflekʃən] *n* 屈,屈曲 | **~al** *a*
fleece [fliːs] *n* 羊毛,羊毛状物
Flegel's disease [ˈfleigəl] (Heine Flegel) 弗莱格尔病,持久性豆状角化过度
Fleischl's test [ˈflaiʃl] (Ernst von Fleischl von Marxow) 弗莱施尔试验(检尿内胆色素)
Fleischmann's hygroma [ˈflaiʃmən] (Godfried Fleischmann) 弗莱施曼水囊瘤(口腔底的颏舌肌外侧的黏液囊膨大)
Fleischner's disease [ˈflaiʃnə] (Felix Fleischner) 费莱希内病(影响手中指骨的骨软骨炎)
Fleitmann's test [ˈflaitmən] (Theodore Fleitmann) 弗莱特曼试验(检砷化物)
flemingen [fleˈmindʒin] *n* 非洲楸荚素
Flemming's center [ˈflemiŋ] (Walther Flemming) 弗莱明中心,生发中心 | ~ solution (fixing fluid) 弗莱明液(固定液)(组织标本固定液,含三氧化铬、四氧化锇、冰醋酸和水)
fleroxacin [fleˈrɔksəsin] *n* 氟罗沙星(一种氟喹诺酮抗生素,具有与环丙沙星〈ciprofloxacin〉类似的作用和用途,口服或静脉输注给药)
flesh [fleʃ] *n* 肉;皮肤 | goose ~ 鸡皮疙瘩(因冷或惊吓时皮乳头勃起) / proud ~ 赘肉
flesh-colo(u)red [ˈfleʃ ˌkʌləd] *a* 肉色的
flesh-eating [ˈfleʃ ˌiːtiŋ] *a* 食肉的
fleshiness [ˈfleʃinis] *n* 多肉,肥胖
fleshly [ˈfleʃli] *a* 肉体的;肉欲的;多肉的;肥胖的
fleshy [ˈfleʃi] *a* 多肉的,肥胖的;肉的,似肉的
fletazepam [fləˈtæzəpæm] *n* 氟乙西泮(骨骼肌松

弛药）

fletcherism [ˈfletʃərizəm] *n*（Horace Fletcher）弗莱彻进食法，细嚼慢咽法（主张将硬质食物完全咀嚼然后随汤液咽下）

fleurette [fluəˈret] *n*【法】小花型细胞（见于成视黄膜细胞瘤和视网膜细胞瘤）

flex [fleks] *vt*, *vi*, *n* 屈曲

Flexibacter [ˌfleksiˈbæktə] *n* 屈挠杆菌属

flexibility [ˌfleksəˈbiləti] *n* 屈曲性；柔性，灵活性 | waxy ~ 蜡样屈曲

flexibilitas [ˌfleksiˈbiləltəs] *n*【拉】屈曲性

flexible [ˈfleksəbl] *a* 易弯的，能屈的

flexile [ˈfleksail] *a* 易弯的，能屈的

fleximeter [flekˈsimitə] *n* 关节屈度计

flexion [ˈflekʃən] *n* 屈，屈曲，俯屈 | **~al** *a*

Flexithrix [ˈfleksiθriks] *n* 柔发菌属

Flexner's bacillus [ˈfleksnə]（Simon Flexner）弗[莱克斯纳]氏痢疾杆菌 | ~ dysentery 菌痢，杆菌[性]痢疾 / ~ serum 抗脑膜炎球菌血清

Flexner-Wintersteiner rosette [ˈfleksnə ˈvintəˌstainə]（Simon Flexner; Hugo Wintersteiner）弗-温玫瑰花结（在成视网膜细胞瘤和某些其他眼瘤中所发现的一种细胞形成，其柱状细胞呈辐射状从明亮的中央核发出，并由一层膜分隔开来，同时也可见到轮辐似的幅条，代表视杆与视锥）

flexor [ˈfleksə] *n*【拉】屈肌 | ~ retinaculum 屈肌支持带

flexorplasty [ˈfleksəˌplæsti] *n* 屈肌成形术

flexuous [ˈfleksjuəs], **flexuose** [ˈfleksjuəus] *a* 曲的，波状的

flexura [flekˈʃuərə]（[复] **flexurae** [flekˈʃuəriː]）*n*【拉】曲

flexure [ˈflekʃə] *n* 曲 | caudal ~, sacral ~ 尾曲，骶曲 / cephalic ~, cranial ~ 头曲，颅曲 / hepatic ~ of colon 结肠右曲 / left ~ of colon, splenic ~ of colon 结肠左曲 / pontine ~, basicranial ~ 脑桥曲 | **flexural** *a*

flicker [ˈflikə] *n* 闪烁

Fliess treatment (therapy) [fliːs]（Wilhelm Fliess）弗利斯疗法（以鼻甲麻醉法治痛经及神经性胃痛）

flight [flait] *n* 飞翔，飞行；奔逸 | ~ of ideas 意念飘忽，思维奔逸（有时见于急性躁狂状态和急性精神分裂症）/ ~ of thought 思维奔逸

Flinders Island spotted fever [ˈflindəz ˈailənd]（Flinders Island 在澳大利亚塔斯马尼亚州的东北部）弗林德斯岛斑点热（澳大利亚夏季发生的一种急性感染，由搏氏立克次体〈Richettsia bonei〉所致，特征为发热、肌痛和头痛，并出现焦痂和皮疹）

Flint's arcade [flint]（Austin Flint）弗林特弓（肾锥体底部的动静脉弓）| ~ law 弗林特定律（一器官的个体发生过程，即其血液供应的种系发生过程）

Flint's murmur [flint]（Austin Flint）弗林特杂音（主动脉口反流时，心尖收缩前期杂音加大）

float [fləut] *n* 漂浮[物] *vt* 使漂浮，使悬浮 *vi* 浮动，漂浮

floatage [ˈfləutidʒ] *n* 漂浮，浮力；漂浮物

floatation [fləuˈteiʃən] *n* 漂浮；浮集[法]，浮选[法]

floaters [ˈfləutəz] [复] *n* 飘游物，悬浮物

floating [ˈfləutiŋ] *a* 浮的，浮动的

floccillation [ˌflɔksiˈleiʃən], **floccilegium** [ˌflɔksiˈliːdʒiəm] *n* 摸空，捉空摸床，撮摸症（谵妄患者）

floccose [ˈflɔkəus] *a* 柔毛状的，絮状的

flocculate [ˈflɔkjuleit] *vt*, *vi* 絮凝，絮状沉淀 | **flocculation** [ˌflɔkjuˈleiʃən] *n* 絮凝[作用]，絮状沉淀法，絮状反应

floccule [ˈflɔkjuːl] *n* 絮片，絮状物；绒球状沉淀法 | toxoid-antitoxin ~ 类毒素抗毒素絮片[块]

flocculent [ˈflɔkjulənt] *a* 絮凝的，含絮状物的 | **flocculence** *n* 絮凝[作用]，絮状沉淀法

flocculoreaction [ˌflɔkjuləuri(ː)ˈækʃən] *n* 絮凝反应，絮状反应

flocculus [ˈflɔkjuləs]（[复] **flocculi** [ˈflɔkjulai]）*n* 絮片，絮状物；绒球 | accessory ~, secondary ~ 副绒球，第二绒球，旁绒球（小脑）| **floccular** *a* 絮状的，絮凝状的

flock [flɔk] *n* 群 *vi* 群集

floctafenine [ˌflɔktəˈfeniːn] *n* 夫洛非宁（镇痛药）

flood [flʌd] *n* 水灾

flooding [ˈflʌdiŋ] *n* 以恐治恐法

Flood's ligament [flʌd]（Valentine Flood）弗勒德韧带（盂肱上韧带）

floor [flɔː] *n* 底部，底；| pelvic ~ 骨盆底

Flor. flores【拉】花

flora [ˈflɔːrə]（[复] **floras** 或 **florae** [ˈflɔːriː]）*n* 区系，菌群；菌丛 | intestinal ~ 肠内菌丛 | **~l** *a*

florantyrone [fləˈræntaiərəun] *n* 夫洛梯隆（促胆汁排泄药）

Florence's crystals [fləˈrɑːns]（Albert Florence）弗洛朗斯结晶（碘作用于精液中所含卵磷脂的液体而产生的结晶）| ~ test (reaction) 弗洛朗斯试验（反应）（检精液）

flores [ˈflɔːriːz] *n*【拉】花；升华制剂 | ~ benzoini 安息香华，苯甲酸 / ~ sulfuris 升华硫

florescence [flɔːˈresns] *n* 开花；开花期；兴盛时期 | **florescent** *a*

Florey unit [ˈflɔːri]（Howard W. Florey）弗洛里单位，牛津单位（Oxford unit，见 unit 项下相应术语）

florid [ˈflɔrid] *a* 红润的，血色好的；鲜红的

florigen [ˈflɔːridʒən] *n* 成花素

florizine [ˈflɔriziːn] *n* 德里辛（见 dericin）

Florschütz's formula [ˈflɔʃits]（Georg Florschütz）弗洛许茨公式（L：⟨2B-L⟩，其中 L 表示身高，B 表示腹围，指数为 5 表示正常，指数低于 5 表示体重过重的程度）

floss [flɔs] *n* 絮状物；绒毛 | **~y** *a*

flotation [fləuˈteiʃən] *n* 浮集[法]，浮选[法]

Flourens's theory(doctrine) [fluːˈrɑːŋz]（Marie J. P. Flourens）弗洛朗斯学说（全部大脑参与一切精神活动）

flourish [ˈflʌriʃ] *vi* 茂盛，繁荣 *vt* 挥舞；炫耀 *n* 茂盛，兴旺

flow [fləu] *n* 流动，流；流量，流速 | blood ~ 血流量 / forced expiratory ~（FEF）用力呼气流量 / effective renal blood ~（ERBF）有效肾血流量 / effective renal plasma ~（ERPF）有效肾血浆流量 / gene ~ 基因流动 / renal plasma ~（RPF）肾血浆流量 / total renal blood ~ 肾血流总量

flower [ˈflauə] *n* 花；[复]升华制剂 | ~s of arsenic 砷华，三氧化二砷 / ~s of benzoin 安息香华，安息香酸 / ~s of camphor 升华樟脑 / ~s of sulfur 升华硫

Flower's index [ˈflauə]（William H. Flower）弗劳尔指数，牙指数（dental index，见 index 项下相应术语）

flowmeter [ˈfləumitə] *n* 流量计 | blood ~ 血流量计

flow tract [ˈfləutrækt] 流道（血液在心腔内流动的道路）

floxacillin [ˌflɔksəˈsilin] *n* 氟氯西林（抗生素类药，主要用于治疗抗青霉素的葡萄球菌感染）

floxuridine [flɔkˈsjuəridin] *n* 氟尿苷（抗肿瘤药）

fl oz fluidounce 液量英两，液量盎司

FLP fronto-laeva posterior 额左后（胎位）

FLT fronto-laeva transversa 额左横（胎位）

flu [fluː] *n* 流行性感冒，流感 | bird ~ 禽流感

fluazacort [fluˈæzəkɔːt] *n* 氟扎可特（抗炎药）

flubendazole [fluˈbendəzəul] *n* 氟苯达唑（抗原虫药）

flucindole [fluˈsindəul] *n* 氟西吲哚（安定药）

flucloronide [fluˈklɔːrənaid] *n* 氟氯奈德（合成糖皮质激素）

flucloxacillin [ˌfluːklɔksəˈsilin] *n* 氟氯西林（即 floxacillin，抗生素类药）

fluconazole [fluːˈkɔnəzəul] *n* 氟康唑（抗真菌药）

flucrilate [ˈflukrileit] *n* 氟克立酯（组织黏合剂）

fluctuate [ˈflʌktjueit] *vi*，*vt* 变动；起伏，波动 | **fluctuant** *a* 呈现不同层次的；波动状的 / **fluctuation** [ˌflʌktjuˈeiʃən] *n*

flucytosine [fluˈsaitəsiːn] *n* 氟胞嘧啶（抗真菌药）

fludalanine [fluˈdæləniːn] *n* 氟氘丙氨酸（抗菌药）

fludarabine phosphate [fluˈdɛərəbin] 磷酸氟达拉滨（抗肿瘤药，用以治疗慢性淋巴细胞白血病）

fludazonium chloride [ˌfludəˈzəuniəm] 氯氟哒唑（局部抗感染药）

fludeoxyglucose F 18 [ˌfluːdiˌɔksiˈgluːkəus] 氟[^{18}F]脱氧葡糖（用于正电子发射体层摄影，以诊断脑功能障碍、心脏病以及各类器官的肿瘤）

fludorex [ˈfludəreks] *n* 氟多雷司（食欲抑制药，止吐药）

fludrocortisone [ˌfluːdrəuˈkɔːtisəun] *n* 氟氢可的松（肾上腺皮质激素类药） | ~ acetate 醋酸氟氢可的松

fluency [ˈflu(ː)ənsi] *n* 流利，流畅

fluent [ˈflu(ː)ənt] *a* 流利的，流畅的 | **~ly** *ad*

flufenamic acid [flufəˈnæmik] 氟芬那酸（消炎镇痛药）

flufenisal [fluˈfenisəl] *n* 氟苯柳（镇痛药）

fluff [flʌf] *n* 绒毛；汗毛 | **~y** *a* 绒毛状的

flügelplatte [ˌfliːgəlˈplʌtə] *n*【德】翼板

Fluhmann's test [ˈfluːmən]（C. F. Fluhmann）弗路曼试验（检雌激素）

fluid [ˈflu(ː)id] *a* 流动的，液体的；流质的 *n* 液体，液 | allantoic ~ 尿囊液 / amniotic ~ 羊膜液，羊水 / ascitic ~ 腹水 / body ~ 体液 / cerebrospinal ~（CSF）脑脊液 / chlorpalladium ~ 氯化钯脱钙液 / decalcifying ~ 脱钙液 / extracellular ~ 细胞外液 / follicular ~ 滤泡液，卵泡液 / intracellular ~ 细胞内液 / labyrinthine ~ 外淋巴 / pericardial ~ 心包液 / seminal ~ 精液 / serous ~ 浆液 / synovial ~ 滑液 / ventricular ~ 脑室液 | **~ic** [flu(ː)ˈidik] *a* 流体性的 / **~ity** [flu(ː)ˈidəti] *n* 流动性，流度

fluidextract [ˌflu(ː)idˈekstrækt] *n* 流浸膏

fluidextractum [ˌflu(ː)ideksˈtræktəm]（[复] **fluidextracta** [ˌflu(ː)ideksˈtræktə]）*n*【拉】流浸膏

fluidify [flu(ː)ˈidifai] *vt* 使成流体 *vi* 流体化；积满液体

fluidism [ˈflu(ː)idizəm] *n* 体液学说

fluidize [ˈflu(ː)idaiz] *vt* 流体化 | **fluidization** [ˌflu(ː)idaiˈzeiʃən，-diˈz-] *n*

fluidounce [ˈflu(ː)idˈauns] *n* 液量盎司

fluidrachm，fluidram [ˌflu(ː)iˈdræm] *n* 液量打兰（相当于 3.697 ml）

fluke [fluːk] *n* 吸虫

flulike [ˈfluːlaik] *a* 流感样的；流感样症状的

flumazenil [ˈfluːmeizəˌnil] *n* 氟马西尼（苯二氮䓬类拮抗药）

flumen [ˈfluːmən] ([复]**flumina** [ˈfluːminə]) *n* 【拉】流,波
flumequine [ˈfluməkwin] *n* 氟甲喹(抗菌药)
flumethasone pivalate [fluˈmeθəˌsəun] 特戊酸氟米松(合成糖皮质激素,局部抗炎药,用于皮肤病)
flumethiazide [ˌflumeˈθaiəzaid] *n* 氟甲噻嗪(利尿药)
flumetramide [fluˈmetrəmaid] *n* 氟美吗酮(肌肉松弛药)
flumizole [ˈflumizəul] *n* 氟咪唑(抗炎药)
flumoxonide [fluˈmɔksənaid] *n* 氟莫奈德(肾上腺皮质类固醇)
flunarizine hydrochloride [fluˈnæriziːn] 盐酸氟桂利嗪(血管扩张药)
flunidazole [fluˈnidəzəul] *n* 氟硝唑(抗原虫药)
flunisolide [fluˈnisəlaid] *n* 氟尼缩松(糖皮质激素) | ~ acetate 醋酸氟尼缩松,醋酸9-去氟肤轻松(抗炎药)
flunitrazepam [ˌfluniˈtræzəpæm] *n* 氟硝西泮(麻醉用安眠、诱导药)
flunixin [fluˈniksin] *n* 氟尼辛(消炎镇痛药) | ~ meglumine 氟尼辛葡胺(消炎镇痛药)
fluocinolone acetonide [ˌfluəˈsinələun] 氟轻松(合成糖皮质激素,局部抗炎药)
fluocinonide [ˌfluəˈsinənaid] *n* 醋酸氟轻松(有消炎止痒和收缩血管作用,局部用于治疗某些皮肤病)
fluocortin butyl [ˌflu(ː)əˈkɔːtin] 氟可丁酯(抗炎药)
fluohydrisone [ˌfluəˈhaidrisəun], **fluohydrocortisone** [ˌfluəˌhaidrəuˈkɔːtisəun] *n* 氟氢可的松
fluor [ˈflu(ː)ɔ] *n*【拉】排出物,溢液;荧光体 | ~ albus 白带
fluorane [ˈfluərein] *n* 荧烷
fluoresce [fluəˈres] *vi* 发荧光
fluorescein [ˌfluəˈresiːn] *n* 荧光素 | ~ isothiocyanate(FITC) 异硫氰酸荧光素 / sodium ~, soluble ~ 荧光素钠,可溶性荧光素
fluoresceinuria [ˌfluəˌresiːˈnjuəriə] *n* 荧光素尿
fluorescence [ˌfluəˈresns] *n* 荧光 | secondary ~ 继发荧光
fluorescent [ˌfluəˈresnt] *a* 荧光的
fluorescin [ˌfluəˈresin] *n* 氢化荧光素
fluoric acid [ˈfluərik] 氟酸
fluoridate [ˈfluərideit] *vt* 向…中加入氟化物 | **fluoridation** [ˌfluəriˈdeiʃən] *n* 加氟作用,氟化[作用]
fluoride [ˈfluəraid] *n* 氟化物 | stannous ~ 氟化亚锡
fluoridize [ˈfluəridaiz] *vt* 涂氟 | **fluoridization** [ˌfluəridaiˈzeiʃən] *n* 涂氟法;氟化[作用]
fluorimeter [ˌfluəˈrimitə] *n* 荧光计 | **fluorimetry** *n* 荧光分析法;荧光测定法
fluorinate [ˈfluərineit] *vt* 用氟处理;使与氟化合 | **fluorination** [ˌfluəriˈneiʃən] *n* 氟化[作用]
fluorine(F) [ˈfluəriːn] *n* 氟(化学元素)
fluoroacetate [ˌfluərəuˈæsiteit] *n* 氟醋酸盐(杀鼠药)
fluoroacetic acid [ˌfluərəuəˈsiːtik] 氟乙酸
fluorocarbon [ˈfluərəuˌkɑːbən] *n* 碳氟化合物(氟碳乳剂溶解氧和二氧化碳,并能取代红细胞制剂用于防治贫血)
fluorochrome [ˈfluərəkrəum] *n* 荧光色素,荧光染料
fluorocyte [ˈfluərəsait] *n* 荧光细胞
fluorodeoxyglucose [ˌfluərəudiˌɔksiˈgluːkəus] *a* 氟脱氧葡糖
fluorodopa F 18 [ˌfluərəuˈdəupə] 氟[^{18}F]多巴(用于大脑正电子发射体层摄影)
fluorography [ˌfluəˈrɔgrəfi] *n* 荧光自显影,荧光X线摄影[术]
fluoroimmunoassay [ˌfluərəuˌimjunəuˈæsei] *n* 荧光免疫测定
fluorometer [ˌfluəˈrɔmitə] *n* 荧光计 | **fluorometric** [ˌfluərəuˈmetrik] *a* 荧光测定的 / **fluorometry** *n* 荧光分析法,荧光测定法
fluorometholone [ˌfluərəuˈmeθələun] *n* 氟米龙(合成糖皮质激素,局部抗炎药)
fluoronaphthyridone [ˌfluərəunæfˈθairidəun] *n* 氟萘立酮(抗生素类药)
fluoronephelometer [ˌfluərəunefiˈlɔmitə] *n* 荧光比浊计,荧光散射浊度计
***p*-fluorophenylalanine** [ˌfluərəuˌfeniˈlæləniːn] *n* 对氟苯丙氨酸
fluorophosphate [ˌfluərəuˈfɔsfeit] *n* 氟磷酸(含氟与磷的有机化合物) | diisopropyl ~ 二异丙基氟磷酸
fluorophotometry [ˌfluərəufəuˈtɔmitri] *n* 荧光光度测定法 | vitreous ~ 玻璃体荧光光度测定法
fluoropyrimidine [ˌfluərəupəˈrimidiːn] *n* 氟嘧啶(具有抗肿瘤作用)
fluoroquinolone [ˌfluərəuˈkwinəuləun] *n* 氟喹诺酮(抗菌药)
fluororadiography [ˌfluərəuˌreidiˈɔgrəfi] *n* 荧光X线摄影[术],间接摄影[术]
fluororoentgenography [ˌfluərəuˌrɔntgəˈnɔgrəfi] *n* 荧光X线摄影[术]
fluoroscope [ˈfluərəskəup] *n* 荧光屏,荧光镜 *vt* 用荧光镜检查 | biplane ~ 双面荧光屏
fluoroscopy [ˌfluəˈrɔskəpi] *n* 荧光屏检查,荧光镜透视检查,X线透视检查 | **fluoroscopical** [ˌfluərəˈskɔpikəl] *a*
fluorosilicate [ˌfluərəuˈsilikeit] *n* 氟硅酸盐,硅氟

化物

fluorosis [ˌfluəˈrəusis] *n* (慢性)氟中毒,斑釉 | chronic endemic ~ 慢性地方性[牙]氟中毒 / dental ~ 牙氟中毒

fluorouracil [ˌfluərə*u*ˈjuərəsil] *n* 氟尿嘧啶,5-氟尿嘧啶(抗肿瘤药)

fluosilic acid [fluəˈsilik] 氟硅酸

fluotracen hydrochloride [ˌfluəˈtreisən] 盐酸氟曲辛(安定药,抗抑郁药)

fluoxetine [fluˈɔksətiːn] *n* 氟西汀(抗抑郁药)

fluoxymesterone [fluˌɔksiˈmestərəun] *n* 氟甲睾酮(雄激素)

flupenthixol [ˌflupenˈθiksɔl] *n* 氟哌噻吨(抗精神病药)

flupentixol [ˌflupenˈtiksɔl] *n* 氟哌噻吨(flupenthixol 的 INN 名)

fluperamide [fluˈperəmaid] *n* 氟哌醇胺(减蠕动药)

fluperolone [fluˈperələun] *n* 氟培龙(糖皮质激素,抗炎药)

fluphenazine [fluˈfenəziːn] *n* 氟奋乃静(安定药) | ~ enanthate 庚酸氟奋乃静(安定药) / ~ hydrochloride 盐酸氟奋乃静(安定药)

fluprednisolone [ˌflupredˈnisələun] *n* 氟泼尼龙(合成糖皮质激素) | ~ valerate 戊酸氟泼尼龙

fluprostenol sodium [fluˈprɔstənɔl] 氟前列醇钠(抗不育症药)

fluquazone [ˈflukwəzəun] *n* 氟喹宗(抗炎药)

flurandrenolide [ˌfluərænˈdrenəlaid] *n* 氟氢缩松(糖皮质激素,抗炎药,用于皮肤病)

flurandrenolone [ˌfluərænˈdrenələun] *n* 氟氢缩松(即 flurandrenolide)

flurazepam hydrochloride [fluəˈræzəpæm] 盐酸氟西泮(催眠药)

flurbiprofen [fluəˈbiprəfen] *n* 氟比洛芬(抗炎药)

flurocitabine [ˌfluərəˈsaitəbiːn] *n* 氟西他滨(抗肿瘤药)

flurogestone acetate [ˌfluərəˈdʒestəun] 醋酸氟孕酮(孕激素)

flurothyl [ˈfluərəθil] *n* 氟替尔(吸入用惊厥药)

fluroxene [fluˈrɔksiːn] *n* 氟乙烯醚(吸入麻醉药)

flush [flʌʃ] *n* 潮红 | atropine ~ 阿托品潮红 / breast ~ 乳房潮红 / hectic ~ 痨病性潮红 / mahogany ~ 红木色潮红(见于大叶性肺炎时一侧面颊) / malar ~ 颧颊潮红

fluspiperone [fluˈspipərəun] *n* 氟司哌隆(安定药)

fluspirilene [fluˈspiəriliːn] *n* 氟司必林(安定药)

flutamide [ˈflutəmaid] *n* 氟他胺(抗雄激素药)

flutiazin [fluˈtaiəzin] *n* 氟替阿嗪(兽用抗炎药)

fluticasone propionate [fluˈtikəˌsəun] 丙酸氟替卡松(合成皮质类固醇,用作消炎止痒药,治疗皮质类固醇反应性皮肤病,用于鼻内治疗变应性鼻炎,并用吸入法治疗哮喘)

flutter [ˈflʌtə] *n* 扑动 | atrial ~, auricular ~ 心房扑动 / diaphragmatic ~ 膈扑动 / impure ~ 不整齐扑动 / mediastinal ~ 纵隔扑动 / pure ~ 整齐扑动

flutter-fibrillation [ˈflʌtə-ˌfibriˈleiʃən] *n* 扑动-纤颤[型](心电图)

fluvastatin sodium [ˈfluːvəˌstætin] 氟伐他汀钠(用于治疗高胆固醇血症)

fluvoxamine [fluˈvɔksəmiːn] *n* 氟伏沙明(选择性 5-羟色胺摄取抑制剂,用作马来酸盐)

flux [flʌks] *n* 流;流量;(血液、体液的)流出,溢出;[助]熔剂,焊媒;通量[物] | bloody ~ 血痢,痢疾 / celiac ~ 食糜泻 / hepatic ~, bilious ~ 肝性泻,胆汁泻 / luminous ~ 光通量 / menstrual ~ 月经 / neutral ~ 中性焊媒 / oxidizing ~ 氧化性焊媒 / reducing ~ 还原性焊媒

fluxion [ˈflʌkʃən] *n* 流动;流出,溢出 | **~al**, **~ary** *a*

fly [flai] *n* 蝇(双翅昆虫) | black ~ 黑蝇(蚋类) / bloodsucking flies 吸血蝇类 / blow ~, bluebottle ~ 丽蝇 / bot ~ 肤蝇(类) / caddis ~ 毛翅蝇 / cheese ~ 酪蝇 / deer ~ 斑虻(即 Chrysops discalis) / drone ~ [绒]蜂蝇(即 Eristalis tenax) / face ~ 秋家蝇(即 Musca autumnalis) / filth ~ 家蝇(即 Musca domestica) / flesh ~ 麻蝇,肉蝇 / fruit ~ 果蝇 / gad ~ 虻 / gold ~ 凯撒绿蝇(即 Lucilia caesar) / green-bottle ~ 绿蝇 / heel ~ 皮下蝇 / horse ~ 马蝇(指虻) / house ~ 家蝇(即 Musca domestica) / latrine ~ 灰腹厕蝇(Frannia scalaris) / mango ~, mangrove ~ 斑虻(即 Chrysops dimidiata) / moth ~ 蛾蝇(指毛蠓) / nose ~, nostril ~ 羊狂蝇(即 Oestrus ovis) / phlebotomus ~ 白蛉 / Russian ~ 斑蝥(即 Lytta) / sand ~ 白蛉 / screwworm ~ 锥蝇,嗜人锥蝇(即 Cochliomyia hominivorax) / Seroot ~ 二带虻(即 Tabanus gratus) / soldier ~ 水虻(即 Hermetia illucens) / Spanish ~ 斑蝥,欧芫青 / stable ~ 厩螫蝇 / tick ~ 蜱蝇 / tsetse ~ 采采蝇 / tumbu ~ 嗜人瘤蝇 / vinegar ~ 果蝇,蜂蝇 / warble ~ 肤蝇(即 Hypoderma)

fly-borne [ˈflai bɔːn] *a* 蝇传播的

flyflap [ˈflaiflæp] *n* 蝇拍 *vi* (用蝇拍)拍苍蝇

Flynn-Aird syndrome [flin ɛəd] (P. Flynn; R. B. Aird) 弗-艾综合征(一种罕见的常染色体显性遗传综合征,神经系统和外胚叶结构异常,其中包括白内障、色素性视网膜炎、近视、龋牙、皮肤萎缩和溃疡形成、周围神经病、共济失调、耳聋以及囊性骨病变)

flypaper [ˈflaiˌpeipə] *n* 粘蝇纸,毒蝇纸

flyswatter [ˈflaiˌswætə] *n* 苍蝇拍

flytrap [ˈflaitræp] *n* 捕蝇器

Fm fermium 镄

F. M. fiat mistura【拉】制成合剂
FMN flavin mononucleotide 黄素单核苷酸
FMN adenylyltransferase [ˌædəˌnilil'trænsfəreis] 黄素单核苷酸腺苷酰[基]转移酶
FMNH$_2$ the reduced form of flavin mononucleotide 黄素单核苷酸的还原型
FNH focal nodular hyperplasia 局灶性结节性增生
FNTC fine needle transhepatic cholangiography 细针经肝[穿刺]胆管造影[术]
foam [fəum] *n* 泡沫;泡沫材料(泡沫塑料,泡沫橡胶)
foamy ['fəumi] *a* 起泡沫的;泡沫似的
focal ['fəukəl] *a* 焦点的;病灶[性]的,灶[性]的
focil ['fəusil], **focile** ['fəusili] *n* 前臂骨;小腿骨
focimeter [fəu'simitə] *n* 焦点计
focus ['fəukəs] ([复]**focuses** 或 **foci** ['fəusai]) *n* 焦点;病灶;疫源地(-s⟨s⟩-) *vt* 使聚焦 *vi* 聚焦 | aplanatic ~ 无球面象差焦点 / conjugate ~ 共轭焦点 / epileptogenic ~ 致癫痫病灶 / principal foci 主焦点 / real ~ 实焦点 / virtual ~ 虚焦点
focusing ['fəukəsiŋ] *n* 聚焦 | isoelectric ~ 等电聚焦
fodrin ['fəudrin] *n* 胞衬蛋白,胞影蛋白
foe- 以 foe-起始的词,同样见 fe-起始的词
Foeniculum [fiː'nikjuləm] *n* 茴香属
Foerster 见 Förster
foetus ['fiːtəs] *n* = fetus | **foetal** ['fiːtl] *a* = fetal
fog [fɔg] *n* 雾;(影像)模糊;再生草 | mental ~ 意识混浊
Fogarty catheter ['fəugəti] (Thomas J. Fogarty) 福格蒂导管(一种尖头气囊导管,用于从血管中去除血栓和栓子) | ~ embolectomy catheter 福格蒂取栓导管
fogging ['fɔgiŋ] *n* 雾视法(眼科中检屈光不正)
fogo ['fəugəu] *n*【葡】火,炎症 | ~ selvagem 野火,巴西天疱疮
foil [fɔil] *n* 箔,叶 | gold ~ 金箔 / platinum ~ 铂箔,白金箔 / tin ~ 锡箔
Foix-Alajouanine syndrome [fwɑː ɑːlɑːʒuɑː'niːn] (Charles Foix; Théophile Alajouanine) 富-阿综合征(一种坏死性脊髓病,特征为脊髓灰质坏死,脊柱管壁增厚及脊髓液异常,症状包括下肢亚急性痉挛性截瘫,进而发展到弛缓性麻痹⟨经常是上行性麻痹⟩,括约肌失控及进行性感觉缺失,1~2年内死亡。亦称亚急性坏死性脊髓灰质炎)
Foix syndrome [fwɑː] (Charles Foix) 富瓦综合征,海绵窦综合征(即 cavernous syndrome,见 syndrome 项下相应术语)
Fol. folia【拉】叶
folacin ['fəuləsin] *n* 叶酸
folate ['fəuleit] *n* 叶酸(阴离子型);叶酸盐
fold [fəuld] *n* 折;折叠;[皱]襞,褶 | alar ~s 翼状襞 / amniotic ~ 羊膜褶 / aryepiglottic ~ 杓状会厌襞 / axillary ~s 腋襞 / bulboventricular ~ 球室襞 / caval ~ 腔静脉褶(胚胎) / cecal ~s 盲肠襞 / cholecystoduodenocolic ~ 胆囊十二指肠结肠襞 / ciliary ~s 睫状褶 / conjunctival ~, palpebral ~, retrotarsal ~ 结膜褶 / costocolic ~ 膈结肠韧带 / duodenojejunal ~ 十二指肠空肠襞,十二指肠上襞 / duodenomesocolic ~ 十二指肠结肠系膜襞,十二指肠下襞 / epicanthal ~, epicanthine ~ 内眦赘皮 / epigastric ~ 腹壁动脉襞,脐外侧襞 / gastric ~s 胃襞 / gastropancreatic ~s 胃胰襞 / genital ~ 生殖褶,生殖嵴 / gluteal ~ 臀沟 / head ~ 头褶 / ileocecal ~ 回盲襞 / ileocolic ~ 回结肠襞 / incudal ~ 砧骨褶 / interureteric ~ 输尿管间襞,输尿管间嵴 / lacrimal ~ 鼻泪管襞 / mammary ~ 乳腺褶 / mesolateral ~ 侧肠系膜褶 / mesonephric ~ 中肾褶,中肾嵴 / mesouterine ~ 子宫系膜襞 / mucobuccal ~, mucosobuccal ~ 颊黏膜襞 / mucosal ~, mucous ~ 黏膜襞 / nail ~ 甲褶 / nasopharyngeal ~ 咽鼓管腭襞 / neural ~, medullary ~ 神经褶 / opercular ~ 前柱褶 / palmate ~s 棕榈状褶 / pancreaticogastric ~s 胃胰襞 / paraduodenal ~ 十二指肠旁襞 / parietocolic ~ 回盲上襞 / parietoperitoneal ~ 襞腹膜褶 / pharyngoepiglottic ~ 咽会厌襞 / primitive ~ 原褶 / proximal nail ~ 甲床沟 / rectal ~s 直肠横襞 / rectouterine ~, rectovesical ~, sacrogenital ~ 直肠子宫襞 / rectovaginal ~ 直肠阴道襞 / salpingopalatine ~ 咽鼓管腭襞 / salpingopharyngeal ~ 咽鼓管咽襞 / semilunar ~ 半月襞 / serosal ~, serous ~ 浆膜襞 / synovial ~ 滑膜皱襞 / tail ~ 尾褶 / triangular ~ 三角襞 / urogenital ~ 尿生殖褶,尿生殖嵴 / vaginal ~s 阴道皱褶 / ventricular ~, vestibular ~ 室襞(假声带) / vocal ~ 声襞,声带
fold [后缀]倍,重
Foley catheter ['fəuli] (Frederic E. B. Foley) 福利导管(一种留置导管,借充以空气或液体的小气球留置在膀胱内)
folia ['fəuliə] folium 的复数
foliaceous [ˌfəuli'eiʃəs] *a* 叶状的
folian ['fəuliən] *a* 福利厄斯突的,锤骨前突的(见 Folius' process)
foliar ['fəuliə] *a* 叶的;叶状的
foliate ['fəulieit] *a* 具叶的;叶状的
foliation [ˌfəuli'eiʃən] *n* 生叶;成层,成片
folic acid ['fəulik] 叶酸,维生素 B_c
folie [fɔ'liː] *n*【法】精神错乱,精神病 | ~ à deux 二联性精神病 / ~ circulaire 循环性精神病 / ~ du doute 疑虑癖,疑虑性强迫症 / ~ du pourquoi 问难癖,疑问性精神病 / ~ gémellaire 孪生精神病 / ~ musculaire 重症舞蹈病 / ~ raisonnante

妄想性精神病

Folin and Wu's method (Otto K. O. Folin;吴宪,中国生化学家)福林-吴宪法(检肌酸酐、肌酸肌酸酐之和、葡萄糖、非蛋白氮、无蛋白血滤液、脲及尿酸)

folinic acid [fəuˈlinik] 亚叶酸,甲酰四氢叶酸(叶酸拮抗药的解毒药,抗贫血药,亦称嗜橙菌因子)

Folin's method [ˈfɔlin] (Otto K. O. Folin) 福林法(检丙酮、血液氨基酸、血液氨基酸氮、氨氮、血糖、肌酸、尿中肌酸、尿中肌酸酐、硫酸酯、无机硫酸盐、尿中蛋白质、尿总酸度、尿总硫酸盐、脲及尿囊素) | ~ reagent 福林试剂(100 g 钨酸钠和 80 ml 85% 的[正]磷酸加 750 ml 水煮沸 2 小时,冷却并稀释至 1 L) / ~ test 福林试验(尿酸定量、尿素定量,检正常尿中糖及氨基酸)

foliole [ˈfəuliəul] *n* 小叶;叶状突

folium [ˈfəuliəm] *n* ([复]**folia** [ˈfəuliə])【拉】| folia of cerebellum 小脑叶 / lingual ~ 叶状乳头 / ~ vermis 蚓叶

Folius muscle [ˈfəuliəs] (Caecilius Folius) 锤骨外侧韧带 | ~ process 福利厄斯突,锤骨前突

folliberin [fəˈlibərin] *n* 促滤泡激素释放激素

follicle [ˈfɔlikl] *n* 滤泡,小囊;卵泡 | aggregated ~s 淋巴集结 / dental ~ 牙囊 / gastric ~s 胃腺(滤泡);胃淋巴小结 / hair ~ 毛囊 / intestinal ~s 肠腺(滤泡) / lenticular ~s 胃淋巴小结 / lingual ~s, lymphatic ~s of tongue, ~s of tongue 舌滤泡 / lymph ~s of stomach 胃淋巴滤泡,胃淋巴滤液 / ovarian ~ 卵[巢滤]泡 / primordial ~ 原始卵泡 / sebaceous ~ 皮脂腺 / solitary ~s 孤立(淋巴)滤泡 / vesicular ovarian ~s 囊状卵泡 | **follicular** [fəˈlikjulə], **folliculate(d)** [fəˈlikjuleit(id)] *a*

folliclis [ˈfɔliklis] *n* 丘疹坏死性结核疹

folliculin [fəˈlikjulin] *n* 雌酮(旧名卵泡素)

folliculitis [fəˌlikjuˈlaitis] *n* 滤泡炎;毛囊炎 | ~ abscedens et suffodiens 头部脓肿性穿凿性毛囊周围炎 / agminate ~ 簇集性毛囊炎 / ~ barbae 须疮 / ~ decalvans 毛囊炎性脱发 / ~ gonorrhoeica 淋病性滤泡炎,尿道腺炎 / gram-negative ~ 革兰阴性菌性毛囊炎 / keloidal ~, ~ keloidalis 瘢痕疙瘩性毛囊炎,头部乳头状皮炎 / ~ nares perforans 穿通性鼻部毛囊炎 / ~ ulerythematosa reticulata 网状红瘢性毛囊炎 / ~ varioliformis 痘疮样痤疮

folliculoma [fəˌlikjuˈləumə] *n* 滤泡瘤,粒层滤泡膜细胞瘤 | ~ lipidique 类脂性滤泡瘤

folliculosis [fəˌlikjuˈləusis] *n* 滤泡增殖,淋巴滤泡增殖

folliculostatin [fəˌlikjuləuˈstætin] *n* 滤泡抑素

folliculus [fəˈlikjuləs] ([复]**folliculi** [fəˈlikjulai]) *n*【拉】滤泡,小囊;卵泡

follistatin [ˈfɔliˌstætin] *n* 滤泡素抑制素

follitropin [ˌfɔliˈtrəupin] *n* 促滤泡素,促卵泡[激]素

following [ˈfɔləuiŋ] *n* 刺激效应(脑电图上所见的一种效应,脑波随着某些反复的感觉刺激时而改变其频率)

follow-up [ˈfɔləu ˌʌp] *n* 随访

Foltz's valve [fɔlts] (Jean C. E. Foltz) 福尔兹瓣(泪小管襞)

foment [fəuˈment] *vt* 热敷,热罨 | **fomentation** [ˌfəumenˈteiʃən] *n* 热敷,热罨;罨剂

fomepizole [fəuˈmepizəul] *n* 甲吡唑(醇脱氢酶抑制剂,用作甲醇或乙二醇中毒的解毒药)

fomes [ˈfəumiːz] ([复]**fomites** [ˈfəumitiːz]) *n*【拉】污染物

fomite [ˈfəumait] *n* 污染物

fomivirsen sodium [fəuˈmivəsin] 福米韦辛钠(抗病毒药,玻璃体内注射给药,治疗巨细胞病毒性视网膜炎伴艾滋病)

fonazine mesylate [ˈfəunəziːn] 甲磺二甲替嗪(5-羟色胺抑制药)

Fonsecaeea [fɔnsiˈsiːə] *n* 着色芽生菌属 | ~ compactum 紧密着色芽生菌 / ~ pedrosoi 裴氏着色芽生菌,裴氏着色霉

fontactoscope [fɔnˈtæktəskəup] *n* 水及空气放射力计

Fontana's markings [fɔnˈtɑːnə] (Felice Fontana) 丰塔纳条纹(神经干切面的横纹) | ~ spaces 虹膜角膜角间隙,虹膜角间隙

fontanel [ˌfɔntəˈnel] *n* 囟[门]

fontanelle [ˌfɔntəˈnel] *n* 囟【门】| anterlor ~, bregmatic ~, frontal ~, quadrangular ~ 前囟 / anterolateral ~, sphenoidal ~ 蝶囟 / cranial ~s 颅囟,囟 / mastoid ~, posterolateral ~, posterotemporal ~ 乳突囟 / occipital ~, posterior ~, triangular ~ 后囟

Fontan procedure [fɔnˈtɑːn] (François M. Fontan) 丰唐手术(功能性矫正三尖瓣闭锁,其法为对右心房和肺动脉施行吻合术,或在右心房和肺动脉之间插入非人造瓣膜,关闭心房间的通道,此法也用于其他选择性先天性疾病)

fonticulus [fɔnˈtikjuləs] ([复]**fonticuli** [fɔnˈtikjulai]) *n*【拉】囟,囟门

food [fuːd] *n* 食物,食品 | isodynamic ~s 等热量食物

foodstuffs [ˈfuːdstʌfs] *n* 食料,食品

foot [fut] ([复]**feet** [fiːt]) *n* 足;呎(旧称),英尺 | athlete's ~ 足癣,皮真菌病 / broad ~ 阔足,阔跖足 / cleft ~ 裂足[畸形] / club ~, reel ~ 畸形足 /dangle ~, drop ~ 下垂足 / end ~ 终纽 / flat ~ 扁平足,平足 / forced ~ 行军足 / Hong Kong ~ 足癣 / mossy ~ 苔状足 / rocker-bottom ~ 摇椅足(先天性凸状外翻足;马蹄内翻足)/ sag ~ 弓下陷足,足弓下陷 / shelter ~ 防空壕足 / spread ~ 阔足,阔跖足 / sucker ~ 吸足,吸盘,吸器 /taut ~ 马蹄状足 / trench ~ 战壕足 / weak ~ 柔弱足(早期扁平足)

foot-candle [fut ˈkændl] *n* 英尺烛光(旧照度单位,即每英尺1流明或等于1.076 4毫辐透,现用lx勒[克斯])

footdrop [ˈfutdrɔp] *n* 足下垂

foot lambert [fut' læmbət] 英尺朗伯(旧亮度单位,见lambert,现用cd/m^2〈坎[德拉]每平方米〉)

footplate [ˈfutpleit] *n* 镫骨底 | floating ~ 游动镫骨底 / stapedial ~ 镫骨底

foot-pound [ˈfut paund] *n* 英尺磅(旧功的单位,现用kg/m〈千克/米〉)

footprint [ˈfutˌprint] *n* 足迹

footprinting [ˈfutˌprintiŋ] *n* 足迹法(测定蛋白质与DNA分子间结合位置的一种技术)

forage¹ [ˈfɔridʒ] *n* 饲料

forage² [fɔˈrɑːʒ] *n*【法】楔形切开(用电流在前列腺上形成一个V形纵沟,以切除其因增生而引起的阻塞)

foram [ˈfɔːræm] *n* 有孔虫(即foraminiferan)

foramen [fəˈreimən] ([复] **foramina** [fəˈræminə]) *n*【拉】孔 | anterior condyloid ~ 舌下神经管 / aortic ~ 主动脉裂孔 / cecal ~ (额骨)盲孔/ cervical ~ 横突孔 / esophageal ~ 食管裂孔 / external auditory ~ 外耳道 / frontal ~ 额骨内侧切迹,额骨内侧孔 / incisive ~ 切牙孔 / innominate ~ 岩浅小神经管内口 / internal auditory ~ 内耳门 / malar ~ 颧面孔 / median incisor ~ 鼻腭神经孔 / pleuroperitoneal ~ 胸腹裂孔;膈裂 / posterior condyloid ~ 髁管 / sphenotic ~ 破裂孔 / thyroid ~ 甲状软骨孔 / transverse ~, vertebroarterial ~ 横突孔 / vena caval ~, venous ~, quadrate ~, right ~ 腔静脉孔 / vertebral ~ 椎孔;横突孔 | **foraminal** [fəˈræminəl], **foraminate** [fəˈræminit] *a* 有孔的,有小孔的

foraminifer [ˌfɔrəˈminifə] *n* 有孔虫

foraminiferal [fəˌræmiˈnifərəl] *a* 有孔的;有孔虫的

foraminiferan [fəˌræmiˈnifərən] *n* 有孔虫

Foraminiferida [fəˌræminiˈferidə] *n* 有孔虫目

foraminiferous [fəˌræmiˈnifərəs] *a* 有孔的

foraminotomy [fəˌræmiˈnɔtəmi] *n* 椎间孔切开术

foraminulum [ˌfɔrəˈminjuləm] ([复] **foraminula** [ˌfɔrəˈminjulə]) *n*【拉】小孔

foration [fəˈreiʃən] *n* 环钻术

Forbes-Albright syndrome [ˈfɔːbz' ɔlbrait] (Anne P. Forbes; Fuller Albright) 福-奥综合征(与妊娠无关的乳溢闭经综合征,通常伴分泌催乳素的垂体瘤)

Forbes' disease [ˈfɔːbz] (Gilbert B. Forbes) 福布斯病,糖原贮积症Ⅲ型

force [fɔːs] *n* 力;势 | catabolic ~ 食物分解热力 / electromotive ~ 电动势 / field ~s 区力(参与早期胚胎个体化过程中的假设力量) / masticatory ~, chewing ~ 咀嚼力 / reserve ~ 潜力,保存力 / rest ~ 安静力 / vital ~ 活力

forceplate [ˈfɔːspleit] *n* 受力板

forceps [ˈfɔːseps] *n* 钳,镊;钳状体 | alligator ~ 鳄嘴钳 / artery ~ 动脉钳 / aural ~ 耳镊 / bone ~ 骨钳 / capsule ~ 晶状体囊镊 / clamp ~ 夹钳;夹具钳 / clip ~ 卡环钳,弹簧钳 / dental ~ 牙钳,拔牙钳 / disk ~ 巩膜钻板镊 / ear ~ 耳镊 / epilating ~ 拔毛镊 / hemostatic ~ 止血钳 / high ~ 高位钳(用于高位产钳分娩) / lithotomy ~ 取石钳 / low ~ 低位钳(用于低位产钳分娩) / ~ major, ~ posterior 胼胝体辐射线枕部 / mid ~ 中位钳(用于中位产钳分娩) / ~ minor, ~ anterior 胼胝体辐射线额部 / mosquito ~ 蚊式止血钳 / roller ~, trachoma ~ 转轴镊,沙眼镊 / tissue ~, thumb ~ 组织镊,按捏镊

forcipate(d) [ˈfɔːsipeit(id)] *a* 钳形的

Forcipomyia [ˌfɔːsipəˈmaijə] *n* 铗蠓属

forcipressure [ˈfɔːsipreʃə] *n* 钳压法(主要用以止血)

Fordyce's disease [ˈfɔːdais] (John A. Fordyce) 福代斯病(①异位皮脂腺,见 ~ granule; ②大汗腺粟粒疹,见Fox-Fordyce disease) | ~ granule (spot) 福代斯粒(斑),异位皮脂腺(见于唇与龈上及颊黏膜内的皮脂腺,呈淡黄白色粟丘疹。亦称福代斯病)

forearm [ˈfɔːrɑːm] *n* 前臂

forebrain [ˈfɔːbrein] *n* 前脑

foreconscious [fɔːˈkɔnʃəs] *a* 前意识的

forefinger [ˈfɔːˌfiŋgə] *n* 示指,食指

forefoot [ˈfɔːfut] ([复] **forefeet** [ˈfɔːfiːt]) *n* 前肢(四肢动物);足前段

foregilding [ˈfɔːgildiŋ] *n* (神经组织)氯金酸钠处理

foregut [ˈfɔːgʌt] *n* 前肠

forehead [ˈfɔrid] *n* 额;前部

forehead-plasty [ˈfɔrid ˌplæsti] *n* 额成形术,额整形术

foreign [ˈfɔrin] *a* 外来的;异质的 | ~ body 异物

forekidney [fɔːˈkidni] *n* 前肾

foreleg [ˈfɔːleg] *n* 前足,前肢(四足动物的)

forelimb [ˈfɔːlim] *n* 前肢,上肢

forelock [ˈfɔːlɔk] *n* 额发,前发

Forel's commissure [fɔˈrel] (Auguste H. Forel) 福雷尔连合(丘脑下部核连合) | ~ decussation 福雷尔交叉(中脑的红脊髓束及红核网状束的

被盖前交叉）/ ~ field 福雷尔区（含有联系丘脑与丘脑下部细的纵行纤维的区域）

forensic [fə'rensik] *a* 法庭的，法医的

foreplay ['fɔːplei] *n* 做爱前奏（性交前挑逗）

fore-pleasure ['fɔːpleʒə] *n* 前期性乐

forerunner ['fɔːˌrʌnə] *n* 先驱者；前征，前兆；祖先

forescattering [ˌfɔː'skætəriŋ] *n* 向前散射

foreskin ['fɔːskin] *n* 包皮 | hooded ~ 头巾状包皮

Forestier's disease [ˌfəuresti'ei] (Jacques Forestier) 福莱斯蒂埃病（前外侧脊柱骨肥厚，尤见于胸区）

forestomach ['fɔːstʌmək] *n* 前胃（反刍类）

foretop ['fɔːtɔp] *n*（马的）额鬃

forewaters ['fɔːwɔːtəz] *n* 前羊水

fork [fɔːk] *n* 叉 | tuning ~ 音叉

forked [fɔːkt] *a* 叉状的，有叉的

form [fɔːm] *n* 形状，形态；变形；型 | accolé ~, appliqué ~ 依附型，依附体（恶性疟原虫早期）/ band ~s 带［状核］型（白细胞）/ involution ~s 退化型（细菌）/ juvenile ~, young ~ 晚幼粒细胞 / racemic ~ 消旋式 / retention ~ 固位形（牙洞）/ ring ~ 环状体（疟原虫小滋养体）/ tooth ~ 牙型

Formad's kidney ['fɔːmæd] (Henry F. Formad) 福马德肾（慢性酒精中毒肾肿大）

formaldehyde [fɔː'mældihaid] *n* 甲醛（消毒防腐药）

formaldehyde dehydrogenase (glutathione) [fɔː'mældihaid diː'haidrədʒəneis ˌgluːtə'θaiəun] 甲醛脱氢酶（谷胱甘肽）

formaldehydogenic [fɔːˌmældiˌhaidəu'dʒenik] *a* 甲醛原的，生甲醛的

formalin ['fɔːməlin] *n* 福尔马林，甲醛溶液

formalinize ['fɔːməlinaiz] *vt* 用甲醛处理

formamidase [fɔː'mæmideis] *n* 甲酰胺酶，芳基甲酰胺酶

formamide ['fɔːməmaid] *n* 甲酰胺

formamidoxim [fɔːˌmæmi'dɔksim] *n* 氨基甲肟

formant ['fɔːmənt] *n* 共振峰

formate ['fɔːmit] *n* 甲酸盐

formate dehydrogenase ['fɔːmeit diː'haidrədʒəneis] 甲酸脱氢酶（亦称甲酸氢裂合酶）

formate hydrogenlyase ['fɔːmeit ˌhaidrədʒən'laieis] 甲酸氢裂合酶，甲酸脱氢酶

formate-tetrahydrofolate ligase ['fɔːmeit ˌtetrəˌhaidrəu'fəuleit 'laigeis] 甲酸四氢叶酸连接酶

formatio [fɔː'meiʃiəu] ([复] **formationes** [fɔːmeiʃi'əuniːz]) *n*【拉】结构

formation [fɔː'meiʃən] *n* 形成；结构 | coffin ~ 柩［状］形成（噬神经细胞作用时，卫星细胞包围死亡的神经细胞）/ Gothic arch ~ 哥特式尖拱结构（见 Henning's sign）/ gray reticular ~ 灰网状质（延髓）/ palisade ~ 栅栏形成（神经胶质瘤的细胞排列）/ reaction ~ 反应形成（心理机制）/ reticular ~ 网状结构（延髓等）/ rouleaux ~ 缗钱状形成，钱串形成（红细胞重叠排列呈钱串状）/ spore ~ 孢子形成，芽胞形成 / white reticular ~ 白网状质（延髓）

formative ['fɔːmətiv] *a* 形成的，构成的，结构的

formazan ['fɔːməzæn] *n* 甲臜

formboard ['fɔːmbɔːd] *n* 形状板（测智力用）

form-class [fɔːm'klɑːs] *n* 形态纲

forme [fɔːm] *n*【法】形状，形态；型 | ~ fruste 顿挫型 / ~ tardive 迟发型

form-family [fɔːm 'fæmili] *n* 形态科

formic ['fɔːmik] *a* 蚁的 | ~ acid 甲酸，蚁酸

Formica [fɔː'maikə] *n* 蚁属

formication [ˌfɔːmi'keiʃən] *n* 蚁走感

formiciasis [ˌfɔːmi'saiəsis] *n* 蚁咬［皮］病

Formicidae [fɔː'misidiː] *n* 蚁科

Formicoidea [ˌfɔmi'kɔidiə] *n* 蚁总科

formilase ['fɔːmileis] *n* 甲酸生成酶

formimino [fɔː'miminəu] *n* 亚胺甲基

formiminoglutamate [fɔːˌmiminəu'gluːtəmeit] *n* 亚胺甲基谷氨酸

formiminoglutamic acid [fɔːˌmiminəugluː'tæmik] 亚胺甲基谷氨酸

5-formiminotetrahydrofolate [fɔːˌmiminəu ˌtetrəˌhaidrəu'fəuleit] *n* 亚胺甲基四氢叶酸

formiminotetrahydrofolate cyclodeaminase [fɔːˌmiminəuˌtetrəˌhaidrəu'fəuleitˌsaikləudiː'æmineis] 亚胺甲基四氢叶酸环化脱氨酶

formiminotransferase [fɔːˌmiminəu'trænsfəreis] *n* 亚胺甲基转移酶（常用于指谷氨酸亚胺甲基转移酶）

formiminotransferase deficiency 亚胺甲基转移酶缺乏症，谷氨酸亚胺甲基转移酶缺乏症

formocortal [fɔːmə'kɔːtəl] *n* 福莫可他（糖皮质激素）

formol ['fɔːmɔl] *n* 甲醛溶液

form-order [fɔːm 'ɔːdə] *n* 形态目

formoterol fumarate [fɔː'mɔtərɔl] 延胡索酸福莫特罗（长效拟交感神经 β 受体激动药，治哮喘，鼻内用药）

formula [ˌfɔːmjulə] ([复] **formulas** 或 **formulae** ['fɔːmjuliː]) *n*【拉】处方；公式，式 | acoustic ~ 声学公式（见 Brenner's formula）/ chemical ~ 化学结构式 / constitutional ~ 构成式，结构式 / dental ~ 牙式，牙公式（以符号表示上下颌牙齿的排列）/ digital ~ 指式，趾式（表示指〈趾〉的相关长度，通常手指为 3 > 4 > 2 > 5 > 1，

或3>2>4>5>1,脚趾为1>2>3>4>5,或2>1>3>4>5) / empirical ~ [经]验方(药);实验式,经验式(一种化学式,如乙烷的实验式为CH_3,而其分子式为C_2H_6) / graphic ~ 图解式 / official ~ 法定处方;法定公式 / paretic ~ 麻痹性痴呆公式(脑脊髓液中所见:压力正常或稍高、中等脑脊液细胞增多、中度蛋白质增高、胶态金试验改变以及脑脊髓液华氏试验〈Wassermann test〉阳性) / rational ~ 示性式,示构式 / structural ~ 结构式 / vertebral ~ 椎骨式(以数字表示各部椎骨,在人类为 C7T12L5S5Cd4 =33)

formulary [ˈfɔːmjuləri] *n* 处方集 | National Formulary (美国)国家处方集

formulate [ˈfɔːmjuleit] *vt* 列成公式,使公式化

formulation [ˌfɔːmjuˈleiʃən] *n* 列成公式,公式化 | American Law Institute ~ 美国法律学会案例集

formyl [ˈfɔːmil] *n* 甲酰基 | ~ phenetidin 甲酰非那替汀(抗菌止痛药)

formylase [ˈfɔːmileis] *n* 甲酰基酶,芳[香]基甲酰胺酶

formylation [fɔːmiˈleiʃən] *n* 甲酰化作用

formylglycinamide ribonucleotide [ˌfɔːmilˈglaisinəmaid ˌraibəuˈnjuːkliətaid] 甲酰甘氨酰胺核苷酸

formylkynurenine [ˌfɔːmilkaiˈnjuərəˌniːn] *n* 甲酰犬尿氨酸

formylkynurenine hydrolase [ˌfɔːmilˌkainjuəˈrenin ˈhaidrəleis] 甲酰犬尿氨酸水解酶,芳[香]基甲酰胺酶

formyloxaluric acid [ˌfɔːmilˌɔksəˈljuərik] 甲酰脲[基]草酸

formylporphyrin [ˌfɔːmilˈpɔːfirin] *n* 甲酰[基]卟啉

formylpteroic acid [ˌfɔːmiltəˈrəuik] 甲酰蝶酸

formyltetrahydrofolate [ˌfɔːmilˌtetrəˌhaidrə*u*ˈfəuleit] *n* 甲酰四氢叶酸

5-formyltetrahydrofolate cyclo-ligase [ˌfɔːmilˌtetrəˌhaidrə*u*ˈfəuleitˌsaikləuˈlaigeis] 5-甲酰四氢叶酸环连接酶(亦称 5, 10-次甲基四氢叶酸合成酶)

formyltetrahydrofolate dehydrogenase [ˌfɔːmilˌtetrəˌhaidrə*u*ˈfəuleit diːˈhaidrədʒəneis] 甲酰四氢叶酸脱氢酶

formyltransferase [ˌfɔːmilˈtrænsfəreis] *n* 转甲酰酶,甲酰基转移酶

Fornet's reaction (ring test) [fɔːˈnei] (Walter G. W. Fornet) 福尔内反应(环试验)(检梅毒)

fornical [ˈfɔːnikəl], **foniceal** [fɔːˈnisiəl] *a* 穹窿的,穹的

fornicate¹ [ˈfɔːnikeit] *vi* 非法性交,私通 | **fornication** [ˌfɔːniˈkeiʃən] *n*

fornicate² [ˈfɔːnikit] *a* 穹窿状的

fornix [ˈfɔːniks] ([复] **fornices** [ˈfɔːnisiːz]) *n* 【拉】穹窿,穹;大脑穹窿

Foroblique [ˌfɔːrəˈblek] *n* 直侧视镜(一种斜向远视系统的商品名,用于广视野膀胱镜)

Forsius-Eriksson syndrome [ˈfɔːsiəs ˈeriksən] (Henrik Forsius; Aldur W. Eriksson) 福-埃综合征(一种X连锁遗传的眼白化病,与内氏〈Nettleship〉型不同的在于男性表现为视网膜中央凹发育不良,轴性近视及红色觉异常;女性表现为颜色辨别力稍有不全及隐性眼球震颤,但在眼底无镶嵌式色素。亦称眼白化病,眼白化病2型,福-埃型眼白化病,阿兰群岛眼病)

Forssell's sinus [ˈfɔːsəl] (Gösta Forssell) 福塞尔窦(被黏膜襞围绕的胃壁内平滑部分,见于X线检查)

Forssman's antibody [ˈfɔːsmən] (John Forssman) 福斯曼抗体(用绵羊红细胞、含有豚鼠肾的盐溶液或含有福斯曼抗原的其他组织注射家兔而产生的抗体) | ~ antigen (lipoid) 福斯曼抗原(类脂)(在各种无关动物中能刺激产生抗绵羊溶血素的嗜异性抗原。亦称F抗原) / ~ carotid syndrome 福斯曼颈动脉综合征(注射少量含嗜异性抗体的血清于豚鼠颈动脉后所产生的神经障碍,包括平衡不稳、沿垂直轴及纵轴的旋转运动、眼球的强迫性偏向以及眼球震颤)

Förster's choroiditis (disease) [ˈfəːstə] (Carl F. R. Förster) 弗尔斯特脉络膜炎(病)(晕状中心性脉络膜炎) | ~ photometer 弗尔斯特光觉计

Förster's diplegia (syndrome, atonic-astatic syndrome) [ˈfəːstə] (Otfrid Förster) 弗尔斯特双瘫(综合征、弛缓性综合征),弛缓性双瘫

Förster's operation [ˈfəːstə] (Otfrid Förster) 弗尔斯特手术(促使白内障加速人工成熟的手术)

fosazepam [fəˈsæzəpæm] *n* 膦西泮(催眠药)

foscarnet sodium [fɔsˈkɑːnet] 膦甲酸钠(抗病毒药,用于治疗免疫受损患者的巨细胞病毒性视网膜炎)

fosfomycin [fɔsfəˈmaisin] *n* 磷霉素(抗生素类药)

fosfomycin tromethamine [ˌfɔsfəˈmaisin] 磷霉素氨丁三醇(抗菌药,用于治尿路感染,口服给药)

fosfonet sodium [ˈfɔsfɔnət] 膦乙酸钠(抗病毒药)

Foshay's reaction [fəuˈʃei] (Lee Foshay) 福谢反应(皮内注射对病人所患的感染具有特异性的抗血清,在注射处呈现中央是略为凸起的水肿,而外围是扩散的红斑,亦称红斑水肿性反应) | ~ serum 福谢血清(抗土拉血清,抗野兔热血清) / ~ test 福谢试验(土拉杆菌皮肤试验,一种诊断土拉杆菌病〈野兔热〉的皮肤试验)

fosinopril sodium [fəu'sinəpril] 福辛普利钠(血管紧张素转化酶抑制药,以片剂形式口服给药,治疗高血压,亦可单独使用或与噻嗪类利尿药结合使用)

fosphenytoin sodium ['fɔsfeni,tɔin] 磷苯妥因钠(抗惊厥药,治疗癫痫,不包括癫痫小发作,静脉或肌内注射)

fospirate ['fɔspireit]) *n* 福司吡酯,磷吡酯(兽用抗蠕虫药)

fossa ['fɔsə] ([复]**fossae** ['fɔsiː]) *n*【拉】窝,凹 | acetabular ~ 髋臼窝 / adipose ~e 脂肪窝 / amygdaloid ~ 扁桃体窝 / anconal ~, anconeal ~ 鹰嘴窝 / antecubital ~ 肘窝 / ~ of anthelix 对耳轮窝 / axillary ~ 腋窝 / canine ~, maxillary ~ 尖牙窝,上颌窝 / cerebral ~ 大脑窝 / cochleariform ~ 鼓膜张肌半管 / condylar ~, condyloid ~ 髁窝 / epigastric ~ 腹上窝(亦称心窝);膀胱上凹 / ethmoid ~ 筛沟 / femoral ~ 股凹,股环/ inferior costal ~ 下肋凹 / inferior duodenal ~ 十二指肠下隐窝 / jugular ~ 颈静脉窝 / nasal ~ 鼻前庭 / oral ~ 口凹,口道 / piriform ~ 梨状隐窝 / superior costal ~ 上肋凹 / superior duodenal ~ 十二指肠上隐窝 / terminal ~ 尿道舟状窝 / tonsillar ~ 扁桃体窝(亦称扁桃体窦) / urachal ~ 膀胱上凹

fossette [fɔ'set]) *n*【法】小窝;角膜深溃疡

fossula ['fɔsjulə] ([复]**fossulae** ['fɔsjuliː]) *n*【拉】小窝

fossulate ['fɔsjuleit] *a* 有小窝的

foster ['fɔstə] *vt* 抚养,领养,寄养;促进;培养

fosterage ['fɔstəridʒ] *n* 领养,寄养;助长,促进

Fothergill's disease (sore throat) ['fɔðəgil] (John Fothergill) 猩红热咽峡炎;三叉神经痛 | ~ neuralgia 三叉神经痛

Fothergill's operation ['fɔðəgil] (William E. Fothergill) 福瑟吉尔手术(治子宫脱垂,见 Manchester's operation)

Fouchet's test [fu'ʃei] (André Fouchet) 富歇试验(检血胆红素)

foudroyant [fuː'drɔiənt, ,fuːdrə'jɔːŋ] *a*【法】暴发性的

foulage [fu'lɑːʒ] *n*【法】搓揉按摩法

foulbrood ['faul,brud] *n* (蜜蜂)幼虫腐臭病

foundation [faun'deiʃən] *n* 基础 | denture ~ 义齿承托区 | **~al** *a* 基础的,基本的

founder ['faundə] *n* 马跛病(马因患蹄叶炎而致跛) | chest ~ 胸肌萎缩性马跛病 / grain ~ 伤食病(马由于过食所致消化不良或胃负担过重)

fourchette [fɔː'ʃet] *n*【法】阴唇系带

Fournier's gangrene (disease) [fuəni'ɛə] (Jean A. Fournier) 富尼埃坏疽(病)(阴囊、阴茎或会阴的急性坏疽性感染) | ~ sign 富尼埃征(①梅毒性皮肤损害的明显分界特征;②军刀状胫) / ~ test 富尼埃试验(令患者依口令由坐位站起,向前走,然后依口令突然停止,再向前走,然后依口令急速向后转,如此即产生共济失调步态)

fovea ['fəuviə] ([复]**foveae** ['fəuviiː]) *n*【拉】凹 | **~te** ['fəuvieit] *a*

foveation [,fəuvi'eiʃən] *n* 成凹,凹形

foveola [fəu'viːələ] ([复]**foveolas** 或 **foveolae** [fəu'viːəliː]) *n*【拉】小凹

foveolate(d) ['fəuviə,leit(id)] *a* 有小凹的

Foville's syndrome [fɔ'viːl] (Achille L. F Foville) 福维尔综合征(类似米亚尔-居布勒〈Millard-Gubler〉综合征,除了眼外展运动麻痹外,尚有协同运动麻痹)

Fowler-Murphy treatment ['faulə 'məːfi] (G. R. Fowler; John B. Murphy) 福勒-墨菲疗法(治腹膜炎,见 Murphy treatment②解)

Fowler's angular incision ['faulə] (George R. Fowler) 福勒直角形切口(用于前外侧剖腹术) | ~ operation 福勒手术(胸膜剥除术) / ~ position 福勒位置(斜坡卧位:病床床头提高 51 ~ 57 cm)

Fowler's solution ['faulə] (Thomas Fowler) 亚砷酸钾溶液

fowlpox ['faulpɔks] *n* 鸟痘,传染性上皮瘤,触染性上皮癌

foxglove ['fɔksglʌv] *n* 洋地黄,毛地黄 | purple ~ 洋地黄,毛地黄

Fox's disease, Fox-Fordyce disease ['fɔks 'fɔːdais] (G. H. Fox; John A. Fordyce) 福克斯病,福克斯-福代斯病(一种瘙痒性丘疹,主要限于腋窝及阴阜,由于大汗腺发炎所致。亦称大汗腺粟粒疹)

F. p. fiat potio【拉】制成饮剂;freezing point 冰点

fp foot-pound 英尺磅

FPG fasting plasma glucose 空腹血糖

F. pil. fiant pilulae【拉】制成丸剂

Fr francium 钫

Fract. dos. fracta dosi【拉】均分[剂]量

fraction ['frækʃən] *n* 部分,成分;分数;馏分;级分 | ~ concentration of gas 气体浓度分数 / ejection ~ 射血分数 / filtration ~ 滤过分数 / mol ~ 摩尔分数 / plasma ~, plasma protein ~ 血浆蛋白组分

fractional ['frækʃənl], **fractionary** ['frækʃənəri] *a* 部分的;分数的,小数的;分馏的;分级的;分段的;分成几份的,分次的

fractionate ['frækʃəneit] *vt* 使分馏;把…分成几部分 | **fractionator** *n* 分馏器

fractionation [frækʃə'neiʃən] *n* 分段,分次;分级[分离] | dose ~ 剂量分割

fractography [fræk'tɔgrəfi] *n* 参差表面描绘术

fracture [ˈfræktʃə] *n* 骨折;折断面 | agenetic ~ 骨发育不全性骨折 / apophyseal ~ 骨突折断 / avulsion ~ 撕脱骨折 / boxers' ~ 拳击者骨折 / bumper ~ 车撞骨折 / bursting ~, tuft ~ 爆裂骨折 / butterfly ~ 蝶形骨折 / buttonhole ~, perforating ~ 钮孔形骨折,穿孔骨折 / capillary ~ 毛细骨折,线状骨折 / chisel ~ 凿开状骨折(桡骨头碎片骨折) / cleavage ~ 剥离骨折 / closed ~, simple ~ 闭合性骨折,单纯骨折 / comminuted ~ 粉碎骨折 / complete ~ 完全骨折 / compression ~, pressure ~ 压缩骨折 / ~ by contrecoup 对冲骨折 / depressed ~ 凹陷骨折 / double ~ 两处骨折,双骨折 / dyscrasic ~ 恶病质骨折 / ~ en coin, V-shaped ~ V 字形骨折/ ~ en rave 骨膜下横骨折 / epiphyseal ~ 骺骨折 / extracapsular ~ 关节囊外骨折 / fissure ~, fissured ~ 坼裂骨折 / greenstick ~, willow ~ 青枝骨折 / impacted ~ 嵌入骨折 / intrauterine ~, congenital ~ 宫内骨折,先天骨折/ linear ~ 线形骨折 / open ~, compound ~ 开放性骨折/ pond ~ 斜边骨折 / spiral ~, torsion ~ 螺旋骨折,扭转骨折 / sprain ~ 扭伤骨折 / transcervical ~ 股骨颈骨折 / transcondylar ~, diacondylar ~ 经髁骨折 | **fractural** [ˈfræktʃərəl] *a*

fracture-dislocation [ˈfræktʃədisləuˈkeiʃən] *n* 骨折脱位

Fraenkel 见 Fränkel

fragiform [ˈfrædʒifɔːm] *a* 草莓样的

fragile [ˈfrædʒail] *a* 脆的,易碎的;虚弱的

fragilitas [frəˈdʒilitəs] *n*【拉】脆性,脆弱 | ~ crinium 脆发[症] / ~ ossium 骨脆症 / ~ unguium 脆甲症

fragility [frəˈdʒiləti] *n* 脆性,脆弱 | capillary ~ 毛细[血]管脆性 / erythrocyte ~, ~ of blood 红细胞脆性,血细胞脆性 / hereditary ~ of bone 遗传性骨脆症,成骨不全

fragilocyte [frəˈdʒiləsait] *n* 脆性红细胞

fragilocytosis [frəˌdʒiləsaiˈtəusis] *n* 脆性红细胞增多

fragment [ˈfrægmənt] *n* 碎片,断片,分段[ˈfrægment] *vt, vi* (使)成碎片;(使)分裂 | Fab ~ Fab 片段(见 Fab) / $F(ab')_2$ ~ $F(ab')_2$ 片段(见 $F(ab')_2$) / Fc ~ Fc 片段(见 Fc) / restriction ~ 限制性片段(由限制性内切核酸酶所产生的一个 DNA 片段)

fragmental [frægˈmentl], **fragmentary** [ˈfrægməntəri] *a* 碎片的,断片的;不完全的;不连续的

fragmentation [ˌfrægmenˈteiʃən] *n* 分裂,破碎;断裂 | ~ of myocardium 心肌断裂

fragmentize [ˈfrægməntaiz] *vt, vi* 裂成碎片,分裂

fragmentography [ˌfrægmənˈtɔgrəfi] *n* 片段谱法 | mass ~ 片段质谱法

fragrance [ˈfreigrəns] *n* 香味;香气

fragrant [ˈfreigrənt] *a* 香的

frail [freil] *a* 脆弱的;虚弱的

frailty [ˈfreilti] *n* 脆弱;虚弱;弱点

fraise [freiz] *n*【法】爪棱钻(一种切开骨成形瓣或扩大环钻开口用的锥形或半球形钻)

frambesin [fræmˈbiːsin] *n* 雅司螺旋体素

framb(o)esia [fræmˈbiːziə] *n* 雅司病(即 yaws) | ~ tropica 雅司病

framb(o)esioma [fræmˌbiːziˈəumə] *n* 雅司瘤

frame [freim] *n* 支架 | occluding ~ 𬌗架,咬合架 / quadriplegic standing ~ 四肢麻痹站立支架 / trial ~ 试镜架(配眼镜验光用)

framework [ˈfreimwəːk] *n* 构架组织;支架 | scleral ~ 巩膜构架组织,巩膜房角组织 / uveal ~ 虹膜角膜角梳状韧带,虹膜梳状韧带

framycetin sulfate [frəˈmaisətin] 硫酸新霉素 B(抗生素类药)

Franceschetti-Jadassohn syndrome [ˌfrɑːntʃeiˈskeiti ˈjɑːdəsəun] (Adolphe Franceschetti; Joset Jadassohn) 弗-亚综合征(一种常染色体显性遗传病,特征为在婴儿期后皮肤开始由石板灰色到棕色的网状色素沉着而无先驱炎症,合并有掌跖角化过度、血管舒缩改变与少汗及牙釉质变黄。亦称内格利〈Naegeli〉色素细胞痣、内格利综合征、内格利色素失禁)

Franceschetti's syndrome [ˌfrɑːntʃeiˈsk eiti] (Adolphe Franceschetti) 弗氏综合征,下颌面骨发育不全

Francis' disease [ˈfrænsis] (Edward Francis) 土拉菌病

Francisella [ˌfrænsiˈselə] (Edward Francis) *n* 弗朗西丝菌属 | ~ novicide 新凶手弗朗西丝菌 / ~ tularensis 土拉热弗朗西丝菌,野兔热弗朗西丝菌

francium(Fr) [ˈfrænsiəm] *n* 钫(化学元素)

François' syndrome [frɑːnˈswɑːz] (Jules François) 法朗索综合征,眼下颌面综合征(即 oculomandibulofacial syndrome,见 syndrome 项下相应术语)

Franco's operation [ˈfrɑːŋkəu] (Pierre Franco) 耻骨上膀胱切开术

frange [frænʒ] *n*【法】纤毛刷

frangible [ˈfrændʒibl] *a* 易碎的;脆弱的 | **frangibility** [ˌfrændʒiˈbiləti] *n* 易碎性;脆弱性

frank [fræŋk] *a* 症状明显的

Frankel Classification [ˈfræŋkəl] (Hans L. Frankel) 弗兰克尔分类法(根据损伤级以下的缺损严重程度将脊髓损伤分成 5 组:A 组——全部感觉和运动功能完全中止;B 组——不完全中止,有一些感觉,但无运动功能;C 组——不完全

中止,有明显的随意运动功能,但处于最低的无用的水平;D组——不完全中止,有一定的对患者有用的随意运动功能;E组——已达到恢复正常功能)

Fränkel's sign [ˈfreŋkəl] (Albert Fränkel) 弗兰克尔征(脊髓痨时,髋关节周围肌张力减弱)

Fränkel's speculum [ˈfreŋkəl] (Bernhard Fränkel) 弗兰克尔窥器(一种鼻镜) | ~ test 弗兰克尔试验(体位引流法检查鼻窦炎)

Fränkel's treatment [ˈfreŋkəl] (Albert Fränkel) 弗兰克尔疗法(应用毒毛旋花子苷K治疗心力衰竭)

Frankenhäuser's ganglion [ˈfrɑːŋkənˌhɔizə] (Ferdinand Frankenhäuser) 弗兰肯豪泽神经节(子宫颈神经节)

Franke's operation [fræŋk] (Felix Franke) 弗兰克手术(肋间神经切除)

Frankia [ˈfræŋkiə] (B. Frank) *n* 弗兰克菌属

Frankiaceae [ˌfræŋkiˈeisiiː] *n* 弗兰克菌科

frankincense [ˈfræŋkinsens] *n* 乳香

Frankl-Hochwart's disease [fræŋkl ˈhɔhvɑːt] (Lathar von Frankl-Hochwart) 弗兰克尔·霍希瓦特病,梅尼埃病样多发性脑神经炎

Franklin glasses [ˈfræŋklin] (Benjamin Franklin) 双焦点眼镜

franklinism [ˈfræŋklinizəm] (Benjamin Franklin) *n* 静电;静电疗法

franklinization [ˌfræŋklinaiˈzeiʃən, -niˈz-] *n* 静电疗法

Frank's operation [fræŋk] (Rudolf Frank) 弗兰克手术(胃造口术的一种方法,即在胃锥体外造一瓣状切口,缝合于胸壁的切口上,并插入一管)

Frank-Starling curve [fræŋkˈstɑːliŋ] (Otto Frank; Ernest H. Starling) 法-斯曲线(心排血量的图解曲线)

Frasera [ˈfreizərə] (John Fraser) *n* 轮叶龙胆属

Fraser syndrome [ˈfreizə] (George R. Fraser) 弗雷泽综合征,隐眼[畸形]综合征(即 cryptophthalmos syndrome,见 syndrome 项下相应术语)

fraternity [frəˈtəːnəti] *n* 一群同职业(或同兴趣、同信仰)的人 | medical ~ 医务界

Frateuria [frəˈtəːriə] (Joseph Frateur) *n* 弗拉托菌属

***F*-ratio** (Sir Ronald A. Fisher) *F* 比率(若干组群的均数之间的方差与组群内的方差之比,用于方差分析〈ANOVA〉*F* 检验) | *F*-test *F* 检验(此检验为方差分析的第一步)

Fraunhofer's lines [ˈfraunhɔfə] (Joseph von Fraunhofer) 弗劳恩霍弗线(太阳光谱的黑线)

Fraxinus [frækˈsainəs] *n* 白蜡树属

Frazier-Spiller operation [ˈfreizə ˈspilə] (Charles H. Frazier; William G. Spiller) 弗雷泽-斯皮勒手术(半月神经节感觉根的分离,借以缓解三叉神经痛)

FRC functional residual capacity 功能残气量

FRCP Fellow of the Royal College of Physicians 皇家内科医师学会会员

FRCP(C) Fellow of the Royal College of Physicians of Canada 加拿大皇家内科医师学会会员

FRCPE Fellow of the Royal College of Physicians of Edinburgh 爱丁堡皇家内科医师学会会员

FRCP(Glasg) Fellow of the Royal College of Physicians and Surgeons of Glasgow *qua* Physician 格拉斯哥皇家内外科医师学会(内科医师)会员

FRCPI Fellow of the Royal College of Physicians in Ireland 爱尔兰皇家内科医师学会会员

FRCS Fellow of the Royal College of Surgeons 皇家外科医师学会会员

FRCS(C) Fellow of the Royal College of Surgeons of Canada 加拿大皇家外科医师学会会员

FRCSEd Fellow of the Royal College of Surgeons of Edinburgh 爱丁堡皇家外科医师学会会员

FRCS(Glasg) Fellow of the Royal College of Physicians and Surgeons of Glasgow *qua* Surgeon 格拉斯哥皇家内外科医师学会(外科医师)会员

FRCSI Fellow of the Royal College of Surgeons in Ireland 爱尔兰皇家外科医师学会会员

FRCVS Fellow of the Royal College of Veterinary Surgeons 皇家兽医外科医师学会会员

freckle [ˈfrekl] *n* 雀斑

Fredet-Ramstedt operation [freˈdei ˈrɑːmʃtet] (Pierre Fredet; Conrad Ramstedt) 幽门肌切开术

free [friː] *a* 自由的;无…的;免费的;游离的

Freeman-Sheldon syndrome [ˈfriːmən ˈʃeldən] (Ernest A. Freeman; Joseph H. Sheldon) 弗-谢综合征,颅腕跗骨发育不良

freemartin [ˈfriːmɑːtin] *n* 双牛间雌,牛殖器不全牝犊(与正常牝犊同时产下,成为联胎)

freeze [friːz] *vi* 结冰;凝固 *vt* 使结冰;使凝固;用冷冻保藏 *n* 结冰;凝固

freeze-cleaving [friːz ˈkliːviŋ] *n* 冷冻蚀刻法

freeze-drying [friːz ˈdraiiŋ] *n* 冷冻干燥法

freeze-etching [friːz ˈefʃiŋ] *n* 冷冻蚀刻法

freeze-fracturing [friːz ˈfræktʃəriŋ] *n* 冷冻断裂法

freezer [ˈfriːzə] *n* 冰箱;冷藏库

freeze-substitution [friːz ˌsʌbstiˈtjuːʃən] *n* 冷冻替代法

Freiberg's infraction(disease) [ˈfraibəːg] (Albert H. Freiberg) 弗赖伯格不全骨折(病)(第二跖骨头骨软骨炎)

Frei's antigen [frai] (Wilhelm S. Frei) 弗赖抗原,性病性淋巴肉芽肿皮试抗原(由性病性淋巴肉芽肿患者腹股沟淋巴结无菌脓液制备的皮肤

试验抗原，现此病病毒可接种于正在发育的鸡胚的卵黄囊内〈卵黄囊抗原，鸡胚抗原〉或接种于鼠脑组织内〈鼠脑抗原〉繁殖）| ~ disease 性病性淋巴肉芽肿 / ~ test 弗赖试验（将患部取得的无菌浓液作皮内注射如形成隆起的红色丘疹，则表示性病性淋巴肉芽肿）

Frejka pillow (pillow splint) [ˈfreikɑː] (Bedrich Frejka) 弗雷卡枕（枕头夹板）（一种治疗用的装置，将枕头楔入婴儿的大腿间，藉以矫正先天性髋关节脱位，维持大腿外展和弯曲）

fremitus [ˈfremitəs] *n*【拉】震颤 | friction ~ 摩擦性震颤 / hydatid ~ 包虫囊震颤 / pericardial ~ 心包震颤 / rhonchal ~, bronchial ~ 鼾性震颤，支气管性震颤 / subjective ~ 自觉性震颤 / tactile ~ 触觉，语颤 / tussive ~ 咳嗽性震颤 / vocal ~, pectoral ~ 语音震颤，胸震颤

frena [ˈfriːnə] frenum 的复数

frenal [ˈfriːnl] *a* 系带的

French [frentʃ] *n* 法制标度单位（见 scale 项下相应术语）

frenectomy [friˈnektəmi] *n* 系带切除术

frenetic [friˈnetik] *a* 极度激动的，疯狂的，精神错乱的

Frenkel's movements (treatment) [ˈfreŋkəl] (Heinrich S. Frenkel) 弗伦克尔运动（疗法）（共济失调矫正法）

frenoplasty [ˌfriːnəuˈplæsti] *n* 系带成形术，系带矫正术

frenosecretory [ˌfriːnəusiˈkriːtəri] *a* 抑制分泌的

frenotomy [friˈnɔtəmi] *n* 系带切开术

frentizole [ˈfrentizəul] *n* 夫仑替唑（免疫调节药）

frenuloplasty [ˈfrenjuləuˌplæsti] *n* 系带成形术，系带矫正术

frenulum [ˈfrenjuləm] ([复]**frenula** [ˈfrenjulə]) *n*【拉】系带

frenum [ˈfriːnəm] ([复] **frenums** 或 **frena** [ˈfriːnə]) *n*【拉】系带

frenzy [ˈfrenzi] *n* 暴怒，狂乱；严重躁狂性兴奋状态

frequency [ˈfriːkwənsi] *n* 频数；频率；相对频率 | audio ~ 声频；音频 / gene ~ 基因频率（在某一群体中，某一等位基因除以这个基因可能出现的等位基因的总数）/ infrasonic ~, subsonic ~ 次声频率 / recombination ~ 重组频率（同源染色体上基因交换频率，由重组体的数目除以后代总数即得）/ ultrasonic ~, supersonic ~ 超声频率

Frerichs' theory [ˈfreiriks] (Friedrich T. Frerichs) 弗雷里克斯学说（尿毒症为碳酸铵中毒）

Fresnel lens [freiˈnel] (Augustin J. Fresnel) 菲涅尔镜片（有若干同心排列的梯形后缩制成的薄镜片，具有较厚镜片的光学性能）

fressreflex [ˈfresriːfleks] *n*【德】吃食反射

fretum [ˈfriːtəm] ([复] **freta** [ˈfriːtə]) *n*【拉】峡；狭窄

freudian [ˈfrɔidjən] (Sigmund Freud) *a* 弗洛伊德学说（或学派）的（关于某些神经病成因的学说）*n* 弗洛伊德学派者

Freud's cathartic method [frɔid] (Sigmund Freud) 弗洛伊德精神发泄法（治精神神经[功能]病）

Freund adjuvant [frɔind] (Jules T. Freund) 弗氏佐剂（水油乳剂佐剂，由于含分枝杆菌，故又称为分枝杆菌佐剂）| ~ complete adjuvant 弗氏完全佐剂（含分枝杆菌的水油乳剂佐剂，即弗氏佐剂）/ ~ incomplete adjuvant 弗氏不完全佐剂（不含分枝杆菌的水油乳剂佐剂）

Freund's anomaly [frɔind] (Wilhelm A. Freund) 弗罗因德异常（因第一肋短缩，胸腔上口狭窄，影响肺尖膨胀）| ~ operation 弗罗因德手术（先天性漏斗胸肋软骨切除术）

Freund's reaction [frɔind] (Hermann W. Freund), **Freund-Kaminer reaction** [frɔind ˈkɑːminə] (Ernst Freund; Gisa Kaminer) 弗罗因德反应，弗罗因德-卡米纳反应（非癌症病人的血清破坏癌细胞，而癌症病人的血清则无溶解效应）

Freyer's operation [ˈfraiə] (Peter J. Freyer) 弗里尔手术（耻骨上前列腺剜出术）

Frey's hairs [frai] (Max von Frey) 弗赖毛（检皮肤压点的敏感性）

Frey's syndrome [frai] (Lucje Frey) 弗赖综合征，耳颞神经综合征（auriculotemporal syndrome，见 syndrome 项下相应术语）

FRF follicle-stimulating hormone releasing factor 促滤泡[激]素释放因子

FRFPSG Fellow of the Royal Faculty of Physicians and Surgeons of Glasgow 格拉斯哥皇家内外科医师学会会员

friable [ˈfraiəbl] *a* 易碎的，脆的 | **friability** [ˌfraiəˈbiləti] *n* 易碎性，脆碎度

Friberg test [ˈfraibəːg] (J. Friberg) 弗赖伯格试验，托盘凝集试验（即 tray agglutination test，见 test 项下相应术语）

fricative [ˈfrikətiv] *a* 摩擦的，由摩擦产生的 *n* 摩擦音

Fricke's bandage [ˈfrikə] (Johann K. G. Fricke) 弗里克绷带（阴囊托带，睾丸炎和附睾炎时用以包扎阴囊）

friction [ˈfrikʃən] *n* 摩擦法

frictional [ˈfrikʃənl] *a* 摩擦的；由摩擦而生的

Friderichsen-Waterhouse syndrome [ˌfridəˈriksən ˈwɔːtəhaus] (Carl Friderichsen; Rupert Waterhouse) 弗-沃综合征（见 Waterhouse-Friderichsen syndrome）

Fridericia's method [ˈfridəritʃiə] (Louis S. Fridericia) 弗里德里恰法(测肺泡二氧化碳张力)

Friedländer's bacillus [ˈfriːdlendə] (Karl Friedländer) 弗里德兰德杆菌 | ~ disease 闭塞性动脉内膜炎 / ~ pneumobacillus 弗里德兰德(肺炎)杆菌,肺炎杆菌 / ~ pneumonia 弗里德兰德杆菌性肺炎

Friedmann's vasomotor syndrome (complex) [ˈfriːdmən] (Max Friedmann) 弗里德曼血管舒缩综合征(源于外伤性进行性亚急性脑炎所致的一系列症状,包括头胀感、头痛、眩晕、不安、失眠、容易疲劳及记忆力缺陷)

Friedman's test, Friedman-Lapham test [ˈfriːdmən ˈlæphæm] (Maurice H. Friedman; Maxwell E. Lapham) 弗里德曼试验,弗里德曼-拉帕姆试验(检孕)

Friedreich's ataxia (tabes) [ˈfriːdraik] (Nikolaus Friedreich) 弗里德赖希共济失调(脊髓痨)(一种遗传性疾病,常始于幼年或少年,脊髓的背侧及外侧硬化,伴有共济失调等。亦称遗传性共济失调) | ~ disease 弗里德赖希病(多发性肌阵挛;弗里德赖希共济失调) / ~ foot 弗里德赖希足(马蹄内翻,趾过伸畸形,见于遗传性共济失调) / ~ sign 弗里德赖希征(①心包粘连时颈静脉在心舒张期突然塌陷;②深吸气时,在肺空洞区上的叩音音调降低)

friente [friˈenti] *n* 伐木工皮炎(大半由于黑穗菌所致)

frigid [ˈfridʒid] *a* 寒冷的;冷淡的;缺乏性感的(指妇女) | **frigidity** [friˈdʒidəti] *n* 寒冷;冷淡;性感缺失(指妇女)

frigolabile [ˌfrigəuˈleibail] *a* 不耐寒的,易受寒冷影响的

frigorific [ˌfrigəˈrifik] *a* 发冷的,引起寒冷的

frigostable [ˌfrigəuˈsteibl], **frigostabile** [ˌfrigəˈsteibail] *a* 耐寒的

frigotherapy [ˌfrigəuˈθerəpi] *n* 冷疗法

fringe [frindʒ] *n* 边,缘;缨;条纹

frit [frit] *n* 釉料(半熔的玻璃质,制假牙)

Fritsch's catheter [fritʃ] (Heinrich Fritsch) 弗里奇导管(见 Bozeman's catheter)

froe- 以 froe-起始的词,同样见以 fre-起始的词

frog [frɔg] *n* 蛙;马蹄叉 | ~ in the throat 轻咽喉炎,声嗄

frog stay [frɔg stei] 马蹄嵴

Fröhlich's syndrome [ˈfrelik] (Alfred Fröhlich) 弗勒赫利希综合征,肥胖生殖无能综合征,肥胖性生殖器退化

Frohn's test (reagent) [frɔn] (Damianus Frohn) 弗龙试剂(检生物碱)

Froin's syndrome [frɔˈæŋ] (Georges Froin) 弗鲁安综合征,分室综合征,脑脊液分隔综合征(脑室液和脊液互相阻断而引起脊液变化,呈黄色,含大量蛋白,凝固较快,见于某些器质性神经疾病)

frolement [frəulˈmɔŋ] *n* 沙沙声(心包疾病时听诊所闻);轻擦按摩法

Froment's paper sign [frɔˈmɔŋ] (Jules Froment) 弗罗芒纸征(用拇食二指夹纸片时拇指远侧屈曲,见于尺神经病变)

Frommann's lines [ˈfrɔmən] (Carl Frommann) 弗罗曼线(有髓神经纤维轴索上的横纹,用硝酸银染色可见)

Frommel-Chiari syndrome [ˈfrɔməl kiˈɑːri] 弗罗梅尔-基阿利综合征(见 Chiari-Frommel syndrome)

Frommel's disease [ˈfrɔməl] (Richard J. E. Frommel) 弗罗梅尔病(一种产后病,可能由于垂体功能障碍或垂体瘤所致,特征为子宫萎缩、乳溢、长期闭经等)

frondose [ˈfrɔndəus] *a* 叶状的;多叶的;具叶的

frons [frɔnz] *n*【拉】额

frontad [ˈfrʌntæd] *ad* 向额[面]

frontal [ˈfrʌntl] *a* 前面的,正面的;额的;额平面的

frontalis [frʌnˈteilis] *a*【拉】额的

frontier [ˈfrʌntjə] *n* 国境;边远地区;[常用复](未经充分研究或利用的科学、文化等方面的)尖端,新领域 | the ~s of medicine 医学尖端

frontipetal [frʌnˈtipətl] *a* 向额的

frontomalar [ˌfrʌntəuˈmeilə] *a* 额颧[骨]的

frontomaxillary [ˌfrʌntəumækˈsiləri, -ˈmæksi-] *a* 额上颌的

frontonasal [ˌfrʌntəuˈneizəl] *a* 额鼻的

fronto-occipital [ˌfrʌntəuɔkˈsipitl] *a* 额枕的

frontoparietal [ˌfrʌntəupəˈraiitl] *a* 额顶[骨]的

frontotemporal [ˌfrʌntəuˈtempərəl] *a* 额颞[骨]的

frontozygomatic [ˌfrʌntəuˌzaigəuˈmætik] *a* 颧额的

Froriep's ganglion [ˈfrɔriːp] (August von Froriep) 弗罗里普神经节,枕神经节

Froriep's induration [ˈfrɔriːp] (Robert Froriep) 纤维性肌炎

frost [frɔst] *n* 霜 | urea ~ 尿素霜,结晶尿汗症(沉淀于皮肤的尿素结晶)

frostbite [ˈfrɔstbait] *n* 冻疮

frost-itch [ˈfrɔst itʃ] *n* 冬令瘙痒

frosty [ˈfrɔsti] *a* 霜冻的;霜状的

froth [frɔθ] *n* 泡,泡沫

frottage [frɔˈtɑːʒ] *n*【法】摩擦[法];摩擦淫(指拥挤中向异性摩擦的性变行为)

frotteur [frɔˈtəː] *n* 摩擦癖者

frotteurism [frɔˈtəːrizəm] *n* 摩擦癖
FRS Fellow of the Royal Society 皇家学会会员
fructan [ˈfrʌktæn] *n* 果聚糖
fructification [ˌfrʌktifiˈkeiʃən] *n* 结实;子实体;结实器官
fructivorous [frʌkˈtivərəs] *a* 果食的
fructofuranose [ˌfrʌktəuˈfjuərənəus] *n* 呋喃果糖
***β*-fructofuranosidase** [ˌfrʌktəuˌfjuərəˈnəusideis] *n* *β*-呋喃果糖苷酶,转化酶
fructokinase [ˌfrʌktəuˈkaineis] *n* 果糖激酶(此酶缺乏为常染色体隐性遗传,可致原发性果糖尿症)
fructolysis [frʌkˈtɔlisis] *n* 果糖分解
fructopyranose [ˌfrʌktəuˈpaiərənəus] *n* 吡喃果糖,果糖
fructosamine [ˌfrʌktəuˈseimin] *n* 果糖胺
fructosan [ˈfrʌktəsæn] *n* 果聚糖
fructosazone [frʌkˈtəusəzəun] *n* 果糖脎
fructose [ˈfrʌktəus] *n* 果糖 | ~ 1, 6- diphosphate 果糖-1, 6-二磷酸 / ~ 6-phosphate 果糖-6-磷酸
fructose-bisphosphatase [ˈfrʌktəus bisˈfɔsfəteis] 果糖二磷酸酶(fructose-1, 6- bisphosphatase 的 EC 命名法)
fructose-1, 6-bisphosphatase [ˈfrʌktəus bisˈfɔsfəteis] 果糖-1, 6-二磷酸酶
fructose-2, 6-bisphosphatase [ˈfrʌktəus bisˈfɔsfəteis] 果糖-2, 6-二磷酸酶
fructose-1, 6-bisphosphatase deficiency 果糖-1, 6-二磷酸酶缺乏症(为一种常染色体隐性遗传病,特点为呼吸暂停、换气过度、低血糖、酮病和乳酸中毒,系由于缺乏肝性果糖-1, 6-二磷酸酶引起的糖原异生受损所致,对新生儿可能是致命的,但患儿过了幼儿期发育即正常)
fructose-1, 6-bisphosphate [ˈfrʌktəus bisˈfɔsfeit] 果糖-1, 6-二磷酸
fructose-2, 6-bisphosphate [ˈfrʌktəus bisˈfɔsfeit] 果糖-2, 6-二磷酸
fructose bisphosphate aldolase [ˈfrʌktəus bisˈfɔsfeit ˈældəleis] 果糖二磷酸醛缩酶(已鉴别出 3 种同工酶:同工酶 A〈主要出现在骨骼肌〉、同工酶 B〈出现在肝、肾、小肠和白细胞〉和同工酶 C〈出现于大脑〉。同工酶 B 常指果糖-1-磷酸醛缩酶,对果糖-1-磷酸有较大的亲和力。缺乏后一种活性为一种常染色体隐性性状,可致遗传性果糖不耐症。亦称醛缩酶)
fructose-2, 6-bisphosphate 2-phosphatase [ˈfrʌktəus bisˈfɔsfeit ˈfɔsfəteis] 果糖-2, 6-二磷酸 2-磷酸酶(亦称果糖-2, 6-二磷酸酶)
fructose-1, 6-diphosphatase [ˈfrʌktəus daiˈfɔsfəteis] 果糖-1, 6-二磷酸酶
fructosemia [ˌfrʌktəuˈsiːmiə] *n* 果糖血[症]
fructose 1-phosphate aldolase [ˈfrʌktəus ˈfɔsfeit ˈældəleis] 果糖-1-磷酸醛缩酶,果糖二磷酸醛缩酶同工酶 B
fructosidase [frʌkˈtəusaideis] *n* 果糖苷酶,*β*-呋喃果糖苷酶,转化酶
fructoside [ˈfrʌktəsaid] *n* 果糖苷
fructosuria [ˌfrʌktəuˈsjuəriə] *n* 果糖尿 | essential ~ 原发性果糖尿症
fructosyl [ˈfrʌktəsil] *n* 果糖基
fructosyltransferase [ˌfrʌktəusilˈtrænsfəreis] *n* 转果糖酶,果糖基转移酶
fructovegetative [ˌfrʌktəuˈvedʒitətiv] *a* 果类植物的
fructuronic acid [ˌfrʌktjuəˈrɔnik] 果糖酮酸
frugivorous [fruˈdʒivərəs] *a* 果食的
fruit [fruːt] *n* 果实
fruitarian [fruːˈtεəriən] *n* 果食者
fruitarianism [fruːˈtεəriənizəm] *n* 果食主义(完全食用果实)
fruit bromelain [fruːtˈbrəuməlein] 果食菠萝蛋白
frusemide [ˈfrʌsimaid] *n* 呋塞米(利尿药)
Frust. frustillatim【拉】制成小块
frustration [frʌsˈtreiʃən] *n* 挫折
fry [frai] *vt*, *vi* 油煎,油炒 *n* 油煎食品
F. s. a. fiat secundum artem【拉】须精巧操作
FSG focal segmental glomerulosclerosis 局灶性节段性肾小球硬化症
FSGS focal segmental glomerulosclerosis 局灶性节段性肾小球硬化症
FSH follicle-stimulating hormone 促滤泡素,促卵泡[激]素
FSH/LH-RH follicle-stimulating hormone and luteinizing hormone releasing-hormone 促滤泡[激]素和促黄体素释放[激]素
FSH-RF follicle-stimulating hormone releasing factor 促滤泡[激]素释放因子
FSH-RH follicle stimulating hormone-releasing hormone 促滤泡[激]素释放[激]素
ft. fiat, fiant【拉】制成,作成;foot, feet 呎,英尺
Ft. mas. div. in pil. fiat massa dividenda in pilulae【拉】制成丸块再分制成丸剂
Ft. pulv. fiat pulvis【拉】制成散剂
5-Fu 5-fluorouracil 氟尿嘧啶,5-氟尿嘧啶(抗肿瘤药)
Fuchs' coloboma [fuks] (Ernst Fuchs) 富克斯脉络膜缺损 | ~ dimples 富克斯角膜凹 / ~ dystrophy 角膜上皮营养不良 / ~ optic atrophy 视神经周边性萎缩 / ~ syndrome 富克斯综合征(单侧角膜异色,角膜沉着物及继发性内障)
fuchsin [ˈfuːksin] *n* 品红,复红 | acid ~ 酸性品红 / basic ~ 碱性品红 / new ~ 新品红
fuchsinophil [fuːkˈsinəfil] *n* 嗜品红细胞 *a* 嗜品

红的
fuchsinophilia [ˌfuːksinəˈfiliə] *n* 嗜品红性
fuchsinophilic [ˌfuːksinəˈfilik], **fuchsinophilous** [ˌfuːksiˈnɔfiləs] *a* 嗜品红的
Fuchs' protein test [fuks] (Hans J. Fuchs) 富克斯蛋白试验(检癌)
fucosan [ˈfjuːkəsæn] *n* 岩藻聚糖
fucose [ˈfjuːkəus] *n* 岩藻糖
α-L-fucosidase [fjuˈkəusiˌdeis, ˈfjuːkəsaiˌdeis] α-L-岩藻糖苷酶(此酶的遗传性缺乏为一种常染色体隐性性状,可致岩藻糖苷病)
fucoside [ˈfjuːkəsaid] *n* 岩藻糖苷
fucosidosis [ˌfjuːkəusaiˈdəusis] *n* 岩藻糖苷贮积症,岩藻糖苷沉积症
fucoxanthin [ˌfjuːkəˈzænθin] *n* 岩藻黄素
FUDR floxuridine (5-fluorouracil deoxyribonucleoside) 氟尿苷(5-氟尿嘧啶脱氧核苷)
FUdR 5-fluorouracil deoxyribonucleoside 5-氟尿嘧啶脱氧核苷
Fuerbringer [ˈfəːbriŋə] 见 Fürbringer
fugacious [fju(ː)ˈgeiʃəs] *a* 暂时的,易变的;易逸的 | **fugacity** [fju(ː)ˈgæsəti] *n* 暂时性,易变性;[易]逸性,[易]逸度
-fugal [构词成分]离,远;驱,逐
-fuge [构词成分]驱除剂
fugitive [ˈfjuːdʒitiv] *a* 短暂的;游走的;过渡的
Fugl-Meyer assessment [ˈfuːgəl ˈmaiə] (A. R. Fugl-Meyer) 富-梅评价(神经性损害后一种对某一部分运动功能的标准化评价)
fugu [ˈfuːguː] *n* 河鲀;河鲀肉
Fugu [ˈfuːguː] *n*【日】河鲀属(旧用河豚属),东方鲀属
fugue [fjuːg] *n*【拉】神游症 | epileptic ~ 癫痫性神游症
fuguism [ˈfuːguizəm], **fuguismus** [ˌfuːguˈizməs] *n* 河鲀中毒(旧用河豚中毒)
fugutoxin [ˌfuːguˈtɔksin] *n* 河鲀毒素(旧用河豚毒素)
Fukala's operation [fuˈkɑːlə] (Vincenz Fukala) 富卡拉手术(晶状体摘除术,治深度近视)
Fukuyama type congenital muscular dystrophy (syndrome) [fukuˈjɑːmɑː] (Yukio Fukuyama) 福山型先天性肌营养不良(综合征)(为一种常染色体隐性遗传型肌萎缩,婴儿尤为明显,肌异常类似迪谢内〈Duchenne〉肌营养不良,患者智力迟钝,伴多小脑回及其他大脑异常)
Fuld's test [fuld] (Ernst Fuld) 富尔德试验(检血清抗胰蛋白酶的能力)
fulgurant [ˈfʌlgjuərənt] *a* 闪电状的,电击状的
fulgurate [ˈfʌlgjuəreit] *vi* 电灼 | **fulguration** [ˌfʌlgjuəˈreiʃən] *n* 电灼疗法
fulgurating [ˈfʌlgjuəreitiŋ] *a* 刺痛的
fuliginous [fjuːˈlidʒinəs] *a* 煤烟状的
Fülleborn's method [ˈfiːləbɔːn] (Friedrich Fülleborn) 菲伦博恩法(检粪中虫卵)
Fuller's operation [ˈfulə] (Eugene Fuller) 富勒手术(精囊切开术)
full-grown [ˈful ˈgrəun] *a* 长足的,长成的,长全的,成熟的
füllkörper [ˈfiːlkəːpə] *n*【德】胀大小体(已变性的神经胶质细胞)
full-length [ˈfulˈleŋθ] *a* 全长的;全身的
fullness [ˈfulnis] *n* 发胀
full-term [ˈfulˈtəːm] *a* 足月的
fulminant [ˈfʌlminənt] *a* 暴发性的
fulminate [ˈfʌlmineit] *vi* 爆炸,暴发 *n* 雷酸盐
fulminating [ˈfʌlmineitiŋ] *a* 暴发性的
fulminic [fʌlˈminik] *a* 爆炸性的 | ~ acid 雷酸,异氰酸
fulvous [ˈfʌlvəs] *a* 黄褐色的;茶色的
fumagillin [ˌfjuːməˈdʒilin] *n* 夫马洁林(抗生素类药)
fumarase [ˈfjuːməreis] *n* 延胡索酸酶
fumarate [ˈfjuːməreit] *n* 延胡索酸盐;延胡索酸,富马酸(阴离子型) | ferrous ~ 富马酸亚铁(抗贫血药)
fumarate hydratase [ˈfjuːməreitˈhaidrəteis] 延胡索酸水合酶(亦称延胡索酸酶)
fumaric acid [fjuːˈmærik] 延胡索酸,富马酸
fumaricaciduria [fjuˌmærikˌæsiˈdjuəriə] *n* 延胡索酸尿[症]
fumarylacetoacetase [ˌfjuːmərilәˌsitəuˈæsiteis] *n* 延胡索酰乙酰乙酸酶(缺乏此酶可致酪氨酸血症,表现为进行性肝肾衰竭)
fumarylacetoacetate [ˌfjuːmərilәˌsiːtəuˈæsiteit] *n* 延胡索酰乙酰乙酸
fumarylacetoacetate hydrolase [ˌfjuːmərilәˌsiːtəuˈæsiteit ˈhaidrəleis] 延胡索酰乙酰乙酸水解酶,延胡索酰乙酰乙酸酶
fume [fjuːm] *n* 烟尘,烟,烟雾 *vi* 冒烟 *vt* 熏
fumigacin [fjuːmiˈgeisin] *n* 烟曲霉酸,烟色箒状菌酸
fumigant [ˈfjuːmigənt] *n* 熏剂
fumigate [ˈfjuːmigeit] *vt* 熏蒸,熏烟 | **fumigation** [ˌfjuːmiˈgeiʃən] *n* 熏烟,熏烟消毒法
fuming [ˈfjuːmiŋ] *a* 熏的,熏蒸的
fumonisin [fjuːˈmɔnisin] *n* 串珠镰刀菌毒性因子
functio [ˈfʌŋkʃiəu] *n*【拉】功能,官能 | ~ laesa 功能丧失
function [ˈfʌŋkʃən] *n* 功能,官能;函数 *vi* (器官等)活动,执行功能 | antixenic ~ 抗异物功能 / cumulative distribution ~ (cdf) 累积分布函数 / distribution ~ 分布函数 / probability density ~ 概率密度函数 / sexual ~ 性功能

functioning [ˈfʌŋkʃəniŋ] *n* 执行功能 | borderline intellectual ~ 临界智能活动(亦称临界精神发育迟缓)

functional [ˈfʌŋkʃənl] *a* 功能的,官能的;起作用的

functionalis [ˌfʌŋkʃiənˈneilis]【拉】*a* 功能的 *n* 功能层

functionating [ˈfʌŋkʃəneitiŋ] *n* 执行功能,行使功能

fundal [ˈfʌndl] *a* 底的

fundament [ˈfʌndəmənt] *n* 基底,基础;原基;臀部,肛门,肛周

fundamental [ˌfʌndəˈmentl] *a* 基本的,基础的

fundectomy [fʌnˈdektəmi] *n* 底部切除术(如子宫底)

fundi [ˈfʌndai] fundus 的所有格和复数

fundic [ˈfʌndik] *a* 底的

fundiform [ˈfʌndifɔːm] *a* 吊带形的

fundoplication [ˌfʌndəupliˈkeiʃən] *n* 胃底折叠术(治反流性食管炎)

Fundulus [ˈfʌndələs] *n* 底鳉属

fundus [ˈfʌndəs] ([复]**fundi** [ˈfʌndai]) *n*【拉】底,基底 | albinotic ~ 白化病眼底 / ~ of bladder, ~ of urinary bladder 膀胱底;膀胱尖 / ~ of gallbladder 胆囊底 / ~ of internal acoustic meatus 内耳道底 / ~ oculi 眼底 / ~ of stomach 胃底 / tessellated ~, tigroid ~ 豹纹状眼底 / ~ of uterus 子宫底 / ~ of vagina 阴道穹窿

funduscope [ˈfʌndəskəup] *n* 眼底镜 | **funduscopy** [ˌfʌnˈdʌskəpi] *n* 眼底镜检查

fundusectomy [ˌfʌndəˈsektəmi] *n* 胃底切除术

fungal [ˈfʌŋgəl] *a* 真菌的,霉菌的

fungate [ˈfʌŋgeit] *vi* 真菌样生长,霉菌样生长

fungemia [fʌnˈdʒiːmiə] *n* 真菌血症,霉菌血症

fungi [ˈfʌŋgai, ˈfʌndʒai] fungus 的复数

fungicide [ˈfʌndʒisaid] *n* 杀真菌药 | **fungicidal** [fʌndʒiˈsaidl] *a* 杀真菌的,杀霉菌的

fungicidin [ˌfʌndʒiˈsaidin] *n* 制真菌素,制霉菌素

fungiform [ˈfʌndʒifɔːm] *a* 真菌样的,蕈状的,蘑菇状的

Fungi Imperfecti [ˈfʌŋdʒai ˌimpəˈfektai] 半知菌类,不[完]全菌纲

fungimycin [fʌndʒiˈmaisin] *n* 真菌霉素

fungistasis [fʌndʒiˈsteisis] *n* 抑制真菌

fungistat [ˈfʌndʒistæt] *n* 抑真菌剂

fungistatic [ˌfʌndʒiˈstætik] *a* 抑制真菌的

fungisterol [fʌnˈdʒistərɔl] *n* 霉[菌]甾醇,霉[菌]固醇

fungitoxic [fʌndʒiˈtɔksik] *a* 毒害真菌的

fungitoxicity [ˌfʌndʒitɔkˈsisəti] *n* 真菌毒性

fungoid [ˈfʌŋgɔid] *a* 似真菌的,蕈状的,蕈样的 | chignon ~ 蕈状发结节病,蕈状球发

fungoma [fəŋˈgəumə] *n* 曲霉肿

fungosity [fʌnˈgɔsəti] *n* 蕈状赘肉

fungous [ˈfʌŋgəs] *a* 真菌的,霉菌的

fungus [ˈfʌŋgəs] ([复]**funguses** 或 **fungi** [ˈfʌŋgai, ˈfʌndʒai]) *n*【拉】真菌,霉菌;蕈;海绵肿 | ~ of the brain, cerebral ~ 脑突出 / chignon ~ 蕈状发结节病,蕈状球发 / club ~ 珊瑚菌 / cutaneous ~ 皮[肤]真菌,皮[癣]霉菌 / fission ~ 裂殖菌 / foot ~ 足霉菌 / imperfect fungi 半知菌类 / kefir fungi 开菲乳真菌 / mosaic ~ 真菌镶嵌现象,蕈状胆甾醇沉积,蕈状胆固醇沉积 / mycelial ~, mold ~, thread ~ 丝状真菌,毛霉菌 / ray ~ 放线菌 / sac ~ 子囊菌 / slime ~ 黏菌虫 / ~ testis 睾丸海绵肿,睾丸蕈样肿 / true ~, proper ~ 真菌 / yeast ~ 酵母菌,酿母菌

funic [ˈfjuːnik] *a* 索的;脐带的

funicle [ˈfjuːnikl] *n* 索;精索;脐带

funicular [fju(ː)ˈnikjulə] *a* 索的;精索的;脐带的

funiculitis [fju(ː)ˌnikjuˈlaitis] *n* 精索炎;脊神经根炎 | endemic ~ 地方性精索炎

funiculoepididymitis [fju(ː)ˌnikjuləuˌepiˌdidiˈmaitis] *n* 精索附睾炎

funiculopexy [fju(ː)ˈnikjuləˌpeksi] *n* 精索固定术

funiculus [fju(ː)ˈnikjuləs] ([复]**funiculi** [fju(ː)ˈnikjulai]) *n*【拉】索;菌丝索 | dorsal ~ (脊髓)后索 / hepatic ~ 胆总管 / ligamentous ~ 韧带索,腕尺侧副韧带 / ventral ~ (脊髓)前索

funiform [ˈfjuːnifɔːm] *a* 索状的

funis [ˈfjuːnis] *n*【拉】索;脐带

funisitis [ˌfjuːniˈsaitis] *n* 脐带炎

funnel [ˈfʌnl] *n* 漏斗 | mitral ~ 二尖瓣漏斗,二尖瓣口纽孔状缩窄 / muscular ~ 肌肉漏斗 / pial ~ 软脑膜漏斗 / vascular ~ 血管漏斗

FUO fever of undetermined origin 发热原因不明

fur [fəː] *n* 舌苔 *vt*, *vi* 生苔

furaltadone [fjuəˈræltədəun] *n* 呋喃他酮(尿路抗菌药)

furan [ˈfjuəræn], **furane** [ˈfjuərein] *n* 呋喃

furanose [ˈfjuərənəus] *n* 呋喃糖

furazolidone [ˌfjuərəˈzɔlidəun] *n* 呋喃唑酮(抗菌药,抗原虫药)

furazolium [ˌfjuərəˈzəuliəm] *n* 呋噻咪唑(抗菌药) | ~ chloride 呋唑氯铵(抗菌药) / ~ tartrate 酒石酸呋噻咪唑(抗菌药)

Fürbringer's sign [ˈfəːbriŋə] (Paul Fürbringer) 弗布林格征(膈下脓肿时,将针刺入脓肿内,则呼吸运动传导至针,由此与膈上脓肿相区别) | ~ test 弗布林格试验(检尿白蛋白)

furca [ˈfəːkə] ([复]**furcae** [ˈfəːkiː]) *n*【拉】叉,牙根叉

furcal [ˈfəːkəl] *a* 分叉的
furcate [ˈfəːkeit] *a* 叉形的,分叉的 *vi* 分成叉形 | **furcation** [fəːˈkeiʃən] *n* 分叉;分叉部,杈(牙根)
furcocercous [ˌfəːkəˈsəːkəs] *a* 有叉尾的
furcula [ˈfəːkjulə] *n*【拉】叉状隆(胚胎期喉内的马蹄形嵴) | **~r** *a*
furfur [ˈfəːfə] ([复]**furfures** [ˈfəːfəriːz]) *n* 皮屑,头屑;糠,麸
furfuraceous [ˌfəːfəˈreiʃəs] *a* 糠状的;皮屑状的
furfuran [ˈfəːfəræn] *n* 呋喃
furfurol [ˈfəːfərɔl], **furfural** [ˈfəːfəræl] *n* 糠醛
furibund [ˈfjuəribʌnd] *a* 狂怒的,狂暴的
furifosmin [ˌfjuəriˈfɔzmin] *n* 呋里膦明(一种与^{99m}Tc标记时的膦,用于心肌灌注成像)
furious [ˈfjuəriəs] *a* 狂怒的
furmethonol [fəˈmeθənɔl] *n* 呋喃他酮(尿路抗菌药)
furobufen [ˌfəːrəˈbjuːfen] *n* 呋罗布芬(抗炎药)
furocoumarin [ˌfjuərəˈkuːmərin] *n* 呋喃并香豆素
furodazole [fəˈrəudəzəul] *n* 呋罗达唑(抗蠕虫药)
furor [ˈfjuərɔː] *n*【拉】狂乱,狂暴,狂怒 | ~ epilepticus 癫痫[性]狂暴
furosemide [fjuəˈrəusəmaid] *n* 呋塞米(利尿药)
furred [fəːd] *a* 有苔的
furrow [ˈfʌrəu] *n* 沟;(面部)皱纹 | digital ~ 指沟(指分节线) / genital ~ 生殖沟 / gluteal ~ 臀沟 / mentolabial ~ 颏唇沟 / nympholabial ~ 阴唇间沟 / primitive ~ 原沟 / scleral ~ 巩膜沟 / skin ~s 皮沟
furry [ˈfəːri] *a* 有舌苔的
fursalan [ˈfəːsələn] *n* 呋沙仑(消毒防腐药)
fursemide [ˈfəːsimaid] *n* 呋塞米(利尿药)
Fürstner's disease [ˈfəːstnə] (Carl Fürstner) 菲斯特内病(假性痉挛性麻痹伴发震颤)
furuncle [ˈfjuərʌŋkl] *n* 疖 | **furuncular** [fjuəˈrʌŋkjulə], **furunculous** [fjuəˈrʌŋkjuləs] *a*
furunculoid [fjuəˈrʌŋkjulɔid] *a* 疖样的
furunculosis [fjuəˌrʌŋkjuˈləusis] *n* 疖病 | ~ blastomycetica, ~ cryptococcica 芽生菌性疖病,隐球菌性疖病
furunculus [fjuəˈrʌŋkjuləs] ([复]**furunculi** [fjuəˈrʌŋkjulai]) *n*【拉】疖
fury [ˈfjuəri] *n* 狂乱,狂暴,狂怒
FUS feline urological syndrome 猫泌尿综合征
fusaridiosis [ˌfjuːsəˌridiˈəusis] *n* 镰刀菌病(马的皮肤真菌病)
fusariotoxicosis [fjuˌsæriəutɔksiˈkəusis] *n* 镰刀菌中毒[症]
Fusarium [fjuːˈsɛəriəm] *n* 镰孢[霉]属,镰刀菌属 | ~ oxysporum 尖孢镰刀菌 / ~ solanae 茄病镰刀菌 / ~ sporotrichiella 拟分枝孢镰刀菌
fusarium [fjuːˈsɛəriəm] ([复]**fusaria** [fjuːˈsɛəriə]) *n* 镰刀菌
fuscin [ˈfʌsin] *n* 视褐质;暗褐菌素
fuscous [ˈfʌskəs] *a* 暗褐色的,深色的
fuseau [fjuːˈzəu] ([复]**fuseaux** [fjuːˈzəuz]) *n*【法】顶生厚壁孢子
fusi [ˈfjuːsai] fusus 的复数
fusible [ˈfjuːzəbl] *a* 易熔的,可熔化的 | **fusibility** [ˌfjuːzəˈbiləti] *n* 熔性,熔度
fusicellular [ˌfjuːsiˈseljulə] *a* 梭形细胞的
fusidate [ˈfjuːsaideit] *n* 梭链孢酸盐
fusidic acid [fjuːˈsidik] 梭链孢酸,夫西地酸(抗生素类药)
fusiform [ˈfjuːzifɔːm] *a* 梭形的,梭状的
Fusiformis [ˌfjuːsiˈfɔːmis] *n* 梭[形杆]菌属 | ~ necrophorus 尸体梭[形杆]菌
fusimotor [ˌfjuːsiˈməutə] *n* 肌梭运动纤维
fusion [ˈfjuːʒən] *n* 熔化,熔合;融合;融合术 | binocular ~ 双眼视象融合 / diaphyseal-epiphyseal ~ 骨干骺融合术 / nerve ~ 神经融合术 / nuclear ~ 核融合 / spinal ~ 脊柱融合术,脊柱制动术
fusional [ˈfjuːʒənl] *a* 熔化的,熔合的;融合的
Fusobacterium [ˌfjuːzəubækˈtiəriəm] *n* 梭杆菌属 | ~ gonidiaformans 微生子梭杆菌(亦称微生子放线菌) / ~ mortiferum 死亡梭杆菌 / ~ naviforme 舟形梭杆菌 / ~ necrophorum 坏死梭杆菌(亦称坏死放线菌) / ~ plauti-vincenti 普-奋梭[形杆]菌(见于坏死溃疡性龈炎〈战壕口炎〉及溃疡坏死性口炎) / ~ russii 拉氏梭杆菌 / ~ varium 变形梭杆菌
fusobacterium [ˌfjuːzəubækˈtiəriəm] *n* 梭杆菌
fusocellular [ˌfjuːsəuˈseljulə] *a* 梭形细胞的
fusospirillary [ˌfjuːsəuˈspaiərilәri] *a* 梭菌螺菌的
fusospirillosis [ˌfjuːsəuˌspaiəriˈləusis] *n* 坏死溃疡性龈炎
fusospirochetal [ˌfjuːsəuˌspaiərəuˈkiːtl] *a* 梭菌螺旋体性的
fusospirochetosis [ˌfjuːsəuˌspaiərəukiˈtəusis] *n* 梭菌螺旋体病,梭菌波体病
fusostreptococcicosis [ˌfjuːsəuˌstreptəukɔksiˈkəusis] *n* 梭菌链球菌病
fustic [ˈfʌstik] *n* 黄桑木
fustigation [ˌfʌstiˈgeiʃən] *n* 鞭击法
fusus [ˈfjuːsəs] ([复]**fusi** [ˈfjuːsai]) *n*【拉】梭形物,梭 | cortical fusi (毛干)皮质梭 / fracture fusi (毛干)折裂梭
Futcher's line [ˈfʌtʃə] (Palmer H. Futcher) 法彻线(见 Voigt's line)
fututrix [fjuˈtjuːtriks] *n* 女子同性恋者
FVC forced vital capacity 用力肺活量
F. vs. fiat venaesectio【拉】放血

G

G gauss 高斯；giga- 吉［咖］；gravida 孕妇；guanine 胍；guanosine 鸟苷

G conductance 电导；gravitational constant 引力常数；Gibbs free energy 吉布斯自由能；G force G力

g gram 克

g standard gravity 标准重力

γ 希腊语的第3个字母；免疫球蛋白G的重链（the heavy chain of IgG）和胎儿血红蛋白的γ链（the γ chains of fetal hemoglobin）的符号；微克（microgram，现为μg）的符号

γ- ［前缀］表示①蛋白电泳中与γ带移行的血浆蛋白质（γ球蛋白）；②连于主要功能基上的第3个碳原子，如γ-氨基丁酸

Ga gallium 镓

GABA γ-aminobutyric acid γ-氨基丁酸（治各型肝昏迷药）

GABAergic ［ˌgæbəˈəːdʒik］ *a* γ-氨基丁酸能的（传送或分泌γ-氨基丁酸的，指神经纤维、突触及其他神经结构）

gabapentin ［gæbəˈpentin］ *n* 加巴喷丁（抗癫痫药）

GABA transaminase ［ˌgæbətrænsˈæmineis］ γ-氨基丁酸转氨酶

G-actin G-肌动蛋白

GAD generalized anxiety disorder 广泛性焦虑症

gadfly ［ˈgædflai］ *n* 虻

gadoleic acid ［ˌgædəˈliik］ 二十碳-9-烯酸

gadolinium（Gd） ［ˌgædəˈliniəm］ *n* 钆（化学元素）

gadopentetate dimeglumine ［ˌgædəˈpentəteit］ 钆喷酸双［甲］葡胺盐（一种顺磁剂，用作颅内损伤或脊柱及有关组织损伤的磁共振成像中的造影剂，静脉内给药）

gaduhiston ［ˌgædjuˈhistən］ *n* 鳕组蛋白

Gadus ［ˈgeidəs］ *n* 【拉】鳕属 | ~ morrhua 鳕［鱼］（其肝可制鱼肝油）

Gaenslen's sign（test） ［ˈgenzlən］（Frederick J. Gaenslen）根斯伦征（试验）（令患者仰卧，一腿保持髋膝屈曲，另一腿悬下床边，由检查者下拉致髋部过度伸展，则患有腰骶关节病的患侧即发生疼痛）

Gaertner 见 Gärtner

Gaffkya ［ˈgæfkiə］（G. T. A. Gaffky） *n* 加夫基球菌属 | ~ tetragena 四联球菌

Gaffky scale（table） ［ˈgæfki］（Georg T. A. Gaffky）加氏计数法（根据痰内结核菌数以表示结核病的预后情况）

GAG glycosaminoglycan 糖胺聚糖

gag ［gæg］ *vt* 使作呕；用张口器使口张开 *vi* 作呕，恶心 *n* 张口器，开口器

gage ［geidʒ］ *n* = gauge

Gaillard-Arlt suture ［geiˈjɑː ɑːlt］（François L. Gaillard；Carl F. R. von Arlt）盖拉德-阿尔特缝术（睑内翻矫正缝术）

gain ［gein］ *n* 获得，增加，获益；增益 *vt* 获得，赢得，增加 *vi* 获得利益；增加，增进（健康等）| antigen ~ 抗原获得，抗原增加 / primary ~ 原发得益（由于防御机制而即减轻忧虑）/ secondary ~ 继发得益（因病而获益，如个人得到关注等）

Gairdner's test ［ˈgɛədnə］（William T. Gairdner）盖尔德纳试验，钱币试验（coin test，见 test 项下相应术语）

Gaisböck's disease，syndrome ［ˈgaisbek］（Felix Gaisböck）应激性红细胞增多

gait ［geit］ *n* 步态 | antalgic ~ 防痛步态 / cerebellar ~，swaying ~ 小脑病步态，摇摆步态 / equine ~ 髋屈步态，马行步态（见于腓神经瘫痪）/ festinating ~ 慌促步态（见于震颤麻痹及其他神经性疾病）/ gluteal ~ 偏臀步态（见于臀中肌瘫痪）/ helicopod ~ 环形步态，螺旋形步态（见于某些癔症性疾病）/ hemiplegic ~ 偏瘫步态 / scissor ~ 剪形步态 / spastic ~ 痉挛步态 / staggering ~ 蹒跚步态（与酒精中毒和巴比土酸盐中毒有关）/ steppage ~ 跨阈步态（见于下位运动神经元损害，例如多神经炎、前运动角质细胞损害以及马尾损害）/ tabetic ~，ataxic ~ 脊髓痨步态，共济失调步态 / waddling ~ 鸭步［态］（进行性肌营养不良的特征）

galact- 见 galacto-

galactacrasia ［ˌgælæktəˈkreisiə］ *n* 乳液异常

galactagogin ［gəˌlæktəˈgɔgin］ *n* 胎盘催乳素

galactagogue ［gəˈlæktəgɔg］ *a* 催乳的 *n* 催乳药

galactan ［gəˈlæktən］ *n* 半乳聚糖

galactemia ［ˌgæləkˈtiːmiə］ *n* 乳血症

galactic ［gəˈlæktik］ *a* 乳液的 *n* 催乳药

galactin ［gəˈlæktin］ *n* 催乳激素

galactischia ［ˌgælækˈtiskiə］ *n* 乳液分泌抑制

galactitol ［gəˈlæktitɔl］ *n* 半乳糖醇，卫矛醇

galact（o）- ［构词成分］乳，乳液

galactoblast ［gəˈlæktəblæst］ *n* 成初乳小体

galactobolic [gəˌlæktəuˈbɔlik] *a* 生乳的
galactocele [gəˈlæktəsiːl] *n* 积乳囊肿;乳性鞘膜积液
galactocerebroside [gəˌlæktəusəˈriːbrəsaid] *n* 半乳糖脑苷脂
galactocerebroside β-galactosidase [gəˌlæktəu-səˈriːbrəsaid gəˌlæktəuˈsaideis] 半乳糖脑苷脂β-半乳糖苷酶,半乳糖神经酰胺酶
galactochloral [gəˌlæktəuˈklɔːrəl] *n* 半乳糖氯醛(安眠药)
galactocrasia [gəˌlæktəuˈkreisiə] *n* 乳液异常
galactogen [gəˈlæktədʒən] *n* 半乳多糖
galactogenous [ˌgælækˈtɔdʒinəs] *a* 生乳的,催乳的
galactogogue [gəˈlæktəgɔg] *a* 催乳的 *n* 催乳药
galactography [ˌgælækˈtɔgrəfi] *n* 乳腺导管造影术
galactokinase [gəˌlæktəuˈkaineis] *n* 半乳糖激酶
galactolipin(e) [gəˌlæktəuˈlaipin], **galactolipid** [gəˌlæktəuˈlipid] *n* 半乳糖脂(脑苷脂)
galactoma [ˌgælækˈtəumə] *n* 积乳囊肿;乳性鞘膜积液
galactometastasis [gəˌlæktəumiˈtæstəsis] *n* 异位泌乳
galactometer [ˌgælækˈtɔmitə] *n* 乳[液]比重计
galactonic acid [ˌgælækˈtɔnik] 半乳糖酸
galactopexic [gəˌlæktəuˈpeksik] *a* 半乳糖固定的
galactopexy [gəˈlæktəˌpeksi] *n* 半乳糖固定(由肝固定半乳糖)
galactophagous [ˌgælækˈtɔfəgəs] *a* 乳食的
galactophlebitis [gəˌlæktəfliˈbaitis] *n* 授乳期静脉炎,股白肿
galactophlysis [gælækˈtɔflisis] *n* 乳性疱疹
galactophore [gəˈlæktəfɔː] *a* 输乳的,排乳的 *n* 乳管
galactophoritis [gəˌlæktəufəˈraitis] *n* 乳管炎
galactophorous [ˌgælækˈtɔfərəs] *a* 输乳的,排乳的
galactophygous [gælækˈtɔfigəs] *a* 回乳的,止乳的
galactoplania [gəˌlæktəuˈpleiniə] *n* 异位泌乳
galactopoiesis [gəˌlæktəupɔiˈiːsis] *n* 乳生成 | **galactopoietic** [gəˌlæktəpɔiˈetik] *a* 生乳的 *n* 催乳药
galactopyra [gəˌlæktəuˈpaiərə] *n* 生乳热
galactopyranose [gəˌlæktəuˈpairənəusˌ-ˈpir-] *n* 吡喃[型]半乳糖
galactorrhea [gəˌlæktəuˈriːə] *n* 乳溢
galactosamine [gəˌlæktəuˈsæmin] *n* 半乳糖胺,2-氨基半乳糖,软骨糖胺
galactosamine-6-sulfate sulfatase [gəˌlæktəu-ˈsæmin ˈsʌlfeit ˈsʌlfəteis] 半乳糖胺-6-硫酸盐硫酸酯酶,*N*-乙酰半乳糖胺-6-硫酸酯酶
galactosan [gəˈlæktəsæn] *n* 半乳聚糖
galactosazone [ˌgælækˈtəusəzəun] *n* 半乳糖脎
galactoschesis [ˌgælækˈtɔskisis] *n* 乳液分泌抑制
galactoscope [gəˈlæktəskəup] *n* 乳酪计,乳脂计
galactose [gəˈlæktəus] *n* 半乳糖
galactose epimerase [gəˈlæktəus iˈpiməreis] 半乳糖差向异构酶,尿苷二磷酸葡萄糖4-差向异构酶
galactosemia [gəˌlæktəuˈsiːmiə] *n* 半乳糖血症(可致低能的遗传性代谢病)
galactose-1-phosphate uridyltransferase [gə-ˈlæktəus ˈfɔsfeit ˌjuəridilˈtrænsfəreis] 半乳糖-1-磷酸尿苷酰转移酶,尿苷二磷酸葡萄糖-己糖-1-磷酸尿苷酰基转移酶
galactose 1-phosphate uridylyltransferase [gə-ˈlæktəus ˈfɔsfeit ˌjuəriˌdililˈtrænsfəreis] 半乳糖-1-磷酸尿苷酰基转移酶,尿苷三磷酸-己糖-1-磷酸尿苷酰基转移酶
galactosialidosis [gəˌlæktəusaiˌæliˈdəusis] *n* 半乳糖唾液酸沉积症
α-galactosidase [gəˌlæktəuˈsaideis] *n* α-半乳糖苷酶 | α- ~ A α-半乳糖苷酶A(缺乏此酶为一种X连锁性状,可致血浆和组织内神经酰胺三己糖苷和其他糖〈神经〉鞘脂的蓄积,可致法布莱〈Fabry〉病。亦称神经酰胺三己糖苷酶) / α- ~ B α-半乳糖苷酶B,α-*N*-乙酰氨基半乳糖苷酶
β-galactosidase [gəˌlæktəuˈsaideis] *n* β-半乳糖苷酶(遗传性缺乏细胞溶酶体中的一种酶〈β-半乳糖苷酶A〉,为一种常染色体隐性性状,可致全身性神经节苷脂沉积症。缺乏另一种酶,可致莫尔基奥〈Morquio〉综合征B型,即黏多糖贮积症IVB。亦称乳糖基神经酰胺酶Ⅱ) / neutral β- ~ 中性β-半乳糖苷酶,乳糖基神经酰胺酶 / neutral β- ~ deficiency 中性β-半乳糖苷酶缺乏症,乳糖基酰基鞘氨醇过多症
galactoside [gəˈlæktəsaid] *n* 半乳糖苷
galactosis [ˌgælækˈtəusis] *n* 乳液生成
galactostasis [gælækˈtɔstəsis], **galactostasia** [gə-ˌlæktəuˈsteisiə] *n* 泌乳停止;乳液积滞
galactosuria [gəˌlæktəuˈsjuəriə] *n* 半乳糖尿
galactosyl [gəˈlæktəsil] *n* 半乳糖基
galactosylceramidase [gəˌlæktəsilsəˈræmideis] *n* 半乳糖[基]神经酰胺酶(此酶的遗传性缺乏,为常染色体隐性遗传,可致克拉贝〈Krabbe〉病)
galactosylceramide [gəˌlæktəsilˈserəmaid] *n* 半乳糖[基]神经酰胺,半乳糖脑苷脂
galactosylceramide β-galactosidase [gəˌlæktə-silˈserəmaid gəˌlæktəuˈsaideis] 半乳糖[基]神经酰胺β-半乳糖苷酶,半乳糖[基]神经酰胺酶
galactosylceramide β-galactosidase deficiency 半乳糖神经酰胺β-半乳糖苷酶缺乏症,克拉贝病(Krabbe disease)

galactosylceramide β-galactosylhydrolase [gəˌlæktəsilˈserəmaid gəˈlæktəsil ˈhaidrəleis] 半乳糖神经酰胺β-半乳糖水解酶,半乳糖神经酰胺酶
galactosylhydroxylysyl glucosyltransferase [gəˌlæktəsilhaiˌdrɔksiˈlaisil ˌgluːkəsilˈtrænsfəreis] 半乳糖[基]羟赖氨酰葡糖基转移酶,前胶原葡糖基转移酶
galactosyltransferase [gəˌlæktəusilˈtrænzfəreis] *n* 半乳糖转移酶
galactotherapy [gəˌlæktəuˈθerəpi] *n* 经乳疗法;乳疗法
galactotoxin [gəˌlæktəuˈtɔksin] *n* 乳毒素
galactotoxism [gəˌlæktəuˈtɔksizəm], **galactoxism** [ˌgælækˈtɔksizəm], **galactoxismus** [gəˌlæktɔkˈsizməs] *n* 乳中毒
galactotrophy [ˌgælækˈtɔtrəfi] *n* 乳营养法
galactowaldenase [gəˌlæktəuˈwældəneis] *n* 半乳糖瓦尔登转化酶,UDP 半乳糖-4-差向异构酶
galactozymase [gəˌlæktəuˈzaimeis] *n* 乳酿酶
galacturia [ˌgæləkˈtjuəriə] *n* 乳糜尿
galacturonic acid [gəˌlæktjuəˈrɔnik] 半乳糖醛酸
galantamine hydrobromide [gəˈlæntəmiːn] 氢溴酸加兰他敏(胆碱酯酶抑制药)
galanthamine hydrobromide [gəˈlænθəmiːn] 氢溴酸加兰他敏(胆碱酯酶抑制药)
gaile [gɑːl] *n*【法】疥疮,疥螨病
galea [ˈgeiliə] *n*【拉】帽;头巾(帽状绷带);帽状腱膜 | ~ aponeurotica 帽状腱膜
Galeati's glands [ˌgæliˈɑːti] (Domenico M. Galeati) 十二指肠腺
galeatus [ˌgæliˈeitəs] *a* 羊膜包胎的
Galeazzi's fracture [ˌgæliˈætzi] (Riccardo Galeazzi) 加莱阿齐骨折(桡骨在腕部之上骨折,伴尺骨远侧端脱位) | ~ sign 加莱阿齐征(先天性髋关节脱位时,患者平卧在平台上,双膝和髋关节弯曲成90°,患侧股骨即显示变短)
galenic [gəˈlenik] *a* 盖仑派医学的(Galenus 或 Galen 所教和所行的古医学说的)
galenicals [gəˈlenikəlz], **galenica** [gəˈlenikə], **galenics** [gəˈleniks] *n* 盖仑制剂,植物制剂
galenism [ˈgeilənizəm] *n* 盖仑学说(一种古医学说,为体液学说和古希腊毕达哥拉斯〈Pythagoras〉的数字学说〈例如4液说、4要素说等〉的混合)
Galen's anastomosis, nerve [ˈgeilən] (Claudius 〈或 Clarissimus〉 Galenus) 盖仑吻合、盖仑神经(喉上、下神经的交通支) | ~ bandage 盖仑绷带(用于头部的六头带) / ~ foramen 心前静脉口(进入右心房) / ~ veins 盖伦静脉,脑静脉干(大脑内静脉与大脑大静脉的总称) / ~ ventricle 喉室
Galeodes araneoides [gæliˈəudiːz əˌreiniˈɔidiːz] 蛛毛蝎
galeophobia [ˌgæliəuˈfəubiə] *n* 猫恐怖,恐猫症
Galeorhinus [ˌgæliəuˈrainəs] *n* 鲨鱼属
Galerina [ˌgæləˈrainə] *n* 丝膜蕈属
galeropia [ˌgæləˈrəupiə], **galeropsia** [ˌgæləˈrɔpsiə] *n* 视力超常
gall[1] [gɔːl] *n* 胆汁;没食子,五倍子 | Aleppo ~, Smyrna ~ 没食子 / ox ~ 牛胆汁
gall[2] [gɔːl] *n* 肿痛;擦伤;磨损
gallacetophenone [gæˌlæsitəuˈfinəun] *n* 没食子苯乙酮(防腐抗菌药)
gallamine triethiodide [ˈgæləmain ˌtraieˈθaiədaid] 戈拉碘铵(肌肉松弛药)
gallate [ˈgæleit] *n* 没食子酸盐
gallbladder [ˈgɔːlblædə] *n* 胆囊 | fishscale ~ 鱼鳞状胆囊 / folded fundus ~ 倒圆锥形帽(胆囊造影时表现的胆囊底折叠现象,即弗里及亚帽〈phrygian cap〉—种胆囊形式) / sandpaper ~ 沙纸状胆囊 / stasis ~ 胆囊淤积 / wandering ~, floating ~, mobile ~ 游动胆囊
gallein [ˈgæliːn] *n* 棓因,焦没食子酚酞
gallic [ˈgælik] *a* 没食子的,五倍子的 | ~ acid 没食子酸,棓酸
gallid [ˈgælid] *a* 禽的
Gallie transplant [ˈgæli] (William E. Gallie) 加利移植物(有阔筋膜条作疝手术缝线)
Galli Mainini test [ˈgæli maiˈnini] (Carlos G. Mainini) 加利·迈尼尼试验(检孕)
Gallionella [ˌgæliəuˈnelə] (Benjamin Gaillon) 加立昂菌属
gallipot [ˈgælipɔt] *n* 药罐(存软膏或糖膏用)
gallisin [ˈgælisin] *n* 加立新(类糊精物质)
gallium(Ga) [ˈgæliəm] *n* 镓(化学元素)
gallnut [ˈgɔːlnʌt] *n* 没食子,五倍子
gallon [ˈgælən] *n* 加仑(容量单位,英制为4.546 L,美制3.785 L)
gallop [ˈgæləp] *n* 奔马律(心脏的一种异常节律)
gallotannic acid [ˌgæləuˈtænik] 没食子鞣酸
Gall's craniology [gɔːl] (Franz J. Gall) 颅相学
gallsickness [ˈgɔːlsiknis] *n* 牛胆病
gallstone [ˈgɔːlstəun] *n* 胆[结]石
GalNAc *N*-acetylgalactosamine *N*-乙酰半乳糖胺
GALT gut-associated lymphoid tissue 肠相关[性]淋巴样组织
Galton's delta [ˈgɔːltən] (Francis Galton) 高尔顿三角(指纹三角) | ~ law 高尔顿定律(每一亲代个体对子代的遗传影响平均占1/4,或〈0.5〉^{2},祖代个体的影响为1/16,或〈0.5〉^{4},曾祖代个体的影响为1/64,或〈0.5〉^{6},余类推) / ~ law of regression 高尔顿退化定律(一般的双亲生一般的儿童,特殊的双亲子代继承双亲的

特性,但不及双亲自身表现那样明显)/ ~ whistle 高尔顿笛(检听觉)

Galv. galvanic 伽伐尼的,流电的

galvanic [gæl'vænik] (Luigi Galvanic) *a* 伽伐尼的,流电的

galvanism ['gælvənizəm] *n* 流电;直流电疗法

galvanize ['gælvənaiz] *vt* 通电流于;电镀 | **galvanization** [ˌgælvənai'zeiʃən, -ni'z-] *n* 直流电疗法;电镀

galvanocautery [ˌgælvənəu'kɔːtəri] *n* [流]电烙器;[流]电烙法

galvanochemical [ˌgælvənəu'kemikəl] *n* [流]电化学的

galvanocontractility [ˌgælvənəuˌkɔntræk'tiləti] *n* 电流收缩性

galvanogustometer [ˌgælvənəugʌs'tɔmitə] *n* [流]电味觉计

galvanolysis [ˌgælvə'nɔlisis] *n* 电解[作用]

galvanometer [ˌgælvə'nɔmitə] *n* 电流计,电流测定器

galvanonervous [ˌgælvənəu'nəːvəs] *a* 流电神经的

galvanopalpation [ˌgælvənəupæl'peiʃən] *n* 电触诊[法]

galvanosurgery [ˌgælvənəu'səːdʒəri] *n* 电外科

galvanotaxis [ˌgælvənəu'tæksis] *n* 趋电性

galvanotherapeutics [ˌgælvənəuˌθerə'pjuːtiks], **galvanotherapy** [ˌgælvənəu'θerəpi] *n* [流]电疗法

galvanotropism [ˌgælvə'nɔtrəpizəm] *n* 向电性

galziekte [gæl'ziːkti] *n* 牛胆病

gam- 见 gamo-

gamasid ['gæməsid] *n* 革螨,蚍蜉

Gamasidae [gə'mæsidiː] *n* 革螨科

Gamasides [gə'mæsidiːz] *n* 革螨类

gamasoidosis [ˌgæməsɔi'dəusls] *n* 禽螨病

Gambian horse disease, trypanosomiasis (sleeping sickness) ['gæmbiən] 冈比亚马锥虫病,冈比亚锥虫病(昏睡病)

gambir ['gæmbiə] *n* 棕儿茶

gambling ['gæmbliŋ] *n* 赌博(当赌博成为强迫性行为或长期性行为时,即变成一种冲动性障碍,称为病理性赌博) | pathological ~ 病理性赌博(一种冲动性控制障碍,包括持久地无法抵抗想去赌博的欲望,终于使个人生活和职业生活遭受严重破坏)

gamboge [gæm'buːʒ] *n* 藤黄

gambogic acid [gæm'bɔdʒik] 藤黄酸

Gambusia [gæm'bjuːsiə] *n* 食蚊鱼属,柳条鱼属 | ~ affinis 食蚊鱼,柳条鱼

gamefar ['gæmifɑː] *n* 扑疟喹,帕马喹(即 pamaquine,抗疟药)

gametangium [gæmi'tændʒiəm] ([复] **gametangia** [gæmi'tændʒiə]) *n* 配子囊

gamete ['gæmiːt] *n* 配子 | **gametic** [gə'metik] *a*

gamet(o)- [构词成分]配子

gametocidal [gə'miːtə'saidl] *a* 杀配子[体]的

gametocide [gə'miːtəsaid] *n* 杀配子[体]剂

gametocyst [gə'miːtəsist] *n* 配子囊

gametocyte [gə'miːtəsait] *n* 配子体,配子母细胞

gametocytemia [gəˌmiːtəusai'tiːmiə] *n* 配子体血症

gametogenesis [gəmiːtəu'dʒenisis] *n* 配子发生 | **gametogenic** [gəˌmiːtəu'dʒenik], **gametogenous** [ˌgæmi'tɔdʒənəs] *a*

gametogony [ˌgæmi'tɔgəni] *n* 配子生殖

gametoid ['gæmitɔid] *a* 配子样的

gametokinetic [ˌgæmitəukai'netik] *a* 刺激配子的,促配子活动的

gametology [ˌgæmi'tɔlədʒi] *n* 配子学 | **gametologist** *n* 配子学家

gametophagia [ˌgæmitəu'feidʒiə] *n* 配子消失

gametophyte [gə'miːtəfait] *n* 配子体 | **gametophytic** [gəˌmiːtə'fitik] *a*

gametotropic [gəˌmiːtə'trɔpik] *a* 向配子的

gamfexine [gæm'feksiːn] *n* 更非辛(抗抑郁药)

Gamgee tissue ['gæmdʒiː] (Joseph S. Gamgee) 加姆基敷料(两层脱脂纱布之间夹一厚层脱脂棉制成的外科敷料)

gamic ['gæmik] *a* 性的,受胎的,受精的

gamma ['gæmə] *n* 希腊语的第 3 个字母(Γ, γ),丙种;微克(现用 microgram);伽马(磁场强度单位,γ=0.1 T 特[斯拉]);灰度[非线性]系数(照相底片显影程度的一种数字表示法)

gamma-aminobutyric acid [əˌmiːnəubju'tirik] γ-氨基丁酸

gammacism ['gæməsizəm] *n* G 发音不正

gamma globulin ['gɑmə 'glɔbjulin] 丙种球蛋白

gammaglobulinopathy [ˌgæməˌglɔbjuliˌnɔpəθi] *n* 丙种球蛋白病,γ-球蛋白病

gammagram ['gæməgræm] *n* γ-线谱

gammagraphic [ˌgæmə'græfik] *a* γ-线图的

Gammaherpesvirinae [ˌgæməˌhəːpiːzvi'rainiː] *n* γ-疱疹病毒亚科

gamma-lactone [ˌgæmə'læktəun] *n* γ-内酯

gammaloidosis [ˌgæməlɔi'dəusis] *n* 淀粉样变性

gamma-pipradol [ˌgæmə 'piprədɔl] *n* γ-哌苯甲醇,阿扎环醇(即 azacyclonol,安定药)

gammopathy [gæ'mɔpəθi] *n* 丙球蛋白病,γ-球蛋白病,免疫球蛋白病 | benign monoclonal ~ 良性单克隆 γ-球蛋白病 / monoclonal ~ 单克隆 γ-球蛋白病,浆细胞恶性增生

Gamna's disease ['gæmnə] (Carlo Gamna) 加姆纳病(脾肿大的一型,伴脾胞膜增厚,并有通常

绕以血原带的小棕色区〈加姆纳结节〉出现,脾髓中含铁色素沉积)

gam(o)- [构词成分]婚配,性,两性交合

gamobium [gəˈməubiəm] *n* 有性世代

gamogenesis [ˌgæməuˈdʒenisis] *n* 有性生殖 | **gamogenetic** [ˌgæməudʒiˈnetik] *a*

gamogony [gæˈmɔgəni] *n* 配子生殖

gamone [ˈgæməun] *n* [交]配素(配子所产生的一种化合物,能促进受精作用)

gamont [ˈgæmɔnt] *n* 配子母体

gamophagia [ˌgæməuˈfeidʒiə] *n* 配子消失

gampsodactyly [ˌgæmpsəuˈdæktili] *n* 爪形足

Gamstorp's disease [ˈgæmstɔːp] (Ingrid Gamstorp) 加姆斯托普病,家族性周期性麻痹Ⅱ型

ganciclovir [gænˈsaikləvir] *n* 更昔洛韦(抗病毒药,用于治疗巨细胞病毒感染,口服给药) | ~ sodium 更昔洛韦钠(用于治疗免疫受损患者的巨细胞病毒性视网膜炎,静脉输注给药)

gangli- 见 ganglio-

ganglia [ˈgæŋgliə] ganglion 的复数

ganglial [ˈgæŋgliəl] *a* 神经节的

gangliated [ˈgæŋgliˌeitid] *a* 有神经节的

gangliectomy [ˌgæŋgliˈektəmi] *n* 神经节切除术

gangliform [ˈgæŋglifɔːm] *a* 神经节状的

gangliitis [ˌgæŋgliˈaitis] *n* 神经节炎

gangli(o)- [构词成分]神经节

ganglioblast [ˈgæŋgliəublæst] *n* 成神经节细胞,神经节母细胞

gangliocyte [ˈgæŋgliəusait] *n* 神经节细胞

gangliocytoma [ˌgæŋgliəusaiˈtəumə] *n* 神经节细胞瘤,神经节瘤

ganglioform [ˈgæŋgliəfɔːm] *a* 神经节状的

ganglioglioma [ˌgæŋgliəuglaiˈəumə] *n* 神经节神经胶质瘤

ganglioglioneuroma [ˌgæŋgliəuˌglaiəunjuəˈrəumə] *n* 神经节胶质神经瘤,神经节瘤

gangliolytic [ˌgæŋgliəuˈlitik] *a* 神经节[传导]阻滞的 *n* 神经节阻滞药

ganglioma [ˌgæŋgliˈəumə] *n* 神经节瘤

ganglion [ˈgæŋgliən] ([复] **ganglions** 或 **ganglia** [ˈgæŋgliə]) *n* 神经节;腱鞘囊肿 | accessory ganglia, intermediate ganglia 副节,中间神经节 / auditory ~ 蜗神经核 / azygous ~ 尾骨球 / basal ganglia 基底核 / cardiac ganglia 心神经节 / carotid ~ 颈动脉神经节 / celiac ganglia 腹腔神经节 / cervicothoracic ~, stellate ~ 颈胸神经节 / cervicouterine ~ 子宫颈神经节 / ciliary ~ 睫状神经节 / coccygeal ~ 尾神经节,尾骨球 / compound ~ 复合性腱鞘囊肿 / diffuse ~ 弥漫性腱鞘囊肿 / ganglia of autonomic plexuses 自主神经丛神经节 / hepatic ~ 肝神经节 / nodose ~ 结状神经节,迷走神经下神经节 / pelvic ganglia 盆神经节 / primary ~ 原发性腱鞘囊肿 / semilunar ~ 半月神经节;[复]腹腔神经节 / simple ~ 单纯性腱鞘囊肿 / spinal ~, dorsal root ~ 脊神经节 / trigeminal ~, ~ of trigeminal nerve 三叉神经节,半月神经节 / tympanic ~ 鼓室神经节 / vestibular ~ 前庭神经节 / wrist ~ 腕部腱鞘囊肿

ganglionated [ˈgæŋgliəˌneitid] *a* 有神经节的

ganglionectomy [ˌgæŋgliəuˈnektəmi] *n* 神经节切除术

ganglioneure [ˈgæŋgliəˌnjuə] *n* 神经节细胞

ganglioneuroblastoma [ˌgæŋgliəuˌnjuərəublæsˈtəumə] *n* 成神经节细胞瘤,成神经节胶质神经瘤

ganglioneuroma [ˌgæŋgliəunjuəˈrəumə], **ganglioneurofibroma** [ˌgæŋgliəuˌnjuərəufaiˈbrəumə] *n* 神经节瘤

ganglionic [ˌgæŋgliˈɔnik] *a* 神经节的

ganglionitis [ˌgæŋgliəuˈnaitis] *n* 神经节炎 | acute posterior ~ 带状疱疹 / gasserian ~ 眼[部]带状疱疹

ganglionostomy [ˌgæŋgliəuˈnɔstəmi] *n* 腱鞘囊肿造口术

ganglioplegic [ˌgæŋgliəuˈpliːdʒik], **ganglionoplegic** [ˌgæŋgliˌɔnəˈpliːdʒik] *a* 神经节[传导]阻滞的 *n* 神经节阻滞药

ganglioside [ˈgæŋgliəsaid] *n* 神经节苷脂 | ~ GM_1 神经节苷脂 GM_1(患全身性神经节苷脂贮积症时,此物质在组织中聚积) / ~ GM_2 神经节苷脂 GM_2(患泰-萨克斯〈Tay-Sachs〉病时,此物质在组织中聚积)

ganglioside sialidase [ˈgæŋgliəˌsaid saiˈælideis] 神经节苷脂唾液酸酶

gangliosidosis [ˌgæŋgliəusaiˈdəusis] ([复] **gangliosidoses** [ˌgæŋgliəusaiˈdəusiːz]) *n* 神经节苷脂贮积症 | adult GM_1 ~ 成人型 GM_1 神经节苷脂贮积症(GM_1 神经节苷脂贮积症中最轻型,特征为十几岁发病、痉挛状态和共济失调,患者能存活到 20 岁以上) / adult GM_2 ~ 成人型 GM_2 神经节苷脂贮积症(GM_2 神经节苷脂贮积症中最轻型,特征为十几岁发病、构音障碍、痉挛状态和共济失调,有时出现精神运动性衰退和色素性视网膜炎,患者能存活到 20 岁以上) / generalized ~ 全身性神经节苷脂贮积症(GM_1 神经节苷脂贮积症中最严重型,特征为出生时发病、粗糙面容、水肿、肝脾肿大、樱桃红点〈50% 的婴儿〉、早期失明、听觉过敏、巨舌、癫痫发作、肾小球上皮肿胀和张力减退,可能有黏多糖尿,2 岁以内死亡) / GM_1 ~ GM_1 神经节苷脂贮积症(即 generalized ~) / GM_2 ~ GM_2 神经节苷脂贮积症,泰-萨病(Tay-Sachs disease) / infantile GM_1 ~ 婴儿型 GM_1 神经节苷脂贮积症(即

generlized ~) / juvenile GM_1 ~ 少年型 GM_1 神经节苷脂贮积症(GM_1 神经节苷脂贮积症中不太严重的一型,特征为出生后 6~12 个月发病、癫痫发作、晚期失明、肾小球上皮肿胀、痉挛状态和共济失调,可能有黏多糖尿,可存活到 3~10 岁) / juvenile GM_2 ~ 少年型 GM_2 神经节苷脂贮积症(GM_2 神经节苷脂贮积症中不太严重的一型,特征为 2~6 岁间发病、听觉过敏、癫痫发作、晚期失明、构音障碍、痉挛状态和共济失调,患者可存活到 5~15 岁)

gangliospore [ˈgæŋgliəspɔː] *n* 节孢子(在真菌的菌丝尖端发生的孢子)

gangliosympathectomy [ˌgæŋgliəuˌsimpəˈθektəmi] *n* 交感神经节切除术

Gangolphe's sign [gɑːnˈgɔlf] (Louis Gangolphe) 冈戈尔夫征(腹腔内有血清血液性渗出液,见于绞窄性疝)

gangosa [gæŋˈgəusə] *n* 【西】毁形性鼻咽炎

gangrene [ˈgæŋgriːn] *n* 坏疽 | anaphylactic ~ 过敏性坏疽(注射抗原〈过敏原〉如血清而引起) / angiosclerotic ~ 血管硬化性坏疽 / circumscribed ~ 局限性坏疽 / cold ~ 寒性坏疽 / diabetic ~, glycemic ~, glykemic ~ 糖尿病[性]坏疽 / dry ~ 干性坏疽 / epidemic ~ 麦角中毒 / fulminating ~ 暴发性坏疽,恶性水肿 / gas ~, gaseous ~, emphysematous ~, mephitic ~ 气性坏疽 / moist ~, humid ~ 湿性坏疽 / oral ~ 走马疳,坏疽性口炎 / static ~, venous ~ 血淤滞性坏疽,静脉性坏疽 / thrombotic ~ 血栓性坏疽 / trophic ~ 营养[神经]性坏疽 | **gangrenous** [ˈgæŋgrinəs] *a* 坏疽性的

gangrenopsis [ˌgæŋgrəˈnɔpsis] *n* 走马疳,坏疽性口炎

gangrenosis [ˌgæŋgriˈnəusis] *n* 坏疽[病]

ganirelix acetate [ˌgæniˈreliks] 醋酸加尼瑞克(垂体激素释放抑制药)

ganja(h) [ˈgændʒə, ˈgɑːndʒə] *n* 印度大麻

ganoblast [ˈgænəblæst] *n* 成釉细胞

Ganser's ganglion [ˈgænsə] (Sigbert J. M. Ganser) 脚间核 | ~ symptom 甘瑟症状(答非所问,见于精神病) / ~ syndrome 甘瑟综合征(答非所问,通常伴遗忘症、定向力障碍、知觉障碍、神游及转换症状)

Gant's clamp [gænt] (Samuel G. Gant) 甘特夹(直角痔夹)

Gant's line [gænt] (Frederick J. Gant) 甘特线(股骨大转子下的假想线) | ~ operation 甘特手术(转子下分离股骨骨干,治髋关节粘连)

gap [gæp] *n* 裂,隙,裂孔,裂隙;间隙,间距 | airborn ~ 气骨导间距,气骨隙 / auscultatory ~, silent ~ 听诊无音间隙(由听诊测血压时的无音间隙) / chromatid ~ 染色单体裂隙 / interocclusal ~ 殆间距,颌间距 / isochromatid ~ 等臂染色单体裂隙

GAPD glyceraldehyde-3-phosphate dehydrogenase 甘油醛-3-磷酸脱氢酶

gape [geip] *vi* 张口;打呵欠;张开,裂开 *n* 张口;呵欠

gapes [ˈgeips] *n* 张开病(由气管比翼线虫引起的幼禽病)

gap-toothed [ˈgæp ˈtuːθt] *a* 两齿间隙缝很大的(如由于掉落一齿所致)

garbanzo [gɑːˈbɑːnzəu] *n*【西】鹰嘴豆

Garcinia [gɑːˈsinjə] *n* 藤黄属

Garcin's syndrome [gɑːˈsei] (Raymond Garcin) 加赛综合征(全部或大部分脑神经单侧麻痹,由于颅底或鼻咽部肿瘤所致)

Gardiner-Brown's test [ˈgɑːdnə braun] (Alfred Gardiner-Brown) 加德纳·布朗试验(检中耳病)

Gardner-Diamond syndrome [ˈgɑːdnə ˈdaiəmənd] (Frank H. Gardner; Louis K. Diamond) 加-戴综合征,痛性淤紫综合征(即 painful bruising syndrome,见 syndrome 项下相应术语)

Gardnerella [ˌgɑːdnəˈrelə] (H. L. Gardner) *n* 加德纳菌属

Gardner's syndrome [ˈgɑːdnə] (Eldon J. Gardner) 加德纳综合征(家族性大肠息肉病、额外牙、头颅纤维性结构不良、骨瘤、纤维瘤和皮脂囊肿);(W. J. Gardner)加德纳综合征(常染色体显性遗传的双侧听神经瘤综合征)

Garel's sign [gəˈrel] (Jean Garel) 加雷尔征(见 Heryng's sign)

Garg. gargarismus【拉】[含]漱液

gargalanesthesia [ˌgɑːgəˌlænisˈθiːzjə] *n* 搔感缺失,痒感缺失

gargalesthesia [ˌgɑːgəlisˈθiːzjə] *n* 搔感,痒感,呵痒感 | **gargalesthetic** [ˌgɑːgəlisˈθetik] *a*

gargarism [ˈgɑːgərizəm] *n* [含]漱液

garget [ˈgɑːgət] *n* 牛乳腺炎

gargle [ˈgɑːgl] *vt, vi* 漱口 *n* [含]漱液;漱口声

gargoylism [ˈgɑːgɔilizəm] *n* 脂肪软骨营养不良(见 Hurler's syndrome)

Garland's curve [ˈgɑːlənd] (George M. Garland) 加兰曲线(见 Ellis' line) | ~ triangle 加兰三角(下背部靠近病侧脊柱处出现三角形叩诊相对清音区,见于渗出性胸膜炎)

garlic [ˈgɑːlik] *n* 大蒜;蒜球茎根

garment [ˈgɑːmənt] *n* 外衣 | pneumatic antishock ~ 充气抗休克外衣

garnet [ˈgɑːnit] *n* 石榴子石

Garré's osteomyelitis (disease, osteitis) [gəˈrei] (Carl Garré) 硬化性非化脓性骨髓炎

Garrod's test [ˈgærəd] (Archibald E. Garrod) 加罗德试验(检尿中血卟啉);(Alfred B. Garrod)

加罗德试验(检血中尿酸)
garrot [ˈgærət] *n* 绞扼止血器
Gärtner's bacillus [ˈgetnə] (August Gärtner) 格特内杆菌,肠炎沙门菌
Gartner's cyst [ˈgɑːtnə] (Hermann T. Gartner) 加特纳囊肿(卵巢冠纵管囊肿) | ~ duct (canal) 卵巢冠纵管
Gärtner's phenomenon [ˈgetnə] (Gustav Gärtner) 格特内现象(举臂至不同高度时,其静脉充盈度指示右心房的压力度) | ~ tonometer 格特内血压计(用加压环套在手指上以测血压)
gas [gæs] *n* 气体 | coal ~ 煤气 / ethyl ~ 四乙基铅 / hemolytic ~ 溶血毒气,胂 / laughing ~ 笑气(麻醉药) / marsh ~ 沼气,甲烷 / mustard ~ 芥子气,二氯二乙硫醚 / noxious ~ 毒气/ olefiant ~ 乙烯阴沟气 / sewer ~ 阴沟气/ sneezing ~ 喷嚏毒气,二苯氯[化]胂 / suffocating ~ 窒息毒气,光气 / sweet ~ 甜气,一氧化碳 / tear ~, lacrimator ~ 催泪气 / vesicating ~ 发疱毒气,二氯二乙硫醚 / war ~ 军用毒气
gaseous [ˈgeisjəs], **gasiform** [ˈgæsifɔːm] *a* 气[体]的
gaseousness [ˈgæsiəsnəs, ˈgæʃəsnəs] *n* 肠气(即 burbulence)
gasify [ˈgæsifai] *vt*, *vi* 成为气体,气化 | **gasification** [ˌgæsifiˈkeiʃən] *n* 气化[作用]
Gaskell's bridge [ˈgæskəl] (Walter H. Gaskell) 加斯克尔桥,希氏(His)束(房室束)
gasket [ˈgæskit] *n* 垫圈,垫片
gaskin [ˈgæskin] *n* 马[大]腿
gasogenic [gæsə*u*ˈdʒenik] *a* 产气的
gasoline, gasolene [ˈgæsəliːn] *n* 汽油
gasometer [gæˈsɔmitə] *n* 气量计,气体定量器 | **gasometric** [ˌgæsə*u*ˈmetrik] *a* 气体定量的 / **gasometry** *n* 气体定量法,气体分析法
gasp [gɑːsp] *n* 喘息
gasproof [ˈgæspruːf] *a* 防毒气的;不透气的
gasserectomy [ˌgæsəˈrektəmi] *n* 半月神经节切除术
gasserian [gəˈsiəriən] (Johann L. Gasser) *a* 加塞的(如 ~〈trigeminal〉 ganglion 加塞神经节,三叉神经半月节)
Gasser's ganglion [ˈgæsə] (Johann L. Gasser) 加塞神经节,三叉神经半月节
Gasser's syndrome [ˈgæsə] (Konrad Joseph Gasser) 加塞综合征,溶血性尿毒症综合征(hemolytic-uremic syndrome, 见 syndrome 项下相应术语)
gaster [ˈgæstə] *n*【希】胃
Gasteromycetes [ˌgæstərə*u*maiˈsiːtiːz] *n* 腹菌纲
Gasterophilus [ˌgæstəˈrɔfiləs] *n* 胃蝇属
gastr- 见 gastro-
gastradenitis [ˌgæstrædiˈnaitis] *n* 胃腺炎
gastralgia [gæsˈtrældʒiə] *n* 胃痛
gastralgokenosis [gæsˌtrælgəkiˈnə*u*sis] *n* 胃空痛
gastramine hydrochloride [ˈgæstrəmin] 盐酸氨乙吡唑,盐酸倍他唑(即 betazole hydrochloride, 诊断胃酸分泌用药)
gastratrophia [ˌgæstrətrə*u*ˈfiːə] *n* 胃萎缩,萎缩性胃炎
gastrectomy [gæsˈtrektəmi] *n* 胃切除术
gastric [ˈgæstrik] *a* 胃的
gastricsin [gæsˈtriksin] *n* 胃亚蛋白酶
gastrin [ˈgæstrin] *n* 促胃液素,胃泌素
gastrinoma [ˌgæstriˈnə*u*mə] *n* 胃泌素瘤
gastritis [gæsˈtraitis] *n* 胃炎 | antral ~, antrum ~ 胃窦炎 / catarrhal ~ 卡他性胃炎 / cirrhotic ~ 硬变性胃炎,皮革状胃 / follicular ~ 滤泡性胃炎,胃腺[泡]炎 / giant hypertrophic ~ 巨大肥厚性胃炎 / phlegmonous ~ 蜂窝织炎性胃炎 / polypous ~ 息肉性胃炎 | **gastritic** [gæsˈtritik] *a*
gastr(o)- [构词成分]胃;腹侧
gastroacephalus [ˌgæstrə*u*eiˈsefələs] *n* 有腹无头寄生畸胎(双胎畸形,其一无头而与另一胎的腹部相联)
gastroadenitis [ˌgæstrə*u*ædiˈnaitis] *n* 胃腺炎
gastroadynamic [ˌgæstrə*u*ˌædaiˈnæmik] *a* 胃无力的
gastroamorphus [ˌgæstrə*u*eiˈmɔːfəs] *n* 腹内寄生畸胎
gastroanastomosis [ˌgæstrə*u*əˌnæstəˈməusis] *n* 胃胃吻合术
gastrocamera [ˌgæstrə*u*ˈkæmərə] *n* 胃内照相机
gastrocardiac [ˌgæstrə*u*ˈkɑːdiæk] *a* 胃心的
gastrocele [ˈgæstrəsiːl] *n* 胃膨出
gastrocnemius [ˌgæstrə*u*ˈniːmiəs] *n* 腓肠肌
gastrocoele [ˈgæstrəsiːl] *n* 原肠
gastrocolic [ˌgæstrə*u*ˈkɔlik] *a* 胃结肠的
gastrocolitis [ˌgæstrə*u*kəˈlaitis] *n* 胃结肠炎
gastrocolostomy [ˌgæstrə*u*kəˈlɔstəmi] *n* 胃结肠吻合术
gastrocolotomy [ˌgæstrə*u*kəˈlɔtəmi] *n* 胃结肠切开术
gastrocutaneous [ˌgæstrə*u*kjuˈteinjəs] *a* 胃皮肤的(如瘘)
gastrocystoplasty [ˌgæstrə*u*ˈsistəˌplæsti] *n* 胃膀胱成形术
gastrodermis [ˌgæstrə*u*ˈdəːmis] *n* 胃皮(无脊椎动物消化道内层)
gastrodiaphane [ˌgæstrə*u*ˈdaiəfein] *n* 胃透照灯
gastrodiaphany [ˌgæstrə*u*daiˈæfəni], **gastrodiaphanoscopy** [ˌgæstrə*u*daiˌæfəˈnɔskəpi] *n* 胃透照镜检查

gastrodidymus [ˌgæstrəu'didiməs] *n* 腹部联胎
gastrodisciasis [ˌgæstrəudis'kaiəsis] *n* 似腹盘吸虫病
Gastrodiscoides [ˌgæstrəudis'kɔidiːz] *n* 似腹盘属 | ~ hominis 人似腹盘吸虫 | **Gastrodiscus** [ˌgæstrəu'diskəs] *n*
gastrodisk ['gæstrədisk] *n* 胚盘
gastroduodenal [ˌgæstrəuˌdju(ː)əu'diːnl] *a* 胃十二指肠的
gastroduodenectomy [ˌgæstrəuˌdju(ː)əudi'nektəmi] *n* 胃十二指肠切除术
gastroduodenitis [ˌgæstrəudju(ː)əudi'naitis] *n* 胃十二指肠炎
gastroduodenoscopy [ˌgæstrəuˌdju(ː)əudi'nɔskəpi] *n* 胃十二指肠镜检查
gastroduodenostomy [ˌgæstrəudju(ː)əudi'nɔstəmi] *n* 胃十二指肠吻合术
gastrodynia [ˌgæstrəu'diniə] *n* 胃痛
gastroenteralgia [ˌgæstrəuˌentə'rældʒiə] *n* 胃肠痛
gastroenteric [ˌgæstrəuen'terik] *a* 胃肠的
gastroenteritis [ˌgæstrəuˌentə'raitis] *n* 胃肠炎 | acute infectious ~ 急性感染性胃肠炎 / eosinophilic ~ 嗜酸细胞性胃肠炎 / Norwalk ~ 诺沃克胃肠炎(由诺沃克病毒所致) / transmissible ~ (T. G. E.) of swine 猪传染性胃肠炎
gastroenteroanastomosis [ˌgæstrəuˌentərəuəˌnæstə'məusis] *n* 胃肠吻合术
gastroenterocolitis [ˌgæstrəuˌentərəukə'laitis] *n* 胃小肠结肠炎
gastroenterocolostomy [ˌgæstrəuˌentərəukə'lɔstəmi] *n* 胃小肠结肠吻合术
gastroenterology [ˌgæstrəuˌentə'rɔlədʒi] *n* 胃肠学 | **gastroenterologist** *n* 胃肠学家
gastroenteropathy [ˌgæstrəuˌentə'rɔpəθi] *n* 胃肠病
gastroenteroplasty [ˌgæstrəu'entərəˌplæsti] *n* 胃肠成形术
gastroenteroptosis [ˌgæstrəuˌentərɔp'təusis] *n* 胃肠下垂
gastroenterostomy [ˌgæstrəuentə'rɔstəmi] *n* 胃肠吻合术
gastroenterotomy [ˌgæstrəuˌentə'rɔtəmi] *n* 胃肠切开术
gastroepiploic [ˌgæstrəuˌepi'pləuik] *a* 胃网膜的
gastroesophageal [ˌgæstrəui(ː)ˌsɔfə'dʒi(ː)əl] *a* 胃食管的
gastroesophagitis [ˌgæstrəui(ː)ˌscfə'dʒaitis] *n* 胃食管炎
gastroesophagostomy [ˌgæstrəui(ː)ˌsɔfə'gɔstəmi] *n* 胃食管吻合术
gastrofiberscope [ˌgæstrəu'faibəskəup] *n* 胃纤维镜
gastrogastrostomy [ˌgæstrəugæs'trɔstəmi] *n* 胃胃吻合术
gastrogavage [ˌgæstrəugə'vɑːʒ] *n* 胃管饲法
gastrogenic [ˌgæstrəu'dʒenik] *a* 胃源性的
gastrograph ['gæstrəgrɑːf, -græf] *n* 胃动描记器
gastrohepatic [ˌgæstrəuhi'pætik] *a* 胃肝的
gastrohepatitis [ˌgæstrəuhepə'taitis] *n* 胃肝炎
gastrohypertonic [ˌgæstrəuhaipə(ː)'tɔnik] *a* 胃张力过度的
gastroileac [ˌgæstrəu'iliæk] *a* 胃回肠的
gastroileitis [ˌgæstrəuili'aitis] *n* 胃回肠炎
gastroileostomy [ˌgæstrəuili'ɔstəmi] *n* 胃回肠吻合术
gastrointestinal [ˌgæstrəuin'testinl] *a* 胃肠的
gastrojejunocolic [ˌgæstrəudʒiˌdʒuːnəu'kɔlik] *a* 胃空肠结肠的
gastrojejunoesophagostomy [ˌgæstrəudʒiˌdʒuːnəui(ː)ˌsɔfə'gɔstəmi] *n* 胃空肠食管吻合术
gastrojejunostomy [ˌgæstrəudʒidʒuː'nɔstəmi] *n* 胃空肠吻合术
gastrokinesograph [ˌgæstrəukai'nesəgrɑːf, -ki'nesəgræf] *n* 胃动描记器
gastrolienal [ˌgæstrəu'laiənəl] *a* 胃脾的
gastrolith ['gæstrəliθ] *n* 胃石
gastrolithiasis [ˌgæstrəuli'θaiəsis] *n* 胃石病
Gastrolobium [ˌgæstrəu'ləubiəm] *n* 豆科植物属
gastrology [gæs'trɔlədʒi] *n* 胃病学 | **gastrologist** *n* 胃病学家
gastrolysis [gæs'trɔlisis] *n* 胃松解术
gastromalacia [ˌgæstrəumə'leiʃiə] *n* 胃软化
gastromegaly [ˌgæstrəu'megəli] *n* 巨胃
gastromelus [gæs'trɔmiləs] *n* 腹部寄生肢畸胎
gastromycosis [ˌgæstrəumai'kəusis] *n* 胃霉菌病
gastromyotomy [ˌgæstrəumai'ɔtəmi] *n* 胃肌切开术,幽门切开术
gastromyxorrhea [ˌgæstrəuˌmiksə'riːə] *n* 胃黏液溢
gastrone ['gæstrəun] *n* 抑胃素
gastronesteostomy [ˌgæstrəuˌnesti'ɔstəmi] *n* 胃空肠吻合术
gastropancreatitis [ˌgæstrəuˌpæŋkriə'taitis] *n* 胃胰[腺]炎
gastroparalysis [ˌgæstrəupə'rælisis] *n* 胃麻痹
gastroparesis [ˌgæstrəupə'riːsis] *n* 胃轻瘫
gastroparietal [ˌgæstrəupə'raiitl] *a* 胃腹壁的
gastropathy [gæs'trɔpəθi] *n* 胃病 | **gastropathic** [ˌgæstrə'pæθik] *a*
gastropericardial [ˌgæstrəuˌperi'kɑːdiəl] *a* 胃心包的
gastroperiodynia [ˌgæstrəuˌperiəu'diniə] *n* 周期

性胃痛

gastroperitonitis [ˌgæstrəuˌperitəˈnaitis] *n* 胃腹膜炎

gastropexy [ˈgæstrəˌpeksi] *n* 胃固定术

Gastrophilus [gæsˈtrɔfiləs] *n* 胃蝇属(即 Gasterophilus)

gastrophotography [ˌgæstrəufəˈtɔgrəfi] *n* 胃内照相术

gastrophotor [ˌgæstrəuˈfəutə] *n* 胃内照相器,胃内照相装置

gastrophrenic [ˌgæstrəuˈfrenik] *a* 胃膈的

gastrophthisis [gæstrəuˈθisis] *n* 增殖性胃壁胞厚;腹病性消瘦

gastroplasty [ˈgæstrəˌplæsti] *n* 胃成形术

gastroplegia [ˌgæstrəuˈpliːdʒiə] *n* 胃麻痹,胃瘫

gastroplication [ˌgæstrəupliˈkeiʃən] *n* 胃折叠术

gastropneumonic [ˌgæstrəunju(ː)ˈmɔnik], **gastropulmonary** [ˌgæstrəuˈpʌlmənəri] *a* 胃[与]肺的

gastropod [ˈgæstrəpɔd] *n* 腹足纲软体动物

Gastropoda [gæsˈtrɔpədə] *n* 腹足纲

gastroptosis [ˌgæstrɔpˈtəusis] *n* 胃下垂

gastropylorectomy [ˌgæstrəuˌpailəˈrektəmi] *n* 胃幽门切除术

gastropyloric [ˌgæstrəupaiˈlɔrik] *a* 胃幽门的

gastroradiculitis [ˌgæstrəurəˌdikjuˈlaitis] *n* 胃神经根炎

gastrorrhagia [ˌgæstrəuˈreidʒiə] *n* 胃出血

gastrorrhaphy [gæsˈtrɔrəfi] *n* 胃缝合术

gastrorrhea [ˌgæstrəuˈriːə] *n* 胃液溢,胃液分泌过多

gastrorrhexis [ˌgæstrəuˈreksis] *n* 胃破裂

gastroschisis [gæsˈtrɔskisis] *n* 腹裂[畸形]

gastroscope [ˈgæstrəskəup] *n* 胃镜 | fiberoptic ~ 光导纤维胃镜 | **gastroscopic** [ˌgæstrəˈskɔpik] *a* 胃镜的;胃镜检查的 / **gastroscopist** [gæsˈtrɔskəpist] *n* 胃镜医师 / **gastroscopy** [gæsˈtrɔskəpi] *n* 胃镜检查[术]

gastroselective [ˌgæstrəusiˈlektiv] *a* 胃选择性的(对调节胃活动的受体有亲和力的)

gastrosia [gæsˈtrəusiə] *n* 胃病 | ~ fungosa 真菌性胃病

gastrosis [gæsˈtrəusis] *n* 胃病

gastrospasm [ˈgæstrəspæzəm] *n* 胃痉挛

gastrospiry [ˈgæstrəˌspaiəri] *n* 吞气症

gastrosplenic [ˌgæstrəuˈsplenik] *a* 胃脾的

gastrostaxis [ˌgæstrəuˈstæksis] *n* 胃渗血

gastrostenosis [ˌgæstrəustiˈnəusis] *n* 胃狭窄

gastrostogavage [gæsˌtrɔstəgəˈvɑːʒ] *n* 胃瘘管饲法

gastrostolavage [gæsˌtrɔstələˈvɑːʒ] *n* 胃瘘注洗法

gastrostoma [ˌgæsˈtrɔstəmə] *n* 胃瘘

gastrostomy [gæsˈtrɔstəmi], **gastrostomosis** [gæsˌtrɔstəˈməusis] *n* 胃造口术

gastrosuccorrhea [ˌgæstrəuˌsʌkəˈriːə] *n* 持续性胃液分泌过多 | digestive ~ 消化性胃液溢,消化期胃液分泌过多

gastrothoracopagus [ˌgæstrəuˌθɔːrəˈkɔpəgəs] *n* 腹胸联胎 | ~ dipygus 双臀腹胸联胎

gastrotome [ˈgæstrətəum] *n* 胃刀

gastrotomy [gæsˈtrɔtəmi] *n* 胃切开术

gastrotonometer [ˌgæstrəutəuˈnɔmitə] *n* 胃内压测量器 | **gastrotonometry** *n* 胃内压测量法

gastrotoxin [ˌgæstrəuˈtɔksin] *n* 胃毒素

Gastrotricha [ˌgæstrəˈtrikə] *n* 腹毛纲

gastrotropic [ˌgæstrəuˈtrɔpik] *a* 亲胃的

gastrotympanites [ˌgæstrəuˌtimpəˈnaitiːz] *n* 胃积气,胃鼓胀

gastrula [ˈgæstrulə] ([复] **gastrulae** [ˈgæstruliː]或 **gastrulas**) *n* 原肠胚

gastrulation [ˌgæstruˈleiʃən] *n* 原肠胚形成

Gatch bed [gætʃ] (Willis D. Gatch) 盖奇床(一种活动靠背床)

gate [geit] *n* 门电路,闸门;(细胞膜)通道 *vi* 选择开关

gatifloxacin [ˌgætiˈflɔksəsin] *n* 加氟沙星(抗菌药)

gating [ˈgeitiŋ] *n* 门控;选通(门电路电子信号的选择);门控作用,闸门作用;感觉门控

gatism [ˈgeitizəm] *n* 大小便失禁

gatophobia [ˌgætəuˈfəubiə] *n* 猫恐怖,恐猫症

gattine [ˈgætiːn] *n* 蚕腐败病

Gaucher's cells [gəuˈʃei] (Phillippe C. E. Gaucher) 戈谢细胞(见于戈谢病的脾等) | ~ disease (splenomegaly) 戈谢病(脾大)(一种葡糖脑苷脂代谢的遗传病,特征为骨髓内有戈谢细胞以及脾、肝肿大、骨畸形等。亦称家族性脾性贫血、角苷脂贮积病、脑苷脂沉积症)

gauge [geidʒ] *n* 表;规,量规;计,计器 *vt* (用量具)量,测量,测定 | catheter ~ 导管径计 | **~able** *a* 可计量的,可测量的 / **~r** *n* 计量器

Gaultheria [gɔːlˈθiəriə] (Jean F. Gaultier) *n* 白珠树属

gauntlet [ˈgɔːntlit] *n* 长手套,防护手套;手套形绷带

gauss [gaus] (Johann K. F. Gauss) *n* 高斯(旧磁通量密度单位,现用 T〈特[斯拉]〉,1 G = 10^{-4} T,符号为 G)

gaussian curve [ˈgauʃən] (J. K. F. Gauss) 高斯曲线(正态分布曲线) | ~ distribution 高斯分布(正态分布)

Gauvain's fluid [gəu'vein] (Ernest A. Gauvain) 戈维恩液(脓胸洗涤液)

gauze [gɔːz] *n* 薄纱,纱布 | absorbable ~ 可吸收纱布 / absorbent ~ 脱脂纱布,吸水纱布 / petrolatum ~ 凡士林纱布 / sterile absorbent ~ 无菌脱脂纱布

gavage [gə'vɑːʒ] *n*【法】管饲法(强制喂食,尤指由管灌入胃内);超量营养疗法

Gavard's muscle [gə'vɑː] (Hyacinthe Gavard) 加瓦尔肌(胃壁斜行肌层)

gay [gei] *a* (男子)同性恋的 *n* 同性恋者

Gay-Lussac's law [ˌgei ljuː'sɑːk] (Joseph L. Gay-Lussac) 盖·吕萨克定律(见 Charles' law)

Gay's glands [gei] (Alexander H. Gay) 肛周腺

Gaza's operation ['gɑːzɑː] (Wilhelm von Gaza) 神经支切断术

gaze [geiz] *vi*, *n* 凝视,注视 | conjugate ~ 共轭凝视,同向性凝视

GBG glycine-rich β glycoprotein 富甘氨酸 β 糖蛋白(B 因子的旧称)

GBGase glycine-rich β glycoproteinase 富甘氨酸 β 糖蛋白酶

GBM glomerular basement membrane 肾小球基膜

GC gas chromatography 气相色谱法,气相层析

g-cal. gram calorie 克卡(小卡)

G-CSF granulocyte colony-stimulating factor 粒细胞集落刺激因子

Gd gadolinium 钆

GDH glutamic acid dehydrogenase 谷氨酸脱氢酶

GDM gestational diabetes mellitus 妊娠糖尿病

GDP guanosine diphosphate 鸟苷二磷酸

Ge germanium 锗

gear [giə] *n* 用具,装备 | cervical ~ 颈托 / head ~ 头帽

Geaster [dʒi'æstə] *n* 地星属

geeldikkop [giːl'dikɔp] *n*【荷】羊蒺藜中毒

Gee's disease, Gee-Herter disease, Gee-Herter-Heubner disease, syndrome [giː 'həːtə 'hɔibnə] (Samuel J. Gee; Christian A. Herter; Otto L. Heubner) 婴儿型乳糜泻

Gee-Thaysen disease ['giː 'θaisən] (S. J. Gee; T. E. H. Thaysen) 成人型乳糜泻

Gegenbauer's cells ['geigənˌbauə] (Carl Gegenbaur) 成骨细胞

gegenhalten [ˌgeigən'hɔltən] *n*【德】非自主抗拒(如可能发生于大脑皮质疾病)

Geigel's reflex ['gaigəl] (Richard Geigel) 盖格尔反射,腹股沟反射(女性与男性提睾反射相似的反射,即打击大腿内前侧引起腹股沟韧带上缘处的肌纤维收缩)

Geiger counter, Geiger-Müller counter ['gaigə-'milə] (Hans W. Geiger; Walther Müller) 盖革(离子)计数器,盖革-米勒[离子]计数器

Geissler's test ['gaislə] (Ernst Geissler) 盖斯勒试验(检尿白蛋白)

Geissler's tube ['gaislə] (Heinrich Geissler) 盖斯勒管(经由稀薄气体,显示放电发光效果的放电管)

Geissospermum [ˌgaisəu'spiːrəm] *n* 夹竹桃属

gel [dʒel] *n* 凝胶;凝胶剂 *vi* 形成凝胶,胶化 | aluminum hydroxide ~ 氢氧化铝凝胶 / aluminum phosphate ~ 磷酸铝凝胶 / corticotropin ~ 促肾上腺皮质激素凝胶

gelase ['dʒeleis] *n* 琼脂酶

gelasmus [dʒi'læsməs] *n* 痴笑,歇斯底里性痴笑

gelastic [dʒi'læstik] *a* 痴笑的

gelate ['dʒeleit] *vi* 形成凝胶

gelatification [dʒeˌlætifi'keiʃən] *n* 凝胶[作用],胶体形成

gelatigenous [ˌdʒelə'tidʒənəs] *a* 产胶的,成胶的

gelatin ['dʒelətin] *n* 明胶 | agar ~ 琼脂明胶 / glycerinated ~ 甘油胶 / Japanese ~ 琼脂,洋粉 / lactose litmus ~ 乳糖石蕊明胶(培养基) / litmus ~ 石蕊明胶(培养基) / litmus whey ~ 石蕊乳清明胶(培养基) / meat extract ~ 肉汁明胶(培养基) / medicated ~ 含药明胶 / silk ~ 丝胶(蛋白) / vegetable ~ 植物胶 / whey ~ 乳清胶 / wort ~ 麦芽汁明胶(培养基) / zinc ~ 锌明胶

gelatinase [dʒi'lætineis] *n* 明胶酶

gelatiniferous [ˌdʒeləti'nifərəs] *a* 产胶的

gelatinize [dʒi'lætinaiz] *vt*, *vi* 凝胶化,胶凝 | **gelatinization** [dʒiˌlætinai'zeiʃən, -ni'z-] *n*

gelatinoid [dʒi'lætinɔid] *a* 胶状的,明胶样的

gelatinolytic [ˌdʒelətinə'litik] *a* 明胶分解的

gelatinosa [ˌdʒeləti'nəusə] *n*【拉】胶状质

gelatinous [dʒi'lætinəs] *a* 凝胶的,胶状的

gelatinum [dʒelə'tainəm] *n*【拉】[白]明胶

gelation [dʒi'leiʃən] *n* 胶凝作用

gelatose ['dʒelətəus] *n* 明胶胨

gelatum [dʒi'leitəm] *n*【拉】凝胶,胶冻

geld [geld] (gelded 或 gelt) *vt* 阉割(动物,尤指阉割马的睾丸)

gelding ['geldiŋ] *n* 阉畜(尤指阉马)

gelidusi [ˌgeili'dusi] *n* 皮里迪西指数(见 pelidisi)

Gélineau's syndrome [ʒeili'nəu] (Jean B. E. Gélineau) 发作性睡病

Gell and Coombs classification [dʒel kuːmz] (Philip G. H. Gell; Robert R. A. Coombs) 杰尔-库姆斯分类法(一种组织损伤的免疫机制分类法,杰尔和库姆斯称之为"变应性反应",包括 4 种类型:Ⅰ型为速发型超敏反应,Ⅱ型为细胞性反应,Ⅲ型为由免疫复合物介导的反应,Ⅳ型为迟发型超敏反应)

gelometer [ɡe'lɔmitə] *n* 凝胶形成计时仪
gelose ['dʒeləus] *n* 琼脂糖
gelosis [dʒi'ləusis] ([复]**geloses** [dʒi'ləusiːz]) *n* 凝块,硬块(尤指肌组织内的凝块)
gelotherapy [ˌdʒeləu'θerəpi], **gelototherapy** [ˌdʒelətəu'θerəpi] *n* 欢笑疗法(引笑以治病)
gelotripsy ['dʒeləˌtripsi] *n* 硬肌缓解术(用按摩使肌组织硬块消散)
Gel. quav. gelatina quavis【拉】任何[一种]凝胶
gelsemine ['dʒelsəmiːn] *n* 钩吻素甲,钩吻碱(中枢神经系统兴奋药,有中毒的副作用,如复视、肌无力、呼吸停止)
Gelsemium [ɡel'semiəm] *n* 钩吻属,断肠草属
gelsolin [dʒel'sɔlin] *n* 凝溶胶蛋白
Gély's suture [ʒei'li] (Jules A. Gély) 惹利缝术(肠管创口连续缝合术)
gemästete [ɡe'meʃtetə] *a*【德】肿大的,肿胀的(指变性区肿胀的星形细胞)
gemcadiol [ˌdʒemkə'daiɔl] *n* 四甲癸二醇(抗高脂蛋白血症药)
gemcitabine hydrochloride [dʒem'sitəbiːn] 盐酸吉西他滨(抗肿瘤药,化疗时用于治胰腺癌,静脉输注给药)
Gemella [dʒi'melə] *n* 孪生球菌属 | ~ haemolysans 溶血孪生球菌
gemellary ['dʒemiləri] *a* 双生子的
gemellipara [ˌdʒemə'lipərə] *n* 双胎产妇
gemellology [ˌdʒemə'lɔlədʒi] *n* 双胎学,双胎研究
gemfibrozil [dʒem'fibrəzil] *n* 吉非贝齐(降血脂药)
geminate ['dʒeminit] *a* 成双的 ['dʒemineit] *vt*, *vi* 成双 | **gemination** [ˌdʒemi'neiʃən] *n* 成双,成对;双生牙,并生牙
geminous ['dʒeminəs] *a* 成双的
geminus ['dʒeminəs] ([复] **gemini** ['dʒeminai]) *n*【拉】双胎,双生子
gemistocyte [dʒə'mistəsait] *n* 饲肥星形细胞 | **gemistocytic** [dʒəˌmistə'sitik] *a*
gemma ['dʒemə] ([复] **gemmae** ['dʒemiː]) *n* 胞芽,芽;芽胞(真菌),芽孢
gemmangioma [ˌdʒemændʒi'əumə] *n* 胚芽血管瘤
gemmate ['dʒemit] *a* 有芽的,出芽生殖的 [dʒe'meit] *vi* 出芽生殖,芽生 | **gemmation** [dʒe'meiʃən] *n* 出芽生殖,芽生
Gemminges [dʒə'mindʒiːz] *n* 芽胞球菌属
gemmule ['dʒemjuːl] *n* 胚芽,芽球;树突棘(神经细胞)芽突;泛子(一种假想的遗传单位,由体细胞脱出而储存在生殖细胞内,以决定某一性状的发生)
gemtuzumab ozogamicin [ɡem'təuzəumæb ˌəuzəuɡə'maisin] 吉妥单抗奥唑霉素(抗肿瘤药)
-gen [构词成分]原
genal ['dʒiːnl] *a* 颊的
gender ['dʒendə] *n* 性;性别
gene [dʒiːn] *n* 基因(遗传的生物单位,位于染色体上特定位点并可进行自身复制) | allelic ~s 等位基因(位于一对染色体内对应位点的基因) / amorphic ~ 无效[等位]基因(见 amorph 及 mutant gene) / cell interaction (CI) ~s 细胞相互作用基因 / codominant ~s 等显性基因 / complementary ~s, reciprocal ~s 互补基因(两对独立的非等位基因,一对不存在,则另一对不表现其效应) / ~ complex 基因复合体 / cumulative ~s 累积基因,多基因 / derepressed ~ 去阻遏基因 / dominant ~ 显性基因(机体内产生一定效应〈表型〉的基因) / H ~, histocompatibility ~ H基因,组织相容性基因 / holandric ~s 全雄基因,限雄基因(存在于 Y 染色体上的非同型部位的基因) / hologynic ~s 全雌基因(位于 X 染色体上的基因) / immune response (Ir) ~s 免疫应答基因 / immune suppressor (Is) ~s 免疫抑制基因 / immunoglobulin ~s 免疫球蛋白基因 / Ir ~s 免疫应答基因(即 immune response ~s) / Is ~s 免疫抑制基因(即 immune suppressor ~s) / leaky ~ 渗漏基因(一种突变基因,见 mutant gene) / lethal ~ 致死基因 / major ~ 主基因 / modifying ~s 修饰基因,修饰因子(modifying factors,见 factor 项下相应术语) / mutant ~ 突变基因(由突变所引起基因物质的缺少、增加或交换,导致基因功能永久可遗传的变异。如果导致基因功能失效,即称无效等位基因〈amorph〉,如果导致阻抑正常活动,即称为反效等位基因〈antimorph〉,如增加正常活动,即称超效等位基因〈hypermorph〉,如稍减弱正常活动,即称渗漏基因〈leaky gene〉或亚效等位基因〈hypomorph〉) / nonstructural ~s 非结构基因(指操纵基因和调节基因) / operator ~ 操纵基因(用作读遗传密码的起点,并通过与阻抑物的相互作用以控制与其相连的结构基因的活动) / pleiotropic ~ 多效基因 / recessive ~ 隐性基因(只有在父母双方均有遗传,即只有在个体是纯合子情况下才表现出来的基因) / regulator ~, regulatory ~ 调节基因(产生阻抑物并通过与操纵基因相互作用控制与其相连的结构基因的活动) / repressed ~ 阻遏基因 / repressor ~ 阻抑基因(即 regulator ~) / sex-conditioned ~, sex-influenced ~ 从性基因(只在一个性别中充分表现出来的基因,如人的秃顶) / sex-limited ~ 限性基因(只在一个性别上产生效应的基因) / sex-linked ~ 性连锁基因(在 X 染色体或 Y 染色体上的基因) / silent ~ 沉默基因(一种第三等位基因,用以说明完全缺乏一种特殊酶活性,例如胆碱酯酶活性) / structural ~ 结构基因(排

列多肽链氨基酸顺序的基因) / sublethal ~ 亚致死基因(使机体的功能受到阻碍或损害的基因) / supplementary ~s 补加基因(两对独立的基因,其互相作用的方式为:其中一对显性基因可以在另一对基因不存在的情况下发挥其功效,可是另一对基因却一定要在前一对基因存在的情况下,才能发挥效能) / suppressor ~ 抑制基因 / syntenic ~s 同线基因 / taster ~ 尝味[者]基因(影响尝苯硫脲苦味能力的基因) / wildtype ~ 野生型基因(突变基因的正常等位基因,有时用 + 符号表示之) / X-linked ~ X 连锁基因(存在于女性 X 染色体上的基因,一般即指性连锁基因,因与 Y 染色体有关的基因尚未显示出遗传性的缺陷)

genealogical [ˌdʒiːnjəˈlɔdʒikəl] *a* 家系的;系统的

genealogy [ˌdʒiːniˈælədʒi] *n* 家系,血统;家系学,系谱学 | **genealogist** *n* 家系学家,系谱学家

geneogenous [ˌdʒiːniˈɔdʒinəs] *a* 先天性的

genera [ˈdʒenərə] genus 的复数

generalization [ˌdʒenərəlaiˈzeiʃən, -liˈz-] *n* 泛化(指条件形成后,非条件刺激物予以刺激也会引起条件反射的现象)

generalize [ˈdʒenərəlaiz] *vi* 泛化,扩散,全身化(指自局部病转变为全身病)

generation [ˌdʒenəˈreiʃən] *n* 生殖;代;世代 | alternate ~ 世代交替 / asexual ~, direct ~, nonsexual ~ 无性世代 / first filial ~ 第一代,第一子代,子$_1$ 代 / parental ~ 亲代 / second filial ~ 第二代,第二子代,子$_2$ 代 / sexual ~ 有性世代 / spontaneous ~ 自然发生,非生物起源;无生源说

generative [ˈdʒenərətiv] *a* 生殖的;发生的

generator [ˈdʒenəreitə] *n* 发生器 | pulse ~ 脉冲发生器

generic [dʒiˈnerik] *a* 属的,非专利的

genesial [dʒiˈniziəl], **genesic** [dʒiˈnesik] *a* 生殖的;发生的

genesiology [dʒiˌniziˈɔlədʒi] *n* 生殖学

genesis [ˈdʒenisis] ([复] **geneses** [ˈdʒenisiːz]) *n* 起源,发生;生殖

genesistasis [ˌdʒeniˈsistəsis] *n* 生殖制止[法] | **genestatic** [ˌdʒenisˈtætik] *a* 制止生殖的

genetic [dʒiˈnetik] *a* 遗传的;发生的;生殖的

genetically modified food 转基因食品

genetics [dʒiˈnetiks] *n* 遗传学 | bacterial ~ 细菌遗传学 / biochemical ~ 生化遗传学 / clinical ~ 临床遗传学 / mathematical ~ 数学遗传学 / molecular ~ 分子遗传学 / population ~ 群体遗传学 / reverse ~ 反求遗传学 | **geneticist** [dʒiˈnetisist] *n* 遗传学家

genetotrophic [dʒiˌnetəˈtrɔfik] *a* 遗传性营养的

genetous [ˈdʒinətəs] *a* 先天的,生来的(始于胎生期的)

Geneva Convention [dʒiˈniːvə] 日内瓦公约(1864 年一种国际协定,在战场上凡负伤者及医护人员均应按中立者对待)

Gengou's phenomenon [ʒɑːnˈguː] (Octave Gengou) 让古现象,补体结合(fixation of the complement,见 fixation 项下相应术语)

genial [dʒiˈnaiəl], **genian** [dʒiˈnaiən] *a* 颏的

genic [ˈdʒenik] *a* 基因的

-genic [构词成分]产生,生产

genicular [dʒəˈnikjulə] *a* 膝的

geniculate [dʒəˈnikjulit], **geniculated** [dʒəˈnikjuleitid] *a* 膝状的

geniculocalcarine [dʒəˌnikjuləuˈkælkərin] *a* 膝状体禽距状的(连接膝状体与禽距或距状沟的)

geniculostriate [dʒəˌnikjuləuˈstraieit] *a* 膝状体纹状体的(连接膝状体核与纹状皮质的)

geniculum [dʒəˈnikjuləm] ([复] **genicula** [dʒəˈnikjulə]) *n*【拉】膝,小膝 | ~ of facial canal 面神经管膝 / ~ of facial nerve 面神经膝

genin [ˈdʒenin] *n* 配基,糖苷配基

geni(o)- [构词成分]颏(同样见以 mento-起始的词)

geniocheiloplasty [ˌdʒiːniəuˈkailəˌplæsti] *n* 颏唇成形术,颏唇整形术

genioglossus [ˌdʒiːniəuˈglɔsəs] *n* 颏舌肌

geniohyoglossus [ˌdʒiːniəuˌhaiəuˈglɔsəs] *n* 颏舌骨舌肌,颏舌肌

geniohyoid [ˌdʒiːniəuˈhaiɔid] *a* 颏舌骨的 *n* 颏舌骨肌

geniohyoideus [ˌdʒiːniəuhaiˈɔidiəs] *n* 颏舌骨肌

genioplasty [ˈdʒiːniəuˌplæsti] *n* 颏成形术

genital [ˈdʒenitl] *a* 生殖的;生殖器的 *n* [复]生殖器

genitalia [ˌdʒeniˈteiliə] [复] *n*【拉】生殖器 | external ~ 外生殖器 / indifferent ~ 未分化生殖器 / internal ~ 内生殖器

genitaloid [ˈdʒenitəlɔid] *a* (定性前)原生殖细胞的

genit(o)- [构词成分]生殖,生殖器

genitocrural [ˌdʒenitəuˈkruərəl], **genitofemoral** [ˌdʒenitəuˈfemərəl] *a* 生殖股的

genitography [ˌdʒeniˈtɔgrəfi] *n* 泌尿生殖窦 X 线造影[术]

genitoinfectious [ˌdʒenitəuinˈfekʃəs] *a* 性病的

genitoplasty [ˈdʒenitəˌplæsti] *n* 生殖器成形术

genitourinary [ˌdʒenitəuˈjuərinəri] *a* 生殖泌尿器的;生殖泌尿的,泌尿生殖的

genius [ˈdʒiːnjəs] ([复] **geniuses** 或 **genii** [ˈdʒiːniai]) *n* 特征;天才,天资 | ~ epidemicus

流行病特征(关于自然条件对流行性传染病影响的学说) / ~ loci (肿瘤转移)部位特征 / ~ morbi 疾病特征

Gennari's line (band, layer, stria, stripe) [dʒeˈnɑːri] (Francisco Gennari) 詹纳里线(带,层,纹,条纹)(楔叶皮质外白带)

gen(o)- [构词成分]生殖,性

genoblast [ˈdʒenəblæst] *n* 受胎卵核;成熟性细胞

genocide [ˈdʒenəusaid] *n* 种族灭绝 | **genocidal** [ˌdʒenəuˈsaidl] *a*

genocopy [ˈdʒenəˌkɔpi] *n* 拟基因型(一个个体的表现型模拟另一基因的表现型,但它的特征是由另外一套明显的基因所决定的)

genodermatology [ˌdʒenəuˌdəːməˈtɔlədʒi] *n* 遗传性皮肤病学

genodermatosis [ˌdʒenəudəːməˈtəusis] *n* 遗传性皮肤病

genome [ˈdʒiːnəum] *n* 基因组(一个染色体上所蕴藏的全部基因) | **genomic** [dʒiˈnɔmik] *a*

genomics [dʒiˈnɔmiks] *n* 基因组学

genopathy [ˈdʒenəupæθi] *n* 基因病

genophobia [ˌdʒenəuˈfəubiə] *n* 性恐怖

genospecies [ˈdʒiːnəuspiːʃiːz] *n* 基因种,基因型群(一群菌种能进行基因转移和基因重组)

genotoxic [ˌdʒenəuˈtɔksik] *a* 基因毒性的(损害 DNA 的)

genotype [ˈdʒenətaip] *n* 基因型(一个个体的全部基因组成,亦指在一个或几个特定位点上的等位基因);属模式种,属典型种 | **genotypic (al)** [ˌdʒenəuˈtipik(əl)] *a* / **genotypically** *ad*

-genous [构词成分]产生,发生;被产生

Gensoul's disease [ʒɑːnˈsuːl] (Joseph Gensoul) 让苏尔病(见 Ludwig's angina)

gentamicin, gentamycia [ˌdʒentəˈmaisin] *n* 艮他霉素,庆大霉素(抗生素类药) | ~ sulfate 硫酸庆大霉素

gentian [ˈdʒenʃiən] *n* 龙胆 | ~ violet 甲紫,龙胆紫(消毒防腐药)

gentianophil [ˈdʒenʃənəufil] *n* 嗜龙胆紫素 *a* 嗜龙胆紫的

gentianophilic [ˌdʒenʃənəuˈfilik], **gentianophilous** [ˌdʒenʃəˈnɔfiləs] *a* 嗜龙胆紫的

gentianophobic [ˌdʒenʃənəuˈfəubik], **gentianophobous** [ˌdʒenʃəˈnɔfəbəs] *a* 拒龙胆紫的

gentianose [ˈdʒeʃənəus] *n* 龙胆三糖

gentiavern [ˈdʒenʃəvəːn] *n* 龙胆紫

gentiopicrin [ˌdʒenʃiəuˈpikrin] *n* 龙胆苦苷

gentiotannic acid [ˌdʒenʃiəuˈtænik] 龙胆鞣酸

gentisate [ˈdʒentiseit] *n* 龙胆酸盐

gentisic acid [dʒenˈtisik] 龙胆酸(解热镇痛药)

gentrogenin [ˌdʒentrəuˈdʒenin] *n* 静特诺皂苷元(见 botogenin)

genu [ˈdʒiːnjuː] ([复]**genua** [ˈdʒenjuə]) *n*【拉】膝;膝状体 | ~ valgum 膝外翻 / ~ varum 膝内翻,弓形腿 | **~al** [ˈdʒenjuəl] *a* 膝的;膝状的

genuclast [ˈdʒenjuklæst] *n* 膝关节粘连松解器

genucubital [ˌdʒenjuˈkjuːbitl] *a* 膝[与]肘的

genufacial [ˌdʒenjuˈfeiʃəl] *a* 膝[与]面的

genupectoral [ˌdʒenjuˈpektərəl] *a* 膝[与]胸的

genus [ˈdʒiːnəs] ([复]**genuses** 或 **genera** [ˈdʒenərə]) *n*【拉】属(生物分类)

geny- [构词成分]颌,颊

-geny [构词成分]世代,起源

genyantralgia [ˌdʒeniænˈtrældʒiə] *n* 上颌窦痛

genyantritis [ˌdʒeniænˈtraitis] *n* 上颌窦炎

genyantrum [ˌdʒeniˈæntrəm] *n* 上颌窦

geo- [构词成分]土,地

geobiology [ˌdʒiːəubaiˈɔlədʒi] *n* 陆地生物学

geochemistry [ˌdʒiːəuˈkemistri] *n* 地球化学

Geocyclus [ˌdʒiːəuˈsaikləs] *n* 丝环菌属

geode [ˈdʒiːəud] *n* 淋巴腔

Geodermatophilus [ˌdʒiːəuˌdəːməˈtɔfiləs] *n* 地嗜皮菌属

geogen [ˈdʒiːədʒən] *n* 地区(致病)因素,风土(致病)因素

geographic [dʒiəˈgræfik] *a* 地理的;地区性的

geomedicine [ˌdʒiːəuˈmedisin] *n* 风土医学

geopathology [ˌdʒiːəupəˈθɔlədʒi] *n* 风土病理学

geophagia [dʒiəˈfeidʒiə], **geophagism** [dʒiˈɔfədʒizəm], **geophagy** [dʒiˈɔfədʒi], **geotragia** [ˌdʒiːəuˈtreidʒiə] *n* 食土癖

geophagist [dʒiˈɔfədʒist] *n* 食土癖者

geophilic [ˌdʒiːəuˈfilik] *a* 亲土的,适土的

Georgi's test [geiˈɔːgi] (Walter Georgo) 格奥尔吉试验(见 Sachs-Georgi test)

geotaxis [ˌdʒiːəuˈtæksis] *n* 趋地性 | **geotactic** [ˌdʒiːəuˈtæktik] *a*

geotrichosis [ˌdʒiːəutraiˈkəusis] *n* 地霉病

Geotrichum [dʒiˈɔtrikəm] *n* 地霉属

geotropic [ˌdʒiːəuˈtrɔpik] *a* 向地的 | **~ally** *ad*

geotropism [dʒiˈɔtrəpizəm] *n* 向地性

Geraghty's test [ˈgerəti] (John T Geraghty) 酚磺酞试验(检肾功能)

geraniol [dʒiˈreiniɔl] *n* 牻牛儿醇;信息素,外激素(电工蜂分泌,发送食物位置的信号)

geratic [dʒiˈrætik] *a* 老年的

Gerbich blood group [ˈgəːbitʃ] (从 1960 年首次观察到的美国先证者得名)格比奇血型(含有红细胞抗原 Ge1、Ge2 和 Ge3 的一种血型,世界大部分地区罕见,但常见于巴布亚新几内亚)

gerbil [ˈdʒəːbil] *n* 沙土鼠(非洲及亚洲西南部传播鼠疫的啮齿动物)

Gerbillus [dʒəː'biləs] *n* 沙土鼠属

GERD gastroesophageal reflux disease 胃食管反流病

Gerdy's fibers [ʒə'di] (Pierre N. Gerdy) 惹迪纤维(手指浅横韧带) | ~ fontanel 惹迪囟,矢囟(矢状缝内) / ~ hyoid fossa 惹迪舌骨窝,颈动脉三角 / ~ interauricular loop 惹迪房间襻(房中隔肌束) / ~ ligament 腋窝悬韧带

gereology [ˌdʒeri'ɔlədʒi], **geratology** [ˌdʒərə'tɔlədʒi] *n* 老年医学,老年病学,老人学

Gerhardt's disease ['gəːhʌt] (Carl A. C. J. Gerhardt) 红斑性肢痛病 | ~ sign (phenomenon) 格哈特征(现象)(见 Biermer's sign) / ~ test (reaction) 格哈特试验(反应)(检尿中丙酮)

Gerhardt-Semon's law ['gəːhʌt 'siːmɔn] (Carl A. C. J. Gerhardt; Felix Semon) 格哈特-西蒙定律(多种神经末梢损害和中枢损害,因影响喉返神经,以致声带的位置介于外展与内收之间,其麻痹并不完全)

Gerhardt's test ['gəːhʌt] (Charles F. Gerhardt) 格哈特试验(检尿中乙酰乙酸、胆色素)

geriatrics [ˌdʒeri'ætriks] *n* 老年医学 | dental ~ 老年口腔医学 | **geriatric** *a* / **geriatrician** [ˌdʒeriə'triʃən], **geriatrist** [ˌdʒeri'ætrist] *n* 老年病学家

geriodontics [ˌdʒeriə*u*'dɔntiks] *n* 老年口腔医学 | **geriodontist** [ˌdʒeriə*u*'dɔntist] *n* 老年口腔医学家

geriopsychosis [ˌdʒeriə*u*sai'kəusis] *n* 老年[期]精神病

Gerlach's network ['gəːlʌh] (Joseph von Gerlach) 格拉赫网(脊髓神经节细胞树状突的一种明显的但不是真的网织) | ~ valve 阑尾瓣

Gerlier's disease [ʒəli'ei] (Felix Gerlier) 惹利埃病(地方性麻痹性眩晕) | ~ syndrome 惹利埃综合征(①地方性麻痹性眩晕;②耳部带状疱疹)

germ [dʒəːm] *n* 病菌;芽胞;胚;胚原基,胚芽 | dental ~ 牙胚 / enamel ~ 釉胚 / hair ~ 毛基质,毛芽 / tooth ~ 牙胚 / wheat ~ 小麦胚(内含生育酚、硫胺、核黄素和其他维生素)

germanium (Ge) [dʒəː'meiniəm] *n* 锗(化学元素)

germerine ['dʒəːməriːn] *n* 胚芽儿碱,计莫林(一种晶体生物碱)

germicidal [ˌdʒəːmi'saidl] *a* 杀菌的

germicide ['dʒəːmisaid] *n* 杀菌剂

germinal ['dʒəːminl] *a* 胚的;生发的;原始的

germinate ['dʒəːmineit] *vi, vt* 出芽,生芽,发芽 | **germination** [ˌdʒəːmi'neiʃən] *n* / **germinative** *a* 出芽的,生发的

germinoma [ˌdʒəːmi'nəumə] *n* 生殖细胞瘤(如精原细胞瘤)

germitrine ['dʒəːmitriːn] *n* 胚芽春,计米特林(从绿藜芦分离的一种抗高血压生物碱)

germline, germ line ['dʒəːmlain] 种系

germogen ['dʒəːmədʒən] *n* 胚原浆

ger(o)- [构词成分]老年,老人

gerocomia [ˌdʒerə*u*'kəumiə], **gerocomy** ['dʒerəˌkəumi] *n* 老年摄生法,老年保健

geroderma [dʒerə*u*'dəːmə], **gerodermia** [dʒerə*u*'dəːmiə] *n* 老年状皮肤,老年样皮肤营养不良 | ~ osteodysplastica 骨发育不良性老年状皮肤(亦称沃尔特·迪斯尼侏儒症〈Walt Disney dwarfism〉)

gerodontics [ˌdʒerə*u*'dɔntiks], **gerodontia** [ˌdʒerə*u*'dɔnʃiə] *n* 老年口腔医学(指老年牙齿问题的诊断、预防和治疗) | **gerodontic** *a* / **gerodontist** [ˌdʒerə*u*'dɔntist] *n* 老年口腔医学家,老年口腔医师

gerodontology [ˌdʒerəudɔn'tɔlədʒi] *n* 老年口腔医学(指老年牙齿问题的研究)

gerokomy [dʒe'rəukəmi] *n* 老年摄生法,老年保健

geromarasmus [ˌdʒerə*u*mə'ræzməs] *n* 老年性消瘦

geromorphism [ˌdʒerə*u*'mɔːfizəm] *n* 早老形象 | cutaneous ~ 皮肤早老形象

gerontal [dʒe'rɔntl] *a* 老年的,老人的

gerontic [dʒə'rɔntik] *a* 老年的,老人的

gerontin [dʒe'rɔntin] *n* 狗肝精碱

geront(o)- [构词成分]老年,老人

gerontology [ˌdʒerɔn'tɔlədʒi] *n* 老年学 | **gerontological** [dʒiˌrɔntə'lɔdʒikəl] *a* / **gerontologist** *n* 老年学家

gerontophile [dʒe'rɔntəfail] *n* 嗜耄癖者,亲老人癖者

gerontophilia [dʒeˌrɔntə*u*'filiə] *n* 嗜耄癖,亲老人癖

gerontopia [ˌdʒerɔn'təupiə] *n* 老年期视力回春,视力再生

gerontotherapeutics [dʒeˌrɔntə*u*ˌθerə'pjuːtiks], **gerontotherapy** [dʒeˌrɔntə*u*'θerəpi] *n* 老年病治疗[学]

gerontotoxon [dʒeˌrɔntə*u*'tɔksɔn], **gerontoxon** [ˌdʒerɔn'tɔksɔn] *n* 老人弓,角膜弓,老人环 | ~ lentis 老年白内障针拨术

geropsychiatry [ˌdʒerəusai'kaiətri] *n* 老年精神病学

Gerota's fascia (capsule) [gei'rəutə] (Dumitru Gerota) 格罗塔筋膜(被膜),肾周筋膜 | ~ method 格罗塔法(淋巴管注射法,即以溶于氯仿或醚而不溶于水的染料如普鲁士蓝注入淋巴管)

Gerson-Herrmannsdorfer diet [ˈgersn ˈhermən-sdɔːfə] (Max B. Gerson; Adolph H. Herrmannsdorfer) 格-赫饮食(少脂及蛋白质无盐饮食,治狼疮及结核病)

Gerstmann-Sträussler syndrome [ˈgɛəstmən ˈstr-auslə] (Josef Gerstamann; E. Sträussler) 格-施综合征(一组罕见的朊病毒病,常染色体显性遗传,但与朊病毒蛋白基因不同的突变有联系,具有认知障碍和运动障碍的共同特征,并在脑内存在多中心性淀粉样斑。共济失调型有进行性小脑性共济失调和痴呆,端脑型有构音困难、痴呆、强直、震颤和反射亢进。伴有神经纤维缠结的格-施综合征,有进行性短时记忆丧失和言语不清。1~5年内死亡)

Gerstmann's syndrome [ˈgɛəstmən] (Josef Gerstmann) 格斯特曼综合征(因优势半球角回病灶所致的手指认识不能、左右定向力障碍、书写不能、计算不能等)

Gerstmann-Sträussler-Scheinker syndrome [ˈgɛə-stmən ˈʃtrauslə ˈʃainkə] (J. Gerstmann; E. Sträusler; I. Scheinker) 格-施-沙综合征(见 Gerstmann-Sträussler syndrome)

gerüstmark [gəˈristmɑːk] *n*【德】骨髓支架(见于坏血病)

gesarol [ˈgesərɔl] *n* 滴滴涕(地地涕)(即 chlorophenothane)

Gesell developmental schedule [geˈzel] (A. Gesell) 格塞尔发育量表(一种测试婴儿发育状态的检查,包括运动、适应、言语、与人关系四方面)

gestaclone [ˈdʒestəkləun] *n* 孕氯酮(孕激素)

gestagen [ˈdʒestədʒən] *n* 促孕激素(如孕酮等)

gestalt [gəˈʃtɑːlt] *n* 格式塔,完形

gestaltism [gəˈʃtɑːltizəm] *n* 格式塔学说,完形心理学(现代心理学的一个派别)

gestation [dʒesˈteiʃən] *n* 妊娠 | exterior ~ 孕外发育 / interior ~ 孕内发育 | **~al** *a*

gestodene [ˈdʒestədiːn] *n* 孕二烯酮(孕激素)

gestonorone caproate [dʒesˈtəunɔrəun] 己酸孕诺酮(孕激素,治子宫内膜癌和良性前列腺增生)

gestosis [dʒesˈtəusis] ([复] **gestoses** [dʒes-ˈtəusiːz]) *n* 妊娠中毒

gestrinone [ˈdʒestrinəun] *n* 孕三烯酮(孕激素)

gesture [ˈdʒestʃə] *n* 手势,手语

GeV gigaelectron volt 吉[咖]电子伏,千兆电子伏(10^9 电子伏)

GFAP glial fibrillary acidic protein 胶质[细胞]原纤维酸性蛋白

GFR glomerular filtration rate 肾小球滤过率

G. G. G. gummi guttae gambiae【拉】藤黄

GGT γ-glutamyltransferase γ-谷氨酰转移酶

GH growth hormone 生长激素,促生长素

GHA gluceptate (glucoheptonate) 葡庚糖酸盐

Ghilarducci's reaction [ˌgiːlɑːˈdutʃi] (Francesco Ghilarducci) 吉拉杜奇反应(置一带电电极于四肢肌肉稍远处可引起肌收缩)

Ghon complex [gɔn] (Anton Ghon) 冈氏复征,原发复合征(primary complex,见 complex 项下相应术语) | ~ focus (primary lesion, tubercle) 冈氏病灶(原发病灶、结核灶)(儿童原发性肺结核的主要实质病变,如伴有一相应淋巴结病灶时,即为原发复合征,或冈氏复征)

Ghon-Sachs bacillus [gɔn zɑːks] (Anton Ghon; Anton Sachs) 冈-萨杆菌,败血梭状芽胞杆菌,败血梭菌

ghost [gəust] *n* 幻影;血影;菌蜕 | red cell ~ 红细胞影(溶血后保持完整的红细胞膜)

GH-RH growth hormone-releasing hormone 生长[激]素释放激素

GI gastrointestinal 胃肠的

Giacomini's band [dʒɑːkəuˈmiːni] (Carlo Giacomini) 贾科米尼带(海马齿状回前带)

Gianelli's sign [dʒɑːˈneli] (Giuseppe Gianelli) 吉阿内利征(见 Tournay's sign)

Giannuzzi's crescents (bodies, cells, demilunes) [dʒɑːˈnuːtsi] (Guiseppe Giannuzzi) 贾努齐新月(体、细胞、半月)(浆液黏液腺中黏液小管周围的浆细胞新月形斑)

Gianoti-Crosti syndrome [dʒɑːˈnɔti ˈkrɔsti] (Fernando Gianoti; Agostino Crosti) 儿童丘疹性肢端皮炎

giantism [ˈdʒaiəntizəm] *n* 巨大畸形;巨型;巨大发育,巨体

Giardia [dʒiːˈɑːdiə] (Alfred Giard) *n* 贾第鞭毛虫属 | ~ lamblia, ~ intestinalis 兰氏贾第鞭毛虫

giardiasis [ˌdʒiɑːˈdaiəsis] *n* 贾第虫病

gibberellin [gibəˈrelin] *n* 赤霉素

gibberish [ˈdʒibəriʃ, ˈgi-] *n* 言语凌乱,结巴语

Gibbon-Landis test [ˈgibɔn ˈlændis] (John H. Gibbon, Jr.; Eugene M. Landis) 吉本-蓝迪斯试验(检外周循环)

Gibbon's hernia (hydrocele) [ˈgibɔn] (Q. V. Gibbon) 吉本疝(水囊肿),水囊肿性巨疝

gibbosity [giˈbɔsəti] *n* 驼背

gibbous [ˈgibəs] *a* 驼背的

Gibbs-Donnan equilibrium [gibz ˈdɔnən] (J. W. Gibbs; Frederick G. Donnan) 吉布斯-道南平衡(见 Donnan equilibrium)

Gibbs' free energy [gibz] (Josiah W. Gibbs) 吉布斯自由能(自由能用热力学函数 $G = H - TS$ 表示,式中 H 为热函,T 为绝对温度,S 为熵) | ~ theorem 吉布斯定理(凡能降低纯分散体表面张力的物质,都集合于其表面)

gibbus [ˈgibəs] *n*【拉】驼背

Gibert's disease [ʒiˈbɛə] (Camille M. Gibert) 玫瑰糠疹,蔷薇糠疹

Gibney's bandage (strapping) [ˈgibni] (Virgil P. Gibney) 吉布尼绷带(贴膏法)(踝固定绷带,一种 12.5 cm 宽黏布条,包裹足和下肢的侧面与后面,固定足于轻度内翻的位置,并露出足背与下肢的前面部分) | ~ perispondylitis 吉布尼椎骨周炎(脊椎肌肉的一种疼痛疾病)

Gibson's murmur [ˈgibsn] (George A. Gibson) 吉布森杂音(占据大部分收缩期与舒张期长时间的隆隆音,通常在左第二肋间的近胸骨处,为动脉导管未闭的征象) | ~ rule 吉布森规律(患肺炎时,若脉压的汞柱毫米数不低于脉搏数者预后良好,反之,则预后不佳)

gid [gid] *n* 蹒跚病(一种家畜脑和脊髓的功能性和器质性疾病)

giddiness [ˈgidinis] *n* 眩晕,头晕

Giemsa's stain [ˈgiːmsə] (Gustav Giemsa) 吉姆萨染剂(染原虫)

Gierke's corpuscles [ˈgiəkə] (Hans P. B. Gierke) 吉尔克小体(神经系统内圆形小体)

Gierke's disease [ˈgiəkə] (Edgar O. K. von Gierke) 糖原贮积症 I 型

Gieson [ˈgiːsn] 见 van Gieson

Gifford's operation [ˈgifəd] (Harold Gifford) 吉福德手术(①限界性角膜切开术;②滴入三氯醋酸于泪囊中破坏泪囊术) | ~ reflex 吉福德反射(尽力使张开的眼睑闭合时的瞳孔收缩) / ~ sign 吉福德征(突眼性甲状腺肿初期,上睑不能外翻)

GIFT gamete intrafallopian transfer 配子输卵管内移植

giga- [构词成分]巨大;吉[咖](10^9,符号为 G)

gigantic [dʒaiˈgæntik] *a* 巨大的 | ~ acid 大曲霉酸,巨酸

gigantism [dʒaiˈgæntizəm, ˈdʒaɪ-] *n* 巨大发育,巨人症 | acromegalic ~ 指端肥大症巨大发育,肢端肥大性巨人症 / cerebral ~ 大脑性巨人症 / eunuchoid ~ 无睾性巨人症,阉性巨人症 / fetal ~ 胎儿巨大发育 / normal ~ 全面性巨大发育,匀称性巨大发育 / pituitary ~, hyperpituitary ~ 垂体性巨人症,垂体分泌过多性巨人症

gigant(o)- [构词成分]巨,巨大

gigantocellular [dʒaiˌgæntəuˈseljulə] *a* 巨细胞的

gigantomastia [dʒaiˌgæntəuˈmæstiə] *n* 巨乳房

gigantosoma [dʒaiˌgæntəuˈsəumə] *n* 巨大发育,巨高身材

Gigartina [ˌdʒaigɑːˈtainə] *n* 杉藻属

Gigli's operation [ˈdʒiːlji] (Leonardo Gigli) 季格利手术(耻骨切开术,用于难产) | ~ wire saw 季格利线锯(钢丝锯,用于耻骨切开术)

gikiyami [ˌgikiˈjɑːmi] *n*【日】七日热(钩端螺旋体病)

gilbert [ˈgilbət] (W. Gilbert) *n* 吉伯(旧磁通势单位,现用 A 安〈培〉,1 Gb = 0.795 775 A)

Gilbert's disease (cholemia, syndrome) [ʒiːlˈbɛə] (Nicolas A. Gilbert) 日尔贝病(胆血症、综合征)(一种家族性遗传性高胆红素血[症],伴轻型间歇性黄疸。亦称体质性肝功能不良、家族性胆血症、家族非溶血性黄疸) | ~ sign 日尔贝征(肝硬化时所呈现的饥尿病,即饥饿时的尿量较饭后为多)

Gilchrist's disease, mycosis [ˈgilkrist] (Thomas C. Gilchrist) 北美芽生菌病

gildable [ˈgildəbl] *a* 易染金色的

gill[1] [gil] *n* 鳃;菌褶

gill[2] [gil] *n* 及尔(旧液量单位,=1/4 品脱,1 英品脱〈UK pt〉= $0.568\ 261 \times 10^{-3}\ m^3$)

Gillenia [dʒiˈliːniə] *n* 美吐根属

Gilles de la Tourette's syndrome (disease) [tuˈret] (Georges Gilles de la Tourette) 图雷特综合征(病),抽动秽语综合征(儿童时期开始的一种面肌抽搐和声带抽搐综合征,逐渐发展到全身急动,伴模仿言语和秽亵言语,以前认为预后不良,但近来表明用丁酰苯治疗有效)

Gillespie's operation [giˈlespi] (James D. Gillespie) 吉莱斯皮手术(在指总伸肌和指中伸肌间作一纵向背侧切口的腕关节离断术)

Gillespie's syndrome [giˈlespi] (Frank D. Gillespie) 吉莱斯皮综合征(一种罕见的常染色体隐性遗传综合征,包括无虹膜、小脑性共济失调和智力迟钝)

Gilliam's operation [ˈgiliəm] (David T. Gilliam) 吉列姆手术(子宫后倾矫正术)

Gillies' flap (graft) [ˈgiliz] (Harold D. Gillies) 扇形唇瓣 | ~ operation 吉利斯手术(睑外翻矫正术)

Gill's operation [gil] (Arthur B. Gill) 吉尔手术(马蹄足矫正术)

Gilmer's splint [ˈgilmə] (Thomas L. Gilmer) 吉尔默夹板(下颌骨折用) | ~ wiring 吉尔默栓结术(一种颌间固定法)

gilt [gilt] *n* 母猪(意欲生育,但从未生产的母猪)

Gil-Vernet technique [dʒil vəːˈnet] (Josep M. Gil-Vernet) 吉尔·弗内特技术(一型输尿管膀胱吻合术;切除正常附着膀胱的两根输尿管,在三角区内向内侧相互接近处再附着)

Gimbernat's ligament [hiːmbəˈnæt] (Antonio de Gimbernat) 陷窝韧带 | ~ reflex ligament 腹股沟反转韧带

ginger [ˈdʒindʒə] *n* 生姜,姜

gingiva [ˈdʒindʒivə, dʒinˈdʒaivə] ([复] **gingivae** [ˈdʒindʒiviː, dʒinˈdʒaiviː]) *n*【拉】牙龈 |

alveolar ~ 牙槽龈 / areolar ~ 蜂窝织龈,蜂窝状龈 / attached ~ 附着龈 / buccal ~ 颊侧龈 / cemental ~ 牙骨质龈 / free ~ 游离龈 / labial ~ 唇侧龈 / lingual ~ 舌侧龈 / marginal ~ 边缘龈 / septal ~ 牙间龈 | **~l** [ˈdʒindʒivəl, dʒinˈdʒaivəl] *a* 龈的 / **~lly** [ˈdʒindʒivəli] *ad* 向龈

gingivalgia [ˌdʒindʒiˈvældʒiə] *n* 龈痛

gingivectomy [ˌdʒindʒiˈvektəmi], **gingivoectomy** [ˌdʒindʒivəˈektəmi] *n* 龈切除术

gingivitis [ˌdʒindʒiˈvaitis] *n* 龈炎 | acute necrotizing ulcerative ~ (ANUG) 急性坏死性溃疡性龈炎 / bismuth ~ 铋毒性龈炎 / "cottonroll" ~ 棉卷龈炎 | desquamative ~ 剥脱性龈炎 / herpetic ~ 疱疹性龈炎 / hyperplastic ~ 增生性龈炎 / marginal ~ 边缘性龈炎 / necrotizing ulcerative ~, fusospirochetal ~, ulceromembranous ~ 坏死溃疡性龈炎,梭菌螺旋体性龈炎,溃疡假膜性龈炎 / phagedenic ~ 崩蚀性龈炎 / scorbutic ~ 坏血病龈炎 / streptococcal ~ 链球菌性龈炎

gingiv(o)- [构词成分]龈

gingivoaxial [ˌdʒindʒivəuˈæksiəl] *a* 龈轴的

gingivobuccoaxial [ˌdʒindʒivəuˌbʌkəˈæksiəl] *a* 龈颊轴的

gingivoglossitis [ˌdʒindʒivəugləˈsaitis] *n* 龈舌炎

gingivolabial [ˌdʒindʒivəuˈleibjəl] *a* 龈唇的

gingivolinguoaxial [ˌdʒindʒivəuˌliŋgwəˈæksiəl] *a* 龈舌轴的

gingivoperiodontitis [ˌdʒindʒivəuˌperiɔdɔnˈtaitis] *n* 龈牙周炎 | necrotizing ulcerative ~ 坏死性溃疡性龈牙周炎

gingivoplasty [ˈdʒindʒivəˌplæsti] *n* 龈成形术

gingivosis [ˌdʒindʒiˈvəusis] *n* 龈变性

gingivostomatitis [ˌdʒindʒivəuˌstəuməˈtaitis] *n* 龈口炎 | herpetic ~ 疱疹性龈口炎 / necrotizing ulcerative ~ 坏死性溃疡性龈口炎

ginglyform [ˈdʒiŋglifɔːm], **ginglymoid** [ˈdʒiŋglimɔid] *a* 屈戌样的

ginglymoarthrodial [ˌdʒiŋglimәuɑːˈθrəudiəl] *a* 屈戌样及摩动[关节]的

ginglymus [ˈdʒiŋgliməs] ([复] **ginglymi** [ˈdʒiŋglimai]) *n* 【拉】屈戌关节

Ginkgo [ˈgiŋkəu] *n* 银杏属 | ~ biloba 银杏

ginkgo [ˈgiŋkəu] *n* 银杏叶

ginseng [ˈdʒinseŋ] *n* 人参

Giordano's sphincter [dʒɔːˈdɑːnəu] (Davide Giordano) 胆总管括约肌

GIP gastric inhibitory polypeptide 肠抑胃肽; glucose-dependent insulinotropic polypeptide 糖依赖性胰岛素释放多肽

Giraldés' organ [hiˈrældeis] (Joachim A. C. C. Giraldés) 旁睾

Girardinus [dʒiˈrɑːdinəs] *n* 鳉属(即 Poecilia) | ~ poeciloides 网纹鳉(即 Poecilia reticulata)

Girard's treatment (method) [dʒiˈrɑːd] (Alfred C. Girard) 纪腊德疗法(法)(皮下注射或口服硫酸阿托品和硫酸士的宁,治晕船病)

girdle [ˈgəːdl] *n* 带,托带,引力带 | limbus ~ 角膜缘带 / pelvic ~, ~ of inferior extremity 骨盆带,下肢带 / shoulder ~, pectoral ~, ~ of superior extremity, thoracic ~ 肩胛带,上肢带

Girdlestone resection (operation) [ˈgəːdəlstəun] (Gathorne R. Girdlestone) 格德尔斯通切除术(手术)(严重髋关节感染时切除股骨头和股骨颈)

Girdner's probe [ˈgəːdnə] (John H. Girdner) 格德纳探子(一种电探子,探深部组织内子弹)

gitaligenin [dʒiˈtæliˌdʒinin] *n* 芰他配基

gitalin [ˈdʒitəlin] *n* 吉他林,洋地黄全苷(用以治充血性心脏衰竭和心律失常,亦称无定形吉他林)

gitaloxin [ˌdʒitəˈlɔksin] *n* 吉他洛辛(强心药)

Gitelman's syndrome [ˈgitəlmən] (H. J. Gitelman) 吉泰尔曼综合征([肾小]球旁细胞肥大综合征,类似巴特〈Bartter〉综合征,但伴有低钙尿症和低镁血症,常见于青少年或成年人)

githagism [ˈgiθədʒizəm] *n* 麦仙翁中毒,瞿麦中毒

gitogenin [dʒiˈtɔdʒinin] *n* 吉托吉宁(一种皂苷配基,制自吉托宁 gitonin)

gitonin [ˈdʒitənin] *n* 吉托宁(一种中性皂苷,获自洋地黄种子)

gitoxigenin [dʒiˈtɔksidʒenin] *n* 羟基洋地黄毒苷元,芰毒苷元

gitoxin [dʒiˈtɔksin] *n* 吉妥辛(一种强心苷)

Gitterfasern [ˈgitəˌfɑːsəːn] *n* 【德】网格纤维,格子纤维

Giuffrida-Ruggieri stigma [dʒuˈfridə ˌrudʒiˈeri] (Vincenzo Giuffrida Ruggieri) 朱夫里达·鲁杰里特征(下颌凹浅表异常)

Givens' method [ˈgivnz] (Maurice H. Givens) 吉文斯法(检消化力)

GIX 二氟二苯三氯乙烷(杀虫剂,DFDT)

gizzard [ˈgizəd] *n* 砂囊(鸟类强有力的肌性胃)

GL greatest length 最大长度(测量卷屈小胚胎的轴)

Gl glucinium 铍

gl. glandula, glandulae【拉】小腺,腺

GL 54 athomin 辣根素

glabella [gləˈbelə] ([复] **glabellae** [gləˈbeliː]), **glabellum** [gləˈbeləm] *n* 眉间 | **~r** [gləˈbelə] *a*

glabellad [gləˈbelæd] *ad* 向眉间

glabrous [ˈgleibrəs] *a* 光滑的,光秃的

glacial [ˈgleisjəl, ˈgleiʃəl] *a* 冰的,冰样的

gladiate [ˈglædieit, -it] *a* 剑形的
gladiolic acid [ˌglædiˈəulik] 剑霉酸
gladiolus [ˌglædiˈəuləs, gləˈdaiələs] *n* 胸骨体
gladiomanubrial [ˌglædiəuməˈnjuːbriəl] *a* 胸骨体[与]胸骨柄的
glair [glɛə] *n* 蛋白,卵白;(蛋白制成的)黏合剂;蛋白状黏液
glairin [ˈglɛərin] *n* 胶素,黏胶质
glairy [ˈglɛəri] *a* 蛋白状的,卵白状的
gland [glænd] *n* 腺 | absorbent ~ 淋巴结 / acid ~s 酸腺 / adrenal ~, suprarenal ~ 肾上腺 / aggregate ~s, agminated ~s 淋巴集结 / aortic ~ 主动脉球 / arteriococcygeal ~ 尾骨球 / brachial ~s 臂淋巴结 / bulbourethral ~, bulbocavernous ~ 尿道球腺 / cardiac ~s 贲门腺 / carotid ~ 颈动脉小球 / celiac ~s 腹腔淋巴结 / circumanal ~s, anal ~s 肛周腺 / coccygeal ~ 尾骨球 / conglobate ~ 淋巴结 / ductless ~ 无管腺,内分泌腺 / endocrine ~s, blood ~s, blood vessel ~s, closed ~s, incretory ~s 内分泌腺 / exocrine ~, coil ~ 外分泌腺 / hemolymph ~s 血淋巴结 / hepatic ~s 胆总管腺 / heterocrine ~s 混合腺 / intercarotid ~ 颈动脉小球 / interstitial ~s 间质腺 / jugular ~ 颈静脉淋巴结 / lymph ~, lymphatic ~ 淋巴结(旧名淋巴腺) / mammary ~, lactiferous ~ 乳腺 / mesenteric ~s 肠系膜淋巴结 / mesocolic ~s 结肠系膜淋巴结 / mucilaginous ~s 滑液绒毛 / ~ of neck 咽扁桃体 / odoriferous ~s of prepuce 包皮腺 / peptic ~s 胃液腺 / pituitary ~ 垂体 / pregnancy ~s 妊娠腺(卵巢滤泡,黄体和胎盘) / prostate ~ 前列腺 / salivary ~s 唾液腺 / splenoid ~ 脾样结节(脾切除后代偿性脾组织结节) / thyroid ~ 甲状腺 / trachoma ~s 沙眼腺(沙眼滤泡) / vascular ~ 血管球;血淋巴结
glandered [ˈglændəd] *a* 患[马]鼻疽的
glanderous [ˈglændərəs] *a* [马]鼻疽的
glanders [ˈglændəz] [复] *n* 鼻疽 | African ~, Japanese ~ 假[性]马鼻疽,兽疫性淋巴管炎
glandes [ˈglændiːz] glans 的复数
glandilemma [ˌglændiˈlemə] *n* 腺被囊
glandula [ˈglændjulə] ([复] **glandulae** [ˈglændjuliː]) *n*【拉】小腺,腺
glandular [ˈglændjulə] *a* 腺的,含腺的;阴茎头的;阴蒂头的
glandule [ˈglændjuːl] *n* 小腺,腺
glandulous [ˈglændjuləs] *a* 腺的
glans [glænz] ([复] **glandes** [ˈglændiːz]) *n*【拉】阴茎头 | ~ clitoridis, ~ of clitoris 阴蒂头 / ~ penis 阴茎头
glanular [ˈglænjulə] *a* 阴茎头的;阴蒂头的
glanuloplasty [ˈglænjuːləuˌplæsti] *n* 阴茎头成形术
Glanzmann's thrombasthenia (disease) [ˈglɑːnzmən] (Edward Glanzmann) 格兰茨曼血小板功能不全(病),遗传性出血素质
glare [glɛə] *n* 炫耀,眩目
glarometer [glɛəˈrɔmitə] *n* 抗眩目测量器
glaserian fissure [gləˈsiəriən] (Johann H. Glaser 〈Glaserius〉) 岩鼓裂
Glasgow Coma Scale [ˈglɑːsgəu] (Glasgow 为苏格兰一城市,该市曾开发各种量表)格拉斯哥昏迷量表(评定神经受损患者对刺激反应的一种标准化方法,对各项反应用数字值表明三种类别〈眼张开、言语反应性和运动反应性〉,然后将三种评分加在一起,最低值即为最差的临床评分) | Glasgow Outcome Scale 格拉斯哥结果量表(在严重头部受伤后,根据重新获得的社会功能总的水平用以叙述其结果的一种量表,患者归入 5 种类别之一:良好恢复,中度残疾,重度残疾,植物人状态或死亡)
Glasgow's sign [ˈglɑːsgəu] (William C. Glasgow) 格拉斯哥征(潜伏性主动脉瘤时,可听出肱动脉收缩期杂音)
glass [glɑːs] *n* 玻片,玻璃;玻璃杯;镜;[复] 眼镜 | bifocal ~es 双焦点眼镜 / contact ~es 接触镜片 / cover ~ 盖片 / crown ~ 冕牌玻璃 / crutch ~es 支柱眼镜 / cupping ~ 吸[疗]杯,吸罐,拔罐 / flint ~ 火石玻璃 / hyperbolic ~es 双曲线玻璃 / object ~ 物镜 / optical ~ 光学玻璃 / quartz ~ 石英玻璃 / snow ~es 雪镜 / soluble ~, water ~ 可溶性玻璃,水玻璃 / sun ~es 太阳眼镜 / test ~ 试管 / trifocal ~es 三焦点眼镜 / watch ~ 表玻璃
glassy [ˈglɑːsi] *a* 玻璃状的
glatiramer acetate [gləˈtirəmə] 醋酸格拉替姆(免疫调节药,用于减少多发性硬化复发,皮下给药)
Glauber's salt [ˈglaubə] (Johann R. Glauber) 格劳伯盐,芒硝,硫酸钠
glaucoma [glɔːˈkəumə] *n* 青光眼 | absolute ~ 绝对期青光眼 / auricular ~ 耳性青光眼 / hemorrhagic ~, apoplectic ~ 出血性青光眼 / ~ imminens 前驱期青光眼 / infantile ~ 婴幼儿型青光眼 / primary ~ 原发性青光眼 / secondary ~ 继发性青光眼 | **~tous** *a*
glaucosis [glɔːˈkəusis] *n* 青光眼盲
glaucosuria [ˌglɔːkəuˈsjuəriə] *n* 青尿症,尿蓝母尿
glaukomflecken [ˈglaukəumˈflekn] *n*【德】青光眼性白内障(即 glaucomatous cataract)
glaze [gleiz] *vt* 给…上釉,上光 *n* 釉料;瓷釉
GLC gas-liquid chromatography 气-液层析
GlcNAc *N*-acetylglucosamine *N*-乙酰葡糖胺
Gleason grade (score) [ˈgliːsən] (Donald F. Gl-

eason) 格列森等级(评分)(局部性前列腺癌等级评定,初生生长和次生长的程度划分1~5级评分,未分化型和破坏型评分最高)

gleet [gliːt] *n* 后淋(慢性淋病性尿道炎) | vent ~ 泄殖腔炎,一穴肛炎 | **~y** *a*

Glénard's disease [glei'nɑː] (Frantz Glénard) 内脏下垂

Glenn-Anderson technique [glen 'ændəsən] (James F. Glenn; E. E. Anderson) 格-安技术(一型输尿管膀胱吻合术,受损的输尿管附着部位在原有位置上再修复)

Glenn operation (procedure, shunt) [glen] (William W. L. Glenn) 格伦手术(操作法、分流术)(先天性紫绀型心脏病的一种手术,包括上腔静脉与右侧肺动脉的吻合)

glenohumeral [ˌgliːnəu'hjuːmərəl] *a* 盂肱的

glenoid ['gliːnɔid] *a* 盂样的;关节盂的

Glenospora [gliː'nɔspərə] *n* 蜂窝孢子菌属

Glenosporella [ˌgliːnəuspɔ'relə] *n* 蜂窝小孢子菌属

Gley's cells [glei] (Marcel E. É. Gley) 格莱细胞(睾丸间质细胞) | ~ glands 甲状旁腺

GLI glucagon-like immunoreactivity 胰高血糖素样免疫反应性

glia ['glaiə] *n* 神经胶质 | ameboid ~ 阿米巴样[神经]胶质细胞 / cytoplasmic ~ 原浆性[神经]胶质细胞 / fibrillary ~ 纤维性[神经]胶质细胞 | **~l** *a*

-glia [后缀]神经胶质

gliacyte ['glaiəsait] *n* 神经胶质细胞

gliadin ['glaiədin] *n* 麦醇溶蛋白

gliamilide [glai'æmilaid] *n* 格列胺脲(口服降血糖药)

gliarase ['glaiəreis] *n* 星状细胞合体

glibenclamide [glai'benkləmaid] *n* 格列本脲(口服降血糖药)

glibornuride [glai'bɔːnjuəraid] *n* 格列波脲(口服降血糖药)

glicentin [glai'sentin] *n* 肠高血糖素,肠升糖素

glicetanile sodium [gli'setənail] *n* 格列他尼钠(口服降血糖药)

gliclazide ['glikləzaid] *n* 格列齐特(降血糖药,用以治疗非胰岛素依赖型糖尿病,口服给药)

glide [glaid] *n* 滑动;滑音 | mandibular ~ 下颌滑动

gliflumide [gli'fluːmaid] *n* 格列氟胺(口服降血糖药)

glimepiride [glai'mepiraid] *n* 格列美脲(降血糖药,用于治疗非胰岛素依赖型糖尿病,口服给药)

gli(o)- [构词成分]胶质

gliobacteria [ˌglaiəubæk'tiəriə] *n* 胶细菌

glioblast ['glaiəublæst] *n* 成(神经)胶质细胞

glioblastoma [ˌglaiəublæs'təumə] *n* 成[神经]胶质细胞瘤,胶质细胞瘤

gliococcus [ˌglaiəu'kɔkəs] *n* 胶球菌

gliocyte ['glaiəusait] *n* [神经]胶质细胞

gliocytoma [ˌglaiəusai'təumə] *n* [神经]胶质细胞瘤

gliofibrillary [ˌglaiəu'faibriləri] *a* [神经]胶质原纤维的

gliogenous [ˌglai'ɔdʒinəs] *a* [神经]胶质原的

glioma [glai'əumə] ([复] **gliomata** [glai'əumətə]) *n* [神经]胶质瘤 | astrocytic ~ 星形细胞瘤 / ~ endophytum 内发神经胶质瘤,内向性视网膜胶质瘤 / ependymal ~ 室管膜神经胶质瘤 / ~ exophytum 外发神经胶质瘤,外向性视网膜胶质瘤 / ganglionic ~ 神经节神经胶质瘤 / peripheral ~ 外周神经胶质瘤,神经鞘瘤 / ~ retinae 视网膜神经胶质瘤,成视网膜细胞瘤 / ~ sarcomatosum [神经]胶质肉瘤 | **~ous** *a*

gliomatosis [ˌglaiəumə'təusis] *n* 神经胶质瘤病

glioneuroma [ˌglaiəunjuə'rəumə] *n* [神经]胶质神经瘤

gliophagia [ˌglaiəu'feidʒiə] *n* 吞噬[神经]胶质作用

gliopil ['glaiəpil] *n* [神经]胶质毡

gliosarcoma [ˌglaiəusɑː'kəumə] *n* [神经]胶质肉瘤 | ~ retinae 视网膜[神经]胶质肉瘤,成视网膜细胞瘤

gliosis [glai'əusis] *n* 神经胶质增生 | basilar ~ 脑底神经胶质增生 / cerebellar ~ 小脑神经胶质增生 / diffuse ~ 弥漫性神经胶质增生 / hemispheric ~, unilateral ~ 大脑半球神经胶质增生 / lobar ~ 脑叶神经胶质增生 / spinal ~ 脊髓神经胶质增生,脊髓空洞症

gliosome ['glaiəsəum] *n* [神经]胶质粒

gliotoxin [ˌglaiəu'tɔksin] *n* 胶霉毒素,曲霉菌素

glipizide ['glipəzaid] *n* 格列吡嗪,吡磺环己脲(口服降血糖药)

Gliricola [glai'rikələ] *n* 长虱属 | ~ porcelli 豚鼠长虱

glischrin ['gliskrin] *n* 菌黏素

glischruria [glis'kruəriə] *n* 菌黏素尿

glissade [gli'seid, gli'sɑːd] *n* 滑动,斜向眼球震颤 | **glissadic** [gli'sædik] *a*

glissonitis [ˌglisə'naitis] *n* 肝纤维囊炎

Glisson's capsule ['glisn] (Francis Glisson) 肝纤维囊,血管周围纤维囊 | ~ cirrhosis 纤维囊性肝硬变 / ~ disease 佝偻病 / ~ sling 格利森悬带(颈项脊柱牵伸悬带) / ~ sphincter 肝胰壶腹括约肌

Gln glutamine 谷氨酰胺

globate [ˈgləubeit] *a* 球状的
globe [gləub] *n* 球;球状物
globi [ˈgləubai] globus 的复数;麻风球
globidiosis [gləˌbidiˈəusis] *n* 球虫病(现名 besnoitiosis)
Globidium [gləˈbidiəm] *n* 球虫属(现名 Besnoitia)
globin [ˈgləubin] *n* 珠蛋白 | ~ zinc insulin injection 珠蛋白锌胰岛素注射液
globinometer [ˌgləubiˈnɔmitə] *n* (氧合)血红蛋白计
globoid [ˈgləubɔid] *a* 球状的 *n* 球状体
globose [ˈgləubəus], **globous** [ˈgləubəs] *a* 球形的,球状的 | **globosity** [gləuˈbɔsəti] *n* 球状,球形
globoside [ˈglɔbəsaid] *n* 红细胞糖苷脂
globotriaosylceramide [ˌgləubəutraiˌeiəsilˈserəmaid] *n* 神经酰胺三己糖苷(即 ceramide trihexoside)
globular [ˈglɔbjulə] *a* 球形的;红细胞的
Globularia [ˌglɔbjuˈlɛəriə] *n* 球花属
globulariacitrin [ˌglɔbjuˌlɛəriəˈsitrin] *n* 芸香苷,芦丁
globule [ˈglɔbjuːl] *n* 小球;小体;球剂 | dentin ~s 牙质小体 / milk ~s 乳脂小球 / myelin ~s 髓小球 / polar ~s 极体
globuli [ˈglɔbjulai] globulus 的复数
globulin [ˈglɔbjulin] *n* 球蛋白 | AC ~, accelerator ~ AC 球蛋白,加速凝血球蛋白(凝血因子Ⅴ) / alpha ~s α 球蛋白 / antidiphtheritic ~ 抗白喉球蛋白 / antihemophilic ~ (AHG) 抗血友病球蛋白(凝血因子Ⅷ) / anti-human ~ serum 抗人球蛋白血清 / antilymphocyte ~ (ALG) 抗淋巴细胞球蛋白 / antithymocyte ~ (ATG) 抗胸腺细胞球蛋白 / beta ~s β 球蛋白 / corticosteroid-binding ~, cortisol-binding ~ (CBG) 皮质类固醇结合球蛋白,皮质醇结合球蛋白 / gamma ~s γ 球蛋白 / hepatitis B immune ~ 乙型肝炎免疫球蛋白 / immune ~, immune human serum ~ 免疫球蛋白,人免疫血清球蛋白 / pertussis immune ~ 百日咳免疫球蛋白 / rabies immune ~ 狂犬病免疫球蛋白 / Rh_0 (D) immune ~ Rh_0 (D) 免疫球蛋白(用于预防 Rh_0 同族致敏作用) / testosterone-estradiol-binding ~ (TEBG) 睾酮-雌二醇结合球蛋白 / tetanus immune ~ 破伤风免疫球蛋白 / thyroxine-binding ~ 甲状腺素结合球蛋白 / vaccinia immune ~ (VIG) 牛痘免疫球蛋白 / varicellazoster immune ~ (VZIG) 水痘-带状疱疹免疫球蛋白 / ~ X 球蛋白 X(产生于肌细胞间隙的球蛋白)
globulinemia [ˌglɔbjuliˈniːmiə] *n* 球蛋白血症
globulinuria [ˌglɔbjuliˈnjuəriə] *n* 球蛋白尿
globulolysis [ˌglɔbjuˈlɔlisis], **globulysis** [gləu-ˈbjuːlisis] *n* [红]细胞溶解 | **globulolytic** [ˌglɔbjuləˈlitik] *a* 溶红细胞的
globulose [ˈglɔbjuləus] *n* 球蛋白脲
globulus [ˈglɔbjuləs] ([复] **globuli** [ˈglɔbjulai]) *n* 【拉】小体;球剂
globus [ˈgləubəs] ([复] **globi** [ˈgləubai]) *n* 【拉】球;球形结构;眼球;麻风球 | ~ abdominalis 腹[部]球[状]感 / ~ hystericus 癔症球,癔症性窒息[感]
Gloeotrichia [ˌgləuiːəuˈtrikiə] *n* 胶刺藻属
glomangioma [gləuˌmændʒiˈəumə] *n* 血管球瘤
glomectomy [gləuˈmektəmi] *n* 球切除术(尤指颈动脉球切除术)
glomera [ˈglɔmərə] glomus 的复数
glomerate [ˈglɔmərit] *a* 聚成球形的
glomerular [gləuˈmerjulə] *a* 小球的(尤指肾小球的);血管小球的
glomeruli [gləuˈmerjulai] glomerulus 的复数
glomerulitis [gləuˌmerjuˈlaitis] *n* 肾小球炎
glomerul(o)- [构词成分]小球,肾小球
glomerulonephritis [gləuˌmerjuləuneˈfraitis] *n* 肾小球肾炎 | acute ~ 急性肾小球肾炎 / chronic ~ 慢性肾小球肾炎 / chronic hypocomplementemic ~ 慢性低补体血性肾小球肾炎(即 membranoproliferative ~) / focal ~ 局灶性肾小球肾炎 / focal embolic ~ 局灶性栓塞性肾小球肾炎 / IgA ~ 免疫球蛋白 A 肾小球肾炎(为一种慢性型,特点为血尿和蛋白尿以及肾小球系膜区的免疫球蛋白 A 沉积,继以肾小球系膜细胞反应性增生。亦称免疫球蛋白 A 肾病) / immune complex ~ 免疫复合物性肾小球肾炎 / lobular ~ 小叶性肾小球肾炎(即 membranoproliferative ~) / lobulonodular ~ 小叶结节性肾小球肾炎(即 membranoproliferative ~) / membranoproliferative ~ 膜增生性肾小球肾炎(一种慢性肾小球肾炎,特征为系膜细胞增生和肾小球毛细管壁不规则增厚。有两种亚型:Ⅰ型特征为内皮下电子致密沉积和典型补体途径激活,Ⅱ型特征为肾小球基膜内重电子致密沉积和涉及 C_3 肾炎因子的替代补体途径激活。此病发生于大龄儿童和青年,病程呈慢性进行性,间有无规律性缓解,最终导致肾衰竭) / membranous ~ 膜性肾小球肾炎 / mesangiocapillary ~ 系膜毛细血管性肾小球肾炎(即 membranoproliferative ~) / nodular ~ 结节性肾小球肾炎(即 membranoproliferative ~) / rapidly progressive ~, malignant ~ 急进性肾小球肾炎,恶性肾小球肾炎 / segmental ~ 节段性肾小球肾炎 / subacute ~ 亚急性肾小球肾炎
glomerulonephropathy [gləuˌmerjuləuneˈfrɔpəθi] *n* 肾小球性肾病
glomerulopathy [gləuˌmerjuˈlɔpəθi] *n* 肾小球

病 | diabetic ~ 糖尿病肾小球病,毛细血管间肾小球硬化症

glomerulosclerosis [gləu|merjuləuskliə'rəusis] *n* 肾小球硬化症,小动脉性肾硬化 | focal segmental ~ 局灶性节段性肾小球硬化症 / intercapillary ~, diabetic ~ 毛细血管间肾小球硬化症,糖尿病肾小球硬化症

glomerulose [gləu'merjuləus] *a* 小球的;血管小球的

glomerulotropin [gləu|merjuləu'trɔpin] *n* 促[肾上腺]小球激素

glomerulotubular [gləu|merjuləu'tju:bjulə] *a* [肾小]球[肾小]管的

glomerulus [gləu'merjuləs] ([复] **glomeruli** [gləu'merjulai]) *n* 小球(由血管或神经纤维组成);肾小球 | coccygeal arterial glomeruli 尾骨球 / glomeruli of kidney, renal glomeruli 肾小球 / nonencapsulated nerve ~ 无被囊神经小球 / olfactory ~ 嗅小球

glomic ['gləumik] *a* 球的(尤指血管球的)

glomoid ['gləumɔid] *a* 血管球状的

glomus ['gləuməs] ([复] **glomera** ['glɔmərə]) *n* 【拉】球(尤指血管球) | carotid ~ 颈动脉球 / coccygeal ~ 尾骨球

glonoinism ['glɔnəuinizəm] *n* 三硝酸甘油酯中毒

gloss- 见 glosso-

glossa ['glɔsə] ([复] **glossas** 或 **glossae** ['glɔsi:]) *n* 【拉】舌

glossagra [glɔ'seigrə] *n* 痛风性舌痛

glossal ['glɔsəl] *a* 舌的

glossalgia [glɔ'sældʒiə] *n* 舌痛

glossanthrax [glɔ'sænθræks] *n* 舌痈

glossectomy [glɔ'sektəmi] *n* 舌切除术

Glossina [glɔ'sainə] *n* 舌蝇属 | ~ morsitans 刺舌蝇 / ~ pallidipes 淡足舌蝇 / ~ palpalis 须舌蝇

glossitis [glɔ'saitis] *n* 舌炎 | ~ areata exfoliativa, benign migratory ~, ~ migrans 地图样舌 / idiopathic ~, parenchymatous ~ 自发性舌炎,主质性舌炎 / median rhomboid ~ 正中菱形舌炎 / parasitic ~ 黑舌[病] / psychogenic ~ 舌灼痛

gloss(o)- [构词成分]舌

glossocele ['glɔsəsi:l] *n* 巨舌,大舌病

glossocinesthetic [|glɔsəusinis'θetik] *a* 舌动感觉的

glossocoma [glɔ'sɔkəmə] *n* 舌退缩

glossodynamometer [|glɔsəu|dainə'mɔmitə] *n* 舌力计

glossodynia [|glɔsəu'diniə] *n* 舌痛 | ~ exfoliativa 剥脱性舌痛

glossoepiglottidean [|glɔsəuepiglɔ'tidiən], **glossoepiglottic** [|glɔsəuepi'glɔtik] *a* 舌会厌的

glossograph ['glɔsəgrɑ:f] *n* 舌动描记器

glossohyal [|glɔsə'haiəl] *a* 舌[与]舌骨的

glossokinesthetic [|glɔsəu|kinis'θetik] *a* 舌动感觉的

glossolalia [|glɔsə'leiliə] *n* 言语不清

glossology [glɔ'sɔlədʒi] *n* 舌学;命名学,名词学

glossomantia [|glɔsəumæn'taiə] *n* 舌象预后

glossoncus [glɔ'sɔŋkəs] *n* 舌肿

glossopalatinus [|glɔsəu|pælə'tainəs] *n* 舌腭肌

glossopathy [glɔ'sɔpəθi] *n* 舌病

glossopexy [|glɔsə'peksi] *n* 唇舌粘连,舌固定

glossopharyngeum [|glɔsəufə'rindʒiəm] *n* 舌咽 | **glossopharyngeal** [|glɔsəu|færin'dʒi:əl, -fə'rindʒi-] *a*

glossopharyngeus [|glɔsəufə'rindʒiəs] *n* 舌咽肌

glossophobia [|glɔsəu'fəubiə] *n* 谈话恐怖,言语恐怖,恐语症

glossophytia [|glɔsəu'fitiə] *n* 黑舌[病]

glossoplasty ['glɔsə|plæsti] *n* 舌成形术

glossoptosis [|glɔsəup'təusis] *n* 舌后坠

glossopyrosis [|glɔsəupaiə'rəusis] *n* 舌灼痛

glossorrhaphy [glɔ'sɔrəfi] *n* 舌缝合术

glossoscopy [glɔ'sɔskəpi] *n* 舌检查

glossospasm ['glɔsəspæzəm] *n* 舌痉挛

glossosteresis [|glɔsəustə'ri:sis] *n* 舌切除术

glossotilt ['glɔsətilt] *n* 牵舌器

glossotomy [glɔ'sɔtəmi] *n* 舌切开术

glossotrichia [glɔsəu'trikiə] *n* 毛舌

glotography [gləu'tɔgrəfi] *n* 声门描记[法]

glottal ['glɔtl] *a* 声门的

glottic ['glɔtik] *a* 声门的;舌的

glottis ['glɔtis] ([复] **glottises** 或 **glottides** ['glɔtidi:z]) *n* 声门 | false ~ 假声门,前庭裂 / intercartilaginous ~, respiratory ~ 软骨间部,呼吸声门 / true ~ 真声门,声门裂

glottitis [glɔ'taitis] *n* 舌炎

glottogram ['glɔtəgræm] *n* 声门图

glottography [glɔ'tɔgrəfi] *n* 声门描记[法]

glottology [glɔ'tɔlədʒi] *n* 舌学;命名学,名词学

glou-glou ['gluglu] *n* 【法】咕噜声,嘈杂声(多指胃肠道内);尖锐声(有时于心脏中听到)

glove [glʌv] *n* 手套

Glover's organism ['glʌvə] (T. J. Glover) 格洛弗菌(一种革兰阳性微生物,从恶性瘤分离)

glow [gləu] *n* 电辉,辉光

Glu glutamic acid 谷氨酸

glucagon ['glu:kəgɔn] *n* 胰升糖素,胰高血糖素(由胰脏 α 细胞所分泌的一种多肽激素,能促进肝糖原的分解而使血糖浓度增高);高血糖素(胰岛素拮抗药)

glucagonoma [|glu:kəgɔ'nəumə] *n* 胰升糖素瘤,

胰高血糖素瘤

glucal [ˈgluːkəl] *n* 己烯糖

glucan [ˈgluːkæn, -kən] *n* 葡聚糖

1, 4-α-glucan branching enzyme [ˈgluːkæn ˈbrɑːntʃiŋ ˈenzaim] 1, 4-α-葡聚糖分支酶(此酶的遗传性缺乏为一种常染色体隐性性状,可致糖原贮积症Ⅳ型。亦称分支酶)

glucan 1, 4-α-glucosidase [ˈgluːkæn gluːˈkəusideis] 葡聚糖1, 4-α-葡糖苷酶(此酶的遗传性缺乏为一种常染色体隐性性状,可致糖原贮积症Ⅱ型。亦称酸性麦芽糖酶,溶酶体α-葡糖苷酶)

glucan transferase [ˈgluːkæn ˈtrænsfəreis] 葡聚糖转移酶

glucaric acid [gluːˈkɑːrik] 葡糖二酸

glucatonia [gluːkəˈtəuniə] *n* 血糖极度降低,胰岛素休克

glucemia [gluːˈsiːmiə] *n* 糖血

gluceptate [gluːˈsepteit] *n* 葡庚糖酸盐(glucoheptonate 的 USAN 缩约词)

glucic acid [ˈgluːsik] 糖酸

glucide [ˈgluːsaid] *n* 糖族(碳水化合物和糖苷的总称);糖精

glucidtemns [ˈgluːsidtems] *n* 淀粉水解物(包括糊精、麦芽糖和葡萄糖)

glucinium [gluːˈsiniəm] *n* 铍(化学元素)

gluciphore [ˈgluːsifɔː] *n* 生甜味基

glucitol [ˈgluːsitɔl] *n* 山梨糖醇

gluc(o)- [构词成分]甘,甜;葡萄糖

glucoamylase [ˌgluːkəuˈæmileis] *n* 葡糖淀粉酶,葡聚糖1, 4-α-葡糖苷酶

glucoascorbic acid [ˌgluːkəuəsˈkɔːbik] 葡[萄]糖型抗坏血酸

glucocerebrosidase [ˌgluːkəuˌseribrəˈsaideis] *n* 葡糖脑苷脂酶

glucocerebroside [ˌgluːkəuˈseribrəsaid] *n* 葡糖脑苷脂

glucocinin [ˌgluːkəuˈsinin] *n* 激糖素

glucocorticoid [ˌgluːkəuˈkɔːtikɔid] *n* 糖皮质激素,糖皮质素 *a* 糖皮质素的

glucofuranose [ˌgluːkəuˈfjuərənəus] *n* 呋喃[型]葡萄糖

glucogenesis [ˌgluːkəuˈdʒenisis] *n* 糖生成 | **glucogenic** [ˌgluːkəuˈdʒenik] *a* 生成糖的

glucohemia [ˌgluːkəuˈhiːmiə] *n* 糖血症

glucoheptonate [ˌgluːkəuˈheptəneit] *n* 葡庚糖酸盐

glucoheptonic acid [ˌgluːkəuhepˈtɔnik] 葡[萄]庚糖酸

glucokinase [ˌgluːkəuˈkaineis] *n* 葡糖激酶;己糖激酶Ⅳ型

glucokinetic [ˌgluːkəukaiˈnetik] *a* 激动糖质的

glucokinin [ˌgluːkəuˈkinin] *n* 激糖素,植物胰岛素

glucolactone [ˌgluːkəuˈlæktəun] *n* 葡萄糖酸内酯

gluconolactone [ˌgluːkənəuˈlæktəun] *n* 葡糖酸内酯(螯合剂)

glucolysis [gluːˈkɔlisis] *n* 糖酵解 | **glucolytic** [gluːkəuˈlitik] *a*

glucometer [gluːˈkɔmitə] *n* 血糖测定仪(用以测定葡萄糖在尿中的比例)

gluconate [ˈgluːˈkəneit] *n* 葡萄糖酸盐 | ferrous ~ 葡萄糖酸亚铁(抗贫血药,用于治疗缺铁性贫血)

gluconeogenesis [ˌgluːkəuni(ː)əuˈdʒenisis] *n* 糖异生 | **gluconeogenetic** [ˌgluːkəuˌni(ː)əudʒiˈnetik] *a*

gluconic acid [gluːˈkɔnik] 葡糖酸

Gluconobacter [ˌgluːkənəuˈbæktə] *n* 葡糖杆菌属

glucopenia [ˌgluːkəuˈpiːniə] *n* 低血糖,血糖过少

glucophenetidin [ˌgluːkəufiˈnetidin] *n* 葡萄糖乙氧苯胺

glucophore [ˈgluːkəfɔː] *n* 生甜味基

glucoprotein [ˌgluːkəuˈprəutiːn] *n* 糖蛋白

glucoproteinase [ˌgluːkəuˈprəutiːneis] *n* 糖蛋白酶

glucopyranose [ˌgluːkəuˈpaiərənəus] *n* 吡喃[型]葡萄糖

glucoregulation [ˌgluːkəuˌregjuˈleiʃən] *n* 糖代谢调节

glucosamine [ˌgluːkəuˈsæmin] *n* 葡糖胺;氨基葡萄糖(药用辅料)

glucosamine-phosphate *N*-acetyltransferase [gluːˈkəusəmiːn ˈfɔsfeit ˌæsitilˈtrænsfəreis] 葡糖胺磷酸 *N*-乙酰基转移酶

glucosan [ˈgluːkəsæn] *n* 葡聚糖

glucosazone [ˌgluːkəuˈseizəun] *n* 葡糖脎

glucose [ˈgluːkəus] *n* 葡萄糖 | liquid ~ 液状葡萄糖 / ~ 1-phosphate 葡糖-1-磷酸 / ~ 6-phosphate 葡糖-6-磷酸

glucose oxidase [ˈgluːkəus ˈɔksideis] 葡糖氧化酶

glucose-6-phosphatase [ˈgluːkəus ˈfɔsfəˌteis] 葡糖-6-磷酸酶(此酶缺乏为一种常染色体隐性性状,可致糖原贮积症Ⅰ型)

glucose-6-phosphatase deficiency 葡糖-6-磷酸酶缺乏症,糖原贮积症Ⅰ型

glucose-6-phosphate dehydrogenase [ˈgluːkəus ˈfɔsfeit diːˈhaidrədʒəneis] 葡糖-6-磷酸脱氢酶(此酶的遗传性缺乏可致患者出现严重溶血危象)

glucose-6-phosphate dehydrogenase (G6PD) deficiency 葡糖-6-磷酸脱氢酶缺乏症(最常见的先天性代谢缺陷,表现为不同程度的溶血性贫血)

glucose-6-phosphate isomerase [ˈgluːkəus ˈfɔsfeit aiˈsɔməreis] 葡糖-6-磷酸异构酶(此酶缺乏为一种常染色体隐性性状,可致溶血性贫血)

glucose-6-phosphate translocase [ˈgluːkəus ˈfɔsfeit trænsˈləukeis] 葡糖-6-磷酸移位酶

glucosidase [gluːˈkəusideis] *n* 葡糖苷酶

α-glucosidase [gluːˈkəusideis] *n* α-葡糖苷酶(亦称麦芽糖酶) | lysosomal ~ 溶酶体 α-葡糖苷酶,葡聚糖-1, 4-α 葡糖苷酶

α-1, 4-glucosidase [gluːˈkəusideis] *n* α-1, 4-葡糖苷酶

α-1, 4-glucosidase deficiency α-1, 4-葡糖苷酶缺乏症,糖原贮积症Ⅱ型

β-glucosidase [gluːˈkəusideis] *n* β-葡糖苷酶

glucoside [ˈgluːkəsaid] *n* 葡糖苷;糖苷 | **glucosidic** [ˌgluːkəˈsidik] *a*

glucosidolytic [ˌgluːkəusaidəˈlitik] *a* 分解糖苷的

glucosin [ˈgluːkəsin] *n* 葡萄糖碱

glucosulfone sodium [ˌgluːkəuˈsʌlfəun] 葡胺苯砜钠(抗麻风药)

glucosum [gluːˈkəusəm] *n*【拉】葡萄糖

glucosuria [ˌgluːkəuˈsjuəriə] *n* 糖尿

glucosyl [ˈgluːkəsil] *n* 葡萄糖基

glucosylceramidase [ˌgluːkəsilsəˈræmideis] *n* 葡糖神经酰胺酶(此酶活性缺乏为一种常染色体隐性性状,可致戈谢〈Gaucher〉病,亦称葡糖脑苷脂酶)

glucosylceramide [ˌgluːkəsilˈserəmaid] *n* 葡糖神经酰胺,葡糖脑苷脂

glucosyltransferase [ˌgluːkəsilˈtrænsfəreis] *n* 葡糖基转移酶

glucothionic acid [ˌgluːkəθaiˈɔnik] 乳腺硫酸糖酯

glucoxylose [ˌgluːkəuˈzailəus] *n* 葡萄木二糖

glucurolactone [ˌgluːkjuərəuˈlæktəun] *n* 葡醛内酯(保肝药)

glucuronate [gluːˈkjuərəneit] *n* 葡糖醛酸(盐、酯或阴离子型)

glucuronic acid [gluːkjuəˈrɔnik] 葡糖醛酸

***β*-glucuronidase** [ˌgluːkjuəˈrɔnideis] *n* *β*-葡糖醛酸糖苷酶(此酶缺乏为一种常染色体隐性性状,可致黏多糖贮积症Ⅶ型,见 Sly's syndrome)

glucuronidate [gluːˈkjuərənideit] *vt* 使葡糖醛酸化

glucuronide [gluːˈkjuərənaid] *n* 葡糖苷酸

glucuronide transferase [gluːˈkjuərənaid ˈtrænsfəreis] 葡糖苷酸转移酶(即 glucuronosyltransferase)

glucuronolactone [ˌgluːkjuəˌrəunəˈlæktəun] *n* 葡糖醛酸内酯;葡醛内酯(保肝药)

glucuronoside [ˌgluːkjuəˈrɔnəsaid] *n* 葡糖苷酸

glucuronosyltransferase [ˌgluːkjuəˌrɔnəsilˈtrænsfəreis] *n* 葡糖苷酰基转移酶(此酶缺乏为一种常染色体隐性性状,可致克-纳〈Crigler-Najjar〉综合征)

glucuronyl transferase [gluːˈkjuərənil ˈtrænsfəreis] 葡糖醛酸基转移酶(此术语为 glucuronosyltransferase 的欠正确名)

glue [gluː] *n* 胶;胶水

Glugea [ˈgluːdʒiə] *n* 格留虫属

Gluge's corpuscles [ˈgluːgə] (Gottlieb Gluge)格路格小体(颗粒状细胞,见于脂变的神经组织)

glutamate [ˈgluːtəmeit] *n* 谷氨酸;谷氨酸盐(酯或根)

glutamate-ammonia ligase [ˈgluːtəmeit əˈməuniə ˈlaigeis] 谷氨酸氨连接酶(亦称谷氨酰胺合成酶)

glutamate-cysteine ligase [ˈgluːtəmeit ˈsistiiːn ˈlaigeis] 谷氨酸半胱氨酸连接酶

glutamate decarboxylase [ˈgluːtəmeit diːkɑːˈbɔksileis] 谷氨酸脱羧酶(此酶缺乏为一种常染色体隐性性状,可致吡多辛〈pyridoxine〉依赖性婴儿惊厥)

glutamate dehydrogenase [NAD(P)$^+$] [ˈgluːtəmeit diːˈhaidrədʒəneis] 谷氨酸脱氢酶[NAD(P)$^+$]

glutamate formiminotransferase [ˈgluːtəmeit fɔːˌmiminəuˈtrænsfəreis] 谷氨酸亚胺甲基转移酶(亦称亚胺甲基转移酶)

glutamic acid [gluːˈtæmik] 谷氨酸

glutamic acid hydrochloride [gluːˈtæmik ˈæsid ˌhaidrəuˈklɔːraid] 盐酸谷氨酸(促胃酸药)

glutamic-oxaloacetic transaminase (GOT) [gluːˈtæmik ˌɔksələuəˈsiːtik trænsˈæmineis] 谷[氨酸]-草[酰乙酸]转氨酶,天冬氨酸转氨酶

glutamic-pyruvic transaminase (GPT) [gluːˈtæmik paiəˈruːvik trænsˈæmineis] 谷[氨酸]-丙[酮酸]转氨酶,丙氨酸转氨酶

glutaminase [gluːˈtæmineis] *n* 谷氨酰胺酶

glutamine [ˈgluːtəmiːn] *n* 谷氨酰胺

glutamine synthetase [ˈglutəmin ˈsinθiteis] 谷氨酰胺合成酶,谷氨酸氨连接酶

glutaminyl [gluːˈtæminil] *n* 谷氨酰胺酰[基]

glutamyl [ˈgluːtəmil] *n* 谷氨酰[基]

γ-glutamylcyclotransferase [ˌgluːtəmilˌsaikləuˈtrænsfəreis] *n* γ-谷氨酰[基]环化转移酶

γ-glutamylcysteine [ˌgluːtəmilˈsistiiːn] *n* γ-谷氨酰[基]半胱氨酸

γ-glutamylcysteine synthetase [ˌgluːtəmilsisˈtiiːn ˈsinθiteis] γ-谷氨酰[基]半胱氨酸合成酶,谷氨酸半胱氨酸连接酶

γ-glutamylcysteine synthetase deficiency γ-谷氨酰[基]半胱氨酸合成酶缺乏症(谷胱甘肽合成的遗传性氨基酸病,由于谷氨酸半胱氨酸连接酶缺乏所致,包括溶血性贫血、脊髓小脑变性、周围神经病变、肌病以及氨基酸尿症)

γ-glutamyltransferase (GGT) [ˌgluːtəmilˈtrænsfəreis] *n* γ-谷氨酰[基]转移酶(此酶缺乏为一种常染色体隐性性状,可致 γ-谷氨酰转肽酶缺乏症)

glutamyl transpeptidase [ˈɡluːtəmil trænsˈpeptideis] 谷氨酰[基]转肽酶,γ-谷氨酰[基]转移酶

γ-glutamyl transpeptidase deficiency γ-谷氨酰转肽酶缺乏症(亦称谷胱甘肽尿)

glutaral [ˈɡluːtəræl] *n* 戊二醛(即 glutaraldehyde) | ~ concentrate 浓缩戊二醛(消毒药)

glutaraldehyde [ˌɡluːtəˈrældihaid] *n* 戊二醛(组织固定剂)

glutargin [ˈɡluːtədʒin] *n* 谷氨酸精氨酸

glutaric acid [ˈɡluːˈtærik] 戊二酸

glutaricacidemia [ɡluːˌtærikˌæsiˈdiːmiə] *n* 戊二酸血[症]

glutaricaciduria [ɡluːˌtærikˌæsiˈdjuəriə] *n* 戊二酸尿[症](为常染色体隐性遗传氨基酸病,特征为蓄积和排泄戊二酸。有两型,Ⅱ型亦称多酰基辅酶 A 脱氢作用缺乏;尿内戊二酸排泄过多)

glutaryl [ˈɡluːtəril] *n* 戊二酰[基],戊二酸单酰[基]

glutaryl-CoA dehydrogenase [ˈɡluːtəril kəuˈei diːˈhaidrədʒəneis] 戊二酸单酰-CoA 脱氢酶(此酶缺乏为一种常染色体隐性性状,可致戊二酸尿Ⅰ型)

glutathione [ˌɡluːtəˈθaiəun] *n* 谷胱甘肽(解毒药)

glutathionemia [ˌɡluːtəˌθaiəˈniːmiə] *n* 谷胱甘肽血[症]

glutathione peroxidase [ˌɡluːtəˈθaiəun pəˈrɔksideis] 谷胱甘肽过氧化物酶(此酶活性缺乏可致新生儿黄疸及溶血性贫血)

glutathione reductase (NADPH) [ˌɡluːtəˈθaiəun riˈdʌkteis] 谷胱甘肽还原酶(NADPH)(此酶缺乏可能是一种遗传性状,与中性粒细胞损害有关,可致免疫应答减弱及蚕豆诱发的溶血性贫血)

glutathione synthase [ˌɡluːtəˈθaiəun ˈsinθeis] 谷胱甘肽合酶,谷胱甘肽合成酶

glutathione synthetase [ˌɡluːtəˈθaiəun ˈsinθiteis] 谷胱甘肽合成酶(先天性谷胱甘肽合成酶缺乏,为一种常染色体隐性性状,可致溶血性贫血和严重酸中毒伴羟脯氨酸血症)

glutathione (GSH) synthetase deficiency 谷胱甘肽合成酶缺乏症

glutathionuria [ˌɡluːtəθaiəˈnjuəriə] *n* 谷胱甘肽尿;γ-谷氨酰[基]转肽酶缺乏症

gluteal [ˈɡluːtiəl] *a* 臀的

glutelin [ˈɡluːtəlin] *n* 谷蛋白

gluten [ˈɡluːtən] *n* 麸质,谷胶,谷蛋白 | ~-casein 麸酪蛋白,谷胶酪蛋白,植物干酪素 | **~ous** [ˈɡluːtənəs] *a*

glutenin [ˈɡluːtənin] *n* 麦谷蛋白

gluteofemoral [ˌɡluːtiəuˈfemərəl] *a* 臀股的

gluteoinguinal [ˌɡluːtiəuˈiŋɡwinl] *a* 臀腹股沟的

glutethimide [ɡluˈteθimaid] *n* 格鲁米特(镇静催眠药)

gluteus [ɡluːˈtiːəs] ([复] **glutei** [ɡluːˈtiːai]) *n* 臀肌

glutin [ˈɡluːtin] *n* 明胶蛋白;麸酪蛋白,谷胶酪蛋白

glutinosity [ˌɡluːtiˈnɔsəti] *n* 黏性

glutinous [ˈɡluːtinəs] *a* 胶状的,黏的

glutitis [ɡluːˈtaitis] *n* 臀肌炎

glutolin [ˈɡluːtəlin] *n* 类副球蛋白

glutoscope [ˈɡluːtəskəup] *n* 凝集检查镜

glutose [ˈɡluːtəus] *n* 人造糖

Gluzinski's test [ɡluˈzinski] (Wladyslaw A. Gluzinski)格卢金斯基试验(①检胆色素;②鉴别胃溃疡与胃癌)

Gly glycine 甘氨酸

glyburide [ˈɡlaibjuraid] *n* 格列本脲(口服降血糖药)

glycal [ˈɡlaikəl] *n* 烯糖(一种未饱和糖,—CH═CH—)

glycan [ˈɡlaikæn] *n* 聚糖(即多糖 polysaccharide)

glycase [ˈɡlaikeis] *n* 麦芽糖糊精酶

glycate [ˈɡlaikeit] *n* 糖基化产物

glycation [ɡlaiˈkeiʃən] *n* 非酶促糖基化

glycemia [ɡlaiˈsiːmiə] *n* 糖血

glycemin [ˈɡlaisəmin] *n* 肝抗胰岛素物质

glycentin [ɡlaiˈsentin] *n* 肠升糖素,肠高血糖素(即 enteroglucagon)

glyceraldehyde [ˌɡlisəˈrældihaid] *n* 甘油醛 | ~-3-phosphate 甘油醛-3-磷酸

glyceraldehyde-3-phosphate dehydrogenase (phosphorylating) [ˌɡlisəˈrældihaid ˈfɔsfeit diːˈhaidrədʒəneis] 甘油醛-3-磷酸脱氢酶(磷酸化)(缩写成 GAPD,亦称磷酸丙糖脱氢酶)

glycerate [ˈɡlisəreit] *n* 甘油酸;甘油酸盐(或酯)

glycerate dehydrogenase [ˈɡlisəreit diːˈhaidrədʒəneis] 甘油酸脱氢酶(此酶缺乏据认为是高草酸尿Ⅱ型和 D-甘油酸血症的原因)

glyceric acid [ɡliˈserik] 甘油酸

D-glycericacidemia [ɡliˈserikˌæsiˈdiːmiə] *n* D-甘油酸血症(可能伴有智力迟钝)

L-glycericaciduria [ɡliˌserikˌæsiˈdjuəriə] *n* L-甘油酸尿[症],原发性高草酸尿Ⅱ型

glyceridase [ˈɡlisərideis] *n* 甘油酯酶,脂酶

glyceride [ˈɡlisəraid] *n* 甘油酯 | **glyceridic** [ˌɡlisəˈridik] *a*

glycerin [ˈɡlisərin], **glycerine** [ˌɡlisəˈriːn, ˈɡli-

səriːn] *n* 甘油
glycerinate [ˈglisərineit] *vt* 用甘油处理,把…保存在甘油中 | **glycerination** [ˌglisəriˈneiʃən] *n*
glycerinated [ˈglisəriˌneitid] *a* 甘油制的;保存在油中的
glycerinum [ˌglisəˈrainəm] *n*【拉】甘油
glycerite [ˈglisərait] *n* 甘油剂 | boroglycerin ~ 硼酸甘油甘油剂 / starch ~ 淀粉甘油剂(表面润滑药) / tannic acid ~ 鞣酸甘油剂(收敛药)
glyceritum [ˌglisəˈraitəm] ([复] **glycerita** [ˌglisəˈraitə]) *n*【拉】甘油剂
glycerogel [ˈglisərədʒel] *n* 甘油凝胶
glycerogelatin [ˌglisərəˈdʒelətin] *n* 甘油明胶,甘油凝胶
glycerol [ˈglisərɔl] *n* 甘油 | ~ boroglycerite 硼酸甘油甘油剂 / ~ phosphate 磷酸甘油
glycerolize [ˈglisərəlaiz] *vt* 甘油化
glycerol kinase [ˈglisərɔl ˈkaineis] 甘油激酶
glycerol-3-phosphate *O*-acyltransferase [ˈglisərɔl ˈfɔsfeit ˌæsilˈtrænsfəreis] 甘油-3-磷酸*O*-酰基转移酶
glycerol-3-phosphate dehydrogenase [ˈglisərɔl ˈfɔsfeit diːˈhaidrədʒəneis] 甘油-3-磷酸脱氢酶
glycerol-3-phosphate dehydrogenase (NAD⁺) [ˈglisərɔl ˈfɔsfeit diːˈhaidrədʒəneis] 甘油-3-磷酸脱氢酶(NAD⁺)
glyceroluria [ˌglisərɔlˈjuəriə] *n* 甘油尿[症]
glycerone [ˈglisərəun] *n* 甘油酮(dihydroxyacetone〈二羟基丙酮〉的正式名,很少用)
glycerone phosphate [ˈglisərəun ˈfɔsfeit] 磷酸甘油酮
glycerophilic [ˌglisərəuˈfilik] *a* 亲甘油的
glycerophosphatase [ˌglisərəuˈfɔsfəteis] *n* 甘油磷酸酶
glycerophosphate [ˌglisərəuˈfɔsfeit] *n* 磷酸甘油
glycerophosphoric acid [ˈglisərəufɔsˈfɔrik] 甘油磷酸,磷酸甘油
glycerose [ˈglisərəus] *n* 甘油糖
glyceryl [ˈglisəril] *n* 甘油基 | ~ monostearate 单硬脂酸甘油酯(乳化剂) / ~ triacetate 三乙酸甘油酯(局部抗真菌药) / ~ trinitrate 硝酸甘油(用于防治心绞痛)
glycidol [ˈglisidɔl], **glycide** [ˈglaisid] *n* 缩水甘油
glycinamide ribonucleotide [glaiˈsinəmaid ˌraibəuˈnjuːkliətaid] 甘氨酰胺核苷酸
glycinate [ˈglaisineit] *n* 甘氨酸盐
glycine (G, Gly) [ˈglaisiːn] *n* 甘氨酸
glycine amidinotransferase [ˈglaisiːn ˌæmiˌdiːnəuˈtrænsfəreis] 甘氨酸脒基转移酶
glycine hydroxymethyltransferase [ˈglaisiːn haiˌdrɔksiˌmeθilˈtrænsfəreis] 甘氨酸羟甲基转移酶(亦称丝氨酸羟甲基转移酶)
glycinemia [ˌglaisiˈniːmiə] *n* 甘氨酸血症
glycine transamidinase [ˈglaisiːn ˌtrænsəˈmidineis] 甘氨酸转脒基酶,甘氨酸脒基转移酶
glycinin [ˈglisinin] *n* 大豆球蛋白
Glyciphagus [glaiˈsifəgəs] *n* 甜食螨属(即 Glycyphagus) | ~ domesticus (~ prunorum)家甜食螨(即 Glycyphagus domesticus)
glyc(o)- [构词成分]甘,甜;糖,葡萄糖;甘油;糖原
glycoaldehyde [ˌglaikəuˈældihaid] *n* 乙醇醛,羟乙醛
glycobiarsol [ˌglaikəubaiˈɑːsɔl] *n* 甘铋胂(抗肠阿米巴药)
glycocalix, glycocalyx [ˌglaikəuˈkæliks] *n* 糖萼(多糖蛋白质复合物),多糖包被
glycochenodeoxycholate [ˌglaikəuˌkiːnəudiːˌɔksiˈkəuleit] *n* 甘氨鹅脱氧胆酸,鹅脱氧胆酰甘氨酸
glycochenodeoxycholic acid [ˌglaikəuˌkiːnəudiːˌɔksiˈkəulik] 甘氨鹅脱氧胆酸,鹅脱氧胆酰甘氨酸
glycocholate [ˌglaikəuˈkɔleit] *n* 甘氨胆酸盐
glycocholic acid [ˌglaikəuˈkəulik] 甘氨胆酸
glycocine [ˈglaikəsin] *n* 甘氨酸
glycoclastic [ˌglaikəuˈklæstik] *a* 糖酵解的
glycocoll [ˈglaikəkɔl] *n* 甘氨酸
glycoconjugate [ˌglaikəuˈkɔndʒugit] *n* 复合糖(如糖脂、糖肽、低聚糖或氨基葡聚糖)
glycocyaminase [ˌglaikəuˈsaiæmineis] *n* 胍基乙酸酶
glycocyamine [ˌglaikəuˈsaiəmin] *n* 胍基乙酸
glycodesoxycholic acid [ˌglaikəudeˌzɔksiˈkəulik] 甘氨脱氧胆酸
glycogelatin [ˌglaikəuˈdʒelətin] *n* 甘油明胶
glycogen [ˌglkəudʒen, ˈglaikəudʒen] *n* 糖原 | hepatic ~ 肝糖原 / tissue ~ 组织糖原(尤指贮存在肌肉内的糖原)
glycogenase [ˈglaikəudʒineis] *n* 糖原酶
glycogenesis [ˌglaikəuˈdʒenisis] *n* 糖原生成,糖生成 | **glycogenetic** [ˌglaikəudʒiˈnetik], **glycogenous** [glaiˈkɔdʒinəs] *a*
glycogenic [ˌglaikəuˈdʒenik] *a* 生糖的,糖原的
glycogenolysis [ˌglaikəudʒiˈnɔlisis] *n* 糖原分解 | **glycogenolytic** [ˌglaikəuˌdʒenəˈlitik] *a*
glycogenosis [ˌglaikəudʒiˈnəusis] *n* 糖原贮积症,糖原病 | brancher deficiency ~ 分支酶缺乏性糖原贮积症,糖原贮积症Ⅳ型 / generalized ~ 全身性糖原病,糖原贮积症Ⅱ型 / hepatophosphorylase deficiency ~ 肝磷酸化酶缺乏性糖原贮积症,糖原贮积症Ⅵ型 / hepatorenal ~ 肝肾型糖

原贮积症,糖原贮积症Ⅰ型 / myophosphorylase deficiency ~ 肌磷酸化酶缺乏性糖原病,糖原贮积症Ⅴ型

glycogen phosphorylase [ˈglaikəudʒən fɔsˈfɔːrileis] 糖原磷酸化酶(此酶缺乏为一种常染色体隐性性状,可致糖原贮积症)

glycogen phosphorylase kinase [ˌglaikəudʒən fɔsˈfɔːrileis ˈkaineis] 糖原磷酸化酶激酶,磷酸化酶激酶

glycogen (starch) synthase [ˈglaikədʒən stɑːtʃˈsinθeis] 糖原(淀粉)合酶

glycogen synthase [ˈglaikəudʒənˈsinθeis] 糖原合酶

[**glycogen-synthase-D**] **phosphatase** [ˈglaikədʒən ˈsinθeis ˈfɔsfəteis] [糖原合酶-D]磷酸酶

glycogen synthetase [ˈglaikəudʒən ˈsinθiteis] 糖原合成酶,糖原合酶

glycogeusia [ˌglaikəuˈdʒjuːsiə] *n* 甜味觉,甜幻觉

glycohemia [ˌglaikəuˈhiːmiə] *n* 糖血症

glycohemoglobin [ˌglaikəuˌhiːməˈgləubin] *n* 糖基化血红蛋白

glycohistechia [ˌglaikəuhisˈtekiə] *n* 组织[内]多糖症

glycol [ˈglaikɔl] *n* 脂肪族二元醇类;乙二醇,甘醇 | polyethylene ~ 聚乙二醇(药用辅料)

glycolaldehyde [ˌglaikɔlˈældihaid] *n* 乙醇醛,羟乙醛

glycolate [ˈglaikəleit] *n* 羟乙酸盐

glycolic acid [glaiˈkɔlik] 羟基乙酸

glycolicaciduria [glaiˌkɔlikˌæsiˈdjuəriə] *n* 羟基乙酸尿[症],原发性高草酸尿Ⅰ型

glycolipid [ˌglaikəuˈlipid] *n* 糖脂

glycoluric acid [ˌglaikəuˈljuərik] 脲乙酸

glycolyl [ˈglaikəlil] *n* 羟乙酰基,乙醇酰基

glycolysis [glaiˈkɔlisis] *n* 糖酵解 | **glycolytic** [ˌglaikəuˈlitik] *a*

glycometabolism [ˌglaikəumeˈtæbəlizəm] *n* 糖代谢 | **glycometabolic** [ˌglaikəumetəˈbɔlik] *a*

glycone [ˈglaikəun] *n* 甘油栓

glyconeogenesis [ˌglaikəuˌni(ː)əuˈdʒenisis] *n* 糖原异生[作用]

glyconnectin [ˌglaikəuˈnektin] *n* 糖连接素

glyconucleoprotein [ˌglaikəuˌnjuːkliəuˈprəutiːn] *n* 糖核蛋白

glycopenia [ˌglaikəuˈpiːniə] *n* 低血糖,血糖过少

glycopeptide [ˌglaikəuˈpeptaid] *n* 糖肽

glycopexis [ˌglaikəuˈpeksis] *n* 糖储藏,糖固定 | **glycopexic** *a*

Glycophagus [glaiˈkɔfəgəs] *n* 甜食螨属(即 Glycyphagus)

glycophenol [ˌglaikəuˈfiːnɔl] *n* 糖精

glycophilia [ˌglaikəuˈfiliə] *n* 血糖敏感症

glycophorin [ˌglaikəuˈfɔːrin] *n* 血型糖蛋白

glycopolyuria [ˌglaikəuˌpɔliˈjuəriə] *n* 糖尿性多尿症

glycoprival [ˌglaikəuˈpraivəl] *a* 无糖的

glycoprotein [ˌglaikəuˈprəutiːn] *n* 糖蛋白 | glycine-rich *β* ~ (GBG) 富甘氨酸 *β* 糖蛋白,B 因子

glycoprotein 4-*β*-galactosyltransferase [ˌglaikəuˈprəutiːn gəˌlæktəusilˈtrænsfəreis] 糖蛋白 4-*β*-半乳糖基转移酶(EC 命名法中称为 *β*-*N*-acetylglucosaminylglycopeptide *β*-1, 4-galactosyltransferase)

glycoprotein sialidase [ˌglaikəuˈprəutiːn saiˈælideis] 糖蛋白唾液酸酶

glycoptyalism [ˌglaikəuˈtaiəlizəm] *n* 糖涎症

glycopyrrolate [ˌglaikəuˈpirəleit], **glycopyrronium bromide** [ˌglaikəupiˈrəunjəm] 格隆溴铵(抗胆碱药,用于治疗消化性溃疡和其他胃肠道紊乱)

glycoregulation [ˌglaikəuˌregjuˈleiʃən] *n* 糖[代谢]调节 | **glycoregulatory** [ˌglaikəˈregjulətəri] *a*

glycorrhachia [ˌglaikəuˈreikiə] *n* 糖脊[髓]液

glycorrhea [ˌglaikəuˈriːə] *n* 糖溢

glycosamine [glaiˈkəusəmiːn] *n* 葡糖胺,氨基葡糖

glycosaminoglycan [ˌglaikəusəˌmiːnəuˈglaikæn] *n* 糖胺聚糖,氨基葡聚糖(缩写为 GAG,以前称黏多糖)

glycosaminolipid [ˌglaikəusæminəˈlipid] *n* 氨基葡糖脂类

glycosecretory [ˌglaikəusiˈkriːtəri] *a* 糖原分泌的

glycosemia [glaikəuˈsiːmiə] *n* 糖血症

glycosene [ˈglaikəsiːn] *n* 反烯糖(一种脱水糖)

glycosialia [ˌglaikəusaiˈeiliə] *n* 糖涎症

glycosialorrhea [ˌglaikəuˌsaiələuˈriːə] *n* 糖涎溢

glycosidase [glaiˈkəusideis] *n* 糖苷酶

glycoside [ˈglaikəsaid] *n* [糖]苷 | cardiac ~ 强心苷 / cyanophoric ~ 氰[基]苷 / sterol ~ 植物甾醇苷 | **glycosidic** [glaikəuˈsidik] *a*

glycosometer [ˌglaikəuˈsɔmitə] *n* 尿糖定量器,尿糖计

glycosphingolipid [ˌglaikəuˌsfiŋgəˈlipid] *n* 糖[神经]鞘脂,鞘糖脂

glycosphingolipidosis [ˌglaikəu ˌsfiŋgəˌlipiˈdəusis] 糖[神经]鞘脂病,法布莱病(Fabry's disease)

glycostatic [ˌglaikəuˈstætik] *a* 糖原恒定的(保持糖浓度恒定)

glycosuria [ˌglaikəuˈsjuəriə] *n* 糖尿 | digestive ~, alimentary ~ 消化性糖尿,饮食性糖尿 / renal ~, benign ~, nondiabetic ~, nonhyperglycemic ~, normoglycemic ~, orthoglycemic ~ 肾性糖尿,良性糖尿,非糖尿病性糖尿,非血糖过高性糖尿,正常血糖性糖尿,体位性糖尿

glycosuric [ˌglaikəuˈsjuərik] *a* 糖尿的,有糖尿的

glycosuric acid [ˌglaikəuˈsjuərik] 糖尿酸

glycosyl [ˈglaikəsil] *n* 糖基

glycosylate [ˈglaikəsileit] *vt* 使(蛋白质)糖基化

glycosylated [glaiˈkəusiˌleitid] *a* 糖基化的

glycosylation [ˌglaikəsiˈleiʃən] *n* 糖基化

glycosylceramidase [ˌglaikəusilsəˈræmideis] *n* 糖基神经酰胺酶

glycosyltransferase [ˌglaikəsilˈtrænsfəreis] *n* 糖基转移酶

glycotaxis [ˌglaikəuˈtæksis] *n* 糖[代谢性]分布

glycotropic [ˌglaikəuˈtrɔpik] *a* 亲糖的,嗜糖的

glycuresis [ˌglaikjuəˈriːsis] *n* 糖尿(一次平常碳水化合物食物后,尿中葡萄糖含量的正常性增加)

glycuronate [glaiˈkjuərəneit] *n* 糖羰酸;糖醛酸

glycuronic acid [ˌglaikjuəˈrɔnik] 糖醛酸

glycuronide [glaiˈkjuərənaid] *n* 糖苷酸

glycuronuria [glaiˌkjuərəuˈnjuəriə] *n* 葡萄糖醛酸尿

glycyl [ˈglisil] *n* 甘氨酰基,氨基乙酰基

glycylglycine [ˌglisilˈglisin] *n* 双甘氨肽,甘氨酰甘氨酸

glycyltryptophan [ˌglisilˈtriptəfæn] *n* 甘氨酰色氨酸(用于胃癌检验)

Glycyphagidae [ˌglaisiˈfædʒidiː] *n* 甜食螨科

Glycyphagus [glaiˈsifəgəs] *n* 甜食螨属 | ~ domesticus 家甜食螨

Glycyrrhiza [ˌglisiˈraizə] *n* 甘草属

glycyrrhiza [ˌglisiˈraizə] *n* 甘草

glycyrrhizic acid [ˌglisiˈraizik] 甘草酸

glycyrrhizin [ˌglisiˈraizin] *n* 甘草皂苷,甘草甜素

glydanile sodium [ˈglaidənail] 格列他尼钠(即 glicetanile sodium,口服降血糖药)

glyhexamide [glaiˈheksəmaid] *n* 格列己脲(口服降血糖药)

glykemia [glaiˈkiːmiə] *n* 糖血症

glymidine sodium [ˈglaimidiːn] 格列嘧啶钠(口服降血糖药)

glyoctamide [glaiˈɔktəmaid] *n* 格列辛脲(口服降血糖药)

glyoxal [glaiˈɔksəl] *n* 乙二醛

glyoxalase [glaiˈɔksəleis] *n* 乙二醛酶

glyoxalin [glaiˈɔksəlin] *n* 咪唑,异吡唑,亚胺唑

glyoxisome [glaiˈɔksisəum] *n* 乙醛酸循环体(即 glyoxosome)

glyoxosome [glaiˈɔksəsəum] *n* 乙醛酸循环体

glyoxylate [glaiˈɔksileit] *n* 乙醛酸盐

glyoxylic acid [ˌglaiɔkˈsilik] 乙醛酸

glyphylline [glaiˈfilin] *n* 双羟丙茶碱,喘定(血管和支气管扩张药,强心利尿药)

Glyptocranium [ˌgliptəuˈkreinjəm] *n* 秘鲁毒蛛属(即 Mastophora) | ~ gasteracanthoides 秘鲁毒蛛(即 Mastophora gasteracanthoides)

Gm Gm 同种异型(在遗传学上指人类 IgG 重链上的同种异型标记,作为简单的孟德尔特征遗传的,发现位于 γ 链的 Fc 和 Fd 片段,同种异型已知有 20 种以上)

gm gram 克

GMC General Medical Council 全国医学总会(英国)

GM-CSF granulocyte-macrophage colony-stimulating factor 粒-巨噬细胞集落刺激因子

Gmelin's test [ˈmeilin] (Leopold Gmelin)格梅林试验(检尿中胆色素)

GMK green monkey kidney cells 绿猴肾细胞(制剂)

GMP guanosine monophosphate 鸟苷[一磷]酸;cyclic GPM 3′, 5′-GMP 环鸟苷酸

gnat [næt] *n* 蚊,蚋 | buffalo ~ 蚋 / eye ~ 眼潜蝇(即 Hippelates pusio) / fungus ~ 食菌蚋 / turkey ~ 火鸡蚋

gnath- 见 gnatho-

gnathalgia [nəˈθældʒiə] *n* 颌痛

gnathic [ˈnæθik] *a* 颌的

gnathion [ˈnæθiɔn] *n* 颏下点,颏顶点

gnathitis [næˈθaitis] *n* 颌炎

gnath(o)- [构词成分]颌

Gnathobdellidae [ˌnæθɔbˈdelidiː] *n* 颚蛭科

gnathocephalus [ˌnæθəuˈsefələs] *n* 有颌无头畸胎

gnathodynamics [ˌnæθəudaiˈnæmiks] *n* 颌力学

gnathodynamometer [ˌnæθəuˌdainəˈmɔmitə] *n* 颌力计 | bimeter ~ 双度颌力计

gnathodynia [ˌnæθəuˈdiniə] *n* 颌痛

gnathography [nəˈθɔgrəfi] *n* 颌力描记[法]

gnathology [nəˈθɔlədʒi] *n* 颌学 | **gnathologic** [ˌnæθəˈlɔdʒik] *a*

gnathoplasty [ˈnæθəˌplæsti] *n* 颌成形术

gnathoschisis [nəˈθɔskisis] *n* 颌裂[畸形]

gnathosoma [ˌnæθəuˈsəumə] *n* 颚体

gnathostat [ˈnæθəstæt] *n* 颌固定器

gnathostatics [ˌnæθəuˈstætiks] *n* 牙模定位法

Gnathostoma [nəˈθɔstəmə] *n* 腭口线虫属 | ~ hispidum 刚棘腭口线虫 / ~ spinigerum 棘腭口线虫 | **Gnathostomum** *n*

Gnathostomatidae [ˌnæθəustəuˈmætidiː] *n* 颚口科

gnathostomatics [ˌnæθəustəuˈmætiks] *n* 口颌生理学

gnathostomiasis [ˌnæθəustəuˈmaiəsis] *n* 腭口线

虫病

gnosia [ˈnəusiə] *n* 认识,感知

gnosis [ˈnəusis] *n* 感悟(指大脑皮质感觉冲动所唤起连系性记忆体系,为大脑皮质功能之一)

gnotobiota [ˌnəutəubaiˈəutə] *n* 悉生区系,定菌区系(指实验动物在受控制的饲养条件下保有的一定的、既知的微动物区系和微生物区系)

gnotobiote [ˌnəutəuˈbaiəut] *n* 悉生生物,定菌生物(在特定条件下饲养的,已知其体内外微动物区系和微植物区系的实验动物) | **gnotobiotic** [ˌnəutəubaiˈɔtik] *a* 悉生的,定菌的

gnotobiotics [ˌnəutəubaiˈɔtiks], **gnotobiology** [ˌnəutəubaiˈɔlədʒi] *n* 悉生生物学,限菌生物学

gnotophoresis [ˌnəutəuˈfɔrisis] *n* 悉生形成,定菌形成 | **gnotophoric** [ˌnəutəuˈfɔrik] *a*

Gn-RH gonadotropin-releasing hormone 促性腺[激]素释放激素,促性腺素释放素

Goa powder [ˈgəuə] 柯桠粉

goatpox [ˈgəutpɔks] *n* 山羊痘疮,山羊天花

Godélier's law [gəudeiˈljei] (Charles P. Godélier)戈德利耶定律(腹膜结核同时有胸膜结核)

Goeckerman treatment [ˈgəukəmən] (William H. Goeckerman)戈克曼疗法(以焦油膏继以紫外线B照射治疗银屑病)

Goetsch's skin reaction (test) [ˈgetʃ] (Emil Goetsch)戈奇皮肤反应(试验)(注射肾上腺素,诊查甲状腺功能亢进)

Goggia's sign [ˈgəudʒɑː] (Carlo P. Goggia)果吉亚征(健康时先叩击然后握捏肱二头肌引起的纤维性收缩可延及整个肌肉,虚弱性疾病如伤寒时,此收缩为局部性的)

goggle [ˈgɔgl] *n* 瞪眼,转眼

goiter [ˈgɔitə] *n* 甲状腺肿 | colloid ~ 胶性甲状腺肿 / cystic ~ 囊性甲状腺肿 / diving ~, plunging ~, wandering ~ 游动性甲状腺肿,移动性甲状腺肿 / endemic ~ 地方性甲状腺肿 / exophthalmic ~, toxic ~ 突眼性甲状腺肿,毒性甲状腺肿(见 Graves' disease) / lingual ~ 甲状舌管囊肿 / lymphadenoid ~ 淋巴结样甲状腺肿

goitre [gɔitə] *n*【法】甲状腺肿

goitrin [ˈgɔitrin] *n* 致甲状腺肿素

goitrogen [ˈgɔitrədʒən] *n* 致甲状腺肿物

goitrogenic [ˈgɔitrəuˈdʒenik] *a* 致甲状腺肿的 | **~ity** [ˌgɔitrəudʒeˈnisəti] *n* 致甲状腺肿性,甲状腺肿发生性(素质) / **goitrogenous** [gɔiˈtrɔdʒinəs] *a*

goitrous [ˈgɔitrəs] *a* 甲状腺肿的

gold (Au) [gəuld] *n* 金 | annealed ~ 煅韧金 / cohesive ~ 黏[性]金 / colloidal ~ 胶态金,胶体金 / Dutch ~ 荷兰金(铜锌合金) / mat ~, crystal ~, crystalline ~, fibrous ~ 团金,晶体金,纤维金 / noncohesive ~ 无黏性金,软金 / radioactive ~ 放射性金,射金 / ~ sodium thiomalate 硫代苹果酸金钠(亦称金硫丁二钠,用于治类风湿关节炎和非播散性红斑狼疮) / ~ sodium thiosulfate, ~ aurothiosulfate 硫代硫酸金钠(用于治类风湿关节炎) / ~ thioglucose 硫葡萄糖金,金硫葡糖(用于治类风湿关节炎)

Goldberg's syndrome [ˈgəuldbəːg] (Morton F. Goldberg)戈德伯格综合征,半乳糖唾液酸沉积症

Goldblatt's clamp [ˈgəuldblæt] (Harry Goldblatt)戈德布拉特夹(肾动脉夹,借以产生实验性高血压) | ~ hypertension 戈德布拉特高血压(肾动脉闭塞性高血压) / ~ kidney 戈德布拉特肾(血流闭塞时的肾,导致肾性高血压)

Goldenhar's syndrome [ˈgəuldənhɑː] (Maurice Goldenhar)戈登哈综合征,眼耳脊椎发育不良

goldenseal [ˌgəuldənˈsiːl] *n* 北美黄莲

Goldflam's disease, Goldflam-Erbdisease [ˈgəultflɑːm ˈɛəb] (Samuel V. Goldflam; Wilhelm H. Erb)重症肌无力

Goldscheider's percussion [ˈgəuldʃaidə] (Johannes K. A. E. A. Goldscheider)戈尔德沙伊德尔叩诊(①阈叩诊 threshold percussion,见 percussion 项下相应术语;②直指叩诊法)

Goldstein rays [ˈgəuldstain] (Eugene Goldstein)戈尔茨坦射线(X线穿过透明物质时所产生的一种射线,亦称S射线)

Goldstein's disease [ˈgəuldstain] (Hyman I. Goldstein)遗传性出血性毛细血管扩张 | ~ hematemesis 戈尔茨坦呕血(由胃毛细血管扩张引起) / ~ hemoptysis 戈尔茨坦咯血(气管支气管毛细管扩张性咯血) / ~ sign 戈尔茨坦征(踇趾与邻趾之间相隔空隙很大,见于呆小病及唐氏〈Down〉综合征)

Goldthwait brace [ˈgəuldθweit] (Joel E. Goldthwait)戈德思韦特支架(一种衬垫3层革裹金属带的骨骼支架,最上部装于乳头线,最下部围绕骨盆) | ~ sign (symptom) 戈德思韦特征(症状)(患者仰卧,检查者一手将患者腿抬高,另一手置于其背下部,然后施力于骨盆的一侧,如患者在腰椎移动之前即感疼痛,则损伤即为骶髂关节扭伤,如腰椎移动后始感疼痛,则损伤在骶髂或腰骶关节内)

golgiosome [ˈgɔldʒiəsəum] *n* 高尔基体,网体

Golgi's complex (apparatus, body) [ˈgɔldʒi] (Camillo Golgi)高尔基复合体(器、体)(细胞内一种复杂的杯状结构,由若干囊泡所组成,囊泡通过细胞膜移行,释放糖蛋白和黏多糖,从而起着内分泌和外分泌的作用) | ~ corpuscle 高尔基小体(在腱内腱与肌肉纤维接合处所见的一种腱梭) / ~ cells 高尔基细胞(见 ~ neurons) / ~ law 高尔基定律(疟疾发作的严重程度取决

于血内疟原虫的数目）/ ~ mixed staining method 高尔基混合染色法（染神经细胞及其全部细胞突）/ ~ type Ⅰ neurons 高尔基Ⅰ型神经元（具有长轴突的锥体细胞，起自中枢神经系统灰质，穿入白质，终于外周。亦称高尔基细胞）/ ~ type Ⅱ neurons 高尔基Ⅱ型神经元（具有短轴突的星形神经元，不离开细胞体所在的灰质，在大脑和小脑皮质内及在视网膜内为数最多。亦称高尔基细胞）/ ~ tendon organ 高尔基腱器（发现于哺乳类肌腱中的一种机械性刺激感受器。亦称神经腱梭）/ ~ theory 高尔基学说（神经元由高尔基细胞轴突和外指细胞轴突的侧支而沟通的）

Goll's column, fasciculas, tract [gɔl]（Friedrich Goll）脊髓薄束 | ~ fibers 戈尔纤维（从薄束核延伸到小脑蚓部）/ ~ nucleus 戈尔核（薄束核，在延髓内）

Goltz's experiment [ˈgəults]（Friedrich L. Goltz）戈尔茨实验（叩击蛙腹可引起蛙心停止跳动）| ~ theory 戈尔茨学说（半规管的作用是传递位置觉，从而为平衡觉提供物质辅助）

Goltz syndrome [gəults]（Robert W. Goltz）戈尔茨综合征，局灶性皮肤发育不良

Gombault-Philippe triangle [gɔmˈbəu fiˈlip]（F. A. A. Gombault; Claudius Philippe）贡博-菲利普三角（脊髓圆锥内，由隔缘束的纤维形成）

Gombault's degeneration (neuritis) [gɔmˈbəu]（François A. A. Gombault）进行性肥大性间质性神经病

gomitoli [gəˈmitəlai] *n* 垂体门脉毛细血管网

Gomori methods, stains [ˈgɔməri]（George Gomori）戈莫里法、染剂（组织学上用以显示酶，尤其是染切片中的磷酸酶及脂酶，亦为显示结缔组织纤维及分泌性颗粒的染色法）

Gompertz formula, law [ˈgɔmpəːts]（Benjamin Gompertz）冈珀茨公式、定律（老年期的死亡危险随几何级数增加：年龄为 *x* 时的死亡率，可按公式 $q_x = q_0 ea^x$ 计算，q_x 是年龄 *x* 时死亡率，q_0 是年龄为 0 时的死亡率，*a* 为常数）

gomphiasis [gɔmˈfaiəsis] *n* 牙松动；牙痛

gomphosis [gɔmˈfəusis] *n* 嵌合；钉状关节

gon- [构词成分]精液，种子；膝

gonacratia [ˌgɔnəˈkreiʃiə] *n* 遗精，精溢

gonad [ˈgəunæd, ˈgɔnæd] *n* 性腺，生殖腺 | indifferent ~ 未分化性腺 / streak ~s 条纹性腺（未发育的性腺结构，见于输卵管下阔韧带中，最常见于特纳〈Turner〉综合征）/ third ~ 第三性腺（肾上腺）| **~al** [gɔˈnædl], **~ial** [gɔˈnædiəl] *a*

gonadarche [ˌgəunəˈdɑːki] *n* 性腺功能初现

gonadectomize [ˌgɔnəˈdektəmaiz] *vt* 性腺切除

gonadectomy [ˌgɔnəˈdektəmi] *n* 性腺切除术

gonadoblastoma [ˌgɔnədəublæsˈtəumə] *n* 成性腺细胞瘤

gonadogenesis [ˌgɔnədəuˈdʒenisis] *n* 性腺发生，生殖腺发生

gonadoinhibitory [ˌgɔnədəuinˈhibitəri] *a* 性腺抑制的

gonadokinetic [ˌgɔnədəukaiˈnetik] *a* 促性腺[活动]的

gonadoliberin [ˌgɔnədəuˈlibərin] *n* 促性腺素释放素

gonadopathy [ˌgɔnəˈdɔpəθi] *n* 性腺病，生殖腺病

gonadopause [gɔˈnædəpɔːz] *n* 性腺功能停止，性腺功能丧失

gonadorelin [ˌgɔnədəuˈrelin] *n* 戈那瑞林（促性激素释放素）| ~ hydrochloride 盐酸戈那瑞林（用以评估性腺功能减退时垂体前叶促性腺细胞的功能性能力，并用以治疗青春期延迟和闭经，皮下或静脉内给药）

gonadotherapy [ˌgɔnədəuˈθerəpi] *n* 性激素疗法，性腺剂疗法

gonadotoxic [ˌgəunədəuˈtɔksik] *a* 性腺毒的

gonadotoxicity [ˌgəunədəutɔkˈsisəti] *n* 性腺毒性；性腺中毒程度

gonadotoxin [ˈgəunədəuˌtɔksin] *n* 性腺毒素

gonadotrope [gɔˈnædətrəup] *n* 促性腺细胞；促性腺物质

gonadotroph [gɔˈnædətrəuf] *n* 促性腺激素细胞；促性腺物质

gonadotropic [ˌgɔnədəuˈtrəupik], **gonadotrophic** [ˌgɔnədəuˈtrɔfik] *a* 促性腺的

gonadotropin [ˌgɔnədəuˈtrəupin], **gonadotrophin** [ˌgɔnədəuˈtrəufin] *n* 促性腺激素，促性腺素 | chorionic ~ 绒毛膜促性腺激素（用以治性腺发育不全）/ human chorionic ~（hCG）人绒毛膜促性腺激素 / human menopausal ~（hMG）人类绝经期促性腺激素 / pregnant mare serum ~, equine ~ 孕马血清促性腺激素，马促性腺激素（用以治隐睾病、不育、垂体性侏儒症等）

gonaduct [ˈgɔnədʌkt] *n* 生殖管

gonagra [gɔˈnægrə] *n* 膝关节痛风

gonalgia [gɔˈnældʒiə] *n* 膝痛

gonane [ˈgəunein] *n* 甾烷

gonangiectomy [ˌgɔnændʒiˈektəmi] *n* 输精管切除术

gonarthritis [ˌgɔnɑːˈθraitis] *n* 膝关节炎

gonarthrocace [ˌgɔnɑːˈθrɔkeisi] *n* 膝白肿

gonarthromeningitis [gɔnˌɑːθrəuˌmeninˈdʒaitis] *n* 膝关节滑膜炎

gonarthrosis [ˌgɔnɑːˈθrəusis] *n* 膝关节病

gonarthrotomy [ˌgɔnɑːˈθrɔtəmi] *n* 膝关节切开术

gonatocele [gɔˈnætəsiːl] *n* 膝瘤

gonecyst [ˈgɔnisist], **gonecystis** [ˌgɔniˈsistis] *n*

精囊
gonecystic [ˌgɔniˈsistik] *a* 精囊的
gonecystitis [ˌgɔnisisˈtaitis] *n* 精囊炎
gonecystolith [ˌgɔniˈsistəliθ] *n* 精囊石
gonecystopyosis [ˌgɔniˌsistəpaiˈəusis] *n* 精囊化脓
goneitis [ˌgɔniˈaitis] *n* 膝关节炎
gonepoiesis [ˌgɔnipɔiˈiːsis] *n* 精液生成,精液分泌 | **gonepoietic** [ˌgɔnipɔiˈetik] *a*
Gongylonema [ˌgɔndʒiləˈniːmə] *a* 筒线虫属 | ~ ingluvicola 嗉囊筒线虫 / ~ neoplasticum 瘤筒线虫 / ~ pulchrum, ~ scutatum 美丽筒线虫
gongylonemiasis [ˌgɔndʒiləniˈmaiəsis] *n* 筒线虫病
gonia [ˈgəuniə] gonion 的复数
gonial [ˈgəuniəl] *a* 下颌角点的
gonidangium [ˌgɔniˈdændʒiəm] *n* 分生体囊;藻胞囊
gonidiospore [gəuˈnidiəspɔː] *n* 分生体孢子;藻胞孢
gonidium [gəuˈnidiəm] ([复] **gonidia** [gəuˈnidiə]) *n* 微生子;藻胞(地衣)
Gonin's operation [gɔˈnæn] (Jules Gonin) 戈南手术(经一巩膜切口在视网膜裂上施行热烙术,治疗视网膜脱离)
goni(o)- [构词成分]角
Goniobasis [ˌgəuniəuˈbeisis] *n* 角蜗属
goniocraniometry [ˌgəuniəuˌkreiniˈɔmitri] *n* 颅角测量法
goniodysgenesis [ˌgəuniəudisˈdʒenisis] *n* 前房角发育不良
gonioma [ˌgɔniˈəumə] *n* 生殖细胞瘤
goniometer [ˌgəuniˈɔmitə] *n* 角度计,测角计;测向器(检迷路病) | finger ~ 手指测角计(测手指指骨间关节的屈伸度) | **goniometry** *n* 测角术;测向术 / **goniometric** [ˌgəuniəˈmetrik] *a* 测角的,测角计的
gonion [ˈgəuniɔn] ([复] **gonia** [ˈgəuniə]) *n* 下颌角点(头颅测量名词,下颌外角上的最下、最后及最外侧之点)
goniophotography [ˌgəuniəufəˈtɔgrəfi] *n* 眼前房角照相术
Goniops [ˈgɔniɔps] *n* 虻蝇属
goniopuncture [ˌgəuniəuˈpʌŋktʃə] *n* 前房角穿刺
gonioscope [ˈgəuniəˌskəup] *n* 前房角镜 | **gonioscopy** [ˌgəuniˈɔskəpi] *n* 前房角镜检查[术]
goniosynechia [ˌgəuniəusiˈnekiə] *n* 前房角粘连
goniotomy [ˌgəuniˈɔtəmi] *n* 前房角切开术
gonitis [gəuˈnaitis] *n* 膝关节炎 | fungous ~ 蕈状膝关节炎 / ~ tuberculosa 结核性膝关节炎
gon(o)- [构词成分]种子,精子,生殖
gonoblennorrhea [ˌgɔnəuˌblenəˈriːə] *n* 眼淋病,淋病性结膜炎
gonocampsis [ˌgɔnəuˈkæmpsis] *n* 膝弯曲
gonocele [ˈgɔnəsiːl] *n* 精液囊肿
gonochorism [gɔˈnɔkərizəm, ˌgɔnəˈkɔːrizəm] *n* 雌雄异体
gonococcemia [ˌgɔnəukɔkˈsiːmiə] *n* 淋球菌[菌]血症
gonococcide [ˌgɔnəuˈkɔksaid], **gonococcocide** [ˌgɔnəuˈkɔkəsaid] *n* 杀淋球菌剂
gonococcus [ˌgɔnəuˈkɔkəs] ([复] **gonococci** [ˌgɔnəuˈkɔk(s)ai]) *n* 淋球菌 | **gonococcal, gonococcic** [ˌgɔnəuˈkɔksik] *a*
gonocyte [ˈgɔnəsait] *n* 性原细胞,生殖母细胞;配子母细胞
gonomery [gɔˈnɔməri] *n* 双亲染色体分立
gononephrotome [ˌgɔnəuˈnefrətəum] *n* 生殖肾节
gonophage [ˈgɔnəfeidʒ] *n* 淋球菌噬菌体
gonophore [ˈgɔnəfɔː] *n* 副生殖器(例如输卵管、子宫、输精管、精囊等)
gonorrhea [ˌgɔnəˈriːə] *n* 淋病 | **~l** *a*
gonosome [ˈgɔnəsəum] *n* 生殖体
gonotokont [ˌgɔnəˈtəukɔnt] *n* 性母细胞
gonotome [ˈgɔnətəum] *n* 生殖节
gony- [构词成分]膝
Gonyaulax [ˌgɔniˈɔːlæks] *n* 膝沟藻属
gonycampsis [ˌgɔniˈkæmpsis] *n* 膝弯曲
gonycrotesis [ˌgɔnikrəˈtiːsis] *n* 膝外翻
gonyectyposis [ˌgɔniˌektiˈpəusis] *n* 膝内翻,弓形腿
gonyocele [ˈgɔniəsiːl] *n* 膝滑膜炎,结核性膝关节炎
gonyoncus [ˌgɔniˈɔŋkəs] *n* 膝瘤
Goodell's sign (law) [guˈdel] (William Goodell) 古德尔征(定律)(子宫颈软,可能妊娠,子宫颈硬,决非妊娠)
Goodman's syndrome [ˈgudmən] (Richard M. Goodman) 古德曼综合征,尖头多指并指[畸形]Ⅳ型,尖头多趾并趾[畸形]Ⅳ型
Goodpasture's stain [gudˈpæstʃə] (Ernest W. Goodpasture) 古德帕斯丘染剂(过氧化酶染色法) | ~ syndrome 古德帕斯丘综合征,肺出血肾炎综合征(肾小球性肾炎咯血综合征,主要发生于青年男性,开始为呼吸道感染、肺浸润、咯血和贫血,继则迅速转为进行性肾病)
Goodsall's rule [ˈgudsɔːl] (David H. Goodsall) 古德索尔法则(肛门瘘分类的准则:凡在肛周区后半部有外口者一般来自肛门后半部,凡在前会阴有外口者一般来自肛门前 1/4)
Good's syndrome [gud] (R. A. Good) 古德综合征(免疫缺陷伴胸腺瘤)
Goormaghtigh's apparatus (cells) (Norbert

Goormaghtigh)[肾小]球旁细胞

goose [guːs] *n* 性病肉芽肿,性病性腹股沟腺炎

Gopalan's syndrome [ˈɡəupəlæn](Coluthur Gopalan)果帕兰综合征(营养不良所致的综合征,有核黄素缺乏的体征,肢体有烧灼感,远心部分有"针刺"感,并有多汗症)

Gordiacea [ˌɡɔːdiˈeisiə] *n* 铁线虫亚纲(即 Nematomorpha)

Gordius [ˈɡɔːdiəs] *n* 铁线虫属 | ~ aquaticus, ~ medinensis 麦地那龙线虫(即 Dracunculus medinensis)/ ~ robustus 粗大铁线虫

Gordon's elementary bodies [ˈɡɔːdn](Mervyn H. Gordon)戈登原始小体(一种微粒,曾被认为是霍奇金〈Hodgkin〉病的病毒性原因,以后证明可以从任何含嗜酸细胞的组织中获得)| ~ test 戈登试验(检脊髓液球蛋白及白蛋白)

Gordon's reflex [ˈɡɔːdn](Alfred Gordon)戈登反射(倒错性屈肌反射)| ~ sign 戈登征,伸指现象(finger phenomenon,见 phenomenon 项下相应术语第一解)

Gordon's syndrome [ˈɡɔːdn](Richard D. Gordon)戈登综合征(一型假性醛固酮减少症,伴高血压和高钾血症,但无盐消耗,据认为是由于肾小管吸收氯化物异常增高所致)

gorget [ˈɡɔːdʒit] *n* 有槽导子(一种切石刀导子)

Gorham's disease [ˈɡɔːrəm](Lemuel W. Gorham)戈勒姆病,骨消失病

gorlic acid [ˈɡɔːlik] 环戊烯十三碳烯酸,大风子油烯酸

Gorlin-Chaudhry-Moss syndrome [ˈɡɔːlin ˈtʃɔːdri mɔs](Robert James Gorlin; Anand P. Chaudhry; Melvin Lionel Moss)戈林-乔德利-莫斯综合征(包括颅骨面骨发育不全、多毛、大阴唇发育不全、牙和眼异常以及动脉导管未闭的综合征。亦称 Gorlin's syndrome)

Gorlin formula [ˈɡɔːlin](Richard Gorlin)戈林公式(通过瓣膜口和压力阶差计算流量而得出心瓣膜口估计区的一种公式)

Gorlin-Goltz syndrome [ˈɡɔːlin ɡəults](Robert James Gorlin; Robert William Goltz)戈林-戈尔茨综合征(即基底细胞痣综合征 basal cell nevus syndrome,见 syndrome 项下相应术语)

Gorlin-Psaume syndrome [ˈɡɔːlin səum](Robert James Gorlin; Jean Psaume)戈林-索姆综合征(即口-面-指(趾)综合征 orofaciodigital syndrome,见 syndrome 项下相应术语)

Gorlin's cyst [ˈɡɔːlin](Roberrt J. Gorlin)戈林囊肿(牙源性钙化囊肿)| ~ sign 戈林征(用舌能碰触鼻尖,常为埃勒斯-当洛〈Ehlers-Danlos〉综合征之征)/ ~ syndrome 戈林综合征(①基底细胞痣综合征;②见 Gorlin-Chaudhry-Moss syndrome)

gorondou [ɡəˈrɔndu] *n* 鼻骨增殖性骨膜炎,根度病,巨鼻[症]

goserelin [ˈɡəusəˌrelin] *n* 戈舍瑞林(戈那瑞林〈gonadorelin〉的类似物,用以治疗前列腺恶性肿瘤,以醋酸戈舍瑞林使用)

Goslee tooth [ˈɡɔzliː](Hart J. Goslee)戈斯利牙(连于金属基的互换牙)

Gosselin's fracture [ɡɔsˈlæn](Léon A. Gosselin)果斯兰骨折(胫骨远侧端的 V 字形骨折,延伸至踝关节)

Gossypium [ɡɔˈsipiəm] *n*【拉】棉属

gossypium [ɡɔˈsipiəm] *n*【拉】棉 | ~ asepticum, ~ depuratum, ~ purificatum 消毒棉,脱脂棉,精制棉

gossypol [ˈɡɔsipɔl] *n* 棉酚(男用避孕药)

GOT glutamic-oxalacetic transaminase 谷[氨酸]-草[酰乙酸]转氨酶

Göthlin's test (index) [ˈɡetlin](Gustaf F. Göthlin)格特林试验(指数)(检毛细血管脆性)

Gottlieb's epithelial attachment [ˈɡɔtliːb](Bernhard Gottlieb)戈特利布上皮附着(指口腔上皮附着于牙齿)

Gottron's papules, sign [ˈɡɔtrɔn](Heinrich Adolf Gottron)戈特隆丘疹、征(指关节背侧的平顶紫色丘疹,为皮肌炎的特征性丘疹)

Gottstein's fibers [ˈɡɔtstain](Jacob Gottstein)戈特施泰因纤维(外毛细胞及与之连结的神经纤维,形成耳蜗内听神经的延伸部分)| ~ basal process 戈特施泰因基底突(连结螺旋器基底膜与外毛细胞间的细基底突)

gotu kola [ˈɡəutjuːˈkəulə] 积雪草;积雪草叶茎制剂(外用促进伤口痊愈,并治麻风损害)

gouge [ɡaudʒ] *n* 圆凿

Gougerot-Blum syndrome [ɡuːʒəˈrəu blum](Henri Gougerot; Paul Blum)古热洛-布洛姆综合征,色素性紫癜性苔藓样皮炎

Gougerot-Carteaud syndrome [ɡuːʒəˈrəu kɑːˈtəu](Henri Gougerot; Alexandre Carteaud)古热洛-卡托综合征,融合性网状乳头瘤病

Gougerot-Nulock-Houwer syndrome [ɡuːʒəˈrəu ˈnilɔk ˈhauwə](H. Gougerot; Nulock; A. W. M. Houwer)古-纳-豪综合征,舍格仑综合征(见 Sjögren's syndrome)

Goulard's extract [ɡuˈlɑː](Thomas Goulard)次醋酸铅溶液 | ~ lotion, ~ water 稀次醋酸铅溶液

Gouley's catheter [ˈɡuli](John W. S. Gouley)古利导管(有沟的金属导尿管)

goundou [ˈɡuːndu] *n* 根度病,鼻骨增殖性骨膜炎,巨鼻[症]

gousiekte [ɡuˈsiːkti] *n*【荷】毒草性心肌炎(羊)

gout [ɡaut] *n* 痛风 | abarticular ~, irregular ~

关节外痛风,非典型痛风 / articular ~, regular ~ 关节痛风,典型痛风 / calcium ~ 钙质性痛风,钙质沉着 / latent ~, masked ~ 潜伏性痛风,隐匿性痛风 / lead ~, saturnine ~ 铅中毒性痛风 / misplaced ~, retrocedent ~ 异位性痛风(关节症状消失,全身症状严重) / oxalic ~ 草酸中毒性痛风,草酸中毒 / rheumatic ~ 风湿性痛风,萎缩性关节炎 / tophaceous ~, chalky ~ 痛风石性痛风,白垩性痛风

gouty [ˈgauti] *a* 患痛风的,痛风性的

governor [ˈgʌvənə] *n* 节制器,调节器

Gowers' column (fasciculus, tract) [ˈgauəz] (William R. Gowers)脊髓小脑前束 | ~ contraction 前叩击收缩 / ~ disease 高尔斯病(跳跃性痉挛) / ~ sign 高尔斯征(①在光照影响下,虹膜有间歇性迅速颤动,见于脊髓痨;②假肥大性肌营养不良的一种体征:患者为从仰卧位站起,须先转为伏卧屈膝,再用双手撑住胫部、膝及大腿才能站起) / ~ solution 高尔斯溶液(硫酸钠、冰醋酸和水的溶液,用于以血细胞计数器镜检数红细胞前稀释血液) / ~ syndrome 高尔斯综合征(血管迷走神经性发作)

Goyrand's hernia [gwɑːˈrɑːn] (Jean G. B. Goyrand)古瓦朗疝(未下降到阴囊的腹股沟疝)

GP general practitioner 全科医师;general paresis 麻痹性痴呆

G6PD glucose-6-phosphate dehydrogenase 葡糖-6-磷酸脱氢酶

GPI general paralysis of the insane 麻痹性痴呆

GPT glutamic-pyruvic transaminase 谷[氨酸]-丙[酮酸]转氨酶

gr grain 格令(英国重量单位)

graafian follicle, vesicle [ˈgrɑːfiən] (Reijnier 〈Regner〉 de Graaf)成熟滤泡

Gracilaria [ˌgræsiˈlɛəriə] *n* 江篱属

gracile [ˈgræsail] *a* 薄的,细的

Gracilicutes [ˌgræsiˈlikjutiːz, grəˈsiliˌkjuːtiːz] *n* 薄壁菌门

Grad. gradatim【拉】渐渐,逐步

gradatim [grəˈdeitim] *ad*【拉】渐渐,逐步

grade [greid] *n* 级,等级;评分等级

Gradenigo's syndrome [grɑːdəˈnigəu] (Giuseppe Gradenigo)格拉代尼戈综合征(中耳化脓性疾病时的第6脑神经麻痹及单侧头痛,为感染直接扩及展神经及三叉神经所致)

gradient [ˈgreidjənt] *n* 阶度,梯度;梯度变化曲线 | ~ of approach 接近梯度(离开阳性刺激的距离和接近该刺激的倾向之间的反向关系) / ~ of avoidance 回避梯度(离开阴性刺激的距离和回避该刺激的倾向之间的反向关系) / axial ~ 中轴阶度(表明身体中轴发展情况与代谢率的关系) / mitral ~ 二尖瓣阶差(舒张期内左心房与左心室之间的压力差) / systolic ~ 收缩期阶差(收缩期内左心室与左心房之间的压力差) / ventricular ~ 心室阶差(不同时期心室电活动的净差,如由代表 QRS 与 T 波区的心电向量代数和测定之)

graduate [ˈgrædjuit, ˈgrædʒuit] *n* 量筒,量杯 | **~d** [ˈgrædjueitid, ˈgrædʒueitid] *a* 有刻度的

graduator [ˈgrædjueitə, ˈgrædʒueitə] *n* 刻度器

Graefe's disease [ˈgreifə] (Albrecht von Graefe)进行性眼肌麻痹 | ~ knife 格雷费刀(线状内障刀) / ~ operation 格雷费手术(内障性晶状体切除术) / ~ sign 格雷费征(突眼性甲状腺肿时,上睑不能随眼球运动而下转)

Gräfenberg's ring [ˈgræfənbəːg] (Ernest Gräfenberg)格雷芬伯格环(一种银丝避孕环)

graft [grɑːft, græft] *n* 移植物,移植片 *vt, vi* 移植 | accordion ~ 成折移植片,手风琴样移植物 / allogeneic ~ 同种移植物 / autochthonous ~, autogenous ~, autologous ~, autoplastic ~ 自体移植物 / autodermic ~, autoepidermic ~ 自皮移植片 / avascular ~ 无血管移植物 / bone ~ 骨移植物 / cable ~ 电缆式神经移植物 / chorioallantoic ~ 绒[毛]膜尿囊移植物 / delayed ~ 迟延移植片 / dermal ~, dermic ~, cutis ~ 皮移植片 / diced cartilage ~ 软骨屑移植物 / double-end ~ 蒂状移植物 / epidermic ~ 表皮移植片 / fascia ~ 筋膜移植物 / fascicular ~ 神经束移植物 / fat ~ 脂肪移植物 / filler ~ 充填移植物 / free ~ 游离移植物 / full-thickness ~ 全厚皮片 / gauntlet ~ 蒂状移植物 / heterodermic ~ 异体皮移植片 / heterologous ~, heteroplastic ~ 异种移植物 / homologous ~, homoplastic ~ 同种[异体]移植物 / hyperplastic ~ 增生性移植物 / implantation ~ 植入移植物 / island ~ 岛状移植物,蒂状移植物 / isogeneic ~, isologous ~, isoplastic ~ 同基因移植物 / jump ~ 迁移移植片 / lamellar ~ 角膜薄层移植物 / nerve ~ 神经移植物 / omental ~ 大网膜移植物 / patch ~ 补钉移植物 / pedicle ~ 蒂状移植物 / penetrating ~ 全层角膜移植物 / pinch ~ 颗粒状移植皮片 / rope ~, tube ~, tunnel ~ 管状移植物 / seed ~ 种子移植物,植入移植物 / sieve ~ 筛状移植片 / skin ~ 皮移植片 / split-skin ~ 分层皮移植片 / split-thickness ~ 中厚皮片 / syngeneic ~ 同基因移植物 / thicksplit ~ 厚断层皮片 / thinsplit ~ 薄断层皮片

grafting [ˈgrɑːftiŋ] *n* 移植[术],嫁接 | skin ~ 皮肤移植术,植皮术

Grahamella [ˌgreiəˈmelə] *n* 格雷汉体属

grahamellosis [ˌgreiəməˈləusis] *n* 格雷汉体病

Graham Little syndrome [ˈgreiəm ˈlitl] (Ernest G. Graham Little)格雷厄姆·利特尔综合征,毛囊扁平苔藓(特征为头皮有疤痕性脱发斑,躯干和四肢有毛囊性栓及毛囊角化病,有时在腋部、

阴阜、躯干与四肢有非疤痕性脱毛)

Graham's law [ˈgreiəm] (Thomas Graham) 格雷厄姆定律(气体通过有孔膜的扩散速度,适与其密度的平方根成反比)

Graham Steell murmur [ˈgreiəm stiːl] (Graham Steell) 格雷厄姆·斯蒂尔杂音(肺动脉高压及二尖瓣狭窄时,肺动脉瓣反流所致的杂音,位于左第三肋间隙近胸骨缘处,沿胸骨往下传导)

Graham's test [ˈgreiəm] (Evarts A. Graham) 格雷厄姆试验(胆囊X线造影检查前,静脉内注射或口服四碘酚酞钠)

grain [grein] *n* 谷粒;喱,格令(英国重量单位,等于0.065 g);[颗]粒,晶粒 | cayenne pepper ~s 克恩辣椒粉状颗粒(尿中棕色尿酸沉淀)

grainage [ˈgreinidʒ] *n* 喱量(英衡制)

grainy [ˈgreini] *a* 粒状的;有细粒的

gram(g) [græm] *n* 克(重量单位)

-gram [构词成分]图,像

gram-equivalent [græm iˈkwivələnt] *n* 克当量

gramicidin [ˌgræmiˈsaidin] *n* 短杆菌肽(抗生素类药)

gramine [ˈgræmin] *n* 芦竹碱,2-二甲氨甲基吲哚

Gramineae [grəˈminiiː] *n* 禾本科

graminin [ˈgræminin] *n* 禾头孢素

graminivorous [græmiˈnivərəs] *a* 草食的

gram-ion [græm ˈaiən] *n* 克离子(1克离子 = 1 mol〈摩尔〉)

grammeter [ˈgræmitə] *n* 克米(功单位)

gram-molecule [græm ˈmɔlikjuːl] *n* 克分子

gram-negative [græm ˈnegətiv] *a* 革兰阴性的

gram-positive [græm ˈpɔzətiv] *a* 革兰阳性的

Gram's method (stain) [græm] (Hans C. J. Gram) 革兰法(染色)(鉴别细菌的一种染色法,先用结晶紫染细菌,加碘液处理,再以乙醇脱色,最后用稀复红复染,凡染后菌体呈紫色者,称革兰阳性菌,凡结晶紫被脱色,而对复染着色者,称革兰阴性菌) | ~ solution 革兰溶液(碘1份、碘化钾2份及水300份组成)

gram-stained [græm ˈsteind] *a* 革兰染色的

grana [ˈgreinə] granum 的复数

granatotannic acid [grəˌneitəuˈtænik] 梨皮鞣酸

granatum [grəˈneitəm] *n*【拉】石榴[树]皮

Grancher's system [grɑːnˈʃei] (Jacques J. Grancher) 格朗歇隔离制(早期使幼儿不接触结核病患者)

grandiose [ˈgrændiəus] *a* 夸大的 | **grandiosity** [ˌgrændiˈɔsəti] *n*

grand mal [grɑːn mɑːl] 大发作

Grandry's corpuscles [ˈgrɑːndri] (M. Grandry) 格朗德里小体,触盘,触觉半月板

Granger line [ˈgreindʒə] (Amedee Granger) 格兰哲曲线(头颅X线片所见,指示交叉沟位置的曲线) | ~ sign 格兰哲征(2岁以下婴儿的X片上如见到侧窦的前壁,则为乳突广泛损坏之征)

granisetron hydrochloride [græˈnisətrɔn] 盐酸格拉司琼(止吐药,与癌症化疗或放疗结合使用,口服或静脉内给药)

Granit's loop [ˈgrɑːnit] (R. A. Granit) 格拉尼特环,γ环路

granoplasm [ˈgrænəplæzəm] *n* 颗粒原生质

granula [ˈgrænjulə] ([复] **granulae** [ˈgrænjuliː]) *n*【拉】粒剂;[颗]粒

granular [ˈgrænjulə] *a* 有细粒的,颗粒状的 | **~ity** [ˌgrænjuˈlærəti] *n* 颗粒性

granulase [ˈgrænjuleis] *n* 谷[淀粉]酶

granulate [ˈgrænjuleit] *vt* 使成颗粒,使成粒状 *vi* 形成颗粒;(伤口愈合时)长出肉芽

granulatio [ˌgrænjuˈleiʃiəu] ([复] **granulationes** [ˌgrænjuˌleiʃiˈəuniːz]) *n*【拉】[颗]粒(粒状小体)

granulation [ˌgrænjuˈleiʃən] *n* 形成颗粒;肉芽形成;制粒法(片剂);[颗]粒 | arachnoidal ~s 蛛网膜粒 / cell ~s 细胞颗粒 / exuberant ~s 赘肉,冗长肉芽 / pyroninophilic ~s 嗜派若宁性颗粒

granule [ˈgrænjuːl] *n* [颗]粒;颗粒剂;颗粒体 | acidophil ~s 嗜酸性粒 / albuminous ~s, cytoplasmic ~s 白蛋白粒,胞质粒 / alpha ~s α-粒(粗大而折光力强的嗜酸性粒,由蛋白质构成,亦称嗜酸性粒;垂体细胞内的嗜酸性粒) / azur ~, azurophil ~, hyperchromatin ~ 嗜苯天青颗粒 / basophil ~s 嗜碱性粒 / beta ~s, amphophil ~s β-粒,两染性粒 / chromatic ~s, chromophilic ~s 染色质粒 / delta ~s δ-粒,淋巴细胞嗜碱性粒 / elementary ~s 血尘 / eosinophil ~s 嗜酸性粒 / epsilon ~s, neutrophil ~s ε-粒,嗜中性粒 / fuchsinophil ~s 嗜品红粒 / gamma ~s γ-粒(见于血液、骨髓和组织中的嗜碱性粒) / iodophil ~s 嗜碘颗粒(见于各种急性传染病的多核白细胞内) / kappa ~ κ-粒,嗜天青颗粒 / meningeal ~s 蛛网膜粒 / metachromatic ~s, polar ~s, volutin ~s 异染[颗]粒 / oxyphil ~s 嗜酸性粒(见 alpha ~s) / thread ~s 线粒体 / zymogen ~s 酶原粒(某些细胞含有酶前体的分泌颗粒,离开细胞之后即具有活性)

granuliform [ˈgrænjulifɔːm] *a* 粒状的

granuloadipose [ˌgrænjuləuˈædipəus] *a* 颗粒状脂变的

granuloblast [ˈgrænjuləublæst] *n* 成粒细胞

granuloblastosis [ˌgrænjuləublæsˈtəusis] *n* 成粒细胞增多症

granulocorpuscle [ˌgrænjuləuˈkɔːpʌsl] *n* 颗粒小体

granulocyte [ˈgrænjuləusait] *n* 粒细胞 | band-form ~ 带形核粒细胞 / segmented ~ 分节核粒

细胞 | **granulocytic** [ˌgrænjuləuˈsitik] *a*

granulocytopathy [ˌgrænjuləusaiˈtɔpəθi] *n* 粒细胞病

granulocytopenia [ˌgrænjuləuˌsaitəuˈpiːniə] *n* 粒细胞减少

granulocytopoiesis [ˌgrænjuləuˌsaitəupɔiˈiːsis] *n* 粒细胞生成,粒细胞发生 | **granulocytopoietic** [ˌgrænjuləuˌsaitəupɔiˈetik] *a*

granulocytosis [ˌgrænjuləusaiˈtəusis] *n* 粒细胞增多

granulofatty [ˌgrænjuləuˈfæti] *a* 颗粒状脂变的

granuloma [ˌgrænjuˈləumə] ([复] **granulomas** 或 **granulomata** [ˌgrænjuˈləumətə]) *n* 肉芽肿 | apical ~ [根]尖肉芽肿 / coccidioidal ~ 球孢子菌病 / eosinophilic ~ 嗜酸细胞肉芽肿,异尖线虫病 / ~ inguinale, ulcerating ~ of the pudenda, venereal ~ 腹股沟肉芽肿,性病肉芽肿 / lipoid ~ 类脂[性]肉芽肿,黄瘤 / lipophagic ~ 耗脂[性]肉芽肿 / paracoccidioidal ~ 副球孢子菌病 / rheumatic ~s 风湿性肉芽肿 / septic ~ 脓性肉芽肿 / silicotic ~ 硅肉芽肿,硅沉着性假结核瘤 / ~ tropicum 热带肉芽肿,雅司病(即 yaws) | **~tous** [ˌgrænjuˈlɔmətəs] *a*

granulomatosis [ˌgrænjuˌləuməˈtəusis] *n* 肉芽肿病 | allergic ~ 变应性肉芽肿病 / ~ disciformis progressiva et chronica 慢性进行性盘状肉芽肿病 / lipophagic intestinal ~ 耗脂性肠肉芽肿病 / lymphomatoid ~ 淋巴瘤样肉芽肿病 / malignant ~ 恶性肉芽肿病,霍奇金(Hodgkin)病 / ~ siderotica 铁质沉着性肉芽肿病

granulomere [ˈgrænjuləumiə] *n* (血小板)颗粒区

granulopenia [ˌgrænjuləuˈpiːniə] *n* 粒细胞减少

granulophilocyte [ˌgrænjuləuˈfiləsait] *n* 网织红细胞

granulophthisis [ˌgrænjuləuˈθaisis] *n* 粒细胞系毁灭

granuloplasm [ˈgrænjuləuplæzəm] *n* 内质,内[胞]浆

granuloplastic [ˌgrænjuləuˈplæstik] *a* 颗粒形成的

granulopoiesis [ˌgrænjuləupɔiˈiːsis] *n* 粒细胞生成 | **granulopoietic** [ˌgrænjuləupɔiˈetik] *a*

granulopoietin [ˌgrænjuləupɔiˈiːtin] *n* 粒细胞生成素

granulopotent [ˌgrænjuləuˈpəutənt] *a* 能形成颗粒的

Granuloreticulosea [ˌgrænjuləuriˌtikjuˈləusiə] *n* 黏网亚纲

granulosa [ˌgrænjuˈləusə] *n* 粒层,粒膜(卵泡内)

granulose [ˈgrænjuləus] *n* 细菌淀粉粒 *a* 颗粒状的

granulosis [ˌgrænjuˈləusis] *n* 颗粒团形成 | ~ rubra nasi 鼻红粒病

granulosity [ˌgrænjuˈlɔsəti] *n* [颗]粒团

granulotherapy [ˌgrænjuləuˈθerəpi] *n* 粒细胞疗法(曾用于治疗传染病,认为静脉内注射碳粒能引起白细胞增多)

granulous [ˈgrænjuləs] *a* 颗粒状的;有颗粒的

granulovacuolar [ˌgrænjuləuˈvækjuələ] *a* 粒状空泡的

granum [ˈgreinəm] ([复] **grana** [ˈgreinə]) *n* 【拉】颗粒;(叶绿体)基粒

grapes [greips] *n* 马体葡萄疮;牛结核

graph [græf, grɑːf] *n* 图,图表;描记器 *vt* 用图表表示

-graph [构词成分]图

graphesthesia [ˌgræfisˈθiːzjə] *n* 皮肤书写觉

graphic [ˈgræfik] *a* 图的,图解的,图示的;记录的

graphite [ˈgræfait] *n* 石墨 | **graphitic** [græˈfitik] *a*

graphitoid [ˈgræfitɔid] *a* 石墨状的

graphitosis [ˌgræfiˈtəusis] *n* 石墨沉着病,石墨肺

Graphium [ˈgræfiəm] *n* 石墨菌属

graph(o)- [构词成分]书写

graphoanalysis [ˌgræfəuəˈnælisis] *n* 书写分析(由笔迹来分析其性格)

graphocatharsis [ˌgræfəukəˈθɑːsis] *n* 书写疏泄法

graphokinesthetic [ˌgræfəuˌkinisˈθetik] *a* 书写运动觉的

graphology [græˈfɔlədʒi] *n* 笔迹学,字体学(研究笔迹作为分析人格的一种方法)

graphomotor [ˌgræfəˈməutə] *a* 书写运动的

graphopathology [ˌgræfəupəˈθɔlədʒi] *n* 书写病理学(研究书写笔迹作为精神或身体疾病的一种指征)

graphorrhea [ˌgræfəˈriːə] *n* 书写错乱

graphoscope [ˈgræfəskəup] *n* 近视弱视矫正器

graphospasm [ˈgræfəspæzəm] *n* 书写痉挛

-graphy [构词成分]书写,记录;摄影

Grashey's aphasia [ˈgræʃi] (Hubert von Grashey)格腊希失语,遗忘性失语(见于急性病及脑震荡)

grass [grɑːs] *n* 草;禾本科植物 | couch ~ 匐匍冰草,偃麦草(Agropyron repens) / scurvy ~ 山萮菜,辣根菜(曾用作治坏血病药)

Grasset-Bychowski sign [grɑːˈsei baiˈkɔfski] (J. Grasset; Zygmunt Bychowski)格-贝征(见 Grasset's phenomenon)

Grasset-Gaussel-Hoover sign [grəˈsei gɔˈsel ˈhuːvə] (Joseph Grasset; Amans Gaussel; Charles F. Hoover)格-戈-胡征(当患者斜卧欲举起瘫腿时,检查者手上所感到健侧腿向下的压力较检

查健康人时所感到的压力为大)

Grasset-Gaussel phenomenon [grəˈsei ɡəˈsel] (Joseph Grasset; Amans Gaussel)格-戈现象(见 Grasset's phenomenon)

Grasset's law [grəˈsei] (Joseph Grasset)格拉塞定律(见 Landouzy-Grasset law) | ~ phenomenon (sign)格拉塞现象(征)(在不全偏瘫时,患者能将两下肢各别举起,而不能同时举起)

grating [ˈɡreitiŋ] *n* 格栅,光栅 | diffraction ~ 衍射光栅(分光镜中用以分隔光的波长)

Gratiola [grəˈtaiələ] *n* 水八角属 | ~ officinalis 水八角(泻药、催吐药及利尿药)

Gratiolet's radiating fibers, optic radiation [grəˌtiəˈlei] (Louis P. Gratiolet)视辐射

grattage [grəˈtɑːʒ] *n*【法】刷除术(如刮除或用硬刷刷去沙眼中的肉芽组织)

grave [greiv] *a* 沉重的

gravedo [greiˈviːdəu] *n*【拉】鼻伤风

gravel [ˈɡrævəl] *n* 沙砾;尿沙

Graves' disease [greivz] (Robert. J. Graves)格雷夫斯病,突眼性甲状腺肿(原因不明的甲状腺疾病,常见于妇女,特征为眼球突出,搏动性甲状腺增大,脉率明显加速,有大量出汗倾向,神经质症状〈其中包括频细肌肉震颤、不安宁和暴躁〉、精神障碍、消瘦以及代谢率增加) | ~ orbitopathy (ophthalmopathy)格雷夫斯眶病(眼病)(见于格雷夫斯病的甲状腺功能障碍性眶病)

grave-wax [ˈɡreivwæks] *n* 尸蜡

gravid [ˈɡrævid] *a* 妊娠的 | **~ity** [grəˈvidəti] *n* 妊娠,[受]孕

gravida [ˈɡrævidə] *n* 孕妇

gravidic [grəˈvidik] *a* 妊娠期的

gravidism [ˈɡrævidizəm] *n* 妊娠[现象]

graviditas [grəˈviditəs] *n* 妊娠,[受]孕 | ~ examnialis 羊膜外妊娠 / ~ exochorialis 绒[毛]膜外妊娠

gravidocardiac [ˌɡrævidəuˈkɑːdiæk] *a* 妊娠心脏病的

gravidopuerperal [ˌɡrævidəupju(ː)ˈəːpərəl] *a* 孕期与产褥期的

gravimeter [ɡræˈvimitə] *n* 比重计,比重测定器

gravimetric(al) [ˌɡræviˈmetrik(əl)] *a* 比重测定的;重量分析的

gravistatic [ˌɡræviˈstætik] *a* 坠积的(由于地心引力所引起的)

gravitation [ˌɡræviˈteiʃən] *n* [万有]引力,重力

gravitative [ˈɡrævitətiv] *a* 重力的;受重力作用的

gravitometer [ˌɡræviˈtɔmitə] *n* 比重计,比重测定器

gravity [ˈɡrævəti] *n* 重力 | specific ~ 比重 / standard ~ 标准重力(符号为 g) / zero ~ 零重量,无重量

Grawitz's tumor [ˈɡrɑːvits] (Paul A. Grawitz)格腊维次瘤(肾上腺样瘤,目前认为系肾实质癌)

gray [grei] *a* 灰色的 *n* [神经]灰质;戈[瑞](辐射吸收剂量单位,缩写为 Gy) | central ~ 中央灰质 / silver ~, steel ~ 苯胺黑

grayanotoxin [ˈɡreiənəuˌtɔksin] *n* 木藜芦毒素,梫木毒素

grease [griːs] *n* 动物脂,脂肪,猪油,豚脂;马踵炎

grease-heel [griːs ˈhiːl] *n* 马踵炎

green [griːn] *a* 绿色的 *n* 绿色(物质或染料) | acid ~ 酸绿 / brilliant ~, ethyl ~ 煌绿,乙基绿 / bromocresol ~ 溴甲酚绿 / light ~ SF yellowish, fast acid ~ N 微黄淡绿 SF,固酸绿 N(酸性染料) / malachite ~, benzaldehyde ~, solid ~, Victoria ~ 孔雀绿,苯醛绿,固体绿,维多利亚绿 / Paris ~ 巴黎绿,乙酰亚砷酸铜(杀虫药)

Greene's sign [griːn] (Charles L. Greene)格林征(胸腔积液时心脏游离缘随呼气运动而向外侧移动,叩诊时可判断出)

Greenfield filter [ˈɡriːnfiːld] (Lazar J. Greenfield)格林费尔德滤器(一种伞形滤器,由 6 根不锈钢支柱组成,支持末端上的小钩固定住开放的腔静脉内的滤器)

Greenfield's disease [ˈɡriːnfiːld] (Joseph G. Greenfield)格林费尔德病,异染性脑白质营养不良(婴儿型)

gregaloid [ˈɡreɡəlɔid] *a* 集合样的,簇聚的(指原生动物的簇聚集落)

Gregarina [ˌɡreɡəˈrainə] *n* 簇虫属

gregarina [ˌɡreɡəˈrainə] ([复] **gregarinae** [ˌɡreɡəˈrainiː]) *n* 簇虫

gregarine [ˈɡreɡərin] *n* 簇虫 *a* 簇虫的 | **gregarinian** [ˌɡreɡəˈriniən] *a*

Gregarinia [ˌɡreɡəˈrainiə] *n* 簇虫亚纲

Gregarinida [ˌɡreɡəˈrainidə] *n* 簇虫目

gregarious [greˈɡɛəriəs] *a* 群集的;群居的;聚生的 | **~ness** *n*

Gregory's mixture [ˈɡreɡəri] (James Gregory)复方大黄散

Greig's syndrome [greg] (David M. Greg)格雷格综合征,两眼间距过远

grenz rays [grents] 跨界[射]线,境界[射]线(见 ray 项下相应术语)

grepafloxacin hydrochloride [ˌɡrepəˈflɔksəsin] 盐酸格帕沙星(抗菌药)

GRF growth hormone releasing factor 生长激素释放因子

GRH growth hormone releasing hormone 生长[激]素释放激素

grid [grid] 滤线栅,栅极;表格 | baby ~ 婴儿发育表[格] / focused ~ 聚光[X 线]滤线栅 /

moving ~ 活动[X线]滤线栅 / parallel ~ 平行[X线]滤线栅 / stationary ~ 静止滤线栅

Griesinger's disease [ˈgriːziŋə] (Wilhelm Griesinger)格里辛格病(钩虫病) | ~ sign (symptom)格里辛格征(症状)(横窦血栓形成时乳突后水肿性肿胀)

Griffith's sign [ˈgrifiθ] (J. Griffith)格里菲思征(向上凝视时下睑不能跟上,见于格富夫斯〈Graves〉眶病)

Grignard's reagent (compound) [griːˈnjɑː] (François A. V. Grignard)格里尼亚试剂(化合物)(含有一种有机基团和一种卤素的镁化合物,此种试剂与许多产生重要产物的物质能起反应)

grind [graind] (ground) *vt* 研磨 *vi* 研磨 *n* 磨;摩擦声

Grindelia [grinˈdiːliə] *n* 胶草属

grinder [ˈgraində] *n* 磨工;研磨机;磨牙,臼齿

grinding [ˈgraindiŋ] *n* 研磨,磨损;磨碎;夜磨牙症;磨牙[法] | selective ~ 选磨 / spot ~ 点磨法

grinding-in [ˈgraindiŋin] *n* 磨正[法]

grindstone [ˈgraindstəun] *n* 磨石;砂轮

grip[1] [grip] *n* 握 | power ~ 紧握

grip[2] [grip] *n* 流行性感冒,流感 | devil's ~ 鬼抓风,流行性胸膜痛 | **~pal** *a*

grippe [grip] *n*【拉】流行性感冒,流感 | ~ aurique 金中毒性多神经炎 / Balkan ~ 巴尔干流感

Griscelli syndrome [ˈgriseli] (Claude Griscelli)格里塞利综合征(常染色体隐性遗传的一种类白化病,特点为黑素过少、频发的化脓性感染、肝脾肿大、中性粒细胞与血小板减少,以及可能有免疫缺陷,亦称色素减退-免疫缺陷病)

Grisel's syndrome [griːˈzel] (P. Grisel)格里塞尔综合征(上呼吸道感染或腺样体切除后寰枢关节半脱位,见于儿童)

griseofulvin [ˌgrisiəuˈfʌlvin] *n* 灰黄霉素(抗生素类药)

griseomycin [ˌgrisiəuˈmaisin] *n* 灰色霉素,原放线菌素 B

griseous [ˈgrisiəs] *a* 灰色的

Grisolle's sign [griˈzɔl] (Augustin Grisolle)格里佐尔征(患区皮肤拉紧时,如皮下能触及丘疹,为天花,反之,如不能触及丘疹,则为麻疹)

gristle [ˈgrisl] *n* 软骨

Gritti's amputation (operation) [ˈgriːti] (Rocco Gritti)格里蒂切断术(包括膝关节的小腿切断术,用髌骨作骨成形瓣盖住股骨断端)

Gritti-Stokes amputation [ˈgriːti stəuks] (Rocco Gritti; William Stokes)格里蒂-斯托克斯切断术(格里蒂切断术的一种改良法,使用卵圆形前皮瓣)

Grocco's sign (triangle, triangular dullness) [ˈgrɔkəu] (Pietro Grocco)格罗科征(三角、三角区浊音)(①胸膜渗出液时,健侧脊柱旁的三角形浊音界;②早期突眼性甲状腺肿时心脏扩大;③肝肿大时肝浊音扩及脊柱中线的左侧)

Groenouw's type Ⅰ corneal dystrophy [ˈgrenəu] (Authur Groenouw)格雷诺Ⅰ型角膜营养不良,颗粒状角膜营养不良 | ~ type Ⅱ corneal dystrophy 格雷诺Ⅱ型角膜营养不良,斑点状角膜营养不良

groin [grɔin] *n* 腹股沟

Gromia [ˈgrɔmiə] *n* 网足虫属

Gromiida [grəˈmaiidə] *n* 网足目

gromwell [ˈgrɔmwəl] *n* 药用紫草

Grönblad-Strandberg syndrome [ˈgrenblæd ˈstrændbəːg] (Ester E. Grönblad; James V. Strandberg)格伦伯莱德-斯特兰伯格综合征(视网膜血管样条纹合并皮肤弹力纤维性假黄瘤)

groove [gruːv] *n* 沟 | alveolingual ~ 牙槽舌沟 / arterial ~s 动脉沟 / atrioventricular ~, auriculoventricular ~ 房室沟,心冠状沟 / basilar ~ 脑桥基底沟 / developmental ~s 发育沟 / free gingival ~ 游离龈沟,龈缘沟 / hamular ~ 翼钩沟 / nasal ~, ~ for nasal nerve 鼻骨筛沟 / nasopharyngeal ~ 鼻咽线/ neural ~, medullary ~ 神经沟,髓沟 / optic ~ 视交叉沟 / primitive ~ 原沟 / radial ~, ~ for radial nerve, musculospinal ~ 桡神经沟 / urethral ~, genital ~ 尿道沟,生殖沟

gross [grəus] *a* 大的,粗的;大体的,肉眼可见的 *n* 过失误差

Grossich's method [ˈgrəusik] (Antonio Grossich)格罗西克法(外科手术中使用的碘酊消毒法)

Grossman's sign [ˈgrəusmən] (Morris Grossman)格罗斯曼征(心脏扩张为肺结核的体征)

Gross's disease [ˈgrəus] (Samuel D. Gross)格罗斯病(成囊直肠;肛门壁囊样扩大伴大便干结潴留)

Gross's method [ˈgrəus] (Oskar Gross)格罗斯法(检胰蛋白酶活力) | ~ test 格罗斯试验(①检粪中胰蛋白酶;②诊断癌的显色反应)

ground-glass [ˈgraund ˈglɑːs] *a* 毛玻璃状的(如肺部含大量液体时 X 线片上所示)

groundhog [ˈgraundhɔg] *n* 美洲旱獭,花白旱獭

group [gruːp] *n* 组,型,群,簇;基;(周期表的)属,族 | alcohol ~ 醇基 / azo ~ 偶氮基 / blood ~ 血型 / CMN ~ CMN 菌群(即梭状芽胞杆菌属〈Clostridium〉,分枝杆菌属〈Mycobacterium〉和诺卡菌属〈Nocardia〉的一群细菌) / coli-aerogenes ~ 大肠产气菌类 / colon-typhoid-dysentery

~ 大肠伤寒痢疾菌群 / complementophil ~ 嗜补体基(在埃利希〈Ehrlich〉侧链学说中,指介体分子上与补体相结合的基) / cytophil ~ 嗜细胞基(在埃利希〈Ehrlich〉侧链学说中,指介体分子与敏感细胞相结合的基团) / diagnosis-related ~s 诊断相关组(按诊断类别分类,由医疗照顾方案〈Medicare〉及其他第三方付款计划作为偿付医院医疗费用的依据) / encounter ~ 交朋友组 / ergophore ~ 作用簇(见 ergophore) / haptophore ~ 结合簇(见 haptophore) / hemorrhagic-septicemia ~ 出血性败血菌群 / methyl ~ 甲基 / osmophore ~ 生臭基,生臭团 / paratyphoid-enteritidis ~, hog cholera ~ 副伤寒肠炎杆菌群,猪霍乱菌群 / peptide ~ 肽基 / prosthetic ~ 辅基 / proteus ~ 变形杆菌群 / saccharide ~ 糖基 / salmonella ~ 沙门菌群 / sapophore ~ 生味基,生味团 / sensitivity ~, sensitivity training ~ 感受性组,感受性训练组(亦称训练组) / sulfonic ~ 磺酸基 / toxophore ~ 毒性簇(见 toxophore) / T ~, T- ~, training ~ 训练组

grouper [ˈgruːpə] *n* 石斑鱼

grouping [ˈgruːpiŋ] *n* 分型,分类 | antigenic structural ~ 抗原结构分型,抗原决定簇 / blood ~ 血型鉴定,血型分型 / haptenic ~ 半抗原

group-specific [ˌgruːp spiˈsifik] *a* 种群特异性的(指血凝素对某一种群是有特异性的,如对某一个血型或某一个微生物)

group-transfer [ˌgruːp ˈtrænsfə] *n* 基团转移(指一种化学反应)

Grove's cell [grəuv] (William R. Grove)格罗夫电池(用稀硫酸及稀硝酸充电的两液直流电池,锌和铂作电极)

Grover's disease [ˈgrəuvə] (R. W. Grover)暂时性棘层松解性皮肤病

growth [grəuθ] *n* 生长;异常生长物(如肿瘤);细胞增生 | absolute ~ 绝对生长 / accretionary ~ 增加生长 / appositional ~ 外积生长,外加生长 / auxetic ~, intussusceptive ~ 细胞增大性生长 / differential ~ 微分生长 / heterogonous ~ 变种生长,对数性生长 / histiotypic ~ 组织型生长 / interstitial ~ 内积生长,内加生长 / multiplicative ~ 细胞增多性生长 / new ~ 新生物,[肿]瘤 / organotypic ~ 器官型生长

grübelsucht [ˈgriːbelsuːkt] *n*【德】疑虑癖,穿凿癖(见于强迫性人格)

Gruber's fossa [ˈgrubə] (Wenaslaus L. Gruber)格鲁伯窝(在胸骨上间隙沿锁骨内端的憩室) | ~ hernia 胃系膜内疝

Gruber's reaction, test, Gruber-Widal reaction, test [ˈgrubə viˈdɑːl] (Max von Gruber; Georges F. I. Widal)格鲁伯反应、试验,格鲁伯-肥达反应、试验(伤寒凝集反应)

Gruber's speculum [ˈgrubə] (Josef Gruber)格鲁伯耳镜 | ~ test 格鲁伯试验(检耳对音的灵敏度)

Gruber's syndrome [ˈgluːbə] (Georg B. O. Gruber)格鲁勃综合征(见 Meckel's syndrome)

Grubyella [gruːbiˈelə] *n* 黄癣菌属(发癣菌属 Trichophyton 的旧称)

Gruentzig balloon catheter [ˈgriːntsig] (Andreas R. Gruentzig)格林齐格气囊导管(用于扩张动脉狭窄)

gruffs [grʌfs] *n* 药滓(药材的)

grume [gruːm] *n* 凝块;黏液 | **grumose** [ˈgruːməus], **grumous** [ˈgruːməs] *a* 凝块的,凝集的

Grünbaum-Widal test [ˈgriːnbaum viˈdɑːl] (A. S. Grünbaum; Georges F. I. Widal)格林包姆-肥达试验(伤寒凝集反应)

grundplatte [gruntˈplɑːtə] *n*【德】基板

Grynfelt-Lesshaft triangle [ˈgrinfelt ˈlesgɑːft] (Joseph C. Grynfelt; Peter F. Lesshaft)格林费尔特-勒斯哈夫特三角(见 Lesshaft's space)

Grynfelt's hernia [ˈgrinfelt] (Joseph C. Grynfelt)格林费尔特疝(先天性腰上三角疝) | ~ triangle 格林费特三角(见 Lesgaft's space)

gryochrome [ˈgraiəkrəum] *n* 粒染[神经]细胞 *a* 粒状染色的

gryphosis [griˈfəusis] *n* [异常]弯曲

gryposis [griˈpəusis] *n*【希】[异常]弯曲 | ~ penis 阴茎下弯畸形

GSC gas-solid chromatography 气固色谱法,气固层析法

GSH reduced glutathione 还原型谷胱甘肽

GSS Gerstmann-Sträussler-Scheinker syndrome 格-施-沙综合征

GSSG oxidized glutathione 氧化型谷胱甘肽

gt. gutta【拉】滴

GTH gonadotropic hormone 促性腺激素

GTN gestational trophoblastic neoplasia 妊娠滋养层瘤形成

GTP guanosine triphosphate 鸟苷三磷酸

GTPase GTP 酶,鸟苷三磷酸酶

GTP cyclohydrolase I [ˌsaikləuˈhaidrəleis] GTP 环水解酶 I(此酶缺乏为一种常染色体隐性性状,可致恶性高苯丙氨酸血症)

gtt. guttae【拉】滴

GTT glucose tolerance test 葡萄糖耐量试验

GU genitourinary 泌尿生殖的

guaco [ˈgwɑːkəu] *n* 瓜柯,南美蛇藤菊,米甘菊(产于南美,可用以治气喘、消化不良、痛风、风湿病及皮肤病)

guaiac [ˈgwaiæk], **guaiacum** [ˈgwaiəkəm] *n* 愈创木脂(用作试剂,检潜血,以前用于治风湿病)

Guaiacum [ˈgwaiəkəm] *n* 愈创木属

guaiacol [ˈgwaiəkɔl] *n* 愈创木酚,甲基邻苯二酚(以前用作祛痰药)
guaifenesin [gwaiˈfenəsin], **guaiphenesin** [gwaiˈfenəsin] *n* 愈创甘油醚(祛痰药)
guaithylline [ˈgwaiθiliːn] *n* 愈创茶碱(支气管扩张药及祛痰药)
guanabenz [ˈgwɑːnəbenz] *n* 胍那苄(抗高血压药)
guanacline sulfate [ˈgwɑːnəkliːn] 硫酸胍那克林(抗高血压药)
guanadrel sulfate [ˈgwɑːnədrel] 硫酸胍那决尔(抗高血压药)
guanase [ˈgwɑːneis] *n* 鸟嘌呤酶
guanazolo [ˌgwɑːnəˈzəuləu] *n* 氮鸟嘌呤,8-氮杂鸟嘌呤(一种具有抑制鼠的某些癌细胞生长的化合物,亦对鹦鹉热病毒有效)
guancidine [ˈgwɑːnsidiːn] *n* 胍西定(抗高血压药)
guanethidine [gwɑːˈneθidiːn] *n* 胍乙啶(肾上腺素能阻滞药) | ~ monosulfate 硫酸呱乙啶(抗高血压药) / ~ sulfate 硫酸呱乙啶(抗高血压药)
guanfacine hydrochloride [ˈgwɑːfəsiːn] 盐酸胍法辛(抗高血压药)
guanidase [ˈgwɑːnideis] *n* 胍酶
guanidine [ˈgwɑːnidin] *n* 胍 | ~ hydrochloride 盐酸胍(治重症肌无力)
guanidine-acetic acid [ˈgwɑːnidin əˈsiːtik] 胍基乙酸
guanidinemia [ˌgwɑːnidiˈniːmiə] *n* 胍血
guanidinium [ˌgwɑːniˈdiniəm], **guanidino** [ˌgwɑːniˈdiːnəu] *n* 胍基
guanidinoacetate [ˌgwɑːniˌdiːnəuˈæsiteit] *n* 胍基乙酸(盐或阴离子型)
guanidinoacetate *N*-methyltransferase [ˌgwɑːniˌdiːnəuˈæsiteit ˌmeθilˈtrænsfəreis] 胍[基]乙酸 *N*-转甲基酶
guanidinoacetic acid [ˌgwɑːnidinəuəˈsiːtik] 胍基乙酸
guanido [ˈgwɑːnidəu] *n* 胍基
guanido-acetic acid [ˌgwɑːnidəu əˈsiːtik] 胍基乙酸
guanidylate [ˌgwɑːniˈdileit] *n* 胍基酸(解离型)
guanine [ˈgwɑːniːn] *n* 鸟嘌呤 | ~ nucleotide 鸟[嘌呤核]苷酸
guanine deaminase [ˈgwɑːnin diːˈæmineis] 鸟嘌呤脱氨酶
guanochlor sulfate [ˈgwɑːnəklɔː] 硫酸胍氯酚(抗高血压药)
guanoctine [gwɑːˈnɔktiːn] *n* 胍诺克汀(抗高血压药)
guanophore [ˈgwɑːnəfɔː] *n* 鸟嘌呤细胞
guanosine [ˈgwɑːnəsin] *n* 鸟苷 | cyclic ~ monophosphate (cyclic GMP, cGMP, 3′, 5′-GMP) 环鸟苷酸 / ~ diphosphate (GDP) 鸟苷二磷酸 / ~ monophosphate (GMP) 鸟苷[一磷]酸
guanoxabenz [gwɑːˈnɔksəbenz] *n* 胍诺沙苄(抗高血压药)
guanoxan sulfate [gwɑːˈnɔksæn] 硫酸胍生(抗高血压药)
guanoxyfen [gwɑːˈnɔksifən] *n* 胍诺西芬(抗高血压药)
guanylate [ˈgwɑːnəleit] *n* 鸟苷酸(解离型)
guanylate cyclase [ˈgwɑːnəleit ˈsaikleis] 鸟苷酸环化酶
guanylate kinase [ˈgwɑːnəleit ˈkaineis] 鸟苷酸激酶
guanylic acid [gwɑːˈnilik] 鸟苷[一磷]酸
guanylyl [gwɑːˈnilil] *n* 鸟苷酰
guarana [gwəˈrɑːnə] *n* 瓜拉那,巴西可可(用作腹泻时的收敛药)
guaranine [gwəˈrɑːnin] *n* 瓜拉那碱(即咖啡因)
guard [gɑːd] *n* 防护装置 | mouth ~ 口腔防护器 / occlusal ~, bite ~, night ~ 护殆器(夜间用牙罩)
Guarea [ˈgweiriə] *n* 楝属
Guarnieri's bodies (corpuscles) [ˌgwɑːniˈeri] (Guiseppi Guarnieri) 瓜尔涅里小体(天花包涵体)
guayule [gwaiˈuːli] *n* 银胶菊
gubernaculum [ˌgjuːbəˈnækjuləm] ([复] **gubernacula** [ˌgjuːbəˈnækjulə]) *n*【拉】引带 | chorda ~ 索引带 / ~ testis 睾丸引带 | **gubernacular** *a*
Gubler-Robin typhus [ˈguːblə rɔˈbæn] (A. M. Gubler; Albert E. C. Robin) 古布勒-罗宾斑疹伤寒(肾型斑疹伤寒)
Gubler's hemiplegia [ˈguːblə] (Adolphe M. Gubler) 古尔勒偏瘫(交叉性偏瘫;癔症性偏瘫) | ~ line 古布勒线(连结脑桥下第5脑神经各根起点的线) / ~ paralysis 交叉性偏瘫 / ~ tumor, sign 古布勒瘤、征(铅中毒时腕背有肿瘤,手伸肌麻痹)
Gudden's commissure [ˈgudən] (Bernhard A. von Gudden) 视上连合,弓状连合,下连合 | ~ law 古登定律(神经切断后近端发生的变性是向细胞的)
Guéneau de Mussy's point [geiˈnəu də miˈsi] (Noel F. O. Guéneau de Mussy) 盖诺德米西点(胸骨左缘第10肋骨末端的水平上压痛最剧烈的一点,为膈胸膜炎的一个症状)
Guenz [ˈgints] 见 Günz
Guenzburg [ˈgintsbəːg] 见 Günzburg
Guérin's fold [geiˈræn] (Alphonse F. M. Guérin)

盖兰襞(偶见于尿道舟状窝的黏膜襞) | ~ fracture 盖兰骨折(双侧上颌横形骨折) / ~ glands 盖兰腺(尿道旁管) / ~ sinus 盖兰窦(尿道舟状窝襞后的憩室) / ~ valve 舟状窝襞

guidance [ˈgaidəns] *n* 导 | condylar ~ 髁导 / incisal ~ 切导

guide [gaid] *n* 导[子];标 | adjustable anterior ~ 可调节的前骀导 / condylar ~ 髁导 / incisal ~ 切导

guideline [ˈgaidlain] *n* 导线(牙科) | clasp ~ 带钩导线,观测导线

guidewire [ˈgɑːdwaiə] *n* 导线

Guidi's canal [ˈgwidi] (Guido Guidi)翼管

Guillain-Barré syndrome [giˈjæn bɑːˈrei] (Georges Guillain; Jean A. Barré)吉兰-巴雷综合征,急性特发性多神经炎

guillotine [ˌgiləˈtiːn, ˈgilətiːn] *n*【法】铡除刀,环状刀(铡除扁桃体或悬雍垂)

Guinard's treatment (method) [giˈnɑː] (Aimé Guinard)古纳尔疗法(碳化钙涂于溃疡型肿瘤)

guinea-pig [ˈgini pig] *n* 豚鼠,天竺鼠,荷兰猪

Guinon's disease [giˈnɔŋ] (Georges Guinon)吉农病(见 Gilles de la Tourette's syndrome)

gulf [gʌlf] *n* 湾

gullet [ˈgʌlit] *n* 食管

Gull's disease [gʌl] (William W. Gull)古尔病(甲状腺萎缩伴黏液水肿)

Gullstrand's slit lamp [ˈgulstrænd] (Allvar Gullstrand)古尔斯特兰德裂隙灯(与角膜显微镜配合使用,作结膜、角膜、虹膜、晶状体及玻璃体的显微研究) | ~ law 古尔斯特兰德定律(斜视时,令患者注视一远距离目标而将头转向一方时,角膜反射转移的方向与头移动的方向相同,即向肌肉较弱的方向移转)

gulonic acid [guˈlɔnik] 古洛糖酸

L-gulonolactone [ˌguːlənəuˈlæktəun] *n* L-古洛糖酸内酯

gulose [ˈgjuːləus] *n* 古洛糖

gum[1] [gʌm] *n* 树胶 | acaroid ~, blackboy ~, Botany Bay ~ 禾木胶 / animal ~ 动物胶 / ~ benjamin, ~ benzoin 安息香(树脂) / blue ~ 桉树 / British ~ 糊精 / ~ camphor 樟脑 / Cape ~ 刺金合欢胶 / ghatti ~, Indian ~ 印度胶 / guar ~ 瓜尔胶 / Kordofan ~ 科多凡树胶(阿拉伯胶最好的一种) / mesquite ~ 甜荚豆胶,墨西哥胶(阿拉伯胶代用品) / ~ opium 阿片 / red ~, eucalyptus ~ 桉胶(用作收敛药,治喉疾患) / ~ senegal 阿拉伯胶 / sterculia ~, karaya ~ 梧桐胶,卡拉牙胶(用作泻药) / ~ thus 松脂,松油脂 / ~ tragacanth 西黄蓍胶 / wattle ~, Australian ~ 澳洲胶(阿拉伯胶最好的代用品)

gum[2] [gʌm] *n* 牙龈 | blue ~ 蓝龈(铅线,见于铅中毒)

gumboil [ˈgʌmbɔil] *n* 龈脓肿

Gumboro disease [ˈgʌmbərəu] (Gumboro 为美国特拉华州一地名)传染性黏液囊病

gumma [ˈgʌmə] ([复] **gummas** 或 **gummata** [ˈgʌmətə]) *n* 树胶样肿 | tuberculous ~, scrofulous ~ 结核性树胶样肿,瘰疬性树胶样肿 | **~tous** *a*

gummate [ˈgʌmeit] *n* 阿拉伯胶酸盐

gummi [ˈgʌmai] *n*【拉】树胶

gummy [ˈgʌmi] *a* 树胶状的;树胶样肿的

Gumprecht's shadows [ˈgumpreʃt] (Ferdinand Gumprecht)古姆普雷希特细胞影(涂片中的破碎而畸形的细胞,常见于淋巴性白血病)

gum-resin [gʌmˈrezin] *n* 胶树脂 | soluble ~ 火棉

guncotton [ˈgʌnˌkɔtn] *n* 火棉

gundo [ˈgundəu] *n* 鼻骨增殖性骨膜炎,根度病,巨鼻[症]

Gunning's splint [ˈgʌniŋ] (Thomas B. Gunning)冈宁夹(下颌骨折用)

Gunning's test (reaction) [ˈgʌniŋ] (Jan W. Gunning)冈宁试验(反应)(检尿丙酮)

Gunn's dots [gʌn] (Robert Marcus Gunn)耿氏小点(斜照时黄斑附近可见到的白点) | ~ pupillary phenomenon, Marcus Gunn's pupillary phenomenon 耿氏瞳孔现象,马库斯·耿氏瞳孔现象,摆动电筒征(即 swinging flashlight sign,见 sign 项下相应术语) / ~ crossing sign 耿氏交叉征(眼底动静脉交叉,提示原发性高血压) / ~ sign 耿氏征(①耿氏交叉征;马库斯·耿氏瞳孔现象;②张口时下颌偏向对侧,则下垂的上睑向上抬,见于耿氏综合征) / ~ syndrome (phenomenon) 耿氏综合征(现象),颌动瞬目综合征(单侧睑下垂,患侧上睑即与下颌联合运动)

Günther disease [ˈginθə] 京塞病,先天性红细胞生成性卟啉症

Günzberg's test [ˈgintsbəːg] (Alfred Günzberg)京茨伯格试验(检胃内容物盐酸)

Günz's ligament [ˈgints] (Justus G. Günz)京茨韧带(部分闭孔膜)

gurgle [ˈgəːl] *n*, *vi* 发咯咯声,发咕噜声 | **gurgling** *n* 咕噜声,气过水声

gurgulio [gəˈgjuːliəu] *n*【拉】腭垂,悬雍垂

gurney [ˈgəːni] *n* 轮床(医院推送患者用)

gusher [ˈgʌʃə] *n* 井喷 | stapidial ~ 镫井喷

Gussenbauer's operation [ˈgusənˌbauə] (Carl Gussenbauer)古森包厄手术(治食管狭窄) | ~ suture 古森包厄缝术(肠道裂隙 8 字形缝术)

gustation [gʌsˈteiʃən] *n* 味觉,尝味 | colored ~ 尝味觉色,色味(联觉)

gustin [ˈgʌstin] *n* 味肽,味多肽

gusto [ˈɡʌstəu] *n* 爱好,趣味
gustometer [ɡʌsˈtɔmitə] *n* 味觉计 | **gustometry** *n* 味觉测量法
gut [ɡʌt] *n* 肠;原肠;肠线 | blind ~ 盲肠 / post-anal ~, tail ~ 肛后肠 / preoral ~ 口前肠,咽底憩室 / primitive ~ 原肠 / ribbon ~ 肠线 / silk-worm ~ 蚕肠线
Guthrie's formula [ˈɡʌθri] (Clyde G. Guthrie)格思里公式(成人理想体重磅数,等于 110 + 〈5.5 × 身高超出 5 英尺的英寸数〉)
Guthrie's muscle [ˈɡʌθri] (George J. Guthrie)尿道括约肌
Gutierrezia [ˌɡutiəˈriːziə] *n* 黄花草属
gutta [ˈɡutə] ([复] **guttae** [ˈɡutiː]) *n*【拉】滴
gutta-percha [ˌɡʌtəˈpəːtʃə] *n* 胶木胶,马来乳胶,古塔波胶
Guttat. guttatim【拉】逐滴地
guttate [ˈɡʌteit] *a* 滴状的
guttatim [ɡʌˈteitim] *ad*【拉】逐滴地
guttation [ɡʌˈteiʃən] *n* 吐水(作用)(植物细胞)
guttering [ˈɡʌtəriŋ] *n* 沟状切除术
gutti [ˈɡʌtai] *n* 藤黄
gut-tie [ˈɡʌttai] *n* 肠绞窄(动物)
Guttmann's sign [ˈɡutmən] (Paul Guttmann)古特曼征(突眼性甲状腺肿时,甲状腺部可听出杂音)
Gutt. quibusd. guttis quibusdam【拉】加数滴
guttur [ˈɡʌtə] *n*【拉】咽喉
guttural [ˈɡʌtərəl] *a* 咽喉的
gutturophony [ˌɡʌtəˈrɔfəni] *n* 喉音
gutturotetany [ˌɡʌtərəuˈtetəni] *n* 喉痉挛性口吃
Gutzeit's test [ˈɡuttsait] (Max A. Gutzeit)古特蔡特试验(检砷)
Guy de Chauliac 见 Chauliac
Guyon's amputation (operation) [ɡiˈjɔn] (Felix J. C. Guyon)居永切断术(踝上切断术) | ~ canal 居永管(位于小鱼际底部) / ~ sign 居永征(浮动诊肾法)
GVH graft-versus-host 移植物抗宿主(病或反应)
Gwathmey's oil-ether anesthesia [ˈɡwæθmiː] (James T. Gwathmey)格瓦思米油醚麻醉(将液状醚与橄榄油的混合液灌入直肠以产生麻醉)
GXT graded exercise test 分级运动试验
Gy gray 戈[瑞](辐射吸收剂量单位)
Gymnamoebia [ˌdʒimnəˈmiːbə] *n* 裸阿米巴纲
gymnasium [dʒimˈneizjəm] ([复] **gymnasiums** 或 **gymnasia** [dʒimˈneizjə]) *n* 体育馆,健身房
gymnastic(al) [dʒimˈnæstik(əl)] *a* 体操的,体育的
gymnastics [dʒimˈnæstiks] *n* 体操,体育 | ocular ~ 眼肌体操,眼保健操 / Swedish ~ 瑞典式体操,矫形体操 / vocal ~ 练音体操(在于使肺扩张、嗓音增强)
Gymnema [dʒimˈniːmə] *n* 武靴叶属(其叶可用于掩盖不良的药味)
gymnemic acid [dʒimˈniːmik] 匙羹藤酸
gymn(o)- [构词成分]裸,裸的
Gymnoascaceae [ˌdʒimnəuæsˈkeisiiː] *n* 裸子囊科
Gymnoascus [ˌdʒimnəˈæskəs] *n* 裸子囊菌属
gymnobacterium [ˌdʒimnəubækˈtiəriəm] ([复] **gymnobacteria** [ˌdʒimnəubækˈtiəriə]) *n* 裸菌(无鞭毛菌)
gymnocarpous [ˌdʒimnəˈkɑːpəs] *a* 裸果的(指真菌)
gymnocyte [ˈdʒimnəsait] *n* 裸细胞,无壁细胞
Gymnodinium [ˌdʒimnəuˈdiniəm] *n* 裸甲藻属
gymnoplast [ˈdʒimnəplæst] *n* 裸质体
gymnosperm [ˈdʒimnəspəːm] *n* 裸子植物 | **~ous** [ˌdʒimnəˈspəːməs] *a* / **~y** [ˌdʒimnəˈspəːmi] *n*
gymnospore [ˈdʒimnəspɔː] *n* 裸孢子
Gymnostomatia [ˌdʒimnəustəuˈmeiʃiə] *n* 裸口虫亚纲
gymnothecium [ˌdʒimnəˈθiːsiəm] *n* 裸囊体(皮真菌)
Gymnothorax [ˌdʒimnəˈθɔːræks] *n* 齿鳝属
gynaec(o)- 见 gynec(o)-
gynaecology 见 gynecology | **gynaecologist** 见 gynecologist
gynander [dʒiˈnændə] *n* 两性体,雌雄同体;男化女子(女性假两性体)
gynandrism [dʒiˈnændrizəm, ɡai-], **gynandria** [dʒiˈnændriə] *n* 两性畸形,雌雄同体性;女子男化(女性假两性畸形)
gynandroblastoma [dʒiˌnændrəublæsˈtəumə] *n* 两性胚细胞瘤
gynandroid [dʒiˈnændrɔid] *n* 男化女子(女性假两性体)
gynandromorph [dʒiˈnændrəmɔːf, ɡai-] *n* 雌雄嵌[合]体,两性体,雌雄同体
gynandromorphism [dʒiˌnændrəˈmɔːfizəm, ɡai-] *n* 雌雄嵌[合]性;两性畸形,雌雄同体性 | bilateral ~ 双侧两性畸形
gynandromorphous [dʒiˌnændrəˈmɔːfəs, ɡai-] *a* 雌雄嵌[合]性的;两性畸形的,雌雄同体的
gynandry [ˈdʒinændri, dʒaiˈnændri] *n* 两性畸形,雌雄同体性;女子男化(女性假两性畸形)
gynatresia [ˌdʒinəˈtriːziə] *n* 阴道闭锁
gyne- 见 gynec(o)-
gynecic [dʒiˈnesik, dʒai-] *a* 女性的
gynecium [ˌdʒiˈniːsiəm, ˌɡai-] *n* 雌蕊群
gynec(o)-, gynaec(o)-, gyne-, gyn(o)- [构词成分]女性,女子
gynecogen [ˈdʒinikədʒən] *n* 促雌素
gynecogenic [ˌdʒinikəˈdʒenik, ˌɡai-] *a* 女性化的

gynecography [ˌdʒiniˈkɔgrəfi] *n* 女生殖器造影[术],妇科X线摄影[术]
gynecoid [ˈdʒinikɔid, ˈgai-] *a* 女性的
gynecology [ˌgainiˈkɔlədʒi, ˌdʒiniˈkɔlədʒi] *n* 妇科学 | **gynecologic(al)** [ˌgainikəˈlɔdʒik(əl), ˌdʒinikəˈlɔdʒik(əl)] / **gynecologist** *n* 妇科学家
gynecomania [ˌdʒinikəuˈmeinjə, ˌgai-] *n* 求雌狂,男子色情狂
gynecomastia [ˌdʒinikəuˈmæstiə, ˌgai-] *n* 男子乳腺发育 | refeeding ~, nutritional ~, rehabilitation ~ 营养性男子乳腺发育 | **gynecomastism** [ˌdʒinikəuˈmæstizəm], **gynecomasty** [ˈdʒinikəu-ˌmæsti], **gynecomazia** [dʒinikəuˈmeizjə] *n*
gynecopathy [ˌdʒiniˈkɔpəθi] *n* 妇科病
gynecophoral [ˌdʒiniˈkɔfərəl] *a* 抱雌的(沟)
gynecotokology [ˌgainikəutəˈkɔlədʒi, ˌdʒi-] *n* 妇产科学
gyneduct [ˈdʒinidʌkt] *n* 中肾旁管
gynephilia [ˌdʒiniˈfiliə] *n* 爱慕女性癖
gynephobia [ˌdʒiniˈfəubjə, ˌdʒai-] *n* 女性恐怖,恐女症
gyneplasty [ˈdʒiniˌplæsti] *n* 女生殖器成形术
gynesin [ˈdʒinisin] *n* 胡卢巴碱,*N*-甲基烟酸内盐
gyn(o)- 见 gynec(o)-
gynogamon [dʒinəˈgæmɔn] *n* 雌[性交]配素
gynogenesis [ˌdʒinəuˈdʒenisis, ˌgai-] *n* 雌核发育
gynoid [ˈdʒainɔid, ˈgai-] *a* 女性的
gynomerogon(e) [ˌdʒinəuˈmerəgɔn] *n* 雌核卵块
gynomerogony [ˌdʒinəuməˈrɔgəni] *n* 雌核卵块发育
gynopathy [dʒiˈnɔpəθi] *n* 妇科病 | **gynopathic** [ˌdʒinəuˈpæθik] *a*
gynophobia [ˌdʒinəuˈfəubjə, ˌdʒai-] *n* 女性恐怖,恐女症
gynoplastics [ˌdʒinəuˈplæstiks], **gynoplasty** [ˈdʒainəˌplæsti] *n* 女生殖器成形术 | **gynoplastic** [ˌdʒinəˈplæstik] *a*
gypsum [ˈdʒipsəm] *n*【拉】石膏,硫酸钙 *vt* 用石膏处理
gyral [ˈdʒaiərəl] *a* 旋转的,回旋的;脑回的
gyrate [dʒaiəˈreit] *vi* 旋转,回旋 [ˈdʒaiərit] *a* 旋转的;回状的,环形的 | **gyratory** [ˈdʒaiərətəri] *a* 旋转的
gyration [dʒaiəˈreiʃən] *n* 旋转,回旋,环旋
gyre [ˈdʒaiə] *n* 脑回,回
gyrectomy [dʒaiəˈrektəmi] *n* 脑回切除术 | frontal ~ 额叶脑回切除术,额叶皮质部分切除术
Gyrencephala [ˌdʒaiərenˈsefələ] *n* 多脑回动物类
gyrencephalic [ˌdʒaiərensəˈfælik] *a* 多脑回的;多脑回动物的
gyr(o)- [构词成分]环,圆;脑回
gyrochrome [ˈdʒaiərəukrəum] *n* 环染细胞(神经细胞)
Gyrodactylus [ˌdʒaiərəuˈdæktiləs] *n* 三代[吸虫]属
gyrometer [dʒaiəˈrɔmitə] *n* 脑回测量器
Gyromitra [ˌdʒaiərəuˈmaitrə] *n* 鹿花蕈属
Gyropus [ˈdʒaiərəpəs] *n* 长兽羽虱属 | ~ ovalis 卵形长兽羽虱
gyrose [ˈdʒaiərəus], **gyrous** [ˈdʒaiərəs] *a* 回状的,环形的
gyrospasm [ˈdʒaiərəspæzəm] *n* (头)回旋痉挛
gyrotrope [ˈdʒaiərətrəup] *n* 电流变向器
gyrus [ˈdʒaiərəs] ([复] **gyri** [ˈdʒaiərai]) *n*【拉】脑回,回 | angular ~ 角回 / annectant gyri 连接回,过渡回 / ascending frontal ~ 中央前回 / ascending parietal ~, postcentral ~ 中央后回 / callosal ~, cingulate ~ 扣带回 / gyri of cerebrum 大脑回 / dentate ~ 齿状回;束状回 / fusiform ~ 梭状回 / hippocampal ~ 海马回 / lingual ~, infracalcarine ~ 舌回 / paracentral ~ 中央旁小叶 / paraterminal ~, subcallosal ~ 终板旁回,胼胝下回 / parietal ~ 顶回 / precentral ~ 中央前回 / preinsular gyri, short gyri of insula 岛短回 / supracallosal ~ 胼胝上回,灰被 / uncinate ~ 钩回

H

H Hauch H 型;henry 亨[利]; histidine 组氨酸; Hounsfield unit 亨斯菲尔德单位;hydrogen 氢; hyperopia 远视

H enthalpy 热函,焓

H_0 null hypothesis 无效假设,零假设

H_1 alternative hypothesis 备择假设

H_a alternative hypothesis 备择假设

h hecto 百; hour 小时

h. hora【拉】小时

h Planck's constant 普朗克常数;height 高度

HA hemadsorbent 红细胞吸附的

Ha hahnium 𨭆

HAA hepatitis-associated antigen 肝炎相关抗原

Haab's degeneration [hɑːb] (Otto Haab) 哈布变性(角膜视网膜变性) | ~ magnet 哈布磁铁(用以吸出眼内金属异物) / ~ reflex 哈布反射(患者坐在暗室内时两侧瞳孔收缩,并对早已存在视野中引起其注意的明亮目标无调节或会聚反应。亦称大脑皮质性瞳孔反射)

HAART highly active antiretroviral therapy 高度活性抗反转录病毒疗法

habena [həˈbiːnə] ([复] **habenae** [həˈbiːniː]) *n*【拉】缰,系带 | **~l** [həˈbiːnəl], **~r** [həˈbiːnə] *a*

habenula [həˈbenjulə] ([复] **habenulae** [həˈbenjuliː]) *n*【拉】缰,系带;松果体缰 | ~ arcuata 弓状系带(耳蜗) / ~ conarii 松果体缰 / ~ pectinata 梳状系带 / ~e perforatae 神经孔 / ~ urethralis 尿道系带(女) | **~r** *a*

Habermann's disease [ˈhɑːbəmɑːn] (Rudolf Habermann) 急性苔藓样糠疹

habit [ˈhæbit] *n* 习惯;习性;癖,瘾;体型,型 | apoplectic ~, full ~ 中风体型 / asthenic ~ 无力体型,衰弱体型 / clamping ~, clenching ~ 紧咬癖,磨牙癖,正中磨牙症 / drug ~ 药[物]瘾 / endothelioid ~, leukocytoid ~ 内皮样型(细胞) / glaucomatous ~ 青光眼型 / leptosomatic ~ 瘦长体型 / opium ~ 阿片瘾 / oral ~ 口腔[不良]习惯(如吮指、吸拇、吮唇、吐舌等使牙合关系改变的习惯) / physiologic ~ 生理习惯 / pycnic ~ 矮胖体型

habitat [ˈhæbitæt] *n* (动植物的)生境,栖息地

habitation [ˌhæbiˈteiʃən] *n* 居住,住处,聚居地

habituation [həˌbitjuˈeiʃən] *n* 习服;习惯性;习惯化;成瘾 | vestibular ~ 前庭习服

habitus [ˈhæbitəs] *n*【拉】姿势;体型 | ~ apoplecticus 中风体型,卒中体型 / Buddha-like ~ 佛样体型(胎儿腹部膨大,如蛙腹) / ~ enteroptoticus 肠下垂体型 / ~ phthisicus [肺]结核体型

Habronema [ˌhæbrəuˈniːmə] *n* 丽线虫属

Habronematidae [ˌhæbrəuniːˈmætidiː] *n* 丽线虫科

habronemiasis [ˌhæbrəuniˈmaiəsis] *n* 丽线虫病 | cutaneous ~ 皮肤丽线虫蚴疮,夏疮(马)

habu [ˈhɑːbuː] *n* 饭匙倩(琉球群岛等地的一种毒蛇);蕲蛇,龟壳花蕲

hachement [æʃˈmɔŋ] *n*【法】掌缘击法(按摩)

hadernkrankheit [ˈhɑːdənkrɑːŋkhait] *n*【德】破布病(侵害捡破布者的疾病,被认为是炭疽或恶性水肿)

Hadfield-Clarke syndrome [ˈhædfiːld klɑːk] (Geoffrey Hadfield; Cecil Clarke) 哈-克综合征(见 Clarke-Hadfield syndrome)

hae- 以 hae-起始的词,同样见以 he-起始的词

Haeckel's law [ˈhekəl] (Ernst H. P. A. Haeckel) 赫格尔定律(重演学说 recapitulation theory,见 theory 项下相应术语)

haem [hiːm] *n* 血红素

haema [ˈhiːmə] *n* 血(可拼写成 hema)

haema- 见 hemat(o)-;同样见以 hema-起始的词

Haemadipsa [ˌhiːməˈdipsə] *n* 山蛭属 | ~ ceylonica 锡兰山蛭 / ~ chiliani 智利山蛭 / ~ japonica 日本山蛭

Haemagogus [ˌheməˈgəugəs] *n* 趋血蚊属

Haemaphysalis [ˌheməˈfisəlis] *n* 血蜱属,盲蜱属 | ~ concinna 嗜群血蜱 / ~ humerosa 硕鼠血蜱 / ~ leachi 犬血蜱 / ~ leporispalustris 野兔血蜱 / ~ punctata 刻点血蜱 / ~ spinigera 距刺血蜱

haemat(o)- 见 hemat(o)-

Haematobia [ˌheməˈtəubiə] *n* 血蝇属 | ~ irritans 扰血蝇

Haematopinus [ˌhemətəuˈpainəs] *n* 血虱属,盲虱属

Haematopota [ˌhiːməˈtɔpətə] *n* 麻虻属

Haematosiphon [ˌhemətəuˈsaifɔn] *n* 鸡臭虫属 | ~ indorus 鸡臭虫

Haematoxylon [ˌhiːməˈtɔksilɔn] *n* 洋苏木属

Haementeria [ˌhemənˈtiəriə] *n* 南美水蛭属

haem(o)- 见 hem(o)-

Haemobartonella [ˌhiːməuˌbɑːtəuˈnelə] *n* 血巴尔通体属 | ~ canis 犬血巴尔通体 / ~ felis 猫血巴尔通体 / ~ muris 鼠血巴尔通体

haemobartonellosis [ˌhiːməuˌbɑːtənəˈləusis] *n* 血巴尔通体病,猫感染性贫血

Haemodipsus [ˌheməuˈdipsəs] *n* 虱属 | ~ ventricosus 兔虱

Haemogregarina [ˌheməuˌgregəˈrainə] *n* 血簇虫属

haemonchosis [ˌhiːmɔŋˈkəusis] *n* 血矛线虫病

Haemonchus [hiːˈmɔnkəs] *n* 血矛线虫属 | ~ contortus 捻转血矛线虫

Haemophilus [hiːˈmɔfiləs] *n* 嗜血杆菌属 | ~ aegyptius 埃及嗜血杆菌 / ~ aphrophilus 嗜泡沫嗜血杆菌 / ~ bronchisepticus 支气管败血性嗜血杆菌 / ~ ducreyi 杜克雷嗜血杆菌 / ~ duplex 结膜炎嗜血杆菌 / ~ haemolyticus 溶血性嗜血杆菌 / ~ influenzae 流感嗜血杆菌 / ~ parainfluenzae 副流感嗜血杆菌 / ~ paraphrophilus 副嗜泡沫嗜血杆菌 / ~ parasuis, ~ suis 副猪嗜血杆菌,猪嗜血杆菌 / ~ pertussis 百日咳嗜血杆菌 / ~ vaginalis 阴道嗜血杆菌

Haemophoructus [ˌheməufəˈrʌktəs] *n* 吸血蝇属

Haemopis [hiˈməupis] *n* 黄蛭属

Haemoproteus [ˌheməuˈprəutiəs] *n* 变形血原虫属

haemorrhage [ˈheməridʒ] *n* = **hemorrhage**

haemorrhagia [ˌhiːməˈreidʒiə] *n*【拉】出血

Haemosporidia [ˌhiːməuspəridiə] *n* 血孢子虫目

Haemosporina [ˌhiːməuspəˈrainə] *n* 血孢子虫亚目

haemozoin [ˌhiːməuˈzəuin] *n* 疟原虫色素

Haenel's symptom [ˈheinəl] (Hans Haenel) 黑内尔症状(脊髓痨患者眼球压觉缺失)

Haeser [ˈheizə] 见 Häser

Haff disease [hæf] 哈夫病(哈夫为波罗的海一海湾,渔民由于摄入工业废水中的砷化氢所致,患者突然发生严重四肢疼痛,重度疲倦以及肌球蛋白尿)

Hafnia [ˈhæfniə] *n* 哈夫尼亚菌属 | ~ alvei 蜂房哈夫尼亚菌

hafnium(Hf) [ˈhæfniəm] *n* 铪(化学元素)

Hagedorn's needles [ˈhɑːgədɔːn] (Werner Hagedorn) 哈格多恩针(外科手术用的扁头针)

Hageman factor [ˈheidʒmən] (Hageman 为患者名)凝血因子Ⅻ

Haglund's disease [ˈhɑːglund] (Sims E. P. Haglund) 黑格隆德病(跟腱黏液囊炎)

Hagner's bag [ˈhægnə] (Francis R. Hagner) 哈格纳袋(前列腺止血袋) | ~ operation 哈格纳手术(作淋病性附睾炎的引流,经切口进入附睾)

Hagner's disease [ˈhɑːgnə] (Hagner 为 19 世纪研究的原先证者家族名) 哈格纳病,肥大性肺性骨关节病

hahnemannian [hɑːnəˈmæniən] (Christian Friedrich Samuel Hahnemann) *a* 哈内曼的,哈内曼疗法的,顺势疗法的 | **hahnemannism** [ˈhɑːniˌmænizəm] *n* 顺势疗法

hahnium [ˈhɑːniəm] *n* 锝(化学元素)

Hahn's sign [hɑːn] (Eugen H. Hahn) 哈恩征(儿童患小脑疾患时,头部持续性向两侧转动)

HAI hemagglutination inhibition 血细胞凝集抑制反应

Haidinger's brushes [ˈhaidiŋə] (Wilhelm von Haidinger) 海丁格内视刷(两个锥形刷状像,通过尼科尔〈Nicol〉棱镜注视时可见到,用于测视力功能)

Hailey-Hailey disease [ˈheili ˈheili] (Hugh Hailey; William H. Heiley) 良性家族性天疱疮

Haines' formula(coefficient) [ˈheinz] (Walter S. Haines) 黑恩斯公式(系数)(计算尿内固形物,即取尿比重的最后两个数,乘以 1.1〈黑恩斯系数〉,所得之积相近于每液量盎司尿中固体的格令〈grain〉数) | ~ reagent 黑恩斯试剂(硫酸铜 2 份,氢氧化钾 7.5 份,甘油 15 份,蒸馏水 150 份) / ~ test 黑恩斯试验(检尿葡萄糖)

hair [hɛə] *n* 毛发,毛;体毛 | auditory ~s 听毛 / bamboo ~ 结节性脆发病,发结节病 / beaded ~ 念珠状发 / club ~ 杵状毛 / exclamation point ~ 感叹号形发(斑脱的特征) / ~s of eyebrow 眉毛 / knotted ~ 结毛症,结节性脆发病 / lanugo ~, wooly ~ 胎毛,毳,柔毛 / pubic ~, ~s of pubis 阴毛 / terminal ~ 终毛,恒久毛,成人毛[发] / twisted ~ 扭发 / vellus ~ 毫毛

hairball [ˈhɛəbɔːl] *n* 毛团,毛粪石(胃肠内)

haircap [ˈhɛəkæp] *n* 杜松苔(一种利尿草药)

haircast [ˈhɛəkɑːst] *n* [胃形]毛粪石(充满胃内,具胃的形状)

hairworm [ˈhɛəwəːm] *n* 毛虫,线虫

Hakim-Adams syndrome [hɑːˈkiːm ˈædəmz] (S. Hakim; R. D. Adams) 哈-亚综合征,正常压脑积水

Hakim's syndrome [hɑːˈkiːm] (S. Hakim) 哈基姆综合征,正常压脑积水

Halarachnidae [ˌhæləˈræknidiː] *n* 喘螨科

halation [həˈleiʃən] *n* 晃眼,耀眼

halazepam [hæˈlæzəpæm] *n* 哈拉西泮(安定药)

halazone [hæləˈzəun] *n* 哈拉宗(一种供水消毒药)

halcinonide [hælˈsinənaid] *n* 哈西奈德(合成糖皮质激素,局部抗炎药)

Haldane chamber(apparatus) [ˈhɔːldein] (John S. Haldane) 霍尔丹室(器)(一种密封室,将动物置于其内进行代谢研究) | ~ effect 霍尔丹效应

(高浓度氧,如在肺部肺泡毛细血管中所发生的,促进二氧化碳和氢离子从血红蛋白中解离,因此氧解离曲线移至左)

Hales's piesimeter [heilz] (Stephen Hales) 黑尔斯压觉计(一种可插入动脉内测定血压的玻璃管)

halfaxial [hæf'æksiəl] *a* 半轴的

half-life ['hɑːf laif] *n* 半衰期(放射性核素的数量因核的衰变而减少到原来数目的一半所需的时间) | biological ~ 生物学半衰期(一个活组织、器官或机体将已引入的放射性物质排出一半所需的时间)

half-retinal [hɑːf 'retinl] *a* 半侧视网膜的

half-time($t_{1/2}$) ['hɑːf taim] *n* 半时值 | plasma iron clearance ~ 血浆铁清除率半时值

half-value ['hɑːf 'væljuː] *a* 半值的(指半值层)

halfway house ['hɑːfwei haus] 中途疗养所(为不需要完全住院,但仍需要照料的精神病患者或戒瘾者所设,直至他们重返社会)

halibut ['hælibət] *n* 庸鲽,大比目鱼

Halicephalobus [ˌhæliˌsefə'ləubəs] *n* 海头叶[线虫]属(亦称微线虫属)

halide ['hælaid] *a* 卤族的 *n* 卤化物

hali-ichthyotoxin [ˌhæli ˌikθiə'tɔksin] *n* 盐渍鱼毒素

halisteresis [həˌlistə'riːsis] *n* 骨软化,骨钙缺乏 | ~ cerea 骨蜡样软化 | **halisteretic** [həˌlistə'retik] *a*

halitosis [ˌhæli'təusis] *n* 口臭

halituous [hə'litjuəs] *a* 蒸湿的

halitus ['hælitəs] *n* 【拉】呼气,哈气 | ~ saturninus 铅中毒性口臭

hallachrome ['hæləkrəum] *n* 红痣素,多巴色素

Hallauer's glasses ['hælauə] (Otto Hallauer) 哈劳尔眼镜(防止蓝线及紫外线透过的灰绿色防护眼镜)

Hall band [hɔːl] (Herbert H. Hall) 霍尔带(一种子宫内避孕装置)

Hallberg effect ['hɔːlbəːg] (J. H. Hallberg) 霍尔伯格效应(超短驻波的波峰和波谷有相反的电学特征)

Hallermann-Streiff-François syndrome ['hɑːləmɑːn ʃtraif frɑːn'swɑː] (W. Hallermann; E. B. Streiff; Jules François) 哈-斯-弗综合征,眼下颌面综合征(即 oculomandibulofacial syndrome, 见 syndrome 项下相应术语)

Hallermann-Streiff syndrome ['hɑːləmɑːn ʃtraif] (Wilhelm Hallermann; Enrico B. Streiff) 哈勒曼-斯特雷夫综合征,眼下颌面综合征(即 oculomandibulofacial syndrome,见 syndrome 项下相应术语)

Haller's arches ['hælə] (Albrecht von Haller) 哈勒弓(腰肋外侧弓;腰肋内侧弓) | ~ aberrant duct 附睾迷管 / ~ circle 视神经血管环 / ~ cones 附睾小叶 / ~ crypt 包皮腺 / ~ fretum (isthmus) 哈勒峡(胎儿心房和心室或主动脉球间的狭窄) / ~ habenula 哈勒系带(腹膜鞘突遗迹) / ~ layer 脉络膜血管层 / ~ line 脊髓前正中裂 / ~ membrane 脉络膜血管层 / ~ plexus 喉丛 / ~ rete 睾丸网 / ~ tripod 腹腔干,腹腔动脉

Hallervorden-Spatz disease ['hɑːləˌfɔːdən ʃpɑːts] (Julius Hallervorden; Hugo Spatz) 哈勒沃登-施帕茨病(一种遗传性疾病,特征为苍白球和黑质的髓鞘数显著减少,伴铁质色素累积,开始小腿进行性强直,舞蹈手足徐动症样运动,构音障碍及进行性精神颓废,常染色体隐性遗传,通常于 10~20 岁发病,30 岁以前死亡)

Hallé's point [æ'lei] (Adrien J. M. N. Hallé) 阿累点(输尿管盆缘点,腹壁上示输尿管经过骨盆上口的点)

hallex ['hæleks] ([复] **hallices** ['hælisiːz]) *n* 【拉】踇趾,踇

Hallion's test [æ'ljɔŋ] (Louis Hallion) 阿利翁试验(见 Tuffier's test)

Hallopeau's acrodermatitis [ælɔ'pəu] (François H. Hallopeau) 连续性肢端皮炎

Hallpike's maneuver ['hɔːlpaik] (Charles S. Hallpike) 霍尔派克手法(检良性体位性眩晕的一种试验)

Hall's disease [hɔːl] (Marshall Hall) 假性脑积水 | ~ facies 霍尔面容(额大面小,见于脑积水) / ~ method 霍尔法(一种人工呼吸法,使患者俯卧,轻压其背部,然后放松,再使患者仰卧,轻压之,这样每分钟做 16 次)

Hall's sign [hɔːl] (Josiah N. Hall) 霍尔征(主动脉瘤时,可由气管感到舒张期震动)

Hall-Stone ring ['hɔːlstəun] (Herbert H. Hall; Martin Lawrence Stone) 哈尔-斯通环(节育环的一种)

hallucal ['hæljukəl] *a* 踇趾的

hallucinant [hə'luːsinənt] *n* 幻觉症患者;幻觉剂 *a* 引起幻觉的

hallucinate [hə'luːsineit] *vt* 使生幻觉

hallucination [həˌluːsi'neiʃən] *n* 幻觉 | auditory ~ 幻听 / depressive ~ 抑郁性幻觉 / gustatory ~ 幻味 / hypnagogic ~ 入睡前幻觉 / lilliputian ~ 小人国[视]幻觉,小形象幻视,微形幻视 / olfactory ~ 幻嗅 / stump ~ 残肢幻觉,幻肢 / tactile ~, haptic ~ 幻触 / visual ~ 幻视 | **hallucinative** [hə'luːsinətiv], **hallucinatory** [hə'luːsinətəri] *a*

hallucinogen [hə'luːsinəˌdʒen] *n* 致幻剂

hallucinogenesis [həˌluːsinə'dʒenisis] *n* 幻觉产

生,幻觉发生 | **hallucinogenic** [həˌluːsinə'dʒenik], **hallucinogenetic** [həˌluːsinədʒi'netik] *a* 致幻觉的 *n* 致幻觉药

hallucinosis [həˌhuːsi'nəusis] *n* 幻觉症 | acute ~, alcoholic ~ 急性幻觉症,酒中毒性幻觉症 / organic ~ 器质性幻觉症 | **hallucinotic** [həˌluːsi'nɔtik] *a*

hallux ['hæləks] ([复] **halluces** ['hæləsiːz]) *n* 【拉】踇趾 | ~ valgus 踇外翻 / ~ varus 踇内翻

Hallwachs effect ['hælvæks] (Franz Hallwachs) 光电效应

halmatogenesis [ˌhælmətə'dʒenisis] *n* 突然变异

halo ['heiləu] ([复] halo⟨e⟩s) *n* 【拉】晕,晕轮 | glaucomatous ~ 青光眼晕轮 / ~ saturninus 铅线 / senile ~ 老年性晕斑

hal(o)- [构词成分]盐

Halobacteriaceae [ˌhæləubækˌtiəri'eisiiː] *n* 嗜盐菌科,盐杆菌科

Halobacterium [ˌhæləubæk'tiəriəm] *n* 盐杆菌属

halobacterium [ˌhæləubæk'tiəriəm] ([复] **halobacteria** [ˌhæləubæk'tiəriə]) *n* 嗜盐菌,盐杆菌

halobetasol propionate [ˌhæləu'beitəsɔl] 丙酸卤倍他索尔(一种极高效能的合成皮质类固醇,局部用于缓解皮质类固醇反应性皮肤病的炎症和瘙痒症)

halobiont [ˌhæləu'baiɔnt] *n* 适盐生物,喜盐生物

Halococcus [ˌhæləu'kɔkəs] *n* 盐球菌属

halodermia [ˌhæləu'dəːmiə] *n* 卤化物皮疹

haloduric [ˌhæləu'djuərik] *a* 耐盐的(细菌)

halofantrine hydrochloride [ˌhælə'fæntriːn] 盐酸卤泛群(抗疟药)

halofenate [ˌhæləu'feneit] *n* 卤芬酯(降血脂药,促尿酸排泄药)

halogen ['hælədʒən] *n* 卤素,卤 | **~ous** [hə'lɔdʒinəs] *a*

halogenate ['hælədʒəneit] *vt* 卤化 | **halogenation** [ˌhælədʒə'neiʃən] *n*

halogenide ['hælədʒənaid] *n* 卤化物

halogeton [ˌhælə'dʒiːtɔn, hə'lɔdʒitɔn] *n* 盐生草(含可溶性草酸盐,有剧毒,可引起呼吸困难、出血和低钙血症)

Halogeton [ˌhælə'giːtən] *n* 盐生草属

haloid ['hælɔid] *a* 卤族的 *n* 卤化物 | ~ acid [氢]卤酸

halometer [hə'lɔmitə] *n* 眼晕测定器;红细胞衍射晕测量器 | **halometry** *n* 眼晕测定法;红细胞衍射晕测量法

halopemide [ˌhæləu'pemaid] *n* 卤培米特(安定药)

haloperidol [ˌhæləu'peridɔl] *n* 氟哌啶醇(安定药)

halophil ['hæləfil] *n* 适盐菌,嗜盐菌

halophile ['hæləfail] *n* 适盐菌,嗜盐菌 *a* 适盐的,嗜盐的 | **halophilic** [ˌhælə'filik], **halophilous** [hæ'lɔfiləs] *a* 适盐的,嗜盐的

halopredone acetate [ˌhælə'priːdəun] 醋酸卤泼尼松(局部抗炎药)

haloprogin [ˌhæləu'prəudʒin] *n* 卤普罗近(合成的局部抗真菌药,治癣)

halosteresis [həˌlɔstə'riːsis] *n* 骨软化,骨钙缺乏

halothane ['hæləθein] *n* 氟烷(麻醉药)

haloxon [hə'lɔksɔn] *n* 哈洛克酮(兽用抗蠕虫药)

halquinol, halquinols ['hælkwinɔl(s)] *n* 哈喹诺(局部抗感染药)

Halsted's mastectomy ['hælsted] (William S. Halsted) 霍尔斯特德乳房切除术(乳房根治术) | ~ operation 霍尔斯特德手术(①腹股沟根治手术;②乳房根治术) / ~ suture 霍尔斯特德缝术(郎贝尔⟨Lembert⟩缝术的改良,包括平行缝一针于创口一侧,而两端穿过他侧后打结)

Haltia-Santavuori disease ['hɑːltiɑː sɑːntɑː'vwəuri] (M. Haltia; Pirkko Santavuori) 霍-桑病(一种罕见的婴儿型神经细胞蜡样质脂褐素病,约 1 岁时开始,表现为脂褐素大量贮积,不能茁壮成长,肌阵挛性发作。肌性张力过低,精神运动性发育迟缓和衰退,失明伴视神经萎缩和小脑共济失调,约 5 年内死亡)

halzoun ['hælzən] *n* 哈尔宗病(叙利亚的一种地方性寄生物性咽病)

Hamamelis [ˌhæmə'miːlis] *n* 金缕梅属

hamamelis [ˌhæmə'miːlis] *n* 北美金缕梅(收敛药)

hamamelose [hæ'mæmiləus] *n* 金缕梅糖

hamarthritis [ˌhæmɑː'θraitis] *n* 全身关节炎

hamartia [hæ'mɑːʃiə] *n* 【希】组织构成缺陷 | **~l** *a*

hamart(o)- [构词成分]缺陷;错构瘤

hamartoblastoma [hæˌmɑːtəblæs'təumɑː] *n* 错构胚细胞瘤

hamartoma [ˌhæmɑː'təumə] *n* 错构瘤

hamartomatosis [ˌhæmɑːtəumə'təusis] *n* 错构瘤病,多发性错构瘤

hamartomatous [ˌhæmɑː'təumətəs] *a* 错构的

hamartoplasia [ˌhæmɑːtəu'pleiziə] *n* 组织增生过多

hamate ['heimeit] *a* 钩状的(如钩骨)

hamatum [hə'meitəm] *a* 钩状的 *n* 钩骨

Hamberger's schema ['hæmbəːgə] (Georg E. Hamberger) 汉布格图式(肋间外肌及软骨间肌为吸气肌,肋间内肌为呼气肌)

Hamburger phenomenon (interchange) ['hæmbəːgə] (Hartog J. Hamburger) 汉布格尔现象(交换)(血细胞和血浆之间的离子交换,碳酸氢

盐从红细胞进入血浆,氯离子从血浆进入红细胞。亦称继发缓冲作用)

Hamilton's bandage [ˈhæmiltən] (Frank H. Hamilton) 汉密尔顿绷带(下颌带) | ~ test 汉密尔顿试验(肩关节脱位后,在肱骨上用直尺可同时触及外侧髁和肩峰)

Hamman-Rich syndrome [ˈhæmən ritʃ] (Louis Hamman; Arnold R. Rich) 哈-里综合征,特发性肺纤维化(即 idiopathic pulmonary fibrosis,见 fibrosis 项下相应术语)

Hamman's disease (syndrome) [ˈhæmən] (Louis Hamman) 哈曼病(综合征)(纵隔积气) | ~ sign 哈曼征(心前区与每次心搏同步发生的摩擦音、咔嗒声或叩音在叩诊时听到,提示急性纵隔炎、纵隔积气及气胸)

Hammarsten's test [ˈhæməstən] (Olof Hammarsten) 汉马斯坦试验(检球蛋白、胆色素)

hammer [ˈhæmə] *n* 锤;锤骨

Hammerschlag's method (test) [ˈhæməʃlɑːɡ] (Albert Hammerschlag) 哈默施拉格法(试验)(检血液比重)

hammock [ˈhæmək] *n* 吊床;吊带

Hammond's disease [ˈhæmənd] (William A. Hammond) 手足徐动症

hamster [ˈhæmstə] *n* 仓鼠

Ham's test [hæm] (Thomas Hale Ham) 哈姆试验,酸化血清试验

hamstring [ˈhæmstriŋ] *n* 腘绳肌腱 | inner ~ 内侧腘绳肌腱 / outer ~ 外侧腘绳肌腱

hamular [ˈhæmjulə] *a* 钩状的

hamulus [ˈhæmjuləs] ([复] **hamuli** [ˈhæmjulai]) *n* 【拉】钩,小钩 | lacrimal ~ 泪钩 / pterygoid ~ 翼钩 / trochlear ~ 滑车棘

hamycin [həˈmaisin] *n* 哈霉素(抗生素类药)

Hancock's amputation (operation) [ˈhænkɔks] (Henry Hancock) 汉考克切断术(手术)(皮罗果夫〈pirogoff〉切断术的改良法,即将部分距骨留在皮瓣上,锯掉跟骨的下面,距骨的切面与其接触)

hand [hænd] *n* 手 | ape ~, monkey ~ 猿[样]手(鱼际肌萎缩) / benediction ~, preacher's ~ 祝福状手(见于尺骨神经麻痹及脊髓空洞症) / claw ~ 爪形手 / cleft ~, lobsterclaw ~, split ~ 分裂手,裂手[畸形],龙虾爪手 / club ~ 畸形手 / dead ~ 呆手(见于使用震动性工具者,由于大量震荡所致) / drop ~ 手垂病,腕下垂 / flat ~ 扁平手 / mirror ~s 一腕双手[畸形] / obstetrician's ~, accoucheur's ~ 助产[士]手 / operaglass ~ 短指手(由慢性关节炎所致的指缩短) / phantom ~ 虚手症,幻手(手截断后的异常感觉,仿佛手仍存在) / skeleton ~ 枯骨状手(手高度萎缩,见于进行性肌萎缩) / spade ~ 铲形手(黏液性水肿和肢端肥大症时厚实方形手) / trench ~ 战壕手病(因冻伤所致) / trident ~ 三叉手,三尖手(软骨发育不全所致) / writing ~ 握笔状手(见于震颤麻痹)

H and E hematoxylin and eosin (stain) 苏木精和伊红(染剂)

handedness [ˈhændidnis] *n* 手偏利(偏于用一侧手工作) | left ~ 左[手]利 / right ~ 右[手]利

handicap [ˈhændikæp] *n* 障碍;残障,严重残疾 | mental ~ 精神残疾

handicapped [ˈhændikæpt] *a* 有生理缺陷的,智力低下的;残疾的

handle [hændl] *n* 柄 | ~ of malleus 锤骨柄

Handley's method [ˈhændli] (William S. Handley) 汉德利法(用长棉花和丝线塞在组织内进行引流,治象皮病)

handpiece [ˈhændpiːs] *n* 手机,机头

Hand-Schüller-Christian disease (syndrome), Hand's disease (syndrome) [hænd ˈʃilə ˈkristʃən] (Alfred Hand; Artur Schüller; Henry A. Christian) 汉-许-克病(综合征)、汉德病(综合征),慢性特发性组织细胞增多症(为眼球突出、尿崩症及膜骨缺损的三联征,有时见于朗格汉斯〈Langerhans〉细胞组织细胞增多症。亦称慢性特发性黄瘤病)

HANE hereditary angioneurotic edema 遗传性血管神经性水肿

Hanger's test [ˈhæŋə] (Franklin M. Hanger) 汉格试验(检肝细胞病)

hangnail [ˈhæŋneil] *n* 逆剥,甲刺,倒刺(指甲上皮剥裂)

Hanhart's syndrome [ˈhɑːnhɑːt] (Ernst Hanhart) 汉哈特综合征(若干变异遗传综合征中的任何一种,主要特点为严重小颌、高鼻根、小睑裂、低位耳及指〈趾〉或肢体〈通常在肘或膝以下〉有不同缺损)

Hannover's canal [ˈhænəuvə] (Adolph Hannover) 汉诺佛管腔(界于晶状体悬韧带前后两部分之间的潜在间隙)

Hanot-Chauffard syndrome [æˈnəuʃəuˈfɑː] (Victor C. Hanot; Anatole M. E. Chauffard) 阿诺-肖法综合征(肥大性肝硬化伴色素沉着和糖尿病)

Hanot's cirrhosis (disease, syndrome) [æˈnəu] (Victor C. Hanot) 阿诺肝硬化(病、综合征)(原发性胆汁性肝硬化;继发性胆汁性肝硬化)

Hansemann macrophages [ˈhɑːnsəmɑːn] (David Paul von Hansemann) 汉泽曼巨噬细胞(见 von Hansemann cell)

Hansen's bacillus [ˈhænsn] (Gerhard H. A. Hansen) 麻风分枝杆菌 | ~ disease 麻风

Hansenula [hænˈsenjulə] *n* 汉逊酵母属 | ~ anomala 异常汉逊酵母

Hanson's unit [ˈhænsn] (Adolph M. Hanson) 汉

森单位(甲状旁腺提出物的生物鉴定单位)

Hantavirus [ˈhæntəˌvaiərəs] (Hantaan 为朝鲜一河名)汉滩病毒属

Hapalochlaena [ˌhæpələuˈkliːnə] *n* 软爪属,章鱼属

haphalgesia [ˌhæfælˈdʒiːziə] *n* 触痛

haphephobia [ˌhæfiˈfəubiə] *n* 被触恐怖,恐触症

hapl(o)- [构词成分] 单纯,单独

haplobacteria [ˌhæpləbækˈtiəriə] *n* 单形细菌

Haplochilus [ˌhæpləˈkailəs] *n* 小鳉鱼属 | ~ panchax 马来小鳉鱼(食按蚊幼虫)

haplodiploidy [ˌhæpləuˈdiplɔidi] *n* 单倍二倍性(某些动物如蜜蜂中所特有的一种遗传系统,从非受精卵发育的雄蜂是单倍体,从受精卵发育的雌蜂是二倍体)

haplodont [ˈhæplədɔnt] *n* 单形牙(牙冠无牙尖或嵴的)

haploid [ˈhæplɔid] *a* 单倍[体]的 *n* 单倍体(指一个个体或细胞只具有单套的同源染色体) | **~y** *n* 单倍性

haploidentical [ˌhæpləuaiˈdentikəl] *a* 单倍同一性的(具有一个单倍型的;具有相同等位基因的)

haploidentity [ˌhæpləuaiˈdentəti] *n* 单倍同一性

haplomycosis [ˌhæpləumaiˈkəusis] *n* 单倍真菌病

haplont [ˈhæplɔnt] *n* 单倍体,单倍性生物

Haplopappus [ˌhæpləuˈpæpəs] *n* 单冠菊属 | ~ gracilis 纤细单冠菊

haplopathy [hæpˈlɔpəθi] *n* 单纯病(无合并症疾病)

haplophase [ˈhæpləfeiz] *n* 单倍期(生殖细胞的生活史中一个时期,其核为单倍体)

haplopia [hæpˈləupiə] *n* 单视

Haplorchis [hæpˈlɔːkis] *n* 单睾吸虫属 | ~ taichui 扇形单睾吸虫

haploscope [ˈhæpləskəup] *n* 视轴计 | mirror ~ 镜面式视轴计

haploscopic [hæpləˈskɔpik] *a* 视轴测定的

haplosis [hæpˈləusis] *n* 减半作用(指在减数分裂过程中染色体减少了一半,形成成熟配子所具有的染色体数)

haplosporangin [ˌhæpləuspəˈrændʒin] *n* 单孢子囊菌素

Haplosporangium [ˌhæpləuspəˈrændʒiəm] *n* 单孢子囊菌属

Haplosporidium [ˌhæpləuspəˈridiəm] *n* 单孢子虫属

haplosporosome [ˌhæpləuˈspɔːrəsəum] *n* 单孢子小体

haplotype [ˈhæplətaip] *n* 单体型,单元型(亲代任何一方〈父或母〉所提供的等位基因)

Hapsburg jaw [ˈhæpsbəːg] (Hapsburg 为欧洲德奥王室家族)哈布斯堡型突颌(一种下突颌,常伴有下唇发育过度性肥厚〈哈布斯堡型唇〉,如哈布斯堡家族中许多成员所见) | ~ lip 哈布斯堡型唇(过度发育的肥厚下唇,常伴哈布斯堡型突颌) / ~ disease 血友病(旧称)

hapten [ˈhæptən] *n* 半抗原 | group A ~ A 簇半抗原 | **haptene** [ˈhæptiːn], **haptin** [ˈhæptin] *n* / **haptenic** [hæpˈtenik] *a*

haptephobia [ˌhæptiˈfəubiə] *n* 被触恐怖,恐触症

haptic(al) [ˈhæptik(əl)] *a* 触觉的

haptics [ˈhæptiks] *n* 触觉学

hapt(o)- [构词成分] 接触,结合

haptocorrin [ˌhæptəuˈkɔːrin] *n* 咕啉结合蛋白,R 蛋白

haptocyst [ˈhæptəsist] *n* 触合小囊

haptoglobin [ˌhæptəˈgləubin] *n* 触珠蛋白

haptometer [hæpˈtɔmitə] *n* 触觉计

haptophil(e) [ˈhæptəfail] *a* 亲结合簇的

haptophore [ˈhæptəfɔː] *n* 结合簇(在埃利希〈Ehrlich〉侧链学说中,指毒素、凝集素、沉淀素、调理素和溶素的分子的特殊基团,借此与抗体、抗原或细胞受体结合,遂能发挥其效能) | **haptophoric** [ˌhæptəˈfɔːrik], **haptophorous** [hæpˈtɔfərəs] *a*

Haptorina [ˌhæptəuˈrainə] *n* 刺钩亚目

Harada's disease, syndrome [hɑːˈrɑːdɑː] (Einosuke Harada) 原田病,原田综合征(见 Vogt-Koyanagi-Harada syndrome)

harara [hɑːˈrɑːrə] *n* 白蛉皮炎

hardener [ˈhɑːdənə] *n* 硬化剂,坚硬剂

hardening [ˈhɑːdəniŋ] *n* 硬化法(使组织变硬便于切片,供显微镜检查用)

Harden-Young ester [ˈhɑːdn jʌŋ] (Arthur Harden; William J. Young) 哈-杨酯,果糖-1,6-二磷酸

harderian [ˈhɑːdəriən] (Johann J. Harder) *a* 哈德的(如 ~ fossa 副泪腺窝,泪阜窝; ~ glands 副泪腺)

harderoporphyria [ˌhɑːdərəuˌpɔːˈfiriə] *n* 粪卟啉病

harderoporphyrin [ˌhɑːdərəuˈpɔːfərin] *n* 粪卟啉

Harder's glands [ˈhɑːdə] (Johann J. Harder) 哈德腺,副泪腺

hardness [ˈhɑːdnis] *n* 硬度;硬性 | permanent ~ 永久硬度 / temporary ~ 暂时硬度

Hardy-Weinberg equilibrium [ˈhɑːdi ˈvainbəːg] (Godfrey H. Hardy; Wilhelm Weinberg) 哈迪-温伯格平衡,遗传平衡 | ~ law 哈迪-温伯格定律(两种等位基因〈*A* 和 *a*〉所决定的 3 种基因型比例,分别为 *p* 和 *q* 频率同时发生,在随机交配群体中将一代一代地保持不变: $AA = p^2$, $Aa = 2_{pq}$, $aa = q^2$。突变、选择、非随机分配、迁移和

遗传漂变能干扰这种平衡)

harelip [ˈhɛəlip] *n* 唇裂 | acquired ~ 后天性唇裂,创伤性唇裂 / double ~ 双侧唇裂 / median ~ 正中唇裂 / single ~ 单唇裂

Hare's syndrome [hɛə] (Edward S. Hare) 黑尔综合征(见 Pancoast's syndrome①解)

harlequin [ˈhɑːlikwin] *n* 花斑眼镜蛇

Harley's disease [ˈhɑːli] (George Harley) 哈利病(间歇性血红蛋白尿)

harmaline [ˈhɑːməliːn] *n* 哈马灵,二氢骆驼蓬缄(一种生物缄,具有致幻性质)

harmonia [hɑːˈməuniə] *n*【拉】平缝

harmony [ˈhɑːməni] *n* 和谐,协调 | functional occlusal ~ 功能性殆协调 / occlusal ~ 殆谐调

harness [ˈhɑːnis] *n* 吊带

Harpagophytum [ˌhɑːpəˈgɔfitəm] *n* 抱器植物属

Harpirhynchus [ˌhɑːpiˈriŋkəs] *n* 鸟喙螨属

harpoon [hɑːˈpuːn] *n* 组织针(活组织检查用)

Harrington instrumentation [ˈhæriŋtən] (Paul R. Harrington) 哈氏器械操作法(一套金属钩和棒,外科用以插入脊柱后部,以事舒展和加压,治疗脊柱侧弯及其他畸形) | ~ rod 哈氏棒

Harrington's solution [ˈhæriŋtən] (Charles Harrington) 哈林顿溶液(手消毒剂,含乙醇、盐酸、水和氯化汞)

Harris hematoxylin stain [ˈhæris] (Downey L. Harris) 哈里斯苏木精染剂(一种细胞核染剂,含苏木精、硫酸铝、一氧化汞和含水乙醇)

Harris lines [ˈhæris] (Henry A. Harris) 哈里斯线(X 线片上见到的长骨骨骺生长延缓的线)

Harrison antinarcotic act 哈里森抗麻醉品法案(美国联邦法律之一,自 1915 年 3 月 1 日起生效,管制成瘾药物如可卡因、吗啡、阿片等的拥有、买卖及处方)

Harrison's groove (curve, sulcus) [ˈhærisn] (Edward Harrison) 哈里森沟(沿胸部下缘的水平凹沟,相当于膈的肋骨附着处,见于小儿晚期佝偻病)

Harris' segregator (separator) [ˈhæris] (Malcolm La Selle Harris) 哈里斯分隔采尿器(分离器)(一种分开收集每个肾脏小便的器械)

Harris' staining method [ˈhæris] (Downey L. Harris) 哈里斯染色法(显示内格里〈Negri〉小体的染色法)

Harris' syndrome [ˈhæris] (Seale Harris) 哈里斯综合征(由于内在因素,如胰腺功能紊乱或胰岛素瘤所致的胰岛素分泌过多,特征为低血糖、体弱、出汗、心动过速等)

Harrower's hypothesis [ˈhærəuə] (Henry R. Harrower) 哈罗尔假设,激素饥饿(hormone hunger,见 hunger 项下相应术语)

harrowing [ˈhærəuiŋ] *n* 神经纤维松解法

Hartel's treatment (method, technic) [ˈhɑːtəl] (Fritz Hartel) 哈特尔[疗]法(针头自口内刺入蝶骨卵圆孔区,注射乙醇治疗三叉神经痛)

Hartley-Krause operation [ˈhɑːtli kraus] (Frank Hartley; Fedor Krause) 哈-克手术(三叉神经节及其根切除术,以缓解三叉神经痛)

Hartmannella [ˌhɑːtmæˈnelə] *n* 哈[特曼]氏变形虫属,哈氏虫属 | ~ haylina 透明哈[特曼]氏变形虫,透明哈氏虫

hartmannelliasis [ˌhɑːtmæneˈlaiəsis] *n* 哈[特曼]氏虫病

Hartmann's curet [ˈhɑːtmən] (Arthur Hartmann) 哈特曼刮匙(增殖腺刮匙) | ~ speculum 哈特曼窥器(一种鼻镜)

Hartmann's (critical) point [ˈhɑːtmən] (Henri Hartmann) 哈特曼点(见 Sudeck's critical point) | ~ pouch 哈特曼囊(胆囊颈部的异常小囊) / ~ procedure (operation, colostomy) 哈特曼手术(结肠造口术)(切除结肠病变部分,把近侧端结肠按结肠造口术引出,远侧残端或直肠用缝线缝合)

Hartnup disease [ˈhɑːtnəp] (Hartnup 为英国先证者家族) 哈特纳普病,H 病(一种先天性代谢病,特征为小脑共济失调、糙皮病样皮肤病及大量氨基酸尿,包括一组具有共同肾重吸收机制的中性单氨单羧基氨基酸;患者长期口服烟酰胺反应良好)

hartshorn [ˈhɑːtshɔːn] *n* 碳酸铵

harveian [ˈhɑːviən] *a* 哈维(William Harvey)的

harvest [ˈhɑːvist] *vt* 采集(从供者取下组织或细胞,保存供移植用)

Häser's formula (coefficient) [ˈheizə] (Heinrich Häser) 海泽尔公式(系数)(计算尿内固形物,即取尿比重的最后两个数,乘以 2.33〈海泽尔系数〉,所得之积相近于 1 升尿中所含固体的格令〈grain〉数)

Hashimoto's thyroiditis (disease, struma) [hɑːʃiˈmɔːtɔː] (Hakaru Hashimoto 桥本) 桥本甲状腺炎(病、甲状腺肿),慢性淋巴细胞性甲状腺炎

hashish [hæˈʃiːʃ] *n* 印度大麻(印度大麻〈Cannabis sativa L.〉的茎和叶制成的麻醉品)

hashishin [hæˈʃiːʃin] *n* [印度]大麻瘾者

hashishism [ˈhæʃiːʃizəm] *n* [印度]大麻瘾

hashitoxicosis [ˌhæʃiˌtɔksiˈkəusis] *n* 桥本中毒症(桥本病患者甲状腺功能亢进)

Hasner's fold, valve [ˈhɑːsnə] (Joseph R. von A. Hasner) 泪襞

Hassall's corpuscles (bodies) [ˈhæsl] (Arthur H. Hassall) 哈索尔小体(胸腺小体,为胸腺早期发育过程中,上皮组织的残遗物)

Hassin's syndrome [ˈhæsin] (George B. Hassin) 哈辛综合征(颈交感神经病变时损害侧的耳翼外突,合并霍纳〈Horner〉综合征)

HAT hypoxathine-aminopterin-thymidine (medium) 次黄嘌呤-氨蝶呤-胸苷(培养基)

Hata's phenomenon [ˈhɑːtɑː] (Sahachiro Hata 秦佐八郎)秦氏现象(投予小量化学药物后感染病情反而加重) | ~ preparation 秦氏制剂(胂凡纳明)

hatch [hætʃ] *vt* 孵出 *vi* 孵化 *n* 孵化

hatchet [ˈhætʃit] *n* 手斧,刮刀(牙科用,亦称斧形挖器) | enamal ~ 釉斧,釉质刮刀

H⁺-ATPase H⁺-transporting ATP synthase H⁺-腺苷三磷酸酶,H⁺-转运腺苷三磷酸合酶

Hauch(H) [hauh] *n*【德】H型,鞭毛型,运动型(指某些菌落)

Haudek's sign (niche) [ˈhɔːdek] (Martin Haudek) 豪德克征(龛)(穿透性胃溃疡的放射照片上可见一向壁外突起的阴影,为铋剂在胃壁的病理性壁龛中停滞所致)

haunch [hɔːntʃ] *n* 臀部

hauptganglion of Küttner [ˈhauptˌgæŋgliən] 屈特纳淋巴结,[颈]二腹肌淋巴结(见 Küttner's ganglion)

Haust. haustus【拉】顿服剂

haustellum [hɔːˈsteləm] ([复] **haustella** [hɔːˈsteiə]) *n* 吸喙

haustorium [hɔːˈstɔriəm] ([复] **haustoria**) [hɔːˈstɔrlə] *n* 吸器

haustral [ˈhɔːstrəl] *a* 袋的(结肠袋的)

haustration [hɔːˈstreiʃən] *n* 袋形成;袋(结肠袋)

haustrum [ˈhɔːstrəm] ([复] **haustra** [ˈhɔːstrə]) *n*【拉】袋 | haustra of colon 结肠袋

haustus [ˈhɔːstəs] *n*【拉】顿服剂 | ~ niger 黑色顿服剂(复方番泻叶浸剂)

haut-mal [əuˈmɑːl] *n*【法】癫痫大发作

Hautmann neobladder [ˈhɔːtmɑːn] (Richard E. Hautmann) 霍特曼新膀胱(从 W 形切开回肠构成的一型原位回肠新膀胱)

HAV hepatitis A virus 甲型肝炎病毒

Haverhill fever [ˈheivəril] 哈弗里尔热(流行性关节炎性红斑,1925 年发生在美国哈弗里尔的一种鼠咬热)

Haverhillia multiformis [ˌheivəˈriliə] 多形哈弗里尔菌(现称念珠状链杆菌)

haversian canal (space) [həˈvəːʃən] (Clopton Havers) 哈弗管(腔),中央管 | ~ glands 哈弗腺,滑膜绒毛 / ~ lamella 哈弗骨板,骨单位骨板(围绕哈弗管的同心性骨板) / ~ system 哈弗系统骨单位(哈弗管及其同心排列的骨板构成密质骨结构的基本单位)

haw [hɔː] *n* 瞬膜;瞬膜综合征(即 haw syndrome,见 syndrome 项下相应术语)

hawk [hɔːk] *vi* 清嗓;咳嗽 *vt* 咳出,咯(痰)

hawkinsin [ˈhɔːkinsin] *n* 霍金素(霍金素尿中排出的一种环氨基酸代谢物,为一种罕见型酪氨酸血症。它由 4-羟苯丙酮酸双加氧酶反应的中间产物,与谷胱甘肽结合形成)

hawkinsinuria [ˌhɔːkinsiˈnjuəriə] *n* 霍金素尿(一种罕见的常染色体显性遗传型酪氨酸血症,伴有 4-羟苯丙酮酸双加氧酶缺陷,表现为尿内排出霍金素)

Hawley retainer (appliance) [ˈhɔːli] (C. A. Hawley) 霍利保持器(矫治器)(一种正牙矫治器)

hawthorn [ˈhɔːθɔːn] *n* 山楂;山楂制剂

hay [hei] *n* 干草,枯草

Hayem's corpuscles [ɑːˈjɑːn] (Georges Hayem) 血小板 | ~ encephalitis 增生性脑炎 / ~ icterus (jaundice) 溶血性贫血 / ~ solution 阿扬溶液(以血细胞计数器镜检红细胞前稀释血液用的一种溶液,含有二氯化汞、氯化钠、硫酸钠和水)

Hayem-Widal syndrome [ɑːjɑːn viˈdɑːl] (Georges Hayem; Georges F. I. Widal) 溶血性贫血

Hayflick's limit [ˈheiflik] (Leonard Hayflick) 海弗利克极限(细胞在死亡前能进行分裂的最大数,大部分人类细胞为 50~60 之间,有些恶性细胞系逃过此极限,成为永生)

Haygarth's nodes (nodosities) [ˈheigɑːθ] (John Haygarth) 海加思结(畸形性关节炎时的关节肿胀)

Hay's test [hei] (Matthew Hay) 海氏试验(检尿内胆汁盐)

Hay-Wells syndrome [hei welz] (R. J. Hay; Robert S. Wells) 海-威综合征(一种常染色体显性遗传综合征,表现为外胚层发育不良、唇腭裂及丝状睑缘粘连,同样表现为牙发育不全、掌跖角皮病、部分无汗症、发稀疏坚硬及耳缺损。亦称 AEC 综合征,睑缘粘连-外胚层发育不良-唇腭裂综合征)

Hazen's theorem [ˈheizn] (Allen Hazen) 黑曾定理(净化公共给水免除每一个伤寒病例的死亡,则可避免其他原因所造成的 2 种或 3 种病例的死亡)

HB hepatitis B 乙型肝炎

Hb hemoglobin 血红蛋白

HBc hepatitis B core (antigen) 乙型肝炎核心(抗原)

HBcAg hepatitis B core antigen 乙型肝炎核心抗原

HbCV *Haemophilus* b conjugate vaccine 嗜血杆菌 b 型结合疫苗

HBE His bundle electrogram 希氏束电图

HBe hepatitis B e(antigen) 乙型肝炎 e(抗原)

HBeAg hepatitis B e antigen 乙型肝炎 e 抗原

HbO_2 oxyhemoglobin 氧合血红蛋白

HbPV *Haemophilus* b polysaccharide vaccine 嗜血杆菌 b 型多糖疫苗

HBs hepatitis B surface (antigen) 乙型肝炎表面

(抗原)
HBsAg hepatitis B surface antigen 乙型肝炎表面抗原
HBV hepatitis B virus 乙型肝炎病毒
HC hospital corps 医务队
HCFA Health Care Financing Administration 卫生保健财政管理局(属美国卫生和人类服务部)
HCG, hCG human chorionic gonadotropin 人绒毛膜促性腺素
HCM hypertrophic cardiomyopathy 肥厚型心肌病
HCP hereditary coproporphyria 遗传性粪卟啉症
Hct hematocrit 血细胞比容
HCV hepatits C virus 丙型肝炎病毒
HD hemodialysis 血液透析
H. d. hora decubitus【拉】就寝时
HDCV human diploid cell(rabies) vaccine 人二倍体细胞(狂犬病)疫苗
HDL high-density lipoprotein 高密度脂蛋白
HDL_1 Lp(a) lipoprotein Lp(a) 脂蛋白,高密度脂蛋白1
HDL_2 高密度脂蛋白2
HDL_3 高密度脂蛋白3
HDL-C high-density-lipoprotein cholesterol 高密度脂蛋白胆固醇
HDN hemolytic disease of the newborn 新生儿溶血病
HDP oxidronate(hydroxymethylene diphosphonate) 奥昔膦酸(羟基甲烯二膦酸)
HDV hepatitis D virus 丁型肝炎病毒
H & E hematoxylin and eosin(stain) 苏木精和伊红(染剂)
He helium 氦
he- 以 he-起始的词,同样见以 hae-起始的词
head [hed] *n* 头;头部;(精子)头 | ~ of blind colon 盲肠 / ~ of condyloid process of mandible 下颌小头 / drum ~ 鼓膜 / floating ~ 胎头浮 / hot cross bun ~ 臀形头 / hourglass ~ 葫芦头,沙漏头 / loaf ~ 尖头[畸形] / ~ of mandible 下颌头;下颌骨髁状突 / medusa ~ 脐周静脉曲张,水母头(见于新生儿及肝硬化病人) / nerve ~ 视神经乳头 / saddle ~ 马鞍形头 / scald ~ 头癣,头皮癣 / steeple ~ ,tower ~ 尖头[畸形] / white ~ 头皮白痂病(黄癣)
headache [ˈhedeik] *n* 头痛 | bilious ~, blind ~, migraine ~, sick ~ 偏头痛 / congestive ~, hyperemic ~ 充血性头痛 / dynamite ~ 炸药性头痛(见于高爆炸药的人员) / helmet ~ 盔形头痛,上半部头痛 / miners' ~ 矿工头痛(硝酸甘油爆炸产生气体所致) / organic ~ 器质性头痛 / puncture ~, lumbar puncture ~, postspinal ~ 腰椎穿刺后头痛 / reflex ~, symptomatic ~ 反射性头痛,症状性头痛 / vaccum ~ 真空性头痛(额窦口阻塞所致)
headband [ˈhedbænd] *n* 束发带;额镜带
headgear [ˈhedgiə], **headcap** [ˈhedkæp] *n* 头帽(用作正牙矫治器口外抗基的阻抗)
headgrit [ˈhedgrit] *n* 羊霍乱
headgut [ˈhedgʌt] *n* 前肠
headrest [ˈhedrest] *n* (牙科诊所等)头靠,头托
Head's zones [hed] (Henry Head) 黑德区(与内脏病有关的皮肤感觉过敏区)
Heaf test [hiːf] (Frederick R. G. Heaf) 希夫试验,艉针结核菌素试验(Sterneedle tuberculin test,见 test 项下相应术语)
heal [hiːl] *vt* 治愈 *vi* (伤口)愈合;痊愈
healing [ˈhiːliŋ] *n* 治疗;愈合 | ~ by first intention 第一期愈合 / ~ by second intention, ~ by granulation 第二期愈合,肉芽性愈合 / mental ~ 心理治疗,精神治疗
health [helθ] *n* 健康 | holistic ~ 整体性保健,全面保健 / mental ~ 精神卫生 / public ~ 公共卫生
health maintenance organization(HMO) 保健组织(一种为自愿参加者在一定地区内提供综合性保健的组织,参加者需预先付款)
healthy [ˈhelθi] *a* 健康的;有益于健康的
hearing [ˈhiəriŋ] *n* 听,听觉,听力 | color ~ 色听,闻声觉色 / double disharmonic ~ 复听 / monaural ~ 单耳听觉 / visual ~ 唇读,视听
hearing loss [hiəriŋˈlɔs] 听力损失,聋 | conductive ~ ~, transmission ~ ~ 传导性聋 / pagetoid ~ ~ 变形性骨炎性聋 / paradoxic ~ ~ 听觉倒错性聋 / sensorineural ~ ~ 感音神经性聋
heart [hɑːt] *n* 心[脏] | abdominal ~ 腹位心 / armored ~, armour ~ 装甲心(心包石灰质沉着) / athletic ~ 运动员心脏(无瓣膜疾病的心脏肥大) / beer ~ 啤酒心(饮啤酒过度引起心脏扩大和肥大) / beriberi ~ 脚气[病]心(缺乏维生素 B_1 所致) / boat-shaped ~ 舟状心(左心室扩张和肥大引起主动脉瓣反流) / bony ~ 骨样心(心或心包有钙化斑点) / bovine ~ 巨心,牛心症 / cervical ~ 颈位心 / chaotic ~ 乱搏心(显示频繁过早收缩) / encased ~ 禁闭心(伴有慢性缩窄性心包炎) / fibroid ~ 纤维心,心纤维变性 / flask-shaped ~ 瓶状心(心包炎伴渗出液时X线所显示) / frosted ~, icing ~ 结霜样心,糖衣心(心包增厚时使心脏外形封冻如饼状) / hairy ~ 绒毛心 / hanging ~ 下垂心 / hypoplastic ~ 发育不全心 / intracorporeal ~ 体内人工心脏 / irritable ~ 易激心,神经性循环衰弱 / left ~, systemic ~ 左心 / lymph ~ 淋巴心(青蛙及鱼类) / myxedema ~ 黏液性水肿心 / paracorporeal ~ 体侧人工心脏 / pear-shaped ~ 梨状心(主动脉瓣及二尖瓣病变时X线所显示) / pectoral ~ 胸前位心 / right ~, pulmonary ~ 右心 / round ~ 圆形心(二尖瓣狭窄及反流时X

线所显示）/ sabot ~, wooden-shoe ~ 木鞋状心 / soldier's ~ 神经性循环衰弱 / tabby cat ~, thrush breast ~, tiger ~, tiger lily ~ 斑纹心（心室壁内表面及乳突状肌上有斑纹，见于严重的脂肪变性）/ three-chambered ~, trilocular ~ 三腔心（一室两房或一房两室）/ tobacco ~ 烟草毒性心 / triatrial ~ 三房心（先天性畸形左心房为横膈分成上下两部分，故为三房）/ wandering ~ 游动心

heartbeat [ˈhɑːtbiːt] *n* 心搏，心跳

heart block [ˈhɑːtblɔk] 心传导阻滞 | atrioventricular ~ ~ 房室传导阻滞 / bundle-branch ~ ~, interventricular ~ ~ 束支传导阻滞，室间传导阻滞 / complete ~ ~ 完全性房室传导阻滞 / sinoatrial ~ ~, sinoauricular ~ ~ 窦房传导阻滞

heartburn [ˈhɑːtbəːn] *n* 胃灼热

heart failure [ˈhɑːt ˈfeiljə] 心力衰竭 | acute congestive ~ ~ 急性充血性心力衰竭 / backward ~ ~ 后向性心力衰竭 / congestive ~ ~ 充血性心力衰竭 / forward ~ ~ 前向性心力衰竭 / left-sided ~ ~, left ventricular ~ ~ 左心室衰竭 / ritgh-sided ~ ~, right ventricular ~ ~ 右心室衰竭

heartthrob [ˈhɑːtθrɔb] *n* 心跳

heartwater [ˈhɑːtwɔːtə] *n* 牛羊水胸病，牛羊水心胸病

heartworm [ˈhɑːtwəːm] *n* 犬恶丝虫

heat [ˈhiːt] *n* 热；发情，性欲发动（雌动物）| atomic ~ 原子热 / conductive ~ 传导热 / convective ~ 对流热 / initial ~ 初热（肌收缩开始时肌内产生之热）/ latent ~ 潜热（被身体吸收，故不觉比前温暖，可能被身体吸收而体温不变的一种热）/ prickly ~ 粟疹，痱子，汗疹 / recovery ~, delayed ~ 恢复热，延迟热（肌肉收缩开始变短时，肌收缩所生之热）/ sensible ~ 显热（被身体吸收后使体温上升的一种热）/ specific ~ 比热 | **~er** *n* 发热器，加热器

Heath's operation [hiːθ] (Christopher Heath) 希思手术（切断下颌骨的升支，治关节强硬）

heating [ˈhiːtiŋ] *n* 加热；供热；暖气［装置］

Heaton's operation [ˈhiːtn] (George Heaton) 希顿手术（腹股沟疝手术）

heatstroke [ˈhiːtˌstrəuk] *n* 中暑

heave [hiːv] *vi* 喘息；呕吐 *n*［复］马气喘病

Hebdom hebdomada【拉】一周，一星期

hebdomad [ˈhebdəmæd] *n* 7 天，一周 | **~al** [hebˈdɔmədl] *a* 一周的；出生后第一周的

Hebeloma [ˌhebəˈləumə] *n* 丝膜蕈属

hebeosteotomy [ˌhebiˌɔstiˈɔtəmi], **hebetomy** [hiˈbetəmi] *n* 耻骨切开术

hebephrenia [ˌhebiˈfriːniə] *n* 青春型精神分裂症 | grafted ~ 嫁接性青春型精神分裂症 | **hebephrenic** [ˈhebifrenik], **hebephreniac** [ˌhebiˈfriːniæk] *a* 青春型精神分裂症的 *n* 青春型精神分裂症患者

Heberden's asthma [ˈhiːbədən] (William Heberden) 心绞痛 | ~ disease 赫伯登病（①小关节风湿病，伴远侧指节间关节内或附近结节；②心绞痛）/ ~ nodes (signs) 赫伯登结节（征）（通常在远侧指节间关节处形成小而硬的结节，因关节软骨刺钙化而成，伴有指节间骨关节炎，遗传为重要病因）/ ~ rheumatism 赫伯登风湿病（指关节风湿病，表现为结节形成）

hebetic [hiˈbetik] *a* 青春期的

hebetude [ˈhebitjuːd] *n* 迟钝，精神迟钝

hebiatrics [ˌhiːbiˈætriks] *n* 青年医学，青年期医学

heboid [ˈhebɔid] *n* 单纯型精神分裂症

heboidophrenia [ˌhebɔidəuˈfriːniə] *n* 单纯型早发痴呆

hebosteotomy [hiˌbɔstiˈɔtəmi], **hebotomy** [hiˈbɔtəmi] *n* 耻骨切开术

Hebra's disease [ˈhiːbrə] (Ferdinand von Hebra) 轻症多形红斑 | ~ prurigo 轻型痒疹

hecatomeric [ˌhekətəˈmerik], **hecatomeral** [ˌhekəˈtɔmərəl] *a* 两分的（指某些神经元）

Hecht's phenomenon [hekt] (Adolf F. Hecht) 黑希特现象（见 Rumpel-Leede phenomenon）

Hecht's test [hekt] (Hugo Hecht) 黑希特试验（检梅毒）

Hecht syndrome, Hecht-Beals syndrome, Hecht-Beals-Wilson syndrome [hekt biːlz ˈwilsən] (F. Hecht; Rodney K. Beals; Ralph V. Wilson) 黑希特综合征，黑-比综合征，黑-比-威综合征（牙关紧闭-假性屈曲指综合征）

Heckathorn's disease [ˈhekəθəun] (Heckathorn 为 20 世纪 70 年代首次观察到的先证者的姓) 赫卡索恩病（一种罕见的血友病 A 变异体，此病的凝血因子Ⅷ水平变动不定，作为 X 连锁隐性性状遗传）

hectic [ˈhektik] *a* 消耗性的，痨病的，潮热的

hect(o)- [构词成分] 百（10^2，符号为 h）

hectogram(me) [ˈhektəugræm] *n* 百克，100g（重量单位）

hectolitre, hectoliter [ˈhektəuˌliːtə] *n* 百升，100 l（容量单位）

hectometre hectometer [ˈhektəuˌmiːtə] *n* 百米，100 m（长度单位）

HED Haut-Einheits-Dosis【德】皮肤单位剂量（Seitz 和 Wintz 制定的 X 线剂量单位）

Hedera [ˈhedərə] *n* 常春藤属

hedonia [hiːˈdəuniə] *n* 异常欢乐

hedonic [hiːˈdɔnik] *a* 异常欢乐的，快感的

hedonics [hiːˈdɔniks] *n* 快感学

hedonism [ˈhiːdənizəm] *n* 享乐主义,求乐论 | **hedonist** [ˈhiːdənist] *n* 享乐主义者

hedratresia [ˌhedrəˈtriːsiə] *n* 肛门闭锁,锁肛

heel [hiːl] *n* 足跟;马蹄后部 | anterior ~ 跖骨垫 / big ~ 巨跟[症] / painful ~ 足跟痛 / prominent ~ 足跟隆突

Heerfordt's syndrome(disease) [ˈhɛəfɔːt] (Christian F. Heerfordt) 黑福特综合征(病)(一种偶见的肉样瘤病,包括腮腺和泪腺增大、前色素层炎、贝尔〈Bell〉麻痹和发热。亦称眼色素层腮腺炎)

hefilcon [həˈfilkɔn] *n* 何费尔康(两种亲水性接触镜材料之一,定名为 A 或 B)

Hefke-Turner sign [ˈhefki ˈtəːnə] (Hans W. Hefke; Vernon C. Turner) 海-特征(X 线片上正常闭孔阴影的轮廓增宽变形,提示髋关节病变。亦称闭孔征)

Hegar's dilators [ˈheigɑː] (Alfred Hegar) 黑加扩张器(以粗细不同的各种探条,扩张宫颈口) | ~ sign 黑加征(子宫下段变软,为妊娠指征)

hEGF human epidermal growth factor 人表皮生长因子

Hegglin's anomaly [ˈheglin] (Robert M. Hegglin) 赫格林异常(见 May-Hegglin anomaly)

Heidenhain's cells [ˈhaidənhain] (Rudolf P. Heidenhain) 海登海因细胞(胃腺的主细胞和壁细胞) | ~ iron hematoxylin stain 海登海因铁苏木精染剂(显示大部分细胞结构如细胞核、染色体、中心粒、纤维线粒体、纤毛等的一种重要的细胞染色法) / ~ law 海登海因定律(腺体分泌总是包含腺体结构的改变) / ~ rods 海登海因杆(肾小管杆状细胞)

Heidenhain's syndrome [ˈhaidənhain] (Adolf Heidenhain) 海登海因综合征(一种进展迅速的变性疾病,表现为皮质性失明、早老性痴呆、构音障碍、共济失调、手足徐动症样运动及全身僵直)

height [hait] *n* 高度 | apex ~ 最大收缩高 / ~ of contour 外形高点 / cusp ~ 牙尖高度 / sitting vertex ~, sitting ~ 顶臀长 / standing ~ 顶踵长

Heilbronner's thigh (sign) [ˈhailbrɔnə] (Karl Heilbronner) 海尔布伦内股(征)(患者在硬褥上仰卧时,如为器质性麻痹,股宽大而扁平,如系癔症性麻痹则无此征)

Heim-Kreysig sign [haim ˈkraizig] (Ernst L. Heim; Friedrich L. Kreysig) 海-克征(粘连性心包炎时,肋间隙与心收缩期呈现陷凹)

Heimlich maneuver [ˈhaimlik] (Henry J. Heimlich) 海姆利希手法(从梗死患者喉中取出食物或其他异物的一种操作法)

Heineke-Mikulicz pyloroplasty (operation) [ˈhainəkə ˈmikjulitʃ] (Walter H. Heineke; Johann von Mikulicz-Radecki) 海-米幽门成形术(手术)(纵向切开幽门,横向缝合切口,以重建幽门管)

Heine-Medin disease [ˈhainə ˈmeidin] (Jacob von Heine; Karl O. Medin) 海-梅病(脊髓灰质炎的主型,侵及中枢神经系统,可能有瘫痪)

Heine's operation [ˈhainə] (Leopold Heine) 海因手术(青光眼睫状体分离术)

Heinig's projection [ˈhainig] (C. F. Heinig) 海尼克投照(一种放射投照,用于锁骨和胸锁关节造影)

Heinz bodies (granules), Heinz-Ehrlich bodies [haints ˈɛəliʃ] (Robert Heinz; Paul Ehrlich) 海因茨体(粒)、海-埃小体(球菌状包涵体,由血红蛋白受氧化破坏并沉淀后形成,见于某些异常的血红蛋白及缺酶的红细胞内,在新鲜血涂片中有折射性,用超活体染色法可显出此球体)

Heisrath's operation [ˈhaisrəθ] (Friedrich Heisrath) 海斯拉思手术(切除睑板皱襞以治沙眼)

Heister's diverticulum [ˈhaistə] (Lorenz Heister) 颈静脉上球 | ~ fold, ~ valve 螺旋襞

HEK human embryo kidney 人胚肾(细胞培养)

Hektoen phenomenon [ˈhektəun] (Ludvig Hektoen) 赫克顿现象(将几种抗原注入具有变应性状态的动物体内,新抗体产生的范围扩大,而且包括产生以前感染过的和免疫过的对应抗体)

HEL human embryo lung 人胚肺(细胞培养)

HeLa cells [ˈhiːlə] 海拉细胞,人宫颈癌传代细胞(首次连续培养的癌细胞株,HeLa 由一患者姓名字首组成,1951 年从其所患的宫颈癌中分离得到,用以研究细胞阶段的生活过程,包括病毒的研究)

Helbing's sign [ˈhelbiŋ] (Carl E. Helbing) 墨尔宾征(由后面看时,跟腱向内侧弯曲,见于扁平足)

helcoid [ˈhelkɔid] *a* 溃疡状的

helcology [helˈkɔlədʒi] *n* 溃疡学

helcoma [helˈkəumə] *n*【希】角膜溃疡

helcosis [helˈkəusis] *n* 溃疡形成

Helcosoma tropicum [ˌhelkəˈsəumə ˈtrɔpikəm] 热带利什曼[原]虫

Held's end bulb [held] (Hans Held) 黑尔德终球(蜗神经一级神经元轴突末端扩大了的突起,与蜗腹侧核二级神经元体形成突触)

Heleidae [həˈliːidiː] *n* 蠓科

helenine [ˈheliniːn] *n* 海仑菌素(一种抗病毒物质)

Helenium [həˈliːniəm] *n* 堆心菊属

helianthin [hiːliˈænθin] *n* 甲基橙,半日花素

heliation [ˌhiːliˈeiʃən] *n* 日光疗法

helical [ˈhelikəl] *a* 螺旋[线]的,螺旋形的

Helicella [ˌhiːliˈselə] *n* 厚壳大蜗牛属

Helicellidae [ˌhiːliˈselidiː] *n* 厚壳大蜗牛科
Helicidae [hiːˈlisidiː] *n* 大蜗牛科
helicin [ˈhelisin] *n* 水杨醛葡萄糖苷
helicine [ˈhelisiːn] *a* 螺旋状的;耳轮的
helic(o)- [构词成分]螺旋,蜗,圈
Helicobactor [ˌhelikəuˈbæktə] *n* 螺旋菌属 | ~ cinaedi 淫乱螺旋菌 / ~ pylori 幽门螺旋菌
helicoid [ˈhelikɔid] *a* 螺旋形的;耳轮状的 *n* 螺旋面,螺旋体
helicopepsin [ˌhelikəuˈpepsin] *n* 螺蛋白酶
helicopod [ˈhelikəˌpɔd] *a* 螺旋形步态的,环形步态的
helicopodia [ˌhelikəuˈpəudiə] *n* 螺旋形步态,环形步态
helicoprotein [ˌhelikəuˈprəutiːn] *n* 螺糖蛋白
helicotrema [ˌhelikəuˈtriːmə] *n* 蜗孔
heliencephalitis [ˌhiːlienˌsefəˈlaitis] *n* 日射性脑炎
heli(o)- [构词成分]日光,日
helioaerotherapy [ˌhiːliəuˌɛərəuˈθerəpi] *n* 日光空气疗法
heliopathia [ˌhiːliəuˈpæθiə] *n* 日光病,日照病
heliosin [ˌhiːliˈəusin] *n* 泽漆新苷(含有角蛋白和多种无机盐类的制剂)
heliosis [ˌhiːliˈəusis] *n* 日射病,中暑
heliotaxis [ˌhiːliəuˈtæksis] *n* 趋日性,趋光性
heliotherapy [ˌhiːliəuˈθerəpi] *n* 日光疗法
Heliotiales [ˌhiːliəuʃiˈeiliːz] *n* 趋光菌目
heliotrope B [ˈhiːliəˌtrəup] 水晶紫(四乙蓝光碱性酚藏花红染色液)
heliotropism [ˌhiːliˈɔtrəpizəm] *n* 向日性
heliox [ˈhiːliɔks] *n* 氦氧混合气(低密度氦氧混合物,减少气道内气流动阻力,用于治疗哮喘、支气管炎和以气道阻力增加为特征的其他疾病)
Heliozoa [ˌhiːliəˈzəuə] *n* 太阳虫纲
heliozoa [ˌhiːliəˈzəuə] *n* 太阳虫
heliozoan [hiːliəˈzəuən] *n*, *a* 太阳虫(的) | **heliozoic** [ˌhiːliəˈzəuik] *a*
helisterine [hiˈlistərin] *n* 蜗牛甾醇
helium(He) [ˈhiːljəm] *n* 氦(化学元素)
Helix [ˈhiːliks] *n* 大蜗牛属
helix [ˈhiːliks] ([复]**helices** [ˈhelisiːz, ˈhiːlisiːz] 或 **helixes**) *n* 螺旋构型,螺旋线;耳轮;蜗牛 | α-helix, alpha ~ α-螺旋 / double ~ 双螺旋
Hellat's sign [ˈhelæt] (Piotr Hellat) 希拉特征(乳突化脓时音叉试验患区骨导较其他部位为短)
hellebore [ˈhelibɔː] *n* 嚏根草;藜芦 | American ~, green ~ 绿藜芦 / black ~ 黑嚏根草 / white ~ 白藜芦
Helleborus [ˌheləˈbəurəs] *n* 嚏根草属
Hellendall's sign [ˈheləndɑːl] (Hugo Hellendall) 黑伦达尔征(见 Cullen's sign)
Heller-Döhle disease [ˈhelə ˈdiːlə] (Arnoid L. G. Heller; Karl G. P. Döhle) 梅毒性主动脉炎
Heller's esophagomyotomy (myotomy, operation) [ˈhelə] (Ernst Heller) 黑勒食管肌切开术(肌切开术、手术),食管贲门肌切开术
Heller's plexus [ˈhelə] (Arnold L. G. Heller) 黑勒丛(肠黏膜下的动脉丛)
Heller's test [ˈhelə] (Johann F. Heller) 海勒试验(检尿白蛋白、尿血、尿葡萄糖)
Hellerwork [ˈheləwək] (Joseph Heller) *n* 海勒健身法(从 Rolfing 法派生的一种健身法,即用深按摩、运动再教育和对话以改进体形排列、建立轻松运动型,促进身心关系的意识;用于缓解肌骨骼疼痛、改进姿势以及增强健康)
Hellin's law [ˈhelin] (Dyonizy Hellin) 海林定律(用以计算多胎妊娠的发生率,每 89 例妊娠中有一例为双胞胎,每 89 × 89 或 7 921 例妊娠中有一例为三胞胎,每 89 × 89 × 89 或 704 969 例中有一例为四胞胎)
Helmholtz's ligament [ˈhelmhɔlts] (Hermann L. F. von Helmholtz) 赫尔姆霍茨韧带(附着于鼓大棘的锤骨前韧带部分) | ~ theory 赫尔姆霍茨学说(听觉学说:每一基底纤维对特定音调作出共振性反应,并刺激位于该纤维的科尔蒂〈Corti〉器的毛细胞,刺激毛细胞而形成的神经冲动,则传至大脑)
helminth [ˈhelminθ] *n* 蠕虫,肠虫
helminthagogue [helˈminθəgɔg] *n* 驱肠虫药
helminthemesis [ˌhelminˈθemisis] *n* 吐虫
helminthiasis [ˌhelminˈθaiəsis] *n* 蠕虫病 | ~ elastica 蠕虫性弹性瘤
helminthic [helˈminθik] *a* 蠕虫的
helminthicide [helˈminθisaid] *n* 杀蠕虫药
helminthism [ˈhelminθizəm] *n* 蠕虫寄生
helminthoid [helˈminθɔid] *a* 蠕虫样的
helminthology [ˌhelminˈθɔlədʒi] *n* 蠕虫学
helminthoma [ˌhelminˈθəumə] *n* 蠕虫瘤
helminthous [helˈminθəs] *a* 蠕虫的
hel(o)- [构词成分] 甲,爪,钉;疣;胼胝
Heloderma [ˌhiːləˈdəːmə] *n* 毒蜥属
heloma [hiˈləumə] *n* 鸡眼,钉胼 | ~ durum 硬鸡眼 / ~ molle 软鸡眼
Helophilus [hiˈlɔfiləs] *n* 棘蝇属
helosis [hiˈləusis] *n* 鸡眼
Helotiales [ˌhiːləuʃiːˈeiliːz] *n* 柔膜菌目
helotomy [hiˈlɔtəmi] *n* 鸡眼切除,钉胼切除
Helvella [helˈvelə] *n* 马鞍菌属
Helvellaceae [ˌhelveˈleisiiː] *n* 马鞍菌科
helvellic acid [helˈvelik] 马鞍菌酸
helvolic acid [helˈvɔlik] 烟曲霉酸
Helweg-Larsen's syndrome [ˈhelveg ˈlɑːsən]

(Hans F. Helweg-Larsen) 黑尔维格·拉森综合征(一种常染色体显性遗传综合征,包括生下后就有无汗症及长大后患迷路炎)
Helweg's bundle(tract) [ˈhelveg] (Hans K. S. Helweg) 橄榄脊髓束
hema [ˈhiːmə] *n* 血液
hema- 见 hem(o)-
hemabarometer [ˌheməbəˈrɔmitə] *n* 血比重计
hemachromatosis [ˌhiːməˌkrəuməˈtəusis] *n* 血色病,血色素沉着[症]
hemachrome [ˈhiːməkrəum] *n* 血色素
hemachrosis [ˌheməˈkrəusis] *n* 血色过浓
hemacyanin [ˌheməˈsaiənin] *n* 血青蛋白,血蓝蛋白
hemacyte [ˈhiːməsait] *n* 血细胞
hemacytometer [ˌhiːməsaiˈtɔmitə] *n* 血细胞计数器 | **hemacytometry** *n* 血细胞计数法
hemacytopoiesis [ˌheməˌsaitəpɔiˈiːsis] *n* 血细胞生成
hemaden [ˈhemədən] *n* 内分泌腺
hemadenology [ˌhemədiˈnɔlədʒi] *n* 内分泌学
hemadostenosis [ˌhemədəustiˈnəusis, ˌhiːm-] *n* 血管狭窄
hemadsorbent [ˌhiːmædˈzɔːbənt] *a* 血细胞吸附的
hemadsorption [ˌhiːmædˈzɔːpʃən] *n* 血细胞吸附(红细胞吸附在其他细胞表面)
hemadynamometry [ˌhiːməˌdainəˈmɔmitri] *n* 血压测量法
hemafacient [ˌheməˈfeiʃənt] *a* 血细胞生成的,生血[细胞]的
hemafecia [ˌheməˈfiːsiə] *n* 便血
hemagglutinate [ˌhiːməˈgluːtineit] *vt* 使血细胞凝集
hemagglutination [ˌhiːməgluːtiˈneiʃən] *n* 血凝反应,血细胞凝集 | indirect ~, passive ~ 间接血凝反应,被动血凝反应 / viral ~ 病毒血凝反应
hemagglutinative [ˌhiːməˈgluːtiˌneitiv] *a* 血凝的,血凝集的
hemagglutinin [ˌhiːməˈgluːtinin] *n* 血凝素 | cold ~ 冷血凝素(接近 4 ℃) / warm ~ 温血凝素(接近 37 ℃)
hemagogic [ˌheməˈgɔdʒik] *a* 通经的,催血的
hemagonium [ˌheməˈgəuniəm] *n* 成血细胞
hemal [ˈhiːməl] *a* 血的,血管的;脊柱腹侧的
hemalexin [ˌheməˈleksin] *n* 血防御素,血补体
hemalum [ˈhiːmələm] *n* 苏木精明矾,矾紫
hemanalysis [ˌhiːməˈnæləsis, ˌhem-] *n* 血液分析
hemangiectasia [ˌhiːmændʒiekˈteisiə], **hemangiectasis** [ˌhiːmændʒiˈektəsis] *n* 血管扩张
hemangi(o)- [构词成分] 血管
hemangioameloblastoma [hiːˌmændʒiəuəˌmeləublæsˈtəumə] *n* 血管性成釉细胞瘤
hemangioblast [hiːˈmændʒiəblæst] *n* 成血管细胞
hemangioblastoma [hiːˌmændʒiəublæsˈtəumə] *n* 成血管细胞瘤
hemangioblastomatosis [hiːˌmændʒiəuˌblæstəuməˈtəusis] *n* 成血管细胞瘤病
hemangioendothelioblastoma [hiːˌmændʒiəuˌendəuˌθiːliəublæsˈtəumə] *n* 成血管内皮细胞瘤
hemangioendothelioma [hiːˌmændʒiəuˌendəuˌθiːliˈəumə] *n* 血管内皮细胞瘤 | benign ~ 良性血管内皮细胞瘤 / malignant ~ 恶性血管内皮细胞瘤,血管肉瘤
hemangioendotheliosarcoma [hiːˌmændʒiəuˌendəuθiːliəusɑːˈkəumə] *n* 血管内皮细胞肉瘤,血管肉瘤
hemangiofibroma [hiːˌmændʒiəufaiˈbrəumə] *n* 血管纤维瘤
hemangioma [hiːˌmændʒiˈəumə] *n* 血管瘤 | ameloblastic ~ 血管性成釉细胞瘤 | capillary ~ 毛细血管瘤,焰色痣 / cavernous ~ 海绵状血管瘤 / strawberry ~, ~ simplex 草莓状血管瘤,单纯性血管瘤,血管痣(亦称草莓状痣)
hemangiomatosis [hiːˌmændʒiəuməˈtəusis] *n* 血管瘤病,多发性血管瘤
hemangiopericyte [hiːˌmændʒiəuˈperisait] *n* 血管外皮细胞,周皮细胞
hemangiopericytoma [hiːˌmændʒiəuˌperisaiˈtəumə] *n* 血管外皮细胞瘤
hemangiosarcoma [hiːˌmændʒiəusɑːˈkəumə] *n* 血管肉瘤
hemaphein [ˈhiːməfiːn] *n* 血褐质 | **hemapheic** [hiːməˈfiːik] *a*
hemapheism [ˌhiːməˈfiːizəm] *n* 血褐质尿症
hemapheresis [ˌhiːməfəˈriːsis] *n* 血液成分单采,血液去除术
hemaphotograph [ˌhiːməˈfəutəgrɑːf, -græf] *n* 血细胞照片
hemapoiesis [ˌhiːməpɔiˈiːsis] *n* 血细胞生成,血生成 | **hemapoietic** [ˌhiːməpɔiˈetik] *a* 生血细胞的,生血的
hemapophysis [ˌhiːməˈpɔfisis] *n* 脉管弓突起
hemarthrosis [ˌhiːmɑːˈθrəusis], **hemarthros** [hiːˈmɑːθrɔs] *n* 关节积血
hemartoma [ˌhiːmɑːˈtəumə] *n* 血管瘤
hemasthenosis [ˌhemæsθiˈnəusis] *n* 血液不良
hemastrontium [ˌhiːmæsˈtrɔnʃiəm] *n* 苏木精锶染剂
hemat- 见 hemo-
hematal [ˈhemətl, ˈhiːm-] *a* 血的;血管的
hematalloscopy [ˌhemætəˈlɔskəpi] *n* 血类辨别法
hematapostema [ˌhiːmætəpɔsˈtiːmə] *n* 血脓肿
hemate [ˈhemeit] *n* 氧化苏木精化合物

hemateikon [ˌheməˈtaikɔn] *n* 血象
hematein [ˈhiːmətiːn] *n* 氧化苏木精
hematemesis [ˌhiːməˈtemisis, ˌhem-] *n* 呕血
hematencephalon [ˌhemætenˈsefəlɔn, ˌhiːm-] *n* 脑出血
hematherapy [ˌhiːməˈθerəpi, ˌhem-] *n* 血液疗法
hemathermal [ˌhiːməˈθəːməl, ˌhem-] **hemathermous** [ˌhiːməˈθəːməs, ˌhem-] *a* 温血的
hemathorax [ˌheməˈθɔːræks, ˌhiːm-] *n* 血胸，胸腔积血
hematic [hiːˈmætik] *a* 血的 *n* 补血药
hematidrosis [ˌhiːmætiˈdrəusis, ˌhem-] *n* 血汗[症]
hematimeter [ˌheməˈtimitə, ˌhiːm-] *n* 血细胞计数器 | **hematimetry** *n* 血细胞计数法
hematin [ˈhemətin, ˈhiːm-] *n* 高铁血红素，正铁血红素；羟高铁血红素
hematinemia [ˌhemətiˈniːmiə, ˌhiːm-] *n* 高铁血红素血症，正铁血红素血症
hematinic [ˌheməˈtinik, ˈhiːm-] *a* 高铁血红素的，正铁血红素的 *n* 补血药
hematinogen [ˌheməˈtinədʒən] *n* 高铁血红素原，正铁血红素原
hematinometer [ˌhemətiˈnɔmitə, ˌhiːm] *n* 血红蛋白计
hematinuria [ˌhiːmətiˈnjuəriə] *n* 高铁血红素尿，正铁血红素尿
hematite [ˈhiːmətait] *n* 赤铁矿
hemat(o)-, haemat(o)- [构词成分]血
hematobilia [ˌhemətəuˈbiliə, ˌhiːm-] *n* 胆道出血
hematoblast [ˈhemətəublæst, ˌhiːm-] *n* 成血细胞 | **~ic** [ˌhemətəuˈblæstik, ˌhiːm-] *a*
hematocatharsis [ˌhemətəukəˈθɑːsis] *n* 清血法
hematocele [ˈhemətəuˌsiːl, ˌhiːm-] *n* 血囊肿，积血，鞘膜积血 | parametric ~, pelvic ~, retrouterine ~ 宫旁血囊肿，盆腔积血 / pudendal ~ 外阴血囊肿 / scrotal ~ 阴囊积血 / vaginal ~ 阴道血囊肿
hematocelia [ˌhemətəuˈsiːliə, ˌhiːm-] *n* 腹腔积血
hematocephalus [ˌhemətəuˈsefələs, ˌhiːm-] *n* 胎头血肿
hematochezia [ˌhemətəuˈkiːziə, ˌhiːm-] *n* 便血
hematochlorin [ˌhemətəuˈklɔːrin, ˌhiːm-] *n* 胎盘绿色素
hematochromatosis [ˌhemətəuˌkrəuməˈtəusis, ˌhiːm-] *n* 血色素沉着[症]，血色病
hematochrome [ˌhemətəuˈkrəum, ˌhiːm-] *n* 血色素
hematochyluria [ˌhemətəukaiˈljuəriə, ˌhiːm-] *n* 血性乳糜尿
hematoclasis [ˌheməˈtɔkləsis, ˌhiːm-] *n* 溶血，血细胞溶解 | **hematoclastic** [ˌhemətəuˈklæstik, ˌhiːm-] *a*
hematocoelia [ˌhemətəuˈsiːliə, ˌhiːm-] *n* 腹腔积血
hematocolpometra [ˌhemətəuˌkɔlpəˈmiːtrə, ˌhiːm-] *n* 阴道子宫积血
hematocolpos [ˌhemətəuˈkɔlpɔs, ˌhiːm-] *n* 阴道积血
hematocrit (Hct) [hiːˈmætəkrit] *n* 血细胞比容；血细胞容量计
hematocryal [ˌheməˈtɔkriəl, ˌhiːmətəuˈkraiəl] *a* 冷血的
hematocrystallin [ˌhemətəuˈkristəlin, ˌhiːm-] *n* 血红蛋白
hematocyanin [ˌhemətəuˈsaiənin, ˌhiːm-] *n* 血蓝蛋白
hematocyst [ˈhiːmətəusist, hiːmæt-], **hematocystis** [ˌhemətəuˈsistis, ˌhiːm-] *n* 血囊肿；膀胱积血
hematocyte [ˈhemətəusait, ˈhiːm-] *n* 血细胞
hematocytoblast [ˌhemətəuˈsaitəblæst, ˌhiːm-] *n* 成血细胞
hematocytolysis [ˌhemətəusaiˈtɔlisis, ˌhiːm-] *n* 溶血，血细胞溶解
hematocytometer [ˌhemətəusaiˈtɔmitə, ˌhiːm-] *n* 血细胞计数器
hematocytopenia [ˌhemətəuˌsaitəuˈpiːniə, ˌhiːm-] *n* 血细胞减少
hematocytosis [ˌhemətəusaiˈtəusis, ˌhiːm-] *n* 血细胞增多
hematocyturia [ˌhemətəusaiˈtjuəriə, ˌhiːm-] *n* 血细胞尿
hematodialysis [ˌhemətəudaiˈælisis, ˌhiːm-] *n* 血液透析
hematodystrophy [ˌhemətəuˈdistrəfi, ˌhiːm-] *n* 血营养障碍
hematoencephalic [ˌhemətəuˌensiˈfælik, ˌhiːm-] *a* 血[与]脑的
hematogen [ˈhemətədʒən, ˈhiːm-] *n* 血生质，血母
hematogenesis [ˌhemətəuˈdʒenisis, ˌhiːm-] *n* 生血，血产生 | **hematogenic** [ˌhemətəuˈdʒenik, ˌhiːm-] *a* 生血的；血源性的
hematogenous [ˌheməˈtɔdʒinəs, ˌhiːm-] *a* 血源性的
hematoglobin [ˌhemətəuˈgləubin], **hematoglobulin** [ˌhemətəuˈglɔbjulin] *n* 血红蛋白
hematoglobinuria [ˌhemətəugləubiˈnjuəriə] *n* 血红蛋白尿
hematogone [ˈhiːmətəgəun, hiːˈmæt-] *n* 原始血细胞，成血细胞
hematohidrosis [ˌhemətəuhiˈdrəusis, ˌhiːm-] *n* 血汗症

hematohistioblast [ˌhemətəuˈhistiəblæst, ˌhiːm-] *n* 成血细胞
hematohiston [ˌhemətəuˈhistɔn] *n* 珠蛋白
hematohyaloid [ˌhemətəuˈhaiəlɔid, ˌhiːm-] *n* 血透明质
hematoid [ˈhiːmətɔid, ˈhem-] *a* 血样的
hematoidin [heməˈtɔidin] *n* 橙色血质
hematokolpos [ˌhemətəuˈkɔlpɔs, ˌhiːm-] *n* 阴道积血
hematokrit [hiːˈmætəkrit] *n* 血细胞比容;血细胞容量计
hematology [ˌhiːməˈtɔlədʒi, ˌheməˈtɔlədʒi] *n* 血液学 | **hematologic(al)** [ˌhiːmətəˈlɔdʒik(əl), ˌhem-] *a* | **hematologist** *n* 血液学家
hematolymphangioma [ˌhemətəuˌlimfændʒiˈəuma, ˌhiːm-] *n* 血管淋巴管瘤
hematolysis [ˌhiːməˈtɔlisis, ˌhem-] *n* 溶血[作用],血细胞溶解 | **hematolytic** [ˌhiːmətəuˈlitik, ˌhem-] *a*
hematoma [ˌhiːməˈtəumə, ˌhem-] ([复] **hematomas** 或 **hematomata** [ˌhiːməˈtəumətə, ˌhem-]) *n* 血肿 | aneurysmal ~ 动脉瘤样血肿,假动脉瘤 / ~ auris 耳血肿 / retrouterine ~ 子宫后血肿 / subdural ~ 硬脑膜下血肿
hematomancy [ˈhemətəmænsi] *n* 验血诊断法,验血预断
hematomanometer [ˌhemətəuməˈnɔmitə, ˌhiːm-] *n* 血压计
hematomediastinum [ˌhemətəuˌmiːdiæsˈtainəm, ˌhiːm-] *n* 纵隔积血
hematometakinesis [ˌhemətəuˌmetəkaiˈniːsis] *n* 血液调动现象,血清调剂现象
hematometer [ˌheməˈtɔmitə, ˌhiːm-] *n* 血红蛋白计
hematometra [ˌhemətəuˈmiːtrə, ˌhiːm-] *n* 子宫积血
hematometry [ˌheməˈtɔmitri, ˌhiːm-] *n* 血成分测定法
hematomole [hiːˈmætəməul] *n* 血肿性胎块
hematomphalocele [ˌhemætɔmˈfæləsiːl] *n* 血脐疝
hematomphalus [ˌhemæˈtɔmfələs] *n* 脐部积血,蓝脐
hematomyelia [ˌhemətəumaiˈiːliə, ˌhiːm-] *n* 脊髓出血
hematomyelitis [ˌhemətəuˌmaiəˈlaitis, ˌhiːm-] *n* 出血性脊髓炎
hematomyelopore [ˌhemətəuˈmaiələpɔː] *n* 出血性脊髓空洞[症]
hematoncometry [ˌhemətɔŋˈkɔmitri] *n* 血容积测量法
hematonephrosis [ˌhemətəuniˈfrəusis, ˌhiːm-] *n* 肾盂积血
hematonic [ˌheməˈtɔnik, ˌhiːm-] *n* 补血药
hematonosis [ˌheməˈtɔnəsis] *n* 血液病
hematopathology [ˌhemətəupəˈθɔlədʒi, ˌhiːm-] *n* 血液病理学
hematopedesis [ˌhemətəupiˈdiːsis] *n* 血液渗出(经皮肤)
hematopenia [ˌhemətəuˈpiːniə, ˌhiːm-] *n* 血液不足
hematopericardium [ˌhemətəuˌperiˈkɑːdiəm, ˌhiːm-] *n* 心包积血
hematoperitoneum [ˌhemətəuˌperitəuˈniːəm, ˌhiːm-] *n* 腹腔积血
hematopexin [ˌhemətəuˈpeksin] *n* 血液结合素,血凝酶(一种结合血红素的血清蛋白)
hematopexis [ˌhemətəuˈpeksis, ˌhiːm-] *n* 血凝固
hematophage [ˈhemətəfeidʒ, ˌhiːm-], **hematophagocyte** [ˌhemətəuˈfægəsait, ˌhiːm-] *n* 噬血细胞细胞
hematophagia [ˌhemətəuˈfeidʒiə, ˌhiːm-], **hematophagy** [ˌheməˈtɔfeidʒ, ˌhiːm-] *n* 吸血;血液寄生;噬细胞作用 | **hematophagous** [ˌheməˈtɔfəgəs, ˌhiːm-] *a*
hematophilia [ˌhemətəuˈfiliə, ˌhiːm-] *n* 血友病
hematophobia [ˌhemətəuˈfəubiə, ˌhiːm-] *n* 血恐怖;恐血症
hematopiesis [ˌhemətəuˈpaiəsis, ˌhiːm-] *n* 血压
hematoplasmopathy [ˌhemətəuplæzˈmɔpəθi, ˌhiːm-] *n* 血浆病
hematoplast [ˈhemətəuplæst, ˌhiːm-] *n* 成血细胞
hematoplastic [ˌhemətəuˈplæstik, ˌhiːm-] *a* 成血的
hematopoiesis [ˌhemətəupɔiˈiːsis, ˌhiːm-] *n* 血细胞生成,血细胞发生,血生成,造血 | extramedullary ~ 髓外造血 | **hematopoietic** [ˌhemətəupɔiˈetik, ˌhiːm-] *a* 生血的,造血的 *n* 补血药
hematopoietin [ˌhemətəupɔiˈetin, ˌhiːm-] *n* 红细胞生成素
hematoporphyria [ˌhemətəupɔːˈfairiə, ˌhiːm-] *n* 血卟啉病,血紫质病
hematoporphyrin [ˌhemətəuˈpɔːfirin, ˌhiːm-] *n* 血卟啉,血紫质
hematoporphyrinemia [ˌhemətəupɔːfiriˈniːmiə, ˌhiːm-] *n* 血卟啉血,血紫质血
hematoporphyrinism [ˌhemətəuˈpɔːfirinizəm, ˌhiːm-] *n* 血卟啉病,血紫质病
hematoporphyrinuria [ˌhemətəuˌpɔːfiriˈnjuəriə, ˌhiːm-] *n* 血卟啉尿
Hematopota [ˌheməˈtɔpətə, ˌhiːm-] *n* 麻[翅]虻属(即 Chrysozona)
hematorrhachis [heməˈtɔrəkis, ˌhiːm-] *n* 椎管内

出血
hematorrhea [ˌhemətəuˈriːə, ˌhiːm-] *n* 大出血
hematosalpinx [ˌhemətəuˈsælpinks, ˌhiːm-] *n* 输卵管积血
hematoscheocele [ˌheməˈtɔskiəsiːl, ˌhiːm-] *n* 阴囊积血
hematoscope [ˈhemətəuskəup, ˌhiːm-] 血分光镜 | **hematoscopy** [ˌheməˈtɔskəpi, ˌhiːm-] *n* 血分光镜检查
hematosepsis [ˌhemətəuˈsepsis, ˌhiːm-] *n* 败血病,败血症
hematoside [ˈhemətəsaid] *n* 血苷脂
hematosin [ˌheməˈtəusin, ˌhiːm-] *n* 高铁血红素,正铁血红素
hematospectrophotometer [ˌhemətəuˌspektrəu-fəˈtɔmitə, ˌhiːm-] *n* 血红蛋白分光光度计
hematospectroscope [ˌhemətəuˈspektrəskəup, ˌhiːm-] *n* 血分光镜 | **hematospectroscopy** [ˌhemətəuspekˈtrɔskəpi, ˌhiːm-] *n* 血分光镜检查
hematospermatocele [ˌhemətəuspəːˈmætəsiːl, ˌhiːm-] *n* 血性精液囊肿
hematospermia [ˌhemətəuˈspəːmiə, ˌhiːm-] *n* 血性精液
hematospherinemia [ˌhemətəuˌsfiəriˈniːmiə, ˌhiːm-] *n* 血红蛋白血[症]
hematosporidia [ˌhemətəuspəˈridiə, ˌhiːm-] *n* 血孢子虫
hematostatic [ˌhemətəuˈstætik, ˌhiːm-] *a* 淤血的
hematosteon [ˌheməˈtɔstiɔn, ˌhiːm-] *n* 骨髓腔积血
hematotherapy [ˌhemətəuˈθerəpi, ˌhiːm-] *n* 血液疗法
hematothermal [ˌhemətəuˈθəːməl, ˌhiːm-] *a* 温血的
hematothorax [ˌhemətəuˈθɔːræks, ˌhiːm-] *n* 血胸
hematotoxic [ˌhemətəuˈtɔksik, ˌhiːm-] **hematoxic** [ˌhiːməˈtɔksik] *a* 血中毒的;毒害血液的
hematotoxicosis [ˌhemətəuˌtɔksiˈkəusis, ˌhiːm-] *n* 血中毒
hematotrachelos [ˌhemətəutrəˈkiːlɔs, ˌhiːm-] *n* 宫颈积血
hematotropic [ˌhemətəuˈtrɔpik, ˌhiːm-] *a* 亲血的,亲血细胞的
hematotympanum [ˌhəmətəuˈtimpənəm, ˌhiːm-] *n* 血鼓室,鼓室积血
hematoxylin [ˌhəməˈtɔksilin, ˌhiːm-] *n* 苏木精 | alum ~ 苏木精明矾,矾紫 / iron ~ 铁苏木精染剂
Hematoxylon [ˌhiːməˈtɔksilɔn] *n* = **Haematoxylon**
hematozemia [ˌhemətəuˈziːmiə, ˌhiːm-] *n* 耗血,缓慢出血
hematozoan [ˌhemətəuˈzəun, ˌhiːm-] *a* 血原虫的 *n* 血原虫
hematozoon [ˌhemətəuˈzəuɔn, ˌhiːm-] ([复] **hematozoa** [ˌhemətəuˈzəuə, ˌhiːm-]) *n* 血原虫 | **hematozoic** [ˌhemətəuˈz-əuik, ˌhiːm-], **hematozoal** [ˌhiːmətəuˈzəuəl] *a*
hematozymosis [ˌhemətəuzaiˈməusis, ˌhiːm-] *n* 血发酵
hematuria [ˌheməˈtjuəriə, ˌhiːm-] *n* 血尿 | endemic ~ 地方性血尿,尿路血吸虫病 / essential ~ 特发性血尿 / renal ~ 肾性血尿 | **hematuresis** [ˌhemətjuəˈriːsis, ˌhiːm-] *n*
hemautograph [hiːˈmɔtəgrɑːf, -græf] *n* 动脉喷血描记图 | **~y** [ˌhemɔˈtɔgrəfi] *n* 动脉喷血描记法
heme [hiːm] *n* 血红素
hemendothelioma [ˌhiːmendəuˌθiːliˈəumə] *n* 血管内皮瘤
Hementaria [ˌhiːmənˈtɛəriə] *n* = **Haementaria**
heme oxygenase (decyclizing) [hiːmˈɔksidʒəneis diːˈsaiklaiziŋ] 血红素加氧酶(解环的)
hemeralope [ˈhemərələup] *n* 昼盲者
hemeralopia [ˌhemərəˈləupiə] *n* 昼盲 | **hemeralopic** [ˌhemərəˈlɔpik] *a*
Hemerocampa [ˌhemerəuˈkæmpə] *n* 杉毒蛾属 | ~ leukostigma 白斑天幕毒蛾
hemerythrin [ˌhiːməˈriθrin] *n* 蚯蚓血红蛋白
heme synthase [hiːmˈsinθeis] 血红素合酶,亚铁螯合酶
hemetaboly [ˌhiːmeˈtæbəli] *n* 血液新陈代谢
hemi- [前缀]半,偏侧,单侧
hemiablepsia [ˌhemiəˈblepsiə] *n* 偏盲
hemiacardius [ˌhemiəˈkɑːdiəs] *n* 半无心畸胎
hemiacephalus [ˌhemiəˈsefələs] *n* 半无脑畸胎,无脑畸胎
hemiacetal [ˌhemiˈæsitæl] *n* 半缩醛
hemiachromatopsia [ˌhemiəˌkrəuməˈtɔpsiə] *n* 偏[侧]色盲
hemiacidrin [ˌhemiˈæsidrin] *n* 溶肾石酸素(含枸橼酸、葡萄糖酸、羟基碳酸镁、枸橼酸镁和碳酸钙,可溶鸟粪石)
hemiageusia [ˌhemiəˈgjuːziə], **hemiageustia** [ˌhemiəˈgjuːstiə] *n* 偏侧味觉缺失,半侧味觉丧失
hemialbumose [ˌhemiˈælbjuməus], **hemialbumin** [ˌhemiˈælbjumin] *n* 半朊
hemialbumosuria [ˌhemiælˌbjuməuˈsjuəriə] *n* 半朊尿
hemialgia [ˌhemiˈældʒiə] *n* 偏侧痛
hemiamaurosis [ˌhemiˌæmɔːˈrəusis] *n* 偏盲
hemiamblyopia [ˌhemiˌæmbliˈəupiə] *n* 半侧弱视
hemiamyosthenia [ˌhemiəˌmaiɔsˈθiːniə] *n* 偏身

肌无力

hemianacusia [ˌhemiˌænəˈkjuːziə] *n* 单侧聋

hemianalgesia [ˌhemiˌænælˈdʒiːzjə] *n* 偏身痛觉缺失

hemianencephaly [ˌhemiˌænenˈsefəli] *n* 偏侧无脑[畸形]

hemianesthesia [ˌhemiˌænisˈθiːzjə] *n* 偏侧感觉缺失 | alternate ~, crossed ~ 交叉性偏侧感觉缺失 / cerebral ~ 大脑性偏侧感觉缺失 / mesocephalic ~, pontile ~ 脑桥性偏侧感觉缺失 / spinal ~ 脊髓性偏侧感觉缺失

hemianopia [ˌhemiəˈnəupiə] *n* 偏盲 | absolute ~ 完全偏盲 / altitudinal ~, horizontal ~ 上下性偏盲 / bilateral ~, binocular ~ 两侧偏盲,双眼偏盲 / bitemporal ~ [两]外侧偏盲,[两]颞侧偏盲 / complete ~ 完全偏盲 / congruous ~ 对称性偏盲,同侧偏盲 / heteronymous ~, crossed ~ 异侧偏盲,交叉偏盲 / homonymous ~, lateral ~ 同侧偏盲,外侧偏盲 / incomplete ~ 不全偏盲 / incongruous ~ 非对称性同侧偏盲 / nasal ~ 鼻侧偏盲,内侧偏盲 / unilateral ~, uniocular ~ 单侧偏盲,单眼偏盲 | **hemianopsia** [ˌhemiəˈnɔpsiə] *n* | **hemianopic** [ˌhemiəˈnəupik], **hemianoptic** [ˌhemiæˈnɔptik] *a*

hemianosmia [ˌhemiæˈnɔzmiə] *n* 偏侧嗅觉缺失,单侧嗅觉丧失

hemiapraxia [ˌhemiəˈpræksiə] *n* 偏侧失用症,单侧运用不能

hemiarthrosis [ˌhemiɑːˈθrəusis] *n* 假性软骨结合,半关节强直症

Hemiascomycetidae [ˌhemiˌæskəumaiˈsiːtidiː] *n* 半子囊菌亚纲

hcmiasomatognosia [ˌhemiəˌsəumətɔgˈnəusis] *n* 偏身辨觉不能

hemiasynergia [ˌhemiæsiˈnəːdʒiə] *n* 偏侧协同运动不能

hemiataxia [ˌhemiəˈtæksiə], **hemiataxy** [ˌhemiəˈtæksi] *n* 偏身共济失调

hemiathetosis [ˌhemiæθiˈtəusis] *n* 偏侧手足徐动症

hemiatrophy [ˌhemiˈætrəfi] *n* 偏侧萎缩 | facial ~ 面偏侧萎缩,半面萎缩 / progressive lingual ~ 进行性偏侧舌萎缩

hemiaxial [ˌhemiˈæksiəl] *a* 半轴的

hemiballismus [ˌhemibæˈlizməs], **hemiballism** [ˌhemiˈbælizəm] *n* 偏侧投掷症

hemibladder [ˌhemiˈblædə] *n* 半膀胱畸形

hemiblock [ˈhemiblɔk] *n* 半支传导阻滞

hemic [ˈhiːmik, ˈhemik] *a* 血的

hemicanities [ˌhemikəˈniʃiiːz] *n* 偏侧灰发症

hemicardia [ˌhemiˈkɑːdiə] *n* 半心畸形 | ~ dextra 右半心畸形(只有右心) / ~ sinistra 左半心畸形(只有左心)

hemicardius [ˌhemiˈkɑːdiəs] *n* 半心畸胎

hemicellulase [ˌhemiˈseljuleis] *n* 半纤维素酶

hemicellulose [ˌhemiˈseljuləus] *n* 半纤维素

hemicentrum [ˌhemiˈsentrəm] *n* 单侧椎[骨]体,半侧椎[骨]体

hemicephalia [ˌhemisiˈfeiliə] *n* 半无脑畸形

hemicephalus [ˌhemiˈsefələs] *n* 半无脑畸胎

hemicerebrum [ˌhemiˈseribrəm] *n* 大脑半球

hemichorea [ˌhemikɔˈriə] *n* 偏侧舞蹈症

hemichromatopsia [ˌhemiˌkrəuməˈtɔpsiə] *n* 偏[侧]色盲

hemichrome [ˈhiːmikrəum] *n* 血色质

hemichromosome [ˌhemiˈkrəuməsəum] *n* 半染色体

hemicolectomy [ˌhemikəˈlektəmi] *n* 结肠部分切除术

hemicorporectomy [ˌhemiˌkɔːpəˈrektəmi] *n* 半体切除术(包括骨盆、外生殖器、直肠下段和肛门)

hemicorticectomy [ˌhemiˌkɔːtiˈsektəmi] *n* 大脑半球皮质切除术

hemicrania [ˌhemiˈkreinjə] *n* 偏头痛;半无脑[畸形]

hemicraniectomy [ˌhemiˌkreiniˈektəmi], **hemicraniotomy** [ˌhemiˌkreiniˈɔtəmi] *n* 偏侧颅骨切除术

hemicraniosis [ˌhemiˌkreiniˈəusis] *n* 偏侧颅骨肥大,单侧颅骨肥厚

hemicycle [ˈhemiˌsaikl] *n* 半圆形

hemidecortication [ˌhemidiˌkɔːtiˈkeiʃən] *n* 偏侧大脑皮质切除

hemidesmosome [ˌhemiˈdezməsəum] *n* 半桥粒(亦称 half desmosome)

Hemidesmus [ˌhemiˈdesməs] *n* 充拔属

hemidiaphoresis [ˌhemiˌdaiəfəˈriːsis] *n* 偏身出汗

hemidiaphragm [ˌhemiˈdaiəfræm] *n* 偏侧膈

hemidrosis [ˌhemaiˈdrəusis] *n* 偏身出汗

hemidysergia [ˌhemidiˈsəːdʒiə] *n* 偏身传出性共济失调

hemidysesthesia [ˌhemiˌdisisˈθiːzjə] *n* 偏身感觉障碍

hemidystrophy [ˌhemiˈdistrəfi] *n* 偏身发育障碍

hemiectromelia [ˌhemiektrəuˈmiːliə] *n* 偏侧缺肢畸形

hemielastin [ˌhemiiˈlæstin] *n* 半弹性硬蛋白

hemiencephalus [ˌhemienˈsefələs] *n* 偏侧无大脑半球畸胎,半脑畸胎

hemiepilepsy [ˌhemiˈepilepsi] *n* 偏身癫痫

hemifacial [ˌhemiˈfeiʃəl] *a* 偏侧[颜]面的,半面的

hemigastrectomy [ˌhemigæsˈtrektəmi] *n* 半胃切除术

hemigeusia [ˌhemiˈgjuːsiə] *n* 半侧味觉丧失

hemigigantism [ˌhemiˈdʒaigæntizəm] *n* 偏侧巨大发育
hemiglossal [ˌhemiˈglɔsəl] *a* 半侧舌的
hemiglossectomy [ˌhemiglɔˈsektəmi] *n* 半舌切除术
hemiglossitis [ˌhemiglɔˈsaitis] *n* 半侧舌炎
hemignathia [ˌhemiˈneiθiə] *n* 半下颌畸形
hemihepatectomy [ˌhemiˌhepəˈtektəmi] *n* 半肝切除术
hemihidrosis [ˌhemihaiˈdrəusis] *n* 偏身出汗
hemihypalgesia [ˌhemiˌhaipælˈdʒiːzjə] *n* 偏身痛觉减退
hemihyperesthesia [ˌhemiˌhaipə(ː)risˈθiːzjə] *n* 偏身感觉过敏
hemihyperhidrosis [ˌhemiˌhaipərhaiˈdrəusis] *n* 偏身多汗
hemihypermetria [ˌhemiˌhaipə(ː)ˈmiːtriə] *n* 偏侧伸展过度
hemihyperplasia [ˌhemiˌhaipə(ː)ˈpleiziə] *n* 偏侧发育过度,偏侧增生
hemihypertonia [ˌhemiˌhaipə(ː)ˈtəuniə] *n* 偏侧肌过度紧张,偏侧肌强直
hemihypertrophy [ˌhemihaiˈpəːtrəfi] *n* 偏侧肥大 | facial ~ 偏侧面肥大
hemihypesthesia [ˌhemiˌhaipisˈθiːzjə], **hemihypoesthesia** [ˌhemiˌhaipəuisˈθiːzjə] *n* 偏身感觉迟钝
hemihypometria [ˌhemiˌhaipəuˈmiːtriə] *n* 偏侧伸展不足
hemihypoplasia [ˌhemiˌhaipəuˈpleiziə] *n* 偏侧发育不全
hemihypotonia [ˌhemiˌhaipəuˈtəuniə] *n* 偏身张力减退
hemi-inattention [ˌhemi inəˈtenʃən] *n* 偏侧忽略,单侧忽略(即 unilateral neglect,见 neglect 项下相应术语)
hemikaryon [ˌhemiˈkæriɔn] *n* 单倍核(含染色体单倍的一种细胞核)
hemiketal [ˌhemiˈkiːtəl] *n* 半缩酮
hemilaminectomy [ˌhemiˌlæmiˈnektəmi] *n* 偏侧椎板切除术
hemilaryngectomy [ˌhemiˌlærinˈdʒektəmi] *n* 半喉切除术
hemilateral [ˌhemiˈlætərəl] *a* 偏侧的
hemilesion [ˌhemiˈliːʒən] *n* 脊髓偏侧损伤
hemilingual [ˌhemiˈliŋgwəl] *a* 半侧舌的
hemimacroglossia [ˌhemiˌmækrəuˈglɔsiə] *n* 舌偏侧肥大
hemimandibulectomy [ˌhemimændibjuˈlektəmi] *n* 半下颌切除术
hemimaxillectomy [ˌhemiˌmæksiˈlektəmi] *n* 半上颌骨切除术
hemimelia [ˌhemiˈmiːliə] *n* 半肢,半肢畸形 | fibular ~ 腓侧半肢畸形 / radial ~ 桡侧半肢畸形 / tibial ~ 胫侧半肢畸形 / ulnar ~ 尺侧半肢畸形
hemimelus [heˈmimeləs] *n* 半肢畸胎
hemin [ˈhiːmin] *n* 氯高铁血红素
heminephrectomy [ˌhemineˈfrektəmi] *n* 肾部分切除术
heminephroureterectomy [ˌhemiˌnefrəujuəˌriːtəˈrektəmi] *n* 肾输尿管部分切除术
hemineurasthenia [ˌhemiˌnjuəræsˈθiːnjə] *n* 偏侧神经衰弱
hemiobesity [ˌhemiəuˈbiːsəti] *n* 偏身肥胖
hemiopalgia [ˌhemiɔˈpældʒiə] *n* 偏侧头眼痛
hemiopia [ˌhemiˈəupiə] *n* 偏盲;一侧视野缺失
hemiopic [ˌhemiˈɔpik] *a* 单眼的;偏盲的
hemipagus [heˈmipəgəs] *n* 胸侧联胎
hemiparalysis [ˌhemipəˈrælisis] *n* 偏瘫,半身不遂
hemiparanesthesia [ˌhemiˌpærænisˈθiːzjə] *n* 偏侧下身麻木
hemiparaplegia [ˌhemiˌpærəˈpliːdʒiə] *n* 偏侧下身麻痹
hemiparesis [ˌhemipəˈriːsis] *n* 轻偏瘫,偏侧不全麻痹
hemiparesthesia [ˌhemiˌpærisˈθiːzjə] *n* 偏身感觉异常
hemiparetic [ˌhemipəˈretik] *a* 轻偏瘫的,偏侧不全麻痹的 *n* 轻偏瘫者,偏侧不全麻痹患者
hemiparkinsonism [ˌhemiˈpɑːkinsənizəm] *n* 偏侧震颤麻痹
hemipelvectomy [ˌhemiˌpelˈvektəmi] *n* 偏侧骨盆切除术
hemipeptone [ˌhemiˈpeptəun] *n* 半[蛋白]胨
hemiphalangectomy [ˌhemiˌfælænˈdʒektəmi] *n* 指部分切除术,趾部分切除术
hemipinic acid [ˌhemiˈpainik] 3,4-二甲氧苯二甲酸
hemipinta [ˌhemiˈpintə] *n* 偏身品他病(品他病的一种罕见型,其色素障碍仅影响身体的一侧)
hemiplacenta [ˌhemipləˈsentə] *n* 半胎盘(使有袋动物的胚胎与母体子宫有暂时性的关连)
hemiplegia [ˌhemiˈpliːdʒiə] *n* 偏瘫 | alternate ~, crossed ~ 交替性瘫痪,交叉性偏瘫 / alternating oculomotor ~ 动眼神经交叉性偏瘫 / capsular ~ 内囊性偏瘫 / cerebral ~ 脑性偏瘫 / contralateral ~ 对侧偏瘫 / faciobrachial ~ 面臂偏瘫 / flaccid ~ 松弛性偏瘫 | **hemiplegic** [ˌhemiˈpliːdʒik] *a*
hemiprostatectomy [ˌhemiˈprɔstəˈtəktəmi] *n* 偏侧前列腺切除术
Hemiptera [hiˈmiptərə] *n* 半翅目 | **hemipterous** [hiˈmiptərəs] *a*

hemipylorectomy [ˌhemiˌpailəˈrektəmi] *n* 幽门部分切除术

hemipyocyanin [ˌhemiˌpaiəˈsaiənin] *n* 半绿脓菌青素,半绿脓菌蓝素

hemipyonephrosis [ˌhemiˌpaiəniˈfrəusis] *n* 偏侧肾盂积脓

hemirachischisis [ˌhemirəˈkiskisis] *n* 隐性脊柱裂

hemisacralization [ˌhemiˌseikrəlaiˈzeiʃən, ˌliˈz-] *n*(第五腰椎)半骶化

hemiscotosis [ˌhemiskəˈtəusis] *n* 偏盲

hemisection [ˌhemiˈsekʃən] *n* 半切除;对切

hemisectomy [ˌhiːmiˈsektəmi] *n* 偏侧根尖切除术

hemiseptum [ˌhemiˈseptəm] *n*【拉】偏侧隔 | ~ cerebri 偏侧透明隔

hemisoantibody [ˌhiːmaisəuˈæntibɔdi] *n* 血同种抗体(与同一物种的另一个体的红细胞起反应的抗体)

hemisomnambulism [ˌhemisɔmˈnæmbjulizəm] *n* 半梦游症(指其行动表现如清醒时的梦游症)

hemisomus [ˌhemiˈsəuməs] *n* 半躯干畸胎

hemisotonic [ˌhemaisəuˈtɔnik] *a* 血液等渗性的

hemispasm [ˈhemispæzəm] *n* 偏侧痉挛,半侧痉挛

hemisphaerium [ˌhemiˈsfiːriəm] ([复] **hemisphaeria** [ˌhemiˈsfiːriə]) *n*【拉】半球 | hemisphaeria bulbi urethrae 尿道球半球

hemisphere [ˈhemisfiə] *n* 半球 | animal ~ 动物半球(已受精的端黄卵经分裂形成的细胞群最接近动物极的半边)/ cerebellar ~ 小脑半球 / cerebral ~ 大脑半球 / dominant ~ 优势半球(如善用右手者为左侧大脑半球,反之亦然)/ vegetal ~ 植物半球(已受精的端黄卵经分裂形成的细胞群最接近植物极的半边) | **hemispheric(al)** [hemiˈsferik(əl)] *a*

hemispherectomy [ˌhemisfiəˈrektəmi] *n* 大脑半球切除术

hemispherium [ˌhemiˈsfiːriəm] ([复] **hemispheria** [ˌhemiˈsfiːriə]) *n*【拉】半球 | ~ cerebelli 小脑半球 / ~ cerebralis, ~ cerebri 大脑半球

hemisphygmia [ˌhemiˈsfigmiə] *n* 倍脉症

Hemispora stellata [heˈmispərə stəˈleitə] *n* 星形半孢子菌

hemispore [ˈhemispɔː] *n* 半孢子

hemistrumectomy [ˌhemistruˈmektəmi] *n* 偏侧甲状腺切除术

hemisyndrome [ˌhemiˈsindrəum] *n* 偏侧综合征(脊髓偏侧损害)

hemiterata [ˌhemiˈterətə] *n* 轻度畸形儿,半畸形者(发育异常,但尚不属畸形者)

hemiteratic [ˌhemitəˈrætik] *a* 轻度畸形的,半畸形的

hemitetany [ˌhemiˈtetəni] *n* 偏身手足搐搦

hemithermoanesthesia [ˌhemiˌθəːməˌænisˈθiːzjə] *n* 偏身热觉缺失,偏侧温度觉缺失

hemithorax [ˌhemiˈθɔːræks] *n* 单侧胸廓,偏侧胸廓

hemithyroidectomy [ˌhemiˌθairɔiˈdektəmi] *n* 偏侧甲状腺切除术

hemitomias [ˌhemiˈtəumiəs] *n* 偏侧无睾[丸]者

hemitonia [ˌhemiˈtəuniə] *n* 偏侧肌紧张,偏侧肌强直

hemitoxin [ˌhemiˈtɔksin] *n* 半毒素

hemitremor [ˌhemiˈtriːmə] *n* 偏身震颤

hemivagotony [ˌhemiveiˈgɔtəni] *n* 偏侧迷走神经紧张症

hemivertebra [ˌhemiˈvəːtibrə] *n* 半脊椎,半椎体;([复] **hemivertebrae** [ˌhemiˈvəːtibriː]) 偏侧脊椎发育不全

hemizona [ˌhemiˈzəunə] *n* 半带(如透明带)

hemizygote [ˌhemiˈzaigəut] *n* 半合子(指一个个体或细胞,只具有决定某一特征的一对基因中的一个者) | **hemizygous** [ˌhemiˈzaigəs], **hemizygotic** [ˌhemizaiˈgɔtik] *a* | **hemizygosity** [ˌhemizaiˈgɔsəti] *n* 半合子状态

hemlock [ˈhemlɔk] *n* 毒茴类毒草(如毒茴、毒芹);铁杉属植物,铁杉 | water ~ 毒芹

hem(o)-, haem(o)-, hema-, haema- [构词成分]血

hemoaccess [ˌhiːməuˈæksəs] *n* 血管入口(动静脉入口)

hemoagglutination [ˌhiːməuəˌgluːtiˈneiʃən] *n* 血凝,血细胞凝集[作用]

hemoagglutinin [ˌhiːməuəˈgluːtinin] *n* 血凝素,血细胞凝集素

hemoalkalimeter [ˌhiːməuˌælkəˈlimitə] *n* 血碱度计

hemobilia [ˌhiːməuˈbiliə] *n* 胆道出血

hemobilinuria [ˌhiːməubailiˈnjuəriə] *n* 血胆素尿

hemoblast [ˈhiːməblæst] *n* 成血细胞

hemoblastosis [ˌhiːməblæsˈtəusis] *n* 生血组织增殖,骨髓组织增殖

hemocatatonistic [ˌhiːməuˌkætətəuˈnistik] *a* 血液内聚性减弱的

hemocatharsis [ˌhiːməukəˈθɑːsis] *n* 清血法

hemocatheresis [ˌhiːməkəˈθerisis] *n* 红细胞破坏 | **hemocatheretic** [ˌhiːməˌkæθəˈretik] *a*

hemocelom [ˌhiːməuˈsiːləm], **hemocele** [ˈhiːməsiːl] *n* 围心腔(胚胎);血腔(如节肢动物)

hemocholecyst [ˌhiːməuˈkəulisist] *n* 胆囊积血(非外伤性出血)

hemocholecystitis [ˌhiːməukəulisisˈtaitis] *n* 出血性胆囊炎

hemochorial [ˌhiːməuˈkɔːriəl] *a* 绒[毛]膜受血的

hemochromatosis [ˌhiːməuˌkrəuməˈtəusis] *n* 血色素沉着

hemochromatotic [ˌhiːməuˌkrəuməˈtɔtik] *a* 血色素沉着的

hemochrome [ˈhiːməkrəum] *n* 血色素

hemochromogen [ˌhiːməuˈkrəumədʒən] *n* 血色原 | hemoglobin ~ 血红蛋白血色原

hemochromometer [ˌhiːməukrəuˈmɔmitə] *n* 血红蛋白计,血色计 | **hemochromometry** *n* 血红蛋白测定法

hemochromoprotein [ˌhiːməuˌkrəuməˈprəutiːn] *n* 血色蛋白

hemocidal [ˌhiːməuˈsaidl] *a* 破坏血细胞的

hemoclasia [ˌhiːməuˈkleisiə] *n* 食后白细胞减少

hemoclasis [hiːˈmɔkləsis] *n* 溶血,血细胞溶解 | **hemoclastic** [hiːməˈklæstik] *a*

hemoclip [ˈhiːməklip] *n* 血管结扎夹,止血夹

hemocoagulin [ˌhiːməukəuˈægjulin] *n* 蛇毒凝血素

hemocoelom [ˌhiːməuˈsiːləm], **hemocoeloma** [ˌhiːməusiːˈləumə] *n* 围心腔(胚胎);血腔(如节肢动物)

hemoconcentration [ˌhiːməuˌkɔnsenˈtreiʃən] *n* 血液浓缩

hemoconia [ˌhiːməˈkəuniə] *n* 血尘

hemoconiosis [ˌhiːməuˌkəuniˈəusis] *n* 血尘病,血尘过多症

hemocrine [ˈhiːməkrin] *a* 血液激素的

hemocrinia [ˌhiːməˈkriniə] *n* 激素血(血内有激素)

hemocrinotherapy [ˌhiːməˌkrinəuˈθerəpi] *n* 自血激素疗法

hemocryoscopy [ˌhiːməukraiˈɔskəpi] *n* 血冰点测定法

hemocrystallin [ˌhiːməuˈkristəlin] *n* 血红蛋白

hemoculture [ˌhiːməuˈkʌltʃə] *n* 血[细菌]培养

hemocuprein [ˌhiːməˈkjuːpriin] *n* 血铜蛋白,超氧物歧化酶

hemocyanin [ˌhiːməuˈsaiənin] *n* 血蓝蛋白 | keyhole-limpet ~ (KLH)钥孔蝛血蓝蛋白(从"钥孔蝛"〈一种软体动物〉提取的血蓝蛋白,常用作哺乳动物实验性抗原,KLH免疫接种可用作急性髓细胞白血病的试验)

hemocyte [ˈhiːməsait] *n* 血细胞

hemocytoblast [ˌhiːməˈsaitəblæst] *n* 成血细胞

hemocytoblastoma [ˌhiːməˌsaitəblæsˈtəumə] *n* 成血细胞瘤,成骨髓细胞瘤

hemocytocatheresis [ˌhiːməˌsaitəkəˈθerisis] *n* 红细胞破坏,红细胞溶解

hemocytogenesis [ˌhiːməˌsaitəˈdʒenisis] *n* 血细胞生成,血生成,造血

hemocytology [ˌhiːməusaiˈtɔlədʒi] *n* 血细胞学

hemocytolysis [ˌhiːməusaiˈtɔlisis] *n* 溶血,血细胞溶解 | **hemocytolytic** [ˌhiːməuˌsaitəˈlitik] *a*

hemocytoma [ˌhiːməusaiˈtəumə] *n* 血细胞瘤

hemocytometer [ˌhiːməusaiˈtɔmitə] *n* 血细胞计数器 | **hemocytometry** *n* 血细胞计数

hemocytophagia [ˌhiːməuˌsaitəˈfeidʒiə] *n* 吞噬血细胞作用 | **hemocytophagic** [ˌhiːməuˌsaitəˈfædʒik] *a* 吞噬血细胞的

hemocytopoiesis [ˌhiːməuˌsaitəpɔiˈiːsis] *n* 血细胞生成,血细胞发生,血生成,造血

hemocytotripsis [ˌhiːməuˌsaitəˈtripsis] *n* 血细胞压碎

hemodiafiltration [ˌhiːməuˌdaiəfilˈtreiʃən] *n* 血液透析滤过

hemodiagnosis [ˌhiːməuˌdaiəgˈnəusis] *n* 验血诊断[法]

hemodialysis [ˌhiːməudaiˈælisis] *n* 血液透析

hemodialytic [ˌhiːməudaiəˈlitik] *a* 血液透析的

hemodialyzer [ˌhiːməuˈdaiəlaizə] *n* 血液透析器(俗称人工肾) | ultrafiltration ~ 超滤血液透析器

hemodiapedesis [ˌhiːməuˌdaiəpiˈdiːsis] *n* 血液渗出(经皮肤)

hemodiastase [ˌhiːməuˈdaiəsteis] *n* 血[液]淀粉酶

hemodilution [ˌhiːməudaiˈljuːʃən] *n* 血液稀释

hemodynamic [ˌhiːməudaiˈnæmik] *a* 血流动力的

hemodynamics [ˌhiːməudaiˈnæmiks] *n* 血流动力学

hemodynamometry [ˌhiːməuˌdainəˈmɔmitri] *n* 血压测定法

hemodystrophy [ˌhiːməuˈdistrəfi] *n* 血营养障碍

hemoendocrinopathic [ˌhiːməuˌendəukrinəˈpæθik] *a* 血内分泌病的

hemoendothelial [ˌhiːməuˌendəuˈθiːliəl] *a* 血内皮的

hemoerythrin [ˌhiːməuiˈriθrin] *n* 蠕虫血红蛋白

hemoferrum [ˌhiːməˈferəm] *n* 氧合血红蛋白

hemofilter [ˌhiːməuˈfiltə] *n* 血液滤过器,滤血器

hemofiltration [ˌhiːməufilˈtreiʃən] *n* 血液滤过 | continuous arteriovenous ~ 连续性动静脉血液滤过

hemoflagellate [ˌhiːməuˈflædʒeleit] *n* 血鞭毛虫

hemofuscin [ˌhiːməuˈfjuːsin] *n* 血褐素,血棕色素

hemogenesis [ˌhiːməuˈdʒenisis] *n* 血细胞生成,血生成,造血

hemogenic [ˌhiːməuˈdʒenik] *a* 生血的;血源性的

hemoglobic [ˌhiːməuˈgləubik] *a* 生血红蛋白的,含血红蛋白的

hemoglobin [ˈhiːməuˌgləubin] *n* 血红蛋白 | ~ A 血红蛋白A(正常成年人血红蛋白) / ~ A_{1c} 血红蛋白 A_{1c}(糖基化血红蛋白A) / ~ A_2 血红

蛋白 A_2(正常成年人血红蛋白)/ ~ C 血红蛋白 C(镰状细胞性贫血患者的血红蛋白)/ ~ carbamate 氨基甲酸血红蛋白 / ~ D 血红蛋白 D(同型结合体轻度贫血)/ deoxygenated ~ 脱氧血红蛋白 / ~ E 血红蛋白 E(异常血红蛋白,东南亚最常见)/ "fast" ~s 快泳血红蛋白 / fetal ~, ~ F 胎儿血红蛋白 / glycosylated ~ 糖基化血红蛋白 / ~ H 血红蛋白 H(引起贫血和血红蛋白过少、红细胞不均、异型红细胞症)/ ~ I 血红蛋白 I(引起镰状化)/ ~ M 血红蛋白 M(因氨基酸的替代使之易于形成正铁血红蛋白血)/ mean corpuscular ~ 红细胞平均血红蛋白量 / muscle ~肌红蛋白 / oxidized ~, oxygenated ~ 氧合血红蛋白 / ~ S 血红蛋白 S(镰状细胞性贫血患者的血红蛋白)/ "slow" ~s 慢泳血红蛋白 | **~ic** [ˌhiːməuɡləu'binik] *a*

hemoglobinated [ˌhiːməu'ɡləubineitid] *a* 含血红蛋白的

hemoglobinemia [ˌhiːməuˌɡləubi'niːmiə] *n* 血红蛋白血症

hemoglobiniferous [ˌhiːməuˌɡləubi'nifərəs] *a* 带血红蛋白的

hemoglobinocholia [ˌhiːməuˌɡrəubinə'kəuliə] *n* 血红蛋白胆汁

hemoglobinogenous [ˌhiːməuˌɡrəubi'nɔdʒinəs] *a* 血红蛋白生成的

hemoglobinolysis [ˌhiːməuˌɡləubi'nɔlisis], **hemoglobinopepsia** [ˌhiːməuˌɡrəubinə'pepsiə] *n* 血红蛋白分解

hemoglobinometer [ˌhiːməuˌɡləubi'nɔmitə] *n* 血红蛋白计 | **hemoglobinometry** *n* 血红蛋白测定法

hemoglobinopathy [ˌhiːməuˌɡləubi'nɔpəθi] *n* 血红蛋白病

hemoglobinophilia [ˌhiːməuˌɡləubinəu'filiə] *n* 嗜血红蛋白性(指微生物) | **hemoglobinophilic** *a* 嗜血红蛋白的

hemoglobinorrhea [ˌhiːməuˌɡrəubinəu'riːə] *n* 血红蛋白溢

hemoglobinous [ˌhiːməu'ɡrəubinəs] *a* 含血红蛋白的

hemoglobinuria [ˌhiːməuˌɡləubi'njuəriə] *n* 血红蛋白尿 | malarial ~ 疟疾性血红蛋白尿,黑水热,黑尿热 / paroxysmal cold ~ 阵发性冷性血红蛋白尿症 / paroxysmal nocturnal ~ (PNH) 阵发性睡眠性血红蛋白尿症 | **hemoglobinuric** *a*

hemogram ['hiːməɡræm] *n* 血象

hemohistioblast [ˌhiːməu'histiəˌblæst] *n* 成血细胞

hemohydraulics [ˌhiːməuhai'drɔːliks] *n* 血液水力学

hemoid ['hiːmɔid] *a* 血样的

hemokinesis [ˌhiːməukai'niːsis, -ki'n-] *n* 血液流动 | **hemokinetic** [ˌhiːməukai'netik, -ki'n-] *a*

hemokonia [ˌhiːmə'kəuniə] *n* 血尘

hemokoniosis [ˌhiːməuˌkəuni'əusis] *n* 血尘病,血尘过多症

hemology [hiː'mɔlədʒi] *n* 血液学

hemolutein [ˌhiːməu'ljuːtiin] *n* 血清黄素

hemolymph ['hiːməˌlimf] *n* 血淋巴;血液(无脊椎动物)

hemolymphadenosis [ˌhiːməlimˌfædi'nəusis] *n* 生血组织增殖,骨髓组织增殖

hemolymphangioma [ˌhiːməlimˌfændʒi'əumə] *n* 血管淋巴管瘤

hemolymphocytotoxin [ˌhiːməˌlimfəuˌsaitə'tɔksin] *n* 血淋巴细胞毒素

hemolysate [hiː'mɔliseit] *n* 溶血产物

hemolysin [hiː'mɔːlisin, ˌhiːmə'laisin] *n* 溶血素 | immune ~ 免疫溶血素(用于补体结合试验)

hemolysis [hiː'mɔlisis] ([复] **hemolyses** [hiː'mɔlisiːz]) *n* 溶血 | biologic ~ 生物性溶血 / immune ~ 免疫溶血 / passive ~ 被动溶血 / siderogenous ~ 铁过多性溶血(引起继发性血色素沉着症) | **hemolytic** [ˌhiːmə'litik] *a*

hemolysoid [hiː'mɔlisɔid] *n* 去毒簇溶血素

hemolysophilic [ˌhiːməˌlaisə'filik] *a* 亲溶血素的

hemolyzable [ˌhiːmə'laizəbl] *a* 可溶血的

hemolyze ['hiːməlaiz] *vt, vi* 引起溶血,使血细胞溶解 | **hemolyzation** [ˌhiːməlai'zeiʃən, -li'z-] *n* 溶血[作用]

hemomanometer [ˌhiːməumə'nɔmitə] *n* 血压计

hemomediastinum [ˌhiːməuˌmiːdiæs'tainəm] *n* 纵隔积血

hemometer [hiː'mɔmitə] *n* 血红蛋白计

hemometra [ˌhiːməu'miːtrə] *n* 子宫积血

hemometry [hiː'mɔmitri] *n* 血成分测定法

hemomyelosis [ˌhiːməuˌmaiə'ləusis] *n* 生血组织增殖,骨髓组织增殖

hemonephrosis [ˌhiːməne'frəusis] *n* 肾盂积血

hemo-opsonin [ˌhiːməu ɔp'səunin] *n* 血调理素,红细胞调理素

hemopathology [ˌhiːməupə'θɔlədʒi] *n* 血液病理学

hemopathy [hiː'mɔpəθi] *n* 血液病 | **hemopathic** [ˌhiːmə'pæθik] *a*

hemoperfusion [ˌhiːməupə(ː)'fjuːʒən] *n* 血液灌流

hemopericardium [ˌhiːməuˌperi'kɑːdiəm] *n* 心包积血

hemoperitoneum [ˌhiːməuˌperitəu'niːəm] *n* 腹腔积血

hemopexin [ˌhiːməu'peksin] *n* 血红素结合蛋白,血液结合素(一种结合血红素的血浆糖蛋白)

hemopexis [ˌhiːməu'peksis] *n* 血凝固
hemophagocyte [ˌhiːməu'fægəsait], **hemophage** [ˌhiːməfeidʒ]*n* 噬血细胞细胞(破坏血细胞的一种吞噬细胞)
hemophagocytosis [ˌhiːməuˌfægəsai'təusis] *n* 噬血细胞吞噬作用
hemophil ['hiːməfil] *a* 嗜血的 *n* 嗜血菌
hemophilia [ˌhiːmə'filiə] *n* 血友病 | ~ A, classical ~ 血友病A,典型血友病(缺乏凝血因子Ⅷ所致) / ~B 血友病B(缺乏凝血因子Ⅸ所致)/ ~ C 血友病C(缺乏凝血因子Ⅺ所致)/ ~ neonatorum 新生儿血友病(新生儿紫癜) / vascular ~ 血管性血友病
hemophiliac [ˌhiːmə'filiæk] *n* 血友病[患]者
hemophilic [ˌhiːmə'filik] *a* 嗜血的;血友病的
hemophilioid [ˌhiːmə'filiɔid] *a* 血友病样的
Hemophilus [hiː'mɔfiləs] *n* 嗜血杆菌属(见 Haemophilus)
hemophilus [hiː'mɔfiləs] *n* 嗜血杆菌
hemophobia [ˌhiːməu'fəubiə] *n* 血恐怖,恐血症
hemophoric [ˌhiːməu'fɔːrik] *a* 带血液的,运送血液的
hemophotograph [ˌhiːməu'fəutəgrɑːf, -græf] *n* 血细胞照片
hemophotometer [ˌhiːməufəu'tɔmitə] *n* 血红蛋白光度测定计
hemophthalmos [ˌhiːmɔf'θælmɔs], **hemophthalmia** [ˌhiːmɔf'θælmiə], **hemophthalmus** [ˌhiːmɔf'θælməs] *n* 眼内渗血
hemophthisis [hiː'mɔfθisis] *n* 贫血,血亏(此术语曾用以表示因血细胞营养不足所致的贫血)
hemopiezometer [ˌhiːməuˌpaii'zɔmitə] *n* 血压计
hemoplasmopathy [ˌhiːməuplæz'mɔpəθi] *n* 血浆病
hemoplastic [ˌhiːməu'plæstik] *a* 成血的
hemopleura [ˌhiːməu'pluərə] *n* 血胸
hemopneumopericardium [ˌhiːməuˌnjuːməuˌperi'kɑːdiəm] *n* 血气心包
hemopneumothorax [ˌhiːməuˌnjuːməu'θɔːræks] *n* 血气胸
hemopoiesis [ˌhiːməupɔi'iːsis] *n* 血细胞生成,血细胞发生,血生成,造血 | **hemopoiesic** [ˌhiːməupɔi'iːsik], **hemopoietic** [ˌhiːməupɔi'etik] *a* 生血的,造血的
hemopoietin [ˌhiːməupɔi'iːtin] *n* 红细胞生成素
hemoporphyrin [ˌhiːməu'pɔːfirin] *n* 血卟啉,血紫质
hemoposia [ˌhiːməu'pəuziə] *n* 饮血(如寄生虫噬血)
hemoprecipitin [ˌhiːməupri'sipitin] *n* 血沉淀素
hemoproctia [ˌhiːməu'prɔkʃiə] *n* 直肠出血
hemoprotein [ˌhiːməu'prəutiːn] *n* 血红素蛋白
hemopsonin [ˌhiːmɔp'səunin] *n* 血调理素,红细胞调理素(使血细胞易被吞噬的调理素)
hemoptysis [hi'mɔptisis] *n* 咯血 | cardiac ~ 心脏病性咯血 / parasitic ~, endemic ~, oriental ~ 寄生虫性咯血,卫氏并殖吸虫病,肺吸虫病 / vicarious ~ 代偿性咯血(正常月经时发生的一种现象) | **hemoptysic** [ˌhiːmɔp'taisik], **hemoptic** [hiː'mɔptik], **hemoptoic** [hiːmɔp'təuik] *a*
hemopyelectasis [ˌhiːməupaii'lektəsis] *n* 肾盂积血扩张
hemopyrrol [ˌhiːməu'pirɔl] *n* 血吡咯
hemorheology [ˌhiːməuri'ɔlədʒi] *n* 血液流变学
hemorrhachis [hi'mɔrəkis] *n* 椎管内出血
hemorrhage ['hemərid3] *n*, *vi* 出血 | alveolar ~ 牙槽出血 / arterial ~ 动脉出血 / capillary ~ 毛细血管出血,渗血 / capsuloganglionic ~ 内外囊神经节出血 / cerebral ~ 脑出血 / dot ~ 视网膜微观动脉瘤(见于糖尿病性视网膜病) / essential ~ 自发性出血 / essential uterine ~ 自发性子宫出血,功能性子宫出血病 / external ~ 外出血 / gravitating ~ 引力性椎管积血 / intermediary ~, intermediate ~ 中间期出血 / internal ~, concealed ~ 内出血,隐匿性出血 / intracranial ~ 颅内出血 / intrapartum ~ 分娩时出血 / massive ~ 大出血 / nasal ~ 鼻出血 / ~ per rhexin 破裂性出血 / petechial ~ 点状[皮下]出血 / postpartum ~ 产后出血 / punctate ~ 点状出血(自毛细管出血到组织内) / splinter ~s 裂片形出血(亚急性细菌性心内膜炎的甲下线状出血)/ unavoidable ~ 难免性出血(前置胎盘剥离出血) / venous ~ 静脉出血 / vicarious ~ 代偿性出血 | **hemorrhagic** [ˌhemə'rædʒik] *a*
hemorrhagenic [ˌhemərə'dʒenik],**hemorrhagiparous** [ˌhemәri'dʒipərəs] *a* 引起出血的
hemorrhagin [ˌhemə'reidʒin] *n* 出血素(在某些蛇毒和其他毒素中的一种溶细胞素,能破坏内皮细胞和血管)
hemorrhaphilia [ˌhemərə'filiə] *n* 血友病
hemorrhea [ˌhemə'riːə] *n* 大出血
hemorrheology [ˌhiːməuri'ɔlədʒi] *n* 血液流变学
hemorrhoid ['hemərɔid] *n* 痔 | external ~ 外痔 / internal ~ 内痔 / lingual ~ 舌静脉曲张 / mixed ~, combined ~, mucocutaneous ~ 混合痔(连结直肠上、下丛的静脉呈曲张性扩大,使内、外痔相连) / prolapsed ~ 脱痔/ strangulated ~ 绞窄性痔 / thrombosed ~ 血栓性痔 | **~al** [ˌhemə'rɔidl] *a*
hemorrhoidectomy [ˌhemərɔi'dektəmi] *n* 痔切除术
hemorrhoidolysis [ˌhemərɔi'dɔlisis] *n* 清痔术,痔灼除术
hemosalpinx [ˌhiːməu'sælpiŋks] *n* 输卵管积血

hemoscope [ˈhiːməskəup] *n* 血分光镜
hemosialemesis [ˌhiːməuˌsaiəˈlemisis] *n* 吐血涎症
hemosiderin [ˌhiːməuˈsidərin] *n* 含铁血黄素
hemosiderinuria [ˌhiːməuˌsidəriˈnjuəriə] *n* 含铁血黄素尿症
hemosiderosis [ˌhiːməuˌsidəˈrəusis] *n* 含铁血黄素沉着症(组织并未受损)
hemosozic [ˌhiːməuˈsəuzik] *a* 防止溶血的,抗溶血的
hemospermia [ˌhiːməuˈspəːmiə] *n* 血性精液
hemosporian [ˌhiːməuˈspɔːriən] *n*, *a* 血孢子虫(的)
Hemosporidia [ˌhiːməuspəˈridiə] *n* = **Haemosporidia**
hemosporidian [ˌhiːməuspəuˈridiən] *n*, *a* 血孢子虫(的)
hemostasis [ˌhiːməuˈsteisis, ˌhiˈmɔstəsis], **hemostasia** [ˌhiːməuˈsteiziə] *n* 止血[法]
hemostat [ˈhiːməstæt] *n* 止血器;止血药
hemostatic [hiːməˈstætik] *a* 止血的 *n* 止血药 | capillary ~ 毛细血管止血药 | **hemostyptic** [ˌhiːməˈstiptik] *a*, *n*
hemotherapy [ˌhiːməuˈθerəpi], **hemotherapeutics** [ˌhiːməuˌθerəˈpjuːtiks] *n* 血液疗法
hemothorax [ˌhiːməuˈθɔːræks] *n* 血胸
hemotonia [ˌhiːməuˈtəuniə] *n* 血液渗性(血液中固体成分的张力)
hemotoxic [ˌhiːməuˈtɔksik] *a* 血中毒的
hemotoxin [ˌhiːməuˈtɔksin] *n* [溶]血毒素(一种具有溶血活性特征的外毒素) | cobra ~ 眼镜蛇溶血毒素
hemotroph(e) [ˈhiːmətrɔf] *n* [母]血营养质 | **hemotrophic** [ˌhiːməuˈtrɔfik] *a* [母]血营养的
hemotropic [ˌhiːməuˈtrɔpik] *a* 亲血的,亲红细胞的
hemotropin [hiːˈmɔtrəpin] *n* 亲血素,血调理素,红细胞调理素
hemotympanum [ˌhiːməuˈtimpənəm] *n* 血鼓室
hemovolumetry [ˌhiːməuvɔˈljuːmitri] *n* 血容量测定法
hemozoic [ˌhiːməˈzəuik] *a* 血原虫的
hemozoin [ˌhiːməuˈzəuin] *n* 疟原虫色素
hemozoon [ˌhiːməuˈzəuɔn] *n* 血原虫
hemp [hemp] *n* 大麻(植物)
hempa [ˈhempə] *n* 氮磷致变物(一种无色液体,具有氨样气味,用作喷气燃料中的除冰剂,用作溶剂,并用作虫疫的化学不育剂。亦称六甲基磷酰胺,缩写为 HMPA)
HEM-PAS [ˈhem pəs] *h*ereditary *e*rythroblastic *m*ultinuclearity with *p*ositive *a*cidified *s*erum 遗传性幼红细胞多核性伴阳性酸化血清(先天性红细胞生成不良性贫血的最常见型)
hempen [ˈhempən] *a* 大麻的;大麻制的
hemuresis [ˌhemjuəˈriːsis] *n* 血尿
henbane [ˈhenbein] *n* 莨菪
Hench-Aldrich test (index) [hentʃ ˈældritʃ] (Philip S. Hench; Martha Aldrich) 亨奇-奥尔德里奇试验(指数)(检唾液的汞结合力)
Hench-Rosenbery syndrome [hentʃ ˈrəuzənbəːg] (Philip S. Hench; Edward F. Rosenberg) 汉-罗综合征,复发性风湿病
Henderson-Hasselbalch equation [ˈhendəsn ˈhæsəlbɑːlh] (Lawrence J. Henderson; Karl A. Hasselbalch) 亨德森-哈塞尔巴赫方程(表示缓冲系统 pH 的一种方程: $pH = pK_a + \log\frac{[A^-]}{[HA]}$ 式中[HA]为游离酸浓度,[A^-]为电离形式的浓度,pK_a 为该酸解离常数〈K_a〉的负对数)
Henderson-Jones disease [ˈhendəsn ˈdʒəunz] (Melvin S. Henderson; Hugh T. Jones) 亨德森-琼斯病(关节腔内或腱鞘囊内有大量软骨性异物的一种骨软骨瘤病)
Henderson-Paterson bodies [ˈhendəsn ˈpætəsn] (William Henderson; Robert Paterson) 软疣小体
Hendersonula [ˌhendəˈsɔnjuːlə] *n* 亨德森真菌属
Henke's space [ˈhenkə] (Philipp J. W. Henke) 汉克间隙(脊柱和咽、食管之间的间隙,内含结缔组织) | ~ triangle (trigone) 汉克三角(介于腹股沟降部、外侧部和直肌外缘间的三角区)
Henle-Coenen test (sign) [ˌhenlə ˈkiːnən] (Adolf R. Henle; Hermann Coenen) 亨勒-克南试验(征)(检侧支循环)
Henle's ampulla [ˈhenlə] (Friedrich G. J. Henle) 输精管壶腹 | ~ fibers 亨勒纤维(存在于某些动脉中外层之间的窗膜纤维,部分为弹性纤维,其余为有核纤维) / ~ fissures 亨勒裂(在心肌纤维间充满结缔组织的间隙) / ~ glands 亨勒腺(睑结膜内的管状腺) / ~ layer 亨勒层(毛囊内根鞘细胞的外层) / ~ ligament 腹股沟镰 / ~ loop 髓襻(细尿管襻,在肾小管髓部的 U 形弯曲) / ~ membrane 亨勒膜(富克斯〈Fuchs〉后界膜;脉络膜基底层) / ~ reaction 亨勒反应(肾上腺髓质细胞用铬盐处理染成暗褐色) / ~ sheath 亨勒鞘(神经内膜,即凯-雷济厄斯〈Key-Retzius〉结缔组织鞘) / ~ sphincter 亨勒括约肌(环绕尿道前列腺部的肌纤维) / ~ spine [耳]道上棘,耳道棘 / ~ tubules 亨勒细管(形成亨勒襻的肾小管直升及下降部分,亦称肾直小管、直细精管)
henna [ˈhenə] *n* 散沫花叶(用作美容剂及发染料,亦用于治肠念珠菌病);棕红色 *a* 棕红色的
Hennebert's sign (test) [enˈbɛə] (Camille Hennebert) 安纳贝尔征(试验)(先天性梅毒迷路炎时,压空气入外耳道,使患侧产生旋转性眼球震

颤,减压时对侧眼球震颤。亦称气压试验)

Henning's sign [ˈheniŋ] (Wilhelm Henning) 赫宁征(胃的角切迹出现形似哥特式尖拱的角畸形,为慢性胃溃疡之征。亦称哥特式尖拱结构)

Henoch-Schönlein purpura (syndrome) [ˈhenɔh ˈʃeinlain] (E. H. Henoch; Johann L. Schönlein) 亨诺赫-舍恩莱因紫癜(综合征)(见 Schönlein-Henoch purpura)

Henoch's chorea [ˈhenɔh] (Edouard H. Henoch) 亨诺赫舞蹈症,痉挛性抽搐(慢性进行性电击样舞蹈症) | ~ purpura (disease) 亨诺赫紫癜(病)(一种舍恩莱因-亨诺赫〈Schönlein-Henoch〉综合征,其特征为急性发作内脏症状,如呕吐、腹胀、血尿及肾绞痛,无关节症状。亦称神经性紫癜)

henogenesis [ˌhenəuˈdʒenisis] *n* 个体发生,个体发育

henpue, henpuye [henˈpuːjiː] *n* 鼻骨增殖性骨膜炎,根度病,巨鼻[症]

henry [ˈhenri] (Joseph Henry) *n* 亨[利](电感单位,符号为 H)

Henry's law [ˈhenri] (William Henry) 亨利定律(气体在液体中的溶解度与该气体的分压成正比)

Henry's melanin test (reaction, melanoflocculation test) [ˈhenri] (Adolf F. G Henry) 亨利黑[色]素试验(反应、黑色素絮状试验),疟疾黑色素试验(诊断疟疾的一种血清絮状反应,用牛眼黑素甲醛悬液加在可疑血清上,是一种非特异性试验,视血清中的优球蛋白增多以及黑素的沉淀而定)

Hensen's body [ˈhensen] (Victor Hensen) 亨森体(螺旋器外毛细胞膜下的圆形高尔基〈Golgi〉网) | ~ canal, ~ duct 连合管 / ~ cell 亨森细胞(覆盖科尔蒂〈Corti〉器最外层的支持细胞) / ~ disk 亨森盘(H 盘,横纹肌盘) / ~ knot, ~ node 亨森结,原结(原线颅端的细胞集团) / ~ line 亨森线(即 M band,见 band 项下相应术语)

Henshaw test [ˈhenʃau] (Russell Henshaw) 亨肖试验(为特定病例选择适当顺势疗法药物的一种辅助试验,当患者血清与按顺势疗法适宜该病例的强化药物接触时,将出现可见的絮凝带)

Hensing's ligament (fold) [ˈhensiŋ] (Frederich W. Hensing) 亨辛韧带(皱襞)(由降结肠上端至腹壁的小浆膜皱襞)

HEP hepatoerythropoietic porphyria 肝性红细胞生成性卟啉病

Hepacivirus [heˈpæsiˌvaiərəs] *n* 丙型肝炎病毒属

Hepadnaviridae [hepˌædnəˈviridiː] *n* 嗜肝 DNA 病毒科

Hepadnavirus [hepˈædnəˌvaiərəs] *n* 嗜肝 DNA 病毒属

hepadnavirus [hepˈædnəˌvaiərəs] *n* 嗜肝 DNA 病毒

hepar [ˈhiːpɑː] *n*【希】肝;动物肝脏(用作药物制剂);肝样或肝脏色物质 | ~ adiposum 脂[肪]肝 / ~ lobatum 分叶肝 / ~ siccatum 肝粉 / ~ sulfuris 硫肝,含硫钾

heparan-α-glucosaminide *N*-acetyltransferase [ˈhepəræn ˌgluːkəuˈsæminaid ˌæsitilˈtrænsfəreis] 类肝素-α-氨基葡糖苷 *N*-乙酰转移酶(此酶缺乏为一种常染色体隐性性状,可致桑菲利波〈Sanfilippo〉综合征 C 型。亦称乙酰辅酶 A-α-氨基葡糖苷-*N*-乙酰转移酶)

heparan *N*-sulfatase [ˈhepəræn ˈsʌlfəteis] 类肝素 *N*-硫酸酯酶(此酶缺乏,为一种常染色体隐性性状,可致桑菲利波〈Sanfilippo〉综合征 A 型)

heparan sulfate [ˈhepəræn] 硫酸类肝素(为若干黏多糖贮积症的蓄积物)

heparan sulfate sulfamidase [ˈhepəræn ˈsʌlfeit sʌlˈfæmideis] 硫酸类肝素磺酰胺酶,类肝素 *N*-硫酸酯酶

heparin [ˈhepərin] *n* 肝素(抗凝药) | ~ sodium 肝素钠

heparinate [ˈhepərineit] *n* 肝素盐

heparinemia [ˌhepəriˈniːmiə] *n* 肝素血

heparinize [ˈhepəriˌnaiz] *vt* 肝素化(利用肝素增加血液凝固时间)

heparitin sulfate [ˈhepəritin] 硫酸乙酰肝素

hepat- 见 hepato-

hepatalgia [ˌhepəˈtældʒiə] *n* 肝痛

hepatatrophia [ˌhepətəˈtrəufiə], **hepatatrophy** [ˌhepəˈtætrəfi] *n* 肝萎缩

hepatectomize [ˌhepəˈtektəmaiz] *vt* 肝切除

hepatectomy [ˌhepəˈtektəmi] *n* 肝切除术

hepatic [hiˈpætik] *a* 肝的;肝状的;肝色的

hepatic lipase [hiˈpætik ˈlaipeis] 肝性脂[肪]酶

hepatic(o)- [构词成分]肝管;肝

hepaticocholangiojejunostomy [hiˌpætikəukəuˌlændʒiəˌdʒidʒuˈnɔstəmi] *n* 肝管胆管空肠吻合术

hepaticocholedochostomy [hiˌpætikəukəuˌledəˈkɔstəmi] *n* 肝管胆总管吻合术

hepaticodochotomy [hiˌpætikəudeˈkɔtəmi] *n* 肝管切开术

hepaticoduodenostomy [hiˌpætikəuˌdju(ː)əudiˈnɔstəmi] *n* 肝管十二指肠吻合术

hepaticoenterostomy [hiˌpætikəuˌentəˈrɔstəmi] *n* 肝管[小]肠吻合术

hepaticogastrostomy [hiˌpætikəugæsˈtrɔstəmi] *n* 肝管胃吻合术

hepaticojejunostomy [hiˌpætikəuˌdʒidʒuːˈnɔstəmi] *n* 肝管空肠吻合术

Hepaticola [ˌhepəˈtikələ] *n* 毛细线虫属(即 Capillaria)

hepaticoliasis [hiˌpætikəuˈlaiəsis] *n* 肝毛细线

虫病

hepaticolithotomy [hiˌpætikəuliˈθɔtəmi] *n* 肝管[切开]取石术

hepaticolithotripsy [hiˌpætikəuˈliθətripsi] *n* 肝管碎石术

hepaticopulmonary [hiˌpætikəuˈpʌlmənəri] *a* 肝肺的

hepaticostomy [hiˌpætiˈkɔstəmi] *n* 肝管造口术

hepaticotomy [hiˌpætiˈkɔtəmi] *n* 肝管切开术

hepatic phosphorylase [hiˈpætik fɔsˈfɔrileis] 肝性磷酸化酶(糖原磷酸化酶的肝同工酶)

hepatic phosphorylase deficiency 肝性磷酸化酶缺乏症,糖原贮积症Ⅵ型

hepatic phosphorylase kinase [hiˈpætik fɔsˈfɔrileis ˈkaineis] 肝性磷酸化酶激酶(磷酸化酶激酶的肝同工酶)

hepatic phosphorylase kinase deficiency 肝性磷酸化酶激酶缺乏症,磷酸化酶 b 激酶缺乏症

hepatin [ˈhepətin] *n* 糖原,动物淀粉

hepatism [ˈhepətizəm] *n* 肝[脏]病(状态)

hepatitis [ˌhepəˈtaitis] ([复] **hepatitides** [ˌhepəˈtitidiːz]) *n* 肝炎 | ~ A 甲型肝炎 / ~B 乙型肝炎 / cholangiolitic ~ 毛细胆管炎性肝炎 / cholangitic ~ 胆管炎性肝炎 / cholestatic ~ 淤胆型肝炎 / chronic active ~, chronic aggressive ~ 慢性活动性肝炎 / chronic interstitial ~ 慢性间质性肝炎,肝硬变 / chronic persisting ~ 慢性迁移性肝炎 / ~ contagiosa canis, canine virus ~ 犬触染性肝炎 / delta ~ 丁型肝炎 / duck virus ~ 鸭病毒性肝炎 / familial ~ 家族性肝炎,进行性豆状核变性 / fulminant ~ 急性重型肝炎 / infectious ~, epidemic ~ 传染性肝炎,流行性肝炎 / long-incubation ~ 长潜伏期肝炎(即乙型肝炎) / lupoid ~ 狼疮样肝炎 / MS-1 ~ MS-1 肝炎(即甲型肝炎) / MS-2 ~ MS-2 肝炎(即乙型肝炎) / neonatal ~, giant cell ~, neonatal giant cell ~ 新生儿肝炎,巨细胞性肝炎,新生儿巨细胞性肝炎 / plasma cell ~ 浆细胞性肝炎 / serum ~, homologous serum ~, inoculation ~ 血清肝炎,同种血清肝炎,接种后肝炎(即乙型肝炎) / short-incubation ~ 短潜伏期肝炎(即甲型肝炎) / subacute ~ 亚急性肝炎 / posttransfusion ~, transfusion ~ 输血后肝炎,输血性肝炎 / viral ~ 病毒性肝炎

hepatization [ˌhepətaiˈzeiʃən, -tiˈz-] *n* 肝样变 | gray ~ 灰色肝样变 / red ~ 红色肝样变 / yellow ~ 黄色肝样变

hepatized [ˈhepətaizd] *a* 肝样变的

hepat(o)- [构词成分]肝

hepatobiliary [ˌhepətəuˈbiljəri] *a* 肝胆的,肝胆管的

hepatoblastoma [ˌhepətəublæsˈtəumə] *n* 肝胚细胞瘤

hepatobronchial [ˌhepətəuˈbrɔŋkiəl] *a* 肝支气管的

hepatocarcinogen [ˌhepətəukɑːˈsinədʒən] *n* 致肝癌物

hepatocarcinogenesis [ˌhepətəu ˌkɑːsinəu ˈdʒenisis] *n* 肝癌发生

hepatocarcinogenic [ˌhepətəuˌkɑːsinəuˈdʒenik] *a* 引起肝癌的

hepatocarcinoma [ˌhepətəuˌkɑːsiˈnəumə] *n* 肝癌,肝细胞癌

hepatocele [hiˈpætəsiːl] *n* 肝突出

hepatocellular [ˌhepətəuˈseljulə] *a* 肝细胞的

hepatocholangeitis [ˌhepətəukəuˌlændʒiˈaitis] *n* 肝胆管炎

hepatocholangiocarcinoma [ˌhepətəukəuˌlændʒiəuˌkɑːsiˈnəumə] *n* 胆管肝细胞癌,胆管肝细胞瘤

hepatocholangioduodenostomy [ˌhepətəukəuˌlændʒiəuˌdju(ː)əudiˈnɔstəmi] *n* 肝管十二指肠吻合术

hepatocholangioenterostomy [ˌhepətəukəuˌlændʒiəuˌentəˈrɔstəmi] *n* 肝管[小]肠吻合术

hepatocholangiogastrostomy [ˌhepətəukəuˌlændʒiəugæsˈtrɔstəmi] *n* 肝管胃吻合术

hepatocholangiostomy [ˌhepətəukəuˌlændʒiˈɔstəmi] *n* 胆管造口[引流]术 | external ~ 胆管造外口术 / internal ~ 胆管造内口术

hepatocholangitis [ˌhepətəuˌkəulænˈdʒaitis] *n* 肝胆管炎

hepatocirrhosis [ˌhepətəusiˈrəusis] *n* 肝硬变

hepatocolic [ˌhepətəuˈkɔlik] *a* 肝结肠的

hepatocuprein [ˌhepətəuˈkjuːprin] *n* 肝铜蛋白,超氧物歧化酶

hepatocystic [ˌhepətəuˈsistik] *a* 肝胆囊的

Hepatocystis [ˌhepətəuˈsistis] *n* 肝囊原虫属

hopatocyto [ˈhepətəsait] *n* 肝细胞

hepatoduodenostomy [ˌhepətəuˌdju(ː)əudiˈnɔstəmi] *n* 肝十二指肠吻合术

hepatodynia [ˌhepətəuˈdiniə] *n* 肝痛

hepatodystrophy [ˌhepətəuˈdistrəfi] *n* 急性黄色肝萎缩

hepatoenteric [ˌhepətəuenˈterik] *a* 肝小肠的

hepatoenterostomy [ˌhepətəuˌentəˈrɔstəmi] *n* 肝肠吻合术

hepatoflavin [ˌhepətəuˈfleivin] *n* 肝核黄素

hepatofugal [ˌhepəˈtɔfjugəl] *a* 离肝的

hepatogastric [ˌhepətəuˈgæstrik] *a* 肝胃的

hepatogenic [ˌhepətəuˈdʒenik], **hepatogenous** [ˌhepəˈtɔdʒinəs] *a* 肝源性的

hepatoglycemia glycogenetica [ˌhepətəuglaiˈsiːmiə ˌglaikəudʒiˈnetikə] 糖元病,糖元贮积症

hepatogram [ˈhepətəgræm] *n* 肝搏动描记波;肝X线[照]片
hepatography [ˌhepəˈtɔgrəfi] *n* 肝脏论;肝搏动描记法;肝X线摄影[术]
hepatoid [ˈhepətɔid] *a* 肝[质]样的
hepatojugular [ˌhepətəuˈdʒʌgjulə] *a* 肝颈静脉的
hepatolenticular [ˌhepətəulenˈtikjulə] *a* 肝豆状核的
hepatolienal [ˌhepətəulaiˈiːnəl] *a* 肝脾的
hepatolienography [ˌhepətəuˌlaiəˈnɔgrəfi] *n* 肝脾X线摄影[术]
hepatolienomegaly [ˌhepətəuˌlaiənəuˈmegəli] *n* 肝脾大
hepatolith [ˈhepətəˌliθ] *n* 肝石(尤指肝内胆结石)
hepatolithectomy [ˌhepətəuliˈθektəmi] *n* 肝石切除术
hepatolithiasis [ˌhepətəuliˈθaiəsis] *n* 肝内胆管结石病
hepatology [ˌhepəˈtɔlədʒi] *n* 肝脏病学,肝脏学 | **hepatologist** *n* 肝脏病学家
hepatolysin [ˌhepəˈtɔlisin] *n* 溶肝素
hepatolysis [ˌhepəˈtɔlisis] *n* 肝细胞溶解 | **hepatolytic** [ˌhepətəuˈlitik] *a* 溶解肝细胞的,溶肝的
hepatoma [ˌhepəˈtəumə] *n* 肝细胞瘤(尤指肝细胞癌) | malignant ~ 肝细胞癌
hepatomalacia [ˌhepətəuməˈleiʃiə] *n* 肝软化
hepatomegalia [ˌhepətəumiˈgeiliə] *n* 肝大 | ~ glycogenica 糖原病,糖原贮积症
hepatomegaly [ˌhepətəuˈmegəli] *n* 肝大 | glycogenic ~ 糖原病,糖原贮积症
hepatomelanosis [ˌhepətəuˌmeləˈnəusis] *n* 肝黑变病
hepatometry [ˌhepəˈtɔmitri] *n* 肝测量法
hepatomphalocele [ˌhepəˈtɔmfələˌsiːl], **hepatomphalos** [ˌhepəˈtɔmfələs] *n* 脐部肝突出
hepatonephric [ˌhepətəuˈnefrik] *a* 肝肾的
hepatonephritis [ˌhepətəuneˈfraitis] *n* 肝肾炎 | **hepatonephritic** [ˌhepətəuneˈfritik] *a*
hepatonephromegaly [ˌhepətəuˌnefrəuˈmegəli] *n* 肝肾大
hepatopancreas [ˌhepətəuˈpæŋkriəs] *n* 肝胰腺
hepatopath [ˈhepətəpæθ] *n* 肝病患者
hepatopathy [ˌhepəˈtɔpəθi] *n* 肝[脏]病
hepatoperitonitis [ˌhepətəuˌperitəˈnaitis] *n* 肝腹膜炎
hepatopetal [ˌhepəˈtɔpitl] *a* 向肝的
hepatopexy [ˌhepətəˈpeksi] *n* 肝固定术
hepatophage [ˈhepətəfeidʒ] *n* 噬肝巨细胞
hepatophlebitis [ˌhepətəufliˈbaitis] *n* 肝静脉炎
hepatophlebography [ˌhepətəufliˈbɔgrəfi] *n* 肝静脉造影[术]
hepatophlebotomy [ˌhepətəufliˈbɔtəmi] *n* 肝血吸出术
hepatopleural [ˌhepətəuˈpluərəl] *a* 肝胸膜的
hepatopneumonic [ˌhepətəunju(ː)ˈmɔnik], **hepatopulmonary** [ˌhepətəuˈpʌlmənəri] *a* 肝肺的
hepatoportal [ˌhepətəuˈpɔːtl] *a* 肝门静脉的
hepatoportoenterostomy [ˌhepətəu ˌpɔːtəˌentəˈrɔstəmi] *n* 肝门肠吻合术
hepatoptosis [ˌhepətəuˈtəusis] *n* 肝下垂;结肠定位(X线时,为肝与横膈之间的结肠定位)
hepatorenal [ˌhepətəuˈriːnl] *a* 肝肾的
hepatorrhagia [ˌhepətəuˈreidʒiə] *n* 肝出血
hepatorrhaphy [ˌhepəˈtɔrəfi] *n* 肝缝合术
hepatorrhea [ˌhepətəuˈriːə] *n* 肝液溢,胆汁分泌过多
hepatorrhexis [ˌhepətəuˈreksis] *n* 肝破裂
hepatoscan [ˈhepətəskæn] *n* 肝闪烁扫描图
hepatoscopy [ˌhepəˈtɔskəpi] *n* 肝检查
hepatosis [ˌhepəˈtəusis] *n* 肝功能病,肝功能障碍 | serous ~ 浆液性肝功能病(肝的静脉闭塞病)
hepatosolenotropic [ˌhepətəusəˌliːnəuˈtrɔpik] *a* 向毛细胆管的
hepatosplenitis [ˌhepətəuspliˈnaitis] *n* 肝脾炎
hepatosplenography [ˌhepətəuspliˈnɔgrəfi] *n* 肝脾X线摄影[术]
hepatosplenomegaly [ˌhepətəuˌspliːnəuˈmegəli] *n* 肝脾大
hepatosplenometry [ˌhepətəuspliˈnɔmitri] *n* 肝脾测量法
hepatosplenopathy [ˌhepətəuspliˈnɔpəθi] *n* 肝脾病
hepatostomy [ˌhepəˈtɔstəmi] *n* 肝造口术
hepatotherapy [ˌhepətəuˈθerəpi] *n* 肝质疗法
hepatotomy [ˌhepəˈtɔtəmi] *n* 肝切开术 | transthoracic ~ 经胸肝切开术
hepatotoxemia [ˌhepətəutɔkˈsiːmiə] *n* 肝原性毒血症
hepatotoxic [ˌhepətəuˈtɔksik], **hepatoxic** [ˌhepəˈtɔksik] *a* 肝细胞毒的
hepatotoxicity [ˌhepətəutɔkˈsisəti] *n* 肝细胞毒性
hepatotoxin [ˌhepətəuˈtɔksin] *n* 肝细胞毒素
hepatotropic [ˌhepətəuˈtrɔpik] *a* 亲肝的
Hepatovirus [ˌhepətəuˈvaiərəs] *n* 肝病毒属
Hepatozoon [ˌhepətəuˈzəuɔn] *n* 肝簇虫属
hepatozoonosis [ˌhepətəuˌzəuəuˈnəusis] *n* 肝簇虫病
hepta-, hept- [构词成分] 七,庚
heptabarbital [ˌheptəˈbɑːbitæl] *n* 庚巴比妥(催眠镇静药)
heptachromic [ˌheptəˈkrəumik] *a* 七色的;能辨

［光谱］七色的，色觉健全的
heptad ［'heptæd］ *n* 七价元素
heptadactyly ［ˌheptə'dæktili］, **heptadactylia** ［ˌheptədæk'tiliə］, **heptadactylism** ［ˌheptə'dæktilizəm］ *n* 七指畸形，七趾畸形
heptadecadienoic acid ［ˌheptəˌdekədaiiː'nəuik］十七碳二烯酸
heptadecanoic acid ［ˌheptəˌdekə'nəuik］十七［烷］酸
heptaene ［'heptəiːn］ *n* 七烯化合物
-heptaene ［构词成分］七烯，庚烯
heptaiodic acid ［ˌheptəai'ɔdik］庚碘酸，过碘酸
heptanal ［ˌheptənl］ *n* 庚醛
heptanoate ［ˌheptə'nəueit］ *n* 庚酸盐
heptanoic acid ［ˌheptə'nəuik］庚酸
heptapeptide ［ˌheptə'peptaid］ *n* 七肽
heptaploid ［'heptəplɔid］ *a* 七倍的 *n* 七倍体（含七组染色体的个体或细胞） | **~y** ［'heptəˌplɔidi］ *n* 七倍性
heptavalent ［'heptəˌveilənt, hep'tævələnt］, **heptatomic** ［ˌheptə'tɔmik］ *a* 七价的
heptoglobin ［ˌheptəu'gləubin］ *n* 庚珠蛋白
heptoglobinemia ［ˌheptəugləubi'niːmiə］ *n* 庚珠蛋白血
heptose ［'heptəus］ *n* 庚糖
heptosuria ［ˌheptəu'sjuəriə］ *n* 庚糖尿
heptozoonosis ［ˌhepətəuˌzəuə'nəusis］ *n* 肝簇虫病
heptylic acid ［hep'tilik］庚酸
herb ［əːb, həːb］ *n* 草，草本；草药 | death's ~ 颠茄叶 / vulnerary ~ 愈创草
herbaceous ［əː-, həː'beiʃəs］ *a* 草的，草本的；草质的
herbal ［'əː-, 'həːbəl］ *a* 草本植物的；草药的 *n* 草药书，本草书
herbalist ［'əː-, 'həːhəlist］ *n* 草本植物学家；草药采集者；草药医生
Herbert's operation ［'həːbət］（Major H. Herbert）赫伯特手术（巩膜楔状瓣移位，以形成过滤性瘢痕，治青光眼） | ~ pits 赫伯特小窝（沙眼边缘滤泡治愈后留下的典型缺损）
herbicide ［'əː-, 'həːbisaid］ *n* 除莠剂
herbivore ［'əː-, 'həːbivɔː］ *n* 食草动物
herbivorous ［əː-, həː'bivərəs］ *a* 草食的，食草的
herborize ［'əː-, 'həːbəraiz］ *vi* 采集植物；收集药草
Herb. recent. herbarium recentium【拉】鲜草
herbalism ［'həːbəlizəm］ *n* 药草学，草本植物学
Herbst's corpuscles ［həːbst］（Ernst F. G. Herbst）赫布斯特小体（在鸭嘴部皮肤内及鸭舌黏膜中所特有的感觉神经终器）
hereditable ［hi'reditəbl］ *a* 可遗传的
hereditary ［hi'reditəri］ *a* 遗传的
heredity ［hi'redəti］ *n* 遗传 | autosomal ~ 常染色体遗传 / sex-linked ~, X-linked ~ 性连锁遗传，X 连锁遗传
heredoataxia ［ˌheridəuə'tæksiə］ *n* 遗传性共济失调
heredobiologic ［ˌheridəubaiə'lɔdʒik］ *a* 遗传内因性的
heredodegeneration ［ˌheridəudiːˌdʒenə'reiʃən］ *n* 遗传性变性，遗传性小脑性共济失调
heredodiathesis ［ˌheridəudai'æθisis］ *n* 遗传素质
heredofamilial ［ˌheridəufə'miljəl］ *a* 家族遗传性的
heredoimmunity ［ˌheridəui'mjuːnəti］ *n* 遗传免疫，先天免疫
heredoinfection ［ˌheridəuin'fekʃən］ *n* 先天传染，胚种传染
heredolues ［ˌheridəu'ljuːiːz］ *n* 遗传梅毒，先天梅毒 | **heredoluetic** ［ˌheridəulju'etik］ *a*
heredopathia ［ˌheridəu'pæθiə］ *n* 遗传病 | ~ atactica polyneuritiformis 多神经炎型遗传性运动失调
heredoretinopathia congenita ［ˌheridəuˌretinəu-'pæθiə kən'dʒenitə］【拉】先天性遗传性视网膜病，遗传性视网膜病
heredosyphilis ［ˌheridəu'sifilis］ *n* 遗传梅毒，先天梅毒 | **heredosyphilitic** ［ˌheridəuˌsifi'litik］ *a* 遗传梅毒的，先天梅毒的 *n* 遗传梅毒患者，先天梅毒患者
heredosyphilology ［ˌheridəuˌsifi'lɔlədʒi］ *n* 遗传梅毒学，先天梅毒学
Hérelle 见 d'Hérelle
Herellea ［hi'reliə］ *n* 赫尔菌属 | ~ vaginicola 阴道赫尔菌
Herff's clamp ［həːf］（Otto von Herff）赫夫夹（一种伤口夹）
Hering-Breuer reflex ［'heriŋ 'brɔiə］（H. E. Hering; Josef R. Breuer）赫-布反射（限制呼吸旅程的神经机制。来自肺内以及或许在其他部分感觉神经末梢的刺激，通过迷走神经，限制常态呼吸的吸气和呼气）
Hering's law ［'heriŋ］（Carl E. K. Hering）赫林定律（①两眼神经支配原理：即两眼的肌肉受同等神经的支配，任何一眼不能单独运动；②任何概念或感觉的明晰程度视其强度与当时所有其他概念或感觉强度的总和之比而定） | ~ test 赫林试验（检实体视觉） / ~ theory 赫林学说（色觉取决于视质的分解和复原，异化产生红、黄、白，复原产生蓝、绿、黑）
Hering's nerve ［'heriŋ］（Heinrich E. Hering）舌咽神经颈动脉窦支 | ~ phenomenon 赫林现象（在死后的短时间内可用听诊器在胸骨下听到

轻杂音)

heritable [ˈheritəbl] *a* 可遗传的 | **heritability** [ˌheritəˈbiləti] *n* 遗传度

Herlitz's disease [ˈhəːlits] (Gillis Herlitz) 赫利兹病,交界大疱性表皮松解

Hermann-Perutz reaction [ˈhəːmænˈpeirut] (Otto Hermann; Alfred Perutz) 赫-佩反应(检梅毒)

Hermansky-Pudlak syndrome [ˈhəːmɑːnski ˈpuːdlæk] (F. Hermanski; P. Pudlak) 赫曼斯基-普德拉克综合征(一种常染色体隐性遗传的酪氨酸酶阳性眼皮肤白化病,伴有继发于血小板缺乏的出血性素质以及网状内皮系统、口腔黏膜和尿中有蜡样物质聚积)

hermaphrodite [həːˈmæfrədait] *n* 两性体,半阴阳体,雌雄同体 | pseudo-~ 假两性体 / true ~ 真两性体

hermaphroditic(al) [həːˌmæfrəˈditik(əl)] *a* 两性同体的,两性畸形的,半阴阳的;雌雄同体的

hermaphroditism [həːˈmæfrədaiˌtizəm] *n* 两性同体,两性畸形,半阴阳;雌雄同体性 | bilateral ~ 双侧两性畸形 / ~ with excess 过余性两性畸形 / false ~, spurious ~ 假两性畸形,假半阴阳 / lateral ~, dimidiate ~ 异侧两性畸形 / protandrous ~ 先男后女两性畸形 / protogynous ~ 先女后男两性畸形 / transverse ~ 内外异性畸形 / true ~ 真两性畸形 / unilateral ~ 单侧两性畸形 | **hermaphrodism** [həːˈmæfrədizəm] *n*

hermaphroditismus [həːˌmæfrədaiˈtizməs] *n* 【拉】两性畸形,半阴阳,阴阳体 | ~ verus 真阴阳体,真两性畸形 / ~ verus bilateralis 双侧真阴阳体,双侧两性畸形 / ~ verus lateralis 单侧真阴阳体,异侧两性畸形 / ~ verus unilateralis 单侧真阴阳体,单侧两性畸形

Hermetia illucens [həːˈmiːʃiə iˈljuːsənz] 光亮扁角水虻(其幼虫可引起人类感染肠蝇蛆病或假蝇蛆病)

hermetic(al) [həːˈmetik(əl)] *a* 密封的,不漏气的

Hermodsson's projection [ˈhəːmədsn] (I. Hermodsson)赫莫德松投照(一种罕见型放射投照,以评估不稳定的肩关节反复脱位,并有些微病情诸如希-萨〈Hill-Sachs〉损害;令患者站立,受患上肢置于背后,其手置于腰椎上,中心射线侧向从下后方向进入肩胛)

hernia [ˈhəːnjə] ([复] **hernias** 或 **herniae** [ˈhəːniiː]) *n* 【拉】疝,突出 | abdominal ~ 腹疝 / acquired ~ 后天性疝 / ~ of bladder 膀胱疝 / concealed ~ 隐匿性疝 / cystic ~ 膀胱疝,膀胱突出 / direct ~ 直疝 / dry ~ 粘连性疝 / duodenojejunal ~ 十二指肠空肠窝疝 / encysted ~ 包绕性腹股沟疝 / femoral ~, crural ~, gluteal ~ 股疝 / foraminal ~ 网膜孔疝 / funicular ~ 精索突出 / hiatal ~, hiatus ~ 食管裂孔疝 / incarcerated ~ 箝闭性疝 / incisional ~ 切口疝(经腹部旧切口的疝) / indirect ~ 斜疝(腹股沟) / infantile ~ 婴儿型疝(腹膜精索突后面的腹股沟斜疝) / inguinal ~ 腹股沟疝 / intermuscular ~, interparietal ~, interstitial ~ 腹壁间层疝 / irreducible ~ 难复性疝 / ischiatic ~ 坐骨孔疝 / ischiorectal ~, perineal ~ 坐骨直肠窝疝,会阴疝 / labial ~ 阴唇疝 / mucosal ~, tunicary ~ 肠壁黏膜[层]突出 / oblique ~ 斜疝 / obturator ~, subpubic ~, thyroidal ~ 闭孔疝 / omental ~ 网膜突出 / ovarian ~ 卵巢突出 / paraperitoneal ~ 腹膜旁疝 / parietal ~ 肠壁疝 / pudendal ~, levator ~ 阴部疝 / ~ of pulp 牙髓息肉,[牙]髓疝 / pulsion ~ 腹压增高性疝,内压性疝 / rectovaginal ~ 直肠突出 / reducible ~ 可复性疝 / retrograde ~, w ~ 逆行性疝(肠突出两个襻,两襻之间的肠段在腹腔内) / retroperitoneal ~ 腹膜后疝 / sciatic ~ 坐骨大孔疝 / scrotal ~ 阴囊[腹股沟]疝 / sliding ~, slip ~, slipped ~, extrasaccular ~, parasaccular ~, ~ par glissement 滑动性疝 / spigelian ~ 半月线疝 / strangulated ~ 绞窄性疝 / synovial ~ 滑膜突出 / tonsillar ~ 小脑扁桃体[枕大孔]突出 / umbilical ~ 脐疝 / uterine ~ 子宫突出 / vaginolabial ~, posterior labial ~ 阴唇阴道突出,阴唇后疝 / ventral ~ 腹壁疝 / vesical ~ 膀胱突出 | **~l**, **herniary** [ˈhəːnjəri] *a*

herniate [ˈhəːnieit] *vi* 疝形成,突出 | **~d** *a* 成疝的,突出的

herniation [ˌhəːniˈeiʃən] *n* 疝出,突出 | ~ of intervertebral disk 椎间盘突出 / ~ of nucleus pulposus 髓核突出 / painful fat ~ 痛性脂肪突出,痛性脂肪疝,压力性丘疹(即 piezogenic papules) / transtentorial ~, uncal ~ 穿小脑幕突出,小脑幕疝

hernioappendectomy [ˌhəːniəuˌæpənˈdektəmi] *n* 疝阑尾切除术

hernioenterotomy [ˌhəːniəuˌentəˈrɔtəmi] *n* 肠疝切开术

hernioid [ˈhəːniɔid] *a* 疝样的

herniolaparotomy [ˌhəːniəuˌlæpəˈrɔtəmi] *n* 剖腹治疝术

herniology [ˌhəːniˈɔlədʒi] *n* 疝学

hernioplasty [ˈhəːniəˌplæsti] *n* 疝根治术,疝整复术

herniopuncture [ˌhəːniəuˈpʌŋktʃə] *n* 疝穿刺术

herniorrhaphy [ˌhəːniˈɔrəfi] *n* 疝修补术

herniotomy [ˌhəːniˈɔtəmi] *n* 疝切开术

heroic(al) [hiˈrəuik(əl)] *a* 英雄的;崇高的;大剂量的

heroin [ˈherəuin] *n* 海洛因,二乙酰吗啡(镇痛药,镇咳药)

heroinism [ˈherəuinizəm], **heroinomania** [ˌherəuˌinəˈmeinje] *n* 海洛因瘾
heroism [ˈherəuizəm] *n* 英雄行为,英雄主义
herpangina [ˌhəːpænˈdʒainə] *n* 疱疹性咽峡炎
herpes [ˈhəːpiːz] *n*【拉;希】疱疹 | ~ corneae 角膜疱疹 / ~ digitalis 指单纯疱疹 / ~ facialis 面疱疹 / ~ febrilis 发热性疱疹 / genital ~, ~ genitalis, ~ progenitalis 生殖器疱疹,包皮疱疹 / ~ gestationis 妊娠疱疹 / ~ labialis 唇疱疹 / ~ simplex 单纯疱疹 / traumatic ~, ~ gladiatorum, wrestler's ~ 外伤性疱疹,格斗性疱疹,摔跤者疱疹 / ~ zoster auricularis 耳带状疱疹 / ~ zoster ophthalmicus, ~ ophthalmicus 眼带状疱疹 / ~ zoster oticus 耳带状疱疹
herpesencephalitis [ˌhəːpiːzenˌsefəˈlaitis] *n* 疱疹脑炎
herpesviral [ˈhəːpiːzˌvaiərəl] *a* 疱疹病毒的
Herpesviridae [ˌhəːpiːzˈvaiəridiː] *n* 疱疹病毒科
herpesvirus [ˈhəːpiːzˌvaiərəs] *n* 疱疹病毒
Herpesvirus hominis [ˈhəːpiːzˌvaiərəs ˈhɔminis] 人疱疹病毒
herpetic [həːˈpetik] *a* 疱疹的;疱疹病毒的
herpetiform [həːˈpetifɔːm] *a* 疱疹样的
herpet(o)- [构词成分] 疱疹;蛇,爬行动物,爬行
herpetology [ˌhəːpəˈtɔlədʒi] *n* 爬虫学,爬行类学 | **herpetologist** *n* 爬虫学家,爬行类学家
Herpetomonas [ˌhəːpiˈtɔmənəs] *n* 匐滴虫属
herpetophobia [həːˌpetəuˈfəubjə] *n* 爬虫恐怖,恐虫症
Herpetosiphon [ˌhəːpitəuˈsaifən] *n* 滑柱菌属
Herpetosoma [həːˌpetəuˈsəumə] *n* 蛇滴虫亚属
Herrick's anemia [ˈherik] (James B. Herrick) 镰状细胞性贫血
Herring bodies [ˈheriŋ] (Percy T. Herring) 赫林体(散见于脑垂体神经部的玻璃样或胶态团块)
herringbone [ˈheriŋbəun] *a* 人字形的
Herrmannsdorfer diet [ˌhəːmænsˈdɔːfə] (Adolf Herrmannsdorfer) 赫氏饮食(少脂及蛋白质无盐饮食,治狼疮及结核病)
Herrmann's syndrome [həːmən] (Christian Herrmann, Junior) 赫尔曼综合征(一种常染色体显性遗传综合征,开始表现为光致肌阵挛发作和进行性聋,以后发展成糖尿病、肾病和精神衰退直至痴呆)
hersage [ɛəˈsɑːʒ] *n*【法】周围神经纤维松解法
Hers' disease [ɛəz] (Henri-Géry Hers) 赫斯病,糖原贮积症Ⅵ型
Herter-Heubner disease [ˈhəːtə ˈhɔibnə] (C. A. Herter; Johann O. L. Heubner) 赫脱-霍伊布内病(婴儿型非热带口炎性腹泻,乳糜泻)
Herter's disease (infantilism) [ˈhəːtə] (Christian A. Herter) 赫脱病(幼稚型)(婴儿型非热带性口炎性腹泻) | ~ test 赫脱试验(检吲哚;检粪臭素)
Hertig-Rock ova [ˈhəːtig rok] (Arthur T. Hertig; John Rock) 赫蒂格-罗克受精卵(自 1938 至 1953 年发现的 34 个受精卵,年龄为 1 ~ 17 天,其中 13 个为程度不等的异常卵,21 个为正常卵,为现存此种早期人类孕体的唯一成组标本)
Hertwig-Magendie phenomenon, sign [ˈhəːtvig mɑːʒæŋˈdiː] (Richard Hertwig; François Magendie) 赫特维希-马让迪现象、征,(眼球)反侧偏斜(skew deviation,见 deviation 项下相应术语)
Hertwig's sheath [ˈhəːtvig] (Richard Hertwig) 赫特维希鞘,根鞘(root sheath,见 sheath 项下相应术语)
hertz(Hz) [həːts] *n* 赫[兹](频率单位,每秒周数)
hertzian waves (rays) [ˈhəːtsiən] (Heinrich R. Hertz) 赫兹电波(类似光波的电波,但波长较长,用于无线电报)
HERV human endogenous retroviruses 人内源性反转录病毒
Herxheimer's fever [ˈhəːkshaimə] (Karl Herxheimer) 赫克斯海默热(有时伴随雅里希-赫克斯海默〈Jarisch-Herxheimer〉反应而来的发热) | ~ fibers(spirals) 赫克斯海默纤维(皮肤黏膜层小螺旋纤维) / ~ reaction 赫克斯海默反应,治疗加重反应(见 Jarisch-Herxheimer reaction)
Heryng's sign [ˈheriŋ] (Teodor Heryng) 赫林征(用电光透照口腔,如系上颌窦积脓,可见眶下部阴影)
herztod [ˈhəːtstəut] *n* 猪应激综合征
Heschl's gyrus (convolutions) [ˈhəʃl] (Richard L. Heschl) 颞横回
hesperanopia [ˌhesperəˈnəupiə] *n* 夜盲症(昼视)
hesperidin [hesˈperidin] *n* 橙皮苷(存在于某些柑橘果中,据报道可减少毛细血管脆性)
Hess capillary test [hes] (Alfred Hess) 黑斯毛细血管试验(检毛细血管脆性)
Hesselbach's hernia [ˈhesəlbɑːh] (Franz K. Hesselbach) 黑塞尔巴赫疝,筛筋膜疝(憩室经筛筋膜突出成疝) | ~ ligament 凹间韧带 / ~ triangle 腹股沟三角
hetacillin [ˌhetəˈsilin] *n* 海他西林(半合成的青霉素,抗生素类药) | ~ potassium 海他西林钾
hetaflur [ˈhetəfluː] *n* 氢氟酸十六胺(防龋药)
hetastarch [ˈhetəstɑːtʃ] *n* 羟乙基淀粉,淀粉羟乙基醚(血浆容量扩充药)
HETE hydroxyeicosatetraenoic acid 羟基二十碳四烯酸
heter- 见 hetero-
heteradelphia [ˌhetərəˈdelfiə] *n* 大小体联胎[畸形]

heteradelphus [ˌhetərəˈdelfəs] *n* 大小体联胎畸胎

heteradenia [ˌhetərəˈdiːniə] *n* 腺组织异常 | **heteradenic** [ˌhetərəˈdenik] *a*

Heterakidae [ˌhetəˈrækidiː] *n* 异刺线虫科

Heterakis [ˌhetəˈreikis] *n* 异刺线虫属 | ~ gallinae 鸡异刺线虫

heteralius [ˌhetəˈreiliəs] *n* 大小迥异联胎畸胎

heterauxesis [ˌhetərɔːkˈziːsis] *n* 不对称发育,异速生长

heteraxial [ˌhetəˈræksiəl] *a* 长短不等轴的,复轴的

heterecious [ˌhetəˈriːʃəs] *a* 异栖的,异种[宿主]寄生性的 | **heterecism** [ˌhetəˈriːsizəm] *n* 异栖,异种[宿生]寄生

heterergic [ˌhetəˈrəːdʒik] *a* 异效的(指两种不同药物具有不同作用,一种有特别的作用,另一种则无)

heteresthesia [ˌhetərisˈθiːzjə] *n* 差异感觉(体表相邻区域皮肤敏感性有差异)

heter(o)- [构词成分] 异,不同;杂

heteroagglutination [ˌhetərəuəˌgluːtiˈneiʃən] *n* 异种凝集反应

heteroagglutinin [ˌhetərəuəˈgluːtinin] *n* 异种凝集素

heteroalbumose [ˌhetərəuˈælbjuməus] *n* 杂脲,异脲,不溶性半[蛋白]脲

heteroalbumosuria [ˌhetərəuˌælbjuməuˈsjuəriə] *n* 杂脲尿

heteroallele [ˌhetərəuəˈliːl] *n* 异点等位基因 | **heteroallelic** *a*

heteroantibody [ˌhetərəuˈæntiˌbɔdi] *n* 异种抗体

heteroantigen [ˌhetərəuˈæntidʒən] *n* 异种抗原

heteroatom [ˌhetərəuˈætəm] *n* 杂原子

heteroautoplasty [ˌhetərəuˈɔːtəplæsti] *n* 自身异位移植

heteroauxin [ˌhetərəuˈɔːksin] *n* 吲哚乙酸,异植物生长素

Heterobasidiomycetidae [ˌhetərəubəˌsidiəumaiˈsiːtidiː] *n* 异担子菌亚纲

Heterobilharzia [ˌhetərəubilˈhɑːziə] *n* 异毕吸虫属 | ~ americana 美洲异毕吸虫

heteroblastic [ˌhetərəuˈblæstik] *a* 异生的

heterocaryon [ˌhetərəuˈkæriɔn] *n* 异核体

heterocellular [ˌhetərəuˈseljulə] *a* 异种细胞的,异型细胞构成的

heterocentric [ˌhetərəuˈsentrik] *a* 复心的,散乱的(指光线)

heterocephalus [ˌhetərəuˈsefələs] *n* 大小[双]头畸胎

heterochiral [ˌhetərəuˈkaiərəl] *a* 左右异向的,左右相反的

Heterochlorida [ˌhetərəuˈklɔːridə] *n* 异鞭目

heterochromatin [ˌhetərəuˈkrəumətin] *n* 异染色质 | constitutive ~ 结构异染色质,组成异染色质 / facultative ~ 功能性异染色质,兼性异染色质

heterochromatinization [ˌhetərəuˌkrəumətinaiˈzeiʃən, -niˈz-] *n* 异染色质化;莱昂化作用(即 lyonization, X 染色体失活) | **heterochromatization** [ˌheterəuˌkrəumətaiˈzeiʃən, -tiˈz-] *n*

heterochromia [ˌhetərəuˈkrəumiə] *n* 异色性 | ~ iridis 虹膜异色 | **heterochromatosis** [ˌhetərəuˌkrəuməˈtəusis] *n*

heterochromosome [ˌhetərəuˈkrəuməsəum] *n* 异染色体(一种性染色体)

heterochromous [ˌhetərəuˈkrəuməs] *a* 异色的

heterochron [ˌhetərəuˈkrəun] *a* 异时值的,不等时值的

heterochronia [ˌhetərəuˈkrəuniə] *n* 异时性;异时发生 | **heterochronic** [ˌhetərəuˈkrɔnik], **heterochronous** [ˌhetəˈrɔkrənəs] *a* 异时[发生]的

heterochthonous [ˌhetəˈrɔkθənəs] *a* 异地发生的

heterochylia [ˌhetərəuˈkailiə] *n* 胃酸突变

heterocinesia [ˌhetərəusiˈniːsiə] *n* 动作倒错,动作异常

heterocladic [ˌhetərəuˈklædik] *a* 异支吻合的(指不同动脉末梢支之间的吻合)

heterocomplement [ˌhetərəuˈkɔmplimənt] *n* 异种补体

heterocrine [ˈhetərəkriːn] *a* 多种分泌的

heterocrisis [ˌhetəˈrɔkrisis] *n* 异常危象

heterocyclic [ˌhetərəuˈsaiklik] *a* 杂环的

heterocytolysin [ˌhetərəusaiˈtɔlisin] *n* 异种细胞溶素

heterocytotoxin [ˌhetərəuˌsaitəuˈtɔksin] *n* 异种细胞毒素

heterocytotropic [ˌhetərəuˌsaitəuˈtrɔpik] *a* 亲异种细胞的(如抗体)

Heterodera radicicola [ˌhetəˈrɔdərə ˌrædiˈsikələ] 住根异皮线虫

heterodermic [ˌhetərəuˈdəːmik] *a* 异体皮肤的(移植)

heterodesmotic [ˌhetərəudesˈmɔtik] *a* 异联的,连结不同部分的(神经纤维)

heterodimer [ˌhetərəuˈdaimə] *n* 杂二聚体

heterodont [ˈhetərədɔnt] *a* 异型牙的

Heterodoxus [ˌhetərəuˈdɔksəs] *n* 异袋鼠虱属

heterodromous [ˌhetəˈrɔdrəməs] *a* 反向运动的,异向的

heterodymus [ˌhetəˈrɔdiməs], **heterodidymus** [ˌhetərəuˈdidiməs] *n* 附头联胎

heteroecious [ˌhetərəuˈiːʃəs] *a* 异寄主的(指需要两种或两种以上寄主才能完成其生活史的,

如某些真菌和昆虫）
heteroeroticism [ˌhetərəuiˈrɔtisizəm] *n* 异体性欲，异体恋 | **heteroerotism** [ˌhetərəuˈerətizəm] *n*
heterofermentation [ˌhetərəuˌfəːmenˈteiʃən] *n* 异型发酵
heterofermenter [ˌhetərəufəːˈmentə] *n* 杂发酵菌（发酵时除产生大量乳酸外，还产生醋酸、乙醇和二氧化碳）
heterogamete [ˌhetərəuˈgæmiːt, ˌhetərəugəˈmiːt] *n* 异形配子 | **heterogametic** [ˌhetərəugəˈmetik] *a*
heterogamety [ˌhetərəuˈgæmiti] *n* 配子异型，异形配子形成
heterogamous [ˌhetəˈrɔgəməs] *a* 具异型配子的 | **heterogamy** [ˌhetəˈrɔgəmi] *n* 配子异形；异配生殖
heteroganglionic [ˌhetərəuˌgæŋgliˈɔnik] *a* 不同神经节的
heterogeneity [ˌhetərəudʒiˈniːəti] *n* 异种性，异质性（遗传学中指由于不同遗传机制产生相同的或类似的表现型）；不均匀性，多相性 | genetic ~ 遗传异质性（一个以上的基因型产生一种特殊的临床或生化表现型） | **heterogenicity** [ˌhetərəudʒiˈnisəti] *n*
heterogeneous [ˌhetərəuˈdʒiːnjəs] *a* 异种的，异质的；异种基因的，不均匀的；多相的
heterogenesis [ˌhetərəuˈdʒenisis], **heterogony** [ˌhetəˈrɔgəni] *n* 异型生殖，异型世代交替；无性世代；自然发生 | **heterogenetic** [ˌhetərəudʒiˈnetik], **heterogonous** [ˌhetəˈrɔgənəs] *a*
heterogenic [ˌhetərəuˈdʒenik] *a*（错发生于）异性的（如妇女长胡须）；异原的，异种的，异型的
heterogenote [ˈhetərəuˌdʒiːnəut] *n* 异基因细胞，杂基因子
heterogenous [ˌhetəˈrɔdʒinəs] *a* 异原的；异种的，异型的
heterogeusia [ˌhetərəuˈgjuːziə] *n* 味觉异常，味觉倒错
heteroglobulose [ˌhetərəuˈglɔbjuləus] *n* 杂球胨，异球胨
heterograft [ˈhetərəgrɑːft] *n* 异种移植物
heterography [ˌhetəˈrɔgrəfi] *n* 书写异常，错写症，异写症 | **heterographic** [ˌhetərəu ˈgræfik] *a*
heterohemagglutination [ˌhetərəu ˌheməˌgluːtiˈneiʃən] *n* 异种血凝反应，异种血细胞凝集［作用］
heterohemagglutinin [ˌhetərəuˌheməˈgluːtinin] *n* 异种血凝素，异种血细胞凝集素
heterohemolysin [ˌhetərəuhiːˈmɔlisin] *n* 异种溶血素
heterohexosan [ˌhetərəuˈheksəsæn] *n* 杂己聚糖
Heterohyrax [ˌhetərəuˈhairæks] *n* 异岩狸属
heteroimmunity [ˌhetərəuiˈmjuːnəti] *n* 异种免疫 | **heteroimmune** [ˌhetərəuiˈmjuːn] *a*
heteroinfection [ˌhetərəuinˈfekʃən] *n* 异种传染，外源性传染
heteroinoculable [ˌhetərəuiˈnɔkjuləbl] *a* 可异体接种的
heteroinoculation [ˌhetərəuiˌnɔkjuˈleiʃən] *n* 异种接种
heterointoxication [ˌhetərəuinˌtɔksiˈkeiʃən] *n* 外源性中毒
heterokaryon [ˌhetərəuˈkæriɔn] *n* 异核体
heterokaryosis [ˌhetərəukæriˈəusis] *n* 异核体形成，异核性，异核现象
heterokeratoplasty [ˌhetərəuˈkerətəuˌplæsti] *n* 异种角膜成形术，异种角膜移植术
heterokinesis [ˌhetərəukaiˈniːsis] *n* 异化分裂（指性染色体）
heterolactic [ˌhetərəuˈlæktik] *a* 杂乳酸的（指细菌性发酵，产生大量乳酸，伴随着乙酸、乙醇和二氧化碳）
heterolalia [ˌhetərəuˈleiliə] *n* 异语症，错语症
heterolateral [ˌhetərəuˈlætərəl] *a* 对侧的
heteroliteral [ˌhetərəuˈlitərəl] *a* 错［字］音的
heterolith [ˈhetərəliθ] *n* 异质肠石（非矿物质组成）
heterologous [ˌhetəˈrɔləgəs] *a* 异组织的（非该部正常组织组成的）；异源的，异种的；异系的，异性的 | **heterology** [ˌhetəˈrɔlədʒi] *n* 异源性，异种性；异系性
heterolysin [ˌhetəˈrɔlisin] *n* 异种溶素
heterolysis [ˌhetəˈrɔlisis] *n* 异种溶解（指细胞）；异种裂解，异裂（指原子间的化学键断裂） | **heterolytic** [ˌhetərəuˈlitik] *a*
heterolysosome [ˌhetərəuˈlaisəsəum] *n* 异型溶酶体
heteromastigote [ˌhetərəuˈmæstigəut] *a* 异鞭毛的
heteromeric [ˌhetərəuˈmerik], **heteromeral** [ˌhetəˈrɔmərəl], **heteromerous** [hetəˈrɔmərəs] *a* 异侧的（神经细胞突）
heterometaplasia [ˌhetərəuˌmetəˈpleisiə] *n* 异形发育
heterometropia [ˌhetərəumiˈtrəupiə] *n* 双眼屈光差异
heteromorphosis [ˌhetərəuməˈfəusis] *n* 异形化，异形形成，形态变异
heteromorphous [ˌhetərəuˈmɔːfəs], **heteromorphic** [ˌhetərəuˈmɔːfik] *a* 异形的，异态的 | **heteromorphism** [hetərəuˈmɔːfizəm] *n* 异态性
Heteronematina [ˌheterəuˌniːməˈtainə] *n* 异眼纽虫亚目

heteronomous [ˌhetəˈrɔnəməs] *a* 受不同规律支配的,异律的;受别人支配的,不自主的

heteronymous [ˌhetəˈrɔniməs] *a* 异名的;异侧的

hetero-osteoplasty [ˌhetərəu ˈɔstiəˌplæsti] *n* 异体骨成形术

hetero-ovular [ˌheterəu ˈəuvjulə] *a* 异卵的,二卵的

heteropagus [ˌhetəˈrɔpəgəs] *n* 非对称联胎,大小体联胎

heteropancreatism [ˌhetərəuˈpæŋkriətizəm] *n* 胰腺功能异常

heteropathy [ˌhetəˈrɔpəθi] *n* 反应性异常;对抗疗法,对症疗法

heteropentosan [ˌhetərəuˈpentəsæn] *n* 杂戊聚糖

heterophagosome [ˌhetərəuˈfægəsəum] *n* 异噬体

heterophagy [ˌhetəˈrɔfədʒi] *n* 异体吞噬,异物吞噬作用

heterophany [ˌhetəˈrɔfəni] *n* 异种表现,不同表现

heterophasia [ˌhetərəuˈfeiziə], **heterophasis** [ˌhetərəuˈfeisis], **heterophemia** [ˌhetərəuˈfiːmiə] *n* 异语症,错语症

heterophil [ˈhetərəfil] *n* 嗜异细胞 *a* 嗜异性的(指对抗原或抗体);异染性的 | **heterophile** [ˈhetərəˌfail, -fil] *a*

heterophilic [ˌhetərəuˈfilik] *a* 嗜异性的(指对抗原或抗体);异染性的

heterophonia [ˌhetərəuˈfəuniə], **heterophony** [ˌhetəˈrɔfəni] *n* 声音异常,发声异常

heterophoralgia [ˌhetərəufəuˈrældʒiə] *n* 隐斜眼痛

heterophoria [ˌhetərəuˈfəuriə] *n* 隐斜 | **heterophoric** *a*

heterophosphatase [ˌhetərəuˈfɔsfəteis] *n* 己糖[磷酸]激酶

heterophthalmia [ˌhetərɔfˈθælmiə], **heterophthalmos** [ˌhetərɔfˈθælmɔs] *n* 两眼轴向不等;两眼异色

heterophthongia [ˌhetərɔfˈθɔndʒiə] *n* 言语异常

Heterophyes [ˌhetəˈrɔfiiːz] *n* 异形吸虫属 | ~ heterophyes 异形异形吸虫 / ~ katsuradai 桂田异形吸虫

heterophyiasis [ˌhetərəufiˈaiəsis], **heterophydiasis** [ˌhetərəufiˈdaiəsis] *n* 异形吸虫病

Heterophyidae [ˌhetərəuˈfaiidiː] *n* 异形吸虫科

heteroplasia [ˌhetərəuˈpleiziə] *n* 发育异常,再生异常

heteroplasm [ˈhetərəplæzəm] *n* 异种组织

heteroplastid [ˌhetərəuˈplæstid] *n* 异种移植物

heteroplasty [ˈhetərəuˌplæsti] *n* 异种移植,异种移植术,异种成形术 | **heteroplastic** [ˌhetərəu-ˈplæstik] *a* 异种移植的,异种成形的

heteroploid [ˈhetərəuˌplɔid] *a* 异倍体的 *n* 异倍体(染色体数异常的个体或细胞) | **~y** [ˈhetərəuˌplɔidi] *n* 异倍性

Heteropoda [ˌhetəˈrɔpədə] *n* 异足蛛属

heteropodal [ˌhetəˈrɔpədl] *a* 异突的(神经细胞)

heteropolymeric [ˌhetərəuˌpɔliˈmerik] *a* 杂聚的

heteropolysaccharide [ˌhetərəuˌpɔliˈsækeraid] *n* 杂多糖

heteroprosopus [ˌhetərəuˈprəusəpəs] *n* 双面畸胎,双面联胎

heteroproteose [ˌhetərəuˈprəutiəus] *n* 杂脲,异脲

heteropsia [ˌhetəˈrɔpsiə] *n* 两眼不等视

heteropsychologic [ˌhetərəuˌsaikəˈlɔdʒik] *a* 非我心理的(指不是自己心理形成的概念)

Heteroptera [ˌhetəˈrɔptərə] *n* 异翅亚目

heteroptics [ˌhetəˈrɔptiks] *n* 视觉异常

heteropyknosis [ˌhetərəupikˈnəusis] *n* 异固缩(某个染色体或染色体中某一区域,其固缩程度与其他部分有所不同的现象) | negative ~ 负异固缩(指固缩浓度较小,染色较浅) / positive ~ 正异固缩(指固缩浓度较高,染色较深)

heteropyknotic [ˌhetərəupikˈnɔtik] *a* 异固缩的 | negatively ~ 负异固缩的 / positively ~ 正异固缩的

heterosaccharide [ˌhetərəuˈsækəraid] *n* 杂多糖

heteroscedasticity [ˌhetərəuskədæsˈtisəti] *n* 方差不齐[性],异方差性

heteroscope [ˈhetərəskəup] *n* 斜视镜,斜视计 | **heteroscopy** [ˌhetəˈrɔskəpi] *n* 斜视镜检查

heteroserotherapy [ˌhetərəuˌsiərəuˈθerəpi] *n* 异体血清疗法

heterosexual [ˌhetərəuˈseksjuəl] *a* 异性的 | **~ity** [ˌhetərəuˌseksjuˈæləti] *n* 异性性欲,异性恋

heterosis [ˌhetəˈrəusis] *n* 杂种优势 | **heterotic** [ˌhetəˈrɔtik] *a*

heterosmia [ˌhetəˈrɔsmiə] *n* 嗅觉异常

heterosome [ˈhetərəsəum] *n* 性染色体,异型染色体

heterospore [ˈhetərəspɔː] *n* 异形孢子 | **heterosporous** [ˌhetəˈrɔspərəs] *a*

heterostimulation [ˌhetərəustimjuˈleiʃən] *n* 异种刺激(用不同种动物的抗原刺激动物)

heterosuggestion [ˌhetərəusəˈdʒestʃən] *n* 他人暗示

heterotaxia [ˌhetərəuˈtæksiə], **heterotaxis** [ˌhetərəuˈtæksis], **heterotaxy** [ˈhetərəuˌtæksi] *n* 内脏异位 | **heterotaxic** [ˌhetərəuˈtæksik] *a*

heterothallism [ˌhetərəuˈθælizəm] *n* 异宗配合,雌雄异株 | **heterothallic** [ˌhetərəuˈθælik] *a*

heterotherapy [ˌhetərəuˈθerəpi] *n* 抗症状疗法

(非特异性疗法)

heterotherm [ˈhetərəuθəːm] *n* 异温动物

heterothermy [ˈhetərəuˌθəːmi] *n* 异温[现象] | **heterothermic** [ˌhetərəuˈθəːmik] *a* 异温的

heterotonia [ˌhetərəuˈtəuniə] *n* 异张性,张力不等 | **heterotonic** [ˌhetərəuˈtɔnik] *a*

heterotopia [ˌhetərəuˈtəupiə], **heterotopy** [ˌhetəˈrɔtəpi] *n* 异位;语音错乱 | **heterotopic** [ˌhetərəuˈtɔpik] *a* 异位的

heterotransplant [ˌhetərəuˈtrænsplɑːnt, -plænt] *n* 异种移植物;异种移植

heterotransplantation [ˌhetərəuˌtrænsˌplɑːnˈteiʃən, -ˌplæn-] *n* 异种移植,异种移植术

Heterotrichida [ˌhetərəuˈtrikidə] *n* 异毛目

Heterotrichina [ˌhetərəutriˈkainə] *n* 异毛亚目

heterotrichosis [ˌhetərəutraiˈkəusis] *n* 毛[发]异色 | ~ superciliorum 眉异色

heterotrichous [ˌhetəˈrɔtrikəs] *a* 异纤毛的,不等纤毛的

heterotrimer [ˌhetərəuˈtraimə] *n* 异三体(至少具有一个与其他相区别的亚单位的三体)

heterotroph [ˈhetərəutrɔf] *n* 异养生物

heterotrophia [ˌhetərəuˈtrəufiə], **heterotrophy** [hetəˈrɔtrəfi] *n* 异养性;营养异常

heterotrophic [ˌhetərəuˈtrɔfik] *a* 异养的;异养生物的

heterotropia [ˌhetərəuˈtrəupiə], **heterotropy** [ˌhetəˈrɔtrəpi] *n* 斜视,斜眼

heterotropic [ˈhetərəuˌtrəupik] *a* 向异性的(属于一种变构酶,受一个或一个以上的效应物分子刺激或抑制)

heterotrypsin [ˌhetərəuˈtripsin] *n* 异种胰蛋白酶

heterotypic(al) [ˌhetərəuˈtipik(əl)] *a* 异型的

heterovaccine [ˌhetərəuˈvæksiːn] *n* 异种疫苗,异种菌苗(用不引起疾病的微生物制成的疫苗,为一种非特异性疗法)

heteroxenous [ˌhetəˈrɔksinəs] *a* 异种[宿主]寄生的,异栖的

heteroxeny [ˌhetəˈrɔksini] *n* 异种[宿主]寄生,异栖

heterozoic [ˌhetərəuˈzəuik] *a* 异种动物的

heterozygosis [ˌhetərəuzaiˈgəusis] *n* 杂合[现象],异型接合(具有不同遗传成分性细胞的结合)

heterozygosity [ˌhetərəuzaiˈgɔsəti] *n* 杂合性,异型结合性(在某一位点上具有不同的等位基因)

heterozygote [ˌhetərəuˈzaigəut] *n* 杂合子,异形合子(指一个个体具有不同的等位基因) | manifesting ~ 显性杂合子(一种女性杂合子的X连锁遗传病) | **heterozygotic** [ˌhetərəuzaiˈgɔtik] *a*

heterozygous [ˌhetərəuˈzaigəs] *a* 杂合的

HETP hexaethyltetraphosphate 六乙基四磷酸,四磷酸六乙酯

Heublein method [ˈhɔiblain] (Arthur C. Heublein) 霍伊布莱因法(每日以低剂量的X线照射全身10~20小时,连续数日,以治癌症)

Heubner-Herter disease [ˈhɔibnəˈhəːtə] (J. O. L. Heubner; Christian A. Herter) 霍-赫病,婴儿型非热带性口炎性腹泻

Heubner's disease (endarteritis) [ˈhɔibnə] (Johann O. L. Heubner) 霍伊布内病(梅毒性大脑动脉内膜炎)

heuristic [hjuəˈristik] *a* 启发的,启发式的 | **~s** *n* 启发式,直观推断

heurteloup [ˈhəːtiluːp, əːtˈluː] (Charles L. S. Heurteloup) *n*【法】吸血器,吸血杯

Heuser's membrane [ˈhɔizə] (Chester Heuser) 霍伊泽膜(胚外体腔膜)

HEW Department of Health, Education, and Welfare (美国)卫生、教育与福利部(现改为HHS)

hex-, hexa- [构词成分] 六

hexabasic [ˌheksəˈbeisik] *a* 六[碱]价的,六元的

hexabiose [ˌheksəˈbaiəus] *n* 己二糖(即二糖)

hexachlorobenzene [ˌheksəklɔːrəuˈbenziːn] *n* 六氯苯(用于有机合成及用作杀真菌药)

hexachlorocyclohexane [ˌheksəˌklɔːrəˌsaikləu-ˈheksein] *n* 六氯环己烷,六氯化苯,六六六(杀虫药)

hexachloroethane [ˌheksəˌklɔːrəuˈeθein] *n* 六氯乙烷(用于牛、羊的抗肝吸虫药)

hexachlorophene [ˌheksəˈklɔːrəfiːn] *n* 六氯酚(皮肤消毒药及在兽医学中用于反刍动物的抗吸虫药)

hexachromic [ˌheksəˈkrəumik] *a* 六色的;辨别六色的

hexacosane [hekˈsækəsein] *n* 二十六烷

hexad [ˈheksæd], **hexade** [ˈhekseid] *n* 六个一组;六价元素,六价基

hexadactyly [ˌheksəˈdæktili], **hexadactylia** [ˌheksədækˈtiliə], **hexadactylism** [ˌheksəˈdæktilizəm] *n* 六指畸形,六趾畸形

hexadecanoate [ˌheksəˌdekəˈnəueit] *n* 十六酸盐,棕榈酸盐

hexadecanoic acid [ˌheksəˌdekəˈnəuik] 十六[烷]酸

hexadimethrine bromide [ˌheksədaiˈmeθriːn] 海美溴铵(肝素拮抗药)

hexaene [ˈheksəiːn] *n* 六烯,己烯

-hexaene [ˈheksəiːn] [构词成分] 六烯,己烯

hexaethyltetraphosphate [ˌheksəˌeθilˌtetrəˈfɔsfeit] *n* 六乙基四磷酸,四磷酸六乙酯

hexafluorenium bromide [ˌheksəfluəˈreniəm]

己芴溴铵(神经肌肉阻断剂,骨骼肌松弛药)

Hexagenia bilineata [ˌheksəˈdʒiːniə baiˌliniˈeitə] 二纹蜉蝣

hexahydric [ˌheksəˈhaidrik] *a* 六氢的

hexahydrohematoporphyrin [ˌheksəˌhaidrəuˌhemətəuˈpɔːfirin] *n* 六氢血卟啉

hexamer [ˈheksəmə] *n* 六聚物;六壳粒(病毒)

hexamethonium [ˌheksəmiˈθəuniəm] *n* 六甲双铵(季铵神经节阻断剂) | ~ bromide 六甲溴铵,溴化六甲双铵(抗高血压药) / ~ chloride 六甲氯铵,氯化六甲双铵(抗高血压药)

hexamethylated [ˌheksəˈmeθileitid] *a* [含]六甲基的

hexamethylenamine [ˌheksəˌmeθiliːnˈæmin] *n* 环六亚甲基四胺,乌洛托品(尿路消毒药)

hexamethylendiamine [ˌheksəˌmeθiliːnˈdaiəmin] *n* 己二胺

hexamethylmelamine (HMM) [ˌheksəˌmeθilˈmeləmiːn] *n* 六甲蜜胺(抗肿瘤药)

hexamethylphosphoramide [ˌheksəˌmeθilfɔsˈfɔrəmaid] *n* 六甲基磷酰胺,氮磷致变物(见 hempa)

hexamine [ˈheksəmin] *n* 环六亚甲基四胺,乌洛托品(尿路消毒药)

Hexamita [hekˈsæmitə] *n* 六鞭虫属

hexamitiasis [hekˌsæmiˈtaiəsis] *n* 六鞭虫病

hexamylose [hekˈsæmiləus] *n* 直链六己糖

hexane [ˈheksein] *n* 己烷

hexanoate [ˌheksəˈnəueit] *n* 己酸盐

hexanoic acid [ˌheksəˈnəuik] 己酸

hexaploid [ˈheksəplɔid] *a* 六倍体的 *n* 六倍体(含六组染色体的个体或细胞) | **~y** [ˈheksəˌplɔidi] *n* 六倍性

Hexapoda [hekˈsæpədə] *n* 六足纲,昆虫纲

hexatomic [ˌheksəˈtɔmik] *a* 六元的,六价的;结合六补体的(免疫学中指具有结合不同菌株六种补体的能力)

hexavaccine [ˌheksəˈvæksiːn] *n* 六联疫苗,六联菌苗(包含有 6 种不同微生物的一种疫苗)

hexavalent [ˌheksəˈveilənt] *a* 六价的

hexavitamin [ˌheksəˈvaitəmin] *n* 六合维生素(含维生素 A、维生素 D、维生素 C、维生素 B_1、维生素 B_2 及烟酰胺)

hexedine [ˈheksidiːn] *n* 海克西定(抗菌药)

hexenmilch [ˈheksənmilh] *n* 【德】新生儿乳,婴乳

hexestrol [hekˈsestrɔl] *n* 己烷雌酚(雌激素类药)

hexethal sodium [ˈheksəθəl] 己巴比妥钠(催眠镇静药)

hexetidine [hekˈsetidiːn] *n* 海克替啶(抗真菌、抗原虫、抗细菌药,治疗阴道炎时主要用作局部抗感染药)

hexhydric [heksˈhaidrik] *a* 六氢的

hexobarbital [ˌheksəˈbɑːbitæl] *n* 海索比妥(镇静、安眠药) | sodium ~ 海索比妥钠 | **hexobarbitone** *n*

hexobendine [ˌheksəuˈbendiːn] *n* 海索苯定(血管扩张药)

hexocyclium methylsulfate [ˌheksəuˈsaikliəm] 己环铵甲硫酸盐,环苯甲哌甲硫酸盐(抗胆碱药,抗消化性溃疡药)

hexokinase [ˌheksəuˈkaineis] *n* 己糖激酶

hexonate [ˈheksəneit] *n* 六烃季铵烟酸酯(神经节阻滞药)

hexone [ˈheksəun] *n* 异己酮

hexonic acid [hekˈsɔnik] 己糖酸

hexosamine [ˈheksəuˌsæmin, hekˈsəusəmin] *n* 己糖胺,氨基己糖

hexosaminidase [ˌheksəusəˈminideis] *n* 己糖胺酶,氨基己糖苷酶

hexosan [ˈheksəsæn] *n* 己聚糖

hexosazone [ˌheksəuˈseizəun] *n* 己糖脎

hexose [ˈheksəus] *n* 己糖 | ~ diphosphate 二磷酸己糖,己糖二磷酸 / ~ monophosphate 磷酸己糖,己糖磷酸

hexosediphosphoric acid [ˌheksəusˌdaifɔsˈfɔrik] 二磷酸己糖,己糖二磷酸

hexosephosphatase [ˌheksəusˈfɔsfəteis] *n* 磷酸己糖酶

hexosephosphate [ˌheksəusˈfɔsfeit] *n* 磷酸己糖,己糖磷酸

hexosephosphate isomerase [ˌheksəusˈfɔsfeit aiˈsɔməreis] 己糖磷酸异构酶,6-磷酸葡糖异构酶

hexose-1-phosphate uridylyltransferase [ˈheksəus ˈfɔsfeit ˌjuəriˌdililˈtrænsfəreis] 己糖-1-磷酸尿苷酰基转移酶,尿苷二磷酸葡萄糖-己糖-1-磷酸尿苷酰基转移酶

hexoside [ˈheksəsaid] *n* 己糖苷

hexosyltransferase [ˌheksəusilˈtrænsfəreis] *n* 己糖基转移酶,转己糖酶

hexoxidase [hekˈsɔksideis] *n* 抗坏血酸氧化酶

hexulose [ˈheksjuləus] *n* 己糖酮

hexuronic acid [ˌheksjuəˈrɔnik] 己糖醛酸

hexyl [ˈheksil] *n* 己基

***n*-hexylamine** [ˌheksiˈlæmiːn] *n* 正己胺

hexylcaine hydrochloride [ˈheksilkein] 盐酸海克卡因(局部麻醉药)

hexylresorcinol [ˌheksilriˈzɔːsinɔl] *n* 己雷琐辛(抗蠕虫药)

Heymann's nephritis [ˈheimɑːn] (Walter Heymann) 海曼肾炎(膜性肾小球肾炎的一种实验模型,对大鼠注射得自肾小管刷状缘的抗原制备诱发,可引起原肾小管的自身免疫反应)

Heynsius' test [ˈhainsius] (Adrian Heynsius) 海

恩修斯试验(检白蛋白)

Hey's amputation (operation) [hei] (William Hey) 海伊切断术(手术)(使跖骨断离跗骨,部分切除第一楔骨) | ~ hernia 包绕性腹股沟疝 / ~ internal derangement 海伊膝关节不全脱位(特征为剧痛并伴肌痉挛) / ~ ligament 阔筋膜镰缘,隐裂孔镰缘 / ~ saw 海伊锯(用以扩大骨内洞口的小锯)

HF Hageman factor 哈格曼因子(凝血因子 XII); high frequency 高频

Hf hafnium 铪

Hfr high frequency of recombination 高频重组

Hg hydrargyrum 汞

Hgb hemoglobin 血红蛋白

HGBV hepatitis GB virus GB 肝炎病毒

HGE human granulocytic ehrichiosis 人类粒细胞性埃利希菌病

HGF hyperglycemic-glycogenolytic factor (glucagon) 高血糖性糖原分解因子(胰高血糖素)

HGG human gamma globulin 人丙球蛋白

HGH, hGH human (pituitary) growth hormone 人(垂体)生长激素

hGHr growth hormone recombinant 生长激素重组体

HGPRT hypoxanthine-guanine phosphoribosyltransferase 次黄嘌呤-鸟嘌呤磷酸核糖基转移酶

HHS Department of Health and Human Services (美国)卫生与人类服务部(前身为 HEW); hepatocyte growth factor 肝细胞生长因子

HHT hydroxyheptadecatrienoic acid 羟基十七碳三烯酸

HI hemagglutination inhibition 血凝抑制反应; hydriodic acid 氢碘酸

5-HIAA 5-hydroxyindoleacetic acid 5-羟基吲哚乙酸

hiation [haiˈeiʃən] *n* 打呵欠

hiatopexia [haiˈeitəuˈpeksiə], **hiatopexy** [haiˈeitəˌpeksi] *n* 生殖道裂孔修复术

hiatus [haiˈeitəs] ([复] **hiatus⟨es⟩**) *n*【拉】裂孔,孔 | adductor ~ 收肌裂孔 / ~ leukemicus 白血病性裂隙(成髓细胞与成熟中性粒细胞之间的过渡型细胞完全缺如或很少,见于急性成髓细胞白血病时) / maxillary ~, ~ of maxillary sinus 上颌窦裂孔 / neural ~ 神经管裂孔 / saphenous ~ 隐静脉裂孔卵圆窝 / tentorial ~ 小脑幕切迹 / venacaval ~ 腔静脉孔 | **hiatal** *a*

Hibbs' frame [hibz] (Russell A. Hibbs) 希布斯支架(治脊柱侧凸时,用以支持牵引石膏背心的支架) | ~ operation 希布斯手术(波特⟨Pott⟩病时脊柱关节固定术)

hibernation [ˌhaibəːˈneiʃən] *n* 冬眠 | artificial ~ 人工冬眠

hibernoma [ˌhaibəˈnəumə] *n* 蛰伏脂肪瘤

hiccup, hiccough [ˈhikʌp, -əp] *n* 呃逆 | epidemic ~ 流行性呃逆(常见于流行性脑炎)

Hickman catheter [ˈhikmən] (R. O. Hickman) 希克曼导管(一型中央静脉导管,用于经静脉系统长期给药,如抗生素、肠外营养或化疗药物;此导管可用于连续给药或间歇性给药,导管可能为单腔或双腔)

Hicks contractions(sign), version [hiks] (John Braxton Hicks) 希克斯收缩(征)、转胎位术(见 Braxton Hicks contraction⟨sign⟩, version)

Hicks' syndrome [hiks] (Eric P. Hicks) 希克斯综合征,遗传性感觉根性神经病变

Hicks version [hiks] (John Braxton Hicks) 希克斯转胎位术(见 Braxton Hicks version)

HIDA hepatobiliary iminodiacetic acid 肝胆管亚氨基二已酸

hidebound [ˈhaidbaund] *a* 绷紧的,包紧的(指硬皮病时的皮肤)

hidradenitis [ˌhaidrædiˈnaitis] *n* 汗腺炎 | ~ axillaris 腋汗腺炎 / ~ suppurativa 化脓性汗腺炎

hidradenocarcinoma [haiˌdrædinəuˌkɑːsiˈnəumə] *n* 汗腺癌,汗腺腺癌

hidradenoid [haiˈdrædinɔid] *a* 汗腺样的,类汗腺的

hidradenoma [ˌhidrædiˈnəumə] *n* 汗腺瘤,汗腺腺瘤 | ~ eruptivum 疹状汗腺瘤

hidr(o)- [构词成分]汗;汗腺

hidroacanthoma [ˌhaidrəuˌækænˈθəumə] *n* 汗腺棘皮瘤 | ~ simplex 单纯性汗腺棘皮瘤

hidroadenoma [ˌhidrəuˌædiˈnəumə] *n* 汗腺瘤,汗腺腺瘤

hidrocystoma [ˌhidrəusisˈtəumə] *n* 汗腺囊瘤

hidrocystomatosis [ˌhidrəuˌsistəuməˈtəusis] *n* 汗腺囊瘤病

hidrolic acid [hiˈdrɔlik] 汗酸

hidropoiesis [ˌhidrəupɔiˈiːsis] *n* 汗生成,汗分泌 | **hidropoietic** [ˌhidrəupɔiˈetik] *a*

hidrorrhea [hidrəuˈriːə] *n* 多汗[症],大汗

hidrosadenitis [ˌhaidrɔsˌædiˈnaitis] *n* 汗腺炎

hidroschesis [hiˈdrɔskisis] *n* 止汗

hidrosis [hiˈdrəusis, hai-] *n* 多汗;出汗

hidrotic [hiˈdrɔtik, hai-] *a* 出汗的,发汗的 *n* 发汗药

hiemal [ˈhaiiməl] *a* 冬季的,冬令的

hieralgia [haiəˈrældʒiə] *n* 骶骨痛

hier(o)- [构词成分]骶骨

hierolisthesis [ˌhaiərəulisˈθiːsis] *n* 骶骨脱位

high-grade [ˈhaiˈgreid] *a* 高度的

Highmore's antrum [ˈhaimɔː] (Nathaniel Highmore) 上颌窦 | ~ body 睾丸纵隔

Higouménaki's sign [hiːguːˈmeinaːkiː] (G. Higouménaki) 锁骨征

hilar [ˈhailə] *a* 门的,肺门的
Hildebrandt's test [ˈhildəbrɑːnt] (Fritz Hildebrandt) 希尔德布兰特试验(检尿中尿胆素)
Hildenbrand's disease [ˈhildənbrɑːnd] (Johann V. von Hildenbrand) 斑疹伤寒
hilifuge [ˈhailifjuːdʒ] *a* [从]肺门放射的(X线阴影)
hilitis [haiˈlaitis] *n* 门炎(尤指肺门炎)
hillock [ˈhilək] *n* 丘,阜 | auricular ~s, 耳丘 / axon ~ 轴丘 / germ ~, germ-bearing ~ [载]卵丘 / seminal ~ 精阜
Hill posterior gastropexy [hil] (Lucius D. Hill) 希尔胃后固定术(一种矫正胃食管的手术)
Hill-Sachs lesion [hil sæks] (Harold A. Hill; Maurice D. Sachs) 希-萨损害(后内肱骨头的一种受压骨折,有时与肩前脱位同时发生,系由肱骨头撞击下颌窝的前缘所致)
Hill's sign [hil] (Leonard E. Hill) 希尔征(股动脉收缩区过度增高)
Hilton's law [ˈhiltən] (John Hilton) 希尔顿定律(分布于某一关节的神经,亦同时分布于运动该关节的各肌及各肌附丽处的皮肤) | ~ muscle 杓会厌肌 / ~ sac 喉小囊 / ~ white line 梳状线,肛门皮肤线
hilus [ˈhailəs] ([复] **hili** [ˈhailai]) *n* 【拉】门 | ~ of(the) kidney 肾门 / ~ of(the) lung 肺门 | **hilum** ([复] **hila** [ˈhailə]) *n*
himantosis [ˌhaimənˈtəusis] *n* 腭垂延长
hinchazon [ˌhintʃəˈzɔn] *n* 【古巴】脚气[病]
hind [haind] (hinder, hindmost 或 hindermost) *a* 后面的,后部的;在后的
hindbrain [ˈhaindbrein] *n* 后脑,菱脑
Hindenlang's test [ˈhidənlɑːŋ] (Karl Hindenlang) 欣登朗试验(检白蛋白)
hindfoot [ˈhaindfut] *n* 足后段(包括距骨和跟骨)
hindgut [ˈhaindgʌt] *n* 后肠
hind-kidney [haindˈkidni] *n* 后肾
hindquarter [ˈhaindkwɔːtə] *n* 后腿部(指四足动物的后肢及其邻近的腰、骨盆和肌肉系统)
Hines-Bannick syndrome [hainz ˈbænik] (Edgar A. Hines; Edwin Bannick) 海-班综合征(低温和不能出汗间歇性发作)
Hines-Brown test [ˈhainz ˈbraun] (Edgar A. Hines; George E. Brown) 海因斯-布朗试验(冷加压试验,即先量血压然后将患者的手浸入冰水,再量血压,若血压过高,则表明有原发性高血压)
hinge-bow [ˈhindʒ bəu] *n* 铰链式面弓
Hinman syndrome [ˈhinmən] (Frank Hinman Jr.) 欣曼综合征(一种精神性障碍,见于儿童,模拟神经源性膀胱,含逼尿肌括约肌协同失调,而无任何神经损害证据。亦称非神经源性神经源性膀胱)
Hinton test [ˈhintən] (William A. Hinton) 欣顿试验(检梅毒)
hip [hip] *n* 髋;髋关节 | ~ pointer 髋挫伤 / snapping ~ 弹响髋,髋关节弹响
Hippelates [ˌhipəˈleitiːz] *n* 潜蝇属 | ~ flavipes 黄潜蝇 / ~ pusio 眼潜蝇
Hippel-Lindau disease [ˈhipəl ˈlindau] (Eugen von Hippel; Arvid Lindau) 希佩尔-林道病(遗传性斑痣性错构瘤病,特征为视网膜和小脑先天性血管瘤病。亦称脑视网膜血管瘤病)
Hippel's disease [ˈhipəl] (Eugen von Hippel) 希佩尔病(主要限于视网膜血管瘤病,当伴有小脑成血管细胞瘤时,即称 von Hippel-Lindau disease, 见 Hippel-Lindau disease)
Hippeutis [haiˈpjuːtis] *n* 圆扁螺属 | ~ cantori 尖口圆扁螺
hippo [ˈhipəu] *n* 吐根
hipp(o)- [构词成分]马
Hippobosca [hipəuˈbɔskə] *n* 虱蝇属 | ~ rufipes 赭虱蝇
Hippoboscidae [ˌhipəuˈbɔskidiː] *n* 虱蝇科
hippoboscid [ˌhipəuˈbɔskid] *a* 虱蝇科的 *n* 虱蝇
hippocampus [ˌhipəuˈkæmpəs] *n* 海马 | ~ major 海马 / ~ minor 禽距 | **hippocampal** *a*
hippocoprosterol [ˌhipəukəˈprɔstərɔl], **hippostercorin** [ˌhipəuˈstəːkərin] *n* 马粪甾醇
Hippocrates [hiˈpɔkrətiːz] *n* 希波克拉底(古希腊名医,被尊为"医学之父") | **hippocratic** [ˌhipəuˈkrætik] *a* 希波克拉底的;希波克拉底医派的
Hippocratic Oath [ˌhipəuˈkrætik əuθ] 希波克拉底誓言
hippocratism [hiˈpɔkrətizəm] *n* 希波克拉底医派(以模仿自然过程为基础,并强调治疗与预后)
hippocratist [hiˈpɔkrətist] *n* 希波克拉底医派者
Hippoglossus [ˌhipəuˈglɔsəs] *n* 庸鲽鱼属
hippolith [ˈhipəliθ], **hippolite** [ˈhipəlait] *n* 马粪石
hippomane [hiˈpɔməni] *n* 尿囊小体
Hippomane [hiˈpɔməni] *n* 吐根属
hippomelanin [ˌhipəuˈmelənin] *n* 马黑[色]素
hippulin [ˈhipjulin] *n* 异马烯雌[甾]酮
hippurase [ˈhipjureis] *n* 马尿酸酶
hippurate [ˈhipjureit] *n* 马尿酸盐
hippuria [hiˈpjuəriə] *n* 马尿酸尿
hippuric [hiˈpjuərik] *a* 马尿的 | ~ acid 马尿酸
hippuricase [hiˈpjuərikeis] *n* 马尿酸酶
hippus [ˈhipəs] *n* 虹膜震颤
hircic acid [ˈhəːsik] 羊脂酸
hircismus [həˈsizməs] *n* 腋窝臭,狐臭
hircus [ˈhəːkəs] ([复] **hirci** [ˈhəːsai]) *n* 【拉】腋毛

Hirschberg's magnet [ˈhirʃbəːg] (Julius Hirschberg) 希尔施贝格电磁铁(吸除眼内铁屑) | ~ method 希尔施贝格法(观察角膜的烛光反射,以测量斜视的偏向)
Hirschberg's sign [ˈhəːʃbəg] (Leonard K. Hirschberg) 赫希伯格征,足收肌反射
Hirschfelder's tuberculin [ˈhəːʃfeldə] (Joseph O. Hirschfelder) 氧化结核菌素
Hirschfeld's canals [ˈhəːʃfeld] (I. Hirschfeld) 牙间管
Hirschfeld's disease [ˈhəːʃfeld] (Felix Hirschfeld) 急性糖尿病
Hirschsprung's disease [ˈhirʃspruŋ] (Harald Hirschsprung) 希尔施普龙病,先天性巨结肠
hirsute [ˈhəːsjuːt] *a* 多毛的
hirsutic acid [həːˈsjuːtik] 多毛真菌酸
hirsuties [həːˈsjuːʃiiːz] *n* 多毛[症]
hirsutism [ˈhəːsjuːtizəm] *n* 多毛症(尤指妇女多毛症)
hirudicide [hiˈruːdisaid] *n* 杀水蛭药 | **hirudicidal** [hiˌrudiˈsaidl] *a* 杀水蛭的
hirudin [hiˈruːdin] *n* 蛭素
Hirudinaria [hiˌruːdiˈnɛəriə] *n* 水蛭属
Hirudinea [ˌhiruˈdiniə] *n* 蛭纲
hirudiniasis [hiˌruːdiˈnaiəsis] *n* 水蛭病
hirudinization [hiˌruːdinaiˈzeiʃən] *n* 水蛭素防凝;水蛭疗法
hirudinize [hiˈruːdinaiz] *vt* 用水蛭素防凝
Hirudo [hiˈruːdəu] ([复]hirudines [hiˈruːdiːnz]) *n* 水蛭属 | ~ aegyptiaca 埃及水蛭 / ~ japonica 日本水蛭 / ~ javanica 爪哇水蛭 / ~ medicinalis 医[用水]蛭 / ~ quinquestriata 澳洲水蛭 / ~ sanguisorba 马蛭 / ~ troctina 欧洲水蛭
hirulog [ˈhirjuːlɔg] *n* 蛭素类似物(试验用作抗凝药)
His histidine 组氨酸
His-Purkinje system [his pəˈkindʒɪ] (Wilhelm His Jr.; Johannes E. Purkinje) 希-普系统(心脏传导系统的一部分,一般特指始于希氏〈His〉束止于心室内浦肯野〈Purkinje〉纤维网末端的那一段)
His's bundle (band) [ˈhis] (Wilhelm His, Jr.) 希氏束(带),房室束 | ~ disease 战壕热 / ~ spindle 主动脉梭
His's bursa [his] (Wilhelm His) 希氏囊(原肠末端的膨大) | ~ canal (duct) 甲状舌管 / ~ perivascular space 希氏血管周隙(脑与脊髓血管外膜和神经胶质血管周界膜之间的空隙) / ~ zones 希氏区(沿胚胎脊髓全长有 4 个增厚束)
Hiss capsule stain [his] (Philip H. Hiss, Jr.) 希斯荚膜染色法(显示细菌荚膜的方法)
hist- 见 histo-
histaffine [hisˈtæfiːn] *a* 亲组织的 *n* 亲组织素
histaminase [hisˈtæmineis] *n* 组胺酶
histamine [ˈhistəmiːn] *n* 组胺(诊断用药) | $\sim_1$ 组胺 1(使血管扩张和平滑肌收缩的组胺细胞受体点,缩写为 H_1) / $\sim_2$ 组胺 2(刺激心率和胃液分泌的组胺细胞受体点,缩写为 H_2) / ~ hydrochloride 盐酸组胺 / ~ phosphate 磷酸组胺(胃液检查用药,血管扩张药,脱敏药) | **histaminic** [ˌhistəˈminik] *a*
histamine-fast [ˈhistəmiːn ˌfaːst] *a* 抗组胺的
histaminemia [hisˌtæmiˈniːmiə] *n* 组胺血[症]
histaminergic [ˌhistəmiˈnəːdʒik] *a* 组胺能的
histaminia [ˌhistəˈminiə] *n* 组胺休克
histanoxia [ˌhistəˈnɔksiə] *n* 组织缺氧[症]
histic [ˈhistik] *a* 组织的
histidase [ˈhistideis], **histidinase** [ˈhistidineis] *n* 组氨酸酶,组氨酸氨-裂解酶
histidine [ˈhistidiːn] *n* 组氨酸 | ~ monohydrochloride 盐酸组氨酸(曾一度用于治消化性溃疡)
histidine ammonia-lyase [ˈhistidiːn] 组氨酸氨-裂合酶(此酶的遗传性缺乏为一种常染色体隐性性状,可致组氨酸血症。亦称组氨酸酶)
histidinemia [ˌhistidiˈniːmiə] *n* 组氨酸血症,组氨酸酶缺乏症(一种遗传性代谢病)
histidinuria [ˌhistidiˈnjuəriə] *n* 组氨酸尿
histidyl [ˈhistidil] *n* 组氨酰[基]
histi(o)- [构词成分]组织
histioblast [ˈhistiəblæst] *n* 成组织细胞
histiocyte [ˈhistiəˌsait] *n* 组织细胞 | cardiac ~ 心肌组织细胞 / sea-blue ~ 海蓝色组织细胞(见 syndrome 项下相应术语) / wandering ~s 游走性组织细胞(一种活动的巨噬细胞) | **histiocytic** [ˌhistiəˈsitik] *a*
histiocytoma [ˌhistiəusaiˈtəumə] *n* 组织细胞瘤 | fibrous ~ 皮肤纤维瘤 / lipoid ~ 纤维黄瘤
histiocytomatosis [ˌhistiəusaiˌtəuməˈtəusis] *n* 组织细胞瘤病
histiocytosis [ˌhistiəusaiˈtəusis] *n* 组织细胞增多症 | acute disseminated ~ X 急性播散性组织细胞增多症 X(见 Letterer-Siwe disease) / sinus ~ 窦性组织细胞增多症 / ~ X 组织细胞增多症 X(一种统称,包含嗜酸性细胞肉芽肿、莱特勒-西韦病〈Letterer-Siwe disease〉、汉-许-克病〈Hand-Schüller-Christian disease〉,并表示三者具有共同的起因)
histiogenic [ˌhistiəuˈdʒenik] *a* 组织原的
histioid [ˈhistiɔid] *a* 蜘蛛网状的;单一组织的(肿瘤);组织样的
histio-irritative [ˌhistiəu ˈiriˌteitiv] *a* 刺激[结缔]组织的
histioma [ˌhistiˈəumə] *n* 组织瘤(如纤维瘤)

histionic [ˌhistiˈɔnik] *a* 组织的
hist(o)- [构词成分]组织
histoblast [ˈhistəblæst] *n* 成组织细胞
histochemistry [ˌhistəuˈkemistri] *n* 组织化学 | **histochemical** [ˌhistəuˈkemikəl] *a*
histochemotherapy [ˌhistəuˌkeməuˈθerəpi] *n* 组织化学疗法
histochromatosis [ˌhistəuˌkrəuməˈtəusis] *n* 组织着色病
histoclastic [ˌhistəuˈklæstik] *a* 破坏组织的(指某些细胞)
histoclinical [ˌhistəuˈklinikəl] *a* 组织临床的
histocompatible [ˌhistəukəmˈpætəbl] *a* 组织相容的 | **histocompatibility** [ˌhistəu kəmˌpætəˈbiləti] *n* 组织相容性(指移植物能被接受并维持其原有功能的性质或状态,由于供者和受者的基因型关系,移植物一般不出现排斥现象)
histocyte [ˈhistəsait] *n* 组织细胞
histodiagnosis [ˌhistəuˌdaiəgˈnəusis] *n* 组织学诊断
histodialysis [ˌhistəudaiˈælisis] *n* 组织断离,组织分解
histodifferentiation [ˌhistəuˌdifərenʃiˈeiʃən] *n* 组织分化
histofluorescence [ˌhistəuˌfluəˈresəns] *n* 组织荧光
histogenesis [ˌhistəuˈdʒenisis], **histogeny** [hisˈtɔdʒini] *n* 组织发生 | **histogenetic** [ˌhistəudʒiˈnetik] *a*
histogenous [hisˈtɔdʒinəs] *a* 组织原的
histogram [ˈhistəgræm] *n* 直方图,柱形图,矩形图(以柱形或矩形表示统计研究中数值分布的图)
histography [hisˈtɔgrəfi] *n* 组织论
histohematin [ˌhistəuˈhemətin] *n* 细胞色素
histohematogenous [ˌhistəuˌheməˈtɔdʒinəs] *a* 组织血原性的
histohydria [ˌhistəuˈhaidriə] *n* 组织含水过多
histohypoxia [ˌhistəuhaiˈpɔksiə] *n* 组织氧过少
histoid [ˈhistɔid] *a* 蜘蛛网状的;单一组织的;组织样的
histoincompatible [ˌhistəuinkəmˈpætəbl] *a* 组织不相容的 | **histoincompatibility** [ˌhistəuˌinkəmˌpætəˈbiləti] *n* 组织不相容性(指移植物不被接受并不具备维持原有功能的性质或状态,由于供者和受者的基因型关系,移植物一般出现排斥现象)
histokinesis [ˌhistəukaiˈniːsis] *n* 组织运动
histology [hisˈtɔlədʒi] *n* 组织学(亦称显微解剖学) | normal ~ 正常组织学 / pathologic ~ 病理组织学 | **histologic(al)** [ˌhistəˈlɔdʒik(əl)] *a* / **histologist** *n* 组织学家

histolysate [hisˈtɔliseit] *n* 组织溶解物
histolysis [hisˈtɔlisis] *n* 组织溶解 | **histolytic** [ˌhistəˈlitik] *a* 溶组织的
histoma [hisˈtəumə] *n* 组织瘤(如纤维瘤)
histometaplastic [ˌhistəuˌmetəˈplæstik] *a* 促组织变形的
Histomonas [ˌhistəˈməunəs] *n* 组织滴虫属
histomoniasis [ˌhistəməˈnaiəsis] *n* 组织滴虫病
histomorphology [ˌhistəumɔːˈfɔlədʒi] *n* 组织形态学
histomorphometric [ˌhistəuˌmɔːfəˈmetrik] *a* 组织形态测定的
histone [ˈhistəun] *n* 组蛋白 | ~ nucleinate 核酸组蛋白
histoneurology [ˌhistəunjuəˈrɔlədʒi] *n* 神经组织学
histonomy [hisˈtɔnəmi] *n* 组织发生律,组织发生法则
histonuria [histəuˈnjuəriə] *n* 组织蛋白尿
histopathology [ˌhistəupəˈθɔlədʒi] *n* 组织病理学,病理组织学
histophagous [hisˈtɔfəgəs] *a* 噬组织的
histophysiology [ˌhistəuˌfiziˈɔlədʒi] *n* 组织生理学
Histoplasma [ˌhistəuˈplæzmə] *n* 组织胞浆菌属 | ~ capsulatum 荚膜组织胞浆菌 / ~ capsulatum var. duboisii 荚膜组织胞浆菌杜氏变种 / ~ farciminosus 马皮疽组织胞浆菌
histoplasmin [ˌhistəuˈplæzmin] *n* (荚膜)组织胞浆菌素,组胞浆菌素
histoplasmoma [ˌhistəuplæzˈməumə] *n* 组织胞浆菌瘤
histoplasmosis [ˌhistəuplæzˈməusis] *n* 组织胞浆菌病 | African ~ 非洲组织胞浆菌病 / ocular ~ 眼组织胞浆菌病
historadiography [ˌhistəuˌreidiˈɔgrəfi] *n* 组织射线照相术
historetention [ˌhistəuriˈtenʃən] *n* 组织[内]贮留
historrhexis [ˌhistəuˈreksis] *n* 组织破碎
history [ˈhistəri] *n* 历史 | case ~ 病历,病史;个案史
histoteliosis [ˌhistəuteliˈəusis] *n* 组织终变(指细胞的最后分化)
histotherapy [ˌhistəuˈθerəpi] *n* 组织疗法(以动物组织治病)
histothrombin [ˌhistəuˈθrɔmbin] *n* 组织凝酶
histotome [ˈhistətəum] *n* 组织切片机
histotomy [hisˈtɔtəmi] *n* 组织切片术
histotoxic [ˌhistəuˈtɔksik] *a* 毒害组织的,组织毒的
histotroph [ˈhistətrəuf] *n* 组织营养质 | **~ic**

[ˌhistəuˈtrɔfik] *a* 促组织生成的;组织营养的
histotropic [ˌhistəuˈtrɔpik] *a* 向组织的
histozoic [ˌhistəuˈzəuik] *a* 组织内寄生的
histozyme [ˈhistəzaim] *n* 马尿酸酶
histrelin acetate [hisˈtrelin] 醋酸组氨瑞林(促性腺激素释放激素的合成制剂,用于治疗中枢性早熟,注射给药)
histrionism [ˈhistriəˌnizəm] *n* 表演症,戏迷症 | **histrionic** [ˌhistriˈɔnik] *a* 演戏状的,表演样的
His-Werner disease [his ˈvəːnə] (Wilhelm His Jr.; Heinrich Werner)战壕热
hitch [hitʃ] *n* 钩子
Hittorf's number [ˈhitɔf] (Johann W. Hittorf)希托夫值,离子导电率 | ~ tube 希托夫管(克鲁克斯〈Crookes〉X 线真空管)
Hitzig's girdle [ˈhitsig] (Eduard Hitzig) 希茨希带(与乳房同高的一环状痛觉缺失区,在第三和第六背神经支配区内,见于脊髓痨早期) | ~ test 希茨希试验(检前庭器)
HIV human immunodeficiency virus 人免疫缺陷病毒
hive [haiv] *n* 风团
hives [haivz] [复] *n* 荨麻疹
HKAFO hip-knee-ankle-foot orthosis 髋大腿矫形器
H^+, K^+-ATPase [eitiːˈpiːeis] H^+, K^+-腺苷三磷酸酶(亦称 H^+/K^+-交换腺苷三磷酸酶)
H^+/ K^+-exchanging ATPase [eksˈtʃændʒiŋ eitiːˈpiːeis] H^+/K^+-交换腺苷三磷酸酶(H^+, K^+-ATPase 的 EC 命名法)
H^+/ K^+-transporting ATPase [trænsˈpɔːtiŋ eitiːˈpiːeis] H^+/K^+-转运腺苷三磷酸酶,H^+, K^+-腺苷三磷酸酶
HL hearing level 听力级
Hl latent hyperopia 隐性远视
HLA human leukocyte antigen 人[类]白细胞抗原
HLHS hypoplastic left heart syndrome 左心发育不全综合征
Hm manifest hyperopia 显性远视
HMDP oxidronate (hydroxymethylene diphosphonate) 奥昔膦酸(羟亚甲基二膦酸)
HMG 3-hydroxy-3-methylglutaryl 3-羟基-3-甲基戊二酰[基]
HMM hexamethylmelamine 六甲蜜胺,六甲三聚氰胺
HMO health maintenance organization 保健组织
HMPA hexamethylphosphoramide 六甲基磷酰胺(见 hempa)
HMPAO hexamethylpropyleneamine oxime 六甲基丙烯胺肟
HMSN hereditary motor and sensory neuropathy 遗传性运动和感觉神经病变
HMWK high-molecular-weight kininogen 高分子量激肽原
HMW-NCF high-molecular-weight neutrophil chemotactic factor 高分子量中性粒细胞趋化因子
HN2 mechlorethamine 氮芥
hnRNA heterogenous nuclear RNA 不均一核 RNA,核内不均一 RNA
Ho holmium 钬(化学元素)
hoarse [hɔːs] *a* 声嘶的,嘶哑的 | **~ness** *n*
hoary [ˈhɔːri] *a* 灰发的,白发的
hobnail [ˈhɔbneil] *n* 平头钉,鞋钉(如 ~ liver 鞋钉状肝,见 liver 项下相应术语)
Hoboken's nodules [ˈhɔbɔkən] (Nicolas von Hoboken) 霍博肯小结(脐动脉外面扩张) | ~ valves 霍博肯瓣(脐动脉襞)
Hochenegg's operation [ˈhɔhəneg] (Julius von Hochenegg) 霍亨内格手术(治直肠癌手术,即将直肠全切除,而保留肛门括约肌)
Hoche's bandelette [ˈhɔhə] (Alfred E. Hoche) 霍赫小带(形成固有束的神经纤维小束)
Hochsinger's phenomenon [ˈhɔksiŋə] (Karl Hochsinger) 霍赫辛格尔现象(手足搐搦时压迫肱二头肌内侧引起握拳现象) | ~ sign 霍赫辛格尔征(①小儿结核的尿蓝母尿;②霍赫辛格尔现象)
hock [hɔk] *n* 后踝(指马或牛) | capped ~ 跟垫,跟盖(马) / curby ~ 后脚硬瘤(马) / spring ~ 弹簧后跟(马)
HOCM hypertrophic obstructive cardiomyopathy 肥大性阻塞性心肌病
hodegetics [ˌhɔdiˈdʒetiks] *n* 医学伦理学
Hodgen splint(apparatus) [ˈhɔdʒən] (John T. Hodgen)霍金夹板(器)(一种金属丝夹板,用于股骨骨折)
Hodge's forceps [ˈhɔdʒ] (Hugh L. Hodge) 霍奇钳(一种产钳) | ~ pessary 霍奇子宫托(子宫后倾子宫托) / ~ planes 霍奇平面(一组与骨盆入口平行的平面)
Hodgkin cycle [ˈhɔdʒkin] (A. L. Hodgkin) 霍奇金循环(可兴奋细胞内在去极化与至钠通透性之间发生的一系列再生循环事件;去极化提高钠通透性,从而使进入细胞的钠〈Na^+〉增多,而 Na^+ 浓度增高又使细胞膜进一步去极化)
Hodgkin's cells [ˈhɔdʒkin] (Thomas Hodgkin) 霍奇金细胞(见 Sternberg-Reed cells) | ~ disease(granuloma) 霍奇金病(肉芽肿)(恶性淋巴瘤的一型,临床特征为无痛的和进行性淋巴结、脾及全身性淋巴组织肿大,其他症状包括厌食、倦怠、体重减轻、发热、盗汗、贫血等) / ~ sarcoma 霍奇金肉瘤(淋巴细胞缺失型霍奇金病)
Hodgson's disease [ˈhɔdʒsn] (Joseph Hodgson) 霍奇森病(主动脉起端部动脉瘤样扩张,常伴心扩张或心肥大)
hodoneuromere [ˌhəudəˈnjuərəmiə] *n* 神经分支节(胚胎)

hoe [həu] *n* 锄(一种切割牙齿的器械)

Hoehne's sign [ˈheinə] (Ottomar Hoehne) 霍内征(分娩时,反复注射催产剂仍不能引起子宫收缩,为子宫破裂之征)

hof [hɔf] *n*【德】核窝(由细胞核凹形围成的胞质区)

Hofbauer cells [ˈhɔfbauə] (J. Isfred I. Hofbauer) 霍夫鲍尔细胞(绒毛膜内大的嗜染细胞,很可能是巨噬细胞)

Hoffa-Lorenz operation [ˈhɔfəˈlɔrənts] (A. Hoffa; Adolf Lorenz) 霍法-洛伦茨手术(见 Lorenz's operation)

Hoffa's disease [ˈhɔfə] (Albert Hoffa) 霍法病(膝关节创伤性脂肪组织增生〈孤立脂肪瘤〉) | ~ operation 霍法手术(见 Lorenz's operation)

Hoffmann's anodyne [ˈhɔfmɑːn] (Friedrich Hoffmann) 霍夫曼止痛药(复方醚酯) | ~ drops 霍夫曼滴剂(醚酯)

Hoffmann's atrophy [ˈhɔfmɑːn] (Johann Hoffmann) 霍夫曼萎缩(见 Werdnig-Hoffmann paralysis) | ~ phenomenon 霍夫曼现象(感觉神经对电刺激反应增强,常测试尺神经) / ~ reflex 霍夫曼反射(指反射,见霍夫曼征②解)/ ~ sign 霍夫曼征(①手足抽搦时,感觉神经对机械刺激应激性增强;②偏瘫时,突然弹压示指、中指或无名指指甲时,拇指末节及其他指的第二、第三指屈曲,亦称指反射和霍夫曼反射)

Hoffmann's duct [ˈhɔfmɑːn] (Moritz Hoffmann) 胰管

Hoffmann-Werdnig syndrome [ˈhɔfmɑːn ˈvəːdnig] (Johann Hoffmann; Guido Werdnig) 霍-韦综合征(见 Werdnig-Hoffmann paralysis)

Hofmann's bacillus [ˈhɔfmɑːn] (Georg von Hofmann-Wellenhof) 假白喉棒状杆菌

Hofmann's violet [ˈhɔfmən] (August W. von Hofmann) 大丽菊紫

Hofmeister's test [ˈhɔfmaistə] (Franz Hofmeister) 霍夫迈斯特试验(检亮氨酸、胨)

Holacanthida [ˌhɔləˈkænθidə] *n* 全射棘目

holagogue [ˈhɔləgɔg] *n* 攻药,剧药

holandric [hɔˈlændrik] *a* 限雄的(遗传方式从雄亲传给雄性子代,由 Y 染色体上的基因遗传的)

holarthritis [ˌhɔlɑːˈθraitis] *n* 全身关节炎

Holden's line [ˈhəuldən] (Luther Holden) 霍尔登线(腹股沟下方,横过髋关节囊的沟)

holder [ˈhəuldə] *n* 支架;柄;持器

holdfast [ˈhəulfɑːst] *n* 固着器;吸盘

holdup [ˈhəuldʌp] *n* 停顿,阻碍

hole [həul] *n* 洞;孔眼 | burr ~s of skull 颅骨穿孔术

holergasia [ˌhɔləˈgeiziə] *n* 重性精神病 | **holergastic** [ˈhɔləˌgæstik] *a*

Holger Nielson method [ˈhəulgə ˈnilsen] (Holger Nielsen) 霍尔格·尼尔森法(人工呼吸)

holism [ˈhəulizəm] *n* 功能整体性 | **holistic** [həuˈlistik] *a*

Hollenhorst plaques [ˈhɔlənhɔːst] (Robert W. Hollenhorst) 霍伦霍斯特斑(视网膜微动脉内粥样栓子含胆固醇结晶,为即将发生的严重心血管疾病警示之征,如卒中、心肌梗死、主动脉瘤或视网膜微动脉阻塞)

hollow [ˈhɔləu] *a* 中空的;凹的

hollow-back [ˈhɔləu bæk] *n* 脊柱前凸

Holmes-Adie syndrome [həumz ˈeidi] (G. M. Holmes; William J. Adie) 霍-埃综合征(见 Adie's syndrome)

Holmes's degeneration [həumz] (Gordon Morgan Holmes) 霍姆斯变性(原发性进行性小脑变性) | ~ phenomenon (sign) 回缩现象(rebound phenomenon, 见 phenomenon 项下相应术语)

Holmes's operation [həumz] (Timothy Holmes) 霍姆斯手术(一种跟骨切除术)

Holmes-Stewart phenomenon [ˈhəumz ˈstjuːət] (G. M. Holmes; James P. Stewart) 回缩现象(rebound phenomenon, 见 phenomenon 项下相应术语)

Holmgren's test [ˈhɔlmgrən] (Alarik F. Holmgren) 霍姆格伦彩线试验(检色觉,即给患者一束彩线,让他在各色彩线中配色)

holmium (Ho) [ˈhɔlmiəm] *n* 钬(化学元素)

hol(o)- [构词成分]全部,完全

holoacardius [ˌhɔləuəˈkɑːdiəs] *n* 无心寄生胎畸胎 | ~ acephalus 无头无心寄生胎畸胎 / ~ acormus 无躯干无心寄生胎畸胎 / ~ amorphus 无定形无心寄生胎畸胎

holoantigen [ˌhɔləuˈæntidʒən] *n* 完全抗原

holoarthric [ˌhəuləuˈɑːθrik] *a* 全节生[产孢]的

Holobasidiomycetes [ˌhəuləubəˌsidiəumaiˈsiːtiːz] *n* 无隔担子菌纲

Holobasidiomycetidae [ˌhəuləubəˌsidiəumaiˈsetidiː] *n* 无隔担子菌亚纲

holoblastic [ˌhɔləuˈblæstik] *a* 全裂的(卵)

holocarboxylase synthetase [ˌhɔləukɑːˈbɔksileis ˈsinθəteis] 全羧化酶合成酶(此酶缺乏也许是一种常染色体隐性性状,可致多羧化酶缺乏症)

holocephalic [ˌhɔləusəˈfælik] *a* 头部完整的[畸胎]

holocrine [ˈhɔləkrin, -rain] *a* 全质分泌的

holodiastolic [ˌhɔləuˌdaiəˈstɔlik] *a* 全舒张[期]的

holoendemic [ˌhɔləuenˈdemik] *a* 全地方病的

holoenzyme [ˌhɔləuˈenzaim] *n* 全酶

hologamy [həˈlɔgəmi] *n* 配子大型;成体配合,整体交配

hologastroschisis [ˌhɔləugæsˈtrɔskisis] *n* 腹壁全裂

hologenesis [ˌhɔləuˈdʒenisis] *n* 泛生学(主张人类源于地球上一切地方)

hologram [ˈhɔləugræm] *n* 全息图

holography [həˈlɔgrəfi] *n* 全息照相术,全息术(用激光把被摄对象的照片以立体的图象记录下来进行研究) | acoustical ~ 声全息照相术

hologynic [ˌhɔləuˈdʒinik] *a* 限雌的(限雌或女性遗传,即通过位于X染色体上的基因遗传的)

holomastigote [ˌhɔləuˈmæstigəut] *a* 遍身鞭毛的,全身有鞭毛的

holomorph [ˈhəuləmɔːf] *n* 全性态(具有所有形式和时期的整个真菌,可能包括一个有性态〈telemorph〉和一个或一个以上无性态〈anamorph〉,不完全真菌时,只有无性态)

holomorphosis [ˌhɔləumɔːˈfəusis] *n* 完全再生

holomyarial [ˌhɔləumaiˈɛəriəl] *a* 全肌型的(指线虫)

holoparasite [ˌhɔləuˈpærəsait] *n* 全寄生物 | **holoparasitic** [ˌhɔləuˌpærəˈsitik] *a*

Holophyra coli [həˈlɔfirəˈkəuli] 结肠小袋[纤毛]虫(即 Balantidium coli)

holophytic [ˌhɔləuˈfitik] *a* 植物式营养的,自养植物的(指某些原虫)

holoprosencephaly [ˌhɔləuˌprɔsenˈsefəli] *n* 前脑无裂畸形(前脑未分裂为半球或叶) | familial alobar ~ 家族性前脑无叶无裂畸形

holorachischisis [ˌhɔləurəˈkiskisis] *n* 脊柱全裂

holorepressor [ˌhɔləuriˈpresə] *n* 全阻抑物(阻抑物原与辅阻抑物结合之后具有活性的阻抑物)

holosaccharide [ˌhɔləuˈsækəraid] *n* 纯多糖

holoschisis [ˌhɔləuˈskaisis] *n* 无丝分裂,直接分裂

Holospora [ˌhɔləuˈspɔːrə] *n* 全孢螺菌属

holosystolic [ˌhɔləusisˈtɔlik] *a* 全收缩[期]的

holothallic [ˌhəuləuˈθælik] *a* 全体殖[产孢]的

holothurin [ˌhəuləˈθjuərin] *n* 海参毒素

Holothyrus [ˌhɔləuˈθairəs] *n* 全壳螨属

holotonia [ˌhɔləuˈtəuniə] *n* 全身肌紧张,全身肌强直 | **holotonic** [ˌhɔləuˈtɔnik] *a*

holotopy [həˈlɔtəpi] *n* 全局关系(一器官的位置对于全身的关系)

holotrichous [həˈlɔtrikəs] *a* 遍生纤毛的,周身有纤毛的

holotype [ˈhɔlətaip] *n* 全型,正模标本(指微生物一个物种或亚种的模式培养)

holoxenic [ˌhɔləˈzenik] *a* 全污染的(指未在特殊实验室条件下饲养的动物)

holozoic [ˌhɔləˈzəuik] *a* 动物式营养的

holozymase [ˌhɔləuˈzaimeis] *n* 全酶

Holten's test [ˈhɔltən] (Cai Holten) 霍尔顿试验,肌酸酐清除率试验(检肾功能)

Holter monitor [ˈhəult] (Norman J. Holter) 霍尔特监护仪(一种非卧床的心电图监护仪)

Holthouse's hernia [ˈhɔlthauz] (Carsten Holthouse) 腹股沟股疝

Holth's operation [hɔlθ] (Sören Holth) 霍尔思手术(用钻孔术作巩膜切除)

Holt-Oram syndrome [həultˈəurəm] (Mary C. Holt; Samuel Oram) 霍-奥综合征(一种严重程度不等的常染色体遗传的心脏疾病,通常有房间隔或室间隔缺损,伴有骨骼畸形〈拇指发育不全及前臂短〉。亦称心-手综合征)

Holzknecht's chromoradiometer [ˈhɔltsknekt] (Guido Holzknecht) 霍尔兹克内希特X线量感色计(测X线剂量) | ~ space 霍尔兹克内希特间隙(X线斜面投影胸透时三个清晰的肺野的中间一个,亦称H间隙、椎前间隙、心后间隙) / ~ stomach 霍尔兹克内希特胃(X线照片显示幽门部位于对角线下端的胃) / ~ unit 霍尔兹克内希特单位(X线剂量的单位,等于红斑量的1/5)

homalocephalus [ˌhɔmələuˈsefələs] *n* 扁平头[畸形]

homaluria [ˌhɔməˈljuəriə] *n* 尿排泄[率]均匀

Homans' operation [ˈhəumənz] (John Homans) 霍曼斯手术(以前常用的治疗象皮肿和其他类型下肢大面积水肿,包括切除皮下组织及内外侧多余皮肤) | ~ sign 霍曼斯征(足被动性背屈时产生疼痛,为腓肠肌深部静脉血栓之征)

homarine [ˈhɔməriːn] *n* 龙虾肌碱

homatropine [həuˈmætrəpin] *n* 后马托品(散瞳药) | ~ hydrobromide 后马托品氢溴酸盐(睫状肌麻痹药,散瞳药) / ~ methylbromide 甲溴后马托品(解痉药,分泌抑制剂,尤用于胃肠道紊乱,口服)

homaxial [həuˈmæksiəl] *a* 等轴的

home [həum] *n* 家;疗养所,养育院 | nursing ~ 老人之家

Homén's syndrome [ˈhəumein] (Ernst A. Homén) 霍门综合征(一种遗传所决定的神经系统疾病,豆状核明显异常,特征为眩晕、运动失调、构语困难、渐进性痴呆及身体僵硬,尤其是小腿)

home(o)- [构词成分]相同,相等,类似

homeobox [ˈhəumiəuˌbɔks] *n* 同源框(任何一类高度保存的DNA顺序,约180碱基对长,把与DNA结合的蛋白质结构区编码。本词原先发现作为同源异形突变中重要的果蝇座位而得名的,但亦在人类中发现,通常是在控制发育的基因中找到)

homeochromatic [ˌhəumiəukrəuˈmætik] *a* 同色的

homeochrome [ˈhəumiəˌkrəum] *a* 同染性的(用于某些涎腺的浆液细胞)

homeocyte [həu'miːəsait] *n* 淋巴细胞
homeograft['həumiəgrɑːft, -græft] *n* 同种移植物
homeokinesis [ˌhəumiəukai'niːsis, -ki'n-] *n* 均等分裂(减数分裂期子细胞得到同等数量和种类的染色质)
homeomorphous [ˌhəumiəu 'mɔːfəs] *a* 同形[态]的,同结构的
homeo-osteoplasty [ˌhəumiəu ˌɔstiəu'plæsti] *n* 同种骨成形术
homeopathy [ˌhəumi'ɔpəθi] *n* 顺势疗法(对患者给予能使健康者产生类似待治疾病症状的药物进行治疗,但药物须用小剂量) | **homeopathic** ['həumiəu'pæθik] *a* / **homeopath** ['həumiəˌpæθ], **homeopathist** [ˌhəumi'ɔpəθist] *n* 顺势医疗者
homeoplasia [ˌhəumiəu'pleizjə] *n* 同质形成,同质新生 | **homeoplastic** [ˌhəumiəu'plæstik] *a* 同质的;同质形成的,同质新生的
homeorrhesis [ˌhəumiəu'riːsis] *n* 生理过程恒定
homeosis [ˌhəumi'əusis] *n* 异位同型形成,同源异形
homeostasis [ˌhəumiəu'steisis] *n* [体内] 稳态,内环境稳定(指有机体经常保持体内环境平衡稳定) | immunologic ~ 免疫自身稳定 | **homeostatic** [ˌhəumiəu'stætik] *a*
homeotherapy [ˌhəumiəu'θerəpi] *n* 顺势疗法(用一种与病原体相似而不相同的物质以治疗或预防疾病)
homeotherm ['həumiəθəːm] *n* 温血动物,恒温动物
homeothermal [ˌhəumiəu'θəːməl] *a* 温血的
homeothermic [ˌhəumiəu'θəːmik] *a* 恒温的;吸热的
homeothermism [ˌhəumiəu'θəːmizəm], **homeothermy** [ˌhəumiəu'θəːmi] *n* 恒温
homeotransplant [ˌhəumiəu'trænsplɑːnt] *n* 同种移植物
homeotransplantation ['həumiəuˌtrænsplɑːn'teiʃən] *n* 同种移植
homeotypic(al) [ˌhəumiəu'tipik(əl)] *a* 同型的(指生殖细胞的第二次成熟分裂)
homergic [həu'məːdʒik] *a* 同效的(指两种药物各自产生相同明显效果)
Homer Wright rosette ['həumə rait] (James Homer Wright) 霍默尔·赖特玫瑰花结(暗肿瘤细胞的一种环形或球形分型,周围是含有嗜中性粒细胞的苍白嗜酸性中心区,但无腔,见于某些成髓细胞瘤、成神经细胞瘤和成视网膜细胞瘤或其他眼科肿瘤)
homicide ['hɔmisaid] *n* 杀人;杀人者
homicidomania [ˌhɔmisaidəu'meinjə] *n* 杀人狂
homiculture ['hɔmiˌkʌltʃə] *n* 人种改良,积极优生学
homidium [hɔ'midiəm] *n* 乙菲啶(杀锥虫药)
hominal ['hɔminəl] *a* 人的,人类的
homing ['həumiŋ] *a* 归巢的(淋巴细胞)
hominid ['hɔminid] *a* 人科(Hominidae)的 *n* 类人类
Hominidae [həu'minidiː] *n* 人科
homininoxious [ˌhɔmini'nɔkʃəs] *a* 有害于人的
hominoid ['hɔminɔid] *a* 人上科的 *n* 人上科动物,类人动物
Hominoidea [ˌhɔmi'nɔidiə] *n* 类人动物总科
homme [ɔm] *n*【法】人 | ~ **rouge** [ɔm'rəuʒ] 大片红斑期(蕈样真菌病的一期,其红斑浸润而连接身体的大片面积)
Homo ['həuməu] *n*【拉】人属 | ~ sapiens 智人
homo- [构词成分]同一,同;[前缀]高,后莫
homoarterenol hydrochloride [ˌhəuməuˌɑːtə'riːnɔl] 盐酸异肾上腺素(血管收缩药)
Homobasidiomycetidae [ˌhəuməubəˌsidiəumai'siːtidiː] *n* 无隔担子菌亚纲
homobiotin [ˌhəuməu'baiətin] *n* 高生物素
homobody ['həuməˌbɔdi] *n* 同体(指含有一个个体基因型决定簇的一种抗体)
homocarnosinase [ˌhəumə'kɑːnəsineis] *n* 高肌肽酶
homocarnosine [ˌhəuməu'kɑːnəsiːn] *n* 高肌肽(人脑的正常成分)
homocarnosinosis [ˌhəuməˌkɑːnəsi'nəusis] *n* 高肌肽病
homocentric [ˌhɔməu'sentrik, ˌhəu-] *a* 同心的,共心的
homochronous [həu'mɔkrənəs] *a* 同龄发生的,同期发生的(各世代同龄的)
homocinchonine [ˌhəuməu'sinkənin] *n* 后莫辛可宁(一种生物碱,辛可宁的异构体)
homocladic [ˌhəuməu'klædik] *a* 同脉吻合的,同支吻合的
homocyclic [ˌhəuməu'siklik] *a* 同素环型的,纯环型的
homocysteine [ˌhəuməusis'tiːin] *n* 高半胱氨酸
homocysteine-tetrahydrofolate methyltransferase [ˌhəuməusis'tiːin ˌtetrəˌhaidrə'fəuleit ˌmeθil'trænsfəreis] 高半胱氨酸-四氢叶酸甲基转移酶,5-甲基四氢叶酸-高半胱氨酸 *S*-甲基转移酶
homocystine [ˌhəuməu'sistin] *n* 高胱氨酸
homocystinemia [ˌhəuməuˌsisti'niːmiə] *n* 高胱氨酸血
homocystinuria [ˌhəuməuˌsisti'njuəriə] *n* 高胱氨酸尿,同型胱氨酸尿症
homocytotropic [ˌhəuməuˌsaitəu'trɔpik] *a* 亲同种细胞的
homodesmotic [ˌhəməudes'mɔtik, ˌhəu-] *a* 同联

的,连接相同部分的(指连接中枢神经系统相同部分的神经纤维)

homodont [ˈhəumədɔnt] *a* 同型牙的

homodromous [hɔˈmɔdrəməs] *a* 同向的,同向运动的

homoe(o)- 见 home(o)-

homoeosis [ˌhəumiˈəusis] *n* 同源异形

homoeroticism [ˌhɔməuiˈrɔtisizəm, ˌhəu-] *n* 同性性欲,同性恋 | **homoerotism** [ˌhɔməuˈerətizəm] *n*, **homoerotic** [ˌhɔməuiˈrɔtik] *a*

homofermentation [ˈhəuməuˌfəːmenˈteiʃən] *n* 纯发酵[作用](通过恩伯顿-迈耶霍夫-帕纳斯〈Embden-Meyerhof-Parnas〉途径,发酵的主要产物为乳酸)

homofermenter [ˌhɔməufəːˈmentə] *n* 纯发酵菌

homogamete [ˌhɔməuˈgæmiːt] *n* 同型配子 | **homogametic** [ˌhɔməugəˈmetik] *a*

homogamy [hɔˈmɔgəmi] *n* 同配生殖 | **homogamous** [hɔˈmɔgəməs], **homogamic** [ˌhɔməuˈgæmik] *a*

homogenate [hɔˈmɔdʒineit] *n* [组织]匀浆

homogeneous [ˌhɔməuˈdʒiːnjəs] *a* 同种的,同质的 | **homogeneity** [ˌhɔməudʒeˈniːəti], **homogenicity** [ˌhɔməudʒiˈnisəti] *n* 同种性,同质性

homogenesis [ˌhɔməuˈdʒenisis] *n* 同型生殖,纯一生殖 | **homogenetic** [ˌhɔməudʒiˈnetik] *a*

homogenic [ˌhɔməuˈdʒenik] *a* 同种的,同型的;同基因的;纯合的

homogenize [hɔˈmɔdʒənaiz] *vt* 使匀浆 | **~r** *n* 匀浆器 / **homogenization** [hɔˌmɔdʒənaiˈzeiʃən, -niˈz-], **homogeneization** [ˌhɔməu ˌdʒiniaiˈzeiʃən, -iˈz-] *n* 匀浆化

homogenote [ˌhəuməuˈdʒiːnəut] *n* 纯基因子,同型基因接合子

homogenous [hɔˈmɔdʒinəs] *a* 同源的,纯系的;同质的 | **homogeny** [hɔˈmɔdʒini] *n* 同型生殖,纯一生殖

homogentisate [ˌhəuməˈdʒentiseit] *n* 尿黑酸,2,5-二羟苯乙酸

homogentisate 1,2-dioxygenase [ˌhəuməˈdʒentiseit daiˈɔksidʒineis] 尿黑酸1,2-双加氧酶(此酶缺乏为一种常染色体隐性性状,可致尿黑酸尿)

homogentisic acid [ˌhəumədʒenˈtisik] 尿黑酸,2,5-二羟苯乙酸

homogentisic acid oxidase [ˌhəuməudʒenˈtisik ˈæsid ˈɔksideis] 尿黑酸氧化酶,尿黑酸1,2-双加氧酶

homogentisic acid oxidase deficiency [ˌhəuməˈdʒənˈtisik] 尿黑酸氧化酶缺乏症,尿黑酸尿

homogentisuria [ˌhəuməuˌdʒentiˈsjuəriə] *n* 尿黑酸尿

homogeny [hɔˈmɔdʒini] *n* 同型生殖,纯一生殖

homoglandular [ˌhəuməuˈglændjulə] *a* 同腺的

homograft [ˈhɔməgrɑːft, -græft] *n* 同种移植物;同种移植

homografting [ˌhɔməuˈgrɑːftiŋ, -ˈgræft-] *n* 同种移植

homoi(o)- 见 home(o)-

homoioplasia [ˌhəumɔiəuˈpleizjə] *n* 同质形成,同质新生

homoiopodal [ˌhəumɔiˈɔpədl] *a* 同突的(指神经细胞)

homoiostasis [ˌhəumɔiˈɔstəsis] *n* 体内平衡,自身稳定(功能)(见 homeostasis)

homoiotherm [həuˈmɔiəθəːm] *n* 温血动物,恒温动物

homoiothermy [həuˈmɔiəˌθəːmi], **homoiothermism** [ˌhəumɔiəuˈθəːmizəm] *n* 体温调节,保持恒温 | **homoiothermic** [ˌhəumɔiəuˈθəːmik], **homoiothermal** [ˌhəumɔiəuˈθəːməl] *a* 恒温的,调温的

homoiotoxin [həuˈmɔiətɔksin] *n* 同种毒素

homokeratoplasty [ˌhəuməuˈkerətəˌplæsti] *n* 同种角膜成形术,同种角膜移植术

homolactic [ˌhəuməuˈlæktik] *a* 纯乳酸的

homolateral [ˌhəuməuˈlætərəl] *a* 同测的

homologen [həuˈmɔlədʒin] *n* 同系[化合]物

homologous [hɔˈmɔləgəs], **homological** [ˌhɔməˈlɔdʒikəl] *a* 同种的,同源的(指鸟羽及鱼鳞、抗原及其特异性抗体、等位基因染色体);同种异体的;同系的(化合物)

homolog(ue) [ˌhɔmələg] *n* 同种组织;同系[化合]物;相应物

homology [hɔˈmɔlədʒi] *n* 同种性,同源性;同系性

homolysin [həuˈmɔlisin] *n* 同种溶素(用同种的个体的抗原注射至另一个体所产生的溶素)

homolysis [həuˈmɔlisis] *n* 同种溶解(指细胞);同一裂解,均裂(指原子间化学键断裂)

homomorphic [ˌhɔməuˈmɔːfik], **homomorphous** [ˌhɔməuˈmɔːfəs] *a* 同形的

homomorphosis [ˌhɔməumɔːˈfəusis] *n* 同形新生

homonomous [hɔˈmɔnəməs] *a* 同律的,同列的,同系的(部分)

homonymous [hɔˈmɔniməs] *a* 同名的;同侧的,同一关系的

homophil [ˈhɔməfil] *n* 嗜同种抗体(只与某一特异性抗原起反应的一种抗体)

homophilic [ˌhɔməuˈfilik] *a* 嗜同种的(与某一特异性抗原有亲和力或起反应的,指抗体)

homophthalic acid [ˌhɔməuˈθælik] 高邻苯二酸,高酞酸

homopiperidinic acid [ˌhɔməupiˌperiˈdinik] 高哌

啶酸
homoplastic [ˌhɔməuˈplæstik] *a* 同种移植的,同种成形的;同型的
homoplasty [ˈhɔməˌplæsti] *n* 同种移植术,同种成形术;同型,相似(指器官相似)
homopolymer [ˌhɔməˈpɔlimə] *n* 同聚物
homopolysaccharide [ˌhəuməˌpɔliˈsækəraid] *n* 同多糖
homorganic [ˌhɔmɔːˈgænik] *a* 同种器官的
homosalate [ˌhəuməˈsæleit] *n* 胡莫柳酯(紫外线遮光剂)
homoscedastic [ˌhɔməuskiˈdæstik] *n* 同方差的
homoscedasticity [ˌhɔməuskidæsˈtisəti] *n* 同方差性,方差齐性
homosexual [ˌhɔməuˈseksjuəl] *a* 同性性欲的,同性恋的 *n* 同性恋者
homosexuality [ˌhɔməuˌseksjuˈæləti] *n* 同性恋 | female ~ 女子同性恋
homospore [ˈhɔməspɔː] *n* 同形孢子
homosporous [həuˈmɔspərəs] *a* 具同形孢子的
homostimulant [ˌhəuməuˈstimjulənt] *a* 同种刺激的 *n* 同种刺激剂(一器官的浸出物作用于原器官)
homostimulation [ˌhəuməuˌstimjuˈleiʃən] *n* 同种刺激法
homothallism [ˌhɔməuˈθælizəm] *n* 同种配合,同种接合 | **homothallic** [ˌhɔməuˈθælik] *a*
homotherm [ˌhəuməuθəːm] *n* 温血动物,恒温动物
homothermal [ˌhəuməuˈθəːməl], **homothermic** [ˌhəuməuˈθəːmik] *a* 恒温的,调温的
homotonia [ˌhɔməuˈtəuniə] *n* 等张性;等渗性
homotonic [ˌhɔməuˈtɔnik] *a* 等张的;等渗的
homotopic [ˌhɔməuˈtɔpik] *a* 同位的
homotransplant [ˌhɔməuˈtrænsplɑːnt, -plænt] *n* 同种移植物;同种移植 | **homotransplantation** [ˌhɔməuˌtrænsplɑːnˈteiʃən, -plæn-] *n* 同种移植
homotropism [hɔˈmɔtrəpizəm] *n* 亲同类性
homotype [ˈhɔmətaip] *n* 同型(身体左右对称的部分,如手) | **homotypic(al)** [ˌhəuməuˈtipik(əl)] *a*
homovanillic acid [ˌhɔməuvəˈnilik] 高香草酸
homoxenous [həuˈmɔksinəs] *n* 单[宿主]寄生的
homozoic [ˌhɔməuˈzəuik] *a* 同种动物的
homozygosis [ˌhəuməuzaiˈgəusis] *n* 纯合[现象],同型接合 | **homozygotic** [ˌhəuməuzaiˈgɔtik] *a*
homozygosity [ˌhəuməuzaiˈgɔsəti] *n* 纯合性(在一定位点上具有一对相同等位基因的情况)
homozygote [ˌhəuməuˈzaigəut] *n* 纯合子(在一定位点上具有一对相同等位基因的个体) | **homozygous** [ˌhəuməuˈzaigəs] *a*
homunculus [həuˈmʌŋkjuləs] ([复] **homunculi** [həuˈmʌŋkjulai]) *n* 【拉】矮人;小人(一度认为精子或卵子预成的微型人)
honey [ˈhʌni] *n* 蜂蜜
honeycomb [ˈhʌnikəum] *n* 蜂窝状物;蜂窝 *a* 蜂窝状的
hood [hud] *n* 突冠;兜状瓣 | tooth ~ 龈裹牙
hoof [huːf] ([复] **hoofs** 或 **hooves** [huːvz]) *n* 蹄
hoof-bound [ˈhuːf baund] *a* (马等) 挛缩足的 *n* 挛缩足
hook [huk] *n* 钩;牵引钩 | blunt ~ 钝钩(臀先露胎儿牵引用) / muscle ~, squint ~ 斜眼钩 / posterior palate ~ 提腭钩 / tracheostomy ~ 气管切开钩
hooked [hukt] *a* 钩状的,有钩的
hooknose [ˈhuknəuz] *n* 鹰鼻
hook-up [ˈhuk ʌp] *n* 缆络(为特殊诊断或治疗所安排的电路、器械及电极)
hookworm [ˈhukwəːm] *n* 钩虫 | American ~, New World ~ 美洲钩虫(即 Necator americanus) / ~ of the dog 犬钩虫(即 Ancylostoma caninum) / European ~, Old World ~ 十二指肠钩虫,十二指肠钩口线虫(即 Ancylostoma duodenale) / ~ of the rat 鼠钩虫(即 Nippostrongylus muris) / ~ of ruminants 反刍类钩虫(即 Bunostomum)
hoolamite [ˈhuləmait] *n* 浮石(测定一氧化碳用的试剂,含发烟硫酸、戊糖苷碘及浮石粉,遇一氧化碳即由淡灰色变成绿色)
hoose [huːz] *n* 蠕虫性支气管炎(牛、羊等)
Hoover's sign [ˈhuːvə] (Charles F. Hoover) 胡佛征(①正常情况或真性麻痹仰卧时,一侧下肢用力压床,则另侧下肢上举,但癔症及诈病无此反应;②吸气时,两侧肋下缘向中移动,见于肺气肿,但在胸腔积液或气胸则仅有一侧移动)
HOP hydroxydaunomycin (doxorubicin), vincristine, and prednisone 多柔比星-长春新碱-泼尼松(联合化疗治癌方案)
Hope's sign [həup] (James Hope) 霍普征(主动脉瘤时出现双重心搏)
Hopkins-Cole test [ˈhɔpkinz kəul] (Frederick G. Hopkins; Sidney W. Cole) 霍普金斯-科尔试验(检蛋白质)
Hoplopsyllus anomalus [ˌhɔpləˈsiləs əˈnɔmələs] 异胄蚤
Hopmann's polyp (papilloma) [ˈhɔpmən] (Carl M. Hopmann) 霍普曼息肉(乳头[状]瘤),鼻息肉
Hoppe-Seyler's test [ˌhɔpə ˈsailə] (Ernst F. I. Hoppe-Seyler) 霍佩-赛勒试验(检血一氧化碳、黄嘌呤)
hops [hɔps] *n* 啤酒花(药用缓解神经系统和失眠症)

hoquizil hydrochloride [ˈhɔkwizil] 盐酸胡喹嗪(支气管扩张药)

Hor. decub. hora decubitus【拉】就寝时

hordein [ˈhɔːdiin] *n* 大麦醇溶蛋白

hordeolum [hɔˈdiːələm] *n*【拉】睑腺炎

hordeum [ˈhɔːdiəm] *n*【拉】大麦

horehound [ˈhɔːhaund] *n* 夏至草(用作祛痰、苦味健胃及驱虫药)

Hor. interm. horis intermediis【拉】在间隔时间内,中间时刻

horizon [həˈraizən] *n* 人胚发育阶段

horizontal [ˌhɔriˈzɔntəl] *a* 水平的 *n* 水平线;水平面

horizontalis [ˌhɔrizɔnˈteilis] *a* 水平的;平行的

hormesis [hɔːˈmiːsis] *n*【希】刺激作用

hormion [ˈhɔːmiən] *n* 蝶枕点

Hormocardiol [ˌhɔːməuˈkɑːdiɔl] *n* 蛙心激素(冠状血管舒张药)

Hormodendrum [ˌhɔːməuˈdendrəm] *n* 着色芽生菌属,单孢枝霉属

hormonagogue [hɔːˈməunəgɔg] *a* 催激素的 *n* 催激素药

hormone [ˈhɔːməun] *n* 激素 | adrenocortical ~, cortical ~ 肾上腺皮质激素 / adrenocorticotropic ~ 促肾上腺皮质激素 / androgenic ~s 雄激素 / anterior pituitary ~ 垂体前叶激素 / chromaffin ~ 肾上腺素 / chromatophorotropic ~ 促黑激素,中叶素 / corpus luteum ~ 黄体激素,孕酮 / corticotropin releasing ~ (CRH) 促肾上腺皮质[激]素,释放[激]素 / estrogenic ~s 雌激素 / follicle-stimulating ~ (FSH) 促卵泡[激]素 / follicle-stimulating hormone releasing ~ (FSH-RH) 促卵泡[激]素释放[激]素 / galactopoietic ~, lactation ~, lactogenic ~, mammotropic ~ 催乳激素 / gonadotropin releasing ~ (GnRH) 促性腺[激]素释放[激]素 / growth ~ (GH), chondrotropic ~, somatotrophic ~, somatotropic ~ 生长激素 / growth hormone releasing ~ (GH-RH) 生长[激]素释放激素 / juvenile ~ 虫卵发育素,咽侧体激素(昆虫) / luteal ~ 黄体激素,孕酮 / luteinizing ~, interstitial cell-stimulating ~ 黄体生成素,促间质细胞激素 / luteinizing hormone releasing ~ (LH-RH) 促黄体素释放素 /luteotropic ~ 促黄体激素 / melanocyte-stimulating ~, melanophore-stimulating ~ 促黑[素细胞]激素 / orchidic ~, testicular ~, testis ~ 睾丸激素(睾酮) / posterior pituitary ~s [垂体]后叶激素 / progestational ~ 孕酮 / P. U. ~ (pregnancy urine ~) 孕尿激素(孕尿中的绒膜促性腺激素) / releasing ~s 释放激素 / somatotropin release inhibiting ~ 生长激素释放抑制激素,生长抑素 / somatotropin releasing ~ (SRH) 生长激素释放激素 / thyroid-stimulating ~ (TSH), thyrotropic ~ 促甲状腺[激]素 / thyrotropin releasing ~ (TRH) 促甲状腺[激]素释放[激]素 | **hormonal** [hɔːˈməunl], **hormonic** [hɔːˈmɔnik] *a*

hormonogen [ˈhɔːmənəˌdʒin] *n* 激素原,前激素

hormonogenesis [ˌhɔːmənəuˈdʒenisis], **hormonopoiesis** [ˌhɔːmənəupɔiˈiːsis], **hormopoiesis** [ˌhɔːməupɔiˈiːsis] *n* 激素生成 | **hormonogenic** [ˌhɔːmənəuˈdʒenik], **hormonopoietic** [ˌhɔːmənəupɔiˈetik], **hormopoietic** [ˌhɔːməupɔiˈetik] *a*

hormonology [ˌhɔːməˈnɔlədʒi] *n* 内分泌学,临床内分泌学

hormonopexic [ˌhɔːmənəuˈpeksik] *a* 激素固定的

hormonoprivia [hɔˌməunəˈpriviə] *n* 激素缺乏

hormonosis [ˌhɔːməuˈnəusis] *n* 激素过多症(如可的松疗法时治疗使用的结果)

hormonotherapy [ˌhɔːmənəuˈθerəpi] *n* 激素疗法,内分泌疗法

horn [hɔːn] *n* 角;角质;角状物 | cicatricial ~ 瘢痕角 / coccygeal ~ 尾骨角 / sacral ~ 骶骨角

horned [hɔːnd] *a* 有角的;角状的

Horner's law [ˈhɔːnə] (Johann F. Horner) 霍纳定律(一般的色盲经健康妇女由男性传于男性) | ~ syndrome (ptosis) 霍纳综合征(上睑下垂)(颈交感神经麻痹时,眼球内陷、上睑下垂、下睑轻度抬高、瞳孔缩小、睑裂变窄、以及受累侧面部无汗、潮红)

Horner's muscle [ˈhɔːnə] (William E. Horner) 睑板张肌(眼轮匝肌的泪囊部)

Horner's sign [ˈhɔːnə] (David A. Horner) 霍纳征(见 Spalding sign)

hornet [ˈhɔːnət] *n* 大黄蜂

hornification [ˌhɔːnifiˈkeiʃən] *n* 角[质]化

hornskin [ˈhɔːnskin] *n* 漆皮(矫形外科用)

Horn's sign [hɔːn] (C. ten Horn) 霍恩征(急性阑尾炎时,牵引右侧精索,引起疼痛)

horny [ˈhɔːni] *a* 角的,角制的,角状的

horopter [həˈrɔptə] *n* 双眼单视界 | **horopteric** [ˌhɔːrɔpˈterik] *a*

horripilation [ˌhɔripəˈleiʃən] *n* 鹅皮,立毛状态;鸡皮疙瘩

horror [ˈhɔrə] *n*【拉】恐惧 | ~ autotoxicus 恐惧自身中毒,自身中毒禁忌(埃利希〈Ehrlich〉等提出的术语,表示正常动物形成自身抗体的拒斥现象,认为此种抗体的形成可能导致抗体产生者自身破坏,这是由于存在于组织中的自身抗体与相应的抗原之间的反应结果所致,现称自身耐受性〈self-tolerance〉)

horsefly [ˈhɔːsflai] *n* 马蝇

horsepox [ˈhɔːspɔks] *n* 马天花,马痘

horseradish [ˈhɔːsrædiʃ] *n* 辣根;似辣根的十字

科形植物;辣根制成的调味品

horseradish peroxidase (HRP) [ˈhɔːsrædiʃ pəˈrɔksiˌdeis] 辣根过氧化物酶(用作生化测定的试剂)

horse-sickness [hɔːsˈsiknis] *n* 马传染病,马疫

Horsley's operation [ˈhɔːsli] (Victor A. H. Horsley) 霍斯利手术(切除皮质运动区以缓解上肢指痉病样和痉挛性运动) | ~ test 霍斯利试验(检葡萄糖) / ~ trephine 霍斯利环钻(一种可拆洗的环钻) / ~ wax(putty) 霍斯利蜡(油灰)(用以填塞小骨髓腔,以控制出血)

Hortega cell [hɔːˈteigə] (Pio del Rio Hortega) 小神经胶质细胞 | ~ method 霍特加法(一种使用碳酸氨银显示小神经胶质细胞的染色法)

hortobezoar [ˌhɔːtəuˈbiːzɔː] *n* 植物粪石

Horton's headache [ˈhɔːtn] (Bayard T. Horton) 丛集性头痛 | ~ arteritis 巨细胞动脉炎 / ~ disease 霍顿病(①丛集性头痛;②巨细胞动脉炎) / ~ syndrome 霍顿综合征(①丛集性头痛;②巨细胞动脉炎)

hortungskörper [ˌhɔːtuŋsˈkəːpə] *n*【德】体内沉积物(人变老的一种现象)

Hor. un. spatio horae unius spatio【拉】一小时后

hospice [ˈhɔspis] *n* 济贫院,晚期患者收容所

hospital [ˈhɔspitəl] *n* 医院 | base ~ 后方医院 / camp ~ 兵站医院 / closed ~ 不开放医院(只许本院医师诊治患者) / cottage ~ 诊疗所,(乡村)小医院 / day ~ 日间医院(见 partial hospitalization) / evacuation ~ 转运医院,后送医院 / field ~ 野战医院 / lyingin ~, maternity ~ 产院 / night ~ 夜间医院(见 partial hospitalization) / teaching ~ 教学医院

hospitalism [ˈhɔspitəlizəm] *n* 医务人员病(由于医院的特殊环境而引起的精神病态);住医院癖,就医癖;(恋母)依赖性抑郁症(anaclitic depression, 见 depression 项下相应术语)

hospitalist [ˈhɔspitəlist] *n* 住院医师

hospitalization [ˌhɔspitəlaiˈzeiʃən, -liˈz-] *n* 住院,入院;住院期 | partial ~ 部分住院[制](对完全不需要全日住院的患者的一种精神治疗方案,医院有一套专门设施或安排,患者可以在白天来治疗,晚上回家〈日间医院 day hospital〉,或者白天在社区,晚上回来接受夜间治疗,并晚上留院〈夜间医院 night hospital〉,或在一周内从事正常活动后于周末来院接受治疗并留院〈周末医院 weekend hospital〉)

hospitalize [ˈhɔspitəlaiz] *vt* (送患者)住院

host [həust] *n* 主人;寄主,宿主(指寄生另一机体的动物或植物,或指接受其他机体器官或组织移植的接受者) | definitive ~, final ~, primary ~ 终宿主,最后宿主,首要宿主 / intermediate ~, alternate ~, intermediary ~, secondary ~ 中间宿主 / paratenic ~ 转续宿主 / ~ of predilection 专嗜宿主,最适宿主 / reservoir ~ 储存宿主

hot [hɔt] *a* 热的,强放射性的

Hotchkiss' operation [ˈhɔtʃkis] (Lucius W. Hotchkiss) 霍奇基斯手术(治颊上皮瘤手术,即切除部分上颌骨和下颌骨,然后自舌及颈的一侧作缺损部的整形手术)

hot line [hɔt lain] 热线(昼夜电话咨询服务,由非专业人员和精神卫生专业人员组成)

Hottentot bustle [ˈhɔtntɔt] 臀脂过多,女臀过肥(Hottentot 为非洲南部的霍屯督人)

hottentotism [ˈhɔtntɔtizəm] *n* 剧烈口吃

hough [hɔk] *n* 后踝(牛,羊等)

Houghton's test [ˈhautən] (E. Mark Houghton) 霍顿试验(检麦角,即将麦角喂白色来克亨鸡,若鸡冠变深色,则麦角有药力)

Hounsfield unit [ˈhaunsfiːld] Sir Godfrey N. Hounsfield 亨斯菲尔德单位(X线衰减单位,用于CT扫描)

Houssay animal [uːˈsai] (Bernardo A. Houssay) 乌赛动物(切除垂体和胰腺的实验动物) | ~ phenomenon 乌赛现象(胰腺切除的实验动物,因垂体切除术可引起低血糖及对胰岛素的过敏性明显增加)

Houston's muscle [ˈhjuːstən] (John Houston) 休斯顿肌,阴茎背静脉压肌(压迫阴茎背静脉的球海绵体肌的肌纤维) | ~ valve 休斯顿瓣,直肠横襞

hoven [ˈhəuvən] *n* 胃气胀

Hoverbed [ˈhɔvəbed] *n* 气垫床(商品名,供烧伤患者用,患者整个身体支撑在一股温暖的无菌气流上,气流即沿床一些开口处向上流动)

Hovius' canal [ˈhəuviəs] (Jacob Hovius) 霍维斯管(某些哺乳动物眼球外壁上的涡静脉间的衔接管) | ~ circle 霍维斯环(一种密切吻合的睫静脉的巩膜内环形排列,见于人类以外的哺乳动物) / ~ plexus 霍维斯静脉丛(睫状体区内与巩膜静脉窦连接的静脉丛)

Howard's method [ˈhauəd] (Benjamin D. Howard) 霍华德法(一种人工呼吸法,患者仰卧,背下置一垫子,使其头部低于腹部,然后将其双臂高举过头,在下端肋骨处作向内及向上来回的加压,每分钟约16次)

Howel-Evans' syndrome [ˈhauəl ˈevənz] (W. Howel-Evans) 豪厄尔·埃文思综合征(5~15岁间出现的弥漫性掌跖角化病,伴晚年食管癌形成)

Howell-Jolly bodies [ˈhauəl ʒɔˈli] (W. H. Howell; Justin M. J. Jolly) 豪厄尔-若利小体(圆形或卵圆形小体,呈淡红或淡蓝色,出现于各种类型的贫血或白血病以及在脾切除后的红细胞内,可能为非正常的红细胞核残片)

Howell's bodies [ˈhauəl] (William H. Howell) 豪厄尔小体(见 Howell-Jolly bodies) | ~ method 豪厄尔法(检血凝时间) / ~ test 豪厄尔试验(检凝血酶原)

Howship's lacunae [ˈhauʃip] (John Howship) 吸收陷窝

Howship-Romberg sign [ˈhauʃipˈrɔmbəːg] (J. Howship; Moritz H. von Romberg)豪-龙征(疼痛沿股内侧传至膝,由于闭孔疝压迫闭孔神经所致)

Hoyne's sign [hɔin] (Archibald L. Hoyne) 霍因征(麻痹性或非麻痹性脊髓灰质炎时引发之征:患者仰卧,抬起双肩时头即后垂)

HP house physician 内科住院医师

HP haptoglobin 结合珠蛋白,触珠蛋白

HPETE hydroperoxyeicosatetraenoic acid 氢过氧化二十碳四烯酸

HPF high-power field 高倍视野

HPG human pituitary gonadotropin 人垂体促性腺激素

HPL, hPL human placental lactogen 人胎盘催乳素

HPLC high-performance liquid chromatography 高效液相层析,高效液相色谱法

HPRT hypoxanthine phosphoribosyltransferase 次黄嘌呤磷酸核糖基转移酶

HPTA hepatopoietin A 肝生成素 A

HPV human papillomavirus 人乳头瘤病毒

HRA high right atrium 高右心房(电描记图)

HRCT high-resolution computed tomography 高分辨力计算体层摄影[术]

HRF histamine releasing factor 组胺释放因子

HRIG human rabies immune globulin 人狂犬病免疫球蛋白

HRP horseradish peroxidase 辣根过氧化物酶

HRSA Health Resources and Services Administration 卫生资源与卫生事业管理局(属美国公共卫生署)

HRT hormone replacement therapy 激素替补疗法

HS house surgeon 外科住院医师

h. s hora somni【拉】就寝时

HSA human serum albumin 人血清白蛋白

HSAN hereditary sensory and autonomic neuropathy 遗传性感觉和自主神经病变

HSAN-Ⅰ hereditary sensory and autonomic neuropathy (type Ⅰ) 遗传性感觉和自主神经病变(Ⅰ型)

HSAN-Ⅱ hereditary sensory and autonomic neuropathy (type Ⅱ) 遗传性感觉和自主神经病变(Ⅱ型)

HSAN-Ⅲ hereditary sensory and autonomic neuropathy (type Ⅲ) 遗传性感觉和自主神经病变(Ⅲ型)

HSF hydrazine sensitive factor 肼敏感因子

HSR homogeneously staining regions 匀染区

HSV herpes simplex virus 单纯疱疹病毒

5-HT 5-hydroxytryptamine 5-羟色胺

Ht total hyperopia 总远视

HTACS human thyroid adenylate cyclase stimulators 人甲状腺腺苷酸环化酶刺激因子

HTC homozygous typing cells 纯合子分型细胞

^{3}H-TdR tritium-labeled thymidine 氚标记胸苷

HTL hearing threshold level 听阈级

HTLV human T-cell leukemia / lymphoma virus 人 T 细胞白血病 / 淋巴瘤病毒

HTLV-1 human T-lymphotropic virus 1 人嗜 T 淋巴细胞病毒 1

HTLV-2 human T-lymphotropic virus 2 人嗜 T 淋巴细胞病毒 2

HTLV-Ⅲ human T-lymphotropic virus type Ⅲ 人嗜 T 淋巴细胞病毒Ⅲ型

H^+-transporting ATP synthase [trænsˈpɔːtiŋ ˈsinθeis] H^+-转运腺苷三磷酸合酶(亦称腺苷三磷酸酶,H^+-腺苷三磷酸酶,线粒体腺苷三磷酸酶)

Hua [ˈhjuːə] *n* 华螺属 | ~ ningpoensis 宁波华螺 / ~ toucheana 触发华螺

huang-qi【汉】黄芪

Hubbard tank [ˈhʌbəd] (Carl Hubbard) 哈伯德浴池(供患者在水下练力的浴池)

Huchard's disease [juːˈʃɑː] (Henri Huchard) 尤夏病(持续性动脉压过高,被认为是引起动脉硬化的原因) | ~ sign (symptom) 尤夏征(症状)(肺水肿时的一种反常叩响)

Huebner-Herter disease [ˈhɔibnə ˈhəːtə] (J. O. L. Huebner; Christian A. Herter) 婴儿型非热带性口炎性腹泻,乳糜泻

Hueck's ligament [hjuːk] (Alexander F. Hueck) 许克韧带(虹膜角膜角小梁网)

Hueter's bandage [ˈhjuːtə] (Karl Hueter) 许特绷带(会阴人字形绷带) | ~ line 许特线(当臂伸展时,连接肱骨上髁与鹰嘴尖的直线) / ~ maneuver 许特手法(插胃管时,用左示指将患者的舌向下及向前压下) / ~ sign 许特征(骨折断片间有纤维组织时,骨振动传递缺乏)

Huët-Pelger nuclear anomaly [ˈhjuet ˈpelgə] (G. J. Huët; Karel Pelger) 许特-佩尔格尔核异常(见 Pelger-Huët nuclear anomaly)

Huggins operation [ˈhʌginz] (Charles B. Huggins) 哈金斯手术(治前列腺癌的睾丸切除术) | ~ test 哈金斯试验(检癌,即取患者血样,以碘乙酸处理并加热,血清白蛋白在健康人结块较快,癌症患者较慢)

Hughes' reflex [hjuːz] (Charles H. Hughes) 休斯反射,男性反射(virile reflex, 见 reflex 项下相应术语的②解)

Hughes-Stovin syndrome [hjuːz ˈstəuvin] (John

P. Hughes; Peter G. I. Stovin) 休斯-斯托文综合征(肺动脉和周围静脉血栓形成,特征为头痛、发热、咳嗽、视神经乳头水肿和咯血)

Hughston's projection [ˈhjuːstən] (J. C. Hughston)休斯顿投照(髌股区放射摄影投照)

Huguenin's edema [igəˈnæŋ] (Gustave Huguenin) 于根南水肿(急性充血性脑水肿)

Huguier's canal [igiˈɛə] (Pierre C. Huguier) 鼓索小管 | ~ circle 于吉埃环(在子宫颈和子宫体结合部附近,由子宫动脉形成的环) / ~ sinus 于吉埃窦(鼓室前庭窗与蜗窗间的凹陷)

Huhner test [ˈhunə] (Max Huhner) 胡讷试验,性交后试验(检精子)

HuIFN human interferon 人干扰素

humankind [ˌhjuːmənˈkaind] *n* 人类

Human's sign [ˈhjuːmən] (J. U. Human) 下颌回缩征(chin-retraction sign, 见 sign 项下相应术语)

humectant [hjuˈmektənt] *a* 致湿的 *n* 致湿物,致湿剂

humectation [ˌhjumekˈteiʃən] *n* 致湿[作用]

humeral [ˈhjuːmərəl] *a* 肱骨的

humeroradial [ˌhjuːmərəuˈreidjəl] *a* 肱桡的

humeroscapular [ˌhjuːmərəuˈskæpjuːlə] *a* 肱[骨]肩胛的

humeroulnar [ˌhjuːmərəuˈʌlnə] *a* 肱尺的

humerus [ˈhjuːmərəs] ([复] **humeri** [ˈhjuːmərai]) *n* 【拉】肱骨 | ~ varus 肱骨内弯

humic [ˈhjuːmik] *a* 腐殖的 | ~ acid 腐殖酸

humidify [hju(ː)ˈmidifai] *vt* 使湿润 | **humidifier** *n* 增湿器,加湿器 / **humidification** [hju(ː)ˌmidifiˈkeiʃən] *n* 湿化,增湿

humidistat [hjuːˈmidistæt] *n* 恒湿器,湿度调节器

humidity [hju(ː)ˈmiditi] *n* 湿气;湿度 | absolute ~ 绝对湿度 / relative ~ 相对湿度

humin [ˈhjuːmin] *n* 腐殖酸;(水解蛋白) 腐黑物

humor [ˈhjuːmə] ([复] **humors, humores** [hjuːˈmɔris]) *n* 液;体液 | aqueous ~ 水状液(眼房水) / crystalline ~ 晶状体;玻璃体 / ocular ~ 眼液(眼房水或玻璃体液) / vitreous ~ 玻璃体;玻璃体液

humoral [ˈhjuːmərəl] *a* 体液的

humoralism [ˈhjuːmərəlizəm], **humorism** [ˈhjuːmərizəm] *n* 体液学说(一种废弃的学说,认为一切疾病都是由体液的变化引起的)

hump [hʌmp] *n* 驼背 | buffalo ~ 水牛背

humpback [ˌhʌmpbæk] *n* 脊柱后凸,驼背

Humphry's ligament [ˈhʌmfri] (George M. Humphry) 半月板股骨前韧带

Humulus [ˈhjuːmjuːləs] *n* 【拉】葎草属 | ~ lupulus 啤酒花

humus [ˈhjuːməs] *n* 【拉】腐殖土,腐殖质

hunchback [ˈhʌntʃbæk] *n* 驼背,脊柱后凸;驼背者 | **~ed** *a* 驼背的

hunger [ˈhʌŋgə] *n* 饥饿 | air ~ 空气饥(一种阵发性痛苦状呼吸困难) / calcium ~ 钙饥饿,缺钙症(在月经期或月经后的剧烈头痛) / chlorine ~ 氯饥饿,血氯离子缺乏(血内氯缺乏所致的渴望食盐) / hormone ~ 激素饥饿,激素缺乏(身体器官缺乏其保持生理功能所需特殊激素的状态)

Hunner's ulcer [ˈhʌnə] (Guy LeRoy Hunner) 亨纳溃疡,全[膀胱]壁纤维变性(慢性间质性膀胱炎的一种损害,危及膀胱壁所有层,黏膜上呈现红褐色斑点)

hunterian [hʌnˈtiəriən] (John Hunter) *a* 亨特的(如 ~ chancre 亨特下疳,硬下疳)

Hunter's canal [ˈhʌntə] (John Hunter) 亨特管,收肌管 | ~ gubernaculum 睾丸引带 / ~ operation 亨特手术(动脉瘤近侧即在第一侧支上方的动脉结扎术)

Hunter's glossitis [ˈhʌntə] (William Hunter) 亨特舌炎,萎缩性舌炎(见于恶性贫血,舌表面及舌缘呈光滑性萎缩)

Hunter's ligament [ˈhʌntə] (William Hunter) 子宫圆韧带 | ~ line [腹]白线

Hunter's syndrome, Hunter-Hurler syndrome [ˈhuntə ˈhuələ] (Charles H. Hunter; Gertrud Hurler) 亨特综合征,亨特-胡尔勒综合征(黏多糖贮积症的一型,临床上类似胡尔勒综合征,但无驼背和角膜混浊,其他症状为色素性视网膜炎、多毛、视神经乳头水肿、视神经萎缩、进行性聋,属于X染色体隐性遗传。亦称黏多糖贮积症Ⅱ型)

Huntington's chorea (disease) [ˈhʌntiŋtən] (George Huntington) 亨廷顿舞蹈症〈病〉(一种罕见的遗传性疾病,特征为慢性遗传性舞蹈症和精神衰退,最终导致痴呆,一般发病后15年即死亡,由常染色体显性遗传) | ~ sign 亨廷顿征(患者仰卧,小腿悬出床边,并令其咳嗽,如瘫痪大腿屈曲小腿伸直,提示瘫痪是由上运动神经元病变引起的)

Hunt's atrophy [hʌnt] (James Ramsay Hunt) 亨特[肌]萎缩(神经性手部小肌萎缩,无感觉障碍) | ~ disease 亨特病(①肌阵挛性小脑协同失调;②见 Ramsay Hunt syndrome ①解) / ~ neuralgia 亨特神经痛(见 Ramsay Hunt syndrome ①解) / ~ paradoxical phenomenon 亨特反常现象(变形性肌张力障碍时,令患者将原向背侧痉挛的足用力向跖侧屈曲,则背侧痉挛加强,若令患者伸足,反见其足向跖侧屈曲) / ~ striatal syndrome 亨特纹状体综合征(①旧纹状体综合征,特征为自动性联合运动麻痹、肌强直及震颤麻痹型节律性震颤,为纹状体的苍白球系统的萎缩或变性所致。亦称苍白球综合征、震颤麻痹综合征;②新纹状体综合征,特征为自动联合

型自发性舞蹈状样运动,为纹状体的新纹状体系统或纹状体苍白球系统的萎缩或变性所致,亦称舞蹈症样综合征;③混合性纹状体综合征,特征为舞蹈症及麻痹震颤的各种合并症状,有手足徐动症、肌张力障碍和进行性豆状核变性) / ~ syndrome 亨特综合征(见 Ramsay Hunt syndrome)

Hunt's method [hʌnt] (Reid Hunt) 亨特法(测甲状腺制剂的活性) | ~ reaction(test) 亨特反应(试验),乙腈反应(小白鼠受甲亢患者的血处理后,增加对乙腈的抵抗力)

Huppert's test [ˈhuːpət] (Hugo Huppert) 赫珀试验(检胆色素)

Hurler-Scheie syndrome [ˈhuələ ˈʃaii] (G. Hurler; Harold G. Scheie) 胡尔勒-沙伊综合征(黏多糖贮积症Ⅰ型3个等位基因疾病之一,其临床特征介于胡尔勒综合征和沙伊综合征之间,系由L-艾杜糖苷酸酶缺乏所致,特征为颏后缩〈小颌症〉,症状包括智力迟钝、侏儒症、多发性骨发育不全、角膜混浊、耳聋、疝、关节强直〈爪形手〉及瓣膜性心脏病。患者可活到18~19岁或20几岁。亦称黏多糖贮积症ⅠH/S型)

Hurler's syndrome (disease) [ˈhuələ] (Gertrud Hurler) 胡尔勒综合征(病)(一种常染色体隐性遗传性疾病,特征为滴水嘴面形、鼻塌陷、体格矮小、耳聋、驼背、精神发育迟缓、角膜混浊等。亦称脂肪软骨营养不良、黏多糖贮积症Ⅰ型)

Hurst disease [həːst] (Edward W. Hurst) 赫斯特病,急性坏死性出血性脑脊髓炎

Hürthle cells [ˈhəːtl] (Karl Hürthle) 许特尔细胞(大嗜酸细胞,有时见于甲状腺内的大细胞) | ~ cell tumor 许特尔细胞瘤(由许特尔细胞组成的一种甲状腺瘤)

Hurtley's test [ˈhəːtli] (William H. Hurtley) 赫特利试验(检乙酰乙酸)

Huschke's canal [ˈhuʃkə] (Emil Huschke) 胡施克管(鼓环管,由鼓环的小结连合而成的通道,一般在童年即已消失) | ~ foramen 胡施克孔(靠近鼓板内端的穿孔,由发育停止所致) / ~ ligaments 胃胰襞 / ~ valve 鼻泪管襞

husk [hʌsk] *n* 蠕虫性气管炎(牛、羊等)

Hutch diverticulum [hʌtʃ] (J. A. Hutch) 哈奇憩室(膀胱黏膜通过输尿管膀胱连接附近壁内的弱点突出,常为长期膀胱内高压引起)

Hutchinson-Gilford disease, syndrome [ˈhʌtʃinsn ˈgilfəd] (Jonathan Hutchinson; Hastings Gilford) 早老症

hutchinsonian [hʌtʃinˈsəuniən] (Jonathan Hutchinson) *a* 哈钦森的

Hutchinson's disease [ˈhʌtʃinsn] (Jonathan Hutchinson) 哈钦森病(①夏令痒疹;②匐行性血管瘤;③泰氏脉络膜炎〈见 Tay's choroiditis〉) | ~ facies 哈钦森面容(眼外肌麻痹的一种特殊表现,眼球固定,眉提高和眼睑下垂) / ~ mask 哈钦森面具感(面部皮肤有一种面具感觉,常为脊髓痨性症状) / ~ patch 哈钦森斑(梅毒性角膜炎时角膜上的红色或橙黄色斑) / ~ pupil 哈钦森瞳孔(一个瞳孔散大,另一个瞳孔不散大) / ~ sign 哈钦森征(①先天性梅毒时的间质性角膜炎及角膜暗红变色;②哈钦森牙;③哈钦森三征) / ~ teeth 哈钦森牙,锯齿形牙(为先天性梅毒征,但不一定由先天梅毒引起) / ~ triad 哈钦森三征(弥漫性间质性角膜炎、耳迷路病及哈钦森牙,见于先天性梅毒)

Hutchison type (syndrome) [ˈhʌtʃisn] (Robert Hutchison)哈奇森型(综合征)(成神经细胞瘤转移至颅内)

Hutinel's disease [iːtiˈnel] (Victor H. Hutinel) 于廷内尔病(小儿结核性心包炎,伴有肝硬变)

Huxley's layer (membrane) [ˈhʌksli] (Thomas H. Huxley) 赫胥黎层(膜)(毛囊的内根鞘层)

huygenian [haiˈdʒeniən] (Christian Huygens〈或 Huyghens〉) *a* 惠更斯的(如 ~ eyepiece 惠更斯目镜)

HVA homovanillic acid 高香草酸

HVL half-value layer 半值层,半价厚度

Hy hyperopia 远视[眼]

hyal [ˈhaiəl] *a* 舌骨的

hyal- 见 hyalo-

hyalin [ˈhaiəlin] *n* 透明蛋白,透明素;包囊质(包虫囊壁的构成物质) | hematogenous ~ 血透明质

hyaline [ˈhaiəliːn] *a* 透明的,玻璃样的

hyalinization [ˌhaiəˈlinaiˈzeiʃən] *n* 玻璃样化,透明化

hyalinosis [ˌhaiəliˈnəusis] *n* 透明变性 | ~ cutis et mucosae 皮肤黏膜透明变性,脂质蛋白沉积病

hyalinuria [ˌhaiəliˈnjuəriə] *n* 透明蛋白尿

hyalitis [ˌhaiəˈlaitis] *n* 玻璃体膜炎;玻璃体炎,玻璃体囊炎 | asteroid ~ 星形玻璃体炎 / ~ punctata 点状玻璃体炎 / ~ suppurativa 化脓性玻璃体炎 | **hyaloiditis** [ˌhaiəlɔiˈdaitis] *n*

hyalo-, hyal- [构词成分] 透明,玻璃体,玻璃液;玻璃样的

hyalogen [haiˈælədʒin] *n* 透明蛋白原

hyalohyphomycosis [ˌhaiələuˌhaifəumaiˈkəusis] *n* 透明丝状菌病,无色丝状菌病

hyaloid [ˈhaiəlɔid] *a* 透明的,玻璃样的

hyaloidin [ˌhaiəˈlɔidin] *n* 玻璃糖质(类似软骨质,但不含硫酸)

hyalomere [ˈhaiələmiə] *n* [血小板]透明区

hyalomitome [ˌhaiələuˈmitəum] *n* 透明质,胞基质

Hyalomma [ˌhaiəˈlɔmə] *n* 璃眼蜱属

hyalomucoid [ˌhaiələuˈmjuːkɔid] *n* 玻璃体黏

液质

hyalonyxis [ˌhaiələuˈniksis] *n* 玻璃体穿刺术

hyalophagia [ˌhaiələuˈfeidʒiə], **hyalophagy** [ˌhaiəˈlɔfədʒi] *n* 食玻璃癖

hyaloplasm [ˈhaiələplæzəm] *n* 透明质,胞基质;轴浆 | nuclear ~ 核透明质,核液,核淋巴 | **hyalotome** [haiˈælətəum] *n*

hyaloserositis [ˌhaiələuˌsiərəˈsaitis] *n* 透明性浆膜炎 | progressive multiple ~ 进行性多发性透明性浆膜炎

hyalosis [ˌhaiəˈləusis] *n* 玻璃体变性 | asteroid ~ 星形玻璃体变性(亦称星形玻璃体炎)

hyalosome [haiˈæləsəum] *n* 拟核仁,透明体

hyalurate [ˌhaiəˈljureit], **hyaluronate** [ˌhaiəˈljurəneit] *n* 透明质酸盐(或酯)

hyaluronate lyase [ˌhaiəˈljurəneit ˈlaieis] 透明质酸裂合酶

hyaluronic acid [ˌhaiəljuˈrɔnik] 透明质酸

hyaluronidase [ˌhaiəljuˈrɔnideis] *n* 透明质酸酶

hyaluronoglucosaminidase [ˌhaiəljuˌrɔnəuˌgluːkəuˈsæminideis] *n* 透明质酸氨基葡糖苷酶

hyaluronoglucuronidase [ˌhaiəljuˌrɔnəuˌgluːkjuəˈrɔnideis] *n* 透明质酸葡糖醛酸酶

hybaroxia [ˌhaibəˈrɔksiə] *n* 高压氧疗法

hybenzate [haiˈbenzeit] *n* 羟苯酰苯酸盐,邻-(4-羟基苯甲酰基)苯甲酸盐 [*O*-(4-hydroxybenzoyl) benzoate 的 USAN 缩约词]

Hybomitra [ˌhaibəuˈmaitrə] *n* 瘤虻属

hybrid [ˈhaibrid] *n* 杂种 *a* 杂种的 | false ~ 假杂种 | **~ism** *n* 杂种性;杂交 / **~ity** [haiˈbridəti] *n* 杂种性

hybridize [ˈhaibridaiz] *vt, vi* 杂交 | **hybridization** [ˌhaibridaiˈzeiʃən, -diˈz-] *n* 杂交;杂化

hybridoma [ˌhaibriˈdəumə] *n* 杂交瘤

hycanthone [haiˈkænθəun] *n* 海恩酮(抗血吸虫药) | ~ mesylate 甲磺海蒽酮

hyclate [ˈhaikleit] *n* 盐酸去氧土霉素 (monohydrochloride hemiethanolate hemihydrate 的 USAN 缩约词)

hydantoic acid [ˌhaidænˈtəuik] 脲乙酸

hydantoin [haiˈdæntəuin] *n* 乙内酰脲

hydantoinate [ˌhaidænˈtəuineit] *n* 乙内酰脲盐

hydathode [ˈhaidəθəud] *n* 排水器,排水孔(植物)

hydatid [ˈhaidətid] *n* 棘球囊,棘球蚴囊,包虫囊;囊 | alveolar ~s 泡状棘球囊 / sessile ~ 睾丸附件

hydatidiform [ˌhaidəˈtidifɔːm] *a* 囊状的;棘球囊状的,包虫囊状的

hydatidosis [ˌhaidətiˈdəusis] *n* 棘球蚴病,包虫病

hydatidostomy [ˌhaidətiˈdɔstəmi] *n* 棘球囊切开引流术

hydatiduria [ˌhaidətiˈdjuəriə] *n* 棘球囊尿

Hydatigena [ˌhaidəˈtidʒenə] *n* 绦虫属,带绦虫属(即 Taenia)

hydatism [ˈhaidətizəm] *n* 腔液音(腔内液体动荡声)

hydatoid [ˈhaidətɔid] *n* 水状液,房水;玻璃体膜 *a* 水状液的,房水的

hydnocarpate [ˌhidnəˈkɑːpeit] *n* 次大风子油酸盐(或酯)

hydnocarpic acid [ˌhidnəˈkɑːpic] 次大风子油酸,环戊烯十一[烷]酸

Hydnocarpus [ˌhidnəˈkɑːpəs] *n* 大风子属

hydr- 见 hydro-

hydracetin [haiˈdræsitin] *n* 乙酰苯肼

hydracid [haiˈdræsid] *n* [氢]卤酸

hydracrylic acid [ˌhaidrəˈkrilik] *β*-羟基丙酸,3-羟基丙酸

hydradenitis [ˌhaidrædiˈnaitis] *n* 汗腺炎

hydradenoma [ˌhaidrædiˈnəumə] *n* 汗腺腺瘤

hydraeroperitoneum [haiˌdrɛərəperitəuˈniːəm] *n* 水气腹(腹腔积水充气)

hydragogue [ˈhaidrəgɔg] *a* 致水泻的 *n* 水泻剂

hydralazine [haiˈdræləziːn] *n* 肼屈嗪(抗高血压药)

hydramine [ˈhaidrəmin] *n* 羟基胺

hydramnios [haiˈdræmniɔs], **hydramnion** [haiˈdræmniɔn] *n* 羊水过多

hydranencephaly [ˌhaidrænenˈsefəli] *n* 积水性无脑畸形

Hydrangea [haiˈdreindʒə] *n* 绣球[花]属,八仙花属

hydrangiography [haiˌdrændʒiˈɔgrəfi] *n* 淋巴管论;淋巴管 X 线造影[术]

hydrangiology [haiˌdrændʒiˈɔlədʒi] *n* 淋巴管学

hydrangiotomy [haiˌdrændʒiˈɔtəmi] *n* 淋巴管切开术

hydrargyri [haiˈdrɑːdʒiri] (hydrargyrum 的所有格) *n*【拉】汞,水银 | ~ bichloridum, ~ chloridum corrosivum 升汞 / ~ iodidum flavum 黄碘化亚汞 / ~ iodidum rubrum [红]碘化汞 / ~ oxidum flavum 黄氧化汞,黄降汞 / ~ salicylas 水杨酸汞

hydrargyria [ˌhaidrɑːˈdʒiriə], **hydrargyrism** [haiˈdrɑːdʒirizəm], **hydrargyrosis** [haiˌdrɑːdʒiˈrəusis] *n* 汞中毒

hydrargyromania [haiˌdrɑːdʒirəuˈmeiniə] *n* 汞中毒性精神病

hydrargyrorelapsing [haiˌdrɑːdʒirəuriˈlæpsiŋ] *a* 汞[中毒]治疗后复发的

hydrargyrum [haiˈdrɑːdʒirəm] *n*【拉】汞,水银 | ~ ammoniatum 氯化氨基汞,白降汞 / ~ chloridum mite 甘汞 / ~ oleatum 油酸汞

hydrarthrosis [ˌhaidrɑːˈθrəusis] *n* 关节积水 | in-

termittent ~ 间歇性关节积水 | **hydrarthrodial** *a*
hydrase [ˈhaidreis] *n* 水化酶
Hydrastis [haiˈdræstis] *n* 黄连属 | ~ canadensis 北美黄连
hydratase [ˈhaidrəteis] *n* 水合酶
hydrate [ˈhaidreit] *n* 水合物,水化物 *vt*, *vi* 水合 | **~d** *a* 水合的,水化的 / **hydration** [haiˈdreiʃən] *n* 水合[作用],水化[作用]
hydraulic [haiˈdrɔːlik] *a* 水力的;水压的,液压的 | **~s** [复] *n* 水力学
hydrazine [ˈhaidrəziːn] *n* 肼,联胺
hydrazinolysis [ˌhaidrəziˈnɔləsis] *n* 肼解[作用]
hydrazoate [ˌhaidrəˈzəueit] *n* 叠氮化物
hydrazoic acid [ˌhaidrəˈzəuik] 叠氮酸
hydrazone [ˈhaidrəzəun] *n* 腙
hydremia [haiˈdriːmiə] *n* 血水分过多[症],稀血症
hydrencephalocele [ˌhaidrenˈsefələsiːl] *n* 积水性脑突出
hydrencephalomeningocele [ˌhaidrenˌsefələuməˈniŋgəsiːl] *n* 积水性脑膜突出
hydrencephalus [ˌhaidrenˈsefələs], **hydrencephaly** [ˌhaidrenˈsefəli] *n* 脑积水
hydrepigastrium [ˌhaidrepiˈgæstriəm] *n* 腹膜腹肌间积水
hydriatrics [ˌhaidriˈætriks] *n* 水疗法 | **hydriatric** *a*
hydric [ˈhaidrik] *a* 氢的,含氢的
hydride [ˈhaidraid] *n* 氢化物
hydrindicuria [ˌhaidrindiˈkjuəriə] *n* 吲哚尿
hydriodic acid [ˌhaidriˈɔdik] 氢碘酸
hydrion [haiˈdraiən] *n* 氢离子
hydr(o)- [构词成分] 水,氢
hydroa [hiˈdrəuə] *n* 水疱,水疱病
hydroadipsia [ˌhaidrəuəˈdipsiə] *n* 不渴[症],渴感缺乏
hydroappendix [ˌhaidrəuəˈpendiks] *n* 阑尾积水
Hydrobiidae [ˌhaidrəuˈbiːidiː] *n* 觿螺科
Hydrobiinae [ˌhaidrəuˈbiːiniː] *n* 觿螺亚科
hydrobilirubin [ˌhaidrəuˌbiliˈruːbin] *n* 氢胆红素
hydroblepharon [ˌhaidrəuˈblefərɔn] *n* 睑水肿
hydrobromic acid [ˌhaidrəuˈbrəumik] 氢溴酸
hydrobromide [ˌhaidrəuˈbrəumaid] *n* 氢溴化物
hydrocaffeic acid [ˌhaidrəukəˈfiːik] 二羟苯丙酸
hydrocalycosis [ˌhaidrəuˌkæliˈkəusis] *n* 肾盏积水
hydrocalyx [ˌhaidrəuˈkæliks] *n* 肾盏积水,肾盏积液
hydrocarbon [ˌhaidrəuˈkɑːbən] *n* 烃,碳氢化合物 | alicyclic ~ 脂环烃 / aliphatic ~脂肪族烃,链烃 / carcinogenic ~ 致癌性烃 / cyclic ~ 环烃 / saturated ~ 饱和烃 / unsaturated ~ 不饱和烃
hydrocarbonism [ˌhaidrəuˈkɑːbənizəm], **hydrocarbarism** [ˌhaidrəuˈkɑːbərizəm] *n* 碳氢化合物中毒
hydrocardia [ˌhaidrəuˈkɑːdiə] *n* 心包积水
hydrocele [ˈhaidrəsiːl] *n* 水囊肿;鞘膜积液 | cervical ~, ~ of neck 颈导管积水,颈导管水囊肿 / chylous ~ 乳糜样水囊肿 / diffused ~ 弥漫性(精索)鞘膜积液 / encysted ~ 包绕性鞘膜积液 / funicular ~ 精索鞘膜积液 / hernial ~ 疝水囊肿 / scrotal ~ 阴囊水囊肿
hydrocelectomy [ˌhaidrəusiˈlektəmi] *n* 水囊肿切除术
hydrocenosis [ˌhaidrəusiˈnəusis] *n* 导液法
hydrocephalocele [ˌhaidrəuˈsefələsiːl] *n* 积水性脑突出
hydrocephaloid [ˌhaidrəuˈsefəlɔid] *a* 脑积水样的 *n* 类脑积水
hydrocephalus [ˌhaidrəuˈsefələs] *n* 脑积水 | communicating ~ 交通性脑积水 / obstructive ~, noncommunicating ~ 梗阻性脑积水 | **hydrocephaly** [ˌhaidrəuˈsefəli] *n* / **hydrocephalic** [ˌhaidrəusəˈfælik], **hydrocephalous** [ˌhaidrəuˈsefələs] *a*
hydrochloric acid [ˌhaidrəuˈklɔːrik] 盐酸,氢氯酸
hydrochloride [ˌhaidrəuˈklɔːraid] *n* 氢氯化物,盐酸化物,盐酸盐
hydrochloroplatinic acid [ˌhaidrəuˌklɔ(ː)rəupləˈtinik] 氯铂酸
hydrochlorothiazide [ˌhaidrəuˌklɔːrəuˈθaiəzaid] *n* 氢氯噻嗪(利尿药)
hydrocholecystis [ˌhaidrəuˌkəuliˈsistis] *n* 胆囊积水,胆囊水肿
hydrocholeresis [ˌhaidrəuˌkəuləˈriːsis] *n* 胆液排泄增多 | **hydrocholeretic** [ˌhaidrəuˌkəuləˈretik] *a*
hydrocholesterol [ˌhaidrəukəˈlestərɔl] *n* 氢化胆甾醇,氢化胆固醇
hydrocinchonidine [ˌhaidrəusinˈkɔnidin] *n* 氢化辛可尼丁
hydrocinnamic acid [ˌhaidrəusiˈnæmik] *n* 氢化桂皮酸,苯基丙酸
hydrocirsocele [ˌhaidrəuˈsəːsəsiːl] *n* 精索静脉曲张水囊肿
hydrocodone [ˌhaidrəuˈkəudəun] *n* 氢可酮(镇咳药) | ~ bitartrate 重酒石酸氢可酮(镇咳药)
hydrocollidine [ˌhaidrəuˈkɔlidin] *n* 氢化可力丁
hydrocolloid [ˌhaidrəuˈkɔlɔid] *n* 水胶体 | irreversible ~ 不可逆性水胶体 / reversible ~ 可逆性水胶体
hydrocolpos [ˌhaidrəuˈkɔlpəs] *n* 阴道积液,阴道积水
hydroconion [ˌhaidrəuˈkəuniən] *n* 喷雾器,喷洒器

hydrocortamate [ˌhaidrəuˈkɔːtəmeit] *n* 氢可他酯 | ~ hydrochloride 盐酸氢可他酯(合成糖皮质激素)

hydrocortisone [ˌhaidrəuˈkɔːtisəun] *n* 氢化可的松,皮质醇(糖皮质激素) | ~ acetate 醋酸氢化可的松 / ~ cyclopentylpropionate, ~ cypionate 氢化可的松环戊丙酸酯 / ~ hemisuccinate 氢化可的松半琥酯 / ~ sodium phosphate 氢化可的松磷酸酯钠 / ~ sodium succinate 氢化可的松琥珀酸酯钠 / ~ valerate 戊酸氢化可的松

hydrocumaric acid [ˌhaidrəukjuːˈmærik] β-苯酚丙酸

hydrocyanic acid [ˌhaidrəusaiˈænik] 氢氰酸,氰化氢

hydrocyanism [ˌhaidrəuˈsaiənizəm] *n* 氢氰酸中毒

hydrocyst [ˈhaidrəusist] *n* 水囊肿

hydrocystadenoma [ˌhaidrəuˌsistædiˈnəumə] *n* 汗腺腺瘤

hydrodelineation [ˌhaidrəudiˌliniˈeiʃən] *n* 注液划区(白内障手术时,用钝针在晶状体核层之间注射液体,以便划出核区)

hydrodiascope [ˌhaidrəuˈdaiəskəup] *n* 散光矫正镜

hydrodictiotomy [ˌhaidrəuˌdiktiˈɔtəmi] *n* 视网膜移位术

hydrodiffusion [ˌhaidrəudiˈfjuːʒən] *n* 水中扩散

hydrodipsia [ˌhaidrəuˈdipsiə] *n* 饮水(习性)

hydrodipsomania [ˌhaidrəuˌdipsəuˈmeinjə] *n* 剧渴性癫狂,发作性狂渴

hydrodissection [ˌhaidrəudiˈsekʃən] *n* 水分离术(将少量液体,通常为等渗性盐溶液,注入晶状体囊,以便从晶状体皮质切除它的前面部分,在囊外手术和晶状体乳化法手术时便于对晶状体核进行操作)

hydrodiuresis [ˌhaidrəuˌdaijuəˈriːsis] *n* 水性多尿

hydrodynamic [ˌhaidrəudaiˈnæmik] *a* 水力的,水压的;流体动力学的 | **~s** *n* 流体动力学

hydroelectric [ˌhaidrəuiˈlektrik] *a* 水电的;水电治疗的

hydroencephalocele [ˌhaidrəuenˈsefələsiːl] *n* 积水性脑突出

hydroflumethiazide [ˌhaidrəuˌflumiˈθaiəzaid] *n* 氢氟噻嗪(利尿药,用于治疗高血压和水肿)

hydrofluoric acid [ˌhaidrəuflu(ː)ˈɔrik] *n* 氢氟酸

hydrofluosilicic acid [ˌhaidrəuˌfluəsiˈlisik] 氟硅酸(饮水氟化剂)

hydrogel [ˈhaidrədʒel] *n* 水凝胶

hydrogen(H) [ˈhaidridʒən, ˈhaidrədʒən] *n* 氢 | arseniuretted ~ 砷化氢,胂 / ~ cyanide 氰化氢 / ~ disulfide 二硫化二氢 / heavy ~ 重氢 / light ~ 轻氢 / ~ monoxide 一氧化氢,水 / ~ peroxide 过氧化氢 / ~ selenide 硒化氢 / ~ sulfide, ~ sulfuretted 硫化氢 | **~ous** [haiˈdrɔdʒinəs] *a* 氢的;含氢的

hydrogenase [ˈhaidrədʒineis] *n* 氢化酶 | fumaric ~ 延胡索酸氢化酶

hydrogenate [ˈhaidrədʒineit, haiˈdrɔdʒineit], **hydrogenize** [ˈhaidrədʒinaiz, haiˈdrɔdʒinaiz] *vt* 氢化 | **hydrogenation** [ˌhaidrəudʒəˈneiʃən] *n* 氢化【作用】

hydrogenlyase [ˌhaidrədʒənˈlaieis] *n* 氢解酶,甲酸脱氢酶

hydrogenoid [haiˈdrɔdʒinɔid] *a* 湿性体质的(顺势疗法的术语)

hydrogenolysis [ˌhaidrədʒəˈnɔlisis] *n* 氢解作用

Hydrogenomonas [haiˌdrəudʒənəˈməunəs] *n* 氢单孢菌属

hydrogymnastic [ˌhaidrəudʒimˈnæstik] *a* 水中运动的 | **~s** *n* 水中运动[治疗]学

hydrohalogen acid [ˌhaidrəuˈhælədʒin] *n* [氢]卤酸

hydrohematonephrosis [ˌhaidrəuˌhemətəuniˈfrəusis] *n* 肾积血尿

hydrohepatosis [ˌhaidrəuˌhepəˈtəusis] *n* 肝积水

hydrohymenitis [ˌhaidrəuˌhaiməˈnaitis] *n* 浆膜炎

hydrokinesitherapy [ˌhaidrəukaiˌniːsiˈθerəpi] *n* 水中运动疗法

hydrokinetic [ˌhaidrəukaiˈnetik] *a* 流体动力的 | **~s** *n* 流体动力学

hydrokollag [ˌhaidrəuˈkɔlæg] *n* 石墨悬液(用于纤毛活动及淋巴引流的实验研究)

hydrol [ˈhaidrɔl] *n* 二聚水分子;玉米糖母液

hydrolabile [ˌhaidrəuˈleibail] *a* (组织内)水分不稳定的 | **hydrolability** [ˌhaidrəuləˈbiləti] *n* (组织内)水分不稳定性

hydrolabyrinth [ˌhaidrəuˈlæbirinθ] *n* 膜迷路积水

hydrolase [ˈhaidrəleis] *n* 水解酶

hydrology [haiˈdrɔlədʒi] *n* 水文学,水理学

hydro-lyase [ˌhaidrəuˈlaieis] *n* 水解酶

hydrolymph [ˈhaidrəlimf] *n* 水淋巴,血淋巴(某些低等动物的水样营养液)

hydrolysate [haiˈdrɔlizeit] *n* 水解[产]物 | protein ~ 蛋白质水解物(用作特殊饮食,或供患者食用)

hydrolysis [haiˈdrɔlisis] ([复] **hydrolyses** [haiˈdrɔlisiːz]) *n* 水解[作用] | **hydrolytic** [ˌhaidrəuˈlitik] *a* 水解的

hydrolyst [ˈhaidrəlist] *n* 水解酶,水解催化剂

hydrolyte [ˈhaidrəlait] *n* 水解质

hydrolyze [ˈhaidrəlaiz] *vt, vi* 水解

hydroma [haiˈdrəumə] *n* 水囊瘤

hydromassage [ˌhaidrəuməˈsɑːʒ] *n* 水按摩,漩水

按摩

hydromel [ˈhaidrəmel] *n* 蜂蜜水；水蜜剂

hydromeningitis [ˌhaidrəuˌmeninˈdʒaitis] *n* 浆液性脑膜炎

hydromeningocele [ˌhaidrəuməˈniŋgəsiːl] *n* 积水性脑膜突出

hydrometer [haiˈdrɔmitə] *n* [液体]比重计 | **hydrometric(al)** [ˌhaidrəuˈmetrik(əl)] *a* 液体比重测定法的 / **hydrometry** *n* 液体比重测定法

hydrometra [ˌhaidrəuˈmiːtrə] *n* 子宫积水

hydrometrocolpos [ˌhaidrəuˌmiːtrəuˈkɔlpəs] *n* 子宫阴道积水

hydromicrocephaly [ˌhaidrəuˌmaikrəuˈsefəli] *n* 积水性小头

hydromorphone [ˌhaidrəuˈmɔːfəun] *n* 氢吗啡酮(麻醉镇痛药) | ~ hydrochloride 盐酸氢吗啡酮(亦称盐酸二氢吗啡酮)

hydromphalus [haiˈdrɔmfələs] *n* 脐积水

hydromyelia [ˌhaidrəumaiˈiːliə] *n* 脊髓积水

hydromyelomeningocele [ˌhaidrəuˌmaiələuməˈniŋgəsiːl], **hydromyelocele** [ˌhaidrəumaiˈeləsiːl] *n* 积水性脊髓膜突出

hydromyoma [ˌhaidrəumaiˈəumə] *n* 水囊性肌瘤

hydronaphthylamine [ˌhaidrəuˌnæfθiˈlæmin] *n* 氢化萘胺(散瞳药)

hydronephrosis [ˌhaidrəuniˈfrəusis] *n* 肾积水 | closed ~ 密闭性肾积水 / opened ~ 开放性肾积水 | **hydronephrotic** [ˌhaidrəuneˈfrɔtik] *a*

hydronium [haiˈdrəuniəm] *n* 水合氢离子

hydro-oligocythemia [ˌhaidrəu ˌɔligəusaiˈθiːmiə] *n* 稀血性红细胞减少

hydropancreatosis [ˌhaidrəuˌpæŋkriəˈtəusis] *n* 胰积水

hydroparacumaric acid [ˌhaidrəuˌpærəkjuːˈmærik] 苯酚丙酸

hydroparotitis [ˌhaidrəuˌpærəˈtaitis] *n* 积水性腮腺炎

hydropenia [ˌhaidrəuˈpiːniə] *n* [体内]缺水 | **hydropenic** [ˈhaidrəˌpiːnik] *a*

hydropericarditis [ˌhaidrəuˌperikɑːˈdaitis] *n* 积水性心包炎

hydropericardium [ˌhaidrəuˌperiˈkɑːdiəm] *n* 心包积液

hydroperinephrosis [ˌhaidrəuˌperiniˈfrəusis] *n* 肾周积水

hydroperion [ˌhaidrəuˈperiən] *n* 卵膜水

hydroperitoneum [ˌhaidrəuˌperitəuˈniːəm], **hydroperitonia** [ˌhaidrəuˌperiˈtəuniə] *n* 腹水

hydroperoxidase [ˌhaidrəpəˈrɔksideis] *n* 氢过氧化物酶

hydroperoxide [ˌhaidrəupəˈrɔksaid] *n* 氢过氧化物，过氧化氢物

hydroperoxy acid [ˌhaidrəuˌpəˈrɔksi] 过氧化氢酸

hydroperoxyeicosatetraenoic acid (**HPETE**) [ˌhaidrəupəˌrɔksiaiˌkəusəˌtetrəiːˈnəuik] 氢过氧化二十碳四烯酸

hydropexis [ˌhaidrəuˈpeksis], **hydropexia** [ˌhaidrəuˈpeksiə] *n* 水固定，水滞留 | **hydropexic** *a*

hydrophagocytosis [ˌhaidrəuˌfægəusaiˈtəusis] *n* 饮液作用

Hydrophiidae [ˌhaidrəˈfaiidiː] *n* 海蛇科

hydrophilia [ˌhaidrəuˈfiliə], **hydrophilism** [haiˈdrɔfilizəm] *n* 吸水性，亲水性

hydrophilic [ˌhaidrəuˈfilik], **hydrophil** [ˈhaidrəfil], **hydrophilous** [haiˈdrɔfiləs] *a* 吸水的，亲水的

hydrophobia [ˌhaidrəuˈfəubjə] *n* 恐水症；恐水；狂犬病 | paralytic ~ 瘫痪型狂犬病

hydrophobic [ˌhaidrəuˈfəubik] *a* 狂犬病的；疏水的 | **~ity** [ˌhaidrəufəuˈbisəti] *n* 疏水性

hydrophorograph [ˌhaidrəuˈfɔːrəgrɑːf, -græf] *n* 液流描记器

hydrophthalmos [ˌhaidrɔfˈθælmɔs] *n* 水眼，眼积水 | ~ anterior 眼前部水眼 / ~ posterior 眼后部水眼 / ~ totalis 全眼球水眼 | **hydrophthalmia** [ˌhaidrɔfˈθælmiə], **hydrophthalmus** [ˌhaidrɔfˈθælməs] *n*

hydrophysometra [ˌhaidrəuˌfaisəuˈmiːtrə] *n* 子宫积水气

hydrophyte [ˈhaidrəufait] *n* 水生植物

hydropic [haiˈdrɔpik] *a* 水肿的

hydropigenous [ˌhaidrəuˈpidʒinəs] *a* 致水肿的，水肿性的

hydroplasma [ˌhaidrəuˈplæzmə] *n* 透明质

hydroplasmia [ˌhaidrəuˈplæzmiə] *n* 血浆变稀症，血浆稀薄

hydropneumatosis [ˌhaidrəuˌnjuːməˈtəusis] *n* 水气肿症，[组织内]水气积贮

hydropneumogony [ˌhaidrəunjuːˈmɔgəni] *n* 关节注气检查法

hydropneumopericardium [ˌhaidrəuˌnjuːməuˌperiˈkɑːdiəm] *n* 水气心包，心包积水气

hydropneumoperitoneum [ˌhaidrəuˌnjuːməuˌperitəuˈniːəm] *n* 水气腹，腹腔积水气

hydropneumothorax [ˌhaidrəuˌnjuːməuˈθɔːræks] *n* 水气胸

hydroponics [ˌhaidrəuˈpɔniks] *n* [植物]溶液栽培学 | **hydroponic** *a* / **hydroponicist** [ˌhaidrəuˈpɔnisisit], **hydroponist** [haiˈdrɔpənist] *n* 溶液栽培学家

hydropotherapy [ˌhaidrəupəuˈθerəpi] *n* 腹水注

射疗法

hydrops [ˈhaidrɔps] *n*【拉;希】积水,水肿 | endolymphatic ~, labyrinthine ~ 内淋巴水肿,(膜)迷路积水 / fetal ~ 胎儿水肿(发生于 Rh 阴性母亲血液中的抗体所致的溶血性疾病) / ~ pericardii 心包积水,水心包 / ~ spurius 假性积水,腹膜假黏液瘤 / ~ tubae 输卵管积水 / ~ tubae profluens 外溢性输卵管积水,间歇性输卵管积水 | **hydropic** [haiˈdrɔpik] *a* / **hydropsy** [ˈhaidrɔpsi] *n*

hydropsychotherapy [ˌhaidrəuˌsaikəuˈθerəpi] *n* 水浴心理疗法,精神病水疗法

hydropyonephrosis [ˌhaidrəuˌpaiəuniˈfrəusis] *n* 肾盂积尿脓

hydroquinone [ˌhaidrəuˈkwinəun], **hydroquinol** [ˌhaidrəuˈkwinəul] *n* 氢醌(脱色药)

hydroquinone-acetic acid [ˌhaidrəuˈkwinəun əˈsiːtik] 尿黑酸

hydrorachis [ˌhaidrəuˈreikis] *n* 椎管积水

hydrorachitis [ˌhaidrəurəˈkaitis] *n* 炎性椎管积水

hydrorrhea [ˌhaidrəuˈriːə] *n* 溢液 | ~ gravidarum 妊娠溢液 / nasal ~ 鼻溢液

hydrosalpinx [ˌhaidrəuˈsælpiŋks] *n* 输卵管积水 | intermittent ~ 间歇性输卵管积水,外溢性输卵管积水

hydrosarcocele [ˌhaidrəuˈsɑːkəsiːl] *n* 睾丸积水肉样肿

hydroscheocele [haiˈdrɔskiəsiːl] *n* 积水性阴囊疝

hydroscope [ˈhaidrəskəup] *n* 检水器,检湿器

hydrosol [ˈhaidrəsɔl] *n* 水溶胶

hydrosoluble [ˌhaidrəuˈsɔljubl] *a* 水溶性的

hydrosphygmograph [ˌhaidrəuˈsfigməgrɑːf, -græf] *n* 水柱[式]脉搏描记器

hydrospirometer [ˌhaidrəuspaiəˈrɔmitə] *n* 水柱[式]肺活量计

hydrostabile [ˌhaidrəuˈsteibail, -bil] *a* (组织内)水分稳定的

hydrostat [ˈhaidrəstæt] *n* 水压调节器

hydrostatics [ˌhaidrəuˈstætiks] *n* 流体静力学 | **hydrostatic(al)** [ˌhaidrəuˈstætik(əl)] *a* 流体静力[学]的

hydrosulfide [ˌhaidrəuˈsʌlfaid] *n* 氢硫化物

hydrosulfuric acid [ˌhaidrəusʌlˈfjuərik] 氢硫酸,硫化氢

hydrosulfurous acid [ˌhaidrəuˈsʌlfərəs] 硫代硫酸

hydrosynthesis [ˌhaidrəuˈsinθisis] *n* 水合成[作用]

hydrosyringomyelia [ˌhaidrəusiˌriŋgəumaiˈiːliə] 脊髓积水空洞症

Hydrotaea [ˌhaidrəuˈtiːə] *n* 齿股蝇属 | ~ meteorica 速跃齿股蝇

hydrotaxis [ˌhaidrəuˈtæksis] *n* 趋水性(指能动的生物体或细胞) | **hydrotactic** [ˌhaidrəuˈtæktik] *a*

hydrotherapy [ˌhaidrəuˈθerəpi], **hydrotherapeutics** [ˌhaidrəuˈθerəˈpjuːtiks] *n* 水疗法 | **hydrotherapeutic** [ˌhaidrəuˌθerəˈpjuːtik] *a*

hydrothermal [ˌhaidrəuˈθəːməl] *a* 热水的,热液的

hydrothermic [ˌhaidrəuˈθəːmik] *a* 热水的(如热水浴)

hydrothionammonemia [ˌhaidrəuˌθaiəˌnæməˈniːmiə] *n* 氢硫化铵血

hydrothionemia [ˌhaidrəuˌθaiəˈniːmiə] *n* 硫化氢血

hydrothionuria [ˌhaidrəuˌθaiəˈnjuəriə] *n* 硫化氢尿

hydrothorax [ˌhaidrəuˈθɔːræks] *n* 胸膜腔积液 | chylous ~ 乳糜胸

hydrotis [haiˈdrəutis] *n* 耳[内]积水

hydrotomy [haiˈdrɔtəmi] *n* 注水解剖术

hydrotropism [haiˈdrɔtrəpizəm] *n* 向水性(指不运动的生物体) | **hydrotropic** [ˌhaidrəuˈtrɔpik] *a*

hydrotubation [ˌhaidrəutjuˈbeiʃən] *n* 输卵管通液术

hydrotympanum [ˌhaidrəuˈtimpənəm] *n* 鼓室积水

hydroureter [ˌhaidrəujuəˈriːtə], **hydroureterosis** [ˌhaidrəujuəˌriːtəˈrəusis] *n* 输尿管积水

hydroureteronephrosis [ˌhaidrəujuəˌriːtərəuniˈfrəusis] *n* 输尿管肾盂积水

hydrouria [ˌhaidrəuˈjuəriə] *n* 稀尿,尿量增多

hydrous [ˈhaidrəs] *a* 含水的

hydrovarium [ˌhaidrəuˈvɛəriəm] *n* 卵巢积水

hydroxide [haiˈdrɔksaid] *n* 氢氧化物 | ferric ~ 氢氧化铁(砷中毒解毒药)

hydroxocobalamin [haiˌdrɔksəukəuˈbæləmin] *n* 羟钴胺,维生素 B_{12a}(具有长效造血作用)

hydroxy [haiˈdrɔksi] *a* 羟[基]的

hydroxy- [前缀]羟[基]

hydroxyacetanilide [haiˌdrɔksiæsiˈtænilaid] *n* 对乙酰氨基酚,扑热息痛(解热镇痛药)

hydroxyacetic acid [haidˌrɔksiəˈsiːtik] 羟乙酸,乙醇酸

hydroxy acid [haiˈdrɔksi] 羟酸

hydroxyacyl CoA [haiˌdrɔksiˈæsil] 羟酰辅酶 A

3-hydroxyacyl-CoA dehydrogenase [haiˌdrɔksiˈæsil diːˈhaidrədʒəneis] 3-羟酰-辅酶 A 脱氢酶,3-羟酰 CoA 脱氢酶

3-hydroxyacyl CoA epimerase [haiˌdrɔksiˈæsil

kəu'ei i'piməreis] 3-羟酰辅酶 A 差向异构酶,3-羟丁酰辅酶 A 差向异构酶

hydroxyacyl coenzyme A [hai,drɔksi'æsil kəu'en-zaim] 羟酰辅酶 A

hydroxyacylglutathione hydrolase [hai,drɔksi-,æsil,glu:tə'θaiəun 'haidrəleis] 羟酰基谷胱甘肽水解酶

hydroxyamphetamine [hai,drɔksiæm'fetəmin] *n* 羟苯丙胺(拟交感神经药、鼻内减轻充血药、加压素及散瞳药) | ~ hydrobromide 氢溴酸羟苯丙胺(肾上腺素能药,散瞳药)

hydroxyanthranilic acid [hai,drɔksi,ænθrə'nilik] 羟基氨基苯甲酸

hydroxyapatite [hai,drɔksi'æpətait] *n* 羟[基]磷灰石

hydroxybenzene [hai,drɔksi'benzi:n] *n* 羟基苯,苯酚

***p*-hydroxybenzoic acid** [hai,drɔksiben'zəuik] 对羟苯甲酸

hydroxybutyrate [hai,drɔksi'bju:tileit] *n* 羟丁酸(盐或阴离子型)

3-hydroxybutyrate dehydrogenase [hai,drɔksi-'bju:tireit di:'haidrədʒəneis] 3-羟丁酸脱氢酶

hydroxybutyric acid [hai,drɔksibju(:)'tirik] 羟丁酸

4-hydroxybutyricaciduria, *γ*-hydroxybutyrica-ciduria [hai,drɔksibju:,tirik,æsi'djuəriə] *n* 4-羟丁酸尿[症],*γ*-羟丁酸尿[症],琥珀酸半醛脱氢酶缺乏症

hydroxybutyryl [hai,drɔksi'bju:tiril] *n* 羟基丁酰[基]

3-hydroxybutyryl-CoA epimerase [hai,drɔksi-'bjutiril kəu'ei i'piməreis] 3-羟丁酰辅酶 A 差向异构酶(亦称 3-羟酰辅酶 A 差向异构酶)

hydroxychloroquine sulfate [hai,drɔksi'klɔ:rə-kwin] 硫酸羟氯喹(抗疟药,红斑狼疮抑制药)

25-hydroxycholecalciferol [hai,drɔksi,kəulikæl-'sifərɔl] *n* 25-羟胆钙化醇,25-羟维生素 D_3

hydroxycholesterol [hai,drɔksikə'lestərɔl] *n* 羟基胆甾醇,羟基胆固醇

hydroxycorticosteroid [hai,drɔksi,kɔ:tikə*u* 'stiə-rɔid] *n* 羟皮质类固醇 | 17- ~ (17-OHCS)17-羟皮质类固醇

17-hydroxycorticosteroid [hai,drɔksi,kɔ:tikə*u*'st-erɔid] *n* 17-羟皮质类固醇,17-羟皮质甾醇

17-hydroxycorticosterone [hai,drɔksi,kɔ:tikə*u*-'sterəun] *n* 17-羟皮质[甾]酮,氢[化]可的松

hydroxydione sodium succinate [hai,drɔksi-'daiəun] 羟二酮琥钠(静脉麻醉药)

hydroxyeicosatetraenoic acid (HETE) [hai-,drɔksiai,kəusətetrəi:'nəuik] 羟基二十碳四烯酸

25-hydroxyergocalciferol [hai,drɔksi,ə:gə*u* kæl-'sifərɔl] *n* 25-羟麦角钙化醇,25-羟维生素 D_2

hydroxyestrin benzoate [hai,drɔksi'i:strin] 苯[甲]酸雌二醇

2-hydroxyethanesulfonate [hai,drɔksi,eθein'sʌl-fəneit] *n* 2-羟乙磺酸盐

2-hydroxyethanesulfonic acid [hai,drɔksi,eθei-nsʌl'fɔnik] 2-羟乙磺酸

hydroxyethanoic acid [hai,drɔksieθə'nəuik] 羟基乙酸

hydroxyethyl cellulose [hai,drɔksi'eθil'seljul-əus] 羟乙基纤维素

hydroxyformobenzoylic acid [hai,drɔksi,fɔ:mə-,benzəu'ilik] 羟甲醛苯甲酰酸

hydroxyglutamic acid [hai,drɔksiglu:'tæmik] 羟谷氨酸

hydroxyglutaric acid [hai,drɔksiglu:'tærik] 羟基戊二酸

hydroxyheptadecatrienoic acid [hai,drɔksi,he-ptə,dekətraii:'nəuik] 羟基十七碳三烯酸

5-hydroxyindoleacetic acid [hai,drɔksi,indəulə-'si:tik] 5-羟基吲哚乙酸

3-hydroxyisobutyryl [hai,drɔksi,aisə*u*'bju:tiril] *n* 3-羟基异丁酰[基]

3-hydroxyisobutyryl-CoA hydrolase [hai,drɔ-ksi,aisə*u*'bju:tiril 'haidrəleis] 3-羟异丁酰-辅酶 A 水解酶,3-羟异丁酰-CoA 水解酶

hydroxyisovaleric acid [hai,drɔksi,aisə*u*və'lerik] 羟基异戊酸

hydroxykynurenine [hai,drɔksi'kainjuərə,ni:n] *n* 羟基犬尿氨酸,羟基犬尿素

hydroxyl [hai'drɔksil] *n* 羟[基],氢氧基 | **~ic** [,haidrɔk'silik] *a*

hydroxylamine [,haidrɔk'siləmi:n] *n* 羟胺(用作还原剂)

hydroxylapatite [hai,drɔksil'æpətait] *n* 羟磷灰石

hydroxylase [hai'drɔksileis] *n* 羟化酶 | 11*β*-~ 11*β*-羟化酶,类固醇 11*β*-单加氧酶 / 17α-~ 17α-羟化酶,类固醇 17α-单加氧酶 / 21-~ 21-羟化酶,类固醇 21-单加氧酶 / 27-~ 27-羟化酶,胆甾烷三醇 26-单加氧酶

11*β*-hydroxylase deficiency 11*β*-羟化酶缺乏症(一种类固醇生成的常染色体隐性遗传病,类固醇 11*β*-单加氧酶缺乏可致典型和非典型先天性肾上腺增生症的一型〈Ⅳ型〉)

17α-hydroxylase deficiency 17α-羟化酶缺乏症(一种类固醇生成的常染色体隐性遗传病,类固醇 17α-单加氧酶缺乏可致先天性肾上腺增生症〈Ⅴ型〉)

18-hydroxylase deficiency 18-羟化酶缺乏症,皮质[甾]酮甲基氧化酶缺乏症

21-hydroxylase deficiency 21-羟化酶缺乏症(一种类固醇生成的常染色体隐性遗传病,类固醇21-单加氧酶缺乏有损于糖皮质激素生成的能力,若严重而又未治疗,则可致命。本症可致若干型先天性肾上腺增生症的一型〈Ⅲ型〉)

hydroxylysine [ˌhaidrɔksiˈlaisiːn] *n* 羟赖氨酸

hydroxylysyl galactosyltransferase [haiˌdrɔksiˈlaisil ɡəˌlæktəsilˈtrænsfəreis] 羟赖氨酰半乳糖[基]转移酶,前胶原半乳糖[基]转移酶

hydroxymandelic acid [haiˌdrɔksimænˈdelik] 对羟苯羟乙酸

hydroxymethyl [haiˌdrɔksiˈmeθil] *n* 羟甲基

hydroxymethylbilane synthase [haiˌdrɔksiˌmeθilˈbilein ˈsinθeis] 羟甲基[原]胆色烷合酶(此酶缺乏为一种常染色体显性性状,可致急性间歇性卟啉症。亦称胆色素原脱氨酶,尿卟啉原Ⅰ合酶)

3-hydroxy-3-methylglutaric acid [haiˌdrɔksiˌmeθilɡluːˈtærik] 3-羟[基]-3-甲[基]戊二酸

3-hydroxy-3-methylglutaricaciduria [haiˌdrɔksiˌmeθilɡluːˌtærikˌæsiˈdjuəriə] *n* 3-羟[基]-3-甲[基]戊二酸尿(亦可写成 *β*-hydroxy-*β*-methylglutaricaciduria)

3-hydroxy-3-methylglutaryl [haiˌdrɔksi ˌmeθilˈɡluːtəril] *n* 3-羟[基]-3-甲[基]戊二酸单酰[基](亦可写成 *β*-hydroxy-*β*-methylglutaryl)

hydroxymethylglutaryl-CoA lyase [haiˌdrɔksiˌmeθilɡluːˈtæril kəuˈei ˈlaieis] 羟甲基戊二酸单酰辅酶A裂合酶(此酶缺乏为一种常染色体隐性性状,可致3-羟(基)-3-甲[基]戊二酸尿)

hydroxymethylglutaryl-CoA reductase (NADPH) [haiˌdrɔksiˌmeθilˈɡluːtəril kəuˈei riˈdʌkteis] 羟甲基戊二酸单酰辅酶A还原酶(NADPH)

hydroxymethylglutaryl-CoA synthase [haiˌdrɔksiˌmeθilˈɡluːtəril kəuˈei ˈsinθeis] 羟甲基戊二酸单酰辅酶A合酶

hydroxymethyltransferase [haiˌdrɔksiˌmeθilˈtrænsfəreis] *n* 羟甲基转移酶,转羟甲酶

hydroxynaphthoic acid [haiˌdrɔksinæfˈθəuik] 羟萘甲酸

hydroxynervone [haiˌdrɔksiˈnəːvəun] *n* 羟烯脑苷脂,羟神经苷脂

4-hydroxy-2-oxoglutarate aldolase [haiˌdrɔksiˌɔksəuˈɡluːtəreit ˈældəleis] 4-羟基-2-酮戊二酸醛缩酶

hydroxyphenamate [haiˌdrɔksiˈfenəmeit] *n* 羟基丁氨酯,奥芬氨酯(弱安定药)

hydroxyphenylaminopropionic acid [haiˌdrɔksiˌfenilˌæminəuprəupiˈɔnik] 酪氨酸

hydroxyphenylethylamine [haiˌdrɔksiˌfenileθiˈlæmin] *n* 酪胺

***p*-hydroxyphenylpyruvate** [haiˌdrɔksiˌfenilˈpaiəruveit] *n* 对羟苯丙酮酸(阴离子型,亦可写成 4-hydroxyphenylpyruvate)

4-hydroxyphenylpyruvate dioxygenase [haiˌdrɔksiˌfenilˈpaiəruveit diːˈɔksidʒəneis] 4-羟苯[基]丙酮酸双加氧酶(此酶的遗传性缺乏,据认为可致酪氨酸代谢症,亦称对羟苯[基]丙酮酸氧化酶)

***p*-hydroxyphenylpyruvate oxidase** [haiˌdrɔksiˌfenilˈpaiəruveit ˈɔksideis] 对羟苯[基]丙酮酸氧化酶,4-羟苯[基]丙酮酸双加氧酶

***p*-hydroxyphenylpyruvic acid** [haiˌdrɔksiˌfenilpaiˈruːvik] 对羟苯丙酮酸(缩写为 PHPP,亦可写成 4-hydroxyphenylpyruvic acid)

hydroxypregnenolone [haiˌdrɔksipreɡˈniːnələun] *n* 羟基孕[甾]烯醇酮

hydroxyprogesterone [haiˌdrɔksiprəuˈdʒestərəun] *n* 羟孕酮 | ~ caproate 羟孕酮己酸酯(合成孕激素)

17*α*-hydroxyprogesterone [haiˌdrɔksiprəˈdʒestərəun] *n* 17*α*-羟孕[甾]酮

17*α*-hydroxyprogesterone aldolase [haiˌdrɔksiprəˈdʒestərəun ˈældəleis] 17*α*-羟孕[甾]酮醛缩酶(此酶活性缺乏称为17, 20-裂合酶缺乏症。亦称17, 20-裂合酶,17, 20-碳链〈裂合〉酶)

hydroxyproline [haiˌdrɔksiˈprəuliːn] *n* 羟脯氨酸

hydroxyprolinemia [haiˌdrɔksiˌprəuliˈniːmiə] *n* 羟脯氨酸血症(一种氨基酸代谢障碍,特征为血浆和尿内有过量的游离羟脯氨酸,系由羟脯氨酸氧化酶缺乏所缺,可伴有精神发育迟缓。亦称4-羟-L-脯氨酸氧化酶缺乏症)

hydroxyproline oxidase [haiˌdrɔksiˈprəuliːn ˈɔksideis] 羟脯氨酸氧化酶(此酶缺乏为一种常染色体隐性性状,可致高羟脯氨酸血症)

2-hydroxypropionic acid [haiˌdrɔksiˌprəupiˈɔnik] 2-羟基丙酸,乳酸

hydroxypropyl cellulose [haiˌdrɔksiˈprəupilˈseljuləus] 羟丙基纤维素

hydroxypropyl methylcellulose [haiˌdrɔksiˈprəupil] 羟丙基甲基纤维素(药用辅料)

hydroxypyruvate [haiˌdrɔksiˈpaiəruveit] *n* 羟基丙酮酸

8-hydroxyquinoline [haiˌdrɔksiˈkwinəˌliːn] 8-羟基喹啉,羟喹啉

hydroxystearic acid [haiˌdrɔksisti ˈærik] 羟硬脂酸

hydroxysteroid [haiˌdrɔksiˈsterɔid] *n* 羟类固醇

3*β*-hydroxy-Δ^5-steroid dehydrogenase [haiˌdrɔksi ˈstiərɔid diːˈhaidrədʒəneis] 3*β*-羟-Δ^{5}类固醇脱氢酶(此酶的遗传性缺乏可引起17-羟基孕烯醇酮在血内聚积,并导致先天性肾上腺增

生症Ⅱ型）

3β-hydroxysteroid dehydrogenase deficiency 3β-羟类固醇脱氢酶缺乏症（一种类固醇生成的常染色体隐性遗传性疾病，可致若干型先天性肾上腺增生症的一型〈Ⅱ型〉）

11β-hydroxysteroid dehydrogenase 11β-羟类固醇脱氢酶

11β-hydroxysteroid dehydrogenase deficiency 11β-羟类固醇脱氢酶缺乏症（此酶缺乏导致皮质醇代谢物排泄过多和肾内盐皮质素过剩，引起钾排泄〈低钾血症〉、钠潴留〈高钠血症〉和高血压）

17β-hydroxysteroid dehydrogenase [haiˌdrɔksi-ˈsterɔid diːˈhaidrədʒəneis] 17β-羟类固醇脱氢酶，睾酮17β-脱氢酶

17β-hydroxysteroid dehydrogenase deficiency 17β-羟类固醇脱氢酶缺乏症（一种类固醇生成的常染色体隐性遗传病，由于缺乏睾丸酶即睾酮17β-脱氢酶所致。特征为男性假两性畸形伴青春期后男性化，有时为男子女性型乳房。血浆睾酮减少，雄烯二酮增加）

18-hydroxysteroid dehydrogenase [haiˌdrɔksi-ˈsterɔid diːˈhaidrədʒəneis] 18-羟类固醇脱氢酶（此酶的活性缺乏称为皮质[甾]酮甲基氧化酶缺乏症Ⅱ型）

hydroxytetracycline [haiˌdrɔksiˌtetrəˈsaiklin] *n* 羟四环素，氧四环素，土霉素

5-hydroxytryptamine (5-HT) [haiˌdrɔksiˈtript-əmiːn] *n* 5-羟色胺

3-hydroxytyramine [haiˌdrɔksiˈtairəmiːn] *n* 3-羟酪胺，多巴胺

hydroxyurea [haiˌdrɔksiˈjuəriə] *n* 羟基脲（抗肿瘤药）

hydroxyvaline [haiˌdrɔksiˈvælin] *n* 羟缬氨酸

25-hydroxyvitamin D [haiˌdrɔksiˈvaitəmin] 25-羟基维生素 D

25-hydroxyvitamin D_3 [haiˌdrɔksiˈvaitəmin] 25-羟基维生素 D_3，25-羟基胆钙化醇

hydroxyzine [haiˈdrɔksiziːn] *n* 羟嗪（安定药，解痉药，抗组胺药）| ~ hydrochloride 盐酸羟嗪，安泰乐 / ~ pamoate 双羟萘酸羟嗪

Hydrozoa [ˌhaidrəuˈzəuə] *n* 水螅纲

hydrozoan [ˌhaidrəuˈzəuən] *n* 水螅，水螅纲生物

hydruria [haiˈdruəriə] *n* 稀尿症，多尿症 | **hydruric** [haiˈdruərik] *a* 多尿的

hyenanchin [ˌhaiəˈnæŋkin] *n* 南非野葛素（其作用类似士的宁）

Hygeia [haiˈdʒi(ː)ə] *n* [希]健康女神（医神 Aesculapius 之女）

hygeiophrontis [ˌhaidʒiəuˈfrɔntis] *n* 疑病[症] | **hygeiophrontistic** [ˌhaidʒiəufrɔnˈtistik] *a*

hygiene [ˈhaidʒiːn] *n* 卫生，卫生学，保健[法] | industrial ~ 工业卫生 / mental ~ 心理卫生，精神卫生 / oral ~ 口腔卫生 / sex ~ 性卫生 / social ~ 社会[心理]卫生 | **hygienic** [haiˈdʒiːnik] *a* 卫生的

hygienics [haiˈdʒiːniks] *n* 卫生学

hygienism [haiˈdʒiːnizəm] *n* 卫生，摄生

hygienist [haiˈdʒiːnist] *n* 卫生学家 | dental ~ 牙科保健员（洁治员）| **hygieist** [haiˈdʒiːist] *n*

hygienization [ˌhaidʒiːnaiˈzeiʃən, -niˈz-] *n* 卫生化

hygieology, hygiology [ˌhaidʒiˈɔlədʒi] *n* 卫生学

hygiogenesis [ˌhaidʒiəuˈdʒenisis] *n* 保健机制

hygrechema [ˌhaigriˈkiːmə] *n* 水音（一种听诊音）

hygremometry [ˌhaigriˈmɔmitri] *n* 血干燥物质测定法（测血红蛋白比例）

hygric [ˈhaigrik] *a* 湿的，潮的

hygr(o)- [构词成分] 湿

hygroblepharic [ˌhaigrəubliˈfærik] *a* 润睑的

hygrograph [ˈhaigrəgrɑːf-, græf] *n* 湿度记录器

hygrology [haiˈgrɔlədʒi] *n* 湿度学

hygroma [haiˈgrəumə] ([复] **hygromas** 或 **hygromata** [haiˈgrəumətə]) *n* 水囊瘤 | ~ colli 颈部水囊瘤 / cystic ~ 水囊状淋巴管瘤 / ~ praepatellare 髌前囊炎 / subdural ~ 硬膜下水囊瘤 | **~tous** [haiˈgrəumətəs] *a*

hygrometer [haiˈgrɔmitə] *n* 湿度计 | hair ~ 毛发湿度计 | **hygrometric** [ˌhaigrəuˈmetrik] *a* 湿度测定的 / hygrometry *n* 湿度测定法

hygromycin [ˌhaigrəuˈmaisin] *n* 潮霉素（抗生素类药）| ~ B 潮霉素 B（抗蠕虫药，用于猪）

hygroscope [ˈhaigrəskəup] *n* 验湿器 | **hygroscopic** [ˌhaigrəuˈskɔpik] *a* 吸湿的，收湿的；湿度器的

hyle [ˈhaili] *n* [希]原质，原始物质

hyle- 见 hyl(o)-

Hylemyia [ˌhailəˈmaiə] *n* 黑蝇属

hylergography [ˌhailəˈgɔgrəfi] *n* 环境（对细胞）影响记录法

hylic [ˌhailik] *a* 物质的；髓质的（指胚胎的原髓组织）

hyl(o)-, hyle- [构词成分] 物质

hylogenesis [ˌhailəuˈdʒenisis], **hylogeny** [haiˈlɔdʒini] *n* 物质生成

hylology [haiˈlɔlədʒi] *n* 原始物质学

hylotropy [haiˈlɔtrəpi] *n* 恒质变形，保组变相（物质改变物理形态，化学成分不变）| **hylotropic** [ˌhailəuˈtrɔpik] *a*

hylozoism [ˌhailəˈzəuizəm] *n* 万物有生论 | **hylozoic** [ˌhailəˈzəuik] *a*

hymecromone [ˌhaimiˈkrəuməun] *n* 羟甲香豆素（利胆药）

hymen [ˈhaimen, -mən] *n* [希]处女膜 | circular ~, annular ~ 环状处女膜 / cribriform ~, fenestrated ~ 筛状处女膜 / denticular ~ 锯齿状

处女膜 / falciform ~ 镰状处女膜 / imperforate ~ 处女膜闭锁 / infundibuliform ~ 漏斗形处女膜 / lunar ~ 半月形处女膜 / septate ~ 中隔处女膜 | **~al** *a*

hymenectomy [ˌhaiməˈnektəmi] *n* 处女膜切除术

hymenitis [ˌhaiməˈnaitis] *n* 处女膜炎

hymenium [haiˈmiːniəm] ([复] **hymeniums** 或 **hymenia** [haiˈmiːniə]) *n* 子实层 | **hymenial** *a*

hymen(o)- [构词成分] 膜;处女膜

hymenolepiasis [ˌhaimənəuleˈpaiəsis] *n* 膜壳绦虫病

Hymenolepididae [ˌhaimənəuˈlepidaidiː] *n* 膜壳【绦虫】科

Hymenolepis [ˌhaimiˈnɔləpis] *n* 膜壳绦虫属 | ~ diminuta 长膜壳绦虫 / ~ fraterna, ~ nanavar. fraterna 鼠型短膜壳绦虫,鼠变异型短膜壳绦虫 / ~ lanceolata 矛形剑带绦虫(即 Drepanidotaenia lanceolata) / ~ nana 短膜壳绦虫

hymenology [ˌhaiməˈnɔlədʒi] *n* 膜学

Hymenomycetes [ˌhaimənəumaiˈsiːtiːz] *n* 层菌纲

Hymenoptera [ˌhaiməˈnɔptərə] *n* 膜翅目(昆虫)

hymenopteran [ˌhaiməˈnɔptərən] *n* 膜翅[目]昆虫 *a* 膜翅昆虫的 | **hymenopterous** [ˌhaiməˈnɔptərəs] *a*

hymenopterism [ˌhaiməˈnɔptərizəm] *n* 膜翅目昆虫螫症,蜂螫症

hymenorrhaphy [ˌhaiməˈnɔrəfi] *n* 处女膜缝合术

Hymenostomatia [ˌhaiminəustəuˈmeiʃiə] *n* 膜口亚纲

Hymenostomatida [ˌhaiminəustəuˈmeitidə] *n* 膜口目

hymenotomy [ˌhaiməˈnɔtəmi] *n* 处女膜切开术

hymenovin [ˌhaiməˈnəuvin] *n* 内酯草(含毒性内酯,可致牛羊胃肠炎)

Hymenoxys [ˌhaiməˈnɔksis] *n* 草本属 | ~ odorata苦草

hyobasioglossus [ˈhaiəuˌbeisiəuˈglɔsəs] *n* 舌骨舌肌底部

hyodeoxycholic acid [ˌhaiəudiːˌɔksiˈkəulik] 猪去氧胆酸,3, 6-二羟基胆烷酸

hyoepiglottic [ˌhaiəuˌepiˈglɔtik], **hyoepiglottidean** [ˌhaiəuˌepiglɔˈtidiən] *a* 舌骨会厌的

hyoglossal [ˌhaiəuˈglɔsəl] *a* 舌骨舌的

hyoglycocholic acid [ˌhaiəuˌglikəˈkəulik] 猪甘氨胆酸

hyoid [ˈhaiɔid] *a* 舌骨的;舌骨形的,(希腊字母)υ形的

hyoscine [ˈhaiəsin] *n* 东莨菪碱

hyoscyamine [ˌhaiəˈsaiəmin] *n* 莨菪碱,天仙子胺(解痉药,散瞳药) | ~ hydrobromide 氢溴酸莨菪碱(作用和用途与阿托品〈atropine〉相似) / ~ sulfate 硫酸莨菪碱(作用和用途与阿托品相似)

Hyoscyamus [ˌhaiəˈsaiəməs] *n* 莨菪属

hyoscyamus [ˌhaiəˈsaiəməs] *n* 莨菪

Hyostrongylus rubidus [ˌhaiəuˈstrɔndʒiləs ˈruːbidəs] 淡红猪圆线虫

hyotaurocholic acid [ˌhaiəuˌtɔːrəˈkəulik] 猪牛磺胆酸

hyothyroid [ˌhaiəuˈθairɔid] *a* 舌骨甲状软骨的

hypacidemia [haiˌpæsiˈdiːmiə] *n* 血酸过少

hypacusis [ˌhaipəˈkjusis], **hypacusia** [ˌhaipəˈkjuːziə] *n* 听觉减退,重听

hypadrenia [ˌhaipəˈdriːniə] *n* 肾上腺功能减退,肾上腺功能不全

hypalbuminemia [ˌhaipælˌbjuːmiˈniːmiə], **hypalbuminosis** [ˌhaipælbjuːmiˈnəusis] *n* 血白蛋白减少

hypalgesia [ˌhaipælˈdʒiːzjə], **hypalgia** [haiˈpældʒiə] *n* 痛觉减退 | **hypalgesic** [ˌhaipælˈdʒiːsik], **hypalgetic** [ˌhaipælˈdʒetik] *a*

hypamnios [haiˈpæmniəs], **hypamnion** [haiˈpæmniən] *n* 羊水过少

hypanakinesia [haiˌpænəkaiˈniːziə], **hypanakinesis** [haiˌpænəkaiˈniːsis] *n* 蠕动缺失,蠕动功能减退

hypaphorine [haiˈpæfərin] *n* 下箴刺桐碱,色氨酸三甲基内盐

hyparterial [ˌhaipɑːˈtiəriəl] *a* 动脉下的

hypaxial [haiˈpæksiəl] *a* 体轴下的

hypazoturia [hiˌpæzəuˈtjuəriə] *n* 尿氮减少

hypemia [haiˈpiːmiə] *n* 贫血

hypenchyme [ˈhaipenkaim] *n* 下胚叶(原肠腔内胚组织)

hypeosinophil [haiˌpiːəˈsinəfil] *n* 次嗜酸细胞 *a* 次嗜酸性的

hyper- [前缀] 过多,超过,上,高,重,过度

hyperabsorption [ˌhaipə(ː)rəbˈsɔːpʃən] *n* 吸收过多

hyperacanthosis [ˌhaipə(ː)ˌrækənˈθəusis] *n* 棘层增厚

hyperacid [ˌhaipə(ː)ˈræsid] *a* 酸过多的

hyperacidaminuria [ˌhaipə(ː)ˌræsidæmiˈnjuəriə] *n* 高氨基酸尿

hyperacidity [ˌhaipə(ː)rəˈsidəti] *n* 酸过多,胃酸过多 | gastric ~ 胃酸过多[症]

hyperactive [ˌhaipə(ː)ˈræktiv] *a* 活动过强的;功能亢进的 | **hyperactivity** [ˌhaipə(ː)rækˈtivəti] *n*

hyperacusis [ˌhaipə(ː)rəˈkjuːsis], **hyperacousia** [ˌhaipə(ː)rəˈkuːziə], **hyperacusia** [ˌhaipə(ː)rəˈkjuːziə] *n* 听觉过敏

hyperacute [ˌhaipə(ː)rəˈkjuːt] *a* 过急性的,超急性的

hyperadenosis [ˌhaipə(ː)ˌrædiˈnəusis] *n* 腺增大
hyperadiposis [ˌhaipə(ː)ˌrædiˈpəusis], **hyperadiposity** [ˌhaipə(ː)ˌrædiˈpɔsəti] *n* 肥胖过度
hyperadrenalemia [ˌhaipə(ː)rədriːnəˈliːmiə] *n* 高肾上腺素血症
hyperadrenalism [ˌhaipə(ː)rəˈdriːnəlizəm], **hyperadrenia** [ˌhaipə(ː)rəˈdriːniə] *n* 肾上腺功能亢进
hyperadrenocorticism [ˌhaipə(ː)rəˌdriːnəuˈkɔːtisizəm] *n* 肾上腺皮质功能亢进
hyperaemia [ˌhaipə(ː)ˈriːmiə] *n* = **hyperemia**
hyperaemization [haipə(ː)ˌriːmaiˈzeiʃən, -miˈz-] *n* = **hyperemization**
hyperaesthesia [ˌhaipə(ː)risˈθiːzjə] *n* = **hyperesthesia** | **hyperaesthetic** [ˌhaipə(ː)risˈθetik] *a* = **hyperesthetic**
hyperaffectivity [ˌhaipə(ː)rəfekˈtivəti] *n* 情感过强 | **hyperaffective** [ˌhaipə(ː)rəˈfektiv] *a*
hyperakusis [ˌhaipə(ː)rəˈkjuːsis] *n* 听觉过敏
hyper-β-alaninemia [ˌhaipə(ː) ˌbeitə ˌæləniˈniːmiə] *n* 血[内]β-丙氨酸过多,高 β-丙氨酸血症(亦称 β-丙氨酸血症)
hyperalbuminemia [ˌhaipə(ː)rælˌbjuːmiˈniːmiə] *n* 高白蛋白血症
hyperalbuminosis [ˌhaipə(ː)rælˌbjuːmiˈnəusis] *n* 白蛋白过多
hyperaldosteronemia [ˌhaipə(ː)rælˌdɔstərəˈniːmiə] *n* 高醛固酮血症
hyperaldosteronism [ˌhaipə(ː)rælˌdɔˈstərəˌnizəm] *n* 醛固酮过多症
hyperaldosteronuria [ˌhaipə(ː)rælˌdɔˌstərəˈnjuəriə] *n* 高醛固酮尿
hyperalgesia [ˌhaipə(ː)rælˈdʒiːzjə] *n* 痛觉过敏 | auditory ~ 听觉性痛觉过敏 / muscular ~ 肌痛觉过敏 | **hyperalgia** [haipə(ː)ˈrældʒiə] *n* / **hyperalgestic** [ˌhaipə(ː)rælˈdʒiːsik], **hyperalgetic** [ˌhaipə(ː)rælˈdʒetik] *a*
hyperalimentation [ˌhaipə(ː)ˌrælimenˈteiʃən] *n* 营养过度 | parenteral ~ 胃肠外高营养,静脉高营养
hyperalimentosis [ˌhaipə(ː)ˌrælimenˈtəusis] *n* 营养过度病
hyperalkalescence [ˌhaipə(ː)ˌrælkəˈlesns], **hyperalkalinity** [ˌhaipə(ː)ˌrælkəˈlinəti] *n* 碱性过度
hyperallantoinuria [ˌhaipə(ː)ræˌlæntəiˈnjuəriə] *n* 尿[内]尿囊素过多
hyperalonemia [ˌhaipə(ː)ˌræləuˈniːmiə] *n* 血盐过多
hyperalphalipoproteinemia [ˌhaipə(ː)ˌrælfəˌlipəuprəutiːˈniːmiə] *n* 高 α 脂蛋白血症
hyperaminoacidemia [ˌhaipə(ː)rəˌminəuˌæsiˈdiːmiə] *n* 高氨基酸血症
hyperaminoaciduria [ˌhaipə(ː)rəˌmiːnəuˌæsiˈdjuəriə] *n* 高氨基酸尿,氨基酸尿
hyper-β-aminoisobutyricaciduria [ˌhaipə(ː)rəˌmiːnəuˌaisəubjuːˌtirikˌæsiˈdjuəriə] *n* 高-β-氨基异丁酸尿,β-氨基异丁酸尿
hyperammonemia [ˌhaipə(ː)ˌræməuˈniːmiə] *n* 高氨血症 | cerebroatrophic ~ 大脑萎缩性高氨血症,雷特综合征(见 Rett syndrome) / congenital ~, type I先天性高氨血症I型,氨甲酰基磷酸合成酶缺乏症 / congenital ~, type II先天性高氨血症II型,鸟氨酸氨甲酰基磷酸缺乏症 | **hyperammoniemia** [ˌhaipə(ː)rəˌməuniˈiːmiə] *n*
hyperammonuria [ˌhaipə(ː)ˌræməuˈnjuəriə] *n* 高氨尿
hyperamylasemia [ˌhaipə(ː)ˌræmileiˈsiːmiə] *n* 高淀粉酶血[症]
hyperanacinesia [ˌhaipə(ː)ˌrænəsaiˈniːziə], **hyperanakinesia** [ˌhaipə(ː)ˌrænəkaiˈniːziə] *n* 蠕动亢进,蠕动过强
hyperandrogenism [ˌhaipə(ː)ˈrændrədʒənizəm] *n* 雄激素过多症
hyperaphia [ˌhaipə(ː)ˈreifiə] *n* 触觉过敏 | **hyperaphic** [ˌhaipə(ː)ˈræfik] *a*
hyperarginemia [ˌhaipe(ː)ˌrɑːdʒiˈniːmiə] *n* 高精氨酸血症
hyperarousal [ˌhaipə(ː)rəˈrauzəl] *n* 觉醒过度
hyperazotemia [ˌhaipə(ː)ˌræzəuˈtiːmiə] *n* 高氮血[症]
hyperazoturia [ˌhaipə(ː)ˌræzəuˈtjuəriə] *n* 高氮尿
hyperbaric [ˌhaipə(ː)ˈbærik] *a* 高压的;高比重的 | **hyperbarism** *n* 高气压病
hyperbasophilic [ˌhaipə(ː)ˌbeisəuˈfilik] *a* 强嗜碱性的
hyperbetalipoproteinemia [ˌhaipə(ː)ˌbeitəˌlipəuˌprəutiːˈniːmiə] *n* 高 β 脂蛋白血症 | familial ~ 家族性高 β 脂蛋白血症,家族性高脂蛋白血症
hyperbicarbonatemia [ˌhaipə(ː)baiˌkɑːbəneiˈtiːmiə] *n* 高重碳酸盐血
hyperbilirubinemia [ˌhaipə(ː)ˌbiliˌruːbiˈniːmiə] *n* 高胆红素血[症] | congenital ~ 先天性高胆红素血[症],克-奈综合征(见 Crigler-Najjar syndrome) / conjugated ~ 结合性高胆红素血[症] / constitutional ~, ~ I 体质性高胆红素血[症],高胆红素血症 I,吉尔伯(Gilbert)综合征 / neonatal ~ 新生儿高胆红素血[症] / unconjugated ~ 非结合性高胆红素血[症]
hyperblastosis [ˌhaipə(ː)blæsˈtəusis] *n* 组织增生
hyperbrachycephaly [ˌhaipə(ː)ˌbrækiˈsefəli] *n*

头部过短[症] | **hyperbrachycephalic** [ˌhaipə(ː)ˌbrækiseˈfælik] *a* 头部过短的(颅指数85.5或以上的)

hyperbradykininemia [ˌhaipə(ː)ˌbrædiˌkainiˈniːmiə] *n* 高缓激肽血症

hyperbradykininism [ˌhaipə(ː)ˌbrædiˈkaininizəm] *n* 缓激肽过多症

hyperbulia [ˌhaipə(ː)ˈbjuːliə] *n* 意志过强

hypercalcemia [ˌhaipə(ː)kælˈsiːmiə] *n* 高钙血症,高血钙 | familial hypocalciuric ~ 家族性低尿钙性高钙血症 / idiopathic ~ 特发性高钙血症(婴儿) | **hypercalcinemia** [ˌhaipə(ː)ˌkælsiˈniːmiə] *n*

hypercalcipexy [ˌhaipə(ː)ˈkælsiˌpeksi] *n* 钙沉积过多

hypercalcitoninemia [ˌhaipə(ː)ˌkælsitəniˈniːmiə] *n* 高降钙素血症

hypercalciuria [ˌhaipə(ː)ˌkælsiˈjuəriə], **hypercalcinuria** [ˌhaipə(ː)ˌkælsiˈnjuəriə] *n* 高钙尿

hypercapnia [ˌhaipə(ː)ˈkæpniə], **hypercarbia** [ˌhaipə(ː)ˈkɑːbiə] *n* 高碳酸血症 | **hypercapnie** [ˌhaipə(ː)ˈkæpnik] *a*

hypercarotenemia [ˌhaipə(ː)ˌkærətiːˈniːmiə], **hypercarotinemia** [ˌhaipə(ː)ˌkærətiˈniːmiə] *n* 高胡萝卜素血症

hypercatabolism [ˌhaipə(ː)kəˈtæbəlizəm] *n* 分解代谢过度 | **hypercatabolic** [ˌhaipəːˌkætəˈbɔlik] *a*

hypercatharsis [ˌhaipə(ː)kəˈθɑːsis] *n* 泻下过度,腹泻过度

hypercathartic [ˌhaipə(ː)kəˈθɑːtik] *a* 导泻过度的,剧泻的

hypercellularity [ˌhaipə(ː)ˌseljuˈlærəti] *n* 细胞过多(如骨髓中) | **hypercellular** [ˌhaipə(ː)ˈseljulə] *a*

hypercementosis [ˌhaipə(ː)ˌsiːmenˈtəusis] *n* 牙骨质增生

hyperchloremia [ˌhaipə(ː)klɔːˈriːmiə] *n* 高氯血症 | **hyperchloremic** [ˌhaipə(ː)klɔːˈriːmik] *a*

hyperchlorhydria [ˌhaipə(ː)klɔːˈhaidriə] *n* 胃酸过多[症]

hyperchloridation [ˌhaipə(ː)ˌklɔːraiˈdeiʃən] *n* 供盐过多

hyperchloriduria [ˌhaipə(ː)ˌklɔːriˈdjuəriə] *n* 尿氯排泄

hyperchloruration [ˌhaipə(ː)ˌklɔːrjuəˈreiʃən] *n* 氯化物过多

hyperchloruria [ˌhaipə(ː)ˌklɔːˈrjuəriə] *n* 高氯尿

hypercholesterolemia [ˌhaipə(ː)kəˌlestərɔˈliːmiə] *n* 高胆固醇血症 | familial ~ 家族性高胆固醇血症,家族性高脂蛋白血症Ⅱ$_a$型 / **hypercholesteremia** [ˌhaipə(ː)kəˌlestəˈriːmiə], **hypercholesterinemia** [ˌhaipə(ː)kəˌlestəriˈniːmiə] *n* / **hypercholesterolemic** [ˌhaipə(ː)kəˌlestərɔˈliːmik], **hypercholesteremic** [ˌhaipə(ː)kəˌlestəˈriːmik] *a*

hypercholesterolia [ˌhaipə(ː)kəˌlestəˈrɔliə] *n* 胆固醇过多

hypercholia [ˌhaipə(ː)ˈkəuliə] *n* 胆汁过多

hyperchondroplasia [ˌhaipə(ː)ˌkɔndrəuˈpleiziə] *n* 软骨增殖过多

hyperchromaffinism [ˌhaipə(ː)krəuˈmæfinizəm] *n* 嗜铬组织功能亢进

hyperchromatin [ˌhaipə(ː)ˈkrəumətin] *n* 深色染色质

hyperchromatism [ˌhaipə(ː)ˈkrəumətizəm], **hyperchromasia** [ˌhaipə(ː)krəuˈmeiziə] *n* 着色过度,染色过深 | **hyperchromatic** [ˌhaipə(ː)krəuˈmætik] *a* 染深色的,浓染的;含染色质多的

hyperchromatopsia [ˌhaipə(ː)ˌkrəuməˈtɔpsiə] *n* 色视症

hyperchromatosis [ˌhaipə(ː)ˌkrəuməˈtəusis] *n* 色素过多;着色过度,染色过深

hyperchromemia [ˌhaipə(ː)krəuˈmiːmiə] *n* 血色指数过高

hyperchromia [ˌhaipə(ː)ˈkrəumiə] *n* 血红蛋白过多;着色过度,染色过深

hyperchromic [ˌhaipə(ː)ˈkrəumik] *a* 深色的,浓染的

hyperchylia [ˌhaipə(ː)ˈkailiə] *n* 胃液过多

hyperchylomicronemia [ˌhaipə(ː)ˌkailəuˌmaikrəuˈniːmiə] *n* 高乳糜微粒血症(亦称乳糜微粒血症) / familial ~ 家族性高乳糜微粒血症,家族性高脂蛋白血症Ⅰ型

hypercinesia [ˌhaipə(ː)siˈniːsiə] *n* 运动过度,运动功能亢进

hypercoagulable [ˌhaipə(ː)kəuˈægjuləbl] *a* 高凝的,凝固性过高的 | **hypercoagulability** [ˌhaipə(ː)kəuˌægjuləˈbiləti] *n* 高凝性

hypercoria [ˌhaipə(ː)ˈkɔːriə] *n* 易饱症

hypercorticalism [ˌhaipə(ː)ˈkɔːtikəlizəm], **hypercorticism** [ˌhaipə(ː)ˈkɔːtisizəm] *n* 肾上腺皮质功能亢进

hypercortisolism [ˌhaipə(ː)ˈkɔːtiˌsəulizəm] *n* 皮质醇增多症,肾上腺皮质功能亢进

hypercreatinemia [ˌhaipə(ː)kriːətiˈniːmiə] *n* 高肌酸血症

hypercrine [ˌhaipə(ː)ˈkrin] *a* 内分泌功能亢进的

hypercrinism [ˌhaipə(ː)ˈkrainizəm], **hypercrinemia** [ˌhaipə(ː)kriˈniːmiə], **hypercrinia** [ˌhaipə(ː)ˈkriniə], **hypercrisia** [ˌhaipə(ː)ˈkriziə] *n* 内分泌过多,内分泌功能亢进

hypercryalgesia [ˌhaipə(ː)ˌkraiælˈdʒiːzjə], **hypercryesthesia** [ˌhaipə(ː)ˌkraiisˈθiːzjə] *n* 冷觉过敏
hypercupremia [ˌhaipə(ː)kjuːˈpriːmiə] *n* 高铜血症
hypercupriuria [ˌhaipə(ː)ˌkjuːpriˈjuəriə] *n* 高铜尿
hypercyanotic [ˌhaipə(ː)ˌsaiəˈnɔtik] *a* 高度发绀的,高度青紫的
hypercyesis [ˌhaipə(ː)saiˈiːsis] *n* 异期复孕(指卵)
hypercythemia [ˌhaipə(ː)saiˈθiːmiə] *n* 红细胞过多症
hypercytochromia [ˌhaipə(ː)ˌsaitəuˈkrəumiə] *n* 血细胞染色过深
hypercytosis [ˌhaipə(ː)saiˈtəusis] *n* 血细胞过多(尤指白细胞)
hyperdactyly [ˌhaipə(ː)ˈdæktili], **hyperdactylia** [ˌhaipə(ː)dækˈtiliə], **hyperdactylism** [ˌhaipə(ː)ˈdæktilizəm] *n* 多指,多趾
hyperdicrotic [ˌhaipə(ː)daiˈkrɔtik] *a* 强二波[脉]的 | **hyperdicrotism** [ˌhaipə(ː)ˈdaikrətizəm] *n* 强二波脉[现象]
hyperdiploid [ˈhaipə(ː)ˌdiplɔid] *a* 超二倍的,多倍的 *n* 超二倍体,多倍体(见 polyploid) | **~y** *n* 多倍性,超二倍性
hyperdipsia [ˌhaipə(ː)ˈdipsiə] *n* 剧渴
hyperdistention [ˌhaipə(ː)disˈtenʃən] *n* 膨胀过度
hyperdiuresis [ˌhaipə(ː)ˌdaijuəˈriːsis] *n* 尿分泌过多,多尿
hyperdontia [ˌhaipə(ː)ˈdɔnʃiə] *n* 牙[数]过多
hyperdynamia [ˌhaipə(ː)daiˈneimiə] *n* 肌活动过多,肌力过度 | ~ uteri 子宫收缩过度 | **hyperdynamic** [ˌhaipə(ː)daiˈnæmik] *a*
hypereccrisia [ˌhaipə(ː)reˈkriziə], **hypereccrisis** [ˌhaipə(ː)ˈrekrisis] *n* 排泄过多 | **hypereccritic** [ˌhaipə(ː)reˈkritik] *a*
hyperechema [ˌhaipə(ː)riːˈkiːmə] *n* 听诊音过强
hyperechoic [ˌhaipə(ː)rəˈkəuik] *a* 高回声的,强回声的
hyperelectrolytemia [haipə(ː)riˌlektrəulaiˈtiːmiə] *n* 高电解质血症
hyperemesis [ˌhaipə(ː)ˈremisis] *n* 剧吐 | ~ gravidarum 妊娠剧吐 / ~ lactentium 乳儿剧吐 | **hyperemetic** [ˌhaipə(ː)riˈmetik] *a*
hyperemia [ˌhaipə(ː)ˈriːmiə] *n* 充血 | active ~, arterial ~, fluxionary ~ 主动性充血,动脉性充血,流动性充血 / collateral ~ 侧支充血 / leptomeningeal ~ 软脑脊膜充血 / passive ~, venous ~ 被动性充血,静脉性充血 | **hyperemic** [haipə(ː)ˈriːmik] *a*
hyperemization [ˌhaipə(ː)ˌriːmaiˈzeiʃən, -miˈz-] *n* 致充血,人工充血法(尤其为了治疗目的而使用)
hyperemotivity [ˌhaipə(ː)ˌriməuˈtivəti] *n* 情感过强
hyperencephalus [ˌhaipə(ː)renˈsefələs] *n* 缺顶露脑畸胎
hyperendemic [ˌhaipə(ː)renˈdemik] *a* 高度地方性的
hyperendocrinism [ˌhaipə(ː)renˈdɔkrinizəm], **hyperendocrinia** [ˌhaipə(ː)ˌrendəuˈkriniə], **hyperendocrisia** [ˌhaipə(ː)ˌrendəuˈkriziə] *n* 内分泌过多,内分泌功能亢进
hyperenergia [ˌhaipə(ː)reˈnəːdʒiə] *n* 精力过盛,活动过度
hypereosinophilia [ˌhaipə(ː)ˌriːəsinəˈfiliə] *n* 嗜酸细胞增多症 | filarial ~ 丝虫性嗜酸细胞增多症,热带嗜酸细胞增多
hyperepinephrinemia [ˌhaipə(ː)ˌrepiˌnefriˈniːmiə] *n* 血肾上腺素过多,高肾上腺素血
hyperepinephry [ˌhaipə(ː)ˌrepiˈnefri] *n* 肾上腺功能亢进
hyperequilibrium [ˌhaipə(ː)ˌriːkwiˈlibriəm] *n* 平衡觉过敏,易晕性
hypererethism [ˌhaipə(ː)ˈreriθizəm] *n* 兴奋过度
hyperergasia [ˌhaipə(ː)rəˈgeisiə] *n* 活动力过强,功能活动亢进
hyperergia [ˈhaipə(ː)ˈrəːdʒiə] *n* 活动力过强,功能活动亢进;超反应性,变应性过强,过敏
hyperergy [ˈhaipə(ː)ˌrəːdʒi] *n* 活动力过强;超反应性,反应性增高 | **hyperergic** [ˌhaipə(ː)ˈrəːdʒik] *a*
hypererythrocythemia [ˌhaipə(ː)riˌriθrəusaiˈθiːmiə] *n* 红细胞过多(症)
hyperesophoria [ˌhaipə(ː)ˌresəˈfəuriə] *n* 上内隐斜
hyperesthesia [ˌhaipə(ː)risˈθiːzjə] *n* 感觉过敏 | acoustic ~, auditory ~ 听觉过敏 / cerebral ~ 大脑性感觉过敏 / gustatory ~ 味觉过敏 / muscular ~ 肌觉过敏 / oneiric ~ 睡梦性感觉过敏 / optic ~ 视觉过敏,光感过敏 / tactile ~ 触觉过敏 | **hyperesthetic** [ˌhaipə(ː)risˈθetik] *a*
hyperestrinism [ˌhaipə(ː)ˈrestrinizəm], **hyperestrogenism** [ˌhaipə(ː)ˈrestrədʒinizəm], **hyperestrogenosis** [ˌhaipə(ː)ˌrestrədʒəˈnəusis] *n* 雌激素过多
hyperestrogenemia [ˌhaipə(ː)ˌrestrədʒiˈniːmiə], **hyperestrinemia** [ˌhaipə(ː)restriˈniːmiə] *n* 高雌激素血症
hypereuryopia [ˌhaipə(ː)ˌrjuəriˈəupiə] *n* 睑裂过大,眼过度开大
hyperevolutism [ˌhaipə(ː)riːˈvɔljuːtizəm] *n* 发

育过度

hyperexcretory [ˌhaipə(ː)reksˈkriːtəri] *a* 排泄过度的

hyperexophoria [ˌhaipə(ː)ˌreksəˈfəuriə] *n* 上外隐斜

hyperexplexia [ˌhaipə(ː)ˌreksˈpleksiə] *n* 肌张力过度

hyperextension [ˌhaipə(ː)reksˈtenʃən] *n* 伸展过度

hyperferremia [ˌhaipə(ː)feˈriːmiə], **hyperferricemia** [ˌhaipə(ː)ˌferiˈsiːmiə] *n* 高铁血症 | **hyperferemic** [ˌhaipə(ː)fəˈriːmik] *a*

hyperfibrinogenemia [ˌhaipə(ː)faiˌbrinəudʒiˈniːmiːə] *n* 高纤维蛋白原血症

hyperfiltration [ˌhaipə(ː)filˈtreiʃən] *n* 超过滤(肾小球滤过率升高,常为早期胰岛素依赖型糖尿病之征)

hyperflexion [ˌhaipə(ː)ˈflekʃən] *n* 屈曲过度

hyperfolliculinemia [ˌhaipə(ː)fəˌlikjuliˈniːmiə] *n* 血滤泡素过多

hyperfolliculinism [ˌhaipə(ː)fəˈlikjulinizəm] *n* 滤泡素过多

hyperfolliculinuria [ˌhaipə(ː)fəˌlikjuliˈnjuəriə] *n* 尿滤泡素过多

hyperfractionation [ˌhaipə(ː)ˌfrækʃəˈneiʃən] *n* 高分割(放射治疗日程安排的细分部分,每次照射减少一定的剂量,但在总的治疗跨距中并不减少,以便在给予等量或较大的总放射剂量时减少副作用)

hyperfunctioning [ˌhaipə(ː)ˈfʌŋkʃəniŋ] *n* 功能亢进

hypergalactia [ˌhaipə(ː)gəˈlækʃiə], **hypergalactosis** [ˌhaipə(ː)ˌgælækˈtəusis] *n* 乳汁[分泌]过多 | **hypergalactous** [ˌhaipə(ː)gəˈlæktəs] *a*

hypergammaglobulinemia [ˌhaipə(ː)ˌgæməˌglɔbjuliˈniːmiə] *n* 高丙球蛋白血症(常见于慢性传染病) | monoclonal ~ 单克隆高丙球蛋白血症,浆细胞恶性增生

hypergasia [ˌhaipə(ː)ˈgeisiə] *n* 活动力减弱

hypergastrinemia [ˌhaipə(ː)ˌgæstriˈniːmiə] *n* 高胃泌素血症

hypergenesis [ˌhaipə(ː)ˈdʒenisis] *n* 发育过度 | **hypergenetic** [ˌhaipə(ː)dʒiˈnetik] *a*

hypergenitalism [ˌhaipə(ː)ˈdʒenitəlizəm] *n* 生殖器发育过度,性腺功能亢进

hypergeusesthesia [ˌhaipə(ː)ˌgjuːsisˈθiːzjə], **hypergeusia** [ˌhaipə(ː)ˈgjuːsiə] *n* 味觉过敏

hypergia [haiˈpəːdʒiə] *n* 活动力减弱;变应性减弱,反应性减弱

hypergigantosoma [ˌhaipə(ː)dʒaiˌgæntəˈsəumə] *n* 极度巨大发育,巨大畸形,巨人症

hyperglandular [ˌhaipə(ː)ˈglændjulə] *a* 腺功能过强的

hyperglobulia [ˌhaipə(ː)gləuˈbjuːliə], **hyperglobulism** [ˌhaipə(ː)ˈglɔbjulizəm] *n* 红细胞过多[症],红细胞增多

hyperglobulinemia [ˌhaipə(ː)ˌglɔbjuliˈniːmiə] *n* 高球蛋白血症

hyperglucagonemia [ˌhaipə(ː)ˌgluːkəgɔˈniːmiə] *n* 高胰增血糖素血症

hyperglycemia [ˌhaipə(ː)glaiˈsiːmiə] *n* 高血糖[症] | **hyperglycemic** *a* 高血糖的 *n* 促血糖增高药

hyperglyceridemia [ˌhaipə(ː)glisəraiˈdiːmiə] *n* 血甘油酯过多,高甘油酯血(通常为甘油三酯) | **hyperglyceridemic** *a*

hyperglycerolemia [ˌhaipə(ː)ˌglisərɔˈliːmiə] *n* 血[内]甘油过多,高甘油血症

hyperglycinemia [ˌhaipə(ː)ˌglaisiˈniːmiə] *n* 高甘氨酸血症(为一种遗传性先天性疾病)

hyperglycinuria [ˌhaipə(ː)ˌglaisiˈnjuəriə] *n* 高甘氨酸尿症

hyperglycistia [ˌhaipə(ː)glaiˈsistiə] *n* 组织糖分过多

hyperglycodermia [ˌhaipə(ː)ˌglaikəuˈdəːmiə] *n* 皮肤糖分过多

hyperglycogenolysis [ˌhaipə(ː)ˌglaikəudʒiˈnɔlisis] *n* 糖原分解过度

hyperglycoplasmia [ˌhaipə(ː)ˌglaikəuˈplæzmiə] *n* 血浆糖分过多

hyperglycorrhachia [ˌhaipə(ː)ˌglaikəuˈreikiə] *n* 脑脊液糖分过多

hyperglycosemia [ˌhaipə(ː)ˌglaikəuˈsiːmiə], **hyperglykemia** [ˌhaipə(ː)glaiˈkiːmiə] *n* 高血糖[症]

hyperglycosuria [ˌhaipə(ː)ˌglaikəuˈsjuəriə] *n* 尿糖过多

hyperglycystia [ˌhaipə(ː)glaiˈsistiə] *n* 组织糖分过多

hypergnosis [ˌhaipə(ː)ˈnəusis] *n* [妄想性]知觉过敏

hypergonadism [ˌhaipə(ː)ˈgəunædizəm] *n* 性腺功能亢进

hypergonadotropic [ˌhaipə(ː)ˌgɔnədəuˈtrɔpik] *a* 促性腺激素过多的

hyperguanidinemia [ˌhaipə(ː)ˌgwænidiˈniːmiə] *n* 高胍血症

hyperhedonia [ˌhaipə(ː)hiˈdəuniə], **hyperhedonism** [ˌhaipə(ː)ˈhiːdənizəm] *n* 快感过盛,过度快感,欣快[症]

hyperhemoglobinemia [ˌhaipə(ː)ˌhiːməuˌgləubiˈniːmiə] *n* 高血红蛋白血症

hyperheparinemia [ˌhaipə(ː)ˌhepəriˈniːmiə] *n* 高肝素血症

hyperhepatia [ˌhaipə(ː)hiˈpætiə] *n* 肝功能亢进 | **hyperhidrosis** [ˌhaipə(ː)haiˈdrəusis] *n* 多汗[症] **hyperhidrotic** [ˌhaipə(ː)haiˈdrɔtik] *a* 多汗的,引起多汗的

hyperhomocysteinemia [ˌhaipə(ː)ˌhəuməusisˌtiːiˈniːmiə] *n* 高半胱氨酸血过多

hyperhormonal [ˌhaipə(ː)ˈhɔːməunəl], **hyperhormonic** [ˌhaipə(ː)hɔːˈmɔnik] *a* 激素过多的

hyperhormonism [ˌhaipə(ː)ˈhɔːməunizəm] *n* 激素过多[症],内分泌功能亢进

hyperhydration [ˌhaipə(ː)haiˈdreiʃən] *n* 水分过多,多水

hyperhydrochloria [ˌhaipə(ː)haidrəuˈklɔːriə], **hyperhydrochloridia** [ˌhaipə(ː)haidrəukləˈridiə] *n* 胃酸过多[症]

hyperhydroxyprolinemia [ˌhaipə(ː)haiˌdrɔksiprəuliˈniːmiə] *n* 高羟脯氨酸血症

hyperhypercytosis [ˌhaipə(ː)ˌhaipə(ː)saiˈtəusis] *n* 中性粒细胞过多性白细胞增多

hyperhypocytosis [ˌhaipə(ː)ˌhaipəusaiˈtəusis] *n* 中性粒细胞过多性白细胞减少

hyperhypophysism [ˌhaipə(ː)haiˈpɔfisizəm] *n* 垂体功能亢进

Hypericum [haiˈperikəm] *n* 金丝桃属 | ~ perforatum 贯叶连翘

hyperidrosis [ˌhaipə(ː)raiˈdrəusis] *n* 多汗[症]

hyperimidodipeptiduria [ˌhaipə(ː)ˌrimidəudaiˌpeptiˈdjuəriə] *n* 高亚氨基二肽尿,氨酰基脯氨酸[二肽]酶缺乏症

hyperimmune [ˌhaipə(ː)riˈmjuːn] *a* 高免疫的(在血清中含有极丰富的特异性抗体)

hyperimmunity [ˌhaipə(ː)riˈmjuːnəti] *n* 高免疫性(比通常相同情况下显示更强的免疫性程度)

hyperimmunization [ˌhaipə(ː)ˌrimjuːnaiˈzeiʃən, -niˈz-] *n* 高免疫[作用](多次注射加强剂量的抗原使产生较高的自动获得性免疫,或注射高免疫丙种球蛋白使产生较高的被动获得性免疫)

hyperimmunoglobulinemia [ˌhaipə(ː)ˌrimjunəu-ˌglɔbjuliˈniːmiə] *n* 高免疫球蛋白血症 | ~ E 高免疫球蛋白 E 血症(伴皮肤无反应性及缺乏抗体反应,如约伯综合征时。见 Job's syndrome)

hyperinflation [ˌhaipə(ː)rinˈfleiʃən] *n* 充气过度

hyperingestion [ˌhaipə(ː)rinˈdʒestʃən] *n* 摄食过度

hyperinsulinar [ˌhaipə(ː)ˈrinsjulinə] *a* 胰岛素[分泌]过多的

hyperinsulinemia [ˌhaipə(ː)ˌrinsjuliˈniːmiə] *n* 高胰岛素血症 | **hyperinsulinemic** *a*

hyperinsulinemic [ˌhaipə(ː)ˌrinsjuliˈniːmik] *a* 高胰岛素血症的

hyperinsulinism [ˌhaipə(ː)ˈrinsjulinizəm] *n* 胰岛素分泌过多;胰岛素休克;高胰岛素血症

hyperinterrenal [ˌhaipə(ː)ˌrintəˈriːnəl] *a* 肾上腺皮质功能亢进的

hyperinterrenopathy [ˌhaipə(ː)ˌrintəriˈnɔpəθi] *n* 肾上腺皮质功能亢进病

hyperinvolution [ˌhaipə(ː)ˌrinvəˈluːʃən] *n* 复旧过度(如妊娠后子宫复旧过度)

hyperiodemia [ˌhaipə(ː)ˌraiəˈdiːmiə] *n* 高碘血症

hyperirritability [ˌhaipə(ː)ˌiritəˈbiləti] *n* 过度应激性,高度过敏

hyperisotonia [ˌhaipə(ː)ˌraisəuˈtəuniə] *n* 高度等张性

hyperisotonic [ˌhaipə(ː)ˌraisəuˈtɔnik] *a* 高渗的

hyperkalemia [ˌhaipə(ː)kəˈliːmiə], **hyperkaliemia** [ˌhaipə(ː)ˌkæliˈiːmiə] *n* 高钾血症 | **hyperkalemic** [ˌhaipə(ː)kəˈliːmik] *a*

hyperkeratinization [ˌhaipə(ː)ˌkerəˌtinaiˈzeiʃən, -niˈz-] *n* 角化过度

hyperkeratosis [ˌhaipə(ː)ˌkerəˈtəusis] ([复]**hyperkeratoses** [ˌhaipəːˌkerəˈtəusiːz]) *n* 角化过度(亦称 perkeratosis) | epidermolytic ~ 表皮松解性角化过度 / ~ follicularis in cutem penetrans, ~ follicularis et parafollicularis in cutem penetrans 真皮穿通性毛囊和毛囊旁角化过度 / ~ lenticularis perstans 持久性豆状角化过度 / ~ of palms and soles 掌跖角化过度[症] / progressive dystrophic ~ 进行性营养不良性角化过度,遗传性残毁性角化瘤 | **hyperkeratotic** [ˌhaipəːˌkerəˈtɔtik] *a*

hyperketonemia [ˌhaipə(ː)ˌkiːtəuˈniːmiə] *n* 高酮血症

hyperketonuria [ˌhaipə(ː)ˌkiːtəuˈnjuəriə] *n* 多酮尿

hyperketosis [ˌhaipə(ː)kiːˈtəusis] *n* 酮过多

hyperkinemia [ˌhaipə(ː)kaiˈniːmiə] *n* 心输出量过多

hyperkinemic [ˌhaipə(ː)kaiˈniːmik] *a* 组织血流增多的 *n* 促组织血流增多剂

hyperkinesia [ˌhaipə(ː)kaiˈniːziə, -kiˈn-] *n* 运动过度 | professional ~ 职业性运动过度,职业性神经功能病

hyperkinesis [ˌhaipə(ː)kaiˈniːsis, -kiˈn-] *n* 运动过度,高动力

hyperkinetic [ˌhaipə(ː)kaiˈnetik, -kiˈn-] *a* 运动过度的

hyperkoria [ˌhaipə(ː)ˈkɔːriə] *n* 易饱症

hyperlactacidemia [ˌhaipə(ː)ˌlæktæsiˈdiːmiə] *n* 高乳酸血症

hyperlactation [ˌhaipə(ː)lækˈteiʃən] *n* 泌乳过多,乳汁过多,泌乳期过久

hyperlecithinemia [ˌhaipə(ː)ˌlesiθiˈnimiə] *n* 高卵磷脂血症

hyperleptinemia [ˌhaipə(ː)ˌleptiˈniːmiə] *n* 高苗条蛋白血症,高减肥蛋白血症

hyperlethal [ˌhaipə(ː)ˈliːθəl] *a* 超致死量的

hyperleukocytosis [ˌhaipə(ː)ˌljuːkəsaiˈtəusis] *n* 白细胞过多

hyperleydigism [ˌhaipə(ː)ˈlaidigizəm] *n* 莱迪希间质细胞(Leydig's cells)功能亢进,雄激素分泌过多

hyperlipemia [ˌhaipə(ː)liˈpiːmiə] *n* 高脂血症 | carbohydrate-induced ~ 碳水化合物引起的高脂血症,高脂蛋白血症Ⅳ型 / combined fat and carbohydrate-induced ~ 联合脂肪和碳水化合物引起的高脂血症,家族性高脂蛋白血症Ⅴ型 / essential familial ~ 原发性家族性高脂血症,家族性高脂蛋白血症Ⅰ型 / familial fat-induced ~ 家族性脂肪引起的高脂血症,家族性高脂蛋白血症Ⅰ型 / idiopathic ~ 特发性高脂血症,家族性高脂蛋白血症Ⅰ型 / mixed ~ 混合高脂血症,家族性高脂蛋白血症Ⅱ$_b$ 和Ⅴ型

hyperleucinemia [ˌhaipə(ː)ˌljuːsiˈniːmiə] *n* 高亮氨酸血症

hyperlipacidemia [ˌhaipə(ː)ˌlipæsiˈdiːmiə] *n* 高脂酸血症,脂酸血

hyperlipasemia [ˌhaipə(ː)ˌlipeiˈsiːmiə] *n* 高脂酶血症(亦称脂酶血)

hyperlipidemia [ˌhaipə(ː)ˌlipiˈdiːmiə] *n* 高脂血症 | familial combined ~ 家族性复合高脂血症,家族性高脂蛋白血症Ⅱ,Ⅱ$_b$ 和Ⅳ型 /mixed ~ 混合高脂血症,家族性高脂蛋白血症Ⅱ$_b$ 型 / multiple lipoprotein-type ~ 复合脂蛋白型高脂血症,家族性高脂蛋白血症Ⅱ和Ⅳ型 | **hyperlipidemic** [ˌhaipə(ː)ˌlipiˈdiːmik] *a*

hyperlipoproteinemia [ˌhaipə(ː)ˌlipəuˌprəutiːˈniːmiə] *n* 高脂蛋白血症 | acquired ~ 获得性高脂蛋白血症 / familial ~ 家族性高脂蛋白血症(有五种类型:Ⅰ型亦称家族性脂蛋白脂酶缺乏症,家族性高乳糜微粒血症,原发性家族性高脂血症,家族性脂肪引起的高脂血症或特发性高脂血症。Ⅱ型有两种亚型:Ⅱ$_a$ 型,亦称低密度脂蛋白受体病,家族性高胆固醇血症,家族性高β脂蛋白血症;Ⅱ$_b$ 型,亦称家族性联合高脂蛋白血症或高脂血症,混合高脂蛋白血症或高脂血症。Ⅲ型亦称宽β脂蛋白病或脂蛋白血症,家族性血β脂蛋白异常症,家族性宽β高脂蛋白血症。Ⅳ型亦称家族性高前β脂蛋白血症,碳水化合物引起的高脂血症。Ⅴ型亦称家族性脂蛋白脂酶缺乏症,家族性高乳糜微粒血症伴高前β脂蛋白血症,联合脂肪和碳水化合物引起的高脂血症,混合高脂蛋白血症或高脂血症) / familial broad-beta ~ 家族性宽β高脂蛋白血症,家族性高脂蛋白血症Ⅲ型 / familial combined ~ 家族性联合高脂蛋白血症,家族性高脂蛋白血症Ⅱ和Ⅱ$_b$ 型 / mixed ~ 混合高脂蛋白血症,家族性高脂蛋白血症Ⅱ$_b$ 和Ⅴ型)

hyperliposis [ˌhaipə(ː)liˈpəusis] *n* 脂肪过多

hyperlithemia [ˌhaipə(ː)liˈθiːmiə] *n* 高锂血症

hyperlithic [ˌhaipə(ː)ˈliθik] *a* 尿酸过多的

hyperlithuria [ˌhaipə(ː)liˈθjuəriə] *n* 高尿酸尿

hyperlordosis [ˌhaipə(ː)lɔˈdəusis] *n* 脊柱前凸过度

hyperlucency [ˌhaipə(ː)ˈljuːsnsi] *n* 过度透亮,过度透光(超射线透射性)

hyperluteinization [ˌhaipə(ː)ˌljuːtiːnaiˈzeiʃən, -niˈz-] *n* 黄体化过度,过度黄体化

hyperlutemia [ˌhaipə(ː)ljuːˈtiːmiə] *n* 高黄体激素血症,高孕酮血症

hyperlysinemia [ˌhaipə(ː)ˌlaisiˈniːmiə] *n* 高赖氨酸血症(亦称L-赖氨酸:NAD氧化还原酶缺乏症,赖氨酸不耐症)

hyperlysinuria [ˌhaipə(ː)ˌlaisiˈnjuəriə] *n* 高赖氨酸尿,赖氨酸尿

hypermagnesemia [ˌhaipə(ː)ˌmægniˈsiːmiə] *n* 高镁血症

hypermania [ˌhaipə(ː)ˈmeinjə] *n* 重[症]躁狂

hypermastia [ˌhaipə(ː)ˈmæstiə] *n* 多乳腺;乳房肥大

Hypermastigida [ˌhaipə(ː)mæsˈtidʒidə] *n* 超鞭毛目

hypermastigote [ˌhaipə(ː)ˈmæstigəut] *n* 超鞭毛虫

hypermature [ˌhaipə(ː)məˈtjuə] *a* 成熟过度的

hypermegasoma [ˌhaipə(ː)ˌmegəˈsəumə] *n* [极度]巨大身体,巨大畸形

hypermelanosis [ˌhaipə(ː)ˌmeləˈnəusis] *n* 黑变病,黑色素沉着病

hypermelanotic [ˌhaipə(ː)ˌmeləˈnɔtik] *a* 黑色素沉着过多的

hypermenorrhea [ˌhaipə(ː)ˌmenəˈriːə] *n* 月经过多

hypermesosoma [ˌhaipə(ː)ˌmesəˈsəumə] *n* 中[等以]上身材

hypermetabolism [ˌhaipə(ː)meˈtæbəlizəm] *n* 高代谢,代谢亢进 | extrathyroidal ~ 非甲状腺性代谢亢进 | **hypermetabolic** [ˌhaipə(ː)-metəˈbɔlik] *a*

hypermetamorphosis [ˌhaipə(ː)ˌmetəˈmɔːfəsis] *n* 思想变化过速,思维奔逸(见于躁狂症);对视觉刺激过分注意

hypermetaplasia [ˌhaipə(ː)metəˈpleiziə] *n* 组织变形过度,间变过度

hypermethioninemia [ˌhaipə(ː)məˌθaiəniˈniːmiə] *n* 高甲硫氨酸血症

hypermetria [ˌhaipə(ː)ˈmiːtriə] *n* 伸展过度,运

动范围过度
hypermetrope [ˌhaipə(ː)ˈmetrəup] *n* 远视者
hypermetropia [ˌhaipə(ː)miˈtrəupiə] *n* 远视[眼] | **hypermetropic** [ˌhaipə(ː)miˈtrɔpik] *a*
hypermicrosoma [ˌhaipə(ː)ˌmaikrəuˈsəumə] *n* [过度]矮小身材(明显的侏儒症)
hypermimia [ˌhaipə(ː)ˈmimiə] *n* 表情过分,表情[运动]过度(讲话时)
hypermineralization [ˌhaipə(ː)ˌminərəlaiˈzeiʃən, -liˈz-] *n* 矿质过多
hypermnesia [ˌhaipə(ː)mˈniːzjə] *n* 记忆过旺,记忆增强 | **hypermnesic** [ˌhaipə(ː)mˈniːsik] *a* 记忆过旺的,记忆增强的;精神活动增强的
hypermodal [ˌhaipə(ː)ˈməudəl] *a* 超众数的(在统计学上,指在变量曲线上位于众数的右方的数值或项目)
hypermorph [ˌhaipə(ː)ˌmɔːf] *n* 上型身材者(躯短肢长身材者);超效等位基因(一种突变基因,功效较强)
hypermotility [ˌhaipə(ː)məuˈtiləti] *n* 运动过度,运动过强
hypermyotonia [ˌhaipə(ː)maiəuˈtəuniə] *n* 肌张力过度
hypermyotrophy [ˌhaipə(ː)maiˈɔtrəfi] *n* 肌肥大
hypernanosoma [ˌhaipə(ː)ˌnænəˈsəumə] *n* 极度矮小(并非绝对侏儒身材)
hypernasality [ˌhaipə(ː)neiˈzæləti] *n* 鼻音过多
hypernatremia [ˌhaipə(ː)nəˈtriːmiə] *n* 高钠血症 | hypodipsic ~ 渴感减退性高钠血症 | **hypernatronemia** [ˌhaipə(ː)ˌnætrəˈniːmiə] *n* | **hypernatremic** [ˌhaipə(ː)nəˈtriːmik] *a*
hypernea [ˌhaipə(ː)ˈniːə] *n* 精神活动亢进,精神活动增强
hyperneocytosis [ˌhaipə(ː)ˌniːəusaiˈtəusis] *n* 幼稚[白]细胞过多性白细胞增多[症]
hypernephritis [ˌhaipə(ː)nəˈfraitis] *n* 肾上腺炎
hypernephroid [ˌhaipə(ː)ˈnefrɔid] *a* 肾上腺样的
hypernephroma [ˌhaipə(ː)neˈfrəumə] *n* 肾上腺样瘤
hyperneurotization [ˌhaipə(ː)njuəˌrɔtaiˈzeiʃən, -tiˈz-] *n* 神经功能加强法(神经移植)
hypernitremia [ˌhaipə(ː)naiˈtriːmiə] *n* 高氮血症
hypernoia [ˌhaipə(ː)ˈnɔiə] *n* 精神活动过度
hypernomic [ˌhaipə(ː)ˈnɔmik] *a* 超规律的,过度的
hypernormal [ˌhaipə(ː)ˈnɔːməl] *a* 超常的
hypernormocytosis [ˌhaipə(ː)ˌnɔːməusaiˈtəusis] *n* 中性粒细胞过多[症]
hypernutrition [ˌhaipə(ː)nju(ː)ˈtriʃən] *n* 营养过度
hyperontomorph [ˌhaipə(ː)ˈrɔntəmɔːf] *n* 甲状腺功能亢进体型者
hyperonychia [ˌhaipə(ː)rɔˈnikiə], **hyperonychosis** [ˌhaipə(ː)ˌrɔniˈkəusis] *n* 甲状腺肥大
hyperope [ˈhaipə(ː)rəup] *n* 远视者
hyperopia [ˌhaipə(ː)ˈrəupiə] *n* 远视[眼] | axial ~ 轴性远视 / curvature ~ 曲度远视 / facultative ~, relative ~ 条件性远视,相对远视 / index ~ 填质性远视(指数远视) / latent ~ 隐性远视(潜伏远视) / manifest ~ 显性远视 / total ~ 总远视(显性远视加隐性远视) | **hyperopic** [ˌhaipə(ː)ˈrɔpik] *a*
hyperorchidism [ˌhaipə(ː)rɔːkidizəm] *n* 睾丸功能亢进
hyperorexia [ˌhaipə(ː)rəuˈreksiə] *n* 食欲过旺,善饥
hyperornithinemia [ˌhaipə(ː)ˌɔːniθiˈniːmiə] *n* 高鸟氨酸血症(血浆内鸟氨酸过多)
hyperorthocytosis [ˌhaipə(ː)ˌrɔːθəusaiˈtəusis] *n* 正比例性白细胞增多[症]
hyperosmia [ˌhaipə(ː)ˈrɔzmiə], **hyperosphresia** [ˌhaipə(ː)rɔsˈfriːziə] *n* 嗅觉过敏
hyperosmolality [ˌhaipə(ː)ˌrɔsməuˈlæləti] *n* [体液]重量渗摩尔浓度过高,高[重量]渗摩尔浓度,高渗透压
hyperosmolarity [ˌhaipə(ː)ˌrɔzməuˈlæriti] *n* 容积渗摩尔浓度过高,高容积渗摩尔浓度
hyperosmotic [ˌhaipə(ː)rɔzˈmɔtik] *a* 高渗的
hyperosteogeny [ˌhaipə(ː)rɔstiˈɔdʒini] *n* 骨发育过度,骨质增生
hyperostosis [ˌhaipə(ː)rɔsˈtəusis] *n* 骨肥厚 | flowing ~ 条纹状骨肥厚 / infantile cortical ~ 婴儿骨外层肥厚 | **hyperostotic** [ˌharpə(ː)rɔsˈtɔtik] *a*
hyperovaria [ˌhaipə(ː)rəuˈvɛəriə], **hyperovarianism** [ˌhaipə(ː)rəuˈvɛəriənizəm], **hyperovarism** [ˌhaipə(ː)ˈrəuvərizəm] *n* 卵巢功能亢进
hyperoxaluria [ˌhaipəːˌrɔksəˈljuəriə] *n* 高草酸尿(亦称草酸尿)
hyperoxemia [ˌhaipə(ː)rɔkˈsiːmiə] *n* 高氧血
hyperoxia [ˌhaipə(ː)ˈrɔksiə] *n* 高氧,氧过多 | **hyperoxic** [ˌhaipə(ː)ˈrɔksik] *a* 氧过多的,含氧量高的
hyperoxidation [ˌhaipə(ː)ˌrɔksiˈdeiʃən] *n* 氧化过度
hyperoxide [ˌhaipə(ː)ˈrɔksaid] *n* 过氧化物
hyperpallesthesia [ˌhaipə(ː)ˌpælisˈθiːzjə] *n* 振动觉过敏
hyperpancreorrhea [ˌhaipə(ː)ˌpæŋkriəuˈriːə] *n* 胰液[分泌]过多
hyperparasite [ˌhaipə(ː)ˈpærəsait] *n* 重寄生物(寄生于寄生虫的寄生物) | second degree ~ 第二级重寄生物 | **hyperparasitic** [ˌhaipə(ː)pærəˈsitik] *a* 重寄生的(在寄生物上寄生的)

hyperparasitism [ˌhaipə(ː)ˈpærəsaitizəm] *n* 重寄生[现象]

hyperparathyroidism [ˌhaipə(ː)ˌpærəˈθairɔidizəm] *n* 甲状旁腺功能亢进[症]

hyperparotidism [ˌhaipə(ː)pəˈrɔtidizəm] *n* 腮腺功能亢进

hyperpathia [ˌhaipə(ː)ˈpæθiə] *n* 痛觉过度

hyperpepsia [ˌhaipə(ː)ˈpepsiə] *n* 胃酸过多性消化不良;消化过速

hyperpepsinemia [ˌhaipə(ː)ˌpepsiˈniːmiə] *n* 高胃蛋白酶血症

hyperpepsinia [ˌhaipə(ː)pepˈsiniə] *n* 胃蛋白酶过多

hyperpepsinuria [ˌhaipə(ː)ˌpepsiˈnjuəriə] *n* 高胃蛋白酶尿

hyperperistalsis [ˌhaipə(ː)ˌperiˈstælsis] *n* 蠕动过强

hyperpermeability [ˌhaipə(ː)ˌpəːmiəˈbiləti] *n* 渗透性过高

hyperpexia [ˌhaipə(ː)ˈpeksiə], **hyperpexy** [ˌhaipə(ː)ˈpeksi] *n* 固定[量]过多(组织)

hyperphagia [ˌhaipə(ː)ˈfeidʒiə] *n* 饮食过多

hyperphalangia [ˌhaipə(ː)fəˈlændʒiə], **hyperphalangism** [ˌhaipə(ː)fəˈlændʒizəm] *n* 多节指,多节趾

hyperphasia [ˌhaipə(ː)ˈfeiziə] *n* 言语过多,多语症

hyperphenylalaninemia [ˌhaipə(ː)feniˌlæləniˈniːmiə] *n* 高苯丙氨酸血症

hyperphonesis [ˌhaipə(ː)fəuˈniːsis] *n* 声响过强(听诊或叩诊音)

hyperphonia [ˌhaipə(ː)ˈfəuniə] *n* 发声过强(如口吃时)

hyperphoria [ˌhaipə(ː)ˈfəuriə] *n* 上隐斜 | **hyperphoric** [ˌhaipəːˈfəurik] *a*

hyperphosphatasemia [ˌhaipə(ː)ˌfɔsfəteiˈsiːmiə] *n* 高磷酸酶血症

hyperphosphatasia [ˌhaipə(ː)ˌfɔsfəˈteiziə] *n* 磷酸酯酶过多

hyperphosphatemia [ˌhaipə(ː)ˌfɔsfəˈtiːmiə] *n* 高磷[酸盐]血症

hyperphosphaturia [ˌhaipə(ː)ˌfɔsfəˈtjuəriə] *n* 高磷[酸盐]尿症

hyperphosphoremia [ˌhaipə(ː)fɔsfəˈriːmiə] *n* 高磷[酸盐]血症

hyperphrasia [ˌhaipə(ː)ˈfreiziə] *n* 多语症

hyperphrenia [ˌhaipə(ː)ˈfriːniə] *n* 精神兴奋过度;精神活动亢进

hyperpigmentation [ˌhaipə(ː)ˌpigmənˈteiʃən] *n* 色素沉着过多,着色过度

hyperpinealism [ˌhaipə(ː)ˈpainiəlizəm] *n* 松果体功能亢进

hyperpipecolatemia [ˌhaipə(ː)ˌpipəˌkɔləˈtiːmiə] *n* 高六氢吡啶羧酸血症

hyperpituitarism [ˌhaipə(ː)piˈtjuːitərizəm] *n* 垂体功能亢进 | **hyperpituitary** [ˌhaipə(ː)piˈtjuːitəri] *a*

hyperplasia [ˌhaipə(ː)ˈpleiziə] *n* 增生,超常增生 | cementum ~ 牙骨质增生 / congenital adrenal ~(CAH) 先天性肾上腺增生,肾上腺[性]性征综合征 / lipoid ~ 类脂组织增生 / neoplastic ~ 瘤性增生 / ovarian stromal ~ 泡膜细胞增生症(卵巢) / Swiss-cheese ~ 瑞士干酪样增生 | **hyperplastic** [ˌhaipə(ː)ˈplæstik] *a*

hyperplasmia [ˌhaipə(ː)ˈplæzmiə] *n* 血浆过多

hyperplasminemia [ˌhaipə(ː)ˌplæzmiˈniːmiə] *n* 高纤维蛋白溶酶血症

hyperploid [ˈhaipə(ː)plɔid] *a* 超倍的 *n* 超倍体(指一个个体或细胞在不平衡的组合中含有多于典型数目的染色体) | **~y** [ˌhaipə(ː)ˈplɔidi] *n* 超倍性

hyperpnea [ˌhaipə(ː)ˈpniːə] *n* 呼吸过度,呼吸增强 | **hyperpneic** [ˌhaipə(ː)ˈpniːik] *a*

hyperpolarization [ˌhaipə(ː)ˌpəuləraiˈzeiʃən, -riˈz-] *n* 超极化

hyperpolypeptidemia [ˌhaipə(ː)ˌpɔliˌpeptiˈdiːmiə] *n* 高多肽血症

hyperponesis [ˌhaipə(ː)pəuˈniːsis] *n* 皮质运动区活动过度 | **hyperponetic** [ˌhaipə(ː)pəuˈnetik] *a*

hyperposia [ˌhaipə(ː)ˈpəuziə] *n* 饮水过多,进液过多(短时期多饮症,参见 polyposia)

hyperpostpituitary [ˌhaipə(ː)ˌpəustpiˈtjuːitəri] *a* 垂体后叶激素过多的

hyperpotassemia [ˌhaipə(ː)ˌpɔtæˈsiːmiə] *n* 高钾血症

hyperpragia [ˌhaipə(ː)ˈpreidʒiə] *n* 精神活动过度 | **hyperpragic** [ˌhaipə(ː)ˈpreidʒik] *a*

hyperpraxia [ˌhaipə(ː)ˈpræksiə] *n* 活动过度,动作过多

hyperprebetalipoproteinemia [ˌhaipə(ː)priːˌbeitəˌlipəˌprəutiːˈniːmiə] *n* 高前β脂蛋白血症 | familial ~ 家族性高前β脂蛋白血症,家族性高脂蛋白血症Ⅳ型

hyperpresbyopia [ˌhaipə(ː)ˌprezbiˈəupiə] *n* 高度老视

hyperproinsulinemia [ˌhaipə(ː)prəuˌinsjuliˈniːmiə] *n* 高胰岛素原血症

hyperprolactinemia [ˌhaipə(ː)prəuˌlæktiˈniːmiə] *n* 高催乳素血症 | **hyperprolactinemic** *a*

hyperprolanemia [ˌhaipə(ː)ˌprəuləˈniːmiə] *n* 高促性腺激素血症

hyperprolinemia [ˌhaipə(ː)ˌprəuliˈniːmiə] *n* 高脯氨酸血症

hyperprolinuria [ˌhaipə(ː)ˌprəuliˈnjuəriə] *n* 高脯氨酸尿
hyperprosexia [ˌhaipə(ː)prəuˈseksiə] *n* 注意过强
hyperprosody [ˌhaipə(ː)ˈprɔsədi] *n* 言语韻调过分
hyperproteinemia [ˌhaipə(ː)prəutiːˈniːmiə] *n* 高蛋白血[症]
hyperproteosis [ˌhaipə(ː)ˌprəutiˈəusis] *n* 蛋白过多,蛋白质摄食过多
hyperpselaphesia [ˌhaipə(ː)ˌpseləˈfiːziə] *n* 触觉过敏
hyperpsychosis [ˌhaipə(ː)saiˈkəusis] *n* 精神活动亢进(伴思维奔逸)
hyperptyalism [ˌhaipə(ː)ˈtaiəlizəm] *n* 多涎[症],唾液[分泌]过多
hyperpyremia [ˌhaipə(ː)paiˈriːmiə] *n* 血碳过多,高碳血
hyperpyrexia [ˌhaipə(ː)paiˈreksiə] *n* 高热 | **hyperpyretic** [ˌhaipə(ː)paiˈretik], **hyperpyrexial** [ˌhaipə(ː)paiˈreksiəl] *a*
hyperreactive [ˌhaipə(ː)ri(ː)ˈæktiv] *a* 反应过度的
hyperreactivity [ˌhaipə(ː)ri(ː)ækˈtivəti] *n* 反应过度性
hyperreactio luteinalis [ˌhaipə(ː)ri(ː)ˈækʃiəu-ˌljuːtiˈneilis] 黄体素反应过度性
hyperreflexia [ˌhaipə(ː)riːˈfleksiə] *n* 反射亢进
hyperreninemia [ˌhaipə(ː)ˌriːniˈniːmiə] *n* 高肾素血症 | **hyperreninemic** *a*
hyperresonance [ˌhaipə(ː)ˈrezənəns] *n* 反响过强
hyperresponsive [ˌhaipə(ː)risˈpɔnsiv] *a* 反应过度的 | **~ness** *n* 反应过度性
hypersalemia [ˌhaipə(ː)sæˈliːmiə] *n* 高盐血症
hypersaline [ˌhaipə(ː)ˈseilain] *a* 多盐的(给以大剂量食盐的治疗法)
hypersalivation [ˌhaipə(ː)ˌsæliˈveiʃən] *n* 多涎[症],唾液[分泌]过多
hypersarcosinemia [ˌhaipə(ː)ˌsɑːkəsiˈniːmiə] *n* 高肌氨酸血症
hypersecretion [ˌhaipə(ː)siˈkriːʃən] *n* 分泌过多 | gastric ~ 胃液分泌过多,胃酸过多[症]
hypersecretory [ˌhaipə(ː)siˈkriːtəri] *a* 分泌过多的
hypersegmentation [ˌhaipə(ː)ˌsegmənˈteiʃən] *n* 分裂过多,分节过多,分叶过多
hypersensibility [ˌhaipəˌsensiˈbiləti] *n* 过敏[性],超敏感性
hypersensitive [ˌhaipə(ː)ˈsensitiv] *a* 过敏的,超敏感的
hypersensitivity [ˌhaipə(ː)ˌsensiˈtivəti] *n* 超敏感性,超敏反应 | contact ~ 接触性超敏反应 / cutaneous basophil ~ 皮肤嗜碱粒细胞超敏反应 / delayed ~(DH), delayed-type ~(DTH) 迟发型超敏反应 / immediate ~ 速发型超敏反应,立即型超敏反应 / tuberculin-type ~ 结核菌素型超敏反应
hypersensitization [ˌhaipə(ː)ˌsensitaiˈzeiʃən, -tiˈz-] *n* 促过敏作用,致敏作用
hyperserotonemia [ˌhaipə(ː)ˌsiərətəuˈniːmiə] *n* 高血清素血症
hypersexuality [ˌhaipə(ː)ˌseksjuˈæləti] *n* 性欲亢进
hypersialosis [ˌhaipə(ː)ˌsaiəˈləusis] *n* 多涎[症],唾液[分泌]过多
hyperskeocytosis [ˌhaipə(ː)ˌskiəsaiˈtəusis] *n* 幼稚[白]细胞过多性白细胞增多[症]
hypersomatatropism [ˌhaipə(ː)səuˌmætəˈtrɔpizəm] *n* 生长激素分泌过多
hypersomia [ˌhaipə(ː)ˈsəumiə] *n* 巨大发育,巨人症
hypersomnia [ˌhaipə(ː)ˈsɔmniə] *n* 睡眠过度
hypersomnolence [ˌhaipə(ː)ˈsɔmnələns] *n* 嗜睡[症]
hypersphyxia [ˌhaipə(ː)ˈsfiksiə] *n* 血循环加速合并高血压
hypersplenism [ˌhaipə(ː)ˈsplenizəm], **hypersplenia** [ˌhaipə(ː)ˈspliːniə] *n* 脾功能亢进
hypersplenotrophy [ˌhaipə(ː)spliˈnɔtrəfi] *n* 脾大
hyperspongiosis [ˌhaipə(ː)ˌspɔndʒiˈəusis] *n* 海绵质增生
hypersteatosis [ˌhaipə(ː)stiəˈtəusis] *n* 皮脂分泌过多,皮脂溢
hyperstereoradiography [ˌhaipə(ː)ˌstiəriəuˌreidiˈɔgrəfi], **hyperstereoskiagraphy** [ˌhaipə(ː)-ˌstiəriəuskaiˈægrəfi] *n* 增距立体X线摄影[术]
hypersthenia [ˌhaipə(ː)ˈsθiːnjə] *n* 体力过盛 | **hypersthenic** [ˌhaipə(ː)ˈsθenik] *a*
hypersthenuria [ˌhaipə(ː)sθiˈnjuəriə] *n* 尿浓缩过度,高渗尿
hyperstimulation [ˌhaipə(ː)stimjuˈleiʃən] *n* 刺激过度
hypersuprarenalemia [ˌhaipə(ː)ˌsjuːprəˌriːnəˈliːmiə] *n* 高肾上腺素血症
hypersuprarenalism [ˌhaipə(ː)ˌsjuːprəˈriːnəlizəm] *n* 肾上腺功能亢进
hypersusceptibility [ˌhaipə(ː)səˌseptiˈbiləti] *n* 感受性过强,过敏性,超易感性
hypersympathicotonus [ˌhaipə(ː)simˌpæθikəu-ˈtəunəs] *n* 交感神经张力过敏
hypertarachia [ˌhaipə(ː)təˈrækiə] *n* 神经兴奋性过度

hypertaurodontism [ˌhaipə(ː)ˌtɔːrəˈdɔntizəm] *n* 超牛牙[症](牙根不分支的牛牙症)

hypertelorism [ˌhaipə(ː)ˈtiːlərizəm] *n* 距离过远 | ocular ~, orbital ~ 两眼距离过远,眼距过宽征(有时伴精神发育不全)

hypertensinase [ˌhaipə(ː)ˈtensineis] *n* 血管紧张素酶

hypertensinogen [ˌhaipə(ː)tenˈsinədʒin] *n* 血管紧张素原

hypertension [ˌhaipə(ː)ˈtenʃən] *n* 高血压,血压过高;张力过强,压力过高 | adrenal ~ 肾上腺[缺血]性高血压 / benign ~, red ~ 良性高血压,红色高血压 / benign intracranial ~ 脑假瘤 / essential ~, primary ~, idiopathic ~ 特发性高血压,原发性高血压 / malignant ~, accelerated ~, pale ~ 恶性高血压 / neuromuscular ~ 神经肌肉张力过强 / portal ~ 门静脉高血压,门静脉血压过高 / pulmonary ~ 肺动脉高压 / renal ~ 肾性高血压 / secondary ~, symptomatic ~ 继发性高血压 / vascular ~ 血管性高血压 | **hypertensive** *a* 高血压的 *n* 致高血压药;高血压患者

hypertensor [ˌhaipə(ː)ˈtensə] *n* 加压药,增[血]压药

hypertetraploid [ˌhaipə(ː)ˈtetrəplɔid] *a* 超四倍体的,高四倍体的 *n* 超四倍体,高四倍体(指一个个体或细胞在不平衡组合中含有多于四倍体的染色体〈4n + x〉)

hyperthecosis [ˌhaipə(ː)θiˈkəusis] *n* 卵泡膜细胞增殖症

hyperthelia [ˌhaipə(ː)ˈθiːliə] *n* 多乳头[畸形]

hyperthermal [ˌhaipə(ː)ˈθəːməl] *a* 高温的,热的

hyperthermalgesia [ˌhaipə(ː)ˌθəːməlˈdʒiːziə] *n* 热觉过敏

hyperthermesthesia [ˌhaipə(ː)ˌθəːmisˈθiːzjə], **hyperthermoesthesia** [ˌhaipə(ː)θəːməuisˈθiːzjə] *n* 热觉过敏

hyperthermia [ˌhaipə(ː)ˈθəːmiə] *n* 体温过高,过热 | malignant ~, ~ of anesthesia 恶性体温过高,麻醉性体温过高 | **hyperthermy** [ˌhaipə(ː)ˈθəːmi] *n*

hyperthrombinemia [ˌhaipə(ː)ˌθrɔmbiˈniːmiə] *n* 高凝血酶血症

hyperthymergasia [ˌhaipə(ː)ˌθaiməˈgeiziə] *n* 情感过盛,情感活泼 | **hyperthymergastic** [ˌhaipə(ː)ˌθaiməˈgæstik] *a*

hyperthymia [ˌhaipə(ː)ˈθaimiə] *n* 情感增盛 | **hyperthymic** *a*

hyperthymism [ˌhaipə(ː)ˈθaimizəm] *n* 胸腺功能亢进

hyperthyroid [ˌhaipə(ː)ˈθairɔid] *a* 甲状腺功能亢进的 *n* 甲状腺功能亢进患者

hyperthyroidism [ˌhaipə(ː)ˈθairɔidizəm] *n* 甲状腺功能亢进 | masked ~ 掩蔽性甲状腺功能亢进 | **hyperthyrea** [ˌhaipə(ː)ˈθairiə], **hyperthyreosis** [ˌhaipə(ː)ˌθairiˈəusis], **hyperthyroidosis** [ˌhaipə(ː)ˌθairɔiˈdəusis] *n*

hyperthyroxinemia [ˌhaipə(ː)θaiˌrɔksiˈniːmiə] *n* 高甲状腺素血症 | familial dysalbuminemic ~ 家族性白蛋白血异常性高甲状腺素血症(一种家族性常染色体显性遗传综合征)

hypertonia [ˌhaipə(ː)ˈtəuniə] *n* 张力过高 | ~ polycythaemica 红细胞增多性高血压 | **hypertonus** [ˌhaipə(ː)ˈtəunəs] *n*

hypertonic [ˌhaipə(ː)ˈtɔnik] *a* 高张的;高渗的 | **~ity** [ˌhaipə(ː)təuˈnisəti] *n* 高张性;高渗性

hypertoxic [ˌhaipə(ː)ˈtɔksik] *a* 剧毒的 | **~ity** [ˌhaipə(ː)tɔkˈsisəti] *n* 剧毒性

hypertransfusion [ˌhaipə(ː)trænsˈfjuʒən] *n* 高灌注

hypertrichosis [ˌhaipə(ː)triˈkəusis] *n* 多毛症 | ~ lanuginosa 多胎毛症 / ~ pinnae auris 耳翼多毛症(耳翼毛异常过度生长,可能是一种X连锁或常染色体显性遗传特性) / ~ universalis 全身性多毛症

hypertriglyceridemia [ˌhaipə(ː)traiˌglisəraiˈdiːmiə] *n* 高甘油三酯血症 | carbohydrate-induced ~ 碳水化合物引起的高甘油三酯血症,家族性高脂蛋白血症Ⅲ型和Ⅳ型 / familial ~ 家族性高甘油三酯血症,家族性高脂蛋白血症Ⅳ型

hypertriploid [ˌhaipə(ː)ˈtriplɔid] *a* 超三倍体的,高三倍体的 *n* 超三倍体,高三倍体(指一个个体或细胞在不平衡组合中含有多于三倍体的染色体〈3n + x〉)

hypertrophy [haiˈpəːtrəfi] *n* 肥大 | adaptive ~ 适应性肥大 / compensatory ~ 代偿性肥大 / complementary ~ 补偿性肥大 / concentric ~ 向心性肥大 / eccentric ~ 离心性肥大,扩张性肥大 / numeric ~ 增数性肥大 / pseudomuscular ~ 假性肌肥大,假肥大性肌营养不良 / quantitative ~ 数量性肥大,增生 / vicarious ~ 替代性肥大 | **hypertrophia** [ˌhaipə(ː)ˈtrəufiə] *n* / **hypertrophic** [ˌhaipə(ː)ˈtrɔfik] *a*

hypertropia [ˌhaipə(ː)ˈtrəupiə] *n* 上斜视

hypertyrosinemia [ˌhaipə(ː)ˌtairəusiˈniːmiə] *n* 高酪氨酸血症

hyperuraturia [ˌhaipə(ː)ˌjuərəˈtjuəriə] *n* 高尿酸尿

hyperuresis [ˌhaipə(ː)rjuəˈriːsis] *n* 多尿症

hyperuricemia [ˌhaipə(ː)ˌrjuəriˈsiːmiə], **hyperuricacidemia** [ˌhaipə(ː)ˌrjuəriˌkæsiˈdiːmiə] *n* 高尿酸血症(亦称尿酸血症) | **hyperuricemic** [ˌhaipə(ː)ˌrjuəriˈsiːmik] *a*

hyperuricosuria [ˌhaipə(ː)ˌjuərikəuˈsjuəriə] *n* 高尿酸尿

hyperuricuria [ˌhaipə(ː)ˌrjuəriˈkjuəriə], **hyperuricaciduria** [ˌhaipə(ː)ˌrjuəriˌkæsiˈdjuəriə] *n* 高尿酸尿

hypervaccination [ˌhaipə(ː)ˌvæksiˈneiʃən] *n* 超接种(对已预先免疫了的动物,再以足够的疫苗进一步接种〈一次或多次〉,使其能对其他动物产生保护性血清)

hypervalinemia [ˌhaipə(ː)væliˈniːmiə] *n* 高缬氨酸血症

hypervascular [ˌhaipə(ː)ˈvæskjulə] *a* 血管过多的

hypervegetative [ˌhaipə(ː)ˌvedʒiˈteitiv] *a* 内脏型的,高自主性功能体型的(内脏功能即自主性神经功能占优势)

hyperventilation [ˌhaipə(ː)ˌventiˈleiʃən] *n* 通气增强,通气过度(过量空气进入肺泡,致二氧化碳张力降低,最终导致碱中毒);过度呼吸(常用于癫痫及手足搐搦时的检验方法) | **hyperventilate** [ˌhaipə(ː)ˈventileit] *vi*, *vt*

hypervigilance [ˌhaipə(ː)ˈvidʒiləns] *n* 警觉过度

hyperviscosity [ˌhaipə(ː)visˈkɔsəti] *n* 高黏滞

hypervitaminosis [ˌhaipə(ː)ˌvaitəmiˈnəusis] *n* 维生素过多[症] | ~ A 维生素 A 过多症 / ~ D 维生素 D 过多症 | **hypervitaminotic** [ˌhaipə(ː)ˌvaitəmiˈnɔtik] *a*

hypervolemia [ˌhaipə(ː)vɔˈliːmiə] *n* 血容量过多 | **hypervolemic** [ˌhaipə(ː)vɔˈliːmik] *a*

hypervolia [ˌhaipə(ː)ˈvɔliə] *n* 水[含]量过多,液量过多

hypesthesia [ˌhaipisˈθiːzjə] *n* 感觉减退 | **hypesthesic** [ˌhaipisˈθiːsik], **hypesthetic** [ˌhaipisˈθetik] *a*

hypha [ˌhaifə]([复] **hyphae** [ˈhaifiː]) *n*【拉】菌丝 | **~l** *a*

hyphedonia [ˌhaiphiˈdəuniə] *n* 快感减少

hyphema [haiˈfiːmə] *n* 前房积血

hyphemia [haiˈfiːmiə] *n* 血量减少,贫血

hyphephilia [ˌhifiˈfiliə] *n* 恋丝织物[色情]癖

hyphidrosis [ˌhaiphaiˈdrəusis] *n* 少汗

Hyphomicrobiaceae [ˌhaifəumaiˌkrəubiːˈeisiiː] *n* 生丝微菌科

Hyphomicrobiales [ˌhaifəumaiˌkrəubiːˈeiliːz] *n* 生丝微菌目

Hyphomicrobium [ˌhaifəumaiˈkrəubiːəm] *n* 生丝微菌属

Hyphomonas [ˌhaifəuˈməunəs] *n* 生丝单胞菌属

Hyphomyces [ˌhaifəuˈmaisiːz] *n* 丝霉菌属 | ~ destruens 毁坏性丝霉菌

Hyphomycetales [ˌhaifəuˌmaisiˈteiliːz] *n* 丝状菌目

hyphomycete [ˌhaifəumaiˈsiːt] *n* 丝状菌

Hyphomycetes [ˌhaifəumaiˈsiːtiːz] *n* 丝状菌纲

hyphomycosis [ˌhaifəumaiˈkəusis] *n* 丝状菌病 | ~ destruens equi 马毁坏性丝状菌病

hyphylline [haiˈfilin] *n* 双羟丙茶碱,喘定(血管和支气管扩张药,强心药,利尿药)

hypisotonic [ˌhaipaisəuˈtɔnik] *a* 低张的;低渗的

hypnagogic [ˌhipnəˈgɔdʒik] *a* 催眠的,安眠的;入睡前的(指幻觉)

hypnagogue [ˈhipnəgɔg] *a* 催眠的 *n* 安眠药,催眠药

hypnalgia [hipˈnældʒiə] *n* 睡眠疼痛

hypnic [ˈhipnik] *a* 催眠的,睡眠的

hypn(o)- [构词成分]睡眠,催眠

hypnoanalysis [ˌhipnəuəˈnæləsis] *n* 催眠[精神]分析

hypnoanesthesia [ˌhipnəuˌænisˈθiːzjə] *n* 催眠麻醉[法]

hypnocinematograph [ˌhipnəuˌsiniˈmætəgrɑːf, -græf] *n* 睡眠动作记录仪

hypnocyst [ˈhipnəsist] *n* 静止囊肿

hypnodontics [ˌhipnəuˈdɔntiks], **hypnodontia** [ˌhipnəuˈdɔnʃiə] *n* 牙科催眠术

hypnogenesis [ˌhipnəuˈdʒenisis] *n* 催眠 | **hypnogenetic** [ˌhipnəudʒiˈnetik], **hypnogenic** [ˌhipnəuˈdʒenik], **hypnogenous** [hipˈnɔdʒinəs] *a*

hypnoid [ˈhipnɔid] *a* 催眠[状态]样的

hypnoidal [hipˈnɔidl] *a* 催眠样的

hypnoidization [ˌhipnɔidaiˈzeiʃən] *n* 催眠样状态

hypnolepsy [ˈhipnəˌlepsi] *n* 发作性睡病

hypnology [hipˈnɔlədʒi] *n* 催眠学

hypnonarcoanalysis [ˌhipnəuˌnɑːkəuəˈnæləsis] *n* 催眠麻醉[精神]分析

hypnonarcosis [ˌhipnəunɑːˈkəusis] 催眠麻醉法

hypnopedia [ˌhipnəuˈpiːdiə] *n* 睡眠中教学,睡眠学习(如听录音)

hypnopompic [ˌhipnəuˈpɔmpik] *a* 半醒前的;睡意朦胧[状态]的

hypnosia [hipˈnəuziə] *n* 嗜眠[症]

hypnosis [hipˈnəusis]([复] **hypnoses** [hipˈnəusiːz]) *n* 催眠术

hypnosophy [hipˈnɔsəfi] *n* 睡眠学

hypnotherapy [ˌhipnəuˈθerəpi] *n* 催眠疗法

hypnotic [hipˈnɔtik] *a* 催眠的;催眠性的 *n* 催眠药,安眠药

hypnotism [ˈhipnətizəm] *n* 催眠状态;催眠术 | **hypnotist** *n* 催眠术士

hypnotization [ˌhipnəutaiˈzeiʃən, -tiˈz-] *n* 诱导催眠

hypnotize [ˈhipnətaiz] *vt* 催眠

hypnotoxin [ˌhipnəu'tɔksin] *n* 催眠毒素
hypnozoite [ˌhipnəu'zəuit] *n* 休眠体
hypo ['haipəu] *n* 皮下注射;皮下注射器;海波,硫代硫酸钠(用作相片定影剂)
hyp(o)- [前缀]下,低,少,减退,迟,在下,逊,不足,次,过少
hypoacidity [ˌhaipəuə'sidəti] *n* 酸过少,胃酸过少
hypoactivity [ˌhaipəuæk'tivəti] *n* 活动减退 | **hypoactive** [ˌhaipəu'æktiv] *a*
hypoacusis [ˌhaipəuə'kjuːsis], **hypoacusia** [ˌhaipəuə'kjuːziə] *n* 听力减退,重听
hypoadenia [ˌhaipəuə'diːniə] *n* 腺功能减退
hypoadrenalemia [ˌhaipəuəˌdriːnə'liːmiə] *n* 低肾上腺素血症
hypoadrenalism [ˌhaipəuə'driːnəlizəm], **hypoadrenia** [ˌhaipəuə'driːniə] *n* 肾上腺功能减退
hypoadrenocorticism [ˌhaipəuəˌdriːnəu'kɔːtisizəm] *n* 肾上腺皮质功能减退
hypoalbuminemia [ˌhaipəuælˌbjuːmi'niːmiə] *n* 低白蛋白血症
hypoalbuminosis [ˌhaipəuælˌbjuːmi'nəusis] *n* 白蛋白过少
hypoaldosteronemia [ˌhaipəuælˌdɔstərə'niːmiə] *n* 低醛固酮血症
hypoaldosteronism [ˌhaipəuæl'dɔstərəˌnizəm] *n* 醛固酮减少症 | isolated ~ 孤立性醛固酮减少症
hypoaldosteronuria [ˌhaipəuælˌdɔstərə'njuəriə] *n* 低醛固酮尿
hypoalgesia [ˌhaipəuæl'dʒiːsiə] *n* 痛觉减退
hypoalimentation [ˌhaipəuˌælimen'teiʃən] *n* 营养不足,进食不足
hypoalkaline [ˌhaipəu'ælkəlain] *a* 碱性不足的 | **hypoalkalinity** [ˌhaipəuˌælkə'linəti] *n*
hypoalonemia [ˌhaipəuˌælə'niːmiə] *n* 低盐血症
hypoalphalipoproteinemia [ˌhaipəuˌælfəˌlipəuˌprəutiː'niːmiə] *n* 低 α 脂蛋白血[症](①血内高密度〈α〉脂蛋白缺乏;②丹吉尔〈Tangier〉病)
hypoaminoacidemia [ˌhaipəuˌæminəuˌæsi'diːmiə] *n* 低氨酸血症
hypoandrogenism [ˌhaipəuæn'drəudʒinizəm] *n* 雄激素缺乏,雄激素不足
hypoazoturia [ˌhaipəuˌæzə'tjuəriə] *n* 低氮尿
hypobaric [ˌhaipəu'bærik] *a* 低压的(气体);低密度的(溶液)
hypobarism [ˌhaipəu'bærizəm] *n* 低气压病
hypobaropathy [ˌhaipəubə'rɔpəθi] *n* 低气压病,高空病
hypobasophilism [ˌhaipəubei'sɔfilizəm] *n* [脑]垂体功能减退
hypobetalipoproteinemia [ˌhaipəu ˌbeitəˌlipəuˌprəutiː'niːmiə] *n* 低 β 脂蛋白血症 | familial ~ 家族性低 β 脂蛋白血症
hypobicarbonatemia [ˌhaipəubaiˌkaːbɔnei'tiːmiə] *n* 低重碳酸盐血症
hypobilirubinemia [ˌhaipəuˌbiliˌruːbi'niːmiə] *n* 低胆红素血症
hypoblast ['haipəblæst] *n* 下胚层,内胚层 | **~ic** [ˌhaipə'blæstik] *a*
hypobranchial [ˌhaipəu'bræŋkiə] *a* 鳃下的
hypobromite [ˌhaipəu'brəumait] *n* 次溴酸盐
hypobromous acid [ˌhaipəu'brəuməs] 次溴酸
hypocalcemia [ˌhaipəukæl'siːmiə] *n* 低钙血症,低血钙
hypocalcemic [ˌhaipəukæl'siːmik] *a* 低钙血症的
hypocalcia [ˌhaipəu'kælsiə] *n* 钙过少,钙不足
hypocalcification [ˌhaipəuˌkælsifi'keiʃən] *n* 钙化不全 | enamel ~ 釉质钙化不全[症]
hypocalcipexy [ˌhaipəu'kælsiˌpeksi] *n* 钙沉积过少 | **hypocalcipectic** [ˌhaipəuˌkælsi'pɔktik] *a*
hypocalciuria [ˌhaipəuˌkælsi'juəriə] *n* 低钙尿
hypocapnia [ˌhaipəu'kæpniə], **hypocarbia** [ˌhaipəu'kɑːbiə] *n* 低碳酸血症 | **hypocapnic** [ˌhaipəu'kæpnik] *a*
hypocatalasemia [ˌhaipəuˌkætəlei'siːmiə] *n* 低过氧化氢酶血
hypocatalasia [ˌhaipəuˌkætə'leiziə] *n* 过氧化氢酶过少[症]
hypocellular [ˌhaipəu'seljulə] *a* 细胞过少的 | **~ity** [ˌhaipəuˌselju'lærəti] *n*
hypocelom [ˌhaipəu'siːləm] *n* 下体腔
hypochloremia [ˌhaipəuklɔː'riːmiə], **hypochloridemia** [ˌhaipəuˌklɔːri'diːmiə] *n* 低氯血症 | **hypochloremic** [ˌhaipəuklɔː'riːmik] *a* **hypochlorhydria** [ˌhaipəuklɔː'haidriə] *n* 胃酸过少[症]
hypochloridation [ˌhaipəuˌklɔːri'deiʃən] *n* [组织]氯过少
hypochlorite [ˌhaipəu'klɔːrait] *n* 次氯酸盐
hypochlorization [ˌhaipəuˌklɔːrai'zeiʃən] *n* [饮食]供盐减少,减盐疗法
hypochlorous acid [ˌhaipəu'klɔːrəs] 次氯酸
hypochloruria [ˌhaipəuklɔː'rjuəriə] *n* 低氯尿
hypocholesterolemia [ˌhaipəukəuˌlestərəu'liːmiə], **hypocholesteremia** [ˌhaipəukəuˌlestə'riːmiə], **hypocholesterinemia** [ˌhaipəukəuˌlestəri'niːmiə] *n* 低胆固醇血症 | **hypocholesterolemic** [ˌhaipəukəuˌlestərəu'liːmik], **hypocholesteremic** [ˌhaipəukəuˌlestə'riːmik] *a*
hypocholia [ˌhaipəu'kəuliə] *n* 胆汁过少
hypocholuria [ˌhaipəukəu'ljuəriə] *n* 低胆汁尿
hypochondria [ˌhaipəu'kɔndriə] *n* 季肋区(hypochondrium 的复数);疑病症 **hypochondriac**

[ˌhaipəuˈkɔndriæk] *a* 疑病症的;季肋部的 *n* 疑病患者

hypochondriasis [ˌhaipəukɔnˈdraiəsis] *n* 疑病症 | **hypochondriacal** [ˌhaipəukɔnˈdraiəkəl] *a*

hypochondrium [ˌhaipəuˈkɔndriəm] ([复] **hypochondria**[ˌhaipəuˈkɔndriə]) *n* 季肋区

hypochondroplasia [ˌhaipəuˌkɔndrəuˈpleiziə] *n* 季肋发育不全,软骨发育不良

hypochordal [ˌhaipəuˈkɔːdəl] *a* 脊索腹侧的

hypochromasia [ˌhaipəukrəuˈmeiziə] *n* 着色不足,染色过浅

hypochromatic [ˌhaipəukrəuˈmætik] *a* 含染色体少的;染浅色的,淡染的

hypochromatism [ˌhaipəuˈkrəumətizəm] *n* 着色不足(尤指细胞核内染色质过少)

hypochromatosis [ˌhaipəuˌkrəuməˈtəusis] *n* 细胞核[染色质]消失,核溶解

hypochromemia [ˌhaipəukrəuˈmiːmiə] *n* 血色指数过低 | idiopathic ~ 特发性低色[指数]性贫血

hypochromia [ˌhaipəuˈkrəumiə] *n* 低色素;着色不足(尤指细胞核内染色质过少) | **hypochromic** *a*

hypochromotrichia [ˌhaipəuˌkrəuməuˈtrikiə] *n* 毛发着色不足

hypochrosis [ˌhaipəuˈkrəusis] *n* 低色性贫血,血红蛋白过少性贫血

hypochylia [ˌhaipəuˈkailiə] *n* 乳糜缺乏

hypocinesia [ˌhaipəusaiˈniːziə], **hypocinesis** [ˌhaipəusaiˈniːsis] *n* 运动减少,少动症

hypocistis [ˌhaipəuˈsistis], **hypocist** [ˈhaipəsist] *n* 大花寄生草汁

hypocitraturia [ˌhaipəuˌsitreiˈtjuəriə] *n* 低枸橼酸尿

hypocitremia [ˌhaipəusiˈtriːmiə] *n* 低枸橼酸血症

hypocitruria [ˌhaipəusiˈtruəriə] *n* 低枸橼酸尿

hypocoagulable [ˌhaipəukəuˈægjuləbl] *a* 低凝固性的 | **hypocoagulability** [ˌhaipəukəuˌægjuləˈbiləti] *n*

hypocoelom [ˌhaipəuˈsiːləm] *n* 下体腔

Hypocomatina [ˌhaipəuˌkəuməˈtainə] *n* 腹纤毛亚目

hypocomplementemia [ˌhaipəuˈkɔmplimenˈtiːmiə] *n* 低补体血症 | **hypocomplementemic** [ˌhaipəuˌkɔmplimenˈtiːmik] *a*

hypocondylar [ˌhaipəuˈkɔndilə] *a* 髁下的

hypocone [ˈhaipəkəun] *n* 次尖(上磨牙的远中舌尖)

hypoconid [ˌhaipəuˈkəunid] *n* 下次尖(下磨牙的远中颊尖)

hypoconulid [ˌhaipəuˈkɔnjulid]*n* 下次小尖(下磨牙的远中尖)

hypocorticalism [ˌhaipəuˈkɔːtikəlizəm], **hypocorticism** [ˌhaipəuˈkɔːtisizəm] *n* 肾上腺皮质功能减退

hypocotyl [ˌhaipəˈkɔtil] *n* 下胚轴(植物)

Hypocrea [ˌhaipəuˈkriːə] *n* 肉座菌属

Hypocreaceae [ˌhaipəukriˈeisiiː] *n* 肉座菌科

Hypocreales [ˌhaipəukriˈeiliːz] *n* 肉座菌目

hypocrine [ˈhaipəkrin] *a* 内分泌功能减退的

hypocrinism [ˌhaipəuˈkrainisəm], **hypocrinia** [ˌhaipəuˈkriniə] *n* 内分泌过少

hypocupremia [ˌhaipəukjuːˈpriːmiə] *n* 低铜血症

hypocyclosis [ˌhaipəusaiˈkləusis] *n* 调视功能减退,调节功能减退

hypocystotomy [ˌhaipəusisˈtɔtəmi] *n* 经会阴膀胱切开术

hypocythemia [ˌhaipəusaiˈθiːmiə] *n* 红细胞减少[症]

hypocytosis [ˌhaipəusaiˈtəusis] *n* 血细胞减少

hypodactyly [ˌhaipəuˈdæktili] *n* 缺指,缺趾

hypodense [ˈhaipəudens] *a* 低致密的(特指 X 线片上的物体或区域,其致密度比其他地方低)

hypoderm [ˈhaipədəːm] *n* 皮下组织 | **~al** [ˌhaipəuˈdəːməl] *a*

Hypoderma [ˌhaipəuˈdəːmə] *n* 皮下蝇属,皮蝇属 | ~ bovis 牛皮下蝇 / ~ lineatum 纹皮下蝇

hypodermatic [ˌhaipəudəːˈmætik] *a* 皮下的

hypodermatoclysis [ˌhaipəudəːməˈtɔklisis] *n* 皮下灌注术,皮下输液

hypodermatomy [ˌhaipəudəːˈmætəmi] *n* 皮下切开术

hypodermiasis [ˌhaipəudəːˈmaiəsis] *n* 皮下蝇蛆病

hypodermic [ˌhaipəuˈdəːmik] *a* 皮下的;皮下注射的 *n* 皮下注射,皮下注射器 | **~ally** *ad*

hypodermis [ˌhaipəuˈdəːmis] *n* 下皮,皮下组织;真皮(昆虫)

hypodermoclysis [ˌhaipəudəːˈmɔklisis] *n* 皮下灌注术,皮下输液

hypodermolithiasis [ˌhaipəuˌdəːməuliˈθaiəsis] *n* 皮下结石[症]

hypodermosis [ˌhaipəudəːˈməusis] *n* 皮下蝇蛆病

hypodiaphragmatic [ˌhaipəuˌdaiəfrægˈmætik] *a* 膈下的

hypodiploid [ˌhaipəuˌdiplɔid] *a* 亚二倍的 *n* 亚二倍体(指一个个体或细胞含有少于二倍体数目的染色体) | **~y** [ˈhaipəuˌdiplɔidi] *n* 亚二倍性

hypodipsia [ˌhaipəuˈdipsiə] *n* 渴感减退 | **hypodipsic** [ˌhaipəuˈdipsik] *a*

hypodontia [ˌhaipəuˈdɔnʃiə] *n* 牙发育不全

hypodynamia [ˌhaipəudaiˈneimiə] *n* 力不足,乏力 | ~ cordis 心力不足 | **hypodynamic** [ˌhaipəudaiˈnæmik] *a*

hypoeccrisia [ˌhaipəueˈkrisiə], **hypoeccrisis** [ˌhaipəuˈekrisis] *n* 排泄过少 | **hypoeccritic** [ˌhaipəu-eˈkritik] *a*

hypoechoic [ˌhaipəuəˈkəuik] *a* 低回声的,弱回声的

hypoelectrolytemia [ˌhaipəuiˌlektrəulaiˈtiːmiə] *n* 低电解质血[症]

hypoemotivity [ˌhaipəuˌiːməuˈtivəti] *n* 情感减弱,情感不足

hypoendocrinism [ˌhaipəuenˈdɔkrinizəm], **hypoendocrinia** [ˌhaipəuˌendəuˈkriniə], **hypoendocrisia** [ˌhaipəuˌendəuˈkriziə] *n* 内分泌过少,内分泌功能减退

hypoeosinophilia [ˌhaipəuˌiːəsinəˈfiliə] *n* 嗜酸细胞减少

hypoepinephrinemia [ˌhaipəuˌepiˌnefriˈniːmiə] *n* 低肾上腺素血症

hypoequilibrium [ˌhaipəuˌiːkwiˈlibriəm] *n* 平衡觉减退

hypoergasia [ˌhaipəuəːˈgeisiə] *n* [功能]活动力减弱

hypoergia [ˌhaipəuˈəːdʒiə] *n* [功能]活动力减弱,反应力过低(对变应原低敏感性)

hypoergy [ˌhaipəuˈəːdʒi] *n* 活动性减弱;低应性,反应性减低 | **hypoergic** *a*

hypoesophoria [ˌhaipəuˌesəˈfəuriə] *n* 下内隐斜

hypoesthesia [ˌhaipəuisˈθiːzjə] *n* 感觉减退 | acoustic ~, auditory ~ 听觉减退 / gustatory ~ 味觉减退 / olfactory ~ 嗅觉减退 / tactile ~ 触觉减退 | **hypoesthetic** [ˌhaipəuisˈθetik] *a*

hypoestrogenemia [ˌhaipəuˌiːstrədʒəˈniːmiə], **hypoestrinemia** [ˌhaipəuˌiːstriˈniːmiə] *n* 低雌激素血症

hypoevolutism [ˌhaipəui(ː)ˈvɔljutizəm] *n* 发育迟缓,发育不良

hypoexophoria [ˌhaipəuˌeksəuˈfəuriə] *n* 下外隐斜

hypoferremia [ˌhaipəufəˈriːmiə] *n* 低铁血症

hypoferrism [ˌhaipəuˈferizəm] *n* (组织)铁过少

hypofertile [ˌhaipəuˈfəːtail] *n* 低生育力的,生殖力减低的 | **hypofertility** [ˌhaipəufəˈtiləti] *a*

hypofibrinogenemia [ˌhaipəufaiˌbrinəudʒiˈniːmiə] *n* 纤维蛋白原

hypofunction [ˌhaipəuˈfʌŋkʃən] *n* 功能减退

hypogalactia [ˌhaipəugəˈlækʃiə] *n* 乳汁减少 | **hypogalactous** [ˌhaipəugəˈlæktəs] *a*

hypogammaglobulinemia [ˌhaipəuˌgæməˌglɔbjuːliˈniːmiə] *n* 低丙球蛋白血症 | acquired ~ 获得性低丙球蛋白血症 / common variable ~ 常见变异型低丙球蛋白血症 / congenital ~ 先天性低丙球蛋白血症 / transient ~ of infancy 婴儿一时性低丙球蛋白血症 / X-linked ~, X-linked infantile ~ X 连锁低丙种球蛋白血症,婴儿 X 连锁低丙球蛋白血症 | **hypogammaglobulinemic** *a*

hypoganglionosis [ˌhaipəuˌgæŋgliəuˈnəusis] *n* 肠肌丛神经节细胞缺乏症

hypogastric [ˌhaipəuˈgæstrik] *a* 腹下部的,下腹的;腹下区的;髂内动脉的

hypogastrium [ˌhaipəuˈgæstriəm] ([复] **hypogastria** [ˌhaipəuˈgæstriə]) *n* 腹下区,耻区

hypogastropagus [ˌhaipəugæsˈtrɔpəgəs] *n* 下腹联胎

hypogastroschisis [ˌhaipəugæsˈtrɔskisis] *n* 下腹裂[畸形]

hypogenesis [ˌhaipəuˈdʒenisis] *n* 发育不全 | polar ~ 极性发育不全(胚胎头尾两极发育不全,可形成畸形) | **hypogenetic** [ˌhaipəudʒiˈnetik] *a*

hypogenitalism [ˌhaipəuˈdʒenitəlizəm] *n* 生殖腺发育不全

hypogeusesthesia [ˌhaipəuˌgjusisˈθiːzjə], **hypogeusia** [ˌhaipəuˈgjuːzjə] *n* 味觉减退

hypoglandular [ˌhaipəuˈglændjulə] *a* 腺功能减退的

hypoglobulia [ˌhaipəugləˈbjuːliə] *n* 红细胞减少[症]

hypoglossal [ˌhaipəuˈglɔsəl] *a* 舌下的

hypoglottis [ˌhaipəuˈglɔtis] *n* 舌下部,舌下;舌下囊肿

hypoglucagonemia [ˌhaipəuˌgluːkəgəˈniːmiə] *n* 低[胰]高血糖素血症

hypoglycemia [ˌhaipəuglaiˈsiːmiə] *n* 低血糖[症] | factitial ~, factitious ~ 假性低血糖 / fasting ~ 空腹性低血糖 / ketotic ~ 酮性低血糖 / leucine-induced ~ 亮氨酸诱导性低血糖 / mixed ~ 混合性低血糖 / reactive ~ 反应性低血糖 | **hypoglycemic** [ˌhaipəuglaiˈsiːmik] *a* 低血糖的 *n* 降血糖药

hypoglycemosis [ˌhaipəuˌglaisiˈməusis] *n* 低血糖症

hypoglycin [ˌhaipəuˈglaisin], **hypoglycine** [ˌhaipəuˈglaisiːn] *n* 降糖氨酸

hypoglycogenolysis [ˌhaipəuˌglaikəudʒiˈnɔlisis] *n* 糖原分解不足

hypoglycorrhachia [ˌhaipəuˌglaikəuˈreikiə] *n* 脑脊液糖分过少

hypognathous [haiˈpɔgnəθəs] *a* 下颌突出的;下颌寄生胎的

hypognathus [haiˈpɔgnəθəs] *n* 下颌寄生胎

hypogonadism [ˌhaipəuˈgəunədizəm] *n* 性腺功能

减退症 | eugonadotropic ~ 正常促性腺素性功能减退症 / hypergonadotropic ~, primary ~ 高促性腺素性功能减退症,原发性性腺功能减退 / hypogonadotropic ~, secondary ~ 低促性腺素性功能减退症,继发性性腺功能减退 | **hypogonadia** [ˌhaipəuɡəu'nædiə] *n*

hypogonadotropic [ˌhaipəuˌɡɔnədəu'trɔpik] *a* 促性腺激素分泌不足的,低促性腺素性的

hypogranulocytosis [ˌhaipəuˌɡrænjuləusai'təusis] *n* 粒细胞过少症

hypohemia [ˌhaipəu'hiːmiə] *n* 贫血

hypohepatia [ˌhaipəuhi'pætiə] *n* 肝功能减退

hypohidrosis [ˌhaipəuhai'drəusis] *n* 少汗症 | **hypohidrotic** [ˌhaipəuhai'drɔtik] *a*

hypohormonal [ˌhaipəuhɔː'məunl], **hypohormonic** [ˌhaipəuhɔː'mɔnik] *a* 激素不足的

hypohormonism [ˌhaipəu'hɔːməunizəm] *n* 激素过少[症],内分泌功能减退

hypohydration [ˌhaipəuhai'dreiʃən] *n* 水分过少,失水

hypohydrochloria [ˌhaipəuˌhaidrəu'klɔːrie] *n* 胃酸过少[症]

hypohypnotic [ˌhaipəuhip'nɔtik] *a* 浅睡眠的,浅催眠的

hypohypophysism [ˌhaipəuhai'pɔfisizəm] *n* 垂体功能减退

hypoidrosis [ˌhaipəui'drəusis] *n* 少汗

hypoimmunity [ˌhaipəui'mjuːnəti] *n* 低免疫性(降低的免疫性)

hypoinsulinemia [ˌhaipəuˌinsjuli'niːmiə] *n* 低胰岛素血症

hypoinsulinism [ˌhaipəu'insjuliˌnizəm] *n* 胰岛素分泌过少

hypointense [ˌhaipəuin'tens] *a* 低强度的(具有比某一物体的强度较低的)

hypoiodidism [ˌhaipəuai'əudidizəm] *n* 碘过少

hypoisotonic [ˌhaipəuˌaisəu'tɔnik] *a* 低渗的

hypokalemia [ˌhaipəukə'liːmiə], **hypokaliemia** [ˌhaipəuˌkæli'iːmiə] *n* 低钾血症 | **hypokalemic** [ˌhaipəukə'liːmik] *a* 低钾血症的 *n* 降血钾药

hypokinemia [ˌhaipəukai'niːmiə] *n* 心排血量过少,心输出量不足

hypokinesia [ˌhaipəukai'niːziə, -ki'n-] *n* 运动减少

hypokinesis [ˌhaipəukai'niːsis, -ki'n-] *n* 运动减少,低动力

hypokinetic [ˌhaipəukai'netik, -ki'n-] *a* 运动减少的

hypolactasia [ˌhaipəulæk'teiziə] *n* 肠乳糖酶缺乏

hypolarynx [ˌhaipəu'læriŋks] *n* 声门下,喉下部

hypolemmal [ˌhaipəu'leməl] *a* 膜下的

hypolethal [ˌhaipəu'liːθəl] *a* 致死量以下的,小于致死量的

hypoleydigism [ˌhaipəu'laidiɡizəm] *n* 莱迪希(Leydig)间质细胞功能减退

hypolipemia [ˌhaipəuli'piːmiə] *n* 低脂血症

hypolipidemic [ˌhaipəuˌlipi'diːmik] *a* 降血脂的;降血脂药

hypolipoproteinemia [ˌhaipəuˌlipəuˌprəutiː'niːmiə] *n* 低脂蛋白血症

hypoliposis [ˌhaipəuli'pəusis] *n* 脂质过少

hypoliquorrhea [ˌhaipəuˌlaikwə'riə] *n* 脑脊液不足

hypolutemia [ˌhaipəuljuː'tiːmiə] *n* 低黄体激素血症,低孕酮血症

hypolymphemia [ˌhaipəulim'fiːmiə] *n* 低淋巴细胞血症

hypomagnesemia [ˌhaipəuˌmæɡni'siːmiə] *n* 低镁血症

hypomania [ˌhaipəu'meinjə] *n* 轻躁狂 | **hypomacin** *a* / **hypomaniac** [ˌhaipəu'meiniæk] *n* 轻躁狂者

hypomastia [haipəu'mæstiə], **hypomazia** [ˌhaipəu'meiziə] *n* 乳腺过小

hypomegasoma [ˌhaipəuˌmeɡə'səumə] *n* 轻度巨大发育,高身材

hypomelancholia [ˌhaipəuˌmelən'kəuliə] *n* 轻性忧郁症

hypomelanosis [ˌhaipəuˌmelə'nəusis] *n* 黑素减少症 | idiopathic guttate ~ 特发性滴状黑素减少症 / ~ of Ito 伊藤黑素减少症,无色性色素失调症

hypomenorrhea [ˌhaipəuˌmenə'riːə] *n* 月经过少

hypomere ['haipəmiə] *n* [肌节]腹侧段;下中胚层,轴外中胚层

hypomesosoma [ˌhaipəuˌmesə'səumə] *n* 中[等以]下身材

hypometabolism [ˌhaipəume'tæbəlizəm] *n* 代谢减退 | **hypometabolic** [ˌhaipəuˌmetə'bɔlik] *a*

hypomethioninemia [ˌhaipəuməˌθaiəni'niːmiə] *n* 低甲硫氨酸血症

hypometria [ˌhaipəu'miːtriə] *n* 伸展不足,运动范围不足

hypomicron [ˌhaipəu'maikrɔn] *n* 亚微粒,次微粒

hypomicrosoma [ˌhaipəuˌmaikrəu'səumə] *n* 矮小身材

hypomineralization [ˌhaipəuˌminərəlai'zeiʃən, -li'z-] *n* 矿质过少

hypomnesis [ˌhaipɔm'niːsis] *n* 记忆减退

hypomodal [ˌhaipəu'məudl] *a* 低于众数的(在统计学上,指在变量曲线上位于众数的左方的数值或项目,即数值小于众数的变量)

hypomorph ['haipəmɔːf] *n* 肢短体高者,下型身材者;亚效等位基因(一种突发基因,其功效较弱) | **~ic** [ˌhaipəu'mɔːfik] *a*

hypomotility [ˌhaipəuməu'tiləti] *n* 运动不足,运动减弱

hypomyotonia [ˌhaipəuˌmaiəu'təuniə] *n* 肌张力减低

hypomyxia [ˌhaipəu'miksiə] *n* 黏液[分泌]减少

hyponanosoma [ˌhaipəuˌneinə'səumə] *n* 过小侏儒[畸形]

hyponasality [ˌhaipəunei'zæləti] *n* 鼻音过少

hyponatremia [ˌhaipəunə'triːmiə] *n* 低钠血症 | depletional ~ 失水失钠性低钠血症 / dilutional ~ 稀释性低钠血症 / hyperlipemic ~ 高脂血性低钠血症

hyponatruria [ˌhaipəunə'truəriə] *n* 钠尿过少,低钠尿

hyponeocytosis [ˌhaipəuˌni(ː)əusai'təusis] *n* 幼稚[白]细胞性白细胞过少[症]

hyponitremia [ˌhaipəunai'triːmiə] *n* 低氮血症

hyponitrous acid [ˌhaipəu'naitrəs] 次氮酸,次硝酸

hyponoia [ˌhaipəu'nɔiə], **hyponea** [ˌhaipəu'niːə] *n* 精神迟钝,精神活动不足

hyponoic [ˌhaipəu'nəuik] *a* 潜意识精神活动的

hyponychial [ˌhaipəu'nikiəl] *a* 甲下的

hyponychium [ˌhaipəu'nikiəm] *n* 甲下皮

hyponychon [hai'pɔnikən] *n* 甲下瘀斑

hypo-orchidia [ˌhaipəu ɔː'kidiə] *n* 睾丸内分泌功能减退

hypo-orchidism [ˌhaipəu 'ɔːkidizəm] *n* 睾丸功能减退

hypo-orthocytosis [ˌhaipəu ˌɔːθəusai'təusis] *n* 正比例性白细胞减少[症]

hypo-osmolality [ˌhaipəu ˌɔzməu'læləti] *n* 低[重量]渗摩尔浓度

hypoosmotic [ˌhaipəuɔz'mɔtik] *a* 低渗的

hypo-ovaria [ˌhaipəu əu'vɛəriə], **hypo-ovarianism** [ˌhaipəu əu'vɛəriənizəm] *n* 卵巢功能减退

hypopallesthesia [ˌhaipəuˌpælis'θiːzjə] *n* 振动觉减退

hypopancreatism [ˌhaipəu'pæŋkriətizəm] *n* 胰腺功能减退

hypopancreorrhea [ˌhaipəuˌpæŋkriəu'riːə] *n* 胰液分泌过少

hypoparathyroid [ˌhaipəuˌpærə'θairɔid] *a* 甲状旁腺功能减退的(亦称甲状旁腺缺失的)

hypoparathyroidism [ˌhaipəuˌpærə'θairɔidizəm], **hypoparathyreosis** [ˌhaipəupærəˌθairi'əusis] *n* 甲状旁腺功能减退[症]

hypopepsia [ˌhaipəu'pepsiə] *n* 消化不良

hypopepsinia [ˌhaipəupep'siniə] *n* 胃蛋白酶过少

hypoperfusion [ˌhaipəupə(ː)'fjuʒən] *n* 灌注不足

hypoperistalsis [ˌhaipəuˌpəri'stælsis] *n* 蠕动迟缓

hypopexia [ˌhaipəu'peksiə], **hypopexy** ['haipəˌpeksi] *n* 固定[量]不足(组织)

hypophalangism [ˌhaipəufə'lændʒizəm] *n* 少节指,少节趾

hypophamine [hai'pɔfəmin] *n* 垂体胺 | alpha ~ α-垂体胺,催产素 / beta ~ β-垂体胺,加压素

hypopharyngoscope [ˌhaipəufə'riŋgəskəup] *n* 下咽镜 | **hypopharyngoscopy** [ˌhaipəuˌfæriŋ'gɔskəpi] *n* 下咽镜检查

hypopharynx [ˌhaipəu'færiŋks] *n* 下咽[部],喉咽[部] | **hypopharyngeal** [ˌhaipəufə'rindʒiːəl] *a*

hypophonesis [ˌhaipəufəu'niːsis] *n* 声响过弱

hypophonia [ˌhaipəu'fəuniə] *n* 发声过弱

hypophoria [ˌhaipəu'fəuriə] *n* 下隐斜

hypophosphatasia [ˌhaipəuˌfɔsfə'teiziə] *n* 低磷酸酯酶症

hypophosphate [ˌhaipəu'fɔsfeit] *n* 连二磷酸盐,低磷酸盐

hypophosphatemia [ˌhaipəuˌfɔsfə'tiːmiə] *n* 低磷[酸盐]血症 | familial ~ 家族性低磷血症(一种X连锁显性遗传的磷酸盐代谢障碍,可能伴有抗维生素D佝偻病) | **hypophosphatemic** [ˌhaipəuˌfɔsfə'tiːmik] *a* / **hypophosphoremia** [ˌhaipəuˌfɔsfəu'riːmiə] *n*

hypophosphaturia [ˌhaipəuˌfɔsfə'tjuəriə] *n* 低磷[酸盐]尿症

hypophosphite [ˌhaipəu'fɔsfait] *n* 次磷酸盐

hypophosphoric acid [ˌhaipəufɔs'fɔrik] 低磷酸

hypophosphorous acid [ˌhaipəu'fɔsfərəs] 次磷酸

hypophrenia [ˌhaipəu'friːniə] *n* 智力薄弱,低能(精神发育迟缓)

hypophrenic [ˌhaipəu'frenik] *a* 低能的;膈下的

hypophrenium [ˌhaipəu'friːniəm] *n* 膈下腔

hypophrenosis [ˌhaipəufri'nəusis] *n* 智力薄弱症

hypophyseal [ˌhaipəu'fiziəl] *a* 垂体的

hypophysectomize [ˌhaipəufi'zektəmaiz] *vt* 切除垂体

hypophysectomy [haiˌpɔfi'sektəmi], **hypophysiectomy** [ˌhaipəufizi'ektəmi] *n* 垂体切除术,垂体摘除术

hypophysial [ˌhaipəu'fiziəl] *a* 垂体的

hypophysioportal, **hypophyseoportal** [ˌhaipəufiziəu'pɔːtl] *a* 垂体门脉的

hypophysioprivic [ˌhaipəuˌfiziəu'privik], **hypophysoprivic** [haiˌpɔfizəu'praivik] *a* 垂体分泌缺乏的

hypophysiotropic, **hypophyseotropic** [ˌhaipəuˌfiziəu'trɔpik] *a* 促垂体的

hypophysis [hai'pɔfisis] ([复] **hypophyses** [hai-

ˈpɔfisiːz]) *n* 垂体 | ~ cerebri [大脑]垂体 / pharyngeal ~ 咽垂体 / ~ sicca 干垂体后叶
hypophysitis [haiˌpɔfiˈsaitis] *n* 垂体炎
hypophysoma [haiˌpɔfiˈzəumə] *n* 垂体瘤
hypopiesia [ˌhaipəupaiˈiːʃə -ˈiːziə] *n* 血压过低，低血压
hypopiesis [ˌhaipəupaiˈiːsis] *n* 压力过低，低压 | **hypopietic** [ˌhaipəupaiˈetik] *a*
hypopigmentation [ˌhaipəuˌpigmenˈteiʃən] *n* 色素减退
hypopigmenter [ˌhaipəuˌpigˈmentə] *n* [皮肤]脱色剂
hypopinealism [ˌhaipəuˈpiniəlizəm] *n* 松果体功能减退
hypopituitarism [ˌhaipəupiˈtju(ː)itərizəm] *n* 垂体功能减退症 | **hypopituitary** [ˌhaipəupiˈtju(ː)itəri] *a*
hypoplasia [ˌhaipəuˈpleiziə] *n* 发育不全，再生不良 | cartilage-hair ~ 软骨毛发发育不良 / enamel ~ 釉质发育不全 / focal dermal ~ 局灶性皮肤发育不良 / oligomeganephronic renal ~ 肾单位稀少巨大症性肾发育不全，肾单位稀少巨大症 / ~ of right ventricle 右心室发育不全 / thymic ~ 胸腺发育不良 | **hypoplastic** [ˌhaipəuˈplæstik] *a* / **hypoplasty** [ˈhaipəˌplæsti] *n*
hypoplasminogenemia [ˌhaipəuˌplæsminəudʒiˈniːmiə] *n* 低纤溶酶原血症
hypoploid [ˈhaipəplɔid] *a* 亚倍的，*n* 亚倍体（属于异倍体，少于正常二倍体数目的染色体，例如人体为 45 个染色体，即 2n − 1）
hypopnea [haiˈpɔpniːə] *n* 呼吸不足，呼吸减弱 | **hypopneic** [ˌhaipɔpˈniːik] *a*
hypoponesis [ˌhaipəupəuˈniːsis] *n* 皮质运动区活动不足
hypoporosis [ˌhaipəupəˈrəusis] *n* 骨痂形成不全
hypoposia [ˌhaipəuˈpəuziə] *n* 饮水过少，进液过少
hypopotassemia [ˌhaipəuˌpəutəˈsiːmiə] *n* 低钾血症 | **hypopotassemic** *a*
hypopotentia [ˌhaipəupəuˈtenʃiə] *n* 电位过低（尤指大脑皮质电活动性减少）
hypopraxia [ˌhaipəuˈpræksiə] *n* 活动减退，动作减退
hypoprosody [ˌhaipəuˈprɔsədi] *n* 言语韵调减少
hypoproteinemia [ˌhaipəuˌprəutiːˈniːmiə] *n* 低蛋白血症 | prehepatic ~ 肝前性低蛋白血症
hypoproteinia [ˌhaipəuˌprəuˈtiːniə] *n* 蛋白过少，蛋白缺乏 | **hypoproteinic** [ˌhaipəuˌprəuˈtiːnik] *a*
hypoproteinosis [ˌhaipəuˌprəutiːˈnəusis] *n* 蛋白[质]缺乏症
hypoprothrombinemia [ˌhaipəuprəuˌθrɔmbiˈniːmiə] *n* 血凝血酶原过少，低凝血酶原血症
hypopselaphesia [ˌhaipɔpˌseləˈfiːziə] *n* 触觉减退
hypopsychosis [ˌhaipəusaiˈkəusis] *n* 思想迟钝
hypopteronosis cystica [ˌhaipəteˈrɔnəusis ˈsistikə] 羽下囊肿病（鸟类）
hypoptyalism [haiˌpɔpˈtaiəlizəm] *n* 唾液[分泌]减少，缺涎症
hypopus [haiˈpəupəs] *n* 休眠体，休眠稚虫（螨类）
hypopyon [haiˈpəupiɔn] *n* 前房积脓
hyporeactive [ˌhaipəuri(ː)ˈæktiv] *a* 反应不足的
hyporeflexia [ˌhaipəuriˈfleksiə] *n* 反射减弱
hyporeninemia [ˌhaipəuˌriːniˈniːmiə] *n* 低肾素血症 | **hyporeninemic** *a*
hyporrhea [ˌhaipəuˈriːə] *n* 轻度出血
hyposalemia [ˌhaipəusəˈliːmiə] *n* 血盐过少，低盐血[症]
hyposalivation [ˌhaipəuˌsæliˈveiʃən] *n* 唾液[分泌]减少，缺涎症
hyposarca [ˌhaipəuˈsɑːkə] *n* 全身水肿，普遍性水肿
hyposcheotomy [haiˌpɔskiˈɔtəmi] *n* 睾丸鞘膜低位穿刺术
hyposcleral [ˌhaipəuˈskliərəl] *a* 巩膜下的
hyposecretion [ˌhaipəusiˈkriːʃən] *n* 分泌过少
hyposensitive [ˌhaipəuˈsensitiv] *a* 敏感减轻的，低敏感的 | **hyposensitivity** [ˌhaipəuˌsensiˈtivəti] *n* 低敏感性
hyposensitize [ˌhaipəˈsensitaiz] *vt* 脱敏 | **hyposensitization** [ˌhaipəuˌsensitaiˈzeiʃən, -tiˈz-] *n* 脱敏作用
hyposexuality [ˌhaipəuˌseksjuˈæləti] *n* 性欲减退
hyposiagonarthritis [ˌhaipəusaiˌægənɑːˈθraitis] *n* 颞下颌关节炎
hyposialadenitis [ˌhaipəuˌsaiəˌlædiˈnaitis] *n* 颌下腺炎
hyposialosis [ˌhaipəuˌsaiəˈləusis] *n* 唾液[分泌]过少
hyposkeocytosis [ˌhaipəuˌskiəusaiˈtəusis] *n* 幼稚[白]细胞性白细胞过少[症]
hyposmia [ˌhaiˈpɔzmiə] *n* 嗅觉减退
hyposmolarity [ˌhaiˌpɔzməˈlærəti] *n* 低容积渗摩尔浓度
hyposmosis [ˌhaipɔzˈməusis] *n* 低渗透，渗透力减弱
hyposomatotropism [ˌhaipəuˌsəumətəuˈtrəupizəm] *n* 生长激素过少症
hyposomia [ˌhaipəuˈsəumiə] *n* 身体发育不全
hyposomnia [ˌhaipəuˈsɔmniə] *n* 失眠[症]
hypospadiac [ˌhaipəuˈspeidiæk] *n* 尿道下裂者
hypospadias [ˌhaipəuˈspeidiəs] *n* 尿道下裂 | balanic ~, balanitic ~, glandular ~ 阴茎头

型尿道下裂 / female ～ 女性尿道下裂 / penoscrotal ～ 阴茎阴囊型尿道下裂 / perineal ～, pseudovaginal ～ 会阴型尿道下裂 | **hypospadia** *n*

hypospermatogenesis [ˌhaipəuˌspəːmətəuˈdʒenəsis] *n* 低精子发生(精子生成异常减少)

hyposphresia [ˌhaipəsˈfriːziə] *n* 嗅觉减退

hyposplenism [ˌhaipəuˈsplenizəm] *n* 脾功能减退[症]

hypostasis [haiˈpɔstəsis] ([复] **hypostases** [haiˈpɔstəsiːz]) *n* [血液]坠积;下位(以一基因或诸基因掩饰或抑制另一基因) | **hypostatic** [ˌhaipəuˈstætik] *a*

hyposteatolysis [ˌhaipəuˌstiəˈtɔlisis] *n* 脂肪分解不全

hyposteatosis [ˌhaipəuˌstiəˈtəusis] *n* 皮脂分泌不足

hyposthenia [ˌhaipɔsˈθiːniə] *n* 衰弱,体力不足 | **hyposthenic** [ˌhaipɔsˈθenik] *a*

hypostheniant [ˌhaipɔsˈθiːniənt] *a* 致衰弱的 *n* 致衰弱剂

hyposthenuria [ˌhaipɔsθiˈnjuəriə] *n* 低渗尿 | tubular ～ 肾小管性低渗尿

Hypostomatia [ˌhaipəustəuˈmeiʃiə] *n* 下口纤毛虫亚纲

hypostome [ˌhaipəstəum] *n* 口下板(口下器)

hypostomia [ˌhaipəuˈstəumiə] *n* 小嘴[畸形]

hypostomial [ˌhaipəuˈstəumiəl] *a* 下口纤毛虫亚纲的

hypostosis [ˌhaipɔsˈtəusis] *n* 骨发育不全

hypostypsis [ˌhaipəuˈstipsis] *n* 轻度收敛 | **hypostyptic** [ˌhaipəuˈstiptik] *a*

hyposulfite [ˌhaipəuˈsʌlfait] *n* 次硫酸盐

hyposuprarenalemia [ˌhaipəuˌsjuːprəˌriːnəˈliːmiə] *n* 低肾上腺素血症

hyposuprarenalism [ˌhaipəuˌsjuprəˈriːnəlizəm] *n* 肾上腺功能减退

hyposympathicotonus [ˌhaipəusimˌpæθikəuˈtəunəs] *n* 交感神经张力减退

hyposynergia [ˌhaipəusiˈnəːdʒiə] *n* 协同[动作]不足

hypotaxia [ˌhaipəuˈtæksiə] *n* 控制力减弱,自制力减弱(如发生于催眠初期)

hypotelorism [ˌhaipəuˈtelərizəm] *n* (两器官间)距离过近 | ocular ～, orbital ～ 两眼距离过近,眼距过窄征

hypotension [ˌhaipəuˈtenʃən] *n* 低血压 | chronic orthostatic ～, chronic idiopathic orthostatic ～, idiopathic orthostatic ～ 慢性直立性低血压,慢性特发性直立性低血压,特发性直立性低血压 / orthostatic ～, postural ～ 直立性低血压,体位性低血压 / vascular ～ 血管性低血药 | **hypotensive** *a* 低血压的 *n* 低血压者

hypotensor [ˌhaipəuˈtensə] *n* 降压药

hypotetraploid [ˌhaipəuˈtetrəplɔid] *a* 亚四倍的 *n* 亚四倍体(指一个个体或细胞在不平衡的组合中,含有少于四倍体数目的染色体〈4n－x〉)

hypothalamic [ˌhaipəuθəˈlæmik] *a* 下丘脑的

hypothalamotomy [ˌhaipəuˌθæləˈmɔtəmi] *n* 下丘脑切断术(治精神病疾患)

hypothalamus [ˌhaipəuˈθæləməs] *n* 下丘脑

hypothenar [haiˈpɔθinə] *n*, *a* 小鱼际(的)

hypothermia [ˌhaipəuˈθəːmiə] *n* 低体温 | endogenous ～ 内源性低体温 | **hypothermic** [ˌhaipəuˈθəːmik], **hypothermal** [ˌhaipəuˈθəːməl] *a* / **hypothermy** [ˌhaipəuˈθəːmi] *n*

hypothesis [haiˈpɔθisis] *n* 假设,假说 | alternative ～ 备择假设(在统计检验时与无效假设〈null hypothesis〉作比较的假设。符号为 H_1 或 H_a) / biogenic amine ～ 生物胺假说(认为抑郁症与在大脑功能上很重要的受体部位缺乏儿茶酚胺特别是去甲肾上腺素有关,并认为情绪高涨与儿茶酚胺过多有关) / cardionector ～ 心动调节结构假说(认为心脏内有两个起搏点或心动调节结构,一个是窦房结〈atrionector〉,支配心房,另一个是房室束〈ventriculonector〉,支配心室) / gate ～ 闸门假说(即闸门学说,见 theory 项下相应术语) / insular ～ 胰岛假说(糖尿病是由于胰岛功能失常所致) / lattice ～ 格子假说,万字格假说(认为抗原抗体反应为多价抗原与二价抗体之间的反应而构成万字格状的抗原－抗体复合物) / null ～ 无效假设,零假设(假定正在研究的效果是不存在的假设) / one gene-one polypeptide chain ～ 一基因一多肽链假说(基因为提供产生一个多肽链密码的 DNA 顺序。以前称为一基因一酶假说〈one gene-one enzyme hypothesis〉或一基因一蛋白假说〈one gene-one protein hypothesis〉。抗体基因是一例外,其可变部位和恒定部位的单个基因重新组合,提供单个多肽的密码) / sliding-filament ～ 滑动细丝假说(牵拉个别肌纤维可增加滑动收缩的蛋白成分〈肌动蛋白和肌球蛋白〉之间形成的张力增强桥的数目,从而加强下一次肌收缩的力量) / unitarian ～ 抗体一元论(认为抗体总是一种单一的变异血清球蛋白,虽然它与同原抗原反应能产生明显的结果,如凝集反应、沉淀反应、补体结合反应等) / wobble ～ 摆动假说(克里克〈F. H. C. Crick〉为解释一种特异的 tRNA 分子如何能够把不同的密码子翻译成 mRNA 模板而提出的一种假说。据此假说,tRNA 反密码子的第三碱基不一定与互补密码子配对〈而前两个碱基则与之配对〉,但能与几种 mRNA 密码子形成碱基配对)

hypothrepsia [ˌhaipəuˈθrepsiə] *n* 营养不良

hypothrombinemia [ˌhaipəuˌθrɔmbiˈniːmiə] *n* 低

凝血酶血症

hypothymergasia [ˌhaipəuˌθaiməgeiziə] *n* 情感低落性整体反应 | **hypothymergastic** [ˌhaipəuˌθaiməˈgæstik] *a*

hypothymia [ˌhaipəuˈθaimiə] *n* 情感减退 | **hypothymic** *a*

hypothymism [ˌhaipəuˌθaimizəm] *n* 胸腺功能减退

hypothyroidation [ˌhaipəuˌθairɔiˈdeiʃən] *n* [促使]甲状腺功能减退[作用]

hypothyroidism [ˌhaipəuˈθairɔidizəm], **hypothyrea** [ˌhaipəuˈθairiə], **hypothyreosis** [ˌhaipəuˌθairiˈəusis], **hypothyroidea** [ˌhaipəuθaiˈrɔidiə], **hypothyrosis** [ˌhaipəuθaiˈrəusis] *n* 甲状腺功能减退症 | **hypothyroid** [ˌhaipəuˈθairɔid] *a* 甲状腺功能减退的 *n* 甲状腺功能减退者

hypotonia [ˌhaipəuˈtəuniə] *n* 张力减退,压力过低 | benign congenital ~ 良性先天性张力减退 / ~ oculi 眼压过低 | **hypotonus** [haiˈpɔtənəs], **hypotony** [haiˈpɔtəni] *n* 张力减退,压力过低

hypotonic [haipəuˈtɔnik] *a* 低张的;低渗的 | **~ity** [ˌhaipəutəˈnisəti] *n* 低张性;低渗性

hypotoxicity [ˌhaipəutɔkˈsisəti] *n* 弱毒性,低毒性

hypotransferrinemia [ˌhaipəutrænsˌferiˈniːmiə] *n* 低转铁蛋白血症

Hypotricha [ˌhaipəuˈtrikə] *n* 腹纤毛亚目

hypotrichiasis [ˌhaipəutriˈkaiəsis] *n* 先天性脱发,先天性秃

Hypotrichida [ˌhaipəuˈtrikidə] *n* 腹纤毛目

hypotrichosis [ˌhaipəutriˈkəusis] *n* 稀毛症

hypotrichous [haiˈpəutrikəs] *a* 下纤毛的(指某些纤毛虫)

hypotriploid [ˌhaipəuˈtriplɔid] *a* 亚三倍的 *n* 亚三倍体(指一个个体或细胞在不平衡的组合中,含有少于三倍体数目的染色体〈3n – x〉)

hypotrophy [haiˈpɔtrəfi] *n* 生活力缺失;半自主生长,亚独立生长

hypotropia [ˌhaipəuˈtrəupiə] *n* 下斜视

hypotryptophanic [ˌhaipəutriptəˈfænik] *a* 色氨酸缺乏的

hypotympanic [ˌhaipəutimˈpænik] *a* 鼓室下的

hypotympanotomy [ˌhaipəuˌtimpəˈnɔtəmi] *n* 下鼓室开放术,鼓室下部切开术

hypotympanum [ˌhaipəuˈtimpənəm] *n* 下鼓室,鼓室下部

hypouremia [ˌhaipəujuəˈriːmiə] *n* 低尿素血症

hypouresis [ˌhaipəujuəˈriːsis] *n* 排尿减少

hypouricemia [ˌhaipəuˌjuəriˈsiːmiə] *n* 低尿酸血症

hypouricosuria [ˌhaipəuˌjuərikəˈsjuəriə] *n* 低尿酸尿

hypouricuria [ˌhaipəuˌjuəriˈkjuəriə] *n* 低尿酸尿

hypourocrinia [ˌhaipəuˌjuərəuˈkriniə] *n* 尿分泌减少,尿量减少

hypovaria [ˌhaipəuˈvɛəriə], **hypovarianism** [ˌhaipəuˈvɛəriənizəm] *n* 卵巢功能减退

hypovegetative [ˌhaipəuˌvedʒiˈteitiv] *a* 躯体型的,低自主性功能体型的(躯体系统比内脏占优势)

hypovenosity [ˌhaipəuviˈnɔsəti] *n* 静脉[系统]发育不全

hypoventilation [ˌhaipəuˌventiˈleiʃən] *n* 通气不足

hypovitaminosis [ˌhaipəuˌvaitəmiˈnəusis] *n* 维生素缺乏[症]

hypovolemia [ˌhaipəuvəˈliːmiə] *n* 血容量不足,低血容量症 | **hypovolemic** *a*

hypovolia [ˌhaipəuˈvəuliə] *n* 水[含]量过少,液量过少

hypoxanthine [ˌhaipəuˈzænθiːn] *n* 次黄嘌呤

hypoxanthine guanine phosphoribosyltransferase (HGPRT) [ˌhaipəuˈzænθiːn ˈgwaːniːn ˌfɔsfəuˌraibəusilˈtrænsfəreis] 次黄嘌呤鸟嘌呤磷酸核糖基转移酶,次黄嘌呤磷酸核糖基转移酶

hypoxanthine oxidase [ˌhaipəˈzænθiːn ˈɔksideis] 次黄嘌呤氧化酶,黄嘌呤氧化酶

hypoxanthine phosphoribosyltransferase (HPRT) [ˌhaipəuˈzænθiːn ˌfɔsfəuˌraibəusilˈtrænsfəreis] 次黄嘌呤磷酸核糖基转移酶(此酶活性缺乏为一种 X 连锁性状,可致莱施-奈恩〈Lesch-Nyhan〉综合征。亦称次黄嘌呤鸟嘌呤磷酸核糖基转移酶)

hypoxanthylic acid [ˌhaipəuzænˈθilik] 次黄[嘌呤核]苷酸,肌苷酸

hypoxemia [ˌhaipɔkˈsiːmiə] *n* 低氧血[症]

hypoxia [haiˈpɔksiə] *n* 低氧,缺氧 | altitude ~ 高空低氧 / anemic ~ 贫血性缺氧 / histotoxic ~ 组织中毒性缺氧 / hypoxic ~ 低氧性缺氧 / stagnant ~ 淤血性缺氧 | **hypoxic** *a*

hypoxia-ischemia [haiˈpɔksiə isˈkiːmiə] 低氧-局部缺血(血供中断时组织内发生的病变,尤见于窒息的胎儿或婴儿)

hypoxidosis [haiˌpɔksiˈdəusis] *n* 低氧症

hypoxyphilia [haiˌpɔksiˈfiliə] *n* 低氧癖

hypromellose [haiˌprəuməˈləus] *n* 羟丙甲纤维素(药用辅料) | ~ phthalate 邻苯二甲酸羟丙甲纤维素

hypsar(r)hythmia [ˌhaisəˈriθmiə] *n* 高度节律失调(指一种脑电图异常,有时见于儿童,通常呈现痉挛或震颤发作〈肌阵挛〉,常与精神发育迟缓有关)

hypsi- [构词成分]高

hypsibrachycephalic [ˌhipsiˌbrækisəˈfælik] *a* 高

阔头的
hypsicephaly [ˌhipsiˈsefəli] *n* 尖头[畸形] | **hypsicephalic** [ˌhipsisəˈfælik] *a*
hypsiconchous [ˌhipsiˈkɔŋkəs] *a* 高眶的
hypsiloid [ˈhipsilɔid] *a* (希腊字母)Υ 字形的
hypsistaphylia [ˌhipsistəˈfiliə] *n* 高狭腭
hypsistenocephalic [ˌhipsiˌstenəusəˈfælik] *a* 高狭头的
hypso- [构词成分]高
hypsocephalous [ˈhipsəˈsefələs] *a* 尖头[畸形]的
hypsochrome [ˈhipsəkrəum] *n* 浅色团,向紫团 | **hypsochromic** [ˌhipsəˈkrəumik] *a*
hypsochromy [ˌhipsəuˈkrəumi] *n* 浅色团作用,向紫(吸收光带向较高频率移动,使色变浅)
hypsodont [ˈhipsədɔnt] *a* 长冠牙的(如食草哺乳动物)
hypsokinesis [ˌhipsəukaiˈniːsis, -kiˈn-] *n* 后仰,后倾(见于震颤麻痹及其他肌震颤性综合征)
hypsonosus [hipˈsəunəsəs] *n* 高空病,高山病
hypsotherapy [ˌhipsəuˈθerəpi] *n* 高地疗法
hypurgia [haiˈpəːdʒiə] *n* 辅助因素,辅助疗法
hyrax [ˈhairæks] *n* 蹄兔 | rock ~ 岩蹄兔 / tree ~ 树蹄兔
hyrtenal [ˈhəːtin] *n* 莲叶桐萜醛
Hyrtl's loop (anastomosis) [ˈhəːtl] (Jozsef Hyrtl) 希尔特尔襻(吻合)(偶见于颏舌骨肌中的左右舌下神经襻形吻合) | ~ recess 鼓室上隐窝 / ~ sphincter 希尔特尔括约肌(一种不完全的肌纤维带,位于肛门约 10cm 以上的直肠壁内。亦称直肠括约肌)
hyssop [ˈhisəp] *n* 海索草
hysteralgia [ˌhistəˈrældʒiə] *n* 子宫痛
hysteratresia [ˌhistərəˈtriːziə] *n* 子宫闭锁
hysterectomy [ˌhistəˈrektəmi] *n* 子宫切除术 | abdominal ~ 腹式子宫切除术 / cesarean ~ 剖宫产子宫切除术/ chemical ~ 化学性子宫内膜破坏法 / subtotal ~, partial ~, supracervical ~, supravaginal ~ 子宫次全切除术,子宫部分切除术,颈上式子宫切除术,阴道上子宫切除术 / total ~, complete ~ 子宫全切除术
hysteresis [ˌhistəˈriːsis] *n* 滞后 | protoplasmic ~ 原生质滞后现象(细胞衰老的一个假设的原因) | **hysteretic** [ˌhistəˈretik] *a*
hystereurynter [ˌhistərjuəˈrintə] *n* 宫口扩张袋(一种宫颈扩张袋)
hystereurysis [ˌhistəˈrjuərisis] *n* 宫口扩张术
hysteria [hisˈtiəriə] *n* 癔症 | anxiety ~ 焦虑性癔症 / canine ~ 犬惊病,犬癔症 / conversion ~ 转换性癔症 / dissociative ~ 分离型癔症 / fixation ~ 固定[病位]性癔症 / ~ major 大发作性癔症,重癔症 / ~ minor 小发作性癔症,轻癔症 / monosymptomatic ~ 单一症状性癔症 | **hysterism** [ˈhistərizəm] *n*
hysteriac [hisˈtiəriæk] *n* 癔症患者
hysteric [hisˈterik] *a* 癔症的 *n* 癔症患者 | **~s** *n* 癔症发作
hysterical [hisˈterikəl] *a* 癔症的
hystericism [hisˈterisizəm] *n* 癔症素质
hysteriform [hisˈterifɔːm] *a* 癔症样的
hyster(o)- [构词成分]子宫;癔症
hysterobubonocele [ˌhistərəubjuˈbɔnəsiːl] *n* 腹股沟子宫疝
hysterocarcinoma [ˌhistərəuˌkɑːsiˈnəumə] *n* 子宫癌
hysterocatalepsy [ˌhistərəuˈkætəˌlepsi] *n* 癔症性僵住[症]
hysterocele [ˌhistərəˌsiːl] *n* 子宫疝
hysterocleisis [ˌhistərəuˈklaisis] *n* 子宫口闭合术
hysterocolpectomy [ˌhistərəukɔlˈpektəmi] *n* 子宫阴道切除术
hysterocolposcope [ˌhistərəuˈkɔlpəskəup] *n* 子宫阴道镜
hysterocystic [ˌhistərəuˈsistik] *a* 子宫膀胱的
hysterocystocleisis [ˌhistərəuˌsistəuˈklaisis] *n* 子宫膀胱缝合术
hysterocystopexy [ˌhistərəuˈsistəˌpeksi] *n* 膀胱子宫腹壁固定术
hysterodynia [ˌhistərəuˈdiniə] *n* 子宫痛
hysteroepilepsy [ˌhistərəuˈepiˌlepsi] *n* 癔症性癫痫
hysteroepileptogenic [ˌhistərəuˌepiˌleptəuˈdʒenik] *a* 致癔症性癫痫的
hysteroerotic [ˌhistərəuiˈrɔtik] *a* 癔症性色情的
hysterogenic [ˌhistərəuˈdʒenik] *a* 致癔症的
hysterogram [ˈhistərəgræm] *n* 子宫 X 线[照]片
hysterograph [ˈhistərəgrɑːf] *n* 子宫收缩描记器 | **~y** [ˌhistəˈrɔgrəfi] *n* 子宫收缩描记术;子宫造影[术]
hysteroid [ˈhistərɔid], **hysteroidal** [ˌhistəˈrɔidl] *a* 癔症样的
hysterolaparotomy [ˌhistərəuˌlæpəˈrɔtəmi] *n* 剖腹子宫切开术
hysterolith [ˈhistərəˌliθ] *n* 子宫石
hysterology [ˌhistəˈrɔlədʒi] *n* 子宫学
hysterolysis [ˌhistəˈrɔlisis] *n* 子宫松解术
hysteromania [ˌhistərəuˈmeinjə] *n* 癔症性躁狂;慕男狂,女子色情狂
hysterometer [ˌhistəˈrɔmitə] *n* 子宫测量器 | **hysterometry** *n* 子宫测量法
hysteromyoma [ˌhistərəumaiˈəumə] *n* 子宫肌瘤
hysteromyomectomy [ˌhistərəuˌmaiəuˈmektəmi] *n* 子宫肌瘤切除术
hysteromyotomy [ˌhistərəumaiˈɔtəmi] *n* 子宫肌

切开术

hysteronarcolepsy [ˌhistərəuˈnɑːkəˌlepsi] *n* 癔症发作性睡病

hysteroneurasthenia [ˌhistərəuˌnjuəræsˈθiːnjə] *n* 癔症性神经衰弱

hysteropathy [ˌhistəˈrɔpəθi] *n* 子宫病

hysterope [ˈhistərəup] *n* 癔症性视力障碍者

hysteropexy [ˈhistərəpeksi], **hysteropexia** [ˌhistərəuˈpeksiə] *n* 子宫固定术

hysteropia [ˌhistəˈrəupiə] *n* 癔症性视力障碍

hysteroptosia [ˌhistərɔpˈtəuziə], **hysteroptosis** [ˌhistərɔpˈtəusis] *n* 子宫下垂,子宫脱垂

hysterorrhaphy [histəˈrɔːrəfi] *n* 子宫固定术;子宫缝合术

hysterorrhexis [ˌhistərəuˈreksis] *n* 子宫破裂

hysterosalpingectomy [ˌhistərəuˌsælpiŋˈdʒektəmi] *n* 子宫输卵管切除术

hysterosalpingography [ˌhistərəuˌsælpiŋˈgɔgrəfi] *n* 子宫输卵管造影术

hysterosalpingo-oophorectomy [ˌhistərəusælˌpiŋgəuˌəuɔfəˈrektəmi] *n* 子宫输卵管卵巢切除术

hysterosalpingostomy [ˌhistərəuˌsælpiŋˈgɔstəmi] *n* 子宫输卵管吻合术

hysteroscope [ˈhistərəˌskəup] *n* 宫腔镜 | **hysteroscopy** [ˌhistəˈrɔskəpi] *n* 宫腔镜检查

hysterospasm [ˈhistərəˌspæzəm] *n* 子宫痉挛

hysterostat [ˈhistərəstæt] *n* 子宫内镭管支持器,宫腔射源装置器

hysterostomatocleisis [ˌhistərəuˌstəumətəuˈklaisis] *n* 宫口闭合术

hysterostomatome [ˌhistərəuˈstəumətəum] *n* 宫口刀

hysterostomatomy [ˌhistərəustəuˈmætəmi] *n* 宫口切开术

hysterosyphilis [ˌhistərəuˈsifilis] *n* 梅毒性癔症(梅毒引起的癔症性神经功能病)

hysterotabetism [ˌhistərəuˈteibitizəm] *n* 癔症脊髓痨

hysterothermometry [ˌhistərəuθəːˈmɔmitri] *n* 子宫温度测量法

hysterotome [ˈhistərətəum] *n* 子宫刀

hysterotomy [ˌhistəˈrɔtəmi] *n* 子宫切开术(常用于取儿术) | abdominal ~ 腹式子宫切开术 / vaginal ~ 阴道式子宫切开术

hysterotrachelectasia [ˌhistərəuˌtreikəlekˈteisiə] *n* 宫颈扩张术

hysterotrachelectomy [ˌhistərəuˌtreikəˈlektəmi] *n* 宫颈切除术

hysterotracheloplasty [ˌhistərəuˈtreikələˌplæsti] *n* 宫颈成形术

hysterotrachelorrhaphy [ˌhistərəuˌtreikəˈlɔːrəfi] *n* 宫颈缝合术

hysterotrachelotomy [ˌhistərəuˌtreikəˈlɔtəmi] *n* 宫颈切开术

hysterotraumatism [ˌhistərəuˈtrɔːmətizəm] *n* 创伤性癔症 | **hysterotraumatic** [ˌhistərəutrɔːˈmætik] *a*.

hysterotubography [ˌhistərəutjuːˈbɔgrəfi] *n* 子宫输卵管造影[术]

hysterovagino-enterocele [ˌhistərəuˌvædʒinəuˈentərəsiːl] *n* 子宫阴道肠疝

Hz hertz 赫[兹]

I

I incisor 切牙; iodine 碘; inosine 肌苷
I electric current 电流; intensity〈of radiant energy〉(辐射能)强度; ionic strength 离子强度
-ia [构词成分]情况
IAB intra-aortic balloon 主动脉内球囊(反搏)
IABP intra-aortic balloon pump 主动脉内球囊泵
IAEA International Atomic Energy Agency 国际原子能机构
IAHA immune adherance hemagglutination assay 免疫粘连血凝测定
iamatology [ˌaiæməˈtɔlədʒi] *n* 药疗学
IAP inhibitor of apoptosis protein 细胞凋亡蛋白的抑制物
IAPP islet amyloid polypeptide 胰岛淀粉样多肽
-iasis [构词成分]病,病态
iathergy [aiˈæθədʒi] *n* 治疗反应性(已免疫的个体在其结核菌素皮肤敏感性经特异性脱敏后,仍存留的免疫状态)
iatraliptic [ˌaiətrəˈliptik] *a* 涂擦法的,擦药疗法的 | **~s** *n*
iatrarchy [ˈaiəˌtrɑːki] *n* 医师监视
iatreusiology [ˌaiətrusiˈɔlədʒi] *n* 治疗学,疗学
iatreusis [ˌaiəˈtruːsis] *n*【希】疗法,治疗
-iatric [构词成分]医疗术的
iatric(al) [aiˈætrik(əl)] *a* 医学的;医师的
-iatrics [构词成分]医疗术
iatr(o)- [构词成分]医师;医学
iatrochemistry [aiˌætrəuˈkemistri] *n* 化学医学[派] | **iatrochemical** *a* / **iatrochemist** *n* 化学医学家
iatrogenesis [aiˌætrəuˈdʒenisis] *n* 医源病发生
iatrogenic [ˌaiætrəuˈdʒenik] *a* 医源性的,受医师影响的
iatrology [ˌaiəˈtrɔlədʒi] *n* 医学
iatromathematical [aiˌætrəuˌmæθiˈmætikəl], **iatromechanical** [aiˌætrəumiˈkænikəl] *a* 物理医学的
iatrophysics [aiˌætrəuˈfiziks] *n* 物理医学[派];物理疗法 | **iatrophysical** *a* 物理医学的 / **iatrophysicist** *n* 物理医学家
iatrotechnics [aiˌætrəuˈtekniks], **iatrotechnique** [aiˌætrəutekˈniːk] *n* 治疗[技]术
-iatry [构词成分]医疗术
IB inclusion body 包涵体
IBC iron-binding capacity 铁结合量
IBF immunoglobulin-binding factor 免疫球蛋白结合因子
ibogaine [iˈbəugəiːn] *n* 伊波加因(一种生物碱,具有抗抑郁和欣快作用)
ibotenic acid [ˌaibəˈtenik] 鹅膏蕈氨酸
IBS irritable bowel syndrome 肠易激综合征
ibufenac [aiˈbjuːfənæk] *n* 异丁芬酸(消炎镇痛药)
ibuprofen [aiˈbjuːprəufen] *n* 布洛芬(消炎镇痛药)
Ibutilide fumarate [iˈbjuːtilaid] 延胡索酸伊布利特(抗心律失常药)
IC inspiratory capacity 深吸气量; irritable colon 激惹性结肠,结肠过敏
-ic [后缀]属于…的,显示…特征的(如 acidic);在化学上用以表示离子或酸,显示两种氧化状态中较高的一种,另一种则以后缀 -ous 表示)
ICAM-1 intercellular adhesion molecule 1 胞间黏附分子 1
ICAM-2 intercellular adhesion molecule 2 胞间黏附分子 2
ICD International Classification of Diseases 国际疾病分类法(世界卫生组织); intrauterine contraceptive device 宫内节育器
ice [ais] *n* 冰 | dry ~ 干冰,碳酸雪,二氧化碳雪
Iceland disease [ˈaislənd] 冰岛病,慢性疲劳综合征,良性肌痛性脑脊髓炎
ich [ik] *n* 白点病(见 ichthyophthiriasis)
ichnogram [ˈiknəgræm] *n* 足印
ichor [ˈaikɔː] *n* 败液 | **~ous** [ˈaikərəs] *a*
ichoremia, **ichorrhemia** [ˌaikəˈriːmiə] *n* 败血病,败血症
ichoroid [ˈaikərɔid] *a* 败液样的
ichorrhea [aikəˈriːə] *n* 败液溢
ichthammol [ˈikθæmɔl] *n* 鱼石脂(用作局部皮肤抗感染药)
ichthyism [ˈikθiizəm], **ichthyismus** [ˌikθiˈizməs] *n* 鱼中毒
ichthy(o)- [构词成分]鱼
ichthyoacanthotoxin [ˌikθiəuəˌkænθəˈtɔksin] *n* 鱼刺毒
ichthyoacanthotoxism [ˌikθiəuəˌkænθəˈtɔksizəm] *n* 鱼刺中毒
ichthyocolla [ˌikθiəuˈkɔlə] *n* 鱼胶

ichthyohemotoxin [ˌikθiəuˌhiːmə'tɔksin] *n* 鱼血毒

ichthyohemotoxism [ˌikθiəuˌhiːmə'tɔksizəm] *n* 鱼血中毒

ichthyoid ['ikθiɔid] *a* 鱼样的

ichthyology [ˌikθi'ɔlədʒi] *n* 鱼类学

ichthyolsulfonate [ˌikθiɔl'sʌlfəneit] *n* 鱼石脂磺酸盐

ichthyolsulfonic acid [ˌikθiɔlsʌl'fɔnik] 鱼石脂磺酸

ichthyootoxin [ˌikθiˌəuə'tɔksin] *n* 鱼卵毒

ichthyootoxism [ˌikθiˌəuə'tɔksizəm] *n* 鱼卵中毒

ichthyophagia [ˌikθiəu'feidʒiə] *n* 食鱼[生活]

ichthyophagous [ˌikθi'ɔfəgəs] *a* 食鱼的 | **ichthyophagy** [ˌikθi'ɔfədʒi] *n* 食鱼[生活]

ichthyophthiriasis [ˌikθiəu'θairiəsis] *n* 白点病，小瓜虫病(海鱼和淡水鱼因感染多子小瓜虫而发生的皮、鳃、眼的脓疱性皮疹)

Ichthyophthirius [ˌikθiəu'θairiəs] *n* 小瓜虫属 | ~ multifiliis 多子小瓜虫

ichthyosarcotoxin [ˌikθiəuˌsɑːkə'tɔksin] *n* 鱼肉毒

ichthyosarcotoxism [ˌikθiəuˌsɑːkə'tɔksizəm] *n* 鱼肉中毒

ichthyosiform [ˌikθi'əusifɔːm] *a* 鱼鳞病样的

ichthyosis [ˌikθi'əusis] *n* 鱼鳞病 | ~ congenita, congenital ~ 先天性鱼鳞病 / ~ hystrix 豪猪状鱼鳞病，高起鱼鳞病 / lamellar ~ 片层状鱼鳞癣 / ~ linearis circumflexa 回旋形线状鱼鳞病 / ~ palmaris et plantaris 掌跖角化病 / ~ uteri 子宫鳞癣 / ~ vulgaris, ~ simplex 寻常性鱼鳞病，单纯鱼鳞病 / X-linked ~ X 连锁鱼鳞病 | **ichthyotic** [ˌikθi'ɔtik] *a*

ichthyotoxic [ˌikθiəu'tɔksik] *a* 鱼毒的

ichthyotoxicology [ˌikθiəuˌtɔksi'kɔlədʒi] *n* 鱼毒学

ichthyotoxicum [ˌikθiəu'tɔksikəm] *n* [鳗]鱼血清毒

ichthyotoxin [ˌikθiəu'tɔksin] *n* 鱼毒

ichthyotoxism [ˌikθiəu'tɔksizəm] *n* 鱼中毒

ick [ik] *n* 白点病(见 ichthyophthiriasis)

ICN International Council of Nurses 国际护士理事会

icon ['aikɔn] *n* 影像，图像；形象

iconography [ˌaikɔ'nɔgrəfi] *n* 影像学；影像塑造术

iconoscope [ai'kɔnəskəup] *n* 光电摄像管

icosahedral [ˌaikəusə'hiːdrəl] *a* 二十面体的

icosanoic acid [ˌaikəusə'nəuik] 二十[烷]酸，花生酸

ICP intracranial pressure 颅内压

ICRP International Commission on Radiological Protection 国际放射防护委员会

ICRU International Commission on Radiological Units and Measurements 国际放射单位与测量委员会

ICS International College of Surgeons 国际外科医师学会

ICSH interstitial cell-stimulating hormone 促间质细胞激素，促黄体生成激素(黄体化激素)

ICSI intracytoplasmic sperm injection 胞质内精子注射

ICT insulin coma therapy 胰岛素昏迷疗法

ictal ['iktl] *a* 发作的

icterepatitis [ˌiktəˌrepə'taitis] *n* 黄疸性肝炎

icteric [ik'terik] *a* 黄疸的

icteritious [ˌiktə'riʃəs] *a* 黄疸的；黄疸色的

icter(o)- [构词成分]黄疸

icteroanemia [ˌiktərəuə'niːmiə] *n* 溶血性黄疸贫血病

icterogenic [ˌiktərəu'dʒenik] *a* 致黄疸的 | **~ity** [ˌiktərədʒi'nisəti] *n* 致黄疸性

icterohematuria [ˌiktərəuˌhemə'tjuəriə] *n* 黄疸血尿 | **icterohematuric** *a*

icterohemoglobinuria [ˌiktərəuˌhiːməuˌgləubi'njuəriə] *n* 黄疸血红蛋白尿

icterohepatitis [ˌiktərəuˌhepə'taitis] *n* 黄疸性肝炎

icteroid ['iktərɔid] *a* 黄疸样的

icterus ['iktərəs] *n* 【拉】黄疸 | chronic familial ~, congenital familial ~, congenital hemolytic ~ 遗传性球形红细胞症 / epidemic catarrhal ~ 流行性卡他性黄疸(一种轻型钩端螺旋体性黄疸) / febrile ~ 发热性黄疸(急性传染性肝炎) / ~ gravis 重黄疸(急性黄色肝萎缩) / ~ gravis neonatorum 新生儿重黄疸(亦称成红白细胞过多病) / ~ infectiosus 钩端螺旋体性黄疸 / ~ intermittens juvenilis 青年间歇性黄疸 / ~ neonatorum 新生儿黄疸 / nuclear ~ 核黄疸 / ~ praecox 早发性黄疸 / ~ simplex 传染性肝炎 / spirochetal ~ 钩端螺旋体性黄疸 / ~ typhoides 伤寒样黄疸(急性黄色肝萎缩)

ictus ['iktəs] ([复] **ictus⟨es⟩**) *n* 【拉】暴发，发作，猝发；搏动，冲击 | ~ cordis 心搏 / ~ epilepticus 癫痫猝发 / ~ immunisatorius 冲击式免疫法，大量免疫法 / ~ sanguinis [脑]溢血猝发，卒中 / ~ solis 日射病，中暑

ICU intensive care unit 重症监护治疗病房，重症监护室

ID intradermal 真皮内的；inside diameter 内径；infective dose 感染剂量

ID_{50} median infective dose 半数感染剂量

id [id] *n* 伊特，私我(精神分析法的术语)；附发疹(全身或局部的无菌性皮疹)

-id [构词成分]形状,形式,型;疹

IDA iminodiacetic acid 亚氨基二乙酸

-idae [后缀]科(动物学)

idarubicin hydrochloride [ˌaidəˈruːbisin] 盐酸伊达比星(蒽环类抗肿瘤药,用于治疗急性髓性白血病,静脉内给药)

IDD, IDDM insulin-dependent diabetes mellitus 胰岛素依赖型糖尿病

-ide [后缀]二元化合物(如 chloride, sulfide 或 carbide)

idea [aiˈdiə] *n* 观念,思想 | autochthonous ~ 自生观念 / compulsive ~, imperative ~ 强迫观念 / dominant ~ 优势观念 / fixed ~ 固定观念 / hyperquantivalent ~ 超价观念 / ~ of reference, referential ~ 牵连观念

ideal [aiˈdiəl] *a* 理想的,观念的 *n* 理想;思想,观念 | ego ~ 自我理想

idealize [aiˈdiəlaiz] *vt* 理想化,观念化 | **idealization** [aiˌdiəlaiˈzeiʃən, -liˈz-] *n*

ideation [ˌaidiˈeiʃən] *n* 观念作用,思想作用 | **~al** *a*

idée [iˈdei] *n*【法】观念 | ~ fixé 固定观念

identification [aiˌdentifiˈkeiʃən] *n* 证明同一,等同;鉴别,鉴定;自居等同(精神分析) | cosmic ~ 自居万物思想,天人合一(妄想)(见于精神分裂症)

identity [aiˈdentəti] *n* 同一性,一致性;认同 | ego ~ 自我一致性

ideodynamism [iˌdiːəuˈdainəmizəm] *n* 意想统制,观念统制,意念行动

ideogenetic [ˌaidiəudʒiˈnetik], **ideogenous** [ˌaidiˈɔdʒinəs] *a* 意想性的,观念性的

ideoglandular [ˌaidiəuˈglændjulə] *a* 意想性腺分泌的,观念性腺分泌的

ideokinetic [aiˌdiːəukaiˈnetik] *a* 意想性动作的,观念性动作的

ideology [ˌaidiˈɔlədʒi] *n* 意识形态;观念学

ideometabolic [ˌaidiəumetəˈbɔlik] *a* 意想性代谢的,观念性代谢的

ideometabolism [ˌaidiəumeˈtæbəlizəm] *n* 意想性代谢,观念性代谢

ideomotion [ˌaidiəˈməuʃən] *n* 意想性动作,观念性动作

ideomotor [ˌaidiəˈməutə] *a* 意想性动作的,观念性动作的

ideomuscular [ˌaidiəuˈmʌskjulə] *a* 意想性肌动作的

ideophrenia [ˌaidiəuˈfriːniə] *n* 观念倒错 | **ideophrenic** [ˌaidiəuˈfrenik]

ideovascular [ˌaidiəuˈvæskjulə] *a* 意想性血管作用的(由观念作用、记忆或幻觉所引起的血管变化)

Ide test (reaction) [iːˈde] (Sobei Ide; Tamao Ide) 井出试验(反应)(检梅毒)

idi(o)- [构词成分]自体,自发,自生;特异

idioagglutinin [ˌidiəuəˈgluːtinin] *n* 自发凝集素

idioblapsis [ˌidiəuˈblæpsis] *n* 自发性食物过敏 | **idioblaptic** *a*

idioblast [ˈidiəblæst] *n* 细胞原体,生原体 | **~ic** [ˌidiəˈblæstik] *a*

idiochromatin [ˌidiəuˈkrəumətin] *n* 性染色质

idiochromidia [ˌidiəukrəuˈmidiə] *n* 核外性染色质,性染色[小]粒

idiochromosome [ˌidiəuˈkrəuməsəum] *n* 性染色体

idiocrasy [ˌidiˈɔkrəsi] *n* 特[异反]应性;特异质 | **idiocratic** [ˌidiəˈkrætik] *a*

idiocy [ˈidiəsi] *n* 白痴 | amaurotic familial ~ 家族黑矇性白痴 / athetosic ~ 手足徐动性白痴,手足徐动症 / cretinoid ~ 呆小病样白痴,呆小病 / developmental ~ 发育性白痴 / genetous ~ 先天性白痴 / intrasocial ~ 合作性白痴(尚能从事一般职业) / mongolian ~ 先天愚型,伸舌样白痴 / moral ~ 悖德白痴 / plagiocephalic ~ 斜颅白痴,颅变形性白痴 / profound ~, absolute ~ 深度白痴 / sensorial ~ 感觉缺陷性白痴

idiogenesis [ˌidiəˈdʒenisis] *n* 自发病,疾病自发

idioglossia [ˌidiəˈglɔsiə] *n* 自解[言]语症 | **idioglottic** [ˌidiəˈglɔtik] *a*

idiogram [ˈiːdiəgræm] *n* 核型模式图

idioheteroagglutinin [ˌidiəuˌhetərəuəˈgluːtinin] *n* 自发异种凝集素

idioheterolysin [ˌidiəuhetəˈrɔlisin] *n* 自发异种溶素

idiohypnotism [ˌidiəuˈhipnətizəm] *n* 自我催眠

idioisoagglutinin [ˌidiəuˌaisəuəˈgluːtinin] *n* 自发同种凝集素

idioisolysin [ˌidiəuaiˈsɔləsin] *n* 自发同种溶素

idiolalia [ˌidiəuˈleiliə] *n* 新语症,语词新作

idiolog [ˈidiəlɔg] *n* 自解词

idiologism [ˌidiˈɔlədʒizəm] *n* 自解[言]语症

idiolysin [ˌidiˈɔləsin] *n* 自发溶素

idiomere [ˈidiəmiə] *n* 染色粒

idiomuscular [idiəuˈmʌskjulə] *a* 肌本身的(收缩)

idioneural [ˌidiəuˈnjuərəl] *a* 神经本身的,神经自身的

idiopathic [ˌidiəˈpæθik], **idiopathetic** [ˌidiəupəˈθætik] *a* 自发的,特发的

idiopathy [ˌidiˈɔpəθi] *n* 自发病,特发病,特发症 | toxic ~ 中毒性自发病,毒性特发症

idiophore [ˈidiəfɔː] *n* 原活质

idiophrenic [ˌidiəuˈfrenik] *a* 脑本身的

idioplasm [ˈidiəplæzəm] *n* 种质

idiopsychologic [ˌidiəuˌsaikəˈlɔdʒik] *a* 自发思想

的,自发心理的

idioreflex [ˌidiəuˈriːfleks] *n* 自发[性]反射

idioretinal [ˌidiəuˈretinəl] *a* 视网膜自感性的

idiosome [ˈidiəˌsəum] *n* 胶粒,微胶粒;核旁体(指精母细胞的中心体及其周围的网体和线粒体)

idiospasm [ˈidiəspæzəm] *n* 局部痉挛

idiosyncrasy [ˌidiəuˈsiŋkrəsi] *n* 特[异反]应性;特异质 | **idiosyncratic** [ˌidiəusiŋˈkrætik] *a*

idiot [ˈidiət] *n* 白痴 | mongolian ~ 先天愚型,伸舌样白痴 / ~ savant [iːdjˈəusɑːvɔŋ]【法】低能特才,学者性"白痴"(指在记忆、数学、音乐方面具有特定才能的低能者)

idiotic [ˌidiˈɔtik] *a* 白痴的,愚蠢的 | **~ally** *ad*

idiotope [ˈidiəˌtəup] *n* 独特位(抗体分子可变区上能被其他抗体识别的特殊部位)

idiotopy [ˈidiəˌtɔpi] *n* 各部关系,各部相关

idiotoxin [ˌidiəuˈkɔksin] *n* 变[态反]应原,特应性毒素

idiotrophic [ˌidiəuˈtrɔfik] *a* 自选食物的

idiotropic [ˌidiəuˈtrɔpik] *a* 自向性的(指人格型)

idiotype [ˈidiətaip] *n* 独特型 | **idiotypic** [ˌidiəu-ˈtipik] *a*

idiovariation [ˌidiəuˌvεəriˈeiʃən] *n* 自发[性]变异,突变

idioventricular [ˌidiəuvenˈtrikjulə] *a* 心室自身的

idiozome [ˈidiəzəum] *n* = **idiosome**

iditol [ˈaiditɔl] *n* 艾杜糖醇

L-iditol 2-dehydrogenase [ˈaiditɔl diːˈhaidrədʒəneis] L-艾杜糖醇 2-脱氢酶(亦称山梨[糖]醇脱氢酶)

IDL intermediate-density lipoprotein 中密度脂蛋白

idose [ˈaldəus] *n* 艾杜糖(一种己醛糖)

idoxuridine [aidɔkˈsuəridiːn] *n* 碘苷(抗病毒药)

IDU idoxuridine 碘苷

iduronate [ˌaidjuˈrɔneit] *n* 艾杜糖醛酸(盐、酯或阴离子型)

Iduronate-2-sulfatase [ˌaidjuˈrɔneit ˈsʌlfəteis] 艾杜糖醛酸-2-硫酸酯酶(此酶缺乏为一种 X 连锁隐性性状,可致亨特〈Hunter〉综合征,即黏多糖贮积症Ⅱ型)

iduronic acid [ˌaidjuˈrɔnik] 艾杜糖醛酸

L-iduronidase [ˌaidjuˈrɔnideis] *n* L-艾杜糖苷酸酶(此酶的遗传性缺乏为一种常染色体隐性性状,可致黏多糖贮积症Ⅰ型)

IEP immunoelectrophoresis 免疫电泳

IF intrinsic factor 内在因子

IFA immunofluorescence assay 免疫荧光测定

IFN interferon 干扰素

ifosfamide [aiˈfɔsfəmaid] *n* 异环磷酰胺(抗肿瘤药)

Ig immunoglobulin 免疫球蛋白(主要有五种:IgA, IgD, IgE, IgG, IgM)

IGF insulin-like growth factor 胰岛素样生长因子

IGIV immune globulin intravenous (human) 免疫球蛋白静脉注射(人)

ignatia [igˈneiʃiə] *n*【拉】吕宋豆(含士的宁和马钱子碱,用作苦补剂)

igniextirpation [ˌigniˌekstəˈpeiʃən] *n* 烙除法

ignioperation [ˌigniˌɔpəˈreiʃən] *n* 热烙手术

ignipuncture [ˈigniˌpʌŋktʃə] *n* 火针术

ignis [ˈignis] *n*【拉】发热;火 | ~ infernalis 麦角中毒

ignisation [ˌignaiˈzeiʃən, -niˈz-] *n* 人工热源照射法

ignotine [ˈignətin] *n* 肌肽

IGT impaired glucose tolerance 糖耐量减低

IH infectious hepatitis 传染性肝炎

IHD ischemic heart disease 缺血性心脏病

IHS Indian Health Service 印第安人保健部(属美国公共卫生署)

IL interleukin 白细胞介素,白介素

il- 见 in-

ILA International Leprosy Association 国际麻风协会

Ile isoleucine 异亮氨酸

ileac [ˈiliæk] *a* 肠梗阻的;回肠的

ileadelphus [ˌiliəˈdelfəs] *n* 髂部联胎

ileal [ˈiliəl] *a* 回肠的

ileectomy [ˌiliˈektəmi] *n* 回肠切除术

ileitis [ˌiliˈaitis] *n* 回肠炎 | distal ~, regional ~, terminal ~ 回肠末端炎,节段性回肠炎

ile(o)- [构词成分]回肠

ileocecal [ˌiliəuˈsiːkəl] *a* 回盲肠的

ileocecocystoplasty [ˌiliəuˌsiːkəuˈsistəˌplæsti] *n* 回肠盲肠膀胱扩大术

ileocecostomy [ˌiliəusiˈkɔstəmi] *n* 回肠盲肠吻合术

ileocecum [ˌiliəuˈsiːkəm] *n* 回盲肠

ileocolic [ˌiliəuˈkɔlik], **ileocolonic** [ˌiliəukəˈlɔnik] *a* 回肠结肠的

ileocolitis [ˌiliəukəˈlaitis] *n* 回肠结肠炎 | tuberculous ~ 结核性回肠结肠炎 / ~ ulcerosa chronica 慢性溃疡性回肠结肠炎

ileocolostomy [ˌiliəukəˈlɔstəmi] *n* 回肠结肠吻合术

ileocolotomy [ˌiliəukəˈlɔtəmi] *n* 回肠结肠切开术

ileocystoplasty [ˌiliəuˈsistəˌplæsti] *n* 回肠膀胱扩大术

ileocystostomy [ˌiliəusisˈtɔstəmi] *n* 回肠膀胱吻合术

ileoileostomy [ˌiliəuˌiliˈɔstəmi] *n* 回肠回肠吻合术

ileoproctostomy [ˌiliəuprɔkˈtɔstəmi], **ileorectostomy** [ˌiliəurekˈtɔstəmi] *n* 回肠直肠吻合术

ileorectal [ˌiliəuˈrektl] *a* 回肠直肠的（如瘘）
ileorrhaphy [ˌiliˈɔrəfi] *n* 回肠缝合术
ileosigmoid [ˌiliəuˈsigmɔid] *a* 回肠乙状结肠的
ileosigmoidostomy [ˌiliəuˌsigmɔiˈdɔstəmi] *n* 回肠乙状结肠吻合术
ileostomy [ˌiliˈɔstəmi] *n* 回肠造口术
ileotomy [ˌiliˈɔtəmi] *n* 回肠切开术
ileotransversostomy [ˌiliəuˌtrænsvəsˈɔstəmi] *n* 回肠横结肠吻合术
ileoureteral [ˌiliəujuəˈriːtərəl] *a* 回肠输尿管的，输尿管回肠的
ileourethral [ˌiliəujuəˈriːθrəl] *a* 回肠尿道的（亦称尿道回肠的）
ileovesical [ˌiliəuˈvesikəl] *a* 回肠膀胱的（亦称膀胱回肠的）
ileovesicostomy [ˌiliəuˌvesiˈkɔstəmi] *n* 回肠膀胱造口术（亦称回肠膀胱吻合术）
ileum [ˈiliəm] *n*【拉】回肠 | duplex ~ 双回肠
ileus [ˈiliəs] *n* 肠梗阻 | adynamic ~, paralytic ~ 无动力性肠梗阻，麻痹性肠梗阻 / dynamic ~, hyperdynamic ~ 动力性肠梗阻（机械性肠梗阻；痉挛性肠梗阻）/ mechanical ~, occlusive ~ 机械性肠梗阻 / spastic ~ 痉挛性肠梗阻 / ~ subparta 孕性肠梗阻
Ilex [ˈaileks] *n* 冬青属
Ilheus encephalitis [iːˈleiuːs]（Ilheus 为巴西一地名，1944 年首次在该地发现此病）伊利乌斯脑炎（巴西蚊子传播的一种病毒性脑炎）| ~ virus 伊利乌斯病毒（黄病毒属的一种虫媒病毒，首先从巴西伊蚊和鳞蚊中分离出来；也见于巴拿马，其宿主可能是鸟，与圣路易斯病毒、日本乙型脑炎病毒和西尼罗河病毒有关）
ilia [ˈiliə] ilium 的复数
iliac [ˈiliæk] *a* 髂的，髂骨的
iliadelphus [ˌiliəˈdelfəs] *n* 髂部联胎
ilicin [ˈilisin] *n* 冬青素
ili(o)- [构词成分] 髂，髂骨
iliococcygeal [ˌiliəukɔkˈsidʒiəl] *a* 髂尾骨的
iliococcygeus [ˌiliəukɔkˈsidʒiəs] *n*【拉】髂尾肌
iliocolotomy [ˌiliəukəˈlɔtəmi] *n* 髂式结肠切开术
iliocostal [ˌiliəuˈkɔstl] *a* 髂肋的
iliofemoral [ˌiliəuˈfemərəl] *a* 髂股的
iliofemoroplasty [ˌiliəuˈfemərəuˌplæsti] *n* 髂股成形术
iliohypogastric [ˌiliəuˌhaipəuˈgæstrik] *a* 髂下腹的
ilioinguinal [ˌiliəuˈiŋgwinl] *a* 髂腹股沟的
iliolumbar [ˌiliəuˈlʌmbə] *a* 髂腰的
iliolumbocostoabdominal [ˌiliəuˌlʌmbəuˌkɔstəuæbˈdɔminl] *a* 髂腰肋腹的
iliometer [ˌiliˈɔmitə] *n* 髂棘测量器
iliopagus [ˌiliˈɔpəgəs] *n* 髂部联胎
iliopectineal [ˌiliəupekˈtiniəl], **iliopubic** [ˌiliəuˈpjuːbik] *a* 髂耻的
iliopelvic [ˌiliəuˈpelvik] *a* 髂盆的
iliopsoas [ˈiliəuˈsəuəs] *n* 髂腰肌
iliosacral [ˌiliəuˈseikrəl] *a* 髂骶的
iliosciatic [ˌiliəusaiˈætik] *a* 髂坐[骨]的
iliospinal [ˌiliəuˈspainl] *a* 髂脊柱的
iliothoracopagus [ˌiliəuˌθɔːrəˈkɔpəgəs] *n* 髂胸联胎
iliotibial [ˌiliəuˈtibiəl] *a* 髂胫的
iliotrochanteric [ˌiliəuˌtrəukænˈterik] *a* 髂转子的
ilioxiphopagus [ˌiliəuzaiˈfɔpəgəs] *n* 髂部剑突联胎
ilium [ˈiliəm]（[复] **ilia** [ˈiliə]）*n*【拉】髂骨
ill [il] *a* 有病的，不健康的 *n* 病 | föhn ~（欧洲）热南风病 / quarter ~ 气肿性炭疽，黑腿病
illacrimation [iˌlækriˈmeiʃən] *n* 泪溢
illaqueation [ilˌækwiˈeiʃən] *n* 倒睫拔除[法]
Illicium [iˈlisiəm] *n*【拉】八角[茴香]属
illinition [iliˈniʃən] *n* 涂擦法
illinium [iˈlinjəm] *n* 钔（元素钷的旧名）
illness [ˈilnis] *n* 病 | compressed-air ~ 潜涵病，减压病 / mental ~ 精神疾患，精神病 / radiation ~ 放射病
ill thrift [il θrift] 不旺盛
illumination [iˌljuːmiˈneiʃən] *n* 照明；照度（符号为 *E*）| axial ~, central ~ 轴心照明，中心照明 / contact ~ 接触照明 / critical ~ 临界照明 / darkfield ~, dark-ground ~ 暗[视]野照明 / focal ~ 焦点照明 / through ~ 透照[法]
illuminator [iˌljuːmiˈneitə] *n* 照明器，映光器
illuminism [iˈljuːminizəm] *n* 通神妄想，通神症，通神性幻觉状态
illusion [iˈljuːʒən] *n* 错觉 | passive ~ 被动错觉 | **~al**, **~ary** *a*
illusive [iˈljuːsiv] *a* 产生错觉的；虚幻的
ILT infectious laryngotracheitis 传染性喉气管炎
IM intramuscular 肌内（注射）
im- [前缀] 见 in-；二价的亚氨基 = NH
ima [ˈaimə] *a*【拉】最下的，最低的
imafen hydrochloride [ˈiməfən] 盐酸苯双咪唑（抗抑郁药）
image [ˈimidʒ] *n* 像，影像，图像；表象，意象 | accidental ~ 意外像，后像 / acoustic ~, auditory ~ 听像，声像 / body ~ 体像 / eidetic ~ 遗觉像 / false ~ 虚像，假像 / heteronymous ~ 远复视像 / homonymous ~ 近复视像 / incidental ~ 副像，残像 / memory ~ 记忆影像 / mental ~ 意象，心象，表象 / mirror ~ 裂隙灯像；镜像 / negative ~ 负像，后像 / real ~, inverted ~ 实像，倒像 / virtual ~, direct ~, erect ~ 虚像，直接像 / visual ~, ocular ~ 视觉像，目像
imagery [ˈimədʒəri] *n* 像；显像术

imaging [ˈimidʒiŋ] *n* 成像 | electrostatic ~ 静电成像 / magnetic resonance ~ (MRI)磁共振成像

imago [iˈmeigəu] ([复] **imagoes, imagines** [iˈmædʒiniːz] *n*【拉】成虫(昆虫);意象(心理)

imagocide [iˈmeigəusaid] *n* 杀成虫剂(尤指杀蚊剂)

imapunga [iməˈpʌŋgə] *n* 非洲牛疫

imatinib mesylate [iˈmætinib] *n* 甲磺伊马尼布(用于治疗慢性髓细胞白血病)

imbalance [imˈbæləns] *n* 不平衡,失调 | autonomic ~, vasomotor ~ 自主神经功能失调,血管运动功能失调 / sympathetic ~ 交感神经功能失调,迷走神经过敏

imbecile [ˈimbisiːl] *n* 痴愚者(智商 25～49) *a* 痴愚的 | moral ~ 悖德痴愚者

imbecilic [ˌimbiˈsilik] *a* 痴愚的

imbecility [ˌimbiˈsiləti] *n* 痴愚 | moral ~ 悖德狂 / phenylpyruvic ~ 苯丙酮酸性精神幼稚症

imbed [imˈbed] *vt* 包埋,植入

imbibe [imˈbaib] *vt* 喝,饮;浸渗,吸收 *vi* 喝,饮;吸收

imbibition [ˌimbiˈbiʃən] *n* 浸渗,吸胀[作用],吸液 | hemoglobin ~ 血红蛋白浸渗

imbricate [ˈimbrikeit] *vt*, *vi* 叠盖 [ˈimbrikit] *a* 叠盖的 | **~d** [ˈimbrikeitid] *a* 叠瓦状的 / **imbrication** [ˌimbriˈkeiʃən] *n* 叠盖

ImD_{50} median immunizing dose 半数免疫剂量

Imerslund-Graesbeck syndrome [ˈiməːslənd ˈgreisbek] (Olga Imerslund; Ralf G. Graesbeck) 维生素 B_{12} 选择性吸收障碍综合征

Imerslund syndrome [ˈiməːslənd] (Olga Imerslund) 伊默斯伦综合征,家族性巨成红细胞贫血

imhoff tank [ˈimhɔf] (Karl Imhoff) 隐化池

imidamine [ˌimiˈdæmin] *n* 安他唑啉(antazoline,抗组胺药,抗心律失常药)

imidazole [ˌimiˈdæzəul] *n* 咪唑,异吡唑

imidazolylethylamine [ˌimiˌdæzəuliˌleθiˈlæmin] *n* 咪唑乙胺,组胺

imide [ˈimid] *n* 酰亚胺

imido- [前缀]亚氨基

imidocarb hydrochloride [iˈmidəukɑːb] 盐酸咪多卡(抗原虫药)

imidodipeptide [ˌimidəudaiˈpeptaid] *n* 亚氨二肽(C 末端氨基酸为亚氨基酸的二肽)

imidodipeptiduria [ˌimidəudaiˌpeptiˈdjuəriə] *n* 亚氨二肽尿[症]

imidogen [iˈmidədʒin] *n* 亚氨基

imiglucerase [ˌimiˈgljuːsəreis] *n* 咪葡糖神经酰胺酶(葡糖神经酰胺酶类似物,由重组 DNA 技术产生,用作酶补充剂,以取代葡糖神经酰胺酶〈葡糖脑苷脂酶〉,用于治疗Ⅰ型戈谢〈Gaucher〉病,静脉滴注给药)

iminazole [ˌimiˈnæzəul] *n* 咪唑,异吡唑

imine [iˈmiːn] *n* 亚胺

imino- [iˈmiːnə] [前缀]亚氨基

imino acid [iˈmiːnə] 亚氨基酸

iminodiacetic acid (IDA) [ˌiminəuˌdaiəˈsiːtik] 亚氨基二乙酸 | hepatobiliary ~ (HIDA) 肝胆管亚氨基二乙酸

iminodipeptide [ˌiminəudaiˈpeptaid] *n* 亚氨基二肽(*N* 末端氨基酸为亚氨基酸的二肽)

iminoglycinuria [iˌmiːnəuˌglaisiˈnjuəriə] *n* 亚氨基甘氨酸尿

iminostilbene [ˌiminəuˈstilbiːn] *n* 亚氨基芪

iminourea [iˌminəjuəˈriə] *n* 胍

imipenem [ˌimiˈpenəm] *n* 亚胺培南(抗菌药)

imipramine [iˈmiprəmiːn] *n* 米帕明(抗抑郁药) | ~ hydrochloride 盐酸米帕明(抗抑郁药)

imiquimod [ˌimiˈkwimɔd] *n* 咪喹莫特(生物反应调节物,局部用于治疗外生殖器和肛周区尖锐湿疣)

Imlach's fat plug [ˈimlæk] (Francis Imlach) 英拉克脂肪块(有时存在于腹股沟外环内角的脂肪小块)

immature [ˌiməˈtjuə] *a* 发育未全的;未成熟的;不完全的 | immaturity [iməˈtjuərəti] *n*

immediate [iˈmiːdjət] *a* 直接的

immedicable [iˈmedikəbl] *a* 不治的,无法可治的

immersion [iˈməːʃən] *n* 沉浸,浸没,浸渍 | homogeneous ~ 同质油浸(显微镜) / oil ~ 油浸法(显微镜) / water ~ 水浸法(显微镜)

immiscible [iˈmisəbl] *a* 不可混和的

immittance [iˈmitəns] *n* 导抗 | acoustic ~ 声导抗

immobile [iˈməubail] *a* 不动的,固定的,稳定的;不变的 | **immobility** [ˌiməuˈbiləti] *n* 不动[性];慢性脑积水病(牛)

immobilize [iˈməubilaiz] *vt* 使不动,使固定 | **immobilization** [iˌməubilaiˈzeiʃən, -liˈz-] *n* 制动术,固定[术]

immobilizer [iˈməubiˌlaizə] *n* 固定器,制动装置 | sternal-occipital-mandibular ~ (SOMI) 胸骨-枕骨-下颌骨组合制动装置(亦称 SOMI orthosis)

immortalization [iˌmɔːtələzeiʃən] *n* 无限增殖化,永生化

immune [iˈmjuːn] *a* 有免疫力的;免疫的 *n* 免疫者

immunifacient [iˌmjuːniˈfeiʃənt] *a* 产生免疫的 *n* 免疫发生剂

immunifaction [iˌmjuːniˈfækʃən] *n* 免疫[法],免疫接种,免疫作用

immunisin [iˈmjuːnizin] *n* 免疫素(抗体)

immunity [iˈmjuːnəti] *n* 免疫[力] | acquired ~,

adaptive ~ 获得性免疫，适应性免疫 / active ~, actual ~ 主动免疫，真正免疫 / adoptive ~ 过继免疫 / antibacterial ~ 抗菌免疫 / antiblastic ~ 抗菌发育免疫 / antitoxic ~ 抗毒素免疫 / antiviral ~ 抗病毒免疫 / artificial ~ 人工免疫 / bacteriolytic ~ 溶菌免疫 / cell-mediated ~ (CMI), cellular ~ 细胞介导免疫，细胞免疫 / concomitant ~ 伴随免疫 / congenital ~ 先天免疫 / cross ~ 交叉免疫 / genetic ~, inherited ~, familial ~ 遗传免疫，家族性免疫 / herd ~, community ~ 群体免疫 / humoral ~ 体液免疫 / innate ~, inherent ~ 先天免疫，固有免疫 / intrauterine ~, placental ~ 宫内免疫，胎盘免疫 / local ~, tissue ~ 局部免疫，组织免疫 / maternal ~ 母体免疫 / maturation ~ 成熟免疫 / mixed ~ 混合免疫 / native ~ 自然免疫，天然免疫 / natural ~ 天然免疫 / nonspecific ~ 非特异性免疫 / opsonic ~ 调理免疫（由于调理素存在而具有的免疫） / passive ~ 被动免疫 / phagocytic ~ 噬细胞免疫 / postoncolytic ~ 溶瘤后免疫 / preemptive ~ 先占免疫（干扰现象） / racial ~ 种系免疫，种族免疫 / residual ~ 残余免疫 / species ~ 种免疫 / specific ~ 特异性免疫 / T cell-mediated ~ (TCMI) T 细胞介导免疫 / toxin-antitoxin ~ 毒素抗毒素免疫

immunization [ˌimju(ː)naiˈzeiʃən, -niˈz-] *n* 免疫[法]，免疫接种，免疫作用 | active ~, isopathic ~ 自动免疫接种，同源免疫接种 / collateral ~ 间接免疫接种 / occult ~ 隐伏免疫作用 / passive ~ 被动免疫接种 / Rh ~, rhesus ~ Rh 免疫[作用]（Rh 致敏） / side-to-side ~ 并排免疫接种，两侧免疫接种（抗原注射至身体一侧，而对应抗体注射至另一侧）

immunizator [ˌimju(ː)naiˈzeitə] *n* 免疫剂

immunize [ˈimju(ː)naiz] *vt* 使免疫

immunoablative [ˌimjunəuˈæblətiv] *a* 免疫消融的

immunoadjuvant [ˌimjunəuˈædʒəvənt] *n* 免疫佐剂

immunoadsorbent [ˌimjunəuədˈsɔːbənt] *n* 免疫吸附剂

immunoadsorption [ˌimjunəu ædˈsɔːpʃən] *n* 免疫吸附

immunoassay [ˌimjunəuˈæsei] *n* 免疫测定 | enzyme ~ (EIA) 酶免疫测定

immunobiology [ˌimjunəubaiˈɔlədʒi] *n* 免疫生物学 | **immunobiological** [ˌmjunəuˌbaiəˈlɔdikəl] *a*

immunoblast [ˌimjunəuˈblæst] *n* 免疫母细胞 | ~**ic** *a*

immunoblot [ˈimjunəuˌblɔt] *n* 免疫印迹[法]（经由抗原-抗体特异性反应分析或鉴定蛋白质的一种技术，或由此产生的印染，如用于蛋白质印迹技术或斑点印迹技术）

immunocatalysis [ˌimjunəukəˈtælisis] *n* 免疫催化作用

immunochemical [ˌimjunəuˈkemikəl] *a* 免疫化学的

immunochemistry [ˌimjunəuˈkemistri] *n* 免疫化学

immunochemotherapy [ˌimjunəuˌkiːməuˈθerəpi] *n* 免疫化学疗法，免疫化疗

immunocompetence [ˌimjunəuˈkɔmpitəns] *n* 免疫活性，免疫适格力 | **immunocompetent** *a*

immunocomplex [ˌimjunəuˈkɔmpleks] *n* 免疫复合物

immunocompromised [ˌimjunəuˈkɔmprəmaizd] *n* 免疫受损的

immunoconglutinin [ˌimjunəukənˈgluːtinin] *n* 免疫胶固素

immunocyte [ˈimjunəsait] *n* 免疫细胞

immunocytoadherence [ˌimjunəuˌsaitəuədˈhiərəns] *n* 免疫细胞粘连

immunocytochemistry [ˌimjunəuˌsaitəuˈkemistri] *n* 免疫细胞化学

immunodefecient [ˌimjunəudiˈfiʃənt] *a* 免疫缺陷的，免疫受损的

immunodeficiency [ˌimjunəudiˈfiʃənsi] *n* 免疫缺陷，免疫缺损（体液抗体介导的或免疫淋巴细胞介导的免疫应答缺陷） | combined ~ 联合免疫缺陷（指体液免疫和细胞免疫都有缺陷） / common variable ~, common variable unclassifiable ~ 普通可变型免疫缺陷，普通可变型不可分类性免疫缺陷 / ~ with hyper-IgM 高免疫球蛋白 M 性免疫缺陷 / severe combined ~ (SCID) 重症联合免疫缺陷 / ~ withshort-limbed dwarfism 短肢侏儒症型免疫缺陷 / ~ with thymoma 胸腺瘤型免疫缺陷

immunodepression [ˌimjunəudiˈpreʃən] *n* 免疫抑制 | **immunodepressive** *a* 抑制免疫的 *n* 免疫抑制剂

immunodermatology [ˌimjunəuˌdəːməˈtɔlədʒi] *n* 免疫皮肤学

immunodetection [ˌimjunəudiˈtekʃən] *n* 免疫检测，免疫闪烁显像（即 immunoscintigraphy）

immunodeviation [ˌimjunəuˌdiːviˈeiʃən] *n* 免疫偏移

immunodiagnosis [ˌimjunəuˌdaiəgˈnəusis] *n* 免疫诊断

immunodiffusion [ˌimjunəudiˈfjuːʒən] *n* 免疫扩散 | radial ~ (RID) 辐射状免疫扩散，单向辐射状扩散

immunodominance [ˌimjunəuˈdɔminəns] *n* 免疫显性

immunodominant [ˌimjunəuˈdɔminənt] *a* 免疫显

性的

immunoelectrophoresis [ˌimjuːnəuiˌlektrəufə'riːsis] *n* 免疫电泳[法] | counter ~, countercurrent ~对流免疫电泳 / cross ~交叉免疫电泳 / reverse ~反向免疫电泳(将抗原与抗体位置倒置的一种免疫电泳技术) / rocket ~火箭免疫电泳

immunoenhancement [ˌimjunəuin'hɑːnsmənt] *n* 免疫促进,免疫增强

immunoferritin [ˌimjunəu'feritin] *n* 免疫铁蛋白

immunofiltration [ˌimjunəufil'treiʃən] *n* 免疫过滤[法]

immunofluorescence [ˌimjunəufluə'resəns] *n* 免疫荧光[法]

immunogen [imjuːnədʒən] *n* 免疫原

immunogenesis [ˌimjunəu'dʒenisis] *n* 免疫发生

immunogenetics [ˌimjunəudʒi'netiks] *n* 免疫遗传学 | **immunogenetic** [ˌimjuːnəudʒi'netik] *a* 免疫遗传的

immunogenic [ˌimjunəu'dʒenik] *a* 免疫源的,致免疫的 | **~ity**[ˌimjunəudʒi'nisəti] *n* 免疫原性

immunoglobulin [ˌimjunəu'glɔbjulin] *n* 免疫球蛋白 | monoclonal ~ 单克隆免疫球蛋白 / secretory ~ 分泌型免疫球蛋白 / thyroid-binding inhibitory ~s(TBII)甲状腺结合抑制性免疫球蛋白 / thyroid-stimulating ~s(TSI)促甲状腺免疫球蛋白(亦称人甲状腺腺苷酸环化酶刺激因子,以前称长效甲状腺刺激素) / TSH-binding inhibitory ~s(TBII)促甲状腺激素结合抑制性免疫球蛋白(亦称 TSH 置换性抗体)

immunoglobulinopathy [ˌimjunəu ˌglɔbjuli'nɔpəθi] *n* 免疫球蛋白病,丙种球蛋白病

immunohematology [ˌimjuːnəuˌhemə'tɔlədʒi] *n* 免疫血液学

immunoheterogeneity [ˌimjunəuˌhetərəudʒi'niːəti] *n* 免疫不均性,免疫多相性,免疫异质性

immunoheterogenous [ˌimjunəuˌhetərəu'dʒiːnəs] *a* 免疫不均的,免疫多相的,免疫异质的

immunohistochemical [ˌimjunəuˌhistəu'kemikəl] *a* 免疫组织化学的

immunohistofluorescence [ˌimjunəuˌhistəuˌfluə'resəns] *n* 免疫组织荧光[法]

immunohistology [ˌimjunəuhis'tɔlədʒi] *n* 免疫组织学 | **immunohistologic** [ˌimjunəuhistə'lɔdʒik] *a*

immunoincompetent [ˌimjunəuin'kɔmpitənt] *a* 无免疫活性的,免疫功能不全的

immunology [ˌimju'nɔlədʒi] *n* 免疫学 | **immunologic(al)** [ˌimjunəu'lɔdʒik(əl)] *a* / **immunologically** [ˌimjunə'lɔdʒikəli] *ad* / **immunologist** *n* 免疫学家

immunolymphoscintigraphy [ˌimjunəuˌlimfəu-sin'tigrəfi] *n* 免疫淋巴闪烁图检查(使用放射标记的单克隆抗体或肿瘤相关抗原特异性的抗体片段,对淋巴结内的转移性肿瘤进行闪烁图检测)

immunomodulation [ˌimjunəuˌmɔdju'leiʃən] *n* 免疫调变

immunomodulator [ˌimjunəu'mɔdjuˌleitə] *n* 免疫调节药

immunoparasitology [ˌimjunəuˌpærəsai'tɔlədʒi] *n* 免疫寄生物学

immunoparesis [ˌimjunəupæ'riːsis] *n* 免疫不全麻痹

immunopathogenesis [ˌimjunəuˌpæθə'dʒenisis] *n* 免疫发病机制

immunopathology [ˌimjunəupə'θɔlədʒi] *n* 免疫病理学 | **immunopathologic** [ˌimjunəu ˌpæθə'lɔdʒik] *a*

immunoperoxidase [ˌimjunəupə'rɔksideis] *n* 免疫过氧化物酶

immunophenotype [ˌimjunəu'fiːnəutaip] *n* 免疫表型(造血肿瘤细胞的一种表型)

immunophenotyping [ˌimjunəu'finəutaipiŋ] *n* 免疫分型

immunophysiology [ˌimjunəuˌfizi'ɔlədʒi] *n* 免疫生理学

immunopotency [ˌimjunəu'pəutənsi] *n* 免疫效价,免疫能力,免疫效能

immunopotentiation [ˌimjunəupəuˌtenʃi'eiʃən] *n* 免疫强化(利用佐剂或免疫刺激剂增强免疫应答)

immunopotentiator [ˌimjunəupəu'tenʃieitə] *n* 免疫强化剂(如疫苗,在注射时产生全身性免疫应答)

immunoprecipitation [ˌimjunəupriˌsipi'teiʃən] *n* 免疫沉淀反应(特异性抗体和抗原相互作用引起的)

immunoproliferative [ˌimjunəuprə'lifərətiv] *a* 免疫增生的(以淋巴细胞增生并产生免疫球蛋白为特征的)

immunoprophylaxis [ˌimjunəuˌprɔfi'læksis] *n* 免疫预防

immunoprotein [ˌimjuːnəu'prəutiːn] *n* 免疫蛋白

immunoradiometry [ˌimjunəuˌreidi'ɔmitri] *n* 免疫放射测定 | **immunoradiometric** [ˌimjunəuˌreidiəu'metrik] *a*

immunoreactant [ˌimjunəuri(ː)'æktənt] *n* 免疫反应物 | glucagon ~s 高血糖素免疫反应物,肠高血糖素

immunoreaction [iˌmjuːnəuri(ː)'ækʃən] *n* 免疫反应(抗原与其抗体之间的反应,或抗原与对抗原致敏的免疫细胞之间的反应)

immunoreactive [ˌimjunəuri(ː)'æktiv] *a* 免疫反应的

immunoreactivity [ˌimjunəuri(ː)æk'tivəti] *n* 免疫反应性 | glucagon-like ~ 胰高血糖素样免疫反应性
immunoregulation [ˌimjunəuˌregju'leiʃən] *n* 免疫调节
immunoresponsiveness [ˌimjunəuris'pɔnsivnis] *n* 免疫应答
immunoscintigraphy [ˌimjunəusin'tigrəfi] *n* 免疫闪烁显像(使用放射标记的单克隆抗体或与损害相关的抗原特异性的抗体片段,对损害进行闪烁显像)
immunoselection [ˌimjunəusi'lekʃən] *n* 免疫选择[法](某些细胞系的生存由于表面抗原性极弱,因此对抗体和(或)免疫淋巴细胞极不敏感)
immunosenescence [ˌimjunəusi'nesns] *n* 免疫衰老(免疫系统随机体年龄增长而减弱和萎缩)
immunosorbent [ˌimjunəu'sɔːbənt] *n* 免疫吸附剂,免疫吸收剂(一种含抗原的不溶性支持物,用以从抗体混合物中吸收同种抗体)
immunostaining [ˌimjunəu'steiniŋ] *n* 免疫染色
immunostimulant [ˌimjunəu'stimjulənt] *a* 免疫刺激的 *n* 免疫刺激剂,免疫兴奋药
immunostimulating [ˌimjunəu'stimjuˌleitiŋ] *a* 免疫刺激的
immunostimulation [ˌimjunəuˌstimju'leiʃən] *n* 免疫刺激[作用]
immunosuppression [ˌimjuːnəusə'preʃən] *n* 免疫抑制(人工防止或减弱免疫应答) | **immunosuppressive** [ˌimjuːnəusə'presiv], **immunosuppressant** [ˌimjuːnəusə'presənt] *a* 免疫抑制的 *n* 免疫抑制药
immunosurgery [iˌmjuːnəu'səːdʒəri] *n* 免疫外科
immunosurveillance [ˌimjunəusə'veiləns] *n* 免疫监视,免疫监督(指免疫系统的监视作用)
immunosympathectomy [ˌimjunəu ˌsimpə'θektəmi] *n* 免疫交感神经破坏法,交感神经免疫去除术(静脉注射交感神经细胞主要蛋白质的抗血清至新生动物,以破坏交感神经节)
immunotherapy [ˌimjuːnəu'θerəpi] *n* 免疫疗法
immunotoxin [ˌimjuːnəu'tɔksin] *n* 免疫毒素(抗毒素)
immunotransfusion [ˌimjuːnəutræns'fjuːʒən] *n* 免疫输血法,免疫输液
immunotropic [ˌimjunəu'trɔpik] *a* 向免疫的,亲免疫的
immunoturbidimetry [ˌimjunəutəːbi'dimətri] *n* 免疫浊度测定法,免疫比浊法
immunprotein [imjun'prəutiːn] *n* 免疫蛋白
IMPA incisal mandibular plane angle 下颌中切牙-下颌平面角
impaction [im'pækʃən] *n* 嵌入,嵌塞;阻生 | ceruminal ~ 耵聍嵌塞 / dental ~ 牙阻生 / fecal ~ 粪便嵌塞
impaludation [ˌimpælju'deiʃən] *n* 疟热疗法
impar ['impɑː] *a* 【拉】奇[数]的,无对的
imparidigitate [imˌpæri'didʒiteit] *a* 奇数指的,奇数趾的
impatent [im'peitənt] *a* 不通的,闭阻的 | **impatency** [im'peitənsi] *n*
impedance [im'piːdəns] *n* 阻抗 | acoustic ~ 声阻抗
imperception [ˌimpə'sepʃən] *n* 知觉缺乏,未感知
imperfect [im'pəːfikt] *a* 不完全的,未完成的,半知的
imperforate [im'pəːfərit] *a* 不通的,无孔的,闭锁的
imperforation [imˌpəːfə'reiʃən] *n* 不通,无孔,闭锁[畸形] | otic ~ 外耳道闭锁
imperialine [im'piəriˌælin] *n* 西贝母碱
impervious [im'pəːvjəs] *a* 不可渗透的,不能透过的
impetiginization [ˌimpiˌtidʒinai'zeiʃən, -ni'z-] *n* 脓疱化,脓疱病发生
impetigo [ˌimpi'taigəu] *n* 【拉】脓疱病 | bullous ~ 大疱性脓疱病 / chronic symmetric ~ 白糠疹 / ~ circinata 环状脓疱病 / ~ contagiosa, ~ vulgaris 触染性脓疱病,寻常脓疱病 / ~ neonatorum 新生儿脓疱病,大疱性脓疱病 / ~ pityroides 糠疹样脓疱病,白糠疹 / staphylococcal ~, staphylococcic ~ 葡萄球菌性脓疱病,大疱性脓疱病 | **impetiginous** [ˌimpi'tidʒinəs] *a*
impetus ['impitəs] *n* 动力;冲动,动能;起始(病)
impf-malaria ['impfməˌlɛəriə] *n* 【德】接种性疟疾
impilation [ˌimpai'leiʃən] *n* 红细胞钱串形成
implacentalia [ˌimplæsən'teiliə] *n* 无胎盘类
implant[1] [im'plɑːnt, -'plænt] *vt* 插入,埋入,移入
implant[2] ['implɑːnt, -plænt] *n* 种植体,植入物,移植片 | dental ~ 牙种植体 / endodontic ~ 根管内种植体 / endometrial ~s 内膜植入片 / endosseous ~, endosteal ~ 骨内种植体 / intraperiosteal ~ 骨膜内种植体 / magnet ~ 磁体种植体 / osseointegrated ~ 骨内整合性植入物 / subperiosteal ~ 骨膜下种植体
implantation [ˌimplɑːn'teiʃən, -plæn-] *n* 种植;植入法,移植术(如皮肤、神经、腱等);植入(胚泡在子宫内的);埋入法,植入法(如药物等) | eccentric ~ 偏心植入(胚泡) / filigree ~ 银网植入法(银网修补腹疝法) / hypodermic ~ 皮下植入法(药物) / interstitial ~ 间质植入(胚泡) / silk ~ 丝线植入法 / superficial ~, central ~, circumferential ~ 表面植入,中心植入,环形植入(胚泡) / teratic ~ 植入性[畸胎]畸形(不完全胎儿与几乎完全胎儿的部分融合)

implantodontics [ˌimplɑːntəˈdɔntiks, -plæn-], **implantodontology** [imˌplɑːntədɔnˈtɔlədʒi, -ˌplæn-] *n* 口腔种植学 | **implantodontist** [imˌplɑːntəˈdɔntist, -ˌplæn-] *n* 口腔种植学家,植牙医师

implantologist [ˌimplɑːnˈtɔlədʒist, -plæn-] *n* 植入学家;口腔种植学家,植牙医师

implantology [ˌimplɑːnˈtɔlədʒi, -plæn-] *n* 植入学 | dental ~, oral ~ 口腔种植学

implosion [imˈpləuʒən] *n* 以恐治恐法(精神病学中用接触恐惧物的方法治疗恐怖症)

impotence [ˈimpətəns], **impotency** [ˈimpətənsi] *n* 阳痿;无能力

impotent [ˈimpətənt] *a* 阳痿的;无能力的

impotentia [ˌimpəˈtenʃiə] *n*【拉】阳痿;无能力 | ~ coeundi 交媾不能 / ~ erigendi 勃起不能 / ~ generandi 生育不能

impregnate [ˈimpregneit] *vt* 使受孕,使受精;浸渗[imˈpregnit] *a* 怀孕的;浸透的 | **impregnation** [ˌimpregˈneiʃən] *n* 受孕,受精;浸渗[作用]

impressio [imˈpresiəu]([复]**impressiones** [imˌpresiˈəuniːz)] *n*【拉】压迹

impression [imˈpreʃən] *n* 压迹;印模(牙);印象;影响 | basilar ~ 扁后脑,扁颅底 / cardiac ~ 心压迹 / ~ of costoclavicular ligament 肋锁韧带压迹 / deltoid ~ of humerus 三角肌粗隆(肱骨) / dental ~ 牙印模 / digastric ~ 二腹肌窝(下颌骨) / digital ~s, digitate ~s 脑压迹 / final ~ 终印模 / hydrocolloid ~ 水胶模 / preliminary ~, primary ~ 初印模 / rhomboid ~ of clavicle 菱形压迹(锁骨),肋锁韧带压迹

imprinting [imˈprintiŋ] *n* 印记,印刻[作用](动物在生命早期敏感发育时期,接触到适当的刺激后,很快学到物种独有的行为模式)

impuberal [imˈpjuːbərəl] *a* 无阴毛的,未成年的

impuberism [imˈpjuːbərizəm] *n* 未成年,前青春期

impulse [ˈimpʌls] *n* 冲动;搏动 | cardiac ~ 心脏冲动 / episternal ~ 胸骨上搏动 / nerve ~, neural ~ 神经冲动

impulsion [imˈpʌlʃən] *n* 冲动;癖 | wandering ~ 神游[症]

imputation [ˌimpjuːˈteiʃən] *n* 归因法(当数据遗漏时,如由于缺乏对调查反应所致,使用统计方法从有效值中评估遗漏值)

Imu [ˈiːmu] *n* 伊姆病(日本阿伊努人患的地方病,因情绪上受打击,而发生精神运动性疾患)

IMV intermittent mandatory ventilation 间歇强制通气

IMViC, imvic indole, methyl red, Voges-Proskauer, citrate 吲哚、甲基红、V-P、枸橼酸(表示大肠杆菌分类试验记忆法)

In indium 铟

in inch 英寸

INA International Neurological Association 国际神经病学协会

inacidity [ˌinəˈsidəti] *n* 无酸

inaction [inˈækʃən] *n* 无行动,不活跃,迟钝,无作用

inactivate [inˈæktiveit] *vt* 灭活,使不活动

inactivation [inˌæktiˈveiʃən] *n* 灭活,失活,灭能[作用],失效 | ~ of complement 补体灭活(破坏补体活性,一般将血清加温至 56 ℃持续 30 分钟即产生) / heat ~ 热灭活(用热破坏生物学活性,如加热到 56 ℃持续 30 分钟即可破坏血清中补体的活性) / X-~ X(染色体)失活(即莱昂化作用 lyonization)

inactivator [inˈæktiveitə] *n* 灭活剂,灭活酶 | anaphylatoxin ~ (AI)过敏毒素抑制剂 / C3b ~ (C3b INA)C3b 灭活因子

inactive [inˈæktiv] *a* 不活跃的,迟钝的;静止的,不活动的;不旋光的 | **inactivity** [ˌinækˈtivəti] *n*

inactose [inˈæktəus] *n* 不旋糖

inadaptation [ˌinədæpˈteiʃən] *n* 不适应

inadequacy [inˈædikwəsi] *n* 不适当,不足;功能不全;闭锁不全,关闭不全

inadequate [inˈædikwit] *a* 不充足的,不适当的;功能不足的,功能不全的

inagglutinable [inəˈgluːtinəbl] *a* 不凝集的

inalimental [ˌinæliˈmentl] *a* 无营养的

inamrinone [inˈæmrinəun] *n* 氨力农(强心药)

inanimate [inˈænimit] *a* 无生命的;无生机的

inanition [ˌinəˈniʃən] *n* 食物不足,营养不足

inapparent [ˌinəˈpærənt] *a* 隐性的,不显性的

inappetence [inˈæpitəns], **inappetency** [inˈæpitənsi] *n* 食欲不振 | **inappetent** *a*

in articulo mortis [in ɑːˈtikjuləu ˈmɔːtis]【拉】濒死,临终时

inarticulate [ˌinɑːˈtikjulit] *a* 无关节的;脱臼的;(言语)无音节的,口齿不清的

inassimilable [ˌinəˈsimiləbl] *a* 不[能]同化的

inattention [ˌinəˈtenʃən] *n* 不注意,疏忽 | selective ~ 选择性忽略(①单侧忽略〈unilateral neglect〉,见 neglect 项下相应术语;②忽视或经筛选去除一些威胁性的、产生焦虑的或认为是次要的刺激)

inaxon [inˈæksɔn] *n* 长轴索细胞

inborn [ˈinbɔːn] *a* 先天的

inbred [inˈbred] *a* 近亲繁殖的,近交的

inbreeding [ˈinˈbriːdiŋ] *n* 近交

incallosal [ˌinkəˈləusəl] *a* 缺胼胝体的

incandescent [ˌinkænˈdesnt] *a* 白炽的,白热的 | **incandescence** [ˌinkænˈdesns] *n*

incapacitant [ˌinkəˈpæsitənt] *n* 失能性毒剂,智能麻醉剂(精神性毒剂,暂时引起嗜睡、头晕、瘫痪等反应)

incapacitate [ˌinkəˈpæsiteit] *vt* 使无能力,使残废

incapacity [ˌinkəˈpæsəti] *n* 无能力 | renal ~ 肾功能不全

incarcerated [inˈkɑːsəreitid] *a* 箝闭的

incarceration [inˌkɑːsəˈreiʃən] *n* 箝闭 | placental ~ 胎盘嵌顿

incarnatio [ˌinkɑːˈneiʃiəu] *n*【拉】入肉 | ~ unguis 嵌甲

incarnative [inˈkɑːnətiv] *a* 肉芽生长的 *n* 生肉芽剂

incasement [inˈkeismənt] *n* 被覆,包装

incendiarism [inˈsendjərizəm] *n* 纵火狂

incertae sedis [inˈsəːtiː ˈsiːdis]【拉】位置未定,地位未确定(指生物分类上)

incest [ˈinsest] *n* 近亲通婚,近亲婚配

inch(in) [intʃ] *n* 英寸

inchacao [intʃəˈkɑːəu] *n*【巴西】脚气[病]

incidence [ˈinsidəns] *n* 发生率,发病率;入射

incident [ˈinsidənt] *n* 事件,事情 *a* 入射的

incidental [ˌinsiˈdentl] *a* 附带的,伴随的,偶见的,偶然的

incidentaloma [ˌinsiˌdentəˈləumə] *n* 偶见瘤(一种无症状瘤,通常为肾上腺瘤,在为某种理由进行诊断造影操作时发现)

incinerate [inˈsinəreit] *vt* 焚化,灰化;火葬 *vi* 烧成灰 | **incineration** [inˌsinəˈreiʃən] *n* 焚化,灰化,火葬;烧灼灭菌

incinerator [inˈsinəreitə] *n* 焚化者;火葬炉

incipient [inˈsipiənt] *a* 初发的,初期的 | **incipience, incipiency** *n*

incisal [inˈsaizəl] *a* 切[开]的

incise [inˈsaiz] *vt* 切,切入,切开 | **~d** *a*

incision [inˈsiʒən] *n* 切口;切开 | celiotomy ~ 腹壁切开 / confirmatory ~ 诊断性切开 / crucial ~ 十字切开 / hockey stick ~ 弯形切口 / lateral-rectus ~ 腹直肌旁切口 / median ~ 正中切口 / paramedian ~ 正中旁切口 / relief ~ 减张切开

incisive [inˈsaisiv] *a* 切的,切入的;切牙的

incisolabial [inˌsaizəuˈleibiəl] *a* 切唇的

incisolingual [inˌsaizəuˈliŋgwəl] *a* 切舌的

incisoproximal [inˌsaizəuˈprɔksiməl] *a* 切邻的

incisor [inˈsaizə] *a* 适于切割的 *n* 切牙 | central ~, first ~, medial ~ 中切牙 / lateral ~, second ~ 侧切牙 / shovel-shaped ~s 铲形切牙

incisura [ˌinsaiˈsjuərə] ([复] **incisurae** [ˌinsaiˈsjuəriː]) *n*【拉】切迹

incisure [inˈsaiʒə] *n* 切迹 | ~ of acetabulum 髋臼切迹 / clavicular ~ of sternum 锁骨切迹(胸骨) / costal ~s of sternum 肋骨切迹(胸骨)/inferior thyroid ~ 甲状软骨下切迹 / inferior vertebral ~, greater vertebral ~ 椎骨下切迹 / palatine ~, pterygoid ~ 翼切迹 / ~ of scapula, semilunar ~ 肩胛切迹 / sternal ~ 颈静脉切迹(胸骨) / superior thyroid ~ 甲状软骨上切迹 / superior vertebral ~, lesser vertebral ~ 椎骨上切迹 / ~ of tentorium of cerebellum 小脑幕切迹 / thoracic ~ 肋弓角 / umbilical ~ 脐[静脉]切迹

incitant [inˈsaitənt] *n* 刺激因素,激发因素(如引起传染病或诱发变应性反应);提神药,精神兴奋药 *a* 刺激的,激发的,兴奋的

incitogram [inˈsaitəgræm] *n* 冲动发放(组织和发动传出冲动的神经状态)

inclinatio [ˌinkliˈneiʃiəu] ([复] **inclinationes** [ˌinkliˌneiʃiˈəuniːz]) *n*【拉】倾斜,斜度 | ~ pelvis 骨盆斜度

inclination [ˌinkliˈneiʃən] *n* 倾斜,斜度 | condylar guidance ~, condylar guide ~ 髁导斜度 / lingual ~ 舌侧倾斜 / pelvic ~, ~ of pelvis 骨盆倾斜度

incline [inˈklain] *vi* 倾斜 *vt* 使倾斜 *n* 斜面,斜度 | pelvic ~, ~ of pelvis 骨盆倾斜度

inclinometer [ˌinkliˈnɔmitə] *n* 眼径计

inclusion [inˈkluːʒən] *n* 内含物,包涵物,包涵,包埋 | cell ~ 细胞包涵物 / dental ~ 牙包埋 / fetal ~ 胎内胎[畸形] / intranuclear ~s包涵体 / leukocyte ~s白细胞包涵体,窦勒包涵体(见 Döhle's inclusion bodies)

incoagulable [ˌinkəuˈægjuləbl] *a* 不凝的,不能凝固的 | **incoagulability** [ˌinkəuˌægjuləˈbiləti] *n* 不凝性

incoherent [ˌinkəuˈhiərənt] *a* 无凝聚力的;不连贯的 | **incoherence** *n*

incombustible [ˌinkəmˈbʌstəbl] *a* 不燃的 *n* 不燃物 | **incombustibility** [ˈinkəmˌbʌstəˈbiləti] *n* 不燃性

incompatibility [ˌinkəmpætəˈbiləti] *n* 不相容性,不适合性;配伍禁忌 | chemical ~ 化学性配伍禁忌 / physiologic ~ 生理性配伍禁忌 / therapeutic ~ 治疗性配伍禁忌

incompatible [ˌinkəmˈpætəbl] *a* 不相容的,配伍禁忌的

incompetence [inˈkɔmpitəns] *n* 不胜任,无能力,不合适;无行为能力,(法律上)无资格;功能不全;关闭不全 | aortic ~ 主动脉瓣关闭不全 / ~ of the cardiac valves 心瓣关闭不全 / ileocecal ~ 回盲瓣关闭不全 / relative ~ 相对性关闭不全 / valvular ~ 瓣关闭不全 | **incompetency** [inˈkɔmpitənsi] *n*

incompetent [inˈkɔmpitənt] *a* 不胜任的,不适合的;无能力的;无行为能力的,(法律上)无资格

的;功能不全的 *n* 无能力者;无行为能力者

incompressible [ˌinkəmˈpresəbl] *a* 不能压缩的,不易压缩的

incongruity [ˌinkɔŋˈgru(ː)iti] *n* 不协调,不一致 | ~ of affect 情感不协调

incontinence [inˈkɔntinəns] *n* 失禁;无节制 | active ~ 自动性失禁 / fecal ~, ~ of the feces, rectal ~ 大便失禁,直肠失禁 / intermittent ~ 间歇性失禁(尿) / overflow ~, paradoxical ~ 充溢性[尿]失禁,反常性[尿]失禁 / passive ~ 被动性失禁 / stress ~ 压力性尿失禁 / urinary ~, ~ of urine 尿失禁

incontinent [inˈkɔntinənt] *a* 失禁的;无节制的

incontinentia [inˌkɔntiˈnenʃiə] *n*【拉】失禁;无节制 | **~al** *vi* 大便失禁 / ~ pigmenti 色素失调症 / ~ pigmenti achromians 无色性色素失调症

inconvertible [ˌinkənˈvəːtəbl] *a* 不可转化的,不可逆的 | **inconvertibility** [ˌinkənˌvəːtəˈbiləti] *n* 不可转化性,不可逆性

incoordinate [ˌinkəuˈɔːdinit] *a* 不协调的 | **incoordination** [ˌinkəuˌɔːdiˈneiʃən] *n* 不协调;动作失调,协调不能

incorporation [inˌkɔːpəˈreiʃən] *n* 掺合,混合;合并,合体,合一(精神分析理论中,指外界对象合并于自己)

incostapedial [ˌinkɔstəˈpiːdiəl] *a* 砧镫[骨]的

increment [ˈinkrimənt] *n* 增加,增大;增值,增量 | absolute ~ 绝对增加 / relative ~ 相对增加 | **~al** [ˌinkriˈmentl] *a*

increscent [inˈkresnt] *a* 增大的

incretin [inˈkriːtin] *n* 肠降血糖素

incretion [inˈkriːʃən] *n* 内分泌

incretodiagnosis [inˌkriːtəuˌdaiəgˈnəusis] *n* 内分泌病诊断法

incretogenous [ˌinkriˈtɔdʒinəs] *a* 内分泌源的,激素源的

incretology [ˌinkriˈtɔlədʒi] *n* 内分泌学

incretopathy [ˌinkriˈtɔpəθi] *n* 内分泌病

incretory [ˈinkritəri] *a* 内分泌的

incretotherapy [inˌkriːtəuˈθerəpi] *n* 内分泌疗法

incross [ˈinkrɔs] *n* 纯合体交配(相同的纯合体之间的交配)

incrustation [ˌinkrʌsˈteiʃən] *n* 结痂;痂

incubate [ˈinkjubeit] *vt*, *vi* 孵育,孵化;(在恒温箱内)温育(早产婴儿);保温(将培养基或反应混合物保持在固定的温度下) *n* 孵育物

incubation [ˌinkjuˈbeiʃən] *n* 孵育,孵化;潜伏期;保温育婴(在恒温箱内温育早产婴儿);保温(将反应混合物保持在特定的温度的过程)

incubative [ˈinkjubeitiv] *a* 孵育的;潜伏期的

incubator [ˈinkjubeitə] *n* 恒温箱(早产婴儿保育箱);孵化器;培养箱(细菌培养器)

incubus [ˈiŋkjubəs]([复] **incubuses** 或 **incubi** [ˈiŋkjubai]) *n* 梦魇,梦魔;沉重精神负担

incudal [ˈiŋkjudl] *a* 砧骨的

incudectomy [ˌiŋkjuˈdektəmi] *n* 砧骨切除术

incudiform [iŋˈkjuːdifɔːm] *a* 砧形的,铁砧形的

incudomalleal [ˌiŋkjudəuˈmæliəl] *a* 砧锤[骨]的

incudomallear [ˌiŋkjudəuˈmæliə], **incudomalleolar** [ˌiŋkjudəuˌmeliˈəulə] *a* 砧锤[骨]的

incudostapedial [ˌiŋkjudəustəˈpiːdiəl] *a* 砧镫[骨]的

incurable [inˈkjuərəbl] *a* 不能治愈的 *n* 患不治之症者 | **incurability** [inˌkjuərəˈbiləti] *n*

incurvate [ˈinkəːveit] *a* 弯曲的,向内弯曲的 *vt*, *vi* 弯曲,向内弯曲 | **incurvation** [ˌinkəːˈveiʃən] *n* 内曲,弯曲

incurve [inˈkəːv] *vt*, *vi* 弯曲,向内弯曲 *n* 弯曲,内弯

incus [ˈiŋkəs] *n* 砧骨

incyclophoria [inˌsaikləuˈfəuriə] *n* 内旋转隐斜

incyclotropia [inˌsaikləuˈtrəupiə] *n* 内旋转斜视

in d. in dies【拉】每日

indacrinic acid [ˌindəˈkrinik] 吲达克林酸(indacrinone 的 INN 名)

indacrinone [ˌindəˈkrainəun] *n* 茚达立酮(促尿酸排泄的利尿药)

indanedione [ˌindeinˈdaiəun] *n* 茚满二酮

indapamide [inˈdæpəmaid] *n* 吲达帕胺(抗高血压药,利尿药)

Indecidua [ˌindiˈsidjuə] *n* 无蜕膜类(动物)

indenization [inˌdenaiˈzeiʃən, -niˈz-] *n* 移生,移地发育

indentation [ˌindenˈteiʃən] *n* 压痕;切迹,凹入

index [ˈindeks]([复] **indexes** 或 **indices** [ˈindisiːz]) *n* 示指;指数;索引 | ACH ~ 臂胸髋指数(根据臂围〈arm girth〉、胸厚〈chest depth〉及髋宽〈hip width〉的测量表示儿童营养状况的指数) / altitudinal ~, height ~, length-height ~ 颅长高指数 / antitryptic ~ 抗胰蛋白酶指数(检癌) / auricular ~ 耳幅高指数 / auriculoparietal ~ 耳顶幅指数/auriculovertical ~ 头耳高指数 / baric ~ 体重身长指数〔100×体重 kg/(身长 cm)^3〕/ basilar ~ 颅槽指数 / biochemical racial ~ 生物化学种族指数(红细胞中有凝集原 A 的人数百分率和有凝集原 B 的人数百分率之比,或血型Ⅱ的人数与血型Ⅲ的人数之比) / body build ~ 体格指数(体重除以身高的平方) / calcium ~ 血钙指数 / cardiothoracic ~ 心胸横径指数(心胸横径比率) / cephalic ~ 颅指数 / color ~ 血色指数 / coronofrontal ~ 冠额指数 / Cumulated Index Medicus 累积医学索引(美国国家医学图书馆年刊) / cytophagic ~ 细胞吞噬指数 / dental ~ 牙指数(牙长度乘 100 再除以鼻基

底线长度）/ generation ~ 各代增长指数（细菌）/ gnathic ~, alveolar ~颌指数，颌突度 / hematopneic ~ 血氧合［作用］指数 / hemophagocytic ~, opsonocytophagic ~ 血吞噬指数，调理吞噬指数 / hemorenal ~, hemorenalsalt ~ 尿血无机盐指数 / length-breadth ~ 颅长阔指数 / leukopenic ~ 白细胞减少指数 / lower leg-foot ~ 小腿足长指数 / Index Medicus 医学索引（美国国家医学图书馆月刊）/ mitotic ~ 有丝分裂指数 / opsonic ~ 调理指数 / sedimentation ~ 血沉指数 / short increment sensitivity ~（SISI）短增量敏感指数 / spleen ~ 脾肿指数（居民中脾肿大的百分率，用于疟疾调查）/ staphylo-opsonic ~ 葡萄球菌调理指数 / stimulation ~（SI）刺激指数 / thoracic ~ 胸径指数 / tuberculo-opsonic ~ 结核菌调理指数 / vertical ~ 颅长高指数 / vital ~ 生命指数，出生死亡比率

indicanemia ［ˌindikəˈniːmiə］ *n* 尿蓝母血

indicanmeter ［ˌindikənˈmiːtə］ *n* 尿蓝母定量器

indicanorachia ［ˌindikənəˈreikiə］ *n* 尿蓝母脑脊液

indicant ［ˈindikənt］ *a* 指示的 *n* 指征

indicanuria ［ˌindikəˈnjuəriə］ *n* 尿蓝母尿

indicarmine ［ˌindiˈkɑːmin］ *n* 靛卡红，靛胭脂

indicate ［ˈindikeit］ *vt* 指示，指出；表明；需要

indicatio ［ˌindiˈkeiʃiəu］ *n*【拉】指征，适应证

indication ［ˌindiˈkeiʃən］ *n* 指示，指征；适应证

indicophose ［ˈindiˌkəufəuz］ *n* 青幻视，蓝幻视

Indiella ［ˌindiˈelə］ *n* 白色足霉菌属

indifférence ［anˌdifeˈrɑːns］ *n*【法】淡漠，漠不关心 | belle ~ ［ˌbelənˌdifeˈrɑːns］泰然漠视（指癔症患者对自己躯体症状采取自满的态度）

indifferent ［inˈdifrənt］ *a* 不关心的，淡漠的；中性的；无亲和力的

indigenous ［inˈdidʒinəs］ *a* 原产的，本土的，土生的

indigested ［ˌindiˈdʒestid, ˌindai-］ *a* 未消化的

indigestible ［ˌindiˈdʒestəbl, ˌindai-］ *a* 不消化的

indigestion ［ˌindiˈdʒestʃən, ˌindai-］ *n* 消化不良 | acid ~ 胃酸过多性消化不良，胃酸过多［症］/ fat ~ 脂肪消化不良，脂肪痢 / gastric ~ 胃消化不良 / intestinal ~ 肠消化不良 / nervous ~ 神经性消化不良 / sugar ~ 糖消化不良 | **indigestive** ［ˌindiˈdʒestiv, ˌindai-］ *a*

indigitation ［inˌdidʒiˈteiʃən］ *n* 套叠

indiglucin ［ˌindiˈgluːsin］ *n* 靛糖

indigo ［ˈindigəu］（［复］**indigo⟨e⟩s**）*n* 靛，靛蓝

Indigofera ［ˌindiˈgɔfərə］ *n* 木蓝属

indigogen ［ˈindigəudʒən］ *n* 靛原，靛白

indigopurpurine ［ˌindigəuˈpəːpjurin］ *n* 靛紫红

indigotic ［ˌindiˈgɔtik］ *a* 靛蓝的，靛青的

indigotin ［ˌindiˈgəutin］ *n* 靛蓝，靛蓝色

indigotindisulfonate sodium ［ˌindiˌgəutindaiˈsʌlfəneit］ 靛蓝二磺酸钠（用于肾功能试验，亦称靛胭脂，可溶性靛蓝）

indinavir sulfate ［inˈdinəvir］ 硫酸印地那韦（会引起未成熟无病毒颗粒形成的一种 HIV 蛋白酶抑制剂，用于治疗人免疫缺陷病毒感染和获得性免疫缺陷综合征，口服给药）

indirect ［ˌindiˈrekt, ˌindaiˈrekt］ *a* 间接的

indirubin ［ˌindiˈruːbin］ *n* 靛红

indirubinuria ［ˌindiˌruːbiˈnjuəriə］ *n* 靛红尿

indiscriminate ［ˌindisˈkriminit］ *a* 无差别的，普遍的

indisposed ［ˌindisˈpəuzd］ *a* 不舒服的，有病的

indisposition ［ˌindispəˈziʃən］ *n* 不舒服，不适，违和

indium（In） ［ˈindiəm］ *n* 铟（化学元素）

individuate ［ˌindiˈvidjueit, -dʒu-］ *vt* 使个体化，使具个性（或特色）| **individuation** ［ˌindiˌvidjuˈeiʃən, -dʒu-］ *n* 个性发生；个体化

indolaceturia ［ˌindəuˌlæsiˈtjuəriə］ *n* 吲哚乙酸尿

indolamine ［inˈdɔləmiːn］ *n* 吲哚胺（吲哚的衍生物，如 5-羟色胺或褪黑激素）

indole ［ˈindəul］ *n* 吲哚

indoleacetic acid ［ˌindəuləˈsiːtik］ 吲哚乙酸

indolent ［ˈindələnt］ *a* 无痛的 | **indolence** ［ˈindələns］ *n*

indologenous ［ˌindəuˈlɔdʒinəs］ *a* 吲哚生成的

indoluria ［ˌindəuˈljuəriə］ *n* 吲哚尿

indomethacin ［ˌindəuˈmeθəsin］ *n* 吲哚美辛（消炎镇痛药）

indophenol ［ˌindəuˈfiːnɔl］ *n* 靛酚

indophenolase ［ˌindəuˈfiːnəuleis］ *n* 靛酚酶

indophenol-oxidase ［ˌindəuˌfiːnɔlˈɔksideis］ *n* 靛酚氧化酶，细胞色素氧化酶

indoprofen ［ˌindəuˈprəufən］ *n* 吲哚洛芬（消炎镇痛药）

indopropionic acid ［ˌindəuprəupiˈɔnik］ 吲哚丙酸

indoramin ［inˈdɔrəmin］ *n* 吲哚拉明（抗高血压药）

indoxole ［inˈdɔksəul］ *n* 吲哚克索（退热、消炎药）

indoxyl ［inˈdɔksil］ *n* 吲哚酚

indoxylemia ［inˌdɔksiˈliːmiə］ *n* 吲哚酚血

indoxylglucuronic acid ［inˌdɔksilgluːkjuəˈrɔnik］ 葡糖吲哚苷酸

indoxylic acid ［ˌindɔkˈsilik］ 羟吲哚酸

indoxyl-sulfate ［inˈdɔksil ˈsʌlfeit］ *n* 硫酸吲哚酚

indoxylsulfonic acid ［inˌdɔksilsʌlˈfɔnik］ 羟吲哚磺酸

indoxyluria ［ˌindɔksiˈljuəriə］ *n* 吲哚酚尿

indriline hydrochloride ［ˈindriliːn］ 盐酸茚屈林（中枢神经系统兴奋药）

induce ［inˈdjuːs］ *vt* 诱导，诱发；感应 | **~d** *a* 人工

的;诱导的;感应的 | **~r** *n* 诱导物,诱导剂
inducible [in'dju:sibl] *a* 可诱导的
inductance [in'dʌktəns] *n* 电感;感应系数
inductile [in'dʌktail] *a* 无延性的
induction [in'dʌkʃən] *n* 诱导;感应 | autonomous ~ 自身感应 / complementary ~ 补偿感应 / somatic ~ 躯体诱导 / spinal ~ 脊髓诱导
inductive [in'dʌktiv] *a* 诱发的;感应的
inductogram [in'dʌktəgræm] *n* X 线【照】片
inductor [in'dʌktə] *n* 诱导者,诱导物;诱导体;感应器,感应机
inductorium [ˌindʌk'tɔ:riəm] *n* 感应器
inductotherm [ˌin'dʌktəθə:m] *n* 感应电热器
inductothermy [in'dʌktəˌθə:mi] *n* 感应电热疗法
induline ['indjuli:n], **indulin** ['indjulin] *n* 引杜林,对氮蒽蓝(染料)
indulinophil [ˌindju'linəfil] *n* 嗜引杜林质 *a* 嗜引杜林的
indulinophilic [ˌindjulinə'filik] *a* 嗜引杜林的
indurate ['indjuəreit] *vt* 使硬化,使硬结 *vi* 变硬 ['indjuərit] *a* 硬化的 | **~d** ['indjuəˌreitid], **indurative** ['indjuərətiv] *a* 硬结的
induration [ˌindjuə'reiʃən] *n* 硬结 | black ~ 黑色硬结(见于肺炎) / brawny ~【组织】硬结 / fibroid ~ 纤维性硬结,硬变 / granular ~ 颗粒性硬结,硬变 / gray ~ 灰色硬结(肺炎时或肺炎后肺组织硬结,但无色素沉着) / laminate ~, parchment ~ 层片硬结(下疳底) / penile ~ 阴茎硬结 / phlebitis ~ 静脉炎性硬结,硬结性蜂窝织炎 / plastic ~ 阴茎海绵体硬结症 / red ~ 红色硬结(间质性肺炎时)
indusium griseum [in'dju:ziəm 'grisiəm]【拉】灰被(胼胝体上回)
indwelling ['indweliŋ] *a* 留置的(指留在器官内的导管以便引流或给药等)
-ine [后缀]生物碱,有机碱,卤素
inebriant [i'ni:briənt] *a* 致醉的 *n* 酩酊剂,致醉剂
inebriate [i'ni:brieit] *vt* 使醉 [i'ni:briit] *a* 酒醉的 *n* 醉汉 | **inebriation** [iˌni:bri'eiʃən] *n* 醉[状]
inebriety [ˌini(:)'braiəti] *n* 醉癖,习惯性酒醉
inedible [in'edibl] *a* 不可食的,不适合食用的
inefficacious [ˌinefi'keiʃəs] *a* 无效的,无效力的,疗效不好的
inefficacy [in'efikəsi] *n* 无效,无效力,无疗效
inelastic [ˌini'læstik] *a* 无弹性的;无适应性的
Inermicapsifer [iˌnə:mi'kæpsifə] *n* 无头虫属
inert [i'nə:t] *a* 无活动力的;惰性的(如惰性气体),不活泼的
inertia [i'nə:ʃjə] *n*【拉】惯性;不活动,无力,惰性 | colonic ~ 结肠无力 / immunological ~ 免疫惰性(母体对胎儿或胎儿对母体的组织相容性抗原发生一种不属免疫耐受性的特殊免疫抑制) / ~ uteri 宫缩乏力
inertial [i'nə:ʃjəl] *a* 惯性的
in extremis [in ek'stri:mis]【拉】濒死,将死,临终时
Inf. infunde【拉】注入,倒入
infancy ['infənsi] *n* 婴儿期
infant ['infənt] *n* 婴儿 | floppy ~ 松软婴儿(见 syndrome 项下相应术语) / immature ~ 不成熟儿 / mature ~ 成熟儿 / newborn ~ 新生儿 / postmature ~, postterm ~ 过熟儿 / premature ~ 早产儿,未成熟儿 / preterm ~ 早产儿 / term ~ 足月儿
infanticide [in'fæntisaid] *n* 杀婴现象,杀婴者
infanticulture [in'fæntiˌkʌltʃə] *n* 育儿法
infantile ['infəntail] *a* 婴儿[期]的,幼稚的
infantilism [in'fæntilizəm] *n* 幼稚症 | cachectic ~ 恶病质性幼稚症 / celiac ~ 粥样泻性幼稚症(乳糜泻) / dysthyroidal ~ 甲状腺功能障碍性幼稚症 / hepatic ~ 肝硬化性幼稚症 / hypophyseal ~, pituitary ~ 垂体性幼稚症 / intestinal ~ 肠性幼稚症(婴儿型非热带性口炎性腹泻) / lymphatic ~ 淋巴[体质]性幼稚症 / myxedematous ~ 黏液水肿性幼稚症 / regressive ~, reversive ~, tardy ~ 迟发幼稚症(成年期发育停顿) / renal ~ 肾性幼稚症 / universal ~ 全身性幼稚症
infantorium [ˌinfən'tɔ:riəm] *n* 婴儿医院
infarct [in'fɑ:kt] *n* 梗死 | anemic ~, pale ~, white ~ 贫血性梗死,白梗死 / bilirubin ~s 胆红素性梗死(尤见于新生儿肾锥体内) / bland ~ 单纯梗死(非感染性梗死) / calcareous ~ 钙盐沉着,石灰质梗死 / embolic ~ 栓子性梗死 / hemorrhagic ~, red ~ 出血性梗死,红梗死 / thrombotic ~ 血栓性梗死 / uric acid ~ 尿酸梗死,尿酸沉着(新生儿肾小管内)
infarctectomy [ˌinfɑ:k'tektəmi] *n* 梗死切除术
infarction [in'fɑ:kʃən] *n* 梗死形成;梗死 | cerebral ~ 脑梗死 / myocardial ~, cardiac ~ 心肌梗死 / pulmonary ~ 肺梗死
infaust ['infaust] *a* 不利的,不良的
infect [in'fekt] *vt* 传染,感染 | **~ed** *a* 传染的,感染的
infectible [in'fektəbl] *a* 能受感染的
infection [in'fekʃən] *n* 传染;感染,侵染;传染病 | airborne ~, aerial ~ 空气传染 / apical ~ [牙]根尖感染 / autochthonous ~ 本地性感染(由环境内,如病房的病原引起的感染) / colonization ~ 定居传染(侵入病菌对组织或在组织内附着和生长的一种传染) / cross ~ 交叉感染,交叉传染 / cryptogenic ~ 隐原性感染 / diaplacental ~ 经胎盘感染 / direct ~, contact ~ 直接传染,接触传染 / droplet ~ 飞沫传染 /

dustborne ~ 尘埃传播传染 / endogenous ~ 内源性感染 / exogenous ~ 外源性感染 / focal ~ 灶性感染 / germinal ~ 胚性传染 / herd ~ 群体传染(流行病学术语,指一大群人或动物发生的传染) / iatrogenic ~ 医源性感染 / indirect ~ 间接传染 / latent ~ 潜在性感染 / mass ~ 重大感染(在血液循环中有大量病原微生物引起的感染) / mixed ~ 混合感染 / nosocomial ~ 医院内感染 / opportunistic ~ 机会性感染 / phytogenic ~ 寄生植物性感染 / pyogenic ~ 脓性感染 / retrograde ~ 逆行性感染(在管腔内与分泌或排泄流向相反的上行感染,如泌尿道感染) / secondary ~ 继发感染,续发感染 / subclinical ~, inapparent ~, silent ~ 亚临床感染,隐性感染,不显性感染(无明显症状的感染,但这种感染是由能产生易于识别的疾病,如脊髓灰质炎或腮腺炎的微生物所引起) / terminal ~, agonal ~ 末期感染,濒死期感染 / vecto-borne ~ 虫传感染 / viral respiratory ~ 病毒性呼吸道感染

infectiosity [inˌfekʃiˈɔsəti] *n* 传染度,感染度

infectious [inˈfekʃəs] *a* 传染性的 | ~ nucleic acid 传染性核酸 | **~ness** *n* 传染性,传染力

infective [inˈfektiv] *a* 传染性的,感染性的 | **infectivity** [ˌinfekˈtivəti] *n* 传染性,感染性,侵染性

infecundity [ˌinfiˈkʌndəti] *n* 不[生]育,无生育力

inferent [ˈinfərənt] *a* 传入的,输入的

inferior [inˈfiəriə] *a* (位置)下方的;下面的

inferiority [inˌfiəriˈɔrəti] *n* 下位;自卑,低劣 | constitutional psychopathic ~ 素质性病态人格性低劣 / psychopathic ~ 病态人格性低劣

inferolateral [ˌinfərəuˈlætərəl] *a* 下侧的

inferomedian [ˌinfərəuˈmiːdjən] *a* 下中的

inferonasal [infiərəuˈneizl] *a* 鼻下的

inferoposterior [ˌinfərəu pɔsˈtiəriə] *a* 下后的

inferotemporal [infiərəuˈtempərəl] *a* 颞下的

infertile [inˈfəːtail] *a* 不孕的,不育的

infertilitas [ˌinfəˈtilitəs] *n* 【拉】不孕,不育

infertility [ˌinfəˈtiləti] *n* 不孕,不育 | primary ~ 原发不孕(患者从未受孕) / secondary ~ 继发不孕(患者曾受孕)

infest [inˈfest] *vt* 侵扰;感染 | **~ation** [ˌinfesˈteiʃən] *n* 侵扰;侵染,感染

infibulation [infibjuːˈleiʃən] *n* 锁阴术,阴部扣锁法

infiltrate [ˈinfiltreit, inˈfiltreit] *vi, vt* 浸润 *n* 渗入物,浸润物 | **infiltrative** [ˈinfilˌtreitiv] *a* 浸润的

infiltration [ˌinfilˈtreiʃən] *n* 浸润 | calcareous ~ 石灰质浸润 / calcium ~ 钙质浸润 / cellular ~ 细胞浸润 / epituberculous ~ 结核灶周围浸润,上部肺结核浸润 / fatty ~, adipose ~ 脂肪浸润 / gray ~, gelatinous 灰色浸润,胶样浸润(结核性胶样肺炎) / paraneural ~ 神经周麻醉 / sanguineous ~ 血【液】浸润 / tuberculous ~ 结核浸润 / urinous ~ 尿浸润,尿外渗

infirm [inˈfəːm] *a* 虚弱的

infirmary [inˈfəːməri] *n* 医务所,医务室,小医院

infirmity [inˈfəːməti] *n* 体弱,虚弱;意志薄弱;虚弱病症

inflammagen [inˈflæmədʒən] *n* 促炎物质

inflammation [ˌinfləˈmeiʃən] *n* 炎症 | acute ~ 急性炎 / adhesive ~ 粘连性炎 / atrophic ~, cirrhotic ~, fibroid ~, sclerosing ~ 萎缩性炎,硬变性炎,纤维性炎,硬化性炎 / catarrhal ~ 卡他性炎 / chronic ~ 慢性炎 / croupous ~ 格鲁布性炎,假膜性炎 / diffuse ~ 弥散性炎 / disseminated ~ 播散性炎 / exudative ~ 渗出性炎 / fibrinous ~ 纤维蛋白性炎 / focal ~ 局灶性炎 / hyperplastic ~, plastic ~, productive ~, proliferous ~ 增生性炎 / interstitial ~ 间质性炎 / metastatic ~转移性炎 / seroplastic ~ 浆液组织形成性炎 / suppurative ~, purulent ~ 化脓性炎,脓性炎

inflammatory [inˈflæmətəri] *a* 炎的,炎性的

inflatable [inˈfleitbl] *a* 可膨胀的

inflate [inˈfleit] *vt* 使充气;使膨胀 *vi* 进行充气;膨胀

inflation [inˈfleiʃən] *n* 充气;膨胀;吹张,吹张法 | **inflator**, **inflater** [inˈfleitə] *n* 吹张器

inflect [inˈflekt] *vt* 内曲

inflection, **inflexion** [inˈflekʃən] *n* 内曲,屈曲

infliximab [inˈfliksimæb] *n* 英昔单抗(一种嵌合人-鼠免疫球蛋白,充作抗肿瘤坏死因子抗体,静脉注射给药,治疗局限性肠炎和类风湿关节炎)

inflorescence [ˌinflɔ(ː)ˈresns] *n* 花序(植物);生殖苞(苔藓)

inflow [ˈinfləu] *n* 流入;流入物 | coronary arterial ~ 冠状动脉流入血流

influent [ˈinfluənt] *a* 流入的 *n* 流入

influenza [ˌinfluˈenzə] *n* 流行性感冒,流感 | ~ A 甲型流感 / Asian ~ 亚洲流感(1957 年发生的甲型流感,据认为起源于中国) / avian ~ 禽流感(即新城疫 Newcastle disease) / ~ B 乙型流感 / ~ C 丙型流感 / endemic ~ 地方性流感,类流感 / epidemic ~ 流行性感冒 / feline ~ 猫流感 / Hong Kong ~ 香港流感(1968 年发生的甲型流感大流行,据认为起源于香港) / pandemic ~ 大流行性流感 / Russian ~ 俄罗斯流感(1978 年发生的甲型流感大流行,据认为起源于前苏联) | **~l** *a*

influenzavirus [ˌinfluˈenzəˌvaiərəs] *n* 流感病毒

influx [ˈinflʌks] *n* 流入,注入;内向通量

infolding [in'fəuldiŋ] *n* 内折
informant [in'fɔːmənt] *n* 病史申述者
information [ˌinfə'meiʃən] *n* 信息 | **~al** *a*
informosome [in'fɔːməsəum] *n* 信息体(mRNA和蛋白质的结合物,见于真核细胞的胞质中)
infra- [前缀]下
infra-axillary [ˌinfrə'æksiləri] *a* 腋下的
infrabulge ['infrəbʌldʒ] *n* 膨出下(牙)
infraciliature [ˌinfrə'siliətʃə] *n* 下层纤毛结构
infraclass ['infrəklɑːs] *n* 下纲(生物分类)
infraclavicular [ˌinfrəklə'vikjulə] *a* 锁骨下的
infraclusion [ˌinfrə'kluːʒən] *n* 低殆,低咬合
infracolic [ˌinfrə'kɔlik] *a* 结肠下的
infraconstrictor [ˌinfrəkən'striktə] *n* 咽下缩肌
infracortical [ˌinfrə'kɔːtikəl] *a* 皮质下的,皮层下的
infracostal [ˌinfrə'kɔstl] *a* 肋骨下的
infracotyloid [ˌinfrə'kɔtilɔid] *a* 髋臼下的
infraction [in'frækʃən] *n* 不全骨折
infradentale [ˌinfrəden'teili] *n* 牙下点,下颌中切牙下槽嵴顶点(头颅测量学名词,在下颌骨中切牙之间齿龈前面的最高点)
infradian [ˌinfrə'diːən, in'freidiːən] *a* 超昼夜的
infradiaphragmatic [ˌinfrəˌdaiəfræg'mætik] *a* 膈下的
infraduction [ˌinfrə'dʌkʃən] *n* 下转,眼下转
infraglenoid [ˌinfrə'gliːnɔid] *a* 关节盂下的
infraglottic [ˌinfrə'glɔtik] *a* 声门下的
infrahyoid [ˌinfrə'haiɔid] *a* 舌骨下的
infrainguinal [ˌinfrə'iŋgwənəl] *a* 腹股沟[韧带]下的
inframalleolar [ˌinfrəmæli'əulə] *a* 踝下的
inframamillary [ˌinfrə'mæmiləri] *a* 乳头下的
inframammary [ˌinfrə'mæməri] *a* 乳房下的
inframandibular [ˌinfrəmæn'dibjulə] *a* 下颌下的
inframarginal [ˌinfrə'mɑːdʒinl] *a* 缘下的
inframaxillary [ˌinfrə'mæksiləri] *a* 上颌下的
infranuclear [ˌinfrə'njuːkliə] *a* 核下的
infraocclusion [infrəə'kluːʒən] *n* 低殆,低咬合
infraorbital [ˌinfrə'ɔːbitl] *a* 眶下的
infrapatellar [ˌinfrəpə'telə] *a* 髌下的
infraplacement [ˌinfrə'pleismənt] *n* 向下移位
infrapopliteal [ˌinfrəpɔp'litiəl] *a* 腘下的
infratympanic [ˌinfrətim'pænik] *a* 鼓室下的
infrapsychic [ˌinfrə'saikik] *a* 精神域以下的;自动性的
infrared ['infrə'red] *a* 红外[线]的,红下的 *n* 红外线,红外区
infrascapular [ˌinfrə'skæpjulə] *a* 肩胛下的
infrasonic [ˌinfrə'sɔnik] *a* 听域下的,次声的,亚声频的,亚声速的
infraspinous [ˌinfrə'spainəs] *a* 冈下的,棘突下的
infrasternal [ˌinfrə'stəːnl] *a* 胸骨下的
infrastructure [ˌinfrə'strʌktʃə] *n* 下部结构 | implant ~ 植入结构(见 substructure 项下相应术语)
infratemporal [ˌinfrə'tempərəl] *a* 颞下的
infratentorial [ˌinfrəten'tɔːriəl] *a* 幕下的
infratonsillar [ˌinfrə'tɔnsilə] *a* 扁桃体下的
infratracheal [ˌinfrə'treikiəl] *a* 气管下的
infratrochlear [ˌinfrə'trɔkliə] *a* 滑车下的
infratubal [ˌinfrə'tjuːbəl] *a* 管下的
infraturbinal [ˌinfrə'təːbinl] *n* 下鼻甲
infraumbilical [ˌinfrəʌm'bilikəl] *a* 脐下的
infravergence [ˌinfrə'vəːdʒəns] *n* 下转(眼)
infraversion [ˌinfrə'vəːʒən] *n* 眼下斜;低位牙;下转(两眼共轭性下转)
infravesical [ˌinfrə'vesikəl] *a* 膀胱下的
infriction [in'frikʃən] *n* 涂擦法(皮肤上涂擦药物)
infundibular [ˌinfʌn'dibjulə], **infundibulate** [ˌinfʌn'dibjulit] *a* 漏斗的
infundibulectomy [ˌinfʌnˌdibju'lektəmi] *n* 动脉圆锥切除术
infundibuliform [ˌinfʌn'dibjulifɔːm] *a* 漏斗状的
infundibuloma [ˌinfʌndibju'ləumə] *n* (下丘脑)漏斗瘤
infundibulopelvic [ˌinfʌnˌdibjuləu'pelvik] *a* 漏斗骨盆的
infundibulum [ˌinfʌn'dibjuləm] ([复] **infundibula** [ˌinfʌn'dibjulə]) *n*【拉】漏斗;动脉圆锥 | crural ~ 股管 / ethmoidal ~ of cavity of nose, ~ of nose 鼻腔筛漏斗 / ethmoidal ~ of ethmoid bone 筛骨筛漏斗 / ~ of fallopian tube, ~ of uterine tube 输卵管漏斗 / ~ of heart 动脉圆锥 / ~ of hypothalamus 下丘脑漏斗 / infundibula of kidney 肾小盏 / ~ of urinary bladder 膀胱底
infuse [in'fjuːz] *vt* 注入;浸渍;泡制(药) *vi* 注;泡,浸 | **~r** *n* 注入器;浸渍器
infusible [in'fjuːzəbl] *a* 不熔的 | **infusibility** [infjuːzə'biləti] *n* 不熔性,难熔性
infusion [in'fjuːʒən] *n* 浸,浸出;浸渍;浸液,浸剂;输注,输液 | cold ~ 冷浸剂 / meat ~ 肉浸液 / saline ~ 盐水输注
infusodecoction [inˌfjuːzəudi'kɔkʃən] *n* 浸煎剂
Infusoria [ˌinfjuː'zɔːriə, -'sɔː-] [复] *n*【拉】纤毛虫类
infusorial [ˌinfjuː'zɔːriəl] *a* 纤毛虫的
infusorian [ˌinfjuː'zɔːriən] *n* 纤毛虫 *a* 纤毛虫的
infusoriotoxin [ˌinfjuːˌzɔːriəu'tɔksin] *n* 杀纤毛虫毒素
infusum [in'fjuːsəm] *n*【拉】浸剂
ingest [in'dʒest] *vt* 摄入,食入,摄食 | **~ion**

[in'dʒestʃən] *n* / **~ive** *a*
ingesta [in'dʒestə] [复] *n*【拉】饮食物
ingestant [in'dʒestənt] *n* 食入物,摄食物
ingluvies [in'gluːviiːz] *n*【拉】嗉囊;瘤胃(反刍类的第一胃)
Ingrassia's process (apophysis) [in'grɑːsiə] (Giovanni F. Ingrassia) 蝶骨小翼 | ~ wings 蝶骨翼(包括大翼及小翼)
ingravescent [ˌingrə'vesnt] *a* 渐重的
ingredient [ˌin'griːdjənt] *n* 组成部分,成分
ingrowing ['inˌgrəuiŋ] *a* 向内长的,长入肌肉内的
ingrown ['ingrəun] *a* 长在内的,向内长的,长入肌肉内的
ingrowth ['ingrəuθ] *n* 向内生长;向内生长物 | epithelial ~ 上皮向内生长
inguen ['iŋgwən] ([复] **inguina** ['iŋgwinə]) *n*【拉】腹股沟(旧名鼠蹊) | **inguinal** ['iŋgwinl] *a*
inguinoabdominal [ˌiŋgwinəuæb'dɔminl] *a* 腹股沟腹的
inguinocrural [ˌiŋgwinəu'kruərəl] *a* 腹股沟股的
inguinodynia [ˌiŋgwinəu'diniə] *n* 腹股沟痛
inguinolabial [ˌiŋgwinəu'leibjəl] *a* 腹股沟阴唇的
inguinoscrotal [ˌiŋgwinəu'skrəutl] *a* 腹股沟阴囊的
inhalant [in'heilənt] *a* 吸入的 *n* 吸入剂,吸入物 | antifoaming ~ 止泡吸入剂(以蒸汽方式吸入,防止肺水肿患者呼吸道泡沫形成)
inhalation [ˌinhə'leiʃən] *n* 吸入;吸入剂 | isoproterenol sulfate ~ 硫酸异丙肾上腺素吸入剂
inhalator ['inhəleitə] *n* 吸入器;人工呼吸器
inhale [in'heil] *vt* 吸入 *vi* 吸气
inhaler [in'heilə] *n* 吸入器;滤气器 | ether ~ 醚吸入器 / H. H. ~ 氧吸入器(治气体中毒患者,为 Henderson 和 Haggard 所发明,故名)
inheritance [in'heritəns] *n* 遗传 | alternative ~ 交替遗传 / amphigonous ~, biparental ~, duplex ~ 双亲遗传 / blending ~ 融合遗传 / codominant ~ 共显性遗传 / complemental ~ 互补遗传 / crisscross ~ 交叉遗传 / cytoplasmic ~ 细胞质遗传 / dominant ~ 显性遗传 / holandric ~ 男性遗传,限雄遗传 / hologynic ~ 女性遗传,限雌遗传 / homochronous ~ 同期遗传 / homotropic ~ 获得性遗传 / intermediate ~ 中间性遗传 / maternal ~ 母体[影响]遗传 / mendelian ~ 孟德尔遗传(见 Mendel's law) / mitochondrial ~ 线粒体遗传 / polygenic ~, quantitative ~ 多基因遗传,数量遗传(由许多基因的积累作用所控制的数量性状的遗传,其中每个基因只有微小的作用) / quasidominant ~ 类显性遗传 / recessive ~ 隐性遗传 / sex-linked ~ 性连锁遗传,伴性遗传
inhibin [in'hibin] *n* 抑制素(睾丸分泌的水溶性激素)
inhibit [in'hibit] *vt* 抑制 *vi* 起抑制作用
inhibition [ˌinhi'biʃən] *n* 抑制 | allogenic ~ 同种抑制 / allosteric ~ 变构性抑制(一种酶抑制) / competitive ~, selective ~ 竞争性抑制,选择性抑制 / contact ~ 接触性抑制 / endproduct ~, feedback ~ 终产物抑制,反馈抑制 / enzyme ~ 酶抑制 / hemagglutination ~ (HI, HAI) 血凝抑制反应,红细胞凝集抑制反应 / noncompetitive ~ 非竞争性抑制 / proactive ~ 前摄抑制(早先学到的东西干扰新学到的东西的记忆,参见 retroactive ~) / reciprocal ~ 交互抑制 / retroactive ~ 倒摄抑制(新学到的东西干扰早先学到的东西的记忆,参见 proactive ~) / uncompetitive ~ 非竞争性抑制
inhibitive [in'hibitiv] *a* 抑制的
inhibitor [in'hibitə] *n* 抑制剂;抑制物 | angiotensin converting enzyme(ACE) ~s血管紧张素转化酶抑制剂 / C̄1̄ ~ (C̄1̄ INH) C̄1̄抑制因子 / carbonic anhydrase ~ 碳酸酐酶抑制剂 / C1 esterase ~ C1 酯酶抑制因子 / cholesterol ~ 胆固醇抑制剂 / cholinesterase ~ 胆碱酯酶抑制剂,抗胆碱酯酶 / membrane attack complex ~ (MACINH) 膜攻击复合物抑制剂,S 蛋白 / monoamine oxidase ~ (MAOI) 单胺氧化酶抑制剂
inhibitory [in'hibitəri] *a* 抑制的
inhibitrope [in'hibitrəup] *n* 抑制倾向者
inhomogeneity [inˌhɔməudʒe'niːiti] *n* 不纯一性,不同质性,不匀一性
inhomogeneous [ˌinˌhɔmə'dʒiːnjəs] *a* 不纯一的,不同质的
iniac ['iniæk], **inial**['iniəl] *a* 枕外隆凸点的
iniad ['iniæd] *ad* 向枕外隆凸点
iniencephalus [ˌinien'sefələs] *n* 枕骨裂脑露畸胎
iniencephaly [ˌinien'sefəli] *n* 枕骨裂脑露畸形
inio-[构词成分] 枕[骨]部
Inocybe [ai'nɔsibi] *n* 锈伞属
inodilator [ˌinəu'daileitə] *n* 纤维扩张剂
iniodymus [ˌini'ɔdiməs] *n* 枕部联胎
inion ['iniən] *n* 枕外隆凸点
iniopagus [ˌini'ɔpəgəs] *n* 枕部联胎
inoperculate [ˌinəu'pəːkjuleit] *a* 无囊盖的(指子囊)
iniops ['iniɔps] *n* 双脸畸胎
initial [i'niʃəl] *a* 初期的,开始的 *n* 原始细胞
initiate [i'niʃieit] *vt* 开始,起始 | **initiator**[i'niʃieitə] *n* 起始物,起始因子;(树脂聚合)引发剂;起始密码子

initiation [iˌniʃi'eiʃən] *n* 开始,起始
initis [i'naitis] *n* 肌炎
inject [in'dʒekt] *vt* 注射,注入
injectable [in'dʒektəbl] *a* 可注射的 *n* 注射物
injected [in'dʒektid] *a* 注入的;充血的
injectio [in'dʒekʃiəu]([复] **injectiones** [inˌdʒekʃi'əuniːz]) *n*【拉】注射;注射液
injection [in'dʒekʃən] *n* 注射;注射剂,注射液,针剂;充血 | adrenal cortex ~ 肾上腺皮质注射剂 / anatomical ~ 解剖[用]注射液 / circumcorneal ~ 角膜周围充血 / coarse ~大血管注射[液] / dextrose ~葡萄糖注射[液] / epifascial ~ 筋膜上注射 / ethiodized oil ~ 乙碘油注射剂 / fine ~ 小血管注射液 / fructose ~ 果糖注射液 / gaseous ~ 气体注射 / gelatin ~ 明胶注射液 / hypodermic ~, subcutaneous ~ 皮下注射 / insulin ~ 胰岛素注射液 / intracutaneous ~, intradermal ~, intradermic ~, endermic ~ 皮内注射 / intramuscular ~ 肌内注射 / intrathecal ~ 鞘内注射 / intravascular ~ 血管[内]注射 / intravenous ~ 静脉注射 / iodinated ^{125}I albumin ~ 碘[^{125}I]化清蛋白注射剂 / iodinated I 131 albumin ~ 碘[^{131}I]化清蛋白注射剂 / iron dextran ~ 葡聚糖铁注射剂 / iron sorbitex ~ 山梨糖醇铁注射剂 / jet ~ 喷射注射 / opacifying ~ 造影注射 / paraperiosteal ~ 骨膜旁注射 / parathyroid ~ 甲状旁腺注射剂 / parenchymatous ~ 主质内注射 / posterior pituitary ~ 垂体后叶注射液 / preservative ~ 防腐性注射剂 / protamine sulfate ~ 硫酸[鱼]精蛋白注射剂 / protein hydrolysate ~ 水解蛋白注射液 / sclerosing ~ 硬化性注射(如将枸橼酸钠注入血管,治静脉曲张及血管瘤等) / sensitizing ~, exciting ~, preparatory ~ 致敏性注射,准备性注射(第一次注射致敏性抗原) / sodium chloride ~ 氯化钠注射液 / sodium pertechnetate [^{99m}Tc] ~ 高锝酸钠锝[^{99m}Tc]注射液 / technetium Tc 99m albumin aggregated ~ 锝[^{99m}Tc]清蛋白聚集注射液 / vasopressin ~ 加压素注射剂(抗利尿药)
injector [in'dʒektə] *n* 注射器
injury ['indʒəri] *n* 损伤,损害 | birth ~ 产伤 / blast ~ 冲击伤 / deceleration ~ 减速性[损]伤 / egg-white ~ 生物素缺乏 / steering-wheel ~ 驾驶盘伤(驾驶员猛撞驾驶盘所致的胸部损伤,有时为心脏挫伤) / whiplash ~ 挥鞭伤(第四和第五颈椎联接处脊柱和脊髓损伤,例如汽车相撞时由于身体的加速和减速过猛所致,因颈椎的活动度较大,上四个颈椎作用如皮鞭,下三个为鞭柄)
inlay ['in'lei] *vt* 嵌入 ['inlei] *n* 嵌体;内置法,嵌入法 | epithelial ~ 上皮嵌体;上皮内置[法] / gold ~, cast ~ 金嵌体 / porcelain ~ 瓷嵌体
inlet ['inlet] *n* 入口 | pelvic ~ 骨盆入口,骨盆上口
inmate ['inmeit] *n* (精神病院等)被收容者;(医院的)住院者
INN International Nonproprietary Names 国际非专利药名,国际非专有药名
innate ['i'neit] *a* 天生的;先天的
inner ['inə] *a* 内部的;内心的;精神的
innervate ['inəːveit] *vt* 使受神经支配
innervation [ˌinəː'veiʃən] *n* 神经支配;神经分布 | double ~ 双重神经支配 / reciprocal ~ 交互神经支配
innidiation [iˌnidi'eiʃən] *n* 移生,移地发育
innocent ['inəsnt] *a* 无害的;良性的
innocuous [i'nɔkjuəs] *a* 无害的;良性的
innominatal [iˌnɔmi'neitl] *a* 无名的(如无名动脉,无名骨)
innominate [i'nɔminit] *a* 未定名的,无名的
innoxious [i'nɔkʃəs] *a* 无害的
innutrition [ˌinju(ː)'triʃən] *n* 营养缺乏 | **innutritious** [ˌinju(ː)'triʃəs] *a*
in(o)- [构词成分]纤维
inoblast ['inəblæst] *n* 成纤维细胞
inoccipitia [iˌnɔksi'pitiə] *n* 枕叶缺失
inochondritis [ˌinəukɔn'draitis] *n* 纤维软骨炎
inoculability [iˌnɔkjulə'biləti] *n* 可接种性
inoculable [i'nɔkjuləbl] *a* 可接种的
inoculate [i'nɔkjuleit] *vt* 接种;预防注射 | **inoculative** *a* / **inoculator**[i'nɔkjuleitə] *n* 接种者;注射者;接种器
inoculation [iˌnɔkju'leiʃən] *n* 接种;预防注射 | curative ~ 治疗接种 / protective ~ 预防接种
inoculum [i'nɔkjuləm]([复] **inocula** [i'nɔkjulə]) *n*【拉】接种物
inocyte ['inəsait] *n* 纤维细胞
inogen ['inədʒən] *n* 肌收缩原
inogenesis [ˌinəu'dʒenisis] *n* 纤维组织形成
inogenous [i'nɔdʒinəs] *a* 纤维组织原的
inoglia [i'nɔgliə] *n* 纤维胶质
inohymenitis [ˌinəuˌhaimə'naitis] *n* 纤维膜炎
inolith ['inəliθ] *n* 纤维石
inomyositis [ˌinəuˌmaiə'saitis] *n* 纤维肌炎
inoperable [in'ɔpərəbl] *a* 不能手术的,不宜手术的
inopexia [ˌinəu'peksiə] *n* 血液自凝性
inophragma [ˌinəu'frægmə] *n* 基膜
inorganic [ˌinɔː'gænik] *a* 无器官的,非器质性的;无机的;无机物的 *n* 无机物
inorganic pyrophosphatase [ˌinɔː'gænik ˌpaiərəu'fɔsfəteis] 无机焦磷酸酶
inosclerosis [ˌinəusklia'rəusis] *n* 纤维组织硬化
inoscopy [i'nɔskəpi] *n* 纤维质消化检查

inosculate [iˈnɔskjuleit] *vi*, *vt* 吻合,连合 | **inosculation** [iˌnɔskjuˈleiʃən] *n*
inose [ˈinəus] *n* 肌醇,环己六醇
inosemia [ˌinəuˈsiːmiə] *n* 肌醇血;纤维蛋白血
inosinate [iˈnəusineit] *n* 肌苷酸盐
inosine [ˈinəsiːn] *n* 肌苷 | ~ monophosphate (IMP) 肌苷酸 / ~ triphosphate (ITP) 肌苷三磷酸
inosinic acid [ˌinəˈsinik] 肌苷酸
inositide [iˈnəusitaid] *n* 肌醇化物
inositis [ˌinəuˈsaitis] *n* 纤维织炎
inositol [iˈnəusitɔl] *n* 肌醇,环己六醇 | ~ niacinate 烟酸肌醇酯(周围血管扩张药) | **inosite** [ˈinəsait] *n*
inosituria [ˌinəusaiˈtjuəriə], **inositoluria** [ˌinəuˌsaitɔˈljuəriə] *n* 肌醇尿
inostosis [ˌinɔsˈtəusis] *n* 骨质再生
inosuria [ˌinəuˈsjuəriə] *n* 纤维蛋白尿
inotagma [ˌinəuˈtægmə] *n* 肌细胞收缩线
inotropic [ˌinəuˈtrɔpik] *a* 影响[肌]收缩力的,变力的 | negatively ~ 减弱肌收缩力的 / positively ~ 增强肌收缩力的
inotropism [iˈnɔtrəpizəm] *n* 肌收缩力变化,变力性
in ovo [inˈəuvəu]【拉】卵内
inpatient [ˈinˌpeiʃənt] *n* 住院病人
input [ˈinput] *n* 输入;输入端
inquest [ˈinkwest] *n* 验尸,检验
inquiline [ˈinkwilain] *n* 寄居物,寓栖动物(指寄居在另一生物体内的一种生物,但不从宿主中摄食营养)
inructation [ˌinrʌkˈteiʃən] *n* 咽气声
insalivate [inˈsæliveit] *vt* 混涎,和涎 | **insalivation** [inˌsæliˈveiʃən] *n* 混涎作用
Insall-Salvati ratio [ˈinsəl sɑːlˈvɑːtiː] (J. N. Insall; E. Salvati) 英-萨比(髌韧带长度与髌骨高度之比)
insalubrious [ˌinsəˈljuːbriəs] *a* 有碍健康的,有碍卫生的 | **insalubrity** [ˌinsəˈljuːbrəti] *n*
insane [inˈsein] *a* 精神错乱的,精神失常的
insanitary [inˈsænitəri] *a* 不卫生的,有害健康的
insanity [inˈsænəti] *n* 精神错乱,精神病 | affective ~, emotional ~ 情感性精神病 / alcoholic ~ 乙醇中毒性精神病 / alternating ~ 更替性精神病,躁狂抑郁性精神病 / anticipatory ~ 先发性精神病 / circular ~, cyclic ~ 循环型精神病 / climacteric ~ 更年期精神病,更年期忧郁症 / communicated ~, simultaneous ~ 感应性精神病 / compound ~ 混合性精神病 / compulsive ~ 强迫性精神病 / consecutive ~ 衔接性精神病 / doubting ~ 猜疑性精神病 / homochronous ~ 同年龄性精神病 / hysteric ~ 癔症性精神病,焦虑性癔症 / manic-depressive ~ 躁狂抑郁性精神病,躁郁病 / moral ~ 悖德精神病 / periodic ~ 周期性精神病,定期精神错乱 / recurrent ~ 间歇性精神病 / toxic ~ 中毒性精神病
inscriptio [inˈskripʃiəu] ([复] **inscriptiones** [inˌskripʃiˈəuniːz]) *n*【拉】划;交切,交叉
inscription [inˈskripʃən] *n* 划;药量记载 | tendinous ~ 腱划
insect [ˈinsekt] *n* 昆虫,虫
Insecta [inˈsektə] *n* 昆虫纲(六足纲)
insectarium [ˌinsekˈtɛəriəm] *n* 昆虫[饲养]室,养虫室
insecticide [inˈsektisaid] *a* 杀昆虫的 *n* 杀昆虫剂 | **insecticidal** [inˌsektiˈsaidl] *a*
insectifuge [inˈsektifjuːdʒ] *n* 驱昆虫剂
insectile [inˈsektail], **insectival** [ˌinsekˈtaivl] *a* [似]昆虫的
Insectivora [ˌinsekˈtivərə] *n* 食虫目(动物)
insectivore [inˈsektivɔː] *n* 食虫目动物
insectivorous [ˌinsekˈtivərəs] *a* 食虫的
insectology [ˌinsekˈtɔlədʒi] *n* 昆虫学
inseminate [inˈsemineit] *vt* 对…施人工授精
insemination [inˌsemiˈneiʃən] *n* 授精 | artificial ~ 人工授精 / donor ~, heterologous ~ 他精人工授精,异配[人工]授精 / homologous ~ 未精人工授精,同配[人工]授精
insenescence [ˌinsəˈnesns] *n* 衰老
insensible [inˈsensəbl] *a* 无感觉的,麻木的;不省人事的 | **insensibility** [inˌsensəˈbiləti] *n* / **insensibly** *ad*
insensitive [inˈsensitiv] *a* 不敏感的 | **insensitivity** [inˌsensiˈtivəti] *n* 不敏感症
insert [inˈsəːt] *vt* 插入,植入,嵌入 *vi* (肌肉)附着 [ˈinsəːt] *n* 插入物,嵌入物;插入片段 | intramucosal ~, mucosal ~ 黏膜内嵌入物 / package ~ 药物说明书
insertio [inˈsəːʃiəu] *n*【拉】附着
insertion [inˈsəːʃən] *n* 插入,植入,嵌入;(肌肉的)附着 | parasol ~ 伞形附着(脐带) / velamentous ~ 帆状附着(脐带)
insheathed [inˈʃiːðd] *a* 包于鞘内的,被包的
insidious [inˈsidiəs] *a* 隐袭的,隐伏的
insight [ˈinsait] *n* 自知力
in situ [inˈsitjuː]【拉】原位
insolation [ˌinsəuˈleiʃən] *n* 日光浴;日射病,中暑 | asphyxial ~ 窒息性日射病 / hyperpyrexial ~ 高热性日射病
insoluble [inˈsɔljubl] *a* 不溶解的 | **insolubility** [inˌsɔljuˈbiləti] *n* 不溶性
insolvable [inˈsɔlvəbl] *a* 不能解决的
insomnia [inˈsɔmniə] *n* 失眠[症] | **~c** [inˈsɔmniæk] *n* 失眠者

insomnic [in'sɔmnik] *a* 失眠的
insomnious [in'sɔmniəs] *a* 失眠的,患失眠症的
insonate [in'səuneit] *vt* 使接受超声波
insorption [in'sɔːpʃən] *n* 内吸渗(指胃肠道的内含物进入循环血液内)
InsP$_3$ insitol 1, 4, 5-triphosphate 肌醇 1, 4, 5-三磷酸
inspect [in'spekt] *vt* 检查,视察 | **~ion** [in'spekʃən] *n* 检查,视察;望诊
inspectionism [in'spekʃənizəm] *n* 窥阴癖,窥淫癖
inspersion [in'spəːʒən] *n* 撒粉法,扑粉法
inspirate ['inspireit] *vt* 吸气(吸入气体或空气)
inspiration [ˌinspə'reiʃən] *n* 吸气
inspirator ['inspəreitə] *n* 吸[入]器
inspiratory [in'spaiərətəri] *a* 吸入的,吸气的
inspire [in'spaiə] *vt* 吸入;注入 *vi* 吸入
inspirium [in'spaiəriəm] *n*【拉】吸[气]
inspirometer [ˌinspaiə'rɔmitə] *n* 吸气测量计
inspissate [in'spiseit] *vt* 蒸浓,浓缩 | **~d** [in'spiseitid] *a* 蒸浓的,浓缩的 / **inspissation** [ˌinspi'seiʃən] *n* 蒸浓法,浓缩法 / **inspissator** *n* 蒸浓器,浓缩器
instability [ˌinstə'biləti] *n* 不稳定性
instar ['instɑː] *n*【拉】龄期(幼虫两次蜕皮之间的时期)
instep ['instep] *n* 足背
instil(l) [in'stil] (-ll-) *vt* 滴注 | **instillation** [ˌinsti'leiʃən] *n* 滴注法
instillator ['instiˌleitə] *n* 滴注器
instinct ['instiŋkt] *n* 本能 | death ~ 死亡本能 / ego ~ 自我本能 / herd ~ 合群本能,群集本能 / mother ~ 母性本能
institute ['institjuːt] *n* 学会,协会;学院,(研究)所;基本原理 | ~ s of medicine 医学基本原理(尤指生理学、病理学及医学教育近缘学科)
institutionalization [ˌinstitjuːʃənəlai'zeiʃən, -li'z-] *n* 收容入院(常为精神病患者);适应收容环境(长期住院的患者过多依赖医院及医院的一套常规制度,因而他们独立活动的意志也就逐渐减少)
instrument ['instrumənt] *n* 仪器,器械;工具 | **~al** [ˌinstru'mentl] *a*
instrumentarium [ˌinstrumen'tɛəriəm] *n* 全套器械,特组器械
instrumentation [ˌinstrumen'teiʃən] *n* 器械用法,器械操作法
insuccation [ˌinsə'keiʃən] *n* 浸渍
insudate [in'sjuːdeit] *n* 蓄积物
insudation [ˌinsju'deiʃən] *n* 蓄积
insufficiency [ˌinsə'fiʃənsi] *n* 不充分,不足;功能不全;关闭不全 | active ~ 肌运动功能不全 / adrenal ~ 肾上腺皮质功能不全 / aortic ~ 主动脉瓣关闭不全 / cardiac ~ 心功能不全 / ~ of the externi 眼外直肌功能不全 / ~ of the eyelids 眼睑功能不全 / gastric ~, gastromotor ~ 胃运动功能不全,胃肌无力 / hepatic ~ 肝功能不全 / ~ of the interni 眼内直肌功能不全 / mitral ~ 二尖瓣关闭不全 / muscular ~ 肌功能不全 / myocardial ~ 心肌功能不全 / parathyroid ~ 甲状旁腺功能减退 / pulmonary ~ 肺动脉瓣关闭不全 / renal ~ 肾功能不全 / thyroid ~ 甲状腺功能减退 / tricuspid ~ 三尖瓣关闭不全 / uterine ~ 子宫功能不全 / ~ of the valves, valvular ~ 心瓣关闭不全 / velopharyngeal ~ 腭咽关闭不全 / venous ~ 静脉功能不全
insufficient [ˌinsə'fiʃənt] *a* 不足的,不够的;功能不全的
insufficientia [ˌinsəˌfiʃi'enʃiə] *n*【拉】功能不全;关闭不全
insufflate ['insəfleit] *vt* 吹入 | **insufflator** *n* 吹入器
insufflation [ˌinsə'fleiʃən] *n* 吹入法,注气法;吹入剂 | cranial ~ 颅内注气 / endotracheal ~ 气管内吹入法(胸内手术时用,使肺充气) / ~ of the lungs 肺吹气法(为人工呼吸用) / perirenal ~ 肾周注气法(为肾上腺 X 线造影用) / tubal ~ 输卵管通气术(见 Rubin's test①解)
insula ['insjulə, -sə-] ([复] **insulae** ['insjuliː, -sə-]) *n*【拉】岛;岛叶
insular ['insjulə, -sə-] *a* 岛的;胰岛的;脑岛的
insularine ['insjulərin, -sə-] *n* 海岛锡生藤碱
insular-pancreatotropic [ˌinsjulə'pæŋkriətəu'trɔpik] *a* 促胰岛的
insulation [ˌinsju'leiʃən] *n* 隔离;绝缘 | ventricular heat ~ 心室热绝缘
insulator ['insjuˌleitə] *n* 绝缘体
insulin ['insjulin, -sə-] *n* 胰岛素 | extended ~ zinc suspension 结晶性胰岛素锌混悬液 / globin zinc ~ injection 珠蛋白锌胰岛素注射液 / ~ injection 胰岛素注射液 / isophane ~ suspension, NPH ~ (Neutral Protamine Hagedorn) 低精蛋白锌胰岛素混悬液,中效低精蛋白锌胰岛素 / prompt ~ zinc suspension 非晶体胰岛素锌混悬液 / protamine zinc ~ suspension 精蛋白锌胰岛素混悬液(长效胰岛素) / regular ~ 普通胰岛素 / three-to-one ~ 3:1 胰岛素混合剂(普通胰岛素与精蛋白锌胰岛素 3:1 混合剂) / ~ zinc suspension 胰岛素锌混悬液
insulinase ['insjulineis] *n* 胰岛素酶
insuline ['insjulain] *n* 胰岛素
insulinemia [ˌinsjuli'niːmiə, -sə-] *n* 胰岛素血症
insulinlipodystrophy [ˌinsjulinˌlipəu'distrəfi, -sə-] *n* 胰岛素性脂肪萎缩

insulinogenesis [ˌinsjuˌlinəuˈdʒenisis, -sə-] *n* 胰岛素生成
insulinogenic [ˌinsjuˌlinəuˈdʒenik, -sə-] *a* 胰岛素源的,胰岛素性的
insulinoid [ˈinsjulinɔid, -sə-] *a* 胰岛素样的 *n* 类胰岛素
insulinoma [ˌinsjuliˈnəumə, -sə-] *n* 胰岛素瘤
insulinopathy [ˌinsjuliˈnɔpəθi] *n* 胰岛素病,胰岛素分泌异常
insulinopenic [ˌinsjulinəuˈpiːnik, -sə-] *a* 胰岛素分泌减少的
insulism [ˈinsjulizəm, -sə-] *n* 胰岛功能亢进,胰岛素过多;胰岛素过多性休克
insulitis [ˌinsjuˈlaitis, -sə-] *n* 胰岛炎
insulogenic [ˌinsjuləuˈdʒenik, -sə-] *a* 胰岛素源的,胰岛素性的
insuloma [ˌinsjuˈləumə, -sə-] *n* 胰岛素瘤
insulopathic [ˌinsjuləu ˈpæθik, -sə-] *a* 胰岛素分泌异常的
insultus [inˈsʌltəs] *n*【拉】发作
insusceptible [ˌinsəˈseptəbl] *a* 不受…影响的 | **insusceptibility** [ˌinsəˌseptəˈbiləti] *n* 不易感受性,无感受性;免疫性
intact [inˈtækt] *a* 未受损的;完整的,无伤的
intake [ˈinteik] *n* 吸入,纳入;摄取[量] | caloric ~ 热量摄取量 / fluid ~ 液体摄取
integration [ˌintiˈgreiʃən] *n* 整合[作用];同化[作用];协调 | biological ~ 生物整合 / primary ~ 初级整合(精神分析,指幼儿意识到自己的身体与心理和周围环境确有区别) / secondary ~ 次级整合(精神分析,初级整合后,心身各部分功能进一步协调统一,以适应社会性活动)
integrator [ˈintiˌgreitə] *n* 积分仪;体表测量计 | bioelectrical ~ 生物电积分仪
integrin [ˈintəgrin] *n* 整合素
integument [inˈtegjumənt] *n* 体被,皮;珠被,包膜 | common ~ 皮,皮肤 | **~ary** [inˌtegjuˈmentəri] *a* 体被的,皮的
integumentum [inˌtegjuˈmentəm] *n*【拉】体被,皮;珠被,包膜
in tela [inˈtiːlə]【拉】组织内
intellect [ˈintilekt] *n* 智力,才智 | **~ion** [ˌintiˈlekʃən] *n* 理解,智力活动 / **~tive** [ˌintiˈlektiv] *a* 智力的,有智力的
intellectual [ˌintiˈlektjuəl] *a* 智力的,理智的
intellectualization [ˌintiˌlektjuəlaiˈzeiʃən, -liˈz-] *n* 理智化
intelligence [inˈtelidʒəns] *n* 智力;(计算机)智能 | artificial ~ 人工智能 / crystallized ~ 晶化智力
intensify [inˈtensifai] *vt* 加强 *vi* 强化 | **intensification** [inˌtensifiˈkeiʃən] *n* 强化[作用];增强
intensimeter [ˌintenˈsimitə] *n* X 线强度计
intensionometer [inˌtensiəˈnɔmitə] *n* X 线强度量计
intensity [inˈtensəti] *n* 强度 | ~ of electric field 电场强度 / luminous ~ 发光强度 / ~ of roentgen rays X 线强度
intensive [inˈtensiv] *a* 加强的,增强的 *n* 加强器;加强剂
intensivist [inˈtensivist] *n* 监护室医师
intention [inˈtenʃən] *n* 意图,意向;愈合(见 healing)
inter- [前缀]间,中间
interaccessory [ˌintərækˈsesəri] *a* 副突间的(椎骨)
interacinar [ˌintəˈræsinə], **interacinous** [ˌintəˈræsinəs] *a* 腺泡间的
interact [ˌintərˈækt] *vi* 相互作用 | **~ive** *a*
interactant [ˌintərˈæktənt] *n* 相互作用物;反应物
interaction [ˌintərˈækʃən] *n* 相互作用,交互作用 | drug ~ 药物相互作用
interagglutination [ˌintərəgluːtiˈneiʃən] *n* 相互凝集反应
interalveolar [ˌintərælˈviələ] *a* 牙槽间的;小泡间的
interangular [ˌintərˈæŋgjulə] *a* 角间的
interannular [ˌintərˈænjulə] *a* 环间的
interarticular [ˌintərɑːˈtikjulə] *a* 关节间的
interarytenoid [ˌintərˌæriˈtiːnɔid] *a* 杓状软骨间的
interatrial [ˌintərˈeitriəl], **interauricular** [ˌintərɔːˈrikjulə] *a* [心]房间的
interbrain [ˈintəbrein] *n* 间脑;丘脑
intercalary [inˈtəːkələri] *a* 插入的,间介的
intercalate [inˈtəːkəleit] *vt* 插入,间介 | **intercalation** [inˌtəːkəˈleiʃən] *n* 插入[作用];嵌入;插语症
intercanalicular [ˌintəˌkænəˈlikjulə] *a* 小管间的
intercapillary [ˌintəˈkæpiləri] *a* 毛细[血]管间的
intercapitular [ˌintəkəˈpitjulə] *a* 小头间的
intercarotic [ˌintəkəˈrɔtik], **intercarotid** [ˌintəkəˈrɔtid] *a* 颈动脉间的
intercarpal [ˌintəˈkɑːpl] *a* 腕骨间的
intercartilaginous [ˌintəˌkɑːtiˈlædʒinəs] *a* 软骨间的
intercavernous [ˌintəˈkævənəs] *a* 腔间的
intercellular [ˌintəˈseljulə] *a* [细]胞间的
intercentral [ˌintəˈsentrəl] *a* 中枢间的
intercerebral [ˌintəˈseribrəl] *a* 脑间的,脑半球间的
interchange [ˌintəˈtʃeindʒ] *vt* 交换,交替 *vi* 交替发生 [ˈintəˌtʃeindʒ] *n* 交换,交替;易位

interchondral [ˌintəˈkɔndrəl] *a* 软骨间的
intercilium [ˌintəˈsiliəm] *n* 眉间
interclavicular [ˌintəkləˈvikjulə] *a* 锁骨间的
interclinoid [intəˈklainɔid] *a* 床突间的
intercoccygeal [ˌintəkɔkˈsidʒiəl] *a* 尾骨间的
intercolumnar [ˌintəkəˈlʌmnə] *a* 柱间的
intercondylar [ˌintəˈkɔndilə], **intercondyloid** [ˌintəˈkɔndilɔid], **intercondylous** [ˌintəˈkɔndiləs] *a* 髁间的
interconversion [ˌintəkənˈvəːʃən] *n* 互变[现象]
intercostal [ˌintəˈkɔstl] *a* 肋间的
intercostohumeral [ˌintəkɔstəuˈhjuːmərəl] *a* 肋间臂的
intercourse [ˈintəkɔːs] *n* 交际,往来;性交 | sexual ~ 性交
intercricothyrotomy [ˌintəˌkraikəuθaiˈrɔtəmi] *n* 喉下部切开术,环甲膜切开术
intercristal [ˌintəˈkristl] *a* 嵴间的
intercritical [ˌintəˈkritikəl] *a* 发作间期的(如痛风)
intercross [ˈintəkrɔs] *n* 互交(杂合体之间的交配)
intercrural [ˌintəˈkruərəl] *a* 股间的,脚间的
intercrystalline [intəˈkristəlain] *a* 晶粒间的
intercurrent [ˌintəˈkʌrənt] *a* 间发的,介入的
intercuspation [ˌintəkʌsˈpeiʃən] *n* 牙尖吻合
intercusping [ˌintəˈkʌspiŋ] *a* 牙尖吻合的
intercutaneomucous [ˌintəkjuˌteiniəuˈmjuːkəs] *a* 皮肤黏膜间的
interdeferential [ˌintəˌdefəˈrenʃəl] *a* 输精管间的
interdental [ˌintəˈdentl] *a* 牙间的
interdentale [ˌintədenˈteili] *n* 中切牙间点
interdentium [ˌintəˈdenʃiəm] *n* 牙间隙
interdependence [ˌintədiˈpendəns], **interdependency** [ˌintədiˈpendənsi] *n* 互相依赖,互相依存 | **interdepedent** *a*
interdialytic [intəˌdaiəˈlitik] *a* 透析间期的(指血液透析疗法之间的时期)
interdigit [ˌintəˈdidʒit] *n* 指间隙,趾间隙
interdigital [ˌintəˈdidʒitl] *a* 指间的,趾间的
interdigitate [intəˈdidʒiteit] *n* 并指,并趾;犬牙交错
interdigitation [ˌintəˌdidʒiˈteiʃən] *n* 并指,并趾;牙间交错
interface [ˈintəfeis] *n* 界面,接触面;(计算机)接口 | dineric ~ 二液界面 / electrospray ~ 电喷雾接口
interfacial [ˌintəˈfeiʃəl] *a* 界面的
interfascicular [ˌintəfəˈsikjulə] *a* 束间的
interfemoral [ˌintəˈfemərəl] *a* 股间的
interfemus [ˌintəˈfiːməs] *n* 【拉】股间,股内侧
interference [ˌintəˈfiərəns] *n* 干预,干涉;干扰[现象];阻碍 | caspal ~ 牙尖阻碍 / occlusal ~s 咬合阻碍 / proactive ~ 前摄干扰(见 inhibition 项下相应术语) / retroactive ~ 倒摄干扰(见 inhibition 项下相应术语)
interfering [ˌintəˈfiəriŋ] *a* 干涉的
interferometer [ˌintəfiəˈrɔmitə] *n* 干涉仪 | **interferometry** *n* 干涉量度学
interferon [ˌintəˈfiərɔn] *n* 干扰素 | ~-α (IFN-α) 干扰素 α / ~-β (IFN-β) 干扰素 β / epithelial ~, fibroblast ~, fibroepithelial ~ 上皮细胞干扰素,成纤维细胞干扰素,纤维上皮细胞干扰素(干扰素 β) / ~-γ (IFN-γ) 干扰素 γ / immune ~ 免疫干扰素(干扰素 γ) / leukocyte ~ 白细胞干扰素(干扰素 α) / type Ⅰ ~ Ⅰ型干扰素(干扰素 α 和干扰素 β) / type Ⅱ ~ Ⅱ型干扰素(干扰素 γ)
interfibrillar [ˌintəˈfaibrilə], **interfibrillary** [ˌintəˈfaibriləri] *a* 原纤维间的
interfibrous [ˌintəˈfaibrəs] *a* 纤维间的
interfilamentous [ˌintəˌfiləˈmentəs] *a* 丝间的
interfilar [ˌintəˈfailə] *a* 网丝间的
interfrontal [ˌintəˈfrʌntl] *a* 额骨间的
interfurca [ˌintəˈfəːkə] ([复] **interfurcae** [ˌintəˈfəːsiː]) *n* 牙根间区
interganglionic [ˌintəˌgæŋgliˈɔnik] *a* 神经节间的
intergemmal [ˌintəˈdʒeməl] *a* 味蕾间的,芽间的
intergenic [ˌintəˈdʒenik] *a* 基因间的
interglobular [ˌintəˈglɔbjulə] *a* 球间的
intergluteal [ˌintəˈgluːtiəl] *a* 臀间的
intergonial [ˌintəˈgəuniəl] *a* 下颌角间的
intergradation [ˌintəgrəˈdeiʃən] *n* 间渡,渐变(指物种间的杂交繁殖) | primary ~ 初级间渡 / secondary ~ 次级间渡
intergrade [ˈintəgreid] *n* 中间级,中间期 | sex ~ 雌雄间体
intergranular [ˌintəˈgrænjulə] *a* [脑]粒细胞间的
intergyral [ˌintəˈdʒaiərəl] *a* 脑回间的
interhemicerebral [ˌintəˌhemiˈseribrəl], **interhemispheric** [ˌintəˌhemiˈsferik] *a* [脑]半球间的
interictal [ˌintəˈriktl] *a* 发作间的
interior [inˈtiəriə] *a* 内部的 *n* 内部
interischiadic [ˌintərˌiskiˈædik] *a* 坐骨间的
interjacent [ˌintəˈdʒeisənt] *a* 处在中间的
interkinesis [ˌintəkaiˈniːsis, -kiˈn-] *n* 分裂间期(减数分裂的第一和第二次分裂之间的短暂间期)
interlabial [ˌintəˈleibjəl] *a* 唇间的
interlace [ˌintəˈleis] *vt*, *vi* 交错,交织

interlamellar [ˌintələˈmelə] *a* 板间的,层间的
interleukin [ˌintəˈljuːkin] *n* 白细胞介素,白介素 | ~-1(IL-1)白细胞介素1 / ~-2(IL-2)白细胞介素2 / ~-3(IL-3)白细胞介素3
interligamentary [ˌintəˌligəˈmentəri], **interligamentous** [ˌintəˌligəˈmentəs] *a* 韧带间的
interlobar [ˌintəˈləubə] *a* 叶间的
interlobitis [ˌintələuˈbaitis] *n* 叶间胸膜炎
interlobular [ˌintəˈlɔbjulə] *a* 小叶间的
interlocking [ˌintəˈlɔkiŋ] *n* [双胎]交锁
intermalleolar [ˌintəməˈliːələ] *a* 踝间的
intermammary [ˌintəˈmæməri] *a* 乳房间的
intermammillary [ˌintəˈmæmiləri] *a* 乳头间的
intermarriage [ˌintəˈmæridʒ] *n* 近亲结婚,血族结婚;异种结婚
intermaxilla [ˌintəmækˈsilə] *n* 上颌间骨
intermaxillary [ˌintəˈmæksiləri] *a* [上]颌间的
intermediary [ˌintəˈmiːdjəri] *a* 中间的 *n* 中间阶段
intermediate [ˌintə(ː)ˈmiːdjət] *a* 中间的 *n* 中间体,媒介物
intermedin [ˌintəˈmiːdin] *n* 垂体中间叶激素(即促黑素细胞激素,为两栖类动物脑下垂体中叶所分泌,故名)
intermediolateral [ˌintəˌmiːdiəuˈlætərəl] *a* 中间[与]外侧的
intermedium [ˌintəˈmiːdjəm] ([复] **intermidiums** 或 **intermedia** [ˌintəˈmiːdjə]) *n* 中间体,媒介物
intermedius [ˌintəˈmiːdiəs] *n* 中间部 *a* 中间的
intermembranous [ˌintəˈmembrənəs] *a* 膜间的
intermeningeal [ˌintəmiˈnindʒiəl] *a* 脑脊膜间的
intermenstrual [ˌintəˈmenstruəl] *a* [月]经间期的,经间的
intermenstruum [ˌintəˈmenstruəm] *n* [月]经间期
intermetacarpal [ˌintəˌmetəˈkɑːpl] *a* 掌骨间的
intermetameric [ˌintəˌmetəˈmerik] *a* 体节间的
intermetatarsal [ˌintəˌmetəˈtɑːsəl] *a* 跖骨间的
intermission [ˌintəˈmiʃən] *n* 间歇;间歇期
intermitotic [ˌintəmaiˈtɔtik] *a* 有丝分裂间期的
intermittent [ˌintəˈmitənt] *a* 间歇的;周期性的 | **intermittence** [ˌintəˈmitəns] *n* 间歇,中止;周期性
intermix [ˌintəˈmiks] *vt, vi* 混合,混杂
intermixture [ˌintəˈmikstʃə] *n* 混合,混合物
intermolecular [ˌintəməuˈlekjulə] *a* 分子间的
intermural [intəˈmjuərəl] *a* 壁间的
intermuscular [ˌintəˈmʌskjulə] *a* 肌间的
intern [ˈintəːn] *n* 实习医师 [inˈtəːn] *vt* 约束,禁闭
internal [inˈtəːnl] *a* 内的,内部的;内在的;体内的,内服的 *n* [复]内脏,内部器官
internalization [inˌtəːnəlaiˈzeiʃən, -liˈz-] *n* 内在化
internarial [ˌintəˈnɛəriəl] *a* 鼻孔间的
internasal [ˌintəˈneizəl] *a* 鼻骨间的
internatal [ˌintəˈneitl] *a* 臀间的
internation [ˌintəˈneiʃən] *n* 约束,禁闭(如对精神病患者)
International Nonproprietary Names 国际非专利药名,国际非专有药名
interne [inˈtəːn, ˈintəːn] *n*【法】实习医师
interneuron [ˌintəˈnjuərɔn] *n* 中间神经元
internist [inˈtəːnist] *n* 内科医师
internode [ˈintənəud] *n* 结间体 | **internodal** [ˌintəˈnəudl] *a* 结间的
internodular [ˌintəˈnɔdjulə] *a* 小结间的,结间的
internship [ˈintəːnʃip] *n* 实习医师职位;实习医师[实习]期
internuclear [ˌintəˈnjuːkliə] *a* 核间的;(视网膜)核层间的
internuncial [ˌintəˈnʌnʃiəl] *a* 联络的(作为沟通神经细胞间或中枢间的媒介)
internus [inˈtəːnəs] *a* 内的,内部的(指位置较接近于器官或腔的中央)
interocclusal [ˌintərɔˈkluːsəl] *a* 耠面间的,咬合面间的
interoceptive [ˌintərəuˈseptiv] *a* 内感受的
interoceptor [ˌintərəuˈseptə] *n* 内感受器
interofection [ˌintərəuˈfekʃən] *n* 对内反应作用(身体对由于交感神经影响的体内内部环境改变的反应)
interofective [ˌintərəuˈfektiv] *a* 对内反应的(指自主神经系统)
interogestate [ˌintərəuˈdʒesteit] *a* 宫内发育的 *n* 宫内发育婴儿
interoinferiorly [ˌintərəu inˈfiəriəli] *ad* 向内下
interolivary [ˌintərˈɔlivəri] *a* [脑]橄榄体间的
interorbital [ˌintərˈɔːbitl] *a* 眶间的
interosseal [ˌintərˈɔsiəl] *a* 骨间的;骨间肌的
interosseous [ˌintərˈɔsiəs] *a* 骨间的
interpalpebral [ˌintəˈpælpibrəl] *a* 睑间的
interpandemic [ˌintəpænˈdemik] *a* 大流行期间的
interparietal [ˌintəpəˈraiitl] *a* 壁间的;顶骨间的
interparoxysmal [ˌintəˌpærəkˈsizməl] *a* 发作间期的
interpediculate [ˌintəpiˈdikjulit] *a* 椎弓根间的,蒂间的
interpeduncular [ˌintəpiˈdʌŋkjulə] *a* [脑]脚间的

interphalangeal [ˌintəfəˈlændʒiəl] *a* 指节间的，趾节间的
interphase [ˈintəfeiz] *n* 分裂间期(两次连续的有丝分裂之间的时期)
interphyletic [ˌintəfaiˈletik] *a* (两型细胞间的)中间型的
interpial [ˌintəˈpaiəl] *a* 软脑膜间的
interplant [ˈintəplɑːnt, -plænt-] *n* 移植体(分离出来的胚胎部分,移植到另一胚胎所提供的相同环境中发育)
interpleural [ˌintəˈpluərəl] *a* 胸膜间的
interpolar [ˌintəˈpəulə] *a* 极间的
interpolation [inˌtəːpəuˈleiʃən] *n* 插入,补入;移植(组织);插植法,内插法(依据观察的数字而决定一系列的中间值)
interpolymer [ˈintəˈpɔlimə] *n* 互聚物
interposition [ˌintəpəˈziʃən] *n* 间位;介植,补植;插补术
interpositum [ˌintəˈpɔzitəm] *a* 【拉】插入的,居间的 *n* 中间帆
interpretation [inˌtəːpriˈteiʃən] *n* 解释,阐明
interprotometamere [ˌintəˌprəutəˈmetəmiə] *n* 原节间组织
interproximal [ˌintəˈprɔksiməl] *a* 邻间的,邻接近端间的
interpubic [ˌintəˈpjuːbik] *a* 耻骨间的
interpupillary [ˌintəˈpjuːpiləri, -ˌlɛəri] *a* 瞳孔间的
interradial [ˌintəˈreidjəl] *a* 射线间的
interrenal [ˌintəˈriːnl] *a* 肾间的
interrenicular [ˌintərəˈnikjulə], **interrenuncular** [ˌintərəˈnʌŋkjulə] *a* 两肾间的
interrupt [ˌintəˈrʌpt] *vt* 中断,阻断,中止 | **~ed** [ˌintəˈrʌptid] *a* / **~ion** [ˌintəˈrʌpʃən] *n*
interscapilium [ˌintəskəˈpiljəm], **interscapulum** [ˌintəˈskæpjuləm] *n* 肩胛间隙
interscapular [intəˈskæpjulə] *a* 肩胛间的
intersciatic [ˌintəsaiˈætik] *a* 坐骨间的
intersectio [ˌintəˈsekʃiəu] ([复] **intersectiones** [ˌintəˌsekʃiˈəuniːz]) *n* 【拉】交切,交叉;交切点
intersection [ˌintəˈsekʃən] *n* 交切,交叉;交切点 | tendinous ~ 腱划
intersegment [ˌintəˈsegmənt] *n* 节间 | **~al** [ˌintəsegˈmentl] *a*
interseptal [ˌintəˈseptl] *a* 隔间的
interseptum [ˌintəˈseptəm] *n* 【拉】隔膜
intersex [ˈintəseks] *n* 雌雄间性,间性;间性体,雌雄间体 | female ~ 雌间性,女性假两性体 / male ~ 雄间性,男性假两性体 / true ~ 真中间性,真两性体
intersexuality [ˌintəˌseksjuˈæləti] *n* 雌雄间性,间性 | **intersexual** [ˌintəˈseksjuəl] *a*
intersolubility [ˌintəˌsɔljuˈbiləti] *n* 互溶性;互溶度
interspace [ˈintəspeis] *n* 间隙 | dineric ~ 两液界面
interspecific [ˌintəspiˈsifik] *a* 种间的
intersphincteric [intəsfiŋkˈterik] *a* 括约肌间的(内外肛门括约肌间的)
interspinal [intəˈspainl], **interspinous** [intəˈspainəs] *a* 棘突间的,棘间的
intersternal [ˌintəˈstəːnl] *a* 胸骨间的
interstice [inˈtəːstis] *n* 小间隙
intestinocystoplasty [inˌtestinəuˈsistəuˌplæsti] *n* 肠膀胱扩大术
interstitial [ˌintəˈstiʃəl] *a* 间隙的;间质的
interstitium [ˌintəˈstiʃiəm] *n* 【拉】小间隙;间质组织
intertarsal [ˌintəˈtɑːsəl] *a* 跗骨间的
intertexture [ˌintəˈtekstʃə] *n* 交织;交织物
intertransverse [ˌintətrænsˈvəːs] *a* 横突间的
intertriginous [ˌintəˈtridʒinəs] *a* 擦烂的
intertrigo [ˌintəˈtraigəu] *n* 擦烂 | ~ labialis 唇间擦烂
intertrochanteric [ˌintəˌtrəukænˈterik] *a* 转子间的
intertubercular [ˌintətju(ː)ˈbəːkjulə], **intertuberous** [ˌintəˈtjuːbərəs] *a* 结节间的
intertubular [ˌintəˈtjuːbjulə] *a* 管间的
interureteric [ˌintəˌjuəriˈterik], **interureteral** [ˌintəjuəˈriːtərəl] *a* 输尿管间的
intervaginal [ˌintəˈvædʒinəl] *a* 鞘间的
interval [ˈintəvəl] *n* 间隔,间距;间期 | atrioventricular ~, auriculoventricular ~ 房室[收缩]间期 / cardioarterial ~, c-a ~ 心搏动脉间期 / confidence ~ 置信区间(一种对未知参数的统计区间计算) / focal ~ 焦间距(前后焦点间的距离) / lucid ~ (神志)清明期 / postsphygmic ~ 脉后间期(心) / P-R ~ P-R 间期(介于 P 波与 QRS 复合波之间的心电图部分) / presphygmic ~ 脉前间期(心) / QRST ~, Q-T ~ Q-T 间期(心电图) / tolerance ~ 容许区间(一种具有特定概率的区间估算) | **~lic** [intə(ː)ˈvælik] *a*
intervalvular [ˌintəˈvælvjulə] *a* 瓣膜间的
intervascular [ˌintəˈvæskjulə] *a* 血管间的
intervene [ˌintəˈviːn] *vi* 干涉,介入
intervenient [ˌintəˈviːniənt] *a* 干涉的,介入的 *n* 介入物
intervention [ˌintəˈvenʃən] *n* 干涉,干预,介入 | crisis ~ (精神病)危机干预;应急性措施 / surgical ~ 外科手术
interventricular [ˌintəvenˈtrikjulə] *a* [心]室间的

intervertebral [ˌintəˈvəːtibrəl] *a* 椎[骨]间的
interview [ˌintəvjuː] *n*, *vt* 面谈,面试;精神检查
intervillous [ˌintəˈviləs] *a* 绒毛间的
intestine [inˈtestin] *n* 肠 | blind ~ 盲肠 / empty ~ 空肠 / iced ~ 糖衣肠,慢性纤维包裹性腹膜炎 / jejunoileal ~ , mesenterial ~ 系膜小肠(指空肠与回肠) / large ~ 大肠 / segmented ~ 结肠 / small ~ 小肠 / straight ~ 直肠 | **intestinal** *a*
intestino-intestinal [inˌtestinəu inˈtestinl] *a* 肠肠的(两个不同部分的肠,如肠肠反射)
intestinum [ˌintesˈtainəm] ([复] **intestina** [ˌintesˈtainə]) *n*【拉】肠
intima [ˈintimə] *n* [血管]内膜 | **~l** *a*
intimitis [ˌintiˈmaitis] *n* 内膜炎
intolerance [inˈtɔlərəns] *n* 不耐受[性] | congenital lactose ~ 先天性乳糖不耐受 / congenital lysine ~ 先天性赖氨酸不耐受,高赖氨酸血症 / congenital sucrose ~ 先天性蔗糖不耐受 / disaccharide ~ 二糖不耐受 / drug ~ 药物不耐性 / hereditary fructose ~ 遗传性果糖不耐受 / lactose ~ 乳糖不耐受[症](亦称二糖不耐受和乳糖酶缺乏症) / lysinuric protein ~ 赖氨酸尿性蛋白不耐受
intorsion [inˈtɔːʃən] *n* 内扭转,内旋
intorter [ˈintɔtə] *n* 内旋肌
intoxation [ˌintɔkˈseiʃən] *n* 中毒
intoxicant [inˈtɔksikənt] *a* 致醉的;使中毒的 *n* 酒类饮料;中毒药
intoxication [inˌtɔksiˈkeiʃən] *n* 中毒;醉[酒] | acid ~ (重度)酸中毒 / alcohol idiosyncratic ~ 特应性醉酒 / alkaline ~ (重度)碱中毒 / anaphylactic ~ 过敏性中毒,过敏性休克 / bongkrek ~ 米酵霉中毒 / intestinal ~ 肠中毒,自体中毒 / roentgen ~ X线中毒,放射病 / serum ~ 血清中毒,血清病 / water ~ 水中毒(水分过度积滞所致的状态)
intra- [前缀] 内,在内
intracanalicular [ˌintrəˌkænəˈlikjulə] *a* 小管内的
intracapsular [ˌintrəˈkæpsjulə] *a* 囊内的
intracardiac [ˌintrəˈkɑːdiæk] *a* 心内的
intracarpal [ˌintrəˈkɑːpl] *a* 腕内的
intracartilaginous [ˌintrəˌkɑːtiˈlædʒinəs] *a* 软骨内的
intracavitary [ˌintrəˈkævitəri, -ˌtεəri] *a* 腔内的
intracelial [ˌintrəˈsiːliəl] *a* 体腔内的
intracellular [ˌintrəˈseljulə] *a* [细]胞内的
intracephalic [ˌintrəsəˈfælik] *a* 脑内的
intracerebellar [ˌintrəˌseriˈbelə] *a* 小脑内的
intracerebral [ˌintrəˈseribrəl] *a* 大脑内的
intraauricular [ˌintrəɔːˈrikjulə] *a* 耳郭内的
intra-abdominal [ˌintrə æbˈdɔmin] *a* 腹内的
intra-acinous [ˌintrə ˈæsinəs] *a* 腺泡内的
intra-alveolar [ˌintrə ælˈviələ] *a* 肺泡内的
intra-appendicular [ˌintrə ˌæpənˈdikjulə] *a* 阑尾内的
intra-arachnoid [ˌintrə əˈræknɔid] *a* 蛛网膜内的
intra-arterial [ˌintrə ɑːˈtiəriəl] *a* 动脉内的
intra-articular [ˌintrə ɑːˈtikjulə] *a* 关节内的
intra-atomic [ˌintrə əˈtɔmik] *a* 原子内的
intra-atrial [ˌintrə ˈeitriəl] *a* 心房内的
intra-aural [ˌintrə ˈɔːrəl] *a* 耳内的
intrabronchial [ˌintrəˈbrɔŋkiəl] *a* 支气管内的
intrabuccal [ˌintrəˈbʌkəl] *a* 口内的,颊内的
intracerebroventricular [ˌintrəˌseribrəuvenˈtrikjulə] *a* 脑室内的
intracervical [ˌintrəˈsəːvikəl] *a* [子宫]颈管内的
intrachondral [ˌintrəˈkɔndrəl], **intrachondrial** [ˌintrəˈkɔndriəl] *a* 软骨内的
intrachordal [ˌintrəˈkɔːdl] *a* 脊索内的
intracisternal [ˌintrəsisˈtəːnl] *a* 脑池内的
intracolic [ˌintrəˈkɔlik] *a* 结肠内的
intracordal [ˌintrəˈkɔːdl] *a* 心内的
intracorporeal [ˌintrəkɔːˈpɔːriəl], **intracorporal** [ˌintrəˈkɔːpərəl] *a* 体内的
intracorpuscular [ˌintrəkɔːˈpʌskjulə] *a* 小体内的
intracostal [ˌintrəˈkɔstl] *a* 肋内[面]的
intracranial [ˌintrəˈkreinjəl] *a* 颅内的
intracrine [ˈintrəkrin] *a* 内分泌的
intracrureus [ˌintrəkruˈriəs] *n* 股间肌
intractable [inˈtræktəbl] *a* 顽固的,难治的
intracutaneous [ˌintrəkju(ː)ˈteinjəs] *a* 皮内的 | **~ly** *ad* 皮内注射
intracystic [ˌintrəˈsistik] *a* 囊内的
intracytoplasmic [ˌintrəˌsaitəuˈplæzmik] *a* 胞质内的
intrad [ˈintræd] *ad* 向内
intradermal [ˌintrəˈdəːməl] *a* 真皮内的;皮内的
intradermoreaction [ˌintrəˌdəːməuri(ː)ˈækʃən] *n* 皮内反应
intradialytic [ˌintrəˌdaiəˈlitik] *a* 透析中的(血液透析时发生的)
intradiscal [ˌintrəˈdiskəl] *a* 椎间盘内的
intraductal [ˌintrəˈdʌktl] *a* 管内的
intraduodenal [ˌintrəˌdju(ː)əuˈdiːnl] *a* 十二指肠内的
intradural [ˌintrəˈdjuərəl] *a* 硬膜内的
intraepidermal [ˌintrəˌepiˈdəːməl] *a* 表皮内的
intraepiphyseal [ˌintrəˌepiˈfiziəl] *a* 骺内的
intraepithelial [ˌintrəˌepiˈθiːliəl] *a* 上皮内的
intraerythrocytic [ˌintrəiˌriθrəuˈsitik] *a* 红细胞内的

intrafascicular [ˌintrəfəˈsikjulə] *a* 束内的
intrafat [ˌintrəˈfæt] *a* 脂肪[组织]内的
intrafetation [ˌintrəfiːˈteiʃən] *n* 胎内[成]胎
intrafilar [ˌintrəˈfailə] *a* 丝内的,网内的
intrafissural [ˌintrəˈfiʃjurəl] *a* 裂内的
intrafistular [ˌintrəˈfistjulə] *a* 瘘管内的
intrafollicular [ˌintrəfəˈlikjulə] *a* 滤泡内的
intrafusal [ˌintrəˈfjuːzəl] *a* 肌梭内的
intragalvanization [ˌintrəˌgælvənaiˈzeiʃən, -niˈz-] *n* 体腔流电疗法
intragastric [ˌintrəˈgæstrik] *a* 胃内的
intragemmal [ˌintrəˈdʒeməl] *a* 蕾内的,芽内的
intragenic [ˌintrəˈdʒenik] *a* 基因内的
intraglandular [ˌintrəˈglændjulə] *a* 腺内的
intraglobular [ˌintrəˈglɔbjulə] *a* 球内的,小球内的;小体内的
intragyral [ˌintrəˌdʒaiərəl] *a* 脑回内的
intrahyoid [ˌintrəˈhaiɔid] *a* 舌骨内的
intraictal [ˌintrəˈiktl] *a* 发作中的,发作期内的
intraintestinal [ˌintrəinˈtestinl] *a* 肠内的
intrajugular [ˌintrəˈdʒʌgjulə] *a* 颈静脉内的(在颈静脉孔、颈静脉突或颈静脉之内的)
intralamellar [ˌintrələˈmelə] *a* 板内的
intralaryngeal [ˌintrələˈrindʒiəl] *a* 喉内的
intralesional [ˌintrəˈliːʒənl] *a* 损害内的
intraleukocytic [ˌintrəˌljuːkəuˈsitik] *a* 白细胞内的
intraligamentous [ˌintrəˌligəˈmentəs] *a* 韧带内的
intralingual [ˌintrəˈliŋgwəl] *a* 舌内的
intralobar [ˌintrəˈləubə] *a* 叶内的
intralobular [ˌintrəˈlɔbjulə] *a* 小叶内的
intralocular [ˌintrəˈlɔkjulə] *a* 小房内的
intraluminal [ˌintrəˈljuːminl] *a* 管腔内的
intramammary [ˌintrəˈmæməri] *a* 乳房内的
intramarginal [ˌintrəˈmɑːdʒinl] *a* 边缘内的
intramastoiditis [ˌintrəˌmæstɔiˈdaitis] *n* 乳突窦炎,乳突腔炎
intramatrical [ˌintrəˈmætrikəl] *a* 基质内的
intramedullary [ˌintrəˈmedələri, -ˌlɛəri] *a* 髓内的(指脊髓内的,延髓内的,骨髓腔内的)
intramembranous [ˌintrəˈmembrənəs] *a* 膜内的
intrameningeal [ˌintrəmiˈnindʒiəl] *a* 脑[脊]膜内的
intramolecular [ˌintrəməuˈlekjulə] *a* 分子内的
intramural [ˌintrəˈmjuərəl] *a* (器官)壁内的
intramuscular [ˌintrəˈmʌskjulə] *a* 肌内的 | **~ly** *ad* 肌内注射
intramyocardial [ˌintrəˌmaiəuˈkɑːdiəl] *a* 心肌内的
intranarial [ˌintrəˈnɛəriəl] *a* 鼻孔内的
intranasal [ˌintrəˈneizəl] *a* 鼻内的
intranatal [ˌintrəˈneitl] *a* 产期内的
intraneural [ˌintrəˈnjuərəl] *a* 神经内的
intranuclear [ˌintrəˈnjuːkliə] *a* 核内的
intraocular [ˌintrəˈɔkjulə] *a* 眼内的
intraoperative [ˌintrəˈɔpərətiv] *a* 手术[期]中的
intraoral [ˌintrəˈɔːrəl] *a* 口内的
intraorbital [ˌintrəˈɔːbitl] *a* [眼]眶内的
intraosseous [ˌintrəˈɔsiəs], **intraosteal** [ˌintrəˈɔstiəl] *a* 骨内的
intraovarian [ˌintrəəuˈvɛəriən] *a* 卵巢内的
intraovular [ˌintrəˈəuvjulə] *a* 卵内的
intrapancreatic [ˌintrəˌpænkriˈætik] *a* 胰内的
intraparenchymatous [ˌintrəˌpærənˈkimətəs] *a* 实质内的
intraparietal [ˌintrəpəˈraiitl] *a* 壁内的;顶内的
intrapartal [ˌintrəˈpɑːtəl] *a* 分娩间期[内]的,产时的
intrapartum [ˌintrəˈpɑːtəm] *a* 产时的
intrapelvic [ˌintrəˈpelvik] *a* 骨盆内的
intrapericardial [ˌintrəˌperiˈkɑːdiəl] *a* 心包内的
intraperineal [ˌintrəˌperiˈniːəl] *a* 会阴内的
intraperitoneal [ˌintrəˌperitəˈniːəl] *a* 腹膜内的
intrapial [ˌintrəˈpiəl] *a* 软膜内的,软膜下的
intraplacental [ˌintrəpləˈsentl] *a* 胎盘内的
intrapleural [ˌintrəˈpluərəl] *a* 胸膜内的
intrapontine [ˌintrəˈpɔntain] *a* 脑桥内的
intraprostatic [ˌintrəprɔsˈtætik] *a* 前列腺内的
intraprotoplasmic [ˌintrəˌprəutəˈplæzmik] *a* 原生质内的
intrapsychic(al) [intrəˈsaikik(əl)] *a* 内心的
intrapulmonary [ˌintrəˈpʌlmənəri] *a* 肺内的
intrapyretic [ˌintrəpaiˈretik] *a* 发热期内的
intrarachidian [ˌintrərəˈkidiən] *a* 脊柱内的
intrarectal [ˌintrəˈrektl] *a* 直肠内的
intrarenal [ˌintrəˈriːnl] *a* 肾内的
intraretinal [ˌintrəˈretin] *a* 视网膜内的
intrascleral [ˌintrəˈskliərəl] *a* 巩膜内的
intrascrotal [ˌintrəˈskrəutl] *a* 阴囊内的
intrasegmental [ˌintrəsegˈmentəl] *a* 节段内的(在一个节段内的,如支气管肺段和脊髓节段)
intrasellar [ˌintrəˈselə] *a* 蝶鞍内的
intraserous [ˌintrəˈsiərəs] *a* 血清内的
intraspinal [ˌintrəˈspainl] *a* 脊柱内的
intrasplenic [ˌintrəˈsplenik, -ˈspliː-] *a* 脾内的
intrasternal [ˌintrəˈstəːnl] *a* 胸骨内的
intrastitial [ˌintrəˈstiʃəl] *a* 细胞内的;纤维内的
intrastromal [ˌintrəˈstrəuməl] *a* 基质内的
intrasynovial [ˌintrəsiˈnəuviəl] *a* 滑膜[腔]内的
intratarsal [ˌintrəˈtɑːsəl] *a* 跗骨内的
intratendinous [ˌintrəˈtendinəs] *a* 腱内的

intratesticular [ˌintrətes'tikjulə] *a* 睾丸内的
intrathecal [ˌintrə'θiːkəl] *a* 鞘内的 | **~ly** *ad* 鞘内注射
intrathenar [ˌintrə'θiːnə] *a* 鱼际间的
intrathoracic [ˌintrəθɔ(ː)'ræsik] *a* 胸内的,胸廓内的
intratonsillar [ˌintrə'tɔnsilə] *a* 扁桃体内的
intratrabecular [ˌintrətrə'bekjulə] *a* 小梁内的
intratracheal [ˌintrə'treikiəl] *a* 气管内的
intratubal [ˌintrə'tjubəl] *a* 管内的(尤指输卵管内的)
intratubular [ˌintrə'tjuːbjulə] *a* 小管内的
intratympanic [ˌintrətim'pænik] *a* 鼓室内的
intraureteral [ˌintrəjuə'riːtərəl] *a* 输尿管内的
intraurethral [ˌintrəjuə'riːθrəl] *a* 尿道内的
intrauterine [ˌintrə'juːtərain] *a* 宫内的
intravaginal [ˌintrə'vædʒinl] *a* 阴道内的
intravasation [inˌtrævə'zeiʃən] *n* 内渗,进入血管(异物)
intravascular [ˌintrə'væskjulə] *a* 血管内的
intravenation [ˌintrəvi'neiʃən] *a* 进入静脉,注入静脉(异物)
intravenous [ˌintrə'viːnəs] *a* 静脉内的 | **~ly** *ad* 静脉注射
intraventricular [ˌintrəven'trikjulə] *a* 心室内的
intraversion [ˌintrə'vəːʒən] *n* 牙弓狭窄
intravertebral [ˌintrə'vəːtibrəl] *a* 脊柱内的
intravesical [ˌintrə'vesikəl] *a* 膀胱内的
intravillous [ˌintrə'viləs] *a* 绒毛内的
intravital [ˌintrə'vaitl] *a* 生活期内的;活体[内]的
intra vitam [ˌintrə'vaitəm] [拉]生活期间
intravitelline [ˌintrəvai'telin] *a* 卵黄内的
intravitreous [ˌintrə'vitriəs] *a* 玻璃体内的
intrazole ['intrəzəul] *n* 吲四唑(抗炎药)
intrinsic [in'trinsik] *a* 内在的,内源性的,固有的;内部的,体内的
intriptyline hydrochloride [in'triptiliːn] 盐酸英曲替林(抗抑郁药)
intro- [前缀]入内,在内
introducer [ˌintrə'djuːsə] *n* 插管器,喉管插入器
introfier ['intrəˌfaiə] *n* 减张剂
introflexion [ˌintrəu'flekʃən] *n* 内屈
introgastric [ˌintrəu'gæstrik] *a* 入胃的
introgression [ˌintrə'grəʃən] *n* 基因渗入 | **introgressive** [ˌintrə'gresiv] *a* **introitus** [in'trəuitəs] [单复同] *n* [拉]入口,口
introjection [ˌintrə'dʒekʃən] *n* 内向投射(一种精神作用,使人视某一事件或特性为私有,而成为自我的一部分,或把对他人的敌意转向自己,造成自我敌对)
intromit [ˌintrəu'mit] *vt* 插入;输入 | **intromission** [ˌintrəu'miʃən] *n*
intron ['intrɔn] *n* 内含子
introrsus [in'trɔːsəs] *a* [拉]内转的,内翻的
introspection [ˌintrəu'spekʃən] *n* 内省,自省 | **introspective** [ˌintrəuspektiv] *a*
introsusception [ˌintrəusə'sepʃən] *n* 套叠,肠套叠
introversion [ˌintrəu'vəːʒən] *n* 内翻,内向;[精神]内向,内倾;牙弓狭窄
introvert [ˌintrəu'vəːt] *vt* 使内向 ['intrəuvəːt] *n* [精神]内向者,内倾[性格]者 ['intrəuvəːt] *a* 内向性格的
intrusion [in'truːʒən] *n* 突入
intubate ['intjubeit] *vt* 插管,插入喉管 | **intubation** [ˌintju'beiʃən] *n* 插管术(尤指喉管插入法)
intubationist [ˌintju'beiʃənist] *n* 插管术者
intubator ['intjubeitə] *n* 插管器,喉管插入器
intumesce [ˌintju(ː)'mes] *vi* 肿大;膨大,隆起
intumescence [ˌintju(ː)'mesns] *n* 肿大;膨大,隆起 | **intumescent** [ˌintju(ː)'mesnt] *a*
intumescentia [ˌintju(ː)mə'senʃiə] ([复] **intumescentiae** [ˌintju(ː)mə'senʃiiː]) *n* [拉]肿大;膨大,隆起
intussusception [ˌintəsə'sepʃən] *n* 套叠,肠套叠;内吸收(把食物吸收到机体内变成新的原生质) | agonic ~, postmortem ~ 濒死肠套叠 / retrograde ~ 逆行性套叠 | **intussusceptive** *a*
intussusceptum [ˌintəsə'septəm] *n* [拉]肠套叠套入部
intussuscipiens [ˌintəsə'sipiəns] *n* [拉]肠套叠鞘部
Inula ['injulə] *n* 旋覆花属(菊科)
inulase [ˌinjuleis], **inulinase** ['injulineis] *n* 菊粉酶
inulin ['injulin] *n* 菊粉,菊糖
inulinase ['injulineis] *n* 菊粉酶
inuloid ['injulɔid] *n* 类菊粉
inunction [i'nʌŋkʃən] *n* 涂擦法;[复]涂擦剂
inunctum [i'nʌŋktəm] *n* 涂擦剂 | ~ mentholis compositum 复方薄荷脑涂擦剂,复方薄荷脑软膏
in utero [in'jutərəu] [拉] 子宫内
InV 印维异型, km[同种]异型(InV 源于病人名,表示人免疫球蛋白 κ 链恒定区上的异型抗原位置,有 3 种异型)
invaccination [inˌvæksi'neiʃən] *n* 偶然接种,意外接种(接种时因疏忽而接种了不是制备疫苗的微生物)
invaginate [in'vædʒineit] *vt, vi* 折入,凹入,内陷,内折;套叠

invagination [inˌvædʒiˈneiʃən] *n* 折入,凹入,内陷,内折;套叠 | basilar ~ 扁后脑,扁颅底
invalid [ˈinvəlid] *a* 有病的,衰弱的 *n* 病弱者,久病衰弱者
invalidism [ˈinvəlidizəm] *n* 病弱,伤残
invalidity [ˌinvəˈlidəti] *n* 无效力;病弱,劳动能力丧失
invasin [inˈveizin] *n* 侵袭素,透明质酸酶
invasion [inˈveiʒən] *n* 侵入,侵害;侵袭;发病,发作
invasive [inˈveisiv] *a* 侵入的,侵害的;侵袭的 | ~**ness** *n* 侵入力,侵袭力
inventory [ˈinvəntri] *n* 调查表 | Millon clinical multiaxial ~ (MCMI) 米伦临床多轴调查表 / Minnesota Multiphasic Personality Inventory (MMPI) 明尼苏达多相人格调查表
invermination [inˌvəːmiˈneiʃən] *n* 蠕虫感染,蠕虫病
inversion [inˈvəːʒən] 转化;内翻;反向,倒向;性倒错;倒位(染色体畸变) | carbohydrate ~ 碳水化物转化,碳水化物水解[作用] / chromosome ~ 染色体倒位 / sexual ~ 性倒错,同性恋 / thermic ~ 体温反常 / ~ of uterus 子宫内翻 / visceral ~ 内脏[左右]易位,内脏反向 | **inversive** [inˈvəːsiv] *a*
inversus [inˈvəːsəs] *a* [拉] 反向的,倒向的
invert [inˈvəːt] *vt* 使颠倒,使内翻,转换;使转化 [ˈinvəːt] *a* 转化的 *n* 性倒错者,同性恋者
invertase [inˈvəːteis] *n* 转化酶
Invertebrata [inˌvəːtiˈbreitə] *n* 无脊椎动物类
invertebrate [inˈvəːtibrit] *n* 无脊椎动物 *a* 无脊椎的
invertin [inˈvəːtin] *n* 转化酶
invertor [inˈvəːtə] *n* 内转肌
invertose [ˈinvətəus] *n* 转化糖
invest [inˈvest] *vt* 包埋,围模
investing [inˈvestiŋ] *n* 包埋,围模
investment [inˈvestmənt] *n* 包埋料,围模料;包埋法,围模法;投资
inveterate [inˈvetərit] *a* 长期形成的,根深蒂固的;慢性顽固性的,绵延难治的
invigorate [inˈvigəreit] *vt* 使强壮,使精力充沛 | **invigoration** [inˌvigəˈreiʃən] *n* 增益精力,滋补 | **invigorat or** *n* 补药
inviscation [ˌinvisˈkeiʃən] *n* 食物混黏液[作用]
in vitro [inˈviːtrəu] [拉] 体外,离体,在试管内
in vivo [inˈviːvəu] [拉] 体内,在活体内
involucre [ˈinvəluːkə] *n* 总苞
involucrum [ˌinvəˈluːkrəm] ([复] **involucra** [ˌinvəˈluːkrə]) *n* 总苞;包壳(死骨的)
involuntary [inˈvɔləntəri] *a* 不随意的
involuntomotory [inˌvɔləntəuˈməutəri] *a* 不随意运动的
involute [ˌinvəˈluːt] *vi* 复旧;退化
involution [ˌinvəˈluːʃən] *n* 内转;复旧;退化 | ~ of uterus 子宫复旧 / senile ~ 老年性退化 | ~**al** *a*
involve [inˈvɔlv] *vt* 累及,牵涉 | ~**d** *a* 累及的 / ~**ment** *n*
in vucuo [inˈvækjuəu] [拉] 真空内
invulnerable [inˈvʌlnərəbl] *a* 不会受伤害的
Io ionium 锾
iobenguane [ˌaiəuˈbengwein] *n* 碘苄胍(诊断用药)
iobenzamic acid [ˌaiəubenˈzæmik] 碘苯扎酸(诊断用胆囊造影剂)
iocarmate meglumine [ˌaiəuˈkɑːmeit] 碘卡葡胺(造影剂,用于腰骶神经根造影、脑室造影和膝关节造影)
iocarmic acid [ˌaiəuˈkəːmik] 碘卡酸(见 iocarmate meglumine)
iocetamic acid [ˌaiəusiˈtæmik] 碘西他酸(口服胆囊造影剂)
iodamide [aiˈəudəmaid] *n* 碘达胺(诊断用造影剂)
Iodamoeba [ˌaiədəˈmiːbə] *n* 嗜碘变形虫属,嗜碘阿米巴属 | ~ buetschlii, ~ williamsi 布氏嗜碘变形虫,布氏嗜碘阿米巴 / ~ suis 猪嗜碘变形虫,猪嗜碘阿米巴
iodate [ˈaiədeit] *vt* 用碘处理,向…加碘 *n* 碘酸盐 | **iodation** [ˌaiəˈdeiʃən] *n* 碘化作用
iod-Basedow [ˌaiəud-ˈbæsidəu] *n* 碘性巴塞多病,碘性甲状腺功能亢进
iodemia [ˌaiəˈdiːmiə] *n* 碘血
iodic [aiˈɔdik] *a* 碘的,含碘的,五价碘的 | ~ acid 碘酸
iodide [ˈaiədaid] *n* 碘化物
iodide peroxidase [ˈaiədaid pəˈrɔksideis] 碘化物过氧化物酶(此酶缺乏为一种常染色体隐性性状,影响有机碘的形成,可致家族性甲状腺肿,亦称甲状腺过氧物酶)
iodimetry [ˌaiəˈdimitri] *n* 碘定量法
iodinate [aiˈəudineit] *vi* 碘化,碘处理 | **iodination** [ˌaiəudiˈneiʃən] *n* 碘化作用
iodine (I) [ˈaiədiːn] *n* 碘 | butanol-extractable ~ 丁醇可提取的碘 / imidecyl ~ 咪癸碘(局部抗感染药) / povidone ~ 聚维酮碘,聚烯吡酮碘,聚乙烯吡咯酮碘(局部抗感染药) / proteinbound ~ 蛋白结合碘 / radioactive ~ 放射性碘
iodinophil [ˌaiəˈdinəfil] *a* 嗜碘的 *n* 嗜碘细胞,嗜碘体
iodinophilous [ˌaiədiˈnɔfiləs] *a* 嗜碘的
iodipamide [ˌaiəˈdipəmaid] *n* 胆影酸(造影剂) | ~ meglumine, ~ methylglucamine 胆影葡胺(静

脉胆道造影剂) / ~ sodium 胆影酸钠(静脉胆道造影剂)

iodism [ˈaiədizəm] *n* 碘中毒

iodixanol [ˌaiəuˈdiksənɔl] *n* 碘克沙醇(一种非离子造影剂,用于血管造影、计算机体层摄影和排泄性尿路造影)

iodize [ˈaiədaiz] *vt* 用碘(或碘化物)处理,加碘

iod(o)- [前缀]碘

iodoacetic acid [aiˌəudəuəˈsiːtik] 碘乙酸

iodoalphionic acid [aiˌɔdəuælfiˈɔnik] 碘阿芬酸(诊断用药)

***m*-iodobenzylguanidine** [ˌaiəudəuˌbenzilˈgwɑːniˌdiːn] *n* 碘苄胍

iodobrassid [aiˌəudəuˈbræsid] *n* 二碘顺芜酸乙酯(碘治疗及造影剂)

iodochlorhydroxyquin [aiˌəudəuˌklɔːhaiˈdrɔksikwin] *n* 氯碘羟喹(抗阿米巴药)

iodocholesterol ^{131}I [aiˌəudəukəˈlestərɔl] 碘[^{131}I]胆甾醇(放射性药品)

iododerma [aiəudəuˈdəːmə] *n* 碘疹

iodoform [aiˈɔdəfɔːm], **iodoformum** [aiəudəuˈfɔːməm] *n* 碘仿,三碘甲烷(局部抗感染药)

iodoformism [aiəudəuˈfɔːmizəm] *n* 碘仿中毒

iodogenic [aiəudəuˈdʒenik] *a* 生碘的

iodoglobulin [aiəudəuˈglɔbjulin] *n* 碘球蛋白

iodogorgoric acid [ˌaiəudəuˈgɔgərik] 二碘酪氨酸

iodohippurate sodium [aiˌəudəuˈhipjuəreit] 碘马尿酸钠(肾功能测定药)

iodolography [aiəudəuˈlɔgrəfi] *n* 碘油造影[术]

iodomethamate sodium [aiˌəudəuˈmeθəmeit] 甲碘吡酮酸钠(造影剂)

iodomethane [aiˌəudəuˈmeθein] *n* 碘代甲烷,甲基碘

iodomethylnorcholesterol [aiˌəudəuˌmeθilˌnɔːkəˈlestərɔl] *n* 碘甲基降胆固醇(碘[^{131}I]-6β-碘甲基降胆固醇,一种碘[^{131}I]标记的胆固醇类似物,用于肾上腺皮质的放射性核素显像。亦称NP-59)

iodometry [ˌaiəˈdɔmitri] *n* 碘定量法,碘量滴定法 | **iodometric** [ˌaiədəuˈmetrik] *a* 碘定量的

iodopanoic acid [aiˌəudəupəˈnɔik] 碘番酸(胆囊造影剂)

iodophenol [aiəudəuˈfiːnɔl] *n* 碘[苯]酚

***p*-iodophenylarsenic acid** [aiˌəudəuˌfenilˈɑːsnik] 对碘苯砷酸

iodophil [aiˈɔdəfil] *a* 嗜碘的 *n* 嗜碘细胞,嗜碘体

iodophilia [aiəudəuˈfiliə] *n* 嗜碘性

iodophor [aiˈɔdəfɔː] *n* 碘附(碘与一种载体如聚乙烯吡咯酮的化合物,兽医用作手术前皮肤消毒剂)

iodophthalein sodium [aiˌəudəuˈθæliːn] 碘酞钠(胆囊造影剂)

iodopsin [ˌaiəˈdɔpsin] *n* 视青质

iodopyracet [aiˌəudəuˈpaiərəset] *n* 碘奥酮(尿路造影剂)

iodoquinol [aiˌəudəuˈkwinɔl] *n* 双碘喹啉(亦称双碘羟喹,抗阿米巴药)

iodo-salicylic acid [aiˌəudəusæliˈsilik] 碘[代]水杨酸

iodosobenzoic acid [ˌaiəˌdəusəubenˈzəuik] 氧碘[代]苯甲酸

iodosulfate [aiəudəuˈsʌlfeit] *n* 碘硫酸盐

iodotherapy [aiəudəuˈθerəpi] *n* 碘疗法

iodothyrine [aiəudəuˈθaiərin] *n* 甲状腺碘质,碘化甲状腺素

iodothyroglobulin [aiəudəuˌθairəuˈglɔbjulin] *n* 碘甲状腺球蛋白

iodothyronine [aiəudəuˈθairəniːn] *n* 碘甲腺原氨酸

iodotyrosine [aiəudəuˈtairəsiːn] *n* 碘酪氨酸

iodotyrosine dehalogenase [aiəudəuˈtairəsiːn diːˈhælədʒəneis] 碘酪氨酸脱卤酶,碘酪氨酸脱碘酶

iodotyrosine deiodinase [aiəudəuˈtairəsiːn diːˈaiədineis] 碘酪氨酸脱碘酶(此酶的先天性缺乏可致碘严重丧失,并导致甲状腺功能减退和甲状腺肿。亦称碘酪氨酸脱卤酶)

iodoventriculography [aiəudəuvenˌtrikjuˈlɔgrəfi] *n* 碘剂脑室造影[术]

iodovolatilization [aiəudəuˌvɔlətilaiˈzeiʃən, -liˈz-] *n* (藻类)放碘作用

iodoxamic acid [aiəudɔkˈsæmik] 碘沙酸(胆囊造影剂)

iodoxybenzoic acid [ˌaiəˌdɔksibenˈzəuik] 二氧碘[代]苯甲酸

iodoxyl [ˌaiəˈdɔksil] *n* 碘多啥,甲碘吡酮酸钠(造影剂)

iodoxyquinoline sulfonic acid [ˌaiəˌdɔksiˈkwinəliːn] 碘羟喹啉磺酸

iodum [aiˈəudəm] *n* [拉]碘

ioduria [ˌaiəˈdjuəriə] *n* 碘尿

iofetamine hydrochloride ^{123}I [ˌaiəuˈfetəmiːn] 盐酸碘[^{123}I]非他胺(用作脑成像剂)

ioglicic acid [ˌaiəuˈglisik] 碘格利酸(造影剂)

ioglycamic acid [ˌaiəuglaiˈsæmik] 碘甘卡酸(胆囊造影剂)

iohexol [ˌaiəuˈheksɔl] *n* 碘海醇(一种非离子水溶性低同渗重摩不透射线造影剂,鞘内或血管内注射给药)

ion [ˈaiən, ˈaiɔn] *n* 离子 | dipolar ~ 偶极离子,两性离子 / gram ~ 克离子,摩尔 / hydrogen ~ 氢离子 / hydronium ~ 水合氢离子

ionic [aiˈɔnik] *a* 离子的 | **~ity** [aiɔˈnisəti] *n* 电

离度,离子性

ionium [ai'əuniəm] *n* 锾(元素钍的放射性核素)

ionization [ˌaiənai'zeiʃən, -ni'z-] *n* 电离,离子化;离子电渗作用 | avalanche ~ 雪崩式电离(因气体倍增而引起离子泛滥)

ionize ['aiənaiz] *vt, vi* 电离,离子化

ionocolorimeter [ˌaiənəuˌkʌlə'rimitə] *n* 氢离子比色计

ionogen [ai'ɔnədʒən] *n* 离子化基团

ionogenic [aiˌɔnə'dʒenik] *a* 离子生成的

ionomer [ai'ɔnəmə] *n* 离聚物,离子交联聚合物

ionometer [ˌaiəu'nɔmitə] *n* 离子计(测量射线量的仪器)

ionone ['aiənəun] *n* 芷香酮,紫罗酮

ionophore ['aiənəˌfɔː, ai'ɔnəfɔː] *n* 离子载体

ionophose ['aiənəuˌfəuz] *n* 紫幻视

ionoscope [ai'ɔnəskəup] *n* (氧化亚氮)酸碱杂质测定器

ionosphere [ai'ɔnəsfiə] *n* 电离层(大气) | **ionospheric** [aiˌɔnə'sferik] *a*

ionotherapy [ˌaiənəu'θerəpi] *n* 电离子透入疗法;紫外线疗法

iopromide [ˌaiəu'prəumaid] *n* 碘普胺(一种非离子低同渗重摩,不透射线造影剂,用于心血管系统成像、排泄性尿路造影和计算机体层摄影时使造影增强;动脉内或静脉内输注)

ion-protein [aiən'prəutiːn] *n* 离子蛋白

iontophoresis [aiˌɔntəufə'riːsis], **iontherapy** [ˌaiən'θerəpi] *n* 电离子透入疗法 | **iontophoretic** [aiˌɔntəfəu'retik] *a*

iontoquantimeter [aiˌɔntəukwæn'timitə], **iontoradiometer** [aiˌɔntəˌreidi'ɔmitə] *n* 离子计(测量射线量的仪器)

IOP intraocular pressure 眼压

iopamidol [ˌaiə'pæmidəul] *n* 碘帕醇(造影剂,用于脊髓造影)

iopanoic acid [ˌaiəpə'nɔik] 碘番酸(胆囊造影剂)

iophendylate [ˌaiə'fendileit] *n* 碘苯酯(脊髓造影剂)

iophenoxic acid [ˌaiəfə'nɔksik] 碘芬酸(胆囊造影剂)

iopydol [ˌaiəu'paidɔl] *n* 碘吡多(造影剂,用于支气管造影)

iopydone [aiə'paidəun] *n* 碘吡酮(支气管造影剂)

ioseric acid [ˌaiəu'siərik] 碘丝酸(造影剂)

iosulamide meglumine [ˌaiə'sʌləmaid] 碘砜葡胺(造影剂)

iosumetic acid [ˌaiəusjuː'metik] 碘琥酸(造影剂)

iota [ai'əutə] *n* 希腊语的第九个字母(Ι, ι)

iotacism [ai'əutəsizəm] *n* 衣(iː)音滥用

iotetric acid [ˌaiəu'tetrik] 碘替酸(造影剂)

iothalamate [ˌaiəu'θæləmeit] *n* 碘酞酸盐 | ~ meglumine 碘酞葡胺 / ~ sodium 碘酞钠

iothalamic acid [ˌaiəu'θæləmik] 碘他拉酸,碘酞酸(造影剂)

iothiouracil [aiəˌθaiəu'juərəsil] *n* 碘硫尿嘧啶(甲状腺抑制药)

iotroxic acid [ˌaiəu'trɔksik] 碘曲西酸(造影剂)

ioversol [ˌaiəu'vəːsɔl] *n* 碘佛醇(一种非离子造影剂,用于血管造影和尿路造影以及用于计算机体层摄影时使造影增强)

ioxaglate [ˌaiɔk'sægleit] *n* 碘克沙酸盐(或酯) | ~ meglumine 碘克沙酸葡胺(用作低同渗重摩不透射线造影剂) / ~ sodium 碘克沙酸钠(用作低同渗重摩不透射线造影剂)

ioxaglic acid [ˌaiɔk'sæglik] 碘克沙酸(一种低同渗重摩不透射线造影剂)

ioxilan [ai'ɔksilæn] *n* 碘昔兰(一种低黏性低同渗重摩非离子造影剂,用于动脉造影、排泄性尿路造影和计算机体层摄影)

IP intraperitoneally 腹膜内; isoelectric point 等电点

IP_3 inositol 1,4,5-triphosphate 肌醇 1, 4, 5-三磷酸

IPAA International Psychoanalytical Association 国际精神分析协会

I-para primipara 初产妇

IPD intermittent peritoneal dialysis 间歇性腹膜透析

ipecac ['ipəkæk] *n* 吐根 | powdered ~ 吐根粉(用于吐根糖浆制剂)

ipecacuanhic acid [ˌipəkæ'kwænik] 吐根酸

ipodate ['aipədeit] *n* 碘泊酸 | ~ calcium 碘泊酸钙(造影剂,用于胆囊造影) / ~ sodium 碘泊酸钠(造影剂,用于胆囊造影)

ipomea [ˌaipə'miːə] *n* 药薯(其根用作泻药)

Ipomoea [ˌaipə'miːə] *n* 番薯属(旋花科)

IPPB intermittent positive pressure breathing 间歇正压呼吸

ipratropium bromide [ˌiprə'trəupiəm] 异丙托溴铵(支气管扩张药)

iprindole [i'prindəul] *n* 伊普吲哚(抗抑郁药)

iproniazid [ˌaiprə'naiəzid] *n* 异丙烟肼(单胺氧化酶抑制药,抗抑郁药,抗结核药)

ipronidazole [ˌaiprəu'naidəzəul] *n* 异丙硝唑(抗原虫药)

iproplatin ['aiprəuˌplætin] *n* 异丙铂(抗肿瘤药)

iproxamine hydrochloride [i'prɔksəmiːn] 盐酸异丙沙明(血管扩张药)

ipsation [ip'seiʃən], **ipsism** ['ipsizəm] *n* 手淫

ipsi- [构词成分] 相同的,同一的

ipsilateral [ˌipsi'lætərəl] *a* 同侧的

IPSP inhibitory postsynaptic potential 抑制性突触后电位

IPV poliovirus vaccine inactivated 灭活脊髓灰质炎病毒疫苗
IQ intelligence quotient 智商,智力商数
Ir iridium 铱
ir- 见 in-
iraser [iˈreisə] (*i*nfra-*r*ed *a*mplification by *s*timulated *e*mission of *r*adiation) *n* 红外激射;红外激射器
irbesartan [ˌirbəˈsɑːtæn] *n* 伊比沙坦(抗高血压药)
IRC inspiratory reserve capacity 补吸气量; International Red Cross 国际红十字会
irid- 见 irido-
iridal [ˈaiəridl] *a* 虹膜的
iridalgia [ˌaiəriˈdældʒiə] *n* 虹膜痛
iridauxesis [ˌiridɔːkˈsiːsis] *n* 虹膜肥厚
iridectasis [ˌiriˈdektəsis] *n* 虹膜开大,瞳孔开大
iridectome [ˌiriˈdektəum] *n* 虹膜刀
iridectomesodialysis [ˌiriˌdektəuˌmiːsəudaiˈælisis] *n* 虹膜分离切除术
iridectomize [ˌiriˈdektəmaiz] *vt* 虹膜切除
iridectomy [ˌiriˈdektəmi] *n* 虹膜切除术 | basal ~ 虹膜基部切除术 / complete ~, total ~ 全虹膜切除术 / optical ~ 光学性虹膜切除术 / peripheral ~, stenopeic ~ 周边虹膜切除术,小孔形虹膜切除术 / preliminary ~, preparatory ~ 准备性虹膜切除术 / therapeutic ~ 治疗性虹膜切除术
iridectopia [ˌiridekˈtəupiə] *n* 虹膜异位
iridectropium [ˌiridekˈtrəupiəm] *n* 虹膜外翻
iridemia [ˌiriˈdiːmiə] *n* 虹膜出血
iridencleisis [ˌiridenˈklaisis] *n* 虹膜箝顿术(降眼压)
iridentropium [ˌiridenˈtrəupiəm] *n* 虹膜内翻
irideremia [ˌiridəˈriːmiə] *n* 无虹膜,虹膜缺失
irides [ˈaiəridiːz, ˈiridiːz] iris 的复数
iridescent [ˌiriˈdesnt] *a* 彩虹色的,晕色的 | **iridescence** [ˌiriˈdesns] *n*
iridesis [aiˈridəsis] *n* 虹膜固定术
iridiagnosis [ˌaiəridaiəgˈnəusis] *n* 虹膜诊断
iridic [aiˈridik], **iridial** [aiˈridiəl], **iridian** [aiˈridiən] *a* 虹膜的
iridic acid [aiˈridik] 鸢尾根酸
iridium(Ir) [aiˈridiəm, iˈridiəm] *n*【拉】铱(化学元素)
iridization [ˌiridaiˈzeiʃən, -diˈz-] *n* 虹视
irid(o)- [构词成分] 虹膜
iridoavulsion [ˌiridəuəˈvʌlʃən] *n* 虹膜撕脱
iridocapsulitis [ˌiridəukæpsjuˈlaitis] *n* 虹膜晶状体囊炎
iridocele [aiˈridəsiːl] *n* 虹膜突出
iridochoroiditis [ˌiridəuˌkɔːrɔiˈdaitis] *n* 虹膜脉络膜炎
iridociliary [ˌiridəuˈsiliˌɛəri] *a* 虹膜睫状体的
iridocoloboma [ˌiridəuˌkɔləˈbəumə] *n* 虹膜缺损,虹膜裂开
iridoconstrictor [ˌiridəukənˈstriktə] *n* 虹膜收缩肌;缩瞳剂
iridocorneosclerectomy [ˌiridəuˌkɔːniəuskliəˈrektəmi] *n* 虹膜角膜巩膜切除术
iridocyclectomy [ˌiridəusaiˈklektəmi] *n* 虹膜睫状体切除术
iridocyclitis [ˌiridəusaiˈklaitis] *n* 虹膜睫状体炎 | heterochromic ~ 异色性虹膜睫状体炎(亦称异色性眼色素层炎)
iridocyclochoroiditis [ˌiridəuˌsaikləuˌkɔːrɔiˈdaitis] *n* 虹膜睫状体脉络膜炎
iridocystectomy [ˌiridəusisˈtektəmi] *n* 虹膜囊切除术
iridocyte [aiˈridəsait] *n* 虹[色]细胞
iridodesis [ˌiriˈdɔdisis] *n* 虹膜固定术
iridodiagnosis [ˌiridəuˌdaiəgˈnəusis] *n* 虹膜诊断
iridodialysis [ˌiridəudaiˈælisis] *n* 虹膜根部断离
iridodiastasis [ˌiridəudaiˈæstəsis] *n* 虹膜根部缺损(虹膜周缘的一种缺损,但未波及瞳孔的边缘,产生临床性的多瞳外貌)
iridodilator [ˌiridəudaiˈleitə] *n* 虹膜扩大肌;虹膜扩大剂
iridodonesis [ˌiridəudəˈniːsis] *n* 虹膜震颤
iridokeratitis [ˌiridəuˌkerəˈtaitis] *n* 虹膜角膜炎
iridokinesis [ˌiridəukaiˈniːsis, -kiˈn-], **iridokinesia** [ˌiridəukaiˈniːziə, -kiˌn-] *n* 虹膜伸缩 | **iridokinetic** [ˌiridəukaiˈnetik, -kiˈn-] *a*
iridoleptynsis [ˌiridəulepˈtinsis] *n* 虹膜薄缩,虹膜萎缩
iridology [ˌiriˈdɔlədʒi] *n* 虹膜学
iridolysis [ˌiriˈdɔlisis] *n* 虹膜松解术
iridomalacia [ˌiridəuməˈleiʃiə] *n* 虹膜软化
iridomesodialysis [ˌiridəuˌmiːsəudaiˈælisis] *n* 虹膜内缘黏着部分离
iridomotor [ˌiridəuˈməutə] *a* 虹膜伸缩的,虹膜运动的
iridoncus [ˌiriˈdɔŋkəs] *n* 虹膜瘤,虹膜肿
iridopathy [ˌiriˈdɔpəθi] *n* 虹膜病
iridoperiphakitis [ˌiridəuˌperifeiˈkaitis] *n* 虹膜晶状体囊炎
iridoplegia [ˌiridəuˈpliːdʒiə] *n* 虹膜麻痹 | accommodation ~ 调节性虹膜麻痹 / complete ~ 完全虹膜麻痹 / sympathetic ~ 交感性虹膜麻痹 | **iridoparalysis** [ˌiridəupəˈrælisis] *n*
iridoptosis [ˌiridɔpˈtəusis] *n* 虹膜脱垂
iridopupillary [ˌiridəuˈpjuːpiləri] *a* 虹膜瞳孔的
iridorhexis [ˌiridəuˈrəksis] *n* 虹膜破裂;虹膜撕裂法

iridoschisis [ˌiriˈdɔskisis] *n* 虹膜缺损;虹膜襞裂症
iridosclerotomy [ˌiridəuskliəˈrɔtəmi] *n* 虹膜巩膜切开术
iridosteresis [ˌiridəustiˈriːsis] *n* 虹膜缺失,虹膜切除术
iridotasis [ˌiriˈdɔtəsis] *n* 虹膜展开术
iridotomy [ˌiriˈdɔtəmi] *n* 虹膜切开术
Iridoviridae [ˌiridəuˈviridiː] *n* 虹彩病毒属
iridovirus [ˌiridəuˈvaiərəs] *n* 虹色病毒
irinotecan hydrochloride [ˌaiərinəuˈtiːkæn] 盐酸伊立替康(DNA 拓扑异构酶抑制剂,用作抗肿瘤药,治疗结肠直肠癌,静脉输注给药)
IRIS International Research Information Service 国际研究情报服务处
Iris [ˈaiəris] *n* 鸢尾属
iris [ˈaiəris] ([复] **irises** 或 **irides** [ˈaiəridiːz]) *n* 虹膜;[蓝旗]鸢尾根 | ~ bombé, umbrella ~ 虹膜膨隆 / Florentine ~ 南欧香菖根 / tremulous ~ 虹膜震颤
irisin [ˈaiərisin] *n* 鸢尾糖,茑尾淀粉
irisopsia [ˌaiəriˈsɔpsiə] *n* 虹视
iritis [ˌaiəˈraitis] *n* 虹膜炎 | ~ catamenialis 经期前虹膜炎 / gouty ~, uratic ~ 痛风虹膜炎 / ~ papulosa 丘疹性虹膜炎 / plastic ~ 成形性虹膜炎 / serous ~ 浆液性虹膜炎 / spongy ~ 海绵状虹膜炎 | **iritic** [aiəˈritik] *a*
iritoectomy [ˌiritəuˈektəmi] *n* 虹膜部分切除术
iritomy [aiˈritəmi] *n* 虹膜切开术
irium [ˈiriəm] *n* 月桂硫酸钠,十二烷硫酸钠
iron(Fe) [ˈaiən] *n* 铁 | ~ acetate 醋酸铁(收敛剂)/ alcoholized ~, pulverized ~ 铁粉 / available ~ (食物)可利用铁,可吸收铁 / ~ citrate green 绿枸橼酸铁(用作肌内注射及皮下注射)/ dialyzed ~ 渗析铁 / ~ glycerophosphate 甘油磷酸铁 / iodobehanate 碘萮树酸铁,碘二十二碳酸铁(曾用于治淋巴结结核、萎黄病、佝偻病等)/ ~ magnesium sulfate 硫酸铁镁(治贫血)/ reduced ~ 还原铁 / ~ sorbitex 山梨醇铁(补血药)/ ~ succinate 琥珀酸铁,丁二酸铁(可用于治胆石病)
irotomy [aiˈrɔtəmi] *n* 虹膜切开术
irradiance [iˈreidjəns] *n* 辐照度
irradiate [iˈreidieit] *vt* (用 X 线或其他放射线)照射,辐照 | **irradiative** *a* 有放射力的 / **irradiator** *n* 辐照器
irradiation [iˌreidiˈeiʃən] *n* 照射;扩散 | graft ~ 移植物照射 / interstitial ~ 间质内照射 / ultraviolet blood ~ 紫外线照血法 / whole-body ~ 全身辐照,全身照射
irradicable [iˈrædikəbl] *a* 不能根除的
irrecoverable [ˌiriˈkʌvərəbl] *a* 不能恢复的;医治不好的
irreducible [ˌiriˈdjuːsəbl] *a* 不能复位的;不能还原的
irregular [iˈregjulə] *a* 不齐的,不规则的
irregularity [iˌregjuˈlærəti] *n* 不齐,不规则 | ~ of pulse 脉律不齐,心律不齐,无节律
irreinoculability [ˌiriiˌnɔkjuləˈbiləti] *n* 再接种不能
irremediable [ˌiriˈmiːdjəbl] *a* 医治不好的
irremovable [iriˈmuːvəbl] *a* 不能切除的
irrespirable [iˈrespirəbl, ˌirisˈpaiərəbl] *a* 不能呼吸的
irresponsible [ˌirisˈpɔnsəbl] *a* 无责任能力的 | **irresponsibility** [ˈirisˌpɔnsəˈbiləti] *n*
irresponsive [ˌirisˈpɔnsiv] *a* 无反应的
irretention [ˌiriˈtenʃən] *n* 失禁(尤指小便)
irretentive [iriˈtentiv] *a* 无保持力的(尤指记忆)
irreversibility [ˌiriˌvəːsəˈbiləti] *n* 不可逆性 | ~ of conduction 传导不可逆性
irreversible [ˌiriˈvəːsəbl] *a* 不可逆的
irrigate [ˈirigeit] *vt* 灌注;冲洗(伤口) | **irrigator** *n* 冲洗器
irrigation [ˌiriˈgeiʃən] *n* 灌注;冲洗,冲洗法;冲洗液 | continuous ~ 连续冲洗法 / mediate ~ 间接冲洗法 / ~ of maxillary sinus 上颌窦冲洗 / sodium chloride ~ 氯化钠冲洗液
irrigoradioscopy [ˌirigəuˌreidiˈɔskəpi], **irrigoscopy** [ˌiriˈgɔskəpi] *n* 灌肠 X 线透视检查,注洗 X 线检查法
irritability [ˌiritəˈbiləti] *n* 易激惹;应激性;过敏 | ~ of the bladder 膀胱过敏 / chemical ~ 化学应激性 / electric ~ 电应激性 / faradic ~ 感应电应激性 / galvanic ~ 流电应激性 / mechanical ~ 机械[刺激]应激性 / muscular ~ 肌应激性 / myotatic ~ 肌牵张应激性 / nervous ~ 神经应激性;神经过敏 / ~ of the stomach 胃过敏 / tactile ~ 接触应激性(细胞)
irritable [ˈiritəbl] *a* 易怒的;应激性的;过敏的
irritant [ˈiritənt] *a* 刺激[性]的;引起发炎的 *n* 刺激剂,刺激物
irritation [ˌiriˈteiʃən] *n* 刺激[作用];兴奋 | cerebral ~ 大脑刺激 / direct ~ 直接刺激 / functional ~ 功能性刺激
irritative [ˈiriteitiv] *a* 刺激的
Irukandji syndrome (sting) [ˌirjuːˈkændʒi] (Irukandji 为澳大利亚昆士兰州土著部落)依鲁坎吉综合征(螫伤)(澳大利亚昆士兰州观察到的临床综合征,由于水母螫伤所致;症状包括可能致命的初期神经肌肉麻痹及存活者中系统性症状,伴肺水肿和感染部位的皮肤溃疡)
IRV inspiratory reserve volume 补吸气量
Irving technique (operation) [ˈəːviŋ] (F. C.

Irving) 欧文技术(手术)(输卵管结扎法,此法将输卵管结扎和截断,其近端缝入子宫肌膜)

IS intercostal space 肋间隙

ISA intrinsic sympathomimetic activity 内在拟交感神经活动

Isaacs' syndrome [ˈaizəks] (H. Isaacs) 艾萨克综合征(进行性肌僵硬和痉挛,伴持续性肌纤维活动,类似神经性肌强直所见)

Isaacs-Mertens syndrome [ˈaizəks ˈmertenz] (H. Isaacs; H. G. Mertens) 艾-梅综合征(见 Isaacs' syndrome)

Isambert's disease [izɑːmˈbɛə] (Emile Isambert) 伊桑贝尔病(急性粟粒性咽喉结核)

isamoxole [ˌaisəˈmɔksəul] *n* 双丁噁胺(平喘药)

isatin [ˈaisətin] *n* 靛红(用作试剂)

isauxesis [ˌisɔːkˈsiːsis] *n* 均等增生,同度发育,等速增长(指个体的一个部分或各部分与整体长得一样快)

ischemia [isˈkiːmiə] *n* 缺血 | myocardial ~ 心肌缺血 | **ischemic** [isˈkemik] *a*

ischesis [isˈkiːsis] *n* 分泌物潴留

ischia [ˈiskiə] ischium 的复数

ischiadelphus [ˌiskiəˈdelfəs] *n* 坐骨联胎

ischialgia [ˌiskiˈældʒiə], **ischias** [ˈiskiəs] *n* 坐骨神经痛

ischiatic [ˌiskiˈætik], **ischiac** [ˈiskiæk], **ischiadic** [ˌiskiˈædik], **ischial** [ˈiskiəl] *a* 坐骨的

ischidrosis [ˌiskiˈdrəusis] *n* 汗闭

ischiectomy [ˌiskiˈektəmi] *n* 坐骨切除术

ischi(o)- [构词成分] 髋,坐骨

ischioanal [ˌiskiəuˈeinl] *a* 坐骨肛门的

ischiobulbar [ˌiskiəuˈbʌlbə] *a* 坐骨尿道球的

ischiocapsular [ˌiskiəuˈkæpsjulə] *a* 坐骨囊韧带的

ischiocele [ˈiskiəsiːl] *n* 坐骨孔疝

ischiococcygeal [ˌiskiəukɔkˈsidʒiəl] *a* 坐骨尾骨的

ischiococcygeus [ˌiskiəukɔkˈsidʒiəs] *n* 坐骨尾骨肌,尾骨肌

ischiodidymus [ˌiskiəuˈdidiməs] *n* 坐骨联胎

ischiodymia [ˌiskiəuˈdimiə] *n* 坐骨联胎畸形

ischiodynia [ˌiskiəuˈdiniə] *n* 坐骨神经痛

ischiofemoral [ˌiskiəuˈfemərəl] *a* 坐骨股骨的

ischiofibular [ˌiskiəuˈfibjulə] *a* 坐骨腓骨的

ischiohebotomy [ˌiskiəuhiˈbɔtəmi] *n* 耻骨坐骨支切开术

ischiomelus [ˌiskiˈɔmiləs] *n* 坐骨寄生肢畸胎

ischionitis [ˌiskiəuˈnaitis] *n* 坐骨结节炎

ischiopagia [ˌiskiəuˈpeidʒiə], **ischiopagy** [ˌiskiˈɔpədʒi] *n* 坐骨联胎畸形

ischiopagus [iskiˈɔpəgəs] *n* 坐骨联胎

ischiopubic [ˌiskiəuˈpjuːbik] *a* 坐骨耻骨的

ischiorectal [ˌiskiəuˈrektl] *a* 坐骨直肠的

ischiosacral [ˌiskiəuˈseikrəl] *a* 坐骨骶骨的

ischiothoracopagus [ˌiskiəuˌθɔːrəˈkɔpəgəs] *n* 坐骨胸部联胎,髂胸联胎

ischiovaginal [ˌiskiəuˈvædʒinl] *a* 坐骨阴道的

ischiovertebral [ˌiskiəuˈvəːtibrəl] *a* 坐骨脊椎的

ischium [ˈiskiəm] ([复] **ischia** [ˈiskiə]) *n* 【拉】坐骨

isch(o)- [构词成分] 闭止,抑制,缺乏

ischogyria [ˌiskəuˈdʒaiəriə] *n* 脑回萎小

ischuria [isˈkjuəriə] *n* 尿闭 | ~ paradoxa 矛盾尿闭,奇异尿闭(患者虽排尿而膀胱仍过度膨胀)/ ~ spastica 痉挛性尿闭 | **ischuretic** [ˌiskjuəˈretik] *a*

ISCP International Society of Comparative Pathology 国际比较病理学会

-ise 见-ize

iseiconia, iseikonia [ˌaisiˈkəuniə] *n* 双眼等像 | **iseiconic** [ˌaisiˈkɔnik] *a*

isethionate [ˌisəˈθaiəneit] *n* 羟乙磺酸盐(2-hydroxyethanesulfonate 的 USAN 缩约词)

isethionic acid [ˌiseθaiˈɔnik] 羟乙磺酸

ISGE International Society of Gastro-Enterology 国际胃肠病学会

ISH International Society of Hematology 国际血液学会

Ishihara's plates [ˌiʃiˈhɑːrə] (Shinobu Ishihara 石原忍) 石原板(假同色板,用于石原试验) | ~ test 石原试验(用一系列同色板检色彩视力)

isinglass [ˈaiziŋglɑːs] *n* 鱼胶 | Japanese ~ 琼脂,洋粉

island [ˈailənd] *n* 岛 | blood ~s 血岛 / cartilage ~s 软骨岛,软骨内骨 / olfactory ~s 嗅岛

islet [ˈailet] *n* 岛;胰岛 | blood ~s 血岛

ISM International Society of Microbiologists 国际微生物学家学会

-ism [后缀]中毒;行为,状态;主义

ISO International Standards Organization 国际标准组织

iso- [前缀]相等,均等;同族,同种;异构

isoadrenocorticism [ˌaisəuəˌdriːnəuˈkɔːtisizəm] *n* 肾上腺皮质功能正常

isoagglutination [ˌaisəuəˌgluːtiˈneiʃən] *n* 同种凝集

isoagglutinin [ˌaisəuəˈgluːtinin] *n* 同种凝集素

isoallele [ˌaisəuəˈliːl] *n* 同等位基因(只能通过特殊测验方法才能区别于正常基因的等位基因)

isoallelism [ˌaisəuəˈliːlizəm] *n* 同等位基因

isoalloxazine [ˌaisəuəˈlɔksəziːn] *n* 异咯嗪

isoamylamine [ˌaisəuˌæmiˈlæmin] *n* 异戊胺

isoamylethylbarbituric acid [ˌaisəuˌæmilˌeθilbɑːbiˈtjuərik] 异戊基乙基巴比妥酸,异戊巴比妥

isoamyl methoxycinnamate [ˌaisəuˈæmilmeˌθɔksiˈsinəmeit] 异戊甲氧肉桂酸(即 amiloxate,防晒药)
isoamyl nitrite [ˌaisəuˈæmil] 亚硝酸异戊酯(抗心绞痛药)
isoanaphylaxis [ˌaisəuˌænəfiˈlæksis] *n* 同种过敏性
isoandrosterone [ˌaisəuænˈdrɔstərəun] *n* 异雄甾酮
isoantibody [aisəuˈæntiˌbɔdi] *n* 同种抗体
isoantigen [ˌaisəuˈæntidʒən] *n* 同种抗原
isoascorbic acid [ˌaisəuəsˈkɔːbik] 异抗坏血酸,阿拉伯糖型抗坏血酸
isobar [ˈaisəubɑː] *n* 同量异位素;等压线 | ~**ic** [ˌaisəuˈbærik] *a* 等比重的;等压的
isobody [ˈaisəuˌbɔdi] *n* 同族体,同种抗体
isobolism [aiˈsɔbəlizəm] *n* 均等兴奋性
isobornyl thiocyanoacetate [ˌaisəuˈbɔːnilˌθaiəuˌsaiənəuˈæsiteit] 异龙脑硫氰醋酸酯,硫氰乙酸萜品酯(灭虱药)
isobucaine hydrochloride [ˌaisəuˈbjuːkein] 盐酸异布卡因(牙科局部麻醉药)
isobutamben [ˌaisəubjuːˈtæmben] *n* 氨苯异丁酯,对氨苯酸异丁酯(局部麻醉药)
isobutane [ˌaisəuˈbjuːtein] *n* 异丁烷
isobutanol [ˌaisəuˈbjuːtənɔl] *n* 异丁醇
isobutyric acid [ˌaisəubju(ː)ˈtirik] 异丁酸
isocaloric [ˌaisəukəˈlɔːrik] *a* 等热量的
isocarboxazid [ˌaisəukɑːˈbɔksəzid] *n* 异卡波肼(单胺氧酶抑制药,抗抑郁药)
isocarveol [ˌaisəuˈkɑːviɔl] *n* 异香芹醇,松香芹醇
isocellobiose [ˌaisəuˌseləˈbaiəus] *n* 异纤维二糖
isocellular [ˌaisəuˈseljulə] *a* 等细胞的,相同细胞[构成]的
isocenter [ˈaisəuˌsentə] *n* 等中心(指最大或最小照射剂量点)
isocholesterol [ˌaisəukəˈlestərɔl], **isocholesterin** [ˌaisəukəˈlestərin] *n* 异胆甾醇,异胆固醇
isochromatic [ˌaisəukrəuˈmætik] *a* 等色的
isochromatophil [ˌaisəukrəuˈmætəfil] *a* 等嗜染的
isochromosome [ˌaisəuˈkrəuməsəum] *n* 等臂染色体
isochronia [aisəuˈkrəuniə], **isochronism** [aiˈsɔkrənizəm] *n* 等时性;等时值(指肌肉与其神经间有相同的时值)
isochronous [aiˈsɔkrənəs], **isochronal** [aiˈsɔkrənl], **isochronic** [ˌaisəuˈkrɔnik] *a* 等时的
isochroous [aiˈsɔkrəuəs] *a* 等色的
isocitrate [ˌaisəuˈsitreit] *n* 异枸橼酸盐
isocitrate dehydrogenase (NAD$^+$) [ˌaisəuˈsitreit diːˈhaidrədʒəneis] 异枸橼酸脱氢酶(NAD$^+$)
isocitrate dehydrogenase (NADP$^+$) [ˌaisəuˈsitreit diːˈhaidrədʒəneis] 异枸橼酸脱氢酶(NADP$^+$)
isocitric acid [ˌaisəuˈsitrik] 异枸橼酸
isocoagulase [ˌaisəukəuˈægjuleis] *n* 同工凝固酶
isocolloid [aisəuˈkɔlɔid] *n* 等相胶体,等相胶质
isocomplement [ˌaisəuˈkɔmplimənt] *n* 同种补体,同族补体
isocomplementophilic [ˌaisəuˌkɔmplimentəuˈfilik] *a* 亲同种补体的
isoconazole [ˌaisəuˈkəunəzəul] *n* 异康唑(抗细菌和抗真菌药)
isocoria [ˌaisəuˈkɔːriə] *n* 瞳孔等大
isocortex [ˌaisəuˈkɔːteks] *n* 同形皮质,新[脑]皮质
isocreatinine [ˌaisəukriˈætinin] *n* 异肌酸酐
isocyanate [ˌaisəuˈsaiəneit] *n* 异氰酸盐
isocyanide [ˌaisəuˈsaiənaid] *n* 胩,异腈,异氰化物
isocyclic [ˌaisəuˈsaiklik, -ˈsik-] *a* 等环的,同素环的(化合物);碳环的(化合物)
isocytolysin [ˌaisəusaiˈtɔlisin] *n* 同种溶细胞素
isocytosis [ˌaisəusaiˈtəusis] *n* 细胞等大(尤指红细胞等大)
isocytotoxin [ˌaisəuˌsaitəuˈtɔksin] *n* 同种细胞毒素
isodactylism [ˌaisəuˈdæktilizəm] *n* 指等长
isodesmosine [ˌaisəuˈdesməsiːn] *n* 异锁链[赖氨]素
isodiagnosis [ˌaisəuˌdaiəgˈnəusis] *n* 血液接种诊断法
isodiametric [ˌaisəuˌdaiəˈmetrik] *a* 等径的
isodimorphism [ˌaisəudaiˈmɔːfizəm] *n* 同二晶[现象] | **isodimorphous** [ˌaisəudaiˈmɔːfəs] *a*
isodispersoid [ˌaisəudisˈpəːsɔid] *n* 等相胶体,等相胶质
isodontic [ˌaisəuˈdɔntik] *a* 同形牙的
isodose [ˈaisəudəus] *n* 同等[辐射]量
isodulcite [ˌaisəuˈdʌlsait] *n* 鼠李糖
isodynamic [ˌaisəudaiˈnæmik] *n* 等力的
isodynamogenic [ˌaisəudaiˌnæməuˈdʒenik] *a* 生力均等的
isoeffect [ˌaisəuiˈfekt] *n* 等效[应]
isoelectric [ˌaisəuiˈlektrik] *a* 等电的,等电势的
isoenergetic [ˌaisəuˌenəˈdʒetik] *a* 等能的
isoenzyme [ˌaisəuˈenzaim] *n* 同工酶
isoerucic acid [ˌaisəuiˈruːsik] 异芥子酸,异二十二碳烯酸
isoetharine [ˌaisəuˈeθəriːn] *n* 异他林(支气管扩张药)
isoeugenol [ˌaisəuˈjuːdʒənɔl] *n* 异丁香油酚,异

丁子香酚

isofebrifugine [ˌaisəuˌfebriˈfjuːdʒiːn] *n* 异[黄]常山碱

isoflupredone acetate [ˌaisəuˈfljupridəun] 异氟泼尼龙醋酸酯(抗炎药)

isoflurane [ˌaisəuˈfljuərein] *n* 异氟醚,异氟烷(吸入麻醉药)

isoflurophate [ˌaisəuˈfluərəfeit] *n* 异氟磷(胆碱酯酶抑制药,缩瞳药)

isogamete [ˌaisəuˈgæmiːt] *n* 同形配子 | **isogametic** [ˌaisəugəˈmetik] *a*

isogamety [ˌaisəuˈgæməti] *n* 同形配子产生

isogamy, isogame [aiˈsɔgəmi] *n* 同配生殖 | **isogamous** [aiˈsɔgəməs] *a*

isogeneic [ˌaisəudʒiˈniːik] *a* 同基因的,同系的,同源的

isogeneric [ˌaisəudʒiˈnəːrik] *a* 同属的(生物)

isogenesis [ˌaisəuˈdʒenisis] *n* 同源,同式发育

isogenic [ˌaisəuˈdʒenik] *a* 同基因的,同源的

isogenous [aiˈsɔdʒinəs] *a* 同源的 | **isogeny** [aiˈsɔdʒəni] *n*

isograft [ˈaisəugrɑːft, -græft] *n* 同系移植物,同基因移植物;同系移植,同型移植

isohemagglutination [ˌaisəuˌheməˌgluːtiˈneiʃən] *n* 同种血细胞凝集[作用],同族血凝反应

isohemagglutinin [ˌaisəuˌheməˈgluːtinin] *n* 同种血细胞凝集素,同族血凝素

isohemolysin [ˌaisəuhiˈmɔlisin] *n* 同种溶血素,同族溶血素

isohemolysis [ˌaisəuhiˈmɔləsis] *n* 同种溶血,同族溶血 | **isohemolytic** [ˌaisəuˌhiːməˈlitik] *a*

isohydric [ˌaisəuˈhaidrik] *a* 等氢离子的

isohypercytosis [ˌaisəuˌhaipəːsaiˈtəusis] *n* 等比例白细胞增多

isohypocytosis [ˌaisəuˌhaipəusaiˈtəusis] *n* 等比例白细胞减少

isoiconia [ˌaisəuaiˈkɔniə] *n* 双侧像相同 | **isoiconic** [ˌaisəuaiˈkɔnik] *a*

isoimmunization [ˌaisəuˌimju(ː)naiˈzeiʃən, -niˈz-] *n* 同种免疫 | Rh ~ Rh 同种免疫作用(Rh 阴性者由于接受 Rh 阳性者的输血,或 Rh 阴性妇女怀有 Rh 阳性胎儿,而产生抗 Rh 凝集素)

isointense [ˌaisəuinˈtens] *a* 等强度的(具有与某一物体的强度相同的)

Isojima test [ˌiːsəuˈdʒiːmə] (S. Isojima) 矶岛试验,精子制动试验(检男性不育因子)

isokinetic [ˌaisəukəˈnetik] *a* 等动力的(指一种操练,在肌肉缩短或伸长时,维持经常的旋力和张力)

isokreatinin [ˌaisəukriˈætinin] *n* 异肌酸酐

isolactose [ˌaisəuˈlæktəus] *n* 异乳糖

isolate [ˈaisəuleit] *vt* 隔离,孤立;分离 *n* 分离菌;隔离群 | **isolated** *a* 隔离的,孤立的;分离的;单一性的

isolation [ˌaisəuˈleiʃən] *n* 隔离;分离;单离 | reverse ~ 反向隔离

isolator [ˈaisəuleitə] *n* 隔离者;隔离物,隔离包 | surgical ~ 外科隔离包,手术隔离包(用透明塑料制成,可分别容纳并隔离患者和医护人员)

isolecithal [ˌaisəuˈlesiθəl] *a* 等[卵]黄的,均[卵]黄的

isolette [ˌaisəˈlet] *n* 早产婴儿保育箱

isoleucine [ˌaisəuˈljuːsiːn] *n* 异亮氨酸

isoleucyl [ˌaisəuˈluːsil] *n* 异亮氨酰[基]

isoleukoagglutinin [ˌaisəuˌljuːkəəˈgluːtinin] *n* 同种白细胞凝集素

isoleukocytosis [ˌaisəuˌljuːkəsaiˈtəusis] *n* 等比例白细胞增多

isologous [aiˈsɔləgəs] *a* 同基因的,同系的

isolog(ue) [ˈaisəulɔg] *n* 同构[异素]体

isolysergic acid [ˌaisəulaiˈsəːdʒik] 异麦角酸

isolysin [aiˈsɔlisin] *n* 同种溶素,同族溶素

isolysis [aiˈsɔləsis] *n* 同种溶解,同族溶解 | **isolytic** [ˌaisəuˈlitik] *a*

isomaltase [ˌaisəuˈmɔːlteis] *n* 异麦芽糖酶,低聚 1, 6-α-葡糖苷酶

isomaltose [ˌaisəuˈmɔːltəus] *n* 异麦芽糖,糊精糖

isomastigote [ˌaisəuˈmæstigəut] *a* 等鞭毛的

isomer [ˈaisəumə] *n* 同分异构[体];同质异能素(原子核物理)

isomerase [aiˈsɔməreis] *n* 异构酶

isomeric [ˌaisəuˈmerik] *a* 同分异构的;同质异能的

isomeride [aiˈsɔməraid] *n* 同分异构体

isomerism [aiˈsɔmərizəm] *n* 异构[现象] | chain ~, muclear ~ 异链[同分]异构,同核异构 / *cis-trans* ~ 顺-反异构,立体异构 / configurative ~ 立体异构 / conformational ~ 构象异构 / constitutional ~ 结构异构 / dynamic ~ 互变异构,同质异性 / functional group ~ [同分]功能基团异构 / geometric ~ 立体异构 / optical ~ 旋光异构 / position ~, substitution ~ 位置异构 / spatial ~, stereochemical ~ 立体异构 / structural ~ 结构异构

isomerization [aiˌsɔməraiˈzeiʃən, -riˈz-] *n* 异构化

isometheptene hydrochloride [ˌaisəuməˈθeptiːn] 盐酸异美汀(拟肾上腺素药,解痉药,血管扩张药)

isometheptene mucate [ˌaisəuməˈθeptiːn ˈmjuːkeit] 半乳糖二酸异美汀(与氯醛比林〈dichloroalphenazone〉和对乙酰氨基酚〈acetaminophen〉合用,治疗血管性和紧张性头痛,口服给药)

isometric(al) [ˌaisəuˈmetrik(əl)] *a* 等长的;非等渗的

isometropia [ˌaisəuməˈtrəupiə] *n* 屈光等同
isometry [aiˈsɔmitri] *n* 等长,等距
isomicrogamete [ˌaisəuˌmaikrəuˈgæmiːt] *n* 同形小配子
isomorphism [ˌaisəuˈmɔːfizəm] *n* 同形性;同晶型
isomorphous [ˌaisəuˈmɔːfəs], **isomorphic** [ˌaisəuˈmɔːfik] *a* 同形的;(异质)同晶的
isomuscarine [ˌaisəuˈmʌskəriːn] *n* 异毒蕈碱
isomylamine hydrochloride [ˌaisəuˈmiləmiːn] 盐酸异戊拉明(平滑肌松弛药)
isonaphthol [ˌaisəuˈnæfθɔl] *n* 异萘酚, β-萘酚
isonephrotoxin [ˌaisəuˌnefrəuˈtɔksin] *n* 同种肾毒素
isoniazid [ˌaisəuˈnaiəzid], **isonicotinoylhydrazine** [ˌaisəuˌnikətinəuilˈhaidrəziːn], **isonicotinylhydrazine** [ˌaisəuˌnikəˌtinilˈhaidrəziːn] *n* 异烟肼(抗结核药)
isonicotinic acid [ˌaisəuˌnikəˈtinik] 异烟酸
isonipecaine [ˌaisəuˈnipikein] *n* 哌替啶,度冷丁(麻醉镇痛药)
isonitrile [ˌaisəuˈnaitrail] *n* 异腈,胩,异氰化物
isonormocytosis [ˌaisəuˌnɔːməusaiˈtəusis] *n* 等比例白细胞正常
iso-oncotic [ˌaisəuɔŋˈkɔtik] *a* 等膨胀压的
iso-osmotic [ˌaisəuɔzˈmɔtik] *a* 等渗的
Isoparorchis trisimilitubis [ˌaisəupəˈrɔːkis traiˌsimilaiˈtjuːbis] 三等管等睾吸虫,三似管等睾吸虫
isopathy [aiˈsɔpəθi] *n* 同源疗法 | **isopathic** [ˌaisəuˈpæθik] *a*
isopatin [aiˈsɔpətin] *n* 无蛋白免疫原
isopentenyl-diphosphate δ-isomerase [ˌaisəuˌpentinil daiˈfɔsfeit aiˈsɔməreis] 异戊烯[基]二磷酸 δ-异构酶
isophagy [aiˈsɔfədʒi] *n* 自溶,自体溶解
isophan [ˈaisəufən] *n* 同型杂种
isophane [ˈaisəufein] *a* 低精蛋白锌的 *n* 低精蛋白锌胰岛素
isophenolization [ˌaisəuˌfiːnəlaiˈzeiʃən, -liˈz-] *n* 异酚处理法(注射异酚使交感神经麻痹或破坏)
isophoria [ˌaisəuˈfəuriə] *n* 两眼视线等平(无上下隐斜)
isopia [aiˈsəupiə] *n* 两眼视力相等
isoplassont [ˌaisəuˈplæsɔnt] *n* 同种物
isoplastic [ˌaisəuˈplæstik] *a* 同基因的,同系的(指组织移植物)
isoprecipitin [ˌaisəupriˈsipitin] *n* 同种沉淀素,同族沉淀素
isopregnenone [ˌaisəuˈpregninəun] *n* 异孕烯酮,6-脱氢[逆]孕酮(人工合成的孕酮)
isoprenaline [ˌaisəuˈprenəli(ː)n] *n* 异丙肾上腺素(见 isoproterenol)
isoprene [ˈaisəupriːn] *n* 异戊二烯
isoprenoid [ˌaisəuˈpriːnɔid] *n* 类异戊二烯
isopropamide [ˌaisəuˈprəupəmaid] *n* 异丙酰胺
isopropamide iodide [ˌaisəuˈprəupəmaid] 异丙碘铵(抗胆碱药,抗消化性溃疡药)
isopropanol [ˌaisəuˈprəupənɔl] *n* 异丙醇
isopropyl [ˌaisəuˈprəupil] *n* 异丙基 | ~ alcohol, ~ rubbing alcohol 异丙醇(消毒剂) / ~ myristate 十四酸异丙酯,肉豆蔻酸异丙酯(药用润滑剂)
isopropylaminoacetic acid [ˌaisəuˌprəupilˌæminəuəˈsiːtik] 异丙氨乙酸,缬氨酸
isopropylarterenol [ˌaisəuˌprəupilˌɑːtəˈriːnɔl] *n* 异丙肾上腺素
isopropyl-benzanthracene [ˌaisəuˌprəupil benzˈænθrəsiːn] *n* 异丙苯并蒽
isoprostane [ˌaisəuˈprɔstein] *n* 异前列烷
isoproterenol [ˌaisəuˌprəutəˈriːnɔl] *n* 异丙肾上腺素(用作拟交感神经药、心兴奋剂及解痉药,亦用于缓解支气管痉挛) | ~ hydrochloride 盐酸异丙肾上腺素(支气管扩张药) / ~ sulfate 硫酸异丙肾上腺素(支气管扩张药)
isopter [aiˈsɔptə] *n* 等视力线
isopyknic [ˌaisəuˈpiknik] *a* 等固缩的,等致密的,等密度的
isopyknosis [ˌaisəupikˈnəusis] *n* 等固缩现象,致密[度]相等(染色体) | **isopyknotic** [ˌaisəupikˈnɔtik] *a* 等固缩的,等致密的
isorhodeose [ˌaisəuˈrəudiəus] *n* 异万年青糖,奎诺糖
isoriboflavin [ˌaisəuˈraibəuˌfleivin] *n* 异核黄素
isorrhea [ˌaisəuˈriə] *n* 水出纳相等,水平衡 | **isorrheic** [ˌaisəuˈriik] *a*
isorrhopic [ˌaisəuˈrɔpik] *a* 等价的,等值的
isorubin [ˌaisəuˈruːbin] *n* 新品红
isosaccharic acid [ˌaisəusəˈkærik] 异葡萄糖二酸
isoscope [ˈaisəuskəup] *n* 眼动测位镜
isosensitization [ˌaisəuˌsensitaiˈzeiʃən, -tizˈ-] *n* 同族致敏作用
isoserine [ˌaisəuˈsiərin] *n* 异丝氨酸
isoserotherapy [ˌaisəuˌsiərəuˈθerəpi] *n* 同病血清疗法,恢复期血清疗法
isoserum [ˌaisəuˈsiərəm] *n* 同病血清
isosexual [ˌaisəuˈseksjuəl] *a* 同性的
isosmotic [ˌaisɔzˈmɔtik] *a* 等渗的 | **~ity** [ˌaisɔzməˈtisəti] *n* 等渗性
isosorbide [ˌaisəuˈsɔːbaid] *n* 异山梨醇(利尿药) | ~ dinitrate 硝酸异山梨酯(冠状动脉扩张药)
isospermotoxin [ˌaisəuˌspəːməuˈtɔksin] *n* 同种精子毒素
Isospora [aiˈsɔspərə] *n* 等孢子球虫属 | ~ belli

贝氏等孢子球虫,大等孢子球虫 / ~ bigemina 二联等孢子球虫 / ~ felis 猫等孢子球虫 / ~ hominis 人等孢子球虫 / ~ lacazei 鸟等孢子球虫 / ~ rivolta 犬等孢子球虫

isospore [ˈaisəuspɔː] *n* 同形孢子

isosporiasis [aiˌsɔspəˈraiəsis] *n* 等孢子球虫病

isosporous [ˌaisəuˈspɔːrəs, aiˈsɔspərəs] *a* 具同形孢子的

isospory [ˈaisəuˌspɔːri, aiˈsɔspəri] *n* 孢子同型

isostere [ˈaisəustiə] *n* 电子等排[体]

isosthenuria [ˌaisɔsθeˈnjuəriə] *n* 等渗尿,等张尿

isostimulation [ˌaisəuˌstimjuˈleiʃən] *n* 同质刺激法

isosulfocyanic acid [ˌaisəuˌsʌlfəusaiˈænik] 异硫氰酸

isothebaine [ˌaisəuˈθiːbeiin] *n* 异蒂巴因,异二甲基吗啡

isotherapy [ˌaisəuˈθerəpi] *n* 同源疗法

isotherm [ˈaisəuθəːm] *n* 等温线,恒温线 | **~al** [ˌaisəuˈθəːməl], **~ic** [ˌaisəuˈθəːmik] *a* 等温[线]的

isothermognosis [ˌaisəuˌθəːməuˈnəusis] *n* 等温感觉(痛、冷、热等刺激均引起温觉)

isothiazine hydrochloride [ˌaisəuˈθaiəziːn] 盐酸二乙异丙嗪(抗震颤麻痹药)

isothiocyanate [ˌaisəuˌθaiəuˈsaiəneit] *n* 异硫氰酸盐 | allyl ~ 异硫氰酸烯丙酯,烯丙基芥子油 / butyl ~ 异硫氰酸丁酯 / phenyl-ethyl ~ 异硫氰酸苯乙酯

isothiocyanic acid [ˌaisəuˌθaiəusaiˈænik] 异硫氰酸

isothipendyl [ˌaisəuˈθaipəndil] *n* 异西喷地,氮异丙嗪(抗组胺药)

isothromboagglutinin [ˌaisəuˌθrɔmbəuəˈgluːtinin] *n* 同种血小板凝集素

isotone [ˈaisəutəun] *n* 同中子异荷素,等中子[异位]素

isotonia [ˌaisəuˈtəuniə] *n* 等张性;等渗性

isotonic [ˌaisəuˈtɔnik] *a* 等张的;等渗的 | **~ity** [ˌaisəutəˈnisəti] *n* 等张性;等渗性

isotope [ˈaisəutəup] *n* 同位素 | radioactive ~ 放射性同位素 / stable ~ 稳定同位素 | **isotopic** [ˌaisəuˈtɔpik] *a* / **isotopy** [aiˈsɔtəpi] *n* 同位素学

isotopology [ˌaisəutəuˈpɔlədʒi] *n* 同位素学

isotoxin [ˌaisəuˈtɔksin] *n* 同种毒素,同族毒素 | **isotoxic** [ˌaisəuˈtɔksik] *a*

isotransplant [ˌaisəuˈtrænsplɑːnt, -plænt] *n* 同系移植物,同基因移植物;同系移植

isotransplantation [ˌaisəuˌtrænsplɑːnˈteiʃən] *n* 同系移植,同基因移植术

isotretinoin [ˌaisəuˈtretinɔin] *n* 异维 A 酸(角质溶解药)

Isotricha [aiˈsɔtrikə] *n* 等[纤]毛虫属

isotrimorphism [ˌaisəutraiˈmɔːfizəm] *n* 同三晶形[现象] | **isotrimorphous** [ˌaisəutraiˈmɔːfəs] *a*

isotron [ˌaisəutrɔn] *n* 同位素分析器

isotropic [ˌaisəuˈtrɔpik], **isotropous** [aiˈsɔtrəpəs] *a* 各向同性的;单折射的,单折光的 | **isotropy** [aiˈsɔtrəpi] *n*

isotropism [aiˈsɔtrəpizəm] *n* 各向同性(现象)

isotype [ˈaisəˌtaip] *n* 同种型(指免疫球蛋白重链或轻链类或亚类) | **isotypic** [ˌaisəuˈtipik] *a*

isotypical [ˌaisəuˈtipikəl] *a* 同种型的(指同一类型的)

isouretin [ˌaisəujuəˈriːtin] *n* 氨基甲肟

isouric acid [ˌaisəuˈjuərik] 异尿酸

isovaleric acid [ˌaisəuvəˈlerik], **isovalerianic acid** [ˌaisəuvəˌliəriˈænik] 异戊酸

isovalericacidemia [ˌaisəuvəˌlerikˌæsiˈdiːmiə] *n* 异戊酸血[症]

isovaleryl [ˌaisəuvəˈleril] *n* 异戊酰[基]

isovaleryl-CoA dehydrogenase [ˌaisəuvəˈleril diːˈhaidrədʒəneis] 异戊酸-CoA 脱氢酶,异戊酰辅酶 A 脱氢酶(此酶缺乏为一种常染色体隐性性状,可致异戊酸血症)

isovalerylglycine [ˌaisəuvəˌlerilˈglaisiːn] *n* 异戊酰甘氨酸

isovolumic [ˌaisəuvəˈljuːmik] *a* 等容的(维持相同容量的)

isoxepac [aiˈsɔksəpæk] *n* 伊索克酸(抗炎药)

isoxicam [aiˈsɔksikəm] *n* 伊索昔康(抗炎药)

isoxsuprine hydrochloride [aiˈsɔksjupriːn] 盐酸异克舒令(血管扩张药)

isozyme [ˈaisəuzaim] *n* 同工酶

isradipine [isˈrædipiːn] *n* 伊拉地平(其作用类似硝苯地平〈nifedipine〉,单独使用或与利尿药噻嗪类配伍治疗高血压,口服给药)

issue [ˈisjuː, ˈiʃjuː] *n* 流出,流出物;脓疮口

IST insulin shock therapy 胰岛素休克治疗

isthmectomy [isˈmektəmi] *n* 峡部切除术(甲状腺肿时)

isthmic [ˈismik], **isthmian** [ˈismiən] *a* 峡的

isthmitis [isˈmaitis] *n* 咽峡炎

isthmoplegia [ˌisməuˈpliːdʒiə], **isthmoparalysis** [ˌisməupəˈrælisis] *n* 咽峡麻痹,咽峡瘫痪

isthmospasm [ˈisməspæzəm] *n* 峡痉挛(如输卵管峡痉挛或咽峡痉挛)

isthmus [ˈisməs]([复] **isthmi** [ˈismai]) *n* 峡 | aortic ~ 主动脉峡 / ~ of auditory tube, ~ of eustachian tube 咽鼓管峡 / ~ of cingulate gyrus, ~ of limbic lobe 扣带回峡 / ~ of fallopian tube 输卵管峡 / ~ of fauces, oropharyngeal ~, pharyngooral ~ 咽峡 / ~ of thyroid gland 甲状腺峡

/ ~ of uterus 子宫峡
ISU International Society of Urology 国际泌尿学会
isuria [ai'sjuəriə] *n* 平均排尿
ITA International Tuberculosis Association 国际结核病协会
itaconic acid [ˌitə'kɔnik] 衣康酸,甲烯基丁二酸
Itard-Cholewa sign [i'tɑː kɔ'leivə] (Jean M. G. Itard; Erasmus R. Cholewa) 伊泰尔-科勒瓦征(耳硬化时鼓膜感觉消失)
Itard's catheter [i'tɑː] (Jean M. G. Itard) 伊塔尔导管(咽鼓管导管)
itate ['aiteit] *n* (乳中)亚硝酸氧化质
itch [itʃ] *n* 痒,痒病 *vi* 发痒 | bakers' ~ 揉面痒病 / barbers' ~ 须癣 / copra ~ 椰子螨皮炎 / Cuban ~ 轻型天花 / dhobie ~ 洗衣工痒病,洗衣员癣 / grain ~ , barley ~, mattress ~, millers' ~, straw ~ 谷痒病 / grocers' ~ 食品店员痒病,杂货商样病 / ground ~, dew ~, miners' ~ 钩虫痒病,着地痒 / jock ~ 股癣 / mad ~ 假狂犬病 / seven-year ~ 疥疮,疥螨病 / swimmers' ~ 游泳者皮炎,尾蚴性皮炎,血吸虫皮炎 / winter ~ 冬令瘙痒
itching ['itʃiŋ] *n* 痒,瘙痒
itchy ['itʃi] *a* 生疥疮的;[发]痒的**-ite** [后缀]矿物,岩石;身体,器官;亚…酸盐(如 phosphite)
iter ['aitə] *n*【拉】导管,通路 | ad infundibulum 漏斗口 / ~ a tertio ad quartum ventriculum 中脑水管 | **~al** ['aitərəl] *a*
iteroparity [ˌitərəu'pærəti] *n* 反复生殖 | **iteroparous** [ˌitə'rɔpərəs] *a*
-ites [后缀]水肿,浮肿
ithylordosis [ˌiθilɔː'dəusis] *n* 脊柱前凸
ithyokyphosis [ˌiθiəukai'fəusis], **ithycyphos** [ˌiθi'saifəus] *n* 脊柱后凸
itinerant [i'tinərənt] *a* 巡回的 *n* 巡回者
-itis ([复]**-itides**) [后缀]炎
Ito nevus ['iːtəu] (Minor Ito) 伊藤痣(亦称肩峰三角肌褐青色痣)
Ito-Reenstierna test ['iːtəu riːn'stiənə] (Hayazo Ito 伊藤隼三; John Reenstierna) 伊藤-林斯蒂尔纳试验(软下疳皮内试验)
ITP idiopathic thrombocytopenic purpura 特发性血小板减少性紫癜; inosine triphosphate 肌苷三磷酸
itraconazole [ˌitrə'kɔnəzəul] *n* 伊曲康唑(抗真菌药)
IU immunizing unit 免疫单位; international unit 国际单位
IUCD, IUD intrauterine contraceptive device 宫内节育器
IUGR intrauterine growth retardation 宫内发育迟缓
IV intravenously 静脉注射
ivain ['aiveiin] *n* 麝蓍草素
ivaol ['aiveiɔl] *n* 麝蓍油
IVC inferior vena cava 下腔静脉
Ivemark's syndrome ['iːvəmɑːk] (Bjön I. I. Ivemark) 伊弗马克综合征(先天性脾脏发育不全,有心脏缺陷及部分内脏转位。亦称无脾综合征)
ivermectin [aivəː'mektin] *n* 伊维菌素(抗寄生虫药)
IVF in vitro fertilization 试管内受精,体外受精
IVIC syndrome ['iːviːk] (Instituto Venezolano de Investigaciones Cientificas 委内瑞拉科学调查研究所) IVIC 综合征(一种罕见的常染色体显性遗传综合征,为内眼肌麻痹、听力损伤和桡骨辐条缺损,从细长拇指到整个上肢畸形不等,首次在委内瑞拉以后在意大利观察到。亦称眼-耳-桡骨综合征)
ivory ['aivəri] *n* 象牙;牙本质
VIP intravenous pyelogram 静脉肾盂造影[照]片; intravenous pyelography 静脉肾盂造影[术]
Ivy loop wiring ['aivi] (Robert H. Ivy) 艾维环状栓结术(栓结邻近两组牙,以供颌间皮圈附着)
IVRT isovolumic relaxation time 等容舒张时间
IVS interventricular septum (of heart) [心]室间隔
ivy ['aivi] *n* 常青藤 | poison ~ 毒漆,毒葛,野葛
Ivy's test (method) ['aivi] (Andrew C. Ivy) 艾维试验(法)(测出血时间,即以标准穿刺刺伤前臂后引起出血持续时间)
Iwanoff's (Iwanow's) cysts [i'wænɔf] (Wladimir P. Iwanoff) 伊凡诺夫囊肿(见 Blessig's cysts)
Ixodes [ik'səudiːz] *n* 硬蜱属 | ~ bicornis 双角硬蜱 / calvepalpus 须硬蜱 / ~ crenulatus, ~ canisuga 草原硬蜱,犬硬蜱 / ~ frequens, ~ ovatus 常见硬蜱,卵形硬蜱 / ~ hexagonus 六角形硬蜱 / ~ holocyclus 全环硬蜱 / ~ pacificus 太平洋硬蜱 / ~ persulcatus 全沟硬蜱 / ~ pilosus 多毛硬蜱 / ~ putus 海鸟硬蜱 / ~ rasus 獾硬蜱 / ~ ricinus 蓖子硬蜱 / ~ rubicundus 浅红硬蜱 / ~ scapularis 肩突硬蜱 / ~ spinipalpus 刺须硬蜱
ixodiasis [ˌiksəu'daiəsis], **ixodism** ['iksədizəm] *n* 蜱病
ixodic [ik'sɔdik] *a* 蜱的
ixodid ['iksədid] *n*, *a* 硬蜱(的)
Ixodidae [ik'sɔdidiː] *n* 硬蜱科
Ixodides [ik'sɔdidiːz] *n* 蜱亚目
Ixodiphagus [ˌiksəu'difəgəs] *n* 食蜱蜂属 | ~ caucurtei 柯氏食蜱蜂
Ixodoidea [ˌiksəu'dɔidiə] *n* 蜱总科
Iyengar yoga [iː'jengɑː] (B. K. S. Iyengar 为印度瑜伽教师) 伊因伽瑜伽(一种瑜伽法,在姿势方面强调正确的身体排列,并使姿势保持相当长的时间,亦可用木制支撑物帮助和支撑姿势)
Izar's reagent ['aizɑː] (Guido Izar) 伊扎试剂(用等量亚油酸和蓖麻油酸配成)
-ize [后缀]使成为,使…化;使…处理;类似于;使接受…活动方式

J

J joule 焦耳

jaagsiekte [jɑːɡ'siːkti], **jaagziekte** [jɑːɡ'ziːkti] *n* 南非羊肺炎

Jaboulay's amputation (operation) [ˌʒɑːbu'lei] (Mathieu Jaboulay) 股盆部分切断术,腹盆间切断术 | ~ button 雅布累钮(肠吻合钮,用于肠吻合术)

Jaccoud's dissociated fever [ʒə'kuː] (Sigismond Jaccoud) 雅库分离性热(脉搏缓慢不整的发热,见于成人结核性脑膜炎) | ~ sign 雅库征(胸骨上切迹的主动脉隆起) / ~ syndrume (arthritis) 雅库综合征(关节炎)(风湿热后,一般在反复发作后发生的慢性关节炎,特征为关节囊和肌腱的纤维化改变,导致类似类风湿关节炎畸形〈尤其是指尺骨偏位〉、关节疼痛,且常出现风湿结节,但骨糜烂不会发生)

jacket ['dʒækit] *n* 背心;甲冠 | plaster-of-Paris ~ 石膏背心 / strait ~ 约束衣

jackscrew ['dʒækskruː] *n* 螺旋正牙器

Jackson appliance (crib) ['jæksn] (Victor Hugo Jackson) 杰克逊矫正器(正牙器)(一种可摘正牙矫正器)

jacksonian epilepsy [dʒæk'səuniən] (John H. Jackson) 杰克逊癫痫(皮质局限性癫痫)

Jackson's law ['dʒæksn] (John H. Jackson) 杰克逊定律(最晚发生的神经功能最早损坏) | ~ rule 杰克逊规律(癫痫发作后,低级神经功能先行恢复) / ~ syndrome 杰克逊综合征(第十、十一和十二脑神经麻痹,软腭、喉、半面舌麻痹,伴胸锁乳突肌及斜方肌麻痹)

Jackson's membrane (veil) ['dʒæksn] (Jabez N. Jackson) 杰克逊膜(帆)(一种细薄帘状或蛛网状附着物〈有人认为是腹膜层〉,从腹侧壁延伸至盲肠,覆盖盲肠,并引起肠梗阻)

Jackson's safety triangle ['dʒæksn] (Chevalier Jackson)杰克逊安全三角(下界为甲状软骨的下边,尖端位于胸骨上切迹内,两边为胸锁乳突肌的内缘,之所以如此命名,是因为气管造口术时可通过此区安全地切开气管) | ~ sign 杰克逊征(气喘病样哮鸣)

Jackson's sign ['dʒæksn] (James Jackson, Jr.) 杰克逊征(肺结核时病灶部位呼气音延长)

Jacobaeus operation [ˌjɑːkə'beiəs] (Hans C. Jacobaeus) 雅科贝厄斯手术(胸膜松解术,用胸腔镜检查和烙术治胸膜粘连)

jacobine ['dʒeikəbin] *n* 贾可宾,千里光碱(一种有毒的生物碱,可引起肝坏死)

Jacob's ladder ['dʒeikəb] (源自《圣经》祖先雅克〈Jacob〉梦中所见的天梯)花葱;花葱制剂(局部用于溃疡,内服用于发热和炎症)

Jacob's membrane ['dʒeikəb] (Arthur Jacob) 雅各布膜,(视网膜)杆体(锥体)层 | ~ ulcer 雅各布溃疡(睑侵蚀性溃疡)

Jacobson's canal ['dʒeikəbsn] (Ludwig L. Jacobson) 鼓室小管 | ~ cartilage 犁鼻软骨 / ~ nerve 鼓室神经 / ~ organ 犁鼻器 / ~ plexus 鼓室丛 / ~ sulcus 鼓室岬沟;颞骨鼓沟

Jacobson's retinitis ['jɑːkɔbsən] (Julius Jacobson) 梅毒性视网膜炎

Jacobsthal's test ['jɑːkɔbztəl] (Erwin W. J. Jacobsthal) 雅各布斯他尔试验(①检梅毒的血清诊断:患者血清与梅毒肝脏乙醇浸出液按 1∶10 混合,用暗视野观察沉淀结果,强阳性有块状沉淀,弱阳性有小脂肪颗粒密聚,阴性呈均匀细小的跳动颗粒;②华氏〈Wassermann〉试验的改良,其补体结合在低温下进行)

Jacod's syndrome (triad) [ʒɑː'kəu] (Maurice Jacod) 雅可综合征(三联征)(单侧盲和眼肌麻痹,伴面偏瘫或三叉神经痛,常由于蝶骨后肿瘤或某一损害造成对第2、第3、第4、第5和第6脑神经损伤所致)

Jacquet's dermatitis (erythema) [ʒɑː'kei] (Leonard M. L. Jacquet) 尿布皮炎

jactatio [dʒæk'teiʃiəu] *n* 【拉】辗转不安 | ~ capitis nocturna 夜间摇头(见于儿童)

jactitation [ˌdʒækti'teiʃən], **jactation** [dʒæk'teiʃən] *n* 辗转不安(指急性病患者)

jaculiferous [ˌdʒækju'lifərəs] *a* 具刺的

Jadassohn-Lewandowsky syndrome ['jɑːdəsəun levɑːn'dɔvski] (Josef Jadassohn; Felix Lewandowsky) 亚-莱综合征,先天性厚甲

Jadassohn-Pellizari anetoderma ['jɑːdəsəun ˌpeli'zɑːri] (Josef Jadassohn; Pietro Pellizari) 亚-佩皮肤松弛(见 Jadassohn's anetoderma)

Jadassohn's anetoderma ['jɑːdəsəun] (Josef Jadassohn) 亚达佐恩皮肤松弛(炎症或荨麻疹性皮疹后发生的原发性皮肤松弛) / ~ sebaceous nevus 皮脂腺痣 / ~ test 亚达佐恩试验,(尿道)冲洗试验(检后尿道病)

Jadelot's lines(furrows) [ʒəd'ləu] (Jean F. N. Jadelot) 惹德洛线(面纹),病容线(幼儿面部表现特定疾病类型的线纹)

Jaeger's chart ['jeigə] (Edward Jaeger von Jastthal) 耶格近视力表 | ~ test types 耶格近距视力标型

Jaffe-Lichtenstein disease ['dʒæfi 'liktənstain] (Henry L. Jaffe; Louis Lichtenstein) 雅-利病(囊性骨纤维瘤病,多发性骨纤维发育不良的一型;特点为骨髓腔扩大而骨皮质薄,腔内充满纤维组织〈纤维瘤〉)

Jaffé's reaction [jɑː'fei] (Max Jaffé) 雅费反应(检肌酸酐) | ~ test 雅费试验(检肌酸酐、葡萄糖及尿蓝母)

jagsiekte [jɑːg'siːkti], **jagziekte** [jɑːg'ziːkti] *n* 见 jaagsiekte

Jakob's disease, Jakob-Creutzfeldt disease ['jɑːkɔb 'krɔitsfelt] (Alfons M. Jakob; Hans G. Creutzfeldt) 见 Creutzfeldt-Jakob disease

Jaksch's anemia(disease) ['jɑːkʃ] (Rudolf von Jaksch) 雅克什贫血(婴儿假白血病性贫血) | ~ test 雅克什试验(检胃酸、尿葡萄糖、黑素、尿酸)

jalap ['dʒæləp] *n* 球根牵牛,药喇叭(其干块根可制泻药)

jalapinolic acid [ˌdʒæləpi'nɔlik] 药喇叭脂酸,11-羟基十六酸

JAMA Journal of the American Medical Association 美国医学会杂志

jamais vu ['ʒɑːme 'vjuː]【法】认旧如新

Janet's disease [ʒɑː'nei] (Pierre M. F. Janet) 惹奈病(精神衰弱) | ~ test 惹奈试验(鉴别功能性和器质性之间的感觉丧失)

Janeway's lesion, spots ['dʒeinwei] (Edward Gamaliel Janeway) 詹韦损害、斑(亚急性细菌性心内膜炎时,手掌和足底常出现小的红斑性或出血性损害)

Janeway's sphygmomanometer ['dʒeinwei] (Theodore C. Janeway) 詹韦血压计

janiceps ['dʒæniseps] *n* 双面联胎 | ~ asymmetros 不对称双面联胎 / ~ parasiticus 寄生性双面联胎

Janin's tetanus [ʒə'næn] (Joseph Janin) 头部破伤风

Jannetta procedure [dʒə'netə] (Peter J. Jannetta) 詹内特手术,微血管减压术

Janošík's embryo ['jɑːnəusik] (Jan Janošík) 雅诺西克胚(具有3个主动脉弓和2个鳃囊的胚)

Jansen's disease ['jɑːnsən] (W. Murk Jansen) 干骺端发育不全 | ~ test 扬森试验(检畸形性髋关节炎)

Jansen's operation ['jɑːnsən] (Albert Jansen) 扬森手术(一种额窦手术)

Jansky-Bielschowsky disease ['jɑːski bil'ʃɔvski] (J. Jansky; Alfred Bielschowski) 扬-比病(晚发婴儿型神经元蜡样脂褐素沉积症)

Janský's classification ['jɑːnski] (Ján Janský) 扬斯基分类(ABO血型分类,用罗马数字Ⅰ到Ⅳ表示之,分别相当于O型、A型、B型和AB型)

Janthinobacterium [ˌdʒænθinəbæk'tiəriəm] *n* 詹森菌属

Janthinosoma [ˌdʒænθinə'səumə] *n* 詹森蚊属 | ~ lutzi 卢[茨]氏詹森蚊 / ~ posticata 胶携詹森蚊

japonic acid [dʒə'pɔnik] 儿茶鞣酸

Jaquet's apparatus [ʒɑː'kei] (Alfred Jaquet) 雅盖记录仪(记录静脉和心脏搏动)

jar [dʒɑː] *n* 缸,罐,瓶 | bell ~ 钟罩(用于实验室真空试验)

jararaca [ˌdʒɑːrɑː'rɑːkə] *n* 巴西具窍蝮蛇

Jarcho-Levin syndrome ['dʒɑːkəu 'levin] (Saul W. Jarcho; Paul M. Levin) 贾-列综合征(一种常染色体隐性遗传病,包括多发性脊椎缺损、胸短、肋骨畸形、指〈趾〉弯曲及并指〈趾〉畸形;有时存在泌尿生殖畸形,通常在婴儿期发生呼吸功能不全造成的死亡。亦称脊椎胸发育不全)

Jarcho's pressometer ['dʒɑːkəu] (Julius Jarcho) 贾科(子宫造影)压力测量器

jargon ['dʒɑːgən] *n* 行话,术语;胡言乱语,杂乱语

jargonaphasia [ˌdʒɑːgɔnə'feiziə] *n* 杂乱性失语[症]

Jarisch-Herxheimer reaction ['jɑːriʃ 'həːkshaimə] (Adolf Jarisch; Karl Herxheimer) 雅里希-赫克斯海默反应(应用抗生素治疗二期梅毒和回归热后2小时内症状加重,但并非所有接受抗生素治疗的人均有此反应)

Jarjavay's muscle [ʒɑːʒɑː'vei] (Jean F. Jarjavay) 尿道压肌

Jarotzky's (Jarotsky's) treatment [jɑː'rɔtski] (Alexander Jarotzky) 雅若茨基疗法(胃溃疡饮食疗法)

Jarvik-7 artificial heart ['dʒɑːvik] (Robert K. Jarvik), 贾维克-7人工心(一种空气驱动的人工心脏,含有两个表面光滑囊样聚氨酯泵,取代心室,具有高温分解的碳盘瓣膜和涤纶覆盖的假体连接心房和大血管;驱动系统中气动动力单位通过搏动空气经过聚氨酯管道驱动线调节血流量)

Jarvis' operation ['dʒɑːvis] (William C. Jarvis) 贾维斯手术(用金属绞勒器切除与下鼻甲相连的肥大组织的蒂)

Jatropha ['dʒætrəfə] *n* 麻风树属

jaundice ['dʒɔːndis] *n* 黄疸 *vt* 使患黄疸病 |

acholuric ~ 无胆色素尿性黄疸 / acholuric familial ~, chronic acholuric ~ 家族性无胆色素尿性黄疸,慢性无胆色素尿性黄疸,遗传性球形红细胞症 / acute febrile ~, acute infectious ~ 急性发热性黄疸,急性传染性黄疸,传染性肝炎 / black ~ 黑色黄疸;新生儿黄疸 / blue ~ 青紫色黄疸,发绀 / epidemic catarrhal ~ 流行性卡他性黄疸 / hematohepatogenous ~ 血肝原性黄疸 / hemolytic ~ 溶血性黄疸,溶血性贫血 / hepatocellular ~ 肝细胞性黄疸 / hepatogenic ~, hepatogenous ~ 肝原性黄疸 / homologous serum ~, human serum ~ 同种血清性黄疸,人血清性黄疸,乙型肝炎 / infectious ~, infective ~ 传染性肝炎;钩端螺旋体性黄疸 / latent ~ 潜伏性黄疸,隐性黄疸 / leptospiral ~, spirochetal ~ 钩端螺旋体性黄疸 / malignant ~ 恶性黄疸(大块性肝坏死) / regurgitation ~ 回流性黄疸 / retention ~ 潴留性黄疸

Javal's ophthalmometer [ʒəˈvæl] (Louis E. Javal) 惹瓦尔检眼计

jaw [dʒɔː] *n* 颌,颌骨 | bird-beak ~, parrot ~ 鹦鹉颌 / crackling ~ 弹响颌 / lower ~ 下颌 / phossy ~ 磷毒性颌骨坏死 / pipe ~ 烟斗颌[病] / upper ~ 上颌

jawbone [ˈdʒɔːbəun] *n* 颌骨

Jaworski's corpuscles (bodies) [jəˈwɔːski] (Walery Jaworski) 雅沃尔斯基小体(螺旋状黏液小体,见于胃酸过多的胃液中) | ~ test 雅沃尔斯基试验(检葫芦胃)

JCV JC virus JC 病毒(一种人多瘤病毒)

Jeanselme's nodules [ʒɑːnˈselm] (Antoine E. Jeanselme) 让塞尔姆小结,关节旁结节(见于梅毒、雅司病等)

jecorize [ˈdʒekəraiz] *vt* 鱼肝油化(如用紫外线照射牛乳)

jecur [ˈdʒiːkə] *n* 【拉】肝

Jeddah ulcer [ˈdʒedə] 皮肤利什曼病(Jeddah 为阿拉伯半岛一城市名)

Jefferson fracture [ˈdʒefəsn] (Sir Geoffrey Jefferson) 杰斐逊骨折(寰椎粉碎骨折) | ~ syndrome 杰斐逊综合征,海绵窦综合征(即 cavernous sinus syndrome,见 syndrome 项下相应术语)

Jeffersonia [ˌdʒefəˈsəuniə] (T. Jefferson) *n* 鲜黄莲属(虎耳草科) | ~ diphylla 北美鲜黄莲(其根可作强壮、利尿、祛痰,大剂量可作催吐药)

jejunal [dʒiˈdʒuːnəl] *a* 空肠的

jejune [dʒiˈdʒuːn] *a* 干燥无味的;缺乏营养的;不成熟的

jejunectomy [ˌdʒidʒuːˈnektəmi] *n* 空肠切除术

jejunitis [ˌdʒidʒuːˈnaitis] *n* 空肠炎

jejun(o)- [构词成分]空肠

jejunocecostomy [dʒiˌdʒuːnəusiˈkɔstəmi] *n* 空肠盲肠吻合术

jejunocolostomy [dʒiˌdʒuːnəukəˈlɔstəmi] *n* 空肠结肠吻合术

jejunoileal [dʒiˌdʒuːnəuˈiliəl] *a* 空肠回肠的

jejunoileitis [dʒiˌdʒuːnəuˌiliˈaitis] *n* 空肠回肠炎

jejunoileostomy [dʒiˌdʒuːnəuˌiliˈɔstəmi] *n* 空肠回肠吻合术

jejunojejunostomy [dʒiˌdʒuːnəuˌdʒidʒuːˈnɔstəmi] *n* 空肠空肠吻合术

jejunorrhaphy [ˌdʒidʒuːˈnɔrəfi] *n* 空肠缝合术

jejunostomy [ˌdʒidʒuːˈnɔstəmi] *n* 空肠造口术

jejunotomy [ˌdʒidʒuːˈnɔtəmi] *n* 空肠切开术

jejunum [dʒiˈdʒuːnəm] *n* 【拉】空肠

Jellinek's sign (symptom) [ˈjelinek] (Stefan Jellinek) 耶利内克征(症状)(甲状旁腺功能亢进时睑缘上常呈褐色色素沉着)

jelly [ˈdʒeli] *n* 胶冻剂;凝胶,胶冻 | cardiac ~ 心胶质(胚胎) / contraceptive ~ 避孕胶冻 / cyclomethycaine sulfate ~ 硫酸环美卡因凝胶(局部麻醉药) / enamel ~ 釉胶质 / glycerin ~ 甘油凝胶 / lidocaine hydrochloride ~ 盐酸利多卡因凝胶(局部麻醉药) / mineral ~, petroleum ~ 矿油凝胶,石油凝胶 / pramoxine hydrochloride ~ 盐酸普莫卡因凝胶(局部麻醉药)

jellyfish [ˈdʒelifiʃ] *n* 海蜇,水母

Jendrassik's maneuver [jenˈdræsik] (Ernst Jendrassik) 晏德拉西克手法(患者两手屈指钩住并用力向外拉,以试膝反射) | ~ sign 晏德拉西克征(外肌群麻痹,格雷夫斯〈Graves〉眶病的一种表现)

jennerization [ˌdʒenəraiˈzeiʃən, -riˈz-] *n* 减毒接种

Jenner's method [ˈdʒenə] (Louis L. Jenner) 詹纳法(用詹纳血液染剂染血细胞的方法)

Jensen's classification [ˈjensən] (Orla Jensen) 晏森分类法(根据细菌对营养的特性分类)

Jensen's disease [ˈjensən] (Edmund Jensen) 晏森病,近视乳头性视网膜脉络膜炎

Jensen's sarcoma (tumor) [ˈjensən] (Carl O. Jensen) 晏森肉瘤(小鼠的一种恶性瘤,可移植于健鼠)

jerk [dʒəːk] *n* 急跳;反射 | biceps ~ 肱二头肌反射 / crossed ~ 交叉性反射 / elbow ~ 肘反射 / jaw ~ (下)颌反射 / quadriceps ~, knee ~ 四头肌反射,膝跳反射 / tendon ~ 腱反应 / triceps surae ~, Achilles ~, ankle ~ 小腿三头肌反射,踝反射

Jervell and Lange-Nielsen syndrome [jeˈvel ˈlɑːŋgə ˈniːlsən] (Anton Jervell; Friedrik Lange-Nielsen) 耶韦尔和朗格-尼尔森综合征(一种常染色体隐性遗传型 Q-T 间期延长综合征,特征为神经性聋和晕厥,有时伴心室颤动并猝死。参见 Romano-Ward syndrome)

Jesionek lamp [je'siənek] (Albert Jesionek) 耶济奥内克灯(一种人工太阳灯)

jessur ['dʒesər] *n* 杰塞尔蝰蛇(孟加拉人对鲁塞尔蝰蛇〈Russell's vipers〉的称呼)

jet [dʒet] *vt*, *vi* 喷出,射出,喷射 *n* 喷射,喷注,喷气;喷嘴,喷射器

Jeuné's syndrome [ʒəːn] (Mathis Jaune) 惹恩综合征,窒息性胸廓营养不良

Jewett nail ['dʒuːət] (Eugene L. Jewett) 朱厄特钉(转子骨折内固定钉)

jhin jhinia [dʒin'dʒiniə] 今今尼亚病(一种模仿性精神病,初见于加尔各答,足底痒,头部有压感,并全身震颤)

jigger ['dʒigə] *n* 沙蚤

Jimson weed ['jimsənwiːd] 曼陀罗

jing【汉】精

jitter ['dʒitə] *n* 颤抖(单纤维肌电描记法中,发生连续放电时的电势间间隔中的变化,通常以连续电势差的平均数表示之)

Jobert's fossa [ʒəu'bɛər] (Antoine J. Jobert de Lamballe) 若贝尔窝(腘区内的窝,上以大收肌为界,下以股薄肌和缝匠肌为界,当膝盖弯曲与大腿用力向外旋时极易见到)

Job's syndrome [dʒəub] (Job 为《旧约》中的人物,身患皮肤病及蒙受其他不幸)约伯综合征(为常染色体隐性遗传的中性粒细胞病,特征为葡萄球菌性寒性脓肿及湿疹,常伴有红发和白肤,以及高免疫球蛋白 E 血症,多见于女孩)

Jocasta complex [dʒəu'kæstə] 柔卡斯塔情结,(母)恋子情结

Jochmann's test ['jɔhmən] (Georg Jochmann) 约赫曼试验(①鉴别结核性脓;②抗胰蛋白酶试验)

jodbasedow [ˌjɔd'bæsidəu] *n* 碘性甲状腺功能亢进

Joest's bodies [jest] (Ernst Joest) 耶斯特小体(见于患博纳〈Borna〉病的动物脑内的核内包涵体)

Joffroy's reflex [ʒɔ'frwɑː] (Alexis Joffroy) 若夫鲁瓦反射(痉挛性麻痹时压臀部即引起臀肌颤搐) | ~ sign 若夫鲁瓦征(突眼性甲状腺肿时患者眼突然向上,前额皱纹即消失)

Johne's bacillus ['jɔnə] (Heinrich A. Johne) 副结核分枝杆菌 | ~ disease 约尼病(牛慢性痢疾)

johnin ['jəunin] *n* 副结核[杆]菌素(类似结核菌素的一种物质,用于产生皮肤反应〈johnin reaction,见 reaction 项下相应术语〉,以诊断牛的约尼〈Johne〉病)

Johnson's test ['dʒɔnsn] (George Johnson) 约翰逊试验(检白蛋白)

Johnson-Stevens disease ['dʒɔnsn 'stiːvnz] (Frank C. Johnson; Albert M. Stevens) 约翰逊-史蒂文斯病(见 Stevens-Johnson syndrome)

joint [dʒɔint] *n* 接合,接缝;关节 *a* 连接的,接合的 *vt* 连接,结合;(从关节处)切断 | amphidiarthrodial ~ 屈戍动关节 / ankle ~ 踝关节 / biaxial ~ 双轴关节 / bilocular ~ 双腔关节 / bleeders' ~, hemophilic ~ 出血性关节,血友病性关节 / cochlear ~, spiral ~ 蜗状关节 / composite ~, compound ~ 复合关节,复关节 / condyloid ~ 髁状关节 / dry ~, fringe ~ 慢性绒毛[增生]性关节炎 / elbow ~ 肘关节 / ellipsoidal ~ 椭圆关节 / false ~ 假关节 / flail ~ 连枷状关节 / gliding ~ 摩动关节 / hinge ~ 屈戍关节 / hip ~ 髋关节 / intercarpal ~ s 腕骨间关节 / knee ~ 膝关节 / ligamentous ~ 韧带联合 / pivot ~, rotary ~, trochoid ~ 车轴关节,旋转关节 / sacrococcygeal ~ 骶尾联合 / saddle ~, sellar ~ 鞍状关节 / spheroidal ~, ball-and-socket ~, enarthrodial ~, multiaxial ~ 球窝关节,杵臼关节 / synovial ~, diarthrodial ~, freely movable ~, through ~ 滑膜关节,动关节

jointed ['dʒɔintid] *a* 有接缝的;有关节的

Jolles' test ['jɔləs] (Adolf Jolles) 约勒斯试验(检尿内胆色素,尿蓝母)

Jolly's bodies [ʒəu'liː] (Justin M. J. Jolly) 若利小体(见 Howell-Jolly bodies)

Jolly's reaction ['jɔli] (Friedrich Jolly) 约利反应(检肌无力,肌肉对感应电刺激的反应消失,但仍有随意收缩力以及对直流电刺激的反应)

Jonas' symptom ['jɔnəs] (Siegfried Jonas) 约纳斯症状(狂犬病时幽门痉挛)

Jones' albumosuria, cylinder, protein [dʒəunz] 见 Bence Jones

Jones' brace [dʒəunz] (Robert Jones) 琼斯支架(一种胸腰骶椎矫形器) / ~ fracture 琼斯骨折(第五跖骨骨干的骨折) / ~ position 琼斯位置(前臂锐屈,治肱骨内侧髁骨折)

Jones' nasal splint [dʒəunz] (John Jones) 琼斯鼻夹(鼻骨骨折用)

Jonnesco's fold [dʒəu'neskəu] (Thoma Jonnesco) 脏壁腹膜褶 | ~ fossa 十二指肠上隐窝,十二指肠空肠隐窝 / ~ operation 交感神经切除术

Jonston's arc ['dʒɔnstən] (Johns Jonston) 斑秃,斑形脱发

Jordans' anomaly ['jɔːdənz] (Godefridus H. W. Jordans) 约旦斯异常(粒细胞、单核细胞,有时为浆细胞和淋巴细胞内存在脂质空泡,有些患者发展成肌营养不良,而另一些患者则患鱼鳞病)

josamycin [dʒəusə'maisin] *n* 交沙霉素(一种大环内酯抗生素,其抗菌作用类似红霉素〈erythromycin〉)

Joseph clamp ['jəusif] (Jacques Joseph) 约瑟夫

夹(鼻手术后使用的夹,用以改善鼻骨构架活动碎片的排列) | ~ knife 约瑟夫刀(用于鼻成形术) / ~ rhinoplasty 约瑟 夫鼻成形术(用锯切除鼻背骨软骨隆起的鼻)

Joseph's disease [ˈjəusif] (Joseph 为亚速尔群岛感染此病的家族)约瑟夫病(见 Azorean disease)

Joubert's syndrome [ʒuːˈber] (Marie Joubert) 儒贝尔综合征(一种常染色体隐性遗传综合征,包括小脑蚓部部分或全部发育不全,伴张力减低、发作性呼吸深快、智力迟钝及眼运动异常;大部分患者于婴儿期死亡)

joule (J) [dʒuːl] (James P. Joule) *n* 焦耳(功或能量单位)

Joule's equivalent [dʒuːl] (James P. Joule) 焦耳当量(热功当量,符号为 J)

Jourdain's disease [ʒuəˈdæn] (Anselme L. B. B. Jourdain) 儒丹病(牙槽脓炎)

juccuya [juˈkuːjə] *n* 溃疡[型]皮肤利什曼病

juga [ˈdʒuːgə] jugum 的复数

jugal [ˈdʒuːgəl] *a* 轭的;颧骨的

jugale [dʒuːˈgeili] *n* 颧点

jugate [ˈdʒuːgeit] *a* 共轭的,联锁的;有隆突的,有嵴的

juglandic acid [dʒuˈglændik] 胡桃皮酸

Juglans [ˈdʒuːglənz] *n* 胡桃属

juglans [ˈdʒuːglənz] *n* 灰胡桃(根皮)

juglone [ˈdʒʌgləun] *n* 胡桃醌,5-羟萘醌

jugomaxillary [ˌdʒuːgəuˈmæksiləri] *a* 颧颌的

jugular [ˈdʒʌgjulə] *a* 颈的;颈静脉的 *n* 颈静脉

jugulate [ˈdʒʌgjuleit] *vt* 顿挫,陡止(疾病的恶化) | **jugulation** [ˌdʒʌgjuˈleiʃən] *n* 顿挫疗法,陡止疗法

jugum [ˈdʒuːgəm] *n*【拉】轭,隆凸 | ~ penis 阴茎钳

juice [dʒuːs] *n* 汁,液 | appetite ~ 食欲液 / cherry ~ 樱桃汁 / gastric ~ 胃液 / intestinal ~ 肠液 / pancreatic ~ 胰液 / press ~ 榨出汁 / raspberry ~ 红覆盆子汁

Jukes [dʒuːks] *n* 朱克斯家族(由美国社会学家 R. L. Dugdale 描述的一个虚构的纽约家族,该家族显示犯罪率高、道德败坏和贫穷,像卡利卡克〈Kallikak〉家族一样用于提出遗传决定的理论)

jump [dʒʌmp] *vi* 跳,跳跃;*n* 跳跃;[复] 舞蹈病,震颤性谵妄

jumper [ˈdʒʌmpə] *n* 跳跃病患者;神经质性跳跃者

jumping [ˈdʒʌmpiŋ] *a* 跳跃的 *n* 跳跃病(见 Gilles de la Tourette's syndrome) | ~ the bite 反殆矫正

junctio [ˈdʒʌŋkʃiəu] ([复] **junctiones** [dʒʌŋkʃiˈəuniːs]) *n*【拉】结合,关节

junction [ˈdʒʌŋkʃən] *n* 连接,接[合]处;接点,[接]界 | dentinocemental ~, cementodentinal ~ 牙本质牙骨质界 / dentinoenamel ~, amelodentinal ~ 釉质牙本质界 / manubrioglad-iolar ~ 胸骨软骨结合 / neuromuscular ~ 神经肌肉接头 / sclerocorneal ~ 角膜巩膜[接]界,角膜巩膜缘 / tendinous **~s** 腱结合 | **~al** *a* 结合的,接合的

junctura [dʒʌŋkˈtjuərə] ([复] **juncturae** [dʒʌŋkˈtjuəriː]) *n*【拉】结合,接合;关节

Jungbluth's vasa propria (vessels) [ˈjuŋbluːt] (Hermann Jungbluth) 荣格布路特固有血管(血管)(早期胚羊膜下滋养血管)

Jüngling's disease [ˈjeŋliŋ] (Otto Jüngling) 肉样瘤病,结节病

Jung's method [juŋ] (Carl G. Jung) 荣格法,精神分析法

Jung's muscle [juŋ] (Karl G. Jung) 耳郭锥状肌

juniper [ˈdʒuːnipə] *n* 杜松(实)

Juniperus [dʒuːˈnipərəs] *n* 桧属,刺柏属

junk [dʒʌŋk] *n* 麻絮敷料;麻醉品(俚语,尤指海洛因)

Junker inhaler (apparatus, bottle) [ˈdʒʌŋkə] (Ferdinand E. Junker) 琼克吸入器(瓶状吸入器,氯仿麻醉时用)

junket [ˈdʒʌŋkit] *n* 乳冻(食品)

Junod's boot [ʒuˈnəu] (Victor T. Junod) 朱诺靴(引血靴)

Jürgensen's sign [ˈjəːgənsən] (Theodor von Jürgensen) 于根森征(急性肺结核听诊时有时可听到细微的捻发音)

jurisprudence [ˌdʒuərisˈpruːdəns] *n* 法学,法理学 | dental ~ 牙[科]法医学 / medical ~ 法医学

jury-mast [ˈdʒuərimɑːst] *n* 正头支柱(脊椎结核病时用以支持头部)

juscul. jusculum【拉】肉汤

jusculum [ˈdʒʌskjuləm] *n*【拉】肉汤

justo major [ˈdʒʌstəu ˈmeidʒə] 大于正常,过大(指 pelvis aequabiliter justo major 均大骨盆)

justo minor [ˈdʒʌstəu ˈmainə] 小于正常,过小(指 pelvis aequabiliter justo minor 均小骨盆)

Justus' test [ˈdʒustus] (J. Justus) 贾斯特斯试验(检梅毒)

jute [dʒuːt] *n* 黄麻;黄麻纤维(以前用作外科敷料)

juvantia [dʒuˈvænʃiə] *n* 佐药,缓和药

juvenile [ˈdʒuːvinail] *a* 青少年的;幼稚的 *n* 青少年;幼畜

juxta- [构词成分]接近,近旁

juxta-articular [ˌdʒʌkstəɑːˈtikjulə] *a* 近关节的,关节旁的

juxtacardiac [ˌdʒʌkstəˈkɑːdiæk] *a* 心旁的

juxtaepiphyseal [ˌdʒʌktəepiˈfiziəl] *a* 近骺的

juxtaglomerular [ˌdʒʌkstəgləuˈmerjulə] *a* 近肾

小球的

juxtallocortex [dʒʌkˌstæləuˈkɔːteks] *n* 中间皮质

juxtamedullary [ˌdʒʌkstəˈmedəˌlɛəri] *a* 近肾髓质的,肾髓质旁的

juxtapulmonary [ˌdʒʌkstəˈpʌlməˌnɛəri] *a* 近肺的,肺旁的

juxtangina [dʒʌksˈtændʒinə] *n* 咽肌炎

juxtapose [ˈdʒʌkstəpəuz] *vt* 把…并列,使并置 ‖

juxtaposition [ˌdʒʌkstəpəˈziʃən] *n* 并列,并置,对合

juxtapyloric [ˌdʒʌkstəpaiˈlɔrik] *a* 近幽门的

juxtaspinal [dʒʌksteˈspainl] *a* 近脊柱的,脊柱旁的

juxtavesical [ˌdʒʌkstəˈvesikəl] *a* 近膀胱的,膀胱旁的

K

K potassium【拉 kalium】钾；kelvin 开（开尔文温标的计量单位）

K equilibrium constant 平衡常数

K_a acid dissociation constant 酸离解常数

K_b base dissociation constant 碱离解常数

K_d dissociation constant 离解常数

K_{eq} equilibrium constant 平衡常数

K_M，K_m Michaelis constant 米氏常数

K_{sp} solubility product constant 溶度积常数

K_w ion product of water 水离子积

k kilo-千

k Boltzmann's constant 玻耳兹曼常数

k kappa 希腊语的第 10 个字母；为两种免疫球蛋白轻链中的一个的符号

kabure [kəˈbuəri] *n* 蚴疹，血吸虫蚴疹

Kader's operation [ˈkɑːdə]（Bronis law Kader）卡德尔手术（胃瓣状造口术）

Kaes-Bekhterev layer [keiz bekˈterev]（Theodor Kaes；Vladimir M. Bekhterev）克斯－别赫捷列夫层（见 Bekhterev's layer）

Kaes' feltwork [keiz]（Theodor Kaes）克斯神经纤维网（在大脑皮质内）| ~line克斯线（大脑皮质外粒层内的薄纤维层）

KAF conglutinogen activating factor（factor I）胶固素原活化因子（因子 I）

Kafka's test（reaction） [ˈkɑːfkə]（Victor Kafka）卡夫卡试验（反应）（检脑脊髓梅毒）

KAFO knee-ankle-foot orthosis 大腿矫形器

Kahlbaum's disease [ˈkɑːlbaum]（Karl L. Kahlbaum）紧张症型精神分裂症，紧张症

Kahler's disease [ˈkɑːlə]（Otto Kahler）多发性骨髓瘤 | ~ law卡勒定律（脊神经升支定律，即脊神经后根的升支支在脊髓内连续从根区通向正中面）

Kahn's test [kɑːn]（Reuben L. Kahn）康氏试验（一种梅毒沉淀反应试验，检梅毒）

kahweol [ˈkɑːwiɔl] *n* 咖啡白脂

kaif [kif] *n*【阿拉伯】梦样舒畅（如用麻醉品后）

kainic acid [ˈkeinik] 红藻氨酸

kain(o)- [构词成分]新

kaiserling [ˈkaizəliŋ] *n* 凯泽林（凯泽林溶液；用凯泽林溶液保存的标本）

Kaiserling's method [ˈkaizəliŋ]（Karl Kaiserling）凯泽林法（博物馆标本的保色法）| ~ solution（fixative）凯泽林溶液（标本固定、保色、保存用）

Kaiserstuhl disease [ˈkaizəʃtul]（Kaiserstuhl 为德国一地区）凯泽斯杜病（二次大战前在德国葡萄园工人中发生的一种慢性砷中毒，由于葡萄上使用含砷的杀虫剂所致）

kak- 以 kak-起始的词，同样见以 cac-起始的词

kakidrosis [ˌkækiˈdrəusis] *n* 臭汗

kakke [ˈkɑːkei] *n*【日】脚气[病]

kakodyl [ˈkækədil] *n* 二甲胂

kakosmia [kæˈkɔzmiə] *n* 恶臭；恶臭[气味]幻觉

kakotrophy [kæˈkɔtrəfi] *n* 营养不良

kala-azar [ˈkɑːlə əˈzɑː] *n* 黑热病，内脏利什曼病 | Mediterranean ~，canine ~，infantile ~ 地中海黑热病，犬利什曼病，婴儿黑热病

kaladana [ˌkæləˈdeinə] *n* 牵牛子

kalafungin [ˌkerləˈfʌndʒin] *n* 卡拉芬净（抗真菌抗生素）

kalagua [kəˈlɑːɡwə] *n* 卡拉瓜（南美产，治肺结核的药物）

kalemia [kəˈliːmiə] **kaliemia** [keiliˈiːmiə] *n* 血钾过多，高钾血[症]

kali [ˈkeilai，ˈkɑːli] *n*【德】钾 | **~arsenicosum** 亚砷酸钾

kaligenous [kæˈlidʒinəs] *a* 产生碳酸钾的

kalimeter [kəˈlimitə] *n* 碱定量器，碳酸定量器

kaliopenia [ˌkeiliəuˈpiːniə] *n* 血钾过少，低钾血[症] | **kaliopenic** [ˌkeiliəuˈpiːnik] *a*

kalium [ˈkeiliəm] *n*【拉】钾

kaliuresis [ˌkeilijuəˈriːsis] *n* 尿钾排泄，尿钾增多 | **kaliuretic** [ˌkeilijuəˈretik] *a* [促]尿钾排泄的 *n* 尿钾排泄药

kallak [ˈkælək] *n* 爱斯基摩[化脓性]皮炎

kallidin [ˈkælidin] *n* 胰激肽，血管舒张素

Kallikak [ˈkælikæk] *n* 卡利卡克家族（美国社会学家 H. H. Goddard 描述的一个虚构的新泽西家族，该家族有两个分支，一个是由非常聪明而有成就的成员组成，另一支则显示智力缺陷、道德败坏、犯罪率高，据此提出一种理论，即这些特性都是由遗传决定的）

kallikrein [kæliˈkriːin] *n* 激肽释放酶 | plasma ~ 血浆激肽释放酶 / tissue ~ 组织激肽释放酶

kallikreinogen [ˌkæliˈkriːnədʒin] *n* 激肽释放酶原

Kallmann's syndrome [ˈkɑːlmɑːn] (Franz J. Kallmann)卡尔曼综合征,促性腺激素分泌不足性无睾症

Kalmia [ˈkælmiə] *n* 山月桂属(其叶用于治梅毒、腹泻及慢性炎症)

Kalmuk idiocy [ˈkælmuk] 伸舌样白痴(一种伴有唐氏〈Down〉综合征的严重精神发育迟缓,Kalmuk 为蒙古族名)

kaluresis [ˌkæljuəˈriːsis] *n* 尿钾排泄,尿钾增多 | **kaluretic** [ˌkæljuəˈretik] *a* [促]尿钾排泄的 *n* 尿钾排泄药

kalymana-bacterium [ˌkæliˈmeinei-bækˈtiəriəm] *n* 性病肉芽肿杆菌

kamala [ˈkæmələ] *n* 卡马拉,吕宋楸荚粉,粗糠柴(曾用作泻药)

Kambin's triangular working zone [ˈkæmbin] (Parviz Kambin)坎宾三角工作区(无明显血管和神经结构的三角区,在显微椎间盘切除术时可安全接近腰盘。前界为脊神经,下界为下一个下椎板的上缘,后界为上关节突的侧缘)

Kaminer's reaction [ˈkæminə] (Gisa Kaminer)卡米纳反应(见 Freund reaction)

Kammerer-Battle incision [ˈkæmərə ˈbætəl] (Frederic Kammerer; William H. Battle)卡–巴切口(经皮肤和浅筋膜作腹部垂直切口,再垂直切开腹直肌鞘前层,将腹直肌向内拉开,在近中线处切开腹直肌鞘后层、浆膜下蜂窝组织和腹膜)

kanamycin [ˌkænəˈmaisin] *n* 卡那霉素(抗生素类药) | ~ sulfate 硫酸卡那霉素

Kanavel's sign [kəˈneivəl] (Allen B. Kanavel)卡纳佛尔征(腱鞘感染时,掌内接近小指基底部 2.5 cm处有一最强压痛点)

kangaroo [ˌkæŋgəˈruː] *n* 袋鼠(尾部的腱可作结扎线)

Kanner's syndrome [ˈkɑːnə] (Leo Kanner)卡纳综合征,孤独症

kansasiin [kænˈzæsiin] *n* 堪萨斯杆菌素(用于过敏性皮肤试验)

Kantor's sign [ˈkæntə] (John L. Kantor)坎特征,线样征(结肠 X 线摄影时,可见一条造影剂通过充盈缺损的线样构型)

kanyemba [ˌkæniˈembə] *n* 坏疽性直肠结肠炎

kaodzera [ˌkeiɔdˈziərə] *n* 罗得西亚锥虫病

kaolin [ˈkeiəlin] *n* 白陶土,高岭土

kaolinosis [ˌkeiəliˈnəusis] *n* 白陶土肺,肺白陶土沉着病

kapha [ˈkɑːfɑː] *n*【梵】黏液

Kaplan-Meier survival curve (method) [ˈkæplən ˈmæiə] 卡普兰–迈耶存活曲线(法)(能由随机调查数据计算出的对存活曲线的相容估计,亦称乘积—限估计,其法亦称积–限法)

Kaplan's test [ˈkæplən] (David M. Kaplan)卡普兰试验(检脊髓液球蛋白及白蛋白)

Kaposi's sarcoma [ˈkæpəuʃi] (Moritz Kaposi Kohn)卡波西肉瘤(皮肤多发性出血性肉瘤) | ~ varicelliform eruption 卡波西水痘样疹(急性痘疮样脓疱病)

kappa [ˈkæpə] *n* 希腊语的第 10 个字母(Κ, κ);卡巴粒(某些草履虫的细胞中含有 DNA,结构复杂而又能自体复制的颗粒)

kara-kurt [ˈkærəˌkuət] *n* 红带毒珠

karaya [kɑːrɑːjə] *n* 卡拉牙胶,梧桐胶

Karell's diet [ˈkærəl] (Philip Kerell)卡列尔饮食(每日饮 800 ml 牛乳,治疗肾炎和心脏病) | ~ treatment(cure)卡列尔疗法(以卧床及卡列尔饮食治心脏病和肾病)

karma [ˈkɑːmə] *n*【梵】行动,行为

Karnofsky scale [kɑːˈnɔfski] (David A. Karnofsky)卡诺夫斯基量表(测定患者执行功能的能力和进行正常活动的能力,评分范围从 0〈患者为无功能者或死亡者〉到 100〈功能完全正常者〉)

Karplus' sign [ˈkɑːplʌs] (Johann P. Karplus)卡普拉斯征(一种语响改变,胸膜腔积液处听诊时,患者发元音 u,而听到的是 a 音)

Karroo syndrome [kəˈruː] 卡罗综合征(见于南非卡罗地区青年中的一种病症,包括高热、消化道紊乱及颈淋巴结有压痛)

Kartagener's syndrome (triad) [kɑːˈtægənə] (Manes Kartagener)卡塔格内综合征(三联征)(右位心〈内脏易位〉、支气管扩张、鼻窦炎)

Karwinskia [kɑːˈwinskiə] *n* 鼠李属

Karyamoebina falcata [ˌkæriæmiˈbainə fælˈkeitə] 镰状丛核变形虫

Karyapsis [ˌkæriˈæpsis] *n* 核接合

karyenchyma [ˌkæriˈenkimə], **karyochylema** [ˌkæriəukaiˈliːmə] *n* 核液

kary(o)- [构词成分]核(见 caryo-)

karyochromatophil [ˌkæriəukrəuˈmætəfil] *a* 核嗜色的,核嗜染性的

karyochrome [ˈkæriəˌkrəum] *n* 核[深]染色细胞

karyochylema [ˌkæriəukaiˈliːmə] *n* 核液,核淋巴

karyoclasis [ˌkæriˈɔkləsis] *n* 核断裂 | **karyoclastic** [ˌkæriəuˈklæstik] *a* 核断裂的;分裂中止的,无丝分裂的

karyocyte [ˈkæriəsait] *n* 有核细胞

karyogamy [ˌkæriˈɔgəmi] *n* 核配[合],[原]核融合 | **karyogamic** [ˌkæriəuˈgæmik] *a*

karyogen [ˈkæriədʒən] *n* 核铁质

karyogenesis [ˌkæriəuˈdʒenisis] *n* 核生成 | **karyogenic** [ˌkæriəuˈdʒenik] *a* 核生成的,生核的

karyogonad [ˌkæriəuˈgəunəd] *n* 小核,生殖核

karyokinesis [ˌkæriəukaiˈniːsis, -kiˈn-] *n* 核分裂

| asymmetrical ~ 不对称核分裂 / hyperchromatic ~ 染色质过多性核分裂 / hypochromatic ~ 染色质过少性核分裂 | **karyokinetic** [ˌkæriəukaiˈnetik, -kiˈn-] *a*

karyoklasis [ˌkæriˈɔkləsis] *n* 核断裂 | **karyoklastic** [ˌkæriəuˈklæstik] *a* 核断裂的;分裂中止的,无丝分裂的

karyolobism [ˌkæriəuˈləubizəm] *n* [细胞]核分叶 | **karyolobic** *a*

karyology [ˌkæriˈɔlədʒi] *n* 核学

karyolymph [ˈkæriəlimf] *n* 核液,核淋巴

karyolysis [ˌkæriˈɔlisis] *n* 核溶解 | **karyolytic** [ˌkæriəuˈlitik] *a* 核溶解的,溶核的

Karyolysus lacertarum [kæriˈɔlisəs læsəˈtɛərəm] 蜥蜴溶核簇虫

karyomastigont [ˌkæriəuˈmæstigɔnt] *n* 核鞭毛

karyomegaly [ˌkæriəuˈmegəli] *n* 核[过]大

karyomere [ˈkæriəˌmiə] *n* 染色粒;染色体泡(只含有一小部分正常核的小泡,常见于不正常的有丝分裂)

karyometry [ˌkæriˈɔmitri] *n* 细胞核测量法,核测定法

karyomicrosome [ˌkæriəuˈmaikrəsəum] *n* 核微粒体

karyomit [ˈkæriəmit] *n* 核网丝;染色体

karyomitome [ˌkæriˈɔmitəum] *n* 核网丝

karyomitosis [ˌkæriəumaiˈtəusis] *n* [细胞]核分裂,有丝分裂 | **karyomitotic** [ˌkæriəumaiˈtɔtik] *a*

karyomorphism [ˌkæriəuˈmɔːfizəm] *n* 核形(尤指白细胞)

karyon [ˈkæriɔn] *n* 细胞核,核

karyonide [ˈkæriənaid] *n* 核系

karyophage [ˈkæriəˌfeidʒ] *n* 噬核细胞;噬核体

karyoplasm [ˈkæriəˌplæzəm] *n* 核质 | **~ic** [ˌkæriəˈplæzmik] *a*

karyoplast [ˈkæriəplæst] *n* 核体

karyoplastin [ˌkæriəuˈplæstin] *n* 副染色质

karyopyknosis [ˌkæriəupikˈnəusis] *n* 核固缩 | **karyopyknotic** [ˌkæriəupikˈnɔtik] *a*

karyoreticulum [ˌkæriəuriˈtikjuləm] *n* 核网

karyorrhexis [ˌkæriəˈreksis] *n* 核碎裂 | **karyorrhectic** *a*

karyosome [ˈkæriəˌsəum] *n* 染色质核仁,核体

karyospherical [ˌkæriəuˈsferikəl] *a* 核球的

karyostasis [ˌkæriˈɔstəsis] *n* 核静止,核静止期 | **karyostatic** [ˌkæriəuˈstætik] *a*

karyota [ˌkæriˈəutə] *n* 有核细胞

karyotheca [ˌkæriəˈθiːkə] *n* 核膜

karyotin [ˈkæriətin] *n* 核染色质,核质

karyotype [ˈkæriətaip] *n* 核型 | **karyotypic** [ˌkæriəuˈtipik] *a*

karyozoic [ˌkæriəuˈzəuik] *a* 核内寄生的

Kasabach-Merritt syndrome [ˈkæsəbæk ˈmerit] (Haig Haigouni Kasabach; Katharine Krom Merritt) 卡萨巴赫－梅里特综合征(发生在婴儿的综合征,表现为皮肤和脾脏巨大血肿,伴血小板减少性紫癜和纤维蛋白原缺乏血症。亦称血管瘤血小板减少综合征)

kasai [kəˈsai] *n* 开赛病(发生在刚果的一种综合征,表现为贫血、皮肤脱色和水肿,所有这些症状可能继发于铁的缺乏)

Kasai operation [kɑːˈsai] (Morio Kasai) 肛门肠吻合术

kasal [ˈkeisəl] *n* 碱性磷酸钠铝(食品添加剂)

Kashin-Bek (Kaschin-Beck) disease [ˈkɑːʃiːn bek] (Nikolai I. Kashin〈或 Kaschin〉; E. V. Bek〈或 Beck〉) 卡－贝病,大骨节病(一种周围关节和脊柱的缓慢进行性慢性致残性变性病,主要发生于儿童,为西伯利亚东部、中国北方和朝鲜的地方病。据认为此病系由摄食分枝孢镰刀菌〈Fusarium sporotrichiella〉污染的谷粒所致。亦称地方性变形性骨关节炎)

Kast's syndrome [kɑːst] (Alfred Kast) 卡斯特综合征(见 Maffucci's syndrome)

kat katal 开特

kat(a)- [前缀]下,向下,在下;依照;对抗

kata [ˈkɑːtə] *n* 小反刍动物瘟疫

katachromasis [ˌkætəˈkrəuməsis] *n* 末期核变(子染色体重组子核的过程)

katadidymus [ˌkætəˈdidiməs] *n* 下身联胎,双上身联胎

katal (kat) [ˈkætəl] *n* 开特(酶活性测量单位,1 开特相当于每秒钟催化 1 摩尔基质的反应速率的酶活性的量)

katalase [ˈkætəleis] *n* 过氧化氢酶,触酶

kataphylaxis [ˌkætəfiˈlæksis] *n* 炎灶趋向性(指抗体、白细胞);[机体]防卫力毁灭

katathermometer [ˌkætəθəˈmɔmitə] *n* 干湿球温度计,卡他温度计

Katayama [ˌkɑːtɑːˈjɑːmə] *n* 钉螺属(即 Oncomelania)

Katayama fever (disease) [ˌkɑːtɑːˈjɑːmə] (Katayama 为日本一河谷,19 世纪首次在此报道) 片山热(病)(一种急性全身性血吸虫病)

Katayama's test [ˌkɑːtɑːˈjɑːmə] (Kunika Katayama 片山国嘉) 片山试验(检碳氧血红蛋白)

katharometer [ˌkæθəˈrɔmitə] *n* 导热析气计

kathepsin [kəˈθepsin] *n* 组织蛋白酶

kathisophobia [ˌkæθisəuˈfəubjə] *n* 静坐恐怖,静坐不能

katholysis [kəˈθɔlisis] *n* 阴极电解法

katine [ˈkeitin] *n* 阿拉伯茶叶碱

kation [ˈkætaiən] *n* 阳离子,阴向离子
katolysis [kəˈtɔlisis] *n* 不完全分解,中间分解(尤指消化过程)
katotropia [ˌkætəˈtrəupiə], **katophoria** [ˌkætəˈfɔːriə] *n* 下隐斜
katzenjammer [ˈkætsenˈjæmə] *n*【德】宿酒病,酒后病
Katz formula [kɑːts] (Johann R. Katz) 卡茨公式[平均血沉率 = $\left(S_1 + \frac{S_2}{2}\right)\Big/2$, 其中 S_1 为 1 小时结束时清液柱高度的毫米数,S_2 则为 2 小时结束时的高度]
Kauffmann-White classification [ˈkɔːfmɑːn hwait] (Fritz Kauffmann; P. B. White) 考-怀分类(血清学鉴定沙门菌属各菌种对 O, H 和 Vi 抗血清的反应的一种分类表)
Kaufman-McKusick syndrome [ˈkɔːfmən məˈkjuːsik] (Robert L. Kaufman; Victor A. McKusick) 考-麦综合征(一种罕见的常染色体隐性遗传性子宫阴道积水病,伴轴后多指〈趾〉畸形、先天性心脏缺损及随后有时为两侧肾盂积水。男性表现症状包括尿道下裂和明显的阴囊缝)
kava kava [ˈkɑːvəˈkɑːvə] 卡瓦根(卡瓦植物麻醉椒根制剂,具有骨骼松弛、抗痉挛、抗焦虑和镇静作用)
Kawasaki disease [ˌkɑːwɑːˈsɑːkiː] 川崎病(一种罕见的综合征,常与儿童有关,亦见之于成人,特征为高热持续 5 天以上、眼周充血、口唇干红、手足发红、肢体肿胀以及指尖脱屑。Kawasaki〈川崎〉为日本东京湾一城市名)
Kawasaki syndrome [ˌkɑːwɑːˈsɑːki] (Tomisaku Kawasaki) 川崎综合征,黏膜皮肤淋巴结综合征(即 mucocutaneous lymph node syndrome,见 syndrome 项下相应术语)
Kayser-Fleischer ring [ˈkaizə ˈflaiʃə] (Bernhard Kayser; Bruno Fleischer) 凯-弗环(角膜外缘的绿色环,见于肝豆状核变性及假硬化)
Kayser's disease [ˈkaizə] (Bernhard Kayser) 肝豆状核变性
Kazanjian forceps [kəˈzænjən] (Varaztad Hovhannes Kazanjian) 卡赞言钳(用以切除鼻背隆凸的切钳) | ~ operation 卡赞言手术(颊沟加深术,改善义齿固位)
kb kilobase 千碱基
kbp kilobase pairs 千碱基对
kcal kilocalorie 千卡
kCi kilocurie 千居里
kcps kilocycles per second 千赫,千周/秒
kD, kDa kilodalton 千道尔顿
Ke Ke 标记(一种抗原标记,以区别人免疫球蛋白 λ 轻链亚型,亦称 Kern)
Kearns-Sayre syndrome [kəːnsˈseiə] (Thomas P. Kearns; George P. Sayre) 卡恩斯-塞尔综合征(进行性眼肌麻痹、视网膜色素变性、肌病、共济失调及心脏传导缺陷,为常染色体显性遗传,于 15 岁前发病)
Keating-Hart's fulguration (method, treatment [ˈkiːtiŋ hɑːt] (Walter V de Keating-Hart) 基廷·哈特疗法(外表癌电灼术)
kebocephaly [ˌkebəˈsefeli] *n* 猴头畸形
ked [ked] *n* 羊蜱蝇
Keegan's operation [ˈkiːgən] (Denis F. Keegan) 基根手术(人工鼻成形术)
keel [kiːl] *n* 幼鸭败血病(幼鸭败血性肠炎,由鸭沙门菌引起)
Keen's operation [kiːn] (William W. Keen) 脐切除术 | ~ sign 基恩征(腓骨波特〈Pott〉骨折时,踝部直径增大)
Kehrer's reflex [ˈkɛərə] (Ferdinand Kehrer) 克勒尔反射(听睑反射,用触觉或温觉刺激外耳道最深部和鼓室,则睑闭)
Kehr's incision [kɛə] (Hans Kehr) 克尔切口(一种大面积腹部切开法) | ~ sign 克尔征(有些脾破裂时,左肩剧痛)
keirospasm [ˈkairəspæzəm] *n* 修面痉挛(理发师职业性神经功能病,表现为手指、手和前臂肌肉痉挛性收缩)
Keith-Flack node [ˈkiːθ ˈflæk] (Arthur Keith; Martin W. Flack) 窦房结
Keith's bundle [kiːθ] (Arthur Keith) 窦房束 | ~ node 窦房结
Keith's low ionic diet [kiːθ] (Norman M. Keith) 基思低离子饮食(治慢性肾炎)
Keith-Wagener-Barker classification [kiːθ ˈwægənə ˈbɑːkə] (Norman M. keith; Henry P. Wagener; N. W. Barker) 基-瓦-巴分类法(根据视网膜病变的高血压及小动脉硬化分类法。第一类,自发性良性高血压,指征为小动脉中度减弱。第二类,持久性高血压,但对健康无明显影响,指征为小动脉减弱更为明确,伴局部狭窄。第三类,伴视网膜、肾、大脑及其他症状的高血压,指征为小动脉明显减弱——棉絮状渗出物和出血。第四类,伴严重神经系统、视觉及其他器官障碍的重度高血压,指征为第三类检眼镜检查征,伴乳头水肿)
kelectome [ˈkiːlektəum] *n* 瘤组织剪钳
Kell blood group [kel] (Kell 为 1946 年首次观察到的先证者的姓) 凯尔血型(包含众多红细胞抗原的血型,尤其是三对交替抗原,系由一个位点复合基因决定的,其中包括无效等位基因,同样亦受 X 染色体调节的,此血型与性连锁慢性肉芽肿病有关。一种抗原 K6 是非洲裔人中比较常见的)
Keller operation [ˈkelə] (Col. William L. Keller)

凯勒手术(为矫正踇外翻所做的手术,即矢状切除第一跖骨头的内侧突,并切除近端踇趾骨的基底部)

Kelling's test [ˈkeliŋ] (Georg Kelling)凯林试验(检胃乳酸、食管憩室、胃癌)

Kellock's sign [ˈkelək] (T. H. Kellock)凯洛克征(一手紧贴乳头下的胸部,一手用力叩诊时肋骨振动增加,为胸腔积液体征)

Kelly's operation [ˈkeli] (Howard A. Kelly)凯利手术(治妇女尿失禁) | ~ sign 凯利征(若用动脉钳拨动输尿管时,可引起其蛇或蠕虫样收缩) / ~ speculum 凯利直肠窥器

keloid [ˈkiːlɔid] *n* 瘢痕疙瘩 | acne ~ 痤疮性瘢痕疙瘩,头部乳头状皮炎 / ~ of gums 龈纤维瘤病

kelosomus [kiːləˈsəuməs] *n* 露脏畸胎

kelotomy [kiˈlɔtəmi] *n* (绞窄性)疝切开术

kelp [kelp] *n* 海藻

kelvin(K) [ˈkelvin] *n* 开(开尔文温标的计量单位)

Kelvin scale [ˈkelvin] (William T. Kelvin)开氏温标,绝对温标

Kempner diet [ˈkempnə] (Walter Kempner)肯普纳饮食(高血压病和慢性肾病饮食)

Kendall's method [ˈkendl] (Edward C. Kendall)肯德尔法(检甲状腺组织中的碘)

Kendall's rank correlation coefficient (tau) [ˈkendl] (Maurice George Kendall)肯德尔秩相关系数(τ)(一种非参数性相关量,计算如下:一组 *n* 次观察数据样本,按变量值以递增次序排列;然后观察另一相应的变量值,在顺序中后一种观察数据的数要超过前一种观察数据中每一个数,并计算之,最后计数的总和乘以 4,除以 *n*〈*n*−1〉,并减 1 而得出 −1 和 +1 之间的值)

Kennedy classification [ˈkenidi] (Edward Kennedy)肯尼迪分类法(部分无牙状态及部分义齿的分类法,根据无牙间隙相对于残存牙的位置所作的分类)

Kennedy's syndrome [ˈkenidi] (Robert Foster Kennedy)肯尼迪综合征(损害侧有眼球后视神经炎、中心盲点和视神经萎缩,对侧视神经乳头水肿,为脑额叶肿瘤向下压迫所致)

Kenny's treatment [ˈkeni] (Elizabeth Kenny)肯尼疗法(用湿热绒布敷裹小儿麻痹患者的背与四肢,俟痛止,施被动运动,而后教以自动运动)

ken(o)- [构词成分]空,空间;以 ken(o)-起始的词,同样见以 cen(o)-起始的词

kenotoxin [ˈkiːnəˌtɔksin] *n* 疲倦毒素(由于肌肉收缩在肌内产生的)

Kent-His bundle [kent his] (A. F. Stanley Kent; Wilhelm His, Jr.)房室束

kentrokinesis [ˌkentrəukaiˈniːsis] *n* 中枢性运动 | **kentrokinetic** [ˌkentrəukaiˈnetik] *a*

Kent's bundle [kent] (Albert F. Stanley Kent)房室肌束(哺乳类及人)

kephal- 见 cephal-

kephalophosphoric acid [ˌkefələufɔsˈfɔrik] 脑磷脂磷酸

Kerandel's sign (symptom) [ˌkerənˈdel] (Jean F. Kerandel)克朗德尔征(症状)(轻听骨隆突处后引起深部感觉过敏并伴疼痛〈常稍后发生〉,见于非洲锥虫病患者)

keraphyllocele [ˌkerəˈfiləsiːl] *n* 角质瘤(马蹄)

kerasin [ˈkerəsin] *n* 角苷脂

keratalgia [ˌkerəˈtældʒiə] *n* 角膜痛

keratan sulfate [ˈkerətæn] 硫酸角质素

keratansulfaturia [ˌkerətænˌsʌlfəˈtjuəriə] *n* 硫酸角质素尿症,莫尔基奥(Morquio)综合征

keratectasia [ˌkerətekˈteiziə] *n* 角膜扩张,角膜突出

keratectomy [ˌkerəˈtektəmi] *n* 角膜切除术(一般治前葡萄肿)

keratic [kəˈrætik] *a* 角的;角蛋白的;角膜的

keratin [ˈkerətin] *n* 角蛋白 | false ~ 假角蛋白

keratinase [ˈkerətineis] *n* 角蛋白酶

keratinize [ˈkerətinaiz] *vi* 角化 | **keratinization** [ˌkerəˌtinaiˈzeiʃən, -niˈz-] *n*

keratinocyte [kəˈrætinəsait] *n* 角质形成细胞

keratinoid [ˈkerətinɔid] *n* 角衣片(一种肠溶片)

keratinophilic [kəˌrætinəuˈfilik] *a* 喜角质的(指真菌)

keratinosome [kəˈrætinəˌsəum] *n* 角蛋白小体(亦称膜被颗粒,奥德兰德〈Odland〉小体)

keratinous [kəˈrætinəs] *a* 角质的;角蛋白的

keratitis [ˌkerəˈtaitis] *n* 角膜炎 | acnerosacea ~ 酒渣鼻角膜炎 / hypopyon ~ 前房积脓性角膜炎 / mycotic ~ 角膜真菌病 / punctate ~ 点状角膜炎 / ribbon-like ~, band ~, ~ bandelette 带状角膜炎 / serpiginous ~ 匐行性角膜炎,匐行性角膜溃疡 / striate ~, alphabet ~ 条状角膜炎 / trachomatous ~ 沙眼性角膜炎,血管翳 / trophic ~, neuroparalytic ~ 营养性角膜炎,神经麻痹性角膜炎

kerat(o)- [构词成分]角质;角膜

keratoacanthoma [ˌkerətəuˌækənˈθəumə] *n* 角化棘皮瘤

keratocele [ˈkerətəsiːl] *n* 角膜后[弹性]层突出

keratocentesis [ˌkerətəusenˈtiːsis] *n* 角膜穿刺术

keratoconjunctivitis [ˌkerətəu kənˌdʒʌŋk tiˈvaitis] *n* 角膜结膜炎 | epidemic ~, shipyard ~, viral ~ 流行性角膜结膜炎,船坞角膜结膜炎,病毒性角膜结膜炎 / flash ~ 闪光性角膜结膜炎 / phlyctenular ~ 泡性角膜结膜炎 / ~ sicca 干燥性角膜结膜炎

keratoconus [ˌkerətəuˈkəunəs] *n* 圆锥角膜
keratocyst [ˈkerətəusist] *n* 角质囊肿
keratocyte [ˈkerətəˌsait] *n* 角膜细胞
keratoderma [ˌkerətəuˈdəːmə] *n* 皮肤角质层;皮肤角化病,角皮病 | ~ blennorrhagicum 脓溢性角皮病 / ~ climactericum 绝经期角皮病,更年期角皮病 / diffuse palmoplantar ~ 弥漫性掌跖角化病 / palmoplantar ~, ~ palmare et plantare 掌跖角皮病 | **keratodermia** [ˌkerətəuˈdəːmiə] *n*
keratodermatocele [ˌkerətəuˈdəːmətəsiːl] *n* 角膜后[弹性]层突出
keratoectasia [ˌkerətəuekˈteiziə] *n* 角膜扩张,角膜突出
keratogenesis [ˌkerətəuˈdʒenisis] *n* 角质生成 | **keratogenetic** [ˌkerətəudʒiˈnetik] *a* 角质生成的,生角质的
keratogenous [ˌkerəˈtɔdʒinəs] *a* 生角质的,角质增生的
keratoglobus [ˌkerətəuˈgləubəs] *n* 球形角膜
keratohelcosis [ˌkerətəuhelˈkəusis] *n* 角膜溃疡
keratohemia [ˌkerətəuˈhiːmiə] *n* 角膜血沉着
keratohyalin [ˌkerətəuˈhaiəlin] *n* 角质透明蛋白,透明角蛋白
keratohyaline [ˌkerətəuˈhaiəlain] *a* 角质性透明的,透明角质性的
keratoid [ˈkerətɔid] *a* 角质样的
keratoiditis [ˌkerətɔiˈdaitis] *n* 角膜炎
keratoiridocyclitis [ˌkerətəuˌiridəusikˈlaitis] *n* 角虹膜睫状体炎
keratoiridoscope [ˌkerətəuaiˈridəskəup] *n* 角虹膜镜
keratoiritis [ˌkerətəuaiˈraitis] *n* 角虹膜炎 | hypopyon ~ 前房积脓性角膜炎
keratoleptynsis [ˌkerətəulepˈtinsis] *n* 结膜遮盖角膜术
keratoleukoma [ˌkerətəuljuːˈkəumə] *n* 角膜白斑
keratolysis [ˌkerəˈtɔlisis] *n* 角质层分离,角质松解离 | pitted ~, ~ plantare sulcatum 窝状角质松解,凹陷性角质松解,足跖沟状角质松解 | **keratolytic** [ˌkerətəuˈlitik] *a* 角质层分离的 *n* 角质软化剂
keratoma [ˌkerəˈtəumə] ([复] **keratomas** 或 **keratomata** [ˌkerəˈtəumətə]) *n* 胼胝,角化瘤;角质瘤(马蹄) | ~ hereditarium multilans 遗传性残毁性角化病 / ~ plantare sulcatum 跖部沟状角化病 / ~ senile 老年角化瘤,光化性角化病
keratomalacia [ˌkerətəuməˈleiʃiə] *n* 角膜软化[症]
keratome [ˈkerətəum] *n* 角膜刀
keratometer [ˌkerəˈtɔmitə] *n* 角膜曲率计 | **keratometric** [ˌkerətəuˈmetrik] *a* 角膜曲率测量的 / **keratometry** *n* 角膜曲率测量[法]
keratomileusis [ˌkerətəumiˈljuːsis] *n* 角膜磨削术
keratomycosis [ˌkerətəumaiˈkəusis] *n* 角膜真菌病,角膜霉菌病 | ~ linguae 黑舌[病]
keratonosus [ˌkerəˈtɔnəsəs] *n* 角膜病
keratonyxis [ˌkerətəuˈniksis] *n* 角膜穿刺
keratopathy [ˌkerəˈtɔpəθi] *n* 角膜病变 | band ~, band-shaped ~ 带状角膜病变
keratophakia [ˌkerətəuˈfeikiə] *n* 角膜透镜移植术
keratoplasty [ˈkerətəˌplæsti] *n* 角膜成形术;角膜移植术 | optic ~ 光学角膜移植术 / tectonic ~ 整复性角膜移植术
keratoprotein [ˌkerətəuˈprəutiːn] *n* 角质蛋白
keratorhexis, keratorrhexis [ˌkerətəuˈreksis] *n* 角膜破裂
keratoscleritis [ˌkerətəuskliəˈraitis] *n* 角巩膜炎
keratoscope [ˈkerətəskəup] *n* 角膜镜 | **keratoscopy** [ˌkerəˈtɔskəpi] *n* 角膜镜检查
keratose [ˈkerətəus] *a* 角质的
keratosis [ˌkerəˈtəusis] ([复] **keratoses** [ˌkerəˈtəusiːz]) *n* 角化病 | actinic ~, solar ~, senile ~ 光线性角化病 / arsenic ~, arsenical ~ 砷角化病 / ~ blennorrhagica 脓溢性角化病 / ~ linguae 舌角化病,舌白斑病 / ~ obturans 阻塞性角化病,耵聍栓塞 / seborrheic ~ 脂溢性角化病 | **keratotic** [ˌkerəˈtɔtik] *a*
keratosulfate, keratosulphate [ˌkerətəuˈsʌlfeit] *n* 硫酸角质素
keratotome [kəˈrætətəum] *n* 角膜刀
keratotomy [ˌkerəˈtɔtəmi] *n* 角膜切开术 | delimiting ~ 限界性角膜切开术
keratotorus [ˌkerətəuˈtɔːrəs] *n* 角膜隆凸
keraunoneurosis [kəˌrɔːnəunjuəˈrəusis] *n* 闪电性神经[功能]病
Kerckring's (Kerkring's) center (ossicle) [ˈkerkriŋ] (Theodorus Kerckring〈或 Kerkring〉) 克尔克林中心(小骨)(有时在16周岁胎儿的枕大孔后缘可见的骨化中心,出生前与其他鳞部联合) | ~ folds (valves) 克尔克林襞(瓣)(环状襞)
kerectasis [kəˈrektəsis] *n* 角膜突出,角膜扩张
kerectomy [kəˈrektəmi] *n* 角膜[部分]切除术
Kergaradec's sign [kergɑːrɑːˈdek] (Jean Alexandre le Jameau, Vicomte de Kergaradec) 凯加拉德克征,子宫杂音
Kerilla [kəˈrilə] *n* 毒海蛇属
kerion [ˈkiəriən] *n* 脓癣
keritherapy [ˌkeriˈθerəpi] *n* 石蜡浴疗法;石蜡疗法
Kerkring 见 Kerckring
Kerley's lines [ˈkəːli] (Peter J. Kerley) 克利线(在X线胸片上水平线性密度为1~2.5 cm,呈阶梯状排列,据认为代表如由于水肿〈二尖瓣狭

窄时〉或纤维化〈矽肺时〉所致的小叶间隔增宽。如在外周特别位于肺底部时,则称为凯利 B 线或肋膈间隔线。如位于中央,则称为凯利 A 线)

kerma [ˈkəːmə] (*k*inetic *e*nergy *r*eleased in *ma*terial) *n* 比释动能(表示每单位质量的被照射基质由非带电粒子转移给带电粒子的动能的计量单位)

kermes [ˈkəːmiːz] *n* 胭脂虫,冬青虫(提供一种红色素,用作染料)

Kern Kern 标记(见 Ke)

kern [kəːn] *n* 核

kernel [ˈkəːnl] *n* 核,仁;原子实,原子核

kernicterus [kəˈniktərəs] *n* 胆红素脑病(通常是重症新生儿黄疸的后遗症)

Kernig's sign [ˈkerniɡ] (Vladimir M. Kernig) 凯尔尼格征(仰卧时,患者容易伸腿,起坐时或大腿屈向腹部仰卧时,则不能伸腿,为一种脑膜炎的体征)

Kernohan's notch [ˈkəːnəhæn] (James W. Kernohan) 坎诺汉切迹(在某些小脑幕疝病例中,脑干对着小脑幕向下移位在大脑脚内造成一条沟)

keroid [ˈkerɔid] *a* 角质样的;角膜样的

kerosene, kerosine [ˈkerəsiːn] *n* 煤油

kerotherapy [ˌkerəuˈθerəpi] *n* 石蜡浴疗法;石蜡疗法

kerril [ˈkeril] *n* 毒海蛇(印度洋产)

Kerr's sign [kəː] (Henry H. Kerr) 克尔征(脊髓损害时躯体平面下的皮肤纹理改变)

Kerteszia [kerˈtiːziə] *n* 按蚊亚属

Keshan disease 克山病(一种致命性充血性心肌病,首次发现于中国克山的儿童)

Kesling appliance [ˈkesliŋ] (Harold D. Kesling) 凯斯林矫正器(用以治疗磨牙症) | ~ spring 凯斯林弹簧(用于固定正牙装置以分隔牙齿,便于放置环带)

Kestenbaum's sign [ˈkestənbaum] (Alfred Kestenbaum) 凯斯顿波姆征(小动脉横穿视神经盘缘的数目减少,可作为视神经萎缩的标准)

ketal [ˈkiːtəl] *n* 缩酮,酮缩醇

ketamine hydrochloride [ˈkiːtəmiːn] 盐酸氯胺酮(全身麻醉药)

ketazocine [kiːˈteizəsiːn] *n* 酮佐辛(镇痛药)

ketazolam [kiːˈteizəlæm] *n* 凯他唑仑(弱安定药)

keten [ˈkiːtən], **ketene** [ˈkiːtiːn] *n* 烯酮类;乙烯酮

kethoxal [kiˈθɔksəl] *n* 凯托沙(抗病毒药)

ketimine [ˈkiːtimiːn] *n* 酮亚胺

ketipramine fumarate [kiːˈtiprəmiːn] 延胡索酸凯替帕明(抗抑郁药)

keto- [前缀]酮[基]

keto acid [ˈkiːtəu] 酮酸

3-ketoacid CoA transferase [ˌkiːtəuˈæsid kəuˈei ˈtrænsfəreis] 3-酮酸辅酶 A 转移酶

keto acid decarboxylase [ˈkiːtəuˈæsid ˌdiːkɑːˈbɔksileis] 酮酸脱羧酶,α-酮酸脱氢酶

α-keto acid dehydrogenase [ˈkiːtəuˈæsid diːˈhaidrədʒəneis] α-酮酸脱氢酶

α-keto acid dehydrogenase deficiency α-酮酸脱氢酶缺乏症(①硫辛酰胺脱氢酶缺乏症;②任何一种 α-酮酸脱氢酶复合物缺乏)

ketoacidemia [ˌkiːtəuˌæsiˈdiːmiə] *n* 酮酸血症

ketoacid-lyase [ˌkiːtəuˌæsidˈlaieis] *n* 酮酸裂合酶

ketoacidosis [ˌkiːtəuˌæsiˈdəusis] *n* 酮酸中毒

ketoaciduria [ˌkiːtəuˌæsiˈdjuəriə] *n* 酮酸尿症 | branched-chain ~ 支链酮酸尿症,枫糖尿病

ketoacyl [ˌkiːtəuˈæsil] *n* 酮酰(酮酸酰基)

3-ketoacyl-CoA thiolase [ˌkiːtəuˈæsil ˈkəuei ˈθaiəleis] 3-酮酰 CoA 硫解酶,3-酮酰辅酶 A 硫解酶,乙酰-CoA *C*-酰基转移酶

α-ketoadipate [ˌkiːtəuəˈdipeit] *n* α-酮己二酸(阴离子型)

α-ketoadipate dehydrogenase [ˌkiːtəuəˈdipeit diːˈhaidrədʒəneis] α-酮己二酸脱氢酶(此酶缺乏可致 α-酮己二酸尿症)

α-ketoadipic acid [ˌkiːtəuəˈdipik] α-酮己二酸(亦可写成 2-ketoadipic acid)

α-ketoadipicacidemia [ˌkiːtəuəˌdipikˌæsiˈdiːmiə] *n* α-酮己二酸血[症]

α-ketoadipicaciduria [ˌkiːtəuəˌdipikˌæsiˈdjuəriə] *n* α-酮己二酸尿[症]

keto-aldehyde [ˌkiːtəuˈældihaid] *n* 酮醛

ketoaminoacidemia [ˌkiːtəuəˌmiːnəuˌæsiˈdiːmiə] *n* 酮氨基酸血症,枫糖尿病

β-ketobutyric acid [ˌkiːtəubjuːˈtirik] β-丁酮酸,乙酰乙酸

ketocaproic acid [ˌkiːtəukəˈprəuik] 己酮酸

ketocholanic acid [ˌkiːtəukəuˈlænik] 酮胆烷酸

ketoconazole [ˌkiːtəuˈkɔnəzəul] *n* 酮康唑(口服抗真菌药)

ketogenesis [ˌkiːtəuˈdʒenisis] *n* 生酮作用 | **ketogenetic** [ˌkiːtəudʒiˈnetik] *a* 生酮的,酮生成的

ketogenic [ˌkiːtəuˈdʒenik] *a* 生酮的

α-ketoglutarate [ˌkiːtəuˈgluːtəreit] *n* α-酮戊二酸(阴离子形式)

α-ketoglutarate dehydrogenase [ˌkiːtəu ˈgluːtəreit diːˈhaidrədʒəneis] α-酮戊二酸脱氢酶

α-ketoglutaric acid [ˌkiːtəugluːˈtærik] α-酮戊二酸

ketoheptose [ˌkiːtəuˈheptəus] *n* 庚酮糖

ketohexokinase [ˌkiːtəuˌheksəuˈkaineis] *n* 己酮糖激酶(此酶的遗传性缺乏可致原发性果糖尿症,亦称果糖激酶)

ketohexonic acid [ˌkiːtəuhekˈsɔnik] 己酮糖酸

ketohexose [ˌkiːtəuˈheksəus] *n* 己酮糖

ketohydroxyestrin [ˌkiːtəuhaiˌdrɔksiˈestrin] *n* 雌酮

α-ketoisovalerate dehydrogenase [ˌkiːtəu ˌais-əuˈvæləreit diːˈhaidrədʒəneis] α-酮异戊酸脱氢酶

ketol [ˈkiːtɔl] *n* 乙酮醇

ketol-isomerase [ˌkiːtɔl-aiˈsɔməreis] *n* 乙酮醇异构酶

ketolysis [kiːˈtɔlisis] *n* 解酮[作用] | **ketolytic** [ˌkiːtəuˈlitik] *a*

ketone [ˈkiːtəun] *n* 酮;甲酮 | dimethyl ~ 二甲酮,丙酮

ketonemia [ˌkiːtəuˈniːmiə] *n* 酮血[症]

ketonic [kiːˈtɔnik] *a* 酮的 | ~ acid 酮酸

ketonization [ˌkiːtəunaiˈzeiʃən, -niˈz-] *n* 酮基化[作用]

ketonuria [ˌkiːtəuˈnjuəriə] *n* 酮尿[症]

ketonurine [ˌkiːtəuˈnjuərin] *n* 食物性酮尿

ketopentose [ˌkiːtəuˈpentəus] *n* 酮戊糖

ketoplasia [ˌkiːtəuˈpleiziə] *n* 酮体生成 | **keto-plastic** [ˌkiːtəuˈplæstik] *a*

ketopregnene [ˌkiːtəuˈpregniːn] *n* 氧代孕烯

ketoprofen [ˌkiːtəuˈprəufən] *n* 酮洛芬(非甾体消炎药)

β-ketoreductase [ˌkiːtəuriˈdʌkteis] *n* β-酮还原酶

9-ketoreductase [ˌkiːtəuriˈdʌkteis] *n* 9-酮还原酶,前列腺素-E_2 9-还原酶

ketorolac tromethamine [ˈkiːtəurəˌlæk] 酮咯酸氨丁三醇(非甾体消炎药,用以短期处理疼痛,肌内或口服给药)

ketose [ˈkiːtəus] *n* 酮糖

ketoside [ˈkiːtəsaid] *n* 酮[糖]苷

ketosis [kiːˈtəusis] *n* 酮病

ketostearic acid [ˌkiːtəustiˈærik] 酮硬脂酸

ketosteroid [ˌkiːtəuˈsterɔid] *n* 甾酮类,酮甾类,酮固醇类

17-ketosteroid reductase [ˌkiːtəuˈsterɔid riˈdʌkt-eis] 17-酮甾类还原酶,睾酮 17 β-脱氢酶($NADP^+$)

ketosuccinic acid [ˌkiːtəusəkˈsinik] 酮丁二酸,草酰乙酸

ketosuria [ˌkiːtəuˈsjuəriə] *n* 酮糖尿

keto-tetrahydrophenanthrene [ˌkiːtəuˌtetrəˌhai-drəufiˈnænθriːn] *n* 酮四氢菲(一种致癌物质)

ketotetrose [ˌkiːtəuˈtetrəus] *n* 酮丁糖

3-ketothiolase, β-ketothiolase [ˌkiːtəuˈθaiəleis] *n* 3-酮硫解酶,β-酮硫解酶,乙酰 CoA *C*-酰基转移酶

β-ketothiolase deficiency β-酮硫解酶缺乏症,α-甲基乙酰乙酸尿[症]

ketotic [kiːˈtɔtik] *a* 酮病的

ketotifen fumarate [ˌkiːtəuˈtaifen] 延胡索酸酮替芬(一种非竞争性 H_1 受体拮抗剂和肥大细胞稳定剂,口服用于长期治疗患特应性气喘儿童,局部用于结膜止痒药,治疗变应性结膜炎)

ketotriose [ˌkiːtəuˈtraiəus] *n* 酮丙糖

ketourine [ˌkiːtəuˈjuərin] *n* 食物性酮尿

ketoxime [kiːˈtɔksaim] *n* 酮肟

Kety-Schmidt method [kiːti ʃmit] (Seymour S. Kety; Carl F. Schmidt)基-施法(测定脑组织血液灌流量的方法)

keV kilo electron volts 千电子伏特

key [kiː] *n* 钥匙;关键;键 | torquing ~ 扭转键(一种正牙器)

keynote [ˈkiːnəut] *n* 同治药性

Key-Retzius connective tissue sheath [ˈkiː ˈr-etsiəs] (Ernst A. H. Key; Magnus G. Retzins) 凯-雷结缔组织鞘(神经内膜) | ~ foramen 第四脑室外侧孔

keyway [ˈkiːwei] *n* 键槽;榫沟

kg kilogram 千克,公斤

kg-cal large calorie 大卡

khellin [ˈkelin] *n* 凯林(抗高血压药,血管扩张药)

kHz kilohertz 千赫[兹]

ki [kiː] *n* 【日】气(即 qi)

kibisitome [kaiˈbisitəum] *n* 晶状体囊刀

Kibrick test [ˈkaibrik] (S. Kibrick)明胶凝集试验

Kidd blood group [kid] (Kidd 为 1951 年首次观察到的先证者的姓)基德血型(主要含有 Jk^a 和 Jk^b 抗原的血型,由等位基因决定;无效等位基因在东亚裔人中最常见)

kidinga pepo [kiˈdingə ˈpiːpəu] 类登革热(发生于桑给巴尔)

kidney [ˈkidni] *n* 肾 | amyloid ~, lardaceous ~, waxy ~ 淀粉样肾 / arteriosclerotic ~ 动脉硬化性肾 / artificial ~ 人工肾 / cake ~, clump ~, lump ~ 饼状肾,团块肾 / cyanotic ~ 淤血肾 / definite ~, hind ~ 后肾 / disk ~ 盘状肾 / doughnut ~ 环状肾 / flea-bitten ~ 蚤咬状肾 / fused ~ 融合肾 / head ~, primordial ~ 前肾 / hypermobile ~, movable ~, wandering ~ 游走肾 / polycystic ~ 多囊肾 / sacciform ~ 囊状肾,扩张肾 / supernumerarv ~ 额外肾

Kiel classification [kiːl] (Kiel 为德国首次发展此分类法的地方)基尔分类法(非霍奇金〈Hodgkin〉淋巴瘤分类法,主要用于欧洲,根据形态学和细胞学分类。以后的分类法为修订的欧美淋巴瘤〈REAL〉分类法)

Kielland's (Kjelland) forceps [ˈkiːlənd] (Ch-ristian Kielland) 基耶兰德钳(一种产钳,用于枕横位时旋转胎头)

Kienböck-Adamson points [ˈkiːnbek ˈædəmsn] (Robert Kienböck; Horatio G. Adamson) 金伯

克-亚当森点(X 线治疗发癣的定位点)
Kienböck disease [ˈkiːnbek] (Robert Kienböck) 金伯克病(腕半月骨慢性进行性骨软骨病;脊髓外伤性空腔形成) / ~ dislocation 金伯克脱位(半月骨脱位) / ~ phenomenon 金伯克现象(脓胸时,病侧膈肌在吸气时上升,呼气时下降)
Kiernan's spaces [ˈkiənən] (Francis Kiernan) 基尔南间隙(肝小叶间淋巴隙)
Kiesselbach's area (space) [ˈkiːsəlbɑːh] (Wilhelm Kiesselbach)基塞尔巴赫区(间隙)(鼻中隔前下方易出血区)
kiestein [kaiˈestiːn] *n* 孕尿翳,孕尿皮(孕妇尿表面有皮样形成)
Kikuchi's lymphadenitis (disease) [kiːˈkuːtʃi] (M. Kikuchi) 菊池淋巴结炎(病)(一种良性自限性淋巴结病综合征,一般在颈内具有女性优势,其特征包括副皮质斑状坏死性损害和明显的组织细胞、浆细胞样单核细胞和免疫母细胞增生,周围为核破裂碎屑。有些人认为是自限性系统性红斑狼疮。亦称组织细胞坏死性淋巴结炎和亚急性坏死性淋巴结炎)
kil [kil] *n* 黑海白黏土(消毒后可作软膏基质,用于皮肤病)
Killian's dehiscence (triangle) [ˈkiliən] (Gustav Killian)基利安裂开(三角)(下缩肌和环咽肌之间的咽壁内的三角区,此区代表一个潜在弱点,为咽食管憩室十分可能所在之处) | ~ operation 基利安手术(切除额窦前壁,除去患病组织,与鼻形成永久性沟通)
Kilian's line [ˈkiliən] (Hermann F. Kilian) 基利安线(骶岬隆凸线)
killeen [ˈkiliːn] *n* 角叉菜
Killian-Freer operation [ˈkiliən ˈfriːə] (Gustav Killian; Otto 〈Tiger〉Freer) 基-弗手术(鼻中隔黏膜下切除术,其中包括切除鼻中隔软骨、犁骨和筛骨垂直板)
Killian's test [ˈkiliən] (John A. Killian) 基利安试验(检糖耐量)
killifish [ˈkilifiʃ] *n* 鳉,花鳉
kilo- [构词成分] 千(k)
kilobar [ˈkiləubɑː] *n* 千巴(旧压强单位,现用 Pa 帕[斯卡])
kilobase (kb) [ˈkiləubeis] *n* 千碱基(用以表示核酸顺序长度的单位)
kilocalorie [ˈkiləuˌkæləri] *n* 千卡,大卡(旧热量单位,现用 J〈焦耳〉)
kilocurie (kCi) [ˌkiləuˈkjuəriə] *n* 千居里(旧放射强度单位,现用 Bq 贝克[勒尔])
kilocycle [ˈkiləusaikl] *n* 千周
kilodalton (kD, kDa) [ˌkiləuˈdɔːltən] *n* 千道尔顿(质量单位)
kilogram (kg) [ˈkiləugræm] *n* 千克,公斤
kilohertz (kHz) [ˈkiləuhəːts] *n* 千赫[兹]
Kiloh-Nevin syndrome [ˈkailəu ˈnevin] (Leslie G. Kiloh; Samuel Nevin) 卡-内综合征(①上睑下垂和进行性外眼肌麻痹患者的眼肌病;②骨间前综合征)(即 anterior interosseous syndrome,见 syndrome 项下相应术语)
kiloliter, kilolitre (kl) [ˈkiləuˌliːtə] *n* 千升
kilomegacycle (kMc) [ˌkiləuˈmegəˌsaikl] *n* 千兆周(用于电磁波频率)
kilometer, kilometre (km) [ˈkiləuˌmiːtə] *n* 千米,公里
kilonem [ˈkiləunem] *n* 千能母(旧营养值单位,相当于 667 卡,现用 J〈焦耳〉)
kilounit [ˌkiləuˈjuːnit] *n* 千单位
kilovolt (kV) [ˈkiləuvəult] *n* 千伏[特]
kilowatt (kW) [ˈkiləuwɔt] *n* 千瓦[特]
kilurane [ˈkiljuərein] *n* 千铀单位(旧放射性能单位,现用 Bq 贝克[勒尔])
Kimberley horse disease [ˈkimbəli] 金伯利马病(西澳大利亚东北部金伯利区的一种马病,亦称踯躅病)
Kimmelstiel-Wilson lesion (nodule) [ˈkiməlstiːl ˈwilsn] (Paul Kimmelstiel; Clifford Wilson) 基-威损害(小结)(一种显微镜可见的球形透明团块,结节型毛细血管间肾小球硬化症时,在肾小球内所见) | ~ syndrome 基-威综合征(结节型毛细血管间肾小球硬化症)
Kimpton-Brown tube [ˈkimptən braun] (Arthur R. Kimpton) 金普顿-布朗管(一种输血管,间接输血用)
kimputu [kiːmˈpuːtu] *n* 【非洲】回归热
Kimura's disease [kiːˈmuːrɑː] (Tetsuji Kimura) 木村病,血管淋巴样增生
kinanesthesia [ˌkinænisˈθiːzjə] *n* 运动觉缺失
kinase [ˈkaineis] *n* 激酶
kindling [ˈkindliŋ] *n* 诱发(脑生理学中的一种改变,系由反复阈下电刺激引起,最后结果可能是致癫痫性改变或者是不太明显的但却是慢性的行为改变)
kindred [ˈkindrid] *n* 家族
kine-, kin(o)- [构词成分] 运动
kinematics [ˌkiniˈmætiks, -kai-] *n* 运动学 | **kinematic(al)** *a*
kinematograph [ˌkiniˈmætəgrɑːf, -græf] *n* 运动描记器
kineplasty [ˈkiniˌplæsti], **kineplastics** [ˌkiniˈplæstiks] *n* 运动成形切断术
kinesalgia [ˌkiniˈsældʒiə], **kinesialgia** [kaiˌniːsiˈældʒiə] *n* 动痛,运动痛
kinescope [ˈkiniskəup] *n* 眼屈光计
kinesia [kiˈniːziə] *n* 晕动病
kinesiatrics [kaiˌniːsiˈætriks] *n* 运动疗法

kinesics [kaiˈniːsiks] *n* 运动学,动力学 | **kinesic** *a* 运动的,动的,动力的
kinesi-esthesiometer [kaiˌniːsiisˌθiːziˈɔmitə] *n* 肌动觉测量器
kinesigenic [kaiˌniːsiˈdʒenik] *a* 运动引起的
kinesimeter [ˌkiniˈsimitə] *n* 运动测量器;皮肤感觉计
kinesin [kaiˈniːsin] *n* 动力蛋白
kinesi(o)- [构词成分] 运动,活动
kinesiodic [kaiˌniːsiˈɔdik] *a* 运动道的(指运动冲动传导的)
kinesis [kaiˈniːsis] *n*【希】运动;动作
-kinesis [后缀]运动, 活动
kinesiology [kiˌniːsiˈɔlədʒi] *n* 运动学
kinesiometer [kiˌniːsiˈɔmitə] *n* 运动测量器;皮肤感觉计
kinesioneurosis [kiˌniːsiəunjuəˈrəusis] *n* 运动[性]神经功能病
kinesiphony [ˌkiniˈsifəni] *n* 蜂音器疗法
kinesitherapy [kiˌniːsiˈθerəpi], **kinesiotherapy** [kiˌniːsiəuˈθerəpy] *n* 运动疗法
kinesodic [ˌkiniˈsɔdik] *a* 运动道的(指运动冲动传导的)
kinesthesia [ˌkinisˈθiːzjə], **kinesthesis** [ˌkinisˈθiːsis] *n* 运动觉, 动觉 | **kinesthetic** [ˌkinisˈθetik] *a*
kinesthesiometer [ˌkinisˌθiːziˈɔmitə] *n* 肌动觉测量器
kinetia [kiˈniːʃiə] kinety 的复数
kinetic [kaiˈnetik, kiˈnetik] *a* 动力[学]的;[运]动的;活动的
kinetics [kiˈnetiks, kai-] *n* 动力学 | **kineticist** [kaiˈnetisist] *n* 动力学家
kinetid [kiˈniːtid] *n* 运动体,动粒(纤毛原虫基本的重复的结构单位)
kinetin [kaiˈniːtin] *n* 激动素,N^6-呋喃甲基腺嘌呤(一种植物生长因子)
kinetism [ˈkinitizəm] *n* [肌肉]运动能力
kinet(o)- [构词成分] 运动
kinetocardiogram [kiˌniːtəuˈkɑːdiəgræm] *n* 心振动图
kinetocardiography [kiˌniːtəuˌkɑːdiˈɔgrəfi] *n* 心振动描记术
kinetochore [kaiˈniːtəkɔː] *n* 动粒(即着丝粒,着丝点)
kinetocyte [kaiˈniːtəsait] *n* 活动细胞,动细胞
kinetodesma [kaiˌniːtəuˈdesmə] ([复] **kinetodesmata** [kaiˌniːtəuˈdesmətə]) *n* 动丝
kinetodesmos [kaiˌniːtəuˈdesmɔs] *n* 动丝
kinetofragment [kiˌniːtəuˈfrægmənt] *n* 动基片
Kinetofragminophorea [kaiˌniːtəuˌfrægminəuˈfɔːriə] *n* 动基片纲
kinetogenic [kiˌniːtəuˈdʒenik] *a* 促动的,引起运动的
kinetographic [kaiˌniːtəuˈgræfik] *a* 描记运动的
kinetoplasm [kiˈniːtəplæzəm] *n* 动质, 动浆
kinetoplast [kiˈniːtəplæst], **kinetonucleus** [kiˌniːtəuˈnjuːkliəs] *n* 动基粒,动核
kinetoplastid [kiˌniːtəuˈplæstid] *a* 动基体目原生动物的
Kinetoplastida [kiˌniːtəuˈplæstidə] *n* 动基体目
kinetoscope [kiˈniːtəskəup] *n* 人体运动电影照相机 | **kinetoscopy** [ˌkiniˈtɔskəpi] *n* 人体运动电影照相术
kinetosis [ˌkiniˈtəusis] ([复] **kinetoses** [ˌkiniˈtəusiːz]) *n* 晕动病
kinetosome [kiˈniːtəsəum] *n* 动体,基体,毛基体
kinetotherapy [kiˌniːtəuˈθerəpi] *n* 运动疗法
kinety [kaiˈniːti] ([复] **kinetia, kineties**) *n* 动体(总体), 动体列(亦称动体系)
kingdom [ˈkiŋdəm] *n* 界(动物,植物,矿物)
Kingella [kiŋˈgelə] (Elizabeth O. King) *n* 金氏菌属 | ~ dentitrificans 脱氮金氏菌 / ~ indologenes 生吲哚金氏菌
Kingsley appliance (plate) [ˈkiŋsli] (Norman W. Kingsley) 金斯莱矫正器(基托) | ~ splint 金斯莱夹板(上颌骨骨折用)
King syndrome [kiŋ] (J. O. King)金氏综合征(恶性体温过高的一型,病人同样显示具有特征的躯体畸形,其中包括身材矮小,特征性面容、脊柱后侧凸、鸡胸、隐睾病、迟发性运动发育、进行性肌病及心血管结构缺损)
King unit [kiŋ] (Earl J. King) 金氏单位(一种磷酸酶效能单位)
kinic acid [ˈkinik] 奎尼酸
kinin [ˈkainin] *n* 激肽 | C2 ~ C2 激肽
kininase [ˈkainineis] *n* 激肽酶 | ~ Ⅰ激肽酶Ⅰ, 丝氨酸羧肽酶 / ~ Ⅱ激肽酶Ⅱ,肽基二肽酶 A
kininogen [kaiˈninəˌdʒən] *n* 激肽原
kink [kiŋk] *n* 扭结,缠结;(颈、背等处的)肌肉痉挛;转折 | ileal ~ 回肠扭结
kinky [ˈkiŋki] *a* 缠结的,扭结的;卷曲的
Kinnier Wilson [ˈkiniərˈwilson] 见 Wilson
kion [ˈkaiːnəu] *n* 奇诺(曾用作收敛药)
kino- [构词成分] 动,运动
kinocentrum [ˌkinəuˈsentrəm, ˌkai-] *n* 中心体
kinocilium [ˌkainəuˈsiljəm] ([复] **kinocilia** [ˌkainəuˈsiliə]) *n* 动纤毛
kinohapt [ˈkainəhæpt] *n* 触觉计
kinology [kiˈnɔlədʒi, kai-] *n* 运动学
kinomometer [ˌkinəuˈmɔmitə, ˌkai-] *n* 指腕动度测量器
kinoplasm [ˈkainəplæzəm] *n* 动质,动浆 | **kinoplastic** [ˌkainəuˈplæstik] *a*

Kinorhyncha [ˌkinəuˈrinkə] *n* 动吻纲
kinosphere [ˈkainəsfiə] *n* 星体
kinotoxin [ˌkainəuˈtɔksin] *n* 疲劳毒素
kinovin [kiˈnəuvin] *n* 奎诺温,金鸡纳[皮]苷
kinship [ˈkinʃip] *n* 家属关系,血缘关系
kion(o)- 以 kion(o)-起始的词,同样见以 ciono-起始的词
kiotome [ˈkaiətəum] *n* 悬雍垂刀
kiotomy [kaiˈɔtəmi] *n* 悬雍垂切除术
Kirchner's diverticulum [ˈkiəknə] (Wilhelm Kirchner) 咽鼓管憩室
Kirk's amputation [kəːk] (Norman T. Kirk) 柯克切断术(在股骨踝上方的一种腱成形性切断术)
Kirlian photography [ˈkiːrliən] (Semyon Kirlian; Valentina Kirliana) 基利安摄影术(对受试者通过高压电流与照相胶片和照相纸接触产生一种周围是发光放射线和晕轮的影像,有些人认为这种影像是一种生物能场,能显示关于受试者身体健康和情绪状态的信息)
Kirmisson's operation [ˌkiəmiːˈsɔŋ] (Edouard Kirmisson) 基尔米松手术(将跟腱移植于腓长肌,治畸形足)
Kirschner wire [ˈkiəʃnə] (Martin Kirschner) 基施纳钢丝(骨骼牵引时用)
Kirstein's method [ˈkiəstain] (Alfred Kirstein) 基尔施泰因法(直接检喉法)
Kisch's reflex [kiʃ] (Bruno Kisch) 基施反射(见 Kehrer's reflex)
kit [kit] *n* 用具包;工具箱;成套用具 | a first-aid ~ 急救药箱,急救包
kitasamycin [ˌkitəsəˈmaisin] *n* 吉他霉素(抗生素类药)
Kitasatoa [ˌkaitəsɑːˈtəuə] *n* 北里杆菌属
Kitasato's filter [kitəˈsɑːtəu] (Shibasaburo Kitasato 北里柴三郎) 北里滤器(素瓷滤器)
kitol [ˈkaiˌtɔl] *n* 鲸醇(加热则产生维生素 A)
Kittel's treatment [ˈkitəl] (M. J. Kittel) 基特尔疗法(用按摩和推拿法以消散沉积在痛风性关节中的尿酸盐)
kj knee jerk 膝反射
Kjeldahl's method (test) [ˈkeldɑːl] (Johan G. C. Kjeldahl) 基耶达法(试验)(检一种有机化合物中的氮量)
Kjelland 见 Kielland
kl Kiloliter 千升
Klapp's creeping treatment [klæp] (Rudolf Klapp) 克拉普爬行疗法(对脊柱侧凸者练习脊柱运动的方法)
Klatskin's tumor [ˈklætskin] (Gerald Klatskin) 克拉斯金瘤,肝门胆管癌
Klebs' disease [klebz] (Theodor A. E. Klebs) 克雷伯病,肾小球肾炎
Klebsiella [ˌklebsiˈelə] (T. A. E. Klebs) *n* 克雷伯杆菌属 | ~ oxytoca 催产克雷伯杆菌 / ~ planticola 植物克雷伯杆菌 / ~ pneumoniae ozaenae, ~ ozaenae 臭鼻肺炎克雷伯杆菌,臭鼻克雷伯杆菌 / ~ pneumoniae rhinoscleromatis, ~ rhinoscleromatis 鼻硬结肺炎克雷伯杆菌,鼻硬结克雷伯杆菌
Klebsielleae [ˌklebsiˈeliiː] *n* 克雷伯杆菌科
Klebs-Löffler bacillus [ˈklebz ˈleflə] (T. A. E. Klebs; Friederich A. J. Löffler) 克-吕杆菌,白喉棒状杆菌,白喉杆菌
kleeblattschädel [ˌkleiblætˈʃeidel] *n*【德】三叶草叶形头颅,苜蓿状颅
Kleine-Levin syndrome [ˈklainəˈlevin] (Willi Kleine; Max Levin) 克莱恩-莱文综合征(周期性嗜睡、贪食,可持续数周,通常发生于青春期男孩)
Klein-Waardenburg syndrome [klain ˈvɑːdənbəːg] (David Klein; Petrus J. Waardenburg) 克-瓦综合征(见 Waardenburg's syndrome②解)
Kleist's sign [klaist] (Karl Kleist) 克莱斯特征(检查者用数个手指轻轻抬起患者手指时,如患者手指钩住检查者手指,提示大脑额叶及丘脑损伤)
Klemm's sign [klem] (Paul Klemm) 克累姆征(慢性阑尾炎时,X 线片上常见右下腹鼓胀)
Klemperer's tuberculin [ˈklempərə] (Felix and Georg Klemperer) 牛结核菌素
klept(o)- [构词成分] 偷窃
kleptolagnia [ˌkleptəˈlægniə] *n* 偷窃性色情狂
kleptomania [ˌkleptəˈmeinjə] *n* 偷窃狂 | ~c [ˌkleptəˈmeiniæk] *n* 偷窃狂者
Klieg eye [kliːg] 电影[性]眼(拍电影时由强烈灯光所引起的眼病)
Klimow's test [ˈklimɔf] (Ivan Alex. Klimow) 克利莫夫试验(检尿血)
Klinefelter's syndrome [ˈklainfeltə] (Harry F. Klinefelter) 克兰费尔特综合征,先天性睾丸发育不全(特征为睾丸小伴细精管透明性变,不同程度的男性化,精子缺乏与不育,尿中促性腺激素排泄增加,患者趋于身高腿长,约一半有男子女性型乳房,主要与性染色体组分为 XXY 型有关)
Kline's test [klain] (Benjamin S. Kline) 克兰试验(检梅毒)
Klippel-Feil sign [kilˈpel fail] (Maurice Klippel; André Feil) 克利佩尔-费尔征(挛缩手指被牵伸时,则拇指屈曲与内收,为锥体束疾患的指征) | ~ syndrome 先天性短颈综合征,短颈畸形(先天性颈椎缺少或融合,使颈部短缩,颈部活动受限)
Klippel's disease [kliˈpel] (Maurice Klippel) 关

节炎性全身假瘫

Klippel-Trénaunay syndrome [kli'pel treinə'nei] (Maurice Klippel; Paul Trénaunay) 克-特综合征(一种罕见的病症,通常累及一肢体,特征为骨及相关软组织肥大、皮肤大血管瘤、持久性鲜红斑痣及皮肤脉管曲张)

Klippel-Trénaunay-Weber syndrome [kli'pel treinə'nei 'webə] (M. Klippel; P. Trénaunay; Frederick P. Weber) 克-特-韦综合征,血管骨肥大综合征(见 Klippel-Trénaunay syndrome)

Klippel-Weil sign [kli'pel vail] (Maurice Klippel; Mathieu P. Weil) 克-魏征(检查者将患者屈曲的手指伸直时,如拇指屈曲与内收,提示锥体束病)

kliseometer [ˌklisi'ɔmitə] *n* 骨盆斜度计

klismaphilia [ˌklizmə'filiə] *n* 灌肠性欲倒错(利用灌肠取得性兴奋)

Kloeckera ['kliːkərə] *n* 克勒克酵母属 | ~ apiculatus 尖端酵母

Klossiella [ˌkilɔsi'elə] *n* 克洛球虫属

Klumpke's paralysis, Klumpke-Dejerine paralysis, syndrome ['klumpkə ˌdəʒə'riːn] (Madame A. Klumpke Dejerine; Joseph J. Dejerine) 克隆普克麻痹,克隆普克-德热里纳麻痹、综合征(臂麻痹的下丛型,臂、手肌肉萎缩性麻痹,由于第八颈神经和第一胸神经损害所致,常发生于臀位娩出的婴儿)

Klüver-Bucy syndrome ['kliːvə 'bjusi] (Heinrich Klüver; Paul Clancy Bucy) 克吕弗-布西综合征(双侧额叶切除后出现的异常行为,表现为用口检查各种物体、运动与情感反应减退、视觉刺激过分注意和性抑制力缺乏)

Kluyvera ['klaivərə] (A. J. Kluyver) *n* 克罗非菌属

Km 同种异型的标记

km kilometer 千米,公里

Knapp's forceps [næp] (Herman J. Knapp) 纳普镊,转轴镊(压碎沙眼小粒镊) | ~ operation 纳普手术(治内障) / ~ streaks (striae) 纳普线(纹)(网状血管样线条,偶见于出血后的视网膜)

Knapp's test [knæp] (Karl Knapp) 克纳普试验(检尿糖、胃中有机酸)

knead [niːd] *vt* 捏,搓,揉;按摩 | ~ing *n* 揉捏法

knee [niː] *n* 膝;膝状物 | ~ of aquaeductus fallopii 面神经管膝 / back ~ 膝反屈,翻膝 / beat ~ 膝蜂窝织炎 / football ~ 足球员膝病 / housemaid's ~ 髌前囊炎 / in ~, knock ~ 膝外翻 / ~ of internal capsule 内囊膝 / locked ~ 膝闭锁 / out ~ 膝内翻,弓形腿 / rugby ~ 橄榄球员膝病(胫骨粗隆骨软骨病) / septic ~ 化脓性膝关节炎

kneecap ['niːkæp] *n* 髌,膝盖骨;护膝

knee-gall ['niː gɔːl] *n* 膝肿(马膝关节背侧腕鞘膨胀)

kneippism ['nipizəm] (Rev. Sebastian Kneipp 为德牧师,于1897年应用此法) *n* 奈普法,践露疗法(应用冷水包括冷水浴和在清晨露水中赤足步行的一种水疗法)

Knemidokoptes [ˌniːmidəu'kɔptiːz] *n* 鸟疥螨属 | ~ gallinae 鸡疥螨

Knies' sign [kniːz] (Max Knies) 克尼斯征(瞳孔不等扩大,为格雷夫斯〈Graves〉眶病的一种表现)

knife [naif] *n* 刀 | cataract ~ 内障刀 / cautery ~ 烙刀 / electric ~, endotherm ~ 电热刀 / hernia ~ 疝刀

Knight brace [nait] (James C. Knight) 奈特支具(最古老的椅背形支具之一,其上下带和直立杆是铝制的)

knismogenic [ˌnisməu'dʒenik] *a* 发痒的

knitting ['nitiŋ] *n* 骨愈合

knob [nɔb] *n* 球形突出物;结,隆凸 | surfers' ~s 冲浪者结节 / synaptic ~s 突触小结,突触小丘

knock [nɔk] *vi, vt* 打,敲,击 *n* 敲击;叩击音 | pericardial ~ 心包叩击音

knock-knee ['nɔkniː] *n* 膝外翻

Knoepfelmacher's butter meal [ˌknepfəl'mɑːhə] (Wilhelm Knoepfelmacher) 克内费尔马赫尔奶油餐(用于小孩喂养)

knokkelkoorts ['nɔkəlkuəts] *n* 印度尼西亚登革热

Knops blood group [nɔps] (Knops 为1970年报道的美国先证者的姓) 诺普斯血型(含有抗原 Kn^a, Kn^b, McC^a, Sl^a, YK^a 的一种血型,这些抗原位于补体受体型1)

knot [nɔt] *n* 结 *vt, vi* 打结 | clove hitch ~ 双眼结 / false ~ 假结(脐带);顺结,十字结 / friction ~, double ~ 双结 / granny ~ 顺结,十字结 / net ~ 染色质核仁,核粒 / primitive ~, protochordal ~ 原结 / reef ~, sailor's ~, square ~ 帆结,水手结,方结,反结 / stay ~ 合结 / surfers' ~s 冲浪者结节 / surgeons' ~, surgical ~ 外科结 / syncytial ~s 合胞体结 / true ~ 真结(脐带)

knuckle ['nʌkl] *n* 指节;膨出部 *vt* 用指节扣打(或压、摩、触) | aortic ~ 主动脉弓节

knuckling ['nʌkliŋ] *n* 球节前突(马)

Kobelt's tubes ['kɔːbelt] (George L. Kobelt) 科贝尔特管(卵巢冠横管) | ~ tubules 科贝尔特小管(①卵巢旁体小管;②旁睾小管)

Kober's test ['kəubə] (Philip A. Kober) 科贝尔试验(检雌激素及牛乳蛋白质)

Kobert's test ['kɔːbɛət] (Eduard R. Kobert) 科贝特试验(检血红蛋白)

KOC kathodal (cathodal) opening contraction 阴极断电收缩

Kocher-Debré-Sémélaigne syndrome [ˈkɔkə dəˈbrei seimeiˈleniə] (Emil Theodor Kocher; Robert Debré; Georges Sémélaigne) 科-德-塞综合征(见 Debré-Sémélaigne syndrome)

kocherization [ˌkɔkeraiˈzeiʃən,-riˈz-] *n* 科赫尔处置(暴露胆总管壶腹)

Kocher's forceps [ˈkɔkə] (Emil T. Kocher) 科赫尔钳(手术时夹持组织或压迫出血组织用) | ~ operation 科赫尔手术(①踝关节切除法;②肱骨喙突下脱位整复法;③舌切除术;④移动十二指肠的一种方法;⑤幽门切除术) / ~ reflex 科赫尔反射(压迫睾丸时的腹肌收缩)

Kochia [ˈkəukiə] *n* 地肤属

Koch's bacillus [kɔk] (Robert Koch) 科赫杆菌(结核杆菌) | ~ phenomenon 科赫现象(结核菌再感染剧烈反应) / ~ postulates 科赫要点(确定病原体的四要点:①在该疾病的每一病人体内须寻出微生物;②微生物在纯培养物内须能生长发育;③纯培养物接种于易感的动物时再产生此病;④从实验致病的动物中须能寻得同样的微生物) / ~ reaction 科赫反应,结核菌素反应(试验) / ~ tuberculin 科赫结核菌素(新结核菌素和旧结核菌素)

Koch's node [kɔk] (Walter Koch) 房室结

Koch-Weeks bacillus (hemophilus) [kɔk wiːks] (Robert Koch; John E. Weeks) 结膜炎嗜血杆菌

Kock ileostomy (procedure) [kɔk] (Nils G. Kock) 科克回肠造口术(手术)(以前最常用的一种可控性回肠膀胱术,有一个科克囊袋) | ~ pouch 科克囊袋,可控性回肠膀胱术(①回肠造口术最常用的可控性回肠膀胱术,其容量为 500 ~ 1 000 ml,并有一个末端回肠套叠制成的瓣;②回肠造口术使用的囊袋的一种改良,用作新膀胱)

Koeberlé's forceps [ˌkiːbəˈlei] (Eugène Koeberlé) 止血钳

Koebner's phenomenon [ˈkəːbnə] (Heinrich Koebner) 科布内现象,同形现象(一种皮肤反应,见于某些皮肤病,如银屑病、扁平苔藓、传染性湿疹样皮炎,表现为在未受累的皮肤上出现典型皮肤病的损害。亦称同形反应)

Koenecke's reaction, test [kiˈnek] 克内克反应、试验(检骨髓功能)

Koerber-Salus-Elschnig syndrome [ˈkəːbə ˈsɑːluːs ˈelʃnik] (Hermann Koerber; Robert Salus; Anton Elschnig) 科-索-埃综合征(见 sylvian syndrome)

Kogoj's pustule [ˈkəugɔi] (Franjo Kogoj)科戈伊脓疱(即科戈伊海绵状脓疱 spongiform pustule of Kogoj)

koha [ˈkɔhə] *n* 隐花青(一种日本药物,据说有促进伤口愈合的功效)

Köhler-Pellegrini-Stieda [kəːlə ˌpeleiˈgriːni ˈstiːdə] (Alban Köhler; Augusto Pellegrini; Alfred Stieda) 克勒-佩莱格利尼-施蒂达病(见 Pellegrini's disease)

Köhler's bone disease [ˈkəːlə] (Alban Köhler) 克勒骨病(①儿童足舟骨病;②第二跖骨病) ~ second disease 克勒第二病(第二跖骨病)

Kohlrausch's folds (valves) [ˈkəulrauʃ] (Otto L. B. Kohlrausch) 科尔劳施褶(瓣),直肠横襞

Kohn's pores [kəun] (Hans kohn) 肺泡间孔

Kohnstamm's phenomenon [ˈkəunstəm] (Oscar F. Kohnstamm) 后继性运动(见 after-movement)

koil(o)- [构词成分]洼,凹

koilocyte [ˈkɔiləuˌsait] *n* 中空细胞

koilocytosis [ˌkɔiləusaiˈtəusis] *n* 中空细胞病

koilocytotic [ˌkɔiləusaiˈtɔtik] *a* 中空细胞的

koilonychia [ˌkɔiləuˈnikiə] *n* 反甲

koilorrhachic [ˌkɔiləuˈrækik] *a* 腰椎后凸的

koilosternia [ˌkɔiləuˈstəːniə] *n* 漏斗[状]胸

koin(o)- 见 cen(o)-第二解

koinonia [kɔiˈnəuniə] *n*【希】联合作用(指细胞)

koinotropy [kɔiˈnɔtrəpi] *n* 向群性(对社会和公共关系有兴趣) | **koinotropic** [ˌkɔinəˈtrɔpik] *a*

kojic acid [ˈkəudʒik] 曲酸

koktigen [ˈkɔktidʒən] *n* 煮沸疫苗

Kölliker's column [ˈkelikə] (Rudolf A. von Kölliker) 肌柱,肌原纤维 | ~ interstitial granules 克利克尔间质粒,肌浆间质粒 / ~ membrane 网状膜(蜗管) / ~ nucleus 中央灰质(脊髓)

Kollmann's dilator [ˈkɔlmən] (Arthur Kollmann) 科尔曼扩张器(可屈尿道扩张器)

Kolmer's test [ˈkəulmə] (John A. Kolmer) 科氏试验(检梅毒和细菌性疾病)

Kolmogorov-Smirnov test [kɔlˈmɔgərɔv ˈsmiənɔv] (Andrei N. Kolmogorov; Nicolai V. Smirnov) 高尔莫哥罗夫-斯米诺夫检验(拟合适度的统计检验,检查样本是否符合特定的理论分布函数,或两种样本是否来自同一群体)

kolp- 以 kolp -起始的词,同样见以 colp- 起始的词

kolypeptic [ˌkəuliˈpeptik] *a* 抑制消化的,调整消化的

kolytic [kəuˈlitik] *a* 抑制的,沉静气质的

Kondoleon's operation [kɔnˈdəuliən] (Emmerich Kondoleon) 康多莱昂手术(切除皮下组织,治象皮病)

König's operation [ˈkenig] (Franz König) 柯尼希手术(治先天性髋脱位) | ~ syndrome 柯尼希综合征(便秘与腹泻交替发生,伴腹痛、鼓胀以及在右髂窝可闻及气过水声)

König's rods [ˈkenig] (Charles J. König) 柯尼希[音]杆(为一系列的钢杆,敲击每一根钢杆即发

出一定音调的律音）

koniocortex [ˌkəuniəuˈkɔːteks] *n* 粒状皮质（大脑感觉区）

koniology [ˌkəuniˈɔlədʒi] *n* 尘埃学

konometer [kəuˈnɔmitə], **konimeter** [kəuˈnimitə] *n* 尘埃计算器，计尘器

koomis [ˈkuːmis] *n* 霉乳酒

kopf-tetanus [kɔpfˈtetənəs] *n* 头部破伤风

kophemia [kəuˈfiːmiə] *n* 辨语聋，听性聋

kopiopia [ˌkəupiˈəupiə] *n* 眼疲劳

Koplik's spots (sign) [ˈkɔplik] (Henry Koplik) 科氏斑（征）（颊黏膜和舌黏膜上出现小而不规则的鲜红斑，中央有蓝白色小点，见于麻疹前驱期）

Kopp's asthma [kɔp] (Johann H. Kopp) 喘鸣性喉痉挛

kopr- 以 kopr-起始的词，同样见以 copr-起始的词

kopratin [ˈkɔprətin] *n* 次高铁血红素

koprosterin [ˌkɔprəˈstiərin] *n* 粪甾醇，粪甾烷醇

Korányi-Grocco triangle [kɔˈrænji ˈgrɔkəu] (Baron F. von Korányi; Pietro Grocco) 科兰伊-格罗科三角（见 Grocco sign①解）

Korányi's auscultation (percussion) [kɔˈrænji] (Baron Friedrich von Korányi) 科兰伊听诊法（叩诊法）（以一手的示指轻敲垂直置于患部的另一手的示指的第二关节）| ～ sign 科兰伊征（叩击胸椎棘突时，背侧段叩诊音增强，为胸腔积液之征）

Korányi's treatment [kɔˈrænji] (Alexander von Korányi) 科兰伊疗法（从前用苯治白血病）

Kordofan gum [ˈkɔːdəfæn] (Kordofan 为苏丹省名) 科尔多凡树胶

koro [ˈkəurəu] *n* 缩阳症（一种特定文化背景下的急性妄想综合征，见于马来人，病人认为阴茎正在缩入腹内而消失，一旦发生，即将死亡）

korocyte [ˈkɔːrəsait] *n* 幼稚[中性]粒细胞，杆状中性粒细胞

koronion [kəˈrəuniɔn] ([复] **koronia** [kəˈrəuniə]) *n* (下颌骨)冠突尖

koroscopy [kəˈrɔspəki] *n* 瞳孔检影法，视网膜镜检查，视网膜检影法

Korotkoff's method [kəˈrɔtkəf] (Nicolai S. Korotkoff) 科罗特科夫法（用听诊法测定血压）| ～ sounds 科罗特科夫音（听诊测血压时听到动脉扩张音）/ ～ test 科罗特科夫试验（检动脉瘤的侧支循环）

Korsakoff's (Korsakov's) psychosis (disease, syndrome) [ˈkɔːsəkəf] (Sergei S. Korsakoff) 科尔萨科夫精神病（病、综合征）（酒毒性精神病，一种慢性型出血性脑上部灰质炎。亦称多神经炎性精神病、精神中毒性脑病、慢性酒毒性谵妄）

Körte-Ballance operation [ˈkiətə ˈbæləns] (Werner Körte; Charles A. Ballance) 科尔特-巴朗斯手术（面神经和舌下神经吻合术）

kosam [ˈkəusəm] *n* 苦参子，鸦胆子（其籽有时用于治腹泻、痢疾及子宫出血）

Koshevnikoff's (Koschewnikow's, Kozhevnikov's) disease, epilepsy [kəˈʃevnikɔf] (Alexei J. Koshevnikoff) 持续性不全癫痫

Kossel's test [ˈkɔsəl] (Albrecht Kossel) 科塞尔试验（检次黄嘌呤）

Köster's nodule [ˈkestə] (Karl Köster) 克斯特尔小结（含有巨细胞的结核结节，四周有双层细胞围绕）

Kostmann's neutropenia (syndrome) [ˈkɔstmɑːn] (Rolf Kostmann) 科斯特曼中性粒细胞减少（综合征），婴儿遗传性粒细胞缺乏症

Kottmann's test (reaction) [ˈkɔtmɑːn] (K. Kottmann) 科特曼试验（反应）（检甲状腺功能）

koumiss [ˈkuːmis] *n* 霉乳酒 | kefir ～ 发酵乳霉乳酒

Kovalevsky's canal [ˌkɔvəˈlevski] (Alexander O. Kovalevsky) 神经肠管

Kowarsky's test [kəˈvɑːski] (Albert Kowarsky) 科瓦尔斯基试验（检尿糖；检糖尿病）

Koyter's muscle [ˈkɔitə] (Volcherus Koyter) 皱眉肌

KP keratic precipitates 角膜后沉着物

Kr krypton 氪

Krabbe's disease (leukodystrophy) [ˈkræbiː] (Knud H. krabbe) 克拉伯病，脑白质营养不良（一种家族型脑白质病，亦称家族性弥漫性婴儿脑硬化、球形细胞脑白质营养不良）

Kraepelin's classification [ˈkreipeilin] (Emil Kraepelin) 克雷佩林分类（辨别精神分裂症及躁狂抑郁性精神病）

krait [kreit] *n* 金环蛇（印度等地产）

Krameria [krəˈmiəriə] (J. G. H. and W. H. Kramer) *n* 拉坦尼属（见 rhatany）

Kraske's operation [ˈkræski] (Paul Kraske) 克拉斯克手术（切除尾骨和部分骶骨以便接近直肠癌）

kratometer [kreiˈtɔmitə] *n* 棱镜矫视器

krauomania [ˌkrɔːəˈmeinjə] *n* 节律性抽搐

kraurosis [krɔːˈrəusis] *n* 干皱 | ～ penis 阴茎干皱症，干燥性龟头炎 / ～ vulvae 外阴干皱

Krause's bulbs, corpuscle [krauz] (Wilhelm J. F. Krause) 克劳泽小体（球状小体）| ～ line, membrane 克劳泽线（膜），Z 盘（横纹肌间线）

Krause's ligament [ˈkrauzə] (Karl F. T. Krause) 骨盆横韧带 | ～ valve 克劳泽瓣（泪囊襞）

Krause's operation [krauz] (Fedor V. Krause) 克劳泽手术（硬膜外切除三叉神经节以治疗三

叉神经痛)

Krause-Wolfe graft [ˈkrauzə ˈvɔlf] (Fedor Krause; John R. Wolfe) 克劳泽-沃尔夫移植片(全层皮移植片)

kreatin [ˈkriːətin] *n* 肌酸

krebiozen [kriˈbaiəzen] *n* 克力生物素(由美国食品及药物管理局鉴定为与肌酸同一物质,据称该物质治癌有效。美国已禁止出售)

Krebs cycle [krebz] (Hans A. Krebs) 三羧酸循环

Krebs' leukocyte index [ˈkrebz] (Carl Krebs) 克雷布斯白细胞指数(中性粒细胞的百分比以淋巴细胞的百分比除之所得的数)

Kremer test [ˈkreimə] (Jan A. M. Kremer) 克雷默试验(即 SCMC test, 见 test 项下相应术语)

kre(o)- [构词成分] 以 kre(o)-起始的词,同样见以 cre(o)- 起始的词

kreotoxicon [ˌkriəˈtɔksikɔn] *n* 肉毒质

kreotoxin [ˌkriəˈtɔksin] *n* 肉毒素

kreotoxism [ˌkriəˈtɔksizəm] *n* 肉中毒

kresofuchsin [ˌkresəˈfuːksin] *n* 甲酚品红

kresol [ˈkresɔl] *n* 甲[苯]酚,煤酚(防腐消毒用)

Kretschmann's space [ˈkretʃmɑːn] (Friedrich Kretschmann) 克雷奇曼间隙(鼓室上隐窝内的凹陷区)

Kretschmer types [ˈkretʃmə] (Ernst Kretschmer) 克雷奇默尔体型(认为体型与人格有关,如瘦长型为类精神分裂人格,矮胖型为和谐人格)

Kretz's granules [krets] (Richard Kretz) 克雷茨粒(肝硬化小结) | ~ paradox 克雷茨奇异现象(正常动物注射中和的毒素-抗毒素混合物不产生不利作用,以前已主动免疫接种过毒素的动物则情况相反)

Kreysig's sign [ˈkraizig] (Friedrich L. Kreysig) 克赖济希征(见 Heim-Kreysig sign)

krimpsiekte [krimpˈziːkti] *n* 子叶中毒病(牛)

kringle [ˈkriŋgl] *n* 三环域,环饼

krinin [ˈkrinin] *n* 激泌素

Krishaber's disease [ˌkriːshəˈbεə] (Maurice Krishaber) 克里萨贝病(一种神经功能病,表现为心动过速、失眠、眩晕、感觉过敏等症状。亦称脑-心综合征)

Krisovski's (Krisowski's) sign [kriˈsɔvski] (Max Krisovski〈或 Krisowski〉) 克列苏夫斯基征(先天性梅毒时,从病人口角放射出瘢痕线)

Kristeller's method (expression, technique) [ˈkristələ] (Samuel Kristeller) 克里斯特勒法(压出法、操作法)(胎儿压出法)

Kromayer's burn [ˈkrəumaiə] (Ernst L. F. Kromayer) 紫外线灼伤 | ~ lamp 克罗迈尔灯(水银石英灯,放出紫外线)

Krompecher's carcinoma (tumor) [ˈkrəumpekə] (Edmund Krompecher) 侵蚀性溃疡

kromskop [ˈkrəumskəup] *n* 【德】原色摄影装置(用于病理标本)

Kronecker's center [ˈkrəunekə] (Karl H. Kronecker) 克罗内克尔中枢(心抑制中枢) | ~ puncture 克罗内克尔穿刺(穿刺心抑制中枢)

Krönig's field (area) [ˈkreinig] (Georg Krönig) 克勒尼希区(肺尖的胸部叩响区) | ~ isthmus 克勒尼希峡(肩上的狭长带状叩响区,并连接胸与背的较大叩响区,位于肺尖〈克勒尼希区〉)

Krönlein's hernia [ˈkreinlain] (Rudolf U. Krönlein) 腹股沟腹膜前疝 | ~ operation 克伦莱因手术(切除眼眶外壁以清除眶内肿瘤)

Krukenberg's hand (arm) [ˈkruːkənbəːg] (Hermann Krukenberg) 克鲁肯贝格手(臂)(前臂叉形残株假手)

Krukenberg's spindle [ˈkruːkənbəːg] (Friedrich E. Krukenberg) 克鲁肯贝格梭(角膜后面垂直梭状棕红色浑浊) | ~ tumor 克鲁肯贝格瘤(一种特殊型卵巢癌,通常从胃肠道癌〈尤其从胃癌〉转移而得,特征为黏液样变性区并有印指环状细胞,亦称黏液细胞癌)

Krukenberg's veins [ˈkruːkənbəːg] (Adolph Krukenberg) 肝中央静脉

Kruse's brush [ˈkruːzə] (Walther Kruse) 克鲁泽刷(细白金丝刷,用以接种培养基表面)

Kruskal-Wallis test [ˈkrʌskæl ˈwælis] (William H. Kruskal; Wilson A. Wallis) 克鲁斯卡尔-沃利斯检验法(顺序数据的非参数性检验,同时比较三组或三组以上,所有数据按数字分级,然后将每一组的分级值加以总和并计算平均数。如果全组都从同一群体抽出的无效假设是真的,则全组的平均值应该是相同的)

kryoscopy [kraiˈɔskəpi] *n* (溶液)冰点测定法,冰点降低测定法

krypt(o)- 以 krypt(o)-起始的词,同样见以 crypt(o)-起始的词

krypton (Kr) [ˈkriptɔn] *n* 氪(化学元素)

17-KS 17-ketosteroid 17-酮甾类

KSC kathodal (cathodal) closing contraction 阴极通电收缩

KST kathodal (cathodal) closing tetanus 阴极通电强直

Kt/V 脲动力学中血液透析一段时间的效率或脲清除率分数的表达式,*K* 为清除率,*t* 为一段时间的量,*V* 为血液透析后脲分布体积

KUB kidney, ureter and bladder 肾、输尿管及膀胱

kubisagari [kuˌbisəˈgɑːri], **kubisgari** [ˌkubisˈgɑːri] *n* 垂头病(日本流行的一种麻痹性眩晕)

Kufs' disease [kuːfs] (H. Kufs) 库夫斯病(青年后期家族性黑矇痴呆)

Kugelberg-Welander syndrome [ˈkuːgəlbəːg

ˈveləndə](Eric K. H. Kugelburg; Lisa Welander)库-韦综合征(一种遗传性青少年型肌萎缩,通常作为常染色体隐性性状遗传,系由脊髓前角损害所致。本征特点为10或20岁内〈主要在2岁和17岁之间〉起病,下肢和骨盆带近端肌肉萎缩和无力,然后累及远端肌肉和肌颤搐。亦称青少年〈脊髓性〉肌萎缩或近端脊髓性肌萎缩)

Kuhlmann's test [ˈkuːlmən](Frederick Kuhlmann)库尔曼智力测验(比奈〈Binet〉智力测验的一种改良,以适合婴儿智力测验)

Kühne's methylene blue [ˈkiːnə](Heinrich Kühne)屈内甲烯蓝(酚溶液内甲烯蓝和无水乙醇的混合物)

Kühne's muscular phenomenon [ˈkiːnə](Wilhelm F. Kühne)屈内肌现象(持续电流通过活肌纤维引起由阳极至阴极的波动)| ~ terminal plates 屈内终板(肌梭内神经运动终板)/ ~ spindle 肌梭

Kuhn's mask [kuːn](Ernst Kuhn)库恩面罩(治疗肺结核的面罩)

Kuhn's tube [kuːn](Franz Kuhn)库恩管(气管内麻醉用)

Kuhnt-Junius disease [ˈkuːnt ˈjuːniəs](Hermann Kuhnt; Paul Junius)库-尤病,盘状黄斑变性

Kuhnt's illusion [kuːnt](Hermann Kuhnt)库恩特视错觉(用单眼看相似间距,似乎颞视野较鼻视野小)

kukuruku [ˌkukuˈruku] *n* 库库鲁库病(尼日利亚库库鲁库地区病,似黄热病)

Kulchitsky's cells [kulˈtʃitski](Nicolai K. Kulchitsky)库尔契茨基细胞(胃肠嗜银细胞)

Kulenkampff's anesthesia [ˈkulənkɑːmpf](Dietrich Kulenkampff)库伦坎普夫麻醉(臂丛阻滞麻醉)

Külz's cast (cylinder) [kilts](Rudolph E. Külz)屈尔茨管型,昏迷[兆]管型(见于糖尿病性昏迷)| ~ test 屈尔茨试验(检β-羟丁酸)

kumiss, kumyss [ˈkuːmis] *n* 霉乳酒

Kümmell's disease (spondylitis), Kümmell-Verneuil disease [ˈkimelˌvɛəˈneiiː](Hermann Kümmell; Aristide A. S. Verneuil)坎梅尔病,坎-韦病,外伤后脊椎炎(脊椎受压骨折)

kundalini [ˌkuːndəˈliːni] *n*【梵】生命力(印度传统中,指位于最低的人体精神心灵力量中心〈chakra〉的精神心灵力量)

Kunkel's syndrome [ˈkuŋkel](Henry George Kunkel)孔凯尔综合征,狼疮样肝炎

Küntscher nail [ˈkintʃə](Gerhard küntscher)金切尔钉(骨髓腔内插钉)

Kupffer's cells [ˈkupfə](Karl W. von Kupffer)普弗细胞(肝星形细胞)

kupramite [ˈkjuprəmait] *n* 防氨面罩

Kupressoff's center [kuˈpresəf](Ivan Kupressoff)库普雷索夫中枢(排尿中枢)

Kurloff's (Kurlov's) bodies [ˈkuələf](Mikhail G. Kurloff)库尔洛夫体(豚鼠淋巴细胞原虫)

Kurthia [ˈkuətiə](Heinrich Kurth)库尔特杆菌属

kurtosis [kəːˈtəusis] *n* 峰度(概率分布的峰度或平顶度)

kuru [ˈkuəru] *n* 库鲁病,新几内亚震颤病(一种由病毒引起的慢性进行性神经系统疾病,仅在新几内亚福雷〈Fore〉族及相邻的土著人中发现,主要症状为躯干与四肢共济失调、震颤及构语障碍)

Kurunegala ulcer [ˌkuəruneiˈgɑːlə] 热带化脓病(Kurunegala 为斯里兰卡一地区名)

Kusnezovia [ˌkuːsniˈzəuviə](S. I. Kusnezov) *n* 库兹涅佐夫菌属

Küss' experiment [kiːs](Emil Küss)屈斯实验(注射阿片和颠茄溶液于膀胱内,若不产生中毒症状,即示膀胱上皮对这些物质无通透性)

Kussmaul-Kien respiration [ˈkusmaul ˈkiːn](Adolf Kussmaul; Alphonse M. J. Kien)库斯莫尔-基恩呼吸,空气饥(air hunger,见 hunger 项下相应术语)

Kussmaul-Landry paralysis [ˈkusmaul ˈlændri](Adolf Kussmaul; Jean B. O. Landry)急性热病性多神经炎

Kussmaul- Maier disease [ˈkusmaul ˈmaiə](Adolf Kussmaul; Rudolf Maier)见 Kussmaul disease

Kussmaul's aphasia [ˈkusmaul](Adolph Kussmaul)库斯莫尔失语(有意识的不语,如精神错乱时)| ~ disease 结节性动脉外膜炎,结节性多动脉炎 / ~ paralysis 急性热病性多神经炎 / ~ pulse 奇脉,逆脉 / ~ respiration 库斯莫尔呼吸,空气饥(air hunger,见 hunger 项下相应术语)/ ~ sign 库斯莫尔征(①吸气时颈静脉出现怒张,见于纵隔心包炎及纵隔瘤;②胃病时由于毒素吸收作用所致的昏迷及惊厥;③奇脉)

Küstner's law [ˈkiːstnə](Otto E. Küstner)屈斯特纳定律(卵巢囊肿扭转方向为其蒂所在侧的对侧,如卵巢囊肿在左侧,其蒂的扭转方向向右,如在右侧,则向左)| ~ sign 屈斯特纳征(卵巢皮样囊肿时可在子宫前方中线上呈现一囊性肿物)

kuttarosome [kʌˈtærəsəum] *n* 并杆小体

Küttner's ganglion [ˈkitnə] 屈特纳淋巴结,颈二腹肌淋巴结(位于内颈静脉上正在二腹肌后腹下的大淋巴结,形成舌的主要淋巴终支)

kV kilovolt 千伏[特]

Kveim test [kvaim](Morten A. Kveim)克韦姆试验(检结节病)

kVp kilovolt peak 千伏峰位

kW kilowatt 千瓦[特]
kwashiorkor [kwɑːʃiˈɔːkə] *n* 夸希奥科,蛋白质缺乏症,恶性营养不良病(为一种严重蛋白缺乏综合征,特征为发育迟缓、皮肤毛发变色、水肿及肝脏病理性变化,包括脂肪浸润、坏死和纤维变性,四肢及背部呈红色,可能脱皮,并有深色斑点,首见于非洲,现全世界主要是热带和亚热带都有发现,此病与营养不良有关) | marasmic ~ 消瘦型恶性营养不良病
kwaski [ˈkwɑːski] *n* 寒战病
kW-hr kilowatt- hour 千瓦[特]小时
kyan(o)- 以 kyan(o)- 起始的词,同样见以 cyano- 起始的词
kyanophane [ˈkaiənəfein] *n* 视青质,视蓝质(视网膜内)
Kyasanur Forest disease [ˈkaiˈæsənur] (Kyasanur Forest 位于印度迈索尔邦〈Mysore State〉,1957 年报道在林业工人和猴中间出现首批病例) 夸赛纳森林病(一种严重出血热,特点为发热、出血表现和皮疹,发生在印度迈索尔邦,系由黄病毒引起,由血蜱属的蜱,尤其是距刺血蜱从贮主猴和田鼠传播给人)
kyestein [kaiˈestiːn] *n* 孕尿翳,孕尿皮(有时在不新鲜的尿表面上见到一种膜,以前认为是孕征)
kyllosis [kiˈləusis] *n* 畸形足
kymatism [ˈkaimətizəm] *n* 肌纤维颤搐
kymocyclograph [ˌkaiməˈsaikləgrɑːf, -græf] *n* 运动描记器
kymogram [ˈkaiməgræm] *n* 记波图
kymograph [ˈkaiməgrɑːf, -græf] *n* 记纹器 记波器 | ~**ic** [ˌkaiməˈgræfik] *a*
kymography [kaiˈmɔgrəfi] *n* 记波法,记波摄影[术] | roentgen ~ X 线记波法,X 线记波摄影[术]
kymotrichous [ˌkaiməˈtrikəs] *a* 卷发的
kynocephalus [ˌkainəˈsefələs] *n* 狗头畸胎
kynurenic acid [ˌkinjuəˈrenik] 犬尿烯酸
kynureninase [ˌkainjuəˈrenineis] *n* 犬尿氨酸酶
kynurenine [kaiˈnjuərəˌniːn, ˈkain-], **kynurenin** [ˌkainjuəˈriːnin] *n* 犬尿氨酸,犬尿素
kynurenine formamidase [kaiˈnjuərəˌniːnfɔːˈmæmideis] 犬尿氨酸甲酰胺酶,芳香基甲酰胺酶
kynurenine 3-hydroxylase [kaiˈnjuərəˌniːn haiˈdrɔksileis] 犬尿氨酸 3-羟化酶,犬尿氨酸 3-单加氧酶
kynurenine 3-monooxygenase [kaiˈnjuərəˌniːn ˌməunəuˈɔksidʒineis] 犬尿氨酸 3-单加氧酶(亦称犬尿氨酸 3-羟化酶)
kyogenic [ˌkaiəˈdʒenik] *a* 引起妊娠的,致孕的
kyphoplasty [ˈkaifəuˌplæsti] *n* 脊柱后凸矫治术
kyphos [ˈkaifəs] *n* 脊柱后凸
kyphoscoliosis [ˌkaifəuˌskɔliˈəusis] *n* 脊柱后凸侧弯
kyphosis [kaiˈfəusis] *n*【希】脊柱后凸 | ~ dorsalis juvenilis 幼年期脊柱后凸 | **kyphotic** [kaiˈfɔtik] *a*
kyphotone [ˈkaifətəun] *n* 驼背矫正器
kyrin [ˈkairin] *n* 三肽
Kyrle's disease [ˈkirlə] (Joseph Kyrle) 基勒病(一种罕见的慢性角化病,其特征为丘疹样皮疹和在毛囊及小汗腺管内角化过度的锥形栓形成,经表皮侵入真皮,引起异物巨细胞反应和疼痛,亦称真皮穿通性毛囊及毛囊旁角化过度)
kyrtorrhachic [ˌkəːtəˈrækik] *a* 腰椎前凸的
kysth(o)- [构词成分] 阴道;以 kysth(o)- 起始的词,同样见以 colp(o)- 起始的词
kyt(o)- 以 kyt(o)- 起始的词,同样见以 cyt(o)- 起始的词

L

L lambert 朗伯; left 左; leucine 亮氨酸; liter 升; lung 肺; light chain 轻链(免疫球蛋白); lumbar vertebrae 腰椎(L1～L5)

L. libra【拉】磅

L- luminance 亮度;self-induction 自感

L_0 limes nul 无毒界量

L＋, L_+ limes tod 致死界量

L- [前缀]左型

l 升(liter)以前的符号

l. ligamentum【拉】韧带

l length 长度

l- levo- 左旋

λ lambda 希腊语的第 11 个字母;波长(wavelength)、衰变常数(decay constant)以及两种免疫球蛋白轻链之一的符号;微米(microliter)以前的符号

La lanthanum 镧

L & A light and accommodation (瞳孔)对光和调节反应

Labarraque's solution [ˈlæbəˈræk] (Antoine G. Labarraque) 拉巴腊克溶液(用等量水稀释的次氯酸钠)

Labbé's triangle [ləˈbei] (Léon Labbé) 拉贝三角(胃三角) | ～ vein 上吻合静脉

label [ˈleibl] *n* 标签,瓶签;标记 *vt* 贴标签;做标记;(用放射性核素)使(元素或原子)示踪 | radioactive ～ 放射性标记

labetalol [ləˈbetələl] *n* 拉贝洛尔(*β* 和 *α* 受体阻滞药,用于治疗高血压) | ～ hydrochloride 盐酸拉贝洛尔

labia [ˈleibiə] labium 的复数

labial [ˈleibjəl] *a* 唇的

labialism [ˈleibiəlizəm] *n* 唇音滥用

labially [ˈleibjəli] *ad* 向唇

labiate [ˈleibieit] *a* 唇形的;有唇的

labichorea [ˌleibikɔˈriə] *n* 唇肌痉挛性口吃

Labidognatha [ˌlæbiˈdɔgnəθə] *n* 钳腭亚目

labile [ˈleibail] *a* 不稳定的,易变的 | ～ acid 不稳定酸 / heat ～ 不耐热的 | **lability** [ləˈbiləti] *n* 不稳定性,易变性

labio- [构词成分]唇

labioalveolar [ˌleibiəuælˈviələ] *a* 唇牙槽的;牙槽唇侧的

labioaxiogingival [ˌleibiəuˌæksiəuˈdʒindʒivəl] *a* 唇牙轴龈的

labiocervical [ˌleibiəuˈsəːvikəl] *a* 唇颈的;唇龈的

labiochorea [ˌleibiəukɔˈriə] *n* 唇舞病,口吃病

labioclination [ˌleibiəuklaiˈnejʃən] *n* 唇侧倾斜(牙)

labiodental [ˌleibiəuˈdentl] *a* 唇牙的 *n* 唇齿音

labiogingival [ˌleibiəuˈdʒindʒivəl] *a* 唇龈的

labioglossolaryngeal [ˌleibiəuˌglɔsəuləˈrindʒiəl] *a* 唇舌喉的

labioglossopharyngeal [ˌleibiəuˌglɔsəufəˈrindʒiəl] *a* 唇舌咽的

labiograph [ˈleibiəˌgrɑːf, -græf] *n* 唇动描记器

labioincisal [ˌleibiəuinˈsaizəl] *a* 唇牙切面的

labiolingual [ˌleibiəuˈliŋgwəl] *a* 唇舌的

labiology [ˌleibiˈɔlədʒi] *n* 唇运动学 | **labiologic** [ˌleibiəuˈlɔdʒik] *a*

labiomancy [ˈleibiəˌmænsi] *n* 唇读,唇谈法

labiomental [ˌleibiəuˈmentl] *a* 唇颏的

labiomycosis [ˌleibiəumaiˈkəusis] *n* 唇真菌病,唇霉菌病

labionasal [ˌleibiəuˈneizəl] *a* 唇鼻的 *n* 唇鼻音

labiopalatine [ˌleibiəuˈpælətin] *a* 唇腭的

labioplacement [ˌleibiəuˈpleismənt] *n* 唇向移位

labioplasty [ˈleibiəˌplæsti] *n* 唇成形术

labiotenaculum [ˌleibiəutiˈnækjuləm] *n* 固唇器

labioversion [ˌleibiəuˈvəːʃən] *n* 唇向错位

labium [ˈleibiəm] ([复] **labia** [ˈleibiə]) *n*【拉】唇;[复]阴唇

labor [ˈleibə] *n* 产程;分娩,生产;阵痛 | atonic ～ 子宫乏力性分娩 / complicated ～ 并发症分娩 / dry ～ 干产 / false ～, mimetic ～ 假[临]产 / habitual premature ～ 习惯性早产 / immature ～ 早产 / induced ～, artificial ～ 引产 / instrumental ～ 器械分娩 / missed ～ 滞留死胎 / multiple ～ 多胎分娩 / obstructed ～ 梗阻性分娩 / postmature ～, postponed ～, delayed ～ 逾期分娩,过期分娩 / precipitate ～ 急产 / premature ～ 早产 / prolonged ～, protracted ～ 滞产 / spontaneous ～ 顺产,自然分娩 / term ～ 足月分娩

laboratorian [ˌlæbərəˈtɔːriən] *n* 检验师,化验员

laboratory [ləˈbɔrətəri, ˈlæbərətəri] *n* 实验室,检验室,化验室

Laborde's forceps [ləˈbɔːd] (Jean B. V. Laborde) 拉博德钳(持舌钳,用于拉博德法以刺激呼

吸) | ~ method 拉博德法(以节奏性牵舌动作刺激呼吸中枢,治疗窒息患者) / ~ sign (test) 拉博德征(试验)(检死征)
labrale [lə'breili] *n* 唇中点,唇缘(人体测量名词) | ~ inferius 下唇中点,下唇缘 / ~ superius 上唇中点,上唇缘
labrocyte ['læbrəsait] *n* 肥大细胞
labrum ['leibrəm] ([复] **labra** ['leibrə]) *n*【拉】唇,缘
laburinine [lə'bjuəriniːn] *n* 金雀花碱,野靛碱
Laburnum [lə'bəːnəm] *n* 金莲花属
laburnum [lə'bəːnəm] *n* 金莲花属植物;金莲花
labyrinth ['læbərinθ] *n* 迷路 | acoustic ~ 听迷路,[耳]蜗 / cortical ~ [肾]皮质迷路 / bony ~, osseous ~ 骨迷路 / ~ of ethmoid, ethmoidal ~, olfactory ~ 筛骨迷路 / membranous ~ 膜迷路 / statokinetic ~, nonacoustic ~ 位觉迷路(前庭及半规管)
labyrinthectomy [ˌlæbərin'θektəmi] *n* 迷路切除术
labyrinthi [ˌlæbə'rinθai] labyrinthus 的复数
labyrinthine [ˌlæbə'rinθain], **labyrinthian** [ˌlæbə'rinθiən] **labyrinthic** [ˌlæbə'rinθik] *a* 迷路的
labyrinthitis [ˌlæbərin'θaitis] *n* 迷路炎 | circumscribed ~ 局限性迷路炎
labyrinthodont [ˌlæbə'rinθədɔnt] *n*, *a* 迷齿亚纲动物(的)
Labyrinthomorpha [ˌlæbəˌrinθə'mɔːfə] *n* 盘蜷门
labyrinthotomy [ˌlæbərin'θɔtəmi] *n* 迷路切开术
Labyrinthulea [ˌlæbərin'θjuːliə] *n* 盘根足虫纲
Labyrinthulida [ˌlæbərin'θjuːlidə] *n* 盘根足虫目
labyrinthus [ˌlæbə'rinθəs] ([复] **labyrinthi** [ˌlæbə'rinθai]) *n*【拉】迷路
lac [læk] ([复] **lacta** ['læktə]) *n*【拉】乳;乳剂;紫胶,虫胶
laccase ['lækeis] *n* 漆酶
Laccifer ['læksifə] *n* 胶蚧属
lacerate ['læsəreit] *vt* 撕裂,裂伤,划破(软组织等);伤害(感情) ['læsərit] *a* 撕碎了的,划破了的 | **~d** *a* 撕裂的 / **lacerable** ['læsərəbl] *a* 可撕裂的,易划破的 / **laceration** [ˌlæsə'reiʃən] *n* 撕裂;撕裂伤
lacertofulvin [ləˌsəːtə'fʌlvin] *n* 蛇黄质
lacertus [lə'səːtəs] *n* [肌]纤维束
Lachesis ['lækisis] *n*【拉;希】饭匙倩属(蝰科)
Lachnospira [ˌlæknəu'spaiərə] *n* 毛螺菌属 | ~ multiparis 多对毛螺菌
lachry- 以 lachry-起始的词,同样见以 lacri- 起始的词
lacis ['leisis] *n*【法】[肾小]球旁细胞
lacmus ['lækməs] *n* 石蕊
lacri- [构词成分]泪
lacrima ['lækrimə] ([复] **lacrimae** ['lækrimiː]) *n*【拉】泪
lacrimal, **lacrymal** ['lækriməl] *a* 泪的
lacrimalin [læ'kriməlin] *n* 促流泪素
lacrimase ['lækrimeis] *n* 泪[腺]酶
lacrimation, **lacrymation** [ˌlækri'meiʃən] *n* 流泪
lacrimator, **lachrymator** ['lækriˌmeitə] *n* 催泪剂
lacrimatory, **lachrymatory** ['lækriməˌtəri] *a* 催泪的
lacrimonasal [ˌlækriməu'neizəl] *a* 泪鼻的
lacrimotome ['lækrimətəum] *n* 泪管刀
lacrimotomy [ˌlækri'mɔtəmi] *n* 泪器切开术
lacta ['læktə] lac 的复数
lactacidemia [lækˌtæsi'diːmiə] *n* 乳酸血
lactacidin [læk'tæsidin] *n* 拉克塔西丁(一种由乳酸与水杨酸组成的食物防腐剂)
lactacidogen [ˌlæktə'sidədʒən] *n* 6-磷酸果糖
lactaciduria [lækˌtæsi'djuəriə] *n* 乳酸尿
lactagogue ['læktəgɔg] *a* 催乳的 *n* 催乳药
lactalbumin [ˌlæktæl'bjumin] *n* 乳白蛋白,乳清蛋白
lactam ['læktəm] *n* 内酰胺
β-lactamase ['læktəmeis] *n* β-内酰胺酶(亦称头孢菌素酶,青霉素酶)
lactamide [læk'tæmid] *n* 乳酰胺
Lactarius [læk'teiriəs] *n* 乳菇属
lactaroviolin [ˌlæktərə'vaiəlin] *n* 乳菇紫素(旧名乳紫林)
lactase ['lækteis] *n* 乳糖酶 | adult ~ deficiency 成人乳糖酶缺乏症,二糖不耐受症Ⅲ / ~ deficiency 乳糖酶缺乏症,乳糖不耐受[症] / intestinal ~ deficiency 肠乳糖酶缺乏症,二糖不耐受症Ⅲ
lactate ['lækteit] *n* 乳酸(阴离子形式) *vi* 分泌乳汁 | lactic acid ~ 乳酸乳酸盐
L-lactate dehydrogenase (**LDH**) ['lækteit diː'haidrədʒəneis] L-乳酸脱氢酶
lactation [læk'teiʃən] *n* 泌乳;泌乳期;哺乳 | **~al** *a*
lacteal ['læktiəl] *a* 乳的 *n* 乳糜管
lactein ['læktiːn] *n* 炼乳
lactenin ['læktinin] *n* 乳抑菌素,乳烃素
lactescence [læk'tesns] *n* 乳状,乳汁状;乳色
lactic ['læktik] *a* 乳的 | ~ acid 乳酸;乳酸制剂
lacticacidemia [ˌlæktikˌæsi'diːmiə] *n* 乳酸血[症]
lacticemia [ˌlækti'siːmiə] *n* 乳酸血
lactiferous [læk'tifərəs], **lactigerous** [læk'tidʒərəs] *a* 生乳的,输乳的
lactifuge ['læktifjuːdʒ] *a* 回乳的,止乳的 *n* 回乳

药,止乳药
lactigenous [læk'tidʒinəs] *a* 生乳的,泌乳的
lactim ['læktim] *n* 内酰亚胺
lactimorbus [ˌlækti'mɔːbəs] *n* 乳毒病
lactin ['læktin] *n* 乳糖
lactinated ['læktiˌneitid] *a* 含乳糖的
lactitol ['læktitɔl] *n* 拉克替醇(甜味药,轻泻药)
lactivorous [læk'tivərəs] *a* 乳食的
lact(o)- [构词成分] 乳,乳酸
Lactobacillaceae [ˌlæktəuˌbæsi'leisiiː] *n* 乳[酸]杆菌科
Lactobacilleae [ˌlæktəubə'siliiː] *n* 乳[酸]杆菌族
lactobacillin [ˌlæktəubə'silin] *n* 乳[酸]杆菌素
Lactobacillus [ˌlæktəubə'siləs] *n* 乳[酸]杆菌属 | ~ acidophilus 嗜酸乳杆菌 / ~ bifidus 双叉乳杆菌 / ~ bulgaricus 保加利亚乳杆菌
lactobacillus [ˌlæktəubə'siləs] ([复] **lactobacilli** [ˌlæktəubə'silai]) *n* 乳[酸]杆菌
Lactobacteriaceae [ˌlæktəubækˌtiəri'eisiiː] *n* 乳[酸]杆菌科(旧名,现称 Lactobacillaceae)
lactobutyrometer [ˌlæktəuˌbjuti'rɔmitə] *n* 乳脂计
lactocele ['læktəsiːl] *n* 乳腺囊肿;乳性鞘膜积液
lactochrome ['læktəkrəum] *n* 核黄素,维生素 B_2
lactoconium [læktə'kəuniəm] *n* 乳微粒
lactocrit ['læktəkrit] *n* 乳脂计
lactodensimeter [ˌlæktəuden'simitə] *n* 乳比重计
lactofarinaceous [ˌlæktəuˌfæri'neiʃəs] *a* 乳和谷粉的
lactoferrin ['læktəuˌferin] *n* 乳铁蛋白,乳铁传递蛋白
lactoflavin ['læktəˌfleivin] *n* 核黄素,维生素 B_2
lactogen ['læktədʒən] *n* 催乳激素 | human placental ~ (hPL) 人胎盘催乳素(亦称绒毛膜生长催乳激素,胎盘生长激素)
lactogenesis [ˌlæktəu'dʒenisis] *n* 通乳,生乳,乳生成 | **lactogenic** *a*
lactoglobulin [ˌlæktəu'glɔbjulin] *n* 乳球蛋白 | immune ~s 免疫乳球蛋白(动物初乳中存在的一种抗体〈免疫球蛋白〉)
lactolin ['læktəlin] *n* 炼乳
lactometer [læk'tɔmitə] *n* 乳比重计
lactone ['læktəun] *n* 内酯;乳酸干馏液
lactonic acid [læk'tɔnik] 半乳糖酸
lacto-ovovegetarian [ˌlæktəu ˌəuvəu ˌvedʒi'tɛəriən] *n* 乳蛋素食者
lactophenin [ˌlæktəu'fiːnin] *n* 乳酸乙氧苯胺(镇静、解热药)
lactophosphate [ˌlæktəu'fɔsfeit] *n* 乳磷酸盐
lactoprecipitin [ˌlæktəupri'sipitin] *n* 乳沉淀素
lactoprotein [ˌlæktəu'prəutiːn] *n* 乳蛋白[质]
lactorrhea [ˌlæktəu'riːə] *n* 乳溢
lactosazone [ˌlæktəu'seizəun] *n* 乳糖脎
lactoscope ['læktəskəup] *n* 乳酪计
lactose ['læktəus] *n* 乳糖 | beta ~ β-乳糖
lactoserum [ˌlæktə'siərəm] *n* [抗]乳血清
lactose synthase ['læktəus 'sinθeis] 乳糖合酶
lactoside ['læktəusaid] *n* 乳糖苷 | ceramide ~ 神经酰胺乳糖苷(亦称胞糖脂 H)
lactosidosis [ˌlæktəusai'dəusis] ([复] **lactosidoses** [ˌlæktəusai'dəusiːz]) *n* 乳糖苷贮积症 | ceramide ~ 神经酰胺乳糖苷贮积症
lactosum [læk'təusəm] *n* 乳糖
lactosuria [ˌlæktəu'sjuəriə] *n* 乳糖尿
lactosylceramide [lækˌtəusil'serəmaid] *n* 乳糖基神经酰胺
lactotherapy [ˌlæktəu'θerəpi] *n* 乳食疗法
lactotoxin [ˌlæktəu'tɔksin] *n* 乳毒素
lactotransferrin [ˌlæktəutræns'ferin] *n* 乳运铁蛋白
lactotrope ['læktəutrəup] *n* 催乳素细胞
lactotroph ['læktəutrəuf] *n* 催乳素细胞
lactotrophin [ˌlæktəu'trəufin], **lactotropin** [ˌlæktəu'trəupin] *n* 催乳素
lactovegetarian [ˌlæktəuˌvedʒi'tɛəriən] *a* 乳与蔬菜的 *n* 乳品素食者
lactovegetarianism [ˌlæktəuˌvedʒə'tɛəriəˌnizəm] *n* 乳品素食主义
lactoyl ['læktəil] *n* 乳酰[基]
lactoylglutathione [ˌlæktəilˌgluːtə'θaiəun] *n* 乳酰谷胱甘肽
lactoylglutathione lyase [ˌlæktəuilˌgluːtə'θaiəun 'laieis] 乳酰谷胱甘肽裂合酶(以前称乙二醛酶 I)
Lactuca [læk'tjuːkə] *n*【拉】莴苣属
lactulose ['læktjuːləus] *n* 乳果糖,半乳糖苷果糖(泻药)
lacuna [lə'kjuːnə] ([复] **lacunae** [lə'kjuːni]) *n*【拉】腔隙,陷窝;缺损,裂隙(如视野中的暗点) | absorption ~ 吸收腔隙 / cerebral lacunae 脑腔隙 / great ~ of urethra, ~ magna 尿道舟状窝 / intervillous ~, trophoblastic ~ 绒毛间腔隙,滋养层腔隙 / parasinoidal lacunae 窦外侧陷窝,窦旁窦 / lacunae of urethra, urethral lacunae 尿道腔隙 / ~ of vesseles 血管腔隙 | ~**r** *a*
lacune [lə'kjuːn] *n* 腔隙,陷窝
lacunule [lə'kjuːnjuːl] *n* 小腔隙,小陷窝
lacus ['leikəs] [单复同] *n*【拉】湖 | ~ lacrimalis 泪湖
LAD left anterior descending 左前降支(冠状动脉);left axis deviation 轴左偏
Ladd's band [læd] (Wiliam E. Ladd) 拉德带(使盲肠附着于右侧腹壁的腹膜带) | ~ procedure

拉德手术(外科切割拉德带以矫正肠旋转不良和梗阻) / ~ syndrome 拉德综合征(先天性十二指肠梗阻,由于盲肠旋转不良形成腹膜带〈拉德带〉所致)

laddergram [ˈlædəgræm] *n* 阶梯图(即 ladder diagram,见 diagram 项下相应术语)

Ladd-Franklin theory [læd ˈfræŋklin] (Christine Ladd- Franklin) 莱德-富兰克林学说(关于色觉的一种学说,即红、绿、蓝刺激物质是由复合性感光分子的适当光波在神经末梢释放的)

Ladendorff's test [ˈlɑːdəndɔf] (August Ladendorff) 拉登多夫试验(检血)

Ladin's sign [ˈleidin] (Louis J. Ladin) 莱丁征(为妊娠之征,宫前壁中线宫体宫颈交界处的环形区,指触有波动感,随妊娠增大)

ladle [ˈleidl] *n* 勺,杓

lae- 以 lae- 起始的词,同样见以 le- 起始的词

Laelaps [ˈliːlæps] *n* 砺螨属(即棘砺螨属 Echinolaelaps)

LAE left atrial enlargement 左心房增大

Laënnec's catarrh [ˌleiəˈnek] (René T. H. Laënnec) 拉埃内克卡他(气喘性支气管炎,痰黏且呈珠形) | ~ cirrhosis 拉埃内克肝硬化(萎缩性门静脉性肝硬变,与慢性饮酒过度有密切关系,在早期由于急性饮酒损伤,肝大可能反映肝细胞的脂肪浸润,并伴坏死和炎症) / ~ disease 拉埃内克病(即拉埃内克肝硬化) / ~ pearls 拉埃内克珠(见于支气管气喘) / ~ sign 拉埃内克征(支气管性气喘患者的痰中出现圆形胶质块〈拉埃内克珠〉)

laetrile [ˈleiətril] *n* 左旋扁桃腈,苦杏仁苷(具有抗肿瘤性质)

laeve [ˈliːvə] *a* 无绒毛的(如平滑绒毛膜 chorion laeve)

laev(o)- 以 laev(o)- 起始的词,同样见以 lev(o)- 起始的词

Lafora's bodies [ləˈfɔːrə] (Gonzalo R. Lafora) 拉福拉体(胞质内包涵体,含糖蛋白和酸性黏多糖的复合物,其广泛沉积见于拉福拉肌阵挛型癫痫) | ~ myoclonic epilepsy (disease) 拉福拉肌阵挛型癫痫(病)(一种缓慢进行的常染色体隐性遗传型癫痫,始于儿童期,特征为间歇性或持续性肌群阵挛发作,导致随意运动困难,智力衰退,有时发展成完全痴呆。拉福拉体存在于各种细胞中,其中包括神经系统、视网膜、心脏、肌肉和肝脏的细胞之中) / ~ sign 拉福拉征(挖鼻孔动作被视为脑脊膜炎的一种早期体征)

Lag. lagena【拉】瓶,壶

lag [læg] *n* 迟滞期;迟滞 | nitrogen ~ 氮迟滞

lagena [ləˈdʒiːnə] *n*【拉】瓶,壶;(蜗管)顶盲端;听壶(低等动物的听器)

lageniform [ləˈdʒenifɔːm] *a* 烧瓶形的,瓶形的

lagging [ˈlægiŋ] *n* 迟延(指细胞分裂后期染色体从赤道板向两极移动的延迟)

Lagochilascaris minor [ˌlægəukaiˈlæskərisˈmainə] 小兔唇蛔虫

lagophthalmos [ˌlægɔfˈθælmɔs], **lagophthalmus** [ˌlægɔfˈθælməs] *n* 兔眼

Lagrange's operation [ləˈgrɑːnʒe] (Pierre F. Lagrange) 巩膜虹膜切除术

la grippe [ləˈgrip] *n*【法】流行性感冒

LAH left anterior hemiblock 左前分支阻滞

laiose [ˈlaiəus] *n* 莱奥糖(糖尿病患者尿中的一种左旋糖)

lake[1] [leik] *vi, vt* 血细胞溶解 *n* 湖 | lacrimal ~ 泪湖 / marginal ~ 缘湖(靠近胎盘边缘,亦称缘窦) / subchorial ~ 绒毛膜下窦(在胎盘边缘,亦称绒毛膜下腔) / venous ~ 静脉湖(常见于老人唇部、耳朵和面部的丘疹或大疱)

lake[2] [leik] *n* 色淀;胭脂红

Lake's pigment [leik] (Richard Lake) 莱克涂剂(一种乳酸、甲醛液、酚和水的混合物,用于喉结核止痛)

laky [ˈleiki] *a* 血细胞溶解的;胭脂红的,深红色的

laliatry [ləˈlaiətri] *n* 言语病学

lallation [ləˈleiʃən] *n* 婴儿样语

Lallemand's bodies [ləlˈmɑːŋ] (Claude F. Lallemand) 拉尔孟体(见 Bence Johnes cylinders)

lalo- [构词成分] 言语

lalognosis [ˌlæləgˈnəusis] *n* 言语理解

lalopathology [ˌlæləupəˈθɔlədʒi] *n* 言语病理学

lalopathy [ləˈlɔpəθi] *n* 言语障碍

lalophobia [ˌlæləˈfəubiə] *n* 谈话恐怖,恐语症

laloplegia [ˌlæləuˈpliːdʒiə] *n* 言语器官麻痹

lalorrhea [ˌlæləuˈriə] *n* 多言癖

Lalouette's pyramid [ˌlæluˈet] (Pierre Lalouette) 甲状腺锥体叶

LAM lymphangiomyomatosis 淋巴管肌瘤病

Lamarck's theory [ləˈmɑːk] (Jean B. P. A. M. de Lamarck) 拉马克学说(认为物种通过不断加强和完善适应性状,便能逐渐转变成新种,而且这些获得性状能遗传给后代)

Lamaze method [ləˈmɑːz] (Fernand Lamaze) 拉马士法(一种准备分娩的心理预防法,包括教育待产妇有关妊娠生理和分娩以及一些促进分娩的技术,如练习呼吸和分娩时屏气)

lambda [ˈlæmdə] *n* 希腊语的第 11 个字母(Λ, λ);人字点

lambdacism [ˈlæmdəsizəm], **lambdacismus** [læmdəˈsizməs] *n* 言语中 r 音发 l 音;l 发音不准

lambdoid [ˈlæmdɔid] *a* 希腊字母 λ 形的;人字形的

lambert [ˈlæmbət] (Johann H. Lambert) *n* 朗伯

(旧亮度单位,现用坎〈德拉〉)
Lambert-Eaton syndrome [ˈlæmbət ˈiːtən] (Edward H. Lambert; Lealdes Mckendree Eaton) 兰伯特-伊顿综合征(见 Eaton-Lambert syndrome)
Lambert's cosine law [ˈlʌmbəːt] (Johann H. Lambert) 朗伯特余弦定律(平行光线对于一吸收面的辐射强度与其入射角余弦成比例)
Lambert's treatment [ˈlæmbə(ː)t] (Alexander Lambert) 兰伯特疗法(戒鸦片瘾)
Lamblia [ˈlæmbliə] (Vilem D. Lambl) *n* 兰[伯]氏鞭毛虫属(即贾第鞭毛虫属 Giardia) | ~ intestinalis 肠兰[伯]氏鞭毛虫(即兰[伯]氏贾第鞭毛虫 Giardia lamblia)
lambliasis [læmˈblaiəsis], **lambliosis** [læmbliˈəusis] *n* 兰[伯]氏鞭毛虫病
Lambotte's treatment [læmˈbɔt] (Albin Lambotte) 兰博特疗法(骨折牵伸疗法)
lame [leim] *a* 跛的,跛行的
lame foliacée [ˈlæm fɔliəˈsei]【法】叶状板(某些痣内含有,亦称 foliate lamina)
lamel [ˈlæməl] *n* 眼片(眼用薄片剂)
lamella [ləˈmelə] ([复] **lamellae** [ləˈmeliː]) *n*【拉】薄片,薄板;片层,板层;眼片(眼用薄片剂) | articular ~ 关节软骨板 / circumferential ~, basic ~ 环板 / concentric ~ 同心板 / enamel lamellae 釉板 / endosteal ~ 骨内板 / interstitial ~, ground ~, intermediate ~ 间骨板 / osseous ~ 骨板 / periosteal ~, peripheral ~ 骨膜板 / vitreous ~ 玻璃层,脉络膜基底层 | **~r** *a* 板的,层的;板状的,层状的
lamellasome [ləˈmeləsəum] *n* 片层体(一种胞质内包涵体)
lamelliform [ləˈmelifɔːm] *a* 薄片形的,片层状的
lamellipodia [ləˌmeliˈpəudiə] ([单] **lamellipodium** [ləˌmeliˈpəudiəm]) *n* 板状伪足
lameness [ˈleimnis] *n* 跛,跛行 | fescue ~, tall fescue ~ 羊茅足
lamin [ˈlæmin] *n* 核纤层蛋白
lamina [ˈlæminə] ([复] **laminae** [ˈlæminiː]) *n*【拉】板,层 | alar ~ 翼板(神经管) / anterior limiting ~ 前界层,前弹性层(角膜) / basal ~ 基底层 / basal ~ of choroid 脉络膜基底层 / basal ~ of ciliary body 睫状体基底层 / cribriform ~ 筛状板 / dental ~, dentogingival ~ 牙板,牙龈板 / episcleral ~ 巩膜上层 / labial ~ 唇板 / palatine ~ of maxilla 上颌腭突 / posterior limiting ~ 后界层,后弹性层(角膜) / proper ~ of mesentery 肠系膜固有层 / ~ of thyroid cartilage 甲状软骨板 / ungual laminae 甲床嵴 / white laminae of cerebellum 小脑髓板 | **~l**, **~r**, **~ry** *a* 板状的,层状的
laminagram [ˈlæminəgræm] *n* [X 线]体层[照]片
laminagraph [ˈlæminəgrɑːf, -græf] *n* [X 线]体层照相机 | **~y** [ˌlæmiˈnægrəfi] *n* [X 线]体层摄影[术]
laminaplasty [ˈlæminəˌplæsti] *n* 断层成形术
Laminaria [ˌlæmiˈnεəriə] *n* 昆布属
laminarin [ˌlæmiˈnεərin] *n* 昆布多糖 | ~ sulfate 硫酸昆布多糖(具有抗血脂和抗凝作用)
laminarinase [ˌlæmiˈnεərineis] *n* 昆布多糖酶
laminate [ˈlæmineit] *vt*, *vi* 分成薄片;分层,成层 | **~d** *a* 层状的,分层的;叠层的,层压的
lamination [ˌlæmiˈneiʃən] *n* 叠合,层压;叠片结构,层压结构
laminectomy [ˌlæmiˈnektəmi] *n* 椎板切除术
laminin [ˈlæminin] *n* 层黏素,层粘连蛋白
laminitis [ˌlæmiˈnaitis] *n* 板炎,蹄叶炎(马)
laminogram [ˈlæminəgræm] *n* [X 线]体层[照]片
laminography [ˌlæmiˈnɔgrəfi] *n* [X 线]体层摄影[术]
laminoplasty [ˈlæminəuˌplæsti] *n* 椎板成形术
Laminosioptes [ˌlæminəusiˈɔptiːz] *n* 鸡雏螨属
Laminosioptidae [ˌlæminəusiˈɔptidiː] *n* 鸡雏螨科
laminotomy [ˌlæmiˈnɔtəmi] *n* 椎板切开术
lamivudine [ləˈmivjudiːn] *n* 拉米夫定(抗病毒药)
lamotrigine [ləˈməutridʒiːn] *n* 拉莫三嗪(抗惊厥药)
lamp [læmp] *n* 灯 | arc ~ 弧光灯 / carbon arc ~ 炭弧灯 / cold quartz mercury vapor ~ (人工)太阳灯,冷光石英水银灯 / mignon ~ 微型灯(用于膀胱镜检查等) / slit ~ 裂隙灯 / tungsten arc ~ 钨弧灯 / ultraviolet ~ 紫外线灯
lampas [ˈlæmpəs] *n* 腭嵴红肿(马)
Lamprocystis [ˌlæmprəˈsistis] *n* 闪囊菌属
Lampropedia [ˌlæmprəˈpediə] *n* 俊片菌属
lamprophonia [ˌlæmprəˈfəuniə] *n* 发声清晰,语音清晰 | **lamprophonic** [ˌlæmprəˈfɔnik] *a*
Lamus [ˈleiməs] *n* 莱末蝽属(现归属锥蝽属 Panstrongylus 和 Triatoma)
lamziekte [ˈlæmziːkti] *n*【荷】牛肉毒中毒症,牛跛足病
lana [ˈlænə] ([复] **lanae** [ˈlæniː]) *n*【拉】羊毛
lanatoside C [ləˈnætəsaid] *n* 毛花苷 C(强心药)
lanaurin [ˈlænɔːrin] *n* 羊毛黄
lance [lɑːns, læns] *n* 柳叶刀,小刀 *vt* 用柳叶刀切割
Lancefield classification [ˈlænsfiːld] (Rebecca C. Lancefield) 兰斯菲尔德分类(根据沉淀素试验将溶血性链球菌进行血清学分类)
lanceolate [ˈlænsiəlit] *a* 柳叶刀形的
Lancereau-Mathieu disease [ˌlɑːŋsəˈrəu ˈmæti-

juː] (Etienne Lancereau; Albert Mathieu) 钩端螺旋体性黄疸

Lancereaux's diabetes [ˌlɑːŋsə'rəu] (Etienne Lancereaux) 郎瑟罗糖尿病(伴有明显消瘦)

lancet ['lænsət] *n* 柳叶刀,小刀

Lancet coefficient ['lɑːnsət, 'læn-] (The Lancet 为英国一家医学期刊名)兰塞特系数,苯酚系数(化合物的消毒能力与苯酚的比较值)

lancinate ['lɑːnsineit, 'læn-] *vt* 撕裂;刺,刀刺 | **lancinating** ['lɑːnsiˌneitiŋ, 'læn-] *a* 刀刺般的;撕裂性的 / **lancination** [ˌlɑːnsi'neiʃən, 'læn-] *n*

Lancisi's nerves, stria [læn'tʃiːsi] (Giovanni M. Lancisi) 胼胝体外侧纵纹与胼胝体内侧纵纹

Landau-Kleffner syndrome ['lɑːndau 'klefnə] (William M. Landau; F. R. Kleffner) 兰-克综合征(一种儿童期癫痫综合征,特征为部分或全身发作,精神运动异常,失语症发展成缄默症。双侧颞区脑电图异常,其棘波像良性罗兰多癫痫棘波。亦称获得性癫痫性失语症)

Landau's color test (reaction) ['lʌndau] (Leopold Landau) 兰道色试验(检梅毒)

landmark ['lænd*m*ɑːk] *n* 界标

Landolt's bodies [lɑːŋ'dɔl] (Edmund Landolt) 朗多尔体(视网膜杆状体和锥体之间的长形小体) | ~ operation 朗多尔手术(用上睑的双蒂或桥式皮瓣形成下睑)

Landouzy-Dejerine dystrophy (atrophy) [lɑːndu'zi deʒə'riːn] (L. T. J. Landouzy; Joseph J. Dejerine) 朗杜齐-德热里纳营养不良(萎缩)(一种良性的肌营养不良,亦称面肩肱型肌营养不良)

Landouzy-Grasset law [lɑːndu'zi grɑː'sei] (L. T. J. Landouzy; Joseph Grasset) 朗杜齐-格拉塞定律(一侧大脑半球病变时,如有瘫痪则头偏向同侧,如有肌痉挛则偏向对侧)

Landouzy's disease [lɑːndu'zi] (Louis T. J. Landouzy) 钩端螺旋体性黄疸 | ~ dystrophy (type) 朗杜齐营养不良(型)(见 Landouzy-Dejering dystrophy)

Landry's paralysis (disease, palsy, syndrome) [lɑːn'driː] (Jean B. O. Landry) 急性热病性多神经炎

Landsteiner's classification ['lændstainə] (Karl Landsteiner) 兰斯泰讷分类(一种 ABO 血型系)

Landström's muscle ['lɑːndstrem] (John Landström) 兰斯特勒姆肌(眼球筋膜内肌纤维)

Lane's bands (kink) [lein] (William A. Lane) 莱恩带(纽结),回肠纽结 | ~ disease 莱恩病(慢性肠停滞,慢性便秘时小肠梗阻) / ~ operation 莱恩手术(一种回肠吻合术) / ~ plates 莱恩[接骨]板(用于固定骨折)

Langdon Down's disease ['læŋdən daun] (John H. Down) 兰登·唐氏病(见 Down syndrome)

Langenbeck's amputation ['lʌŋənbek] (Bernhard R. K. von Langenbeck) 朗根贝克切断术(从外向内切瓣) | ~ incision 朗根贝克切口(在半月状线上与腹直肌肌纤维平行的切开法) / ~ triangle 朗格贝克三角(股骨颈三角)

Langer-Giedion syndrome ['læŋəzidi'ɔː] (Leonard O. Langer; A. Giedion) 朗-吉综合征(一种遗传性疾病,特征为精神发育迟缓、小头、多发性外生骨疣、球状鼻特殊面容、发稀少、锥形骺、松弛多余皮肤、关节松弛以及其他异常)

Langerhans cells (corpuscles) ['lʌŋəhɑːnz] (Paul Langerhans) 朗格汉斯细胞(表皮生发层深部的星形细胞;角膜细胞间隙中不规则的游走细胞) | ~ islands (areas, bodies, islets) 胰岛 / ~ layer 表皮粒层

Langer's axillary arch ['lʌŋə] (Carl R. von Edenberg von Langer) 朗格腋弓 | ~ lines 皮纹(线) / ~ muscle 朗格肌(臂弓)

Lange's operation ['lʌŋə] (Fritz Lange) 丝线植入法(人工腱移植术)

Lange's solution ['lʌŋə] (Carl Lange) 胶态金溶液 | ~ test (reaction) 朗格试验(反应)(①检脑脊液蛋白-球蛋白,以诊断脑脊髓梅毒,亦称胶态金试验、金反应;②检尿内丙酮)

Langhans cells ['lʌŋhɑːnz] (Theodor Langhans) 朗汉斯细胞,多角形细胞(表皮)(构成细胞滋养层的多面形上皮细胞;结核性结节巨细胞) | ~ layer, ~ stria 细胞滋养层

Langley's ganglion ['læŋli] (John N. Langley) 兰利神经节(某些动物神经细胞在下颌腺门的集结) | ~ granules 兰利粒(分泌浆液腺的细胞粒) / ~ nerves 立毛神经

laniary ['læniəri] *a* 适于撕裂的,短刀形的(指犬牙)

Lankesterella ranarum [læŋˌkestə'relə rə'nɛərəm] (Edwin R. Lankester) 蛙兰[克]氏球虫

Lankesteria culicis [ˌlæŋkis'tiəriə' kjulisis] 蚊兰[克]氏原虫

Lannelongue's foramina [lɑːnə'lɔːg] (Odilon M. Lannelongue)兰内龙格孔,右房最小静脉孔

Lannois-Gradenigo syndrome [lə'nwɑː grədə'niːgəu] 拉-格综合征(见 Gradenigo's syndrome)

lanoceric acid [ˌlænə'serik] 羊毛蜡酸

lanolin ['lænəlin] *n* 羊毛脂 | anhydrous ~ 无水羊毛脂

lanosterol [lə'nɔstərɔl] *n* 羊毛甾固醇

lansoprazole [læn'səuprəzəul] *n* 兰索拉唑(抗溃疡药)

Lanterman-Schmit incisures ['lʌntmæn ʃmit] (A. J. Lanterman; Henry D. Schmit) 兰-施切迹

（即 incisures of Lanterman，见 Lanterman's incisures）

anterman's incisures（clefts）［'lʌntmæn］（A. J. Lanterman）兰特曼切迹（裂）（神经元髓鞘上通向神经鞘细胞体的细胞质通道，在鞘内呈斜线形或条状）

anthanic［'lænθənik］*a* 无症状的（疾病）

anthanin［'lænθənin］*n* 嗜酸染色质

anthanum（La）［'lænθənəm］*n* 镧（化学元素）

anuginous［lə'njudʒinəs］*a* 覆以胎毛的

anugo［lə'njugəu］*n*【拉】胎毛

anum［'leinəm］*n* 羊毛脂

anz's operation［lɑːnts］（Otto Lanz）兰茨手术（治象皮病）｜～ point 兰茨点（表明阑尾位置的点，位于两髂前上棘的连线上，距右棘 1/3 处）

AO left anterior oblique 左前斜位

AP leucocyte adhesion protein 白细胞粘连蛋白；leukocyte alkaline phosphatase 白细胞碱性磷酸酶；lyophilized anterior pituitary（tissue）冻干垂体前叶（组织）

apactic［lə'pæktik］*a* 泻下的，致泻的

aparectomy［ˌlæpə'rektəmi］*n* 腹壁部分切除术

apar（o）-［构词成分］腰，胁腹，腹

aparocele［'læpərəusiːl］*n* 腹［壁］疝

aparocholecystotomy［ˌlæpərəuˌkəulisis'tɔtəmi］*n* 剖腹胆囊造口术

aparocolectomy［ˌlæpərəukə'lektəmi］*n* 剖腹结肠切除术，结肠切除术

aparocolostomy［ˌlæpərəukə'lɔstəmi］*n* 剖腹结肠造口术

laparocolotomy［ˌlæpərəukə'lɔtəmi］*n* 剖腹结肠切开术

laparocystectomy［ˌlæpərəusis'tektəmi］*n* 剖腹囊肿切除术

laparocystidotomy［ˌlæpərəuˌsisti'dɔtəmi］*n* 剖腹膀胱切开术

laparocystotomy［ˌlæpərəusis'tɔtəmi］*n* 宫外胎儿取出术；剖腹囊肿切开术

laparoenterostomy［ˌlæpərəuˌentə'rɔstəmi］*n* 剖腹肠造口术

laparoenterotomy［ˌlæpərəuˌentə'rɔtəmi］*n* 剖腹肠切开术

laparogastroscopy［ˌlæpərəugæs'trɔskəpi］*n* 剖腹胃检查法

laparogastrostomy［ˌlæpərəugæs'trɔstəmi］*n* 剖腹胃造口术

laparogastrotomy［ˌlæpərəugæs'trɔtəmi］*n* 剖腹胃切开术

laparohepatotomy［ˌlæpərəuˌhepə'tɔtəmi］*n* 剖腹肝切开术

laparohysterectomy［ˌlæpərəu ˌhistə'rektəmi］*n* 剖腹子宫切除术

laparohystero-oophorectomy［ˌlæpərəuˌhistərəuˌəuɔfə'rektəmi］*n* 剖腹子宫卵巢切除术

laparohysterosalpingo-oophorectomy［ˌlæpərəuˌhistərəusælˌpiŋgəuˌəuɔfə'rektəmi］*n* 剖腹子宫输卵管卵巢切除术

laparohysterotomy［ˌlæpərəuˌhistə'rɔtəmi］*n* 剖腹子宫切开术

laparoileotomy［ˌlæpərəuˌili'ɔtəmi］*n* 剖腹回肠切开术

laparomonodidymus［ˌlæpərəuˌmɔnəu'didiməs］*n* 双上身畸胎

laparomyitis［ˌlæpərəumai'aitis］*n* 腹肌炎

laparomyomectomy［ˌlæpərəuˌmaiə'mektəmi］*n* 剖腹肌瘤切除术

laparonephrectomy［ˌlæpərəune'frektəmi］*n* 剖腹肾切除术

laparorrhaphy［ˌlæpə'rɔrəfi］*n* 腹壁缝合术

laparosalpingectomy［ˌlæpərəuˌsælpiŋ'dʒektəmi］*n* 剖腹输卵管切除术

laparosalpingo-oophorectomy［ˌlæpərəusælˌpiŋgəuˌəuɔfə'rektəmi］*n* 剖腹输卵管卵巢切除术

laparosalpingotomy［ˌlæpərəuˌsælpiŋ'gɔtəmi］*n* 剖腹输卵管切开术

laparoscope［'læpərəskəup］*n* 腹腔镜｜**laparoscopy**［ˌlæpə'rɔskəpi］*n* 腹腔镜检查［术］

laparoscopic［ˌlæpərəu'skɔpik］*a* 腹腔镜的；腹腔镜检查的

laparosplenectomy［ˌlæpərəuspli'nektəmi］*n* 剖腹脾切除术

laparosplenotomy［ˌlæpərəuspli'nɔtəmi］*n* 剖腹脾切开术

laparotomaphilia［ˌlæpəˌrɔtəmə'filiə］*n* 剖腹手术癖

laparotome［'læpərətəum］*n* 剖腹刀

laparotomy［ˌlæpə'rɔtəmi］*n* 剖腹术

laparotyphlotomy［ˌlæpərəutif'lɔtəmi］*n* 剖腹盲肠切开术

Lapicque's constant［lə'piːk］（Louis Lapicque）拉皮克常数（将无感电阻换算为直流电当量所使用的数值 0.37）｜～ law 拉皮克定律（神经时值与神经纤维直径成反比）

Lapidus operation［'læpidəs］（Paul W. Lapidus）拉皮德斯手术（矫正踇外翻手术）

lapinize［'læpinaiz］*vt* 使…兔化｜**lapinization**［ˌlæpinai'zeiʃən，-ni'z-］*n* 兔化法（将病毒通过家兔传代作为减轻病毒毒性的方法）

lapis［'læpis］*n*【拉】石｜～ albus 白石（硅氟化钙）/ ～ calaminaris 炉甘石，异极石 / ～ imperialis，～ infernalis，～ lunaris 硝酸银

Laplace's law［lɑː'plɑːs］（Pierre Simon de Laplace）拉普拉定律（心室壁张力与室内压和内径成正比，与室壁厚度成反比）

lapsus [ˈlæpsəs] *n*【拉】下垂,滑落;失误 | ~ calami 笔误 / ~ linguae 失言 / ~ memoriae 失忆,遗忘

lapyrium chloride [ləˈpiəriəm] 拉匹氯铵(表面活性剂)

Larat's treatment [ləˈræ] (Jules L. F. A. Larat) 拉腊疗法(电疗白喉性腭麻痹)

lard [lɑːd] *n* 豚脂,猪油 | benzoinated ~ 安息香豚脂,苯甲酸豚脂

lardacein [lɑːˈdeisiːn] *n* 豚脂状蛋白

lardaceous [lɑːˈdeiʃəs] *a* 豚脂状的;含有豚脂状蛋白的

Lardennois' button [ˌlɑːdənˈwɑː] (Henri Lardennois) 拉德努瓦钮(一种肠吻合钮)

large [lɑːdʒ] *a* 大的 | ~ for gestational age infant 大于胎龄儿

laricic acid [ləˈrisik] 落叶松酸

larithmics [ləˈriθmiks] *n* 人口学(人口数量的研究)

Larix [ˈlɛəriks] *n*【拉】落叶松属

larixin [ləˈriksin] *n* 落叶松酸

larkspur [ˈlɑːkspəː] *n* 飞燕草子(灭虱药)

Laron dwarf [ləˈrɔn] (Zvi Laron) 拉伦侏儒(由于合成胰岛素样生长因子 I 的能力受损而致的骨骼生长迟缓的侏儒) | ~ syndrome (dwarfism) 拉伦综合征(侏儒症)(骨骼生长迟缓的常染色体隐性遗传综合征,由于受损不能合成胰岛素样生长因子 I 所致,通常因生长激素受体缺损之故)

Larrey's amputation (operation) [lɑːˈrei] (Dominique J. Larrey) 拉雷切断术(肩关节肱骨断离术) | ~ bandage 拉雷绷带(多头胶边绷带) / ~ cleft 胸肋三角 / ~ spaces 胸肋三角隙

Larsen's disease, Larsen-Johansson disease [ˈlɑːsn jəuˈhɑːnsn] (Christian M. F. S. Larsen; Sven Johansson) 拉尔逊病、拉尔逊-约翰逊病(一种髌骨病,X 线显示髌骨下极副骨化中心形成)

Larsen's syndrome [ˈlɑːsn] (Loren J. Larsen) 拉尔逊综合征(腭裂,扁平面容,多处关节先天性脱位和足畸形)

larva [ˈlɑːvə] ([复] **larvae** [ˈlɑːviː]) *n*【拉】幼体,幼虫(昆虫),蚴(蠕虫) | cutaneous ~ migrans 皮肤幼虫移行症/ ~ currens 肛周匍行症,类圆线虫病 / ~ migrans 幼虫移行症 / ocular ~ migrans 眼幼虫移行症 / visceral ~ migrans 内脏幼虫移行症 | **~l** *a* 幼虫的,蚴的;隐蔽的,潜在的

larvate [ˈlɑːveit], **larvaceous** [lɑːˈveiʃəs] *a* 隐蔽的,潜在的(指病或病的症状)

larvicide [ˈlɑːvisaid] *n* 杀幼虫剂,杀蚴剂 *vt* 对…施杀幼虫剂 | Panama ~ 杀按蚊幼虫剂 | **larvicidal** [ˌlɑːviˈsaidəl] *a*

larviposition [ˌlɑːvipəˈziʃən] *n* 产幼虫[现象]

larvivorous [lɑːˈvivərəs], **larviphagic** [ˌlɑːviˈfeidʒik] *a* 食幼虫的(尤指食孑孓的鱼)

laryngalgia [ˌlærinˈgældʒiə] *n* 喉痛

laryngeal [ləˈrindʒiəl, ˌlærinˈdʒi(ː)əl] *a* 喉的

laryngectomee [ˌlærinˈdʒektəmiː], **laryngect** [ˈlærindʒekt] *n* 喉切除患者

laryngectomy [ˌlærinˈdʒektəmi] *n* 喉切除术

laryngemphraxis [ˌlærindʒemˈfræksis] *n* 喉梗阻,喉阻塞

laryngendoscope [ˌlærinˈdʒendəskəup] *n* 喉[内]镜

larynges [ləˈrindʒiːz] larynx 的复数

laryngismus [ˈlærinˈdʒizməs] *n* 喉痉挛 | ~ paralyticus 麻痹性喉痉挛,喘鸣症(马) / ~ stridulus 喘鸣性喉痉挛 | **laryngismal** *a*

laryngitis [ˌlærinˈdʒaitis] *n* 喉炎 | croupous ~ 格鲁布性喉炎 / diphtheritic ~ 白喉性喉炎 / ~ stridulosa 喘鸣性喉痉挛 | **laryngitic** [ˌlærinˈdʒitik] *a*

laryng(o)- [构词成分] 喉

laryngocele [ləˈriŋgəsiːl] *n* 喉膨出 | ventricular ~ 喉室膨出

laryngocentesis [ləˌriŋgəusenˈtiːsis] *n* 喉穿刺术

laryngofissure [ləˌriŋgəˈfiʃə], **laryngofission** [ləˌriŋgəˈfiʃən] *n* 喉裂开术,喉正中切开术

laryngogram [ləˈriŋgəgræm] *n* 喉 X 线[照]片

laryngograph [ləˈriŋgəgrɑːf] *n* 喉动描记器 | **~y** [ˌlæriŋˈgɔgrəfi] *n* 喉描记[法];喉 X 线摄影术

laryngohypopharynx [ləˌriŋgəuˌhaipəuˈfæriŋks] *n* 喉[下]咽部(包括咽下部的后壁、梨状隐窝和喉的毗连部分)

laryngology [ˌlæriŋˈgɔlədʒi] *n* 喉科学 | **laryngological** [ləˌriŋgəˈlɔdʒikəl] *a* / **laryngologist** *n* 喉科学家

laryngomalacia [ləˌriŋgəuməˈleiʃiə] *n* 喉[软骨]软化

laryngometry [ˌlæriŋˈgɔmitri] *n* 喉测量法

laryngoparalysis [ləˌriŋgəupəˈrælisis] *n* 喉麻痹

laryngopathy [ˌlæriŋˈgɔpəθi] *n* 喉病

laryngophantom [ˌlæriŋgəuˈfæntəm] *n* 喉模型

laryngopharyngeal [ləˌriŋgəufəˈrindʒiːəl] *a* 喉咽的

laryngopharyngectomy [ləˌriŋgəuˌfærinˈdʒektəmi] *n* 喉咽切除术

laryngopharyngeus [ləˌriŋgəufəˈrindʒiəs] *n* 咽下缩肌

laryngopharyngitis [ləˌriŋgəuˌfærinˈdʒaitis] *n* 喉咽炎

laryngopharynx [ləˌriŋgəuˈfæriŋks] *n* 喉咽

aryngophony [ˌlæriŋˈgɔfəni] *n* 喉听诊音
aryngophthisis [ˌlæriŋˈgɔfθisis] *n* 喉结核
aryngoplasty [ləˈriŋgəˌplæsti] *n* 喉成形术
aryngoplegia [ləˌriŋgəuˈpliːdʒiə] *n* 喉麻痹
aryngoptosis [ləˌriŋgəuˈtəusis] *n* 喉下垂
aryngopyocele [ləˌriŋgəuˈpaiəsiːl] *n* 喉脓囊肿
aryngorhinology [ləˌriŋgəuraiˈnɔlədʒi] *n* 鼻喉科学
aryngorrhagia [ˌlæriŋgəuˈreidʒiə] *n* 喉出血
aryngorrhaphy [ˌlæriŋˈgɔrəfi] *n* 喉缝合术
aryngorrhea [ˌlæriŋgəuˈriːə] *n* 喉黏液溢
aryngoscleroma [ləˌriŋgəuskliəˈrəumə] *n* 喉硬结病
aryngoscope [ləˈriŋgəskəup] *n* 喉镜
aryngoscopy [ˌlæriŋˈgɔskəpi] *n* 喉镜检查[法] | direct ~ 直接喉镜检查[法] / indirect ~, mirror ~ 间接喉镜检查[法] / suspension ~ 仰垂喉镜检查,悬吊喉镜检查 | **laryngoscopic(al)** [ləˌriŋgəuˈskɔpik(əl)] *a* / **laryngoscopist** *n* 喉镜检查专家
laryngospasm [ləˈriŋgəˌspæzəm] *n* 喉痉挛
laryngostasis [ˌlæriŋˈgɔstəsis] *n* 喉阻塞,格鲁布,哮吼
laryngostat [ləˈriŋgəstæt] *n* 喉镭疗支持器,喉施镭器
laryngostenosis [ləˌriŋgəustiˈnəusis] *n* 喉狭窄
laryngostomy [ˌlæriŋˈgɔstəmi] *n* 喉造口术,喉切开术
laryngostroboscope [ləˌriŋgəuˈstrəubəskəup] *n* 喉动态镜
laryngotome [ləˈriŋgətəum] *n* 喉刀
laryngotomy [ˌlæriŋˈgɔtəmi] *n* 喉切开术 | complete ~ 全喉切开术 / inferior ~ 喉下部切开术,环甲膜切开术 / median ~ 喉正中切开术,甲状软骨切开术 / superior ~, subhyoid ~, thyrohyoid ~ 喉上部切开术,甲状舌骨膜切开术
laryngotracheal [ləˌriŋgəuˈtreikiəl] *a* 喉气管的
laryngotracheitis [ləˌriŋgəuˌtreikiˈaitis] *n* 喉气管炎 | avian ~, infectious ~ 鸟喉气管炎,传染性喉气管炎
laryngotracheobronchitis [ləˌriŋgəuˌtreikiəubrɔŋˈkaitis] *n* 喉气管支气管炎
laryngotracheobronchoscopy [ləˌriŋgəuˌtreikiəubrɔŋˈkɔskəpi] *n* 喉气管支气管镜检查
laryngotracheoscopy [ləˌriŋgəuˌtreikiˈɔskəpi] *n* 喉气管镜检查,经口气管镜检查
laryngotracheotomy [ləˌriŋgəuˌtreikiˈɔtəmi] *n* 喉气管切开术
laryngovestibulitis [ləˌriŋgəuvesˌtibjuˈlaitis] *n* 喉前庭炎
laryngoxerosis [ləˌriŋgəuziəˈrəusis] *n* 喉干燥[症]
larynx [ˈlæriŋks] ([复] **larynges** [ləˈrindʒiːz]) *n* 喉 | artificial ~ 人工喉 / cleft ~ 喉裂
lasalocid [ləˈsæləsid] *n* 拉沙洛西(家禽抗球虫药)
lasanum [ˈlæsənəm] *n* 产科椅
lase [leiz] *vi* 放射激光
Lasègue's disease [ləˈseig] (Ernest C. Lasègue) 拉塞格病(迫害狂) | ~ sign (syndrome) 拉塞格征(综合征)(坐骨神经痛时,当膝伸展时髋部弯曲疼痛,但当膝屈曲时无痛,此与髋关节病引起的病痛有别)
laser [ˈleizə] (*l*ight *a*mplification by *s*timulated *e*mission of *r*adiation) *n* 激光,激光器 | argon ~ 氩激光器(用于光凝固) / carbon-dioxide ~ 二氧化碳激光器(用于切除和切开组织并使之汽化) / dye ~ 染料激光器(用于光动力疗法) / helium-neon ~ 氦-氖激光器(用作激光器在不可见光波长操作时的导向光束) / ion ~ 离子激光器 / krypton ~ 氪激光器(用于光凝固) / neodymium: yttrium-aluminum-garnet (Nd: YAG) ~ 钕:钇-铝-石榴子石激光器(用于光凝固和光挥发)
LASIK laser-assisted in-situ keratomileusis 激光辅助原位角膜磨削术
Lasiohelea [ˌlæsiəˈhiːliə] *n* 蠛蠓属
Lassa fever, virus [ˈlɑːsə] (Lassa 为尼日利亚一城市,拉沙热于 1959 年首次报道)拉沙热、病毒(分别见 fever, virus 项下相应术语)
Lassar's paste [ˈlʌsə] (Oscar Lassar) 拉萨尔糊[剂](氧化锌水杨酸糊[剂]) | ~ plain zinc paste 拉萨尔单纯锌糊[剂](氧化锌糊[剂])
lassitude [ˈlæsitjuːd] *n* 无力,倦怠
latah [ˈlɑːtə] *n* 拉塔病(一种文化特异性综合征,主要见于马来人和其他东南亚人,表现为极其受暗示、模仿言语、模仿行动、秽亵言语、混乱和自动服从症)
latanoprost [ləˈtænəˌprɔst] *n* 拉坦前列素(抗青光眼药)
Latarjet's nerve [lɑːtɑːˈʒei] (André Latarjet) 拉塔泽神经(迷走神经前干的远端部分,其走向沿胃小弯)
latebra [ˈlætibrə] *n* 【拉】卵黄心
lateroconal [ˌletərəuˈkɔnəl] *a* 锥体旁的
Lat. dol. lateri dolenti 【拉】朝向痛侧
latency [ˈleitənsi] *n* 潜伏期;潜伏,隐伏
latent [ˈleitənt] *a* 潜伏的,潜在的;隐性的
latentiation [leiˌtenʃiˈeiʃən] *n* 潜伏化(在药理学上,指对一种生物活性化合物进行化学改变,以影响它的吸收、分布等,被改变了的化合物口服后通过生物学过程转变为有活性的化合物)
laterad [ˈlætəræd] *ad* 侧向
lateral [ˈlætərəl] *a* 侧的,外侧的;旁边的
lateralis [ˌlætəˈreilis] *a* 【拉】侧的,外侧的

laterality [ˌlætəˈræləti] *n* 偏利,偏侧性(指惯用一侧器官〈手、足、耳、眼〉) | crossed ~ 交叉偏利 / dominant ~ 同侧偏利

lateritious [ˌlætəˈriʃəs], **latericeous** [ˌlætəˈriʃəs] *a* 红砖灰状的,土红色的

latero- [构词成分]侧,旁

lateroabdominal [ˌlætərəuæbˈdɔminl] *a* 腹旁的

laterodeviation [ˌlætərəuˌdiːviˈeiʃən] *n* 侧向偏斜,侧偏

lateroduction [ˌlætərəuˈdʌkʃən] *n* 侧转,侧展(眼)

lateroflexion [ˌlætərəuˈflekʃən] *n* 侧屈,旁屈

lateroposition [ˌlætərəupəˈziʃən] *n* 偏侧变位

lateropulsion [ˌlætərəuˈpʌlʃən] *n* 侧步,横行

laterotorsion [ˌlætərəuˈtɔːʃən] *n* 侧旋,外旋(眼)

lateroversion [ˌlætərəuˈvəːʃən] *n* 侧倾(如子宫)

latex [ˈleiteks] ([复] **latexes** 或 **latices** [ˈleitisiːz]) *n*【拉】乳汁,胶乳(植物)

Latham's circle [ˈleiθəm] (Peter M. Latham) 莱瑟姆圈(心包浊音区)

lathe [leið] *n* 车床 | dental ~ 牙医车床

lathyrism [ˈlæθirizəm] *n* 山黧豆中毒 | **lathyritic** [ˌlæθiˈritik] *a*

lathyrogen [ˈlæθirədʒən] *n* 致山黧豆中毒物,山黧豆中毒因子 | **lathyrogenic** [ˌlæθirəˈdʒenik] *a* 致山黧豆中毒的

Lathyrus [ˈlæθərəs] *n* 山黧豆属

latices [ˈlætisiːz] latex 的复数

latissimus [ləˈtisiməs] *a*【拉】最阔的

latitude [ˈlætitjuːd] *n* 纬度;地区 | **latitudinal** [ˌlætiˈtjuːdinl] *a*

latrine [ləˈtriːn] *n* 坑厕,沟厕

latrodectism [ˌlætrəuˈdektizəm] *n* 毒蛛中毒

Latrodectus [ˌlætrəuˈdektəs] *n* 毒蛛属

LATS long-acting thyroid stimulator 长效甲状腺刺激物

LATS-p LATS protector 长效甲状腺刺激物保护物

lattice [ˈlætis] *n* 格子;晶格,点阵;网络

latus[1] [ˈleitəs] *a* 阔的

latus[2] [ˈleitəs] ([复] **latera** [ˈleitərə]) *n*【拉】胁腹

Latzko's cesarean section [ˈlɑːtskəu] (Wilhelm Latzko) 腹膜外剖腹产术

Lauber's disease [ˈləubə] (Hans Lauber) 罗勃病,白点状眼底

laudable [ˈlɔːdəbl] *a* 值得称赞的;健康的

laudanum [ˈlɔːdənəm] *n* 阿片酒,阿片酊

laugh [lɑːf] *vi*[大]笑;发笑 *n* 笑,笑声 | canine ~, sardonic ~ 痉笑

laughter [ˈlɑːftə] *n* 笑,大笑 | compulsive ~, forced ~, obsessive ~ 强制性痴笑(精神分裂症的一种症状)

Laugier's hernia [ˌləuʒiˈɛə] (Stanislas Laugier) 洛日埃疝(陷窝韧带股疝) | ~ sign 洛日埃征(桡骨茎突和尺骨茎突在同一水平上,见于桡骨下端骨折)

Laumonier's ganglion [ləuˌmɔniˈɛə] (Jean B. P. N. R. Laumonier) 颈动脉神经节,颈动脉丛神经节

Launois-Cléret syndrome [ləuˈnwɑː kleiˈrei] (Pierre-Emile Launois; M. Cléret) 肥胖性生殖器退化

laurate [ˈlɔːreit] *n* 月桂酸盐(酯或阴离子型)

laurel [ˈlɔrəl] *n* 月桂树,月桂;桂冠,荣誉

Laurence-Biedl syndrome, Laurence-Moon-Biedl syndrome [ˈlɔrənsmuːn ˈbiːdl] (John Z. Laurence; R. C Moon; Arthur Biedl) 劳-比综合征,劳-穆-比综合征(肥胖、生殖功能减退、色素性视网膜炎、智能缺陷等综合征)

Laurence-Moon syndrome [ˈlɔrəns muːn] (John Z. Laurence; Robert C . Moon) 劳-穆综合征(一种常染色体隐性疾患,特征为精神发育迟缓、色素性视网膜病、性腺功能减退和痉挛性截瘫)

laureth 9 [ˈlɔreθ] 聚乙二醇单十二醚(杀精子剂和表面活性剂)

lauric acid [ˈlɔrik], **laurostearic acid** [ˌlɔrəusti ˈærik] 月桂酸

laurocerasus [ˌlɔrəˈserəsəs] *n* 月桂樱[树]

Lauth's canal, sinus [laut] (Ernst A. Lauth) 巩膜静脉窦

Lauth's ligament [laut] (Thomas Lauth) 寰椎横韧带

Lauth's violet [lɔːθ] (Charles Lauth) 盐酸硫堇

LAV lymphadenopathy-associated virus 淋巴结病相关病毒

lavage [læˈvɑːdʒ] *vt* 灌洗(肠、胃等);洗(伤口) *n*【法】灌洗;洗出去 | ~ of the blood, blood ~, systemic ~ 血液毒素洗出去 / ether ~ (腹腔内)乙醚洗法 / gastric ~ 洗胃 / intestinal ~ 肠道清洗 / peritoneal ~ 腹腔灌洗 / pleural ~ 胸膜腔灌洗

Lavandula [ləˈvændjulə] *n*【拉】熏衣草属

lavation [læˈveiʃən] *n* 灌洗,洗出法

Lavdovski's nucleoid [lævˈdɔvski] (Mikhail D. Lavdovski) 中心体

lave [leiv] *vt* 洗,冲洗 *vi* 洗 | **~ment** *n* 灌洗,洗出法

lavender [ˈlævəndə] *n* 熏衣草[花]

Laveran' bodies, corpuscles [lævˈræn] (Charles Louis Alphonse Laveran) 莱佛兰体,疟原虫

laveur [ləˈvəː] *n*【法】灌洗器

law [lɔː] *n* 法律;法则,定律,规则 | all-or-none ~ 全或无定律(心肌受刺激,将收缩至极限,或全

不收缩) / ~ of avalanche 雪崩定律,爆发定律(外周的单一感觉可能引起脑内多种感觉) / ~ of average localization 平均定位定律(内脏疼痛在活动性最小的脏器内定位最准确) / biogenetic ~ 生物发生律(个体发生重演种系发生;recapitulation theory, 见 theory 项下相应术语) / ~ of contrary innervation 拮抗神经支配定律(见 Meltzer's law) / ~ of denervation 神经去除定律(去除神经的结构对化学刺激的敏感性增高) / ~ of diffusion 扩散[定]律(神经中枢建立的任何活动,对全身均可有扩散式的影响) / ~ of the heart 心脏定律(心脏每次收缩所释放的能量是构成肌壁的纤维长度的简单函数) / ~ of independent assortment 独立分配定律(减数分裂时,每对基因各自独立分离) / ~ of segregation 分离定律(每代中①纯显性,②按显性三隐性一的比例产生子代的显性,与③纯隐性的比率为 1∶2∶1)

lawn [lɔːn] *n* 菌苔

Lawrence-Seip syndrome [ˈlɔrəns saip] (Robert Daniel Lawrence; Martin Fredrik Seip) 劳-赛综合征,全身脂肪营养不良

lawrencium(Lw) [lɔːˈrensiəm] *n* 铹(化学元素)

lawsone [ˈlɔːsəun] *n* 散沫花素

Lawsonia [lɔːˈsəuniə] *n* 散沫花属

lax [læks] *a* 松弛的;易通便的;腹泻的

laxation [lækˈseiʃən] *n* 松弛;排粪,轻泻

laxative [ˈlæksətiv] *a* 轻泻的 *n* 轻泻药 | bulk ~ 容积性泻药

laxator [lækˈseitə] *n* 松弛肌

laxity [ˈlæksəti] *n* 松弛,无紧张;轻泻[性]

layer [ˈleiə] *n* 层 | ambiguous ~ 疑层(大脑皮质第二层) / bacillary ~ [视网膜]杆体(锥体)层 / basal ~ 脉络膜基底层;基底层 / basement ~ 基层,基膜 / cerebral ~ 脑层(视网膜第五至第九层) / circular ~ of eardrum, circular ~ of tympanic membrane 鼓膜环层 / columnar ~ 杆体(锥体)层;套层 / compact ~ 致密层(蜕膜) / cuticular ~ 表皮层(柱状上皮细胞) / deep ~ of triangular ligament 尿生殖膈上筋膜 / germ ~, blastodermic ~ 胚层 / germinative ~ of epidermis 表皮生发层 / granule ~ 小脑粒层 / half-value ~ 半值层,半价厚度 / horny ~ of epidermis 表皮角质层 / ~ of rods and cones 视杆视锥层 / trophic ~, vegetative ~ 滋养层,内胚层 / yellow ~ 血沉棕黄层

layette [leiˈet] *n* 新生儿衣被

lazaretto [ˌlæzəˈretəu] *n* 传染病院,隔离病院;检疫留验站

lb libra【拉】磅

LBBB left bundle branch block 左束支传导阻滞

LBW low birth weight 低出生体重

LCA left coronary artery 左冠状动脉; leukocyte common antigen 白细胞共同抗原

LCAD deficiency long-chain acyl-CoA dehydrogenase deficiency 长链酰基辅酶 A 脱氢酶缺乏症

LCAT lecithin-cholesterol acyltransferase 卵磷脂-胆固醇酰基转移酶

LCAT deficiency lecithin-cholesterol acyltransferase deficiency 卵磷脂-胆固醇酰基转移酶缺乏症

LCIS lobular carcinoma in situ 原位小叶癌

LD lethal dose 致死量; light difference 光差; late deceleration 晚期减速

LD_{50} median lethal dose 半数致死量

LDA left dorsoanterior 背左前(胎位)

LDH L-lactate dehydrogenase L-乳酸脱氢酶

LDL low-density lipoproteins 低密度脂蛋白; loudness discomfort level 响度不适级

LDL-C low-density-lipoprotein cholesterol 低密度脂蛋白胆固醇

L-dopa levodopa 左旋多巴

LDP left dorsoposterior 背左后(胎位)

LE left eye 左眼; lupus erythematosus 红斑狼疮

leach [liːtʃ] *vt* 沥滤(液体);滤取,滤去 *vi* 滤掉 *n* 沥滤;沥滤器 | **~able** *a* 可沥滤的,可滤去(或滤取)的

leaching [ˈliːtʃiŋ] *n* 沥滤[法],沥取[法],浸沥[法]

lead¹ [liːd] *n* 导联,导程 | bipolar ~ 双极导联 / esophageal ~ 食管导程 / precordial ~s 心前区导联 / unipolar ~ 单极导联 / vector ~ 向量导联 / ventricular ~ 心室(起搏)电极

lead² [led] *n* 铅 | ~ acetate, sugar of ~ 醋酸铅,铅糖(试剂、收敛剂) / ~ arsenate 砷酸铅(杀虫剂) / black ~ 黑铅,石墨 / ~ chloride 氯化铅(试剂) / ~ chromate 铬酸铅,铬黄,贡黄(染剂) / ~ monoxide 一氧化铅,密陀僧(试剂) / ~ nitrate 硝酸铅(试剂) / radioactive ~ [放]射铅 / red ~ 红铅,四氧化铅,铅丹 / white ~ 铅白,碳酸铅白,碱式碳酸铅

leaf [liːf] ([复]**leaves** [liːvz]) *n* 叶 | beladonna ~ 颠茄叶 / betel ~ 蒌叶

leaflet [ˈliːflit] *n* 小叶(尤指心瓣的尖)

leafy [ˈliːfi] *a* 叶状的

leakage [ˈliːkidʒ] *n* 漏;漏出;漏出物;漏失量 | duodenal stump ~ 十二指肠残端漏

Leão's spreading depression [leiˈɑː] (A. A. P. Leão) 雷阿扩张性阻抑(从大脑皮质记录的正常电节律的阻抑,同时从刺激区或皮质损坏区向外扩张,扩散率十分接近偏头痛的视觉先兆。亦称扩散性阻抑)

learning [ˈləːniŋ] *n* 学习 | insight ~ 顿悟学习,洞察学习 / latent ~ 潜伏学习(指动物未加以强化的学习,如予以强化或奖赏,效果就明显)

leash [liːʃ] *n* 索

leben [ˈlebən] *n*【阿拉伯】发酵乳饮料

Leber's congenital amaurosis [leiˈbɔː] (Theodor Leber) 莱伯先天性黑矇(一种常染色体隐性遗传性疾病,出生时或出生后双目即告失明,常伴有视神经萎缩和视网膜血管变细等症状,此型较少见) | ~ optic atrophy 莱伯视神经萎缩(男性遗传性疾病,主要症状为双侧性进行性视神经萎缩,出现于20岁左右,被认为是X连锁遗传特性) / ~ corpuscle 莱伯小体(胸腺小体) / ~ disease 莱伯病(见莱伯视神经萎缩及莱伯先天性黑矇) / ~ plexus 莱伯静脉丛(在睫状体区内与巩膜静脉窦相连)

Lebistes [liˈbistiːz] *n* 虹鳉属 | ~ reticulatus 虹鳉(普通称为"百万鱼",食孑孓)

Leboyer method (technique) [ləbɔːˈjei] (Frederick Leboyer) 勒博耶分娩法(此法基于这样一种理论,认为分娩时使用暴力会导致婴儿情绪创伤,影响儿童的性格及其一生,故此法强调分娩必需轻巧协调和有节制,轻柔地处理婴儿)

lecanopagus [ˌlekəˈnɔpəgəs] *n* 腰下联胎

Lecat's gulf [ləˈkɑː] (Claude N. Lecat) 勒卡湾(尿道球膨大)

leche de higuerón [ˈleitʃei dei ˌiːgeiˈrɔn]【西】野无花果乳汁(驱虫药)

lechopyra [ˌlekəˈpaiərə] *n* 产褥热

lechuguille [leitʃuːˈgiːjə] *n* 龙舌兰

-lecithal [构词成分] 卵黄

lecithal [ˈlesiθəl] *a* 卵黄的

lecithalbumin [ˌlesiˈθælbjumin] *n* 卵磷脂白蛋白

lecithid [ˈlesiθid] *n* 蛇毒溶血卵磷脂 | cobra ~ 蝮蛇毒溶血卵磷脂

lecithin [ˈlesiθin] *n* 卵磷脂

lecithinase [ˈlesiθineis] *n* 卵磷脂酶 | ~ A 卵磷脂酶A(磷酸脂酶 A_1 和磷酸脂酶 A_2) / ~ B 卵磷脂酶B(溶血磷酸脂酶) / ~ C 卵磷脂酶C(磷酸脂酶C) / ~ D 卵磷脂酶D(磷酸脂酶D)

lecithin-cholesterol acyltransferase (LCAT) [ˈlesiθin kəˈlestərɔl ˌæsilˈtrænsfəreis] 卵磷脂-胆固醇酰基转移酶,磷脂酰胆固醇 *O*-酰基转移酶 | familial ~ deficiency 家族性卵磷脂-胆固醇酰基转移酶缺乏症

lecithin-cholesterol acyltransferase (LCAT) deficiency 卵磷脂胆固醇酰基转移酶缺乏症(一种常染色体隐性遗传病,由于LCAT不能酯化血浆胆固醇所致;胆固醇和磷脂酰胆碱在血浆和组织内蓄积,从而导致角膜混浊、贫血和蛋白尿症。各类脂蛋白显示异常)

lecithinemia [ˌlesiθiˈniːmiə] *n* 卵磷脂血症

lecith(o)- [构词成分] 卵黄

lecithoblast [ˈlesiθəˌblæst] *n* 成卵黄细胞

lecithoprotein [ˌlesiθəuˈprəutiːn] *n* 卵磷脂蛋白

lecithovitellin [ˌlesiθəuvaiˈtelin] *n* 卵黄悬胶液

Leclanché's cell [ˌleklənˈʃei] (Georges Leclanché) 勒克朗谢电池(一种电动势电池)

lectin [ˈlektin] *n* 凝集素(在凝集红细胞时,表现了血型的特异性,亦称外源凝集素)

lectotype [ˈlektətaip] *n* 选型(细菌培养物等)

Lecythophora [ˌleisiˈθɔfərə] *n* 暗色孢属

ledbänder [ˈledbendə] *n*【德】宾格内带(见Büngner's bands)

Le Dentu's suture [lə dɔŋˈtjuː] (Jean François-Auguste Le Dentu) 勒当屠缝术(腱分裂缝术)

Lederer's anemia (disease) [ˈledərə] (Max Lederer) 莱德勒贫血(病)(急性溶血性贫血的一种)

Leduc's current [ləˈduk] (Stéphane A. N. Leduc) 勒杜克电流(等强断续直流)

LeDuc technique (implantation) [ləˈduːk] (A. LeDuc) 勒迪克技术(植入法)(一种输尿管的肠管吻合术)

leech [liːtʃ] *n* 水蛭,蛭,蚂蟥 *vt* 用水蛭给…抽血 | American ~ 美洲水蛭(即北美巨蛭 Macrobdella decora) / artificial ~ 人工吸血器,人工水蛭 / land ~ 山蛭(即山蛭属 Haemadipsa) / medicinal ~ 医用水蛭,医蛭(即 Hirudo medicinalis)

leeches [ˈliːtʃəs] [复] *n* 腐霉病

leeching [ˈliːtʃiŋ] *n* 水蛭吸血法

Lee's ganglion [liː] (Robert Lee) 宫颈神经节

Leeuwenhoekia [ˌljuːenˈhəukiə] (Antonj van Leeuwenhoek) *n* 里汶恙螨属

leflunomide [ləˈfluːnəumaid] *n* 来氟米特(抗风湿药)

Le Fort amputation [ləˈfɔː] (Léon-Clement Le Fort) 勒福切断术(皮罗果夫〈Pirogoff〉切断术的一种改良法,即将跟骨横锯而非直锯) | ~ fracture 勒福骨折(双侧上颌横形骨折) / ~ operation 勒福手术,阴道闭合术(沿中线将阴道前后壁连在一起,以修复子宫脱垂) / ~ sound 勒福探子(带有联结线形探条的螺旋头,用于通过紧缩的尿道狭窄) / ~ suture 勒福缝术(用于缝合腱断裂)

left-handed [ˈleft ˈhændid] *a* 左手的;善用左手的,左利的;向左旋转的

leg [leg] *n* 腿,小腿 | badger ~ 獾腿(两腿长短不等) / baker ~ 膝外翻 / bandy ~ 膝内翻 / bayonet ~ 枪刺形腿 / black ~ 黑腿病,气肿性炭疽 / bow ~ 弓形腿,膝内翻 / deck ~s, tropical ~ 甲板腿,热带腿(热带乘船旅行者的下肢水肿) / elephant ~ 象皮病 / milk ~ 股白肿 / red ~ 蛙腿红肿病 / restless ~s 多动腿(小腿麻痛感,不断活动可以消除) / rider's ~ 骑马者腿病(内收肌劳损) / scissor ~ 剪形腿 /

white ～ 股白肿
Legal's disease [leiˈgɑːl] (Emmo Legal) 莱加尔病(咽鼓室炎性头痛) | ～ test 莱加尔试验(检丙酮及吲哚)
Legg's disease, Legg-Calvé-Perthes disease, Legg-Calvé-Perthes-Waldenström disease [ˈleg kəlˈvei ˈpɑːtəz] (Arthur T. Legg; Jacques Calvé; Georg C. Perthes; Johan H. Waldenström) 股骨小头骺骨软骨病,幼年变形性骨软骨炎
leghemoglobin [ˌlegˌhiːməuˈgləubin] *n* 豆血红蛋白
Legionella [ˌliːdʒəˈnelə] *n* 军团杆菌属(1976年在费城美国退伍军人大会上首次确认的疾病中分离的一属细菌) | ～ pneumophila 嗜肺性军团杆菌
legionella [ˌliːdʒəˈnelə] ([复] legionellae) [ˌliːdʒəˈneliː] *n* 军团杆菌
Legionellaceae [ˌliːdʒəneˈleisiiː] *n* 军团杆菌科
legionellosis [ˌliːdʒəneˈləusis] *n* 军团杆菌病
legionnaires' disease [ˌliːdʒəˈnɛəz] 军团病(见 disease 项下相应术语)
legume [ˈlegjuːm, ləˈgjuːm] *n* 豆, [豆]荚
legumelin [ˌlegjuːˈmiːlin] *n* 豆白蛋白,豆清蛋白
legumin [ləˈgjuːmin] *n* 豆球蛋白
leguminivorous [ləˌgjuːmiˈnivərəs] *a* 豆食的
Leguminosae [ləgjuːˈminəsiː] *n* 豆科
leguminous [ləˈgjuːminəs] *a* 豆科的
leiasthenia [ˌlaiæsˈθiːnjə] *n* 平滑肌无力
Leichtenstern's encephalitis (type) [ˈlaiʃtənstəːn] (Otto M. Leichtenstern) 出血性脑炎 | ～ sign (phenomenon) 莱希登斯坦征(现象)(脑脊髓膜炎时,轻叩四肢骨,病人迅即退缩)
Leigh disease, syndrome [liː] (Archibald Denis Leigh) 利氏病、综合征,亚急性坏死性脑脊髓病
Leiner's disease [ˈlainə] (Karl Leiner) 脱屑性红皮病 | ～ test 莱内试验(检酪蛋白)
leio- [构词成分] 平滑
leiodermia [ˌlaiəuˈdəːmiə] *n* 滑泽皮
leiodystonia [ˌlaiəudis'təuniə] *n* 平滑肌张力障碍
Leiognathus bacoti [laiˈɔgnəθəs bəˈkɔti] 巴[科特]氏刺脂螨(即巴[科特]氏禽刺螨 Ornithonyssus bacoti)
leiomyoblastoma [ˌlaiəuˌmaiəublæsˈtəumə] *n* 成平滑肌瘤,上皮样平滑肌瘤
leiomyofibroma [ˌlaiəuˌmaiəufaiˈbrəumə] *n* 平滑肌纤维瘤
leiomyoma [ˌlaiəumaiˈəumə] *n* 平滑肌瘤 | epithelioid ～, bizarre ～ 上皮样平滑肌瘤(亦称成平滑肌瘤) / ～ uteri 子宫平滑肌瘤 / vascular ～ 血管平滑肌瘤
leiomyomatosis [ˌlaiəuˌmaiəuməˈtəusis] *n* 平滑肌瘤病 | ～ peritonealis disseminata 播散性腹膜平滑肌瘤病
leiomyosarcoma [ˌlaiəuˌmaiəusɑːˈkəumə] *n* 平滑肌肉瘤
leiotrichous [laiˈɔtrikəs] *a* [毛]发滑泽的
leiphemia [laiˈfiːmiə] *n* 血液缺乏
leip(o)- 以 leip(o)-起始的词,同样见 lip(o)-起始的词
Leishman-Donovan body [ˈliːʃmən ˈdɔnəvən] (William B. Leishman; Charles Donovan) 利-杜小体,无鞭毛体
Leishmania [liːʃˈmeiniə] (William B. Leishman) *n* 利什曼[原]虫属 | ～ aethiopica, ～ tropica aethiopica 埃塞俄比亚利什曼原虫,埃塞俄比亚热带利什曼原虫 / ～ braziliensis, ～ brasiliensis 巴西利什曼原虫 / ～ braziliensis braziliensis 巴西利什曼原虫巴西亚种 / ～ braziliensis guyanensis 巴西利什曼原虫圭亚那亚种 / ～ braziliensis panamensis 巴西利什曼原虫巴拿马亚种 / ～ donovani 杜[诺凡]氏利什曼原虫 / ～ donovani chagasi 杜氏利什曼原虫恰加斯亚种 / ～ donovani donovani 杜氏利什曼原虫杜氏亚种 / ～ donovani infantum, ～ infantum 杜氏利什曼原虫婴儿亚种,婴儿利什曼原虫 / ～ major, ～ tropica major 大型利什曼原虫,大型热带利什曼原虫 / ～ mexicana 墨西哥利什曼原虫 / ～ mexicana amazonensis 墨西哥利什曼原虫亚马逊亚种 / ～ mexicana mexicana 墨西哥利什曼原虫墨西哥亚种 / ～ peruviana 秘鲁利什曼原虫 / ～ pifanoi, ～ mexicana pifanoi 玻氏利什曼原虫,玻氏墨西哥利什曼原虫 / ～ tropica, ～ nilotica 热带利什曼原虫,尼罗河利什曼原虫
leishmania [liːʃˈmeiniə] *n* 利什曼[原]虫
leishmanial [liːʃˈmeiniəl] *a* 利什曼原虫的;锥体虫的
leishmaniasis [ˌliːʃməˈnaiəsis] *n* 利什曼病 | American ～ 美洲利什曼病(新大陆型利什曼病) / canine ～ 犬利什曼病(婴儿型内脏利什曼病) / cutaneous ～ 皮肤利什曼病 / diffuse cutaneous ～, anergic cutaneous ～, ～ tegmentaria diffusa 弥漫性皮肤利什曼病 / infantile ～ 婴儿利什曼病(婴儿型内脏利什曼病) / mucocutaneous ～ 黏膜皮肤利什曼病 / New World ～ 新大陆型利什曼病 / Old World ～ 旧大陆型利什曼病 / post-kala-azar dermal ～ 黑热病后皮肤利什曼病 / ～ recidivans, lupoid ～ 复发性利什曼病,狼疮样利什曼病 / rural ～ 农村型利什曼病 / urban ～ 城区型利什曼病 / visceral ～ 内脏利什曼病,黑热病
leishmanicidal [ˌliːʃməniˈsaidl] *a* 杀利什曼[原]虫的
leishmanid [ˈliːʃmənid] *n* 利什曼结节
leishmanin [ˈliːʃmənin] *n* 利什曼原虫素(用于皮肤试验,检皮肤利什曼病)

leishmaniosis [ˌliːʃməniˈəusis] *n* 利什曼病
leishmanoid [ˈliːʃmənɔid] *a* 类利什曼病的 *n* 利什曼疹,利什曼斑,皮肤利什曼斑 | dermal ~, post-kala-azar dermal ~ 皮肤利什曼斑,黑热病后皮肤利什曼斑(即黑热病后皮肤利什曼病)
Leishman's chrome cells [ˈliːʃmən] (William B. Leishman) 利什曼色素细胞(黑水热时所见的嗜碱性粒性白细胞) | ~ stain 利什曼染剂(曙红和亚甲蓝溶液)
leistungskern [ˈlaistuŋskən] *n*【德】功能核心(细胞)
Leksell apparatus [ˈleksəl] (Lars Leksell) 莱克塞尔定位器(用于立体定位外科的莱克塞尔技术) | ~ technique 莱克塞尔技术(一种立体定位技术,使用弧形制导系统和立方体形支架使头部定位,并标以三维定向的 X, Y 和 Z 坐标)
Lelaps [ˈliːlæps] *n* 棘蛎螨属(即 Echinolaelaps) | ~ echidninus 毒棘蛎螨(即 Echinolaelaps echidninus)
Leloir's disease [liːlˈwɑː] (Henri C. Leloir) 盘状红斑狼疮
lema [ˈliːmə] *n* 睑皮脂
Lembert's suture [læmˈbɛə] (Antoine Lembert) 间断浆肌层缝合
lemic [ˈliːmik] *a* 疫病的
Lemierre syndrome [ləmiˈɛə] (André Lemierre) 勒米埃综合征(颈内静脉血栓性静脉炎,伴感染继发扩散,由于急性口咽感染所致。亦称咽峡后脓毒症)
Lemieux-Neemeh syndrome [ləˈmjuːˈneimei] (Guy Lemieus; Jean A. Neemeh) 勒-内综合征(一种常染色体显性遗传综合征,包括进行性神经性肌萎缩,伴进行性聋)
lemma [ˈlemə] *n* 膜,衣,鞘
-lemma [构词成分]鞘,膜
lemmoblast [ˈleməblæst] *n* 成神经膜细胞
lemmoblastic [ˌleməuˈblæstik] *a* 成神经膜的
lemmocyte [ˈleməsait] *n* 神经膜细胞
lemniscus [lemˈniskəs] ([复] **lemnisci** [lemˈnisai]) *n*【拉】丘系(蹄系) | lateral ~ 外侧丘系 / medial ~ 内侧丘系 / optic ~ 视束 / spinal ~ 脊髓丘系 / trigeminal ~ 三叉丘系
lemography [liˈmɔgrəfi] *n* 疫病论,疫病论文集
lemology [liˈmɔlədʒi] *n* 传染病学(尤指疫病学)
lemon [ˈlemən] *n* 柠檬树;柠檬
lemoparalysis [ˌliːməupəˈrælisis] *n* 食管麻痹,食管瘫痪
lemostenosis [ˌleməustiˈnəusis] *n* 食管狭窄,咽狭窄
Lempert's fenestration operation [ˈlempəːt] (Julius Lempert) 兰珀特开窗术(用于治耳硬化症,即在外半规管钻上一小窗,然后在瘘管上置一层皮瓣,只要新通道保持畅通,听力即有明显改善)
LEMS Lambert-Eaton myasthenic syndrome 兰伯特-伊顿肌无力综合征(见 Eaton-Lambert syndrome)
lemur [ˈlemə] *n* 狐猴
Lemuridae [leˈmjuridiː] *n* 狐猴亚目
Lenard rays [leˈnɑːd] (Philipp Lenard) 勒纳射线(通过放电管外的阴极射线)
Lenègre's disease [ləˈnegrə] (Jean Lenègre) 勒内格尔病(获得性完全性心传导阻滞,由于传导系统原发性变性所致)
length(*l*) [leŋθ] *n* 长,长度 | crown-heel ~ 顶踵长(系人胚、胎儿、婴儿的颅最高点至足跟的长度,类同成人的立高) / crown-rump ~ 顶臀长(系人胚、胎儿、婴儿的颅最高点至臀部的长度,类同成人的坐高) / focal ~ 焦距 / foot ~ 足长度(估计胎儿的年龄) / greatest ~ 最大长度(测量早期胚胎) / wave ~ 波长
leniceps [ˈleniseps] *n* 短柄产钳
leniquinsin [ˌleniˈkwinsin] *n* 来尼喹新(抗高血压药)
lenitive [ˈlenitiv] *a* 润泽的,缓和的 *n* 润泽药
Lennert's classification [ˈlenərt] (K. Lennert) 伦诺分类法(见 Kiel classification) | ~ lymphoma 伦诺淋巴瘤(一型非霍奇金〈Hodgkin〉淋巴瘤,伴有大量上皮样组织细胞,常累及骨髓,对化疗反应常不佳)
Lennhoff's index [ˈlenhɔf] (Rudolf Lennhoff) 伦霍夫指数(躯干长腹围指数,即胸骨切迹至耻骨联合的距离除以最大腹围乘上 100 所得之数) | ~ sign 伦霍夫征(深吸气时,最后一根肋骨下及肝包虫囊上方出现的横沟)
Lennox-Gastaut syndrome [ˈlenɔks gæsˈtəu] (W. G. Lennox; Henri J. P. Gastaut) 伦-格综合征(一种非典型失神性癫痫,特征为弥漫性慢棘波,常伴有弛缓性强直性或阵挛性癫痫发作以及智力迟钝;可能有其他神经病学异常或多发性癫痫发作型。与典型的失神性癫痫不同,非典型的失神性癫痫可能持续到成年期。亦称癫痫小发作变型)
Lennox syndrome [ˈlenɔks] (William G. Lennox) 伦诺克斯综合征(见 Lennox-Gastaut syndrome)
lenperone [ˈlenpərəun] *n* 仑哌隆(安定药)
lens [lenz] *n* 透镜,镜片;晶状体 | achromatic ~ 消色差透镜 / acrylic ~ 丙烯透镜 / aplanatic ~ 消球差透镜 / apochromatic ~ 全消色差透镜 / biconcave ~ 双凹镜片 / bicylindrical ~ 双柱镜片 / bifocal ~ 双焦点镜片 / bispherical ~ 双球面透镜 / cataract ~ [白]内障镜片 / concave ~ 凹球镜片 / concavo-convex ~ 凹凸镜片 / contact ~ 接触镜片 / convex ~ 凸球镜片 / crystal-

line ~ 晶状体 / immersion ~ 浸没透镜 / iseikonic ~ 眼像平衡透镜 / orthoscopic ~ 无畸透镜 / periscopic ~ 周视镜片 / planoconcave ~ 平凹镜片 / planoconvex ~ 平凸镜片 prosthetic ~, artificial ~ 人工晶状体 / toric ~ 复曲面透镜 / trial ~ 试镜片

lensometer [lenˈzɔmitə] *n* 镜片计

lente [lent] *a* 长效的

lentectomize [lenˈtektəmaiz] *vt* 切除晶状体

lentectomy [lenˈtektəmi] *n* 晶状体切除术

lenticel [ˈlentisel] *n* 舌根腺

lenticonus [ˌlentiˈkəunəs] *n* 圆锥晶状体

lenticula [lenˈtikjulə] *n*【拉】豆状核

lenticular [lenˈtikjulə] *a* 透镜的,透镜状的;晶状体的;豆状核的

lenticulo-optic [lenˌtikjuləu ˈɔptik] *a* 豆状核丘脑的

lenticulostriate [lenˌtikjuləuˈstraiit] *a* 豆状核纹状体的

lenticulothalamic [lenˌtikjuləuθəˈlæmik] *a* 豆状核丘脑的

lentiform [ˈlentifɔːm] *a* 透镜状的;豆状的

lentigines [lenˈtidʒiniːz] lentigo 的复数

lentiginosis [lenˌtidʒiˈnəusis] *n* 着色斑病,雀斑样痣病 | progressive cardiomyopathic ~ 进行性心肌病性着色斑病(见 Moynahan's syndrome ①解)

lentiginous [lenˈtidʒinəs] *a* 着色斑的,雀斑样痣的

lentiglobus [ˌlentiˈgləubəs] *n* 球形晶状体

lentigo [lenˈtaigəu] ([复] **lentigines** [lenˈtidʒiniːz]) *n*【拉】雀斑痣 | ~ maligna, malignant ~ 恶性雀斑样痣 / nevoid ~ 痣样雀斑,雀斑样痣;斑痣 / senile ~, ~ senilis 老年性雀斑样痣 / ~ simplex 单纯性雀斑痣; / solar ~ 日光斑;老年性雀斑样痣

lentitis [lenˈtaitis] *n* 晶状体炎

Lentivirinae [ˌlentiviˈrainiː] *n* 慢病毒亚科

Lentivirus [ˈlentiˌvaiərəs] *n* 慢病毒属

lentivirus [ˈlentiˌvaiərəs] *n* 慢病毒

lentula [ˈlentʃuːlə] *n* 根管糊剂螺旋形输送器(即 lentulo)

lentulo [ˈlentʃuːləu, lenˈtuːləu] *n* 根管糊剂螺旋形输送器(用于牙根管疗法)

Lenz's syndrome [lents] (Widukind D. Lenz) 伦茨综合征(一种 X 连锁性状遗传综合征,包括单侧或双侧眼小或无眼畸胎、指〈趾〉异常、窄肩、双拇指及其他骨骼异常;牙、泌尿生殖器及心血管缺陷也可能发生)

leontiasis [ˌliːənˈtaiəsis] *n* 狮面(瘤型麻风) | ~ ossea, ~ ossium 骨性狮面(亦称巨头)

Leontodon [liˈɔntədɔn] *n* 狮齿菊属,蒲公英属

Leopold's law [ˈleiəpɔld] (Christian G. Leopold) 利奥波德定律(胎盘附着于子宫后壁时,输卵管则会聚于前壁,胎盘如附着于子宫前壁,则卧位时输卵管转向后方,与宫体轴平行)

Leo's test [ˈleiəu] (Hans Leo) 莱奥试验(检游离盐酸)

leotropic [ˌliːəˈtrɔpik] *a* 左蟠的,左旋的

leper [ˈlepə] *n* 麻风病人,麻风患者

lepidic [liˈpidik] *a* 鳞屑的;胚层的

lepid(o)- [构词成分] 鳞,鳞屑

Lepidoptera [ˌlepiˈdɔptərə] *n* 鳞翅目

Lepiota [ˌlepiˈəutə] *n* 伞菌属

lepirudin [ˌlepiˈruːdin] *n* 来匹芦定(蛭素的重组型,用作抗凝药,用于肝素诱发的血小板减少症和相关的血栓栓塞性疾病,静脉给药)

lepocyte [ˈlepəsait] *n* 有壁细胞

Leporipoxvirus [ˌlepəriˈpɔksˌvaiərəs] *n* 兔痘病毒属

lepothrix [ˈlepəθriks] *n* 腋毛菌病,结节性毛菌病

lepra [ˈleprə] *n* 麻风;银屑病(19 世纪中叶以前用法)

leprechaunism [ˈlepreˌkɔːnizəm] *n* 矮妖精貌综合征(面貌如传说中的矮妖精,内分泌严重紊乱)

leprid [ˈleprid], **lepride** [ˈlepraid] *n* 麻风疹

leprology [leˈprɔlədʒi] *n* 麻风学 | **leprologist** *n* 麻风学家

leproma [leˈprəumə] *n* 麻风结节,麻风瘤 | **~tous** *a*

lepromin [ˈleprəmin] *n* 麻风菌素

leprosarium [ˌlepreˈsɛəriəm], **leprosary**, **leprosery** [ˈleprəsəri] *n* 麻风病院,麻风病人隔离区

leprostatic [ˌlepreˈstætik] *a* 抑制麻风菌的 *n* 制麻风[菌]药

leprosy [ˈleprəsi] *n* 麻风 | borderline ~, dimorphous ~, intermediate ~ 界线类麻风,双型性麻风,中间型麻风 / borderline lepromatous ~ 偏瘤型界线类麻风 / borderline tuberculoid ~ 偏结核样型界线类麻风 / indeterminate ~, uncharacteristic ~ 未定类麻风 / lazarine ~ 残毁性麻风 / lepromatous ~ 瘤型麻风 / rat ~, murine ~ 鼠麻风 / reactional ~ 反应性麻风 / tuberculoid ~ 结核样型麻风 / water-buffalo ~ 水牛麻风 | **leprotic** [leˈprɔtik] *a*

leprous [ˈleprəs] *a* 麻风的;患麻风的

leptandra [lepˈtændrə] *n* 黑根,北美草本威灵仙(用作泻药)

leptazol [ˈleptəzɔl] *n* 戊四氮(中枢兴奋药)

leptin [ˈleptin] *n* 苗条蛋白,减肥蛋白

leptinemia [ˌleptiˈniːmiə] *n* 苗条蛋白血症,减肥蛋白血症,高苗条蛋白血症,高减肥蛋白血症

lept(o)- [构词成分] 薄,细,狭,软
leptocephalus [ˌleptəuˈsefələs] *n* 狭长头者
leptocephaly [ˌleptəu ˈsefəli] *n* 狭长头 | **leptocephalic** [ˌleptəusəˈfelik], **leptocephalous** [ˌleptəuˈsefələs] *a*
leptochromatic [ˌleptəukrəuˈmætik] *a* 细染色质网的
Leptocimex [ˌleptəuˈsaimeks] *n* 细臭虫属(即臭虫属 Cimex) | ~ boueti 卜氏细臭虫(即卜氏臭虫 Cimex boueti)
Leptoconops [ˌleptəuˈkəunəps] *n* 细蠓属
leptocyte [ˈleptəsait] *n* 薄红细胞
leptocytosis [ˌleptəusaiˈtəusis] *n* 薄红细胞增多
leptodactyly [ˌleptəuˈdæktili] *n* 细长指,细长趾 | **leptodactylous** [ˌleptəuˈdæktiləs] *a*
Leptodera pellio [lepˈtəudərəˈpeliəu] 生殖器小杆线虫
leptodontous [ˌleptəuˈdɔntəs] *a* 细长牙的
leptokurtic [ˌleptəuˈkəːtik] *a* 峰态的
leptomeningeal [ˌleptəuməˈnindʒiəl] *a* 柔脑膜的
leptomeninges [ˌleptəuməˈnindʒiːz] leptomeninx 的复数
leptomeningioma [ˌleptəuməˌnindʒiˈəumə] *n* 柔脑膜瘤
leptomeningitis [ˌleptəuˌmeninˈdʒaitis] *n* 柔脑膜炎 | ~ interna 内层柔脑膜炎 / sarcomatous ~ 肉瘤性柔脑膜炎
leptomeningopathy [ˌleptəuˌmeniŋˈgɔpəθi] *n* 柔脑膜病
leptomeninx [ˌleptəuˈmeniŋks] ([复] **leptomeninges** [ˌleptəuməˈnindʒiːz]) *n* 柔脑膜
Leptomitus [lepˈtɔmitəs] *n* 细丝菌属(Absidia 的旧名)
leptomonad [ˌleptəuˈməunæd] *a* 细滴虫的 *n* 细滴虫
Leptomonas [ˌleptəuˈməunəs] *n* 细滴虫属
leptomonas [ˌleptəuˈməunəs] *n* 细滴虫
Leptomyxida [ˌleptəuˈmiksidə] *n* 细胶丝目
leptonema [ˌleptəuˈniːmə] *n* 细线,细线期(原指细线状的染色体,加以引伸,指这一时期)
leptonomorphology [ˌleptənəumɔːˈfɔlədʒi] *n* 膜形态学
leptopellic [ˌleptəuˈpelik] *a* 狭骨盆的
leptophonia [ˌleptəuˈfəuniə] *n* 声弱 | **leptophonic** [ˌleptəuˈfɔnik] *a*
leptoprosope [lepˈtɔprəsəup] *n* 窄面人
leptoprosopia [ˌleptəuprəˈsəupiə] *n* 窄面(长颅) | **leptoprosopic** [ˌleptəuprəˈsəupik] *a*
Leptopsylla [ˌleptəˈsilə] *n* 细蚤属 | ~ segnis, ~ musculi 缓慢细蚤
leptorrhine [ˈleptərain] *a* 窄鼻的(鼻指数在 48 以下)
leptoscope [ˈleptəskəup] *n* 测膜镜
leptosomatic [ˌleptəusəuˈmætik] *a* 瘦长型的
leptosome [ˈleptəsəum] *n* 瘦长型者
Leptosphaeria [ˌleptəuˈsfiəriə] *n* 钩端球体属
Leptospira [ˌleptəˈspaiərə] *n* 钩端螺旋体属 | ~ australis, ~ interrogans serogroup australis 澳大利亚钩端螺旋体,澳大利亚问号血清型钩端螺旋体 / ~ autumnalis, ~ interrogans serogroup autumnalis 秋季热钩端螺旋体,秋季问号血清型钩端螺旋体 / ~ bataviae, ~ interrogans serogroup bataviae 巴达维亚钩端螺旋体,巴达维亚问号血清型钩端螺旋体 / ~ biflexa 双曲钩端螺旋体 / ~ canicola, ~ interrogans serogroup canicola 犬钩端螺旋体,犬型问号血清型钩端螺旋体 / ~ grippotyphosa, ~ interrogans serogroup grippotyphosa 流感伤寒钩端螺旋体,流感伤寒型问号血清型钩端螺旋体 / ~ hebdomidis, ~ interrogans serogroup hebdomidis 七日热钩端螺旋体,七日热问号血清型钩端螺旋体 / ~ hyos 猪钩端螺旋体 / ~ icterohaemorrhagiae, ~ interrogans serogroup icterohaemorrhagiae 出血性黄疸钩端螺旋体,出血性黄疸问号血清型钩端螺旋体 / ~ illini 伊林钩端螺旋体 / ~ interrogans 问号钩端螺旋体 / ~ pomona, ~ interrogans serogroup pomona 波摩那钩端螺旋体,波摩那问号血清型钩端螺旋体 / ~ pyrogenes, ~ interrogans serogroup pyrogenes 致热钩端螺旋体,致热问号血清型钩端螺旋体
leptospira [ˌleptəˈspaiərə], **leptospire** [ˈleptəspaiə] *n* 钩端螺旋体 | **leptospiral** *a*
Leptospiraceae [ˌleptəuspaiəˈreisiiː] *n* 钩端螺旋体科
leptospirosis [ˌleptəuspaiəˈrəusis] *n* 钩端螺旋体病 | benign ~, anicteric ~ 良性钩端螺旋体病 / ~ icterohemorrhagica 出血性黄疸钩端螺旋体病,钩端螺旋体性黄疸
leptospiruria [ˌleptəuspiˈrjuərə] *n* 钩端螺旋体尿
leptostaphyline [ˌleptəˈstæfilain] *a* 窄腭的(腭指数为 79.9 或少于 79.9)
leptotene [ˈleptətiːn] *n* 细线期(减数分裂的一个时期,染色体呈细长如线)
Leptothrix [ˈleptəθriks] *n* 纤发菌属
leptothrix [ˈleptəθriks] *n* 纤发菌
Leptotrichia [ˌleptəuˈtrikiə] *n* 纤毛菌属 | ~ buccalis 颊纤毛菌
leptotrichosis [ˌleptəutriˈkəusis] *n* 纤毛菌病 | ~ conjunctivae 结膜纤毛菌病 | **leptothricosis** [ˌleptəuθraiˈkəusis] *n*
Leptotrombidium [ˌleptəutrɔmˈbidiəm] *n* 纤恙螨亚属
Leptus [ˈleptəs] *n*【拉】蚬,恙虫属(旧名) | ~

akamushi 红恙螨(即 Trombicula akamushi)

Lerch's percussion [ləːtʃ] (Otto Lerch) 落槌叩诊

Leredde syndrome [lə'red] (Emile Leredde) 勒雷德综合征(用力时严重呼吸困难,合并晚期肺气肿和急性发热性支气管炎反复发作,见于先天性梅毒患儿)

leresis [lə'riːsis] *n* 冗谈,饶舌

lergotrile ['ləːgətrail] *n* 麦角腈(泌乳素抑制剂) | ~ mesylate 甲磺麦角腈(抗震颤麻痹药)

Leriche's disease [lə'riːʃ] (René Leriche) 外伤后骨质疏松[症] | ~ syndrome 勒里施综合征(主动脉末端梗阻引起的综合征,一般见于男性,特征为髋、股或腿部在活动时疲劳,股动脉搏动缺失和阳萎,下肢经常苍白和冰冷)

Léri's sign ['leiri] (André Léri) 莱里征(偏瘫侧手及腕被动屈曲时,肘部无正常屈曲运动)

Lermoyez's syndrome [ˌləːmɔi'jei] (Marcel Lermoyez) 莱穆瓦耶综合征(耳鸣、耳聋、随之发生眩晕,眩晕发生后即消失)

les local excitatory state 局部刺激状态

lesbian ['lezbiən] *a* 女子同性恋的 *n* 女子同性恋 | ~**ism** *n*

Lesch-Nyhan syndrome [leʃ 'naiən] (Michael Lesch; William L. Nyhan, Jr.) 莱施-奈恩综合征(一种罕见的 X 连锁遗传嘌呤代谢病,由于次黄嘌呤磷酸核糖基转移酶缺乏所致,特征为身体和精神发育迟缓、有咬指咬唇的强迫性自残行为、舞蹈手足徐动症、痉挛性大脑性麻痹及肾功能损害,另为鸟嘌呤合成过度,由此而引起高尿酸血和尿酸尿)

Leser-Trélat sign ['leizə 'triːlə] (Edmund Leser; Ulysse Trélat, Jr.) 莱泽-特雷拉征(突然发生脂溢性角化病,并迅速变大增多,可能是内脏尤其是胃肠道恶性肿瘤的体征)

lesion ['liːʒən] *n* 损害,损伤 | coin ~ 钱币形损害(指瘤) / gross ~ 肉眼损害 / histologic ~ 组织损害(一种显微镜可见损害) / impaction ~ 嵌塞损害,碰撞损害 / indiscriminate ~ 散在性损害 / initial syphilitic ~ 下疳 / local ~ 局部损害 / peripheral ~ 神经末梢损害 / primary ~ 原发病灶 / ring-wall ~ 环状(出血性)损害(见于恶性贫血) / systemic ~ 器官系统损害 / total ~ 全部损害 / trophic ~ 营养性损害 / wire-loop ~ 线圈损害(播散性红斑狼疮时)

lesionectomy [ˌliːʒə'nektəmi] *n* 病灶切除术(用于治疗癫痫)

Lesser's test ['lesə] (Fritz Lesser) 累塞尔试验(含碘的分泌物用甘汞处理时变成黄色)

Lesshaft's space (triangle) ['leshɑːft] (Peter F. Lesshaft) 勒斯哈夫特间隙(三角)(斜方形:前界外斜肌,后界背阔肌,上界后锯肌,下界内斜肌,常为脓头出现或疝发生之处)

LET linear energy transfer 传能线密度

let-down ['let daun] *n* 射乳 | milk ~ 射乳

lethal ['liːθəl] *a* 致死的 | ~**ity** [li'θæləti] *n* 致死率

lethargic [le'θɑːdʒik] *a* 昏睡的,嗜睡的;冷淡的

lethargus [li'θɑːgəs] *n* 非洲昏睡病

lethargy ['leθədʒi] *n* 嗜睡;淡漠 | African ~ 非洲昏睡病,非洲锥虫病 / hysteric ~ 癔症性嗜睡 / induced ~ (催眠)诱导性迷睡 / lucid ~ 清醒呆滞

lethe ['liːθi(ː)] *n* 【希】记忆缺失,完全遗忘 | ~**ral** ['liːθərəl] *a*

letimide hydrochloride ['letimaid] 盐酸来替米特(镇痛药)

letrozole ['letrəzəul] *n* 来曲唑(抗肿瘤药,治疗绝经后妇女晚期乳腺癌,口服给药)

Letterer-Siwe disease ['letərə 'sivə] (Erich Letterer; Sture A. Siwe) 莱特勒-西韦病(婴儿非类脂网状内皮组织增殖,很可能是一种常染色体隐性遗传特性,其特征为出血性倾向、湿疹样皮疹、肝脾肿大和淋巴结肿大、进行性贫血)

leukocyte elastase ['ljuːkəsait i'læsteis] 白细胞弹性蛋白酶(α_1-抗胰蛋白酶缺乏时发生的肺气肿是由于白细胞弹性蛋白酶对肺组织损伤所致。亦称嗜中性细胞弹性蛋白酶)

leukocytospermia [ˌljuːkəˌsaitəu'spəːmiə] *n* 白细胞精液(精液中白细胞过多)

Leu leucine 亮氨酸

leucemia [ljuː'siːmiə] *n* 白血病

leucine (Leu, L) ['ljuːsi(ː)n] *n* 亮氨酸

leucine aminopeptidase (LAP) ['ljuːsinˌæminəu'peptideis] 亮氨酸氨肽酶

leucinethylester [ˌljuːsinˌeθil'estə] *n* 亮氨酸乙酯

leucinimide [ljuː'siniˌmaid] *n* 环缩二亮氨酸

leucinosis [ljuːsi'nəusis] *n* 亮氨酸过多[症],亮氨酸病

leucinuria [ˌljuːsi'njuəriə] *n* 亮氨酸尿

leucismus [ljuː'sizməs] *n* 白变 | ~ pilorum [头]发白变

leucitis [ljuː'saitis] *n* 巩膜炎

leuc(o)- [构词成分] 白(见 leuko-)

leucocyte ['ljuːkəsait] *n* 白细胞

leucocytopenia [ˌljuːkəsaitəu'piːniə] *n* 白细胞减少

leucocytosis [ˌljuːkəsai'təusis] *n* 白细胞增多

Leucocytozoon [ˌljuːkəˌsaitə'zəuən] *n* 白细胞球虫属

leucocytozoonosis [ˌljuːkəuˌsaitəuˌzəuəu'nəusis] *n* 白细胞球虫病(家禽的一种急性疟疾样原虫病)

leucofluorescein [ˌljuːkəuˌfluə'resiːn] *n* 白荧光

素,无色荧光素

Leucoium [ljuːˈkəuiəm] *n*【拉;希】雪片莲属(石蒜科)

leucomycin [ˌljuːkəuˈmaisin] *n* 柱晶白霉素,吉他霉素(抗生素类药)

Leuconostoc [ˌljuːkəuˈnɔstɔk] *n* 明串珠菌属,白联珠菌属 | ~ cremoris, ~ citrovorum 乳脂明串珠菌,噬枸橼酸明串珠菌 / ~ dextranicum 葡聚糖明串珠菌 / ~ lactis 乳明串珠菌 / ~ mesenteroides 肠系膜样明串珠菌 / ~ oenos 酒明串珠菌

leucopterin [ljuːˈkɔptərin] *n* 白蝶呤

leucosin [ˈljuːkəsin] *n* 谷白蛋白

Leucothrix [ˈljuːkəuθriks] *n* 亮发菌属

leucotomy [ljuːˈkɔtəmi] *n* 脑白质切断术

Leucotrichaceae [ˌljuːkəuˌtriˈkeisiiː] *n* 亮发菌科

leucovorin [ljuːˈkɔvərin] *n* 亚叶酸(抗贫血药) | ~ calcium 亚叶酸钙

leucyl [ˈljuːsil] *n* 亮氨酰[基]

leucyl aminopeptidase(LAP) [ˈljuːsil əˌminəuˈpeptideis] 亮氨酰氨肽酶(亦称细胞溶胶氨肽酶)

Leudet's tinnitus(bruit, sign) [leˈdei] (Théodor E. Leudet) 勒代耳鸣(耳鸣杂音、征)(由耳内部肌肉不随意收缩所产生)

leu-enkephalin [ˌljuːenˈkefəlin] *n* 亮氨酸脑啡肽、亮脑啡肽

leukapheresis [ˌljuːkəfəˈriːsis] *n* 白细胞去除术

leukemia [ljuːˈkiːmiə] *n* 白血病 | acute nonlymphocytic ~(ANLL) 急性非淋巴细胞白血病 / acute promyelocytic ~ 急性早幼粒细胞白血病 / adult T-cell ~ 成人 T 细胞白血病 / aleukemic ~, aleukocythemic ~ 白细胞不增多白血病,非白血性白血病 / basophilic ~ 嗜碱粒细胞白血病 / bovine ~ 牛白血病 / chronic granulocytic ~, chronic myelocytic ~ 慢性粒细胞白血病 / eosinophilic ~ 嗜酸粒细胞白血病 / granulocytic ~ 粒细胞白血病 / hair-cell ~ 多毛细胞白血病 / hemoblastic ~, hemocytoblastic ~ 成血细胞白血病 / lymphatic ~, lymphoblastic ~, lymphocytic ~, lymphogenous ~, lymphoid ~ 淋巴白血病,淋巴细胞白血病 / lymphosarcoma cell ~ 淋巴肉瘤细胞白血病 / mast-cell ~ 肥大细胞白血病 / megakaryoblastic ~ 巨核细胞白血病,出血性血小板增多 / megakaryocytic ~ 巨核细胞白血病,出血性血小板增多 / micromyeloblastic ~ 小原粒型白血病 / monocytic ~ 单核细胞白血病 / myeloblastic ~ 原始粒细胞白血病 / myelocytic ~, myelogenous ~, myeloid granulocytic ~ 髓细胞白血病,骨髓粒细胞白血病 / myelomonocytic ~ 粒-单核细胞型白血病 / plasmacytic ~ 浆细胞白血病 / promyelocytic ~ 前髓细胞白血病 / stem cell ~, blast cell ~, embryonal ~, undifferentiated cell ~ 干细胞白血病,未分化细胞白血病 | **leukemic** *a*

leukemid [ljuːˈkiːmid] *n* 白血病疹

leukemogen [ljuːˈkiːmədʒən] *n* 致白血病物质

leukemogenesis [ljuːˌkiːməuˈdʒənisis] *n* 白血病生成

leukemogenic [ljuːˌkiːməuˈdʒenik] *a* 致白血病的

leukemoid [ljuːˈkiːmɔid] *a* 白血病样的,类白血病的

leukencephalitis [ˌljuːkenˌsefəˈlaitis] *n* 白质脑炎

leukexosis [ˌljuːkekˈsəusis] *n* 死白细胞聚集

leukin [ˈljuːkin] *n* 白细胞[杀菌]素

leuk(o)- [构词成分] 白,白细胞

leukoagglutinin [ˌljuːkəuəˈgluːtinin] *n* 白细胞凝集素

leukoblast [ˈljuːkəblæst] *n* 成白细胞 | granular ~ 前髓细胞,早幼粒细胞

leukoblastosis [ˌljuːkəblæsˈtəusis] *n* 白细胞组织增生

leukocidin [ˌljuːkəuˈsaidin] *n* 杀白细胞素

leukocoria [ˌljuːkəuˈkɔːriə] *n* 白瞳[症],瞳孔泛白

leukocrit [ˈljuːkəukrit] *n* 白细胞比容

leukocyte [ˈljuːkəsait] *n* 白细胞 | agranular ~s 无粒白细胞 / basophilic ~ 嗜碱白细胞 / endothelial ~ 内皮性白细胞 / eosinophilic ~ 嗜酸粒细胞,嗜伊红白细胞 / granular ~s(granulocytes) 粒性白细胞,粒细胞 / heterophilic ~s 嗜异性白细胞 / hyaline ~ 单核细胞 / lymphoid ~s 淋巴细胞,无粒白细胞 / mast ~ 肥大细胞,嗜碱粒细胞 / motile ~ 运动性白细胞 / neutrophilic ~ 中性粒细胞,中性白细胞 / nongranular ~s 无粒白细胞(包括淋巴细胞和单核细胞) / nonmotile ~ 非动性白细胞 / polymorphonuclear ~ 多形核白细胞 / polynuclear neutrophilic ~ 多形核中性粒细胞 / transitional ~ 单核细胞(旧称) | **leukocytic** [ˌljuːkəˈsitik], **leukocytal** [ˌljuːkəˈsaitl] *a*

leukocythemia [ˌljuːkəsaiˈθiːmiə] *n* 白血病

leukocytoblast [ˌljuːkəˈsaitəblæst] *n* 成白细胞

leukocytogenesis [ˌljuːkəˌsaitəuˈdʒenisis] *n* 白细胞形成

leukocytoid [ˈljuːkəˌsaitɔid] *a* 白细胞样的

leukocytology [ˌljuːkəsaiˈtɔlədʒi] *n* 白细胞学

leukocytolysin [ˌljuːkəsaiˈtɔlisin] *n* 白细胞溶素

leukocytolysis [ˌljuːkəsaiˈtɔlisis] *n* 白细胞溶解 | venom ~ 蛇毒性白细胞溶解 | **leukocytolytic** [ˌljuːkəˌsaitəˈlitik] *a* 白细胞溶解的 *n* 致白细胞溶解剂

leukocytoma [ˌljuːkəsaiˈtəumə] *n* 白细胞瘤

leukocytometer [ˌljuːkəsaiˈtɔmitə] *n* 白细胞计数器

leukocytopenia [ˌljuːkəsaitəuˈpiːniə] *n* 白细胞减少

leukocytophagy [ˌljuːkəsaiˈtɔfədʒi] *n* 吞噬白细胞现象(网状内皮系统的组织细胞吞噬和破坏白细胞的现象)

leukocytoplania [ˌljuːkəˌsaitəuˈpleiniə] *n* 白细胞游出

leukocytopoiesis [ˌljuːkəˌsaitəupɔiˈiːsis] *n* 白细胞生成

leukocytosis [ˌljuːkəsaiˈtəusis] *n* 白细胞增多 | absolute ~ 绝对性白细胞增多 / agonal ~, terminal ~ 濒死期白细胞增多 / basophilic ~ 嗜碱白细胞增多 / mononuclear ~ 单核细胞增多 / neutrophilic ~ 中性粒细胞增多 / pathologic ~ 病理性白细胞增多 / physiologic ~ 生理性白细胞增多 / pure ~ 单纯性白细胞增多 / relative ~ 比较性白细胞增多 / toxic ~ 中毒性白细胞增多 | **leukocytotic** [ˌljuːkəsaiˈtɔtik] *a*

leukocytotactic [ˌljuːkəˌsaitəuˈtæktik] *a* 白细胞趋向性的,诱白细胞的

leukocytotaxis [ˌljuːkəˌsaitəuˈtæksis] *n* 白细胞趋向性

leukocytotherapy [ˌljuːkəˌsaitəuˈθerəpi] *n* 白细胞疗法

leukocytotoxicity [ˌljuːkəˌsaitəutɔkˈsisəti] *n* 白细胞毒性,白细胞毒力

leukocytotoxin [ˌljuːkəˌsaitəuˈtɔksin] *n* 白细胞毒素

leukocytotropic [ˌljuːkəˌsaitəuˈtrɔpik] *a* 白细胞趋向性的,诱白细胞的

Leukocytozoon [ˌljuːkəˌsaitəˈzəuɔn] *n* 白细胞虫属

leukocyturia [ˌljuːkəsaiˈtjuəriə] *n* 白细胞尿

leukoderivative [ˌljuːkəudiˈrivətiv] *n* 白色衍生物

leukoderma [ˌljuːkəˈdəːmə] *n* 白斑病 | ~ acquisitum centrifugum 离心性获得性白斑病 / ~ colli 颈部白斑病 | **~tous** [ˌljuːkəˈdəːmətəs], **leukodermic** [ˌljuːkəˈdəːmik] *a* / **leukodermia** [ˌljuːkəˈdəːmiə] *n*

leukodextrin [ˌljuːkəuˈdekstrin] *n* 无色糊精

leukodystrophy [ˌljuːkəuˈdistrəfi] *n* 脑白质营养不良 | globoid ~, globoid cell ~ 球样细胞性脑白质营养不良 / hereditary cerebral ~, sudanophilic ~ 遗传性脑白质营养不良,嗜苏丹性脑白质营养不良,家族性脑中叶硬化 / metachromatic ~ 异染性脑白质营养不良(一种脑白质病,遗传方式属常染色体隐性,其特征为在神经和非神经组织中鞘脂类〈硫脂类〉积聚,中枢神经系统中髓磷脂弥漫性缺失。亦称异染性白质脑病,异质性白质脑病,硫脂沉积症) / spongiform ~ 海绵状脑白质营养不良

leukoedema [ˌljuːkəui(ː)ˈdiːmə] *n* 白色水肿

leukoencephalitis [ˌljuːkəuenˌsefəˈlaitis] *n* 白质脑炎;饲料中毒(马) | acute hemorrhagic ~ 急性出血性白质脑炎 / ~ periaxialis concentrica 同中心性轴周白质脑炎

leukoencephalomalacia [ˌljuːkəuenˌsəfələuməˈleiʃiə] *n* 白质脑软化;饲料中毒(马)

leukoencephalopathy [ˌljuːkəuenˌsefəˈlɔpəθi] *n* 白质脑病 | metachromatic ~ 异染性白质脑病(见 leukodystrophy 项下相应术语) / progressive multifocal ~ 进行性多灶性白质脑病 / subacute sclerosing ~ 亚急性硬化性白质脑病,亚急性硬化性全脑炎 | **leukoencephaly** [ˌljuːkəuenˈsefəli] *n*

leukoerythroblastic [ˌljuːkəuiˌriθrəuˈblæstik] *a* 成白红细胞的

leukoerythroblastosis [ˌljuːkəuiˌriθrəublæsˈtəusis] *n* 成白红细胞增多病(亦称成白红细胞性贫血、骨髓病性贫血)

leukogram [ˈljuːkəgræm] *n* 白细胞象

leukokeratosis [ˌljuːkəuˌkerəˈtəusis] *n* 黏膜白斑病

leukokinesis [ˌljuːkəukaiˈniːsis] *n* 白细胞移动 | **leukokinetic** [ˌljuːkəukaiˈnetik] *a*

leukokinetics [ˌljuːkəukaiˈnetiks] *n* 白细胞动态学

leukokinin [ˌljuːkəuˈkainin] *n* 白细胞激肽

leukokoria [ˌljuːkəuˈkɔːriə] *n* 白瞳[症],瞳孔泛白

leukokraurosis [ˌljuːkəukrɔːˈrəusis] *n* 外阴干皱

leukolymphosarcoma [ˌljuːkəuˌlimfəusɑːˈkəumə] *n* 淋巴肉瘤细胞性白血病,白血病性肉瘤

leukolysin [ˌljuːkəˈlaisin, ljuːˈkɔlisin] *n* 白细胞溶素

leukolysis [ljuːˈkɔlisis] *n* 白细胞溶解 | **leukolytic** [ˌljuːkəˈlɪtɪk] *a*

leukoma [ljuːˈkəumə] ([复] **leukomata** [ˌljuːˈkəumətə]) *n* 角膜白斑 | adherent ~ 粘连性角膜白斑 | **~tous** [ljuˈkəumətəs] *a*

leukomaine [ˌljuːkəˈmein] *n* 蛋白碱 | **leukomainic** [ˌljuːkəˈmeinik] *a*

leukomainemia [ˌljuːkəmeiˈniːmiə] *n* 蛋白碱血

leukomalacia [ˌljuːkəuməˈleiʃiə] *n* 脑白质软化 | periventricular ~ (PVL) 室周脑白质软化

leukomonocyte [ˌljuːkəuˈmɔnəsait] *n* 淋巴细胞

leukomyelitis [ˌljuːkəuˌmaiəˈlaitis] *n* 脊髓白质炎

leukomyelopathy [ˌljuːkəuˌmaiəˈlɔpəθi] *n* 脊髓白质病

leukomyoma [ˌljuːkəumaiˈəumə] *n* 白色肌瘤,脂

肌瘤
leukon [ˈljuːkɔn] *n* 白细胞系
leukonecrosis [ˌljuːkəuneˈkrəusis] *n* 白色坏疽
leukonychia [ˌljuːkəuˈnikiə] *n* 白甲
leukopathia [ˌljuːkəuˈpæθiə] *n* 白斑病 ǀ ~ punctata reticularis symmetrica 对称性网点状白斑病，特发性点状黑素过少症 ǀ **leukopathy** [ljuːˈkɔpəθi] *n*
leukopedesis [ˌljuːkəupiˈdiːsis] *n* 白细胞渗出
leukopenia [ˌljuːkəuˈpiːniə] *n* 白细胞减少 ǀ basophil ~, basophilic ~ 嗜碱白细胞减少 / congenital ~ 先天性中性粒细胞减少 / malignant ~, pernicious ~ 恶性白细胞减少，粒细胞缺乏症 ǀ **leukopenic** *a*
leukophagocytosis [ˌljuːkəuˌfægəsaiˈtəusis] *n* 吞噬白细胞现象（见 leukocytophagy）
leukophyl(l) [ˈljuːkəfil] *n* 叶白[色]素（可转为原叶绿素）
leukophyte [ˈljuːkəufait] *n* 白化植物（不含叶绿素的一种藻，即无色藻）
leukoplakia [ˌljuːkəuˈpleikiə] *n* 白斑 ǀ ~ buccalis 颊白斑 / ~ lingualis 舌白斑 / oral ~ 口腔白斑[症] / speckled ~ 颗粒性白斑 / ~ vulvae 外阴白斑，外阴干皱 ǀ **leukoplasia** [ˌljuːkəuˈpleiziə] *n*
leukoplastid [ˌljuːkəˈplæstid], **leukoplast** [ˈljuːkəplæst] *n* 白色体
leukopoiesis [ˌljuːkəpɔiˈiːsis] *n* 白细胞生成 ǀ **leukopoietic** [ˌljuːkəpɔiˈetik] *a*
leukopoietin [ˌljuːkəupɔiˈiːtin] *n* 白细胞生成素；粒细胞生成素
leukoprecipitin [ˌljuːkəupriˈsipitin] *n* 白细胞沉淀素（对白细胞抗原具有特异性的一种沉淀素）
leukoprophylaxis [ˌljuːkəuprɔfiˈlæksis] *n* 白细胞预防法（通过人工的方法增加血中白细胞数以便获得对外科感染的免疫性）
leukopsin [ljuːˈkɔpsin] *n* 视白质
leukorrhagia [ˌljuːkəˈreidʒiə] *n* 白带过多
leukorrhea [ˌljuːkəˈriə] *n* 白带 ǀ menstrual ~, periodic ~ 经期白带 ǀ **~l** *a*
leukosarcoma [ˌljuːkəsɑːˈkəumə] *n* 白血病性肉瘤
leukosarcomatosis [ˌljuːkəsɑːˌkəuməˈtəusis] *n* 白血病性肉瘤病
leukoscope [ˈljuːkəskəup] *n* 色盲测验器
leukosis [ljuːˈkəusis] ([复] **leukoses** [ljuːˈkəusiːz]) *n* 白血病，造白细胞组织增生 ǀ avian ~, fowl ~ 禽类白血病 / lymphoid ~ 淋巴样白血病 / myeloblastic ~ 成髓细胞白血病 / myelocytic ~ 髓细胞白血病
leukospermia [ˌljuːkəuˈspəːmiə] *n* 白细胞精液
leukotaxin(e) [ˌljuːkəˈtæksin] *n* 白细胞诱素（组织损伤时出现的一种晶体含氮多肽，可从炎症渗出液中分出，能促进白细胞增多，增高毛细管渗透性和促使白细胞渗出）
leukotaxis [ˌljuːkəˈtæksis] *n* 白细胞趋向性 ǀ **leukotactic** *a* 白细胞趋向性的，诱白细胞的
leukotherapy [ˌljuːkəuˈθerəpi] *n* 白细胞疗法 ǀ preventive ~ 预防性白细胞疗法（见 leukoprophylaxis）
Leukothrix [ˈljuːkəuθriks] *n* 亮发菌属
leukothrombin [ˌljuːkəuˈθrɔmbin] *n* 白细胞凝血酶
leukotome [ˈljuːkətəum] *n* 脑白质切断器
leukotomy [ljuːˈkɔtəmi] *n* 脑白质切断术 ǀ transorbital ~ 经眼眶白质切断术
leukotoxic [ˌljuːkəˈtɔksik] *a* 毒害白细胞的
leukotoxicity [ˌljuːkətɔkˈsisəti] *n* 白细胞毒性（对白细胞有毒性）
leukotoxin [ˌljuːkəˈtɔksin] *n* 白细胞毒素
Leukotrichaceae [ˌljuːkəutriˈkeisiiː] *n* 亮发菌科
leukotrichia [ˌljuːkəˈtrikiə] *n* 白发
leukotriene [ˌljuːkəuˈtraiiːn] *n* 白细胞三烯，白三烯（一类具有生物活性的化合物，其功能为调节变态反应和炎症反应，白三烯 A，B，C，D 和 E 加上下标表明分子中的双键数。有些〈LTB_4〉促进白细胞运动，有些〈LTC_4，LTD_4 和 LTE_4〉构成过敏性慢反应物质，从而引起支气管收缩以及其他变态反应）
leukourobilin [ˌljuːkəjuərəˈbailin] *n* 白色尿胆素
leukovirus [ˈljuːkəuˌvaiərəs] *n* 白血病病毒
Leunbach's paste [ˌlɔiənˈbɑːh]（Jonathan H. Leunbach）洛因巴赫糊（以前曾用于注入子宫引起流产）
leupeptin [ˌljuːˈpeptin] *n* 亮肽素
leuprolide acetate [ljuːˈprəulaid] 醋酸亮丙利特（一种合成的促性腺激素释放激素类似物，用作抗肿瘤药，姑息性治疗晚期前列腺癌，亦用于治疗子宫内膜异位症和中枢性性早熟。皮下和肌内给药）
leuprorelin acetate [ˌljuːprəuˈrelin] 醋酸亮丙瑞林（leuprolide acetate 的 INN 和 BAN 名）
Levaditi's method [ˌlevəˈdiːtiː]（Constantin Levaditi）列瓦迪提[染色]法（使用还原银显示切片中梅毒螺旋体之法）ǀ ~ stain 列瓦迪提染剂（染螺旋体）
levalbuterol hydrochloride [ˌlevælˈbjuːtərɔl] 盐酸左沙丁胺醇（支气管扩张药）
levallorphan tartrate [ˌlevəˈlɔːfæn] 酒石酸左洛啡烷（吗啡拮抗药）
levamfetamine [ˌlivæmˈfetəmiːn] *n* 左苯丙胺（食欲抑制药）ǀ ~ succinate 琥珀酸左苯丙胺 ǀ **levamphetamine** *n*
levamisole hydrochloride [liˈvæmisəul] 盐酸左

旋咪唑(抗蠕虫药,也是免疫增强剂,用于癌症以刺激免疫反应)

levan [ˈlevæn] *n* 果聚糖

levansucrase [ˌlevænˈsuːkreis] *n* 蔗糖-6-果糖基转移酶,果聚糖蔗糖酶

levarterenol [ˌlevɑːtəˈriːnɔl] *n* 去甲肾上腺素(升压药) | ~ bitartrate 重酒石酸去甲肾上腺素(血管加压药)

levator [ləˈveitə] ([复] **levators** 或 **levatores** [ˌlevəˈtɔːriːz]) *n* 提肌;骨片提拉器

level [ˈlevl] *n* 水平,等级,浓度 | confidence ~ 置信度 / ~s of consciousness 意识程度,神志清醒程度,意识水准 / isoelectric ~ 等电位(心电图基线) / significance ~, ~ of significance, α-~ 显著性水平(统计检测无效假设时用)

levetiracetam [ˌlevətaiˈræsətæm] *n* 左乙拉西坦(抗惊厥药,口服给药,用作辅剂治疗成人癫痫的部分发作)

levicellular [ˌleviˈseljulə] *a* 平滑细胞的

levidulinose [liˈvidjulinəus] *n* 甘露三糖

levigation [ˌleviˈgeiʃən] *n* 研磨,研碎,研末

Lévi-Lorain dwarf [leiˈviː ləuˈrei] (E. L. Lévi; Paul J. Lorain) 莱-洛侏儒(垂体性侏儒) | ~ infantilism(syndrome) 莱-洛幼稚型(综合征)(垂体性幼稚型)

Levin's tube [ləˈvin] (Abraham L. Levin) 列文管(经鼻胃肠管)

Lévi's syndrome [ˈleivi] (E. Léopold Lévi) 阵发性甲状腺功能亢进

levitation [ˌleviˈteiʃən] *n* (躯体)飘浮感;(严重烧伤患者的)支持系统

lev(o)- [构词成分]左,向左;左旋

levmetamfetamine [ˌlevmetæmˈfetəmiːn] *n* 左去氧麻黄碱(用作鼻减轻充血剂,吸入使用)

levobetaxolol hydrochloride [ˌlevəubeiˈtæksəlɔl] 盐酸左倍他洛尔(β 受体阻滞药,局部用于结膜,治疗高眼压症和青光眼)

levobunolol hydrochloride [ˌlevəuˈbjuːnəulɔl] 盐酸左布诺洛尔(β 受体阻滞药,局部用于结膜,治疗青光眼和高眼压症)

levobupivacaine hydrochloride [ˌlevəubjuːˈpivəkein] 盐酸左布比卡因(局部麻醉药,用于外科手术时的局部浸润麻醉、周围神经传导阻滞和硬膜外麻醉,亦用于术后疼痛处理)

levocabastine hydrochloride [ˌlevəuˈkæbəstiːn] 盐酸左卡巴斯汀(抗组胺药,局部用于结膜,治疗季节性变应性结膜炎)

levocardia [ˌliːvəuˈkɑːdiə] *n* 左位心 | isolated ~ 孤立性左位心 / mixed ~ 混合性左位心

levocardiogram [ˌliːvəuˈkɑːdiəgræm] *n* 左心电图

levocarnitine [ˌliːvəuˈkɑːnitiːn] *n* 左卡尼汀(用于治疗原发性系统性卡尼汀〈carnitine〉缺乏症,口服给药)

levoclination [ˌliːvəuklaiˈneiʃən, -kliˈn-] *n* 左旋(眼)

levodopa [ˌliːvəuˈdəupə] *n* 左旋多巴,左多巴(抗胆碱药,抗震颤麻痹药)

levoduction [ˌliːvəuˈdʌkʃən], **levocycloduction** [ˌliːvəuˌsaikləuˈdʌkʃən] *n* 左旋(眼)

levofloxacin [ˌlevəuˈflɔksəsin] *n* 左氧氟沙星(抗菌药)

levofuraltadone [ˌliːvəufjuəˈræltədəun] *n* 左呋喃他酮(抗菌药,抗原虫药)

levogram [ˈlevəgræm] *n* 左心电图;轴左偏心电图(表明左心室肥大)

levogyral [liːvəuˈdʒaiərəl] *a* 左旋的

levogyration [ˌliːvəudʒaiəˈreiʃən] *n* 左旋

levomepromazine [ˌliːvəuməˈprəuməziːn] *n* 左美丙嗪(即甲氧异丁嗪 methotrimeprazine,镇痛药,安定药)

levomethadyl acetate [ˌliːvəuˈmeθədil] 左醋美沙朵(麻醉止痛药,用于治海洛因瘾)

levonordefrin [ˌliːvəuˈnɔːdifrin] *n* 左旋异肾上腺素(血管收缩药)

levonorgestrel [ˌliːvəunɔːˈdʒestrel] *n* 左炔诺孕酮(与雌激素组分结合,用作口服避孕药)

levopropoxyphene napsylate [ˌliːvəuprəˈpɔksifiːn ˈnæpsileit] 萘磺酸左丙氧吩(镇咳药)

levopropylcillin potassium [ˌliːvəuˌprəupilˈsilin] 左普匹西林钾(抗菌药)

levorotary [ˌliːvəuˈrəutəri], **levorotatory** [ˌliːvəuˈrəutəˌtəri] *a* 左旋的

levorotation [ˌliːvəurəuˈteiʃən] *n* 左旋

levorphanol tartrate [liˈvɔːfənəul] 酒石酸左啡诺(麻醉性镇痛药)

levotartaric acid [ˌliːvəutɑːˈtærik] 左旋酒石酸

levothyroxine sodium [ˌliːvəuθaiˈrɔksiːn] 左甲状腺素钠(甲状腺激素)

levotorsion [ˌliːvəuˈtɔːʃən] *n* 左旋(眼)

levoversion [ˌliːvəuˈvəːʃən] *n* 左转,左旋

levoxadrol hydrochloride [liːˈvɔksədrɔl] 盐酸左噁屈尔(局部麻醉药,平滑肌松弛药)

Levret's forceps [ləˈvrei] (André Levret) 利夫雷产钳(一种改良的原始产钳) | ~ law 利夫雷定律(前置胎盘的脐带为边缘性附着)

Lev's disease [lev] (Maurice Lev) 列夫病(获得性完全性心传导阻滞,由于心脏骨骼硬化所致)

levulan [ˈlevjulən] *n* 果聚糖

levulin [ˈlevjulin] *n* 块茎糖,多缩左旋糖

levulinic acid [ˌlevjuˈlinik] 乙酰丙酸

levulosan [ˌlevjuˈləusən] *n* 果聚糖(如菊粉)

levulosazone [ˌlevjuˈləusəzəun] *n* 果糖脎

levulose [ˈlevjuləus] *n* 果糖

levulosemia [ˌlevjuləˈsiːmiə] *n* 果糖血[症]
levulosuria [ˌlevjuləˈsjuəriə] *n* 果糖尿
levurid(e) [ˈlevjurid] *n* 念珠菌疹
Levy-Hollister syndrome [ˈliːvi ˈhɔlistə] (Walter J. Levy; David W. Hollister) 莱-霍综合征，泪-耳-牙-指(趾)综合征(即 lacrimo-auriculo-dento-digital syndrome，见 syndrome 项下相应术语)
Lévy-Roussy syndrome [leiˈviː ruˈsiː] (Gabrielle Lévy; Gustave Roussy) 雷维-罗西综合征(见 Roussy-Lévy syndrome)
Lewandowsky-Lutz disease [levɑːnˈdɔvski luːts] (F. Lewandowsky; Wilhelm Lutz) 莱-鲁病，疣状表皮发育不良
Lewandowsky's nevus elasticus [levɑːnˈdɔvski] (Felix Lewandowsky) 莱万多夫斯基弹力纤维痣，结缔组织痣
Lewis blood group [ˈljuːis] (Lewis 为 1946 年首次报道的英国先证者的姓) 刘易斯血型，依附于红细胞表面的血浆糖脂决定的一种血型。该血型依据显性独立 *Le* 基因，但与 A 和 B 的 H 前体寡糖相互作用。*Le/le* 提供"双负"血型 Le(a－b－)，而不伴 H 的 *Le* 产生 Le^a，即血型 Le(a＋b－)，伴 H 的则产生 Le^bH，即血型 Le(a－b＋)
lewisite [ˈlju(ː)isait] *n* (W. Lee Lewis) 刘易斯毒气(一种致命的军用毒气)
Lewisohn's method [ˈlju(ː)isn] (Richard Lewisohn) 刘易逊法(血内加枸橼酸钠的一种间接输血法)
Lewis-Pickering test [ljuːis ˈpikəriŋ] (T. Lewis; George W. Pickering) 刘-皮试验(使用迅速升温的方法，使待检部分产生血管扩张，以检外周循环状况)
Lewis' reaction [ljuːis] (Thomas Lewis) 刘易斯反应，风团潮红反应(即 wheal and flare reaction，见 reaction 项下相应术语)
Lewy bodies [ˈleivi] (Frederic H. Lewy) 雷维小体(向心性多层的圆形小体，见于震颤麻痹病人的中脑一些神经元的胞质液泡内)
Leyden jar [ˈlaidən] 莱登瓶(用作电流的电容器或聚电器)
Leyden-Möbius dystrophy, type [ˈlaidən ˈmiːbiəs] (E. V. von Leyden; Paul J. Möbius) 肢带肌营养不良(进行性肌营养不良)
Leyden's ataxia [ˈlaidən] (Ernst V. von Leyden) 假脊髓痨 | ~ crystals 莱登晶体(嗜酸粒细胞破碎后晶体，亦称气喘晶体，白细胞晶体) / ~ disease 莱登病(周期性呕吐)
leydigarche [ˌlaidiˈgɑːki] *n* 睾丸功能开始
Leydig's cells [ˈlaidiʃ] (Franz von Leydig) 莱迪希细胞(①睾丸间质细胞，亦称间介细胞；②不排出黏液于上皮表面的黏液细胞) | ~ aplasia 睾丸间质细胞发育不全 / ~ cylinders 莱迪希圆柱体(被原生质所隔开的肌纤维束) / ~ duct 中肾管
Lf (limes flocculating) 絮状反应限量
LFA left frontoanterior 额左前(胎位)
LFA-1 leukocyte function-associated antigen 1 白细胞功能相关抗原 1
LFA-2 leukocyte function-associated antigen 2 白细胞功能相关抗原 2
LFA-3 leukocyte function-associated antigen 3 白细胞功能相关抗原 3
L-form L-型，L-相变种(L phase variant)
LFP left frontoposterior 额左后(胎位)
LFT left frontotransverse 额左横(胎位)
LGB laparoscopic gastric banding 腹腔镜胃环束术
LH luteinizing hormone 黄体化激素，黄体生成素，促黄体素
Lhermitte's sign [ˈlɛəmit] (Jean Lhermitte) 莱尔米特征(当病人将头向前屈曲时，发生突然的、短暂的电击样休克感觉向下扩散到全身，主要见于多发性脑脊髓硬化、脊髓变性及颈髓损伤)
LH-RH luteinizing hormone-releasing hormone 促黄体素释放素
Li lithium 锂
LIA leukemia-associated inhibitory activity 白细胞相关抑制活性
liability [ˌlaiəˈbiləti] *n* 易患性
-liberin [构词成分]释放素
liberomotor [ˌlibərəˈməutə] *a* 随意运动的
libidinal [liˈbidinəl] *a* 性欲的，色情的；力必多的
libidinous [liˈbidinəs] *a* 好色的
libido [liˈbiːdəu, liˈbaidəu] ([复] **libidines** [liˈbidiniːz]) *n* 【拉】性欲；欲望；力必多，欲力 | bisexual ~ 两性性欲 / ego ~ 自爱欲，恋己癖
Libman-Sacks disease (syndrome) [ˈlibmən ˈsæks] (Emanuel Libman; Benjamin Sacks) 利伯曼-萨克斯病(综合征)，非典型性疣状心内膜炎
Libman's sign [ˈlibmən] (Emanuel Libman) 利伯曼征(乳突骨尖部剧烈触痛，但无压痛)
libra (L.) [ˈliːbrə, ˈlaibrə] *n* ([复] **librae** [ˈliːbriː, ˈlai-]) 【拉】磅
library [ˈlaibrəri] *n* 文库(在遗传学上指一套克隆的 DNA 片断，这些片断一起代表整个基因组或者由某一特别组织转录的基因群。亦称 DNA 文库)
lice [lais] louse 的复数
Liceida [liˈsaidə] *n* 无丝目
license, licence [ˈlaisəns] *n* 执照
licentiate [laiˈsenʃiit] *n* 执照持有人；开业证持有人
lichen [ˈlaikən] *n* 地衣；苔藓 | ~ chronicus simplex, ~ simplex chronicus 慢性单纯性苔藓、神

经性皮炎 / ~ nitidus 光泽苔藓 / ~ obtusus corneus 角质性钝头苔藓 / ~ planus 扁平苔藓 / ~ ruber moniliformis 念珠状红苔藓 / ~ sclerosus et atrophicus 硬化萎缩性苔藓 / ~ scrofulosorum, ~ scrofulosus 瘰疬性苔藓 / ~ spinulosus, ~ pilaris 小棘苔藓,毛发苔藓 / ~ striatus 条纹状苔藓 / ~ tropicus 热带苔藓,粟疹 / ~ urticatus 荨麻疹性苔藓,丘疹性荨麻疹 | **~ous** [ˈlaikinəs], **~ose** [ˈlaikinəus] *a*

lichenase [ˈlaikəneis] *n* 地衣多糖酶,昆布多糖酶

lichenification [ˌlaikənifiˈkeiʃən] *n* 苔藓样变,苔藓化

licheniformin [laiˌkeniˈfɔːmin] *n* 地衣形菌素

lichenin [ˈlaikənin] *n* 地衣淀粉

lichenoid [ˈlaikənɔid] *a* 苔藓样的

Lich-Gregoir technique [lik grəˈgwɑː] (R. Lich; W. Gregoir) 利-格技术(见 Lich technique)

Lich technique [lik] (R. Lich, Jr.) 利克技术(一型输尿管膀胱吻合术,将输尿管从依附于膀胱处切除,再重新将输尿管依附于膀胱内造成的黏膜下隧道)

Lichtenstein repair [ˈliːktənˌstain] (Irving L. Lichtenstein) 列克登斯坦修复术(无张力疝修复术)

Lichtheimia [likˈθaimiə] *n* 毛霉菌属(犁头霉属 Absidia 的旧名)

Lichtheim's aphasia [ˈliʃthaim] (Ludwig Lichtheim) 利希特海姆失语(可重复他人语言,但无自发说话能力) | ~ disease 利希特海姆病(亚急性脊髓混合变性) / ~ plaque 利希特海姆斑(恶性贫血时大脑白质的变性区) / ~ sign 利希特海姆征(皮质性失语患者不能言语,但能用手指示意) / ~ syndrome 利希特海姆综合征(亚急性脊髓混合变性) / ~ test 利希特海姆测验(检查失语症)

Licnophorina [ˌliknəufəuˈrainə] *n* 簸箕虫亚目

licorice [ˈlikəris] *n* 甘草

lid [lid] *n* 睑 | granular ~s 沙眼

lidamidine [laiˈdæmidiːn] *n* 利达脒(止泻药)

lidamine [ˈlaidəmiːn] *n* 利达明(止泻药)

Liddell and Sherrington reflex [liˈdel ˈʃeriŋtən] (Edward G. T. Liddell; Sir Charles S. Sherrington) 牵张反射

Liddle syndrome [ˈlidəl] (Grant W. Liddle) 利德尔综合征(一种罕见的常染色体显性遗传综合征,特征为高血压伴肾重吸收钠过多、钾丢失以及肾素和醛固酮活性低)

lidocaine [ˈlaidəkein] *n* 利多卡因(局部麻醉及抗心律失常药) | ~ hydrochloride 盐酸利多卡因(局部麻醉药)

lidofenin (HIDA) [ˌlaidəuˈfenin] *n* 利多苯宁酸(测肝功能)

lidoflazine [ˌlaidəuˈfleiziːn] *n* 利多氟嗪(冠状动脉扩张药)

lie [lai] *n* 产式 | longitudinal ~ 纵产式 / transverse ~ 横产式

lie² [lai] *n* 谎言 | white ~ 不怀恶意的谎言

Lieben's test (reaction) [ˈliːbən] (Adolf Lieben) 李本试验(反应)(检尿丙酮)

Lieberkühn's ampulla [ˈliːbəkwiːn] (Johann N. Lieberkühn) 利贝屈恩壶腹(肠绒毛内乳糜管壶腹) | ~ glands (crypts, follicles) 肠腺

Liebermann-Burchard test (reaction) [ˈliːbəmɑːn ˈbəːkhɑːd] (Carl T. Liebermann; H. Burchard) 李-伯试验(反应)(检胆固醇:胆固醇氯仿混合液中加入浓缩于醋酐的硫酸后即产生蓝绿色)

Liebermann's test [ˈliːbəmɑːn] (Leo von S. Liebermann) 李伯曼试验(检蛋白质)

Liebermeister's furrow [ˈliːbəmaistə] (Carl von Liebermeister) 肋压迹 | ~ grooves 利贝迈斯特沟(肝表面上的发育沟) / ~ rule 利贝迈斯特规律(发热性心动过速时,体温每升高 1 ℃,脉率每分钟约增加 8 次)

Liebig's test [ˈliːbig] (Justus von Liebig) 利比希试验(检胱氨酸) | ~ theory 利比希学说(易氧化的烃类为动物提供热能的食物)

lien [ˈlaiən] *n*【拉】脾 | ~ mobilis 游动脾 | **~al** [laiˈiːnəl] *a*

lienculus [laiˈenkjuləs] *n* 副脾

lienectomy [ˌlaiəˈnektəmi] *n* 脾切除术

lienitis [ˌlaiəˈnaitis] *n* 脾炎

lien(o)- [构词成分]脾

lienocele [laiˈiːnəsiːl] *n* 脾疝

lienography [ˌlaiiˈnɔgrəfi] *n* 脾造影[术]

lienomalacia [laiˌiːnəuməˈleiʃiə] *n* 脾软化

lienomedullary [laiˌiːnəuˈmedələri] *a* 脾骨髓的

lienomyelogenous [laiˌiːnəumaiəˈlɔdʒinəs] *a* 脾骨髓原的

lienomyelomalacia [laiˌiːnəumaiələuməˈleiʃiə] *n* 脾骨髓软化

lienopancreatic [laiˌiːnəuˌpæŋkriˈætik] *a* 脾胰的

lienopathy [ˌlaiiˈnɔpəθi] *n* 脾病

lienorenal [laiˌiːnəˈriːnəl] *a* 脾肾的

lienotoxin [laiˌiːnəuˈtɔksin] *n* 脾毒素

lientery [ˈlaiəntəri] *n* 消化不良性腹泻 | **lienteric** [ˌlaiənˈterik] *a*

lienunculus [ˌlaiəˈnʌŋkjuləs] *n* 副脾

Liepmann's apraxia [ˈliːpmɑːn] (Hugo C. Liepmann) 利普曼运用不能(四肢并不麻痹,却不能作协调运动)

Liesegang's phenomenon (striae, waves) [ˈliːzəgʌŋ] (Ralph E. Liesegang) 利泽甘现象(纹、波)(两种电解质在溶胶中扩散和遇合时所

形成的环状、波状、纹状沉淀)

Lieskeela [liːskiːˈelə] (Lieske) *n* 利斯克菌属 | ~ bifida 双歧利斯克菌

Lieutaud's triangle (body) [ljuˈtɔː] (Joseph Lieutaud) 膀胱三角 | ~ uvula (luette) 膀胱悬雍垂

LIF left iliac fossa 左髂窝; leukocyte inhibitory factor 白细胞抑制因子

life [laif] ([复] **lives** [laivz]) *n* 生命;寿命;生活 | animal ~ 动物;动物性生活 / intellectual ~, mental ~, psychic ~ 精神生活 / intrauterine ~, uterine 宫内寿命,宫内存活 / vegetative ~ 植物;植物性生活

life-span [ˈlaifˈspæn] *n* 寿命;平均生命期

lifetime [ˈlaiftaim] *n* 寿命,平均寿命

lifibrate [liˈfaibreit] *n* 利贝特(抗高血脂药)

lig. ligament, ligamentum 韧带

ligament [ˈligəmənt] *n* 韧带 | accessory ~ 副韧带 / broad ~ 阔韧带 / cardinal ~ 主韧带,基本韧带 / check ~s of axis 翼状韧带 / cotyloid ~ 髋关节盂缘,髋臼唇 / crural ~ 腹股沟韧带 / spring ~ 跟舟跖侧韧带 / triangular ~ of linea alba 白线支座 | **~ous** [ˌligəˈmentəs] *a*

ligamentopexy [ˌligəˌmentəuˈpeksi], **ligamentopexis** [ˌligəˈmentəuˈpeksis] *n* 圆韧带固定术,吊宫术

ligamentum [ˌligəˈmentəm] ([复] **ligamenta** [ˌligəˈmentə]) *n* 【拉】韧带

ligand [ˈlaigənd, ˈligənd] *n* 配体(能和某一结构的互补位置相结合的分子,如氧是血红蛋白的配合基)

ligase [ˈlaigeis, ˈligeis] *n* 连接酶

ligate [ˈlaigeit] *vt* 结扎

ligation [laiˈgeiʃən] *n* 结扎[术],[结]扎法 | pole ~ 两极扎法(甲状腺) / tubal ~ 输卵管结扎[术]

ligature [ˈligətʃuə] *n* 结扎线,缚线;[结]扎法 | chain ~ 锁链样扎法 / elastic ~ 弹性结扎线 / interlacing ~, interlocking ~ 交叉扎法 / kangaroo ~ 袋鼠腱结扎线 / lateral ~ 侧扎法 / occluding ~ 闭塞性扎法 / provisional ~ 临时结扎线 / soluble ~ 可溶化结扎线 / suboccluding ~ 轻闭塞性扎法 / terminal ~ 末端扎法 / thread-elastic ~ (牙列矫形)弹性结扎线

Ligg. ligaments, ligamenta 韧带

light[1] [lait] *n* 光,光线 | actinic ~ 光化性光 / ~ difference 光差 / diffused ~ 弥散光 / idioretinal ~ 视网膜自发光感 / infrared ~ 红外线 / intrinsic ~ 内在光感(视网膜) / ~ minimum 最低度光觉 / polarized ~ 偏振光 / reflected ~ 反射光 / refracted ~ 折射光 / ultraviolet ~ 紫外线

light[2] [lait] *a* 轻的;晕眩的;易消化的;淡食的;浅[色]的

lightening [ˈlaitniŋ] *n* 胎儿下降感(产前数星期子宫下降所致的感觉)

Lightwood's syndrome [ˈlaitwuːd] (Reginald Lightwood) 赖特伍德综合征,肾小管性酸中毒

Lignac syndrome [liːˈnjɑːk] (George O. E. Lignac), **Lignac-Fanconi syndrome** [liːˈnjɑːk fɑːŋˈkəuni] (G. O. E. Lignac; Guido Fanconi) 利尼亚克综合征,利-范综合征(①见 Fanconi syndrome ②解; ②胱氨酸病)

ligneous [ˈligniəs] *a* 木的,木质的;木样的

Lignières' test (reaction) [liːˈnjɛə] (José Lignières) 利尼埃尔试验(反应)(一种结核菌素皮肤反应)

lignin [ˈlignin] *n* 木素

lignocaine [ˈlignəkein] *n* 利多卡因(局部麻醉药,抗心律失常药)

lignocellulose [ˌlignəˈseljuləus] *n* 木质纤维素

lignocerate [ˌlignəusiəreit] *n* 木蜡酸(盐、酯或阴离子型)

lignoceric acid [ˌlignəˈserik] 木蜡酸

lignum [ˈlignəm] *n* 【拉】木 | ~ sanctum, ~ vitae 愈创木

ligroin(e) [ˈligrəuin] *n* 石油英,轻石油

likelihood [ˈlaiklihud] *n* 似然[性];似然值

Liley chart [ˈlili] (Sir (Albert) William Liley) 利利图表(利用光谱仪测量羊水胆红素水平针对孕龄标绘的图表,以估计由于 Rh 同种免疫所致的胎儿溶血严重程度。图表分成 3 个区,测量下降在区 1 内,提示无病或轻度疾病,而下降在区 3 内,则提示严重疾病,伴随着即将来临的胎儿死亡)

Lilienthal's probe [ˈliliənˌθæl] (Howard Lilienthal) 利连撒尔探子(检弹探子)

limb [lim] *n* 肢,四肢 | anacrotic ~ (脉波)升脚,升支 / lower ~ 下肢 / pectoral ~, thoracic ~ 上肢 / pelvic ~ 下肢 / phantom ~ 幻肢 / upper ~ 上肢

limberneck [ˈlimbənek] *n* 鸡垂颈病

limbus [ˈlimbəs] ([复] **limbi** [ˈlimbai]) *n* 【拉】缘 | ~ of cornea 角膜缘 | **limbic** [ˈlimbik], **limbal** [ˈlimbəl] *a* 缘的

lime [laim] *n* 石灰,氧化钙,酸柚,枸橼 | ~ arsenate 砷酸石灰(杀昆虫剂) / chlorinated ~ 氯化石灰,含氯石灰,漂白粉 / slaked ~ 熟石灰,消石灰,氢氧化钙 / soda ~ 碱石灰 / sulfurated ~ 硫化石灰

limen [ˈlaimən] ([复] **limina** [ˈliminə]) *n* 【拉】阈 | ~ of insula 岛阈 / ~ of twoness 两触点区别阈,两点阈

limes [ˈlaimiːz] *n* 界量,限量 | ~ dose 限量(指 L_+ dose, Lo dose, Lf dose 和 Lr dose,见 dose 项

下各相关术语）

liminal [ˈliminəl] *a* 易觉的；阈的；阈限的

liminometer [ˌlimiˈnɔmitə] *n* 反射阈计

limit [ˈlimit] *n* 限度，界限，范围，极限 | assimilation ~, saturation ~ 同化限度，饱和限度 / audibility ~ 可听限度 / ~ of flocculation 絮状限度（用以表示毒素、类毒素和抗毒素的强度的术语）/ ~ of perception 视觉限度 / quantum ~ 量子限，最短波长

limitans [ˈlimitənz] *n*【拉】界膜

limitation [ˌlimiˈteiʃən] *n* 限界，限制，限度，局限 | eccentric ~ 偏心性限界（指视野）/ genetic ~ 遗传限度（指所有细胞必需依其所属特殊种类的标准发生反应）

limitative [ˈlimiteitiv] *a* 限制［性］的

limit dextrinase [ˈdekstrineis] 极限糊精酶，低聚-1, 6-葡糖苷酶

limitrophic [ˌlimiˈtrɔfik] *a* 控制营养的

Limnatis [limˈneitis] *n* 软水蛭属 | ~ nilotica 尼罗河水蛭（亦称埃及水蛭 Hirudo aegyptiaca）

limnology [limˈnɔlədʒi] *n* 湖沼学

limo [ˈlaiməu] *n*【拉】柠檬

limonene [ˈliməniːn] *n* 柠檬烯，柠烯

limonis [laiˈməunis] *a*【拉】柠檬的

limonite [ˈlimənait] *n* 褐铁矿

limophthisis [laiˈmɔfθisis] *n* 饥饿性虚损

limosis [laiˈməusis] *n* 善饥症

limotherapy [ˌlaiməuˈθerəpi] *n* 饥饿疗法

limp [limp] *vi*, *n* 跛行

limpet [ˈlimpət] *n* 蝛 | keyhole ~ 钥孔蝛

linamarin [ˌlinəˈmɛərin] *n* 亚麻苦苷

lincomycin [ˌliŋkəuˈmaisin] *n* 林可霉素（抗生素类药）| ~ hydrochloride 盐酸林可霉素（抗生素类药）

linctus [ˈliŋktəs], **lincture** [ˈliŋktʃə] *n* 舐剂，药糖剂

lindane [ˈlindein] *n* 林旦（抗寄生虫药）

Lindau's disease, Lindau-von Hippel disease [ˈlindau fəun ˈhipəl] (Arvid Lindau; Eugen von Hippel) 林道病、林道-冯·希佩尔病（见 Hippel-Lindau disease）

Lindau's disease [ˈlindau] (Arvid Lindau) 林道病（见 Hippel-Lindau disease）| ~ tumor 林道瘤（成血管细胞瘤）

Lindbergh pump [ˈlindbəːg] (Charles A. Lindbergh) 林白泵（一种灌注泵，用于长期保存离体器官）

Lindemann's cannula [ˈlindəmən] (August Lindemann) 林德曼套管（输血套管）| ~ method 林德曼法（输血法）

linden [ˈlindən] *n* 椴

line [lain] *n* 线；界线；系；家系；血统 | abdominal ~ 腹线 / adrenal ~, white adrenal ~ 肾上腺性白线（腹部手指划痕后发生的白线，见于肾上腺功能不良）/ atropic ~ 眼旋转轴平面方向线 / base ~ 底线 / base-apex ~ 底尖线，折光角等分线 / blood ~ 血统 / blue ~ 蓝线，铅线（慢性铅中毒）/ cell ~ 细胞系（指原代细胞培养以后的传代培养物）/ established cell ~ 确立细胞株 / lead ~ 蓝线，铅线（铅中毒）/ lower lung ~ 肺下界线 / mammary ~ 乳头线 / median ~ 正中线，中线 / primitive ~ 原线，原条 / recessional ~s 退缩线 / ~ of sight 视线 / visual ~ 视线，视轴

linea [ˈliniə] ([复] **lineae** [ˈliniiː]) *n*【拉】线

lineage [ˈliniidʒ] *n* 谱系 | cell ~ 细胞谱系

linear [ˈliniə] *a* 线的，直线的；线形的；线性的

Lineola [liniːˈəulə] *n* 线丝菌属

liner [ˈlainə] *n* 衬里，衬垫 | cavity ~ 龋洞分离剂，护洞剂，洞衬剂

Lineweaver-Burk equation [ˈlainwiːvə bəːk] (Hans Lineweaver; Dean Burk) 莱因威弗-伯克方程式（为米凯利斯-门顿〈Michaelis-Menten〉酶动力学方程式的重排；$1/v = (K_m/V_{max})(1/[S]) + 1/V_{max}$，其中，$v$ 为反应常数，[S] 为底物浓度，V_{max} 为最大速度，K_m 为米氏〈Michaelis〉常数。如果酶反应按照米凯利斯-门顿动力学进行，则 $1/v$ 对 1/[S] 的标绘将为一直线，见 Lineweaver-Burk plot）| ~ plot 莱因威弗-伯克图（为米凯利斯-门顿〈Michaelis-Menten〉方程式的双倒数变换图，其中 $1/v$ 作为 1/[S] 的函数作图。当 x-截距在 $-1/K_m$，y-截距在 $1/V_{max}$ 时，可得一条直线）

linezolid [liˈnezəulid] *n* 利奈佐列（合成抗菌药）

lingua [ˈliŋgwə] ([复] **linguae** [ˈliŋgwiː]) *n*【拉】舌 | ~ frenata 结舌，舌系带短缩/ ~ geographica 地图样舌 / ~ nigra, ~ villosa nigra 黑舌［病］/ ~ plicata 裂缝舌

lingual [ˈliŋgwəl] *a* 舌的 | **~ly** *ad* 向舌

linguale [liŋˈgweili] *n* 舌点（下颌联合舌面上端的一点）

lingualis [liŋˈgweilis] ([复] **linguales** [liŋˈgweiliz]) *a*【拉】舌的

Linguatula [liŋˈgwætjulə] *n* 舌形虫属 | ~ serrata, ~ rhinaria 鼻腔舌形虫，锯齿状舌形虫

linguatuliasis [liŋˌgwætjuˈlaiəsis], **linguatulosis** [liŋˌgwætjuˈləusis] *n* 舌形虫病

linguatulid [liŋˈgwætjulid] *n* 舌形虫

Linguatulidae [liŋgwəˈtjuːlidiː] *n* 舌形虫科

linguiform [ˈliŋgwifɔːm] *a* 舌形的

lingula [ˈliŋgjulə] ([复] **lingulae** [ˈliŋgjuliː]) *n*【拉】小舌 | **~r** *a*

lingulate [ˈliŋgjulit] *a* 舌形的，舌状的

lingulectomy [ˌliŋgjuˈlektəmi] *n* 肺小舌切除术，

肺舌叶切除术
lingu(o)- [构词成分]舌
linguoaxial [ˌliŋgwəˈæksiəl] *a* 舌轴的
linguoaxiogingival [ˌliŋgwəˌæksiəuˈdʒindʒivəl] *a* 舌轴龈的
linguocervical [ˌliŋgwəˈsəːvikəl] *a* 舌颈的,舌龈的
linguoclination [ˌliŋgwəuklaiˈneiʃən] *n* 舌侧倾斜
linguoclusion [ˌliŋgwəˈkluːʒən] *n* 舌侧错殆,舌侧错位咬合
linguodental [ˌliŋgwəˈdentəl] *a* 舌牙的,舌齿的 *n* 舌齿音
linguodistal [ˌliŋgwəˈdistəl] *a* 舌侧远中的
linguogingival [ˌliŋgwəuˈdʒindʒivəl] *a* 舌龈的
linguoincisal [ˌliŋgwəuinˈsaizəl] *a* 舌牙切面的,舌切的
linguomesial [ˌliŋgwəˈmiːzjəl] *a* 舌侧近中的
linguo-occlusal [ˌliŋgwəuə ˈkluːzəl] *a* 舌殆的
linguopapillitis [ˌliŋgwəuˌpæpiˈlaitis] *n* 舌乳头炎
linguoplacement [ˌliŋgwəˈpleismənt] *n* 舌向移位,舌侧移位
linguopulpal [ˌliŋgwəˈpʌlpəl] *a* 舌侧髓的
linguoversion [ˌliŋgwəˈvəːʃən] *n* 舌向移位,舌向错位
liniment [ˈlinimənt] *n* 搽剂 | camphor ~ 樟脑搽剂 / medicinal soft soap ~ 药用软皂搽剂
linimentum [ˌliniˈmentəm] *n* 【拉】搽剂,擦剂
linin [ˈlainin] *n* 核丝
lining [ˈlainiŋ] *n* 衬里;衬料
linitis [liˈnaitis] *n* 胃蜂窝织炎 | ~ plastica 皮革样胃,硬变性胃炎
linkage [ˈliŋkidʒ] *n* 键;键合;连接,结合;连锁(在遗传学上指等位基因存在于同一染色体上) | sex ~ 性连锁
linked [liŋkt] *a* 连接的,结合的
linker [linkə] *n* 连接体,接头,衔接物
linn(a)ean [liˈniːən] *a* (Carolus Linnaeus)林奈的,林奈分类系统的
Linognathus [liˈnɔgnəθəs] *n* 长颚虱属
linoleate [liˈnəulieit] *n* 亚油酸(盐、酯或阴离子型) | ethyl ~ 亚油酸乙酯
linoleic acid [ˌlinəˈtiːik], **linolic acid** [liˈnəulik] 亚油酸
linolein [liˈnəuliːn] *n* 亚麻油脂
linolenate [liˈnəulәneit] *n* 亚麻酸(盐,酯或阴离子型)
linolenic acid [ˌlinəˈliːnik] 亚麻酸
linseed [ˈlinsiːd] *n* 亚麻子
Linser's method [ˈlinsə] (Paul Linser)林泽尔法(注射氯化汞治静脉曲张)
Linstowiidae [linstəˈwaiidiː] *n* 连士[绦虫]科
lint [lint] *n* 绒布(外科敷料)
lintin [ˈlintin], **lintine** [ˈlintiːn] *n* 脱脂绒布
Linton shunt [ˈlintən] (Robert R. Linton)林顿分流术,脾肾静脉分流术
Linum [ˈlainəm] *n* 亚麻属
linum [ˈlainəm] *n* 亚麻子
lio- 以 lio-起始的词,同样见以 leio-起始的词
liothyronine [ˌlaiəˈθairəniːn] *n* 碘塞罗宁(甲状腺激素) | ~ sodium 碘塞罗宁钠
liotrix [ˈlaiətriks] *n* 复方甲状腺素,三碘合剂(三碘甲腺原氨酸钠与左甲状腺素钠按重量 1∶4 的合剂)
lip [lip] *n* 唇;(伤口的)边缘 | cleft ~ 唇裂
lipacidemia [ˌlipæsiˈdiːmiə] *n* 脂酸血
lipaciduria [ˌlipæsiˈdjuəriə] *n* 脂酸尿
liparocele [liˈpærəsiːl] *n* 阴囊脂瘤;脂肪疝
liparodyspnea [ˌlipərəuˈdispniːə] *n* 肥胖性呼吸困难
liparoid [ˈlipərɔid] *a* 脂肪的,脂肪样的
lipase [ˈlaipeis, ˈlipeis] *n* 脂肪酶 | acid ~ 酸性脂肪酶 / pancreatic ~ 胰脂肪酶,三酰甘油脂肪酶 | **lipasic** [laiˈpeisik] *a* 脂酶的;分解脂肪的
lipasemia [ˌlipeiˈsiːmiə] *n* 脂酶血,高脂酶血症
lipasuria [ˌlipeiˈsjuəriə] *n* 脂酶尿
lipectomy [liˈpektəmi] *n* 脂肪切除术
lipedema [ˌlipiˈdiːmə] *n* 脂肪水肿(皮下脂肪过多兼水肿)
lipemia [liˈpiːmiə], **lipidemia** [ˌlipiˈdiːmiə] *n* 脂血[症] | **lipemic** [liˈpiːmik] *a*
lipese [ˈlipiːs] *n* 合脂酶
lipid [ˈlipid, ˈlaipid] *n* 脂质,类脂 | ~ A 脂质 A | ~**ic** [liˈpidik] *a* / **lipide** [ˈlipaid, ˈlaipaid] *n*
lipidase [ˈlipideis] *n* 脂质酶(统称)
lipidol [ˈlipidɔl] *n* 脂醇
lipidolysis [ˌlipiˈdɔlisis] *n* 脂类分解 | **lipidolytic** [ˌlipidəˈlitik] *a* 分解脂类的
lipidosis [ˌlipiˈdəusis] *n* 脂肪沉积,脂沉积症 | cerebroside ~ 脑苷脂沉积症,戈谢病(Gaucher disease) / galactosylceramide ~ 半乳糖[基]神经酰胺脂沉积症,克拉贝病(Krabbe's disease) / glucosylceramide ~ 葡糖神经酰胺脂沉积症,戈谢病(Gaucher's disease) / hereditary dystopic ~ 遗传性异位脂沉积症,法布莱病(Fabry's disease) / sphigomyelin ~ 鞘磷脂沉积症,尼-皮病(Niemann-Pick disease) / sulfatide ~ 硫脂沉积症,异染性脑白质营养不良
lipidtemns [ˈlipidtəmz] *n* 脂肪分解产物(如甘油和脂肪酸)
lipiduria [ˌlipiˈdjuəriə] *n* 脂肪尿
lipin [ˈlipin] *n* 脂质
lip(o)- [构词成分]脂,脂肪
lipoadenoma [ˌlipəuˌædiˈnəumə] *n* 脂肪腺瘤

lipoamide [ˌlipəuˈæmaid] *n* 硫辛酰胺

lipoamide dehydrogenase [ˌlipəuˈæmaid diːˈhaidrədʒəneis] 硫辛酰胺脱氢酶(dihydrolipoamide dehydrogenase〈二氢硫辛酰胺脱氢酶〉的不正确名)

lipoamide dehydrogenase deficiency 硫辛酰胺脱氢酶缺乏症(一种常染色体隐性遗传氨基酸病,特征为新生儿起病,蓄积和排泄乳酸、丙酮酸和α-酮戊二酸,支链受损及幼儿期即死亡)

lipoarthritis [ˌlipəuɑːˈθraitis] *n* 关节脂肪组织炎

lipoatrophy [ˌlaipəuˈætrəfi] *n* 脂肪萎缩;脂肪营养不良 | insulin ~ 胰岛素性脂肪萎缩(胰岛素反复注射处的局限性脂肪萎缩)

lipoblast [ˈlipəblæst] *n* 成脂肪细胞

lipoblastic [ˌlipəuˈblæstik] *a* 成脂肪细胞的

lipoblastoma [ˌlipəublæsˈtəumə] *n* 成脂肪细胞瘤

lipoblastomatosis [ˌlipəuˌblæstəuməˈtəusis] *n* 成脂肪细胞瘤病(多发性成脂细胞发生,局部扩散,但无转移倾向)

lipocaic [ˌlipəuˈkeiik] *n* 胰抗脂肪肝因素

lipocardiac [ˌlipəuˈkɑːdiæk] *a* 脂肪心的

lipocatabolic [ˌlipəuˌkætəˈbɔlik] *a* 脂肪分解代谢的

lipocele [ˌlipəsiːl] *n* 脂肪突出,脂肪疝

lipocellulose [ˌlipəuˈseljuləus] *n* 脂肪纤维素

lipoceratous [ˌlipəuˈserətəs] *a* 尸蜡[样]的

lipocere [ˈlipəsiə] *n* 尸蜡

lipochondria [ˌlipəuˈkɔndriə] *n* 脂粒体

lipochondrodystrophy [ˌlipəuˌkɔndrəuˈdistrəfi] *n* 脂肪软骨营养不良

lipochondroma [ˌlipəukɔnˈdrəumə] *n* 脂肪软骨瘤

lipochrome [ˈlipəkrəum] *n* 脂色素

lipochromemia [ˌlipəukrəuˈmiːmiə] *n* 脂色素血[症]

lipochromogen [ˌlipəuˈkrəumədʒən] *n* 脂色素原

lipoclasis [liˈpɔkləsis] *n* 脂肪分解 | **lipoclastic** [ˌlipəˈklæstik] *a* 分解脂肪的

lipocorticoid [ˌlipəˈkɔːtikɔid] *n* 脂肪[肾上腺]皮质激素类(尤指肝内)

lipocortin [ˌlipəuˈkɔːtin] *n* 脂皮质蛋白

lipocyanine [ˌlipəˈsaiənin] *n* 脂蓝质

lipocyte [ˈlipəsait] *n* 脂细胞;贮脂细胞(肝内)

lipodieresis [ˌlipəudaiˈiərisis] *n* 脂肪分解 | **lipodieretic** [ˌlipəudaiiəˈretik] *a* 分解脂肪的

lipodystrophia [ˌlipəudisˈtrəufiə] *n*【拉】脂肪营养不良,脂肪代谢障碍 | ~ intestinalis 肠性脂肪营养不良 / ~ progressiva 进行性脂肪营养不良

lipodystrophy [ˌlipəuˈdistrəfi] *n* 脂肪营养不良,脂质营养不良 | intestinal ~ 肠性脂肪营养不良 / partial ~ , progressive ~ 部分脂肪营养不良,进行性脂肪营养不良 / total ~ , congenital progressive ~ , generalized ~ , progressive congenital 全身性脂肪营养不良,先天性进行性脂肪营养不良

lipofection [ˌlipəuˈfekʃən] *n* 脂[质]转染

lipoferous [liˈpɔfərəs] *a* 带脂肪的;嗜苏丹的

lipofibroma [ˌlipəufaiˈbrəumə] *n* 脂肪纤维瘤

lipofuscin [ˌlipəuˈfʌsin] *n* 脂褐素,脂褐质

lipofuscinosis [ˌlipəuˌfʌsiˈnəusis] *n* 脂褐素沉积症 | neuronal ceroid ~ 神经元蜡样脂褐素沉积症

lipogenesis [ˌlipəuˈdʒenisis] *n* 脂肪生成 | **lipogenic** [ˌlipəuˈdʒenik], **lipogenetic** [ˌlipəudʒiˈnetik] *a* 脂肪生成的,生脂肪的

lipogenous [liˈpɔdʒinəs] *a* 生脂肪的

lipogranuloma [ˌlipəugrænjuˈləumə] *n* 脂肪肉芽肿

lipogranulomatosis [ˌlipəuˌgrænjuləuməˈtəusis] *n* 脂肪肉芽肿病

lipohemarthrosis [ˌlipəuˌhemɑːˈθrəusis] *n* 关节积脂血病

lipohemia [ˌlipəuˈhiːmiə] *n* 脂血[症]

lipohistiodieresis [ˌlipəuˌhistiəudaiˈiərisis] *n* 组织内脂肪消失

lipohyalin [ˌlipəuˈhaiəlin] *n* 透明素脂质,透明质脂肪

lipohypertrophy [ˌlipəuhaiˈpəːtrəfi] *n* 脂肪增生(皮下脂肪增生) | insulin ~ 胰岛素性脂肪增生(胰岛素注射时皮下脂肪局限性增生,由于胰岛素的生脂肪作用所致)

lipoic acid [liˈpəuik] 硫辛酸

lipoid [ˈlipɔid] *a* 脂样的,类脂的 *n* 脂质,类脂 | acetone-insoluble ~s 丙酮不溶性脂质(梅毒补体结合试验时用作抗原) / anisotropic ~ 双折射脂质 | **~al** [liˈpɔidl] *a* 脂样的,类脂的

lipoidemia [ˌlipɔiˈdiːmiə] *n* 脂血[症]

lipoidic [liˈpɔidik] *a* 脂样的,类脂的

lipoidolytic [liˌpɔidəuˈlitik] *a* 分解脂类的

lipoidosis [ˌlipɔiˈdəusis] *n* 脂质贮积病,脂[质]沉积[症] | arterial ~ 动脉脂沉积症,动脉粥样硬化 / cerebroside ~ 脑苷脂沉积症,戈谢病(Gaucher's disease) / cholesterol ~ 胆固醇沉积症,汉-许-克病(Hand-Schüller-Christian disease) / ~ cutis et mucosae 皮肤黏膜脂沉积症,脂质蛋白沉积症 / phosphatide ~ 磷脂沉积症 / renal ~ 肾[脏]脂沉积症,脂性肾病

lipoidproteinosis [ˌlipɔidˌprəutiːˈnəusis] *n* 类脂蛋白质沉积症

lipoidsiderosis [ˌlipɔidsidəˈrəusis] *n* 类脂铁质沉积症

lipoiduria [ˌlipɔiˈdjuəriə] *n* 脂尿

lipolipoidosis [ˌlipəuˌlipɔiˈdəusis] *n* 脂肪类脂沉积症

lipolysis [liˈpɔlisis] *n* 脂肪分解,脂解[作用] |

lipolytic [ˌlipəu'litik] *a*

lipoma [li'pəumə] ([复] **lipomas** 或 **lipomata** [li'pəumətə]) *n* 脂肪瘤 | diffuse ~ 弥漫性脂肪瘤,弥漫性脂肪过多症 / fetal fat cell ~ 胎儿性脂肪细胞脂肪瘤,蛰伏脂瘤 / telangiectatic ~ 毛细管扩张性脂肪瘤,血管脂肪瘤 | **~tous** [li'pəumətəs] *a*

lipomatoid [li'pəumətɔid] *a* 脂肪瘤样的

lipomatosis [ˌlipəumə'təusis] *n* 脂肪瘤样病,脂肪过多症

lipomeningocele [ˌlipəumə'niŋgəsiːl] *n* 脂性脑膜膨出

lipomeria [ˌlaipə'miəriə] *n* 先天性缺肢

lipometabolism [ˌlipəume'tæbəlizəm] *n* 脂肪代谢 | **lipometabolic** [ˌlipəuˌmetə'bɔlik] *a*

lipomicron [ˌlipəuˌmaikrɔn] *n* 血脂粒

lipomucopolysaccharidosis [ˌlipəuˌmjuːkəuˌpɔlisækəri'dəusis] *n* 脂黏多糖贮积病,黏脂沉积病Ⅰ型

lipomyelomeningocele [ˌlipəuˌmaiələuməˈniŋgəsiːl] *n* 脂性脊髓脊膜膨出

lipomyohemangioma [ˌlipəuˌmaiəuhiˌmændʒi'əumə] *n* 脂肌血管瘤

lipomyoma [ˌlipəumai'əumə] *n* 脂肌瘤

lipomyxoma [ˌlipəumik'səumə] *n* 黏液脂瘤

liponephrosis [ˌlipəuni'frəusis] *n* 脂性肾变病

liponeurocyte [ˌlipəu'njuərəsait] *n* 脂神经细胞

Liponyssus [ˌlipəu'nisəs] *n* 刺脂螨属(即禽刺螨属 Ornithonyssus) | ~ bacoti 巴氏刺脂螨(即巴氏禽刺螨 Ornithonyssus bacoti) / ~ bursa 囊形刺脂螨(即囊禽刺螨 Ornithonyssusbursa) / ~ sylviarum 林刺脂螨(即林禽刺螨 Ornithonyssus sylviarum)

lipopathy [li'pɔpəθi] *n* 脂质代谢病

lipopenia [ˌlipəu'piːniə] *n* 脂肪减少 | **lipopenic** *a*

lipopeptid [ˌlipəu'peptid] *n* 脂肽

lipopexia [ˌlipəu'peksiə] *n* 脂肪蓄积 | **lipopexic** [ˌlipəu'peksik], **lipopectic** [ˌlipəu'pektik] *a*

lipophage ['lipəfeidʒ] *n* 噬脂细胞

lipophagia [ˌlipəu'feidʒiə] *n* 噬脂[性];脂肪耗失,脂肪分解 | ~ granulomatosis 噬脂性肉芽肿,肠性脂肪营养不良

lipophagy [li'pɔfədʒi] *n* 噬脂[性];脂肪耗失,脂肪分解 | **lipophagic** [ˌlipəu'feidʒik] *a*

lipophanerosis [ˌlipəuˌfænə'rəusis] *n* 脂粒显现

lipophil ['lipəfil] *a* 亲脂的 *n* 亲脂体

lipophilia [ˌlipə'filiə] *n* 亲脂性;肥胖倾向 | **lipophilic** [ˌlipə'filik] *a*

lipophillin [ˌlipəu'filin] *n* 亲脂蛋白

lipophore ['lipəfɔː] *n* 黄色素细胞

lipoplasty [ˌlipəu'plæsti] *n* 脂肪整复(见 liposuction)

lipopolysaccharide [ˌlipəuˌpɔli'sækəraid] *n* 脂多糖

lipoprotein [ˌlipə'prəutiːn, ˌlaipə'prəutiːn] *n* 脂蛋白 | familial ~ deficiency 家族性脂蛋白缺乏症 / familial high-density ~ (HDL) deficiency 家族性高密度脂蛋白缺乏症,丹吉尔病(Tangier disease) / high-density ~ (HDL)高密度脂蛋白(亦称 α-脂蛋白) / intermediate-density ~ (IDL)中密度脂蛋白 / low-density ~ (LDL)低密度脂蛋白(亦称 β-脂蛋白) / Lp(a) ~ Lp(a)脂蛋白(亦称 HDL_1 和下沉前 β-脂蛋白) / very low-density ~ (VLDL)极低密度脂蛋白(亦称前 β-脂蛋白) / ~ X X 脂蛋白(一种异常低密度脂蛋白,游离胆固醇含量高和蛋白含量异常,见于胆汁淤积病人)

lipoproteinemia [ˌlipəuˌprəutiː'niːmiə] *n* 脂蛋白血症

lipoprotein lipase [ˌlipəuˌprəutiːn 'lipeis, 'laipeis] 脂蛋白脂肪酶(此酶的遗传性缺乏可致家族性高脂蛋白血症Ⅰ型)

lipoprotein lipase (LPL) deficiency, familial 家族性脂蛋白脂肪酶缺乏症,家族性高脂蛋白血症Ⅰ型和Ⅴ型

lipoproteinosis [ˌlipəuˌprəutiː'nəusis] *n* 脂蛋白沉积症

liporhodin [ˌlipə'rəudin] *n* 脂红质

liposarcoma [ˌlipəusɑː'kəumə] *n* 脂肪肉瘤

liposis [li'pəusis] *n* 脂肪过多症

liposoluble [ˌlipəu'sɔljubl] *a* 脂溶的

liposome ['lipəsəum] *n* 脂质体

lipostomy [lai'pɔstəmi] *n* 无口[畸形]

liposuction [ˌlipəu'sʌkʃən] *n* 脂肪抽吸[术](通过高压真空装置,由切口经皮下将插管插入,手术除去局限性脂肪沉积)

lipoteichoic acid [ˌlipəutai'kəuik] *n* 脂磷壁酸

lipotroph ['lipətrɔf] *n* 促脂肪增多细胞

lipotrophy [li'pɔtrəfi] *n* 脂肪增多 | **lipotrophic** [ˌlipə'trɔfik] *a*

lipotropic [ˌlipə'trɔpik] *a* 促脂肪代谢的,抗脂肪肝的 *n* 促脂解剂,抗脂肪肝剂

lipotropin [ˌlipə'trəupin, ˌlaipə'trəupin] *n* 促脂解素

β-lipotropin [ˌlipə'trəupin] *n* β-促脂解素

lipotropism [li'pɔtrəpizəm], **lipotropy** [li'pɔtrəpi] *n* 亲脂性;抗脂肪肝现象

lipotuberculin [ˌlipəutju(ː)'bəːkjulin] *n* 类脂结核菌素(在溶液或乳剂内含有分枝杆菌脂肪组分的一种结核菌素制剂)

lipovaccine [ˌlipə'væksiːn] *n* 类脂菌苗(在植物油中混悬微生物所制备的一种菌苗,能使抗原物质延缓吸收)

lipovitellin [ˌlipəvaiˈtelin] *n* 卵黄脂磷蛋白
lipoxanthine [ˌlipəˈzænθin] *n* 脂黄质
lipoxin [liˈpɔksin] *n* 脂毒素
lipoxygenase [liˈpɔksidʒəneis], **lipoxidase** [liˈpɔksideis] *n* 脂加氧酶,脂[肪]氧化酶
lipoxysm [liˈpɔksizəm] *n* 油酸中毒
lipoyl [ˈlipɔil] *n* 硫辛酰[基]
lipoyl transacetylase [ˈlipɔil trænsˈæsitileis] 硫辛酰转乙酰酶,二氢硫辛酰胺乙酰[基]转移酶
lippa [ˈlipə] *n* 睑缘炎
lipping [ˈlipiŋ] *n* 唇状[X线]阴影;唇状突出
lippitude [ˈlipitjuːd] *n* 睑缘炎
lip-reading [ˈlipˌriːdiŋ] *n* (聋者从他人嘴唇的动作了解话意的)读唇
Lipschütz bodies [ˈlipʃjits] (Benjamin Lipschütz) 利普许茨体(核内包涵体,见于单纯性疱疹) | ~ cell 中心细胞 / ~ ulcer(disease)急性外阴溃疡
lipsotrichia [ˌlipsəˈtrikiə] *n* 脱发,脱毛
lipuria [liˈpjuəriə] *n* 脂肪尿 | **lipuric** [liˈpjuərik] *a*
Liq. liquor 液体;液
liquefacient [ˌlikwiˈfeiʃənt] *a* 液化的 *n* 解凝剂
liquefaction [ˌlikwiˈfækʃən] *n* 液化 | **liquefactive** *a*
liquid [ˈlikwid] *a* 液体的,液态的 *n* 液体
liquiform [ˈlikwifɔːm] *a* 液状的
liquogel [ˈlikwədʒel] *n* 液胶体,液状凝胶
liquor [ˈlikə] ([复] **liquors, liquores** [laiˈkwɔːriːz]) *n* 液体;液
liquorice [ˈlikəris] *n* 甘草
liquorrhea [ˌlaikwəˈriə] *n* [体]液排出过多,液溢
Lisch nodules [liʃ](Karl Lisch) 列希结节(神经纤维瘤病时发生的虹膜错构瘤)
Lisfranc's amputation [lisˈfrɑːŋ] (Jacques Lisfranc)利斯弗朗切断术(①肩关节切断术;②跖跗关节切断术) | ~ joint 跗跖关节 / ~ ligament 利斯弗朗韧带(楔跖韧带) / ~ tubercle 斜角肌结节
lisinopril [laiˈsinəpril] *n* 赖诺普利(依那普利〈enalapril〉激活型的赖氨酸衍生物,一种血管紧张素转换酶抑制剂,用于治疗高血压)
lisp [lisp] *vi, vt, n* 牙语,咬舌发音(如将 s, z 读作 th)
lisping [ˈlispiŋ] *n* 牙语,咬舌发音
Lissauer's paralysis [ˈlisauə] (Heinrich Lissauer)利索厄麻痹(卒中型麻痹性痴呆) | ~ tract (column, marginal zone)背外侧束
Lissencephala [ˌlisenˈsefələ] *n* 缺脑回动物类(脑回甚少或无的胎盘动物)
lissencephalia [ˌlisensəˈfeiliə], **lissencephaly** [ˌlisenˈsefəli] *n* 无脑回[畸形]
lissencephalic [ˌlisensəˈfælik] *a* 缺脑回的(动物);缺脑回动物的;无脑回[畸形]的
lissive [ˈlisiv] *a* [促]肌肉弛缓的,解痉挛的
list [list] *n* 表,一览表;目录;名单 | critical ~ 病危名单 / essential drug ~ 基本药物目录 / sick ~ 病人名单,病人册
Listeria [lisˈteriə] (Joseph Lister) *n* 利斯特菌属 | ~ monocytogenes 产单核细胞利斯特菌 | **listerial** *a* 利斯特菌的 / **Listerella** [ˌlistəˈrelə] *n*
listeriosis [lisˌteriˈəusis], **listerellosis** [ˌlistərəˈləusis] *n* 利斯特菌病
listerism [ˈlistərizəm] *n* 防腐无菌法
Lister's tubercle [ˈlistə] (Baron J. Lister)利斯特结节,桡骨背侧结节
Listing's law [ˈlistiŋ] (Johann B. Listing)利斯廷定律(当眼球运动离静止位置时,在第二位置的转动角,与眼围绕垂直于视线第一第二位置的固定轴上转动时相同) | ~ plane 利斯廷平面(垂直于眼前后轴的横垂直面)
Liston's forceps [ˈlistən] (Robert Liston)利斯顿钳(剪骨钳) | ~ knives 利斯顿刀(长刃切断九) / ~ operation 利斯顿手术(上颌骨切除术) / ~ splint 利斯顿夹板(股骨骨折用)
lisp [lisp] *vi, vt, n* 牙语,咬舌发音(如将 s, z 读作 th)
Listrophoridae [ˌlistrəuˈfɔːridiː] *n* 牦螨科
-lith [构词成分]石,结石
lithagogectasia [ˌliθəgəudʒekˈteiziə] *n* 尿道扩张取石术
lithagogue [ˈliθəgɔg] *a* 排石的,驱石的 *n* 驱石剂
lithangiuria [ˌliθændʒiˈjuəriə] *n* 尿路结石
litharge [ˈliθɑːdʒ] *n* 密陀僧,一氧化铅
lithate [ˈliθeit] *n* 尿酸盐
lithecbole [liˈθekbəli] *n* 结石排出
lithectasy [liˈθektəsi] *n* 尿道扩张取石术
lithectomy [liˈθektəmi] *n* 切[开取]石术(尤指膀胱切开取石术)
lithemia [liˈθiːmiə] *n* 尿酸[盐]血症 | **lithemic** *a*
lithia [ˈliθiə] *n* 氧化锂
-lithiasis [构词成分]结石
lithiasis [liˈθaiəsis] *n* 结石[病] | **lithiasic** [ˌliθiˈæsik] *a* 结石病的
lithic [ˈliθik] *a* 结石的,锂的
lithic acid [ˈliθik] 尿酸
lithium(Li) [ˈliθiəm] *n* 锂(化学元素) | ~ bromide 溴化锂(中枢神经系统抑制药) / ~ carbonate 碳酸锂(治躁狂抑郁性精神病药)
lith(o)- [构词成分]石,结石
lithocenosis [ˌliθəusiˈnəusis] *n* 碎石清除术
lithocholate [ˌliθəuˈkəuleit] *n* 石胆酸(盐、酯或阴离子型)
lithocholic acid [ˌliθəˈkəulik] 石胆酸

lithocholylglycine [ˌliθəuˌkəulilˈglaisiːn] *n* 石胆酰甘氨酸
lithocholyltaurine [ˌliθəuˌkəulilˈtɔːriːn] *n* 石胆酰牛磺酸
lithoclast [ˈliθəklæst] *n* 碎石器
lithoclysmia [ˌliθəˈklizmiə] *n* [膀胱]灌药溶石法
lithocystotomy [ˌliθəusisˈtɔtəmi] *n* 膀胱切开取石术
lithodialysis [ˌliθəudaiˈælisis] *n* 溶石术;碎石术
lithogenesis [ˌliθəuˈdʒenisis] *n* 结石形成,结石发生 | **lithogenous** [liˈθɔdʒinəs] *a* 结石形成的,成结石的
lithogenic [ˌliθəuˈdʒenik] *a* 结石生成的,促结石形成的
lithokelyphopedion [ˌliθəuˌkelifəˈpiːdiən] *n* 胎膜胎儿石化
lithokelyphos [ˌliθəˈkelifɔs] *n* 胎膜石化
lithokonion [ˌliθəˈkəuniən] *n* 碎石器
litholabe [ˈliθəlæb] *n* 持石器
litholapaxy [liˈθɔləˌpæksi] *n* 碎石洗出术
lithology [liˈθɔlədʒi] *n* 结石学
litholysis [liˈθɔlisis] *n* 结石溶解
litholyte [ˈliθəlait] *n* 溶石液灌注器
litholytic [ˌliθəˈlitik] *a* 溶石的 *n* 溶石剂
lithometer [liˈθɔmitə] *n* 结石测定器
lithomoscus [ˌliθəˈmɔskəs] *n* 牛胎石化
lithomyl [ˈliθəmil] *n* 膀胱碎石器
lithonephria [ˌliθəˈnefriə] *n* 肾石病
lithonephritis [ˌliθəuneˈfraitis] *n* 结石性肾炎
lithonephrotomy [ˌliθəuneˈfrɔtəmi] *n* 肾石切除术
lithontriptic [ˌliθɔnˈtriptik] *a* 碎石的
lithopedion [ˌliθəˈpiːdiən] *n* 石胎
lithophone [ˈliθəfəun] *n* 听石探杆
lithoscope [ˈliθəskəup] *n* 膀胱石镜
lithotome [ˈliθətəum] *n* 切石刀
lithotomy [liˈθɔtəmi] *n* 切[开取]石术(尤指膀胱切开取石术) | bilateral ~ 两侧切石术,横行切石术 / median ~ , prerectal ~ 正中切石术,直肠前切石术 / perineal ~ 经会阴切石术 / rectal ~ , rectovesical ~ 经直肠切石术 / suprapubic ~ , high ~ 耻骨上切石术,高位切石术 / vaginal ~ , vesicovaginal ~ 经阴道切石术 | **lithotomic** [ˌliθəˈtɔmik] *a* / **lithotomist** *n* 切石术者
lithotony [liˈθɔtəni] *n* 造瘘取石术
lithotresis [ˌliθəˈtriːsis] *n* 结石钻孔术
lithotripsy [ˈliθəˌtripsi] *n* 碎石术 | **lithotriptic** [ˌliθəˈtriptik] *a* 碎石术的,碎石的
lithotripter [ˌliθəuˈtriptə] *n* 碎石器
lithotriptoscope [ˌliθəˈtriptəskəup] *n* 碎石膀胱镜
lithotriptoscopy [ˌliθəutripˈtɔskəpi] *n* 膀胱镜碎石术
lithotrite [ˈliθətrait], **lithotriptor** [ˈliθəˌtriptə] *n* 碎石器
lithotrity [liˈθɔtriti] *n* 碎石术
lithotroph [ˈliθətrəuf] *n* 无机营养菌
lithous [ˈliθəs] *a* 石的,结石的
lithoxiduria [ˌliθɔksiˈdjuəriə] *n* 黄嘌呤尿
lithuresis [ˌliθjuəˈriːsis] *n* 石尿症
lithureteria [ˌliθjuərəˈtiəriə] *n* 输尿管结石病
lithuria [liˈθjuəriə] *n* 石尿
litmocidin [ˌlitməˈsaidin] *n* 石蕊样放线菌素,变色放线菌素
litmus [ˈlitməs] *n* 石蕊
Litomosoides [ˌlitəuməˈsɔidiːz] *n* 丝虫属 | ~ carinii 棉鼠丝虫
litre [ˈliːtə] *n* [法]升
Litten's diaphragm phenomenon (sign) [ˈlitən] (Moritz Litten)利滕膈现象(征)(呼吸时胸廓下部可移动的水平凹陷)
litter [ˈlitə] *n* 担架;同窝仔(多产动物一胎所生的仔)
litterol [ˈlitərɔl] *a* 沿岸的
Little's area [ˈlitl] (James L. Little)利特尔区(见 Kiesselbach's area)
Little's disease [ˈlitl] (William J. Little)利特尔病(四肢先天性痉挛性强直,从出生之日起即有,为一种大脑痉挛性瘫痪,由于锥体束缺乏发育所致,可能伴有各种疾病,包括产伤、胎儿缺氧,或母亲在妊娠期生病,在临床上,此病特点为肌无力、步行困难等。亦称痉挛性双瘫)
Littre's crypts [ˈlitr] (Alexis Littre)包皮腺 | ~ glands 包皮腺;男尿道腺 / ~ hernia 憩室疝 / ~ operation 利特雷手术(腹股沟部结肠切开术)
littritis [liˈtraitis] *n* 尿道腺炎
Litzmann's obliquity [ˈlitsmən] (Karl K. T. Litzmann)利次曼倾斜(后头盆倾势不均)
liveborn [ˈlaivbɔːn] *a* 活产的
livedo [liˈviːdəu] *n* 【拉】青斑
livedoid [ˈlividɔid] *a* 青斑样的
liver [ˈlivə] *n* 肝 | albuminoid ~ , amyloid ~ , lardaceous ~ , waxy ~ 淀粉样肝 / biliary cirrhotic ~ 胆汁性肝硬变 / brimstone ~ 硫[黄]色肝 / bronze ~ 青铜色肝 / cirrhotic ~ 硬变肝 / degraded ~ 分叶肝 / frosted ~ , icing ~ , sugar-icing ~ 糖衣肝,结霜样肝(慢性增生性肝周炎) / hobnail ~ 鞋钉状肝,结节性肝硬变,萎缩性门脉性肝硬变(肝表面由于硬化而形成鞋钉状点) / infantile ~ 小儿胆汁性肝硬变 / iron ~ 铁沉着肝 / nutmeg ~ 肉豆蔻肝 / pigmented ~ 肝色素沉着 / sago ~ 西米肝,淀粉样肝 /

stasis ~ 淤血肝 / wandering ~ 游动肝
liver phosphorylase [ˈlivə fɔsˈfɔrileis] 肝磷酸化酶(糖原磷酸化酶的肝同工酶)
liver phosphorylase deficiency 肝磷酸化酶缺乏症,糖原贮积症Ⅵ型
liver phosphorylase kinase [ˈlivəfɔsˈfɔrileis ˈkaineis] 肝磷酸化酶激酶(磷酸化酶激酶的肝同工酶)
liver phosphorylase kinase deficiency 肝磷酸化酶激酶缺乏症,磷酸化酶 b 激酶缺乏症
liverwort [ˈlivəwəːt] *n* 苔类植物,地钱
livetin [ˈlaivətin] *n* 卵黄蛋白
livid [ˈlivid] *a* 青紫的(由于挫伤或充血而呈现)
lividity [liˈvidəti] *n* 绀,青紫 | postmortem ~ 尸斑
Livierato's sign [ˌliːviəˈrɑːtəu] (Panagino Livierato)利韦拉托征(沿剑突脐线叩击前腹,可刺激腹部交感神经而引起血管收缩)
Livingston's triangle [ˈliviŋstən] (Edward M. Livingston)利文斯顿三角(髂耻脐三角,阑尾炎时,触诊敏感区)
Livi's index [ˈlivi] (Rodolfo Livi) 利维指数($100 \times \sqrt[3]{P/6}$,其中 P = 体重〈g〉 × 身高〈cm〉)
livor [ˈlaivə] ([复] **livores** [laiˈvɔriːz] *n*【拉】绀,青紫;尸斑 | ~ mortis 尸斑
lixiviate [likˈsivieit] *vt* 浸滤,浸提 | **lixiviation** [ˌliksiviˈeiʃən] *n*
lixivium [likˈsiviəm] *n*【拉】浸滤液
Lizars' operation [ˈlaizəz] (John Lizars)利扎斯手术(一种上颌骨切除术)
LLL left lower lobe (of the lung) 左下叶(肺)
LM light minimum 最小明视光度;linguomesial 舌侧近中的
LMA left mentoanterior 颏左前(胎位)
LMF lymphocyte mitogenic factor 淋巴细胞致有丝分裂因子
lm lumen 流明(光通量单位)
LMP left mentoposterior 颏左后(胎位);last menstrual period 末次月经
LMT left mentotransverse 颏左横(胎位)
LMWK low-molecular-weight kininogen 低分子量激肽原
ln natural logarithm 自然对数
LNPF lymph node permeability factor 淋巴结通透性因子
LOA left occipitoanterior 枕左前(胎位)
Loa [ˈləuə] *n* 罗阿[丝虫]属 | ~ loa 罗阿丝虫,眼丝虫
load [ləud] *n* 负载,负荷;装载,充填 | glucose ~ 糖负荷 / occlusal ~ 䫌[面]负荷
loading [ˈləudiŋ] *n* 负荷(试验)(如组氨酸负荷试验) | over ~ 超负荷
LOAEL lowest observed adverse effect level 最低明显有害效应剂量
loaiasis [ˌləuəˈaiəsis] *n* 罗阿丝虫病
lobar [ˈləubə] *a* 叶的
lobate [ˈləubeit] *a* 有叶的,叶状的
lobation [ləuˈbeiʃən] *n* 叶状形成 | renal ~ 肾叶形成(X 线片上出现肾表面小切迹,提示肾叶的位置)
lobe [ləub] *n* 叶 | azygos ~ 奇叶(右肺) / ~s of cerebrum 大脑叶 / hepatic ~s, ~s of liver 肝叶 / ~s of lung 肺叶 / optic ~s 视叶(四叠体)
lobectomy [ləuˈbektəmi] *n* 叶切除术(切除甲状腺、肝、脑或肺的一叶)
Lobelia [ləuˈbiːliə] *n* 半边莲属
lobelia [ləuˈbiːljə] *n* 北美山梗菜,祛痰菜
lobeline [ˈlɔbəliːn] *n* 洛贝林(呼吸中枢兴奋药,目前用于戒烟制剂)
lobendazole [ləuˈbendəzəul] *n* 洛苯达唑(兽用抗蠕虫药)
lobi [ˈləubai] lobus 的复数
lobite [ˈləubait] *a* 限于一叶的
lobitis [ləuˈbaitis] *n* 叶炎(尤指肺叶炎)
Loboa loboi [ləuˈbəuəˈləubɔi] 罗布菌,罗布芽生菌(为瘢痕疙瘩性芽生菌病的致病因子)
lobocyte [ˈləubəsait] *n* 分叶核白细胞
lobomycosis [ˌləubəumaiˈkəusis] *n* 瘢痕疙瘩性芽生菌病
lobopodium [ˌləubəˈpəudiəm] ([复] **lobopodia** [ˌləubəˈpəudiə]) *n* 叶状假足
Lobo's disease [ˈləubəu] (Jorge Lobo)洛伯病,瘢痕疙瘩性芽生菌病
Lobosea [ləuˈbəusiə] *n* 叶足纲
lobotomy [ləuˈbɔtəmi] *n* 叶切断术(精神外科学中指脑叶纤维切断术) | frontal ~ , prefrontal ~ 额叶切断术,前额叶切断术,前额叶白质切断术 / transorbital ~ 经眼眶额叶切断术,经眼眶白质切断术
Lobstein's disease (syndrome) [ˈlɔbstain] (Johann F. G. C. M. Lobstein)成骨不全 | ~ ganglion 洛布斯坦神经节(内脏大神经节)
lobulated [ˈlɔbjuˌleitid] *a* 分成小叶的
lobulation [ˌlɔbjuˈleiʃən] *n* 分成小叶,小叶状 | portal ~ 门小叶形成
lobule [ˈlɔbjuːl] *n* 小叶 | **lobular** [ˈlɔbjulə], **lobulate** [ˈlɔbjuleit] *a*
lobulose [ˈlɔbjuləus], **lobulous** [ˈlɔbjuləs] *a* 小叶的
lobulus [ˈlɔbjuləs] ([复] **lobuli** [ˈlɔbjulai]) *n*【拉】小叶
lobus [ˈləubəs] ([复] **lobi** [ˈləubai]) *n*【拉】叶
local [ˈləukəl] *a* 局部的,局限的
localization [ˌləukəlaiˈzeiʃən, -liˈz-] *n* 定位[作

用];局部化,局限化;前定位 | cerebral ~ 大脑[中枢]定位 / germinal ~ 胚区定位 / selective ~, elective ~(细菌)选择性定位

localized [ˈləukəlaizd] *a* 局限的

localizer [ˈləukəˌlaizə] *n* (眼内异物)定位器

locator [ləuˈkeitə] *n* 定位器 | electroacoustic ~ 电声[异物]定位器

Loc. dol. loco dolenti【拉】用于痛处

lochia [ˈləukiə] *n*【希】恶露(产后一二周阴道排泄物) | ~ alba, ~ purulenta 白色恶露 / ~ sanguinolenta 脓性恶露 / ~ cruenta, ~ rubra 红恶露,血性恶露 | ~l *a*

lochiocolpos [ˌləukiəˈkɔlpəs] *n* 阴道积恶露

lochiocyte [ˈləukiəsait] *n* 恶露细胞

lochiometra [ˌləukiəˈmiːtrə] *n* 子宫积恶露

lochiometritis [ˌləukiəumiˈtraitis], **lochometritis** [ˌləukəumiˈtraitis] *n* 产后子宫炎

lochiorrhea [ˌləukiəˈriːə], **lochiorrhagia** [ˌləukiəˈreidʒiə] *n* 恶露过多

lochioschesis [ˌləukiˈɔskisis], **lochiostasis** [ˌləukiˈɔstəsis] *n* 恶露潴留

loci [ˈləusai] locus 的复数

Locke's solution (fluid) [lɔk] (Frank S. Locke) 洛克[溶]液(一种氯化钠、氯化钙、氯化钾、碳酸氢钠和葡萄糖溶液,用于生理实验,维持哺乳动物心脏搏动)

lockjaw [ˈlɔkdʒɔː] *n* 牙关紧闭

Lockwood's ligament [ˈlɔkwud] (Charles B. Lockwood)洛克伍德韧带(眼球悬韧带)

loc(o)- [构词成分]地点,部位

loco [ˈləukəu] ([复] **loco⟨e⟩s**) *n*【西】洛苛草,疯草;洛苛草中毒;洛苛草中毒的家畜 *vt* 用疯草毒害

locoism [ˈkəukəizəm] *n* 洛苛草中毒

locomotion [ˌləukəˈməuʃən] *n* 行进,行动,运动 | brachial ~ 臂运动,臂力摆荡 | **locomotive** [ˈləukəˌməutiv, ləukəˈməutiv] *a* 行动的,运动的 / **locomotory** [ˌləukəˈməutəri] *a*

locomotor [ˌləukəˈməutə] *a* 运动的;运动器官的

locomotorium [ˌləukəməuˈtɔːriəm] *n* 运动器 | **locomotorial** *a*

locoregional [ˌləukəuˈriːdʒənəl] *a* 局部区域的

locoweed [ˈləukəuwiːd] *n* 洛苛草

loculate [ˈlɔkjuleit] *a* 分为小腔的

Loculoascomycetidae [ˌlɔkjuləˌæskəmaiˈsiːtidiː] *n* 腔菌亚纲

loculus [ˈlɔkjuləs] ([复] **loculi** [ˈlɔkjulai]) *n*【拉】小腔 | **locular** [ˈlɔkjulə] *a*

locum [ˈləukəm] *n*【拉】地点,部位 | ~ tenens, ~ tenent 代理开业医师

locus [ˈləukəs] ([复] **loci** [ˈləusai]) *n*【拉】位置,部位;基因座,位点(在遗传学上指基因在染色体上的特殊位置) | ~ ceruleus, ~ cinereus, ~ ferrugineus 蓝斑 / complex ~ 复合座位,基因综合体 / H-2 ~ H-2 位点(小鼠的主要组织相容性位点,具有至少 33 种以上同种异体抗原特异性的 20 多个等位基因,推测由两个基因团 H-2k和 H-2D 组成,H-2k 紧靠着着丝粒) / heteromorphic ~ 异形位点(以两个或两个以上的等位形式存在的位点) / ~ minoris resistentiae 最小抵抗部 / operator ~ 操纵基因 / ~ ruber 红核

lodoxamide tromethamine [ləuˈdɔksəmiːn] 洛草氨酸氨丁三醇(平喘药和抗过敏药)

Loeb's deciduoma [ləub] (Leo Loeb)洛勃蜕膜瘤(通过孕酮作用在豚鼠子宫内产生类似胎盘母体部的瘤样结构) | ~ decidual reaction 洛勃蜕膜反应(在黄体发育正常时,子宫黏膜可因玻璃珠或其他刺激物的存在而形成蜕膜瘤)

Loeffler 见 Löffler

Loefflerella [ˌlefləˈrelə] *n* 吕弗勒菌属(旧名,现归入假单胞菌属 Pseudomonas)

LOEL lowest observed effect level 最低明显效应剂量

loempe [ˈlempi] *n* 脚气[病]

Loevit's cell [ˈliːfit] (Moritz Loevit)成红细胞,有核红细胞

Loewi's test (reaction, symptom) [ˈleivi] (Otto Loewi) 勒维试验(反应、症状)(于眼结膜囊内滴入 3 滴 1∶1 000 的氯化肾上腺素,5 分钟后再滴 3 滴,如有糖尿病、胰腺功能不全及甲状腺功能亢进时,便引起瞳孔扩大)

löffleria [lefˈliəriə] (F. A. J. Löffler) *n* 隐性白喉,无症状白喉,非典型白喉

Löffler's coagulated serum medium [ˈləːflə] (Friederich A. J. Löffler)勒夫勒凝固血清培养基(用于分离白喉杆菌) | ~ serum 勒夫勒血清(含葡萄糖和血清的肉汤,即勒夫勒凝固血清或培养基) / ~ alkaline methylene blue stain 勒夫勒碱性甲烯蓝染剂(用以显示白喉杆菌颗粒的一种简单染剂)

Löffler's endocarditis (disease) [ˈləːflə] (Wilhelm Löffler)缩窄性心内膜炎 | ~ syndrome (eosinophilia, pneumonia) 勒夫勒综合征(嗜酸细胞增多、肺炎),单纯性肺嗜酸细胞浸润症(特征为暂时性肺浸润的一种疾病,伴血内嗜酸白细胞增加)

Löfgren's syndrome [ˈləːfgrən] (Sven H. Löfgren)勒夫格伦综合征(结节性红斑,结合肺门淋巴结双侧腺病,见于作为结节病的一种表现)

logadectomy [ˌlɔgəˈdektəmi] *n* 结膜切除术

logaditis [ˌlɔgəˈdaitis] *n* 巩膜炎

logagnosia [ˌlɔgəgˈnəuziə] *n* 言语不能,失语[症]

logagraphia [ˌlɔgəˈgræfiə] *n* 书写不能,失写[症]

logamnesia [ˌlɔgæm'niːzjə] *n* 感觉性失语,记言不能
logaphasia [ˌlɔgə'feizjə] *n* 表达性失语症
logasthenia [ˌlɔgæs'θiːniə] *n* 言语理解困难
loge [ləuʒ] *n*【法】小屋,小室,小亭 | ~ de Guyon 居永管(即 Guyon's canal)
log(o)- [构词成分]词,言语
logoclonia [ˌlɔgə'klɔniə], **logoklony** ['lɔgəˌklɔni] *n* 言语痉挛,痉语[症]
logogram ['lɔgəugræm] *n* 疾病鉴诊图
logokophosis [ˌlɔgəukəu'fəusis] *n* 词聋,听觉性失语
logomania [ˌlɔgəu'meinjə] *n* 多语症
logopathy [lɔ'gɔpəθi] *n* (中枢性)言语障碍
logopedics [ˌlɔgəu'piːdiks] *n* 言语矫治学,言语矫正法 | **logopedia** [ˌlɔgəu'piːdiə] *n*
logoplegia [ˌlɔgəu'pliːdʒiə] *n* 发音器麻痹,语器麻痹
logorrhea [ˌlɔgəu'riːə] *n* 多语症
logoscope ['lɔgəskəup] *n* 疾病鉴诊器,症状鉴别器 | **logoscopy** [lə'gɔskəpi] *n* 疾病鉴诊器用法
logospasm ['lɔgəspæzəm] *n* 痉语
-logy [后缀] 学,论;言语
logwood ['lɔgwuːd] *n* 洋苏木
Löhlein-Baehr lesion ['ləːleinbεə] (Max H. F. Löhlein; George Baehr)勒-贝损害(细菌性心内膜炎时发生的一种局灶性肾小球坏死和透明化损害,此过程被认为是局灶性栓塞性肾小球肾炎)
Lohnstein's saccharimeter ['lɔːnstain] (Theodor Lohnstein)洛恩斯坦尿糖定量器(一种进行尿糖定量发酵试验的仪器)
loiasis [ləu'aiəsis] *n* 罗阿丝虫病
loimic ['lɔimik] *a* 疫病的
loimographia [ˌlɔimə'greifiə] *n* 疫病论
loimology [lɔi'mɔlədʒi] *n* 疫病学,传染病学
loin [lɔin] *n* 腰[部]
Lolium ['ləuliəm] *n* 黑麦草属 | ~ temulentum 毒麦
Lombardi's sign [lɔm'bɑːdi] (Antonio Lombardi) 伦巴迪征(在第七颈椎及头三根胸椎棘突区出现静脉曲张,见于早期肺结核)
lomefloxacin [ˌləumə'flɔksəsin] *n* 洛美沙星(抗菌药)
lometraline hydrochloride [ləu'metrəliːn] 盐酸洛美曲林(安定药,抗震颤麻痹药)
lomofungin [ləumə'fʌndʒin] *n* 洛蒙真菌素,洛蒙霉素
lomosome ['ləuməsəum] *n* 缘饰体(真菌)
lomustine [ləu'mʌstiːn] *n* 洛莫司汀(抗肿瘤药)
Lonchocarpus [ˌlɔŋkə'kɑːpəs] *n* 醉鱼豆属(豆科)
long-chain-fatty-acid-CoA ligase [lɔŋ tʃein 'fæti 'æsid kəu'ei 'laigeis] 长链脂肪酸辅酶 A 连接酶(亦称酰基辅酶 A 合成酶)
longevity [lɔn'dʒevəti] *n* 长寿
longilineal [ˌlɔndʒi'liniəl] *a* 细长形的,长形的;细长[体]型的
longimanous [ˌlɔndʒi'mænəs] *a* 长手的
longipedate [ˌlɔndʒi'pedeit] *a* 长脚的
longiradiate [ˌlɔndʒi'reidieit] *a* 长放线状的,长突的
longissimus [lɔn'dʒisiməs] *a*【拉】最长的 *n* 最长肌
longitudinal [ˌlɔndʒi'tjuːdinəl] *a* 纵[向]的
longitudinalis [ˌlɔŋdʒiˌtjuːdi'neilis] *a*【拉】纵的 *n* 纵肌
longitypical [ˌlɔndʒi'tipikəl] *a* 细长形的,长形的
Long's formula (coefficient) [lɔŋ] (John H. Long)朗氏公式(系数)(尿液比重的最后两个数字乘以 2.6〈朗氏系数〉所得之积,接近于 1 L 尿中固体的 G〈格令,grain〉数)
long-term ['lɔŋtəːm] *a* 长期的
longus ['lɔŋgəs] *a*【拉】长的 *n* 长肌
loop [luːp] *n* 袢,环,套圈 | archoplasmic ~ 假膜 / capillary ~s 毛细血管袢 / ~ of hypoglossal nerve 颈袢 / lenticular ~ 豆状核袢 / peduncular ~ 脑脚袢 / platinum ~ 铂环,白金耳 / subclavian ~ 锁骨下袢 / ventricular ~ 室袢(胚心早期 U 形袢)
loopful ['luːpful] *n* 铂环量,菌环量
loopogram ['luːpəugræm] *n* [肠]袢造影[照]片
loopography [luː'pɔgrəfi] *n* [肠]袢造影[术]
loosening ['luːsniŋ] *n* 松散(在精神病学中指一种思维障碍,表现为观念联想减少,变得支离破碎,因而缺乏逻辑性,见于精神分裂症)
Looser-Milkman syndrome ['ləuzə'milkmən] (Emil Looser; Louis A. Milkman)卢-米综合征(见 Milkman's syndrome)
Looser's transformation zones ['ləuzə] (Emil Looser)卢塞变形区,假骨折线(骨 X 线片所见的暗线,据认为系表示某些骨病发生的疲劳骨折病理性治愈期)
LOP left occipitoposterior 枕左后(胎位)
loperamide hydrochloride [ləu'perəmaid] 盐酸洛哌丁胺(减蠕动药)
loph(o)- [构词成分]脊,丛
lophodont ['lɔfədɔnt] *a* 脊牙型的
Lophomonadina [ˌlɔfəuˌməunə'dainə] *n* 缨滴虫亚目
Lophomonas [ˌlɔfəu'məunəs] *n* 缨滴虫属
Lophophora [lə'fɔfərə] *n* 魔根属 | ~ williamsii 魔根,威廉斯仙人球
lophophorine [lə'fɔfəriːn] *n* 魔根碱

Lophotrichea [ˌləufəˈtrikiə] *n* 偏端丛毛菌类
lophotrichous [ləˈfɔtrikəs] *a* 偏端丛毛的
lopinavir [ləuˈpinəvir] *n* 洛匹那韦(一种 HIV 蛋白酶抑制剂,抗病毒药,与利托那韦〈ritonavir〉联合用于治疗人免疫缺陷病毒感染,口服给药)
loracarbef [ˌlɔːrəˈkɑːbef] *n* 氯碳头孢(抗生素类药)
Lorain-Lévi dwarfism(syndrome) [lɔˈrei leiˈviː] (P. J. Lorain; E. L. Lévi) 洛兰-勒维侏儒症(综合征),垂体性幼稚型
Lorain's infantilism (disease, type) [lɔˈrei] (Paul J. Lorain)垂体性幼稚型
lorajmine hydrochloride [lɔːˈrædʒmiːn] 盐酸劳拉义明(抗心律失常药)
loratadine [ləˈrætədiːn] *n* 氯雷他定(抗组胺药)
lorazepam [lɔːˈræzəpæm] *n* 劳拉西泮(抗焦虑药)
lorbamate [lɔːˈbɑːmeit] *n* 劳氨酯(肌肉松弛药)
lorcainide hydrochloride [lɔːˈkeinaid] 盐酸劳卡尼(抗心律失常药)
lordoscoliosis [ˌlɔːdəuˌskɔliˈəusis] *n* 脊柱前侧凸
lordosis [lɔːˈdəusis] *n* 脊柱前凸 | **lordotic** [lɔːˈdɔtik] *a*
Lorenz's operation [ˈlɔrənts] (Adolf Lorenz)洛伦茨手术(治先天性髋关节脱位,包括脱位还原及使股骨头固定于残余髋臼,直至臼形成为止) | ~ osteotomy 洛伦茨截骨术(股骨颈 V 型截骨术) / ~ sign 洛伦茨征(脊柱关节强直,尤指胸腰段,偶见于早期结核)
Loreta's operation [lɔˈriːtə] (Pietro Loreta)洛雷塔手术(胃切开术以扩张幽门)
lorica [ləuˈraikə] ([复] **loricae** [ləuˈraikiː]) *n* 甲[壳]
loricate [ˈlɔːrikeit] *a* 有甲[壳]的
losartan potassium [ləuˈsɑːtæn] 氯沙坦钾(血管紧张素Ⅱ受体拮抗药,用作抗高血压药,口服给药)
loss [lɔ(ː)s] *n* 丧失,丢失 | hearing ~ 听力丧失
Lossen's rule(law) [ˈlɔsən] (Herman F. Lossen) 洛森规律(定律)(血友病仅由女性遗传,而由男性继承)
LOT left occipitotransverse 枕左横(胎位)
Lot. lotio【拉】洗液,洗剂
lota [ˈləutə] *n* 品他病(即 pinta)
loteprednol [ˌləutəˈprednɔl] *n* 氯替泼诺(一种皮质类固醇,局部用于结膜,治疗季节性变应性结膜炎、术后炎症和眼炎症性疾患)
lotio [ˈləuʃiəu] *n*【拉】洗液,洗剂
lotion [ˈləuʃən] *n* 洗液,洗剂 | amphotericin B ~ 两性霉素 B 洗液(外用抗真菌药) / benzyl benzoate-chlorophenothane-benzocaine ~ 苯甲酸苄酯-滴滴涕-苯佐卡因洗液(外用杀疥螨药和灭虱药) / betamethasone dipropionate ~ 二丙酸倍他米松洗液(外用糖皮质激素) / betamethasone valerate ~ 戊酸倍他米松洗液(抗炎药) / dimethisoquin hydrochloride ~ 盐酸奎尼卡因洗液(用作局部麻醉药以止痛、止痒及皮肤烧伤) / flurandrenolide ~ 氟氢缩松洗液,丙酮缩氟氢羟龙洗液(外用糖皮质激素) / hydrocortisone ~ 氢化可的松洗液(外用抗炎药,治胆固醇反应的皮病) / lindane ~, gamma benzene hexachloride ~ 林旦洗液,γ-六六六洗液(外用灭虱药和杀疥螨药) / methylbenzethonium chloride ~ 甲苄索氯铵洗液(局部抗感染药) / nystatin ~ 制霉菌素洗液(外用抗真菌药) / selenium sulfide ~ 二硫化硒洗液(外用抗真菌药,治花斑癣,亦可用作角质层分离剂以及治疗头皮、皮脂溢性皮炎和头皮屑) / white ~ 白色洗液,含硫洗液(表面收敛和保护剂)
Lotus [ˈləutəs] *n* 百脉根属,牛角化属
louchettes [luˈʃet] *n*【法】斜视矫正[眼]镜
Lou Gehrig disease [ˈluːˈgerig] (Lou Gehrig 为美国棒球运动员,死于此病)卢·盖里格病(肌萎缩侧索硬化)
Louis-Bar syndrome [luː(ː)ˈiːbɑː] (Denise Louis-Bar)毛细血管扩张性共济失调综合征
Louis's angle [ˈlu(ː)iː] (Pierre C. A. Louis)胸骨角 | ~ law 路易定律(①肺结核一般始于左肺;②任何部位的结核必伴之以在肺内定位)
loupe [luːp] *n*【法】放大镜 | corneal ~ 角膜放大镜(检角膜)
louse [laus] ([复] **lice** [lais]) *n* 虱 | biting ~ 啮毛虱,禽虱(食毛目虱的统称) / body ~, clothes ~ 体虱,衣虱 / chicken ~ 鸡虱,鸡皮刺螨 / crab ~, pubic ~ 阴虱 / head ~ 头虱 / sucking ~ 吸吮虱(虱目虱的统称)
lousewort [ˈlauswəːt] *n* 虱子草
lousicide [ˈlausisaid] *n* 灭虱剂
lousiness [ˈlauzinis] *n* 多虱,虱病
lousy [ˈlauzi] *a* 多虱的
lovastatin [ˈləuvəˌstætin] *n* 洛伐他汀(一种胆固醇生物合成抑制剂,用于治疗高胆固醇血症)
Löwenberg's canal(scala) [ˈleivənbəːg] (Benjamin B. Löwenberg)勒文伯格管(阶)(蜗管) | ~ forceps 勒文伯格钳(增殖体钳)
Löwenstein's culture medium [ˈleivənstain] (Ernst Löwenstein)勒文斯坦培养基(培养血内结核杆菌)
Löwenthal's tract [ˈleivəntəl] (Wilhelm Löwenthal)顶盖脊髓束
lowering [ˈləuəriŋ] *n* 减少 | vapor pressure ~ 蒸气压减少
Lower's rings [ˈləuə] (Richard Lower)心纤维环 | ~ tubercle 静脉间结节
Löwe's ring [ˈleivə] (Karl F. Löwe)勒弗环(视野

内由黄斑所致的环)

Lowe's syndrome(disease) [ləu] (Charles U. Lowe)洛氏综合征(病),眼脑肾综合征(oculocerebrorenal syndrome,见 syndrome 项下相应术语)

Lowe-Terrey-MacLachlan syndrome [ləu 'tɛəri mək'læklən] (C. U. Lowe; Mary Terrey; Elsie A. MacLachlan) 洛-特-麦综合征,眼脑肾综合征(即 oculocerebrorenal syndrome,见 syndrome 项下相应术语)

low-grade ['ləu 'greid] *a* (热度)低的;低级的(指恶性等级)

Löwitt's bodies, lymphocytes ['leivit] (Moritz Löwitt)淋巴原细胞

Lowman balance board ['ləumən] (Charles LeRoy Lowman)娄曼平底足平衡板(矫正平脚)

Lown-Ganong-Levine syndrome [laun 'gænən lə'vain] (Bernard Lown; William F. Gauong; Samuel A. Levine)朗-甘-莱综合征,短 P-R 综合征(一种预激综合征〈preexcitation syndrome〉,特征为心电图异常,短 P-R 间期,QRS 复合波正常,伴房性心动过速)

Lowsley operation ['ləuzli] (Oswald S. Lowsley)洛斯利手术(修复单纯性尿道上裂的一种手术,包括闭合裂开的尿道,劈开龟头,将修复的尿道深埋于软组织中,使尿道口处于正常的位置)

Lowy's test ['ləui] (Otto Lowy)娄伊试验(检癌)

loxapine ['lɔksəpiːn] *n* 洛沙平(三环类抗精神病药) | ~ succinate 琥珀酸洛沙平(用以治疗精神分裂症,口服)

loxarthron [lɔks'ɑːθrɔn], **loxarthrosis** [ˌlɔksɑː'θrəusis] *n* 关节斜弯

loxia ['lɔksiə] *n* 斜颈,捩颈

loxophthalmus [ˌlɔksɔf'θælməs] *n* 斜视,斜眼

Loxosceles [lɔk'sɔsəliːz] *n* 花蛛属 | ~ laeta 棕花蛛 / ~ reclusa 褐皮花蛛

Loxoscelidae [ˌlɔksɔ'selidiː] *n* 花蛛科

loxoscelism [lɔk'sɔsəlizəm] *n* 棕花蛛咬中毒 | viscerocutaneous ~ 内脏皮肤型棕花蛛咬中毒

loxotomy [lɔk'sɔtəmi] *n* 卵圆形切断术

Loxotrema ovatum [ˌlɔksə'triːmə əu'veitəm] 横川后殖吸虫(即 Metagonimus yokogawai)

lozenge ['lɔzindʒ] *n*【法】锭剂,糖锭

Lp(a) lipoprotein little A antigen 脂蛋白(a)抗原

LPF low-power field 低倍视野

LPH left posterior hemiblock 左后半支传导阻滞

LPN licensed practical nurse 有照护士

LPS lipopolysaccharide 脂多糖

LPV lymphotropic papovavirus 亲淋巴乳[头]多[瘤]空[泡]病毒

LRD living related donor 活体亲属供者

LSA left sacroanterior 骶左前(胎位);Licentiate of Society of Apothecaries 领有药学会开业证书者

LScA left scapuloanterior 肩左前(胎位)

LScP left scapuloposterior 肩左后(胎位)

LSD lysergic acid diethylamide 麦角二乙胺(致幻药)

LSO lumbosacral orthosis 腰骶支具

LSP left sacroposterior 骶左后(胎位)

L-spine limbar spine 腰椎

LST left sacrotransverse 骶左横(胎位)

LT lymphotoxin 淋巴毒素

LTB_4, LTC_4, etc. 各种白细胞三烯的符号(见 leukotriene)

LTF lymphocyte transforming factor 淋巴细胞转化因子

LTR long terminal repeats 长末端重复(序列)

Lu lutetium 镥

Lubarsch's crystals ['lubɑːʃ] (Otto Lubarsch)鲁巴尔希结晶(存于睾丸内,类似精液结晶)

lubb [lʌb] *n* 路布(摹拟第一心音)

lubb-dupp [lʌb 'dʌp] *n* 路布杜普(摹拟第一和第二心音)

lubricant ['ljuːbrikənt] *a* 润滑的 *n* 润滑剂,滑润剂

lubricate ['ljuːbrikeit] *vt* 使润滑 *vi* 起润滑作用 | **lubrication** [ljuːbri'keiʃən] *n* 润滑[作用] / **lubricator** *n* 润滑剂;润滑器

Lucae's probe ['luːkei] (August Lucae)路卡探子(耳按摩探子,治疗卡他性中耳炎)

lucanthone hydrochloride [lu'kænθəun] 盐酸硫恩酮(抗血吸虫药)

Lucas' sign ['ljuːkəs] (Richard C. Lucas)鲁卡斯征(佝偻病早期腹胀)

Lucatello's sign [ˌlukə'teləu] (Luigi Lucatello)路卡太洛征(甲状腺功能亢进患者腋下体温比口腔体温高 0.2~0.3 ℃)

Luciani's triad [ˌlutʃi'æni] (Luigi Luciani)路恰尼三征(无力、张力缺乏和起立不能,为小脑疾病 3 个主要症状)

Lucibacterium [ˌljuːsaibæk'tiːəriəm] *n* 射光杆菌属

lucid ['ljuːsid] *a* 神志清醒的 | ~ **ity** [ljuː'sidəti] *n* 清醒度(神志)

lucidification [ljuːˌsidifi'keiʃən] *n* 清明化,透明化(胞质)

luciferase [ljuː'sifəreis] *n* 荧光素酶

luciferin [ljuː'sifərin] *n* 荧光素

lucifugal [ljuː'sifjugəl] *a* 避光的,离光的

Lucilia [luː'siliə] *n* 绿蝇属 | ~ caesar 恺撒绿蝇 / ~ cuprina 铜绿蝇 / ~ illustris 亮绿蝇 / ~ regina 暗伏绿蝇(即 Phormia regina) / ~ sericata 丝光绿蝇(即 Phaenicia sericata)

Lucio leprosy ['luːʃəu] (R. Lucio)露西奥麻风(一种皮肤呈弥漫性瘤型浸润的麻风) | ~ phe-

nomenon 露西奥现象(发生于弥漫性瘤型麻风的局部加剧反应)
lucipetal [lju:ˈsipətl] *a* 趋光的,向光的
lucium [ˈlju:siəm] *n* 稀土金属元素混合物
lückenschädel [ˈlikənʃeidəl] *n*【德】颅盖缺裂
Lücke's test [ˈlikə] (George A. Lücke) 吕克试验(检马尿酸)
lucotherapy [ˌlju:kəuˈθerəpi] *n* 光线疗法
Luc's operation [luk] (Henri Luc) 路克手术(见 Caldwell-Luc operation)
Ludloff's sign [ˈludlɔf] (Karl Ludloff) 路德洛夫征(坐位时股三角底部肿胀和瘀斑,同时举腿不能,为股骨大转子骨骺创伤性分离之征)
Ludwig's angina [ˈludvig] (Wilhelm F. von Ludwig) 路德维希咽峡炎(脓性颌下腺炎,通常由链球菌感染所致)
Ludwig's angle [ˈludvig] (Daniel Ludwig) 胸骨角
Ludwig's ganglion [ˈludvig] (Karl F. W. Ludwig) 路德维希神经节(与心丛相连,接近心右房的神经节) | ~ theory 路德维希学说(泌尿学说,即尿是由肾小球过滤过程而形成,再吸收是由于扩散过程在泌尿管内发生)
Luer's syringe [ˈluə] 路厄注射器(一种玻璃注射器,静脉内和皮下注射用)
lues [ˈlju:i:z] *n*【拉】梅毒 | **luetic** [lju(:)ˈetik] *a*
luetin [ˈlju:ətin] *n* 梅毒螺旋体素
luette [ljuˈet] *n*【法】悬雍垂
Luft's disease [luft] (Rolf Luft) 勒夫特病(横纹肌代谢亢进病,由于线粒体数量及类型异常而产生细胞呼吸过盛所致,特征为多汗、虚弱无力、进行性软弱和基础代谢率异常增高)
lug [lʌg] *n* 支托
Lugol's caustic [luˈgɔl] (Jean G. A. Lugol) 卢戈尔腐蚀剂(一份碘和碘化钾溶于二份水中) | ~ iodine(iodine solution) 卢戈尔碘(碘溶液)(浓碘溶液)
luic [ˈlju:ik] *a* 梅毒的
Lukes-Collins classification [lu:ks ˈkɔlinz] (L. J. Lukes; R. D. Collins) 路-科分类法(根据假定的细胞来源的一种非霍奇金〈non-Hodgkin〉淋巴瘤分类法,强调 B 细胞、T 细胞和淋巴细胞性淋巴瘤之间的区别,B 细胞和 T 细胞型有若干亚型,可依据恶性等级排列)
lukewarm [ˈlju:kwɔ:m] *a* 微温的
LUL left upper lobe 左上叶(肺)
luliberin [lju:ˈlibərin] *n* 促黄体素释放[激]素
lumbago [lʌmˈbeigəu] *n* 腰痛 | ischemic ~ 缺血性腰痛
lumbar [ˈlʌmbə] *a* 腰的
lumbarization [ˌlʌmbəraiˈzeiʃən, -riˈz-] *n* 腰椎化
lumbo- [构词成分]腰
lumboabdominal [ˌlʌmbəuæbˈdɔminəl] *a* 腰腹的
lumbocolostomy [ˌlʌmbəukəˈlɔstəmi] *n* 腰部结肠造口术
lumbocolotomy [ˌlʌmbəukəˈlɔtəmi] *n* 腰部结肠切开术
lumbocostal [ˌlʌmbəuˈkɔstəl] *a* 腰肋的
lumbocrural [ˌlʌmbəuˈkruərəl] *a* 腰股的
lumbodorsal [ˌlʌmbəuˈdɔ:səl] *a* 腰背的
lumbodynia [ˌlʌmbəuˈdiniə] *n* 腰痛
lumboiliac [ˌlʌmbəuˈiliæk] *a* 腰髂的
lumboinguinal [ˌlʌmbəuˈiŋgwinəl] *a* 腰腹股沟的
lumbosacral [ˌlʌmbəuˈseikrəl] *a* 腰骶的
lumbrical [ˈlʌmbrikəl] *a* 蚯蚓的,蚓状的 *n* 蚓状肌
lumbricide [ˈlʌmbrisaid] *n* 驱蛔虫药
lumbricoid [ˈlʌmbrikɔid] *a* 蚯蚓状的(一般指蛔虫)
lumbricosis [ˌlʌmbriˈkəusis] *n* 蛔虫病
Lumbricus [ləmˈbrikəs] *n*【拉】蚯蚓属
lumbricus [ləmˈbrikəs] ([复] **lumbrici** [ˈlʌmbrisai]) *n*【拉】蛔虫;蚯蚓
lumbus [ˈlʌmbəs] *n*【拉】腰[部]
lumen [ˈlju:min] ([复] **lumens** 或 **lumina** [ˈlju:minə]) *n* 腔;流明(光通量单位) | residual ~ 遗腔,残留腔(垂体中的颅颊囊残余)
lumichrome [ˈlju:mikrəum] *n* 光色素
lumiflavin [ˌlju:miˈfleivin] *n* 光黄素
luminal [ˈlju:minl] *a* 腔的
luminalis [ˌlju:miˈneilis] *a* 腔的
luminance (L) [ˈlju:minəns] *n* 亮度
luminescence [ˌlju:miˈnesns] *n* 发光 | **luminescent** *a*
luminiferous [ˌlju:miˈnifərəs] *a* 发光的
luminophore [ˈlju:minəfɔ:] *n* 发光团;发光体
luminosity [ˌlju:miˈnɔsəti] *n* 发光度,明度;发光体
luminous [ˈlju:minəs] *a* 发光的
lumirhodopsin [ˌlu:mirəˈdɔpsin] *n* 光视紫红[质]
lump [lʌmp] *n* 块,肿块
lumpectomy [lʌmˈpektəmi] *n* 肿块切除术(手术切除乳腺癌仅可触知的病灶,亦称 tylectomy;手术切除肿块)
lumps [lʌmps] [复] *n* 羽下囊肿病(鸟类)
Lumsden's center [ˈlʌmzdən] (Thomas W. Lumsden) 呼吸调节中枢
lunacy [ˈlju:nəsi] *n* 疯狂,精神错乱
lunare [lju:ˈnɛəri] *n* 月骨
lunate(d) [ˈlju:neit(id)] *a* 月状的,半月形的
lunatic [ˈlju:nətik] *a* 精神错乱的 *n* 精神病患者
lunatomalacia [ljuˌneitəuməˈleiʃiə] *n* 月骨软化

Lund-Browder classification [lʌnd braud] (C. C. Lund; N. C. Browder)伦-布分类(一种儿童烧伤程度的分类)

lune [ljuːn] *n* 月牙形,半月形

lung [lʌŋ] *n* 肺 | arc-welder ~ 电弧焊工肺,肺铁末沉着病,铁尘肺 / artificial ~ 人工肺(即氧合器 oxygenator) / black ~, coalminer's ~, miners' ~ 矿工肺,炭末沉着病,炭肺 / book ~, book-~ 书肺(某些蛛形纲动物的呼吸气管) / brown ~ 棕色肺(即棉尘肺) / cardiac ~ 心力衰竭性肺充血 / drowned ~ 溺水肺(指肺不张) / eosinophilic ~ 嗜酸[细胞]性肺,热带嗜酸细胞增多症 / farmer's ~, harvester's ~, thresher's ~ 农民肺,脱粒工[尘]肺(吸入发霉草灰尘引起的肺病) / hyperlucent ~ 单侧肺气肿 / iron ~ 铁肺(德林克〈Drinker〉人工呼吸器的俗名) / masons' ~ 肺石末沉着病 / pigeon-breeder's ~, bird-breeder's ~ 养鸽者肺,养鸟者肺(对鸟粪产生获得性过敏所致的一种呼吸道疾病,可能导致肺纤维变性) / shock ~ 休克肺,成人呼吸窘迫综合征 / silofiller's ~ 地窖装填工肺(一种罕见的急性支气管炎,因吸入氮氧化物所致) / trench ~ 战壕肺(第一次世界大战时见于战壕,特征为急促呼吸发作) / vanishing ~ 消失肺,肺泡消失肺 / wet ~ 湿肺,肺积水,肺水肿 / white ~ 白肺(婴儿梅毒性肺炎)

lungmotor [ˈlʌŋməutə] *n* 肺充气机

lungworm [ˈlʌŋwəːm] *n* 肺蠕虫(如肺吸虫)

lunula [ˈljuːnjulə] ([复] **lunulae** [ˈljuːnjuliː]) *n* 【拉】弧影 | ~ of nail 甲弧影 / lunulae of semilunar valves 半月瓣弧影

lupeose [ˈljuːpiəus] *n* 羽扇豆糖,水苏四糖

lupiform [ˈljuːpifɔːm] *a* 狼疮状的;粉瘤状的

lupinosis [ljuːpiˈnəusis] *n* 羽扇豆中毒(指家畜等)

Lupinus [ˈljuːpinəs] *n* 羽扇豆属

lupoid [ˈljuːpɔid] *a* 狼疮状的 *n* 类狼疮(一种肉样瘤)

lupus [ˈljuːpəs] *n* 狼疮 | chilblain ~ erythematosus 冻疮样红斑狼疮 / cutaneous ~ erythematosus 皮肤红斑狼疮 / discoid ~ erythematosus (DLE) 盘状红斑狼疮 / drug-induced ~ 药物性狼疮 / ~ erythematosus(LE) 红斑狼疮 / hypertrophic ~ erythematosus 增殖性红斑狼疮 / neonatal ~, transient neonatal systemic ~ erythematosus 新生儿狼疮,新生儿暂时性系统性红斑狼疮 / systemic ~ erythematosus(SLE) 系统性红斑狼疮 / ~ tumidus 肿胀性狼疮 / ~ vulgaris 寻常狼疮

Luque instrumentation [ˈluːkei] (Eduardo R. Luque)卢克器械用法(矫正脊柱侧凸的一种方法,使用金属杆和丝在腰区施行前脊柱融合术) | ~ rod 卢克杆(一种坚硬的具有波状轮廓的不锈钢杆,用于卢克器械用法)

Luschka's bursa [ˈluʃkɑː] (Hubert von Luschka)咽扁桃体 | ~ crypts 卢施卡隐窝(胆囊黏膜) / ~ duct 卢施卡管(胆囊腺管) / ~ gland 尾骨球 / ~ muscles 卢施卡肌(含有肌组织的子宫骶韧带)

Lust's phenomenon (sign) [luːst] (Franz A. Lust)卢斯特现象(征)(轻叩腓骨头正下方的腓总神经,足背屈外展,提示痉挛倾向。亦称腓神经现象和腓骨征)

lusus naturae [ˈljuːsəs nəˈtjuəriː]【拉】先天畸形

lute [ljuːt] *n* 封泥 *vt* 密封

luteal [ˈljuːtiəl] *a* 黄体的

luteectomy [ˌljuːtiˈektəmi] *n* 黄体切除术

lutein [ˈljuːtiin] *n* 黄体素;脂色素 | serum ~ 血清黄体素 | **~ic** [ˌljuːtiˈinik] *a* 黄体素的,黄体的;黄体化的

luteinization [ˌljuːtiinaiˈzeiʃən, -niˈz-] *n* 黄体化

Lutembacher's syndrome (complex, disease) [ˈluːtəmˌbɑːhə] (René Lutembacher)鲁藤巴赫综合征(病)(二尖瓣狭窄伴有房间隔缺损)

luteohormone [ˌljuːtiəˈhɔːməum] *n* 孕酮,黄体酮

luteoid [ˈljuːtiɔid] *n* 类黄体素

luteolysin [ˌljuːtiˈɔlisin] *n* 黄体溶素,溶黄体素 | uterine ~ 子宫黄体溶素,前列腺素 $F_{2\alpha}$

luteolysis [ˌljuːtiˈɔlisis] *n* 黄体溶解

luteolytic [ˌljuːtiəuˈlitik] *a* 黄体溶解的 *n* 促黄体溶解药

luteoma [ˌljuːtiˈəumə] *n* 黄体瘤

luteose [ˈljuːtiəus] *n* 淡黄青霉多糖

luteotroph [ˈljuːtiəuˌtrəuf] *n* 催乳细胞

luteotropic [ˌljuːtiəˈtrɔpik], **luteotrophic** [ˌljuːtiəˈtrɔfik] *a* 促黄体的

luteotropin [ˌljuːtiəˈtrəupin], **luteotrophin** [ˌljuːtiəˈtrəufin] *n* 催乳激素

lutetium(Lu) [ljuːˈtiːʃiəm] *n* 镥(化学元素)

Lutheran blood group [ˈluːθərən] (Lutheran 为 1945 年首次报道的先证者的姓)卢瑟兰血型(一种复合血型系统,包括抗原 Lu^a 和 Lu^b,有点类似 Kell 血型,具有成对交替抗原和无效等位基因,但同样受到显性独立分离阻抑物的影响)

lutropin [ˈljuːtrɔpin] *n* 促黄体素

lututrin [ˈluːtjutrin] *n* 卵黄素,黄体弛子宫素(子宫弛缓药,治功能性痛经)

Lutzomyia [ˌluːtzəˈmaiə] *n* 罗蛉属

Lutz-Splendore-Almeida disease [luːts splenˈdɔːrei ɑːlˈmeidɑː] (Adolfo Lutz; Alfonso Splendore; Floriano Paulo de Almeida)卢-斯-艾病,副球孢子菌病

Luys' body syndrome [ljuˈiːz] (Jules B. Luys) 吕伊斯体综合征(偏身颤搐) | ~ nucleus 吕伊斯核(底丘脑核)

Luys' segregator(separator) [ljuˈiːz] (Georges Luys)吕伊斯分[隔采]尿器
lux(lx) [lʌks] *n* 勒[克司](照度单位)
luxate [ˈlʌkseit] *vt* 使脱位
luxatio [lʌkˈseiʃiəu] *n*【拉】脱位 | ~ coxae congenita 先天性髋脱位 / ~ erecta 直举性肱骨脱位 / ~ imperfecta 挨伤 / ~ perinealis 股骨会阴部脱位
luxation [lʌkˈseiʃən] *n* 脱位
luxuriant [lʌgˈzjuəriənt] *a* 过盛的,过多的 | **luxuriance** [lʌgˈzjuəriəns] *n* 过多;杂种旺势
luxury [ˈlʌkʃəri] *n* 过度
luxus [ˈlʌksəs] *n*【拉】过盛,过多
LVAD left ventricular assist device 左心室辅助装置
LVEDP left ventricular end-diastolic pressure 左心室舒张末期压
LVEDV left ventricular end-diastolic volume 左心室舒张末期容积
LVET left ventricular ejection time 左心室射血时间
LVH left ventricular hypertrophy 左心室肥大
LVN licensed vocational nurse 有照职业护士
Lw lawrencium 铹
lx lux 勒[克司](照度单位)
lyase [ˈlaieis] *n* 裂合酶
17, 20-lyase deficiency 17, 20-裂合酶缺乏症(由于缺乏 17α-羟孕〈甾〉酮醛缩酶所致的一种类固醇生成病)
lycanthropy [laiˈkænθrəpi], **lycomania** [ˌlaikəˈmeinjə] *n* 变兽妄想
lycetamine [laiˈsiːtəmiːn] *n* 氨棕己胺(局部抗菌药)
Lychnis githago [ˈlikis giˈθeigəu] 毒莠草,麦仙翁(即 Agrostemma githago)
lycine [ˈlaisiːn] *n* 甜菜碱
lycopene [ˈlaikəpiːn] *n* 番茄红素
lycopenemia [ˌlaikəpiˈniːmiə] *n* 番茄红素血
Lycoperdaceae [ˌlaikəupəːˈdeisiiː] *n* 马勃科
Lycoperdales [ˌlaikəpəˈdeiliːs] *n* 马勃目
Lycoperdon [ˌlaikəˈpəːdən] *n* 马勃属
lycoperdonosis [ˌlaikəˌpəːdəˈnəusis] *n* 马勃[孢子]病
Lycopodium [ˌlaikəˈpəudjəm] *n* 石松属
lycopodium [ˌlaikəˈpəudjəm] *n* 石松子(孢子)
lycorexia [ˌlaikəˈreksiə] *n* 狼样贪食,极度善饥
lycorine [ˈlikərin] *n* 石蒜碱
Lycoris [ˈlikəris] *n* 石蒜属
Lycosa tarentula [laiˈkəusə təˈrentjulə] 欧狼蛛
Lycosidae [laiˈkəusidiː] *n* 狼蛛科
lydimycin [lidiˈmaisin] *n* 利地霉素(抗真菌抗生素)
lye [lai] *n* 碱液,灰汁
Lyell's disease, syndrome [ˈlaiəl] (Alan Lyell)莱尔病、综合征,毒性表皮坏死松解
lying-in [ˌlaiiŋ ˈin] ([复]**lyings-in** 或 **lying-ins**) *n* 产褥期,产后期 *a* 产褥期的,产后的
Lyme disease (arthritis) [laim] (1975 年首次在美国康涅狄州 Old Lyme 报道)莱姆病(关节炎)(由博氏疏螺旋体〈Borrelia burgdorferi〉引起的复发性多系统性疾病,大部分病例开始为游走性慢性红斑〈直径至少 5 cm〉,继以各种不同表现,其中包括肌痛、大关节关节炎并累及神经和心血管系统) | ~ borreliosis 莱姆疏螺旋体病(一些由博氏疏螺旋体引起的并有相同表现的疾病的统称,其中包括莱姆病、慢性萎缩性肢端皮炎、班伐尔特〈Bannwarth〉综合征和游走性慢性红斑)
Lymnaea [limˈniːə] *n* 椎实螺属
lymph [limf] *n* 淋巴,淋巴液;浆,苗 | animal ~ 动物苗;动物淋巴 / aplastic ~, corpuscular ~ 非机化性淋巴,非成形性淋巴 / bovine ~, calf ~ 牛痘苗,牛痘浆 / croupous ~ 假膜性淋巴 / euplastic ~, fibrinous ~ 机化性淋巴,纤维蛋白性淋巴 / glycerinated ~ 甘油[化]痘浆 / humanized ~ 人痘浆 / inflammatory ~ 炎性淋巴 / intravascular ~ 淋巴管内淋巴 / plastic ~ 成形性淋巴,机化性淋巴 / vaccine ~ 痘苗、痘浆
lympha [ˈlimfə] *n*【拉】淋巴
lymphaden [ˈlimfədən] *n* 淋巴结
lymphadenectasis [limˌfædiˈnektəsis] *n* 淋巴结膨大
lymphadenectomy [limˌfædiˈnektəmi] *n* 淋巴结切除术
lymphadenhypertrophy [limˌfædənhaiˈpəːtrəfi] *n* 淋巴结肥大
lymphadenia [ˌlimfəˈdiːniə] *n* 淋巴组织增生 | ~ ossea 多发性骨髓瘤
lymphadenitis [limˌfædiˈnaitis] *n* 淋巴结炎 | caseous ~, paratuberculous ~ 干酪性淋巴结炎,异处结核性淋巴结炎 / nonbacterial regional ~, regional ~ 非细菌性区域性淋巴结炎,猫抓病,猫抓热 / tuberculous ~ 结核性淋巴结炎
lymphadenocele [limˈfædinəuˌsiːl] *n* 淋巴结囊肿
lymphadenocyst [limˈfædinəuˌsist] *n* 淋巴结囊肿
lymphadenogram [limˈfædinəuˌgræm] *n* 淋巴结造影[照]片
lymphadenography [limˌfædiˈnɔgrəfi] *n* 淋巴结造影[术]
lymphadenoid [limˈfædinɔid] *a* 淋巴结样的(组织)
lymphadenoleukopoiesis [limˌfædinəuˌljuːkəpɔiˈiːsis] *n* 淋巴组织性白细胞生成
lymphadenoma [ˌlimfædiˈnəumə] *n* 淋巴[组

织]瘤
lymphadenopathy [limˌfædiˈnɔpəθi] *n* 淋巴结病 | angioimmunoblastic ~, angioimmunoblastic ~ with dysproteinemia (AILD) 血管免疫母细胞淋巴结病,血管免疫母细胞淋巴结病伴异常蛋白血症(亦称免疫母细胞淋巴结病) / dermatopathic ~ 皮肤病性,淋巴结病 / giant follicular ~ 巨滤泡性淋巴结病,巨滤泡性淋巴瘤 / immunoblastic ~ 免疫母细胞淋巴结病,血管免疫母细胞淋巴结病 / tuberculous ~ 结核性淋巴结病,结核性淋巴结炎
lymphadenosis [limˌfædiˈnəusis] *n* 淋巴组织增生 | aleukemic ~ 非白血病性淋巴组织增生 / ~ benigna cutis 皮肤良性淋巴组织增生 / leukemic ~ 白血病性淋巴组织增生,慢性淋巴细胞性白血病
lymphadenotomy [limˌfædiˈnɔtəmi] *n* 淋巴结切开术
lymphadenovarix [limˌfædinəuˈvɛəriks] *n* 淋巴结增大
lymphagogue [ˈlimfəgɔg] *n* 利淋巴药,催淋巴剂
lymphangeitis [ˌlimfændʒiˈaitis] *n* 淋巴管炎
lymphangial [limˈfændʒiəl] *a* 淋巴管的
lymphangiectasia [limˌfændʒiekˈteiziə] *n* 淋巴管扩张 | intestinal ~ 肠淋巴管扩张
lymphangiectasis [limˌfændʒiˈektəsis] *n* 淋巴管扩张 | **lymphangiectatic** [limˌfændʒiekˈtætik] *a*
lymphangiectomy [limˌfændʒiˈektəmi] *n* 淋巴管切除术
lymphangiitis [limˌfændʒiˈaitis] *n* 淋巴管炎
lymphangioadenography [limˌfændʒiəuˌædiˈnɔgrəfi] *n* 淋巴系造影[术]
lymphangioendothelioma [limˌfændʒiəuˌendəuθiːliˈəumə] *n* 淋巴管内皮瘤
lymphangiofibroma [limˌfændʒiəufaiˈbrəumə] *n* 淋巴管纤维瘤
lymphangiogram [limˈfændʒiəgræm] *n* 淋巴管造影[照]片
lymphangiography [limˌfændʒiˈɔgrəfi] *n* 淋巴管造影[术] | pedal ~ 足淋巴管造影[术]
lymphangioitis [limˌfændʒiəuˈaitis] *n* 淋巴管炎
lymphangioleiomyomatosis [limˌfændʒiəuˌlaiəuˌmaiəuməˈtəusis] *n* 淋巴管平滑肌瘤病,淋巴管肌瘤病
lymphangiology [limˌfændʒiˈɔlədʒi] *n* 淋巴管学
lymphangioma [limˌfændʒiˈəumə] *n* 淋巴管瘤 | cavernous ~ 海绵状淋巴管瘤 / ~ circumscriptum 局限性淋巴管瘤,曲张性淋巴管瘤 / cystic ~ 囊状淋巴管瘤 / fissural ~ 胎缝性淋巴管瘤 / ~ simplex 单纯性淋巴管瘤
lymphangiomyomatosis (LAM) [limˌfændʒiəuˌmaiəuməˈtəusis] *n* 淋巴管肌瘤病
lymphangion [limˈfændʒiɔn] *n* 淋巴管
lymphangiophlebitis [limˌfændʒiəufliˈbaitis] *n* 淋巴管静脉炎
lymphangioplasty [limˈfændʒiəˌplæsti] *n* 淋巴管成形术
lymphangiosarcoma [limˌfændʒiəusɑːˈkəumə] *n* 淋巴管肉瘤
lymphangioscintigraphy (LAS) [limˌfændʒiəusinˈtigrəfi] *n* 淋巴管闪烁造影[术]
lymphangiotomy [limˌfændʒiˈɔtəmi] *n* 淋巴管切开术
lymphangitis [ˌlimfænˈdʒaitis] *n* 淋巴管炎 | gummatous ~ 树胶肿性淋巴管炎(即屠宰工人帚霉病 cladiosis) | **lymphangitic** [ˌlimfænˈdʒitik] *a*
lymphapheresis [ˌlimfəfəˈriːsis] *n* 淋巴细胞去除术
lymphatic [limˌfætik] *a* 淋巴的;淋巴[素]质的 *n* 淋巴管
lymphaticostomy [limˌfætiˈkɔstəmi] *n* 淋巴管造口术
lymphatism [ˈlimfətizəm] *n* 淋巴体质;淋巴质,黏液质
lymphatitis [ˌlimfəˈtaitis] *n* 淋巴系炎
lymphatogenous [ˌlimfəˈtɔdʒinəs] *a* 淋巴生成的
lymphatology [ˌlimfəˈtɔlədʒi] *n* 淋巴学
lymphatolysin [ˌlimfəˈtɔlisin] *n* 淋巴组织溶素
lymphatolysis [ˌlimfəˈtɔlisis] *n* 淋巴组织破坏,淋巴组织溶解 | **lymphatolytic** [ˌlimfətəˈlitik] *a* 溶解淋巴组织的
lymphatome [ˈlimfətəum] *n* 淋巴组织切除器
lymphectasia [ˌlimfekˈteiziə] *n* 淋巴性扩张;淋巴管扩张
lymphedema [ˌlimfi(ː)ˈdiːmə] *n* 淋巴水肿 | congenital ~ 先天性淋巴水肿 / ~ praecox 早发型淋巴水肿 / ~ tarda 迟发型淋巴水肿(35 岁后发生)
lymphemia [limˈfiːmiə] *n* 淋巴性白血病
lymphenteritis [ˌlimfentəˈraitis] *n* 浆液性肠炎
lymphepithelioma [ˌlimfepiˌθiːliˈəumə] *n* 淋巴上皮瘤,淋巴上皮癌
lymphization [ˌlimfaiˈzeiʃən, -fiˈz-] *n* 淋巴生成
lymphnoditis [ˌlimfnəuˈdaitis] *n* 淋巴结炎
lymph(o)- [构词成分] 淋巴
lymphoblast [ˈlimfəblæst] *n* 淋巴母细胞,原淋巴细胞 | **~ic** [ˌlimfəˈblæstik] *a*
lymphoblasthemia [ˌlimfəblæstˈhiːmiə] *n* 淋巴母细胞增多[症]
lymphoblastoma [ˌlimfəblæsˈtəumə] *n* 淋巴母细胞瘤 | **~tous** *a*
lymphoblastomatosis [ˌlimfəˌblæstəuməˈtəusis] *n* 淋巴母细胞瘤病

lymphoblastomid [ˌlimfəˈblæstəumid] *n* 淋巴母细胞瘤疹

lymphoblastosis [ˌlimfəblæsˈtəusis] *n* 淋巴母细胞增多[症]

lymphocele [ˈlimfəuˌsiːl] *n* 淋巴囊肿

lymphocerastism [ˌlimfəusiˈræstizəm] *n* 淋巴细胞生成

lymphocinesia [ˌlimfəusaiˈniːziə] *n* 内淋巴流动(半规管);淋巴循环

Lymphocryptovirus [ˌlimfəuˈkriptəˌvaiərəs] *n* 淋巴隐病毒属

lymphocyst [ˈlimfəusist] *n* 淋巴囊肿

lymphocystis [ˌlimfəuˈsistis] *n* 淋巴囊肿(海洋鱼和淡水鱼的一种常见慢性非致命性疾病,系淋巴囊肿病毒所致)

Lymphocystivirus [ˌlimfəuˈsistiˌvaiərəs] *n* 淋巴囊肿病毒属

lymphocytapheresis [ˌlimfəuˌsaitəfəˈriːsis] *n* 淋巴细胞去除术

lymphocyte [ˈlimfəsait] *n* 淋巴细胞 | amplifier T-~ 放大性 T 淋巴细胞,强化性 T 淋巴细胞 / B-~s,"bursa-equivalent" ~s, thymus-independent ~s B[淋巴]细胞,[腔上]囊依赖淋巴细胞,非胸腺依赖淋巴细胞(亦称 B 细胞) / cytotoxic T ~s (CTL)细胞毒性 T 淋巴细胞 / large granular ~s 大颗粒淋巴细胞 / T-~s, thymusdependent ~s T 淋巴细胞,胸腺依赖淋巴细胞(亦称 T 细胞) | **lymphocytic** [ˌlimfəˈsitik] *a*

lymphocythemia [ˌlimfəsaiˈθiːmiə] *n* 淋巴细胞增多[症]

lymphocytoblast [ˌlimfəˈsaitəblæst] *n* 成淋巴细胞,原始淋巴细胞

lymphocytoma [ˌlimfəsaiˈtəumə] *n* 假淋巴瘤;淋巴细胞瘤 | ~ cutis 皮肤淋巴细胞瘤 | **~tous** *a*

lymphocytomatosis [ˌlimfəˌsaitəuməˈtəusis] *n* 淋巴细胞瘤病

lymphocytopenia [ˌlimfəˌsaitəuˈpiːniə] *n* 淋巴细胞减少

lymphocytopheresis [ˌlimfəuˌsaitəufəˈriːsis] *n* 淋巴细胞去除术

lymphocytopoiesis [ˌlimfəˌsaitəupɔiˈiːsis] *n* 淋巴细胞发生 | **lymphocytopoietic** [limfəˌsaitəupɔiˈetik] *a*

lymphocytorrhexis [ˌlimfəˌsaitəˈreksis] *n* 淋巴细胞破裂

lymphocytosis [ˌlimfəsaiˈtəusis] *n* 淋巴细胞增多 | acute infectious ~ 急性传染性淋巴细胞增多症 | **lymphocytotic** [ˌlimfəsaiˈtɔtik] *a*

lymphocytotoxicity [ˌlimfəˌsaitəutɔkˈsisəti] *n* 淋巴细胞毒性

lymphocytotoxin [ˌlimfəˌsaitəˈtɔksin] *n* 淋巴细胞毒素

lymphoduct [ˈlimfədʌkt] *n* 淋巴管

lymphoepithelioma [ˌlimfəˌepiˌθiːliˈəumə] *n* 淋巴上皮瘤,淋巴上皮癌

lymphoganglin [ˌlimfəuˈgæŋglin] *n* 淋巴结激素(一种假定的激素)

lymphogenesis [ˌlimfəuˈdʒenisis] *n* 淋巴生成

lymphogenous [limˈfɔdʒinəs] *a* 成淋巴的;淋巴源的

lymphoglandula [ˌlimfəuˈglændjulə] ([复] **lymphoglandulae** [ˌlimfəuˈglændjuliː]) *n* 淋巴结

lymphogonia [ˌlimfəuˈgəuniə] *n* 淋巴原细胞

lymphogram [ˈlimfəgræm] *n* 淋巴系造影[照]片

lymphogranuloma [ˌlimfəuˌgrænjuˈləumə] *n* 淋巴肉芽肿 | ~ malignum 恶性淋巴肉芽肿,霍奇金(Hodgkin)病 / ~ venereum, ~ inguinale 性病淋巴肉芽肿,腹股沟淋巴肉芽肿,第五性病

lymphogranulomatosis [ˌlimfəuˌgrænjuləuməˈtəusis] *n* 淋巴肉芽肿病;霍奇金(Hodgkin)病 | benign ~ 良性淋巴肉芽肿病,肉样瘤病 / ~ cutis 皮肤淋巴肉芽肿病(霍奇金病皮肤表现) / ~ inguinalis 腹股沟淋巴肉芽肿 / ~ maligna 恶性淋巴肉芽肿病,霍奇金病

lymphography [limˈfɔgrəfi] *n* 淋巴系造影[术]

lymphohistiocytic [ˌlimfəuˌhistiəˈsitik] *a* 淋巴组织细胞的(淋巴细胞与组织细胞的)

lymphohistiocytosis [ˌlimfəuˌhistiəusaiˈtəusis] *n* 淋巴组织细胞增多症

lymphohistioplasmacytic [ˌlimfəuˌhistiəuˌplæsməˈsitik] *a* 淋巴组织浆细胞的(淋巴细胞,组织细胞与浆细胞的)

lymphoid [ˈlimfɔid] *a* 淋巴样的;淋巴组织样的;淋巴的,淋巴系统的

lymphoidectomy [ˌlimfɔiˈdektəmi] *n* 淋巴组织切除术

lymphoidocyte [limˈfɔidəsait] *n* 淋巴样细胞,成血细胞

lymphoidotoxemia [limˌfɔidəutɔkˈsiːmiə] *n* 淋巴毒血症

lymphokentric [ˌlimfəuˈkentrik] *a* 刺激淋巴细胞生成的 | ~ acid 淋巴细胞生长酸

lymphokine [ˈlimfəkain] *n* 淋巴因子

lymphokinesis [ˌlimfəukaiˈniːsis, -kiˈn-] *n* 内淋巴流动(半规管);淋巴循环

lymphology [limˈfɔlədʒi] *n* 淋巴学

lympholysis [limˈfɔlisis] *n* 淋巴细胞溶解 | cell-mediated ~ (CML) 细胞介导淋巴细胞溶解

lympholytic [ˌlimfəuˈlitik] *a* 淋巴细胞溶解的

lymphoma [limˈfəumə] *n* 淋巴瘤 | African ~ 非洲淋巴瘤(即伯基特淋巴瘤 Burkitt's lymphoma) / convoluted T-cell ~ 卷曲核 T 细胞淋巴瘤 / cutaneous T-cell ~ 皮肤 T 细胞淋巴瘤 / ~ cutis

皮肤淋巴瘤 / diffuse ~ 弥漫型淋巴瘤(亦称淋巴肉瘤) / follicular ~ 滤泡型淋巴瘤 / follicular center cell ~ 滤泡中心细胞淋巴瘤 / giant follicle ~, giant follicular ~ 巨滤泡型淋巴瘤 / granulomatous ~ 肉芽肿性淋巴瘤,霍奇金(Hodgkin)病 / histiocytic ~ 组织细胞淋巴瘤(亦称网状细胞肉瘤) / lymphoblastic ~ 淋巴细胞淋巴瘤 / malignant ~ of cattle, bovine malignant ~ 牛恶性淋巴瘤 / Mediterranean ~ 地中海淋巴瘤,α-重链病 / mixed lymphocytichistiocytic ~ 淋巴细胞-组织细胞混合性淋巴瘤 / nodular ~ 结节型淋巴瘤 / non-Hodgkin's ~s 非霍奇金淋巴瘤 / plasmacytoid lymphocytic ~ 浆细胞样淋巴细胞淋巴瘤 / pleomorphic ~ 多形淋巴瘤 / poorly-differentiated lymphocytic ~ 低分化淋巴细胞淋巴瘤 / small B-cell ~ 小 B 细胞淋巴瘤 / small lymphocytic T-cell ~ 小淋巴细胞性 T 细胞淋巴瘤 / T-cell ~s T 细胞淋巴瘤 / U-cell(undefined) ~ 不明细胞淋巴瘤 / undifferentiated ~ 未分化淋巴瘤(亦称多形性淋巴瘤) / well-differentiated lymphocytic ~ 高分化淋巴细胞淋巴瘤(亦称淋巴细胞瘤)

lymphomatoid [limˈfəumətɔid] *a* 淋巴瘤样的

lymphomatosis [ˌlimfəuməˈtəusis] *n* 淋巴瘤病

lymphomatous [limˈfəumətəs] *a* 淋巴瘤的

lymphomyxoma [ˌlimfəumikˈsəumə] *n* 淋巴黏液瘤

lymphonodulus [ˌlimfəˈnɔdjuləs] ([复] **lymphonoduli** [ˌlimfəˈnɔdjulai]) *n*【拉】淋巴小结

lymphonodus [ˌlimfəˈnəudəs] ([复] **lymphonodi** [ˌlimfəˈnəudai]) *n*【拉】淋巴结

lymphopathia [ˌlimfəˈpæθiə] *n* 淋巴[组织]病,淋巴肉芽肿 | ~ venereum 性病性淋巴肉芽肿,腹股沟淋巴肉芽肿

lymphopathy [limˈfɔpəθi] *n* 淋巴[组织]病 | ataxic ~ 共济失调性淋巴[组织]病

lymphopenia [ˌlimfəuˈpiːniə] *n* 淋巴细胞减少

lymphoplasia [ˌlimfəuˈpleiziə] *n* 淋巴组织形成 | cutaneous ~ 皮肤淋巴组织形成,皮肤淋巴细胞瘤

lymphoplasm [ˈlimfəplæzəm] *n* 海绵质

lymphoplasmapheresis [ˌlimfəuˌplæzməfəˈriːsis] *n* 淋巴细胞与血浆去除术

lymphoplasmia [ˌlimfəuˈplæzmiə] *n* 红细胞失色症

lymphoplasty [ˈlimfəˌplæsti] *n* 淋巴管成形术

lymphopoiesis [ˌlimfəupɔiˈiːsis] *n* 淋巴组织生成;淋巴细胞生成 | **lymphopoietic** [ˌlimfəupɔiˈetik] *a*

lymphoproliferative [ˌlimfəuprəuˈlifərətiv] *a* 淋巴组织增生的

lymphoreticular [ˌlimfəuriˈtikjulə] *a* 淋巴网状内皮细胞的

lymphoreticulosis [ˌlimfəuriˌtikjuˈləusis] *n* 淋巴网状内皮细胞增生[症] | benign ~ 良性淋巴网状内皮细胞增生[症],猫抓病

lymphorrhage [ˈlimfəreidʒ] *n* 淋巴细胞集积(在肌内)

lymphorrhea [ˌlimfəˈriːə], **lymphorrhagia** [ˌlimfəˈreidʒiə] *n* 淋巴溢

lymphorrhoid [ˈlimfərɔid] *n* 肛周淋巴管扩张,淋巴管痔

lymphosarcoleukemia [ˌlimfəuˌsɑːkəuljuːˈkiːmiə] *n* 淋巴肉瘤细胞性白血病

lymphosarcoma [ˌlimfəusɑːˈkəumə] *n* 淋巴肉瘤 | fascicular ~, sclerosing ~ 硬化性淋巴肉瘤

lymphosarcomatosis [ˌlimfəuˌsɑːkəuməˈtəusis] *n* 淋巴肉瘤病

lymphoscintigraphy [ˌlimfəusinˈtigrəfi] *n* 淋巴系闪烁造影[术](检测淋巴结转移性肿瘤) | radiocolloid ~ 放射性胶体淋巴系闪烁造影[术]

lymphosporidiosis [ˌlimfəuspəˌridiˈəusis] *n* 淋巴孢子虫病,兽疫性淋巴管炎

lymphostasis [limˈfɔstəsis] *n* 淋巴淤滞

lymphotaxis [ˌlimfəˈtæksis] *n* 淋巴细胞趋向性

lymphotism [ˈlimfətizəm] *n* 淋巴组织发育障碍

lymphotome [ˈlimfətəum] *n* 增殖体切除器

lymphotoxemia [ˌlimfəutɔkˈsiːmiə] *n* 淋巴毒血症

lymphotoxin [ˌlimfəˈtɔksin] *n* 淋巴毒素

lymphotrophy [limˈfɔtrəfi] *n* 淋巴营养性

lymphotropic [ˌlimfəuˈtrɔpik] *a* 亲淋巴的

lymphous [ˈlimfəs] *a* 淋巴的;含淋巴的

lymph-vascular [limfˈvæskjulə] *a* 淋巴管的

Lynchia maura [ˈlinkiə ˈmɔːrə] 拟虱蝇(即 Pseudolynchia canariensis)

Lynch's incision [lintʃ] (Robert C. Lynch)林奇切口(额窦手术外切口) | ~ operation 林奇手术(切除额窦并除去额窦底及其内容物,此手术在额窦扩展黏液囊肿、鞘膜积脓和肿瘤病情时施行)

lynestrenol [liˈnestrinɔl] *n* 利奈孕酮(孕激素类药)

Lynxacarus [liŋkˈsækərəs] *n* 牦螨属

-lysis [构词成分]溶解,分解,分离,破坏,缓解,减少,减轻,松解,释放

lyo- [构词成分] 溶解

lyochrome [ˈlaiəkrəum] *n* 黄素

lyogel [ˈlaiədʒel] *n* 水凝胶,多液凝胶

Lyon hypothesis [ˈlaiən] (Mary F. Lyon)莱昂假说(在胚胎发育的早期,所有哺乳动物的体细胞中 X 染色体多于一个时,所有 X 染色体均以随机方式失活,成为性染色质)

lyonization [ˌlaiənaiˈzeiʃən, -niˈz-] (Mary F. Lyon) *n* 莱昂作用(指细胞中 X 染色体多于一个时,X 染色体以随机方式失活的过程或状况,亦称异染质化,X 染色体失活。同样见 Lyon hypothesis)

lyonized [ˈlaiənaizd] *a* 莱昂化的(根据莱昂假说,指细胞中失活的 X 染色体)

lyophil [ˈlaiəfil] *n* 亲液物;亲液胶体,亲媒胶体

lyophile [ˈlaiəfail] *n* 亲液物;亲液胶体,亲媒胶体 *a* 亲液的,亲媒的

lyophilic [ˌlaiəuˈfilik] *a* 亲液的,亲媒的

lyophilize [laiˈɔfilaiz] *vt* 冻干 | **lyophilization** [laiˌɔfilaiˈzeiʃən, -iˈz-] *n* 冻干[保藏]法,冷冻干燥

lyophilizer [laiˈɔfilaizə] *n* 冻干器,冷冻干燥器

lyophobe [ˈlaiəfəub] *n* 疏液物;疏液胶体 | **lyophobic** [ˌlaiəˈfəubik] *a* 疏液的;疏媒的(胶体)

lyosol [ˈlaiəsɔl] *n* 水溶胶,液体溶胶

lyosorption [ˌlaiəuˈsɔːpʃən] *n* 溶媒吸附[作用],吸收溶剂[作用]

lyotropic [ˌlaiəuˈtrɔpik] *a* 易溶的

Lyperosia irritans [ˌlaipəˈrəusiə ˈiritəns] 扰角蝇(即扰血蝇 Haematobia irritans)

Lyponyssus [ˌlaipəˈnisəs] *n* 刺脂螨属(即禽刺螨属 Ornithonyssus)

lypressin [laiˈpresin] *n* 赖氨加压素(治尿崩症用的制尿药)

lyra [ˈlaiərə] *n*【拉;希】琴,琴形物

lyre [ˈlaiə] *n* 琴,琴形物

Lys lysine 赖氨酸

lysate [ˈlaiseit] *n* [细胞]溶解产物,溶胞产物;溶成剂(用人工消化方法从动物器官中获得的药物制剂)

lysatin [ˈlisətin] *n* 溶解素(原由 Drechsel 测定为源于酪蛋白的一种要素,后来证明是赖氨酸和精氨酸的混合物)

lyse [laiz] *vt, vi* 溶解,溶化

lysemia [laiˈsiːmiə] *n* 血液分解

lysergic acid [liˈsəːdʒik] 麦角酸 | ~ diethylamide (LSD) 麦角二乙胺(致幻药)

lysergide [ˈlaisədʒaid] *n* 麦角二乙胺(致幻药)

lysidin [ˈlisidin] *n* 甲咪唑啉(用作尿酸溶剂) | ~ bitartrate 重酒石酸甲咪唑啉

lysimeter [laiˈsimitə] *n* 溶度测定器,溶度计

lysin [ˈlaisin] *n* 溶素,溶解素 | beta ~ β 溶素(某些动物血清中一种较耐热的杀菌性成分,在 56 ~ 60 ℃, 30 ~ 40 分钟时并不失活) / immune ~ 免疫溶素(一种溶细胞性抗体,与细胞性抗原相互作用,以便介导补体溶解细胞的作用)

lysine [ˈlaisiːn] *n* 赖氨酸

lysine carboxypeptidase [ˈlaisiːn kɑːˌbɔksiˈpeptideis] 赖氨酸羧肽酶(亦称精氨酸羧肽酶,激肽酶 I)

lysine dehydrogenase [ˈlaisiːn diːˈhaidrədʒəneis] 赖氨酸脱氢酶(此酶的遗传性缺乏可致先天性赖氨酸不耐受)

lysine ketoglutarate reductase [ˈlaisiːn ˌkiːtəu-ˈgljuːtəreit riˈdʌkteis] 赖氨酸酮戊二酸还原酶,酵母氨酸脱氢酶($NADP^+$, L-赖氨酸形成的)

lysine-ketoglutarate reductase deficiency 赖氨酸酮戊二酸还原酶缺乏症,高赖氨酸血症

L-lysine: NAD oxidoreductase [ˈlaisiːn ˌɔksidəuriˈdʌkteis] L-赖氨酸:NAD 氧化还原酶,赖氨酸脱氢酶

L-lysine: NAD oxidoreductase deficiency L-赖氨酸:NAD 氧化还原酶缺乏症,先天性赖氨酸不耐受

lysinogen [laiˈsinədʒən] *n* 溶素原

lysinogenesis [ˌlaisinəuˈdʒenisis] *n* 溶素生成

lysinosis [ˌlisiˈnəusis] *n* 肺棉屑沉着病,棉屑肺

lysinuria [ˌlaisiˈnjuəriə] *n* 赖氨酸尿

lysis [ˈlaisis] *n* 溶解,分解;松解术;渐退,消散(指症状);溶胞[作用] | hot-cold ~ 冷却溶解(物质经培养后置于室温下过夜而引起的溶解)

lys(o)- [构词成分]溶解,溶化

lysocephalin [ˌlaisəuˈsefəlin] *n* 溶血脑磷脂

lysochrome [ˈlaisəkrəum] *n* 溶色素,脂肪染色剂

lysocythin [ˌlaisəuˈsaiθin] *n* 溶细胞素

lysogen [ˈlaisədʒən] *n* 溶素原

lysogenesis [ˌlaisəˈdʒenisis] *n* 溶素生成,致溶解性溶源现象 | **lysogenic** [laisəˈdʒenik] *a* 生成溶素的,引起溶解的;溶源性的

lysogenicity [ˌlaisəudʒiˈnisəti], **lysogeny** [laiˈsɔdʒini] *n* 致溶解性;产噬菌体;溶源性,溶源现象

lysokinase [ˌlaisəuˈkaineis] *n* 溶解激酶

lysolecithin [ˌlaisəuˈlesiθin] *n* 溶血卵磷脂

lysophosphatidate [ˌlaisəuˌfɔsfəˈtaideit] *n* 溶血磷脂酸(阴离子型)

lysophosphatide [ˌlaisəuˈfɔsfətaid] *n* 溶血磷脂

lysophosphatidic acid [ˌlaisəuˌfɔsfəˈtidik] 溶血磷脂酸

lysophospholipase [ˌlaisəuˌfɔsfəuˈlaipeis, -ˈlip-] *n* 溶血磷脂酶

lysophospholipid [ˌlaisəuˌfɔsfəuˈlipid] *n* 溶血磷脂

lysosomal [ˌlaisəˈsəuməl] *a* 溶酶体的

lysosomal α-glucosidase [ˌlaisəuˈsəuməl gluːˈkəusideis] 溶酶体 α-葡糖苷酶,葡聚糖 1, 4-α-葡糖苷酶

lysosomal α-glucosidase deficiency 溶酶体 α-葡糖苷酶缺乏症,糖原贮积症 Ⅱ 型

lysosome [ˈlaisəsəum] *n* 溶酶体 | primary ~ 初级溶酶体 / secondary ~ 次级溶酶体 | **lysosomal** [ˌlaisəˈsəuməl] *a*

lysostaphin [ˌlaisəuˈstæfin] *n* 溶葡萄球菌素

lysotype [ˈlaisətaip] *n* 噬菌体型
lysozyme [ˈlaisəzaim] *n* 溶菌酶
lysozymuria [ˌlaisəuzaiˈmjuəriə] *n* 溶菌酶尿
lyssa [ˈlisə] *n*【希】狂犬病,瘈咬病;舌中隔 | **lyssic** [ˈlisik] *a* 狂犬病的
Lyssavirus [ˈlisəˌvaiərəs] *n* 狂犬病病毒属
lyss(o)- [构词成分] 狂犬病
lyssodexis [ˌlisəuˈdeksis] *n* 狂犬咬伤
lyssoid [ˈlisɔid] *a* 狂犬病样的
lyssophobia [ˌlisəuˈfəubjə] *n* 狂犬病恐怖,瘈咬病恐怖
Lyster tube [ˈlistə] (William J. L. Lyster) 利斯特管(玻璃管内含次氯酸钙,饮水消毒用)
lysyl [ˈlaisil] *n* 赖氨酰[基]
lysyl hydroxylase [ˈlaisil haiˈdrɔksileis] 赖氨酰羟化酶(此酶活性缺乏为一种常染色体隐性性状,可致埃勒斯-当洛〈Ehlers-Danlos〉综合征Ⅵ型,在EC命名法中称前胶原-赖氨酸5-双加氧酶)
lysyl oxidase [ˈlaisil ˈɔksideis] 赖氨酰氧化酶(此酶活性缺乏以及在埃勒斯-当洛〈Ehlers-Danlos〉综合征Ⅸ型〈X连锁遗传皮肤松垂〉和门克斯〈Menkes〉综合征时发生伴随的生理结果,似乎继发于铜代谢或运输的缺乏)
lyterian [laiˈtiəriən] *a* (病势)渐退的,消散的
lytic [ˈlitik] *a* 溶解的,溶素的;松解的;渐退的
Lytta [ˈlitə] *n* 芫青属 | ~ vesicatoria 西班牙芫青(亦称 Cantharis vesicatoria)
lytta [ˈlitə] *n* 狂犬病
lyxonic acid [likˈsɔnik] 来苏糖酸
lyxose [ˈliksəus] *n* 来苏糖
lyze [laiz] *vt*, *vi* 溶解,溶化

M

M mega- 百万,兆(10^6); methionine 甲硫氨酸; molar[1] 摩尔浓度; molar[2] 磨牙; morgan 摩[尔根]; mucoid (colony) 黏液状(菌落); myopia 近视;第一心音低频成分

M. misce 混合; mistura 合剂

M mutual inductance 互感; molar mass 摩尔量; molar[1] 摩尔浓度

M_1 mitral valve closure 二尖瓣关闭

M_r relative molecular mass 相对分子量

m median 中位数; meter 米; milli- 毫

m. minim 量滴; musculus【拉】肌[肉]

m mass 质量; molal (重量)摩尔的

m- meta- 间[位]

β_2-m β_2 微球蛋白

μ mu 希腊语的第 12 个字母; linear attenuation coefficient 线性衰减系数; population mean 总体均数; micro- 微; micron 微米; electrophoretic mobility 电泳泳动度; 重链 IgM

MA Master of Arts 文学硕士; mental age 智力年龄,心理年龄; meter angle 米角,公尺角

mA milliampere 毫安[培]

μA microampere 微安[培]

MAA macroaggregated albumin 大颗粒聚清蛋白

MAC membrane attack complex 攻膜复合物

Mac. macerare【拉】浸渍,浸软

Mac-1 Mac-1 糖蛋白

Macaca [məˈkækə] *n* 猕猴属 | ~ cynomulgus 南美猕猴 / ~ mulatta 猕猴,罗猴,恒河猴

macaque [məˈkɑːk] *n* 猕猴

MacCallum's patch [məˈkæləm] (William G. MacCallum) 麦卡勒姆斑(心内膜深层的肉芽组织片,系风湿热时心肌中阿孝夫〈Aschoff〉小结广泛融合形成) | ~ plaques 麦卡勒姆斑(风湿性心脏病时,常见于左心房内心内膜下损害引起的不规则增厚)

MacConkey's agar, broth [məˈkɔnki] (Alfred T. MacConkey) 麦康基琼脂(肉汤)(分离大肠菌类用,亦称麦康基胆盐琼脂)

mace [meis] *n* 肉豆蔻衣

macerate [ˈmæsəreit] *vt*, *vi*. 浸软,浸渍 | **maceration** [ˌmæsəˈreiʃən] *n* / **macerative** *a* / **macerator** [ˈmæsəreitə] *n* 浸渍器

Macewen's operation [məˈkjuːən] (William Macewen) 麦克尤恩手术(①股骨髁上楔形切骨治膝外翻;②疝根治术) | ~ sign 麦克尤恩征(脑积水及脑脓肿时,叩诊额骨、颞骨和顶骨接缝后的颅骨,则反响叩音较正常强) / ~ triangle 麦克尤恩三角(颞骨乳突窝)

Machado-Joseph disease [məˈʃɑːdəu ˈdʒəusif] 神经系统亚速尔病(发现于亚速尔群岛后裔的家族,Machado 和 Joseph 为受患家族)

Mache unit [ˈmɑːʃə] (Heinrich Mache) 马谢单位(溶液中镭射气浓度单位)

machine [məˈʃiːn] *n* 机器,机械 | heart-lung ~ 心肺机

Macht's test [mækt] (David I. Macht) 麦克特试验(检血清对白羽扇豆苗生长的效果,恶性贫血及其他不正常血液的血清可使其苗生长缓慢)

macies [ˈmeiʃiiːz] *n*【拉】消瘦

MAC INH membrane attack complex inhibitor 膜攻击复合体抑制剂

macintosh [ˈmækintɔʃ] (Charles Macintosh) *n* 橡皮防水布,不透水布(曾用作外科敷料)

macis [ˈmeisis] *n*【拉】肉豆蔻衣

MacKay-Marg electronic tonometer [məˈkei mɑːg] (Ralph S. Mackay; Elwin Marg) 麦-马电子眼压计(带有平芯直接放在角膜上测量眼内压的电子压平眼压计)

Mackenrodt's ligament [ˈmʌkənrɔt] (Alwin K. Mackenrodt) 直肠子宫襞 | ~ operation 马肯罗特手术(阴道式圆韧带固定术,用以矫正子宫后移位)

Mackenzie's disease [məˈkenzi] (James Mackenzie) 麦肯齐病,X 病(X disease,见 disease 项下相应术语)

Mackenzie's syndrome [məˈkenzi] (Stephen Mackenzie) 麦肯齐综合征(即 Jackson's syndrome)

Maclagan's thymol turbidity test [məkˈlɑːgən] (Noel F. Maclagan) 麦克拉根麝香草酚混浊度试验(检肝代谢紊乱)

MacLean-Maxwell disease [məkˈlein ˈmækswəl] (Charles M. MacLean; James L. Maxwell) 麦克莱恩-马克斯韦尔病(跟骨的一种慢性疾病,特征为跟骨后三分之一肿大,并有压痛)

MacLeod's capsular rheumatism [məkˈlaud] (Roderick MacLeod) 麦克劳德关节囊风湿病(一种类风湿关节炎,有渗出液进入滑液囊、黏液囊及关节囊鞘中)

Macleod's syndrome [məˈklaud] (William Mathieson Macleod) 麦克劳德综合征(单侧透明肺综

合征,见 Swyer-James syndrome)
MacMunn's test [mək'mʌn] (Charles A. MacMunn) 麦克莫恩试验(检尿蓝母)
MacQuarrie's test [mə'kwɔri] (F. W. MacQuarrie) 麦夸里试验(以铅笔及纸,试一般机械操作能力)
Macracanthorhynchus [ˌmækrəˌkænθə'riŋkəs] *n* 巨吻棘头虫属 | ~ hirudinaceus 猪巨吻棘头虫
macradenous [mæ'krædinəs] *a* 巨腺的
macrencephaly [ˌmækrən'sefəli], **macrencephalia**[məˌkrensə'feiliə] *n* 巨脑
macr(o)- [构词成分]巨,大,长
macroabrasion [ˌmækrəuə'breiʒən] *n* 巨磨损
macroadenoma [ˌmækrəuˌædə'nəumə] *n* 巨腺瘤(直径超过 10 mm 的一种垂体腺瘤)
macroaggregate [ˌmækrə'ægrigeit] *n* 大集合物
macroaleuriospore [ˌmækrəuə'ljuəriəspɔː] *n* 大粉状孢子,大侧生孢子
macroamylase [ˌmækrəu'æmileis] *n* 巨淀粉酶,大分子淀粉酶
macroamylasemia [ˌmækrəuæmilə'siːmiə] *n* 巨淀粉酶血症 | **macroamylasemic** *a*
macroanalysis [ˌmækrəuə'nælisis] *n* 常量分析
Macrobdella [ˌmækrəu'delə] *n* 巨蛭属 | ~ decora 北美巨蛭
macrobiota [ˌmækrəubai'əutə] *n* 大生物区[系]
macrobiotic [ˌmækrəubai'ɔtik] *a* 大生物区的;长寿的,延年的 | **~s** *n* 长寿法(如通过节食方式)
macroblast ['mækrəblæst] *n* 大成红细胞
macroblepharia [ˌmækrəubli'fɛəriə] *n* 巨睑
macrobrachia [ˌmækrəu'breikiə] *n* 巨臂
macrocardius [ˌmækrəu'kɑːdiəs] *n* 巨心畸胎
macrocephaly [ˌmækrəu'sefəli], **macrocephalia** [ˌmækrəusə'feiliə], **macrocephalus** [ˌmækrəu'sefələs] *n* 大头[畸形] | **macrocephalous** [ˌmækrəu'sefələs], **macrocephalic** [ˌmækrəu-sə'fælik] *a*
macrocheilia, **macrochilia** [ˌmækrəu'kailiə] *n* 巨唇[症]
macrocheiria, **macrochiria** [ˌmækrəu'kaiəriə] *n* 巨手
macrochemistry [ˌmækrəu'kemistri] *n* 常量化学(可以用肉眼观察化学反应的化学) | **macrochemical** *a*
macroclitoris [ˌmækrəu'klitəris] *n* 巨阴蒂
macrocnemia [ˌmækrɔk'niːmiə] *n* 巨小腿
macrocolon [ˌmækrəu'kəulən] *n* 巨结肠
macroconidium [ˌmækrəukə'nidiəm] ([复] **macroconidia** [ˌmækrəukə'nidiə]) *n* 大分生孢子
macrocornea [ˌmækrəu'kɔːniə] *n* 大角膜
macrocosm ['mækrəkɔzəm] *n* 宏观世界;大宇宙
macrocrania [ˌmækrəu'kreiniə] *n* 巨颅
macrocyclic [ˌmækrəu'siklik] *a* 大环的(大环有机化合物的,一般含有 15 个以上的原子)
macrocyst ['mækrəusist] *n* 巨囊;大包囊,产囊体
macrocytase [ˌmækrəu'saiteis] *n* 巨噬细胞溶解酶
macrocyte ['mækrəusait] *n* 大红细胞,巨红细胞 | **macrocytic**[ˌmækrəu'sitik] *a*
macrocythemia [ˌmækrəusai'θiːmiə], **macrocytosis**[ˌmækrəusai'təusis] *n* 大红细胞血症,大红细胞
macrodactyly [ˌmækrəu'dæktili], **macrodactylia**[ˌmækrəudæk'tiliə] *n* 巨指,巨指畸形,巨趾,巨趾畸形
macrodontia [ˌmækrəu'dɔnʃiə], **macrodontism** [ˌmækrəu'dɔntizəm] *n* 巨牙,巨牙症 | **macrodontic**[ˌmækrəu'dɔntic], **macrodont**[ˌmækrə-dɔnt] *a*
macrodystrophia [ˌmækrəudis'trəufiə] *n* 营养异常性巨大发育 | ~ lipomatosa progressiva 进行性脂瘤性巨大发育
macroelement [ˌmækrəu'elimənt] *n* 大量元素
macroencephaly [ˌmækrəuen'sefəli] *n* 巨脑
macroerythroblast [ˌmækrəui'riθrəublæst] *n* 大成红细胞
macroesthesia [ˌmækrəuis'θiːzjə] *n* 物体巨大感,触物显大症
macrofauna [ˌmækrəu'fɔːnə] *n* 大动物区系(某一地区能用肉眼看到的动物)
macroflora [ˌmækrəu'flɔːrə] *n* 大植物区系(某一地区能用肉眼看到的植物)
macrogamete [ˌmækrəu'gæmiːt] *n* 大配子
macrogametocyte [ˌmækrəugə'miːtəsait] *n* 大配子母细胞
macrogamont [ˌmækrəu'gæmɔnt] *n* 大配子母细胞
macrogenesy [ˌmækrəu'dʒenisi] *n* 巨大发育,巨人症
macrogenia [ˌmækrəu'dʒeniə] *n* 巨颏畸形
macrogenitosomia [ˌmækrəuˌdʒenitəu'səumiə] *n* 巨生殖器 | ~ precox 早熟性巨生殖器
macrogingivae [ˌmækrəu'dʒindʒiviː] *n* 龈纤维瘤病
macroglia [mæ'krɔgliə] *n* 大胶质
macroglobulin [ˌmækrəu'glɔbjulin] *n* 巨球蛋白
macroglobulinemia [ˌmækrəuˌglɔbjuli'niːmiə] *n* 巨球蛋白血症
macroglossia [ˌmækrəu'glɔsiə] *n* 巨舌[症]
macrognathia [ˌmækrəu'neiθiə] *n* 巨颌[症]
macrogol ['mækrəgɔl] *n* 聚乙二醇,碳蜡
macrography [mæ'krɔgrəfi], **macrographia** [ˌmækrəu'greifiə] *n* 巨大字体

macrogyria [ˌmækrəuˈdʒaiəriə] *n* 巨脑回
macrohematuria [ˌmækrəuˌhiːməˈtjuəriə] *n* 肉眼血尿
macrolabia [ˌmækrəuˈleibiə] *n* 巨唇
macrolecithal [ˌmækrəuˈlesiθəl] *a* 巨[卵]黄的
macroleukoblast [ˌmækrəuˈljuːkəblæst] *n* 巨成白细胞
macrolide [ˈmækrəlaid] *n* 大环内酯
macrolymphocyte [ˌmækrəuˈlimfəsait] *n* 大淋巴细胞
macrolymphocytosis [mækrəuˌlimfəsaiˈtəusis] *n* 大淋巴细胞增多
macromania [ˌmækrəuˈmeinjə] *n* 夸大狂,夸大妄想;显大性妄想(指外界物体或自己肢体显大)
macromastia [ˌmækrəuˈmæstiə], **macromazia** [ˌmækrəuˈmeiziə] *n* 乳房过大
macromelia [ˌmækrəuˈmiːliə] *n* 巨肢
macromelus [mæˈkrɔmiləs] *n* 巨肢畸胎
macromere [ˈmækrəmiə] *n* 大[分]裂球
macromethod [ˈmækrəˌmeθəd] *n* 大体方法,肉眼方法;常量法
macromimia [ˌmækrəuˈmimiə] *n* 模仿过分
macromineral [ˌmækrəuˈminərəl] *n* 大量矿物质,大量元素
macromolecule [ˌmækrəuˈmɔlikjuːl] *n* 高分子,大分子 | **macromolecular** [ˌmækrəuməuˈlekjulə] *a*
Macromonas [ˌmækrəuˈməunəs] *n* 大单胞菌属,大极毛硫细菌属
macromonocyte [ˌmækrəuˈmɔnəusait] *n* 巨单核细胞
macromyeloblast [ˌmækrəuˈmaiələblæst] *n* 巨成髓细胞
macronematous [ˌmækrəuˈnemətəs] *a* 粗大菌丝体的
macronodular [ˌmækrəuˈnɔdjulə] *a* 巨结的
macronormoblast [ˌmækrəuˈnɔːməblæst] *n* 巨成红细胞
macronucleus [ˌmækrəuˈnjuːkliəs] *n* 大核,滋养核 | **macronuclear** *a*
macronutrient [ˌmækrəuˈnjuːtriənt] *n* 常量营养物(需要相当数量的一种必需营养物,如钙、氯化物、镁、磷、钾和钠)
macronychia [ˌmækrəuˈnikiə] *n* 巨[指]甲
macro-orchidism [ˌmækrəuˈɔːkidizəm] *n* 巨睾丸
macro-ovalocyte [ˌmækrəuˈəuvələusait] *n* 大卵形红细胞
macropathology [ˌmækrəupəˈθɔlədʒi] *n* 大体病理学,肉眼病理学
macropenis [ˌmækrəuˈpiːnis] *n* 巨阴茎
macrophage [ˈmækrəfeidʒ] *n* 巨噬细胞 | alveolar ~ 肺泡巨噬细胞(亦称尘细胞) / armed ~s 武装巨噬细胞 / fixed ~ 固定巨噬细胞 / free ~, inflammatory ~ 游走巨噬细胞,炎症巨噬细胞 | **macrophagus** [mæˈkrɔfəgəs] *n* / **macrophagic** [ˌmækrəˈfædʒik] *a*
macrophagocyte [ˌmækrəuˈfægəsait] *n* 巨噬细胞
macrophallus [ˌmækrəuˈfæləs] *n* 巨阴茎
macrophthalmia [ˌmækrɔfˈθælmiə] *n* 大眼球 | **macrophthalmous** *a*
macropia [mæˈkrəupiə] *n* 视物显大症
macroplasia [ˌmækrəuˈpleiziə], **macroplastia** [ˌmækrəuˈplæstiə] *n* 过度发育
macropodia [ˌmækrəuˈpəudiə] *n* 巨足
macropolycyte [ˌmækrəuˈpɔlisait] *n* 大多核白细胞
macroprolactinoma [ˌmækrəuprəuˌlæktiˈnəumə] *n* 巨催乳激素瘤
macropromyelocyte [ˌmækrəuprəuˈmaiələsait] *n* 巨前髓细胞
macroprosopia [ˌmækrəuprəˈsəupiə] *n* 巨面
macropsia [mæˈkrɔpsiə] *n* 视物显大症
macrorhinia [ˌmækrəuˈriniə] *n* 巨鼻
macroscelia [ˌmækrəuˈsiːliə] *n* 巨腿
macroscopic [ˌmækrəuˈskɔpik] *a* 肉眼可见的,目视的
macroscopy [mæˈkrɔskəpi] *n* 肉眼检查,粗视检查 | **macroscopical** [ˌmækrəuˈskɔpikəl] *a* 肉眼检查的;肉眼可见的,目视的
macroshock [ˈmækrəuˌʃɔk] *n* 强电流休克(心脏病学使用的术语,表示电流通过完整皮肤两个区域的中到高电平电流;约 100 mA 就能引起心室纤颤)
macrosigmoid [ˌmækrəuˈsigmɔid] *n* 巨乙状结肠,乙状结肠扩张
macrosis [mæˈkrəusis] *n* 巨大;体积增加
macrosmatic [ˌmækrɔsˈmætik] *a* 嗅觉敏锐的
macrosomatia [ˌmækrəusəˈmeiʃiə] *n* 巨体 | ~ adiposa congenita 先天肥胖性巨体 | **macrosomia** [ˌmækrəuˈsəumiə] *n*
macrosplanchnic [ˌmækrəuˈsplæŋknik] *a* 巨脏的,巨腹的
macrospore [ˈmækrəspɔː] *n* 大孢子
macrosteatosis [ˌmækrəuˌstiːəˈtəusis] *n* 大脂肪变性
macrostereognosia [ˌmækrəuˌstiəriəuˈnəuʒə] *n* 物体巨大感
macrostomia [ˌmækrəuˈstəumiə] *n* 巨口,巨口畸形,大口畸形
macrostructural [ˌmækrəuˈstrʌktʃərəl] *a* 大体构造的,巨大结构的
macrotia [mæˈkrəuʃiə] *n* 大耳畸形
macrotome [ˈmækrətəum] *n* 大切片刀
macrotooth [ˈmækrətuːθ] ([复] **macroteeth**

[ˈmækrəti:θ]) *n* 巨牙
macrovasculature [ˌmækrəuˈvæskjulətʃə] *n* 大血管 | **macrovascular**[ˌmækrəuˈvæskjulə] *a*
macula [ˈmækjulə] ([复] **maculas** 或 **maculae** [ˈmækjuli:]) *n*【拉】斑;斑疹 | acoustic ~e 位觉斑 / false ~ 假性黄斑 / ~ lutea retinae 视网膜黄斑 / Mongolian ~ 胎斑(初生时青紫斑) | **~r** *a*
maculate [ˈmækjulit] *a* 有斑点的 | **maculation** [ˌmækjuˈleiʃən] *n* 成斑[点]
macule [ˈmækju:l] *n* 斑
maculocerebral [ˌmækjuləuˈseribrəl] *a* 黄斑[与]脑的
maculopapule [ˌmækjuləuˈpæpju:l] *n* 斑丘疹 | **maculopapular** *a*
maculopathy [ˌmækjuˈlɔpəθi] *n* 黄斑病变 | bull's eye ~ 牛样眼黄斑病变(视网膜黄斑环形区色素增加,伴变性,见于某些中毒状态、斑状角膜营养不良、施塔加特〈Stargardt〉病及其他病)
maculovesicular [ˌmækjuləuviˈsikjulə] *a* 斑疹水疱的
MacWilliam's test [məkˈwiljəm] (John A. MacWilliam) 麦克威廉试验(检尿白蛋白)
mad [mæd] *a* 患狂犬病的
madarosis [ˌmædəˈrəusis] *n* 睫毛脱落;眉毛脱落
MADD multiple acyl CoA dehydrogenation deficiency 多酰基辅酶 A 脱氢作用缺乏,戊二酸尿Ⅱ型
madder [ˈmædə] *n* 欧茜草[根]
Maddox prism [ˈmædɔks] (Ernest E. Maddox) 马多克斯棱镜(两个棱镜以其基底相连,用以测眼球的扭转力) | ~ rods 马多克斯杆(一套平行的圆柱状玻璃杆,检隐斜视)
Madelung's deformity [ˈmɑ:dəluŋ] (Otto W. Madelung) 曲腕畸形 | ~ disease 马德隆病(①曲腕畸形;②弥漫性对称性颈脂肪瘤) / ~ neck 马德隆颈(弥漫性对称性颈脂肪瘤)
Madurella [ˌmædjuˈrelə] *n* 马杜拉分枝菌属
maduromycosis [məˌdjuərəmaiˈkəusis] *n* 足分枝菌病
maedi [ˈmaiθə] *n* 绵羊肺腺瘤病(由病毒引起的冰岛绵羊慢性进行性肺病)
MAF macrophage activating factor 巨噬细胞活化因子
mafenide [ˈmæfənaid] *n* 磺胺米隆(磺胺类抗菌药) | ~ acetate 醋酸磺胺米隆(局部抗感染药) / ~ hydrochloride 盐酸磺胺米隆(局部抗感染药)
Maffucci's syndrome [məˈfu:tʃi] (Angelo Maffucci) 马富奇综合征(内生软骨瘤病合并多发性皮肤或内脏血管瘤)
mafilcon A [məˈfilkɔn] 马费尔康 A(亲水性接触镜材料)
Mag. magnus【拉】大的
MAG3 mertiatide 巯替肽
magaldrate [ˈmægəldreit] *n* 镁加铝(抗酸药)
mageiric [məˈdʒaiərik] *a* 烹调的,饮食的
magenblase [ˌmɑ:gənˈblɑ:zə] *n*【德】胃泡(在胃 X 线片上,造影餐明亮区上方的暗区,显示胃上部有气体积存)
Magendie-Hertwig sign [məʒæŋˈdi: ˈhə:tviʃ] (François Magendie; Richard Hertwig) (眼球)反向偏斜
Magendie's foramen [məʒæŋˈdi:] (François Magendie) 第四脑室正中孔 | ~ law 马让迪定律(见 Bell's law) / ~ solution 马让迪液(硫酸吗啡注射液) / ~ spaces 马让迪隙(蛛网膜下池)
magenstrasse [ˌmɑ:gənˈʃtrɑ:sə] *n*【德】胃路,胃道,胃管
magenta [məˈdʒentə] *n* 品红,复红 | acid ~ 酸性品红 / basic ~ 碱性品红 / ~ O 副品红
magersucht [ˈmɑ:gəzuht] *n*【德】消瘦症
maggot [ˈmægət] *n* 蛆 | Congo floor ~ 黄燥蝇蛆(刚果地板蛆) / rat-tail ~ 蜂蝇蛆(长尾蛆) / sheep ~ 丝光绿蝇蛆(羊蝇蛆)
Magill forceps [məˈgil] (Sir Ivan W. Magill) 麦氏钳(一种角钳,用于在直视下引导气管导管进入喉或引导鼻胃管进入食管;亦用于放置咽填塞物并取出异物) | ~ intubating forceps 麦氏插管钳
magistral [ˈmædʒistrəl] *a* 按处方配制的
Magitot's disease [ˌmɑ:ʒiˈtɔ:] (Emile Magitot) 马吉托病(牙槽骨膜炎)
magma [ˈmægmə] *n* 乳浆剂;糊状黏质 | bentonite ~ 皂黏土乳[浆] / bismuth ~ 铋乳[浆] / dihydroxyaluminum aminoacetate ~ 氨乙酸二羟铝乳浆剂 / magnesia ~ 镁乳[浆] / ~ reticulare 网状黏质
Magnan's movement [ˈmɑ:njɑ:ŋ] (Valentin J. J. Magnan) 马尼安运动(麻痹性痴呆病人舌外伸时的前后伸缩动作) | ~ symptom (sign) 马尼安症状(征)(慢性可卡因中毒时,皮内觉有圆体)
magnesemia [ˌmægniˈsi:miə] *n* 镁血[症]
magnesia [mægˈni:ʃə, -ʒə] *n* 苦土,氧化镁;氢氧化镁 | ~ alba 白苦土,碳酸镁 / ~ calcinata 煅镁,氧化镁 / ~ carbonata 碳酸镁 / ~ usta 煅镁,氧化镁
magnesite [mægˈni:sait] *n* 菱镁矿,碳酸镁
magnesium (Mg) [mægˈni:zjəm] *n* 镁 | ~ chloride 氯化镁(试剂、以前用作轻泻药) / ~ hydroxide 氢氧化镁(轻泻药及抗胃酸药) / ~ oxide 氧化镁(抗胃酸药) / ~ peroxide 过氧化镁(抗胃酸药) / ~ stearate 硬脂酸镁(撒粉及片剂润滑剂) / ~ sulfate 硫酸镁(泻药) / ~ trisili-

cate 三硅酸镁(抗胃酸药)
magnesuria [ˌmægnəˈsjuːriə] *n* 高镁尿
magnet [ˈmægnit] *n* 磁铁,磁体,磁石 | permanent ~ 永[久]磁铁 / temporary ~ 暂时磁铁
magnetic [mægˈnetik] *a* 磁的;有磁性的
magnetism [ˈmægnitizəm] *n* 磁力,磁性;磁学 | animal ~ 动物磁力(Mesmer 所主张的一种假设的力量,可传至他人进行治疗性催眠术)
magnetize [ˈmægnitaiz] *vt, vi* 磁化 | **magnetization** [ˌmægnitaiˈzeiʃən, -tiˈz-] *n*
magnetocardiograph [mægˌniːtəuˈkɑːdiəgrɑːf, -græf] *n* 心磁波描记器
magnetoconstriction [mægˌniːtəukənˈstrikʃən] *n* 磁性伸缩
magnetoelectricity [mægˌniːtəuˌilekˈtrisəti] *n* 磁电
magnetoencephalograph [mægˌniːtəuenˈsefələgrɑːf] *n* 脑磁波描记器
magnetoinduction [mægˌniːtəuinˈdʌkʃən] *n* 磁感应
magnetology [ˌmægniˈtɔlədʒi] *n* 磁学
magnetometer [ˌmægniˈtɔmitə] *n* 磁强计;地磁仪
magneton [ˈmægnitɔn] *n* 磁子
magnetotherapy [mægˌniːtəuˈθerəpi] *n* 磁疗法
magnetron [ˈmægnitrɔn] *n* 磁控[电子]管
magnetropism [mægˈnetrəpizəm] *n* 应磁性,向磁性
magnicellular [ˌmægniˈseljulə] *a* 大细胞性的
magnification [ˌmægnifiˈkeiʃən] *n* 放大;放大率;放大倍数
magnifier [ˈmægnifaiə] *n* 放大器;放大[透]镜
magnocellular [ˌmægnəuˈseljulə] *a* 大细胞性的
Magnolia [mægˈnəuljə] *n* 木兰属
magnolia [mægˈnəuliə] *n* 木兰皮
magnum [ˈmægnəm] *a*【拉】大的 *n* 头状骨
Mahaim fibers [meiˈheim] (Ivan Mahaim) 马海姆纤维(心脏的特化组织,将传导系统的成分直接连接室间隔)
Maher's disease [ˈmeihə] (James J. E. Maher) 阴道周组织炎
Mahler's sign [ˈmɑːlə] (Richard A. Mahler) 马勒尔征(血栓形成时,脉数不断增多,而体温并不随之上升)
ma huang 麻黄
maidenhead [ˈmeidnhed] *n* 处女膜
Maier's sinus [ˈmaiə] (Rudolf Maier) 迈尔窦(泪囊憩室)
maim [meim] *vt* 残伤,使残废 *n* 残伤,残废
main [mɛn] *n*【法】手 | ~ d'accoucheur 助产[士]手 / ~ de tranchées 战壕手病 / ~ en crochet 钩针手(第三、四指屈曲手) / ~ en griffe 爪形手 / ~ en lorgnette 短指手 / ~ en pince 钳形手,手裂[畸形],裂手[畸形] / ~ en singe 猴手 / ~ en squelette 枯骨状手 / ~ fourché 龙虾爪手,手裂[畸形],裂手[畸形] / ~ succulente 腊肠样手
Mainini [maiˈnini] 见 Galli Mainini
maintainer [meinˈteinə] *n* 保持器 | space ~ 缺隙保持器;分牙器
maintenance [ˈmeint(ə)nəns] *n* 保持,维持;保养 | airway ~ 维持气道通畅
maisin [ˈmeizin] *n* 玉蜀黍蛋白
maisonneuve [ˌmeizɔˈnev] *n* 尿道刀(见 Maisonneuve's urethrotome)
Maisonneuve's amputation [ˌmeizɔˈnev] (Jules G. F. Maisonneuve) 梅松纳夫切断术(先切破骨,然后切除软组织部分) | ~ bandage 梅松纳夫绷带(一种巴黎石膏绷带) / ~ urethrotome 梅松纳夫尿道刀(直达狭窄处方始露出的一种尿道刀)
Maissiat's band (ligament, tract) [ˌmeisiˈɑː] (Jacques H. Maissiat) 髂胫带,髂胫束
maize [meiz] *n* 玉蜀黍,玉米
maizenate [ˈmeizəneit] *n* 玉米酸盐
Majocchi's disease (purpura) [məˈjɔki] (Domenico Majocchi) 毛细[血]管扩张性环状紫癜
majoon [məˈjun] *n* 印度大麻
makr(o)- 以 makr(o)-起始的词,同样见以 macr(o)-起始的词
mal [mɑːl] *n*【法】病 | ~ de caderas (南美)马锥虫病 / ~ de Cayemme 象皮病 / ~ comitial 癫痫 / grand ~, haut ~ 大发作 / ~ de Meleda 梅勒达病(见于 Meleda 岛上居民的掌跖角化病) / ~ de mer 晕船 / ~ morado 旋盘尾丝虫皮炎(皮肤呈蓝色或淡紫红色,尤见于躯干和上肢) / ~ perforant 足部穿通性溃疡 / petit ~ 小发作 / ~ del pinto 品他病(即 pinta)
mal- [前缀]不良,异常
mala[1] [ˈmeilə] *n*【拉】颊;颧骨
mala[2] [ˈmʌlə] *n*【梵】废物,排泄物
malabsorption [ˌmæləbˈsɔːpʃən] *n* 吸收不良 | congenital lactose ~ 先天性乳糖吸收不良,二糖不耐症Ⅱ / congenital sucrose-isomaltose ~ 先天性蔗糖-异麦芽糖吸收不良,二糖不耐症Ⅰ / familial glucose-galactose ~ 家族性葡糖-半乳糖吸收不良
Malacarne's pyramid [ˌmæləˈkɑːnei] (Michele V. G. Malacarne) 马拉卡内锥体(小脑蚓锥体后端) | ~ space (antrum) 马拉卡内隙(窦)(后穿质)
malacia [məˈleiʃiə] *n* 软化 | metaplastic ~ 囊状纤维性骨炎 / myeloplastic ~ 成骨不全 / porotic ~ 骨痂形成性软化
-malacia [构词成分]软化

malacic [mə'leisik] *a* 软化的
malac(o)- [构词成分]软化,软
malacoma [ˌmælə'kəumə] *n* 软化
malacoplakia [ˌmæləkəu'pleikiə] *n* 软斑病(指空腔器官的黏膜) | ~ vesicae 膀胱软斑病
malacosarcosis [ˌmæləkəusɑː'kəusis] *n* 肌软化
malacosis [ˌmælə'kəusis] *n* 软化
malacosteon [ˌmælə'kɔstiɔn] *n* 骨软化
malacotic [ˌmælə'kɔtik] *a* 软化的;软的(指牙)
malactic [mə'læktik] *a* 软化的,润滑的 *n* 润滑药
maladie [ˌmælə'diː] *n*【法】[疾]病 | ~ bleue 蓝色病,紫绀病 / ~ bronzéo 流行性血红蛋白尿;艾迪生(Addison)病 / ~ de Capdepont 牙本质生长不全 / ~ des jambes 足病(见于美国路易斯安那州的稻农,可能为脚气病) / ~ de Nicolas et Favre 性病性淋巴肉芽肿 / ~ de plongeurs 海葵皮炎 / ~ de Roger 罗杰病(见 Roger's disease) / ~ du sommeil 昏睡病,非洲锥虫病 / ~ destics 抽搐病(见 Gilles de la Tourette syndrome)
maladjusted [ˌmælə'dʒʌstid] *a* 调节得不好的;适应不良的 | **maladjustment** *n* 失调;(社会生活)适应不良
malady ['mælədi] *n* 病
malagma [mə'lægmə] *n*【希】润滑剂,泥罨剂
malaise [mæ'leiz] *n*【法】不适,欠爽
malakoplakia [ˌmæləkəu'pleikiə] *n* 软斑病(指空腔器官的黏膜)
malalignment, malalinement [ˌmælə'lainmənt] *n* 排列不齐(指牙)
malar ['meilə] *a* 颊的;颧骨的 *n* 颧骨
malaria [mə'lɛəriə] *n* 疟[疾] | algid ~, cold ~ 寒冷型疟 / bilious remittent ~ 黄疸弛张疟 / cerebral ~ 脑型疟 / falciparum ~, malignant tertian ~, pernicious ~, subtertian ~ 恶性疟 / hemolytic ~ 溶血性疟,黑水热 / hemorrhagic ~ 出血性疟 / induced ~, therapeutic ~ 诱发热 / ovale ~ 卵形(疟原虫)疟 / quartan ~ 三日疟 / quotidian ~ 日发疟 / tertian ~ 间日疟 / transfusion ~ 输血疟 / vivax ~, benign tertian ~ 间日疟原虫疟,间日疟,良性间日疟 | **~l**, **~n**, **malarious** *a*
malariacidal [məˌlɛəriə'saidl] *a* 杀疟原虫的
malariology [məˌlɛəri'ɔlədʒi] *n* 疟疾学 | **malariologist** *n* 疟疾学家
malariometry [məˌlɛəri'ɔmitri] *n* 疟疾统计
malariotherapy [məˌlɛəriəu'θerəpi], **malariatherapy**[məˌlɛəriə'θerəpi] *n* 疟热疗法
malaris [mə'lɛəris] *a*【拉】颊的;颧骨的
Malassezia [ˌmælə'siːziə] (Louis C. Malassez) *n* 马拉塞菌属,糠疹癣菌 | ~ furfur, ~ macfadyani, ~ tropica 糠秕马拉塞菌
Malassez's disease [ˌmælə'seiz] (Louis C. Malassez) 马拉塞病(睾丸囊肿) | ~ rest 牙周上皮剩余(一种在牙周膜中赫特维希〈Hertwig〉鞘的上皮剩余,有时发展成牙囊肿)
malassimilation [ˌmæləˌsimi'leiʃən] *n* 同化不全,同化不良
malate ['meileit, 'mæleit] *n* 苹果酸(阴离子型)
malate dehydrogenase ['meileit, 'mæleit diː'haidrədʒəneis] 苹果酸脱氢酶(亦称苹果酸-NAD 脱氢酶)
malate dehydrogenase (oxaloacetate-decarboxylating) (NADP⁺) ['meileit, 'mæleit diː'haidrədʒəneis] 苹果酸脱氢酶(草酰乙酸脱羧)(NADP⁺)
malathion [ˌmælə'θaiɔn] *n* 马拉硫磷(杀虫药)
malaxate ['mæləkseit] *vt* 捏,揉(如制药丸) | **malaxation**[ˌmælək'seiʃən] *n* 揉捏法
maldevelopment [ˌmældi'veləpmənt] *n* 发育不良
maldigestion [ˌmældi'dʒestʃən] *n* 消化不良
male [meil] *a* 男性的,雄性的 *n* 男性,男子,雄性生物
maleate ['mælieit] *n* 马来酸盐,马来酸酯
maleic acid [mə'liːik] 马来酸
malemission [ˌmæli'miʃən] *n* 射精不良
Malerba's test [mə'ləːbə] (Pasquale Malerba) 马莱尔巴试验(检丙酮)
maleruption [ˌmæli'rʌpʃən] *n* 错位长出(牙)
malethamer [mə'leθəmə] *n* 马来他姆(减螨动药)
4-maleylacetoacetate [ˌmæliələˌsiːtəu'æsiteit] *n* 4-马来酰乙酰乙酸
maleylacetoacetate isomerase ['meili-, 'mæliiləˌsiːtəu'æsiteit ai'sɔməreis] 马来酰乙酰乙酸异构酶
malformation [ˌmælfɔː'meiʃən] *n* 畸形 | **malformed**[ˌmæl'fɔːmd] *a*
malfunction [mæl'fʌŋkʃən] *vi* 功能失常 *n* 功能障碍,功能不良
Malgaigne's amputation [mæl'gein] (Joseph F. Malgaigne) 马尔盖尼切断术(距骨下切断术) | ~ hooks 马尔盖尼钩(髌钩) / ~ luxation 马尔盖尼脱位(牵引肘,桡骨头半脱位) / ~ triangle 颈动脉上三角
Malherbe's calcifying epithelioma [mɑː'lɛəb] (Albert Malherbe) 马莱伯钙化上皮瘤,毛母质瘤
maliasmus [ˌmæli'æsməs] *n* 鼻疽
malic acid ['mælik, 'meilik] 苹果酸
malic enzyme ['meilik, 'mælik] 苹果酸酶
malignancy [mə'lignənsi], **malignance** [mə'lignəns] *n* 恶性;恶性肿瘤,癌
malignant [mə'lignənt] *a* 恶性的(指肿瘤)
malignin [mə'lignin] *n* 毒曲菌素

malignogram [məˈlignəgræm] *n* 癌发生图
mali-mali [ˈmɑːliˈmɑːli] *n* 麻立病(菲律宾的一种痉跳病)
malinger [məˈliŋgə] *vi* 诈病 | **~er** [məˈliŋgərə] *n* 诈病者
malingering [məˈliŋgəriŋ] *n* 诈病
malinterdigitation [ˌmælintəˌdidʒiˈteiʃən] *n* 异常牙尖间𬌗
malleable [ˈmæliəbl] *a* (金属)有展性的 | **malleability** [ˌmæliəˈbiləti] *n* 展性
mallear [ˈmæliə], **malleal** [ˈmæliəl] *a* 锤骨的
malleation [ˌmæliˈeiʃən] *n* 锤击样[手肌]颤搐
mallein [ˈmæliːn] *n* [马]鼻疽菌素
malleoidosis [ˌmæliɔiˈdəusis] *n* 类鼻疽
malleoincudal [ˌmæliəuˈiŋkjudəl] *a* 锤骨砧骨的
malleolus [məˈliːələs] ([复] **malleoli** [məˈliːəlai]) *n* 【拉】踝 | external ~, lateral ~, outer ~ 外踝 / inner ~, internal ~, medial ~ 内踝 | **malleolar** *a*
Malleomyces [ˌmæliəˈmaisiːz] *n* 鼻疽杆菌属 | ~ mallei 鼻疽杆菌 / ~ pseudomallei, ~ whitmori 假鼻疽杆菌,惠特莫尔鼻疽杆菌
malleotomy [ˌmæliˈɔtəmi] *n* 踝切离术;锤骨切开术
mallet [ˈmælit] *n* 锤,槌
malleus [ˈmæliəs] ([复] **mallei** [ˈmæliai]) *n* 【拉】锤骨;[马]鼻疽
mallochorion [ˌmæləˈkɔːriɔn] *n* 原绒[毛]膜
Mallophaga [mæˈlɔfəgə] *n* 食毛目(蛃)
Mallory's bodies [ˈmæləri] (Frank B. Mallory) 马洛里小体(①营养性肝硬变时肝细胞内透明的内质网;②猩红热时皮肤上皮细胞及淋巴间隙内的原虫样小体) | ~ acid fuchsin, orange G, and aniline blue stain, ~ triple stain 马洛里酸性品红、橙黄 G 及苯胺蓝染剂,马洛里三重染剂(染结缔组织和分泌粒) / ~ phosphotungstic acid-hematoxylin stain 马洛里磷钨酸苏木精染剂(染细胞核与胞浆的细微结构以及结缔组织纤维)
Mallory-Weiss syndrome [ˈmæləri wais] (G. K. Mallory; Soma Weiss) 马洛里-魏斯综合征(典型者在严重呕吐或干呕数小时或数天之后出现呕血或黑粪,纵行位于食管胃连接处或略低的部位可查出一处或多处胃黏膜裂缝样撕裂伤)
mallotoxin [ˈmæləˌtɔksin] *n* 楸毒素,粗糠柴毒素
Mallotus [məˈləutəs] *n* 野桐属,楸属
mallow [ˈmæləu] *n* 锦葵
Mall's formula [mæl] (Franklin P. Mall) 马尔公式(胎龄〈天数〉等于从头顶至臀部胎长毫米数的平方根 ×100)
malnourished [ˌmælˈnʌriʃt] *a* 营养不良的
malnutrition [ˌmælnjuːˈtriʃən] *n* 营养不良 | malignant ~, protein ~ 恶性营养不良,蛋白质营养不良(见 kwashiorkor)
malocclusion [ˌmæləˈkluːʒən] *n* 错𬌗 | closed-bite ~ 短面错𬌗,紧咬合 / open-bite ~ 开𬌗,开位错𬌗
malonate-semialdehyde dehydrogenase (acetylating) [ˈmæləneit ˌsemiˈældihaid diːˈhaidrədʒəneis əˈsetileitiŋ] 丙二酸半醛脱氢酶(乙酰化的)
malonic acid [məˈlɔnik] 丙二酸
malonyl [ˈmælənil] *n* 丙二酰[基]
malonyl CoA [ˈmælənil kəuˈei] 丙二酸单酰辅酶 A
malonyl coenzyme A [ˈmælənil kəuˈenzaim] 丙二酸单酰辅酶 A
malperfusion [ˌmælpə(ː)ˈfjuːʒən] *n* 灌注异常
Malpighia [mælˈpigiə] (Marcell Malpighi) *n* 金虎尾属
malpighian bodies (corpuscles) of kidney [mælˈpigiən] (Marcello Malpighi) 肾小体 | ~ bodies (corpuscles) of spleen 脾淋巴滤泡,脾淋巴小结 / ~ cell 角[质]化细胞 / ~ glomeruli 肾小球 / ~ layer, ~ rete 表皮生发层 / ~ stigma 马尔皮基小孔(脾静脉上小静脉的入口) / ~ tuft 肾小球
Malpighi's pyramids [mælˈpigi] (Marcello Malpighi) 肾锥体 | ~ vesicles 肺泡
malposed [mælˈpəuzd] *a* 错位的
malposition [ˌmælpəˈziʃən] *n* 错位 | ~ of great arteries 大动脉错位
malpractice [mælˈpræktis], **malpraxis** [mælˈpræksis] *n* 治疗失当,医疗差错;过失行为,违法行为
malpresentation [ˌmælprezenˈteiʃən] *n* 先露异常(胎儿产式异常)
malrotation [ˌmælrəuˈteiʃən] *n* 旋转不良 | ~ of intestine 肠旋转不良
malt [mɔ(ː)lt] *n* 麦芽
maltase [ˈmɔːlteis] *n* 麦芽糖酶
malthusian [mælˈθjuːzjən] (Thomas R. Malthus) *a* 马尔萨斯的 | ~ law 马尔萨斯人口论(一种说明人口增加的速度,超过人口赖以为生的物质增加速度的假设) | **~ism** *n* 马尔萨斯人口论
maltobiose [ˌmɔːltəuˈbaiəus] *a* 麦芽糖
maltodextrin [ˌmɔːltəuˈdekstrin] *n* 麦芽[糖]糊精
maltoflavin [ˌmɔːltəuˈfleivin] *n* 麦芽黄素
maltol [ˈmɔːltɔl] *n* 落叶松皮素
MALToma [mɔːlˈtəumə] *n* 黏膜相关[性]淋巴样组织瘤
maltosazone [ˌmɔːltəuˈseizəun] *n* 麦芽糖脎
maltose [ˈmɔːltəus] *n* 麦芽糖
maltoside [ˈmɔːltəsaid] *n* 麦芽[糖]苷

maltosuria [ˌmɔːltəuˈsjuəriə] *n* 麦芽糖尿
maltotriose [ˌmɔːltəuˈtraiəus] *n* 麦芽三糖
maltum [ˈmæltəm] *n*【拉】麦芽
malturned [mælˈtəːnd] *a* 错扭转的(指以中央轴扭转的牙齿)
malum [ˈmeiləm] *n*【拉】[疾]病
malunion [mæˈljuːnjən] *n* 畸形愈合
Malus [ˈmeiləs] *n* 海棠属
Malva [ˈmælvə] *n*【拉】锦葵属
malvaria [mælˈvɛəriə] *n* 紫红因子尿
Maly's test [ˈmɑːli] (Richard L. Maly) 马利试验(检胃液游离盐酸、胃内容物游离盐酸)
mamanpian [məˌmɑːnpiˈɑːŋ] *n* 初发雅司疹
mamba [ˈmɑːmbə] *n* 窄头眼镜蛇
mamelon [ˈmæmələn] *n*【法】切缘结节;乳头状物
mamilla [mæˈmilə] ([复] **mamillae**[mæˈmiliː]) *n*【拉】乳头;乳头状物
mamillaria [ˌmæmiˈlɛəriə] *n* 深层粟疹
mamillary [ˈmæmiləri] *a* 乳头的,乳头状的
mamillated [ˈmæmileitid] *a* 乳头状的;有乳头的;乳头状突起的 | **mamillation** [ˌmæmiˈleiʃən] *n* 乳头形成;乳头状隆凸
mamilliform [məˈmilifɔːm] *a* 乳头状的
mamilliplasty [məˈmiliˌplæsti] *n* 乳头成形术
mamillitis [ˌmæmiˈlaitis] *n* 乳头炎
mamma [ˈmæmə] ([复] **mammae**[ˈmæmiː]) *n*【拉】乳房 | accessory ~e, supernumerary ~e 额外乳房 / ~ areolata 乳晕 / ~ masculina, ~ virilis 男性乳房
mammal [ˈmæməl] *n* 哺乳动物 | **~ian**[mæˈmeiljən] *a*, *n*
mammalgia [məˈmældʒiə] *n* 乳房痛
Mammalia [mæˈmeiljə] *n* 哺乳纲
mammalogy [mæˈmælədʒi] *n* 哺乳动物学 | **mammalogist** *n* 哺乳动物学家
mammaplasty [ˈmæməˌplæsti] *n* 乳房成形术 | reduction ~ 乳房复位成形术
mammary [ˈmæməri] *a* 乳房的
mammatroph [ˈmæmətrəuf] *n* 催乳细胞
mammectomy [məˈmektəmi] *n* 乳房切除术
mammiferous [mæˈmifərəs] *a* 有乳房的;哺乳类的
mammiform [ˈmæmifɔːm] *a* 乳房形的
mammiliplasty [məˈmiliˌplæsti] *n* 乳头成形术
mammilla [mæˈmilə] ([复] **mammillae** [mæˈmiliː]) *n*【拉】乳头 | **mammillary** [ˈmæmiləri] *a*
Mammillaria [ˌmæmiˈlɛəriə] *n* 鸡冠仙人掌属
mammillate(d) [ˈmæmileit(id)] *a* 乳头状的;有乳头的;乳头状突起的 | **mammillation** [ˌmæmiˈleiʃən] *n* 乳头形成;乳头状隆凸
mammilliform [məˈmilifɔːm] *a* 乳头形的
mammillitis [ˌmæmiˈlaitis] *n* 乳头炎 | bovine ulcerative ~ 牛溃疡性乳头炎
mammiplasia [ˌmæmiˈpleiziə] *n* 乳房组织增生
mammitis [mæˈmaitis] *n* 乳腺炎
mamm(o)- [构词成分]乳房,乳腺
mammogen [ˈmæmədʒən] *n* [垂体]激乳腺素,乳腺发育激素
mammogenesis [ˌmæməˈdʒenisis] *n* 乳腺发育
mammogram [ˈmæməgræm] *n* 乳房X线[照]片
mammography [mæˈmɔgrəfi] *n* 乳房X线照相术
mammoplasia [ˌmæməˈpleiziə] *n* 乳房组织增生 | adolescent ~ 青年期乳房组织增生
mammoplasty [ˈmæməˌplæsti] *n* 乳房成形术
mammose [məˈməus] *a* 大乳房的;有乳头的
mammosometatrope [ˌmæməsəuˈmætətrəup], **mammosometatroph**[ˌmæməsəuˈmætətrəuf] *n* 促乳生长激素细胞(分泌生长激素和催乳激素的腺垂体嗜酸性细胞)
mammotomy [mæˈmɔtəmi] *n* 乳房切开术
mammotroph [ˈmæmətrəuf] *n* 促乳激素细胞
mammotrophic [ˌmæməˈtrɔfik] *a* 激乳腺的
mammotropic [ˌmæməˈtrɔpik] *a* 激乳腺的
mammotropin [məˈmɔtrəpin] *n* 催乳激素
Man. manipulus【拉】一把,少量
manaca [ˈmænəkə] *n* 番茉莉(治痛风和风湿病)
management [ˈmænidʒmənt] *n* 处理;治疗
Manchester operation [ˈmæntʃistə] (Manchester 为英国一港市)曼彻斯特手术(一种子宫脱垂手术,包括扩张宫颈和刮宫术,修补阴道前壁,切断宫颈阴道部,缩短主要韧带及后阴道会阴缝术)
manchette [mænˈʃet] *n*【法】尾管(精子颈部)
manchineel [ˌmænkiˈniːl] *n* 马疯木
mancinism [ˈmænsainizəm] *n* 左利,善用左手
mandama [mænˈdæmə] *n* 蟾皮病
mandelate [ˈmændəleit] *n* 扁桃酸盐(或酯)
mandelic acid [mænˈdelik] 扁桃酸(尿路抗菌药)
mandible [ˈmændibl] *n* 下颌骨 | **mandibular** [mænˈdibjulə] *a*
mandibula [mænˈdibjulə] ([复] **mandibulae** [mænˈdibjuliː]) *n*【拉】下颌骨
mandibulectomy [mænˌdibjuˈlektəmi] *n* 下颌骨切除术
mandibulopharyngeal [mænˌdibjuləfəˈrindʒiəl] *a* 下颌[骨]咽的
Mandragora [mænˈdrægərə] *n*【拉】毒参茄属
mandrake [ˈmændreik] *n* 毒参茄;普达非伦根,北美鬼臼根
mandrel [ˈmændrəl], **mandril** [ˈmændril] *n* 夹轴

针(牙科器械上的)
mandrin [ˈmændrin] *n* 导管导子,管心针
maneuver [məˈnuːvə] *n* 手法,操作法
mangafodipir trisodium [ˌmæŋgəˈfəudipir] 锰福地匹三钠(一种离子顺磁性药剂,含有锰〈Ⅱ〉联于螯合剂福地匹〈fodipir〉;此药剂增加磁共振成像〈MRI〉时组织的信号强度,增强获得的影像,并用于检测和评估肝损害,静脉内给药)
manganate [ˈmæŋgəneit] *n* 锰酸盐
manganese(Mn) [ˌmæŋgəˈniːz, ˈmæŋgəniːz] *n* 锰 | ~ butyrate 丁酸锰(曾用以治皮肤病) / ~ glycerophosphate 甘油磷酸锰(曾用作补血药及神经强壮药) / ~ hypophosphite 次磷酸锰(用作营养素及曾用作补血药)
manganic [mæŋˈgænik] *a* 锰的,三价锰的 | ~ acid 锰酸
manganism [ˈmæŋgənizəm] *n* 锰中毒
manganite [ˈmæŋgənait] *n* 亚锰酸盐
manganous [ˈmæŋgənəs] *a* 亚锰的,二价锰的 | ~ acid 亚锰酸
manganum [ˈmæŋgənəm] *n*【拉】锰
mange [meindʒ] *n* (家畜的)疥癣 | demodectic ~, follicular ~ 犬毛囊蠕螨病 / sarcoptic ~ 兽疥癣
mango [ˈmæŋgəu] *n* 杧果
Mangoldt's epithelial grafting [ˈmɑːŋgəult] (Heinrich von Mangoldt) 曼戈尔特上皮移植术(用剃刀从表皮切下上皮组织覆盖伤口)
mangosteen [ˈmæŋgɔstiːn] *n* 倒捻子(收敛药)
mangostin [ˈmæŋgɔstin] *n* 倒捻子素
mania [ˈmeinjə] *n*【希】躁狂症,狂 | acute hallucinatory ~ 急性幻觉性躁狂 / akinetic ~ 无动性躁狂 / ~ à potu 震颤性谵妄 / dancing ~ 舞蹈狂 / doubting ~ 疑虑癖,疑虑性强迫症 / puerperal ~ 产后躁狂 / reasoning ~ 推理狂 / transitory ~ 暂时性躁狂 / unproductive ~ 缄默性躁狂
-mania [构词成分]狂
maniac [ˈmeiniæk] *a* 躁狂的 *n* 躁狂者
maniacal [məˈnaiəkəl] *a* 躁狂的
manic [ˈmeinik] *a* 躁狂的
manic-depressive [ˈmeinik diˈpresiv] *a* 躁狂抑郁的 *n* 躁狂抑郁症患者
manifestation [ˌmænifesˈteiʃən] *n* 表现
manifold [ˈmænifəuld] *n* 歧管,支管
Manihot [ˈmænihɔt] *n* 木薯属
manikin [ˈmænikin] *n* 人体模型
maniloquism [məˈniləkwizəm] *n* [手]指语
maniluvium [ˌmæniˈljuːviəm] *n* 手浴
manioc [ˈmæniɔk] *n* 木薯
Manip. manipulus【拉】一把,少量
maniphalanx [ˌmæniˈfeilənks] *n* 手指骨
manipulation [məˌnipjuˈleiʃən] *n* 手法治疗;控制,操纵;操作法;推拿[术] | conjoined ~ 双手操作法 / genetic ~ 基因操作,基因人工操纵(即遗传工程)
manipulus [məˈnipjuləs] *n*【拉】一把,少量
manna [ˈmænə] *n*【拉】甘露,木蜜
mannan [ˈmænən] *n* 甘露聚糖(见于植物中)
Mann-Bollman fistula [ˈmæn ˈbɔlmən] (Frank C. Mann; Jesse L. Bollman) 曼-博尔曼瘘(在一段分离的肠管做一个人工开口,其近端缝合于腹壁,而远端则与十二指肠或小肠的其他部分做端边吻合,用于动物实验)
manner [ˈmænə] *n* 方式 | ~ death 死亡方式(如自杀或意外事故)
mannerism [ˈmænərizəm] *n* 装相
manninotriose [ˌmæninəˈtraiəus] *n* 甘露三糖,木蜜三糖
mannitan [ˈmænitæn] *n* 一缩甘露醇
mannitic acid [ˈmænitik] 甘露酸
mannitol [ˈmænitɔl] *n* 甘露[糖]醇(利尿药以及用于肾功能诊断性试验) | ~ hexanitrate 甘露六硝酯(血管扩张药) | **mannite** [ˈmænait] *n*
mannitose [ˈmænitəus] *n* 甘露糖
Mannkopf's sign (symptom) [ˈmɑːnkɔpf] (Emil W. Mannkopf) 曼科普夫征(症状)(压迫痛点,则脉数增加,诈痛时不增加)
mannocarolose [ˌmænəuˈkærələus] *n* 甘露多糖
mannohydrazone [ˌmænəuˈhaidrəzəun] *n* 甘露糖腙
mannoketoheptose [ˌmænəuˌkiːtəuˈheptəus] *n* 甘露庚糖
mannonic acid [məˈnɔnik] 甘露糖酸
mannopyranose [ˌmænəuˈpaiərənəus] *n* 甘露吡喃糖,甘露糖
mannosaccharic acid [ˌmænəusəˈkærik] 甘露糖二酸
mannosamine [məˈnəusəmiːn] *n* 甘露糖胺
mannosan [ˈmænəsən] *n* 甘露聚糖
mannosazone [məˈnəusəzəun] *n* 甘露糖脎
mannose [ˈmænəus] *n* 甘露糖
mannose-1-phosphate guanylyltransferase (GDP) [ˈmænəus ˈfɔsfeit ˌgwɑːnililˈtrænsfəreis] 甘露糖-1-磷酸鸟苷酰转移酶(GDP)
mannose-6-phosphate isomerase [ˈmænəus ˈfɔsfeit aiˈsɔməreis] 甘露糖-6-磷酸异构酶(亦称磷酸甘露糖异构酶)
***α*-mannosidase** [ˈmænəsideis] *n* *α*-甘露糖苷酶(此酶溶酶体缺乏为一种常染色体隐性性状,可致甘露糖苷过多症)
***β*-mannosidase** [ˈmænəsideis] *n* *β*-甘露糖苷酶
mannoside [ˈmænəsaid] *n* 甘露糖苷
mannosidosis [ˌmænəsiˈdəusis] *n* 甘露糖苷贮

积症

mannosidostreptomycin [ˌmænəuˌsaidəuˌstreptəu'maisin] *n* 甘露糖链霉素,链霉素 B

mannosocellulose [mæˌnəusəˌseljuləus] *n* 甘露糖纤维素

Mann's sign [mæn] (John D. Mann) 曼氏征(①突眼性甲状腺肿时两眼不在同一水平线上;②外伤性神经官能症时,头皮对恒定电流的阻抗减弱)

mannuronic acid [ˌmænjuə'rɔnik] 甘露糖醛酸

Mann-Whitney test [mæn 'hwitni] (Henry Berthold Mann; Donald Ransom Whitney) 曼-惠试验,秩和检验(即 rank sum test,见 test 项下相应术语)

Mann-Williamson ulcer ['mæn 'wiljəmsn] (Frank C. Mann; Carl S. Williamson) 曼-威廉森溃疡(实验动物行胃切除术或胃肠吻合术后产生的进行性消化性溃疡)

manoeuvre [mə'nuːvə] *n* = **maneuver**

manometer [mə'nɔmitə] *n* 检压计,[液体]压力计 | aneroid ~ 无液压力计 | **manometric** [ˌmænə'metrik] *a* 测压计的;测压的;随压力变化的 | **manometry** *n* 测压法

manoptoscope [mæ'nɔptəskəup] *n* 主视检查器(测眼优势)

manoscopy [mæ'nɔskəpi] *n* 气体密度检查法

Man. pr. mane primo【拉】清晨

manquea [mɑːn'keiɑː] *n*【西】南美幼牛放线菌病(特点为腿部脓肿形成)

mansa ['mænsə] *n* 洋蕺菜根

Mansonella [ˌmænsə'nelə] *n* 曼森线虫属 | ~ ozzardi 奥[扎尔德]氏曼森线虫 / ~ perstans 常现曼森线虫 / ~ streptocerca 链尾曼森线虫

mansonellosis [ˌmænsənə'ləusis], **mansonelliasis** [ˌmænsənə'laiəsis] *n* 曼森线虫病

Mansonia [mæn'səuniə] *n* 曼蚊属

Mansoniini [ˌmænsəni'aini] *n* 曼蚊族

Mansonioides [ˌmænsəni'ɔidiːz] *n* 曼蚊亚属 | ~ annulifera 多环曼蚊

Manson's hemoptysis ['mænsən] (Sir Patrick Manson) 曼森咯血(寄生虫性咯血) | ~ schistozomiasis (disease) 曼森血吸虫病(病)(感染曼[森]氏血吸虫的吸虫,该吸虫主要寄生在肠系膜上、下静脉,但迁移将虫卵沉积于小静脉内,主要是大肠小静脉内。在肝内的虫卵可导致周围纤维化、肝脾肿大和腹水)

mantle ['mæntl] *n* 包膜,外层;[大脑]皮质 / chordomesodermal ~ 中胚层索膜 / myoepicardial ~ 心肌心外膜套

Mantoux conversion [mɑːŋ'tuː] (Charles Mantoux) 芒图转化,结核菌素试验阳转(由结核菌素试验阴性转化为结核菌素试验阳性) | ~ reversion 芒图逆转,结核菌素试验阴转(结核菌素试验阳性随时间消逝变为结核菌素试验阴性,见于用卡介苗免疫者,芒图逆转表明需再接种卡介苗) / ~ test (reaction) 芒图试验(反应)(皮内注射 0.1 ml 结核菌素,连续注射其逐渐增加的浓度直到反应发生为止。亦称结核菌素皮内试验)

manual ['mænjuəl] *a* 手的,手工的,用手的

manubrium [mə'njuːbriəm] ([复] **manubria** [mə'njuːbriə]) *n*【拉】柄 | ~ of malleus 锤骨柄 / ~ of sternum 胸骨柄

manudynamometer [ˌmænjuˌdainə'mɔmitə] *n* 器械冲力计

manufacture [ˌmænju'fæktʃə] *n* 生产,制造

manus ['meinəs] *n*【拉】手

manyplies ['meniˌplaiz] *n* 重瓣胃(反刍类的第三胃)

manzanita [ˌmænzə'nitə] *n*【西】美熊果

Manz's glands [mɑːnts] (Wilhelm Manz) 曼茨腺,球结膜囊状腺(睑缘上的腺性凹陷)

Manzullos's test [mæn'zuləu] (Alfredo Manzullo) 曼佐罗试验,亚碲酸钾试验(检白喉)

MAO monoamine oxidase 单胺氧化酶

MAOI monoamine oxidase inhibitor 单胺氧化酶抑制剂

MAP mean arterial pressure 平均动脉压

map [mæp] *n* 图,图型 | fate ~ 囊胚发育图(表示将来胚胎正常发育) / genetic ~ 基因图(示基因在染色体上的直线排列) / linkage ~ 连锁图(示基因在同一染色体上的相对位置和距离)

maple ['meipəl] *n* 枫树,槭树

mapping ['mæpiŋ] *n* 定位图;标测 | endocardial ~ 心内膜标测

maprotiline [mə'prəutiliːn] *n* 马普替林(抗抑郁药)

Marañón's sign (reaction) [mɑː'rɑːnjɔn] (Gregorio Marañón) 马拉尼翁征(反应)(刺激喉头皮肤引起的一种血管舒缩反应,见于突眼性甲状腺肿) | ~ syndrome 马拉尼翁综合征(包括脊柱侧凸、扁平足及卵巢功能不全的综合征)

Maranta [mə'ræntə] *n* 竹芋属

marasmoid [mə'ræzmɔid] *a* 消瘦样的

marasmus [mə'ræzməs] *n* 重度消瘦型营养不良 | enzootic ~ 地方性牛羊消瘦病,丛林病 / nutritional ~ 消瘦性恶性营养不良病 | **marasmic** [mə'ræzmik], **marantic** [mə'ræntik], **marasmatic** [ˌmærəz'mætik] *a* 消瘦的,消耗的

marble ['mɑːbl] *n* 大理石

marbleization [ˌmɑːbəlai'zeiʃən, -li'z-] *n* 大理石状纹理

Marburg disease (hemorrhagic fever) ['mɑː-

burk]（Marburg 为德国一城市，1967 年首次报道此病）马尔堡病（出血性热）（见 disease 项下相应术语）| ~ virus 马尔堡病毒（见 virus 项下相应术语）

marc [mɑːk] *n*【法】浸渍渣，残渣

march [mɑːtʃ] *n* 前进，进行（电活动经过运动皮质的进行）| cortical ~，epileptic ~ 皮质性进行，癫痫性进行（见 jacksonian ~）/ jacksonian ~ 杰克逊进行（异常电活动从大脑皮质一个区扩展到邻近区，为杰克逊癫痫的特征）

Marchand's adrenals（organs） [ˈmɑːʃənd]（Felix J. Marchand）马尔尚肾上腺（器官）（阔韧带内的副肾上腺）| ~ cell 马尔尚细胞（外膜细胞，周皮细胞）

marche [mɑːʃ] *n*【法】步态 | ~ a petite pas [əpəˈtiːpɑː] 短小步态（见于某些帕金森综合征和脑动脉硬化病人）

Marchesani's syndrome [mɑːkəˈsɑːni]（Oswald Marchesani）马克萨尼综合征（一种常染色体显性或隐性性状遗传的先天性结缔组织病，特征为短头、短指〈趾〉、身材矮小、胸廓宽大及肌肉系统发达、关节活动度减少、球形晶状体、晶状体异位、近视及青光眼。亦称先天性中胚叶增生性营养不良，球形晶状体-短矮畸形综合征）

Marchiafava-Bignami disease [ˌmɑːkiəˈfɑːvə biːˈnjɑːmi]（Ettore Marchiafava；Amico Bignami）马基法瓦-比恩亚米病（胼胝体进行性变性）

Marchiafava-Micheli disease（syndrome） [ˌmɑːkiəˈfɑːvə miˈkeili]（Ettore Marchiafava；F. Micheli）阵发性睡眠性血红蛋白尿症

Marchi's balls [ˈmɑːki]（Vittorio Marchi）马尔基小球（髓鞘质变性时所产生的节片，呈椭圆形或卵圆形，用马尔基法染色后呈褐色）| ~ globules 马尔基小体（经马尔基法染色的髓鞘分解球，见于脊髓变性）/ ~ method 马尔基法（显示变性神经纤维的染色法，先将组织在重铬酸钾溶液中固定，以防止正常髓鞘纤维被锇酸着色）/ ~ reaction 马尔基反应（神经髓鞘用锇酸处理后不能褪色的反应）/ ~ tract 顶盖脊髓束

marcid [ˈmɑːsid] *a* 消瘦的，消耗的

marcov [ˈmɑːkɔv] *n* 消瘦，消耗

Marcus Gunn [ˈmɑːkəs gʌn] 见 Gunn

marcy [ˈmɑːsi] *n* 马尔西病毒（伴有无热型病毒性腹泻的病毒）

Maréchal's test，Maréchal-Rosin test [ˌmɑːreiˈʃɑːl ˈrɔːzin]（Louis E. Maréchal；Heinrich Rosin）马雷夏尔试验、马雷夏尔-罗辛试验（检尿内胆色素）

Marek's disease [ˈmɑːrek]（Josef Marek）马雷克病（鸡的淋巴增生性疾病）

marennin [məˈrenin] *n* 马瑞尼蠔绿

marenostrin [ˌmærəˈnɔstrin]（源自拉丁 Mare Nostrum 我们的海，即地中海）*n* 地中海蛋白（见 pyrin）

Marey's law [mɑːˈrei]（Etienne J. Marey）马雷定律（血压升高时，脉率减慢）

marfanoid [ˈmɑːfənɔid] *a* 马方（Marfan）综合征的

Marfan's puncture（epigastric puncture，method） [mɑːˈfɑːŋ]（Bernard-Jean A. Marfan）马方穿刺（上腹部穿刺、法）（穿刺心包）| ~ sign 马方征（患伤寒病时、舌面有苔，舌尖呈红色三角，此现象极罕见）/ ~ syndrome 马方综合征（一种先天性结缔组织病，特征为指、趾极为细长，两侧晶状体异位，心血管异常〈一般为升主动脉扩张〉以及其他身体缺陷，系常染色体显性遗传）

margaric acid [mɑːˈgærik] 十七[烷]酸

margarid [ˈmɑːgərid] *a* 珠状的

margarine [ˌmɑːdʒəˈriːn，ˈmɑːgəriːn] *n* 人造奶油，珠脂

margaritoma [ˌmɑːgəriˈtəumə] *n* 珠光瘤，胆脂瘤

margarone [ˈmɑːgərɔn] *n* 软脂酮，十七[烷]酮，棕榈酮

Margaropus [mɑːˈgærəpəs] *n* 巨肢蜱属 | ~ annulatus 具环牛蜱（即 Boophilus annulatus）/ ~ winthemi 巨肢蜱

margin [ˈmɑːdʒin] *n* [边]缘；界限 | ciliary ~ of iris 虹膜睫状缘 / dentate ~ 齿状线，梳状线，肛门皮肤线 | **~al** *a* [边]缘的；界限的

marginate [ˈmɑːdʒineit] *vt* 加边于 [ˈmɑːdʒinit] *a* 有边缘的 | **margination** [ˌmɑːdʒiˈneiʃən] *n* 边缘；着边，壁立（炎症初期时，白细胞黏着于血管壁）

marginoplasty [mɑːˈdʒinəˌplæsti] *n* 睑缘成形术

margo [ˈmɑːgəu]（[复] **margines** [ˈmɑdʒiniːz]）*n*【拉】缘

mariahuana，mariajuana [ˌməriəˈhwɑːnə] *n* 大麻

mariculture [ˌmæriˈkʌltʃə] *n* 海产养殖

Marie-Bamberger disease [məˈriː ˈbɑːmbəːgə]（Pierre Marie；Eugen Bamberger）肥大性肺性骨关节病

Marie-Foix sign [məˈriː fwɑː]（Pierre Marie；Charles Foix）马-福征（横压跗骨或用力屈曲足趾时，即使下肢不能随意运动，小腿也会回缩）

Marie's ataxia [məˈriː]（Pierre Marie）遗传性小脑性共济失调 | ~ disease 马里病（①肢端肥大症；②肥大性肺性骨关节病）/ ~ hypertrophy 马里肥大（骨膜炎所致的关节软组织肥大）/ ~ sign 马里征（突眼性甲状腺肿时，身体或四肢震颤）/ ~ syndrome 马里综合征（①垂体分泌异常性肢端巨大症；②肥大性肺性骨关节病）

Marie-Strümpell disease, spondylitis [mə'riː 'strimpəl] (Pierre Marie; Adolf von Strümpell) 强直性脊柱炎

Marie-Tooth disease [mə'riː 'tuːθ] (Pierre Marie; Howard H. Tooth) 进行性神经性[腓骨]肌萎缩

marigold ['mærigəuld] *n* 金盏花

marihuana, mariguana, marijuana [ˌmæri'*h*wɑːnə] *n* 大麻

Marinesco-Sjögren syndrome [mæri'neskəu 'ʃəugren] (G. Marinesco; Karl G. T. Sjögren) 马-舍综合征(为常染色体隐性性状遗传的综合征,包括小脑性共济失调、精神和躯体生长发育迟缓、先天性白内障、咀嚼无力、薄脆甲及头发稀少且角化不全)

Marinesco's sign, succulent hand [ˌmæri'neskəu] (Georges Marinesco) 马里内斯科征、浮胀手(手皮肤青紫和冷厥并有水肿,见于脊髓空洞症。亦称腊肠样手)

marinobufagin [ˌmærinəu'bjuːfədʒin] *n* 海蟾蜍毒素

marinotherapy [ˌmærinə*u*'θerəpi] *n* 海滨治疗,海滨疗养

Marion's disease [məri'ɔn] (Jean B. C. G. Marion) 马里翁病(由于膀胱颈肌层肥厚或泌尿道丛状开大肌纤维缺如所致的先天性后尿道阻塞)

Mariotte's experiment [ˌmæri'ɔt] (Edme Mariotte) 马里奥特实验(检眼盲点) | ~ law 马里奥特定律(见 Boyle's law) / ~ spot 盲点

mariposia [ˌmæri'pəuziə] *n* 饮[用]海水

marisca [mə'riskə] ([复] **mariscae**[mə'riskiː]) *n* 痔 | ~l *a*

maritonucleus [ˌmæritə'njuːkliəs] *n* 受精卵核

Marjolin's ulcer [ˌmɑːʒəu'læn] (Jean N. Marjolin) 瘢痕癌

mark [mɑːk] *n* 标记;斑点;标志,特征;*vt* 表示…的特征 | beauty ~ 美人斑 / birth ~ 胎记,胎痣 / pock ~ 痘痕 / portwine ~ 葡萄酒色痣,烟色痣莓 / raspberry ~, strawberry ~ 莓状痣,海绵状血管瘤

marker ['mɑːkə] *n* 标记,标志 | cell-surface ~ 细胞表面标记(在特殊类型细胞表面上的抗原决定簇) / genetic ~ 遗传标记(用以研究群体中基因的分布和连锁分析)

marking ['mɑːkiŋ] *n* 斑纹,记号

Marlow' test ['mɑːləu] (Frank W. Marlow) 马尔洛试验(检隐斜视)

marma ['mɑːmə] *n* 马尔玛(古代印度对于人体一重要部位的称呼,这个部位如受伤害,即可致严重后果或死亡)

marmoration [ˌmɑːmə'reiʃən] *n* 大理石状纹理

marmoreal [mɑː'mɔːriəl], **marmorean** [mɑː'mɔːriən] *a* 大理石的,大理石状的

marmot ['mɑːmət] *n* 土拨鼠

Marmota [mɑː'məutə] *n* 旱獭属

Maroteaux-Lamy syndrome [mərə'tɔː lə'mi] (Pierre Maroteaux; M. Lamy) 马洛托-拉梅综合征(黏多糖贮积症的一种,为常染色体隐性遗传,十分类似胡尔勒〈Hurler〉综合征,只是面部畸形不十分显著,关节僵硬最小,智力未受损伤。亦称黏多糖贮积症Ⅵ型)

Marriott's method ['mæriət] (William McKim Marriott) 马里奥特法(检碱储量)

marrow ['mærəu] *n* 髓(尤指骨髓) | bone ~ 骨髓 / depressed ~ 骨髓功能减退 / fat ~, yellow (bone) ~ 黄骨髓 / red (bone) ~ 红骨髓 / spinal ~ 脊髓

marrowbrain ['mærəubrein] *n* 末脑;脑脊髓

marrubiin [mə'ruːbiin] *n* 夏至草苦素

Marrubium [mə'ruːbiəm] *n* 夏至草属

mars [mɑːz] *n*【拉】铁

Marsdenia [mɑːz'diːniə] *n* 牛猕菜属

Marshall Hall 见 Hall

Marshall-Marchetti-Krantz operation ['mɑːʃəl mɑː'keti krænts] (Victor F. Marshall; Andrew A. Marchetti; Kermit E. Krantz) 马-马-克手术(矫治压力性尿失禁手术,将尿道前部、膀胱颈和膀胱缝于耻骨后面)

Marshall's fold ['mɑːʃəl] (John Marshall) 左腔静脉襞 | ~ vein 左房斜静脉

marshmallow ['mɑːʃˌmeləu, -ˌmæləu] *n* 药蜀葵;药蜀葵制剂(治咳嗽等)

Marsh's disease ['mɑːʃ] (Henry Marsh) 突眼性甲状腺肿

Marsh's test ['mɑːʃ] (James Marsh) 马什试验(检砷或锑)

marsupial [mɑː'sjuːpjəl] *a* 有袋[类]的;袋状的 *n* 有袋类(动物)

Marsupialia [mɑːˌsjupi'eiliə] *n* 有袋目

marsupialization [mɑːˌsjuːpjəlai'zeiʃən, -li'z-] *n* 袋形缝术

marsupium [mɑː'sjuːpjəm] ([复] **marsupia** [mɑː'sjuːpiə]) *n*【拉】阴囊;袋(指动物的育儿袋或卵袋) | marsupia patellaris 翼状襞

Marteiliida [ˌmɑːti'laiidə] *n* 闭合孢子虫目(即 Occlusosporida)

martial [mɑːʃəl] *a* 含铁的,铁的

Martin-Bell syndrome ['mɑːtin bel] (J. Purdon Martin; Julia Bell) 马-贝综合征,脆性 X[染色体]综合征(即 fragil X syndrome,见 syndrome 项下相应术语)

Martinotti's cell [ˌmɑːti'nɔti] (Giovanni Martinotti) 马尔提诺蒂细胞(大脑皮质多形层内的梭形细胞)

Martin's bandage [ˈmɑːtin] (Henry A. Martin) 马丁绷带(薄弹性橡胶绷带) | ~ disease 马丁病(过劳性足骨膜关节炎) / ~ operation 马丁手术(阴囊水囊肿根治手术)

Martorell's syndrome [mɑːtəˈrel] (Fernando Martorell Otzet) 马托雷尔综合征,无脉病

masc mass concentration 质量浓度

maschaladenitis [ˌmæskəˌlædiˈnaitis] *n* 腋腺炎

maschaloncus [ˌmæskəˈlɔŋkəs] *n* 腋窝瘤

masculation [ˌmæskjuˈleiʃən] *n* 男征发生

masculine [ˈmæskjulin] *a* 男性的,雄性的 | **masculinity** [ˌmæskjuˈlinəti] *n* 男子本性,男性

masculinize [ˈmæskjulinaiz] *vt* 男性化 | **masculinization** [ˌmæskjulinaiˈzeiʃən, -niˈz-] *n*

masculinovoblastoma [ˌmæskjuliˌnəuvəublæsˈtəumə] *n* 男化卵巢瘤,卵巢类脂质细胞瘤

masculonucleus [ˌmæskjuləˈnjuːkliəs] *n* 雄胚质,雄性原核

maser [ˈmeizə] (*m*icrowave *a*mplification by *s*timulated *e*mission of *r*adiation) *n* 微波激射器;微波激射,脉泽

mash [mæʃ] *n* 醪液

mask [mɑːsk] *n* 口罩,面罩,面具 *vt* 掩盖;掩蔽 | BLB ~ BLB 面罩(由 Boothby, Lovelace 和 Bulbulian 设计的飞行员用供氧面具,亦用于临床) / death ~ 尸体面模 / ecchymotic ~ 瘀斑状面色 / meter ~ 氧量计面具(飞行员用) / ~ of pregnancy 妊娠面斑 / tabetic ~ 脊髓痨性面具感

masker [ˈmɑːskə] *n* 掩蔽器 | tinnitus ~ 耳鸣掩蔽器

masochism [ˈmæsəkizəm] *n* 受虐癖 | **masochist** [ˈmæsəkist] *n* 受虐癖者 / **masochistic** [ˌmæsəˈkistik] *a*

masoprocol [məˈsəuprəkɔl] *n* 马索罗酚(抗肿瘤药,治疗光线性角化病)

Mas. pil. massa pilularum【拉】丸块

mass [mæs] *n* 质,物质;块,丸块,团;质量(符号为 *m*) | achromatic ~ 非染色质 / appendiceal ~, appendix ~ 阑尾块 / atomic ~ 原子质量 / body cell ~ 体细胞总量 / electronic ~ 电子质量 / ferrous carbonate ~ 碳酸亚铁丸块 / injection ~ 注射物质(一种悬液或溶液,一般有色,注入血管或其他组织间隙,使之显示,便于解剖或切割) / inner cell ~ 内细胞群 / intermediate ~ 中间块,丘脑间粘连 / intermediate cell ~ 中间细胞群,肾节 / lean body ~ 瘦体重,无脂肪体 / mercury ~, blue ~ 汞丸块,蓝丸块 / pill ~, pilular ~ 丸块 / tigroid ~es 虎斑(小体) / ventrolateral ~ 腹外侧块(胚胎)

massa [ˈmæsə] ([复] **massae** [ˈmæsiː]) *n*【拉】质,物质;块,丸,团

massage [ˈmæsɑːʒ, məˈsɑːʒ] *n*, *vt* 按摩[术] | auditory ~ 鼓膜按摩 / cardiac ~, heart ~ 心脏按压 / electrovibratory ~ 电震颤按摩 / hydropneumatic ~ 水气按摩 / tremolo ~ 机械震颤按摩 / vapor ~ 蒸汽变压按摩[法] / vibratory ~ 振动按摩[法]

massasauga [ˌmæsəˈsɔːgə] *n* 侏响尾蛇

Masselon's spectacles [ˌmæsəˈlɔŋ] (Miche J. Masselon) 马塞龙眼镜,睑垂镜,上睑下垂矫正眼镜

masseter [mæˈsiːtə] *n* 咬肌 | **~ic** [ˌmæsiˈterik] *a*

Masset's test [məˈsei] (Alfred A. Masset) 马塞试验(检尿内胆色素)

masseur [mæˈsəː] *n*【法】男按摩员;按摩器

masseuse [mæˈsəːz] *n*【法】女按摩员

massicot [ˈmæsikɔt] *n* 铅黄,铅丹,一氧化铅

massive [ˈmæsiv] *a* 大块的,整块的;大量的

Masson stain [mɑːˈsɔː] (C. L. Pierre Masson) 马松染剂(一种三色染剂,染结缔组织)

massotherapy [ˌmæsəuˈθerəpi] *n* 按摩疗法

MAST military or medical antishock trousers 军用或医用抗休克裤

mastadenitis [ˌmæstædiˈnaitis] *n* 乳腺炎

mastadenoma [ˌmæstædiˈnəumə] *n* 乳腺瘤

Mastadenovirus [mæstˈædinəuˌvaiərəs] *n* 乳腺腺病毒属

mastalgia [mæsˈtældʒiə] *n* 乳腺痛

mastatrophy [mæsˈtætrəfi], **mastatrophia** [ˌmæstəˈtrəufiə] *n* 乳腺萎缩

mastauxe [mæsˈtɔːksi] *n* 乳房增大

mastectomy [mæsˈtektəmi] *n* 乳房切除术 | extended radical ~ 乳房扩大根除术 / modified radical ~ 乳房改良根治术 / radical ~ 乳房根治术 / segmental ~, partial ~ 乳腺区段切除术 / simple ~, total ~ 单纯乳房切除术,乳房全切除术 / subcutaneous ~ 皮下乳腺切除术

Master "2-step" exercise test [ˈmɑːstə] (Arthur M. Master) 马斯特二级梯运动试验(检冠状动脉供血不足:一种心电图试验,被试者反复上下梯阶,每级高 22.5 cm,其运动量〈登梯数〉依年龄、体重及性别而定其标准,于运动刚停止时以及然后于 2 分钟与 6 分钟后立即各作心电图一次)

masthelcosis [ˌmæsθəlˈkəusis] *n* 乳房溃疡,乳腺溃疡

mastic [ˈmæstik] *n* 洋乳香,熏陆香

masticate [ˈmæstikeit] *vt*, *vi* 咀嚼 | **mastication** [ˌmæstiˈkeiʃən] *n* / **masticator** *n* 咀嚼器官

masticatory [ˈmæstikeitəri] *a* 咀嚼的;咀嚼器官的 *n* 咀嚼剂

mastiche [ˈmæstiki] *n*【拉】洋乳香、熏陆香

mastichic acid [mæˈstikik] 熏陆香脂酸

Mastigomycotina [ˌmæstigəuˌmaikəuˈtainə] *n* 鞭

毛[真]菌亚门
mastigont ['mæstigɔnt] *n* 鞭毛
Mastigophora [ˌmæsti'gɔfərə] *n* 鞭毛纲
mastigophoran [ˌmæsti'gɔfərən] *n* 鞭毛虫 | **mastigophorous** *a*
Mastigoproctus [ˌmæstigəu'prɔktəs] *n* 鞭蝎属
mastigote ['mæstigəut] *n* 鞭毛虫
mastitis [mæs'taitis] *n* 乳腺炎 | gargantuan ~ 乳房巨大性乳腺炎 / parenchymatous ~, glandular ~ 实质性乳腺炎 / puerperal ~ 产褥期乳腺炎 / retromammary ~, submammary ~ 乳腺周炎 / stagnation ~ 乳汁潴留性乳腺炎
mast(o)- [构词成分]乳房;乳突
mastocarcinoma [ˌmæstəuˌkɑːsi'nəumə] *n* 乳[房]癌
mastoccipital [ˌmæstɔk'sipitl] *a* 乳突枕骨的
mastochondroma [ˌmæstəukɔn'drəumə], **mastochondrosis** [ˌmæstəukɔn'drəusis] *n* 乳房软骨瘤
mastocyte ['mæstəsait] *n* 肥大细胞
mastocytoma [ˌmæstəusai'təumə] *n* 肥大细胞瘤
mastocytosis [ˌmæstəusai'təusis] *n* 肥大细胞增生病 | diffuse ~, diffuse cutaneous ~ 弥漫性肥大细胞增生病,弥漫性皮肤肥大细胞增生病 / systemic ~ 系统性肥大细胞增生病
mastodynia [ˌmæstəu'diniə] *n* 乳痛症
mastogram ['mæstəgræm] *n* 乳房 X 线[照]片
mastography [mæs'tɔgrəfi] *n* 乳房 X 线摄影[术]
mastoid ['mæstɔid] *a* 乳头状的;乳突的 *n* 乳突
mastoidal [mæs'tɔidl] *a* 乳突的
mastoidale [ˌmæstɔi'deili] *n* 乳突尖
mastoidalgia [ˌmæstɔi'dældʒiə] *n* 乳突痛
mastoidea [mæs'tɔidiə], **mastoideum** [mæs'tɔidiəm] *n* 乳突部(颞骨)
mastoidectomy [ˌmæstɔi'dektəmi] *n* 乳突切除术
mastoideocentesis [mæsˌtɔidiəusen'tiːsis] *n* 乳突穿刺术
mastoiditis [ˌmæstɔi'daitis] *n* 乳突炎 | ~ externa 外乳突炎,乳突骨膜炎 / ~ interna 内乳突炎、乳突气房炎 / sclerosing ~ 硬化型乳突炎 / silent ~ 隐性乳突炎,无症状乳突炎
mastoidoplasty ['mæstɔidəˌplæsti] *n* 乳突成形术
mastoidotomy [ˌmæstɔi'dɔtəmi] *n* 乳突切开术
mastoidotympanectomy [mæsˌtɔidəuˌtimpə'nektəmi] *n* 根治乳突切除术,乳突根治术
mastomenia [ˌmæstəu'miːniə] *n* 乳房倒经
Mastomys ['mæstəumis] *n* 非洲小啮齿动物属
mastoncus [mæs'tɔŋkəs] *n* 乳房瘤,乳腺瘤
masto-occipital [ˌmæstəu ɔk'sipitl] *a* 乳突枕骨的
mastoparietal [ˌmæstəupə'raiitl] *a* 乳突顶骨的
mastopathy [mæs'tɔpəθi], **mastopathia** [ˌmæstəu'pæθiə] *n* 乳腺病,乳房病
mastopexy ['mæstəpeksi] *n* 乳房固定术
Mastophora [mæs'tɔfərə] *n* 秘鲁毒蛛属 | ~ gasteracanthoides 秘鲁毒蛛
mastoplasia [ˌmæstəu'pleiziə], **mastoplastia** [ˌmæstəu'plæstiə] *n* 乳房组织增生
mastoplasty ['mæstəˌplæsti] *n* 乳房成形术
mastoptosis [ˌmæstəp'təusis] *n* 乳房下垂
mastorrhagia [ˌmæstəu'reidʒiə] *n* 乳腺出血
mastoscirrhus [ˌmæstəu'skirəs] *n* 乳腺硬癌
mastosis [mæs'təusis] ([复] **mastoses** [mæs'təusiːz]) *n* 乳房病,乳腺病
mastosquamous [mæstəu'skweiməs] *a* 乳突鳞部的
mastostomy [mæs'tɔstəmi] *n* 乳房切开引流术
mastotic [mæs'tɔtik] *a* 乳房病的,乳腺病的
mastotomy [mæs'tɔtəmi] *n* 乳房切开术
masturbate ['mæstəbeit] *vi*, *vt* 行手淫 | **masturbation** [ˌmæstə'beiʃən] *n* 手淫 / **masturbator** *n* 手淫者
Masugi's nephritis [mɑː'suːgi] (Matazo Masugi) 马杉肾炎(即肾毒性血清肾炎 nephrotoxic serum nephritis,见 nephritis 项下相应术语)
masurium [mə'sjuəriəm] *n* 钨(元素锝的旧名)
MAT multifocal atrial tachycardia 多源性房性心动过速
Matas' band ['mætəs] (Rudolph Matas) 马塔斯带(铝质带,用以暂时关闭大血管,检侧支循环情况) | ~ operation 动脉瘤内缝术 / ~ test 马塔斯试验(检侧支循环)
matching ['mætʃiŋ] *n* 配合 | ~ of blood 配血,血液配合 / cross ~ 交叉配血 / HLA ~ HLA 配型
maté [mə'tei] *n* 巴拉圭茶,冬青茶
Mátéfy test (reaction) [mə'teifi] (László Mátéfy) 马太菲试验(反应)(早期诊断肺结核血清试验)
mater ['meitə] *n* 【拉】脑膜,脊膜 | dura ~ 硬膜 / pia ~ 软膜
materia [mə'tiəriə] ([复] **materiae** [mə'tiəriiː]) *n* 【拉】物质 | ~ medica 药物学;药物
material [mə'tiəriəl] *a* 物质的 *n* 物质;原料,材料 | base ~ 基质 / cross-reacting ~ (CRM) 交叉反应物质(突变型顺反子所产生的一种蛋白质) / genetic ~ 遗传物质 / raw ~ 原料 / tissue equivalent ~ 组织等效物质,组织等效材料
materies [mə'tiəriiːz] *n* 【拉】物质 | ~ morbi 致病物质 / ~ peccans 病因物,致病物质
maternal [mə'təːnl] *a* 母亲的;母系的;母性的
maternity [mə'təːnəti] *n* 母性;产院
maternohemotherapy [məˌtəːnəuˌhiːməu'θerəpi] *n* 母血疗法(注射母血至婴儿,过去曾用此法企图将麻疹、脊髓灰质炎等免疫力从母亲转

移给儿童）

Mathieu procedure [mɑːti'juː]（P. Mathieu）马蒂尤手术（手术矫治远端尿道的尿道下裂，即使用尿道周围组织，在阴茎头内做一个切口，并将阴茎头一起在缺损上缝合）

Mathieu's disease [məti'juː]（Albert Mathieu）钩端螺旋体性黄疸

matico [mə'tiːkəu] *n* 马替可［叶］，狭叶胡椒［叶］（以前用作收敛、止血药）

mating ['meitiŋ] *n* 交配 | assortative ~，assorted ~，assortive ~，nonrandom ~ 选择性交配，非随机交配 / backcross ~ 回交，逆代杂交 / random ~ 随机交配，随机配种

matlazahuatl [mətˌlɑːzə'*h*wɑːtl] *n* 地方性斑疹伤寒（墨西哥）

matrass ['mætrəs] *n*（长颈）卵形瓶

matrical ['mætrikəl]，**matricial** [mə'triʃəl] *a* 基质的，基层的，母质的

Matricaria [ˌmætri'kɛəriə] *n*【拉】母菊属

matricaria [ˌmætri'kɛəriə] *n* 母菊

matrilineal [ˌmætri'liniəl] *a* 母系的

matrix ['meitriks]（［复］**matrixes** 或 **matrices** ['meitrisiːz]）*n*【拉】基质；基体；模床；基架；成型片；树脂基质；牙瓷料 | amalgam ~ 汞合金成型片 / fluid ~ 液体基质 / hair ~ 毛基质 / interterritorial ~ 区间基质 / nail ~ 甲床 / territorial ~ 区基质（软骨）

matroclinous [ˌmætrə'klainəs]，**matriclinous** [ˌmætri'klainəs] *a* 母传的，偏母的（母性遗传特征的）

matrocliny [ˌmætrə'klaini] *n* 偏母遗传

matte [mæt] *a* 无光泽的

matter ['mætə] *n* 物质；脓 *vi* 化脓，出脓 | gelatinous ~ 胶质 / gray ~ of nervous system 灰质 / radiant ~ 辐射质 / white ~ of nervous system 白质

Mattox maneuver ['mætəks]（Kenneth L. Mattox）麦托克斯手法（使腹内脏活动并使其内侧反射以暴露肾上腺主动脉，藉以修复创伤性外伤）

maturant ['mætʃurənt] *n* 催脓药

maturate ['mætjureit, -tʃu-] *vi*, *vt* 成熟；化脓 | **maturation** [ˌmætju'reiʃən, -tʃu-] *n* 成熟；化脓

mature [mə'tjuə, -'tʃu] *a* 成熟的；成年人的

maturity [mə'tjuərəti, -'tʃuə-] *n* 成熟，成年；成熟期，发身期 | fetal ~ 胎儿成熟度

Matut. matutinus【拉】晨间

matutinal [ˌmætju(ː)'tainl, mə'tjuːtinl] *a* 晨间的，早晨的

matzoon [mæt'zjuːn] *n* 乳冻（一种发酵乳）

Mauchart's ligament ['mauʃɑːt]（Burkhard D. Mauchart）翼状韧带

Maumené's test [məum'nei]（Edme J. Maumené）莫默内试验（检尿葡萄糖）

Maunoir's hydrocele ['məunwɑː]（Jean P. Maunoir）颈导管水囊肿

Maurer's dots (clefts, spots, stippling) ['maurə]（Georg Maurer）毛雷尔小点（裂、点、点彩）（恶性疟的红细胞内红色不规则小点）

Mauriac's syndrome [ˌmɔːri'æk]（Pierre Mauriac）莫里阿克综合征（侏儒症、肝大、肥胖、迟缓性性成熟伴糖尿病）

Mauriceau's lance [ˌmɔːri'səu]（François Mauriceau）莫里索柳叶刀（切胎尖刀）| ~ maneuver 莫里索手法（臀先露时胎头后出娩出法）

Mauthner's cell ['mautnə]（Ludwig Mauthner）毛特讷细胞（在鱼类和两栖类后脑中分出毛特讷纤维的大细胞）| ~ fiber 毛特讷纤维（从鱼类和两栖类的后脑延伸到脊髓尾端的轴索，是尾部兴奋的最后共同路径）/ ~ membrane (sheath) 轴膜 / ~ test 毛特讷试验（检色盲）

mauve [məuv] *n*, *a* 紫红色（的）

mauvein ['məuviːn] *n* 苯胺紫（指示剂）

mawseed ['mɔːsiːd] *n* 罂粟子

Maxcy's disease ['mæksi]（Kenneth F. Maxcy）马克西病（美国东南部地方性斑疹伤寒）

maxilla [mæk'silə]（［复］**maxillas** 或 **maxillae** [mæk'siliː]）*n* 上颌骨 | inferior ~ 下颌骨 | **maxillary** [mæk'siləri, 'mæksi-] *a*

maxillectomy [ˌmæksi'lektəmi] *n* 上颌骨切除术

maxillitis [ˌmæksi'laitis] *n* 上颌骨炎

maxillodental [mækˌsiləu'dentl] *a* 上颌牙的

maxilloethmoidectomy [ˌmæksiləuˌeθmɔi'dektəmi] *n* 上颌窦筛窦切除术

maxillofacial [mækˌsiləu'feiʃəl] *a* 上颌面的

maxillojugal [mækˌsiləu'dʒuːgəl] *a* 上颌颧的

maxillolabial [mækˌsiləu'leibjəl] *a* 上颌唇的

maxillomandibular [mækˌsiləumæn'dibjulə] *a* 上下颌的

maxillopalatine [mækˌsiləu'pælətain] *a* 上颌腭的

maxillopharyngeal [mækˌsiləufə'rin'dʒiːəl] *a* 上颌咽的

maxillotomy [ˌmæksi'lɔtəmi] *n* 上颌骨切开术

maximal ['mæksiməl] *a* 最大的，最高的

maximize ['mæksimaiz] *vt* 把…增加到最大限度 | **maximization** [ˌmæksimai'zeiʃən, -mi'z-] *n*

maximum ['mæksiməm]（［复］**maxima** ['mæksimə]）*n* 最大［量］，最高［量］，最大限度 *a* 最大的 | tubular ~ 肾小管最大排泄量，肾小管排泄最高限

maxwell ['mækswel]（James C. Maxwell）*n* 麦克斯韦（旧磁通量单位，现用韦［伯］〈Wb〉）

Maxwell's ring ['mækswel]（Patrick W. Maxwell）马克斯韦尔环（一种类似勒韦〈Löwe〉环，但较纤细而微弱）｜ ~ spot 视网膜黄斑

Maydl's operation [ˈmeidl]（Karel Maydl）梅德尔手术（①结肠造口术，将结肠牵出切口，在下面垫一玻璃棒，保持其位置直至粘连形成；②导输尿管入直肠中，用于膀胱外翻）

mayer [ˈmeiə]（Julius R. von Mayer）*n* 迈尔（比热容单位，1 mayer = 10^3 J〈kg · K〉）

Mayer-Rokitansky-Küster-Hauser syndrome [ˈmaiə ˌrɔkiˈtʌnski ˈkiːstə ˈhauzə]（August F. J. K. Mayer; Karl F. von Rokitansky; Hermann Küster; G. A. Hauser）迈-罗-屈-豪综合征（副中肾管发育缺陷，先天性阴道缺失及子宫未成熟〈典型者仅有双角残留物〉，而输卵管、卵巢、女性第二性征及生长均正常）

Mayer's hemalum [ˈmeiə]（Paul Mayer）迈尔苏木精明矾染剂（由氧化苏木精、明矾、麝香草脑和90％乙醇的水溶液制成的染剂）｜ ~ muchematein 迈尔明矾苏木精染剂（使黏液着色的特殊染剂）

Mayer's test [ˈmeiə]（Ferdinand F. Mayer）迈尔试验（检生物碱）｜ ~ reagent 迈尔试剂（碘化汞钾试剂）

May-Hegglin anomaly [mai ˈheglin]（Richard May; Robert M. Hegglin）梅-赫异常（一种血细胞形态学常染色体显性遗传性疾病，特征为蓝色含RNA胞质包涵体，类似大多数粒细胞中的窦勒〈Döhle〉小体，伴有异常大的而颗粒形成不良的血小板，有时伴有血小板减小，通常无其他明显特征）

mayhem [ˈmeihem] *n* 伤残，残废

mayidism [ˈmeiaidizəm] *n* 糙皮病，蜀黍红斑，陪拉格

Mayo Robson 见 Robson

Mayor's scarf [mεə]（Mathias L. Mayor）梅尔三角巾（固定上肢）

Mayo's operation [ˈmeiəu]（William J. Mayo and Charles H. Mayo）梅奥手术（①切除胃幽门端，缝合十二指肠和胃，再施行一独立性后侧胃空肠吻合术；②脐疝根治术时腹肌腱膜折叠缝术；③静脉曲张的皮下治疗法）｜ ~ sign 梅奥征（下颌肌肉松弛，指示麻醉已达到深度）

Mayo's vein [ˈmeijəu]（W. J. Mayo）幽门前静脉

maytansine [meiˈtænsiːn] *n* 美登素，美坦新（抗肿瘤药）

mayweed [ˈmeiwiːd] *n* 臭甘菊

May-White syndrome [mei hwait]（Duane L. May; Harry H. White）梅-怀综合征（一种罕见的常染色体显性遗传综合征，表现为肌阵挛、小脑性共济失调和耳聋）

maza [ˈmæzə] *n*【希】胎盘

maze [meiz] *n* 迷津（用于测验实验动物学习和记忆能力）

mazic [ˈmeizik] *a* 胎盘的

mazindol [ˈmeizindɔl] *n* 马吲哚（食欲抑制药）

maz(o)- [构词成分]乳房，乳腺；同样见以 mamm(o)-和 mast(o)-起始的词

mazodynia [ˌmeizəˈdiniə] *n* 乳房痛

mazopexy [ˈmeizəˌpeksi] *n* 乳房固定术

mazoplasia [ˌmeizəˈpleiziə] *n* 乳房组织增生

Mazzini's test [məˈzini]（L. Y. Mazzini）梅齐尼试验（一种诊断梅毒用的絮状试验）

Mazzoni's corpuscles [mæˈdzəuni]（Vittorio Mazzoni）马佐尼小体（感觉神经末梢，类似克劳泽〈Krause〉小体）

Mazzotti reaction [məˈzɔti]（Luis Mazzotti）马佐蒂反应（一系列不良反应，可能是严重的或可能很少危及生命，盘尾丝虫病时服用乙胺嗪所致，最常见的为强烈瘙痒症，但有时全身性表现为发热、不适、淋巴结肿大、嗜酸粒细胞增多、关节痛、心动过速和低血压；如眼内出现无数微丝蚴，则可能失明）｜ ~ test 马佐蒂试验（检盘尾丝虫病）

MB Medicinae Baccalaureus【拉】医学士

Mb megabase 兆碱基

m. b. misce bene【拉】混合均匀，混匀

MBP mannose-binding protein 甘露糖结合蛋白；major basic protein 主要碱性蛋白；myelin basic protein 髓磷脂碱性蛋白

MBq megabecquerel 兆贝克［勒尔］

mbundu [əmˈbuːnduː] *n* 姆本杜毒（一种西非洲的毒物，得自马钱科植物）

MC Magister Chirurgiae【拉】外科硕士；Medical Corps 军医队

mC millicoulomb 毫库［仑］

μC microcoulomb 微库［仑］

MCA 3-methylcholanthrene 3-甲基胆蒽

MCAD deficiency medium-chain acyl-CoA dehydrogenase deficiency 中链酰基辅酶 A 脱氢酶缺乏症

McArdle's disease (syndrome) [məˈkɑːdl]（Brian McArdle）麦卡德尔病（综合征），糖原贮积症Ⅴ型

McBride operation [mækˈbraid]（Earl D. McBride）麦克布赖德手术（为矫正踇外翻而切除第一跖骨头的内侧突手术）

McBurney's incision [mækˈbəːni]（Charles McBurney）麦克伯尼切口（髂前上棘内按腹外斜肌肌纤维方向切口，入内则按肌纤维方向分别切开腹内斜肌和腹横肌）｜ ~ operation 麦克伯尼手术（腹股沟疝根治手术）／ ~ point 麦克伯尼点（急性阑尾炎压痛点）／ ~ sign 麦克伯尼征（距脐到髂前上棘三分之二的点有压痛，为阑尾炎之征）

McCarthy's reflex [məˈkɑːθi]（Daniel J. McCarthy）麦卡锡反射（轻触眶上神经时眼轮匝肌收缩）

McClure-Aldrich test [məˈkluə ˈɔːldritʃ] (William B. McClure; Charles A. Aldrich) 麦克卢尔-奥尔德里奇试验(皮内注射 0.8% 氯化钠溶液,中毒时氯化钠吸收速度〈亦即肿块消失的速度〉较正常者慢)

McCune-Albright syndrome [məˈkjuːn ˈɔːlbrait] (Donovan J. McCune; Fuller Albright) 麦-奥综合征(见 Albright syndrome)

MCD mean of consecutive difference 连续差平均值

McDonald's maneuver [məkˈdɔnəld] (Ellice McDonald) 麦克唐纳法(测量腹围以推算孕期) | ~ rule 麦克唐纳规律(从耻骨连合上缘到宫底的腹围长度厘米数除以 3.5,即孕期的阴历月数,只适用于妊娠 6 个月后)

MCE myocardial contrast echocardiography 心肌心脏超声造影[术]

MCF macrophage chemotactic factor 巨噬细胞趋化因子

Mcg Mcg 标记(区别人免疫球蛋白 λ 轻链亚型的一种抗原标记)

mcg microgram 微克

McGill operation [məˈgil] (Arthur F. McGill) 麦吉尔手术,耻骨上经膀胱前列腺切除术

McGinn-White sign [məkˈgin *h*wait] (Sylvester McGinn; Paul D. White) 麦克金-怀特征(Ⅲ导联呈 Q 波及末段倒置的 T 波,Ⅱ导联 S-T 段与 T 波低位及胸导联 V_2 与 V_3 的 T 波倒置,为严重性肺栓塞引起右心室扩张的心电图所显示者,外加急性肺源性心脏病的临床体征)

MCH mean corpuscular hemoglobin 平均红细胞血红蛋白量

MCHB Maternal and Child Health Bureau 妇幼保健处(属卫生资源与卫生事业管理局)

MCHC mean corpuscular hemoglobin concentration 平均红细胞血红蛋白浓度

MCi megacurie 兆居里

mCi millicurie 毫居里

μCi microcurie 微居里

mCi-hr millicurie-hour 毫居里-小时

MCI/MI a mixture of methylchloroisothiazolinone and methylisothiazolinone 甲氯异噻唑啉酮-甲基异噻唑啉酮合剂

McKusick-Kaufman syndrome [məˈkjuːsik ˈkaufmən] (Victor A. McKusick; Robert L. Kaufman) 麦-考综合征(见 Kaufman-McKusick syndrome)

McLean's formula (index) [məkˈlein] (Franklin C. McLean) 麦克莱恩公式(指数)(计算肾脏排脲指数,即

$$\frac{\text{每 24 小时脲克数}\sqrt{\text{每升尿内脲克数}\times 8.96}}{\text{体重/千克}\times\langle\text{每升血内脲克数}\rangle^2}$$
)

McLeod phenotype [məˈkləud] (McLeod 为 1961 年首次观察到的先征者的姓)麦克劳德表型(一种罕见的血液表型,为 X 连锁遗传,凯尔〈Kell〉血型几种抗原表现很弱,患者有时有贫血状况,称为麦克劳德综合征) | ~ syndrome 麦克劳德综合征(见于一些个体具有麦克劳德血液表型的一种综合征,特征为轻度溶血性贫血伴刺状红细胞、血清肌酸酐磷酸激酶增高以及有时为肌肉萎缩和神经系统缺陷。少数病例为 X 连锁型慢性肉芽肿病)

MCMI Millon clinical multiaxial inventory 米伦临床多轴调查表

McMurray's sign [məkˈmʌri] (Thomas P. McMurray) 麦氏征(用手活动膝部时听到软骨的咔嗒声,提示半月板损伤) | ~ test 麦氏试验(检半月板撕裂)

McNaughten 见 M'Naughten

MCP membrane cofactor protein 膜辅因子蛋白

McPheeters' treatment [məkˈfiːtəz] (Herman O. McPheeters) 麦克菲特斯疗法(治静脉曲张性溃疡,即用橡皮海绵缚于溃疡处,并指令患者尽量多走路)

Mcps megacycles per second 兆周/秒

M-CSF macrophage colony-stimulating factor 巨噬细胞集落刺激因子

MCT mean circulation time 平均循环时间

MCV mean corpuscular volume 平均红细胞体积

MD Medicinae Doctor【拉】医学博士

Md mendelevium 钔

MDA methylenedioxyamphetamine 亚甲基二氧苯丙胺;mento-dextra anterior 颏右前(胎位)

MDF myocardial depressant factor 心肌抑制因子

MDMA 3,4-methylenedioxymethamphetamine 3,4-亚甲基二氧去氧麻黄碱

MDP mento-dextra posterior 颏右后(胎位);methylene diphosphonate 亚甲基二膦酸

MDS myelodysplasia 脊髓发育不良

MDT mento-dextra transversa 颏右横(胎位)

2-ME 2-mercaptoethanol 2-巯基乙醇

Me methyl 甲基

meal [miːl] *n* 膳食,餐;粗粉 | bismuth ~ 铋餐 / butter ~ 奶油餐(一种含奶油、糖、奶的浓缩食物) / liver ~ 肝粉 / motor test ~ 胃肠运动试餐(X 线检查) / opaque ~ 造影餐,不透光餐 / retention ~ 滞留(试验)餐 / test ~ 试餐,试[验]食

mealworm [ˈmiːlwəːm] *n* 粉[蛀]虫

mean [miːn] *n* 均数;算术平均数;均值 | arithmetic ~ 算术平均数 / geometric ~ 几何平均数 / population ~ 总体均数 / sample ~ 样品平均[值]

Mean's sign [miːn] (James H. Mean) 米氏征(突眼性甲状腺肿时向上凝视可见眼球迟滞)

measles [ˈmiːzlz] *n* 麻疹;(家畜)囊尾蚴病 | bastard ~, German ~ 风疹 / black ~, hemorrhagic ~ 黑麻疹,出血性麻疹 / pork ~ 猪囊尾蚴病 / three-day ~ 三日麻疹,风疹
measly [ˈmiːzli] *a* 含囊尾蚴的,米珠的
measure [ˈmeʒə] *n* 测量;度量;量
meatal [miˈeitl] *a* 道的
meatitis [ˌmiːəˈtaitis] *n* 尿道口炎
meatometer [ˌmiːəˈtɔmitə] *n* 尿道口计
meatoplasty [ˈmiːətəˌplæsti] *n* 耳道成形术
meatorrhaphy [ˌmiːəˈtɔrəfi] *n* 尿道口缝合术
meatoscope [miˈætəskəup] *n* 尿道口镜
meatoscopy [ˌmiːəˈtɔskəpi] *n* 尿道口镜检查 | ureteral ~ 输尿管口镜检查
meatotome [miˈætətəum], **meatome** [ˈmiːətəum] *n* 尿道口刀
meatotomy [ˌmiːəˈtɔtəmi] *n* 尿道口切开术
meatus [miˈeitəs] ([复] **meatus⟨es⟩**) *n*【拉】道 | external acoustic ~, external auditory ~ 外耳道 / fish-mouth ~ 鱼口式尿道口 / internal acoustic ~, internal auditory ~ 内耳道 / urinary ~ 尿道外口
mebendazole [miˈbendəzəul] *n* 甲苯达唑(抗蠕虫药)
mebeverine hydrochloride [miˈbevəriːn] 盐酸美贝维林(平滑肌松弛药)
mebrofenin(BrIDA) [ˈmiːbrəuˌfenin] *n* 甲溴菲宁(一种亚氨基二乙酰⟨IDA⟩三甲基溴取代的类似物,与^{99m}Tc 络合用于肝胆成像和肝功能研究,静脉内给药)
mebutamate [miˈbjutəmeit] *n* 美布氨酯(抗高血压药)
mecamine [ˈmekəmin] *n* 美加明(抗高血压药)
mecamylamine hydrochloride [ˌmekəˈmiləmin] 盐酸美卡拉明(神经节阻断药,用作抗高血压药)
MeCbl methylcobalamin 甲钴胺
meCCNU semustine 司莫司汀
mechanical [miˈkænikəl] *a* 机械的,力学的
mechanicoreceptor [miˌkænikəuriˈseptə] *n* 机械[性刺激]感受器
mechanicotherapeutics [miˌkænikəuˌθerəˈpjuːtiks], **mechanicotherapy** [miˌkænikəuˈθerəpi] *n* 力学疗法,机械疗法
mechanics [miˈkæniks] *n* 力学,机械学 | animal ~ 动物力学,生物力学,生物机械学 / body ~ 躯体力学 / developmental ~ 实验胚胎学
mechanism [ˈmekənizəm] *n* 机械结构,机构;机制;机械论(认为生命现象乃基于控制整个无机界的同一物理及化学定律) | countercurrent ~ 逆流机制(肾脏浓缩尿的机制,它取决于亨勒⟨Henle⟩袢和直小管的解剖排列) / defense ~, escape ~ 防御机制,防卫机制,逃避机制(一种表现精神紧张减少的心理机制) / ~ of labor 分娩机制 / mental ~ 心理机制 / neutralizing ~ 中和机制(一种中和梦境的心理机制) / oculogyric ~ 眼动机制(与眼球运动有关的一系列神经中枢) / outgoing ~ 表示机构,表达机构(用言语、书写或手势以说明文字或表达思想的器械) / pingpong ~ 乒乓机制(一底物与酶起反应并离解成一产物的过程,依附在酶上有一个功能簇,在另一次反应中,改变了的酶将所依附的功能簇转变成另一个底物,形成另一个产物并释放出原来形式的酶) / somatic ~ 躯体机构 / splanchnic ~ 内脏机构
mechanist [ˈmekənist] *n* 机械论者(认为生命所有现象仅是物理和化学性的)
mechan(o)- [构词成分]机械
mechanocyte [ˈmekənəsait] *n* 成纤维细胞
mechanogymnastics [ˌmekənəudʒimˈnæstiks] *n* 器械体操
mechanology [ˌmekəˈnɔlədʒi] *n* 机械学
mechanoreceptor [ˌmekənəuriˈseptə] *n* 机械[性刺激]感受器
mechanosensory [ˌmekənəuˈsensəri] *a* 机械性感觉的
mechanotherapy [ˌmekənəuˈθerəpi] *n* 力学疗法,机械疗法
mechanothermy [ˌmekənəˈθəːmi] *n* 按摩生热法,力学热疗法
mechlorethamine hydrochloride [ˌmeklɔˈreθəmiːn] 盐酸氮芥(抗肿瘤药)
Mechnikov 见 Metchnikoff
mecillinam [miˈsilinəm] *n* 美西林(抗生素类药)
mecism [ˈmiːsizəm] *n* 过长
mecistocephalic [miˌsistəusəˈfælik], **mecistocephalous** [miˌsistəuˈsefələs] *a* 长头的(颅指数小于 71)
Mecistocirrhus [miˌsistəuˈsirəs] *n* 长刺线虫属 | ~ digitatus 指形长刺线虫
meckelectomy [ˌmekəˈlektəmi] *n* 蝶腭神经节切除术
Meckel's band (ligament) [ˈmekəl] (Johann F. Meckel ⟨Senior⟩) 梅克尔带(韧带)(锤骨前韧带的一部分) | ~ cavity (space) 梅克尔腔,三叉腔(含半月神经节的硬膜腔) / ~ ganglion 蝶腭神经节
Meckel's cartilage (rod) [ˈmekəl] (Johann F. Meckel ⟨Junior⟩) 麦克尔软骨(棒)(第一鳃弓软骨,鼓室下颌软骨) | ~ diverticulum 麦克尔憩室(卵黄管的遗迹) / ~ plane 麦克尔平面(通过耳点和牙槽中点的平面) / ~ syndrome 麦克尔综合征(为常染色体隐性遗传,最常见的特征为前额倾斜、后脑膜膨出、多指⟨趾⟩畸形及多囊

肾,死于围生期。亦称头颅异常和内脏囊肿)

meclizine hydrochloride [ˈmekliziːn] 盐酸美克洛嗪(抗组胺药,用作止吐药)

meclocycline sulfosalicylate [ˌmekləuˈsaikliːn] 磺基水杨酸甲氯环素(一种四环素抗生素,用于治疗寻常痤疮,局部用药)

meclofenamate [miˌkləufəˈnæmeit] *n* 甲氯芬那酸(为甲氯芬那酸的结合型,用作 meclofenamate sodium〈甲氯芬那酸钠〉,以治骨关节炎和类风湿关节炎)

meclofenamic acid [miˌkləufəˈnæmik] 甲氯芬那酸(非甾体消炎药)

meclofenoxate [miˌkləufəˈnɔkseit] *n* 甲氯芬酯(此药据称在氧浓度减少时有助于细胞代谢)

mecloqualone [ˌmekləˈkwɔləun] *n* 甲氯喹酮(催眠镇静药)

mecobalamine [ˌmikə*u*ˈbæləmiːn] *n* 甲钴胺(抗贫血药)

mecocephalic [ˌmikə*u*səˈfælik] *a* 长头的

meconate [ˈmekəneit] *n* 袂康酸盐

meconic acid [miˈkɔnik] 袂康酸

meconiorrhea [miˌkəuniəˈriːə] *n* 胎粪溢

meconism [ˈmekənizəm] *n* 阿片癖,阿片中毒

meconium [miˈkəunjəm] *n* 胎粪

mecrylate [miˈkrileit] *n* 美克立酯(外科用组织黏合剂)

mecystasis [miˈsistəsis] *n* 等张性[肌纤维]长度增加

MED minimal effective dose 最小有效量;minimal erythema dose 最小红斑量

medazepam hydrochloride [miˈdæzəpæm] 盐酸美达西泮(弱安定药)

Medex [ˈmedeks]【法】(**médecin extension**) *n* 军医召募方案(召募原军队卫生员进行培训使之成为助理医师的方案)

medi [ˈmaiθə] *n* 见 maedi

media [ˈmiːdjə] *n*【拉】medium 的复数;中间;[血管]中膜

mediad [ˈmiːdiæd] *ad* 向中

medial [ˈmiːdjəl] *a* 内侧的,近中的;中层的

medialecithal [ˌmiːdiəˈlesiθəl] *a* 中[卵]黄的

medialis [ˌmiːdiˈeilis] *a*【拉】内侧的,近中的

median [ˈmiːdjən] *a* 中央的,正中的 *n* 中线;正中;中[位]数

medianus [ˌmiːdiˈeinəs] *a*【拉】正中的

mediaometer [ˌmiːdiəˈɔmitə] *n* 眼介质屈光计

mediastina [ˌmiːdiəsˈtainə] mediastinum 的复数

mediastinal [ˌmiːdiəsˈtainl] *a* 纵隔的

mediastinitis [ˌmiːdiæstiˈnaitis] *n* 纵隔炎 | fibrous ~, indurative ~ 纤维性纵隔炎,硬化性纵隔炎

mediastinogram [ˌmiːdiəsˈtainəgræm] *n* 纵隔 X 线[照]片

mediastinography [ˌmiːdiˌæstiˈnɔgrəfi] *n* 纵隔 X 线摄影[术]

mediastinopericarditis [ˌmiːdiˌæstinə*u*ˌperikɑːˈdaitis] *n* 纵隔心包炎

mediastinoscope [ˌmiːdiəˈstainəskəup] *n* 纵隔镜 | **mediastinoscopic** [ˌmiːdiˌæstinəˈskɔpik] *a* 纵隔镜的;纵隔镜检查的 / **mediastinoscopy** [ˌmiːdiˌæstiˈnɔskəpi] *n* 纵隔镜检查术

mediastinotomy [ˌmiːdiˌæstiˈnɔtəmi] *n* 纵隔切开术

mediastinum [ˌmiːdiəsˈtainəm]([复] **mediastina** [ˌmiːdiəsˈtainə]) *n*【拉】纵隔

mediastinus [ˌmiːdiəsˈtainəs] *n*【拉】(内外科)助理医师

mediate [ˈmiːdieit] *vi* 居间 [ˈmiːdiət] *a* 间接的,居间的

mediation [ˌmiːdiˈeiʃən] *n* 间介[作用],居间[作用] | chemical ~ 化学间介作用

mediator [ˈmiːdieitə] *n* 间介器,传递器;介质,介体

medic [ˈmedik] *n* 医学生

medicable [ˈmedikəbl] *a* 可治疗的

Medicago [ˌmediˈkeigəu] *n* 苜蓿属

Medicaid [ˈmedikeid] *n* 医疗补助方案(美国联邦、州和地方税收中拨款补助低收入的人支付住院和医疗费用的方案)

medical [ˈmedikəl] *a* 医学的,医疗的;内科的

medicament [meˈdikəmənt] *n* 药物,药剂

medicamentosus [ˌmedikəmenˈtəusəs] *a*【拉】药物的,药剂的

medicamentous [ˌmedikəˈmentəs] *a* 药物的,药剂的

Medicare [ˈmedikεə] *n* 医疗照顾方案(美国社会保障局对 65 岁以上老年人提供医疗保健的方案)

medicaster [ˈmediˌkæstə] *n* 庸医

medicate [ˈmedikeit] *vt* 用药治疗,投药;加药,使含药 | **~d** *a* 含药[物]的,药制的 / **medicative** *a* 加入药物的;医药的,药用的,医治的

medication [ˌmediˈkeiʃən] *n* 加药;药疗法,投药法;药物,药剂 | conservative ~ 补养药疗法 / dialytic ~ 渗透药疗法,矿泉饮料法 / hypodermatic ~ 皮下投药法 / ionic ~ 离子透药疗法 / sublingual ~ 舌下投药法 / substitutive ~ 代替[药]疗法 / transduodenal ~ 十二指肠内投药法

medicator [ˈmediˌkeitə] *n* 涂药器

medicephalic [ˌmidisəˈfælik] *a* 头正中[静脉]的

medicinal [meˈdisinl] *a* 医药的,药用的,医治的

medicine [ˈmedis*i*n] *n* 药品,药物;医学;内科学 | aviation ~ 航空医学 / Chinese herbal ~ 中草药 / clinical ~ 临床医学 / comparative ~ 比较医

学 / compound ~ 复方药物 / domestic ~ 家庭医疗 / dosimetric ~ 剂量学 / emergency ~ 急诊医学 / environmental ~ 环境医学 / experimental ~ 实验医学 / family ~ 家庭医学 / folk ~ 民间医药 / forensic ~, legal ~ 法医学 / geriatric ~ 老年医学 / group ~ 联合医疗(如联合诊所) / holistic ~ 整体医学(把人当作一个不可分割的有机整体的医学) / Indian ~ 印第安医学(北美的一种民间医学) / internal ~ 内科学 / mental ~ 精神病学 / nuclear ~ 核医学 / oral ~ 口腔医学,口腔内科学 / patent ~ 成药,专卖药(指不要处方就能买到的现成药) / physical ~ 物理医学,理疗学 / preclinical ~ 基础医学 / preventive ~ 预防医学 / proprietary ~ 特许专卖药 / psychologic ~ 精神病学,心理医学 / psychosomatic ~ 心身医学 / rational ~ 合理医学 / social ~ 社会医学 / socialized ~, state ~ 国家公费医疗 / space ~ 宇宙医学 / sports ~ 运动医学 / static ~ 饮食医学(以饮食、排泄量和体重的关系为医疗的根据) / suggestive ~ 暗示疗法 / traditional Chinese ~ (TCM) 中医 / tropical ~ 热带病学,热带医学 / veterinary ~ 兽医学

medico [ˈmedikəu] *n* 医生

medicochirurgic [ˌmedikəukaiˈrəːdʒik] *a* 内外科的

medicodental [ˌmedikəuˈdentl] *a* 内科与牙科的

medicolegal [ˌmedikəuˈliːgəl] *a* 法医学的

medicomechanical [ˌmedikəumiˈkænikəl] *a* 药物与机械[治疗]的

medicophysics [ˌmedikəuˈfiziks] *n* 医学物理学

medicopsychology [ˌmedikəusaiˈkɔlədʒi] *n* 医学心理学 | **medicopsychological** [ˌmedikəuˌsaikəˈlɔdʒikəl] *a*

medicosocial [ˌmedikəuˈsəuʃəl] *a* 医学社会的

medicotopographical [ˌmedikəuˌtəupəˈgræfikəl] *a* 临床[与]局部解剖学的

medicozoological [ˌmedikəuzəuəˈlɔdʒikəl] *a* 医用动物学的

medicus [ˈmedikəs] ([复] **medici** [ˈmedisai]) *n* 【拉】医师(尤指内科医师)

medifrontal [ˌmiːdiˈfrʌntl] *a* 额中部的

Medin's disease [ˈmeidiːn] (Oskar Medin) 脊髓灰质炎

mediocarpal [ˌmiːdiəuˈkɑːpl] *a* 腕骨间的,腕骨中部的

medioccipital [ˌmiːdiɔkˈsipitl] *a* 枕中[部]的

mediolateral [ˌmiːdiəuˈlætərəl] *a* 中间外侧的,中侧的

medionecrosis [ˌmiːdiəuneˈkrəusis] *n* 中层坏死,中膜坏死 | ~ of aorta 主动脉中层坏死

mediotarsal [ˌmiːdiəuˈtɑːsəl] *a* 跗中部的

mediscalenus [ˌmiːdiskəˈliːnəs] *n* 中斜角肌

medisect [ˈmiːdisekt] *vt* 正中切开

meditation [ˌmediˈteiʃən] *n* 沉思;默念 | transcendental ~ (印度教的)超脱静坐(默念一段祷文使身心放松的方法)

medium [ˈmiːdjəm] ([复] **mediums** 或 **media** [ˈmiːdjə]) *n* 方法;介质;培养基 *a* 中间的 | active ~ 活性介质 / clearing ~ 透明介质,澄清剂 / contrast ~ 造影剂,对比剂 / culture ~ 培养基 / disperse ~, dispersion ~, dispersive ~ 分散媒,分散介质 / HAT ~ HAT 培养基(含次黄嘌呤 hypoxanthine,氨蝶呤 aminopterin 和胸苷 thymidine 的组织培养基,用于体细胞融合实验) / mounting ~ 封固剂 / nutrient ~ 营养培养基 / radiolucent ~ 透射线造影剂 / radiopaque ~ 不透射线造影剂 / refracting media 屈光介质 / separating ~ 分离介质,分离剂

medius [ˈmiːdiəs] *a* 【拉】中间的

MEDLARS [ˈmedlɑːz] (*MED*ical *L*iterature *A*nalysis and *R*etrieval *S*ystem) 医学文献分析和检索系统(美国国家医学图书馆的一个计算机化文献目次系统,由此产生医学索引〈Index Medicus〉)

MEDLINE [ˈmedlain] (*MED*LARS on-*line*) 联机医学文献分析和检索系统(一种计算机化的文献目次检索系统,是 MEDLARS 的联机部分)

medorrhea [ˌmedəˈriːə] *n* 尿道溢,后淋

medrogestone [medrəˈdʒestəun] *n* 美屈孕酮(孕激素类药)

medronate disodium [ˈmedrəneit] 亚甲膦酸二钠(药物佐剂)

medroxyprogesterone acetate [meˌdrɔksiprəuˈdʒestərəun] 醋酸甲羟孕酮(孕激素类药)

medrysone [ˈmedrisəun] *n* 甲羟松(合成糖皮质激素)

medulla [məˈdʌlə] ([复] **medullas** 或 **medullae** [məˈdʌliː]) *n* 【拉】髓质;延髓;骨髓 | adrenal ~, suprarenal ~ 肾上腺髓质 / ~ oblongata 延髓 / spinal ~ 脊髓 | **~ry** [məˈdʌləri, ˈmedəˌlɛəri] *a* 髓的;脊髓的

medullated [ˈmedəleitid] *a* 有髓[鞘]的

medullation [ˌmedəˈleiʃən] *n* 髓鞘形成;骨髓生成;髓形成

medullectomy [ˌmedəˈlektəmi] *n* 髓质切除术

medullitis [ˌmedəˈlaitis] *n* 骨髓炎;脊髓炎

medullization [ˌmedəlaiˈzeiʃən, -liˈz-] *n* [骨]髓形成,[骨]髓化

medull(o)- [构词成分] 髓

medulloadrenal [məˌdʌləuəˈdriːnl], **medulliadrenal** [məˌdʌliəˈdriːnl] *a* 肾上腺髓质的

medulloarthritis [məˌdʌləuɑːˈθraitis] *n* 关节骨髓炎

medulloblast [mə'dʌləublæst] *n* 髓母细胞,成神经管细胞
medulloblastoma [məˌdʌləublæs'təumə] *n* 髓母细胞瘤,成神经管细胞瘤
medulloencephalic [məˌdʌləuensi'fælik] *a* 脑脊髓的
medulloepithelioma [məˌdʌləuˌepiˌθiːli'əumə] *n* 髓上皮瘤
medulloid ['medələid] *n* 类[肾上腺]髓质素
medullosuprarenoma [məˌdʌləuˌsjuːprəriː'nəumə] *n* 肾上腺髓质瘤,嗜铬细胞瘤
medullotherapy [məˌdʌləu'θerəpi] *n* 脊髓疗法(狂犬病的预防疗法)
medusa [mi'djuːzə] *n* 水母,海蜇
medusocongestin [miˌdjuːsəukən'dʒestin] *n* 水母毒素
Mees' line [miːz] (R. A. Mees) 米士线(指甲上出现一条或多条白色横行条纹,与砷中毒和其他微量元素中毒有关,见于麻风、败血症、主动脉夹层动脉瘤和急慢性肾衰竭)
mefenamic acid [ˌmefə'næmik] 甲芬那酸(消炎镇痛药)
mefenorex hydrochloride [mə'fenəreks] 盐酸美芬雷司(食欲抑制药)
mefexamide [mə'feksəmaid] *n* 美非沙胺(中枢神经系统兴奋药)
mefloquine hydrochloride ['mefləkwin] 盐酸甲氟喹(抗疟药)
mefruside ['mefrusaid] *n* 美夫西特(降压利尿药)
MEG magnetoencephalograph 脑磁波描记器
mega- [构词成分]巨,大(见 megalo-);兆,百万(10^6)
megabase (Mb) ['megbeis] *n* 兆碱基
megabecquerel (MBq) [ˌmegəbekə'rel] *n* 兆贝克[勒尔](放射性强度单位,10^6 Bq)
megabladder [ˌmegə'blædə] *n* 巨膀胱,膀胱扩张
megacalycosis [ˌmegəˌkæli'kəusis] *n* 巨肾盏
megacalyx [ˌmeg'keiliks, -kæ-] *n* 巨肾盏
megacardia [ˌmegə'kɑːdiə] *n* 心肥大
megacaryoblast [ˌmegə'kæriəblæst] *n* 原巨核细胞
megacaryocyte [ˌmegə'kæriəˌsait] *n* 巨核细胞
megacecum [ˌmegə'siːkəm] *n* 巨盲肠
megacephaly [ˌmegə'sefəli] *n* 巨头 | **megacephalic** [ˌmegəse'fælik], **megacephalous** [ˌmegə'sefələs] *a*
megacholedochus [ˌmegəkə'ledəkəs] *n* 巨总胆管(总胆管异常扩大)
megacolon [ˌmegə'kəulən] *n* 巨结肠
megacurie (MCi) [ˌmegə'kjuəri] *n* 兆居里(旧放射单位,$=10^6$ Ci,现用贝克[勒尔]〈Bq〉)
megacycle ['megəˌsaikl] *n* 兆周(一百万周)
megacystis [ˌmegə'sistis] *n* 巨膀胱,膀胱扩张
megadontia [ˌmegə'dɔnʃiə], **megadontism** [ˌmegə'dɔntizəm] *n* 巨牙 | **megadont** ['megədɔnt], **megadontic** [ˌmegə'dɔntik] *a*
megaduodenum [ˌmegəˌdju(ː)əu'diːnəm] *n* 巨十二指肠
megadyne ['megəˌdain] *n* 兆达因(旧功的单位,$=10^6$ dyn,现用牛[顿]〈N〉)
megaesophagus [ˌmegəi(ː)'sɔfəgəs] *n* 巨食管,食管扩张
megagametophyte [ˌmegəgə'miːtəfait] *n* 大配子体
megahertz (MHz) ['megəhəːts] *n* 兆赫[兹](10^6 Hz, 10^6 周/s)
megakaryoblast [ˌmegə'kæriəblæst] *n* 原巨核细胞
megakaryocyte [ˌmegə'kæriəsait] *n* 巨核细胞
megakaryocytic [ˌmegəˌkæriə'sitik] *a* 巨核细胞的
megakaryocytopoiesis [ˌmegəˌkæriəuˌsaitəupɔi'iːsis] *n* 巨核细胞生成
megakaryocytosis [ˌmegəˌkæriəsai'təusis] *n* 巨核细胞增多症
megakaryophthisis [ˌmegəˌkæriə'θaisis] *n* (骨髓)巨核细胞缺乏症
megalakria [ˌmegə'lækriə] *n* 肢端肥大症
megalecithal [ˌmegə'lesiθəl] *a* 多[卵]黄的
megalencephalon [ˌmegəlen'sefələn], **megalencephaly** [ˌmegəlen'sefəli] *n* 巨脑
megalgia [me'gældʒiə] *n* 剧痛(如在肌风湿病时)
megal(o)- [构词成分]巨,大
megaloblast ['megələuˌblæst] *n* 巨成红细胞,巨幼细胞 | **~ic** [ˌmegələu'blæstik] *a*
megaloblastoid [ˌmegələu'blæstɔid] *a* 巨成红细胞样的,巨幼细胞样的
megalobulbus [ˌmegələu'bʌlbəs] *n* 十二指肠冠过大(X 线片)
megalocardia [ˌmegələu'kɑːdiə] *n* 心肥大
megalocaryocyte [ˌmegələu'kæriəsait] *n* 巨核细胞
megalocephaly [ˌmegələu'sefəli], **megalocephalia** [ˌmegələusə'feiliə] *n* 巨头 | **megalocephalic** [ˌmegələusə'fælik] *a*
megaloceros [ˌmegə'lɔsərəs] *n* 有角畸胎
megalocheiria [ˌmegələu'kaiəriə] *n* 巨手
megaloclitoris [ˌmegələu'klitəris] *n* 巨阴蒂
megalocornea [ˌmegələu'kɔːniə] *n* 巨角膜,球形角膜
megalocystis [ˌmegələu'sistis] *n* 巨膀胱,膀胱

扩张
megalocyte [ˈmegələsait] *n* 巨红细胞
megalocytosis [ˌmegələusaiˈtəusis] *n* 巨红细胞症
megalodactyly [ˌmegələuˈdæktili], **megalodactylia** [ˌmegələudækˈtiliə], **megalodactylism** [ˌmegələuˈdæktilizəm] *n* 巨指,巨趾 | **megalodactylous** [ˌmegələuˈdæktiləs] *a*
megalodontia [ˌmegələuˈdɔnʃiə] *n* 巨牙
megaloesophagus [ˌmegələui(ː)ˈsɔfəgəs] *n* 巨食管,食管扩张
megalogastria [ˌmegələuˈgæstriə] *n* 巨胃
megaloglossia [ˌmegələuˈglɔsiə] *n* 巨舌
megalographia [ˌmegələuˈgræfiə], **megalography** [ˌmegəˈlɔgrəfi] *n* 巨大字体
megalohepatia [ˌmegələuhiˈpætiə] *n* 巨肝,肝肿大
megalokaryocyte [ˌmegələuˈkæriəsait] *n* 巨核细胞
megalomania [ˌmegələuˈmeinjə] *n* 夸大狂 | **~c** [ˌmegələuˈmeiniæk] *a* 夸大狂的 *n* 夸大狂者
megalomelia [ˌmegələuˈmiːliə] *n* 巨肢
megalomicin potassium phosphate [ˌmegələuˈmaisin] 美加米星 A 磷酸二氢钾(抗生素类药)
megalonychia [ˌmegələuˈnikiə] *n* 巨[指]甲
megalopenis [ˌmegələuˈpiːnis] *n* 巨阴茎
megalophallus [ˌmægələuˈfæləs] *n* 巨阴茎
megalophthalmos [ˌmegəlɔfˈθælmɔs] *n* 巨眼 | anterior ~ 巨角膜,球形角膜 | **megalophthalmus** [ˌmegəlɔfˈθælməs] *n*
megalopia [ˌmegəˈləupiə], **megalopsia** [ˌmegəˈlɔpsiə] *n* 视物显大症
megaloplastocyte [ˌmegələuˈplæstəˌsait] *n* 巨血小板
megalopodia [ˌmegələuˈpəudiə] *n* 巨足
Megalopyge [ˌmegələuˈpidʒi] *n* 绒蠹属 | ~ opercularis 壳盖绒蠹
megaloscope [ˈmegələskəup] *n* 放大镜,扩大镜
megalosplenia [ˌmegələuˈspliːniə] *n* 巨脾,脾[肿]大
megalospore [ˈmegələˌspɔː] *n* 大孢子;大孢子癣菌
Megalosporon [ˌmegəˈlɔspərɔn] *n* 大孢子癣菌属
megalosporon [ˌmegəˈlɔspərɔn] *n* 大孢子癣菌
megalosyndactyly [ˌmegələusinˈdæktili] *n* 巨并指,巨并趾
megalothymus [ˌmegələuˈθaiməs] *n* 巨胸腺,胸腺肥大
megaloureter [ˌmegələujuəˈriːtə] *n* 巨输尿管(没有明显原因的先天性输尿管扩张,亦称先天性或原发性巨输尿管、原发性输尿管张力缺乏和输尿管神经肌发育异常) | congenital ~, primary ~ 先天性巨输尿管,原发性巨输尿管(即巨输尿管) / reflux ~ 反流性巨输尿管(输尿管扩张伴膀胱输尿管反流现象)
megalourethra [ˌmægələujuːˈriːθrə] *n* 巨尿道
-megaly [构词成分]大,增大[症],肿大
megapolycalicosis [ˌmegəˌpɔliˌkæliˈkəusis] *n* 巨肾盏
megaprosopous [ˌmegəˈprɔsəpəs] *a* 巨面的
megarectum [ˌmegəˈrektəm] *n* 巨直肠,直肠扩张
Megarhinini [ˌmegəˈrainini] *n* 巨蚊族
Megarhinus [megəˈrainəs] *n* 巨蚊属
megascopic [ˌmegəsˈkɔpik] *a* 肉眼可见的,根据肉眼观察的
Megaselia [ˌmegəˈsiːliə] *n* 巨沟蝇属
megaseme [ˌmegəsiːm] *n* 巨眶(眶指数为 89 或超过 89)
megasigmoid [ˌmegəˈsigmɔid] *n* 巨乙状结肠,乙状结肠扩张
megasoma [ˌmegəˈsəumə] *n* 巨体,身材高大
Megasphaera [ˌmegəˈsfiːrə] *n* 巨球型菌属
megasporangium [ˌmegəspɔːˈrændʒiəm] ([复] **megasporangia** [ˌmegəspɔːˈrændʒiə]) *n* 大孢子囊
megaspore [ˈmegəspɔː] *n* 大孢子;大分生孢子 | **megasporic** [megəˈspɔːrik] *a*
megathrombocyte [ˌmegəˈθrɔmbəusait] *n* 巨血小板
Megatrichophyton [ˌmegəˌtraiˈkɔfitɔn] *n* 巨毛癣菌属
Megatrypanum [ˌmegəˈtripənəm] *n* 巨锥虫亚属
megaunit [ˈmegəˌjuːnit] *n* 兆单位,100 万国际单位(IU)(10^6 倍于标准单位)
megaureter [ˌmegəjuəˈriːtə] *n* 巨输尿管,输尿管扩张
megavitamin [ˌmegəˈvaitəmiːn] *n* 大剂量维生素
megavolt (MV) [ˈmegəvəult] *n* 兆伏[特](10^6 V)
megavoltage [ˈmegəˌvɔltidʒ] *n* 兆伏数(10^6 V),巨电压(电离放射疗法时大于 1 兆伏的电压)
megestrol acetate [məˈdʒestrɔl] 甲地孕酮(黄体激素,抗肿瘤药)
Méglin's point [meiˈglæn] (J. A. Méglin) 梅格兰点,腭孔点(腭神经自腭大孔出现之点)
meglumine [ˈmegluminː] *n* 葡甲胺(用以制备某些不透 X 线的造影剂) | ~ diatrizoate 泛影葡胺(尿路、心血管造影剂) / ~ iodipamide 胆影葡胺(胆道造影剂) / ~ iothalamate 碘酞葡胺(脑血管、尿路、周围动脉造影剂)
meglutol [ˈmegljutɔl] *n* 美格鲁托(抗高脂蛋白血症药)
megohm [ˈmegəum] *n* 兆欧[姆](10^6 Ω)

megophthalmos [megɔf'θælmɔs] *n* 巨眼,牛眼
megoxycyte [me'gɔksisait] *n* 巨嗜酸细胞
megoxyphil [me'gɔksifil] *n* 巨粒嗜酸粒细胞
megrim ['miːgrim] *n* 偏头痛
MEGX monoethylglycinexylidide 单乙基甘氨酸二甲代苯胺
mehlnährschaden [ˌmeilnεə'ʃɑːdən] *n*【德】谷粉营养障碍(一种营养缺乏综合征,类似夸希奥科病 kwashiorkor)
meibomian cyst [mai'bəumiən] (Heinrich Meibom) 迈博姆囊肿(睑板腺囊肿,霰粒肿) | ~ foramen 舌盲孔 / ~ glands 睑板腺 / ~ stye 迈博姆睑腺炎(睑板腺炎)
meibomianitis [maiˌbəumiə'naitis], **meibomitis** [ˌmaibə'maitis] *n* 睑板腺炎
Meige's disease ['meʒə] (Henri Meige) 梅热病(见 Milroy's disease) | ~ syndrome 梅热综合征(①Milroy's disease;②眼睑痉挛-口下颌张力障碍综合征。亦称勃鲁盖尔〈Brueghel〉综合征)
Meigs' capillaries [megz] (Arthur V. Meigs) 梅格斯毛细管(心肌毛细管) | ~ test 梅格斯试验(检乳脂)
Meigs' syndrome, Meigs-Salmon syndrome [megz'sælmən] (J. V. Meigs; Udall J. Salmon) 梅格斯综合征,梅-沙综合征(腹水和水胸伴卵巢纤维瘤和其他盆腔肿瘤)
meio- [构词成分]减少,不足,减缩
meiogenic [ˌmaiəu'dʒenik] *a* 致减数分裂的,引起减数分裂的
meiosis [mai'əusis] ([复] **meioses** [mai'əusiːz]) *n*【希】减数分裂 | **meiotic** [mai'ɔtik] *a*
Meirowsky phenomenon [mai'rɔfski] (Emil Meirowsky) 迈洛夫斯基现象(黑色素颜色变深现象:黑色素经过长波紫外线照射后也许由于氧化作用其颜色在数秒钟内开始变深,数分钟到数小时内完成)
Meissner's corpuscles ['maisnə] (Georg Meissner) 触觉小体(乳头内) | ~ ganglion 迈斯纳神经节(肠黏膜下丛神经节) / ~ plexus 黏膜下神经丛
mel [mel] *n*【拉】蜂蜜,蜜浆
melagra [mə'lægrə] *n* 肢痛(肢肌肉痛)
Melaleuca [ˌmelə'luːkə] *n* 白千层属
melalgia [mə'lældʒiə] *n* 肢痛(肢神经痛)
melancholia [ˌmelən'kəuljə] *n* 忧郁症 | affective ~ 情感性忧郁症 / agitated ~ 激越性忧郁症 / ~ with delirium 谵妄性忧郁症 / involutional ~ 衰老期忧郁症,更年期忧郁症 / recurrent ~ 周期性忧郁症 / ~ religiosa 宗教性忧郁症 / ~ simplex 单纯性忧郁症 / stuporous ~, ~ attonita 木僵性忧郁症 | **~c** [ˌmelən'kəuliæk] *a* 忧郁症的 *n* 忧郁症患者
melancholic [ˌmelən'kɔlik] *a* 忧郁的;忧郁症的 *n* 忧郁症患者
melancholy ['melənkəli] *n* 忧郁,忧郁症 *a* 忧郁的
melanemesis [ˌmelə'nemisis] *n* 黑色呕吐
melanemia [ˌmelə'niːmiə] *n* 黑血[症]
mélangeur [ˌmeilɑːn'ʒəː] *n*【法】血液混合管
Melania [mə'leiniə] *n* 川蜷螺属
melanic [mə'lænik] *a* 黑变病的,黑色素沉着病的
melanicterus [ˌmelə'niktərəs] *n* 黑色黄疸
melaniferous [ˌmelə'nifərəs] *a* 含黑素的
melanin ['melənin] *n* 黑[色]素 | artificial ~, factitious ~ 人造黑素
melanism ['melənizəm] *n* 黑化,黑变病,黑[色]素沉着病 | industrial ~ 工业黑化(由于捕食动物的选择压力,栖息在煤灰漫布区域里的生物群体逐渐黑化,未黑化的个体被吃掉,只有具备黑化基因型的个体能成活并繁殖) / metallic ~ 银质沉着病 | **melanistic** [ˌmelə'nistik] *a*
melanize ['melənaiz] *vt* 使黑素过多,使产生黑变病 | **melanization** [ˌmelənai'zeiʃən, -ni'z-] *n*
melan(o)- [构词成分]黑
melanoacanthoma [ˌmelənəuˌækæn'θəumə] *n* 黑棘皮瘤
melanoameloblastoma [ˌmelənəuəˌmeləublæs'təumə] *n* 黑[色]素成釉细胞瘤
melanoblast ['melənəuˌblæst] *n* 成黑[色]素细胞,黑[色]素母细胞
melanoblastoma [ˌmelənəublæsˌtəumə] *n* 成黑[色]素细胞瘤,恶性黑素瘤
melanoblastosis [ˌmelənəublæs'təusis] *n* 成黑[色]素细胞增多症
melanocarcinoma [ˌmelənəuˌkɑːsi'nəumə] *n* 黑[素]癌
melanocyte ['melənəuˌsait] *n* 黑[色]素细胞 | dendritic ~ 树突状黑素细胞 | **melanocytic** [ˌmelənəu'sitik] *a*
melanocytoma [ˌmelənəusai'təumə] *n* 黑[色]素细胞瘤 | compound ~ 复合性黑素细胞瘤 / dermal ~ 真皮黑素细胞瘤(蓝痣;细胞性蓝痣)
melanocytosis [ˌmelənəusai'təusis] *n* 黑[色]素细胞增多,黑[色]素细胞增生病 | oculodermal ~ 眼、皮肤黑素细胞增生病(即太田痣 nevus of Ota)
melanoderma [ˌmelənəu'dəːmə] *n* 黑皮病 | parasitic ~ 寄生性黑皮病 / senile ~ 老年黑皮病
melanodermatitis [ˌmelənəuˌdəːmə'taitis] *n* 黑皮炎 | ~ toxica lichenoides 中毒性苔藓样黑皮炎
melanodermic [ˌmelənəu'dəːmik] *a* 黑皮的
melanoepithelioma [ˌmelənəuˌepiθiːli'əumə] *n* 黑[色]素上皮瘤,恶性黑瘤

melanoflocculation [ˌmelənəuˌflɔkjuˈleiʃən] *n* 黑[色]素絮凝反应(检疟疾)
melanogen [məˈlənəudʒən] *n* 黑[色]素原
melanogenesis [ˌmelənəuˈdʒenisis] *n* 黑[色]素发生 | **melanogenic** [ˌmelənəuˈdʒenik] *a*
melanoglossia [ˌmelənəuˈglɔsiə] *n* 黑舌[病]
melanoid [ˈmelənɔid] *a* 黑[色]素样的 *n* 类黑[色]素,人造黑素
Melanolestes [ˌmelənəuˈlestiːz] *n* 小墨蝽 | picipes 刺唇蝽
melanoleukoderma [ˌmelənəuˌljuːkəˈdəːmə] *n* 黑白皮病,黑白斑(如慢性砷中毒时) | ~ colli 颈部黑白皮病,颈部梅毒白斑病
melanoma [ˌmeləˈnəumə] ([复] **melanomas** 或 **melanomata** [ˌmeləˈnəumətə]) *n* 黑[色]素瘤 | acral-lentiginous ~, subungual ~ 肢端雀斑样痣黑[色]素瘤,甲下黑[色]素瘤 / amelanotic ~ 无黑[色]素性黑[色]素瘤 / benign juvenile ~, juvenile ~ 良性幼年黑[色]素瘤,幼年黑[色]素瘤 / lentigo maligna ~ 恶性雀斑样痣黑[色]素瘤 / malignant ~ 恶性黑[色]素瘤 / nodular ~ 结节性黑[色]素瘤 / superficial spreading ~ 浅表扩张性黑[色]素瘤 | **~tous** *a*
melanomatosis [ˌmeləˌnəuməˈtəusis] *n* 黑[色]素瘤病
melanonychia [ˌmelənəuˈnikiə] *n* 黑甲
melanophage [ˈmelənəufeidʒ] *n* 噬黑[色]素细胞
melanophore [ˈmelənəufɔː] *n* 载黑[色]素细胞
melanophorin [ˌmeləˈnɔfərin] *n* 黑[色]素细胞刺激素
melanoplakia [ˌmelənəˈpleikiə] *n* 黏膜黑斑
melanoprecipitation [ˌmelənəupriˌsipiˈteiʃən] *n* 黑[色]素沉淀反应(检疟疾)
melanoptysis [ˌmeləˈnɔptisis] *n* 咳黑痰(如炭末沉着病时)
melanosarcoma [ˌmelənəusɑːˈkəumə] *n* 黑[色]素肉瘤
melanosarcomatosis [ˌmelənəusɑːˌkəuməˈtəusis] *n* 黑[色]素肉瘤病
melanoscirrhus [ˌmelənəuˈskirəs] *n* 黑硬癌,黑[色]素癌
melanosis [ˌmeləˈnəusis] *n* 黑变病,黑[色]素沉着病 | ~ coli 结肠黑[色]素沉着病 / ~ sclerae 巩膜黑变病 / tar ~ 焦油性黑变病
melanosome [ˈmelənəusəum] *n* 黑[色]素体,黑[色]素小体(黑[色]素细胞内含黑[色]素的颗粒)
melanotic [ˌmeləˈnɔtik] *a* 黑色素的;黑变病的,黑[色]素沉着病的
melanotrichia [ˌmelənəuˈtrikiə] *n* 毛黑变,黑毛发 | ~ linguae 黑舌[病]
melanotroph [ˈmelənəuˌtrəuf] *n* 促黑[色]素激素细胞
melanotropic [ˌmelənəuˈtrɔpik] *a* 向黑[色]素的
melanotropin [ˈmelənəuˌtrəupin] *n* 促黑[素细胞]激素,促黑素
melanous [ˈmelənəs] *a* 黑发的,黑肤的,面黝黑的
melanthin [məˈlænθin] *n* 毛茛籽皂素
melanuria [ˌmeləˈnjuəriə], **melanuresis** [ˌmelənjuəˈriːsis] *n* 黑尿 | **melanuric** [ˌmeləˈnjuərik] *a*
melanurin [ˌmeləˈnjuərin] *n* 尿黑质
melarsoprol [məˈlɑːsəprəul] *n* 美拉胂醇(抗锥虫药)
melasma [məˈlæzmə] *n* 黑斑病(亦称黄褐斑,妊娠面斑) | ~ addisonii, ~ suprarenale 艾迪生[黑斑]病,肾上腺性黑斑病(即 Addison's disease)
melatonin [ˌmeləˈtəunin] *n* 褪黑[激]素(松果体的激素)
Meleda disease [ˈmelədɑː] 梅勒达病,家族性掌跖角化过度[症](梅勒达为亚德里亚海东部一小岛名)
melena [məˈliːnə] *n* 黑粪;呕黑 | ~ neonatorum 新生儿黑粪症 / ~ spuria 假性黑粪症 / ~ vera 真性黑粪症
Meleney's ulcer (chronic undermining ulcer) [məˈliːni] (Frank Lamont Meleney) 梅勒尼溃疡(慢性穿凿性溃疡)(进行性协同性坏疽) | ~ synergistic gangrene 梅勒尼协同性坏疽(进行性协同性坏疽)
melengestrol acetate [melənˈdʒestrɔl] 醋酸美仑孕酮(孕激素,抗肿瘤药)
melenic [məˈliːnik] *a* 黑粪的
meletin [ˈmelətin] *n* 槲皮素,槲皮黄素,栎精
melezitose [məˈlezitəus] *n* 松三糖
meli- [构词成分]蜜,糖
-melia [构词成分]肢
melibiase [ˌmeliˈbaieis] *n* 蜜二糖酶
melibiose [ˌmeliˈbaiəus] *n* 蜜二糖
melicera [ˌmeliˈsiərə], **meliceris** [ˌmeliˈsiəris] *n* 蜜样囊 *a* 黏稠的,糖浆状的
melicitose [məˈlisitəus] *n* 松三糖
melilotic acid [ˌmeliˈlɔtik] 黄木犀酸,邻羟苯丙酸
melilotoxin [ˌmeliləˈtɔksin] *n* 草木犀毒素,双香豆素
Melilotus [ˌmeliˈləutəs] *n* 草木犀属
melioidosis [ˌmiːliɔiˈdəusis] *n* 类鼻疽
Melissa [məˈlisə] *n* 蜜蜂花属,滇荆芥属
melissic acid [miˈlisik] 蜂花酸,三十[烷]酸
melissophobia [məˌlisəuˈfəubiə] *n* 蜂恐怖,蜂螯

恐怖
melissotherapy [məˌlisəuˈθerəpi] *n* 蜂毒疗法
melitensis [ˌmeliˈtensis] *n* 波状热,布鲁[杆]菌病
melitin [ˈmelitin] *n* 波状热菌素,布鲁菌素
melitis [məˈlaitis] *n* 颊炎
melit(o)- [构词成分]蜜,糖
melitoptyalism [ˌmelitəˈtaiəlizəm] *n* 糖涎(涎内含葡萄糖分泌)
melitoptyalon [ˌmelitəˈtaiələn] *n* 糖涎(涎内产生的葡萄糖)
melitose [ˈmelitəus], **melitriose** [ˌmeˈlitraiəus] *n* 蜜三糖,棉子糖
melitracen hydrochloride [ˌmeliˈtreisən] 盐酸美利曲辛(抗抑郁药)
Melittangium [ˌmeliˈtændʒiəm] *n* 蜂窝囊菌属
melituria [ˌmeliˈtjuəriə] *n* 糖尿[症] | ~ inosita 肌醇糖尿 | **melituric** [ˌmeliˈtjuərik] *a*
melizame [ˈmelizeim] *n* 四唑氧酚(甜味剂)
melizitose [məˈlizitəus] *n* 松三糖
Melkersson-Rosenthal syndrome [ˈmelkəsən ˈrəuzentɑːl] (Ernst Gustaf Melkersson; Curt Rosenthal) 梅-罗综合征(见 Melkersson's syndrome)
Melkersson's syndrome [ˈmelkəsən] (Ernst Gustaf Melkersson) 梅克逊综合征(为常染色体显性遗传综合征,通常始于儿童期或青春期,主要特征为慢性非炎性面部水肿〈通常局限于口唇〉及复发性外周性面部麻痹,有时有舌裂。伴有眼部症状,可包括兔眼、眼部烧灼感、睑松垂、眼睑水肿、角膜混浊、眼球后神经炎及双侧复发性眼球突出)
mellitic acid [meˈlitik] 苯六[羧]酸,苯六甲酸
mellitum [məˈlaitəm] ([复] **melliti** [məˈlaitai]) *n* 【拉】蜜剂
mellituria [ˌmeliˈtjuəriə] *n* 糖尿[症]
mel(o)-¹ 【希】[构词成分]肢
mel(o)-² 【希】[构词成分]颊
Melochia pyramidata [məˈləukiə piˌræmiˈdeitə] 锥状马松子
melodidymus [ˌmeləˌdidiməs] *n* 额外肢畸胎
Meloidae [məˈləuidiː] *n* 斑蝥科
melomelus [məˈləmiləs] *n* 赘肢畸胎
meloncus [məˈləŋkəs] *n* 颊瘤
melonoplasty [məˈlənəˌplæsti] *n* 颊成形术
Melophagus [məˈləfəgəs] *n* 蜱蝇属 | ~ ovinus 羊蜱蝇
meloplasty [ˈmeləˌplæsti] *n* 颊成形术
melorheostosis [ˌmeləˌriəsˈtəusis] *n* 肢骨纹状肥大
melosalgia [ˌmeləˈsældʒiə] *n* 下肢痛
meloschisis [məˈləskisis] *n* 颊横裂
Melopsittacus [ˌmeləuˈsitəkəs] *n* 鹦鹉属
melotia [məˈləuʃiə] *n* 颊耳畸形
Melotte's metal [meˈlɔt] (George W. Melotte) 梅洛特合金(铋铅锡软合金,有时用于牙科)
melotus [miˈləutəs] *n* 颊耳畸胎
meloxicam [məˈlɔksikəm] *n* 美洛昔康(非甾体消炎药,用于治疗骨关节炎,口服给药)
melphalan [ˈmelfələn] *n* 美法仑(抗肿瘤药)
melting [ˈmeltiŋ] *n* 熔解;解链
Meltzer-Lyon test (method) [ˈmeltsə ˈlaiən] (S. J. Meltzer; B. B. Vincent Lyon) 梅尔泽-莱昂试验(法)(检胆管病)
Meltzer's law [ˈmeltsə] (Samuel J. Meltzer) 梅尔泽定律(拮抗神经支配定律,即所有生命活动均经常受两种相反的力量控制,一方面是增强或引起作用,另一方面则为抑制) | ~ method (anesthesia) 梅尔泽法(麻醉)(含麻醉性蒸汽的空气通过气管内导管的吹入用法,用于胸外科手术)
MEM macrophage electrophoretic mobility (test) 巨噬细胞电泳泳动度(试验)
member [ˈmembə] *n* 肢,肢体
memberment [ˈmembəmənt] *n* 各部配列式(体内各部配置情形)
membra [ˈmembrə] membrum 的复数
membrana [memˈbreinə] ([复] **membranae** [meˈbreiniː]) *n* 【拉】膜
membranaceous [ˌmembrəˈneiʃəs] *a* 膜性的,膜状的
membranate [ˈmembrəneit] *a* 膜性的
membrane [ˈmembrein] *n* 膜 | adventitious ~ 异位膜 / alveolodental ~ 牙周膜 / anal ~ 肛膜,肛板 / basement ~ 基膜 / birth ~s 衣胞(即羊膜及绒毛膜) / buccopharyngeal ~ 颊咽膜(咽颅底筋膜;口咽膜) / chorioallantoic ~ 绒[毛]膜尿囊 / cloacal ~ 泄殖腔膜,一穴肛膜 / costocoracoid ~ 喙锁筋膜 / cyclitic ~ 睫状体炎性假膜 / enamel ~ 釉膜;牙护膜 / endoneural ~ 神经鞘,神经膜 / exocoelomic ~ 胚外体腔膜 / false ~, accidental ~ 假膜 / germinal ~ 胚膜 / glassy ~ 玻璃膜;基底层/ gradocol ~s 超滤膜(应用在超滤法中的一种薄膜) / ground ~ 基膜 / haptogen ~ 凝膜(蛋白质组成的膜) / homogeneous ~ 均质膜(胎盘绒毛的) / interspinal ~ 棘间膜,棘(突)间韧带 / ion-selective ~ 离子选择膜 / keratogenous ~ 甲床 / meconic ~ 胎肛膜 / medullary ~ 骨内膜 / mucous ~ 黏膜 / nictitating ~ 瞬膜 / oral ~ 口膜,咽颅底筋膜 / ovular ~ 卵黄膜 / proligerous ~ [载]卵丘/ prophylactic ~, pyophylactic ~ 防脓膜 / purpurogenous ~ 眼色素上皮层 / slit ~ 裂孔膜,裂隙滤过膜 / striated ~ 透明带 / submucous ~ 黏膜下组织 / tarsal ~ 睑板 / tympanic ~ 鼓膜 / unit ~ 单位膜 / vitreous ~ 玻璃体膜;透明膜(毛根);脉络膜基底层;角膜后界层

membranectomy [ˌmembrəˈnektəmi] *n* 膜切除术
membranelle [ˌmembrəˈnel] *n* 微膜,小膜
membraniform [memˈbreinifɔːm] *a* 膜样的,膜状的
membranin [ˈmembrənin] *n* 膜蛋白
membranocartilaginous [ˌmembrənəuˌkɑːtiˈlædʒinəs] *a* 膜[与]软骨性的
membranoid [ˈmembrənɔid] *a* 膜样的
membranolysis [ˌmembreiˈnɔləsis] *n* 膜溶解
membranous [memˈbreinəs, ˈmembrənəs] *a* 膜的,膜性的,膜样的
membrum [ˈmembrəm]([复] **membra** [ˈmembrə]) *n*【拉】肢,肢体 | ~ inferius 下肢 / ~ muliebre 阴蒂 / ~ superius 上肢 / ~ virile 阴茎
memory [ˈmeməri] *n* 记忆;存储,存储器 | anterograde ~ 远事记忆,顺行性记忆 / coast ~ 热带性遗忘 / echoic ~ 回声记忆 / iconic ~ 映象记忆,瞬时形象记忆 / immunologic ~ 免疫记忆(指免疫系统对第二次接触抗原的应答能力比第一次更快且更强) / kinesthetic ~ 动觉记忆 / long-term ~ 长时记忆 / screen ~ 映幕记忆,掩蔽性记忆(用以掩蔽其他不愉快或痛苦的回忆) / short-term ~ 短时记忆 / visual ~, eye ~ 视觉记忆
memotine hydrochloride [ˈmemətiːn] 盐酸美莫汀(抗病毒药)
MEN multiple endocrine neoplasia 多发性内分泌瘤病
Menacanthus [ˌmenəˈkænθəs] *n* 食毛虱属
menacme [məˈnækmi] *n* 经潮期
menadiol [ˌmenəˈdaiɔl] *n* 甲萘氢醌(止血药)
menadione [ˌmenəˈdaiəun] *n* 甲萘醌(止血药) | ~ sodium bisulfite 甲萘醌亚硫酸氢钠(止血药) | **menaphthone** [məˈnæfθəun] *n*
menalgia [məˈnældʒiə] *n* 痛经
menaquinone [ˌmenəˈkwinəun] *n* 甲基萘醌类(亦称维生素 K_2)
menarche [məˈnɑːki] *n* 月经初潮 | **menarchal** [məˈnɑːkəl], **menarcheal**, **menarchial** [məˈnɑːkiəl] *a*
Mendel-Bekhterev reflex (sign), Mendel's reflex, Mendel's dorsal reflex of foot [ˈmendəl bekˈterjev](Kurt Mendel; V. M. Bekhterev) 孟德尔-别赫捷列夫反射(征)、孟德尔反射、孟德尔足背反射(轻叩足背时,通常引起第二到第五趾向背侧屈曲,但在某些器质性神经病变时,则导致足趾向跖侧屈曲)
Mendeleev's (Mendeléeff's) law [ˌmendəˈlejəf](Dimitri I. Mendeleev) 周期律 | ~ table 周期表
mendelevium(Md) [ˌmendəˈliːviəm] *n* 钔(化学元素)
mendelian [menˈdiːljən](Gregor J. Mendel) *a* 孟德尔的 | ~ characters 孟德尔性状(在遗传学中指动物或植物所显示各别的特殊的性状,这些性状取决于生物体的基因组成,可能是隐性的,也可能是显性的) / ~ law 孟德尔定律(见 Mendel's law)
mendelism [ˈmendəlizəm] *n* 孟德尔遗传学说(见 mendelian characters 及 Mendel's law)
mendelizing [ˈmendəˌlaiziŋ] *a* 孟德尔[遗传]方式的
Mendel's law [ˈmendəl](Gregor J. Mendel) 孟德尔定律(遗传律,即在某一特征或性状上,子代的特征并非介于父母之间,而是从父母中之一遗传得来,现今孟德尔定律常以独立分配定律〈law of independent assortment〉及分离定律〈law of segregation〉表示之)
Mendelsohn's test [ˈmendəlsəun](Martin A. Mendelsohn) 门德尔松试验(检心肌效率,即根据运动所致心跳加速及复原时间的快慢而测定之)
Mendelson's syndrome [ˈmendəlsən](Curtis L. Mendelson) 门德尔松综合征,肺部酸吸入综合征
Mendel's test [ˈmendəl](Felix Mendel) 孟德尔试验(见 Mantoux test)
Mendocutes [mənˈdɔkjutiːz, ˌmendəuˈkjuːtiːz] *n* 疵壁细菌门
Mendosicutes [ˌmendəuˈsikjutiːz, ˌmendəusiˈkjuːtiːz] *n* 疵壁细菌门
Ménétrier's disease [ˌmeineitriˈɛə](Pierre Ménétrier) 梅内特里耶病,巨大肥厚性胃炎
Menge's pessary [ˈmeŋgə](Karl Menge) 门格子宫托(环状有柄子宫托)
Mengo encephalomyelitis [ˈmengəu](Mengo 为乌干达一地区,1948 年首次在此地区见到此病)门戈脑脊髓炎 | ~ virus 门戈病毒(脑心肌炎病毒)
menhidrosis [ˌmenhiˈdrəusis], **menidrosis** [ˌmeniˈdrəusis] *n* 月经代偿性出汗,出汗倒经
Ménière's disease (syndrome) [ˌmeniˈɛə](Prosper Ménière) 梅尼埃病(综合征),耳性眩晕病
meningeal [məˈnindʒiəl] *a* 脑脊膜的
meningematoma [məˌnindʒeməˈtəumə] *n* 硬脑[脊]膜血肿
meningeocortical [məˌnindʒiəˈkɔːtiːkəl] *a* 脑膜脑皮质的
meningeoma [məˌnindʒiˈəumə] *n* 脑[脊]膜瘤
meningeorrhaphy [məˌnindʒiˈɔrəfi] *n* 脑[脊]膜缝合术
meninges [məˈnindʒiːz](meninx 的复数) *n*【希】脑脊膜
meninghematoma [məˌnindʒheməˈtəumə] *n* 硬

脑[脊]膜血肿

meninginitis [ˌmenindʒiˈnaitis] *n* 软膜蛛网膜炎，柔脑[脊]膜炎

meningioma [məˌnindʒiˈəumə] *n* 脑[脊]膜瘤 | angioblastic ~ 成血管细胞性脑[脊]膜瘤，成血管细胞瘤

meningiomatosis [məˌnindʒiˌəuməˈtəusis] *n* 多发性脑[脊]膜瘤，脑[脊]膜[纤维]瘤病

meningism [məˈnindʒizəm], **meningismus** [ˌmeninˈdʒisməs] *n* 假性脑[脊]膜炎

meningitis [ˌmeninˈdʒaitis]（[复] **meningitides** [ˌmeninˈdʒitidiːz]）*n* 脑[脊]膜炎 | African ~ 非洲脑膜炎，昏睡病 / cerebral ~ 脑膜炎 / cerebrospinal ~（CSM）脑脊膜炎 / epidemic cerebrospinal ~，meningococcic ~ 流行性脑脊髓膜炎，脑膜炎球菌性脑膜炎 / external ~ 硬脑[脊]膜外层炎 / gummatous ~ 树胶肿性脑膜炎 / internal ~ 硬脑[脊]膜内层炎 / mumps ~ 流行性腮腺炎性脑膜炎 / posterior ~ 后[颅凹]脑膜炎 / purulent ~ 化脓性脑膜炎 / simple ~ 单纯性脑膜炎 / spinal ~ 脊膜炎 / sterile ~ 无菌性脑膜炎 / torula ~，torular ~ 串酵母菌性脑膜炎 / tubercular ~，tuberculous ~ 结核性脑膜炎 / viral ~，aseptic ~，acute aseptic ~，benign lymphocytic ~，lymphocytic ~ 病毒性脑膜炎，无菌性脑膜炎，急性无菌性脑膜炎，良性淋巴细胞性脑膜炎，淋巴细胞性脑膜炎 | **meningitic** [ˌmeninˈdʒitik] *a*

mening(o)- [构词成分]脑膜，脊膜

meningoarteritis [məˌniŋgəuˌɑːtəˈraitis] *n* 脑膜动脉炎

meningoblastoma [məˌniŋgəublæsˈtəumə] *n* 成脑[脊]膜细胞瘤

meningocele [məˈniŋgəsiːl] *n* 脑[脊]膜膨出 | spurious ~ 假性脑膜膨出

meningocephalitis [məˌniŋgəuˌsefəˈlaitis], **meningocerebritis** [məˌniŋgəuseriˈbraitis] *n* 脑膜脑炎

meningococcemia [məˌniŋgəukɔkˈsiːmiə] *n* 脑膜炎球菌血症 | acute fulminating ~ 急性暴发型脑膜炎球菌败血症

meningococcic [məˌniŋgəuˈkɔksik], **meningococcal** [məˌniŋgəuˈkɔkəl] *a* 脑膜炎球菌的

meningococcidal [məˌniŋgəukɔkˈsaidl] *a* 杀脑膜炎球菌的

meningococcin [məˌniŋgəuˈkɔksin] *n* 脑膜炎球菌素

meningococcosis [məˌniŋgəukɔˈkəusis] *n* 脑膜炎球菌病

meningococcus [məˌniŋgəuˈkɔkəs]（[复] **meningococci** [məˌniŋgəuˈkɔksai]）*n* 脑膜炎球菌

meningocortical [məˌniŋgəuˈkɔːtikəl] *a* 脑膜皮质的

meningocyte [məˈniŋgəsait] *n* 脑膜[组织]细胞

meningoencephalitis [məˌniŋgəuenˌsefəˈlaitis] *n* 脑膜脑炎 | eosinophilic ~ 嗜酸性脑膜脑炎，嗜酸性脑膜炎 / mumps ~ 腮腺炎性脑膜脑炎 / primary amebic ~ 原发性阿米巴脑膜脑炎 / syphilitic ~ 梅毒性脑膜脑炎，全身性麻痹症，麻痹性痴呆

meningoencephalocele [məˌniŋgəuenˈsefələsiːl] *n* 脑脑膜膨出

meningoencephalomyelitis [məˌniŋgəuenˌsefələuˌmaiəˈlaitis] *n* 脑脊膜脑脊髓炎

meningoencephalomyelopathy [məˌniŋgəuenˌsefələuˌmaiəˈlɔpəθi] *n* 脑脊膜脑脊髓病

meningoencephalopathy [məˌniŋgəuenˌsefəˈlɔpəθi] *n* 脑膜脑病

meningofibroblastoma [məˌniŋgəuˌfaibrəublæsˈtəumə] *n* 脑[脊]膜成纤维细胞瘤，脑[脊]膜瘤

meningogenic [məˌniŋgəuˈdʒenik] *a* 脑膜源性的

meningoma [ˌmeninˈgəumə] *n* 脑[脊]膜瘤

meningomalacia [məˌniŋgəuməˈleiʃiə] *n* 脑膜软化

meningomyelitis [məˌniŋgəuˌmaiəˈlaitis] *n* 脊膜脊髓炎

meningomyelocele [məˌniŋgəuˈmaiələsiːl] *n* 脊膜脊髓膨出，脊髓脊膜膨出

meningomyeloencephalitis [məˌniŋgəuˌmaiələuenˌsefəˈlaitis] *n* 脑脊膜脑脊髓炎

meningomyeloradiculitis [məˌniŋgəuˌmaiələurəˌdikjuˈlaitis] *n* 脊膜脊髓神经根炎

meningo-osteophlebitis [məˌniŋgəu ˌɔstiəufliˈbaitis] *n* 骨膜骨静脉炎

meningopathy [ˌmeninˈgɔpəθi] *n* 脑[脊]膜病

meningopneumonitis [məˌniŋgəunjuːməuˈnaitis] *n* 脑膜肺炎

meningopolyneuritis [məˌniŋgəuˌpɔlinjuəˈraitis] *n* 脑膜多神经炎（神经根神经炎、无菌性脑膜炎和脑神经炎三联征）

meningorachidian [məˌniŋgəurəˈkidiən] *a* 脊膜脊髓的

meningoradicular [məˌniŋgəurəˈdikjulə] *a* 脑[脊]膜神经根的

meningoradiculitis [məˌniŋgəurəˌdikjuˈlaitis] *n* 脑[脊]膜神经根炎

meningorecurrence [məˌniŋgəuriˈkʌrəns] *n* [梅毒]脑膜再发（抗梅毒治疗诱发的梅毒性脑膜炎）

meningorrhagia [məˌniŋgəuˈreidʒiə] *n* 脑[脊]膜出血

meningorrhea [məˌniŋgəuˈriːə] *n* 脑[脊]膜渗血

meningosis [ˌmeninˈgəusis] *n* [骨间]膜性附着

meningothelioma [məˌniŋgəuˌθiːliˌəumə] *n* 脑[脊]膜瘤

meningovascular [məˌniŋɡəuˈvæskjulə] *a* 脑[脊]膜血管的
meninguria [ˌmeninˈɡjuəriə] *n* 膜片尿
meninx [ˈmiːniŋks]([复] **meninges** [miˈnindʒiːz]) *n*【希】脑[脊]膜
meniscal [məˈniskəl] *a* 半月板的
meniscectomy [ˌmeniˈsektəmi] *n* 半月板切除术
menischesis [ˌmeniˈskiːsis] *n* 经闭,闭经
menisci [məˈnisai] meniscus 的复数
meniscitis [ˌmeniˈsaitis] *n* 半月板炎
meniscocyte [məˈniskəsait] *n* 新月形红细胞,镰状红细胞
meniscocytosis [məˌniskəsaiˈtəusis] *n* 新月形红细胞症,镰状红细胞性贫血
meniscosynovial [məˌniskəusiˈnəuviəl] *a* 半月板滑膜的
Meniscus [miˈniskəs] *n* 半月菌属
meniscus [məˈniskəs]([复] **meniscuses** 或 **menisci** [məˈnisai]) *n*【拉】关节盘;半月板;凹凸透镜 | articular ~, joint ~ 关节半月板 / converging ~ 会聚透镜,正透镜 / diverging ~ 分散透镜,负透镜 / negative ~ 负透镜,凸凹透镜 / positive ~ 正透镜,凹凸透镜 / tactile menisci 触盘,触觉半月板
menispermine [ˌmeniˈspəːmiːn] *n* 印防已碱
Menispermum [ˌmeniˈspəːməm] *n* 蝙蝠葛属
Menkes' disease, syndrome [ˈmeŋkəz](John H. Menkes)门克斯病、综合征(遗传性铜吸收异常,特点为大脑严重变性及动脉病变,导致在婴儿期死亡,头发稀疏脆弱并在显微镜下呈卷缩状,系 X 连锁隐性性状遗传。亦称扭结发综合征,钢发综合征)
men(o)- [构词成分]月经
menolipsis [ˌmenəˈlipsis] *n* 停经
menometrorrhagia [ˌmenəuˌmetrəˈreidʒiə] *n* 月经频多
menopause [ˈmenəpɔːz] *n* 绝经[期] | artificial ~ 人工绝经 / ~ praecox 早期绝经 | **menopausal** [ˌmenəˈpɔːzəl] *a*
menoplania [ˌmenəˈpleiniə] *n* 异位月经,代偿性月经
menorrhagia [ˌmenəˈreidʒiə] *n* 月经过多
menorrhalgia [ˌmenəˈrældʒiə] *n* 经痛,痛经
menorrhea [ˌmenəˈriːə] *n* 行经,月经;月经过多 | **~l** *a*
menoschesis [məˈnɔskisis] *n* 闭经
menostasia [ˌmenəuˈsteiziə], **menostasis** [ˌmenəuˈsteisis] *n* 闭经
menostaxis [ˌmenəuˈstæksis] *n* 月经淋漓
menotropins [ˌmenəˈtrəupinz] *n* 尿促性素(绝经期后人尿中的提取物,亦称促卵泡激素,绝经期促性腺激素)
menouria [ˌmenəuˈjuəriə] *n* 月经尿
mens [menz] *n*【拉】精神,意志;心
mensis [ˈmensis]([复] **menses** [ˈmensiːz]) *n*【拉】月经
menstrual [ˈmenstruəl] *a* 月经的
menstruant [ˈmenstruənt] *n* 有月经者
menstruate [ˈmenstrueit] *vi* 行经
menstruation [ˌmenstruˈeiʃən] *n* 月经,行经 | anovular ~, anovulatory ~, nonovulational ~ 无排卵性月经,不排卵性月经 / delayed ~ 初经迟延 / difficult ~ 月经困难,痛经 / infrequent ~ 月经稀少 / regurgitant ~, retrograde ~ 逆行月经 / scanty ~ 月经过少 / suppressed ~ 闭经 / vicarious ~ 代偿性月经,异位月经 | **menstruous** [ˈmenstruəs] *a*
menstruum [ˈmenstruəm] *n* 溶媒
mensual [ˈmensjuəl] *a* 按月的,每月的
mensurable [ˈmenʃurəbl] *a* 可量的
mensuration [ˌmensjuəreiʃən] *n* 测量,测诊
mentagrophyton [ˌmentəˈɡrɔfitən] *n* 须疮菌(现名须发癣菌 Trichophyton mentagrophytes)
mental¹ [ˈmentl] *a* 精神的,智力的,心理的;精神病的
mental² [ˈmentl] *a* 颏的
mentalis [menˈteilis] *a*【拉】颏的 *n* 颏肌
mentality [menˈtæləti] *n* 智力,智能;心态,心性
mentation [menˈteiʃən] *n* 精神活动,精神作用
Mentha [ˈmenθə] *n*【拉】薄荷属 | ~ canadensis 加拿大薄荷,野薄荷 / ~ piperita 欧薄荷 / ~ pulegium 欧亚薄荷 / ~ spicata, ~ viridis 留兰香,绿薄荷
menthol [ˈmenθɔl] *n* 薄荷醇,薄荷脑,薄醇(局部止痒药)
menthyl [ˈmenθil] *n* 薄荷酯,薄荷基,薄基
menticide [ˈmentisaid] *n* 精神摧毁,洗脑
mentimeter [menˈtimitə] *n* 智力测验器
ment(o)- [构词成分]颏
mentoanterior [ˌmentəuænˈtiəriə] *n* 颏前位(胎位)
mentolabial [ˌmentəuˈleibjəl] *a* 颏唇的
menton [ˈmentɔn] *n* 颏下点
mentoplasty [ˈmentəuˌplæsti] *n* 颏成形术
mentoposterior [ˌmentəupɔsˈtiəriə] *n* 颏后位(胎位)
mentotransverse [ˌmentəutrænsˈvəːs] *n* 颏横位(胎位)
mentula [ˈmentjulə] *n*【拉】阴茎
mentulagra [ˌmentjuˈlæɡrə] *n* 阴茎异常勃起;痛性阴茎勃起
mentulate [ˈmentjulit] *a* 巨阴茎的
mentum [ˈmentəm] *n*【拉】颏
Menyanthes [ˌmeniˈænθiːz] *n* 睡菜属

Menzel's ataxia [ˈmentsel] (P. Menzel) 门泽尔共济失调(成年型橄榄体脑桥小脑萎缩的旧称,现认为是一型弗里德赖希〈Friedreich〉共济失调)
meobentine sulfate [ˌmiːəuˈbentiːn] 硫酸甲氧苯汀(抗心律失常的心抑制药)
MEP maximum expiratory pressure 最大呼气压
mepacrine hydrochloride [ˈmepəkrin] 盐酸米帕林(抗疟药)
mepartricin [məˈpɑːtrisin] *n* 美帕曲星(抗真菌和抗原虫药)
mepazine acetate [ˈmepəziːn] 乙酸密哌嗪(安定药)
mepenzolate bromide [məˈpenzəleit] 溴美喷酯(口服抗胆碱药)
meperidine hydrochloride [məˈperidiːn] 盐酸哌替啶(镇痛药)
mephenamine [məˈfenəmiːn] *n* 邻甲苯海拉明(即奥芬那君 orphenadrine,解痉药)
mephenesin [məˈfenisin] *n* 美芬新(骨骼肌松弛药)
mephenoxalone [ˌmefəˌnɔksələun] *n* 美芬诺酮(安定药)
mephentermine sulfate [məˈfentəmiːn] 硫酸美芬丁胺(肾上腺素能药,用作血管加压药,升压药)
mephenytoin [məˈfenitəuin] *n* 美芬妥英(抗惊厥药,抗癫痫药)
mephitic [məˈfitik] *a* 污气的,臭气的
mephitis [məˈfaitis] *n*【拉】臭气
mephobarbital [ˌmefəˈbɑːbitæl] *n* 甲苯比妥(抗惊厥及镇静药)
mepivacaine hydrochloride [məˈpivəkein] 盐酸甲哌卡因(局部麻醉药)
meprednisone [məˈprednisəun] *n* 甲泼尼松(合成糖皮质激素)
meprobamate [məˈprəubəmeit, ˌmeprəˈbæmeit] *n* 甲丙氨酯(安定药) | isopropyl ~ 异丙安宁(即卡立普多 carisoprodol,安定药,肌肉松弛药)
meprylcaine hydrochloride [ˈmeprilkein] 盐酸美普卡因(局部麻醉药)
mepyramine [məˈpirəmiːn] *n* 美吡拉敏(抗感染药)
mepyrapone [meˈpaiərəpəun] *n* 甲双吡丙酮,甲吡酮(即美替拉酮 metyrapone,用于下丘脑垂体功能试验)
mEq., meq. milliequivalent 毫[克]当量
mequidox [ˈmekwidɔks] *n* 美喹多司(抗菌药)
MER the mathanol extraction residue of BCG 卡介苗甲醇提取残留物
meradimate [meˈrædimeit] *n* 美拉地酯(防晒药)
meralgia [məˈrældʒiə] *n* 股痛 | ~ paresthetica 感觉异常性股痛
meralluride [məˈræljuraid] *n* 美拉鲁利(汞利尿药)
merbromin [məˈbrəumin] *n* 汞溴红(消毒防腐药)
mercaptan [məˈkæptæn] *n* 硫醇
mercaptide [məˈkæptaid] *n* 硫醇盐
2-mercaptoethanol [məˌkæptəˈeθənɔl] *n* 2-巯基乙醇
***β*-mercaptoethylamine** [məˌkæptəuˈeθiləˌmiːn] *n* *β*-巯基乙胺
mercaptol [məˈkæptɔl] *n* 缩硫醇
mercaptomerin [ˌməkæpˈtɔmərin] *n* 硫汞林(利尿药)
6-mercaptopurine (6-MP) [məˌkæptəˈpjuəriːn] *n* 巯嘌呤,6-巯基嘌呤(抗肿瘤药)
mercapturic acid [məˌkæpˈtjuərik] 硫醚氨酸
Merchant's projection [ˈməːtʃənt] (A. C. Merchant) 莫强特投照(一种膝关节轴向 X 线片摄取,令患者仰卧,膝在台端上屈曲成 45°,下肢靠拢,线管调至水平线下成 30°角,胶片置于胫骨上,与光束垂直)
Mercier's bar (valve) [məsiˈei] (Louis A. Mercier) 输尿管间襞,输尿管间嵴 | ~ catheter 梅尔西埃导管(弯头软导管,用于前列腺增生病人)
Meriones [meriˈəuniːz] *n* 沙鼠属
mercocresols [ˌməːkəˈkriːsɔlz] *n* 汞克利索(灭菌药)
mercupurin [məːˈkjuːpərin] *n* 汞罗茶碱,汞茶碱(mercurophylline 的旧名,利尿药)
mercuramide [məːˈkjuərəmaid] *n* 汞撒利(利尿药)
mercurammonium [məˌkjuərəˈməuniəm] *n* 氨基汞 | ~ chloride 氯化氨基汞,白降汞
mercurate [ˈməːkjureit] *vt* 使汞化,用汞处理
mercurial [məːˈkjuəriəl] *a* 水银的,汞的 *n* 汞制剂
Mercurialis [məˌkjuəriˈeilis] *n* 山靛属 | ~ annua 法国山靛(曾用作利尿、抗梅毒药)
mercurialism [məːˈkjuəriəlizəm] *n* 汞中毒,水银中毒
mercurialize [məːˈkjuəriəlaiz] *vt* 用汞剂治疗 | **mercurialization** [məːˌkjuəriəlaiˈzeiʃən, -liˈz-] *n* (持续小量)汞剂治疗,汞剂化
mercurialized [məːˈkjuəriəlaizd] *a* 用汞剂治疗的;含汞的
mercuric [məːˈkjuərik] *a* 汞的,二价汞的 | ~ benzoate 苯甲酸汞(曾用于治疗梅毒) / ~ chloride 氯化汞(消毒防腐药) / ~ cyanide 氰化汞(曾用于治疗梅毒) / ~ oxycyanide 氧氰化汞(曾用作抗菌和抗梅毒药) / red ~ iodide 红碘

化汞(曾用作抗菌药) / ~ salicylate 水杨酸汞(曾用于治疗梅毒) / yellow ~ oxide 黄氧化汞,黄降汞(眼科用局部抗感染药)
mercurophylline [ˌməːkjurə'filin] *n* 汞罗茶碱(利尿药)
mercurous ['məːkjurəs] *a* 亚汞的,一价汞的 | ~ chloride 氯化亚汞,甘汞(消毒防腐药) / yellow ~ iodide 黄碘化亚汞(曾用于治疗梅毒)
mercury ['məːkjuri] *n* 汞,水银 | ammoniated ~ 氯化氨汞(局部抗感染药) / ~ bichloride, ~ perchloride 氯化汞,升汞(曾用于治疗梅毒,现用作消毒剂) / ~ with chalk 汞白垩(治阴虱病) / French ~ 法国山靛(曾用作利尿、抗梅毒药) / mild ~ chloride 甘汞,氯化亚汞(消毒防腐药)
-mere [构词成分]节段,部分
merergasia [ˌmerə'geiziə] *n* 轻精神病 | **merergastic** [ˌmerə'gæstik] *a*
merethoxylline procaine [ˌmerə'θɔksiliːn] 汞乙氧茶碱普鲁卡因(用于治疗继发于充血性心力衰竭和肾病综合征所致的水肿)
Meretoja type familial amyloid polyneuropathy (syndrome) [meirei'təujə] (J. Meretoja) 梅莱托耶型家族性淀粉样蛋白多神经病(芬兰型家族性淀粉样蛋白多神经病)
meridian [mə'ridiən] *n* 子午线,经线;经络(针灸) *a* 子午线的,经线的 | ~ of cornea 角膜子午线 / ~s of eyeball 眼球子午线
meridianus [məˌridi'einəs] ([复] **meridiani** [məˌridi'einai]) *n*【拉】子午线,经线
meridional [mə'ridiənl] *a* 子午线的,经线的
merisis ['merisis] *n* [细胞]分裂性增大
merism ['merizəm] *n* 节构造
meristem ['meristem] *n* 分生组织 | **~atic** [ˌmeristi'mætik] *a*
meristic [mə'ristik] *a* 对称[排列]的
meristoma [ˌmeri'stəumə] *n* 分生组织瘤
Merkel-Ranvier cells ['məːkəl rɑːnvi'ɛə] (F. S. Merkel; Louis A. Ranvier) 梅-郎细胞(表皮基层的明细胞,含有儿茶酚胺颗粒,类似黑素细胞)
Merkel's cells (corpuscles, disks, tactile cells) ['məːkəl] (Friedrich S. Merkel) 梅克尔细胞(小体、盘、触觉细胞),触盘,触觉半月板
Merkel's filtrum ['məːkəl] (Karl L. Merkel) 喉室沟 | ~ muscle 角环肌
merlin ['məːlin] *n* 膜突样蛋白(一种细胞骨架蛋白,充当肿瘤抑制基因,蛋白编码的基因中的缺损为神经纤维瘤病 2 型的原因。亦称神经鞘瘤蛋白)
mermithid ['məːmiθid] *a* 索虫科的
Mermithidae [mə'miθidiː] *n* 索虫科
Mermithoidea [ˌməːmi'θɔidiə] *n* 索虫总科
mero- [构词成分]部分,局部;股
meroacrania [ˌmerəuə'kreinjə] *n* 部分无颅[畸形]
meroanencephaly [ˌmerəuˌænən'sefəli] *n* 部分无脑[畸形]
meroblastic [ˌmerə'blæstik] *a* 部分分裂的,不全[卵]裂的
merocoxalgia [ˌmiːrəukɔk'sældʒiə] *n* 髋股痛
merocrine ['merəkrin] *a* 局质分泌的
merocyst ['merəusist] *n* 裂殖子囊
merocyte ['merəsait] *n* 剩余精核
merodiastolic [ˌmerəudaiə'stɔlik] *a* 部分舒张[期]的
meroergasia [ˌmerəuəː'geiziə] *n* 轻精神病
merogamy [mə'rɔgəmi] *n* 配子小型;小体配合
merogastrula [ˌmerə'gæstrulə] *n* 偏裂卵原肠胚
merogenesis [ˌmerə'dʒenisis] *n* 卵裂 | **merogenetic** [ˌmerədʒi'netik] *a*
merogenic [ˌmerə'dʒenik] *a* 卵裂的,节裂的
merogony [mə'rɔgəni] *n* 卵片发育,[无核]卵块发育 | diploid ~ 二倍卵片发育 / parthenogenetic ~ 单性卵片发育 | **merogonic** [ˌmerə'gɔnik] *a*
meromelia [ˌmerə'miːliə] *n* 残肢
meromicrosomia [ˌmerəuˌmaikrəu'səumiə] *n* 部分躯干过小,部分体小
meromorphosis [ˌmerəumɔː'fəusis] *n* 再生不全,复原不全
meromyarial [ˌmerəumai'ɛəriəl], **meromyarian** [ˌmerəumai'ɛəriən] *a* 少肌型的
meromyosin [ˌmerə'maiəsin] *n* 酶解肌球蛋白
meronecrosis [ˌmiərəune'krəusis], **meronecrobiosis** [ˌmiərəuˌnekrəubai'əusis] *n* 细胞坏死
meront ['merɔnt] *n* 子黏变体,分裂体
meropenem [ˌmerəu'penəm] *n* 美罗培南(广谱抗生素)
meropia [mə'rəupiə] *n* 部分失明,部分盲
merorachischisis [ˌmiərərə'kiskisis] *n* 部分脊柱裂,脊柱不全裂
merosmia [mə'rɔsmiə] *n* 嗅觉减退
merosporangium [ˌmerəuspə'rændʒiəm] *n* 柱孢子囊
merostotic [ˌmerɔs'tɔtik] *a* 骨段的,部分骨段的
merotomy [mə'rɔtəmi] *n* 分节,节裂(尤指细胞)
merozoite [ˌmerə'zəuait] *n* 裂殖子;裂体性孢子
merozygote [ˌmerə'zaigəut] *n* 部分合子
mersalyl ['məːsəlil] *n* 汞撒利(利尿药)
Merseburg triad ['mɛəzəbuəg] 梅尔泽堡三征(突眼性甲状腺肿的特征,即甲状腺肿、突眼及心动过速。梅尔泽堡为德国一地名)
mertiatide ['məːtiəˌtaid] *n* 巯替肽(与 ^{99m}Tc 络合,用于功能性和解剖肾成像)
Merulius [mə'ruliəs] *n* 干朽真菌属

merycism ['merisizəm], **merycismus** [ˌmeri'sizməs] *n* 反刍

Merzbacher-Pelizaeus disease ['mɛətsbʌhə ˌpeili'zaiəs] (Ludwig Merzbacher; Friedrich Pelizaeus) 家族性脑中叶硬化

MESA microsurgical epididymal sperm aspiration 显微外科附睾精子抽吸[术]

mesad ['miːsæd] *ad* 向中线,向中

mesal ['miːsəl] *a* 正中的;中线的

mesalamine [mə'sæləmiːn] *n* 美沙拉明(消炎药。5-氨基水杨酸,柳氮磺吡啶的活性代谢产物,用于预防和治疗炎性肠病和溃疡性直肠炎,口服或直肠注射给药)

mesalazine [mə'sæləziːn] *n* 美沙拉秦(mesalamine 的 INN 和 BAN 名)

mesameboid [ˌmesə'miːbɔid] *n* 成血细胞

mesangiocapillary [meˌsændʒiəu'kæpiˌlɛəri] *a* 系膜毛细血管的

mesangiolysis [meˌsændʒi'ɔlisis] *n* 系膜溶解

mesangium [me'sændʒiəm] *n* 血管系膜 | **mesangial** *a* 系膜的

mesaraic [ˌmesə'reiik] *a* 肠系膜的

mesarteritis [ˌmesɑːtə'raitis] *n* 动脉中层炎

mesaticephalic [meˌsætisə'fælik] *a* 中脑的;中型头的

mesatikerkic [məˌsæti'kəːkik] *a* 中等肱桡指数的(肱桡指数在 75 ~80 之间)

mesatipellic [məˌsæti'pelik], **mesatipelvic** [məˌsæti'pelvik] *a* 中型骨盆的

mesaxon [mə'sæksɔn] *n* 轴[突]系膜

mescal [mes'kɑːl] *n*【墨】威廉斯仙人球;龙舌兰酵汁,龙舌兰酒

mescaline ['meskəliːn] *n* 麦司卡林,仙人球毒碱;三甲氧苯乙胺

mescalism ['meskəlizəm] *n* 仙人球瘾

meseclazone [mi'sekləzəun] *n* 美西拉宗(抗炎药)

mesectic [me'sektik] *a* 正常血氧的(血氧分解曲线正常)

mesectoblast [me'zektəblæst] *n* 中外胚层,外中胚层

mesectoderm [me'zektədəːm] *n* 中外胚层

mesencephalitis [ˌmezenˌsefə'laitis] *n* 中脑炎

mesencephalohypophyseal, **mesencephalohypophysial** [ˌmezenˌsefələuhaipəu'fiziəl] *a* 中脑垂体的

mesencephalon [ˌmezen'sefəlɔn], **mesencephal** [me'sensifəl] *n* 中脑 | **mesencephalic** [mezensə'fælik] *a*

mesencephalotomy [ˌmezenˌsefə'lɔtəmi] *n* 中脑切开术

mesenchyma [ˌmez'eŋkimə], **mesenchyme** ['mezəŋkaim] *n* 间充质 | **mesenchymal** [ˌmez'eŋkiməl] *a*

mesenchymoma [ˌmezənkai'məumə] *n* 间叶瘤,间充质瘤

mesenterectomy [ˌmezəntə'rektəmi] *n* 肠系膜切除术

mesenteric [ˌmezən'terik] *a* 肠系膜的

mesenteriolum [məˌsentə'raiələm] *n* 小肠系膜 | ~ appendicis vermiformis, ~ processus vermiformis 阑尾系膜

mesenteriopexy [ˌmezən'teriəˌpeksi] *n* 肠系膜固定术

mesenteriorrhaphy [ˌmezənˌteri'ɔrəfi] *n* 肠系膜缝合术

mesenteriplication [ˌmeʒənˌteriplai'keiʃən] *n* 肠系膜折术

mesenteritis [ˌmezəntə'raitis] *n* 肠系膜炎

mesenterium [ˌmezən'tiəriəm] *n* 肠系膜

mesenteron [me'zentərɔn] *n* 中肠 | **~ic** [meˌzentə'rɔnik] *a*

mesentery ['mezəntəri] *n* 肠系膜 | caval ~ 腔静脉系膜 / common ~, dorsal common ~ 背侧总肠系膜 / dorsal ~ 背肠系膜,背侧总肠系膜 / ~ of vermiform appendix 阑尾炎膜

mesentoderm [mi'zentədəːm] *n* 中内胚层

mesentomere [mi'zentəmiə] *n* 中内裂球

mesentorrhaphy [ˌmezən'tɔrəfi] *n* 肠系膜缝合术

mesepithelium [ˌmezepi'θiːljəm] *n* 间皮

MeSH [meʃ] *M*edical *S*ubject *H*eadings 医学主题词(美国国家医学图书馆出版的词汇,为 MEDLARS 所采用)

mesh [meʃ] *n* 筛眼,筛孔;网眼

meshwork ['meʃwəːk] *n* 网 | trabecular ~ 小梁网

mesiad ['miːziæd] *ad* 向中线,向中

mesial ['miːziəl] *a* 正中的;近中的 | **~ly** *ad* 向中线

mesien ['miːziən] *a* 正中面的

mesi(o)- [构词成分]近中

mesiobuccal [ˌmiːziəu'bʌkəl] *a* 近中颊[侧]的

mesiobucco-occlusal [ˌmiːziəuˌbʌkəuɔ'kluːzəl] *a* 近中颊殆面的

mesiobuccopulpal [ˌmiːziəuˌbʌkəu'pʌlpl] *a* 近中颊髓的

mesiocervical [ˌmiːziəu'səːvikəl] *a* 近中颈的;近中龈的

mesioclination [ˌmiːziəuklai'neiʃən, -kli-] *n* 近中倾斜(牙)

mesioclusion [ˌmiːziə'kluʒən] *n* 近中殆

mesiodens ['miːziədənz] ([复] **mesiodentes** [ˌmiːziəu'dentiːz]) *n* 正中额外牙

mesiodistal [ˌmiːziəu'distl] *a* 近中远中的

mesiogingival [ˌmiːziəuˈdʒindʒivəl] *a* 近中龈的
mesioincisodistal [ˌmiːziəuinˌsaisəuˈdistl] *a* 近中切远中的
mesiolabial [ˌmiːziəuˈleibjəl] *a* 近中唇[侧]的
mesiolabioincisal [ˌmiːziəuˌleibiəuinˈsaizəl] *a* 近中唇切的
mesiolingual [ˌmiːziəuˈliŋgwəl] *a* 近中舌侧的
mesiolinguoincisal [ˌmiːziəuˌliŋgwəuinˈsaizəl] *a* 近中舌切的
mesiolinguo-occlusal [ˌmiːziəuˌliŋgwəu ɔˈkluːzəl] *a* 近中舌侧殆面的
mesiolinguopulpal [ˌmiːziəuˌliŋgwəuˈpʌlpl] *a* 近中舌[侧]髓的
mesion [ˈmiːziɔn] *n* 正中面
mesio-occlusal [ˌmiːziəuɔˈkluːzəl] *a* 近中殆面的
mesio-occlusion [ˌmiːziəuɔˈkluːʒən] *n* 近中殆
mesio-occlusodistal [ˌmiːziəu ɔˌkluːsəuˈdistl] *a* 近中殆远中的
mesiopulpal [ˌmiːziəuˈpʌlpl] *a* 近中髓的
mesiopulpolabial [ˌmiːziəuˌpʌlpəuˈleibiəl] *a* 近中髓唇的
mesiopulpolingual [ˌmiːziəupʌlpəˈliŋgwəl] *a* 近中髓舌[侧]的
mesioversion [ˌmiːziəuˈvəːʒən] *n* 近中错位
mesiris [meˈsaiəris] *n* 虹膜中层
mesitylene [miˈsitiliːn] *n* 均三甲苯,1, 3, 5-三甲苯
mesitylenic acid [miˌsitiˈlenik] 二甲基苯甲酸
mesityluric acid [miˌsitiˈljuərik] 二甲基苯甲酰甘氨酸
mesmerism [ˈmezmərizəm] (Franz A. Mesmer) *n* 催眠术 | **mesmeric** [mezˈmerik] *a*
mesmerize [ˈmezməraiz] *vt* 对…施催眠术,催眠 | **mesmerization** [ˌmezməraiˈzeiʃən, -riˈz-] *n* 施催眠术
mesna [ˈmeznə] *n* 美司钠(一种巯基化合物,与尿毒素抗肿瘤药如异环磷酰胺〈ifosfamide〉或环磷酰胺〈cyclophosphamide〉合用,口服或静脉内给药,因它可使这些药物的代谢产物失活,从而减少对膀胱的损伤)
mes(o)- [前缀]正中,中间;中位;内消旋
meso-aortitis [ˌmesəu ˌeiɔːˈtaitis, ˌmez-] *n* 主动脉中层炎
mesoappendicitis [ˌmesəuəˌpendiˈsaitis, ˌmez-] *n* 阑尾系膜炎
mesoappendix [ˌmesəuəˈpendiks, ˌmez-] *n* 阑尾系膜
mesoarium [ˌmesəˈɛəriəm, ˌmez-] *n* 卵巢系膜 | **mesoarial** [ˌmesəˈɛəriəl, ˌmez] *a*
mesobacterium [ˌmesəubækˈtiəriəm, ˌmez-] ([复] **mesobacteria** [ˌmesəubækˈtiəriə, ˌmez-]) *n* 中型细菌
mesobilin [ˌmesəuˈbailin, ˌmez-] *n* 中胆色素
mesobilirubin [ˌmesəubiliˈruːbin, ˌmez] *n* 中胆红素
mesobilirubinogen [ˌmesəuˌbiliruˈbinədʒən, ˌmez-] *n* 中胆红素原,四氢中胆红素,中胆色烷
mesobiliviolin [ˌmesəubiliˈvaiəlin, ˌmez-] *n* 中胆紫素
mesoblast [ˈmesəublæst, ˈmez-] *n* 中胚层 | **~ic** [ˌmesəuˈblæstik, ˌmez-] *a*
mesoblastema [ˌmesəublæsˈtiːmə, ˌmez-] *n* 中胚层细胞
mesobronchitis [ˌmesəubrɔŋˈkaitis, ˌmez-] *n* 支气管中层炎
mesocardia [ˌmesəuˈkɑːdiə, ˌmez-] *n* 中位心
mesocardium [ˌmesəuˈkɑːdiəm, ˌmez-] *n* 心系膜 | arterial ~ 动脉性心系膜 / dorsal ~ 背心系膜 / lateral ~ 侧心系膜,肺嵴 / venous ~ 静脉性心系膜 / ventral ~ 腹心系膜
mesocarpal [ˌmesəuˈkɑːpl, ˌmez-] *a* 腕骨间的
mesocaval [ˌmesəuˈkeivəl, ˌmez-] *a* 肠系膜腔静脉的(有关或连接肠系膜上静脉和下腔静脉的)
mesocecum [ˌmesəuˈsiːkəm, ˌmez-] *n* 盲肠系膜 | **mesocecal** *a*
mesocephalic [ˌmesəusəˈfælik, ˌmez-] *a* 中脑的;中型头的(颅指数在 76.0～80.9 之间)
mesocephalon [ˌmesəuˈsefəlɔn, ˌmez-] *n* 中脑
Mesocestoides [ˌmesəusesˈtɔidiːz, ˌmez-] *n* 中殖孔[绦虫]属
Mesocestoididae [ˌmesəusesˈtɔididiː, ˌmez-] *n* 中殖孔[绦虫]科
mesochondrium [ˌmesəuˈkɔndriəm, ˌmez-] *n* 软骨基质
mesochoroidea [ˌmesəukɔːˈrɔidiə, ˌmez-] *n* 脉络[膜]中层
mesococcus [ˌmesəuˈkɔkəs, ˌmez-] ([复] **mesococci** [ˌmesəuˈkɔksai, ˌmez-]) *n* 中型球菌
mesocolon [ˌmesəuˈkəulən, ˌmez-] *n* 结肠系膜 | ascending ~, right ~ 升结肠系膜 / descending ~, left ~ 降结肠系膜 / sigmoid ~, iliac ~, pelvic ~ 乙状结肠系膜 / transverse ~ 横结肠系膜 | **mesocolic** [ˌmesəˈkɔlik, ˌmez-] *a*
mesocolopexy [ˌmesəˈkəuləˌpeksi, ˌmez-] *n* 结肠系膜固定术
mesocoloplication [ˌmesəuˌkəuləplaiˈkeiʃən, ˌmez-] *n* 结肠系膜折术
mesocord [ˈmesəkɔːd, ˈmez-] *n* 脐带系膜
mesocornea [ˌmesəuˈkɔːniə, ˌmez-] *n* 角膜中层,角膜固有质
mesocortex [ˌmezəuˈkɔːteks, ˌmez-] *n* 中间皮质(亦称 juxtallocortex)
mesocranial [ˌmesəuˈkreinjəl, ˌmez-], **mesoc-**

ranic [ˌmesəuˈkreinik, ˌmez-] *a* 中型头的(颅指数在 75 ~ 79.9 之间)

Mesocricetus [ˌmesəukraiˈsiːtəs] *n* 仓鼠属 | ~ aurius 金仓鼠

mesocuneiform [ˌmesəuˈkjuːniifɔːm, ˌmez-] *n* 第二楔骨

mesocyst [ˈmesəsist, ˌmez-] *n* 胆囊系膜

mesocytoma [ˌmesəusaiˈtəumə, ˌmez-] *n* 结缔组织瘤

mesoderm [ˈmesədəːm, ˈmez-] *n* 中胚层 | extraembryonic ~ 胚外中胚层 / gastral ~ 原肠中胚层 / peristomal ~ 口缘中胚层 / splanchnic ~ 脏壁中胚层 | **~al** [ˌmesəˈdəːməl, ˌmez-], **~ic** [ˌmesəˈdəːmik, ˌmez-] *a*

mesodiastolic [ˌmesəuˌdaiəˈstɔlik, ˌmez-] *a* 舒张期中的

mesodont [ˈmesədɔnt, ˈmez-] *a* 中型牙的(牙指数在 42 ~ 44 之间)

mesodontic [ˌmesəuˈdɔntik, ˌmez-] *n* 中型牙的

mesodontism [ˌmesəuˈdɔntizəm, ˌmez-] *a* 中型牙(或牙指数在 42 ~ 44 之间)

mesoduodenum [ˌmesəuˌdju(ː)əuˈdiːnəm, ˌmez-] *n* 十二指肠系膜(胚胎早期) | **mesoduodenal** *a*

mesoepididymis [ˌmesəuˌepiˈdidimis, ˌmez-] *n* 附睾系膜

mesoesophagus [ˌmesəui(ː)ˈsɔfəgəs, ˌmez-] *n* 食管系膜

mesogastrium [ˌmesəuˈgæstriəm, ˌmez-] **mesogaster** [ˌmesəuˈgæstə, ˌmez-] *n* 胃系膜 | **mesogastric** *a*

Mesogastropoda [ˌmezəugæsˈtrɔpədə] *n* 中腹足目

mesoglea [ˌmesəuˈgliːə, ˌmez-] *n* 中胶层,中胶质

mesoglia [miˈsɔgliə] *n* 少突(神经)胶质,间[神经]胶质;小神经胶质 | **~l** *a*

mesoglioma [ˌmesəuglaiˈəumə, ˌmez-] *n* 间[神经]胶质瘤,少突[神经]胶质瘤

mesogluteus [ˌmesəuˈglutiəs, ˌmez-] *n* 臀中肌 | **mesogluteal** *a*

mesognathous [məˈsɔgnəθəs], **mesognathic** [ˌmesɔgˈneiθik] *a* 中型颌的(颌指数在 98 ~ 103 之间)

Mesogonimus [ˌmesəˈgɔniməs, ˌmez-] *n* 中殖[吸虫]属 | ~ heterophyes 异形异形吸虫(即 Heterophyes heterophyes)

mesohemin [ˌmesəuˈhiːmin, ˌmez-] *n* 中氯化血红素

mesohyloma [ˌmesəuhaiˈləumə, ˌmez-] *n* 间皮瘤

mesohypoblast [ˌmesəuˈhaipəblæst, ˌmez-] *n* 中内胚层

mesoileum [ˌmesəuˈiliəm] *n* 回肠系膜

***meso*-inositol** [ˌmesəu iˈnəusitɔl, ˌmez-] *n* 肌醇,内消旋肌醇

mesojejunum [ˌmesəudʒiˈdʒuːnəm, ˌmez-] *n* 空肠系膜

mesolecithal [ˌmesəuˈlesiθəl, ˌmez-] *a* 中[等卵]黄的

mesology [meˈsɔlədʒi] *n* 生态学

mesolymphocyte [ˌmesəuˈlimfəsait, ˌmez-] *n* 中型淋巴细胞

mesomelic [ˌmesəuˈmelik, ˌmez-] *a* 肢中部的

mesomere [ˈmesəumiə, ˌmez-] *n* 中[分]裂球;中段(中胚层)

mesomeric [ˌmesəuˈmerik, ˌmez-] *a* 内消旋的;中介的

mesomerism [miˈsɔmərizəm] *n* 稳变异构[现象],缓变异构[现象];中介[现象]

mesometrium [ˌmesəuˈmiːtriəm, ˌmez-] *n* 子宫系膜;子宫肌层

mesomorph [ˈmesəumɔːf, ˈmez-] *n* 中胚层体型者;中型身材者 | **~y** *n* 中胚层体型;中型身材 / **~ic** [ˌmesəˈmɔːfik, ˌmez-] *a*

mesomucinase [ˌmesəuˈmjuːsineis, ˌmez-] *n* 中黏蛋白酶

mesomula [məˈsɔmjulə] *n* 中实肠胚

meson [ˈmiːzɔn, ˈmesɔn] *n* 正中面;介子(中电子) | **~ic** [miːˈzɔnik, meˈsɔnik] *a*

mesonasal [ˌmesəuˈneizəl, ˌmez-] *a* 鼻中部的

mesonephroma [ˌmesəuniˈfrəumə, ˌmez-] *n* 中肾瘤(卵巢)

mesonephros [ˌmesəuˈnefrɔs, ˌmez-] ([复] **mesonephroi** [ˌmesəuˈnefrɔi, ˌmez-]), **mesonephron** [ˌmesəuˈnefrɔn, ˌmez-] *n* 中肾 | **mesonephric** *a*

meso-omentum [ˌmesəu əuˌmentəm, ˌmez-] *n* 网膜系膜

meso-ontomorph [ˌmesəu ˈɔntəmɔːf, ˌmez-] *n* 矮胖体型者

mesopallium [ˌmesəuˈpæliəm, ˌmez-] *n* 旧[大脑]皮质,原[大脑]皮质

mesopexy [ˈmesəuˌpeksi, ˈmez-] *n* 肠系膜固定术

mesophile [ˈmesəfai, ˈmez-] *n* 嗜[常]温菌

mesophilic [ˌmesəˈfilik, ˌmez-] *a* 嗜[常]温的,适温的(指细菌)

mesophlebitis [ˌmesəufliˈbaitis, ˌmez-] *n* 静脉中层炎

mesophragma [ˌmesəuˈfrægmə, ˌmez-] *n* M 线(横纹肌)

mesophryon [miˈsɔfriɔn] *n* 眉间

mesophyll [ˈmesəufil, ˈmez-] *n* 叶肉 | **~ic** [ˌmesəuˈfilik, ˌmez-], **~ous** [ˌmesəuˈfiləs, ˌmez-] *a*

mesopia [meˈsəupiə] *n* 暮视,中等照明视力 |

mesopic [me'sɔpik] *a*
mesopneumon [ˌmesəu'njuːmɔn, ˌmez-] *n* 肺系膜,胸膜连系
mesoporphyrin [ˌmesəu'pɔːfirin, ˌmez-] *n* 中卟啉
mesoprosopic [ˌmesəuprə'sɔpik, ˌmez-] *a* 中型[颜]面的
mesopsychic [ˌmesəu'saikik, ˌmez-] *a* 精神发育中期的
mesopulmonum [ˌmesəupʌl'məunəm, ˌmez-] *n* 肺系膜
mesorachischisis [ˌmesəurə'kiskisis, ˌmez-] *n* 脊柱不全裂
mesorchium [mə'sɔːkiəm] *n* 睾丸系膜 | **mesorchial** *a*
mesorectum [ˌmesəu'rektəm, ˌmez-] *n* 直肠系膜
mesoretina [ˌmesəu'retinə, ˌmez-] *n* 视网膜中层
mesoridazine [ˌmesəu'ridəziːn, ˌmez-] *n* 美索达嗪(强安定药) | ~ besylate, ~ benzenesulfonate 苯磺美索达嗪
mesoropter [ˌmesəu'rɔptə, ˌmez-] *n* 眼球正位
mesorrhaphy [me'zɔrəfi] *n* 肠系膜缝合术
mesorrhine ['mezərain] *a* 中型鼻的(鼻指数在48~53之间)
mesosalpinx [ˌmesəu'sælpiŋks, ˌmez-] *n* 输卵管系膜
mesoscapula [ˌmesəu'skæpjulə, ˌmez-] *n* 肩胛冈
mesoseme ['mesəusiːm, ˌmez-] *a* 中型眶的(眼眶指数在83~89之间)
mesosigmoid [ˌmesəu'sigmɔid, ˌmez-] *n* 乙状结肠系膜
mesosigmoiditis [ˌmesəuˌsigmɔi'daitis, ˌmez-] *n* 乙状结肠系膜炎
mesosigmoidopexy [ˌmesəusig'mɔidəˌpeksi, ˌmez-] *n* 乙状结肠系膜固定术
mesoskelic [ˌmesəu'skelik, ˌmez-] *a* 中型腿的
mesosoma [ˌmesəu'səumə, ˌmez-] *n* 中等身材 | **~tous** *a*
mesosome ['mesəusəum, 'mez-] *n* 间体(某些细菌细胞膜的向内陷入部分,各种间体与DNA复制以及与蛋白质分泌有关)
mesostaphyline [ˌmesəu'stæfilain, ˌmez-] *a* 中型腭的(腭指数在80~84.9之间)
mesostenium [ˌmesəu'stiːniəml, ˌmez-] *n* 小肠系膜
mesosternum [ˌmesəu'stəːnəm, ˌmez-] *n* 胸骨体
mesostroma [ˌmesəu'strəumə, ˌmez-] *n* 中基质
mesosyphilis [ˌmesəu'sifilis, ˌmez-] *n* 二期梅毒
mesosystolic [ˌmesəusis'tɔlik, ˌmez-] *a* 收缩中期的
mesotarsal [ˌmesəu'tɑːsəl, ˌmez-] *a* 跗骨间的
***meso*-tartaric acid** [ˌmesəu tɑː'tærik, ˌmez-] 内消旋酒石酸,中酒石酸
mesotaurodontism [ˌmesəuˌtɔːrrəu'dɔntizəm, ˌmez-] *n* 中牛牙
mesotendineum [ˌmesəuten'diniəm, ˌmez-] **mesotendon** [ˌmesəu'tendən, ˌmez-], **mesotenon** [ˌmesəu'tenən, ˌmez-] *n* 腱系膜
mesothelioma [ˌmesəuˌθiːli'əumə, ˌmez-] ([复] **mesotheliomas** 或 **mesotheliomata** [ˌmesəuˌθiːli'əumətə, ˌmez-]) *n* 间皮瘤
mesothelium [ˌmesəu'θiːljəm, ˌmez-] ([复] **mesothelia** [ˌmesəu'θiːljə, ˌmez-]) *n* 间皮 | **mesothelial** *a*
mesothenar [məzɔ'θiːnə] *n* 拇收肌
mesothorium [ˌmesə'θɔːriəm] *n* 新钍(用以治癌)
mesotocin [ˌmesəu'tɔsin, ˌmez-] *n* 中催产素,8-异亮催产素
mesotron ['mesəutrɔn] *n* 介子(中电子) | **~ic** [ˌmesəu'trɔnik] *a*
mesotropic [ˌmesəu'trɔpik, ˌmez-] *a* 腔中央的
mesotympanum [ˌmesəu'timpənəm, ˌmez-] *n* 中鼓室
mesouranic [ˌmesəujuə'rænik, ˌmez-] *a* 中型腭的(见 mesuranic)
mesovarium [ˌmesəu'vɛəriəm, ˌmez-] *n* 卵巢系膜
mesoxalic acid [meˌzɔk'sælik] 丙酮二酸
Mesozoa [ˌmesəu'zəuə] *n* 中生动物(一群小的寄生物,与原生动物和后生动物的关系尚未明确)
mesquite [mə'skiːt] *n* 牧豆树
message ['mesidʒ] *n* 信息
messenger ['mesindʒə] *n* 信使 | second ~ 第二信使(环腺苷酸或环鸟苷酸,为激素作用的介体,主要位于细胞质膜上)
mesterolone [məs'terələun] *n* 美睾酮(雄激素类药)
mestranol ['mestrənɔl] *n* 美雌醇(雌激素类药)
mesuprine hydrochloride ['mesjuprin] 盐酸美舒令(血管扩张药,平滑肌松弛药)
mesuranic [ˌmezjuə'rænik] *a* 中型腭的(上颌牙槽指数在110.0~114.9之间)
mesylate ['mesileit] *n* 甲磺酸盐(methanesulfonate的USAN缩约词)
Met methionine 甲硫氨酸
met [met] *n* 梅脱(测机体产热的一个单位:在静坐时产生的代谢热,每小时每平方米身体面积为209 kJ〈千焦〉)
meta- [前缀]变,转;后,旁,次;间[位];偏[位]
meta-analysis [ˌmetə ə'nælisis] *n* 元分析
meta-arthritic [ˌmetə ɑː'θritik] *a* 关节炎后的
metabasis [mə'tæbəsis] ([复] **metabases** [mə'tæbəsiːz]) *n* 疾病转变;转移,迁徙(病理过程

由身体的一个区向另一个区部位的转移或变化）

metabiosis [ˌmetəbaiˈəusis] *n* 代谢共栖

metabolimeter [ˌmetəbəˈlimitə] *n* 代谢计 | **metabolimetry** *n* 基础代谢测量法

metabolism [meˈtæbəlizəm] *n* 新陈代谢，代谢；生物转化 | ammonotelic ~ 排铵代谢 / basal ~ 基础代谢 / endogenous ~ 内源性代谢 / energy ~ 能量代谢 / excess ~ of exercise 运动过量代谢 / exogenous ~ 外源性代谢 / inborn error of ~ 先天性代谢缺陷 / intermediary ~ 中间代谢 / urotelic ~ 排尿素代谢 / uricotelic ~ 排尿酸代谢 | **metabolic** [ˌmetəˈbɔlik] *a*

metabolite [məˈtæbəlait] *n* 代谢[产]物 | essential ~ 主要代谢产物

metabolize [məˈtæbəlaiz] *vt, vi* 产生代谢变化，引起代谢 | **metabolizable** [məˈtæbəˌlaizəbl] *a* 可代谢的

metabolon [məˈtæbəlɔn] *n* 蜕变中间物质

metaboreceptor [məˌtæbəuriˈseptə] *n* 代谢受体

metabromsalan [ˌmetəˈbrɔmsələn] *n* 美溴沙仑（消毒防腐药）

metabutethamine hydrochloride [ˌmetəbjuˈteθəmin] 盐酸美布他明（牙科用局部麻醉药）

metabutoxycaine hydrochloride [ˌmetəbjuˈtɔksikein] 盐酸美布卡因（牙科用局部麻醉药）

metacarpal [ˌmetəˈkɑːpl] *a* 掌的 *n* 掌骨

metacarpectomy [ˌmetəkɑːˈpektəmi] *n* 掌骨切除术

metacarpophalangeal [ˌmetəˌkɑːpəufəˈlændʒiəl] *a* 掌指的

metacarpus [ˌmetəˈkɑːpəs]（[复] **metacarpi** [ˌmetəˈkɑːpai]）*n* 掌

metacele [ˈmetəsiːl] *n* 第四脑室后部，后室；后体腔

metacentric [ˌmetəˈsentrik] *a* 具中间着丝粒的（指着丝粒位于中央部位的染色体，因此两臂的长度相等）

metacercaria [ˌmetəsəːˈkɛəriə]（[复] **metacercariae** [ˌmetəsəːˈkɛəriiː]）*n* [后]囊蚴

metachemistry [ˌmetəˈkemistri] *n* 原子结构化学；超级化学 | **metachemical** [ˌmetəˈkemikəl] *a*

metachromasia [ˌmetəkrəuˈmeiziə], **metachromatism** [ˌmetəˈkrəumətizəm], **metachromia** [ˌmetəˈkrəumiə] *n* 异染性，变色反应性，变色现象

metachromatic [ˌmetəkrəuˈmætik], **metachromic** [ˌmetəˈkrəumik] *a* 异染性的

metachromatin [ˌmetəˈkrəumətin] *n* 异染质

metachromatophil [ˌmetəkrəuˈmætəfil] *n* 嗜异染细胞

metachromophil [metəˈkrəuməfil], **metachromophile** [ˌmetəˈkrəuməfail] *a* 嗜异染的

metachromosome [ˌmetəˈkrəuməsəum] *n* 后期染色体

metachronous [məˈtækrənəs] *a* 异时的

metachrosis [ˌmetəˈkrəusis]（[复] **metachroses** [metəˈkrəusiːz]）*n* 变色功能，变色（指动物）

metachysis [miˈtækisis] *n* 输血

metacinesis [ˌmetəsaiˈniːsis] *n* 中期分裂（有丝分裂时子星体互相分离）

metacoele [ˈmetəsiːl] *n* 第四脑室后部，后室；后体腔

metacoeloma [ˌmetəsiːˈləumə] *n* 后体腔

metacone [ˈmetəkəun] *n* 后尖（上磨牙的远中颊尖）

metaconid [ˌmetəˈkɔnid] *n* 下后尖（下磨牙的近中舌尖）

metaconule [ˌmetəˈkɔnjuːl] *n* 后小尖（哺乳动物上磨牙的上后尖与原尖之间的小尖，有时也见于人）

metacortandracin [ˌmetəkɔːˈtændrəsin] *n* 泼尼松（即 prednisone，合成糖皮质激素）

metacortandralone [ˌmetəkɔːˈtændrələun] *n* 泼尼松龙（即 prednisolone，合成糖皮质激素）

metacresol [ˌmetəˈkriːsɔl] *n* 间甲酚（最强防腐剂）| ~ acetate 醋酸间甲酚酯（用于真菌感染）/ ~ purple, ~ sulfonphthalein 甲酚紫，间甲酚磺酞

metacyesis [ˌmetəsaiˈiːsis] *n* 宫外妊娠，宫外孕

metaduodenum [ˌmetədju(ː)əuˈdiːnəm] *n* 后十二指肠

metafemale [ˌmetəˈfiːmeil] *n* 超雌（性染色体异常，雌性中核型为 XXX，亦称 X 三体）

metagaster [ˌmetəˈgæstə] *n* 后肠管

metagastrula [ˌmetəˈgæstrulə] *n* 后原肠胚

metagelatin [ˌmetəˈdʒelətin] *n* 变性明胶（用草酸处理过的明胶）

metagenesis [ˌmetəˈdʒenisis] *n* 世代交替 | **metagenetic** [ˌmetədʒiˈnetik] *a*

metagglutinin [ˌmetəˈglutinin] *n* 部分凝集素，变性凝集素

metaglobulin [ˌmetəˈglɔbjulin] *n* 纤维蛋白原

metagonimiasis [ˌmetəˌgɔniˈmaiəsis] *n* 后殖吸虫病

Metagonimus [ˌmetəˈgɔniməs] *n* 后殖吸虫属 | ~ yokogawai, ~ ovatus 横川后殖吸虫

metagranulocyte [ˌmetəˈgrænjuləsait] *n* 晚幼粒细胞

metagrippal [ˌmetəˈgripl] *a* 流感后遗的

metahemoglobin [ˌmetəˌhiːməuˈgləubin] *n* 高铁血红蛋白

metaicteric [ˌmetəikˈterik] *a* 黄疸后的

metainfective [ˌmetəinˈfektiv] *a* 传染后的
metaiodobenzylguanidine (**MIBG**) [ˌmetəˌaidəuˌbenzilˈgwɑːnidiːn] *n* 碘苄胍(一种以 ^{123}I 或 ^{131}I 标记的去甲肾上腺素类似物,被神经内分泌细胞所吸收,并在激素储存囊内浓缩,用于肾上腺髓质显像及嗜铬细胞瘤定位)
metakinesis [ˌmetəkaiˈniːsis] *n* 中期分裂;中期
metal [ˈmetl] *n* 金属 | alkali ~ 碱金属 / alkaline earth ~s 碱土金属 / bell ~ 钟铜(锡铜合金)
metalbumin [meˈtælbjumin] *n* 变清蛋白
metaldehyde [meˈtældəhaid] *n* 聚乙醛(曾用作消毒药)
metallaxis [ˌmetəˈlæksis] *n*【希】[器官]变形
metallergy [meˈtælədʒi] *n* 变型变态反应(机体经特异性致敏后,能与其他抗原反应,其临床表现与对原致敏抗原的反应相同)
metallesthesia [ˌmetəlisˈθiːzjə] *n* 金属[触]觉
metallic [miˈtælik] *a* 金属的;金属制的
metallize [ˈmetəlaiz] *vt* 敷金属 | **~d** *a* / **metallization** [ˌmetəlaiˈzeiʃən, -liˈz-] *n* 敷金属[法]
metallizing [ˈmetəlaiziŋ] *n* 敷金属的
metallocarboxypeptidase [məˌtæləukɑːˌbɔksiˈpeptideis] *n* 金属羧肽酶
metallocyanide [məˌtæləuˈsaiənaid] *n* 氰化金属
metalloendopeptidase [məˌtæləuˌendəuˈpeptideis] *n* 金属内肽酶
metalloenzyme [məˌtæləuˈenzaim] *n* 金属酶
metalloflavoprotein [məˌtæləuˌfleivəuˈprəutiːn] *n* 金属黄素蛋白
Metallogenium [məˌtæləuˈdʒiːniəm] *n* 生金菌属
metalloid [ˈmetəlɔid] *n* 非金属;类金属 *a* 金属样的
metallophilic [məˌtæləuˈfilik] *a* 嗜金属的(指细胞)
metalloplastic [məˌtæləuˈplæstik] *a* 金属修补术的
metalloporphyrin [məˌtæləuˈpɔːfirin] *n* 金属卟啉
metalloprotein [məˌtæləuˈprəutiːn] *n* 金属蛋白
metalloproteinase [miˌtæləuˈprəutiːneis] *n* 金属蛋白酶 | matrix ~ 间质金属蛋白酶
metalloscopy [ˌmetəˈlɔskəpi] *n* 金属反应检查[法]
metallotherapy [məˌtæləuˈθerəpi] *n* 金属疗法
metallurgy [meˈtælədʒi] *n* 冶金学,冶金术 | **metallurgic(al)** [metəˈləːdʒik(əl)] *a*
metal-sol [ˈmetl ˌsɔl] *n* 金属溶胶
metamer [ˈmetəmə] *n* 位变异构体,同质异性体
metamere [ˈmetəmiə] *n* 体节;节
metamerism [miˈtæmərizəm] *n* 位变异构[现象],同质异性;分节(一种结构类型系列重复排列成节) | **metameric** [ˌmetəˈmerik] *a*
metamonad [ˌmetəˈməunæd] *n* 鞭毛虫类
metamorphopsia [ˌmetəmɔːˈfɔpsiə] *n* 视物变形症 | ~ varians 变易性视物变形症
metamorphose [ˌmetəˈmɔːfəuz] *vt*, *vi* 变形;变质
metamorphosis [ˌmetəˈmɔːfəsis] *n* 变态 | fatty ~ 脂肪变态 / ovulational ~ 排卵变态 / retrograde ~, retrogressive ~ 退行性变态 / revisionary ~ 返祖性组织变态,退化 / tissue ~ 组织变态 / viscous ~, platelet ~, structural ~ 黏性变态,血小板变态,结构变态 | **metamorphotic** [ˌmetəmɔːˈfɔtik], **metamorphic** [ˌmetəˈmɔːfik] *a*
metamyelocyte [ˌmetəˈmaiələsait] *n* 晚幼粒细胞
metanephrine [ˌmetəˈnefrin] *n* 间甲肾上腺素,3-*O*-甲基肾上腺素
metanephrogenic [ˌmetəˌnefrəuˈdʒenik] *a* 生后肾的
metanephros [ˌmetəˈnefrɔs] ([复] **metanephroi** [ˌmetəˈnefrɔi]), **metanephron** [metəˈnefrɔn] *n* 后肾 | **metanephric** [ˌmetəˈnefrik] *a*
metaneutrophil [ˌmetəˈnjuːtrəfi] *a* 中性异染的
metanucleus [ˌmetəˈnjuːkliəs] *n* 成熟期卵核
metapeptone [ˌmetəˈpeptəun] *n* 变性[蛋白]胨
metaphase [ˈmetəfeiz] *n* [分裂]中期(细胞分裂)
metaphosphate [ˌmetəˈfɔsfeit] *n* 偏磷酸盐
metaphosphoric acid [ˌmetəfɔsˈfɔrik] 偏磷酸
metaphrenia [ˌmetəˈfriːniə] *n* 精神变态
metaphysis [miˈtæfisis] ([复] **metaphyses** [miˈtæfisiːz]) *n* 干骺端 | **metaphyseal**, **metaphysial** [ˌmetəˈfiziəl] *a*
metaphysitis [ˌmetəfiˈsaitis] *n* 干骺端炎
metaplasia [ˌmetəˈpleizjə] *n* [组织]转化,化生,组织变形 | agnogenic myeloid ~ 特发性骨髓外化生(原因不明的骨髓外造血,亦称非白血病性骨髓组织增生,成白红细胞性贫血) / ~ pulp 牙髓转化 | **metaplastic** [ˌmetəˈplæstik] *a* [组织]转化的,化生的;后成质的
metaplasis [meˈtæpləsis] *n* 完全发育期
metaplasm [ˈmetəplæzəm] *n* 后成质,滋养质,副浆 | **~ic** [ˌmetəˈplæzmik] *a*
metapneumonic [ˌmetənju(ː)ˈmɔnik] *a* 肺炎后的
metapodialia [ˌmetəˌpəudiˈeiliə] *n* 掌跖骨(掌骨与跖骨的合称)
metapophysis [ˌmetəˈpɔfisis] *n* 椎骨乳状突
metaprotein [ˌmetəˈprəutiːn] *n* 变性蛋白
metaproterenol sulfate [ˌmetəprəuˈterinɔl] 硫酸异丙喘宁,硫酸间羟喘息定(β 肾上腺素能药,支气管扩张药)
metapsychics [ˌmetəˈsaikiks] *n* 心理玄学,心灵学(研究意识范围以外的心理现象的学科)

metapsychology [ˌmetəsaiˈkɔlədʒi] *n* 心理玄学，心灵学（研究心理作用和心理“结构”的各种哲理，靠逻辑推理，而未为实验或观察所证实；在精神分析中此种哲理涉及心理过程的心理分域〈潜意识、自我、超自我〉和经济学〈精神能力或兴奋的量〉）

metapyrone [ˌmetəˈpaiərəun] *n* 甲双吡丙酮，甲吡酮（即美替拉酮 metyrapone，用于下丘脑垂体功能试验）

metaraminol [ˌmetəˈræminɔl] *n* 间羟胺，间羟基去甲麻黄碱（升压药）

metarchon [meˈtɑːkɔn] *n* 害虫诱惑剂

metargon [meˈtɑːgɔn] *n* 重氩

metarhodopsin [ˌmetərəˈdɔpsin] *n* 变视紫质

metarsenic acid [metˈɑːsnik] 偏砷酸

metarteriole [ˌmetɑːˈtiəriəul] *n* 后微动脉

metarubricyte [ˌmetəˈrubrisait] *n* 正染性幼红细胞，晚幼红细胞

metasaccharic acid [ˌmetəsəˈkærik] 甘露糖二酸

metasomatome [ˌmetəˈsəumətəum] *n* 原椎［骨］间凹痕

metastable [ˌmetəsteibl] *a* 亚稳的（相对稳定的，非完全安定的）

metastannic acids [ˌmetəˈstænik] 偏锡酸

metastasectomy [meˌtæstəˈsektəmi] *n* 转移瘤切除术，转移灶切除术

metastasis [məˈtæstəsis]（［复］ **metastases** [məˈtæstəsiːz]）*n* 转移，迁徙；［复］转移瘤，转移灶 | biochemical ~ 生物化学性转移，代谢性转移 / calcareous ~ 钙质转移 / paradoxical ~，retrograde ~ 逆行转移 | **metastatic** [ˌmetəˈstætik] *a*

metastasize [məˈtæstəsaiz] *vi* 转移，迁徙

metasternum [ˌmetəˈstəːnəm] *n* 剑突（胸骨）

Metastrongylidae [ˌmetəstrɔnˈdʒilidiː] *n* 后圆线虫科

Metastrongylus [ˌmetəˈstrɔndʒiləs] *n* 后圆线虫属 | ~ elongatus 长后圆线虫

metasynapsis [ˌmetəsiˈnæpsis]，**metasyndesis** [ˌmetəsinˈdiːsis] *n* 衔接联合（染色体）

metasyncrisis [ˌmetəˈsinkrisis] *n* 废物排除

metasyphilis [ˌmetəˈsifilis] *n* 变性梅毒（先天梅毒的一种，有全身障碍而没有梅毒疹）；终期梅毒，四期梅毒（脊髓痨或麻痹性痴呆）

metasyphilitic [ˌmetəsifiˈlitik] *a* 梅毒后的；变性梅毒的；终期梅毒的

metatarsal [ˌmetəˈtɑːsəl] *a* 跖的 *n* 跖骨

metatarsalgia [ˌmetətɑːˈsældʒiə] *n* 跖［骨］痛

metatarsectomy [ˌmetətɑːˈsektəmi] *n* 跖骨切除术

metatarsophalangeal [ˌmetəˌtɑːsəufəˈlændʒiəl] *a* 跖趾的

metatarsus [ˌmetəˈtɑːsəs] *n* 跖；跗基节（昆虫腿的跗节的最后一节）

metathalamus [ˌmetəˈθæləməs] *n* 后丘脑

Metatheria [ˌmetəˈθiːəriə] *n* 后兽亚纲

metatherian [ˌmetəˈθiːəriən] *n* 后兽亚纲的动物

metathesis [meˈtæθəsis] *n* 病变移植；复分解［作用］，置换［作用］，易位［作用］ | **metathetic** [ˌmetəˈθetik] *a*

metathrombin [ˌmetəˈθrɔmbin] *n* 变性凝血酶，无活力凝血酶

metatroph [ˈmetətrɔf] *n* 腐物寄生菌

metatrophia [metəˈtrəufiə] *n* 营养不良性萎缩；饮食改变

metatrophic [ˌmetəˈtrɔfik] *a* 腐物寄生的，嗜有机质的

metatrophy [miˈtætrəfi] *n* 营养不良性萎缩；饮食改变；腐物寄生性营养

metatypic(al) [ˌmetəˈtipik(əl)] *a* 异型的，变型的（指肿瘤）

metavanadate [ˌmetəˈvænədeit] *n* 偏钒酸盐

metavanadic acid [ˌmetəvəˈnædik] 偏钒酸

metaxalone [məˈtæksələun] *n* 美他沙酮（平滑肌松弛药）

metaxenia [ˌmetəˈziːniə] *n* 果实直感（见 xenia）；孕势（ectogony 的误用名，见 ectogony）

metaxeny [məˈtæksəni] *n* 转换寄生

Metazoa [ˌmetəˈzəuə] *n* 后生动物门，多细胞动物门（原生动物以外的一切动物均属之）

metazonal [ˌmetəˈzəunəl] *a* 附肌带后的，附肌带下的

metazoon [ˌmetəˈzəuɔn]（［复］ **metazoa** [ˌmetəˈzəuə]）*n* 后生动物（有时指多细胞动物） | **metazoal** [ˌmetəˈzəuəl] *a* | **metazoan** [ˌmetəˈzəuən] *a*，*n*

Metchnikoff's law [ˈmetʃnikɔf]（Elie Metchnikoff）梅契尼可夫定律（身体一旦受到细菌侵袭时，多形核白细胞和大单核细胞很快变为具有保护作用的吞噬细胞） | ~ theory 梅契尼可夫学说（认为细菌和其他有害成分在体内由吞噬细胞附着和破坏，有害物质和吞噬细胞之间的相互作用产生炎症）

Metchnikovellida [ˌmetʃnikəˈvelidə] *n* 异型目

metecious [məˈtiːʃəs] *a* 异栖的，异种［宿主］寄生性的

metencephalon [ˌmetenˈsefəlɔn]（［复］ **metencephala** [ˌmetenˈsefələ]），**metencephal** [meˈtensifəl] *n* 后脑 | **metencephalic** [meˌtensiˈfælik] *a*

metencephalospinal [ˌmetensefələuˈspainl] *a* 后脑脊髓的

met-enkephalin [ˌmet enˈkefəlin] *n* 甲硫氨酸脑啡肽

meteorism [ˈmiːtjərizəm] *n* 鼓胀,腹中积气
meteoropathology [ˌmiːtjərəupəˈθɔlədʒi] *n* 气候病理学
meteoropathy [ˌmiːtjəˈrɔpəθi] *n* 气候病
meteororesistant [ˌmiːtjərəuriˈzistənt] *a* 对气候不敏感的
meteorosensitive [ˌmiːtjərəˈsensitiv] *a* 对气候敏感的
meteorotropism [ˌmiːtjəˈrɔtrəpizəm] *n* 气候影响性[反应] | **meteorotropic** [ˌmiːtjərəˈtrɔpik] *a* 受气候影响的
metepencephalon [ˌmetepenˈsefələn] *n* 末脑
meter[1] [ˈmiːtə] *n* 米,公尺(符号为 m)
meter[2] [ˈmiːtə] *n* 计,表,量器 *vi* 用表测量(或计量);计量(或按规定量)供给 | dosage ~ 放射量计 / flicker ~ 闪变光度计/ light ~ 光计 / peak flow ~ 最大流量计(测定用力呼气早期气流量的仪器) / rate ~ 速率计(一种辐射测定仪,其放射发射量与瞬时辐射强度〈放射性发射率〉成正比)
-meter [构词成分]计,表,量器
metergasis [ˌmetəˈgeisis] *n* 功能变化,机能变化
metestrus [məˈtestrəs], **metestrum** [məˈtestrəm] *n* 动情后期
metformin hydrochloride [metˈfɔːmin] 盐酸甲福明(口服降血糖药)
methacholine [ˌmeθəˈkəuliːn] *n* 醋甲胆碱 | ~ bromide 溴醋甲胆碱(用法与氯醋甲胆碱同) / ~ chloride 氯醋甲胆碱(胆碱能药,主要治心血管系统疾病)
methacrylate [meˈθækrileit] *n* 甲基丙烯酸酯(用于医药和牙科);甲基丙烯酸树脂
methacrylic acid [ˌmeθəˈkrilik] 甲基丙烯酸
methacycline [ˌmeθəˈsaiklin] *n* 美他环素(抗生素类药) | ~ hydrochloride 盐酸美他环素(抗菌药)
methadone hydrochloride [ˈmeθədɔn] 盐酸美沙酮(镇痛药)
methadyl acetate [ˈmeθədil] 醋美沙朵(麻醉镇痛药)
methallenestril [ˌmeθæliˈnestril] *n* 美沙雌酸(雌激素类药)
methallibure [meˈθælibjuə] *n* 美他硫脲(用作猪垂体前叶激活剂)
methamphetamine [ˌmeθæmˈfetəmiːn] *n* 去氧麻黄碱(中枢兴奋药,升压药) | ~ hydrochloride 盐酸去氧麻黄碱(中枢兴奋药)
methanal [ˈmeθənæl] *n* 甲醛
methandriol [meˈθændriɔl] *n* 美雄醇(雄激素,同化激素类药)
methandrostenolone [meˌθændrəuˈstenələun] *n* 美雄酮(雄激素,同化激素类药)
methane [ˈmeθein] *n* 甲烷,沼气
methanesulfonate [ˌmeθeinˈsʌlfəneit] *n* 甲磺酸盐(或酯)
methanesulfonic acid [ˌmeθeinsʌlˈfɔnik] 甲磺酸
Methanobacteriaceae [ˌmeθənəubækˌtiːriˈeisiiː] *n* 甲烷杆菌科
Methanobacterium [ˌmeθənəubækˈtiəriəm] *n* 甲烷杆菌属
Methanococcus [ˌmeθənəuˈkɔkəs] *n* 甲烷球菌属
methanogen [ˌmeθənəuˈdʒən] *n* 产甲烷菌
methanogenic [ˌmeθənəuˈdʒenik] *a* 产甲烷的
methanol [ˈmeθənɔl] *n* 甲醇,木醇(溶媒,溶剂)
methanolysis [ˌmeθəˈnɔlisis] *n* 甲醇分解
Methanomonadaceae [ˌmeθənəuˌməunəˈdeisiiː] *n* 甲烷单胞菌科(即甲基球菌科 Methylococcaceae)
Methanomonas [ˌmeθənəuˈməunəs] *n* 甲烷单胞菌属
Methanosarcina [ˌmeθənəusɑːˈsainə] *n* 甲烷八叠球菌属
methantheline bromide [məˈθænθilin] 溴甲胺太林(抗胆碱能药)
methapyrilene [ˌmeθəˈpiriliːn] *n* 美沙吡林(抗组胺药)
methaqualone [məˈθækwələun] *n* 甲喹酮(催眠镇静药) | ~ hydrochloride 盐酸甲喹酮(催眠镇静药)
metharbital [məˈθɑːbitæl] *n* 美沙比妥(抗惊厥药,抗癫痫药)
methazolamide [meθəˈzəuləmaid] *n* 醋甲唑胺(碳酸酐酶抑制药,治青光眼药)
methdilazine [meθˈdailəziːn] *n* 甲地嗪(抗组胺药,止痒药) | ~ hydrochloride 盐酸甲地嗪(抗组胺药,止痒药)
methectic [meˈθektik] *a* 各级智力的
methemalbumin [ˌmethemælˈbjuːmin] *n* 高铁白蛋白(亦称假高铁血红蛋白)
methemalbuminemia [ˌmethemælˌbjuːmiˈniːmiə] *n* 高铁白蛋白血症
metheme [ˈmethiːm] *n* 高铁血红素
methemoglobin [metˌhiːməuˈgləubin] *n* 高铁血红蛋白
methemoglobinemia [ˌmethiːməuˌgləubiˈniːmiə] *n* 高铁血红蛋白血症 | **methemoglobinemic** [ˌmethiːməuˌgləubiˈniːmik] *a* 高铁血红蛋白血症的 *n* 致高铁血红蛋白血症药
methemoglobin reductase (NADH) [metˌhiːməuˈgləubin riˈdʌkteis] 高铁血红蛋白还原酶(NADH),细胞色素-b_5 还原酶
methemoglobin reductase (NADPH) [metˌhiːməuˈgləubin riˈdʌkteis] 高铁血红蛋白还原酶(NADPH)

methemoglobinuria [ˌmethiːməuˌgləubiˈnjuəriə] *n* 高铁血红蛋白尿

methenamine [meθˈenæmin] *n* 乌洛托品(尿路抗菌药) | ~ hippurate 马尿酸乌洛托品(尿路抗菌药) / ~ mandelate 孟德立酸乌洛托品(尿路抗菌药)

methenolone [miˈθenələun] *n* 美替诺龙(同化激素类药) | ~ acetate 醋酸美替诺龙 / ~ enanthate 庚酸美替诺龙

5,10-methenyltetrahydrofolate [ˌmeθənilˈtətrəˌhaidrəuˈfəuleit] *n* 5,10-次甲基四氢叶酸

methenyltetrahydrofalate cyclohydrolase [ˌmeθənilˌtetrəˌhaidrəuˈfəuleitˌsaikləuˈhaidrəleis] 次甲基四氢叶酸环化脱水酶

5,10-methenyltetrahydrofolate synthetase [ˌmeθənilˌtetrəˌhaidrəuˈfəuleit ˈsinθəteis] 5,10-次甲基四氢叶酸合成酶,5-甲酰四氢叶酸环连接酶

methestrol diproprionate [ˈmeθestrɔl] 二丙酸美雌酚(即 promethestrol dipropionate,雌激素类药)

methetoin [meˈθetəuin] *n* 美替妥英(抗惊厥药,用于治疗癫痫)

methexenyl [meˈθeksinil] *n* 环己巴比妥(即海索比妥 hexobarbital,催眠镇静药)

methicillin sodium [meθiˈsilin] 甲氧西林钠(抗菌药)

methilepsia [ˌmeθiˈlepsiə] *n* 酒狂

methimazole [meˈθiməzəul] *n* 甲巯咪唑(抗甲状腺药)

methine [ˈmeθain] *n* 次甲基(即 methylidyne)

methiocarb [məˈθaiəukɑːb] *n* 灭虫威,灭梭威(杀虫剂)

methiodal sodium [meˈθaiədl] 碘甲磺钠(尿路造影剂)

methionic acid [ˌmeθaiˈɔnik] 甲二磺酸

methionine [məˈθaiəniːn] *n* 甲硫氨酸(一种天然氨基酸,为饮食的必需成分);蛋氨酸(氨基酸类药)

methionine adenosyltransferase [məˈθaiəniːn əˌdenəsilˈtrænsfəreis] 甲硫氨酸腺苷基转移酶

methionine synthase [məˈθaiəniːnˈsinθeis] 甲硫氨酸合酶

methionyl [məˈθaiənil] *n* 甲硫氨酰[基]

methisazone [məˈθisəzəun] *n* 美替沙腙(抗病毒药)

methixene hydrochloride [məˈθiksiːn] 盐酸美噻吨(平滑肌松弛药)

methocarbamol [ˌmeθəuˈkɑːbəmɔl] *n* 美索巴莫(骨骼肌松弛药)

method [ˈmeθəd] *n* 方法,法 | A. B. C. (alum, blood, clay) ~ A. B. C. 法(明矾、血、黏土沉淀清洁法) / absorption ~ 吸收法(从特异性免疫血清中分离和选择性去除凝集素) / acid hematin ~ 酸性高铁血红素测定法(检血红蛋白) / autoclave ~ 压热器法(检血钙及血脲) / brine flotation ~ 盐水浮集法(检卵浓度) / cathartic ~ 渲泻法,泻法(一种治疗精神神经病法,即用适当的引导问题,使病人从模糊不清和无形恐惧中恢复到完全清醒) / closed-plaster ~ 石膏固定法(治创伤、哆开骨折及骨髓炎) / cubicle ~ 分间隔离法(治疗接触传染病患者) / direct ~ 直接(眼底检查)法 / direct aeration ~ 直接灌气法(检血脲) / direct centrifugal flotation ~ 直接离心浮集法(检钩虫卵) / flash ~ 快速牛奶消毒法 / flotation ~ 浮集法,浮选法(检粪中虫卵) / gasometric ~ 气体定量法(检脲) / gold number ~ 金值法(胶体金试验,检脑脊液球蛋白) / holding ~ 持久牛奶消毒法 / Japanese ~ 日本裱片方法 / lime ~ 石灰发生甲醛气法 / panoptic ~ 全染法,全显法 / permutit ~ 人造浮石法(检尿氨) / probit ~ 概率度法(测定半数致死量) / rhythm ~ 安全期避孕法 / turbidity ~ 比浊法(检白蛋白) / uranium acetate ~ 乙酸铀法(检磷) / urease ~s 脲酶法

methodism [ˈmeθədizəm] *n* 方法医学 | **methodist** *n* 方法医学派(根据少数简单法则和理论治病的古代医学派);方法医学派者

methodology [ˌmeθəˈdɔlədʒi] *n* 方法论,方法学 | **methodologic(al)** [ˌmeθədəˈlɔdʒik(əl)] *a* / **methodologist** *n* 方法论者,方法学者

methohexital [ˌmeθəˈheksitæl] *n* 美索比妥(催眠镇静药) | ~ sodium 美索比妥钠(静脉用全身麻醉药)

methopholine [ˌmeθəuˈfəulin] *n* 甲氧夫啉(镇痛药)

methopromazine maleate [ˌmeθəuˈprəuməziːn] 马来酸美索丙嗪(中枢抑制药)

methotrexate (MTX) [ˌmeθəˈtrekseit] *n* 甲氨蝶呤(抗肿瘤药)

methotrimeprazine [ˌmeθətraiˈmeprəziːn] *n* 甲氧异丁嗪(镇痛药,供肌内注射,亦称左美丙嗪 levomepromazine)

methoxamine hydrochloride [məˈθɔksəmiːn] 盐酸甲氧明(肾上腺素能药,用作血管加压药)

methoxsalen [məˈθɔksələn] *n* 甲氧沙林(紫外线照射促使白癜风再着色,对银屑病产生光毒性反应,亦用作促晒黑药和防晒药)

methoxychlor [məˈθɔksiklɔː] *n* 甲氧氯,甲氧滴滴涕(杀虫药)

methoxyflurane [məˌθɔksiˈfluərein] *n* 甲氧氟烷(吸入性麻醉药)

methoxyl [məˈθɔksil] *n* 甲氧基

methoxyphenamine hydrochloride [məˌθɔksi-

ˈfenəmiːn] 盐酸甲氧那明(肾上腺素能药,主要用作支气管扩张药)

methoxypromazine maleate [məˌθɔksiˈprəuməziːn] 马来酸美索丙嗪(中枢抑制药)

8-methoxypsoralen [məˌθɔkisˈsɔrələn] *n* 甲氧沙林(见 methoxsalen)

methphenoxydiol [ˌmeθfeˌnɔksiˈdaiɔl] *n* 愈创木酚甘油醚(即 guaifenesin)

methscopolamine bromide [ˌmeθskəˈpɔləmiːn] 甲溴东莨菪碱(抗胆碱能药)

methsuximide [ˌmeθˈsʌksimaid] *n* 甲琥胺(抗惊厥药,用于治疗癫痫小发作和精神运动性癫痫)

methyclothiazide [ˌmeθikləˌθaiəzaid] *n* 甲氯噻嗪(利尿药,用于治疗高血压和水肿)

methyene [ˈmeθiːn] *n* 亚甲基

methyl [ˈmeθil, ˈmiːθail] *n* 甲基 | ~ chloride 氯甲烷(局部喷雾麻醉药) / ~ iodide 碘甲烷(局部麻醉药) / ~ methacrylate 甲基丙烯酸甲酯(有时用于外科和牙科手术) / ~ salicylate 水杨酸甲酯,冬绿油(风湿性疾病、腰痛、坐骨神经痛时用作表面搽剂) / ~ sulfonate 磺酸甲酯(一种无腐蚀性、无毒性晶状防腐剂)

methylacetic acid [ˌmeθiləˈsiːtik] 丙酸

***α*-methylacetoacetic acid** [ˌmeθiləˌsiːtəuəˈsiːtik] *α*-甲基乙酰乙酸

***α*-methylacetoaceticaciduria** [ˌmeθiləˌsiːtəuəˌsiːtikˌæsiˈdjuəriə] *n* *α*-甲基乙酰乙酸尿[症]

***α*-methylacetoacetyl** [ˌmeθiləˌsiːtəuˈæsətiːl] *n* *α*-甲基乙酰乙酰基

***α*-methylacetoacetyl CoA-*β*-ketothiolase** [ˌmeθiləˌsiːtəuˈæsitil ˌkiːtəuˈθaiəleis] *α*-甲基乙酰乙酰基辅酶 A-*β*-酮硫解酶,乙酰-CoA 酰基转移酶

***α*-methylacetoacetyl CoA thiolase** [ˌmeθiləˌsiːtəuˈæsətiːl kəuˈei ˈθaiəleis] *α*-甲基乙酰乙酰基辅酶 A 硫解酶(此酶缺乏为一种常染色体隐性性状,可致 *α*-甲基乙酰乙酸尿症)

methylal [ˈmeθiləl] *n* 甲缩醛,甲醛缩二甲醇(催眠麻醉药,在某些化学反应时似甲醛)

methylamine [ˌmeθiləˈmiːn, ˌmeθiˈlæmiːn] *n* 甲胺(一种气体尸碱)

methyl-aminoacetic acid [ˌmeθilˌæminəuəˈsiːtik] 甲[基]甘氨酸,肌氨酸

methylamino acid [ˌmeθilˈæminəu] 甲基氨基酸

methylarsinate [ˌmeθiˈlɑːsineit] *n* 甲[基]砷酸盐

methyl-arsinic acid [ˌmeθilˈɑːsinik] 甲基砷酸

***N*-methyl-D-aspartate (NMDA)** [ˈmeθil əsˈpɑːteit] *N*-甲基-D-天冬氨酸(一种神经递质,类似谷氨酸,见于中枢神经系统,合成制备用于实验研究谷氨酸递质的兴奋机制)

methylate [ˈmeθileit] *n* 甲醇盐 *vi* 甲基化,加甲基 | **~d** 甲基化的 / **methylation** [ˌmeθiˈleiʃən] *n* 甲基化(作用)

methylatropine nitrate [ˌmeθiˈlætrəpin] 甲硝阿托品(抗胆碱能药)

methylaurin [meθilˈɔːrin] *n* 甲[基]蔷薇色酸

methylazoxymethanol [ˌmeθilæˌzɔksiˈmeθənɔl] *n* 甲基氧化偶氮甲醇(经肠道细菌水解苏铁苷〈cycasin〉后形成的一种致癌物质)

methylbenzethonium chloride [ˌmeθilˌbenziˈθəunjəm] 甲苄索氯铵(消毒防腐药)

methylcellulose [ˌmeθilˈseljuləus] *n* 甲基纤维素(用作药品制剂中的悬浮、增黏、赋形剂,口服用作泻药,在某些眼科手术中局部用于结膜以保护和润滑角膜)

methylchloroformate [ˌmeθilˌklɔːrəuˈfɔːmeit] *n* 氯甲酸甲酯(一种催泪性毒气)

methylchloroisothiazolinone [ˌmeθilˌklɔːrəuˌaisəuθaiəˈzəulinəun] *n* 甲氯异噻唑啉酮(见 methylisothiazolinone)

3-methylcholanthrene [ˌmeθilkəuˈlænθriːn] *n* 3-甲[基]胆蒽

methylcobalamin [ˌmeθilkəuˈbæləmin] *n* 甲钴胺

methylcreosol [ˌmeθilˈkriəsɔl] *n* 甲基木溜油酚,甲基甲氧甲酚

3-methylcrotonic acid [ˌmeθilkrəuˈtɔnik] 3-甲基巴豆酸,3-甲基丁烯酸

methylcrotonoyl-CoA carboxylase [ˌmeθilkrəuˈtɔnəil kɑːˈbɔksileis] 甲基巴豆酰-CoA 羧化酶,甲基巴豆酰辅酶 A 羧化酶(此酶的遗传性缺陷可致 *β*-甲基巴豆酰甘氨酸尿症)

3-methylcrotonyl [ˌmeθilˈkrəutəˌnil] *n* 3-甲基巴豆酰

3-methylcrotonyl CoA carboxylase deficiency 3-甲基巴豆酰 CoA 羧化酶缺乏症(亦称 *β*-甲基巴豆酰甘氨酸尿症)

3-methylcrotonylglycine [ˌmeθilˌkrəutənilˈglaisiːn] *n* 3-甲基巴豆酰甘氨酸

***β*-methylcrotonylglycinuria** [ˌmeθilˌkrəutənilˌglisiˈnjuəriə] *β*-甲基巴豆酰甘氨酸尿症(患者可能出现精神发育迟缓、中枢神经系统功能障碍和肌萎缩)

methylcytosine [ˌmeθilˈsaitəsin] *n* 甲基胞嘧啶

methyldichlorarsin [ˌmeθilˌdaikləˈrɑːsin] *n* 甲基二氯砷(一种致命的糜烂性毒气)

methyldihydromorphinone [ˌmeθildaiˌhaidrəˈmɔːfinəun] *n* 甲氢吗啡酮,甲基二氢吗啡酮

methyldopa [ˌmeθilˈdəupə] *n* 甲基多巴(抗高血压药)

methyldopate hydrochloride [ˌmeθilˈdəupeit] 盐酸甲基多巴乙酯(抗高血压药,静脉输液)

methylene [ˈmeθiliːn] *n* 亚甲基 | ~ blue 亚甲蓝(解毒药) / ~ chloride, ~ dichloride, ~ bichloride 二氯甲烷(曾用作小手术麻醉药)

methylenedioxyamphetamine (MDA) [ˌmeθiliːndaiˌɔksiæmˈfetəmiːn] *n* 亚甲基二氧苯丙胺（本品具有致幻性质，被广泛滥用，造成依赖性）

3，4-methylenedioxymethamphetamine (MDMA) [ˌmeθiliːndaiˌɔksiˌmeθæmˈfetəmiːn] *n* 3，4-亚甲基二氧去氧麻黄碱（本品具有致幻性质，被广泛滥用。俗称迷魂药〈ecstasy〉）

5，10-methylenetetrahydrofolate [ˌmeθiliːnˌtetrəˌhaidrəuˈfəuleit] *n* 5，10-亚甲四氢叶酸

methylenetetrahydrofolate dehydrogenase (NADP⁺) [ˌmeθiliːnˌtetrəˌhaidrəuˈfəuleit diːˈhaidrədʒəneis] 亚甲四氢叶酸脱氢酶（NADP⁺）

5，10-methylenetetrahydrofolate reductase ($FADH_2$) [ˌmeθiliːnˌtetrəˌhaidrəuˈfəuleit riˈdʌkteis] 5，10-亚甲四氢叶酸还原酶（$FADH_2$）（此酶缺乏为一种常染色体隐性性状，可致高胱氨酸尿症）

methylenetetrahydrofolate (THF) reductase deficiency 亚甲四氢叶酸还原酶缺乏症（主要临床征象是中枢神经系统损害）

methylenophil [ˌmeθiˈliːnəfil] *n* 嗜亚甲蓝质 *a* 嗜亚甲蓝的

methylenophilous [ˌmeθiliːˈnɔfiləs] *a* 嗜亚甲蓝的

methylergonovine maleate [ˌmeθilˌəːgəuˈnəuviːn] 马来酸甲麦角新碱（催产药）

methylglucamine [ˌmeθilˈgluːkəmiːn] *n* 甲葡糖胺，甲基葡胺

3-methylglutaconic acid [ˌmeθilgluːtəˈkɔnik] 3-甲基戊烯二酸

3-methylglutaconicaciduria [ˌmeθilˌgluːtəˌkɔnikˌæsiˈdjuəriə] *n* 3-甲基戊烯二酸尿[症]

3-methylglutaconyl [ˌmeθilˌgluːtəˈkɔnil] *n* 3-甲基戊烯二酸单酰[基]

methylglutaconyl-CoA hydratase [ˌmeθilˌgluːtəˈkɔnil kəuˈei ˈhaidrəteis] 甲基戊烯二酸单酰辅酶A水化酶（此酶缺乏为一种常染色体隐性性状，可致3-甲基戊烯二酸尿症）

3-methylglutaric acid [ˌmeθilgluːˈtærik] 3-甲基戊二酸

methylglyoxal [ˌmeθilglaiˈɔksəl] *n* 甲基乙二醛，丙酮醛

methylglyoxalase [ˌmeθilglaiˈɔksəleis] *n* 甲基乙二醛酶，乳酰谷胱甘肽裂合酶

methylglyoxalidin [ˌmeθilˌglaiɔkˈsælidin] *n* 甲咪唑啉（抗风湿药）

methylguanidine [ˌmeθilˈgwænidin] *n* 甲[基]胍

methylguanidinoacetic acid [ˌmeθilˌgwænidinəuəˈsiːtik] 甲基胍[基]乙酸，肌酸

methylhexaneamine [ˌmeθilhekˈseinəmiːn]，**methylhexamine** [ˌmeθilˈheksəmiːn] *n* 甲己胺

3-methylhistidine [ˌmeθilˈhistidiːn] *n* 3-甲基组氨酸

methylhydantoic acid [ˌmeθilˌhaidænˈtəuik] 甲基脲乙酸

methylhydantoin [ˌmeθilhaiˈdæntəuin] *n* 甲内酰脲，甲脲乙醇酸酐

methylhydroxybenzoic acid [ˌmeθilhaiˌdrɔksibenˈzəuik] 甲[基]对羟苯甲酸，甲基水杨酸

methylic [meˈθilik] *a* 甲[基]的

methylidyne [miːˈθilidain] *n* 次甲基（亦称 methine）

methylindol [ˌmeθilˈindəul] *n* 甲苯吲哚，粪臭素

methylisothiazolinone [ˌmeθilˌaisəuθaiəˈzəulinəun] 甲基异噻唑啉酮（一种防腐剂，与甲氧异噻唑啉酮〈methylchloroisothiazolinone〉合用，用作广谱抗真菌和抗生素药，用于化妆品、游泳池杀虫剂及各种工业制剂，为接触变应性的常见病因，高浓度时可致化学烧伤）

methylmaleic acid [ˌmeθilməˈliːik] 甲基顺丁烯二酸，柠康酸

methylmalonic acid [ˌmeθilməˈlɔnik] 甲基丙二酸

methylmalonicacidemia [ˌmeθilməˌlɔnikˌæsiˈdiːmiə] *n* 甲基丙二酸血[症]（①为一种常染色体隐性遗传氨基酸病，特征为血内和尿内甲基丙二酸过多，亦称甲基丙二酸尿；②血内甲基丙二酸过多）

methylmalonicaciduria [ˌmeθilməˌlɔnikˌæsiˈdjuəriə] *n* 甲基丙二酸尿[症]（①尿内甲基丙二酸过多；②甲基丙二酸血）

methylmalonyl [ˌmeθilˈmælənil] *n* 甲基丙二酸单酰[基]

methylmalonyl-CoA epimerase [ˌmeθilˈmælənil kəuˈei iˈpiməreis] 甲基丙二酸单酰-CoA 差向异构酶，甲基丙二酸单酰辅酶A差向异构酶（亦称甲基丙二酸单酰-CoA 消旋酶）

methylmalonyl-CoA mutase [ˌmeθilˈmælənil kəuˈei ˈmjuːteis] 甲基丙二酸单酰-CoA 变位酶，甲基丙二酸单酰辅酶A变位酶（此酶缺乏为一种常染色体隐性性状，可致甲基丙二酸血症）

methylmalonyl-CoA racemase [ˌmeθilˈmælənil kəuˈei ˈreisimeis] 甲基丙二酸单酰-CoA 消旋酶，甲基丙二酸单酰辅酶A消旋酶，甲基丙二酸单酰-CoA 差向异构酶

methylmercaptan [ˌmeθilməˈkæptən] *n* 甲硫醇

methylmethacrylate [ˌmeθilmeˈθærileit] *n* 甲基丙烯酸甲酯（见 methyl 项下相应术语）

methylmorphine [ˌmeθilˈmɔːfiːn] *n* 甲基吗啡，可待因

Methylococcaceae [ˌmeθiləukɔkˈkeisiiː] *n* 甲基球菌科

Methylococcus [ˌmeθiləuˈkɔkəs] *n* 甲基球菌属

Methylomonadaceae [ˌmeθiləuˌməunəˈdeisiiː] *n*

甲基单胞菌科(即甲基球菌科 Methylococcaceae)

Methylomonas [ˌmeθiləuˈməunəs] *n* 甲基单胞菌属(旧称甲烷单胞菌属 Methanomonas)

3-methyl-2-oxobutanoate dehydrogenase (lipoamide) [ˈmeθil ˌɔksəuˌbjuːtəˈnəueit diːˈhaidrədʒəneis ˌlipəuˈæmaid] 3-甲基-2-酮丁酸脱氢酶(硫辛酰胺)(亦称 α-酮异戊酸脱氢酶)

methylparaben [ˌmeθilˈpærəbən] *n* 羟苯甲酯(抗真菌药,用作药物制剂的防腐药)

methylparafynol [ˌmeθilˌpærəˈfainɔl], **methylpentynol** [ˌmeθilˈpɔntinɔl] *n* 甲戊炔醇(催眠镇静药)

methylpentose [ˌmeθilˈpentəus] *n* 甲基戊糖

methylphenidate hydrochloride [ˌmeθilˈfenideit] 盐酸哌甲酯(中枢兴奋药)

methylphenylhydrazine [ˌmeθilˌfiːnilˈhaidrəzin] *n* 甲[基]苯肼

methylphenyl levulosazone [ˌmeθilˈfenil ˌlevjuˈləuseizəun] 果糖甲苯脎

methylprednisolone [ˌmeθilˈprednisələun] *n* 甲泼尼龙(合成糖皮质激素) | ~ acetate 醋酸甲泼尼龙 / ~ hemisuccinate 半琥珀酸甲泼尼龙 / ~ sodium phosphate 磷钠甲泼尼龙 / ~ sodium succinate 琥钠甲泼尼龙

methylprotocatechuic acid [ˌmeθilˌprəutəuˈkætitʃuːik] 4-羟基-3-甲氧基苯甲酸,香草酸

methylpurine [ˌmeθilˈpjuərin] *n* 甲[基]嘌呤

methylpyrapone [ˌmeθilˈpaiərəpəun] *n* 甲双吡丙酮,甲吡酮(即美替拉酮 metyrapone,用于下丘脑垂体功能试验)

4-methyl-1H-pyrazole [ˌmeθilˈ paiərəzəul] 甲吡唑(解毒药)

methylpyridine [ˌmeθilˈpiridin] *n* 甲[基]吡啶

methylquinoline [ˌmeθilˈkwinəlin] *n* 甲[基]喹啉

methylrosaniline chloride [ˌmeθilrəuˈzænilin] 甲紫(消毒防腐药)

10-methylstearic acid [ˌmeθilstiˈærik] 10-甲基硬脂酸,结核菌硬脂酸

methylsuccinic acid [ˌmeθilsəkˈsinik] 甲基琥珀酸,焦酒石酸

methyltestosterone [ˌmeθiltesˈtɔstərəun] *n* 甲睾酮(雄激素类药)

5-methyltetrahydrofolate [ˌmeθilˌtetrəˌhaidrəuˈfəuleit] *n* 5-甲基四氢叶酸

5-methyltetrahydrofolate-homocysteine *S*-methyltransferase [ˌmeθilˌtetrəˌhaidrəuˈfəuleitˌhəuməuˈsistiːin ˌmeθilˈtrænsfəreis] 5-甲基四氢叶酸-高半胱氨酸 *S*-甲基转移酶(此酶活性降低可致高胱氨酸尿症,伴发育迟缓和神经异常,以及低蛋氨酸血症)

methyltheobromine [ˌmeθilˌθiəˈbrəumiːn] *n* 甲基可可豆碱,咖啡因

methylthionine chloride [ˌmeθilˈθaiənin] 亚甲蓝(解毒药)

methylthiouracil [ˌmeθilˌθaiəˈjuərəsil] *n* 甲硫氧嘧啶(抗甲状腺药)

methyltransferase [ˌmeθilˈtrænsfəreis] *n* 甲基转移酶

5-methyluracil [ˌmeθilˈjuərəsil] *n* 5-甲基尿嘧啶,胸腺嘧啶

methyluramine [ˌmeθiljuəˈræmin] *n* 甲[基]胍

methylxanthine [ˌmeθilˈzænθin] *n* 甲基黄嘌呤

methynodiol diacetate [meˌθinəˈdaiəul] 双醋甲异炔诺醇(孕激素)

methyprylon [ˌmeθiˈprailɔn] *n* 甲乙哌酮(催眠镇静药)

methysergide [ˌmeθiˈsəːdʒaid] *n* 美西麦角(5-羟色氨拮抗药,具有直接血管收缩作用) | ~ maleate 马来酸美西麦角(镇痛药,治疗某些患者的血管性偏头痛)

metiamide [miˈtaiəmaid] *n* 甲硫米特(组胺拮抗药)

metiapine [miˈtaiəpiːn] *n* 甲硫平(安定药,治精神分裂症)

metipranolol hydrochloride [ˌmetiˈprænəlɔl] 盐酸美替洛尔(一种非选择性 β 受体阻滞药,局部用于结膜,治疗青光眼和高眼压症)

metizoline hydrochloride [miˈtizəliːn] 盐酸美替唑啉(拟肾上腺素药,具有血管收缩作用)

metmyoglobin [mətˌmaiəuˈgləubin] *n* 高铁肌红蛋白

metoclopramide hydrochloride [ˌmetəˈkləuprəmaid] 盐酸甲氧氯普胺(镇吐药)

metocurine iodide [ˌmetəuˈkjuəriːn] 碘甲筒箭毒(骨骼肌松弛药)

metoestrus [məˈtestrəs], **metoestrum** [məˈtestrəm] *n* 动情后期

metogest [ˈmetəudʒest] *n* 16, 16-二甲诺龙(一种激素)

metolazone [məˈtəuləzəun] *n* 美托拉宗(利尿药,用于治疗高血压和水肿)

metonymy [məˈtɔnimi] *n* 换喻语言,近似性代语(一种语言障碍,见于精神分裂症) | **metonymic(al)** [ˌmetəˈnimik(əl)] *a*

metopagus [məˈtɔpəgəs] *n* 额部联胎

metopic [miˈtɔpik] *a* 额的

metopimazine [ˌmetəuˈpiməziːn] *n* 美托哌丙嗪(镇吐药)

metopion [məˈtəupjən] *n* 额中点

metopism [ˈmetəpizəm] *n* 囟门不闭

metop(o)- [构词成分]额

metopodynia [ˌmetəpəuˈdiniə] *n* 额痛

metopon [ˈmetəpɔn] *n* 美托酮(镇痛药)

metopopagus [ˌmetəˈpɔpəgəs] *n* 额部联胎

metoposcopy [ˌmetəˈpɔskəpi] *n* 相额术
metoprine [ˈmetəupriːn] *n* 氯苯氨啶(抗肿瘤药)
metoprolol [miˈtəuprələul] *n* 美托洛尔(β受体阻滞药,治高血压)
metoprolol tartrate [ˌmetəuˈprəulɔl] 酒石酸美托洛尔(心脏选择性β受体阻滞药,用于治疗高血压、慢性心绞痛和心肌梗死)
Metorchis [meˈtɔːkis] *n* 次睾吸虫属
metoserpate hydrochloride [ˌmetəuˈsəːpeit] 盐酸美托舍酯(兽用镇静药)
metoxeny [məˈtɔksəni] *n* 转换寄生 | **metoxenous** [məˈtɔksənəs] *a*
metra [ˈmiːtrə] *n*【希】子宫
metra- 见 metro-
metralgia [miˈtrældʒiə] *n* 子宫痛
metraterm [ˈmiːtrətəːm] *n* 子宫末段,小宫(绦虫)
metratonia [ˌmiːtrəˈtəuniə] *n* 子宫无力,宫张力缺乏
metratrophia [ˌmiːtrəˈtrəufiə] *n* 子宫萎缩
metre [ˈmiːtə] *n* 米,公尺(即 meter)
metrechoscopy [ˌmetrəˈkɔskəpi] *n* 量听望联[合]诊法
metrectasia [ˌmiːtrekˈteiziə] *n* 子宫扩张(指非怀孕子宫)
metrectomy [miˈtrektəmi] *n* 子宫切除术
metrectopia [ˌmiːtrekˈtəupiə] *n* 子宫异位,子宫移位
metreurynter [ˌmiːtruəˈrintə] *n* 宫颈扩张袋
metreurysis [miˈtruərisis] *n* 宫颈扩张术
metria [ˈmiːtriə] *n* 产后子宫炎
metric [ˈmetrik] *a* 米的,公尺的;(以米)测量的;公制的,米制的
metrical [ˈmetrikəl] *a* 测量的,度量的
metrifonate, metriphonate [ˌmetriˈfəuneit] *n* 美曲膦酯(杀虫药)
metriocephalic [ˌmetriəusəˈfælik] *a* 中型头的(头长高指数在 72 ~ 77 之间)
metritis [məˈtraitis] *n* 子宫炎 | ~ dissecans, dissecting ~ 分割性子宫炎 / puerperal ~ 产褥期子宫炎
metrizamide [məˈtrizəmaid] *n* 甲泛葡胺(造影剂)
metrizoate sodium [ˌmetriˈzəueit] 甲泛影酸钠(诊断性造影剂)
metr(o)- [构词成分]子宫;同样见 hyster(o)-
metrocarcinoma [ˌmiːtrəuˌkɑːsiˈnəumə] *n* 子宫癌
metrocele [ˈmiːtrəsiːl] *n* 子宫疝
metrocolpocele [ˌmiːtrəuˈkɔlpəsiːl] *n* 子宫阴道突出
metrocystosis [ˌmiːtrəusisˈtəusis] *n* 子宫囊肿形成
metrocyte [ˈmiːtrəsait] *n* 母细胞
metrodynia [ˌmiːtrəuˈdiniə] *n* 子宫痛
metroendometritis [ˌmiːtrəˌendəumiˈtraitis] *n* 宫体内膜炎,宫肌层内膜炎
metrofibroma [ˌmiːtrəufaiˈbrəumə] *n* 子宫纤维瘤
metrogenous [məˈtrɔdʒinəs] *a* 子宫源的
metrography [məˈtrɔgrəfi] *n* 子宫 X 线摄影[术],子宫 X 线造影[术]
metroleukorrhea [ˌmiːtrəuˌljuːkəˈriːə] *n* 子宫白带
metrology [miˈtrɔlədʒi] *n* 度量衡学,计量学;度量衡制,计量制
metrolymphangitis [ˌmiːtrəuˌlimfænˈdʒaitis] *n* 子宫淋巴管炎
metromalacia [ˌmiːtrəuˌməˈleiʃiə], **metromalacoma** [ˌmiːtrəumæləˈkəumə] *n* 子宫软化
metromenorrhagia [ˌmiːtrəuˌmenəˈreidʒiə] *n* 月经过多
metronidazole [ˌmetrəˈnaidəzəul] *n* 甲硝唑(抗毛滴虫及阿米巴药)
metronoscope [məˈtrɔnəskəup] *n* 眼肌失调矫正器
metroparalysis [ˌmiːtrəupəˈrælisis] *n* 子宫麻痹
metropathia [ˌmiːtrəuˈpæθiə] *n* 子宫病 | ~ hemorrhagica 功能性子宫出血病,自发性子宫出血
metropathy [məˈtrɔpəθi] *n* 子宫病 | syncytiotrophoblastic ~ 合胞体滋养层子宫病,合胞体细胞子宫内膜炎 | **metropathic** [ˌmiːtrəuˈpæθik] *a*
metroperitoneal [ˌmiːtrəuˌperitəuˈniːəl] *a* 子宫腹膜的,子宫腹腔相通的
metroperitonitis [ˌmiːtrəuˌperitəuˈnaitis] *n* 子宫腹膜炎
metrophlebitis [ˌmiːtrəufliˈbaitis] *n* 子宫静脉炎
metroplasty [ˌmiːtrəˈplæsti] *n* 子宫成形术
metropolis [məˈtrɔpəlis] *n* 产地,生地(指特殊菌种滋生地)
metroptosis [ˌmiːtrəˈtəusis] *n* 子宫下垂,子宫脱垂
metrorrhagia [ˌmiːtrəˈreidʒiə] *n* 子宫不规则出血 | **metrorrhagic** [ˌmiːtrəˈrædʒik] *a*
metrorrhea [ˌmiːtrəˈriːə] *n* 子宫液溢
metrorrhexis [ˌmiːtrəˈreksis] *n* 子宫破裂
metrosalpingitis [ˌmiːtrəuˌsælpinˈdʒaitis] *n* 子宫输卵管炎
metrosalpingography [ˌmiːtrəuˌsælpiŋˈgɔgrəfi] *n* 子宫输卵管造影[术]
metroscope [ˈmiːtrəskəup] *n* 子宫镜
metrostasis [məˈtrɔstəsis] *n* 定长状态(肌纤维活动时原长度不变)

metrostaxis [ˌmiːtrəuˈstæksis] *n* 子宫渗血
metrostenosis [ˌmiːtrəustiˈnəusis] *n* 子宫狭窄
metrotherapy [ˌmetrəuˈθerəpi] *n* 测算疗法(如精确测算损伤关节随意运动的增加程度,使病人了解其进步的情况)
metrotomy [məˈtrɔtəmi] *n* 子宫切开术
metrotoxin [ˌmiːtrəuˈtɔksin] *n* 子宫毒素(由孕妇子宫产生的物质,能抑制卵巢功能)
metrotubography [ˌmiːtrəutjuˈbɔgrəfi] *n* 子宫输卵管造影[术]
-metry [构词成分]测定,定量,测量
M. et sig. misce et signa【拉】混合及写明用法
Mett's(Mette) method [met] (Emil L. P. Mett 〈Mette〉)梅特法(检验胃蛋白酶活力) | ~ test 梅特试验(测验胃蛋白酶) / ~ tubes 梅特管(检胃蛋白酶活力)
metula [ˈmetjulə] *n* 梗基
meturedepa [ˌmetjuəriˈdipə] *n* 美妥替哌(抗肿瘤药)
metyrapone [meˈtirəpəun] *n* 美替拉酮(用于下丘脑垂体功能试验) | ~ tartrate 酒石酸美替拉酮
metyrosine [miˈtaiərəsiːn] *n* 甲基酪氨酸(抗高血压药)
Meulengracht's diet [ˈmɔiləngræht] (Einar Meulengracht)莫伊伦格腊赫特饮食(胃溃疡饮食) | ~ method 莫伊伦格腊赫特法(检血清胆色素)
MeV megaelectron volt 兆电子伏[特]
mevalonate [meˈvæləneit] *n* 甲羟戊酸
mevalonate kinase [məˈvæləneit ˈkaineis] 甲羟戊酸激酶(此酶缺乏可致甲羟戊酸尿症)
mevalonic acid [ˌmevəˈlɔnik] 甲羟戊酸
mevalonicaciduria [ˌmevəˌlɔnikˌæsiˈdjuəriə] *n* 甲羟戊酸尿[症](一种遗传性氨基酸病,由于甲羟戊酸激酶缺乏所致,特征为尿内大量排泄甲羟戊酸,伴发育延迟、张力减退、肝脾肿大、不能茁壮成长等临床症状)
mexiletine hydrochloride [ˈmeksilətiːn] 盐酸美西律(口服抗心律失常药,其结构和作用与利多卡因〈lidocaine〉相类似,用于治疗室性心律失常)
mexrenoate potassium [meksˈrenəeit] 孕甲酯丙酸钾(醛固酮拮抗药)
Meyer-Archambault loop [ˈmaiə ɑːʃɑːmˈbəu] (A. Meyer; La Salle Archambault)麦-阿袢(见 Meyer's loop)
Meyer-Betz disease [ˈmaiə bets] (Friedrich Meyer-Betz)麦耶·贝茨病(一种罕见的病因不明的家族病,特点为肌红蛋白尿发作,可能由于极度劳累或某种感染促使肌肉不同程度的压痛、肿胀及软弱无力,可能伴有慢性弥漫性肌病或营养不良。亦称特发性或家族性肌红蛋白尿)
Meyer-Schwickerath and Weyers syndrome [ˈmaiə ˈʃvikərɑːt ˈvaiə] (Gerhard R. E. Meyer-Schwickerath; Helmut Weyers)麦-魏综合征,眼牙指发育不良,眼牙趾发育不良
Meyer's disease [ˈmaiə] (Hans W. Meyer)麦耶病(咽部腺样体增殖)
Meyer's line [ˈmaiə] (Georg H. von Meyer)麦耶线(跗趾轴线) | ~ organ 麦耶器官(舌后部两侧轮廓乳头区) / ~ sinus 麦耶窦(外耳道底鼓膜前的小凹)
Meyer's loop [ˈmaiə] (Adolf B. Meyer)麦耶襻(视辐射某些纤维在向后转向前环绕侧脑室下角所形成的襻)
Meynert's bundle, fasciculus, tract [ˈmainət] (Theodor H. Meynert)后屈束 | ~ cells 迈内特细胞(大脑皮质距状裂内孤独的锥体细胞) / ~ commissure 迈内特连合(视上背侧或上方连合)
Meynet's nodes [meiˈnei] (Paul C. H. Meynet)迈内结(风湿病时,关节囊及腱内的小结,尤见于儿童)
mezerein [məˈziəriːin] *n* 欧瑞香素,密执毒素
mezereum [miˈziəriəm], **mezereon** [miˈziəriən] *n* 紫花欧瑞香
mezlocillin [ˌmezləˈsilin] *n* 美洛西林(抗生素类药)
μF microfarad 微法[拉]
M. flac. membrana flaccida【拉】松弛膜,鼓膜松弛部
M. ft. mistura fiat【拉】制成合剂
Mg magnesium 镁
mg milligram 毫克
mγ milligamma (milli-microgram, micromilligram 或 nanogram)毫微克,纳克
μg microgram 微克
μγ microgamma(micro-microgram 或 picogram)微,微克,皮克
mgm milligram 毫克(旧符号)
MGUS monoclonal gammopathy of undetermined significance 意义未定的单克隆 γ-球蛋白病
3-MH 3-methylhistidine 3-甲基组氨酸
MHA-TP microhemagglutination assay-*Treponema-pallidum* 梅毒螺旋体微量血细胞凝集测定
MHC major histocompatibility complex 主要组织相容性复合体
MHD minimum hemolytic dose 最小溶血量
mho [məu] *n* 姆[欧](旧电导单位)
MHz megahertz 兆赫[兹]
MI myocardial infarction 心肌梗死
miana [maiˈænə] *n* 回归热(指中东地区)
Mianeh bug [ˈmiənei] 波斯锐缘蜱(Mianeh 为伊

朗城市名）

mianserin hydrochloride [miːˈænsərin] 盐酸米安色林(5-羟色胺抑制药,抗组胺药)

miasma [miˈæzmə, maiˈæzmə], **miasm** [ˈmaiəzəm] *n* 瘴毒,瘴气 | **miasmatic** [ˌmiəzˈmætik, maiəzˈmætik], **miasmic** [maiˈæzmik] *a*

Mibelli's porokeratosis [miˈbeli] (Vittorio Mibelli)汗孔角化病

MIBG, miBG iobenguane(*m*-iodobenzylguanidine) 碘苄胍(间碘苄基胍)

MIBI sestamibi 赛司米比(诊断用药)

mibolerone [maiˈbəulərəun] *n* 米勃酮(雄激素类药,同化激素)

mica [ˈmaikə] *n*【拉】云母;小片,小粒 | **~ceous** [maiˈkeiʃəs] *a* 云母的;碎屑状的

mication [maiˈkeiʃən] *n* 急促动作(如瞬目)

micatosis [ˌmaikəˈtəusis] *n* 云母屑肺,云母尘肺

mice [mais] mouse 的复数

micelle [maiˈsel], **micella** [maiˈselə] ([复] **micellae** [maiˈseliː]) *n* 胶粒,胶束;微团 | **micellar** *a*

Michaelis' constant [miˈkeilis] (Leonor Michaelis)米氏常数(表示酶反应速度为最大速度一半时的底物浓度)

Michaelis-Gutmann bodies [miˈkeilis ˈgutmən] (Leonor Michaelis; C. Gutmann)米-古小体(见于膀胱软斑病灶内的小体)

Michaelis-Menten equation [miˈkeilis ˈmentən] (Leonor Michaelis; Maude Lenore Menten)米-门方程式(酶动力学的基本方程式: $V=\frac{V_{max}[S]}{K_m+[S]}$,其中 V 为酶催化反应的"起始速度",[S]为底物,V_{max}为最大速度,K_m 为米氏常数)

Michaelis' rhomboid [miˈkeiliz] (Gustav A. Michaelis)米氏菱形区(髂后上棘小凹、臀肌线和髂后上棘末端沟形成的盆腔后侧上方的菱形区)

Michel's aplasia [miˈʃel] (E. M. Michel)米歇尔未发育(内耳未发育导致米歇尔聋) | ~ deafness 米歇尔聋(由于内耳全部未发育而引起的先天性聋)

miconazole nitrate [miˈkɔnəzəul] 硝酸咪康唑(抗真菌药)

micra [ˈmaikrə] micron 的复数

micracoustic [ˌmaikrəˈkuːstik] *a* 听弱声的 *n* 弱声助听器

micranatomy [ˌmaikrəˈnætəmi] *n* 显微解剖学;组织学

micrangium [maiˈkrændʒiəm] *n* 微血管(一般指毛细血管)

micranthine [maiˈkrænθin] *n* 小花芫碱

micrencephalon [ˌmaikrenˈsefələn] *n* 脑过小

micrencephaly [ˌmaikrenˈsefəli], **micrencephalia** [ˌmaikrensiˈfeiliə] *n* 脑过小 | **micrencephalous** [ˌmaikrənˈsefələs] *a*

micrergy [ˈmaikrədʒi] *n* 显微操作术

micr(o)- [构词成分]小,细,微

microabrasion [ˈmaikrəuəˌbreiʒən] *n* 微磨损[症](使用一种磨损化合物去除微量牙釉质以纠正釉质缺损)

microabscess [ˌmaikrəuˈæbsis] *n* 微脓疡(仅在显微镜下能看到的极小脓肿)

microadenoma [ˌmaikrəuˌædiˈnəumə] *n* 微腺瘤

microadenomectomy [ˌmaikrəuˌædinəuˈmektəmi], **microadenectomy** [ˌmaikrəuˌædiˈnektəmi] *n* 微腺切除术

microadenopathy [ˌmaikrəuˌædiˈnɔpəθi] *n* 细淋巴管病

microaerobic [ˌmaikrəuεəˈrəubik] *a* 微需氧的,微量需氧的

microaerophile [ˌmaikrəuˈεərəfail] *n* 微[量]需氧菌,微需氧微生物

microaerophilic [ˌmaikrəuˈεərəˌfilik], **microaerophilous** [ˌmaikrəuˌεəˈrɔfiləs] *a* 微需氧的,微量需氧的

microaerotonometer [ˌmaikrəuˌεərəutəuˈnɔmitə] *n* 微量血气计

microaggregate [ˌmaikrəuˈægrigeit] *n* 微聚集体

microalbuminuria [ˌmaikrəuˌælbjumiˈnjuəriə] *n* 微白蛋白尿[症](尿内白蛋白排出量过稀,以致无法用常规方法测得,常见于胰岛素依赖型糖尿病超过滤时)

microaleuriospore [ˌmaikrəuəˈljuəriəspɔː] *n* 小粉状孢子

microammeter [ˌmaikrəuˈæmitə] *n* 微安[培]计

microampere (μA) [ˌmaicrəuˈæmpεə] *n* 微安[培]

microanalysis [ˌmaikrəuəˈnæləsis] *n* 微量分析

microanastomosis [ˌmaikrəuəˌnæstəˈməusis] *n* 微吻合术

microanatomy [ˌmaikrəuəˈnætəmi] *n* 组织学(尤指器官学)

microaneurysm [ˌmaikrəuˈænjuərizəm] *n* 微动脉瘤

microangiopathy [ˌmaikrəuˌændʒiˈɔpəθi] *n* 微血管病 | diabetic ~ 糖尿病性微血管病 | **microangiopathic** [ˌmaikrəuˌændʒiəuˈpæθik] *a*

microangioscopy [ˌmaikrəuˌændʒiˈɔskəpi] *n* 毛细管显微镜检查

Microascaceae [ˌmaikrəuæsˈkeisiiː] *n* 微子囊菌科

Microascales [ˌmaikrəuæsˈkeiliːz] *n* 微子囊菌目

Microascus [ˌmaikrəuˈæskəs] *n* 微子囊菌属
Microbacterium [ˌmaikrəubækˈtiəriəm] *n* 微杆菌属,小细菌属 | ~ flavum 黄色微杆菌 / ~ lacticum 乳酸微杆菌
microbacterium [ˌmaikrəubækˈtiəriəm] ([复] **microbacteria** [ˌmaikrəubækˈtiəriə]) *n* 微杆菌;微生物
microbalance [ˈmaikrəuˌbæləns] *n* 微量天平
microbar [ˈmaikrəbɑː] *n* 微巴(旧压强单位, = 10^{-6}巴,现用 Pa 帕〈斯卡〉)
microbe [ˈmaikrəub] *n* 微生物 | **microbial** [maiˈkrəubiəl], **microbic** [maiˈkrəubik] *a* / **microbian** [maiˈkrəubiən] *a*, *n*
microbicide [maiˈkrəubisaid] *n* 杀微生物剂 | **microbicidal** [maiˌkrəubiˈsaidl] *a* 杀微生物的
microbioassay [ˌmaikrəuˌbaiəuˈæsei] *n* 微生物测定
microbiology [ˌmaikrəubaiˈɔlədʒi] *n* 微生物学 | **microbiologic(al)** [ˌmaikrəubaiəˈlɔdʒikəl] *a* / **microbiologist** *n* 微生物学家
microbiophotometer [ˌmaikrəuˌbaiəufəuˈtɔmətə] *n* 微生物浊度计
microbiota [ˌmaikrəubaiˈəutə] *n* 微生物区系,微生物丛
microbiotic [ˌmaikrəubaiˈɔtik] *a* 微生物区系的;微生物的
Microbispora [ˌmaikrəubaiˈspɔːrə] *n* 小双孢菌属
microblast [ˈmaikrəblæst] *n* 小成红血细胞(直径为 5 μm 或更小者)
microblepharia [ˌmaikrəubliˈfɛəriə], **microblepharism** [ˌmaikrəuˈblefərizəm], **microblepharon** [maikrəuˈblefərɔn], **microblephary** [ˌmaikrəuˈblefəri] *n* 小[眼]睑
microbody [ˌmaikrəˈbɔdi] *n* 微体(细胞)
microbrachia [ˌmaikrəuˈbreikiə] *n* 细臂,臂过小
microbrachius [ˌmaikrəuˈbreikiəs] *n* 细臂者
microbrenner [ˌmaikrəuˈbrenə] *n* 尖头电烙器
microbubble [ˈmaikrəuˌbʌbl] *n* 微泡
microburet [ˌmaikrəubjuəˈret] *n* 微量滴定管
microcalcification [ˌmaikrəuˌkælsifiˈkeiʃən] *n* 微钙化作用
microcalcificectomy [ˌmaikrəuˌkælsifiˈsektəmi] *n* 微钙化切除
microcalix, **microcalyx** [ˌmaikrəuˈkæliks] *n* 微肾盏
microcalorie, **microcalory** [ˌmaikrəuˈkæləri] *n* 小卡(使 1 ml 蒸馏水从 0 ℃上升到 1 ℃所需的热量)
microcannula [ˈmaikrəuˌkænjulə] *n* 微套管,微插管
microcardia [ˌmaikrəuˈkɑːdiə] *n* 心过小
microcaulia [ˌmaikrəuˈkɔːliə] *n* 小阴茎
microcentrum [ˌmaikrəuˈsentrəm] *n* 中心体
microcephalus [ˌmaikrəuˈsefələs] *n* 小头者
microcephaly [ˌmaikrəuˈsefəli], **microcephalia** [ˌmaikrəusəˈfeiliə], **microcephalism** [ˌmaikrəuˈsefəlizəm] *n* 小头,小头畸形 | **microcephalic** [ˌmaikrəusəˈfælik], **microcephalous** [ˌmaikrəuˈsefələs] *a*
microcheilia [ˌmaikrəuˈkailiə] *n* 小唇
microcheiria [ˌmaikrəuˈkaiəriə] *n* 小手畸形
microchemistry [ˌmaikrəuˈkemistri] *n* 微量化学 | **microchemical** *a*
microcinematography [ˌmaikrəuˌsiniməˈtɔgrəfi] *n* 显微电影术
microcirculation [ˌmaikrəuˌsəːkjuˈleiʃən] *n* 微循环(直径小于 100 μm 的微细血管中的血液循环)
microcirculatory [ˌmaikrəuˈsəːkjulətəri] *a* 微循环的
microclimate [ˌmaikrəuˈklaimit] *n* 微小气候(如指病媒昆虫的气候环境)
microclyster [ˌmaikrəuˈklistə] *n* 微量灌肠(小量直肠灌法)
microcnemia [ˌmaikrəuˈniːmiə] *n* 小腿过短
Micrococcaceae [ˌmaikrəukəˈkeisiiː] *n* 微球菌科
Micrococcus [ˌmaikrəuˈkɔkəs] *n* 微球菌属
micrococcus [ˌmaikrəuˈkɔkəs] ([复] **micrococci** [ˌmaikrəuˈkɔksai]) *n* 微球菌
microcolon [ˌmaikrəuˈkəulən] *n* 小结肠
microcolony [ˈmaikrəuˌkɔləni] *n* 小菌落,微菌落
microconcentration [ˌmaikrəuˌkɔnsənˈtreiʃən] *n* 微浓缩
microconidium [ˌmaikrəukəuˈnidiəm] ([复] **microconidia** [ˌmaikrəukəuˈnidiə]) *n* 小分生孢子
microcoria [ˌmaikrəuˈkɔːriə] *n* 小瞳孔
microcornea [ˌmaikrəuˈkɔːniə] *n* 小角膜
microcoulomb (μC) [ˌmaikrəuˈkuːlɔm] *n* 微库[仑](电量单位, -10^{-6}C)
microcoustic [ˌmaikrəuˈkuːstik] *a* 听弱声的 *n* 弱声助听器
microcrania [ˌmaikrəuˈkreiniə] *n* 小颅,颅过小(颅腔直径减少,而相对地面部过大)
microcrystal [ˌmaikrəuˈkristl] *n* 微晶
microcrystalline [ˌmaikrəuˈkristəlain, -lin] *a* 微晶的,细晶质的
microcurie (μCr) [ˌmaikrəuˈkjuəri] *n* 微居里(旧放射性强度单位, = 10^{-6}居里,或放射性物质在每秒内有 3.7×10^4 次核蜕变)
microcurie-hour (μC-hr) [ˌmaikrəuˈkjuəri ˌauə] *n* 微居里 1 小时(旧照射剂量单位,相当于在每秒 3.7×10^4 次原子蜕变的放射性物质下照射 1 小时的剂量)

Microcyclus [ˌmaikrəuˈsaikləs] *n* 微环菌属
microcyst [ˈmaikrəsist] *n* 微包囊
Microcystis [ˌmaikrəuˈsistis] *n* 微囊藻属
microcystometer [ˌmaikrəusisˈtɔmitə] *n* 袖珍膀胱内压测量器
microcytase [ˌmaikrəuˈsaiteis] *n* 小噬细胞消化酶
microcyte [ˈmaikrəsait] *n* 小红细胞(直径为 5 μm 或更小者) | **microcytic** [ˌmaikrəuˈsitik] *a*
microcythemia [ˌmaikrəusaiˈθiːmiə], **microcytosis** [ˌmaikrəusaiˈtəusis] *n* 小红细胞症
microcytotoxicity [ˌmaikrəuˌsaitəutɔkˈsisəti] *n* 微量细胞毒[性]
microdactyly [ˌmaikrəuˈdæktili], **microdactylia** [ˌmaikrəudækˈtiliə] *n* 小形指,小形趾
microdensitometer [ˌmaikrəuˌdensiˈtɔmitə] *n* 显微光密度计
microdermatome [ˌmaikrəuˈdəːmətəum] *n* 微[植]皮刀
microdetermination [ˌmaikrəudiˌtəːmiˈneiʃən] *n* 微量测定[法]
microdiskectomy [ˌmaikrəudisˈkektəmi] *n* 显微椎间盘切除术 | arthroscopic ~ 关节镜显微椎间盘切除术
microdissection [ˌmaikrəudiˈsekʃən] *n* 显微切割
microdont [ˈmaikrəudɔnt], **microdontous** [ˌmaikrəuˈdɔntəs] *a* 小牙的(牙指数在 42 以下)
microdontia [ˌmaikrəuˈdɔnʃiə], **microdentism** [ˌmaikrəuˈdentizəm], **microdontism** [ˌmaikrəuˈdɔntizəm] *n* 小牙,小牙症 | **microdontic** *a*
microdosage [ˈmaikrəuˌdəusidʒ] *n* 微小剂量
microdose [ˈmaikrədəus] *n* 微量,小量
microdrepanocytic [ˌmaikrəuˌdrepənəuˈsitik] *a* 小镰状细胞的
microdrepanocytosis [ˌmaikrəuˌdrepənəusaiˈtəusis] *n* 小镰状细胞病,镰状红细胞珠蛋白生成障碍性贫血[病]
microdysgenesia [ˌmaikrəudisdʒəˈniːziə] *n* 微发生不全(海马和小脑周围区神经元些微异常,见于癫痫病例)
microecology [ˌmaikrəuiˈkɔlədʒi] *n* 微观生态学(寄生物生态学的分支,研究寄生物与其宿主提供的环境之间的关系)
microecosystem [ˌmaikrəuˌiːkəuˈsistim] *n* 微生态系(自然的或为实验目的在实验室建立的微型生态系统)
microelectrode [ˌmaikrəuiˈlektrəud] *n* 微电极
microelectronics [ˌmaikrəuilekˈtrɔniks] *n* 微电子学 | **microelectronic** *a* 微电子[学]的
microelectrophoresis [ˌmaikrəuiˌlektrəufəˈriːsis] *n* [显]微电泳,微量电泳 | **microelectrophoretic** [ˌmaikrəuiˌlektrəufəˈretik] *a*
microelement [ˌmaikrəuˈelimənt] *n* 微量元素
Microellobosporia [ˌmaikrəuˌeləbɔˈspɔːriə] *n* 小荚孢囊菌属
microembolus [ˌmaikrəuˈembələs] ([复] **microemboli** [ˌmaikrəuˈembəlai]) *n* 微栓子
microencephaly [ˌmaikrəuenˈsefəli] *n* 脑过小
microenvironment [ˌmaikrəuinˈvaiərənmənt] *n* 微环境
microerythrocyte [ˌmaikrəuiˈriθrəsait] *n* 小红细胞
microestimation [ˌmaikrəuˌestiˈmeiʃən] *n* 微量测定[法]
microevolution [ˌmaikrəuˌiːvəˈljuːʃən] *n* 微观进化(从短期角度探讨生物进化的历程,常涉及物种的分化)
microfarad (μF) [ˌmaikrəuˈfærəd] *n* 微法[拉](电容单位,$=10^{-6}$ F)
microfauna [ˌmaikrəuˈfɔːnə] *n* 微动物区系(某一地区的仅在显微镜下能看到的极小的动物)
microfibril [ˌmaikrəuˈfaibril] *n* 微原纤维
microfilament [ˌmaikrəuˈfiləmənt] *n* 微丝(直径约 60 Å,见于细胞质基质)
microfilaremia [ˌmaikrəuˌfiləˈriːmiə] *n* 微丝蚴血症
microfilaria [ˌmaikrəufiˈlɛəriə] *n* 微丝蚴 | ~ bancrofti 班[克罗夫特]氏微丝蚴 / ~ diurna 昼现微丝蚴 / ~ streptocerca 旋盘尾微丝蚴
microfilm [ˈmaikrəfilm] *n* 显微胶片,小型胶片 *vt* 摄制显微胶片
microfilter [ˌmaikrəuˌfiltə] *n* 微滤器
microflora [ˌmaikrəuˈflɔːrə] *n* 微生物区系
microfluorometry [ˌmaikrəuˌfluəˈrɔmitri] *n* 显微荧光测定法(即细胞光度测定法 cytophotometry)
microfracture [ˌmaikrəuˈfræktʃə] *n* 小骨折
microgamete [ˌmaikrəuˈgæmiːt] *n* 小配子,雄配子
microgametocyte [ˌmaikrəugəˈmiːtəsait] *n* 小配子体,小配子细胞
microgametophyte [ˌmaikrəugəˈmiːtəfait] *n* 小配子体
microgamma [ˌmaikrəuˈgæmə] *n* 微微克,皮克(10^{-12} g,即 picogram)
microgamont [ˌmaikrəuˈgæmɔnt] *n* 小配子母细胞
microgamy [maiˈkrɔgəmi] *n* 小型配子结合
microgastria [ˌmaikrəuˈgæstriə] *n* 小胃,胃过小
microgenesis [ˌmaikrəuˈdʒenisis] *n* 矮小发育,发育过小
microgenia [ˌmaikrəuˈdʒeniə] *n* 小颏
microgenitalism [ˌmaikrəuˈdʒenitəlizəm] *n* 小生殖器,生殖器过小
microglia [maiˈkrɔgliə] *n* 小胶质[细胞] | **~l** *a*

microgliocyte [maiˈkrɔgliəusait], **microgliacyte** [maiˈkrɔgliəsait] *n* 小神经胶质细胞
microglioma [ˌmaikrəuglaiˈəumə] *n* 小神经胶质细胞瘤
microgliomatosis [ˌmaikrəuˌglaiəuməˈtəusis] *n* 小神经胶质细胞瘤病,脑网状细胞肉瘤
microglobulin [ˌmaikrəuˈglɔbjulin] *n* 微球蛋白
β_2-microglobulin [ˌmaikrəuˈglɔbjulin] *n* β_2-微球蛋白
microglossia [ˌmaikrəuˈglɔsiə] *n* 小舌
micrognathia [ˌmaikrəuˈneiθiə] *n* 小颌[症],小颌畸形
microgonioscope [ˌmaikrəuˈgəuniəskəup] *n* 前房角镜
microgram(μg) [ˈmaikrəgræm] *n* 微克(10^{-6}g)
micrograph [ˈmaikrəgrɑːf, -græf] *n* 微动描记器;显微照片 | electron ~ 电子显微照片
micrographia [ˌmaikrəuˈgræfiə] *n* 字体过小,细小字体
micrography [maiˈkrɔgrəfi] *n* 显微镜描记法;显微镜检查 | **micrographic** [ˌmaikrəuˈgræfik] *a*
microgyria [ˌmaikrəuˈdʒaiəriə] *n* 小脑回,多小脑回
microgyrus [ˌmaikrəuˈdʒaiərəs]([复] **microgyri** [ˌmaikrəuˈdʒaiərai]) *n* 小脑回
microhematocrit [ˌmaikrəuhiːˈmætəkrit] *n* 微量血细胞比容(用毛细管及高速离心机快速测定血细胞比容)
microhematuria [ˌmaikrəuˌhiːməˈtjuəriə] *n* 显微镜血尿
microhepatia [ˌmaikrəuhiˈpætiə] *n* 小肝
microhistology [ˌmaikrəuhisˈtɔlədʒi] *n* 显微组织学
microhm [ˈmaikrəum] *n* 微欧[姆](百万分之一欧姆)
microincineration [ˌmaikrəuinˌsinəˈreiʃən] *n* 微量灰化法(组织灰化后,从其灰烬中辨别其成分)
microinfarct [ˌmaikrəuˈinfɑːkt] *n* 微梗死
microinjector [ˌmaikrəuinˈdʒektə] *n* 微量注射器
microinterlock [ˌmaikrəuˈintəˌlɔk] *n* 微交锁
microinvasion [ˌmaikrəuinˈveiʒən] *n* 微管侵袭(指恶性细胞微小蔓延侵入原位癌邻近组织) | **microinvasive** [ˌmaikrəuinˈveisiv] *a*
microkeratome [ˌmaikrəuˈkerətəum] *n* 微角膜刀
microkinematography [ˌmaikrəuˌkiniməˈtɔgrəfi] *n* 显微电影摄影[术]
microlaminectomy [ˌmaikrəuˌlæmiˈnektəmi] *n* 椎板显微切除术
microlaparoscopy [ˌmaikrəuˌlæpəˈrɔskəpi] *n* 显微腹腔镜检查[术] | **microlaparoscopic** [ˌmaikrəuˌlæpərəˈskɔpik] *a*
microlaryngoscopy [ˌmaikrəuˌlæriŋˈgɔskəpi] *n* 显微喉镜检查
microleakage [ˌmaikrəuˈliːkədʒ] *n* 微漏(微量液体、碎屑和细菌漏入牙修复体或它的黏固粉与洞制备的邻近表面之间的显微间隙,也可能通过牙本质进入牙髓)
microlecithal [ˌmaikrəuˈlesiθəl] *a* 小[卵]黄的
microlentia [ˌmaikrəuˈlenʃiə] *n* 小晶状体
microlesion [ˌmaikrəuˈliːʒən] *n* 小损害,微小损伤
microleukoblast [ˌmaikrəuˈljuːkəblæst] *n* 成髓细胞,原[始]粒细胞
microliter(μl) [ˈmaikrəuˌliːtə] *n* 微升(千分之一毫升,或百万分之一升)
microlith [ˈmaikrəliθ] *n* 小结石,细石
microlithiasis [ˌmaikrəuliˈθaiəsis] *n* 微结石症 | ~ alveolaris pulmonum, pulmonary alveolar ~ 肺泡微结石症
micrology [maiˈkrɔlədʒi] *n* 显微学
microlymphoidocyte [ˌmaikrəulimˈfɔidəsait] *n* 小淋巴样细胞
micromandible [ˌmaikrəuˈmændibl] *n* 小颌,下颌过小
micromanipulation [ˌmaikrəuməˌnipjuˈleiʃən] *n* 显微操作
micromanipulator [ˌmaikrəuməˈnipjuˌleitə] *n* 显微操作器(一种显微镜附件)
micromanometer [ˌmaikrəuməˈnɔmitə] *n* 微量[液体]测压计 | **micromanometric** [ˌmaikrəumænəˈmetrik] *a* 微量[液体]测压的
micromastia [ˌmaikrəuˈmæstiə], **micromazia** [ˌmaikrəuˈmeiziə] *n* 乳房过小
micromaxilla [ˌmaikrəumækˈsilə] *n* 小上颌骨,上颌骨过小
micromegalopsia [ˌmaikrəuˌmegəˈlɔpsiə] *n* 视物显大显小交替症
micromelia [ˌmaikrəuˈmiːliə] *n* 细肢,小肢,四肢短小[畸形]
micromelus [maiˈkrɔmələs] *n* 细肢者,小肢者
micromere [ˈmaikrəmiə] *n* 小[分]裂球
micrometabolism [ˌmaikrəumeˈtæbəlizəm] *n* 微体[新陈]代谢
micrometastasis [ˌmaikrəumiˈtæstəsis] *n* 微转移 | **micrometastatic** [ˌmaikrəuˌmetəˈstætik] *a*
micrometeorology [ˌmaikrəuˌmiːtjəˈrɔlədʒi] *n* 微气象学,地面气象学
micrometer¹ [maiˈkrɔmitə] *n* 测微计 | diffraction ~ 眼晕测定器;红细胞折光晕测量器 / eyepiece ~, ocular ~ [接]目镜测微计 / filar ~ 螺旋测微计 / stage ~ (显微镜)镜台测微计
micrometer²(μm) [ˈmaikrəuˌmiːtə] *n* 微米(10^{-6}m)
micromethod [ˌmaikrəuˈmeθəd] *n* 微量法,微量

测定[法]

micrometry [maiˈkrɔmitri] *n* 测微法 | **micrometric(al)** [ˌmaikrəuˈmetrik(ə)l] *a*

micromicro- [前缀]微微(10^{-12},现改用皮[可] pico-,符号为 p)

micromicrocurie [ˌmaikrəuˌmaikrəuˈkjuəri] *n* 微微居里,皮居里(10^{-6} μCi,或 10^{-12} Ci)

micromicron [ˌmaikrəuˈmaikrɔn] *n* 微微米,皮米(10^{-6} μm,或 10^{-9} mm,或 10^{-12} m)

micromolar(μM) [ˌmaikrəuˈməulə] *a* 微摩尔的

micromolecular [ˌmaikrəuməuˈlekjulə] *a* 小分子的

Micromonospora [ˌmaikrəuməˈnɔspərə] *n* 小单孢菌属,单孢丝菌属 | ~ keratolyticum 溶角质小单孢菌 / ~ purpurea 紫色小单孢菌

Micromonosporaceae [ˌmaikrəuməuˌnɔspəˈreisiiː] *n* 小单孢菌科

micromonosporin [ˌmaikrəuməˈnɔspərin] *n* 单孢丝菌素,小单孢菌素

Micromyces [maiˈkrɔmisiːz] *n* 小霉菌属

micromyelia [ˌmaikrəumaiˈiːliə] *n* 小脊髓

micromyeloblast [ˌmaikrəuˈmaiələblæst], **micromyelolymphocyte** [ˌmaikrəuˌmaiələuˈlimfəsait] *n* 小成髓细胞,小骨髓淋巴细胞

micron(μ) [ˈmaikrɔn]([复] **microns** 或 **micra** [ˈmaikrə]) *n* 微米(10^{-3} mm,或 10^{-6} m,现为 micrometer 取代,符号为 μm)

microne [ˈmaikrəun] *n* 微粒(10^{-5} ~ 10^{-3} cm)

microneedle [ˌmaikrəuˈniːdl] *n* 显微操作针

Micronema [ˌmaikrəuˈniːmə] *n* 微线虫属

micronematous [ˌmaikrəuˈnemətəs] *a* 微丝的,微线体的

microneme [ˈmaikrəniːm] *n* 微丝,微线体,短丝

microneurography [ˌmaikrəunjuəˈrɔgrəfi] *n* 微神经学(用微电极研究个体神经纤维或纤维束的传导)

microneurosurgery [ˌmaikrəuˌnjuərəuˈsəːdʒəri] *n* 显微神经外科[学]

micronize [ˈmaikrənaiz] *vt* 微粉化

micronodular [ˌmaikrəuˈnɔdjulə] *a* 小结的

micronormoblast [ˌmaikrəuˈnɔːməblæst] *n* 小幼红细胞

micronucleus [ˌmaikrəuˈnjuːkliəs] *n* 小核,微核(纤毛虫细胞中形状较小的生殖核,区别于大形的营养核);核仁 | **micronuclear** [ˌmaikrəuˈnjuːkliə] *a*

micronutrient [ˌmaikrəuˈnjuːtriənt] *n* 微量营养

micronychia [ˌmaikrəuˈnikiə], **micronychosis** [ˌmaikrəuniˈkəusis] *n* 指甲过小,趾甲过小

micro-orchidia [ˌmaikrəuɔːˈkidiə], **micro-orchidism** [ˌmaikrəuˈɔːkidizəm] *n* 小睾丸

microorganism [ˌmaikrəuˈɔːgənizəm] *n* 微生物 | **microorganic** [ˌmaikrəuɔːˈgænik], **~al** [ˌmaikrəuɔːgəˈnizməl] *a*

microparasite [ˌmaikrəuˈpærəsait] *n* 微寄生物,寄生性微生物 | **microparasitic** [ˌmaikrəuˌpærəˈsitik] *a*

micropathology [ˌmaikrəupəˈθɔlədʒi] *n* 显微病理学;微生物病理学

micropenis [ˌmaikrəuˈpiːnis] *n* 小阴茎

microperfusion [ˌmaikrəupə(ː)ˈfjuːʒən] *n* 微量灌注

microphage [ˈmaikrəfeidʒ], **microphagocyte** [ˌmaikrəuˈfægəsait], **microphagus** [maiˈkrɔfəgəs] *n* 小噬细胞

microphakia [ˌmaikrəuˈfeikiə] *n* 小晶状体

microphallus [ˌmaikrəuˈfæləs] *n* 小阴茎

microphone [ˈmaikrəfəun] *n* 扩音器,传声器;微音器 | cardiac catheter- ~ 心音导管

microphonia [ˌmaikrəuˈfəuniə] *n* 声弱症

microphonic [ˌmaikrəˈfɔnik] *a* 传声的 *n* 耳蜗微音电位 | cochlear ~s 耳蜗微音效应,耳蜗微音电位

microphonograph [ˌmaikrəuˈfəunəgrɑːf] *n* 微音传声器(聋者学话用)

microphotograph [ˌmaikrəuˈfəutəgrɑːf] *n* 显微照片 | **~ic** [ˌmaikrəuˌfəutəˈgræfik] *a* / **~y** [ˌmaikrəufəˈtɔgrəfi] *n* 显微摄影术

microphthalmia [ˌmaikrɔfˈθælmiə] *n* 小眼,小眼畸形,小眼球

microphthalmos [ˌmaikrɔfˈθælməs] *n* 小眼

microphthalmoscope [ˌmaikrɔfˈθælməskəup] *n* 显微眼底镜

microphthalmus [ˌmaikrɔfˈθælməs] *n* 小眼,眼过小;小眼者

microphysics [ˌmaikrəuˈfiziks] *n* 微粒物理学

microphyte [ˈmaikrəfait] *n* 微[生]植物 | **microphytic** [ˌmaikrəuˈfitik] *a*

micropia [maiˈkrəupiə] *n* 视物显小症

micropinocytosis [ˌmaikrəuˌpainəusaiˈtəusis] *n* 微胞饮作用

micropipet(te) [ˌmaikrəupiˈpet] *n* 微量吸移管,微量移液管

micropituicyte [ˌmaikrəupiˈtju(ː)sait] *n* 小垂体[后叶]细胞

microplasia [ˌmaikrəuˈpleiziə] *n* 矮小,侏儒症

microplastocyte [ˌmaikrəuˈplæstəsait] *n* 小血小板

microplethysmography [ˌmaikrəuˌpleθisˈmɔgrəfi] *n* 微差体积描记法

micropodia [ˌmaikrəuˈpəudiə] *n* 小足,足过小

micropolariscope [ˌmaikrəupəuˈlæriskəup] *n* 偏振[光]显微镜

micropolygyria [ˌmaikrəuˌpɔliˈdʒaiəriə] *n* 小脑回,多小脑回

Micropolyspora [ˌmaikrəuˌpɔliˈspɔːrə] *n* 小多孢菌属 | ~ faeni 费[恩]氏小多孢菌

micropore [ˈmaikrəpɔː] *n* 微孔

microprecipitation [ˌmaikrəupriˌsipiˈteiʃən] *n* 微量沉淀[反应]

micropredation [ˌmaikrəuprəˈdeiʃən] *n* 依附寄生

micropredator [ˌmaikrəuˈpredətə] *n* 依附寄生物

microprint [ˈmaikrəprint] *n* 显微印制卡

microprobe [ˈmaikrəprəub] *n* [显]微探子(显微手术用) | laser ~ 激光[显]微探子,激光显微刀(显微手术用)

microprojection [ˌmaikrəuprəˈdʒekʃən] *n* 显微投影

microprojector [ˌmaikrəuprəˈdʒektə] *n* 显微投影器

microprolactinoma [ˌmaikrəuprəuˈlæktiˈnəumə] *n* 小泌乳素瘤,小催乳激素瘤

microprosopus [ˌmaikrəuprəˈsəupəs] *n* 小面者(胎儿)

micropsia [maiˈkrɔpsiə] *n* 视物显小症 | **microptic** [maiˈkrɔptik] *a*

micropuncture [ˈmaikrəuˌpʌŋktʃə] *n* 微穿刺;微穿刺术

micropus [maiˈkrəupəs] *n* 小足者

micropyle [ˈmaikrəpail] *n* 卵孔,珠孔 | **micropylar** [ˌmaikrəuˈpailə] *a*

microradiogram [ˌmaikrəuˈreidiəgræm] *n* 显微放射照片,X线放大摄影[照]片

microradiography [ˌmaikrəuˌreidiˈɔgrəfi] *n* 显微放射摄影[术],X线放大摄影[术]

microrchidia [ˌmaikrɔːˈkidiə] *n* 小睾丸

microrefractometer [ˌmaikrəuˌriːfrækˈtɔmitə] *n* 显微折射计

microrespirometer [ˌmaikrəuˌrespiˈrɔmitə] *n* 微量呼吸计

microrhinia [ˌmaikrəuˈriniə] *n* 小鼻

microroentgen (μR) [ˌmaikrəuˈrɔntjən, ˌmaikrəuˈrentgən] *n* 微伦琴(百万分之一伦琴)

microscelous [maiˈkrɔskələs] *a* 短腿的

Microscilla [ˌmaikrəuˈsilə] *n* 微颤菌属

microscler [ˈmaikrəskliə] *a* 长形的

microscope [ˈmaikrəskəup] *n* 显微镜 | acoustic ~ 声学显微镜 / beta ray ~ β[射]线显微镜 / binocular ~ 双目显微镜,双筒显微镜 / capillary ~ 毛细血管显微镜 / color-contrast ~ 色对比显微镜 / comparison ~ 比较显微镜 / compound ~ 复式显微镜 / dark-field ~ 暗视野显微镜 / electron ~ 电[子显微]镜 / epic ~ 不透明显微镜 / fluorescence ~ 荧光显微镜 / hypodermic ~ 皮下显微镜 / infrared ~ 红外光显微镜 / integrating ~ 累计显微镜 / interference ~ 干涉显微镜 / ion ~ 离子显微镜 / laser ~ 激光显微镜 / light ~ 光学显微镜 / operating ~ 手术显微镜 / phase ~, phase-contrast ~ 相差显微镜 / polarizing ~ 偏振光显微镜 / projection X-ray ~ 投影[式]X线显微镜 / rectified polarizing ~ 校正偏振光显微镜 / reflecting ~ 反射显微镜 / scanning ~, scanning electron ~ 扫描显微镜,扫描电[子显微]镜 / schlieren ~ 纹影显微镜(显示标本中折射率的差异) / simple ~ 单式显微镜 / slit lamp ~ 裂隙灯显微镜 / stereoscopic ~ 实体显微镜,双目显微镜 / stroboscopic ~ 动态显微镜 / transmission electron ~ 透射电子显微镜,透视电镜 / trinocular ~ 三目显微镜 / ultra ~ 超显微镜 / ultrasonic ~ 超声显微镜 / ultraviolet ~ 紫外光显微镜 / X-ray ~ X线显微镜

microscopic [ˌmaikrəsˈkɔpik] *a* 显微的,用显微镜可见的;显微镜的,显微镜检查的

microscopical [ˌmaikrəsˈkɔpikəl] *a* 微观的,用显微镜可见的;显微镜的,显微镜检查的

microscopist [maiˈkrɔskəpist] *n* 显微镜学家,显微镜工作者

microscopy [maiˈkrɔskəpi] *n* 显微镜检查,显微术 | clinical ~ 临床显微镜检查 / electron ~ 电子显微镜术 / fluorescence ~ 荧光显微术 / fundus ~ 眼底显微镜检查 / immunofluorescent ~ 免疫荧光显微术 / television ~ 电视显微术

microsecond (μs) [ˈmaikrəuˌsekənd] *n* 微秒(百万分之一秒)

microsection [ˌmaikrəuˈsekʃən] *n* 显微切片

microseme [ˈmaikrəsiːm] *a* 小眼型的(眼眶指数在83或83以下)

microshock [ˈmaikrəuˌʃɔk] *n* 弱电流休克(心脏病学使用的术语,表示直接用于心肌组织的低电平电流;小到0.1 mA就能引起心室纤颤)

Microsiphonales [ˌmaikrəuˌsaifəˈneiliːz] *n* 发癣菌目

microslide [ˈmaikrəslaid] *n* 显微镜玻片,载玻片

microsmatic [ˌmaikrɔsˈmætik] *a* 嗅觉减退的

microsoma [ˌmaikrəuˈsəumə] *n* 矮小(身材矮小,但非侏儒)

microsome [ˈmaikrəsəum] *n* 微粒体 | **microsomal** [ˌmaikrəuˈsəuməl] *a*

microsomia [ˌmaikrəuˈsəumiə], **microsomatia** [ˌmaikrəusəˈmeiʃiə] *n* 矮小(身材)

microspectrophotometer [ˌmaikrəuˌspektrəufəˈtɔmitə] *n* 显微分光光度计

microspectroscope [ˌmaikrəuˈspektrəskəup] *n* 显微分光镜

microsphere [maikrəˈsfiə] *n* 微球

microspherocyte [ˌmaikrəuˈsfiərəsait] *n* 小球形红细胞
microspherocytosis [ˌmaikrəuˌsfiərəsaiˈtəusis] *n* 小球形红细胞症
microspherolith [ˌmaikrəuˈsfiərəliθ] *n* 小球状石
microsphygmia [ˌmaikrəuˈsfigmiə], **microsphygmy** [ˌmaikrəuˈsfigmi] *n* 微脉,细脉
Microspira [ˌmaikrəuˈspaiərə] *n* 小螺旋菌属
Microspironema [ˌmaikrəuˌspaiərəˈniːmə] *n* 密螺旋体属
microsplanchnic [ˌmaikrəuˈsplæŋknik], **microsplanchnous** [ˌmaikrəuˈsplæŋknəs] *a* 小内脏型的(体型)
microsplenia [ˌmaikrəuˈspliːniə] *n* 小脾,脾过小 | **microsplenic** [ˌmaikrəuˈspliːnik] *a*
Microspora [maiˈkrɔspərə] *n* 微孢子门
microsporangium [ˌmaikrəuspəˈrændʒiəm], ([复] **microsporangia** [ˌmaikrəuspəˈrændʒiə]) *n* 小孢子囊
microspore [ˈmaikrəspɔː] *n* 小孢子 | **microsporic** [ˌmaikrəuˈspɔːrik] *a*
Microsporea [ˌmaikrəuˈspɔːriə] *n* 微孢子纲
microsporid [maiˈkrɔspərid] *n* 小孢子菌疹
Microsporida [ˌmaikrəuˈspɔːridə] *n* 微孢子目
microsporidan [ˌmaikrəuˈspɔːridən] *n* 微孢子虫;微孢子门原虫 *a* 微孢子门原虫的
Microsporidia [ˌmaikrəuspəˈridiə] *n* 微孢子目
microsporidia [ˌmaikrəuspəˈridiə] *n* 微孢子虫
microsporidian [ˌmaikrəuspəˈridiən] *n* 微孢子虫;微孢子目原虫 *a* 微孢子目原虫的
Microsporon [maiˈkrɔspərɔn] *n* 小孢子菌属
microsporophyll [ˌmaikrəˈspɔːrəfil] *n* 小孢子叶
microsporosis [ˌmaikrəuspəˈrəusis] *n* 小孢子菌病
Microsporum [maiˈkrɔspərəm] *n* 小孢子菌属 | ~ audouini 奥杜安小孢子菌 / ~ canis, ~ felineum, ~ lanosum 犬小孢子菌,猫小孢子菌,羊毛状小孢子菌 / ~ furfur 糠秕小孢子菌 / ~ gypseum 石膏样小孢子菌
microstat [ˈmaikrəstæt] *n* 显微镜[载物]台
microsteatosis [ˌmaikrəuˌstiːəˈtəusis] *n* 小脂肪变性
microsthenic [ˌmaikrəuˈsθenik] *a* 肌力弱的
microstomia [ˌmaikrəuˈstəumiə] *n* 小口,小口畸形
microstrabismus [ˌmaikrəustrəˈbizməs] *n* 微斜视
microsurgery [ˌmaikrəuˈsəːdʒəri] *n* 显微外科 | **microsurgical** [ˌmaikrəuˈsəːdʒikəl] *a*
microsyringe [ˌmaikrəuˈsirindʒ] *n* 微量注射器
Microtatobiotes [ˌmaikrəuˌteitəubaiˈəutiːz] *n* 最小微生物纲(包含立克次体目、病毒目)
microtechnic [ˌmaikrəuˈteknik] *n* 显微技术
microthelia [ˌmaikrəuˈθiːliə] *n* 小乳头
Microthoracina [ˌmaikrəuθɔːˈræsinə] *n* 小胸虫亚目
microthrombosis [ˌmaikrəuθrɔmˈbəusis] *n* 小血栓形成
microthrombus [ˌmaikrəuˈθrɔmbəs] *n* 微血栓
microtia [maiˈkrəuʃiə] *n* 小耳,小耳畸形
microtiter [ˌmaikrəuˈtaitə] *n* 微量滴定
microtome [ˈmaikrətəum] *n* 切片机(将组织切成薄片,供显微镜研究用) | freezing ~ 冷冻切片机 / rocking ~ 摇动切片机 / rotary ~ 轮转切片机 / sliding ~ 滑动切片机
microtomy [maiˈkrɔtəmi] *n* 组织切片术
microtonometer [ˌmaikrəutəuˈnɔmitə] *n* 微测压计(测定动脉血液中氧和二氧化碳张力)
microtransfusion [ˌmaikrəutrænsˈfjuːʒən] *n* 少[量]输血
microtrauma [ˌmaikrəuˈtrɔːmə] *n* 轻[外]伤,微伤
Microtrombidium akamushi [ˌmaikrəutrɔmˈbidiəm ækəˈmuʃiː] 红恙螨(即 Trombicula akamushi)
microtron [ˈmaikrətrɔn] *n* 电子回旋加速器
microtropia [ˌmaikrəuˈtrəupiə] *n* 微斜视
microtubule [ˌmaikrəuˈtjuːbjuːl] *n* 微管(许多能运动的细胞,尤其是红细胞胞质基质内的长而空的柱状结构,在有丝分裂纺锤体中发现有微管) | subpellicular ~ 表膜下微管
Microtus [maiˈkrəutəs] *n* 田鼠属 | ~ montebelli 野田鼠
microtus [maiˈkrəutəs] *n* 小耳者,耳过小者
microunit(μU) [ˈmaikrəˌjuːnit] *n* 微单位(百万分之一〈10^{-6}〉标准单位)
microvascular [ˌmaikrəuˈvæskjulə] *a* 微血管的,微脉管的
microvasculature [ˌmaikrəuˈvæskjulətʃə] *n* 微脉管系统
microvasculopathy [ˌmaikrəuˌvæskjuˈlɔpəθi] *n* 微血管系统病
microvessel [ˈmaikrəuˌvesəl] *n* 微血管
microvillus [ˌmaikrəuˈviləs] ([复] **microvilli** [ˌmaikrəuˈvilai]) *n* 微绒毛(细胞游离表面的微小突起)
microviscosimeter [ˌmaikrəuˌviskəuˈsimitə] *n* 微量黏度计
microvivisection [ˌmaikrəuˌviviˈsekʃən] *n* 显微活体解剖
microvolt(μV) [ˈmaikrəvəult] *n* 微伏[特](百万分之一伏特)
microvoltometer [ˌmaikrəuvəulˈtɔmitə] *n* 微电位计,微伏计

microvolumetry [ˌmaikrəuvɔˈljuːmitri] *n* 微容量计数法
microwatt(μW) [ˈmaikrəwɔt] *n* 微瓦[特](百万分之一瓦特)
microwave [ˈmaikrəweiv] *n* 微波
microxycyte [maiˈkrɔksisait], **microxyphil** [maiˈkrɔksifil] *n* 小嗜酸细胞
microzoaria [ˌmaikrəuzəuˈɛəriə] *n* 微生物(统称)
microzoon [ˌmaikrəuˈzəuɔn] ([复] **microzoa** [ˌmaikrəuˈzəuə]) *n* 微[生]动物
micrurgy [ˈmaikrəːdʒi] *n* 显微手术,显微操作术 | **micrurgic** [maiˈkrəːdʒik] *a* 显微操作的
Micruroides [ˌmaikruəˈrɔidiːz] *n* 拟小尾眼镜蛇属
Micrurus [maiˈkruərəs] *n* 小尾眼镜蛇属,珊瑚毒蛇属
miction [ˈmikʃən] *n* 排尿
micturate [ˈmiktjuəreit] *vi* 排尿 | **micturition** [ˌmiktjuəˈriʃən] *n*
MID minimum infective dose 最小感染量
midabdomen [midˈæbdəmən] *n* 中腹,中腹部
midaflur [ˈmaidəfljuː] *n* 咪达氟(镇静药)
midaxilla [ˌmidækˈsilə] *n* 腋窝中点,腋中
midazolam [ˈmideizəˌlæm] *n* 咪达唑仑(苯〈并〉二氮䓬类安定药) | ~ maleate 马来酸咪达唑仑(苯〈并〉二氮䓬类镇静药,用于诱导麻醉,静脉内给药)
midbody [ˈmidˌbɔdi] *n* 中体,中间体(有丝分裂后期纺锤体赤道区形成的颗粒体;亦指躯干中区)
midbrain [ˈmidˌbrein] *n* 中脑
midcarpal [midˈkɑːpl] *a* 腕骨间的
Middeldorpf's triangle (splint) [ˈmidəldɔːpf] (Albrecht T. Middeldorpf) 米德尔多夫三角(夹板)(三角形夹板,用于肱骨骨折)
middiastolic [ˌmiddaiəˈstɔlik] *a* 中1/3舒张期的
middlepiece [ˈmidlpiːs] *n* 中段(精子头和尾之间的部分)
midepigastrium [ˈmidˌepiˈgæstriəm] *n* 腹中上部
midface [ˈmidˌfeis] *n* 面中部(包括鼻、鼻根和眉间)
midfoot [ˈmidfut] *n* 足中段(包括舟骨、骰骨和楔骨部分)
midfrontal [midˈfrʌntl] *a* 额中[部]的
midge [midʒ] *n* 蠓,蚋 | owl ~ 白蛉
midget [ˈmidʒit] *n* 躯体矮小,正常侏儒
midgetism [ˈmidʒitizəm] *n* 侏儒症
midgut [ˈmidˌgʌt] *n* 中肠
mid-line [ˈmidlain] *n* 中线
midoccipital [ˌmidɔkˈsipitl] *a* 枕中[部]的
midodrine hydrochloride [ˈmaidəudriːn] 盐酸米多君(升压药)
midpain [ˈmidˌpein] *n* 经间痛
midperiphery [ˌmidpeˈrifəri] *n* 视网膜赤道部
midpiece [ˈmidpiːs] *n* 补体中段(在早期免疫学说中指豚鼠血清的优球蛋白部分,相当于补体的C1部分);[尾]中段
midplane [ˈmidˌplein] *n* 正中平面(盆腔中段平面)
midriff [ˈmidrif] *n* 膈
midsection [midˈsekʃən] *n* 正中切开
midsternum [midˈstəːnəm] *m* 胸骨体
midstream [ˈmidstriːm] *n* 中流;中段
midtarsal [midˈtɑːsəl] *a* 跗骨间的
midtegmentum [ˌmidtegˈmentəm] *n* 被盖中部
midwife [ˈmidwaif] ([复] **midwives** [ˈmidwaivz]) *n* 助产士,接生员 | **~ry** [ˈmidwifəri] *n* 助产学,产科学
Mierzejewski effect [ˌmiəziˈjefski] (Jan L. Mierzejewski) 米尔泽耶夫斯基效应(脑灰质及白质的不对称性发育,灰质过多)
Miescheria [miːˈʃiəriə] (J. F. Miescher) *n* 米舍尔肉孢子虫属
Miescher's granuloma [ˈmiːʃə] (Guido Miescher) 米舍尔肉芽肿(光线性肉芽肿) | ~ granulomatous cheilitis 米舍尔肉芽肿唇炎
Miescher's tubule, tube [ˈmiːʃə] (Johann F. Miescher) 米舍尔小管、管,肉孢子虫囊
MIF melanocyte-stimulating hormone inhibiting factor 促黑[素细胞]激素抑制因子; migration inhibiting factor 移动抑制因子
mifepristone [ˌmifəˈpristəun] *n* 米非司酮(抗孕激素药)
miglitol [ˈmiglitɔl] *n* 米格列醇(抗糖尿病药)
migraine [ˈmiːgrein, ˈmaigrein] *n* 偏头痛 | abdominal ~ 腹型偏头痛 / fulgurating ~ 闪电状偏头痛 / ophthalmic ~ 眼型偏头痛 / ophthalmoplegic ~ 眼肌麻痹性[周期性]偏头痛 | **migrainous** [ˈmaigreinəs] *a*
migraineur [ˌmiːgreiˈnəː] *n* 【法】偏头痛病人
migrainoid [ˈmaigrənɔid] *a* 类偏头痛的
migrate [maiˈgreit] *vi* 迁移;移动;移行,游走 | **migration** [maiˈgreiʃən] *n*
migrateur [ˌmiːgrəˈtəː] *n* 【法】流浪癖者
migratory [ˈmaigrətəri] *a* 迁移的;移动的;移行的,游走的
Migula's classification [ˈmigulə] (Walter Migula) 米古拉细菌分类法
Mikania [miˈkeiniə] (J. G. Mikan) 薇甘菊属
Mikulicz's cells [ˈmikjulitʃ] (Johann von Mikulicz-Radecki) 米库利奇细胞,鼻硬结细胞(内含鼻硬结杆菌,亦称泡沫细胞) | ~ angle 米库利奇角(由两平面形成的角,一经股骨骺长轴,另一经股骨干长轴,该角正常为130°,亦称偏角或偏倾角) / ~ clamp 米库利奇结肠夹(钳)(袋形

缝术后压碎结肠近段和远段之间的中隔所使用的夹) / ~ disease (syndrome) 米库利奇病(综合征)(原指泪腺及涎腺慢性良性炎症性肿大,有人扩大此病范围,即泪腺及涎腺肿大,伴其他疾病如 Sjögren 综合征、结节病、红斑狼疮、白血病及结核病,并称之为米库利奇综合征) / ~ drain 米库利奇引流敷料 / ~ operation 米库利奇手术(①胸锁乳突肌切除术,治疗斜颈;②见 Heineke-Mikulicz pyloroplasty;③跗骨切除术;④分期肠切除术) / ~ pad 米库利奇垫(纱布折成的垫,用于外科手术)

milammeter [mi'læmitə] *n* 毫安[培]计

Milch's method ['miltʃ] 米尔奇法(前肩关节脱位闭合复位术)

mildew ['mildjuː] *n* 霉;植物霉病

milenperone [mi'lenpərəun] *n* 咪仑哌隆(安定药)

Miles' operation [mailz] (William E. Miles) 迈尔斯手术(腹部会阴直肠癌切除术)

milfoil ['milfɔil] *n* 洋蓍草

milia ['miliə] milium 的复数

Milian's erythema [miː'ljɑːn] (Gaston A. Milian) 米利安红斑(注射胂凡纳明后 7 ~ 9 天所引起的猩红热样疹,伴不适和发热) | ~ sign 米利安征(头部及面部的皮下炎症不犯耳部,而皮肤病可犯耳部)

miliaria [ˌmili'ɛəriə] *n* 痱 | ~ crystallina, ~ alba 白痱 / ~ rubra 红痱

miliary ['miliəri] *a* 粟粒状的,粟粒性的

milieu [mi'ljuː] *n*【法】周围,环境 | ~ extérieur 外环境 / ~ intérieur 内环境(指细胞周围的血液和淋巴)

Miliolina [ˌmiliə'lainə] *n* 粟虫亚目

milipertine [mili'pəːtiːn] *n* 米利哌汀(安定药)

military ['militəri] *a* 军事的

milium ['miliəm] ([复] **milia** ['miliə]) *n*【拉】粟丘疹 | colloid ~ 胶样粟丘疹 / milia neonatorum 新生儿粟丘疹

milk [milk] *n* 乳,奶;牛奶;乳状物;乳剂 | acidophilus ~ 酸乳 / adapted ~ 适应乳(适于婴儿消化的) / certified ~ 给证牛乳 / condensed ~ 炼乳 / diabetic ~ 低乳糖乳 / dialyzed ~ 透析乳 / fortified ~ 强化乳(加乳脂或蛋白的乳) / grade A ~ 甲级乳 / homogenized ~ 匀脂乳 / laboratory ~ 配方乳 / litmus ~ 石蕊乳(细菌培养基) / metallized ~ 金属强化乳 / modified ~ 加工乳(使成分与人乳近似) / perhydrase ~ 过氧化氢乳 / skimmed ~ 脱脂乳 / uviol ~ 紫外线消毒乳 / vegetable ~ 植物合成乳 / virgin's ~ 铅乳(碱式醋酸铅与牛乳合成的洗剂) / witch's ~ 新生儿乳,婴乳

milking ['milkiŋ] *n* 挤奶;挤出(从管道中挤出,如用手指沿尿道向外挤压)

milk-leg ['milkleg] *n* 股白肿;产后髂股栓塞性静脉炎

Milkman's syndrome ['milkmæn] (Louis A. Milkman) 米尔克曼综合征(一种全身性骨病,特征为长扁骨内有多发性透明吸收带)

milkpox ['milkpɔks] *n* 乳白痘,类天花

milksick ['milksik] *n* 白蛇根中毒

milkweed ['milkwiːd] *n* 马利筋(马利筋属〈Asclepias〉的任何植物)

milkwort ['milkwɔːt] *n* 远志(远志属〈Polygala〉的任何植物)

milky ['milki] *a* 乳汁的;牛奶的;乳状的;乳色的

Millard-Gubler syndrome (paralysis) [mi'jɑː 'gublə] (Auguste L. J. Millard; Adolphe M. Gubler) 米亚尔-居布勒综合征(麻痹)(影响身体一侧肢体及对侧面神经的交叉性麻痹,伴眼外展运动麻痹,系脑桥梗死所致)

Millard's test ['miləd] (Henry B. Millard) 米勒德试验(检白蛋白)

Millar's asthma ['milə] (John Millar) 喘鸣性喉痉挛

Miller-Abbott tube ['milə 'æbət] (T. Grier Miller; William O. Abbott) 米-艾管(一种双腔肠管,用于治疗小肠梗阻,有时亦用于诊断)

Miller-Dieker syndrome ['milə 'diːkə] (James Q. Miller; H. Dieker) 米-迪综合征(一种常染色体隐性遗传综合征,特征为无脑回[畸形]、小头[畸形]、精神发育迟缓、面部呈畸形以及有时为多指(趾)畸形、隐睾[症]、心脏损害、肾脏缺损和胃肠系统缺损。亦称无脑回综合征)

Miller-Fisher syndrome ['milə 'fiʃə] (C. Miller Fisher) 米-费综合征(见 Fisher's syndrome)

Miller syndrome ['milə] (Marvin Miller) 米勒综合征(广泛性面部和肢体缺陷综合征,特征为颧骨发育不全、斜下睑裂、小颌、唇腭裂、杯形耳、下睑外翻、轴后肢缺乏及并指〈趾〉畸形。心脏缺陷和耳聋并不常见。本综合征可能是常染色体隐性性状。亦称轴后肢体面骨骨发育不全)

milli- [前缀]毫,千分之一(符号为 m)

milliammeter [mili'æmitə], **milliamperemeter** [ˌmili'æmpɛəmitə] *n* 毫安[培]计

milliampere (mA) [ˌmili'æmpɛə] *n*【法】毫安[培](千分之一安培)

milliampere-minute [ˌmili'æmpɛə 'minit] *n* 毫安[培]分(电量单位,每分钟输出 1 mA 电流)

millibar ['milibɑː] *n* 毫巴(千分之一巴)

millicoulomb (mC) [ˌmili'kuːlɔm] *n* 毫库仑(电量单位,$=10^{-3}$ C)

millicurie (mCi) ['miliˌkjuəri] *n* 毫居里(旧放射能量单位,$=10^{-3}$ Ci,或放射性物质量单位,其核蜕变数为每秒 3.7×10^{7} 次)

millicurie-hour [ˈmiliˌkjuəri ˌhauə] *n* 毫居里小时(累积放射能量单位)
milliequivalent(mEq) [ˌmiliiˈkwivələnt] *n* 毫[克]当量
milligamma [ˌmiliˈgæmə] *n* 毫微克,纳克(即 nanogram, ng)
milligram(mg) [ˈmiligræm] *n* 毫克(千分之一克)
Millikan rays [ˈmilikən] (Robert A. Millikan)宇宙线
Millikan-Siekert syndrome [ˈmiləkən ˈsiːkəːt] (Clark H. Millikan; Robert G. Siekert)米-西综合征,椎动脉及基底动脉功能不全
millilambert [ˈmiliˌlæmbət] *n* 毫朗伯(旧亮度单位,千分之一朗伯,现用 cd 坎[德拉])
milliliter(ml) [ˈmiliˌliːtə] *n* 毫升(千分之一升)
millimeter(mm) [ˈmiliˌmiːtə] *n* 毫米(千分之一米)
millimicr(o)- [前缀]毫微,纳(用 10^{-9} 来表示,现由前缀 nano-所取代,符号为 n)
millimicrocurie [ˌmiliˌmaikrəuˈkjuəri] *n* 毫微居里,纳居里(10^{-9}Ci, nCi)
millimicrogram [ˌmiliˈmaikrəgræm] *n* 毫微克,纳克(10^{-9}g, ng)
millimicroliter [ˌmilimaiˈkrɔliːtə] *n* 毫微升,纳升(10^{-9}L, nl)
millimicrometer [ˌmilimaiˈkrɔmitə] *n* 毫微米,纳米(10^{-9}m, nm)
millimolar(mM) [ˌmiliˈməulə] *a* 毫摩尔的
millimole(mmol) [ˈmiliməul] *n* 毫摩尔,毫模
milling-in [ˈmiliŋ-in] *n* 研磨
Millin operation [ˈmilin] (Terence J. Millin)米林手术(以前根治性耻骨后前列腺切除术常用方法)
millinormal [ˌmiliˈnɔːməl] *a* 毫当量的,千分之一当量的
millions [ˈmiljənz] *n* 食孑孓鱼,百万鱼
milliosmole(mOsm) [ˌmiliˈɔzməul, -ˈɔs-] *n* 毫渗模,毫渗量,毫渗摩尔
millipede [ˈmilipiːd] *n* 千足虫
milliphot [ˈmilifɔt] *n* 毫辐透(旧照度单位, =0.001 ph,约 1 英尺烛光)
millirad(mrad) [ˈmiliræd] *n* 毫拉德(旧辐射剂量单位, $=10^{-3}$rad)
millirem(mrem) [ˈmilirem] *n* 毫雷姆(旧吸收剂量单位)
milliroentgen(mR) [ˈmilirɔntjən, ˈmilirentgən] *n* 毫伦琴(剂量单位, $=10^{-3}$伦琴)
millisecond(ms) [ˈmiliˌsekənd] *n* 毫秒(千分之一秒)
milliunit(mU) [ˈmiliˌjuːnit] *n* 毫单位(千分之一单位)
millivolt(mV) [ˈmilivəult] *n* 毫伏(特)(千分之一伏特)
Millon's test(reaction, reagent) [ˈmilɔn] (Auguste N. E. Millon)米隆试验(反应、试剂)(检蛋白质及含氮化合物)
Mills' disease [milz] (Charles K. Mills)米尔斯病,上行性偏瘫(最终发展成四肢麻痹,其病因不明)
Mills-Reincke phenomenon [milz ˈrainkə] (Hiram F. Mills; J. J. Reincke)米尔斯-赖因克现象(净化用水后一切疾病的死亡率均降低)
milphae [ˈmilfiː], **milphosis** [milˈfəusis] *n* 眉毛脱落;睫毛脱落
milrinone [ˈmilrinəun] *n* 米力农(强心药)
Milroy's disease(edema) [ˈmilrɔi] (William F. Milroy)米尔罗伊病(水肿)(先天性遗传性下肢淋巴水肿)
Milton's edema [ˈmiltən] (John L. Milton)血管神经性水肿
milzbrand [ˈmiltsbrɑːnt] *n* 炭疽(anthrax 的旧称)
Mima polymorpha [ˈmiːmə ˌpɔliˈmɔːfə] 多形模仿菌(即醋酸钙不动杆菌 Acinetobacter calcoaceticus)
mimbane hydrochloride [ˈmimbein] 盐酸米姆本(镇痛药)
mimesis [miˈmiːsis, mai-] *n* 模仿,模拟;拟态;疾病模仿 | **mimetic** [miˈmetik, mai-] *a*
-mimetic [构词成分]拟
mimetism [ˈmimitizəm] *n* 拟态,模仿性
mimic [ˈmimik] *a* 模仿的,模拟的;拟态的;模仿疾病的
mimicry [ˈmimikri] *n* 模仿;拟态(一种动物和另一种动物的外表的相似性)
mimmation [miˈmeiʃən] *n* m 音滥用
mimosis [miˈməusis, mai] *n* 模拟;拟态;疾病模仿
min. minimum【拉】最小,最低,极小;最低点;最小量,最低量,最低数
Minamata disease [ˌmiːnɑːˈmɑːtɑː] 水俣病(烷基汞中毒所致的一种严重的神经疾病,其特征一般为周围及口周感觉异常、共济失调、构语困难和周边视觉丧失,并导致严重永久性神经病和精神病或死亡。1953～1958 年间日本水俣湾海洋食物含大量烷基汞化合物,食用后即得此病)
mind [maind] *n* 精神;意识;意识形态
mineral [ˈminərəl] *n* 矿[物]质;无机物 *a* 矿[物]质的;无机的 | ~ acid 矿物酸;无机酸
mineralize [ˈminərəlaiz] *vt* 使矿物化;使含无机化合物 | **mineralization** [ˌminərəlaiˈzeiʃən, -riˈz-] *n* 矿化[作用];供给矿质[法]
mineralocorticoid [ˌminərələuˈkɔːtikɔid] *n* 盐皮

质[激]素

Minerva jacket [mi'nəːvə] (Minerva 为罗马智慧女神,此背心酷似她的盔甲,故名)密涅瓦背心(一种煅石膏背心,包括躯干和头,耳、面在外,用于颈椎骨折和斜颈手术后)

mini- [构词成分]极小的,微型的

minify ['minifai] *vt* 缩减,缩小 | **minification** [ˌminifi'keiʃən] *n*

minilaparoscopy [ˌminiˌlæpə'rɔskəpi] *n* 小型腹腔镜检查[术] | **minilaparoscopic** [ˌminiˌlæpərə'skɔpik] *a*

minilaparotomy [ˌminiˌlæpə'rɔtəmi] *n* 小切口开腹术

minim(m.) ['minim] *n* 量滴(旧液量单位,=1/60 液量打兰,或 0.061 6 ml);微小物 *a* 微小的,最小的

minimal ['miniməl] *a* 最低限度的,最小的

minimum ['miniməm] ([复] **minima** ['minimə]) *n*【拉】最小[量],最低[量] *a* 最小的,最低的 | ~ audibile, ~ audible [最小]听阈 / ~ cognoscibile 最小辨视阈 / ~ legibile 最小明视阈 / light ~, ~ visibile 最小明视光度 / ~ sensibile 意识阈,知觉阈 / ~ separable 最小辨距阈

Minin light ['minin] (A. V. Minin)米宁灯(一种治疗用灯,所发出的光可作紫光与紫外线治疗)

minipill ['minipil] *n* 小丸剂(仅含孕酮的避孕丸)

miniplate ['minipleit] *n* 小骨板

Minisporida [ˌmini'spɔːridə] *n* 小孢子目

minium ['miniəm] *n*【拉】铅丹,四氧化铅,红铅

Minkowski-Chauffard syndrome [min'kɔvski ʃəu'fɑː] (Oskar Minkowski; Anatole-Marie-Emile Chauffard)遗传性球形红细胞症

Minkowski's figure [min'kɔvski] (Oskar Minkowski)明科夫斯基值(用数字表示纯肉食时尿中葡萄糖与氮之比,禁食时为 2.8∶1) | ~ method 明科夫斯基法(用气体扩张结肠后,进行肾触诊检查)

minocycline [minəu'saiklain, -kliːn] *n* 米诺环素(抗生素类药) | ~ hydrochloride 盐酸米诺环素(抗生素类药)

Minor's disease ['minɔː] (Lazar S. Minor)米诺尔病(中央性脊髓出血) | ~ sign 米诺尔征(坐骨神经痛病人由坐位起立时,以健侧支撑身体,一手置于背后,弯曲患腿,并以健腿保持平衡)

Minot-Murphy diet(treatment) ['mainət 'məːfi] (George R. Minot; William P. Murphy)米诺特–墨菲饮食疗法(食物中加生肝或肝精治恶性贫血)

Minot-von Willebrand syndrome ['mainɔt fɔn 'vilibrɑːnt] (Francis Minot; Erick A. von Willebrand)迈诺特–冯·维勒布兰特综合征(见Wille-brand's disease)

minoxidil [mi'nɔksidil] *n* 米诺地尔(抗高血压药)

mint ['mint] *n* 薄荷 | wild ~ 北美野薄荷,加拿大薄荷

minute [mai'njuːt] *a* 微小的 *n* 微[小]体 | double ~s 双微体(无着丝粒染色体断片,为基因放大所创造,并新近才被整合成染色体;双微体是肿瘤标记,提示实体性肿瘤,预后不良)

minuthesis [mi'njuːθisis] *n*【希】感觉器疲劳

MIO minimal identifiable odor 最低可嗅度

mi(o)- [构词成分]减少,不足,减缩

miocardia [ˌmaiəu'kɑːdiə] *n* 心收缩

miodidymus [ˌmaiəu'didiməs] *n* 枕联双头畸胎

miolecithal [ˌmaiəu'lesiθəl] *a* 少[卵]黄的

mionectic [ˌmaiəu'nektik] *a* 低氧的,少氧的(血)

miophone ['maiəfəun] *n* 肌音听测器

mioplasmia [ˌmaiəu'plæzmiə] *n* 血浆减少

miopragia [ˌmaiəu'preidʒiə] *n* 功能减弱

miopus ['maiəpəs] *n* 单面双头畸胎

miosis [mai'əusis] *n* 瞳孔缩小,缩瞳;成熟分裂,减数分裂;(疾病)减退期 | spastic ~, irritative ~ 痉挛性瞳孔缩小,刺激性瞳孔缩小 | **miotic** [mai'ɔtik] *a* 缩瞳的;减数分裂的 *n* 缩瞳药

miostagmin [ˌmaiəu'stægmin] *n* 微滴(感染动物血清中的一种假设的物质,能与抗原结合降低此混合物的表面张力)

MIP maximum inspiratory pressure 最大吸气压

miracidium [ˌmaiərə'sidiəm] ([复] **miracidia** [ˌmaiərə'sidiə]) *n* 毛蚴,纤毛幼虫

miraculin [mi'rækjulin] *n* 改味糖蛋白

mire [miə] *n*【法】梯形目标(检眼计臂上数字之一,其影像反射到角膜上,影像改变即可测量散光程度)

mirincamycin hydrochloride [mi'rinkəˌmaisin] *n* 盐酸米林霉素(抗菌药和抗疟药)

MIRL membrane inhibitor of reactive lysis 活性溶胞作用的膜抑制蛋白

mirror ['mirə] *n* 镜,反光镜 | concave ~ 凹面[反光]镜 / convex ~ 凸面[反光]镜 / frontal ~, head ~ 额镜,头镜 / mouth ~, dental ~ 口腔镜 / nasographic ~ 鼻通气检验镜 / plane ~ 平面[反光]镜

mirtazapine [mir'tæzəpiːn] *n* 米氮平(抗抑郁药)

miryachit [mi'riətʃit] *n*【俄】西伯利亚痉跳病

mis-action [mis 'ækʃən] *n* 行为失检,错误行为(由于自我的正常压抑失去效力所致)

misanthropia [ˌmisæn'θrəupiə], **misanthropy** [mis'ænθrəpi] *n* 嫌人症

miscarriage [mis'kæridʒ] *n* 流产

miscarry [mis'kæri] *vi* 流产

misce(M.) ['misiː] *vt*【拉】混合,混和

miscegenation [ˌmisidʒiˈneiʃən] *n* 异族通婚
miscible [ˈmisibl] *a* 能溶和的,可混合的
misclassification [ˌmisklæsifiˈkeiʃən] *n* 分类错误
misdiagnosis [ˌmisˌdaiəgˈnəusis] *n* 误诊
miserere mei [ˌmizəˈrɛəri ˈmeii]【拉】肠扭转;肠绞痛
misidentification [ˌmisaiˌdentifiˈkeiʃən] *n* 错误认同,错认(不能正确认同病人所知的人和物,由于精神模糊或记忆丧失所致) | delusional ~ 妄想性错认(错误认为人或物身心均已改变所致)
mismatch [misˈmætʃ] *vt*, *n* 失配,失调,错配
mis(o)- [构词成分]厌恶,憎恨
misogamy [miˈsɔgəmi] *n* 厌婚症,婚姻嫌忌 | **misogamist** [miˈsɔgəmist] *n* 厌恶婚姻者
misogyny [miˈsɔdʒini] *n* 厌女症,女人嫌忌
misoneism [ˌmaisəuˈniːizəm] *n* 厌新[症] | **misoneist** *n* 厌新者
misonidazole [ˌmaisəuˈnidəzəul] *n* 米索硝唑(抗滴虫、抗原虫药)
misoprostol [ˌmaisəˈprɔstɔl] *n* 米索前列醇(合成的前列腺素 E_1 类似物,口服治疗由于长期使用非甾体消炎药物疗法所引起的胃刺激)
missense [ˈmisˌsens] *n*, *a* 错义(的)
missexual [misˈseksjuəl] *a* 性平衡失调的
mist. mistura【拉】合剂
mistletoe [ˈmisəltəu] *n* 槲寄生,槲寄生属植物
mistranslate [ˌmistrænsˈleit] *vt* 错译 | **mistranslation** [ˌmistrænsˈleiʃən] *n*
mistura(M.) [misˈtjuərə] *n*【拉】合剂 | ~ cretae 白垩合剂 / ~ glycyrrhizae composita 复方甘草合剂,棕色合剂 / ~ oleobalsamica 油香树脂合剂 / ~ pectoralis 祛痰合剂,舒胸合剂
MIT monoiodotyrosine 一碘酪氨酸
Mit. mitte【拉】送,发
mitapsis [miˈtæpsis] *n* 染色质粒融合
Mitchella [miˈtʃelə] (John Mitchell) *n* 挛果藤属
mitchella [miˈtʃelə] *n* 挛果藤(曾用作子宫收缩药)
Mitchell operation [ˈmitʃəl] (Charles L. Mitchell)米切尔手术(为矫正跗外翻而对第一跖骨做远侧骨切除手术)
Mitchell's disease [ˈmitʃəl] (Silas W. Mitchell)红斑性肢痛症 | ~ treatment 米切尔疗法(通过绝对卧床休息、按摩、电疗等治疗神经衰弱、癔症等)
mite [mait] *n* 螨 | auricular ~ 耳螨 / bird ~, chicken ~, poultry ~ 鸟螨,鸡螨(即鸡皮刺螨 Dermanyssus gallinae) / borrowing ~ 疥螨 / cheese ~ 长食酪螨(即 Tyrophagus longior) / copra ~ 长粉螨(即卡氏食酪螨 Tyrophagus castellani) / depluming ~ 弃羽螨(即鸡疥螨 Knemidokoptes gallinae) / face ~ 脸螨(即毛囊蠕螨 Demodex folliculorum) / flour ~ 粉螨,蛘螨(即粗脚食酪螨 Tyrophagus farinae) / fowl ~ 鸡螨 / hair follicle ~ 毛囊螨(即毛囊蠕螨 Demodex folliculorum) / harvest ~ 秋蚲 / itch ~ 疥螨 / kedani ~ 红恙螨(即 Trombicula akamushi) / louse ~, straw ~ 虱螨 / mange ~ 兽疥螨 / meal ~ 蛘螨 / mouse ~ 鼠螨 / mower's ~, red ~ 恙螨 / onion ~ 洋葱螨(即 Acarus rhyzoglypticus hyacinthi) / rat ~ 鼠螨,刺脂螨 / scab ~ 痒螨 / spider ~ 革螨 / spinning ~ 刺螨(即苜蓿苔螨 Bryobia praetiosa) / tropical fowl ~ 囊禽刺螨(即 Ornithonyssus bursa) / tropical rat ~ 热带鼠螨(即柏氏禽刺螨 Ornithonyssus bacoti)
mitella [maiˈtelə] *n*【拉】臂吊带,臂悬带
mithramycin [ˌmiθrəˈmaisin] *n* 普卡霉素(即 plicamycin,抗肿瘤抗生素)
mithridatism [ˈmiθriˌdeitizəm] *n* 人工耐毒法(日常服用逐渐增量的毒物而获得对毒物的耐受性)
miticidal [ˌmaitiˈsaidl] *a* 杀螨的,杀疥虫的
miticide [ˈmaitisaid] *n* 杀螨药,杀疥虫药
mitigate [ˈmitigeit] *vt*, *vi* 缓和;镇静;减轻 | **mitigation** [ˌmitiˈgeiʃən] *n* / **mitigative** [ˈmitigətiv], **mitigatory** [ˈmitigətəri] *a* / **mitigator** [ˈmitigeitə] *n* 缓和剂
mitis [ˈmaitis] *a*【拉】轻的,缓和的
mito- [构词成分]线
mitocarcin [ˌmaitəuˈkɑːsin] *n* 米托卡星(抗肿瘤抗生素)
mitochondrial ATPase [ˌmaitəuˈkɔndriəl eitiːˈpiːeis] 线粒体腺苷三磷酸酶,H^+-转运腺苷三磷酸合酶
mitochondrion [ˌmaitəˈkɔndriən] ([复] **mitochondria** [ˌmaitəˈkɔndriə]) *n* 线粒体(细胞质中的一种细胞器) | **mitochondrial** [ˌmaitəˈkɔndriəl] *a*
mitocromin [ˌmaitəˈkrəumin] *n* 丝裂霉素(抗肿瘤抗生素)
mitogen [ˈmaitədʒən] *n* 丝裂原,促[细胞]分裂原;促细胞分裂剂
mitogenesia [ˌmaitəudʒiˈniːziə] *n* 有丝分裂发生
mitogenesis [ˌmaitəuˈdʒenisis] *n* 有丝分裂发生;促有丝分裂[作用] | **mitogenetic** [ˌmaitəudʒiˈnetik] *a*
mitogenic [ˌmaitəuˈdʒenik] *a* 促有丝分裂的
mitokinetic [ˌmaitəukaiˈnetik, -kiˈn-] *a* 有丝分裂动能的
mitomalcin [ˌmaitəuˈmælsin] *n* 米托马星(抗肿瘤抗生素)
mitome [ˈmaitəum] *n* 原生质网,胞质网丝
mitomycin [ˌmaitəuˈmaisin] *n* 丝裂霉素(抗肿瘤

抗生素)
mitoplasm [ˈmaitəˌplæzəm] *n* 核染质
mitoschisis [maiˈtɔskisis] *n* 有丝分裂,[间接]核分裂
mitosin [ˈmaitəsin] *n* [核]分裂激素
mitosis [maiˈtəusis] ([复] **mitoses** [maiˈtəusiːz]) *n* 有丝分裂(细胞间接分裂的一种方法) | heterotypic ~ 异型有丝分裂 / homeotypic ~ 同型有丝分裂 / pathologic ~ 病理性有丝分裂 / pluripolar ~, multicentric ~ 多极有丝分裂 | **mitotic** [maiˈtɔtik] *a*
mitosome [ˈmaitəsəum] *n* 纺锤剩体(从在先的有丝分裂的纺锤体纤维中所形成的小体)
mitosper [ˈmaitəspə] *n* 米托司培(抗肿瘤药)
mitospore [ˈmaitəspɔː] *n* 有丝分裂孢子
mitotane [ˈmaitətein] *n* 米托坦(抗肿瘤药)
mitoxantrone hydrochloride [ˌmaitəuˈzæntrəun] 盐酸米托蒽醌(一种蒽二酮族抗肿瘤药,静脉内给药,治疗急性非淋巴细胞白血病)
mitral [ˈmaitrəl] *a* 僧帽状的;僧帽瓣的,左房室瓣的,二尖瓣的
mitralism [ˈmaitrəlizəm] *n* 二尖瓣病素质
mitralization [ˌmaitrəlaiˈzeiʃən, -liˈz-] *n* 二尖瓣狭窄阴影(X 线片上)
Mitrofanoff procedure [miːˈtrəufɑːnɔf] (Paul Mitrofanoff)米特罗芬诺夫手术,阑尾膀胱造口术
Mitsuda antigen [ˈmitsuˌdɑː] (Kensuke Mitsuda 健辅光田)光田抗原,麻风菌素 | ~ reaction 光田反应,麻风菌素晚期反应(皮内注射麻风菌素后 3~4 周,在注射部位出现丘疹结节损害,这表示对麻风杆菌的细胞免疫,而不是感染麻风杆菌) / ~ test 光田试验,麻风菌素试验(即 lepromin test,见 test 项下相应术语)
mittelschmerz [ˈmitəlʃmεəts] *n*【德】经间痛
mittor [ˈmitə] *n* 神经传器,神经元接头
mivacurium chloride [ˌmaivəˈkjuəriəm] 米库氯铵(一种短时间非去极化神经肌肉阻滞药,静脉内给药,用作全身麻醉的辅助剂,便于气管插管及在机械通气时促使骨骼肌松弛)
mix [miks] *vt, vi* 混合;配制,调制 | **~ed** *a* 混合性的
mixidine [ˈmiksidiːn] *n* 米克昔定(冠状血管扩张药)
mixoscopia [ˌmiksəˈskəupiə] *n* 性交窥视癖
mixotroph [ˈmiksətrɔf] *n* 兼养微生物
mixotrophic [ˌmiksəˈtrɔfik] *a* 混合营养的,兼养的
mixture [ˈmikstʃə] *n* 合剂,混合物 | A. C. E. ~ ACE 合剂(乙醇、氯仿、乙醚混合而成) / brown ~ 棕色合剂,复方甘草合剂(镇咳祛痰药) / chalk ~ 白垩合剂 / expectorant ~, pectoral ~ 祛痰合剂 / racemic ~ 消旋[混合]物 / T.-A. ~, toxin-antitoxin ~ 毒素抗毒素合剂 / triple dye-soap ~ 三重染料肥皂合剂
Miyagawanella [ˌmiːjɑːˌgɑːwɑːˈnelə] (Yoneji Miyagawa 宫川米次) *n* 宫川体属
Miyasato disease [ˌmiːjɑːˈsɑːtəu] (Miyasato 为先证者的姓) α_2 抗血纤维蛋白酶缺乏症
MK monkey lung 猴肺(细胞培养)
MKS meter-kilogram-second system 米千克秒制
ml milliliter 毫升
μl microliter 微升
MLA mento-laeva anterior 颏左前(胎位); Medical Library Association 医学图书馆协会
MLBW moderately low birth weight (infant) 中等低出生体重(儿)
MLC mixed lymphocyte culture 混合淋巴细胞培养
MLD median lethal dose 半数致死量; minimum lethal dose 最小致死量
MLNS mucocutaneous lymph node syndrome 黏膜皮肤淋巴结综合征
MLP mento-laeva posterior 颏左后(胎位)
MLR mixed lymphocyte reaction 混合淋巴细胞反应
MLT mento-laeva transversa 颏左横(胎位)
MM mucous membranes 黏膜
mM millimolar 毫摩尔
μM micromolar 微摩尔
mm millimeter 毫米
mμ millimicron 毫微米
μm micrometer 微米
mμCi millimicrocurie 毫微居里(10^{-9} Ci, 见 nanocurie)
μμCi micromicrocurie 微微居里(10^{-12} Ci, 见 picocurie)
MMF mycophenolate mofetil 霉酚酸酯(免疫抑制药)
mmHg millimeter of mercury 毫米汞柱
MMIHS megacystis-microcolon-intestinal hypoperistalsis syndrome 巨膀胱-小结肠-肠蠕动迟缓综合征
mmol millimole 毫摩尔,毫模
MMPI Minnesota Multiphasic Personality Inventory 明尼苏达多相人格调查表
MMR measles-mumps-rubella (vaccine) 麻疹-腮腺炎-风疹(疫苗)
Mn manganese 锰
M'Naghten (McNaughten) rule [məkˈnɔːtən] 麦克诺登原则(精神病患者不负刑事责任的原则。M'Naghten 为英国一精神病患者,1843 年病发时杀人,法庭判其无罪。此原则现仍在美国司法中沿用)
mnemism [ˈniːmizəm] *n* [细胞]记忆印迹学说(见 mnemic theory,见 theory 项下相应术语)
mnemonic [ni(ː)ˈmɔnik], **mnemic** [ˈniːmik] *a* 记忆的

mnemonics [ni(ː)ˈmɔniks] *n* 记忆术;记忆力培养法

mnemotechnics [ˌniːməˈtekniks] *n* 记忆术

MO Medical Officer 医官

Mo molybdenum 钼

Mobilina [ˌməubiˈlainə] *n* 游动亚目

mobility [məuˈbiləti] *n* 可动性,移动性;移动度,迁移率 | electrophoretic ~ 电泳迁移率

mobilization [ˌməubilaiˈzeiʃən, -liˈz-] *n* 活动法,松动术;动员 | stapes ~ 镫骨松动术(治聋)

mobilometer [ˌməubiˈlɔmitə] *n* 淌度计(量液体的稠度)

Mobiluncus [ˌməubiˈlʌŋkəs] *n* 游动钩菌属

Mobin-Uddin filter [ˈməubin ˈuːdin] (Kazi Mobin-Uddin)莫宾·乌定滤器(一种伞形滤器,由6条连接至毂的不锈钢辐条组成,并有一层有孔的浸透肝素的硅胶膜所覆盖)

Möbius' disease [ˈmiːbiəs] (Paul J. Möbius)默比乌斯病(周期性偏头痛兼眼肌麻痹) | ~ sign 默比乌斯征(突眼性甲状腺肿时,左右眼球不能聚合于一定位置) / ~ syndrome 默比乌斯综合征(脑神经运动核发育不全或先天萎缩,特征为先天性双侧面瘫,兼有单侧或双侧眼外展肌麻痹,有时伴脑神经特别是动眼神经、三叉神经和舌下神经受累及肢体异常)

MOCA methotrexate, vincristine, cyclophosphamide, and doxorubicin 甲氨蝶呤-长春新碱-环磷酰胺-多柔比星(联合化疗治癌方案)

moccasin [ˈmɔkəsin] *n* 噬鱼蝮蛇

mocezuelo [ˌməusiˈzweiləu] *n* 【墨】新生儿牙关紧闭,新生儿破伤风

mock-up [ˈmɔkʌp] *n* 模型机(供试验或教学用)

modafinil [məuˈdæfiˌnil] *n* 莫达非尼(中枢兴奋药)

modal [ˈməudl] *a* (统计学中)众数的

modaline [ˈmɔdəliːn] *n* 莫达林(抗抑郁药)

modality [məuˈdæləti] *n* 治疗方式;药征;用药程式(顺势疗法派所用的名词);感觉体(如味觉) | ~ of sensation 感觉型

mode [məud] *n* 方式;众数(在统计学上指在一个变异曲线中频率最高的值) | ~ of cardiac pacing 起搏方式

model [ˈmɔdl] *n* 模式,模型 *vt, vi* 作模型 | animal ~ 动物模型

modeling [ˈmɔdliŋ] *n* 造型(一种行为矫正法,指导病人模仿他人的行为)

moderator [ˈmɔdəreitə] *n* 缓和器;减速器;减速剂(核化学和核物理学中的一种物质,如石墨或铍,以减缓亚原子粒子流或辐射)

modification [ˌmɔdifiˈkeiʃən] *n* 矫正,改变;修饰 | behavior ~ 行为矫正,行为改变 / racemic ~ 外消旋[变]体

modifier [ˈmɔdifaiə] *n* 修饰基因

modioliform [ˌməudiˈəulifɔːm] *a* 轴状的,毂状的

modiolus [məuˈdaiələs] *n* 【拉】蜗轴,口角轴

Mod. praesc. modo praescripto 【拉】依指示方式

modulation [ˌmɔdjuˈleiʃən] *n* 调节,调变 | antigen ~ 抗原调变

modulator [ˌmɔdjuˈleitə] *n* 调制器,调幅器;调质

modulus [ˈmɔdjuləs] ([复] **moduli** [ˈmɔdjulai]) *n* 模数 | elastic ~, ~ of elasticity 弹性模数

MODY maturity-onset diabetes of youth 青年成熟期突发型糖尿病

Moebius [ˈmiːbiəs] 见 Möbius

Moeller-Barlow disease [ˈmelə bɑːləu] (J. O. L. Moeller; Thomas Barlow)默勒-巴洛病(佝偻病时骨膜下血肿)

Moeller's glossitis [ˈmelə] (Julius O. L. Moeller)默勒舌炎,慢性舌乳头炎,光滑舌

Moeller's reaction [ˈmelə] (Afred Moeller)默勒反应(鼻内结核菌素反应)

Moenckeberg [ˈmenkibəːg] 见 Mönckeberg

moenomycins [ˌməuənəuˈmaisinz] [复] *n* 默诺霉素(见 bambermycins)

Moentjang tina 桐油中毒

Moe plate [məu] (John H. Moe)莫氏板(股骨转子间骨折内固定的一种不锈钢板)

Moerner-Sjöqvist method (test) [ˈməːnə ˈsjekvist] (Carl T. Moerner; John A. Sjöqvist)默尔纳-斯耶克维斯特法(试验)(检尿中脲)

moexipril hydrochloride [məuˈeksiˌpril] 盐酸莫昔普利(抗高血压药)

mofetil [ˈməufitil] *n* 莫非替尔(2-⟨4-morpholinyl⟩ ethyl 的 USAN 缩约词)

mogi- [构词成分]困难

mogiarthria [mɔdʒiˈɑːθriə] *n* 发声困难

mogilalia [mɔdʒiˈleiliə] *n* 出语困难,口吃

mogiphonia [mɔdʒiˈfəuniə] *n* 发声困难

Mohrenheim's fossa [ˈmɔrənhaim] (J. J. F. von Mohrenheim)锁骨下窝

Mohr's test [mɔə] (Francis Mohr)莫尔试验(检胃内容物的盐酸)

Mohr syndrome [mɔr] (Otto L. Mohr)莫尔综合征(一种常染色体隐性遗传病,特征为短指⟨趾⟩、指⟨趾⟩弯曲、多指⟨趾⟩、并指⟨趾⟩及双侧踇趾多并畸形,颅、面、舌、腭及下颌骨异常,并有发作性神经肌肉紊乱。亦称口-面-指⟨趾⟩综合征Ⅱ型)

Mohs hardness number [məuz] (Friedrich Mohs)莫氏硬度值

Mohs' technique (chemosurgery, surgery) [məuz] (Frederic Edward Mohs)莫氏技术(化学外科、外科)(一种切除皮肤瘤的化学外科术)

moiety [ˈmɔiəti] *n* 等分,一半;一部分 | carbohydrate ~ 碳水化物部分 / corrin ~ 咕啉部分

mol [məul] *n* 摩尔,克分子,模

molal(*m*) [ˈməuləl] *a* [重量]摩尔的,[重量]克分子的,重模的 | **~ity** [məuˈlæləti] *n* 重量摩尔浓度,重量克分子浓度,重模浓度

molar[1](M, *M*) [ˈməulə] *a* [容积]摩尔的,[容积]克分子的,容模的 *n* 摩尔浓度,克分子浓度 | **~ity** [məuˈlæriti] *n* 容积摩尔浓度,容积克分子浓度,容模浓度

molar[2](M) [ˈməulə] *n* 磨牙 | impacted ~ 阻生磨牙 / mulberry ~ 桑葚状磨牙 / sixth-year ~ 第一恒磨牙,六岁磨牙 / third ~ 第三磨牙 / twelfth-year ~ 第二恒磨牙,十二岁磨牙

molariform [məuˈlærifɔːm] *a* 磨牙形的

molaris [məuˈleiris] *a* 宜磨的 *n* 磨牙 | ~ tertius 第三磨牙

molasses [məˈlæsiz] *n* 糖蜜 | sugarhouse ~ 糖浆 / West India ~ 西印度糖蜜

molc molar concentration 容积摩尔浓度,容积克分子浓度,容模浓度

mold[1] [məuld] *n* 模型,铸模 *vt* 定型 | ear ~ 耳模

mold[2] [məuld] *n* 霉,霉菌 *vt*, *vi* 发霉 | slime ~ 黏菌 / white ~ 白霉

molding [ˈməuldiŋ] *n* 塑型,造型;(分娩时)胎头变形 | border ~, tissue ~ 边缘整塑,组织整塑 / compression ~ 压迫塑型 / injection ~ 注入整塑

moldy [ˈməuldi] *a* 发霉的

mole[1] [məul] *n* 胎块;痣 | blood ~ 血性胎块 / false ~ 假胎块 / fleshy ~ 肉样胎块 / hairy ~ 毛痣 / hydatid ~, hydatidiform ~, cystic ~, vesicular ~ 葡萄胎 / invasive ~, malignant ~, metastasizing ~ 侵袭性葡萄胎,恶性葡萄胎,绒[毛]膜腺瘤 / pigmented ~ 色[素]痣 / stone ~ 石化胎块 / true ~ 真性胎块 / tubal ~ 输卵管胎块

mole[2](mol) [məul] *n* 摩尔,克分子[量],克模

molecular [məuˈlekjulə] *a* 分子的 | **~ity** [məuˌlekjuˈlærəti] *n* 分子性,分子状态;分子数

molecule [ˈmɔlikjuːl] *n* 分子 | cell interaction (CI) ~s, CI ~s 细胞相互作用因子(细胞相互作用基因的产物) / diatomic ~ 二原子分子 / hexatomic ~ 六原子分子 / monatomic ~ 单原子分子 / nonpolar ~ 无极分子 / polar ~ 有极分子 / tetratomic ~ 四原子分子 / triatomic ~ 三原子分子

molilalia [ˌmɔliˈleiliə] *n* 出语困难,口吃

molimen [məˈlaimən] ([复] **molimina** [məˈliminə]) *n*【拉】功能紧张,违和

molindone hydrochloride [məˈlindəun] 盐酸吗茚酮(抗精神病药)

Molisch's test (reaction) [ˈmɔliʃ] (Hans Molisch)莫利希试验(反应)(检尿葡萄糖、尿蛋白质)

mollescuse [mɔˈleskjuːs] *n* 软化

Mollicutes [ˌmɔliˈkjutiːz] *n* 柔膜体纲

mollin [ˈmɔlin] *n* 软皂脂(一种含甘油肥皂脂肪的外用润滑基质)

mollities [mɔˈliʃiiːz] *n*【拉】软化

Moll's glands [mɔl] (Jacob A. Moll)睫毛腺,结膜睫毛腺

mollusc [ˈmɔləsk] *n* 软体动物

Mollusca [mɔˈlʌskə] *n* 软体动物门

molluscacidal [mɔˌlʌskəˈsaidl] *a* 灭螺的,灭软体动物的

molluscacide [mɔˈlʌskəsaid], **molluscicide** [mɔˈlʌsisaid] *n* 灭螺剂,软体动物杀灭剂

Molluscipoxvirus [mɔˈlʌskipɔksˌvaiərəs] *n* 软体动物痘病毒属

molluscum [mɔˈlʌskəm] *n*【拉】软疣 | ~ contagiosum 触染性软疣 | **molluscous** [mɔˈlʌskəs] *a*

mollusk [ˈmɔləsk] *n* 软体动物

Moloney test (reaction) [məˈləuni] (Peter J. Moloney)莫洛尼试验(反应)(测对白喉类毒素的迟发型敏感性:皮内注射 0.1 ml 1∶10 的白喉类毒素至前臂内侧,12 ~ 24 小时红肿硬结大于 12 mm 者为阳性。亦称类毒素反应)

molting [ˈməultiŋ] *n* 蜕皮;换羽

Mol wt, mol wt molecular weight 分子量

molybdate [mɔˈlibdeit] *n* 钼酸盐

molybdenosis [mɔˌlibdiˈnəusis] *n* [慢性]钼中毒

molybdenum(Mo) [mɔˈlibdinəm] *n* 钼(化学元素)

molybdic [mɔˈlibdik] *a* 钼的,六价钼的

molybdic acid [mɔˈlibdik] 钼酸

molybdoenzyme [mɔˌlibdəuˈenzaim] *n* 钼酶

molybdoflavoprotein [mɔˌlibdəuˈfleivəuˌprəutiːn] *n* 钼黄素蛋白

molybdoprotein [mɔˌlibdəuˈprəutiːn] *n* 钼蛋白

molybdopterin [ˌmɔlibˈdɔptərin] *n* 钼蝶呤

molybdous [mɔˈlibdəs] *a* 亚钼的,四价钼的

momentum [məuˈmentəm] ([复] **momentums** 或 **momenta** [məuˈmentə]) *n*【拉】冲力;力量;动量

mometasone furoate [mɔˈmetəˌsəun] 糠酸莫米松(合成皮质类固醇,局部用于缓解皮质类固醇反应性皮病时的炎症及瘙痒症)

monacid [mɔˈnæsid] *a* 一元酸的,一价酸的

monad [ˈmɔnæd] *n* 单胞[原]虫,单胞[球]菌;一价物,一价基;单体,单倍体数(减数分裂时四体的一部分) | **~ic(al)** [mɔˈnædik(əl)] *a*

Monadidae [mɔˈnædidiː] *n* 纤毛滴虫属

monadin [ˈmɔnədin] *n* 纤毛滴虫
Monadina [ˌmɔnəˈdainə] *n* 纤毛滴虫属
Monakow's syndrome [mɔˈnɑːkɔv] (Constantin von Monakow)莫纳科夫综合征(脉络膜前动脉闭塞时损伤的对侧出现偏瘫,有时伴偏身麻木和偏盲)/ ~ theory 莫纳科夫学说,神经功能联系不能 / ~ tract (bundle, fasciculus) 红核脊髓束
Monaldi's drainage [mɔˈnældi] (V. Monaldi)莫纳迪引流法(用吸引引流法引流肺结核空洞)
monamide [mɔˈnæmid] *n* 一酰胺
monamine [mɔˈnæmin] *n* 一元胺,单胺
monaminergic [mɔˌnæmiˈnəːdʒik] *a* 单胺能的
monamino acid [mɔˈnæminəu] 一氨基酸
monangle [ˈmɔnæŋgl] *a* 单角形的 *n* 单角器(牙科)
monarthric [mɔˈnɑːθrik], **monarticular** [ˌmɔnɑːˈtikjulə] *a* 单关节的
monarthritis [ˌmɔnɑːˈθraitis] *n* 单关节炎 | ~ deformans 变形性单关节炎
Monas [ˈməunəs] *n* 单胞菌属;滴虫属
monaster [mɔˈnæstə] *n* 单星体(有丝分裂前期结束时出现)
monathetosis [ˌmɔnæθiˈtəusis] *n* 单肢[手足]徐动症
monatomic [ˌmɔnəˈtɔmik] *a* 一价的;一价碱的;一原子的
monauchenos [mɔˈnɔːkinəs] *n* 单颈联胎,单颈双头畸胎
monaural [mɔˈnɔːrəl] *a* 单耳的
monavalent [mɔˈnævələnt] *a* 一价的,单价的
monavitaminosis [ˌmɔnəˌvaitəmiˈnəusis] *n* 单维生素缺乏病
monaxon [mɔˈnæksɔn] *n* 单轴神经元 | ~ic [ˌmɔnækˈsɔnik] *a*
Mönckeberg's arteriosclerosis (calcification, degeneration, mesarteritis, sclerosis) [ˈmenkəbəːg] (Johann G. Mönckeberg)门克伯格动脉硬化(钙化、变性、动脉中层炎、硬化)(动脉中层硬化,伴有钙质广泛沉着)
Mondini's cochlea [mɔnˈdiːni] (C. Mondini)蒙迪尼耳蜗(蒙迪尼畸形时所见的畸形耳蜗) | ~ deafness 蒙迪尼聋(科尔蒂〈Corti〉器发育不全所致的先天性聋,伴骨迷路和膜迷路部分不发育,导致耳蜗变平)/ ~ deformity (malformation) 蒙迪尼畸形(畸形耳蜗,伴骨迷路和膜迷路发育不全或不发育,如蒙迪尼聋时所见)
Mondonesi reflex [ˌmɔndəˈneizi] (Filippo Mondonesi)蒙多内西反射,眼球颜面反射(bulbomimic reflex,见 reflex 项下相应术语)
Mondor's disease [ˈmɔndɔː] (Henri Mondor)蒙道尔病(胸壁浅表血栓性静脉炎)
monecious [məˈniːʃəs] *a* 雌雄同株的;雌雄同体的
monensin [məˈnensin] *n* 莫能星,莫能菌素(兽用抗细菌、抗真菌和抗原虫的抗生素)
moner [ˈməunə] *n* 无核原生质团
Monera [məuˈniərə] *n* 无核原虫类,原核原虫类
monerula [məˈnerjulə] ([复] **monerulae** [məˈnerjuliː]) *n* 无核裂卵
monesia [məˈniːziə] *n* 【拉】巴西金叶树浸膏(收敛健胃药)
monesthetic [ˌmɔnisˈθetik] *a* 单感觉的
monestrous [mɔˈnestrəs] *a* 一次动情[期]的,单动情性的(每年仅有一次求偶期的)
Monge's disease [məunˈʒei] (Carlos Monge)蒙热病,慢性高山病
mongolian [mɔŋˈgəuljən] *a* 先天愚型的,伸舌样白痴的
mongolism [ˈmɔŋgəlizəm] *n* 先天愚型,伸舌样白痴(即唐氏综合征,见 Down syndrome) | translocation ~ 易位先天愚型,易位伸舌样白痴(见 syndrome 项下 translocation Down syndrome)
mongoloid [ˈmɔŋgəlɔid] *a* 先天愚型样的 *n* 先天愚型样者
Moniezia [ˌmɔniˈiːziə] *n* 蒙尼茨[绦虫]属
monilated [ˈmɔniˌleitid] *a* 念珠状的
monilethrix [məˈniliθriks] *n* 念珠状发
Monilia [məˈniliə] *n* 念珠菌属(旧名,现称 Candida);丛梗孢属
Moniliaceae [məˌniliˈeisiiː] *n* 丛梗孢科;念珠菌科
monilial [məˈniliəl] *a* 念珠菌的
Moniliales [məˌniliˈeiliːz] *n* 丛梗孢目;念珠菌目
moniliasis [mɔniˈlaiəsis], **moniliosis** [məˌniliˈəusis] *n* 念珠菌病
moniliform [məˈnilifɔːm] *a* 念珠形的
Moniliformis [məˌniliˈfɔːmis] *n* 念珠棘虫属
moniliid [məˈniliid] *n* 念珠菌疹
monitor [ˈmɔnitə] *n* 放射量探测器;监护员;(病人)监护仪 *vt, vi* 检验;监护 | bubble ~ 气泡监测器
monitory [ˈmɔnitəri] *a* 警告的,起始的(指病的早期体征)
monkey [ˈmʌŋki] *n* 猴 | rhesus ~ 罗猴,恒河猴,猕猴(即 Macaca mulatta)
monkeypox [ˈmʌŋkipɔks] *n* 猴痘
monkshood [ˈmʌŋkshud] *n* 乌头
Monneret's pulse [mɔnəˈrei] (Jules A. E. Monneret)蒙讷雷脉(迟软而洪,见于黄疸时)
mon(o)- [构词成分]单,一
monoacid [ˌmɔnəˈæsid] *a* 一价酸的,一元酸的 *n* 一元酸
monoacylglycerol [ˌmɔnəuˌæsilˈglisərɔl] *n* 单酰

甘油

monoacylglycerol lipase [ˌmɔnəuˌæsil'glisərɔl 'laipeis] 单酰甘油脂[肪]酶

monoamide [ˌmɔnəu'æmaid] *n* 一酰胺

monoamine [ˌmɔnəuə'miːn, -'æmin] *n* 单胺

monoamine oxidase (MAO) [ˌmɔnəuə'miːn 'ɔksideis] 单胺氧化酶,胺氧化酶(含黄素)

monoaminergic [ˌmɔnəuˌæmi'nəːdʒik] *a* 单胺能的

monoaminodicarboxylic acid [ˌmɔnəuˌæminəudaikɑːbɔk'silik] 一氨基二羧酸

monoaminodiphosphatide [ˌmɔnəuˌæminəudai'fɔsfətaid] *n* 一氨二磷脂

monoaminomonocarboxylic acid [ˌmɔnəuæminəuˌmɔnəukɑːbɔk'silik] 一氨基一羧基酸

monoaminomonophosphatide [ˌmɔnəuˌæminəuˌmɔnə'fɔsfətaid] *n* 一氨一磷脂

monoamnionic [ˌmɔnəuˌæmni'ɔnik] *a* 单羊膜的,一卵性的

monoamniotic [ˌmɔnəuˌæmni'ɔtik] *a* 单羊膜的

monoanesthesia [ˌmɔnəuˌænis'θiːzjə] *n* 单麻木,局部麻木

monoarticular [ˌmɔnəuɑː'tikjulə] *a* 单关节的

monoatomic [ˌmɔnəuə'tɔmik] *a* 单原子的

monobacillary [ˌmɔnəubə'siləri], **monobacterial** [ˌmɔnəubæk'tiəriəl] *a* 单杆菌的,一种杆菌的

monobactam [ˌmɔnəu'bæktæm] *n* 单菌霉素

monobasic [ˌmɔnəu'beisik] *a* 一价碱的,一元碱的 | ~ acid 一元酸

monobenzone [ˌmɔnə'benzəun] *n* 莫诺苯宗(脱色剂)

monoblast ['mɔnəublæst] *n* 原单核细胞

monoblastoma [ˌmɔnəublæs'təumə] *n* 原单核细胞瘤

monoblepsia [ˌmɔnəu'blepsiə] *n* 单眼视[症];单色视[觉]

monobrachia [ˌmɔnəu'breikiə] *n* 单臂畸形

monobrachius [ˌmɔnəu'breikiəs] *n* 单臂畸胎

monobromated [ˌmɔnəu'brəumeitid] *a* 一溴化的

monobromophenol [ˌmɔnəuˌbrəumə'fiːnɔl] *n* 一溴酚,一溴苯酚

monocalcic [ˌmɔnəu'kælsik] *a* 一钙的

monocarboxylic acid [ˌmɔnəuˌkɑːbɔk'silik] 一元羧酸

monocardian [mɔnəu'kɑːdiən] *a* 单腔心的(如鲨鱼)

monocelled ['mɔnəuseld], **monocellular** [ˌmɔnəu'seljulə] *a* 单细胞的

monocephalus [ˌmɔnəu'sefələs] *n* 单头联胎

Monocercomonoides [ˌmɔnəuˌsəːkəməu'nɔidiːz] *n* 类单鞭滴虫属

monochloride [ˌmɔnəu'klɔːraid] *n* 一氯化物

monochloroacetic acid [ˌmɔnəuˌklɔ(ː)rəuə'siːtik] 一氯乙酸,一氯醋酸

monochlorothymol [ˌmɔnəuˌklɔːrə'θaimɔl] *n* 氯麝酚(抗菌药)

monochord ['mɔnəukɔːd] *n* 单音[测听]弦

monochorea [ˌmɔnəukɔ'riə] *n* 单[肢]舞蹈症,局部舞蹈症

monochorionic [ˌmɔnəuˌkɔːri'ɔnik], **monochorial** [ˌmɔnəu'kɔːriəl] *a* 单绒[毛]膜的(双胎)

monochroic [ˌmɔnəu'krəuik] *a* 单色的

monochromacy [ˌmɔnəu'krəuməsi] *n* 全色盲,单色视觉

monochromasy [ˌmɔnəu'krəuməsi] *n* 全色盲,单色视觉

monochromat [ˌmɔnəu'krəumæt] *n* 全色盲者

monochromatic [ˌmɔnəukrəu'mætik] *a* 单色的单色光的;单染色的

monochromatism [ˌmɔnəu'krəumətizəm] *n* 全色盲,单色视觉 | cone ~ 锥体全色盲 / rod ~ 杆体全色盲

monochromatophil [ˌmɔnəukrəu'mætəfil] *a* 单染色的 *n* 单染细胞

monochromatopsis [ˌmɔnəuˌkrəumə'tɔpsis] *n* 全色盲,单色视觉

monochromophilic [ˌmɔnəuˌkrəumə'filik] *a* 单染色的

monocle ['mɔnɔkl] *n* 单[片]眼镜;单眼绷带 | ~d *a*

monoclinic [ˌmɔnəu'klinik] *a* 单斜晶[系]的

monoclonal [ˌmɔnəu'kləunl] *a* 单细胞系的;单克隆的

monocontaminated [ˌmɔnəukən'tæmiˌneitid] *a* 单种[菌]感染的;单种[污染物]污染的

monocontamination [ˌmɔnəukənˌtæmi'neiʃən] *n* 单种[菌]感染(动物实验时);单种[污染物]污染

monocorditis [ˌmɔnəukɔː'daitis] *n* 单声带炎

monocranius [ˌmɔnəu'kreiniəs] *n* 单头联胎

monocrotaline [ˌmɔnəu'krəutəliːn] *n* 一野百合碱,单猪屎豆碱

monocrotism [mə'nɔkrətizəm] *n* 单波脉[现象] | **monocrotic** [ˌmɔnəu'krɔtik] *a* 单波[脉]的

monocular [mə'nɔkjulə] *a* 单眼的;单目镜的(显微镜)

monoculus [mə'nɔkjuləs] *n* 单眼绷带;独眼畸胎

monocyclic [ˌmɔnəu'saiklik] *a* 单环的,一环的

monocyesis [ˌmɔnəusai'iːsis] *n* 单胎妊娠

Monocystis [ˌmɔnəu'sistis] *n* 单囊胞虫属;单房簇虫属

monocytangina [ˌmɔnəusai'tændʒinə] *n* 传染性单核细胞增多症

monocyte [ˈmɔnəsait] *n* 单核细胞 | **monocytic** [ˌmɔnəˈsitik] *a* 单核细胞的;单核细胞系的
monocytoid [ˌmɔnəˈsaitɔid] *a* 单核细胞样的
monocytopenia [ˌmɔnəusaitəˈpiːniə] *n* 单核细胞减少[症]
monocytopoiesis [ˌmɔnəuˌsaitəupɔiˈiːsis] *n* 单核细胞发生
monocytosis [ˌmɔnəusaiˈtəusis] *n* 单核细胞增多
monodactyly [ˌmɔnəuˈdæktili], **monodactylia** [ˌmɔnəudækˈtiliə], **monodactylism** [mɔnəuˈdæktilizəm] *n* 先天性单指,先天性单趾
monodal [mɔˈnəudl] *a* 高频电导联的
monodermal [ˌmɔnəuˈdəːməl] *a* 单层的,单生殖细胞层的(指肿瘤)
monodermoma [ˌmɔnəudəˈməumə] *n* 单胚叶瘤
monodiplopia [ˌmɔnəudiˈpləupiə] *n* 单眼复视
Monodontus [ˌmɔnəuˈdɔntəs] *n* 单齿虫属
monoecious [məˈniːʃəs] *a* 雌雄同体的,雌雄同株的 | **monoecism** [məˈniːsizəm] *n*
monoester [ˌmɔnəuˈestə] *n* 单酯
monoethanolamine [ˌmɔnəuˌeθəˈnəuləmiːn] *n* 单乙醇胺(表面活性剂) | ~ oleate 油酸单乙醇胺(硬化药)
monoethylglycinexylidide (MEGX) [ˌmɔnəuˌeθilˌglaisinˈzailidaid] *n* 单乙基甘氨酸二甲代苯胺(利多卡因〈lidocaine〉的主要活性代谢物,由肝内产生,测定利多卡因转换成 MEGX,用以评估肝功能)
monofilm [ˈmɔnəfilm] *n* 单[层]分子膜
monogametic [ˌmɔnəugəˈmetik] *a* 单型配子的
monogamy [məˈnɔgəmi] *n* 一夫一妻制;单配性(指动物的交配) | **monogamous** [məˈnɔgəməs], **monogamic** [mɔnəˈgæmik] *a* 单配的
monoganglial [ˌmɔnəˈgæŋgliəl] *a* 单神经节的
monogastric [ˌmɔnəˈgæstrik] *a* 单腹的,单胃的
monogen [ˈmɔnəudʒən] *n* 一价元素;单种血清
monogenesis [ˌmɔnəuˈdʒenisis] *n* 单性生殖,无性生殖;一元发生说(认为一切生物皆源于单一细胞) | **monogenetic** [ˌmɔnəudʒiˈnetik] *a* 一元发生的;无性生殖的
monogenic [ˌmɔnəuˈdʒenik] *a* 单基因的
monogerminal [ˌmɔnəuˈdʒəːminl] *a* 单胚性的,一卵生的
monoglyceride [ˌmɔnəuˈglisəraid] *n* 单酸甘油酯,甘油单酯
monoglyceride acyltransferase [ˌmɔnəuˈglisəraid ˌæsilˈtrænsfəreis] 单酰甘油酯酰基转移酶,2-酰基甘油-*O*-酰基转移酶
monograph [ˈmɔnəgrɑːf] *n* 专著,专题著作;专论 | **~ic** [ˌmɔnəˈgræfik] *a* 专题性的,专著的
monohormonal [ˌmɔnəuhɔːˈməunl] *a* 单激素的
monohybrid [ˌmɔnəuˈhaibrid] *n* 单基因杂种
monohydrate [ˌmɔnəuˈhaidreit] *n* 一水合物,一水化物 | **~d** *a* 一水化物的,一羟[基]的
monohydric [ˌmɔnəuˈhaidrik] *a* 一氢的
monoideism [ˌmɔnəuˈaidiizəm] *n* 单一意念,单一观念
monoinfection [ˌmɔnəuinˈfekʃən] *n* 单菌性传染
monoiodotyrosine [ˌmɔnəuaiˌəudəˈtaiərəsiːn] *n* 一碘酪氨酸
monokaryon [ˌmɔnəuˈkæriɔn] *n* 单核
monokaryote [ˌmɔnəuˈkæriəut] *n* 单倍体核细胞
monokaryotic [ˌmɔnəuˌkæriˈɔtik] *a* 单核的;单倍体核细胞的
monoketoheptose [ˌmɔnəukiːtəuˈheptəus] *n* 庚酮糖
monokine [ˈmɔnəkain] *n* 单核因子
monolayer [ˈmɔnəˌleiə, ˌmɔnəˈleiə] *n* 单分子层;单层细胞 *a* 单层的
monolene [ˈmɔnəliːn] *n* 烃油
monolepsis [ˌmɔnəuˈlepsis] *n* 单亲遗传(只有一个亲本的性状传于子代)
monolocular [ˌmɔnəuˈlɔkjulə] *a* 单腔的,单房的
monolog(ue) [ˈmɔnəlɔg] *n* (使别人无法插嘴的)滔滔不绝言语
monomania [ˌmɔnəuˈmeinjə] *n* 单狂,偏狂 | **~c** [ˌmɔnəuˈmeiniæk] *n* 单狂者,偏狂者 / **~cal** [ˌmɔnəuməˈnaiəkəl] *a* 单狂的,偏狂的
monomaxillary [ˌmɔnəuˈmæksiləri] *a* 单颌的
monomelic [ˌmɔnəuˈmelik] *a* 单肢的
monomer [ˈmɔnəmə] *n* 单体(比较简单的分子单位)
monomeric [ˌmɔnəˈmerik] *a* 单体的;单基因的
monometallic [ˌmɔnəumiˈtælik] *n* 一金属的,单金属的
monomethylhydrazine [ˌmɔnəuˌmeθilˈhaidrəziːn] *n* 单甲基肼(在鹿花菌属〈Gyromitra〉许多菌蕈中发现的一种毒素,充当吡哆醇的拮抗物,食用后 6 小时以上即发生头痛、头晕、不适、呕吐,有时发展成谵妄、昏迷和惊厥)
monomicrobic [ˌmɔnəumaiˈkrəubik] *a* 单微生物的,一种细菌的
monomolecular [ˌmɔnəuməuˈlekjulə] *a* 单分子的
monomoria [ˌmɔnəuˈmɔːriə] *n* 单狂,偏狂
monomorphic [ˌmɔnəuˈmɔːfik], **monomorphous** [ˌmɔnəuˈmɔːfəs] *a* 单形的
monomorphism [ˌmɔnəuˈmɔːfizəm] *n* 单形现象,单态现象
monomphalus [məˈnɔmfələs] *n* 脐部联胎
monomyoplegia [ˌmɔnəuˌmaiəˈpliːdʒiə] *n* 单肌麻痹,单肌瘫[痪]
monomyositis [ˌmɔnəuˌmaiəˈsaitis] *n* 单肌炎

Mononchus [mə'nɔŋkəs] *n* 单齿[线虫]属
mononephrous [ˌmɔnə*u*'nefrəs] *a* 单肾的
mononeural [ˌmɔnə*u*'njuərəl] *a* 单神经的
mononeuric [ˌmɔnə*u*'njuərik] *a* 单神经元的
mononeuritis [ˌmɔnə*u*njuə'raitis] *n* 单神经炎 | ~ multiplex 多发性单神经炎,多神经炎
mononeuropathy [ˌmɔnə*u*njuə'rɔpəθi] *n* 单神经病 | cranial ~ 单脑神经病
mononoea [ˌmɔnə*u*'niːə] *n* 单一思想
mononuclear [ˌmɔnə*u*'njuːkliə] *a* 单核的 *n* 单核细胞
mononucleate [ˌmɔnə*u*'njuːklieit] *a* 单核的
mononucleosis [ˌmɔnə*u*ˌnjuːkli'əusis] *n* 单核细胞增多[症] | cytomegalovirus ~ 巨细胞病毒性单核细胞增多症 / infectious ~ 传染性单核细胞增多症 / post-transfusion ~ 输血后单核细胞增多[症](即 postperfusion syndrome,见 syndrome 项下相应术语)
mononucleotide [ˌmɔnə*u*'njuːkliətaid] *n* 单核苷酸 | flavin ~ (FMN) 黄素单核苷酸
monooctanoin [ˌmɔnə*u*ˌɔktə'nəuin] *n* 单辛酸(一种半合成甘油衍生物,用于溶解胆总管和肝内胆管的胆固醇结石,经导管连续输注给药)
mono-osteitic [ˌmɔnə*u*ˌɔsti'itik] *a* 单骨炎的
mono-ovular [ˌmɔnə*u*'ɔvjulə] *a* 单卵的
monooxygenase [ˌmɔnə*u*'ɔksidʒiˌneis] *n* 单加氧酶 | unspecific ~ 非特异性单加氧酶
monoparesis [ˌmɔnə*u*pə'riːsis] *n* 单肢轻瘫
monoparesthesia [ˌmɔnə*u*ˌpæris'θiːzjə] *n* 单肢感觉异常
monopathy [mə'nɔpəθi] *n* 单病,局部病
monopenia [ˌmɔnə*u*'piːniə] *n* 单核[白]细胞减少症
monophagia [ˌmɔnə*u*'feidʒiə], **monophagism** [mə'nɔfədʒizəm] *n* 偏食(嗜食一种食物);单食(日进一餐)
monophasia [ˌmɔnə*u*'feiziə] *n* 单语症(只能讲单个词或短语的失语症)
monophasic [ˌmɔnə*u*'feizik] *a* 单相的
monophenol monooxygenase [ˌmɔnə*u*'fiːnɔl ˌmɔnə*u*'ɔksidʒiˌneis] 单酚单加氧酶
monophenyl oxidase [ˌmɔnə*u*'fenil 'ɔksideis] 单苯基氧化酶,单酚单加氧酶
monophosphate [ˌmɔnə*u*'fɔsfeit] *n* 一磷酸盐
monophthalmus [ˌmɔnɔf'θælməs] *n* 独眼畸胎
monophyletic [ˌmɔnə*u*fai'letik] *a* 一元的(起于或源自单细胞型的) | **monophyletism** [ˌmɔnə*u* 'failətizəm] *n* 一元论(monophyletic theory,见 theory 项下相应术语) | **monophyletist** [ˌmɔnə*u*'failətist] *n* 一元论者
monophyodont [ˌmɔnə*u*'faiədɔnt] *a* 单套牙的(恒牙)

monopia [mə'nəupiə] *n* 独眼[畸形]
monoplasmatic [ˌmɔnə*u*plæz'mætik] *a* 单质的
monoplast ['mɔnə*u*plæst] *n* 单细胞
monoplegia [ˌmɔnə*u*'pliːdʒiə] *n* 单瘫 | **monoplegic** [ˌmɔnə*u*'pliːdʒik] *a*
monoploid ['mɔnəplɔid] *a* 单倍的 *n* 单倍体,一倍体(细胞仅含有一组染色体的个体) | **~y** *n* 单倍性,一倍性
monopodia [ˌmɔnə*u*'pəudiə] *n* 单足[畸形] | **~l** *a*
monopoiesis [ˌmɔnə*u*pɔi'iːsis] *n* 单核细胞生成
monopolar ['mɔnəˌpəulə] *a* 单极的
monops ['mɔnəps] *n* 独眼畸胎
monopsychosis [ˌmɔnə*u*sai'kəusis] *n* 单狂,偏狂
Monopsyllus [ˌmɔnə*u*'siləs] *n* 单蚤属 | ~ anisus 不等单蚤,横滨角叶蚤
monoptychial [ˌmɔnə*u*'taikiəl] *a* 单层的(指腺体细胞成单层排列在基膜上)
monopus ['mɔnəpəs] *n* 单足畸胎
monorchid [mɔ'nɔːkid], **monorchis** [mɔ'nɔːkis] *n* 单睾丸者
monorchism ['mɔnəkizəm], **monorchia** [mɔ'nɔːkiə], **monorchidism** [mɔ'nɔːkidizəm] *n* 单睾症,单睾丸[畸形] | **monorchidic** [ˌmɔnə'kidik] *a* 单睾丸的
Monorchotrema [mɔˌnɔːkəu'triːmə] *n* 单睾孔[吸虫]属
monorecidive [ˌmɔnə*u*ri'sidiv] *n* 再发性下疳
monorhinic [mɔnə'rinik] *a* 单鼻孔的
monosaccharide [ˌmɔnə*u*'sækəraid], **monosaccharose** [ˌmɔnə*u*'sækərəus], **monose** ['mɔnəus] *n* 单糖
monosexual [ˌmɔnə*u*'seksjuəl] *a* 单性的
monosodium glutamate [ˌmɔnə*u*'səudjəm 'gluːtəmeit] 谷氨酸钠,谷氨酸单钠(治肝昏迷药)
monosome ['mɔnəsəum] *n* 单染色体;单核糖体
monosomian [ˌmɔnə*u*'səumiən] *n* 单体联胎
monosomy [mɔnə'səumi] *n* 单体性(正常二倍体的染色体中有一对缺少一个成员〈$2n-1$〉) | **monosomic** [ˌmɔnə'səumik] *a* 单体的 *n* 单体,单体生物
monospasm ['mɔnə*u*spæzəm] *n* 局部痉挛,单处痉挛
monospecific [ˌmɔnə*u*spi'sifik] *a* 单一特异性的
monospermy ['mɔnə*u*ˌspəːmi] *n* 单精入卵 | **monospermic** [ˌmɔnə*u*'spəːmik] *a*
Monosporium [ˌmɔnə*u*'spɔːriəm] *n* 单孢子菌属 | ~ apiospermum 梨形单孢子菌
Monostoma [ˌmɔnə*u*'stəumə], **Monostomum** [ˌmɔnə*u*'stəuməm] *n* 单盘[吸虫]属
monostotic [ˌmɔnɔs'tɔtik] *a* 单骨性的
monostratal [ˌmɔnə*u*'streitl] *a* 单层的

monostratified [ˌmɔnəuˈstrætifaid] *a* 单层[排列]的

monosubstituted [ˌmɔnəuˈsʌbstiˌtjuːtid] *a* 一原子置换的,单基置换的

monosymptom [ˌmɔnəuˈsimptəm] *n* 单症状 | **~atic** [ˌmɔnəuˌsimptəˈmætik] *a*

monosynaptic [ˌmɔnəusiˈnæptik] *a* 单突触的

monosyphilid [ˌmɔnəuˈsifilid], **monosyphilide** [ˌmɔnəuˈsifilaid] *n* 单发[性]梅毒疹

monoterminal [ˌmɔnəuˈtəːminl] *a* 单极的(仅用单一电极作治疗,以地线为第二电极)

Monothalamida [ˌmɔnəuθəˈlæmidə] *n* 单室目

monotherapy [ˌmɔnəuˈθerəpi] *n* 单一疗法(用单一药物治病)

monothermia [ˌmɔnəuˈθəːmiə] *n* 体温[全日]恒定

monothetic [ˌmɔnəuˈθetik] *a* 单一原则的

monothioglycerol [ˌmɔnəuˌθaiəuˈglisərɔl] *n* 硫代甘油(用作药物制剂的防腐剂)

monotic [mɔˈnɔtik] *a* 单耳的

monotocous [məˈnɔtəkəs] *a* 单胎分娩的

Monotremata [ˌmɔnəuˈtriːmətə] *n* 单孔目

monotreme [ˈmɔnəutriːm] *n* 单孔类 | **monotrematous** [ˌmɔnəuˈtremətəs] *a*

monotricha [məˈnɔtrikə] *n* 单鞭毛菌,偏端单毛菌

monotrichous [məˈnɔtrikəs], **monotrichic** [ˌmɔnəuˈtrikik] *a* 单鞭毛的,偏端单毛的

monotropic [ˌmɔnəuˈtrɔpik] *a* 单亲的,单嗜的(仅影响一种特殊细菌或一种组织的)

monounsaturated [ˌmɔnəuʌnˈsætʃəreitid] *a* 单不饱和的

monoureide [ˌmɔnəuˈjuəriid] *n* 一酰脲,一脲化物

monovalent [ˌmɔnəuˈveilənt] *a* 一价的,单价的 | **monovalence**, **monovalency** *n*

monovular [mɔˈnɔvjulə] *a* 单卵的

monovulatory [mɔˈnɔvjulətəri] *a* 排单卵的

monoxenic [ˌmɔnəuˈzenik] *a* 单种菌[感染]的(实验动物)

monoxenous [məˈnɔksənəs] *a* 单栖的,单[宿主]寄生的 | **monoxeny** [məˈnɔksəni] *n*

monoxide [mɔˈnɔksaid, məˈnɔksaid] *n* 一氧化物

monoxygenase [mɔˈnɔksidʒəneis] *n* 单氧合酶

monozygosity [ˌmɔnəuzaiˈgɔsəti] *n* 单合子发育[状态],单卵发育[状态]

monozygotic [ˌmɔnəuzaiˈgɔtik] *a* 单合子的,单卵的

monozygous [ˌmɔnəuˈzaigəs] *a* 单合子的,单卵的

Monro-Kellie doctrin [mənˈrəu ˈkeli] (A. Monro (Secundus); George Kellie) 门-凯学说(中枢神经系统及其伴随的液体封闭在坚硬的容器内,其总容量倾向于保持恒定;一个成分如脑、血液或脑脊液的容量增加必将增高其他成分之一的压力并减少其容量)

Monro-Richter line [mənˈrəu ˈriktə] (Alexander Monro; August G. Richter) 门-里线(自脐至左髂前上棘的线)

Monro's bursa [mənˈrəu] (Alexander Monro 〈Secundus〉) 鹰嘴腱内囊 | ~ foramen 室间孔 / ~ line 门罗线(从脐至髂前上棘的直线) / ~ sulcus 丘脑下部沟,下丘脑沟

mons [mɔnz] ([复] **montes** [ˈmɔntiːz]) *n*【拉】山,阜 | ~ pubis, ~ veneris 阴阜 / ~ ureteris 输尿管阜

Monsonia [mɔnˈsəuniə] *n* 多蕊老鹳草属(若干种在医学上用作收敛药并用于痢疾)

monster [ˈmɔnstə] *n* 畸胎;[噬菌体]畸形体 | acardiac ~ 无心畸胎 / autositic ~ 自养[畸]胎 / celosomian ~ 露脏畸胎 / compound ~ 复体畸胎 / cyclopic ~ 独眼畸胎 / double ~, twin ~ 双畸胎,联胎 / emmenic ~ 行经畸胎(行经女婴) / endocymic ~ 胎内寄生胎 / hair ~ 多毛畸胎 / monoaxial ~ 单轴畸胎 / parasitic ~ 寄生畸胎 / polysomatous ~ 多体畸胎 / single ~ 单体畸胎 / sirenoform ~ [无足]并腿畸胎 / triplet ~ 三体畸胎,三联胎

monstricide [ˈmɔnstrisaid] *n* 畸胎毁除术

monstrosity [mɔnˈstrɔsəti] *n* 畸形;畸胎

monstrous [ˈmɔnstrəs] *a* 畸形的

monstrum [ˈmɔnstrəm] ([复] **monstra** [ˈmɔnstrə]) *n*【拉】畸胎

montage [munˈtɑːʒ] *n* 组合,安装(头皮上一排电极组合,在某一区或整个脑多处部位作若干次同时脑电图记录)

montanic acid [mɔnˈtænik] 褐煤酸

Monteggia's dislocation [mɔnˈtedʒə] (Giovanni B. Monteggia) 蒙特吉亚脱位(使股骨头接近髂前上棘的髋关节脱位) | ~ fracture 蒙特吉亚骨折(尺骨骨干骨折兼桡骨头脱位)

montelukast sodium [ˌmɔntəˈluːkæst] 孟特鲁卡钠(一种白三烯拮抗剂,用作平喘药,预防和长期治疗哮喘,口服给药)

montes [ˈmɔntiːz] mons 的复数

Montgomery's follicles [məntˈgʌməri] (William F. Montgomery) 蒙哥马利滤泡(见 Naboth's follicles) | ~ glands, ~ tubercles 乳晕腺

monticulus [mɔnˈtikjuləs] ([复] **monticuli** [mɔnˈtikjulai]) *n*【拉】小山 | ~ cerebelli 小脑小山

mood [muːd] *n* 心境,情绪 | pure ~ 内向心境(如忧虑、抑郁或愉快)

mood-congruent [muːd kənˈgruːənt] *a* 心境协调

的(精神病特征)

mood-incongruent [muːd ˌinkən'gruːənt] *a* 心境不协调的(精神病特征)

Moon's teeth (molars) [muːn] (Henry Moon) 穆恩磨牙(先天性梅毒患者的第一磨牙,小而呈圆顶形)

Mooren's ulcer ['murən] (Albert Mooren) 莫伦溃疡,蚕食性角膜溃疡(角膜慢性匐行性溃疡)

Moore's fracture [muə] (Edward M. Moore) 穆尔骨折(桡骨下端骨折兼尺骨头脱位)

Moore's lightning streaks [muə] (Robert F. Moore) 穆尔光纹(光的垂直闪动,类似闪电,有时见于两眼转动时周边视野,本病为良性)

Moore's syndrome [muə] (Matthew T. Moore) 腹型癫痫

Moore's test [muə] (John Moore) 穆尔试验(检右旋糖或任何碳水化合物)

Moorhead foreign body locator ['muəhed] (John J. Moorhead) 穆尔黑德[金属]异物探索器

MOPP mechlorethamine, vincristin, procarbazine, and prednisone 氮芥-长春新碱-丙卡巴肼-泼尼松(联合化疗治癌方案)

Morand's foot [mɔ'rɑːn] (Sauveur F. Morand) 莫朗足(八趾足) | ~ foramen 舌盲孔 / ~ spur 禽距

morantel tartrate [mə'ræntəl] 酒石酸莫仑太尔(兽用抗蠕虫药)

Morax-Axenfeld conjunctivitis ['mɔːræks 'æksənfelt] (Victor Morax; Theodor Axenfeld) 莫-阿结膜炎(结膜炎嗜血杆菌所致的一种结膜炎,亦称双杆菌结膜炎) | ~ diplococcus (bacillus, hemophilus) 结膜炎嗜血杆菌,结膜炎莫拉菌

Moraxella [ˌmɔːræk'selə] (Victor Morax) *n* 莫拉菌属 | ~ bovis 牛莫拉菌,牛嗜血杆菌 / ~ lacunata 结膜炎莫拉菌,结膜炎嗜血杆菌 / ~ liquefaciens 液化莫拉菌

morbid ['mɔːbid] *a* 疾病的,病态的

morbidity [mɔː'bidəti] *n* 病态,成病,发病;发病率

morbidostatic [ˌmɔːbidə'stætik] *a* 阻止疾病的

morbific(al) [mɔː'bifik(əl)], **morbigenous** [mɔː'bidʒənəs] *a* 致病的

morbilli [mɔː'bilai] *n*【拉】麻疹

morbilliform [mɔː'bilifɔːm] *a* 麻疹样的

Morbillivirus [mɔː'biliˌvaiərəs] *n* 麻疹病毒属

morbillous [mɔː'biləs] *a* 麻疹的

morbus ['mɔːbəs] *n*【拉】[疾]病 | ~ coxae senilis 老年性髋关节病 / ~ moniliformis 念珠状病,念珠状红苔藓

MORC Medical Officers Reserve Corps 军医预备队

morcellation [ˌmɔːsə'leiʃən], **morcellement** [ˌmɔːsəl'mɔŋ] *n* 分碎术

mordant ['mɔːdənt] *a* 剧烈的,腐蚀的;媒染的 *n* 媒染剂;腐蚀剂

Mor. dict. more dicto【拉】用法口授

Morel ear [mɔ'rel] (Benoit A. Morel) 莫雷尔耳(耳畸形发育,其特征为耳轮、对耳轮和舟状窝发育异常,耳大而光滑,沟折不显,边缘菲薄) | ~ syndrome 莫雷尔综合征(额骨肥厚、肥胖、头痛、神经障碍及有精神病的倾向)

Morel-Kraepelin disease [mɔ'rel 'kreipəlin] (B. A. Morel; Emil Kraepelin) 精神分裂症

Morelli's test (reaction) [mɔ'reli] (F. Morelli) 莫雷利试验(反应)(鉴别渗出液与漏出液)

mores ['mɔːriːz] *n*【拉】风俗,习惯

Moreschi's phenomenon [mɔ'reski] (Carlo Moreschi) 莫雷斯基现象,补体结合现象(fixation of complement,见 fixation 项下相应术语)

Morestin's operation (method) [ˌmɔres'tæn] (Hippolyte Morestin) 莫雷斯坦手术(法)(股骨髁内分离的膝关节断离术)

Moretti's test [mɔ'reti] (E. Moretti) 莫雷蒂试验(检伤寒的一种尿色泽反应)

Morgagni-Adams-Stokes syndrome [mɔ'gɑːnji 'ædəmz stəuks] (Giovanni B. Morgagni; Robert Adams; Wiliam Stokes) 莫-亚-斯综合征(见 Adams-Stokes disease)

morgagnian [mɔ'gɑːniən] *a* 莫尔加尼(Giovanni B. Morgagni)的

Morgagni's appendix [mɔ'gɑːni] (Giovanni B. Morgagni) 莫尔加尼附件(①睾丸附件;②卵巢冠囊状附件) | ~ caruncle 莫尔加尼小阜(前列腺中叶) / columns of Morgagni 莫尔加尼柱(肛柱) / crypt of Morgagni 莫尔加尼隐窝(①尿道舟状窝;②肛窦) / ~ foramen 莫尔加尼孔(①胸膜裂孔;②舌盲孔) / fossa of Morgagni 莫尔加尼窝(尿道舟状窝) / frenum of Morgagni 莫尔加尼系带(回盲瓣系带) / ~ glands 莫尔加尼腺(男尿道腺) / ~ globules 莫尔加尼球(晶状体外层内圆形细胞碎片,为成熟白内障的征象) / ~ hernia 莫尔加尼疝(先天性胸骨后膈疝,组织经莫尔加尼突出进入胸腔) / lacunae of Morgagni 莫尔加尼陷窝(男尿道陷窝) / ~ nodules 莫尔加尼小结(主动脉半月瓣小结) / ~ prolapse 莫尔加尼脱垂(喉小囊黏膜和黏膜下层的慢性炎性增生) / ~ tubercle 莫尔加尼结节(①嗅球;②乳腺乳晕表面小结节之一,由浅表大皮脂腺产生) / ~ valves 莫尔加尼瓣(肛瓣) / ~ ventricle 莫尔加尼室(喉室)

morgan ['mɔːgən] (Thomas H. Morgan) *n* 摩[尔根](染色体图距单位,符号为 M)

Morganella [mɔːgə'nelə] (H. de R. Morgan) *n* 摩根菌属 | ~ morganii 摩氏摩根菌

Morgan's bacillus ['mɔːgən] (Harry de R. Morgan) 摩根[变形]杆菌

Morgan's line [ˈmɔːgən] 摩尔根线(变位性皮炎时,下睑继发性皮皱)

morgue [mɔːg] *n*【法】停尸室,太平间

moria [ˈmɔːriə] *n*【希】[儿]童样痴呆,诙谐状痴呆

moribund [ˈmɔ(ː)ribʌnd] *a* 濒死的

moricizine hydrochloride [mɔˈrisiziːn] 盐酸莫雷西嗪(抗心律失常药)

Moringa [məˈriŋgə] *n* 辣木属

Morison's pouch [ˈmɔrisn] (James R. Morison) 莫里森陷凹(肝下的腹膜陷凹,肝下方至右肾右侧,向下至横结肠系膜)

Morita therapy [mɔˈriːtə] (Shomei Morita) 森田疗法(坐禅疗法)

Moritz reaction [ˈmɔrits] (Friedrich H. L. Moritz) 莫里茨反应(试验)(见 Rivalta's reaction)

Mörner's body [ˈməːnə] (Carl A. H. Mörner) 核白蛋白 | ~ reagent 梅尔肉尔试剂(福尔马林1份、蒸馏水45份、浓硫酸55份组成的溶液,用于检酪氨酸试验) / ~ test 梅尔内尔试验(①检酪氨酸;②硝基氢氰酸盐试验,检半胱氨酸)

morning glory [ˈmɔːniŋˈglɔri] 牵牛花

moron [ˈmɔːrɔn] *n* 愚鲁(智商为 50 ~ 69) | **~ic** [mɔˈrɔnik] *a* / **~ity** [məˈrɔnəti], **~ism, morosis** [məˈrəusis] *n* 愚鲁

Moro's reaction (test) [ˈmɔːrəu] (Ernst Moro) 莫罗反应(试验)(用 5 ml 旧结核菌素与 5 g 无水羊毛脂配成的软膏在皮肤区敷贴,以后出现苍白或红色丘疹,此种试验业已被其他结核菌素皮上试验所取代) / ~ reflex, ~ embrace reflex 莫罗反射、莫罗拥抱反射(将婴儿置于桌上,重击其任一侧的桌面,婴儿手臂突然伸出作拥抱状。亦称惊吓反射)

-morph [构词成分] 形态,形

morphallaxis [mɔːfəˈlæksis] ([复]**morphallaxes** [ˌmɔːfəˈlæksiːz]) *n* 变形再生 | **morphallactic** *a*

morphea [məˈfiːə] *n* 硬斑病(亦称局限性硬皮病) | generalized ~ 泛发性硬斑病 / guttate ~ 滴状硬斑病(亦称白点病) / linear ~, ~ linearis 线状硬斑病

morpheme [ˈmɔːfiːm] *n* 语素,词素

morphina [mɔːˈfinə] ([复]**morphinae** [mɔːˈfiniː]) *n*【拉】吗啡

morphine [ˈmɔːfiːn] *n* 吗啡 | dimethyl ~ 二甲基吗啡,蒂巴因(thebaine) / ~ hydrochloride 盐酸吗啡(麻醉镇痛药,英国和德国常用) / ~ sulfate 硫酸吗啡(麻醉镇痛药,美国常用) | **morphia** [ˈmɔːfjə], **morphium** [ˈmɔːfiəm] *n* / **morphinic** [mɔːˈfinik] *a*

morphinism [ˈmɔːfinizəm] *n* 吗啡瘾,吗啡中毒 | **morphinistic** [ˌmɔːfiˈnistik] *a*

morphinist [ˈmɔːfinist] *n* 吗啡瘾者,吗啡中毒者

morphinium [mɔːˈfiniəm] *n*【拉】吗啡

morphinization [ˌmɔːfinaiˈzeiʃən, -niˈz-] *n* 吗啡作用,吗啡影响

morphinomania [ˌmɔːfinəuˈmeinjə], **morphiomania** [ˌmɔːfiəuˈmeinjə] *n* 吗啡瘾;吗啡狂

morph(o)- [构词成分] 形态,形

morphodifferentiation [ˌmɔːfəuˌdifəˌrenʃiˈeiʃən] *n* 形态分化

morphogen [ˈmɔːfədʒən] *n* 形态发生素

morphogenesis [ˌmɔːfəuˈdʒenisis], **morphogenesia** [ˌmɔːfəudʒiˈniːziə], **morphogeny** [mɔːˈfɔdʒini] *n* 形态发生 | **morphogenetic** [ˌmɔːfəudʒiˈnetik] *a*

morphography [mɔːˈfɔgrəfi] *n* 形态论

morphology [mɔːˈfɔlədʒi] *n* 形态学 | **morphologic(al)** [ˌmɔːfəˈlɔdʒik(əl)] / **morphologist** *n* 形态学家

morpholysis [mɔːˈfɔlisis] *n* 形态残毁,形态崩坏

morphometry [mɔːˈfɔmitri] *n* 形态计量法

morphon [ˈmɔːfɔn] *n* 单体[形态]

morphophyly [mɔːˈfɔfili] *n* 成形发育

morphophysics [ˌmɔːfəuˈfiziks] *n* 形态物理学

morphoplasm [ˈmɔːfəˌplæzəm] *n* 成形质

morphosis [mɔːˈfəusis] *n*【希】形态构成 | **morphotic** [mɔːˈfɔtik] *a*

-morphous [构词成分] 形态,形

morpio [ˈmɔːpiəu], **morpion** [ˈmɔːpiən] ([复]**morpiones** [ˌmɔːpiˈəuniːz]) *n*【拉】阴虱

Morquio's sign [mɔːˈkiːəu] (Louis Morquio) 莫尔基奥征(脊髓灰质炎的体征,即病人仰卧,除非下肢被动屈曲,则躯干不能抬起至坐位) | ~ syndrome(disease) 莫尔基奥综合征(病)(一种罕见的黏多糖贮积症,病孩开始走路时变得明显,特征为严重侏儒症,尤其躯干矮小、短颈、胸骨隆凸、膝外翻、扁平足及鸭步态,与胡尔勒〈Hurler〉综合征相对照,精神发育迟缓无或轻微,面部畸形不太显著,角膜混浊以及耳聋程度轻微,除或许有主动脉瓣病以外,无心血管变化,为常染色体隐性遗传。亦称黏多糖贮积症Ⅳ型,硫酸角质素尿)

Morquio-Ullrich disease [mɔːˈkiːəu ˈulrik] (Louis Morquio; Otto Ullrich) 莫-乌病(见 Morquio's syndrome)

morrhua [ˈmɔːrjuə] *n*【拉】鳕鱼

morrhuate [ˈmɔːrjueit] *n* 鱼肝油酸盐

morrhuic acid [ˈmɔːrjuik] *n* 鱼肝油酸

morrhuin [ˈmɔːrjuin] *n* 鳕肝尸胺

Morris syndrome [ˈmɔris] (John McLean Morris) 莫里斯综合征(完全性雄激素抗性)

mors [mɔːz] *n*【拉】死亡 | ~ thymica 胸腺病性死亡

morsal [ˈmɔːsəl] *a* 狢面的
Mor. sol. more solito【拉】照常规
morsulus [ˈmɔːsjuləs] *n* 锭剂
morsus [ˈmɔːsəs] *n*【拉】咬,螫 | ~ diaboli 输卵管缴 / ~ humanus 人咬伤
mortal [ˈmɔːtl] *a* 致死的
mortality [mɔːˈtæləti] *n* 死亡率 | actual ~ 实际死亡率(一百万人寿保险者经过一百年的死亡数) / annual actual ~ 每年实际死亡率(每一百个人寿保险者的死亡数) / perinatal ~ 围生期死亡率 / tabular ~ 图表死亡率(寿命图表中表示每一千个人寿保险者的预期死亡率)
mortalogram [mɔːˈtæləgræm] *n* 死亡率图
mortar [ˈmɔːtə] *n* 研钵
mortician [mɔːˈtiʃən] *n* 殡仪业者
Mortierella [mɔːtiəˈrelə] *n* 被孢霉属
Mortierellaceae [ˌmɔːtiəreˈleisiiː] *n* 被孢霉科
mortification [ˌmɔːtifiˈkeiʃən] *n* 坏疽
mortinatality [ˌmɔːtineiˈtæləti] *n* 死产率
Morton's cough [ˈmɔːtn] (Richard Morton)莫顿咳(肺结核的剧咳,引起呕吐,因而损失营养)
Morton's neuralgia (disease, foot, metatarsalgia, toe) [ˈmɔːtən] (Thomas G. Morton)莫顿神经痛(病、足、跖骨痛、趾)(一型足痛,由于跖骨头压迫跖神经分支引起的跖骨痛,长期压迫可能导致神经瘤形成) | ~ neuroma 莫顿神经瘤(由于莫顿神经痛引起的神经瘤) / ~ test 莫顿试验(检跖骨痛)
Morsler's diabetes [ˈmɔslə] (Karl F. Morsler)莫斯勒糖尿病(肌醇尿性糖尿病) | ~ sign 莫斯勒征(急性成髓细胞白血病时有胸骨压痛)
mortuary [ˈmɔːtjuəri] *n* 停尸室,太平间 *a* 丧葬的;死亡的
morula [ˈmɔːrulə] *n* 桑葚胚 | **~r** *a* 桑葚胚的;桑葚状的 / **~tion** [ˌmɔːruˈleiʃən] *n* 桑葚胚形成
moruloid [ˈmɔːrulɔid] *a* 桑葚样的 *n* 桑葚状菌落
Morvan's disease [ˈmɔːvæn] (Augustin M. Morvan)莫旺病(脊髓空洞症;见莫旺综合征②) | ~ syndrome 莫旺综合征(①脊髓空洞症;②脊髓空洞症的表现,特征为双手皮下组织增厚,使手变得松软、肿胀、青紫和冰冷,伴手指尖无痛性溃疡及手与前臂感觉异常和萎缩。亦称无痛性瘭疽,莫旺病)
mosaic [məuˈzeiik] *n* 嵌合体(在遗传学上指由单一合子内不同基因型组成的具有两种或两种以上细胞群的个体;在胚胎学上指某些生物种〈如海胆〉受精卵的情况,此时早期细胞所生成的细胞质可决定将来身体某些部分的发育);花斑病,花叶病(在植物病理学上,一种病毒性疾病,其特征为叶成斑状)
mosaicism [məuˈzeiisizəm] *n* 镶嵌性(在遗传学上指由单一合子内不同基因型所组成的两个或两个以上细胞群的个体同时存在的状态) | erythrocyte ~ 红细胞镶嵌性
Moschcowitz's disease [ˈmɔskəwits] (Eli Moschcowitz)莫斯科维茨病(血栓形成性血小板减少性紫癜) | ~ test(sign)莫斯科维茨试验(征)(检动脉硬化症,以埃斯马赫〈Esmarch〉驱血带阻断下肢血流5分钟后松去,正常者下肢颜色于数秒内即恢复,但动脉硬化者的下肢颜色甚慢恢复。亦称充血试验)
Moschcowitz's operation [ˈmɔskəwits] (Alexis V. Moschcowitz)莫斯科维茨手术(经由腹股沟修复股疝手术)
Mosenthal's test [ˈmɔzənθəl] (Herman O. Mosenthal)莫森索尔试验(检肾功能)
Moser's serum [ˈmɔːzə] (Paul Moser)莫塞尔血清,猩红热链球菌免疫血清(由猩红热患者血中的链球菌免疫马后所制备的抗链球菌血清)
Mosetig-Moorhof bone wax (filling) [mɔˈsetiʃ ˈmɔːhɔf] (Albert von Mosetig-Moorhof)莫塞堤·莫尔霍夫骨蜡(填料)(无菌骨空隙蜡填料)
Mosler's diabetes [ˈmɔslə] (Karl F. Mosler)莫斯勒糖尿病(肌醇尿性糖尿病)
mOsm milliosmol 毫渗模,毫渗量,毫渗摩尔
mosquito [məsˈkiːtəu] ([复] **mosquitoes**) *n* 蚊 | anautogenous ~ 非自生蚊 / arygamous ~ 旷生蚊 / autogenous ~ 自生蚊 / house ~ 家蚊 / steyogamous ~ 局生蚊 / tiger ~ 虎斑蚊,埃及伊蚊
mosquitocidal [məsˌkiːtəuˈsaidl] *a* 灭蚊的
mosquitocide [məsˈkiːtəusaid] *n* 杀蚊剂
moss [mɔs] *n* 藓,苔藓植物 | Ceylon ~ 锡兰苔,石花菜 / Iceland ~ 冰岛苔,冰岛衣 / Irish ~, pearl ~, salt rock ~ 角叉菜,爱兰苔 / juniper ~ 杜松苔
Mosse's syndrome [ˈmɔsə] (Max Mosse)莫塞综合征(真性红细胞增多症伴肝硬化)
Mosso's ergograph [ˈmɔsəu] (Angelo Mosso)莫索测指力器(记录手指屈曲力和频率) | ~ sphygmomanometer 莫索血压计
Moss's classification [mɔs] (William L. Moss)莫斯分类(一种用罗马数字Ⅰ—Ⅳ表示的ABO血型分类法,Ⅰ,Ⅱ,Ⅲ,Ⅳ分别相当于AB,A,B和O血型)
Motais' operation [mɔˈteiz] (Ernst Motais)莫泰手术(睑下垂手术,即将眼球上直肌肌腱的中部移植到上睑)
moth [mɔθ] *n* 蛾,蠹 | brown-tail ~ 褐尾蠹(即Euproctis chrysorrhoea) / flannel ~ 绒蛾 / io ~ 巨斑刺蛾(即Automeris io) / meal ~ 大斑粉螟 / tussock ~ 白斑天幕毒蛾(即Hemerocampa leucostigma)
mother [ˈmʌðə] *n* 母亲;母体 | ~ of vinegar 醋

母,醋酸杆菌,醋母杆菌

motile [ˈməutail, ˈməutil] *a* 能动的 | **motility** [məuˈtiləti] *n* 能动性,能动力

motilin [məuˈtilin] *n* 促胃动素(由肠嗜铬细胞分泌一种多肽激素,能促进胃肠活动,并刺激胃蛋白酶分泌)

motion [ˈməuʃən] *n* 运动;活动 | systolic anterior ~ 收缩期前向活动 / ventricular wall ~ 室壁运动

motivate [ˈməutiveit] *vt* 促动,激发,诱导;成为…的动机 | **motivation** [ˌməutiˈveiʃən] *n* 动机

motive [ˈməutiv] *n* 动机,目的

motoceptor [ˈməutəˌseptə] *n* 运动感受器(指肌感受器)

motofacient [ˌməutəuˈfeiʃənt] *a* 促动的,发动的

motoneuron [ˌməutəuˈnjuərən] *n* 运动神经元

motor [ˈməutə] *n* 运动原(指影响或产生运动的肌肉、运动神经或中枢);传动器(假肢部件) *a* 运动的 | plastic ~ 成形传动器(指截肢残端组织用于使假肢获得活动)

motorgraphic [ˌməutəˈgræfik] *a* 描记运动的

motorial [məuˈtɔːriəl] *a* 运动的;运动中枢的;运动器官的

motoricity [ˌməutəˈrisəti] *n* 运动力

motorium [məuˈtɔːriəm] *n*【拉】运动中枢;运动器官;意志(在心理学上,为指导有目的活动的心理功能)

motorius [məuˈtɔːriəs] *n*【拉】运动神经

motorogerminative [ˌməutərəˈdʒəːmineitiv] *a* 动胚的,成肌的(指中胚层的一部分)

motorpathy [məuˈtɔːpəθi] *n* 运动疗法,体操疗法

MOTT mycobacteria other than tubercle bacilli 非结核杆菌的分枝杆菌

mottling [ˈmɔtliŋ] *n* 斑[状阴]影,斑点状阴影

Mott's law of anticipation [mɔt] (Fredrick W Mott)莫特提前出现律(后代精神病者比上代精神病者发病年龄提早,目前证明此定律并非真实)

mouche [muːʃ] ([复]**mouches**) *n*【法】斑点;蝇 | ~s volantes 飞蝇幻视

moulage [muːˈlɑːʒ] *n*【法】蜡模[型]

mould [məuld] *n*, *vt* 见 mold

moulding [ˈməuldiŋ] *n* (分娩时)胎头变形;塑型 | ~ of head 胎头变形

mounding [ˈmaundiŋ] *n* 肌耸起,肌耸肿(肌受击时所产生)

Mounier-Kuhn syndrome [muːniˈei kjuːn] (Pierre Mounier-Kuhn)莫尼埃-库恩综合征,气管支气管扩大

mount [maunt] *vt* 支固;制作标本和载片,置标本于载片上,封固(显微镜的)载片 *n* 底座;(显微镜的)载片

mountant [ˈmauntənt] *n* 封固剂(如天然树脂、多聚物或甘油,将标本包埋其中,以便显微镜研究)

mounting [ˈmauntiŋ] *n* 装片,封固,封片;装置,上殆架 | split cast ~ 分模装置(一种牙模型)

Mount-Reback syndrome [maunt ˈriːbæk] (L. A. Mount; S. Reback)蒙-里综合征(一种罕见的常染色体显性遗传病,特征为舞蹈手足徐动症阵发性发作和张力障碍性运动,伴角膜上凯-弗〈Kayser-Flelscher〉环。儿童期及青年期发病,并不影响意识改变。亦称阵发性或家族性阵发性舞蹈手足徐动症)

Mount's syndrome [maunt] (Lester A. Mount) 蒙特综合征(见 Mount-Reback syndrome)

mourning [ˈmɔːniŋ] *n* 悲伤,哀悼;哀悼仪式

mouse [maus] ([复]**mice** [mais]) *n* 小鼠;游动小体 | C. F. W ~ (cancer-free white mouse)无癌小鼠 / joint ~ 关节内游动体,关节鼠 / nude ~, nu / nu ~ 裸鼠,无胸腺小鼠 / peritoneal ~ 腹膜腔游动体 / pleural ~ 胸膜鼠(胸膜炎时纤维组织造成的异物,见于 X 线检查)

mousepox [ˈmauspɔks] *n* [小]鼠痘,传染性缺肢畸形

mouth [mauθ] *n* 口 | Ceylon sore ~ 热带性口炎性腹泻 / denture sore ~ 义齿性口腔痛 / dry ~ 口干燥 / glassblowers' ~ (吹玻璃者)腮腺增大 / tapir ~ 貘状口,突唇口,撅嘴 / trench ~ 战壕口炎,坏死性溃疡性龈炎 / white ~ 鹅口疮,霉菌性口炎

mouth-to-mouth [ˈmauθ tə ˈmauθ] *a* 口对口的(指人工呼吸法)

mouthwash [ˈmauθwɔʃ] *n* 漱口药

movement [ˈmuːvmənt] *n* 运动,活动;排粪 | active ~ 主动运动 / ameboid ~ 阿米巴运动,变形运动 / angular ~ 角动(指两骨间的角度发生改变) / associated ~ 联合运动(如眼) / automatic ~ 自动性运动 / border ~ 边缘性运动 / border tissue ~ 周边组织性运动 / bowel ~ 肠运动,排粪 / ciliary ~ 纤毛运动 / excessive ~ 运动过度,运动功能亢进 / fetal ~ 胎动 / free mandibular ~ 下颌自由运动 / functional mandibular ~s 下颌功能性运动 / hinge ~ 铰链式运动 / intermediary ~s, intermediate ~ 颌中运动 / opening ~ 张开[口]运动 / passive ~ 被动运动 / pendular ~ 摆[摇运]动(消化时小肠的一种运动) / posterior opening ~ 后部张开[口]运动 / rapid eye ~ (REM) 快速眼动(见于作梦睡眠) / saccadic eye ~ 眼扫视运动 / scissors ~ 剪式运动(一种瞳孔反射运动,表示不规则散光) / segmentation ~ 节段运动(消化时小肠运动方式之一) / sleep ~ 睡眠运动(植物的一种感性运动) / vermicular ~s 蠕动

mover [ˈmuːvə] *n* 原动力 | prime ~ 原动力;原

动肌

moxa [ˈmɔksə] *n*【日】灸料,艾,灼烙剂

moxalactam [ˌmɔksəˈlæktæm] *n* 拉氧头孢(抗生素类药)

moxazocine [mɔkˈseizəsiːn] *n* 莫沙佐辛(镇痛药,镇咳药)

moxibustion [ˌmɔksiˈbʌstʃən] *n* [艾]灸术

moxifloxacin [ˌmɔksiˈflɔksəsin] *n* 莫氟沙星(抗菌药)

moxnidazole [mɔksˈnidəzəul] *n* 吗硝唑(抗原虫药,抗滴虫药)

moyamoya [ˈmɔiəˌmɔiə] *n*【日】烟雾阴影(动脉造影照片所见)

Moynahan's syndrome [ˈmɔinəhən] (E. J. Moynahan)莫伊纳罕综合征(①多发性对称性着色斑、先天性左房室瓣狭窄、侏儒、生殖器发育不全和精神发育迟缓,亦称进行性心肌病性着色斑病;②一种家族性先天性综合征,包括头皮上毛发生长迟缓、癫痫、精神发育迟缓和脑电图异常)

Moynihan's cream [ˈmɔinjən] (Berkeley G. A. Moynihan)莫伊尼汉乳膏(敷伤用) | ~ test 莫伊尼汉试验(检葫芦胃)

Mozart ear [ˈməutsɑːt] (Wolfgang A. Mozart 为奥地利作曲家,据报道他患有此耳畸形)莫扎特耳(对耳轮脚和耳轮脚先天性融合)

6-MP 6-mercaptopurine 6-巯基嘌呤,巯基嘌呤(抗肿瘤药)

mp melting point 熔点

MPD maximum permissible dose 最大容许剂量

MPH Master of Public Health 公共卫生硕士

MPO myeloperoxidase 髓过氧化物酶

MPS mononuclear phagocyte system 单核吞噬细胞系统;mucopolysaccharidosis 黏多糖贮积症

MR mitral regurgitation 二尖瓣反流

mR milliroentgen 毫伦琴

μR microroentgen 微伦琴

MRA Medical Record Administrator 医疗档案管理员,病案管理员;magnetic resonance angiography 磁共振血管造影[术]

MRACP Member of Royal Australasian College of Physicians 澳大利西亚皇家内科医师学会会员

mrad millirad 毫拉德

MRC Medical Reserve Corps 军医预备队

MRCP Member of the Royal College of Physicians 皇家内科医师学会会员

MRCPE Member of the Royal College of Physicians of Edinburgh 爱丁堡皇家内科医师学会会员

MRCP (Glasg) Member of the Royal College of Physicians and Surgeons of Glassgow *qua* Physician 格拉斯哥皇家内外科医师学会(内科医师)会员

MRCPI Member of the Royal College of Physicians of Ireland 爱尔兰皇家内科医师学会会员

MRCS Member of the Royal College of Surgeons 皇家外科医师学会会员

MRCSEd Member of the Royal College of Surgeons of Edinburgh 爱丁堡皇家外科医师学会会员

MRCSI Member of the Royal College of Surgeons of Ireland 爱尔兰皇家外科医师学会会员

MRCVS Member of the Royal College of Veterinary Surgeons 皇家外科兽医学会会员

MRD minimum reacting dose 最小反应剂量

MRDM malnutrition-related diabetes mellitus 营养不良相关性糖尿病

mrem millirem 毫雷姆

MRF melanocyte-stimulating hormone releasing factor 促黑[素细胞]激素释放因子

MRI magnetic resonance imaging 磁共振成像

MRL Medical Record Librarian 病案管理员(现称 Medical Record Administrator)

mRNA messenger RNA 信使 RNA

MRSA methicillin-resistant *Staphylococcus aureus* 抗甲氧西林金黄色葡萄球菌

MS Master of Science 理科硕士; Master of Surgery 外科硕士; mitral stenosis 二尖瓣狭窄; multiple sclerosis 多发性硬化

ms millisecond 毫秒

μs microsecond 微秒

MSE Mental Status Examination 精神状态检查

msec millisecond 毫秒

MSG monosodium glutamate 谷氨酸钠,谷氨酸单钠(治肝昏迷药)

MSH melanocyte-stimulating hormone 促黑[素细胞]激素,促黑素

MSL midsternal line 胸骨中线

MSLT multiple sleep latency test 多发性睡眠潜伏期试验

MS/MS tandem mass spectrometry 串联质谱分析法

MSUD maple syrup urine disease 枫糖尿病

MT Medical Technologist 医学技术员; membrana tympani 鼓膜

MTD maximum tolerated dose 最大耐受剂量

mtDNA mitochondrial DNA 线粒体 DNA

MTX methotrexate 甲氨蝶呤(抗肿瘤药)

Mu Mache unit 马谢单位(镭射气浓度单位)

mU milliunit 毫单位

mu [mjuː] *n* 希腊语的第 12 个字母(M, μ);微米

m. u. mouse unit 小鼠单位(雌激素的生物鉴定单位)

μU microunit 微单位

MUAP motor unit action potential 运动单位动作电位

Muc. mucilago【拉】胶浆,黏浆

mucase [ˈmjuːkeis] *n* 黏多糖酶

Mucha-Habermann disease [ˈmuːkə ˈhɑːbəmən] (Viktor Mucha; Rudolf Habermann) 急性苔藓样糠疹
Mucha's disease [ˈmuːkə] (Viktor Mucha) 急性苔藓样糠疹
Much-Holzmann reaction [muh ˈhɔltsmən] (Hans Much; V. Holzmann) 穆赫-霍尔兹曼反应(见 Much's reaction)
Much's granules [muh] (Hans C. R. Much) 穆赫粒(结核病痰中的粒状及杆状结核菌,不能以染抗酸菌的常法染之,但可用革兰法染色,可视为变性的结核菌) | ~ reaction 穆赫反应(眼镜蛇毒对红细胞的溶血作用有抑制的反应,据报道此反应见于精神分裂症及躁郁症,但未被以后的研究所证实。亦称精神性反应)
muci- [构词成分] 黏蛋白;黏液
mucic acid [ˈmjuːsik] 黏酸,半乳糖二酸
mucicarmine [ˌmjuːsiˈkɑːmin] *n* 黏蛋白卡红,黏蛋白胭脂红
mucicarminophilic [ˌmjuːsiˌkɑːminəuˈfilik] *a* 嗜黏蛋白卡红的,嗜黏蛋白胭脂红的
muciferous [mjuːˈsifərəs] *a* 分泌黏液的,生黏液的
mucification [ˌmjuːsifiˈkeiʃən] *n* 黏液化
muciform [ˈmjuːsifɔːm] *a* 黏液样的
mucigen [ˈmjuːsidʒən] *n* 黏蛋白原
mucigenous [mjuːˈsidʒinəs] *a* 生黏液的
mucigogue [ˈmjuːsigɔg] *a* 催黏液的,促黏液分泌的 *n* 催黏液剂,黏液分泌促进剂
mucihematein [ˌmjuːsiˈhiːmətiin] *n* 黏蛋白氧化苏木精
mucilage [ˈmjuːsilidʒ] *n* 胶浆,黏液;胶浆剂 | acacia ~ 阿拉伯胶浆(药物悬浮剂) / tragacanth ~ 西黄蓍胶浆(保护剂)
mucilaginous [ˌmjuːsiˈlædʒinəs] *a* 胶浆性的,胶黏的,黏性的
mucilago [ˌmjuːsiˈlɑːgəu] *n* 【拉】胶浆,黏浆
mucilloid [ˈmjuːsilɔid] *n* 胶浆剂 | psyllium hydrophilic ~ 车前子亲水胶浆(用于治单纯性便秘)
mucin [ˈmjuːsin] *n* 黏蛋白 | gastric ~ 胃黏蛋白(治消化性溃疡)
mucinase [ˈmjuːsineis] *n* 黏多糖酶
mucinoblast [mjuːˈsinəblæst] *n* 成黏液细胞
mucinogen [mjuːˈsinədʒən] *n* 黏蛋白原
mucinoid [ˈmjuːsinɔid] *a* 黏蛋白样的 *n* 类黏蛋白
mucinolytic [ˌmjuːsinəuˈlitik] *a* 黏蛋白分解的
mucinosis [ˌmjuːsiˈnəusis] *n* 黏蛋白沉积症 | follicular ~ 毛囊皮脂腺黏蛋白沉积症 / papular ~ 丘疹性黏蛋白沉积症
mucinous [ˈmjuːsinəs] *a* 黏蛋白的,黏蛋白状的
mucinuria [ˌmjuːsiˈnjuəriə] *n* 黏蛋白尿
muciparous [mjuːˈsipərəs] *a* 分泌黏液的,生黏液的
mucitis [mjuːˈsaitis] *n* 黏膜炎
Muckle-Wells syndrome [ˈmʌkl welz] (Thomas James Muckle; Michael Vernon Wells) 默-韦综合征(一种常染色体显性遗传,特征为淀粉样变性,累及肾脏,引起肾炎、复发性荨麻疹、耳聋和四肢疼痛)
muc(o)- [构词成分] 黏液
mucoantibody [ˌmjuːkəuˈæntibɔdi] *n* 黏液抗体(在黏膜表面与黏液相混的局部抗体,一般是 IgA)
mucocartilage [ˌmjuːkəuˈkɑːtilidʒ] *n* 黏液软骨
mucocele [ˈmjuːkəsiːl] *n* 黏液囊肿;黏液息肉 | suppurating ~ 化脓性黏液囊肿
mucociliary [ˌmjuːkəuˈsiliəri] *a* 黏液纤毛的
mucoclasis [mjuːˈkɔkləsis] *n* 黏膜毁除术
mucocolitis [ˌmjuːkəukɔˈlaitis] *n* 黏液性结肠炎
mucocolpos [ˌmjuːkəuˈkɔlpɔs] *n* 阴道黏液蓄积
mucocutaneous [ˌmjuːkəukju(ː)ˈteinjəs] *a* 黏膜[与]皮肤的
mucocyst [ˈmjuːkəsist] *n* 黏液囊
mucocyte [ˈmjuːkəsait] *n* 黏液变细胞(胞质呈黏液变性的少突神经胶质细胞)
mucoderm [ˈmjuːkədəːm] *n* 黏膜固有层 | **~al** [ˌmjuːkəuˈdəːməl] *a*
mucoenteritis [ˌmjuːkəuentəˈraitis] *n* 黏液性肠炎(肠易激综合征 irritable bowel syndrome 的旧称)
mucoepidermoid [ˌmjuːkəuˌepiˈdəːmɔid] *a* 黏液表皮样的
mucofibrous [ˌmjuːkəuˈfaibrəs] *a* 黏液纤维的
mucoflocculent [ˌmjuːkəuˈflɔkjulənt] *a* 含黏液细丝的
mucogingival [ˌmjuːkəuˈdʒindʒivəl] *a* 黏膜龈的
mucogingivitis [ˌmjuːkəuˌdʒindʒiˈvaitis] *n* 黏膜龈炎
mucoglobulin [ˌmjuːkəuˈglɔbjulin] *n* 黏球蛋白
mucoid [ˈmjuːkɔid] *a* 黏液样的 *n* 类黏蛋白
mucoitin sulfate [mjuːˈkəuitin] 硫酸黏多糖,硫酸黏液素
mucoitin sulfuric acid [mjuːˈkəuitin] 硫酸黏多糖,硫酸黏液素
mucolemma [ˌmjuːkəuˈlemə] *n* 黏蛋白膜
mucolipid [ˌmjuːkəuˈlipid] *n* 黏脂质
mucolipidosis [ˌmjuːkəuˌlipiˈdəusis] *n* 黏脂贮积症 | ~ Ⅰ 黏脂贮积症Ⅰ型(亦称脂黏多糖病) / ~ Ⅱ 黏脂贮积症Ⅱ型(亦称Ⅰ-细胞病,包涵体纤维细胞病) / ~ Ⅲ 黏脂贮积症Ⅲ型(亦称假胡尔勒〈Hurler〉多种营养不良) / ~ Ⅳ 黏脂贮积症Ⅳ型(特征为早期角膜混浊、精

神运动性阻滞及溶酶体贮积,据称属常染色体隐性遗传)

mucolytic [ˌmjuːkəuˈlitik] *a* 溶解黏液的 *n* 黏液溶解药

mucomembranous [ˌmjuːkəuˈmembrənəs] *a* 黏膜的

muconic acid [mjuːˈkɔnik] 己二烯二酸,黏康酸

mucoperichondrium [ˌmjuːkəuˌperiˈkɔndriəm] *n* 黏膜[性]软骨膜 | **mucoperichondrial** [ˌmjuːkəuˌperiˈkɔndriəl] *a*

mucoperiosteal [ˌmjuːkəuˌperiˈɔstiəl] *a* [含]黏膜骨膜的

mucoperiosteum [ˌmjuːkəuˌperiˈɔstiəm] *n* 黏膜骨膜

mucopolysaccharidase [ˌmjuːkəuˌpɔliˈsækəraideis] *n* 黏多糖酶

mucopolysaccharide [ˌmjuːkəuˌpɔliˈsækəraid] *n* 黏多糖

mucopolysaccharidosis [ˌmjuːkəupɔliˌsækəriˈdəusis] ([复] **mucopolysaccharidoses** [ˌmjuːkəuˌpɔliˌsækəriˈdəusiːz]) *n* 黏多糖贮积症 | ~ Ⅰ, MPS Ⅰ 黏多糖贮积症Ⅰ型(原指胡尔勒综合征 Hurler's syndrome,现包括以 α-L-艾杜糖苷酸酶缺乏、尿中排泄硫酸皮肤素和硫酸乙酰肝素为特征的任何病) / ~ ⅠH, MPS ⅠH 黏多糖贮积症 H 型(即胡尔勒综合征 Hurler syndrome) / ~ ⅠH/S, MPS ⅠH/S 黏多糖贮积症ⅠH/S 型(即胡-沙综合征 Hurler-Scheie syndrome) / ~ IS, MPS ⅠS 黏多糖贮积症 IS 型(即沙伊综合征 Scheie syndrome) / ~ Ⅱ, MPS, Ⅱ 黏多糖贮积症Ⅱ型(即亨特综合征 Hunter syndrome) / ~ Ⅲ, MPS Ⅲ 黏多糖贮积症Ⅲ型(即桑菲利波综合征 Sanfilippo syndrome) / ~ Ⅳ, MPS Ⅳ 黏多糖贮积症Ⅳ型(即莫尔基奥综合征 Morquio syndrome) / ~ Ⅴ, MPS Ⅴ 黏多糖贮积症Ⅴ型(为沙伊综合征 Scheie syndrome 的前称,现归入黏多糖贮积症 S 型) / ~ Ⅵ, MPS Ⅵ 黏多糖贮积症Ⅵ型(即马-拉综合征 Maroteaux-Lamy syndrome) / ~ Ⅶ 黏多糖贮积症Ⅶ型(即斯赖综合征 Sly syndrome)

mucopolysacchariduria [ˌmjuːkəuˌpɔliˌsækəriˈdjuəriə] *n* 黏多糖尿

mucoprotein [ˌmjuːkəuˈprəutiːn] *n* 黏蛋白

mucopurulent [ˌmjuːkəuˈpjuərulənt] *a* 黏液脓性的

mucopus [ˈmjuːkəpʌs] *n* 黏液性脓

Mucor [ˈmjuːkə] *n*【拉】毛霉属,毛霉菌属 | ~ corymbifer 伞状毛霉 / ~ mucedo 蜂毛霉 / ~ pusillus 微小毛霉 / ~ racemosus 总头毛霉,葡萄状毛霉 / ~ ramosus 分枝状毛霉 / ~ rhizopodiformis 根足状毛霉

Mucoraceae [ˌmjuːkəˈreisiiː] *n* 毛霉科

mucoraceous [ˌmjuːkəˈreiʃəs] *a* 毛霉的

Mucorales [ˌmjuːkəˈreiliːz] *n* 毛霉目

mucorin [ˈmjuːkərin] *n* 毛霉蛋白

mucormycosis [ˌmjuːkəmaiˈkəusis] *n* 毛霉病

mucosa [mjuːˈkəusə] ([复] **mucosas** 或 **mucosae** [mjuːˈkəusiː]) *n* 黏膜 | **~l** *a*

mucosanguineous [ˌmjuːkəusæŋˈgwiniəs] *a* 黏液血性的

mucosectomy [ˌmjuːkəuˈsektəmi] *n* 黏膜切除术

mucosedative [ˌmjuːkəuˈsedətiv] *a* 润滑黏膜的

mucoserous [ˌmjuːkəuˈsiərəs] *a* 黏液浆液性的

mucosin [mjuːˈkəusin] *n* 黏精,黏膜素

mucositis [ˌmjuːkəuˈsaitis] *n* 黏膜炎 | ~ necroticans agranulocytica 粒细胞缺乏性坏死性黏膜炎

mucosity [mjuːˈkɔsəti] *n* 黏性

mucosocutaneous [mjuːˌkəusəukju(ː)ˈteinjəs] *a* 黏膜皮肤的

mucostatic [ˌmjuːkəuˈstætik] *a* 抑制黏液分泌的

mucosulfatidosis [ˌmjuːkəuˌsʌlfətiˈdəusis] *n* 黏硫脂病,多硫酸酯酶缺乏症

mucotome [ˈmjuːkətəum] *n* 植黏膜刀,黏膜刀

mucous [ˈmjuːkəs] *a* 黏液的,分泌黏液的

mucoviscidosis [ˌmjuːkəuˌvisiˈdəusis] *n* 黏液黏稠病

mucro [ˈmjuːkrəu] ([复] **mucrones** [mjuːˈkrəuniːz]) *n*【拉】尖,突 | ~ baseos cartilaginis arytaenoideae (杓状软骨)声带突 / ~ cordis 心尖 / ~ sterni 剑突(胸骨)

mucronate [ˈmjuːkrənit], **mucronated** [ˈmjuːkrəneitid] *a* 棘状的,具短尖的(叶端)

mucroniform [mjuːˈkrɔnifɔːm] *a* 棘状的,具短尖的

Mucuna [mjuːˈkjuːnə] *n* 黎豆属,油麻藤属

mucus [ˈmjuːkəs] *n*【拉】黏液

Mueller [ˈmilə] 见 Müller

Muellerius [miˈleriəs] *n* 米[勒]氏线虫属

muffle [ˈmʌfl] *vt* 包裹;抑压 *n* 烘炉

muffler [ˈmʌflə] *n* 消声器

MUGA multiple gated acquisition(scanning)多次闸门探测(扫描)

muguet [muˈgwei] *n*【法】霉菌性口炎,鹅口疮

mugwort [ˈmʌgwəːt] *n* 艾蒿;艾蒿制剂(内服用于胃肠病和用作补药,亦用于顺势疗法和中医)

Muirhead's treatment [ˈmjuəhed] (Archibald L. Muirhead)米尔黑德疗法(注入最大可耐量的肾上腺素及口服肾上腺皮质治艾迪生〈Addison〉病)

Muir-Torre syndrome [ˈmjuə ˈtɔri] (E. G. Muir; Douglas P. Torre)缪-托综合征(见 Torre's syndrome)

mular [ˈmjuːlə] *a* 骡的(本词亦用于人类某种秘鲁疣,因与骡的此病特征相似)

mulatto [mju(ː)ˈlætəu] ([复] **mulattoes**) *n* 黑白混血儿
mulberry [ˈmʌlbəri] *n* 桑树,桑葚
Mulder's angle [ˈmʌldə] (Johannes Mulder)穆尔德角(坎珀尔〈Camper〉面线与自鼻根至蝶枕缝连接线交叉所形成的角)
Mulder's test [ˈmʌldə] (Gerardus J. Mulder)穆尔德试验(检葡萄糖、蛋白质)
Mules' operation [mjuːlz] (Philip H. Mules)米尔斯手术(眼球内容剜出,插入人工玻璃体)
muliebria [ˌmjuːliˈebriə] *n*【拉】女生殖器
muliebrity [ˌmjuːliˈebrəti] *n* 女子特性,女性;男子女性征
mull [mʌl] *n* 软布(曾用于手术) | plaster ~ 硬膏布
muller [ˈmʌlə] *n* 平底乳钵(研磨器)
Müller-Haeckel law [ˈmilə ˈhekəl] (Fritz Müller; Ernst H. Haeckel)生物发生律(biogenetic law,见 law 项下相应术语)
müllerian [miˈliəriən] 米勒(Johannes P. Müller)的(如 ~ duct 中肾旁管)
müllerianoma [miˌliəriəˈnəumə] *n* 米勒管瘤
Müllerius [miˈleriəs] *n* 米[勒]氏线虫属 | ~ capillaris 毛细米[勒]氏线虫
Müller-Jochmann test [ˈmilə ˈjɔkmən] (Edward Müller; George Jochmann)米勒-约克曼试验(①鉴别结核性脓;②抗胰蛋白酶试验)
Müller's capsule [ˈmilə] (Johannes P. Müller)肾小球囊 | ~ duct(canal) 中肾旁管 / ~ maneuver(experiment) 米勒手法(实验)(呼气时声门关闭,再强吸气,荧光镜透视检查时用以产生胸内负压,而让胸腔内血管充血,有助于识别食管血管曲张及区别血管与非血管的结构) / ~ tubercle 窦结节(中肾管及中肾旁管向下生长而突出于生殖窦中)
Müller's fibers (cells, radial cells) [ˈmilə] (Heinrich Müller)米勒纤维(细胞、放射状细胞)(视网膜内神经胶质的支持纤维,亦称支柱纤维) | ~ muscle 睫状肌环状纤维;眼眶肌
Müller's fluid (liquid) [ˈmilə] (Hermann F. Müller)米勒液(溶液)(一种组织硬固液,含有重铬酸钾、硫酸钠和水)
Müller's sign [ˈmilə] (Friedrich von Müller)米勒征(主动脉瓣关闭不全的一种体征:悬雍垂搏动,扁桃体与腭帆发红,与心搏同时出现)
Müller's test [ˈmilə] (Edward Müller)米勒试验(检胱氨酸及结核性脓)
Müller's test (reaction) [ˈmilə] (Rudolf Müller)米勒试验(反应)(检梅毒)
multangular [məlˈtæŋgulə] *a* 多角的
multi- [构词成分] 多,多数
multiallelic [ˌmʌltiəˈlelik] *a* 多等位基因的
multiarticular [ˌmʌltiɑːˈtikjulə] *a* 多关节的
multibacillary [ˌmʌltiˈbæsiˌləri] *a* 多种杆菌的
multicapsular [ˌmʌltiˈkæpsjulə] *a* 多囊的,多被膜的
multicell [ˈmʌltisel] *n* 多细胞体
multicellular [ˌmʌltiˈseljulə] *a* 多细胞的;多空隙的
multicellularity [ˌmʌltiˌseljuˈlærəti] *n* 多细胞性
multicentric [ˌmʌltiˈsentrik] *a* 多中心的 | **~ity** [ˌmʌltisenˈtrisəti] *n* 多中心性
Multiceps [ˈmʌltiseps] *n* 多头绦虫属 | ~ multiceps 多头绦虫 / ~ serialis 链形多头绦虫
multicontaminated [ˌmʌltikənˈtæmineitid] *a* 多种[菌]感染的,多种[污染物]污染的
multicuspid [ˌmʌltiˈkʌspid], **multicuspidate** [ˌmʌltiˈkʌspideit] *a* 多尖的
multicystic [ˌmʌltiˈsistik] *n* 多囊的
multidentate [ˌmʌltiˈdenteit] *a* 多牙的;多牙状突起的
multielectrode [ˌmʌltiiˈlektrəud] *n* 多电极
multifactorial [ˌmʌltifækˈtɔːriəl] *a* 多因子的,多因素的;多遗传因子的
multifarious [ˌmʌltiˈfɛəriəs] *a* 多种多样的
multifid [ˈmʌltifid] *a* 多裂的
multifidus [mʌlˈtifidəs] *n*【拉】多裂肌
multifocal [ˌmʌltiˈfəukəl] *a* 多[病]灶的;多疫源地的
multiform [ˈmʌltifɔːm] *a* 多形的,多态的 | **~ity** [ˌmʌltiˈfɔːməti] *n*
multiganglionic [ˌmʌltiˌgæŋgliˈɔnik] *a* 多[神经]节的
multigenic [ˌmʌltiˈdʒenik] *a* 多基因的
multigesta [ˌmʌltiˈdʒestə] *n* 经[产]孕妇
multiglandular [ˌmʌltiˈglændjulə] *a* 多腺性的
multigravida [ˌmʌltiˈgrævidə] *n* 经孕妇 | grand ~ 多孕妇(妊娠 6 次或 6 次以上的孕妇)
multihallucalism [ˌmʌltiˈhæləkəlizəm], **multihallucism** [ˌmʌltiˈhæləsizəm] *n* 多踇[趾]畸形
multi-infection [ˌmʌltiinˈfekʃən] *n* 多菌传染
multilateral [ˌmʌltiˈlætərəl] *a* 多边的
multilineal [ˌmʌltiˈliniəl] *a* 多线的
multilobar [ˌmʌltiˈləubə] *a* 多叶的
multilobular [ˌmʌltiˈlɔbjulə] *a* 多小叶的
multilocular [ˌmʌltiˈlɔkjulə] *a* 多腔的,多房的
multimammae [ˌmʌltiˈmæmiː] *n* 多乳房[畸形]
multimer [ˈmʌltimə] *n* 多聚体,多体
multimodal [ˌmʌltiˈməudl] *a* 多峰的
multinodular [ˌmʌltiˈnɔdjulə] *a* 多小结的
multinucleate [ˌmʌltiˈnjuːkliit], **multinuclear** [ˌmʌltiˈnjuːkliə] *a* 多核的
multipara [mʌlˈtipərə] ([复] **multiparas** 或

multiparae [mʌlˈtipəriː]) *n* 经产妇 | grand ~ 多产妇(妊娠6次或6次以上,而且胎儿都能存活)
multiparity [ˌmʌltiˈpærəti] *n* 经产;多胎产
multiparous [mʌlˈtipərəs] *a* 经产的;多胎产的,多胞胎的
multipartial [ˌmʌltiˈpɑːʃəl] *a* 多型的(血清)
multiple [ˈmʌltipl] *a* 多发的;多重的 *n* 倍数
multiplex [ˈmʌltipleks] *a* 复合的,多样的;多重的
multiplication [ˌmʌltipliˈkeiʃən] *n* 倍增 | countercurrent ~ 逆流倍增
multiplicitas [ˌmʌltiˈplisitəs] *n* 多重[畸形],过多[畸形] | ~ cordis 多心畸形
multipolar [ˌmʌltiˈpəulə] *a* 多极的
multipollicalism [ˌmʌltiˈpɔlikəlizəm] *n* 多拇[指]畸形
multirooted [ˌmʌltiˈruːtid] *a* 多根的(磨牙)
multirotation [ˌmʌltirəuˈteiʃən] *n* 变异旋光
multisensitivity [ˌmʌltiˌsensiˈtivəti] *n* 多敏感性(对不止一种抗原〈变应原〉有变态反应)
multisensory [ˌmʌltiˈsensəri] *a* 多种感觉[并用]的(指中枢神经系统某些神经元,能对一种以上的感觉输入起反应)
multisynaptic [ˌmʌltisiˈnæptik] *a* 多突触的
multiterminal [ˌmʌltiˈtəːminl] *a* 多端钮的,多末端的
multituberculate [ˌmʌltitju(ː)ˈbəːkjulit] *a* 多结节的
multiplet [ˈmʌltiplet] *n* 多样冲动,复合冲动,多冲动发放
multivalent [ˌmʌltiˈveilənt] *a* 多价的 *n* 多价
Multivalvulida [ˌmʌltiˌvælvjuˈlaidə] *n* 多壳目
multivariate [ˌmʌltiˈvɛərieit] *a* 多变量的
mummification [ˌmʌmifiˈkeiʃən] *n* 干尸化,木乃伊化,干性坏疽
mummy [.ˈmʌmi] *n* 木乃伊,干尸
mummying [ˈmʌmiiŋ] *n* 木乃伊样裹身
mumps [mʌmps] [复] *n* 流行性腮腺炎 | iodine ~ 碘中毒性腮腺炎
mumu [ˈmuːmuː] *n* 精索水肿(可兼发阴囊、附睾、睾丸肿胀)
Münchausen's syndrome [menˈʃauzən] 闵希豪生综合征(以著名夸张故事《吹牛男爵历险记》中的主人公冯·闵希豪生男爵得名,表现为幻想性虚构病史,到处求医或住院癖)
Münchmeyer's disease [ˈminʃmaiə] (Ernst Münchmeyer)明希迈尔病(弥漫性进行性骨化性多肌炎)
munity [ˈmjuːniti] *n* 易感性
Munk's disease [muŋk] (Fritz Munk)脂性肾变病
Munro Kerr cesarean section [mənˈrəu kəː(r)] (John M. Munro Kerr)芒罗·克尔剖宫产术(经膀胱子宫襞横向切开子宫下段,但不使膀胱移位) / ~ incision 芒罗·克尔切口(为剖宫产术所作的子宫下段横向切口) / ~ maneuver 芒罗·克尔手法(确定产妇骨盆和胎头的比例)
Munro's microabscess (abscess) [mənˈrəu] (William J. Munro)芒罗微脓肿(脓肿)(固缩多形核白细胞的小灶性集合,位于角化不全的角质层中,为活动性银屑病的主要组织学特征,亦见于皮脂溢性皮炎和莱特尔〈Reiter〉病)
Munro's point [mənˈrəu] (John. C. Munro)芒罗点(脐至左髂前上棘的直线中点,为腹腔穿刺点)
Munson's sign [ˈmʌnsən] (Edward S. Munson)蒙生征(患者眼球向下转动时下睑异常突出,系角膜曲度异常〈圆锥形角膜〉所引起)
MUP motor unit potential 运动单位电位
mupirocin [mjuˈpirəsin] *n* 莫匹罗星(从荧光假单胞菌〈Pseudomonas fluorescens〉发酵衍生的一种抗菌药,对葡萄球菌和非肠性链球菌有效,局部用于治疗脓疱病)
mural [ˈmjuərəl] *a* 壁的,腔壁的
muralium [mjuːˈreiliəm] ([复] **muralia** [mjuːˈreiliə]) *n* 壁
muramic acid [mjuˈræmik] 胞壁酸
muramidase [mjuˈræmideis] *n* 胞壁质酶,溶菌酶
Murchison-Pel-Ebstein fever [ˈməːtʃisn pel ˈebstain] (Charles Murchison; Pieter K. Pel; Wilhelm Ebstein)默基森-佩尔-埃布斯坦热(霍奇金〈Hodgkin〉病患者的一型热病,其特征为多日的不规则性发热,间以周期性体温正常)
Murex [ˈmjuəreks] *n* 紫螺属 | ~ purpurea 紫螺
murexide [mjuəˈreksaid] *n* 骨螺紫,紫脲酸铵,红紫酸铵
murexine [mjuəˈreksin] *n* 骨螺毒素
muriatic [ˌmjuəriˈætik] *a* 氯化物的,盐的 | ~ acid 盐酸,氢氯酸
Muricidae [mjuːˈrisidiː] *n* 骨螺科
Muridae [ˈmjuridiː] *n* 鼠科
muriform [ˈmjuərifɔːm] *a* 砖格状的(在细菌学中用以描述具有横膈和纵隔的芽胞)
Murimyces [ˌmjuəriˈmaisiːz] *n* 鼠胸膜肺炎菌属(现归入支原体属 Mycoplasma)
murine [ˈmjuərin] *a* 鼠的
murivirus [ˌmjuəriˈvaiərəs] (*m*ild *u*pper *r*espiratory + *virus*) *n* 鼻病毒(现称 rhinovirus)
murmur [ˈməːmə] *n* 杂音 | accidental ~ 偶发性杂音 / amphoric ~ 空瓮性呼吸音 / aortic ~ 主动脉瓣杂音 / attrition ~ 摩擦杂音(由心包炎引起) / bellows ~ 风箱[状杂]音 / blood ~, hemic ~ 血性杂音 / cardiopulmonary ~, cardio-

respiratory ~ 心肺杂音,心搏呼吸杂音 / crescendo ~ 渐强性杂音 / deglutition ~ 吞咽杂音 / diastolic ~ 舒张期杂音 / hour-glass ~ 沙漏样杂音 / humming-top ~ 地牛音,静脉哼鸣 / machinery ~ 机器样杂音 / obstructive ~, direct ~ 阻塞性杂音,直接杂音 / organic ~ 器质性杂音 / pulmonic ~ 肺动脉瓣杂音 / systolic ~ 收缩期杂音 / to-and-fro ~, seesaw ~ 往返性杂音 / vesicular ~ 肺泡呼吸音

muromonab-CD3 [ˌmjuərəˈməunæb] 莫罗单抗-CD3(一种鼠单克隆抗人 T 细胞 CD3 抗原的抗体,用作免疫抑制剂,治疗肾移植的急性同种异体移植物排斥,静脉内给药)

Murphy button [ˈməːfi] (John B. Murphy)墨菲钮(肠吻合钮) | ~ method 墨菲法(①动脉缝合术;②直肠滴注法;③腹膜炎的一种疗法,见墨菲疗法) / ~ percussion 墨菲叩诊,四指叩诊 / ~ sign 墨菲征(胆囊病的一种触诊体征,当医生手指在病人右肋弓下的肝缘下深压时,病人不能深吸气) / ~ test 墨菲试验(病人坐时,双手交臂前胸,检查者以拇指置于病人第十二肋骨下部并作短促戳击,以测定深部压痛及肌肉强直。亦称墨菲肾脏冲击诊) / ~ treatment 墨菲疗法(①胸膜腔内注射氮使肺萎陷治疗肺结核;②腹膜炎的一种疗法:置病人于斜卧位,以利于从腹部引流至骨盆内,然后用生理盐水缓慢冲洗结肠)

Murray Valley encephalitis (disease) [ˈməːri ˈvæli] 墨累山谷脑炎(病)(1950 年和 1951 年流行于澳洲墨累山谷的一种病毒性脑炎,以后证明是 20 世纪 20 年代澳大利亚 X 脑炎的复发,由一种感染鸟和蚊的黄病毒所致,流行病很少发生,儿童感染此病最为严重) | Murray Valley encephalitis virus 墨累山谷脑炎病毒(黄病毒属的蚊传病毒,抗原上与日本脑炎病毒有关,为墨累山谷脑炎的病原体)

murrina [muːˈriːnə] *n*【西】马锥虫病

Murri's disease [ˈmuəri] (Augusto Murri)间歇性血红蛋白尿,阵发性血红蛋白尿

Mus [mʌs] *n*【拉】鼠属 | ~ alexandrinus 屋顶鼠,埃及鼠 / ~ decumanus, ~ norvegicus 褐鼠,沟鼠 / ~ musculus 小家鼠 / ~ rattus 黑鼠

Musca [ˈmʌskə] *n*【拉】蝇属 | ~ autumnalis 秋家蝇 / ~ domestica 家蝇 / ~ domestica nebulo 户蝇 / ~ domestica vicina 舍蝇 / ~ luteola 黄燥蝇,黄火蝇 / ~ sorbens 山蝇,山市家蝇 / ~ vomitoria 反吐丽蝇(即 Calliphora vomitoria)

musca [ˈmʌskə] ([复] **muscae** [ˈmʌskiː]) *n*【拉】蝇 | ~e hispanicae 斑蝥,芫青 / ~e volitantes 飞蚊症,飞蝇,幻视

muscacide [ˈmʌskəsaid] *a* 杀蝇的 *n* 杀蝇剂

muscardine [ˈmʌskədiːn] *n* 白僵病,蚕硬化病

muscarine [ˈmʌskəri(ː)n] *n* 毒蝇碱 | **muscarinic** [ˌmʌskəˈrinik] *a*

muscarinism [ˈmʌskərinizəm] *n* 毒蝇碱中毒

muscegenetic [mʌsidʒiˈnetik] *a* 引起飞蝇幻视的

muscicide [ˈmʌsisaid] *a* 杀蝇的 *n* 杀蝇剂

Musci [ˈmʌski] *n*【拉】苔藓

Muscidae [ˈmʌsidiː] *n* 蝇科

muscimol [ˈmʌskimɔl] *n* 蝇蕈醇,氨甲基羟异噁唑(在捕蝇蕈属〈Amanita〉各蕈种中发现的一种神经毒素,化学结构和作用与鹅膏氨蕈氨酸〈ibotenic acid〉相似)

Muscina [məˈsainə] *n* 腐蝇属

muscle [ˈmʌsl] *n* 肌[肉] | agonistic ~ 主动肌 / antagonistic ~ 对抗肌,拮抗肌 / antigravity ~s 抗引力肌 / appendicular ~ 肢体肌 / cardiac ~ 心肌 / congenerous ~s 协同肌(若干肌肉唤起同一动作) / epimeric ~ 上段[中胚层]肌 / extrinsic ~ 外附肌 / hamstring ~s 腘绳肌群 / hypaxial ~s, subvertebral ~s 轴下肌,椎下肌 / hypomeric ~ 下段[中胚层]肌 / inspiratory ~s 吸[气]肌 / intrinsic ~ 内附肌 / involuntary ~ 不随意肌 / iridic ~s 虹膜肌 / nonstriated ~, smooth ~, unstriated ~ 平滑肌 / striated ~, striped ~ 横纹肌 / voluntary ~ 随意肌 / visceral ~, organic ~ 脏腑肌 / yoked ~s 共轭肌

muscle phosphofructokinase [mʌsl ˌfɔsfəuˌfrʌktəuˈkaineis] 肌磷酸果糖激酶(6-磷酸果糖激酶的肌同工酶)

muscle phosphofructokinase deficiency 肌磷酸果糖激酶缺乏症,糖原贮积症Ⅶ型

muscle phosphorylase [ˈmʌsl fɔsˈfɔrileis] 肌磷酸化酶(糖原磷酸化酶的肌同工酶)

muscle phosphorylase deficiency 肌磷酸化酶缺乏症,糖原贮积症Ⅴ型

musculamine [ˌmʌskjuˈlæmin] *n* 肌胺

muscular [ˈmʌskjulə] *a* 肌[肉]的;肌肉发达的,壮健的 | **~ity** [ˌmʌskjuˈlærəti] *n* 肌肉发达,壮健

muscularis [ˌmʌskjuˈlɛəris] *a*【拉】肌的 *n* 肌层

muscularize [ˈmʌskjuləraiz] *vi* 肌化,肌组织化

musculation [ˌmʌskjuˈleiʃən] *n* 肌肉系统;肌活动

musculature [ˈmʌskjulətʃə] *n* 肌肉系统

musculi [ˈmʌskjulai] musculus 的复数

musculoaponeurotic [ˌmʌskjuləuˌæpənjuəˈrɔtik] *a* 肌腱膜的

musculocutaneous [ˌmʌskjuləukju(ː)ˈteinjəs], **musculodermic** [ˌmʌskjuləuˈdəːmik] *a* 肌皮的

musculoelastic [ˌmʌskjuləuiˈlæstik] *a* 肌[与]弹性组织的

musculointestinal [ˌmʌskjuləuinˈtestinl] *a* 肌[与]肠的

musculomembranous [ˌmʌskjuləuˈmembrənəs]

a 肌性膜性的

Musculomyces [ˌmʌskjuləuˈmaisiːz] *n* 肌丝菌属(现归入支原体属 Mycoplasma)

musculophrenic [ˌmʌskjuləuˈfrenik] *a* 肌膈的

musculoprecipitin [ˌmʌskjuləupriˈsipitin] *n* 肌沉淀素(用以区别各种肉类)

musculoskeletal [ˌmʌskjuləuˈskelitl] *a* 肌[与]骨骼的

musculospiral [ˌmʌskjuləuˈspaiərəl] *a* 肌螺旋的

musculospiralis [ˌmʌskjuləuspaiˈreilis] *n* 桡神经

musculotendinous [ˌmʌskjuləuˈtendinəs] *a* 肌腱的

musculotonic [ˌmʌskjuləuˈtɔnik] *a* 肌收缩力的

musculotropic [ˌmʌskjuləuˈtrɔpik] *a* 向肌性的(对肌组织有特别亲和或影响力的)

musculus [ˈmʌskjuləs] ([复] **musculi** [ˈmʌskjulai]) *n*【拉】肌[肉](详见附录)

mushbite [ˈmʌʃbait] *n* 蜡秴片法,咬蜡法

mushroom [ˈmʌʃrum] *n* 蕈,蘑菇

musicogenic [ˌmjuːzikəuˈdʒenik] *a* 音乐性的

musicotherapy [ˌmjuːzikəuˈθerəpi] *n* 音乐疗法

Musset's sign [mjuːˈse] (Louis C. A. de Musset 法国诗人,死于主动脉瓣关闭不全)缪塞征(头节律性跳动,见于主动脉瘤及主动脉瓣关闭不全)

mussitation [ˌmʌsiˈteiʃən] *n* 无声嗫语(口唇蠕动,但不出声)

mustard [ˈmʌstəd] *n* 芥子;芥属植物 | black ~, brown ~ 黑芥(内服催吐药及外用抗刺激剂) / nitrogen ~s 氮芥类(有些用于治癌) / L-phenylalanine ~ 左旋苯丙氨酸氮芥(即美法仑 melphalan,抗肿瘤药) / uracil ~ 尿嘧啶氮芥,尿嘧啶芥(即乌拉莫司汀 uramustine,抗肿瘤药) / white ~, yellow ~ 白芥(用途与黑芥同)

Mustard operation [ˈmʌstəd] (William Thornton Mustard)默斯塔德手术(大血管转位时,为纠正解剖缺陷利用心包组织造一个心房内挡板)

mutable [ˈmjuːtəbl] *a* 可变的,易变的 | **mutability** [ˌmjuːtəˈbiləti] *n* 可突变性,易变性

mutacism [ˈmjuːtəsizəm] *n* 无音字母不正确发音;m 音滥用

mutafacient [ˌmjuːtəˈfeiʃənt] *a* 诱变的

mutagen [ˈmjuːtədʒən] *n* 致突变原,诱变剂,诱变因素 | **~ic** [ˌmjuːtəˈdʒenik] *a* 诱变的

mutagenesis [ˌmjuːtəˈdʒenisis] *n* 诱变,诱发突变,突变发生

mutagenicity [ˌmjuːtədʒiˈnisəti] *n* 诱变性

mutant [ˈmjuːtənt] *a* 变异的 *n* 突变株,突变体,突变型

mutarotase [ˌmjuːtəˈrəuteis] *n* 变旋酶

mutarotation [ˌmjuːtərəuˈteiʃən] *n* 变旋[现象]

mutase [ˈmjuːteis] *n* 变位酶

mutate [mjuːˈteit] *vt*, *vi* 变异,突变

mutation [mju(ː)ˈteiʃən] *n* 突变(生物的遗传物质发生可遗传的变异) | auxotrophic ~ 营养缺陷性突变 / chromosomal ~ 染色体[性]突变 / frameshift ~ 移码突变 / genomic ~ 染色体组突变(改变个体正常染色体数目的突变) / induced ~ 诱导突变(由于实验性人工引入的外来因素而引起的突变) / missense ~ 错义突变(指(DNA 上的遗传密码或 mRNA 上的密码子的突变,引起了编码的错乱,导致产生不同氨基酸) / natural ~ 自然突变(未涉及任何已知外界因素所出现的遗传突变) / nonsense ~ 无义突变(一个密码子的变化导致这个密码子无法形成一个氨基酸) / ploidic ~ 倍增性突变(基因组突变的一种,染色体数目增加一个单倍组) / point ~ 点突变(染色体上的一种突变,形态上无明显变化) / silent ~ 同义突变,缄默突变 / somatic ~ 体细胞突变(发生在体细胞中的突变,为嵌合体的出现提供基础) | **~al** *a*

mute [mjuːt] *a* 哑的 *n* 哑人 | deaf ~ 聋哑人

mutein [ˈmjuːtiːn] *n* 突变蛋白质

mutilate [ˈmjuːtileit] *vt* 使断肢;致残废 | **mutilation** [ˌmjuːtiˈleiʃən] *n* (肢体或器官)残毁,残缺

Mutisia [mjuˈtiziə] *n* 帚菊木属 | ~ viciaefolia 巢菜叶帚菊木

mutism [ˈmjuːtizəm] *n* 哑症,缄默症 | akinetic ~ 运动不能性缄默症 / deaf ~ 聋哑症 / elective ~ 选择性缄默症(儿童的一种精神障碍) / hysterical ~ 癔症性缄默症

muton [ˈmjuːtɔn] *n* 突变子(DNA 分子链上能够引起突变的最小单位)

mutualism [ˈmjuːtʃuəlizəm, ˈmjuːtjuəlizəm] *n* 共生,互利共栖(不同种类的两种生物彼此得到一定利益的共生) | **mutualist** *n* 共生生物,共栖生物

muzolimine [mjuːˈzəulimiːn] *n* 莫唑胺(利尿药,降压药)

muzzle [ˈmʌzl] *n* 口套(狗,马)

MV¹ Medicus Veterinarius【拉】兽医

MV² megavolt 兆伏[特]; minute volume 每分钟容积

Mv mendelevium 钔

mV millivolt 毫伏[特]

μV microvolt 微伏[特]

M-VAC methotrexate, vinblastine, doxorubicin, and cisplatin 甲氨蝶呤-长春碱-多柔比星-顺铂(联合治疗移行细胞癌方案)

MVP mitral valve prolapse 二尖瓣脱垂

MW molecular weight 分子量

μW microwatt 微瓦[特]

Mx Medex 军医召募方案

My myopia 近视[眼]

my mayer 迈尔(比热容单位)

myalgia [mai'ældʒiə] *n* 肌痛 | ~ abdominis 腹肌痛 / ~ capitis 头肌痛,头痛 / ~ cervicalis 颈肌痛,斜颈,捩颈 / epidemic ~ 流行性肌痛,流行性胸膜痛 / lumbar ~ 腰痛 | **myalgic** *a*

myasis [mai'eisis] *n* 蝇蛆病

myasthenia [ˌmaiæs'θiːniə] *n* 肌无力 | angiosclerotic ~ 血管硬化性肌无力 / ~ gravis, ~ gravis pseudoparalytica 重症肌无力 | **myasthenic** [ˌmaiæs'θenik] *a*

myatonia [ˌmaiə'təuniə], **myatony** [mai'ætəni] *n* 肌弛缓,肌张力缺失

myatrophy [mai'ætrəfi] *n* 肌萎缩

myautonomy [ˌmaiɔː'tɔnəmi] *n* 肌[动]反应延缓

mycelioid [mai'siːliɔid] *a* 菌丝状的,菌丝样的

mycelium [mai'siːliəm] ([复] **mycelia** [mai'siːliə]) *n* 菌丝体 | **mycelial** [mai'siːliəl], **mycelian** [mai'siːliən] *a*

mycete ['maisiːt] *n* 真菌,霉菌

mycethemia [ˌmaisi'θiːmiə] *n* 真菌血症

mycetismus [ˌmaisə'tizməs], **mycetism** ['maisətizəm] *n* 真菌中毒

mycet(o)- 见 myc(o)-

mycetogenic [maiˌsiːtəu'dʒenik], **mycetogenous** [ˌmaisi'tɔdʒinəs] *a* 真菌所致的,真菌原的

mycetoma [ˌmaisi'təumə] *n* 足菌肿 | actinomycotic ~ 放线菌性足菌肿 / eumycotic ~ 真菌性足菌肿

Mycetozoida [ˌmaisiːtəu'zɔidə], **Mycetozoa** [maiˌsiːtəu'zəuə] *n* 黏菌虫类

mycid ['maisid] *n* 皮真菌疹,霉菌疹

myc(o)-, mycet(o)- [构词成分] 真菌,霉菌

mycoagglutinin [ˌmaikəuə'gluːtinin] *n* 真菌凝集素,霉菌凝集素

mycobacteria [ˌmaikəubæk'tiəriə] mycobacterium 的复数

Mycobacteriaceae [ˌmaikəubækˌtiəri'eisiiː] *n* 分枝杆菌科

mycobacteriosis [ˌmaikəubækˌtiəri'əusis] *n* 分枝杆菌病

Mycobacterium [ˌmaikəubæk'tiəriəm] *n* 分枝杆菌属 | ~ avium-intracellulare 鸟-胞内分枝杆菌 / ~ bovis 牛型结核菌 / ~ butyricum 乳酪分枝杆菌 / ~ leprae 麻风分枝杆菌,麻风杆菌 / ~ lepraemurium 鼠麻风分枝杆菌 / ~ marinum 海分枝杆菌 / ~ paratuberculosis 副结核分枝杆菌 / ~ phlei 草分枝杆菌 / ~ smegmatis 耻垢分枝杆菌 / ~ tuberculosis 结核分枝杆菌,结核杆菌

mycobacterium [ˌmaikəubæk'tiəriəm] ([复] **mycobacteria** [ˌmaikəubæk'tiəriə]) *n* 分枝杆菌 | anonymous mycobacteria, atypical mycobacteria 无名分枝杆菌,非典型分枝杆菌,非结核分枝杆菌 / Group Ⅰ-Ⅳ mycobacteria Ⅰ-Ⅳ 类分枝杆菌,非结核分枝杆菌

mycobactin [ˌmaikəu'bæktin] *n* 分枝杆菌生长素

Mycocandida [ˌmaikəu'kændidə] *n* 念珠菌属

Mycocentrospora [ˌmaikəusen'trɔspərə] *n* 中孢真菌属

mycocidin [ˌmaikəu'saidin] *n* 杀枝曲菌素

Mycococcus [ˌmaikəu'kɔkəs] *n* 芽生球菌属

Mycoderma [ˌmaikəu'dəːmə] *n* 生膜菌属 | ~ aceti 醋生膜菌,化醋菌 / ~ dermatitidis 皮炎生膜菌,皮炎芽生菌 / ~ immite 粗球孢子菌

mycoderma [ˌmaikəu'dəːmə] *n* 黏膜

mycodermatitis [ˌmaikəuˌdəːmə'taitis], **mycodermomycosis** [ˌmaikəuˌdəːməmai'kəusis] *n* 念珠菌病

mycoflora [ˌmaikəu'flɔːrə] *n* 真菌区系;真菌志(在某一特定地区内存在的或具有特征的真菌数目和品种)

mycohemia [ˌmaikəu'hiːmiə] *n* 真菌血症,霉菌血症

mycolic acid [mai'kɔlik] 分枝菌酸

mycology [mai'kɔlədʒi] *n* 真菌学 | **mycologic (al)** [ˌmaikəu'lɔdʒik(əl)] *a* / **mycologist** *n* 真菌学家

mycomyringitis [ˌmaikəuˌmirin'dʒaitis] *n* 真菌性鼓膜炎,鼓膜真菌病

Myconostoc [ˌmaikəu'nɔstɔk] *n* 裂殖真菌属

mycopathology [ˌmaikəupə'θɔlədʒi] *n* 真菌病理学

mycophage ['maikəfeidʒ] *n* 真菌噬菌体

mycophagy [mai'kɔfədʒi] *n* 蘑菇食用;噬[真]菌[作用]

mycophenolate mofetil [ˌmaikəu'fenəuleit] 霉酚酸酯(一种免疫抑制药,与环孢素和皮质类固醇结合使用,防止异基因肾肝心脏移植的排斥反应,口服或静脉输注给药)

mycophenolic acid [ˌmaikəufi'nɔlik] 麦考酚酸,霉酚酸(抗肿瘤药)

Mycoplana [ˌmaikəu'pleinə] *n* 支动杆菌属

Mycoplasma [ˌmaikəu'plæzmə] *n* 支原体属 | ~ fermentans 发酵支原体 / ~ gallisepticum 鸡败血支原体 / ~ granularum 颗粒支原体 / ~ hominis 人支原体 / ~ hyorhinis 猪鼻炎支原体 / ~ mycoides 蕈状支原体 / ~ orale, ~ pharyngis 口腔支原体,咽支原体 / ~ pneumoniae 肺炎支原体 / ~ salivarium 唾液支原体

mycoplasma [ˌmaikəu'plæzmə] ([复] **mycoplasmas** 或 **mycoplasmata** [ˌmaikəu'plæzmətə]) *n* 支原体,类菌质体 | T ~ T 支原体,小支原体(T 代表 tiny) / T-strain ~ T 株支原体,解脲脲原体 | **~l** *a*

Mycoplasmas [ˌmaikəu'plæzməz] *n* 支原体目

Mycoplasmataceae [ˌmaikəuˌplæzmə'teisiiː] *n* 支

原体科
Mycoplasmatales [ˌmaikəuˌplæzməˈteiliːz] *n* 支原体目
mycoplasmosis [ˌmaikəuplæzˈməusis] *n* 支原体病,支原菌病
mycoprecipitin [ˌmaikəupriˈsipitin] *n* 真菌沉淀素,霉菌沉淀素
mycoproteination [ˌmaikəuˌprəutiːˈneiʃən] *n* 死菌接种,菌蛋白接种
mycopus [ˈmaikəpəs] *n* 脓性黏液
mycorrhiza [ˌmaikəˈraizə] *n* 菌根 | **~l** *a*
mycose [ˈmaikəus] *n* 海藻糖
mycoside [ˈmaikəsid] *n* 海藻糖苷
mycosis [maiˈkəusis] *n* 真菌病,霉菌病,肉芽肿病 | cutaneous ~ 皮真菌病,皮霉菌病 / ~ fungoides 蕈样肉芽肿病 / ~ intestinalis 肠真菌病,肠炭疽 / ~ leptothrica 纤毛菌病 / splenic ~ 脾真菌病,铁质沉着性脾大
-mycosis [构词成分] 真菌病,霉菌病
mycostasis [maiˈkɔstəsis] *n* 真菌制阻
mycostat [ˈmaikəstæt] *n* 制霉[菌]药
mycosterol [maiˈkɔstərɔl] *n* 真菌甾醇,酵母甾醇
mycotic [maiˈkɔtik] *a* 真菌病的,霉菌病的
Mycotoruloides [ˌmaikəuˌtɔrəˈlɔidiːz] *n* 念珠菌属
mycotoxicosis [ˌmaikəuˌtɔksiˈkəusis] *n* 真菌[毒素]中毒症
mycotoxin [ˌmaikəuˈtɔksin] *n* 真菌毒素
mycotoxinization [ˌmaikəuˌtɔksinaiˈzeiʃən, -niˈz-] *n* 真菌毒素接种
mycteric [mikˈterik] *a* 鼻腔的
mycteroxerosis [ˌmiktərəuziəˈrəusis] *n* 鼻腔干燥
mydaleine [maiˈdeiliin] *n* 腐脏尸胺
mydatoxine [ˌmaidəˈtɔksin] *n* 腐脏毒胺
mydriasis [miˈdraiəsis] *n*【希】瞳孔开大(生理性开大);瞳孔散大(疾病性散大);瞳孔扩大(药物性扩大) | alternating ~, bounding ~, springing ~ 交替性瞳孔开大
mydriatic [ˌmidriˈætik] *a* 瞳孔开大的,散瞳的 *n* 扩瞳药,散瞳药
myectomy [maiˈektəmi] *n* 肌[部分]切除术
myectopia [ˌmaiekˈtəupiə], **myectopy** [maiˈektəpi] *n* 肌异位
myelacephalus [ˌmaiələˈsefələs] *n* 下级无头畸胎
myelalgia [ˌmaiəˈlældʒiə] *n* 脊髓痛
myelanalosis [ˌmaiəˌlænəˈləusis] *n* 脊髓痨
myelapoplexy [ˌmaiəˈlæpəpleksi] *n* 脊髓出血
myelasthenia [ˌmaiəlæsˈθiːniə] *n* 脊髓性神经衰弱
myelatelia [ˌmaiələˈtiːliə] *n* 脊髓发育不全
myelatrophy [ˌmaiəˈlætrəfi] *n* 脊髓萎缩
myelauxe [ˌmaiəˈlɔːksi] *n* 脊髓肥大
myelemia [ˌmaiəˈliːmiə] *n* 髓细胞性血症,骨髓性白血病
myelencephalitis [ˌmaiəlenˌsefəˈlaitis] *n* 脑脊髓炎
myelencephalon [ˌmaiəlenˈsefəlɔn] *n* 末脑;脑脊髓
myelencephalospinal [ˌmaiəlenˌsefələuˈspainl] *a* 脑脊髓的
myeleterosis [ˌmaiəˌletəˈrəusis] *n* 脊髓病变
myelin [ˈmaiəlin] *n* 髓磷脂,髓鞘质 | **~ic** [ˌmaiəˈlinik] *a*
myelinated [ˈmaiəliˌneitid] *a* 有髓[鞘]的
myelinization [ˌmaiəlinaiˈzeiʃən, -niˈz-], **myelination** [ˌmaiəliˈneiʃən] *n* 髓鞘形成
myelinoclasis [ˌmaiəliˈnɔkləsis] *n* 髓鞘破坏,髓鞘消失,脱髓鞘病变 | acute perivascular ~ 急性血管周围脱髓鞘病,急性播散性脑脊髓炎 / central pontine ~ 中心性脑桥髓鞘破坏 / postinfection perivenous ~ 传染病后静脉周围脱髓鞘病,传染病后脑脊髓病
myelinogenesis [ˌmaiəˌlinəuˈdʒenisis] *n* 髓鞘形成
myelinogenetic [ˌmaiəˌlinəudʒiˈnetik] *a* 生髓[鞘]的
myelinogeny [ˌmaiəliˈnɔdʒini] *n* (神经纤维)髓鞘形成
myelinolysin [ˌmaiəliˈnɔlisin] *n* 溶髓鞘质素
myelinolysis [ˌmaiəliˈnɔlisis] *n* 髓鞘破坏,髓鞘脱失 | central pontine ~ 中心性脑桥髓鞘破坏
myelinopathy [ˌmaiəliˈnɔpəθi] *n* 髓鞘质病
myelinosis [ˌmaiəliˈnəusis] *n* 脂肪分解性髓磷脂生成
myelinotoxic [ˌmaiəlinəuˈtɔksik] *a* 对髓鞘有毒性的;致脱髓鞘的
myelinotoxicity [ˌmaiəlinəutɔkˈsisəti] *n* 髓鞘毒性
myelitis [ˌmaiəˈlaitis] *n* 脊髓炎 | acute ~ 急性脊髓炎 / apoplectiform ~ 突发性脊髓炎,卒中性脊髓炎 / ascending ~ 上行性脊髓炎 / bulbar ~ 延髓炎 / central ~ 中心性脊髓炎,脊髓灰质炎 / cornual ~ 脊髓灰质角炎 / descending ~ 下行性脊髓炎 / focal ~ 局灶性脊髓炎 / interstitial ~, sclerosing ~ 间质性脊髓炎,硬化性脊髓炎 / systemic ~ 系统性脊髓炎 | **myelitic** [ˌmaiəˈlitik] *a*
myel(o)- [构词成分] 髓,脊髓
myeloablation [ˌmaiələuæbˈleiʃən] *n* 重度骨髓抑制 | **myeloablative** [maiələuˈæblətiv] *a*
myeloarchitecture [ˌmaiələuˈɑːkiˌtektʃə] *n* 脑皮质[神经]纤维结构;(脊髓与脑干)神经束结构
myeloblast [ˈmaiələuˌblæst] *n* 原粒细胞
myeloblastemia [ˌmaiələublæsˈtiːmiə] *n* 原粒细

胞血症

myeloblastoma [ˌmaiələublæs'təumə] *n* 原粒细胞瘤

myeloblastomatosis [ˌmaiələuˌblæstəumə'təusis] *n* 原粒细胞瘤病

myeloblastosis [ˌmaiələublæs'təusis] *n* 原粒细胞过多症,原粒细胞血症;原粒细胞白血病

myelocele ['maiələusiːl] *n* 脊髓突出

myeloclast ['maiələuklæst] *n* 破髓鞘细胞

myelocone ['maiələukəun] *n* 脑脂尘

myelocyst ['maiələusist] *n* 脊髓囊肿

myelocystic [ˌmaiələu'sistik] *a* 髓性[及]囊性的;脊髓囊肿的

myelocystocele [ˌmaiələu'sistəsiːl] *n* 脊髓囊肿状突出;脊髓脊膜突出

myelocystomeningocele [ˌmaiələuˌsistəumə'niŋgəsiːl] *n* 脊髓脊[髓]膜囊肿状突出,脊髓脊膜突出

myelocyte ['maiələusait] *n* 中幼粒细胞;神经系统灰质细胞

myelocythemia [ˌmaiələusai'θiːmiə] *n* 髓细胞血症

myelocytic [ˌmaiələu'sitik] *a* 髓细胞的

myelocytoma [ˌmaiələusai'təumə] *n* 髓细胞瘤,慢性粒细胞白血病;骨髓瘤

myelocytomatosis [ˌmaiələuˌsaitəumə'təusis] *n* 髓细胞瘤病

myelocytosis [ˌmaiələusai'təusis] *n* 髓细胞增多症,髓细胞血症

myelodysplasia [ˌmaiələudis'pleiziə] *n* 脊髓发育不良,骨髓增生异常 | **myelodysplastic** [ˌmaiələudis'plæstik] *a*

myeloencephalic [ˌmaiələuˌensi'fælik] *a* 脑脊髓的

myeloencephalitis [ˌmaiələuenˌsefə'laitis] *n* 脑脊髓炎 | eosinophilic ~ 嗜酸细胞性脑脊髓炎 / epidemic ~ 流行性脑脊髓炎,流行性脑灰质炎

myeloencephalopathy [ˌmaiələuenˌsefə'lɔpəθi] *n* 脑脊髓病

myelofibrosis [ˌmaiələufai'brəusis] *n* 骨髓纤维化[症] | osteosclerosis ~ 骨硬化性骨髓纤维化[症],骨髓硬化

myelofugal [ˌmaiə'lɔfjugəl] *a* 离脊髓的

myelogenesis [ˌmaiələu'dʒenisis] *n* 骨髓发生;髓鞘发生

myelogenous [ˌmaiə'lɔdʒinəs], **myelogenic** [ˌmaiələu'dʒenik] *a* 骨髓性的

myelogeny [ˌmaiə'lɔdʒini] *n* 髓鞘发生

myelogone ['maiələugəun], **myelogonium** [ˌmaiələu'gəuniəm] *n* 髓原细胞 | **myelogonic** [ˌmaiələu'gəunik] *a*

myelogram ['maiələugræm] *n* 脊髓造影[照]片;骨髓细胞分类[计数]像

myelography [ˌmaiə'lɔgrəfi] *n* 脊髓造影[术] | oxygen ~ 脊髓氧造影[术]

myeloid ['maiəlɔid] *a* 骨髓的;脊髓的;髓细胞样的

myeloidin [ˌmaiə'lɔidin] *n* 类髓磷脂(视网膜色素细胞内)

myeloidosis [ˌmaiəlɔi'dəusis] *n* 骨髓组织增生

myelokentric [ˌmaiələu'kentrik] *a* 促髓细胞形成的

myelolipoma [ˌmaiələuli'pəumə] *n* 髓脂瘤

myelolymphangioma [ˌmaiələulimˌfændʒi'əumə] *n* 象皮病

myelolysis [ˌmaiə'lɔlisis] *n* 髓鞘质分解 | **myelolytic** [ˌmaiələu'litik] *a*

myeloma [ˌmaiə'ləumə]([复]**myelomas** 或 **myelomata** [ˌmaiə'ləumətə]) *n* 骨髓瘤 | endothelial ~ 内皮[细胞]性骨髓瘤 / multiple ~, plasma-cell ~ 多发性骨髓瘤,浆细胞性骨髓瘤

myelomalacia [ˌmaiələumə'leiʃiə] *n* 脊髓软化

myelomatoid [ˌmaiə'ləumətɔid] *a* 骨髓瘤样的

myelomatosis [ˌmaiələumə'təusis] *n* 骨髓瘤[病],多发性骨髓瘤

myelomenia [ˌmaiələu'miːniə] *n* 脊髓倒经

myelomeningitis [ˌmaiələuˌmenin'dʒaitis] *n* 脊髓脊膜炎

myelomeningocele [ˌmaiələumə'niŋgəsiːl] *n* 脊髓脊膜膨出

myelomere ['maiələumiə] *n* 髓节

myelomonocyte [ˌmaiələu'mɔnəsait] *n* 骨髓单核细胞,髓细胞

myelomyces [ˌmaiə'lɔmisiːz] *n* 髓样癌

myeloneuritis [ˌmaiələunjuə'raitis] *n* 脊髓神经炎

myelonic [ˌmaiə'lɔnik] *a* 脊髓的,髓样的

myelo-opticoneuropathy [ˌmaiələuˌɔptikəunjuə'rɔpəθi] *n* 脊髓视神经病 | subacute ~ 亚急性脊髓视神经病

myelopathy [ˌmaiə'lɔpəθi] *n* 脊髓病;骨髓病 | **myelopathic** [ˌmaiələu'pæθik] *a*

myeloperoxidase (MPO) [ˌmaiələupə'rɔksideis] *n* 髓过氧化物酶

myeloperoxidase (MPO) deficiency 髓过氧化物酶缺乏症

myelopetal [ˌmaiə'lɔpitl] *a* 向脊髓的

myelophage ['maiələuˌfeidʒ] *n* 噬髓鞘质细胞

myelophthisic(al) [ˌmaiələu'θaisik(əl)] *a* 脊髓痨的;骨髓痨的

myelophthisis [ˌmaiə'lɔfθisis] *n* 脊髓痨;骨髓痨,全骨髓萎缩

myeloplast ['maiələuplæst] *n* 骨髓白细胞

myeloplax ['maieləˌplæks], **myeloplaque** [mai-

ˈeləplæk] *n* 骨髓多核巨细胞

myeloplegia [ˌmaiələuˈpliːdʒiə] *n* 脊髓麻痹,脊髓瘫痪

myelopoiesis [ˌmaiələupɔiˈiːsis] *n* 骨髓组织生成,骨髓细胞生成 | ectopic ~, extramedullary ~ 异位性骨髓组织生成

myelopoietic [ˌmaiələupɔiˈetik] *a* 骨髓组织生成的,骨髓细胞生成的

myelopore [ˈmaiələupɔː] *n* 脊髓孔

myeloproliferative [ˌmaiələuprəuˈlifəreitiv] *a* 骨髓增生的,骨髓增殖的

myeloradiculitis [ˌmaiələurəˌdikjuˈlaitis] *n* 脊髓神经根炎

myeloradiculodysplasia [ˌmaiələurəˌdikjuləudisˈpleiziə] *n* 脊髓神经根发育异常

myeloradiculopathy [ˌmaiələurəˌdikjuˈlɔpəθi] *n* 脊髓神经根病

myelorrhagia [ˌmaiələuˈreidʒiə] *n* 脊髓出血

myelosarcoma [ˌmaiələusɑːˈkəumə] *n* 骨髓肉瘤

myelosarcomatosis [ˌmaiələusɑːˌkəuməˈtəusis] *n* 骨髓肉瘤病

myeloschisis [ˌmaiəˈlɔskisis] *n* 脊髓裂

myeloscintogram [ˌmaiələuˈsintəgræm] *n* 脊髓闪烁图

myelosclerosis [ˌmaiələuskliəˈrəusis] *n* 骨髓硬化症

myeloscope [ˈmaiələuˌskəup] *n* 椎管镜

myeloscopy [ˌmaiəˈlɔskəpi] *n* 椎管镜检查[术]

myelosis [ˌmaiəˈləusis] *n* 骨髓组织增生;脊髓瘤形成;脊髓[变性]病 | aleukemic ~, nonleukemic ~, chronic nonleukemic ~ 非白血病性骨髓组织增生,慢性非白血病性骨髓增生,特发性骨髓外化生 / funicular ~ 索性脊髓[变性]病

myelospongium [ˌmaiələuˈspɔndʒiəm] *n* 髓管网

myelosuppression [ˌmaiələusəˈpreʃən] *n* 骨髓抑制

myelosuppressive [ˌmaiələusəˈpresiv] *a* 骨髓抑制的 *n* 骨髓抑制药

myelosyphilis [ˌmaiələuˈsifilis] *n* 脊髓梅毒

myelosyphilosis [ˌmaiələuˌsifiˈləusis] *n* 梅毒性脊髓病

myelosyringosis [ˌmaiələuˌsiriŋˈgəusis] *n* 脊髓空洞症

myelotherapy [ˌmaiələuˈθerəpi] *n* 骨髓疗法

myelotome [ˈmaiələtəum] *n* 脊髓切片器;脊髓刀

myelotomy [ˌmaiəˈlɔtəmi] *n* 脊髓切开术 | commissural ~ 脊髓连合部切开术

myelotoxic [ˈmaiələuˌtɔksik] *a* 骨髓中毒的;骨髓病性的 | **~ity** [ˌmaiələutɔkˈsisəti] *n* 骨髓中毒性

myelotoxin [ˌmaiələuˈtɔksin] *n* 骨髓细胞毒素

myenteron [maiˈentərɔn] *n* 肠肌层 | **myenteric** [ˌmaienˈterik] *a*

Myerson's sign [maiərsən] (Abraham Myerson) 迈尔森征(帕金森〈Parkinson〉病的一种体征,叩击额肌,即引起睑痉挛)

myesthesia [ˌmaiisˈθiːzjə] *n* 肌[肉感]觉

myiasis [maiˈaiəsis] *n* 蝇蛆病 | creeping ~ 匐行蝇蛆病,游走性蝇蛆病 / cutaneous ~, dermal ~, ~ dermatosa 皮肤蝇蛆病 / intestinal ~ 肠蝇蛆病 / ~ linearis 线状蝇蛆病,匐行蝇蛆病,游走性蝇蛆病 / traumatic ~ 创伤性蝇蛆病

myiocephalon [ˌmaiaiəuˈsefəlɔn], **myiocephalum** [ˌmaiaiəuˈsefələm] *n* 角膜穿孔性虹膜脱出

myiodesopsia [ˌmaiaiəudiˈsɔpsiə] *n* 飞蝇幻视

myiosis [maiˈjəusis] *n* 蝇蛆病

myitis [maiˈaitis] *n* 肌炎

myk(o)- 以 myk(o)-起始的词,同样见以 myc(o)-起始的词

mylohyoid [ˌmailəuˈhaiɔid] *a* 下颌舌骨的,磨牙舌骨的

mylopharyngeal [ˌmailəufəˈrindʒiəl] *a* 下颌咽的,磨牙咽的

my(o)- [构词成分] 肌

myoadenylate deaminase [ˌmaiəuˈædinileit, ˌmaiəuəˈdenileit diːˈæmineis] 肌腺苷酸脱氨酶

myoadenylate deaminase deficiency 肌腺苷酸脱氨酶缺乏症

myoalbumin [ˌmaiəuælˈbjumin] *n* 肌清蛋白,肌白蛋白

myoarchitectonic [ˌmaiəuˌɑːkitekˈtɔnik] *a* 肌结构的

myoasthenia [ˌmaiəuæsˈθiːniə] *n* 肌无力

myoatrophy [ˌmaiəuˈætrəfi] *n* 肌萎缩

Myobia [maiˈəubiə] *n* 肉螨属

Myobiidae [ˌmaiəuˈbiːidiː] *n* 肉螨科

myoblast [ˈmaiəblæst] *n* 肌原细胞 | **~ic** [ˌmaiəuˈblæstik] *a*

myoblastoma [ˌmaiəublæsˈtəumə] *n* 肌原细胞瘤 | granular cell ~ 颗粒细胞肌原细胞瘤 | **myoblastomyoma** [ˌmaiəuˌblæstəumaiˈəumə] *n*

myobradia [ˌmaiəuˈbreidiə] *n* 肌反应迟钝

myocardiac [ˌmaiəuˈkɑːdiæk] *a* 心肌的;(非炎性)心肌病的

myocardial [ˌmaiəuˈkɑːdiəl] *a* 心肌的

myocardiogram [ˌmaiəuˈkɑːdiəgræm] *n* 心肌运动[描记]图

myocardiograph [ˌmaiəuˈkɑːdiəgrɑːf] *n* 心肌运动描记器

myocardiolysis [ˌmaiəuˌkɑːdiˈɔlisis] *n* 心肌破坏

myocardiopathy [ˌmaiəuˌkɑːdiˈɔpəθi] *n* (非炎性)心肌病 | alcoholic ~ 乙醇性心肌病 / chagasic ~ 恰加斯心肌病

myocardiorrhaphy [ˌmaiəuˌkɑːdiˈɔrəfi] *n* 心肌缝合术
myocardiosis [ˌmaiəukɑːdiˈəusis] *n* (非炎性)心肌病
myocarditis [ˌmaiəukɑːˈdaitis] *n* 心肌炎 | acute bacterial ~ 急性细菌性心肌炎 / acute isolated ~, idiopathic ~ 急性孤立性心肌炎,特发性心肌炎 / fibrous ~ 纤维性心肌炎,慢性间质性心肌炎 / fragmentation ~ 断裂性心肌炎 / rheumatic ~ 风湿性心肌炎 | **myocarditic** [ˌmaiəukɑːˈditik] *a*
myocardium [ˌmaiəuˈkɑːdiəm] *n* 心肌,心肌膜
myocardosis [ˌmaiəukɑːˈdəusis] *n* (非炎性)心肌病
myocele [ˈmaiəsiːl] *n* 肌突出
myocelialgia [ˌmaiəuˌsiːliˈældʒiə] *n* 腹肌痛
myocelitis [ˌmaiəusiːˈlaitis] *n* 腹肌炎
myocellulitis [ˌmaiəuˌseljuˈlaitis] *n* 肌蜂窝织炎
myoceptor [ˈmaiəˌseptə] *n* 肌感受器(终板)
myocerosis [ˌmaiəusiˈrəusis] *n* 肌蜡样变性
myochorditis [ˌmaiəukɔːˈdaitis] *n* 声带肌炎
myochosis [ˌmaiəuˈkəusis] *n* 肌皱缩
myochrome [ˈmaiəkrəum] *n* 肌色素
myocinesimeter [ˌmaiəusiniˈsimitə] *n* 肌收缩计
myoclonia [ˌmaiəuˈkləuniə] *n* 肌阵挛[症] | ~ epileptica 癫痫性肌阵挛 / ~ fibrillaris multiplex 多发性纤维性肌阵挛,肌纤维颤搐 / fibrillary ~ 纤维颤动性肌阵挛 / pseudoglottic ~ 假性声门肌阵挛,呃逆
myoclonus [maiˈɔklənəs] *n* 肌阵挛 | ~ multiplex 多发性肌阵挛 / palatal ~ 软腭阵挛 | **myoclonic** [ˌmaiəuˈklɔnik] *a*
myocoele [ˈmaiəsiːl] *n* 肌节腔
myocolpitis [ˌmaiəukɔlˈpaitis] *n* 阴道肌层炎
myocomma [ˌmaiəuˈkɔmə] *n* 肌节;肌[节间]隔,肌障(胎)
Myocoptes [ˌmaiəuˈkɔptiːz] *n* 牦螨属
myocrismus [ˌmaiəuˈkrismэs] *n* 肌音(收缩声)
myoctonine [maiˈɔktənin] *n* 牛扁碱,肉乌头碱
myoculator [maiˈɔkjuˌleitə] *n* 眼肌运动矫正器
myocyte [ˈmaiəsait] *n* 肌细胞;肌丝层(原虫外胞质内层)
myocytolysis [ˌmaiəusaiˈtɔlisis] *n* 肌细胞破坏,肌纤维破坏 | focal ~ of heart 灶性心肌纤维破坏
myocytoma [ˌmaiəusaiˈtəumə] *n* 肌细胞瘤
myodegeneration [ˌmaiəudiˈdʒenəˈreiʃən] *n* 肌变性
myodemia [ˌmaiəuˈdiːmiə] *n* 肌脂肪变性
myodesopsia [ˌmaiəudeˈsɔpsiə] *n* 飞蝇幻视
myodiastasis [ˌmaiəudaiˈæstəsis] *n* 肌分离
myodiopter [ˌmaiəudaiˈɔptə] *n* 睫状肌屈光度
myodynamic [ˌmaiəudaiˈnæmik] *a* 肌力的
myodynamics [ˌmaiəudaiˈnæmiks] *n* 肌动力学(肌肉活动的生理学)
myodynamometer [ˌmaiəuˌdainəˈmɔmitə] *n* 肌力计
myodynia [ˌmaiəuˈdiniə] *n* 肌痛 | hysterical ~ 癔症性肌痛(一般在卵巢区)
myodystonia [ˌmaiəudisˈtəuniə], **myodystony** [ˌmaiəuˈdistəni] *n* 肌张力障碍
myodystrophia [ˌmaiəudisˈtrəufiə] *n* 肌营养不良,肌营养障碍;肌强直性营养不良 | ~ fetalis 胎儿性肌营养不良,先天性肌发育不全
myodystrophy [ˌmaiəuˈdistrəfi] *n* 肌营养不良,肌营养障碍
myoedema [ˌmaiəui(ː)ˈdiːmə] *n* 肌水肿;肌耸起
myoelastic [ˌmaiəuiˈlæstik] *a* 肌弹性的
myoelectric(al) [ˌmaiəuiˈlektrik(əl)] *a* 肌电的
myoendocarditis [ˌmaiəuˌendəukɑːˈdaitis] *n* 心肌[心]内膜炎
myoepithelioma [ˌmaiəuˌepiθiːliˈəumə] *n* 肌上皮瘤
myoepithelium [ˌmaiəuˌepiˈθiːljəm] *n* 肌上皮 | **myoepithelial** *a*
myofascial [ˌmaiəuˈfæʃiəl] *a* 肌筋膜的
myofascitis [ˌmaiəufəˈsaitis] *n* 肌筋膜炎
myofiber [ˌmaiəuˈfaibə] *n* 肌纤维
myofibril [ˌmaiəuˈfaibril] *n* 肌原纤维 | **~lar** [ˌmaiəuˈfaibrilə] *a*
myofibrilla [ˌmaiəufaiˈbrilə] ([复] **myofibrillae** [ˌmaiəufaiˈbriliː]) *n* 肌原纤维
myofibroblast [ˌmaiəuˈfaibrəblæst] *n* 肌成纤维细胞
myofibroma [ˌmaiəufaiˈbrəumə] *n* 肌纤维瘤,平滑肌瘤
myofibromatosis [ˌmaiəuˌfaibrəuməˈtəusis] *n* 肌纤维瘤病
myofibrosis [ˌmaiəufaiˈbrəusis] *n* 肌纤维变性,肌纤维化 | ~ cordis 心肌纤维变性
myofibrositis [ˌmaiəuˌfaibrəuˈsaitis] *n* 肌纤维鞘炎;肌束膜炎
myofilament [ˌmaiəuˈfiləmənt] *n* 肌丝(在横纹肌原纤维中)
myofunctional [ˌmaiəuˈfʌŋkʃənl] *a* 肌功能的,肌机能的
myogelosis [ˌmaiəudʒiˈləusis] *n* 肌硬结
myogen [ˈmaiədʒin] *n* 肌浆蛋白
myogenesis [ˌmaiəuˈdʒenisis] *n* 肌生成,肌发生 | **myogenetic** [ˌmaiəudʒiˈnetik] *a*
myogenic [ˌmaiəuˈdʒenik], **myogenous** [maiˈɔdʒinəs] *a* 生肌的;肌[源]性的
myoglia [maiˈɔgliə] *n* 肌胶质
myoglobin [ˌmaiəuˈgləubin] *n* 肌红蛋白
myoglobinuria [ˌmaiəuˌgləubiˈnjuəriə] *n* 肌红蛋

白尿

myoglobulin [ˌmaiəuˈglɔbjulin] *n* 肌球蛋白(已被 myosin 替代)

myoglobulinuria [ˌmaiəuˌglɔbjuliˈnjuəriə] *n* 肌球蛋白尿(已被 myosinuria 替代)

myognathus [maiˈɔgnəθəs] *n* 下颌寄生畸胎

myogram [ˈmaiəgræm] *n* 肌动[描记]图

myograph [ˈmaiəgrɑːf] *n* 肌动描记器 ǀ **~ic** [ˌmaiəˈgræfik] *a* 肌动描记的 / **~y** [maiˈɔgrəfi] *n* 肌动描记[法];肌学;肌组织 X 线摄影[术]

myohematin [ˌmaiəuˈhemətin] *n* 肌色质,肌高铁血红素

myohemoglobin [ˌmaiəuˌhiːməuˈgləubin] *n* 肌红蛋白

myohypertrophia [ˌmaiəuˌhaipə(ː)ˈtrəufiə] *n* 肌肥大 ǀ ~ kymoparalytica 麻痹性肌营养障碍,麻痹性肌肥大

myoid [ˈmaiɔid] *a* 肌样的 *n* 肌样质,肌样体 ǀ cone ~ 锥体肌样部 / rod ~ 杆体肌样部 / visual cell ~ 视[觉]细胞肌样部

myoidem [maiˈɔidem], **myoidema** [ˌmaiɔiˈdiːmə] *n* 肌水肿;肌耸起

myoideum [maiˈɔidiəm] *n* 肌肉组织

myoidism [maiəuˈidizəm] *n* 自发性肌收缩

***mya*-inositol** [ˌmaiəu iˈnəusitɔl] *n* 肌醇

myo-inositol-1 (or 4)-monophosphatase [ˌmaiəu iˈnəusitɔl ˌmɔnəuˈfɔsfəteis] 肌醇-1(或 4)-一磷酸[酯]酶

myoischemia [ˌmaiəuisˈkiːmiə] *n* 肌局部缺血

myokerosis [ˌmaiəukiˈrəusis] *n* 肌蜡样变性

myokinase [ˌmaiəuˈkaineis] *n* 肌激酶,腺苷酸激酶

myokinesimeter [ˌmaiəukiniˈsimitə] *n* 肌收缩计

myokinesis [ˌmaiəukaiˈniːsis, -kiˈn-] *n* 肌运动,肌位移(尤指肌纤维的位移) ǀ **myokinetic** [ˌmaiəukaiˈnetik, -kiˈn-] *a*

myokinin [ˌmaiəuˈkinin] *n* 肌碱

myokymia [ˌmaiəuˈkimiə] *n* 肌纤维颤搐

myolemma [ˌmaiəuˈlemə] *n* 肌纤维膜,肉膜

myolin [ˈmaiəlin] *n* 肌[纤维]素

myolipoma [ˌmaiəuliˈpəumə] *n* 肌脂瘤

myology [maiˈɔlədʒi], **myologia** [ˌmaiəˈləudʒiə] *n* 肌学 ǀ **myologic(al)** [ˌmaiəˈlɔdʒik(əl)] *a*

myolysis [maiˈɔlisis] *n* 肌溶解 ǀ ~ cardiotoxica 中毒性心肌溶解 / nodular ~ 小结性[舌]肌溶解

myoma [maiˈəumə] ([复]**myomas** 或 **myomata** [maiˈəumətə]) *n* 肌瘤 ǀ ball ~ 球形肌瘤 / myoblastic ~ 肌原细胞瘤 / ~ previum 前置肌瘤,子宫平滑肌瘤 / ~ sarcomatodes 肉瘤化肌瘤,平滑肌肉瘤 / ~ striocellulare 横纹肌瘤 / ~ telangiectodes 血管扩张性肌瘤,血管平滑肌瘤 ǀ **~tous** [maiˈɔmətəs] *a*

myomagenesis [maiˌəuməˈdʒenisis] *n* 肌瘤形成,肌瘤发生

myomalacia [ˌmaiəuməˈleiʃiə] *n* 肌软化

myomatectomy [ˌmaiəuməˈtektəmi] *n* 肌瘤切除术

myomatosis [ˌmaiəuməˈtəusis] *n* 肌瘤病,多发性肌瘤

myomectomy [ˌmaiəuˈmektəmi] *n* 肌瘤切除术,子宫肌瘤切除术;肌[部分]切除术

myomelanosis [ˌmaiəuˌmeləˈnəusis] *n* 肌黑变

myomere [ˈmaiəmiə] *n* 肌节

myometer [maiˈɔmitə] *n* 肌收缩计,肌力计

myometritis [ˌmaiəumiˈtraitis] *n* 子宫肌[层]炎

myometrium [ˌmaiəuˈmiːtriəm] *n* 子宫肌层 ǀ **myometrial** *a*

myomohysterectomy [ˌmaiəuməuˌhistəˈrektəmi] *n* 肌瘤子宫切除术

myomotomy [ˌmaiəuˈmɔtəmi] *n* 肌瘤切开术

myon [ˈmaiɔn] *n* 肌,肌单位

myonecrosis [ˌmaiəuneˈkrəusis] *n* 肌坏死 ǀ clostridial ~ 气性坏疽

myoneme [ˈmaiəniːm] *n* 肌纤丝(原虫)

myonephropexy [ˌmaiəuˈnefrəpeksi] *n* 肌式肾固定术

myoneural [ˌmaiəuˈnjuərəl] *a* 肌神经的

myoneuralgia [ˌmaiəunjuəˈrældʒiə] *n* 肌神经痛

myoneure [ˈmaiənjuə] *n* 肌神经细胞

myonosus [maiˈɔnəsəs] *n* 肌病

myonymy [maiˈɔnimi] *n* 肌命名法

myopachynsis [ˌmaiəupəˈkinsis] *n* 肌肥大

myopalmus [ˌmaiəuˈpælməs] *n* 肌颤搐

myoparalysis [ˌmaiəupəˈrælisis], **myoparesis** [ˌmaiəuˈpærisis] *n* 肌麻痹,肌瘫痪

myopathy [maiˈɔpəθi], **myopathia** [ˌmaiəuˈpæθiə] *n* 肌病 ǀ **myopathic** [ˌmaiəuˈpæθik] *a*

myope [ˈmaiəup] *n* 近视者

myopectineal [ˌmaiəupekˈtiniəl] *a* 肌耻骨的

myopericarditis [ˌmaiəuperikɑːˈdaitis] *n* 心肌心包炎

myophage [ˈmaiəfeidʒ] *n* 噬肌细胞

myophagism [maiˈɔfədʒizəm] *n* 肌萎缩

myophone [ˈmaiəfəum] *n* 肌音听诊器

myophosphorylase [ˌmaiəufɔsˈfɔrileis] *n* 肌磷酸化酶

myophosphorylase deficiency 肌磷酸化酶缺乏症,糖原贮积症 V 型

myopia(M) [maiˈəupiə] *n* 近视[眼] ǀ chromic ~ 远距色盲 / curvature ~ 曲率性近视 / index ~ 指数性近视(屈光性近视) / prodromal ~ 前驱期近视 ǀ **myopic** [maiˈɔpik] *a*

myoplasm [ˈmaiəplæzəm] *n* 肌质,肌浆
myoplasty [ˈmaiəˌplæsti] *n* 肌成形术 | **myoplastic** [ˌmaiəuˈplæstik] *a*
myopolar [ˌmaiəuˈpəulə] *a* 肌极的
Myoporum [ˌmaiəuˈpəurəm] *n* 苦槛蓝属
myoprotein [ˌmaiəuˈprəutiːn] *n* 肌蛋白[质]
myopsis [maiˈɔpsis] *n* 飞蝇幻视
myopsychic [ˌmaiəuˈsaikik] *a* 肌[与]精神的(指肌肉活动的记忆影像)
myopsychopathy [ˌmaiəusaiˈkɔpəθi], **myopsychosis** [ˌmaiəusaiˈkəusis] *n* 精神性肌病(肌病伴精神障碍)
myoreceptor [ˌmaiəuriˈseptə] *n* 肌感受器
myorrhaphy [maiˈɔrəfi] *n* 肌缝合术
myorrhexis [ˌmaiəuˈreksis] *n* 肌断裂
myosalgia [ˌmaiəuˈsældʒiə] *n* 肌痛
myosalpingitis [ˌmaiəuˌsælpinˈdʒaitis] *n* 输卵管肌[层]炎
myosalpinx [ˌmaiəuˈsælpiŋks] *n* 输卵管肌层
myosan [ˈmaiəsən] *n* 变性肌凝蛋白
myosarcoma [ˌmaiəusɑːˈkəumə] *n* 肌肉瘤
myoschwannoma [ˌmaiəuʃvʌˈnəumə] *n* 神经鞘瘤
myosclerosis [ˌmaiəuskliəˈrəusis] *n* 肌硬化
myoscope [ˈmaiəskəup] *n* 肌缩观测器;眼肌矫正器
myoseism [ˈmaiəsaizəm] *n* 肌颤搐
myoseptum [ˌmaiəuˈseptəm] *n* 肌节;肌(节间)隔,肌障
myoserum [ˌmaiəuˈsiərəm] *n* 肌汁,肉汁
myosin [ˈmaiəsin] *n* 肌球蛋白 | vegetable ~ 自主性肌球蛋白
myosin ATPase 肌球蛋白 ATP 酶,肌球蛋白腺苷三磷酸酶(亦称肌动球蛋白)
myosinogen [ˌmaiəuˈsinədʒən] *n* 肌浆蛋白,肌蛋白
myosinuria [ˌmaiəusiˈnjuəriə] *n* 肌球蛋白尿
myosis [maiˈəusis] *n* 瞳孔缩小,缩瞳
myositis [ˌmaiəuˈsaitis] *n* 肌炎 | epidemic ~ 流行性肌炎,流行性胸膜痛 / primary multiple ~, acute disseminated ~ 原发性多发性肌炎,急性播散性肌炎,假毛线虫病 / progressive ossifying ~ 进行性骨化性肌炎 / rheumatoid ~ 类风湿肌炎,纤维织炎 / trichinous ~ 旋毛虫性肌炎 | **myositic** [ˌmaiəuˈsitik] *a*
myospasia [ˌmaiəuˈspeiziə] *n* 肌阵挛
myospasm [ˈmaiəspæzəm] *n* 肌痉挛
myospasmia [ˌmaiəuˈspæzmiə] *n* 肌痉挛病
myospherulosis [ˌmaiəuˌsfiərjuˈləusis] *n* 肌小球增多(一种炎症性巨细胞反应,与伤口上局部使用油性软膏中的四环素有关)
myosteoma [maiˌɔstiˈəumə] *n* 肌骨瘤
myosthenic [ˌmaiɔsˈθenik] *a* 肌力的
myosthenometer [ˌmaiəusθeˈnɔmitə] *n* 肌力测量器
myostroma [ˌmaiəuˈstrəumə] *n* 肌基质
myostromin [ˌmaiəuˈstrəumin] *n* 肌基质蛋白
myosuria [ˌmaiəuˈsjuəriə] *n* 肌球蛋白尿
myosuture [ˌmaiəuˈsjuːtʃə] *n* 肌缝术
myosynizesis [ˌmaiəuˌsiniˈziːsis] *n* 肌粘连
myotactic [ˌmaiəuˈtæktik] *a* 肌[触]觉的
myotamponade [ˌmaiəuˈtæmpəneid] *n* 胸肌填塞法
myotasis [maiˈɔtəsis] *n* 肌伸张 | **myotatic** [ˌmaiəuˈtætik] *a*
myotenontoplasty [ˌmaiəutiˈnɔntəˌplæsti] *n* 肌腱成形术
myotenositis [ˌmaiəuˌtenəˈsaitis] *n* 肌腱炎
myotenotomy [ˌmaiəutiˈnɔtəmi] *n* 肌腱切断术
myotherapy [ˌmaiəuˈθerəpi] *n* 肌疗法
myothermic [ˌmaiəuˈθəːmik] *a* 肌温的
myotic [maiˈɔtik] *a* 缩瞳的 *n* 缩瞳药
myotility [ˌmaiəuˈtiləti] *n* 肌收缩力
myotome [ˈmaiətəum] *n* 肌力;生肌节;同神经肌丛
myotomic [ˌmaiəuˈtɔmik] *a* 生肌节的
myotomy [maiˈɔtəmi] *n* 肌切开术
myotone [ˈmaiətəun] *n* 肌强直,肌强直性痉挛
myotonia [ˌmaiəuˈtəuniə] *n* 肌强直 | ~ acquisita 后天性肌强直 / ~ atrophica 萎缩性肌强直 / ~ congenita, ~ hereditaria 先天性肌强直 / ~ dystrophica 营养不良性肌强直 / ~ neonatorum 新生儿肌强直 | **myotonic** [ˌmaiəuˈtɔnik] *a* 肌强直的;肌紧张的
myotonoid [maiˈɔtənɔid] *a* 肌强直样的
myotonometer [ˌmaiəutəuˈnɔmitə] *n* 肌张力测量器
myotonus [maiˈɔtənəs] *n* 肌强直,肌强直性痉挛
myotony [maiˈɔtəni] *n* 肌强直
myotrophy [maiˈɔtrəfi] *n* 肌营养 | **myotrophic** [ˌmaiəuˈtrɔfik] *a* 增加肌重量的;肌营养的
myotropic [ˌmaiəuˈtrɔpik] *a* 亲肌的,向肌的
myotubular [ˌmaiəuˈtjuːbjulə] *a* 肌管的
myotubule [ˌmaiəuˈtjuːbjuːl], **myotube** [ˈmaiətjuːb] *n* 肌管
myovascular [ˌmaiəuˈvæskjulə] *a* 肌血管的
myrcene [ˈməːsiːn] *n* 月桂烯,桂叶烯
myria- [构词成分] 无数;万($=10^4$)
myriachit [miˈriətʃit] *n* 【俄】西伯利亚痉跳病
Myriangiales [ˌmiriˌændʒiˈeiliːz] *n* 多腔菌目
myriapod [ˈmiriəpɔd] *n* 多足虫(指蜈蚣、千足虫)
Myriapoda [ˌmiriˈæpədə] *n* 多足纲
myrica [miˈraikə] *n* 蜡果杨梅(根皮)

myricin [ˈmirisin] *n* 蜂蜡素,软脂酸蜂酯;杨梅脂
myricyl [ˈmirisil] *n* 蜂花基
myringa [miˈriŋgə] *n*【拉】鼓膜
myringitis [ˌmirinˈdʒaitis] *n* 鼓膜炎 | bullous ~ 大疱性鼓膜炎
myring(o)- [构词成分] 鼓膜
myringodectomy [miˌriŋgəuˈdektəmi], **myringectomy** [ˌmirinˈdʒektəmi] *n* 鼓膜切除术
myringodermatitis [miˌriŋgəuˌdəːməˈtaitis] *n* 鼓膜外层炎
myringomycosis [miˌriŋgəumaiˈkəusis] *n* 鼓膜真菌病,真菌性鼓膜炎 | ~ aspergillina 鼓膜曲霉病
myringoplasty [miˈriŋgəˌplæsti] *n* 鼓膜成形术
myringorupture [miˌriŋgəuˈrʌptʃə] *n* 鼓膜破裂
myringostapediopexy [miˌriŋgəustəˈpiːdiəuˌpeksi] *n* 鼓膜镫骨固定术
myringotome [miˈriŋgətəum] *n* 鼓膜刀
myringotomy [ˌmiriŋˈgɔtəmi] *n* 鼓膜切开术
myrinx [ˈmairiŋks, ˈmiriŋks] *n* 鼓膜
myristate [miˈristeit, ˈmiː-] *n* [肉]豆蔻酸,[肉]豆蔻酸盐(或酯) | isopropyl ~ 豆蔻酸异丙酯
Myristica [miˈristikə] *n* 肉豆蔻属
myristica [miˈristikə] *n* 肉豆蔻
myristic acid [miˈristik] 豆蔻酸
myristicene [miˈristisiːn] *n* 肉豆蔻萜
myristicol [miˈristikɔl] *n* 肉豆蔻脑
myristin [miˈristin] *n* 豆蔻酸甘油酯
myrmecia [məːˈmiːʃiə] *n* 蚁冢状疣
myronate [ˈmairəneit] *n* 黑芥子硫苷酸盐 | potassium ~ 黑芥子硫苷酸钾
myronic acid [maiˈrɔnik] 黑芥子硫苷酸
myrosin [ˈmairəsin], **myrosinase** [maiˈrəusineis] *n* 葡糖硫苷酶
myrotheciotoxicosis [ˌmairəuˌθiːsiəuˌtɔksiˈkəusis] *n* 漆斑[真]菌[毒素]中毒症
Myrothecium [ˌmairəuˈθiːsiəm] *n* 漆斑[真]菌属
Myroxilon [maiˈrɔksəlɔn] *n* 妥鲁树属
myrrh [məː] *n* 没药;没药树;没药树脂 | **~ic** [ˈməːrik] *a* 没药的;没药树[脂]的
myrrholin [ˈməːrəlin] *n* 没药林(没药与脂肪等量混合剂,用作木溜油的赋形剂)
myrtenol [ˈməːtinɔl] *n* 桃金娘烯醇,香桃木醇
myrtiform [ˈməːtifɔːm] *a* 桃金娘形的
myrtle [ˈməːtl] *n* 桃金娘
Myrtus [ˈməːtəs] *n* 桃金娘属 | ~ communis, L. (Myrtaceae) 桃金娘(其叶用作防腐剂和收敛剂)
mysophilia [ˌmaisəˈfiliə] *n* 恋秽癖,嗜污癖
mysophobia [ˌmaisəˈfəubjə] *n* 污秽恐怖,极端好洁癖 | **mysophobic** *a*
mysophobiac [ˌmaisəˈfəubiæk] *n* 污秽恐怖者
mystin [ˈmistin] *n* 米斯廷(含甲醛及亚硝酸钠的牛奶防腐剂)
mytacism [ˈmaitəsizəm] *n* m 音滥用
mythomania [ˌmiθəˈmeinjə] *n* 谎语癖;神话癖,奇异故事癖
mythophobia [ˌmiθəˈfəubjə] *n* 神话恐怖,奇异故事恐怖
mytilocongestin [ˌmitiləukənˈdʒestin] *n* 蛤贝充血毒[素]
mytilotoxin [ˌmitiləuˈtɔksin] *n* 蛤贝毒,淡菜毒
mytilotoxism [ˌmitiləuˈtɔksizəm] *n* 蛤贝中毒,淡菜中毒
myxadenitis [ˌmiksædiˈnaitis] *n* 黏液腺炎
myxadenoma [ˌmiksædiˈnəumə] *n* 黏液腺瘤
myxameba [ˌmiksəˈmiːbə] *n* 黏液阿米巴
myxangitis [ˌmiksænˈdʒaitis], **myxangoitis** [ˌmiksæŋgəˈaitis] *n* 黏液[腺]管炎
myxasthenia [ˌmiksæsˈθiːniə] *n* 黏液分泌功能衰弱,黏液[分泌]不足
myxedema [ˌmiksiˈdiːmə] *n* 黏液水肿 | congenital ~ 先天性黏液水肿,呆小病 / infantile ~ 婴儿黏液水肿 / operative ~ 手术性黏液水肿,甲状腺切除后黏液水肿 | **~tous** [ˌmiksiˈdemətəs] *a*
myxedematoid [ˌmiksiˈdemətɔid] *a* 黏液水肿样的
myxidiotie [mikˈsidiəti], **myxidiocy** [mikˈsidiəsi] *n* 黏液水肿性白痴
Myxidium [mikˈsidiəm] *n* 两极虫属
myxiosis [ˌmiksiˈəusis] *n* 黏液排泄
myx(o)- [构词成分] 黏液
myxoadenoma [ˌmiksəuˌædiˈnəumə] *n* 黏液腺瘤
Myxobacterales [ˌmiksəubæktəˈreiliːz] *n* 黏液菌目,黏细菌目
myxoblastoma [ˌmiksəublæsˈtəumə] *n* 成黏液细胞瘤
Myxobolus [ˌmiksəˈbəuləs] *n* 黏液丸虫属 | ~ cyprini 鱼痘黏液丸虫 / ~ pfeifferi 发否黏液丸虫
myxochondrofibrosarcoma [ˌmiksəuˌkɔndrəuˌfaibrəusɑːˈkəumə] *n* 黏液软骨纤维肉瘤
myxochondroma [ˌmiksəukɔnˈdrəumə] *n* 黏液软骨瘤
myxochondrosarcoma [ˌmiksəuˌkɔndrəusɑːˈkəumə] *n* 黏液软骨肉瘤
Myxococcaceae [ˌmiksəukəˈkeisiiː] *n* 黏液球菌科,黏球菌科
Myxococcus [ˌmiksəuˈkɔkəs] *n* 黏液球菌属,黏球菌属
myxocystitis [ˌmiksəusisˈtaitis] *n* 膀胱黏膜炎
myxocystoma [ˌmiksəusisˈtəumə] *n* 黏液[样]囊瘤

myxocyte [ˈmiksəsait] *n* 黏液细胞
myxoenchondroma [ˌmiksəuˌenkɔnˈdrəumə] *n* 黏液软骨瘤
myxoendothelioma [ˌmiksəuˌendəuˌθiːliˈəumə] *n* 黏液内皮瘤
myxofibroma [ˌmiksəufaiˈbrəumə] *n* 黏液纤维瘤
myxofibrosarcoma [ˌmiksəuˌfaibrəusɑːˈkəumə] *n* 黏液纤维肉瘤
Myxogastria [ˌmiksəuˈgæstriə] *n* 黏腹菌亚纲
myxoglioma [ˌmiksəuglaiˈəumə] *n* 黏液神经胶质瘤
myxoglobulosis [ˌmiksəuˌglɔbjuˈləusis] *n* 黏液球囊肿(阑尾)
myxoid [ˈmiksɔid] *a* 黏液样的
myxoinoma [ˌmiksəuiˈnəumə] *n* 黏液纤维瘤
myxolipoma [ˌmiksəuliˈpəumə] *n* 黏液脂瘤
myxoma [mikˈsəumə] ([复] **myxomas** 或 **myxomata** [mikˈsəumətə]) *n* 黏液瘤 | enchondromatous ~ 软骨黏液瘤 / erectile ~ 血管性黏液瘤 | **~tous** *a*
myxomatosis [ˌmiksəuməˈtəusis] *n* (多发性)黏液瘤病;黏液瘤变性 | ~ cuniculi, infectious ~ 传染性黏液瘤病(由病毒引起的一种兔类传染病)
Myxomycetes [ˌmiksəumaiˈsiːtiːz] *n* 黏菌纲
myxomyoma [ˌmiksəumaiˈəumə] *n* 黏液肌瘤
myxoneurosis [ˌmiksəunjuəˈrəusis] *n* 黏液[分泌]神经功能病 | intestinal ~ 肠黏液神经功能病,黏液性结肠炎
myxopapilloma [ˌmiksəuˌpæpiˈləumə] *n* 黏液乳头瘤
myxopoiesis [ˌmiksəupɔiˈiːsis] *n* 黏液生成
myxorrhea [ˌmiksəˈriːə] *n* 黏液溢
myxosarcoma [ˌmiksəusɑːˈkəumə] *n* 黏液肉瘤 | **~tous** *a*
Myxosoma [ˌmiksəuˈsəumə] *n* 黏体虫属
myxosporan [ˌmiksəuˈspɔːrən] *n* 黏孢子原虫
myxospore [ˈmiksəspɔː] *n* 黏孢子
Myxosporea [ˌmiksəuˈspɔːriə] *n* 黏孢子纲
Myxosporidia [ˌmiksəuspəˈridiə] *n* 黏孢子目,胶孢子目
myxovirus [ˈmiksəuˌvaiərəs] *n* 黏液病毒
Myxozoa [ˌmiksəuˈzəuə] *n* 黏原虫门
myxozoan [ˌmiksəuˈzəuən] *n*, *a* 黏原虫(的)
myzesis [maiˈziːsis] *n* 吸,吮
Myzomyia [ˌmaizəˈmaijə] *n* 迈蚊亚属(按蚊的一亚属)
Myzorhynchus [ˌmaizəˈriŋkəs] *n* 吻蚊亚属(按蚊的一亚属)

N

N newton 牛[顿];nitrogen 氮;normal(solution)当量(溶液)

N normal 当量;number 数;Avogadro's number 阿伏伽德罗数;neutron number 中子数;population size(统计学中的)群体大小

N-[前缀]基

N_A Avogadro's number 阿伏伽德罗数

n nano-纳[诺];refractive index 屈光指数,屈光率;neutron 中子

n. nervus【拉】神经

n chromosome number (单倍体)染色体数;refractive index 屈光指数,屈光率;samplesize (统计学中的)样本大小

n- normal 正[链]的

n_D refractive index 屈光指数,屈光率

ν nu 希腊语第 13 个字母;自由度(degrees of freedom)、频率(frequency)、中微子(neutrino)和运动黏度(kinematic viscosity)的符号

NA Nomina Anatomica 解剖学名词;numerical aperture 数值孔径

Na sodium(【拉】natrium)钠

nabidrox [ˈnæbidrɔks] *n* 庚苯吡醇(抗高血压药)

nabilone [ˈnæbiləun] *n* 大麻隆(弱安定药和止吐药)

nabothian [nəˈbəuθiən] *a* 纳博特的(见 Naboth)

Naboth's follicles (cysts, glands, ovules, vesicles) [nəˈbɔt] (Martin Naboth)纳博特滤泡(囊、腺、卵状小体),子宫颈腺囊肿(宫颈黏膜上的腺体腔闭塞所致)

nabumetone [nəˈbjuːməˌtəun] *n* 萘丁美酮(非甾体消炎药,用于治疗骨关节炎和类风湿关节炎,口服给药)

nacreous [ˈneikriəs], **nacrous** [ˈneikrəs] *a* 真珠色的,具珠光的

NAD nicotinamide-adenine dinucleotide 烟酰胺腺嘌呤二核苷酸;no appreciable disease 无明显疾病

NAD⁺ the oxidized form of NAD 氧化型,烟酰胺腺嘌呤二核苷酸,二磷酸吡啶核苷酸(DPN⁺)

NADH the reduced form of NAD 还原型烟酰胺腺嘌呤二核苷酸,还原型二磷酸吡啶核苷酸(DPNH)

NADH cytochrome b_5 reductase [ˈsaitəkrəum riˈdʌkteis] NADH 细胞色素 b_5 还原酶,细胞色素 b_5 还原酶

NADH dehydrogenase (ubiquinone) [diːˈhaidrədʒəneis juˈbikwinəun] NADH 脱氢酶(泛醌)

NADH methemoglobin reductase [metˈhiːməuˌgləubin riˈdʌkteis] NADH 高铁血红蛋白还原酶,细胞色素 b_5 还原酶

NADH oxidase [ˈɔksideis] NADH 氧化酶,NADH 过氧化物酶

NADH peroxidase [pəˈrɔksideis] *n* NADH 过氧化物酶

NADH-Q reductase [riˈdʌkteis] NADH-Q 还原酶,NADH 脱氧酶(泛醌)

nadide [ˈneidaid] *n* 辅酶 I(解毒药)

NAD⁺ kinase [ˈkaineis] NAD⁺ 激酶

nadolol [neiˈdəulɔl] *n* 纳多洛尔(β 受体阻滞药)

NADP nicotinamide-adenine dinucleotide phosphate 烟酰胺腺嘌呤二核苷酸磷酸

NADP⁺ the oxidized form of NADP 氧化型烟酰胺腺嘌呤二核苷酸磷酸,三磷酸吡啶核苷酸(TPN⁺)

NADPH the reduced form of NADP 还原型烟酰胺腺嘌呤二核苷酸磷酸,还原型三磷酸吡啶核苷酸(TPNH)

NADPH-cytochrome P-450 reductase [ˈsaitəkrəum riˈdʌkteis] NADPH-细胞色素 P-450 还原酶,NADPH-高铁血红蛋白还原酶

NADPH-ferrihemoprotein reductase [ˌferiˌhiːməuˈprəutiːn riˈdʌkteis] NADPH-高铁血红蛋白还原酶(亦称 NADPN-细胞色素 P-450 还原酶)

NADPH methemoglobin reductase [metˈhiːməuˌgləubin riˈdʌkteis] NADPH 高铁血红蛋白还原酶(此酶在红细胞内,其生理意义不明)

NADPH oxidase [ˈɔksideis] NADPH 氧化酶(此酶系统的遗传性缺陷导致慢性肉芽肿病)

NAD(P)⁺ transhydrogenase (AB specific) [trænsˈhaidrədʒəneis spəˈsifik] NAD(P)⁺ 转氢酶(AB 特异性的)(此来自心脏的酶,其 NAD⁺ 为 A 特异性的,NADP⁺ 则为 B 特异性的)

NAD⁺ synthase (glutamine-hydrolyzing) [ˈsinθeis ˈgluːtəmiːn ˈhaidrəuˌlaiziŋ] NAD⁺ 合酶(谷氨酰胺水解的)

Naegeli's law [ˈneigəli] (Otto Naegeli)内格利定律(嗜酸粒细胞数目,如有正常数目的一半,或正常或较正常为多时,均不可能是伤寒,即使出现少数嗜酸粒细胞,诊断时亦应特别谨慎) | ~

leukemia 内格利白血病,急性髓细胞单核细胞白血病

Naegeli's syndrome [ˈneigəliː] (Oskar Naegeli) 内格利综合征(内格利色素细胞痣,见 Franceschetti-Jadassohn syndrome) | ~ incontinentia pigmenti 内格利色素失禁(见 Franceschetti-Jadassohn syndrome)

Naegleria [neiˈgliːriə] (F. P. O. Naegler) *n* 纳格勒[原虫]属 | ~ fowleri 福[勒]氏纳格勒原虫,福[勒]氏纳格勒阿米巴(可引起原发性阿米巴脑膜脑炎)

naegleriasis [ˌneigliˈraiəsis] *n* 纳格勒阿米巴病

naepaine [ˈniːpein] *n* 纳衣卡因(其盐酸盐用于眼科局部麻醉药)

naev(o)- [构词成分]以 naev(o)-起始的词,同样见于以 nev(o)-起始的词

nafarelin acetate [ˌnæfəˈrelin] 醋酸那法瑞林(促性腺激素释放激素的合成制剂,用于治疗中枢性早熟,通过鼻喷雾剂给药)

nafcillin sodium [næfˈsilin] 萘夫西林钠(抗生素类药)

nafemostat mesylate [nəˈfæməustæt] 甲磺萘莫司他(蛋白酶抑制药,用于治疗急性胰腺炎,并用作血液滤过时的抗凝药)

nafenopin [nəˈfenəpin] *n* 萘酚平(降血脂药)

Naffziger's operation [ˈnæfzigə] (Howard C. Naffziger) 纳夫济格手术(切除眼眶上壁和外壁,以治眼球突出) | ~ syndrome 纳夫济格综合征,前斜角肌综合征(scalenus syndrome,见 syndrome 项下相应术语)

nafomine malate [ˈnæfəmiːn] 苹果酸萘甲羟胺(肌肉松弛药)

nafoxidine hydrochloride [næˈfɔksidiːn] 盐酸萘福昔定(雌激素拮抗药,用于治疗乳腺癌)

nafronyl oxalate [ˈnæfrənil] 草酸萘呋胺酯(血管扩张药,用于治疗外周血管和脑血管疾患)

naftalofos [ˈnæftəˌləufɔs] *n* 萘酞磷(兽用抗蠕虫药)

naftifine hydrochloride [ˈnæftifiːn] 盐酸萘替芬(抗真菌药)

nagana [nəˈgɑːnə] *n* 非洲锥虫病

naganol [ˈnægənɔl] *n* 舒拉明钠(suramin sodium,抗锥体虫病药)

Nägele's obliquity [ˈneigələ] (Franz K. Nägele) 内格勒倾斜(前头盆倾势不匀,前顶骨对准产道的胎头位置,顶骨间直径对骨盆上口是斜位) | ~ pelvis 内格勒骨盆(偏斜骨盆) / ~ rule 分娩日期规律(预产期的计算法,自最后一次月经的第一天减去 3 个月再加 7 天)

Nägeli's maneuver (method, treatment) [ˈneigəli] (Otto Nägeli) 内格利手法(法、疗法)(治疗鼻出血时,将一手置于枕部下方,另一手置于颌下,将病人头部向上牵拉,以止鼻出血)

Nagel's test [ˈnɑːgəl] (Willibald A. Nagel) 纳格尔试验(检色彩视力)

Nageotte bracelets [nɑːˈʒjɔːt] (Jean Nageotte) 纳热奥特带(在朗〈飞〉氏〈Ranvier〉结轴索上覆盖环棘之带) | ~ cell 纳热奥特细胞(脑脊液中的一种细胞,患病时数目大量增多)

Nager acrofacial dysostosis (syndrome) [nɑːˈʒer] (Félix R. Nager) 纳杰肢端面骨发育不全(一种先天性疾病,下颌骨面骨发育不全,伴肢体畸形,其中有桡骨缺如、桡尺骨连结、拇指发育不全或缺如)

Nager-de Reynier syndrome [nɑːˈʒer dəreiniˈei] (F. R. Reynier; Jean P. de Reynier) 纳-德综合征(见 Nager acrofaial dysostosis)

Nagler effect [ˈnɑːglə] (Joseph Nagler) 纳格勒效应(置于高频率电场的充气管可作引起单向电流的整流器)

Nagler's reaction (test) [ˈnæglə] (F. P. O. Nagler) 纳格勒反应(试验)(人血清中加入产气荚膜〈梭状芽胞〉杆菌毒素后产生混浊,表示血清中有该菌存在,出现不透明现象是由于该毒素的卵磷脂酶的作用,抗血清则可抑制此反应)

naiad [ˈnaiæd] 若虫,稚虫

nail [neil] *n* 甲,爪;钉 | double-edge ~s 双缘甲 / eggshell ~ 蛋壳状甲 / fracture ~ 骨折钉 / hippocratic ~ 杵状指 / ingrown ~ 嵌甲 / parrot beak ~ 鹦鹉嘴状指甲 / pitted ~ 点状凹陷甲 / spoon ~ 匙状甲 / turtleback ~ 龟背甲

nailbed [ˈneilbed] *n* 甲床

nail-biting [ˈneilˌbaitiŋ] *n* 咬甲癖

nailing [ˈneiliŋ] *n* 插钉术 | intramedullary ~, marrow ~, medullary ~ 骨髓腔内插钉术

Nairobi eye [naiəˈrəubi] (Nairobi 为肯尼亚首都) 内罗毕眼,班蝥汁性结膜炎 | ~ sheep disease 内罗毕绵羊病(一种绵羊和山羊传染病,表现为急性出血性胃肠炎,绿色水样腹泻,黏液脓性鼻涕和呼吸困难)

naïve [nɑːˈiːv] *a* 幼稚的;以前未接触治疗的,首次用于实验的

Nairovirus [ˌnairəuˈvaiərəs] *n* 内罗病毒属(包括克里米亚-刚果出血热病毒和内罗毕绵羊病病毒)

Naja [ˈneidʒə] *n* 眼镜蛇属

naja [ˈnɑːdʒə] *n* 【阿拉伯】眼镜蛇(其毒液亦是顺势疗法的制剂)

Na^+, K^+-ATPase [eitiːˈpiːeis] Na^+, K^+-ATP 酶(EC 命名法中称为 Na^+/ K^+-exchanging ATPase)

Na^+/Ka^+ transporting ATPase [trænsˈpɔːtiŋ eitiːˈpiːeis] Na^+/Ka^+ 转运 ATP 酶,Na^+, Ka^+-ATP 酶

Nakayama's reagent [nɑːkɑː'jɑːmɑː] (M. Nakayama)中山试剂(氯化铁 0.4 g,浓盐酸 1 ml 和 95% 乙醇 99 ml) | ~ test 中山试验(检胆色素)

naked ['neikid] *a* 裸体的,无掩饰的,裸露的 | **~ly** *ad* / **~ness** *n*

Na^+/K^+-exchanging ATPase [eks'tʃændʒiŋ eiti:'pi:eis] Na^+/K^+-交换 ATP 酶(Na^+, K^+-ATPase 的 EC 命名法)

nalbuphine hydrochloride ['nælbjufiːn] 盐酸纳布啡(类阿片拮抗药)

nalidixate sodium [næli'dikseit] 萘啶酸钠(抗菌药)

nalidixic acid [ˌnæli'diksik] 萘啶酸,萘啶酮酸(抗菌药,用于治疗尿路感染)

nalmefene hydrochloride ['nælməˌfiːn] 盐酸纳美芬(类阿片拮抗药)

nalmexone hydrochloride [næl'meksəun] 盐酸纳美酮(吗啡拮抗药)

nalorphine ['næləfiːn, næ'lɔːfiːn] *n* 烯丙吗啡(吗啡拮抗药)

naloxone hydrochloride [næ'lɔksəun] 盐酸纳洛酮(类阿片拮抗药)

naltrexone hydrochloride [næl'treksəun] 盐酸纳曲酮(类阿片拮抗药)

name [neim] *n* 名,名称 | British Approved Name (BAN)英国通用药名(英国药典委员会批准的非专利药名) / generic ~ 类名(化学);非专有名;属名(生物学) / International Nonproprietary Name(INN)国际非专利药名 / nonproprietary ~ 非专利药名 / proprietary ~ 专利药名 / systemic ~ 系统名[称],学名(根据化合物的化学结构而定的物质的名称) / trivial ~ 通用名(在化学命名法中不反映化学结构的物质的名称,许多通用名都是半系统名) / United States Adopted Name(USAN)美国采用药名(美国药物命名委员会采用的非专利商标名称)

NAMI National Alliance for the Mentally Ill 全国精神病患者联盟

NAN *N*-acetylneuraminic acid *N*-乙酰神经氨酸

NANBH non-A, non-B hepatitis 非甲非乙型肝炎

nandrolone ['nændrələun] *n* 诺龙(雄激素,同化激素类药) | ~ cyclotate 双环辛烯酸诺龙 / ~ decanoate 癸酸诺龙 / ~ phenpropionate 苯丙酸诺龙

nanism ['neinizəm] *n* 矮小,侏儒症 | muliberey ~ 肌肝脑眼侏儒症(本词表示肌〈*mu*scle〉、肝〈*li*ver〉、脑〈*br*ain〉、眼〈*ey*e〉缺陷) / pituitary ~ 垂体性侏儒症,垂体性幼稚型 / renal ~ 肾性侏儒症 / senile ~ 早老性侏儒症,早老症 / symptomatic ~ 症状性侏儒症(伴骨化、出牙和性功能发育不全)

Nannizzia [nə'niziə] *n* 奈尼兹皮真菌属

nann(o)- 见 nan(o)-

Nannocystis [ˌnænəu'sistis] *n* 侏囊菌属

Nannomonas [ˌnænəu'məunəs] *n* 唾窦锥虫亚属

nano- [构词成分] 矮,小;纳[诺],毫微(10^{-9})

nanocephaly [ˌneinəu'sefəli], **nanocephalia** [ˌnænəusə'feiliə] *n* 小头[畸形] | **nanocephalous** [ˌneinəu'sefələs] *a* 小头的,头小的

nanocormia [ˌneinəu'kɔːmiə] *n* 小躯干

nanocurie(nCi) [ˌneinəu'kjuəri] *n* 纳居里,毫微居里(旧放射性强度单位,$=10^{-9}$Ci)

nanogram(ng) ['neinəgræm] *n* 纳克,毫微,克(重量单位,$=10^{-9}$g)

nanoid ['neinɔid] *a* 矮小的,侏儒样的

nanoliter(nL) [ˌneinəu'liːtə] *n* 纳升,毫微升(容量单位,$=10^{-9}$L)

nanomelia [ˌneinəu'miːliə] *n* 小肢,短肢 | **nanomelous** [nei'nɔmiləs] *a*

nanomelus [nei'nɔmiləs] *n* 小肢者,短肢者

nanometer(nm) [ˌneinəu'miːtə] *n* 纳米,毫微米(长度单位,$=10^{-9}$m)

nanophthalmia [ˌnænɔf'θælmiə], **nanophthalmos** [ˌnænɔf'θælmɔs] *n* 小眼

Nanophyetus [nei'nəufaiitəs] *n* 隐孔吸虫属

nanoplankton [ˌneinəu'plæŋktɔn] *n* 微小浮游生物,微型浮游生物

nanosecond(ns) [ˌnænəu'sekənd] *n* 纳秒,毫微秒(10^{-9}s)

nanosomia [ˌneinəu'səumiə], **nanosoma** [ˌneinəu'səumə] *n* 矮小,侏儒症

nanosomus [neinəu'səuməs] *n* 矮小,侏儒

nanounit(nU) [ˌneinəu'juːnit] *n* 纳单位,毫微单位(10^{-9}U)

nanous ['neinəs] *a* 矮小的

nanukayami [ˌnɑːnjukə'jɑːmi] *n* 七日热(一种钩端螺旋体病)

nanus ['neinəs] *n*【拉】侏儒,矮人

NAP nasion, point A, pogonion 鼻根点、A 点和颏点(连接而成面凸角)

nape [neip] *n* 项,颈背

napelline [nei'pelin] *n* 欧乌头碱,苦乌头碱

napex ['neipeks] *n* 枕下部

naphazoline hydrochloride [næ'fæzəliːn] *n* 盐酸萘甲唑林(血管收缩药)

naphtalin ['næftəlin] *n* 萘

naphtalinum [ˌnæftə'lainəm], **naphthalinum** [ˌnæfθə'lainəm] *n*【拉】萘

naphtha ['næfθə] *n*【拉】石油精,石脑油 | ~ aceti, vinegar ~ 醋酸乙酯,乙酸乙酯 / wood ~ 甲醇

naphthalene ['næfθəliːn] *n* 萘

naphthamine ['næfθəmin] *n* 乌洛托品(尿路消毒药)

naphthionic acid [næfθi'ɔnik] 氨基萘磺酸(其钠

盐用作止血药)
naphthol [ˈnæfθɔl] *n* 萘酚
naphtholate [ˈnæfθəleit] *n* 萘酚化物
naphtholcarboxylic acid [ˌnæfθəlˌkɑːbɔkˈsilik] 萘酚羧酸
naphtholdisulfonic acid [ˌnæfθəldaisʌlˈfɔnik] 二磺酸萘酚
naphtholism [ˈnæfθəlizəm] *n* 萘酚中毒
naphtholsulfonic acid [ˌnæfθəlsʌlˈfɔnik] 磺酸萘酚
naphtholum [næfˈθəuləm] *n*【拉】萘酚
naphthoresorcine [ˌnæfθəuriˈsɔːsin] *n* 萘酚雷琐辛
naphthyl [ˈnæfθil] *n* 萘基 | ~ alcohol, phenol ~ 萘酚 / ~ benzoate 苯甲酸萘酚(即苯佐萘酚〈benzonaphthol〉,肠道抗菌药) / ~ lactate 乳酸萘酯,*β*-萘酚乳酸酯 / ~ phenol 萘酚
naphthylamine [næfˈθiləmiːn] *n* 萘胺
naphthylaminosulfonic acid [ˌnæfθilˌæminəusʌlˈfɔnik] 氨基萘磺酸
naphthylmercapturic acid [ˌnæfθilˌməːkæpˈtjuərik] 萘硫醇尿酸
naphthylpararosaniline [ˌnæfθilˌpærərəuˈsænilin] *n* 萘基玫瑰苯胺
naphtol [ˈnæftəl] *n* 萘酚
napiform [ˈneipifɔːm] *n* 芜菁状的,大头菜形的
napkin [ˈnæpkin] *n* 餐巾;尿布
NAPNES National Association for Practical Nurse Education and Services 全国经验护士教育与服务协会
nappy [ˈnæpi] *n* 尿布
naprapath [ˈnæprəpæθ] *n* 推拿疗病者
naprapathy [nəˈpræpəθi] *n* 推拿疗病派
naproxen [nəˈprɔksən] *n* 萘普生(非甾体消炎药,用于治疗骨关节炎和类风湿关节炎,也可作为萘普生钠使用)
naproxol [nəˈprɔksəul] *n* 萘普索(抗炎、解热、镇痛药,用于治疗类风湿关节炎,口服)
napsylate [ˈnæpsileit] *n* 萘磺酸盐(2-naphthalene sulfonate 的 USAN 缩约词)
NAPT National Association of Poetry Therapy 全国诗疗法协会
naranol hydrochloride [ˈnɑːrənəul] 盐酸萘拉诺(安定药)
narasin [ˈnɑːrəsin] *n* 甲基盐霉素(兽用抗球虫药和生长刺激剂)
Narath's operation [ˈnɑːrət] (Albert Narath)纳拉特手术(门静脉阻塞时,将网膜固定于腹壁皮下组织,以建立侧支循环)
naratriptan hydrochloride [ˌnærəˈtriptæn] 盐酸那拉曲坦(一种选择性血清素受体激动药,用于治疗急性偏头痛,口服给药)
narcissism [ˈnɑːsisizəm](源自希腊神话中的人物 Narcissus,他热恋水中自己的人影) *n* 自恋,影恋 | primary ~ 原发性自恋 / secondary ~ 继发性自恋
Narcissus [nɑːˈsisəs] *n* 水仙属
narcissus [nɑːˈsisəs] *n* 水仙
narcissistic [ˌnɑːsiˈsistik] *n* 自恋的
narc(o)- [构词成分]麻木,麻醉
narcoanalysis [ˌnɑːkəuəˈnæləsis] *n* 麻醉分析
narcohypnia [ˌnɑːkəuˈhipniə] *n* 乍醒麻木
narcohypnosis [ˌnɑːkəuhipˈnəusis] *n* 麻醉[药]催眠
narcolepsy [ˈnɑːkəˌlepsi] *n* 发作性睡病 | **narcoleptic** [ˌnɑːkəˈleptik] *a*
narcoma [nɑːˈkəumə] *n* 麻醉性昏睡
narcose [ˈnɑːkəus] *a* 昏糊的,麻醉[状态]的
narcosine [ˈnɑːkəsiːn] *n* 那可丁(镇咳药)
narcosis [nɑːˈkəusis] ([复] **narcoses** [nɑːˈkəusiːz]) *n* 麻醉 | basal ~, basis ~ 基础麻醉 / insufflation ~ 吹入麻醉 / intravenous ~ 静脉麻醉[法] / medullary ~ 脊髓麻醉 / rausch ~ 酩酊麻醉,浅乙醚麻醉
narcostimulant [ˌnɑːkəuˈstimjulənt] *a* 麻醉[与]兴奋性的
narcosynthesis [ˌnɑːkəuˈsinθisis] *n* 精神综合法,精神分析法,[精神]麻醉分析
narcotic [nɑːˈkɔtik] *a* 麻醉的 *n* 麻醉性镇痛药
narcotico-acrid [nɑːˌkɔtikəuˈækrid] *a* 麻辣的
narcotico-irritant [nɑːˌkɔtikəuˈiritənt] *a* 麻醉刺激性的
narcotile [ˈnɑːkətail] *n* 乙基氯,氯乙烷
narcotine [ˈnɑːkətiːn] *n* 那可丁(镇咳药)
narcotism [ˈnɑːkətizəm] *n* 麻醉[法];麻醉品嗜好,麻醉剂成瘾
narcotize [ˈnɑːkətaiz] *vt* 使麻醉 | **narcotization** [ˌnɑːkəutaiˈzeiʃən, -tiˈz-] *n*
narcous [ˈnɑːkəs] *a* 昏糊的,麻醉[状态]的
nard [nɑːd] *n* 甘松香,甘松
naris [ˈnɛəris] ([复] **nares** [ˈnɛəriːz]) *n* 鼻孔 | anterior ~, external ~ 前鼻孔 / posterior nares, internal nares 后鼻孔 | **narial** [ˈnɛəriəl], **narine** [ˈnɛəriːn] *a*
Narthecium [nɑːˈθiːsiəm] *n* 纳西菜属
nasal [ˈneizəl] *a* 鼻的;鼻音的 *n* 鼻音;鼻骨 | **~ity** [neiˈzæləti] *n* 鼻音性 / **~ly** *ad* 以鼻音
nasalis [neiˈzeilis] *a*【拉】鼻的
nascent [ˈnæsnt, ˈneisnt] *a* 初生的,新生的 | **nascence** [ˈnæsns], **nascency** [ˈnæsnsi] *n* 发生,起源
NASH nonalcoholic steatohepatitis 非酒精性脂肪肝炎
nasioiniac [ˌneiziəuˈiniæk] *a* 鼻根枕外隆凸的

nasion [ˈneiziɔn] *n* 鼻根;鼻根点 | **nasial** [ˈneiziəl] *a*

nasitis [neiˈzaitis] *n* 鼻炎

Nasmyth's membrane [ˈnæsmiθ] (Alexander Nasmyth)原发性釉护膜,釉小皮

NAS-NRC National Academy of Sciences-National Research Council 国家科学院-国家研究委员会

nas(o)- [构词成分]鼻

nasoantral [ˌneizəuˈæntrəl] *a* 鼻上颌窦的

nasoantritis [ˌneizəuænˈtraitis] *n* 鼻上颌窦炎

nasoantrostomy [ˌneizəuænˈtrɔstəmi] *n* 鼻上颌窦造口术

nasobronchial [ˌneizəuˈbrɔŋkiəl] *a* 鼻支气管的

nasobuccal [ˌneizəuˈbʌkəl] *a* 鼻颊的

nasociliary [ˌneizəuˈsiliəri] *a* 鼻睫的

nasoethmoidal [ˌneizəueθˈmɔidəl] *a* 鼻筛[骨]的,筛鼻[骨]的

nasofrontal [ˌneizəuˈfrʌntl] *a* 鼻额的

nasogastric [ˌneizəuˈgæstrik] *a* 鼻胃的

nasograph [ˈneizəgrɑːf, -græf] *n* 鼻描记器

nasolabial [ˌneizəuˈleibjəl] *a* 鼻唇的

nasolacrimal [ˌneizəuˈlækriməl] *a* 鼻泪的

nasomanometer [ˌneizəuməˈnɔmitə] *n* 鼻压计

nasonnement [ˌneizɔnˈmɔŋ] *n*【法】鼻音

naso-oral [ˌneizəuˈɔːrəl] *a* 鼻口的

nasopalatine [ˌneizəuˈpælətiːn] *a* 鼻腭的

nasopharyngeal [ˌnaizəufəˈrindʒiəl] *a* 鼻咽的

nasopharyngitis [ˌneizəuˌfærinˈdʒaitis] *n* 鼻咽炎

nasopharyngolaryngoscope [ˌneizəufəˌriŋgəuləˈriŋgəskəup] *n* 鼻咽喉镜

nasopharyngoscope [ˌneizəufəˈriŋgəskəup] *n* 电[光]鼻咽镜

nasopharynx [ˌneizəuˈfæriŋks] *n* 鼻咽

nasorostral [ˌneizəuˈrɔstrəl] *a* 鼻蝶[骨]嘴的

nasoscope [ˈneizəskəup] *n* [电光]鼻镜,鼻窥器

nasoseptal [ˌneizəuˈseptl] *a* 鼻中隔的

nasoseptitis [ˌneizəusepˈtaitis] *n* 鼻中隔炎

nasosinusitis [ˌneizəuˌsainjuˈsaitis] *n* 鼻鼻窦炎

nasospinale [ˌneizəuspaiˈneili] *n* 鼻下点,前鼻棘点

nasoturbinal [ˌneizəuˈtəːbinəl] *a* 鼻鼻甲的

Nassellarida [ˌnæsəˈlɛəridə] *n* 罩笼虫目

Nassulida [neiˈsulidə] *n* 篮口目

Nassulidea [ˌneisuˈlidiə] *n* 篮口总目

Nassulina [neiˈsulinə] *n* 篮口亚目

nastic [ˈnæstik] *a* 感性的(指树叶或植物其他部分对外界刺激的一种反应,与来自刺激的方向无关)

nastinic acid [næsˈtinik] 分支菌脂酸

nasus [ˈneisəs] *n*【拉】鼻

natal [ˈneitl] *a* 分娩的,生产的;臀的

natality [neiˈtæləti] *n* 出生率

nataloin [neiˈtæləin] *n* 纳塔尔芦荟素

natamycin [ˌnætəˈmaisin] *n* 那他霉素(抗生素类药)

natant [ˈneitənt] *a* 漂浮的,浮游的

nateglinide [nəˈteglinaid] *n* 那格尼特(抗糖尿病药)

nates [ˈneitiːz] natis 的复数

natimortality [ˌneitimɔːˈtæləti] *n* 死产率

National Formulary (美国)国家处方集

natis [neitis]([复]**nates** [ˈneitiːz]) *n*【拉】臀

natremia [nəˈtriːmiə] *n* 钠血[症]

natrium [ˈneitriəm] *n*【拉】钠

natriuresis [ˌneitrijuəˈriːsis], **natruresis** [ˌnætruːˈriːsis] *n* 尿钠排泄,尿钠增多 | **natriuretic** [ˌneitrijuəˈretik], **natruretic** [ˌnætruːˈretik] *a* (促)尿钠排泄的 *n* 尿钠排泄药

natron [ˈneitrən] *n* 天然碳酸钠,苏打

natrum [ˈneitrəm] *n* 钠

naturopath [ˈneitʃərəpæθ] *n* 自然医[术]士

naturopathy [ˌneitʃəˈrɔpəθi] *n* 自然医术(不用药物,利用空气、阳光、水、热等自然因素进行治疗) | **naturopathic** [ˌneitʃərəuˈpæθik] *a*

Nauheim bath [ˈnauhaim] 瑙海姆水浴(在德国瑙海姆地方,病人浸入含有碳酸盐的温水内进行浴疗) | ~ treatment 瑙海姆疗法(见 Schott's treatment)

Naumanniella [nauˌmæniˈelə] *n* 瑙曼菌属

Naunyn-Minkowski method [ˈnaunin minˈkəuski] (Bernard Naunyn; Oscar Minkowski) 瑙宁-明可斯基法(用气体扩张结肠后,进行肾触诊检查)

nausea [ˈnɔːsjə] *n* 恶心 | ~ gravidarum 妊娠期恶心 / ~ marina, ~ navalis 航海性恶心,晕船 | **~nt** [ˈnɔːsiənt] *a* 使恶心的 *n* 恶心药

nauseate [ˈnɔːsieit] *vt, vi* (使)恶心,作呕;(使)厌恶 | **nauseation** [ˌnɔːsiˈeiʃən] *n*

nauseating [ˈnɔːsieitiŋ] *a* 令人作呕的;令人厌恶的 | **~ly** *ad*

nauseous [ˈnɔːsjəs] *a* 恶心的,致恶心的

navel [ˈneivəl] *n* 脐 | blue ~ 蓝脐,脐部积血(见 Cullen's sign) / enamel ~ 釉结

navicula [nəˈvikjulə] *n*【拉】舟状窝

navicular [nəˈvikjulə] *a* 舟状的

navicularthritis [nəˌvikjuləˈθraitis] *n* 舟骨关节炎(指马前足)

Nb niobium 铌

N. B., NB, n. b. nota bene【拉】注意,留心

NBS National Bureau of Standards 国家标准局

NBT nitroblue tetrazolium 四唑氮蓝(见 test 项下相应术语)

NBTE nonbacterial thrombotic endocarditis 非细菌

性血栓性心内膜炎
NCF neutrophil chemotactic factor 中性粒细胞趋化因子
NCHS National Center for Health Statistics 全国卫生统计中心
NCI National Cancer Institute 国立癌症研究所
nCi nanocurie 纳居里(10^{-9}Ci)
NCMH National Committee for Mental Hygiene 全国精神卫生委员会
NCN National Council of Nurses 全国护士理事会
NCRP, NCRPM National Committee on Radiation Protection and Measurements 全国辐射防护与测量委员会
NCV nerve conduction velocity 神经传导速度
Nd neodymium 钕
NDA National Dental Association 全国牙科协会
nDNA nuclear DNA 核 DNA,核脱氧核糖核酸
NDV Newcastle disease virus 新城鸡瘟病毒
Nd:YAG neodymium: yttrium-aluminum-garnet 钕:钇-铝-石榴子石(激光器)
Ne neon 氖
near-sight [ˈniəsait] *n* 近视
nearsighted [ˈniəˈsaitid] *a* 近视的 | **~ness** *n*
nearthrosis [ˌniɑːˈθrəusis] *n* 人造关节;假关节
nebenagglutinin [ˌneibənəˈgluːtinin] *n* 副凝集素,部分凝集素
nebenkern [ˌneibənˈkəːn] *n*【德】副核
nebramycin [ˌnebrəˈmaisin] *n* 尼拉霉素(抗生素类药)
nebula [ˈnebjulə] ([复] **nebulae** [ˈnebjuliː] 或 **nebulas**) *n*【拉】薄翳,角膜云翳;(尿的)混浊;喷雾剂 | ~ epinephrinae hydrochloridi 盐酸肾上腺素喷雾(剂) | **~r** *a*
nebularine [nebjuˈlɛərin] *n* 水粉蕈素
nebulize [ˈnebjulaiz] *vt* 喷雾,喷洒 | **nebulization** [ˌnebjulaiˈzeiʃən, -liˈz-] *n* 雾化;喷雾治疗 / **nebulizer** [ˈnebjulaizə] *n* 雾化器
nebulous [ˈnebjuləs], **nebulose** [ˈnebjuləus] *a* 星云的,星云状的;模糊不清的
Necator [niˈkeitə] *n* 板口线虫属 | ~ americanus 美洲板口线虫,美洲钩虫
necatoriasis [niˌkeitəuˈraiəsis] *n* 板口线虫病
necessity [niˈsesəti] *n* 必需品 | pharmaceutic(al) ~ 调剂辅助剂,调剂用剂(如防腐剂、溶媒、软膏基质、矫味剂等)
neck [nek] *n* 颈 | ~ of ankle bone 距骨颈 / bull ~ 公牛颈(颈淋巴结肿大,如恶性白喉时) / Nithsdale ~ 甲状腺肿 / ~ of urinary bladder 膀胱颈 / uterine ~, ~ of uterus 子宫颈 / webbed ~ 蹼状颈 / wry ~ 斜颈,捩颈
necrectomy [nekˈrektəmi] *n* 坏死[物]切除术
necremia [nekˈriːmiə] *n* 血[细胞]活力丧失
necrencephalus [ˌnekrenˈsefələs] *n* 脑软化
necr(o)- [构词成分] 坏死,尸体
necrobacillosis [ˌnekrəuˌbæsiˈləusis] *n* 坏死杆菌病
necrobiosis [ˌnekrəubaiˈəusis] *n* 渐进性坏死 | ~ lipoidica diabeticorum, ~ lipoidica 糖尿病脂质渐进性坏死,脂质渐进性坏死 | **necrobiotic** [ˌnekrəubaiˈɔtik] *a*
necrocytosis [ˌnekrəusaiˈtəusis] *n* 细胞坏死
necrocytotoxin [ˌnekrəusaitəuˈtɔksin] *n* 坏死细胞毒素
necrogenic [ˌnekrəuˈdʒenik], **necrogenous** [neˈkrɔdʒinəs] *a* 死质性的,坏死源的
necrohormone [ˌnekrəuˈhɔːməun] *n* 坏死激素
necrology [neˈkrɔlədʒi] *n* 死亡统计;死亡统计学 | **necrologic(al)** [ˌnekrəuˈlɔdʒik(əl)] *a* / **necrologist** *n* 死亡统计学家
necrolysis [neˈkrɔlisis] *n* 坏死松解 | toxic epidermal ~ 中毒性表皮坏死松解症
necromania [ˌnekrəuˈmeiniə] *n* 恋尸狂,恋尸癖
necrometer [neˈkrɔmitə] *n* 尸体测量器
necromimesis [ˌnekrəumaiˈmiːsis] *n* 死亡妄想;装死
necronectomy [ˌnekrəuˈnektəmi] *n* 坏死(组织)切除术
necrophagous [neˈkrɔfəgəs] *a* 食尸的,食腐肉的
necrophilia [ˌnekrəuˈfiliə], **necrophilism** [neˈkrɔfilizəm], **necrophily** [neˈkrɔfili] *n* 恋尸癖;奸尸 | **necrophilic** [ˌnekrəuˈfilik], **necrophilous** [neˈkrɔfiləs] *a* 恋尸癖的;食腐的
necrophobia [ˌnekrəuˈfəubjə] *n* 死亡恐怖;尸体恐怖
necropneumonia [ˌnekrəunju(ː)ˈməunjə] *n* 肺坏疽
necropsy [ˈnekrɔpsi], **necroscopy** [neˈkrɔskəpi] *n* 尸体剖检,验尸
necrosadism [ˌnekrəuˈseidizəm] *n* 残毁尸体色情[狂]
necroscopy [nəˈkrɔskəpi] *vt* 尸体剖检
necrose [ˈnekrəus] *vt*, *vi* (使)发生坏死
necrosin [ˈnekrəsin] *n* 坏死素
necrosis [neˈkrəusis] ([复] **necroses** [neˈkrəusiːz]) *n* 坏死 | aseptic ~ 无菌性坏死 / bacillary ~ 坏死杆菌病 / central ~ 中心性坏死 / cheesy ~, caseous ~ 干酪样坏死 / coagulation ~, ischemic ~ 凝固性坏死,缺血性坏死 / colliquative ~, liquefaction ~ 液化性坏死 / dry ~ 干性坏死 / focal ~ 局灶性坏死 / hyaline ~ 透明坏死,玻璃样坏死 / massive hepatic ~ 大块肝坏死(旧称急性黄色萎缩) / medial ~ 主动脉中层坏死 / mercurial ~ 汞中毒性坏死 / moist ~ 湿性坏死 / mummification ~ 干性坏疽 / pe-

ripheral ~ (肝小叶)周围性坏死 / phosphorus ~ 磷中毒性坏死 / pressure ~ 压迫性坏死 / ~ progrediens 进行性坏死,进行性腐肉形成 / progressive emphysematous ~ 气性坏疽 / simple ~ 单纯性坏死 / subcutaneous fat ~ (新生儿)皮下脂肪坏死(假硬化病) / superficial ~ 表层坏死 | **necrotic** [neˈkrɔtik] *a*

necrospermia [ˌnekrəuˈspəːmiə], **necrozoospermia** [ˌnekrəuˌzəuəˈspəːmiə] *n* 死精症(精液中的精子死亡或不活动) | **necrospermic** *a*

necrotizing [ˈnekrəˌtaiziŋ] *a* 引起坏死的,坏死性的

necrotomy [neˈkrɔtəmi] *n* 尸体解剖;死骨切除 | osteoplastic ~ 骨成形性死骨切除

necrotoxin [ˌnekrəuˈtɔksin] *n* 坏死毒素

Nectria [ˈnektriə] *n* 丛赤壳属

Necturus [nekˈtjuːrəs] *n* 泥螈属

NED no evidence of disease 无疾病迹象

nedocromil [ˌnedəuˈkrəumil] *n* 奈多罗米(非甾体消炎药,吸入用药,预防气道炎症和支气管收缩,治疗支气管哮喘)

needle [ˈniːdl] *n* 针 *vt* 用针缝;用针刺 | aneurysm ~ 动脉瘤针(用于结扎血管) / aspirating ~ 吸液针 / cataract ~ 内障针 / discission ~ 截囊针 / hypodermic ~ 皮下注射针 / knife ~ 刀针(用于白内障和其他眼科手术) / ligature ~ 结扎针 / stop ~ 有档针

needlescopic [ˌniːdiˈskɔpik] *a* 针状内镜的

Neef's hammer [neif] (Christopher E. Neef) 内夫锤(电流启闭锤)

Neelsen [ˈniːlsən] 见 Ziehl-Neelsen

neem [niːm] *n* 印楝

neencephalon [ˌniːenˈsefələn] *n* 新脑(大脑皮质及其所属)

NEFA nonesterified fatty acids 非酯化脂肪酸

nefazodone hydrochloride [nəˈfeizəudəun] 盐酸萘法唑酮(抗抑郁药)

nefluorophotometer [niˌfluərəufəuˈtɔmitə] *n* 荧光比浊计,荧光散射浊度计(即 fluoronephelometer)

nefopam hydrochloride [ˈnefəpæm] *n* 盐酸奈福泮(镇痛药,肌肉松弛药)

negativism [ˈnegətivizəm] *n* 违拗症

negatol [ˈnegətɔl] *n* 间甲酚磺酸-甲醛缩聚物(杀寄生虫药,杀菌和抑菌药,局部用于子宫颈)

negatoscope [ˈnegətəskəup] *n* 看片灯,读片灯(看 X 线片)

negatron [ˈnegətrɔn] *n* 负电子,阴电子

neglect [niˈglekt] *vt*, *n* 忽视,忽略;疏忽 | unilateral ~ 单侧忽略(偏侧失用症,不能注意身体整饰和一侧的刺激而不是另一侧,通常由于如卒中后中枢神经系统损害所致,亦称选择性忽略)

Negri bodies [ˈneigri] (Adelchi Negri) 内氏小体(见于狂犬病动物的神经细胞内和细胞突中的卵圆形或圆形包涵体)

Negri-Jacod syndrome [ˈneigri ʒɑːˈkəu] (Silvio Negri; Maurice Jacod) 内-雅综合征(见 Jacod's syndrome)

Negro's phenomenon [ˈneigrəu] (Camillo Negro) 内格罗现象,齿轮现象(cogwheel phenomenon,见 phenomenon 项下相应术语)

NEI National Eye Institute 国立眼科研究所

neighborwise [ˈneibəwaiz] *a*, *ad* 邻向(形容被移植的胚细胞或组织的可塑性行为,适于新的异常部位)

Neill-Mooser bodies [niːl ˈmuːsə] (Mather H. Neill; H. Mooser) 尼尔-穆塞体(充满立克次体的大单核细胞,见于接种鼠型斑疹伤寒的实验动物的阴囊肿胀炎性渗出物中) | ~ reaction 豚鼠阴囊肿胀反应(实验动物接种鼠型斑疹伤寒立克次体后的反应,在阴囊肿胀的炎性渗出物中含有充满立克次体的大单核细胞)

Neisser-Doering phenomenon [ˌnaisə ˈdeiriŋ] (Ernst Neisser; Hans Doering) 奈瑟-德林现象(抗溶血物质所致的人类血清正常溶血作用的抑制现象,有时见于肾硬变及动脉硬化)

Neisseria [naiˈsiəriə] *n* 奈瑟菌属 | ~ catarrhalis 卡他奈瑟菌,黏膜炎奈瑟菌 / ~ flavescens 浅黄色奈瑟菌 / ~ gonorrhoeae 淋病奈瑟菌,淋[病双]球菌 / ~ lactamica 乳酰胺奈瑟菌 / ~ meningitidis 脑膜炎奈瑟菌 / ~ mucosa 黏液奈瑟菌 / ~ sicca 干燥奈瑟菌 / ~ subflava 微黄色奈瑟菌

Neisseriaceae [naiˌsiəriˈeisiiː] *n* 奈瑟菌科

neisserial [naiˈsiəriəl] *a* 奈瑟菌属的

Neisser's diplococcus [ˈnaisə] (Albert L. S. Neisser) 奈瑟双球菌,淋[病双]球菌 | ~ syringe 奈瑟尿道注射器(用于淋病)

Neisser-Wechsberg phenomenon [ˈnaisə ˈveksbəːg] (Max Neisser; Friedrich Wechsberg) 奈瑟-韦克伯格现象,补体转向现象,补体偏向现象(complement deviation,见 deviation 项下相应术语) | ~ test 奈瑟-韦克伯格试验,杀菌试验(测定病人血液杀菌力的一种试验)

nekton [ˈnektɔn] *n* 自游生物

Nélaton's catheter [neiləˈtɔːn] (Auguste Nélaton) 内拉通导管,软导管(一种用橡皮做的软导管) | ~ line 内拉通线(髂前上棘至坐骨结节的线) / ~ operation 内拉通手术(肩关节切断术) / ~ probe 内拉通探杆,缶头探子 / ~ sphincter 内拉通括约肌(直肠内的肌束,位于与前列腺相同的高度)

nelavane [ˈneləvæn] *n* 非洲锥虫病

nelfinavir mesylate [nelˈfinəviə] 甲磺奈非那韦(HIV 蛋白酶抑制剂,可致未成熟尚未感染的病

毒颗粒形成,用于治疗人免疫缺陷病毒感染,口服给药)

Nelson's syndrome [ˈnelsən] (Don H. Nelson) 纳尔逊综合征(库欣〈Cushing〉综合征患者两侧肾上腺切除后发生的一种产生 ACTH 的垂体肿瘤,特征为肿瘤侵袭性生长和皮肤色素沉着过度)

nem [nem] (由德文 Nahrungs Einheit Milch 字首组成)*n* 奶牧(儿童食物的营养价值单位,相当于1 g 母乳的营养价)

nema [ˈniːmə] *n*【希】线虫

nemaline [ˈneməliːn] *a* 线样的,杆状的

nemathelminth [ˌneməˈθelminθ] *n* 线虫

Nemathelminthes [ˌneməθəlˈminθiːz] *n* 线形动物门

nemathelminthiasis [ˌneməˌθelminˈθaiəsis] *n* 线虫病

nematicide [neˈmætisaid] *a* 杀线虫的 *n* 杀线虫剂

nematization [ˌnemətaiˈzeiʃən, -tiˈz-] *n* 线虫感染

nemat(o)- [构词成分]线,线虫

nematoblast [ˈnemətəblæst] *n* 精子细胞

Nematocera [ˌneməˈtɔsərə] *n* 长角亚目(昆虫)

nematocide [ˈnemətəsaid] *a* 杀线虫的 *n* 杀线虫剂

nematocyst [ˈnemətəsist] *n* 刺丝囊(腔肠动物类的一种小刺毛)

Nematoda [ˌneməˈtəudə] *n* 线虫纲

nematode [ˈnemətəud] *n* 线虫

nematodesma [ˌniːmətəuˈdezmə] ([复] **nematodesmata** [ˌniːmətəuˈdezmətə]) *n* 丝带,线带(某些纤毛原生动物的器官。亦称丝泡,线泡)

nematodiasis [ˌnemətəuˈdaiəsis] *n* 线虫病

Nematodirus [ˌnemətəˈdairəs] *n* 细颈线虫属

nematoid [ˈnemətɔid] *a* 线形的;线虫的

nematology [ˌneməˈtɔlədʒi] *n* 线虫学 | **nematologist** *n* 线虫学家

Nematomorpha [ˌnemətəuˈmɔːfə] *n* 线形[虫]纲

nematosis [ˌneməˈtəusis] *n* 线虫寄生,线虫病

nematospermia [ˌnemətəuˈspəːmiə] *n* 长尾精虫

Nemertea [neˈməːtiə], **Nemertina** [neməˈtainə] *n* 纽形动物门

nemertean [neməˈtiən] *a* 纽形动物的 *n* 纽形动物

nemic [ˈnemik] *a* 线虫的

Nencki's test [ˈnentski] (Marcellus von Nencki) 能斯基试验(检吲哚)

ne(o)- [构词成分]新

neoadjuvant [ˌniːəuˈædjuvənt] *n* 新佐剂(本词用以表示在必要的第2次治疗方式之前的预先癌治疗〈通常为化学治疗和放射治疗〉)

neoantigen [ˌni(ː)əuˈæntidʒən] *n* 新生抗原(存在于肿瘤细胞中的一种核内抗原,如T抗原)

neoantimosan [ˌni(ː)əuænˈtiməsən] *n* 锑波芬,福锑(治血吸虫病药)

neoarsphenamine [ˌni(ː)əuɑːsˈfenəmiːn] *n* 新胂凡纳明,九一四(以前用作抗梅毒药)

neoarthrosis [ˌni(ː)əuɑːˈθrəusis] *n* 人造关节;假关节

neobiogenesis [ˌni(ː)əuˌbaiəuˈdʒenisis] *n* 新生物发生,新生源说(认为生命曾一再从无机物产生)

neobladder [ˌniːəu ˈblædə] *n* 新膀胱

neocerebellum [ˌni(ː)əuˌseriˈbeləm] *n* 新小脑

neocinchophen [ˌni(ː)əuˈsiŋkəfən] *n* 新辛可芬(镇痛、解热、促尿酸尿药)

neocinetic [ˌni(ː)əusaiˈnetik] *a* 新[成]运动区的

neocortex [ˌni(ː)əuˈkɔːteks] *n* 新[大脑]皮质

neocyte [ˈni(ː)əusait] *n* 未成熟白细胞

neocytosis [ˌni(ː)əusaiˈtəusis] *n* 未成熟白细胞血症

neodarwinism [ˌni(ː)əuˈdɑːwinizəm] *n* 新达尔文学说(认为物种的进化主要是自然选择,从而排除获得性性状遗传)

neodiathermy [ˌni(ː)əuˈdaiəˌθəːmi] *n* 短波透热法,短波透热电疗法

neodymium [ˌni(ː)əuˈdimiəm] *n* 钕(化学元素)

neoencephalon [ˌni(ː)əuenˈsefəlɔn] *n* 新脑(指大脑皮质及其所属)

neoendorphin [ˌniːəu enˈdɔːfin, -ˈendɔːfin] *n* 新内啡肽

neofetal [ˌni(ː)əuˈfiːtl] *a* 幼胎的

neofetus [ˌni(ː)əuˈfiːtəs] *n* 幼胎(约第八周胎儿)

neoformation [ˌni(ː)əufɔːˈmeiʃən] *n* 新生物,赘生物

neoformative [ˌni(ː)əuˈfɔːmətiv] *a* 新生的

neogala [niˈɔgələ] *n* 初乳

Neogastropoda [ˌniːəu gæsˈtrɔpədə] *n* 新腹足纲

neogenesis [ˌni(ː)əuˈdʒenisis] *n* 新生 | **neogenetic** [ˌni(ː)əudʒiˈnetik] *a*

neogermitrine [ˌni(ː)əuˈdʒəːmitriːn] *n* 新吉密春(绿藜芦的生物碱之一)

neoglottis [ˌni(ː)əuˈglɔtis] *n* 新声门(手术再造的声门,亦称假声门 pseudoglottis) | **neoglottic** *a*

neoglycogenesis [ˌni(ː)əuˌglaikəuˈdʒenisis] *n* 糖原异生[作用]

Neogregarinida [ˌni(ː)əuˌgregəˈrainidə] *n* 新簇目

neo-hippocratism [ˌni(ː)əuhiˈpɔkrətizəm] *n* 新希波克拉底医派(强调观察与临床医学)

neohymen [ˌni(ː)əuˈhaimen] *n* 假膜

neointima [ˌniːəu ˈintimə] *n* 新内膜

neokinetic [ˌni(ː)əukaiˈnetik, -kiˈn-] *a* 新[成]运

动区的

neolallia [ˌni(ː)əuˈlæliə], **neolallism** [ˌni(ː)əuˈlælizəm] *n* 新语症(如精神分裂症患者说话时加入许多新词)

neologism [ni(ː)ˈɔlədʒizəm] *n* 语词新作(精神病患者或谵妄病患者所作无意义的语句)

neomembrane [ˌni(ː)əuˈmembrein] *n* 假膜

neomin [ˈniːəmin] *n* 新霉素(即 neomycin)

neomorph [ˈniːəmɔːf] *n* 新形体,新形态(进化过程中刚获得的部分或器官);新效等位基因(一个突变基因引起与正常基因不相同的新的质效应)

neomorphism [ˌni(ː)əuˈmɔːfizəm] *n* 新[形体]形成

neomort [ˈniːəu mɔːt] *n* 新尸体(刚死后的尸体)

neomycin [ˌni(ː)əuˈmaisin] *n* 新霉素(抗生素类药) | ~ palmitate 棕榈酸新霉素 / ~ sulfate 硫酸新霉素

neon [ˈniːɔn] *n* 氖(化学元素)

neonatal [ˌni(ː)əuˈneitl] *a* 新生[期]的(产后开头四周内的),新生儿的

neonate [ˈni(ː)əneit] *a* 新生的 *n* 新生儿

neonatology [ˌni(ː)əuneiˈtɔlədʒi] *n* 新生儿学 | **neonatologist** *n* 新生儿学家

neontology [ˌniːɔnˈtɔlədʒi] *n* 近代生物学

neopallium [ˌni(ː)əuˈpæliəm] *n* 新[大脑]皮质

neophrenia [ˌni(ː)əuˈfriːniə] *n* 儿童期精神病

neoplasia [ˌni(ː)əuˈpleiziə] *n* 瘤形成 | multiple endocrine ~ (MEN) 多发性内分泌瘤病

neoplasm [ˈni(ː)əuplæzəm] *n* 新生物,赘生物,[肿]瘤 | histoid ~ 组织样瘤 / organoid ~ 器官样瘤

neoplastic [ˌni(ː)əuˈplæstik] *a* 新生物的,赘生的,[肿]瘤的;瘤形成的

neoplastigenic [ˌni(ː)əuplæstiˈdʒenik] *a* 引起[肿]瘤的

Neopsylla [niːˈɔpsillə] *n* 新蚤属

neopterin [niˈɔptərin] *n* 新蝶呤

neoquassin [ˌni(ː)əuˈkwæsin] *n* 新苦楝素,新苦木苦素

neorectum [ˌniːəu ˈrektəm] *n* 新直肠

Neorickettsia [ˌni(ː)əuriˈketsiə] *n* 新立克次体属

Neoschoengastia [ˌni(ː)əuʃeinˈgæstiə] *n* 新棒恙螨属 | ~ americana 美洲新棒恙螨

Neospora [niˈɔspərə] *n* 新孢子属

Neosporidia [ˌni(ː)əuspəˈridiə] *n* 新孢子亚纲

neosporosis [ˌniːəu spəˈrəusis] *n* 新孢子病

neostigmine [ˌni(ː)əuˈstigmin] *n* 新斯的明(一种胆碱能药,用于重症肌无力) | ~ bromide 溴新斯的明 / ~ methylsulfate 甲基硫酸新斯的明

neostomy [niˈɔstəmi] *n* [器官]造口术

neostriatum [ˌni(ː)əustraiˈeitəm] *n* 新纹状体

Neostrongylus [ˌniːəu ˈstrɔndʒilus] *n* 新圆线虫属

neoteny [niˈɔtini] *n* 幼体性熟,幼态持续

Neotestudina [ˌniːəu ˌtestuːˈdainə] *n* 新龟甲形菌属

neothalamus [ˌni(ː)əuˈθæləməs] *n* 新丘脑

Neotoma [niˈɔtəmə] *n* 林鼠属 | ~ lepida 荒漠林鼠

Neotrombicula [ˌniːəu trɔmˈbikjulə] *n* 新恙螨属

neotype [ˈni(ː)əutaip] *n* 新型[菌株];新模标本

neourethra [ˌniːəu juəˈriːθrə] *n* 新尿道

neovagina [ˌniːəu vəˈdʒainə] *n* 新阴道

neovascularization [ˌni(ː)əuˌvæskjuləraiˈzeiʃən, -riˈz-] *n* 新血管形成;血管再生

nepenthe [neˈpenθi], **nepenthes** [neˈpenθiːz] *n* (古希腊人用的)忘忧药

nepenthic [neˈpenθik] *a* 忘忧的

Nepeta [ˈnepətə] *n* 假荆芥属

nepetalactone [ˌnepətəˈlæktəun] *n* 假荆芥内酯

nephel(o)- [构词成分]云,雾,浑浊

nephelometer [ˌnefiˈlɔmitə] *n* 比浊计,浊度计 | photoelectric ~ 光电比浊计 | **nephelometry** *n* 浊度测定法,比浊法

nephelopia [ˌnefiˈləupiə] *n* 角膜翳性视力障碍,角膜混浊性视力障碍

nephelopsychosis [ˌnefiləusaiˈkəusis] *n* 恋云癖

nephradenoma [ˌnefrædiˈnəumə] *n* 肾腺瘤

nephralgia [neˈfrældʒiə] *n* 肾痛 | **nephralgic** *a*

nephrapostasis [ˌnefrəˈpɔstəsis] *n* 肾脓肿

nephratonia [ˌnefrəˈtəuniə]; **nephratony** [neˈfrætəni] *n* 肾弛缓

nephrauxe [neˈfrɔːksi] *n* 肾增大,肾胀大

nephrectasia [ˌnefrekˈteiziə], **nephrectasis** [neˈfrektəsis], **nephrectasy** [neˈfrektəsi] *n* 肾扩张,囊状肾

nephrectomize [neˈfrektəmaiz] *vt*, *vi* 肾切除

nephrectomy [neˈfrektəmi] *n* 肾切除术 | abdominal ~, anterior ~ 经腹肾切除术 / lumbar ~, posterior ~ 经腰肾切除术 / paraperitoneal ~ 腹膜旁肾切除术

nephredema [ˌnefriˈdiːmə] *n* 肾盂积水,肾充血

nephrelcosis [ˌnefrelˈkəusis] *n* 肾溃疡

nephremia [neˈfriːmiə] *n* 肾充血

nephric [ˈnefrik] *a* 肾的

nephridium [neˈfridiəm] *n* 肾管(胚胎) | **nephridial** [neˈfridiəl] *a*

nephritic [neˈfritik] *a* 肾炎的;肾的 *n* 治肾病药

nephritis [neˈfraitis] ([复] **nephritides** [neˈfritidiːz]) *n* 肾炎 | acute ~, croupous ~ 急性肾炎 / Balkan ~ 巴尔干肾炎(一种十分缓慢的进行性间质性肾炎,亦称巴尔干肾病) / chloroazotemic ~ 氯氮血症性肾炎/ degenerative ~ 变性肾炎,肾变病 / glomerulocapsular ~ 肾小球被

膜性肾炎 / lipomatous ~ 脂肪瘤性肾炎 / lupus ~ 狼疮肾炎 / nephrotoxic serum ~ 肾毒性血清肾炎(由于注射抗肾抗原的异种抗体后所产生的一种抗体介导肾小球性肾炎的动物模型) / nephrotoxic ~ 肾毒性肾炎/ potassium-losing ~ 失钾性肾炎 / ~ of pregnancy 妊娠期肾炎 / productive ~ 增殖性肾炎 / salt-losing ~ 失盐性肾炎 / saturnine ~ 铅毒性肾炎 / transfusion ~ 输血性肾炎 / tubal ~, tubular ~ 肾小管肾炎 / vascular ~ 肾硬化,肾硬变

nephritogenic [niˌfritəuˈdʒenik] *a* 致肾炎的

nephr(o)- [构词成分]肾

nephroabdominal [ˌnefrəuæbˈdɔminl] *a* 肾腹的

nephroangiosclerosis [ˌnefrəuˌændʒiəuskliəˈrəusis] *n* 肾血管硬化

nephroblastoma [ˌnefrəublæsˈtəumə] *n* 肾母细胞瘤

nephroblastomatosis [ˌnefrəu blæsˌtəuməˈtəusis] *n* 肾母细胞瘤病

nephrobronchial [ˌnefrəu ˈbrɔŋkiəl] *a* 肾支气管的

nephrocalcinosis [ˌnefrəuˌkælsiˈnəusis] *n* 肾钙质沉着症

nephrocapsectomy [ˌnefrəukæpˈsektəmi], **nephrocapsulectomy** [ˌnefrəukæpsjuˈlektəmi] *n* 肾被膜剥除术

nephrocapsulotomy [ˌnefrəuˌkæpsjuˈlɔtəmi] *n* 肾被膜切开术

nephrocardiac [ˌnefrəuˈkɑːdiæk] *a* 肾心[脏]的

nephrocele [ˈnefrəsiːl] *n* 肾突出

nephrocolic [ˌnefrəuˈkɔlik] *a* 肾结肠的 *n* 肾绞痛

nephrocolonic [ˌnefrəu kəˈlɔnik] *a* 肾结肠的

nephrocolopexy [ˌnefrəuˈkəuləˌpeksi] *n* 肾结肠固定术

nephrocoloptosis [ˌnefrəuˌkəulɔpˈtəusis] *n* 肾结肠下垂

nephrocutaneous [ˌnefrəu kju(ː)ˈteinjəs] *a* 肾皮肤的

nephrocystanastomosis [ˌnefrəuˌsistəˌnæstəˈməusis] *n* 肾膀胱吻合术

nephrocystitis [ˌnefrəusisˈtaitis] *n* 肾膀胱炎

nephrocystosis [ˌnefrəusisˈtəusis] *n* 肾囊肿形成

nephroerysipelas [ˌnefrəuˌeriˈsipiləs] *n* 肾炎性丹毒

nephrogastric [ˌnefrəuˈgæstrik] *a* 肾胃的

nephrogenic [ˌnefrəuˈdʒenik], **nephrogenous** [neˈfrɔdʒinəs] *a* 肾源性的,肾发生的

nephrogram [ˌnefrəgræm] *n* 肾图,肾造影[照]片

nephrography [neˈfrɔgrəfi] *n* 肾造影[术]

nephrohemia [ˌnefrəuˈhiːmiə] *n* 肾充血

nephrohydrosis [ˌnefrəuhaiˈdrəusis] *n* 肾盂积水

nephrohypertrophy [ˌnefrəuhaiˈpəːtrəfi] *n* 肾肥大

nephroid [ˈnefrɔid] *a* 肾形的,肾样的

nephrolith [ˈnefrəliθ] *n* 肾石

nephrolithiasis [ˌnefrəuliˈθaiəsis] *n* 肾结石

nephrolithotomy [ˌnefrəuliˈθɔtəmi] *n* 肾切开取石术

nephrology [neˈfrɔlədʒi] *n* 肾脏病学 | **nephrologist** *n* 肾脏病学家

nephrolysine [neˈfrɔlisin] *n* 溶肾素,肾毒素

nephrolysis [neˈfrɔlisis] *n* 肾溶解;肾松解术 | **nephrolytic** [ˌnefrəuˈlitik] *a*

nephroma [neˈfrəumə] *n* 肾瘤 | embryonal ~ 胚胎性肾瘤

nephromalacia [ˌnefrəuməˈleiʃiə] *n* 肾软化

nephromegaly [ˌnefrəuˈmegəli] *n* 巨肾,肾肥大

nephromere [ˈnefrəmiə] *n* 肾节,原肾节

nephron [ˈnefrɔn] *n* 肾单位 | lower ~ 下部肾单位

nephroncus [neˈfrɔŋkəs] *n* 肾瘤

nephronia [nəˈfrəuniə] *n* 肾病 | lobar ~ 大叶性肾病,急性肾盂肾炎

nephronophthisis [ˌnefrɔˈnɔfθisis] *n* 肾消耗病 | familial juvenile ~ 家族性幼年型肾消耗病(亦称髓质囊肿病)

nephro-omentopexy [ˌnefrəu əuˈmentəˌpeksi] *n* 肾网膜固定术

nephroparalysis [ˌnefrəupəˈrælisis] *n* 肾麻痹

nephropathia [ˌnefrəuˈpæθiə] *n* 肾病

nephropathy [neˈfrɔpəθi] *n* 肾病 | analgesic ~ 镇痛剂肾病(由于服用大量含有非那西丁镇痛药所致) / Balkan ~ 巴尔干肾病(见 nephritis 项下相应术语) / gouty ~ 痛风性肾病 / hypazoturic ~ 低氮尿性肾病 / hypochloruric ~, dropsical ~ 低氯尿性肾病,水肿性肾病 / IgA ~ IgA 肾病 / membranous ~ 膜性肾病 / reflux ~ 反流性肾病 | **nephropathic** [ˌnefrəuˈpæθik] *a*

nephropexy [ˈnefrəˌpeksi] *n* 肾固定术

nephrophagiasis [ˌnefrəufəˈdʒaiəsis] *n* 肾毁蚀病(寄生虫所致)

nephrophthisis [neˈfrɔfθisis] *n* 肾结核;肾消耗病

nephropoietic [ˌnefrəupɔiˈetik] *a* 生成肾组织的

nephropoietin [ˌnefrəupɔiˈiːtin] *n* 生肾素,促肾组织生成素

nephroptosis [ˌnefrɔpˈtəusis], **nephroptosia** [ˌnefrɔpˈtəusiə] *n* 肾下垂

nephropyelitis [ˌnefrəuˌpaiəˈlaitis] *n* 肾盂肾炎

nephropyelography [ˌnefrəuˌpaiəˈlɔgrəfi] *n* 肾盂造影[术]

nephropyelolithotomy [ˌnefrəuˌpaiələuliˈθɔtəmi] *n* 剖肾肾盂石切除术,剖肾肾盂取石术

nephropyeloplasty [ˌnefrəuˈpaiələuˌplæsti] *n* 肾盂成形术
nephropyosis [ˌnefrəupaiˈəusis] *n* 肾化脓
nephrorosein [ˌnefrəuˈrəuziin] *n* 尿红素
nephrorrhagia [ˌnefrəuˈreidʒiə] *n* 肾出血
nephrorrhaphy [neˈfrɔrəfi] *n* 肾缝合术
nephrosclerosis [ˌnefrəuskliəˈrəusis] *n* 肾硬化 | arteriolar ~, intercapillary ~ 小动脉性肾硬化症,毛细管间性肾硬化 / benign ~, hyaline arteriolar ~ 良性肾硬化 / malignant ~, hyperplastic arteriolar ~ 恶性肾硬化 / senile ~ 老年性肾硬化 | **nephroscleria** [ˌnefrəuˈskliəriə] *n*
nephroscope [ˈnefrɔskəup] *n* 肾镜
nephroscopy [niˈfrɔskəpi] *n* 肾镜检查
nephrosis [neˈfrəusis] ([复] **nephroses** [neˈfrəusiːz]) *n* 肾病 | larval ~ 隐性肾病(临床表现为蛋白尿) / lipid ~ 脂性肾病
nephrosonephritis [neˌfrəusəuneˈfraitis] *n* 肾变病肾炎 | hemorrhagic ~, Korean hemorrhagic ~ 出血性肾变病肾炎,流行性出血热
nephrosonography [ˌnefrəusəuˈnɔgrəfi] *n* 肾超声波检查,肾声像图检查
nephrospasis [ˌnefrəuˈspæsis] *n* 悬垂肾
nephrosplenopexy [ˌnefrəuˈsplinəˌpeksi] *n* 肾脾固定术
nephrostogram [neˈfrɔstəugræm] *n* 肾造瘘术图(肾内注射造影剂后放射摄影检查肾造瘘术)
nephrostolithotomy [ˌnifrəustəuliˈθɔtəmi] *n* 肾造口取石术
nephrostoma [ˌnefrəuˈstəumə], **nephrostome** [ˈnefrəstəum] *n* 肾孔(胚胎)
nephrostomy [neˈfrɔstəmi] *n* 肾造口术
nephrotic [neˈfrɔtik] *a* 肾变病的,肾病的
nephrotome [ˈnefrətəum] *n* 肾节,原肾节,中板
nephrotomogram [ˌnefrəuˈtəuməgræm] *n* 肾体层摄影[照]片
nephrotomography [ˌnefrəutəˈmɔgrəfi] *n* 肾体层摄影[术]
nephrotomy [neˈfrɔtəmi] *n* 肾切开术 | abdominal ~ 经腹肾切开术 / anatrophic ~ 防萎缩肾切开术 / lumbar ~ 经腰肾切开术
nephrotoxic [ˌnefrəuˈtɔksik] *a* 肾中毒的 | **~ity** [ˌnefrəutɔkˈsisəti] *n* 中毒性肾损害
nephrotoxin [ˌnefrəuˈtɔksin] *n* 肾毒素,溶肾素
nephrotresis [ˌnefrəuˈtriːsis] *n* 肾造口术
nephrotropic [ˌnefrəuˈtrɔpik] *a* 向肾性的
nephrotuberculosis [ˌnefrəutju(ː)ˌbəːkjuˈləusis] *n* 肾结核
nephrotyphoid [ˌnefrəuˈtaifɔid] *n* 肾型伤寒
nephrotyphus [ˌnefrəuˈtaifəs] *n* 肾型斑疹伤寒(伴血尿)
nephroureterectomy [ˌnefrəujuəˌriːtəˈrektəmi] *n* 肾-输尿管切除术
nephroureterocystectomy [ˌnefrəujuəˌriːtərəusisˈtektəmi] *n* 肾输尿管膀胱切除术
nephroureteroscopy [ˌnefrəujuəˌriːtəˈrɔskəpi] *n* 肾输尿管镜检查,输尿管肾镜检查
nephrozymase [ˌnefrəuˈzaimeis] *n* 肾酿酶
nephrozymosis [ˌnefrəuzaiˈməusis] *n* 肾发酵病
nephrydrosis [ˌnefriˈdrəusis] *n* 肾盂积水 | **nephrydrotic** [ˌnefriˈdrɔtik] *a*
neptunium [nepˈtjuːniəm] *n* 镎(化学元素)
nequinate [neˈkwineit] *n* 奈喹酯(禽类抑球虫药)
Neri's sign [ˈneiri] (Vincenzo Neri) 内里征(①器质性偏瘫之征,患者仰卧,患腿被动上举时,患侧膝自行屈曲。②患者站立,躯干前屈,则引起患侧膝屈曲,见于腰骶和髋骶部的损害)
Nerium [ˈniːriəm] *n* 夹竹桃属
Nernst equation [nernst] (Walther Hermann Nernst) 能斯脱方程式(电化学反应所产生的电压方程式:

$$E = E^0 - \frac{RT}{zF}\ln Q$$

式中 E 为所产生的电压,E^0 为该反应的标准还原电位,R 为气体常数,T 为绝对温度,z 为反应中转移的电子数,F 为法拉第常数,Q 为反应商,ln 为自然对数。该式还可得出可扩散离子穿过膜的浓度所产生的膜电位,在此情况下,E^0 为零,z 为离子电荷,Q 为膜两侧浓度比) | ~ potential 能斯脱电位(在膜中经膜孔可扩散的离子,其浓度梯度穿过膜所产生的电压,而相反电荷的离子则不能穿过此膜,见 Nernst equation)
nerol [ˈnirɔl] *n* 橙花醇
neroli [ˈniərəli] *n* 橙花油
nerve [nəːv] *n* 神经(详见附录) | accelerator ~s 加速神经 / afferent ~, centripetal ~, esodic ~ 传入神经,向中神经 / anabolic ~ 促同化神经 / autonomic ~s 自主神经 / cranial ~s 脑神经,颅神经 / crotaphitic ~ 上颌神经 / depressor ~ 降压神经 / efferent ~, exodic ~, centrifugal ~ 传出神经,离中神经 / eighth cranial ~, eighth ~ 第八脑神经,听神经 / eleventh cranial ~, eleventh ~ 第十一脑神经,副神经 / fifth cranial ~, fifth ~ 第五脑神经,三叉神经 / first cranial ~s, first ~s 第一脑神经,嗅神经 / fourth cranial ~, fourth ~ 第四脑神经,滑车神经 / gangliated ~ 有节神经,交感神经 / inhibitory ~ 抑制神经 / motor ~ 运动神经 / ninth cranial ~, ninth ~ 第九脑神经,舌咽神经 / pain ~ 痛觉神经 / pilomotor ~s 立毛神经 / second cranial ~, second ~ 第二脑神经,视神经 / seventh cranial ~, seventh ~ 第七脑神经,面神经 / sixth cranial ~ sixth ~ 第六脑神经,展神经 / somatic ~s 体干神经 / sudomotor ~s 泌汗神经 / sympathetic ~

交感神经 / tenth cranial ~, tenth ~ 第十脑神经,迷走神经 / third cranial ~, third ~ 第三脑神经,动眼神经 / twelfth cranial ~, twelfth ~ 第十二脑神经,舌下神经 / vasoconstrictor ~ 血管收缩神经 / vasodilator ~ 血管舒张神经 / vasomotor ~ 血管舒缩神经,血管运动神经 / vasosensory ~ 血管感觉神经

nerveless [ˈnəːvlis] *a* 没有劲的,无力的;无神经的

nervi [ˈnəːvai] nervus 的复数

nervimotility [ˌnəːviməuˈtiləti] *n* 神经运动力

nervimotion [ˌnəːviˈməuʃən] *n* 神经[兴奋性]运动

nervimotor [ˌnəːviˈməutə] *a* 运动神经的

nervimuscular [ˌnəːviˈmʌskjulə], **nervomuscular** [ˌnəːvəuˈmʌskjulə] *a* 神经肌肉的

nervonate [nəːˈvɔneit] *n* 神经酸,二十四[碳]烯酸(盐、酯或阴离子型)

nervone [ˈnəːvəun] *n* 神经苷脂,烯脑苷脂

nervonic acid [nəːˈvɔnik] 神经酸,二十四[碳]烯酸

nervous [ˈnəːvəs] *a* 神经的;神经质的 | ~**ness** *n* 神经质

nervous breakdown [ˈnəːvəs ˈbreikdaun] 神经崩溃,精神崩溃

nervus [ˈnəːvəs] ([复] **nervi** [ˈnəːvai]) *n*【拉】神经(详见附录)

nesidiectomy [neˌsidiˈektəmi] *n* 胰岛切除术

nesidioblast [neˈsidiəuˌblæst] *n* 成胰岛细胞

nesidioblastoma [neˌsidiəublæsˈtəumə] *n* 成胰岛细胞瘤

nesidioblastosis [neˌsidiəublæsˈtəusis] *n* 胰岛细胞增殖症

nesiritide [nəˈsiritaid] *n* 奈西利肽(重组人脑钠尿肽制剂,用于治疗急性失代偿性充血性心力衰竭,静脉内给药)

Nesokia [nəˈsəukiə] *n* 地鼠属

nesslerize [ˈnesləraiz] *vt* 用奈氏(Nessler)试剂处理 | **nesslerization** [ˌneslərai'zeiʃən, -riˈz-] *n* 奈氏试剂处理法

Nessler's reagent(solution, test) [ˈneslə] (A. Nessler) 奈[斯勒]氏试剂(溶液、试验)(5% 碘化钾、2.5% 氯化汞和 16% 氢氧化钾的水溶液,检验水中氨量)

nest [nest] *n* 巢,穴 | bird's ~s 心内膜袋 / cancer ~s 癌细胞巢 / cell ~ 细胞巢 / swallow's ~ 小脑禽巢

nested [ˈnestəd] *a* 巢状的,网状的,嵌套的

nesteostomy [ˌnestiˈɔstəmi] *n* 空肠造口术

nestotherapy [ˌnestəuˈθerəpi], **nestitherapy** [ˌnestiˈθerəpi], **nestiatria** [ˌnestiˈeitriə] *n* 饥饿疗法

net¹ [net] *n* 网;网状物 | achromatic ~ 无色网 / chromidial ~ 核外染色质网 / nerve ~ 神经网

net² [net] *a* 纯净的 *n* 净数,净重,净值

nethalide [ˈneθəlaid] *n* 萘心定(即丙萘洛尔 pronethalol, β 受体阻滞药)

Netherton's syndrome [ˈneθətən] (Earl Weldon Netherton) 内塞顿综合征(一种先天性综合征,包括层板状鱼鳞病或迂回线状鱼鳞病、毛发缺失、特异反应性素质,有时为精神发育迟缓和氨基酸尿,一般认为是常染色体隐性遗传)

netilmicin sulfate [ˌnetilˈmaisin] 硫酸奈替米星(抗菌药)

nettle [ˈnetl] *n* 荨麻

Nettleship-Falls type ocular albinism [ˈnetəlʃip fɔːlz] (Edward Nettleship; Harold F. Falls) 内-福型眼白化病,X 连锁(内氏〈Nettleship〉型)眼白化病

network [ˈnetwəːk] *n* 网,网状物,网状构造;网络 | cell ~ 原生质网,胞质网丝 / idiotype-anti-idiotype ~ 独特型-抗独特型网络(B 细胞的一种调节机制) / neurofibrillar ~ 神经原纤维网 / peritarsal ~ 眼睑淋巴管网/ subpapillary ~ 乳头下毛细血管网(皮肤) / venous ~ 静脉网

neu [njuː] *n* 神经鞘,神经膜

Neubauer-Fischer test [ˈnɔibauə ˈfiʃə] (Otto Neubauer) 甘氨酰色氨酸试验(检胃癌)

Neubauer's artery [ˈnɔibauə] (Johann E. Neubauer) 甲状腺最下动脉

Neuberg ester [ˈnɔibəg] (Carl Neuberg) 诺勃酯,果糖-6-磷酸

Neuber's treatment [ˈnɔibə] (Gustav A. Neuber) 诺伊贝尔疗法(用碘仿甘油治疗骨关节结核) | ~ tubes 诺伊贝尔管(骨引流管)

Neufeld nail [ˈnjuːfeld] (Alonzo J. Neufeld) 纽菲尔德钉(用于股骨转子间骨折的内部固定)

Neufeld's phenomenon [ˈnɔifeld] (Fred Neufeld) 诺伊菲尔德现象(肺炎球菌溶解于胆盐溶液中) | ~ reaction(test) 诺伊菲尔德反应(试验)(肺炎球菌与特异性免疫血清相混时,除有凝集反应外,该菌周围部膨大。亦称肺炎球菌荚膜肿胀反应)

Neumann's cells [ˈnɔimən] (Ernst Neumann) 诺伊曼细胞(骨髓内的有核红细胞) | ~ sheath 诺伊曼鞘,牙质小管鞘

Neumann's law [ˈnɔimən] (Franz E. Neumann) 诺伊曼定律(类似成分的化合物其分子热量相等)

Neumann's method [ˈnɔimən] (Heinrich Neumann) 诺伊曼法(骨膜下注射可卡因及肾上腺素,为耳部手术局部麻醉法)

neurad [ˈnjuəræd] *ad* 向神经

neuradynamia [ˌnjuərədaiˈneimiə] *n* 神经衰弱

neuragmia [njuə'rægmiə] *n* 神经撕除术
neural ['njuərəl] *a* 神经的
neuralgia [njuə'rældʒə] *n* 神经痛 | cranial ~ 脑神经痛 / geniculate ~, otic ~ 膝状节神经痛,耳神经痛 / hallucinatory ~ 幻觉性神经痛 / naso-ciliary ~ 鼻睫神经痛 / peripheral ~ 周围神经痛 / postherpetic ~ 带状疱疹[后]神经痛 / red ~ 红斑性肢痛病 / reminiscent ~ 回忆性神经痛,痕迹性神经痛 / sciatic ~ 坐骨神经痛 / sphenopalatine ~ 蝶腭神经痛 / stump ~ 残肢神经痛 / trigeminal ~, trifacial ~ 三叉神经痛 | **neuralgic** *a*
neuralgiform [njuə'rældʒifɔːm] *a* 神经痛样的
neuraminic acid [ˌnjuərə'minik] 神经氨[糖]酸,甘露糖胺丙酮酸
neuraminidase [ˌnjuərə'minideis] *n* 神经氨酸酶,唾液酸酶
neuranagenesis [ˌnjuərænə'dʒenisis] *n* 神经再生
neurapophysis [ˌnjuərə'pɔfisis] *n* 神经突
neurapraxia [ˌnjuərə'præksiə] *n* 神经失用症,功能性麻痹
neurarchy ['njuərɑːki] *n* 神经控制[作用]
neurarthropathy [ˌnjuərɑː'θrɔpəθi] *n* 神经性关节病
neurasthenia [ˌnjuəræs'θiːniə] *n* 神经衰弱 | angioparalytic ~, angiopathic ~, pulsating ~ 血管麻痹性神经衰弱,搏动感性神经衰弱 / cardiac ~, cardiovascular ~ 神经性循环衰弱 / grippal ~ 流感后神经衰弱 / obsessive ~ 强迫性神经衰弱,精神衰弱 | **neurasthenic** [ˌnjuəræs'θenik] *a* 神经衰弱的 *n* 神经衰弱者
neurastheniac [ˌnjuəræs'θiːniæk] *n* 神经衰弱患者
neuratrophia [ˌnjuərə'trəufiə], **neuratrophy** [ˌnjuə'rætrəfi] *n* 神经萎缩,神经营养不良 | **neuratrophic** [ˌnjuərə'trɔfik] *a* 神经萎缩的,神经营养不良的 *n* 神经萎缩者
neuraxis [njuə'ræksis] *n* 轴突,轴索;中枢神经系统 | **neuraxial** [ˌnjuə'ræksiəl] *a* 轴索的
neuraxon [njuə'ræksɔn] *n* 轴突,轴索
neure ['njuə] *n* 神经元
neurectasia [ˌnjuərek'teiziə] *n* 神经牵伸术
neurectomy [njuə'rektəmi] *n* 神经切除术 | gastric ~ 迷走神经切断术 / opticociliary ~ 视神经睫状神经切除术
neurectopia [ˌnjuərek'təupiə], **neurectopy** [njuə'rektəpi] *n* 神经异位
neuregulin [njuə'regjulin] *n* 神经调节蛋白
neurenteric [ˌnjuəren'terik] *a* 神经管[与]原肠的
neurepithelium [ˌnjuərepi'θiːljəm] *n* 神经上皮 | **neurepithelial** *a*
neurergic [njuə'rəːdʒik] *a* 神经作用的
neurexeresis [ˌnjuərek'serəsis] *n* 神经抽出术
neurhypnology [ˌnjuəhip'nɔlədʒi] *n* 催眠学
neuriatry [njuə'raiətri] *n* 神经病治疗学
neuridine ['njuəridiːn] *n* 精胺,脑胺
neurilemma [ˌnjuəri'lemə] *n* 神经鞘,神经膜 | **~l** [ˌnjuəri'leməl], **~tic** [ˌnjuərilə'mætik], **~tous** [ˌnjuəri'lemətəs] *a*
neurilemmitis [ˌnjuərilə'maitis] *n* 神经鞘炎
neurilemmoma [ˌnjuərilə'məumə] *n* 神经鞘瘤
neurilem(m)oma [ˌnjuərilə'məumə] *n* 神经鞘瘤 | acoustic ~ 听神经[鞘]瘤
neurility [njuə'riləti] *n* 神经性能
neurimotility [ˌnjuərimәu'tiləti] *n* 神经运动力
neurimotor [ˌnjuəri'məutə] *a* 运动神经的
neurine ['njuərin] *n* 神经[毒]碱
neurinoma [ˌnjuəri'nəumə] *n* 神经鞘瘤 | acoustic ~ 听神经[鞘]瘤
neurite ['njuərait] *n* 轴突
neuritis [njuə'raitis] *n* 神经炎 | adventitial ~ 神经鞘炎 / alcoholic ~ 酒毒[中毒]性神经炎 / brachial ~ 神经痛性肌萎缩 / central ~, parenchymatous ~ 中心性神经炎,实质性神经炎 / dietetic ~, endemic ~ 脚气病,地方性神经炎 / disseminated ~, multiple ~ 播散性神经炎,多神经炎 / fallopian ~ 骨管性面神经炎 / interstitial hypertrophic ~ 肥大性间质性神经炎,进行性肥大性间质性神经病 / intraocular ~ 眼内神经炎,视神经网膜部神经炎 / jake ~ 姜酒性神经炎,姜酒中毒性麻痹 / pressure ~ 压迫性神经炎 / radiation ~ 放射性神经炎 / radicular ~ 神经根炎 / retrobulbar ~, orbital optic ~, postocular ~ 球后视神经炎/ sciatic ~ 坐骨神经炎,坐骨神经痛 / serum ~ 血清神经炎,血清神经病(serum neuropathy,见 neuropathy 项下相应术语) / shouldergirdle ~ 神经痛性肌萎缩 | **neuritic** [njuə'ritik] *a*
neur(o)- [构词成分]神经
neuroacanthocytosis [ˌnjuərəuəˌkænθəusai'təusis] *n* 神经刺状红细胞增多,舞蹈样运动刺状红细胞增多(见 choreoacanthocytosis)
neuroallergy [ˌnjuərəu'ælədʒi] *n* 神经变[态反]应性
neuroamebiasis [ˌnjuərəuˌæmi'baiəsis] *n* 神经型阿米巴病,阿米巴性神经炎
neuroanastomosis [ˌnjuərəuəˌnæstə'məusis] *n* 神经吻合术
neuroanatomy [ˌnjuərəuə'nætəmi] *n* 神经解剖学
neuroarthropathy [ˌnjuərəuɑː'θrɔpəθi] *n* 神经性关节病
neuroastrocytoma [ˌnjuərəuˌæstrəusai'təumə] *n* 神经星形细胞瘤
neurobehavioral [ˌnjuərəubi'heivjərəl] *a* 神经行为的
neurobiologist [ˌnjuərəubai'ɔlədʒist] *n* 神经生物

学家

neurobiology [ˌnjuərəubaiˈɔlədʒi] *n* 神经生物学

neurobiotaxis [ˌnjuərəuˌbaiəuˈtæksis] *n* 神经生物趋向性

neuroblast [ˈnjuərəblæst] *n* 成神经细胞

neuroblastoma [ˌnjuərəublæsˈtəumə] *n* 成神经细胞瘤

neuroborreliosis [ˌnjuərəu bəˌreliˈəusis] *n* 神经疏螺旋体病

neurocanal [ˌnjuərəukəˈnæl] *n* 神经管(椎管)

neurocardiac [ˌnjuərəuˈkɑːdiæk] *a* 神经心脏的

neurocentrum [ˌnjuərəuˈsentrəm] *n* 髓椎体(胚胎) | **neurocentral** *a*

neuroceptor [ˈnjuərəˌseptə] *n* 神经受体

neuroceratin [ˌnjuərəuˈserətin] *n* 神经角蛋白

neurochemistry [ˌnjuərəuˈkemistri] *n* 神经化学

neurochitin [ˌnjuərəuˈkaitin] *n* 神经壳质

neurochondrite [ˌnjuərəuˈkɔndrait] *n* 胚神经弓(胚胎)

neurochorioretinitis [ˌnjuərəuˌkɔriəuˌretiˈnaitis] *n* 视神经脉络膜视网膜炎

neurochoroiditis [ˌnjuərəuˌkɔːrɔiˈdaitis] *n* 视神经脉络膜炎

neurocirculatory [ˌnjuərəuˈsəːkjulətəri] *a* 神经[与]循环系统的

neurocladism [njuəˈrɔklədizəm] *n* 神经分支新生

neuroclonic [ˌnjuərəuˈklɔnik] *a* 神经性阵挛的

neurocoele [ˈnjuərəsiːl] *n* 神经管腔(脑室和脊髓管腔的统称)

neurocommunications [ˌnjuərəukəˌmjuːniˈkeiʃənz] *n* 神经通信学(神经学的分支,研究神经系统内信息的传递与整合)

neurocranium [ˌnjuərəuˈkreinjəm] *n* 脑颅 | **neurocranial** *a*

neurocrine [ˈnjuərəkrain] *a* 神经内分泌的;神经性分泌的 *n* 神经分泌[作用]

neurocrinia [ˌnjuərəuˈkriniə] *n* 神经性分泌作用

neurocristopathy [ˌnjuərəukrisˈtɔpəθi] *n* 神经嵴病

neurocutaneous [ˌnjuərəukju(ː)ˈteinjəs] *a* 神经[与]皮肤的;皮神经的

neurocysticercosis [ˌnjuərəuˌsistisəˈkəusis] *n* 神经型囊尾蚴病(中枢神经系统感染猪肉绦虫的蚴型〈囊尾蚴〉,临床表现十分多变,取决于囊虫的位置和数目,其中包括癫痫发作,脑积水以及许多其他神经功能障碍,常伴有特征性的损害,用计算机体摄影及磁共振成像可见之)

neurocyte [ˈnjuərəsait] *n* 神经细胞

neurocytology [ˌnjuərəusaiˈtɔlədʒi] *n* 神经细胞学

neurocytolysin [ˌnjuərəusaiˈtɔlisin] *n* 溶神经细胞素

neurocytoma [ˌnjuərəuˈsaitəumə] *n* 神经细胞瘤,神经上皮瘤

neurodealgia [ˌnjuərəudiˈældʒiə] *n* 视网膜痛

neurodeatrophia [ˌnjuərəudiəˈtrəufiə] *n* 视网膜萎缩

neurodegenerative [ˌnjuərəudiˈdʒenərətiv] *a* 神经变性的

neurodendrite [ˌnjuərəuˈdendrait], **neurodendron** [ˌnjuərəuˈdendrɔn] *n* 树突

neuroderm [ˈnjuərədəːm] *n* 神经外胚层

neurodermatitis [ˌnjuərəuˌdəːməˈtaitis] *n* 神经性皮炎 | exudative ~, nummular ~ 渗出性神经性皮炎,钱币状神经性皮炎,钱币状湿疹

neurodevelopmental [ˌnjuərəu diˌvelɔpˈmentəl] *a* 神经发育的

neurodiagnosis [ˌnjuərəuˌdaiəgˈnəusis] *n* 神经病诊断

neurodin [njuəˈrəudin] *n* 纽罗丁,镇神定,乙酰基对羟基苯乌拉坦(止神经痛及解热药)

neurodynamic [ˌnjuərəudaiˈnæmik] *a* 神经动力的,神经能的

neurodynia [ˌnjuərəuˈdiniə] *n* 神经痛

neuroectoderm [ˌnjuərəuˈektədəːm] *n* 神经外胚层 | **~al** [ˌnjuərəuˌektəuˈdəːməl] *a*

neuroeffector [ˌnjuərəuiˈfektə] *a* 神经效应器的(指连接点)

neuroelectricity [ˌnjuərəuilekˈtrisəti] *n* 神经电

neuroelectrotherapeutics [ˌnjuərəuˌilektrəuˌθerəˈpjuːtiks] *n* 神经病电疗法

neuroencephalomyelopathy [ˌnjuərəuenˌsefələuˌmaiəˈlɔpəθi] *n* 神经脑脊髓病

neuroendocrine [ˌnjuərəuˈendəukrin] *a* 神经内分泌的

neuroendocrinology [ˌnjuərəuˌendəukriˈnɔlədʒi] *n* 神经内分泌学

neuroendoscope [ˌnjuərəuˈendəˌskəup] *n* 神经内镜

neuroendoscopy [ˌnjuərəu enˈdɔskəpi] *n* 神经内镜检查术

neuroenteric [ˌnjuərəuenˈterik] *a* 神经管[与]原肠的

neuroepidermal [ˌnjuərəuˌepiˈdəːməl] *a* 神经表皮的

neuroepithelioma [ˌnjuərəuˌepiˌθiːliˈəumə] *n* 神经上皮瘤

neuroepithelium [ˌnjuərəuˌepiˈθiːljəm] *n* 神经上皮 | **neuroepithelial** *a*

neurofiber [ˌnjuərəuˈfaibə] *n* 神经纤维 | afferent ~s 传入[神经]纤维 / association ~s 联络[神经]纤维 / commissural ~s 连合[神经]纤维 / efferent ~s 传出[神经]纤维 / postganglionic ~s

节后[神经]纤维 / preganglionic ~s 节前[神经]纤维 / projection ~s 投射[神经]纤维 / somatic ~s 躯体[神经]纤维 / tangential ~s 切线[神经]纤维 / viseral ~s 内脏[神经]纤维

neurofibra [ˌnjuərəuˈfaibrə] ([复] **neurofibrae** [ˌnjuərəuˈfaibriː]) *n*【拉】神经纤维 | ~e afferentes 传入[神经]纤维 / ~e associationes 联络[神经]纤维 / ~e commissurales 连合[神经]纤维 / ~e efferentes 传出[神经]纤维 / ~e postganglionares 节后[神经]纤维 / ~e preganglionares 节前[神经]纤维 / ~e projectiones 投射[神经]纤维 / ~e somaticae 躯体[神经]纤维 / ~e tangentiales 切线[神经]纤维 / ~e viscerales 内脏[神经]纤维

neurofibril [ˌnjuərəuˈfaibril] *n* 神经原纤维 | **~lar** [ˌnjuərəufaiˈbrilə] *a*

neurofibrilla [ˌnjuərəufaiˈbrilə] ([复] **neurofibrillae** [ˌnjuərəufaiˈbriliː]) *n*【拉】神经原纤维

neurofibroma [ˌnjuərəufaiˈbrəumə] *n* 神经纤维瘤

neurofibromatosis [ˌnjuərəuˌfaibrəuməˈtəusis] *n* 神经纤维瘤病,多发性神经纤维瘤

neurofibromin [ˌnjuərəuˈfaɪbrəumin] *n* 神经纤维瘤蛋白

neurofibrosarcoma [ˌnjuərəuˌfaibrəu saːˈkəumə] *n* 神经纤维肉瘤

neurofilament [ˌnjuərəuˈfiləmənt] *n* 神经微丝

neurofixation [ˌnjuərəufikˈseiʃən] *n* 神经固定

neurogangliitis [ˌnjuərəuˌgæŋgliˈaitis] *n* 神经节炎

neuroganglion [ˌnjuərəuˈgæŋgliən] *n* 神经节

neurogastric [ˌnjuərəuˈgæstrik] *a* 胃神经的

neurogen [ˈnjuərədʒin] *n* 介质,传递质;神经原质

neurogenesis [ˌnjuərəuˈdʒenisis] *n* 神经发生 | **neurogenetic** [ˌnjuərəudʒiˈnetik] *a*

neurogenetics [ˌnjuərəudʒiˈnetiks] *n* 神经遗传学(研究对神经系统的遗传影响,其中包括神经系统的胚胎发育以及有遗传碱基的神经障碍)

neurogenic [ˌnjuərəuˈdʒenik] *a* 发生神经的;神经原[性]的 | **~ally** *ad*

neurogenous [njuəˈrɔdʒinəs] *a* 神经原[性]的

neuroglia [njuəˈrɔgliə] *n* 神经胶质 | interfascicular ~ 束间神经胶质 | **~l** [njuəˈrɔgliəl], **~r** [njuəˈrɔgliə] *a*

neurogliocyte [njuəˈrɔgliəˌsait] *n* 神经胶质细胞

neurogliocytoma [njuəˌrɔgliəusaiˈtəumə] *n* 神经胶质细胞瘤

neuroglioma [ˌnjuərəuglaiˈəumə] *n* 神经胶质瘤

neurogliosis [njuəˌrɔgliˈəusis], **neurogliomatosis** [ˌnjuərəuˌglaiəuməˈtəusis] *n* 神经胶质瘤病

neuroglycopenia [ˌnjuərəuˌglaikəuˈpiːniə] *n* 神经低血糖症

neurogram [ˈnjuərəgræm] *n* 神经印迹

neurography [njuəˈrɔgrəfi] *n* 神经论,神经学

neurohistology [ˌnjuərəuhisˈtɔlədʒi] *n* 神经组织学

neurohormone [ˌnjuərəuˈhɔːməun] *n* 神经激素 | **neurohormonal** *a*

neurohumor [ˌnjuərəuˈhjuːmə] *n* 神经元介质,神经体液(神经元内形成的一种化学物质,能激活或改变邻近神经元、肌肉或腺体的功能) | **~al** *a*

neurohumoralism [ˌnjuərəuˈhjuːmərəlizəm] *n* 神经元介质说(自主神经对末梢器官的作用是由已激活的神经末端释放化学物质的介质〈即neurohumor〉所致的)

neurohypnology [ˌnjuərəuhipˈnɔlədʒi] *n* 催眠学 | **neurohypnologist** *n* 催眠学家

neurohypophysectomy [ˌnjuərəuˌhaipəufiˈzektəmi] *n* 垂体神经部切除术,垂体后叶切除术

neurohypophysis [ˌnjuərəuhaiˈpɔfisis] *n* 神经垂体,垂体神经部,脑下垂体后叶 | **neurohypophyseal**, **neurohypophysial** [ˌnjuərəuˌhaipəuˈfiziəl] *a*

neuroid [ˈnjuərɔid] *a* 神经样的

neuroimaging [ˈnjuərəu ˌimədʒiŋ] *n* 神经成像

neuroimmunology [ˌnjuərəuˌimjuˈnɔlədʒi] *n* 神经免疫学 | **neuroimmunologic** [ˌnjuərəuˌimjunəˈlɔdʒik] *a*

neuroinduction [ˌnjuərəuinˈdʌkʃən] *n* 神经感应,精神暗示

neuroinflammation [ˌnjuərəuˌinfləˈmeiʃən] *n* 神经炎症

neuroinidia [ˌnjuərəuiˈnidiə] *n* 神经细胞营养不良

neurokeratin [ˌnjuərəuˈkerətin] *n* 神经角蛋白

neurokinet [ˌnjuərəuˈkinet] *n* 神经叩击器

neurokinin [ˌnjuərəuˈkainin] *n* 神经激肽

neurokyme [ˌnjuərəkaim] *n* 神经能

neurolabyrinthitis [ˌnjuərəuˌlæbirinˈθaitis] *n* 神经迷路炎

neurolathyrism [ˌnjuərəuˈlæθirizəm] *n* 山黧豆中毒

neurolemma [ˌnjuərəuˈlemə] *n* 神经鞘,神经膜

neurolemmitis [ˌnjuərəuleˈmaitis] *n* 神经鞘炎

neurolemmoma [ˌnjuərəuleˈməumə] *n* 神经鞘瘤

neuroleptanalgesia [ˌnjuərəuˌleptænælˈdʒiːziə] *n* 神经安定镇痛术 | **neuroleptanalgesic** *a* 神经安定镇痛的 *n* 神经安定镇痛药

neuroleptanesthesia [ˌnjuərəuˌleptænisˈθiːziə] *n* 安定麻醉[法] | **neuroleptanesthetic** [ˌnjuərəuˌleptænisˈθetik] *a* 安定麻醉的 *n* 安定麻醉剂

neuroleptic [ˌnjuərəuˈleptik] *a* 抑制精神的,神经

安定的 *n* 精神安定药

neurolinguistics [ˌnjuərəuliŋˈgwistiks] *n* 神经语言学

neurolipomatosis [ˌnjuərəuliˌpəuməˈtəusis] *n* 神经脂瘤病 | ~ dolorosa 痛性肥胖症

neurology [njuəˈrɔlədʒi] *n* 神经病学 | **neurologic(al)** [ˌnjuərəˈlɔdʒik(əl)] *a* / **neurologist** *n* 神经病学家 / **neurologia** [ˌnjuərəuˈləudʒiə] *n*

neurolues [ˌnjuərəuˈljuːiːz] *n* 神经梅毒

neurolymphomatosis [ˌnjuərəuˌlimfəuməˈtəusis] *n* 神经淋巴瘤病

neurolysin [njuəˈrɔlisin] *n* 溶神经素

neurolysis [njuəˈrɔlisis] *n* 神经松解术;神经疲惫;神经组织崩解 | **neurolytic** [ˌnjuərəuˈlitik] *a* 松解神经的;破坏神经的;神经疲惫的

neuroma [njuəˈrəumə] ([复] **neuromas** 或 **neuromata** [njuəˈrəumətə]) *n* 神经瘤 | fascicular ~, medullated ~ 有髓[鞘]神经瘤 / ganglionar ~, ganglionated ~, ganglionic ~ 神经[节]细胞性神经瘤 / multiple ~ 多发性神经瘤,神经瘤病 / myelinic ~ 有髓[鞘]神经瘤 / plexiform ~ 丛状神经瘤 / ~ telangiectodes, nevoid ~ 毛细血管扩张性神经瘤,痣样神经瘤 | **~tous** [njuəˈrɔmətəs] *a*

neuromalacia [ˌnjuərəuməˈleiʃiə], **neuromalakia** [ˌnjuərəuməˈleikiə] *n* 神经软化

neuromatosis [ˌnjuərəuməˈtəusis] *n* 神经瘤病

neuromechanism [ˌnjuərəuˈmekənizəm] *n* 神经结构

neuromediator [ˌnjuərəuˈmiːdieitə] *n* 神经介质

neuromeningeal [ˌnjuərəumiˈnindʒiəl] *a* 神经脑[脊]膜的

neuromere [ˈnjuərəmiə] *n* 菱脑节;神经管节

neurometrics [ˌnjuərəuˈmetriks] *n* 神经测量法(一种计算机辅助的测定脑功能的方法,即通过对诸如脑电图这样一些试验的结果进行定量分析,或通过对诱发电位进行测定)

neuromimesis [ˌnjuərəumaiˈmiːsis] *n* 模仿病 | **neuromimetic** [ˌnjuərəumaiˈmetik] *a* 模仿病的;模仿神经冲动的 *n* 神经冲动模仿物

neuromittor [ˌnjuərəuˈmitə] *n* 神经传导器,神经元接头

neuromodulation [ˌnjuərəuˌmɔdjuˈleiʃən] *n* 神经调制

neuromodulator [ˌnjuərəuˈmɔdjuleitə] *n* 神经调质(除神经递质以外的一种物质,由某一神经元释放并将信息传递给邻近的或远处的神经元,增强或阻遏它们的活动。神经肽常常是神经调质)

neuromotor [ˌnjuərəuˈməutə] *a* 神经[肌]运动的

neuromuscular [ˌnjuərəuˈmʌskjulə], **neuromyal** [ˌnjuərəuˈmaiəl], **neuromyic** [ˌnjuərəuˈmaiik] *a* 神经肌肉的

neuromyasthenia [ˌnjuərəuˌmaiæsˈθiːniə] *n* 神经肌无力 | epidemic ~ 流行性神经肌无力(亦称良性肌痛性脑脊髓炎和冰岛病)

neuromyelitis [ˌnjuərəuˌmaiəˈlaitis] *n* 神经脊髓炎

neuromyopathy [ˌnjuərəumaiˈɔpəθi] *n* 神经肌病 | carcinomatous ~ 癌性神经肌病 | **neuromyopathic** [ˌnjuərəuˌmaiəuˈpæθik] *a*

neuromyositis [ˌnjuərəuˌmaiəuˈsaitis] *n* 神经肌炎

neuromyotonia [ˌnjuərəuˌmaiəuˈtəuniə] *n* 神经性肌强直

neuron [ˈnjuərɔn] *n* 神经元 | central ~ 中枢神经元 / intercalary ~, internuncial ~ 中间神经元 / long ~ 轴索 / projection ~ 投射神经元(传递神经元) / pyramidal ~ 锥体细胞 / short ~ 短轴索 | **~e** [ˈnjuərəun] *n* / **~al** [ˈnjuərənəl], **~ic** [njuəˈrɔnik] *a*

neuronagenesis [ˌnjuərəunəˈdʒenisis] *n* 神经元发育不全

neuronatrophy [ˌnjuərɔˈnætrəfi] *n* 神经元萎缩,神经元硬化病

neuronephric [ˌnjuərəuˈnefrik] *a* 肾[与]神经系统的

neuronevus [ˌnjuərəuˈniːvəs] *n* 神经痣

neuronin [ˈnjuərənin] *n* 轴索蛋白

neuronitis [ˌnjuərəuˈnaitis] *n* 神经元炎

neuronopathy [ˌnjuərəuˈnɔpəθi] *n* 神经元病

neuronophage [njuəˈrɔnəfeidʒ] *n* 噬神经细胞

neuronophagia [ˌnjuərɔnəuˈfeidʒiə], **neuronophagy** [ˌnjuərɔˈnɔfədʒi] *n* 噬神经细胞作用

neuronosis [ˌnjuərəuˈnəusis] *n* 神经病

neuronotropic [njuəˌrɔnəuˈtrɔpik] *a* 亲神经元的,向神经元的

neuronymy [njuəˈrɔnimi] *n* 神经命名法

neurooncology [ˌnjuərəuɔnˈkɔlədʒi] *n* 神经肿瘤学

neuro-ophthalmology [ˌnjuərəu ˌɔfθælˈmɔlədʒi] *n* 神经眼科学,眼神经学

neuro-otology [ˌnjuərəuəuˈtɔlədʒi] *n* 神经耳科学,耳神经学

neuropacemaker [ˌnjuərəuˈpeismeikə] *n* 神经起搏器(减轻由于神经损伤所致的疼痛的一种植入装置)

neuropapillitis [ˌnjuərəuˌpæpiˈlaitis] *n* 视神经乳头炎,视神经炎

neuroparalysis [ˌnjuərəupəˈrælisis] *n* 神经性麻痹 | **neuroparalytic** [ˌnjuərəuˌpærəˈlitik] *a*

neuropath [ˈnjuərəpæθ] *n* 神经病患者

neuropathogenesis [ˌnjuərəuˌpæθəˈdʒenisis] *n*

神经病发病机制，神经病发生
neuropathogenicity [ˌnjuərəuˈpæθəudʒiˈnisiti] *n* 致神经病性，神经发病性
neuropathology [ˌnjuərəupəˈθɔlədʒi] *n* 神经病理学 | **neuropathologist** *n* 神经病理学家
neuropathy [njuəˈrɔpəθi] *n* 神经病 | progressive hypertrophic interstitial ~ 进行性肥大性间质性神经病，肥大性间质性神经炎 / serum ~ 血清神经病（注射异种蛋白后 2 ~ 8 天引起颈神经或臂丛的神经异常）| **neuropathic** [ˌnjuərəˈpæθik] *a*
neuropeptide [ˌnjuərəuˈpeptaid] *n* 神经肽
neurophage [ˈnjuərəfeidʒ] *n* 噬神经细胞
neuropharmacology [ˌnjuərəuˌfɑːməˈkɔlədʒi] *n* 神经药理学 | **neuropharmacological** [ˌnjuərəufɑːməkəˈlɔdʒikəl] *a*
neurophilic [ˌnjuərəuˈfilik] *a* 亲神经的，向神经的
neurophonia [ˌnjuərəuˈfəuniə] *n* 神经性叫喊（有时类似某些动物的叫声）
neurophthalmology [ˌnjuərɔfθælˈmɔlədʒi] *n* 神经眼科学
neurophthisis [ˌnjuəˈrɔfθisis] *n* 神经组织消耗
neurophysin [ˌnjuərəuˈfaisin] *n* 后叶激素运载蛋白，神经垂体素运载蛋白
neurophysiology [ˌnjuərəuˌfiziˈɔlədʒi] *n* 神经生理学
neuropil [ˈnjuərəpil], **neuropile** [ˈnjuərəpail], **neuropilem** [njuərəuˈpailəm] *n* 神经毡，神经纤维网
neuroplasm [ˈnjuərəuplæzəm] *n* 神经胞质，神经浆 | **~ic** [ˌnjuərəuˈplæzmik] *a*
neuroplasty [ˈnjuərəˌplæsti] *n* 神经成形术
neuroplexus [ˌnjuərəuˈpleksəs] *n* 神经丛
neuropodium [ˌnjuərəuˈpəudiəm]（[复] **neuropodia** [ˌnjuərəuˈpəudiə]），**neuropodion** [ˌnjuərəuˈpəudiɔn] *n* 神经终丝
neuropore [ˈnjuərəpɔː] *n* 神经孔（胚胎）
neuropotential [ˌnjuərəupəuˈtenʃəl] *n* 神经电位，神经能
neuroprobasia [ˌnjuərəuprəˈbeiziə] *n* 沿神经蔓延（指病毒活动）
neuroprotectant [ˌnjuərəuprəˈtektənt] *a* 神经保护的
neuropretection [ˌnjuərəuprəˈtekʃən] *n* 神经保护（保护神经中毒性）
neuroprotective [ˌnjuərəuprəˈtektiv] *a* 神经保护的
neuropsychiatry [ˌnjuərəusaiˈkaiətri] *n* 神经精神病学 | **neuropsychiatric** [ˌnjuərəuˌsaikiˈætrik] *a* | **neuropsychiatrist** *n* 神经精神病学家
neuropsychic [ˌnjuərəuˈsaikik] *a* 神经精神的
neuropsychology [ˌnjuərəusaiˈkɔlədʒi] *n* 神经心理学 | **neuropsychological** [ˌnjuərəusaikəˈlɔdʒikəl] *a*
neuropsychometric [ˌnjuərəuˌsaikəuˈmetrik] *a* 神经心理测量的
neuropsychopathy [ˌnjuərəusaiˈkɔpəθi] *n* 神经精神病
neuropsychopharmacology [ˌnjuərəuˌsaikəuˌfɑːməˈkɔlədʒi] *n* 神经精神药理学
neuroradiology [ˌnjuərəuˌreidiˈɔlədʒi] *n* 神经系放射学
neurorelapse [ˌnjuərəuriˈlæps], **neurorecidive** [ˌnjuərəuˌresiˈdiːv], **neurorecurrence** [ˌnjuərəuriˈkʌrəns] *n* 神经梅毒复发
neuroretinitis [ˌnjuərəuˌretiˈnaitis] *n* 视神经[视]网膜炎
neuroretinopathy [ˌnjuərəuˌretiˈnɔpəθi] *n* 视神经[视]网膜病
neuroroentgenography [ˌnjuərəuˌrɔntgəˈnɔgrəfi] *n* 神经系放射学
neurorrhaphy [njuəˈrɔrəfi] *n* 神经缝合术
Neurorrhyctes hydrophobiae [ˌnjuərəuˈriktiːz ˌhaidrəuˈfəubiiː] 狂犬病包涵体，内格里小体（见 Negri bodies）
neurosarcocleisis [ˌnjuərəuˌsɑːkəuˈklaisis] *n* 神经移入肌肉术（治神经痛）
neurosarcoma [ˌnjuərəusɑːˈkəumə] *n* 神经肉瘤
neuroschistosomiasis [ˌnjuərəuˌskistəusəuˈmaiəsis] *n* 神经血吸虫病（影响中枢神经系统的血吸虫病，常由日本血吸虫所致）
neuroscience [ˌnjuərəuˈsaiəns] *n* 神经科学
neuroscientist [ˌnjuərəuˈsaiəntist] *n* 神经科学家
neurosclerosis [ˌnjuərəuskliəˈrəusis] *n* 神经硬化
neurosecretion [ˌnjuərəusiˈkriːʃən] *n* 神经分泌[作用] | **neurosecretory** [ˌnjuərəusiˈkriːtəri] *a*
neurosegmental [ˌnjuərəusegˈmentl] *a* 神经节段的
neurosensory [ˌnjuərəuˈsensəri] *a* 感觉神经的，感音神经性的
neurosis [njuəˈrəusis]（[复] **neuroses** [njuəˈrəusiːz]）*n* 神经症 | accident ~ [意外]事故性神经症 / anxiety ~ 焦虑性神经症 / cardiac ~ 心脏神经功能病，神经性循环衰弱 / combat ~ 战争神经症 / expectation ~ 期待性焦虑症 / obsessional ~ 强迫性神经症 / occupation ~，craft ~，professional ~ 职业性神经症 / vegetative ~ 自主性神经症，肢痛症，红皮水肿性多神经病
neuroskeletal [ˌnjuərəuˈskelitl] *a* 神经[与]骨骼肌的

neuroskeleton [ˌnjuərəuˈskelitn] *n* 内骨骼
neurosome [ˈnjuərəsəum] *n* 神经细胞[胞]体;神经微粒
neurospasm [ˈnjuərəspæzəm] *n* 神经性痉挛
neurosplanchnic [ˌnjuərəuˈsplæŋknik] *a* 脑脊髓[与]交感神经系统的
neurospongioma [ˌnjuərəuˌspɔndʒiˈəumə] *n* 神经胶质瘤
neurospongium [ˌnjuərəuˈspɔndʒiəm] *n* 神经海绵质,神经胶质;神经纤维网
Neurospora [njuəˈrɔspərə] *n* 链孢霉属
neurostatus [ˌnjuərəuˈsteitəs] *n* 神经系统状态(记录病史时)
neurosteroid [ˌnjuərəuˈsterɔid] *n* 神经类固醇(脑内产生的类固醇)
neurosthenia [ˌnjuərəuˈsθiːniə] *n* 神经能过旺
neurosurgeon [ˌnjuərəuˈsəːdʒən] *n* 神经外科医师
neurosurgery [ˌnjuərəuˈsəːdʒəri] *n* 神经外科[学]
neurosurgical [ˌnjuərəuˈsəːdʒikəl] *a* 神经外科的
neurosuture [ˌnjuərəuˈsjuːtʃə] *n* 神经缝合术
neurosyphilis [ˌnjuərəuˈsifilis] *n* 神经梅毒 | ectodermogenic ~ 外胚层性神经梅毒 / meningeal ~ 脑膜神经梅毒 / meningovascular ~ 脑膜血管性神经梅毒 / mesodermogenic ~ 中胚层性神经梅毒 / paretic ~ 麻痹性神经梅毒,麻痹性痴呆 / tabetic ~ 脊髓痨性神经梅毒,脊髓痨
neurotagma [ˌnjuərəuˈtægmə] *n* 神经细胞[线状]排列
neurotendinous [ˌnjuərəuˈtendinəs] *a* 神经[与]腱的
neurotensin [ˌnjuərəuˈtensin] *n* 神经降压肽(一种十三肽,最初从牛丘脑提出,可引起血管扩张和低血压)
neuroterminal [ˌnjuərəuˈtəːminəl] *n* 神经终器
neurothele [ˌnjuərəuˈθiːli] *n* 神经乳头(真皮)
neurotic [njuəˈrɔtik] *a* 神经功能病的,神经[官能]症的;神经过敏的,神经质的 *n* 神经过敏者,神经质者 | **~ism** [njuəˈrɔtisizəm] *n* 神经过敏症
neurotigenic [njuəˌrɔtiˈdʒenik] *a* 致神经功能病的,致神经[官能]症的
neurotization [ˌnjuərɔtiˈzeiʃən] *n* 神经再生;神经植入术
neurotmesis [ˌnjuərɔtˈmiːsis] *n* 神经断伤
neurotology [ˌnjuərəuˈtɔlədʒi] *n* 神经耳科学,耳神经学
neurotome [ˈnjuərətəum] *n* 神经刀;菱脑节
neurotomography [ˌnjuərəutəˈmɔgrəfi] *n* 神经[X线]体层摄影[术]
neurotomy [njuəˈrɔtəmi] *n* 神经切断术;神经解剖 | radiofrequency ~ 射频神经切断术 / retrogasserian ~ 半月神经节后根切断术
neurotonia [ˌnjuərəuˈtəuniə] *n* 神经张力不稳定;神经牵伸术
neurotonic [ˌnjuərəuˈtɔnik] *a* 对神经有牵伸作用的;使神经强壮的 *n* 神经强壮剂
neurotonometer [ˌnjuərəutəuˈnɔmitə] *n* 皮肤紧张度计
neurotony [njuəˈrɔtəni] *n* 神经牵伸术
neurotoxia [ˌnjuərəuˈtɔksiə] *n* 神经中毒症(把神经衰弱看作一种中毒)
neurotoxic [ˌnjuərəuˈtɔksik] *a* 神经中毒的,毒害神经的 | **~ity** [ˌnjuərəutɔkˈsisəti] *n* 神经中毒性
neurotoxin [ˌnjuərəuˈtɔksin] *n* 神经毒素
neurotransducer [ˌnjuərəutrænsˈdjuːsə] *n* 神经传导器(合成和释放激素的一种神经元,起到神经系统和垂体之间功能性连接的作用)
neurotransmission [ˌnjuərəutrænsˈmiʃən] *n* 神经传递
neurotransmitter [ˌnjuərəutransˈmitə] *n* 神经递质
neurotrauma [ˌnjuərəuˈtrɔːmə] *n* 神经外伤
neurotrophasthenia [ˌnjuərəuˌtrəufæsˈθiːniə] *n* 神经营养不足
neurotrophin [ˈnjuərəuˌtrəufin] *n* 神经营养蛋白
neutrophil elastase [ˈnjuːtrəfiliˈlæsteis] 嗜中性细胞弹性蛋白酶,白细胞弹性蛋白酶
neurotrophy [njuəˈrɔtrəfi] *n* 神经营养 | **neurotrophic** [ˌnjuərəuˈtrɔfik] *a* **neurotropic** [ˌnjuərəuˈtrɔpik] *a* 向神经的,亲神经的
neurotropism [njuəˈrɔtrəpizəm], **neurotropy** [njuəˈrɔtrəpi] *n* 向神经性,亲神经性;神经趋向性
neurotrosis [ˌnjuərəuˈtrəusis] *n* 神经外伤
neurotubule [ˌnjuərəuˈtjuːbjul] *n* 神经微管,神经小管
neurovaccine [ˌnjuərəuˈvæksin], **neurovariola** [ˌnjuərəuvəˈraiələ] *n* 兔脑疫苗,兔脑痘苗(在家兔脑内生长的病毒制备的疫苗)
neurovaricosis [ˌnjuərəuˌværiˈkəusis] *n* 神经纤维曲张
neurovascular [ˌnjuərəuˈvæskjulə] *a* 神经血管的
neurovegetative [ˌnjuərəuˈvedʒitətiv] *a* 自主性神经系统的
neurovirulence [ˌnjuərəuˈvirjuləns] *n* 神经毒力(指病原体毒害神经的能力)
neurovirulent [ˌnjuərəuˈvirjulənt] *a* 神经毒力的
neurovirus [ˌnjuərəuˈvaiərəs] *n* 神经病毒(经神经组织传代而改变的一种疫苗病毒)
neurovisceral [ˌnjuərəuˈvisərəl] *a* 脑脊髓[与]交

感神经系统的

neurula [ˈnjuərulə] *n* 神经胚

neurulation [ˌnjuəruˈleiʃən] *n* 神经胚形成

neururgic [njuəˈrəːdʒik] *a* 神经活动的,神经作用的

neurypnology [ˌnjuəripˈnɔlədʒi] *n* 催眠学

Neursser's granules [ˈnɔisə] (Edmund von Neusser) 诺伊瑟粒(白细胞核周的嗜碱性小粒)

neuter [ˈnjuːtə] *a* 无性的;无性生殖的

neutral [ˈnjuːtrəl] *a* 中立的;中性的;无作用的

neutralism [ˈnjuːtrəlizəm] *n* 中立;种间共处(两种不同种而共存的生物之间无相互作用)

neutrality [nju(ː)ˈtræləti] *n* 中性,中和性;无作用[性]

neutralization [ˌnjuːtrəlaiˈzeiʃən, -liˈz-] *n* 中和作用,中和反应 | viral ~ 病毒中和[作用](抗体或抗体加补体使病毒失去感染力的作用)

neutramycin [ˌnjuːtrəˈmaisin] *n* 中性霉素(获自龟裂链霉菌的一种抗菌物质)

neutretto [njuːˈtretəu] *n* 中介子

neutrino [njuːˈtriːnəu] *n* 中微子

neutroclusion [ˌnjuːtrəˈkluːʒən] *n* 中性𬌗,中性咬合

neutrocyte [ˈnjuːtrəsait] *n* 中性粒细胞,中性白细胞

neutrocytopenia [ˌnjuːtrəuˌsaitəuˈpiːniə] *n* 中性白细胞减少[症],中性粒细胞减少[症]

neutrocytophilia [ˌnjuːtrəuˌsaitəuˈfiliə], **neutrocytosis** [ˌnjuːtrəusaiˈtəusis] *n* 中性白细胞增多[症],中性粒细胞增多[症]

neutroflavine [ˌnjuːtrəuˈfleivin] *n* 吖啶黄

neutron [ˈnjuːtrɔn] *n* 中子 | epithermal ~ 超热能中子 / fast ~ 快中子 / intermediate ~ 中能中子 / slow ~ 慢中子;热[能]中子 / thermal ~ 热(能)中子

neutropenia [ˌnjuːtrəuˈpiːniə] *n* 中性粒细胞减少[症],中性白细胞减少[症] | chronic benign ~ of childhood 儿童慢性良性中性粒细胞减少症 / chronic hypoplastic ~ 慢性再生不良性中性粒细胞减少症 / congenital ~ 先天性中性粒细胞减少症(亦称先天性白细胞缺乏症,先天性白细胞减少) / familial benign chronic ~ 家族性良性慢性中性粒细胞减少症 / idiopathic ~, malignant ~ 恶性中性粒细胞减少,粒细胞缺乏症 / primary splenic ~, hypersplenic ~ 原发性脾性中性粒细胞减少 / transitory neonatal ~ 新生儿一过性中性粒细胞减少症(可能为同种免疫型)

neutrophil [ˈnjuːtrəfil] *n* 中性粒细胞 *a* 嗜中性的 | filamented ~ 连丝核中性粒细胞 / giant ~ 大多核白细胞 / juvenile ~ 晚幼粒细胞 / nonfilamented ~ 无连丝核中性粒细胞 / rod ~, stab ~ 杆状核中性粒细胞,带状核粒细胞

neutrophilia [ˌnjuːtrəuˈfiliə] *n* 中性细胞增多[症],中性粒细胞增多[症]

neutrophilic [ˌnjuːtrəuˈfilik] *a* 嗜中性的(可用中性染剂着色的);非嗜血性的(指蚊)

neutrophilopenia [ˌnjuːtrəuˌfiləuˈpiːniə] *n* 中性粒细胞减少[症],中性白细胞减少[症]

neutropism [ˈnjuːtrəpizəm] *n* 向神经性,亲神经性

neutrotaxis [ˌnjuːtrəuˈtæksis] *n* 中性粒细胞趋向性,中性白细胞趋向性

nevi [ˈniːvai] nevus 的复数

nevirapine [nəˈvirəpiːn] *n* 奈韦拉平(人免疫缺陷病毒-1〈HIV-1〉反转录酶非核苷抑制剂,与其他抗反转录病毒结合使用,治疗 HIV-1 感染,口服给药)

nev(o)- [构词成分]痣,胎痣

nevoblast [ˈniːvəublæst] *n* 成痣细胞

nevocarcinoma [ˌniːvəuˌkɑːsiˈnəumə] *n* 痣癌,黑色素癌

nevocyte [ˈniːvəusait] *n* 痣细胞 | **nevocytic** [niːvəuˈsitik] *a*

nevoid [ˈniːvɔid] *a* 痣样的

nevolipoma [ˌniːvəuliˈpəumə] *n* 痣脂瘤,脂瘤痣

nevoxanthoendothelioma [ˌniːvəuˌzænθəuˌendəuˌθiːliˈəumə] *n* 痣黄色内皮瘤

Nevskia [ˈnevskiə] *n* 涅瓦河菌属(涅瓦河〈Neva〉为俄罗斯河名)

nevus [ˈniːvəs] ([复] **nevi** [ˈniːvai]) *n*【拉】痣 | bathing trunk ~ 游泳裤式痣 / blue rubber bleb ~ 蓝色橡皮疱样痣 / chromatophore ~ of Naegeli 内格利色素细胞痣(见 Franceschetti-Jadassohn syndrome) / dysplastic ~ 发育不良性痣 / giant congenital pigmented ~, giant hairy ~, giant pigmented ~ 巨大先天性色素痣,巨大色痣,巨大色素痣 / halo ~ 晕痣 / hepatic ~ 肝斑痣,肝出血性梗死 / ~ of Ito, ~ fuscoceruleus acromiodeltoideus 伊藤痣,肩峰三角肌褐青色痣 / junction ~, junctional ~ 交界痣 / ~ of Ota, Ota's ~, ~ fuscoceruleus ophthalmomaxillaris 太田痣,眼上颌部褐青色痣 / spider ~, stellar ~ 蜘蛛痣,蛛状痣 / strawberry ~ 草莓状痣,海绵状血管瘤 / verrucoid ~ 疣状痣

newborn [ˈnjuːbɔːn] *a* 新生的 *n* 新生儿

Newcastle disease [ˈnjuːkɑːsl] 纽卡斯尔病,新城疫(鸡的病毒性肺炎及脑脊髓炎,此疫病可传至人类。Newcastle 为英国港市名)

newt [njuːt] *n* 水螈

newton [ˈnjuːtn] *n* 牛[顿](力的单位,符号为 N)

Newton's law [ˈnjuːtn] (Isaac Newton) 牛顿定律,万有引力定律 | ~ rings 牛顿环、牛顿圈(由于光波作用,透明薄膜〈如肥皂泡〉表面上所见的彩色环)

nexeridine hydrochloride [nekˈseridiːn] 盐酸奈西利定(镇痛药)

nexin [ˈneksin] *n* 连接素(连接纤毛和鞭毛内外层成对的微管)

nexus [ˈneksəs] [单复同] *n* 结合,接合;结合膜,融合膜(缝隙连接)

Nezelof's syndrome [ˈnezilɔf] (C. Nezelof) 纳泽洛夫综合征(一组异质的免疫缺陷病,表现为细胞免疫力极度缺乏,体液免疫缺乏则程度不一。免疫球蛋白水平可能正常或增加,但抗体对免疫的反应可能缺乏。患者对低度或机会致病菌如白念珠菌、卡氏肺囊虫和巨细胞病毒的感染高度敏感。常染色体隐性遗传和 X 连锁遗传均有报道。亦称伴免疫球蛋白的细胞免疫缺陷)

NF National Formulary 国家处方集

NF1 neurofibromatosis 1 神经纤维瘤病 1

NF2 neurofibromatosis 2 神经纤维瘤病 2

NFLPN National Federation for Licensed Practical Nurses 全国有照护士联合会

ng nanogram 纳克(10^{-9}g)

n'gana [nəˈgɑːnə] *n* 非洲锥虫病

NGF nerve growth factor 神经生长因子

NHC National Health Council 全国卫生理事会

NHLBI National Heart, Lung, and Blood Institute 国立心肺和血液研究所

NHMRC National Health and Medical Research Council 全国卫生与医学研究委员会

NHS National Health Service 国家卫生局(英国)

NH_2-terminal 氨基末端(见 N-terminal)

Ni nickel 镍

NIA National Institute on Aging 国立衰老研究所

NIAAA National Institute on Alcohol Abuse and Alcoholism 全国酗酒和酒精中毒研究所

niacin [ˈnaiəsin] *n* 烟酸,尼克酸,抗糙皮病维生素,维生素 PP

niacinamide [ˌnaiəsiˈnæmaid] *n* 烟酰胺,尼克酰胺,抗糙皮病维生素

NIAID National Institute of Allergy and Infectious Diseases 国立变态反应与传染病研究所

nialamide [naiˈæləmaid] *n* 尼亚拉胺(抗抑郁药)

NIAMSD National Institute of Arthritis and Musculoskeletal and Skin Diseases 国立关节炎、肌骨骼病和皮肤病研究所

nib [nib] *n* 尖头,尖端(牙科充填器的工作部位)

nibroxane [naiˈbrɔksein] *n* 硝溴生(局部用抗微生物药)

nicabazin [naiˈkɑːbəzin] *n* 尼卡巴净(抗球虫药,用于家禽)

niccolum [ˈnikələm] *n*【拉】镍

nicergoline [naiˈsəːgəliːn] *n* 尼麦角林(血管扩张药)

niche [nitʃ] *n* 壁龛,龛,龛影(如 X 线片所见或肉眼所见器官上的凹陷);小境 | ecologic(al) ~ 生态小境(生物体在其群落或生态系统中所占的地位) / enamel ~ 釉隙

NICHHD National Institute of Child Health and Human Development 国立儿童健康与人类发展研究所

nick [nik] *n* 断口,缺口,切口

nickel [ˈnikl] *n* 镍 *vt* 把…镀镍 | ~ carbonyl 羰基镍(用于工业,可能产生严重肺水肿和呼吸困难)

nicking [ˈnikiŋ] *n* 血管局部缩窄,血管凹痕(动脉性高血压时视网膜血管局部收缩)

Nicklès' test [niːˈklei] (François J. J. Nicklès) 尼克累试验(鉴别蔗糖与葡萄糖)

niclosamide [niˈkləusəmaid] *n* 氯硝柳胺(抗蠕虫药)

Nicoladoni's sign [ˌnikələˈdəuni] (Carl Nicoladoni) 尼克拉唐尼征(见 Branham's sign)

Nicolas-Favre disease [nikɔˈlɑːˈfɑːvr] (Joseph Nicolas; M. Favre) 性病性淋巴肉芽肿

Nicollela [nikəˈlelə] (Charles J. H. Nicolle) *n* 尼科尔[原]虫属

Nicol prism [ˈnikɔl] (William Nicol) 尼科尔棱镜(两块冰洲石胶合在一起,把光线裂分为二,一部分〈普通光〉全部折射,另一部分〈极光〉则通过)

Nicotiana [ˌnikəʃiˈeinə] *n* 烟草属

nicotinamide [ˌnikəˈtinəmaid] *n* 烟酰胺,尼克酰胺 | ~ adenine dinucleotide (NAD) 烟酰胺腺嘌呤二核苷酸(以前亦称辅酶 I,二磷酸吡啶核苷酸) / ~ adenine dinucleotide phosphate (NADP) 烟酰胺腺嘌呤二核苷酸磷酸(以前亦称辅酶 Ⅱ,三磷酸吡啶核苷酸) / ~ mononucleotide (NMN) 烟酰胺单核苷酸

nicotinamidemia [ˌnikətiˌnæmiˈdiːmiə] *n* 烟酰胺血[症]

nicotinate [ˌnikəˈtineit] *n* 烟酸,尼克酸(解离型) | ~ ribonucleotide 烟酸核[糖核]苷酸

nicotine [ˈnikəti(ː)n] *n* 烟碱,尼古丁

nicotinic acid [ˌnikəˈtinik] 烟酸,尼克酸

nicotinism [ˈnikətinizəm] *n* 烟碱中毒

nicotinolytic [ˌnikətinəuˈlitik] *a* 解烟碱[毒]的

nicotinuric acid [ˌnikətiˈnjuərik] 烟酰甘氨酸,烟尿酸

β-nicotyrine [niˈkəutairin] *n* 烟碱烯,β-烟碱烯,二烯烟碱,尼可他因

nicoumalone [naiˈkuːmələun] *n* 新抗凝(即醋硝香豆素 acenocoumarin,抗凝药)

nictate [ˈnikteit], **nictitate** [ˈniktiteit] *vi* 瞬眼,眨眼 | **nictation** [nikˈteiʃən], **nictitation** [ˌniktiˈteiʃən] *n*

NIDA National Institute on Drug Abuse 国立药物滥用研究所

nidation [naiˈdeiʃən] *n* 着床(孕卵在子宫内)

NIDCR National Institute of Dental and Craniofacial Research 国立牙科和颅面研究所

NIDD non-insulin-dependent diabetes 非胰岛素依赖型糖尿病

NIDDK National Institute of Diabetes and Digestive and Kidney Diseases 国立糖尿病、消化系疾病和肾病研究所

NIDDM non-insulin-dependent diabetes mellitus 非胰岛素依赖型糖尿病

NIDR National Institute of Dental Research 国立牙科研究所

nidus [ˈnaidəs]([复]**niduses** 或 **nidi** [ˈnaidai]) *n*【拉】巢,核;病灶;发源地 | ~ avis, ~ hirundinis 小脑禽巢 | **nidal** [ˈnaidl] *a*

NIEHS National Institute of Environmental Health Sciences 国立环境卫生科学研究所

Nielsen method [ˈniːlsen](Holger Nielsen)尼尔森法(人工呼吸)

Niemann-Pick cells [ˈniːmənˈpik](Albert Niemann; Ludwig Pick)尼曼-皮克细胞(尼曼-皮克病患者骨髓和脾内所含圆形、卵圆形或多边形细胞)

Niemann's disease (splenomegaly), Niemann-Pick disease [ˈniːmənˈpik](Albert Niemann; Ludwig Pick)尼曼病(脾大)、尼曼-皮克病(一种遗传性疾病,其特征为肝脾肿大,皮肤呈棕黄色,神经系统受累及,肝、脾、肺、淋巴结、骨髓内有泡沫样网状细胞或组织细胞,此等细胞贮存磷脂,主要是卵磷脂和鞘髓磷脂。亦称类脂组织细胞增多症、鞘脂沉积病、鞘髓磷脂沉积病)

Niewenglowski's ray [njevenˈglɔvski](Gaston H. Niewenglowski)涅温格洛夫斯基线(物质受阳光照射后所发出的光线)

nifedipine [naiˈfedipiːn] *n* 硝苯地平(冠状动脉扩张药)

nifungin [naiˈfʌndʒin] *n* 尼芬净(抗生素类药)

nifuradene [naiˈfjuərədiːn] *n* 硝呋拉定(抗菌药)

nifuraldezone [ˌnaifjuəˈrældizəun] *n* 硝呋地腙(抗菌药)

nifuratel [naiˈfjuərətəl] *n* 硝呋太尔(抗菌、抗真菌、抗滴虫药)

nifuratrone [naiˈfjuərətrəun] *n* 硝呋隆(抗菌药)

nifurdazil [naiˈfjuədəzil] *n* 硝呋达齐(抗菌药)

nifurimide [naiˈfjuərimaid] *n* 硝呋米特(抗菌药)

nifurmerone [naiˈfjumərəun] *n* 硝呋美隆(抗真菌药)

nifuroxime [ˌnaifjuəˈrɔksim] *n* 硝呋醛肟(抗真菌药,抗原虫药)

nifurpirinol [ˌnaifjuˈpiərinɔl] *n* 硝呋吡醇(抗菌药)

nifurquinazol [ˌnaifjuˈkwinəzɔl] *n* 硝呋奎唑(抗菌药)

nifursemizone [ˌnaifjuˈsemizəun] *n* 硝呋米腙(抗原虫药,对组织滴虫属有效,用于家禽)

nifursol [ˈnaifjusɔl] *n* 硝呋索尔(抗原虫药,对组织滴虫属有效,用于家禽)

nifurtimox [naiˈfjutimɔks] *n* 硝呋替莫(抗锥虫药)

nightmare [ˈnaitmεə] *n* 梦魇

nightshade [ˈnaitʃeid] *n* 茄属植物 | deadly ~ 颠茄叶

NIGMS National Institute of General Medical Sciences 国立综合医学科学研究所

nigra [ˈnaigrə] *n*【拉】黑质 | **~l** *a*

nigrescent [naiˈgresnt] *a* 发黑的,转黑的 | **nigrescence** [naiˈgresns] *n*

nigricans [ˈnaigrikəns] *a*【拉】微黑的

nigrities [naiˈgriʃiiːz] *n*【拉】发黑,黑变 | ~ linguae 黑舌[病]

nigrosin [ˈnaigrəsin] *n* 苯胺黑

nigrostriatal [ˌnaigrəustraiˈeitəl] *a* 黑质纹状体的(指一束神经纤维)

NIH National Institutes of Health 国立卫生研究院

nihilism [ˈnaihilizəm] *n* 虚无妄想;虚无主义 | therapeutic ~ 治疗的虚无主义

nikethamide [niˈkeθəmaid] *n* 尼可刹米(中枢兴奋药)

Nikiforoff's method [ˌniːkiˈfɔrɔf](Mikhail Nikiforoff)尼基弗罗夫法(固定血片法,即将血片放入无水醇、纯乙醚或等量的醇和乙醚中 5 ~ 15 分钟)

Nikolsky's sign [niˈkɔlski](Petr V. Nikolsky)尼科尔斯基征(表皮层轻擦即容易剥离,见于寻常天疱疮)

nilutamide [naiˈljuːtəmaid] *n* 尼鲁米特(非甾体抗雄激素药,用作抗肿瘤药,结合一些降低睾酮水平措施,如双侧睾丸切除术,以治疗前列腺癌,口服给药)

nimazone [ˈniməzəun] *n* 尼马宗,腈胺唑酮(抗炎药)

Nimeh's method [ˈniːmi](William Nimeh)尼梅法(一种测肝脾体积的方法,分别在肝区和脾区拍出的平片上测定之)

NIMH National Institute of Mental Health 国立精神卫生研究所

nimidane [ˈnimidein] *n* 尼米旦(兽用杀螨药)

nimodipine [naiˈməudipiːn] *n* 尼莫地平(血管扩张药)

NINCDS National Institute of Neurological and Communicative Disorders and Stroke 国立神经障碍、语言交往障碍和卒中研究所

NINDS National Institute of Neurological Disorders and Stroke 国立神经障碍和卒中研究所

NINR National Institute for Nursing Research 国立护理研究所

niobium(Nb) [naiˈəubiəm] *n* 铌(化学元素)

NIOSH National Institute of Occupational Safety and Health 国立职业安全与卫生研究所
nip [nip] (-pp-) *vt*, *vi*, *n* 夹,钳,捏,咬
Nipah virus [ˈniːpə] (Nipah 为马来西亚吉隆坡附近一村名,该病毒首次在此分离)尼伯病毒(一种副黏病毒,为尼伯脑炎的病原体)
niperyt [ˈnaipərit] *n* 戊四硝酯,硝酸戊四醇酯(即 pentaerythritol tetranitrate,口服抗心绞痛药)
niphablepsia [ˌnifəˈblepsiə], **niphotyphlosis** [ˌnifəutifˈləusis] *n* 雪盲
nipper [ˈnipə] *n* 夹,钳,镊子
nipple [ˈnipl] *n* 乳头;橡皮奶头
Nippostrongylus [ˌnipəuˈstrɔŋdʒiləs] *n* 日圆线虫属 | ~ brasiliensis 巴西日圆线虫 / ~ muris 鼠日圆线虫
niridazole [niˈridəzəul] *n* 尼立达唑(抗血吸虫药)
nisbuterol mesylate [nisˈbjuːtərɔl] 甲磺尼司特罗(支气管扩张药)
nisin [ˈnaisin] *n* 乳酸链球菌肽
nisobamate [ˌnaisəuˈbɑːmeit] *n* 尼索氨酯(弱安定药,镇静药和催眠药)
nisoldipine [naiˈsɔldipiːn] *n* 尼索地平(钙通道阻滞药,用于治疗高血压,口服给药)
nisoxetine [niˈsɔksətiːn] *n* 尼索西汀(抗抑郁药)
Nissen fundoplication (operation) [ˈnisen] (Rudolf Nissen) 尼森胃底折叠术(手术)(胃底围绕远端食管完全包裹起来的一型手术)
Nissen operation [ˈnisən] (Rudolph Nissen)尼森手术(即胃底折术)
Nissl bodies (granules, substance) [ˈnisl] (Franz Nissl)尼[斯尔]氏体,虎斑小体(组成神经细胞浆中网状组织的大颗粒,可被碱性染料染色,其主要成分为核糖核蛋白) | ~ degeneration 尼[斯尔]氏变性(神经断离后神经细胞所起的变性) / ~ method of staining 尼[斯尔]氏染色法(染神经细胞体)
nisterime acetate [naiˈstiəriːm] 尼司特林醋酯(雄激素)
nisus [ˈnaisəs] *n*【拉】努力,奋发
nit [nit] *n* 虮,虱卵
Nitabuch's stria (layer, zone) [ˈniːtəbuh] (Raissa Nitabuch)尼塔布赫纹(层、带)(胎盘发育中的一层类纤维蛋白,沿蜕膜表面发生,滋养层与蜕膜在此消失)
nitarsone [naiˈtɑːsəun] *n* 硝苯胂酸(抗原虫药,对组织滴虫属有效,用于家禽)
nitavirus [ˌnaitəˈvaiərəs] (*n*uclear *i*nclusion *t*ype *A*) *n* 尼他病毒,A 型核包涵体病毒
niter [ˈnaitə] *n* 硝石,硝酸钾(即 niter)
nithiamide [naiˈθaiəmaid] *n* 醋胺硝唑(兽用抗生素)
niton [ˈnaitɔn] *n* 氡,镭射气
nitramine [naiˈtræmin] *n* 硝[基]胺
nitramisole hydrochloride [naiˈtræmisəul] 盐酸硝拉咪唑(抗蠕虫药)
nitratase [ˈnaitrəteis] *n* 硝酸盐酶
nitrate [ˈnaitreit] *n* 硝酸盐,硝酸酯 *vt* 使硝化
nitrate reductase [ˈnaitreit riˈdʌkteis] 硝酸盐还原酶(细菌培养中的硝酸盐还原试验,对鉴定肠杆菌科、分枝杆菌和某些厌氧菌是有用的,亦称硝酸盐酶)
nitration [naiˈtreiʃən] *n* 硝化[作用]
nitrazepam [naiˈtræzəpæm] *n* 硝西泮(苯二氮䓬类安定药,用作抗惊厥和催眠药)
nitre [ˈnaitə] *n* 硝石,硝酸钾 | cubic ~ 硝酸钠
nitremia [naiˈtriːmiə] *n* 氮血[症]
nitrendipine [naiˈtrendipiːn] *n* 尼群地平(钙通道阻滞药,用作抗高血压药,口服给药)
nitric [ˈnaitrik] *a* [含]氮的 | ~ oxide 一氧化氮
nitric acid [ˈnaitrik] 硝酸
nitridation [ˌnaitriˈdeiʃən] *n* 氮化[作用]
nitride [ˈnaitraid] *n* 氮化物
nitrify [ˈnaitrifai] *vt*, *vi* 硝化 | **nitrification** [ˌnaitrifiˈkeiʃən] *n* 硝化[作用] / **nitrifier** [ˈnaitrifaiə] *n* 硝化菌
nitrifying [ˈnaitrifaiiŋ] *a* 硝化的
nitrilase [ˈnaitrileis] *n* 腈水解酶
nitrile [ˈnaitril] *n* 腈
nitrilotriacetic acid [ˌnaitriləutraiəˈsiːtik] 次氮基三乙酸(一种螯合剂,见于合成的去污剂中,此酸大量使用系肾癌和膀胱癌的基因外致癌物质)
nitrite [ˈnaitrait] *n* 亚硝酸盐(或酯)
nitritoid [ˈnaitritɔid] *a* 亚硝酸盐样的
nitrituria [ˌnaitriˈtjuəriə] *n* 亚硝酸盐尿
nitro- [前缀]硝基
nitro-amine [ˈnaitrəu əˌmiːn] *n* 硝[基]胺
nitroaniline [ˌnaitrəuˈæniliːn] *n* 硝基苯胺
nitro-anisol [ˌnaitrəuˈænisɔl] *n* 硝基茴香醚
Nitrobacter [ˌnaitrəuˈbæktə] *n* 硝化杆菌属(亦称硝化囊菌属)
Nitrobacteraceae [ˌnaitrəuˌbæktəˈreisiiː] *n* 硝化杆菌科
nitrobacterium [ˌnaitrəubækˈtiəriəm] ([复] **nitrobacteria** [ˌnaitrəubækˈtiəriə]) *n* 硝化菌
nitrobenzene [ˌnaitrəuˈbenziːn], **nitrobenzol** [ˌnaitrəuˈbenzɔl] *n* 硝基苯
nitroblue tetrazolium [ˈnaitrəbluːˌtetrəˈzəuliəm] 四唑氮蓝
nitrocellulose [ˌnaitrəuˈseljuləus] *n* 硝化纤维素,火棉 | **nitrocellulosic** [ˌnaitrəuseljuˈlɔsik] *a*
Nitrococcus [ˌnaitrəuˈkɔkəs] *n* 硝化球菌属
nitrocycline [ˌnaitrəuˈsaikliːn] *n* 硝环素
Nitrocystis [ˌnaitrəuˈsistis] *n* 硝化囊菌属,硝化杆

菌属

nitroferrocyanic acid [ˌnaitrəuˌferəusaiˈænik] *n* 亚硝基铁氰酸

nitrofuran [ˌnaitrəuˈfjuərən] *n* 硝基呋喃

nitrofurantoin [ˌnaitrəufjuəˈræntɔin] *n* 呋喃妥因(尿路抗菌药)

nitrofurazone [ˌnaitrəuˈfjuərəzəun] *n* 呋喃西林(局部抗菌药)

nitrogen [ˈnaitrədʒən] *n* 氮 | alloxuric ~ 嘌呤氮 / amide ~ 酰胺氮 / ~ dioxide 二氧化氮 / ~ monoxide 氧化亚氮,笑气 / ~ mustards 氮芥 / nomadic ~ (大气)游离氮 / nonprotein ~ 非蛋白氮 / ~ pentoxide 硝酸酐,五氧化二氮 / ~ peroxide, ~ tetroxide 过氧化氮,四氧化二氮 / rest ~ 余氮

nitrogenase [ˈnaitrədʒəneis] *n* 固氮酶

nitrogen-fixing [ˈnaitrədʒənˈfiksiŋ] *a* 固氮的(指细菌)

nitrogenization [ˌnaitrəudʒənaiˈzeiʃən, -niˈz-] *n* 氮化[作用],充氮[作用]

nitrogenous [naiˈtrɔdʒinəs] *a* 含氮的

nitroglycerin [naitrəuˈglisərin] *n* 硝酸甘油(抗心绞痛药)

nitrohydrochloric acid [ˌnaitrəuˌhaidrəuˈklɔːrik] 王水

nitromannite [ˌnaitrəuˈmænait] *n* 甘露六硝酯(即 mannitol hexanitrate,抗心绞痛药)

nitromersol [ˌnaitrəuˈməːsɔl] *n* 硝甲酚汞(消毒防腐药)

nitrometer [naiˈtrɔmitə] *n* 氮定量器,量氮器

nitromethane [ˌnaitrəuˈmeθein] *n* 硝基甲烷

nitromifene citrate [naiˈtrəumifiːn] 枸橼酸硝米芬(雌激素拮抗药)

nitromuriatic acid [ˌnaitrəuˌmjuəriˈætik] 王水

nitron [ˈnaitrɔn] *n* 硝酸灵;镭射气分子量

nitronaphthalene [ˌnaitrəuˈnæfθəliːn], **nitronaphthalin** [ˌnaitrəuˈnæfθəlin] *n* 硝基萘

nitrophenol [ˌnaitrəuˈfiːnɔl] *n* 硝基(苯)酚

2-nitropropane [ˌnaitrəuˈprəupein] *n* 2-硝基丙烷(用作溶剂、火箭推进剂和汽油添加剂,致癌)

nitropropiol [ˌnaitrəuˈprəupiɔl] *n* (邻)硝基苯丙烯酸

nitroprotein [ˌnaitrəuˈprəutiːn] *n* 硝基蛋白,硝化蛋白

nitroprussic acid [ˌnaitrəuˈprʌsik] 亚硝基铁氰酸

nitroprusside [ˌnaitrəuˈprʌsaid] *n* 硝普盐

nitrosaccharose [ˌnaitrəuˈsækərəus] *n* 硝化蔗糖,硝糖

nitrosalol [ˌnaitrəuˈsælɔl] *n* 硝基萨罗,硝基水杨酸苯酯

nitrosamine [naiˈtrəusəmiːn] *n* 亚硝胺

nitrosate [ˈnaitrəseit] *vt*, *vi* 亚硝基化

nitrosation [ˌnaitrəuˈseiʃən] *n* 亚硝基化

nitroscanate [ˌnaitrəuˈskæneit] *n* 硝硫氰酯(兽用抗蠕虫药)

nitrose [ˈnaitrəus] *n* 硝酸类(硝酸及亚硝酸的统称)

nitrosification [naiˌtrəusifiˈkeiʃən] *n* 亚硝化[作用](氨氧化成亚硝酸盐)

nitrosifying [niˈtrəusiˌfaiiŋ] *a* 亚硝化的

nitroso- [前缀] 亚硝基

nitrosobacterium [naiˌtrəusəubækˈtiəriəm] ([复] **nitrosobacteria** [naiˌtrəusəubækˈtiəriə]) *n* 亚硝化菌

Nitrosococcus [ˌnaitrəusəuˈkɔkəs]) *n* 亚硝化球菌属

Nitrosocystis [naiˌtrəusəuˈsistis] *n* 亚硝化囊菌属

***N*-nitrosodimethylamine** [naiˌtrəusəudaiˈmeθiləˌmiːn] *n* *N*-亚硝基二甲胺(一种黄色液体亚硝胺,曾用于火箭燃料,用作抗氧化剂及其他用途,致癌。亦称二甲基亚硝胺)

***N*-nitrosodiphenylamine** [naiˌtrəusəudaiˈfeniləˌmiːn] *n* *N*-亚硝基二苯胺(一种二环亚硝胺,橡胶硫化时用作加速剂,致癌。亦称二苯亚硝胺)

Nitrosogloea [naiˌtrəusəuˈgliːə] *n* 亚硝化胶菌属

nitroso-indol [naiˌtrəusəu ˈindɔl] *n* 亚硝基吲哚

Nitrosolobus [naiˌtrəusəuˈləubəs] *n* 亚硝化叶菌属 | ~ multiformis 多形亚硝化叶菌

Nitrosomonas [ˌnaitrəusəuˈməunəs] *n* 亚硝化单胞菌属

Nitrosospira [naiˌtrəusəuˈspaiərə] *n* 亚硝化螺菌属

nitrososubstitution [naiˌtrəusəuˌsʌbstiˈtjuːʃən] *n* 亚硝基取代[作用]

nitrosourea [naiˌtrəusəuˈjuəriə] *n* 亚硝基脲

Nitrospina [ˌnaitrəuˈspainə] *n* 硝化脊菌属 | ~ gracilis 硝化薄脊菌

nitrosugars [ˌnaitrəuˈʃugəz] *n* 硝化糖类,硝基糖类

nitrosyl [ˈnaitrəsil] *n* 亚硝酰基

nitrous [ˈnaitrəs] *a* 亚硝的 | ~ oxide 氧化亚氮,笑气(麻醉药)

nitrous acid [ˈnaitrəs] 亚硝酸

nitroxanthic acid [ˌnaitrəuˈzænθik] 苦味酸,三硝基酚

nitroxyl [naiˈtrɔksil], **nitryl** [ˈnaitril] *n* 硝酰基

Nitzschia [ˈnitʃiə] *n* 菱形藻属

nivazol [ˈnaivəzɔl] *n* 尼伐可醇(糖皮质激素)

nivemycin [ˌnivəˈmaisin] *n* 新霉素

nivimedone sodium [niˈvaimidəun] 尼维美酮钠(抗过敏药)

nizatidine [niˈzeitidiːn] *n* 尼扎替丁(组胺 H_2 受体阻滞药,用于治疗十二指肠溃疡)

nl nanoliter 纳升(10^{-9}L)
NLN National League for Nursing 全国护理联合会
Nm. nux moschata【拉】肉豆蔻
nm nanometer 纳米(10^{-9} m)
NMA National Medical Association 全国医学协会
NMDA *N*-methyl-D-aspartate *N*-甲基-D-天冬氨酸
NMN nicotinamide mononucleotide 烟酰胺单核苷酸
NMR nuclear magnetic resonance 核磁共振
NMRI Naval Medical Research Institute 海军医学研究所
NMS neuroleptic malignant syndrome 神经安定药恶性综合征
nn. nervi【拉】神经
NND *New and Nonofficial Drugs*《非法定新药集》(美国医学会以前出版的年刊)
No nobelium 锘
No. numero【拉】号码,数目
Noack's syndrome [ˈnəuɑːk] (Margot Noack) 诺亚克综合征,尖头、多及并指畸形Ⅰ型,尖头、多及并趾畸形Ⅰ型
NOAEL no observed adverse effect level 无毒性有害效应剂量
nobelium(No) [nəuˈbeliəm] *n* 锘(化学元素)
Nobel prize [ˈnəubel] (Alfred B. Nobel) 诺贝尔奖金
Noble's position [ˈnəubl] (Charles P. Noble) 诺布尔位置(患者站立,上身向前屈,以手臂支撑,用于检查肾脏)
Nocardia [nəuˈkɑːdiə] (Edmond I. É. Nocard) *n* 诺卡菌属 | ~ asteroides 星形诺卡菌 / ~ brasiliensis 巴西诺卡菌 / ~ farcinica 皮疽诺卡菌 / ~ madurae 马杜拉诺卡菌
Nocardiaceae [nəuˌkɑːdiˈeisiiː] *n* 诺卡菌科
nocardial [nəuˈkɑːdiəl] *a* 诺卡[放线]菌的
nocardin [nəuˈkɑːdin] *n* 诺卡[放线]菌素
nocardioform [nəuˈkɑːdiəˌfɔːm] *a* 诺卡型的(一种分裂成细菌型或球菌型的短暂的菌丝体)
Nocardiopsis [nəuˌkɑːdiˈɔpsis] *n* 诺卡土壤菌属
nocardiosis [nəukɑːdiˈəusis], **nocardiasis** [ˌnəukɑːˈdaiəsis] *n* 诺卡菌病
Nocard's bacillus [nɔˈkɑː] (Edmond I. É. Nocard) 诺卡菌,鼠伤寒沙门菌
nocebo [nəuˈsiːbəu] *n*【拉】非特异性不良副作用
Nochtia [ˈnɔktiə] *n* 小线虫属 | ~ nochti 猴胃线虫
noci- [构词成分]伤害
nociassociation [ˌnəusiəˌsəusiˈeiʃən] *n* 伤害性联合反应(如外科手术时)
nociception [ˌnəusiˈsepʃən] *n* 伤害感受
nociceptive [ˌnəusiˈseptiv] *a* 感受伤害的(指感受神经元对疼痛感觉而言)
nociceptor [ˌnəusiˈseptə] *n* 伤害性感受器
nocifensor [ˌnəusiˈfensə] *n* 防伤害系统,伤害防卫系统
noci-influence [ˌnəusiˈinfluəns] *n* 伤害性影响
nociperception [ˌnəusipəˈsepʃən] *n* 伤害性知觉
nocodazole [nəuˈkəudəzəul] *n* 诺考达唑,噻氨酯哒唑(抗肿瘤药)
Noct. nocte【拉】[在]夜间
noctalbuminuria [ˌnɔktælˌbjuːmiˈnjuəriə] *n* 夜蛋白尿[症]
noctambulism [nɔkˈtæmbjulizəm], **noctambulation** [ˌnɔktæmbjuˈleiʃən] *n* 梦行[症] | **noctambulic** [ˌnɔktæmˈbjuːlik] *a* / **noctambulist** [nɔkˈtæmbjulist] *n* 梦行者
noctiphobia [ˌnɔktiˈfəubjə] *n* 黑夜恐怖
Noct. maneq. nocte maneque【拉】早晚(晚上和早晨)
nocturia [nɔkˈtjuəriə] *n* 夜尿
nocturnal [nɔkˈtəːnl] *a* 夜间的,夜发的,夜间活动的
nocuous [ˈnɔkjuəs] *a* 有害的,有毒的
node [nəud] *n* 结,结节 | hemal ~s, hemolymph ~s 血淋巴结 / lymph ~ 淋巴结 / sentinel ~, signal ~ 前哨淋巴结,信号淋巴结(锁骨上肿大的淋巴结,常是腹部肿瘤第一个体征) / singer's ~, teacher's ~ 声带结节,结节性声带炎 / triticeous ~ 麦粒软骨 | **nodal** [ˈnəudl] *a*
nodi [ˈnəudai] nodus 的复数
nodose [ˈnəudəus] *a* 有结的,结节状的 | **nodosity** [nəuˈdɔsəti] *n* 结节性,结节状;结节
nodoventricular [ˌnəudəuvenˈtrikjulə] *a* 结室的(连接房室结与心室的)
nodular [ˈnɔdjulə] *a* 小结的,结的;小结状的,结节性的
Nodularia [ˌnɔdjuˈleiriə] *n* 节球藻属
nodulated [ˈnɔdjuleitid] *a* 有结的,有小结的
nodulation [ˌnɔdjuˈleiʃən] *n* 小结形成,小结化
nodule [ˈnɔdjuːl] *n* 结,小结;结节 | aggregate ~s 淋巴集结,集合淋巴小结 / apple jelly ~s 苹果酱状结节(狼疮) / juxta-articular ~s 关节旁结节 / lentiform ~ 豆状突 / lymphatic ~s 淋巴小结 / milkers' ~s 挤奶者结节 / pearly ~ 珠样小结(牛型结核病的一种小结) / primary ~ 初级淋巴小结(无生发中心) / pulp ~ 髓石 / secondary ~s 次级淋巴小结(生发中心) / singers' ~, teachers' ~ 声带小结(结节性声带炎时) / ~s tabac 含铁结节 / triticeous ~ 麦粒软骨 / ~ of vermis 蚓部小结 / vestigial ~ 残遗结节,耳郭结节
nodulous [ˈnɔdjuləs] *a* 有节的,结节的
nodulus [ˈnɔdjuləs] ([复] **noduli** [ˈnɔdjulai]) *n*【拉】结,小结
nodus [ˈnəudəs] ([复] **nodi** [ˈnəudai]) *n*【拉】

结,结节

NOEL no observed effect level 无毒性效应剂量

noematachograph [nəuˌiːməˈtækəgrɑːf] *n* 思考速度描记器

noematachometer [nəuˌiːmətəˈkɔmitə] *n* 思考速度测验器

noematic [ˌnəuiːˈmætik] *a* 思考的,思想的;心理过程的

noesis [nəuˈiːsis] *n*【希】认识,识别;智力 | **noetic** [nəuˈetik] *a*

noeud [njuː] *n*【法】结,结节

nogalamycin [nəuˌgæləˈmaisin] *n* 诺拉霉素(抗肿瘤抗生素)

Noguchia [nɔˈguːtʃiə] *n* (Hideyo Noguchi 野口英世)野口菌属 | ~ cuniculi 兔野口菌 / ~ granulosis 颗粒性野口菌 / ~ simiae 猩猩野口菌,猿野口菌

Noguchi's culture medium [nɔˈguːtʃi] (Hideyo Noguchi 野口英世)野口(组织)培养基(含有无菌的新鲜的兔肾组织,用于培养螺旋体) | ~ reaction 野口反应(①华氏〈Wassermann〉反应的一种改良法:抗原用狗和牛的肝、心提取的脂类物质,用人红细胞,溶血素用家兔抗人正常红细胞的抗血清,抗原和溶血素在溶液中迅速失效,故用一定长度滤纸〈0.5 mm 方块〉分别浸渍后以干燥形式保存之;②全身麻痹和脊髓痨时所见的一种反应) / ~ luetin reaction 野口梅毒螺旋体素反应(此法目前已不再使用) / ~ reagent 野口试剂(丁酸 10 份和 0.9% 氯化钠溶液 90 份) / ~ test 野口试验(①见野口反应;②检球蛋白)

noise [nɔiz] *n* 噪声

noiseless [ˈnɔizlis] *a* 无噪声的

noisome [ˈnɔisəm] *a* 有害的,有毒的;恶臭的

noli-me-tangere [ˌnəulai miː ˈtændʒəri] *n*【拉】侵蚀性溃疡

nolinium bromide [nəuˈliniəm] 诺利溴铵(抗分泌和抗溃疡药)

noma [ˈnəumə] *n* 走马疳,坏疽性口炎 | ~ vulvae 阴部走马疳,腐蚀性外阴炎

nomen [ˈnəumən] ([复] **nomina** [ˈnəuminə]) *n*【拉】名词 | nomina generalia 普通[解剖]名词,一般[解剖]名词

nomenclature [nəuˈmenklətʃə, ˈnəumenˌkleitʃə] *n* 命名法;名称,名词,术语;术语表 | binomial ~ 双[命]名法

nomifensine maleate [ˌnɔmiˈfensiːn] 马来酸诺米芬新(中枢神经系统兴奋药,用作抗抑郁药)

Nomina Anatomica [ˈnəuminə ænəˈtɔmikə] 解剖学名词(国际解剖学名词委员会采用,现为解剖学术语 Terminologia Anatomica [TA]〈1998〉所取代)

nom(o)- [构词成分]法规,惯例

nomogenesis [ˌnəuməˈdʒenisis] *n* 循规进化说

nomogram [ˌnɔməgræm], **nomograph** [ˈnɔməgrɑːf, -græf] *n* 列线图,计算图

nomography [nəuˈmɔgrəfi] *n* 列线图解法 | **nomographic** [ˌnɔməˈgræfik, ˌnəuməˈgræfik] *a*

nomotopic [ˌnəuməˈtɔpik] *a* 正位发生的

non- [前缀]不,非,无

nona [ˈnəunə] *n* 南欧嗜眠性脑炎

nonacosane [ˌnəunəˈkəusein] *n* 二十九[碳]烷

nonadherent [ˌnɔnədˈhiərənt] *a* 非粘连的

nonan [ˈnəunæn] *a* 第九日[再发]的

nonantigenic [ˌnɔnæntiˈdʒenik] *a* 非抗原性的

nonapeptide [ˌnɔnəˈpeptaid] *n* 九肽

nonaqueous [ˌnɔnˈeikwiəs] *a* 非水[性]的

non compos mentis [nɔn ˈkɔmpəs ˈmentis]【拉】精神不健全

nonconductor [ˌnɔnkənˈdʌktə] *n* 非导体

nondepolarizer [ˌnɔndiːˈpəuləraizə] *n* 非去极化剂,非退极化剂

non-disjunction [ˌnɔndisˈdʒʌŋkʃən] *n* 不分离(细胞分离中期,成对染色体不互相分开的现象,结果一个子细胞得到两个染色体,而另一个则缺了这一染色体)

noneffective [ˌnɔniˈfectiv] *a* 无效力的

nonelastic [ˌnɔniˈlæstik] *a* 无弹性的

nonelectrolyte [ˌnɔniˈlektrəulait] *n* 非电解质,不电离质

nonentity [nɔnˈentəti] *n* 不存在

nonessential [ˌnɔniˈsenʃəl] *a* 非本质的,不重要的,非必需的

nonesterified fatty acid [ˌnɔnesˈterifaid] 游离脂肪酸,非酯化脂肪酸

nonexistence [ˌnɔnigˈsistəns] *n* 不存在 | **nonexistent** [ˌnɔnigˈsistənt] *a*

nongranulocyte [nɔnˈgrænjuləusait] *n* 非粒性白细胞

nonheme [ˈnɔnhiːm] *a* 非血红素的(指蛋白质内的铁)

nonhomogeneity [nɔnˌhɔməudʒeˈniːəti] *n* 非同种性,非纯一性;非同质性,非均匀性

nonigravida [ˌnəuniˈgrævidə] *n* 第九次孕妇

noninfectious [ˌnɔninˈfekʃəs] *a* 非传染性的

noninflammable [ˌnɔninˈflæməbl] *a* 不燃的

non-inflammatory [ˌnɔninˈflæmətəri] *a* 非炎性的

non-invasive [ˌnɔn inˈveisiv] *a* 非侵害的,非侵袭的;非侵入性的,非介入性的

noninvolution [ˌnɔninvəˈluːʃən] *n* 复旧不能(如子宫的)

nonipara [nəuˈnipərə] *n* 九产妇

nonmetal [ˌnɔnˈmetl] *n* 非金属

nonmyelinated [nɔn'maiəliˌneitid], **nonmedullated** [nɔn'medəleitid] *a* 无髓[鞘]的

Nonne-Apelt reaction (phase, test) ['nɔnə 'ɑːpelt] (Max Nonne; F. Apelt) 农内-阿佩尔特反应(期、试验)(取 2 ml 脑脊液与等量中性的饱和硫酸铵溶液混合,3 分钟后与另一个只含有脑脊液的试管比较,若无差异或仅有微弱乳光出现,则为阴性反应,若显现乳白色或混浊则为阳性期 1,表示液内有大量球蛋白,而知有神经疾病,正常液仅用热和乙酸处理,就变成混浊,称为阳性期 2)

Nonne-Milroy disease ['nɔnə 'milrɔi] (Max Nonne; William F. Milroy) 农内-米尔罗依病(见 Milroy disease)

Nonne-Milroy-Meige syndrome ['nɔnə 'milrɔi 'meʒə] (Max Nonne; William F. Milroy; Henri Meige) 农内-米尔罗伊-迈热综合征(见 Milroy's disease)

Nonne's syndrome ['nɔnə] (Max Nonne) 农内综合征(遗传性小脑性共济失调) | ~ test 农内试验(检脑脊液球蛋白过多)

non-neuronal [ˌnɔnjuə'rəunəl] *a* 非神经元的

non-nucleated [nɔn'njuːkliˌeitid] *a* 无核的

nonocclusion [ˌnɔnə'kluːʒən] *n* 开殆,无殆

nonoliguric [nɔnˌɔli'gjuərik] *a* 非少尿的

nononcogenic [ˌnɔnɔŋkəu'dʒenik] *a* 非致瘤的

nonopaque [ˌnɔnəu'peik] *a* 透 X 线的,透光的

nonoperative [nɔn'ɔpərətiv] *a* 非手术[治疗]的

nonose ['nɔnəus] *n* 壬糖

nonoxynol [nəu'nɔksinəul] *n* 壬苯醇醚,壬苯聚醇,对壬基苯氧聚乙氧乙醇(即 nonylphenoxy polyethoxyethanol,壬苯聚醇 4,15 和 30 为非离子化表面活性药,壬苯聚醇 9 用作杀精子药,壬苯聚醇 10 用作药物表面活性药)

nonparametric [ˌnɔnpærə'metrik] *a* 非参数的

nonparous [nɔn'pærəs] *a* 未经产的

nonphotochromogen [ˌnɔnfəutəu'krəumədʒən] *n* 非光照产色菌

nonpolar [nɔn'pəulə] *a* 非极性的

nonproductive ['nɔnprə'dʌktiv] *a* 不能生产的;非生产性的;(咳嗽)干咳的

nonproprietary [ˌnɔnprəu'praiətəri] *a* 非专有的,非专利的

nonprotein ['nɔn'prəutiːn] *n* 非蛋白质

nonradiable [nɔn'reidiəbl] *a* 不透放射线的

non repetat. non repetatur【拉】不要重复,不要重配

nonresponder [nɔnri'spɔndə] *n* 非应答者(指人或动物接种某一病毒后在受到该病毒攻击时未显示免疫应答)

nonrotation [ˌnɔnrəu'teiʃən] *n* 未[能]旋转

nonsaponifiable [nɔnsəˌpɔni'faiəbəl] *a* 非皂化的(指脂类)

nonsecretor [ˌnɔnsi'kriːtə] *n* 非分泌型者(指具有 A 或 B 血型,而其唾液和其他分泌液中不含有特殊的〈A 或 B〉物质的人)

nonself ['nɔnself] *a* 非自身的(在免疫学中指外来的抗原)

nonseptate [nɔn'septeit] *a* 无中隔的,无间隔的

non sequitur [nɔn 'sekwitə]【拉】不根据前提的推理

nonsexual [ˌnɔn'seksjuəl] *a* 无性别的,无性的

non-smoker [ˌnɔn 'sməukə] *n* 非吸烟者

nonspecific [ˌnɔnspi'sifik] *a* 非特异性的

non-suppurative [nɔn'sʌpjuərətiv] *a* 非化脓性的

nonsurgical [nɔn'səːdʒikəl] *a* 非外科的

nonsyndromic [ˌnɔnsin'drɔmik] *a* 非综合征的

nontaster [nɔn'teistə] *n* 味盲(指对一种特殊试验物质如用于某些遗传研究的苯硫脲不能尝出苦味的人)

nonunion [nɔn'juːnjən] *n* (骨)不连接

nonvalent [nɔn'veilənt] *a* 无价的,惰性的

nonviable [nɔn'vaiəbl] *a* 不能生活的,不能存活的

nonyl ['nəunil] *n* 壬[烷]基

Noonan's syndrome ['nuːnən] (Jacqueline Anne Noonan) 努南综合征(蹼颈、上睑下垂、性腺功能减退、先天性心脏病及身材矮小,即无性腺发育不全的特纳〈Turner〉综合征的表型,在女性特纳综合征确认之前称之为男性特纳综合征)

noopsyche ['nəuəˌsaiki] *n* 理智,智力精神

Noorden treatment ['nɔːdən] (Carl H. von Noorden) 诺尔登疗法,燕麦食疗法(oatmeal treatment,见 treatment 项下相应术语)

noothymopsychic [ˌnəuəˌθaiməu'saikik] *a* 理智情感的

nootropic [ˌnəuə'trɔpik] *a* 向精神的,亲精神的(对器质性受损的认知或对神经系统的功能有积极影响的,指某些药物)

nopalin G ['nəupælin] 蓝曙红

NOPHN National Organization for Public Health Nursing 全国公共卫生护理组织

noradrenaline [ˌnɔːrə'drenəliːn] *n* 去甲肾上腺素(升压药)

noradrenergic [ˌnɔːrədrə'nəːdʒik] *a* 去甲肾上腺素能的

noramidopyrine [nɔːˌræmidəu'paiəriːn] *n* 安乃近(解热镇痛药)

norandrostenolone [nɔːˌrændrəu'stenələun] *n* 去甲雄甾烯醇酮,诺龙(即南诺龙 nandrolone,雄激素,同化激素类药)

nordauism [nɔː'dauizəm] *n* 诺道病(见 Nordau's disease)

Nordau's disease [ˈnɔːdau] (Max S. Nordau) 诺尔道病,变质症,精神变质(指身体、精神的衰退或变质)

nordefrin hydrochloride [nɔːˈdefrin] 盐酸异肾上腺素(肾上腺素能药,具有明显的中枢兴奋作用,需要收缩血管时常使用左旋异肾上腺素 levonordefrin)

no-reflow [nəuˈriːfləu] *n* 无回流(见 phenomenon 项下相应术语)

norepinephrine [ˌnɔːrepiˈnefrin] *n* 去甲肾上腺素 | ~ bitartrate 重酒石酸去甲肾上腺素

norethandrolone [ˌnɔːreθˈændrələun] *n* 诺乙雄龙,乙诺酮(合成雄激素)

norethindrone [nɔːˈreθindrəun] *n* 炔诺酮(孕激素) | ~ acetate 醋炔诺酮

norethisterone [ˌnɔːreˈθistərəun] *n* 炔诺酮(孕激素)

norethynodrel [ˌnɔːreˈθainədrəl] *n* 异炔诺酮(孕激素)

norfloxacin [nɔːˈflɔksəsin] *n* 诺氟沙星(一种抗菌有机酸,对耐青霉素的淋病奈瑟菌有效,口服给药)

norflurane [nɔːˈfluːrein] *n* 诺氟烷(吸入麻醉药)

norgestimate [nɔːˈdʒestimeit] *n* 诺孕酯(孕激素)

norgestomet [nɔːˈdʒestəmit] *n* 诺孕美特(孕激素)

norgestrel [nɔːˈdʒestrəl] *n* 炔诺孕酮(高效孕激素,与雌激素合用作为口服避孕药)

norhyoscyamine [nɔːˌhaiəuˈsaiəmiːn] *n* 去甲莨菪碱

norleucine [nɔːˈljuːsiːn] *n* 正亮氨酸,正白氨酸

norm [nɔːm] *n* 标准,规格,准则;定额;平均数;常模,正常

norma [ˈnɔːmə] *n*【拉】外观(颅)

normal [ˈnɔːməl] *a* 正常的,正规的,标准的;正[链]的;规度的;当量的 *n* 正常物;正常状态(或数量、程度等);标准 | **~ly** *ad* / **normality** [nɔːˈmæləti] *n* 正常状态;规度;当量浓度

normalize [ˈnɔːməlaiz] *vt* 使正常化,使标准化,使规度化 | **normalization** [ˌnɔːməlaiˈzeiʃən, -liˈz-] *n*

normergy [nɔːˈməːdʒi] *n* 反应正常 | **normergic** [nɔːˈməːdʒik] *a*

normetanephrine [nɔˌmetəˈnefrin] *n* 去甲变肾上腺素,去甲-3-*O*-甲基肾上腺素

norm(o)- [构词成分]正常,标准

normoblast [ˈnɔːməˌblæst] *n* 正成红细胞,幼红细胞,晚幼红细胞 | basophilic ~, early ~ 嗜碱性正成红细胞,早幼红细胞 / orthochromatic ~, acidophilic ~, eosinophilic ~, late ~, oxyphilic ~ 正染性正成红细胞,晚幼红细胞 / polychromatic ~, intermediate ~ 多染性正成红细胞,中幼红细胞 | **~ic** [ˌnɔːməˈblæstik] *a*

normoblastosis [ˌnɔːməublæsˈtəusis] *n* 正成红细胞过多[症]

normocalcemia [ˌnɔːməukælˈsiːmiə] *n* 血钙正常 | **normocalcemic** [ˌnɔːməukælˈsiːmik] *a*

normocapnia [ˌnɔːməuˈkæpniə] *n* 血碳酸正常 | **normocapnic** *a*

normocholesterolemia [ˌnɔːməukəˌlestərəuˈliːmiə] *n* 血胆固醇正常 | **normocholesterolemic** *a*

normochromasia [ˌnɔːməukrəuˈmeiziə] *n* 正常染色反应;血[细胞]色正常

normochromia [ˌnɔːməuˈkrəumiə] *n* 血[细胞]色正常 | **normochromic** *a*

normochromocyte [ˌnɔːməuˈkrəuməsait] *n* 正[常]色红细胞

normocrinic [ˌnɔːməuˈkrinik] *a* 正常分泌的,内分泌[作用]正常的

normocyte [ˈnɔːməsait] *n* [正常]红细胞 | **normocytic** [ˌnɔːməˈsitik] *a*

normocytosis [ˌnɔːməusaiˈtəusis] *n* 血细胞正常

normoerythrocyte [ˌnɔːməuiˈriθrəusait] *n* [正常]红细胞

normoglycemia [ˌnɔːməuglaiˈsiːmiə] *n* 血糖量正常 | **normoglycemic** *a*

normokalemia [ˌnɔːməukəˈliːmiə] *n* 血钾正常 | **normokalemic** *a*

normolineal [ˌnɔːməuˈliniəl] *a* 正[常]线的

normolipidemic [ˌnɔːməuˌlipiˈdiːmik] *a* 脂血正常的,血脂正常的

normomastic [ˌnɔːməuˈmæstik] *a* 正洋乳香的

normo-orthocytosis [ˌnɔːməuˌɔːθəusaiˈtəusis] *n* 等比例白细胞增多(白细胞总数增多,百分率正常)

normoproteinemia [ˌnɔːməuˌprəutiːˈniːmiə] *n* 血蛋白正常

normosexual [ˌnɔːməuˈseksjuəl] *a* 正常性欲的

normoskeocytosis [ˌnɔːməuˌskiəusaiˈtəusis] *n* 正数未成熟白细胞症(血象左移)

normospermia [ˌnɔːməuˈspɜːmiə] *n* 精子正常 | **normospermic** [ˌnɔːməuˈspɜːmik] *a*

normosthenuria [ˌnɔːməusθəˈnjuəriə] *n* 尿比重正常;排尿正常

normotension [ˌnɔːməuˈtenʃən] *n* 压力正常;张力正常;血压正常 | **normotensive** *a* 压力正常的;张力正常的;血压正常的 *n* 血压正常者

normothermia [ˌnɔːməuˈθəːmiə] *n* 正常体温 | **normothermic** *a*

normotonia [ˌnɔːməuˈtəuniə] *n* 张力正常 | **normotonic** [ˌnɔːməuˈtɔnik] *a*

normotrophic [ˌnɔːməuˈtrɔfik] *a* 发育正常的

normouricemia [ˌnɔːməuˌjuəriˈsiːmiə] *n* 血[内]

尿酸正常 | **normouricemic** *a*

normouricuria [ˌnɔːməuˌjuəri'kjuəriə] *n* 尿[内]尿酸正常 | **normouricuric** *a*

normovolemia [ˌnɔːməuvə'liːmiə] *n* 血量正常 | **normovolemic** *a*

norpseudoephedrine [nɔːpsjudəui'fedriːn] *n* 去甲麻黄碱(神经系统兴奋药)

Norrie's disease ['nɔːri] (Gordon Norrie) 诺里病(一种先天性 X 连锁遗传病,包括视网膜异常而引起两侧失明,以后可能发生智力迟钝和耳聋。亦称遗传性眼球萎缩)

Norris's corpuscles ['nɔris] (Richard Norris) 诺里斯小体(血清中无色透明小体)

norsulfazole [nɔː'sʌlfəzəul] *n* 磺胺噻唑(磺胺类药)

Northern blot technique (blot analysis, blot hybridization, blot test) ['nɔːθən] (类似 Southern blot technique 的诙谐式造词) RNA 印迹技术(印迹分析,印迹杂交,印迹试验)(类似塞慎〈Southern〉印迹技术的一种技术,但在被插入 DNA 的 RNA 碎片上进行,尼龙膜代之以硝化纤维素滤器)

nortriptyline hydrochloride [nɔː'triptiliːn] 盐酸去甲替林(抗抑郁药)

nortropinon [nɔː'trəupinɔn] *n* 去甲托品酮

Norwalk gastroenteritis ['nɔːwɔːk] (Norwalk 为美国俄亥俄州一城市) 诺沃克胃肠炎(诺沃克病毒所致的胃肠炎) | ~ virus 诺沃克病毒(见 virus 项下相应术语)

nosazontology [nɔˌsæzɔn'tɔlədʒi] *n* 病因学

noscapine ['nɔskəpiːn] *n* 那可丁(镇咳药) | ~ hydrochloride 盐酸那可丁

nose [nəuz] *n* 鼻;鼻状物 *vt* 闻出 *vi* 嗅,闻(at, about) | brandy ~ 酒渣鼻,红斑痤疮 / cleft ~ 鼻裂[畸形] / hammer ~, potato ~ 鼻赘,肥大性酒渣鼻 / saddle ~, saddle-back ~, swayback ~ 鞍鼻

nosebleed ['nəuzbliːd] *n* 鼻出血,鼻衄

nosegay ['nəuzgei] *n* 花束,束

Nosema [nəu'siːmə] *n* 微孢子虫属,小孢子虫属;脑胞内原虫属,脑炎微孢子虫属(即 Encephalitozoon) | ~ apis 蜜蜂微粒子虫 / ~ bombycis 蚕微粒子虫 / ~ cuniculi 兔微粒子虫(即 Encephalitozoon cuniculi)

nosematosis [nəuˌsiːmə'təusis] *n* 微粒子虫病,小孢子虫病;脑胞内原虫病,脑炎微孢子虫病(即 encephalitozoonosis)

nosencephalus [ˌnəusen'sefələs] *n* 颅脑不全畸胎

nosepiece [nəuz'piːs] *n* (显微镜的)物镜旋座

nosetiology [ˌnɔsiːti'ɔlədʒi] *n* 病因学,病原学

nosiheptide [ˌnəusi'heptaid] *n* 诺西肽,诺肽菌素(兽用生长刺激剂)

nos(o)- [构词成分]疾病

nosochthonography [ˌnɔsɔkθəu'nɔgrəfi] *n* 疾病地理学

nosocomial [ˌnɔsə'kəumiəl] *a* 医院的

nosodes ['nɔsəud] *n* 病质药(疾病产物,用于治疗)

nosogenesis [ˌnɔsəu'dʒenisis], **nosogeny** [nəu'sɔdʒini] *n* 发病机制,发病机理

nosogenic [ˌnɔsəu'dʒenik] *a* 致病的,病原的

nosogeography [ˌnɔsəudʒi'ɔgrəfi] *n* 疾病地理学

nosographer [nəu'sɔgrəfə] *n* 病情学家

nosography [nəu'sɔgrəfi] *n* 病情学

nosohemia [ˌnɔsəu'hiːmiə] *n* 血液病

nosointoxication [ˌnɔsəuinˌtɔksi'keiʃən] *n* 病质中毒

nosology [nəu'sɔlədʒi] *n* 疾病分类学 | **nosologic(al)** [ˌnɔsə'lɔdʒik(əl)] *a*

nosomania [ˌnɔsəu'meinjə] *n* 疑病妄想,疑病症

nosometry [nəu'sɔmitri] *n* 发病率计算法

nosomycosis [ˌnɔsəumai'kəusis] *n* 真菌病,霉菌病

nosonomy [nəu'sɔnəmi] *n* 疾病分类法

nosoparasite [ˌnɔsəu'pærəsait] *n* 病情寄生物,病时寄生物

nosophilia [ˌnɔsəu'filiə] *n* 患病癖,罹病癖

nosophobe ['nɔsəfəub] *n* 疾病恐怖者

nosophobia [ˌnɔsəu'fəubjə] *n* 疾病恐怖,患病恐怖

nosophyte ['nɔsəfait] *n* 植物性病原体

nosopoietic [ˌnɔsəupɔi'etik] *a* 发病的,病源性的

Nosopsyllus [ˌnɔsəu'siləs] *n* 病蚤属 | ~ fasciatus 具带病蚤

nosotaxy ['nɔsəˌtæksi] *n* 疾病分类[法]

nosotherapy [ˌnɔsəu'θerəpi] *n* 以病治病法

nosotoxic [ˌnɔsəu'tɔksik] *a* 中毒病的 | **~ity** [ˌnoθoutək'ɐisəti] *n* 中毒病性

nosotoxicosis [ˌnɔsəuˌtɔksi'kəusis] *n* 中毒病

nosotoxin [ˌnɔsəu'tɔksin] *n* 疾病毒素

nosotrophy [nəu'sɔtrəfi] *n* 病人护养法

nosotropic [ˌnɔsəu'trɔpik] *a* 抗病的,针对疾病的

nostalgia [nɔs'tældʒiə] *n* 怀乡症,思家症 | **nostalgic** [nɔs'tældʒik] *a*

nostomania [ˌnɔstəu'meiniə] *n* 怀乡狂,思家狂

nostril ['nɔstril] *n* 鼻孔

nostrum ['nɔstrəm] *n*【拉】秘方

nota bene ['nəutə 'biːni]【拉】注意,留心

notalgia [nəu'tældʒiə] *n* 背痛

notancephalia [ˌnəutænsə'feiliə] *n* 无后颅[畸形]

notanencephalia [ˌnəutənensə'feiliə] *n* 无小脑[畸形]

notch [nɔtʃ] *n* 切迹 | acetabular ~, cotyloid ~ 髋臼切迹 / auricular ~ 耳前切迹 / dicrotic ~, aortic ~ 降中峡 / gastric ~ 角切迹(胃) / marsupial ~ 小脑后切迹 / trigeminal ~ 三叉神经压迹 | **~ed** [ˈnɔtʃt] *a* 切迹状的,有缺口的

Notechis [nəuˈtekis] *n* 虎蛇属 | ~ scutatus 虎蛇

notencephalocele [ˌnəutenˈsefələˌsiːl] *n* 后脑突出

notencephalus [ˌnəutenˈsefələs] *n* 后脑突出畸胎

Nothnagel's bodies [ˈnɔtnəgəl] (Carl W. H. Nothnagel)诺特纳格尔小体(直径为15~60 μm的卵形或圆形小体,见于肉食者的粪便内) | ~ syndrome 诺特纳格尔综合征(大脑脚病灶所致的一侧眼动神经麻痹伴小脑性共济失调) / ~ type 诺特纳格尔型(肢端感觉异常)

not(o)- [构词成分]背,脊

notochord [ˈnəutəkɔːd] *n* 脊索

notochordoma [ˌnəutəukɔːˈdəumə] *n* 脊索瘤

Notoedres [ˌnəutəuˈedriːz] *n* 耳螨属 | ~ cati 猫耳螨

Notoedric [ˌnəutəuˈedrik] *a* 耳螨的,耳螨引起的

notogenesis [ˌnəutəuˈdʒenisis] *n* 脊索形成

notomelus [nəuˈtɔmiləs] *n* 背肢畸胎(背部寄生肢)

not-self [ˈnɔtself] *n* 非自身(此术语表示对机体自己来说是外来的抗原成分,机体通过体液免疫或细胞介导免疫排除这种非自身抗原)

notum [ˈnəutəm] *n* 背部;背板(节肢动物)

noumenon [ˈnuːminən, ˈnau-] *n* 本体,实体 | **noumenal** [ˈnuːmənəl, ˈnau-] *a*

nourish [ˈnʌriʃ] *vt* 养育;滋养;怀抱(希望等) | **~ing** *a* 滋养的,富于营养的 / **~ment** *n* 营养;营养品,食物

nousic [ˈnuːsik] *a* 智力的

novelty [ˈnɔvəlti] *n* 新颖,新奇

novobiocin [ˌnəuvəuˈbaiəsin] *n* 新生霉素(抗生素类药) | ~ calcium 新生霉素钙 / ~ sodium 新生霉素钠

novoscope [ˈnəuvəskəup] *n* 叩听诊器

Novy's rat disease [ˈnəuvi] (Frederick G. Novy) 诺维鼠病(在实验鼠中发现的一种病毒性疾病)

noxa [ˈnɔksə] ([复] **noxae** [ˈnɔksiː]) *n*【拉】害因,病因,病原

noxious [ˈnɔkʃəs] *a* 有害的,有毒的

nozzle [ˈnɔzl] *n* 嘴,喷嘴,吹口

Np neptunium 镎

NP-59 iodomethylnorcholesterol 碘甲基降胆固醇

NPA National Perinatal Association 全国围生期协会

NPN nonprotein nitrogen 非蛋白氮

NPO nil per os【拉】禁食

NRC normal retinal correspondence 正常视网膜对应

NREM non-rapid eye movements 非快眼动(睡眠)

ns nanosecond 纳秒(10^{-9} s)

NSAIA nonsteroidal anti-inflammatory analgesic 非甾体消炎镇痛药

NSAID nonsteroidal anti-inflammatory drug 非甾体消炎药

NSCLC non-small cell lung carcinoma (or cancer) 非小细胞肺癌

NSNA National Student Nurse Association 全国护士生协会

NSR normal sinus rhythm 正常窦性节律

NST nonstress test 无应激试验

N-terminal [ˈtəːminl] *n* N末端,氨基末端(多肽链的氨基〈NH_2〉末端,通常写在左侧)

NTP normal temperature and pressure 正常温度与压力;National Toxicology Program 国家毒理学计划

nu nanounit 纳单位(10^{-9}U)

nu [njuː] *n* 希腊语的第12个字母(N, ν)

nubecula [njuˈbekjulə] *n* 薄翳,角膜翳;尿微混浊[症];位觉砂,耳石

nubile [ˈnjuːbail] *a* (指女子)适合结婚的,可以结婚的 | **nubility** [njuːˈbiləti] *n* (女子)适合结婚,适婚性

nucha [ˈnjuːkə] ([复] **nuchae** [ˈnjuːkiː]) *n*【拉】项,颈背 | **~l** *a*

nucin [ˈnjuːsin] *n* 胡桃素,胡桃皮酸

nucis [ˈnjuːsis] *a* 核果的

Nuck's canal, diverticulum [ˈnuk] (Anton Nuck) 腹膜鞘突

nuclear [ˈnjuːkliə] *a* [原子]核的,核心的

nuclease [ˈnjuːklieis] *n* 核酸酶 | purine ~ 嘌呤核酸酶

nucleate [ˈnjuːkliit] *a* 有核的 [ˈnjuːklieit] *vt, vi* 成核[心],使集结 | **~d** [ˈnjuklieitid] *a* 有核的 / **nucleation** [ˌnjuːkliˈeiʃən] *n* 成核[现象];核晶过程,核子作用

nuclei [ˈnjuːkliai] nucleus 的复数

nucleic acid [njuːˈkliːik] 核酸 | infectious ~ ~ 感染性核酸

nucleide [ˈnjuːkliaid] *n* 核酸金属化物

nucleiform [ˈnjuːkliifɔːm] *a* 核状的

nuclein [ˈnjuːkliin] *n* 核素,核质

nucleinic acid [njuːkliˈinik] 核酸

nucle(o)- [构词成分]核

nucleocapsid [ˌnjuːkliəuˈkæpsid] *n* 核壳体,核蛋白壳,壳包核酸,病毒粒子

nucleochylema [ˌnjuːkliəukaiˈliːmə] *n* 核汁,核液

nucleochyme [ˈnjuːkliəkaim] *n* 核液,核淋巴

nucleocytoplasmic [ˌnjuːkliəuˌsaitəuˈplæzmik] *a* 核[与]质的

nucleofugal [ˌnjuːkliˈɔfjugəl] *a* 离核的

nucleoglucoprotein [ˌnjuːkliəuˌgluːkəuˈprəutiːn] *n* 核糖蛋白
nucleohistone [ˌnjuːkliəuˈhistəun] *n* 核组蛋白
nucleohyaloplasm [ˌnjuːkliəuhaiˈæləplæzəm] *n* 核透明质,核丝
nucleoid [ˈnjuːkliɔid] *a* 拟核的,核样的 *n* 核状小体(红细胞中心);拟核,类核;病毒核心(病毒的遗传物质〈核酸〉,位于病毒粒子的中心)
nucleokeratin [ˌnjuːkliəuˈkerətin] *n* 核角蛋白
nucleolar [njuːˈkliːələ] *a* 核仁的
nucleole [ˈnjuːkliəul] *n* 核仁
nucleoli [njuːˈkliːəlai] nucleolus 的复数
nucleoliform [ˌnjuːkliˈɔlifɔːm], **nucleoloid** [ˈnjuːkliəlɔid] *a* 核仁样的
nucleolin [njuːˈkliːəlin] *n* 核仁素
nucleolinus [ˌnjuːkliəuˈlainəs] *n* 核仁内粒,核点
nucleololus [ˌnjuːkliˈɔləuləs] *n* 核仁小斑
nucleolonema [ˌnjuːkliˌəuləuˈniːmə], **nucleoloneme** [ˌnjuːkliˈəulәniːm] *n* 核仁丝,核仁线
nucleolonucleus [ˌnjuːkliəuləuˈnjuːkliəs] *n* 核仁小斑
nucleolus [njuːˈkliələs] ([复] **nucleoli** [njuːˈkliːəlai]) *n*【拉】核仁 | chromatin ~, false ~, nucleinic ~ 染色质核仁,核粒
nucleolymph [ˈnjuːkliəlimf] *n* 核液,核淋巴
nucleomicrosome [ˌnjuːkliəuˈmaikrəusəum] *n* 核微粒体
nucleon [ˈnjuːkliɔn] *n* 核子
nucleonic [ˌnjuːkliˈɔnik] *a* 核的;核子的
nucleonics [ˌnjuːkliˈɔniks] *n* 核子学
nucleopetal [ˌnjuːkliˈɔpitəl] *a* 向核的
nucleophaga [ˌnjuːkliˈɔfəgə] *n* 噬核菌
nucleophagocytosis [ˌnjuːkliəuˌfægəusaiˈtəusis] *n* 噬核现象
nucleophile [ˈnjuːkliəfail] *n* 亲核物质 | **nucleophilic** [ˌnjuːkliəuˈfilik] *a* 亲核的
nucleophosphatase [ˌnjuːkliəuˈfɔsfəteis] *n* 核酸磷酸酶
nucleoplasm [ˈnjuːkliəplæzəm] *n* 核质,核浆 | ~**ic** [ˌnjuːkliəuˈplæzmik] *a*
nucleoplasmin [ˌnjuːkliəuˌplæzmin] *n* 核质蛋白
nucleoprotamine [ˌnjuːkliəuprəuˈtæmin] *n* 核精蛋白,鱼精蛋白
nucleoprotein [ˌnjuːkliəuˈprəutiːn] *n* 核蛋白 | deoxyribose ~ 脱氧核糖核蛋白 / ribose ~ 核糖核蛋白
nucleoreticulum [ˌnjuːkliəuriˈtikjuləm] *n* 核网
nucleosidase [ˌnjuːkliəuˈsaideis] *n* 核苷酶
nucleoside [ˈnjuːkliəˌsaid] *n* 核苷
nucleoside-diphosphate kinase [ˈnjuːkliəsaid daiˈfɔsfeit ˈkaineis] 二磷酸核苷激酶
nucleoside monophosphate kinase [ˈnjuːkliəˌsaid ˌmɔnəuˈfɔsfeit ˈkaineis] 核苷酸激酶
nucleoside-phosphate kinase [ˈnjukliəsaid ˈfɔsfeit ˈkaineis] 磷酸核苷激酶
nucleoside phosphorylase [ˈnjuːkliəˌsaid fɔsˈfɔːrileis] 核苷磷酸化酶
nucleosin [ˈnjuːkliəsin] *n* 胸腺生成素
nucleosis [ˌnjuːkliˈəusis] *n* 核增生
nucleosome [ˈnjuːkliəˌsəum] *n* 核小体
nucleospindle [ˌnjuːkliəuˈspindl] *n* 核纺锤体
nucleotherapy [ˌnjuːkliəuˈθerəpi] *n* 核素疗法
nucleotidase [ˌnjuːkliəˈtaideis] *n* 核苷酸酶
5′-nucleotidase [ˌnjuːkliəˈtaideis] *n* 5′-核苷酸酶
nucleotide [ˈnjuːkliətaid] *n* 核苷酸 | cyclic ~s 环核苷酸
nucleotide cyclase [ˈnjuːkliətaid ˈsaikleis] 核苷酸环化酶
nucleotide polymerase [ˈnjuːkliətaid pɔˈliməreis] 核苷酸聚合酶
nucleotidyl [ˌnjuːkliəuˈtaidil] *n* 核苷酸[基]
nucleotidylexotransferase [ˌnjuːkliəˌtaidilˌeksəuˈtrænsfəreis] *n* 核苷酸外转移酶,DNA 核苷酸外转移酶
nucleotidyltransferase [ˌnjuːkliəuˌtaidilˈtrænsfəreis] *n* 核苷酸转移酶
nucleotoxin [ˌnjuːkliəuˈtɔksin] *n* 核毒素
nucleus [ˈnjuːkliəs] ([复] **nucleuses** 或 **nuclei** [ˈnjuːkliai]) *n* 核;[细]胞核;环 | ambiguous ~ 疑核 / ~ of atom, atomic ~ 原子核 / auditory nuclei 听神经核 / basal ~ 下橄榄核;[复]基底神经节 / caudate ~ 尾核 / daughter ~ 子核 / diploid ~ 二倍体核 / fertilization ~ 受精核,合核 / free ~ 游离核 / germ ~, germinal ~ 原核,前核 / gonad ~ 生殖核,小核 / gray ~ 灰质(脊髓) / haploid ~ 单元核,单倍核,减数核 / ~ intercalatus 闰核(在迷走神经的背核和舌下神经核之间的一群神经细胞) / large cell auditory ~ 前庭神经外侧核 / reproductive ~ 生殖核,小核 / somatic ~, trophic ~ 巨核,大核,滋养核 / triangular ~ 楔束核
nuclide [ˈnjuːklaid] *n* [原子]核素 | radioactive ~ 放射性核素 | **nuclidic** [njuːˈklidik] *a*
nudophobia [ˌnjudəuˈfəubjə] *n* 裸体恐怖
Nuel's space [niːˈel] (Jean P. Nuel) 纽尔间隙(耳蜗指细胞长突之间的间隙)
nufenoxole [ˌnjuːfiˈnɔksəul] *n* 奴芬克索(抗蠕动药)
NUG necrotizing ulcerative gingivitis 坏死性溃疡性龈炎
Nuhn's glands [nun] (Anton Nuhn) 舌尖腺
nullipara [nəˈlipərə] *n* 未产妇
nulliparity [ˌnʌliˈpærəti] *n* 未经产

nulliparous [nəˈlipərəs] *a* 未经产的
numb [nʌm] *a* 麻木的,感觉缺失的 *vt* 使麻木
number [ˈnʌmbə] *n* 数,值 | acetyl ~ 乙酰值 / atomic ~ 原子序数 / chromosome ~ 染色体数 / CT ~s CT 值(在 CT 扫描时,在标度上为每一个像素定的衰减值,水为 0,密度骨为 +1 000,空气为 −1 000) / dibucaine ~ 地布卡因值(表示用地布卡因在血清样品上抑制胆碱酯酶的百分数,用以鉴别正常和异常血清胆碱酯酶表型。正常的或一般的约为 80,中间的约 60,异常的或非典型的约为 20) / hydrogen ~ 氢值 / iodine ~ 碘值 / isotopic ~ 同位素数 / polar ~ 极性值 / saponification ~ 皂化值 / thiocyanogen ~ 硫氰酸值 / transport ~ 迁移数 / wave ~ 波数
numbness [ˈnʌmnəs] *n* 麻木
nummular [ˈnʌmjulə] *a* 钱币形的;碟形的;钱串状的
nunnation [nʌˈneiʃən] *n* n 音滥用
nurse [nəːs] *n* 护士 *vt* 喂奶;护理,照料;培育 *vi* 喂奶,吃奶;看护病人 | charge ~, head ~ 护士长 / clinical ~ specialist 临床护理专家 / clinician ~ 临床护士 / community ~, district ~ 地段护士 / dry ~ 保姆,(婴儿)保育员 / general duty ~ 普通护士 / graduate ~, trained ~ 毕业护士 / hospital ~ 病室护士 / licensed practical ~ 有照护士 / monthly ~ 产褥护士 / occupational health ~ 职业卫生护士 / practical ~ 经验护士(未经护校毕业而有实际经验的人员) / private ~, private duty ~ 私人护士,私人值班护士 / probationer ~ 护生 / public health ~, community health ~, visiting ~ 公共卫生护士,社区保健护士,访视护士 / Queen's ~ 地段护士(英国) / registered ~ 注册护士 / scrub ~ 手术助理护士 / special ~ 私人护士,特约护士;专门护士 / student ~ 护生 / wet ~ 奶妈,乳母
nurse-midwife [nəːs ˈmidwaif] *n* 助产护士
nurse-midwifery [nəːs ˈmidwifəri, nəːsˈmidwaifiri] *n* 助产护士学
nursery [ˈnəːsri] *n* 婴儿室;托儿所 | day ~, day care ~ 日托托儿所
nursing [ˈnəːsiŋ] *n* 保育;喂乳[法],护理[法]
nursling [ˈnəːsliŋ] *n* 乳婴,婴儿
nurture [ˈnəːtʃə] *n* 营养物;养育;环境因素 *vt* 给…营养物;养育
Nussbaum's experiment [ˈnusbaum] (Moritz Nussbaum) 努斯鲍姆实验(结扎动物肾动脉,使肾小球与血液循环分离)
Nussbaum's narcosis [ˈnusbaum] (Johann N. Nussbaum) 努斯鲍姆麻醉法(用醚或氯仿作全身麻醉前,先注射吗啡)
nut [nʌt] *n* 核果,坚果 | betel ~ 槟榔
nutation [njuˈteiʃən] *n* 章动,点头(尤指不随意性点头)
nutatory [ˈnjutətəri] *a* 点头的
nutgall [ˈnʌtgɔːl] *n* 没食子,五倍子
nutmeg [ˈnʌtmeg] *n* 肉豆蔻
nutraceuticals [ˌnjuːtrəˈsjuːtikəlz] *n* 功能性食品
nutrilite [ˈnjuːtrilait] *n* 微量营养素
nutriment [ˈnjuːtrimənt] *n* 营养;营养品,食物 | **~al** [ˌnjuːtriˈmentl] *a* 有营养的,滋养的
nutriology [ˌnjuːtriˈɔlədʒi] *n* 营养学
nutrition [nju(ː)ˈtriʃən] *n* 营养;营养品;肠道喂养 | adequate ~ 适量营养 / total parenteral ~ 胃肠道外全面营养 | **~al** *a* 营养的
nutritionist [nju(ː)ˈtriʃənist] *n* 营养学家
nutritious [nju(ː)ˈtriʃəs] *a* 有营养的,滋养的
nutritive [ˈnjuːtritiv] *a* 营养的,滋养的
nutriture [ˈnjuːtritʃə] *n* 营养状况
nutrix [ˈnjuːtriks] *n* 奶妈,乳母
nutrose [ˈnjuːtrəus] *n* 钠酪蛋白
Nuttallia [nəˈtæliə] (George H. F. Nattall) *n* 纳脱原虫属(即巴贝虫属 Babesia) | ~ equi 马纳脱原虫,马巴贝虫,马梨浆虫 / ~ gibsoni 犬纳脱原虫
nux [nʌks] *n* 【拉】核果,坚果 | ~ moschata 肉豆蔻 / ~ vomica 马钱子,番木鳖(苦味健胃及中枢兴奋药)
nvCJD new variant Crentzfeldt-Jakob disease 新变异型克-雅病
nyacyne [ˈnaiəsain] *n* 新霉素(即 neomycin)
nyad [ˈnaiæd] *n* 稚虫,若虫,蛹
nyctalbuminuria [ˌniktelˌbjuːmiˈnjuəriə] *n* 夜蛋白尿
nyctalgia [nikˈtældʒiə] *n* 夜痛(睡时痛)
nyctalope [ˈniktələup] *n* 夜盲者
nyctalopia [ˌniktəˈləupiə] *n* 夜盲[症](昼视) | **nyctalopic** [ˌniktəˈlɔpik] *a*
nyctaphonia [ˌniktəˈfəuniə] *n* 夜间失声
nycterine [ˈniktərain] *a* 夜间的,夜发的
nyct(o)- [构词成分]夜
nyctohemeral [ˌniktəuˈhemərəl], **nycterohemeral** [ˌniktərəˈhemərəl] *a* 昼夜的
nyctophilia [ˌniktəuˈfiliə] *n* 嗜夜癖
nyctophobia [ˌniktəuˈfəubjə] *n* 黑夜恐怖,黑暗恐怖,恐夜症
nyctophonia [ˌniktəuˈfəuniə] *n* 白昼失声(夜能发声)
nyctotyphlosis [ˌniktəutifˈləusis] *n* 夜盲症(昼视)
nycturia [nikˈtjuəriə] *n* 夜尿症
NYD not yet diagnosed 尚未诊断
Nyhus classification [ˈnaihəs] (Lloyd M. Nyhus) 奈赫斯分类法(根据对腹股沟管内环的损坏或腹股沟三角内缺损的一种腹股沟疝分类法)

nylestriol [nai'lestriɔl] *n* 羟炔雌醚(雌激素)
nylidrin hydrochloride ['nilidrin] 盐酸布酚宁(周围血管扩张药)
nymph [nimf] *n* 若虫,蛹
nympha ['nimfə] ([复] **nymphae** ['nimfiː]) *n* 【拉】小阴唇
nymphectomy [nim'fektəmi] *n* 小阴唇切除术
nymphitis [nim'faitis] *n* 小阴唇炎
nympho- [构词成分]小阴唇
nymphocaruncular [ˌnimfəukə'rʌŋkjulə] *a* 小阴唇处女膜痕的
nymphohymeneal [ˌnimfəuhai'meniəl] *a* 小阴唇处女膜的
nymphomania [ˌnimfəu'meinjə] *n* 慕男狂 | **~c** [ˌnimfəu'meiniæk] *a* 慕男狂的 *n* 慕男狂者
nymphoncus [nim'fɔŋkəs] *n* 小阴唇肿
nymphotomy [nim'fɔtəmi] *n* 小阴唇切开术;阴蒂切开术
Nyssen-van Bogaert syndrome ['naisen vɑːn 'bəugɛət] (René Nyssen; Ludo van Bogaert) 奈森-范博格特综合征,异染性脑白质营养不良(成年型)
Nyssorhynchus [ˌnisəu'riŋkəs] *n* 刺蚊亚属(按蚊属)
nystagmic [nis'tægmik] *a* 眼球震颤的
nystagmograph [nis'tægməgrɑːf] *n* 眼球震颤描记器,眼震[颤]描记仪
nystagmoid [nis'tægmɔid], **nystagmiform** [nis'tægmifɔːm] *a* 眼球震颤样的
nystagmus [nis'tægməs] *n* 眼球震颤,眼震[颤] | aural ~ 耳源性眼球震颤 / caloric ~ 温热性眼球震颤 / end-position ~ 终位性眼球震颤 / fixation ~ 凝视性眼球震颤 / head ~ 旋转性头震颤(动物) / lateral ~ 摆动性眼球震颤 / ocular ~ 眼性眼球震颤 / palatal ~ 腭震颤,腭帆提肌痉挛 / paretic ~ 不全麻痹性眼球震颤 / rhythmical ~, resilient ~, jerking ~ 律动性眼球震颤 / undulatory ~, vibratory ~, oscillating ~ 振动性眼球震颤 / vestibular ~, labryrinthine ~ 前庭性眼球震颤,迷路性眼球震颤 / visual ~ 视觉性眼球震颤
nystagmus-myoclonus [nis'tægməs mai'ɔklənəs] *n* 眼球震颤肌阵挛症
nystatin ['nistətin] *n* 制霉菌素(抗生素类药)
nystaxis [nis'tæksis] *n* 眼球震颤,眼震
Nysten's law [nis'tɑːŋ] (Pierre H. Nysten) 奈斯当定律(尸僵定律,即尸僵最先出现于咀嚼肌,次为脸部和颈部肌肉,再则为上躯干和手臂肌肉,最后为腿和足肌肉)
nyxis ['niksis] *n* 穿刺术

O

O oxygen 氧；ohne Hauch O 型［菌］
O. octarius【拉】品脱；oculus【拉】眼
o- ortho 正邻
o omicron 希腊语的第 15 个字母
Ω 希腊语大写字母 omega；ohm 欧姆
ω omega 希腊语第 24 个字母；角频率（angular frequency）或角速度（angular velocity）的符号
ω- 末位的（离主要功能基最远的碳原子的符号，如 ω-oxidation）
OA ocular albunism 眼白化病 | OA1 ocular albunism, type 1 眼白化病 1 型 / OA2 ocular albunism, type 2 眼白化病 2 型（见 Forsius-Eriksson syndrome）
OAE otoacoustic emission 耳声发射
OAF osteoclast activating factor 破骨细胞激活因子
oaf［əuf］*n* 白痴；精神发育不全者
oak［əuk］*n* 栎树，橡树 | poison ~ 槲叶毒葛
oakum［'əukəm］*n* 麻絮（过去用于制作外科敷料）
OAP vincristine, ara-C, and prednisone 长春新碱-阿糖胞苷-泼尼松（联合化疗治癌方案）
oari(o)- 以 oari(o)-起始的词，同样见以 oophor(o)-和 ovari(o)-起始的词
oasis［əu'eisis］（［复］**oases**［əu'eisiːz］）*n*（沙漠中的）绿洲；健岛（病变区中的健康组织）
OAT ornithine aminotransferase 鸟氨酸转氨酶
oat［aut］*n* 燕麦
oath［əuθ］*n* 誓言 | ~ of Hippocrates, hippocratic ~ 希波克拉底誓言（关于医生道德的一段誓词）
oatmeal［'əutmiːl］*n* 燕麦片 | colloidal ~ 胶体燕麦片（皮肤病学制剂中用作润滑剂）
OB obstetrics 产科学
obcecation［ˌɔbsi'keiʃən］*n* 部分盲
obducent［ɔb'djuːsnt］*a* 覆盖的
obduction［ɔb'dʌkʃən］*n* 尸体解剖，尸体剖验
obedience［ə'biːdjəns］*n* 服从 | passive ~ 被动服从
obedient［ə'biːdjənt］*a* 服从的
O'Beirne's sphincter［əu'bɛən］（James O'Beirne）奥贝恩括约肌（在乙状结肠与直肠连接处的大肠壁内的环状肌纤维）
obeliad［əu'biːliæd］*ad* 向顶孔间点
obelion［əu'biːliən］*n* 顶孔间点 | **obeliac**［əu'biːliæk］*a*
Obermayer's test［'ɔːbəˌmaiə］（Friedrich Obermayer）奥伯梅尔试验（检尿蓝母）
Obermüller's test［'ɔːbəmilə］（Kuno Obermüller）奥伯米勒试验（检胆固醇）
Ober's operation［'əubə］（Frank R. Ober）奥伯手术（关节囊切开术）| ~ test（sign）奥伯试验（征）（患者卧于左侧，左大腿与小腿均屈曲，检查者提患者右腿使之外展并伸直，若检查者突然放手，患者右腿仍保持原位而不落，则有股筋膜张肌挛缩及阔筋膜挛缩的现象）
Oberst's method［'ɔːbəst］（Maximilian Oberst）奥伯斯特法（皮下结缔组织内注射盐水或蒸馏水所产生的局部麻醉法）
obese［əu'biːs］*a* 过度肥胖的，肥大的
obesitas［əu'biːsitəs］*n*【拉】肥胖，多脂
obesity［əu'biːsəti］*n* 肥胖［症］| adult-onset ~, hypertrophic ~ 成年型肥胖症 / exogenous ~, alimentary ~, simple ~ 外源性肥胖症，饮食性肥胖症，单纯性肥胖症 / hyperinsulinar ~ 胰岛功能亢进性肥胖症 / hyperinterrenal ~ 肾上腺皮质功能亢进性肥胖症 / hyperplasmic ~ 原生质增生性肥胖症 / hypogonad ~ 性腺功能减退性肥胖症 / hypoplasmic ~ 原生质减少性肥胖症 / hypothyroid ~ 甲状腺功能减退性肥胖症 / life-long ~, hyperplastic-hypertrophic ~ 终身性肥胖症 / morbid ~ 病态肥胖症
obesogenous［əubiː'sɔdʒinəs］*a* 致肥胖的
Obesumbacterium［əuˌbiːsəmbæk'tiəriəm］*n* 脂肝菌属
obex［'əubeks］*n*【拉】闩（脑）
obidoxime chloride［əubi'dɔksiːm］双复磷（胆碱酯酶复活药，解毒药）
objective［əb'dʒektiv］*a* 客观的；真实的；对象的，他觉的 *n* 目标，目的；物镜 | achromatic ~ 消色差物镜 / apochromatic ~ 全消色差物镜 / dry ~ 干物镜 / flat field ~ 平视野物镜 / fluorite ~ 萤石物镜 / immersion ~ 油［浸物］镜 / semiapochromatic ~ 半复消色差物镜
obliquity［ə'blikwəti］*n* 倾斜，斜度 | ~ of pelvis 骨盆斜度
obliquus［əb'laikwəs］*a*【拉】斜的，倾斜的 *n* 斜肌
obliterate［ə'blitəreit］*vt* 涂抹；消灭，使消失
obliteration［əˌblitə'reiʃən］*n* 消灭，消失（因疾病、变性、外科手术、照射法等使之完全消除）|

cortical ~ 脑皮质消失,皮质色素缺乏(大脑皮质区神经节细胞消失)
oblongatal [ˌɔblɔŋ'geitl] *a* 延髓的
obmutescence [ˌɔbmjuː'tesns] *n* 失音,失声 | **obmutescent** *a*
obnubilation [ɔbˌnjuːbi'leiʃən] *n* 神志不清,意识混浊
O'Brien akinesia [əu'braiən] (Cecil S. O'Brien) 奥布赖恩运动不能(直接在第七脑神经眶支上注射麻醉液所产生的眼轮匝肌麻痹,使眼球有较佳的外露)
observer [əb'zəːvə] *n* 观察者 | participant ~ 参与观察者
observerscope [əb'zəːvəskəup] *n* 双臂内镜(两人用内镜),示教窥镜
obsession [əb'seʃən] *n* 强迫症,强迫观念 | **obsessive** [əb'sesiv] *a* 强迫[症]的
obsessive-compulsive [əb'sesiv kəm'pʌlsiv] *a* 强迫观念与行为的
obsolescent [ˌɔbsəu'lesnt] *a* 逐渐被废弃的,逐渐过时的;废退的 | **obsolescence** *n*
obsolete ['ɔbsəliːt] *a* 已废弃的;已不用的;(器官)不明显的;不发育的,废退的
obstetrics [əb'stetriks] *n* 产科学 | **obstetric(al)** *a* 产科学的,产科的 / **obstetrician** [ˌɔbste'triʃən] *n* 产科医师
obstinacy ['ɔbstinəsi] *n* (病痛等)难治
obstinate ['ɔbstinit] *a* 难治的
obstipation [ˌɔbsti'peiʃən] *n* 顽强便秘
obstruct [əb'strʌkt] *vt* 妨碍,阻塞
obstruction [əb'strʌkʃən] *n* 阻塞,梗阻 | false colonic ~ 假性结肠梗阻 / intestinal ~ 肠梗阻 / laryngeal ~ 喉阻塞
obstructive [əb'strʌktiv] *a* 妨碍的;引起阻塞的,阻塞性的 | **~ly** *ad*
obstruent ['ɔbstruənt] *a* 梗阻的,阻塞的 *n* 止泻药
obtundation [ˌɔbtən'deiʃən] *n* 意识模糊
obtundent [ɔb'tʌndənt] *a* 使感觉迟钝的;止痛的 *n* 缓和药,安抚药
obturate ['ɔbtjuəreit] *vt* 封闭,充填,填塞
obturation [ˌɔbtjuə'reiʃən] *n* 充填,填塞;闭塞(肠梗阻的一种) | canal ~ 根管充填
obturator ['ɔbtjuəˌreitə] *n* 【拉】充填器,填塞器,充填体;闭孔肌;闭孔
OCA oculocutaneous albunism 眼皮肤白化病
occipital [ɔk'sipit] *a* 枕骨的,枕部的
occipitalis [ɔkˌsipi'teilis] *a* 枕的;枕骨的 *n* 【拉】枕部
occipitalization [ɔkˌsipitəlai'zeiʃən,-li'z-] *n* 寰枕骨性接合,寰[椎]枕骨化
occipitoanterior [ɔkˌsipitəuæn'tiəriə] *a* 枕前位(胎位)
occipitoatloid [ɔkˌsipitəu'ætlɔid] *a* 枕寰的
occipitoaxoid [ɔkˌsipitəu'æksɔid] *a* 枕枢的
occipitobasilar [ɔkˌsipitəu'bæsilə] *a* 枕部颅底的
occipitobregmatic [ɔkˌsipitəubreg'mætik] *a* 枕部前囟的
occipitocalcarine [ɔkˌsipitəu'kælkərain] *a* 枕叶禽距的
occipitocervical [ɔkˌsipitəu'səːvikəl] *a* 枕颈的
occipitofacial [ɔkˌsipitəu'feiʃəl] *a* 枕[部颜]面的
occipitofrontal [ɔkˌsipitəu'frʌntl] *a* 枕额的
occipitofrontalis [ɔkˌsipitəufrʌn'teilis] *a* 枕额的 *n* 枕额肌
occipitomastoid [ɔkˌsipitəu'mæstɔid] *a* 枕乳突的
occipitomental [ɔkˌsipitəu'ment] *a* 枕颏的
occipitoparietal [ɔkˌsipitəupə'raiitl] *a* 枕顶的
occipitoposterior [ɔkˌsipitəupɔs'tiəriə] *a* 枕后位(胎位)
occipitotemporal [ɔkˌsipitəu'tempərəl] *a* 枕颞的
occipitothalamic [ɔkˌsipitəuθə'læmik] *a* 枕叶丘脑的
occlude [ɔ'kluːd] *vt* 闭塞,闭合 *vi* 殆,咬合
occluder [ɔ'kluːdə] *n* 殆器,咬合器
occlusal [ɔ'kluːsəl] *a* 闭合的;殆[面]的,咬合[面]的
occlusion [ɔ'kluːʒən] *n* 闭塞,阻塞,闭合;吸留;殆,咬合 | abnormal ~ 异常殆 / acentric ~, eccentric ~ 非正[中]殆 / anatomic ~ 解剖性咬合 / anterior ~, protrusive ~ 前殆,前伸殆 / capsular ~ 肾被囊[肾]固定术 / centric ~, central ~ 正中殆 / coronary ~ 冠状动脉闭塞 / distal ~, postnormal ~ 远中殆,错后殆 / edge-to-edge ~, end-to-end ~ 对刃殆 / enteromesenteric ~ 肠肠系膜栓塞 / functional ~ 功能性殆 / labial ~ 唇[向]殆 / mesial ~, prenormal ~ 近中殆,错前殆 / normal ~, neutral ~ 正常殆,中性殆 / ~ of pupil 瞳孔膜闭 / retrusive ~ 后退殆 / traumatic ~, hyperfunctional 创伤性殆,过用殆 / traumatogenic ~ 致创伤性殆 | **occlusive** [ɔ'kluːsiv] *a*
occlusocervical [ɔˌkluːsəu'səːvikəl] *a* 殆颈的,咬合颈的
occlusometer [ˌɔklu'sɔmitə] *n* 殆力计,咬合力计,下颌动力计
occlusorehabilitation [ɔˌkluːsəuˌriːhəˌbili'teiʃən] *n* 殆关系恢复法,咬合关系恢复法
Occlusosporida [ɔˌkluːsəu'spɔːridə] *n* 闭合孢子虫目
occult [ɔ'kʌlt] *a* 隐的,隐伏的,潜隐的
occupancy ['ɔkjupənsi] *n* 存留期间(指用一种特殊方法给予的单位量的物质,在被排出或破坏之前,存留于身体或占有身体某一部分的期间)

OCD obsessive-compulsive disorder 强迫障碍
oceanic [ˌəuʃiˈænik] *a* 海洋的
Oceanospirillum [ˌəuʃiˌeinəuspiˈriləm] *n* 海洋螺菌属
ocellus [əuˈseləs] ([复] **ocelli** [əuˈselai]) *n* 【拉】单眼(昆虫及其他无脊椎动物的);眼点(昆虫复眼内的);眼样色斑 | **ocellar** *a*
ochlesis [ɔkˈliːsis] *n* 拥挤病
ochlophobia [ˌɔkləuˈfəubjə] *n* 人群恐怖,恐群症
ochratoxicosis [ˌəukrəˌtɔksiˈkəusis] *n* 赭曲[毒素]中毒症
ochratoxin [ˈəukrəˌtɔksin] *n* 赭曲毒素
Ochrobium [əuˈkrəubiəm] *n* 赭菌属 | ~ tectum 遮盖赭菌
ochrometer [əuˈkrɔmitə] *n* 毛细管血压计
Ochromonadidae [ˌɔkrəməˈnædidiː] *n* 赭球虫科
Ochromyia [ˌəukrəˈmaijə] *n* 瘤蝇属(即 Cordylobia)
ochronosis [ˌəukrəˈnəusis], **ochronosus** [ˌəukrəˈnəusəs] *n* 褐黄病 | **ochronotic** [ˌəukrəˈnɔtik] *a*
Ochsner's muscle [ˈɔksnə] (Albert J. Ochsner)奥克斯纳肌(胆总管口末端十二指肠肌的肌增厚) | ~ ring 奥克斯纳环(入胆总管的胰管口环形黏膜增厚) / ~ treatment 奥克斯纳疗法(禁食、抽胃液、肛门插管排气以减少肠蠕动,促使腹膜粘连的一种阑尾炎疗法)
Ocimum [ˈɔsiməm] *n* 罗勒属
ocrylate [ˈɔkrileit] *n* 奥克立酯(组织黏合剂)
OCT ornithine carbamoyltransferase 鸟氨酸氨甲酰基转移酶; oxytocin challenge test 催产素激惹试验
octa- [构词成分]八
octabenzone [ˌɔktəˈbenzəun] *n* 奥他苯酮(防晒药)
octacosane [ˌɔktəˈkəusein] *n* 二十八[碳]烷
octacosanol [ˌɔktəkəuˈseinɔl] *n* 二十八[烷]醇
octadecanoate [ˌɔktəˌdekəˈnəueit] *n* 十八酸盐,硬脂酸盐(stearate 的系统名)
octadecanoic acid [ˌɔktəˌdekəˈnəuik] 十八[烷]酸,硬脂酸
octamethyl pyrophosphoramide [ˌɔktəˈmeθil ˌpaiərəufɔsˈfɔrəmaid] 八甲磷胺(胆碱酯酶抑制药,用作杀虫药)
octamylose [ɔkˈtæmiləus] *n* 八聚淀粉糖
octan [ˈɔktən] *a* 每八日[再发]的
octane [ˈɔktein] *n* 辛烷
octanoic acid [ˌɔktəˈnəuik] 辛酸(抗真菌药)
octapeptide [ˌɔktəˈpeptaid] *n* 八肽
octaploid [ˈɔktəplɔid] *a* 八倍体的 *n* 八倍体(具有八组染色体的个体或细胞) | ~**y** *n* 八倍性
octarius [ɔkˈtɛəriəs] *n* 【拉】品脱(一加仑的八分之一,英制 1 pt = 0.568 L,美制 1 pt = 0.55 L)
octavalent [ˌɔktəˈveilənt] *a* 八价的
octave [ˈɔktiv, ˈɔkteiv] *n* 倍频程,八度音
octazamide [ɔkˈteizəmaid] *n* 奥他酰胺(镇痛药)
octet [ˈɔktet] *n* 八隅体,八角体(指一组相同的或相似的物体,如一个原子核外壳的八个电子群)
octicizer [ˌɔktiˈsaizə] *n* 2-乙基己二苯酯磷酸(药物制剂的增塑剂)
octigravida [ˌɔktiˈgrævidə] *n* 第八次孕妇
octinoxate [ɔkˈtinɔkseit] *n* 奥克丁酯(防晒药)
octipara [ɔkˈtipərə] *n* 八产妇
octisalate [ˌɔktiˈsæleit] *n* 辛水杨酸(防晒药)
octocrylene [ˈɔktəuˌkriliːn] *n* 奥克立林(防晒药)
octodrine [ˈɔktədriːn] *n* 奥托君(肾上腺素能药,具有血管收缩和局部麻醉作用)
octofollin [ˌɔktəˈfɔlin] *n* 辛[烷]雌酚,苯雌酚
Octomitus [ɔkˈtɔmitəs] *n* 微小鞭毛虫属(即六鞭虫属 Hexamita) | ~ hominis 人微小鞭毛虫(即人毛滴虫 Trichomonas hominis)
Octomyces etiennei [ˌɔktəuˈmaisiːz etiˈenei] 酵母菌样丝状菌
octopamine [ˌɔktəˈpæmiːn] *n* 酚乙醇胺(升压药)
octopus [ˈɔktəpəs] *n* 章鱼 | blue-ringed ~ 蓝环章鱼
octose [ˈɔktəus] *n* 辛糖
octoxynol 9 [ɔkˈtɔksinɔl] 辛苯昔醇-9(药物制剂时用作表面活性剂,亦称辛基苯氧聚乙氧基乙醇)
octreotide [ɔkˈtriːətaid] *n* 奥曲肽(一种合成的生长激素〈somatostatin〉类似物,其作用与生长激素相同,但药效时间长,其醋酸盐用作治疗佐剂,以便姑息性治疗伴有胃肠道内分泌肿瘤的腹泻以及姑息性治疗胰腺瘤时高胰岛素血症的症状,肢端肥大症时用以减少生长激素分泌) | ~ acetate 醋酸奥曲肽
octriptyline phosphate [ɔkˈtriptiliːn] 磷酸奥克替林(抗抑郁药)
octyl [ˈɔktil] *n* 辛基 | ~ methoxycinnamate 甲氧基肉桂酸辛酯(即 octinoxate) / ~ salicylate 水杨酸辛酯(即 octisalate)
octylphenoxy polyethoxyethanol [ˌɔktilfiˈnɔksi ˌpɔlieˌθɔksiˈeθənɔl] 辛基苯氧聚乙氧基乙醇,辛苯昔醇-9
ocufilcon [ˌɔkjuˈfilkɔn] *n* 奥费尔康(三种亲水接触镜材料 A、B 或 C 任何一种)
ocular [ˈɔkjulə] *a* 眼的 *n* 目镜
oculentum [ˌɔkjuˈlentəm] ([复] **oculenta** [ˌɔkjuˈlentə]) *n* 眼膏
oculi [ˈɔkjulai] oculus 的复数
oculist [ˈɔkjulist] *n* 眼科医师
oculistics [ˌɔkjuˈlistiks] *n* 眼科治疗学
ocul(o)- [构词成分]眼
oculocephalogyric [ˌɔkjuləuˌsefələuˈdʒaiərik] *a*

眼头运动(反射)的
oculocutaneous [ˌɔkjuləukju(ː)ˈteinjəs] *a* 眼[与]皮的
oculofacial [ˌɔkjuləuˈfeiʃəl] *a* 眼面的
oculogyration [ˌɔkjuləudʒaiəˈreiʃən] *n* 眼球转动
oculogyria [ˌɔkjuləuˈdʒaiəriə] *n* 眼球转动 | **oculogyric** *a*
oculomandibulodyscephaly [ˌɔkjuləumænˌdibjuləˈdiˈsefəli] *n* 眼下颌颅面骨畸形
oculometroscope [ˌɔkjuləuˈmetrəskəup] *n* 转动检眼镜
oculomotor [ˌɔkjuləuˈməutə] *a* 眼球运动的,动眼的
oculomotorius [ˌɔkjuləuməuˈtɔːriəs] *n*【拉】动眼神经
oculomycosis [ˌɔkjuləumaiˈkəusis] *n* 眼真菌病
oculonasal [ˌɔkjuləuˈneizəl] *a* 眼鼻的
oculopathy [ˌɔkjuˈlɔpəθi] *n* 眼病 | pituitarigenic ~ 垂体性眼病
oculopupillary [ˌɔkjuləuˈpjuːpiləri] *a* 瞳孔的
oculoreaction [ˌɔkjuləuri(ː)ˈækʃən] *n* 眼反应
oculospinal [ˌɔkjuləuˈspain] *a* 眼[与]脊髓的
oculozygomatic [ˌɔkjuləuˌzaigəˈmætik] *a* 眼颧的
oculus [ˈɔkjuləs] ([复] **oculi** [ˈɔkjulai]) *n*【拉】眼
OD[1] oculus dexter【拉】右眼
OD[2] optical density 光密度;Doctor of Optometry 视力测定术博士,验光术博士;outside diameter 外径;overdose 过量
ODA occipito-dextra anterior 枕右前(胎位)
odaxesmus [ˌəudækˈsezməs] *n* 龈痒;咬舌,唇舌咬破(癫痫发作时)
odaxetic [ˌəudækˈsetik] *a* 龈痒的;咬舌的
ODC orotidine 5ˈ-phosphate decarboxylase 乳清酸核苷 5ˈ-磷酸脱羧酶
odd [ɔd] *a* 奇数的;单只的;带零头的;临时的;额外的;奇特的 | **~ly** *ad*
Oddi's muscle (sphincter) [ˈɔdiː] (Ruggero Oddi)奥迪括约肌(胆道口括约肌,或当壶腹存在时,表示此肌与肝胰管壶腹括约肌组合)
odditis [ɔˈdaitis] *n* 胆道口括约肌炎
odogenesis [ˌɔdəˈdʒenisis] *n* 神经分支新生
odograph [ˈəudəgrɑːf,-græf] *n* 自动计程仪;计步器
odon-eki [ˌəudɔn ˈeki] *n*【日】黄疸疫,传染性黄疸(一种类似螺旋体黄疸的疾病)
odontalgia [ˌɔdɔnˈtældʒiə] *n* 牙痛 | **odontalgic** *a*
odontectomy [ˌɔdɔnˈtekəmi] *n* 牙切除术,拔牙
odontiatria [ɔˌdɔntiˈætriə] *n* 牙科[治疗]学
odontiatrogenic [ɔˌdɔntiˌætrəˈdʒenik] *a* 牙科医源性的
odontic [ɔˈdɔntik] *a* 牙的
odont(o)- [构词成分]牙,齿
odontoameloblastoma [ɔˌdɔntəuˌæmələublæsˈtəumə] *n* 成牙釉质细胞瘤,釉质母细胞牙瘤
odontoblast [ɔˈdɔntəblæst] *n* 成牙质细胞 | **~ic** [ɔˌdɔntəˈblæstik] *a*
odontoblastoma [ɔˌdɔntəblæsˈtəumə] *n* 成牙质细胞瘤
odontobothrion [ɔˌdɔntəuˈbɔθriən] *n* 牙槽
odontobothritis [ɔˌdɔntəubɔˈθraitis] *n* 牙槽炎
odontoclamis [ɔˌdɔntəuˈkleimis] *n* 龈裹牙
odontoclast [ɔˈdɔntəklæst] *n* 破牙质细胞
odontogen [ɔˈdɔntədʒən] *n* 牙质原
odontogenesis [ɔˌdɔntəuˈdʒenisis] *n* 牙发生,牙生成 | ~ imperfecta 牙生长不全 | **odontogeny** [ˌɔdɔnˈtɔdʒini] *n* / **odontogenetic** [ɔˌdɔntəudʒiˈnetik] *a*
odontogenic [ɔˌdɔntəuˈdʒenik] *a* 生牙的;牙源性的
odontogenous [ˌɔdɔnˈtɔdʒinəs] *a* 牙源性的
odontogram [ɔˈdɔntəgræm] *n* 牙面描记图
odontograph [ɔˈdɔntəgrɑːf,-græf] *n* 牙面描记器 | **~y** [ˌɔdɔnˈtɔgrəfi] *n* 牙体形态学;牙面描记法
odontoiatria [ɔˌdɔntəuaiˈætriə] *n* 牙科[治疗]学,牙医学
odontoid [ɔˈdɔntɔid] *a* 牙样的,牙形的
odontolith [ɔˈdɔntəliθ] *n* 牙垢,牙积石
odontolithiasis [ɔˌdɔntəuliˈθaiəsis] *n* 牙垢症,牙石症
odontology [ˌɔdɔnˈtɔlədʒi] *n* 牙科学 | **odontological** [ˌɔdɔntəuˈlɔdʒikəl] *a* / **odontologist** *n* 牙医师
odontolysis [ɔdɔnˈtɔlisis] *n* 牙质崩解,牙质吸收
odontoma [ɔdɔnˈtəumə] *n* 牙瘤 | composite ~ 复质牙瘤 / coronal ~, coronary ~ 连冠牙瘤 / radicular ~ 连根牙瘤
odontonomy [ˌɔdɔnˈtɔnəmi] *n* 牙科学名词,牙名词学
odontopathy [ˌɔdɔnˈtɔpəθi] *n* 牙病 | **odontopathic** [ɔˌdɔntəuˈpæθik] *a*
odontoperiosteum [ɔˌdɔntəuˌperiˈɔstiəm] *n* 牙周膜
odontophobia [ɔˌdɔntəuˈfəubjə] *n* 恐牙症,牙科手术恐怖症
odontoplasty [ɔˈdɔntəˌplæsti], **odontorthosis** [ɔˌdɔntɔːˈθəusis] *n* 正牙学,正牙法
odontoprisis [ɔˌdɔntəuˈpraisis] *n* 磨牙,咬牙,牙摩擦
odontoradiograph [ɔˌdɔntəuˈreidiəugrɑːf,-græf] *n* 牙 X 线[照]片
odontoschism [ɔˈdɔntəskizəm] *n* 牙裂,牙裂隙

odontoscopy [ˌɔdɔnˈtɔskəpi] *n* 牙印检查
odontoseisis [ɔˌdɔntəuˈsaisis] *n* 牙松动
odontosis [ˌɔdɔnˈtəusis] *n* 出牙;牙发生
Odontostomatida [ˌɔdɔntəuˌstəuməˈtaidə] *n* 齿口目
odontotechny [ɔˈdɔntəˌtekni] *n* 牙科技术学,牙医学
odontotheca [ɔˌdɔntəuˈθiːkə] *n* 牙囊
odontotomy [ˌɔdɔnˈtɔtəmi] *n* 牙造洞术,牙切开术
odontotripsis [ɔˌdɔntəuˈtripsis] *n* 牙磨损,牙磨耗症
odorant [ˈəudərənt] *n* 臭气物质 *a* 臭的;香的
odoratism [ˌəudəˈreitizəm] *n* 香[豌]豆中毒(实验动物)
odoriferous [ˌəudəˈrifərəs] *a* 散发气味的,有香气的,香的;发臭味的,臭的
odorimeter [ˌəudəˈrimitə] *n* 气味测量计 | **odorimetry** *n* 气味测量法
odoriphore [əuˈdɔːrifɔː] *n* 生臭基,生臭团
odorivector [ˌəudəriˈvektə] *n* 发香质
odorography [ˌəudəˈrɔgrəfi] *n* 气味论
odorous [ˈəudərəs] *a* 有气味的;香的;臭的
odo(u)r [ˈəudə] *n* 气味;香气;臭气 | butcher shop ~ 肉店气味(黄热病患者发出的气味) / minimal identifiable ~ 最小嗅分辨阈 | **~less** *a* 没有气味的
ODP occipito-dextra posterior 枕右后(胎位)
ODT occipito-dextra transversa 枕右横(胎位)
O'Dwyer's tubes [əuˈdwaiə] (Joseph P. O'Dwyer) 奥德外耶管(插管套管)
odynacusis [ˌəudinəˈkuːsis] *n* 听音痛,听声痛
-odynia [构词成分] 痛
odyn(o)- [构词成分] 痛
odynometer [ˌəudiˈnɔmitə] *n* 痛觉计
odynophagia [ˌɔdinəuˈfeidʒiə], **odynphagia** [ˌəudinˈfeidʒiə]*n* 吞咽痛
oe-以 oe-起始的词,同样见以 e-起始的词
Oeciacus [iːˈsaiəkəs] *n* 燕臭虫属
oedema [i(ː)ˈdiːmə] *n* 水肿(即 edema)
oedipism [ˈiːdipizəm] *n* 眼自伤(即 edipism)
Oedipus complex [ˈiːdipəs] (Oedipus 为希腊传说中的人物,由养父母抚养,以后违心地杀父娶母)俄迪浦斯情结,恋母情结
Oehler's symptom [ˈiːlə] (Johannes Oehler) 厄勒症状(间歇性跛行症时足部发冷及苍白)
Oehl's muscle [ɔːl] (Eusebio Oehl)奥勒肌(左房室瓣腱索内的肌纤维)
Oenanthe [iːˈnænθi] *n* 水芹属
oenanthol [iːˈnænθɔl] *n* 庚醛
oenanthylic acid [iːnænˈθilik] 庚酸
oersted [ˈəːsted] (Hans C. Oersted) 奥[斯特](旧磁场强度单位,现用安[培]每米,1 Oe ≙ 79.577 47A/m)
Oertel's treatment [ˈəːtəl] (Max J. Oertel) 厄特尔疗法(运动节食疗法以治心脏病等)
oesophageal [iːˌsɔfəˈdʒi(ː)əl] *a* 食管的(即 esophageal)
oesophag(o)- 以 oesophag(o)-起始的词,同样见以 esophag(o)-起始的词
oesophagostomiasis [iːˌsɔfəgəustəˈmaiəsis] *n* 结节线虫病
Oesophagostomum [iːˌsɔfəˈgɔstəməm] *n* 结节线虫属 | ~ bifurcum, ~ apiostomum, ~ brumpti 猴结节线虫 / ~ brevicaudum, ~ suis 短尾结节线虫 / ~ columbianum 哥伦比亚结节线虫 / ~ dentatum 有齿结节线虫 / ~ longicaudum 长尾结节线虫 / ~ radiatum, ~ inflatum 辐射结节线虫,牛结节线虫 / ~ stephanostomum 猩猩结节线虫
oesophagus [iːˈsɔfəgəs] *n* 食管,食道(即 esophagus)
oestr- 以 oestr-起始的词,同样见以 estr-起始的词
Oestreicher's reaction [ˈiːstraiʃə] (A. Oestreicher) 伊斯特赖歇尔反应,黄嘌呤醇反应(xanthydrol reaction, 见 reaction 项下相应术语)
oestriasis [esˈtraiəsis] *n* 狂蝇蛆病
Oestridae [ˈestrədiː] *n* 狂蝇科
oestrogen [ˈiːstrədʒən, ˈes-] *n* 雌激素(即 estrogen)
oestrone [ˈiːstrəun, ˈes-] *n* 雌酮(即 estrone)
Oestrus [ˈestrəs] *n* 狂蝇属 | ~ ovis, ~ hominis 羊狂蝇,人体狂蝇
oestrus [ˈiːstrəs, ˈes-], **oestrum** [ˈiːstrəm, ˈes-] *n* 动情期(即 estrus, estrum) | **oestrous** [ˈiːstrəs, ˈes-], **oestrual** [ˈiːstruəl, ˈes-] *a* (即 estrous, estrual)
OFD oral-facial-digital 口-面-指(趾)(综合征)
office [ˈɔfis] *n* 办公室,办事处;职务 | admission ~ 入院处
ofloxacin [əˈflɔksəsin] *n* 氧氟沙星(广谱抗菌药)
Ogata's method [ɔˈgɑːtə] (M. Ogata, 绪方正清) 绪方[氏]法(击胸以刺激呼吸的一种方法)
ogee [ˈəudʒiː] *n*, *a* S 形曲线(的)
Ogilvie's syndrome [ˈəugilvi] (William H. Ogilvie)奥吉尔维综合征(一种类似梗阻引起的结肠膨胀,但无机械性梗阻的证据,常由于交感神经供应缺陷所致。亦称假性结肠梗阻)
ogive [ˈəudʒaiv] *n* S 形曲线(用于生物统计学)
ogo [ˈəugəu] *n* 毁形性鼻咽炎
Ogston's line [ˈɔgstn] (Alexander Ogston) 奥格斯顿线(从股骨结节至髁间切迹的线) | ~ operation 奥格斯顿手术(①膝外翻的股骨内髁切除术;②矫正扁平足弓的跗骨楔状切除术)

OGTT oral glucose tolerance test 口服葡萄糖耐量试验
Oguchi's disease [ɔ'gutʃi] (Chuta Oguchi, 小口忠太)小口[氏]病(见于日本的一种先天性夜盲症)
Ohara's disease [ɔ'hɑːrə] (Hachiro Ohara 大原八郎)大原[氏]病(日本兔热病)
OH-Cbl hydroxocobalamin 羟钴胺,维生素 B_{12a}
17-OHCS 17-hydroxycorticosteroid 17-羟皮质类固醇
ohm(Ω) [əum] *n* 欧[姆](电阻单位)
ohmammeter ['əumæ,miːtə] *n* 欧安计
ohmmeter ['əum,miːtə] *n* 欧姆计
Ohm's law [əum] (George S. Ohm)欧姆定律(电流强度的改变与电动势成正比,与电阻成反比)
ohne Hauch ['ɔːne hauh]【德】O 型(菌)
OI osteogenesis imperfecta 成骨不全
OIC osteogenesis imperfecta congenita 先天性成骨不全
-oid [后缀]…样的,…状的,如…的
Oidiomycetes [əu,idiəumai'siːtiːz] *n* 念珠菌类,卵丝真菌类
oidiomycosis [əu,idiəumai'kəusis] *n* 念珠菌病 | **oidiomycotic** [əu,idiəumai'kɔtik] *a*
Oidium [əu'idiəm] *n* 卵状菌属(旧名),念珠菌属;粉孢属
oidium [əu'idiəm] *n* 粉孢子
OIH orthoiodohippurate 邻碘马尿酸盐
oikoid ['ɔikɔid] *n* 红细胞基质
oikosite ['ɔikəsait] *n* 定居寄生物
oil [ɔil] *n* 油 | almond ~ 扁桃[仁]油 / bergamot ~ 香柠檬油,香柑油 / betula ~, wintergreen ~ 桦木油,冬绿油,水杨酸甲酯 / cade ~ 杜松焦油 / camphorated ~ 樟脑油,樟脑擦剂 / caraway ~ 藏茴香油,贲蒿油 / castor ~, ricinus ~ 蓖麻油 / cedar ~ 香柏油,红桧油 / cinnamon ~, cassia ~ 桂皮油 / citronella ~ 香茅油,雄刈萱油 / cod liver ~ 鱼肝油 / coriander ~ 芫荽油,胡荽油 / corn ~ 玉蜀黍油 / cottonseed ~ 棉籽油 / ~ of dill 莳萝油 / drying ~ 干性油 / empyreumatic ~ 干馏油,焦油 / eucalyptus ~ 桉油 / fixed ~, expressed ~, fatty ~ 不挥发油,脂肪油 / halibut liver ~ 庸鲽鱼肝油,大比目鱼肝油 / iodized ~ 碘[化]油(子宫及输卵管 X 线摄影的造影剂) / light white mineral ~ 轻质液状石蜡 / linseed ~, flaxseed ~ 亚麻油 / ~ of male fern 绵马油 / mineral ~ 矿物油,石油;液体石蜡 / ~ of mirbane 硝基苯 / myrcia ~, bay ~ 玉桂油 / myristica ~, nutmeg ~ 肉豆蔻油 / nondestearinated cod liver ~ 硬脂鱼肝油 / olive ~, sweet ~ 齐墩果油,橄榄油 / orange ~ 橙皮油 / peanut ~, arachis ~, groundnut ~ 花生油 / peppermint ~ 欧薄荷油 / pine ~ 松油 / sesame ~, gingilli ~ 麻油,芝麻油 / spearmint ~ 绿薄荷油 / ~ of spike 宽叶熏衣草油 / sweet birch ~ 香桦油,水杨酸甲酯 / theobroma ~ 可可豆油,可可脂 / volatile ~, distilled ~, essential ~ 挥发油 / white mineral ~ 液状石蜡
oily ['ɔili] *a* [含]油的;油状的;浸透油的
oinomania [,ɔinəu'meinjə] *n* 震颤谵妄;纵酒狂;间发性酒狂
ointment ['ɔintmənt] *n* 软膏[剂],油膏 | anthralin 蒽林软膏,蒽三酚软膏(局部抗湿疹药) / bacitracin ~ (枯草)杆菌肽软膏(表面抗菌素) / benzocaine ~, ethyl aminobenzoate ~ 苯佐卡因软膏,氨基苯甲酸乙酯软膏(局部麻醉药) / blue ~ 蓝[色]软膏,弱汞软膏 / chloramphenicol ophthalmic ~ 氯霉素眼膏 / compound resorcinol ~ 复方雷琐辛软膏(局部抗真菌药及角质层分离剂) / hydrocortisone acetate ~ 醋酸氢化可的松软膏(表面肾上腺皮质类固醇) / hydrophilic ~ 亲水性软膏 / ichthammol ~ 鱼石脂软膏(皮肤科制剂) / mild (strong) mercurial ~ 弱(强)汞软膏(表面杀寄生物药) / neomycin sulfate ~ 硫酸新霉素软膏(表面抗细菌药) / thimerosal ~ 硫柳汞软膏(抗菌药) / zinc (oxide) ~ 氧化锌软膏(外用收敛药及保护剂)
Oken's body (corpus) ['ɔːkən] (Lorenz Oken) 中肾 | ~ canal 中肾管
OIT osteogenesis imperfecta tarda 迟缓性成骨不全
O. L. oculus laevus【拉】左眼
Ol. oleum【拉】油
-ol [后缀]醇,酚
OLA occipito-laeva anterior 枕左前(胎位)
olamine ['ɔləmiːn] *n* 乙醇胺,氨基乙醇,胆胺(ethanolamine 的 USAN 缩约词)
olanzapine [əu'lænzəpiːn] *n* 奥氮平(多巴胺受体阻滞药,治疗精神分裂症,并短期治疗双相型障碍躁狂发作,口服给药)
Oldfield's syndrome ['əuldfiːld] (Michael C. Oldfield)奥尔德菲尔德综合征(家族性结肠息肉病,伴有广泛性皮脂囊肿)
Olea ['əuliə] *n* 齐墩果属,洋橄榄属
olea ['əuliə] *n*【拉】齐墩果,洋橄榄;油(oleum 的复数)
oleaginous [,əuli'ædʒinəs] *a* 油脂性的,油状的
oleander [,əuli'ændə] *n* 夹竹桃
oleandomycin phosphate [,əuli'ændə,maisin] 磷酸竹桃霉素(抗生素类药)
oleandrin [,əuli'ændrin] *n* 夹竹桃苷(强心药)
oleandrism [,əuli'ændrizəm] *n* 夹竹桃中毒
oleanol [əu'liːənɔl] *n* 鱼肝油醇
olease ['əulieis] *n* 油酸酶
oleaster [,əuli'æstə] *n* 野生橄榄;胡颓子属植物
oleate ['əulieit] *n* 油酸盐;油酸制剂

olecranal [əuˈlekrənl] *a* 鹰嘴的
olecranarthritis [əuˌlekrənɑːˈθraitis] *n* 肘关节炎
olecranarthrocace [əuˌlekrənɑːˈθrɔkəsi] *n* 肘关节结核
olecranarthropathy [əuˌlekrənɑːˈθrɔpəθi] *n* 肘关节病
olecranoid [əuˈlekrənɔid] *a* 鹰嘴状的
olecranon [əuˈlekrənɔn] *n* 鹰嘴
olefin [ˈəuləfin] *n* 烯[属]烃
olefinic acid [ˌəuləˈfinik] 烯脂酸
oleic [əuˈliːik] *a* 油的 | ~ acid 油酸
olein [ˈəuliin] *n* 甘油三油酸酯,[三]油酸甘油酯
olenitis [əuleˈnaitis] *n* 肘关节炎
ole(o)- [构词成分]油
oleoarthrosis [ˌəuliəuɑːˈθrəusis] *n* 关节注油疗法
oleochrysotherapy [ˌəuliəuˌkrisəuˈθerəpi] *n* 金油疗法
oleocreosote [ˌəuliəuˈkriːəsəut] *n* 油酸木溜油
oleodipalmitin [ˌəuliəudaiˈpælmitin] *n* 一油二棕榈脂,甘油二软脂酸油酸酯
oleodistearin [ˌəuliəudaiˈstiərin] *n* 一油二硬脂,甘油二硬脂酸油酸酯
oleogranuloma [ˌəuliəuˌgrænjuˈləumə], **oleoma** [ˌəuliˈəumə] *n* 石蜡瘤
oleoinfusion [ˌəuliəuinˈfjuːʒən] *n* 油浸剂
oleomargarine [ˌəuliəuˈmɑːdʒərin] *n* 人造奶油,珠脂
oleometer [ˌəuliˈɔmitə] *n* 油纯度计
oleonucleoprotein [ˌəuliəuˌnjuːkliəˈprəutiːn] *n* 油核蛋白,脂酪蛋白
oleopalmitate [ˌəuliəuˈpælmiteit] *n* 油棕榈酸盐
oleoperitoneography [ˌəuliəuˌperitəuniˈɔgrəfi] *n* 碘油腹膜[X线]造影[术]
oleoresin [ˌəuliəuˈrezin] *n* 油树脂 | aspidium ~ 绵马油树脂(驱肠虫药,治肠绦虫感染) / capsicum ~ 辣椒油树脂,辣椒浸膏(刺激剂和祛风药)
oleoresina [ˌəuliəuriˈzainə] ([复] **oleoresinae** [ˌəuliəuriˈzainiː]) *n*【拉】油树脂
oleosaccharum [ˌəuliəuˈsækərəm] *n* 油糖剂
oleostearate [ˌəuliəuˈstiəreit] *n* 油硬脂酸盐
oleosus [ˌəuliˈəusəs] *a*【拉】油润的,油滑的
oleotherapy [ˌəuliəuˈθerəpi] *n* 油疗法
oleothorax [ˌəuliəuˈθɔːræks] *n* [人工]油胸
oleotine [ˌəuliˈəutain] *n* 人造奶油(一种加蛋白胨的油脂)
oleovitamin [ˌəuliəuˈvaitəmin] *n* 维生素油剂 | ~ A 维生素 A 油 / ~ A and D 维生素 A、D 油 / ~ D_2 钙化[甾]醇 / ~ D_3 活化 7-脱氢胆固醇 / synthetic ~ D 合成维生素 D 油
oleoyl [əuˈliːəil] *n* 油酰
oleum [ˈəuliəm] ([复] **olea** [ˈəuliə]) *n*【拉】油
olfact [ˈɔlfækt] *n* 嗅阈值,嗅觉系数(气味单位,最小可嗅量,即物质在溶液中发出的气味可为大多数正常人嗅知的最小浓度)
olfactant [ɔlˈfæktənt] *n* 加臭剂,添味剂
olfactie [ɔlˈfæktiː], **olfacty** [ɔlˈfækti] *n* 嗅距单位(按嗅觉计测定管的距离)
olfaction [ɔlˈfækʃən] *n* 嗅,嗅觉 | **olfactory** *a*
olfactism [ɔlˈfæktizəm] *n* 嗅联觉,牵连嗅觉(指其他感觉刺激引起嗅觉)
olfactology [ˌɔlfækˈtɔlədʒi] *n* 嗅觉学
olfactometer [ˌɔlfækˈtɔmitə] *n* 嗅觉计 | **olfactometric** [ˌɔlfæktəuˈmetrik] *a* 嗅觉测量法的 / **olfactometry** *n* 嗅觉测量法
olfactus [ɔlˈfæktəs] *n* 嗅敏度单位
oligakisuria [ˌɔligækiˈsjuəriə] *n* 尿次[数]减少
oligemia [ˌɔliˈdʒiːmiə] *n* 血量减少 | **oligemic** *a*
oligergasia [ˌɔligəˈgeiziə] *n* 整体反应欠缺(即精神发育不全或低能)
oligergastic [ˌɔligəˈgæstik] *n* (脑)发育不全性精神障碍
olig(o)- [构词成分]少,缺少
oligoamnios [ˌɔligəuˈæmniɔs] *n* 羊水过少
oligoanalgesia [ˌɔligəuˌænəlˈdʒiːziə] *n* 镇痛缺乏(使用镇痛药次数过少或剂量不足以镇痛)
oligoanuria [ˌɔligəuəˈnjuəriə] *n* 少尿,无尿症
oligoarthritis [ˌɔligəuɑːˈθraitis] *n* 少关节炎
oligoasthenospermia [ˌɔligəuˌæsθənəuˈspɜːmiə] *n* 少精子活力不足
oligoastrocytoma [ˌɔligəuˌæstrəusaiˈtəumə] *n* 少星形细胞瘤
oligoblast [ˈɔligəublæst] *n* 成少突神经胶质细胞
oligocardia [ˌɔligəuˈkɑːdiə] *n* 心动过缓
oligochromasia [ˌɔligəukrəuˈmeiziə] *n* 染色过浅,着色不足
oligochromemia [ˌɔligəukrəuˈmiːmiə] *n* 血红蛋白过少
oligoclonal [ˌɔligəuˈkləunəl] *a* 少克隆的
oligocystic [ˌɔligəuˈsistik] *a* 少囊的
oligocythemia [ˌɔligəusaiˈθiːmiə] *n* 红细胞减少[症] | **oligocythemic** [ˌɔligəusaiˈθemik] *a* / **oligocytosis** [ˌɔligəusaiˈtəusis] *n*
oligodactyly [ˌɔligəuˈdæktili] *n* 少指[畸形],少趾[畸形]
oligodendrocyte [ˌɔligəuˈdendrəsait] *n* 少突神经胶质细胞
oligodendroglia [ˌɔligəudenˈdrɔgliə], **oligodendria** [ˌɔligəuˈdendriə] *n* 少突神经胶质
oligodendroglioma [ˌɔligəuˌdendrəuglaiˈəumə], **oligodendroblastoma** [ˌɔligəuˌdendrəublæsˈtəumə] *n* 少突神经胶质瘤,成少突神经胶质细胞瘤
oligodipsia [ˌɔligəuˈdipsiə] *n* 渴感过少

oligodontia [ˌɔligəu'dɔnʃiə] *n* 少牙[畸形]
oligodynamic [ˌɔligəudai'næmik] *a* 微量活动的，微量作用的
oligoencephalon [ˌɔligəuen'sefələn] *n* 脑过小
oligoerythrocythemia [ˌɔligəuiˌriθrəusai'θiːmiə] *n* 红细胞减少[症]
oligogalactia [ˌɔligəugə'lækʃiə] *n* 乳汁减少
oligogenic [ˌɔligəu'dʒenik] *a* 寡基因的，少基因的（指某些遗传性状）
oligogenics [ˌɔligəu'dʒeniks] *n* 节[制生]育
oligoglia [ˌɔli'gɔgliə] *n* 少突神经胶质
oligoglobulia [ˌɔligəuglɔ'bjuːliə] *n* 红细胞减少[症]
oligo-1, 4-1, 4-glucantransferase [ˌɔligəuˌgluːkæn'trænsfəreis] *n* 低聚-1, 4-1, 4-葡聚糖转移酶
oligo-1, 6-glucosidase ['ɔligəu gluː'kəusideis] 低[聚]-1, 6-葡糖苷酶（α-dextrinase 的 EC 命名法）
oligoglucoside [ˌɔligəu'gluːkəsaid] *n* 低聚葡糖苷
oligohemia [ˌɔligəu'hiːmiə] *n* 血量减少
oligohydramnios [ˌɔligəuhai'dræmniɔs] *n* 羊水过少
oligohydruria [ˌɔligəuhai'drjuəriə] *n* 尿过浓，尿[中]水分过少
Oligohymenophorea [ˌɔligəuˌhaiminəu'fɔriə] *n* 寡膜纲
oligohypermenorrhea [ˌɔligəuˌhaipəːˌmenə'riːə] *n* 稀发月经过多（月经稀而量多）
oligohypomenorrhea [ˌɔligəuˌhaipəuˌmenə'riːə] *n* 稀发月经过少（月经稀而量少）
oligolecithal [ˌɔligəu'lesiθəl] *a* 少[卵]黄的
oligoleukocythemia [ˌɔligəuˌljuːkəsai'θiːmiə], **oligoleukocytosis** [ˌɔligəuˌljuːkəsai'təusis] *n* 白细胞减少
oligomeganephronia [ˌɔligəuˌmegəni'frəuniə] *n* 先天性肾单位减少症伴代偿肥大 | **oligomeganephronic** [ˌɔligəuˌmegəne'frɔnik] *a*
oligomenorrhea [ˌɔligəuˌmenə'riːə] *n* 月经稀发
oligomer ['ɔligəmə] *n* 低聚物，低聚体
oligometallic [ˌɔligəumi'tælik] *a* 少量金属的
oligomorphic [ˌɔligəu'mɔːfik] *a* 少数发育型的（指微生物）
oligonatality [ˌɔligəunei'tæləti] *n* 低出生率
oligonecrospermia [ˌɔligəuˌnekrəu'spəːmiə] *n* 精子死灭[及]过少
oligonephronia [ˌɔligəunə'frəuniə] *n* 肾发育不良
oligonitrophilic [ˌɔligəuˌnaitrəu'filik] *a* 嗜微量氮的
oligonucleotide [ˌɔligəu'njukliətaid] *n* 低[聚]核苷酸，寡核苷酸
oligo-ovulation [ˌɔligəu ˌəuvju'leiʃən] *n* 排卵过少
oligopeptide [ˌɔligəu'peptaid] *n* 寡肽
oligophosphaturia [ˌɔligəuˌfɔsfə'tjuəriə] *n* 尿磷酸盐减少，低磷酸盐尿
oligophrenia [ˌɔligəu'friːniə] *n* 智力发育不全，精神幼稚病 | moral ~ 悖德狂 / phenylpyruvic ~, ~ phenylpyruvica 苯丙酮酸性精神幼稚病，苯丙酮尿性智力发育不全 / polydystrophic ~ 多种营养不良性智力发育不全 | **oligophrenic** [ˌɔligəu'frenik] *a* 智力发育不全的，精神幼稚病的 *n* 智力发育不全者，精神幼稚病患者
oligoplasmia [ˌɔligəu'plæzmiə] *n* 血浆减少
oligoplastic [ˌɔligəu'plæstik] *a* 少胞质的，细胞浆过少的
oligopnea [ˌɔligɔ'pniːə] *n* 肺换气不足
oligoposia [ˌɔligəu'pəuziə], **oligoposy** [ˌɔli'gɔpəsi] *n* 饮料[摄取]过少
oligoptyalism [ˌɔligəu'taiəlizəm] *n* 唾液[分泌]减少
oligopyrene [ˌɔligəu'paiəriːn], **oligopyrous** [ˌɔligəu'paiərəs] *a* 少核质的，少染色质的
oligosaccharide [ˌɔligəu'sækəraid] *n* 低聚糖，寡糖
oligosialia [ˌɔligəusai'eiliə] *n* 唾液[分泌]过少，缺涎症
oligosideremia [ˌɔligəuˌsidə'riːmiə] *n* 血铁减少，低铁血
oligospermia [ˌɔligəu'spəːmiə], **oligospermatism** [ˌɔligəu'spəːmətizəm] *n* 精子减少[症]，少精液症
Oligosporidia [ˌɔligəuspə'ridiə] *n* 少孢子虫亚目
oligosynaptic [ˌɔligəusi'næptik] *a* 少突触的
Oligotrichida [ˌɔligəu'trikidə] *n* 寡毛目
Oligotrichina [ˌɔligəutri'kainə] *n* 寡毛亚目
oligotrophy [ˌɔli'gɔtrəfi], **oligotrophia** [ˌɔligəu'trəufiə] *n* 营养不足，营养过少 | **oligotrophic** [ˌɔligəu'trɔfik] *a*
oligozoospermatism [ˌɔligəuˌzouou'spəːmətizəm], **oligozoospermia** [ˌɔligəuˌzəuəu'spəːmiə] *n* 精子减少，精液缺乏
oliguria [ˌɔli'gjuəriə], **oliguresis** [ˌɔligjuə'riːsis] *n* 少尿 | **oliguric** [ˌɔli'gjuərik] *a*
olisthetic [əulis'θetik] *a* 滑脱的
olisthy, olisthe [əu'lisθi] *n* 滑脱（关节）
oliva [əu'laivə]（[复] **olivae** [əu'laiviː]）*n*【拉】橄榄体 | ~ cerebellaris [小脑]齿状核
olivary ['ɔlivəri] *a* 橄榄状的
olive ['ɔliv] *n* [洋]橄榄；橄榄体 | inferior ~ 下橄榄体 / spurge ~ 紫花欧瑞香 / superior ~ 上橄榄体
Oliver's sign ['ɔlivə]（William S. Oliver）气管牵引感（见于主动脉弓动脉瘤）

Oliver's test [ˈɔlivə] (George Oliver) 奥利佛试验(检白蛋白、糖、吗啡、胆汁酸)
olivifugal [ˌɔliˈvifjugəl] *a* 离橄榄体的
olivipetal [ˌɔliˈvipətl] *a* 向橄榄体的
olivopontocerebellar [ˌɔliveuˌpɔntəuˌseriˈbelə] *a* 橄榄体脑桥小脑的
Ollier's disease [ˌɔliˈɛə] (Léopold L. X. E. Ollier) 内生软骨瘤病 | ~ law 奥利埃定律(两平行骨在其端点由韧带相连时,若其中之一停止生长,则另一的生长亦受阻)/ ~ layer 生骨层(骨膜最内层)
Ollier-Thiersch graft [ˌɔliˈɛə tiəʃ] (L. L. X. E. Ollier; Karl Thiersch) 奥利埃-蒂尔施移植物(有表皮及一小部真皮的薄条皮移植片)
Ollulanus [ˌɔljuˈlænəs] *n* 线虫属
Ol. oliv. oleum olivae【拉】齐墩果油,[洋]橄榄油
olopatadine hydrochloride [ˌəuləuˈpætədiːn] 盐酸奥洛帕定(抗组胺药〈H_1 受体拮抗药〉,用于治疗变应性结膜炎,局部用于结膜)
olophonia [ˌɔləˈfəuniə] *n* 器官性发声不良
OLP occipito-laeva posterior 枕左后(胎位)
Olpitrichum [ɔlpiˈtrikəm] *n* 念珠菌属
olsalazine sodium [ɔlˈsæləziːn] 奥沙拉秦钠(用于治疗溃疡性结肠炎,口服给药)
Olshausen's operation [ˈɔlshauzən] (Robert von Olshausen) 奥尔斯豪森手术(将子宫固定或缝合于腹壁,治子宫后倾)
Olshevsky tube [ɔlˈʃevski] (Dimitry E. Olshevsky) 奥尔舍夫斯基管(一种 X 线管,仅使较强射线透过靶并屏护管内其余部分)
OLT occipito-laeva transversa 枕左横(胎位)
o. m. omni mane【拉】每晨
-oma [后缀]瘤
omacephalus [ˌəuməˈsefələs] *n* 头不全无上肢畸胎
omagra [əuˈmeigrə] *n* 肩[关节]痛风
omalgia [əuˈmældʒiə] *n* 肩痛
omarthritis [ˌəumɑːˈθraitis] *n* 肩关节炎
omasal [əuˈmeisəl] *a* 重瓣胃的
omasitis [ˌəuməˈsaitis] *n* 重瓣胃炎
omasum [əuˈmeisəm] *n*【拉】重瓣胃(反刍类的第三胃)
Ombrédanne's operation [ɔːmbreiˈdæn] (Louis Ombrédanne) 翁布雷丹手术(①治疗尿道下裂;②经越阴囊的睾丸固定术)
ombrophore [ˈɔmbrəfɔː] *n* 碳酸水淋浴器
OMD Doctor of Oriental Medicine 东方医学博士
omega [ˈəumigə] *n* 希腊语的第 24 个即最后一个字母(Ω, ω) | ~ melancholicum 忧郁症皱眉面容(眉间皮肤皱纹似希腊字母 ω)
omega peptidase [əuˈmiːgə ˈpeptideis] ω-肽酶
omeire [əuˈmairi] *n* 乳酒(西南非洲一种用乳酿成的酒)
Omenn's syndrome [ˈəumen] (Gilbert S. Omenn) 奥曼综合征,组织细胞性髓性网状细胞增生病
omenta [əuˈmentə] omentum 的复数
omental [əuˈmentl] *a* 网膜的
omentectomy [ˌəumenˈtektəmi] *n* 网膜切除术
omentitis [ˌəumenˈtaitis] *n* 网膜炎
omentopexy [əuˈmentəˌpeksi], **omentofixation** [əuˌmentəufikˈseiʃən] *n* 网膜固定术
omentoplasty [əuˈmentəˌplæsti] *n* 网膜成形术
omentoportography [əuˌmentəupɔːˈtɔgrəfi] *n* 网膜门静脉造影[术]
omentorrhaphy [ˌəumenˈtɔrəfi] *n* 网膜缝合术
omentosplenopexy [əuˌmentəuˈspliːnəˌpeksi] *n* 网膜脾固定术
omentotomy [ˌəumenˈtɔtəmi] *n* 网膜切开术
omentovolvulus [əuˌmentəuˈvɔlvjuləs] *n* 网膜扭转
omentum [əuˈmentəm] ([复] **omenta** [əuˈmentə]) *n*【拉】网膜 | colic ~, gastrocolic ~, greater ~, ~ majus 胃结肠韧带,大网膜 / gastrohepatic ~, ~ minus 小网膜 / gastrosplenic ~, splenogastric ~ 胃脾韧带 / lesser ~ 肝胃韧带;小网膜 / pancreaticosplenic ~ 胰脾韧带
omentumectomy [əuˌmentəˈmektəmi] *n* 网膜切除术
omeprazole [əuˈmeprəzəul] *n* 奥美拉唑(一种取代的苯并咪唑,用作胃酸分泌抑制剂,治疗症状性胃食管反流病,口服给药)
omicron [əuˈmaikrɔn, ˈɔmi-] *n* 希腊语的第 15 个字母(Ο, ο)
ommatidium [ˌəuməˈtidiəm] *n* 小眼(节肢动物的复眼)
Ommaya reservoir [ɔˈmaijɑː] (Ayub Khan Ommaya) 奥马耶贮器(植入帽状腱膜下方的一种装置,以便通过置于侧脑室的导管取出液体或滴注药物)
ommochrome [ˈɔməkrəum] *n* 眼色素(某些动物的色氨酸代谢产物)
Omn. bih. omni bihora【拉】每 2 小时
Omn. hor. omni hora【拉】每小时
omnifarious [ˌɔmniˈfɛəriəs] *a* 各种各样的
omnipotence [ɔmˈnipətəns] *n* 全能 | ~ of thought 全能妄想
omnivorous [ɔmˈnivərəs] *a* 杂食的
Omn. noct. omni nocte【拉】每夜
om(o)- [构词成分]肩
omocephalus [ˌəuməuˈsefələs] *n* 头不全无上肢畸胎
omoclavicular [ˌəuməu kləˈvikjulə] *a* 肩锁的

omodynia [ˌəuməuˈdiniə] *n* 肩痛
omohyoid [ˌəuməuˈhaiɔid] *a* 肩胛舌骨的
omophagia [ˌəuməuˈfeidʒiə] *n* 生食癖 | **omophagist** [ˌəuˈmɔːfədʒist] *n* 生食癖者 / **omophagous** [əuˈmɔːfəgəs], **omophagic** [ˌəuməuˈfædʒik] *a*
omoplata [ˌəuməuˈplætə] *n* 肩胛骨
omosternum [ˌəuməuˈstəːnəm] *n* 胸锁关节间软骨
OMPA octamethyl pyrophosphoramide 八甲磷胺(杀虫药)
omphalectomy [ˌɔmfəˈlektəmi] *n* 脐切除术
omphalelcosis [ˌɔmfəlelˈkəusis] *n* 脐溃疡
Omphalia [ɔmˈfeiliə] *n* 脐菇属
omphalic [ɔmˈfælik] *a* 脐的
omphalitis [ɔmfəˈlaitis] *n* 脐炎 | ~ of birds 禽脐炎
omphal(o)- [构词成分] 脐
omphaloangiopagus [ˌɔmfələuˌændʒiˈɔpəgəs] *n* 脐血管联胎 | **omphaloangiopagous** *a*
omphalocele [ˈɔmfələuˌsiːl] *n* 脐膨出
omphalochorion [ˌɔmfələuˈkɔːriɔn] *n* 脐绒毛膜(绒[毛]膜卵黄囊胎盘)
omphalodidymus [ˌɔmfələuˈdidiməs] *n* 腹部联胎
omphalogenesis [ˌɔmfələuˈdʒenisis] *n* 脐形成
omphaloischiopagus [ˌɔmfələuiskiˈɔpəgəs] *n* 脐坐骨联胎
omphaloma [ˌɔmfəˈləumə], **omphaloncus** [ˌɔmfəˈlɔŋkəs] *n* 脐瘤
omphalomesenteric [ˌɔmfələuˌmesənˈterik], **omphalomesaraic** [ˌɔmfələumesəˈreiik] *a* 脐肠系膜的
omphalopagus [ˌɔmfəˈlɔpəgəs] *n* 脐部联胎
omphalophlebitis [ˌɔmfələufliˈbaitis] *n* 脐静脉炎;(幼小动物患的)脐炎
omphalorrhagia [ˌɔmfələˈreidʒiə] *n* 脐出血
omphalorrhea [ˌɔmfələˈriːə] *n* 脐液溢
omphalorrhexis [ˌɔmfələˈreksis] *n* 脐破裂
omphalos [ˈɔmfəlɔs] *n* 脐;中心点
omphalosite [ˈɔmfələˌsait] *n* 脐营养[无心]畸胎
omphalotomy [ˌɔmfəˈlɔtəmi] *n* 断脐术
omphalus [ˈɔmfələs] *n* 脐
Om. quar. hor. omni quadrante hora【拉】每一刻钟,每 15 分钟
omunono [ˌɔmjuˈnəunəu] *n* 雅司病(即 yaws)
o. n. omni nocte【拉】每夜
onanism [ˈəunənizəm] *n* 手淫;性交中断
onaye [əuˈnɑːji] *n* 棕色毒毛旋花子素
onch(o)- 见 onc(o)-²
Onchocerca [ˌɔŋkəuˈsəːkə] *n* 盘尾[丝虫]属 | ~ cervicalis 马颈盘尾丝虫 / ~ gibsoni 吉[布逊]氏盘尾丝虫,牛盘尾丝虫 / ~ volvulus, ~ caecutiens 旋盘尾丝虫
onchocerciasis [ˌɔŋkəusəˈkaiəsis], **onchocercosis** [ˌɔŋkəusəˈkəusis] *n* 盘尾丝虫病
onchocercoma [ˌɔŋkəusəːˈkəumə] *n* 盘尾丝虫瘤
Onciola [ɔŋˈsaiələ] *n* 棘头虫属 | ~ canis 犬棘头虫
onc(o)-¹ [构词成分]肿瘤,肿胀,肿块
onc(o)-² [构词成分]钩
Oncocerca [ˌɔŋkəuˈsəːkə] *n* 盘尾[丝虫]属
oncocyte [ˈɔnkəˌsait] *n* 嗜酸瘤细胞 | **oncocytic** [ˌɔnkəuˈsitik] *a*
oncocytoma [ˌɔŋkəusaiˈtəumə] *n* 大嗜酸粒细胞瘤(甲状腺)
oncocytosis [ˌɔŋkəusaiˈtəusis] *n* 嗜酸瘤细胞化生
oncodnavirus [ɔnˈkɔdnəˌvaiərəs] *n* 致肿瘤 DNA 病毒,致癌 DNA 病毒
oncofetal [ˌɔnkəuˈfiːtl] *a* 癌胚的
oncogene [ˈɔŋkədʒiːn] *n* 癌基因
oncogenesis [ˌɔŋkəuˈdʒenisis] *n* 瘤形成,瘤发生 | **oncogenetic** [ˌɔŋkəudʒiˈnetik] *a*
oncogenic [ˌɔŋkəuˈdʒenik] *a* 致瘤的
oncogenicity [ˌɔŋkəudʒiˈnisəti] *n* 致瘤性
oncogenous [ɔŋˈkɔdʒinəs] *a* 瘤源性的;致瘤的
oncoides [ɔŋˈkɔidiːz] *n* 膨大,隆起
oncolipid [ˌɔŋkəuˈlipid] *n* 肿瘤脂质
oncology [ɔŋˈkɔlədʒi] *n* 肿瘤学 | **oncologic** [ˌɔŋkəˈlɔdʒik] *a* / **oncologist** *n* 肿瘤学家
oncolysate [ɔnˈkɔliseit] *n* 肿瘤溶解剂
oncolysis [ɔŋˈkɔlisis] *n* 瘤细胞溶解,溶瘤作用 | **oncolytic** [ˌɔŋkəuˈlitik] *a*
oncoma [ɔŋˈkəumə] *n* [肿]瘤
Oncomelania [ˌɔŋkəumiˈleiniə] *n* 钉螺属
oncometer [ɔŋˈkɔmitə] *n* 器官体积测量器
oncornavirus [ɔnˈkɔnəˌvaiərəs] *n* 致肿瘤 RNA 病毒,致癌 RNA 病毒
oncosis [ɔŋˈkəusis] *n* 肿瘤病
oncosphere [ˈɔŋkəsfiə] *n* 六钩蚴,钩球蚴
oncotherapy [ˌɔŋkəuˈθerəpi] *n* 肿瘤治疗
oncothlipsis [ˌɔŋkəuˈθlipsis] *n* 肿瘤压迫
oncotic [ɔŋˈkɔtik] *a* 膨胀的,膨胀引起的
oncotomy [ɔŋˈkɔtəmi] *n* 肿块切开术
oncotropic [ˌɔŋkəuˈtrɔpik] *a* 亲瘤的,向瘤的(对肿瘤细胞具有特殊亲和力或吸引力的)
Oncovirinae [ˌɔŋkəuviˈrainiː] *n* 肿瘤病毒亚科
oncovirus [ˈɔnkəuˌvaiərəs] *n* 肿瘤病毒,致癌病毒
ondansetron hydrochloride [ɔnˈdænsətrɔn] 盐酸昂丹司琼(镇吐药,用于术后或结合癌症化疗或放疗时预防恶心和呕吐,口服或静脉内给药)
Ondine's curse [ɔnˈdiːn] (Ondine 为德国神话中

的海仙女）原发性肺泡换气不足
ondometer [ɔn'dɔmitə] *n* 波数计
-one [后缀]酮
oneiric [əu'naiərik] *a* 梦的，梦样的
oneirism [əu'naiərizəm] *n* 梦样状态，醒梦状态，梦幻症
oneir(o)- [构词成分]梦
oneiroanalysis [əuˌnaiərəuə'næləsis] *n* 梦态[精神]分析（药物催眠后发掘其意识和潜意识人格）
oneirodynia [əuˌnaiərəu'diniə] *n* 梦魇，噩梦
oneirogenic [ˌəunairəu'dʒenik] *a* 致梦的，引起梦的
oneirogmus [ˌəunai'rɔgməs] *n* 梦遗[精]
oneiroid ['əunairɔid] *a* 梦样的
oneirology [ˌəunai'rɔlədʒi] *n* 梦学
oneirophrenia [əuˌnaiərəu'friːniə] *n* 梦呓性精神病，梦状精神分裂症
oneiroscopy [ˌəunai'rɔskəpi] *n* 析梦，（精神病）析梦诊断
onion ['ʌnjən] *n* 洋葱
oniric [əu'naiərik] *a* 梦的，梦样的
onirogenic [ˌəunairəu'dʒenik] *a* 致梦的，引起梦的
oniroid ['əunairɔid] *a* 梦样的
onium ['əunjəm] *n* 鎓（指氮有最大同价原子时的阳离子，如铵离子 NH_4^+，其化合物包括甜菜碱、胆碱和氧化胺）
onkinocele [ɔn'kinəsiːl] *n* 腱鞘肿
onlay ['ɔnlei] *n* 高嵌体（放在器官或组织表面上的移植物）
onobaio [ˌəunə'beijəu] *n* 欧博克箭毒（非洲欧博克〈Obok〉的一种强力箭毒，对心脏有抑制作用）
onomatology [ˌɔnəumə'tɔlədʒi] *n* 命名学，名词学
onomatomania [ˌɔnəuˌmætəu'meinjə] *n* 强迫性观念插入，称名癖
onomatophobia [ˌɔnəuˌmætəu'fəubjə] *n* 名称恐怖，姓名恐怖
onomatopoeia [ˌɔnəˌmætə'piːə] *n* 新语症，词语创新（模仿声音形成无意义的词语，如见于某些精神分裂症患者）| **onomatopoiesis** [ˌɔnəˌmætəpɔi'iːsis] *n*
onset ['ɔnset] *n* 起病，开始，病发作 | at the ~ 起病时
Ontjom ['ɔntjɔm] *n* 发酵花生饼（爪哇及苏门答腊人做的饼，有时会引起中毒，其中一个体征为黄疸）
ontogeny [ɔn'tɔdʒəni]，**ontogenesis** [ˌɔntəu'dʒenisis] *n* 个体发育 | **ontogenic** [ˌɔntəu'dʒenik]，**ontogenetic** [ˌɔntəudʒi'netik] *a*

onyalai [ˌəuni'æleii]，**onyalia** [ˌəuni'æliə] *n* 奥尼赖病（血小板减少性紫癜的一型，见于非洲）
onychatrophia [ˌəunikə'trəufiə]，**onychatrophy** [ˌɔnik'ætrəfi] *n* 甲萎缩
onychauxis [ˌɔni'kɔːksis] *n* 甲肥厚
onychectomy [ˌɔni'kektəmi] *n* 甲切除术
onychia [əu'nikiə]，**onychitis** [ˌɔni'kaitis] *n* 甲床炎
onych(o)- [构词成分]甲，爪
onychoclasis [ˌɔni'kɔkləsis] *n* 甲折断
onychocryptosis [ˌɔnikəukrip'təusis] *n* 嵌甲
onychodystrophy [ˌɔnikəu'distrəfi] *n* 甲营养不良
onychogenic [ˌɔnikəu'dʒenik] *a* 生甲的，长甲的
onychogram [ɔ'nikəgræm] *n* 指甲毛细管搏动图
onychograph [ɔ'nikəgrɑːf, -græf] *n* 指甲毛细管搏动描记器
onychogryphosis [ˌɔnikəugri'fəusis]，**onychogryposis** [ˌɔnikəugri'pəusis] *n* 甲弯曲，钩甲，弯甲症
onychoheterotopia [ˌɔnikəuˌheterəu'təupiə] *n* 指甲异位，趾甲异位
onychoid ['ɔnikɔid] *a* 指甲样的
onycholysis [ˌɔni'kɔlisis] *n* 甲剥离，甲脱离
onychomadesis [ˌɔnikəumə'diːsis] *n* 无甲，甲缺乏
onychomalacia [ˌɔnikəumə'leiʃiə] *n* 甲软化，软甲
onychomycosis [ˌɔnikəumai'kəusis] *n* 甲真菌病，甲癣 | dermatophytic ~ 甲癣
onycho-osteodysplasia [ˌɔnikəu ˌɔstiəudis'pleiziə] *n* 甲-骨发育不良（亦称关节-甲发育不良、甲-髌骨综合征）
onychopathology [ˌɔnikəupə'θɔlədʒi] *n* 指甲病理学，趾甲病理学
onychopathy [ˌɔni'kɔpəθi] *n* 甲病 | **onychopathic** [ˌɔnikəu'pæθik] *a*
onychophagia [ˌɔnikəu'feidʒiə]，**onychophagy** [ˌɔni'kɔfədʒi] *n* 咬甲癖 | **onychophagist** [ˌɔni'kɔfədʒist] *n* 咬甲癖者
onychoptosis [ˌɔnikɔ'ptəusis] *n* 甲脱落
onychorrhexis [ˌɔnikəu'reksis] *n* 脆甲症，甲脆折
onychoschizia [ˌɔnikəu'skiziə] *n* 甲裂
onychosis [ˌɔni'kəusis] *n* 甲病
onychotillomania [ˌɔnikəuˌtilə'meinjə] *n* 剔甲癖
onychotomy [ˌɔni'kɔtəmi] *n* 甲切开术
onym ['ɔnim] *n* 术语
O'nyong-nyong [əu'niɔŋ niɔŋ] *n* 奥尼翁-尼翁（一种急性非致命性发热性疾病，系由按蚊传播的甲病毒所致，见于乌干达、肯尼亚、坦桑尼亚、马拉维和塞内加尔。临床上类似登革热和基孔

肯雅病〈chikungunya〉,特征为淋巴结炎、关节痛和极痒的麻疹样皮疹,亦称翁尼翁-尼翁热)
onyx [ˈɔniks] *n*【希】爪甲,甲;眼前房积脓
onyxis [ɔˈniksis] *n* 嵌甲
oo- [构词成分]卵,蛋
ooblast [ˈəuəblæst] *n* 成卵细胞
oocenter [ˌəuəˈsentə] *n* 卵中心体
oocephalus [ˌəuəˈsefələs] *n* 卵形头者
oocinesia [ˌəuəsiˈniːziə] *n* 卵核分裂
oocinete [ˌəuəˈsiniːt] *n* 动合子(见 ookinete)
oocyan [ˌəuəˈsaiən], **oocyanin** [ˌəuəˈsaiənin] *n* 胆绿素,蛋壳青素
oocyesis [ˌəuəsaiˈiːsis] *n* 卵巢妊娠
oocyst [ˈəuəsist] *n* 卵囊,卵袋
oocytase [ˌəuəˈsaiteis] *n* 溶卵酶,卵细胞溶[解]酶
oocyte [ˈəuəsait] *n* 卵母细胞
oocytin [ˌəuəˈsaitin] *n* 促[卵]受精膜生成素
oogamy [əuˈɔgəmi] *n* 异配生殖 | **oogamous** [əuˈɔgəməs] *a*
oogenesis [ˌəuəˈdʒenisis] *n* 卵子发生 | **oogenetic** [ˌəuədʒiˈnetik] *a*
oogenic [ˌəuəˈdʒenik] *a* 生卵的
oogonium [ˌəuəˈgəuniəm] ([复] **oogoniums** 或 **oogonia** [ˌəuəˈgəuniə]) *n* 卵原细胞
ookinesis [ˌəuəkiˈniːsis] *n* 卵核分裂
ookinete [ˌəuəkiˈniːt] *n* 动合子(蚊体内疟原虫的授精型)
oolemma [ˌəuəˈlemə] *n* 卵黄膜;透明带
Oomycetes [ˌəuə*u*maiˈsiːtiːz] *n* 卵菌纲
oophagy [ə*u*ˈɔfədʒi], **oophagia** [ˌəuəˈfeidʒiə] *n* 卵食[生活](指昆虫)
oophoralgia [ˌəuɔfəˈrældʒiə] *n* 卵巢痛
oophorectomize [ˌəuɔfəˈrektəmaiz] *vt* 卵巢切除
oophorectomy [ˌəuɔfəˈrektəmi] *n* 卵巢切除术
oophoritis [ˌəuɔfəˈraitis] *n* 卵巢炎
oophor(o)- [构词成分]卵巢
oophorocystectomy [əuˌɔfərə*u*sisˈtektəmi] *n* 卵巢囊肿切除术
oophorocystosis [əuˌɔfərə*u*sisˈtəusis] *n* 卵巢囊肿形成
oophorogenous [əuˌɔfəˈrɔdʒinəs] *a* 卵巢源的,卵巢性的
oophorohysterectomy [əuˌɔfərə*u*ˌhistəˈrektəmi] *n* 卵巢子宫切除术
oophoroma [əuˌɔfəˈrəumə] *n* 卵巢瘤
oophoron [əuˈɔfərɔn] *n* 卵巢
oophoropathy [əuˌɔfəˈrɔpəθi] *n* 卵巢病
oophoropexy [əuˈɔfərə*u*ˌpeksi] *n* 卵巢固定术
oophoroplasty [əuˈɔfərə*u*ˌplæsti] *n* 卵巢成形术
oophorosalpingectomy [əuˌɔfərə*u*ˌsælpinˈdʒektəmi] *n* 卵巢输卵管切除术,输卵管卵巢切除术
oophorosalpingitis [əuˌɔfərə*u*ˌsælpinˈdʒaitis] *n* 卵巢输卵管炎
oophorostomy [əuˌɔfəˈrɔstəmi] *n* 卵巢[囊肿]造口[引流]术
ooplasm [ˈəuəplæzəm] *n* 卵质,卵浆
ooporphyrin [ˌəuəˈpɔːfirin] *n* 卵壳[原]卟啉
oorhodein [ˌəuəˈrəudiːn] *n* 蛋红素,卵红素
oosome [ˈəuəsəum] *n* 卵小体,生殖细胞决定体
oosperm [ˈəuəspəːm] *n* 受精卵
oosphere [ˈəuəsfiə] *n* 卵球
Oospora [əuˈɔspərə] *n* 卵孢子菌属 | ~ catenata, ~ fragilis 链状卵孢子菌,脆弱卵孢子菌 / ~ lactis 乳卵孢子菌 / ~ tozenri 黑色卵孢子菌
oosporangium [ˌəuəspəˈrændʒiəm] *n* 卵孢子鞘,卵孢子囊
oospore [ˈəuəspɔː] *n* 卵孢子 | **oosporic** [ˌəuəˈspɔrik] *a*
ootheca [əuəˈθiːkə] *n* 卵囊,卵鞘;卵巢 | **~l** *a*
oothec(o)-以 oothec(o)-起始的词,同样见以 oophor(o)-和 ovari(o)-起始的词
ootherapy [ˌəuəˈθerəpi] *n* 卵巢制剂疗法
ootid [ˈəuətid] *n* 卵细胞
ootype [ˈəuətaip] *n* 卵模(腔)
ooxanthine [ˌəuəˈzænθin] *n* 卵壳黄素
oozooid [ˌəuəˈzəuɔid] *n* 卵生体
oozy [ˈuːzi] *a* 渗出的,分泌出的;有黏液的
opacification [ə*u*ˌpæsifiˈkeiʃən] *n* 浑浊化(指角膜或晶状体);不透光
opacity [ə*u*ˈpæsəti] *n* 混浊,不透明;不透 X 线,不透光;不透明区,浊斑
opalescent [ˌəupəˈlesnt] *a* 乳光的,乳色的 | **opalescence** [ˌəupəˈlesns] *n*
opalescin [ˌəupəˈlesin] *n* 乳光蛋白
opalgia [əuˈpældʒiə] *n* 面神经痛
Opalina [ˌəupəˈlainə] *n* 扁纤毛虫属,蛙片虫属 | ~ ranarum 蛙扁纤毛虫
Opalinata [ˌəupəlaiˈneitə] *n* 蛙片亚门
Opalinatea [ˌəupəliˈneitiə] *n* 蛙片纲
opaline [ˈəupəliːn] *a* 乳光的,蛋白石的
opalinid [ˌəupəˈlinid] *n*, *a* 蛙片亚门原虫(的)
Opalinida [ˌəupəˈlinidə] *n* 蛙片目
opalisin [əuˈpælisin] *n* 人乳光蛋白
opaque [ə*u*ˈpeik] *a* 不透 X 线的,不透光的,不透明的
opeidoscope [əuˈpaidəskəup] *n* 喉声振动检查器
opening [ˈəupniŋ] *n* 孔,口;开始,开端 | ~ in adductor magnus muscle 大[内]收肌孔 / aortic ~ in diaphragma 主动脉裂孔 / ~ to lesser sac of peritoneum 网膜孔 / ovarian ~ of uterine tube 输卵管腹腔口 / ~ for vena cava 腔静脉孔 / ~ of

vermiform appendix 阑尾口

operability [ˌɔpərə'biləti] *n* 可手术性;手术率

operable ['ɔpərəbl] *a* 可行手术的

operant ['ɔperənt] *n* 操作人员

operate ['ɔpəreit] *vi* 操作;运转;起作用,奏效;动手术 *vt* 操作,开动;对…施行手术 *n* 受过实验性手术者(与正常对照者进行比较)

operating ['ɔpəreitiŋ] *a* 手术的;工作的

operation [ˌɔpə'reiʃən] *n* 操作;作用;手术 | cosmetic ~ 整容术/ equilibrating ~ 平衡手术(对麻痹性眼肌的直接对抗肌施行腱切断术)/ Indian ~ 印度式手术(额部皮瓣鼻成形术)/ interval ~ 间期手术(在疾病两次急性发作的间期所施行的手术,如对阑尾炎)/ Italian ~, tagliacotian ~ 意大利式手术(臂部皮瓣鼻成形术)/ magnet ~ 磁铁(吸金属异物)术(用强力磁铁吸出眼球内的铁片或钢片)/ major ~ 大手术/ mastoid ~ 乳突切除术/ mika ~ 米卡手术(尿道球部造瘘术,藉以达到避孕的目的)/ open ~ 开放性手术/ plastic ~ 成形手术/ radical ~ 根治手术/ shelf ~ 加盖术/ shelving ~ 支架手术(先天性髋脱位手术)

operative ['ɔpərətiv] *a* 操作的;起作用的;手术的

operator ['ɔpəreitə] *n* 操作人员,操纵员;手术者;操纵基因

operatory ['ɔpərəˌtɔri] *n* (为患者提供治疗的)牙科操作区

opercula [əu'pəːkjulə] operculum 的复数

opercular [əu'pəːkjulə] *a* 盖的

operculectomy [əuˌpəːkju'lektəmi] *n* 牙黏膜盖切除术(用于未长出牙)

operculitis [əuˌpəːkju'laitis] *n* (牙)冠周炎

operculum [əu'pəːkjuləm] ([复] **opercula** [əu'pəːkjulə]) *n* 【拉】盖,岛盖;盖(昆虫),厣(软体动物),鳃盖(鱼) | frontal ~ 岛盖额部/ frontoparietal ~ 岛盖顶部/ occipital ~ 枕盖/ temporal ~ 岛盖颞部/ trophoblastic ~ 滋养层盖

operon ['ɔpərɔn] *n* 操纵子(指由一个操纵基因和紧密相连的若干结构基因所组成的染色体)

ophiasis [əu'faiəsis] *n* 【希】匐行性脱发,蛇行性脱发

Ophidia [ɔ'fidiə] *n* 蛇亚目

ophidic [ɔ'fidik] *a* 蛇的

ophidism ['ɔfidizəm], **ophidiasis** [ˌəufi'daiəsis] *n* 蛇咬中毒

Ophiophagus hannah [ˌəufi'ɔfəgəs 'hænə] (印度)扁颈眼镜蛇

ophiotoxemia [ˌəufiətɔk'siːmiə], **ophitoxemia** [ˌəufitɔk'siːmiə] *n* 蛇咬中毒

Ophryoglenina [ˌɔfriəugli'nainə] *n* 睫杆亚目

ophryon ['ɔfriɔn] *n* 印堂,眉间中点

ophryosis [ˌɔfri'əusis] *n* 眉痉挛

ophthalmagra [ˌɔfθæl'mægrə] *n* 眼骤痛

ophthalmalgia [ˌɔfθæl'mældʒiə] *n* 眼痛

ophthalmatrophia [ˌɔfθælmə'trəufiə] *n* 眼萎缩

ophthalmectomy [ˌɔfθæl'mektəmi] *n* 眼球摘除术

ophthalmencephalon [ˌɔfθælmen'sefəlɔn] *n* 视脑(视网膜、视神经及脑内视觉器官的总称)

ophthalmia [ɔf'θælmiə] *n* 眼炎 | actinic ray ~ 光化性眼炎 / catarrhal ~, mucous ~ 卡他性眼炎,黏膜性眼炎(严重型单纯性结膜炎) / Egyptian ~ 沙眼 / electric ~, flash ~ 电光性眼炎 / granular ~ 粒性结膜炎 / jequirity ~ 相思豆(中毒性)眼炎 / ~ neonatorum 新生儿眼炎,新生儿眼脓溢 / purulent ~ 脓性眼炎,睑脓溢 / scrofulous ~ 瘰疬性眼炎(结核性角膜结膜炎) / spring ~ 春季卡他性眼炎 / strumous ~ 小泡性角膜结膜炎 / sympathetic ~, migratory ~, transferred ~ 交感性眼炎,移动性眼炎(亦称交感性眼色素层炎)

ophthalmiac [ɔf'θælmiæk] *n* 眼炎患者

ophthalmiatrics [ˌɔfθælmi'ætriks] *n* 眼病治疗学,眼科治疗学

ophthalmic [ɔf'θælmik] *a* 眼的

ophthalmitis [ˌɔfθæl'maitis] *n* 眼炎 | **ophthalmitic** [ˌɔfθæl'mitik] *a*

ophthalm(o)- [构词成分]眼

ophthalmoblennorrhea [ɔfˌθælməuˌblenə'riːə] *n* 脓性眼炎

ophthalmocele [ɔf'θælməsiːl] *n* 眼球突出

ophthalmocopia [ɔfˌθælməu'kəupiə] *n* 眼疲劳,视力衰弱

ophthalmodesmitis [ɔfˌθælməudez'maitis] *n* 眼腱炎

ophthalmodiaphanoscope [ɔfˌθælməudaiə'fænəskəup] *n* 眼透照镜

ophthalmodiastimeter [ɔfˌθælməuˌdaiəs'timitə] *n* 眼距计,眼距测量器

ophthalmodonesis [ɔfˌθælməudəu'niːsis] *n* 眼颤动

ophthalmodynamometer [ɔfˌθælməudainə'mɔmitə] *n* 视网膜血管血压计;辐辏近点计 | **ophthalmodynamometry** *n* 视网膜血管血压测定法;辐辏近点测定法

ophthalmodynia [ɔfˌθælməu'diniə] *n* 眼痛

ophthalmoeikonometer [ɔfˌθælməuˌaikə'nɔmitə] *n* 眼影像计

ophthalmograph [ɔf'θælməgrɑːf] *n* 眼球运动照相机

ophthalmography [ˌɔfθæl'mɔgrəfi] *n* 眼球运动照相法;眼科专著

ophthalmogyric [ɔfˌθælməu'dʒaiərik] *a* 眼球转

动的,眼动的

ophthalmoleukoscope [ɔfˌθælməuˈljuːkəskoup] *n* 旋光色觉镜

ophthalmolith [ɔfˈθælməliθ] *n* 眼石,泪石

ophthalmology [ˌɔfθælˈmɔlədʒi] *n* 眼科学 | **ophthalmologic(al)** [ˌɔfθælməˈlɔdʒik(əl)] *a* | **ophthalmologist** *n* 眼科医生,眼科学家

ophthalmomalacia [ɔfˌθælməuməˈleiʃiə] *n* 眼球软化

ophthalmometer [ˌɔfθælˈmɔmitə] *n* 检眼计,[眼]屈光计 | **ophthalmometry** *n* 眼屈光测量法

ophthalmometroscope [ɔfˌθælməˈmetrəskəup] *n* 检眼屈光镜

ophthalmomycosis [ɔfˌθælməumaiˈkəusis] *n* 眼真菌病

ophthalmomyiasis [ɔfˌθælməˈmaijəsis] *n* 眼[羊狂蝇]蛆病

ophthalmomyitis [ɔfˌθælməumaiˈaitis], **ophthalmomyositis** [ɔfˌθælməumaiəˈsaitis] *n* 眼肌炎

ophthalmomyotomy [ɔfˌθælməumaiˈɔtəmi] *n* 眼肌切开术

ophthalmoneuritis [ɔfˌθælməunjuəˈraitis] *n* 眼神经炎

ophthalmoneuromyelitis [ɔfˌθælməuˌnjuərəumaiəˈlaitis] *n* 视神经脊髓炎

ophthalmopathy [ˌɔfθælˈmɔpəθi] *n* 眼病

ophthalmophacometer [ɔfˌθælməufeiˈkɔmitə] *n* 晶状体屈光计

ophthalmophantom [ɔfˌθælməˈfæntəm] *n* 模型眼;眼球固定器(动物实验)

ophthalmophlebotomy [ɔfˌθælməufliˈbɔtəmi] *n* 眼静脉切开术

ophthalmophthisis [ˌɔfθælˈmɔfθisis] *n* 眼球皱缩,眼球软化

ophthalmoplasty [ɔfˈθælməˌplæsti] *n* 眼成形术

ophthalmoplegia [ɔfˌθælməˈpliːdʒiə] *n* 眼肌麻痹 | basal ~ 颅底性眼肌麻痹 / exophthalmic ~ 突眼性眼肌麻痹 / fascicular ~ 脑桥束性眼肌麻痹 | **ophthalmoplegic** *a*

ophthalmoptosis [ɔfˌθælmɔˈptəusis] *n* 眼球突出

ophthalmoreaction [ɔfˌθælməuri(ː)ˈækʃən] *n* 眼反应

ophthalmorrhagia [ɔfˌθælməˈreidʒiə] *n* 眼出血

ophthalmorrhea [ɔfˌθælməˈriːə] *n* 眼渗血

ophthalmorrhexis [ɔfˌθælməˈreksis] *n* 眼球破裂

ophthalmoscope [ɔfˈθælməskəup] *n* 检眼镜,眼底镜 | binocular ~ 双目检眼镜,立体检眼镜 / direct ~ 直接检眼镜 / indirect ~ 间接检眼镜 | **ophthalmoscopic** [ɔfˌθælməˈskɔpik] *a*

ophthalmoscopy [ˌɔfθælˈmɔskəpi] *n* 检眼镜检查[法] | direct ~ 检眼镜直接检查[法] / indirect ~ 检眼镜间接检查[法] / medical ~ 检眼镜诊断法 / metric ~ 检眼镜屈光检查[法]

ophthalmospectroscope [ɔfˌθælməˈspektrəskəup] *n* 分光检眼镜

ophthalmospectroscopy [ɔfˌθælməuspekˈtrɔskəpi] *n* 分光检眼法

ophthalmostasis [ˌɔfθælˈmɔstəsis] *n* 眼球固定法

ophthalmostat [ɔfˈθælməstæt] *n* 眼球固定器

ophthalmostatometer [ɔfˌθælməustəˈtɔmitə] *n* 眼球突出计

ophthalmosteresis [ɔfˌθælməustəˈriːsis] *n* 无眼,眼缺失

ophthalmosynchysis [ɔfˌθælməˈsinkisis] *n* 眼内渗液

ophthalmothermometer [ɔfˌθælməuθəˈmɔmitə] *n* 眼温度计

ophthalmotomy [ˌɔfθælˈmɔtəmi] *n* 眼球切开术

ophthalmotonometer [ɔfˌθælməutəuˈnɔmitə] *n* 眼压计 | **ophthalmotonometry** *n* 眼压测量法

ophthalmotoxin [ɔfˌθælməˈtɔksin] *n* 眼毒素

ophthalmotrope [ɔfˈθælmətrəup] *n* 眼肌模型

ophthalmotropometer [ɔfˌθælməutrəˈpɔmitə] *n* 眼转动计,斜视计 | **ophthalmotropometry** *n* 眼转动测量法,斜视测量法

ophthalmovascular [ɔfˌθælməˈvæskjulə] *a* 眼血管的

ophthalmoxerosis [ɔfˌθælməuziəˈrəusis] *n* 眼干燥,干眼病

ophthalmoxyster [ɔfˌθælmɔkˈsistə] *n* 结膜刮匙

-opia [构词成分]眼,视力

opian [ˈəupiən], **opianine** [əuˈpaiənin] *n* 那可丁(镇咳药)

opianic acid [ˌəupiˈænik] 阿片酸,二甲氧苯醛酸

opiate [ˈəupiit] *n* 阿片制剂(亦指任何诱发睡眠的药物)

Opie paradox [ˈəupi] (Eugene L. Opie)奥皮奇异现象(坏死性局部过敏反应,具有保护性机制作用)

opilação [ˌəupiləˈsɑːəu] *n*【葡】南美锥虫病

opilation [ˌəupiˈleiʃən] *n* 南美锥虫病

opinionated [əˈpinjəneitid] *a* 固执己见的,武断的

opioid [ˈəupiɔid] *n* 阿片样物质(指任何一种合成麻醉剂) *a* 类阿片的,阿片样的(指天然存在的肽,如脑啡肽)

opiomania [ˌəupiəˈmeinjə] *n* 阿片瘾

opiomaniac [ˌəupiəˈmeiniæk] *n* 阿片瘾者

opiophagism [ˌəupiˈɔfədʒizəm], **opiophagy** [əupiˈɔfedʒi] *n* [吞]阿片瘾

opipramol hydrochloride [əuˈpiprəmɔl] 盐酸奥匹哌醇(抗抑郁药)

opisthe [əu'pisθi] *n* 后子体,后端子代(原生动物通过横裂所产生的后端的子体)
opisthenar [ə'pisθənɑː] *n* 手背
opisthencephalon [əˌpisθen'sefələn] *n* 小脑
opisthiobasial [əˌpisθiəu'beisiəl] *a* 颅后点[与]颅底点的
opisthion [ə'pisθiən] *n* 颅后点(枕骨大孔后缘的中点)
opisthionasial [əˌpisθiəu'neiziəl] *a* 颅后点[与]鼻根中点的
opisth(o)- [构词成分] 背,后面
opisthocranion [əˌpisəu'kreiniən] *n* 颅后最远点
opisthogenia [əˌpisθəu'dʒiːniə] *n* 缩颏,退缩颏
opisthognathism [ˌəupis'θəunəθizəm] *n* [退]缩颌,后退颌
opisthomastigote [ˌəupisθəu'mæstigəut] *n* 后鞭毛体
opisthoporeia [əˌpisθəupə'raiə] *n* 反步症,退行症,后冲步态
Opisthorchis [ˌəupis'θɔːkis] *n* 后睾[吸虫]属 | ~ felineus 猫后睾吸虫 / ~ noverca 犬后睾吸虫 / ~ sinensis 华支睾吸虫(即 Clonorchis sinensis) / ~ viverrini 麝猫后睾吸虫
opisthorchosis [ˌəupisθɔː'kəusis], **opisthorchiasis** [ˌəupisθɔː'kaiəsis] *n* 后睾吸虫病
opisthotic [ˌəupis'θɔtik] *a* 耳后的
opisthotonoid [ˌəupis'θɔtənɔid] *a* 角弓反张样的
opisthotonos [ˌəupis'θɔtənɔs], **opisthotonus** [ˌəupis'θɔtənəs] *n* 角弓反张
Opitz-Frias syndrome ['əupits 'friːəs] (J. M. Opitz; Jaime L. Frias) 奥-弗综合征(见 Opitz's syndrome)
Opitz's disease ['ɔːpits] (Hans Opitz) 奥皮茨病,血栓静脉炎性脾大
Opitz's syndrome ['əupits] (John M. Opitz) 奥皮茨综合征(一种常染色体显性遗传综合征,包括器官距离过远和疝,男性者表现为尿道下裂、隐睾病及叉形阴囊。心脏异常、喉气管畸形、肛门闭锁、肾缺损、肺发育不全以及下斜睑裂亦可能存在。亦称 G 综合征,器官距离过远-尿道下裂综合征)
opium ['əupjəm] *n* 阿片,鸦片 | denarcotized ~, deodorized ~ 除臭阿片 / granulated ~ 粒状阿片,阿片粒 / lettuce ~ 毒莴苣浓汁 / powdered ~ 阿片粉
opobalsamum [ˌəupə'bælsəməm] *n* 麦加香脂
opocephalus [ˌəupəu'sefələs] *n* 无口鼻独眼并耳畸胎
opodeldoc [ˌɔpəu'deldɔk] *n* 肥皂樟脑搽剂
opodidymus [ˌəupəu'didiməs], **opodymus** [əu'pɔdiməs] *n* 双面畸胎
opossum [ə'pɔsəm] *n* 负鼠

opotherapy [ˌəupəu'θerəpi] *n* 液汁疗法(尤指器官制剂疗法)
Oppenheim's disease (syndrome) ['ɔpənhaim] (Hermann Oppenheim) 先天肌弛缓 | ~ sign (reflex) 奥本海姆征(反射)(向下摩胫骨内侧则拇趾背屈,见于锥体束疾病)
opponens [ə'pəunenz] *a*【拉】对向的 *n* 对向肌
opponent [ə'pəunənt] *a* 对立的,对抗的
opportunist ['ɔpətjuːnist] *n* 机会致病菌 | **~ic** [ˌɔpətjuː'nistik] *a* 机会性的,机会致病性的
OPRT orotate phosphoribosyltransferase 乳清酸磷酸核糖基转移酶
-opsia [构词成分] 视力
opsialgia [ˌɔpsi'ældʒiə] *n* 膝状神经节神经痛,面神经痛
opsigenes [ɔp'sidʒeniːz] *n* 智牙
opsin ['ɔpsin] *n* 视蛋白
opsinogen [ɔp'sinədʒən] *n* 调理素原
opsinogenous [ˌɔpsi'nɔdʒinəs] *a* 产生调理素的
opsiometer [ˌɔpsi'ɔmitə] *n* 视力计
opsiuria [ˌɔpsi'juəriə] *n* 饥尿[症]
opsoclonia [ˌɔpsə'kləuniə], **opsoclonus** [ˌɔpsə'kləunəs] *n* 视性眼阵挛
opsogen ['ɔpsədʒən] *n* 调理素原
opsomania [ˌɔpsəu'meinjə] *n* 美味癖,珍馐癖
opsoniferous [ˌɔpsə'nifərəs] *a* 含调理素的
opsonify [ɔp'sɔnifai] *vt* 受调理[素作用] | **opsonification** [ɔpˌsɔnifi'keiʃən] *n* 调理作用,调理素作用
opsonin ['ɔpsənin] *n* 调理素(指能使细菌和其他细胞易被吞噬的一种抗体,亦指能使细菌易被吞噬的一种非抗体物质) | immune ~ 免疫调理素(在体内或体外与同种抗原相结合后能使一种颗粒性抗原对吞噬作用敏感的一种抗体) | **opsone** ['ɔpsəun] *n* / **opsonic** [ɔp'sɔnik] *a*
opsonist ['ɔpsənist] *n* 调理素专家
opsonize ['ɔpsənaiz] *vt* 受调理[素作用] | **opsonization** [ˌɔpsənai'zeiʃən, -ni'z-] *n* 调理作用,调理素作用
opsonocytophagic [ˌɔpsənəusaitəu'fædʒik] *a* 调理素细胞吞噬的(指血液在有血清调理素和同种白细胞时的吞噬活性)
opsonogen [ɔp'sɔnədʒən] *n* 调理素原
opsonology [ˌɔpsə'nɔlədʒi] *n* 调理素学
opsonometry [ˌɔpsə'nɔmitri] *n* 调理素定量法
opsonophilia [ˌɔpsənəu'filiə] *n* 亲调理素性 | **opsonophilic** *a* 亲调理素的
opsonophoric [ˌɔpsənəu'fɔrik] *a* 带调理素的;调理素簇的
opsonotherapy [ˌɔpsənəu'θerəpi] *n* 调理素疗法(应用菌苗疗法增强血液的调理素的作用)
optesthesia [ˌɔptis'θiːzjə] *n* 视觉

optic [ˌɔptik] *a* 眼的;视力的
optical [ˈɔptikəl] *a* 眼的;视力的;视觉的;光学的 | **~ly** *ad*
optician [ɔpˈtiʃən] *n* 眼镜师
opticianry [ɔpˈtiʃənri] *n* 眼科光学
opticist [ˈɔptisist] *n* 光学家
opticochiasmatic [ˌɔptikəuˌkaiæzˈmætik] *a* 视交叉的
opticociliary [ˌɔptikəuˈsiliəri] *a* 视[神经]睫状神经的
opticokinetic [ˌɔptikəukaiˈnetik, -kiˈn-] *a* 眼运动的
opticonasion [ˌɔptikəuˈneisiən] *n* 视神经孔鼻根间径(视神经孔后缘至鼻根中点间的距离)
opticopupillary [ˌɔptikəuˈpju:piləri] *a* 视神经瞳孔的
optics [ˈɔptiks] *n* 光学 | fiber ~ 纤维光学
optimal [ˈɔptiməl] *a* 最适的,最佳的
optimeter [ɔpˈtimitə] *n* 视力计
optist [ˈɔptist] *n* 验光师
opt(o)-[构词成分]视,视力
optoblast [ˈɔptəblæst] *n* 成视细胞(视网膜内)
optochiasmic [ˌɔptəukaiˈæzmik] *a* 视交叉的
optogram [ˈɔptəgræm] *n* 视网膜像
optokinetic [ˌɔptəukaiˈnetik, -kiˈn-] *a* 视觉运动的
optomeninx [ˌɔptəuˈmi:niŋks] *n* 视网膜
optometer [ɔpˈtɔmitə] *n* 视力计
optometrist [ɔpˈtɔmitrist] *n* 验光师
optometry [ɔpˈtɔmitri] *n* 视力测定法,验光(法) | **optometric(al)** [ˌɔptəˈmetrik(əl)] *a*
optomyometer [ˌɔptəumaiˈɔmitə] *n* 眼肌力计
optophone [ˌɔptəfəun] *n* 光声机(变光波为声波)
optotype [ˈɔptətaip] *n* 试视力字体
OPV polivirus vaccine live oral 口服脊髓灰质炎病毒活疫苗
OR operating room 手术室
ora[1] [ˈəurə] ([复] **orae** [ˈəuri:]) *n*【拉】缘 | ~ serrata retinae 视网膜锯齿缘
ora[2] os 的复数
orad [ˈəuræd, ˈɔ:-] *ad* 向口
oral [ˈɔ:rəl] *a* 口的;口头的;口服的 | **~ly** *ad*
orale [ɔ:ˈreili] *n* 切牙颌内缝终点
orality [ɔ:ˈræləti] *n* 口欲性欲,口欲色情(据心理分析学说,一切感觉、冲动和个性品质均源于性心理发育的口欲期)
oralogy [ɔ:ˈrælədʒi] *n* 口腔学
Oramorph [ˈɔ:reˌmɔ:f] *n* 硫酸吗啡(morphine sulfate)制剂的商品名
orange [ˈɔrindʒ] *n* 橙,柑;橙色,橙黄,橘黄 | ethyl ~ 乙橙 / ~ G, wool ~ 橙黄 G,毛橙 / methyl ~, gold ~, ~ Ⅲ甲橙,金橙,橙黄Ⅲ,半日花素 / victoria ~ 维多利亚橙黄(组织学上用作染色剂)
orangeophil [ɔˈrændʒiəfil] *a* 嗜橙黄的 *n* 嗜橙黄细胞(亦称 α-嗜酸细胞)
orangutan [əuˈræŋu:ˌtæn] *n* 猩猩(常用作实验研究)
Orbeli phenomenon (effect) [ɔ:ˈbeili] (Leon A. Orbeli)奥尔别利现象(效应)(当神经-肌肉准备反应由于疲劳而减弱时,刺激交感神经可使肌肉收缩亢进)
orbicular [ɔ:ˈbikjulə] *a* 环状的,圆的
orbiculare [ɔ:ˌbikjuˈlɛəri] *n*【拉】豆状突(砧骨)
orbiculus [ɔ:ˈbikjuləs] ([复] **orbiculi** [ɔ:ˈbikjulai]) *n*【拉】小环,盘
orbit [ˈɔ:bit] *n* 眶;轨道 | **~al** *a*
orbita [ˈɔ:bitə] ([复] **orbitae** [ˈɔ:biti:]) *n*【拉】眶
orbitale [ˌɔ:biˈteili] *n* 眶最下点(眶下缘最低点)
orbitalis [ˌɔ:biˈteilis] *a*【拉】眶的
orbitography [ˌɔ:biˈtɔgrəfi] *n* 眶造影[术](用 X 线摄影和计算机体层摄影使眶及其内容物显影)
orbitonasal [ˌɔ:bitəuˈneizəl] *a* 眶鼻的
orbitonometer [ˌɔ:bitəuˈnɔmitə] *n* 眶压计 | **orbitonometry** *n* 眶压测量法
orbitopagus [ˌɔ:biˈtɔpəgəs] *n* 眶部联胎(寄生胎在眼眶部)
orbitopathy [ˌɔ:biˈtɔpəθi] *n* 眶病
orbitostat [ˈɔ:bitəstæt] *n* 眶轴计
orbitotemporal [ˌɔ:bitəuˈtempərəl] *a* 眶颞的
orbitotomy [ˌɔ:biˈtɔtəmi] *n* 眶切开术
Orbivirus [ˈɔ:biˌvaiərəs] *n* 环状病毒属
orbivirus [ˈɔ:biˌvaiərəs] *n* 环状病毒
orcein [ˈɔ:siin, ɔ:ˈsi:in] *n* 地衣红,苔红素
orchectomy [ɔ:ˈkektəmi] *n* 睾丸切除术
orchella [ɔ:ˈʃelə] *n* 地衣紫,海石蕊紫
orchialgia [ɔ:kiˈældʒiə] *n* 睾丸痛
orchic [ˈɔ:kik] *a* 睾丸的
orchichorea [ˌɔ:kikɔˈriə] *n* 睾丸颤搐
orchidalgia [ˌɔ:kiˈdældʒiə] *n* 睾丸痛
orchidectomy [ˌɔ:kiˈdektəmi] *n* 睾丸切除术
orchidic [ɔ:ˈkidik] *a* 睾丸的
orchiditis [ˌɔ:kiˈdaitis] *n* 睾丸炎
orchid(o)- [构词成分]睾丸
orchidocelioplasty [ˌɔ:kidəuˈsi:liəuˌplæsti] *n* 隐睾移植术(移入腹腔)
orchidoepididymectomy [ˌɔ:kidəuˌepiˌdidiˈmektəmi] *n* 睾丸附睾切除术
orchidometer [ˌɔ:kiˈdɔmitə] *n* 睾丸测量器 | Prader ~ 普雷德睾丸测量器(一串睾丸形塑料模型,根据其体积标以立方厘米,用作测量睾丸在生殖器发育中的大小)
orchidoncus [ˌɔ:kiˈdɔŋkəs] *n* 睾丸瘤

orchidopathy [ˌɔːkiˈdɔpəθi] *n* 睾丸病
orchidopexy [ˈɔːkidəˌpeksi] *n* 睾丸固定术
orchidoplasty [ˈɔːkidəˌplæsti] *n* 睾丸成形术
orchidoptosis [ˌɔːkidɔˈptəusis] *n* 睾丸下垂
orchidorrhaphy [ˌɔːkiˈdɔrəfi] *n* 睾丸缝合术，睾丸固定术
orchidotherapy [ˌɔːkidəuˈθerəpi] *n* 睾丸制剂疗法
orchidotomy [ˌɔːkiˈdɔtəmi] *n* 睾丸切开术
orchiectomy [ˌɔːkiˈektəmi] *n* 睾丸切除术
orchiencephaloma [ˌɔːkienˌsefəˈləumə] *n* 睾丸脑状癌，胚胎性癌
orchiepididymitis [ˌɔːkiˌepiˌdidiˈmaitis] *n* 睾丸附睾炎
orchilytic [ˌɔːkiˈlitik] *a* 溶睾丸组织的，破坏睾丸组织的
orchi(o)- [构词成分]睾丸
orchiocatabasis [ˌɔːkiəukəˈtæbəsis] *n* 睾丸下降
orchiocele [ˈɔːkiəˌsiːl] *n* 睾丸突出；阴囊疝；睾丸瘤
orchiococcus [ˌɔːkiəuˈkɔkəs] *n* 睾丸炎[双]球菌
orchiodynia [ˌɔːkiəuˈdiniə] *n* 睾丸痛
orchiomyeloma [ˌɔːkiəuˌmaiəˈləuma] *n* 睾丸髓样瘤，睾丸浆细胞瘤
orchioncus [ˌɔːkiˈɔŋkəs] *n* 睾丸瘤
orchioneuralgia [ˌɔːkiəunjuəˈrældʒiə] *n* 睾丸[神经]痛
orchiopathy [ˌɔːkiˈɔpəθi] *n* 睾丸病
orchiopexy [ˌɔːkiəuˈpeksi], **orchiorrhaphy** [ˌɔːkiˈɔrəfi] *n* 睾丸固定术，睾丸缝合术
orchioplasty [ˈɔːkiəˌplæsti] *n* 睾丸成形术
orchioscheocele [ˌɔːkiˈɔskiəˌsiːl] *n* 睾丸阴囊疝，阴囊疝瘤
orchioscirrhus [ˌɔːkiəuˈskirəs] *n* 睾丸硬变
orchiotomy [ˌɔːkiˈɔtəmi] *n* 睾丸切开术
Orchis [ˈɔːkis] *n* 红门兰属
orchis [ˈɔːkis] *n*【希】睾丸
orchitis [ɔːˈkaitis] *n* 睾丸炎 | **orchitic** [ɔːˈkitik] *a*
orchitolytic [ˌɔːkitəuˈlitik] *a* 溶睾丸组织的，破坏睾丸组织的
orchotomy [ɔːˈkɔtəmi] *n* 睾丸切开术
orcinol [ˈɔːsinɔl], **orcin** [ˈɔːsin] *n* 地衣酚，5-甲基间苯二酚
order [ˈɔːdə] *n* 目(生物分类)；命令，指令；医嘱 *vt* 命令，指令；开医嘱
orderly [ˈɔːdəli] *n* 男护理员
Ord's operation [ɔːd] (William M. Ord)奥德手术(新形成的关节粘连的剥离术)
ordure [ˈɔːdjuə] *n* 排泄物，粪便
orectic [ɔˈrektik] *a* 开胃的，促食欲的
oreoselinum [ˌɔːriəsiˈlainəm] *n*【拉】防葵
orexia [əuˈreksiə], **orexis** [əuˈreksis] *n* 食欲
orexigenic [əuˌreksiˈdʒenik] *a* 开胃的
oreximania [əuˌreksiˈmeinjə] *n* 多食癖，贪食癖
orf [ɔːf] *n* 羊触染性深脓疱(由病毒引起，可传染给人)；羊痘，羊天花
Orfila museum [ˌɔːfiˈlɑː] (Mathieu J. B. Orfila)奥尔菲拉解剖学博物馆(在巴黎医学院)
organ [ˈɔːgən] *n* 器官，器 | acoustic ~, spiral ~ 听器，螺旋器 / cement ~ 牙骨质器 / genital ~s, reproductive ~s 生殖器 / parenchymal ~, parenchymatous ~ 主质器官，实质器官 / primitive fat ~ 肩胛间腺 / rudimentary ~ 原基，始基；残遗器官，残余器官 / segmental ~ 分节器(前肾、中肾和后肾的合称) / sense ~s, sensory ~s 感觉器 / ~ of shock, shock ~ 休克器官(过敏性休克时发生反应的器官) / target ~ 靶器官(受特殊激素影响的器官) / vestigial ~ 残遗器官 / ~ of vision, visual ~ 视器
organa [ˈɔːgənə] organum 和 organon 的复数
organacidia [ˌɔːgənəˈsidiə] *n* 有机酸症，有机酸存在(如胃内)
organella [ˌɔːgəˈnelə] ([复] **organellae** [ˌɔːgəˈneliː]) *n*【拉】细胞器；小器官
organelle [ˌɔːgəˈnel] *n* 细胞器；小器官
organic [ɔːˈgænik] *a* 器官的，器的；有生命的；有机体的；有机的；器质性的 | ~ acid 有机酸
organicism [ɔːˈgænisizəm] *n* 器质病说(认为一切症状均由器质性疾病所致)；机体说(认为身体每一器官均有其特殊构造) | **organicist** [ɔːˈgænisist] *n* 器质病说者
organism [ˈɔːgənizəm] *n* 生物[体]；[有]机体 | nitrifying ~s 硝化菌 / nitrosifying ~s 亚硝化菌 / pleuropneumonia-like ~s (PPLO)类胸膜肺炎菌
organization [ˌɔːgənaiˈzeiʃən, -niˈz-] *n* 组织，组构，有机体；机化(血栓或坏死组织) | columnar ~ 柱状组构
organize [ˈɔːgənaiz] *vt* 组织，构成；使有机化，使成有机体 *vi* 成有机体
organizer [ˈɔːgənaizə] *n* 组织导体，组织中心，组织者(胚胎的一部分，对于另一部分具有形态建成刺激作用，可促使后者分化) | nucleolar ~, nucleolus ~ 核仁组织导体，核仁组成中心
organ(o)- [构词成分]器官，有机
organochlorine [ˌɔːgənəuˈklɔːriːn] *n* 有机氯
organofaction [ˌɔːgənəuˈfækʃən] *n* 器官形成
organoferric [ˌɔːgənəuˈferik] *a* 有机铁的
organogel [ɔːˈgænədʒel] *n* 有机凝胶
organogen [ɔːˈgænədʒən] *n* 有机物元素
organogenesis [ˌɔːgənəuˈdʒenisis], **organogeny** [ˌɔːgəˈnɔdʒeni] *n* 器官发生 | **organogenetic**

[ˌɔːgənəudʒiˈnetik] *a*
organogenic [ˌɔːgənəuˈdʒenik] *a* 器官原的,器官性的
organography [ɔːgəˈnɔgrəfi] *n* 器官 X 线摄影[术] | **organographic** [ˌɔːgənəuˈgræfik] *a*
organoid [ˈɔːgənɔid] *a* 器官样的 *n* 类器官 | cytoplasmic ~s 胞浆类器官,细胞器
organoleptic [ˌɔːgənəuˈleptik] *a* 传入感觉器的;特殊感觉的
organology [ˌɔːgəˈnɔlədʒi] *n* 器官学 | **organologic(al)** [ˌɔːgənəˈlɔdʒik(əl)] *a* / **organologist** *n* 器官学专家
organoma [ˌɔːgəˈnəumə] *n* 器官瘤(如皮样囊肿)
organomegaly [ˌɔːgənəuˈmegəli] *n* 内脏巨大
organomercurial [ˌɔːgənəuməːˈkjuəriəl] *a* 有机汞的(指含汞的有机化合物,如利尿的硫汞灵)
organometallic [ɔːgənəumiˈtælik] *a* 有机金属的
organon [ˈɔːgənɔn] ([复] **organa** [ˈɔːgənə]) *n* 【希】器官,器
organonomy [ˌɔːgəˈnɔnəmi] *n* 有机生活论,有机生活规律
organopathy [ˌɔːgəˈnɔpəθi] *n* 器官病
organopexy [ˌɔːgənəuˈpeksi], **organopexia** [ˌɔːgənəuˈpeksiə] *n* 器官固定术(尤指子宫)
organophilism [ɔːgəˈnɔfilizəm] *n* 亲器官性 | **organophilic** [ˌɔːgənəuˈfilik] *a* 亲器官的
organophosphate [ˌɔːgənəuˈfɔsfeit] *n* 有机磷酸盐
organophosphorus [ˌɔːgənəuˈfɔsfərəs] *n* 有机磷
organoscopy [ˌɔːgəˈnɔskəpi] *n* 内脏镜检查
organotaxis [ˌɔːgənəuˈtæksis] *n* 趋器官性
organotherapy [ˌɔːgənəuˈθerəpi] *n* 器官疗法,内脏制剂疗法
organotrope [ɔːˈgænətrəup] *n* 亲器官剂
organotrophic [ˌɔːgənəuˈtrɔfik] *a* 器官营养的;有机营养的(指细菌)
organotropism [ˌɔːgəˈnɔtrəpizəm], **organotropy** [ˌɔːgəˈnɔtrəpi] *n* 亲器官性 | **organotropic** [ˌɔːgənəuˈtrɔpik] *a* 亲器官的
organ-specific [ˈɔːgən spiˈsifik] *a* 器官特异性的(局限于某一特殊器官,或仅对某一特殊器官有作用,如器官特异性抗原)
organule [ˈɔːgənjul] *n* 感觉终器,感觉末梢(如味蕾)
organum [ˈɔːgənəm] ([复] **organa** [ˈɔːgənə]) *n*【拉】器官,器
orgasm [ˈɔːgæzəm] *n* 性欲高潮,性乐高潮 | **orgasmic** [ɔːˈgæzmik], **orgastic** [ɔːˈgæstik] *a*
orgotein [ˈɔːgətiːn] *n* 奥古蛋白,肝蛋白(从血细胞、肝等产生的一种有协同作用的物质,由小牛肝提取,作为铜锌混合螯合物,具有抗炎性质,曾用作抗风湿药)
orientation [ˌɔːrienˈteiʃən] *n* 定向力
orifice [ˈɔrifis] *n* 孔;口,管口 | abdominal ~ of uterine tube 输卵管腹腔口 / aortic ~ 主动脉口 / atrioventricular ~, auriculoventricular ~ 房室口 / cardiac ~ 贲门 / duodenal ~ of stomach 幽门 / external ~ of uterus 子宫外口 / hymenal ~ 处女膜口,阴道口 / pilosebaceous ~s 毛囊皮脂腺口,毛囊口 / pulmonary ~ 肺动脉口 / root canal ~, canal ~ 牙根管口 / vesicourethral ~, internal ~ of urethra 尿道内口 | **orificial** [ˌɔriˈfiʃəl] *a*
orificialist [ɔriˈfiʃəlist] *n* 管口外科医师
orificium [ˌɔriˈfiʃiəm] ([复] **orificia** [ˌɔriˈfiʃiə]) *n*【拉】口,管口
origin [ˈɔridʒin] *n* 起源;起因,起端
orinotherapy [ɔːˌrainəuˈθerəpi] *n* 高山疗法
ormetoprim [ɔːˈmetəprim] *n* 奥美普林(抗菌药)
Ormond's disease [ˈɔːmən] (John K. Ormond) 奥蒙德病,腹膜后纤维变性
Orn ornithine 鸟氨酸
ornidazole [ɔːˈnidəzəul] *n* 奥硝唑(抗感染药)
ornithine [ˈɔːniθiːn, -θin] *n* 鸟氨酸
ornithine aminotransferase [ˈɔːniθiːn əˌminəuˈtrænsfəreis] 鸟氨酸转氨酶(此酶缺乏为一种常染色体隐性性状,可致脉络膜和视网膜环状萎缩。在 EC 命名法中称为 ornithine-oxo-acid transaminase)
ornithine carbamoyltransferase [ˈɔːniθiːn ˌkɑːbəˌmɔilˈtrænsfəreis] 鸟氨酸氨甲酰基转移酶(亦称鸟氨酸转氨甲酰酶,缩写为 OCT)
ornithine carbamoyltransferase (OCT) deficiency 鸟氨酸氨甲酰基转移酶缺乏症(一种 X 连锁氨基酸病,其特征性体征包括高氨血症、神经异常及乳清酸尿症。亦称鸟氨酸转氨甲酰酶缺乏症)
ornithine decarboxylase [ˈɔːniθiːn ˌdiːkɑːˈbɔksileis] 鸟氨酸脱羧酶
ornithine-keto-acid aminotransferase [ˈɔːniθiːn ˈkiːtəuˈæsid əˌminəuˈtrænsfəreis] 鸟氨酸酮酸转氨酶,鸟氨酸转氨酶
ornithinemia [ˌɔːniθiˈniːmiə] *n* 鸟氨酸血[症],高尿氨酸血[症]
ornithine-oxo-acid transaminase [ˈɔːniθin ˈɔksəu ˈæsid trænsˈæmineis] 鸟氨酸氧[代]酸转氨酶(ornithine aminotransferase 的 EC 命名法)
ornithine transcarbamoylase (OTC) [ˈɔːniθiːn ˌtrænskɑːbəˈmɔileis], **ornithine transcarbamylase (OTC)** [trænskɑːˈbæmileis] 鸟氨酸转氨甲酰酶,鸟氨酸氨甲酰转移酶
Ornithodoros [ˌɔːniˈθɔdərəs] *n* 钝缘蜱属 | ~ coriaceus 皮革钝缘蜱
Ornithonyssus [ˌɔːniθəˈnisəs] *n* 禽刺螨属 | ~

bacoti 柏氏禽刺螨(热带鼠螨) / ~ bursa 囊禽刺螨 / ~ sylviarum 林禽刺螨

ornithosis [ˌɔːni'θəusis] *n* 鸟疫,饲鸟病(可传染人,称鹦鹉热,鸟类的一种病毒性疾病)

ornithuric acid [ˌɔːni'θjuərik] 鸟尿酸

oro-[1] [构词成分] 口

oro-[2] [构词成分] 血清(见 orrho-)

oro-immunity [ɔːrəui'mjuːnəti] *n* 血清免疫,被动免疫

orokinase [ˌɔːrəu'kineis] *n* 唾液淀粉激酶,唾涎致活酶

orolingual [ˌɔːrəu'liŋgwəl] *a* 口舌的

oromandibular [ˌəurəumæn'dibjulə] *a* 口下颌[骨]的

oromaxillary [ˌɔːrəu'mæksiləri] *a* 口上颌的

oromeningitis [ˌɔːrəuˌmenin'dʒaitis] *n* 浆膜炎

oronasal [ˌɔːrəu'neizəl] *a* 口鼻的

oropharynx [ˌɔːrəu'færiŋks] *n* 口咽[部]

Oropsylla [ˌɔːrəu'silə] *n* 山蚤属 | ~ idahoensis 爱达荷山蚤 / ~ montana 蒙大拿山蚤 / ~ silantiewi 谢氏山蚤,长须山蚤,旱獭山蚤

orosomucoid [ˌɔːrəsəu'mjuːkɔid] *n* 血清类黏蛋白,α_1-酸性糖蛋白

orotate ['ɔːrəteit] *n* 乳清酸(解离型)

orotate phosphoribosyltransferase (OPRT) ['ɔːrəteit ˌfɔsfəuˌraibəusil'trænsfəreis] 乳清酸磷酸核糖基转移酶

orotherapy [ˌɔːrəu'θerəpi] *n* 乳清疗法;血清疗法

orotic acid [ɔː'rɔtik] 乳清酸

oroticaciduria [ɔːˌrɔtikˌæsi'djuəriə] *n* 乳清酸尿

orotidine [ɔː'rɔtidiːn] *n* 乳清酸核苷

orotidine 5′-phosphate decarboxylase (ODC) [ɔː'rɔtidiːn 'fɔsfeit ˌdiːkɑː'bɔksileis] 乳清酸核苷 5′-磷酸脱羧酶(缺乏 ODC 活性为一种常染色体隐性性状,可致乳清酸尿Ⅱ型)

orotidylate [əˌrɔti'dileit] *n* 乳清酸核苷酸(解离型)

orotidylate decarboxylase [ɔːˌrɔti'dileit ˌdiːkɑː'bɔksileis] 乳清酸核苷酸脱羧酶,乳清酸核苷 5′-磷酸脱羧酶

orotidylic acid [əˌrɔti'dilik] 乳清酸核苷酸(磷酸化乳清酸核苷,一般指乳清酸核苷 5′-磷酸)

Oroya fever [ɔ'rɔiə] 奥罗亚热(巴尔通体病急性发热贫血阶段,奥罗亚为秘鲁地名)

orpanoxin [ˌɔːpə'nɔksin] *n* 奥帕诺辛(抗炎药)

orphenadrine [ɔː'fenədrin] *n* 奥芬那君(解痉药) | ~ citrate 枸橼酸奥芬那君(骨骼肌松弛药) / ~ hydrochloride 盐酸奥芬那君(抗震颤麻痹药)

orpiment ['ɔːpimənt] *n* 雌黄,三硫化二砷

orrho- [构词成分] 血清;浆液

orrhoimmunity [ˌɔːrəui'mjuːnəti] *n* 血清免疫,被动免疫

orrhology [ɔː'rɔlədʒi] *n* 血清学

orrhomeningitis [ˌɔːrəuˌmenin'dʒaitis] *n* 浆膜炎

orrhoreaction [ˌɔːrəuri(ː)'ækʃən] *n* 血清反应

orrhotherapy [ˌɔːrəu'θerəpi] *n* 血清疗法 | **orrhotherapeutic** [ɔːrəuˌθerə'pjuːtik] *a*

orris ['ɔris] *n* 香菖(做牙粉、香水等用)

Orr treatment (method, technique) [ɔː] (Hiram W. Orr)奥尔疗法(治哆开骨折及骨髓炎)

orsellinic acid [ɔsə'linik] 苔色酸,4,6-二羟-2-甲苯甲酸

Orsi-Grocco method ['ɔːsi 'grɔkəu] (Francesco Orsi; Pietro Grocco)奥西-格罗科法(心脏的触叩诊)

orthergasia [ˌɔːθə'geiziə] *n* 功能正常

orthesis [ɔː'θiːsis] ([复] **ortheses** [ɔː'θiːsiːz]) *n* 整直法,矫正法

orthetics [ɔː'θetiks] *n* 矫正器修配学 | **orthetic** *a* 整直的,矫正的 / **orthetist** ['ɔːθətist] *n* 矫正器修配者,整直师

ortho- [构词成分] 直的,正的,正常的;正,原,邻(化学)

ortho-acid [ˌɔːθəu 'æsid] *n* 正酸,原酸

orthoarsenic acid [ˌɔːθəu'ɑːsnik] 砷酸

orthoarteriotony [ˌɔːθəuˌɑːtiəri'ɔtəni] *n* 正常[动脉]血压

orthobiosis [ˌɔːθəubai'əusis] *n* 正常生活

orthoboric acid [ˌɔːθəu'bɔːrik] 硼酸

orthocephalic [ˌɔːθəusə'fælik], **orthocephalous** [ˌɔːθəu'sefələs] *a* 正颅型的 | **orthocephaly** [ˌɔːθəu'sefəli] *n* 正颅型,正头型

orthochorea [ˌɔːθəukɔ'riə] *n* 立位舞蹈症

orthochromatic [ˌɔːθəukrəu'mætik] *a* 正染的;正色的(指一种照相乳剂,除红色外对任何颜色都敏感的)

orthochromia [ˌɔːθəu'krəumiə] *n* 血色正常,正[常]血色(血红蛋白含量正常)

orthochromophil [ˌɔːθəu'krəuməfil] *a* (中性染剂)正染性的

orthocresol [ˌɔːθəu'kriːsɔl] *n* 邻甲酚

orthocytosis [ˌɔːθəusai'təusis] *n* 血细胞全熟,血细胞正常

orthodactylous [ˌɔːθəu'dæktiləs] *a* 直指的,直趾的

orthodentin [ˌɔːθəu'dentin] *n* 直型牙本质,正牙质(见于哺乳动物的牙齿)

orthodeoxia [ˌɔːθəudiː'ɔksiə] *n* 直立低氧血症

orthodiagram [ˌɔːθəu'daiəgræm] *n* 矫形 X 线[照]片

orthodiagraph [ˌɔːθəu'daiəgrɑːf] *n* 矫形用 X 线机

orthodiascope [ˌɔːθəu'daiəskəup] *n* 矫形用 X 线透视机 | **orthodiascopy** [ˌɔːθəudai'æskəpi] *n* 矫形 X 线透视

orthodichlorobenzene [ˌɔːθəudaiˌklɔ(ː)rəˈbenziːn] *n* 邻二氯苯(用作喷雾杀虫剂)
orthodigita [ˌɔːθəuˈdidʒitə] *n* 指矫形术,趾矫形术
orthodontics [ˌɔːθəuˈdɔntiks], **orthodontia** [ˌɔːθəuˈdɔnʃiə], **orthodontology** [ˌɔːθəudɔnˈtɔlədʒi] *n* 口腔正畸学 | **orthodontic** *a* 正畸的 | **orthodontist** *n* 口腔正畸学家
orthodromic [ˌɔːθəuˈdrɔmik] *a* 顺行的,顺向传导的(神经纤维)
orthogenesis [ˌɔːθəuˈdʒenisis] *n* 定向进化,定向进化学说(认为进化的过程是固定的,向预定的方向演变) | **orthogenetic** [ˌɔːθəudʒiˈnetik] *a*
orthogenics [ˌɔːθəuˈdʒeniks] *n* 优生学
orthoglycemic [ˌɔːθəuglaiˈsiːmik] *a* 血糖正常的
Orthognatha [ɔːˈθɔgnəθə] *n* 直颚蛛亚目
orthognathia [ˌɔːθɔgˈnæθiə] *n* 正颌学 | **orthognathic** [ˌɔːθɔgˈneiθik] *a* 正颌学的;直颌的,正颌的
orthognathous [ɔːˈθɔgnəθəs] *a* 直颌的 | **orthognathism** [ˌɔːθɔgˈneisizəm] *n*
orthogonal [ɔːˈθɔgənl] *a* 互相垂直的,直角的,正交的;矩形的
orthograde [ˈɔːθəgreid] *a* 直体步行的(指两足动物)
orthohydroxybenzoic acid [ˌɔːθəuhaiˌdrɔksibenˈzəuik] 邻羟基苯甲酸,水杨酸
orthoiodohippurate [ˌɔːθəuˌaiədəuˈhipjureit] *n* 邻碘马尿酸盐
orthomelic [ˌɔːθəuˈmiːlik] *a* 肢体矫形的
orthometer [ɔːˈθɔmitə] *n* 突眼比较计
orthomolecular [ˌɔːθəuməuˈlekjulə] *a* 正分子的
orthomorphia [ˌɔːθəuˈmɔːfiə] *n* 矫形术
Orthomyxoviridae [ˌɔːθəuˌmiksəuˈviridiː] *n* 正黏病毒科
orthomyxovirus [ˌɔːθəuˈmiksəuˌvaiərəs] *n* 正黏病毒
orthoneutrophil [ˌɔːθəuˈnjuːtrəfil] *a* (中性染剂)正染性的
ortho-oxybenzoic acid [ˌɔːθəu ˌɔksibenˈzəuik] 邻羟基苯甲酸,水杨酸
orthopaedics [ˌɔːθəuˈpiːdiks] *n* 矫形外科学,矫形学 | **orthopedic** *a* 矫形的,矫形外科的
orthopantograph [ˌɔːθəuˈpæntəˌgrɑːf, -græf] *n* 曲面全颌摄片,全景 X 线片
Orthopantomograph [ˌɔːθəuˈpæntəməugrɑːf, -græf] *n* 曲面体层全颌摄影机(商品名,用于曲面体层摄影〈pantomography〉的仪器)
orthopercussion [ˌɔːθəupəˈkʌʃən] *n* 直指叩诊法
orthophenanthrolene [ˌɔːθəufiˈnænθrəliːn] *n* 邻二氮杂菲(指示剂)
orthophenolase [ˌɔːθəuˈfiːnəleis] *n* 邻酚酶
orthophony [ɔːˈθɔfəni] *n* 发声正常
orthophoria [ˌɔːθəˈfɔːriə] *n* 位置正常,正位;视轴正常,直视 | asthenic ~ 眼肌衰弱性直视 | **orthophoric** [ɔːθəˈfɔːrik] *a*
orthophosphate [ˌɔːθəuˈfɔsfeit] *n* 正磷酸盐
orthophosphoric acid [ˌɔːθəufɔsˈfɔrik] 正磷酸
orthophrenia [ˌɔːθəuˈfriːniə] *n* 精神正常
orthopia [ɔːˈθəupiə] *n* 斜视预防,斜视矫正
orthoplastocyte [ˌɔːθəuˈplæstəsait] *n* 正常血小板
orthoplessimeter [ˌɔːθəupliˈsimitə] *n* 直位叩诊板
orthopnea [ˌɔːθɔˈpniːə] *n* 端坐呼吸 | **orthopneic** [ˌɔːθɔˈpniːik] *a*
orthopod [ˈɔːθəpɔd] *n* 矫形外科医师
Orthopoxvirus [ˈɔːθəuˌpɔksˌvaiərəs] *n* 正痘病毒属
orthopoxvirus [ˈɔːθəuˌpɔksˌvaiərəs] *n* 正痘病毒
orthopraxy [ˈɔːθəpræksi], **orthopraxis** [ˌɔːθəuˈpræksis] *n* 机械矫形术
orthopsychiatry [ˌɔːθəusaiˈkaiətri] *n* 行为精神病学 | **orthopsychiatric** [ˌɔːθəuˌsaikiˈætrik] *a* / **orthopsychiatrist** *n* 行为精神病学家
Orthoptera [ɔːˈθɔptərə] *n* 直翅目
orthoptics [ɔːˈθɔptiks] *n* 视轴矫正法 | **orthoptic** *a* 视轴矫正的 | **orthoptist** *n* 视轴矫正师
orthoptoscope [ɔːˈθɔptəskəup] *n* 视轴矫正器
orthorhombic [ˌɔːθəuˈrɔmbik] *a* 正交[晶]的,斜方[晶]的
orthoroentgenography [ˌɔːθəuˌrɔntgeˈnɔgrəfi] *n* 矫形 X 线[术]
orthorrhachic [ˌɔːθəuˈrækik] *a* 直腰椎的
orthoscope [ˈɔːθəskəup] *n* 水层检眼镜(用一层水中和角膜屈光,检眼用) | **orthoscopy** [ɔːˈθɔskəpi] *n* 水层检眼镜检查
orthosis [ɔːˈθəusis] ([复] **orthoses** [ɔːˈθəusiːz]) *n* 整直器,矫正器
orthoskiagraph [ˌɔːθəuˈskaiəgrɑːf, -græf] *n* 矫形用 X 线摄影机 | **~y** [ˌɔːθəuskaiˈægrəfi] *n* 矫形 X 线[术]
orthostatic [ˌɔːθəˈstætik] *a* 直立的,直体的
orthostatism [ˈɔːθəˌstætizəm] *n* 直立位,直立姿势
orthostereoscope [ˌɔːθəuˈstiəriəskəup] *n* 矫形用立体 X 线机
orthosympathetic [ˌɔːθəuˌsimpəˈθetik] *a* [正]交感神经的(与副交感〈颅骶〉部分相对)
orthotast [ˈɔːθətæst] *n* 正骨器
orthoterion [ˌɔːθəuˈtiəriɔn] *n* 牵伸器,牵引器
orthotherapy [ˌɔːθəuˈθerəpi] *n* 矫形疗法
orthotics [ɔːˈθɔtiks] *n* 整直学,矫正学,矫形器 | **orthotic** *a* 整直的,矫正的 / **orthotist**

[ˈɔːθətist] *n* 整直师,矫正师,矫正器修配者

ortho-tolueno-azo-beta-naphthol [ˌɔːθəu ˌtɔlju-ˈiːnəu ˌæzəu ˌbeitə ˈnæfθɔl] 邻甲苯偶氮-β-萘酚(一种用于加工柑橘果的有毒染料)

orthotonos [ɔːˈθɔtənɔs], **orthotonus** [ɔːˈθɔtənəs] *n* 挺直性痉挛,身体强直

orthotopic [ˌɔːθəuˈtɔpik] *a* 常位的,正位的

orthotyphoid [ˌɔːθəuˈtaifɔid] *n* [正]伤寒

orthovoltage [ˌɔːθəuˈvɔltidʒ] *n* 常压,中压,平压(X线治疗时电压为30~400 kV)

orthropsia [ɔːˈθrɔpsiə] *n* 暮视[症]

orthuria [ɔːˈθjuəriə] *n* 尿次[数]正常

Ortner's syndrome [ˈɔːtnə] (Norbert Ortner)奥特纳综合征(喉麻痹伴心脏病,由于主动脉与扩张的肺动脉之间的喉返神经压迫所致)

Ortolani's click (sign) [ɔːtəuˈlɑːni] (Marius Ortolani)奥托拉尼卡嗒音(征)(髋关节先天脱位时,当大腿外展屈曲时听到的卡嗒音)

Oryza [əuˈraizə] *n*【拉;希】稻属

oryzenin [əuˈraizənin] *n* 米谷蛋白

O. S. oculus sinister【拉】左眼

Os osmium 锇

os¹ [ɔs] ([复] **ora** [ˈɔrə]) *n*【拉】口 | external ~ of uterus 子宫外口,子宫口

os² [ɔs] ([复] **ossa** [ˈɔsə]) *n*【拉】骨(详见附录)

osamine [ˈəusəmiːn] *n* 糖胺(如葡萄糖胺)

OSAS obstructive sleep apnea syndrome 阻塞性睡眠呼吸暂停综合征

osazone [ˈəusəzəun] *n* 脎

oscedo [ɔˈsiːdəu] *n*【拉】呵欠

oscheal [ˈɔskiəl] *a* 阴囊的

oscheitis [ˌɔskiˈaitis] *n* 阴囊炎

oschelephantiasis [ˌɔskəlifənˈtaiəsis] *n* 阴囊象皮病

osche(o)- [构词成分] 阴囊

oscheocele [ˈɔskiəˌsiːl] *n* 阴囊瘤;阴囊肿大

oscheohydrocele [ˌɔskiəuˈhaidrəsiːl] *n* 阴囊[鞘膜]水囊肿

oscheolith [ˈɔskiəliθ] *n* 阴囊石

oscheoma [ˌɔskiˈəumə], **oscheoncus** [ˌɔskiˈɔŋkəs] *n* 阴囊瘤

oscheoplasty [ˈɔskiəˌplæsti] *n* 阴囊成形术

oschitis [ˌɔsˈkaitis] *n* 阴囊炎

Oscillaria [ˌɔsiˈlɛəriə] *n* 颤藻属

oscillation [ˌɔsiˈleiʃən] *n* 振荡,振动,摆动 | bradykinetic ~ 缓慢摆动(见于流行性脑炎)

oscillator [ˈɔsiˌleitə] *n* 振荡器

oscillo- [构词成分] 振动,震动,摆动

oscillogram [ɔˈsiləgræm] *n* 示波图

oscillograph [ɔˈsiləgrɑːf, -græf] *n* 示波器 | **~ic** [ɔˌsiləˈgræfik] *a*

oscillometer [ˌɔsiˈlɔmitə] *n* 示波计 | **oscillometric** [ˌɔsiləuˈmetrik] *a* 示波的,示波计的 / **oscillometry** *n* 示波测量法

oscillopsia [ˌɔsiˈlɔpsiə] *n* 振动幻视

oscilloscope [ɔˈsiləskəup] *n* 示波器 | **oscilloscopic** [ɔˌsiləuˈskɔpik] *a*

Oscillospira [ˌɔsiləuˈspaiərə] *n* 颤螺菌属

Oscillospiraceae [ˌɔsiləuspaiəˈreisiiː] *n* 颤螺菌科

oscine [ˈɔsin] *n* 异东莨菪醇

Oscinis pallipes [ˈɔsinis ˈpælipiːz] 套膜蝇(即Hippelates pallipes)

oscitate [ˈɔsiteit] *vi* 呵欠 | **oscitation** [ˌɔsiˈteiʃən] *n*

osculant [ˈɔskjulənt] *a* 中间型的

osculum [ˈɔskjuləm] ([复] **oscula** [ˈɔskjulə]) *n*【拉】小口,细孔

-ose [后缀] 糖

Osgood-Haskins test [ˈɔzgud ˈhæzkinz] (Edwin E. Osgood; Howard D. Haskins)奥-哈试验(检白蛋白)

Osgood-Schlatter disease [ˈɔzgudˈʃlætə] (Robert B. Osgood; Carl Schlatter)奥斯古德-施莱特病(胫骨粗隆骨软骨病,亦称青年期胫骨骨突炎)

OSHA Occupational Safety and Health Administration 职业安全与卫生管理局

-osis [后缀] 病,病态(同样见-sis)

Osler's disease [ˈəuzlə] (William Osler)奥斯勒病(①真性红细胞增多;②遗传性出血性毛细血管扩张) | ~ nodes 奥斯勒结(小而高起的肿胀压痛区,约豌豆大,呈蓝色,但有时呈淡红或红色,偶有变白的中心,最常见于指尖或趾尖、大小鱼际或足底,为亚急性细菌性心内膜炎的特征性病变) / ~ phenomenon 奥斯勒现象(血小板离开血循环后即凝集) / ~ sign 奥斯勒征(① 恶性心内膜炎时,手足皮肤上呈现痛性红斑小肿胀;②奥斯勒结) / ~ triad 奥斯勒三征(毛细血管扩张、毛细血管脆性增加和遗传性出血性素质)

Osler-Vaquez disease [ˈəuzlə vəˈkei] (William Osler; Louis H. Vaquez)真性红细胞增多

Osler-Weber-Rendu disease [ˈəuzləˈwebə rɔŋˈdjuː] (William Osler; Frederick P. Weber; Henri J. L. M. Rendu)奥斯勒-韦伯-朗迪病,遗传性出血性毛细血管扩张

Oslo meal (breakfast) [ˈɔzləu] 奥斯陆早餐(供学童用的一种餐食,奥斯陆为挪威首都)

osmate [ˈɔzmeit] *n* 锇酸盐

osmatic [ɔzˈmætik] *a* 嗅觉的;有嗅觉的,嗅觉正常的(指动物种类)

osmazome [ˈɔzməzəum] *n* 肉香质

osmesis [ɔzˈmiːsis] *n*【希】嗅

osmesthesia [ˌɔzmisˈθiːzjə] *n* 嗅觉

osmic [ˈɔzmik] *a* 锇的
osmicate [ˈɔzmikeit] *vt* 用锇酸染色,加锇酸
osmics [ˈɔzmiks] *n* 嗅觉学
osmidrosis [ˌɔzmiˈdrəusis] *n* 臭汗,腋臭
osmification [ˌɔzmifiˈkeiʃən] *n* 锇(或锇酸)处理
osmiophilic [ˌɔzmiəuˈfilik] *a* 嗜锇(或嗜锇酸)的,亲锇(或亲锇酸)的
osmiophobic [ˌɔzmiəuˈfəubik] *a* 厌锇(或厌锇酸)的,疏锇(或疏锇酸)的
osmium(O_s) [ˈɔzmiəm] *n* 锇(化学元素) | ~ tetroxide 四氧化锇(制组织标本时用作固定液)
osm(o)[1]- [构词成分] 嗅,嗅觉
osm(o)[2]- [构词成分] 渗透
osmoceptor [ˈɔzməˌseptə] *n* 渗[透]压感受器;嗅觉感受器
osmolality [ˌɔzməuˈlæləti] *n* 同渗重摩,重量摩尔渗透压浓度
osmolar [ɔzˈməulə] *a* 摩尔渗透压的
osmolarity [ˌɔzməuˈlærəti] *n* 同渗容摩,摩尔渗透压浓度
osmole [ˈɔzməul] *n* 渗摩,渗透压摩尔(用摩尔表示的渗透压单位)
osmology [ɔzˈmɔlədʒi] *n* 嗅觉学;渗透学
osmolute [ˈɔzməˌljuːt] *n* 渗质
osmometer [ɔzˈmɔmitə] *n* 渗透压计;嗅觉计
osmonosology [ˌɔzməunəuˈsɔlədʒi] *n* 嗅觉障碍学
osmophilic [ˌɔzməˈfilik] *a* 趋渗的,易渗的
osmophobia [ˌɔzməuˈfəubiə] *n* 臭气恐怖,恐臭症
osmophore [ˈɔzməfɔː] *n* 生臭基,生臭团
osmoreceptor [ˌɔzməuriˈseptə] *n* 渗透压感受器;嗅觉感受器
osmoregulation [ˌɔzməuˌregjuˈleiʃən] *n* 渗透调节 | **osmoregulatory** [ˌɔzməuˈregjulətəri] *a* 调节渗透的
osmoscope [ˈɔzməskəup] *n* 嗅镜,助嗅器
osmose [ˈɔzməus] *vt, vi* 渗透
osmosis [ɔzˈməusis] *n* 渗透[作用] | **osmotic** [ɔzˈmɔtik] *a* | **osmotically** *ad*
osmosology [ˌɔzməuˈsɔlədʒi] *n* 渗透学
osmostat [ˈɔzməˌstæt] *n* 渗透压稳定器
osmotaxis [ˌɔzməuˈtæksis] *n* 趋渗性
osmotherapy [ˌɔzməuˈθerəpi] *n* 渗透疗法
osmyl [ˈɔzmil] *n* 气味,臭
osone [ˈəusəun] *n* 邻酮醛糖
osphresi(o)- [构词成分] 嗅,嗅觉
osphresiology [ˌɔsfriziˈɔlədʒi] *n* 嗅觉学
osphresiometer [ˌɔsfriziˈɔmitə] *n* 嗅觉计,嗅觉测量器
osphresis [ɔsˈfriːsis] *n* 嗅觉 | **osphretic** [ɔsˈfretik] *a*
osphyarthrosis [ˌɔsfiɑːˈθrəusis] *n* 髋关节炎
osphyomyelitis [ˌɔsfiəuˌmaiəˈlaitis] *n* 腰髓炎
osphyotomy [ˌɔsfiˈɔtəmi] *n* 腰部切开术
ossa [ˈɔsə] os 的复数(见 os[2])
ossature [ˈɔsətʃə] *n* 骨骼
ossein [ˈɔsiin] *n* 骨胶原
osselet [ˈɔsilet] *n* 马膝骨赘
osseoalbumoid [ˌɔsiəuˈælbjumɔid] *n* 骨硬蛋白
osseoaponeurotic [ˌɔsiəuæpənjuəˈrɔtik] *a* 骨[与]腱膜的
osseocartilaginous [ˌɔsiəukɑːtiˈlædʒinəs] *a* 骨软骨的
osseofibrous [ˌɔsiəuˈfaibrəs] *a* 骨[与]纤维组织的
osseointegration [ˌɔsiəuˌintəˈgreiʃən] *n* 骨整合
osseomucin [ˌɔsiəuˈmjuːsin] *n* 骨黏素
osseomucoid [ˌɔsiəuˈmjuːkɔid] *n* 骨[类]黏蛋白
osseosonometer [ˌɔsiəusəuˈnɔmitə] *n* 骨导听力计 / **osseosonometry** *n* 骨导听力检查
osseous [ˈɔsiəs] *a* 骨的,骨性的
ossicle [ˈɔsikl] *n* 小骨 | epactal ~s, intercalcar ~s 缝间骨 / sphenoturbinal ~s 蝶骨甲 | **ossicular** [ɔˈsikjulə], **ossiculate** [ɔˈsikjulit] *a*
ossicula [ɔˈsikjulə] ossiculum 的复数
ossiculectomy [ˌɔsikjuˈlektəmi] *n* 听小骨切除术
ossiculoplasty [ˌɔsikjuləˈplæsti] *n* 听骨链成形术
ossiculotomy [ˌɔsikjuˈlɔtəmi] *n* 听小骨切开术
ossiculum [ɔˈsikjuləm] ([复] **ossicula** [ɔˈsikjulə]) *n* 【拉】小骨
ossidesmosis [ˌɔsidesˈməusis] *n* 骨[与]腱形成;腱骨化
ossiferous [ɔˈsifərəs] *a* 生骨的
ossific [ɔˈsifik] *a* 骨化的,成骨的
ossification [ˌɔsifiˈkeiʃən] *n* 骨化 | cartilaginous ~, endochondral ~ 软骨内成骨 / metaplastic ~ 化生性骨化 / perichondral ~ 软骨膜[下]骨化
ossifluence [ɔˈsifluəns] *n* 骨软化
ossiform [ˈɔsifɔːm] *a* 骨样的
ossify [ˈɔsifai] *vt, vi* 骨化,成骨
ossifying [ˈɔsiˌfaiiŋ] *a* 骨化的
ossiphone [ˈɔsifəun] *n* 骨导助听器
ostalgia [ɔsˈtældʒiə] *n* 骨痛
ostarthritis [ˌɔstɑːˈθraitis] *n* 骨关节炎
osteal [ˈɔstiəl] *a* 骨的,骨性的
ostealbumoid [ˌɔstiˈælbjumɔid] *n* 骨硬蛋白
ostealgia [ˌɔstiˈældʒiə] *n* 骨痛
osteameba [ˌɔstiəˈmiːbə] *n* 骨小体
osteanabrosis [ˌɔstiænəˈbrəusis] *n* 骨萎缩
osteanagenesis [ˌɔstiˌænəˈdʒenisis] *n* 骨再生
osteanaphysis [ˌɔstiəˈnæfisis] *n* 骨再生
ostearthritis [ˌɔstiɑːˈθraitis] *n* 骨关节炎

ostearthrotomy [ˌɔstiɑːˈθrɔtəmi] *n* 骨关节端切除术
ostectomy [ɔsˈtektəmi], **osteectomy** [ˌɔstiˈektəmi] *n* 骨切除术
osteectopia [ˌɔstiekˈtəupiə], **osteectopy** [ˌɔstiˈektəpi] *n* 骨异位
ostein [ˈɔstiin] *n* 骨胶原
osteite [ˈɔstiait] *n* 骨化中心
osteitis [ˌɔstiˈaitis] *n* 骨炎 | carious ~, necrotic ~ 骨髓炎 / caseous ~ 干酪样骨炎,结核性骨疽 / central ~ 骨内膜炎 / condensing ~, formative ~, sclerosing ~ 致密性骨炎,骨质增生性骨炎,硬化性骨炎 / ~ fibrosa cystica, ~ fibrosa cystica generalisata 囊性纤维性骨炎,全身性囊性纤维性骨炎 / productive ~ 增生性骨炎,骨质象牙化 / secondary hyperplastic ~ 继发性增殖性骨炎,肥大性肺性骨关节病
ostembryon [ɔsˈtembriɔn] *n* 胎儿石化,石胎
ostempyesis [ˌɔstempaiˈiːsis] *n* 骨化脓
oste(o)- [构词成分] 骨
osteoacusis [ˌɔstiəuəˈkuːsis] *n* 骨传导
osteoanagenesis [ˌɔstiəuˌænəˈdʒenisis] *n* 骨再生,成骨,骨发育
osteoanesthesia [ˌɔstiəuænisˈθiːzjə] *n* 骨感觉缺失,骨无感觉
osteoaneurysm [ˌɔstiəuˈænjuərizəm] *n* 骨内动脉瘤
osteoarthritis [ˌɔstiəuɑːˈθraitis] *n* 骨关节炎 | hyperplastic ~ 增殖性骨关节炎,肥大性肺性骨关节病 | **osteoarthritic** [ˌɔstiəuɑːˈθritik] *a*
osteoarthropathy [ˌɔstiəuɑːˈθrɔpəθi] *n* 骨关节病 | hypertrophic pneumic ~, hypertrophic pulmonary ~, pulmonary ~, secondary hypertrophic ~ 肥大性肺性骨关节病
osteoarthrosis [ˌɔstiəuɑːˈθrəusis] *n* 骨关节病(非炎性慢性关节炎)
osteoarthrotomy [ˌɔstiəuɑːˈθrɔtəmi] *n* 骨关节端切除术
osteoarticular [ˌɔstiəuɑːˈtikjulə] *a* 骨关节的
osteoblast [ˈɔstiəˌblæst] *n* 成骨细胞 | **~ic** [ˌɔstiəuˈblæstik] *a*
osteoblastoma [ˌɔstiəublæsˈtəumə] *n* 成骨细胞瘤
osteocachexia [ˌɔstiəukəˈkeksiə] *n* 骨性恶病质,慢性骨病 | **osteocachectic** [ˌɔstiəukəˈkektik] *a*
osteocalcin [ˌɔstiəuˈkælsin] *n* 骨钙素(一种维生素 K 依赖性钙结合骨蛋白,骨内最丰富的非胶原蛋白,血清浓度增加是病态骨更新增加的标志)
osteocamp [ˈɔstiəkæmp] *n* 切骨矫形器
osteocampsia [ˌɔstiəuˈkæmpsiə], **osteocampsis** [ˌɔstiəuˈkæmpsis] *n* 骨屈曲(如佝偻病时)
osteocartilaginous [ˌɔstiəukɑːtiˈlædʒinəs] *a* 骨软骨的
osteocele [ˈɔstiəsiːl] *n* 阴囊骨瘤,睾丸骨瘤;骨性疝
osteocementum [ˌɔstiəusiˈmentəm] *n* 骨样牙骨质
osteochondral [ˌɔstiəuˈkɔndrəl] *a* 骨软骨的;骨[与骨]关节软骨的
osteochondritis [ˌɔstiəukɔnˈdraitis] *n* 骨软骨炎
osteochondrodysplasia [ˌɔstiəuˌkɔndrəudisˈpleiziə] *n* 骨软骨发育不良
osteochondrodystrophia [ˌɔstiəuˌkɔndrəudisˈtrəufiə], **osteochondrodystrophy** [ˌɔstiəukɔndrəuˈdistrəfi] *n* 骨软骨营养不良
osteochondrofibroma [ˌɔstiəuˌkɔndrəufaiˈbrəumə] *n* 骨软骨纤维瘤
osteochondrolysis [ˌɔstiəukɔnˈdrɔlisis] *n* 骨软骨脱离,剥脱性骨软骨炎
osteochondroma [ˌɔstiəukɔnˈdrəumə] *n* 骨软骨瘤
osteochondromatosis [ˌɔstiəuˌkɔndrəuməˈtəusis] *n* 骨软骨瘤病
osteochondromyxoma [ˌɔstiəuˌkɔndrəumikˈsəumə] *n* 骨软骨黏液瘤
osteochondropathia [ˌɔstiəuˌkɔndrəuˈpæθiə] *n* 骨软骨病
osteochondropathy [ˌɔstiəuˌkɔnˈdrɔpəθi] *n* 骨软骨病 | polyglucose (dextran) sulfate-induced ~ 硫酸缩合葡萄糖(葡聚糖)引起的骨软骨病
osteochondrophyte [ˌɔstiəuˈkɔndrəfait] *n* 骨软骨瘤
osteochondrosarcoma [ˌɔstiəuˌkɔndrəusɑːˈkəumə] *n* 骨软骨肉瘤
osteochondrosis [ˌɔstiəukɔnˈdrəusis] *n* 骨软骨病
osteochondrous [ˌɔstiəuˈkɔndrəs] *a* 骨软骨的
osteoclasia [ˌɔstiəuˈkleiziə] *n* 折骨术(骨的吸收和破坏)
osteoclasis [ˌɔstiˈɔkləsis], **osteoclasty** [ˈɔstiəˌklæsti] *n* 折骨术(外科的骨折或再骨折)
osteoclast [ˈɔstiəˌklæst] *n* 破骨细胞;折骨器 | **~ic** [ˌɔstiəuˈklæstik] *a* 折骨器的;破坏骨的
osteoclastoma [ˌɔstiəuklæsˈtəumə] *n* 破骨细胞瘤
osteocomma [ˌɔstiəuˈkɔmə] *n* 单骨,骨件
osteocope [ˈɔstiəˌkəup] *n* 骨剧痛(常为梅毒骨病症状) | **osteocopic** [ˌɔstiəˈkɔpik] *a*
osteocranium [ˌɔstiəˈkreinjəm] *n* 骨颅(在骨化期的胎儿头颅)
osteocystoma [ˌɔstiəusisˈtəumə] *n* 骨囊瘤
osteocyte [ˈɔstiəsait] *n* 骨细胞
osteodentin [ˌɔstiəuˈdentin] *n* 骨性牙质
osteodentinoma [ˌɔstiəudentiˈnəumə] *n* 骨牙

质瘤
osteodermia [ˌɔstiəu'dəːmiə] *n* 皮[肤]骨化
osteodesmosis [ˌɔstiəudes'məusis] *n* 骨[与]腱形成;腱骨化
osteodiastasis [ˌɔstiəudai'æstəsis] *n* 骨分离
osteodynia [ˌɔstiəu'diniə] *n* 骨痛
osteodysplasty [ˌɔstiəudis'plæsti] *n* 骨发育异常
osteodystrophia [ˌɔstiəudis'trəufiə] *n* 骨营养不良 | ~ cystica 囊性骨营养不良 / ~ fibrosa 纤维性骨营养不良
osteodystrophy [ˌɔstiəu'distrəfi] *n* 骨营养不良 | renal ~ 肾性骨营养不良症
osteoectasia [ˌɔstiəuek'teiziə] *n* 骨膨胀症 | familial ~ 家族性骨膨胀症,青少年骨外层变形肥厚
osteoectomy [ˌɔstiəu'ektəmi] *n* 骨切除术
osteoenchondroma [ˌɔstiəuˌenkɔn'drəumə] *n* 骨软骨瘤
osteoepiphysis [ˌɔstiəui'pifisis] *n* 骨骺
osteofibrochondrosarcoma [ˌɔstiəuˌfaibrəuˌkɔndrəusɑː'kəumə] *n* 骨纤维软骨肉瘤
osteofibroma [ˌɔstiəufai'brəumə] *n* 骨纤维瘤,纤维骨瘤
osteofibromatosis [ˌɔstiəuˌfaibrəumə'təusis] *n* 骨纤维瘤病 | cystic ~ 囊性骨纤维瘤病
osteofluorosis [ˌɔstiəufluə'rəusis] *n* 骨氟中毒(骨骼变化,一般包括骨软化和骨硬化,由于慢性摄入过量氟化物所致)
osteogen ['ɔstiədʒen] *n* 成骨质
osteogenesis [ˌɔstiəu'dʒenisis] *n* 骨生成,骨发生 | ~ imperfecta (OI) 成骨不全 / ~ imperfecta cystica 囊性成骨不全 | **osteogenetic** [ˌɔstiəudʒi'netik] *a* | **osteogeny** [ˌɔsti'ɔdʒəni] *n*
osteogenic [ˌɔstiəu'dʒenik], **osteogenous** [ˌɔsti'ɔdʒinəs] *a* 成骨的
osteogram ['ɔstiəgræm] *n* 椎骨图
osteography [ˌɔsti'ɔgrəfi] *n* 骨论
osteohalisteresis [ˌɔstiəuhəˌlistə'riːsis] *n* 骨质缺乏
osteohemachromatosis [ˌɔstiəuˌheməˌkrəumə'təusis] *n* 骨血色素沉着[症](动物)
osteohydatidosis [ˌɔstiəuˌhaidəti'dəusis] *n* 骨棘球蚴病
osteoid ['ɔstiɔid] *a* 骨样的 *n* 类骨质
osteoinduction [ˌɔstiəuin'dʌkʃən] *n* 诱导骨生成
osteolathyrism [ˌɔstiəu'læθirizəm] *n* 香[豌]豆中毒性骨病(实验动物)
osteolipochondroma [ˌɔstiəuˌlipəukɔn'drəumə] *n* 骨脂软骨瘤
osteolipoma [ˌɔstiəuli'pəumə] *n* 骨脂瘤
osteology [ˌɔsti'ɔlədʒi], **osteologia** [ˌɔstiə'lɔdʒiə] *n* 骨学 | **osteological** [ˌɔstiə'lɔdʒikəl] *a* | **osteologist** [ɔsti'ɔlədʒist] *n* 骨学家
osteolysis [ˌɔsti'ɔlisis] *n* 骨质溶解 | **osteolytic** [ˌɔstiəu'litik] *a* 溶骨的
osteoma [ˌɔsti'əumə] ([复] **osteomas** 或 **osteomata** [ˌɔsti'əumətə]) *n* 骨瘤 | cavalryman's ~ 骑士骨瘤(股长收肌附着处的骨瘤) / compact ~ 密质骨瘤 / giant osteoid ~ 巨大骨样骨瘤,成骨细胞瘤
osteomalacia [ˌɔstiəumə'leiʃiə], **osteomalacosis** [ˌɔstiəumælə'kəusis] *n* 骨软化症 | **osteomalacic** [ˌɔstiəumə'leisik] *a*
osteomatoid [ˌɔsti'əumətɔid] *a* 骨瘤样的
osteomatosis [ˌɔstiəumə'təusis] *n* 骨瘤病
osteomere ['ɔstiəmiə] *n* 单骨,骨件
osteometry [ˌɔsti'ɔmitri] *n* 骨测量法
osteomiosis [ˌɔstiəumai'əusis] *n* 骨碎裂
osteomyelitis [ˌɔstiəuˌmaiə'laitis] *n* 骨髓炎 | conchiolin ~ 珍珠工骨髓炎(骨髓内有矿尘沉着) / typhoid ~ 伤寒性骨髓炎 / ~ variolosa 天花性骨髓炎 | **osteomyelitic** [ˌɔstiəuˌmaiə'litik] *a*
osteomyelodysplasia [ˌɔstiəuˌmaiələudis'pleisiə] *n* 骨髓发育不良
osteomyelography [ˌɔstiəumaiə'lɔgrəfi] *n* 骨髓X线摄影[术]
osteomyxochondroma [ˌɔstiəuˌmiksəukɔn'drəumə] *n* 骨黏液性软骨瘤,骨软骨黏液瘤
osteon ['ɔstiɔn], **osteone** ['ɔstiəun] *n* 骨单位(骨密质构造的基本单位)
osteonecrosis [ˌɔstiəune'krəusis] *n* 骨坏死
osteonectin [ˌɔstiəu'nektin] *n* 骨连接素(一种结合胶原和钙的磷蛋白,用作矿化的调节剂,存在于骨内和血小板内)
osteoneuralgia [ˌɔstiəunjuə'rældʒiə] *n* 骨神经痛
osteonosus [ˌɔsti'ɔnəsəs] *n* 骨病
osteo-odontoma [ˌɔstiəu ˌɔdɔn'təumə] *n* 釉质牙瘤
osteopath ['ɔstiəpæθ] *n* 骨疗法医士,按骨术医士
osteopathia [ˌɔstiəu'pæθiə] *n* 骨病
osteopathology [ˌɔstiəupə'θɔlədʒi] *n* 骨病理学
osteopathy [ˌɔsti'ɔpəθi] *n* 骨病;骨疗法,按骨术,整骨术 | disseminated condensing ~ 播散性致密性骨病,全身脆性骨硬化 / hunger ~, alimentary ~ 饥饿性骨病,营养不良性骨病 / myelogenic ~ 骨髓性骨病 | **osteopathic** [ˌɔstiəu'pæθik] *a*
osteopecilia [ˌɔstiəupə'siliə] *n* [全身]脆弱性骨硬化
osteopedion [ˌɔstiəu'piːdiɔn] *n* 胎儿石化,石胎
osteopenia [ˌɔstiəu'piːniə] *n* 骨质稀少,骨质减少 | **osteopenic** [ˌɔstiəu'penik] *a*
osteoperiosteal [ˌɔstiəuˌperi'ɔstiəl] *a* 骨骨膜的
osteoperiostitis [ˌɔstiəuˌperiɔs'taitis] *n* 骨骨膜炎

| alveolodental ~ 牙槽骨骨膜炎,牙周炎
osteopetrosis [ˌɔstiəupiˈtrəusis] *n* 骨硬化病
osteophage [ˈɔstiəfeidʒ] *n* 噬骨细胞
osteophagia [ˌɔstiəuˈfeidʒiə] *n* 食骨癖
osteophlebitis [ˌɔstiəufliˈbaitis] *n* 骨静脉炎
osteophone [ˈɔstiəfəun] *n* [骨导]助听器
osteophony [ˌɔstiˈɔfəni] *n* 骨导音,骨传导
osteophore [ˈɔstiəfɔː] *n* 碎骨钳
osteophyma [ˌɔstiəuˈfaimə] *n* 骨赘
osteophyte [ˈɔstiəˌfait] *n* 骨赘 | **osteophytic** [ˌɔstiəˈfitik] *a*
osteophytosis [ˌɔstiəufaiˈtəusis] *n* 骨赘病
osteoplaque [ˈɔstiəplæk] *n* 骨层
osteoplast [ˈɔstiəplæst] *n* 成骨细胞
osteoplastic [ˌɔstiəuˈplæstik] *a* 成骨的;骨成形的 | **osteoplasty** [ˈɔstiəˌplæsti] *n* 骨成形术,骨整形术
osteoplastica [ˌɔstiəuˈplæstikə] *n* 囊状纤维性骨炎
osteopoikilosis [ˌɔstiəuˌpɔikiˈləusis] *n* 全身脆性骨硬化 | **osteopoikilotic** [ˌɔstiəuˌpɔikiˈlɔtik] *a*
osteoporosis [ˌɔstiəupəˈrəusis] *n* 骨质疏松[症] | **osteoporotic** [ˌɔstiəupəˈrɔtik] *a*
osteopsathyrosis [ˌɔstiɔpˌsæθiˈrəusis] *n* 骨脆症,成骨不全
osteoradionecrosis [ˌɔstiəuˌreidiəuneˈkrəusis] *n* 放射性骨坏死
osteorrhagia [ˌɔstiəuˈreidʒiə] *n* 骨出血
osteorrhaphy [ˌɔstiˈɔrəfi] *n* 骨缝合术
osteosarcoma [ˌɔstiəusɑːˈkəumə] *n* 骨肉瘤 | **~tous** [ˌɔstiəusɑːˈkəumətəs] *a*
osteosarcomatosis [ˌɔstiəusɑːˌkəuməˈtəusis] *n* 骨肉瘤病(多发性骨肉瘤同时发生;同步多中心骨肉瘤)
osteosclerosis [ˌɔstiəuskliəˈrəusis] *n* 骨硬化 | **osteosclerotic** [ˌɔstiəuskliəˈrɔtik] *a*
osteoscope [ˈɔstiəskəup] *n* X线测骨器
osteoseptum [ˌɔstiəuˈseptəm] *n* 骨性[鼻]中隔
osteosis [ˌɔstiˈəusis] *n* 骨质生成,骨化病 | parathyroid ~ 甲状旁腺性骨化病,囊性纤维性骨炎
osteostixis [ˌɔstiəuˈstiksis] *n* 骨穿刺术
osteosuture [ˈɔstiəsjuːtʃə] *n* 骨缝合术
osteosynovitis [ˌɔstiəuˌsinəˈvaitis] *n* 骨滑膜炎
osteosynthesis [ˌɔstiəuˈsinθisis] *n* 骨缝合术,骨接合术
osteotabes [ˌɔstiəuˈteibiːz] *n* 骨髓痨,骨耗病
osteotelangiectasia [ˌɔstiəuteˌlændʒiekˈteiziə] *n* 毛细血管扩张性骨肉瘤
osteothrombophlebitis [ˌɔstiəuˌθrɔmbəufliˈbaitis] *n* 骨血栓静脉炎
osteothrombosis [ˌɔstiəuθrɔmˈbəusis] *n* 骨内[静脉]血栓形成
osteotome [ˈɔstiəˌtəum] *n* 骨凿
osteotomoclasis [ˌɔstiəutəˈmɔkləsis], **osteotomoclasia** [ˌɔstiəuˌtəuməˈkleiziə] *n* 折骨矫形术
osteotomy [ˌɔstiˈɔtəmi] *n* 截骨术,切骨术 | block ~ 大块切骨术 / cuneiform ~ 楔形切骨术 / cup-and-ball ~ 杵臼样切骨术 / hinge ~ 铰链样切骨术,屈戌状切骨术 / pelvic ~ 耻骨切开术 / subtrochanteric ~ 转子下切骨术 / transtrochanteric ~ 经转子切骨术
osteotribe [ˈɔstiəˌtraib], **osteotrite** [ˈɔstiəˌtrait] *n* 骨锉
osteotrophy [ˌɔstiˈɔtrəfi] *n* 骨营养
osteotylus [ˌɔstiˈɔtiləs] *n* 骨痂
osteotympanic [ˌɔstiəutimˈpænik] *a* 颅鼓[室]的,颅骨耳鼓的,骨鼓的
Ostertagia [ˌɔstəˈteidʒiə] (Robert von Ostertag) *n* 胃线虫属
osthexia [ɔsˈθeksiə], **osthexy** [ˈɔsθeksi] *n* 骨化异常
ostiole [ˈɔstiəul] *n* 小孔,孔口 | **ostiolar** *a*
ostitis [ɔsˈtaitis] *n* 骨炎
ostium [ˈɔstiəm] ([复] **ostia** [ˈɔstiə]) *n* 【拉】口,门口 | **ostial** [ˈɔstiəl] *a*
ostomate [ˈɔstəmeit] *n* 造口者(曾受肠造口术或输尿管造口术者)
ostomy [ˈɔstəmi] *n* 造口术,造瘘术,吻合术
ostosis [ɔsˈtəusis] *n* 骨生成,骨发生
ostraceous [ɔsˈtreiʃəs] *a* 蠔壳状的,蛎壳状的
ostracosis [ˌɔstrəˈkəusis] *n* 蠔壳状(骨)变性
ostreasterol [ˌɔstriˈæstərɔl] *n* 牡蛎甾醇
ostreotoxism [ˌɔstriəuˈtɔksizəm] *n* 牡蛎中毒,蠔中毒
Ostrum-Furst syndrome [ˈɔstrəm fəːst] (Herman W. Ostrum; William Furst) 奥-弗综合征(先天性颈部骨性联接、扁颅底及施普伦格〈Sprengel〉畸形)
Oswaldocruzia [ɔzˌwɑːldəuˈkruːziə] (G. Oswaldo Cruz) *n* 渥氏线虫属
OT old term in anatomy 解剖学旧名词; old tuberculin 旧结核菌素
otacoustic [ˌəutəˈkuːstik] *a* 助听的
otalgia [əuˈtældʒiə] *n* 耳痛 | geniculate ~ 膝状神经节耳痛 / reflex ~ 反射性耳痛 / tabetic ~ 脊髓痨性耳痛 | **otagra** [əuˈtægrə] *n* / **otalgic** [əu ˈtældʒik] *a* 耳痛的 *n* 耳痛药
otaphone [ˈəutəfəun] *n* 助听器
OTC over the counter 非处方药(指根据法律不需要处方即可出售的药物); ornithine transcarbamoylase 鸟氨酸转氨甲酰酶
OTD organ tolerance dose 器官耐受量(放射量)
otectomy [əuˈtektəmi] *n* 耳组织切除术(指内耳

和中耳）
othelcosis [ˌəuthelˈkəusis] *n* 耳溃疡;耳化脓
othematoma [ˌəuthiːməˈtəumə] *n* 耳血肿
othemorrhea [ˌəutheməˈriːə] *n* 耳出血
othygroma [ˌəuthaiˈgrəumə] *n* 耳水瘤
otiatrics [ˌəutiˈætriks], **otiatry** [əuˈtaiətri] *n* 耳病治疗学 | **otiatric** [ˈəutiˈætrik] *a*
otic [ˈəutik] *a* 耳的
oticodinia [ˌəutikəuˈdinjə], **oticodinosis** [ˌəutikəudiˈnəusis] *n* 耳病性眩晕
otiobiosis [ˌəutiəubaiˈəusis] *n* 耳蜱病
Otiobius [əutiˈəubiəs] *n* 耳蜱属,残喙蜱属
otitis [əuˈtaitis] *n* 耳炎 | ~ externa 外耳炎 / furuncular ~ 外耳道疖 / ~ interna 内耳炎 / ~ media 中耳炎 / mucosis ~, mucosus ~ 黏液链球菌性耳炎 | **otitic** [əuˈtitik] *a*
ot(o)- [构词成分]耳
otoacariasis [ˌəutəuˌækəˈraiəsis] *n* 耳螨病
otoantritis [ˌəutəuænˈtraitis] *n* 鼓窦炎
otobiosis [ˌəutəubaiˈəusis] *n* 耳蜱病
Otobius [əuˈtəubiəs] *n* 耳蜱属,残喙蜱属
otoblennorrhea [ˌəutəuˌblenəˈriːə] *n* 耳黏液溢
otocariasis [ˌəutəukəˈraiəsis] *n* 耳螨病
Otocentor [ˌəutəuˈsentə] *n* 暗眼蜱属(即 Anocentor) | ~ nitans 明暗眼蜱(即 Anocentor nitans)
otocephalus [ˌəutəuˈsefələs] *n* 无下颌并耳畸胎
otocephaly [ˌɔtəuˈsefəli] *n* 无下颌并耳畸形
otocerebritis [ˌəutəuseriˈbraitis] *n* 中耳[炎]性脑炎
otocleisis [ˌəutəuˈklaisis] *n* 耳道闭合
otoconite [əuˈtɔkənait] *n* 位觉砂,耳石
otoconium [ˌəutəuˈkəunjəm] ([复] **otoconia** [ˌəutəuˈkəunia]) *n*【拉】位觉砂,耳石
otocranium [ˌəutəuˈkreinjəm] *n* 耳颅 | **otocranial** *a*
otocyst [ˈəutəsist] *n* 听泡(胚胎);听囊(低等动物) | **~ic** [ˌəutəuˈsistik] *a*
Otodectes [ˌəutəuˈdektiːz] *n* 耳螨属
otodynia [ˌəutəuˈdiniə] *n* 耳痛
otoencephalitis [ˌəutəuenˌsefəˈlaitis] *n* 中耳[炎]性脑炎
otoganglion [ˌəutəuˈgæŋgliən] *n* 耳神经节
otogenous [əuˈtɔdʒinəs], **otogenic** [ˌəutəuˈdʒenik] *a* 耳源性的
otography [əuˈtɔgrəfi] *n* 耳论,耳学
otohemineurasthenia [ˌəutəuˌhemiˌnjuəræsˈθiːniə] *n* 神经衰弱性单耳听力减退
otolaryngology [ˌəutəuˌlæriŋˈgɔlədʒi] *n* 耳鼻咽喉[科]学 | **otolaryngologist** *n* 耳鼻咽喉[科]学家
otolith [ˈəutəliθ], **otolite** [ˈəutəlait] *n* 位觉砂,耳石 | **~ic** [ˌəutəˈliθik] *a*
otolithiasis [ˌəutəuliˈθaiəsis] *n* 耳石病
otology [əuˈtɔlədʒi] *n* 耳科学 | **otologic** [ˌəutəˈlɔdʒik] *a* / **otologist** *n* 耳科医师,耳科学家
otomastoiditis [ˌəutəuˌmæstɔiˈdaitis] *n* 耳乳突炎
otomucormycosis [ˌəutəuˌmjuːkəmaiˈkəusis] *n* 耳毛霉病
otomyasthenia [ˌəutəuˌmaiæsˈθiːniə] *n* 耳肌无力性听力减退,听肌无力
Otomyces [ˌəutəuˈmaisiːz] *n* 耳真菌属 | ~ hageni, ~ purpureus 人耳真菌
otomycosis [ˌəutəumaiˈkəusis] *n* 耳真菌病,耳癣 | ~ aspergillina 耳曲霉病
otomyiasis [ˌəutəuˈmaijəsis] *n* 耳蛆病
otoncus [əuˈtɔŋkəs] *n* 耳[肿]瘤
otonecrectomy [ˌəutəunəˈkrektəmi] *n* 耳坏死组织切除术
otoneuralgia [ˌəutəunjuəˈrældʒiə] *n* 耳神经痛
otoneurasthenia [ˌəutəuˌnjuəræsˈθiːniə] *n* 耳病性神经衰弱
otoneurology [ˌəutəunjuəˈrɔlədʒi] *n* 耳神经科学 | **otoneurologic** [ˌɔtəuˌnjuərəˈlɔdʒik] *a*
otopathy [əuˈtɔpəθi] *n* 耳病
otopharyngeal [ˌəutəufəˈrindʒiəl] *a* 耳咽的
otophone [ˈəutəfəun] *n* 助听器;耳听诊管
otopiesis [ˌəutəuˈpaiisis] *n* 鼓膜内陷;内耳受压症
otoplasty [ˈəutəˌplæsti] *n* 耳成形术
otopolypus [ˌəutəuˈpɔlipəs] *n* 耳息肉
otopyorrhea [ˌəutəupaiəˈriːə] *n* 耳脓溢
otopyosis [ˌəutəupaiˈəusis] *n* 耳化脓
otor [ˈəutə] *a* 耳的
otorhinolaryngology [ˌəutəuˌrainəuˌlæriŋˈgɔlədʒi] *n* 耳鼻咽喉[科]学
otorhinology [ˌəutəuraiˈnɔlədʒi] *n* 耳鼻科学
otorrhagia [ˌəutəuˈreidʒiə] *n* 耳出血
otorrhea [ˌəutəuˈriːə] *n* 耳漏 | cerebrospinal fluid ~ 脑脊液耳漏
otosalpinx [ˌəutəuˈsælpiŋks] *n* 咽鼓管
otoscleronectomy [ˌəutəuˈskliərəuˈnektəmi], **otosclerectomy** [ˌəutəuskliəˈrektəmi] *n* 硬化听骨切除术
otosclerosis [ˌəutəuskliəˈrəusis] *n* 耳硬化 | **otosclerotic** [ˌəutəuskliəˈrɔtik] *a*
otoscope [ˈəutəskəup] *n* 耳镜 | **otoscopy** [əuˈtɔskəpi] *n* 耳镜检查
otosis [əuˈtəusis] *n* 错听
otospongiosis [ˌəutəuˌspɔndʒiˈəusis] *n* 耳硬化症
otosteal [əuˈtɔstiəl] *a* 耳骨的
otosteon [əuˈtɔstiɔn] *n* 位觉砂,耳石;听小骨
ototomy [əuˈtɔtəmi] *n* 耳切开术

ototoxic [ˌəutəuˈtɔksik] *a* 耳毒性的(对第八脑神经或听觉及平衡器官有毒性作用的) | **~ity** [ˌəutəutɔkˈsisəti] *n*
Otto disease [ˈɔtəu] (Adolph W. Otto) 奥托病(髋臼骨关节突出;〈髋〉关节内陷) | ~ pelvis 奥托骨盆(骨盆的髋臼内陷,使股骨头突入骨盆腔内)
Ott's test [ɔt] (Isaac Ott) 奥特试验(检尿核白蛋白)
OU oculus uterque【拉】每眼
ouabain [wɑːˈbeiin] *n* 哇巴因,毒毛花苷 G(强心药)
Ouchterlony technique [ˈɔkteˌləuni] (Oryan T. G. Ouchterlony) 二维双向扩散
Oudin current [uˈdæn] (Paul Oudin) 奥丁电流(高压的高频电流,用于透热疗法) | ~ resonator 奥丁共振器(连接在高频电流源上的线圈,用于电疗法)
oulectomy [uˈlektəmi] *n* 瘢痕切除术;龈切除术
oulitis [uˈlaitis] *n* 龈炎
oulonitis [ˌuləˈnaitis] *n* 牙髓炎
oulorrhagia [ˌuləˈreidʒiə] *n* 龈出血
ounce(oz) [auns] *n* 盎司,英两(常衡 =1/16 磅,或 28.349 5 g;药衡 =1/12 磅,或 31.103 g) | fluid ~ (fl oz) 流质英两(药衡 =8 液量打兰,或合 29.57 ml)
-ous [前缀]具有…的,充满…的;亚…的
outbalance [autˈbæləns] *vt* 重于,重量超过
outbreak [ˈautbreik] *n* [突然]发生,暴发,流行,发作
outbreeding [ˈautbriːdiŋ] *n* 杂交繁殖,远系繁殖,远交(完全不相关的个体的交配)
outburst [ˈautbəːst] *n* 爆发 | delirious ~ 谵妄型爆发
outgrowth [ˈautgrəuθ] *n* 长出,派出;旁枝;赘疣
outlet [ˈautlet] *n* 出口 | pelvic ~ 骨盆出口,骨盆下口 / transvers ~ 出口横径
outlier [ˈautlaiə] *n* 无关项(在统计学中指一项观察离资料的中心题太远,以致被认为是一项明显的错误,应该从资料中去掉,而不管是否能找出此偏差的原因)
outpatient [ˈautˌpeiʃənt] *n* 门诊病人
outpocketing [autˈpɔkitiŋ] *n* 外包缝合法
outpouching [ˈautpautʃiŋ] *n* 凸出,外突
outpour [autˈpɔː] *vt*, *vi* (使)泻出,(使)倾泻 | [ˈautpɔː] *n*
output [ˈautput] *n* 产量,产品;排出量,输出量;排泄物 | cardiac ~ 心排血量,心输出量 / energy ~ 能[量]排出量 / stroke ~ 每搏输出量 / urinary ~ 尿排出量
ova [ˈəuvə] ovum 的复数
oval [ˈəuvəl] *a* 卵圆的,卵形的
ovalbumin [əuˈvælbjumin] *n* 卵白蛋白,卵清蛋白
ovalocytary [ˌəuvələuˈsaitəri] *a* 卵形红细胞的
ovalocyte [ˈəuvələuˌsait] *n* 卵形红细胞
ovalocytosis [əuˌvæləsaiˌtəusis] *n* 卵形红细胞症
ovarialgia [əuˌvεəriˈældʒiə] *n* 卵巢痛
ovarian [əuˈvεəriən] *a* 卵巢的,卵巢性的
ovariectomy [ˌəuvəriˈektəmi] *n* 卵巢切除术
ovari(o)- [构词成分]卵巢
ovariocele [əuˈvεəriəˌsiːl] *n* 卵巢突出
ovariocentesis [əuˌvεəriəusenˈtiːsis] *n* 卵巢穿刺术
ovariocyesis [əuˌvεəriəusaiˈiːsis] *n* 卵巢妊娠
ovariodysneuria [əuˌvεəriəudisˈnjuəriə] *n* 卵巢神经痛
ovariogenic [əuˌvεəriəˈdʒenik] *a* 卵巢源的,卵巢性的
ovariohysterectomy [əuˌvεəriəuˌhistəˈrektəmi] *n* 卵巢子宫切除术,子宫卵巢切除术
ovariopathy [əuˌvεəriˈɔpəθi] *n* 卵巢病
ovariopexy [əuˌvεəriəˈpeksi] *n* 卵巢固定术
ovariorrhexis [əuˌvεəriəˈreksis] *n* 卵巢破裂
ovariosalpingectomy [əuˌvεəriəuˌsælpinˈdʒektəmi] *n* 卵巢输卵管切除术,输卵管卵巢切除术
ovariostomy [əuˌvεəriˈɔstəmi] *n* 卵巢囊肿造口引流术
ovariotestis [əuˌvεəriəuˈtestis] *n* 卵睾体,两性生殖腺(卵巢睾丸并存)
ovariotherapy [əuˌvεəriəuˈθerəpi] *n* 卵巢制剂疗法
ovariotomy [əuˌvεəriˈɔtəmi] *n* 卵巢切开术,卵巢切除术;卵巢肿瘤切除术 | abdominal ~ 剖腹卵巢切除术 / vaginal ~ 阴道式卵巢切除术
ovariotubal [əuˌvεəriəuˈtjuːbəl] *a* 卵巢输卵管的
ovaritis [ˌəuvəˈraitis] *n* 卵巢炎
ovarium [əuˈvεəriəm] ([复] **ovaria** [əuˈvεəriə]) *n*【拉】卵巢
ovarotherapy [ˌəuvərəuˈθerəpi] *n* 卵巢制剂疗法
ovary [ˈəuvəri] *n* 卵巢 | adenocystic ~ 腺囊肿性卵巢 / oyster ~ 牡蛎状卵巢(一般见于水泡状胎块)
ovaserum [ˌəuvəˈsiərəm] *n* 抗卵蛋白血清
ovate [ˈəuveit] *a* 卵[圆]形的(叶)
OVD occlusal vertical dimension 殆垂直距离
overact [ˌəuvərˈækt] *vi* 活动过度
overaction [ˌəuvərˈækʃən] *n* 活动过度,作用过度
overactive [ˌəuvərˈæktiv] *a* 活动过度的
overactivity [ˌəuvərˌækˈtivəti] *n* 活动过度,过度活跃
overage [ˌəuvərˈeidʒ] *a* 过老的;超龄的
overall [ˈəuvərɔːl] *a* 全面的;综合的 *ad* 总的说来 *n* 宽大的罩衫;[复]工装裤 | operating ~s 手术

外套

overbite [ˈəuvəbait] *n* 覆𬌗,覆咬合 | horizontal ~ 平覆𬌗 / vertical ~ 直覆𬌗

overclosure [ˌəuvəˈkləuʒə] *n* 超闭合(牙),咬合过度 | reduced interarch distance ~ 𬌗间距离减少的咬合过度

overcompensation [ˌəuvəˌkɔmpenˈseiʃən] *n* 过度代偿,过度补偿

overcorrection [ˌəuvəkəˈrekʃən] *n* 矫正过度(指使用过强的镜片矫正视力缺陷)

overdenture [ˌəuvəˈdentʃə] *n* 外托牙,覆盖托牙

overdetermination [ˌəuvədiˌtəːmiˈneiʃən] *n* 多因素决定(在精神分析上指梦或症状的每一成分是多种因素的结果)

overdevelop [ˌəuvədiˈveləp] *vt* 过度发展;发育过度;使显影过度 | **~ment** *n*

overdosage [ˌəuvəˈdəusidʒ] *n* 超剂量

overdose [ˈəuvədəus] *n* 过量(用药) [ˈəuvəˈdəus] *vt* 使…服药过量

overdrive [ˈəuvədraiv] *n* 超速(用药物或电起搏器增加心率,以克服异位性心律)

overdue [ˈəuvəˈdjuː] *a* 迟到的,延误的;过度的;期待已久的

overeat [ˌəuvərˈiːt] *vi* 吃得过饱,暴食

overage [ˌəuvərˈeidʒ] *a* 过老的;超龄的

overall [ˈəuvərɔːl] *a* 全面的;综合的 *ad*

overfatigue [ˌəuvəfəˈtiːg] *vt* 使疲劳过度 *n* 过度疲劳

overfeeding [ˈəuvəˈfiːdiŋ] *n* 喂养过度

overgrafting [ˌəuvəˈgrɑːftiŋ,-ˈgræf-] *n* 覆盖移植[法]

overgrowth [ˈəuvəgrəuθ] *n* 生长过度,肥大,增生

overhydration [ˌəuvəhaiˈdreiʃən] *n* (体内)水分过多

overinflation [ˌəuvərinˈfleiʃən] *n* 膨胀过度 | nonobstructive pulmonary ~ 非阻塞性肺膨胀过度,代偿性肺气肿 / obstructive pulmonary ~ 阻塞性肺膨胀过度,局限性阻塞性肺气肿

overjet [ˈəuvədʒet], **overjut** [ˈəuvədʒʌt] *n* 覆盖,平覆盖

overlap [ˌəuvəˈlæp] *vt*, *vi* (与…)重叠 [ˈəuvəlæp] *n* 重叠,交错 | horizontal ~ 横重叠(牙),水平覆盖 / vertical ~ 纵重叠(牙),垂直覆盖,覆𬌗

overlay[1] [ˌəuvəˈlei] *vt* 在…上铺(或盖,涂) [ˈəuvəlei] *n* 增加,续加;高嵌体(牙) | emotional ~, psychogenic ~ 情绪性症状加重,精神性症状加重

overlie [ˌəuvəˈlai] *vt* 躺在…上面;覆在…上面;压在…上面;压得…闷死

overproductivity [ˌəuvəˌprɔdʌkˈtivəti] *n* 精神过旺

overreaching [ˌəuvəˈriːtʃiŋ] *n* 交突致伤(马的后蹄踢前蹄)

overreact [ˌəuvəri(ː)ˈækt] *vi* 过度反应;反作用过强

overresponse [ˌəuvərisˈpɔns] *n* 反应过度

overriding [ˌəuvəˈraidiŋ] *n* (骨折端)重叠,架叠

oversensitive [ˌəuvəˈsensitiv] *a* 过分敏感的,过于灵敏的

oversexed [ˌəuvəˈsekst] *a* 性欲过度的

overstain [ˈəuvəˈstein] *vt* 染色过度

overstrain [ˌəuvəˈstrein] *vt*, *vi* 过度紧张,过度劳累 [ˈəuvəstrein] *n* 紧张过度,用力过度,伤力

overstress [ˈəuvəstres] *n* 紧张过度

overtoe [ˈəuvətəu] *n* 跗内翻

overtransfusion [ˌəuvətrænsˈfjuːʒən] *n* 输血过多,输液过多

overventilation [ˌəuvəˌventiˈleiʃən] *n* 换气过度(肺)

ovi [ˈəuvai] *n* 卵,蛋(ovum 的所有格) | ~ albumin 卵白,卵清,蛋清 / ~ vitellus 卵黄

ovi- 见 ovo-

ovicidal [ˌəuviˈsaidl] *a* 杀卵的

ovicide [ˈəuvisaid] *n* 杀卵剂,灭卵剂

oviduct [ˈəuvidʌkt] *n* 输卵管 | **oviducal** [ˌəuviˈdjuːkəl], **oviductal** [ˌəuviˈdʌktəl] *a*

oviferous [əuˈvifərəs] *a* 产卵的

oviform [ˈəuvifɔːm] *a* 卵形的

ovigenesis [ˌəuviˈdʒenisis] *n* 卵[子]发生 | **ovigenetic** [ˌəuvidʒiˈnetik] *a*

ovigenic [ˌəuviˈdʒenik], **ovigenous** [əuˈvidʒinəs] *a* 生卵的

ovigerm [ˈəuvidʒəːm] *n* 原卵,胚卵

ovination [ˌəuviˈneiʃən] *n* 羊痘接种

ovine [ˈəuvain] *a* 羊的

ovinia [əuˈviniə] *n* 羊天花,羊痘

oviparous [əuˈvipərəs] *a* 卵生的 | **oviparity** [ˌəuviˈpærəti] *n*

oviposit [ˌəuviˈpɔzit] *vi* 产卵 | **~ion** [ˌəuvipəˈziʃən] *n* / **~or** *n* (昆虫)产卵器,产卵管

ovisac [ˈəuvisæk] *n* 囊状卵泡

ovist [ˈəuvist] *n* 卵原论者(认为未发育的胚胎预先形成存在于卵内)

ovium [ˈəuviəm] *n* 成熟卵

ov(o)-, ovi- [构词成分]卵,蛋

ovocenter [ˈəuvəˌsentə] *n* 卵中心体

ovocyte [ˈəuvəsait] *n* 卵母细胞

ovoflavin [ˌəuvəˈfleivin] *n* 核黄素,维生素 B_2

ovogenesis [ˌəuvəˈdʒenisis] *n* 卵[子]发生

ovoglobulin [ˌəuvəˈglɔbjulin] *n* 卵球蛋白

ovogonium [ˌəuvəˈgəuniəm] *n* 卵原细胞

ovoid [ˈəuvɔid] *a* 卵[圆]形的; *n* 卵形体(疟原

虫);卵形物 | **~al** [ˈəuvɔidəl] *a*

ovolactovegetarian [ˌəuvəuˌlæktəuˌvedʒiˈtɛəriən] *n* 乳蛋素食者,乳蛋素食主义者

ovolactovegetarianism [ˌəuvəuˌlæktəuˌvedʒiˈtɛəriənizəm] *n* 乳蛋素食主义

ovolysin [əuˈvɔlisin] *n* 溶卵白素

ovolytic [ˌəuvəˈlitik] *a* 溶卵白的

ovomucin [ˌəuvəˈmjuːsin] *n* 卵黏蛋白

ovomucoid [ˌəuvəˈmjuːkɔid] *n* 卵类黏蛋白

ovoplasm [ˈəuvəplæzəm] *n* 卵[细胞]质

ovoprecipitin [ˌəuvəupriˈsipitin] *n* 卵[白]沉淀素

ovoserum [ˌəuvəˈsiərəm] *n* 卵[白蛋白抗]血清(用卵白蛋白免疫的动物的血清,该血清能沉淀同种动物的卵白蛋白)

ovotestis [ˌəuvəuˈtestis] *n* 卵精巢,卵睾体,两性生殖腺(卵巢睾丸并存)

ovotherapy [ˌəuvəuˈθerəpi] *n* 卵巢制剂疗法

ovotransferrin [ˌəuvəutrænsˈferin] *n* 卵转铁蛋白

ovovegetarian [ˌəuvəuˌvedʒiˈtɛəriən] *n* 蛋品素食者,蛋品素食主义者

ovovegetarianism [ˌəuvəuˌvedʒiˈtɛəriənizəm] *n* 蛋品素食主义

ovoverdin [ˌəuvəˈvəːdin] *n* 虾卵绿蛋白,龙虾子青蛋白

ovovitellin [ˌəuvəuvaiˈtelin] *n* 卵黄磷蛋白

ovoviviparous [ˌəuvəuviˈvipərəs] *a* 卵胎生的 | **ovoviviparity** [ˌəuvəuˌviviˈpærəti] *n*

ovula [ˈɔvjulə] ovulum 的复数

ovular [ˈəuvjulə] *a* 原卵的;卵状小体的

ovulase [ˈəuvjuleis] *n* 卵酶,卵分裂酶

ovulate [ˈəuvjuleit] *vi* 排卵

ovulation [ˌəuvjuˈleiʃən] *n* 排卵 | amenstrual ~ 无月经排卵 / paracyclic ~, supplementary ~ 周期外排卵 | **ovulatory** [ˈəuvjulətəri] *a*

ovule [ˈəuvjuːl] *n* 原卵,卵泡内卵;卵状小体,小卵;胚珠,幼籽 | graafian ~s 卵泡原卵 / primitive ~, primordial ~ 原卵

ovulogenous [ˌəuvjuˈlɔdʒinəs] *a* 生小卵的;小卵性的

ovulum [ˈɔvjuləm] ([复] **ovula** [ˈɔvjulə]) *n*【拉】原卵,卵泡内卵;卵状小体,小卵

ovum [ˈəuvəm] ([复] **ova** [ˈəuvə]) *n*【拉】卵,卵子 | alecithal ~, oligolecithal ~ 无黄卵,少黄卵 / blighted ~ 萎缩卵,枯萎卵 / cleidoic ~ 有壳卵(爬行类、鸟类)/ macrolecithal ~ 多黄卵 / miolecithal ~, microlecithal ~ 少黄卵 / permanent ~ 永久卵,能受精卵 / primitive ~, primordial ~ 原卵

Owen's lines [ˈəuin] (Richard Owen) 欧文线(纵切面上所见之线,为牙冠牙质深部内球间隙的分界层,亦称外廓线)

Owren's disease [ˈəuren] (Paul A. Owren) 奥伦病,[凝血]因子V缺乏

ox- 见 oxy-

oxacid [ɔksˈæsid] *n* 含氧酸

oxacillin sodium [ˌɔksəˈsilin] 苯唑西林钠(抗生素类药)

oxalaldehyde [ˌɔksəlˈældihaid] *n* 乙二醛

oxalate [ˈɔksəleit] *n* 草酸盐

oxalated [ˈɔksəˌleitid] *a* 草酸盐处理的,草酸盐抗凝的

oxalation [ˌɔksəˈleiʃən] *n* 草酸盐处理

oxalemia [ˌɔksəˈliːmiə] *n* 草酸盐血

oxalic acid [ɔkˈsælik] 草酸,乙二酸

oxalism [ˈɔksəlizəm] *n* 草酸中毒

oxaloacetate [ˌɔksələˈæsiteit] *n* 草酰乙酸盐(或酯);草酰乙酸(阴离子形式)

oxaloacetic acid [ˌɔksələəˈsiːtik] 草酰乙酸,丁酮二酸

oxalosis [ˌɔksəˈləusis] *n* 草酸盐沉积症,原发性高草酸盐尿症

oxaluria [ˌɔksəˈljuəriə] *n* 草酸尿

oxaluric acid [ˌɔksəˈljuərik] 草尿酸,脲基乙酮酸

oxalyl [ˈɔksəlil] *n* 乙二酰[基],草酰[基]

oxalylurea [ˌɔksəliˈljuəriə] *n* 草酰脲,乙二酰脲

oxamic acid [ɔkˈsæmik] 草氨酸,草酰一胺

oxamide [ɔkˈsæmid] *n* 草酰胺

oxamniquine [ɔkˈsæmnikwin] *n* 奥沙尼喹(抗血吸虫药)

oxanamide [ɔkˈsænəmaid] *n* 奥沙那胺(安定药)

oxandrolone [ɔkˈsændrələun] *n* 氧雄龙(雄激素,同化激素类药)

oxantel pamoate [ˈɔksəntel] 双羟萘酸奥克太尔(抗蠕虫药)

oxaprozin [ˌɔksəˈprəuzin] *n* 奥沙普秦(消炎药)

oxarbazole [ɔkˈsɑːbəzəul] *n* 奥沙巴唑(平喘药)

oxatomide [ɔkˈseitəmaid] *n* 奥沙米特(抗过敏药,平喘药)

oxazepam [ɔkˈsæzipæm] *n* 奥沙西泮(安定药)

oxethazaine [ɔkˈseθəzein] *n* 奥昔卡因(局部麻醉药)

oxetorone fumarate [ɔkˈsetərəun] 延胡索酸奥昔托隆(镇痛药,对治偏头痛特别有效)

oxfendazole [ɔksˈfendəzəul] *n* 奥芬达唑(抗蠕虫药)

oxgall [ˈɔksgɔːl] *n* 牛胆汁

oxibendazole [ˌɔksiˈbendəzəul] *n* 奥苯达唑(兽用抗蠕虫药)

oxiconazole nitrate [ˌɔksiˈkɔnəzɔl] 硝酸奥昔康唑(抗真菌药)

oxidant [ˈɔksidənt] *n* 氧化剂

oxidase [ˈɔksideis] *n* 氧化酶 | direct ~ (oxygenase), primary ~ 直接氧化酶(加氧酶) / indirect

~（peroxidase）间接氧化酶（过氧物酶）
oxidate [ˈɔksideit] *vt* 使氧化
oxidation [ˌɔksiˈdeiʃən] *n* 氧化[作用] | **oxidative** [ˈɔksideitiv] *a*
oxidation-reduction [ˌɔksiˈdeiʃən riˈdʌkʃən] *n* 氧化还原作用
oxide [ˈɔksaid] *n* 氧化物 | arsenous ~ 三氧化二砷 / stannic ~ 氧化锡，二氧化锡
oxidize [ˈɔksidaiz] *vt, vi* 氧化 | **~r** *n* 氧化剂
oxidopamine [ˌɔksiˈdəupəmiːn] *n* 羟多巴胺（抗青光眼药）
oxidoreductase [ˌɔksidəuriˈdʌkteis] *n* 氧化还原酶
oxidosis [ˌɔksiˈdəusis] *n* 酸中毒
oxidronate（HDP，HMDP） [ˌɔksiˈdrəuneit] *n* 奥昔膦酸（用于骨显影）
oxifungin hydrochloride [ˌɔksiˈfʌndʒin] 盐酸奥昔芬净（抗真菌药）
oxilorphan [ˌɔksiˈlɔːfæn] *n* 奥昔啡烷（麻醉药拮抗药）
oxim(e) [ˈɔksim] *n* 肟
oximeter [ɔkˈsimitə] *n* 血氧计 | **oximetry** *n* 血氧定量法
oximinotransferase [ɔkˌsiminəuˈtrænsfəreis] *n* 转肟酶，肟基转移酶
oxine [ɔkˈsiːn] *n* 羟喹啉
oxiperomide [ˌɔksiˈperəmaid] *n* 奥哌咪酮（安定药）
oxiramide [ɔkˈsirəmaid] *n* 奥昔拉米（心抑制药，具有抗心律失常作用）
oxirane [ˈɔksirein] *n* 环氧乙烷
oxisuran [ˌɔksiˈsjuərən] *n* 奥昔舒仑（抗肿瘤药）
oxmetidine mesylate [ɔksˈmetidiːnˈmesileit] 甲磺奥美替丁（组胺 H_2 受体拮抗药）
oxo- 氧[代]（在正式命名法中取代 keto-所采用的前缀，如 oxoglutarate 取代 ketoglutarate，带有以 keto-为前缀的术语是美国的常用形式）
3-oxoacid CoA-transferase [ˌɔksəuˈæsid kəuˈei ˈtrænsfəreis] 3-氧[代]酸辅酶 A 转移酶（亦称 3-酮酸辅酶 A 转移酶）
oxo-acid-lyase [ˌɔksəu ˌæsid ˈlaieis] 氧[代]酸裂合酶
oxogestone phenpropionate [ˌɔksəuˈdʒestəun] 奥索孕酮苯丙酸酯（孕激素）
oxoglutarate dehydrogenase（lipoamide） [ˌɔksəuˈgluːtəreit diːˈhaidrədʒəneis ˌlipəuˈæmaid] 酮戊二酸脱氢酶（硫辛酰胺）（α-ketoglutarate dehydrogenase 的 EC 命名法）
2-oxoglutaric acid [ˌɔksəugluːˈtærik] 2-酮戊二酸（即 α-ketoglutaric acid）
2-oxoisovalerate dehydrogenase（lipoamide） [ˌɔksəuˌaisəuˌvæləreit diːˈhaidrədʒəneis] 2-氧[代]异戊酸脱氢酶（硫辛酰胺）（即 α-酮异戊酸脱氢酶〈硫辛酰胺〉α-ketoisovalerate dehydrogenase〈lipoamide〉）
oxolinic acid [ˌɔksəuˈlinik] 奥索利酸（抗菌药）
oxonium [ɔkˈsəunjəm] *n* 氧鎓，鉾（四价氧）
oxophenarsine hydrochloride [ˌɔksəufiˈnɑːsin] 盐酸氧芬胂（一种胂剂，具有杀螺旋体和抗锥虫作用，很少用于治疗梅毒和锥虫病）
5-oxoprolinase（ATP-hydrolyzing） [ˌɔksəuˈprəulineis] 5-羟脯氨酸酶（ATP 水解的）（亦称焦谷氨酸酶）
5-oxoproline [ˌɔksəuˈprəuliːn] *n* 5-羟脯氨酸（亦称焦谷氨酸）
5-oxoprolinuria [ˌɔksəuˌprəuliˈnjuəriə] *n* 5-羟脯氨酸尿（亦称焦谷氨酸尿）
oxosteroid [ˌɔksəuˈsterɔid] *n* 类固醇酮
oxozone [ˈɔksəzəun] *n* 双氧气
oxpentifylline [ˌɔkspinˈtifiliːn] *n* 己酮可可碱（血管扩张药）
oxprenolol hydrochloride [ɔksˈprenəlɔl] 盐酸氧烯洛尔（β 受体阻滞药）
oxtriphylline [ɔksˈtrifiliːn] *n* 胆茶碱（利尿药，支气管扩张药）
oxy- [构词成分]尖锐，锐敏；氧化，氧（有时用羟）
oxyacetic acid [ˌɔksiəˈsiːtik] 羟乙酸，乙醇酸
oxyachrestia [ˌɔksiəˈkrestiə] *n* 神经元内血糖不足
oxyacid [ˌɔksiˈæsid] *n* 含氧酸
oxyacoia [ˌɔksiəˈkɔiə] *n* 听觉锐敏，听觉亢进
oxyamygdalic acid [ˌɔksiəmigˈdælik] 苯酚羟乙酸，对羟苯羟乙酸
oxybenzene [ˌɔksiˈbenziːn] *n* 酚，苯酚
oxybenzoic acid [ˌɔksibenˈzəuik] 邻羟苯甲酸，水杨酸
oxybenzone [ˌɔksiˈbenzəun] *n* 羟苯甲酮（防晒药）
oxyblepsia [ˌɔksiˈblepsiə] *n* 视觉锐敏，视觉亢进
oxybutynin chloride [ˌɔksiˈbjuːtinin] 氯化奥昔布宁（抗胆碱药，对平滑肌有直接抗痉挛作用）
oxybutyria [ˌɔksibjuˈtiriə]，**oxybutyricacidemia** [ˌɔksibjuˌtirikˌæsiˈdiːmiə] *n* 羟丁酸尿，羟丁酸血
oxybutyric acid [ˌɔksibjuːˈtirik] 羟丁酸
oxycalorimeter [ˌɔksikæləˈrimitə] *n* 耗氧热量计
oxycanthine [ɔksiˈkænθin] *n* 刺檗碱
oxycephaly [ˌɔksiˈsefəli]，**oxycephalia** [ˌɔksisəˈfeiliə] *n* 尖形头，尖头[畸形] | **oxycephalic** [ˌɔksisəˈfælik]，**oxycephalous** [ˌɔksiˈsefələs] *a*
oxychloride [ˌɔksiˈklɔːraid] *n* 氯氧化物
oxychlorosene [ˌɔksiˈklɔːrəsiːn] *n* 奥昔氯生（局部抗感染药）| ~ sodium 奥昔氯生钠（局部抗感染药）
oxycholine [ˌɔksiˈkəulin] *n* 羟基胆碱，毒蕈碱

oxychromatic [ˌɔksikrəuˈmætik] *a* 嗜酸染色的
oxychromatin [ˌɔksiˈkrəumətin] *n* 嗜酸染色质
oxycinesia [ˌɔksisaiˈniːziə] *n* 动时痛
oxyclozanide [ˌɔksiˈkləuzənaid] *n* 羟氯扎胺(抗蠕虫药)
oxycodone hydrochloride [ˌɔksiˈkəudəun] 盐酸羟考酮(麻醉性镇痛药)
oxycyanide [ˌɔksiˈsaiənaid] *n* 氧氰化物
oxydendron [ˌɔksiˈdendrən] *n* 酸浆树
oxydesis [ˌɔksiˈdiːsis] *n* (血)结酸力 | **oxydetic** [ˌɔksiˈdetik] *a*
oxydoreductase [ˌɔksidəuriˈdʌkteis] *n* 氧化还原酶
oxyecoia [ˌɔksiiˈkɔiə] *n* 听觉锐敏,听觉亢进
oxyesthesia [ˌɔksiisˈθiːzjə] *n* 感觉锐敏,感觉亢进
oxyetherotherapy [ˌɔksiˌiːθərəuˈθerəpi] *n* 氧醚疗法(过去用于治肺部感染及百日咳)
oxygen (O) [ˈɔksidʒən] *n* 氧 | ~ acid 含氧酸 / excess ~ 超耗氧(超过身体静止状态需要量所用的氧量)
oxygenase [ˌɔksidʒiˌneis] *n* 氧合酶,加氧酶
oxygenate [ɔkˈsidʒineit] *vt* 氧合,充氧 | **oxygenation** [ˌɔksidʒiˈneiʃən] *n* 氧合,充氧[作用] / **oxygenator** [ˌɔksidʒiˈneitə] *n* 氧合器
oxygenic [ˌɔksiˈdʒenik], **oxygenous** [ɔkˈsidʒinəs] *a* 氧的,含氧的
oxygeusia [ˌɔksiˈgjuːziə] *n* 味觉锐敏,味觉亢进
oxyhematoporphyrin [ˌɔksiˌhemətəuˈpɔːfirin] *n* 氧血卟啉
oxyheme [ˈɔksihiːm], **oxyhemochromogen** [ˌɔksiˌhiːməuˈkrəumədʒən] *n* 血红素,正铁血红素,高铁血红素
oxyhemocyanine [ˌɔksiˌhiːməuˈsaiənin] *n* 氧合血蓝蛋白,氧合血青蛋白
oxyhemoglobin [ˌɔksiˌhiːməuˈgləubin] *n* 氧合血红蛋白
oxyhemogram [ˌɔksiˈhiːməgræm] *n* 血氧谱
oxyhemograph [ˌɔksiˈhiːməgrɑːf, -græf] *n* 血氧测定器
oxyhydrocephalus [ˌɔksiˌhaidrəuˈsefələs] *n* 尖头脑积水
oxyhyperglycemia [ˌɔksiˌhaipəglaiˈsiːmiə] *n* 陡急高血糖,快速血糖过多(此病有轻微糖尿,口服葡糖耐量曲线为每 100 ml 升高 180 ~ 200 mg,但摄入葡糖后 2.5 小时即可回复至空腹时的血糖值)
oxyiodide [ˌɔksiˈaiədaid] *n* 氧碘化物
oxykrinin [ɔksiˈkrinin] *n* 促胰液素
oxylalia [ɔksiˈleiliə] *n* 言语急促
oxydase [ɔksiˈleis] *n* 氧化酶
oxymetazoline hydrochloride [ˌɔksimeˈtæzəliːn] 盐酸羟甲唑啉(血管收缩药)
oxymetholone [ˌɔksiˈmeθələun] *n* 羟甲烯龙(雄激素,同化激素类药)
oxymetry [ɔkˈsimitri] *n* 血氧定量法
Oxymonadida [ˌɔksiməuˈnædidə] *n* 锐滴虫目
Oxymonas [ˌɔksiˈməunəs] *n* 锐滴虫属
oxymorphone hydrochloride [ˌɔksiˈmɔːfəun] 盐酸羟吗啡酮(镇痛药)
oxymyoglobin [ˌɔksiːmaiəuˈgləubin] *n* 氧合肌红蛋白
oxymyohematin [ˌɔksiˌmaiəuˈhemətin] *n* 氧化肌细胞色素
oxynaphthoic acid [ˌɔksinæfˈθəuik] 羟萘甲酸
oxynervon [ˌɔksiˈnəːvɔn] *n* 羟基神经苷脂,羟基烯脑苷脂
oxyneurine [ˌɔksiˈnjuərin] *n* 甜菜碱
oxynitrilase [ˌɔksiˈnaitrileis] *n* 醇腈[醛化]酶,氧腈酶,苦杏仁腈酶
oxyntic [ɔkˈsintik] *a* 泌酸的
oxyntomodulin [ɔkˌsintəuˈmɔdjulin] *n* 胃泌酸调节素(肠高血糖素的主要形式)
oxyopia [ˌɔksiˈəupiə] *n* 视觉锐敏,视觉亢进
oxyopter [ˌɔksiˈɔptə] *n* 视度(视力的一种单位)
oxyosis [ˌɔksiˈəusis] *n* 酸中毒
oxyosmia [ˌɔksiˈɔsmiə], **oxyosphresia** [ˌɔksiɔsˈfriːziə] *n* 嗅觉锐敏,嗅觉亢进
oxyparaplastin [ˌɔksiˌpærəˈplæstin] *n* 嗜酸副染色质
oxypathia [ˌɔksiˈpeiθiə] *n* 感觉锐敏,感觉亢进
oxyperitoneum [ˌɔksiˌperitəuˈniːəm] *n* 人工氧腹,腹腔注氧
oxypertine [ˌɔksiˈpəːtiːn] *n* 奥昔哌汀(抗抑郁药)
oxyphenbutazone [ˌɔksifənˈbjuːtəzəun] *n* 羟布宗(消炎镇痛药)
oxyphencyclimine hydrochloride [ˌɔksifənˈsaiklimiːn] 盐酸羟苄利明(抗胆碱药,用于治消化性溃疡和胃肠道痉挛)
oxyphenisatin [ˌɔksifiˈnaisətin] *n* 酚丁(泻药) | ~ acetate 双醋酚丁(泻药)
oxyphenonium bromide [ˌɔksifiˈnəuniəm] 奥芬溴铵(副交感神经阻滞药)
oxyphenylacetic acid [ˌɔksiˌfeniləˈsiːtik] 对羟苯乙酸
oxyphenylethylamine [ˌɔksiˌfeniˌleθiˈlæmin] *n* 酪胺
oxyphil [ˈɔksifil] *n* 嗜酸[性]细胞,许特尔(Hürthle)细胞 *a* 嗜酸[性]的
oxyphilic [ˌɔksiˈfilik], **oxyphilous** [ɔkˈsifiləs] *a* 嗜酸[性]的
oxyphonia [ˌɔksiˈfəuniə] *n* 尖音
oxyphorase [ˈɔksiˌfɔreis] *n* 带氧酶

Oxyphotobacteria [ˌɔksiˌfəutəubækˈtiəriə] *n* 带氧发光菌纲
oxyplasm [ˈɔksiplæzəm] *n* 嗜酸[性]胞质
oxypropionic acid [ˌɔksiˌprəupiˈɔnik] α-羟基丙酸,乳酸
oxyproteic acid [ˌɔksiprəuˈtiːik] 氧蛋白酸(肽类)
oxyproteinic acid [ˌɔksiprəuˈtiːinik] 羟基蛋白酸
oxypurinase [ˌɔksiˈpjuərineis] *n* 羟嘌呤酶,氧嘌呤酶
oxypurine [ˌɔksiˈpjuərin] *n* 羟基嘌呤
oxypurinol [ˌɔksiˈpjuərinɔl] *n* 奥昔嘌醇(黄嘌呤氧化酶抑制剂)
oxyquinoline [ˌɔksiˈkwinəliːn] *n* 羟喹啉(在杀真菌剂制备中用作制菌剂和制真菌剂,并用作消毒剂,也用作螯合剂) | ~ sulfate 硫酸羟喹啉(在药物制剂时用作络合剂,也用作局部防腐消毒药)
oxyrenin [ˌɔksiˈriːnin] *n* 氧肾素,氧高血压蛋白原酶
oxyrhine [ˈɔksirain] *a* 尖鼻的
oxysalt [ˈɔksisɔːlt] *n* 含氧酸盐
oxysantonin [ˌɔksiˈsæntənin] *n* 氧山道年
Oxyspirura [ˌɔksispaiəˈruːrə] *n* 尖旋尾线虫属 | ~ mansoni 曼氏尖旋尾线虫
oxytalan [ɔkˈsitələn] *n* 耐酸纤维(一种结缔组织纤维,存在于牙周膜和牙龈中)
oxytalanolysis [ɔkˌsitələˈnɔlisis] *n* 耐酸纤维溶解
oxytetracycline [ˌɔksiˌtetrəˈsaiklain] *n* 土霉素(抗生素类药) | ~ calcium 土霉素钙(抗菌药) / ~ hydrochloride 盐酸土霉素(抗细菌及抗立克次体药)
oxytocia [ɔksiˈtəusiə] *n* 分娩急速 | **oxytocic** [ɔksiˈtəusik] *a* 催产的 *n* 催产药,催生药
oxytocin [ˌɔksiˈtəusin] *n* 催产素,缩宫素(子宫收缩药)
oxytoluic acid [ˌɔksitəˈljuik] 甲基水杨酸
Oxytropis [ˌɔksiˈtrəupis] *n* 棘豆属
oxytropism [ɔkˈsitrəpizəm] *n* 向氧性(活细胞对氧刺激的反应)
oxytuberculin [ˌɔksitju(ː)ˈbəːkjulin] *n* 氧化结核菌素
oxyuria [ˌɔksiˈjuəriə], **oxyuriasis** [ˌɔksijuəˈraiəsis], **oxyuriosis** [ˌɔksiˌjuəriˈəusis] *n* 蛲虫病
oxyuricide [ˌɔksiˈjuərisaid] *n* 杀蛲虫药
oxyurid [ɔksiˈjuərid] *n*, *a* 蛲虫(的)
Oxyuridae [ˌɔksiˈjuəridiː] *n* 尖尾科,蛲虫科
oxyurifuge [ˌɔksiˈjuərifjuːdʒ] *n* 驱蛲虫药
Oxyuris [ˌɔksiˈjuəris] *n* 尖尾线虫属,蛲虫属 | ~ equi 马尖尾线虫 / ~ incognita 未定尖尾线虫(大约为住根异皮线虫) / ~ vermicularis 蠕形住肠线虫,蛲虫(即 Enterobius vermicularis)
oxyuroid [ɔksiˈjuərɔid] *a* 蛲虫的
Oxyuroidea [ˌɔksijuəˈrɔidiə] *n* 尖尾总科,蛲虫总科
oyster [ˈɔistə] *n* 牡蛎,蚝
Oz Oz 标记(一种抗原标记,以区别人免疫球蛋白 λ 轻链亚型)
oz ounce 英两
ozena [əuˈziːnə] *n* 臭鼻症 | ~ laryngis 臭鼻性喉症,萎缩性喉炎 | **ozenous** [ˈəuzinəs] *a*
ozolinone [əuˈzəulinəun] *n* 奥唑林酮(利尿药)
ozonator [ˈəuzəˌneitə] *n* 臭氧发生器
ozone [ˈəuzəun] *n* 臭氧 | ~-ether 臭氧乙醚(乙醚、过氧化氢、醇合剂,用作防腐剂及治百日咳和糖尿病) | **ozonic** [əuˈzɔnik], **ozonous** [ˈəuzənəs] *a* 臭氧的;含臭氧的
ozonide [ˈəuzənaid] *n* 臭氧化物
ozonize [ˈəuzənaiz] *vt* 使臭氧化 *vi* 变成臭氧 | **ozonization** [ˌəuzəunaiˈzeiʃən, -niˈz-] *n* 臭氧作用 / **~r** *n* 臭氧施放器(将臭氧用于伤口、瘘管等)
ozonolysis [ˌəuzəuˈnɔlisis] *n* 臭氧分解
ozonometer [ˌəuzəuˈnɔmitə] *n* 臭氧计
ozonophore [əuˈzəunəfɔː] *n* 原浆粒(细胞的);红细胞
ozonoscope [əuˈzəunəskəup] *n* 臭氧检验器
ozonosphere [əuˈzəunəsfiə] *n* 臭氧层
ozostomia [ˌəuzəˈstəumiə] *n* 口臭[症]

P

P para 对[位]; peta-秭; phosphate group 磷酸基; phosphorus 磷; poise 泊; posterior 后的; premolar 前磨牙; pupil 瞳孔
P_1 paremtal generation 亲代
P_2 pulmonic second sound 肺动脉瓣第二音
Pco_2 carbon dioxide partial pressure or tension 二氧化碳分压
P_1 orthophosphate 正磷酸盐
Po_2 oxygen partial pressure or tension 氧分压
p pico-皮[可]; proton 质子; the short arm of a chromosome 染色体短臂
p power 功率; pressure 压; probability 概率
***p*-** para-[2] 对[位]
Π 希腊语大写字母 pi,在数学上用以表示乘积
π pi,希腊语第 16 个字母,数学上为圆周率的符号,约为 3.141 592 653 6; osmotic pressure 渗透压
Φ phi,希腊语第 21 个字母
Ψ psi,希腊语第 23 个字母;pseudouridine 假尿[嘧啶核]苷
PA posteroanterior 后前[位]的;physician assistant 助理医师;pulmonary artery 肺动脉
Pa protactinium 镤;pascal 帕[斯卡]
Paas's disease [pɑːz] (H. R. Paas)帕斯病(一种家族性疾病,主征为骨骼畸形,如髋外翻、指趾过短、脊柱侧凸、脊椎炎等)
PAB, PABA para-aminobenzoic acid 对氨基苯甲酸
PAC premature atrial complex 期前心房复合波
paca [ˈpɑːkə, ˈpæ-] *n* 无尾刺豚鼠
pacchionian depressions [ˌpækiˈəuniən] (Antonio Pachioni) 颗粒小凹 | ~ foramen 膈孔(蝶鞍) / ~ granulation (bodies, glandes) 蛛网膜粒
pacemaker [ˈpeismeikə] *n* 起搏点;起搏器;定步物 | artificial ~ 人工心脏起搏器 / asynchronous ~ 非同步起搏器 / cardiac ~ 起搏点,窦房结 / cilium ~ 纤毛运动调节器 / demand ~ 按需型起搏器 / ectopic ~ 异位起搏点(窦房结以外的心起搏点) / external ~ 体外起搏器 / implanted ~ 埋藏式起搏器 / radio-frequency ~ 射频起搏器 / synchronous ~ 同步起搏器 / wandering ~ 游走节律点
pachismus [pəˈkizməs] *n* 肥厚
pachonychia [ˌpækəuˈnikiə] *n* 甲肥厚
pachy- [构词成分]厚,硬,肥,粗
pachyacria [ˌpækiˈeikriə] *n* 肢软部肥厚
pachyblepharon [ˌpækiˈblefərɔn], **pachyblepharosis** [ˌpækiˌblefəˈrəusis] *n* 睑缘肥厚
pachycephaly [ˌpækiˈsefəli], **pachycephalia** [ˌpækisəˈfeiliə] *n* 颅骨肥厚 | **pachycephalic** [ˌpækisəˈfælik], **pachycephalous** [ˈpækiˈsefələs] *a*
pachycheilia [ˌpækiˈkailiə] *n* 唇肥厚
pachychromatic [ˌpækikrəuˈmætik] *a* 粗染色质线的
pachycolpismus [ˌpækikɔlˈpizməs] *n* 肥厚性阴道炎
pachydactyly [ˌpækiˈdæktili], **pachydactylia** [ˌpækidækˈtiliə] *n* 指肥大,趾肥大
pachyderma [ˌpækiˈdəːmə] *n* 皮肥厚,厚皮
pachydermatocele [ˌpækidəːˈmætəsiːl] *n* 神经瘤性象皮病
pachydermatous [ˌpækiˈdəːmətəs], **pachydermic** [ˌpækiˈdəːmik] *a* 厚皮的
pachydermoperiostosis [ˌpækiˌdəːməˌperiɔsˈtəusis] *n* 厚皮性骨膜病
pachyemia [ˌpækiˈiːmiə], **pachyhemia** [ˌpækiˈhiːmiə] *n* 血液浓缩 | **pachyhematous** [ˌpækiˈhemətəs] *a*
pachyglossia [ˌpækiˈglɔsiə] *n* 舌肥厚,厚舌
pachygnathous [pəˈkignəθəs] *a* 巨颌的
pachygyria [ˌpækiˈdʒaiəriə] *n* 巨脑回
pachyleptomeningitis [ˌpækiˌleptəuˌmeninˈdʒaitis] *n* 硬软脑膜炎,硬软脊膜炎
pachymeningitis [ˌpækiˌmeninˈdʒaitis] *n* 硬脑膜炎,硬脊膜炎 | external ~ 硬脑膜外层炎,硬脊膜外层炎 / internal ~ 硬脑膜内层炎,硬脊膜内层炎
pachymeningopathy [ˌpækiˌmeniŋˈgɔpəθi] *n* 硬脑膜病,硬脊膜病
pachymeninx [ˌpækiˈmiːniŋks] ([复] **pachymeninges** [ˌpækimiˈnindʒiːz]) *n* 硬脑膜,硬脊膜
pachymeter [pəˈkimətə] *n* 厚度测量仪
pachymucosa [ˌpækimjuːˈkəusə] *n* 黏膜肥厚
pachynema [ˌpækiˈniːmə] *n* 粗线期(有丝分裂的 DNA 合成后期,染色质呈粗的纽丝状)
pachynesis [ˌpækiˈniːsis] *n* 线粒体粗肿
pachynsis [pəˈkinsis] *n* 【希】肥厚 | **pachyntic** [pəˈkintik] *a*
pachyonychia [ˌpækiəuˈnikiə] *n* 甲肥厚

pachyostosis [ˌpækiɔsˈtəusis] *n* 骨肥厚
pachypelviperitonitis [ˌpækiˌpelviˌperitəuˈnaitis] *n* 肥厚性盆腔腹膜炎
pachyperiosteoderma [ˌpækiperiˌɔstiəˈdəːmə] *n* 厚皮性骨膜病
pachyperiostitis [ˌpækiˌperiɔsˈtaitis] *n* 肥厚性骨膜炎
pachyperitonitis [ˌpækiperitəuˈnaitis] *n* 肥厚性腹膜炎
pachypleuritis [ˌpækipluəˈraitis] *n* 肥厚性胸膜炎,纤维胸;胸膜纤维化
pachypodous [pəˈkipədəs] *a* 足肥厚的
pachyrhizid [ˌpækiˈraizid] *n* 豆薯苷
pachysalpingitis [ˌpækiˌsælpinˈdʒaitis] *n* 肥厚性输卵管炎,实质性输卵管炎(亦称输卵管主质炎)
pachysalpingo-ovaritis [ˌpækisælˌpiŋgəu ˌəuvəˈraitis] *n* 肥厚性输卵管卵巢炎
pachysomia [ˌpækiˈsəumiə] *n* 躯体肥厚
pachytene [ˈpækitiːn] *n* 粗线期(生殖细胞减数分裂过程中,接在联会〈synapsis〉后的阶段,同源染色体线变短、变粗及相互扭缠)
pachyvaginalitis [ˌpækiˌvædʒinəˈlaitis] *n* 肥厚性鞘膜炎
pachyvaginitis [ˌpækiˌvædʒiˈnaitis] *n* 肥厚性阴道炎 | cystic ~ 囊性肥厚性阴道炎,气肿性阴道炎
pacing [ˈpeisiŋ] *n* 定速,调速;起搏 | cardiac ~ 心脏起搏 / burst ~ 短阵快速起搏
Pacini's corpuscles [pəˈtʃiːni], **pacinian corpuscles** [pəˈsiniən] (Filippo Pacini) 环层小体
Paci's operation [ˈpɑːtʃi] (AgostinoPaci) 帕奇手术(先天性髋脱位手术)
pack [pæk] *n* 包,捆;[包]裹法;塞子,填塞物 | cold ~ 冷裹法 / dry ~ 干裹法 / full ~ 全身裹法 / half ~ 半身裹法 / hot ~ 热裹法 / one sheet ~ 一块被单裹法 / periodontal ~ 牙周塞治剂 / three-quarters ~ 3/4 裹法(上至腋部) / wet ~, wet-sheet ~ 湿裹法
packer [ˈpækə] *n* 填塞器(将敷料填塞子宫、阴道等用)
packing [ˈpækiŋ] *n* 包装;(用纱布、棉花等)填塞;填料,填塞物;包扎法,[包]裹法 | nasal ~ 鼻填塞术
paclitaxel [ˌpækliˈtæksəl] *n* 紫杉酚(从太平洋短叶紫杉〈Taxus brevifolia〉中分离,用于研究性治疗卵巢癌和黑素瘤)
pad [pæd] *n* 垫,托;纱布垫 | abdominal ~ 腹部垫(吸收腹部伤口排出物) / dinner ~ 缓餐垫 / fat ~ 颊脂垫;髌后脂垫 / gum ~s 龈垫 / kidney ~ 肾托 / knuckle ~s 指拐垫,指节垫 / periarterial ~ 动脉周[围]垫,近血管球体 / sucking ~, suctorial ~ 吸吮垫,颊脂垫体,颊脂体
Padgett's dermatome [ˈpædʒet] (Earl C. Padgett) 帕杰特植皮刀
padimate A [ˈpædimeit] 帕地马酯 A〈防晒药〉
padimate O [ˈpædimeit] 帕地马酯 O〈防晒药〉
pae- 以 pae-起始的词,同样见以 pe-起始的词
Paecilomyces [piːˌsiləuˈmaisiːz] *n* 类青霉菌属,拟青霉菌属
Paederus [ˈpiːdərəs] *n* 毒隐翅虫属,隐翅虫属
paed(o)- 见 ped(o)-
PAF platelet activating factor 血小板激活因子
PAF-acether [əˈsiːθə] 血小板激活因子-乙酰乙酯
PAGE polyacrylamide gel electrophoresis 聚丙烯酰胺凝胶电泳
Page kidney [peidʒ] (Irwin H. Page) 佩吉肾(被膜下血肿压迫肾造成高血压,一般见于腹背扭伤后)
Pagenstecher's circle [ˈpɑːgənˈstekə] (Alexander Pagenstecher) 帕根斯特赫尔环(在腹壁上表明移动性腹部肿瘤位置的点联起来,形成一个环,环的中心即为肿瘤的附着点) | ~ ointment 帕根斯特赫尔软膏(含黄氧化汞) / ~ linen thread 帕根斯特赫尔亚麻线(用作缝线)
pagetic [pəˈdʒetik] *a* 畸形性骨炎的
pagetoid [ˈpædʒitɔid] *a* 畸形性骨炎样的
Paget's abscess [ˈpædʒit] (James Paget) 佩吉特脓肿(再发性脓肿) | ~ cells 佩吉特细胞(见于乳头佩吉特病的变性细胞) / ~ disease 佩吉特病(①畸形性骨炎;②乳头乳晕湿疹样癌,常伴输乳管癌和深部乳腺癌,常发生于中年妇女) / ~ quiet necrosis 佩吉特静性坏死(长骨干表层局部坏死和死骨片形成) / ~ test 佩吉特试验(中心最硬的即肿瘤,中心不硬的是囊肿)
pagon [ˈpægɔn] *n* 冰内生物
pagophagia [ˌpeigəuˈfeidʒiə] *n* 食冰癖(也许与缺铁有关)
pagoplexia [ˌpeigəuˈpleksiə] *n* 冻疮
-pagus [构词成分]联胎
PAH, PAHA para-aminohippuric acid 对氨基马尿酸(检肾功能)
Pahvant Valley fever, plague [ˈpɑːvənt] 土拉菌病,兔热病(Pahvant 为美国犹他州的一个山谷)
PAI plasminogen activator inhibitor 纤溶酶原激活物抑制剂
pain [pein] *n* 痛,疼痛, | aching ~ 酸痛 / bearing-down ~ 坠痛(分娩第二期) / boring ~, terebrant ~, terebrating ~ 锥痛 / bursting ~ 撕裂痛 / central ~ 中枢性痛 / dilating ~s (子宫)扩张期痛 / expulsive ~s 娩出期痛 / false ~s 假阵痛 / gas ~s 胀痛 / girdle ~ 束带样痛 / growing ~s 发育期痛 / homotopic ~ 同位痛,损伤处痛 / ideogenous ~ 意念性疼痛 / imperative ~

强迫性[疼]痛(精神衰弱) / labor ~s 阵痛,分娩痛 / lancinating ~ 刀刺性痛 / lightning ~s, fulgurant ~, shooting ~s 闪痛,射痛(脊髓痨) / middle ~, intermenstrual ~ 经间痛 / mind ~ 精神性痛 / phantom limb ~ 假性肢痛,幻肢痛 / postprandial ~ 食后腹痛 / premonitory ~s 先兆阵痛 / psychic ~ 精神性疼痛 / psychogenic ~ 精神性疼痛 / referred ~, heterotopic ~ 牵涉痛,异位痛 / root ~ 神经根痛 / soul ~ 精神性痛 / spot ~s 斑点状痛 / starting ~s 睡眠早期痛 / wandering ~ 游走性痛

painkiller [ˈpeinkilə] *n* 止痛药

paint [peint] *n* 涂料,涂剂 | antiseptic ~ 抗体护层(指分泌在黏膜表面上的免疫球蛋白 A,防止同种抗原的物质侵入,起到局部保护作用)

pair [pɛə] *n* 对,偶;二联律(在心脏病学中,指两个连续期前收缩) | base ~ 碱基对(由氢键结合起来的两对〈鸟嘌呤和胞嘧啶,腺嘌呤和胸腺嘧啶〉中任何一对嘌呤和嘧啶的配对组成 DNA,在组成 RNA 时,尿嘧啶代替胸腺嘧啶) / buffer ~ 缓冲偶 / ion ~ 离子对

pairing [ˈpɛəriŋ] *n* 配对,成对 | base ~ 碱基配对(嘌呤与嘧啶通过氢键形成碱基对,见 pair) / somatic ~ 体细胞(染色体)配对

pajaroello [pəhərəuˈeljəu] *n* 皮革钝缘蜱(即 Ornithodoros coriaceus)

Pajot's hook [pɑːˈʒɔː] (Charles Pajot)帕若钩(用于胎儿断头术) | ~ law 帕若定律(一个实体若容纳在另一个具有平滑壁的体中,必趋于适合该平滑壁的形状,此定律支配着分娩时胎儿的旋转运动) / ~ maneuver 帕若手法(顺骨盆入口的轴作产钳牵引术,一手握住产钳扣锁处向下拉至骨盆底,另一手作水平面牵引) / ~ method 帕若法(用帕若钩断胎头法)

pakurin [ˈpækjurin] *n* 帕库林(一种箭毒,对心脏可产生与洋地黄相似的作用)

palae(o)- 以 palae(o)-起始的词,同样见 pale(o)-起始的词

palaeocerebellum [ˌpæliəuˌseriˈbeləm] *n* 旧小脑

palaeocortex [ˌpæliəuˈkɔːteks] *n* 旧皮质

palata [pæˈleitə] palatum 的复数

palatable [ˈpælətəbl] *a* 可口的,美味的

palate [ˈpælit] *n* 腭 | artificial ~ 假腭 / cleft ~ 腭裂 / falling ~ 垂腭 / gothic ~ 尖腭 / pendulous ~ 腭垂,悬雍垂 / primary ~, premaxillary ~ 初腭 / secondary ~ 继发腭 | **palatal** [ˈpælətl], **palatine** [ˈpælətain] *a*

palategraph [ˈpælitgrɑːf, -græf] *n* 腭动描记器

palatiform [pəˈlætifɔːm] *a* 腭形的

palatitis [ˌpæləˈtaitis] *n* 腭炎

palat(o)- [构词成分]腭

palatoglossal [ˌpælətəuˈglɔsəl] *n* 腭舌的

palatognathous [ˌpæləˈtɔgnəθəs] *a* 腭裂的

palatograph [ˈpælətəgrɑːf, -græf] *n* 腭动描记器 | **~y** [ˌpæləˈtɔgrəfi] *n* 腭动描记术

palatomaxillary [ˌpælətəuˈmæksiləri] *a* 腭上颌的

palatomyograph [ˌpælətəuˈmaiəgrɑːf, -græf] *n* 腭肌运动描记器,腭动描记器 | **~y** [ˌpælətəumaiˈɔgrəfi] *n* 腭动描记法

palatonasal [ˌpælətəuˈneizəl] *a* 腭鼻的

palatopagus [ˌpæləˈtɔpəgəs] *n* 腭[对称]联胎

palatopharyngeal [ˌpælətəufəˈrinˈdʒiəl] *a* 腭咽的

palatoplasty [ˈpælətəˌplæsti] *n* 腭成形术

palatoplegia [ˌpælətəuˈpliːdʒiə] *n* 腭麻痹

palatoproximal [ˌpælətəuˈprɔksiməl] *a* 腭[舌]邻面的(上颌牙)

palatorrhaphy [ˌpæləˈtɔrəfi] *n* 腭裂修复术

palatosalpingeus [ˌpælətəusælˈpindʒiəs] *n* 腭帆张肌

palatoschisis [ˌpæləˈtɔskisis] *n* 腭裂

palatostaphylinus [ˌpælətəuˌstæfiˈlainəs] *n* 腭悬雍垂肌

palatouvularis [ˌpælətəuˌjuːvjuˈlɛəris] *n* 腭垂肌,悬雍垂肌

palatum [ˌpæˈleitəm]([复] **palata** [pæˈleitə]) *n* 【拉】腭

paleencephalon [ˌpælienˈsefəlɔn], **paleoencephalon** [ˌpæliəuenˈsefəlɔn] *n* 旧脑,原脑(除大脑皮质及其附件以外的大脑全部)

pale(o)- [构词成分]老,古,旧

paleocerebellum [ˌpæliəuˌseriˈbeləm] *n* 旧小脑 | **paleocerebellar** *a*

paleocortex [ˌpæliəuˈkɔːteks] *n* 旧皮质

paleogenesis [ˌpæliəuˈdʒenisis] *n* 重演性发生(祖代的特征重现于以后各代) | **paleogenetic** [ˌpæliəudʒiˈnetik] *a*

paleokinetic [ˌpæliəukaiˈnetik], **paleocinetic** [ˌpæliəusaiˈnetik] *a* 古旧运动的(指纹状体所控制的自动性联合运动)

paleoneurology [ˌpæliəunjuəˈrɔlədʒi] *n* 古神经病学

paleontology [ˌpæliɔnˈtɔlədʒi] *n* 古生物学

paleopallium [ˌpæliəuˈpæljəm] *n* 旧皮质

paleopathology [ˌpæliəupəˈθɔlədʒi] *n* 古生物病理学

paleosensation [ˌpæliəsenˈseiʃən] *n* 旧感觉(指痛觉及温度感觉)

paleostriatum [ˌpæliəustraiˈeitəm] *n* 旧纹状体,原纹状体 | **paleostriatal** *a*

paleothalamus [ˌpæliəuˈθæləməs] *n* 旧丘脑,原丘脑

pali-, palin- [构词成分]重复,向后

Palicourea [ˌpælikəuˈjuəriə] *n* 巴柯树属

palikinesia [ˌpælikaiˈniːziə], **palicinesia** [ˌpælisaiˈniːziə] *n*（病态）重复动作
palilalia [ˌpæliˈleiliə] *n* 言语重复
palin- 见 pali-
palindrome [ˈpælindrəum] *n* 回文对称（在遗传学上一种顺读和倒读都一样的 DNA 或 RNA 顺序）
palindromia [ˌpælinˈdrəumiə] *n*（病的）复发，再发 | **palindromic** [ˌpælinˈdrɔmik] *a*
palinesthesia [ˌpælinisˈθiːzjə] *n*（全身麻醉的）复苏，苏醒
palingenesis [ˌpælinˈdʒenisis] *n* 再生；重演性发生（祖代的特征重现于以后各代）
palingraphia [ˌpælinˈgreifiə] *n*（病态）重复书写
palinmnesis [ˌpæliˈniːsis] *n*（往事）回忆
palinopsia [ˌpæliˈnɔpsiə] *n* 视象存留，视后象稽延持续
palinphrasia [ˌpælinˈfreiziə]，**paliphrasia** [ˌpæliˈfreiziə] *n*（病态）重复言语
palisade [ˌpæliseid] *n* 栅栏（指某些细菌染色涂片上细胞的排列）
palivizumab [ˌpæliˈvizjumæb] *n* 帕利单抗（由重组 DNA 技术产生的人源化单克隆抗体，针对呼吸道合胞病毒〈RSV〉，用作易感的婴儿和儿童被动免疫药，肌内注射）
palladium [pəˈleidiəm] *n* 钯（化学元素）；钯制剂（顺势疗法的钯制剂）
pallanesthesia [ˌpælænisˈθiːzjə] *n* 振动觉缺失
pallesthesia [ˌpælisˈθiːzjə] *n* 振动觉 | **pallesthetic** [ˌpælisˈθetik] *a*
pallhypesthesia [ˌpælhaipisˈθiːzjə] *n* 振动［感］觉减退
pallial [ˈpæliəl] *a*（大脑）皮质的
palliate [ˈpælieit] *vt* 减轻，缓和（痛苦、疾病等）| **palliation** [ˌpæliˈeiʃən] *n*
palliative [ˈpæliətiv, -ˌeitiv] *a* 减轻的，缓和的，治标的，姑息的 *n* 姑息剂，治标剂
pallid [ˈpælid] *a* 无血色的，病状的
pallidal [ˈpælidəl] *a* 苍白球的
pallidectomy [ˌpæliˈdektəmi] *n* 苍白球切除术
pallidin [ˈpælidin] *n* 梅毒螺旋体悬液（用先天性梅毒死婴肺制备的悬液，用于梅毒的皮肤试验）
pallidoansection [ˌpælidəuænˈsekʃən] *n* 苍白球豆状核襻切除术
pallidoansotomy [ˌpælidəuænˈsɔtəmi] *n* 苍白球豆状核襻切开术
pallidofugal [ˌpæliˈdɔfjugəl] *a* 离苍白球的
pallidoidosis [ˌpælidɔiˈdəusis] *n* 兔梅毒
pallidotomy [ˌpæliˈdɔtəmi] *n* 苍白球切开术
pallidum [ˈpælidəm] *n*【拉】苍白球 | ~ Ⅰ 内侧苍白球 / ~ Ⅱ 外侧苍白球
pallium [ˈpæliəm] *n*【拉】大脑皮质
palmellin [pælˈmelin] *n* 胶群藻色素
pallor [ˈpælə] *n* 苍白，灰白
palm[1] [pɑːm] *n* 棕榈
palm[2] [pɑːm] *n* 掌，手掌，掌面 | handball ~ 手球员掌（一种掌部挫伤）
palma [ˈpælmə]（［复］**palmae** [ˈpælmiː]）*n*【拉】掌；棕榈
Palmaceae [ˌpɑːlˈmeisiiː] *n* 棕榈科
Palmae [ˈpɑːlmiː] *n* 棕榈科
palmanesthesia [ˌpælmænisˈθiːzjə] *n* 振动觉缺失
palmar [ˈpælmə] *a* 掌的
palmaris [pælˈmeiris] *a* 掌的 *n* 掌肌
palmature [ˈpælmətʃə] *n* 蹼指
Palmaz [pɑːlˈmɑːz]（Julio C. Palmaz）帕尔马支架（一种血管内支架）
palmesthesia [ˌpælmisˈθiːzjə] *n* 振动觉 | **palmesthetic** [ˌpælmisˈθetik] *a*
palmital [ˈpælmitl] *n* 棕榈醛，软脂醛
palmitate [ˈpælmiteit] *n* 棕榈酸，软脂酸；棕榈酸盐
palmitic acid [pælˈmitik] 棕榈酸
palmitin [ˈpælmitin] *n* 棕榈酸甘油酯
palmitoleate [ˌpælmiˈtəulieit] *n* 棕榈油酸盐（酯或阴离子型）
palmitoleic acid [ˌpælmitəuˈliːik] 棕榈油酸
palmitone [ˈpælmitəun] *n* 棕榈酮，软脂酮
palmitoyl [ˌpælmiˈtəuil] *n* 棕榈酰，软脂酰
palmus [ˈpælməs] *n* 心悸；痉跳病
palp [pælp] *n*［触］须，触器（昆虫）| **~al** *a*
palpable [ˈpælpəbl] *a* 可触知的
palpate[1] [ˈpælpeit] *vt*（诊断时的）摸，触，按
palpate[2] [ˈpælpeit] *a* 有触器的，有触须的
palpation [pælˈpeiʃən] *n* 触诊，扪诊 | bimanual ~ 双手触诊 / light touch ~ 轻触诊
palpatometry [ˌpælpəˈtɔmitri] *n* 痛压测验法
palpatopercussion [ˌpælpətəupəːˈkʌʃən] *n* 触叩诊
palpebra [ˈpælpibrə]（［复］**palpebrae** [ˈpælpibriː]）*n*【拉】眼睑 | ~ inferior 下睑 / ~ superior 上睑 / ~ tertius 第三睑，瞬膜 | **~l** [ˈpælpibrəl] *a*
palpebralis [ˌpælpəˈbreilis] *a*【拉】眼睑的
palpebrate [ˈpælpibreit] *vi* 霎眼，瞬目 *a* 有睑的
palpebration [ˌpælpiˈbreiʃən] *n* 霎眼；霎眼过频，瞬目过多
palpebritis [ˌpælpiˈbraitis] *n* 睑缘炎
palpitate [ˈpælpiteit] *vi* 心悸 | **palpitant** [ˈpælpitənt] *a* / **palpitation** [ˌpælpiˈteiʃən] *n*
palpus [ˈpælpəs]（［复］**palpi** [ˈpælpi]）*n* 须肢；［触］须
PALS periarterial lymphoid sheath 围动脉淋巴鞘

Pal's stain [pɑːl] (Jocob Pal) 帕尔染剂(染有髓神经)
palsy [ˈpɔːlzi] *n* 麻痹,瘫痪 *vt* 使瘫痪 | birth ~ 产伤麻痹 / brachial ~ 上肢麻痹,臂丛麻痹 / crossed ~, transverse ~ 交叉性麻痹 / crossed leg ~ 交腿性麻痹 / diver's ~ 潜水员麻痹,潜水员病,减压病 / facial ~ 面神经麻痹,面瘫 / hammer ~ 锤手麻痹 / printer's ~ 印刷工麻痹,锑毒性麻痹 / scrivener's ~ 书写麻痹,书写痉挛 / shaking ~ 震颤麻痹 / spastic bulbar ~ 痉挛性延髓性麻痹 / wasting ~ 消瘦性麻痹,脊髓性肌萎缩
Paltauf's dwarf [ˈpɑːltauf] (Arnold Paltauf) 垂体性矮小 | ~ nanism (dwarfism) 淋巴[体质]性侏儒症
paludism [ˈpælj*u*dizəm] *n* 疟疾
2-PAM pralidoxime 解磷定(解有机磷中毒药)
L-PAM L-phenylalanine mustard L-苯丙氨酸氮芥(抗肿瘤药)
pamabrom [ˈpæməbrɔm] *n* 帕马溴(轻度利尿药,用于缓解经前症状的制剂)
pamaquine [ˈpæməkwin] *n* 帕马喹(抗疟药) | ~ naphthoate 双羟萘酸帕马喹(作为抗疟药现主要被伯氨喹〈primaquine〉所取代)
pamatolol sulfate [ˌpæməˈtəulɔl] 硫酸帕马洛尔(β 受体阻滞药)
pamidronate (APD) [ˌpæmiˈdrəuneit] *n* 帕米膦酸(与 ^{99m}Tc 络合,用于骨成像)
pamoate [ˈpæm*ə*ueit] *n* 双羟萘酸盐,双羟水杨酸盐
pampiniform [pæmˈpinifɔːm] *a* 蔓状的,卷须状的
pampinocele [pæmˈpinəsiːl] *n* 精索静脉曲张
pamplegia [pæmˈpliːdʒiə] *n* 全麻痹,全瘫
PAN polyarteritis nodosa 结节性多动脉炎
Pan [pæn] *n* 灵长属(包括黑猩猩和大猩猩在内的一类灵长类动物)
pan- [前缀]全,全部,总,泛
panacea [ˌpænəˈsiə] *n* 万灵药;万应药 | **~n** *a*
panacinar [pænˈæsinə] *a* 全腺泡的
panagglutinable [ˌpænəˈgluːtinəbl] *a* 泛凝集的,全可凝集的(能被同种内任何型血清所凝集的,例如指能被所有型的人血清凝集的红细胞)
panagglutination [ˌpænəˌgluːtiˈneiʃən] *n* 泛凝集[反应],全凝集[反应]
panagglutinin [ˌpænəˈgluːtinin] *n* 泛凝集素,全凝集素
panangiitis [ˌpænændʒiˈaitis] *n* 全血管炎,血管诸层炎
pananxiety [ˌpænængˈzaiəti] *n* 泛焦虑症
panaris [ˈpænəris] *n* 甲沟炎,瘭疽 | analgesic ~ 无痛性瘭疽(见 Morvan's syndrome②解)
panarteritis [ˌpænɑːtəˈraitis] *n* 全身动脉炎;全动脉炎,动脉诸层炎
panarthritis [ˌpænɑːˈθraitis] *n* 全关节炎,全身关节炎
Panas' operation [pəˈnɑː] (Photinos Panas) 帕纳手术(上睑下垂手术)
panasthenia [ˌpænæsˈθiːniə] *n* 神经衰弱
panatrophy [pæˈnætrəfi] *n* 全身萎缩
panautonomic [pænˌɔːtəuˈnɔmik] *a* 全自主神经系统的
Panax [ˈpeinæks] *n* 人参属 | ~ ginseng 人参 / ~ pseudo-ginseng 三七,田三七,参三七
panblastic [pænˈblæstik] *a* 全胚层的
panbronchiolitis [pænˌbrɔŋkiəuˈlaitis] *n* 全细支气管炎
pancarditis [ˌpænkɑːˈdaitis] *n* 全心炎,心包[心]肌[心]内膜炎
panchontee [pænʃɔnˈtiː] *n* 印度乳胶
panchrest [ˈpænkrest] *n* 万应药
panchromatic [ˌpænkrəuˈmætik] *a* 全色的,泛色的(指照相乳剂)
panchromia [pænˈkrəumiə] *n* 全染性
Pancoast's suture [ˈpæŋkəust] (Joseph Pancoast) 潘科斯特缝合术(一种成形缝合术)
Pancoast's syndrome [ˈpæŋkəust] (Henry. K. Pancoast) 潘科斯特综合征(①肺尖部有 X 线阴影、臂神经痛、臂手肌萎缩以及霍纳〈Horner〉综合征,见于肺尖附近的肿瘤,由于臂丛累及所致;②一个或一个以上肋骨后部的骨质溶解,有时亦累及相应的脊椎) | ~ tumor 肺上沟瘤
pancolectomy [ˌpænkəuˈlektəmi] *n* 全结肠切除术
pancolitis [ˌpænkəuˈlaitis] *n* 全结肠炎
pancreas [ˈpæŋkriəs] ([复] **pancreata** [ˈpæŋkriətə]) *n* 胰 | accessory ~ 副胰 / annular ~ 环状胰腺 / dorsal ~ 背胰 / lesser ~ 胰钩突 / ventral ~ 腹胰 | **pancreatic** [ˌpæŋkriˈætik] *a*
pancreatalgia [ˌpæŋkriəˈtældʒiə], **pancrealgia** [ˌpæŋkriˈældʒiə] *n* 胰痛
pancreatectomy [ˌpæŋkriəˈtektəmi] *n* 胰切除术
pancreatic elastase Ⅱ [ˌpæŋkriˈætik iˈlæsteis] 胰弹性蛋白酶Ⅱ
pancreatic lipase [ˌpæŋkriˈætik ˈlaipeis] 胰脂肪酶
pancreatic(o)- [构词成分]胰管
pancreaticoduodenal [ˌpæŋkriˌætikəuˌdju(ː)əuˈdiːnl] *a* 胰十二指肠的
pancreaticoduodenostomy [ˌpæŋkriˌætikəuˌdju(ː)əudiːˈnɔstəmi] *n* 胰管十二指肠吻合术
pancreaticoenterostomy [ˌpæŋkriˌætikəuˌentəˈrɔstəmi] *n* 胰管小肠吻合术
pancreaticogastrostomy [ˌpæŋkriˌætikəugæsˈtr-

ɔstəmi] *n* 胰管胃吻合术
pancreaticojejunostomy [ˌpæŋkriˌætikəuˌdʒidʒuˈnɔstəmi] *n* 胰空肠吻合术
pancreaticosplenic [ˌpæŋkriætikəuˈsplenik] *a* 胰脾的
pancreatin [ˈpæŋkriətin] *n* 胰酶制剂(助消化药)
pancreatism [ˈpæŋkriətizəm] *n* 胰活动
pancreatitis [ˌpæŋkriəˈtaitis] *n* 胰腺炎 | calcareous ~ 结石性胰腺炎 / centrilobar ~ 小叶中心性胰腺炎 / perilobar ~ 小叶周围性胰腺炎
pancreat(o)- [构词成分]胰
pancreatoblastoma [ˌpæŋkriətəublæsˈtəumə] *n* 胰胚细胞瘤(一种罕见的恶性胰腺瘤,原因不明,通常侵犯儿童)
pancreatoduodenectomy [ˌpæŋkriətəuˌdju(:)əu-diˈnektəmi] *n* 胰头十二指肠切除术
pancreatoduodenostomy [ˌpæŋkriətəuˌdju(:)-əudiˈnɔstəmi] *n* 胰管十二指肠吻合术
pancreatoenterostomy [ˌpæŋkriətəuˌentəˈrɔstəmi] *n* 胰管小肠吻合术
pancreatogenous [ˌpæŋkriəˈtɔdʒinəs], **pancreatogenic** [ˌpæŋkriətəuˈdʒenik] *a* 胰发生的,胰源性的
pancreatogram [ˌpæŋkriˈætəgræm] *n* 胰造影[照]片
pancreatography [ˌpæŋkriəˈtɔgrəfi] *n* 胰造影[术] | endoscopic retrograde ~ 内镜逆行胰管造影[术]
pancreatoid [pæŋˈkriːətɔid] *a* 胰样的
pancreatolipase [ˌpæŋkriətəuˈlipeis] *n* 胰脂酶
pancreatolith [ˌpæŋkriˈætəliθ] *n* 胰石
pancreatolithectomy [ˌpæŋkriətəliˈθektəmi] *n* 胰石切除术
pancreatolithiasis [ˌpæŋkriətəliˈθaiəsis] *n* 胰石病
pancreatolithotomy [ˌpæŋkriətəliˈθɔtəmi] *n* 胰切开取石术
pancreatolysis [ˌpæŋkriəˈtɔlisis] *n* 胰组织破坏 | **pancreatolytic** [ˌpæŋkriətəuˈlitik] *a* 破坏胰组织的
pancreatoncus [ˌpæŋkriəˈtɔnkəs] *n* 胰瘤
pancreatopathy [ˌpæŋkriəˈtɔpəθi] *n* 胰病
pancreatoscopy [ˌpæŋkriəˈtɔskəpi] *n* 胰管内镜检查
pancreatotomy [ˌpæŋkriəˈtɔtəmi], **pancreatomy** [pæŋkriˈætəmi] *n* 胰切开术
pancreatotropic [ˌpæŋkriətəuˈtrɔpik], **pancreatropic** [ˌpæŋkriəˈtrɔpik] *a* 向胰[腺]的,促胰[腺]的
pancreectomy [ˌpæŋkriˈektəmi] *n* 胰切除术
pancrelipase [ˌpæŋkriˈlaipeis] *n* 胰脂肪酶
pancreolithiasis [ˌpæŋkriəuliˈθaiəsis] *n* 胰石病
pancreolithotomy [ˌpæŋkriəuliˈθɔtəmi] *n* 胰切开取石术
pancreolysis [ˌpæŋkriˈɔlisis] *n* 胰组织破坏 | **pancreolytic** [ˌpæŋkriəuˈlitik] *a* 破坏胰组织的
pancreopathy [ˌpæŋkriˈɔpəθi] *n* 胰病
pancreoprivic [ˌpæŋkriəuˈprivik] *a* 无胰的
pancreotherapy [ˌpæŋkriəuˈθerəpi] *n* 胰制剂疗法
pancreotropic [ˌpæŋkriəuˈtrɔpik] *a* 向胰[腺]的,促胰[腺]的
pancreozymin [ˈpæŋkriəuˌzaimin] *n* 促胰酶素(十二指肠分泌的一种激素,能促使胰酶分泌)
pancuronium bromide [ˌpænkjuˈrəuniəm] 泮库溴铵(非去极化性骨骼肌松弛药)
pancystitis [ˌpænsisˈtaitis] *n* 全膀胱炎
pancytolysis [ˌpænsaiˈtɔlisis] *n* 全血细胞溶解
pancytopenia [ˌpænsaitəuˈpiːniə] *n* 全血细胞减少
pancytosis [ˌpænsaiˈtəusis] *n* 全血细胞增多
pandemic [pænˈdemik] *a* 大流行的 *n* 大流行病 | **~ity** [ˌpændeˈmisəti] *n* 大流行状态
Pander's islands [ˈpændə] (Heinrich C. Pander) 潘德尔血岛(在胚脏壁中由小球样物质组成的微红黄素,发育成为血液及血管) | ~ layer 中胚层脏壁层 / ~ nucleus 丘脑下核
pandiculation [ˌpændikjuˈleiʃən] *n* 伸体呵欠,欠伸
Pándy's test (reaction) [ˈpændi] (Kálmán Pándy)潘迪试验(反应)(检脑脊液球蛋白)
panel [ˈpænl] *n* 名簿,名单;专门小组;英国保险医师名簿
panelectroscope [ˌpæniˈlektrəskəup] *n* 通用电光[窥]镜(检身体各种器官,如胃、直肠、尿道等)
panencephalitis [ˌpænenˌsefəˈlaitis] *n* 全脑炎 | subacute sclerosing ~ 亚急性硬化性全脑炎
panendography [ˌpænenˈdɔgrəfi] *n* 广视野膀胱镜描记检查法
panendoscope [pænˈendəskəup] *n* 广视野内镜;广视野膀胱镜 | **panendoscopy** [ˌpænənˈdɔskəpi] *n* 全上消化道内镜检查[术];广视野膀胱镜检查[术]
panepizootic [pænˌepizəuˈɔtik] *a* 兽疫大流行的 *n* 大流行动物病
panesthesia [ˌpænisˈθiːzjə] *n* 全部感觉,总感觉 | **panesthetic** [ˌpænisˈθetik] *a*
Paneth's cells [ˈpɑːneit] (Josef Paneth)帕内特细胞(肠腺的嗜酸细胞)
pang [pæŋ] *n* 剧痛,猝然刺痛 | breast ~ 心绞痛 / brow ~ 眶上神经痛;偏头痛
pangamic acid [pænˈgæmik] 泮加酸,泛配子酸(维生素 B_{15})
pangen [ˈpændʒin] *n* 胚芽;泛子(生命力最小

单位）
pangenesis [pæn'dʒenisis] *n* 泛生论（生殖时母体每一个细胞均为微粒的一种学说）
panglossia [pæn'glɔsiə] *n* 饶舌，多辩
Pangonia [pæn'gəuniə] *n* 剧虻属
panhematopenia [pæn͵hemətəu'pi:niə] *n* 各型血细胞减少
panhematopoietic [pæn͵hemətəupɔi'etik] *a* 全造血系的
panhemocytophthisis [͵pænhi:məusai'tɔfθisis] *n* 各型血细胞变性，各型血细胞形成不全
panhydrometer [͵pænhai'drɔmitə] *n* 通用[液体]比重计
panhyperemia [͵pænhaipə:'ri:miə] *n* 全身充血，全身多血
panhypogammaglobulinemia [pæn͵haipəugæmə͵glɔbju:li'ni:miə] *n* 全丙球蛋白过少血症
panhypogonadism [pæn͵haipə'gəunədizəm] *n* 全性腺功能减退
panhypopituitarism [pæn͵haipəupi'tju:itərizəm] *n* 全垂体功能减退症
panhysterectomy [͵pænhistə'rektəmi] *n* 全子宫切除术
panhystero-oophorectomy [pæn͵histərəu͵əuɔfə'rektəmi] *n* 全子宫卵巢切除术
panhysterosalpingectomy [pæn͵histərəu͵sælpin'dʒektəmi] *n* 全子宫输卵管切除术
panhysterosalpingo-oophorectomy [pæn͵histərəu͵sælpiŋgəu͵əuɔfə'rektəmi] *n* 全子宫输卵管卵巢切除术
panic ['pænik] *n* 恐慌，惊恐；极度焦虑 | acute homosexual ~, homosexual ~ 急性同性恋惊恐反应，同性恋惊恐反应（一种极度焦虑反应，无意识恐惧被认为是同性恋者或屈从于同性恋冲动所诱发）
panic-stricken ['pænik͵strikən] *a* 惊慌失措的
panicum ['pænikəm] *n* 黍属
panimmunity [͵pæni'mju:nəti] *n* 全免疫，泛免疫，多种免疫（对几种细菌和病毒感染都具有免疫性）
Panizza's plexuses [pæ'nidzə]（Bartolomeo Panizza）帕尼扎丛（包皮系带外侧窝内的两个淋巴管丛）
panleukopenia [͵pænlju:kəu'pi:niə] *n* 全白细胞减少症，猫传染性粒细胞缺乏症，猫肠炎，猫瘟
panmeristic [͵pænmə'ristik] *a* 泛生的
panmixis [pæn'miksis], **panmixia** [pæn'miksiə] *n* 随机婚配；随机交配
panmural [pæn'mju:rəl] *a* 全壁的
panmyeloid [pæn'maiəlɔid] *a* 全骨髓的
panmyelopathy [͵pænmaiə'lɔpəθi], **panmyelopathia** [͵pænmaiələu'pæθiə] *n* 全骨髓病
panmyelophthisis [pæn͵maiə'lɔfθisis] *n* 全骨髓萎缩，全骨髓再生障碍，再生障碍性贫血
panmyelosis [͵pænmaiə'ləusis] *n* 全骨髓增生
Panner's disease ['pænə]（Hans J. Panner）潘纳病（肱骨小头的骨软骨病）
panneurosis [͵pænjuə'rəusis] *n* 泛神经症（包括焦虑、转换症状、强迫症和恐怖症）
panniculalgia [pə͵nikju'lældʒiə] *n* 脂膜痛，脂肪痛
panniculectomy [pə͵nikju:'lektəmi] *n* 脂膜切除术
panniculitis [pə͵nikju'laitis] *n* 脂膜炎 | LE ~, lupus ~ 红斑狼疮性脂膜炎，狼疮性脂膜炎，深部红斑狼疮 / relapsing febrile nodular nonsuppurative ~ 复发性发热性结节性非化脓性脂膜炎（亦称结节性非化脓性脂膜炎）/ subacute nodular migratory ~ 亚急性结节性游走性脂膜炎
panniculus [pə'nikjuləs]（[复] **panniculi** [pə'nikjulai]）*n*【拉】膜
pannus ['pænəs] *n*【拉】血管翳，角膜翳；关节翳；脂膜
panodic [pə'nɔdik] *a* 四周放射的，多向传导的（神经）
panophobia [͵pænə'fəubiə] *n* 泛恐怖症
panophthalmitis [͵pænɔfθæl'maitis], **panophthalmia** [͵pænɔf'θælmiə] *n* 全眼球炎
panoptic [pæ'nɔptik] *a* 全染[色]的
panorama [͵pænə'rɑ:mə] *n* 全景；概观；概论 | **panoramic** [͵pænə'ræmik] *a*
panosteitis [͵pænɔsti'aitis], **panostitis** [͵pænɔs'taitis] *n* 全骨炎
panotitis [͵pænəu'taitis] *n* 全耳炎
panphobia [pæn'fəubjə] *n* 泛恐怖症
panplegia [pæn'pli:dʒiə] *n* 全麻痹，全瘫
panproctocolectomy [pæn͵prɔktəukəu'lektəmi] *n* 全直肠结肠切除术
panretinal [pæn'retinəl] *a* 泛视网膜的
Pansch's fissure ['pʌnʃ]（Adolf Pansch）顶间沟
pansclerosis [͵pænskliə'rəusis] *n* 全硬化
panseptum [pæn'septəm] *n* 全鼻中隔
pansinusectomy [͵pænsainə'sektəmi] *n* 全鼻窦切除术
pansinusitis [͵pænsainə'saitis], **pansinuitis** [͵pænsainə'aitis] *n* 全鼻窦炎
panspermatist [pæn'spə:mətist] *n* 泛生说者（亦称 panspermist，参见 panspermy）
panspermia [pæn'spə:miə], **panspermatism** [pæn'spə:mətizəm] *n* 病原普遍存在说；生物发生，生源说（见 biogenesis）
panspermy [pæn'spə:mi] *n* 泛生说（认为大气充满看不见的动植物胚芽或生殖体）| **panspermic** *a*
pansphygmograph [pæn'sfigməgrɑ:f] *n* 心脉搏

胸[运]动描记器

pansporoblast [ˌpæn'spɔːrəblæst] *n* 泛成孢子细胞,泛孢子母细胞

Pansporoblastina [ˌpænspɔːˌrəublæs'tainə] *n* 泛成孢子虫亚目

Panstrongylus [pæn'strɔndʒiləs] *n* 锥蝽属 | ~ geniculatus 弯节锥蝽 / ~ infestans 骚扰锥蝽(即 Triatoma infestans) / ~ megistus 大锥蝽

pantachromatic [ˌpæntəkrəu'mætik] *a* 全消色差的

pantalgia [pæn'tældʒiə] *n* 全身痛

pantamorphia [ˌpæntə'mɔːfiə] *n* 全畸形

pantamorphic [ˌpæntə'mɔːfik] *a* 全畸形的,无形体的

pantanencephaly [ˌpæntənen'sefəli] *n* 全无脑(胎儿)

pantankyloblepharon [pænˌtæŋkiləu'blefərɔn] *n* 全睑球粘连

pantatrophia [ˌpæntə'trəufiə], **pantatrophy** [pæn'tætrəfi] *n* 全身营养不良,全身萎缩

pantetheine [ˌpænti'θiːin] *n* 泛硫乙胺,泛酰巯基乙胺

panthenol ['pænθənɔl] *n* 泛醇(维生素类药)

pantherapist [pæn'θerəpist] *n* 综合治疗医师

panthodic [pæn'θɔdik] *a* 四周放射的,多向传导的(神经)

panting ['pæntiŋ] *n* 喘气,气促(呼吸困难)

pant(o)- [构词成分]全,全部,总,泛

pantochromism [ˌpæntəu'krəumizəm] *n* 多色[现象]

pantogamy [pæn'tɔgəmi] *n* 杂交,自由交配

pantograph ['pæntəgrɑːf, -græf] *n* 缩放仪,比例绘图仪

pantoic acid [pæn'təuik] 泛解酸

pantomography [ˌpæntəu'mɔgrəfi] *n* 曲面断层摄影[术](亦称全景 X 线摄影[术]) | **pantomographic** [pænˌtəumə'græfik] *a*

pantomorphia [ˌpæntəu'mɔːfiə] *n* 全对称;多形性(如阿米巴)

pantomorphic [ˌpæntəu'mɔːfik] *a* 一切形态的,多形的

pantophobia [ˌpæntəu'fəubjə] *n* 泛恐怖症 | **pantophobic** *a*

pantoprazole sodium [pæn'təuprəzəul] 泮托拉唑钠(抗溃疡药)

pantoscopic [ˌpæntəu'skɔpik] *a* 双光的(眼镜)

pantothen ['pæntəθən] *n* 泛酸

pantothenate [pæn'təuθəneit] *n* 泛酸盐

pantothenic acid [ˌpæntə'θenik] 泛酸

pantothenol [ˌpæntə'θiːnɔl] *n* 泛醇;右泛醇

pantoyltaurine [ˌpæntɔil'tɔːri(ː)n] *n* 泛磺酸

pantropic [pæn'trɔpik], **pantotropic** [ˌpæntəu'trɔpik] *a* 泛向的(对许多组织有亲和力的;对三个胚胎层中任何一个胚层的衍生物均侵袭的)

panturbinate [pæn'təːbineit] *n* 全鼻甲

Panum's area ['pɑːnuːm] (Peter L. Panum) 视网膜融合区

panus ['peinəs] *n* (非化脓性)淋巴结炎

panuveitis [ˌpænjuvi'aitis] *n* 全葡萄膜炎

panzerherz ['pænzəhəːz] *n*【德】装甲心(心包石灰质沉着)

panzootic [ˌpænzəu'ɔtik] *a* 动物大流行的

PAP peroxidase-antiperoxidase 过氧化酶-抗过氧化酶; placental alkaline phosphatase 胎盘碱性磷酸酶

pap [pæp] *n* 面包糊,软食[物]

papain [pə'peiin, -'pai-] *n* 木瓜蛋白酶;木瓜蛋白酶消化剂

Papanicolaou's stain [ˌpɑːpə'niːkəˌlau] (George N. Papanicolaou) 巴帕尼科拉乌染剂(取自呼吸道、消化道或生殖泌尿道各种身体分泌物的染色涂片法,检查其中脱落细胞,以检测是否有恶性过程) | ~ test (smear) 巴帕尼科拉乌试验(涂片)(一种表皮脱落细胞学染色法,以检查和诊断各种病况,尤用于妇女生殖道恶性和恶性前病况的检查和诊断,亦用于评价内分泌功能及诊断诸如呼吸道和肺、胃肠道、泌尿道、乳房等器官的恶性变化)

Papaver [pə'pæva] *n* 罂粟属

Papaveraceae [ˌpæpəvə'reisiiː] *n* 罂粟科

papaverine [pə'pævərin] *n* 罂粟碱 | ~ hydrochloride 盐酸罂粟碱(平滑肌松弛药)

papaw [pə'pɔː] *n* 番木瓜

papaya [pə'paiə] *n* 番木瓜;番木瓜汁

papayotin [pə'paiətin] *n* 番木瓜酶,番木瓜蛋白酶

paper ['peipə] *n* 纸;论文;考卷 | alkanin ~ 紫草素试纸 / amboceptor ~ 介体试纸 / articulating ~, occluding ~ 咬合纸,船纸 / azolitmin ~ 石蕊素试纸 / biuret ~ 双缩脲试纸 / filter ~ 滤纸 / litmus ~ 石蕊试纸 / niter ~, asthma ~, saltpeter ~ 硝石纸(用作艾或哮喘时吸入用) / test ~ 试纸 / turmeric ~ 姜黄[试]纸

papery ['peipəri] *a* (薄或硬)似纸的

papescent [pə'pesənt] *a* 面包糊状的

Papez circuit [pə'pez] (James W. Papez) 帕佩士回路(边缘系统包括海马、大脑穹窿、乳头体、丘脑前核和扣带回的一种神经元回路,与情绪的体验以及对情绪的反应有关)

papilliform [pə'pilifɔːm] *a* 乳头状的

papilla [pə'pilə] ([复] **papillae** [pə'piliː]) *n*【拉】乳头;乳头状突起 | acoustic ~ 螺旋器 / bile ~ 胆汁乳头,十二指肠大乳头 / optic ~ 视

神经乳头 / palatine ~ 腭(前)乳头,切牙乳头

papillary [pəˈpiləri] *a* 乳头的,乳头状的;乳突的

papillate [ˈpæpileit] *a* 乳头状的

papillectomy [ˌpæpiˈlektəmi] *n* 乳头切除术(肾)

papilledema [ˌpæpili(ː)ˈdiːmə] *n* 视[神经]盘水肿

papilliferous [ˌpæpiˈlifərəs] *a* 有乳头的

papillitis [ˌpæpiˈlaitis] *n* 视[神经]盘炎;乳头炎 | necrotizing ~, necrotizing renal ~ 肾乳头坏死

papilloadenocystoma [pəˌpiləuˌædinəusisˈtəumə] *n* 乳头状腺囊瘤

papillocarcinoma [pəˌpiləuˌkɑːsiˈnəumə] *n* 乳头状癌

papilloma [ˌpæpiˈləumə] ([复] **papillomas** 或 **papillomata** [ˌpæpiˈləumətə]) *n* 乳头状瘤 | ~**tous** [ˌpæpiˈləumətəs] *a*

papillomatosis [ˌpæpiˌləuməˈtəusis] *n* 乳头状瘤病 | confluent and reticulate ~ 融合性网状乳头状瘤病

Papillomavirinae [ˌpæpiˌləuməviˈrainiː] *n* 乳头瘤病毒亚科

Papillomavirus [ˌpæpiˈləuməˌvaiərəs] *n* 乳头瘤病毒属

papillomavirus [ˌpæpiˈləuməˌvaiərəs] *n* 乳头瘤病毒

Papillon-Lefèvre syndrome [ˌpæpiˈjɔn ləˈfei] (M. M. Papillon; Paul Lefèvre) 帕皮永-勒菲弗综合征(掌跖角化病伴牙周病)

papilloretinitis [pəˌpiləuretiˈnaitis] *n* 乳头视网膜炎

papillosphincterotomy [ˌpæpiləuˌsfiŋktəˈrɔtəmi] *n* (十二指肠)乳头括约肌切开术

papillotome [ˈpæpiləˌtəum] *n* 乳头切开刀

papillotomy [ˌpæpiˈlɔtəmi] *n* 乳头括约肌切开[术]

Papin's digester [pəˈpæn] (Denis Papin) 帕宾热压浸渍器

Papio [ˈpeipiˌəu] *n* (西非)狒狒属

papoid [ˈpæpɔid] *n* 番木瓜消化酶(商业制剂)

Papovaviridae [pəˌpəuvəˈviridiː] *n* 乳多空病毒科,乳头多瘤空泡病毒科

papovavirus [pəˈpəuvəˌvaiərəs] (*pa*pilloma *po*lyoma *va*cuolating agent + *virus*) *n* 乳多空病毒,乳头多瘤空泡病毒 | lymphotropic ~ (LPV) 亲淋巴乳多空病毒

Pappenheim's stain [ˈpʌpənhaim] (Artur Pappenheim) 帕彭海姆染剂(用以鉴别红细胞嗜碱粒及核碎片)

pappose [ˈpæpəus] *a* 有软毛的;有冠毛的(菊科)

pappus [ˈpæpəs] *n* 软毛,柔毛,胎毛;冠毛(植物)

paprika [pæˈprikə] *n* 辣椒;辣椒粉

Pap test (smear) [pæp] 巴氏试验(涂片)(见 Papanicolaou's test)

papulation [ˌpæpjuˈleiʃən] *n* 丘疹形成

papule [ˈpæpjuːl] *n* 丘疹 | dry ~ 干丘疹(下疳丘疹) / moist ~, mucous ~ 湿丘疹,尖锐湿疣,性病湿疣 / pearly penile ~s 珍珠样阴茎丘疹 / piezogenic ~s, painful piezogenic pedal ~s 压力性丘疹,痛性压力性足部丘疹(亦称痛性脂肪突出) / prurigo ~ 丘疹性痒疹 / split ~s 裂开丘疹 | **papula** [ˈpæpjulə] *n* | **papular** *a*

papuloerythematous [ˌpæpjuləuˌeriˈθemətəs] *a* 丘疹性红斑的

papuloid [ˈpæpjulɔid] *a* 丘疹样的,丘疹的

papulopustular [ˌpæpjuləuˈpʌstjulə] *a* 丘疹脓疱的

papulosis [ˌpæpjuˈləusis] *n* 丘疹病 | lymphomatoid ~ 淋巴瘤样丘疹病 / malignant atrophic ~ 恶性萎缩性丘疹病

papulosquamous [ˌpæpjuləuˈskweiməs] *a* 丘疹鳞屑的

papulovesicular [ˌpæpjuləuviˈsikjulə] *a* 丘疱疹的

Paquelin's cautery [ˌpɑːkiˈlæn] (Claude A. Paquelin) 巴圭林烙器(此器有一白金点,烙术时使用)

par [pɑː] *n*【拉】对,双

para [ˈpære] *n* 产次(指产过能存活的婴儿者称之,用数序表示分娩可存活婴儿的妊娠次数,如 para 0〈0 产〉, para 1〈1 产〉, para 2〈2 产〉等,其数序不指多胎分娩的婴儿数)

para^{-1}**, par-** [前缀]类,副,拟;旁,周;倒错,错乱,异常

para^{-2} [前缀]对[位](化学);副,仲(化学)

paraactinomycosis [ˌpærəˌæktinəumaiˈkəusis] *n* 假放线菌病

paraadventitial [ˌpærəˌædvənˈtiʃəl] *a* 旁外膜的

para-agglutinin [ˌpærə əˈgluːtinin] *n* 副凝集素

para-albuminemia [ˌpærə ælˌbjuːmiˈniːmiə] *n* 副白蛋白血症,双白蛋白血症,拟清蛋白血症

para-aminobenzenesulfonamide [ˌpærə ˌæminəu-ˌbenziːnsʌlˈfɔnəmaid] *n* 对氨基苯磺酰胺,氨苯磺胺

para-aminobenzoate [ˌpærə ˌæminəuˈbenzəueit] *n* 对氨基苯甲酸盐

para-aminobenzoic acid [ˌpærə ˌæminəubenˈzəuik] 对氨基苯甲酸

para-aminohippurate [ˌpærə ˌæminəuˈhipjuəreit] *n* 对氨基马尿酸盐

para-aminohippuric acid [ˌpærə ˌæminəuhiˈpjuərik] 对氨马尿酸

para-aminosalicylic acid [ˌpærə ˌæminəuˌsæliˈsilik] 对氨水杨酸

para-analgesia [ˌpærə ˌænælˈdʒiːzjə] *n* 下身痛觉

缺失

para-anesthesia [ˌpærə ˌænis'θiːzjə] *n* 下身感觉缺失

para-aortic [ˌpærə ei'ɔːtik] *a* 主动脉旁的

para-appendicitis [ˌpærə əˌpendi'saitis] *n* 阑尾旁炎

parabanic acid [ˌpærə'bænik] 仲班酸,乙二酰脲

Parabasalidea [ˌpærəˌbeisə'lidiə] *n* 副基总目

parabiont [pə'ræbiɔnt], **parabion** [pə'ræbiɔn] *n* 联体者,间生体者(组成联体生活的单个机体)

parabiosis [ˌpærəbai'əusis] *n* 并生,联体生活(联体的双生或用外科手术方法将两个实验动物做成联体);间生态(神经的传导性和兴奋性暂受阻抑) | dialytic ~ 渗析性联体生活 / vascular ~ 血管性联体生活 | **parabiotic** [ˌpærəbai'ɔtik] *a*

parablast ['pærəblæst] *n* 副胚层 | **~ic** [ˌpærə'blæstik] *a*

parablepsia [pærə'blepsiə] *n* 错视

parabola [pə'ræbələ] *n* 抛物线

parabolic(al) [ˌpærə'bɔlik(əl)] *a* 抛物线[状]的

paraboloid [pə'ræbəlɔid] *n* 抛物面

parabolus [pə'ræbələs] ([复] **paraboli** [pə'ræbəlai]) *n* 贫病救助员

parabulia [ˌpærə'bjuːliə] *n* 意向倒错

paracarbinoxamine [ˌpærəˌkɑːbi'nɔksəmin] *n* 氯苯吡醇胺,吡氯苄氧胺(即卡比沙明 carbinoxamine,抗组胺药)

paracardiac [ˌpærə'kɑːdiæk] *a* 心旁的

paracarmine [ˌpærə'kɑːmin] *n* 副卡红,副胭脂红

paracasein [ˌpærə'keisiːn] *n* 衍酪蛋白,副酪蛋白

paracellular [ˌpærə'seljulə] *a* 旁细胞的

paracellulose [ˌpærə'seljuləus] *n* 副纤维素

paracelsian [ˌpærə'selsiən] *a* 帕拉塞尔苏斯(Paracelssus)的

paracenesthesia [ˌpærəˌsiːnis'θiːzjə] *n* 自身感觉异常,一般感觉不佳

paracentesis [ˌpærəsen'tiːsis] *n* [放液]穿刺术 | abdominal ~ 腹腔穿刺[术] / aqueous ~ 角膜穿刺术 | **paracentetic** [ˌpærəsen'tetik] *a*

paracentral [ˌpærə'sentrəl] *a* 旁中央的,近中心的

paracephalus [ˌpærə'sefələs] *n* 头不全畸胎

paracerebellar [ˌpærəseri'belə] *a* 小脑侧部的

paracervix [ˌpærə'səːviks] *n* 子宫颈旁组织

paracetaldehyde [pəˌræsi'tældihaid] *n* 三聚乙醛

paracetamol [pəˌræsi'tæmɔl] *n* 对乙酰氨基酚(解热镇痛药)

parachloralose [ˌpærə'klɔːrələus] *n* 聚氯醛糖

parachloramine [ˌpærə'klɔːrəmin] *n* 氯苯甲嗪(即美克洛嗪 meclozine,抗组胺药)

parachlorometaxylenol [ˌpærəˌklɔːrəuˌmetə'zailənɔl] *n* 对氯间二甲苯酚,氯二甲酚

parachlorophenol [ˌpærəˌklɔːrə'fiːnɔl] *n* 对氯酚(抗菌药) | camphorated ~ 樟脑对氯酚

paracholera [ˌpærə'kɔlərə] *n* 副霍乱

paracholesterin [ˌpærəkə'lestərin] *n* 副胆固醇,衍胆甾醇

parachordal [ˌpærə'kɔːdəl] *a* 脊索旁的

Parachordodes [ˌpærəkɔː'dəudiːz] *n* 拟绳铁线虫属

parachromatin [ˌpærə'krəumətin] *n* 副染色质,副核染质

parachromatism [ˌpærə'krəumətizəm], **parachromatopsia** [ˌpærəˌkrəumə'tɔpsiə] *n* 色盲

paracinesia [ˌpærəsai'niːsiə], **paracinesis** [ˌpærəsai'niːsis] *n* 运动倒错

paraclinical [ˌpærə'klinikəl] *a* 产生临床症状体征的

paracnemis [ˌpærək'niːmis], **paracnemidion** [ˌpærəkniː'midiən] *n* 腓骨

Paracoccidioides brasiliensis [ˌpærəkɔkˌsidi'ɔidiːz brəˌsili'ensis] 巴西副球孢子菌

paracoccidioidomycosis [ˌpærəkɔkˌsidiˌɔidəumai'kəusis] *n* 副球孢子菌病

Paracoccus [ˌpærə'kɔkəs] *n* 副球菌属

paracolitis [ˌpærəkɔ'laitis] *n* 结肠周炎

Paracolobactrum [ˌpærəˌkəulə'bæktrəm] *n* 副大肠菌属

paracolpitis [ˌpærəkɔl'paitis] *n* 阴道周[组织]炎

paracolpium [ˌpærə'kɔlpiəm] *n* 阴道周组织

paracone ['pærəkəun] *n* 上前尖,上颌磨牙近中颊尖

paraconid [ˌpærə'kəunid] *n* 下前尖,下颌磨牙近中颊尖

paracortex [ˌpærə'kɔːteks] *n* 副皮质(胸腺依赖区)

paracousis [ˌpærə'kuːsis] *n* 听觉倒错,错听

paracoxalgia [ˌpærəkɔk'sældʒiə] *n* 类髋关节痛

paracresol [ˌpærə'kriːsɔl] *n* 对甲酚

paracrine ['pærəkrin] *n* 旁分泌

paracrystals [ˌpærə'kristlz] [复] *n* 酝晶,不全晶体(如烟草花叶病病毒的晶体)

paracusis [ˌpærə'kuːsis], **paracusia** [ˌpærə'kuːziə] *n* 误听

paracystic [ˌpærə'sistik] *a* 膀胱旁的

paracystitis [ˌpærəsis'taitis] *n* 膀胱周炎

paracystium [ˌpærə'sistiəm] *n* 膀胱周组织

paracytic [ˌpærə'sitik] *a* 异常细胞的;细胞旁的

paradental [ˌpærə'dentl] *a* 牙科的;牙周的,牙旁的

paradentitis [ˌpærəden'taitis] *n* 牙周炎

paradentium [ˌpærə'denʃiəm] *n* 牙周组织

paradentosis [ˌpærədenˈtəusis] *n* 牙周病
paraderm [ˈpærədəːm] *n* 生胚卵黄
paradesmose [ˌpærəˈdesməus] *n* 副连丝
paradidymis [ˌpærəˈdidimis] *n* 旁睾 | **paradidymal** *a* 旁睾的;睾丸旁的
paradimethylaminobenzaldehyde [ˌpærədaiˌmeθiləˌmiːnəubenˈzældihaid] *n* 对二甲氨基苯甲醛
paradiphenylbiuret [ˌpærədaiˌfenilˈbaijuəret] *n* 对二苯基双缩脲
paradipsia [ˌpærəˈdipsiə] *n* 渴感倒错
paradox [ˈpærədɔks] *n* 反论,奇论,相矛盾,奇异现象
paradoxic(al) [ˌpærəˈdɔksik(əl)] *a* 反论的,反常的,自相矛盾的,奇异的,逆理的 | **~ly** *ad* / **~ness** *n*
paradysentery [ˌpærəˈdisəntri] *n* 副痢疾,类痢疾
paraeccrisis [ˌpærəˈekrisis] *n* 分泌障碍;排泄障碍
paraepilepsy [ˌpærəepiˈlepsi] *n* 局限性癫痫小发作
paraequilibrium [ˌpærəˌiːkwiˈlibriəm] *n* 平衡感觉障碍,前庭性眩晕
paraesophageal [ˌpærəi(ː)ˌsɔfəˈdʒi(ː)əl] *a* 食管周围的
parafalx [ˌpærəˈfælks] *a* 镰周的(近大脑镰或近小脑镰的)
Par. aff. pars affecta【拉】患部,损伤部
paraffin [ˈpærəfin] *n* 石蜡 *vt* 用石蜡涂(或浸透) | chlorinated ~ 氯化石蜡 / hard ~ 固体石蜡,硬石蜡 / liquid ~ 液状石蜡 / pliable ~ 石蜡敷糊(裹灼伤或其他伤口用) / white soft ~ 白凡士林,白软石蜡
paraffinoma [ˌpærəfiˈnəumə] *n* 石蜡瘤
Parafilaria [ˌpærəfiˈlɛəriə] *n* 副丝虫属 | ~ multipapillosa 多乳头副丝虫
paraflocculus [ˌpærəˈflɔkjuləs] *n* 旁绒球(小脑)
paraformaldehyde [ˌpærəfɔːˈmældihaid] *n* 多聚甲醛,仲甲醛
Parafossarulus [ˌpærəfɔˈsærələs] *n* 沼螺属 | ~ sinensis 中华沼螺
parafrenal [ˌpærəˈfriːnəl] *a* 系带旁的
parafunction [ˈpærəˌfʌŋkʃən] *n* 功能异常,功能倒错 | **~al** [ˌpærəˈfʌŋkʃənl] *a*
paragammacism [ˌpærəˈgæməsizəm] *n* g, k, ch 发音障碍或发音不正
paraganglioma [ˌpærəˌgæŋgliˈəumə] *n* 副神经节瘤 | medullary ~ 嗜铬细胞瘤 / nonchromaffin ~ 非嗜铬性副神经节瘤,化学感受组织瘤
paraganglion [ˌpærəˈgæŋgliən] ([复] **paraganglia** [ˌpærəˈgæŋgliə]) *n* 节旁体,副神经节,嗜铬体
paragelatose [ˌpærəˈdʒelətəus] *n* 衍明胶脲
paragenitalis [ˌpærəˌdʒeniˈteilis] *n* 副生殖器(旁睾或卵巢旁体)
parageusia [ˌpærəˈgjuːziə] *n* 味觉倒错;味觉异常 | **parageusic** [ˌpærəˈgjuːsik] *a*
paragglutination [ˌpærəˌgluːtiˈneiʃən] *n* 副凝集反应,类属凝集反应,组凝集反应,族凝集反应
paraglobulin [ˌpærəˈglɔbjulin] *n* 副球蛋白
paraglobulinuria [ˌpærəˌglɔbjuliˈnjuəriə] *n* 副球蛋白尿
paraglossia [ˌpærəˈglɔsiə], **paraglossitis** [ˌpærəglɔˈsaitis] *n* 舌下[组织]炎
paragnathus [pæˈrægnəθəs] *n* 颌旁寄生胎
paragnosis [ˌpærəgˈnəusis] *n* 死后诊断
paragonimiasis [ˌpærəˌgɔniˈmaiəsis], **paragonimosis** [ˌpærəˌgɔniˈməusis] *n* 并殖吸虫病
Paragonimus [ˌpærəˈgɔniməs] *n* 并殖吸虫属 | ~ africanus 非洲并殖吸虫 / ~ kellicotti 猫肺并殖吸虫 / ~ westermani, ~ ringeri 卫[斯特曼]氏并殖吸虫,肺吸虫
Paragordius [ˌpærəˈgɔːdiəs] *n* 拟铁线虫属
paragrammatism [ˌpærəˈgræmətizəm] *n* 语法倒错性言语障碍
paragranuloma [ˌpærəˌgrænjuˈləumə] *n* 类肉芽肿
paragraphia [ˌpærəˈgræfiə] *n* 书写倒错,错写
parahemophilia [ˌpærəˌhiːməˈfiliə] *n* 副血友病(由于凝血因子 V 缺乏所致)
parahepatic [ˌpærəhiˈpætik] *a* 肝旁的
parahepatitis [ˌpærəˌhepəˈtaitis] *n* 肝周炎
paraheredity [ˌpærəhiˈredəti] *n* 假遗传(指性状不是从母细胞遗传给子细胞,而是通过外来的介质从受影响的细胞传给正常细胞)
parahippocampal [ˌpærəˌhipəuˈkæmpəl] *a* 海马旁的
parahormone [ˌpærəˈhɔːməun] *n* 副激素
parahypnosis [ˌpærəhipˈnəusis] *n* 睡眠异常
parahypophysis [ˌpærəhaiˈpɔfisis] *n* 副垂体
parainfectious [ˌpærəinˈfekʃəs] *a* 副传染性的
parainsulin [ˌpærəˈinsjulin] *n* 类胰岛素
parakeratinized [ˌpærəˈkerətiˌnaizd] *a* 角化不全的
parakeratosis [ˌpærəˌkerəˈtəusis] *n* 角化不全 | ~ scutularis, ~ ostracea 发痂性角化不全,蛎壳状角化不全 / ~ variegata 多样性类银屑病,网状类银屑病
parakinesia [ˌpærəkaiˈniːziə, -kiˈn-] *n* 运动倒错 | **parakinetic** [ˌpærəkaiˈnetik, -kiˈn-] *a*
paralactic acid [ˌpærəˈlæktik] 副乳酸,右旋乳酸
paralalia [ˌpærəˈleiliə] *n* 言语障碍,构音倒错,错语症 | ~ literalis 字音倒错,构音倒错
paralambdacism [ˌpærəˈlæmdəsizəm] *n* l 发音

不正

paralbumin [ˌpærælˈbjuːmin] *n* 副清蛋白,副白蛋白,拟清蛋白

paraldehyde [pæˈrældihaid] *n* 副醛,三聚乙醛(催眠镇静药)

paraldehydism [pæˈrældiˌhaidizəm] *n* 三聚乙醛中毒

paralepsy [ˈpærəˌlepsi] *n* 情绪突变,心境突变,精神猝变

paralexia [ˌpærəˈleksiə] *n* 错读[症] | **paralexic** *a*

paralgesia [ˌpærælˈdʒiːsiə], **paralgia** [pæˈrældʒiə] *n* 痛觉异常 | **paralgesic** [ˌpærælˈdʒiːsik] *a*

paralinin [ˌpærəˈlainin] *n* 核基质,核液,核淋巴

parallagma [ˌpærəˈlægmə] *n*【希】骨移位

parallax [ˈpærəlæks] *n* 视差 | binocular ~ 双眼视差 / crossed ~, heteronymous ~ 交叉性视差,异侧性视差 / direct ~, hemonymous ~ 直接性视差,同侧性视差 | **parallactic** [ˌpærəˈlæktik] *a*

parallelism [ˈpærəˌlelizəm] *n* 平行论(认为心理活动与脑活动是并行的,并不相互影响)

parallelometer [ˌpærəleˈlɔmitə] *n* 平行线面测量器

parallergy [pæˈrælədʒi], **parallergia** [ˌpærəˈləːdʒiə] *n* 副变[态反]应性 | **parallergic** [ˌpærəˈləːdʒik] *a*

paralogia [ˌpærəˈləudʒiə] *n* 逻辑倒错,推理倒错(推理能力损害) | thematic ~ 主题性逻辑倒错

paralogism [pəˈrælədʒizəm] *n* 逻辑倒错,推理倒错(精神病患者使用无意义的或不合逻辑的语言) | **paralogistic** [pəˌræləˈdʒistik] *a*

paralogy [pəˈrælədʒi] *n* 貌似(解剖上的相似)

paralyse [ˈpærəlaiz] *vt* 使麻痹,使瘫痪

paralysis [pəˈrælisis] ([复] **paralyses** [pəˈrælisiːz]) *n* 麻痹,瘫痪 | ~ agitans 震颤麻痹 / alternate ~, alternating ~ 交叉性偏瘫 / ambigus-accessorius ~ 疑核副神经核性麻痹 / anesthesia ~ 麻醉后麻痹 / association ~, bulbar ~ 联合麻痹,延髓性麻痹 / asthenobulbospinal ~, bulbospinal ~ 无力性延髓脊髓性麻痹,重症肌无力 / birth ~ 产伤麻痹 / conjugate ~ 同向性麻痹,同向运动麻痹(眼肌) / essential ~ 自发性麻痹,急性脊髓前角灰质炎 / facial ~ 面神经麻痹,面瘫 / flaccid ~ 松弛性瘫痪 / general ~, general ~ of the insane 全身麻痹症,麻痹性痴呆 / histrionic ~ 表情性麻痹(部分面肌麻痹) / immunological ~ 免疫麻痹(对特异性抗原的免疫应答缺乏) / incomplete ~ 不全麻痹,轻瘫 / infantile ~ 婴儿麻痹,脊髓灰质炎 / lead ~ 铅毒性麻痹 / mimetic ~ 表情肌麻痹,面肌麻痹,面瘫 / peroneal ~ 腓神经麻痹,交腿性麻痹 / vasomotor ~ 血管舒缩神经麻痹

paralysor [ˈpærəˌlaizə] *n* 麻痹剂,阻化剂,阻滞剂

paralyssa [ˌpærəˈlisə] *n* 蝙蝠咬恐水病(见于中南美洲)

paralytic [ˌpærəˈlitik] *a* 麻痹的,瘫痪的 *n* 麻痹者,瘫痪病人

paralytogenic [ˌpærəˌlitəuˈdʒenik] *a* 致麻痹的

paralyzant [ˈpærəˌlaizənt] *a* 致麻痹的 *n* 麻痹剂,阻化剂

paralyze [ˈpærəlaiz] *vt* 使麻痹,使瘫痪 | **paralyzation** [ˌpærəlaiˈzeiʃən, -liz-] *n* / **paralyzer**, **paralyzor** *n* 麻痹剂,阻化剂,阻滞剂

paramagnetic [ˌpærəmægˈnetik] *a* 顺磁的 | **paramagnetism** [ˌpærəˈmægnitizəm] *n* 顺磁性

paramania [ˌpærəˈmeinjə] *n* 情感反常(为情感倒错〈parathymia〉的一种)

paramastigote [ˌpærəˈmæstigəut] *a* 副鞭毛的

paramastitis [ˌpærəmæsˈtaitis] *n* 乳腺周炎

paramastoid [ˌpærəˈmæstɔid] *a* 乳突旁的,乳突周的

paramastoiditis [ˌpærəˌmæstɔiˈdaitis] *n* 乳突周炎

parameatal [ˌpærəmiˈeitl] *a* 开口周围的,通道周围的

paramecin [ˌpærəˈmiːsin] *n* 草履虫素

Paramecium [ˌpærəˈmiːsiəm] *n* 草履虫属 | ~ coli 结肠草履虫,结肠小袋虫

paramecium [ˌpærəˈmiːsiəm] ([复] **paramecia** [ˌpærəˈmiːsiə]) *n* 草履虫

paramedian [ˌpærəˈmiːdiən] *a* 正中旁的

paramedic [ˈpærəˌmedik] *n* 急救医士

paramedical [ˌpærəˈmedikəl] *a* 关系医学的,与医学有关的;医务辅助人员的

paramenia [ˌpærəˈmiːniə] *n* 月经障碍

parameningococcus [ˌpærəmiˌniŋgəuˈkɔkəs] *n* 类脑膜炎球菌,副脑膜炎球菌

parameniscitis [ˌpærəmeniˈsaitis] *n* 半月板周炎

parameniscus [ˌpærəmiˈniskəs] *n* 半月板周部

paramesial [ˌpærəˈmiːsiəl] *a* 正中旁的

parameter [pəˈræmitə] *n* 参数(本身不能用直接法精确测定的一种数量或函数,例如血压和脉率是心血管功能的参数,血液内和尿内的葡萄糖浓度是糖代谢的参数)

paramethadione [ˌpærəmeθəˈdaiəun] *n* 甲乙双酮(抗癫痫药)

paramethasone [ˌpærəˈmeθəsəun] *n* 帕拉米松 | ~ acetate 醋酸帕拉米松,醋酸对氟米松(用作糖皮质激素,具有抗炎和抗变应性作用)

Parametorchis [ˌpærəməˈtɔːkis] *n* 副次睾吸虫属

parametric [ˌpærəˈmetrik] *a* 子宫旁的;参数的

parametritis [ˌpærəmiˈtraitis] *n* 子宫旁[组织]炎 | **parametritic** [ˌpærəmiˈtritik] *a*

parametrium [ˌpærəˈmiːtriəm] *n* 子宫旁组织 | **parametrial** *a* 子宫旁组织的；子宫旁的
paramidoacetophenone [pæˌræmidəuæsitəuˈfiːnəun] *n* 对氨苯乙酮
paramimia [ˌpærəˈmimiə] *n* 表情倒错
paramitome [ˌpærəˈmaitəum] *n* 透明质，丝间质
paramnesia [ˌpæræmˈniːziə] *n* 记忆倒错
Paramoeba [ˌpærəˈmiːbə] *n* 副变形虫属
paramolar [ˌpærəˈməulə] *n* 磨牙旁额外牙
Paramonostomum parvum [ˌpærəməuˈnɔstəməm ˈpɑːvəm] 鸡拟单口吸虫
Paramphistomatidae [ˌpæræmˌfistəumæˈtaidiː] *n* 同端盘[吸虫]科
Paramphistomatoidea [ˌpæræmfisˌtəuməˈtɔidiə] *n* 同端盘[吸虫]科
paramphistome [pəˈræmfistəum] *n* 同端盘吸虫
paramphistomiasis [pæˌræmfistəuˈmaiəsis] *n* 同盘吸虫病
Paramphistomum [ˌpæræmˈfistəuməm] *n* 同盘[吸虫]属 | ~ cervi 鹿同盘吸虫
paramucin [ˌpærəˈmjuːsin] *n* 副黏蛋白
paramusia [ˌpærəˈmjuːziə] *n* 歌唱倒错，错唱
paramutable [ˌpærəˈmjuːtəbl] *a* 可发生副突变的
paramutagenic [ˌpærəˌmjuːtəˈdʒenik] *a* 副突变原的
paramutation [ˌpærəmjuˈteiʃən] *n* 副突变（在杂合体中某一基因影响同一座位上另一等位基因的表现）
paramyelin [ˌpærəˈmaiəlin] *n* 衍髓磷脂，副髓磷脂
paramyloidosis [pəˌræmilɔiˈdəusis] *n* 副淀粉样变性
paramylum [pəˈræmiləm] *n* 副淀粉
paramyoclonus [ˌpærəmaiˈɔklənəs] *n* 肌阵挛[状态]
paramyosin [ˌpærəˈmaiəsin] *n* 副肌球蛋白
paramyosinogen [ˌpærəˌmaiəuˈsinədʒən] *n* 副肌球蛋白原
paramyotonia [ˌpærəˌmaiəuˈtəuniə] *n* 副肌强直
paramyotonus [ˌpærəmaiˈɔtənəs], **paramyotone** [ˌpærəˈmaiətəun] *n* 副肌强直[状态]
Paramyxa [ˌpærəˈmiksə] *n* 无孔属
Paramyxea [ˌpærəˈmiksiə] *n* 无孔纲
Paramyxida [ˌpærəˈmiksidə] *n* 无孔目
Paramyxoviridae [ˌpærəˌmiksəuˈviridiː] *n* 副黏病毒科
Paramyxovirus [ˌpærəˈmiksəuˌvaiərəs] *n* 副黏病毒属
paramyxovirus [ˌpærəˈmiksəuˌvaiərəs] *n* 副黏病毒
paranalgesia [ˌpærænælˈdʒiːzjə] *n* 下身痛觉缺失
Paranaplasma [pæˌrænəˈplæzmə] *n* 类无形体属
paranea [ˌpærəˈniːə] *n* 妄想狂，偏执狂
paraneoplastic [ˌpærəˌniːəuˈplæstik] *a* 副肿瘤性的
paranephric [ˌpærəˈnefrik] *a* 肾旁的；肾上腺的
paranephritis [ˌpærəneˈfraitis] *n* 肾上腺炎；肾周炎
paranephroma [ˌpærəneˈfrəumə] *n* 肾上腺样瘤
paranephros [ˌpærəˈnefrɔs] *n* 肾上腺
paranesthesia [ˌpærænisˈθiːzjə] *n* 下身感觉缺失
paraneural [ˌpærəˈnjuərəl] *a* 神经旁的
parangi [pəˈrændʒi] *n* 雅司病（即 yaws）
para-nitrosulfathiazole [ˌpærə ˌnaitrəuˌsʌlfəˈθaiəzəul] *n* 对硝基磺胺噻唑（抗菌药，用于治疗非特异性溃疡性结肠炎和直肠炎）
paranoia [ˌpærəˈnɔiə] *n* 偏执狂 | acute hallucinatory ~ 急性幻觉性偏执狂 / litigious ~ 诉讼偏执狂 / querulous ~ 诉怨偏执狂 | **paranoic** [ˌpærəˈnəuik] *a*
paranoiac [ˌpærəˈnɔiæk] *a* 妄想狂的，偏执狂的 *n* 妄想狂者，偏执狂者
paranoid [ˈpærənɔid] *a* 类妄想狂的，类偏[执]狂的
paranoidism [ˌpærəˈnɔidizəm] *n* 类妄想狂状态，类偏[执]狂状态
paranomia [ˌpærəˈnəumiə] *n* 命名错误（见于失语症）
Paranoplocephala [ˌpærənəupləuˈsefələ] *n* 副裸头[绦虫]属
paranormal [ˌpærəˈnɔːməl] *a* 超正常的，超自然的
paranosis [ˌpærəˈnəusis] *n* 因病获益，疾病获益 | **paranosic** *a*
paranucleolus [ˌpærənjuːˈkliːələs] *n* 副核仁
paranucleus [ˌpærəˈnjuːkliəs] *n* 副核 | **paranuclear** *a* 核旁的；副核的
paraomphalic [ˌpærəɔmˈfælik] *a* 脐旁的
paraoperative [ˌpærəˈɔpərətiv] *a* 辅助手术的（如器械与手套的管理、消毒等）
paraoral [ˌpærəˈɔːrəl] *a* 非经口（给药）的
paraortic [ˌpæreiˈɔːtik] *a* 主动脉旁的
paraosmia [ˌpærəˈɔsmiə] *n* 嗅觉倒错
paraoxon [ˌpærəˈɔksən] *n* 对氧磷（有机磷杀虫剂）
paraoxonase [ˌpærəˈɔksəneiz] *n* 对氧磷酶
parapancreatic [ˌpærəˌpæŋkriˈætik] *a* 胰旁的
paraparesis [ˌpærəˈpærisis] *n* 轻截瘫
parapedesis [ˌpærəpeˈdiːsis] *n* 胆汁移行倒错（胆色素移行于毛细血管内）
paraperitoneal [ˌpærəˌperitəuˈniːəl] *a* 腹膜旁的
parapertussis [ˌpærəpəˈtʌsis] *n* 副百日咳，轻百日咳

parapestis [ˌpærəˈpestis] *n* 轻鼠疫
parapharyngeal [ˌpærəfəˈrindʒiəl] *a* 咽旁的
paraphasia [ˌpærəˈfeiziə] *n* 错语[症] | **paraphasic** [ˌpærəˈfeisik] *a*
paraphasis [pəˈræfəsis] *n* 终脑顶突(动物)
paraphemia [ˌpærəˈfiːmiə] *n* 错语性失语症
paraphenylenediamine [ˌpærəˌfeniliːnˈdaiəmiːn] *n* 对苯二胺(染发剂)
paraphia [pəˈreifiə] *n* 触觉倒错
paraphilia [ˌpærəˈfiliə] *n* 性变态 | **~c** [ˌpærəˈfiliæk] *a* 性变态的 *n* 性变态者
paraphimosis [ˌpærəfaiˈməusis] *n* 嵌顿包茎(包茎包皮退缩,引起龟头痛性肿胀)
paraphobia [ˌpærəˈfəubjə] *n* 轻[度]恐怖
paraphonia [ˌpærəˈfəuniə] *n* 声音变调 | ~ puberum 青春期(男性)声音变调
paraphora [pəˈræfərə] *n* 轻度精神障碍
paraphrasia [ˌpærəˈfreizjə] *n* 言语无序,言语倒错
paraphrenia [ˌpærəˈfriːniə] *n* 妄想痴呆,妄想症 | **paraphrenic** [ˌpærəˈfriːnik] *a* 妄想痴呆的 *n* 妄想痴呆患者
paraphrenitis [ˌpærəfriˈnaitis] *n* 膈周[组织]炎
paraphronia [ˌpærəˈfrəuniə] *n* 性情变易,性格变易
paraphysis [pəˈræfisis] *n* 脑旁体;侧丝 | **paraphyseal** [ˌpærəˈfiziəl] *a*
parapineal [ˌpærəˈpainiəl] *a* 松果体旁的(指某些蜥蜴)
paraplasm [ˈpærəplæzəm] *n* 透明质;副质;异常增生物 | **~ic** [ˌpærəˈplæzmik] *a*
paraplastic [ˌpærəˈplæstik] *a* 异常增生的
paraplastin [ˌpærəˈplæstin] *n* 副网质,副网素(副染色质样物质)
paraplegia [ˌpærəˈpliːdʒiə] *n* 截瘫 | flaccid ~ 弛缓性截瘫 / senile ~, tetanoid ~ 老年性截瘫,破伤风样截瘫 / ~ superior 上肢截瘫 | **paraplegic** [ˌpærəˈpliːdʒik], **paraplectic** [ˌpærəˈplektik] *a*
paraplegiform [ˌpærəˈpledʒifɔːm] *a* 截瘫样的
parapleuritis [ˌpærəpluəˈraitis] *n* 胸壁炎,胸壁胸膜炎
paraplexus [ˌpærəˈpleksəs] *n* 侧脑室脉络丛
parapneumonia [ˌpærənju(ː)ˈməunjə] *n* 类肺炎,副肺炎
parapneumonic [ˌpærənju(ː)ˈmɔnik] *a* 副肺炎的
parapodium [ˌpærəˈpəudiəm] *n* 站立支架(瘫痪儿童用)
parapophysis [ˌpærəˈpɔfisis] *n* (椎骨)副横突(动物)
parapoplexy [pəˈræpəˌpleksi] *n* 类卒中,类中风
Parapoxvirus [ˌpærəˈpɔksvaiərəs] *n* 副痘病毒属
parapoxvirus [ˌpærəˈpɔksvaiərəs] *n* 副痘病毒
parapraxia [ˌpærəˈpræksiə], **parapraxis** [ˌpærəˈpræksis] *n* 动作倒错;失误动作
paraproctitis [ˌpærəprɔkˈtaitis] *n* 直肠周炎
paraproctium [ˌpærəˈprɔkʃiəm] *n* 直肠周组织,直肠旁组织
paraprofessional [ˌpærəprəˈfeʃənl] *n* 辅助性专业人员;有关的卫生专业人员 *a* 辅助专职人员的
paraprostatitis [ˌpærəprɔstəˈtaitis] *n* 前列腺周炎
paraprotein [ˌpærəˈprəutiːn] *n* 副蛋白
paraproteinemia [ˌpærəprəutiːˈniːmiə] *n* 异常蛋白血[症],副蛋白血[症],病变蛋白血[症]
parapsis [pəˈræpsis], **parapsia** [pəˈræpsiə] *n* 触觉倒错
parapsoriasis [ˌpærəsəˈraiəsis] *n* 副银屑病 | ~ guttata, guttate ~ 滴状副银屑病 / poikilodermic ~, poikilodermatous ~ 皮肤异色病性副银屑病 / retiform ~, ~ varigata 网状副银屑病,多样性副银屑病 / ~ varioliformis acuta 急性痘疮样副银屑病,急性苔藓样糠疹 / ~ varioliformis chronica 慢性痘疮样副银屑病,慢性苔藓样糠疹
parapsychology [ˌpærəsaiˈkɔlədʒi] *n* 心灵学,心灵心理学(研究传心术、超人视力等)
parapyknomorphous [ˌpærəˌpiknəuˈmɔːfəs] *a* 轻度致密排列的,轻度密列的(指某些神经细胞)
parapyle [ˈpærəpail] *n* 星状旁口
parapyramidal [ˌpærəpiˈræmidl] *a* 锥体旁的
paraquat [ˈpæreiˈkwæt] *n* 百草枯,对草快(除莠剂)
pararabin [pəˈrærəbin] *n* 副阿拉伯胶素
parareaction [ˌpærəri(ː)ˈækʃən] *n* 偏执反应,妄想反应(指偏执狂及类偏狂状态)
pararectal [ˌpærəˈrektəl] *a* 直肠旁的
parareducine [ˌpærəriˈdjuːsin] *n* 副还原碱,副蛋白碱(尿内发现的一种蛋白毒碱)
parareflexia [ˌpærəriˈfleksiə] *n* 反射紊乱
pararenal [ˌpærəˈriːnl] *a* 肾旁的
pararhizoclasia [ˌpærəˌraizəuˈkleiziə] *n* 牙根周溃坏
pararhotacism [ˌpærəˈrəutəsizəm] *n* r 发音不正
pararosaniline [ˌpærərəuˈzænilin] *n* 副品红 | ~ pamoate 双羟萘酸副品红(抗血吸虫药)
pararosolic acid [ˌpærərəuˈzɔlik] 玫瑰色酸,玫红酸
pararrhythmia [ˌpærəˈriθmiə] *n* 并行心律,两律性心律失常
pararthria [pəˈrɑːθriə] *n* 发声障碍
Parasaccharomyces [ˌpærəˌsækərəuˈmaisiːz] *n* 类酵母菌属
parasacral [ˌpærəˈseikrəl] *a* 骶骨旁的

parasalpingeal [ˌpærəsælˈpindʒiəl] *a* 输卵管旁的,输卵管周的
parasalpingitis [ˌpærəˌsælpinˈdʒaitis] *n* 输卵管周炎
parascapular [ˌpærəˈskæpjulə] *a* 肩胛周的
Parascaris [pæˈræskəris] *n* 副蛔虫属 | ~ equorum 马副蛔虫
parascarlatina [ˌpærəˌskɑːləˈtiːnə], **parascarlet** [ˌpærəˈskɑːlit] *n* 婴儿玫瑰疹,幼儿急疹,猝发疹
parasecretion [ˌpærəsiˈkriːʃən] *n* 分泌紊乱,分泌异常,分泌过多
parasellar [ˌpærəˈselə] *a* 蝶鞍旁的
parasexual [ˌpærəˈseksjuəl] *a* 准性的,超性的
parasexuality [ˌpærəˌseksjuˈæləti] *n* 性欲倒错,性欲异常,性变态
parasigmatism [ˌpærəˈsigmətizəm] *n* s 及 z 发音不正
parasinoidal [ˌpærəsaiˈnɔidl] *a* 窦旁的
parasite [ˈpærəsait] *n* 寄生虫,寄生物;寄生胎 | accidental ~, incidental ~ 偶然寄生物 / allantoic ~ 尿囊寄生物 / celozoic ~ 体腔寄生物 / diheteroxenic ~ 二宿主性寄生物 / eurytrophic ~ 广食性寄生物 / facultative ~ 兼性寄生物(能独立生存的寄生物) / malarial ~ 疟原虫 / obligatory ~ 专性寄生物(不能独立生存的寄生物) / spurious ~ 假性寄生物 / stenotrophic ~ 狭食性寄生物 / teratoid ~ 寄生[畸]胎
parasitemia [ˌpærəsaiˈtiːmiə] *n* 寄生物血症(尤指血内疟原虫)
parasitic(al) [ˌpærəˈsitik(əl)] *a* 寄生物的,寄生的
parasiticide [ˌpærəˈsitisaid] *a* 杀寄生物的 *n* 杀寄生物药 | **parasiticidal** [ˌpærəˌsitiˈsaidəl] *a*
parasitifer [ˌpærəˈsitifə] *n* 宿主
parasitism [ˈpærəˌsaitizəm] *n* 寄生;寄生物感染
parasitization [ˌpærəˌsaitaiˈzeiʃən, -ˌsi-;-tiˈz-] *n* 寄生物感染
parasitize [ˈpærəsaitaiz] *vt* 寄生于
parasitogenic [ˌpærəˌsaitəuˈdʒenik, -ˌsi-] *a* 寄生物原的,寄生物所致的
parasitoid [ˈpærəˌsaitɔid] *a* 寄生物样的
parasitology [ˌpærəsaiˈtɔlədʒi] *n* 寄生物学,寄生虫学 | **parasitological** [ˌpærəsaitəˈlɔdʒikəl] *a* | **parasitologist** *n* 寄生物学家,寄生虫学家
parasitosis [ˌpærəsaiˈtəusis] ([复] **parasitoses** [ˌpærəsaiˈtəusiːz]) *n* 寄生物病,寄生虫病
parasitotropic [ˌpærəˌsaitəuˈtrɔpik], **parasitotrope** [ˌpærəˈsaitətrəup] *a* 亲寄生物的
parasitotropy [ˌpærəsaiˈtɔtrəpi], **parasitotropism** [ˌpærəsaiˈtɔtrəpizəm] *n* 亲寄生物性
parasoma [ˌpærəˈsəumə] *n* 副核
parasomnia [ˌpærəˈsɔmniə] *n* 深眠状态
paraspadias [ˌpærəˈspeidiəs] *n* 尿道旁裂
paraspasm [ˈpærəspæzəm] *n* 两侧痉挛
paraspasmus [ˌpærəˈspæzməs] *n* 两侧痉挛 | ~ facial 面部两侧痉挛
paraspecific [ˌpærəspiˈsifik] *a* 类特异性的,旁特异性的[作用]
parasplenic [ˌpærəˈsplenik] *a* 脾旁的
parasternal [ˌpærəˈstəːnl] *a* 胸骨旁的
parasthenia [ˌpæræsˈθiːniə] *n* 功能异常
parastruma [ˌpærəˈstruːmə] *n* 甲状旁腺肿
parasuicide [ˌpærəˈsjuisaid] *n* 自杀企图(一种表面上自杀企图,如服毒或自残,但死亡并不是目的)
parasympathetic [ˌpærəˌsimpəˈθetik] *a* 副交感[神经]的
parasympathicotonia [ˌpærəsimˌpæθikəuˈtəuniə] *n* 副交感神经过敏,迷走神经过敏
parasympathin [ˌpærəˈsimpəθin] *n* 副交感神经素
parasympatholytic [ˌpærəˌsimpəθəuˈlitik] *a* 副交感神经的,副交感神经阻滞的 *n* 抗副交感神经药,副交感神经阻滞药
parasympathomimetic [ˌpærəˌsimpəθəumiˈmetik] *a* 拟副交感神经的,类副交感神经的 *n* 拟副交感神经药,类副交感[神经]药
parasynanche [ˌpærəˈsinæŋki] *n* 腮腺炎;喉肌炎
parasynapsis [ˌpærəsiˈnæpsis], **parasyndesis** [ˌpærəsinˈdiːsis] *n* 平行联会(染色体)
parasynovitis [ˌpærəˌsinəˈvaitis] *n* 滑液囊周炎
parasyphilis [ˌpærəˈsifilis], **parasyphilosis** [ˌpærəˌsifiˈləusis] *n* 终期梅毒,四期梅毒 | **parasyphilitic** [ˌpærəˌsifiˈlitik] *a*
parasystole [ˌpærəˈsistəli] *n* 并行收缩
paratarsium [ˌpærəˈtɑːsiəm] *n* 跗旁组织
paratartaric acid [ˌpærətɑːˈtærik] 消旋酸
parataxis [ˌpærəˈtæksis] *n* 互补性,趋旁位性 | **paratactic** *a*
paratenic [ˌpærəˈtenik] *a* 旁栖的(中间宿主)
paratenon [ˌpærəˈtenən] *n* 腱旁组织
paratereseomania [ˌpærətəˌriːsiəuˈmeinjə] *n* 窥视癖,窥阴癖,窥淫癖
parathion [ˌpærəˈθaiɔn] *n* 对硫磷,E 六〇五,一六〇五(有机磷杀虫剂)
parathormone [ˌpærəˈθɔːməun] *n* 甲状旁腺激素
parathymia [ˌpærəˈθaimiə] *n* 情感倒错
parathyrin [ˌpærəˈθairin] *n* 甲状旁腺素
parathyroid [ˌpærəˈθairɔid] *a* 甲状旁腺的 *n* 甲状旁腺 | ~**al** [ˌpærəθaiˈrɔidl] *a*
parathyroidectomize [ˌpærəˌθairɔiˈdektəmaiz] *vt* 切除甲状旁腺
parathyroidectomy [ˌpærəˌθairɔiˈdektəmi] *n* 甲状旁腺切除术

parathyroidin [ˌpærəθaiˈrɔidin] *n* 甲状旁腺提取物
parathyroidoma [ˌpærəˌθairɔiˈdəumə] *n* 甲状旁腺瘤
parathyropathy [ˌpærəθaiˈrɔpəθi] *n* 甲状旁腺病
parathyroprival [ˌpærəˌθairəuˈpraivəl], **parathyroprivic** [ˌpærəˌθairəuˈprivik], **parathyroprivous** [ˌpærəθaiˈrɔprivəs] *a* 甲状旁腺缺失的，无甲状旁腺的
parathyroprivia [ˌpærəθairəuˈpraiviə] *n* 甲状旁腺缺失状态
parathyrotoxicosis [ˌpærəˌθairəutɔksiˈkəusis] *n* 甲状旁腺中毒症
parathyrotropic [ˌpærəˌθairəuˈtrɔpik], **parathyrotrophic** [ˌpærəˌθairəuˈtrɔfik] *a* 促甲状旁腺的
paratoloid [ˌpærəˈtəulɔid], **paratoloidin** [ˌpærətəuˈlɔidin] *n* 结核菌素
paratonia [ˌpærəˈtəuniə] *n* 伸展过度
paratope [ˌpærətəup] *n* 对位，互补位(抗体分子上与抗原表位相结合的部位) | **paratopic** [ˌpærəˈtɔpik] *a*
paratose [ˈpærətəus] *n* 泊雷糖(一种不常见的糖，是沙门菌菌体抗原的一种多糖)
paratrachoma [ˌpærətrəˈkəumə] *n* 类沙眼
paratrophic [ˌpærəˈtrɔfik] *a* 活物寄生的，嗜活质的
paratrophy [pəˈrætrəfi] *n* 营养不良，营养障碍；(活物)寄生性营养
paratuberculosis [ˌpærətju(ː)ˌbəːkjuˈləusis] *n* 类结核；副结核 | **paratuberculous** [ˌpærətju(ː)ˈbəːkjuləs] *a*
paratype [ˈpærətaip] *n* 副型(细菌)；对位型，互补型(一类或一族相关的对位)
paratyphlitis [ˌpærətifˈlaitis] *n* 盲肠旁炎
paratyphoid [ˌpærəˈtaifɔid] *a* 伤寒样的 *n* 副伤寒
paratypic(al) [ˌpærəˈtipik(əl)] *a* 副型的，异型的
paraumbilical [ˌpærəʌmbiˈlaikəl] *a* 脐旁的
paraungual [ˌpærəˈʌŋgwəl] *a* 甲旁的
paraurethra [ˌpærəjuəˈriːθrə] *n* 副尿道
paraurethral [ˌpærəjuəˈriːθrəl] *a* 尿道旁的
paraurethritis [ˌpærəˌjuəriˈθraitis] *n* 尿道旁炎，尿道周炎
parauterine [ˌpærəˈjuːtərain] *a* 子宫旁的
paravaccinia [ˌpærəvækˈsiniə] *n* 副牛痘[疹]
paravaginal [ˌpærəˈvædʒinəl] *a* 阴道旁的
paravaginitis [ˌpærəˌvædʒiˈnaitis] *n* 阴道旁炎，阴道周炎
paravenous [ˌpærəˈviːnəs] *a* 静脉旁的
paravertebral [ˌpærəˈvəːtibrəl] *a* 脊柱旁的，椎旁的
paravesical [ˌpærəˈvesikəl] *a* 膀胱旁的，膀胱周的
paravisceral [ˌpærəˈvisərəl] *a* 内脏旁的
paravitaminosis [ˌpærəˌvaitəmiˈnəusis] *n* 类维生素缺乏病
paraxial [pæˈræksiəl] *a* 轴旁的
paraxon [pæˈræksɔn] *n* 轴索侧支，旁轴索
Parazoa [pærəˈzəuə] *n* 侧生动物
parazone [ˈpærəzəun] *n* 明带(在釉柱层内，见于牙的横切面)
parbendazole [pæˈbendəzəul] *n* 帕苯达唑(兽用抗蠕虫药)
parconazole hydrochloride [pæˈkəunəzəul] 盐酸帕康唑(抗真菌药)
parectasis [pæˈrektəsis], **parectasia** [ˌpærekˈteiziə] *n* 膨胀过度
parectropia [ˌpærekˈtrəupiə] *n* (精神性)运用不能，失用症
paregoric [ˌpærəˈgɔrik] *n* 阿片樟脑酊，复方樟脑酊
paregorism [ˈpærəˌgɔrizəm] *n* 阿片樟脑酊瘾
pareidolia [ˌpæraiˈdəuliə] *n* 幻想性视错觉
parelectronomic [ˌpærilektrəuˈnɔmik] *a* 无电反应的
parelectronomy [ˌpærilekˈtrɔnəmi] *n* 电反应降低
pareleidin [pæreˈliːidin] *n* 副角蛋白(副油粒蛋白)
parencephalia [ˌpærensəˈfeiliə] *n* 脑不全[畸形] | **parencephalous** [ˌpærenˈsefələs] *a*
parencephalocele [ˌpærenˈsefələusiːl] *n* 小脑突出
parencephalon [ˌpærenˈsefəlɔn] *n* 小脑
parenchyma [pəˈreŋkimə] *n*【希】实质 | ~ of lens 晶状体质 / ~ of testis 睾丸实质 | **~l**, **~tous** [ˌpæreŋˈkimətəs] *a*
parenchymatitis [ˌpæreŋˌkiməˈtaitis] *n* 实质炎
parenchymula [ˌpæreŋˈkimjulə] *n* 实胚
Parendomyces [ˌpærendeuˈmaisiːz] *n* 皮内真菌亚属
parent [ˈpɛərənt] *n* 父，母，[复]双亲；祖先；(动植物的)亲本；母体
parentage [ˈpɛərəntidʒ] *n* 出身，家系，系谱；父母的身分
parental [pəˈrentl] *a* 父(或母)的；父母的，双亲的；亲本的，亲代的
parenteral [pæˈrentərəl, pə-] *a* 肠胃外的，不经肠的，非肠道的(采取消化道以外的其他途径，如皮下、肌内、静脉内注射) | **~ly** *ad*
parepididymis [ˌpærepiˈdidimis] *n* 旁睾
parepigastric [ˌpærepiˈgæstrik] *a* 上腹旁的
parergasia [ˌpærəˈgeiziə] *n* 动作倒错；乖戾精神反应

parergastic [ˌpærəˈgæstik] *n* 乖戾精神病
paresis [ˈpærisis] ([复] **pareses** [ˈpærisiːz]) *n* 轻瘫;全身麻痹症,麻痹性痴呆 | galloping ~ 奔马型全身麻痹 / general ~ 麻痹性痴呆 / juvenile ~ 少年型全身麻痹 / stationary ~ 静止型全身麻痹 | **paretic** [pəˈretik] *a*
paresthesia [ˌpærisˈθiːziə] *n* 感觉异常 | **paresthetic** [ˌpærisˈθetik] *a*
parfocal [pɑːˈfəukəl] *a* 正焦点的
pargyline hydrochloride [ˈpɑːgiliːn] 盐酸帕吉林(抗高血压药)
Parham band [ˈpɑːrəm] (F. W. Parham) 帕勒姆带,金属带(固定长骨折断处)
parhedonia [ˌpɑːhiˈdəuniə] *n* 快感倒错(生殖器的)
parhormone [pɑːˈhɔːməun] *n* 类激素,副激素(指任何影响其他器官或组织功能的身体代谢产物,例如二氧化碳)
parica [ˈpærikə] *n* 帕立卡(巴西麻醉性鼻烟)
paricalcitol [ˌpæriˈkælsitɔl] *n* 帕立西托(一种维生素 D 合成类似物,用于防治继发于慢性肾衰竭的甲状旁腺功能亢进[症],静脉内给药)
paricine [pəˈrisin] *n* 杷日辛,杷日素(一种喹啉生物碱)
paries [ˈpɛəriːz] ([复] **parietes** [pəˈraiitiːz]) *n* 【拉】壁
parietal [pəˈraiitl] *a* 壁的;顶骨的
parietitis [pəˌraiiˈtaitis] *n* (器官)壁层炎
parietofrontal [pəˌraiitəuˈfrʌntl] *a* 顶额的
parietography [pəˌraiiˈtɔgrəfi] *n* 脏壁 X 线摄影[术] | gastric ~ 胃壁造影[术],胃壁 X 线摄影[术]
parieto-occipital [pəˌraiitəuɔkˈsipitl] *a* 顶枕的
parietosphenoid [pəˌraiitəuˈsfiːnɔid] *a* 顶蝶的
parietosplanchnic [pəˌraiətəuˈsplænknik] *a* 壁脏的
parietosquamosal [pəˌraiitəuskwəˈməusəl] *a* 顶鳞的
parietotemporal [pəˌraiitəuˈtempərəl] *a* 顶颞的
parietovisceral [pəˌraiitəuˈvisərəl], **parietosplanchnic** [pəˌraiitəuˈsplæŋknik] *a* 壁[与内]脏的
Parinaud's oculoglandular syndrome (conjunctivitis) [pəriˈnɔː] (Henri Parinaud) 帕里诺眼淋巴结综合征(结膜炎)(纤毛菌性结膜炎,经常为一侧,一般为滤泡型,继之耳前淋巴结触痛和肿大,常由于感染纤毛菌所致,或可能伴有其他疾病,如猫抓热、腹股沟淋巴肉芽肿、土拉菌病) | ~ syndrome (ophthalmoplegia) 帕里诺综合征(眼肌麻痹)(两眼同向向上运动麻痹,但无会聚性麻痹,与中脑损害有关,例如松果体肿瘤)
pari passu [ˈpɑːriˈpɑːsu] 【拉】一致,按同一比例,按同一程度
paristhmitis [ˌpærisˈmaitis] *n* 扁桃体炎
parity[1] [ˈpærəti] *n* 同等,相等;类似,相同
parity[2] [ˈpærəti] *n* 产次(见 para);经产状况(指妇女产过存活婴儿的状况)
Parker's fluid [ˈpɑːkə] (George H. Parker) 帕克液(甲醛和乙醇的混合固定液)
Parkes Weber syndrome [pɑːksˈveibə] (Frederick Parkes Waber) 巴克斯·韦伯综合征(见 Sturye-Weber syndrome)
Parkhill screws [ˈpɑːkhil] (Clayton Parkhill) 帕克希尔螺旋[夹](固定骨折用)
parkinsonism [ˈpɑːkinsənizəm] *n* 帕金森综合征 | postencephalitic ~ 脑炎后帕金森综合征,帕金森综合征(震颤麻痹综合征) | **parkinsonian** [ˌpɑːkinˈsəuniən] *a* 帕金森的(如 ~ syndrome 帕金森综合征〈震颤麻痹综合征〉);帕金森综合征的
Parkinson's disease [ˈpɑːkinsn] (James Parkinson) 帕金森病(震颤麻痹) | ~ facies (sign) 帕金森面容(征)(一种呆板的假面状面容,瞬目少,为帕金森神经功能障碍特有之征)
Park's aneurysm [pɑːk] (Henry Park) 帕克动脉瘤(两个静脉与一个扩张动脉所形成的动静脉瘤)
paroccipital [ˌpærɔkˈsipitl] *a* 枕骨旁的
parodontal [ˌpærəuˈdɔntl] *a* 牙旁的
parodontid [ˌpærəuˈdɔntid] *n* 龈瘤
parodontitis [ˌpærəudɔnˈtaitis] *n* 牙周炎
parodontium [ˌpærəuˈdɔnʃiəm] *n* 牙周组织,牙周膜
parodontopathy [ˌpærəudɔnˈtɔpəθi] *n* 牙周病(非炎性牙周组织病)
parodontosis [ˌpærəudɔnˈtəusis] *n* 牙周病(非炎性退化性牙周组织病)
parolivary [pæˈrɔlivəri] *a* 橄榄体旁的
paromomycin [ˈpærəməuˌmaisin] *n* 巴龙霉素(抗生素类药) | ~ sulfate 硫酸巴龙霉素(抗阿米巴药)
paromphalocele [ˌpærɔmˈfæləsiːl] *n* 脐旁疝
Parona's space [pɑːˈrəunɑː] (Francesco Parona) 帕罗纳间隙(前臂的旋前方肌和深屈腱之间的间隙,腕上约 5 cm,与腱鞘和掌中间隙直接相邻)
paroniria [pærəˈnaiəriə] *n* 魇梦,噩梦
paronychia [ˌpærəˈnikiə] *n* 甲沟炎 | **~l** *a*
paroophoric [ˌpærəuəuˈfɔrik] *a* 卵巢旁的
paroophoritis [ˌpærəuɔfəˈraitis] *n* 卵巢旁体炎;卵巢旁[组织]炎
paroophoron [ˌpærəuˈɔfərɔn] *n* 卵巢旁体
parophthalmia [ˌpærɔfˈθælmiə] *n* 眼周[组织]炎
parophthalmoncus [ˌpærɔfθælˈmɔŋkəs] *n* 眼旁肿瘤

paropsis [pəˈrɔpsis] *n* 视觉异常,视觉障碍
parorchidium [ˌpærɔːˈkidiəm] *n* 睾丸异位
parorchis [pəˈrɔːkis] *n* 附睾
parorexia [ˌpærəˈreksiə] *n* 食欲倒错,异食癖
parosmia [pæˈrɔzmiə], **parosphresia** [ˌpærɔsˈfriːziə], **parosphresis** [ˌpærɔsˈfriːsis] *n* 嗅觉倒错
parosteal [pæˈrɔstiəl] *a* 骨旁的,骨膜外面的
parosteitis [ˌpærɔstiˈaitis], **parostitis** [ˌpærɔsˈtaitis] *n* 骨周炎
parosteosis [ˌpærɔstiˈəusis], **parostosis** [ˌpærɔsˈtəusis] *n* 骨膜外组织骨化
parotic [pəˈrɔtik] *a* 耳旁的
parotid [pəˈrɔtid] *a* 耳旁的 *n* 腮腺
parotidean [pəˌrɔtiˈdiən] *a* 腮腺的
parotidectomy [pəˌrɔtiˈdektəmi] *n* 腮腺切除术
parotidoscirrhus [pəˌrɔtidəuˈskirəs], **parotidosclerosis** [pəˌrɔtidəuskliəˈrəusis] *n* 腮腺硬化
parotin [ˈpærətin, pəˈrəutin] *n* 腮腺素
parotitis [ˌpærəˈtaitis] *n* 腮腺炎 | celiac ~ 腹病性腮腺炎 / epidemic ~ 流行性腮腺炎 | **parotiditis** [pəˌrɔtiˈdaitis] *n* / **parotitic** [ˌpærəˈtitik] *a*
parous [ˈpærəs] *a* 经产的
parovarian [ˌpærəuˈvɛəriən] *a* 卵巢旁的;卵巢冠的
parovariotomy [ˌpærəuˌvɛəriˈɔtəmi] *n* 卵巢冠切除术
parovaritis [ˌpærəuvəˈraitis] *n* 卵巢冠炎
parovarium [ˌpærəuˈvɛəriəm] *n* 卵巢冠
paroxetine hydrochloride [pəˈrɔksətiːn] 盐酸帕洛西汀(一种选择性5-羟色胺重摄取抑制药,用于治疗抑郁症、强迫症和社交焦虑症,口服给药)
paroxysm [ˈpærəksizəm] *n* 发作,阵发 | **~al** [ˌpærəkˈsizməl] *a*
Parrot's atrophy of the newborn [pəˈrɔː] (Jules M. Parrot) 帕罗新生儿萎缩,原发性婴儿萎缩(或消瘦) | ~ disease (pseudoparalysis) 梅毒性假麻痹 / ~ sign (node) 帕罗征(结节)(①捏颈部皮肤时瞳孔散大,见于脑膜炎;②患先天梅毒的婴儿其头颅外骨板上的骨结节呈臀形) / ulcer 帕罗溃疡(见于鹅口疮)
Parry-Romberg syndrome [ˈpæri ˈrɔmberg] (C. H. Parry; Meritz. H. Romberg) 面部偏瘫侧萎缩
Parry's disease [ˈpæri] (Caleb H. Parry) 突眼性甲状腺肿
pars [pɑːz] ([复] **partes** [ˈpɑːtiːz]) *n* 【拉】部,部分
Parsons' disease [ˈpɑːsnz] (James Parsons) 突眼性甲状腺肿
pars planitis [pɑːz plæˈnaitis] 扁平部睫状体炎
part [pɑːt] *n* 部分;(身体的)部位
Part. aeq. partes aequales 【拉】等分
partal [ˈpɑːtl] *a* 分娩的
Parthenium [pɑːˈθiːniəm] *n* 银胶菊属
parthenocarpy [ˈpɑːθinəuˌkɑːpi] *n* 单性结实
parthenogenesis [ˌpɑːθinəuˈdʒenisis], **parthogenesis** [pɑːθəˈdʒenisis] *n* 孤雌生殖
parthenophobia [ˌpɑːθinəuˈfəubjə] *n* 处女恐怖
partial [ˈpɑːʃəl] *a* 部分的,不完全的 | **~ly** *ad*
partialism [ˈpɑːʃəlizəm] *n* 偏爱(一种性变态,特征为偏爱性交对方身体某一部分)
particle [ˈpɑːtikl] *n* 颗粒,粒子,微粒,质点 | C ~ C 颗粒(一种无感染性的 RNA 病毒,推测是所有活细胞的正常存在的病毒,而且推测它是各种类型癌肿的致病原因) / viral ~ 病毒颗粒,病毒体
particulate [pəˈtikjulit] *a* 微粒的,颗粒的;粒子组合的 *n* 微粒,颗粒
partigen [ˈpɑːtidʒən] *n* 部分抗原(抗原结构的一种假说,认为抗原是部分抗原的混合物)
partimute [ˈpɑːtimjuːt] *n* 聋哑;聋哑者
partimutism [ˌpɑːtiˈmjuːtizəm] *n* 聋哑症
partinium [pɑːˈtiniəm] *n* 铝钨合金
partition [pɑːˈtiʃən] *n* 分隔,分配;隔壁,隔膜 *vt* 分隔 | oropharyngeal ~ 口咽分隔器
partitioning [pɑːˈtiʃəniŋ] *n* 分隔 | gastric ~ 分胃术(一种胃成形术,用于治肥胖症,亦称胃分隔)
partogram [ˈpɑːtəgræm] *n* 产程图
partricin [pɑːˈtrisin] *n* 帕曲星(抗生素类药)
parturient [pɑːˈtjuəriənt] *a* 临产的,分娩的 *n* 产妇
parturifacient [ˌpɑːtjuəriˈfeiʃənt] *a* 催产的 *n* 催产药
parturiometer [ˌpɑːtjuəriˈɔmitə] *n* 分娩力计
parturition [pɑːtjuəˈriʃən] *n* 分娩
partus [ˈpɑːtəs] *n* 【拉】分娩,生产
Part. vic. partitis vicibus 均分剂量
parulis [pəˈrulis] *n* 龈脓肿
parumbilical [pærʌmbiˈlaikəl] *a* 脐旁的
paruria [pəˈrjuəriə] *n* 排尿异常
parvicellular [ˌpɑːviˈseljulə] *a* 小细胞的
Parvobacteriaceae [ˌpɑːvəubækˌtiəriˈeisiiː] *n* 短小杆菌科
parvocellular [ˌpɑːvəuˈseljulə] *a* 小细胞的
parvoline [ˈpɑːvəlin] *n* 衍腐肉毒碱,二乙基吡啶
parvoviral [ˈpɑːvəuˌvairəl] *a* 小病毒的
Parvoviridae [ˌpɑːvəuˈviridiː] *n* 细小病毒科
Parvovirinae [ˌpɑːvəuˌviˈraini] *n* 小病毒科
Parvovirus [ˈpɑːvəuˌvaiərəs] *n* 细小病毒属
parvovirus [ˈpɑːvəuˌvaiərəs] *n* 细小病毒

parvule [ˈpɑːvjuːl] *n* 小丸,小粒

Paryphostomum [ˌpæriˈfɔstəuməm] *n* 缘口[吸虫]属

PAS *P*-aminosalicylic acid 对氨水杨酸; periodic acid-Schiff 过碘酸-希夫(染剂)

PASA *P*-aminosalicylic acid 对氨水杨酸

pascal(Pa) [pæsˈkæl, ˈpæskəl] *n* 帕斯卡,帕(压强单位,1Pa = 1N/m^2)

Pascal's law [pɑːsˈkɑːl] (Blaise Pascal) 帕斯卡尔定律(液体在任何点所受的压力,必向各方向均等地传递)

Paschen's bodies (corpuscles, granules) [ˈpʌʃən] (Enrique Paschen) 帕兴体(小体、粒)(天花、牛痘时组织细胞内的包涵体)

Paschutin's degeneration [pəˈʃutin] (Viktor V. Paschutin) 帕舒廷变性(见于糖尿病)

PASG pneumatic antishock garment 充气抗休克服

paspalism [ˈpæspəlizəm] *n* 雀稗中毒

Paspalum [ˈpæspələm] *n* 雀稗属

paspalum [ˈpæspələm] *n* 雀稗

passage [ˈpæsidʒ] *n* 道,通道;通过;排便;传代 | blind ~ 盲传(将传染性接种物接种至实验动物、鸡胚或组织培养后,在未表现明显病变前连续传代) / false ~ 假通道,瘘 / serial ~ 连续传代(将含有传染因子的组织、渗出液或其他材料接种至实验动物连续传代)

Passavant's bar (cushion, pad, ridge) [ˈpʌsəvənt] (Philip G. Passvant) 帕萨万特隆起(垫,嵴)(吞咽时由腭咽括约肌收缩引起的咽后壁隆起,腭裂患者说话时也有此隆起)

passenger [ˈpæsindʒə] *n* 过客(如过客病毒 ~ virus);娩出物(分娩时的胎儿或胎膜)

passer [ˈpɑːsə] *n* 传递者,传送器 | foil ~ 传箔器(将金箔通过退火焰或从退火盘传送到备填洞,使之坚实,亦称持箔器)

Passiflora [ˌpæsiˈflɔrə] *n* 西番莲属

passivate [ˈpæsiveit] *vt* 使钝化 | **passivation** [ˌpæsiˈveiʃən] *n* 钝化[作用]

passive [ˈpæsiv] *a* 被动的

passivism [ˈpæsivizəm] *n* 被动性性倒错,受鸡奸

passivity [pæˈsivəti] *n* 被动性;受支配妄想

Past. Pasteurella 巴斯德菌属

pasta [ˈpæstə] ([复] **pastae** [ˈpæstiː]) *n*【拉】糊剂,泥膏剂

paste [peist] *n* 糊,糊状物,糊剂,泥膏剂 *vt* 用浆糊粘贴 | bipp ~ 铋泼糊,铋碘仿石蜡糊 / zinc oxide ~ 氧化锌糊 / zipp ~ 氧化锌碘仿糊(含氧化锌、碘仿、液状石蜡)

paster [ˈpeistə] *n* 贴片(贴在双焦点镜上的圆形或椭圆形部分,视近物时用之)

pastern [ˈpæstən] *n* 骹(马足的第一、二趾骨所占据的部分)

Pasteur-Chamberland filter [pɑːsˈtəːʃɑːmbəˈlɑːŋ] (Louis Pasteur; Charles E. Chamberland) 巴-尚滤柱(一种素瓷滤器)

Pasteurella [ˌpæstəˈrelə] *n* 巴斯德菌属 | ~ haemolytica 溶血性巴斯德菌 / ~ multocida, ~ septica 多杀巴斯德菌,出血败血性巴斯德菌 / ~ pestis 鼠疫巴斯德菌,鼠疫杆菌 / ~ pseudotuberculosis 假结核性巴斯德菌 / ~ tularensis 土拉巴斯德菌,野兔热杆菌

Pasteurellaceae [ˌpæstərəˈleisiiː] *n* 巴斯德菌科

Pasteurelleae [ˌpæstəˈreliiː] *n* 巴斯德菌族

pasteurellosis [ˌpæstərəˈləusis] *n* 巴斯德菌病

Pasteuria [pæsˈtəːriə] *n* 巴斯德芽菌属

Pasteuriaceae [pæsˌtəːriˈeisiiː] *n* 巴斯德芽菌科

pasteurization [ˌpæstəraiˈzeiʃən, -riˈz-] *n* 巴[斯德]氏消毒法,低热消毒法

pasteurize [ˈpæstəraiz] *vt* 施行巴[斯德]氏消毒 | **~r** *n* 巴[斯德]氏消毒器

Pasteur's effect (reaction) [pɑːsˈtəː] (Louis Pasteur) 巴斯德效应(反应)(氧存在,则葡萄糖利用糖酵解率减少以及乳酸盐积累受到组织或微生物的抑制) | ~ solution (culture medium, fluid, liquid) 巴斯德溶液(用于真菌培养) / ~ theory 巴斯德学说(认为疾病发作而获得的免疫力是由于疾病微生物生长所必需的物质耗竭所致)

Pastia's sign (lines) [ˈpæstiə] (C. Pastia) 帕斯蒂阿征(线)(猩红热时在肘前窝、腹股沟区以及腕部体表折痕出现出血性线纹,始见于皮疹初起,脱屑后仍存在)

pastil [ˈpæstil], **pastille** [pæsˈtiːl] *n* 锭剂,软锭剂;芳香熏剂;射线测验纸碟

PAT paroxysmal atrial tachycardia 阵发性房性心动过速

Patau's syndrome [pɑːˈtəu] (Klaus Patau) 帕陶综合征,13 三体综合征(即 trisomy 13 syndrome,见 syndrome 项下相应术语)

patch [pætʃ] *n* 斑 | cottonwool ~es 棉絮斑(棉团斑) / herald ~ 前驱斑(玫瑰糠疹的初期病灶) / mucous ~ 黏膜斑,扁头湿疣 / salmon ~ 粉黄色斑(梅毒患者的角膜内) / shagreen ~ 鲨革样斑 / smoker's ~ 吸烟斑,黏膜白斑病 / soldiers' ~es 乳色斑(心包) / white ~ 白斑

patchouli [pəˈtʃuːli] *n* 绿叶刺蕊草(主要用于香料)

patefaction [ˌpætiˈfækʃən] *n* 割开,开放

Patein's albumin [pəˈtæn] (Patein) 醋溶性白蛋白

patella [pəˈtelə] *n* 髌骨 | floating ~ 浮游髌骨 / slipping ~ 移位髌骨 | **~r** *a*

patellapexy [pəˈteləˌpeksi] *n* 髌骨固定术

Patella's disease [pəˈtelə] (Vincenzo Patella) 帕

太拉病(结核病患者于纤维性狭窄后的幽门狭窄)

patellectomy [ˌpætiˈlektəmi] *n* 髌骨切除术

patelliform [pəˈtelifɔːm] *a* 髌样的

patellofemoral [pəˌteləuˈfemərəl] *a* 髌股的

patellometer [ˌpætiˈlɔmitə] *n* 膝盖反射计

patency [ˈpeitənsi] *n* 开放,未闭

patent [ˈpeitənt] *a* 开放的,不闭的;明显的;专利的 *n* 专利权

paternal [pəˈtəːnl] *a* 父系的,父本的

Paterson-Brown Kelly syndrome [ˈpætəsn braun ˈkeli] (D. R. Paterson; Adam Brown Kelly) 帕特森-布朗·凯利综合征(见 Plummer-Vinson syndrome)

Paterson-Kelly syndrome [ˈpætəsn ˈkeli] (D. R. Paterson; Adam B. Kelly) 帕特森-凯利综合征(见 Plummer-Vinson syndrome)

Paterson's bodies, nodules [ˈpætəsn] (Robert Paterson) 软疣小体

Paterson's syndrome [ˈpætəsn] (Donald R. Paterson) 帕特森综合征(见 Plummer-Vinson syndrome)

Patey's operation [ˈpeiti] (David Howard Patey) 佩蒂手术(改良式根治性乳房切除术)

path [pɑːθ] *n* 道,径 | condyle ~ 髁道 / generated occlusal ~ 动殆道 / incisor ~ 切道 / ~ of insertion 就位道 / ionization ~ 电离道(电离辐射通过物质时产生的离子对的轨迹,亦称电离径迹) / milled-in ~s 磨道 / occlusal ~ 殆道

pathema [pəˈθiːmə] ([复] **pathemas** 或 **pathemata** [pəˈθemətə]) *n* 【希】疾病

pathergasia [ˈpæθəˌgeiziə] *n* [变态]精神病 | minor ~s 轻性精神病(或神经症)

pathergization [ˌpæθədʒaiˈzeiʃən] *n* 过敏反应化

pathergy [ˈpæθədʒi], **pathergia** [pəˈθəːdʒiə] *n* 过敏反应性,多种反应性,泛应性,多价变态反应 | **pathergic** *a*

pathfinder [ˈpɑːθˌfaində] *n* 尿道狭窄探针,牙根管探针;探索者;开拓者

path(o)- [构词成分] 病

pathoamine [ˌpæθəˈæmin] *n* 尸毒,尸碱,动物性生物碱

pathoanatomical [ˌpæθəuˌænəˈtɔmikəl] *a* 病理解剖的

pathoanatomy [ˌpæθəuəˈnætəmi] *n* 病理解剖学

pathobiology [ˌpæθəubaiˈɔlədʒi] *n* 病理生物学

pathobolism [pəˈθɔbəlizəm] *n* 代谢异常,病理性代谢

pathoclisis [ˌpæθəuˈklisis] *n* 特异感受性,特异亲和性

pathocrinia [ˌpæθəuˈkriniə] *n* 分泌功能异常 | **pathocrine** [ˈpæθəkrin] *a*

pathodontia [ˌpæθəˈdɔnʃiə] *n* 牙病学,牙科病理学

pathoformic [ˌpæθəˈfɔːmik] *a* 病初的(指精神障碍开始时的症状)

pathogen [ˈpæθədʒin] *n* 病原体,致病菌,病原菌

pathogenesis [ˌpæθəˈdʒenisis] *n* 发病机制 | drug ~ 药物发病机制 | **pathogenesy** [ˌpæθəˈdʒenisi], **pathogeny** [pəˈθɔdʒini] *n* / **pathogenetic** [ˌpæθədʒiˈnetik] *a*

pathogenic [pæθəˈdʒenik] *a* 致病的,病源的

pathogenicity [ˌpæθədʒiˈnisəti] *n* 致病性,病源性

pathoglycemia [ˌpæθəuglaiˈsiːmiə] *n* 血糖异常

pathognomonic [pəˌθɔgnəˈmɔnik], **pathognostic** [ˌpæθəgˈnɔstik] *a* 特殊病征的,特定的,能确定诊断的(病征)

pathognomy [pəˈθɔgnəmi] *n* 病征学

pathography [pəˈθɔgrəfi] *n* 病情记录

pathoklisis [ˌpæθəuˈklisis] *n* 特异感受性,特异亲和性

pathologic [ˌpæθəˈlɔdʒik] *a* 病理的 | **~al** *a* 病理学的;病理的

pathologicoanatomic [ˌpæθəˌlɔdʒikəuænəˈtɔmik] *a* 病理解剖的

pathology [pəˈθɔlədʒi] *n* 病理学 | general ~ 病理学总论 / internal ~, medical ~ 内科病理学 / mental ~ 精神病理学 / solidistic ~ 固体病理学 / special ~ 病理学各论 / surgical ~ 外科病理学 | **pathologist** [pəˈθɔlədʒist] *n* 病理学家

patholysis [pəˈθɔlisis] *n* 疾病消除

pathomaine [ˈpæθəmein] *n* 尸毒碱

pathomania [pæθəˈmeinjə] *n* 悖德狂,悖德精神病(无谵妄性躁狂)

pathometabolism [ˌpæθəuməˈtæbəlizəm] *n* 病理性代谢

pathometer [pəˈθɔmitə] *n* 发病率记录器

pathomimesis [ˌpæθəumaiˈmiːsis], **pathomimia** [ˌpæθəuˈmimiə], **pathomimicry** [ˌpæθəˈmimikri] *n* 疾病模仿,模仿病;诈病,装病

pathomorphism [ˌpæθəuˈmɔːfizəm], **pathomorphology** [ˌpæθəumɔːˈfɔlədʒi] *n* 病理形态学

pathoneurosis [ˌpæθəunjuəˈrəusis] *n* 病位性神经症,躯体[性]神经功能病

pathonomia [pæθəuˈnəumiə], **pathonomy** [pəˈθɔnəmi] *n* 疾病规律学,病律论

patho-occlusion [ˌpæθəu ɔˈkluːʒən] *n* 错殆,错位咬合

pathophilia [ˌpæθəuˈfiliə] *n* 疾病适应性

pathophobia [ˌpæθəuˈfəubiə] *n* 疾病恐怖,恐病症

pathophoresis [ˌpæθəufəˈriːsis] *n* 疾病传播 | **pathophoric** [ˌpæθəˈfɔrik], **pathophorous**

[pə'θɔfərəs] *a* 传播疾病的
pathophysiology [ˌpæθəuˌfizi'ɔlədʒi] *n* 病理生理学
pathopoiesis [ˌpæθəupɔi'iːsis] *n* 致病[作用];罹病性
pathopsychology [ˌpæθəusai'kɔlədʒi] *n* 病理心理学
pathopsychosis [ˌpæθəusai'kəusis] *n* 器质性精神病(如脑肿病、脑炎等引起的精神病)
pathoroentgenography [ˌpæθəuˌrɔntge'nɔgrəfi], **pathoradiography** [ˌpæθəuˌreidi'ɔgrəfi] *n* X 线病理学,病理 X 线学
pathosis [pə'θəusis] *n* 病态
pathotropism [pə'θɔtrəpizəm] *n* 亲病灶性(药物传到病区的倾向)
pathway ['pɑːθwei] *n* 径路,路径,途径 | biosynthetic ~ 生物合成途径 / internuncial ~(神经)联系路径 / pentose phosphate ~ 戊糖磷酸途径 / reentrant ~ 折返径路(心过早搏动或异位搏动联结成正常搏动的机制)
-pathy [构词成分] 病;痛苦;疗法
patient ['peiʃənt] *n* 病人,患者
Patrick's test(sign) ['pætrik] (Hugh T. Patrick) 帕特里克试验(征)(患者仰卧,大腿与膝均弯曲,外踝放到另一腿的膝盖上,压被试腿的膝盖,若引起疼痛,则表明有髋关节炎)
patrilineal [ˌpætri'liniəl] *a* 父系的
patrimony ['pætriməni] *n* 遗产 | **patrimonial** [ˌpætri'məunjəl] *a* 祖传的
patroclinous [ˌpætrə'klainəs] *a* 父系遗传的,父传的,偏父的
patrogenesis [ˌpætrə'dʒenisis] *n* 雄核发育;孤雄生殖
patten ['pætn] *n* 屐(髋关节病患者用)
pattern ['pætən] *n* 型式,模型,图型,范型 | action ~ 动作模式 / behavior ~ 行为模式 / muscle ~ 肌范型 / occlusal ~ 𬌗型 / startle ~ 惊骇反应型式 / stimulus ~ 刺激模式 / wax ~ 蜡型
patulin ['pætjulin] *n* 展青霉素
patulous ['pætjuləs] *a* 扩展的,开放的,膨胀的
pauci- [构词成分] 少
pauciarticular [ˌpɔːsiɑː'tikjulə] *a* 少关节的
paucibacillary [ˌpɔːsibə'siləri] *a* 含菌少的
paucine ['pɔːsin] *n* 巴柯碱(获自非洲植物 pauco 的坚果)
paucisynaptic [ˌpɔːsisi'næptik] *a* 少突触的
paucity ['pɔːsəti] *n* 少量,缺乏
Paul-Bunnell-Davidsohn test [pɔːlbʌ'nel 'deividsn] (J. R. Paul; W. W. Bunnell; Israel Davidsohn) 保-邦-戴试验(异嗜性抗体吸收试验)
Paul-Bunnell test(reaction) [pɔːl bʌ'nel] (John R. Paul; Walls W. Bunnel) 保罗-邦内尔试验(反应),嗜异性凝集试验(试验血内是否有嗜异性抗体存在的一种方法,用以证实临床诊断和血液学诊断传染性单核细胞增多症,此试验的依据是,传染性单核细胞增多症病人的灭活血清可凝集绵羊红细胞,亦称嗜异性抗体反应)
Paullinia [pɔː'liniə] *n* 香无患子属
Paul-Mixter tube [pɔːl 'mikstə] (Frank T. Paul; Samuel J. Mixter) 保罗-米克斯特管(肠引流管,暂时性肠减压用)
Paul's test [pɔːl] (Gustav Paul) 保罗试验(将可疑的脓疹之脓擦入已被划破的兔眼中,如果是天花性或牛痘性脓,则该兔可在 36 ~ 48 小时内发生结合膜上皮增生) | ~ treatment 保罗疗法(将淋巴液用于皮肤,治慢性风湿病)
paunch [pɔːntʃ] *n* 瘤胃(见 rumen)
pause [pɔːz] *n* 中止,暂停,间歇 *vi* 中止,暂停 | compensatory ~ 代偿性间歇(心室过早收缩后的间歇)
Pautrier's microabscess (abscess) [pɔːtri'ei] (Lucien M. A. Pautrier) 波特利埃小脓肿(脓肿)(界线分明的真菌病细胞聚集,位于 T-细胞淋巴瘤和蕈样肉芽肿的非海绵形成的表皮内囊泡中)
pavé [pɑː'vei, 'pævei] *n*【法】铺面(一种微膜状细胞器)
pavementing ['peivməntiŋ] *n* 铺壁(白细胞附着在损伤部位的血管壁上)
pavilion [pə'viljən] *n* 馆;分馆式病房;扩张部;耳郭 | ~ of the ear 耳郭 / ~ of the oviduct 输卵管伞 / ~ of the pelvis 骨盆扩张部,骨盆上部
pavlovian conditioning [pæv'lɔviən] (I. P. Pavlov) 巴甫洛夫条件反射,经典条件反射
Pavlov's method ['pɑːvlɔv] (Ivan P. Pavlov) 巴甫洛夫法(唾液条件反射) | ~ pouch 巴甫洛夫小胃(用于实验性研究胃生理学) / ~ stomach 巴甫洛夫胃(狗胃的一部分,和胃的其他部分相通而分离,借一瘘管开口于腹壁,以研究胃分泌)
pavor ['peivə] *n*【拉】惊,惊悸 | ~ diurnus 昼惊(小儿午睡时惊悸) / ~ nocturnus 夜惊,梦惊
Pavy's disease ['peivi] (Frederick W. Pavy) 周期性蛋白尿
paw [pɔː] *n* 爪 | monkey ~ 猿状手(正中神经损害所致的情况,拇指不能内收及外展,无法与其余手指接触)
Pawlik's triangle (trigone) ['pɑːvlik] (Karel J. Pawlik) 帕弗利克三角(阴道三角)
PAWP pulmonary artery wedge pressure 肺动脉楔压
pawpaw ['pɔːpɔː] *n* 番木瓜,万寿果
Paxillus [pæk'siləs] *n* 桩菇属
Payr's clamp [paiə] (Erwin Payr) 派尔夹(一种挤压夹,用于胃、肠和结肠切除) | ~ disease 派

尔病(便秘,伴左上腹疼痛,由于横结肠和降结肠之间的粘连而扭结并阻塞所致,亦称脾曲综合征) / ~ method 派尔法(血管吻合法)
pazoxide [pə'zɔksaid] *n* 帕佐昔特(抗高血压药)
PB *Pharmacopoeia Britannica*《英国药典》
Pb plumbum 铅
PBG porphobilinogen 胆色素原
PBI protein-bound iodine 蛋白结合碘
PC phosphocreatine 磷酸肌酸(有时用于表示 phosphatidylcholine 磷脂酰胆碱)
P. C. pondus civile【拉】常衡制(英制)
p. c. post cibum【拉】饭后,食后
PCA passive cutaneous anaphylaxis 被动皮肤过敏反应
PCB polychlorinated biphenyl 多氯化联[二]苯
PcB near point of convergence to the intercentral base line 从近集合点至中枢间底线
PCE pseudocholinesterase 假胆碱酯酶
PCEC purified chick embryo cell vaccine 纯化鸡胚胎细胞疫苗
PCG phonocardiogram 心音图
pCi picocurie 皮居里(10^{-12} Ci)
Pco_2 二氧化碳分压(carbon dioxide partial pressure 或 tension)的符号,亦可写成 PCO_2, pCO_2, pCO_2
PCOS polycystic ovary syndrome 多囊卵巢综合征
PCP phencyclidine hydrochloride 盐酸苯环利定
PCR polymerase chain reaction 聚合酶链反应
PCT porphyria cutanea tarda 迟发性皮肤卟啉病
PCV packed cell volume 血细胞比容,血细胞压积
PCWP pulmonary capillary wedge pressure 肺毛细[血]管楔压
PD interpupillary distance 瞳孔间距离; prism diopter 棱镜屈光度; peritoneal dialysis 腹膜透析
Pd palladium 钯
PDA patent ductus arteriosus 动脉导管未闭; posterior descending(coronary) artery(冠状)后降动脉(冠状动脉后室间支)
PE phosphatidylethanolamine 磷脂酰乙醇胺
PEA pulseless electrical activity 无脉电活动
pea [piː] ([复] **peas⟨e⟩** [piːz]) *n* 豌豆
peak [piːk] *n* 峰 *a* 最高的,高峰的 | kilovolt ~ kV 峰值(X 线机使用的)
Péan's clamp (forceps) [pei'æn] (Jules É, Péan) 佩昂(止血)钳 | ~ operation 佩昂手术(手术进行时结扎血管的髋关节切断术)
pearl [pəːl] *n* 珠,珍珠;小珠(药),珠剂;痰珠(早期支气管哮喘发作所见的圆形硬块痰) | epidermic ~s, epithelial ~s 上皮珠 / gouty ~ 痛风珠(痛风病人耳软骨上的尿酸钠结石)
pearlash ['pəːlæʃ] *n* 珍珠灰,粗碳酸钾
PEARS porcine epidemic abortion and respiratory syndrome 猪流行性流产和呼吸综合征
pear-shaped ['pɛəʃeipt] *a* 梨状的
Pearson's product-moment correlation coefficient ['piəsn] (Karl Pearson) 皮尔逊积矩相关系数(即积矩系数 product moment coefficient,见 coefficient 项下相应术语)
Pearson's syndrome ['piəsn] (H. A. Pearson) 皮尔逊综合征(一种罕见的先天性综合征,表现为难治性成铁粒红细胞性贫血,伴骨髓前体空泡形成和外分泌胰腺功能不全;大多数患儿在婴儿期死亡,除非输血)
peau [pəu] *n*【法】皮,皮肤 | ~ de changrin [pəu də ʃɑː'grein]【法】鲨革样皮 / ~ d'orange [pəu də'rɑːndʒ]【法】橘皮状皮肤,橘皮
pebble ['pebl] *n* 小石,水晶,水晶透镜
pébrine [pe'briːn] *n*【法】(蚕)微粒子病
pecazine ['piːkəziːn] *n* 哌卡嗪(即密哌嗪 mepazine,安定药)
peccant ['pekənt] *a* 有病的,不健康的,致病的
peccatiphobia [ˌpekəti'fəubjə] *n* 犯罪恐怖
pechyagra [ˌpeki'eigrə] *n* 肘痛风
pecil(o)- 以 pecil(o)-起始的词,同样见以 poikil(o)-起始的词
Pecquet's cistern (reservoir) [pe'kei] (Jean Pecquet)乳糜池 | ~ duct 胸[导]管
pectase ['pekteis] *n* 果胶酶
pecten ['pektən] ([复] **pectines** ['pektiniːz]) *n* 梳,栉;肛梳;栉膜(动物)
pectenine ['pektinin] *n* 仙人梳碱
pectenitis [ˌpekti'naitis] *n* 肛梳炎
pectenosis [ˌpekti'nəusis] *n* 肛梳(纤维)硬结
pectenotomy [ˌpekti'nɔtəmi] *n* 肛梳切开术
pectic acid ['pektik] 果胶酸
pectin ['pektin] *n* 果胶 | pectic, pectinous ['pektinəs] *a*
pectinase ['pektineis] *n* 果胶酶
pectinate (d) ['pektineit (id)], **pectiniform** [pek'tinifɔːm] *a* 梳状的,栉状的
Pectinatus [ˌpekti'neitəs] *n* 梳状菌属
pectineal [pek'tiniəl] *a* 耻骨的
pectization [ˌpektai'zeiʃən, -ti'z-] *n* 胶凝[作用]
Pectobacterium [ˌpektəubæk'tiəriəm] *n* 果胶杆菌属(亦称欧文菌属 Erwinia)
pectolytic [ˌpektə'litik] *a* 果胶溶解的
pectora ['pektərə] pectus 的复数
pectoral ['pektərəl] *a* 胸的;祛痰的,舒胸的
pectoralgia [ˌpektə'rældʒiə] *n* 胸痛,胸肌痛
pectoralis [ˌpektə'reilis] *a*【拉】胸的
pectoriloquy [ˌpektə'riləkwi] *n* 胸语音 | aphonic ~ 低音胸语音 / whispered ~, whispering ~ 耳语音
pectorophony [ˌpektə'rɔfəni] *n* 语音增强
pectose ['pektəus] *n* 果胶糖
pectous ['pektəs] *a* 果胶的,含果胶的,果胶状的

pectunculus [pek'tʌŋkjuləs] *n* 小梳(在中脑水管中)
pectus ['pektəs]([复] **pectora** ['pektərə]) *n*【拉】胸
pedal ['pedl] *a* 足的,脚的
pedarthrocace [ˌpiːdɑː'θrɔkəsi] *n* 儿童关节疡
pedatrophia [ˌpiːdə'trɔfiə] *n* 儿童消瘦
pederast ['pedəræst] *n* 好男色者
pederasty ['pedəræsti] *n* 鸡奸
pederin ['pedərin] *n* 岬毒素
pederosis [ˌpiːdə'rəusis] *n* 娈童色情(鸡奸儿童)
pedes ['piːdiːz] pes 的复数
pedi- 见 ped(o)-[2]
pedia- [构词成分] 儿童
pediadontia [ˌpiːdiə'dɔnʃiə], **pediadontology** [ˌpiːdiədɔn'tɔlədʒi] *n* 儿童牙科学 | pediadontist [ˌpiːdiə'dɔntist] *n* 儿童牙科学家
pedialgia [ˌpedi'ældʒiə] *n* 足底痛,足神经痛
pediatrician [ˌpiːdiə'triʃən], **pediatrist** [ˌpiːdi'ætrist] *n* 儿科医师,儿科学家
pediatrics [ˌpiːdi'ætriks], **pediatry** ['piːdiˌætri] *n* 儿科学 | **pediatric** [ˌpiːdi'ætrik] *a*
pedication [ˌpedi'keiʃən] *n* 鸡奸,男色
pedicel ['pedisəl] *n* 蒂;花梗 | **pedicellate** [pe'disilit], **pedicellated** ['pedisəˌleitid] *a* 有蒂的
pedicellaria [ˌpedisə'lɛəriə] *n* 叉棘(棘皮动物),叉刺
pedicellation [ˌpedisə'leiʃən] *n* 蒂生成
pedicle ['pedikl] *n* 蒂(如肿瘤的蒂);花梗 | ~ of vertebral arch 椎弓根
pedicled ['pedikld] *a* 有蒂的
pedicular [pi'dikjulə] *a* 虱的
pediculate [pi'dikjulit] *a* 有蒂的
pediculation [piˌdikju'leiʃən] *n* 虱传染;蒂形成
pediculi [pi'dikjulai] pediculus 的复数
pediculicide [pi'dikjulisaid] *a* 灭虱的 *n* 灭虱药
Pediculidae [ˌpedi'kjuːlidiː] *n* 虱科
Pediculoides [piˌdikju'lɔidiːz] *n* 虱螨属(现名 Pyemotes) | ~ ventricosus 袋形虱螨(即 Pyemotes ventricosus)
pediculosis [piˌdikju'ləusis] *n* 虱病
pediculous [pi'dikjuləs] *a* 有虱的
Pediculus [pi'dikjuləs] *n* 虱属 | ~ humanis capitis 头虱 / ~ humanis corporis 衣虱,体虱 / ~ inguinalis, ~ pubis 阴虱
pediculus [pi'dikjuləs]([复] **pediculi** [pi'dikjulai]) *n* 虱;蒂
pedicure ['pedikjuə] *n* 足疗法;手足医
pedigree ['pedigriː] *n* 系谱
pediluvium [ˌpedi'ljuːviəm] *n* 足浴
Pediococcus [ˌpiːdiəu'kɔkəs] *n* 片球菌属
pediodontia [ˌpiːdiəu'dɔnʃiə] *n* 儿童牙科学
pedionalgia [ˌpiːdiəu'nældʒiə] *n* 足底痛,跖痛
pedipalpa [ˌpedi'pælpə] *n* 须肢目
pediphalanx [ˌpedi'feilæŋks] *n* [足]趾
pedistibulum [ˌpedi'stibjuləm] *n*【拉】镫骨
peditis [pi'daitis] *n* 蹄骨炎(马)
ped(o)-[1], **paed(o)-** [构词成分] 儿童
ped(o)-[2], **pedi-** [构词成分]足
pedobarograph [ˌpiːdəu'bærəgrɑːf, -græf] *n* 足压记录仪
pedobarography [ˌpiːdəubɔ'rɔgrəfi] *n* 足压测量
pedodontics [ˌpiːdəu'dɔntiks], **pedodontia** [ˌpiːdəu'dɔnʃiə] *n* 儿童口腔医学 | **pedodontist** *n* 儿童口腔医学家
pedodynamometer [ˌpedəudainə'mɔmitə] *n* 脚力测定器
pedogamy [pi'dɔgəmi] *n* 同配生,同系交配
pedogenesis [ˌpiːdəu'dʒenisis] *n* 幼体生殖
pedograph ['pedəgrɑːf, -græf] *n* 脚印
pedology [pi'dɔlədʒi] *n* 儿童发育学 | **pedologic(al)** [ˌpiːdə'lɔdʒik(əl)] *a* / **pedologist** *n* 儿童发育学家
pedometer [pi'dɔmitə] *n* 步数计,计步器
Pedomicrobium [ˌpiːdəumai'krəubiəm] *n* 土微菌属
pedomorphism [ˌpiːdəu'mɔːfizəm] *n* 稚态,幼稚形态 | **pedomorphic** *a*
pedopathy [pi'dɔpəθi] *n* 足病,脚病
pedophilia [ˌpiːdə'filiə] *n* 恋童癖(在精神病学中指成人对儿童的性欲而言) | **pedophilic** *a* 爱儿童的;恋童癖的
pedophobia [ˌpiːdə'fəubjə] *n* 儿童恐怖
pedorthics [pi'dɔːθiks] *n* 足整直法,足矫正法(按处方设计、制造、安装和修改鞋及有关足的装置以减轻足和肢的疼痛或残疾的情况) | **pedorthic** *a* 足整直的,足矫正的 / **pedorthist** [pi'dɔːθist] *n* 足整直师,足矫正师
peduncle [pi'dʌŋkl] *n* 脚,蒂,茎 | cerebral ~ 大脑脚 / ~ of flocculus 绒球脚 / olfactory ~ 嗅[叶]脚 / pineal ~, ~ of pineal body 松果体脚 | **peduncular** [pi'dʌŋkjulə] *a*
pedunculated [pi'dʌŋkjuleitid] *a* 有脚的,有蒂的
pedunculotomy [piˌdʌŋkju'lɔtəmi] *n* 大脑脚切断术
pedunculus [pi'dʌŋkjuləs] *n*【拉】脚,蒂,茎
peel [piːl] *vt* 去皮 *vi* 脱皮 *n* 皮,果皮 | bitter orange ~ 苦橙皮 / lemon ~ 柠檬皮
peenash ['piːnæʃ] *n* 鼻蝇蛆病
PEEP positive end-expiratory pressure 呼气末正压通气
PEF peak expiratory flow 呼气流量峰值
PEFR peak expiratory flow rate 呼气流速峰值

PEG pneumoencephalography 气脑造影术；polyethylene glycol 聚乙二醇

peg [peg] *n* 钉 | rete ~s 表皮突，钉突

PEG-ADA PEG-adenosine deaminase 聚乙二醇-腺苷脱氨酶（见 pegademase）

pegademase [peg'ædəmeis] *n* 聚乙二醇-腺苷脱氨酶（从牛肠取得的腺苷脱氨酶〈adenosine deaminase〉与聚乙二醇〈polyethylene glycols〉共价结合，用于严重免疫缺陷患者腺苷脱氨酶缺乏症的替补疗法，肌内给药）

PEG-adenosine deaminase (PEG-ADA) 聚乙二醇-腺苷脱氨酶（见 pegademase）

Peganum ['pegənəm] *n* 骆驼蓬属

pegaspargase [peg'æspɑːgeis] *n* 培门冬酶（抗肿瘤药）

peginterferon alfa-2b [ˌpegˌintə'fiərɔn] PEG α-2b 干扰素（为重组 α-2b 干扰素和聚乙二醇-腺苷脱鞍酶〈PEG〉的一种共价结合物，前一部分造成生物活性；本品为生物反应调节物，皮下给药，治疗丙型肝炎慢性感染）

peglicol 5-oleate [pi'glaikɔl] 聚乙二醇 5-油酸酯（制药时用作乳化剂，亦称 polyoxyl 5-oleate）

pegology [pi'gɔlədʒi] *n* 矿泉学（尤指药用矿泉）

pegoterate [ˌpegəu'tereit] *n* 培高特酯（药用辅料）

pegoxol 7-stearate [pe'gɔksəul] 聚乙二醇 7-硬脂酸酯（制药时用作乳化剂）

pegylated ['pegəˌleitid] *a* 带有 PEG 的（带有聚乙二醇-腺苷脱氨酶〈PEG〉的，指某些药物）

peinotherapy [ˌpainəu'θerəpi] *n* 饥饿疗法

pelade [pe'læd] *n*【法】斑秃

peladophobia [ˌpelədəu'fəubjə] *n* 秃发恐怖

pelage ['pelidʒ, pə'lɑːʒ] *n*【法】毛发

pelagic [pe'lædʒik] *a* 海洋的，海栖的

pelagism ['pelədʒizəm] *n* 晕船

Pelamis ['peləmis] *n* 海蛇属 | ~ bicolor 双色海蛇

pelargonic acid [ˌpelɑː'gɔnik] 壬酸

Pel-Ebstein fever (disease, pyrexia) [pel 'ebʃtain]（Pieter K. Pel; Wilhelm Ebstein）佩-埃热（病、发热）（一种周期热，偶见于霍奇金〈Hodgkin〉病）| ~ symptom 慢性间歇热（霍奇金病）

Pelecypoda [ˌpeli'sipədə] *n* 斧足类

Pelger-Huët nuclear anomaly ['pelgə 'hjuet]（Karel Pelger; G. J. Huët）佩-许核异常（本症共有两型，一为遗传型缺陷，影响中性粒细胞的细胞核正常分叶，另一型为非遗传性的，其表现症状与遗传型相仿，在某些贫血和白血病中可以看到）

Pelger's nuclear anomaly ['pelgə]（Karel Pelger）佩尔格尔核异常（白细胞中的多形核细胞的核异常，这是一种人类遗传性疾病）

pelidisi [ˌpeli'disi] *n*（从拉丁文 pondus decies linearis divisus sidentis 创造出来的词）皮里迪西指数（用坐高〈cm〉除以 10×体重〈g〉的立方根即得出小儿营养状况的指数：90 或 90 以下为营养不足，95 ~ 100 为营养良好，101 或 101 以上为营养过多）

pelidnoma [ˌpelid'nəumə] *n* 青紫斑

peliosis [ˌpiːli'əusis] *n*［希］紫癜

Pelizaeus-Merzbacher disease [ˌpeili'zaiəs 'məːzbəhə]（Friedrich Pelizaeus; Ludwig Merzbacher）佩利措伊斯-梅茨巴赫病，家族性中叶性硬化（一种家族型脑白质病）

pellagra [pə'leigrə] *n* 糙皮病 | **~l** [pə'lægrəl] *a*

pellagragenic [pəˌlægrə'dʒenik] *a* 致糙皮病的

pellagramin [pə'lægrəmin] *n* 烟酸

pellagrazein [ˌpelə'greiziin], **pellagrocein** [ˌpelə'grəusiin] *n* 蜀黍毒碱

pellagrin [pə'leigrin, pə'lægrin] *n* 糙皮病患者

pellagroid [pə'lægrɔid] *n* 类糙皮病

pellagrology [ˌpelə'grɔlədʒi] *n* 糙皮病学 | **pellagrologist** *n* 糙皮病学家

pellagrosis [ˌpelə'grəusis] *n* 糙皮病（糙皮病皮肤综合征，特征为皮肤色素沉着、红斑及角化过度）

pellagrous [pə'lægrəs], **pellagrose** [pə'lægrəus] *a* 糙皮病的

pellant ['pelənt] *a* 去垢的，清除的

pellate ['peleit] *vt* 清除，排除

Pellegrini's disease [ˌpelei'griːni], **Pellegrini-Stieda disease** [ˌpelei'griːni 'stiːdə]（Augusto Pellegrini; Alfred Stieda）佩莱格利尼病，佩莱格利尼-施蒂达病（外伤引起的一种病，其特征为膝内、外侧韧带上部半月状骨质形成）

pellet ['pelit] *n* 小丸，小糖丸

pellicle ['pelikl] *n* 表膜 | **pellicular** [pe'likjulə], **pelliculous** [pe'likjuləs] *a*

Pellizzi's syndrome [pe'liːzi]（G. B. Pellizzi）松果体综合征（即 epiphyseal syndrome，见 syndrome 项下相应术语）

pellote [pei'jəutə] *n* 拍约他，仙人球膏（制自墨西哥仙人球的麻醉剂）

pellucid [pe'ljuːsid, pə-] *a* 透明的，清澈的

pel(o)-［构词成分］泥

Pelobiontida [ˌpiːləubai'ɔntidə] *n* 泥生目

Pelodera [ˌpelau'diərə] *n* 小杆线虫属

Pelodictyon [ˌpiːləu'diktiən] *n* 暗网菌属

pelohemia [ˌpiːləu'hiːmiə] *n* 血液浓缩

peloid ['piːlɔid] *a* 泥样的（治疗用，如用作裹法、浴疗）

pelology [pi'lɔlədʒi] *n* 泥土学

Pelomyxa [ˌpiːləu'miksə] *n* 多核变形虫属 | ~

carolinensis 卡罗林多核变形虫
Pelonema [ˌpiːləuˈniːmə] *n* 暗线菌属
Pelonemataceae [ˌpiːləuˌniːməˈteisiiː] *n* 暗线菌科
Peloploca [piˈlɔpləkə] *n* 暗辫菌属
Peloplocaceae [ˌpiːləupləˈkeisiiː] *n* 暗辫菌科
Pelosigma [ˌpiːləuˈsigmə] *n* 暗屈曲菌属
pelosine [piˈləusin] *n* 比比林,甘蜜树皮碱
pelotherapy [ˌpiːləuˈθerəpi], **pelopathy** [piˈlɔpəθi] *n* 泥疗法
Pel's crises [pel] (Pieter K. Pel) 脊髓痨性眼危象
pelta [ˈpeltə] *n* 小盾
peltate [ˈpelteit] *a* 盾形的
peltation [pelˈteiʃən] *n* 血清防护(抗血清或疫苗接种后的防护作用)
pelves [ˈpelviːz] pelvis 的复数
pelvic [ˈpelvik] *a* 骨盆的
pelvicaliceal, pelvicalyceal [ˌpelviˌkæliˈsiːəl] *a* 肾盂肾盏的
pelvicellulitis [ˌpelviˌseljuˈlaitis] *n* 盆腔蜂窝织炎
pelvicephalography [ˌpelviˌsefəˈlɔgrəfi] *n* 骨盆胎头 X 线测量术
pelvicephalometry [ˌpelviˌsefəˈlɔmitri] *n* 骨盆胎头测量法
pelvifemoral [ˌpelviˈfemərəl] *a* 骨盆股骨的
pelvifixation [ˌpelvifikˈseiʃən] *n* 盆腔器官固定术
pelvilithotomy [ˌpelviliˈθɔtəmi], **pelviolithotomy** [ˌpelviəuliˈθɔtəmi] *n* 肾盂切开取石术
pelvimeter [pelˈvimitə] *n* 骨盆测量器
pelvimetry [pelˈvimitri] *n* 骨贫测量 | combined ~ 骨盆(内外径)合并测量法 / digital ~ 骨盆指量法 / external ~ 骨盆外径测量法 / instrumental ~ 骨盆器械测量法/internal ~ 骨盆内测量
pelviography [ˌpelviˈɔgrəfi] *n* 盆腔 X 线摄影[术]
pelvioileoneocystostomy [ˌpelviəuˌiliəuˌniəusisˈtɔstəmi] *n* 肾盂回肠膀胱吻合术
pelvioneostomy [ˌpelviəuniˈɔstəmi] *n* 输尿管肾盂吻合术
pelvioperitonitis [ˌpelviəuˌperitəuˈnaitis] *n* 盆腔腹膜炎
pelvioplasty [ˈpelviəuˌplæsti] *n* 骨盆成形术;肾盂成形术
pelvioradiography [ˌpelviəuˌreidiˈɔgrəfi] *n* 盆腔 X 线摄影[术]
pelvioscope [ˈpelviəskəup] *n* 骨盆检查器
pelvioscopy [ˌpelviˈɔskəpi] *n* 盆腔检查
pelviostomy [ˌpelviˈɔstəmi] *n* 肾盂造口术
pelviotomy [ˌpelviˈɔtəmi] *n* 骨盆切开术;肾盂切开术
pelviperitonitis [ˌpelviˌperitəuˈnaitis] *n* 盆腔腹膜炎
pelvirectal [ˌpelviˈrektəl] *a* 骨盆直肠的
pelviroentgenography [ˌpelviˌrɔntgeˈnɔgrəfi], **pelviradiography** [ˌpelviˌreidiˈɔgrəfi] *n* 盆腔 X 线摄影[术]
pelvis [ˈpelvis] ([复] **pelvises** 或 pelves [ˈpelviːz]) *n*【拉】骨盆,盂,肾盂 | false ~, greater ~, large ~ 假骨盆,大骨盆/giant ~ 均大骨盆/infantile ~, juvenile ~ 婴儿样骨盆/lesser ~, small ~, true ~ 小骨盆,真骨盆/renal ~ 肾盂/spider ~ 蜘蛛样肾盂
pelvisacrum [pelviˈseikrəm] *n* [骨]盆骶骨 | **pelvisacral** *a*
pelviscope [ˈpelviskəup] *n* 骨盆[外形]X 线检查器
pelviscopy [pelˈviskəpi] *n* 盆腔检查;肾盂 X 线透视检查
pelvisection [ˌpelviˈsekʃən] *n* 骨盆切开术
pelvisternum [ˌpelviˈstəːnəm] *n* 耻骨联合软骨
pelvitherm [ˈpelviθəːm] *n* 骨盆器官热疗器
pelvitomy [pelˈvitəmi] *n* 骨盆切开术
pelvitrochanterian [ˌpelviˌtrəukænˈtiəriən] *a* 骨盆转子的
pelviureteral [ˌpelvijuəˈriːtərəl] *a* 肾盂输尿管的
pelviureteroradiography [ˌpelvijuəˌriːtərəˌreidiˈɔgrəfi] *n* 肾盂输尿管造影[术]
pelvocaliceal [ˌpelvəuˌkæliˈsiːəl] *a* 肾盂肾盏的
pelvocaliectasis [ˌpelvəuˌkæliˈektəsis] *n* 肾盂积水
pelvoscopy [pelˈvɔskəpi] *n* 肾盂检查术
pelvospondylitis [ˌpelvəuˌspɔndiˈlaitis] *n* 骨盆部脊椎炎 | ~ ossificans 骨化性骨盆部脊椎炎,类风湿性脊椎炎
pelyc(o)- 以 pelyc(o)- 起始的词,同样见以 pelvi-和 pyelo-起始的词
PEM protein-energy malnutrition 蛋白能量性营养不良
pemerid nitrate [ˈpemərid] 硝酸哌美立特(镇咳药)
pemirolast potassium [pəˈmirəuˌlæst] 吡嘧司特钾(一种肥大细胞稳定剂,抑制炎症介质从肥大细胞和嗜伊红细胞释放,并抑制I型超敏反应;局部用于结膜,预防伴有变应性结膜炎的瘙痒症)
pemoline [ˈpeməliːn] *n* 匹莫林(中枢神经系统兴奋药)
pemphigoid [ˈpemfigɔid] *a* 天疱疮样的 *n* 类天疱疮 | benign mucosal ~, benign mucous membrane ~ 良性黏膜类天疱疮 / cicatricial ~ 瘢痕性类天疱疮 / localized bullous ~, localized chronic ~ 局限性大疱性类天疱疮,局限性慢性类天疱疮

pemphigus [ˈpemfigəs] *n* 天疱疮 | benign ~ vegetans 良性增生型天疱疮 / Brazilian ~, South American ~, wildfire ~ 巴西天疱疮,南美天疱疮,野火天疱疮(即 fogo selvagem)

pempidine tartrate [ˈpempidiːn] 酒石酸潘必啶(抗高血压药)

PEN pharmacy equivalent name 药物等同名称

Peña procedure [ˈpeinjɑː] (Alberto Peña) 矢状后肛门直肠成形术

penatin [ˈpenətin] *n* 点青霉素

penbutolol sulfate [penˈbjuːtələl] 硫酸喷布洛尔(抗肾上腺素能药,β 受体阻滞药)

penciclovir [penˈsaikləuvir] *n* 喷昔洛韦(一种抗病毒化合物,抑制人类疱疹病毒 1 和 2 型的病毒性 DNA 合成和复制,用于治疗复发性唇疱疹,局部用药)

pendelluft [ˈpendəlˌluːft] *n*【德】摆动呼吸(空气在肺内来回流动,结果造成无效腔通气增加)

Pende's sign [ˈpendə] (Nicola Pende) 潘德征(指鼻试验时臂回缩现象,见于小脑疾病)

Pendred's syndrome [ˈpendred] (Vaughan Pendred) 彭德莱综合征(童年中期出现的一种遗传性综合征,表现为先天性双侧神经性聋,伴甲状腺肿形成,而无甲状腺功能减退,其主要生化特点是甲状腺素生物合成有部分缺陷)

pendulous [ˈpendjuləs] *a* 悬垂的,下垂的

pendulum [ˈpendjuləm] *n* 摆 | **pendular** [ˈpendjulə] *a* 摆动的

penectomy [piˈnektəmi] *n* 阴茎切除[术]

penetrability [ˌpenitrəˈbiləti] *n* 可穿透性

penetrable [ˈpenitrəbl] *a* 能透过的

penetrance [ˈpenitrəns] *n* 外显率(在遗传学上指基因与其相应有关遗传性状的表现的个体的比率)

penetrating [ˈpenitreitiŋ] *a* 穿透的;渗透的

penetration [ˌpeniˈtreiʃən] *n* 穿透术;穿透 | egg 精子穿卵

penetrology [ˌpeniˈtrɔlədʒi] *n* 透射学

penetrometer [ˌpeniˈtrɔmitə] *n* [X 线]透度计,[X 线]硬度计

penfluridol [penˈfluridɔl] *n* 五氟利多(安定药)

-penia [构词成分] 缺乏,不足,减少

penial [ˈpiːniəl] *a* 阴茎的

penicidin [ˌpeniˈsaidin] *n* 潘尼西丁(即棒曲霉素)

penicillamine [ˌpenisiˈlæmin] *n* 青霉胺(抗类风湿关节炎药)

penicilli [ˌpeniˈsilai] penicillus 的复数

penicilliary [ˌpeniˈsiliəri] *a* 毛笔形的,帚形的

penicillic acid [ˌpeniˈsilik] 青霉酸

penicillin [ˌpeniˈsilin] *n* 青霉素 | aluminum ~ 青霉素铝 / benzyl ~ potassium 青霉素钾,苄青霉素钾 / benzyl ~ sodium 青霉素钠,苄青霉素钠 / clemizole ~ 克咪西林,氯咪唑青霉素,氯苄咪唑青霉素 / dimethoxyphenyl ~ sodium 甲氧苯青霉素钠 / ~ G 青霉素,苄青霉素 / isoxazolyl ~ 异噁唑青霉素 / ~ N 青霉素 N,头孢菌素 N(即阿地西林 adicillin) / ~ O 青霉素 O,丙烯硫甲青霉素 / ~ O potassium 青霉素 O 钾 / ~ O sodium 青霉素 O 钠 / potassium phenoxymethyl ~ 苯氧甲基青霉素钾,青霉素 V 钾 / ~ V benzathine 苄星青霉素 V / ~ V hydrabamine 哈胺青霉素 V,海巴明青霉素 V / ~ V potassium 青霉素 V 钾

penicillinase [ˌpeniˈsilineis] *n* 青霉素酶

penicillin-fast [ˌpeniˈsilin fɑːst] *a* 抗青霉素的,耐青霉素的

penicilliosis [ˌpenisiliˈəusis] *n* 青霉病(肺部感染)

Penicillium [ˌpeniˈsiliəm] ([复] **penicillia** [ˌpeniˈsiliə]) *n* 青霉属 | ~ chrysogenum 产黄青霉 / ~ citrinum 桔青霉 / ~ glaucum, ~ crustaceum 灰绿青霉,皮壳青霉 / ~ notatum 特异青霉,点青霉 / ~ uticale, ~ patulum 展青霉

penicilloyl-polylysine [ˌpeniˈsiləilˌpɔliˈlaisiːn] *n* 青霉噻唑酰-聚赖氨酸(由聚赖氨酸和青霉烯酸制备,青霉素过敏者在皮内注射后 20 分钟内出现疹块和红斑反应)

penicillus [ˌpeniˈsiləs] ([复] **penicilli** [ˌpeniˈsilai]) *n*【拉】笔毛(脾内微动脉丛)

Peniculina [piˌnikjuˈlainə] *n* 咽膜亚目

peniculus [piˈnikjuləs] ([复] **peniculi** [piˈnikjulai]) *n* 毛撮(见于某些纤毛原虫口腔的左壁)

penillamine [ˌpeniˈlæmin] *n* 青霉酸衍胺

penilloaldehyde [ˌpeniləuˈældihaid] *n* 青霉醛

penis [ˈpiːnis] ([复] **penises** 或 **penes** [ˈpiː-niːz]) *n*【拉】阴茎 | clubbed ~ (勃起时)杵状阴茎弯曲 / webbed ~ 蹼状阴茎 | **penile** [ˈpiːnail] *a*

penischisis [piːˈniskisis] *n* 阴茎裂

penitis [piːˈnaitis] *n* 阴茎炎

penniform [ˈpenifɔːm], **pennate** [ˈpeneit] *a* 羽状的

Penn seroflocculation reaction [pen] (Harry S. Penn) 佩恩血清絮状反应(检癌)

pennyroyal [ˌpeniˈrɔiəl] *n* 薄荷类植物

penoplasty [ˈpiːnəuˌplæti] *n* 阴茎成形术

penoscrotal [ˌpiːnəuˈskrəutl] *a* 阴茎阴囊的

Penrose drain [ˈpenrəuz] (Charles B. Penrose) 卷烟式引流

pent-, penta- [构词成分] 五

penta [ˈpentə] *n* 五氯[苯]酚

pentabasic [ˌpentəˈbeisik] *a* 五元的；五价的
pentachlorophenol [ˌpentəˌkləurəˈfenɔl] *n* 五氯[苯]酚
pentachromic [ˌpentəˈkrəumik] *a* 五色的，五色觉的
pentacyclic [ˌpentəˈsaiklik，-ˈsik-] *a* 五环的
pentad [ˈpentæd] *n* (构成一组的)五个；五年；五天；五价物
pentadactyl [ˌpentəˈdæktil] *a* 五指的，五趾的
pentaene [ˈpentəiːn] *n* 五烯
pentaerythritol [ˌpentəiˈriθritɔl]，**pentaerythrityl** [ˌpentəiˈriθritil] *n* 季戊四醇 | ~ tetranitrate 戊四硝酯，硝酸戊四醇酯，四硝季戊四醇(抗心绞痛药)
pentagastrin [ˌpentəˈgæstrin] *n* 五肽胃泌素
pentalogy [penˈtælədʒi] *n* 五联症
pentamer [ˈpentəmə] *n* 五聚物(化学)；五壳粒(病毒)
pentamethazene [ˌpentəˈmeθəziːn] *n* 氮戊溴铵(即 azamethonium，抗高血压药)
pentamethylenediamine [ˌpentəˌmeθiliːnˈdaiəmiːn] *n* 五甲烯二胺，尸胺
pentamethylenetetrazol [ˌpentəˌmeθiliːnˈtetrəzɔl] *n* 戊四氮，五甲烯四氮唑(中枢兴奋药)
pentamethylmelamine [ˌpentəˌmeθilˈmeləmiːn] *n* 五甲蜜胺(正在研究的抗肿瘤药)
pentamidine [penˈtæmidiːn] *n* 喷他脒(抗感染药)
pentane [ˈpentein] *n* 戊烷
pentanoic acid [ˌpentəˈnəuik] 戊酸
pentapeptide [ˌpentəˈpeptaid] *n* 五肽
pentapiperide methylsulfate [ˌpentəˈpaipəraid] 甲硫酸戊哌立特(抗胆碱药)
pentapiperium methylsulfate [ˌpentəpaiˈperiəm] 甲硫酸戊哌铵(抗胆碱能药)
pentaploid [ˈpentəplɔid] *a* 五倍的 *n* 五倍体(指一个体或细胞具有五组染色体) | **~y** *n* 五倍性
pentapyrrolidinium bitartrate [ˌpentəpiˌrəuliˈdiniəm] 酒石酸戊双吡铵，喷托铵酒石酸盐(神经节阻滞药，用作抗高血压药)
pentasomy [ˌpentəˈsəumi] *n* 五染色体性
pentastarch [ˈpentəˌstaːtʃ] *n* 喷他淀粉(用作白细胞去除术中的佐剂，以增加红细胞沉降率)
Pentastoma [penˈtæstəmə] *n* 舌形虫属，五口虫属
pentastome [ˈpentæstəum] *n* 舌形虫，五口虫
pentastomiasis [ˌpentəstəuˈmaiəsis] *n* 舌形虫病，五口虫病
pentastomid [ˌpentəˈstəumid] *n* 舌形虫
Pentastomida [ˌpentəˈstəumidə] *n* 舌形虫纲
pentatomic [ˌpentəˈtɔmik] *a* 五原子的，五元的
Pentatrichomonas [ˌpentəˌtrikəˈməunəs] *n* 五鞭毛滴虫属
pentavaccine [ˌpentəˈvæksiːn] *n* 五联疫苗，五联菌苗(含有 5 种微生物的疫苗，例如含伤寒杆菌、副伤寒杆菌甲和乙、霍乱弧菌和布鲁菌的死菌苗)
pentavalent [ˌpentəˈveilənt] *a* 五价的
pentazocine [penˈtæzəsiːn] *n* 喷他佐辛(镇痛药) | ~ hydrochloride 盐酸喷他佐辛 / ~ lactate 乳酸喷他佐辛
pentdyopent [pentˈdaiəpent] *n* 525 物质(在一些疾病的尿内发现的一种血色素分解产物，当怀疑某一器官有病时，若尿内无此物质，则可认为是对肝病的否定)
pentene [ˈpentiːn] *n* 戊烯
pentetate calcium trisodium [ˈpentiteit] 喷替酸钙钠(用作螯合剂，治疗钚中毒)
pentetic acid [penˈtiːtik] 喷替酸(螯合剂)
penthienate bromide [penˈθaiəneit] 喷噻溴铵(抗胆碱能药，主要用于治疗胃溃疡)
penthrit [ˌpenθrit] *n* 硝酸戊四醇酯，四硝季戊四醇，戊四硝酯(抗心绞痛药)
pentizidone sodium [penˈtizidəun] 戊齐酮钠(抗菌药)
pentobarbital [ˌpentəuˈbɑːbitæl] *n* 戊巴比妥(催眠镇静药) | ~ sodium 戊巴比妥钠(安眠药，用作镇静、抗惊厥、麻醉前给药等)
pentobarbitone [ˌpentəuˈbaːbitəun] *n* 戊巴比妥(催眠镇静药)
pentolinium tartrate [ˌpentəuˈliniəm] 酒石酸喷托铵(神经节阻滞药，用作抗高血压药)
pentone [ˈpentəun] *n* 缬烯炔
pentosan [ˈpentəsæn] *n* 戊聚糖 | methyl ~ 甲基戊聚糖
pentosazone [penˈtəusəzəun] *n* 戊糖脎
pentose [ˈpentəus] *n* 戊糖
pentosemia [ˌpentəuˈsiːmiə] *n* 戊糖血[症]
pentosenucleic acid [ˌpentəusnjuːˈkliːik] 戊糖核酸
pentosidase [penˈtɔsideis] *n* 戊糖苷酶
pentoside [ˈpentəsaid] *n* 戊糖苷
pentostatin [ˌpentəuˈstætin] *n* 喷司他丁(实验性用于治疗对 α-干扰素无反应的毛细胞白血病。亦称去氧助间型霉素)
pentosuria [ˌpentəuˈsjuəriə] *n* 戊糖尿症 | **pentosuric** *a*
pentosyl [ˈpentəsil] *n* 戊糖基
pentosyltransferase [ˌpentəsilˈtrænsfəreis] *n* 戊糖基转移酶，转戊糖酶
pentoxide [penˈtɔksaid] *n* 五氧化物
pentoxifylline [ˌpentɔkˈsifilin] *n* 己酮可可碱(冠状血管扩张药)
pentrinitrol [ˌpentraiˈnaitrəul] *n* 戊硝醇(血管扩

张药)
pentulose [ˈpentjuləus] *n* 酮戊糖
pentylenetetrazol [ˌpentiliːnˈtetrəzɔl] *n* 戊四氮,戊四唑(中枢兴奋药)
penumbra [pəˈnʌmbrə] *n* 半影(①有部分照明的阴影区,它围绕本影〈umbra〉;②在 X 线摄影时结构边缘周围的模糊区) | ischemic ~ 局部缺血性半影(围绕重度局部缺血区的中度局部缺血性脑组织区,血液流入此区可能得到加强,以防止脑梗死扩散)
Penzoldt-Fisher test [ˈpenzɔld ˈfiʃə] (Franz Penzoldt; Emil Fisher) 彭佐尔德-费希尔试验(检苯酚)
Penzoldt's test, reagent [ˈpenzɔld] (Franz Penzoldt) 彭佐尔德试验、试剂(检丙酮、尿葡萄糖)
peotillomania [ˌpiːəutiləuˈmeinjə] *n* 抚阳癖;假性手淫
peotomy [piˈɔtəmi] *n* 阴茎切除术
PEP phospho*enol*pyruvate 磷酸烯醇丙酮酸; preejection period 射血前期
peplomer [ˈpepləumə] *n* (病毒)包膜子粒,膜粒
peplos [ˈpepləs] *n* 包膜(病毒外面所包被的一层脂蛋白质外膜)
pepo [ˈpiːpəu] *n* 南瓜子
peppermint [ˈpepəmint] *n* 薄荷
Pepper's syndrome (type) [ˈpepə] (William Pepper) 佩珀综合征(型)(右肾上腺发生成神经细胞瘤时,其子瘤大多局限于肝)
pepsic [ˈpepsik] *a* 消化的;胃蛋白酶的
pepsin [ˈpepsin] *n* 胃蛋白酶
pepsinate [ˈpepsineit] *vt* 胃蛋白酶处理
pepsinia [pepˈsiniə] *n* 胃蛋白酶分泌
pepsiniferous [ˌpepsiˈnifərəs] *a* 生成胃蛋白酶的,分泌胃蛋白酶的
pepsinogen [pepˈsinədʒin] *n* 胃蛋白酶原
pepsinogenous [ˌpepsiˈnɔdʒinəs] *a* 生成胃蛋白酶的
pepsinuria [ˌpepsiˈnjuəriə] *n* 胃蛋白酶尿
pepsitensin [ˌpepsiˈtensin] *n* 胃酶解血管紧张肽
pepstatin [pepˈstætin] *n* 胃蛋白酶抑制剂(治胃溃疡)
peptic [ˈpeptik], *a* 消化的;胃蛋白酶的
peptid [ˈpeptid] *n* 肽
peptidase [ˈpeptideis], **peptase** [ˈpepteis] *n* 肽酶
peptide [ˈpeptaid] *n* 肽 | corticotropin-like intermediate lobe ~ (CLIP) 中间叶促皮质样肽 / *N*-formylmethionyl ~s *N*-甲酰甲硫氨酰肽 / vasoactive intestinal ~ (VIP) 血管活性肠肽,血管活性肠多肽
peptide hydrolase [ˈpeptaid ˈhaidrəleis] 肽水解酶,肽酶
peptidergic [ˌpeptriˈdəːdʒik] *a* 肽能的
peptidoglycan [ˌpeptidəuˈglaikən] *n* 肽聚糖
peptidyl-dipeptidase [ˈpeptidil daiˈpeptideis] 肽基-二肽酶
peptidyl-dipeptidase A [ˈpeptidil daiˈpeptideis] 肽基-二肽酶 A(亦称二肽酰羧肽酶 I)
peptinotoxin [ˌpeptinəuˈtɔksin] *a* 胃消化毒素
peptization [ˌpeptaiˈzeiʃən, -tiˈz-] *n* 胶溶[作用]
Peptococcaceae [ˌpeptəukɔˈkeisiiː] *n* 消化球菌科
Peptococcus [ˌpeptəuˈkɔkəs] *n* 消化球菌属 | ~ anaerobius 厌氧消化球菌 / ~ asaccharolyticus 不解糖消化球菌 / ~ constellatus 星群消化球菌 / ~ magnus 大消化球菌
peptogenic [ˌpeptəuˈdʒenik], **peptogenous** [pepˈtɔdʒinəs] *a* 生胃蛋白酶的;生胨的;助消化的
peptohydrochloric acid [ˌpeptəuˌhaidrəˈklɔrik] 胃蛋白酶盐酸
peptolysis [pepˈtɔlisis] *n* 胨分解[作用] | **peptolytic** [peptəuˈlitik] *a* 胨分解的 *n* 解胨剂
peptone [ˈpeptəun] *n* [蛋白]胨 | casein ~, milk ~ 酪[蛋白]胨 | **peptonic** [pepˈtɔnik] *a* 胨的,含胨的
peptonize [ˈpeptənaiz] *vt* 使胨化
peptonoid [ˈpeptənɔid] *n* 类胨
peptonuria [ˌpeptəuˈnjuəriə] *n* 胨尿
Peptostreptococcus [ˌpeptəuˌstreptəuˈkɔkəs] *n* 消化链球菌属 | ~ anaerobius 厌氧消化链球菌 / ~ lanceolatus 矛形消化链球菌 / ~ micros 微小消化链球菌 / ~ parvulus 短小消化链球菌 / ~ productus 产生消化链球菌
peptotoxin [ˌpeptəuˈtɔksin] *n* 胨毒素
per [强 pəː; pə] *prep* 【拉】经,由;每
per- [前缀] 完全,彻底,非常;(化学)高,过,全
per anum [pəː ˈeinəm] 【拉】由肛
peracephalus [ˌpəːrəˈsefələs] *n* 无上体畸胎
peracetate [pəːˈræsitit] *n* 过醋酸盐
peracetic acid [pəːrəˈsiːtik] 过氧乙酸(强氧化剂)
peracid [pəːˈræsid] *n* 过酸,高酸
peracidity [ˌpəːrəˈsidəti] *n* 过酸性,高酸性
peracute [ˌpəːrəˈkjuːt] *a* 极急性的,甚剧的
Peranema [ˌperəˈniːmə] *n* 袋鞭虫属
perarticulation [ˌpəːrɑːtikjuˈleiʃən] *n* 动关节
perborate [pəːˈbɔːreit] *n* 过硼酸盐
perboric acid [pəːˈbɔːrik] 过硼酸
percentile [pəˈsentail, pəˈsentil] *a* 百分率的 *n* 百分位数
percept [ˈpəːsept] *n* 感觉,知觉;知觉对象
perception [pəˈsepʃən] *n* 知觉 | depth ~ 深度知觉 / extrasensory ~ (ESP) 超感官知觉 / facial ~ 面部定向知觉 / stereognostic ~ 实体知觉 | **~al** *a*

perceptive [pə'septiv] *a* 知觉的

perceptivity [pəːsep'tivəti] *n* 知觉,感知力;感受性

perceptorium [ˌpəːsep'tɔːriəm] *n* 感觉中枢

perchlorate [pəː'klɔːreit] *n* 高氯酸盐,过氯酸盐

perchloric acid [pəː'klɔːrik] 高氯酸,过氯酸

perchloride [pəː'klɔːraid] *n* 高氯化物

perchlormethane [ˌpəːklɔː'meθein] *n* 四氯化碳

perchlormethylformate [ˌpəːklɔːˌmeθil'fɔːmeit] *n* 双光气,聚光气(一种毒气)

perchloroethylene [pəːˌklɔːrə'eθiliːn] *n* 四氯乙烯(抗蠕虫药)

percine ['pəːsin] *n* 鲈精蛋白

percipient [pə'sipiənt] *a* 知觉的 *n* 感觉者,感知者

percolate ['pəːkəleit] *vt*, *vi* 渗漉,渗滤 *n* 渗漉液,渗出液,滤出液 | **percolation** [ˌpəːkə'leiʃən] *n* 渗漉法,渗滤

percolator ['pəːkəˌleitə] *n* 渗漉器,渗滤器

percomorph ['pəːkəmɔːf] *n*, *a* 鲈形类鱼(的)(其肝油富有维生素 A 和 D)

per contiguum [pəːkɔn'tigjum]【拉】接触,相邻

per continuum [pəːkɔn'tinjum]【拉】连续

percuss [pəː'kʌs] *vt* 敲,叩,击;叩诊

percussible [pəː'kʌsəbl] *a* 可以叩知的

percussion [pəː'kʌʃən] *n* 拍击法叩击;叩诊 | auscultatory ~ 听叩诊 / bimanual ~ 双手叩诊 / coin ~ 钱币叩诊(见 test 项下相应术语) / deep ~ 重叩诊 / drop ~, drop stroke ~ 落槌叩诊 / finger ~ 指叩诊 / immediate ~, direct ~ 直接叩诊(即不用叩诊板) / mediate ~, pleximetric ~ 间接叩诊(即使用叩诊板) / piano ~ 四指叩诊 / slapping ~ 拍叩[诊] / strip ~ 带条叩诊 / threshold ~ 阈叩诊(以手指轻叩玻璃叩诊棒,该棒的一端套一橡皮帽,置于一肋间,棒与胸壁成一角度而与欲定界的脏器边缘相平行,此法使叩诊振动局限于一小区域) / topographic ~ 定界叩诊

percussive [pəː'kʌsiv] *a* 叩诊的

percussopunctator [pəːˌkʌsəu'pʌŋkteitə] *n* 多尖刺针,梅花针

percussor [pəː'kʌsə] *n* 叩诊器

percutaneous [ˌpəːkju(ː)'teinjəs] *a* 经皮的

percuteur [ˌpəːku'təː] *n*【法】叩诊器

pereirine [pə'riːrin] *n* 拍雷林(美洲热带树树皮的一种生物碱,用作解疟、解热和补药)

perencephaly [ˌpəːren'sefəli] *n* 孔洞脑

perennial [pə'renjəl] *a* 多年生的,常年性的

Pereyra procedure (colposuspension) [pə'reirɑː] (Armand J. Pereyra) 佩雷拉操作(阴道悬吊术)(一型膀胱颈悬吊术,类似布尔赫〈Burch〉操作;缝线圈或其他材料插入膀胱颈附近的尿道旁组织,并依附于腹筋膜)

Perez's sign [pei'reiθ] (Jorje Perez) 佩雷兹征(患者将双臂举起再放下时,则在胸骨可听到摩擦音,为纵隔瘤和主动脉弓动脉瘤之征)

perfect ['pəːfikt] *a* 完全的(指真菌)

perfection [pə'fekʃən] *n* 尽善尽美;完成;改善 | **~ism** *n* 至善主义(一种人格特征,树立不可能达到的标准,最终导致沮丧和自我谴责)

perfilcon A [pəː'filkɔn] 泼费尔康 A (一种亲水性接触镜材料)

perflation [pə'fleiʃən] *n* 吹气引流法,吹入法;自然通气

perflubron [pəː'fluːbrɔn] *n* 全氟溴烷(一种溴化氟碳,用作造影剂,用于胃肠道磁共振成像,口服给药)

perfluorochemical [pəːˌfluːrərəu'kemikəl] *n* 全氟化学物质

perflutren [pəː'fluːtrən] *n* 全氟特伦(一种氟碳,诊断心脏病学和放射学中用作超声成像剂)

perforans ['pəːfərənz] *a*【拉】穿通的(肌或神经) | ~ manus 指深屈肌

perforate ['pəːfəreit] *vt*, *vi* 穿孔 ['pəːfərit] *a* 穿孔的 | **perforated** *a*

perforation [ˌpəːfə'reiʃən] *n* 穿孔

perforative ['pəːfəreitiv] *a* 能穿孔的

perforator ['pəːfəˌreitə] *n* 穿孔器

perforatorium [ˌpəːfərə'tɔːriəm] *n* 穿孔器,顶体(精子)

perforin ['pəːfərin] *n* 穿孔素

performance [pə'fɔːməns] *n* 作业,操作;性能;行为表现 | myocadial ~ 心肌工作能力

perfrication [ˌpəːfrai'keiʃən] *n* (用软膏)涂擦,擦药法

perfrigeration [pəˌfridʒə'reiʃən] *n* 冻疮

perfusate [pə'fjuːzeit] *n* 灌注液

perfuse [pə(ː)'fjuːz] *vt* 洒;灌注;使充满 | **perfusion** [pə(ː)'fjuːʒən] *n* 洒;灌注;灌注液

perfusionist [pə(ː)'fjuːʒənist] *n* 灌注者(心肺分流术时操作心肺机的技术人员)

pergolide mesylate ['pəːgəlaid 'mesileit] 甲磺培高利特(多巴胺激动药)

perhexiline maleate [pə'heksiliːn] 马来酸哌克昔林(冠状动脉扩张药)

peri- [前缀]周围,周

periacetabular [ˌperiˌæsə'tæbjulə] *a* 髋臼周围的

periacinal [ˌperi'æsinl], **periacinous** [ˌperi'æsinəs] *a* 腺泡周的

periadenitis [ˌperiˌædi'naitis] *n* 腺周炎

periadventitial [ˌperiˌædven'tiʃəl] *a* 外膜周的

perialienitis [ˌperiˌeiljə'naitis] *n* 异物周炎

periampullary [ˌperi'æmpuˌləri] *a* 壶腹周围的

perianal [ˌperi'einl] *a* 肛周的

periangiitis [ˌperiændʒiˈaitis] *n* 血管周炎
periangiocholitis [ˌperiˌændʒiəukəuˈlaitis] *n* 胆管周炎
periangioma [ˌperiændʒiˈəumə] *n* 血管周瘤
perianth [ˈperiænθ] *n* 花被(包括花萼和花冠)
periaortic [ˌperieiˈɔːtik] *a* 主动脉周的
periaortitis [ˌperiˌeiɔːˈtaitis] *n* 主动脉周炎
periapex [ˌperiˈeipeks] *n* 根尖周组织(牙)
periapical [ˌperiˈæpikəl] *a* 根尖周的
periappendicitis [ˌperiəˌpendiˈsaitis] *n* 阑尾周炎
periappendicular [ˌperiˌæpenˈdikjulə] *a* 阑尾周的
periapt [ˈperiæpt] *n* 祛病符,护身符,避邪符
periaqueductal [ˌperiˌækwiˈdʌktl] *a* 水管周[围]的
periarterial [ˌperiɑːˈtiəriəl] *a* 动脉周的
periarteritis [ˌperiɑːtəˈraitis] *n* 动脉外膜炎、动脉周炎
periarthric [ˌperiˈɑːθrik], **periarticular** [ˌperiɑːˈtikjulə] *a* 关节周的
periarthritis [ˌperiɑːˈθraitis] *n* 关节周围炎
periatrial [ˌperiˈeitriəl] *a* 心房周的
periauricular [ˌperiɔːˈrikjulə] *a* 耳郭周的;心房周的
periaxial [ˌperiˈæksiəl] *a* 轴周的
periaxillary [ˌperiˈæksiləri] *a* 腋窝周的
periaxonal [ˌperiˈæksɔnl] *a* 轴突周的
periblast [ˈperiblæst] *n* 胚周区,胚周层
peribronchial [ˌperiˈbrɔŋkiəl] *a* 支气管周的
peribronchiolar [ˌperibrɔŋkiˈəulə] *a* 细支气管周的
peribronchiolitis [ˌperiˌbrɔŋkiəuˈlaitis] *n* 细支气管周炎
peribronchitis [ˌperibrɔŋˈkaitis] *n* 支气管周炎
peribulbar [ˌperiˈbʌlbə] *a* 眼球周的
peribursal [ˌperiˈbəːsəl] *a* 黏液囊周的
pericaliceal, **pericalyceal** [ˌperiˌkæliˈsiːəl] *a* 肾盏周的
pericallosal [ˌperikəˈləusəl] *n* 胼胝体周的
pericanalicular [ˌperiˌkænəˈlikjulə] *a* 小管周的
pericapillary [ˌperiˈkæpiˌləri] *a* 毛细管周的
pericapsular [ˌperiˈkæpsjulə] *a* 囊周的,关节囊周的
pericardial [ˌperiˈkɑːdiəl], **pericardiac** [ˌperiˈkɑːdiæk] *a* 心包的
pericardiectomy [ˌperiˌkɑːdiˈektəmi], **pericardectomy** [ˌperikɑːˈdektəmi] *n* 心包切除术
pericardiocentesis [ˌperiˌkɑːdiəusenˈtiːsis], **pericardicentesis** [ˌperiˌkɑːdisenˈtiːsis] *n* 心包穿刺术
pericardiolysis [ˌperiˌkɑːdiˈɔlisis] *n* 心包松解术
pericardiomediastinitis [ˌperiˌkɑːdiəuˌmiːdiæstiˈnaitis] *n* 心包纵隔炎
pericardiophrenic [ˌperiˌkɑːdiəuˈfrenik] *a* 心包膈的
pericardiopleural [ˌperiˌkɑːdiəuˈpluərəl] *a* 心包胸膜的
pericardiorrhaphy [ˌperiˌkɑːdiˈɔrəfi] *n* 心包缝合术
pericardioscopy [ˌperiˌkɑːdiˈɔskɔpi] *n* 心包镜检查
pericardiostomy [ˌperiˌkɑːdiˈɔstəmi] *n* 心包造口术
pericardiotomy [ˌperiˌkɑːdiˈɔtəmi], **pericardotomy** [ˌperikɑːˈdɔtəmi] *n* 心包切开术
pericarditis [ˌperikɑːˈdaitis] *n* 心包炎 | adhesive ~ 粘连性心包炎 / carcinomatous ~ 癌性心包炎 / constrictive ~ 缩窄性心包炎 / ~ externa et interna 内外层心包炎 / ~ villosa 绒毛状心包炎,绒毛心 | **pericarditic** [ˌperikɑːˈditik] *a*
pericardium [ˌperiˈkɑːdiəm] ([复] **pericardia** [ˌperiˈkɑːdiə]) *n* 心包 | adherent ~ 粘连性心包 / bread-and-butter ~ 黄油面包状心包,纤维蛋白性心包 / fibrous ~ 心包纤维层(壁层) / parietal ~ 心包壁层 / serous ~ 心包浆膜层(脏层) / shaggy ~ 粗糙心包 / visceral ~, cardiac ~ 心包脏层(心外膜)
pericarp [ˈperikɑːp] *n* 果皮
pericaryon [ˌperiˈkæriɔn] *n* 核周体
pericecal [ˌperiˈsiːkəl] *a* 盲肠周[围]的
pericecitis [ˌperisiˈsaitis] *n* 盲肠周炎
pericellular [ˌperiˈseljulə] *a* 细胞周的
pericemental [ˌperisiˈmentl] *a* 牙周膜的
pericementitis [ˌperiˌsiːmenˈtaitis] *n* 牙周膜炎 | apical ~ 根尖牙周膜炎,根尖脓肿
pericementoclasia [ˌperisiˌmentəuˈkleiziə] *n* 牙周膜溃坏
pericementum [ˌperisiˈmentəm] *n* 牙周膜
pericentral [ˌperiˈsentrəl] *a* 中枢周[围]的
pericentriolar [ˌperiˌsentriˈəulə] *a* 中心粒周的
pericephalic [ˌperisəˈfælik] *a* 头周的
pericholangitis [ˌperiˌkəulænˈdʒaitis] *n* 胆管周围炎
pericholecystitis [ˌperiˌkəulisisˈtaitis] *n* 胆囊周炎 | gaseous ~ 气肿性胆囊炎
perichondritis [ˌperikɔnˈdraitis] *n* 软骨膜炎
perichondrium [ˌperiˈkɔndriəm] *n* 软骨膜 | **perichondrial** *a*
perichondroma [ˌperikɔnˈdrəumə] *n* 软骨膜瘤
perichord [ˈperikɔːd] *n* 脊索膜 | **~al** [ˌperiˈkɔːdl] *a*
perichoroidal [ˌperikɔːˈrɔidl], **perichorioidal** [ˌperiˌkɔːriˈɔidl] *a* 脉络膜周的,脉络膜外的

perichrome [ˈperikrəum] *n* 周染细胞(一种神经细胞,在此细胞内尼氏〈Nissl〉体成行排列在细胞膜下)
periclasia [ˌperiˈkleiziə] *n* 牙周溃坏
pericolic [ˌperiˈkɔlik] *a* 结肠周的
pericolitis [ˌperikɔˈlaitis] *n* 结肠周炎 | ~ dextra 升结肠周炎 / membranous ~ 膜性结肠周炎 / ~ sinistra 降结肠周炎 | **pericolonitis** [ˌperiˌkəuləˈnaitis] *n*
pericolpitis [ˌperikɔlˈpaitis] *n* 阴道周炎
periconchal [ˌperiˈkɔŋkəl] *a* 耳甲周的
periconchitis [ˌperikɔŋˈkaitis] *n* 眶骨膜炎
pericorneal [ˌperiˈkɔːniəl] *a* 角膜周的
pericoronal [ˌperiˈkɔrənl] *a* (牙)冠周的
pericoronitis [ˌperiˌkɔrəˈnaitis] *n* 冠周炎
pericoxitis [ˌperikɔkˈsaitis] *n* 髋关节周炎
pericranitis [ˌperikreiˈnaitis] *n* 颅骨膜炎
pericranium [ˌperiˈkreinjəm] ([复] **pericrania** [periˈkreinjə]) *n* 颅骨膜 | **pericranial** *a*
pericryptal [ˌperiˈkriptəl] *a* 隐窝周的
pericycle [ˌperiˈsaikl] *n* 中柱鞘(植物)
pericystic [ˌperiˈsistik] *a* 囊周的;膀胱周的
pericystitis [ˌperisisˈtaitis] *n* 囊周炎;膀胱周炎
pericystium [ˌperiˈsistiəm] *n* 囊周膜
pericyte [ˈperisait] *n* 周细胞
pericytial [ˌperiˈsaiʃəl] *a* 细胞周的
pericytoma [ˌperisaiˈtəumə] *n* 周皮细胞瘤
peridectomy [ˌperiˈdektəmi] *n* 球结膜环状切除术
perideferentitis [ˌperiˌdefərənˈtaitis] *n* 输精管周炎
peridendritic [ˌperidenˈdritik] *a* 树状突周的
peridens [ˈperidens] *n* 牙周牙,牙弓外牙
peridental [ˌperiˈdentl] *a* 牙周的,牙周膜的
peridentium [ˌperiˈdenʃiəm] *n* 牙周组织
periderm [ˈperidəːm] *n* 周皮; | ~**al** [ˌperiˈdəːməl], ~**ic** [ˌperiˈdəːmik] *a*
peridesmic [ˌperiˈdezmik] *a* 韧带周的;韧带膜的
peridesmitis [ˌperidezˈmaitis] *n* 韧带膜炎
peridesmium [ˌperiˈdezmiəm] *n* 韧带膜
perididymis [ˌperiˈdidimis] *n* 睾丸鞘膜
perididymitis [ˌperiˌdidiˈmaitis] *n* 睾丸鞘膜炎
peridium [pəˈridiəm] ([复] **peridia** [pəˈridiə]) *n* 包被
peridiverticular [ˌperiˌdaivəːˈtikjulə] *a* 憩室周的
peridiverticulitis [ˌperiˌdaivətikjuˈlaitis] *n* 憩室周炎
peridontium [ˌperiˈdɔnʃiəm] *n* 牙周组织
peridontoclasia [ˌperiˌdɔntəuˈkleiziə] *n* 牙周组织溃坏
periductal [ˌperiˈdʌktl], **periductile** [ˌperiˈdʌktail] *a* 导管周的
periduodenitis [ˌperiˌdju(ː)əudiˈnaitis] *n* 十二指肠周炎
peridural [ˌperiˈdjuərəl] *a* 硬膜外的
peridurogram [ˌperiˈdjuərəgræm] *n* 硬膜外造影[照]片
peridurography [ˌperidjuəˈrɔgrəfi] *n* 硬膜外造影[术]
periencephalitis [ˌperienˌsefəˈlaitis] *n* 脑表层炎
periencephalography [ˌperienˌsefəˈlɔgrəfi] *n* 脑膜造影[术]
periencephalomeningitis [ˌperienˌsefələuˌmeninˈdʒaitis] *n* 脑皮质脑膜炎
perienteric [ˌperienˈterik] *a* 肠周的
perienteritis [ˌperiˌentəˈraitis] *n* 肠周炎,肠腹膜炎
perienteron [ˌperiˈentərɔn] *n* 肠周腔(胚)
periependymal [ˌperieˈpendiməl] *a* 室管膜周的
periepithelioma [ˌperiˌepiθiːliˈəumə] *n* 周皮上皮瘤,肾上腺皮质癌
periesophageal [ˌperiiːˈsɔfədʒiəl] *a* 食管周的
periesophagitis [ˌperiiːˌsɔfəˈdʒaitis] *n* 食管周炎
perifascicular [ˌperifəˈsikjulə] *a* 束周的(神经或肌纤维束周的)
perifistular [ˌperiˈfistjulə] *a* 瘘管周的
perifocal [ˌperiˈfəukəl] *a* 病灶周的
perifollicular [ˌperifəˈlikjulə] *a* 滤泡周的(一般指毛囊周的)
perifolliculitis [ˌperifəˌlikjuˈlaitis] *n* 毛囊周围炎 | ~ capitis abscedens et suffodiens 头部脓肿性穿掘性毛囊周围炎 / superficial pustular ~ 浅表性脓疱性毛囊周围炎
perifornical [ˌperiˈfɔːnikəl] *a* 穹窿周的
perifusate [ˌperiˈfjuːseit] *n* 周围灌注液
perifuse [ˌperiˈfjuːz] *vt* 周围灌注(将悬浮的器官器、细胞、细胞簇或组织所有表面灌注洗液)
perifusion [ˌperiˈfjuːʒən] *n* 周围灌注
perigangliitis [ˌperigæŋgliˈaitis] *n* 神经节周炎
periganglionic [ˌperiˌgæŋgliˈɔnik] *a* 神经节周[围]的
perigastric [ˌperiˈgæstrik] *a* 胃周的
perigastritis [ˌperigæsˈtraitis] *n* 胃周炎,胃腹膜炎
perigemmal [ˌperiˈdʒeməl] *a* 味蕾周的
periglandular [ˌperiˈglændjulə] *a* 腺周的
periglandulitis [ˌperiˌglændjuˈlaitis] *n* 腺周炎
periglial [ˌperiˈglaiəl] *a* 神经胶质细胞周的
periglossitis [ˌperiglɔˈsaitis] *n* 舌周炎
periglottic [ˌperiˈglɔtik] *a* 舌周的
periglottis [ˌperiˈglɔtis] *n* 舌黏膜
perigraft [ˈperigræft] *a* 移植物周围的
perihepatic [ˌperihiˈpætik] *a* 肝周的
perihepatitis [ˌperiˌhepəˈtaitis] *n* 肝周炎 | ~

chronica hyperplastica 慢性增生性肝周炎,糖衣肝,结霜样肝 / gonococcal ~ 淋球菌性肝周炎

perihernial [ˌperiˈhəːnjəl] *a* 疝周的

perihilar [ˌperiˈhailə] *a* 门周的(如肺门周围的)

peri-insular [ˌperiˈinsjulə] *a* 岛周的(尤指脑岛周围的)

peri-islet [ˌperi ˈailit] *a* 胰岛周围的

perijejunitis [ˌperiˌdʒidʒuːˈnaitis] *n* 空肠周炎

perikaryon [ˌperiˈkæriɔn] ([复] **perikarya** [ˌperiˈkæriə]) *n* 核周体

perikeratic [ˌperikəˈrætik] *a* 角膜周的

perikyma [ˌperiˈkaimə] ([复] **perikymata** [ˌperiˈkaimətə]) *n* 釉面横纹(恒牙)

perilabyrinth [ˌperiˈlæbərinθ] *n* 迷路周组织

perilabyrinthitis [ˌperiˌlæbərinˈθaitis] *n* 迷路周炎

perilaryngeal [ˌperiləˈrindʒiəl] *a* 喉周的

perilaryngitis [ˌperiˌlærinˈdʒaitis] *n* 喉周炎

perilemma [ˌperiˈlemə] *n* 外膜

perilenticular [ˌperilenˈtikjulə] *a* 晶状体周的(眼)

perilesional [ˌperiˈliːʒənl] *a* 损害周围的,病灶周围的

periligamentous [ˌperiˌligəˈmentəs] *a* 韧带周的

Perilla [pəˈrilə] *n* 紫苏属

perilobar [ˌperiˈləubə] *a* 叶周的

perilobulitis [ˌperilɔbjuˈlaitis] *n* 肺小叶周炎

perilymph [ˈperilimf], **perilympha** [ˌperiˈlimfə] *n* 外淋巴(内耳骨迷路与膜迷路之间的液体)

perilymphadenitis [ˌperiˌlimfædiˈnaitis] *n* 淋巴结周炎

perilymphangeal [ˌperilimˈfændʒiəl] *a* 淋巴管周的

perilymphangitis [ˌperiˌlimfænˈdʒaitis] *n* 淋巴管周炎

perilymphatic [ˌperilimˈfætik] *a* 外淋巴的;淋巴管周的

perimandibular [ˌperimænˈdibjulə] *a* 下颌骨周的

perimastitis [ˌperimæsˈtaitis] *n* 乳腺周炎,乳腺间质炎

perimeatal [ˌperimiːˈeitəl] *a* 道周的

perimedullary [ˌperiˈmedələri] *a* 髓周的(延髓或骨髓)

perimeningitis [ˌperiˌmeninˈdʒaitis] *n* 硬脑膜炎,硬脊膜炎

perimenopause [ˌperiˈmenəpɔːs] *n* 围绝经期 | **perimenopausal** [ˌperiˌmenəuˈpɔːzəl] *a*

perimeter [pəˈrimitə] *n* 周,周边,周界线;周长;视野计 | bed ~ 床边视野计 / dental ~ 牙周计

perimetric [ˌperiˈmetrik] *a* 视野计的;子宫周的;子宫外膜的 | **~al** *a*

perimetritis [ˌperimiˈtraitis] *n* 子宫外膜炎,子宫浆膜炎 | **perimetritic** [ˌperimiˈtritik] *a*

perimetrium [ˌperiˈmiːtriəm] *n* 子宫外膜,子宫浆膜

perimetrosalpingitis [ˌperiˌmetrəuˌsælpinˈdʒaitis] *n* 子宫输卵管周炎 | encapsulating ~ 包围性子宫输卵管周炎

perimetry [pəˈrimitri] *n* 视野检查法

perimolysis [ˌperiˈmɔlisis] *n* 牙冠硬质崩解

perimycin [periˈmaisin] *n* 真菌霉素,表霉素

perimyelis [ˌperiˈmaiəlis] *n* 髓周膜,骨内膜

perimyelitis [ˌperiˌmaiəˈlaitis] *n* 骨内膜炎;脊髓膜炎

perimyelography [ˌperiˌmaiəˈlɔgrəfi] *n* 脊髓周造影[术]

perimylolysis [ˌperimiˈlɔlisis] *n* 牙冠硬质崩解

perimyocarditis [ˌperiˌmaiəukɑːˈdaitis] *n* 心包心肌炎

perimyoendocarditis [ˌperiˌmaiəuˌendəukɑːˈdaitis] *n* 心包[心]肌[心]内膜炎,全心炎

perimyositis [ˌperiˌmaiəuˈsaitis] *n* 肌周炎

perimysiitis [ˌperiˌmisiˈaitis], **perimysitis** [ˌperimiˈsaitis] *n* 肌束膜炎

perimysium [ˌperiˈmisiəm] ([复] **perimysia** [periˈmisiə]) *n* 肌束膜 | **perimysial** [ˌperiˈmisiəl] *a*

perinatal [ˌperiˈneitl] *a* 围生期的(医学统计学上认为开始于妊娠完成28周,及终止于产后1~4周不等)

perinatology [ˌperinəˈtɔlədʒi] *n* 围生医学 | **perinatologist** *n* 围生医学家,围生期医生

perindopril [pəˈrindəupril] *n* 培哚普利(抗高血压药)

perineal [ˌperiˈniːəl] *a* 会阴的

perineocele [ˌperiˈniːəsiːl] *n* 会阴疝

perineometer [ˌperiniˈɔmitə] *n* 会阴收缩力计

perineoplasty [ˌperiˈniːəˌplæsti] *n* 会阴成形术

perineorrhaphy [ˌperiniˈɔrəfi] *n* 会阴修复术

perineoscrotal [ˌperiniːəuˈskrəutl] *a* 会阴阴囊的

perineotomy [ˌperiniˈɔtəmi] *n* 会阴切开术

perineovaginal [ˌperiˌniːəuˈvædʒinəl] *a* 会阴阴道的

perineovaginorectal [ˌperiˌniːəuˌvæˌdʒinəuˈrektl] *a* 会阴阴道直肠的

perineovulvar [ˌperiˌniːəuˈvʌlvə] *a* 会阴外阴的

perinephric [ˌperiˈnefrik] *a* 肾周围的

perinephritis [ˌperineˈfraitis] *n* 肾周围炎 | **perinephritic** [ˌperineˈfritik] *a*

perinephrium [ˌperiˈnefriəm] *n* 肾周膜,肾外膜 | **perinephrial** *a*

perineum [ˌperiˈniːəm] ([复] **perinea** [ˌperiˈniːə]) *n* 会阴

perineural [ˌperiˈnjuərəl] *a* 神经周的
perineuritis [ˌperinjuəˈraitis] *n* 神经束膜炎 | **perineuritic** [ˌpərinjuəˈritik] *a*
perineurium [ˌperiˈnjuəriəm] *n* 神经束膜 | **perineurial** *a*
perinodal [ˌperiˈnəudəl] *a* 结节周[围]的
perinuclear [ˌperiˈnjuːkliə] *a* 核周的
periocular [ˌperiˈɔkjulə] *a* 眼周的
period [ˈpiəriəd] *n* 期,时期 | absolute refractory ~ 绝对不应期(指神经或肌纤维对刺激不能反应) / child-bearing ~ 育龄期 / G_1 ~ DNA 合成前期 / G_2 ~ DNA 合成后期 / gestational ~ 妊娠期 / half-life ~ 半衰期(放射性物质) / lag ~ 迟滞期,延缓期(细菌培养) / latency ~ 潜伏期;性成熟前期 / latent ~ 潜伏期 / M ~ 有丝分裂期 / menstrual ~, monthly ~ 月经期 / postsphygmic ~, ~ of isometric relaxation 脉搏后期,等长舒张期(心) / presphygmic ~, ~ of isometric contraction 脉搏前期,等长收缩期(心) / quarantine ~ 检疫期,留验期 / refractory ~ 不应期 / relative refractory ~ 相对不应期 / S ~ DNA 合成期 / safe ~ 安全期(避孕) / silent ~ 静止期,和缓期 / sphygmic ~, ejection ~ 脉搏期,射血期(心室)
periodate [pəˈraiədeit] *n* 过碘酸盐,高碘酸盐
periodic [ˌpiəriˈɔdik] *a* 周期性的,间发性的,定期的
periodic acid [ˌperaiˈɔdik] 过碘酸,高碘酸
periodicity [ˌpiəriəˈdisəti] *n* 周期性,间发性 | filarial ~ 丝虫周期性 / lunar ~ (生殖现象的)月周期性 / malarial ~ 疟疾周期性
periodontal [ˌperiɔˈdɔntl] *a* 牙周的,牙周膜的
periodontics [ˌperiɔˈdɔntiks], **periodontia** [ˌperiɔˈdɔnʃiə] *n* 牙周病学 | **periodontic** *a* **periodontist** *n* 牙周病学家
periodontitis [ˌperiɔdɔnˈtaitis] *n* 牙周炎 | apical ~ 根尖牙周炎
periodontium [ˌperiɔˈdɔnʃiəm] *n* 牙周组织,牙周膜,牙槽骨膜
periodontoclasia [ˌperiɔdɔntəuˈkleiziə] *n* 牙周溃坏
periodontology [ˌperiɔdɔnˈtɔlədʒi] *n* 牙周病学
periodontopathy [ˌperiɔdɔnˈtɔpəθi] *n* 牙周病
periodontosis [ˌperiɔdɔnˈtəusis] *n* 牙周变性
periomphalic [ˌperiɔmˈfælik] *a* 脐周的
perionychia [ˌperiɔˈnikiə] *n* 甲周脓炎,甲周炎
perionychium [ˌperiɔˈnikiəm] *n* 甲周皮,甲周表皮
perionyx [ˌperiˈəuniks] *n* [指]甲上皮残遗(胎儿)
perioophoritis [ˌperiˌəuɔfəˈraitis] *n* 卵巢周炎
perioophorosalpingitis [ˌperiəuˌɔfərəuˌsælpinˈdʒaitis] *n* 卵巢输卵管周炎
perioothecitis [periˌəuəθiˈsaitis] *n* 卵巢周炎
perioperative [ˌperiˈɔpərətiv] *a* 手术前后的,手术期间的(自住院手术至出院)
periophthalmic [ˌperiɔfˈθælmik] *a* 眼周的
periophthalmitis [ˌperiˌɔfθælˈmaitis], **periophthalmia** [ˌperiɔfˈθælmiə] *n* 眼周[组织]炎
periople [ˈperiˌɔpl] *n* 蹄外膜
perioptometry [ˌperiɔpˈtɔmitri] *n* 视野检查法
perioral [ˌperiˈɔːrəl] *a* 口周的
periorbit(a) [ˌperiˈɔːbit(ə)] *n* 眶骨膜
periorbital [ˌperiˈɔːbitəl] *a* 眶周的;眶骨膜的
periorbititis [ˌperiˌɔːbiˈtaitis] *n* 眶骨膜炎
periorchitis [ˌperiɔːˈkaitis] *n* 睾丸鞘膜炎
periorchium [ˌperiˈɔːkiəm] *n* 睾丸鞘膜
periost [ˈperiɔst] *n* 骨膜
periosteal [ˌperiˈɔstiəl] *a* 骨膜的
periosteitis [ˌperiɔstiˈaitis] *n* 骨膜炎
periosteoedema [ˌperiˌɔstiəui(ː)ˈdiːmə], **periosteodema** [ˌperiˌɔstiəuˈdiːmə] *n* 骨膜水肿
periosteoma [ˌperiɔstiˈəumə] *n* 骨膜瘤
periosteomyelitis [ˌperiˌɔstiəuˌmaiəˈlaitis], **periosteomedullitis** [ˌperiˌɔstiəuˌmedjuˈlaitis] *n* 全骨炎;骨膜骨髓炎
periosteophyte [ˌperiˈɔstiəfait] *n* 骨膜骨赘
periosteorrhaphy [ˌperiˌɔstiˈɔrəfi] *n* 骨膜缝合术
periosteosis [ˌperiˌɔstiˈəusis] *n* 骨膜瘤形成
periosteotome [ˌperiˈɔstiətəum] *n* 骨膜刀
periosteotomy [ˌperiˌɔstiˈɔtəmi] *n* 骨膜切开术
periosteum [ˌperiˈɔstiəm] *n* 骨外膜 | alveolar ~ 牙槽骨外膜,牙周膜 | **periosteous** *a*
periostitis [ˌperiɔsˈtaitis] *n* 骨膜炎
periostoma [ˌperiɔsˈtəumə] *n* 骨膜瘤
periostomedullitis [ˌperiˌɔstəuˌmedjuˈlaitis] *n* 全骨炎;骨膜骨髓炎
periostosis [ˌperiɔsˈtəusis] *n* 骨膜骨赘形成 | hyperplastic ~ 婴儿骨外层肥厚
periostosteitis [ˌperiɔsˌtɔstiˈaitis] *n* 骨膜骨炎
periostotome [ˌperiˈɔstətəum] *n* 骨膜刀
periostotomy [ˌperiɔsˈtɔtəmi] *n* 骨膜切开术
periotic [ˌperiˈɔtik] *a* 耳周的(尤指内耳周的) *n* 耳周骨
periovaritis [ˌperiˌəuvəˈraitis] *n* 卵巢周炎
periovular [ˌperiˈəuvjulə] *a* 卵周的
peripachymeningitis [ˌperiˌpækiˌmeninˈdʒaitis] *n* 硬脑膜外周炎,硬脊膜外周炎
peripancreatic [ˌperiˌpæŋkriˈætik] *a* 胰周的
peripancreatitis [ˌperiˌpæŋkriəˈtaitis] *n* 胰周炎
peripapillary [ˌperiˈpæpiləri] *a* 视乳头周[围]的
peripartum [ˌperiˈpɑːtəm] *n* 分娩前后,围生期
peripatellar [ˌperipəˈtelə] *a* 髌骨周的

peripatetic [ˌperipəˈtetik] *a* 逍遥的,游走的
peripelvic [ˌperiˈpelvik] *a* 肾盂周的
peripenial [ˌperiˈpiːniəl] *a* 阴茎周的
peripericarditis [ˌperiˌperikɑːˈdaitis] *n* 心包周炎
periphacitis [ˌperifəˈsaitis], **periphakitis** [ˌperifəˈkaitis] *n* 晶状体囊炎
peripharyngeal [ˌperifəˈrindʒiəl] *a* 咽周的
peripherad [pəˈrifəræd] *ad* 向外周,向周围,向末梢
peripheral [pəˈrifərəl], **peripheric** [ˌperiˈferik] *a* 外周的,周围的,末梢的 | **~ly** *ad*
peripheralis [pəˌrifəˈreilis] *a*【拉】外周的,周围的,末梢的
peripheraphose [pəˈrifərəfəus] *n* 外周性影幻视
periphericus [ˌperiˈferikəs] *a*【拉】外周的,周围的,末梢的
pripherocentral [pəˌrifərəuˈsentrəl] *a* 外周中枢性的
peripheroceptor [pəˌrifərəuˈseptə] *n* 外周感受器
pripheromittor [pəˌrifərəuˈmitə] *n* 周围传器,外周传器
peripherophose [pəˈrifərəfəuz] *n* 外周性光幻视
periphery [pəˈrifəri] *n* 外周,周围
periphlebitis [ˌperifliˈbaitis] *n* 静脉周炎 | **periphlebitic** [ˌperifliˈbitik] *a*
periphoria [ˌperiˈfəuriə] *n* 旋向隐斜视,旋转隐斜视
periphrastic [ˌperiˈfræstik] *a* 啰嗦话的,赘语的(常见于精神分裂症患者的言语和书写)
periphrenitis [ˌperifriˈnaitis] *n* 膈周炎
Periplaneta [ˌperipləˈniːtə] *n* 大蠊属
periplasm [ˈperiplæzəm] *n* 周质,胞质 | **~ic** [ˌperiˈplæsmik] *a*
peripleural [ˌperiˈpluərəl] *a* 胸膜周的
peripleuritis [ˌperipluəˈraitis] *n* 胸膜周炎
periplocin [ˌperiˈpləusin] *n* 杠柳苷,萝摩毒苷(强心药,作用同洋地黄)
periplocymarin [ˌperipləuˈsaimərin] *n* 杠柳苦苷,萝摩苦苷
periplogenin [ˌperiˈplɔdʒinin] *n* 杠柳苷元,萝摩毒苷元
peripneumonia [ˌperinju(ː)ˈməunjə], **peripneumonitis** [ˌperiˌnjuːməuˈnaitis] *n* 肺胸膜炎,胸膜肺炎
peripolar [ˌperiˈpəulə] *a* 极周的
peripolesis [ˌperipəˈliːsis] *n* 周边运动,集合现象(淋巴细胞聚集在巨噬细胞周围的现象)
periporitis [ˌperipəˈraitis] *n* 汗孔周炎
periportal [ˌperiˈpɔːtl] *a* 门静脉周的
periproctic [ˌperiˈprɔktik] *a* 直肠周的
periproctitis [ˌperiprɔkˈtaitis] *n* 直肠周炎
periprostatic [ˌperiprɔsˈtætik] *a* 前列腺周的
periprostatitis [ˌperiˌprɔstəˈtaitis] *n* 前列腺周炎
periprosthetic [ˌperiprɔsˈθetik] *a* 假体周的
peripyema [ˌperipaiˈiːmə] *n* 牙周脓溢
peripylephlebitis [ˌperiˌpailifliˈbaitis] *n* 门静脉周炎
peripyloric [ˌperipaiˈlɔːrik] *a* 幽门周的
periradicular [ˌperirəˈdikjulə] *a* 根周的(尤指牙根周围的)
perirectal [ˌperiˈrektl] *a* 直肠周的
perirectitis [ˌperirekˈtaitis] *n* 直肠周炎
perirenal [ˌperiˈriːnl] *a* 肾周的
perirhinal [ˌperiˈrainl] *a* 鼻周的
perirhizoclasia [ˌperiˌraizəuˈkleisiə] *n* (牙)根周溃坏
perisalpingitis [ˌperiˌsælpinˈdʒaitis] *n* 输卵管周炎
perisalpingo-ovaritis [ˌperiˌsælpiŋgəu ˌəuvəˈraitis] *n* 输卵管卵巢周炎
perisalpinx [ˌperiˈsælpiŋks] *n* 输卵管腹膜
perisclerium [ˌperiˈskliəriəm] *n* 骨化软骨膜
periscopic [ˌperiˈskɔpik] *a* 大角度的,周视的(指显微透镜和眼镜透镜)
perisigmoiditis [ˌperiˌsigmɔiˈdaitis] *n* 乙状结肠周炎
perisinuous [ˌperiˈsinjuəs] *a* 窦周的
perisinusitis [ˌperiˌsainəˈsaitis], **perisinuitis** [ˌperiˌsainjuˈaitis] *n* 窦周炎
perisinusoidal [ˌperiˌsainəˈsɔidəl] *a* 窦周的
perispermatitis [ˌperiˌspəːməˈtaitis] *n* 精索周炎
perisplanchnic [ˌperiˈsplæŋknik] *a* 内脏周的
perisplanchnitis [ˌperisplæŋkˈnaitis] *n* 内脏周炎
perisplenic [ˌperiˈsplenik] *a* 脾周的
perisplenitis [ˌperispliˈnaitis] *n* 脾周炎
perispondylic [ˌperispɔnˈdilik] *a* 椎骨周的
perispondylitis [ˌperiˌspɔndiˈlaitis] *n* 椎骨周炎
Perisporiaceae [ˌperiˌspɔːriˈeisiiː] *n* 暗绒菌科
Perissodactyla [pəˌrisəuˈdæktilə] *n* 奇蹄目
perissodactylous [pəˌrisəuˈdæktiləs] *a* 奇[数]指的,奇[数]趾的
peristalsis [ˌperiˈstælsis] ([复] **peristalses** [ˌperiˈstælsiːz]) *n* 蠕动 | mass ~ 集团蠕动 / retrograde ~, reversed ~ 逆蠕动 | **peristaltic** [ˌperiˈstæltik] *a* / **peristaltically** *ad*
peristaltin [ˌperiˈstæltin] *n* 波希鼠李苷
peristaphyline [ˌperiˈstæfilain, -lin] *a* 悬雍垂周的
peristasis [pəˈristəsis] *n* 环境;初期淤滞(炎症变化的一个阶段)
peristomal [ˌperiˈstəuməl] *a* 口周的
peristomatous [ˌperiˈstəumətəs] *a* 口周的
peristome [ˈperistəum], **peristoma** [periˈst-

əumə] *n* 围口部；壳口，口缘（原生动物）| **peristomial** [ˌperiˈstəumiəl] *a*
peristrumitis [ˌperistruˈmaitis] *n* 甲状腺肿周炎
peristrumous [ˌperiˈstruməs] *a* 甲状腺肿周的
perisylvian [ˌperiˈsilviən] *a* 西尔维厄斯裂周的，大脑外侧沟周的
perisynovial [ˌperisiˈnəuviəl] *a* 滑膜周的
perisyringitis [ˌperiˌsirinˈdʒaitis] *n* 汗腺管周炎 | ~ chronica nasi 鼻红粒病
perisystolic [ˌperisisˈtɔlik] *a*（心）收缩前期的；（心）收缩前的
peritectomy [ˌperiˈtektəmi] *n* 球结膜环状切除术
peritendineum [ˌperitenˈdiniəm] *n* 腱束膜
peritendinitis [ˌperiˌtendiˈnaitis], **peritenonitis** [ˌperiˌtenəˈnaitis], **peritenontitis** [ˌperiˌtenənˈtaitis] *n* 腱鞘炎
peritendinous [ˌperiˈtendinəs] *a* 腱鞘周的
peritenon [ˌperiˈtenɔn] *n* 腱鞘
peritenoneum [ˌperiˌtenəuˈniːəm] *n* 腱鞘
perithecium [ˌperiˈθiːsiəm] *n* 子囊壳 | **perithecial** *a*
perithelioma [ˌperiˌθiːliˈəumə] *n* 周皮瘤，血管外皮细胞瘤
perithelium [ˌperiˈθiːljəm] *n* 周皮 | **perithelial** *a*
perithoracic [ˌperiθɔːˈræsik] *a* 胸周的
perithyroiditis [ˌperiˌθairɔiˈdaitis], **perithyreoiditis** [ˌperiˌθairiɔiˈdaitis] *n* 甲状腺囊炎
peritomist [pəˈritəmist] *n* 包皮环切术者
peritomize [pəˈritəmaiz] *vt* 球结膜环状切开；包皮环切
peritomy [pəˈritəmi] *n* 球结膜环状切开术；包皮环切术
peritone(o)- [构词成分]腹膜
peritoneal [ˌperitəuˈniːəl] *a* 腹膜的
peritonealgia [ˌperiˌtəuniˈældʒiə] *n* 腹膜痛
peritonealize [ˌperitəuˈniːəlaiz] *vt* 用腹膜被覆
peritoneocentesis [ˌperiˌtəuniəusenˈtiːsis] *n* 腹腔穿刺[术]
peritoneoclysis [ˌperiˌtəuniəuˈklaisis] *n* 腹[膜]腔输液术
peritoneography [ˌperitəuniˈɔgrəfi] *n* 腹膜造影[术]
peritoneomuscular [ˌperitəuˌniːəuˈmʌskjulə] *a* 腹膜肌的
peritoneopathy [ˌperitəuniˈɔpəθi] *n* 腹膜病
peritoneopericardial [ˌperitəuˌniːəuˌperiˈkɑːdiəl] *a* 腹膜心包的
peritoneopexy [ˌperiˈtəuniəˌpeksi] *n* 腹膜固定术（经阴道固定子宫）
peritoneoplasty [ˌperiˈtəuniəˌplæsti] *n* 腹膜成形术
peritoneoscope [ˌperiˈtəuniəˌskəup] *n* 腹腔镜 | **peritoneoscopy** [ˌperiˌtəuniˈɔskəpi] *n* 腹腔镜检查
peritoneotome [ˌperitəuˈniːətəum] *n*（脊神经）腹膜区
peritoneotomy [ˌperiˌtəuniˈɔtəmi] *n* 腹膜切开术
peritoneovenous [ˌperitəuˌniːəˈviːnəs] *a* 腹腔静脉的（指腹腔静脉分流术）
peritoneum [ˌperitəuˈniəm] *n* 腹膜 | abdominal ~, parietal ~ 腹膜壁层 / intestinal ~, visceral ~ 腹膜脏层
peritonism [ˈperitənizəm] *n* 假性腹膜炎
peritonitis [ˌperitəuˈnaitis] *n* 腹膜炎 | encysted ~ 包围性腹膜炎 / general ~ 弥漫性腹膜炎 / meconium ~ 胎粪性腹膜炎 / silent ~ 潜伏性腹膜炎
peritonization [ˌperitəunaiˈzeiʃən, -niˈz-] *n* 腹膜被覆术，腹膜成形术
peritonize [ˈperitənaiz] *vt* 用腹膜被覆
peritonsillar [ˌperiˈtɔnsilə] *a* 扁桃体周的
peritonsillitis [ˌperiˌtɔnsiˈlaitis] *n* 扁桃体周炎
peritracheal [ˌperiˈtreikiəl] *a* 气管周的
peritrich [ˈperitrik] *n* 缘毛虫 *a* 围口纤毛的
Peritrichia [ˌperiˈtrikiə] *n* 缘毛亚纲
Peritrichida [ˌperiˈtrikidə] *n* 围口纤毛目
peritrichous [pəˈritrikəs], **peritrichal** [piˈritrikəl], **peritrichic** [ˌperiˈtrikik] *a* 周毛的（指细菌细胞）；围口纤毛的（指纤毛虫）
peritrochanteric [ˌperiˌtrəukænˈterik] *a* 转子周的
perituberculosis [ˌperitju(ː)ˌbəːkjuˈləusis] *n* 类结核；副结核
perityphlic [ˌperiˈtiflik] *a* 盲肠周的
perityphlitis [ˌperitifˈlaitis] *n* 盲肠周炎
periumbilical [ˌperiˌʌmbiˈlaikəl] *a* 脐周的
periungual [ˌperiˈʌŋgwəl] *a* 甲周的
periureteral [ˌperijuəˈriːtərəl], **periureteric** [ˌperiˌjuəriˈterik] *a* 输尿管周的
periureteritis [ˌperijuˌriːtəˈraitis] *n* 输尿管周围炎
periurethral [ˌperijuəˈriːθrəl] *a* 尿道周的
periurethritis [ˌperiˌjuəriˈθraitis] *n* 尿道周炎
periuterine [ˌperiˈjuːtərain] *a* 子宫周的
periuvular [ˌperiˈjuːvjulə] *a* 悬雍垂周的
perivaginal [ˌperiˈvædʒinəl] *a* 阴道周的
perivaginitis [ˌperiˌvædʒiˈnaitis] *n* 阴道周炎
perivascular [ˌperiˈvæskjulə] *a* 血管周的
perivascularity [ˌperiˌvæskjuˈlærəti] *n* 血管周浸润[状态]
perivasculitis [ˌperiˌvæskjuˈlaitis] *n* 血管周炎
perivenous [ˌperiˈviːnəs] *a* 静脉周的
periventricular [ˌperivenˈtrikjulə] *a*（心、脑）室周的

perivertebral [ˌperiˈvəːtibrəl] *a* 椎骨周的
perivesical [ˌperiˈvesikəl] *a* 膀胱周的
perivesicular [ˌpeririˈsikjulə] *a* 精囊周的
perivesiculitis [ˌperiviˌsikjuˈlaitis] *n* 精囊周炎
perivisceral [ˌperiˈvisərəl] *a* 内脏周的
perivisceritis [ˌperiˌvisəˈraitis] *n* 内脏周炎
perivitelline [ˌperivaiˈtelin] *a* 卵黄周的
perixenitis [ˌperizeˈnaitis] *n* (组织或器官内)异物周炎
perkeratosis [ˌpəːkerəˈtəusis] *n* 牲畜 X 病,牲畜皮肤角化症
Perkinsea [pəˈkinsiə] *n* 拍琴纲
Perkinsida [pəˈkinsidə] *n* 拍琴目
perlapine [ˈpəːləpiːn] *n* 哌拉平(催眠药)
perlèche [pəˈleʃ] *n*【法】传染性口角炎
Perlia's nucleus [ˈpəːliə] (Richard Perlia) 佩利阿核(动眼神经内侧核)
Perlman syndrome [ˈpəːlmən] (M. Perlman) 珀尔曼综合征(一种罕见的致死性综合征,包含肾发育不良、肾母细胞病、胎儿巨大发育和朗格汉斯〈Langerhans〉岛肥大,伴有高胰岛素症。本征可能由常染色体隐性遗传而遗传的)
Perls' anemia bodies [pəːls] (Max Perls) 珀尔斯贫血性小体(恶性贫血患者血中一种小而活动的杆状小体) | ~ test(stain) 珀尔斯试验(染色)(检含铁血黄素)
perlsucht [ˈpəːlzuht] *n*【德】牛(肠系膜和腹膜)结核病
permanence [ˈpəːmənəns] *n* 永久[性],持久[性]
permanganate [pəːˈmæŋgənit] *n* 高锰酸盐
permanganic acid [ˌpəːmænˈgænik] 高锰酸,过锰酸
permeability [ˌpəːmjəˈbiləti] *n* 通透性 | glomerular ~ 肾小球通透性
permeable [ˈpəːmjəbl] *a* 可渗透的,可透过的 *ad*
permease [ˈpəːmieis] *n* 通透酶
permeate [ˈpəːmieit] *vt, vi* 渗透,透过 | **permeation** [ˌpəːmiˈeiʃən] *n*
permethrin [pəˈmeθrin] *n* 扑灭司林(局部杀虫药)
permselectivity [ˌpəːmsəlekˈtivəti] *n* 选择通透性(限制大分子通透肾小球毛细管壁)
perna [ˈpəːnə] *n* 全氯萘
pernasal [pəˈneizəl] *a* 经鼻的
perneiras [pɛəˈneirəs] *n* 脚气[病](巴西人对beriberi 的称呼)
perniciosiform [pəːˌniʃiˈəusifɔːm] *a* 恶性样的,似乎恶性的
pernicious [pəːˈniʃəs] *a* 有害的,恶性的
pernio [ˈpəːniəu] *n*【拉】冻疮
pero- [构词成分]残缺,不全
perobrachius [ˌpiːrəuˈbreikiəs] *n* 臂不全畸胎
perocephalus [ˌpiːrəuˈsefələs] *n* 头不全畸胎
perochirus [ˌpiːrəuˈkairəs] *n* 手不全畸胎
perocormus [ˌpiːrəuˈkɔːməs] *n* 躯干不全畸胎
perodactylus [ˌpiːrəuˈdæktiləs] *n* 指不全畸胎,趾不全畸胎
peromelia [ˌpiːrəuˈmiːliə] *n* 四肢不全
peromelus [piˈrɔmiləs] *n* 四肢不全畸胎,缺肢畸胎
Peromyscus [ˌpiːrəuˈmiskəs] *n* 鼠属
peronarthrosis [ˌperənɑːˈθrəusis] *n* 鞍状关节
perone [pəˈrəuni] *n* 腓骨 | **~al** [ˌperəˈniəl] *a* 腓骨的,腓侧的
peronealis [pəːrəuniˈeilis] *a* 腓骨的,腓侧的
peroneotibial [ˌperəˌniəuˈtibiəl] *a* 胫腓骨的
peronia [piˈrəuniə] *n* 发育不全性畸形,残缺
Peronosporales [ˌperənəuspɔˈreiliːz] *n* 斜尖状孢子菌目
Per. op. emet. peracta operatione emetici【拉】催吐药作用过去后
peropus [ˈpiːrəpəs] *n* 下肢不全畸胎
peroral [pəˈrɔːrəl] *a* 经口的,由口的,口服的
per os [pəː ɔs]【拉】口服,经口
perosis [pəˈrəusis] *n* 骨短粗病(鸡) | **perotic** [pəˈrɔtik] *a*
perosomus [ˌpiːrəuˈsəuməs] *n* 躯干不全畸胎
perosplanchnia [ˌpiːrəuˈsplæŋkniə] *n* 内脏不全[畸形]
perosseous [pəˈrɔsiəs] *a* 经骨的
peroxidase [pəˈrɔksideis] *n* 过氧化物酶
peroxide [pəˈrɔksaid] *n* 过氧化物
peroxisome [pəˈrɔksisəum] *n* 过氧化物酶体;微体
peroxy- [前缀]过氧
peroxyacetic acid [pəˌrɔksiəˈsiːtik] 过氧乙酸(消毒防腐药)
peroxydol [pəˈrɔksidɔl] *n* 过硼酸钠
perphenazine [pəˈfenəziːn] *n* 奋乃静(强安定药,用作抗精神病药,亦用作止吐药)
per primam intentionem [pəː ˈpraimәm intenʃiˈəunəm]【拉】由第一期愈合
per rectum [pəː ˈrektəm]【拉】经直肠
Perrin-Ferraton disease [ˈperæn ˌferəˈtɔn] (Maurice Perrin; Louis Ferraton) 弹响髋,髋关节弹响
Perroncito's apparatus (spirals) [ˌpərɔnˈtʃiːtəu] (Aldo Perroncito) 佩朗契托器(神经复生时的末端线网)
Perry bag [ˈperi] (Murie Perry) 佩里袋(一种回肠造瘘袋)
persalt [ˈpəːsɔːlt] *n* 过酸盐
per saltam [pəː ˈsæltəm]【拉】一跃,骤发

per secundam intentionem [pəː siˈkundəm intenʃiˈəunəm] 由第二期愈合

perseverate [pə(ː)ˈsevəreit] *vi* 患持续言语症；患持续动作症

perseveration [pə(ː)ˌsevəˈreiʃən] *n* 持续言语；持续动作 | clonic ~ 持续性阵挛 / tonic ~ 持续性强直（姿势） | **perseverative** [pə(ː)ˈsevəreitiv] *a*

persistence [pəːˈsistəns] *n* 坚持，持续，持久性；（视觉等）暂留 | ~ of vision 视觉暂留

persister [pəˈsistə] *n* 耐药株（在细菌学上指对药物一般毒性浓度表现抗性的微生物，而非遗传学上的抗性）

persona [pəːˈsəunə]（[复] **personae** [pəːˈsəuniː]）*n* 人格面具，伪装人格

personalistics [ˌpəːsənəˈlistiks] *n* 人格论

personality [ˌpəːsəˈnæləti] *n* 人格；个性 | affective ~ (disorder) 情感性人格（障碍），环性气质 / alternating ~ 交替性人格 / antisocial ~ (disorder) 反社会型人格（障碍）/ avoidant ~ (disorder) 回避人格（障碍）/ borderline ~ (disorder) 边缘型人格（障碍）/ compulsive ~ 强迫性人格 / cycloid ~ (disorder), cyclothymic ~ (disorder) 循环型人格（障碍），环性气质 / dependent ~ (disorder) 依赖型人格（障碍）/ double ~, dual ~ 双重人格 / epileptoid ~ (disorder) 癫痫型人格（障碍），间歇性暴发性障碍 / explosive ~ 暴发型人格，暴躁性格，间歇性暴发性障碍 / histrionic ~ (disorder), hysterical ~ 表演型人格（障碍），癔症性人格 / inadequate ~（适应能力）不足型人格，缺陷人格 / multiple ~ 多重人格 / narcissistic ~ (disorder) 自恋型人格（障碍）/ obsessive ~, obsessive-compulsive ~ (disorder) 强迫性人格（障碍）/ passive-aggressive ~ (disorder) 被动-攻击性人格（障碍）/ psychopathic ~ 变态人格，病态人格 / sadistic ~ (disorder) 虐待狂人格（障碍）/ schizoid ~, seclusive ~, shut-in ~ 分裂样人格，孤僻人格 / schizotypal ~ (disorder) 分裂型人格（障碍）/ sociopathic ~ 社会病态人格，反社会人格 / split ~ 人格分裂

personalize [ˈpəːsənəlaiz] *vt* 使个人化；使人格化 | **personalization** [ˌpəːsənəlaiˈzeiʃən, -liˈz-] *n*

personification [pə(ː)ˌsɔnifiˈkeiʃən] *n* 拟人化，人格化；化身，体现；典型

personology [ˌpəːsəˈnɔlədʒi] *n* 人格学 | **personologic** [ˌpəːsənəˈlɔdʒik] *a*

perspiratio [ˌpəːspəˈreiʃiəu] *n*【拉】出汗；汗

perspiration [ˌpəːspəˈreiʃən] *n* 出汗；汗 | insensible ~ 不显汗 / sensible ~ 显汗

perspiratory [pəsˈpaiərətəri] *a* 出汗的

perspire [pəsˈpaiə] *vi*, *vt* 出汗

persuasion [pəˈsweiʒən] *n* 说服，说服力；说服，劝导（心理治疗）

persulfate [pəˈsʌlfeit] *n* 过硫酸盐

persulfide [pəˈsʌlfaid] *n* 过硫化物

persulfuric acid [ˌpəːsʌlˈfjuərik] 过硫酸

pertechnetate [pə(ː)ˈteknəteit] *n* 高锝酸盐

Perthes' disease [ˈpəːtiːz] (Georg C. Perthes) 佩尔特斯病（骨骺的骨软骨病） | ~ incision 佩尔特斯切口（暴露胆囊用）/ ~ test 佩尔特斯试验（检静脉曲张侧支循环）

Pertik's diverticulum [ˈpəːtik] (Otto Pertik) 佩尔提克憩室（过深的咽隐窝）

per tubam [pəː ˈtjuːbəm]【拉】由管

pertubation [ˌpəːtjuˈbeiʃən] *n* 输管卵灌气法

pertucin [pəːˈtjuːsin] *n* 穿孔假胞菌素

pertussis [pəˈtʌsis] *n* 百日咳 | **pertussal** [pəˈtʌsəl] *a*

pertussoid [pəˈtʌsɔid] *a* 百日咳样的 *n* 百日咳样咳嗽

pervade [pəːˈveid] *vt* 蔓延，渗透，遍及 | **pervasion** [pəːˈveiʒən] *n*

per vaginam [pəː vəˈdʒainəm]【拉】由阴道，经阴道

perversion [pəˈvəːʃən] *n* 倒错，乖常，颠倒；性反常行为（精神病学） | sexual ~ 性欲倒错，性变态

perversity [pəˈvəːsəti] *n* 反常

perversive [pəˈvəːsiv] *a* 反常的，造成反常的

pervert [pəːˈvəːt] *vt* 使反常；误用 [ˈpəːvəːt] *n* 反常者；性欲倒错者，性欲反常者

pervigilium [ˌpəːviˈdʒiljəm] *n* 失眠[症]

pes [piːz]（[复] **pedes** [ˈpiːdiːz]）*n*【拉】足，脚

pessary [ˈpesəri] *n* 子宫托，阴道环；阴道栓[剂] | cup ~ 杯状子宫托 / diaphragm ~ 膈状子宫托 / doughnut ~ 环状子宫托 / lever ~ 杠杆子宫托 / ring ~ 环状子宫托 / stem ~ 有柄子宫托

pessimism [ˈpesimizəm] *n* 悲观，悲观主义 | therapeutic ~ 医疗悲观主义（不相信药物治疗） | **pessimist** *n* 悲观论者

pessimum [ˈpesiməm] *n* 劣性（指刺激过强或过频）

pest [pest] *n* 有害动物，害虫；鼠疫，瘟疫 | chicken ~, fowl ~ 家禽疫，鸡瘟

peste [pest] *n*【法】瘟疫 | ~ des petits ruminants (PPR) 小反刍动物疫（一种高度致命的绵羊和山羊病毒性疾病，在中非和西非以及中东流行，由麻疹病毒属〈Morbillivirus〉病毒所致，特征为发热、坏死性口炎和肺炎。亦称 pest of small ruminants，口炎-肺肠炎综合征）

pesticemia [ˌpestiˈsiːmiə] *n* 鼠疫菌血症；败血性鼠疫

pesticide [ˈpestisaid] *n* 杀虫药

pestiferous [pesˈtifərəs] *a* 致疫的,传疫的

pestilence [ˈpestiləns] *n* 疫病;疫病流行

pestilent [ˈpestilənt] *a* 致命的,有害的;传染性的

pestilential [ˌpestiˈlenʃəl] *a* 疫病的

pestis [ˈpestis] *n*【拉】鼠疫,瘟疫 | ~ ambulans, ~ minor 轻鼠疫,不卧床鼠疫 / ~ bubonica 腺鼠疫,腹股沟淋巴结鼠疫 / ~ fulminans, ~ major 暴发性鼠疫,重鼠疫,/ ~ siderans 电击状鼠疫,败血性鼠疫 / ~ variolosa 天花

Pestivirus [ˈpestiˌvaiərəs] *n* 瘟病毒属

pestle [ˈpesl, ˈpestl] *n* 研棒,杵 *vt, vi* (用杵)捣,研碎

pestology [pesˈtələdʒi] *n* 鼠疫学

PET position emission tomography 正电子发射体层摄影[术]

peta- [构词成分] 秭(10^{15})

-petal [构词成分] 求,向,趋

petalo- [构词成分] 花瓣,叶

petalobacteria [ˌpetələubækˈtiəriə] *n* 瓣菌

petechia [piˈtiːkiə] ([复] **petechiae** [piˈtiːkiiː]) *n*【拉】出血点,瘀点 | **petechial** *a*

Peterman test [ˈpiːtəmən] (Mynie G. Peterman) 彼德曼试验,梅毒玻片试验(诊断梅毒的一种血清学试验,0.05 ml 灭活的患者血清与 0.01 ml 稀释的牛心抗原混匀,在载玻内置 37 ℃灭活 10 分钟后,镜检结果)

Peters' anomaly [ˈpeitəz] (Albert Peters) 彼得斯畸形(眼前房周围结构内发育缺陷,特征为角膜浑浊,有时虹膜、晶状体和角膜粘连,常伴有其他缺陷,诸如侏儒症和精神发育迟缓)

Petersen's bag [ˈpeitəsən] (C. F. Petersen) 彼得逊袋(施行耻骨上膀胱切开术时用的直肠吹张袋)

Peters' ovum [ˈpeitəz] (Hubert Peters) 彼得斯卵(胎)(受精 13~14 天的卵)

pethidine [ˈpeθidin] *n* 哌替啶(麻醉镇痛药) | ~ hydrochloride 盐酸哌替啶

petiolate(d) [ˈpetiəleit(id)], **petioled** [ˈpetiəuld] *a* 有柄的

petiole [ˈpetiəul] *n* 柄,茎 | epiglottic ~ 会厌软骨柄

petiolus [piˈtaiələs] *n*【拉】柄,茎

petit mal [pəˈtiːˈmɑːl]【法】(癫痫)小发作

Petit's canal [pəˈtiː] (Fransçois P. Du Petit) 小带间隙,悬器隙 | ~ sinus 主动脉窦

Petit's hernia [pəˈtiː] (Jean L. Petit) 腰三角疝 | ~ ligament 子宫骶韧带 / ~ triangle 腰三角

Petit's law [pəˈtiː] (Alexis T. Petit) 波替定律(一切元素的原子其热容量都相等)

Petrén's diet (treatment) [peiˈtren] 佩特伦饮食(疗法)(曾用于治糖尿病,含极少量蛋白质和碳水化合物,以及含大量脂肪,主要是奶油)

Pétrequin's ligament [peitrˈkæn] (Joseph P. E. Pétrequin) 佩特尔坎韧带(下颌关节囊前面增厚部)

petrichloral [ˌpetriˈklɔːrəl] *n* 培曲氯醛(催眠镇静药)

Petri dish [ˈpeitri, ˈpiː-] (Julius R. Petri) 皮氏培养皿 | ~ plate 皮氏平碟(一种佩特里细菌培养皿) / ~ test (reaction) 皮氏试验(反应)(检蛋白质)

Petriellidium [ˌpetriəˈlidiəm] *n* 彼得利壳菌属(假性阿利什利菌属〈Pseudoalleschesia〉的旧称)

petrifaction [ˌpetriˈfækʃən], **petrification** [ˌpetrifiˈkeiʃən] *n* 石化;石人化,僵化,发呆 | **petrifactive** *a*

pétrissage [ˌpeitriˈsɑːʒ] *n*【法】揉捏法

petroccipital [ˌpetrɔkˈsipitl] *a* 岩枕的

petrolatoma [ˌpetrəuləˈtəumə] *n* 液状石蜡瘤

petrolatum [ˌpetrəuˈleitəm], **petrolate** [ˈpetrəleit] *n* [黄]软石蜡,[黄]凡士林,石油凝胶

petroleum [piˈtrəuljəm] *n* 石油

petrolization [ˌpetrəlaiˈzeiʃən, -liˈz-] *n* 石油洒播法,石油治蚊法,石油杀孑孓法

petromastoid [ˌpetrəuˈmæstɔid] *a* 岩[部]乳[突]的 *n* 耳外骨

petro-occipital [ˌpetrəuɔkˈsipitl] *a* 岩枕的

petropharyngeus [ˌpetrəufəˈrindʒiəs] *n* 岩咽肌

petrosal [piˈtrəusəl] *a* 岩部的(颞骨)

petrosalpingostaphylinus [ˌpetrəusælˌpiŋgəuˌstæfiˈlainəs] *n* 腭帆提肌

petrosectomy [ˌpetrəuˈsektəmi] *n* 岩锥切除术

petroselinic acid [ˌpetrəusəˈlinik] 岩芹酸

petrositis [ˌpetrəuˈsaitis] *n* 岩锥炎

petrosomastoid [piˌtrəusəˈmæstɔid] *a* 岩[锥]乳[突]的 *n* 耳外骨

petrosphenoid [ˌpetrəuˈsfiːnɔid] *a* 岩[锥]蝶[骨]的

petrosphere [ˈpetrəsfiə] *n* 地壳

petrosquamosal [ˌpetrəuskweiˈməusəl], **petrosquamous** [ˌpetrəuˈskweiməs] *a* 岩鳞[部]的

petrostaphylinus [ˌpetrəuˌstæfiˈlainəs] *n* 腭帆提肌

petrous [ˈpetrəs] *a* 岩石样的,石状的

petrousitis [ˌpetrəsˈaitis] *n* 岩锥炎,(颞骨)岩部炎

Petruschky's litmus whey [peˈtruʃki] (Johannes Petruschky) 佩特鲁希基石蕊乳清(用石蕊染成深紫红色的乳清,用作培养基) | ~ spinalgia 佩特鲁希基脊痛(支气管淋巴结结核时引起的肩胛间区压痛)

Pette-Döring panencephalitis [ˈpetə ˈderiŋ] (Heinrich W. Pette; Gerhard Döring) 彼-窦全脑

炎(亚急性脑炎的一型,特征为累及大脑的灰质和白质,基底神经节为多发部位)

Pettenkofer's test [ˈpetənkɔfə] (Max J. von Pettenkofer) 佩滕科弗试验(检尿胆汁酸) | ~ theory 佩滕科弗学说(认为流行病〈例如伤寒〉是在地下水处于低水位时发生,致病菌并不直接自患者传播至健康人,但经过干燥的土壤而成熟)

Petzetaki's test (reaction) [ˌpetseiˈtɑːki] 佩泽塔基试验(反应)(检伤寒)

Peucedanum [pjuˈsedənəm] *n* 前胡属

Peucetia [pjuˈsiːtiə] *n* 山猫蛛属 | ~ viridans 山猫蛛

Peutz-Jeghers syndrome [pəːtz ˈdʒegəz] (J. L. A. Peutz; Harold Jeghers) 波伊茨-耶格综合征,色素沉着息肉综合征(特征为胃肠道息肉〈通常为小肠错构瘤〉合并皮肤与黏膜的大量黑色素沉着,常见并发症为胃肠道出血及肠套叠,为常染色体显性性状遗传)

pexic [ˈpeksik] *a* 固定的(指组织有固定力的)

pexin [ˈpeksin] *n* 凝乳酶

pexinogen [pekˈsinədʒən] *n* 凝乳酶原

pexis [ˈpeksis], **pexia** [ˈpeksiə] *n* 固定;固定术

-pexy [构词成分] 固定,固定术

Peyer's patches (glands, insulae, plaques) [ˈpajə] (Johann C. Peyer) 派尔集合淋巴结(小肠黏膜下淋巴组织集结)

peyote [peiˈjəutiː], **peyotl** [peiˈjəutl] *n* 拍约他,仙人球膏(制自墨西哥仙人球的一种兴奋剂)

Peyronie's disease [peirɔˈniː] (François de la Peyronie) 佩罗尼病(阴茎海绵体硬结,产生纤维性痛性阴茎勃起,亦称阴茎纤维性海绵体炎)

Peyrot's thorax [peiˈrəu] (Jean J. Peyrot) 佩罗胸(斜卵圆形胸,见于大量胸膜渗出物)

Pezizales [ˌpeziˈzeiliːz] *n* 盘菌目

Pfannenstiel's incision [ˈfænənstiːl] (Hermann J. Pfannenstiel) 普芬南施蒂尔切口(下腹部横切口)

Pfeifferella [ˌfaifəˈrelə] *n* 发否菌属,鼻疽杆菌属 | ~ mallei 鼻疽发否杆菌,鼻疽杆菌

Pfeiffer's bacillus [ˈfaifə] (Richard F. J. Pfeiffer) 发否杆菌,流感嗜血杆菌 | ~ law 发否定律(注射能抗某一疾病的免疫血清于另一动物体内,能破坏该病的病原菌) / ~ phenomenon (reaction) 霍乱弧菌溶菌现象(霍乱弧菌被注射到已被免疫了的豚鼠腹腔内,即丧失活动能力,并随之溶解,如溶菌血清注入正常豚鼠腹腔也可得到同样结果)

Pfeiffer's disease, glandular fever [ˈfaifə] (Emil Pfeiffer) 传染性单核白细胞增多[症]

Pflüger's law [ˈfliːgə] (Edward F. W. Pflüger) 弗吕格定律(极兴奋法则,极收缩法则,即阴极电紧张时神经兴奋,阳极电紧张时神经兴奋消失,在相反条件下则否) | ~ cords 卵巢管;涎液小管 / ~ tubes 卵巢管

pfropfhebephrenia [ˌpfrɔpfhiːbiˈfriːniə] *n* 嫁接性青春型精神分裂症

pfropfschizophrenia [ˌpfrɔpfskizəuˈfriːniə] *n* 嫁接性精神分裂症

Pfuhl-Jaffé sign [ful ˈjɑːfi] (Eduard Pfuhl; Max Jaffé) 富-雅征(脓气胸时,用力吸气,脓液才可从试探性穿刺针孔或切口流出,真性气胸时则需呼气方使脓液流出)

Pfuhl's sign [ful] (Adam Pfuhl) 富尔征(穿刺放液术时,如该渗出液的流出随吸气而增加则为膈下脓肿,如减少则为脓气胸,但膈膜麻痹时则无此差别)

PG prostaglandin 前列腺素; *Pharmacopoeia Germanica*《德国药典》

pg picogram 皮克(10^{-12}g)

PGD preimplantation genetic diagnosis 植入前遗传诊断

PGD_2, PGE_2, $PGF_{2\alpha}$, PGI_2, etc. 各种前列腺素的符号:前列腺素 D_2,前列腺素 E_2,前列腺素 $F_{2\alpha}$,前列环素等

Ph Pharmacopeia 药典; phenyl 苯基

pH 氢离子指数,pH 值

PHA phytohemagglutinin 植物凝集素

phacitis [fəˈsaitis] *n* 晶状体炎

phac(o)- [构词成分] 晶状体,透镜;痣

phacoanaphylaxis [ˌfækəuˌænəfiˈlæksis] *n* 晶状体蛋白过敏性

phacocele [ˈfækəsiːl] *n* 晶状体突出

phacocyst [ˈfækəsist] *n* 晶状体囊

phacocystectomy [ˌfækəusisˈtektəmi] *n* 晶状体囊[部分]切除术(治白内障)

phacocystitis [ˌfækəusisˈtaitis], **phacohymenitis** [ˌfækəuˌhaiməˈnaitis] *n* 晶状体囊炎

phacoemulsification [ˌfækəuiˌmʌlsifiˈkeiʃən] *n* 晶状体乳化法(一种晶状体摘除术)

phacoerysis [ˌfækəueˈriːsis] *n* 晶状体针吸术

phacoglaucoma [ˌfækəuglɔːˈkəumə] *n* 晶状体性青光眼

phacoid [ˈfækɔid] *a* 透镜状的

phacoiditis [ˌfækɔiˈdaitis] *n* 晶状体炎

phacoidoscope [fəˈkɔidəskəup] *n* 晶状体镜

phacolysin [fəˈkɔlisin] *n* 晶状体溶素(一种晶状体白蛋白,治早期白内障)

phacolysis [fəˈkɔlisis] *n* 晶状体刺开术;晶状体溶解

phacolytic [ˌfækəuˈlitik] *a* 晶状体溶解的

phacoma [fəˈkəumə] *n* 晶状体瘤

phacomalacia [ˌfækəuməˈleiʃiə] *n* 晶状体软化,软内障

phacomatosis [ˌfækəuməˈtəusis] *n* 斑痣性错构瘤病
phacometachoresis [ˌfækəuˌmetəkəˈriːsis], **phacometecesis** [ˌfækəuˌmetəˈsiːsis] *n* 晶状体移位
phacometer [fəˈkɔmitə] *n* 检镜片计,晶状体屈光度计
phacopalingenesis [ˌfækəuˌpælinˈdʒenisis] *n* 晶状体再生
phacoplanesis [ˌfækəupləˈniːsis] *n* 晶状体游动
phacosclerosis [ˌfækəuskliəˈrəusis] *n* 晶状体硬化(一种硬内障)
phacoscope [ˈfækəskəup] *n* 晶状体镜 | **phacoscopy** [fəˈkɔskəpi] *n* 晶状体镜检查
phacoscotasmus [ˌfækəuskəˈtæzməs] *n* 晶状体混浊
phacotherapy [ˌfækəuˈθerəpi] *n* 日光疗法,日光浴
phacotoxic [ˌfækəuˈtɔksik] *a* 晶状体毒性的
phacozymase [ˌfækəuˈzaimeis] *n* 晶状体酶
Phaenicia [feniˈʃiə] *n* 绿蝇属 | ~ cuprina 铜绿蝇 / ~ sericata 丝光绿蝇
phae(o)- 以 phae(o)-起始的词,同样见以 pheo-起始的词
Phaeocalpida [ˌfiːəuˈkælpidə] *n* 暗瓮目
Phaeoconchida [ˌfiːəuˈkɔnkidə] *n* 暗贝目
Phaeocystida [ˌfiːəuˈsistidə] *n* 暗囊目
Phaeodarea [ˌfiːəuˈdɛəriə] *n* 稀孔虫纲
Phaeodendrida [ˌfiːəuˈdendridə] *n* 暗树目
phaeodium [ˌfiːəuˈdiːəm] *n* 暗块(某些海洋浮游生物原虫具有的褐色小球和碎片,也写成 pheodium)
Phaeogromida [ˌfiːəuˈgrɔmidə] *n* 暗天目
phaeohyphomycosis [ˌfiːəuˌhaifəumaiˈkəusis] *n* 暗色丝孢霉病
Phaeosphaerida [ˌfiːəuˈsfiəridə] *n* 暗球目
phaeosporotrichosis [ˌfiːəuˌspɔːrəutriˈkəusis] *n* 暗色丝孢霉病
phage [feidʒ] *n* 噬菌体
-phage [构词成分] 噬,食
phagedena [ˌfædʒiˈdiːnə] *n* 崩蚀性溃疡,蚀疮 | **phagedenic** [ˌfædʒiˈdenik] *a*
phagelysis [ˈfeidʒlaisis] *n* 噬菌体溶解作用
-phagia, -phagy [构词成分] 噬,食
phag(o)- [构词成分] 吞噬
phagocaryosis [ˌfægəukæriˈəusis] *n* 核噬作用
phagocytable [ˈfægəuˌsaitəbl] *a* 可被吞噬的
phagocyte [ˈfægəusait] *n* 吞噬细胞 | alveolar ~s 肺泡吞噬细胞;尘细胞 / endothelial ~ 内皮吞噬细胞,内皮细胞 / globuliferous ~ 血细胞吞噬细胞 / melaniferous ~ 血色素吞噬细胞 / mobile ~ 游走吞噬细胞 / sessile ~ 固定吞噬细胞 | **phagocytic** [ˌfægəuˈsitik] *a*
phagocytin [ˌfægəuˈsaitin] *n* 吞噬素,吞噬细胞素(中性粒细胞内的一种杀菌物质)
phagocytize [ˈfægəuˌsaitaiz, -ˌsi-] *vt* 吞噬(对某物显示吞噬活性)
phagocytoblast [ˌfægəuˈsaitəblæst] *n* 成[吞]噬细胞
phagocytolysis [ˌfægəusaiˈtɔlisis] *n* [吞]噬细胞溶解 | **phagocytolytic** [ˌfægəusaitəuˈlitik] *a*
phagocytose [ˌfægəuˈsaitəus] *vt* 吞噬(包围及破坏细菌及其他异物)
phagocytosis [ˌfægəusaiˈtəusis] *n* 吞噬[作用] | induced ~ 诱发性吞噬作用 / spontaneous ~ 自发吞噬作用 / surface ~ 表面吞噬作用 | **phagocytotic** [ˌfægəusaiˈtɔtik] *a*
phagodynamometer [ˌfægəuˌdainəˈmɔmitə] *n* 嚼力计
phagokaryosis [ˌfægəuˌkæriˈəusis] *n* 核吞噬作用(细胞核的吞噬作用)
phagology [fəˈgɔlədʒi] *n* 噬菌体学 | **phagological** [ˌfægəuˈlɔdʒikəl] *a*
phagolysis [fəˈgɔlisis] *n* 吞噬细胞溶解 | **phagolytic** [ˌfægəuˈlitik] *a*
phagolysosome [ˌfægəuˈlaisəsəum] *n* 吞噬溶酶体
phagomania [ˌfægəuˈmeinjə] *n* 贪食癖
phagophobia [ˌfægəuˈfəubjə] *n* 进食恐怖,恐食症
phagoplasm [ˈfeigəplæsm] *n* 吞噬浆
phagosome [ˈfægəsəum] *n* 吞噬体
phagotroph [ˈfægətrɔf] *n* 营养吞噬体(动物式营养微生物)
phagotrophic [ˌfægəˈtrɔfik] *a* 吞噬营养的,动物式营养的
phagotype [ˈfægətaip] *n* 噬菌体型
-phagy [构词成分] 噬,食
phakitis [fəˈkaitis] *n* 晶状体炎
phak(o)- 以 phak(o)-起始的词,同样见以phac(o)-起始的词
phakoma [fəˈkəumə] *n* 晶状体瘤
phakomatosis [ˌfækəuməˈtəusis] *n* 斑痣性错构瘤病
phalacrosis [ˌfæləˈkrəusis] *n* 秃[发]病,脱发
phalang(o)- [构词成分] 指骨,趾骨
phalangeal [fəˈlændʒiəl] *a* 指骨的,趾骨的
phalangectomy [ˌfælənˈdʒektəmi] *n* 指骨切除术,趾骨切除术
phalanges [fæˈlændʒiːz] phalanx 的复数
phalangette [ˌfælənˈdʒet] *n* 末节指骨,末节趾骨 | drop ~ 末节指骨下垂
phalangitis [ˌfælənˈdʒaitis] *n* 指骨炎,趾骨炎
phalangization [ˌfæləndʒaiˈzeiʃən, -dʒi-] *n* 假指成形术

phalangophalangeal [fəˌlæŋgəufəˈlændʒiəl] *a* 二节指骨之间的,二节趾骨之间的
phalangosis [ˌfælænˈgəusis] *n* 多行睫,倒睫
phalanx [ˈfælæŋks] ([复] **phalanges** [fæˈlændʒiːz]) *n* 指骨,趾骨 | ungual ~ 末节指骨,末节趾骨
Phalen's maneuver [ˈfeilən] (George S. Phalen) 费伦手法(检查腕管综合征:握紧充分屈曲或伸展的患侧手腕 30 ~ 60 秒,或置血压计袖袋于患臂,充气至收缩压与舒张压之间的点 30 ~ 60 秒,腕管即缩小)
Phallales [fəˈleiliːz] *n* 鬼笔目
phallalgia [fæˈlældʒiə] *n* 阴茎痛
phallanastrophe [ˌfælæˈnæstrəfi] *n* 阴茎上曲
phallaneurysm [fæˈlænjuərizəm] *n* 阴茎动脉瘤
phallectomy [fæˈlektəmi] *n* 阴茎切除术
phalli [ˈfælai] phallus 的复数
phallic [ˈfælik] *a* 阴茎的
phalliform [ˈfælifɔːm] *a* 阴茎状的
phallin [ˈfælin] *n* 毒菌溶血苷(制自条蕈)
phallitis [fæˈlaitis] *n* 阴茎炎
phall(o)- [构词成分] 阴茎
phallocampsis [ˌfæləuˈkæmpsis] *n* 阴茎弯曲
phallocrypsis [ˌpæləuˈkripsis] *n* 阴茎退缩,缩阴
phallodynia [ˌfæləuˈdiniə] *n* 阴茎痛
phalloid [ˈfælɔid] *a* 阴茎样的
phalloidin(e) [fəˈlɔidin] *n* 鬼笔[毒]环肽
phalloncus [fæˈlɔŋkəs] *n* 阴茎肿
phalloplasty [ˈfæləˌplæsti] *n* 阴茎成形术
phallorrhagia [ˌfæləuˈreidʒiə] *n* 阴茎出血
phallorrhea [ˌfæləuˈriːə] *n* 阴茎溢液(男性淋病)
phallotomy [fæˈlɔtəmi] *n* 阴茎切开术
phallotoxin [ˌfæləuˈtɔksin] *n* 鬼笔毒素
Phallus [ˈfæləs] *n* 鬼笔属
phallus [ˈfæləs] ([复] **phalluses** 或 **phalli** [ˈfælai]) *n* 阴茎;(胚胎的)初阴
phaner(o)- [构词成分] 显,明
phanerogam [ˈfænərəugæm] *n* 显花植物
phanerogenic [ˌfænərəuˈdʒenik], **phanerogenetic** [ˌfænərəudʒiˈnetik] *a* 原因明显的
phaneroplasm [ˈfænərəplæzəm] *n* 明体,明质
phaneroscope [ˈfænərəskəup] *n* 皮肤透照镜
phanerosis [ˌfænəˈrəusis] *n* 显现,显形
phanerosterol [ˌfænəˈrɔstərəl] *n* 显花植物甾醇
phantasia [fænˈteiziə] *n* 幻想,空想
phantasm [ˈfæntæzəm] *n* 幻象,幻觉
phantasmatology [ˌfæntæzməˈtɔlədʒi], **phantasmology** [ˌfæntæzˈmɔlədʒi] *n* 幻象学
phantasmatomoria [fænˌtæzmətəˈmɔːriə] *n* 童样幻想,幻想性童样痴呆
phantasy [ˈfæntəsi] *n* 幻想,空想
phantogeusia [ˌfæntəˈgjuːziə] *n* 幻味觉(口中有异味觉,一般为金属味或咸味)
phantom [ˈfæntəm] *n* 幻象,幻觉;人体模型 | eyeball ~ 眼球模型
phantosmia [fænˈtɔzmiə] *n* 嗅幻觉
phanurane [ˈfænjuːrein] *n* 烯睾丙内酯(即坎利酮 canrenone,醛甾酮拮抗药)
pha(o)- 以 pha(o)-起始的词,同样见以 phe(o)-起始的词
phar, pharm pharmacy 药学,药剂学;药房;pharmaceutical 药的,制药的;药学的;pharmacopeia 药典
Phar B Pharmaciae Baccalaureus【拉】药学学士
Phar C Pharmaceutical Chemist 药物化学家
pharcidous [ˈfɑːsidəs] *a* 皱纹的
Phar D Pharmaciae Doctor【拉】药学博士
Phar G Graduate in Pharmacy 药学毕业生
Phar M Pharmaciae Magister【拉】药学硕士
pharm 见 phar
pharmacal [ˈfɑːməkəl] *a* 药的,药物的;药学的
pharmaceutic [fɑːməˈsjuːtik] *a* 药学的;制药的;药用的
pharmaceutical [fɑːməˈsjuːtikəl] *a* 药的,制药的;药学的 *n* 药品,药剂
pharmaceutics [fɑːməˈsjutiks] *n* 药剂学;药学制剂
pharmaceutist [ˌfɑːməˈsjuːtist], **pharmacist** [ˈfɑːməsist] *n* 药师,调剂员;药商
pharmaco- [构词成分] 药,药学
pharmacoangiography [ˌfɑːməkəuændʒiˈɔgrəfi] *n* 药物性血管造影[术](应用血管扩张药和血管收缩药操纵血液流动以增强显影的血管造影)
pharmacochemistry [ˌfɑːməkəuˈkemistri] *n* 药物化学
pharmacodiagnosis [ˌfɑːməkəuˌdaiəgˈnəusis] *n* 药物诊断
pharmacodynamics [ˌfɑːməkəudaiˈnæmiks] *n* 药效学 | **pharmacodynamic** *a* 药效的
pharmacoeconomics [ˌfɑːməkəuˌekəˈnɔmiks] *n* 药物经济学(研究关于药物疗法费用的经济因素,其中包括这些因素对卫生保健制度和社会的影响)
pharmacoendocrinology [ˌfɑːməkəuˌendəukriˈnɔlədʒi] *n* 药物内分泌学
pharmacogenetics [ˌfɑːməkəudʒiˈnetiks] *n* 药物遗传学
pharmacognosy [ˌfɑːməˈkɔgnəsi], **pharmacognostics** [ˌfɑːməkɔgˈnɔstiks] *n* 生药学
pharmacography [ˌfɑːməˈkɔgrəfi] *n* 药物记载学
pharmacokinetics [ˌfɑːməkəukaiˈnetiks, -kiˈn-] *n* 药物动力学
pharmacology [ˌfɑːməˈkɔlədʒi] *n* 药理学 |

pharmacologic(al) [ˌfɑːməkəˈlɔdʒik(əl)] *a* | **pharmacologist** *n* 药理学家
pharmacomania [ˌfɑːməkəuˈmeinjə] *n* 药物癖
pharmacometrics [ˌfɑːməkəuˈmetriks] *n* 药物测量学
pharmacon [ˈfɑːməkən] *n* 药,药物
pharmaco-oryctology [ˌfɑːməkəu ˌɔrikˈtɔlədʒi] *n* 矿物药物学
pharmacopedia [ˌfɑːməkəˈpiːdiə], **pharmacopedics** [ˌfɑːməkəˈpiːdiks] *n* 制药学
pharmacopeia [ˌfɑːməkəˈpiːə] *n* 药典 | ~l *a*
pharmacophilia [ˌfɑːməkəuˈfiliə] *n* 嗜药癖
pharmacophobia [ˌfɑːməkəuˈfəubjə] *n* 药物恐怖,恐药症
pharmacophore [ˈfɑːməkəˌfɔː] *n* 药效基团
pharmacopoeia [ˌfɑːməkəˈpiːə] *n* 药典 | ~l *a*
pharmacopsychosis [ˌfɑːməkəusaiˈkəusis] *n* 药物性精神病
pharmacoroentgenography [ˌfɑːməkəuˌrɔntgeˈnɔgrəfi], **pharmacoradiography** [ˌfɑːməkəuˌreidiˈɔgrəfi] *n* 药物 X 线检查法
pharmacotherapeutics [ˌfɑːməkəuˌθerəˈpjuːtiks] *n* 药物治疗学
pharmacotherapy [ˌfɑːməkəuˈθerəpi] *n* 药物疗法
pharmacy [ˈfɑːməsi] *n* 药学;药剂学;制药,配药;药房 | chemical ~ 药物化学 / galenic ~ 植物药学
Pharm D Doctor of Pharmacy 药学博士
pharyngalgia [ˌfærinˈgældʒiə] *n* 咽痛
pharyngeal [ˌfærinˈdʒiːəl, fəˈrindʒi-], **pharyngal** [fəˈriŋgəl] *a* 咽的
pharyngectasia [ˌfærindʒekˈteisiə] *n* 咽扩张,咽突出
pharyngectomy [ˌfærinˈdʒektəmi] *n* 咽[部分]切除术
pharyngemphraxis [ˌfærindʒemˈfræksis] *n* 咽阻塞
pharyngeus [ˌfærinˈdʒiːəs] *a*【拉】咽的
pharyngismus [ˌfærinˈdʒizməs], **pharyngism** [ˈfærindʒizəm] *n* 咽肌痉挛
pharyngitic [ˌfærinˈdʒitik] *a* 咽炎的
pharyngitid [fəˈrindʒaitid] *n* 咽炎疹
pharyngitis [ˌfærinˈdʒaitis] *n* 咽炎 | acute ~, catarrhal ~ 急性咽炎,卡他性咽炎 / croupous ~, membranous ~ 格鲁布性咽炎,膜性咽炎 / follicular ~, glandular ~ 滤泡性咽炎,腺性咽炎
pharyng(o)- [构词成分] 咽
pharyngoamygdalitis [fəˌriŋgəuəˌmigdəˈlaitis] *n* 咽扁桃体炎
pharyngocele [fəˈriŋgəsiːl] *n* 咽突出
pharyngoceratosis [fəˌriŋgəuˌserəˈtəusis] *n* 咽角化病
pharyngoconjunctivitis [fəˌriŋgəukənˌdʒʌŋktiˈvaitis] *n* 咽结膜炎
pharyngodynia [fəˌriŋgəuˈdiniə] *n* 咽痛
pharyngoepiglottic [fəˌriŋgəuˌepiˈglɔtik], **pharyngoepiglottidean** [fəˌriŋgəuˌepiglɔˈtidiən] *a* 咽会厌的
pharyngoesophageal [fəˌriŋgəui(ː)ˈsɔfəˌdʒi(ː)əl] *a* 咽食管的
pharyngoglossal [fəˌriŋgəuˈglɔsəl] *a* 咽舌的
pharyngoglossus [fəˌriŋgəuˈglɔsəs] *n* 咽舌肌
pharyngokeratosis [fəˌriŋgəuˌkerəˈtəusis] *n* 咽角化病
pharyngolaryngeal [fəˌriŋgəuləˈrindʒiəl] *a* 咽喉的
pharyngolaryngitis [fəˌriŋgəuˌlærinˈdʒaitis] *n* 咽喉炎
pharyngolith [fəˈriŋgəliθ] *n* 咽石
pharyngology [ˌfæriŋˈgɔlədʒi] *n* 咽科学
pharyngolysis [ˌfæriŋˈgɔlisis] *n* 咽[肌]麻痹,咽瘫
pharyngomaxillary [fəˌriŋgəuˈmæksiləri] *a* 咽颌的
pharyngomycosis [fəˌriŋgəumaiˈkəusis] *n* 咽真菌病
pharyngonasal [fəˌriŋgəuˈneizəl] *a* 咽鼻的
pharyngo-oral [fəˌriŋgəu ˈɔːrəl] *a* 咽口的
pharyngopalatine [fəˌriŋgəuˈpælətain] *a* 咽腭的
pharyngopathy [ˌfæriŋˈgɔpəθi] *n* 咽病
pharyngoperistole [fəˌriŋgəupəˈristəli] *n* 咽狭窄
pharyngoplasty [fəˌriŋgəˌplæsti] *n* 咽成形术
pharyngoplegia [ˌfæriŋgəuˈpliːdʒiə], **pharyngoparalysis** [fəˌriŋgəupəˈrælisis] *n* 咽[肌]麻痹,咽瘫
pharyngorhinitis [fəˌriŋgəuraiˈnaitis] *n* 咽鼻炎
pharyngorhinoscopy [fəˌriŋgəuraiˈnɔskəpi] *n* 鼻咽镜检查[法]
pharyngorrhagia [ˌfæriŋgəˈreidʒiə] *n* 咽出血
pharyngorrhea [ˌfæriŋgəˈriːə] *n* 咽黏溢液
pharyngosalpingitis [fəˌriŋgəuˌsælpinˈdʒaitis] *n* 咽咽鼓管炎
pharyngoscleroma [fəˌriŋgəuskliəˈrəumə] *n* 咽硬结
pharyngoscope [fəˈriŋgəskəup] *n* 咽镜,咽窥器 | **pharyngoscopy** [ˌfæriŋˈgɔskəpi] *n* 咽镜检查
pharyngospasm [fəˌriŋgəspæzəm] *n* 咽痉挛
pharyngostenosis [fəˌriŋgəustiˈnəusis] *n* 咽狭窄
pharyngostoma [ˌfæriŋˈgɔstəmə] *n* 咽部造口
pharyngostome [fəˈriŋgəuˌstəum] *n* 咽部造口
pharyngostomy [ˌfæriŋˈgɔstəmi] *n* 咽造口术
pharyngotherapy [fəˌriŋgəuˈθerəpi] *n* 咽病疗法

（尤指传染病时鼻咽冲洗法）

pharyngotome [fəˈriŋɡətəum] *n* 咽刀

pharyngotomy [ˌfæriŋˈɡɔtəmi] *n* 咽切开术 | external ~ 咽外切开术 / internal ~ 咽内切开术 / lateral ~ 咽侧切开术

pharyngotonsillitis [fəˌriŋɡəuˌtɔnsiˈlaitis] *n* 咽扁桃体炎

pharyngotyphoid [fəˌriŋɡəuˈtaifɔid] *n* 咽型伤寒

pharyngoxerosis [fəˌriŋɡəuziəˈrəusis] *n* 咽干燥

pharynx [ˈfæriŋks] *n*【希】咽

phase [feiz] *n* 阶段;相;期 | anal ~ 肛欲期(精神分析,儿童性心理发育的第二期) / alpha ~ 动情期(卵巢周期) / apophylactic ~ 易感受期(见 negative ~) / beta ~ 黄体期(卵巢周期) / continuous ~ 连续相,分散媒,分散介质 / ~ of decline 衰退期 / disperse ~, internal ~ 分散相,内相 / erythrocytic ~ 红细胞内期(疟原虫) / estrin ~ 动情增殖期,增生期 / exponential ~ 指数(生长)期(指细菌,即对数期,见 logarithmic ~) / external ~ 外相,分散媒,分散介质 / genital ~ 性器恋期(精神分析,性心理成熟期) / hematic ~ 血相(一种液晶相) / inductive ~ 诱导期(从接触抗原后到出现可测出的免疫应答以前的这段时间) / lag ~ 迟滞期,延缓期 / latency ~ 潜伏期;性成熟前期 / logarithmic ~ 对数期(细菌繁殖速度最快的时期) / meiotic ~, reduction ~ 减数期(染色体) / negative ~ 阴性期(注射相应抗原后,血液抗体量暂时性下降) / oral ~ 口欲期(精神分析,儿童性心理发育最早期) / phallic ~ 阳具期(精神分析,指婴儿性心理发育的第三期) / postmeiotic ~ 减数后期(染色体) / premeiotic ~, prereduction ~ 减数前期(染色体) / smectic ~ 近晶相(一种液晶相) / stance ~ 静止负重相 / stationary ~ 静止相,稳定期(细菌) / swing ~ 摆动负重相 / synaptic ~ 染色体联会期

phasein [ˈfeisiːn] *n* 菜豆凝集素(能使红细胞凝集)

phaseolamin [fəˌsiːəˈlɑːmin] *n* 菜豆素

phaseolin [fəˈsiːəlin] *n* 菜豆球蛋白,菜豆素

phaseolunatin [ˌfeisiəˈljunətin] *n* 亚麻苦苷,棉豆苷

Phaseolus [ˌfeiːziˈəuləs] *n* 菜豆属

phasin [ˈfeisin] *n* 菜豆凝集素

phasmid [ˈfæzmid] *n* 尾感器;尾感器线虫

Phasmidia [fæzˈmidiə] *n* 尾感器亚纲

PhB British Pharmacopoeia 英国药典

PhD Philosophiae Doctor【拉】哲学博士

Phe phenylalanine 苯丙氨酸

phellandrene [fəˈlændriːn] *n* 水芹烯

Phelps' operation [felps] (Abel M. Phelps) 费尔普斯手术(畸形足手术)

phemfilcon A [ˈfemfilkɔn] 非姆费尔康 A(一种亲水性接触镜材料)

-phemia [构词成分]说话方式

Phemister graft [ˈfemist] (Dallus Burton Phemister) 费密斯特移植物(一种骨移植物) | ~ operation 费密斯特手术(使用骨松质的外置移植物,不用内固定,以治疗稳定但不连的骨折)

phemitone [ˈfemitəun] *n* 甲苯巴比妥(抗惊厥及镇静药)

phen- [前缀]苯[基]

phenacaine hydrochloride [ˈfenəkein] *n* 盐酸非那卡因(用于结膜表面麻醉药)

phenacemide [fiˈnæsimaid] *n* 苯乙酰脲(精神运动性癫痫和癫痫大发作时用作抗惊厥药)

phenacetin [fiˈnæsitin] *n* 非那西丁(解热镇痛药)

phenacetolin [ˌfenəˈsetəlin] *n* 非那西托林(一种指示剂)

phenaglycodol [ˌfenəˈɡlaikədɔl] *n* 非那二醇(安定药)

phenakistoscope [ˌfiːnəˈkistəskəup] *n* 频闪观测器,动态镜

phenanthrene [fiˈnænθriːn] *n* 菲

phenanthroline [fiˈnænθrəliːn] *n* 二氮菲,邻二氮杂菲

phenantoin [ˈfenənˌtəuin] *n* 3-甲基苯乙妥因(即美芬妥英 mephenytoin,抗惊厥药)

phenate [ˈfiːneit] *n* 酚盐

phenazocine hydrobromide [fiˈnæzəsiːn] 氢溴酸非那佐辛(合成的麻醉性镇痛药)

phenazone [ˈfenəzəun] *n* 非那宗(解热镇痛药)

phenazopyridine hydrochloride [ˌfenəzəuˈpiridiːn] 盐酸非那吡啶(泌尿道镇痛药,从前用作泌尿道抗菌药)

phenbutazone sodium glycerate [fenˈbjuːtəzəun] 甘油保泰松钠(抗炎药)

phencyclidine hydrochloride [fenˈsaiklidiːn] 盐酸苯环利定(兽用强效镇痛药和麻醉药)

phendimetrazine tartrate [ˌfendaiˈmetrəziːn] 酒石酸苯甲曲秦(食欲抑制药,口服给药)

phene [fiːn] *n* 表型性状(由基因所控制的遗传表型性状的泛称)

phenelzine sulfate [ˈfenəlzin] 硫酸苯乙肼(单胺氧化酶抑制剂,用作抗抑郁药)

phenethicillin [fiˌneθiˈsilin] *n* 非奈西林(抗生素类药)

phenethylbiguanide [feˌneθilˈbaiɡwɑːnaid] *n* 苯乙双胍(即 phenformin,降血糖药)

phenetidin [fiˈnetidin] *n* 非那替丁,氨基苯乙醚

phenetidinuria [fiˌnetidiˈnjuəriə] *n* 非那替丁尿,氨基苯乙醚尿

phenetole [ˈfenitɔl] *n* 乙氧苯,苯乙醚

phenformin hydrochloride [fenˈfɔːmin] 盐酸苯

乙双胍(口服降血糖药,美国已不再使用)
phengophobia [ˌfengəuˈfəubjə] *n* 畏光,羞明
phenic acid [ˈfiːnik] 石炭酸,苯酚
phenindamine tartrate [fiˈnindəmiːn] 酒石酸苯茚胺(抗组胺药)
phenindione [ˌfeninˈdaiəun] *n* 苯茚二酮(抗凝血药)
pheniramine maleate [fəˈnirəmin] 马来酸非尼拉敏(抗组胺药)
phenmetrazine hydrochloride [fenˈmetrəziːn] 盐酸芬美曲秦(中枢神经系统兴奋药,食欲抑制药)
phen(o)- [构词成分]显出,表现;[前缀]苯酚,苯基
phenobarbital [ˌfiːnəuˈbɑːbitəl] *n* 苯巴比妥(抗惊厥及镇静催眠药) | ~ sodium 苯巴比妥钠 | **phenobarbitone** [ˌfiːnəuˈbɑːbitəun] *n*
phenocopy [ˈfiːnəˌkɔpi] *n* 表型模拟(一种环境条件引起的表型,与某一特定基因所产生的表型相似);表型模拟者;表型模拟特征
phenodeviant [ˌfiːnəuˈdiːviənt] *n* 表型偏差体
phenodin [ˈfiːnədin] *n* 羟高铁血红素(治卟啉病药)
phenogenetics [ˌfiːnəudʒiˈnetiks] *n* 表型遗传学
phenol [ˈfiːnɔl] *n* 酚,石炭酸 | liquefied ~ 液化酚 / ~ red 酚红,酚磺酞(肾功能诊断药) / ~ salicylate 水杨酸苯酯 | **~ic** [fiˈnɔlik] *a*
phenolase [ˈfiːnəleis] *n* 酚酶
phenolate [ˈfiːnəleit] *vt* 用酚消毒 *n* 酚盐
phenolated [ˈfiːnəˌleitid] *a* 加酚的,含酚的
phenolemia [ˌfiːnɔˈliːmiə] *n* 酚血[症]
phenolization [ˌfiːnəlaiˈzeiʃən,-liˈz-] *n* 酚处置,石炭酸处置
phenology [fiˈnɔlədʒi] *n* 物候学 | **phenological** [ˌfiːnəˈlɔdʒikəl] *a* / **phenologist** *n* 物候学家
phenolphthalein [ˌfiːnɔlˈθæliːn] *n* 酚酞(泻药)
phenol sulfatase [ˈfiːnɔl ˈsʌlfəteis] 苯硫酸[酯]酶,芳基硫酸酯酶
phenolsulfonphthalein [ˌfiːnɔlˌsʌlfəunˈθæliːn] *n* 酚磺酞(肾功能测定药)
phenoltetrachlorophthalein [ˌfiːnɔlˌtetrəˌklɔːrəˈθæliːn] *n* 四氯酚酞(肝功能试剂)
phenoltetraiodophthalein [ˌfiːnɔlˌtetrəˌaiədəuˈθæliːn] *n* 四碘酚酞(其钠盐用作肝功能试剂及胆囊造影剂)
phenoluria [ˌfiːnɔˈljuəriə] *n* 酚尿,石炭酸尿
phenom [ˈfiːnɔm] *n* 同型种
phenomenology [fiˌnɔmiˈnɔlədʒi] *n* 现象学(精神病理学的一个分科)
phenomenon [fiˈnɔminən]([复] **phenomena** [fiˈnɔminə]) *n* 现象 | abstinence ~ 脱瘾现象 / anaphylactoid ~ 类过敏性现象,假过敏反应 / aqueous-influx ~, glass-rod ~ 房水输入现象,玻璃棒现象 / arm ~ 臂现象(见 Pool's phenomenon) / blanching ~. 转白现象(见 Schultz-Charlton reaction) / cheek ~ 颊反射现象(见于脑膜炎) / cogwheel ~ 齿轮现象(张力过度的肌肉受到被动性牵扯时,即产生抵抗,这种抵抗现象有时呈现为不规则的跳动) / fixation ~ 结合现象(补体结合〈fixation of the complement〉,见 fixation 项下相应术语) / finger ~ 伸指现象(半身不遂时)(①加压豌豆骨时,全部手指或拇指及示指伸展,亦称戈登〈Gordon〉征;②苏克现象,见 Souques' phenomenon) / hip-flexion ~ 屈髋现象(截瘫患者起卧时,瘫痪髋关节屈曲) / interference ~ 干扰现象(①一药物干扰另一药物的疗效;②同时感染另一可能有关或可能无关的病毒以干扰某一病毒的复制或毒力,亦称先占免疫) / jaw-winking ~ 眨眼动颌现象(见 Gunn's syndrome) / LE ~ 红斑狼疮现象(形成红斑狼疮细胞的过程) / no-reflow ~ 无回流现象(大脑血流量在长时间全脑局部缺血后得以恢复时,最初为充血,继之血液灌注逐渐下降,直至几乎无血流量) / orbicularis ~ 眼轮匝肌现象(见 Westphal-Piltz phenomenon) / prezone ~, prozone ~ 前带现象,前区现象(见 prozone) / psi ~ 精神现象 / radial ~ 桡神经现象(手指向掌侧弯曲时,腕部不能随意地向背侧弯曲) / rash-extinction ~ 红疹消退现象(见 Schultz-Charlton reaction) / rebound ~ 回缩现象(使患者屈肘,而后紧握其腕部强使伸直,如突然松握,则患者前臂向其身体回缩,为小脑病灶的体征) / reclotting ~ 触变性,摇溶性 / second set ~ 二次现象(第二次移植同样的异体组织后,移植物加速和加强排斥,亦称二次排斥) / shot-silk ~ 闪缎样现象(视网膜) / toe ~ 伸趾现象(见 Babinski's reflex) / tongue ~ 舌现象(轻吹舌头可引起舌收缩及出现深度下陷,见于手足搐搦) / zone ~ 界现象,(区)带现象(沉淀反应时,上清液中可以有三种不同的区带:抗体过剩带、等价带和抗原过剩带)
phenon [ˈfiːnɔn] *n* 同型种
phenopropazine hydrochloride [ˌfiːnəuˈprəupəziːn] 盐酸二乙异丙嗪,盐酸普罗吩胺(即 ethopropazine hydrochloride,抗震颤麻痹药)
phenothiazine [ˌfiːnəuˈθaiəziːn] *n* 酚噻嗪(抗蠕虫药)
phenotype [ˈfiːnətaip] *n* 表型(个体可见的性状,由于基因型和环境因素共同制约的);表型相同者 | Bombay ~ 孟买表型(ABO 血型系基因与另一位点的罕见的隐性基因相互作用后产生的罕见的表现型,表现为 H 抗原完全缺失,血细胞中没有 A、B 和 H 抗原,而血清含抗 A、抗 B 和抗 H 抗原) | **phenotypic(al)** [ˌfiːnəuˈtipik(əl)] *a*
phenoxide [feˈnɔksaid] *n* 苯氧化物,[苯]酚盐

phenoxy- [前缀]苯氧基
phenoxybenzamine hydrochloride [fiˌnɔksiˈbenzəmiːn] 盐酸酚苄明,盐酸苯氧苄胺(血管扩张药,用作抗高血压药)
phenozygous [fiˈnɔzigəs] *a* 突颧的
phenprocoumon [fenˈprəukumən] *n* 苯丙香豆素(抗凝血药)
phenpromethamine hydrochloride [ˌfenprəu-ˈmeθəmiːn] 盐酸苯丙甲胺(血管收缩药)
phenpropionate [fenˈprəupiəneit] *n* 苯丙酸盐;苯丙酸酯(3-phenylpropionate 的 USAN 缩约词)
phensuximide [fenˈsʌksimaid] *n* 苯琥胺(抗癫痫药)
phentermine [ˈfentəːmiːn] *n* 芬特明(食欲抑制药) | ~ hydrochloride 盐酸芬特明(食欲抑制药)
phentolamine [fenˈtɔləmiːn] *n* 酚妥拉明(血管扩张药) | ~ hydrochloride 盐酸酚妥拉明 / ~ mesylate 甲磺酸酚妥拉明
phenyl [ˈfenil, ˈfiːnil] *n* 苯基 | ~ carbinol 苄醇,苯甲醇 / ~ salicylate 水杨酸苯酯
phenylacetic acid [ˌfeniləˈsiːtik] 苯乙酸
phenylacetylurea [ˌfenilˌæsitiljuəˈriə] *n* 苯乙酰脲(抗癫痫药)
phenylalanine [ˌfeniˈlæləni(ː)n] *n* 苯丙氨酸
phenylalanine hydroxylase [ˌfeniˈlælənin haiˈdrɔksileis] 苯丙氨酸羟化酶,苯丙氨酸 4-单加氧酶
phenylalanine hydroxylase deficiency 苯丙氨酸羟化酶缺乏症,苯丙酮尿症
phenylalaninemia [ˌfeniˌlæləniˈniːmiə] *n* 苯丙氨酸血症,高苯丙氨酸血症
phenylalanine 4-monooxygenase [ˌfeniˈlælənin-ˌmɔnəuˈɔksidʒəneis] 苯丙氨酸 4-单加氧酶(此酶缺乏可致高苯丙氨酸血症)
phenylalanyl [ˌfeniˈlælənil] *n* 苯丙氨酰[基]
***N*-phenylanthranilic acid** [ˌfenəlˌænθrəˈnilik] *N*-苯氨茴酸,邻苯氨基苯甲酸
phenylbenzimidazole sulfonic acid [ˌfenilˌbenziˈmidəzəul sʌlˈfɔnik] 苯基苯并咪唑磺酸(即 ensulizole)
phenylbutazone [ˌfenilˈbjuːtəzəun] *n* 保泰松(消炎镇痛药)
phenylcarbinol [ˌfenilˈkɑːbinɔl] *n* 苄醇,苯甲醇(局部麻醉药,消毒防腐药)
phenyldimethylpyrazolon [ˌfenildaiˌmeθilpaiˈreizəlɔn] *n* 苯二甲基吡唑酮,安替比林(解热镇痛药)
phenylene [ˈfiːniliːn] *n* 亚苯基
***p*-phenylenediamine** [ˌpærəˌfenəliːnˈdaiəmiːn] 对苯二胺(用作染发、服装和织品的染料,用作摄影的显影剂,本品为强变应原,可致接触性皮炎和支气管哮喘)
phenylephrine hydrochloride [ˌfeniˈlefrin] 盐酸去甲肾上腺素(拟肾上腺素药,用作血管收缩药和升压药)
phenylethylbarbituric acid [ˌfeniˌleθilbɑːbiˈtjuərik] 苯基乙基巴比土酸,苯巴比妥(催眠镇静药)
phenylglycolic acid [ˌfenilglaiˈkɔlik] 苯乙醇酸,杏仁酸
phenylglycuronic acid [ˌfenilˌglaikjuˈrɔnik] 苯葡萄糖醛苷酸
phenylhydrazine [ˌfenilˈhaidrəzin] *n* 苯肼
phenylic [fiːˈnilik] *a* 苯基的 | ~ acid 酚,苯酚,石炭酸
phenylindanedione [ˌfenilinˈdeindiəun] *n* 苯茚二酮(抗凝血药)
phenylketonuria (PKU) [ˌfenilˌkiːtəuˈnjuəriə] *n* 苯[丙]酮尿症(即高苯丙氨酸血症Ⅰ型,亦称 PKU1) | atypical ~ 非典型性苯丙酮尿症(即高苯丙氨酸血症Ⅴ型) / maternal ~ 母体苯丙酮尿(患苯丙酮尿症孕妇的宫内发育〈与孕妇的基因型无关〉,可导致经常流产,在存活的非苯丙酮尿症后代中可致精神发育迟缓、小头畸形、低出生体重等) / ~ Ⅱ 苯丙酮尿Ⅱ型(即高苯丙氨酸血Ⅳ型) / ~ Ⅲ 苯丙酮尿症Ⅲ型(即高苯丙氨酸血症Ⅴ型) | **phenylketonuric** *a*
phenyllactic acid [ˌfeniˈlæktik] 苯乳酸
phenylmercuric [ˌfenilməːˈkjuərik] *n* 苯汞基 | ~ acetate 醋酸苯汞(消毒防腐药) / ~ nitrate 硝酸苯汞(消毒防腐药)
phenylmethanol [ˌfenilˈmeθənɔl] *n* 苄醇,苯甲醇(局部麻醉药,消毒防腐药)
phenylpropanolamine hydrochloride [ˌfenilˌprupəˈnɔlæmin] 盐酸苯丙醇胺(血管收缩药,中枢神经系统兴奋药,减食欲药)
phenylpropylmethylamine hydrochloride [ˌfenilˌprəupilˌmeθiˈlæmiːn] 盐酸苯丙甲胺(血管收缩药)
phenylpyruvic acid [ˌfenilpaiˈruvik] 苯丙酮酸
phenylpyruvicaciduria [ˌfenilpaiˌruvikˌæsiˈdjuəriə] *n* 苯丙酮尿
phenylthiourea [ˌfenilˌθaiəjuəˈriːə], **phenylthiocarbamide** [ˌfenilˌθaiəkɑːˈbæmid] *n* 苯硫脲(用于遗传学研究,人们对这种化合物的味觉的显性性状是遗传的,约 70% 的人能尝出它的苦味,其余的人则尝不出)
phenyltoloxamine citrate [ˌfeniltəˈlɔksəmiːn] 枸橼酸苯托沙敏(抗组胺药)
phenyramidol hydrochloride [ˌfeniˈræmidɔl] 盐酸非尼拉朵(镇痛药,骨骼肌松弛药)
phenytoin [ˈfenitəuin] *n* 苯妥英(抗惊厥药,心脏抑制药,抗癫痫药) | ~ sodium 苯妥英钠

phe(o)- [构词成分]棕色,暗褐色,暗黑色;同样见以 phae(o)-起始的词
pheochrome [ˈfiːəkrəum] *a* 嗜铬的
pheochromoblast [ˌfiːəˈkrəuməblæst] *n* 成嗜铬细胞
pheochromoblastoma [ˌfiːəˌkrəuməblæsˈtəumə] *n* 成嗜铬细胞瘤
pheochromocyte [ˌfiːəˈkrəuməsait] *n* 嗜铬细胞
pheochromocytoma [ˌfiːəˌkrəuməsaiˈtəumə] *n* 嗜铬细胞瘤
pheomelanin [ˌfiːəuˈmelənin] *n* 含硫型黑[色]素
pheophytin [ˌfiːəˈfaitin] *n* 脱镁叶绿素
pheresis [fəˈriːsis] *n* 去除术(从供者抽血,分离并保留一部分〈如血浆、白细胞等〉,剩下的再输回给供者。它包括血浆去除术、白细胞去除术等,称apheresis更加恰当)
pheromone [ˈferəməun] *n* 信息素,外激素(由一个体释放而影响同种生物的行为的化合物) | alarm ~ 警报信息素(蚯蚓对有害的刺激分泌出一种黏液,为同种其他生物所回避)
phetharbital [feˈθɑːbitəl] *n* 非沙比妥(抗惊厥药)
PhG Graduate in Pharmacy 药学毕业生; ***Pharmacopoeia Germanica***《德国药典》
phi [fai] *n* 希腊语的第21个字母(Φ,φ)
phial [ˈfaiəl] *n* 管形瓶,小药瓶
phialoconidium [ˌfaiələukəˈnidiəm] *n* 瓶分生孢子
phialide [ˈfaiəlaid] *n* 瓶梗
Phialophora [ˌfaiəˈlɔfərə] *n* 瓶霉属 | ~ verrucosa 疣状瓶霉
phialophore [ˈfaiələfɔː] *n* 瓶梗托
phialospore [ˈfaiələspɔː] *n* 瓶梗孢子
-phil, -phile [构词成分]嗜,亲
philagrypnia [ˌfailəˈgripniə] *n* 少睡习惯
Philasterina [ˌfilæstəˈrainə] *n* 嗜海星亚目
-philia [构词成分](不正常的)癖好;嗜,亲
philiater [fiˈlaiətə] *n* 医学爱好者
-philic [构词成分]嗜…的,亲…的
Philippe-Gombault tract [fiˈlip gɔmˈbəu] (Claudius Philippe; François A. A. Gombault)菲利普-贡博束(见 Gombault-Philippe triangle)
Philip's glands [ˈfilip] (Robert W. Philip)菲利普淋巴结(患结核儿童锁骨上部的淋巴结肿大)
Phillyrea [fiˈliːriə] *n* 连翘属
phillyrin [ˈfilirin] *n* 连翘苷(具有抗疟作用)
philosophic(al) [ˌfiləˈsɔfik(əl)] *a* 哲学家的;哲学上的
philosophy [fiˈlɔsəfi] *n* 哲学;人生观;(某一学科的)基本原理
philothion [ˌfailəˈθaiɔn] *n* 谷胱甘肽
philter, philtre [ˈfiltə] *n* 春药,催情药 *vt* 用春药迷惑,使兴奋
philtrum [ˈfiltrəm] ([复] **philtra** [ˈfiltrə]) *n* 人中(上唇中央部);春药,催情药
phimosiectomy [faiˌməusiˈektəmi] *n* 包皮环切术
phimosis [faiˈməusis] *n*【希】包茎 | ~ vaginalis 阴道闭锁 | **phimotic** [faiˈmɔtik] *a*
phlebalgia [fliˈbældʒiə] *n* 静脉痛
phlebanesthesia [ˌflebænisˈθiːzjə] *n* 静脉[注射]麻醉法
phlebangioma [ˌflebændʒiˈəumə] *n* 静脉瘤
phlebarteriectasia [ˌflebɑːˌtiəriekˈteizjə] *n* 动静脉扩张
phlebasthenia [ˌflebæsˈθiːniə] *n* 静脉壁无力
phlebectasia [ˌflebekˈteizjə], **phlebectasis** [fliˈbektəsis] *n* 静脉扩张
phlebectomy [fliˈbektəmi] *n* 静脉切除术
phlebectopia [ˌflebekˈtəupiə], **phlebectopy** [fliˈbektəpi] *n* 静脉异位
phlebemphraxis [ˌflebemˈfræksis] *n* 静脉梗阻
phlebexairesis [ˌflebekˈsaiərəsis] *n* 静脉抽出术
phlebismus [fliˈbizməs] *n* 阻塞性静脉膨胀
phlebitis [fliˈbaitis] *n* 静脉炎 | adhesive ~, plastic ~, proliferative ~ 粘连性静脉炎 / obliterating ~, obstructive ~ 闭塞性静脉炎 / productive ~ 静脉硬化 | **phlebitic** [fliˈbitik] *a*
phleb(o)- [构词成分]静脉
phleboclysis [fliˈbɔklisis] *n* 静脉输液法 | drip ~, slow ~ 点滴静脉输液法
phlebofibrosis [ˌflebəufaiˈbrəusis] *n* 静脉纤维变性
phlebogenous [fliˈbɔdʒinəs] *a* 静脉原的
phlebogram [ˈflebəgræm] *n* 静脉造影[照]片;静脉搏动描记图
phlebograph [ˈflebəgrɑːf] *n* 静脉搏动描记器
phlebography [fliˈbɔgrəfi] *n* 静脉造影[术];静脉搏动描记法;静脉论
phleboid [ˈflebɔid] *a* 静脉样的
phlebolith [ˈflebəliθ] *n* 静脉石
phlebolithiasis [ˌflebəuliˈθaiəsis] *n* 静脉石病
phlebology [fliˈbɔlədʒi] *n* 静脉学
phlebomanometer [ˌflebəuməˈnɔmitə] *n* 静脉血压计
phlebometritis [ˌflebəumiˈtraitis] *n* 子宫静脉炎
phlebonarcosis [ˌflebəunɑːˈkəusis] *n* 静脉[注射]麻醉法
phlebopexy [ˈflebəˌpeksi] *n* 静脉固定术
phlebophlebostomy [ˌflebəufliˈbɔstəmi] *n* 静脉静脉吻合术
phlebophthalmotomy [ˌflebɔfθælˈmɔtəmi] *n* 眼静脉切开术
phlebopiezometry [ˌflebəuˌpaiəˈzɔmitri] *n* 静脉压检查法

phleboplasty [ˈflebəˌplæsti] *n* 静脉成形术
phleborheography [ˌflebəuriˈɔgrəfi] *n* 静脉流变描记法(用于诊断深静脉血栓形成)
phleborrhagia [ˌflebəuˈreidʒiə] *n* 静脉出血
phleborrhaphy [fliˈbɔrəfi] *n* 静脉缝合术
phleborrhexis [ˌflebəuˈreksis] *n* 静脉破裂
phlebosclerosation [ˌflebəuˌskliərəˈzeiʃən] *n* 静脉硬化法
phlebosclerosis [ˌflebəuskliəˈrəusis] *n* 静脉硬化
phlebosis [fliˈbəusis] *n* (非炎性)静脉病
phlebostasis [fliˈbɔstəsis], **phlebostasia** [ˌflebəˈsteizjə] *n* 静脉止血法;静脉淤滞法(上止血带)
phlebostenosis [ˌflebəustiˈnəusis] *n* 静脉狭窄
phlebothrombosis [ˌflebəuθrɔmˈbəusis] *n* 静脉血栓形成
phlebotome [ˈflebətəum] *n* 静脉刀
phlebotomist [fliˈbɔtəmist] *n* 静脉切开者,静脉切开医师;放血者,放血医师
phlebotomize [fliˈbɔtəmaiz] *vt, vi* 放血,行静脉切开放血术
Phlebotomus [fliˈbɔtəməs] *n* 白蛉属 | ~ argentipes 银足白蛉 / ~ chinensis 中华白蛉 / ~ intermedius 中间白蛉 / ~ macedonicum 马其顿白蛉 / ~ major wui 硕大白蛉吴氏亚种 / ~ mongolensis 蒙古白蛉 / ~ noguchi 野口白蛉 / ~ papatasii 巴浦白蛉(传染白蛉热) / ~ perniciosus 恶毒白蛉 / ~ sergenti 司氏白蛉 / ~ verrucarum 疣肿白蛉
phlebotomy [fliˈbɔtəmi] *n* 静脉切开术,放血术 | bloodless ~ 静脉淤滞法(上止血带)
Phlebovirus [ˈflebəuˌvaiərəs] *n* 白蛉热病毒;白蛉病毒属
phlegm [flem] *n* 黏液(旧时体液学说的四液之一);黏痰
phlegmasia [flegˈmeiziə] *n*【希】炎[症],热 | thrombotic ~ 血栓性静脉炎,股白肿 | **phlegmonosis** [ˌflegməuˈnəusis] *n*
phlegmatic(al) [flegˈmætik(əl)] *a* 黏液质的;迟钝的,冷淡的
phlegmon [ˈflegmən] *n* 蜂窝[组]织炎 | **~ous** *a*
phlegmona [ˈflegmənə] *n*【拉】蜂窝织炎
Phleum [ˈfliːəm] *n* 梯牧草属
phlobaphene [ˈfləubəfiːn] *n* 鞣酐,鞣红
phloem [ˈfləuem] *n* 韧皮部
phlogistic [flɔˈdʒistik] *a* 炎的,炎性的
phlogisticozymoid [flɔˌdʒistikəuˈzaimɔid] *n* 炎性类酶
phlogiston [flɔˈdʒistən] *n* 燃素(假设的易燃物质所含的成分)
phlog(o)- [构词成分]炎
phlogocyte [ˈflɔgəsait] *n* 浆细胞
phlogocytosis [ˌflɔgəusaiˈtəusis] *n* (血内)浆细胞增多
phlogogen [ˈflɔgədʒən] *n* 致炎[物]质,酿炎物
phlogogenic [ˌflɔgəuˈdʒenik], **phlogogenous** [flɔˈgɔdʒinəs] *a* 致炎的
phlogotherapy [ˌflɔgəuˈθerəpi] *n* 非特异疗法
phlogotic [fləˈgətik] *a* 炎的,炎性的
phloretic acid [fləˈretik] 根皮酸,β-苯酚丙酸
phlorhizin [fləˈraizin], **phloridzin** [fləˈridzin], **phlorizin** [fləˈraizin] *n* 根皮苷
phlorhizin hydrolase [fləˈraizin] 根皮苷水解酶,糖基神经酰胺酶
phlorhizinize [fləˈraizinaiz], **phloridzinize** [fləˈridzinaiz] *vt* 根皮苷处理
phloroglucin [ˌflɔrəˈglusin], **phloroglucinol** [ˌfləərəˈglusinɔl] *n* 间苯三酚,藤黄酚,根皮酚
phlorol [ˈflɔrɔl] *n* 邻乙基[苯]酚
phlorose [ˈflɔrəus] *n* 根皮糖,葡萄糖
phlorrhizin [fləˈraizin] *n* 根皮苷
phloryl [ˈflɔril] *n* 木溜油精
phloxine [ˈflɔksin] *n* 焰红染料(对癌细胞有破坏作用)
phlyctena [flikˈtiːnə] ([复] **phlyctenae** [flikˈtiːniː]), **phlycten** [ˈfliktən] *n* 水泡(灼伤所致);小[水]疱(内含淋巴,见于结膜) | **phlyctenar** [ˈfliktinə] *a*
phlyctenoid [ˈfliktinɔid] *a* 水泡样的;小疱样的
phlyctenosis [ˌfliktiˈnəusis] *n* 小泡病,小水疱病
phlyctenotherapy [ˌfliktinəuˈθerəpi] *n* 水疱浆疗法
phlyctenula [flikˈtenjulə] ([复] **phlyctenulae** [flikˈtenjuliː]) *n*【拉】小[水]疱
phlyctenule [ˈfliktənjuːl] *n* 小(水)疱(角膜或结膜的溃烂小结) | **phlyctenular** [flikˈtenjulə] *a* 小疱[形成]的
phlyctenulosis [ˌfliktənjuˈləusis] *n* 小水疱病
phobia [ˈfəubiə] *n* 恐怖症 | simple ~ 单纯恐怖症(包括孤独恐怖、广场恐怖、动物恐怖、高处恐怖等) / social ~ 社交恐怖症(如在公共场所言语或表现恐怖、使用公厕恐怖、在公共场所进食恐怖) | **phobic** *a*
phobophobia [fəubəuˈfəubjə] *n* 恐怖[体验]恐怖(精神衰弱时对自己的恐怖体验感到恐怖)
Phocas' disease [fəˈkɑːz] (B. G. Phocas)福卡斯病(慢性结节性乳腺炎,伴有许多小结节)
phocomelia [ˌfəukəˈmiːliə] *n* 短肢,先天性无臂,海豹肢畸形(臂腿缺如,手足直接与躯干相连)
phocomelus [fəˈkɔmiləs] *n* 短肢畸胎,海豹肢畸胎
Phoma [ˈfəumə] *n* 茎点霉属,疱霉属
phomopsin [fəuˈmɔpsin] *n* 拟茎点霉毒素

Phomopsis [fəu'mɔpsis] *n* 拟茎点霉属
phon [fəun] *n* 昉(响度单位)
phonacoscope [fəu'nækəskəup] *n* 叩听诊器
phonacoscopy [ˌfəunə'kɔskəpi] *n* 叩听诊法
phonal ['fəunəl] *a* 音的,声音的
phonarteriogram [ˌfəunɑːˈtiəriəgræm] *n* 动脉音图
phonarteriographic [ˌfəunɑːˌtiəriə'græfik] *a* 动脉音描记法的;动脉音图的
phonarteriography [ˌfəunɑːˌtiəri'ɔgrəfi] *n* 动脉音描记法
phonasthenia [ˌfəunæs'θiːniə] *n* 发声无力
phonation [fə'neiʃən] *n* 发声 | subenergetic ~ 发声过弱 / superenergetic ~ 发声过强 | **phonatory** ['fəunətəri] *a*
phonautograph [fəu'nɔːtəgrɑːf] *n* 语声描记器
phone [fəun] *n* 单音
phoneme ['fəuniːm] *n* 音素
phonendoscope [fə'nendəuskəup] *n* 扩音听诊器
phonendoskiascope [fəˌnendəu'skaiəskəup] *n* X线透视扩音听诊器
phonetic [fəu'netik] *a* 语声的,语音的
phonetics [fəu'netiks] *n* 语声学,语音学
phoniatrician [ˌfəuniə'triʃən] *n* 语音矫正师
phoniatrics [ˌfəuni'ætriks] *n* 语音矫正法
phonic ['fəunik] *a* 声音的,语音的
phonism ['fəunizəm] *n* 音联觉(指由于光、嗅、味觉等刺激或思想引起的声音感觉)
phon(o)- [构词成分]音,声
phonoangiography [ˌfəunəuˌændʒi'ɔgrəfi] *n* 血管音描记法
phonoauscultation [ˌfəunəuɔːskʌl'teiʃən] *n* 音叉听诊法
phonocardiogram [ˌfəunəu'kɑːdiəgræm] *n* 心音图
phonocardiograph [ˌfəunəu'kɑːdiəgrɑːf, -græf] *n* 心音描记器 | **~y** [ˌfəunəuˌkɑːdi'ɔgrəfi] *n* 心音描记法 / **~ic** [ˌfəunəuˌkɑːdiə'græfik] *a* 心音图的;心音描记的
phonocatheter [ˌfəunəu'kæθitə] *n* 检音导管
phonocatheterization [ˌfəunəuˌkæθitərai'zeiʃən, -ri'z-] *n* 检音导管插入[术]
phonoelectrocardioscope [ˌfəunəuiˌlektrəu'kɑːdiəskəup] *n* 心音心电直视描记器
phonogram ['fəunəgræm] *n* 录声片,录音片(如录心音);声图
phonology [fəu'nɔlədʒi] *n* 语声学,语音学
phonomania [ˌfɔnə'meinjə] *n* 杀人狂
phonomassage [ˌfəunəu'mæsɑːʒ] *n* 音波按摩法(用以治耳病)
phonometer [fəu'nɔmitə] *n* 声强度计
phonomyoclonus [ˌfəunəumai'ɔklənəs] *n* 有音肌阵挛
phonomyogram [ˌfəunəu'maiəgræm] *n* 肌音图
phonomyography [ˌfəunəumai'ɔgrəfi] *n* 肌音描记法
phonopathy [fəu'nɔpəθi] *n* 发声器官病,发音器官病
phonophobia [ˌfəunə'fəubjə] *n* 高声恐怖,声响恐怖,恐响症
phonophore ['fəunəfɔː] *n* 听[小]骨
phonophotography [ˌfəunəufə'tɔgrəfi] *n* 声波照相术
phonopneumomassage [ˌfəunəuˌnjuːməu'mæsɑːʒ] *n* 音波[空气]按摩法(中耳)
phonopsia [fəu'nɔpsiə] *n* 音幻视,闻声见色
phonoreception [ˌfəunəuri'sepʃən] *n* 声感受,感声
phonoreceptor [ˌfəunəuri'septə] *n* 声感受器
phonorenogram [ˌfəunəu'riːnəgræm] *n* 检音肾动脉搏动图
phonoscope ['fəunəskəup] *n* 心音波照相器;内脏叩听器 | **phonoscopy** [fəu'nɔskəpi] *n* 心音波照相检查;内脏叩听检查
phonoselectoscope [ˌfəunəusi'lektəskəup] *n* 高音听诊器
phonostethograph [ˌfəunəu'steθəgrɑːf] *n* 听诊录音机
phorbol ['fɔːbɔl] *n* 佛波醇 | ~ ester 佛波酯(强力辅致癌物,常在研究中使用以增强用致癌物诱发遗传突变或肿瘤)
-phore [构词成分]带有…的,携带者
-phoresis [构词成分]移动,透入;传递
phoria ['fəuriə] *n* 隐斜
phoriascope ['fəuriəskəup] *n* 隐斜视矫正镜
Phormia ['fɔːmiə] *n* 伏蝇属 | ~ regina 伏蝇
phoroblast ['fɔrəblæst] *n* 成纤维细胞
phorocyte ['fɔrəsait] *n* 结缔组织细胞
phorocytosis [ˌfɔrəsai'təusis] *n* 结缔组织细胞增生
phorologist [fə'rɔlədʒist] *n* 疫源探查者
phorology [fə'rɔlədʒi] *n* 带菌[者]学
phorometer [fə'rɔmitə] *n* 隐斜测量计 | **phorometry** [fə'rɔmitri] *n* 隐斜测量[法]
phoront ['fɔːrɔnt] *n* 帚体
phoro-optometer [ˌfəurə ɔp'tɔmitə] *n* 综合屈光检查仪
phoropter [fɔ'rɔptə] *n* 视力检查仪
phoroscope ['fəurəskəup] *n* 固定试眼架
phorotone ['fəurətəun] *n* 眼肌操练器
phorozoon [ˌfəurə'zəuɔn] *n* 无性世代,无性体
phose [fəuz] *n* (主观的)光觉,色觉;光幻觉,色幻觉

phosgene [ˈfɔzdʒiːn] *n* 光气,碳酰氯
phosgenic [fɔzˈdʒenik] *a* 发光的
phosis [ˈfəusis] *n* (主观的)光觉产生,色觉产生;光幻觉产生,色幻觉产生
phosphagen [ˈfɔsfədʒən] *n* 磷酸原(一组高能磷酸化合物,包括磷酸肌酸和磷酸精氨酸)
phosphagenic [ˌfɔsfəˈdʒenik] *a* 生成磷酸盐的
phosphaminase [fɔsˈfæmineis] *n* 氨基磷酸酶
phosphatase [ˈfɔsfəteis] *n* 磷酸酶 | acid ~ 酸性磷酸酶 / alkaline ~ 碱性磷酸酶
phosphate [ˈfɔsfeit] *n* 磷酸盐,磷酸酯 | acid ~ 酸式磷酸盐 / arginine ~ 磷酰精氨酸 / calcium ~ 磷酸钙 / carbamyl ~ 氨甲酰磷酸 / creatine ~ 磷酸肌酸 / dibasic magnesium ~ 磷酸氢镁(缓泻药) / earthy ~ 土金属磷酸盐 / guanidine ~ 磷酸胍 / polyestradiol ~ 聚磷酸雌二醇(雌激素,用于治疗前列腺癌) / soluble ferric ~ 可溶性磷酸铁(补血药) / stellar ~ 星状磷酸盐 / tribasic magnesium ~, trimagnesium ~ 磷酸镁(抗胃酸药) / triose ~ 丙糖磷酸,磷酸丙糖
phosphated [ˈfɔsfeitid] *a* 含磷酸盐的
phosphatemia [ˌfɔsfəˈtiːmiə] *n* 磷酸盐血
phosphatese [ˈfɔsfətiːs] *n* 磷酸酯合成酶
phosphatic [fɔsˈfætik] *a* 磷酸盐的,含磷酸盐的
phosphatidate [ˌfɔsfəˈtaideit] *n* 磷脂酸;磷脂酸盐(酯或根)
phosphatidate cytidylyltransferase [ˌfɔsfəˈtaideit ˌsaitidililˈtrænsfəreis] 磷脂酸胞苷酰转移酶
phosphatidate phosphatase [ˌfɔsfəˈtaideitˈfɔsfəteis] 磷脂酸磷酸[酯]酶
phosphatide [ˈfɔsfətaid] *n* 磷脂
phosphatidic acid [ˌfɔsfəˈtaidik] 磷脂酸
phosphatidosis [ˌfɔsfətiˈdəusis] ([复] **phosphatidoses** [ˌfɔsfətiˈdəusiːz]) *n* 磷脂沉积[症]
phosphatidyl [ˌfɔsfəˈtaidil] *n* 磷脂酰
phosphatidylcholine (PC) [ˌfɔsfəˌtaidilˈkəuliːn] *n* 磷脂酰胆碱(亦称卵磷脂)
phosphatidylcholine-sterol *O*-acyltransferase [ˌfɔsfəˌtaidilˈkəulinˈsterɔl ˌæsilˈtrænsfəreis] 磷脂酰胆碱-甾醇 *O*-酰基转移酶(此酶缺乏为常染色体隐性性状,称为卵磷脂-胆甾醇酰基转移酶〈LCAT〉缺乏症。亦称卵磷脂-胆甾醇酰基转移酶)
phosphatidylethanolamine (PE) [ˌfɔsfəˌtaidilˌeθənɔˈlæmiːn] *n* 磷脂酰乙醇胺
phosphatidylinositol (PI) [ˌfɔsfəˌtaidiliˈnəusitɔl] *n* 磷脂酰肌醇
phosphatidylinositol deacylase [ˌfɔsfəˌtaidiliˈnəusitɔl diːˈæsileis] 磷脂酰肌醇脱酰[基]酶
1-phosphatidylinositol phosphodiesterase [ˌfɔsfəˌtaidiliˈnəusitɔl ˌfɔsfədaiˈestəreis] 1-磷脂酰肌醇磷酸二酯酶
phosphatidylserine [ˌfɔsfəˌtaidilˈsiərin] *n* 磷脂酰丝氨酸
phosphatoptosis [ˌfɔsfətɔpˈtəusis] *n* 磷酸盐沉着
phosphaturia [ˌfɔsfəˈtjuəriə] *n* 磷酸盐尿;磷酸盐沉着 | **phosphaturic** *a*
phosphene [ˈfɔsfiːn] *n* 光幻视 | accommodation ~ 调节性光幻视
phosphide [ˈfɔsfaid] *n* 磷化物
phosphine [ˈfɔsfiːn] *n* 磷化氢,膦;碱性染革黄棕
phosphite [ˈfɔsfait] *n* 亚磷酸盐
phosphoamidase [ˌfɔsfəˈæmideis] *n* 磷酰胺酶
phosphoarginine [ˌfɔsfəˈɑːdʒinin] *n* 磷酸精氨酸
phosphocarnic acid [ˌfɔsfəˈkɑːnik] 磷肉酸
phosphocozymase [ˌfɔsfəukəuˈzaimeis] *n* 辅酶Ⅱ,烟酰胺腺嘌呤二核苷酸磷酸
phosphocreatine (PC) [ˌfɔsfəuˈkriətin] *n* 磷酸肌酸
phosphodiester [ˌfɔsfəudaiˈestə] *n* 磷酸二酯
phosphodiesterase [ˌfɔsfədaiˈestəreis] *n* 磷酸二酯酶
phospho*enol*pyruvate [ˌfɔsfəˌiːnɔlˈpaiəruveit] *n* 磷酸烯醇丙酮酸
phospho*enol*pyruvate carboxykinase (GTP) [ˌfɔsfəˌiːnɔlˈpaiəruveit kɑːˌbɔksiˈkaineis] 烯醇丙酮酸磷酸羧激酶(GTP)(在线粒体或细胞溶质中,此酶缺乏为一种常染色体隐性性状,可致婴儿低血糖)
phosphoesterase [ˌfɔsfəˈestəreis] *n* 磷酸酯酶,磷酸酶
phosphoethanolamine [ˌfɔsfəˌeθəˈnɔləmiːn] *n* 磷酸乙醇胺
phosphofructaldolase [ˌfɔsfəfrʌkˈtældəleis] *n* 磷酸果糖醛缩酶,果糖二磷酸醛缩酶
phosphofructokinase [ˌfɔsfəˌfrʌktəˈkaineis] *n* 磷酸果糖激酶
phosphofructokinase 1 [ˌfɔsfəˌfrʌktəˈkaineis] *n* 磷酸果糖激酶 1, 6-磷酸果糖激酶
phosphofructokinase 2 [ˌfɔsfəˌfrʌktəˈkaineis] *n* 磷酸果糖激酶 2, 6-磷酸果糖-2-激酶
6-phosphofructokinase [ˌfɔsfəˌfrʌktəˈkaineis] *n* 6-磷酸果糖激酶(此肌同工酶缺乏为一种常染色体隐性性状,可致糖原贮积病Ⅶ型。亦称磷酸果糖激酶 1)
6-phosphofructo-2-kinase [ˌfɔsfəˌfrʌktəˈkaineis] *n* 6-磷酸果糖-2-激酶(亦称磷酸果糖激酶 2)
phosphoglobulin [ˌfɔsfəuˈglɔbjulin] *n* 磷酸球蛋白
phosphoglucokinase [ˌfɔsfəuˌgluːkəuˈkaineis] *n* 磷酸葡糖激酶
phosphoglucomutase [ˌfɔsfəuˌgluːkəuˈmjuːteis] *n* 葡糖磷酸变位酶

phosphogluconate [ˌfɔsfəˈgluːkəneit] *n* 磷酸葡糖酸

phosphogluconate 2-dehydrogenase (decarboxylating) [ˌfɔsfəuˈgluːkəneit diːˈhaidrədʒəneis] 磷酸葡糖酸 2-脱氢酶(脱羧)

6-phosphogluconolactonase [ˌfɔsfəˌgluːkənəuˈlæktəneis] *n* 6-磷酸葡糖酸内酯酶

phosphoglucoprotein [ˌfɔsfəˌgluːkəuˈprəutiːn] *n* 磷糖蛋白

phosphoglucose isomerase [ˌfɔsfəuˈgluːkəus aiˈsɔməreis] 磷酸葡糖异构酶,葡糖-6-磷酸异构酶

3-phosphoglyceraldehyde [ˌfɔsfəuˌglisəˈrældihaid] *n* 3-甘油醛磷酸,3-磷酸甘油醛

phosphoglycerate [ˌfɔsfəuˈglisəreit] *n* 磷酸甘油酸

phosphoglycerate kinase [ˌfɔsfəuˈglisəreitˈkaineis] 磷酸甘油酸激酶(此酶缺乏为一种 X 连锁性状,可致溶血性贫血、精神发育迟缓、行为异常和神经系统异常)

phosphoglycerate mutase [ˌfɔsfəuˈglisəreitˈmjuːteis] 磷酸甘油酸变位酶

phosphoglyceric acid [ˌfɔsfəugliˈserik] *n* 磷酸甘油酸

phosphoglyceride [ˌfɔsfəuˈglisəraid] *n* 磷酸甘油酯

phosphoglyceromutase [ˌfɔsfəuˌglisərəuˈmjuːteis] *n* 磷酸甘油酸变位酶

phosphoglycoprotein [ˌfɔsfəˌglaikəuˈprəutiːn] *n* 磷糖蛋白

phosphoguanidine [ˌfɔsfəuˈgwænidiːn] *n* 磷酸胍

phosphohexoisomerase [ˌfɔsfəuˌheksəuaiˈsɔməreis] *n* 磷酸己糖异构酶

phosphohexokinase [ˌfɔsfəuˌheksəuˈkaineis] *n* 磷酸己糖激酶

phosphoinositide [ˌfɔsfəiˈnəusitaid] *n* 磷酸肌醇

phosphoketolase [ˌfɔsfəuˈkiːtəleis] *n* 磷酸酮醇酶

phospholamban [ˌfɔsfəuˈlæmbæn] *n* 肌浆网磷酸受钙蛋白(一种分子量为 22 000 肌浆网的膜结合多肽,在磷酸化作用时通过环腺苷酸依赖性蛋白激酶,激活钙泵,促使肌浆网吸收和贮存钙,从而导致心肌舒张)

phospholipase [ˌfɔsfəuˈlipeis] *n* 磷脂酶

phospholipid [ˌfɔsfəuˈlipid], **phospholipin** [ˌfɔsfəuˈlipin] *n* 磷脂

phospholipidemia [ˌfɔsfəulipiˈdiːmiə] *n* 磷脂血

phosphomannomutase [ˌfɔsfəˌmænəuˈmjuːteis] 磷酸甘露糖变位酶

phosphomannose isomerase [ˌfɔsfəuˈmæməusaiˈsɔməreis] 磷酸甘露糖异构酶,甘露糖-6-磷酸异构酶

phosphomolybdic acid [ˌfɔsfəuməˈlibdik] 磷钼酸

phosphomonoester [ˌfɔsfəuˌmɔnəˈestə] *n* 磷酸单酯

phosphomonoesterase [ˌfɔsfəuˌmɔnəuˈestəreis] *n* 磷酸单酯酶

phosphomutase [ˌfɔsfəuˈmjuːteis] *n* 磷酸变位酶,转磷酸酶

phosphonate [ˌfɔsfəneit] *n* 膦酸盐(阴离子或酯)

phosphonecrosis [ˌfɔsfəuneˈkrəusis] *n* 磷毒性颌骨坏死

phosphonic acid [fɔsˈfɔnik] 膦酸

phosphonium [fɔsˈfəuniəm] *n* 鏻(根)

phosphonuclease [ˌfɔsfəuˈnjuːklieis] *n* 核苷酸酶

phosphopenia [ˌfɔsfəuˈpiːniə] *n* (体内)磷质减少

phosphoprotein [ˌfɔsfəuˈprəutiːn] *n* 磷蛋白

phosphoprotein phosphatase [ˌfɔsfəuˈprəutiːn ˈfɔsfəteis] 磷蛋白磷酸酶(亦称蛋白磷酸酶)

phosphoptomaine [ˌfɔsfəuˈtəumein] *n* 磷尸碱

phosphopyruvate carboxykinase [ˌfɔsfəuˈpaiəruveit kɑːˌbɔksiˈkaineis] 磷酸丙酮酸羧基激酶,磷酸烯醇丙酮酸羧基激酶(GTP)

phosphopyruvate hydratase [ˌfɔsfəˈpaiəruveit ˈhaidrəteis] 磷酸丙酮酸水合酶(亦称烯醇酶)

phosphor [ˈfɔsfə] *n* 磷光体;黄磷

phosphorate [ˈfɔsfəreit] *vt* 与磷化合,含磷 | **~d** *a*

phosphorescence [ˌfɔsfəˈresns] *n* 磷光 | **phosphorescent** *a* 发磷光的

phosphoretted [ˈfɔsfəˌretid] *a* 与磷化合的,含磷的

phosphoriboisomerase [ˌfɔsfəuˌraibəuaiˈsɔməreis] *n* 磷酸核糖异构酶,核糖-5-磷酸异构酶

phosphoribokinase [ˌfɔsfəuˌraibəuˈkaineis] *n* 磷酸核糖激酶

phosphoribosylamine [ˌfɔsfəuˌraibəuˈsiləmiːn] *n* 磷酸核糖胺

phosphoribosylpyrophosphate [ˌfɔsfəuˌraibəusilˌpairəuˈfɔsfeit] *n* 磷酸核糖焦磷酸

phosphoribosylpyrophosphate synthetase [ˌfɔsfəuˌraibəusilˌpaiərəuˈfɔsfeit ˈsinθiteis] 磷酸核糖焦磷酸合成酶,核糖磷酸焦磷酸激酶

phosphoribosyltransferase [ˌfɔsfəuˌraibəusilˈtrænsfəreis] *n* 转磷酸核糖基酶,磷酸核糖基转移酶

phosphoribulokinase [ˌfɔsfəuˌraibjuləuˈ kaineis] *n* 磷酸核酮糖激酶

phosphoric [fɔsˈfɔrik] *a* 磷的 | ~ acid 磷酸

phosphoric acid, diluted [fɔsˈfɔrik] 稀磷酸(用作药物制剂的溶媒和口服胃酸化药)

phosphoric acid, glacial [fɔsˈfɔrik] 冰磷酸,偏磷酸

phosphorism [ˈfɔsfərizəm] *n* 慢性磷中毒
phosphorized [ˈfɔsfəraizd] *a* 含磷的
phosphorolysis [ˌfɔsfəˈ rɔlisis] *n* 磷酸解
phosphoroscope [ˈfɔsfərəuskəup] *n* 磷光测定器,磷光镜
phosphorous [ˈfɔsfərəs] *a* 亚磷的
phosphorous acid [ˈfɔsfərəs] 亚磷酸
phosphorpenia [ˌfɔsfəˈpiːniə] *n* (体内)磷质减少
phosphoruria [ˌfɔsfəˈrjuəriə] *n* 磷尿
phosphorus (P) [ˈfɔsfərəs] *n* 磷(化学元素) | radioactive ~, ^{32}P, labelled ~ 放射性磷, ^{32}磷, 标志磷
phosphoryl [ˈfɔsfəril] *n* 磷酰[基]
phosphorylase [fɔsˈfɔːrileis] *n* 磷酸化酶 | hepatic ~ deficiency 肝磷酸化酶缺乏症,糖原贮积症Ⅵ型 / muscle ~ deficiency 肌磷酸化酶缺乏症,糖原贮积症Ⅴ型
phosphorylase kinase [fɔsˈfɔːrileisˈkaineis] 磷酸化酶激酶(肝内缺乏此酶为一种 X 连锁隐性性状,可致磷酸化酶 *b* 激酶缺乏症)
phosphorylase *b* kinase [fɔsˈfɔrileisˈkaineis] 磷酸化酶 *b* 激酶,磷酸化酶激酶
phosphorylase *b* kinase deficiency 磷酸化酶 *b* 激酶缺乏症(一种 X 连锁糖原贮积症,由于肝内磷酸化酶激酶缺乏所致,其特征在受患男性为肝大,有时为空腹性低血糖和某种程度的生长迟缓,但一般为良性。它的分类,作为糖原贮积症的一种特殊类型,一直是有争议的,曾包括在Ⅵ型内,并称为Ⅷ型和〈以前称为〉Ⅸ型)
[**phosphorylase**] **phosphatase** [fɔsˈfɔːrileis ˈfɔsfəteis] [磷酸化酶]磷酸酶
phosphorylate [ˈfɔsfərileit] *vt* 磷酸化
phosphorylation [ˌfɔsfəriˈleiʃən] *n* 磷酸化[作用] | oxidative ~ 氧化磷酸化[作用] / substrate-level ~ 底物水平磷酸化[作用]
phosphorylysis [ˌfɔsfəˈrilisis] *n* 磷酸分解[作用]
phosphosugar [ˌfɔsfəˈʃugə] *n* 磷糖
phosphotransacetylase [ˌfɔsfəuˌtrænsəˈsetileis] *n* 磷酸转乙酰酶,磷酸乙酰基转移酶
phosphotransferase [ˌfɔsfəuˈtrænsfəreis] *n* 磷酸转移酶
phosphotriose [ˌfɔsfəuˈtraiəus] *n* 丙糖磷酸,磷酸丙糖
phosphotungstate [ˌfɔsfəuˈtʌŋsteit] *n* 磷钨酸盐
phosphotungstic acid [ˌfɔsfəuˈtʌŋstik] 磷钨酸
phosphovitellin [ˌfɔsfəuvaiˈtelin] *n* 卵黄高磷蛋白
phosphuresis [ˌfɔsfjuəˈriːsis] *n* 磷[酸盐]尿排泄 | **phosphuretic** [ˌfɔsfjuəˈretik] *a* 促磷[酸盐]尿排泄的
phosphuret [ˈfɔsfjuret] *n* 磷化物
phosphuretted [ˌfɔsfjuˌretid] *a* 与磷化合的,含磷的
phosphuria [fɔsˈfjuəriə] *n* 磷酸盐尿;磷酸盐沉着
phosvitin [fɔsˈvaitin] *n* 卵黄高磷蛋白
photalgia [fəuˈtældʒiə] *n* 光痛(如眼痛)
photallochromy [fəuˈtæləˌkrəumi] *n* 光照变色性
photaugiaphobia [fəuˌtɔːdʒiəˈfəubjə] *n* 光耀恐怖;闪光恐怖
phot(e) [fəut] *n* 辐透,厘米烛光(照度单位)
photechy [ˈfəutəki] *n* 辐射感应性
photerythrous [ˌfəutiˈriθrəs] *a* 仅感红光的
photesthesis [ˌfəutisˈθiːsis] *n* 光觉;[对]光敏感,畏光
photic [ˈfəutik] *a* 光的,感光的
photism [ˈfəutizəm] *n* 色、光联觉,色、光幻觉(伴有听觉、味觉、嗅觉或触觉的一种色觉)
phot(o)- [构词成分]光
photoablation [ˌfəutəuæbˈleiʃən] *n* 光挥发[作用](由激光器发射紫外线照射而引起的组织发光)
photoactinic [ˌfəutəuækˈtinik] *a* [发出]光化射线的;能产生光化作用的
photoactive [ˌfəutəuˈæktiv] *a* 光敏的
photoaging [ˌfəutəuˈeidʒiŋ] *a* 光照老化的
photoallergen [ˌfəutəuˈæləːdʒin] *n* 光变应原
photoallergy [ˌfəutəuˈælədʒi] *n* 光变应性,对光过敏 | **photoallergic** [ˌfəutəuəˈləːdʒik] *a*
photoautotroph [ˌfəutəuˈɔːtətrəuf] *n* 光能自养生物
photoautotrophic [ˌfəutəuˌɔːtəˈtrɔfik] *a* 光能自养的
photobacteria [ˌfəutəubækˈtiəriə] *n* 发光细菌
Photobacterium [ˌfəutəubækˈtiəriəm] *n* 发光菌属
photobacterium [ˌfəutəubækˈtiəriəm] *n* 发光菌
photobiologic(al) [ˌfəutəuˌbaiəˈlɔdʒik(əl)] *a* 光生物学的
photobiology [ˌfəutəubaiˈɔlədʒi] *n* 光生物学,生物光学
photobiotic [ˌfəutəubaiˈɔtik] *a* 需光生成的,感光生存的
photocatalysis [ˌfəutəukəˈtælisis] *n* 光催化[作用] | **photocatalytic** [ˌfəutəuˌkætəˈlitik] *a*
photocatalyst [ˌfəutəuˈkætəlist], **photocatalyzer** [ˌfəutəuˈkætəˌlaizə] *n* 光催化剂,光触媒
photoceptor [ˌfəutəuˈseptə] *n* 光感受器
photochemistry [ˌfəutəuˈkemistri] *n* 光化学 | **photochemical** *a*
photochemotherapy [ˌfəutəuˌkeməˈθerəpi] *n* 光化学疗法
photochromogen [ˌfəutəuˈkrəumədʒən] *n* 光照

产色菌

photochromogenicity [ˌfəutəuˌkrəuməudʒeˈnisəti] *n* 光照产色性 | **photochromogenic** [ˌfəutəu-ˌkrəuməuˈdʒenik] *a* 光照产色的

photocoagulation [ˌfəutəukəuˌægjuˈleiʃən] *n* 光凝固[术](用于视网膜病等)

photoconvulsive [ˌfəutəukənˈvʌlsiv] *a* 光致惊厥的,光致发作的

photocutaneous [ˌfəutəukjuːˈteinjəs] *n* 光照性皮肤[变化]的

photodermatitis [ˌfəutəuˌdəːməˈtaitis] *n* 光照性皮炎

photodermatosis [ˌfəutəuˌdəːməˈtəusis] *n* 光照性皮肤病

photodetector [ˌfəutəudiˈtektə] *n* 光检测器

photodisruption [ˌfəutəudisˈrʌpʃən] *n* 光致破裂(由激光引起分子快速电离所致的组织破裂)

photodromy [fəuˈtɔdrəmi] *n* 光动现象(趋光或避光的现象,如悬浮液中的粒子)

photodynamic [ˌfəutəudaiˈnæmik] *a* 光动力的

photodynamics [ˌfəutəudaiˈnæmiks] *n* 光动力学

photodynesis [ˌfəutəudaiˈniːsis] *n* 光致[胞质]流动

photodynia [ˌfəutəuˈdiniə] *n* 光痛

photodysphoria [ˌfəutəudisˈfəuriə] *n* 羞明,畏光

photoelectric [ˌfəutəuiˈlektrik] *a* 光电的

photoelectron [ˌfəutəuiˈlektrɔn] *n* 光电子

photoelement [ˌfəutəuˈelimənt] *n* 光元素

photoerythema [ˌfəutəuˌeriˈθiːmə] *n* 光照性红斑

photoesthetic [ˌfəutəuisˈθetik] *a* 光感的,感光的

photofluorogram [ˌfəutəuˈfluərəgræm] *n* 荧光 X 线[照]片

photofluorography [ˌfəutəuˌfluəˈrɔgrəfi] *a* 荧光 X 线摄影[术] | **photofluorographic** [ˌfəut-əuˌfluərəuˈgræfik] *a* 荧光摄影的

photofluoroscope [ˌfəutəufluˈɔrəskəup] *n* 荧光 X 线摄影机

photogastroscope [ˌfəutəuˈgæstrəskəup] *n* 胃内照相器,胃内照相装置

photogene [ˌfəutədʒiːn] *n* 后像,余像

photogenic [ˌfəutəuˈdʒenik] *a* 光所致的,光源性的;发光的

photoglottography [ˌfəutəugləˈtɔgrəfi] *n* 光声门描记法

photography [fəˈtɔgrəfi] *n* 摄影术

photohalide [ˌfəutəuˈhælaid] *n* 感光性卤化物

photohematachometer [ˌfəutəuˌhemətəˈkɔmitə] *n* 血流速度照相器

photohenric [ˌfəutəuˈhenrik] *a* 光亨[利]的

photoheterotroph [ˌfəutəuˈhetərətrəuf] *n* 光能异养生物

photoheterotrophic [ˌfəutəuˌhetərəuˈtrɔfik] *a* 光能异养的

photohmic [fəuˈtəumik] *a* 光欧[姆]的

photoinactivation [ˌfəutəuinˌæktiˈveiʃən] *n* 光照灭活(用光对某一物质,例如补体,进行灭活)

photokinesis [ˌfəutəukaiˈniːsis, -kiˈn-] *n* 趋光性,感光运动 | **photokinetic** [ˌfəutəukaiˈnetik, -kiˈn-] *a*

photokymograph [ˌfəutəuˈkaiməgrɑːf, -græf] *n* 光转筒记录器,记录照相机

photolethal [ˌfəutəuˈliːθəl] *a* 光线致死的

photology [fəuˈtɔlədʒi] *n* 光学

photoluminescence [ˌfəutəuˌljuːmiˈnesns] *n* 光致发光

photolysis [fəuˈtɔlisis] *n* 光解[作用] | **photolytic** [ˌfəutəuˈlitik] *a*

photolyte [ˈfəutəlait] *n* 光解物

photoma [fəuˈtəumə] *n* 闪光

photomagnetic [ˌfəutəumægˈnetik] *a* 光磁的

photomagnetism [ˌfəutəuˈmægnitizəm] *n* 光磁性

photometer [fəuˈtɔmitə] *n* 光度计 | flicker ~ 闪光光度计,闪变光度计

photomethemoglobin [ˌfəutəumetˌhiːməuˈgl-əubin] *n* 光变性血红蛋白(光作用于高铁血红蛋白的产物)

photometry [fəuˈtɔmitri] *n* 光度学,光度术 | flicker ~ 闪光光度术,闪变光度术

photomicrograph [ˌfəutəuˈmaikrəgrɑːf, -græf] *n* 显微照片 *vt* 拍摄显微照片 | ~**ic** [ˌfəutəum-aikrəˈgræfik] *a* 显微摄影的 / ~**y** [ˌfəutəum-aiˈkrɔgrəfi] *n* 显微摄影[术]

photomicroscope [ˌfəutəuˈmaikrəskəup] *n* 照相显微镜,显微摄影镜

photomicroscopy [ˌfəutəumaiˈkrɔskəpi] *n* 显微摄影[术]

photomorphogenesis [ˌfəutəuˌmɔːfəuˈdʒenisis] *n* 光形态发生作用

photomyoclonic [ˌfəutəuˌmaiəuˈklɔnik] *n* 光致肌阵挛的

photomyogenic [ˌfəutəuˌmaiəuˈdʒenik] *n* 光致肌阵挛的

photon [ˈfəutɔn] *n* 光子

photoncia [fəˈtɔnsiə] *n* 光源[性]肿

photone [ˈfəutəun] *n* 光幻视

photo-onycholysis [ˌfəutəu ˌəuniˈkɔlisis] *n* 光甲松解,光甲剥离

photo-ophthalmia [ˌfəutəu ɔfˈθælmiə] *n* 光照性眼炎

photoparoxysmal [ˌfəutəuˌpærəkˈsizməl] *a* 光致发作的

photopathy [fəˈtɔpəθi] *n* 光源[性]病;光刺激反应性

photoperceptive [ˌfəutəupəˈseptiv] *a* 光感受的,

感光的,光觉的

photoperiod [ˌfəutəuˈpiəriəd] *n* 光周期(一个生物每天需要光照的时间) | **~ic** [ˌfəutəupiəriˈɔdik] *a* / **~ism** [ˌfəutəuˈpiəriədizəm] *n* 光周期现象,光周期性(动物和植物对于光周期发生一定反应的生理反应) / **~icity** [ˌfəutəupiəriəˈdisəti] *n* 光周期性

photopharmacology [ˌfəutəuˌfɑːməˈkɔlədʒi] *n* 光药理学

photopheresis [ˌfəutəufəˈriːsis] *n* 光去除术,光提取法(一种治疗皮肤T细胞淋巴瘤技术,服用光敏性化学药品如甲氧沙林〈methoxsalen〉后,血液脱离患者,经紫外线放射源循环,然后输回。据认为治疗效果可刺激宿主免疫系统)

photophilic [ˌfəutəuˈfilik] *a* 嗜光的

photophobia [ˌfəutəuˈfəubjə] *n* 畏光 | **photophobic** [ˌfəutəuˈfəubik] *a*

photophore [ˈfəutəfɔː] *n* 透照灯,内腔照明器(检鼻、喉)

photophosphorylation [ˌfəutəuˌfɔsfəriˈleiʃən] *n* 光合磷酸化[作用]

photophthalmia [ˌfəutɔfˈθælmiə] *n* 光照性眼炎

photopia [fəuˈtəupiə] *n* 光适应 | **photopic** [fəuˈtɔpik] *a*

photopigment [ˌfəutəuˈpigmənt] *n* 感光色素(一种色素,如视色素,光存在时并不稳定)

photoplethysmograph [ˌfəutəupliˈθismәgrɑːf, -græf] *n* 光体积描记仪

photoplethysmography [ˌfəutəuˌpleθizˈmɔgrəfi] *n* 光体积描记法

photoproduct [ˈfəutəˌprɔdʌkt] *n* 光合物

photoprotection [ˌfəutəuprəˈtekfən] *n* 光照保护法(用光照保护细胞)

photopsia [fəuˈtɔpsiə], **photopsy** [fəuˈtɔpsi] *n* 闪光感

photopsin [fəuˈtɔpsin] *n* 光视蛋白(视网膜锥的蛋白成分,和视网膜结合形成光化色素)

photoptarmosis [ˌfəutəutɑːˈməusis] *n* 感光喷嚏

photoptometer [ˌfəutɔpˈtɔmitə] *n* 光觉计

photoptometry [ˌfəutɔpˈtɔmitri] *n* 光觉测定[法]

photoradiation [ˌfəutəuˌreidiˈeiʃən] *n* 光辐射,光动力疗法

photoradiometer [ˌfəutəˌreidiˈɔmitə] *n* X线[辐射]量计

photoreaction [ˌfəutəuri(ː)ˈækfən] *n* 光反应

photoreactivation [ˌfəutəuri(ː)ˌæktiˈveiʃən] *n* 光复活[作用]

photoreceptor [ˌfəutəuriˈseptə] *n* 光感受器,感光器 | **photoreception** [ˌfəutəuriˈsepʃən] *n* 光感受作用(检辐射能,一般波长为3 900~7 700Å,在可见光的范围) / **photoreceptive** *a* 感光的

photorespiration [ˌfəutəuˌrespəˈreiʃən] *n* 光呼吸[作用]

photoretinitis [ˌfəutəuretiˈnaitis] *n* 光照性视网膜炎

photoreversal [ˌfəutəuriˈvəːsəl] *n* 光逆转[作用]

photoscan [ˈfəutəskæn] *n* 光扫描图

photoscanner [ˌfəutəuˈskænə] *n* 光扫描器

photoscope [ˈfəutəskəup] *n* 透视镜(荧光屏) | **photoscopy** [fəuˈtɔskəpi] *n* [X线]透视检查

photosensitive [ˌfəutəuˈsensitiv] *a* 光敏感的,感光的 | **photosensitivity** [ˌfəutəuˌsensiˈtivəti] *n* 光敏感性,感光性,光过敏

photosensitize [ˌfəutəuˈsensitaiz] *vt* 使感光 | **photosensitization** [ˌfəutəuˌsensitaiˈzeiʃən, -tiˈz-] *n* 感光过敏[作用],光致敏[作用],光感作用

photosensitizer [ˌfəutəuˈsensitaizə] *n* 光敏[化]剂

photostable [ˈfəutəˌsteibl] *a* 不感光的,耐光的

photostethoscope [ˌfəutəuˈsteθəskəup] *n* 光波显音器(用以记录胎儿心搏)

photosynthesis [ˌfəutəuˈsinθəsis] *n* 光合作用 | **photosynthetic** [ˌfəutəusinˈθetik] *a* 光合的

phototaxis [ˌfəutəuˈtæksis] *n* 趋光性(指细胞和微生物在光影响下的活动) | **phototactic** [ˌfəutəuˈtæktik] *a* 趋光的

phototherapy [ˌfəutəuˈθerəpi] *n* 光疗,光疗法

photothermy [ˈfəutəθəːmi] *n* 辐射热作用,光热作用 | **photothermal** [ˌfəutəuˈθəːməl] *a* 辐射热的,光热的

phototimer [ˈfəutəutaimə] *n* 照相计时器

phototonus [fəˈtɔtənəs] *n* 光紧张(原生质受光影响所致的一种刺激状态) | **phototonic** [ˌfəutəˈtɔnik] *a*

phototoxic [ˌfəutəuˈtɔksik] *a* 光毒的 | ~**ity** [ˌfəutəutɔkˈsisəti] *n* 光毒性

phototoxis [ˌfəutəuˈtɔksis] *n* 光线损害,射线损害,辐射损害

phototransduction [ˌfəutəutrænsˈdʌkʃən] *n* 光转导,视转导

phototrophic [ˌfəutəuˈtrɔfik] *a* 光营养的

phototropism [fəuˈtɔtrəpizəm] *n* 向光性;光色互变[现象] | **phototropic** [ˌfəutəuˈtrɔpik] *a* 向光的

phototurbidometric [ˌfəutəutəːbidəˈmetrik] *a* 光电比浊[计]的

photoxylin [fəˈtɔksilin] *n* 木髓火棉

photronreflectometer [ˌfəutrɔnˌriːflekˈtɔmitə] *n* 光电反射计

photuria [fəˈtjuəriə] *n* 发光尿

PHPPA *p*-hydroxyphenylpyruvic acid 对羟苯丙酮酸
Phragmidiothrix [fræg'midiəθriks] *n* 三股菌属
Phragmobasidiomycetes [ˌfrægməubəˌsidiəumai'siːtiːz] *n* 栅担子菌纲
Phragmobasidiomycetidae [ˌfrægməubəˌsidiəumai'setidiː] *n* 栅担子菌亚纲
phragmoplast ['frægməplæst] *n* 成膜体(有丝分裂时,在其内形成中体的桶状纺锤体)
phren [fren] *n*【希】膈;精神,意志
phrenalgia [fri'nældʒiə] *n* 膈痛;精神性痛
phrenectomy [fri'nektəmi] *n* 膈切除术;膈神经切除术
phrenemphraxis [ˌfrenem'fræksis] *n* 膈神经压轧术
phrenetic [fri'netik] *a* 躁狂的,精神错乱的 *n* 躁狂患者
phrenic ['frenik] *a* 膈的;精神的
phrenicectomized [ˌfreni'sektəmaizd] *a* 膈神经切除的
phrenicectomy [ˌfreni'sektəmi] *n* 膈神经切除术
phreniclasia [ˌfreni'kleiziə], **phreniclasis** [ˌfreni'kleisis] *n* 膈神经压轧术
phrenicoexeresis [ˌfrenikəuek'serisis], **phrenicoexairesis** [ˌfrenikəuek'sairisis] *n* 膈神经抽出术
phreniconeurectomy [ˌfrenikəunjuə'rektəmi] *n* 膈神经切除术
phrenicotomy [ˌfreni'kɔtəmi] *n* 膈神经切断术
phrenicotripsy [ˌfrenikəu'tripsi] *n* 膈神经压轧术
phrenitis [fri'naitis] *n* 脑炎;谵妄;膈炎
phren(o)- [构词成分]膈;膈神经;精神,意志
phrenocardia [ˌfrenəu'kɑːdiə] *n* 心血管神经衰弱
phrenocolic [ˌfrenəu'kɔlik] *a* 膈结肠的
phrenocolopexy [ˌfrenəu'kəuləpeksi] *n* 膈结肠固定术
phrenodynia [ˌfrenəu'diniə] *n* 膈痛
phrenogastric [ˌfrenəu'gæstrik] *a* 膈胃的
phrenoglottic [ˌfrenəu'glɔtik] *a* 膈声门的
phrenograph ['frenəgrɑːf, -græf] *n* 膈动描记器
phrenohepatic [ˌfrenəuhi'pætik] *a* 膈肝的
phrenology [fri'nɔlədʒi] *n* 颅相学,骨相学 | **phrenological** [ˌfrenə'lɔdʒikəl] *a* / **phrenologist** *n* 颅相学者,骨相学者
phrenopericarditis [ˌfrenəuˌperikɑː'daitis] *n* 膈心包炎
phrenoplegia [ˌfrenəu'pliːdʒiə] *n* 膈瘫痪
phrenoptosis [ˌfrenɔp'təusis] *n* 膈下垂
phrenosin ['frenəsin] *n* 羟脑苷脂
phrenosine ['frenəsiːn] *n* 羟脑苷脂
phrenosinic acid [frenəu'sinik] 脑羟酸,羟二十四酸
phrenospasm ['frenəspæzəm] *n* 膈痉挛
phrenosplenic [ˌfrenəu'splenik] *a* 膈脾的
phrenosterol [ˌfrenəu'sterɔl] *n* 脑甾醇
phrenotropic [ˌfrenəu'trɔpik] *a* 向精神的,作用于精神的
phrictopathic [ˌfriktəu'pæθik] *a* 寒战的
phronema [frə'niːmə] *n* 联想中枢部(指大脑皮质部分)
phrynin ['frainin] *n* 蟾毒,蟾蜍毒素
phrynoderma [ˌfrinə'dəːmə] *n* 蟾皮病,毛囊角化过度
phrynolysin [frai'nɔlisin] *n* 蟾溶素,蟾毒素
phthalate ['θæleit] *n* 邻苯二甲酸盐,酞酸盐
phthalein ['θæliin] *n* 酞 | alphanaphthol ~ α-萘酚酞 / orthocresol ~ 邻甲酚酞
phthaleinometer [ˌθælii'nɔmitə] *n* 酞定量器,酞量计
phthalic acid ['θælik] 酞酸,苯二酸
phthalin ['θælin] *n* 还原酞,酞灵
phthalylsulfacetamide [ˌθælilˌsʌlfə'setəmaid], **phthalylsulfonazole** [ˌθælilsʌl'fɔnəzəul] *n* 酞磺醋胺(肠道抗菌药)
phthalylsulphathiazole [ˌθælilˌsʌlfə'θaiəzəul] *n* 酞磺胺噻唑(肠道抗菌药)
phthinoid ['θainɔid] *a* 痨病样的
phthiocerol [ˌθaiə'siərɔl] *n* 结核菌醇
phthiocol ['θaiəkɔl] *n* 结核萘醌,2-羟-3-甲基-1,4-萘醌(由结核分枝杆菌产生的一种抗菌素,具有维生素 K 活性)
phthiotic acid [θai'ɔtik] 结核菌酸
phthiriasis [θi'raiəsis] *n* 虱病 | ~ inguinalis, pubic ~ 阴虱病
Phthirus ['θirəs] *n* 阴虱属 | ~ pubis 阴虱
phthisic ['θaisik] *a* 痨病的 *n* 痨病患者;气喘(俗名)
phthisical ['θaisikəl] *a* 痨病的
phthisicky ['θaisiki] *a* 气喘的,患气喘病的
phthisiogenesis [ˌθaisiəu'dʒenisis] *n* 致痨,成痨,痨病发生
phthisiogenetic [ˌθaisiəudʒi'netik], **phthisiogenic** [ˌθaisiəu'dʒenik] *a* 致痨病的,痨病发生的
phthisiology [ˌθaisi'ɔlədʒi] *n* 痨病学,肺痨学,结核病学
phthisiotherapeutical [ˌθaisiəuˌθerə'pjuːtikəl] *a* 痨病治疗的
phthisiotherapeutist [ˌθaisiəuˌθerə'pjuːtist], **phthisiotherapist** [ˌθaisiəu'θerəpist] *n* 痨病治疗学家
phthisiotherapy [ˌθaisiəu'θerəpi], **phthisiotherapeutics** [ˌθaisiəuˌθerə'pjuːtiks] *n* 痨病

治疗
phthisis [ˈθaisis] ([复] **phthises** [ˈθaisiːz]) *n* 痨病;肺痨,肺结核 | abdominal ~ 腹痨(肠及肠系膜淋巴结结核) / bacillary ~ 杆菌性痨病,结核病 / black ~, colliers' ~, miner's ~ 炭末沉着病,炭肺 / diabetic ~ 糖尿病性肺结核 / dorsal ~ 脊椎结核 / essential ~ (of the eye) 特发性眼痨,眼球软化 / flax dressers' ~ 亚麻沉着病 / glandular ~ 淋巴结结核 / grinders' ~ 硅肺结核 / Mediterranean ~ 波状热,布鲁[杆]菌病 / ocular ~ 眼痨,眼球软化 / potters' ~ 硅肺结核 / pulmonary ~ 肺结核 / stone cutters' ~ 石末沉着病,石末肺
phyco- [构词成分] 藻
phycobilin [ˌfaikəuˈbilin] *n* 藻胆[色]素
phycochrome [ˈfaikəkrəum] *n* 藻色素;蓝绿藻
phycochromoprotein [ˌfaikəuˌkrəuməuˈprəutiːn] *n* 藻色蛋白
phycocyanin [ˌfaikəuˈsaiənin] *n* 藻蓝蛋白
phycocyanogen [ˌfaikəusaiˈænədʒin] *n* 藻蓝蛋白原
phycoerythrin [ˌfaikəuˈeriθrin] *n* 藻红蛋白
phycology [faiˈkɔlədʒi] *n* 藻类学 | **phycologist** *n* 藻类学家
phycomycete [ˌfaikəuˈmaisiːt] *n* 藻菌 | **phycomycetous** [ˌfaikəumaiˈsiːtəs] *a*
Phycomycetes [ˌfaikəumaiˈsiːtiːz], **Phycomycetae** [ˌfaikəumaiˈsiːtiː] *n* 藻菌纲
phycomycosis [ˌfaikəumaiˈkəusis] *n* 藻菌病 | cerebral ~ 脑藻菌病 / ~ entomophthorae 鼻藻菌病 / subcutaneous ~ 皮下藻菌病 | **phycomycetosis** [ˌfaikəumaisiˈtəusis] *n*
phygogalactic [ˌfaigəugəˈlæktik] *a* 止乳的
phyla [ˈfailə] phylum 的复数
phylacagogic [faiˌlækəˈgɔdʒik] *a* 促成防御素的(能诱发形成防御素或保护性抗体的)
phylactic [faiˈlæktik] *a* 防御的,防御作用的
phylactotransfusion [faiˌlæktəutrænsˈfjuːʒən] *n* 防御输液,免疫输液
phylaxin [faiˈlæksin] *n* 防御素(保护机体防止感染及感染后果的物质,有两种防御素,御菌素和毒素防御素)
phylaxiology [faiˌlæksiˈɔlədʒi] *n* 防御[素]学
phylaxis [faiˈlæksis] *n*【希】防御作用
phyletic [faiˈletik] *a* 门的(生物分类);系统发育的,种系发生的 | **~ally** *ad*
Phyllacanthina [ˌfiləkænˈθainə] *n* 叶棘虫亚目
Phyllanthus [fiˈlænθəs] *n* 叶下珠属 | ~ engleri 恩格叶下珠,毒叶下珠
phyllidea [fiˈlidiə] *n* 吸叶(绦虫)
phyll(o)- [构词成分] 叶
Phyllobacterium [ˌfiləubækˈtiəriəm] *n* 叶杆菌属
phyllochlorin [ˌfiləuˈklɔːrin] *n* 叶绿素蛋白
phyllode [ˈfiləud] *a* 叶状的(指肿瘤切面)
phyllodes [ˈfiləudiːz] *a* 叶状的
phylloerythrin [ˌfiləuˈeriθrin] *n* 叶赤素
phyllolith [ˈfiləliθ] *n* 叶石(见于肾结核的空洞内)
Phyllopharyngidea [ˌfiləufærinˈdʒidiə] *n* 叶咽总目
phylloporphyrin [ˌfiləuˈpɔːfirin] *n* 叶卟啉
phyllopyrrole [ˌfiləˈpirəul] *n* 叶吡咯
phylloquinone [ˌfiləuˈkwinəun] *n* 叶绿醌,维生素 K_1
phylloxanthine [filɔkˈsænθin] *n* 叶黄素
phylobiology [ˌfailəubaiˈɔlədʒi] *n* 种系生物学
phylogeny [faiˈlɔdʒini], **phylogenesis** [ˌfailəˈdʒenisis] *n* 系统发育,种系发生(生物种族的发展史) | **phylogenetic** [ˌfailəudʒiˈnetik], **phylogenic** [ˌfailəˈdʒenik] *a*
phylum [ˈfailəm] ([复] **phyla** [ˈfailə]) *n*【拉】门(生物分类)
phyma [ˈfaimə] ([复] **phymata** [ˈfaimətə]) *n*【希】(皮肤)肿块,(皮肤)结块,肿瘤
phymatoid [ˈfaimətɔid] *a* 肿块样的,肿瘤样的
phymatorhusin [ˌfaimətəˈrusin], **phymatorrhysin** [ˌfaimətəˈrisin] *n* 肿瘤黑[色]素
phymatosis [ˌfaiməˈtəusis] *n* 肿块病,肿瘤病
Physalia [faiˈseiliə] *n* 僧帽水母属
physaliform [faiˈsælifɔːm] *a* 气泡样的
physaliphore [faiˈsælifɔː] *n* 细胞内空泡;空泡细胞
physaliphorous [ˌfisəˈlifərəs], **physaliferous** [ˌfisəˈlifərəs] *a* 含空泡的
physalis [faiˈsælis] ([复] **physalides** [faiˈsælidiːz]) *n* 空泡细胞
physallization [ˌfisəlaiˈzeiʃən, -liˈz-] *n* 泡沫形成,成泡[作用]
Physaloptera [ˌfisəˈlɔptərə] *n* 泡翼线虫属 | ~ caucasica 高加索泡翼线虫 / ~ mordens 咬泡翼线虫 / ~ rara 稀泡翼线虫 / ~ truncata 截尾泡翼线虫
physalopteriasis [ˌfisəlɔptəˈraiəsis] *n* 泡翼线虫病
Physalopteridae [ˌfisəlɔpˈteridiː] *n* 泡翼[线虫]属
Physarida [fiˈsɑːridə] *n* 无钙目
physeal [ˈfiziəl] *a* 生长的,长骨体生长部的
physiatrics [ˌfiziˈætriks], **physiatry** [ˈfiziˌætri] *n* 物理医学与康复[学],物理治疗学,理疗学 | **physiatrist** [ˌfiziˈætrist], **physiatrician** [ˌfiziəˈtriʃən] *n* 理疗医师,理疗学家
physic [ˈfizik] *n* 医学,药物(尤指泻药) *vt* 给…服(泻)药;治愈

physical [ˈfizikəl] *a* 物质的;身体的,躯体的,体格的;自然的,物理的 *n* 体格检查

physician [fiˈziʃən] *n* 医师,内科医师 | ~ assistant 助理医师 / attending ~ 主治医师 / chief ~ 主任医师 / emergency ~ 急症医师 / family ~ 家庭医师 / house ~, resident ~ 住院医师

physicist [ˈfizisist] *n* 物理学家

Physick's operation [ˈfizik] (Philip S. Physick) 菲西克手术(用切割镊作虹膜圆片切除,以造一个人工瞳孔) | ~ pouches 菲西克囊(直肠瓣之间的炎症性小囊,有黏液性排出物)

physicochemical [ˌfizikəuˈkemikəl] *a* 物理化学的

physicogenic [ˌfizikəuˈdʒenik] *a* 身体原[因]的;物理原[因]的

physicotherapeutics [ˌfizikəuˌθerəˈpjuːtiks], **physicotherapy** [ˌfizikəuˈθerəpi] *n* 物理治疗,理疗

physics [ˈfiziks] *n* 物理学

physinosis [ˌfiziˈnəusis] *n* 物理原[因]病

physio- [构词成分] 自然;生理

physiochemistry [ˌfiziəuˈkemistri] *n* 生理化学 | **physiochemical** [ˌfiziəuˈkemikəl] *a*

physiocracy [ˌfiziˈɔkrəsi] *n* 自然疗法

physiogenesis [ˌfiziəˈdʒenisis] *n* 胚胎学

physiognomy [ˌfiziˈɔgnəmi] *n* 面相法;容貌;面容诊断 | **physiognomic(al)** [ˌfiziəˈnɔmik(əl)] *a*

physiognosis [ˌfiziɔgˈnəusis] *n* 面容诊断法

physiologic(al) [ˌfiziəˈlɔdʒik(əl)] *a* 生理学的,生理的 | **~ally** *ad*

physiologicoanatomical [ˌfiziəˌlɔdʒikəuˌænəˈtɔmikəl] *a* 生理解剖学的

physiology [ˌfiziˈɔlədʒi] *n* 生理学 | general ~ 普通生理学 / morbid ~, pathologic ~ 病理生理学 / special ~ 生理学各论,器官生理学 | **physiologist** *n* 生理学家

physiolysis [ˌfiziˈɔlisis] *n* 自然分解

physiomedicalism [ˌfiziəuˈmedikəlizəm] *n* 草药医派 | **physiomedical** [ˌfiziəuˈmedikəl] *a*

physiometry [ˌfiziˈɔmitri] *n* 生理功能测定

physioneurosis [ˌfiziəunjuəˈrəusis] *n* 躯体[性]神经功能病,躯体神经症

physionomy [ˌfiziˈɔnəmi] *n* 自然规律学

physiopathic [ˌfiziəuˈpæθik] *a* 躯体[性]神经功能病的;非精神性神经功能障碍的

physiopathologic [ˌfiziəuˌpæθəˈlɔdʒik] *a* 病理生理的

physiopathology [ˌfiziəupəˈθɔlədʒi] *n* 病理生理学

physiophyly [ˌfiziˈɔfili] *n* [身体]功能进化

physiotherapy [ˌfiziəuˈθerəpi] *n* 物理疗法,理疗 | **physiotherapeutic** [ˌfiziəuˌθerəˈpjuːtik] *a* / **physiotherapeutist** [ˌfiziəuˌθerəˈpjuːtist], **physiotherapist** [ˌfiziəuˈθerəpist] *n* 理疗医师,理疗学家

physique [fiˈziːk] *n* 体格,体型

physis [ˈfaisis] *n* 长骨体生长部

physo- [构词成分] 气,空气

physocele [ˈfaisəsiːl] *n* 气瘤;疝气囊

Physocephalus [ˌfaisəˈsefələs] *n* 膨首线虫属

physocephaly [ˌfaisəˈsefəli] *n* 头气肿

physohematometra [ˌfaisəuˌhemətəuˈmiːtrə] *n* 子宫积血气

physohydrometra [ˌfaisəuhaidrəuˈmiːtrə] *n* 子宫积水气

physometra [ˌfaisəuˈmiːtrə] *n* 子宫积气

Physopsis [faiˈsɔpsis] *n* 瓶形螺亚属

physopyosalpinx [ˌfaisəuˌpaiəuˈsælpiŋks] *n* 输卵管积脓气

Physostigma [ˌfaisəuˈstigmə] *n* 毒扁豆属

physostigmine [ˌfaisəuˈstigmiːn] *n* 毒扁豆碱(拟胆碱药,缩瞳药)

physostigminism [ˌfaisəuˈstigminizəm] *n* 毒扁豆碱中毒

phytagglutinin [ˌfaitəˈgluːtinin] *n* 植物凝血[毒]素

phytalbumin [faiˈtælbjumin] *n* 植物白蛋白

phytalbumose [faiˈtælbjuməus] *n* 植物蛋白脲

phytanate [ˈfaitəneit] *n* 植烷酸盐(或阴离子型)

phytanic acid [faiˈtænik] 植烷酸

phytanic acid α-hydroxylase [faiˈtænik] 植烷酸 α-羟化酶(此酶缺乏为一种常染色体隐性性状,是雷弗素姆〈Refsum〉病的原因)

phytase [ˈfaiteis] *n* 肌醇六磷酸酶,植酸酶(旧称)

phytate [ˈfaiteit] *n* 肌醇六磷酸,植酸(phytic acid 的阴离子形式)

-phyte [构词成分] 植物;附长物,赘生物

phytic acid [ˈfaitik] 植酸,肌醇六磷酸

phytin [ˈfaitin] *n* 非丁,肌醇六磷酸钙镁,植酸钙镁

phyt(o)- [构词成分] 植物

phytoalexin [ˌfaitəuəˈleksin] *n* 植物抗毒素

phytoanaphylactogen [ˌfaitəuˌænəfiˈlæktədʒən] *n* 植物过敏原(来源植物的、能诱发过敏反应的抗原)

phytobezoar [ˌfaitəuˈbiːzɔː] *n* 植物石

phytochemistry [ˌfaitəuˈkemistri] *n* 植物化学

phytochinin [ˌfaitəuˈkinin] *n* 植物促代谢素(由某些草叶分离的一种物质,据说类似胰岛素,对碳水化合物代谢有作用)

phytocholesterol [ˌfaitəukəˈlestərɔl] *n* 植物甾醇

phytochrome [ˈfaitəkrəum] *n* (植物)光敏色素

phytodemic [ˌfaitəuˈdemik] *n* 植物流行病

phytodetritus [ˌfaitəudiˈtraitəs] *n* 植物腐质,植物碎屑
phytoflagellate [ˌfaitəuˈflædʒileit] *n* 植鞭毛虫
phytogenesis [ˌfaitəˈdʒenisis], **phytogeny** [faiˈtɔdʒini] *n* 植物发生 | **phytogenetic(al)** [ˌfaitəudʒiˈnetik(əl)] *a*
phytogenous [faiˈtɔdʒinəs], **phytogenic** [ˌfaitəˈdʒenik] *a* 植物源的,植物性生长的
phytoglobulin [ˌfaitəuˈglɔbjulin] *n* 植物球蛋白
phytohemagglutinin [ˌfaitəuˌheməˈgluːtinin] *n* 植物凝集素
phytohormone [ˌfaitəuˈhɔːməun] *n* 植物激素
phytoid [ˈfaitɔid] *a* 植物样的
phytol [ˈfaitɔl] *n* 叶绿醇(用于制备维生素 E 及维生素 K_1)
Phytolacca [ˌfaitəuˈlækə] *n* 商陆属
Phytomastigophora [ˌfaitəuˌmæstiˈgɔfərə] *n* 植鞭毛纲
Phytomastigophorea [ˌfaitəuˌmæstiˌgɔfəˈriːə] *n* 植鞭毛纲
phytomastigophorean [ˌfaitəuˌmæstiˌgɔfəˈriːən] *n* 植鞭毛虫
phytomedicine [ˌfaitəuˈmedisin] *n* 药草制剂;药草学,草本植物学
phytomelin [ˌfaitəuˈmelin] *n* 芦丁,路丁,芸香苷
phytomitogen [ˌfaitəuˈmaitədʒən] *n* 植物有丝分裂原(植物中提取的、能使人细胞进行有丝分裂的物质)
Phytomonadina [ˌfaitəumɔnəˈdainə] *n* 植滴虫目
Phytomonas [faiˈtɔmənəs] *n* 植物单胞菌属
phytonadione [ˌfaitəunəˈdaiəun], **phytomenadione** [ˌfaitəuˌmenəˈdaiəun] *n* 植物甲萘醌,维生素 K_1(止血药)
phytone [ˈfaitəun] *n* 植物蛋白胨
phytonosis [faiˈtɔnəsis] *n* 植物原[因]病
phytoparasite [ˌfaitəuˈpærəsait] *n* 寄生植物
phytopathogenic [ˌfaitəuˌpæθəˈdʒenik] *a* 致植物病的
phytopathology [ˌfaitəupəˈθɔlədʒi] *n* 植物病理学;植物原[因]病病理学
phytopathy [faiˈtɔpəθi] *n* 植物病
phytophagous [faiˈtɔfəgəs] *a* 食植物的,素食的
phytopharmacology [ˌfaitəuˌfɑːməˈkɔlədʒi] *n* 植物药理学
phytopharmacy [ˌfaitəuˈfɑːməsi] *n* 植物药剂学
phytophotodermatitis [ˌfaitəuˌfəutəudəːməˈtaitis] *n* 植物光皮炎
phytoplankton [ˌfaitəuˈplæŋktən] *n* 浮游植物
phytoplasm [ˈfaitəplæzəm] *n* 植物原浆,植物原生质
phytoprecipitin [ˌfaitəupriˈsipitin] *n* 植物沉淀素
phytosensitinogen [ˌfaitəuˌsensiˈtinədʒən] *n* 植物致敏原,植物过敏原
phytosis [faiˈtəusis] *n* 植物寄生病
phytosterol [faiˈtɔstərɔl], **phytosterin** [faiˈtɔstərin] *n* 植物甾醇,植物固醇
phytosterolemia [faiˌtɔstərəˈliːmiə] *n* 植物甾醇血[症],谷甾醇血[症]
phytosterolin [ˌfaitəuˈstiərəlin] *n* 植物甾醇苷
phytotherapy [ˌfaitəuˈθerəpi] *n* 植物药疗法
phytotoxic [ˌfaitəuˈtɔksik] *a* 植物毒性的;抑制植物生长的 | **~ity** [ˌfaitəutɔkˈsisəti] *n* 植物毒性
phytotoxin [ˌfaitəuˈtɔksin] *n* 植物毒素
phytotrichobezoar [ˌfaitəutraikəuˈbiːzɔː] *n* 植物毛粪石
phytotron [ˈfaitətrɔn] *n* 植物人工气候室(研究植物生长用)
phytovitellin [ˌfaitəuvaiˈtelin] *n* 植物卵黄磷蛋白
phytoxylin [faiˈtɔksilin] *n* 植木胶(类似火棉胶的物质)
PI phosphatidylinositol 磷脂酰肌醇
pI 某一物质在等电点的 pH 值
pi [pai] *n* 希腊语的第 16 字母(Π, π);圆周率(π)
pia [ˈpaiə] *a*【拉】柔的,软的 | ~ mater 软膜
pia-arachnitis [ˌpaiə ˌəræk'naitis], **piarachnitis** [ˌpaiəræk'naitis] *n* 软膜蛛网膜炎,柔脑膜炎
pia-arachnoid [ˌpaiə əˈræknɔid], **piarachnoid** [ˌpaiəˈræknɔid] *n* 软膜蛛网膜,柔脑膜
pia-glia [paiə ˈglaiə] *n* 软膜神经胶[质]层
pia-intima [ˈpaiə ˈintimə] 软膜神经胶[质]层(即 pia-glia)
pial [ˈpaiəl], **piamatral** [ˌpaiəˈmeitrəl] *a* 软膜的
pia mater [ˈpai ˈmeitə] 软膜 | ~ ~ encephali 软脑膜 / ~ ~ spinalis 软脊膜
pian [piˈɑːn] *n*【法】雅司病(即 yaws) | ~ bois 森林雅司病(良性型利什曼病,有时侵袭鼻黏膜,见于圭亚那和哥斯达黎加的森林区) / hemorrhagic ~ 出血性疣,秘鲁疣
piarhemia [ˌpaiəˈhiːmiə] *n* 脂血[症]
piastrinemia [paiˌæstriˈniːmiə] *n* 血小板增多[症]
piblokto [piˈblɔktəu] *n* 匹勃罗柯托病(主要在因纽特妇女中的一种文化特异综合征,表现为赤身裸体在雪地中尖叫、奔跑,有时有自杀或杀人倾向)
pica [ˈpaikə] *n*【拉】异食癖(见于孕妇、缺铁及缺锌患者和营养不良的儿童)
Pichia [ˈpitʃiə] *n* 毕赤酵母属
pick [pik] *n* 铤,牙签
pickling [ˈpikliŋ] *n* 酸浸;浸渍(以清洁金属的表面)
Pick's bodies [pik] (Arnold Pick) 皮克体(皮克

病患者神经元中所见的胞质内微丝状包涵体)| ~ disease 皮克病,局限性脑萎缩,脑叶萎缩

Pick's cells [pik] (Ludwig pick) 皮克细胞(见 Niemann-Pick cells) | ~ disease 皮克病(见 Niemann-Pick disease)

Pick's disease, syndrome [pik] (Friedel Pick) 皮克病、综合征(腹水和纤维化肝病,伴缩窄性心包炎,亦称心包性假性肝硬变)

pickwickian syndrome [pik'wikiən] (从狄更斯〈Dickens〉小说《匹克威克外传》〈Pickwick Papers〉中对胖孩的描写而得名)匹克威克综合征(肥胖、嗜眠、肺换气不足和红细胞增多综合征)

pico- [构词成分] 皮[可],微微(10^{-12})

picocurie(pCi) [ˌpaikəu'kjuəri] *n* 皮居里,微微居里(旧放射性单位, $=10^{-12}$Ci)

picogram(pg) ['paikəgræm] *n* 皮克,微微克(10^{-12}g)

picopicogram [ˌpaikəu'paikəgræm] *n* 皮皮克(10^{-12}pg,或 10^{-24}g)

Picornaviridae [piˌkɔːnə'viridiː] *n* 小核糖核酸病毒科,小 RNA 病毒科

picornavirus [pai'kɔːnəˌvaiərəs] (pico + *r*ibo*nu*cleic acid + *vir*us) *n* 小核糖核酸病毒,小 RNA 病毒

picounit [ˌpaikəu'juːnit] *n* 皮单位(10^{-12}U)

picramic acid [pai'kræmik] 氨基苦味酸

Picrasma [pai'kræzmə] *n* 苦树属

picrate ['pikreit] *n* 苦味酸盐

picric acid ['pikrik] 苦味酸,三硝基酚

picrin ['pikrin] *n* 紫花洋地黄苦素

picr(o)- [构词成分] 苦

picrocarmine [ˌpikrəu'kɑːmin] *n* 苦味酸卡红,苦胭脂红

picrogeusia [ˌpikrəu'gjuːsiə] *n* 苦味异常

picrol ['pikrɔl] *n* 皮克罗尔,二碘雷琐辛一磺酸钾

picronigrosin [ˌpikrəu'naigrəsin] *n* 苦味酸苯胺黑(苦味酸与苯胺黑的醇溶液,用作染剂)

picropodophyllin [ˌpikrəuˌpɔdə'filin] *n* 普达非伦苦素,鬼臼苦素

Picrorrhiza [ˌpikrə'raizə] *n* 胡黄连属

picrosaccharometer [ˌpikrəuˌsækə'rɔmitə] *n* 糖尿定量器

picrosclerotine [ˌpikrəu'skliərətin] *n* 麦角苦碱

picrosulfuric acid [ˌpikrəusʌl'fjuərik] 苦硫酸

picrotoxin [ˌpikrəu'tɔksin] *n* 印防己毒素,苦味毒(中枢兴奋药)

picrotoxinism [ˌpikrəu'tɔksinizəm] *n* 印防己毒素中毒

pictograph ['piktəgrɑːf, -græf] *n* 剪影儿童视力表

PID pelvic inflammatory disease 盆腔炎

PIE pulmonary interstitial emphysema 间质性肺气肿

piebald ['paibɔːld] *a* 斑驳病的,花斑的

piebaldism [pai'bɔːldizəm] *n* 斑驳病,花斑;部分白花病

piece [piːs] *n* 片,段 | end ~ [尾]末段 / principal ~, chief ~ 主段(精子尾的主要部分) / secretory ~ 分泌片,分泌成分(分泌 IgA 的糖肽成分) / Y- ~ Y 型管

pied [paid] *a* 斑驳的,杂色的

piedra [pi'eidrə] *n* 毛结节菌病 | black ~ 黑色毛结节菌病 / white ~ 白色毛结节菌病

Piedraia [ˌpaiə'draiə] *n* 毛孢子菌属

Piedraiaceae [ˌpaiədri'eisiiː] *n* 毛孢子菌科

pier [piə] *n* 桥基,基牙(亦称中间桥基)

Pierre Robin syndrome [pi'jɛərəu'bæn] (Pierre Robin) 皮埃尔·罗班综合征(小颌、腭裂及舌下垂,无咽反射)

Piersol's point ['piəsɔl] (George A. Piersol) 皮索尔点(示膀胱口的位置)

piesesthesia [paiˌiːzis'θiːzjə], **piezesthesia** [ˌpaiizis'θiːzjə] *n* 压觉

piesimeter [paii'simitə] *n* 压力计(测皮肤对压力的敏感度)

-piesis [构词成分] 压

piez(o)- [构词成分] 压

piezallochromy [ˌpaii'zæləkrəumi] *n* 压致变色,压碎变色

piezocardiogram [paiˌiːzəu'kɑːdiəgræm] *n* 心动压力图

piezochemistry [paiˌiːzəu'kemistri] *n* 压力化学

piezoelectric [paiˌiːzəui'lektrik] *a* 压电的 | **~ity** [paiˌiːzəuilek'trisəti] *n* 压电[现象]

piezometer [ˌpaiə'zɔmitə] *n* 压力计,压觉计;眶压计

PIF prolactin inhibiting factor 催乳素抑制因子; proliferation inhibitory factor 增生抑制因子

pifarnine [pi'fɑːniːn] *n* 哌法宁(抗胃溃疡药)

pigeon ['pidʒin] *n* 鸽子 | ~ breast, ~ chest 鸡胸

pigeon-breasted ['pidʒin ˌbrestid], **pigeonchested** ['pidʒinˌtʃestid] *a* 鸡胸的

pigeonpox ['pidʒənpɔks] *n* 鸽痘,鸡痘

pigeon-toed ['pidʒin təud] *a* 足内翻的

pigment ['pigmənt] *n* 色素;色料;涂剂 | bile ~ 胆色素 / ceroid ~ 蜡样色素(鼠肝硬变色素) / lipochrome ~ 脂色素 / malarial ~ 疟色素 / melanotic ~ 黑[色]素 / wear and tear ~s 衰竭色素,脂色素 | **~al** [pig'mentl], **~ary** ['pigmentəri] *a*

pigmentation [ˌpigmən'teiʃən] *n* 色素沉着,着色 | carotinoid ~ 胡萝卜素类沉着,皮橙色病 / malarial ~ 疟色素沉着

pigmented ['pigməntid] *a* 色素沉着的,着色的

pigmentogenesis [ˌpigməntəuˈdʒenisis] *n* 色素生成

pigmentogenic [ˌpigməntəuˈdʒenik] *a* 色素生成的,产生色素的

pigmentolysin [ˌpigmənˈtɔlisin] *n* 色素溶素

pigmentolysis [ˌpigmənˈtɔlisis] *n* 色素溶解

pigmentophage [pigˈmentəfeidʒ] *n* 噬色细胞

pigmentophore [pigˈmentəfɔː] *n* 输色素细胞

pigmentum [pigˈmentəm] *n*【拉】涂剂;色素

Pignet's formula (index, standard) [piːˈnjei] (Maurice-Charles-Joseph Pignet) 比内公式(F=H-〈C+W〉,H 表示身高〈cm〉,C 为最大呼气时的胸围〈cm〉,W 为体重〈kg〉,当 F 少于 10,此人被列为非常强壮,10~15 为强壮,15~20 为良好,20~25 为尚可,25~30 为衰弱,30 以上为非常衰弱)

piitis [paiˈaitis] *n* 软膜炎

pikromycin [pikrəuˈmaisin] *n* 苦霉素

Pil. pilula, pilulae【拉】药丸,丸剂

Pila [ˈpailə] *n* 球螺属 | ~ conica 锥球螺 / ~ polita 光球螺

pila [ˈpailə] ([复] **pilae** [ˈpailiː]) *n*【拉】柱(如骨内小梁)

pilar [ˈpailə], **pilary** [ˈpiləri] *a* 毛的,毛发的

pilaster [piˈlæstə] *n* 壁柱

pilch [piltʃ] *n* 尿布垫

Pilcher bag [ˈpiltʃə] (Lewis S. Pilcher) 皮尔彻袋(附有导尿管的前列腺止血袋)

pile [pail] *n* 堆;电堆;核反应堆;[复]痔 *vt, vi* 堆积,积累 | esophageal ~ 食管静脉曲张 / muscular ~肌电堆 / prostatic ~ 前列腺静脉曲张 / sentinel ~ 前哨痔 / thermoelectric ~ 热电堆 / voltaic ~ 伏打电堆

pileus [ˈpailiəs] *n*【拉】胎头羊膜;菌盖,菌伞

pili [ˈpailai] pilus 的复数

pilial [ˈpailiəl] *a* 毛发的

piliate [ˈpailieit] *a* 有菌毛的(指细菌)

Pilidae [ˈpilidiː] *n* 球螺科

piliferous [paiˈlifərəs] *a* 有毛的

piliform [ˈpailifɔːm] *a* 毛样的

Pilimelia [ˌpiliˈmeliə] *n* 发仙菌属

pilimiction [ˌpailiˈmikʃən], **pilimictio** [ˌpailiˈmikʃiəu] *n* 毛尿症

pilin [ˈpailin] *n* 菌毛素,菌毛蛋白

Pilisuctorina [ˌpiliˌsʌktəuˈrainə] *n* 毛吸管虫亚目

pill [pil] *n* 药丸,丸剂 | A. B. S. ~ ABS 丸,芦荟素颠茄士的宁丸 / blue ~ 蓝色丸,汞丸 / chalybeate ~s 红色补丸 / compound cathartic ~ 复方泻丸 / enteric ~ 肠溶丸剂 / hexylresorcinol ~s 已基间苯二酚丸,已基雷琐辛丸 / radio ~ 遥测丸,遥测囊(即 telemetering capsule,见 capsule 项下相应术语)

pillar [ˈpilə] *n* 支柱,柱,脚 | ~ of diaphragm 膈脚

pillbox [ˈpilbɔks] *n* 药丸盒

pillet [ˈpilit] *n* 小药丸,小糖丸

pillion [piˈljən] *n* 暂用假腿

pillow [ˈpiləu] *n* 枕

pill-rolling [pilˈrəuliŋ] *n* 滚丸(动作)(一种手的帕金森震颤)

pil(o)- [构词成分] 毛,发

pilobezoar [ˌpailəˈbiːzɔː] *n* 毛团,毛粪石

pilocarpine [ˌpailəˈkɑːpin] *n* 毛果芸香碱(缩瞳药,用于治疗青光眼) | ~ hydrochloride 盐酸毛果芸香碱 / ~ nitrate 硝酸毛果芸香碱

Pilocarpus [ˌpailəˈkɑːpəs] *n* 毛果芸香属

pilocystic [ˌpailəˈsistik] *a* 囊样含毛的(指某些皮样瘤)

pilocytic [ˌpailəˈsitik] *a* 纤维状细胞的

piloerection [ˌpailəuiˈrekʃən] *n* 竖毛

pilojection [ˌpailəuˈdʒekʃən] *n* 射毛[疗]法(用气枪将毛射入动脉瘤的囊内,作为囊内血栓的核心,用以治颅内囊状动脉瘤)

piloleiomyomas [ˌpailəuˌlaiəumaiˈəuməs] *n* 毛平滑肌瘤

pilology [paiˈlɔlədʒi] *n* 毛发学

pilomatricoma [ˌpailəuˌmeitriˈkəumə], **pilomatrixoma** [ˌpailəuˌmeitrikˈsəumə] *n* 毛母质瘤

pilomotor [ˌpailəuˈməutə] *a* 毛发运动的(指竖毛)

pilonidal [ˌpailəˈnaidl] *a* 藏毛的

pilose [ˈpailəus] *a* 被毛的,多毛的 | **pilosity** [paiˈlɔsəti] *n* 细毛被;多毛

pilosebaceous [ˌpailəusiˈbeiʃəs] *a* 毛囊皮脂腺的

Piltz's reflex [ˈpilts] (Jan Piltz) 注意性瞳孔反射 | ~ sign 皮尔茨征(注意性瞳孔反射;见 Westphal-Piltz phenomenon)

Piltz-Westphal phenomenon [pilts ˈvestfʌl] (Jan Piltz; A. K. O. Westphal) 皮尔茨-韦斯特法尔现象(见 Westphal-Piltz phenomenon)

pilula [ˈpiljulə] ([复] **pilulae** [ˈpiljuliː]) *n*【拉】丸剂

pilular [ˈpiljulə] *a* 药丸状的;药丸的,丸剂的

pilule [ˈpiljuːl] *n* 小丸剂,小糖丸

pilus [ˈpailəs] ([复] **pili** [ˈpailai]) *n*【拉】毛,发;[复]菌毛(亦称伞毛,纤毛) | ~ cuniculatus ([复] pili cuniculati) 内生毛 / F ~ F 菌毛,性菌毛,致育纤毛 / ~ incarnatus recurvus ([复] pili incarnati recurvi) 反曲性内嵌毛 / pili multigemini 多生毛,多生发

pimaric acid [piˈmærik] 海松酸

pimelic acid [piˈmelik] 庚二酸

pimelitis [ˌpimiˈlaitis] *n* 脂肪组织炎

pimel(o)- [构词成分] 脂肪

pimeloma [ˌpimeˈləumə] *n* 脂[肪]瘤
pimelopterygium [ˌpiməlǝutǝˈridʒiəm] *n* 脂肪性翼状胬肉
pimelorthopnea [ˌpiməˌlɔːθɔˈpniːə] *n* 肥胖性端坐呼吸(躺下时则难以呼吸)
pimelosis [ˌpiməˈləusis] *n* 脂肪化;肥胖[病]
pimeluria [ˌpiməˈljuəriə] *n* 脂尿症
Pimenta [piˈmentə] *n* 玉桂属,香椒属
pimenta [piˈmentə] *n* 玉桂子,香椒(牙买加胡椒)
piminodine esylate [piˈminədiːn] 乙磺酸匹米诺定(麻醉止痛药)
pimozide [ˈpaiməzaid] *n* 匹莫齐特(抗精神病药)
Pimpinella [ˌpimpiˈnelə] *n* 茴芹属
pimpinellin [ˌpimpiˈnelin] *n* 茴芹苦素
pimple [ˈpimpl] *n* 丘疹,小脓疱
pimply [ˈpimpli], **pimpled** [ˈpimpld] *a* 有丘疹的,多脓疱的
pin [pin] *n* 钉 | intramedullary ~ 髓内钉
Pinaceae [paiˈneisiiː] *n* 松科
pinacyanole [ˌpinəˈsaiənəul] *n* 松柏氰醇
Pinard's maneuver [piˈnɑː] (Adolphe Pinard) 比纳手法(臀先露分娩时足牵引手法)
pince-ciseaux [pæns siˈzəu] *n*【法】镊剪,有刃镊(用于虹膜切开术)
pincement [pænsˈmɔŋ] *n*【法】拧按法
pincers [ˈpinsəz] *n* 镊子,钳子;正中乳切牙(马)
pincette [pænˈset] *n*【法】小钳子,小镊子
pinch [pintʃ] *vt*, *n* 捏,拧,夹
Pindborg tumor [ˈpindbɔːg] (Jens J. Pindborg) 牙源性钙化上皮瘤
pindolol [ˈpindələl] *n* 吲哚洛尔(β 受体阻滞药)
pindone [ˈpindəun] *n* 哌酮(茚满二酮抗凝药,杀鼠药)
pine¹ [pain] *n* 松树、松木 | white ~ 白松(复方白松糖浆的成分)
pine² [pain] *n* 地方性牛羊消瘦病
pineal [ˈpiniəl] *a* 松果体的;松果状的
pinealectomy [ˌpiniəˈlektəmi] *n* 松果体切除术
pinealism [ˈpiniəlizəm] *n* 松果体功能障碍
pinealoblastoma [ˌpiniələublæsˈtəumə], **pineoblastoma** [ˌpiniəublæsˈtəumə] *n* 成松果体细胞瘤
pinealocyte [ˈpiniələsait] *n* 松果体细胞
pinealoma [ˌpiniəˈləumə], **pinealocytoma** [ˌpiniələusaiˈtəumə], **pineocytoma** [ˌpiniəusaiˈtəumə] *n* 松果体瘤
pinealopathy [ˌpiniəˈlɔpəθi] *n* 松果体病
pinene [ˈpainiːn] *n* 蒎烯
pinguecula [piŋˈgwekjulə], **pinguicula** [piŋˈgwikjulə] *n* 睑裂斑
piniform [ˈpinifɔːm] *a* 圆锥形的
pining [ˈpainiŋ] *n* 地方性牛羊消瘦病
pink [piŋk] *n* 石竹;石竹花;粉红色 *a* 粉红色的
pinkeye [ˈpiŋkai] *n* 红眼(急性触染性结膜炎)
Pinkus disease [ˈpinkus] (Felix Pinkus) 光泽苔藓
pinledge [ˈpinlidʒ] *n* 针架(牙结构内一种平台或肩台,准备钻针孔用)
pinna [ˈpinə] ([复] **pinnae** [ˈpiniː]) *n*【拉】耳郭;翼;羽 | **~l** [ˈpinl] *a*
pinnaglobin [ˌpinəˈgləubin] *n* 江瑶珠蛋白(一种楔形软体动物江瑶的棕色呼吸色素)
pinocarveol [ˌpainəˈkɑːviɔl] *n* 松香芹醇
pinocyte [ˈpinəsait, ˈpai-] *n* 胞饮细胞,饮液细胞
pinocytic [ˌpinəuˈsitik, ˌpai-] *a* 胞饮细胞的;胞饮的
pinocytosis [ˌpainəusaiˈtəusis, ˌpi-] *n* 胞饮(细胞通过吸液小体的形成,把液体小滴摄入的作用) | **pinocytotic** [ˌpainəusaiˈtɔtik, ˌpi-] *a*
pinosome [ˈpainəsəum, ˈpi-] *n* 胞饮泡,饮液体,胞饮小体(胞饮作用中,细胞膜凹陷围拢后形成的充满液体的空泡,亦称吞噬体)
Pinoyella [ˌpainəˈjelə] *n* 发癣菌属,毛癣菌属(即 Trichophyton) | ~ simii 猴发癣菌,猴毛癣菌(即 Trichophyton simii)
Pins' sign [pins] (Emil Pins) 平斯征(心包渗液时在左肩胛下角叩诊可闻及气管呼吸音及浊音)
pint(pt) [paint] *n* 品脱(旧容量单位,美国制为 16 液量盎司,473.17 ml,英国制为 20 液量盎司,568.25 ml)
pinta [ˈpiːntə] *n* 品他病(美洲热带地方密螺旋体性皮肤病)
pintado [piːnˈtɑːdəu] *n* 品他病患者
pintid [ˈpintid] *n* 品他疹
pinus [ˈpainəs] *n*【拉】松属
pinworm [ˈpinwəːm] *n* 蛲虫
pi(o)- [构词成分] 脂,脂肪;同样见 lip(o) 起始的词
pioepithelium [ˌpaiəepiˈθiːljəm] *n* 含脂上皮,脂变上皮
pioglitazone hydrochloride [ˌpaiəuˈglitəzəun] 盐酸吡格列酮(降血糖药)
pion [ˈpaiɔn] *n* π 介子
pionemia [ˌpaiəˈniːmiə] *n* 脂血[症]
Piophila [paiˈɔfilə] *n* 酪蝇属 | ~ casei 酪蝇,细蝇
piorthopnea [ˌpaiɔːθɔˈpniːə] *n* 肥胖性端坐呼吸(躺下时呼吸困难)
pioscope [ˈpaiəskəup] *n* 乳脂计
Piotrowski's sign(reflex) [ˌpiəˈtrɔvski] (Alexander Piotrowski) 皮奥特罗夫斯基征(反射)(叩诊胫骨前肌时引起足向背屈及外旋现象,当此反射过多时,即表明中枢神经系统的器质性疾

病,亦称胫前肌征或胫前肌反射)

PIP$_1$ phosphatidylinositol 4-phosphate 磷脂酰肌醇4-磷酸

PIP$_2$ phosphatidylinositol 4, 5 -biphosphate 磷脂酰肌醇4, 5-二磷酸

pipamazine [paiˈpæməziːn] *n* 匹哌马嗪(止吐药)

pipamperone [piˈpæmpirəun] *n* 匹泮哌隆(安定药,用以治疗精神分裂症)

pipazethate hydrochloride [piˈpæziθeit] 盐酸匹哌氮酯(非麻醉性镇咳药)

pipecolic acid [ˌpipəˈkəulik] 哌可酸,2-六氢吡啶羧酸

pipecuronium bromide [ˌpipəkjuˈrəniəm] *n* 哌库溴铵(神经肌肉阻断药)

pipenzolate bromide [paiˈpenzəleit] 溴哌喷酯(抗胆碱能药)

Piper [ˈpaipə] *n* 胡椒属

piperacetazine [ˌpaipərəˈsetəziːn] *n* 哌西他嗪(抗精神病药)

piperacillin sodium [paiˈperəˌsilin] 哌拉西林钠(抗菌药)

piperazidine [ˌpaipəˈræzidiːn] *n* 哌嗪(即 piperazine,抗蠕虫药)

piperazine [ˈpaipərəziːn, piˈperəziːn] *n* 哌嗪(抗蠕虫药) | ~ citrate 枸橼酸哌嗪,驱蛔灵 / ~ edetate calcium 哌嗪依地酸钙 / ~ estrone sulfate 哌嗪雌酮硫酸酯,硫酸哌嗪雌酮(雌激素类药) / ~ phosphate 磷酸哌嗪

piperic acid [paiˈperik, pi-] 胡椒酸

piperidine [paiˈperidiːn, pi-] *n* 哌啶,六氢吡啶

piperidione [ˌpaipəriˈdaiəun] *n* 乙哌双酮(即地海哌酮 dihyprylone,镇静药,镇咳药)

piperidolate hydrochloride [ˌpaipəˈridəleit] 盐酸哌立度酯(抗胆碱药,解痉药)

piperine [ˈpaipəriːn, pi-] *n* 胡椒碱(杀虫药)

piperism [ˈpaipərizəm, pi-] *n* 胡椒中毒

piperocaine hydrochloride [ˈpaipərəkein] 盐酸哌罗卡因(局部麻醉药)

piperonyl butoxide [paiˈperənil bjuˈtɔksaid] 胡椒基丁醚(一种增效剂,与除虫菊酯〈pyrethrins〉结合,用于杀虫剂和灭虱剂)

piperoxan hydrochloride [ˌpaipəˈrɔksæn] 盐酸哌罗克生(α 受体阻滞药)

pipet(te) [piˈpet, pai-] *n* 吸(量)管,移液管,滴管 *vt* (用移液管)移液

pipitzahoac [paiˌpitzəhəuˈæk] *n* 墨西哥菊根(用作泻药)

pipobroman [ˌpaipəˈbrəumən] *n* 哌泊溴烷(抗肿瘤药)

piposulfan [pipəˈsʌlfən] *n* 哌泊舒凡(抗肿瘤药)

pipotiazine palmitate [ˌpipəuˈtaiəziːn] 棕榈酸哌泊塞嗪(安定药)

pipoxolan hydrochloride [piˈpɔksələn] 盐酸哌泊索仑(肌肉松弛药)

pipradrol hydrochloride [ˈpaiprədrɔl] 盐酸哌苯甲醇(中枢神经系统兴奋药)

piprozolin [ˌiprəuˈzəulin] *n* 哌普唑林(利胆药)

Piptadenia [ˌpiptəˈdiːniə] *n* 豆属

Piptocephalus [ˌpiptəuˈsefələs] *n* 头珠霉属

piquizil hydrochloride [ˈpikwizil] 盐酸哌喹齐尔(支气管扩张药)

piqûre [piˈkuə] *n*【法】穿刺(尤指糖尿穿刺)

pirandamine hydrochloride [piəˈrændəmiːn] 盐酸吡喃达明(抗抑郁药)

pirbenicillin sodium [piˌbeniˈsilin] 吡苄西林钠(抗菌药)

pirbuterol acetate [piˈbjuːtərəul] 醋酸吡布特罗(支气管扩张药)

pirbuterol hydrochloride [piˈbjuːtərɔl] 盐酸吡布特罗(支气管扩张药)

Pirenella [ˌpaiərəˈnelə] *n* 小塔螺属 | ~ conica 锥形小塔螺(异形吸虫的中间宿主)

pirenzepine hydrochloride [ˌpirənˈzipiːn] 盐酸哌仑西平(胃酸过多和消化性溃疡时用于抑制胃液分泌)

pirfenidone [piˈfenidɔn] *n* 吡非尼酮(抗炎、解热药)

piriform [ˈpirifɔːm] *a* 梨状的,梨形的

Pirogoff's amputation [ˌpirəˈgɔf] (Nikolai I. Pirogoff) 皮罗果夫切断术(一种在踝部的切断术) | ~ angle 静脉角(颈内静脉和锁骨下静脉连接而形成之角) / ~ triangle 舌下舌骨三角

pirolate [ˈpirəleit] *n* 匹罗酯(平喘药)

pirolazamide [ˌpirəˈleizəmaid] *n* 吡拉酰胺(抗心律失常药)

piroplasm [ˈpairəplæzm] *n* 梨浆虫

Piroplasma [ˌpairəˈplæzmə] *n* 梨浆虫属(现名巴贝虫属 Babesia)

Piroplasmia [ˌpairəplæzˈmiːə] *n* 梨浆虫亚纲

piroplasmid [ˌpairəˈplæzmid] *a*, *n* 梨浆虫(的)

Piroplasmida [ˌpairəˈplæzmidə] *n* 梨浆虫目

piroplasmosis [ˌpairəplæzˈməusis] *n* 梨浆虫病,巴贝虫病

piroxantrone hydrochloride [ˌpirəuˈzæntrəun] 盐酸吡罗蒽醌(一种细胞毒性化合物,可致 DNA 链断裂和交联,研究性地用于治疗乳腺癌)

piroxicam [piˈrɔksikæm] *n* 吡罗昔康(抗炎药)

pirprofen [piˈprəufən] *n* 吡洛芬(抗炎药)

Pirquet's reaction(cutireaction, test) [pəˈkei] (Clemens F. von Pirquet) 皮尔盖反应(皮肤反应、试验),划痕试验(加 2 小滴旧结核菌素在皮肤上轻微划痕后 24 ~ 48 小时出现红肿疹块,阳性试验表示以前有感染,但不能区分临床疾病)

pis [piː] *n*【法】排尿

piscicide [ˈpisisaid] *n* 杀鱼剂
Piscidia [piˈsidiə] *n* 毒鱼豆属 | ~ erythrina 牙买加毒鱼豆
piscidin [piˈsaidin] *n* 牙买加毒鱼豆素
pisiform [ˈpaisifɔːm] *a* 豌豆状的 *n* 豌豆骨
pisiformis [ˌpaisiˈfɔːmis] *a*【拉】豌豆形的;豌豆大小的
Piskacek's sign [ˈpiskətʃek] (Ludwig Piskacek) 皮斯卡切克征(宫体在妊娠时呈不对称增大)
piss [pis] *vi*, *vt* 撒尿,小便 *n* 尿,小便
pistil [ˈpistil] *n* 雌蕊
piston [ˈpistən] *n* 活塞(如注射器活塞)
Pisum [ˈpaisəm] *n* 豌豆属
PIT plasma iron turnover 血浆铁转换
pit [pit] *n* 窝,凹,点隙;痘凹;纹孔 | anal ~ 肛凹,肛窝 / arm ~ 腋窝 / basilar ~ 底凹(齿冠) / chrome ~s 铬蚀性溃疡,铬溃疡 / costal ~ 下肋凹 / gastric ~s 胃小凹 / nasal ~, olfactory ~ 鼻窝,嗅窝 / postanal ~ 尾小凹 / ~ of stomach 胸口,胃窝
pita [ˈpiːtə] *n* 迭瓦癣
pitch[1] [pitʃ] *n* 沥青;树脂,松脂 *vt* 用沥青涂 | black ~, naval ~ 黑[色]松脂 / Burgundy ~ (挪威)云杉脂,白树脂 / Canada ~ 加拿大松脂 / liquid ~ 普通松焦油 / mineral ~ 沥青
pitch[2] [pitʃ] *n* 音调
pitchblende [ˈpitʃblend] *n* 沥青铀矿
pith [piθ] *n* 髓 *vt* 刺毁脑脊髓
pithecoid [ˈpiθikɔid] *a* 猿样的
pithiatic [ˌpiθiˈætik] *a* 可说服治疗的(指癔症)
pithiatism [piˈθaiətizəm] *n* (可说服治疗的)暗示病;说服疗法(治疗神经和精神疾病)
pithiatry [piˈθaiətri] *n* 说服疗法 | **pithiatric** [ˌpiθiˈætrik] *a*
pithing [ˈpiθiŋ] *n* 脑脊髓刺毁法
pithode [ˈpaiθəud] *n* 核纺锤体
Pithomyces [ˌpiθəuˈmaisiːz] *n* 髓霉属
pithomycotoxicosis [ˌpɪθəuˌmaɪkəuˌtɔksɪˈkəusɪs] *n* 髓霉菌毒素中毒[症]
Pitres' rule (law) [piˈtres] (Jean A. Pitres) 彼特尔规律(定律)(掌握多种语言的患者患获得性失语症时,最先最完整恢复的是受伤前最经常使用的语言,不论该种语言是否为其母语) | ~ sign 彼特尔征(脊髓痨时,阴囊及睾丸感觉过敏)
pitta [ˈpitə] *n*【梵】胆汁(根据印度生命科学为构成身体三大要素之一)
pitted [ˈpitid] *a* 有凹痕的;有纹孔的
pitting [ˈpitiŋ] *n* 凹痕,凹陷,凹入;纹孔
pituicyte [piˈtju(ː)isait] *n* 垂体[后叶]细胞
pituita [piˈtju(ː)itə] *n*【拉】(稠)黏液
pituitarigenic [piˌtju(ː)itəriˈdʒenik] *a* 垂体源[性]的
pituitarism [piˈtju(ː)itərizəm] *n* 垂体功能障碍
pituitarium [piˌtju(ː)iˈtɛəriəm] *n*【拉】垂体
pituitary [piˈtjuːitəri] *a* 垂体的;(稠)黏液的 *n* 垂体 | anterior ~腺垂体,垂体前叶 / pharyngeal ~ 咽垂体 / posterior ~ 垂体后叶 / whole ~全垂体
pituitary-adrenal [piˌtjuːitəriəˈdriːnl] *a* 垂体肾上腺的
pituitectomy [piˌtju(ː)iˈtektəmi] *n* 垂体切除术
pituitous [piˈtju(ː)itəs] *a* (稠)黏液的
pituitrism [piˈtju(ː)itrizəm] *n* 垂体功能障碍
pityriasis [ˌpitiˈraiəsis] *n* 糠疹 | ~ alba, ~ simplex 白糠疹,单纯糠疹 / ~ capitis 头皮糠疹 / ~ linguae 地图样舌 / ~ rosea 玫瑰糠疹 / ~ rubra pilaris 毛发红糠疹
pityroid [ˈpitirɔid] *a* 糠状的
Pityrosporum [ˌpitiˈrɔspərəm] *n* 糠秕孢子菌属 | ~ orbiculare 环状糠秕孢子菌 / ~ ovale 卵状糠秕孢子菌 | **Pityrosporon** [ˌpitiˈrɔspərɔn] *n*
pivalate [ˈpivəleit] *n* 特戊酸盐,三甲基醋酸(或酯)(trimethylacetate 的 USAN 缩约词)
pivalic acid [paiˈvælik] 特戊酸,三甲基醋酸
pivampicillin hydrochloride [piˌvæmpiˈsilin] 盐酸匹氨西林(抗菌素类药)
pivmecillinam [ˌpivməˈsilinəm] *n* 匹莫西林(抗生素类药)
pivot [ˈpivət] *n* 枢轴;桩冠 | occlusal ~ 船面桩
pivotal [ˈpivətl] *a* 枢轴的
pix [piks] *n*【拉】焦油,沥青
pixel [ˈpiksəl] *n* 像素(电视显示屏表示单位的二维区)
pizotyline [piˈzəutiliːn] *n* 苯噻啶(抗抑郁药,5-羟色胺抑制药,偏头痛特效药)
pizzle [ˈpizəl] *n* (动物)阴茎
PJRT permanent junctional reciprocating tachycardia 持续性交接区折返性心动过速
PJT paroxysmal junctional tachycardia 阵发性交接区心动过速
PK pyruvate kinase 丙酮酸激酶
pK_a酸的电离常数(K_a)的负对数;当缓冲系统的 pK_a 值和 pH 值相等时,缓冲力最大
PKU, PKU1 phenylketonuria 苯丙酮尿症
placebo [pləˈsiːbəu] *n* 安慰剂,无效[对照]剂;安慰治疗
placement [ˈpleismənt] *n* 放置,安排 | linqual ~ (牙向)舌移位
placenta [pləˈsentə] ([复]**placentas** 或 **placentae** [pləˈsentiː]) *n* 胎盘 | adherent ~ 粘连胎盘 / battledore ~ 球拍状胎盘 / bilobate ~, bilobed ~, bipartite ~, dimidiate ~, duplex ~ 双叶胎盘 / choriovitelline ~, yolk-sac ~ 绒[毛]膜卵黄囊胎盘,卵黄囊胎盘 / deciduate

~, deciduous ~蜕膜胎盘 / fundal ~ 宫底胎盘 / horseshoe ~ 马蹄形胎盘 / multilobate ~, multilobed ~ 多叶胎盘 / ~ percreta 穿透性胎盘 / ~ praevia 前置胎盘 / retained ~, incarcerated ~ 胎盘留滞,牢固胎盘 / trilobate ~, tripartite ~, triplex ~ 三叶胎盘 / zonary ~, zonular ~ 环状胎盘 | **~l** *a*

Placentalia [ˌplæsənˈteiliə] *n* 有胎盘类,胎盘动物类

placentation [ˌplæsənˈteiʃən] *n* 胎盘形成

placentin [pləˈsentin] *n* (牛)干胎盘粉

placentitis [ˌplæsənˈtaitis] *n* 胎盘炎

placentogenesis [pləˌsentəˈdʒenisis] *n* 胎盘发生

placentogram [pləˈsentəgræm] *n* 胎盘造影[照]片

placentography [ˌplæsənˈtɔgrəfi] *n* 胎盘造影[术] | indirect ~ 间接胎盘造影[术]

placentoid [pləˈsentɔid] *a* 胎盘样的

placentology [ˌplæsənˈtɔlədʒi] *n* 胎盘学 | **placentologist** *n* 胎盘学家

placentolysin [ˌplæsənˈtɔlisin] *n* 胎盘溶素

placentoma [ˌplæsənˈtəumə] *n* 胎盘瘤

placentopathy [ˌplæsənˈtɔpəθi] *n* 胎盘病

Placido's disk [ˈplɑːsidəu] (A. Placido)角膜镜

placode [ˈplækəud] *n* 基板 | dorsolateral ~s 背外侧基板 / epibranchial ~s 腮背基板

placoderm [ˈplækədəːm] *n* 盾皮鱼

Placodermi [ˈplækəˌdəːmi] *n* 盾皮鱼纲

placoid [ˈplækɔid] *a* 板状的

plafond [plaːˈfɔːn] *n*【法】胫骨下关节面

plagiocephaly [ˌpleidʒiəˈsefəli], **plagiocephalism** [ˌpleidʒiəˈsefəlizəm] *n* 斜形头 | **plagiocephalic** [ˌpleidʒiəsəˈfælik] *a*

plague [pleig] *n* 鼠疫 | ambulatory ~, larval ~ 轻鼠疫,不卧床鼠疫 / bubonic ~, glandular ~ 腺鼠疫,腹股沟淋巴结鼠疫 / premonitory ~ 前驱[轻]鼠疫 / pneumonic ~ 肺鼠疫 / septicemic ~, siderating ~ 败血性鼠疫,电击状鼠疫 / white ~ 结核[病]

plakins [ˈpleikinz] *n* 血小板溶素

plana [ˈpleinə] planum 的复数

planarian [pləˈnɛəriən] *n* 涡虫

planchet [ˈplæntʃit] *n* 金属盘(存放放射性样本)

Planck's constant [plɑːŋk] (Max K. E. L. Planck)普郎克常数,量子常数(h = 6.625 × 10^{-34} J/s) | ~ theory 普郎克学说,量子论(quantum theory,见 theory 项下相应术语)

Planctomyces [ˌplænktəuˈmaisiːz] *n* 浮游菌属

plane [plein] *n* 平面 | auriculoinfraorbital ~, eye-ear ~ 眼耳平面 / bite ~, occlusal ~, ~ of occlusion 𬌗平面 / cove ~ 波动面(心电图) / datum ~ 基准水平面 / guide ~ 导面 / horizontal ~ 水平面,横剖面 / median ~, midsagittal ~ 正中矢状平面 / mesiodistal ~ 近中远中平面 / nasion-postcondylare ~ 髁鼻平面 / principal ~ 主[轴]平面 / ~ of regard 注视平面 / sagittal ~ 矢面 / spinous ~ 棘突平面 / transpyloric ~ 幽门平面(躯干横切面) / vertical ~ 垂直面,矢状面

planigram [ˈplænigræm] *n* X 线体层[照]片,X 线断层[照]片

planigraphy [pləˈnigrəfi] *n* X 线体层摄影[术],X 线断层摄影[术]

planimeter [pləˈnimitə] *n* 面积计

planing [ˈpleiniŋ] *n* [皮肤]整平法(用于消除瘢痕、纹身、色痣等)

planithorax [ˌplæniˈθɔːræks] *n* 胸部平面图

plankton [ˈplæŋktən] *n* 浮游生物 | **~ic** [plæŋkˈtɔnik] *a*

planning [ˈplæniŋ] *n* 计划,规划 | family ~ 计划生育

Planobispora [ˌpleinəubaiˈspɔːrə] *n* 浮游双孢菌属

planocellular [ˌpleinəuˈseljulə] *a* 扁平细胞的

Planococcus [ˌplænəuˈkɔkəs] *n* 浮游球菌属

planoconcave [ˌpleinəuˈkɔnkeiv] *a* 平凹的

planoconvex [ˌpleinəuˈkɔnveks] *a* 平凸的

planocyte [ˈplænəsait] *n* 游走细胞

planogram [ˈpleinəgræm] *n* X 线体层[照]片,X 线断层[照]片

planography [pləˈnɔgrəfi] *n* X 线体层摄影[术],X 线断层摄影[术]

Planomonospore [ˌpleinəuməˈnɔspɔːrə] *n* 浮游单孢菌属

planorbid [pləˈnɔːbid] *n* 扁卷螺 *a* 扁卷螺的

Planorbidae [pləˈnɔːbidiː] *n* 扁卷螺科

Planorbis [pləˈnɔːbis] *n* 扁卷螺属

planotopokinesia [ˌplænəuˌtɔpəukaiˈniːziə] *n* 空间定位障碍

plantaginis semen [plænˈtædʒinisˈsiːmən]【拉】车前子

Plantago [plænˈteigəu] *n* 车前属

plantalgia [plænˈtældʒiə] *n* 足底痛

planta pedis [ˈplæntəˈpiːdiːz]【拉】足底,跖(亦称足底区)

plantar [ˈplæntə] *a* 足底的,跖的

plantaris [plænˈtɛəris] *a*【拉】足底的,跖的 *n* 跖肌

plantation [plænˈteiʃən] *n* 植入,栽植(如牙或其他组织的植入)

plantigrade [ˈplæntigreid] *a* 跖行的

planula [ˈplænjulə] *n* 二胚层胚;浮浪幼体(腔肠动物) | invaginate ~ 原肠胚

planum [ˈpleinəm] ([复] **plana** [ˈpleinə]) *n*

【拉】平面
planuria [pleiˈnjuriə] *n* 异位排尿
plaque [plɑːk] *n*【法】斑块 | bacterial ~, dental ~ 菌斑,牙斑 / fibromyelinic ~s 纤维髓磷脂斑 / opaline ~ 乳光斑,梅毒黏膜斑 / senile ~s 老年斑
-plasia [构词成分] 生长,发育,形成
plasm [ˈplæzəm] *n* 浆,血浆;原生质,原浆 | germ ~ 种质(亲代传递给子代的遗传物质)
-plasm [构词成分] 浆,原生质
plasma [ˈplæzmə] *n* 浆,血浆;原生质,原浆 | albumose ~, peptone ~ 脘血浆,胨血浆 / antihemophilic human ~抗血友病性人血浆 / blood ~ 血浆 / isoimmune ~同族免疫血浆 / muscle ~肌浆 / normal human ~正常人血浆 / pooled ~混合血浆 / salt ~中性盐血浆 / seminal ~精液浆
plasmablast [ˈplæzməblæst] *n* 成浆细胞,浆母细胞
plasmacyte [ˈplæzməsait] *n* 浆细胞 | **plasmacytic** [ˌplæzməˈsitik] *a*
plasmacytoma [ˌplæzməsaiˈtəumə] *n* 浆细胞瘤 | multiple ~ of bone 多发性骨髓瘤(即 multiple myeloma)
plasmacytosis [ˌplæzməsaiˈtəusis] *n* 浆细胞增多[症]
plasmagel [ˈplæzmədʒel] *n* 原生质凝胶
plasmagene [ˈplæzmədʒiːn] *n* 细胞质基因 | **plasmagenic** [ˌplæzməˈdʒenik] *a*
plasmahaut [ˈplæzməhaut] *n*【德】胞质膜
plasmal [ˈplæzməl] *n* 体液素,浆醛
plasmalemma [ˌplæzməˈlemə] *n* 细胞膜
plasmalogen [plæzˈmælədʒən] *n* 缩醛磷脂
plasmapheresis [ˌplæzməfəˈriːsis] *n* 血浆去除术,血浆置换
plasmarrhexis [ˌplæzməˈreksis] *n* 胞质溶解
plasmatherapy [ˌplæzməˈθerəpi] *n* 血浆疗法
plasmatic [plæzˈmætik] *a* 浆的,血浆的;原生质的,原浆的
plasmatogamy [ˌplæzməˈtɔgəmi] *n* 胞质融合
plasmatorrhexis [ˌplæzmətəˈreksis] *n* 细胞破裂,胞质破裂
plasmatosis [ˌplæzməˈtəusis] *n* 胞质液化
plasmic [ˈplæzmik] *a* 浆的,血浆的;原生质的,原浆的;富于原生质的
plasmid [ˈplæzmid] *n* 质粒 | conjugative ~ 转移性质粒(接合时从一个细菌细胞转移到另一个细菌细胞的质粒) / F ~ F 质粒(存在于 F^+ 细菌细胞中的转移性质粒) / F' ~ F' 质粒(一种杂种 F 质粒,也含有一段宿主染色体) / R ~ R 质粒(亦称抗性质粒,抗性因子)
plasmin [ˈplæzmin] *n* 纤维蛋白溶酶,纤溶酶
plasminic acid [plæzˈminik] 胞浆素酸
plasminogen [plæzˈminədʒən] *n* 纤维蛋白溶酶原,纤溶酶原(纤维蛋白溶解药)
plasminogen activator [plæzˈminədʒənˈæktiˌveitə] 纤溶酶原激活物,纤溶酶原激活药
plasm(o)- [构词成分] 血浆,浆,胞质
plasmocyte [ˈplæzməsait] *n* 浆细胞
plasmocytoma [ˌplæzməsaiˈtəumə] *n* 浆细胞瘤
plasmodesm [ˈplæzmədezm], **plasmodesma** [ˌplæzməˈdezmə] *n* 胞间连丝
plasmodesmata [ˌplæzməˈdezmətə] *n* 胞间连丝(plasmodesm 或 plasmodesma 的复数)
plasmodia [plæzˈməudiə] plasmodium 的复数
plasmodial [plæzˈməudiəl] *a* 疟原虫的;原形体的;合胞体的
plasmodiblast [plæzˈməudiblæst] *n* 滋养层
plasmodicidal [ˌplæzməudiˈsaidl] *a* 杀疟原虫的
plasmodicide [plæzˈməudisaid] *n* 杀疟原虫药
Plasmodiidae [ˌplæzməuˈdaiidiː] *n* 疟原虫科
Plasmodiophora brassicae [ˌplæzməudaiˈɔfərəˈbræsikiː] 甘蓝根肿菌
Plasmodiophorea [ˌplæzməuˌdaiəuˈfəuriə] *n* 原质纲
Plasmodiophorida [ˌplæzməuˌdaiəuˈfɔːridə] *n* 原质目
plasmoditrophoblast [plæzˌməudaiˈtrɔfəblæst] *n* 合胞体滋养层
Plasmodium [plæzˈməudiəm] *n* 疟原虫属 | ~ falciparum 恶性疟原虫 / ~ malariae 三日疟原虫 / ~ ovale 卵形疟原虫 / ~ vivax 间日疟原虫
plasmodium [plæzˈməudiəm] ([复] **plasmodia** [plæzˈməudiə]) *n* 疟原虫;原形体,原质团;合胞体 | exoerythrocytic ~红细胞外型疟原虫
Plasmodroma [ˌplæzməˈdrəumə] *n* 质走亚门
plasmogamy [plæzˈmɔgəmi] *n* 原生质融合,胞质配合
plasmogen [ˈplæzmədʒən] *n* 原生质,原浆
plasmoid [ˈplæsmɔid] *n* 类浆(细胞的一种异常蛋白成分)
plasmology [plæzˈmɔlədʒi] *n* 原生质学,原浆学
plasmolysis [plæzˈmɔlisis] *n* 质壁分离(植物细胞由于渗透压作用而失水,致使细胞质脱离细胞壁而收缩) | **plasmolytic** [ˌplæzməˈlitik] *a*
plasmolyze [ˈplæzməlaiz] *vt*, *vi* 胞质皱缩,质壁分离 | **plasmolyzable** [ˌplæzməˈlaizəbl] *a* / **plasmolyzability** [ˌplæzməˌlaizəˈbiləti] *n* 胞质皱缩性,质壁分离性
plasmoma [plæzˈməumə] *n* 浆细胞瘤
plasmon [ˈplæzmɔn] *n* 细胞质基因组,胞质团
plasmonucleic acid [ˌplæzməunjuːˈkliːik] 胞浆核酸,核糖核酸
plasmoptysis [plæzˈmɔptisis] *n* 胞质逸出
plasmorrhexis [ˌplæzməˈreksis] *n* 红细胞[浆]迸

出,红细胞破碎

plasmoschisis [plæzˈmɔskisis] *n* 胞质分裂;红细胞分裂

plasmosin [ˈplæzməsin] *n* 胞质蛋白

plasmosome [ˈplæzməsəum] *n* 真核仁,核小体;[复]线粒体

plasmotomy [plæzˈmɔtəmi] *n* 原质团分割

plasmotrophoblast [ˌplæzməuˈtrɔfəblæst] *n* 合胞体滋养层

plasmotropism [plæzˈmɔtrəpizəm] *n* 原浆破坏 | **plasmotropic** [ˌplæzməuˈtrɔpik] *a*

plasome [ˈplæzəum] *n* 微胶粒(原生质的假设单位)

plasson [ˈplæsɔn] *n* 无核细胞原浆,全能原浆

-plast [构词成分] 原始细胞

plastein [ˈplæstiːn] *n* 改制蛋白,[合成]类蛋白

plaster [ˈplɑːstə, ˈplæ-] *n* 石膏;硬膏剂,膏药 | adhesive ~ 橡皮膏,绊创膏 / belladonna ~ 颠茄硬膏 / dental ~ 牙科石膏 / diachylon ~, lead ~ 铅硬膏,油酸铅硬膏

plaster of Paris [ˈpæris] (Paris 为法国巴黎,19 世纪初期生产石膏之地)煅石膏,干燥硫酸钙

plastic [ˈplæstik, ˈplɑːstik] *a* 成形的,整形的,整复的;可塑的 *n* [常用复]塑料,塑料制品

plasticity [plæsˈtisəti] *n* 成形性;可塑性(生物对环境的适应性)

plasticize [ˈplæstisaiz] *vt, vi* 成为可塑 | **~r** *n* 成形剂,增塑剂

plastid [ˈplæstid] *n* 质体(任何基本的结构单位,如细胞;细胞内除核和中心体以外的细胞器,例如淀粉体)

plastidogenetic [plæsˌtidəudʒiˈnetik] *a* 质体形成的,细胞形成的

plastin [ˈplæstin] *n* 网质,网素(指核丝或透明质);海绵质

plastiosome [ˈplæstiəsəum] *n* 线粒体

plastochondria [ˌplæstəˈkɔndriə] *n* 粒状线粒体,粒体

plastocont, plastokont [ˈplæstəkənt] *n* 杆状线粒体

plastodynamia [ˌplæstəudaiˈneimiə] *n* 发育力

plastogamy [plæsˈtɔgəmi] *n* 胞质融合,胞质配合

plastogel [ˈplæstədʒel] *n* 塑性凝胶

plastomere [ˈplæstəmiə] *n* 质体区,线粒体区

plastoquinone [ˌplæstəuˈkwinəun] *n* 质体醌

plastosome [ˈplæstəsəum] *n* 线粒体

plastron [ˈplæstrən] *n*【法】胸板(胸骨与肋软骨的合称)

-plasty [构词成分] 成形术,整形术,整复术

plate [pleit] *n* 板;托基,基托;平皿 | alar ~, dorsolateral ~ 翼板 / anal ~ 肛膜,肛板 / bite ~ 颌板,颌托 / blood ~s 血小板 / clinoid ~ 床板(在蝶鞍后) / cortical ~ 外板 / cough ~ 咳皿(培养百日咳杆菌) / deck ~, dorsal ~, roof ~ 顶板 / die ~ 成型板 / foot ~ 底板(镫骨) / streak ~ 划线培养平皿

plateau [plæˈtəu] ([复] **plateaus** 或 **plateaux** [plæˈtəuz]) *n* 坪 | tibial ~ 胫骨坪(胫骨接近股骨髁内外侧的骨面) / ventricular ~ 心室坪(心室压曲线的最高段)

platelet [ˈpleitlit] *n* 血小板 | blood ~ 血小板

plateletpheresis [ˌpleitlitfəˈriːsis] *n* 血小板去除术

platform [ˈplætfɔːm] *n* 平台,台

platinectomy [ˌplætiˈnektəmi] *n* 镫骨足板切除术

plating [ˈpleitiŋ] *n* 平皿接种;骨折镶片法;电镀

platinic [pləˈtinik] *a* [正]铂的,四价铂的

platinochloric acid [ˌplætinəuˈklɔːrik] 氯铂酸

platinode [ˈplætinəud] *n* 铂极

platinosis [ˌplætiˈnəusis] *n* 铂中毒

platinous [ˈplætinəs] *a* 亚铂的,二价铂的

platinum(Pt) [ˈplætinəm] *n* 铂(化学元素) | ~ chloride 氯化铂 / ~ diamminodichloride 顺氯氨铂,顺铂(抗肿瘤药)

platy- [构词成分] 阔,扁平

platybasia [ˌplætiˈbeisiə] *n* 扁颅底,扁后脑,后颅[骨]凹陷症

platycelous [ˌplætiˈsiːləs] *a* 前凹后凸的

platycephaly [ˌplætiˈsefəli] *n* 扁头 | **platycephalic** [ˌplætisəˈfælik], **platycephalous** *a*

platycnemia [ˌplætikˈniːmiə] *n* 扁胫骨(左、右侧扁) | **platycnemic** *a*

Platycodon [ˌplætiˈkəudɔn] *n* 桔梗属

platycoria [ˌplætiˈkɔːriə] *n* 瞳孔开大

platycrania [ˌplætiˈkreinjə] *n* 扁颅

platycyte [ˈplætisait] *n* 扁平细胞

platyglossal [ˌplætiˈglɔsəl] *a* 阔舌的

platyhelminth [ˌplætiˈhelminθ] *n* 扁虫,扁形动物

Platyhelminthes [ˌplætihelˈminθiːz] *n* 扁形动物门

platyhieric [ˌplætihaiˈerik] *a* 阔骶[骨]的

platyknemia [ˌplætikˈniːmiə] *n* 扁胫骨

platykurtic [ˌplætiˈkəːtik] *n* 峰态扁平,低峰态

platymeria [ˌplætiˈmiriə] *n* 扁股骨 | **platymeric** [ˌplætiˈmirik] *a*

platymorphia [ˌplætiˈmɔːfiə] *n* 扁型眼,浅型眼 | **platymorphic** [ˌplætiˈmɔːfik] *a*

platymyarial [ˌplætimaiˈɛəriəl], **platymyarian** [ˌplætimaiˈɛəriən] *a* 扁肌型的

platymyoid [ˌplætiˈmaiɔid] *a* 扁肌样的

Platynosomum [ˌplætinəuˈsəuməm] *n* 平体[吸虫]属,扁体[吸虫]属

platyopia [ˌplætiˈəupiə] *n* 阔面 | **platyopic** [ˌplætiˈɔpik] *a*

platypellic [ˌplætiˈpelik], **platypelloid** [ˌplætiˈpelɔid] *a* 阔骨盆的,扁平的
platyphylline [ˌplætiˈfilin] *n* 阔叶千里光碱,狗舌草碱
platypnea [pləˈtipniːə] *n* 平卧呼吸(端坐时所致的呼吸困难在平卧时得以缓解)
platypodia [ˌplætiˈpəudiə] *n* 扁平足
Platyrrhina [ˌplætiˈrainə] *n* 阔鼻科
platyrrhine [ˈplætirain] *a* 阔鼻的
platysma [pləˈtizmə] *n*【希】[颈]阔肌 | ~l *a*
platyspondylisis [ˌplætispɔnˈdilisis], **platyspondylia** [ˌplætispɔnˈdiliə] *n* 扁椎骨
Platysporina [ˌplætispəˈrainə] *n* 扁孢子亚目
platystaphyline [ˌplætisˈtæfilain] *a* 阔腭的
platystencephaly [ˌplætistenˈsefəli], **platystencephalia** [ˌplætiˌstensiˈfeiliə], **platystencephalism** [ˌplætiˌstenˈsefəlizəm] *n* 扁长头 | **platystencephalic** [ˌplætistensəˈfælik] *a*
platytrope [ˈplætitrəup] *n* 对侧部,两侧对称部
plauracin [ˈplɔːrəsin] *n* 普劳拉星(抗生素类药,兽用生长刺激剂)
Plaut's angina(ulcer) [plaut] (Hugo C. Plaut) 坏死性溃疡性龈口炎,坏死性溃疡性龈炎
Playfair's treatment [ˈpleifɛə] (William S. Playfair)普莱费尔疗法(休息与进食疗法)
Plectomycetes [ˌplektəumaiˈsiːtiːz] *n* 不整子囊菌纲,锤形菌纲
plectron [ˈplektrɔn] *n* 锤型(某些杆菌在孢子形成期所呈现的形式)
plectrum [ˈplektrəm] *n* 悬雍垂;锤骨;颞骨茎突
PLED periodic lateralized epileptiform discharge 周期性一侧性癫痫样放电
pledge [pledʒ] *n* 誓言,保证 *vt* 保证 | Nightingale ~ 南丁格尔誓言(护理专业的道德准则誓言)
pledget [ˈpledʒit] *n* 小拭子
plegaphonia [ˌplegəˈfəuniə] *n* 叩喉听诊法
-plegia [构词成分]麻痹,瘫痪
pleiades [ˈplaiədiːz] *n* 淋巴结肿块
pleio- 见 pleo-
pleiochloruria [ˌplaiəukləˈrjuəriə] *n* 尿氯过多
pleionexia [ˌplaiəˈneksiə] *n* 贪婪癖;贪氧性
pleiotropy [plaiˈɔtrəpi], **pleiotropia** [ˌplaiəˈtrəupiə], **pleiotropism** [plaiˈɔtrəpizəm] *n* 多向性(亲多种组织);多效性(单一基因制约多种性状的作用) | **pleiotropic** [ˌplaiəˈtrɔpik] *a*
Pleistophora [plaisˈtɔːfərə] *n* 泛成孢子虫属
plektron [ˈplektrɔn] *n*【希】锤型(见 plectron)
pleniloquence [pliˈniləkwəns] *n* 多言症,多言癖
pleo- [构词成分]过多,增多,多
pleochroism [ˌpli(ː)ˈɔkrəizəm], **pleochromatism** [ˌpli(ː)əˈkrəumətizəm] *n* 多色[现象],多向色性 | **pleochroic** [ˌpli(ː)əˈkrəuik], **pleochromatic** [ˌpli(ː)əkrəuˈmætik] *a*
pleocytosis [ˌpli(ː)əsaiˈtəusis] *n* 脑脊液[淋巴]细胞增多
pleokaryocyte, pleocaryocyte [ˌpli(ː)əˈkæriəsait] *n* 多核细胞
pleomastia [ˌpli(ː)əˈmæstiə], **pleomazia** [ˌpli(ː)əˈmeiziə] *n* 多乳房[畸形] | **pleomastic** *a*
pleomorphism [pli(ː)əˈmɔːfizəm] *n* 多形性 | **pleomorphic, pleomorphous** *a* 多形的
pleonasm [ˈpli(ː)ənæzəm] *n* 赘余畸形
pleonectic [ˌpli(ː)əˈnektik] *a* 贪氧的,多氧的(指血液的含氧量超过正常)
pleonexia [ˌpli(ː)əˈneksiə], **pleonexy** [ˌpli(ː)əˈneksi] *n* 贪婪癖;贪氧性
pleonosteosis [ˌpli(ː)əˌnɔstiˈəusis] *n* 骨化过早,骨化过度
pleonotia [pli(ː)əˈnəuʃiə] *n* 多耳[畸形]
pleoptics [pliˈɔptiks] *n* 增视疗法
plerocercoid [ˌplirəˈsəːkɔid] *n* 全尾蚴,裂头蚴
plerosis [pliˈrəusis] *n* 补复,修复(如病后补复失去的组织)
Plesch's percussion [ˈpleiʃ] (Johann Plesch) *n* 普累施叩诊,铅笔叩诊,肋间叩诊(叩打肋间部,避免肋骨振动,用作叩诊板的手指第一指间关节屈成直角) | ~ test 普累施试验(检未闭动脉导管)
Plesiomonas [ˌpliːsiəˈməunəs] *n* 毗邻单胞菌属
plesiomorphism [ˌpliːsiəˈmɔːfizəm] *n* 形态相似 | **plesiomorphous** *a*
plessesthesia [ˌplesisˈθiːzjə] *n* 触叩诊
plessigraph [ˈplesigrɑːf] *n* 划界叩诊板
plessimeter [pleˈsimitə] *n* 叩诊板;皮像板,透皮玻片 | **plessimetric** [ˌplesiˈmetrik] *a*
plessor [ˈplesə] *n* 叩诊槌
plethora [ˈpleθərə] *n* 多血质;多血[症] | **plethoric** [pliˈθɔrik] *a* / **plethorically** *ad*
plethysmogram [pliˈθizməgræm] *n* 体积描记图
plethysmograph [pliˈθizməgrɑːf] *n* 体积描记器 | ~**ic** [pliˌθizməˈgræfik] *a* / ~**y** [ˌpliθizˈmɔgrəfi] *n* 体积描记法
pleura [ˈpluərə] ([复] **pleurae** [ˈpluəriː]) *n* 胸膜 | cervical ~ 胸膜顶 / costal ~ 肋胸膜,肋椎部(胸膜) / diaphragmatic ~ 膈胸膜,膈部(胸膜) / mediastinal ~ 纵隔胸膜,纵隔部(胸膜) / parietal ~ 胸膜壁层 / pulmonary ~, visceral ~ 肺胸膜,胸膜脏层 | ~**l** *a*
pleuracentesis [ˌpluərəsenˈtiːsis] *n* 胸腔穿刺术
pleuracotomy [ˌpluərəˈkɔtəmi] *n* 胸膜切开术,胸膜腔切开术
pleuralgia [pluəˈrældʒiə] *n* 胸膜痛 | **pleuralgic** [pluəˈrældʒik] *a*
pleuramnion [pluəˈræmniɔn] *n* 体壁羊膜

pleurapophysis [ˌpluərəˈpɔfisis] *n* 椎骨侧突,椎肋(颈椎或腰椎)
pleurectomy [pluəˈrektəmi] *n* 胸膜切除术
pleurisy [ˈpluərisi] *n* 胸膜炎 | adhesive ~, dry ~ 粘连性胸膜炎,干性胸膜炎 / blocked ~ 阻断性胸膜炎 / encysted ~ 包裹性胸膜炎 / exudative ~, wet ~, ~ with effusion 渗出性胸膜炎,湿性胸膜炎 / plastic ~ 成形性胸膜炎 / pulmonary ~, visceral ~ 肺胸膜炎,胸膜脏层炎 | **pleuritis** [pluəˈraitis] *n* | **pleuritic** [pluəˈritik] *a*
pleuritogenous [ˌpluəriˈtɔdʒinəs] *a* 致胸膜炎的
pleur(o)- [构词成分]胸膜
pleurobronchitis [ˌpluərəubrɔŋˈkaitis] *n* 胸膜支气管炎
pleurocele [ˈpluərəsiːl] *n* 胸膜突出,胸膜疝
pleurocentesis [ˌpluərəusenˈtiːsis] *n* 胸腔穿刺术
pleurocentrum [ˌpluərəuˈsentrəm] *n* 单侧椎[骨]体,半侧椎[骨]体
Pleuroceridae [ˌpluərəuˈseridiː] *n* 肋角螺科
pleurocholecystitis [ˌpluərəuˌkəulisisˈtaitis] *n* 胸膜胆囊炎
pleuroclysis [pluəˈrɔklisis] *n* 胸膜腔灌洗术
pleurocutaneous [ˌpluərəukjuˈteinjəs] *a* 胸膜皮肤的
pleurodesis [ˌpluəˈrɔdisis] *n* 胸膜固定术
pleurodont [ˈpluərədɔnt] *n* 连骨牙
pleurodynia [ˌpluərəˈdiniə] *n* 胸膜痛;肋肌痛 | epidemic ~ 流行性胸痛
pleuroesophageal [ˌpluərəuiːˌsɔfəˈdʒiəl] *a* 胸膜食管的
pleuroesophageus [ˌpluərəuiːsəuˈfeidʒiəs] *a* 【拉】胸膜食管的
pleurogenous [pluəˈrɔdʒinəs], **pleurogenic** [ˌpluərəˈdʒenik] *a* 胸膜原[性]的
pleurography [pluəˈrɔgrəfi] *n* 胸膜腔 X 线摄影[术]
pleurohepatitis [ˌpluərəuˌhepəˈtaitis] *n* 胸膜肝炎
pleurolith [ˈpluərəliθ] *n* 胸膜石
pleurolysis [pluəˈrɔlisis] *n* 胸膜松解术
pleuromelus [ˌpluərəˈmiːləs] *n* 胸部多肢畸胎
Pleuromonas [ˌpluərəˈməunəs] *n* 侧滴毛虫属
pleuron [ˈpluərɔn] ([复] **pleura** [ˈpluərə]) *n* 侧板(昆虫)
Pleuronematina [ˌpluərəuˌniːməˈtainə] *n* 口帆亚目
pleuroparietopexy [ˌpluərəupəˈraiətəˌpeksi] *n* 胸膜胸壁固定术
pleuropericardial [ˌpluərəuˌperiˈkɑːdiəl] *a* 胸膜心包的
pleuropericarditis [ˌpluərəuˌperikɑːˈdaitis] *n* 胸膜心包炎
pleuroperitoneal [ˌpluərəuˌperitəuˈniːəl] *a* 胸膜腹膜的
pleuropneumonia [ˌpluərəunju(ː)ˈməunjə] *n* 胸膜肺炎
pleuropneumonia-like [ˌpluərəunju(ː)ˈməunjəˌlaik] *a* 类胸膜肺炎的(指一种滤过性微生物)
pleuropneumonolysis [ˌpluərəuˌnjuːməˈnɔlisis] *n* 胸膜肺松解术
pleuropulmonary [ˌpluərəuˈpʌlmənəri] *a* 胸膜肺的
pleurorrhea [ˌpluərəˈriːə] *n* 胸膜腔渗液
pleuroscopy [pluəˈrɔskəpi] *n* 胸膜腔镜检查
pleurosomus [ˌpluərəˈsəuməs], **pleurosoma** [ˌpluərəˈsəumə] *n* 体侧露脏畸胎(肠突出及一侧上肢发育不全)
Pleurostomatida [ˌpluərəustəˈmætidə] *n* 侧口目
pleurothotonos [ˌpluərəˈθɔtənɔs], **pleurothotonus** [ˌpluərəˈθɔtənəs] *n* 侧弓反张
pleurotin [pluəˈrəutin] *n* 灰侧耳菌素(对疖的葡萄球菌和结核杆菌有效)
pleurotome [ˈpluərətəum] *n* 肺节(由一脊神经后根的传入纤维分布的肺区)
pleurotomy [pluəˈrɔtəmi] *n* 胸膜切开术
pleurotyphoid [ˌpluərəˈtaifɔid] *n* 胸膜型伤寒(急性胸膜炎并发伤寒)
pleurovisceral [ˌpluərəˈvisərəl] *a* 胸膜内脏的
plexal [ˈpleksəl] *a* (血管、淋巴、神经等)丛的
plexectomy [plekˈsektəmi] *n* 丛切除术
plexiform [ˈpleksifɔːm] *a* 丛状的
pleximeter [plekˈsimitə], **plexometer** [plekˈsɔmitə] *n* 叩诊板;皮像板,透皮玻片 | **pleximetric** [ˌpleksiˈmetrik] *a* | **pleximetry** [plekˈsimitri] *n* 板叩诊[法];皮像板检查
plexitis [plekˈsaitis] *n* 神经丛炎
plexogenic [ˈpleksəˌdʒenik] *a* 丛原的
plexopathy [plekˈsɔpəθi] *n* 丛病 | lumbar ~ 腰丛病
plexor [ˈpleksə] *n* 叩诊槌
plexus [ˈpleksəs] ([复] **plexus** 或 **plexuses**) *n* (血管、淋巴、神经等)丛 | cardiac ~ 心丛 / carotid ~ 颈内动脉丛 / celiac ~ 腹腔丛;腹腔淋巴丛 / choroid ~ of third ventricle 第三脑室脉络丛 / common carotid ~ 颈总动脉丛 / crural ~ 股丛 / deferential ~ 输精管丛 / epigastric ~, solar ~ 腹腔丛 / hemorrhoidal ~ 直肠丛 / hypogastric ~ 腹下丛 / inferior choroid ~ 第四脑室脉络丛 / lateral ~ 侧脑室脉络丛 / spermatic ~ 精索丛 / vidian ~ 翼管神经丛
-plexy [构词成分]发作,中风
plica [ˈplaikə] ([复] **plicae** [ˈplaisiː]) *n* 【拉】[皱]襞,褶

plicadentin [ˌplaikəˈdentin] *n* 放射状牙质
plicamycin [ˌplaikəˈmaisin] *n* 普卡霉素(抗肿瘤抗生素,以前称 mithramycin)
plicate [ˈplaikit], **plicated** [ˈplaikeitid] *a* 有襞的,折襞的,具褶的
plicatic acid [pliˈkætik] 大侧柏酸
plication [plaiˈkeiʃən] *n* 折襞,折叠术
plicotomy [plaiˈkɔtəmi] *n* (鼓膜)襞切断术
pli courbe [pliː kuːb]【法】角回(即 gyrus angularis)
pliers [ˈplaiəz] *n* 钳子,镊
Plimmer's bodies [ˈplimə] (Henry G. Plimmer) 普林默小体(癌细胞内小包涵体) | ~ salt 酒石酸锑钠
plinth [plinθ], **plint** [plint] *n* 操练椅
-ploid [构词成分]倍体
ploidy [ˈplɔidi] *n* 倍性
plombage [plɔmˈbɑːʒ] *n*【法】充填术(用甲基丙烯酸甲酯球充填一部分胸部,作为人工气胸时注射空气的代用品)
plombierung [plɔmˈbiːruŋ] *n*【德】充填术(如患骨髓炎时,用碘仿制剂充填骨缺损部)
plop [plɔp] *n* 扑落音 | tumor ~ 肿瘤扑落音(心脏舒张早期发出的声音,由一个带蒂房性瘤的运动引起,但极易与开放性锐声或第三心音相混淆)
plosive [ˈpləusiv] *n*, *a* 爆破音(的)
plot [plɔt] *vt* 标绘;制图,作图 *n* 图,图表
plotolysin [ˌpləutəˈlaisin] *n* 鲇毒溶血素
plotospasmin [ˌpləutəˈspæzmin] *n* 鲇毒痉挛素
Plotosus [pləuˈtəusəs] *n* 鳗尾鲇属
plototoxin [ˌpləutəˈtɔksin] *n* 鲇毒,鲇毒质
PLP proteolipid protein 蛋白脂质蛋白
PLT primed lymphocyte typing 致敏淋巴细胞定型; *p*sittacosis-*l*ymphogranuloma venereum-*t*rachoma (group of organisms) 鹦鹉热-性病性淋巴肉芽肿-沙眼(菌群)
plug [plʌg] *n* 塞,栓;充填剂,填料 | ear ~ 耳塞 / epithelial ~ 上皮栓 / mucous ~ 宫颈黏液塞 / vaginal ~, copulation ~ 阴道塞 / yolk ~ 卵黄栓
plugger [ˈplʌgə] *n* (牙科用的)充填器 | amalgam ~ 汞合金充填器 / backaction ~, reverse ~ 回力充填器 / foot ~ 足形充填器
Plugge's test [ˈplugə] (Pieter C. Plugge) 普拉吉试验(检酚)
plumage [ˈpluːmidʒ] *n* 羽
plumbage [plumˈbɑːʒ] *n* 充填术
plumbagin [plʌmˈbeidʒin] *n* 白花丹素,蓝茉莉素,5-羟基维生素 K_3
plumbago [plʌmˈbeigəu] *n* 石墨 | **plumbaginous** [plʌmˈbædʒinəs] *a*
plumbeous [ˈplʌmbiəs] *a* [似]铅的;含铅的
plumbic [ˈplʌmbik] *a* 铅的,四价铅的
plumbiferous [plʌmˈbifərəs] *a* 含铅的,产铅的
plumbism [ˈplʌmbizəm] *n* 铅中毒
plumbotherapy [ˌplʌmbəuˈθerəpi] *n* 铅疗法
plumbous [ˈplʌmbəs] *a* 亚铅的,二价铅的
plumbum [ˈplʌmbəm] *n*【拉】铅(化学元素)
plume [pluːm] *n* 羽毛,羽状物
plumelet [ˈpluːmlit] *n* 小羽毛
plumericin [ˌpluməˈraisin] *n* 鸡蛋花素(有灭菌作用)
Plummer's disease [ˈplʌmə] (Henry S. Plummer) *n* 普卢默病(单纯性甲状腺腺瘤毒性形成,成为甲状腺功能亢进) | ~ sign 普卢默征(突眼性甲状腺肿时不能踏上椅子或上阶梯)
Plummer-Vinson syndrome [ˈplʌmə ˈvinsn] (Henry S. Plummer; Porter P. Vinson) 普卢默-文森综合征(吞咽困难,伴舌炎、低血色素性贫血、脾肿大及口、咽和食管上端萎缩。亦称缺铁性吞咽困难)
plumose [ˈpluːməus] *a* 有羽毛的,羽毛状的
plumula [ˈplʌmjulə] *n* 胚芽;细沟(中脑水管上壁)
plumy [ˈpluːmi] *a* 绒毛[状]的,有羽毛的
pluri- [构词成分]多数,多
pluriceptor [ˌpluəriˈseptə] *n* 多簇受体
pluricytopenia [ˌpluəriˌsaitəuˈpiːniə] *n* 多种血细胞减少(再生障碍性贫血)
pluridyscrinia [ˌpluəridisˈkriniə] *n* 多种分泌障碍
pluriglandular [ˌpluəriˈglændjulə] *a* 多腺性的
plurigravida [ˌpluəriˈgrævidə] *n* 经产孕妇
plurilocular [ˌpluəriˈlɔkjulə] *a* 多腔的,多房的
plurimenorrhea [ˌpluəriˌmenəˈriːə] *n* 多次行经
plurinatality [ˌpluərineiˈtæləti] *n* 高产率
plurinuclear [ˌpluəriˈnjuːkliə] *a* 多核的
pluriorificial [pluəriˌɔːriˈfiʃəl] *a* 多孔的
pluripara [pluəˈrɪpərə] *n* 经产妇(多于一次生产者)
pluriparity [ˌpluəriˈpærəti] *n* 经产,多产次
pluripolar [ˌpluəriˈpəulə] *a* 多极的
pluripotentiality [ˌpluəripəˌtenʃiˈæləti] *n* 多能性(指胚细胞发育的能力或可能的多种发育途径) | **pluripotential** [ˌpluəripəˈtenʃəl], **pluripotent** [pluəˈripətənt] *a* 多能的
pluriresistant [ˌpluəririˈzistənt] *a* 抗多种药的
pluritissular [ˌpluəriˈtisjulə] *a* 多种组织的
plurivisceral [ˌpluəriˈvisərəl] *a* 多种内脏的,多种器官的
plus [plʌs] *prep* 加,加上 *a* 正的;(菌丝体)阳性的 *n* 正号,加号
plutonium(Pu) [pluːˈtəunjəm] *n* 钚(化学元素)

Pm promethium 钷
PMB polymorphonuclear basophil leukocytes 嗜碱性多形核白细胞
PME polymorphonuclear eosinophil leukocytes 嗜酸性多形核白细胞
PMI point of maximal impulse 最强心尖搏动点
P mitrale [piː maiˈtreili] 二尖瓣 P 波型(在心电描记法中一型异常宽阔有切迹的 P 波,表明大左心房去极化延长,常与二尖瓣病有关)
PMM pentamethylmelamine 五甲蜜胺
PMMA polymethyl methacrylate 聚甲基丙烯酸甲酯
PMN polymorphonuclear 多形核的;polymorphonuclear neutrophil 多形核嗜中性粒细胞
PMR proportionate mortality ratio 比例死亡率
PMSG pregnant mare serum gonadotropin 孕马血清促性腺激素
-pnea [构词成分]呼吸
pne(o)- [构词成分]呼吸;以 pneo-起始的词,同样见以 spiro-(2)起始的词
pneogaster [ˈniːəˌgæstə] *n* 呼吸道
pneogram [ˈniːəgræm] *n* 呼吸描记图
pneograph [ˈniːəgrɑːf] *n* 呼吸描记器
pneometer [niˈɔmitə] *n* 呼吸计,呼吸[气]量计,肺量计
pneoscope [ˈniːəskəup] *n* 呼吸描记器
PNET peripheral neuroectodermal tumor 周围神经外胚层瘤;primitive neuroectodermal tumor 原始神经外胚层瘤
pneuma- 见 pneumat(o)-
pneumal [ˈnjuːməl] *a* 肺的
pneumarthrogram [nju(ː)ˈmɑːθrəgræm] *n* 关节充气造影[照]片
pneumarthrography [ˌnjumɑːˈθrɔgrəfi] *n* 关节充气造影[术]
pneumarthrosis [ˌnjuːmɑːˈθrəusis] *n* 关节积气;关节充气术
pneumascope [ˈnjuːməskəup] *n* 呼吸描记器
pneumathemia [ˌnjuːməˈθiːmiə] *n* 气血症,气栓
pneumatic [nju(ː)ˈmætik] *a* 空气的,气的;呼吸的;充气的;气动的
pneumatics [nju(ː)ˈmætiks] *n* 气体力学
pneumatinuria [ˌnjuːmətiˈnjuəriə] *n* 气尿
pneumatism [ˈnjuːmətizəm] *n* 精气论,精气学说
pneumatist [ˈnjuːmətist] *n* 精气论者
pneumatization [ˌnjuːmətaiˈzeiʃən, -tiˈz-] *n* 气腔形成(尤指在颞骨内形成)
pneumatized [ˈnjuːmətaizd] *a* 充气的,含有气腔的
pneumat(o)-, pneuma- [构词成分]气,气体;呼吸
pneumatocardia [ˌnjuːmətəuˈkɑːdiə] *n* 心[腔]积气
pneumatocele [nju(ː)ˈmætəsiːl] *n* 肺膨出;气瘤,气囊 | extracranial ~, ~ cranii 头皮下气瘤(颅骨骨折后) / intracranial ~ 颅腔积气
pneumatocephalus [ˌnjuːmətəuˈsefələs] *n* 颅腔积气
pneumatodyspnea [ˌnjuːmətəudisˈpniːə] *n* 气肿性呼吸困难
pneumatogram [nju(ː)ˈmætəgræm] *n* 呼吸描记图
pneumatograph [nju(ː)ˈmætəgrɑːf, -græf] *n* 呼吸描记器
pneumatology [ˌnjuːməˈtɔlədʒi] *n* 气体[治疗]学;气体力学
pneumatometer [ˌnjuːməˈtɔmitə] *n* 呼吸计,呼吸[气]量计 | **pneumatometry** *n* 呼吸[气]量测定[法]
pneumatophore [nju(ː)ˈmætəfɔː] *n* 气囊,浮囊;救生氧气袋,氧气囊
pneumatorrhachis [ˌnjuːməˈtɔrəkis] *n* 椎管积气
pneumatoscope [ˌnju(ː)ˈmætəskəup] *n* 口腔听诊器
pneumatosis [ˌnjuːməˈtəusis] *n* 积气[症]
pneumatotherapy [ˌnjuːmətəuˈθerəpi] *n* 气体疗法 | cerebral ~ 气脑疗法
pneumaturia [ˌnjuːməˈtjuəriə] *n* 气尿
pneumatype [ˈnjuːmətaip] *n* 呼气像(用以诊断鼻阻塞)
pneumectomy [njuːˈmektəmi] *n* 肺部分切除术
pneumencephalography [ˌnjuːmenˌsefəˈlɔgrəfi] *n* 气脑造影[术]
pneum(o)- [构词成分]肺;气;呼吸
pneumoalveolography [ˌnjuːməuˌælviəˈlɔgrəfi] *n* 肺泡 X 线摄影[术],肺泡 X 线造影[术]
pneumoamnios [ˌnjuːməuˈæmniɔs] *n* 羊水积气
pneumoangiogram [ˌnjuːməuˈændʒiəgræm] *n* 肺血管造影[照]片
pneumoangiography [ˌnjuːməuˌændʒiˈɔgrəfi] *n* 肺血管造影[术]
pneumoarthrography [ˌnjuːməuɑːˈθrɔgrəfi] *n* 关节充气造影[术]
pneumobacillus [ˌnjuːməubəˈsiləs] *n* 肺炎杆菌
pneumobilia [ˌnjuːməuˈbiliə] *n* 气性胆汁,胆道积气
pneumobulbar [ˌnjuːməuˈbʌlbə], **pneumobulbous** [ˌpjuːməuˈbʌlbəs] *a* 肺延髓的
pneumocardial [ˌnjuːməuˈkɑːdiəl] *a* 肺心的
pneumocardiograph [ˌnjuːməuˈkɑːdiəgrɑːf, -græf] *n* 肺心描记器 / **~y** [ˌnjuːməuˌkɑːdiˈɔgrəfi] *n* 肺心描记法
pneumocele [ˈnjuːməˌsiːl] *n* 肺膨出;气瘤;气囊
pneumocentesis [ˌnjuːməusenˈtiːsis] *n* 肺穿刺术

pneumocephalon [ˌnjuːməuˈsefələn], **pneumocephalus** [ˌnjuːməuˈsefələs] *n* 颅腔积气
pneumocholecystitis [ˌnjuːməuˌkəulisisˈtaitis] *n* 气肿性胆囊炎
pneumochysis [nju(ː)ˈmɔkisis] *n* 肺水肿
pneumococcemia [ˌnjuːməukɔkˈsiːmiə] *n* 肺炎球菌血症
pneumococcidal [ˌnjuːməukɔkˈsaidl] *a* 杀肺炎球菌的
pneumococcolysis [ˌnjuːməukɔˈkɔlisis] *n* 肺炎球菌溶解
pneumococcosis [ˌnjuːməukɔˈkəusis] *n* 肺炎球菌病
pneumococcosuria [ˌnjuːməuˌkɔkəˈsjuəriə] *n* 肺炎球菌尿
pneumococcus [ˌnjuːməˈkɔkəs] ([复] **pneumococci** [ˌnjuːməˈkɔk(s)ai]) *n* 肺炎球菌 | **pneumococcal** [ˌnjuːməˈkɔkəl], **pneumococcic** [ˌnjuːməˈkɔksik] *a*
pneumocolon [ˌnjuːməˈkəulən] *n* 气结肠,结肠积气
pneumoconiosis [ˌnjuːməuˌkɔniˈəusis] *n* 肺尘埃沉着病 | talc ~ 肺滑石沉着病,滑石肺
pneumocrania [ˌnjuːməˈkreinjə], **pneumocranium** [ˌnjuːməˈkreinjəm] *n* 颅腔积气
pneumocystiasis [ˌnjuːməusisˈtaiəsis] *n* 肺囊虫病,间质性浆细胞性肺炎
pneumocystic [ˌnjuːməˈsistik] *a* 肺囊虫的,肺囊虫所致的
Pneumocystis [ˌnjuːməˈsistis] *n* 肺囊虫属 | ~ carinii 卡氏肺囊虫
pneumocystis [ˌpjuːməuˈsistis] *n* 肺囊虫,肺孢子虫
pneumocystography [ˌnjuːməusisˈtɔgrəfi] *n* 膀胱充气造影[术]
pneumocystosis [ˌnjuːməusisˈtəusis] *n* 肺孢子虫病(间质性浆细胞性肺炎)
pneumocystotomography [ˌnjuːməuˌsistəutəˈmɔgrəfi] *n* 膀胱充气体层摄影[术]
pneumocyte [ˈnjuːməsait] *n* 肺细胞
pneumoderma [ˌnjuːməuˈdəːmə] *n* 皮下气肿
pneumodograph [nju(ː)ˈmɔdəgrɑːf] *n* (鼻)呼吸气量描记器
pneumodynamics [ˌnjuːməudaiˈnæmiks] *n* 呼吸动力学
pneumoempyema [ˌnjuːməuˌempaiˈiːmə] *n* 气脓胸
pneumoencephalitis [ˌpjuːməuenˌsefəˈlaitis] *n* 肺脑炎,纽卡斯尔(Newcastle)病,新城疫 | avian ~ 禽肺脑炎,纽卡斯尔病,新城疫
pneumoencephalocele [ˌnjuːməuenˈsefələsiːl] *n* 颅腔积气
pneumoencephalography (**PEG**) [ˌnjuːməu-enˌsefəˈlɔgrəfi] *n* 气脑造影[术]
pneumoencephalomyelogram [ˌnjuːməuenˌsefələumaiˈeləgræm] *n* 气脑脊髓造影[照]片
pneumoencephalomyelography [ˌnjuːməuen-ˌsefələuˌmaiəˌlɔgrəfi] *n* 气脑脊髓造影[术]
pneumoencephalos [ˌnjuːməuenˈsefəlɔs] *n* 脑积气,气脑
pneumoenteritis [ˌnjuːməuˌentəˈraitis] *n* 肺肠炎
pneumofasciogram [ˌnjuːməuˈfæsiəgræm] *n* 筋膜间隙充气造影[照]片
pneumogalactocele [ˌnjuːməugəˈlæktəsiːl] *n* 气乳瘤
pneumogastric [ˌnjuːməˈgæstrik] *a* 肺胃的
pneumogastrography [ˌnjuːməugæsˈtrɔgrəfi] *n* 胃充气造影[术]
pneumogastroscopy [ˌnjuːməugæsˈtrɔskəpi] *n* 充气胃镜检查
pneumogram [ˈnjuːməgræm] *n* 呼吸描记图;充气[照]片
pneumograph [ˈnjuːməgrɑːf, -græf] *n* 呼吸描记器
pneumography [nju(ː)ˈmɔgrəfi] *n* 肺解剖学;呼吸描记法;注气造影[术] | cerebral ~ 脑室注气造影[术] / retroperitoneal ~ 腹膜后注气造影[术]
pneumogynogram [ˌnjuːməuˈgainəgræm] *n* 女生殖器充气 X 线[照]片
pneumohemia [ˌnjuːməˈhiːmiə] *n* 气血症,气栓
pneumohemopericardium [ˌnjuːməuˌhiːməuˌp-eriˈkɑːdiəm] *n* 气血心包,心包积气血
pneumohemothorax [ˌnjuːməuˌhiːməˈθɔːræks] *n* 气血胸
pneumohydrometra [ˌnjuːməuˌhaidrəˈmiːtrə] *n* 子宫积气水
pneumohydropericardium [ˌnjuːməuˌhaidrəuˌp-eriˈkɑːdiəm] *n* 气水心包,心包积气水
pneumohydrothorax [ˌnjuːməuˌhaidrəˈθɔːræks] *n* 气水胸
pneumokidney [ˈnjuːməˌkidni] *n* 肾盂充气造影术
pneumokoniosis [ˌnjuːməuˌkɔniˈəusis] *n* 肺尘埃沉着病
pneumolith [ˈnjuːməliθ] *n* 肺石
pneumolithiasis [ˌnjuːməuliˈθaiəsis] *n* 肺石病
pneumology [nju(ː)ˈmɔlədʒi] *n* 肺病学
pneumolysis [nju(ː)ˈmɔlisis] *n* 肺松解术
pneumomalacia [ˌnjuːməuməˈleiʃiə] *n* 肺软化
pneumomassage [ˌnjuːməuməˈsɑːʒ] *n* (鼓膜)空气按摩法
pneumomediastinogram [ˌnjuːməuˌmiːdiæsˈtai-nəgræm] *n* 纵隔充气造影[照]片
pneumomediastinography [ˌnjuːməuˌmiːdiˌæsti-

ˈnɔgrəfi] *n* 纵隔充气造影[术]

pneumomediastinum [ˌnjuːməuˌmiːdiæsˈtainəm] *n* 纵隔积气

pneumomelanosis [ˌnjuːməuˌmeləˈnəusis] *n* 肺黑变病

pneumometer [nju(ː)ˈmɔmitə] *n* 呼吸计,呼吸[气]量计

pneumomycosis [ˌnjuːməumaiˈkəusis] *n* 肺真菌病,肺霉菌病

pneumomyelography [ˌnjuːməuˌmaiəˈlɔgrəfi] *n* 气脊髓造影[术]

pneumonectasis [ˌnjuːməˈnektəsis], **pneumonectasia** [ˌnjuːməunekˈteiziə] *n* 肺气肿

pneumonectomy [ˌnjuːməˈnektəmi] *n* 全肺切除术

pneumonedema [ˌnjuːməuni(ː)ˈdiːmə] *n* 肺水肿

pneumonemia [ˌnjuːməˈniːmiə] *n* 肺充血

pneumonere [ˈnjuːməniə] *n* 肺终芽

pneumonia [nju(ː)ˈməunjə] *n* 肺炎 | apex ~, apical ~ 肺尖炎,肺尖部肺炎 / aspiration ~ 吸入性肺炎 / atypical ~ 非典型肺炎 / caseous ~, cheesy ~ 干酪样肺炎 / central ~, core ~ 中央肺炎 / cerebral ~ 脑型肺炎 / croupous ~ 格鲁布性肺炎 / dermal ~ 皮内注射性肺炎(向家兔皮肤内注射肺炎双球菌引起的肺炎) / desquamative ~, parenchymatous ~ 脱屑性肺炎,实质性肺炎 / double ~ 双侧肺炎 / giant cell ~ 巨细胞性肺炎 / hypostatic ~ 坠积性肺炎 / lipid ~, lipoid ~, oil-aspiration ~ 脂质性肺炎,油吸入性肺炎 / lobar ~ 大叶性肺炎 / lobular ~ 小叶[性]肺炎,支气管肺炎 / plague ~ 鼠疫性肺炎,肺鼠疫 / pneumocystis ~, Pneumocystis carinii ~ 肺囊虫性肺炎,肺孢子虫病,间质性浆细胞性肺炎 / transplantation ~ 移植肺炎 / woolsorter's ~ 毛工肺炎,炭疽性肺炎 | **pneumonic** [nju(ː)ˈmɔnik] *a* 肺的;肺炎的

pneumonitis [ˌnjuːməuˈnaitis] *n* 肺炎,局限性肺炎 | aspiration ~ 吸入性肺炎 / feline ~ 猫肺炎 / mouse ~ 鼠肺炎 / pneumocystis ~ 肺囊虫性肺炎,间质性浆细胞性肺炎

pneumon(o)- [构词成分]肺

pneumonocele [nju(ː)ˈmɔnəsiːl] *n* 肺膨出;气瘤;气囊

pneumonocentesis [nju(ː)ˌməunəusenˈtiːsis] *n* 肺穿刺术

pneumonocirrhosis [nju(ː)ˌməunəusiˈrəusis] *n* 肺硬变

pneumonococcus [ˌnjuːmənəuˈkɔkəs] *n* 肺炎[双]球菌

pneumonoconiosis, pneumonokoniosis [nju(ː)-ˌməunəukəniˈəusis] *n* 肺尘埃沉着病

pneumonocyte [nju(ː)ˈmɔnəsait] *n* 肺细胞

pneumonoenteritis [nju(ː)ˌməunəuˌentəˈraitis] *n* 肺肠炎

pneumonograph [nju(ː)ˈmɔnəgrɑːf] *n* 肺X线[照]片 / **~y** [ˌnjuːməˈnɔgrəfi] *n* 肺X线造影[术]

pneumonolipoidosis [nju(ː)ˌməunəuˌlipɔiˈdəusis] *n* 脂质性肺炎

pneumonolysis [ˌnjuːməˈnɔlisis] *n* 肺松解术 | extrapleural ~ 胸膜外肺松解术 / intrapleural ~ 胸膜内肺松解术

pneumonomelanosis [nju(ː)ˌməunəumeləˈnəusis] *n* 肺黑变病

pneumonometer [ˌnjuːməˈnɔmitə] *n* 呼吸计,呼吸[气]量计(一种肺量计)

pneumonomoniliasis [nju(ː)ˌməunəuˌməuniˈlaiəsis] *n* 肺念珠菌病

pneumonomycosis [nju(ː)ˌməunəumaiˈkəusis] *n* 肺真菌病,肺霉菌病

pneumonopaludism [nju(ː)ˌməunəˈpæljudizəm] *n* 肺型疟疾,疟性肺炎硬变

pneumonopathy [ˌnjuːməˈnɔpəθi] *n* 肺病 | eosinophilic ~ 嗜酸细胞性肺病

pneumonopexy [nju(ː)ˈməunəˌpeksi] *n* 肺固定术

pneumonophthisis [ˌnjuːmənɔfˈθaisis] *n* 肺结核

pneumonopleuritis [nju(ː)ˌməunəupluəˈraitis] *n* 肺胸膜炎

pneumonoresection [nju(ː)ˌməunəuriːˈsekʃən] *n* 肺部分切除术

pneumonorrhagia [nju(ː)ˌməunəˈreidʒiə] *n* 肺出血

pneumonorrhaphy [ˌnjuːməˈnɔrəfi] *n* 肺缝合术

pneumonosis [ˌnjuːməˈnəusis] *n* 肺病

pneumonotherapy [nju(ː)ˌməunəuˈθerəpi] *n* 肺病疗法

pneumonotomy [ˌnjuːməˈnɔtəmi] *n* 肺切开术

Pneumonyssoides [ˌnjuːməuniˈsɔidiːz] *n* 类肺刺螨属

Pneumonyssus [ˌnjuːməˈnisəs] *n* 肺刺螨属

pneumopaludism [ˌnjuːməˈpæljudizəm] *n* 肺型疟疾,疟性肺尖硬变

pneumoparotitis [ˌnjuːməuˌpærəuˈtaitis] *n* 呼吸性腮腺炎

pneumopathy [nju(ː)ˈmɔpəθi] *n* 肺病

pneumopericardium [ˌnjuːməuˌperiˈkɑːdiəm] *n* 心包积气

pneumoperitoneum [ˌnjuːməuˌperitəuˈniːəm] *n* 气腹 | **pneumoperitoneal** [ˌnjuːməuˌperitəuˈniːəl] *a*

pneumoperitonitis [ˌnjuːməuˌperitəuˈnaitis] *n* 气性腹膜炎

pneumopexy [ˈnjuːməˌpeksi] *n* 肺固定术

pneumophagia [ˌnjuːmə'feidʒiə] *n* 吞气症
pneumophone ['njuːməfəun] *n* 中耳压力计
pneumophonia [ˌnjuːmə'fəuniə] *n* 肺性发声(表现为呼吸声的发声困难)
pneumoplasty ['njuːməuˌplæsti] *n* 肺整复术
pneumopleuritis [ˌnjuːməupluə'raitis] *n* 肺胸膜炎
pneumopleuroparietopexy [ˌnjuːməuˌpluərəupə'raiətəˌpeksi] *n* 肺胸膜壁层固定术
pneumoprecordium [ˌnjuːməupriː'kɔːdjəm] *n* 心前间隙积气
pneumopreperitoneum [ˌnjuːməupriːˌperitəu'niːəm] *n* 腹膜前腔积气;腹膜前腔充气术
pneumopyelography [ˌnjuːməuˌpaii'lɔgrəfi] *n* 肾盂充气造影[术]
pneumopyopericardium [ˌnjuːməuˌpaiəˌperi'kɑːdiəm] *n* 气脓心包,心包积脓气
pneumopyothorax [ˌnjuːməuˌpaiə'θɔːræks] *n* 气脓胸
pneumorachicentesis [ˌnjuːməuˌreikisen'tiːsis] *n* 椎管穿刺注气法
pneumorachis [ˌnjuːməu'reikis] *n* 脊髓积气,椎管注气法(一种 X 线检查法)
pneumoradiography [ˌnjuːməuˌreidi'ɔgrəfi] *n* X 线充气造影[术]
pneumoresection [ˌnjuːməuriː'sekʃən] *n* 肺部分切除术
pneumoretroperitoneum [ˌnjuːməuˌretrəuˌperitəu'niːəm] *n* 腹膜后腔积气,腹膜后气肿
pneumoroentgenogram [ˌnjuːməurɔnt'genəgræm] *n* X 线充气造影[照]片
pneumoroentgenography [ˌnjuːməuˌrɔntge'nɔgrəfi] *n* X 线充气造影[术]
pneumorrhagia [ˌnjuːmə'reidʒiə] *n* 肺出血
pneumoscrotum [ˌpjuːməu'skrəutəm] *n* 阴囊积气
pneumosepticemia [ˌnjuːməuˌsepti'siːmiə] *n* 肺炎败血症
pneumoserosa [ˌnjuːməusi'rəusə] *n* 关节腔充气[透视]法
pneumoserothorax [ˌnjuːməuˌsiərə'θɔːræks] *n* 浆液气胸
pneumosilicosis [ˌnjuːməuˌsili'kəusis] *n* 硅肺
pneumosinus dilatans [ˌnjuːməu'sainəs dai'leitəns] 蝶窦异常扩张
pneumotachometer [ˌnjuːməutæ'kɔmitə] *n* 呼吸速度测定器
pneumotachygraph [ˌnjuːməu'tækigrɑːf], **pneumotachograph** [ˌnjuːməu'tækəgrɑːf] *n* 呼吸速率计
pneumotaxic [ˌnjuːmə'tæksik] *a* 调节呼吸的
pneumotherapy [ˌnjuːməu'θerəpi] *n* 气体疗法;肺病治疗
pneumothermomassage [ˌnjuːməuˌθəːməumə'sɑːʒ] *n* 压缩热气按摩法
pneumothorax [ˌnjuːməu'θɔːræks] *n* 气胸 | artificial ~, induced ~, therapeutic ~ 人工气胸[术] / clicking ~ 卡嗒音气胸(每次心搏动时,患者感到有卡嗒音) / closed ~ 闭合性气胸 / diagnostic ~ 诊断性气胸 / open ~ 开放性气胸 / tension ~, pressure ~ 张力性气胸
pneumotomography [ˌnjuːməutə'mɔgrəfi] *n* X 线充气体层摄影[术]
pneumotomy [nju(ː)'mɔtəmi] *n* 肺切开术
pneumotropism [nju(ː)'mɔtrəpizəm] *n* 亲肺性 | **pneumotropic** [ˌnjuːmə'trɔpik] *a* 亲肺的;亲肺炎球菌的
pneumotympanum [ˌnjuːməu'timpənəm] *n* 鼓室积气
pneumotyphoid [ˌnjuːməu'taifɔid] *n* 肺型伤寒
pneumotyphus [ˌnjuːməu'taifəs] *n* 肺炎伤寒(肺炎与伤寒并发)
pneumouria [ˌnjuːməu'juəriə] *n* 气尿
pneumoventriculi [ˌnjuːməuven'trikjulai], **pneumoventricle** [ˌnjuːməu'ventrik] *n* 脑室积气
pneumoventriculography [ˌnjuːməuvenˌtrikju'lɔgrəfi] *n* 脑室充气造影[术]
Pneumovirinae [ˌnjuːməuvi'rainiː] *n* 肺病毒亚科
Pneumovirus ['njuːməuˌvaiərəs] *n* 肺病毒属
pneusis ['njuːsis] *n* 【希】呼吸
PNH paroxysmal nocturnal hemoglobinuria 阵发性睡眠性血红蛋白尿症
PO per os 【拉】经口
Po_2 氧分压(oxygen partial pressure or tension)的符号,也可写成 pO_2, pO_2
Po polonium 钋
POA pancreatic oncofetal antigen 胰癌胚抗原
Poa ['pəuə] *n* 早熟禾属
Pocill. pocillum 【拉】小杯
pock [pɔk] *n* 痘疱
pocket ['pɔkit] *n* 袋,囊 | gingival ~, supragingival ~ 龈袋 / infra-bony ~, intra-alveolar ~, intrabony ~, subcrestal ~ 骨下袋,骨内袋
pockety ['pɔkiti] *a* 囊形的,有囊状特征的
pockmark ['pɔkmɑːk] *n* 痘痕
Pocul. poculum 【拉】杯
poculum ['pɔkjuləm] *n* 【拉】杯
pod- 见 podo-
podagra [pəu'dægrə] *n* 足痛风 | **~l**, **podagric**, **podagrous** ['pɔdəgrəs] *a*
podalgia [pəu'dældʒiə] *n* 足痛(如由痛风或风湿病所致)
podalic [pəu'dælik] *a* 足的,脚的
Podangium [pəu'dændʒiəm] *n* 足囊黏菌属

podarthritis [ˌpɔdɑːˈθraitis] *n* 足关节炎
podedema [ˌpɔdiˈdiːmə] *n* 足水肿
podencephalus [ˌpɔdenˈsefələs] *n* 有茎露脑畸胎
podgy [ˈpɔdʒi] *a* 矮胖的
podiatry [pəuˈdaiətri] *n* 足医术 / **podiatrist** *n* 足医 | **podiatric** [ˌpəudiˈætrik] *a*
podium [ˈpəudiəm] ([复] **podia** [ˈpəudiə]) *n* 【拉】足,吸足
pod(o)- [构词成分]足,脚
podocyte [ˈpɔdəsait] *n* 足细胞(肾小球内)
pododemodicosis [ˌpəudəuˌdeməudiˈkəusis] *n* 足蠕[形]螨病
pododerm [ˈpɔdədəːm] *n* 蹄部真皮
pododynamometer [ˌpɔdəˌdainəˈmɔmitə] *n* 腿肌力计;足力计
pododynia [ˌpɔdəˈdiniə] *n* 足[底]神经痛
podofilox [pəuˈdɔfilɔks] *n* 波多非洛(一种鬼臼毒素制剂,或化学合成或从植物提取液精制,局部用于治疗尖锐湿疣)
podogram [ˈpɔdəgræm] *n* 足印
podograph [ˈpɔdəgrɑːf] *n* 足印器
podology [pəuˈdɔlədʒi] *n* 足医术
podophyllin [ˌpɔdəˈfilin] *n* 鬼臼树脂(腐蚀药,泻药)
podophyllotoxin [ˌpɔdəˌfiləˈtɔksin] *n* 鬼臼毒素,鬼臼脂素,足叶草毒素(抗肿瘤药)
Podophyllum [ˌpɔdəˈfiləm] *n* 鬼臼属
podophyllum [ˌpɔdəˌfiləm] *n* 鬼臼(根)
podopompholyx [ˌpəudəˈpɔmfəliks] *n* 跖汗疱,足底汗疱
Podostroma [ˌpəudəuˈstrəumə] *n* 肉座菌属
podotrochilitis [ˌpɔdətrəkiˈlaitis] *n* 马舟骨炎
podotrochlosis [ˌpəudəutrɔkˈləusis] *n* 舟骨状病
poe- 以 poe-起始的词,同样见以 pe-起始的词
Poecilia [piːˈsiliə] *n* 鳉属(柳条鱼) | ~ reticulata 网纹鳉
poecil(o)- 以 poecil(o)-起始的词,同样见以 poikil(o)-起始的词
Poehl's test [pel] (Alexander V. von Poehl) 珀尔试验(检霍乱弧菌)
POEMS syndrome polynewopathy, organmegaly, endocrinopathy, M-protein, skin changes syndrome POEMS 综合征
pogoniasis [ˌpəugəuˈnaiəsis] *n* 多须;妇女生须
pogonion [pəˈgəuniən] *n* 颏前点
pOH 表示溶液中氢氧离子近似浓度的符号
Pohl's test [pɔl] (Julius H. Pohl) 波尔试验(检球蛋白)
poi [pɔi] *n* 夏威夷芋泥饼(变态反应的婴儿食用)
-poiesis [构词成分]产生,生,造
-poietin [构词成分]促血细胞生成素
poikilergasia [ˌpɔikiləˈgeiziə] *n* 精神病体质
poikilionia [pɔiˌkiliˈəuniə] *n* 血(无机)离子浓度变异
poikil(o)- [构词成分]异,变,不规则
poikiloblast [ˈpɔikiləuˌblæst] *n* 异形成红细胞
poikilocarynosis [ˌpɔikiləuˌkæriˈnəusis] *n* 异形细胞形成
poikilocyte [ˈpɔikiləuˌsait] *n* 异形红细胞
poikilocytosis [ˌpɔikiləusaiˈtəusis], **poikilocythemia** [pɔiˌkiləsaiˈθiːmiə] *n* 异形红细胞症
poikilodentosis [ˌpɔikiləudenˈtəusis] *n* 斑釉[症]
poikiloderma [ˌpɔikiləuˈdəːmə] *n* 皮肤异色病 | ~ vasculare atrophicans 血管萎缩性皮肤异色病
poikilodermatomyositis [ˌpɔikiləuˌdəːmətəumaiəˈsaitis] *n* 异色性皮肌炎
poikilonymy [ˌpɔikiˈlɔnimi] *n* 名称混乱
poikiloplastocyte [ˌpɔikiləuˈplæstəsait] *n* 异形血小板
poikiloploid [ˈpɔikiləuˌplɔid] *a* 异倍性的,异倍体的 *n* 异倍体(指一个个体具有不同的细胞,其染色体的数目也不相同) | **~y** [ˈpɔikiləuˌplɔidi] *n* 异倍性
poikilosmosis [ˌpɔikilɔzˈməusis] *n* 变渗压(细胞或组织对直接环境调节其渗透压浓度的过程) | **poikilosmotic** [ˌpɔikilɔzˈmɔtik] *a*
poikilostasis [ˌpɔikiləuˈsteisis] *n* 变异停滞(身体状态〈内环境〉保持稳定)
poikilotherm [pɔiˈkiləˌθəːm] *n* 变温动物,冷血动物
poikilothermy [ˌpɔikiləuˈθəːmi], **poikilothermism** [ˌpɔikiləuˈθəːmizəm] *n* 变温[性];温度变化适应性 | **poikilothermal, poikilothermic** *a* 变温的(动物);能适应温度变化的
poikilothrombocyte [pɔiˌkiləˈθrɔmbəsait] *n* 异形血小板
poikilothymia [ˌpɔikiləuˈθaimiə] *n* 心情变异
point [pɔint] *n* 点,尖;根管尖 *vi* (脓肿等)出现脓头 | ~ A A 点,上颌牙槽座点(X 线照相头颅测量名词,在外侧头部摄片上测定,亦称切牙骨下点) / ~ of an abscess 脓肿现头 / alveolar ~ (上)牙槽中点 / apophysiary ~ 鼻下点;棘突压痛点 / ~ Ar(下颌)关节突点(即 articulare) / ~ B B 点,下颌牙槽座点(X 线照相头颅测量名词,在外侧头部摄片上测定,亦称颏上点) / ~ Ba 颅底点(即 basion) / ~ Bo (枕骨)髁后点(即 Bolton ~) / boiling ~ 沸点 / cardinal ~s 方位基点;骨盆主点 / critical ~ 临界点 / ~ of incidence 投射点,入射点 / isoelectric ~ 等电点 / leak ~ 泄漏点,阈值(指血糖) / melting ~ 熔点 / mental ~ 颏点 / paper ~ 纸尖,纸捻 / principal ~s 方位基点 / thermal death ~ 杀菌温度 / trigger ~ 扳机点(身体受压力或其他刺激时出现特

殊感觉或症状的点)/ vaccine ~ 痘苗点(一小骨片或羽毛,一端沾有牛痘浆)/ vital ~ 生命点(延髓内呼吸中枢,刺穿此点即引起死亡)

pointer [ˈpɔintə] *n* 指示针,指示器;(骨隆突)挫伤 | hip ~ 髋部挫伤

pointillage [ˌpwɑːntiˈjɑːʒ] *n*【法】指尖按摩法

Poirier's glands [pwɑːriˈɛə] (Paul Poirier) 普瓦里埃腺(甲状腺峡上缘圆锥状韧带上的淋巴结) | ~ line 普瓦里埃线(从鼻额角至人字缝尖上方的连线)

poise(P) [pɔiz] *n* 泊(黏度单位)

Poiseuille's law [pwɑːˈzəːjə] (Jean L. M. Poiseuille)泊肃叶定律(管内流量:①与沿着管内长度的压力下降成正比,与管的半径的四次幂成正比;②与管的长度和流体黏度成反比) | ~ space 泊肃叶间隙(血管腔的边缘部,没有液体流动,如靠近血管内壁,红细胞实际上并不移动,而排成一层,液体的内层在此层上滑动)

poison [ˈpɔizn] *n* 毒,毒药,毒物 | acrid ~ 苛烈性毒,刺激性毒 / acronarcotic ~, acrosedative ~ 刺激麻醉性毒 / arrow ~ 箭毒 / fatigue ~ 疲劳毒素 / fugu ~, puffer ~ 河豚毒素 / gonyaulax ~, clam ~, mussel ~, shellfish ~ 蛤贝毒 / hemotropic ~ 亲红细胞毒 / mitotic ~ 有丝分裂抑制剂(阻抑细胞分裂的毒物) / muscle ~ 肌毒 / toot ~ 毒空木毒 / vascular ~ 血管毒 / whelk ~ 蛾螺毒

poisoning [ˈpɔizniŋ] *n* 中毒 | akee ~ 阿吉中毒,(西非)荔枝果中毒 / arsenic ~ 砷中毒 / blood ~ 败血病 / broom ~ 金雀花中毒 / carbon monoxide ~ 一氧化碳中毒 / dural ~ 铝镁合金中毒 / fish ~ 鱼肉中毒 / food ~ 食物中毒 / fugu ~, puffer ~, tetraodon ~ 河豚中毒 / milk ~(牛羊)震颤病;乳毒病(人) / O_2 ~ 氧中毒,换气过度 / tobacco ~ 烟草中毒 / trinitrotoluene ~, T. N. T. ~ 三硝基甲苯中毒 / whelk ~ 蛾螺中毒

poison ivy [ˈpɔizən ˈaivi] 毒葛

poison oak [ˈpɔizən ˈəuk] 槲叶毒葛

poisonous [ˈpɔiznəs] *a* 有毒的

poison sumac [ˈpɔizən ˈsuːmæk] 毒漆树,美国毒漆

Poisson distribution [pwɑːˈsɔːn] (Siméon D. Poisson) 泊松分布(描述事件计数如放射性衰变或血细胞计数按时间或空间随机分布的概率分布)

poitrinaire [ˌpwɑːtriˈnɛə] *n*【法】(慢性)胸肺病患者

pokeweed [ˈpəukwiːd], **pokeroot** [ˈpəukruːt] *n* 美洲商陆

polacrilin [ˌpɔləˈkrilin] *n* 宝拉利林(异丁烯酸树脂及二乙烯苯,一种合成阴离子交换树脂,以氢或游离酸形式补充,为药用辅料)

Poland's syndrome(anomaly) [ˈpəulənd] (Alfred Poland)波伦综合征(异常)(一侧胸大肌胸肋头缺失,同时并指或并趾[畸形])

polar [ˈpəulə] *a* 极的

polarimeter [ˌpəuləˈrimitə] *n* 偏振计,旋光计 | **polarimetric** [pəuˌlæriˈmetrik] *a* 测定偏振的,测定旋光的 / **polarimetry** *n* 偏振测定[法],旋光测量法

polariscope [pəuˈlæriskəup] *n* 偏振[光]镜,旋光镜 | **polariscopic** [ˌpəulərіˈskɔpik] *a* 偏振镜的,旋光镜的;偏振镜检查的,旋光镜检查的 | **polariscopy** [ˌpəuləˈriskəpi] *n* 偏振镜检查,旋光镜检查

polaristrobometer [pəuˌlæristrəˈbɔmitə] *n* 精密旋光计,精密偏振计

polarity [pəuˈlærəti] *n* 极性;极性现象 | dynamic ~ 机能极性(神经细胞)

polarization [ˌpəulәraiˈzeiʃən, -riˈz-] *n* 极化;偏振[化] | circular ~ 圆偏振 / elliptical ~ 椭圆偏振 / plane ~ 平面偏振,线偏振 / rotatory ~ 旋偏振

polarize [ˈpəuləraiz] *vt*, *vi* 极化;偏振化 | **polarizable** *a* 可极化的 | **~r** *n* 偏振器、偏振镜

polarogram [pəuˈlærəgræm] *n* 极谱

polarograph [pəuˈlærəgrɑːf, -græf] *n* 极谱仪 | **~ic** [pəuˌlærəˈgræfik] *a* 极谱法的 | **~y** [ˌpəuləˈrɔgrəfi] *n* 极谱法

polaroplast [pəuˈlærəplæst] *n* 极胞体(微孢子虫的细胞器)

poldine methylsulfate [ˈpɔldin] 甲硫酸泊尔定(抗胆碱能药)

pole [pəul] *n* 极,磁极,电极 | anterior ~ of lens 晶状体前极 / negative ~ 负极,阴极 / positive ~ 正极,阳极 / twin ~ 孖极,双极(神经细胞) / vegetal ~, vegetative ~, vitelline ~ 自主性极,卵黄极

Polemonium [ˌpɔləˈməuniəm] *n* 花葱属

poli [ˈpəulai] polus 的复数

policapram [ˌpɔliˈkeiprəm] *n* 聚己酰胺(片剂黏合剂)

policeman [pəˈliːsmən] *n* 淀帚(一端包有橡皮的玻璃棒,在化学分析时用作搅拌棒)

policlinic [ˌpɔliˈklinik] *n* 市立(医院)门诊部;综合门诊所,分科门诊所

polidocanol [ˌpɔlidəuˈkeinɔl] *n* 聚桂醇

poliencephalitis [ˌpɔlienˌsefəˈlaitis] *n* 脑灰质炎

poliencephalomyelitis [ˌpɔlienˌsefələumaiəˈlaitis] *n* 脑脊髓灰质炎

polifeprosan 20 [ˈpɔliˈfeprəusæn] 聚苯丙生 20

polio [ˈpəuliəu] *n* 脊髓灰质炎

poli(o)- [构词成分]灰质

poliocidal [ˌpəuliəuˈsaidl] *a* 杀脊髓灰质炎病毒的

polioclastic [ˌpəuliəuˈklæstik] *a* 破坏(神经系统)灰质的(指脊髓灰质炎、流脑和狂犬病的病毒);向神经的,亲神经的

poliodystrophy [ˌpəuliəuˈdistrəfi], **poliodystrophia** [ˌpəuliəudisˈtrəufiə] *n* 脑灰质萎缩,脑灰质营养不良症

polioencephalitis [ˌpəuliəuenˌsefəˈlaitis] *n* 脑灰质炎 | acute bulbar ~ 急性延髓灰质炎,急性延髓性麻痹 / inferior ~ 脑下部灰质炎,延髓性麻痹 / posterior ~ 脑后部灰质炎,第四脑室后部灰质炎

polioencephalomalacia [ˌpəuliəuenˌsefələuməˈleiʃiə] *n* 脑灰质软化(牛羊等高度致命性疾病,亦称假脑软化,大脑皮质坏死)

polioencephalomeningomyelitis [ˌpəuliəuenˌsefələuməˌniŋgəuˌmaiəˈlaitis] *n* 脑脊髓灰质脑脊膜炎

polioencephalomyelitis [ˌpəuliəuenˌsefələuˌmaiəˈlaitis] *n* 脑脊髓灰质炎

polioencephalopathy [ˌpəuliəuenˌsefəˈlɔpəθi] *n* 脑灰质病

polioencephalotropic [ˌpəuliəuenˌsefələuˈtrɔpik] *a* 亲脑灰质的;向神经的,亲神经的

poliomyelencephalitis [ˌpəuliəuˌmaiəlenˌsefəˈlaitis] *n* 脑脊髓灰质炎

poliomyeliticidal [ˌpəuliəuˌmaiəˈlaitiˌsaidl] *a* 杀脊髓灰质炎病毒的

poliomyelitis [ˌpəuliəuˌmaiəˈlaitis] *n* 脊髓灰质炎 | acute anterior ~ 急性脊髓前角灰质炎 / acute lateral ~ 急性脊髓侧角灰质炎 / ascending ~ 上行性脊髓灰质炎 / bulbar ~ 延髓型脊髓灰质炎 / cerebral ~ 脑型脊髓灰质炎,脑灰质炎 / postinoculation ~ 接种后脊髓灰质炎 / postvaccinal ~ 种痘后脊髓灰质炎,接种疫苗后脊髓灰质炎

poliomyeloencephalitis [ˌpəuliəuˌmaiələuenˌsefəˈlaitis] *n* 脑脊髓灰质炎

poliomyelopathy [ˌpəuliəuˌmaiəˈlɔpəθi] *n* 脊髓灰质病

polioneuromere [ˌpəuliəuˈnjuərəmiə] *n* 脊髓灰质原节

polioplasm [ˈpɔliəˌplæzəm] *n* 网质(细胞内)

poliosis [ˌpɔliˈəusis] *n* 白发[症],灰发[症]

polioviral [ˈpəuliəuˌvaiərəl] *a* 脊髓灰质炎病毒的

poliovirus [ˈpəuliəuˌvaiərəs] *n* 脊髓灰质炎病毒 | ~ muris 鼠脊髓灰质炎病毒

polipropene [ˌpɔliˈprəupiːn] *n* 1-丙烯同聚物(片剂赋形剂)

polishing [ˈpɔliʃiŋ] *n* 打光,磨光;[复]磨下物(如 rice ~s 米糠,富含维生素 B)

polisography [ˌpɔliˈsɔgrəfi] *n* 多次[曝光]X 线摄影[术]

Politano-Leadbetter technique [ˌpɔliˈtɑːnəu ˈledbetə] (Victor A. Politano; Wayland F. Leadbetter)波-莱技术(一型输尿管膀胱吻合术,即将输尿管切除对膀胱的附着,并以更内和更正的位置再附着)

politzerization [ˌpɔlitsəraiˈzeiʃən, -riˈz-] (Adam Politzer) *n* 中耳吹气法,咽鼓管吞咽吹气法 | negative ~ 中耳(负压)吸液法

Politzer's bag [ˈpɔlitsə] (Adam Politzer) 波利策袋(咽鼓管吹气囊) | ~ cone (鼓膜)光锥 / ~ speculum 波利策耳镜 / ~ test 波利策试验(检一侧耳聋:将音叉置于鼻孔前,吞咽时只有正常侧耳方能听到) / ~ treatment 波利策疗法(患者作吞咽运动时吹气入鼻孔,以治中耳病)

polkissen [pəulˈkisən] *n* 【德】[肾小]球旁细胞

poll [pəul] *n* 后头(尤指动物头的后部)

pollakidipsia [ˌpɔləkiˈdipsiə] *n* 频渴,渴感过频

pollakiuria [ˌpɔləkiˈjuəriə], **pollakisuria** [ˌpɔləkiˈsjuəriə] *n* 频尿

pollantin [pɔˈlæntin] *n* 花粉抗毒素(曾用于治枯草热)

polled [pəuld] *a* 无角的(指培育无角之牛,研究其遗传性状)

pollen [ˈpɔlən] *n* 花粉

pollenarium [ˌpɔliˈnɛəriəm] *n* 储花粉室

pollenogenic [ˌpɔlinəˈdʒenik] *a* 花粉引起的

pollenosis [ˌpɔləˈnəusis] *n* 花粉症

pollex [ˈpɔleks] ([复] **pollices** [ˈpɔlisiːz]) *n* 【拉】拇指,拇 | **pollical** *a*

pollicization [ˌpɔlisaiˈzeiʃən, -siˈz-] *n* 拇指化[术]

pollination [ˌpɔliˈneiʃən] *n* 授粉[作用],传粉[作用]

pollinium [pəuˈliniəm] *n* 花粉块

pollinosis [ˌpɔliˈnəusis] *n* 花粉症

pollodic [pəˈlɔdik] *a* 四周放射的,多向传导的(神经)

pollutant [pəˈljuːtənt] *n* 污染物

pollution [pəˈljuːʃən] *n* 污染;遗精 | air ~ 空气污染 / diurnal ~, ~ nimiae 昼遗[精]

pollybeak [ˈpɔliˌbiːk] *n* 鹦嘴[畸形]

polocytes [ˈpəuləsaits] *n* 极体

polonium(Po) [pəˈləuniəm] *n* 钋(化学元素)

poloxalene [pɔˈlɔksəliːn] *n* 泊洛沙林,聚羟亚烃(一种液体泊洛沙姆〈poloxamer〉,作药剂的表面活性剂)

poloxalkol [pɔˈlɔksælkɔl] *n* 泊洛沙姆 188,聚羟亚烃 188(即 poloxamer 188)

poloxamer [pɔˈlɔksəmə] *n* 泊洛沙姆,聚羟亚烃(聚羟乙烯聚羟丙烯共聚物,可以作表面活性剂、乳化剂或稳定剂) | ~ 182L 泊洛沙姆 188L,聚羟亚烃 182L(食品添加剂和药物辅助剂) / ~ 188 泊洛沙姆 188,聚羟亚烃 188(口服

泻药)/ ~ 331 泊洛沙姆 331,聚羟亚烃 331(食品添加剂)

polster [ˈpəulstə] *n* (如在管壁上的)小膨出

poltophagy [pɔlˈtɔfədʒi] *n* 嚼烂,细嚼

polus [ˈpəuləs] ([复] **poli** [ˈpəulai]) *n*【拉】极

poly [ˈpɔli] *n* 多形核白细胞

poly- [构词成分]多,多数

poly A polyadenylate 聚腺苷酸盐(酯或阴离子型);polyadenylic acid 聚腺苷酸

polyacid [ˌpɔliˈæsid] *a* 多[价]酸的 *n* 多元酸

polyacoustic [ˌpɔliəˈkuːstik] *a* 扩音的,扩声的

polyacrylamide [ˌpɔliəˈkriləmaid] *n* 聚丙烯酰胺

polyacrylonitrile [ˌpoliəˌkriləuˈnaitril] *n* 聚丙烯腈(用作血液透析器膜)

polyadenia [ˌpɔliəˈdiːniə] *n* 假白血病

polyadenitis [ˌpɔliˌædiˈnaitis] *n* 多腺炎 | malignant ~ 腺鼠疫,腹股沟淋巴结鼠疫

polyadenoma [ˌpɔliˌædiˈnəumə] *n* 多腺瘤

polyadenomatosis [ˌpɔliˌædinəuməˈtəusis] *n* 多腺瘤病

polyadenopathy [ˌpɔliˌædiˈnɔpəθi] *n* 多腺病

polyadenosis [ˌpɔliˌædiˈnəusis] *n* 多腺病(尤指内分泌腺体的)

polyadenous [ˌpɔliˈædənəs] *a* 多腺的(多内分泌的;多腺性的)

polyadenylate [ˌpɔliəˈdenileit] *n* 聚腺苷酸盐(酯或阴离子型)

polyadenylated [ˌpɔliəˈdenileitid] *a* 有聚腺苷酸尾的

polyadenylation [ˌpɔliəˌdeniˈleiʃən] *n* 聚腺苷酸化[作用]

polyadenylic acid [ˌpɔliˌædəˈnilik] 聚腺苷酸

polyagglutinability [ˌpɔliəˌgluːtinəˈbiləti] *n* 多[种可]凝集性

polyagglutination [ˌpɔliəˌgluːtiˈneiʃən] *n* 多红细胞凝集

polyalcoholism [ˌpɔliˈælkəhɔlizəm] *n* 混合乙醇中毒

polyalgesia [ˌpɔliælˈdʒiːzjə] *n* 多处痛觉

polyalveolar [ˌpɔliəlˈviːələ] *a* 多小泡的(如肺叶)

polyamine [ˌpɔliˈæmiːn] *n* 多胺

polyandry [ˌpɔliˈændri] *n* (一妻)多夫配合;(一雌)多雄配合 | **polyandric** *a*

Polyangiaceae [ˌpɔliˌændʒiˈeisiiː] *n* 多囊黏菌科

polyangiitis [ˌpɔliˌændʒiˈaitis] *n* 多血管炎,多脉管炎

Polyangium [ˌpɔliˈændʒiəm] *n* 多囊黏菌属

poly A polymerase [ˈpɔli ei pəˈliməreis] 聚腺苷酸聚合酶,聚核苷酸腺苷酰[基]转移酶

polyarteritis [ˌpɔliˌɑːtəˈraitis] *n* 多动脉炎

polyarthric [ˌpɔliˈɑːθrik], **polyarticular** [ˌpɔliɑːˈtikjulə] *a* 多关节的

polyarthritis [ˌpɔliɑːˈθraitis] *n* 多关节炎 | chronic villous ~ 慢性多关节滑膜炎 / ~ destruens 类风湿关节炎 / tuberculous ~ 结核性多关节炎,肥大性肺性骨关节病 / vertebral ~ 椎骨多关节炎

polyase [ˈpɔlieis] *n* 多糖酶,聚合酶

Polya's operation [ˈpɔljɑː] (Jenö 〈Eugene〉 Polya)波尔亚手术(次全胃切除术后,胃空肠吻合术)

polyatomic [ˌpɔliəˈtɔmik] *a* 多原子的

polyauxotroph [ˌpɔliˈɔːksətrəuf] *n* 多营养缺陷体,多重营养缺陷型(需要多种生长因子的有机体,尤指一种突变体) | **~ic** [ˌpɔliɔːksəˈtrɔfik] *a* 多养的

polyavitaminosis [ˌpɔlieiˌvaitəmiˈnəusis] *n* 多种维生素缺乏病

polyaxon [ˌpɔliˈæksɔn] *n* 多轴突[神经]细胞

polyaxonic [ˌpɔliækˈsɔnik] *a* 多轴突的

polyazin [ˌpɔliˈæzin] *n* 多氮化合物

polybasic [ˌpɔliˈbeisik] *a* 多碱[价]的,多元的

polyblast [ˈpɔliblæst] *n* 多母细胞,多原始细胞(阿米巴样游走的单核噬细胞,见于炎性渗出物中,本词现与 free macrophage 同义)

polyblennia [ˌpɔliˈbleniə] *n* 黏液分泌过多

polycarbophil [ˌpɔliˈkɑːbəfil] *n* 聚卡波非(导泻药)

polycellular [ˌpɔliˈseljulə] *a* 多细胞的;多空隙的

polycentric [ˌpɔliˈsentrik] *a* 多中心的;具多着丝点的,具多着丝粒的 | **~ity** [ˌpɔlisenˈtrisəti] *n*

polyceptor [ˌpɔliˈseptə] *n* 多受体(能结合若干不同补体的一种介体)

polycheiria [ˌpɔliˈkaiəriə] *n* 多手[畸形]

polychemotherapy [ˌpɔliˌkeməuˈθerəpi] *n* 综合化学疗法

polychloruria [ˌpɔlikləˈrjuəriə] *n* 尿氯增多,多氯尿

polycholia [ˌpɔliˈkəuliə] *n* 胆汁分泌过多

polychondritis [ˌpɔlikɔnˈdraitis] *n* 多软骨炎

polychondropathy [ˌpɔlikɔnˈdrɔpəθi], **polychondropathia** [ˌpɔliˌkɔndrəuˈpæθiə] *n* 多软骨病

polychrest [ˈpɔlikrest] *a* 有多种用途的 *n* 万应药

polychromasia [ˌpɔlikrəuˈmeiziə] *n* 多染[色]性;多染[性]细胞增多

polychromate [ˌpɔliˈkrəumeit] *n* 多色觉者,正常色觉者

polychromatic [ˌpɔlikrəuˈmætik] *a* 多色的

polychromatocyte [ˌpɔlikrəuˈmætəsait] *n* 多染[性]细胞

polychromatocytosis [ˌpɔlikrəuˌmætəsaiˈtəusis] *n* 多染[性]细胞增多[症]

polychromatophil [ˌpɔlikrəuˈmætəfil], **polych-**

romophil [ˌpɔliˈkrəuməfil] *n* 多染[性]细胞 *a* 多染[色]性的

polychromatophilia [ˌpɔliˌkrəumətəˈfiliə], **polychromatia** [ˌpɔlikrəuˈmeiʃiə], **polychromophilia** [ˌpɔlikrəuməˈfiliə] *n* 多染[色]性;多染[性]细胞增多 | **polychromatophilic** [ˌpɔliˌkrəumətəˈfilik] *a* 多染[色]性的

polychromatosis [ˌpɔliˌkrəuməˈtəusis] *n* 多染[性]细胞增多

polychrome [ˈpɔlikrəum] *a* 多色的

polychromemia [ˌpɔlikrəuˈmiːmiə] *n* 血色质增多

polychromic [ˌpɔliˈkrəumik] *a* 多色的

polychylia [ˌpɔliˈkailiə] *n* 乳糜过多

polyclinic [ˌpɔliˈklinik] *n* 综合门诊所,分科门诊所;综合医院,分科医院

polyclonal [ˌpɔliˈkləunl] *a* 多细胞系的,多细胞株的,多克隆的

polyclonia [ˌpɔliˈkləuniə] *n* 多肌阵挛病

polycoria [ˌpɔliˈkɔːriə] *n* 多瞳;储备质过多

polycrotism [pɔˈlikrətizəm] *n* 多波脉[现象] | **polycrotic** [ˌpɔliˈkrɔtik] *a*

polycyclic [ˌpɔliˈsaiklik, -ˈsik-] *a* 多环的

polycyesis [ˌpɔlisaiˈiːsis] *n* 多胎妊娠

polycystic [ˌpɔliˈsistik] *a* 多囊的

Polycystinea [ˌpɔlisisˈtiniə] *n* 多孔虫纲

polycystoma [ˌpɔlisisˈtəumə] *n* 多囊瘤(尤指乳腺)

polycyte [ˈpɔlisait] *n* 多核白细胞

polycythemia [ˌpɔlisaiˈθiːmiə] *n* 红细胞增多[症] | ~ hypertonica 高血压性红细胞增多症 / ~ vera, myelopathic ~, primary ~, ~ rubra, splenomegalic ~ 真性红细胞增多症,红细胞增多[症],骨髓病性红细胞增多,原发性红细胞增多,脾大性红细胞增多

polydactyly [ˌpɔliˈdæktili], **polydactylia** [ˌpɔlidækˈtiliə], **polydactylism** [pɔliˈdæktilizəm] *n* 多指[畸形],多趾[畸形]

polydentia [ˌpɔliˈdenʃiə] *n* 多牙,额外牙

polydeoxyribonucleotide [ˌpɔlidiːˌɔksiˌraibəuˈnjuːkliətaid] *n* 聚脱氧核[糖核]苷酸,脱氧核糖核酸

polydeoxyribonucleotide synthase (ATP) [ˌpɔlidiːˌɔksiˌraibəuˈnjuːkliətaidˈsinθiteis] 聚脱氧核[糖核]苷酸合酶(亦称 DNA 连接酶,聚核苷酸连接酶)

polydimethylsiloxane [ˌpɔlidaiˌmeθilsaiˈlɔksein] *n* 聚二甲基硅氧烷

polydioxanone [ˌpɔlidaiˈɔksənəun] *n* 聚二噁烷(用作可吸收缝线材料)

polydipsia [ˌpɔliˈdipsiə] *n* 烦渴,多饮

polydispersoid [ˌpɔlidisˈpəːsɔid] *n* 多分散胶体(含有不同分散度的胶体)

polydrug [ˈpɔlidrʌg] *n* 多种药物

polydyscrinia [ˌpɔlidisˈkriniə] *n* 多种分泌障碍

polydysplasia [ˌpɔlidisˈpleiziə] *n* 多种发育障碍 | hereditary ectodermal ~ 遗传性外胚层发育障碍(先天性外胚层缺陷)

polydysspondylism [ˌpɔlidiˈspɔndilizəm] *n* 多脊髓畸形症

polydystrophy [ˌpɔliˈdistrəfi] *n* 多[处]营养不良,多[处]营养障碍 | **polydystrophic** [ˌpɔlidisˈtrɔfik] *a*

polyelectrolyte [ˌpɔliiˈlektrəulait] *n* 聚电解质

polyembryoma [ˌpɔliˌembriˈəumə] *n* 多胚瘤

polyembryony [ˌpɔliemˈbriːəni] *n* 多胚[现象]

polyemia [ˌpɔliˈiːmiə] *n* 多血[症]

polyendocrine [ˌpɔliˈendəukrain, -krin-] *a* 多[种]内分泌腺的

polyendocrinoma [ˌpɔliˌendəukraiˈnəumə] *n* 多[种]内分泌腺腺瘤病

polyendocrinopathy [ˌpɔliˌendəukriˈnɔpəθi] *n* 多[种]内分泌腺病

polyene [pəˈliːn, ˈpɔliiːn] *n* 多烯,聚烯

polyerg [ˈpɔliəːg] *n* 多能血清(单种血清而作用于异种抗原)

polyergic [ˌpɔliˈəːdʒik] *a* 多能的,多方面作用的

polyester [ˌpɔliˈestə] *n* 聚酯

polyesthesia [ˌpɔliisˈθiːzjə] *n* 多处感觉,一物多感[症],复觉 | **polyesthetic** [ˌpɔliisˈθetik] *a*

polyestradiol phosphate [ˌpɔliˌestrəˈdaiɔl, ˌpɔliesˈtreidiɔl] 聚磷酸雌二醇(雌激素,用于治疗前列腺癌)

polyestrous [ˌpɔliˈestrəs] *a* 多次动情[期]的

polyethadene [ˌpɔliˈeθədiːn] *n* 聚依他定(抗酸药)

polyether [ˌpɔliˈiːθə] *n* 聚醚,多醚(用作印模材料)

polyethylene [ˌpɔliˈeθiliːn] *n* 聚乙烯 | ~ glycol 聚乙二醇(药用辅料)

polyferose [ˌpɔliˈferəus] *n* 多糖铁(补血药)

polyfolliculinic [ˌpɔlifəˌlikjuˈlinik] *a* 卵泡素过多的

Polygala [pəˈligələ] *n* 远志属

polygalactia [ˌpɔligəˈlækʃiə] *n* 泌乳过多

polygalacturonase [ˌpɔligəlækˈtjuərəneis] *n* 多聚半乳糖醛酸酶

polygalic acid [ˌpɔliˈgælik] 远志酸,美远志酸

polygalin [pəˈligəlin] *n* 美远志皂苷元

polygamy [pəˈligəmi] *n* 多婚(多配偶的性关系,一妻多夫或一夫多妻);多配性(一雌多雄或一雄多雌) | **polygamous** [pəˈligəməs] *a*

polyganglionic [ˌpɔliˌgæŋgliˈɔnik] *a* 多神经节的;多淋巴结的

polygeline [ˌpɔliˈdʒeliːn] *n* 聚明胶肽(血容量减少时用作血浆增容剂)
polygen [ˈpɔlidʒən] *n* 多种价元素;多簇抗原(具有两个或两个以上抗原特异性〈抗原决定簇〉的复合抗原,经接种到动物体内后,每一决定簇能刺激机体产生一种特异性抗体)
polygene [ˈpɔlidʒiːn] *n* 多基因(一群非等位基因相互作用,以同一方式制约同一性状,以致其作用是累加的) | **polygenic** [ˌpɔliˈdʒenik] *a*
polygenesis [ˌpɔliˈdʒenisis] *n* 多元发生 | **polygenetic** [ˌpɔlidʒiˈnetik] *a*
polyglactin 910 [ˌpɔliˈglæktin] 聚格拉丁 910(用作可吸收缝线)
polyglandular [ˌpɔliˈglændjulə] *a* 多腺的
polyglucoside [ˌpɔliˈgluːkəusaid] *n* 聚葡糖苷
polyglycolic acid [ˌpɔliglaiˈkɔlik] 聚乙醇酸(制外科缝线用)
polyglyconate [ˌpɔliˈglikəneit] *n* 聚葡糖酸盐(用作可吸收缝线材料)
polygnathus [pəˈlignəθəs] *n* 颌部寄生胎
polygon [ˈpɔligɔn] *n* 多边形,多角形
Polygonatum [ˌpɔligəˈneitəm] *n* 黄精属
polygram [ˈpɔligræm] *n* 多种波动[描记]图
polygraph [ˈpɔligrɑːf, -græf] *n* 多道[生理]记录仪(如同时描记各种生理反应,如呼吸运动、脉波、血压及心理电流反射,俗名测谎器) | **~ic** [ˌpɔliˈgræfik] *a*
polygyny [pəˈlidʒini] *n* 一夫多妻(配合);一雄多雌(配合) | **polygynous** *a*
polygyria [ˌpɔliˈdʒaiəriə] *n* 多回脑,脑回过多
polyhedral [ˌpɔliˈhedrəl] *a* 多面体的
polyhexose [ˌpɔliˈheksəus] *n* 聚己糖
polyhidrosis [ˌpɔlihaiˈdrəusis, -hi-] *n* 多汗[症]
polyhistiocytoma [ˌpɔliˌhistiəusaiˈtəumə] *n* 多组织细胞瘤,小细胞骨肉瘤
polyhybrid [ˌpɔliˈhaibrid] *n* 多性杂种
polyhydramnios [ˌpɔlihaiˈdræmniəs] *n* 羊水过多
polyhydric [ˌpɔliˈhaidrik] *a* 多羟[基]的
polyhydruria [ˌpɔlihaiˈdrjuriə] *n* 尿液过淡,淡尿
Polyhymenophorea [ˌpɔliˌhaimənəuˈfɔːriə] *n* 多膜纲
polyhypermenorrhea [ˌpɔliˌhaipəːˌmenəˈriːə] *n* 月经频繁[量]过多,月经频发
polyhypomenorrhea [ˌpɔliˌhaipəuˌmenəˈriːə] *n* 月经频繁[量]过少
polyidrosis [ˌpɔliaiˈdrəusis, -iˈd-] *n* 多汗[症]
polyinfection [ˌpɔliinˈfekʃən] *n* 混合感染
polyionic [ˌpɔliaiˈɔnik] *a* 多离子的
polyisoprenoid [ˌpɔliˈaisəupriˌnɔid] *n* 类聚异戊二烯
polykaryocyte [ˌpɔliˈkæriəsait] *n* 多核细胞
polykinety [ˌpɔliˈkainiti] *n* 多动体列(一排紧密排列的纤毛,以逆时针的螺旋形下降至围口纤毛原生动物的漏斗)
polylactic acid [ˌpɔliˈlæktik] 聚乳酸(用作牙拔除部位的外科敷裹材料,用于预防术后牙槽骨炎)
polylecithal [ˌpɔliˈlesiθəl] *a* 多[卵]黄的
polyleptic [ˌpɔliˈleptik] *a* 多次复发的
polylogia [ˌpɔliˈləudʒə] *n* 多言症
polylysine [ˌpɔliˈlaisin] *n* 聚赖氨酸
polymacon [ˌpɔliˈmeikɔn] *n* 多美康(一种亲水性接触镜材料)
polymastia [ˌpɔliˈmæstiə], **polymazia** [ˌpɔliˈmeiziə] *n* 多乳房
polymastic [ˌpɔliˈmæstik] *a* 多乳房的
Polymastigida [ˌpɔliˌmæstiˈgaidə] *n* 多鞭毛[虫]目
polymastigote [ˌpɔliˈmæstigəut] *a* 多鞭毛的
polymelia [ˌpɔliˈmiːliə] *n* 多肢[畸形]
polymelus [pəˈliməlәs] *n* 多肢畸胎
polymenorrhea [ˌpɔliˌmenəˈriːə], **polymenia** [ˌpɔliˈmiːniə] *n* 月经频发
polymer [ˈpɔlimə] *n* 多聚体 | addition ~ 加聚物 / condensation ~ 缩聚物
polymerase [ˈpɔliməreis, pəˈli-] *n* 聚合酶,多聚酶
polymeria [ˌpɔliˈmiriə] *n* 多肢体[畸形]
polymeric [ˌpɔliˈmerik] *a* 聚合的
polymerid [pəˈlimərid] *n* 聚合物
polymerism [pəˈlimərizəm] *n* 聚合[现象]
polymerize [pəˈliməraiz] *vt, vi* 聚合 | **polymerization** [ˌpɔliməraiˈzeiʃən, -riˈz-] *n* 聚合[作用]
polymetacarpia [ˌpɔliˌmetəˈkɑːpiə] *n* 多掌骨[畸形]
polymetaphosphate [ˌpɔliˌmetəˈfɔsfeit] *n* 多聚偏磷酸
polymetatarsia [ˌpɔliˌmetəˈtɑːsiə] *n* 多跖骨[畸形]
polymethyl [ˌpɔliˈmeθil] *n* 聚甲基 | ~ methacrylate(PMMA) 聚甲基丙烯酸甲酯
polymethylmethacrylate [ˌpɔliˌmeθilmeˈθækrileit] *n* 聚甲基丙烯酸甲酯
polymicrobial [ˌpɔlimaiˈkrəubiəl], **polymicrobic** [ˌpɔlimaiˈkrəubik] *a* 多种微生物的
polymicrogyria [ˌpɔliˌmaikrəuˈdʒaiəriə] *n* 多小脑回
polymicrolipomatosis [ˌpɔliˌmaikrəuˌlipəuməˈtəusis] *n* 多发性[皮下]小脂瘤
polymicrotome [ˌpɔliˈmaikrətəum] *n* 多片切片机
Polymnia [pəˈlimniə] *n* 杯苞菊属
polymorph [ˈpɔlimɔːf] *n* 多形核白细胞
polymorphic [ˌpɔliˈmɔːfik] *a* 多形的,多型的,多

形态的

polymorphism [ˌpɔliˈmɔːfizəm] *n* 多形性,多型性;多态性,多态现象 | balanced ~ 平衡多态现象 / genetic ~ 遗传多态现象 / restriction fragment length ~ (RFLP) 限制性[内切酶]片段长度多态性(在分子遗传学中指 DNA 序列的一种多态性,可依据一种特定的限制性内切酶消化所产生的 DNA 片段长度的不同而检出之)

polymorphocellular [ˌpɔliˌmɔːfəˈseljulə] *a* 多形细胞的

polymorphocyte [ˌpɔliˈmɔːfəsait] *n* 多形核细胞

polymorphonuclear [ˌpɔliˌmɔːfəˈnjuːkliə] *a* 多形核的 *n* 多形核白细胞 | filament ~ 丝连多形核白细胞 / nonfilament ~ 非丝连多形核白细胞

polymorphous [ˌpɔliˈmɔːfəs] *a* 多形的,多型的,多形态的

polymyalgia [ˌpɔlimaiˈældʒiə] *n* 多肌痛

polymyarian [ˌpɔlimaiˈɛəriən] *a* 多肌型的

polymyoclonus [ˌpɔlimaiˈɔklənəs] *n* 肌阵挛病;多肌阵挛

polymyopathy [ˌpɔlimaiˈɔpəθi] *n* 多肌病

polymyositis [ˌpɔliˌmaiəˈsaitis] *n* 多肌炎,多发性肌炎 | trichinous ~ 毛线虫性多发性肌炎,毛线虫病

polymyxin [ˌpɔliˈmiksin] *n* 多黏菌素 | ~ B sulfate 硫酸多黏菌素 B

polynesic [ˌpɔliˈniːsik] *a* 多灶性的

polyneural [ˌpɔliˈnjuərəl], **polyneuric** [ˌpɔliˈnjuərik] *a* 多神经性的

polyneuralgia [ˌpɔlinjuəˈrældʒiə] *n* 多神经痛

polyneuritis [ˌpɔlinjuəˈraitis] *n* 多神经炎 | ~ cerebralis menieriformis 梅尼埃病样多发性脑神经炎 / endemic ~ 地方性多神经炎,脚气[病] / Jamaica ginger ~ 姜酒中毒性多神经炎 / ~ potatorum 酒毒性多神经炎 | **polyneuritic** [ˌpɔlinjuəˈritik] *a*

polyneuromyositis [ˌpɔliˌnjuərəuˌmaiəˈsaitis] *n* 多神经肌炎

polyneuropathy [ˌpɔlinjuəˈrɔpəθi] *n* 多神经病

polyneuroradiculitis [ˌpɔliˌnjuərəurəˌdikjuˈlaitis] *n* 多神经根炎

polynuclear [ˌpɔliˈnjuːkliə], **polynucleated** [ˌpɔliˈnjuːkliˌeitid] *a* 多核的;多形核的

polynucleate [ˌpɔliˈnjuːkliit] *a* 多核的

polynucleolar [ˌpɔlinjuːˈkliːələ] *a* 多核仁的

polynucleotidase [ˌpɔliˈnjuːkliətaideis] *n* 多核苷酸酶

polynucleotide [ˌpɔliˈnjuːkliətaid] *n* 多核苷酸

polynucleotide adenylyltransferase [ˌpɔliˈnjuːkliətaid ˌædinililˈtrænfəreis] 多核苷酸腺苷酰[基]转移酶(亦称聚腺苷酸聚合酶)

polynucleotide phosphorylase [ˌpɔliˈnjuːkliətaid fɔsˈfɔːrileis] 多核苷酸磷酸化酶,聚核[糖核]苷酸核苷酸基转移酶

polyodontia [ˌpɔliəuˈdɔnʃiə] *n* 多牙,额外牙

polyol [ˈpɔliɔl] *n* 多羟基化合物(亦称多元醇)

polyol dehydrogenase [ˈpɔliɔl diːˈhaidrədʒəneis] 多元醇脱氢酶,L-艾杜糖醇 2-脱氢酶

polyoma [ˌpɔliˈəumə] *n* 多瘤(由多瘤病毒所致的小鼠腮腺瘤)

Polyomavirinae [ˌpɔliˌəuməviˈrainiː] *n* 多瘤病毒亚科

Polyomavirus [ˌpɔliˌəuməˌvaiərəs] *n* 多瘤病毒属

polyomavirus [ˌpɔliˈəuməˌvaiərəs] *n* 多瘤病毒

polyonychia [ˌpɔliəˈnikiə] *n* 多甲[畸形]

polyopia [ˌpɔliˈəupiə] *n* 视物显多症 | binocular ~ 双眼视物显多症,复视 / ~ monophthalmica 单眼视物显多症,单眼复视 | **polyopsia** [ˌpɔliˈɔpsiə], **polyopy** [ˈpɔliˌəupi] *n*

polyorchidism [ˌpɔliˈɔːkidizəm], **polyorchism** [ˌpɔliˈɔːkizəm] *n* 多睾症

polyorchis [ˌpɔliˈɔːkis] *n* 多睾者

polyostotic [ˌpɔliɔsˈtɔtik] *a* 多骨的

polyotia [ˌpɔliˈəuʃiə] *n* 多耳,畸形

polyovular [ˌpɔliˈəuvjulə] *a* 多卵的

polyovulatory [ˌpɔliˈəuvjulətəri] *a* 多排卵的

polyoxyethylene 50 stearate [ˌpɔliˌɔksiˈeθiliːn] 聚氧乙烯 50 硬脂酸酯(亦称聚乙二醇 50 硬脂酸酯)

polyoxyl [ˌpɔliˈɔksil] *n* 聚乙二醇 | ~ 5 oleate 聚乙二醇 5-油酸酯 / ~ 10 oleate ether 聚乙二醇 10-油醚 / ~ 50 stearate 聚乙二醇 50-硬脂酸酯,聚氧乙烯 50-硬脂酸酯

polyp [ˈpɔlip] *n* 息肉 | adenomatous ~ 腺瘤性息肉 / cardiac ~ 心腔内息肉 / choanal ~s 后鼻孔息肉 / endometrial ~s 子宫内膜息肉 / gelatinous ~ 胶状息肉,黏液瘤 / hydatid ~ 囊状息肉 / juvenile ~s, retention ~s 幼年性息肉,滞留息肉 / ~s of larynx 喉息肉 / lymphoid ~s 淋巴样息肉 / nasal ~s 鼻息肉

polypapilloma tropicum [ˌpɔliˌpæpiˈləumə ˈtrɔpikəm] *n* 雅司病(即 yaws)

polyparasitism [ˌpɔliˈpærəsitizəm] *n* 多类寄生虫感染

polyparesis [ˌpɔlipəˈriːsis] *n* 麻痹性痴呆,全身麻痹症

polypathia [ˌpɔliˈpæθiə] *n* 多病同发

polypectomy [ˌpɔliˈpektəmi] *n* 息肉切除[术]

polypeptidase [ˌpɔliˈpeptideis] *n* 多肽酶

polypeptide [ˌpɔliˈpeptaid] *n* 多肽 | gastric inhibitory ~ (GIP) 抑胃多肽 / pancreatic ~ 胰多肽 / vasoactive intestinal ~ (VIP) 血管活性肠多肽

polypeptidemia [ˌpɔliˌpeptiˈdiːmiə] *n* 多肽血[症]

polypeptidorrhachia [ˌpɔliˌpeptidəˈreikiə] *n* 多肽脑脊液症
polyperiostitis [ˌpɔliˌperiɔsˈtaitis] *n* 多骨膜炎
polyphagia [ˌpɔliˈfeidʒiə] *n* 多食
polyphalangia [ˌpɔlifəˈlændʒiə], **polyphalangism** [ˌpɔlifəˈlændʒizəm] *n* 多指骨[畸形],多趾骨[畸形]
polypharmaceutic [ˌpɔlifɑːməˈsjuːtik] *a* 复方的,多味药的
polypharmacy [ˌpɔliˈfɑːməsi] *n* 复方药剂,多味药剂;给药过多
polyphase [ˈpɔlifeiz] *a* 多相的;多型胶体的(具有若干型胶体的)
polyphasic [ˌpɔliˈfeizik] *a* 多相的;有不同颗粒的(分散相内有不同颗粒的)
polyphenic [ˌpɔliˈfenik] *a* 多向性的;多效性的
polyphenol oxidase [ˌpɔliˈfiːnɔl ɔksideis] 多酚氧化酶
polyphobia [ˌpɔliˈfəubjə] *n* 多种事物恐怖,多样恐怖
polyphosphoinositide [ˌpɔliˌfɔsfəuiˈnəusitaid] *n* 多磷酸肌醇
polyphrasia [ˌpɔliˈfreiziə] *n* 多言[症]
polyphyletic [ˌpɔlifaiˈletik] *a* 多元的,多系的,多源的
polyphyletism [ˌpɔliˈfailətizəm] *n* 多元说,多系学说,多源论(polyphyletic theory,见 theory 项下相应术语) | **polyphyletist** *n* 多元说者
polyphyodont [ˌpɔliˈfaiədɔnt] *a* 多套牙的,多次换牙的
polypi [ˈpɔlipai] polypus 的复数
polypiform [pəˈlipifɔːm] *a* 息肉状的
polypionia [ˌpɔlipaiˈəuniə] *n* 肥胖,多脂
polyplasmia [ˌpɔliˈplæzmiə] *n* 血浆过多
polyplastic [ˌpɔliˈplæstik] *a* 多种构造的;多种变形的,多塑性的
polyplastocytosis [ˌpɔliˌplæstəusaiˈtəusis] *n* 血小板增多
Polyplax [ˈpɔliplæks] *n* 鳞虱属
polyplegia [ˌpɔliˈpliːdʒiə] *n* 多肌麻痹
polypleurodiaphragmotomy [ˌpɔliˌpluərəuˌdaiəfrægˈmɔtəmi] *n* 多肋切断膈切开术
polyploid [ˈpɔliplɔid] *a* 多倍的 *n* 多倍体(一个个体或细胞具有两组以上的同源染色体) | **~y** *n* 多倍性
polypnea [ˌpɔliˈpni(ː)ə] *n* 呼吸急促,气促
polypneic [ˌpɔlipˈniːik] *a* 呼吸加速的
polypodia [ˌpɔliˈpəudiə] *n* 多足[畸形]
polypoid [ˈpɔlipɔid] *a* 息肉状的,息肉样的
polypoidosis [ˌpɔlipɔiˈdəusis] *n* 息肉状腺瘤病
polyporin [pəˈliparin] *n* 多孔菌素
polyporous [pəˈliparəs] *a* 多孔的
Polyporus [pəˈliparəs] *n* 多孔菌属
polyposia [ˌpɔliˈpəuziə] *n* 饮水过多,进液过多(长时期多饮症,参见 hyperposia)
polyposis [ˌpɔliˈpəusis] *n* 息肉病 | familial ~, ~ coli, familial intestinal ~, multiple familial ~ 家族性息肉病,结肠息肉病,家族性肠息肉病,多发性家族性息肉病 / ~ gastrica, ~ ventriculi 胃息肉病
polypotome [pəˈlipətəum] *n* 息肉刀
polypotrite [pəˈlipətrait] *n* 息肉夹碎器
polypous [ˈpɔlipəs] *a* 息肉的,息肉状的
polypragmasy [ˌpɔliˈprægməsi] *n* 复方药剂,多味药剂;给药过多
polypropylene [ˌpɔliˈprəupiˌliːn] *n* 聚丙烯(医学用途包括制造外科铸模和膜氧合器用的半透膜)
polyptychial [ˌpɔliˈtaikiəl] *a* 多层的,复层的(指腺体)
polypus [ˈpɔlipəs]([复] **polypi** [ˈpɔlipai]) *n* 【拉】息肉 | ~ angiomatodes 血管瘤性息肉 / ~ cysticus, ~ hydatidosus 囊状息肉 / ~ telangiectodes 血管扩张性息肉
polyradiculitis [ˌpɔlirəˌdikjuˈlaitis] *n* 多神经根炎
polyradiculoneuritis [ˌpɔlirəˌdikjuləunjuəˈraitis] *n* 多神经根神经炎
polyradiculoneuropathy [ˌpɔlirəˌdikjuləunjuəˈrɔpəθi] *n* 多神经根神经病
polyradiculopathy [ˌpɔlirəˌdikjuˈlɔpəθi] *n* 多神经根病变
polyribonucleotide [ˌpɔliˌraibəuˈnjuːkliətaid] *n* 聚核[糖核]苷酸
polyribonucleotide nucleotidyltransferase [ˌpɔliˌraibəuˈnjuːkliətaid ˌnjuːkliəˌtaidilˈtrænsfəreis] 聚核[糖核]苷酸核苷酸基转移酶(亦称聚核苷酸磷酸化酶)
polyribosome [ˌpɔliˈraibəsəum] *n* 多核糖体(由一条信使 RNA 和许多核糖体串联在一起形成的复合结构)
polyrrhea [ˌpɔliˈriːə] *n* 液溢
polysaccharide [ˌpɔliˈsækəraid] *n* 多糖 | bacterial ~s 细菌多糖 / capsular ~ 荚膜多糖(特异性荚膜物质) / gastric ~ 胃黏液多糖 / immune ~s 免疫多糖(能作为特异性抗原的多糖) / pneumococcus ~ 肺炎球菌多糖 / O-specific ~ O-特异多糖(脂多糖的杂多糖链的可变部分) | **polysaccharose** [ˌpɔliˈsækərəus] *n*
polysarcia [ˌpɔliˈsɑːsiə] *n* 多脂,肥胖 | **polysarcous** [ˌpɔliˈsɑːkəs] *a*
polyscelia [ˌpɔliˈsiːliə] *n* 多腿[畸形]
polyscelus [pəˈlisələs] *n* 多腿畸胎
polyscope [ˈpɔliskəup] *n* [电光]透照镜
polysensitivity [ˌpɔliˌsensiˈtivəti] *n* 多种敏感性

polysensory [ˌpɔliˈsensəri] *a* 多种感觉能的（指大脑皮质和皮质下区的某些神经元）

polyserositis [ˌpɔlisiərəˈsaitis] *n* 多浆膜炎 | familial recurrent ~, periodic ~, recurrent ~ 家族性地中海热

polysialia [ˌpɔlisaiˈeiliə] *n* 多涎，唾液分泌过多

polysialic acid [ˌpɔlisaiˈælik] 多涎酸，多唾液酸

polysiloxane [ˌpɔliˈsailɔksein] *n* 聚硅氧烷

polysinusectomy [ˌpɔliˌsainəˈsektəmi] *n* 多鼻窦切除术

polysinusitis [ˌpɔlisainəˈsaitis], **polysinuitis** [ˌpɔliˌsainjuˈaitis] *n* 多鼻窦炎

polysomaty [ˌpɔliˈsəumәti] *n* 体细胞多倍性 | **polysomatic** [ˌpɔlisəuˈmætik] *a*

polysome [ˈpɔlisəum] *n* 多核糖体，多核[糖核]蛋白体（见 polyribosome）

polysomia [ˌpɔliˈsəumiə] *n* 多体[畸形]

polysomnography [ˌpɔlisɔmˈnɔgrəfi] *n* 多导睡眠描记法（评估睡眠障碍有可能的生物学原因）

polysomus [ˌpɔliˈsəuməs] *n* 多体畸胎

polysomy [ˌpɔliˈsəumi] *n* 多体性（由于染色体不分离所致的一种特别的染色体过多现象） | **polysomic** *a* 多体[畸形]的 *n* 多体性者

polysorbate [ˌpɔliˈsɔːbeit] *n* 聚山梨酯（表面活性剂）

polyspermia [ˌpɔliˈspəːmiə], **polyspermism** [ˌpɔliˈspəːmizəm] *n* 精液过多；多精入卵

polyspermy [ˌpɔliˈspəːmi] *n* 多精入卵

polyspike [ˈpɔlispaik] *a* 多[波]峰的（指脑电波的复合波）

polysplenia [ˌpɔliˈspliniə] *n* 多脾

polystichia [ˌpɔliˈstikiə] *n* 多列睫

polystyrene [ˌpɔliˈstaiəriːn] *n* 聚苯乙烯

polysulfide [ˌpɔliˈsʌlfaid] *n* 多硫化[合]物

polysulfone [ˌpɔliˈsʌlfəun] *n* 聚砜（用作血液透析器膜）

polysuspensoid [ˌpɔlisəsˈpensɔid] *n* 多度悬胶[体]

polysynaptic [ˌpɔlisiˈnæptik] *a* 多突触的

polysyndactyly [ˌpɔlisinˈdæktili] *n* 多指并指[畸形]，多趾并趾[畸形]

polysynovitis [ˌpɔliˌsinəˈvaitis] *n* 多滑膜炎

polysyphilide [ˌpɔliˈsifilaid] *n* 多梅毒疹

polytef [ˈpɔlitef] *n* 聚四氟乙烯（亦称 polytetrafluoroethylene, PTFE）

polytendinitis [ˌpɔliˌtendiˈnaitis] *n* 多腱炎

polytendinobursitis [ˌpɔlitendinəubəːˈsaitis] *n* 多腱滑囊炎

polytene [ˈpɔlitiːn] *a* 多染色线的，多线的

polytenosynovitis [ˌpɔliˌtenəuˌsinəuˈvaitis] *n* 多腱鞘炎

polyteny [ˌpɔliˈtiːni] *n* 多染色线[现象]，多线性（染色线在染色体中的复制现象，不分裂成明显的子染色体）

polytetrafluoroethylene (**PTFE**) [ˌpɔliˌtetrəˌfluərəˈeθiliːn] 聚四氟乙烯（即 polytef）

polythelia [ˌpɔliˈθiːliə], **polythelism** [ˌpɔliˈθiːlizəm] *n* 多乳头[畸形]

polythene [ˈpɔliθiːn] *n* 聚乙烯

polythetic [ˌpɔliˈθetik] *a* 多原则的（指分类学）

polythiazide [ˌpɔliˈθaiəzaid] *n* 泊利噻嗪（利尿降压药）

polytocous [pəˈlitəkəs] *a* 多胎分娩的

polytomogram [ˌpɔliˈtɔməgræm] *n* 多轨迹 X 线体层[照]片

polytomography [ˌpɔlitəˈmɔgrəfi] *n* 多轨迹体层摄影[术] | **polytomographic** [ˌpɔliˌtəuməˈgræfik] *a*

polytrauma [ˌpɔliˈtrɔːmə] *n* 多发性损伤（发生一个以上身体系统的损伤）

polytrichia [ˌpɔliˈtrikiə], **polytrichosis** [ˌpɔlitriˈkəusis] *n* 多毛[症]

Polytrichum [pəˈlitrikəm] *n* 金发藓属

polytrophia [ˌpɔliˈtrəufiə], **polytrophy** [pəˈlitrəfi] *n* 营养过度 | **polytrophic** [ˌpɔliˈtrɔfik] *a*

polytropic [ˌpɔliˈtrɔpik], **polytropous** [pəˈlitrəpəs] *a* 多嗜的，多亲的（亲多种组织或细菌的）

polyunguia [ˌpɔliˈʌŋgwiə] *n* 多甲[畸形]

polyunsaturated [ˌpɔliʌnˈsætʃəreitid] *a* 多不饱和的

polyurethane [ˌpɔliˈjuərəθein] *n* 聚乌拉坦（牙科用作沟封闭剂）

polyuria [ˌpɔliˈjuəriə] *n* 多尿 | **polyuric** *a*

polyvalent [ˌpɔliˈveilənt] *a* 多价的 | **polyvalence** *n*

polyvinyl [ˌpɔliˈvainil] *n* 聚乙烯，乙烯聚合体

polyvinylacetate [ˌpɔliˌvainiˈlæsiteit] *n* 聚乙酸乙烯酯

polyvinylbenzene [ˌpɔliˌvainilˈbenziːn] *n* 聚苯乙烯

polyvinylchloride [ˌpɔliˌvainilˈklɔːraid] *n* 聚氯乙烯

polyvinylpyrrolidone [ˌpɔliˌvainilpiˈrɔlidəun] *n* 聚乙烯吡咯酮，聚烯吡酮（即聚维酮 povidone）

polyzoospermia [ˌpɔliˌzəuəuˈspəːmiə] *n* 多游动精子

Pomatiopsis [pəuˌmætiˈɔpsis] *n* 仿圆口螺属 | ~ cicinnatiensis 辛辛那提仿圆口螺 / ~ lapidaria 石栖仿圆口螺

pomatum [pəˈmeitəm], **pomade** [pəˈmeid] *n* 香膏剂，发膏剂，头油

POMC pro-opiomelanocortin 阿片促黑激素皮质素原

pomegranate [ˈpɔmˌgrænit] *n* 石榴

Pomeroy technique (operation) [ˈpɔmərɔi] (Ralph H. Pomeroy)波默罗伊技术(手术)(一种输卵管结扎法,即从子宫角约 5 cm 处将输卵管襻拉起,并结扎,然后将结扎的襻切除)

POMP prednisone, vincristine, methotrexate, and 6-mercaptopurine 泼尼松-长春新碱-甲氨蝶呤-6-巯基嘌呤(联合化疗治癌方案)

Pompe's disease [ˈpɔmpə] (Johann C. Pompe)糖原贮积症Ⅱ型

pompholyhemia [ˌpɔmfəliˈhiːmiə] *n* 气泡血症

pompholyx [ˈpɔmfəliks] *n* 汗疱疹

pomum adami [ˈpəumən əˈdɑːmi]【拉】喉结,喉隆凸

ponceau B [pɔnˈsəu] 丽春红 B,比布里希猩红 | ~ 3B 丽春红 3B,猩红

Poncet's disease [pɔnˈsei] (Antonin Poncet)蓬塞病(结核性风湿病) | ~ operation 蓬塞手术(会阴切开术;会阴尿道造口术) / ~ rheumatism 结核性风湿病

Pond. pondere【拉】按重量

ponderal [ˈpɔndərəl] *a* 重量的

pondostatural [ˌpɔndəˈstætʃərəl] *a* 体重[与]身材的

ponesiatrics [pəuˌniːsiˈætriks] *n* 活动训练[疗]法(用示波器、肌电描记器等查出误指的神经生理反应,以便识别和纠正之)

Ponfick's shadow [ˈpɔnfik] (Clemens E. Ponfick)红细胞影

Pongidae [pɔndʒidiː] *n* 猩猩科

Pongo [ˈpɔŋgəu] *n* 猩猩属

pon(o)- [构词成分]疲劳;疼痛

ponograph [ˈpəunəgrɑːf, -græf] *n* 疲劳描记器

ponos [ˈpəunəs] *n* 婴儿黑热病(地中海型内脏利什曼病)

pons [pɔnz] ([复] **pontes** [ˈpɔntiːz]) *n*【拉】桥;脑桥 | **pontile** [ˈpɔntiːl], **pontine** [ˈpɔntiːn] *a*

pons-oblongata [ˌpɔnz ɔblɔŋˈgeitə] *n* 脑桥延髓

Pontiac fever [ˈpɔntiæk] 庞蒂亚克热(见 fever 项下相应术语)

pontibrachium [ˌpɔntiˈbreikiəm] *n* 脑桥臂

pontic [ˈpɔntik] *n* 桥体(牙)

ponticulus [pɔnˈtikjuləs] ([复] **ponticuli** [pɔnˈtikjulai]) *n*【拉】小桥,前桥 | **ponticular** *a*

pontil [ˈpɔntil] *a* 脑桥的

pontile [ˈpɔntail, ˈpɔntiːl] *a* 脑桥的

pontine [ˈpɔntain, ˈpɔntiːn] *a* 脑桥的

pontis [ˈpɔntis] pons 的所有格

pont(o)- [构词成分]脑桥

pontobulbar [ˌpɔntəuˈbʌlbə] *a* 脑桥延髓的

pontobulbia [ˌpɔntəuˈbʌlbiə] *n* 脑桥延髓空洞症

pontocerebellar [ˌpɔntəuˌseriˈbelə] *a* 脑桥小脑的

pontocerebellum [ˌpɔntəuˌseriˈbeləm] *n* 脑桥小脑,新小脑

pontomedullary [ˌpɔntəuˈmedʌləri] *a* 脑桥延髓的

pontomesencephalic [ˌpɔntəuˌmesənsəˈfælik] *a* 脑桥中脑的

pontoon [pɔnˈtuːn] *n* 小肠襻

pontopeduncular [ˌpɔntəupiˈdʌŋkjulə] *a* 脑桥小脑脚的

pool [puːl] *n* 池,库;淤血 *vt* (几分血液或血浆)混合 | gene ~ 基因库(某一群体中所有成员具有的基因总数) / metabolic ~ 代谢池,代谢库(身体内变异及反应物质的总质量,有无数物质连续不断地往来其间)

pooled [puːld] *a* 混合的,集合的

Pool-Schlesinger sign [puːl ˈʃleiziŋə] (E. H. Pool; Hermann Schlesinger) 普尔-施勒辛格尔征(见 Schlesinger's sign)

Pool's phenomenon [puːl] (Eugene H. Pool)普尔现象(①见 Schlesinger's sign; ②臂现象:前臂伸展,举臂至头上方后,臂肌即收缩,以致引起臂丛牵张,见于手术后手足抽搦)

poplar [ˈpɔplə] *n* 杨属植物,白杨

poples [ˈpɔpliːs] *n*【拉】腘 | **popliteal** [pɔpˈlitiəl] *a*

poppy [ˈpɔpi] *n* 罂粟

population [ˌpɔpjuˈleiʃən] *n* 人口,人数;全体居民,总体;群体,种群 | genetic ~ 同类群,混交群体(即 deme)

Populus [ˈpɔpjuləs] *n* 杨属

POR problem-oriented record 面向问题记录(见 record项下相应术语)

poractant alfa [pɔːˈæktænt ˈælfə] 卟拉坦阿尔法(猪肺表面活性剂提出物,含有 99% 极性脂质疏水蛋白,通过气管内导管滴注给药,治疗新生儿呼吸窘迫综合征)

poradenitis [ˌpɔurædiˈnaitis] *n* 淋巴肉芽肿,淋巴结炎 | ~ nostras, subacute inguinal ~, ~ venerea 性病性淋巴肉芽肿 | **poradenia** [ˌpɔurəˈdiːniə] *n*

poradenolymphitis [pəuˌrædinəulimˈfaitis] *n* 性病性淋巴肉芽肿

Porak-Durante syndrome [pəuˈræk djuˈrɑːnt] (Charles Porak; Gustave Durante)波-杜综合征,隐性遗传型成骨不全(Ⅱ型)

poral [ˈpɔːrəl] *a* 孔的,有孔的

porcelain [ˈpɔːsəlin] *n* 瓷,瓷料;瓷器 *a* 瓷制的 | **porcel(l)aneous** [ˌpɔːsəˈleiniəs] *a* 瓷的,瓷状的

porcine [ˈpɔːsain] *a* 猪的

pore [pɔː] *n* 孔,门 | biliary ~ 胆总管 / birth ~ 出生孔,子宫末段(绦虫) / gustatory ~, taste ~

味孔 / slit ~s 裂孔(亦称滤隙) / sweat ~, ~ of sweat duct 汗孔

porencephalia [ˌpɔːrensiˈfeiliə], **porencephaly** [ˌpɔːrenˈsefəli] *n* 脑穿通畸形;孔洞脑 | **porencephalic** [ˌpɔːrensiˈfælik], **porencephalous** [ˌpɔːrenˈsefələs] *a*

porencephalitis [ˌpɔːrenˌsefəˈlaitis] *n* 穿通性脑炎;孔洞脑炎

porfimer sodium [ˈpɔːfimə] 卟吩姆钠(一种血卟啉衍生物,在光动力学疗法中用作光致敏药,治疗食管癌和非小细胞肺癌,静脉内给药)

porfiromycin [ˌpɔːfirəuˈmaisin] *n* 泊非霉素(抗肿瘤抗生素)

Porges-Meier test (reaction) [ˈpɔːgəsˈmaiə] (Otto Porges; Georg Meier)波格斯-迈尔试验(反应)(检梅毒:取1%卵磷脂生理盐水乳液与等量血清混合,静置5小时,随后加患者血清,如为梅毒患者,卵磷脂沉淀)

Porges-Salomon test [ˈpɔːgəs ˈzʌlɔmɔn] (Otto Porges; Hugo Salomon)波格斯-扎洛蒙试验(检梅毒:取1%甘氨胆酸钠溶液与等量患者清亮的新鲜血清混合,如为梅毒血清,液体表面有絮状物形成)

pori [ˈpəurai] porus 的复数

Porifera [pəˈrifərə] *n* 多孔动物门(海绵动物门)

porin [ˈpɔːrin] *n* 外膜蛋白

poriomania [ˌpɔːriəuˈmeinjə] *n* 漂泊癖,漂游狂

porion [ˈpəuriən] *n* 耳点(外耳门上缘中点;切牙管后缘中点)

por(o)- [构词成分]管,通道,开口,孔;骨痂,结合

porocarcinoma [ˌpɔːrəuˌkɑːsiˈnəumə] *n* 汗管癌

porocele [ˈpɔːrəsiː] *n* 厚硬性阴囊疝

porocephaliasis [ˌpɔːrəuˌsefəˈlaiəsis], **porocephalosis** [ˌpɔːrəuˌsefəˈləusis] *n* 蛇舌状虫病

Porocephalida [ˌpɔːrəusiˈfælidə] *n* 蛇舌状虫目

Porocephalidae [ˌpɔːrəusiˈfælidiː] *n* 蛇舌状虫科

Porocephalus [ˌpɔːrəuˈsefələs] *n* 蛇舌状虫属,洞头虫属 | ~ armillatus 腕带蛇舌状虫(即 Armillifer armillatus) / ~ constrictus 狭缩蛇舌状虫 / ~ denticulatus 锯齿蛇舌状虫(鼻腔舌形虫蚴)

porofocon [ˌpɔːrəuˈfəukɔn] *n* 包罗福康(疏水性接触镜材料之一,以 A 或 B 表示之)

porokeratosis [ˌpɔːrəuˌkerəˈtəusis] *n* 汗孔角化病 | disseminated superficial actinic ~ 播散性浅表光线性汗孔角化病 | **porokeratotic** [ˌpɔːrəuˌkerəˈtɔtik] *a*

poroma [pəˈrəumə] *n* 汗孔瘤 | eccrine ~ 小汗腺汗孔瘤

poropathy [pəˈrɔpəθi] *n* 毛孔透药疗法

poroplastic [ˌpɔːrəuˈplæstik] *a* 多孔柔韧的

porosis [pəˈrəusis] *n* 骨痂形成;空洞形成 | cerebral ~ 孔洞脑[畸形]

porosity [pəˈrɔsəti] *n* 多孔[性];孔隙率

porotic [pəˈrɔtik] *a* 促结缔组织生长的,促骨痂形成的

porotomy [pəˈrɔtəmi] *n* 尿道口切开术

porous [ˈpɔːrəs] *a* 多孔的;能渗透的 |

porphin [ˈpɔːfin] *n* 卟吩

porphobilinogen [ˌpɔːfəubaiˈlinədʒən] *n* 胆色素原

porphobilinogen deaminase [ˌpɔːfəubaiˈlinədʒən diːˈæmineiz] 胆色素原脱氨酶,羟甲基[原]胆色烷合酶

porphobilinogen synthase [ˌpɔːfəubaiˈlinədʒən ˈsinθeis] 胆色素原合酶(此酶遗传性缺乏可致卟啉症,类似急性间歇性卟啉病。亦称 δ-氨基-γ-酮戊酸脱水酶)

porphobilinogenuria [ˌpɔːfəubaiˌlinəudʒəˈnjuəriə, -bi-] *n* 胆色素原尿

porphyran [ˈpɔːfirən] *n* 金属卟啉

porphyria [pɔːˈfiriə, pɔːˈfairiə], **porphyrism** [ˈpɔːfirizəm] *n* 卟啉病

porphyrin [ˈpɔːfirin] *n* 卟啉

porphyrinemia [ˌpɔːfiriˈniːmiə] *n* 卟啉血

porphyrinogen [ˌpɔːfiˈrinədʒən] *n* 卟啉原,还原卟啉

porphyrinopathy [ˌpɔːfiriˈnɔpəθi] *n* 卟啉代谢病

porphyrinuria [ˌpɔːfiriˈnjuəriə], **porphyruria** [ˌpɔːfiˈrjuəriə] *n* 卟啉尿

porphyrismus [ˌpɔːfiˈrisməs] *n* 卟啉病性精神障碍

Porphyromonas [ˌpɔːfirəuˈməunəs] *n* 卟啉单胞菌属

porphyropsin [ˌpɔːfiˈrɔpsin] *n* 视紫[质]

porphyroxine [ˌpɔːfiˈrɔksin] *n* 阿片紫碱

porphyryl [ˈpɔːfiril] *n* 初卟啉,去铁血红素

porridge [ˈpɔridʒ] *n* 麦片粥,粥

Porro's cesarean section [ˈpɔːrəu] (Edoardo Porro)波罗剖腹产术,剖腹产子宫切除术

port [pɔːt] *n* 口,孔

porta [ˈpɔːtə] ([复] **portae** [ˈpɔːtiː]) *n*【拉】门 | ~ of lung 肺门 / ~ of spleen 脾门

portacaval [ˌpɔːtəˈkeivəl] *a* 门[静脉与]腔静脉的

portacid, porte-acid [pɔːtˈæsid] *n* 移酸滴管

portal [ˈpɔtl] *n* 门,入口 *a* 门的(尤指肝门的);门静脉的 | ~ of entry 侵入门户(细菌或其他致病因子入侵机体的途径) / hepatic ~ 肝门

portcaustic [pɔːtˈkɔːstik], **portecaustique** [ˌpɔːtkɔːˈstiːk] *n* 腐蚀药把持器

porte-aiguille [ˌpɔːt eiˈgiːl] *n*【法】(外科医师用的)持针器

porte-ligature [ˌpɔːt ˈligətʃə] *n* 深部结扎器,缚线把持器

porte-meche [pɔːt ˈmeʃ] *n* 【法】填塞条器

porte-noeud [pɔːt ˈne] *n* 【法】瘤蒂结扎器

porte-polisher [pɔːt ˈpɔliʃə] *n* 握柄磨光器

Porter-Silber chromogens [ˈpɔːtə ˈsilbə] (Curt C. Porter; Robert H. Silber) 波-西色原(17-羟皮质类固醇与二羟丙酮侧链,在波-西反应中反应积极) | ~ reaction 波-西反应(某些17-羟皮质类固醇〈波-西色原〉的二羟丙酮侧链与酸中苯肼的反应,产生一种黄色;为肾上腺皮质功能的指数,现主要被免疫测定技术所取代)

Porter's sign [ˈpɔːtə] (William H. Porter) 波特尔征,气管牵引感(见于主动脉弓动脉瘤)

Porter's test [ˈpɔːtə] (William H. Porter) 波特试验(检过量尿酸、尿蓝母)

Porteus maze test [ˈpɔːtiəs] (Stanley D. Porteus) 鲍德斯迷津试验(检智力)

portio [ˈpɔːʃiəu] ([复] **portiones** [ˌpɔːʃiˈəuniːz]) *n* 【拉】部,部分

portion [ˈpɔːʃən] *n* 部,部分

portligature [ˌpɔːtˈligətʃə] *n* 深部结扎器,缚线把持器

portoenterostomy [ˌpɔːtəuentəˈrɔstəmi] *n* 肝门肠吻合术

portogram [ˈpɔːtəgræm], **portovenogram** [ˌpɔːtəuˈviːnəgræm] *n* 门静脉造影[照]片

portography [pɔːˈtɔgrəfi], **portovenography** [ˌpɔːtəuviˈnɔgrəfi] *n* 门静脉造影[术]

portojejunostomy [ˌpɔːtəuˌdʒidʒjuːˈnɔstəmi] *n* 门空肠吻合术,肝门肠吻合术

portosystemic [ˌpɔːtəusisˈtemik] *a* 门体循环的(连接门静脉和体静脉循环的)

Portuguese man-of-war [pɔːtjuˈgiːs, ˈpɔːtʃəgiːz] 僧帽水母

porus [ˈpəurəs] ([复] **pori** [ˈpəurai]) *n* 【拉】孔,门

Posada's mycosis, Posada-Wernicke disease [pəˈsɑːdə ˈvəːniki] (Alejandro Posada; Robert Wernicke) 球孢子菌病

posed [pəuzd] *a* (牙)位置的 | normally ~, regularly ~ 正常位置的

-posia [构词成分]饮

position [pəˈziʃən] *n* 位置;姿势;(胎)位 *vt* 给…定位 | anatomical ~ 解剖位置 / coiled ~ 蜷腿位置 / dorsal ~ 背卧位,仰卧位 / dorsal elevated ~ 头高背卧位 / dorsal inertia ~ 惯性背卧位 / dorsal recumbent ~ 屈膝背卧位 / English ~, left lateral recumbent ~, obstetrical ~ 左侧偃卧位,分娩卧位 / horizontal ~ 平仰卧位 / jack-knife ~ 折刀状卧位(仰卧,肩部垫高,腿屈曲) / knee-chest ~ 膝胸卧位 / knee-elbow ~, genucubital ~ 膝肘卧位,膝胸卧位 / kneeling-squatting ~ 蹲位 / lithotomy ~, dorsosacral ~ 膀胱切石卧位,切会阴卧位 / prone ~ 俯卧位,伏卧位 / semiprone ~ 半俯卧位 / semireclining ~ 半卧位,半坐位 / supine ~ 仰卧位,背卧位 / trans ~ 反式构型,反式排列 | **~al** *a* | **~er** *n* 矫正固位器(牙)

positive [ˈpɔzətiv] *a* 正的,阳性的

positrocephalogram [ˌpɔzitrəˈsefələugræm] *n* 阳电子脑瘤定位[描记]图

positron [ˈpɔzitrɔn] *n* 阳电子,正电子

Posner's test (reaction) [ˈpɔsnə] (Carl Posner) 波斯纳试验(反应)(检尿中白蛋白来源)

posology [pəuˈsɔlədʒi] *n* 剂量学 | **posologic** [ˌpəusəˈlɔdʒik] *a*

post [pəust] *n* 杆,柱

post- [前缀]在后,后

postabortal [pəustəˈbɔːtl] *a* 流产后的

postaccessual [pəustækˈseʃuəl] *a* 阵发[发作]后的

postacetabular [ˌpəustæsəˈtæbjulə] *a* 髋臼后的

postacidotic [ˌpəustæsiˈdɔtik] *a* 酸中毒后的

postadolescence [ˌpəustædəuˈlesns] *n* 壮年期 | **postadolescent** *a* 壮年期的 *n* 壮年人

postalbumin [ˌpəustˈælbjumin] *n* 后清蛋白,后白蛋白(一种血清蛋白)

postanal [pəustˈeinəl] *a* 肛门后的

postanesthetic [ˌpəustænisˈθetik] *a* 麻醉后的

postapoplectic [ˌpəustæpəˈplektik] *a* 卒中后的

postaurale [ˌpəustɔːˈreili] *n* 耳郭后点(人体测量学名词)

postauricular [ˌpəustɔːˈrikjulə] *n* 耳郭后的

postaxial [pəustˈæksiəl] *a* 轴后的

postbrachial [pəustˈbreikiəl] *a* 臂后部的

postbrachium [pəustˈbreikiəm] *n* 四叠体下臂

postbuccal [pəustˈbʌkəl] *a* 颊后的

postbulbar [pəustˈbʌlbə] *a* 球后的;延髓后的;十二指肠球部后的

postcapillary [ˌpəustˈkæpiləri] *a* 后毛细管的 *n* 后毛细管,毛细静脉

postcardiotomy [ˌpəustˌkɑːdiˈɔtəmi] *a* 心脏切开术后的

postcatheterization [pəustˌkæθəˌtəraiˈzeiʃən] *a* 插导管术后的

postcava [pəustˈkeivə] *n* 下腔静脉 | **~l** *a*

postcecal [pəustˈsiːkəl] *a* 盲肠后的

postcentral [pəustˈsentrəl] *a* 中央后的,中枢后的

postcentralis [ˌpəustsenˈtreilis] *n* 【拉】中央后沟

postcesarean [ˌpəustsi(ː)ˈzɛəriən] *a* 剖腹产后的

postcibal [pəustˈsaibl] *a* 食后的

post cibum [pəust ˈsaibəm] 【拉】饭后,食后

postcisterna [ˌpəustsis'təːnə] *n* 大池,小脑延髓池
postclavicular [ˌpəustklə'vikjulə] *a* 锁骨后的
postclimacteric [ˌpəustklai'mæktərik] *a* 更年[期]后的;经绝后的
postcoital [pəust'kɔitəl] *a* 性交后的
postcondylar [pəust'kɔndilə] *a* 髁后的
postcondylare [ˌpəustkɔndi'lɛə] *n* (枕骨)髁后点
postconnubial [ˌpəustkə'njuːbiəl] *a* 婚后的
postconvulsive [ˌpəustkən'vʌlsiv] *a* 惊厥后的,抽搐后的
postcordial [pəust'kɔːdiəl] *a* 心后的
postcornu [pəust'kɔːnju] *n* 后角(侧脑室)
postcranial [pəust'kreinjiəl] *a* 颅后的,颅下的
postcubital [pəust'kjuːbitl] *a* 肘后的,前臂背侧的
postcyclodialysis [pəustˌsaiklədai'ælisis] *a* 睫状体分离术后的
postdevelopmental [ˌpəustdiˌveləp'mentl] *a* 发育期后的
postdiastolic [ˌpəustdaiəs'tɔlik] *a* 舒张期后的
postdicrotic [ˌpəustdai'krɔtik] *a* 重波后的
postdigestive [ˌpəustdi'dʒəstiv] *a* 消化后的
postdiphtheric [ˌpəustdif'θerik], **postdiphtheritic** [ˌpəustdifθi'ritik] *a* 白喉后的
postdormitum [pəust'dɔːmitəm] *n* 半醒状态 | **postdormital** *a*
postdysenteric [ˌpəustdisen'terik] *a* 痢疾后的
postecdysis [pəust'ekdisis] *n* 蜕皮后期
postembryonic [ˌpəustembri'ɔnik] *a* 胚后期的
postencephalitic [ˌpəustenˌsefə'litik] *a* 脑炎后的
postepileptic [ˌpəustepi'leptik] *a* 癫痫发作后的
posteriad [pɔs'tiəriæd] *ad* 向体躯后面
posterior [pɔs'tiəriə] *a* 后的,后面的
posterity [pɔs'terəti] *n* 后代
poster(o)- [构词成分]后部,在后
posteroanterior [ˌpɔstərəuæn'tiəriə] *a* 后前[位]的
posteroclusion [ˌpɔstərə'kluːʒən] *n* 后殆,远中殆
posteroexternal [ˌpɔstərəueks'təːnl] *a* 后外的
posteroinferior [ˌpɔstərəuin'fiəriə] *a* 后下的
posterointernal [ˌpɔstərəuin'təːnl] *a* 后内的
posterolateral [ˌpɔstərəu'lætərəl] *a* 后外侧的
posteromedial [ˌpɔstərəu'miːdiəl] *a* 后中的
posteromedian [ˌpɔstərəu'miːdiən] *a* 后正中的
posteroparietal [ˌpɔstərəupə'raiitl] *a* 顶骨后部的
posterosuperior [ˌpɔstərəusjuː'piəriə] *a* 后上的
posterotemporal [ˌpɔstərəu'tempərəl] *a* 颞骨后部的
posterula [pɔs'terjulə] *n*【拉】后鼻腔(鼻甲与鼻后孔之间的腔隙)
postesophageal [pəusti(ː)ˌsɔfə'dʒiːəl] *a* 食管后的
postethmoid [pəust'eθmɔid] *a* 筛骨后的
postexed [pəus'tekst] *a* 后屈的
postexion [pəus'tekʃən] *n* 后屈
postfebrile [pəust'fiːbrail] *a* 发热后的
postganglionic [ˌpəustgæŋgli'ɔnik] *a* (神经)节后的
postglenoid [pəust'gliːnɔid] *a* 关节盂后的
postglomerular [ˌpəustgləu'merjulə] *a* 肾小球后的
postgrippal [pəust'gripl] *a* 流行性感冒后的
posthemiplegic [ˌpəusthemi'pliːdʒik] *a* 偏瘫后的
posthemorrhage [pəust'hemərid ʒ] *n* 继发性出血
posthemorrhagic [pəustˌhemə'rædʒik] *a* 出血后的
posthepatic [ˌpəusthi'pætik] *a* 肝后的
posthepatitic [ˌpəusthepə'titik] *a* 肝炎后的
postherpetic [ˌpəusthəː'petik] *a* 带状疱疹后的
posthetomy [pɔs'θetəmi] *n* 包皮环切术
posthioplasty ['pɔsθiəˌplæsti] *n* 包皮成形术
posthitis [pɔs'θaitis] *n* 包皮炎
posth(o)- [构词成分]包皮
postholith ['pɔsθəliθ] *n* 包皮垢石
posthumous ['pɔstjuməs, -tʃu] *a* 死后的;遗腹的
posthyoid [pəust'haiɔid] *a* 舌骨后的
posthypnotic [ˌpəusthip'nɔtik] *a* 催眠后的
posthypoglycemic [pəustˌhaipəuglai'siːmik] *a* 低血糖后的
posthypophysis [ˌpəusthai'pɔfisis] *n* 垂体后叶
posthypoxic [ˌpəusthi'pɔksik] *n* 低氧后的,氧过少后的
postictal [pəus'tiktl] *a* 发作后的(如急性癫痫发作)
posticus [pɔs'taikəs] *a*【拉】后的,后面的
postinfarction [ˌpəustin'fɑːkʃən] *a* 梗死后的(尤指心肌梗死后的)
postinfluenzal [ˌpəustinflu'enzəl] *a* 流行性感冒后的
postischial [pəust'iskiəl] *a* 坐骨后的
postligation [ˌpəustlai'geiʃən] *a* (血管)结扎后的
postlingual [pəust'liŋgwəl] *a* 学语后的;舌后的
postmalarial [ˌpəustmə'lɛəriəl] *a* 疟疾后的
postmastectomy [ˌpəustmæs'tektəmi] *a* 乳房切除术后的
postmastoid [pəust'mæstɔid] *a* (颞骨)乳突后的
postmature [ˌpəustmə'tjuə] *a* 过度成熟的(如婴儿)
postmaturity [ˌpəustmə'tjuərəti] *n* 过度成熟(指

婴儿)
postmaximal [pəust'mæksiməl] *a* 最高度后的
postmeatal [ˌpəustmi'eitl] *a* 道后的,管口后的
postmediastinum [ˌpəustmiːdiæs'tainəm] *n* 后纵隔 | **postmediastinal** [ˌpəustmiːdiæs'tainl] *a* 纵隔后的;后纵隔的
postmeiotic [ˌpəustmai'ɔtik] *a* 减数分裂后的
postmenopausal [ˌpəustmenə'pɔːzəl] *a* 绝经后的
postmenstrua [pəust'menstruə] *n* 经后期
postmeridian [pəustmə'ridiən] *a* 午后的,午后发生的
postmesenteric [ˌpəustmesən'terik] *a* 肠系膜后的,肠系膜后部的
postminimus [pəust'minimǝs] *n* 副生小指,副生小趾
postmiotic [ˌpəustmai'ɔtik] *a* 减数分裂后的
postmitotic [ˌpəustmai'tɔtik] *a* 有丝分裂期后的
postmortal [pəust'mɔːtl] *a* 死后的
postmortem [pəust'mɔːtam] *a* 死后的 *n* 尸体解剖,验尸
post mortem [pəust 'mɔːtəm]【拉】死后
postnares [pəust'nɛəriːs] *n* 后鼻孔 | **postnarial** *a*
postnasal [pəust'neizəl] *a* 鼻后的
postnatal [pəust'neitl] *a* 出生后的,生后的,产后的
postnecrotic [ˌpəustne'krɔtik] *a* 坏死后的
postneuritic [ˌpəustnjuə'ritik] *a* 神经炎后的
postnuptial [ˌpəust'nʌpʃəl] *a* 婚后的
postocular [pəust'ɔkjulə] *a* 眼球后的
postoperative [pəust'ɔpərətiv] *a* 手术后的 | ~**ly** *ad*
postoral [pəust'ɔːrəl] *a* 口后的
postorbital [pəust'ɔːbitl] *a* 眶后的
postpalatine [pəust'pælətain] *a* 腭后的,腭骨后的
postpaludal [pəust'pæljudəl] *a* 疟疾后的
postparalytic [ˌpəustpærə'litik] *a* 麻痹后的
postpartal [pəust'pɑːtəl] *a* 产后的
postpartum [ˌpəust'pɑːtəm] *a* 产后的
post partum [pəust'pɑːtəm]【拉】产后
postpharyngeal [pəustfə'rindʒiəl] *a* 咽后的
postpituitary [pəustpi'tjuːitəri] *a* 垂体后叶的
postprandial [pəust'prændiəl] *a* 饭后的,食后的
postpuberal [pəust'pjuːbərəl], **postpubertal** [pəust'pjuːbətl], **postpubescent** [ˌpəustpju(ː)'besnt] *a* 青春期后的
postpuberty [pəust'pjuːbəti], **postpubescence** [ˌpəustpju(ː)'besns] *n* 少壮时期,青春期后时期
postpycnotic [ˌpəustpik'nɔtik] *a* 固缩后的(指红细胞)
postradiation [ˌpəustreidi'eiʃən] *a* 照射后的,放射后的
postrenal [pəust'riːnəl] *a* 肾后的
postrolandic [ˌpəustrəu'lændik] *a* 中央沟后的
postsacral [pəust'seikrəl] *a* 骶骨后的,骶骨下的
postscapular [pəust'skæpjulə] *a* 肩胛骨后的
postscarlatinal [ˌpəustskɑːlə'tiːnl] *a* 猩红热后的
Post sing. sed. liq. post singulas sedes liquidas【拉】每次稀便后
postsinusoidal [ˌpəustsainə'sɔidəl] *a* 窦状隙后的
postsphenoid [pəust'sfiːnɔid] *n* 后蝶骨(结合后的蝶骨)
postsphenoidal [ˌpəustsfə'nɔidəl] *a* 后蝶骨的
postsphygmic [pəust'sfigmik] *a* 脉波后的
postsplenectomy [ˌpəustspli'nektəmi] *a* 脾切除术后的
postsplenic [pəust'splenik] *a* 脾后的
poststenotic [ˌpəuststi'nɔtik] *a* 狭窄后的
poststertorous [pəust'stəːtərəs] *a* (麻醉)鼾息期后的
post-streptococcal [pəust ˌstreptəu'kɔkəl] *a* 链球菌感染后的
postsylvian [pəust'silviən] *a* 大脑侧裂后的
postsynaptic [ˌpəustsi'næptik] *a* 突触后的
post-tarsal [pəust 'tɑːsəl] *a* 睑板后的;跗骨后的
postterm [pəust'təːm] *a* 过期的(指妊娠或新生儿)
post-tibial [pəust 'tibiəl] *a* 胫骨后的
post-transcriptional [ˌpəust træns'kripʃənl] *a* 转录后的
post-traumatic [ˌpəust trɔː'mætik] *a* 外伤后的
post-tussis [pəust 'tʌsis] *a*【拉】咳后的
post-typhoid [pəust 'taifɔid] *a* 伤寒后的
posture ['pɔstʃə] *n* 姿势,体位 | fetal ~ 胎势 | **postural** *a*
posturing ['pɔstʃəriŋ] *n* 姿势 | catatonic ~ 紧张性姿势(见于精神分裂症)
posturography [ˌpɔstʃə'rɔgrəfi] *n* 姿势描记[法]
postuterine [pəust'juːtərain] *a* 子宫后的
postvaccinal [pəust'væksinl] *a* 接种后的
postvaccinial [ˌpəustvæk'siniəl] *a* 种痘后的
postvenereal [ˌpəustvə'niriəl] *a* 性交后的
postvital [pəust'vaitl] *a* 死后[染色]的
postwar ['pəust'wɔː] *a* 战后的
postzone ['pəustzəun] *n* 后带(见 zone of antigen excess)
postzoster [pəust'zɔstə] *a* 带状疱疹后的
postzygotic [ˌpəustzai'gɔtik] *a* (受精完成并形成)合子后的

potable [ˈpəutəbl] *a* 可饮的 *n* 饮料

pot AGT potential abnormality of glucose tolerance 葡萄糖耐量潜在异常

Potain's apparatus [pəuˈtein] (Pierre C. E. Potain) 波坦吸引器 | ~ sign 波坦征(①主动脉扩张时,在主动脉弓上叩诊,其浊音界超越胸骨柄至右侧第三肋软骨处;②金属音色)

Potamon [ˈpɔtəmən] *n* 溪蟹属

potash [ˈpɔtæʃ] *n* 钾碱,碳酸钾 | caustic ~ 苛性钾,氢氧化钾 / sulfurated ~ 含硫钾,硫化钾

potassa [pəˈtæsə] *n*【拉】氢氧化钾

potassemia [ˌpɔtəˈsiːmiə] *n* 高钾血[症]

potassic [pəˈtæsik] *a* 含钾的

potassiomercuric [pəˌtæsiəuməːˈkjuərik] *a* 含钾汞的 | ~iodide 碘化钾汞

potassium(K) [pəˈtæsjəm] *n* 钾 | ~ aspartate and magnesium aspartate 天冬氨酸钾和天冬氨酸镁(用作营养物) / ~ bicarbonate 碳酸氢钾 / ~ bromide 溴化钾(镇静药) / ~ chloride 氯化钾(电解质补充剂) / ~ glucaldrate 葡铝酸钾(抗酸药) / ~ gluconate 葡萄糖酸钾(电解质补充剂,用以预防和治疗低钾血症) / ~ hydroxide 氢氧化钾,苛性钾 / ~ metaphosphate 聚偏磷酸钾(药物制剂中用作缓冲剂) / ~ permanganate 高锰酸钾(消毒防腐药) / ~ phenoxymethyl penicillin 苯氧甲基青霉素钾,青霉素 V 钾 / ~ sorbate 山梨酸钾(药物制剂中用作防腐剂)

potation [pəuˈteiʃən] *n* 饮(酒);(酒类)饮料

potato [pəˈteitəu]([复]**potatoes**) *n* 马铃薯

potency [ˈpəutənsi] *n* 力,效力,能力(尤指性交能力、药物的效能和效力、胚胎的发育能力) | prospective ~ 预定潜能(胚胎) / reactive ~ 反应能力(胚胎) | **potence** [ˈpəutəns] *n*

potent [ˈpəutənt] *a* 有力的;有效力的;有性交能力的

potentia [pəuˈtenʃiə] *n*【拉】力,能力

potential [pəuˈtenʃəl] *n* 电位,电势;潜力,潜势 | action ~ 动作电位 / after- ~ 后电位 / bioelectric ~ 生物电位 / biotic ~ 生物潜能 / cochlear ~ 蜗电位 / decalcification ~, caries-producing ~ 脱钙潜势,生龋潜势 / demarcation ~ 损伤电位 / electrode ~ 电极电位 / evoked cortical ~s 皮质激发电位 / excitatory postsynaptic ~(EPSP) 兴奋性突触后电位 / inhibitory postsynaptic ~ (IPSP) 抑制性突触后电位 / generator ~ 发生器电位 / negative after- ~ 负后电位 / negative summating ~ 负总和电位 / pacemaker ~ 起搏点电位 / positive after- ~ 正后电位 / receptor ~ 感受器电位 / redox ~ 电极电位;氧化还原电位,氧还电位 / reproductive ~ 生殖潜能,生物潜能 / resting ~ 静息电位,休止电位 / spike ~ 锋电位 / standard electrode ~, standard reduction ~ ($E°$) 标准电极电位,标准还原电位($E°$) / transmembrane ~ (跨)膜电位 / zeta ~ Z 电位

potentiate [pəˈtenʃieit] *vt* 增强,强化(预先或同时使用另一药物以增强药物的效能) | **potentialization** [pəuˌtenʃəlaiˈzeiʃən, -liˈz-], **potentiation** [pəuˌtenʃiˈeiʃən] *n* / **potentiator** *n* 增效剂

potentiometer [pəˌtenʃiˈɔmitə] *n* 电位计;分压器

potentization [pəuˌtentiˈzeiʃən] *n* 增强,强化

potification [ˌpəutifiˈkeiʃən] *n* 饮水淡化法(如海水淡化)

potion [ˈpəuʃən] *n* 剂量;饮剂

potocytosis [ˌpəutəusaiˈtəusis] *n* 细胞摄液作用,细胞饮液作用

potomania [ˌpəutəuˈmeinjə] *n* [饮]酒狂;震颤性谵妄

Pottenger's sign [ˈpɔtəndʒə] (Francis M. Pottenger)波顿格征(①肺炎及胸膜炎触诊时的肋间肌僵硬;②轻触诊时,有不同程度的阻力,表明:实质器官,若与中空器官比较;肺和胸膜病灶,若与正常器官比较)

Potter's syndrome [ˈpɔtə] (Edith L. Potter)波特综合征(一种罕见病征,有其典型面容,伴肾脏发育不全及其他缺陷,表现为面部扁平,眼距增宽,内眦赘皮,下睑下皱褶,耳大、低位及下垂,小颌及颏下皮肤皱褶,骨畸形如畸形足及关节挛缩亦属常见,婴儿出生后不久即死亡)

Potter treatment [ˈpɔtə] (Caryl A. Potter)波特疗法(治小肠瘘)

Potter version [ˈpɔtə] (Irving W. Potter)波特倒转术(臀先露分娩时徒手进行子宫腔内胎儿倒转术)

Pott's abscess [pɔt] (Percivall Pott)波特脓肿(脊椎结核病脓肿) | ~ aneurysm 波特动脉瘤(动静脉瘤性静脉曲张) / ~ disease 波特病(脊柱结核) / ~ fracture 波特骨折(腓骨下端骨折,同时胫骨下部关节亦有严重损伤,通常是内踝部分破裂,或内外侧韧带破裂) / ~ paraplegia, ~ paralysis 波特截瘫(脊柱骨疽性或脊椎结核性截瘫)

Potts operation [pɔts] (Willis J. Potts)波茨手术(主动脉肺动脉吻合术,作为先天性肺动脉瓣狭窄的一种姑息疗法)

potus [ˈpəutəs] *n*【拉】饮剂

pouch [pautʃ] *n* 囊,窝,陷凹 | abdominovesical ~ 腹壁膀胱陷凹 / branchial ~ 鳃囊 / craniobuccal ~, craniopharyngeal ~ 颅颊囊,颅咽囊 / ileocecal ~ 回盲隐窝 / laryngeal ~ 喉小囊 / paracystic ~ 膀胱旁窝 / pararectal ~ 直肠旁窝(直肠子宫陷凹侧部) / paravesical ~, obturator ~ 膀胱旁窝,闭孔囊 / pharyngeal ~, visceral ~ 咽囊 / rectouterine ~, rectovaginal ~ 直肠子宫陷凹,直肠阴道陷凹 / uterovesical ~, vesicouterine ~ 膀胱子宫陷凹

pouchitis [pautʃ'aitis] *n* 囊炎(黏膜发炎)

poudrage [pu'drɑːʒ] *n*【法】撒布;撒粉法,施用粉剂 | pleural ~ 胸膜撒粉法(用粉剂促使胸膜粘连)

poultice ['pəultis] *n* 泥罨剂,泥敷剂 *vt* 敷泥罨剂 | mustard ~ 芥子泥罨

pound(lb) [paund] *n* 磅(重量单位,1 常衡磅 = 453.592 g,药剂磅 = 373.242 g)

Poupart's ligament [pu'pɑː] (François Poupart) 腹股沟韧带 | ~ line 普帕尔线(腹壁上经腹股沟韧带中点的垂直线)

poverty ['pɔvəti] *n* 贫乏,缺少 | emotional ~ 情感贫乏 / ~ of movement 运动缺乏(见于震颤麻痹患者)

povidone ['pəuvidəun] *n* 聚维酮(血容量补充药)

povidone-iodine (PVP-I) ['pəuvidəun 'aiədain] 聚维酮碘(局部抗感染药)

Powassan encephalitis [pəu'wɑːsæn] (Powassan 为加拿大安大略省一城市,1958 年首次在该地观察到此病)波瓦生脑炎(病毒性脑炎的一型,由蜱传病毒所致,十分类似俄罗斯春夏型脑炎) | ~ virus 波瓦生病毒(黄病毒属的一种蜱传病毒,可致美国和加拿大东部地区脑炎)

powder ['paudə] *n* 粉,粉末;粉剂,散剂 | bleaching ~ 漂白粉 / compound chalk ~ 复方白垩散(治腹泻) / compound licorice ~ 复方甘草散 / dusting ~ 撒粉,扑粉 / impalpable ~ 极细粉 / ipecac and opium ~ 阿片吐根散 / sodium bicarbonate and calcium carbonate ~, Sippy ~ No. 1 碳酸氢钠碳酸钙散,一号西皮散 / sodium bicarbonate and magnesium oxide ~, Sippy ~ No. 2 碳酸氢钠氧化镁散,二号西皮散 / tolnaftate ~ 发癣退散,癣退散(局部抗真菌药)

power ['pauə] *n* 力,能力;功率;放大率;幂,乘方 | candle ~ 烛光 / carbon dioxide-combining ~, CO_2-combining ~ 二氧化碳结合力 / resolving ~ 分辨力

pox [pɔks] *n* 痘 | Kaffir ~ 轻型天花,乳白痘,类天花

Poxviridae [ˌpɔks'viridiː] *n* 痘病毒科

poxvirus ['pɔksˌvaiərəs] *n* 痘病毒

PP punctum proximum【拉】近点(调节近点)

PP_1 pyrophosphate 焦磷酸(盐或酯)

PPD purified protein derivative (of tuberculin) 纯蛋白衍生物(结核菌素)

ppg picopicogram 皮皮克(10^{-24} g)

PPLO pleuropneumonia-like organisms 类胸膜肺炎菌

ppm parts per million 百万分之几

PPR peste des petits ruminants 小反刍动物疫

Ppt precipitate 沉淀物;prepared 制备的,精制的

P pulmonale [piː ˌpʌlmə'neili] 肺性 P 波(在心电描记法中的一型,在 Ⅱ, Ⅲ 及 aV_F 导联中的高峰 P 波,表明右心房扩大,常与肺病有关)

PR prosthion 牙槽中点;pulmonic regurgitation 肺动脉回流;punctum remotum【拉】远点(调节远点)

Pr presbyopia 老视;prism 棱镜;praseodymium 镨

PRA panel-reactive antibody 组反应性抗体

practice ['præktis] *n* 实践,实行;练习,实习;行医,医业,开业 | contract ~ 特约医疗 / family ~ 家庭医疗 / general ~ 综合医疗 / group ~ 集体医疗 / panel ~ 保险医业

practitioner [præk'tiʃənə] *n* 行医者,医师 | general ~ 全科医师 / nurse ~ 开业护士

practolol ['præktələl] *n* 普拉洛尔(β 受体阻滞药)

Prader-Willi syndrome ['prɑːdə'vilə] (Andrea Prader; Heinrich Willi) 普拉德-威利综合征(一种先天性病征,特征为圆面、杏型眼、斜视、前额低、性腺功能减退、贪食、早期肌张力减退、不能茁壮成长及智力迟钝)

prae- 见 pre-

praecox ['priːkɔks] *a*【拉】早发的

praeputium [pri'pjuːʃiəm] *n*【拉】包皮

praevia ['priːviə], **praevius** ['priːviəs] *a*【拉】前置的,在前的

pragmatagnosia [ˌprægmətəg'nəuziə] *n* 物体认识不能,物体失认

pragmatamnesia [ˌprægmətæm'niːziə] *n* 物体记忆不能,物体遗忘

pralidoxime [ˌpræli'dɔksiːm] *n* 解磷定(胆碱酯酶再活化剂) | ~ chloride 氯解磷定(解毒药) / ~ iodide 碘解磷定(解毒药) / ~ mesylate 甲磺解磷定(解毒药)

pramipexole dihydrochloride [ˌpræmi'peksɔl] 二盐酸普拉克索(一种非麦角多巴胺激动药,用作抗运动障碍药,治疗帕金森〈Parkinson〉病,口服给药)

pramocaine hydrochloride ['preiməukein] 盐酸普莫卡因(pramoxine hydrochloride 的 INN 和 BAN 名)

pramoxine hydrochloride [prei'mɔksiːn] 盐酸普拉莫辛(局部麻醉药,局部用于皮肤和直肠黏膜,暂时缓解皮肤和直肠疾患有关的疼痛和瘙痒症)

prandial ['prændiəl] *a* 膳食的

pranolium chloride [prei'nəuliəm] 普拉氯铵(具有抗心律失常作用的心抑制药)

praseodymium(Pr) [ˌpreiziəu'dimiəm] *n* 镨(化学元素)

Prasinomonadida [ˌpreisinəuməˈnædidə] *n* 溪滴虫目

P. rat. aetat. pro ratione aetatis【拉】与年龄成正比

pratique [prɑːˈtiːk] *n*【法】(海港)检疫证书
Pratt's test [præt] (Joseph H. Pratt) 普腊特试验(检肾功能)
Prausnitz-Küstner reaction (test) [ˈprausnits ˈkistnə] (Carl W. Prausnitz; Heinz Küstner) 普劳斯尼茨-屈斯特纳反应(试验)(检人体的反应素〈IgE〉的皮肤反应。皮内注射特应性人体的血清,在非特应性人体身上即产生过敏性反应,经 12 小时或更长时间后注射抗原子同一部位,在被转移的血清中存在反应素〈IgE〉抗体,即导致典型的风疹块和潮红反应。由于有传播血清肝炎的危险性,而且血清 IgE 现在可用 RAST 和 RIST 测定,故此试验不再使用)
pravastatin sodium [ˈprævə ˌstætin] 普伐他汀钠(抗高脂血症药)
praxiology [ˌpræksiˈɔlədʒi] *n* 人类行为学
praxis [ˈpræksis] *n* 行为
prazepam [ˈpræzəpæm] *n* 普拉西泮(肌肉松弛药,安定药)
praziquantel [ˌpreiziˈkwɔntəl] *n* 吡喹酮(抗蠕虫药)
prazosin hydrochloride [ˈpreizəsin] 盐酸哌唑嗪(口服抗高血压药)
pre- [前缀]在前
preadaptation [ˌpriːædæpˈteiʃən] *n* 预先适应,前适应
preadipocyte [priːˈædipəˌsait] *n* 前脂肪细胞(脂肪细胞的前体)
preadult [ˌpriːˈædʌlt] *a* 成年期前的
preagonal [priːˈægənl], **preagonic** [priːəˈgɔnik] *a* 濒死前的
prealbumin [priːælˈbjuːmin] *n* 前清蛋白,前白蛋白(即 transthyretin)
prealbuminuric [ˌpriːˌælbjumiˈnjuərik] *a* 蛋白尿前期的
preanal [priːˈeinəl] *a* 肛门前的
preanesthesia [ˌpriːænisˈθiːzjə] *n* 前驱麻醉,准备麻醉 | **preanesthetic** [ˌpriːænisˈθetik] *a* 前驱麻醉的 *n* 前驱麻醉药
preantiseptic [ˌpriːæntiˈseptik] *a* 防腐法[发现]以前的(时期)
preantral [priːˈæntrəl] *a* (成为囊状卵泡前的)卵泡的
preaortic [ˌpriːeiˈɔːtik] *a* 主动脉前的
preaseptic [ˌpriːeiˈseptik] *a* 无菌外科以前的(时期)
preataxic [ˌpriːəˈtæksik] *a* 共济失调前的
preaurale [ˌpriːɔːˈreili] *n* 耳郭前点(头颅测量名词,自耳郭后点之直线,垂直于耳郭的长轴,与耳郭基底相遇之点)
preauricular [ˌpriːɔːˈrikjulə] *a* 耳前的
preaxial [priːˈæksiəl] *a* 轴前的
prebacillary [priːˈbæsiləri] *a* 细胞感染前的
prebacteriological [ˌpriːbækˌtiəriəˈlɔdʒikəl] *a* 细菌学发展以前的
prebase [ˈpriːbeis] *n* 舌根前部
prebeta-lipoprotein [ˌpriːˌbeitəˌ lipəuˈprəutiːn] *n* 前 β-脂蛋白 | sinking ~ 下沉前 β-脂蛋白,Lp(a)脂蛋白
prebetalipoproteinemia [ˌpriːˌbeitəˌlipəuˌprəutiːˈniːmiə] *n* 前 β-脂蛋白血症,高前 β-脂蛋白血症
prebiotic [ˌpriːbaiˈɔtik] *a* 生物[出现]前的
prebladder [priːˈblædə] *n* 膀胱口前腔(在前列腺囊内膀胱口前的宽腔)
prebrachium [priːˈbreikiəm] *n* 四叠体上臂(上丘臂)
precancer [ˈpriːkænsə] *n* 初癌,前期癌
precancerosis [ˌpriːkænsəˈrəusis] *n* 初癌状态,前期癌状态
precancerous [priːˈkænsərəs] *a* 癌前的,癌变前的
precapillary [priːˈkæpiləri] *n* 前毛细血管,后小动脉
precarcinogen [ˌpriːkɑːˈsinədʒən] *n* 前致癌物,前致癌剂(本身不具致癌作用,但进入动物体后能转变为致癌因子的物质)
precarcinomatous [ˌpriːkɑːsiˈnɔmətəs] *a* 癌前期的
precardiac [priːˈkɑːdiæk] *a* 心前的
precardium [priːˈkɑːdiəm] *n* 心口,心窝,心前区
precartilage [priːˈkɑːtilidʒ] *n* 前软骨(胚胎软骨组织)
precava [priˈkeivə] *n* 上腔静脉
precaval [priːˈkeivəl] *a* 上腔静脉的
precementum [ˌpriːsiˈmentəm] *n* 前期牙骨质
precentral [priːˈsentrəl] *a* 中央前的,中枢前的
prechordal [priːˈkɔːdəl] *a* 脊索前的
precipitable [priˈsipitəbl] *a* 可沉淀的 | **precipitability** [priˌsipitəˈbiləti] *n* 沉淀度,沉淀性
precipitant [priˈsipitənt] *n* 沉淀剂
precipitate [priˈsipiteit] *vt* 使沉淀 *vi* 沉淀 [priˈsipitit] *n* 沉淀,沉淀物 | keratic ~s 角膜后沉着物 / sweet ~ 甜味沉淀[物],甘汞 / white ~ 白色沉淀[物],白降汞,氯化氨基汞 | **precipitating** *a* 沉淀的 / **precipitator** *n* 沉淀器
precipitation [priˌsipiˈteiʃən] *n* 沉淀[反应] | group ~ 类属沉淀反应,组沉淀反应,族沉淀反应(一组密切相关的微生物所具有共同的抗原能被特异性抗血清的沉淀素沉淀的现象)
precipitin [priˈsipitin] *n* 沉淀素 | heat ~ 加热沉淀素
precipitinogen [priˌsipiˈtinədʒən] *n* 沉淀原,沉淀素原 | **~ic** [priːsipitinəuˈdʒenik] *a* / **precipi-**

togen [pri'sipitədʒən] *n*
precipitoid [pri'sipitɔid] *n* 类沉淀素
precirrhosis [ˌpriːsi'rəusis] *n* 前期肝硬变
precision [pri'siʒən] *n* 精确性;精密度(在统计学上亦可称为可靠性、可重复性和再现性)
preclavicular [ˌpriːklə'vikjulə] *a* 锁骨前的
preclinical [priː'klinikəl] *a* 临证前期的(临床症状表现前的);临床前的
preclival [priː'klaivəl] *a* (小脑)斜坡前的
preclotting [priː'klɔtiŋ] *n* 预凝血(植入前使患者血液通过一种针织人造血管的间隙,利用纤维蛋白和血小板配置在间隙内,使植入物不易为血液透过,植入后受者的纤维性向内生长物取代纤维蛋白-血小板网)
precocity [pri'kɔsəti] *n* 早熟,过早发育
precoid ['priːkɔid] *a* 类早发痴呆的
precollagenous [ˌpriːkə'lædʒinəs] *a* 前胶原的
precoma [priː'kəumə] *n* 前驱昏迷
precommissure [priː'kɔmisjuə] *n* 前连合
preconditioning [priːkən'diʃəniŋ] *n* 预适应,预处理 | ischemic ~ 缺血预适应,缺血预处理
preconscious [priː'kɔnʃəs] *a* 前意识的
preconvulsant [ˌpriːkən'vʌlsənt], **preconvulsive** [ˌpriːkən'vʌlsiv] *a* 惊厥前的,抽搐前的
precordialgia [ˌpriːkɔːdi'ældʒiə] *n* 心口痛,心前痛
precordium [priː'kɔːdjəm] ([复] **precordia** [priː'kɔːdjə]) *n* 心口,心窝,心前区 | **precordial** *a*
precornu [priː'kɔːnju] *n* 侧脑室前角
precostal [priː'kɔstl] *a* 肋骨前的
precritical [priː'kritikəl] *a* 危象前的
precuneal [priː'kjuːniəl] *a* 楔叶前的
precuneus [priː'kjuːnjəs] *n* 楔前叶 | **precuneate** [priː'kjuːnieit] *a*
precursor [pri(ː)'kəːsə] *n* 先质,前体
predation [pri'deiʃən] *n* 捕食,掠食(指生物体)
predator ['predətə] *n* 捕食者,捕食动物
predentin [priː'dentin] *n* 前期牙本质,前牙本质
prediabetes [ˌpriːdaiə'biːtiːz] *n* 前驱糖尿病
prediastole [ˌpriːdai'æstəli] *n* (心)舒张前期 | **prediastolic** [ˌpriːdaiə'stɔlik] *a* (心)舒张前期的;(心)舒张前的
predicrotic [ˌpriːdai'krɔtik] *a* 重波前的
predigest [ˌpriːdi'dʒest, ˌpriːdai'dʒest] *vt* 预先消化 | **~ion** [ˌpriːdi'dʒestʃən, ˌpriːdai'dʒestʃən] *n*
predispose [ˌpriːdis'pəuz] *vt*, *vi* (使)倾向于;易感染(或接受) | **predisposing** *a* 素因性的,造成素因的 / **predisposition** [ˌpriːˌdispə'ziʃən] *n* 素因,素质
prediverticular [priːˌdaivəː'tikjulə] *a* 憩室前的
prednicarbate [ˌpredni'kaːbeit] *n* 泼尼卡酯(合成皮质类固醇,皮质类固醇反应性皮肤病时局部用于缓解炎症和瘙痒症)
prednimustine [ˌpredni'mʌstiːn] *n* 泼尼莫司汀(抗肿瘤药)
prednisolone [pred'nisələun] *n* 泼尼松龙(糖皮质激素) | ~ acetate 泼尼松龙醋酸酯 / ~ sodium phosphate 泼尼松龙磷酸钠 / ~ sodium succinate for injection 注射用泼尼松龙琥珀酸钠 / ~ succinate 泼尼松龙琥珀酸酯 / ~ tebutate, ~ butylacetate 泼尼松龙叔丁乙酯
prednisone ['prednisəun] *n* 泼尼松(糖皮质激素)
predormitum [pri'dɔːmitəm] *n* 睡前期,半睡期 | **predormital** *a* 睡前的 / **predormitium** [ˌpriːdɔː'miʃiəm] *n*
preeclampsia [ˌpriːe'klæmpsiə] *n* 先兆子痫
preejection [ˌpriːi'dʒekʃən] *n* 排出前的,射出前的
preelacin [priː'eləsin] *n* 前变性弹力蛋白,前弹力素
preembryo [priː'embriəu] *n* 胚前期(表示受精卵发育植入前阶段,受精后头两周发生)
preepiglottic [ˌpriːepi'glɔtik] *a* 会厌前的
preeruptive [ˌpriːi'rʌptiv] *a* [发]疹前的
pre-erythrocytic [ˌpriː iˌriθrəu'sitik] *a* 红细胞前期的
preexcitation [priːˌeksai'teiʃən] *n* 预激(心室部分过早兴奋);预激综合征(见 Wolff-Parkinson-White syndrome) | ventricular ~ 室性预激综合征(见 Wolff-Parkinson-White syndrome)
preflagellate [priː'flædʒeleit] *a* 鞭毛期前的
preformation [ˌpriːfɔː'meiʃən] *n* 预先形成;先成说,预成说(早期生理学家认为完全成形的动植物原是以微小形式存在于生殖细胞之中) | **~ist** *n* 先成说者
prefrontal [priː'frʌntl] *a* 额叶前部的 *n* 筛骨中心部
prefunctional [priː'fʌŋkʃənl] *a* 功能前的
preganglionic [ˌpriːgæŋgli'ɔnik] *a* [神经]节前的
pregenital [priː'dʒenitl] *a* 性前期的(生殖器发育前的)
preglomerular [ˌpriːgləu'merjulə] *a* 肾小球前的
Pregl's test ['preigl] (Fritz Pregl)普雷格尔试验(检肾功能)
pregnancy ['pregnənsi] *n* 妊娠,怀孕;怀孕期 | cervical ~ 宫颈妊娠 / combined ~, heterotopic ~ 复妊娠,异位妊娠 / cornual ~ 宫角妊娠 / ectopic ~, extrauterine ~ 异位妊娠,子宫外妊娠,宫外孕 / exochorial ~ 绒毛膜外妊娠 / false

~, spurious ~ 假妊娠 / hysteric ~, nervous ~, phantom ~ 精神[因素]性假妊娠 / incomplete ~ 未足月妊娠 / interstitial ~, intramural ~, mural ~, parietal ~ 输卵管子宫间妊娠 / intraligamentary ~ 阔韧带内妊娠 / molar ~ 葡萄胎妊娠 / precocious ~ 幼女妊娠 / sarcofetal ~ 胎及葡萄胎妊娠 / sarcohysteric ~ 葡萄胎假妊娠 / stump ~ 残端妊娠 / tubal ~, fallopian ~, oviductal ~ 输卵管妊娠 / tuboligamentary ~, mesenteric ~ 输卵管阔韧带妊娠

pregnane [ˈpregnein] *n* 孕[甾]烷

pregnanediol [ˌpregneinˈdaiɔl] *n* 孕二醇

pregnanetriol [ˌpregneinˈtraiɔl] *n* 孕三醇

pregnant [ˈpregnənt] *a* 妊娠的,有孕的 | fall ~ 怀孕

pregnene [ˈpregniːn] *n* 孕[甾]烯

pregneninolone [ˌpregniːˈninələun] *n* 孕烯醇酮

pregnenolone succinate [pregˈniːnələun] 琥珀酸孕烯诺龙(糖皮质激素,用以治疗类风湿关节炎)

pregonium [priːˈgəuniəm] *n* 下颌角前凹(前颏点)

pregranular [priːˈgrænjulə] *a* 颗粒期前的

pregravidic [ˌpriːgrəˈvidik] *a* 妊娠前的

prehallux [priːˈhælʌks] *n* 蹈前骨

preheat [ˈpriːˈhiːt] *vt* 预热

prehemiplegic [ˌpriːhemiˈpliːdʒik] *a* 偏瘫前的

prehensile [priːˈhensail] *a* 抓握的,捕捉的

prehension [priˈhenʃən] *n* 领会,理解,抓握,捕捉

prehepatic [ˌpriːhiːˈpætik] *a* 肝前的,肝病前的

prehepaticus [ˌpriːhiˈpætikəs] *n* 前肝间质,初肝间质(指胚胎)

Prehn's sign [prein] (D. T. Prehn) 普雷恩征(附睾睾丸炎时提托阴囊可缓解疼痛,但睾丸扭转时则否)

prehormone [priːˈhɔːməun] *n* 前激素

prehyoid [priːˈhaiɔid] *a* 舌骨前的

prehypophysis [ˌpriːhaiˈpɔfisis] *n* 垂体前叶 | **prehypophyseal**, **prehypophysial** [ˌpriːhaipəuˈfiziəl] *a*

preictal [priːˈiktl] *a* 发作前的(如急性癫痫发作)

preicteric [priːikˈterik] *a* 黄疸出现前的(肝病期)

preimmunization [priːˌimjuːnaiˈzeiʃən, -niˈz-] *n* 预先免疫;幼时免疫接种(幼儿期进行人工免疫,如用卡介苗免疫)

preinduction [ˌpriːinˈdʌkʃən] *n* 隔代诱发,前代影响

preinvasive [priːinˈveisiv] *a* 侵袭前的,蔓延前的

Preiser's disease [ˈpraizə] (Georg K. F. Preiser) 普赖泽病(外伤后腕舟骨骨质疏松及萎缩)

Preisz-Nocard bacillus [prais nəuˈkɑːd] (Hugo von Preisz; E. I. E. Nocard) 假结核棒状杆菌

prekallikrein [priːˌkæliˈkriːin] *n* 前激肽释放酶,激肽释放酶原

prelacrimal [priːˈlækriməl] *a* 泪囊前的

prelacteal [priːˈlæktiəl] *a* 哺乳前的

prelaryngeal [ˌpriːlærinˈdʒiːəl] *a* 喉前的

preleukemia [priːljuːˈkiːmiə] *n* 白血病前期 | **preleukemic** [priːljuːˈkiːmik] *a*

prelimbic [priːˈlimbik] *a* 缘前的(尤指卵圆窝缘前的)

prelingual [priːˈliŋgwəl] *a* 学语前的

prelipoid [priːˈlipɔid] *a* 类脂前[阶段]的 *n* 前类脂

pre-β-lipoprotein [ˌpriːbeitəˌlipəuˈprəutiːn] *n* 前β-脂蛋白

preload [ˈpriːləud] *n* 前负荷(舒张末期心脏的机械性状态)

prelocalization [ˌpriːˌləukəlaiˈzeiʃən, -liˈz-] *n* 前定位

prelocomotion [ˌpriːləukəˈməuʃən] *n* 行走前运动(幼儿)

prelum [ˈpriːləm] *n* 【拉】压,加压;加压器

premalignant [ˌpriːməˈlignənt] *a* 恶化前的,癌[症]前期的

premaniacal [ˌpriːməˈnaiəkəl] *a* 躁狂[发作]前的

premarital [priːˈmæritl] *a* 婚前的

premature [ˌpreməˈtjuə, priːməˈtjuə] *a* 早熟的,早产的,早现的 *n* 早产儿 | **prematurity** *n* 早熟

premaxilla [ˌpriːmækˈsilə] *n* 前颌;切牙骨

premaxillary [priːˈmæksiləri, -mækˈsi-] *a* 颌骨前的;切牙骨的 *n* 切牙骨

premedical [priˈmedikəl] *a* 医预科的

premedicant [priːˈmedikənt] *n* 前驱药,术前用药

premedication [ˌpriːmediˈkeiʃən] *n* 麻醉前用药,术前用药法

premeiotic [ˌpriːmaiˈɔtik] *a* 减数分裂前的

premenarche [ˌpriːmiˈnɑːki] *n* 初经前期 | **premenarchal** [ˌpriːmiˈnɑːkəl], **premenarcheal** [ˌpriːmiˈnɑːkiəl] *a*

premenopause [ˌpriːmenəˈpɔːz] *n* 绝经前期

premenstruum [priːˈmenstruəm] ([复] **premenstrua** [priːˈmenstruə]) *n* 【拉】经前期 | **premenstrual** *a* [月]经[期]前的

premie [ˈpriːmi] *n* 早产婴儿

premitotic [ˌpriːmaiˈtɔtik] *a* 有丝分裂前的

premolar(P) [ˌpriːˈməulə] *n* 前磨牙 *a* 磨牙前的

premonition [ˌpriːməˈniʃən] *n* 预感,先兆,预兆 | **premonitory** [priˈmɔnitəri] *a*

premonocyte [priːˈmɔnəsait] *n* 前单核细胞,幼单核细胞

premorbid [priˈmɔːbid] *a* 发病前的
premortal [priːˈmɔːtl] *a* 死前的
premunition [ˌpriːmjuːˈniʃən] *n* 相对免疫,传染[病后]免疫
premunitive [priːˈmjuːnitiv] *a* 预防接种的;传染[病后]免疫的
premyeloblast [priːˈmaiələblæst] *n* 前成髓细胞,原成髓细胞
premyelocyte [priːˈmaiələˌsait] *n* 前髓细胞,早幼粒细胞
prenarcosis [ˌpriːnɑːˈkəusis] *n* 先驱麻醉
prenarcotic [ˌpriːnɑːˈkɔtik] *a* 麻醉[产生]前的
prenares [priˈnɛəriːz] *n* [前]鼻孔
prenasale [ˌpriːneiˈzeili] *n* 鼻尖点,鼻前点(头颅测量名词)
prenatal [priːˈneitl] *a* 产前的,出生前的
preneoplastic [ˌpriːni(ː)əuˈplæstik] *a* 肿瘤[发生]前的
prenylamine [preˈniləmiːn] *n* 普尼拉明(冠状动脉扩张药)
preoccupation [priːˌɔkjuˈpeiʃən] *n* 先占;全神贯注
preoperative [ˌpriːˈɔpərətiv] *a* 手术前的
preoptic [priːˈɔptik] *a* 视交叉前的
preoral [priːˈɔːrəl] *a* 口前的
preoxygenation [priːˌɔksidʒiˈneiʃən] *n* 预充氧[呼吸]法(预防减压病)
prepalatal [priːˈpælətl] *a* 腭前的
preparalytic [ˌpriːpærəˈlitik] *a* 麻痹前的
preparation [ˌprepəˈreiʃən] *n* 制备;制剂,制品;标本 | allergenic protein ~s 变应原性蛋白制剂(用于变应性病的诊断、预防和脱敏) / cavity ~ 洞制[备]法 / corrosion ~ 腐蚀标本 / heart-lung ~ 心肺制备 / impression ~ 按压标本,印片标本
prepartal [priːˈpɑːtl], **prepartum** [priːˈpɑːtəm] *a* 分娩前的;产前的
prepatellar [ˌpriːpəˈtelə] *a* 髌前的
prepatent [priːˈpeitənt] *a* 显露前的,潜伏期的
preperception [ˌpriːpəˈsepʃən] *n* 预觉,预感
preperforative [priːˈpəːfəreitiv] *a* 穿孔前的
preperitoneal [ˌpriːperitəuˈniːəl] *a* 腹膜前的,腹膜外的
prephthisis [priːˈθaisis] *n* 初期肺结核,早期肺结核
preplacental [ˌpriːpləˈsentl] *a* 胎盘形成前的
preponderance [priˈpɔndərəns] *n* 优势 | ventricular ~ 心室优势(两侧心室发育不称) | **preponderant** *a* 占优势的
prepotency [priˈpəutənsi] *n* 优性,优先遗传,遗传优势(一个个体具有较其他个体更强的传递某一特殊性状于下一代的能力) | **prepotent** *a*
prepotential [ˌpriːpəuˈtenʃəl] *n* 前电位
preprandial [priːˈprændiəl] *a* 食前的
preprohormone [ˌpriːprəuˈhɔːməun] *n* 前激素原
preproinsulin [ˌpriːprəuˈinsjulin] *n* 前胰岛素原
preprophage [priːˈprəufeidʒ] *n* 早期前噬菌体
preproprotein [ˌpriːprəuˈprəutiːn] *n* 前蛋白原
preprosthetic [ˌpriːprɔsˈθetik] *a* 修复[术]前的,前假体的
preprotein [priːˈprəutiːn] *n* 前蛋白
prepuberty [priːˈpjuːbəti], **prepubescence** [ˌpriːpjuːˈbesns] *n* 青春期前时期,青春前期 | **prepuberal** [priːˈpjuːbərəl], **prepubertal** [priːˈpjuːbətl], **prepubescent** [ˌpriːpjuːˈbesnt] *a* 青春期前的
prepuce [ˈpriːpjuːs] *n* 包皮 | redundant ~ 包皮过长 | **preputial** [priˈpjuːʃəl] *a*
preputioplasty [priːˈpjuʃiəuˌplæsti] *n* 包皮成形术
preputiotomy [priˌpjuːʃiˈɔtəmi] *n* 包皮切开术
preputium [priˈpjuːʃiəm] *n* 包皮 | ~ clitoris 阴蒂包皮 / ~ penis 阴茎包皮
prepyloric [ˌpriːpaiˈlɔːrik] *a* 幽门前的
prerectal [priːˈrektl] *a* 直肠前的
prerenal [priːˈriːnl] *a* 肾前的
prerennin [priːˈrenin] *n* 前凝乳酶,凝乳酶原
prereproductive [ˌpriːriprəˈdʌktiv] *a* 童年期的,青春期前的
preretinal [priːˈretinl] *a* 视网膜前的
presacral [priːˈseikrəl] *a* 骶骨前的,骶前的
presby- [构词成分]老,老年
presbyatrics [ˌprezbiˈætriks, ˌpres-] *n* 老年医学,老年病学
presbycardia [ˌprezbiˈkɑːdiə, ˌpres-] *n* 老年心脏病
presbycusis [ˌprezbiˈkjuːsis, ˌpres-], **presbyacusia** [ˌprezbiəˈkjuːsiə, ˌpres-] *n* 老年聋
presbyesophagus [ˌprezbii(ː)ˈsɔfəgəs, ˌpres-] *n* 老年性食管(指食管运动功能的改变,由于年老而发生退化性变化的结果所致)
presbyope [ˈprezbiəup, ˈpres-] *n* 老视者
presbyophrenia [ˌprezbiəˈfriːniə, ˌpres-] *n* 老年性精神障碍,老年精神病态
presbyopia [ˌprezbiˈəupiə, ˌpres-], **presbytia** [prezˈbiʃiə, pres-], **presbytism** [ˈprezbitizəm, ˈpres-] *n* 老视 | **presbyopic** [ˌprezbiˈɔpik, ˌpres-] *a*
prescapula [priːˈskæpjulə] *n* 肩胛骨上部
prescapular [priːˈskæpjulə] *a* 肩胛骨前的;肩胛骨上部的
presclerotic [ˌpriːskliəˈrɔtik] *a* 硬化前的
prescribe [prisˈkraib] *vt*, *vi* 开处方

prescription [pris'kripʃən] *n* 处方,药方 | shot-gun ~ 散弹式处方(一种包括多种药物的不合理的处方,期望其中有一二种药物能奏效)
presecretin [priːsi'kriːtin] *n* 前促胰液素
presegmenter [ˌpriːseg'mentə] *n* 裂殖前体(疟原虫)
presenile [priː'siːnail] *a* 早老的 | **presenility** [ˌpriːsi'niləti] *n*
presenium [priː'siːniəm] *n* 老年前期
presentation [ˌprezen'teiʃən] *n* 呈现,显示;先露(产式);传递 | antigen ~ 抗原传递(巨噬细胞的活动,即摄取和部分消化抗原,然后将其表面上已加工的抗原传递给B淋巴细胞和T淋巴细胞) / breech ~, pelvic ~ 臀先露 / footling ~ 足先露 / head ~ 头先露 / longitudinal ~, polar ~ 纵产位 / oblique ~ 斜产位 / parietal ~ 顶先露 / placental ~ 前置胎盘 / transverse ~, torso ~, trunk ~ 横产位 / vertex ~ 顶先露
preseptal [priː'septəl] *a* 隔前的
preservation [ˌprezəː'veiʃən] *n* 保藏,保存,防腐 | myocardial ~ 心肌保护
preservative [pri'zəːvətiv] *a* 防腐的 *n* 防腐剂
presinusoidal [ˌpriːsainə'sɔidəl] *a* 窦状隙前的
presomite [priː'səumait] *n* 体节前胚胎
prespermatid [priː'spəːmətid] *n* 前精细胞,次级精母细胞
presphenoid [priː'sfiːnɔid] *n* 蝶骨前部
presphenoidal [ˌpriːsfə'nɔidəl] *a* 蝶骨前部的
presphygmic [priː'sfigmik] *a* 脉波前的
prespinal [priː'spainl] *a* 棘前的
prespondylolisthesis [priːˌspɔndiləulis'θisis] *n* 初期脊椎前移
pressometer [pre'sɔmitə] *n* 压力测量器
pressor ['presə] *a* 加压的,增压的
pressoreceptive [ˌpresəuri'septiv], **pressosensitive** [ˌpresəu'sensitiv] *a* 压力感受的
pressoreceptor [ˌpresəuri'septə] *n* 压力感受器
pressure (P) ['preʃə] *n* 压力,压 | after ~ 后压觉,残余压觉 / arterial ~ 动脉(血)压 / atmospheric ~ 大气压 / back ~ 反压,回压 / blood ~ 血压 / central venous ~ (CVP) 中心静脉压 / cerebrospinal ~ 脑脊液压 / diastolic ~ 舒张压 / occlusal ~ 殆压 / partial ~ 分压 / positive endexpiratory ~ (PEEP) 呼气末正压(通气) / pulmonary capillary wedge ~ 肺毛细血管楔压 / selection ~ 选择压力(决定某等位基因频率的某基因所产生的效应) / systolic ~ 收缩压
presubiculum [ˌpriːsju'bikjuləm] *n* (海马)下脚前部,海马回钩前部
presumptive [pri'zʌmptiv] *a* 推定的,假定的;预期的,预定的
presuppurative [priː'sʌpjuərətiv] *a* 化脓前的
presylvian [priː'silviən] *a* 大脑侧裂前支的
presymptom [priː'simptəm] *n* 先兆,前驱症状
presymptomatic [ˌpriːsimptə'mætik] *a* 症状发生前的
presynaptic [ˌpriːsi'næptik] *a* 突触前的
presystole [priː'sistəli] *n* (心)收缩前期 | **presystolic** [ˌpriːsis'tɔlik] *a* (心)收缩期前的
pretarsal [priː'tɑːsəl] *a* 跗骨前的;睑板前的
pretectal [priː'tektəl] *a* 顶盖前的
pretectum [priː'tektəm] *n* 顶盖前区(即 pretectal area)
prethrombotic [priːθrɔm'bɔtik] *a* 血栓形成前的
prethyroid [priː'θairɔid] *a* 甲状腺前的,甲状软骨前的
prethyroideal [ˌpriːθai'rɔidiəl], **prethyroidean** [ˌpriːθai'rɔidiən] *a* 甲状腺前的;甲状软骨前的
pretibial [priː'tibiəl] *a* 胫骨前的,胫前的
pretracheal [priːtrə'kiːəl] *a* 气管前的
pretragal [priː'treigəl] *a* 耳屏前的
pretuberculosis [ˌpriːtju(ː)ˌbəːkju'ləusis] *n* 初期结核病
pretuberculous [ˌpriːtju(ː)'bəːkjuləs] *a* 结核发生前的
pretympanic [ˌpriːtim'pænik] *a* 鼓室前的
preurethritis [ˌpriːjuəri'θraitis] *n* 前尿道炎
prev AGT previous abnormality of glucose tolerance 葡萄糖耐量既往异常
prevalent ['prevələnt] *a* 流行的 | **prevalence** ['prevələns] *n* 患病率
prevention [pri'venʃən] *n* 预防
preventive [pri'ventiv] *a* 预防的 *n* 预防措施;预防药
preventorium [ˌpriven'tɔːriəm] *n* 防病疗养院(尤指防痨疗养院)
preventriculus [ˌpriːven'trikjuləs] *n* 贲门
prevertebral [pri'vəːtibrəl] *a* 椎骨前的
prevesical [priː'vesikəl] *a* 膀胱前的
previable [priː'vaiəbl] *a* 还不能生活的(指不能在子宫外生存的胎儿)
previtamin [priː'vaitəmin] *n* 前维生素(维生素先质) | ~H 胡萝卜素
Prévost's law [prei'vɔ] (Jean L. Prévost) 普雷沃定律(一侧大脑有病时,头偏向病侧) | ~ sign 普雷沃征(偏瘫时头与眼球联合偏斜)
Prevotella [ˌpriːvəu'telə] (André R. Prévot) *n* 普雷沃菌属
Preyer's reflex ['praiə] (Thierry W. Preyer) 普赖厄反射(由听觉刺激产生的耳不随意运动) | ~ test 普赖厄试验(检血一氧化碳)
prezone ['priːzəun] *n* 前带,前区(见 prozone)
prezygapophysis [ˌpriːzaigə'pɔfisis] *n* 椎骨上关

节突

prezygotic [priːzaiˈgɔtik] *a* 合子形成前的

prezymogen [priˈzaimədʒən] *n* 前酶原

PRF prolactin releasing factor 催乳素释放因子

priapism [ˈpraiəpizəm] *n* 阴茎异常勃起 | secondary ~ 继发性阴茎异常勃起

priapitis [ˌpraiəˈpaitis] *n* 阴茎炎

priapus [praiˈeipəs] *n* 阴茎

Price-Jones curve (method) [ˈprais ˈdʒəunz] (Cecil Price-Jones)普赖斯·琼斯曲线(法)(表示红细胞大小变化的图解曲线)

prick [prik] *vt* 刺;刺伤,刺痛 *vi* 刺;(感到)刺痛 *n* 刺孔;轻刺

pricking [ˈprikiŋ] *n* 刺;刺痛感

prickle [ˈprikl] *n* 刺;刺痛[感]

prickly [ˈprikli] *a* 多刺的;针刺般痛的

Priessnitz compress (bandage) [ˈpriːsnits] (Vincenz Priessnitz)冷湿敷布

Priestley's mass [ˈpriːstli] (Joseph Priestley)普里斯特利物质(前牙上的绿色沉淀物)

prilocaine hydrochloride [ˈpriləkein] 盐酸丙胺卡因(局部麻醉药)

primaquine phosphate [ˈpriməkwin] 磷酸伯氨喹(抗疟药)

primary [ˈpraiməri] *a* 初级的,初期的;原发的

primate [ˈpraimeit] *n* 灵长类

Primates [praiˈmeitiːz] *n* 灵长目

primed [praimd] *a* 预处理的,已接触抗原的(指免疫系统的细胞已处在被某一抗原特异性地激活的状态)

prime mover [ˈpraim ˈməuvə] 原动肌肉

primer [ˈpraimə] *n* 底料;引物,引子 | cavity ~ 牙洞底料

primeverose [praiˈmevərəus] *n* 樱草糖

primidone [ˈprimidəun] *n* 扑米酮(抗癫痫药)

primigravid [ˌpraimiˈgrævid] *a* 初孕的,初次妊娠的

primigravida [ˌpraimiˈgrævidə] *n* 初孕妇

primipara [praiˈmipərə] ([复] **primiparae** [praiˈmipəriː]) *n* 初产妇

primiparity [ˌpraimiˈpærəti] *n* 初产

primiparous [praiˈmipərəs] *a* 初产的

primite [ˈpraimait] *n* 簇虫前胞

primitiae [praiˈmiʃiiː] *n*【拉】前羊水,初羊水

primitive [ˈprimitiv] *a* 初级的,原始的

primordial [praiˈmɔːdiəl] *a* 原始的

primordium [praiˈmɔːdiəm] ([复] **primordia** [praiˈmɔːdiə]) *n*【拉】原基,始基

primrose [ˈprimrəuz] *n* 报春花,樱草;月见草 | evening ~ 月见草,夜来香;月见草制剂(口服用于特应性湿疹和乳腺痛)

Primula [ˈpraimjulə] *n* 报春花属

primverose [ˈprimvərəuz] *n* 樱草糖,报春花糖

princeps [ˈprinseps] *a*【拉】主要的,首要的

principle [ˈprinsəpl] *n* 原则,原理;成分,要素,物质 | active ~ 有效成分 / antianemia ~, hematinic ~ 抗贫血物质 / follicle-stimulating ~ 促卵泡成熟[激]素,绒[毛]膜促性腺激素 A / immediate ~, organic ~, proximate ~ 直接成分,有机成分,近似成分 / luteinizing ~ 促黄体生成激素,绒[毛]膜促性腺激素 B / pleasure ~ 快乐原则,唯乐原则 / reality ~ 现实原则,唯实原则 / ultimate ~ 化学元素

Pringle's disease [ˈpriŋgl] (John J. Pringle)皮脂腺腺瘤

Prinos [ˈprainɔs] *n* 冬青属

Prinzmetal's angina [ˈprintsmetəl] (Myron Prinzmetal)普林兹梅塔尔心绞痛(变异型心绞痛,血管痉挛性心绞痛)

prion [ˈpraiɔn] *n* 普里昂(又称朊粒)

prism [ˈprizəm] *n* 方晶,棱晶;棱镜 | enamel ~ 釉柱

prisma [ˈprizmə] ([复] **prismata** [ˈprizmətə]) *n*【希】棱晶;棱镜

prismatic [prizˈmætik] *a* 棱晶的,棱晶形的

prismoid [ˈprizmɔid] *a* 棱晶样的

prismoptometer [ˌprizmɔpˈtɔmitə], **prisoptometer** [ˌprizɔpˈtɔmitə] *n* 三棱镜视力计

prismosphere [ˈprizməsfiə] *n* 棱球镜

PRK photorefractive keratectomy 光性屈光性角膜切削术

PRL, Prl prolactin 催乳素 p. r. n. pro re nata【拉】需要时,必要时

Pro proline 脯氨酸

pro- [前缀]前,原;前体

proaccelerin [prəuækˈselərin] *n* 前加速因子,前加速素(凝血因子 V,亦称促凝血球蛋白原,易变因子)

proacrosomal [ˌprəuækrəuˈsəuməl] *a* 原顶体的

Proactinomyces [ˌprəuæktinəuˈmaisiːz] *n* 原放线菌属

proactinomycin [prəuˌæktinəuˈmaisin] *n* 原放线菌素

proactivator [prəuˈæktiveitə] *n* 激活剂前体(在酶的作用下能转化为激活剂的物质) | C3 ~ (C3PA)C3 激活剂前体,B 因子

proadifen hydrochloride [prəuˈædifən] 盐酸普罗地芬(非特异性增效药)

proal [ˈprəuəl] *a* 向前运动的

proamnion [prəuˈæmniən] *n* 前羊膜

proapoptotic [ˌprəuˌæpɔpˈtɔtik] *a* 促[细胞]凋亡的

proarrhythmia [ˌprəuəˈriθmiə] *n* 致心律失常(药物引起的或药物加重的心律失常)

proarrhythmic [ˌprəuə'riθmik] *a* 前心律失常的(引起或加重心律失常的)

proatlas [prəu'ætləs] *n* 前寰椎

proazamine [prə'æzəmiːn] *n* 异丙嗪(抗组胺药)

probability [ˌprɔbə'biləti] *n* 可能性;概率,几率 | significance ~ 显著性概率,P 值

probacteriophage [ˌprəubæk'tiəriəfeidʒ] *n* 前噬菌体

proband ['prəubænd] *n* 先证者(指一个家系中最先发现受影响的个人,男性为 propositus,女性为 proposita)

probang ['prəubæŋ] *n* 除鲠器,食管探子 | ball ~ 球头除鲠器 / bristle ~, horse hair ~ 马鬃除鲠器 / sponge ~ 海绵除鲠器

probarbital [prəu'bɑːbitæl] *n* 普鲁比妥(催眠镇静药)

probation [prə'beiʃən] *n* 检验,鉴定;试用,见习 | **~al**, **~ary** *a* 试用的 | **~er** *n* 见实生;实习护士

probe [prəub] *n* 探子,探针 | blood flow ~ 血流量探测器 / bullet ~ 检弹探子 / drum ~ 声探子 / electric ~, telephonic ~ 电声探子 / eyed ~ 有孔探子 / fiberoptic ~ 纤维光导探子 / lacrimal ~ 泪管探子 / meerschaum ~ 海泡石探子(检铅弹) / oligonucleotide ~ 寡核苷酸探针 / pocket ~ 袋探子 / root canal ~ 根管探子 / scissors ~ 长剪探子 / uterine ~ 子宫探子 / vertebrated ~ 有节探子 / wire ~ 钢丝探子

probenecid [prə'benisid] *n* 丙磺舒(促尿酸排泄药,抗痛风药)

probit ['prɔbit] *n* 概率单位(由百分率变换来的一种变量,主要用于半数效量的统计分析)

proboscis [prəu'bɔsis] *n* 吻,吻突

probucol ['prəubjukəul] *n* 普罗布考(抗胆固醇血症药)

procainamide hydrochloride [prə'keinəmaid] 盐酸普鲁卡因胺(抗心律失常药)

procaine ['prəukein] *n* 普鲁卡因(局部麻醉药) | ~ amide hydrochloride 盐酸普鲁卡因胺(即 procainamide hydrochloride) / ~ hydrochloride 盐酸普鲁卡因

procallus [prə'kæləs] *n* 前驱胼胝,胼胝前肉芽组织

procarbazine hydrochloride [prə'kɑːbəziːn] 盐酸丙卡巴肼(抗肿瘤药)

procarboxypeptidase [ˌprəukɑːˌbɔksi'peptideis] *n* 羧肽酶原

procarcinogen [ˌprəukɑː'sinədʒən] *n* 前致癌物

procaryon [prəu'kæriɔn] *n* 原核

procaryosis [ˌprəukæri'əusis] *n* 原核状态

Procaryotae [prəuˌkæri'əutiː] *n* 原核生物界

procaryote [prəu'kæriəut] *n* 原核生物(指细菌) | **procaryotic** [ˌprəukæri'ɔtik] *a*

procatarctic [ˌprəukə'tɑːktik] *a* 素因性的(指病因)

procatarxis [ˌprəukə'tɑːksis] *n* 素因,素质

procaterol hydrochloride [prəu'kætərɔl] 盐酸丙卡特罗(支气管扩张药)

Procavia [prəu'keiviə] *n* 岩蹄兔属

procedure [prə'siːdʒə] *n* 过程;步骤,程序,操作 | periodic acid / Schiff ~ 过碘酸 / 席夫法 / push-back ~ 推后操作(见 technique 项下相应术语) / V-Y ~ V-Y 法(修补皮肤缺损的一种方法)

procelous [prəu'siːləs] *a* 前凹的

procentriole [prəu'sentriəul] *n* 原中心粒

procephalic [ˌprəusə'fælik] *a* 头前部的

procercoid [prəu'səːkɔid] *n* 前尾蚴,原尾蚴

process ['prɔses, 'prəuses] *n* 过程;方法;突,突起 *vt* 加工,处理 | A. B. C. ~ A. B. C. 法(明矾、血、黏土沉淀清洁法,即 A. B. C. method) / acromial ~, acromion ~ 肩峰 / floccular ~ 绒球(小脑) / folian ~ 锤骨前突 / malar ~ 颧突(上颌骨) / palpebral ~ 泪腺睑部 / sucker ~ 吸盘,吸足 / synovial ~ 滑膜[皱]襞 / temporal ~ of mandible 下颌状冠突 / vermiform ~ 阑尾 / xiphoid ~ 剑突

processor ['prəusesə] *n* 信息处理机 | biological signal ~ 生物信息处理仪

processus [prəu'sesəs] ([复] **processus** [prəu'sesəs]) *n*【拉】突

procheilon [prəu'kailɔn] *n* 唇尖,(上)唇结节

Prochlorophyta [ˌprəuklɔrəu'faitə] *n* 原绿藻门

prochlorpemazine [ˌprəuklɔː'pemәziːn] *n* 甲哌氯丙嗪,丙氯拉嗪(即 prochlorperazine,止吐药)

prochlorperazine [ˌprəuklɔː'perəziːn] *n* 丙氯拉嗪(止吐药) | ~ edisylate 乙二磺酸丙氯拉嗪(止吐药,安定药) / ~ maleate 马来酸丙氯拉嗪(止吐药,安定药)

prochondral [prəu'kɔndrəl] *a* 软骨形成前的

prochordal [prəu'kɔːdəl] *a* 脊索前的

prochoresis [ˌprəukə'riːsis] *n* (食物)推进(运动)

prochorion [prəu'kɔːriɔn] *n* 前绒毛

Prochownick's method [prəu'kɔvnik] (Ludwig Prochownick) 普罗霍夫尼克法(新生儿窒息时的人工呼吸法,即使其头向后仰,同时压迫其胸壁)

prochromatin [prəu'krəumətin] *n* 前染色质(指构成真核仁的物质)

prochromosome [prəu'krəuməsəum] *n* 前染色体(在静止核中所见的类似染色体的构造)

prochymosin [prəu'kaiməsin] *n* 前凝乳酶,凝乳酶原

procidentia [ˌprəusai'denʃiə] *n*【拉】脱垂

procinonide [prəu'sinənaid] *n* 普西奈德(肾上腺皮质类固醇)
procoagulant [ˌprəukəu'ægjulənt] *a* 促凝血的 *n* 前凝血质
procollagen [prəu'kɔlədʒən] *n* 前胶原
procollagen C-endopeptidase [prəu'kɔlədʒən ˌendəu'peptideis] 前胶原C端内肽酶
procollagen C-proteinase [prəu'kɔlədʒən 'prəu-tiːneis] 前胶原C端蛋白酶,前胶原C端内肽酶
procollagen galactosyltransferase [prəu'kɔlə-dʒən gəˌlæktəsil'trænsfəreis] 前胶原半乳糖基转移酶
procollagen glucosyltransferase [prəu'kɔlədʒən ˌgluːkəsil'trænsfəreis] 前胶原葡糖基转移酶
procollagen-lysine 5-dioxygenase [prəu'kɔlə-dʒən 'laisiːn dai'ɔksidʒəneis] 前胶原-赖氨酸5-双加氧酶(lysyl hydroxylase 的 EC 命名法)
procollagen N-endopeptidase [prəu'kɔlədʒən endəu'peptideis] 前胶原N端内肽酶
procollagen N-proteinase [prəu'kɔlədʒən 'prəu-tiːneis] 前胶原N端蛋白酶,前胶原N端内肽酶
procollagen peptidase [prəu'kɔlədʒən 'peptide-is] 前胶原肽酶(特别用于表示前胶原N端内肽酶和前胶原C端内肽酶)
procollagen-proline dioxygenase [prəu'kɔlə-dʒən 'prəuliːn dai'ɔksidʒəneis] 前胶原-脯氨酸双加氧酶(prolyl 4-hydroxylase 的 EC 命名法)
procollagen-proline 3-dioxygenase [prəu'kɔlə-dʒən 'prəupliːn dai'ɔksidʒəneis] 前胶原-脯氨酸3-双加氧酶(prolyl 3-hydroxylase 的 EC 命名法)
proconceptive [ˌprəukən'septiv] *a* 助[受]孕的 *n* 助孕药
proconvertin [ˌprəukən'vəːtin] *n* 前转变素,原转变素,转变加速因子前体(凝血因子Ⅶ)
procreate ['prəukrieit] *vt, vi* 生殖,生育 | **procreation** [ˌprəukri'eiʃən] *n* / **procreative** *a* 生殖的,能生殖的
proctalgia [prɔk'tældʒiə] *n* 肛部痛 | ~ fugax 痉挛性肛部痛
proctatresia [ˌprɔktə'triːziə] *n* 肛门闭锁
proctectasia [ˌprɔktek'teiziə] *n* 直肠扩张
proctectomy [prɔk'tektəmi] *n* 直肠切除术
proctencleisis [ˌprɔkten'klaisis] *n* 直肠狭窄
procteurynter ['prɔktjuːˌrintə] *n* 直肠扩张器
procteurysis [prɔk'tjuərisis] *n* 直肠扩张术
proctitis [prɔk'taitis] *n* 直肠炎 | epidemic gangrenous ~ 流行性坏疽性直肠炎 / radiation ~, factitious ~ 放射性直肠炎,人工性直肠炎(如对子宫颈或子宫进行放射治疗所致)
proct(o)- [构词成分]直肠,肛部
proctocele ['prɔktəsiːl] *n* 直肠突出
proctoclysis [prɔk'tɔklisis] *n* 直肠滴注法
proctococcypexy [ˌprɔktəu'kɔksiˌpeksi] *n* 直肠尾骨固定术
proctocolectomy [ˌprɔktəukəu'lektəmi] *n* 直肠结肠切除术
proctocolitis [ˌprɔktəukɔ'laitis] *n* 直肠结肠炎
proctocolonoscopy [ˌprɔktəuˌkəulə'nɔskəpi] *n* 直肠结肠镜检查
proctocolpoplasty [ˌprɔktəu'kɔlpəˌplæsti] *n* 直肠阴道瘘成形术
proctocystoplasty [ˌprɔktəu'sistəˌplæsti] *n* 直肠膀胱成形术
proctocystotomy [ˌprɔktəusis'tɔtəmi] *n* 直肠膀胱切开术
proctod(a)eum [ˌprɔktə'diːəm] *n* 肛凹;肛道 | **proctod(a)eal** *a*
proctodone ['prɔktədəun] *n* 后肠激素(昆虫)
proctodynia [ˌprɔktəu'diniə] *n* 肛部痛
proctogenic [ˌprɔktəu'dʒenik] *a* 直肠性的
proctography [prɔk'tɔgrəfi] *n* 直肠造影术
proctology [prɔk'tɔlədʒi] *n* 直肠病学 | **proctologic(al)** [ˌprɔktə'lɔdʒik(əl)] *a* / **proctologist** *n* 直肠病学家
proctoparalysis [ˌprɔktəupə'rælisis], **proctoplegia** [ˌprɔktəu'pliːdʒiə] *n* 直肠[肛门]麻痹
proctoperineoplasty [ˌprɔktəuˌperi'niːəˌplæsti], **proctoperineorrhaphy** [ˌprɔktəuˌperini'ɔrəfi] *n* 直肠会阴成形术,直肠会阴缝合术
proctopexy ['prɔktəˌpeksi] *n* 直肠固定术
proctoplasty ['prɔktəˌplæsti] *n* 直肠成形术
proctopolypus [ˌprɔktəu'pɔlipəs] *n* 直肠息肉
proctoptosis [ˌprɔktɔp'təusis] *n* 脱肛,直肠脱垂
proctorrhagia [ˌprɔktə'reidʒiə] *n* 直肠出血
proctorrhaphy [prɔk'tɔrəfi] *n* 直肠缝合术
proctorrhea [ˌprɔktə'riːə] *n* 肛液溢
proctoscope ['prɔktəskəup] *n* 直肠镜 | **proctoscopic** [ˌprɔktəu'skɔpik] *a* 直肠镜的;直肠镜检查的 / **proctoscopy** [prɔk'tɔskəpi] *n* 直肠镜检查[术]
proctosigmoid [ˌprɔktəu'sigmɔid] *n* 直肠乙状结肠
proctosigmoidectomy [ˌprɔktəuˌsigmɔi'dektəmi] *n* 直肠乙状结肠切除术
proctosigmoiditis [ˌprɔktəuˌsigmɔi'daitis] *n* 直肠乙状结肠炎
proctosigmoidopexy [ˌprɔktəusig'mɔidəˌpeksi] *n* 直肠乙状结肠固定术
proctosigmoidoscope [ˌprɔktəusig'mɔidəskəup] *n* 直肠乙状结肠镜
proctosigmoidoscopy [ˌprɔktəuˌsigmɔi'dɔskəpi] *n* 直肠乙状结肠镜检查[术]
proctospasm ['prɔktəspæzəm] *n* 直肠痉挛

proctostasis [prɔkˈtɔstəsis] *n* 直肠积粪
proctostenosis [ˌprɔktəustiˈnəusis] *n* 直肠狭窄
proctostomy [prɔkˈtɔstəmi] *n* 直肠造口术
proctotome [ˈprɔktətəum] *n* 直肠刀
proctotomy [prɔkˈtɔtəmi] *n* 直肠切开术 | external ~ 直肠外切开术 / internal ~ 直肠内切开术
proctotoreusis [ˌprɔktəutəˈruːsis], **proctotresia** [ˌprɔktəuˈtriːziə] *n* 锁肛穿孔术
proctovalvotomy [ˌprɔktəuvælˈvɔtəmi] *n* 直肠瓣切开术
procumbent [prəuˈkʌmbənt] *a* 伏卧的
procurement [prəˈkjuəmənt] *n* 取得,获得 | organ ~ 器官切取
procursive [prəuˈkəːsiv] *a* 前奔的
procurvation [ˌprəukəːˈveiʃən] *n* 前弯,前屈
procuticle [prəuˈkjuːtikl] *n* 前表皮(某些甲壳动物和节肢动物的外骨骼层)
procyclidine hydrochloride [prəˈsaiklidiːn] 盐酸丙环定(抗胆碱能药,用作骨骼肌松弛药,治疗震颤麻痹)
prodigiosin [prəuˌdidʒiˈəusin] *n* 灵杆菌素
prodolic acid [prəuˈdɔlik] 普罗度酸(抗炎药)
prodroma [ˈprɔdrəmə, prəuˈdrəumə] ([复]**prodromata** [prəuˈdrəumətə]) *n* 前驱症状
prodrome [ˈprəudrəum] *n* 前驱症状 | **prodomal** [prəuˈdrəuməl, ˈprɔdrəməl], **prodromic** [prəuˈdrɔmik] *a*
pro-drug [ˈprəu drʌg] *n* 前药
product [ˈprɔdʌkt] *n* 产品,产物 | cleavage ~ 分解产物,分裂产物 / contact activation ~ 接触性活化产物(凝血因子Ⅶ和Ⅵ相互作用的产物,其功能为在内源性凝血激酶形成时激活凝血因子Ⅸ) / decay ~ 衰变产物(亦称子体) / end ~ 最终产物 / fibrinolytic split ~ 溶纤维蛋白性裂解产物(纤维蛋白原片段或由纤维蛋白溶酶降解的纤维蛋白) / fission ~ 核裂产物 / primary gene ~ 一级基因产物(特异性蛋白质或多肽分子,常为酶)
production [prəˈdʌkʃən] *n* 产生,生成 | endogenous heat ~ 内源性产热
productive [prəˈdʌktiv] *a* 生产的;产生新组织的(炎症);生痰的(咳嗽)
proecdysis [prəuˈekdisis] *n* 蜕皮前期
proemial [prəuˈiːmiəl] *a* 前驱的
proencephalon [ˌprəuenˈsefələn] *n* 前脑
proencephalus [ˌprəuenˈsefələs] *n* 裂额露脑畸胎
proenzyme [prəuˈenzaim] *n* 酶原
proerythroblast [ˌprəuiˈriθrəblæst] *n* 原红细胞
proerythrocyte [ˌprəuiˈriθrəsait] *n* 前红细胞
proestrogen [prəuˈestrədʒən] *n* 前雌激素
proestrus [prəuˈestrəs], **proestrum** [prəuˈestrəm] *n* 动情前期,发情前期
Proetz's test [ˈprəuts] (Arthur W. Proetz)普雷茨试验(嗅敏度试验)
profadol hydrochloride [ˈprəufədəul] 盐酸普罗法朵(麻醉性镇痛药)
-profen [后缀]表示布洛芬(ibuprofen)型(丙酸衍生物)的一种抗炎药
profenamine [prəˈfenəmiːn] *n* 普鲁吩胺(即ethopropazine,抗震颤麻痹药)
proferment [prəuˈfəːmənt] *n* 前酶,酶原
professional [prəˈfeʃənl] *a* 职业的,职业性的
professionalize [prəˈfeʃənəlaiz] *vt* 使职业化,使专业化
Professional Standards Review Organization 职业标准评定组织(见 PSRO)
Profeta's immunity [prəuˈfeitə] (Giuseppe Profeta)普罗费塔免疫(梅毒患者的某些子女被认为对梅毒感染有免疫) | ~ law 普罗费塔定律(梅毒患者所生子女对梅毒具有免疫性)
profibrinolysin [ˌprəufaibriˈnɔlisin] *n* 纤维蛋白溶酶原,纤维溶酶原
Profichet's syndrome (disease) [ˌprəufiˈʃei] (Georges C. Profichet)普罗菲歇综合征(病)(大关节附近皮下结石,伴有溃疡、萎缩及神经方面的症状)
profile [ˈprəufail] *n* 外形,全貌,轮廓,侧面图 | antigenic ~ 抗原全貌,抗原轮廓(一种组织或细胞的全部抗原内容和结构)
profilin [prəuˈfilin] *n* 抑制蛋白
profilometry [ˌprəufiˈlɔmətri] *n* 剖面测定 | urethral pressure ~ 尿道压力剖面测定
proflavine [prəuˈfleivin] *n* 原黄素(消毒防腐药)
profluvium [prəuˈfluviəm] *n*【拉】溢出,流出
profondometer [ˌprəufənˈdɔmitə] *n* 深部异物计,异物定位器
profundaplasty [prəˈfʌndəˌplæsti], **profundoplasty** [prəˈfʌndəuˌplæsti] *n* 股深动脉成形术
profundity [prəˈfʌndəti] *n* 深度
profundus [prəˈfʌndəs] *a*【拉】深的
profusion [prəˈfjuːʒən] *n* 丰富,大量
progamous [ˈprɔgəməs] *a* 受精前的(卵)
progaster [ˈprəugæstə] *n* 原肠
progastrin [prəuˈgæstrin] *n* 前[促]胃液素
progenia [prəuˈdʒiːniə] *n* 凸颌
progenital [prəuˈdʒenitl] *a* 生殖器外面的,外阴的
progenitive [prəuˈdʒenitiv] *a* 生殖的,有生殖力的
progenitor [prəuˈdʒenitə] *n* 先祖,祖先,祖代(如 ~ cells 远祖细胞,前期细胞)
progeny [ˈprɔdʒini] *n* 子孙,后裔;后代,子代
progeria [prəuˈdʒiəriə] *n* 早老症(亦称早老性侏儒症)

progestagen [prəuˈdʒestədʒən] *n* 结合孕激素(孕激素类)
progestational [ˌprəudʒesˈteiʃənl] *a* 孕前的,促孕的
progesteroid [prəuˈdʒestərɔid] *n* 类孕酮;孕酮类(包括孕酮和有类似作用的化合物)
progesterone [prəuˈdʒestərəun] *n* 黄体酮,孕酮(孕激素类药)
progestin [prəuˈdʒestin] *n* 孕激素(类);孕酮,黄体酮
progestogen [prəuˈdʒestədʒən] *n* 孕激素
progestomimetic [prəuˌdʒestəumaiˈmetik] *a* 拟孕酮的,类孕酮的
proglossis [prəuˈglɔsis] *n* 舌尖
proglottid [prəuˈglɔtid], **proglottis** [prəuˈglɔtis]([复]**proglottides** [prəuˈglɔtidiːz]) *n* 节片(绦虫)
proglumide [prəuˈgluːmaid] *n* 丙谷胺(抗胆碱药)
prognathism [ˈprɔgnəθizəm], **prognathia** [prɔgˈneiθiə] *n* 凸颌畸形,下颌前突
prognathometer [ˌprɔgnəˈθɔmitə] *n* 颌凸测量器,颌凸计
prognathous [ˈprɔgnəθəs], **prognathic** [prɔgˈnæθik] *a* 凸颌的
prognose [prɔgˈnəus] *vt* 预测(疾病的过程和结局)
prognosis [prɔgˈnəusis] *n* 预后
prognostic [prəgˈnɔstik] *a* 预后的 *n* 预后性症状
prognosticate [prəgˈnɔstikeit] *vt* 预测(疾病的结局) | **prognostication** [prəgˌnɔstiˈkeiʃən] *n*
prognostician [ˌprɔgnɔsˈtiʃən] *n* 预后专家
progoitrin [prəˈgɔitrin] *n* 前致甲状腺肿素,致甲状腺肿素原
progonoma [ˌprəugəˈnəumə] *n* 突变瘤 | melanotic ~ 黑素突变瘤,黑素沉着性神经外胚层瘤
programming [ˈprəuˌgræmiŋ] *n* 程序设计,程序编制 | neurolinguistic ~ 神经语言学程序设计
progranulocyte [prəuˈgrænjuləˌsait] *n* 前髓细胞,早幼粒细胞
progravid [prəuˈgrævid] *a* 孕前的,黄体期的
progression [prəuˈgreʃən] *n* 前进,进展;步态 | backward ~ 后退(见于某些神经疾病的动作) / cross-legged ~ 交叉步态 / metadromic ~ 奔走步态(流行性脑炎后遗症的症状,患者难以缓步,却能疾走)
progressive [prəuˈgresiv] *a* 进行性的
proguanil hydrochloride [prəˈgwænil] 盐酸氯胍(抗疟药)
prohormone [prəuˈhɔːməun] *n* 激素原
proinflammatory [prəuinˈflæmətəri] *a* 能促进炎症的
proinsulin [prəuˈinsjulin] *n* 胰岛素原
pro-invasin [ˌprəu inˈveisin] *n* 前侵袭素(透明质酸酶的前体)
projecting [prəˈdʒektiŋ] *a* 凸出的,突出的 | spikes ~ 钉突样改变
projection [prəˈdʒekʃən] *n* 投射,投影 | eccentric ~ 牵涉性(感觉)投射 / erroneous ~ 投影错误(由于眼肌无力或麻痹所致) / thalamocortical ~s 丘脑皮质投射
prokallikrein [prəuˌkæliˈkriːin] *n* 激肽释放酶原,前激肽释放酶
prokaryon [prəuˈkæriɔn] *n* 原核;原核生物(指细菌)
prokaryosis [ˌprəukæriˈəusis] *n* 原核状态
Prokaryotae [prəuˌkæriˈəutiː] *n* 原核生物界
prokaryote [prəuˈkæriəut] *n* 原核生物 | **prokaryotic** [ˌprəukæriˈɔtik] *a* 原核的;原核生物的
prokinetic [ˌprəukiˈnetik] *a* 促动的(如促胃肠蠕动的药物)
prolabium [prəuˈleibiəm] *n* 前唇
prolactin (PRL, Prl) [prəuˈlæktin] *n* 促乳素
prolactinoma [prəuˌlæktiˈnəumə] *n* 促乳素瘤
prolactoliberin [prəuˌlæktəuˈlibərin] *n* 促乳素释放素
prolactostatin [prəuˌlæktəuˈstætin] *n* 促乳素抑制素
prolamin [prəuˈlæmin] *n* 谷醇溶蛋白
prolan [ˈprəulæn] *n* 绒[毛]膜促性腺激素(~ A 为促卵泡素,绒膜促性腺激素 A, ~ B 为促黄体生成素,绒膜促性腺激素 B)
prolapse [ˈprəulæps] *n* 脱垂,脱出 [prəuˈlæps] *vi*, *vt* 脱垂,下垂 | anal ~, ~ of anus 脱肛 / ~ of the cord 脐带脱垂 / frank ~ 子宫全部脱垂 / ~ of the iris 虹膜脱出 / rectal ~, ~ of rectum 直肠脱垂,脱肛
prolapsus [prəuˈlæpsəs] *n*【拉】脱垂,脱出
prolepsis [prəuˈlepsis] *n* 提早发作 | **proleptic** *a*
proleukocyte [prəuˈljuːkəsait] *n* 前白细胞
prolidase [ˈprəulideis] *n* 氨酰基脯氨酸二肽酶
prolidase deficiency [ˈprəulideis] 氨酰基脯氨酸二肽酶缺乏症(一种常染色体隐性遗传性氨基酸病,由于氨酰基脯氨酸二肽酶缺乏所致。临床表现包括慢性皮肤损害、运动或认知发育受损、反复感染和骨骼畸形)
proliferate [prəuˈlifəreit] *vi*, *vt* 增生,增殖;多育 / **proliferation** [prəuˌlifəˈreiʃən] *n* / **proliferative, proliferous** [prəuˈlifərəs] *a*
prolific [prəuˈlifik] *a* 多产的,多育的,繁殖的
proligerous [prəuˈlidʒərəs] *a* 多育的,繁殖的
prolinase [ˈprəulineis] *n* 脯氨酰氨基酸二肽酶
proline (Pro, P) [ˈprəuliːn] *n* 脯氨酸
proline dehydrogenase [ˈprəuliːn diːˈhaidrədʒ-

əneis] 脯氨酸脱氢酶(此酶缺乏为一种常染色体隐性性状,是高脯氨酸血症Ⅰ型的原因。亦称脯氨酸氧化酶)

proline dipeptidase [ˈprəuliːn daiˈpeptideis] 脯氨酸二肽酶,氨酰基脯氨酸二肽酶

prolinemia [ˌprəuliˈniːmiə] *n* 脯氨酸血

proline oxidase [ˈprəuliːn ˈɔksideis] 脯氨酸氧化酶,脯氨酸脱氢酶

proline racemase [ˈprəuliːn ˈreisəmeis] 脯氨酸消旋酶

prolintane hydrochloride [prəuˈlintein] 盐酸普罗林坦(抗抑郁药)

prolinuria [ˌprəuliˈnjuriə] *n* 脯氨酸尿,高脯氨酸尿

prolyl [ˈprəulil] *n* 脯氨酰

prolyl dipeptidase [ˈprəulil daiˈpeptideis] 脯氨酰二肽酶,脯氨酰氨基酸二肽酶

prolyl 3-hydroxylase [ˈprəulil haiˈdrɔksileis] 脯氨酰 3-羟化酶(在 EC 命名法中称 procollagen-proline 3-dioxygenase)

prolyl 4-hydroxylase [ˈprəulil haiˈdrɔksileis] 脯氨酰 4-羟化酶(在 EC 命名法中称 procollagen-proline dioxygenase)

prolymphocyte [prəuˈlimfəsait] *n* 幼淋巴细胞

promanide [ˈprəumənaid] *n* 葡胺苯砜钠(即 glucosulfone sodium,抗麻风药)

promastigote [prəuˈmæstigəut] *n* 前鞭毛体,前鞭毛型

promazine hydrochloride [ˈprəuməziːn] 盐酸丙嗪(抗精神病药)

promegakaryocyte [ˌprəumegəˈkæriəsait] *n* 幼巨核细胞

promegaloblast [prəuˈmegələuˌblæst] *n* 原巨成红细胞,原巨红细胞

prometaphase [prəuˈmetəfeiz] *n* 前中期(指有丝分裂时期,一般自细胞核膜解体时起)

promethazine hydrochloride [prəuˈmeθəziːn] 盐酸异丙嗪(抗组胺药,具有镇静、止吐作用)

promethestrol dipropionate [prəuˈmeθestrɔl] 丙甲雌酚二丙酸酯(亦称美雌酚二丙酸酯 methestrol dipropionate,合成雌激素)

promethium (**Pm**) [prəˈmiːθiəm] *n* 钷(化学元素)

promine [ˈprəumiːn] *n* 生长促进素,促细胞素(促进细胞的分裂和生长)

prominence [ˈprɔminəns] *n* 隆凸,凸 | tubal ~ 咽鼓管圆枕,咽鼓管隆凸

prominentia [ˌprɔmiˈnenʃiə] ([复] **prominentiae** [ˌprɔmiˈnenʃiiː]) *n* 【拉】隆凸,凸

promitosis [ˌprəumaiˈtəusis] *n* 原有丝分裂

promonocyte [prəuˈmɔnəsait] *n* 幼单核细胞

promontorium [ˌprɔmənˈtɔːriəm] ([复] **promontoria** [ˌprɔmənˈtɔːriə]) *n* 【拉】岬

promontory [ˈprɔməntəri] *n* 岬

promote [prəˈməut] *vt* 促进,助长 | **~r, promotor** *n* 助催化剂,促催化剂;启动子,启动区(位于调节基因和操纵基因之间的一段 DNA 或染色体);助癌剂

promotion [prəˈməuʃən] *n* 促进,助长

promoxolane [prəˈmɔksəlein] *n* 普罗索仑(骨骼肌松弛药、安定药)

promyelocyte [prəuˈmaiələsait] *n* 早幼粒细胞

pronate [ˈprəuneit] *vt* 使…旋前,内转;使伏卧 *vi* 俯卧 | **pronation** [prəuˈneiʃən] *n* 旋前;伏卧,俯卧

pronatoflexor [prəuˌneitəuˈfleksə] *n* 旋前屈肌

pronator [prəuˈneitə] *n* 【拉】旋前肌

prone [prəun] *a* 旋前的;伏的,俯的

pronephros [prəuˈnefrɔs] ([复] **pronephroi** [prəuˈnefrɔai]), **pronephron** [prəuˈnefrɔn] *n* 原肾

pronethalol [prəuˈneθəlɔl], **pronetalol** [prəuˈnetəlɔl] *n* 丙萘洛尔(β 受体阻滞药)

prong [prɔŋ] *n* 尖头(如牙根)

pronograde [ˈprəunəgreid] *a* 俯身步行的(行走时身体与地面平行)

pronometer [prəuˈnɔmitə] *n* 前臂旋转计

pronormoblast [prəuˈnɔːməblæst] *n* 原红细胞

pronucleus [prəuˈnjuːkliəs] *n* 原核,前核 | female ~ 卵原核,雌原核 / male ~ 精原核,雄原核

pro-opiocortin [prəu ˌəupiəuˈkɔːtin] *n* 阿片皮质素原

pro-opiomelanocortin (**POMC**) [prəu ˌəupiəuˌmelənəuˈkɔːtin] (*pro-* + endogenous *opio*ids + *melano*cyte stimulating hormone + *corti*cotropin + *-in*) *n* 阿片促黑激素皮质素原(分子量为 31 000原激素,为 ACTH、促脂素、促黑〈细胞〉激素和内源性类阿片活性肽〈内啡肽和脑啡肽〉的前体)

pro-otic [prəu ˈɔtik] *a* 耳前的

prop [prɔp] *n* 支柱;支持物,支器 | mouth ~ 牙垫

propafenone hydrochloride [ˌprəupəˈfiːnəun] 盐酸普罗帕酮(抗心律失常药)

propagate [ˈprɔpəgeit] *vt* 繁殖;传播 *vi* 繁殖 | **propagative** *a*

propagation [ˌprɔpəˈgeiʃən] *n* 繁殖;传播

propagule [ˈprɔpəgjuːl] *n* 繁殖体

propane [ˈprəupein] *n* 丙烷

propanidid [prəˈpænidid] *n* 丙泮尼地(短效麻醉药)

propanoic acid [ˌprəupəˈnəuik] 丙酸(propionic acid 的系统名)

propanolide [prəˈpænəlaid] *n* 丙内酯,β-丙内酯(消毒药)
propantheline bromide [prəˈpænθəliːn] 溴丙胺太林(抗胆碱药)
proparacaine hydrochloride [prəˈpærəkein] 盐酸丙美卡因(局部麻醉药,结膜局部应用)
propatyl nitrate [ˈprəupətil] 丙帕硝酯(冠状动脉扩张药)
propene [ˈprəupiːn] *n* 丙烯
2-propenenitrile [ˌprəupiːnˈnaitrail] *n* 2-丙烯腈,丙烯腈
propenyl [prəˈpiːnil] *n* 丙烯基
propepsin [prəuˈpepsin] *n* 前胃蛋白酶,胃蛋白酶原
propeptone [prəuˈpeptəun] *n* 前蛋白胨,半胨
propeptonuria [ˌprəupeptəˈnjuəriə] *n* 前蛋白胨尿,半胨尿
properdin [ˈprəupədin] *n* 备解素,p 因子
properitoneal [ˌprəuperitəuˈniːəl] *a* 腹膜外的,腹膜前的
property [ˈprɔpəti] *n* 性质,特性 | colligative ~ 依数性(指溶液的性质)
prophage [ˈprəufeidʒ] *n* 原噬菌体
prophase [ˈprəufeiz] *n* [分裂]前期(指有丝分裂和减数分裂过程的最早一个时期)
prophenpyridamine [ˌprəufənpiˈridəmiːn] *n* 非尼拉敏(即 pheniramine,抗组胺药)
prophylactic [ˌprɔfiˈlæktik] *a* 预防的 *n* 预防用药
prophylaxis [ˌprɔfiˈlæksis] ([复] **prophylaxes** [ˌprɔfiˈlæksiːz]) *n* 预防 | causal ~ 病因预防 / dental ~, oral ~ 牙病预防,口腔病预防
propicillin [ˌprəupiˈsilin] *n* 丙匹西林(即左普匹西林钾 levopropylcillin potassium,抗生素类药)
propidium iodide [prəuˈpidiəm] 碘化丙啶(一种染双链核酸的荧光嵌入染剂,常用于分析细胞 DNA 含量)
propiodal [prəˈpaiədl] *n* 安妥碘(碘制剂)
propiolactone [ˌprəupiəˈlæktəun] *n* 丙内酯,β-丙烯内酯(消毒药)
propiomazine hydrochloride [ˌprəupiəˈmeiziːn] 盐酸丙酰马嗪(镇静药,分娩时用作止吐药)
propionate [ˈprəupiəneit] *n* 丙酸盐
propionate carboxylase [ˈprəupiəneit kɑːˈbɔksileis] 丙酸羧化酶,丙酰-CoA 羧化酶
Propionibacteriaceae [ˌprəupiˌɔnibækˌtiəriˈeisiiː] *n* 丙酸杆菌科
Propionibacterium [ˌprəupiˌɔnibækˈtiəriəm] *n* 丙酸杆菌属 | ~ acnes 痤疮丙酸杆菌 / ~ freudenreichii 费氏丙酸杆菌 / ~ granulosum 颗粒丙酸杆菌 / ~ jensenii 詹氏丙酸杆菌
propionibacterium [ˌprəupiˌɔnibækˈtiəriəm] *n* 丙酸杆菌
propionic acid [ˌprəupiˈɔnik] 丙酸
propionicacidemia [ˌprəupiˌɔnikæsiˈdiːmiə] *n* 丙酸血
propionitrile [ˌprəupiəuˈnaitril] *n* 丙腈,乙基氰
propionyl [ˈprəupiənil] *n* 丙酰[基]
propionyl-CoA carboxylase [ˈprəupiənil kɑːˈbɔksileis] 丙酰-CoA 羧化酶,丙酰辅酶 A 羧化酶(此酶活性缺乏为一种常染色体隐性性状,可致丙酸血症)
propiram fumarate [ˈprəupiræm] 延胡索酸丙吡兰(镇痛药)
proplasmacyte [prəuˈplæzməsait] *n* 幼浆细胞
proplasmin [prəuˈplæzmin] *n* 前纤维蛋白溶酶,纤维蛋白溶酶原
proplastid [prəuˈplæstid] *n* 前质体,原质体
propofol [ˈprəupəufɔl] *n* 丙泊酚(麻醉药)
propons [ˈprəupɔns] *n* 前桥,小桥
proporphyrinogen oxidase [prəupɔːfiˈrinədʒən, prəupɔːˈfrinədʒən ˈɔksideis] 原卟啉原氧化酶
proportion [prəˈpɔːʃən] *n* 比,比率,比例 | mutant ~ 突变体比例 / ~ of aged population 老年人口比例
propositus [prəˈpɔzitəs] ([复] **propositi** [prəˈpɔsitai]) *n* 先证者(见 proband)
propoxycaine hydrochloride [prəˈpɔksikein] 盐酸丙氧卡因(局部麻醉药)
propoxyphene [prəˈpɔksifiːn] *n* 丙氧芬,右丙氧芬(镇痛药) | ~ hydrochloride 盐酸丙氧芬(镇痛药) / ~ napsylate 萘磺酸丙氧芬(镇痛药)
propranolol [prəˈprænəlɔl] *n* 普萘洛尔(β受体阻滞药) | ~ hydrochloride 盐酸普萘洛尔(抗心律失常药,抗高血压药)
proprietary [prəˈpraiətəri] *n* 专卖药,专利药 *a* 专有的,专卖的
proprioception [ˌprəupriəuˈsepʃən] *n* 本体感受
proprioceptive [ˌprəupriəuˈseptiv] *a* 本体感受的
proprioceptor [ˌprəupriəuˈseptə] *n* 本体感受器
propriodcntium [ˌprəupriəuˈdenʃiəm] *n* 牙固有组织
propriospinal [ˌprəupriəuˈspainl] *a* 脊髓固有的
proprotein [prəuˈprəutiːn] *n* 前蛋白
proptometer [prəuˈtɔmitə] *n* 突眼计
proptosis [prɔpˈtəusis] *n* 突出,前垂(尤指眼)
propulsion [prəˈpʌlʃən] *n* 前冲步态,慌促步态 | **propulsive** *a*
propyl [ˈprəupil] *n* 丙基 | ~ gallate 没食子酸丙酯,棓酸丙酯(抗氧化剂) | **~ic** [prəˈpilik] *a*
propylene [ˈprəupiliːn] *n* 丙烯 | ~ glycol 1, 2-丙二醇(用作致湿剂和溶剂)
propylhexedrine [ˌprəupilˈheksədriːn] *n* 丙己君(血管收缩药,使鼻黏膜减轻充血)
propyliodone [ˌprəupiˈlaiədəun] *n* 丙碘酮(支气

管造影剂）

propylparaben [ˌprəupil'pærəbən] *n* 羟苯丙酯（抗真菌药，药物制剂时用作防腐药）

propylthiouracil [ˌprəupilˌθaiə'juərəsil] *n* 丙硫氧嘧啶（抗甲状腺药）

proquazone ['prəukwəzəun] *n* 普罗喹宗（抗炎药）

pro re nata (p. r. n.) [prəu riː 'neitə]【拉】需要时，必要时

prorenin ['prəuriːnin] *n* 前肾素，前血管紧张肽原酶

prorennin [prə*u*'renin] *n* 前凝乳酶，凝乳酶原

prorenoate potassium [prə*u*'renəeit] 丙利酸钾（醛甾酮拮抗药）

proro- [构词成分]突出的前端

Prorocentrum [ˌprəurə*u*'sentrəm] *n* 原甲藻属

Prorodontina [prə*u*ˌrəudɔn'tainə] *n* 前管亚目

proroxan hydrochloride [prə*u*'rɔksən] 盐酸普罗克生（抗肾上腺素能〈α 受体阻滞〉药）

prorsad ['prɔːsæd] *ad* 向前，前向

prorubricyte [prə'rubrisait] *n* 嗜碱性正成红细胞，早幼红细胞

proscillaridin [prə*u*si'læridin] *n* 海葱次苷（强心药）

prosecretin [ˌprəusi'kriːtin] *n* 前促胰液素

prosection [prə*u*'sekʃən] *n*（示教）解剖

prosector [prə*u*'sektə] *n*【拉】（示教）解剖员

prosencephalon [ˌprɔsen'sefəlɔn] *n* 前脑

prosimian [prə*u*'simiən] *n* 原猿，原猴

pros(o)- [前缀] 前，前部

prosoc(o)ele ['prɔsəsiːl] *n* 前脑腔

prosodemic [ˌprɔsə'demik] *a*（以个人接触的方式）缓渐流行的（指疾病）

prosody ['prɔsədi] *n* 语调，语韵；韵律学

prosogaster ['prɔsəˌgæstə] *n* 前肠

prosopagnosia [ˌprɔsəpæg'nəusiə] *n* 面容失认[症]

prosopalgia [ˌprɔsə'pældʒiə] *n* 三叉神经痛 | **prosopalgic** *a*

prosopantritis [ˌprɔsəpæn'traitis] *n* 额窦炎

prosopectasia [ˌprɔsəpek'teiziə] *n* 巨面

prosophenosia [ˌprɔsəfi'nəusiə] *n* 面容失认

Prosopis [prəu'səupis] *n* 豆胶树属

prosoplasia [ˌprɔsə'pleisiə] *n*（组织）分化异常；进行性分化

prosop(o)- [构词成分]面，面部

prosopoanoschisis [ˌprɔsəpə*u*ə'nɔskisis] *n* 面斜裂

prosopodiplegia [ˌprɔsəpə*u*dai'pliːdʒiə] *n* 面肢双瘫（面和一侧下肢瘫痪）

prosopodysmorphia [ˌprɔsəpə*u*dis'mɔːfiə] *n* 单侧面萎缩，半面萎缩

prosoponeuralgia [ˌprɔsəpə*u*njuə'rældʒiə] *n* 面部神经痛

prosopopagus [ˌprɔsə'pɔpəgəs] *n* 面部联胎

prosopoplegia [ˌprɔsəpə*u*'pliːdʒiə] *n* 面神经麻痹，面瘫 | **prosopoplegic** *a*

prosoposchisis [ˌprɔsə'pɔskisis] *n* 面裂[畸形]

prosopospasm [prə'səupəspæzəm] *n* 面肌痉挛

prosoposternodymus [ˌprɔsəpe*u*stəːnə'diməs] *n* 面胸骨联胎畸形

prosopothoracopagus [ˌprɔsəpə*u*ˌθɔːrə'kɔpəgəs] *n* 面胸联胎

prostacyclin [ˌprɔstə'saiklin] *n* 前列环素

prostacyclin synthase [ˌprɔstə'saiklin 'sinθeis] 前列环素合酶，前列腺素 I 合酶

prostaglandin [ˌprɔstə'glændin] *n* 前列腺素 | ~ D_2（PGD_2）前列腺素 D_2 / ~ E_1（PGE_1）前列腺素 E_1（用作前列地尔 alprostadil）/ ~ E_2（PGE_2）前列腺素 E_2（即非专利药名地诺前列酮 dinoprostone）/ ~ F_{2x}（PGF_{2x}）前列腺素 F_{2x}（即非专利药名地诺前列素 dinoprost）/ ~ F_{2x}（PGF_{2x}）tromethamine 前列腺素 F_{2x} 缓血酸胺盐（即地诺前列素氨丁三醇盐 dinoprost tromethamine）/ ~ G_2（PGG_2）前列腺素 G_2 / ~ H_2（PGH_2）前列腺素 H_2 / ~ I_2（PGI_2）前列腺素 I_2（即前列环素 prostacyclin）

prostaglandin-D synthase [ˌprɔstə'glændin 'sinθeis] 前列腺素-D 合酶（亦称内过氧化物-D-异构酶，前列腺素-H_2 D-异构酶）

prostaglandin endoperoxide synthase [prɔstə'glændin ˌendəupe'rɔksaid 'sinθeis] 前列腺素内过氧化物合酶

prostaglandin-E_2 9-reductase [ˌprɔstə'glændin ri'dʌkteis] 前列腺素-E_2 9-还原酶

prostaglandin-E synthase [ˌprɔstə'glændin 'sinθeis] 前列腺素-E 合酶（亦称内过氧化物-E-异构酶，前列腺素-H_2 E-异构酶）

prostaglandin-H_2 D-isomerase [ˌprɔstə'glændin ai'sɔməreis] 前列腺素-H_2 D-异构酶，前列腺素-D 合酶

prostaglandin-H_2 E-isomerase [ˌprɔstə'glændin ai'sɔməreis] 前列腺素-H_2 E-异构酶，前列腺素-E 合酶

prostaglandin-I synthase [ˌprɔstə'glændin 'sinθeis] 前列腺素-I 合酶（此酶主要在血管壁的内皮内起作用。亦称前列环素合酶）

prostaglandin synthase [ˌprɔstə'glændin 'sinθeis] 前列腺素合酶，前列腺素内过氧化物合酶

prostalene ['prɔstəliːn] *n* 前列他林，前列烯（一种前列腺素）

prostanoid ['prɔstənɔid] *n* 前列腺素类（化合物）

prostata ['prɔstətə] *n* 前列腺

prostatalgia [ˌprɔstəˈtældʒiə] *n* 前列腺痛
prostatauxe [ˌprɔstəˈtɔːksi] *n* 前列腺肥大
prostate [ˈprɔsteit] *n*, *a* 前列腺(的) | **prostatic** [prɔsˈtætik] *a*
prostatectomy [ˌprɔstəˈtektəmi] *n* 前列腺切除术 | perineal ~ 经会阴前列腺切除术 / retropubic prevesical ~ 耻骨后膀胱前前列腺切除术 / suprapubic transvesical ~ 耻骨上经膀胱前列腺切除术 / transurethral ~ 经尿道前列腺切除术
prostatelcosis [ˌprɔstətelˈkəusis] *n* 前列腺溃疡
prostaticovesical [prɔsˌtætikəuˈvesikəl] *a* 前列腺膀胱的
prostaticovesiculectomy [prɔsˌtætiˈkəuviˌsikjuˈlektəmi] *n* 前列腺精囊切除术
prostatism [ˈprɔstətizəm] *n* 前列腺病态 | vesical ~ 膀胱(尿潴留)性前列腺病态 | **prostateria** [ˌprɔstəˈtiəriə] *n*
prostatisme [prɔstəˈtiːzəm] *n*【法】前列腺病态 | ~ sans prostate 非前列腺肥大性前列腺病态
prostatitis [ˌprɔstəˈtaitis] *n* 前列腺炎 | **prostatitic** *a*
prostatocystectomy [ˌprɔstətəusisˈtektəmi] *n* 前列腺膀胱切除术,膀胱前列腺切除术
prostatocystitis [ˌprɔstətəusisˈtaitis] *n* 前列腺膀胱炎
prostatocystotomy [ˌprɔstətəusisˈtɔtəmi] *n* 前列腺膀胱切开术
prostatodynia [ˌprɔstətəuˈdiniə] *n* 前列腺痛症
prostatography [ˌprɔstəˈtɔgrəfi] *n* 前列腺 X 线摄影[术]
prostatolith [prɔsˈtætəliθ] *n* 前列腺石
prostatolithotomy [ˌprɔstətəuliˈθɔtəmi] *n* 前列腺石切除术
prostatomegaly [ˌprɔstətəuˈmegəli] *n* 前列腺肥大
prostatometer [ˌprɔstəˈtɔmitə] *n* 前列腺测量器
prostatomyomectomy [ˌprɔstətəuˌmaiəuˈmektəmi] *n* 前列腺肌瘤切除术
prostatorrhea [ˌprɔstətəˈriːə] *n* 前列腺液溢
prostatotomy [ˌprɔstəˈtɔtəmi], **prostatomy** [prɔsˈtætəmi] *n* 前列腺切开术
prostatotoxin [ˌprɔstətəuˈtɔksin] *n* 前列腺毒素
prostatovesical [ˌprɔstətəuˈvesikəl] *a* 前列腺膀胱的,膀胱前列腺的
prostatovesiculectomy [ˌprɔstətəuviˌsikjuˈlektəmi] *n* 前列腺精囊切除术
prostatovesiculitis [ˌprɔstətəuviˌsikjuˈlaitis] *n* 前列腺精囊炎
prostaxia [prəˈstæksiə] *n* 体内蛋白质[分散]稳定
prosternation [ˌprəustəˈneiʃən] *n* 躯干前曲症
prostheca [prɔsˈθiːkə] ([复] **prosthecae** [prɔsˈθiːkiː]) *n* 菌柄(原核细胞的附器);臼叶(某些昆虫的可动性上颚附器)
Prosthecochloris [prɔsˌθiːkəˈklɔːris] *n* 突柄绿菌属
Prosthecomicrobium [prɔsˌθiːkəmaiˈkrəubiəm] *n* 突柄微菌属
prosthesis [prɔsˈθiːsis] ([复] **prostheses** [prɔsˈθiːsiːz]) *n* 修复术;假体(用人造器具代替人体缺损的部分,如假眼、假牙、假肢等) | Cape Town ~ 开普敦修复术(开普敦大学发展起来的一种主动脉瓣代替物,结合心肺分流术插入之) / dental ~ 假牙修复术 / maxillofacial ~ 颌面修复术 / ocular ~ 义眼 | **prosthetic** [prɔsˈθetik] *a* 修复的;假体的
prosthetics [prɔsˈθetiks] *n* 修复学,装补学(假体、假眼、假牙) | dental ~ 口腔修复学 | **prosthetist** [ˈprɔsθətist] *n* 修复学家
prosthion(PR) [ˈprɔsθiɔn] *n* 牙槽中点
prosthodontics [ˌprɔsθəˈdɔntiks], **prosthodontia** [ˌprɔsθəˈdɔnʃiə] *n* 口腔修复学 | **prosthodontic** *a* / **prosthodontist** *n* 口腔修复学家
Prosthogonimus [ˌprɔsθəˈgɔniməs] *n* 前殖吸虫属 | ~ macrorchis 巨睾前殖吸虫
prosthokeratoplasty [ˌprɔsθəˈkerətəˌplæsti] *n* 假角膜修复术,假角膜成形术
Prostomatina [prəˈstəuməˈtainə] *n* 前口亚目
prostrate [ˈprɔstreit] *a* 俯卧的,平卧的;衰竭的,疲惫的 [prɔsˈtreit] *vt* 使俯卧;使平卧;使衰竭,使疲惫
prostration [prɔsˈtreiʃən] *n* 俯卧,平卧;衰竭,虚脱 | heat ~ 中暑衰竭,中暑虚脱 / nervous ~ 神经衰弱
prot- 见 proto-
protactinium(Pa) [ˌprəutækˈtiniəm] *n* 镤(化学元素)
protagon [ˈprəutəgɔn] *n* 初磷脂
protal [ˈprəutl] *a* 先天的;最先的;最初的
protalbumose [prəuˈtælbjuməus] *n* 原朊,初朊
protaminase [prəuˈtæmineis] *n* 鱼精蛋白酶,羧肽酶 B
protamine [ˈprəutəmi(ː)n] *n* 鱼精蛋白 | ~ sulfate 硫酸鱼精蛋白(肝素拮抗药)
Protaminobacter [ˌprəutəˌmainəuˈbæktə] *n* 精蛋白杆菌属
protan [ˈprəutæn] *n* 红色觉变常者;红色盲基因,第一色盲基因(指患有红色盲或红色弱的个体) *a* 红色觉变常的
protandry [prəuˈtændri] *n* 雄性先熟(动物),雄蕊先熟(植物) | **protandrous** [prəuˈtændrəs] *a*
protanomal [ˌprəutəˈnɔməl] *n* 红色弱者,第一色弱者
protanomaly [ˌprəutəˈnɔməli] *n* 红色觉变常(亦

称红色弱或第一色弱) | **protanomalous** [ˌprəutəˈnɔmələs] *a*

protanope [ˈprəutənəup] *n* 红色盲者

protanopia [ˌprəutəˈnəupiə], **protanopsia** [ˌprəutəˈnɔpsiə] *n* 红色盲,第一色盲 | **protanopic** [ˌprəutəˈnɔpik] *a*

Protea [ˈprəutiə] *n*【拉】南非山龙眼属

protean [ˈprəutiən] *a* 变形的 *n* 朊;变态朊(一种不溶的衍生朊)

proteantigen [ˌprəutiˈæntidʒən] *n* 蛋白抗原

protease [ˈprəutieis] *n* 蛋白[水解]酶 | figtree ~ 无花果蛋白酶

protectant [prəˈtektənt] *a* 保护的,防护的 *n* 保护剂,防护剂

protectin [prəˈtektin] *n* 保护素

protection [prəˈtekʃən] *n* 保护,防护

protective [prəˈtektiv] *a* 保护的,防护的 *n* 保护剂,防护剂

protector [prəˈtektə] *n* (催化)保护质;保护器,保护装置 | LATS ~ 长效甲状腺刺激物保护剂

Proteeae [prəˈtiːiiː] *n* 变形杆菌族

proteid(e) [ˈprəutiːd] *n* 蛋白质 | **proteidic** [ˌprəutiˈidik] *a*

proteidin [ˈprəutiːdin] *n* 蛋白溶菌素 | pyocyanase ~ 绿脓菌蛋白溶菌素

proteidogenous [ˌprəutiːˈdɔdʒinəs] *a* 生蛋白[质]的

protein [ˈprəutiːn] *n* 蛋白质 | alcohol-soluble ~ 醇溶蛋白 / allosteric ~ 变构蛋白,别构蛋白 / amyloid A (AA) ~ 淀粉样 A 蛋白,AA 蛋白 / amyloid light chain (AL) ~ 淀粉样轻链蛋白,AL 蛋白 / ~ C 蛋白 C,补体蛋白 / C4 binding ~ C4 结合蛋白,补体 4 结合蛋白 / carrier ~ 载体蛋白(在体外或在体内与半抗原结合的蛋白,使半抗原能激发免疫应答) / cationic ~s 阴离子蛋白 / conjugated ~ 结合蛋白 / cord ~s 脐蛋白 / C-reactive C-反应蛋白 / denatured ~ 变性蛋白 / derived ~ 衍生蛋白 / encephalitogenic ~ 致脑炎蛋白,髓磷脂碱性蛋白 / fibrillar ~ 纤维状蛋白 / ~ hydrolysate 蛋白质水解产物 / immune ~s 免疫蛋白(免疫球蛋白) / incomplete ~, partial ~ 不完全蛋白 / iron-sulfur ~ 铁硫蛋白质 / M ~ M 蛋白质(一种与大肠杆菌细胞膜有关的膜结合载体蛋白) / myelin basic ~ (MBP) 髓磷脂碱性蛋白 / myeloma ~ 骨髓瘤蛋白 / native ~ 天然蛋白 / plasma ~s 血浆蛋白 / racemized ~ 消旋蛋白 / ~ S 蛋白 S(一种维生素 K 依赖性血浆蛋白) / S ~ S 蛋白质(一种补体系统调节蛋白) / serum ~s 血清蛋白 / serum amyloid A (SAA) ~ 血清淀粉样 A 蛋白,SSA 蛋白 / staphylococcal ~ A 葡萄球菌蛋白 A / whole ~ 全蛋白(未分裂的蛋白) | **~aceous** [ˌprəutiiˈneiʃəs] *a*

proteinase [ˈprəutiːneis] *n* 蛋白酶 | clothes-moth ~ 衣蠹蛋白酶

protein disulfide-isomerase [ˈprəutiːn daiˈsʌlfaid aiˈsɔməreis] 蛋白质二硫化物异构酶(亦称二硫化物异构酶)

proteinemia [ˌprəutiːˈniːmiə] *n* 蛋白血症 | broad-beta ~ 宽-β[脂]蛋白血症 / floating-beta ~ 漂浮-β[脂]蛋白血症,宽-β 脂蛋白病

protein-glutamine γ-glutamyltransferase [ˈprəutiːn ˈgluːtəmiːnˌgluːtəmilˈtrænsfəreis] 蛋白质-谷氨酰胺 γ-谷氨酰基转移酶(亦称转谷氨酰胺酶)

proteinic [prəuˈtiːnik, ˌprəutiˈinik] *a* 蛋白[质]的

protein kinase [ˈprəutiːn ˈkaineis] 蛋白激酶

proteinochrome [ˌprəuˈtiːnəkrəum] *n* 蛋白色素

proteinochromogen [ˌprəutiːnəˈkrəumədʒən] *n* 蛋白色素原

proteinogen [ˌprəutiˈinədʒən] *n* 蛋白原

proteinogenous [ˌprəutiːˈnɔdʒinəs] *a* 生蛋白的

proteinogram [prəuˈtiːnəgræm] *n* (血清)蛋白谱

proteinology [ˌprəutiːˈnɔlədʒi] *n* 蛋白[质]学

proteinosis [ˌprəutiːˈnəusis] *n* 蛋白沉积症 | lipid ~ 脂质蛋白沉积症

proteinotherapy [ˌprəutiːnəuˈθerəpi] *n* 蛋白疗法

proteinphobia [ˌprəutiːnˈfəubjə] *n* 蛋白食恐怖,荤食恐怖

protein phosphatase [ˈprəutiːn ˈfɔsfəteis] 蛋白磷酸酶,磷蛋白磷酸酶

proteinpolysaccharide [ˌprəutiːnˌpɔliˈsækəraid] *n* 蛋白多糖(结缔组织基质的成分)

protein-tyrosine kinase [ˈprəutiːn ˈtairəsiːn ˈkaineis] 蛋白-酪氨酸激酶(此酶活性存在于某些膜蛋白内,为某些致癌基因的产物)

protein-tyrosine-phosphatase [ˈprəutiːn ˈtairəsiːn ˈfɔsfəteis] 蛋白-酪氨酸-磷酸酶(此酶活性调节蛋白-酪氨酸激酶的活性,从而可能减少或抑制细胞生长和肿瘤发生)

proteinuria [ˌprəutiːˈnjuəriə] *n* 蛋白尿 | accidental ~, adventitious ~ 偶发性蛋白尿 / cardiac ~ 心脏性蛋白尿 / colliquative ~ 溶化性蛋白尿 / cyclic ~, ~ of adolescence 周期性蛋白尿,青春期蛋白尿 / effort ~, athletic ~ 用力性蛋白尿,运动性蛋白尿 / emulsion ~ 乳剂性蛋白尿 / orthostatic ~ 直立性蛋白尿 / postural ~ 体位性蛋白尿 | **proteinuric** *a*

proteoclastic [ˌprəutiəˈklæstik] *a* 裂蛋白的

proteoglycan [ˌprəutiəˈglaikæn] *n* 蛋白聚糖

Proteoglypha [ˌprəutiˈɔglifə] *n* 前牙类,沟牙类(毒蛇)

proteohormone [ˌprəutiəuˈhɔːməun] *n* 蛋白激素

proteolipid [ˌprəutiəˈlipid], **proteolipin** [ˌprəu-

tiə'lipin] *n* 蛋白脂质

proteolysin [ˌprəuti'ɔlisin] *n* 蛋白分解素,蛋白水解素

proteolysis [ˌprəuti'ɔlisis] *n* 蛋白酶解,蛋白水解 | **proteolytic** [ˌprəutiə'litik] *a* 蛋白水解的 *n* 蛋白水解药

proteome ['prəutiəum] *n* 蛋白质组(从基因组内编码的信息中产生完整的一套蛋白质)

proteometabolism [ˌprəutiəume'tæbəlizəm] *n* 蛋白代谢 | **proteometabolic** [ˌprəutiəuˌmetə'bɔlik] *a*

proteomics [ˌprəuti'əumiks] *n* 蛋白质组学(在各种不同条件下定性和定量研究蛋白质基因组,其中包括蛋白质表达、蛋白质修饰、蛋白质定位和蛋白质功能,以及蛋白质-蛋白质相互作用,作为理解生物过程的一种方法)

Proteomyces [ˌprəutiəu'maisiːz] *n* 毛孢子菌属

proteopepsis [ˌprəutiəu'pepsis] *n* 蛋白消化 | **proteopeptic** *a*

proteopexy ['prəutiəˌpeksi] *n* 蛋白固定 | **proteopexic** [ˌprəutiəu'peksik], **proteopectic** [ˌprəutiəu'pektik] *a*

proteophilic [ˌprəutiəu'filik] *a* 嗜蛋白的(指某些细菌)

proteose ['prəutiəus] *n* 脲(蛋白质的不完全分解物)

Proteosoma [ˌprəutiəu'səumə] *n* 变幻虫属

proteosotherapy [ˌprəutiəusəu'θerəpi] *n* 脲疗法

proteosuria [ˌprəutiəu'sjuəriə] *n* 脲尿

proteotherapy [ˌprəutiəu'θerəpi] *n* 蛋白[质]疗法

proteotoxin [ˌprəutiəu'tɔksin] *n* 蛋白毒素(细菌蛋白和宿主血清相互作用而形成的毒性蛋白质,例如过敏毒素);内毒素

proter ['prəutə] *n* 前子体,前端细胞(原生动物横裂后形成的前端的子体)

Proteroglypha [ˌprəutərə'glifə] *n* 前牙类,沟牙类(毒蛇)

Proteromonadida [ˌprəutəˌrəuməu'nædidə] *n* 原滴虫目

Proteromonas [ˌprəutərə'məunəs] *n* 原滴虫属

proteuria [ˌprəuti'juəriə] *n* 蛋白尿[症] | **proteuric** *a*

Proteus ['prəutiəs, -tjuːs] *n* 变形杆菌属 | ~ hydrophilus 嗜水变形杆菌 / ~ inconstans 无定形杆菌,无恒变形杆菌 / ~ melanovogenes 嗜水气单胞菌 / ~ mirabilis 奇异变形杆菌 / ~ morgani 摩根变形杆菌 / ~ penneri 羽状变形杆菌 / rettgeri 雷特格变形杆菌 / ~ vulgaris 普通变形杆菌

proteus ['prəutiəs] ([复] **protei** ['prəutiai]) *n* 变形杆菌

Proteus syndrome ['prəutiəs] (Proteus 为希腊神话中的海神,善于以多变的形状出现)普鲁透斯综合征(一种罕见的先天性疾患,具有多种表现,包括手足部分巨大症伴掌跖肥厚、痣、偏侧肥大、皮下肿瘤、巨头和其他头颅畸形,以及腹部和骨盆脂肪过多,病因不明,虽然起源是遗传的,据推测可能为常染色体显性遗传)

prothallus [prəu'θæləs] *n* 原叶体(植物)

prothipendyl hydrochloride [prəu'θaipendil] 盐酸丙硫喷地(抗组胺药,镇静药)

prothrombin [prəu'θrɔmbin] *n* 凝血酶原(凝血因子Ⅱ)

prothrombinase [prəu'θrɔmbineis] *n* 凝血酶原酶,促凝血酶原激酶 | extrinsic ~ 外源性促凝血酶原激酶 / intrinsic ~ 内源性促凝血酶原激酶

prothrombinogenic [prəuˌθrɔmbinəu'dʒenik] *a* 促凝血酶原(凝血因子Ⅱ)的

prothrombinopenia [prəuˌθrɔmbinəu'piːniə] *n* 凝血酶原减少[症]

prothyl ['prəuθil] *n* 玄质,始质(见 protyl)

prothymia [prəu'θimiə] *n* 精神活泼

prothymocyte [prəu'θaiməsait] *n* 前胸腺细胞

protide ['prəutaid] *n* 蛋白质

protidemia [ˌprəuti'diːmiə] *n* 蛋白血[症]

protiodide [prəu'taiədaid] *n* 低碘化物,亚碘化物

protirelin [prəu'tairəlin] *n* 普罗瑞林(促甲状腺素释放药)

protist ['prəutist] *n* 原生生物 | eukaryotic ~, higher ~ 真核原生生物 / prokaryotic ~, lower ~ 原核原生生物

Protista [prəu'tistə] *n*【希】原生生物

protistology [ˌprəutis'tɔlədʒi] *n* 原生物学,微生物学 | **protistologist** *a* 原生物学家,微生物学家

protium(^{1}H) ['prəutjəm] *n* 氕(氢的同位素)

prot(o)- [构词成分]原,原始,第一,初

protoalbumose [ˌprəutəu'ælbjuməus] *n* 原脲,初脲

protoanemonin [ˌprəutəuə'nemənin] *n* 原白头翁素

protobiology [ˌprəutəubai'ɔlədʒi] *n* 原生物学(研究比细菌还微小的生命类型,如病毒)

protobios [ˌprəutəu'baiɔs], **protobe** ['prəutəub] *n* 噬菌体

protoblast ['prəutəblæst] *n* 胚细胞,裸细胞;卵核;原[分]裂球 | **~ic** [ˌprəutəu'blæstik] *a*

protobrochal [ˌprəutəu'brəukəl] *a* 卵发育初期的

Protocalliphora [ˌprəutəukə'lifərə] *n* 原丽蝇属

protocaryon [ˌprəutəu'kæriɔn] *n* 原核,初核

protocatechuic acid [ˌprəutəuˌkæti'tʃuːik] 原儿茶酸(平喘消炎药)

protochloride [ˌprəutəu'klɔːraid] *n* 低氯化物,亚

氯化物

protochlorophyll [ˌprəutəuˈklɔːrəfil] *n* 原叶绿素

protochondral [ˌprəutəuˈkɔndrəl] *a* 前软骨的

protochondrium [ˌprəutəuˈkɔndriəm] *n* 前软骨

Protociliata [ˌprəutəuˌsiliˈeitə] *n* 原纤毛亚纲

protociliate [ˌprəutəˈsiliit] *n* 原纤毛虫

Protociliatia [ˌprəutəˌsiliˈeiʃiə] *n* 原纤毛虫亚纲

Protococcidiida [ˌprəutəuˌkɔksiˈdaiidə] *n* 原球孢子菌目

protocol [ˈprəutəkɔl] *n* 科学实验报告;原始记录(尸体剖检、实验或病案时用)

protocone [ˈprəutəkəun] *n* 原尖(上磨牙的近中颊尖)

protoconid [ˌprəutəuˈkəunid] *n* 下原尖(下磨牙的近中颊尖)

protocooperation [ˌprəutəukəuˌɔpəˈreiʃən] *n* 原始互助,基本互助(指生物与生物之间)

protocoproporphyria [ˌprəutəuˌkɔprəpɔːˈfiriə] *n* 原粪卟啉病(指胆汁及粪内原卟啉与粪卟啉过多)

protodiastolic [ˌprəutəuˌdaiəsˈtɔlik] *a* 舒张初期的(即直接在第二心音后)

protoduodenum [ˌprəutəudju(ː)əuˈdiːnəm] *n* 前十二指肠,十二指肠头(从幽门到十二指肠乳头部)

protoelastose [ˌprəutəuiˈlæstəus] *n* 原弹性蛋白脲,半弹性硬蛋白

protofibril [ˌprəutəuˈfaibril] *n* 初原纤维

protogaster [ˈprəutəuˌgæstə] *n* 原肠

protoglobulose [ˌprəutəuˈglɔbjuləus] *n* 原球蛋白脲

protogonocyte [ˌprəutəuˈgəunəsait] *n* 原生殖细胞,原性[原]细胞

protogyny [prəˈtɔdʒini] *n* 雌性先熟(动物),雌蕊先熟(植物) | **protogynous** [prəˈtɔdʒinəs] *a*

protoheme [ˈprəutəhiːm] *n* 血红素

protohemin [ˌprəutəuˈhemin] *n* 氯化血红素

protohydrogen [ˌprəutəuˈhaidrədʒən] *n* 氕(氢的同位素)

protoiodide [ˌprəutəˈaiədaid] *n* 低碘化物,亚碘化物

protokylol hydrochloride [ˌprəutəˈkailɔl] 盐酸普罗托醇(肾上腺素能药,支气管扩张药)

Protomastigida [ˌprəutəumæsˈtidʒidə] *n* 原鞭毛[虫]目

protomere [ˈprəutəmiə] *n* 原粒,胶粒,微胶粒

protomerite [ˌprəutəˈmiərait] *n* (簇虫)前节

protometer [prəuˈtɔmitə] *n* 突眼计,眼球突出测量器

Protominobacter [prəuˈtɔminəˌbæktə] *n* 原胺菌属

Protomonadina [ˌprəutəuˌmɔnəuˈdainə] *n* 原鞭毛[虫]目

proton [ˈprəutɔn] *n* 质子 | **protonic** [prəuˈtɔnik] *a*

protonephridium [ˌprəutəunəˈfridiəm] *n* 原肾管

protonephron [ˌprəutəuˈnefrɔn], **protonephros** [ˌprəutəuˈnefrɔs] *n* 原肾,前肾

protoneuron [ˌprəutəuˈnjuərɔn] *n* 第一神经元(在周围反射弧中);初神经元(低等动物)

protonitrate [ˌprəutəuˈnaitreit] *n* 低硝酸盐

proto-oncogene [ˌprəutəu ˈɔŋkədʒiːn] *n* 原癌基因

protopathic [ˌprəutəuˈpæθik] *a* 粗觉的,原始感觉的

protopectin [ˌprəutəuˈpektin] *n* 原果胶

protophyllin [ˌprəutəuˈfilin] *n* 原叶绿素,氢化叶绿素

Protophyta [ˌprəutəuˈfaitə] *n* 原生植物类

protophyte [ˈprəutəfait] *n* 原生植物

protophytology [ˌprəutəufaiˈtɔlədʒi] *n* 原生植物学

protopine [ˈprəutəpin] *n* 普托品,原阿片碱,前阿片碱

protoplasia [prəutəuˈpleisiə] *n* 初期组织形成

protoplasm [ˈprəutəuplæzəm] *n* 原生质,原浆 | functional ~ 动质,动浆 / superior ~ 内质网 / totipotential ~ 全能原生质,全能原浆 | **~ic** [ˌprəutəuˈplæzmik], **~atic** [ˌprəutəuplæzˈmætik] *a*

protoplast [ˈprəutəplæst] *n* 原生质体 | **~ic** [ˌprəutəuˈplæstik] *a*

protoporphyria [ˌprəutəupɔːˈfiriə] *n* 原卟啉病 | erythrohepatic ~, erythropoietic ~ 红细胞肝性原卟啉病,红细胞生成性原卟啉病

protoporphyrin [ˌprəutəuˈpɔːfirin] *n* 原卟啉

protoporphyrinogen [ˌprəutəuˌpɔːfiˈrinədʒən] *n* 原卟啉原

protoporphyrinogen oxidase [ˌprəutəupɔːfiˈrinədʒən ˈɔksideis] 原卟啉原氧化酶(此酶的遗传性缺乏为一种常染色体显性性状,是混合性卟啉症的原因)

protoporphyrinuria [ˌprəutəuˌpɔːfiriˈnjuəriə] *n* 原卟啉尿

protoproteose [ˌprəutəuˈprəutiəus] *n* 原脲,初脲

protopsis [prəuˈtɔpsis] *n* 眼球突出

protosalt [ˈprəutəsɔːlt] *n* 低盐,低价金属盐

protospasm [ˈprəutəspæzəm] *n* 先兆痉挛(皮质性癫痫早期轻痉挛)

Protospirura [ˌprəutəuspaiˈruːrə] *n* 原旋线虫属 | ~ gracilis 细原旋线虫

protospore [ˈprəutəuspɔː] *n* 原孢子

Protosteliia [ˌprəutəustiˈaiiə] *n* 原星亚纲

Protosteliida [ˌprəutəustiˈlaiidə] *n* 原星目

protostoma [ˌprəutəuˈstəumə] *n* 胚孔
Protostomatida [ˌprəutəustəuˈmætidə] *n* 原口目
protostome [ˈprəutəstəum] *n* 原口动物
Protostomia [ˌprəutəuˈstəumiə] *n* 原口动物类
Protostrongylidae [ˌprəutəustrɔnˈdʒilidiː] *n* 原圆线虫科
Protostrongylus [ˌprəutəuˈstrɔndʒiləs] *n* 原圆线虫属 | ~ rufescens 红色原圆线虫
protosulfate [ˌprəutəuˈsʌlfeit] *n* 低硫酸盐
protosyphilis [ˌprəutəuˈsifilis] *n* 初期梅毒
Prototheca [ˌprəutəuˈθiːkə] *n* 原藻属
protothecosis [ˌprəutəuθiˈkəusis] *n* 原藻病
Prototheria [ˌprəutəuˈθiəriə] *n* 原兽亚纲
prototoxoid [ˌprəutəuˈtɔksɔid] *n* 强性类毒素，强亲和性类毒素(见 protoxoid)
prototroph [ˈprəutətrəuf] *n* 原养型 | **~ic** [ˌprəutəuˈtrɔfik] *a*
prototropy [prəˈtɔtrəpi] *n* 质子移变[作用]，质子转移[作用]
Prototunicatae [ˌprəutəuˌtjuːniˈkeitiː] *n* 原囊壁类
prototype [ˈprəutətaip] *n* 原型
protoveratrine [ˌprəutəuˈverətriːn] *n* 原藜芦碱
protovertebra [ˌprəutəuˈvəːtibrə] *n* 体节；原椎[骨]
protoxide [prəuˈtɔksaid] *n* 低氧化物，亚氧化物
protoxoid [prəuˈtɔksɔid], **protoxeoid** [prəuˈtɔksiɔid] *n* 前类毒素，强性类毒素，强亲和性类毒素(一种对抗毒素的亲和力比毒素还强的类毒素)
Protozoa [ˌprəutəuˈzəuə] *n* 原生动物门
protozoa [ˌprəutəuˈzəuə] protozoon 的复数 | **~l** *a* 原生动物的，原虫的
protozoacide [ˌprəutəuˈzəuəsaid] *a* 杀原生动物的，杀原虫的 *n* 杀原生动物药，杀原虫药
protozoagglutinin [ˌprəutəuˌzəuəˈgluːtinin] *n* 原虫凝集素(在原虫感染时血内形成的凝集素，能与入侵的原虫发生凝集反应)
protozoan [ˌprəutəuˈzəuən] *n*, *a* 原生动物(的)，原虫(的) | **protozoon** [ˌprəutəuˈzəuɔn] *n* ([复] **protozoa** [ˌprəutəuˈzəuə]) *n* | **protozoic** *a*
protozoiasis [ˌprəutəuzəuˈaiəsis], **protozoosis** [ˌprəutəuzəuˈəusis] *n* 原虫病
protozoology [ˌprəutəuzəuˈɔlədʒi] *n* 原生动物学
protozoophage [ˌprəutəuˈzəuəfeidʒ] *n* 噬原虫细胞
protozootherapy [ˌprəutəuˌzəuəuˈθerəpi] *n* 原生动物病疗法，原虫病疗法
protraction [prəˈtrækʃən] *n* (颌)前伸 | mandibular ~ 下颌前伸 / maxillary ~ 上颌前伸
protractor [prəˈtræktə] *n* 钳取器
protransglutaminase [prəuˌtrænzgluːˈtæmineis] *n* 转谷氨酰胺酶原
protriptyline hydrochloride [prəuˈtriptiliːn] 盐酸普罗替林(抗抑郁药)
protrusio [prəˈtruːziəu] *n*【拉】前突，突出 | ~ acetabuli 髋臼前突，(髋)关节内陷
protrusion [prəˈtruːʒən] *n* 前突，突出 | bimaxillary ~ 双颌前突 / intrapelvic ~ 骨盆内前突，(髋)关节内陷
protrusive [prəˈtruːsiv] *a* 突出的
protrypsin [prəuˈtripsin] *n* 前胰蛋白酶，胰蛋白酶原
protuberance [prəˈtjuːbərəns] *n* 隆凸 | ~ of chin 颏隆凸 / laryngeal ~ 喉结 / palatine ~ 腭圆枕，腭隆凸 / transverse occipital ~ 枕骨圆枕 / tubal ~ 咽鼓管圆枕，咽鼓管隆凸
protuberant [prəˈtjuːbərənt] *a* 隆凸的
protuberantia [prətjuːbəˈrænʃiə] *n*【拉】隆凸
protyl(e) [ˈprəutil] *n* 玄质，始质(一种假想中的物质，认为一切化学元素均由此形成)
pro-UK prourokinase 尿激酶原
prourokinase (pro-UK) [ˌprəujuərəuˈkaineis] *n* 尿激酶原(用作治疗性血栓溶解，亦称单链尿激酶型纤溶酶原激活物)
proventriculus [ˌprəuvenˈtrikjuləs] *n* 前胃(指鸟胃腺体部和某些无脊椎动物〈如昆虫〉前肠的一部分)
provertebra [prəˈvəːtibrə] *n* 体节
Providencia [ˌprɔviˈdensiə] (Providence 在美国罗得岛) *n* 普罗维登斯菌属(以前划入变形杆菌属)〈Proteus〉的一种，即无恒变形杆菌) | ~ alcalifaciens 产碱普罗维登斯菌(亦称无恒变形杆菌亚群 A) / ~ rettgeri 雷氏普罗维登斯菌(亦称雷氏变形杆菌) / ~ stuartii 斯氏普罗维登斯菌(亦称无恒变形杆菌亚群 B)
proving [ˈpruːviŋ] *n* 药力试验
provirus [prəuˈvaiərəs] *n* 前病毒，原病毒(动物病毒的染色体组，与宿主细胞的染色体整合，从而复制所有的子细胞)
provisional [prəˈviʒənl] *a* 临时的，暂时性的
provitamin [prəuˈvaitəmin] *n* 维生素原，前维生素(一种维生素的前身，前维生素 A 为胡萝卜素，麦角甾醇称为前维生素 D)
provocation [ˌprɔvəˈkeiʃən] *n* 刺激，激发[作用] | bronchial ~ 支气管激发
provocative [prəˈvɔkətiv] *a* 刺激的，激发的(指激发症状、反射、反应或疗效的出现)
Prowazek-Greeff bodies [prɔˈvɑːtseik greif] (S. J. M. von Prowazek; Carl R. Greeff) 普-格小体，沙眼小体
Prowazek's bodies [prɔˈvɑːtseik] (Stanislas J. M. von Prowazek) 普罗瓦泽克小体(①沙眼小

体;②天花及牛痘小体)

proxazole [ˈprɔksəzəul] *n* 普罗沙唑,胺丙噁二唑(平滑肌松弛药,消炎镇痛药) | ~ citrate 枸橼酸普罗沙唑,枸橼酸胺丙噁二唑

Pro-X dipeptidase [daiˈpeptideis] 脯氨酰氨基酸二肽酶(亦称脯氨酰二肽酶)

proxemics [prɔkˈsiːmiks] *n* 空间关系学,距离效应学(研究人际间相互作用的空间距离的效应以及人际间相互关系定向的影响)

proximad [ˈprɔksimæd] *ad* 向近侧,向近端

proximal [ˈprɔksiməl] *a* 接近的,邻近的,近端的

proximalis [ˌprɔksiˈmeilis] *a*【拉】接近的,邻近的

proximate [ˈprɔksimit] *a* 邻近的,近似的

proximity [prɔkˈsiməti] *n* 接近,近似

proximoataxia [ˌprɔksiməuəˈtæksiə] *n* 近端运动失调,近端共济失调

proximobuccal [ˌprɔksiməuˈbʌkəl] *a* 邻颊的(后牙)

proximoceptor [ˌprɔksiməuˈseptə] *n* 触觉感受器

proximolabial [ˌprɔksiməuˈleibiəl] *a* 邻唇的(前牙)

proximolingual [ˌprɔksiməuˈliŋgwəl] *a* 邻舌的(牙)

prozone [ˈprəuzəun] *n* 前带(在凝集或沉淀反应时,抗体浓度相对高的区不产生反应。当抗体浓度低于前区时,则产生反应。此现象可能只因抗体过剩,或可能因封闭抗体或血清中有非特异性抑制物所致) | **prozonal** [ˈprəuzənl] *a* 附肌带前的;前带的

prozymogen [prəuˈzaimədʒən] *n* 前酶原

PrP prion protein 普里昂蛋白[质]

PRPP phosphoribosylpyrophosphate 磷酸核糖焦磷酸

PRU peripheral resistance unit 外周阻力单位

pruinate [ˈpruːineit] *a* 霜状的,霜掩状的

Prunella [pruˈnelə] *n* 夏枯草属

prunin [ˈpruːnin] *n* 野黑樱素(用于胸部及神经性疾病)

Prunus [ˈpruːnəs] *n*【拉】李属 | ~ americana 美国刺李 / ~ amygdala 苦扁桃(树) / ~ armeniaca 杏(树) / ~ domestica 杏梅,洋李 / ~ laurocerasus 月桂樱(树) / ~ persica 桃(树) / ~ serotina 黑野樱 / ~ spinosa 黑刺李 / ~ virginiana [黑]野樱桃(树)

prurigo [pruəˈraigəu] *n*【拉】痒疹 | ~ agria 重痒疹 / ~ mitis 轻痒疹 / ~ simplex 单纯痒疹 / summer ~ 夏令痒疹 | **pruriginous** [pruəˈridʒinəs] *a*

pruritogenic [ˌpruəritəuˈdʒenik] *a* 引起瘙痒的

pruritus [pruəˈraitəs] *n* 瘙痒[症] | essential ~ 自发性瘙痒 / ~ hiemalis 冬令瘙痒 / senile ~ 老年瘙痒 / symptomatic ~ 症状性瘙痒(如伴有黄疸) / ~ valvae 外阴瘙痒,外阴干皱 | **pruritic** [pruəˈritik] *a*

Prussak's fibers [ˈpruːsɑːk] (Alexander Prussak) 普鲁萨克纤维(自锤骨短突末端至鼓切迹的两根短纤维) | ~ pouch (space) 鼓膜上隐窝

prussiate [ˈprʌʃit, ˈprʌsieit] *n* 氰化物

prussic acid [ˈprʌsik] 氢氰酸

Prymnesiida [ˌprimniˈsaiidə] *n* 定鞭目

PS phosphatidylserine 磷脂酰丝氨酸; pulmonary stenosis 肺动脉瓣狭窄

ps per second 每秒

PSA prostate-specific antigen 前列腺特异性抗原

psalis [ˈseilis] *n*【希】(脑)穹窿

psalterium [sælˈtiəriəm] *n* 海马连合;反刍胃 | **psalterial** *a*

Psalydolytta [ˌsælidəˈlitə] *n* 链芫菁属

Psamminida [səˈminidə] *n* 无线目

psamm(o)- [构词成分]沙

psammocarcinoma [ˌsæməuˌkɑːsiˈnəumə] *n* 沙癌

psammoma [sæˈməumə] *n* 沙样瘤

psamommatous [sæˈməumətəs] *a* 沙瘤样的

psammosarcoma [ˌsæməusɑːˈkəumə] *n* 沙肉瘤

psammotherapy [ˌsæməuˈθerəpi] *n* 沙浴疗法

psammous [ˈsæməs] *a* 沙的

psauoscopy [sɔːˈɔskəpi] *n* 摩动诊法

P_{450} SCC cholesterol monooxygenase (side-chain cleaving) 胆固醇单加氧酶(侧链裂解的)

pselaphesia [seləˈfiːziə] *n* 触觉

psellism [ˈselizəm] *n* 口吃,讷吃

pseudacousma [ˌpsjuːdəˈkuːzmə], **pseudacousis** [ˌpsjuːdəˈkuːsis] *n* 听幻觉

pseudactinomycosis [psjuːˌdæktinəumaiˈkəusis] *n* 假放线菌病

pseudagraphia [ˌpsjuːdəˈgreifiə] *n* 假性失写[症]

pseudalbuminuria [ˌpsjuːdælˌbjuːmiˈnjuəriə] *n* 假蛋白尿,偶发性蛋白尿

Pseudallescheria [ˌpsjuːdæləsˈkiəriə] *n* 假性阿利什利菌属 | ~ boydii 波伊德假性阿利什利菌

pseudallescheriasis [ˌpsjuːdæleskəˈraiəsis] *n* 假性阿利什利菌病

Pseudamphistomum [ˌpsjuːdæmˈfistəuməm] *n* 伪端盘吸虫属 | ~ truncatum 截形伪端盘吸虫

pseudangina [ˌpsjuːdænˈdʒainə] *n* 假心绞痛

pseudankylosis [ˌpsjuːdæŋkiˈləusis] *n* 假[性]关节强硬

pseudaphia [ˌpsjuːˈdeifiə] *n* 触幻觉

pseudarrhenia [ˌpsjuːdəˈriːniə] *n* 女性假两性畸形

pseudarthritis [ˌpsjuːdɑːˈθraitis] *n* 假[性]关节炎

pseudarthrosis [ˌpsjuːdɑːˈθrəusis] *n* 假关节
Pseudechis porphyriacus [sjuːˈdekis pɔˈfiriəkəs] 澳洲黑蛇
pseudencephalus [ˌpsjuːdenˈsefələs] *n* 假脑畸胎
pseudesthesia [ˌpsjuːdisˈθiːzjə] *n* 假感觉,幻觉;联觉,牵连感觉
pseudinoma [ˌpsjuːdiˈnəumə] *n* 假瘤,假性瘤,幻想瘤;假纤维瘤
pseud(o)- [构词成分]假,伪
pseudoacanthosis [ˌpsjuːdəuˌækənˈθəusis] *n* 假性棘皮症 | ~ nigricans 假性黑[色]棘皮症
pseudoacephalus [ˌpsjuːdəueiˈsefələs] *n* 假无头畸胎
pseudoactinomycosis [ˌpsjuːdəuˌæktinəumaiˈkəusis] *n* 假放线菌病
pseudoagglutination [ˌpsjuːdəuəˌgluːtiˈneiʃən] *n* 假凝集反应,假血凝反应
pseudoagraphia [ˌpsjuːdəuəˈgræfiə] *n* 假性失写[症]
pseudoainhum [ˌpsjuːdəuˈeihəm] *n* 假箍趾病(指趾、肢体和躯干周围存在环状结构,先天性发生,最严重表现为子宫内自行断离,亦见于大量遗传性和非遗传性疾病)
pseudoalbuminuria [ˌpsjuːdəuˌælbjumiˈnjuəriə] *n* 假蛋白尿,偶发性蛋白尿
pseudoalleles [ˌpsjuːdəuəˈliːlz] *n* 拟等位基因(此基因看来似乎是等位的,其位点虽不同,但是紧密相连;形成杂合子的等位基因,很像野生型,而不像任何一种的突变型) | **pseudoallelic** [ˌpsjuːdəuəˈlelik] *a*
pseudoallelism [ˌpsjuːdəuˈælilizəm] *n* 拟等位现象
pseudoalveolar [ˌpsjuːdəuælˈviələ] *a* 假牙槽的
Pseudoamphistomum [ˌpsjuːdəuæmˈfistəməm] *n* 伪端盘吸虫属
pseudoanaphylaxis [ˌpsjuːdəuˌænəfiˈlæksis] *n* 假过敏反应,假过敏症(注射已用琼脂、高岭土、淀粉及其他物质处理过的血清或注射其他非特异性蛋白引起的类似过敏反应的一种反应) | **pseudoanaphylactic** *a* 假过敏性的
pseudoanemia [ˌpsjuːdəuəˈniːmiə] *n* 假贫血
pseudoaneurysm [ˌpsjuːdəuˈænjuərizəm] *n* 假动脉瘤
pseudoangina [ˌpsjuːdəuænˈdʒainə] *n* 假心绞痛
pseudoankylosis [ˌpsjuːdəuˌæŋkiˈləusis] *n* 假[性]关节强硬
pseudoanodontia [ˌpsjuːdəuˌænəˈdɔnʃiə] *n* 假无牙,埋伏牙
pseudoantagonist [ˌpsjuːdəuænˈtægənist] *n* 假拮抗肌
pseudoapoplexy [ˌpsjuːdəuˈæpəˌpleksi] *n* 假卒中(似中风,但无脑出血情况)
pseudoappendicitis [ˌpsjuːdəuəˌpendiˈsaitis] *n* 假阑尾炎
pseudoarthrosis [ˌpsjuːdəuɑːˈθrəusis] *n* 假关节
pseudoasthma [ˌpsjuːdəuˈæsmə] *n* 假气喘,假性哮喘,阵发性呼吸困难
pseudoathetosis [ˌpsjuːdəuˌæθiˈtəusis] *n* 假[性]手足徐动症
pseudoatrophoderma colli [ˌpsjuːdəuˌætrəfəuˈdəːmə ˈkɔli] 颈部假性皮萎缩
pseudobacillus [ˌpsjuːdəubəˈsiləs] *n* 假杆菌
pseudobacterium [ˌpsjuːdəubækˈtiəriəm] *n* 假[无芽胞杆]菌
pseudobasedow [ˌpsjuːdəuˈbæsidəu] *n* 假性毒性甲状腺肿,类巴塞多病
pseudobronchiectasis [ˌpsjuːdəuˌbrɔŋkiˈektəsis] *n* 假支气管扩张
pseudobulbar [ˌpsjuːdəuˈbʌlbə] *a* 假延髓病的,似延髓病的
pseudocartilage [ˌpsjuːdəuˈkɑːtilidʒ] *n* 假软骨,软骨样组织
pseudocartilaginous [ˌpsjuːdəuˌkɑːtiˈlædʒinəs] *a* 假软骨的
pseudocast [ˌpsjuːdəkɑːst] *n* 假管型(一种尿中的沉积物,类似真管型,为黏液丝或棉线等黏着而成)
pseudocele [ˌpsjuːdəsiːl] *n* 透明隔腔
pseudocephalocele [ˌpsjuːdəuˈsefələsiːl] *n* 假性脑突出(非先天性的,由于头颅损伤或疾病所致)
pseudochancre [ˌpsjuːdəuˈʃæŋkə] *n* 假下疳
pseudocholecystitis [ˌpsjuːdəuˌkəulisisˈtaitis] *n* 假胆囊炎(由于食物过敏反应引起的类似胆囊炎症状)
pseudocholesteatoma [ˌpsjuːdəuˌkəulistiəˈtəumə] *n* 假胆脂瘤(慢性中耳炎症时的鼓室内)
pseudocholinesterase (PCE) [ˌpsjuːdəuˌkəuliˈnestəreis] *n* 假胆碱酯酶
pseudochorea [ˌpsjuːdəukɔˈriə] *n* 假性舞蹈症
pseudochromesthesia [ˌpsjuːdəuˌkrəumisˈθiˌzjə] *n* 假色觉,色幻觉
pseudochromidrosis [ˌpsjuːdəuˌkrəumiˈdrəusis] *n* 假色汗[症](产色素细菌作用所致)
pseudochromosome [ˌpsjuːdəuˈkrəuməsəum] *n* 假染色体,拟染色体(精母细胞中的杆状高尔基〈Golgi〉体)
pseudochylothorax [ˌpsjuːdəuˌkailəuˈθɔːræks] *n* 假乳糜胸,乳糜样渗漏液
pseudochylous [ˌpsjuːdəuˈkailəs] *a* 假乳糜的(似乳糜,但不含脂肪)
pseudocirrhosis [ˌpsjuːdəusiˈrəusis] *n* 假[肝]硬变 | pericardial ~ of the liver, pericarditic ~ 心

包炎性假肝硬变
pseudoclaudication [ˌpsjuːdəuklɔːdiˈkeiʃən] *n* 假跛行
pseudoclonus [ˌpsjuːdəuˈkləunəs] *n* 假阵挛,短时阵挛
pseudocoarctation [ˌpsjuːdəuˌkəuɑːkˈteiʃən] *n* 假缩窄,假缩小(X线造影所见的一种主动脉扭结,可能是一种主动脉弓异常) | ~ of the aorta 主动脉假缩窄
pseudocoele [ˈpsjuːdəsiːl] *n* 透明隔腔
pseudocoelom [ˌpsjuːdəuˈsiːləm] *n* 假体腔
pseudocoelomate [ˌpsjuːdəuˈsiːləmeit] *a* 有假体腔的 *n* 假体腔动物
pseudocolloid [ˌpsjuːdəuˈkɔlɔid] *n* 假胶体(一种黏液样物质,有时见于卵巢囊内) | ~ of lips 唇假胶体,唇黏膜皮脂腺肿大
pseudocoloboma [ˌpsjuːdəuˌkɔləˈbəumə] *n* 假虹膜缺损
pseudocolony [ˌpsjuːdəuˈkɔləni] *n* 假菌落,假集落
pseudocoma [ˌpsjuːdəuˈkəumə] *n* 假性昏迷,闭锁综合征(即 locked-in syndrome,见 syndrome 项下相应术语)
pseudocopulation [ˌpsjuːdəuˌkɔpjuˈleiʃən] *n* 假[性]抱合,拟交配
pseudo-corpus luteum [ˌpsjuːdəuˈkɔːpəs ˈljuːtiəm] 假黄体
pseudocowpox [ˌpsjuːdəuˈkaupɔks] *n* 假牛痘,挤乳员结节
pseudocoxalgia [ˌpsjuːdəukɔkˈsældʒiə] *n* 假[性]髋关节痛(股骨小头骨骺骨软骨病)
pseudocrisis [ˌpsjuːdəkraisis] *n* 假极期,假[热度]骤退
pseudocroup [ˌpsjuːdəuˈkruːp] *n* 假格鲁布(喘鸣性喉痉挛;胸腺性气喘)
pseudocyanin [ˌpsjuːdəuˈsaiənin] *n* 假异花[青]色苷
pseudocyesis [ˌpsjuːdəusaiˈiːsis] *n* 假孕
pseudocylindroid [ˌpsjuːdəusiˈlindrɔid] *n* 假圆柱状体
pseudocyst [ˌpsjuːdəsist] *n* 假性囊肿
pseudodementia [ˌpsjuːdəudiˈmenʃiə] *n* 假性痴呆
pseudodextrocardia [ˌpsjuːdəuˌdekstrəuˈkɑːdiə] *n* 假右位心
pseudodiabetes [ˌpsjuːdəuˌdaiəˈbiːtiːz] *n* 假性糖尿病,亚临床型糖尿病
pseudodiastolic [ˌpsjuːdəuˌdaiəˈstɔlik] *a* 假舒张[期]的
pseudodiphtheria [ˌpsjuːdəudifˈθiəriə] *n* 假白喉
pseudodisease [ˌpsjuːdəudiˈziːz] *n* 假病(一种隐性疾病,若不用诊断鉴定,对患者来说,此病在其一生不会明显表现出来)
pseudodiverticulum [ˌpsjuːdəuˌdaivəːˈtikjuləm] *n* 假憩室
pseudodominant [ˌpsjuːdəuˈdɔminənt] *n* 拟显性
pseudodysentery [ˌpsjuːdəuˈdisəntri] *n* 假痢疾
pseudoedema [ˌpsjuːdəui(ː)ˈdiːmə] *n* 假水肿
pseudoembryonic [ˌpsjuːdəuˌembriˈɔnik] *a* 假胚的
pseudoemphysema [ˌpsjuːdəuˌemfiˈziːmə] *n* 假气肿
pseudoencephalomalacia [ˌpsjuːdəuenˌsefələuməˈleiʃiə] *n* 假脑软化(牛、羊等致命性疾病)
pseudoendometritis [ˌpsjuːdəuˌendəumiˈtraitis] *n* 假[性]子宫内膜炎
pseudoeosinophil [ˌpsjuːdəuˌiːəˈsinəfil] *a* 假[性]嗜酸性的
pseudoephedrine [ˌpsjuːdəuiˈfedrin] *n* 伪麻黄碱,假麻黄碱 | ~ hydrochloride 盐酸伪麻黄碱(减轻鼻充血药,支气管扩张药)
pseudoepilepsy [ˌpsjuːdəuˈepilepsi] *n* 假性癫痫,假癫痫发作
pseudoepiphysis [ˌpsjuːdəuiˈpifisis] *n* 假骺
pseudoesthesia [ˌpsjuːdəuisˈθiːzjə] *n* 假感觉,幻觉
pseudoexfoliation [ˌpsjuːdəueksˌfəuliˈeiʃən] *n* 假表皮脱落,假鳞皮样脱落
pseudoexophoria [ˌpsjuːdəuˌeksəˈfəuriə] *n* 假性外隐斜视
pseudoexophthalmos [ˌpsjuːdəuˌeksɔfˈθælmɔs] *n* 假眼球突出,假突眼
pseudoextrophy [ˌpsjuːdəuˈekstrəfi] *n* 假膀胱外翻
pseudofarcy [ˌpsjuːdəˌfɑːsi] *n* 假性马皮疽,兽疫性淋巴管炎
pseudofluctuation [ˌpsjuːdəuˌflʌktjuˈeiʃən] *n* 假波动
pseudofolliculitis [ˌpsjuːdəufəˌlikjuˈlaitis] *n* 假毛囊炎(亦称须癣,须部假毛囊炎)
pseudofracture [ˌpsjuːdəuˈfræktʃə] *n* 假骨折
pseudofructose [ˌpsjuːdəuˈfrʌktəus] *n* 假果糖
pseudoganglion [ˌpsjuːdəuˈgæŋgliən] *n* 假神经节
pseudogene [ˈpsjuːdəudʒiːn] *n* 假基因(一种 DNA 序列,在碱基顺序上类似活动基因,但不被转录)
pseudogestation [ˌpsjuːdəudʒesˈteiʃən] *n* 假妊娠
pseudogeusesthesia [ˌpsjuːdəuˌgjuːsisˈθiːzjə] *n* 味幻觉,假味觉
pseudogeusia [ˌpsjuːdəuˈgjuːziə] *n* 味幻觉
pseudoglanders [ˌpsjuːdəuˈglændəz] *n* 假[马]鼻疽,假鼻疽溃疡性淋巴管炎

pseudoglioma [ˌpsjuːdəuglaiˈəumə] *n* 假神经胶质瘤

pseudoglobulin [ˌpsjuːdəuˈglɔbjulin] *n* 假球蛋白

pseudoglottis [ˌpsjuːdəuˈglɔtis] *n* 假声门 | **pseudoglottic** *a*

pseudoglucosazone [ˌpsjuːdəuˌgluːkəˈseizəun] *n* 假葡萄糖脎

pseudogonorrhea [ˌpsjuːdəuˌgɔnəˈriːə] *n* 假淋病,非淋球菌性尿道炎

pseudogout [ˈpsjuːdəgaut] *n* 假[性]痛风

pseudographia [ˌpsjuːdəuˈgræfiə] *n* 假性书写

pseudogynecomastia [ˌpsjuːdəuˌgainikəuˈmæstiə] *n* 假性[男子]女性型乳房

pseudohallucination [ˌpsjuːdəuhəˌluːsiˈneiʃən] *n* 假性,幻觉

pseudohaustration [ˌpsjuːdəuhɔːsˈtreiʃən] *n* 假结肠袋(造影片上出现水肿黏膜岛有规律地排列在溃疡深部的肌层之间,类似结肠壁正常的袋形结构)

pseudohelminth [ˌpsjuːdəuˈhelminθ] *n* 假蠕虫

pseudohemagglutination [ˌpsjuːdəuˌheməˌgluːtiˈneiʃən] *n* 假血凝反应(由于缗钱状形成所致的红细胞聚集)

pseudohematuria [ˌpsjuːdəuˌhiːməˈtjuəriə] *n* 假血尿

pseudohemophilia [ˌpsjuːdəuːˌhiːməˈfiliə] *n* 假血友病

pseudohemoptysis [ˌpsjuːdəuhiːˈmɔptisis] *n* 假咯血

pseudohereditary [ˌpsjuːdəuhiˈreditəri] *a* 假[性]遗传的,拟遗传的

pseudohermaphrodite [ˌpsjuːdəuhəˈmæfrədait] *n* 假两性体,假半阴阳体 | female ~ 女性假两性体 / male ~ 男性假两性体

pseudohermaphroditism [ˌpsjuːdəuhəˈmæfrədaitizəm] *n* 假两性畸形 | female ~ 女假两性畸形 / male ~ 男假两性畸形 | **pseudohermaphrodism** [ˌpsjuːdəuhəˈmæfrədizəm] *n*

pseudohernia [ˌpsjuːdəuˈhəːnjə] *n* 假疝

pseudoheterotopia [ˌpsjuːdəuˌhetərəuˈtəupiə] *n* 假异位

pseudohydrocephalus [ˌpsjuːdəuˌhaidrəuˈsefələs] *n* 假脑积水

pseudohydronephrosis [ˌpsjuːdəuˌhaidrəuniˈfrəusis] *n* 假肾盂积水(肾旁囊肿)

pseudohyoscyamine [ˌpsjuːdəuhaiəˈsaiəmin] *n* 假莨菪碱,去甲莨菪碱

pseudohypacusis [ˌpsjuːdəuˌhaipəˈkjuːsis] *n* 假听觉减退,功能性听力丧失

pseudohyperkalemia [ˌpsjuːdəuˌhaipə(ː)kæˈliːmiə] *n* 假血钾过多,假高血钾症

pseudohypertension [ˌpsjuːdəuˌhaipə(ː)ˈtenʃən] *n* 假高血压(由血压计读出,尤见于老年患者,由于动脉壁顺应性丧失所致)

pseudohypertriglyceridemia [ˌpsjuːdəuˌhaipətraiˌglisəriˈdiːmiə] *n* 假高甘油三醇血症

pseudohypertrichosis [ˌpsjuːdəuˌhaipə(ː)triˈkəusis] *n* 假多毛[症](出生后胎毛不脱)

pseudohypertrophy [ˌpsjuːdəuhaiˈpəːtrəfi] *n* 假性肥大 | muscular ~ 假性肌肥大 | **pseudohypertrophic** [ˌpsjuːdəuˌhaipə(ː)ˈtrɔfik] *a*

pseudohypha [ˌpsjuːdəuˈhaifə] *n* 假菌丝

pseudohypoaldosteronism [ˌpsjuːdəuˌhaipəuælˈdɔstiərəunizəm] *n* 假性醛固酮减少[症]

pseudohyponatremia [ˌpsjuːdəuˌhaipəunəˈtriːmiə] *n* 假低钠血[症]

pseudohypoparathyroidism [ˌpsjuːdəuˌhaipəuˌpærəˈθairɔidizəm] *n* 假性甲状旁腺功能减退症

pseudohypophosphatasia [ˌpsjuːdəuˌhaipəuˌfɔsfəˈteiziə] *n* 假磷酸酶过少[症]

pseudohypothyroidism [ˌpsjuːdəuˌhaipəuˈθairɔidizəm] *n* 假性甲状腺功能减退[症]

pseudoicterus [ˌpsjuːdəuˈiktərəs] *n* 假黄疸

pseudoinfarction [ˌpsjuːdəuinˈfɑːkʃən] *n* 假心肌梗死

pseudointima [ˌpsjuːdəuˈintimə] *n* 假内膜

pseudoion [ˌpsjuːdəuˈaiən] *n* 假离子

pseudoisochromatic [ˌpsjuːdəuˌaisəukrəuˈmætik] *a* 假同色的,假等色的

pseudoisocyanin [ˌpsjuːdəuˌaisəuˈsaiənin] *n* 假异花[青]色苷

pseudojaundice [ˌpsjuːdəuˈdʒɔːndis] *n* 假黄疸

pseudokeratin [ˌpsjuːdəuˈkerətin] *n* 假角蛋白

pseudolamellar [ˌpsjuːdəuləˈmelə] *a* 假板层的

pseudoleukemia [ˌpsjuːdəuˌljuːˈkiːmiə] *n* 假白血病 | ~ cutis 皮肤假白血病 / ~ lymphatica 淋巴性假白血病 / myelogenous ~ 骨髓性假白血病 | **pseudoleukocythemia** [ˌpsjuːdəuˌljuːkəusaiˈθiːmiə] *n*

pseudolipoma [ˌpsjuːdəuliˈpəumə] *n* 假脂瘤,神经病性水肿

pseudolithiasis [ˌpsjuːdəuliˈθaiəsis] *n* 假结石病

pseudologia [ˌpsjuːdəuˈləudʒiə] *n* 谎言癖 | ~ fantastica 幻想性谎言癖

pseudoluxation [ˌpsjuːdəulʌkˈseiʃən] *n* 假脱位

pseudolymphoma [ˌpsjuːdəulimˈfəumə] *n* 假性淋巴瘤(亦称淋巴细胞瘤)

Pseudolynchia [ˌpsjuːdəuˈlintʃiə] *n* 拟虱蝇属 | ~ canariensis, ~ maurah 拟虱蝇,鸽虱蝇

pseudomalfunction [ˌpsjuːdəumælˈfʌŋkʃən] *n* 假功能不良(在心脏起搏术语中,指起搏器明显功能不良,实际上由于一种人为现象造成,如心

电描记法分析时出现机械性错误）

pseudomalignancy [ˌpsjuːdəuməˈlignənsi] *n* 假恶性[病]

pseudomamma [ˌpsjuːdəuˈmæmə] *n* 假乳房（见于卵巢皮样囊肿上）

pseudomania [ˌpsjuːdəuˈmeinjə] *n* 假躁狂；虚构性自罪[症]；谎言癖

pseudomasturbation [ˌpsjuːdəuˌmæstəˈbeiʃən] *n* 假性手淫，抚阳癖

pseudomegacolon [ˌpsjuːdəuˈmegəˌkəulən] *n* 假巨结肠

pseudomelanoma [ˌpsjuːdəuˌmeləˈnəumə] *n* 假黑素瘤

pseudomelanosis [ˌpsjuːdəuˌmeləˈnəusis] *n* 假黑变病

pseudomelia [ˌpsjuːdəuˈmiːliə] *n* 幻肢 | ~ paraesthetica 感觉异常性幻肢

pseudomembrane [ˌpsjuːdəuˈmembrein] *n* 假膜 | **pseudomembranous** *a*

pseudomembranelle [ˌpsjuːdəuˈmembrənel] *n* 假微膜

pseudomeningitis [ˌpsjuːdəuˌmeninˈdʒaitis] *n* 假性脑膜炎

pseudomenstruation [ˌpsjuːdəuˌmenstruˈeiʃən] *n* 假月经

pseudomethemoglobin [ˌpsjuːdəumethiːməuˈgləubin] *n* 假正铁血红蛋白，正铁血白蛋白

pseudomicrocephalus [ˌpsjuːdəuˌmaikrəuˈsefələs] *n* 假性小头者

pseudomilium [ˌpsjuːdəuˈmiliəm] *n* 假粟粒疹，胶状粟粒疹

pseudomonad [ˌpsjuːdəuˈməunæd] *n* 假单胞菌

Pseudomonadaceae [ˌpsjuːdəuˌmɔnəˈdeisiiː] *n* 假单胞菌科

Pseudomonadales [ˌpsjuːdəuˌməunəˈdeiliːz] *n* 假单胞菌目

Pseudomonadineae [ˌpsjuːdəuˌməunəˈdainiiː] *n* 假单胞菌亚目

Pseudomonas [ˌpsjuːdəuˈməunəs] *n* 假单胞菌属 | ~ acidovorans 食酸假单胞菌 / ~ aeruginosa 铜绿假单胞菌，绿脓杆菌 / ~ alcaligenes 产碱假单胞菌 / ~ cepacia, ~ multivorans 葱头假单胞菌，多食假单胞菌 / ~ diminuta 缺陷假单胞菌 / ~ fluorescens 荧光假单胞菌 / ~ mallei 鼻疽假单胞菌 / ~ maltophila 嗜麦芽假单胞菌 / ~ pertucinogena 穿孔假单胞菌（亦称百日咳博代菌Ⅳ相）/ ~ pickettii, ~ thomasii 皮氏假单胞菌，托氏假单胞菌 / ~ polycolor 多色假单胞菌 / ~ pseudoalcaligenes 类产碱假单胞菌 / ~ pseudomallei 类鼻疽假单胞菌 / ~ putida, ~ eisenbergii 恶臭假单胞菌，艾氏假单胞菌，/ ~ putrefaciens 腐败假单胞菌（亦称腐败互生单胞菌）/ ~ pyocyanea 铜绿假单胞菌，绿脓杆菌 / ~ reptilivora 爬虫假单胞菌 / ~ septica 败血假单胞菌 / ~ stutzeri, ~ stanieri 施氏假单胞菌，斯氏假单胞菌 / ~ syncyanea 产蓝假单胞菌 / ~ testosteroni 睾丸酮假单胞菌 / ~ vesicularis 泡囊假单胞菌（亦称泡囊棒状杆菌）

Pseudomonilia [ˌpsjuːdəuməˈniliə] *n* 假念珠菌属

pseudomonillethrix [ˌpsjuːdəuməuˈniləθriks] *n* 假念珠形发

pseudomorphine [ˌpsjuːdəuˈmɔːfiːn] *n* 假吗啡，脱氢吗啡

pseudomotor [ˌpsjuːdəuˈməutə] *a* 假运动的

pseudomucin [ˌpsjuːdəuˈmjuːsin] *n* 假黏蛋白

pseudomucinous [ˌpsjuːdəuˈmjuːsinəs] *a* 假黏蛋白的

pseudomyiasis [ˌpsjuːdəumaiˈaiəsis] *n* 假蝇蛆病

pseudomyopia [ˌpsjuːdəumaiˈəupiə] *n* 假性近视

pseudomyxoma [ˌpsjuːdəumikˈsəumə] *n* 假黏液瘤 | ~ peritonei 腹膜假黏液瘤（亦称假性积水）

pseudonarcotic [ˌpsjuːdəunɑːˈkɔtik] *a* 假麻醉的

pseudonarcotism [ˌpsjuːdəuˈnɑːkətizəm] *n* 假麻醉[状态]

pseudoneoplasm [ˌpsjuːdəuˈni(ː)əuplæzəm] *n* 假瘤；幻想瘤

pseudoneuritis [ˌpsjuːdəunjuəˈraitis] *n* 假视神经炎

pseudoneuroma [ˌpsjuːdəunjuəˈrəumə] *n* 假神经瘤

pseudoneuronophagia [ˌpsjuːdəunjuəˌrəunəˈfeidʒiə] *n* 假性噬神经细胞现象

Pseudonocardia [ˌpsjuːdəunəuˈkɑːdiə] *n* 假诺卡菌属

pseudonucleolus [ˌpsjuːdəunjuːˈkliːələs] *n* 假核仁，染色质核仁，核粒

pseudonystagmus [ˌpsjuːdəunisˈtægməs] *n* 假眼球震颤

pseudo-obstruction [ˌpsjuːdəu əbsˈtrʌkʃən] *n* 假梗阻 | intestinal ~ 假肠梗阻

pseudo-ochronosis [ˌpsjuːdəu ˌəukrəˈnəusis] *n* 假褐黄病

pseudo-optogram [ˌpsjuːdəu ˈɔptəgræm] *n* 假视网膜像

pseudo-osteomalacia [ˌpsjuːdəu ˌɔstiəuməˈleiʃiə] *n* 假性骨软化（骨盆）

pseudo-ovum [ˌpsjuːdəu ˈəuvəm] *n* 假卵（见于卵巢粒层细胞瘤）

pseudopannus [ˌpsjuːdəuˈpænəs] *n* 假角膜翳（有时见于触染性软疣）

pseudopapilla [ˌpsjuːdəupəˈpilə] *n* 假乳头

pseudopapillary [ˌpsjuːdəuˌpæpiˈlɛəri] *a* 假乳

头的
pseudopapilledema [ˌpsjuːdəuˌpæpiliˈdiːmə] *n* 假视神经乳头水肿
pseudoparalysis [ˌpsjuːdəupəˈrælisis] *n* 假麻痹,假瘫 | ~ agitans 震颤[性假]麻痹 / arthritic general ~ 关节炎性全身假瘫 / congenital atonic ~ 先天肌无力性假麻痹,先天肌弛缓
pseudoparaphrasia [ˌpsjuːdəuˌpærəˈfreiziə] *n* 假性言语无序,假性言语倒错
pseudoparaplegia [ˌpsjuːdəupærəˈpliːdʒiə] *n* 假截瘫
pseudoparasite [ˌpsjuːdəuˈpærəsait] *n* 假寄生物
pseudoparesis [ˌpsjuːdəupəˈriːsis] *n* 假性全身麻痹
pseudopelade [ˌpsjuːdəuˈpiːleid] *n* 假性斑秃
pseudopellagra [ˌpsjuːdəupəˈlægrə] *n* 假性糙皮病
pseudopeptone [ˌpsjuːdəuˈpeptəun] *n* 假蛋白胨,类卵黏蛋白
pseudopericardial [ˌpsjuːdəuˌperiˈkɑːdiəl] *a* 假心包的
pseudoperitonitis [ˌpsjuːdəuˌperitəuˈnaitis] *n* 假腹膜炎
pseudoperoxidase [ˌpsjuːdəupəˈrɔksideis] *n* 假过氧化物酶
pseudophakia [ˌpsjuːdəuˈfeikiə] *n* 假晶状体[症] / ~ fibrosa 纤维性假晶状体[症]
pseudophotesthesia [ˌpsjuːdəuˌfəutisˈθiːzjə] *n* 光联觉,连带光觉
pseudophthisis [psjuːˈdɔfθaisis] *n* 假痨病(非结核性痨病)
Pseudophyllidea [ˌpsjuːdəufiˈlidiə] *n* 假叶目
pseudophyllidean [ˌpsjudəufiˈlidiən] *a* 假叶目绦虫的
pseudoplasm [ˌpsjuːdəplæzəm] *n* 假瘤,自消瘤
pseudoplasmodium [ˌpsjuːdəuplæzˈməudiəm] *n* 假原质团
pseudoplegia [ˌpsjuːdəuˈpliːdʒiə] *n* 癔病性麻痹;假麻痹,假瘫
pseudopneumonia [ˌpsjuːdəunju(ː)ˈməuniə] *n* 假肺炎
pseudopodiospore [ˌpsjuːdəuˈpəudiəspɔː] *n* 伪足孢子,变形虫样孢子
pseudopodium [ˌpsjuːdəuˈpəudiəm] ([复] **pseudopodia** [ˌpsjuːdəuˈpəudiə]), **pseudopod** [ˈpsjuːdəpɔd] *n* 假足,伪足
pseudopoliomyelitis [ˌpsjuːdəuˌpɔliəumaiəˈlaitis] *n* 假脊髓灰质炎(由肠病毒而不是由脊髓灰质炎病毒所致)
pseudopolycythemia [ˌpsjuːdəuˌpɔlisaiˈθiːmiə] *n* 假性红细胞增多
pseudopolymelia [ˌpsjuːdəuˌpɔliˈmiːliə] *n* 多肢幻觉,多处幻觉(除手足幻觉外,还包括鼻、乳头和阴茎头的幻觉) | ~ paraesthetica 感觉异常性多肢幻觉,多处感觉倒错
pseudopolyp [ˌpsjuːdəuˈpɔlip] *n* 假息肉
pseudopolyposis [ˌpsjuːdəuˌpɔliˈpəusis] *n* 假息肉病
pseudoporphyria [ˌpsjuːdəupɔːˈfiriə] *n* 假性卟啉病
pseudopregnancy [ˌpsjuːdəuˈpregnənsi] *n* 假妊娠,假孕;子宫内膜经前期
pseudoprognathism [ˌpsjuːdəuˈprɔgnəθizəm] *n* 假凸颌[畸形](由于错殆造成牙排列改变所致)
pseudoproteinuria [ˌpsjuːdəuˌprəutiːˈnjuəriə] *n* 假性蛋白尿,偶发性蛋白尿
pseudopseudohypoparathyroidism [ˌpsjuːdəuˌpsjuːdəuhaipəuˌpærəˈθairɔidizəm] *n* 假性假甲状旁腺功能减退症
pseudopsia [psjuːˈdɔpsiə] *n* 视错觉,假视觉,视幻觉
pseudopsychosis [ˌpsjuːdəusaiˈkəusis] *n* 假精神病,甘塞综合征(见 Ganser syndrome)
pseudopterygium [ˌpsjuːdəutəˈridʒiəm] *n* 假性翼状胬肉
pseudoptosis [ˌpsjuːdəuˈptəusis] *n* 假性上睑下垂
pseudoptyalism [ˌpsjuːdəuˈtaiəlizəm] *n* 假流涎(由于咽下困难所致)
pseudopuberty [ˌpsjuːdəuˈpjuːbəti] *n* 假青春期(第二性征和副生殖器官的发育并不伴有青春期促性腺激素水平)
pseudorabies [ˌpsjuːdəuˈreibiːz] *n* 假性狂犬病 | bovine ~ 牛假性狂犬病
pseudoreaction [ˌpsjuːdəuri(ː)ˈækʃən] *n* 假反应,假阳性反应(皮内试验中的一种皮肤反应,并非对试验中的特异性蛋白质的反应,而由于用于产生毒素培养基中的蛋白质所引起)
pseudoreduction [ˌpsjuːdəuriˈdʌkʃən] *n* 拟减数(由于联会,染色体数目明显减半)
pseudoreminiscence [ˌpsjuːdəuremiˈnisns] *n* 假[性]回忆,虚谈症
pseudoretinitis pigmentosa [ˌpsjuːdəuˌretiˈnaitis ˌpigmənˈtəusə] 假性色素性视网膜炎
pseudorheumatism [ˌpsjuːdəuˈruːmətizəm] *n* 假风湿病
pseudorickets [ˌpsjuːdəuˈrikits] *n* 假佝偻病,肾病性骨营养不良
pseudorinderpest [ˌpsjuːdəuˈrindəpest] *n* 小反刍动物疫
pseudorosette [ˌpsjuːdəurəuˈzet] *n* 假玫瑰体
pseudosarcoma [ˌpsjuːdəusɑːˈkəumə] *n* 假性肉瘤
pseudosarcomatous [ˌpsjuːdəusɑːˈkəumətəs] *a*

假肉瘤的

pseudoscarlatina [ˌpsjuːdəuˌskɑːlə'tiːnə] *n* 假猩红热(由败血性中毒所致)

pseudosclerema [ˌpsjuːdəuskliə'riːmə] *n* 假硬化病(新生儿皮下脂肪组织坏死)

pseudosclerosis [ˌpsjuːdəuskliə'rəusis] *n* 假硬化症 | spastic ~ 痉挛性假硬化症

pseudoscrotum [ˌpsjuːdəu'skrəutəm] *n* 假阴囊

pseudoseizure [ˌpsjuːdəu'siːʒə] *n* 假癫痫发作(类似癫痫发作,但纯系心理性原因,缺少癫痫的脑电图特征,患者可凭意志的动作加以停止。亦称假癫痫,癔症性癫痫)

pseudosmia [psjuː'dɔzmiə] *n* 假嗅觉,嗅幻觉

pseudosolution [ˌpsjuːdəusə'ljuːʃən] *n* 假溶液(有时指胶体溶液)

pseudostoma [psjuː'dɔstəmə] *n* 假孔(在染银色的内皮细胞间)

pseudostrabismus [ˌpsjuːdəustrə'bisməs] *n* 假性斜视

pseudostrophanthin [ˌpsjuːdəuːstrə'fænθin] *n* 假毒毛旋花子苷

pseudostructure [ˌpsjuːdəu'strʌktʃə] *n* 网状基质(见于活体染色法后的红细胞)

pseudotabes [ˌpsjuːdəu'teibiːz] *n* 假[性]脊髓痨

pseudotetanus [ˌpsjuːdəu'tetənes] *n* 假破伤风

pseudothrill [ˌpsjuːdəθril] *n* 假震颤

pseudotoxin [ˌpsjuːdəu'tɔksin] *n* (颠茄)假毒素(取自颠茄叶)

pseudotrachoma [ˌpsjuːdəutrə'kəumə] *n* 假沙眼

pseudotrichinosis [ˌpsjuːdəuˌtriki'nəusis] *n* 假毛线虫病,皮肌炎

pseudotrismus [ˌpsjuːdəu'trisməs] *n* 假牙关紧闭

pseudotropine [psjuː'dɔtrəpin] *n* 假托品(托品的分解产物)

pseudotruncus arteriosus [ˌpsjuːdəu'trʌnkəs ɑːˌtiəri'əusəs] 假性动脉干(法洛〈Fallot〉四联征中最严重型)

pseudotubercle [ˌpsjuːdəu'tjuːbəːkl] *n* 假结核结节

pseudotuberculoma [ˌpsjuːdəutjuːˌbəːkju'ləumə] *n* 假结核瘤 | ~ silicoticum 硅沉着性假结核瘤

pseudotuberculosis [ˌpsjuːdəutjuːˌbəːkjuː'ləusis] *n* 假结核病 | ~ hominis streptothrica 链丝菌[性假结核]病

pseudotumor [ˌpsjuːdəu'tjuːmə] *n* 假性肿瘤 | ~ cerebri 假脑瘤

pseudotyphus [ˌpsjuːdəu'taifəs] *n* 假斑疹伤寒

pseudouremia [ˌpsjuːdəujuə'riːmiə] *n* 假尿毒症(见于肾小球性肾炎及高血压脑病时)

pseudouridine [ˌpsjuːdəu'juəridin] *n* 假尿苷

pseudovacuole [ˌpsjuːdəu'vækjuːəul] *n* 假空泡(某些红细胞内)

pseudovalve ['psjuːdəvælv] *n* 假瓣膜

pseudoventricle [ˌpsjuːdəu'ventrikl] *n* 透明隔腔,第五脑室

pseudovermicule [ˌpsjuːdəu'vəːmikjuːl], **pseudovermiculus** [ˌpsjuːdəuvəː'mikjuləs] *n* 假孕虫(疟原虫发育中的一个时期)

pseudovertigo [ˌpsjuːdəu'vəːtigəu] *n* 假性眩晕(类似眩晕,但无旋转感觉的一种头晕,在众多可能的原因中有换气过度、直立性低血压和恐慌病)

pseudovirion [ˌpsjuːdəu'vaiəriɔn] *n* 假病毒[粒子](由寄主细胞的 DNA 和病毒的外壳所组成的颗粒)

pseudovoice ['psjuːdəvɔis] *n* 假喉音

pseudovomiting [ˌpsjuːdəu'vɔmitiŋ] *n* 假呕吐(反胃)

pseudoxanthine [ˌpsjuːdəu'zænθin] *n* 假黄嘌呤

pseudoxanthoma [ˌpsjuːdəuzæn'θəumə] *n* 假黄色瘤 | ~ elasticum 弹性假黄色瘤(亦称弹性痣)

pseudozooglea [ˌpsjuːdəuˌzəuə'gliːə] *n* 假菌胶团

psi [psai] *n* 希腊语的第 23 个字母(Ψ, *ψ*)

psi pounds per square inch 每平方英寸磅数

psicofuranine [ˌsaikə'fjuərənin] *n* 狭霉素 C,阿洛酮糖腺苷(一种核苷抗生素,具有抗菌、抗肿瘤作用)

psilocin ['sailəsin] *n* 二甲-4-羟色胺(致幻药)

Psilocybe [ˌsailəu'saibi] *n* 裸盖菇属

psilocybin [ˌsailə'saibin] *n* 赛洛西宾(致幻药)

psittacine ['sitəsain] *a* 鹦鹉的

psittacosis [ˌsitə'kəusis] *n* 鹦鹉热

PSM presystolic murmur 收缩前期杂音

PSMA prostate-specific membrane antigen 前列腺特异性膜抗原

psoas ['səuəs] *n* 腰[大]肌

psodymus ['sɔdiməs] *n* 腰部联胎

psoitis [səu'aitis] *n* 腰[大]肌炎

psomophagia [ˌsəumə'feidʒiə], **psomophagy** [səu'mɔfədʒi] *n* 囫囵吞咽,不细嚼吞咽

psoralen ['sɔrələn] *n* 补骨脂素

psorenteritis [ˌsɔrentə'raitis] *n* 疥状肠变化

Psorergates [ˌsɔrər'geitiːz] *n* 生疥螨属

psoriasiform [ˌsɔri'æsifɔːm] *a* 银屑病样的

psoriasis [sɔ'raiəsis] *n* 银屑病 | ~ annularis, ~ annula, ~ circinata 环状银屑病 / ~ arthropathica 关节病性银屑病 / ~ buccalis 颊黏膜白斑[病] / ~ discoidea 盘状银屑 / ~ figurata 图状银屑病 / ~ guttata, guttate ~ 滴状银屑病 / ~ gyrata 回状银屑病 / ~ linguae 舌白斑[病] / ~

palmaris et plantaris, volar ~ 掌跖银屑病 / ~ pustular ~ 脓疱性银屑病 / ~ rupioides 蛎壳状银屑病 / ~ universalis 全身性银屑病 | **psoriatic** [ˌsɔriˈætik] *a* 银屑病的 *n* 银屑病患者

Psorobia [səuˈrəubiə] *n* 生疥螨属

Psorophora [səˈrɔfərə] *n* 鳞蚊属

psorophthalmia [ˌsɔrɔfˈθælmiə] *n* 疥状睑缘炎，溃疡性睑缘炎

Psoroptes [səˈrɔptiːz] *n* 痒螨属 | ~ cuniculi 兔痒螨 / ~ equi 马痒螨

psoroptic [səˈrɔptik] *a* 痒螨的

Psoroptidae [səuˈrɔptidiː] *n* 痒螨科

PSP phenolsulfonphthalein 酚磺酞，酚红

PSRO Professional Standards Review Organization 职业标准评定组织（美国地区、州或社区的医生及有关的保健工作者的组织，建立的目的在于检查通过医疗照顾方案〈Medicare〉、医疗补助方案〈Medicaid〉以及妇幼保健方案〈Maternal and Child Health Program〉所支付的保健服务情况，保证所提供的服务在医务上是必要的，是符合职业标准的，而且是最经济、最适当的机构所提供的）

PSVT paroxysmal supraventricular tachycardia 阵发性室上性心动过速

psychalgia [saiˈkældʒiə], **psychalgalia** [ˌsaikælˈgeiliə] *n* 精神痛苦；精神性疼痛 | **psychalgic** [saiˈkældʒik] *a*

psychanalysis [ˌsaikəˈnælisis] *n* 精神分析，心理分析

psychanopsia [saikəˈnɔpsiə] *n* 精神性盲

psychasthene [ˈsaikəsθiːn] *n* 精神衰弱者

psychasthenia [ˌsaikəsˈθiːniə] *n* 精神衰弱

psychataxia [ˌsaikəˈtæksiə] *n* 精神失调（表现为注意力涣散、情绪激动等）

psyche [ˈsaiki] *n*【希】精神，心灵，心理

psychedelia [ˌsaikiˈdiːljə] *n* 致幻药

psychedelic [ˌsaikiˈdelik] *a* 致幻觉的 *n* 致幻药

psychergograph [saiˈkəːgəgrɑːf] *n* 心理反应描记器

psychiatry [saiˈkaiətri] *n* 精神病学 | biological ~ 生物精神病学（着重研究生物化学、神经病学以及药理学方面的原因和治疗方法）/ community ~ 社区精神病学 / cross-cultural ~, transcultural ~ 跨文化精神病学（研究比较不同社会、国家和文化对精神病态和心理健康的影响）/ descriptive ~ 描述性精神病学（观察和研究各种可见、可触、可听的外界因素）/ dynamic ~ 动力精神病学 / existential ~ 存在主义精神病学（以 Kierkegaard, Heidegger, Jaspers 等人的存在主义〈existential philosophy〉为基础的精神病学，该主义认为一个人应对自己的存在负责）/ forensic ~ 司法精神病学 / organic ~ 器质性精神病学；生物精神病学 / orthomolecular ~ 正分子精神病学（此精神病学所依据的理论是：精神疾病是由于脑的分子环境失调所致，认为只有恢复正常体内如维生素一类物质的最适水平才能治愈）| **psychiatrics** [ˌsaikiˈætriks] *n* / **psychiatrist** *n* 精神病学家 / **psychiatric(al)** [ˌsaikiˈætrik(əl)]

psychic(al) [ˈsaikik(əl)] *a* 精神的，心理的

psychics [ˈsaikiks] *n* 心理学；心灵学

psychism [ˈsaikizəm] *n* 心灵论（认为所有动物有一种液体扩散于全身因而获得生命）

psych(o)- [构词成分]精神，心理

psychoacoustics [ˌsaikəuəˈkuːstiks] *n* 心理声学

psychoactive [ˌsaikəuˈæktiv] *a* 对精神起作用的（如精神作用药物）

psychoalgalia [ˌsaikəuælˈgeiliə] *n* 精神痛苦；精神性疼痛

psychoanaleptic [ˌsaikəuˌænəˈleptik] *a* [促]精神兴奋的 *n* 精神兴奋药（抗抑郁药）

psychoanalysis [ˌsaikəuəˈnæləsis] *n* 精神分析，心理分析 / **psychoanalyst** [ˌsaikəuˈænəlist] *n* 精神分析学家 | **psychoanalytic(al)** [ˌsaikəuænəˈlitik(əl)] *a* | **psychoanalytically** *ad*

psychoanalyze [ˌsaikəuˈænəlaiz] *vt* 用精神分析法医治或研究

psychoauditory [ˌsaikəuˈɔːditəri] *a* 精神性听觉的

psychobiology [ˌsaikəubaiˈɔlədʒi] *n* 精神生物学，生物心理学 | **psychobiological** [ˌsaikəubaiəˈlɔdʒikəl] *a*

psychocatharsis [ˌsaikəukəˈθɑːsis] *n* 精神疏泄，心理疏泄

psychocentric [ˌsaikəuˈsentrik] *a* 精神中枢的，心理中枢的

psychochemistry [ˌsaikəuˈkemistri] *n* 精神化学

psychochrome [ˈsaikəkrəum] *n* 精神色觉

psychochromesthesia [ˌsaikəuˌkrəumisˈθiːzjə] *n* 色联觉（如闻声觉色）

psychocortical [ˌsaikəuˈkɔːtikəl] *a* 精神皮质的，心理皮质的

psychocutaneous [ˌsaikəukjuːˈteinjəs] *a* 精神[与]皮肤[病]的，心理[与]皮肤[病]的

psychodelic [ˌsaikəuˈdelik] *a* 致幻觉的 *n* 致幻药

psychodiagnosis [ˌsaikəuˌdaiəgˈnəusis], **psychodiagnostics** [ˌsaikəudaiəgˈnɔstiks] *n* 心理[测验]诊断法

Psychodidae [saiˈkəudidiː] *n* 毛蠓科

psychodometer [ˌsaikəuˈdɔmitə] *n* 心理活动测时器 / **psychodometry** *n* 心理活动测时法

Psychodopygus [ˌsaikəudəˈpaigəs] *n* 毛蛉属

psychodrama [ˌsaikəuˈdrɑːmə] *n* 心理剧，精神表演疗法（使精神病患者表演他们各自在日常生

活中相冲突情况的一种治疗方法）

psychodynamics [ˌsaikəudaiˈnæmiks] *n* 精神动力学 | **psychodynamic** *a*

psychodysleptic [ˌsaikəudisˈleptik] *a* 致幻觉的 *n* 致幻药

psychogalvanometer [ˌsaikəuˌgælvəˈnɔmitə] *n* 精神流电计，心理流电计

psychogenesis [ˌsaikəuˈdʒenisis] *n* 精神发生，心理发生 | **psychogenetic** [ˌsaikəudʒiˈnetik] *a*

psychogenic [ˌsaikəuˈdʒenik], **psychogenous** [saiˈkɔdʒinəs] *a* 精神性的，心因性的

psychogeriatrics [ˌsaikəuˌdʒeriˈætriks] *n* 老年精神病学

psychogogic [ˌsaikəuˈgɔdʒik] *a* 促进精神[作用]的

psychogram [ˈsaikəgræm] *n* 心理记录表；心理性视幻象

psychograph [ˈsaikəgrɑːf] *n* 心理记录表；心理记录

psychokinesia [ˌsaikəukaiˈniːziə] *n* 精神激动（由于精神抑制缺陷所致）

psychokinesis [ˌsaikəukaiˈniːsis] *n* 精神冲动；精神激动 | **psychokinetic** [ˌsaikəukaiˈnetik] *a*

psychokym [ˈsaikəkim] *n* 精神元气，神经元气

psycholagny [ˈsaikəuˌlægni] *n* 意淫

psycholepsy [ˌsaikəuˈlepsi] *n* 精神猝变，情绪猝变

psycholeptic [ˌsaikəuˈleptik] *a* 抑制精神的 *n* 精神抑制药（安定药）

psycholinguistics [ˌsaikəuliŋˈgwistiks] *n* 心理语言学

psychologize [saiˈkɔlədʒaiz] *vi* 研究心理学；从心理学的观点推究 *vt* 用心理学分析

psychology [saiˈkɔlədʒi] *n* 心理学 | abnormal ~ 变态心理学 / analytic ~, analytical ~ 分析心理学，精神分析学 / behavioristic ~ 行为主义心理学 / child ~ 儿童心理学 / clinical ~ 临床心理学 / cognitive ~ 认知心理学 / constitutional ~ 素质心理学 / depth ~ 深蕴心理学，精神分析学 / gestalt ~ 格式塔心理学，完形心理学 / hormic ~ 策动心理学 | **psychologist** *n* 心理学家 | **psychologic(al)** [ˌsaikəˈlɔdʒik(əl)] *a* | **psychologically** *ad*

psychometer [saiˈkɔmitə] *n* 心理测量器；智力测验器

psychometrics [ˌsaikəuˈmetriks] *n* 心理测量学；心理测量

psychometry [saiˈkɔmitri] *n* 心理测量；智力测验 | **psychometric(al)** [ˌsaikəuˈmetrik(əl)] *a* 心理测量的；心理测量学的 | **psychometrician** [saiˌkɔməˈtriʃən] *n* 心理测量医师，心理测量学家

psychomotor [ˌsaikəuˈməutə] *a* 精神运动性的

psychoneural [ˌsaikəuˈnjuərəl] *a* 精神神经的，心理神经的

psychoneuroendocrinology [ˌsaikəuˌnjuərəuˌendəukriˈnɔlədʒi] *n* 精神神经内分泌学

psychoneuroimmunology [ˌsaikəuˌnjuərəuˌimjuːˈnɔlədʒi] *n* 精神神经免疫学

psychoneurosis [ˌsaikəunjuəˈrəusis]（[复] **psychoneuroses** [ˌsaikəunjuəˈrəusiːz]）*n* 精神神经[功能]病，神经症 | defense ~ 防御性精神神经病 | **psychoneurotic** [ˌsaikəunjuəˈrɔtik] *a* 精神神经[功能]病的 *n* 精神神经[功能]病患者

psychonomy [saiˈkɔnəmi] *n* 心理规律学

psychopath [ˈsaikəpæθ] *n* 精神变态者，变态人格者，病态人格者 | sexual ~ 性欲性精神变态者

psychopathia [ˌsaikəuˈpæθiə] *n* 精神变态，变态人格，病态人格 | ~ sexualis 性欲性精神变态，性变态，性倒错

psychopathic [ˌsaikəuˈpæθik] *a* 精神变态的，变态人格的 *n* 精神变态者

psychopathology [ˌsaikəupəˈθɔlədʒi] *n* 精神病理学 | **psychopathological** [ˌsaikəupæθəˈlɔdʒikəl] *a* / **psychopathologist** *n* 精神病理学家

psychopathy [saiˈkɔpəθi] *n* 精神病态，变态人格，病态人格

psychopharmacology [ˌsaikəuˌfɑːməˈkɔlədʒi] *n* 精神药理学 | **psychopharmacologic(al)** [ˌsaikəufɑːməkəˈlɔdʒik(əl)] *a*

psychophylaxis [ˌsaikəufiˈlæksis] *n* 精神病预防，心理卫生

psychophysics [ˌsaikəuˈfiziks] *n* 精神物理学 | **psychophysical** *a* | **psychophysicist** *n* 精神物理学家

psychophysiology [ˌsaikəuˌfiziˈɔlədʒi] *n* 精神生理学 | **psychophysiologic(al)** [ˌsaikəuˌfiziəˈlɔdʒik(əl)] *a*

psychoplasm [ˈsaikəplæzəm] *n* 精神原质，精神元气；玄质，始质（见 protyl）

psychoplegia [ˌsaikəuˈpliːdʒiə] *n* 急性痴呆，精神麻痹

psychoplegic [ˌsaikəuˈpliːdʒik] *a* 抑制精神的 *n* 精神抑制药（安定药）

psychopneumatology [ˌsaikəuˌnjuːməˈtɔlədʒi] *n* 心身学；心灵学

psychoprophylaxis [ˌsaikəuˌprɔfiˈlæksis] *n* 精神病预防，心理卫生 | **psychoprophylactic** [ˌsaikəuˌprɔfiˈlæktik] *a*

psychoreaction [ˌsaikəuri(ː)ˈækʃən] *n* 精神[病]性（血清）反应（见 Much's reaction）

psychorrhexis [ˌsaikəuˈreksis] *n* 精神崩溃

psychosedation [ˌsaikəusiˈdeiʃən] *n* 精神镇静[法]

psychosedative [ˌsaikəuˈsedətiv] *a* 精神镇静的 *n* 精神镇静药

psychosensory [ˌsaikəuˈsensəri], **psychosensorial** [ˌsaikəusenˈsɔːriəl] *a* 精神[性]感觉的,心理感觉的

psychosexual [ˌsaikəuˈseksjuəl] *a* 性心理的

psychosine [ˈsaikəˌsiːn] *n* 鞘氨醇半乳糖苷

psychosis [saiˈkəusis] ([复] **psychoses** [saiˈkəusiːz]) *n* 精神病 | affective ~ 情感性精神病 / alcoholic ~ 酒精中毒性精神病 / bipolar ~ 双相性精神病,双相性精神障碍 / brief reactive ~ 短暂反应性精神病(对生活中令人悲痛的事件的一种反应,出现一系列精神病症状:思维不连贯、妄想、幻觉、混乱或紧张型行为,起病突然,但不到一个月即消失) / involutional ~ 更年期精神病 / manic ~ 躁狂性精神病 / manicdepressive ~ 躁狂抑郁性精神病,躁郁病 / schizoaffective ~ 分裂情感性精神病 / symbiotic ~, symbiotic infantile ~ 共生性精神病,婴儿与母共生性精神病(见于 2~4 岁儿童,他们与抚养人关系不正常,表现为强烈的分离焦虑、严重的退化、不会说实用的话和孤独症;现包括在儿童期综合性精神发育障碍之列) / unipolar ~ 单相性精神病,重性抑郁症

psychosocial [ˌsaikəuˈsəuʃəl] *a* 精神社会的,心理社会的

psychosolytic [saiˌkəusəˈlitik] *a* 抗精神病的 *n* 抗精神病药(强安定药)

psychosomatic [ˌsaikəusəuˈmætik] *a* 身心的,心身的

psychosomaticist [ˌsaikəusəuˈmætəsist] *n* 身心医学家

psychosomimetic [saiˌkəusəumaiˈmetik] *a* 拟精神病的 *n* 拟精神病药,致幻药

psychostimulant [ˌsaikəuˈstimjulənt] *a* 精神刺激的 *n* 精神兴奋药

psychosurgery [ˌsaikəuˈsəːdʒəri] *n* 精神外科 | **psychosurgical** [ˌsaikəuˈsəːdʒikəl] *a*

psychotechnics [ˌsaikəuˈtekniks] *n* 心理技术学(用心理学方法研究社会问题及其他问题)

psychotherapeutics [ˌsaikəuˌθerəˈpjuːtiks] *n* 精神治疗,心理治疗 | **psychotherapeutic** *a*

psychotherapy [ˌsaikəuˈθerəpi] *n* 精神治疗,心理治疗 | brief ~ 短暂心理治疗 / existential ~ 存在主义心理治疗(以 Kierkegaard, Herdegger, Jaspers 等人的存在主义〈existential philosophy〉为基础的治疗,其重点不在于合理思考,而在于目前的相互作用和情感体验上) / group ~ 集体心理治疗 / personologic ~ 人格心理治疗 / supportive ~ 支持性心理治疗

psychotic [saiˈkɔtik] *a* [患]精神病的 *n* 精神病患者

psychotogenic [saiˌkɔtəˈdʒenik] *a* 致精神病的

psychotomimetic [saiˌkɔtəumaiˈmetik] *a* 拟精神病的 *n* 拟精神病药,致幻药

psychotonic [ˌsaikəuˈtɔnik] *a* [促]精神兴奋的 *n* 精神兴奋药(抗抑郁药)

psychotropic [ˌsaikəuˈtrɔpik] *a* 亲精神的(常指影响精神状态的药物)

psychr(o)- [构词成分]冷,寒冷

psychroalgia [ˌsaikrəuˈældʒiə] *n* 冷痛

psychroesthesia [ˌsaikrəuisˈθiːzjə] *n* 冷觉;寒冷感,感冷

psychrolusia [ˌsaikrəuˈluːziə] *n* 冷水浴

psychrometer [saiˈkrɔmitə] *n* 干湿球湿度计 | sling ~ 手摇干湿球湿度计

psychrophile [ˈsaikrəfail] *n* 嗜冷生物

psychrophilic [ˌsaikrəuˈfilik] *a* 嗜冷的(指细菌)

psychrophore [ˈsaikrəfɔː] *n* 冷却导管,尿道施冷管

psychrotherapy [ˌsaikrəuˈθerəpi] *n* 冷疗[法]

psyllium [ˈsiliəm] *n* 欧车前

PT prothrombin time 凝血酶原时间

Pt platinum 铂

PTA plasma thromboplastin antecedent 血浆凝血激酶前质(凝血因子Ⅺ); pure tone average 纯音听阈均值

ptarmic [ˈtɑːmik] *a* 引嚏的

ptarmus [tɑːmɔs] *n* 痉挛性喷嚏

PTC plasma thromboplastin component 血浆凝血激酶组分(凝血因子Ⅸ); phenylthiocarbamide 苯硫脲

PTCA percutaneous transluminal coronary angioplasty 经皮腔内冠状动脉成形术

PteGlu pteroylglutamate or pteroylglutamic acid 蝶酰谷氨酸

PTEN pentaerythritol tetranitrate 硝酸戊四醇酯,戊四硝酯

pteridine [ˈteridin] *n* 蝶啶

Pteridophyta [ˌteriˈdɔfitə] *n* 蕨类植物门

pteridophyte [təˈridəfait] *n* 蕨类植物

pterin [ˈterin] *n* 蝶呤

pterion [ˈteriən] *n* 翼点(额、顶、颞骨与蝶骨大翼交接之点,在眶骨外角突后面约 3 cm 处)

pternalgia [təˈnældʒiə] *n* 跟痛

pteroic acid [təˈrəuik] 蝶酸

pteropterin [teˈrɔptərin] *n* 蝶罗呤,蝶酰三谷氨酸(亦称干酪乳杆菌发酵因子)

pteroylglutamate [ˌterɔilˈgluːtəmeit] *n* 蝶酰谷氨酸,叶酸(阴离子型)

pteroylglutamic acid (**PteGlu**) [ˌterɔilgluːˈtæmik] 蝶酰谷氨酸,叶酸

pteroylpolyglutamate [ˌterɔilˌpɔliˈgluːtəmeit] *n* 蝶酰多聚谷氨酸盐

pteroyltriglutamic acid [ˌterɔiltraiglu:ˈtæmik] 蝶酰三谷氨酸(即 pteropterin)
pterygium [təˈridʒiəm] *n*【希】翼状胬肉 | **pterygial** *a*
pterygoid [ˈterigɔid] *a* 翼状的
pterygomandibular [ˌterigəumænˈdibjulə] *a* 翼突下颌的
pterygomaxillary [ˌterigəuˈmæksiləri] *a* 翼突上颌的
pterygopalatine [ˌterigəuˈpælətin] *a* 翼突腭的
PTFE polytetrafluoroethylene 聚四氟乙烯
PTH parathyroid hormone 甲状旁腺[激]素
Pthirus [ˈθirəs] *n* 阴虱属
ptilosis [taiˈləusis] *n* 睫毛脱落;鸵鸟毛尘肺
ptomaine [ˈtəumein, təuˈmein] *n* 尸碱,尸毒,肉毒胺
ptomainemia [ˌtəumeiˈni:miə] *n* 尸碱血
ptomainotoxism [ˌtəumeinəuˈtɔksizəm] *n* 尸碱中毒
ptomatine [ˈtəumətin] *n* 尸碱,尸毒,肉毒胺
ptomatopsia [ˌtəuməˈtɔpsiə], **ptomatopsy** [ˌtəuməˈtɔpsi] *n* 尸体剖检
ptomatropine [təuˈmætrəpin] *n* 尸阿托品
ptosed [təust] *a* 下垂的
ptosis [ˈtəusis] *n* 下垂;上睑下垂 | ~ adiposa, false ~ 脂肪性上睑下垂,假上睑下垂 / waking ~, morning ~ 清晨上睑下垂 | **ptotic** [ˈtɔtik] *a*
-ptosis [构词成分]下垂
PTRA percutaneous transluminal renal angioplasty 经皮腔内肾动脉成形术
PTSD posttraumatic stress disorder 创伤后应激障碍
PTT partial thromboplastin time 部分促凝血酶原激酶时间;activated partial thromboplastin time 活化部分促凝血酶原激酶时间
ptyalagogue [taiˈæləgɔg] *a* 催涎的 *n* 催涎药
ptyalectasis [ˌtaiəˈlektəsis] *n* 涎管扩张
ptyalin [ˈtaiəlin] *n* 唾液淀粉酶
ptyalinogen [ˌtaiəˈlinədʒən] *n* 唾液淀粉酶原
ptyalism [ˈtaiəlizəm] *n* 多涎
ptyalith [ˈtaiəliθ] *n* 涎石
ptyalize [ˈtaiəlaiz] *vt* 催涎
ptyal(o)- [构词成分]涎,唾液
ptyalocele [taiˈæləsi:l] *n* 涎[液]囊肿 | sublingual ~ 舌下囊肿
ptyalogenic [ˌtaiələuˈdʒenik] *a* 涎原的,涎性的
ptyalography [ˌtaiəˈlɔgrəfi] *n* 涎管[X 线]造影[术]
ptyalolithiasis [ˌtaiələuliˈθaiəsis] *n* 涎石症
ptyalolithotomy [ˌtaiələuliˈθɔtəmi] *n* 涎石切除术
ptyaloreaction [ˌtaiələuri(:)ˈækʃən] *n* 涎反应
ptyalorrhea [ˌtaiələˈri:ə] *n* 涎分泌过多,流涎
ptyalose [ˈtaiələus] *n* 涎糖,麦芽糖
ptyocrinous [taiˈɔkrinəs] *a* 粒性分泌的,离泌的(指单细胞腺体如杯状细胞的分泌)
Pu plutonium 钚
pubarche [pju(:)ˈba:ki] *n* 阴毛初现
puberal [ˈpju:bərəl] *a* 青春期的
pubertas [pju(:)ˈbɔ:təs] *n*【拉】青春期 | ~ praecox 性早熟
puberty [ˈpju:bə(:)ti] *n* 青春期 | delayed ~ 青春期延迟 | **pubertal** *a*
puberulic acid [pju(:)ˈberulik] 软毛青霉酸
puberulonic acid [pju(:)ˌberuˈlɔnik] *n* 软毛青霉酮酸
pubes [ˈpju:bi:z] *n* pubis 的复数;阴毛;阴阜;耻骨区
pubescence [pju(:)ˈbesns] *n* 青春期;有毛 | **pubescent** *a*
pubic [ˈpju:bik] *a* 耻骨的
pubioplasty [ˈpju:biəˌplæsti] *n* 耻骨成形术
pubiotomy [ˌpju:biˈɔtəmi] *n* 耻骨切开术
pubis [ˈpju:bis] ([复] **pubes** [ˈpju:bi:z]) *n*【拉】耻骨
pubisure [ˈpju:bisjuə] *n* 阴毛
pubococcygeal [ˌpju:bəukɔkˈsidʒiəl] *a* 耻骨尾骨的,耻骨尾骨肌的
pubococcygeus [ˌpju:bəukɔkˈsidʒiəs] *a* 耻骨尾骨的
pubofemoral [ˌpju:bəuˈfemərəl] *a* 耻骨股骨的
puboprostatic [ˌpju:bəuprɔsˈtætik] *a* 耻骨前列腺的
puborectal [ˌpju:bəuˈrektl] *a* 耻骨直肠的,耻骨直肠肌的
puborectalis [ˌpju:bəurekˈteilis] *a* 耻骨直肠的
pubotibial [ˌpju:bəuˈtibiəl] *a* 耻骨胫骨的
pubovesical [ˌpju:bəuˈvesikəl] *a* 耻骨膀胱的
PUBS percutaneous umbilical blood sampling 经皮脐血抽样
pudendagra [ˌpju:denˈdægrə] *n* 阴部痛
pudendum [pju(:)ˈdendəm] ([复] **pudenda** [pju(:)ˈdendə]) *n*【拉】阴部 | female ~ 女阴 | **pudendal**, **pudic** [ˈpju:dik] *a*
puericulture [ˈpjuəriˌkʌltʃə] *n* 育儿法
puericulturist [ˌpjuəriˈkʌltʃərist] *n* 育儿专家
puerile [ˈpjuərail] *a* 童年的,儿童的,幼稚的
puerpera [pju(:)ˈə:pərə] *n* 产妇
puerperalism [pju(:)ˈə:pərəlizəm] *n* 产褥病
puerperant [pju(:)ˈə:pərənt] *a* 分娩的,产后的 *n* 产妇
puerperium [ˌpju:əˈpiəriəm] *n*【拉】产褥期 | **puerperal** [pju(:)ˈə:pərəl] *a*
PUFA polyunsaturated fatty acid 多不饱和脂肪酸
puff [pʌf] *n* 吹气音;疏松(染色体上) | chromo-

some ~s 染色体疏松(昆虫巨唾腺染色体中RNA和DNA合成的活性位点)/ veiled ~ 微哑吹气音(一种肺动脉瓣杂音)
puffer [ˈpʌfə] *n* 河鲀,河豚
puffer fish [ˈpʌfə fiʃ] 河鲀,河豚
puffing [ˈpʌfiŋ] *n* 疏松部(染色体上的)
pulegone [ˈpjuːligəun] *n* 长叶薄荷酮
Pulex [ˈpjuːleks] *n*【拉】蚤属 | ~ cheopis 印度客蚤,鼠疫蚤(即 Xenopsylla cheopis)/ ~ irritans, ~ dugesi 人蚤,扰蚤,长喙蚤/ ~ penetrans 穿皮蚤(即穿皮潜蚤 Tunga penetrans)/ ~ serraticeps 犬栉头蚤(即 Ctenocephalides canis)
pulex [ˈpjuːleks] ([复] **pulices** [ˈpjuːlisiːz]) *n*【拉】蚤
Pulheems [ˈpʌlhiːmz] (英国武装部队记录征募新兵身体和精神状态的)体检分类法(P为 physical capacity 体力,U为 upper limbs 上肢,L为 lower limbs 下肢,H为 hearing〈acuity〉听敏度,EE为 eyesight 视力〈视敏度〉,M为 mental capacity 心理能量,S为 stability〈emotional〉〈情绪〉稳定)
pulicicide [pjuːˈlisisaid] *n* 灭蚤药
Pulicidae [pjuːˈlisidiː] *n* 蚤科
pull [pul] *vt* 牵拉肌肉
Pullularia [ˌpʌljuˈlɛəriə] *n* 芽霉菌属 | ~ pullulans 产糖芽霉菌
pullulate [ˈpʌljuleit] *n* 出芽,生芽,发芽 | **pullulation** [ˌpʌljuˈleiʃən] *n*
pulmo [ˈpʌlməu] ([复] **pulmones** [pʌlˈməuniːz]) *n*【拉】肺
pulmo- [构词成分] 肺
pulmoaortic [ˌpʌlməueiˈɔːtik] *a* 肺[与]主动脉的
pulmogram [ˈpʌlməgræm] *n* 肺X线[照]片
pulmolith [ˈpʌlməliθ] *n* 肺石
pulmometer [pʌlˈmɔmitə] *n* 肺容量计 | **pulmometry** *n* 肺容量测定法
pulmonary [ˈpʌlmənəri], **pulmonal** [ˈpʌlmənl] *a* 肺的
Pulmonata [ˌpʌlməˈneitə] *n* 肺螺亚纲
pulmonectomy [ˌpʌlməuˈnektəmi] *n* 肺切除术
pulmones [pʌlˈməuniːz] pulmo 的复数;左右肺
pulmonic [pʌlˈmɔnik] *a* 肺的;肺动脉的
pulmonitis [ˌpʌlməuˈnaitis] *n* 肺炎
pulmon(o)- [构词成分]肺
pulmonohepatic [ˌpʌlmənəuhiˈpætik] *a* 肺肝的
pulmonology [ˌpʌlməˈnɔlədʒi] *n* 肺病学(研究肺的解剖、生理和病理的科学) | **pulmonologist** *n* 肺病学家
pulmonoperitoneal [ˌpʌlmənəuˌperitəuˈniəl] *a* 肺[与]腹膜的
pulmotor [ˈpʌlməutə] *n* 自动供氧人工呼吸器
pulp [pʌlp] *n* 髓 | coronal ~ 冠髓 / dead ~, devitalized ~, necrotic ~, nonvital ~ 坏死性牙髓,失活髓 / digital ~ 指垫,趾垫 / exposed ~ 露髓 / mummified ~ 干尸化牙髓 / red ~, splenic ~ 红髓,脾髓 / wood ~ 木纸浆 | **~al** *a*
pulpa [ˈpʌlpə] ([复] **pulpae** [ˈpʌlpiː]) *n*【拉】髓
pulpalgia [pʌlˈpældʒiə] *n* 牙髓痛
pulpectomy [pʌlˈpektəmi] *n* 牙髓摘除术
pulpefaction [ˌpʌlpiˈfækʃən], **pulpation** [pʌlˈpeiʃən] *n* 成髓,髓化
pulpiform [ˈpʌlpifɔːm] *a* 髓样的
pulpitis [pʌlˈpaitis] ([复] **pulpitides** [pʌlˈpitidiːz]) *n* 牙髓炎 | anachoretic ~ 细菌性牙髓炎 / hypertrophic ~ 肥大性牙髓炎
pulpless [ˈpʌlplis] *a* 无髓的(牙)
pulpoaxial [ˌpʌlpəuˈæksiəl] *a* 髓轴的
pulpobuccoaxial [ˌpʌlpəuˌbʌkəuˈæksiəl] *a* 髓颊轴的
pulpodistal [ˌpʌlpəuˈdistl] *a* 髓远中的
pulpodontics [ˌpʌlpəuˈdɔntiks], **pulpodontia** [ˌpʌlpəuˈdɔnʃiə] *n* 牙髓病学
pulpolabial [ˌpʌlpəuˈleibjəl] *a* 髓唇的
pulpolingual [ˌpʌlpəuˈliŋgwəl] *a* 髓舌的
pulpolinguoaxial [ˌpʌlpəuˌliŋgwəuˈæksiəl] *a* 髓舌轴的
pulpomesial [ˌpʌlpəuˈmiːziəl] *a* 髓近中的
pulpotomy [pʌlˈpɔtəmi] *n* 牙髓切断术
pulpy [ˈpʌlpi], **pulpous** [ˈpʌlpəs] *a* 髓样的
pulque [ˈpʌlki] *n* 龙舌兰汁酒
pulsate [ˈpʌlseit] *vi* 搏动(如心脏)
pulsatile [ˈpʌlsətail] *a* 搏动的
pulsatilla [ˌpʌlsəˈtilə] *n* 洋白头翁
pulsation [pʌlˈseiʃən] *n* 搏动(如心脏) | expansile ~ 扩张性搏动 / suprasternal ~ 胸骨上搏动
pulsative [ˈpʌlsətiv] *a* 搏动的
pulsator [pʌlˈseitə] *n* 搏动式人工呼吸器
pulsatory [ˈpʌlsətəri] *a* 能搏动的
pulse [pʌls] *n* 脉搏;脉冲 | abdominal ~, epigastric ~ 腹部(主动脉)脉搏 / abrupt ~ 促脉 / anacrotic ~ 升线一波脉 / anadicrotic ~ 升线二波脉 / anatricrotic ~ 升线三波脉 / bigeminal ~, coupled ~ 二联脉 / catadicrotic ~ 降线二波脉 / catatricrotic ~ 降线三波脉 / dicrotic ~ 二波脉,重搏脉 / entopic ~ 闪光感性心搏 / equal ~ 均脉 / frequent ~ 数脉 / full ~ 洪脉 / infrequent ~ 稀脉,迟脉 / intermittent ~, dropped-beat ~ 间歇脉 / jerky ~, sharp ~, vibrating ~ 急冲脉 / monocrotic ~ 单波脉 / nail ~ 甲部搏动 / paradoxical ~ 奇脉 / pistor-shot ~ 射击脉,弹射脉 / plateau ~ 丘状脉,徐脉 / polycrotic ~ 多波脉 / quadrigeminal ~ 四联脉 / quick ~,

short ~ 促脉,短脉 / running ~ 奔逸脉,颤脉 / tricrotic ~ 三波脉 / trigeminal ~ 三联脉 / trip-hammer ~, water-hammer ~ 水冲脉 / undulating ~ 波状脉 / vermicular ~ 蠕动脉 / wiry ~ 弦脉 | ~**less** *a* 无脉的

pulsion [ˈpʌlʃən] *n* 推出,压出

pulsus [ˈpʌlsəs] ([复] **pulsus**) *n*【拉】脉搏

pultaceous [pʌlˈteiʃəs] *a* 髓样的

pulv. pulvis【拉】散剂,粉剂

pulverize [ˈpʌlvəraiz] *vt* 粉碎,研碎 | **pulverization** [ˌpʌlvəraiˈzeiʃən] *n* 粉碎,研末

pulverulent [pʌlˈverjulənt] *a* 粉的,粉状的,粉样的 | **pulverulence** *n*

pulvinar [pʌlˈvainə] *n*【拉】丘脑枕

pulvinate [ˈpʌlvineit] *a* 枕状的,垫状的

pulvis [ˈpʌlvis] *n*【拉】散剂,粉剂

pumice [ˈpʌmis], **pumex** [ˈpjuːmeks] *n* 浮石粉(牙科用作研磨剂)

pump [pʌmp] *n* 泵,唧筒 *vt* 压出,抽吸(液体或气体) | air ~ 排气泵,抽气泵 / blood ~ 血泵(通过体外循环装置的管道推动血液) / breast ~ 吸乳器 / calcium ~ 钙泵 / cardiac balloon ~ 心脏气囊泵 / infusion-withdrawal ~ 输液吸液泵 / peristaltic ~ 蠕动泵 / sodium ~, sodium-potassium ~, Na^+-K^+ ~ 钠泵,钠-钾泵 / stomach ~ 胃泵,胃吸引器

pumpkin [ˈpʌmpkin] *n* 西葫芦

pump-oxygenator [pʌmp ɔksidʒineitə] *n* 泵式充氧器(一般用作体外循环的血液充氧,以便心脏手术时使心肺得到缓解)

puna [ˈpuːnə] *n* 高山病

punch [pʌntʃ] *n* 打孔凿,钻孔器 | kidney ~ 肾脏冲击诊 / pin ~ 牙针钻孔器 / plate ~ 托板打孔凿,穿板器 / rubber dam ~ 橡皮障钻孔器

punchdrunk [ˈpʌntʃdrʌŋk] *a* 拳击手酩酊样的(脑病) *n* 拳击手痴呆,拳击手外伤性脑病

punched-out [ˈpʌntʃtaut] *n* 凿缘(凿孔状边缘)

puncta [ˈpʌŋktə] punctum 的复数

punctal [ˈpʌnktəl] *a* 点的,泪点的

punctate [ˈpʌŋkteit] *a* 点状的 | **punctation** [pʌŋkˈteiʃən] *n*

punctiform [ˈpʌŋktifɔːm] *a* 点状的(细菌学中指极细小的菌落)

punctio [ˈpʌŋkʃiəu] *n*【拉】穿刺[术]

punctograph [ˈpʌŋktəgrɑːf] *n* (异物)定位 X 线摄影机

punctual [ˈpʌŋktjuəl, ˈpʌŋktʃuəl] *a* 点状的

punctuation [ˌpʌŋktjuˈeiʃən, ˌpʌŋktʃuˈeiʃən] *n* 小点,点

punctum [ˈpʌŋktəm] ([复] **puncta** [ˈpʌŋktə]) *n*【拉】点,尖

punctumeter [pʌŋkˈtʌmitə] *n* 眼调节计

punctura [pʌŋkˈtjuərə] *n*【拉】穿刺[术]

puncturatio [ˌpʌŋktjuəˈreiʃiəu] *n*【拉】穿刺

puncture [ˈpʌŋktʃə] *n* 穿刺[术];刺伤 *vt* 刺,刺穿 *vi* 被刺穿 | cisternal ~, cranial ~, intracisternal ~, suboccipital ~ 小脑延髓池穿刺 / diabetic ~ 糖尿穿刺 / epigastric ~ 上腹部穿刺 / exploratory ~ 试探穿刺 / heat ~ 发热穿刺(穿刺动物脑底引起发热) / lumbar ~ 腰椎穿刺 / spinal ~ 椎管穿刺 / splenic ~ 脾穿刺 / sternal ~ 胸骨穿刺 / thecal ~ 脊椎[膜]穿刺 / tonsil ~ 扁桃体穿刺 / ventricular ~ 脑室穿刺

pungent [ˈpʌndʒənt] *a* 刺激味的

punizin [ˈpjuːnizin] *n* 紫螺紫素

Punnett square [ˈpʌnit] (Reginald Crundall Punnett) 庞纳特方格(见 checkerboard)

Puntius [ˈpʌnitəs] *n* 须鲃属 | ~ javanicus 爪哇须鲃

PUO pyrexia of unknown origin 原因不明发热

pupa [ˈpjuːpə] ([复] **pupas** 或 **pupae** [ˈpjuːpiː]) *n*【拉】蛹 | ~**l** *a*

pupil(P) [ˈpjuːpil] *n* 瞳孔 | bounding ~ 弹跃性瞳孔(交替性瞳孔散大和缩小现象) / cat's-eye ~ 猫眼状瞳孔(瞳孔细长) / keyhole ~ 钥孔状瞳孔 / pinhole ~ 针孔状瞳孔 / skew ~s 斜瞳孔 / stiff ~ 强直性瞳孔 / tonic ~ 紧张性瞳孔 | ~**lary** [ˈpjuːpiləri] *a*

pupilla [pjuːˈpilə] ([复] **pupillae** [pjuːˈpiliː]) *n*【拉】瞳孔

pupillatonia [ˌpjuːpiləˈtəuniə] *n* 瞳孔反应消失

Pupillidae [pjuːˈpilidiː] *n* 虹蛹螺科

pupill(o)- [构词成分]瞳孔

pupillograph [pjuːˈpiləgrɑːf, -græf] *n* 瞳孔描记器(检查瞳孔反应)

pupillometer [ˌpjuːpiˈlɔmitə] *n* 瞳孔计 | **pupillometry** *n* 瞳孔测量[法]

pupillomotor [ˌpjuːpiləuˈməutə] *a* 瞳孔运动的

pupilloplegia [ˌpjuːpiləuˈpliːdʒiə] *n* 瞳孔反应消失

pupilloscope [pjuːˈpiləskəup] *n* 瞳孔反应检查器;视网膜镜

pupilloscopy [ˌpjuːpiˈlɔskəpi] *n* 视网膜镜检查

pupillostatometer [pjuːˌpiləustəˈtɔmitə] *n* 瞳孔距离计

pupillotonia [ˌpjuːpiləuˈtəuniə] *n* 瞳孔紧张症

purblind [ˈpəːblaind] *a* 半盲的

Purdy's method [ˈpəːdi] (Charles W. Purdy) 珀迪法(离心定量测定白蛋白、氯化物、硫酸盐等) | ~ test 珀迪试验(检白蛋白)

pure [pjuə] *a* 纯的

purgación [ˌpuəgəsiˈɔn] *n*【西】淋病

purgation [pəːˈgeiʃən] *n* 催泻,通便

purgative [ˈpəːgətiv] *a* 催泻的 *n* 泻药

purge [pəːdʒ] *vt*, *vi* 净化;催泻 *n* 净化;泻药
puric [ˈpjuərik] *a* 脓的;嘌呤的
puriform [ˈpjuərifɔːm] *a* 脓样的
purify [ˈpjuərifai] *vt* 使净化;精制
purification [ˌpjuərifiˈkeiʃən] *n* 净化 | blood ~ 血液净化
purinase [ˈpjuərineis] *n* 嘌呤酶
purine [ˈpjuəri(ː)n] *n* 嘌呤 | amino ~ 氨基嘌呤 / methyl ~s 甲基嘌呤
purinemia [ˌpjuəriˈniːmiə] *n* 嘌呤血[症] | **purinemic** *a*
purine-nucleoside phosphorylase [ˈpjuəriːn ˈnjuːkliəsaid fɔsˈfɔːrileis] 嘌呤-核苷磷酸化酶(此酶活性缺乏为一种常染色体隐性性状,可致细胞免疫缺陷)
purinolytic [ˌpjuərinəˈlitik] *a* 分解嘌呤的
purinometer [ˌpjuəriˈnɔmitə] *n* 尿嘌呤定量器
purity [ˈpjuərəti] *n* 纯度
Purkinje-Sanson mirror images [pəˈkindʒi sɑːŋˈsɔŋ] (J. E. Purkinje; Louis J. Sanson) 浦肯野-桑松镜像(见 Purkinje's images)
Purkinje's cells [pəˈkindʒi] (Johannes E, von Purkinje) 浦肯野细胞(存于小脑皮质中层内) | ~ fibers 浦肯野纤维(在心内膜下组织内的心肌纤维,其稠密的网形成窦房结和房室结) / ~ images 浦肯野[影]像(在角膜前面和晶状体前后面的三个投射像,两个前面像是虚像,非倒像,一个后面像是实像、倒像,用于研究晶状体面在调节时的运动) / ~ network 浦肯野网,心内膜下支 / ~ phenomenon 浦肯野现象(若照光的强度减低时,同等明亮但颜色不同的区域成为明亮不同的现象) / ~ shift 浦肯野转移(最强视力区随着照光的强度减少在光谱中从黄区移至紫区) / ~ vesicle 浦肯野泡,胚泡,生发泡(未成熟卵的核)
purohepatitis [ˌpjuərəuˌhepəˈtaitis] *n* 脓性肝炎,肝脓肿
puromucous [ˌpjuərəˈmjuːkəs] *a* 黏液脓性的
puromycin [ˌpjuərəuˈmaisin] *n* 嘌罗霉素(抗生素类药) | ~ hydrochloride 盐酸嘌罗霉素
puron [ˈpjuərɔn] *n* 氧嘌呤
purple [ˈpəːpl] *n* 紫色,紫 *a* 紫[色]的 | bromcresol ~ 溴甲酚紫(测氢离子浓度) / tyrian ~, royal ~ 泰尔红紫,皇紫(一种古代的紫色染料) / visual ~ 视紫质,视紫红质
Purpura [ˈpəːpjurə] *n* 荔枝螺属
purpura [ˈpəːpjurə] *n* 紫癜 | allergic ~ 变应性紫癜 / anaphylactoid ~ 过敏性紫癜 / ~ hyperglobulinemica 高球蛋白血症性紫癜(反复发生紫癜并伴有血清中丙球蛋白增多) / idiopathic ~ 特发性紫癜 / malignant ~ 恶性紫癜,流行性脑脊膜炎 / nonthrombocytopenic ~ 血小板不减少性紫癜,血小板正常性紫癜 / thrombocytopenic ~, thrombopenic ~ 血小板减少性紫癜
purpurate [ˈpəːpjureit] *n* 红紫酸盐
purpureaglycoside [pəːˌpjuəriəˈglaikəsaid] *n* 紫花洋地黄苷(一种强心苷)
purpuric [pəːˈpjuərik] *a* 紫癜的
purpuric acid [pəˈpjuːrik] 红紫酸
purpuriferous [ˌpəːpjuˈrifərəs], **purpuriparous** [ˌpəːpjuˈripərəs] *a* 生紫色的
purpurin [ˈpəːpjurin] *n* 羟基茜草素,紫红素,1,2,4-三羟蒽醌(用作核染剂);尿紫素
purpurine [ˈpəːpjuriːn] *n* 荔枝螺素; = purpurin
purpurinuria [ˌpəːpjuriˈnjuəriə] *n* 尿紫素尿
purpurogenous [ˌpəːpjuˈrɔdʒinəs] *a* 生视紫质的
purr [pəː] *n* 猫喘音,鸣呜
purring [ˈpəːriŋ] *a* 猫喘音样的
purshianin [pəːˈʃaiənin] *n* 波希鼠李苷(有导泻作用)
pursuit [pəˈsjuit] *n* 跟随,跟踪 | ~ test 跟随试验
Purtilo's syndrome [pəːˈtiləu] (David T. Purtilo) X-连锁淋巴细胞增生综合征
Purtscher's disease (angiopathic retinopathy) [ˈpuətʃə] (Otmar Purtscher) 普尔夏病(血管性视网膜病变)(外伤性视网膜血管病,伴有水肿、出血和渗出物,一般为胸部挤压伤之后出现)
puru [ˈpuru] *n* 雅司病(马来西亚土名,即 yaws)
purulent [ˈpjuərulənt] *a* 脓性的,化脓性的 | **purulence**, **purulency** *n*
puruloid [ˈpjuərulɔid] *a* 脓样的
pus [pʌs] *n* 脓 | anchovy sauce ~ 果酱色脓 / blue ~ 蓝脓 / burrowing ~ 钻穿性脓 / cheesy ~ 稠脓,干脓 / curdy ~ 凝乳样脓 / ichorous ~ 败液性脓,稀臭脓 / laudable ~, ~ bonum et laudabile 黄稠脓,无毒脓 / sanious ~ 血性臭脓
Pusey's emulsion [ˈpjuːsi] (William A. Pusey) 普西乳剂(治婴儿湿症)
pussy [ˈpʌsi] *a* 多脓的,似脓的
pustula [ˈpʌstjulə] ([复] **pustulae** [ˈpʌstjuliː]) *n*【拉】脓疱
pustulant [ˈpʌstjulənt] *a* 起脓疱的 *n* 起脓疱剂
pustulate [ˈpʌstjuleit] *vt*, *vi* 脓疱形成 [ˈpʌstjulit] *a* 生脓疱的 | **pustulation** [ˌpʌstjuˈleiʃən] *n*
pustule [ˈpʌstjuːl] *n* 脓疱 | multilocular ~ 多房性脓疱 / spongiform ~ 海绵状脓疱 / unilocular ~ 单房性脓疱 | **pustular** *a*
pustulosis [ˌpʌstjuˈləusis] *n* 脓疱病 | ~ palmaris et plantaris, palmoplantar ~ 掌跖脓疱病 / ~ vacciniformis acuta, ~ varioliformis acuta 急性痘疮样脓疱病
putamen [pjuːˈteimən] *n*【拉】壳(豆状核)
Putnam type, Putnam-Dana syndrome [ˈput-

nəm ˈdeinə] (James J. Putnam; Charles L. Dana) 普特南型、普特南-达纳综合征(亚急性脊髓混合变性)
putrefaction [ˌpjuːtriˈfækʃən] *n* 腐败[作用],腐化[作用] | **putrefactive** *a*
putrefy [ˈpjuːtrifai] *vt, vi* 腐败,腐化
putrescent [pjuːˈtresnt] *a* 腐败的,腐化的 | **putrescence** *n*
putrescine [pjuːˈtresin] *n* 腐胺
putrid [ˈpjuːtrid] *a* 腐败的,恶臭的 | **~ity** [pjuːˈtridəti] *n*
putrilage [ˈpjuːtrilidʒ] *n* 腐败物,腐质
putromaine [pjuːˈtrəumein] *n* 腐败毒(在活体内食物分解产生的)
Puussepp's operation [ˈpusep] (Lyudvig M. Puussepp) 普塞普手术(分裂脊髓中央管,治脊髓空洞症) | ~ reflex 普塞普反射(刺激足底后外侧,小趾即外展,为锥体外束和锥体束损害之征)
PUVA psoralen plus ultraviolet A 补骨脂素加紫外线A(一种内服补骨脂素,外用紫外线A照射的疗法,治疗各种皮肤病)
PVC polyvinyl chloride 聚氯乙烯;postvoiding cystogram 排尿后膀胱造影[照]片;premature ventricular contraction 室性期前收缩,室性早搏;pulmonary venous congestion 肺静脉充血
PVL periventricular leukomalacia 室周脑白质软化
PVP polyvinylpyrrolidone 聚乙烯吡咯酮,聚烯吡酮,聚维酮
PVP-I povidone-iodine 聚维酮碘,聚烯吡酮碘,聚乙烯吡咯酮碘
PVS persistent vegetative state 持续性植物状态
PWA person with AIDS 艾滋病患者
PWM pokeweed mitogen [美洲]商陆丝裂原
pyarthrosis [ˌpaiɑːˈθrəusis] *n* 关节积脓(急性化脓性关节炎)
Pycnanthemum [pikˈnænθiməm] *n* 密花薄荷属
pycnemia [pikˈniːmiə] *n* 血浓缩
pycnidium [pikˈnidiəm] *n* 分生孢子器
pycn(o)- 以 pycn(o)- 起始的词,同样见以 pykn(o)- 起始的词
pyecchysis [paiˈekisis] *n* 脓溢出
pyelectasis [ˌpaiəlekˈteisis], **pyelectasia** [ˌpaiəlekˈteizjə] *n* 肾盂扩张
pyelic [paiˈelik] *a* 肾盂的
pyelitis [ˌpaiəˈlaitis] *n* 肾盂炎 | calculous ~ 结石性肾盂炎 / defloration ~ 处女膜破裂性肾盂炎 / encrusted ~ (溃疡)结痂性肾盂炎 / ~ granulosa 肉芽性肾盂炎 / ~ gravidarum 妊娠期肾盂炎 / hematogenous ~ 血源性肾盂炎 | **pyelitic** [ˌpaiəˈlitik] *a*
pyel(o)- [构词成分]肾盂
pyelocaliceal, pyelocalyceal [ˌpaiələuˌkæliˈsiːəl] *a* 肾盂肾盏的
pyelocaliectasis [ˌpaiələuˌkæliˈektəsis] *n* 肾盂肾盏扩张
pyelocutaneous [ˌpaiələukju(ː)ˈteiniəs] *a* 肾盂皮的
pyelocystitis [ˌpaiələusisˈtaitis] *n* 肾盂膀胱炎
pyelocystostomosis [ˌpaiələuˌsistəustəˈməusis], **pyelocystanastomosis** [ˌpaiələuˌsistəˌnæstəˈməusis] *n* 肾盂膀胱吻合术
pyeloduodenal [ˌpaiələuˌdjuːəuˈdiːnəl] *a* 肾盂十二指肠的
pyelofluoroscopy [ˌpaiələuˌfluːəˈrɔskəpi] *n* 肾盂X线透视检查
pyelogram [ˈpaiələgræm] *n* 肾盂X线[照]片,肾盂造影[照]片 | dragon ~ 龙形肾盂造影[照]片(见于多囊肾) | **pyelograph** [ˈpaiələgrɑːf, -græf] *n*
pyelography [ˌpaiəˈlɔgrəfi] *n* 肾盂造影[术] | air ~ 肾盂充气造影[术] / intravenous ~, ~ by elimination, excretion ~ 排泄性尿路造影[术] / lateral ~ 侧位肾盂造影[术] / respiration ~ 呼吸法肾盂造影[术] / retrograde ~, ascending ~ 逆行肾盂造影[术],上行性肾盂造影[术]
pyeloileocutaneous [ˌpaiələuˌiliəukju(ː)ˈteinjəs] *a* 肾盂回肠皮肤的
pyelointerstitial [ˌpaiələuˌintəˈstiʃəl] *a* 肾盂间质的
pyelolithotomy [ˌpaiələuliˈθɔtəmi] *n* 肾盂切开取石术
pyelometry [ˌpaiəˈlɔmitri] *n* 肾盂测量法
pyelonephritis [ˌpaiələuneˈfraitis] *n* 肾盂肾炎
pyelonephrosis [ˌpaiələuniˈfrəusis] *n* 肾盂肾病
pyelopathy [ˌpaiəˈlɔpəθi] *n* 肾盂病
pyelophlebitis [ˌpaiələufliˈbaitis] *n* 肾盂静脉炎
pyeloplasty [ˈpaiələˌplæsti] *n* 肾盂成形术
pyeloplication [ˌpaiələuplaiˈkeiʃən] *n* 肾盂折术
pyeloscopy [ˌpaiəˈlɔskəpi] *n* 肾盂镜检查术
pyelosinus [ˌpaiələuˈsainəs] *a* 肾盂肾窦的
pyelostomy [ˌpaiəˈlɔstəmi] *n* 肾盂造瘘术
pyelotomy [ˌpaiəˈlɔtəmi] *n* 肾盂切开术
pyeloureterectasis [ˌpaiələujuəˌriːtəˈrektəsis] *n* 肾盂输尿管扩张
pyeloureteritis [ˌpaiələujuəˌriːtəˈraitis] *n* 肾盂输尿管炎
pyeloureterography [ˌpaiələujuəˌriːtəˈrɔgrəfi] *n* 肾盂输尿管造影[术]
pyeloureterolysis [ˌpaiələujuəˌriːtəˈrɔlisis] *n* 肾盂输尿管松解术
pyeloureteroplasty [ˌpaiələujuəˈriːtərəˌplæsti] *n* 肾盂输尿管成形术
pyelovenous [ˌpaiələuˈviːnəs] *a* 肾盂肾静脉的

pyemesis [pai'emisis] *n* 吐脓,呕脓
pyemia [pai'iːmiə] *n* 脓血症 | cryptogenic ~ 隐源性脓血症 / portal ~ 化脓性门静脉炎 | **pyemic** *a*
Pyemotes [ˌpaiə'məutiz] *n* 蒲螨属 | ~ ventricosus 球腹蒲螨,袋形虱螨
pyencephalus [ˌpaien'sefələs] *n* 脑脓肿
pyesis [pai'iːsis] *n* 化脓[症]
pygal ['paigəl] *a* 臀的
pygalgia [pai'gældʒiə] *n* 臀痛
pygeum ['pidʒiəm] *n* 非洲李制剂(用于治疗与良性前列腺增生有关的排尿问题)
pygmalionism [pig'meiliənizəm] *n* 爱偶像癖,爱雕像癖
pygmy ['pigmi] *n* 矮小者,侏儒
pyg(o)- [构词成分]臀
pygoamorphus ['paigəuə'mɔːfəs] *n* 无体形臀部寄生胎
pygodidymus [ˌpaigəu'didiməs] *n* 臀部联胎
pygomelus [pai'gɔmiləs] *n* 臀肢畸胎,臀部寄生肢畸胎
pygopagus [pai'gɔpəgəs] *n* 臀联双胎,臀部联体儿 | ~ parasiticus 臀部寄生胎(不对称性臀部联胎)
pygopagy [pai'gɔpədʒi] *n* 臀部联胎畸形
pygostyle ['paigəustail] *n* 尾综骨(亦称犁状骨)
pyic ['paiik] *a* 脓的
pyin ['paiin] *n* 脓蛋白,脓素
pyknemia [pik'niːmiə] *n* 血浓缩
pyknic ['piknik] *a* 矮胖型的
pykn(o)- [构词成分]致密,浓厚,浓缩;快速
pyknocyte ['piknəsait] *n* 固缩红细胞(变型收缩状红细胞,常见于溶血性疾患,也偶见于足月婴儿)
pyknocytoma [ˌpiknəusai'təumə] *n* 嗜酸粒细胞瘤
pyknocytosis [ˌpiknəusai'təusis] *n* 固缩红细胞增多[症]
pyknodysostosis [ˌpiknəuˌdisɔs'təusis] *n* 致密性骨发育不全
pyknoepilepsy [ˌpiknəu'epiˌlepsi] *n* 癫痫小发作
pyknometer [pik'nɔmitə] *n* 比重计,比重瓶 | **pyknometry** *n* 比重测定法
pyknomorphous [ˌpiknəu'mɔːfəs], **pyknomorphic** [ˌpiknəu'mɔːfik] *a* 致密排列的,密形的
pyknophrasia [ˌpiknəu'freiziə] *n* 言语重浊
pyknoplasson [ˌpiknəu'plæsən] *n* 致密[全能]原浆
pyknosis [pik'nəusis] *n*【希】核固缩(尤指细胞变性,此时细胞核收缩,染色质缩合成致密的无结构的块状物质) | **pyknotic** [pik'nɔtik] *a* 封闭的(将孔封闭);核固缩的
pyle- [构词成分]门静脉
pylephlebectasis [ˌpailifli'bektəsis] *n* 门静脉扩张
pylephlebitis [ˌpailifli'baitis] *n* 门静脉炎 | adhesive ~ 粘连性门静脉炎,门静脉血栓静脉炎
Pyle's disease [pail] (Edwin Pyle) 派尔病,干骺端发育不良
pylethrombophlebitis [ˌpailiˌθrɔmbəufli'baitis] *n* 门静脉血栓静脉炎
pylethrombosis [ˌpailiθrɔm'bəusis] *n* 门静脉血栓形成
pylic ['pailik] *a* 门静脉的
pylometer [pai'lɔmitə] *n* 输尿管梗阻测量器
pylon ['pailən] *n* 暂用假肢
pyloralgia [ˌpailə'rældʒiə] *n* 幽门痛
pylorectomy [ˌpailə'rektəmi] *n* 幽门切除术
pyloric [pai'lɔːrik] *a* 幽门[部]的
pyloristenosis [paiˌlɔːristi'nəusis] *n* 幽门狭窄
pyloritis [ˌpailə'raitis] *n* 幽门炎
pylor(o)- [构词成分]幽门
pylorodiosis [paiˌlɔːrəudai'əusis] *n* 幽门扩张术
pyloroduodenitis [paiˌlɔːrəuˌdju(ː)əudi'naitis] *n* 幽门十二指肠炎
pylorogastrectomy [paiˌlɔːrəugæs'trektəmi] *n* 幽门胃切除术
pyloromyotomy [paiˌlɔːrəumai'ɔtəmi] *n* 幽门肌切开术
pyloroplasty [pai'lɔːrəˌplæsti] *n* 幽门成形术
pyloroscopy [ˌpailə'rɔskəpi] *n* 幽门镜检查
pylorospasm [pai'lɔːrəspæzəm] *n* 幽门痉挛
pylorostenosis [paiˌlɔːrəusti'nəusis] *n* 幽门狭窄
pylorostomy [ˌpailə'rɔstəmi] *n* 幽门造口术
pylorotomy [ˌpailə'rɔtəmi] *n* 幽门切开术
pylorus [pai'lɔːrəs] ([复] **pylori** [pai'lɔːrai]) *n*【希】幽门
py(o)- [构词成分]脓
pyoarthrosis [ˌpaiəuɑː'θrəusis] *n* 关节积脓
pyoblennorrhea [ˌpaiəuˌblenə'riːə] *n* 脓液溢
pyocalix [ˌpaiəu'keiliks] *n* 肾盏积脓
pyocele ['paiəusiːl] *n* 鞘膜积液
pyocelia [ˌpaiəu'siːliə] *n* 腹腔积脓
pyocephalus [ˌpaiəu'sefələs] *n* 脑室积脓
pyochezia [ˌpaiəu'kiːziə] *n* 脓性粪
pyocin ['paiəsin] *n* 脓菌素
pyococcus [ˌpaiəu'kɔkəs] *n* [化]脓球菌 | **pyococcic** [ˌpaiə'kɔksik] *a*
pyocolpocele [ˌpaiəu'kɔlpəsiːl] *n* 阴道脓囊肿
pyocolpos [ˌpaiəu'kɔlpəs] *n* 阴道积脓
pyoculture ['paiəˌkʌltʃə] *n* 脓液培养法
pyocyanase [ˌpaiəu'saiəneis] *n* 绿脓菌酶
pyocyanic [ˌpaiəusai'ænik] *a* 绿脓的,绿脓菌的

pyocyanin [ˌpaiəuˈsaiənin] *n* 绿脓菌素
pyocyanogenic [ˌpaiəusaiənəuˈdʒenik] *a* 产生绿脓菌素的
pyocyanosis [ˌpaiəuˌsaiəˈnəusis] *n* 绿脓菌病
pyocyst [ˈpaiəsist] *n* 脓囊肿
pyocystis [ˌpaiəuˈsistis] *n* 膀胱积脓
pyocyte [ˈpaiəsait] *n* 脓细胞,中性粒细胞
pyoderma [ˌpaiəuˈdəːmə] *n* 脓皮病 | chancriform ~, ~ chancriforme faciei 下疳样脓皮病,面部下疳样脓皮病 / ~ faciale 面部脓皮病 / ~ gangrenosum 坏疽性脓皮病 / ~ vegetans 增生性脓皮病 | **pyodermia** [ˌpaiəuˈdəːmiə] *n* / **pyodermic** *a*
pyofecia [ˌpaiəuˈfiːsiə] *n* 脓性粪
pyogenesis [ˌpaiəˈdʒenisis] *n* 生脓,脓生成 | **pyogenic** [ˌpaiəˈdʒenik] *a* 生脓的
pyogenin [paiˈɔdʒinin] *n* 脓细胞素(脓细胞内的化合物)
pyogenous [paiˈɔdʒinəs] *a* 生脓的
pyohemia [ˌpaiəuˈhiːmiə] *n* 脓毒症,脓血症
pyohemothorax [ˌpaiəuˌhiːməuˈθɔːræks] *n* 脓血胸
pyohydronephrosis [ˌpaiəuˌhaidrəuniˈfrəusis] *n* 脓性肾积水
pyoid [ˈpaiɔid] *a* 脓样的 *n* 脓样物质(无菌无毒性的)
pyolabyrinthitis [ˌpaiəuˌlæbirinˈθaitis] *n* 脓性迷路炎
pyometra [ˌpaiəuˈmiːtrə], **pyometrium** [ˌpaiəuˈmiːtriəm] *n* 子宫积脓
pyometritis [ˌpaiəumiˈtraitis] *n* 化脓性子宫炎
pyomyoma [ˌpaiəumaiˈəumə] *n* 脓肌瘤
pyomyositis [ˌpaiəumaiəˈsaitis] *n* 脓性肌炎
pyonephritis [ˌpaiəuneˈfraitis] *n* 脓性肾炎
pyonephrolithiasis [ˌpaiəuˌnefrəuliˈθaiəsis] *n* 脓性肾石病
pyonephrosis [ˌpaiəuniˈfrəusis] *n* 肾积脓 | **pyonephrotic** [ˌpaiəuniˈfrɔtik] *a*
pyonychia [ˌpaiəuˈnikiə] *n* 甲沟脓炎
pyo-ovarium [ˌpaiəu əuˈvɛəriəm] *n* 卵巢积脓
pyopericarditis [ˌpaiəuˌperikɑːˈdaitis] *n* 脓性心包炎
pyopericardium [ˌpaiəuˌperiˈkɑːdiəm] *n* 心包积脓
pyoperitoneum [ˌpaiəuˌperitəuˈniːəm] *n* 腹[膜]腔积脓
pyoperitonitis [ˌpaiəuˌperitəuˈnaitis] *n* 脓性腹膜炎
pyophagia [ˌpaiəuˈfeidʒiə] *n* 吞脓
pyophthalmia [ˌpaiɔfˈθælmiə], **pyophthalmitis** [ˌpaiɔfθælˈmaitis] *n* 脓性眼炎
pyophylactic [ˌpaiəufiˈlæktik] *a* 防止生脓的
pyophysometra [ˌpaiəuˌfaisəˈmiːtrə] *n* 子宫积脓气
pyoplania [ˌpaiəuˈpleiniə] *n* 脓扩散
pyopneumocholecystitis [ˌpaiəuˌnjuːməuˌkəulisisˈtaitis] *n* 脓气性胆囊炎
pyopneumocyst [ˌpaiəuˈnjuːməsist] *n* 脓气囊肿
pyopneumohepatitis [ˌpaiəuˌnjuːməuˌhepəˈtaitis] *n* 脓气性肝炎
pyopneumopericardium [ˌpaiəuˌnjuːməuˌperiˈkɑːdiəm] *n* 脓气心包
pyopneumoperitoneum [ˌpaiəuˌnjuːməuˌperitəuˈniːəm] *n* 脓气腹[腔]
pyopneumoperitonitis [ˌpaiəuˌnjuːməuˌperitəuˈnaitis] *n* 脓气性腹膜炎
pyopneumothorax [ˌpaiəuˌnjuːməuˈθɔːræks] *n* 脓气胸
pyopoiesis [ˌpaiəupɔiˈiːsis] *n* 脓生成,生脓 | **pyopoietic** [ˌpaiəupɔiˈetik] *a*
pyoptysis [paiˈɔptisis] *n* 咯脓
pyopyelectasis [ˌpaiəupaiiˈlektəsis] *n* 脓性肾盂扩张
pyorrhea [ˌpaiəˈriə] *n* 脓溢 | **~l** *a*
pyorubin [ˌpaiəˈruːbin] *n* 绿脓菌红素
pyosalpingitis [ˌpaiəuˌsælpinˈdʒaitis] *n* 脓性输卵管炎
pyosalpingo-oophoritis [ˌpaiəusælˌpiŋgəu əuˌɔfəˈraitis], **pyosalpingo-oothecitis** [ˌpaiəusælˌpiŋgəu ˌəuəθiˈsaitis] *n* 脓性输卵管卵巢炎
pyosalpinx [ˌpaiəuˈsælpiŋks] *n* 输卵管积脓
pyosapremia [ˌpaiəusəˈpriːmiə] *n* 脓毒败血病
pyosclerosis [ˌpaiəuskliəˈrəusis] *n* 脓性硬化
pyosemia [ˌpaiəuˈsiːmiə] *n* 脓性精液[症],精液含脓
pyosepticemia [ˌpaiəuˌseptiˈsiːmiə] *n* 脓毒败血病
pyosin [ˈpaiəsin] *n* 脓胞素
pyospermia [ˌpaiəuˈspəːmiə] *n* 脓性精液[症],精液含脓
pyostatic [ˌpaiəuˈstætik] *a* 抑制[化]脓的 *n* 制[化]脓药,抑[化]脓药
pyostomatitis [ˌpaiəuˌstəuməˈtaitis] *n* 脓性口炎
pyotherapy [ˌpaiəuˈθerəpi] *n* 脓液疗法
pyothorax [ˌpaiəuˈθɔːræks] *n* 脓胸
pyotoxinemia [ˌpaiəutɔksiˈniːmiə] *n* 脓毒素血[症]
pyoumbilicus [ˌpaiəuʌmˈbilikəs] *n* 脓脐
pyourachus [ˌpaiəuˈjuərəkəs] *n* 脐尿管积脓
pyoureter [ˌpaiəujuəˈriːtə] *n* 输尿管积脓
pyovesiculosis [ˌpaiəuviˌsikjuːˈləusis] *n* 精囊积脓

pyoxanthine [ˌpaiəuˈzænθin] *n* 绿脓黄质
pyoxanthose [ˌpaiəuˈzænθəus] *n* 半绿脓青素
pyrabrom [ˈpirəbrɔm] *n* 吡拉布隆碱(抗组胺药)
pyracin [ˈpairəsin] *n* 吡拉辛(一种维生素 B_6 代谢产物)
Pyralis [ˈpirəlis] *n* 螟蛾科 | ~ farinalis 粉螟
pyramid [ˈpirəmid] *n* 锥体(本词常单独使用表示延髓锥体) | ~ of cerebellum 蚓锥体 / ~s of kidney, renal ~s 肾锥体 / ~ of light 光锥 / ~ of thyroid 甲状腺锥体叶 / ~ of tympanum (鼓室)锥隆起 | **~al** [piˈræmidl] *a* 锥[体]状的,锥体的
pyramidale [paiˌræmiˈdeili] *n* 三角骨
pyramidalis [paiˌræmiˈdeilis] *a*【拉】锥状的 *n* 锥状肌
pyramides [piˈræmidiːz] pyramis 的复数
pyramidotomy [ˌpirəmiˈdɔtəmi] *n* 锥体束切断术
pyramis [ˈpirəmis] ([复] **pyramides** [piˈræmidiːz]) *n*【希】锥体
pyran [ˈpaiəræn] *n* 吡喃
pyranisamine maleate [ˌpaiərəˈnisəmiːn] 马来酸吡拉敏(见 pyrilamine maleate)
pyranose [ˈpaiərənəus, ˈpirə-] *n* 吡喃糖
pyranoside [ˌpaiəˈrænəsaid, piˈr-] *n* 吡喃糖苷
pyrantel [piˈræntəl] *n* 噻嘧啶(抗蠕虫药) | ~ pamoate 双羟萘酸噻嘧啶,抗虫灵 / ~ tartrate 酒石酸噻嘧啶
pyranyl [ˈpaiərənil] *n* 吡喃基,氧[杂]芑基
pyrathiazine hydrochloride [ˌpirəˈθaiəziːn] 盐酸帕拉噻嗪(抗组胺药)
pyrazinamide [ˌpirəˈzinəmaid] *n* 吡嗪酰胺(抗结核药)
pyrazine [ˈpaiərəziːn] *n* 吡嗪
pyrazofurin [ˌpirəzəˈfjuərin] *n* 吡唑呋林(抗肿瘤药)
pyrazolone [piˈræzələun] *n* 吡唑啉酮(有抗炎、镇痛和解热作用)
pyrectic [paiˈrektik] *a* 致热的 *n* 致热因素
pyrene [ˈpaiəriːn] *n* 芘,嵌二萘
pyrenemia [ˌpaiərəˈniːmiə] *n* 有核红细胞血症
Pyrenochaeta [ˌpairənəuˈkiːtə] *n* 刺壳孢菌属
pyrenoid [ˈpaiərənɔid] *n* 淀粉核
pyrenolysis [ˌpaiərəˈnɔlisis] *n* 核仁溶解
Pyrenomycetes [paiˌriːnəumaiˈsiːtiːz] *n* 核菌纲
pyretherapy [ˌpaiərəˈθerəpi] *n* 发热疗法,治疗性发热;热病治疗法
pyrethrin [ˌpaiəˈriːθrin, -ˈre-] *n* 除虫菊酯
pyrethroid [paiˈreθrɔid] *n* 拟除虫菊酯
pyrethron [ˌpairəθrɔn] *n* 除虫菊酮
Pyrethrum [paiˈriːθrəm] *n* 除虫菊属
pyrethrum [paiˈriːθrəm] *n* 除虫菊
pyretic [paiˈretik] *a* 发热的,发烧的
pyreticosis [paiˌretiˈkəusis] *n* 热病
pyret(o)- [构词成分]热,发热
pyretogen [paiˈretədʒən] *n* 热原质,致热原
pyretogenesis [ˌpaiərətəuˈdʒenisis] *n* 热发生,发热 | **pyretogenetic** [ˌpaiərətəudʒiˈnetik] *a*
pyretogenic [ˌpaiərətəuˈdʒenik] *a* 致热的
pyretogenous [ˌpaiərəˈtɔdʒinəs] *a* 热原的(体温增高引起的);致热的
pyretography [ˌpaiərəˈtɔgrəfi] *n* 热病论
pyretology [ˌpaiərəˈtɔlədʒi] *n* 热病学
pyretolysis [ˌpaiərəˈtɔlisis] *n* 退热,热消退
pyretotherapy [ˌpaiərətəuˈθerəpi] *n* 发热疗法,治疗性发热;热病治疗法
pyretotyphosis [ˌpaiərətəutaiˈfəusis] *n* 热性谵妄
pyrexia [paiˈreksiə] *n* 发热 | **pyrexial, pyrexic** *a* / **pyrexy** [ˈpaireksi] *n*
pyrexiogenic [paiˌreksiəˈdʒenik] *a* 致热的
pyridostigmine bromide [ˌpiridəuˈstigmiːn] 溴吡斯的明(拟胆碱药,治疗重症肌无力,并用作肌肉松弛药)
pyridoxal [ˌpiriˈdɔksəl] *n* 吡哆醛,维生素 B_6
pyridoxamine [ˌpiriˈdɔksəmiːn] *n* 吡哆胺,维生素 B_6
pyridoxic acid [ˌpiriˈdɔksik] 吡哆酸
pyridoxine [ˌpiriˈdɔksi(ː)n] *n* 吡哆辛,吡哆醇,维生素 B_6 | ~ hydrochloride 盐酸吡哆醇(用于防治维生素 B_6 缺乏病)
pyriform [ˈpirifɔːm] *a* 梨状的,梨形的
pyrilamine maleate [piˈriləmiːn] 马来酸吡拉敏(亦称马来酸美吡拉敏 mepyramine maleate, 抗组胺药)
pyrimethamine [ˌpiriˈmeθəmiːn] *n* 乙胺嘧啶(抗疟药)
pyrimidine [paiˈrimidiːn] *n* 嘧啶
pyrimidine-nucleoside phosphorylase [pəˈrimidiːn ˈnjuːkliəsaid fɔsˈfɔrileis] 嘧啶核苷磷酸化酶
pyrin [ˈpairin] *n* 哌啉(一种 781-氨基酸蛋白,对此蛋白编码的基因突变可引起家族性地中海热。亦称地中海蛋白)
pyrinoline [piˈrinəliːn] *n* 吡诺林(抗心律失常的心抑制药)
pyrithiamine [ˌpiriˈθaiəmiːn] *n* 吡啶硫胺素,抗硫胺素(一种硫胺代谢对抗物)
pyrithyldione [paiˈriθildiəun] *n* 吡乙二酮(催眠镇静药)
pyr(o)- [构词成分]火,热;焦,焦性
pyroarsenic acid [ˌpaiərəuˈɑːsnik] 焦砷酸
pyroborate [ˌpaiərəuˈbɔːreit] *n* 焦硼酸盐
pyroboric acid [ˌpaiərəuˈbɔːrik] 焦硼酸
pyrocatechin [ˌpaiərəuˈkætikin], **pyrocatechol**

[ˌpaiərəuˈkætikɔl] *n* 焦儿茶酚,邻苯二酚
pyrocinchonic acid [ˌpaiərəusiŋˈkɔnik] 焦辛可宁酸
pyrocitric acid [ˌpaiərəuˈsaitrik] 焦枸橼酸,焦柠檬酸,柠康酸
pyrodextrin [ˌpaiərəuˈdekstrin] *n* 焦糊精
pyrogallic acid [ˌpaiərəuˈgælik] 焦棓酸,焦性没食子酸
pyrogallol [ˌpaiərəuˈgælɔl] *n* 焦棓酚
pyrogen [ˈpaiərədʒən] *n* 热原,致热物,致热原 | bacterial ~ 细菌性热原质 / endogenous ~, leukocytic ~ 内源性致热原,白细胞致热原 / exogenous ~ 外源性致热原
pyrogenetic [ˌpaiərəudʒiˈnetik], **pyrogenic** [ˌpaiərəuˈdʒenik], **pyrogenous** [paiˈrɔdʒinəs] *a* 致热的
pyroglobulin [ˌpaiərəuˈglɔbjulin] *n* 热球蛋白(一种因加热而沉淀的血清球蛋白)
pyroglobulinemia [ˌpaiərəuˌglɔbjuliˈniːmiə] *n* 热球蛋白血[症]
pyroglutamate [ˌpaiərəuˈgluːtəmeit] *n* 焦谷氨酸,5-羟脯氨酸
pyroglutamic acid [ˌpaiərəugluːˈtæmik] 焦谷氨酸,5-羟脯氨酸
pyroglutamicaciduria [ˌpaiərəugluːˌtæmikˌæsiˈdjuəriə] *n* 焦谷氨尿[症],5-羟脯氨酸尿[症]
pyrolagnia [ˌpaiərəuˈlægniə] *n* 纵火色情,火场色情
pyroligneous [ˌpaiərəuˈligniəs] *a* 焦木的 | ~ acid 焦木酸
pyrolusite [ˌpaiərəuˈljuːsait] *n* 软锰矿,二氧化锰
pyrolysis [paiəˈrɔlisis] *n* 热分解,高温分解 | **pyrolytic** [ˌpaiərəuˈlitik] *a* | **pyrolytically** *ad*
pyromania [ˌpaiərəuˈmeinjə] *n* 纵火狂 | erotic ~ 纵火色情,火场色情
pyrometer [paiˈrɔmitə] *n* 高温计
pyrone [ˈpaiərəun] *n* 吡喃酮
pyronin [ˈpaiərənin] *n* 哌洛宁,焦宁 | ~ B 派洛宁 B(碱性染料) / ~ G 派洛宁 G(碱性染料) | **pyronine** [ˈpaiərəniːn] *n*
pyroninophilia [ˌpaiərəˌninəuˈfiliə] *n* 嗜派洛宁性,嗜焦宁性(对派洛宁有较高亲和力,有时在浆细胞和网状内皮细胞中可见)
pyroninophilic [ˌpaiərəˌninəˈfilik] *a* 嗜哌洛宁的,嗜焦宁的
pyronyxis [ˌpaiərəuˈniksis] *n* 火针术
pyrophobia [ˌpaiərəuˈfəubjə] *n* 火焰恐怖,恐火症
pyrophosphatase [ˌpaiərəuˈfɔsfəteis] *n* 焦磷酸酶
pyrophosphate [ˌpaiərəuˈfɔsfeit] *n* 焦磷酸 | stannous ~ 焦磷酸亚锡(骨扫描用药)
pyrophosphokinase [ˌpaiərəuˌfɔsfəˈkaineis] *n* 焦磷酸激酶
pyrophosphoric acid [ˌpaiərəuˌfɔsˈfɔrik] 焦磷酸
pyrophosphotransferase [ˌpaiərəuˌfɔsfəˈtrænsfəreis] *n* 焦磷酸转移酶,二磷酸转移酶
Pyroplasma [ˌpaiərəuˈplæzmə] *n* 梨浆虫属,巴贝虫属(即 Babesia)
pyropuncture [ˈpaiərəˌpʌŋktʃə] *n* 火针术
pyroracemic acid [ˌpaiərəurəˈsiːmik] 丙酮酸
pyroscope [ˈpaiərəskəup] *n* 测热辐射器
pyrosis [paiˈrəusis] *n* 胃灼热
Pyrosoma [ˌpaiərəˈsəumə] *n* 梨浆虫属,巴贝虫属(即 Babesia)
pyrosulfuric acid [ˌpaiərəusʌlˈfjuərik] 焦硫酸,一缩二硫酸
pyrotartaric acid [ˌpaiərəutɑːˈtɑːrik] 焦酒石酸,甲基琥珀酸
pyrotic [paiˈrɔtik] *a* 苛性的,腐蚀的;胃灼热的
pyrotoxin [ˌpaiərəuˈtɔksin] *n* 热期毒素(在发热期产生的毒素);热毒素(许多细菌甚至包括一些普通非致病菌的一种毒性成分,注入机体引起发热和虚损)
pyrovalerone hydrochloride [pirəuˈvælərəun] 盐酸吡咯戊酮(中枢神经系统兴奋药)
pyroxamine maleate [piˈrɔksəmiːn] 马来酸吡咯沙敏(抗组胺药)
pyroxylin [paiˈrɔksilin] *n* 火棉,硝酸纤维素
pyrrobutamine phosphate [ˌpirəuˈbjuːtəmin] 磷酸吡咯他敏(抗组胺药)
pyrrocaine [ˈpirəkein] *n* 吡咯卡因(局部麻醉药) | ~ hydrochloride 盐酸吡咯卡因(牙科用局部麻醉药)
pyrrole [ˈpirəul, piˈrəul] *n* 吡咯
pyrrolidine [piˈrɔlidin] *n* 吡咯烷,四氢化吡咯
pyrroline [ˈpirəlin] *n* 吡咯啉,二氢吡咯 | Δ^1- ~ 5-carboxylate Δ^1-二氢吡咯 5-羧酸
1-pyrroline-5-carboxylate dehydrogenase [ˈpirəliːn kɑːˈbɔksileit diːˈhaidrədʒəneis] 1-二氢吡咯-5-羧酸脱氢酶(此酶缺乏为一种常染色体隐性性状,是高脯氨酸血症Ⅱ型的原因)
pyrroline-5-carboxylate reductase [ˈpirəliːn kɑːˈbɔksileit riˈdʌkteis] 二氢吡咯-5-羧酸还原酶
pyrroline 5-carboxylate synthase [ˈpirəliːn kɑːˈbɔksileit ˈsinθeis] 二氢吡咯 5-羧酸合酶
pyrrolizidine [pairəuˈlizidiːn] *n* 双吡咯烷(存在于各种植物中的任何一类生物碱,可致反刍动物肝细胞毒综合征)
pyrrolnitrin [pirəulˈnaitrin] *n* 吡咯尼群(抗真菌抗生素)
pyrroloporphyria [ˌpirələupɔˈfiriə] *n* 急性间歇性卟啉病
pyrroporphyrin [ˌpirəuˈpɔːfirin] *n* 焦卟啉

pyruvate [ˈpaiəruveit] *n* 丙酮酸(盐、酯或阴离子型,在生物化学中本词与 pyruvic acid 可互换使用)

pyruvate carboxylase [ˈpaiəruveit kɑːˈbɔksileis] 丙酮酸羧化酶(此酶缺乏为一种常染色体隐性性状,可致婴儿严重的精神运动性阻滞和乳酸性酸中毒)

pyruvate decarboxylase [ˈpaiəruveit ˌdiːkɑːˈbɔksileis] 丙酮酸脱羧酶(亦称 α-羧化酶;以前称丙酮酸脱氢酶〈硫辛酰胺〉)

pyruvate dehydrogenase (lipoamide) [ˈpaiəruveit diːˈhaidrədʒəneisliˈpəuəmaid] 丙酮酸脱氢酶(硫辛酰胺)(此酶缺乏可致乳酸血症、共济失调、精神运动性阻滞及有时为乳酸性酸中毒)

pyruvate dehydrogenase complex [ˈpaiəruveit diːˈhaidrədʒəneis ˈkɔmpleks] 丙酮酸脱氢酶复合物(此复合物中任何成分缺乏,可导致乳酸血症、共济失调和精神运动迟缓)

[pyruvate dehydrogenase (lipoamide)] kinase [ˈpaiəruveit diːˈhaidrədʒəneis ˌlipəuˈæmaid ˈkaineis] [丙酮酸脱氢酶(硫辛酰胺)]激酶

[pyruvate dehydrogenase (lipoamide)] phosphatase [ˈpaiəruveit diːˈhaidrədʒəneis ˌlipəuˈæmaid ˈfɔsfəteis] [丙酮酸脱氢酶(硫辛酰胺)]-磷酸酶(此酶缺乏可致代谢性酸中毒,伴血清内高浓度乳酸、丙酮酸和游离脂肪酸)

pyruvate kinase (PK) [ˈpaiəruveit ˈkaineis] 丙酮酸激酶(红细胞内此酶活性缺乏为一种常染色体隐性性状,可致溶血性贫血)

pyruvate kinase (PK) deficiency, erythrocyte 红细胞丙酮酸激酶缺乏症(此酶缺乏为一种常染色体隐性性状,其临床特征与其他溶血性疾病无明显区别)

pyruvemia [ˌpaiəruˈviːmiə] *n* 丙酮酸血[症]

pyruvic acid [paiəˈruːvik ˈæsid] 丙酮酸

6-pyruvoyltetrahydropterin synthase [paiəˌruːvɔilˌtetrəhaiˈdrɔptərin ˈsinθeis] 6-丙酮酰四氢蝶呤合酶(此酶缺乏为一种常染色体隐性性状,可致恶性高苯丙氨酸血症)

pyrvinium pamoate [pəːˈvinjəm ˈpæməeit] 恩波维铵(即 pyrvinium embonate,抗蛲虫药)

Pythiaceae [ˌpiθiˈeisiiː] *n* 腐霉科

pythiosis [ˌpiθiˈəusis] *n* 腐霉病(主要侵犯马、牛等)

Pythium [ˈpiθiəm] *n* 腐霉属

pythogenesis [ˌpaiθəˈdʒenisis] *n* 腐生;腐化

pythogenic [ˌpaiθəˈdʒenik] *a* 腐化的,腐败的

pythogenous [paiˈθɔdʒinəs] *a* 腐生的

pyuria [paiˈjuəriə] *n* 脓尿 | miliary ~ 粟粒性脓尿

PZD partial zona dissection 部分解剖区

PZI protamine zinc insulin [鱼]精蛋白锌胰岛素

Q

Q ubiquinone 泛醌
Q electric charge 电荷; heat 热力; reaction quotient 反应系数
Q_{10} temperature coefficient 温度系数; ubiquinone 泛醌
Q̇ rate of blood flow 血流率
q 染色体长臂(the long arm of a chromosome)的符号
q. quaque【拉】每
q electric charge 电荷; ubiquinone 泛醌(统计学上)备择事件的概率(probability of alternative event)的符号
Q angle (Q 代表 quadriceps) Q 角
q. d. quaque die【拉】每日
Q fever (Q 代表 query) Q 热(见 fever)
q. h. quaque hora【拉】每小时
qi【汉】气
q. i. d. quater in die【拉】每日 4 次
qi gong【汉】气功
q. l. quantum libet【拉】任意量
QNS Queen's Nursing Sister(of Queen's Institute of District Nursing)女王护士长(皇家地区护理学会)
qns quantity not sufficient 量不足
q. p. quantum placeat【拉】任意量
q. q. h. quaque quarta hora【拉】每 4 小时
Qq. hor. quaque hora【拉】每小时
QS_2 electromechanical systole 电机械收缩
q. s. quantum satis【拉】适量,足量
q-sort [ˈkjuːsɔːt] *n* q 分类,q 选择(一种人格鉴定法,表示受试者〈或实验者〉对一套标准化描述的符合程度)
q. suff. quantum sufficit【拉】适量,足量
qt quart 夸脱
quack [kwæk] *n* 庸医,江湖医 *a* 庸医的,冒充内行医病的
quackery [ˈkwækəri] *n* 江湖医术
quacksalver [ˈkwækˌsælvə] *n* 庸医,江湖医
quadrangle [ˈkwɔdræŋgl] *n* 四角形,四边形;四角器(牙科) | **quadrangular** [kwɔˈdræŋgjulə] *a* 四角形的
quadrant [ˈkwɔdrənt] *n* 四分之一圆;四分体;象限 | **~al** [kwɔˈdræntl] *a*
quadrantanopia [ˌkwɔdrəntəˈnəupiə], **quadrantanopsia** [ˌkwɔdrəntəˈnɔpsiə] *n* 象限盲
quadrantectomy [ˌkwɔdrəˈtektəmi] *n* 四分之一切除术(一种部分乳房切除术,包括整块切除四分之一乳房组织的肿瘤及胸大肌筋膜及在其上面的皮肤)
quadrate [ˈkwɔdreit] *a* 方的,正方形的;长方形的 *n* 正方形;长方形
quadratipronator [kwɔˌdreitiprəˈneitə] *n* 旋前方肌
quadratus [kwɔˈdreitəs] *a*【拉】方的,方形的 *n* 方肌
quadr(i)- [前缀]四,四倍
quadribasic [ˌkwɔdriˈbeisik] *a* 四元的,四碱价的
quadriceps [ˈkwɔdriseps] *n* 四头肌 *a* 四头的 | **quadricipital** [ˌkwɔdriˈsipitl] *a*
quadricepsplasty [ˈkwɔdrisepsˌplæsti] *n* 股四头肌成形术
quadriceptor [ˌkwɔdriˈseptə] *n* 四簇介体
quadricuspid [ˌkwɔdriˈkʌspid] *a* 四尖的 *n* 四尖牙
quadridentate [ˌkwɔdriˈdenteit] *n* 四配位体
quadridigitate [ˌkwɔdriˈdidʒiteit] *a* 四指[畸形]的,四趾[畸形]的
quadrigeminum [ˌkwɔdriˈdʒeminəm] ([复] **quadrigemina** [ˌkwɔdriˈdʒeminə]) *n*【拉】四叠体 | **quadrigeminal, quadrigeminus** *a* 四叠的,四联的;四叠体的
quadrigeminy [ˌkwɔdriˈdʒeməni] *n* 四叠体;四联律
quadrilateral [ˌkwɔdriˈlætərəl] *a* 四边形的 *n* 四边形;四边形物
quadrilocular [ˌkwɔdriˈlɔkjulə] *a* 四腔的,四房的
quadripara [kwɔˈdripərə] *n* 四产妇
quadriparesis [ˌkwɔːdripəˈriːsis] *n* 四肢轻瘫
quadripartite [ˌkwɔdriˈpɑːtait] *a* 四部的,四分的
quadriplegia [ˌkwɔdriˈpliːdʒiə] *n* 四肢瘫痪 | **quadriplegic** *a*, *n*
quadripolar [ˌkwɔdriˈpəulə] *a* 四极的
quadrisect [ˈkwɔdrisekt] *vt* 切为四份 | **~ion** [ˌkwɔdriˈsekʃən] *n* 四分切
quadritubercular [ˌkwɔdritju(ː)ˈbəːkjulə] *a* 四结节的;四尖的
quadrivalent [ˌkwɔdriˈveilənt] *a* 四价的 *n* 四价体(减数分裂中四个联会的同源染色体的总称) | **quadrivalence** [ˌkwɔdriˈveiləns], **quadriva-**

lency [ˌkwɔdriˈveiləsi] *n* 四价
quadroon [kwɔˈdruːn] *n* 混血儿
quadruped [ˈkwɔdruped] *a* 四足的 *n* 四足动物 | **quadrupedal** [kwɔˈdruːpidl] *a* 四足的;四足动物的
quadrupl. quadruplicato【拉】四倍
quadruplet [ˈkwɔdruplit] *n* 四胎
quadruplex [ˈkwɔdrupleks] *a* 四倍的,四重的 *n* 四显性组合,四式型四显性组合
Quain's degeneration [kwein] (Richard Quain) 奎因变性(心肌纤维变性) | ~ fatty heart 奎因脂肪心(心肌脂肪变性)
quale [ˈkweili] ([复]**qualia** [ˈkweiliə]) *n* 性质,性状(尤指感觉或其他意识过程的性质)
qualimeter [kwəˈlimitə] *n* [X 线]透度计,[X 线]硬度计
qualitative [ˈkwɔlitətiv, -tei-], **qualitive** [ˈkwɔlitiv] *a* 性质的,定性的;品质的
quality [ˈkwɔləti] *n* 质,质量;性质;品质 | ~ of life 生命质量
quanta [ˈkwɔntə] quantum 的复数
quantal [ˈkwɔntəl] *a* 量子的(表示一种全或无的反应)
quantasome [ˈkwɔntəsəum] *n* 量子[换能]体,光能转化体(叶绿体基粒中一种有光合作用活性的颗粒,形状扁而椭圆形,轴长 100 Å 和 200 Å,内含叶绿素)
quantatrope [ˈkwɔntətrəup] *n* 光能转化体部位
quantile [ˈkwɔntail] *n* 分位数,分位点
quantimeter [kwɔnˈtimitə] *n* [X 线]量计
quantitative [ˈkwɔntitətiv, -tei-], **quantitive** [ˈkwɔntitiv] *a* 量的,数量的;定量的 | **~ly** *ad*
quantity [ˈkwɔntəti] *n* 量,数量;定量 | an unknown ~ 未知量(数学中以字母 X 表示);难以预测的人(或事),尚待查明的人(或事)
Quant's sign [kwɔnt] (C. A. J. Quant) 宽特征(枕骨 T 字形凹陷,有时见于佝偻病)
quantum [ˈkwɔntəm] ([复]**quanta** [ˈkwɔntə]) *n*【拉】量;量子(能的单位量) | ~ of light 光量子
quantum libet [ˈkwɔntəm ˈlaibət]【拉】任意量
quantum satis [ˈkwɔntəm ˈsætis]【拉】适量,足量
quantum sufficit [ˈkwɔntəm ˈsʌfisit]【拉】适量,足量
quarantine [ˈkwɔrəntiːn] *n* 检疫,留验;检疫站;检疫期 *vt* 对…进行检疫
quart(qt) [kwɔːt] *n* 夸脱(1/4 加仑〈946 ml〉)
quartan [ˈkwɔːtən] *a* 每第四日(复发)的 *n* 三日疟 | double ~ 复三日疟 / triple ~ 日发三日疟
quartation [kwɔːˈteiʃən] *n* (硝酸)析银法
quarter [ˈkwɔːtə] *n* (马的)蹄侧
quartile [ˈkwɔːtail] *n* 四分值;四分线;四分位数
quartipara [kwɔːˈtipərə] *n* 四产妇
quartisect [ˈkwɔːtisekt] *vt* 切为四份
quartisternal [ˌkwɔːtiˈstəːnəl] *a* 胸骨第四节的
quartz [kwɔːts] *n* 石英,水晶
quasi- [前缀]类似,准,半
quasidiploid [ˌkwɑːziˈdiplɔid] *n* 准二倍体
quasidominance [ˌkwɑːziˈdɔminəns] *n* 类显性,准显性(隐性性状直接传递,每代必然连续出现,类似显性遗传) | **quasidominant** *a*
quasispecies [ˌkwɑːziˈspiːʃiːz] *n* 准种(病毒基因组)
quassation [kwɔˈseiʃən] *n* 压碎,细碎
Quassia [ˈkwɔʃiə] *n* 苦木属
quassia [ˈkwɔʃiə] *n* 苦木,美洲苦木
quassin [ˈkwɔʃin] *n* 苦木素
Quat., quat. quattuor【拉】四
quater in die [ˈkwɔtə in ˈdiːei]【拉】每日四次
quaternary [kwəˈtəːnəri] *a* 第四的;四元的,四价的
Quatrefages' angle [ˌkɑːtrəˈfɑːʒə] (Jean L. A. de Quatrefages de Bréau) 卡特尔法日角,顶角(parietal angle,见 angle 项下相应术语)
quazepam [ˈkwɑːzəpæm] *n* 夸西泮(镇静催眠药)
quazodine [ˈkweizədiːn] *n* 夸唑定(强心药,支气管扩张药)
quebrachitol [keiˈbrætʃitɔl] *n* 白坚木醇,肌醇甲醚,橡醇
Queckenstedt's sign(phenomenon, test) [ˈkwekənˌʃtet] (Hans H. G. Queckenstedt) 奎肯施泰特征(现象、试验)(正常时,压颈静脉脑脊液压迅速上升,脊椎管内阻塞时,压颈静脉脑脊液压不受影响)
quenching [ˈkwentʃiŋ] *n* 熄灭,猝灭 | dilution ~ 稀释熄灭 / fluorescence ~ 荧光猝灭(测定抗原与抗体的一级相互作用的一种技术)
Quénu-Mayo operation [keiˈnjuˈmei əu] (Eduard A. V. A. Quénu; William J. Mayo) 凯努-梅奥手术(切除直肠及其相邻的淋巴结以治癌)
Quénu-Muret sign [keiˈnju muˈre] (E. A. V. A. Quénu; Paul L. Muret) 凯努-穆雷征(动脉瘤时,压迫肢的主要动脉,然后在其末梢部穿刺,若血液流出,则侧支循环可能已建立)
Quénu's hemorrhoidal plexus [keiˈnjuː] (E. A. V. A Quénu) 凯努痔丛(直肠静脉丛)
quenuthoracoplasty [ˌkwiːnjuːˈθɔrəkəuˌplæsti] (E. A. V. A. Quénu) 凯努胸廓成形术(脓胸时,分离肋骨,以促使胸壁收缩)
quercetin [ˈkwəːsitin] *n* 槲皮素(用于降低异常的毛细血管脆性) | ~-3-rutinoside 槲皮素-3-芸香苷,芦丁

quercitannic acid [ˌkwəːsiˈtænik] 白槲鞣酸
Quercus [ˈkwəːkəs] *n*【拉】槲属,栎属
Quervain [kεəˈvæn] 见 de Quervain
Quetelet's rule [ˌketiˈlei] (Lambert A. J. Quetelet)凯特累规律(身长超过 100 cm 的数,为成年人体重应有的千克数)
quetiapine fumarate [kweˈtaiəpiːn] 延胡索酸奎他阿平(一种二苯并地平衍生物,为脑内多发性神经递质受体的拮抗剂,用作抗精神病药,治疗精神分裂症和其他精神障碍,口服给药)
Queyrat's erythroplasia [keiˈrɑː] (Louis Auguste Queyrat)凯腊增殖性红斑(原位鳞状细胞癌,在阴茎头、心冠状沟或包皮上出现局限的光滑的红斑丘疹,形成脱屑或浅在性溃疡)
quick [kwik] *a* 快的,迅速的;活的;(孕妇)有胎动感的
quicken [ˈkwikən] *vi* 胎动;(孕妇)进入胎动期
quickening [ˈkwikəniŋ] *n* 胎动感
quick-freeze [ˈkwik ˌfriːz] *vt*, *vi* 速冻 *n* 速冻
quicklime [ˈkwiklaim] *n* 生石灰
Quick's test [kwik] (Armand J. Quick)奎克试验(①检肝功能;②检凝血酶原时间、血友病及黄疸)
quidding [ˈkwidiŋ] *n* 咀嚼病(马将食物吃入口中,反复咀嚼然后吐出的一种病。亦称吐草症)
quigila [ˈkwidʒilə] *n* 奎吉拉病(南美洲似麻风的传染病)
quill [kwil] *n* 卷片(树皮)
quillaia [kwiˈleijə] *n* 皂树皮
quillaic acid [kwiˈleiik] 皂树酸
Quillaia [kwiˈleijə] *n* 皂树属
quina [ˈkwainə] *n* 金鸡纳皮;金鸡纳
quinacrine hydrochloride [ˈkwinəkrin] 盐酸喹吖因(亦称盐酸米帕林 mepacrine hydrochloride 抗疟药、抗原虫药和抗蠕虫药)
quinalbarbitone [ˌkwinəlˈbɑːbitəun] *n* 司可巴比妥(催眠药)
quinaldic acid [kwiˈnældik] *n* 2-喹啉酸,喹啉-2-羧酸
quinaldinic acid [ˌkwinəlˈdinik] 2-喹啉酸,喹啉-2-羧酸
quinapril hydrochloride [ˈkwinəˌpril] 盐酸喹那普利(抗高血压药)
quinazoline [kwiˈnæzəulin] *n* 喹唑啉
quinbolone [ˈkwinbələun] *n* 奎勃龙(雄激素,同化激素类药)
Quincke's disease, edema [ˈkwiŋkə] (Heinrich I. Quincke)血管神经性水肿 | ~ meningitis 急性无菌性脑膜炎 / ~ pulse (sign) 昆克脉搏(征)(有多种方法可引起皮肤颜色红白交替,如压指甲端时见于甲床或指甲根的皮肤,由于乳头层下动静脉丛的搏动所致,有时见于主动脉瓣闭锁不全和其他疾病,但在某种情况下也可能见于正常人,原来曾认为是由毛细管搏动引起,故称毛细管脉搏) / ~ puncture 腰椎穿刺
quinestrol [kwiˈnestrɔl] *n* 炔雌醚(雌激素)
quinethazone [kwiˈneθəzəun] *n* 喹乙宗(利尿、降压药)
quinfamide [ˈkwinfəmaid] *n* 喹法米特(抗阿米巴药)
quingestanol acetate [kwinˈdʒestənɔl] 醋酸奎孕醇(孕激素类药)
quingestrone [kwinˈdʒestrəun] *n* 奎孕酮(孕激素)
quinic acid [ˈkwinik] 奎尼酸
quinidine [ˈkwinidin] *n* 奎尼丁(抗心律失常药) | ~ gluconate 葡萄糖酸奎尼丁 / ~ polygalacturonate 奎尼丁聚半乳糖醛酸盐 / ~ sulfate 硫酸奎尼丁(抗心律失常药)
quinine [ˈkwinin, kwiˈniːn, ˈkwainain] *n* 奎宁(抗疟药) | ~ and urea hydrochloride 盐酸奎宁脲,盐酸奎宁盐酸脲复盐(硬化药,局部麻醉药) / ~ bismuth iodide 碘化铋奎宁(从前用于治梅毒) / ~ bisulfate 重硫酸奎宁(从前用于治各种眼病) / ~ dihydrochloride 二盐酸奎宁(治重症疟疾) / ~ ethylcarbonate 碳酸乙酯奎宁,优奎宁(用法同硫酸奎宁) / ~ hydrobromide 氢溴酸奎宁(从前用于治甲状腺功能亢进及肺炎球菌性肺炎) / ~ hydrochloride 盐酸奎宁(用法同硫酸奎宁) / ~ salicylate 水杨酸奎宁(从前用作解热药和抗风湿药) / ~ sulfate 硫酸奎宁(抗疟药) / ~ tannate 鞣酸奎宁(从前用于治百日咳和腹泻)
quininic acid [kwiˈninik] 奎宁酸
quininism [ˈkwininizəm] *n* 奎宁中毒,金鸡纳中毒
quinoid [ˈkwinɔid] *n* 醌型,醌式
quinoline [ˈkwinəliːn] *n* 喹啉
quinolinic acid [ˌkwinəuˈlinik] 喹啉酸
quinolone [ˈkwinəuləun] *n* 喹诺酮
quinometry [kwiˈnɔmitri] *n* 奎宁标准规定
quinone [kwaiˈnəun, ˈkwinəun] *n* 苯醌,醌
quinonoid [ˈkwinənɔid] *a* 醌型的
quinotannic acid [ˌkwinəˈtænik] 奎鞣酸,金鸡纳鞣酸
quinovic acid [kwiˈnəuvik] 奎诺酸
quinovin [kwiˈnəuvin] *n* 奎诺温,金鸡纳[皮]苷
quinovose [ˈkwinəvəus] *n* 鸡纳糖,异鼠李糖,6-脱氧葡萄
quinoxin [kwiˈnɔksin] *n* 奎诺克辛,亚硝基酚
Quinq. quinque【拉】五
Quinquaud's sign [kæŋˈkəu] (Charles E. Quinquaud)坎科征(醇中毒时患者手指震颤)
quinquecuspid [ˌkwiŋkwiˈkʌspid] *a* 五尖的 *n* 五

尖牙

quinquetubercular [ˈkwiŋkwitju(ː)ˈbəːkjulə] *a* 五结节的,五尖的

quinquevalent [ˌkwiŋkwiˈveilənt] *a* 五价的 | **quinquevalence, quinquevalency** *n*

quinquina [kinˈkiːnə] *n* 金鸡纳[树]皮

quinsy [ˈkwinzi] *n* 扁桃体周脓肿 | lingual ~ 化脓性舌扁桃体炎

Quint. quintus【拉】第五的

quint- [前缀]五,第五

quintan [ˈkwintən] *a* 每第五日[复发]的(如五日热)

quintessence [kwinˈtesns] *n* 精华;浓浸膏

quintile [ˈkwintail] *n* 五分值,五分线

quintipara [kwinˈtipərə] *n* 五产妇

quintisternal [ˌkwintiˈstəːnəl] *a* 胸骨第五节的

Quinton-Scribner shunt [ˈkwintən ˈskribnə] (Wayne E. Quinton; Belding H. Scribner)奎-斯分流术(一种为血液透析而建立的动静脉分流,包括由 U 形硅橡胶管及其特氟隆〈Teflon〉管尖组成的外通道,插在桡动脉和头静脉之间)

quintuplet [ˈkwintjuplit, kwinˈtju-] *n* 五胎

quinupristin [kwiˈnjupristin] *n* 奎奴普丁(抗菌药)

quisqualic acid [kwisˈkwɔlik] 使君子氨酸

quittor [ˈkwitə] *n* 马蹄疽 | simple ~ 单纯性马蹄疽

quoad vitam [ˈkwəuæd ˈvaitæm]【拉】关于生命

quod vide [kwɔd ˈvaidiː]【拉】参阅,参照

Quotid. quotidie【拉】每日

quotidian [kwɔˈtidiən] *a* 每日的,日发的 *n* 日发疟

quotient [ˈkwəuʃənt] *n* 商数,系数 | achievement ~ 能力商数,成绩商数(儿童学习进展程度与其能力之比) / albumin ~ 白蛋白商(血浆和全血白蛋白比值) / caloric ~ 热量商数(在代谢过程中,发出热量〈以卡计〉除以氧气消耗量〈以 mg 计〉所得之商数) / conceptual ~ 受孕率 / D:N ~ D/N(葡萄糖和尿氮比值) / growth ~ 生长商数(全部食物能量中用于生长的商数) / intelligence ~ 智力商数(病人智力年龄,除以实足年龄,再乘以100) / protein ~ 蛋白商(血浆球蛋白量除以蛋白量所得之商) / rachidian ~, spinal ~ 脑脊液压系数(见 Ayala's quotient) / reaction ~ 反应系数 / respiratory ~ 呼吸商(呼出的二氧化碳量与肺吸入的氧气量在每单位时间的比率)

q. v. quantum vis【拉】适量;quod vide【拉】参照,参阅

R

R arginine 精氨酸；organic radical 有机基；Rankine scale 兰氏温标；rate 率；respiratory exchange ratio 呼吸商；Réaumure scale 列氏温标；resistance 电阻；respiration 呼吸；rhythm 节律；right 右［侧］的；roentgen 伦琴；rough(colony)粗糙型(菌落)

R. remotum【拉】远的

R resistance 电阻；gas constant 气体常数

***R*-** rectus【拉】右的

℞ recipe 取(用于处方)

R_A，R_{AW} airway resistance 气道阻力

R_e Reynold number 雷诺数

R_f 比移(在纸色谱法或薄层色谱法中，溶质点从原点移动的距离表示一部分溶剂前沿移动的距离)

r ring chromosome 环形染色体；drug resistance 耐药性；伦琴(roentgen)的符号(旧名，现用 R 代替)

r 相关系数(correlation coefficient)、半径距离(distance radius)和抗药性(drug resistance)的符号

r_s Spearman's rank correlation coefficient 斯皮尔曼秩相关系数

ρ rho 希腊语第 17 个字母；相关系数(correlation coefficient)、质量密度(mass density)和电荷密度(electric charge density)的符号

Ra radium 镭

Raabe's test [ˈrɑːbə] (Gustav Raabe)拉贝试验(检尿白蛋白)

rabbetting [ˈræbitiŋ] *n* 骨折断端交锁

rabbia [ˈræbiə] *n* 狂犬病

rabbit [ˈræbit] *n* 兔 | Watanabe heritable hyperlipidemic(WHHL) ~ 华坦内比可遗传的高脂血兔(兔的突变种，患低密度脂蛋白受体缺乏症，类似人家族性高胆固醇血症，用于研究脂蛋白代谢和动脉粥样化形成)

rabbitpox [ˈræbitpɔks] *n* 兔痘

rabelaisin [ˌræbiˈleiisin] *n* 腊贝来辛(心脏兴奋药)

rabeprazole sodium [rəˈbepreizəul] 雷贝拉唑钠(一种质子泵抑制剂，用于抑制胃酸分泌，治疗腐蚀性或溃疡性食管反流疾病以及治疗以胃酸大量分泌为特点的疾病，口服给药)

rabicidal [ˌreibiˈsaidl] *a* 杀狂犬病病毒的

rabid [ˈræbid] *a* 狂怒的；患狂犬病的

rabies [ˈreibiːz, -biiːz] *n* 狂犬病 | dumb ~ 早瘫性狂犬病 / furious ~ 狂暴性狂犬病 / paralytic ~ 麻痹性狂犬病(通常为一种上行性脊髓麻痹) | **rabic** [ˈræbik] *a*

rabiform [ˈreibifɔːm] *a* 狂犬病状的

Rabson-Mendenhall syndrome [ˈræbsən ˈmendənhɔːl] (S. M. Rabson; E. W. Mendenhall)拉布森-门登豪尔综合征(一种罕见的综合征，见于儿童，特征为胰岛素受体基因的突变或其他缺陷，具有重度胰岛素抗性和黑棘皮症，此外尚有浓发、齿和甲异常以及松果腺增生)

race [reis] *n* 人种；种族；亚种，族(遗传学)；属，类 | the ~ 人类

racemase [ˈreisimeis] *n* 消旋酶

racemate [ˈreisimeit] *n* 消旋物

raceme [reiˈsiːm] *n* 总状花序；消旋物

racemic [rəˈsiːmik] *a* 总状花的；消旋的

racemization [ˌreisimaiˈzeiʃən, -miˈz-] *n* 消旋化

racemose [ˈræsiməus] *a* 葡萄状的，蔓状的

racephedrine hydrochloride [reiˈsefədrin] *n* 盐酸消旋麻黄碱(拟交感神经药)

racephenicol [ˌreisiˈfenikɔl] *n* 消旋甲砜霉素(抗菌药)

racer [ˈreisə] *n* 游蛇属黑蛇

rachial [ˈreikiəl] *a* 脊柱的

rachialbuminimeter [ˌreikiælˌbjuːmiˈnimitə] *n* 脑脊液白蛋白定量器 | **rachialbuminimetry** *n* 脑脊液白蛋白定量法

rachialgia [ˌreikiˈældʒiə] *n* 脊柱痛

rachianesthesia [ˌreikiænisˈθiːzjə]，**rachianalgesia** [ˌreikiˌænælˈdʒiːziə] *n* 脊髓麻醉[法]

rachicentesis [ˌreikisenˈtiːsis]，**rachiocentesis** [ˌreikiəusenˈtiːsis] *n* 椎管穿刺，腰椎穿刺

rachidial [rəˈkidiəl]，**rachidian** [rəˈkidiən] *a* 脊柱的

rachigraph [ˈreikigrɑːf] *n* 脊柱描记器

rachilysis [rəˈkilisis] *n* 弯脊矫正术

rachi(o)- [构词成分]脊柱

rachiocampsis [ˌreikiəuˈkæmpsis] *n* 脊柱弯曲

rachiochysis [ˌreikiˈɔkisis] *n* 椎管积液

rachiodynia [ˌreikiəuˈdiniə] *n* 脊柱痛

rachiokyphosis [ˌreikiəukaiˈfəusis]，**rachiocyphosis** [ˌreikiəusaiˈfəusis] *n* 脊柱后凸，驼背

rachiometer [ˌreikiˈɔmitə] *n* 脊柱弯度计

rachiomyelitis [ˌreikiəuˌmaiəˈlaitis] *n* 脊髓炎

rachiopagus [ˌreikiˈɔpəgəs]，**rachipagus** [rəˈkipəgəs] *n* 脊柱联胎

rachiopathy [ˌreikiˈɔpəθi] *n* 脊柱病

rachioscoliosis [ˌreikiəuˌskəuli'əusis] *n* 脊柱侧凸
rachiotome ['reikiətəum] *n* 椎骨刀,脊椎刀
rachiotomy [ˌreiki'ɔtəmi] *n* 脊柱切开术
rachiresistance [ˌreikiri'zistəns] *n* 脊髓麻醉[药]抗拒性
rachiresistant [ˌreikiri'zistənt] *a* 抗脊髓麻醉的
rachis ['reikis] *n* 脊柱,脊椎
rachisagra [ˌreiki'sægrə] *n* 脊柱猝痛,脊柱痛风
rachischisis [rə'kiskisis] *n* 脊柱裂 | ~ partialis 脊柱不全裂 / ~ posterior 脊柱后裂,脊柱裂 / ~ totalis 脊柱全裂
rachisensibility [ˌreikiˌsensi'biləti] *n* 脊髓麻醉过敏[性]
rachisensible [ˌreiki'sensəbl] *a* 脊髓麻醉过敏的
rachitis [ræ'kaitis, rə'kaitis] *n* 佝偻病;脊柱炎 | ~ fetalis annularis 胎性环状佝偻病 / ~ fetalis micromelica 胎性小肢性佝偻病 / ~ tardia 迟发佝偻病 | **rachitic** [rə'kitik] *a* 佝偻病的
rachitism ['rækitizəm] *n* 佝偻病体质
rachitogenic [rəˌkitəu'dʒenik] *a* 佝偻病源的,引起佝偻病的
rachitome ['rækitəum] *n* 椎管刀
rachitomy [rə'kitəmi] *n* 椎管切开术
racial ['reiʃəl] *a* 种族的;人种的
raclopride ['rækləupraid] *n* 雷氯必利(抗精神病药)
RAD right axis deviation 轴右偏(心电图)
rad [ræd] *n* 拉德(radiation absorbed dose 的首字母缩拼词,旧辐射吸收剂量单位,每 1 g 组织吸收 100 尔格的能,现用戈瑞〈Gy〉, 1 rad = 10^{-2} Gy); 弧度(radian 的缩写词)
rad. radix【拉】根
radarkymography [ˌreidəkai'mɔgrəfi] *n* 雷达计波摄影
radarscope ['reidəskəup] *n* 雷达显示器,雷达示波器
radectomy [rei'dektəmi] *n* 牙根[部分]切除术
Rademacher's system ['rɑːdəˌmʌhə] (Johann G. Rademacher)拉德马赫尔体制(认为每一病都有特效药)
Radfordia [ræd'fɔːdiə] *n* 雷螨属
radiability [ˌreidiə'biləti] *n* X 线可透性
radiable ['reidiəbl] *a* 可透 X 线的,X 线可检的
radiad ['reidiæd] *ad* 向桡侧
radial ['reidjəl] *a* 放射的,辐射状的;桡骨的
radialis [ˌreidi'eilis] *a*【拉】桡骨的,桡侧的
radian ['reidjən] *n* 弧度
radiance ['reidjəns], **radiancy** ['reidjənsi] *n* 发光,辐射性能,辐射率
radiant ['reidjənt] *a* 放射的,辐射的;发出辐射热的
radiate ['reidieit] *vt* 辐射,放射 *vt* 发射,辐射 *a* 有射线的,辐射状的
radiathermy [reiˌdaiə'θəːmi] *n* 短波透热法
radiatio [reidi'eiʃiəu] ([复] **radiationes** [reidiˌeiʃi'əuniːz]) *n* 辐射线(解剖学名词)
radiation [ˌreidi'eiʃən] *n* 放射,辐射;辐射线(解剖);辐射能,放射线;放射(疗法) | acoustic ~, auditory ~, thalamotemporal ~ 听辐射线 / adaptive ~ 适应辐射 / alpha ~, α-~ α[射线]辐射 / background ~ 本底放射,本底辐射 / braking ~ 轫致辐射 / ~ of corpus callosum 胼胝体辐射线 / corpuscular ~s 微粒放射,微粒辐射 / gamma ~, γ-~ γ 射线;γ 线 / heterogeneous ~ 不均匀放射,复色放射 / homogeneous ~ 均匀放射,单色放射 / interstitial ~ 组织内放射(疗法) / mitogenetic ~, mitogenic ~ 促有丝分裂辐射 / monochromatic ~ 单色辐射 / occipitothalamic ~, optic ~ 枕叶丘脑辐射线,视辐射线 / pyramidal ~ 锥体辐射线 / thalamic ~ 视丘辐射线 / white ~ 连续辐射 | **~al**, **radiative** ['reidieitiv] *a* 放射的;辐射的
radiation-proof [ˌreidi'eiʃən'pruːf] *a* 防辐射的
radical ['rædikəl] *a* 根治性的;基的,根的,基团的 *n* 基,根,基团(化学上主要指原子团) | acid ~ 酸根,酸基 / alcohol ~ 醇基 / color ~ 色基,发色团,生色团 / free ~ 自由基
radices ['reidisiːz] radix 的复数
radiciform [rə'disifɔːm] *a* 根状的;牙根状的
radicle ['rædikl] *n* 小根,细根(指血管或神经);根,基,原子团;胚根(植物)
radicotomy [ˌrædi'kɔtəmi] *n* 神经根切断术
radicula [rə'dikjulə] *n*【拉】小根,细根(血管或神经)
radiculalgia [rəˌdikju'lældʒiə] *n* 神经根痛
radicular [rə'dikjulə] *a* 根的
radiculectomy [rəˌdikju'lektəmi] *n* 根切除术(尤指脊神经根切除术)
radiculitis [rəˌdikju'laitis] *n* 神经根炎
radiculoganglionitis [rəˌdikjuləuˌgæŋgliə'naitis] *n* 脊神经根神经节炎
radiculomedullary [rəˌdikjuləu'medʌˌləri] *a* 脊髓脊神经根的
radiculomeningomyelitis [rəˌdikjuləuməˌniŋgəuˌmaiə'laitis] *n* 脊髓脊膜脊神经根炎
radiculomyelopathy [rəˌdikjuləuˌmaiə'lɔpəθi] *n* 脊髓脊神经根病
radiculoneuritis [rəˌdikjuləunjuə'raitis] *n* 神经根神经炎(急性热病性多神经炎)
radiculoneuropathy [rəˌdikjuləunjuə'rɔpəθi] *n* 神经根神经病
radiculopathy [rəˌdikju'lɔpəθi] *n* 神经根病
radiectomy [ˌreidi'ektəmi] *n* 牙根切除术
radiferous [rei'difərəs] *a* 含镭的

radii [ˈreidiai] radius 的复数
radio- [构词成分]放射,辐射;桡骨
radioactinium [ˌreidiəuækˈtiniəm] *n* 放射性锕,射锕
radioaction [ˌreidiəuˈækʃən] *n* 放射性,辐射性;放射现象
radioactive [ˌreidiəuˈæktiv] *a* 放射性的,放射的
radioactivity [ˌreidiəuækˈtivəti] *n* 放射性,辐射性;放射现象 | artificial ~, induced ~ 人工放射性;人工放射现象
radioactor [ˌreidiəuˈæktə] *n* 镭疗器
radioallergosorbent [ˌreidiəuˌælәgəuˈsɔːbənt] *a* 放射变应原吸附的
radioanaphylaxis [ˌreidiəuˌænəfiˈlæksis] *n* 放射过敏反应,放射过敏症(对 X 线或其他辐射能的过敏性反应)
radioautogram [ˌreidiəuˈɔːtəgræm] *n* 放射自显影[照]片
radioautograph [ˌreidiəuˈɔːtəgrɑːf] *n* 放射自显影[照]片 | **~ic** [ˌreidiəuˌɔːtəuˈgræfik] *a* 放射自显影的 / **~y** [ˌreidiəuɔːˈtɔgrəfi] *n* 放射自显影[术],自体放射摄影[术]
radiobe [ˈreidiəub] *n* 放射凝集
radiobicipital [ˌreidiəubaiˈsipitl] *n* 桡骨[与]肱二头肌的
radiobiology [ˌreidiəubaiˈɔlədʒi] *n* 放射生物学 | **radiobiological** [ˌreidiəuˌbaiəˈlɔdʒikəl] *a* / **radiobiologist** *n* 放射生物学家
radiochemotherapy [ˌreidiəuˌkiːməuˈθerəpi] *n* 放射化学治疗,化学放射治疗
radiocalcium [ˌreidiəuˈkælsiəm] *n* 放射性钙,射钙
radiocarbon [ˌreidiəuˈkɑːbən] *n* 放射性碳,射碳
radiocarcinogenesis [ˌreidiəuˌkɑːsinəuˈdʒenisis] *n* 放射性致癌形成,放射致癌
radiocardiogram [ˌreidiəuˈkɑːdiəgræm] *n* 心放射图;放射心电图
radiocardiography [ˌreidiəuˌkɑːdiˈɔgrəfi] *n* 心放射描记法;放射心电描记法
radiocarpal [ˌreidiəuˈkɑːpl] *a* 桡腕的
radiocarpus [ˌreidiəuˈkɑːpəs] *n* 桡侧腕屈肌
radiochemistry [ˌreidiəuˈkemistri] *n* 放射化学 | **radiochemical** *a*
radiochemy [ˌreidiəuˈkemi] *n* 放射[化学]效应
radiochroism [ˌreidiəuˈkrəuizəm] *n* 放射吸收性
radiocinematograph [ˌreidiəuˌsiniˈmætəgrɑːf] *n* X 线电影摄影机
radiocolloids [ˌreidiəuˈkɔlɔids] *n* 放射胶质
radiocurable [ˌreidiəuˈkjuərəbl] *a* 可放射治疗的,可经放射治愈的
radiocystitis [ˌreidiəusisˈtaitis] *n* 放射性膀胱炎
radiode [ˈreidiəud] *n* 镭插入器
radiodense [ˈreidiəuˌdens] *a* 不透 X 线的,不透射线的
radiodensity [ˌreidiəuˈdensəti] *n* 放射密度
radiodermatitis [ˌreidiəudəːməˈtaitis] *n* 放射性皮炎
radiodiagnosis [ˌreidiəuˌdaiəgˈnəusis] *n* 放射诊断,X 线诊断
radiodiagnostics [ˌreidiəuˌdaiəgˈnɔstiks] *n* 放射诊断学,X 线诊断学
radiodiaphane [ˌreidiəuˈdaiəfein] *n* 镭透照镜
radiodigital [ˌreidiəuˈdidʒitl] *a* 桡骨手指的
radiodontics [ˌreidiəuˈdɔntiks] *n* 牙放射学 | **radiodontist** *n* 牙放射学家
radioecology [ˌreidiəui(ː)ˈkɔlədʒi] *n* 放射生态学
radioelectrocardiogram [ˌreidiəuˌilektrəuˈkɑːdiəgræm] *n* 无线电心电图
radioelectrocardiograph [ˌreidiəuiˌlektrəuˈkɑːdiəgrɑːf] *n* 无线电心电描记器 | **~y** [ˌreidiəuiˌlektrəuˌkɑːdiˈɔgrəfi] *n* 无线电心电描记法
radioelement [ˌreidiəuˈelimənt] *n* 放射[性]元素
radioencephalogram [ˌreidiəuenˈsefələˌgræm] *n* 放射脑电图
radioepidermitis [ˌreidiəuˌepidəːˈmaitis] *n* 放射性表皮炎
radioepithelitis [ˌreidiəuˌepiθiːˈlaitis] *n* 放射性上皮炎
radiofrequency [ˌreidiəuˈfriːkwənsi] *n* 射频
radiogen [ˈreidiədʒən] *n* 放射物[质],放射源
radiogenesis [ˌreidiəuˈdʒenisis] *n* 射线产生,射线生成
radiogenic [ˌreidiəuˈdʒenik] *a* 放射所致的,放射原的,致辐射的
radiogold [ˈreidiəuˌgəuld] *n* 放射性金,射金
radiogram [ˈreidiəugræm] *n* 放射照片,X 线[照]片
radiograph [ˈreidiəugrɑːf, -græf] *n* 放射照片,X 线[照]片 | bite-wing ~ 殆翼 X 线[照]片 / lateral oblique jaw ~ 侧斜位颌 X 线[照]片 / lateral skull ~ 侧头颅 X 线[照]片 / maxillary sinus ~ 上颌窦 X 线[照]片(即瓦特位观〈Water's view〉X 线[照]片) / panoramic ~ 全景 X 线[照]片 / submental vertex ~ 颏下顶 X 线[照]片
radiography [ˌreidiˈɔgrəfi] *n* X 线摄影[术],放射摄影[术] | digital ~ 数字 X 线摄影[术] / double contrast ~ 双对比 X 线摄影[术] / mucosal relief ~ 黏膜皱襞 X 线摄影[术] / selective ~ 选择性 X 线摄影[术],居民抽检 X 线摄影[术] | **radiographic** [ˌreidiəuˈgræfik] *a* 放射摄影的,X 线摄影的
radiohumeral [ˌreidiəuˈhjuːmərəl] *a* 桡[骨]肱[骨]的

radioimmunity [ˌreidiəuiˈmjuːnəti] *n* 放射免疫
radioimmunoassay [ˌreidiəuiˌmjuːnəuˈæsei] *n* 放射免疫测定
radioimmunodetection [ˌreidiəuˌimjuːnəudiˈtekʃən] *n* 放射免疫检测,免疫闪烁显像(即 immunoscintigraphy)
radioimmunodiffusion [ˌreidiəuiˌmjuːnəudiˈfjuːʒən] *n* 放射免疫扩散[法]
radioimmunoelectrophoresis [ˌreidiəuiˌmjuːnəuiˌlektrəufəˈriːsis] *n* 放射免疫电泳[法]
radioimmunoimaging [ˌreidiəuˌimjuːməuˈiməgiŋ] *n* 放射免疫显像,免疫闪烁显像(即 immunoscintigraphy)
radioimmunoprecipitation [ˌreidiəuiˌmjuːnəupriˌsipiˈteiʃən] *n* 放射免疫沉淀[法]
radioimmunoscintigraphy [ˌreidiəuˌimjuːnəusinˈtigrəfi] *n* 放射免疫闪烁显像,免疫闪烁显像(即 immunoscintigraphy)
radioimmunosorbent [ˌreidiəuˌimjunəuˈsɔːbənt] *a* 放射免疫吸附的
radioiodine [ˌreidiəuˈaiəudiːn] *n* 放射性碘,射碘
radioiron [ˌreidiəuˈaiən] *n* 放射性铁,射铁
radioisotope [ˌreidiəuˈaisəutəup] *n* 放射性同位素 | carrier-free ~ 无载体放射性同位素
radiokymography [ˌreidiəukaiˈmɔgrəfi] *n* X 线记波摄影[术],X 线描记法
radiolabel [ˌreidiəuˈleibəl] *n* 放射性标记 *vt* 使带有放射性标记
radiolabeled [ˌreidiəuˈleibəld] *a* 放射性标记的
Radiolaria [ˌreidiəuˈlɛəriə] *n* 放射虫纲
radiolarian [ˌreidiəuˈlɛəriən] *n* 放射虫
radiolead [ˌreidiəuˈled] *n* 放射性铅,射铅
radiolesion [ˌreidiəuˈliːʒən] *n* 放射性损害
radioligand [ˌreidiəuˈlaigənd, ˌreidiəuˈligənd] *n* 放射性配体(一种放射性标记物质,如抗原,用于定量检测一个未标记的物质)
radiology [ˌreidiˈɔlədʒi] *n* 放射学 | **radiologic(al)** [ˌreidiəuˈlɔdʒik(əl)] *a* / **radiologist** *n* 放射学家
radiolucent [ˌreidiəuˈljuːsnt] *a* 透射线的,可透 X 线的 | **radiolucency** [ˌreidiəuˈljuːsnsi] *n* 透射线性,可透 X 线性
radiolus [reiˈdiːələs] *n* 【拉】探子
radiometallography [ˌreidiəuˌmetəˈlɔgrəfi] *a* 放射金相学,射线金相学
radiometer [ˌreidiˈɔmitə] *n* 辐射计;放射量计,放射量测定器 | pastille ~ 纸碟式放射量计 / photographic ~ 照相纸式放射量计 | **radiometry** *n* 放射测量学,辐射度学
radiomicrometer [ˌreidiəumaiˈkrɔmitə] *n* 显微辐射计,辐射微量计
radiomimetic [ˌreidiəumaiˈmetik] *a* 类放射的,拟放射的
radiomuscular [ˌreidiəuˈmʌskjulə] *a* 桡动脉[至]肌的,桡神经[至]肌的
radiomutation [ˌreidiəumjuˈteiʃən] *n* 放射性突变
radion [ˈreidiɔn] *n* 放射粒[子]
radionecrosis [ˌreidiəuneˈkrəusis] *n* 放射性坏死
radioneuritis [ˌreidiəunjuəˈraitis] *n* 放射性神经炎
radionitrogen [ˌreidiəuˈnaitrədʒən] *n* 放射性氮,射氮
radionuclide [ˌreidiəuˈnjuːklaid] *n* 放射性核素
radiopacity [ˌreidiəuˈpæsəti], **radioopacity** [ˌreidiəuəuˈpæsəti] *n* 不透 X 线性,不透射线性
radiopalmar [ˌreidiəuˈpælmə] *a* 桡骨手掌的,桡动脉手掌的
radiopaque [ˈreidiəupeik] *a* 不透 X 线的,不透射线的
radioparent [ˌreidiəuˈpɛərənt] *a* 可透 X 线的,可透射线的 | **radioparency** *n* X 线可透性,射线可透性
radiopathology [ˌreidiəupəˈθɔlədʒi] *n* 放射病理学
radiopelvimetry [ˌreidiəupelˈvimitri] *n* 骨盆 X 线测量术
radiopharmaceutical [ˌreidiəuˌfɑːməˈsjuːtikəl] *a* 放射药剂学的 *n* 放射性药品
radiopharmacy [ˌreidiəuˈfɑːməsi] *n* 放射药剂学
radiophobia [ˌreidiəuˈfəubjə] *n* 放射[线]恐怖,射线恐怖
radiophosphorus [ˌreidiəuˈfɔsfərəs] *n* 放射性磷,射磷
radiophotography [ˌreidiəufəˈtɔgrəfi] *n* X 线摄影[术],放射摄影[术]
radiophylaxis [ˌreidiəufiˈlæksis] *n* 放射反应防御作用(先以小剂量照射,从而缓和继续大量照射的反应)
radiophysics [ˌreidiəuˈfiziks] *n* 放射物理学
radioplastic [ˌreidiəuˈplæstik] *a* X 线器官模型的
radiopotassium [ˌreidiəupəˈtæsjəm] *n* 放射性钾,射钾
radiopotentiation [ˌreidiəupəˌtenʃiˈeiʃən] *n* 放射增强[作用]
radiopraxis [ˌreidiəuˈpræksis] *n* 放射疗法,射线疗法
radioprotectant [ˌreidiəuprəuˈtektənt] *a* 辐射防护的 *n* 防辐射药
radioprotector [ˌreidiəuprəuˈtektə] *n* 防辐射药
radiopulmonography [ˌreidiəuˌpʌlməˈnɔgrəfi] *n* 放射肺换气率测定法
radioreaction [ˌreidiəuri(ː)ˈækʃən] *n* 放射反应
radioreceptor [ˌreidiəuriˈseptə] *n* 放射感受器;放

射受体
radioresistant [ˌreidiəuri'zistənt] *a* 抗放射性的 | **radioresistance** *n* 抗放射性,放射抵抗性
radioresponsive [ˌreidiəuris'pɔnsiv] *a* 放射有效的,对放射有反应的
radiosclerometer [ˌreidiəuskliə'rɔmitə] *n* [X线]透度计,[X线]硬度计
radioscope ['reidiəskəup] *n* 放射镜,X线透视屏,放射探测仪
radioscopy [ˌreidi'ɔskəpi] *n* 放射检查,荧光屏检查,X线透视检查 | **radioscopic** [ˌreidiə'skɔpik] *a*
radiosensitive [ˌreidiəu'sensitiv] *a* 放射敏感的 | **radiosensitivity** [ˌreidiəuˌsensi'tivəti], **radiosensibility** [ˌreidiəuˌsensi'biləti], **~ness** *n* 放射敏感性
radiosensitizer [ˌreidiəu'sensiˌtaizə] *n* 放射增敏剂
radiosodium [ˌreidiəu'səudjəm] *n* 放射性钠,射钠
radiostereoscopy [ˌreidiəuˌstiəri'ɔskəpi] *n* X线立体透视检查
radiostrontium [ˌreidiəu'strɔnʃiəm] *n* 放射性锶,射锶
radiosulfur [ˌreidiəu'sʌlfə] *n* 放射性硫,射硫
radiosurgery [ˌreidiəu'səːdʒəri] *n* 放射外科学,镭外科学
radiotelemetry [ˌreidiəuti'lemitri] *n* 无线电遥测术(测各种因子,由无线电波将特殊资料从测量的物体发送到记录器)
radiotellurium [ˌreidiəute'ljuəriəm] *n* 放射性碲,射碲
radiothanatology [ˌreidiəuˌθænə'tɔlədʒi] *n* 放射死因学(研究放射能对死组织的效应)
radiotherapy [ˌreidiəu'θerəpi], **radiotherapeutics** [ˌreidiəuˌθerə'pjuːtiks] *n* 放射疗法,放射治疗 | **radiotherapist** [ˌreidiəu'θerəpist] *n* 放射治疗学家
radiothermy ['reidiəuˌθəːmi] *n* 热放射疗法;短波透热[法]
radiothorium [ˌreidiəu'θɔːriəm] *n* 放射性钍,射钍
radiotomy [ˌreidi'ɔtəmi] *n* X线体层摄影[术]
radiotoxemia [ˌreidiəutɔk'siːmiə] *n* 放射性毒血症
radiotoxicity [ˌreidiəutɔk'sisəti] *n* 放射性毒性
radiotracer [ˌreidiəu'treisə] *n* 放射性示踪物
radiotransparency [ˌreidiəutræns'pɛərənsi] *n* X线可透性,放射线可透性
radiotransparent [ˌreidiəutræns'pɛərənt] *a* X线可透的,射线可透的,透射线的
radiotropic [ˌreidiəu'trɔpik] *a* 放射影响的
radiotropism [ˌreidi'ɔtrəpizəm] *n* 向放射性,向辐射性
radioulnar [ˌreidiəu'ʌlnə] *a* 桡[骨]尺[骨]的
radisectomy [ˌreidi'sektəmi] *n* 牙根切断术
radish ['rædiʃ] *n* 萝卜;萝卜根(用于治支气管炎和消化不良)
radium (Ra) ['reidjəm] *n* 镭(化学元素)
radius ['reidjəs]([复]**radii** ['reidiai]) *n* 半径;桡骨;辐射线(解剖) | radii of lens 晶状体辐射线
radix ['reidiks]([复]**radixes** 或 **radices** ['reidisiːz]) *n*【拉】根
radon (Rn) ['reidɔn] *n* 氡(化学元素)
Radovici's sign [rɑːdəu'viːsi](André Radovici)腊多维西征,掌颏反射
RAE right atrial enlargement 右心房增大
Raeder's syndrome, paratrigeminal syndrome ['reidə](Johan G. Raeder)雷德综合征、三叉神经旁综合征(面部单侧阵发性神经痛伴交感神经麻痹〈Horner 综合征〉,亦称三叉神经旁综合征)
raffinase ['ræfineis] *n* 棉子糖酶
raffinose ['ræfinəus] *n* 棉子糖
rafoxanide [rə'fɔksənaid] *n* 雷复尼特(兽用抗蠕虫药)
rage [reidʒ] *n* 激怒,暴怒 | sham ~ 假怒(见于去除大脑皮质的动物,亦见于胰岛素低血糖或一氧化碳中毒患者)
ragocyte ['rægəusait][*Ragg*(*r*heumatoid serum *agg*lutinator) + *-cyte*] *n* 类风湿(血清凝集者)细胞(在类风湿关节炎的关节中发现的一种多形核白细胞,其胞质包含物摄入凝集的 IgG、类风湿因子、纤维蛋白和补体,亦称 RA 细胞)
ragweed ['rægwiːd] *n* 豚草
ragwort ['rægwɔːt] *n* 千里光,狗舌草 | tansy ~ 雅各布千里光(即 Senecio jacobea)
raigan ['reiigæn] *n*【汉】雷丸(中药用作驱肠虫药)
Raillietina [ˌreiljə'tainə] *n* 瑞列绦虫属 | ~ madagascariensis 马达加斯加瑞列绦虫
raillietiniasis [ˌreiljəti'naiəsis] *n* 瑞列绦虫病
Raimiste's sign [rai'miːstə](Johann M. Raimister)雷米斯特征(检查者将患者的手和臂扶持于垂直位,如手正常,放松时手仍保持垂直;如有轻瘫,手迅即由腕部下垂)
Rainey's corpuscles, tubes, tubule ['reini](George Rainey)雷尼小体,肉孢子虫囊
RAIU radioactive iodine uptake 放射性碘摄取
raking ['reikiŋ] *n* 搜集,搜索 | back ~ 肛掏粪(指动物)
rale [rɑːl] *n* 啰音 | amphoric ~ 空瓮音 / atelectatic ~, border ~, marginal ~ 肺缘啰音,肺膨

胀不全音 / bronchial ~ 支气管啰音 / bubbling ~ 沸泡音 / cavernous ~ 空洞音 / clicking ~ 卡嗒音 / collapse ~ 萎陷肺啰音 / consonating ~, metallic ~ 谐和啰音,金属啰音 / crepitant ~, vesicular ~ 捻发音 / dry ~ 干啰音 / extrathoracic ~ 胸外啰音 / gurgling ~ 咕噜音 / guttural ~ 咽喉音 / ~ indux 实变初期啰音 / laryngeal ~ 喉音 / moist ~ 湿啰音/ mucous ~, ~ muqueux 黏液性音 / pleural ~ 胸膜啰音,胸膜摩擦音 / ~ redux, ~ de retour 消散期啰音 / sibilant ~, whistling ~ 飞箭音,笛音 / sonorous ~ 鼾音 / subcrepitant ~, crackling ~ 细捻发音 / tracheal ~ 气管啰音

Ralfe's test [rælf] (Charles H. Ralfe) 拉尔夫试验(检尿丙酮及尿胨)

raloxifene hydrochloride [ræ'lɔksifiːn] 盐酸雷洛昔芬(雌激素激活剂)

Ralstonia [rɔːl'stəuniə] *n* 罗尔斯通菌属 | ~ pickettii 皮氏罗尔斯通菌

raltitrexed disodium [ˌrælti'treksəd] 雷替曲赛二钠(一种叶酸喹唑啉类似物,可抑制胸苷酸合酶,用作抗肿瘤药,治疗晚期结肠直肠癌,静脉内给药)

ramal ['reiməl] *a* 支的,分支的

Raman effect ['rɑːmən] (Chandrasekhara V. Raman) 拉曼效应(当某物质受到单色光辐照时,此物质散射的光谱中,除含有与入射辐射相同波长的光谱线外,还含有其他光谱线,即随原线移动而原辐射波长已改变了的伴线)

RAMC Royal Army Medical Corps 皇家陆军医疗队

ramex ['reimeks] *n* 【拉】精索静脉曲张

rami ['reimai] ramus 的复数

Ramibacterium [ˌreimibæk'tiəriəm] *n* 分枝乳酸杆菌属

ramification [ˌræmifi'keiʃən] *n* 分支;支状分布

ramify ['ræmifai] *vt, vi* 分支,分叉;成岔状

ramipril [rə'mipril] *n* 雷米普利(抗高血压药)

ramisection [ˌræmi'sekʃən], **ramicotomy** [ˌræmi'kɔtəmi], **ramisectomy** [ˌræmi'sektəmi] *n* 神经支切断术

ramitis [rə'maitis] *n* 神经根炎

Rammstedt ['rɑːmstet] 见 Ramstedt

ramollissement [ˌrɑːmɔliːs'mɔŋ] *n* 【法】软化

Ramond's sign [rə'mɔŋ] (Louis Ramond) 拉蒙征(骶棘肌强直为胸膜积液之征,积液呈脓性时则强直消失)

Ramon's flocculation, flocculation test [rə'mɔŋ] (Gaston Ramon) 拉蒙絮状反应,絮状试验(测定白喉毒素及抗毒素的一种定量沉淀反应试验:一组试管以毒素〈如白喉毒素〉量不变,加抗毒素,其量渐增,出现絮状沉淀之管,表明此管含有完全中和的毒素和抗毒素的混合剂,最初出现絮状沉淀之管称为终点)

Ramón y Cajal [rə'mɔn iː kə'hɑːl] 见 Cajal

ramose [rə'məus] *a* 分支的

rampart ['ræmpɑːt] *n* 垒,阜 | maxillary ~ 上颌阜

Ramsay Hunt paralysis ['ræmsi hʌnt] (James Ramsay Hunt) 拉姆齐·亨特麻痹(〈亨特〉幼年型震颤麻痹) | ~ syndrome 拉姆齐·亨特综合征(①带状疱疹累及面神经和听神经,伴有同侧面部麻痹及外耳与鼓膜疱疹性水疱,可能伴有耳鸣、眩晕及听觉障碍。亦称膝状神经痛、耳带状疱疹和亨特病或亨特神经痛;②〈亨特〉幼年型震颤麻痹;进行性小脑协同失调;③进行性小脑协同失调)

Ramsden's eyepiece ['ræmzdən] (Jesse Ramsden) 拉姆斯登目镜(由两个平凸镜片组成的一种正目镜,其凸面彼此朝向对方)

Ramstedt operation ['rɑːmstet] (Wilhelm C. Ramstedt) 拉姆施泰特手术(见 Fredet-Ramstedt operation)

ramulus ['ræmjuləs] ([复] **ramuli** ['ræmjulai]) *n* 【拉】小支

ramus ['reiməs] ([复] **rami** ['reimai]) *n* 【拉】支

rancid ['rænsid] *a* 酸败的 | **~ity** [ræn'sidəti] *n* 酸败[作用]

rancidify [ræn'sidifai] *vt, vi* (使)酸败(尤指脂肪的腐败)

Randall's plaques ['rædəl] (Alexander Randall) 肾钙斑(在肾乳头顶端内有小钙凝结,突出表面并成为尿盐沉积的集中点)

Randolph's test ['rændɔlf] (Nathaniel A. Randolph) 伦道夫试验(检尿胨)

random ['rændəm] *a* 任意的;随机的

randomize ['rændəmaiz] *vt* 随机取样,随机化 | **randomization** [ˌrændəmai'zeiʃən, -mi'z-] *n*

range [reindʒ] *n* 排,行,范围;区域;幅度 | ~ of accommodation 调节范围 / ~ of audibility 可听域

ranimycin [ræni'maisin] *n* 雷尼霉素(抗生素类药)

ranine ['reinin] *a* 蛙的;舌下囊肿的,舌下面的;舌下静脉的

ranitidine [rei'naitidiːn] *n* 雷尼替丁(组胺 H_2 受体拮抗药,盐酸雷尼替丁用于治疗胃食管反流)

rank [ræŋk] *n* 列,排;等级 *vi* 列为

Ranke's angle ['rʌnkə] (Hans R. Ranke) 兰克角(颅骨水平面与牙槽缘中心及鼻额缝中心间线所成的角)

Ranke's complex ['rʌnkə] (Karl E. Ranke) 兰克复征,原发复征(即 primary complex,见 complex 项下相应术语) | ~ formula 兰克公式(表示比重之数 − 1 000 × 0. 52 − 5. 406 之值,接近于每升

浆液中所含白蛋白的克数) / ~ stages 兰克结核病分期(分①原发病灶,②结核杆菌全身性播散,③孤立器官结核病,主要指肺)

ranula [ˈrænjulə] *n*【拉】舌下囊肿 | pancreatic ~ 胰管[潴留]囊肿 | **~r** *a*

Ranunculaceae [rəˌnʌŋkjuˈleisiiː] *n* 毛茛科

ranunculin [rəˈnʌŋkjulin] *n* 毛茛苷

Ranunculus [rəˈnʌŋkjuləs] *n* 毛茛属

Ranvier's crosses [rɑːnviˈɛə] (Louis A. Ranvier) 郎飞十字(郎飞结内暗色十字形痕迹,用硝酸银染色后纵切开时可见到) | nodes of ~ 郎飞结(有髓神经纤维绞扼所致的结,约每隔 1 mm 有一个,这些部位无髓鞘,轴索周围仅是施万〈Schwann〉细胞突) / ~ segments 郎飞节(郎飞结之间神经纤维的髓质部分) / ~ tactile disks 郎飞触觉盘(神经纤维的末端,在格朗德里〈Grandry〉小体之间透明质内的杯状体内)

RAO right anterior oblique 右前斜位

Raoult's law [rəˈəul] (François M. Raoult) 腊乌尔定律(关于冰点:溶于一定溶剂的相同电解质冰点的下降与溶质的分子浓度成正比;关于蒸气压:①液体溶液中挥发性物质的蒸气压等于该物质的 mol/L 分数乘以纯蒸气压;②当非挥发的非电解质溶于溶剂时,该溶剂蒸气压的下降等于溶质 mol/L 分数乘以纯溶剂的蒸气压)

rape¹ [reip] *n* 强奸

rape² [reip] *n* 芸苔,油菜

raphae [ˈreifiː] raphe 的复数

raphania [rəˈfeiniə] *n* 野萝卜子中毒

Raphanus [rəˈfænəs] *n* 萝卜属

raphe [ˈreifi] *n* 缝 | abdominal ~ [腹]白线 / amniotic ~ 羊膜缝 / anococcygeal ~ 肛尾缝 / lateral palpebral ~ 睑外侧缝 / ~ of perineum 会阴缝 / ~ of pharynx 咽缝 / ~ of pons 脑桥缝 / pterygomandibular ~ 翼突下颌缝,颊咽[肌]缝 / ~ of scrotum 阴囊缝

raphes [ˈreifiːz] raphe 的所有格单数

Rappaport Classification [ˈræpəpɔːt] (Henry Rappaport) 拉帕波特分类法(一种根据组织学标准的非霍奇金〈non-Hodgkin〉淋巴瘤分类法,其形成的种类为结节状淋巴瘤和弥漫性淋巴瘤,此法已被路-科〈Lukes-Collins〉分类法所替代)

rapport [ræˈpɔː] *n*【法】关系(融洽)(病人与医师间)

rapture of the deep 氮麻醉(nitrogen narcosis 的俗称)

raptus [ˈræptəs] *n*【拉】情感爆发

rarefy [ˈrɛərifai] *vt, vi* 稀少,稀薄,稀疏 | **rarefaction** [ˌrɛəriˈfækʃən] *n*

RAS renal artery stenosis 肾动脉狭窄;renin-angiotensin system 肾素-血管紧张素系统

Ras. rasurae【拉】碎片,锉屑

rash [ræʃ] *n* 疹 | brown-tail ~ 褐尾蠹皮炎 / butterfly ~ 蝶形疹 / cable ~ 卤蜡粉刺,氯萘痤疮 / caterpillar ~ 毛虫疹,蛾虫疹 / diaper ~ 尿布疹 / drug ~ 药物疹,药疹 / heat ~ [红]粟疹,痱子,汗疹 / hydatid ~ 包虫囊疹 / lily ~ 水仙皮炎 / nickel ~ 镍疹 / rose ~ 蔷薇疹,玫瑰疹 / wandering ~ 地图样舌

Rashkind balloon atrial septostomy [ˈræʃkind] (W. J. Rashkind) 拉什金德球囊房中隔造口术,球囊房中隔造口术

rasion [ˈreiʒən] *n* 锉刮,锉磨(对药物)

Rasmussen's aneurysm [ˈræsməsn] (Fritz W. Rasmussen) 腊斯默森动脉瘤(结核性空洞壁动脉扩张,常破裂引起出血)

rasp [rɑːsp] *n* 锉 *vt, vi* 粗锉

raspatory [ˈræspətəri] *n* 骨锉,骨刮,刮骨刀

raspberry [ˈrɑːzbəri] *n* 红莓,红覆盆子

RAST radioallergosorbent test 放射变应原吸附试验(见 test 项下相应术语)

Rastelli operation [rɑːsˈteli] (Glan C. Rastelli) 拉斯泰利手术(矫正室中隔大缺损伴肺动脉瓣狭窄、漏斗状狭窄和瓣膜狭窄的一种手术,置一心室内贴片,致使血液流经中隔缺损,并流出主动脉,并置一人造瓣膜以确立右心室和肺动脉之间的连续性)

rasura [rəˈsjuərə] *n*【拉】碎片,锉屑

rat [ræt] *n* 鼠 | BBr ~ BBr 鼠(用作糖尿病 I 型模型的株) / black ~ 黑鼠 / brown ~ 棕鼠,褐鼠,沟鼠 / Egyptian ~, roof ~ 埃及鼠,屋顶鼠 / Long-Evans ~ 朗-埃文斯鼠(罗彻斯特大学培育的鼠株) / Sprague-Dawley ~ 斯普雷格-道利鼠(斯普雷格-道利动物公司培育的白鼠株) / white ~, albino ~ 白鼠 / Wistar ~ 威斯塔鼠(威斯塔研究所培育的白鼠株) / wood ~ 森林鼠

rate [reit] *n* 率,比率;速度,速率 | attack ~ 发病率 / basal metabolic ~ 基础代谢率 / birth ~ 出生率 / case fatality ~ 病死率 / circulation ~ 循环率 / death ~, mortality ~ 死亡率 / DEF ~ 乳牙龋数率(D 表示需补龋乳牙数〈decayed〉, E 表示需拔龋乳牙数〈extraction〉, F 表示已补乳牙数〈filled〉) / dose ~ 剂量率 / erythrocyte sedimentation ~ 红细胞沉降率(简名血沉) / fetal death ~ 胎儿死亡率(一年内胎儿死亡数与该年活产与胎儿死亡数的比率) / fatality ~, lethality ~ 病死率,致死率 / glomerular filtration ~ (GFR)肾小球滤过率 / heart ~ 心率 / incidence ~ 发病率,(疾病)发生率 / morbidity ~, case ~, sickness ~ 患病率 / mutation ~ 突变率 / oocyst ~ 卵囊率(蚊) / output exposure ~ 输出量照射率 / parasite ~ 寄生虫率 / perinatal mortality ~ 围生期死亡率 / puerperal mortality ~ 产后死亡率 / pulse ~ 脉搏率 / respiration ~ 呼吸率 / sedimentation ~ 沉降速度,沉降率 /

sporozoite ~ 子孢子率 / stillbirth ~ 死产率

Rathke's pouch [ˈrʌtkə] (Martin H. Rathke)拉特克囊,神经颊囊,颅颊囊 | ~ column 拉特克柱(脊索前端两块软骨) / ~ cysts 拉特克囊肿(垂体中间叶内含胶体的小囊肿) / ~ trabecula 颅小梁 / ~ tumor 颅咽管瘤

raticide [ˈrætisaid] *n* 杀鼠药

ratio [ˈreiʃiəu] *n* 比,比率 | A-G ~, albumin-globulin ~ 白蛋白球蛋白比率(各种肾病) / arm ~ (染色体)臂比(染色体的长臂与短臂的长度之比) / birth-death ~ 出生死亡比率,生命指数 / body-weight ~ 体重率(体重克数除以身高厘米数) / cell-color ~ 红细胞色素比率 / concentration ~ 浓度比率 / D-N ~, dextrose-nitrogen ~, G-N ~, glucose-nitrogen ~ 糖氮比率(尿) / fetal death ~ 胎儿死亡比率(一年内胎儿死亡与该年活产数的比率) / grid ~ 栅[条]比[率] / hand ~ 手长宽度比率 / ketogenic-antiketogenic ~ 生酮抗生酮比率(体内形成葡萄糖的物质和形成脂肪酸的物质之比) / lecithin-sphingomyelin ~ (L/S ~) 卵磷脂与鞘磷脂比值 / nucleocytoplasmic ~, nucleoplasmic ~, karyoplasmic ~ 核质比率 / nutritive ~ 营养比率 / proportionate mortality ~ (PMR)死亡率比例 / respiratory exchange ~, expiratory exchange ~ 呼吸商(respiratory quotient,见 quotient 项下相应术语) / sex ~ 两性比率,性[别]比率 / standardized morbidity ~ (SMR)标准化发病率比 / standardized mortality ~ (SMR)标准化死亡率比 / stimulation ~ (SR) 刺激率 / therapeutic ~, curative ~ 治疗比率 / urea excretion ~ 尿素清除率(尿内每小时清除尿素的毫克数与100 ml 血内毫克数的比率,正常比率为 50) / zeta sedimentation ~ (ZSR)Z 血沉比积(一种测量法,可与红细胞沉降率〈即血沉 ESR〉相比较,有一点除外,即不受贫血影响。血样在一种仪器〈zetafuge〉中离心,产生紧密与分散的受控循环过程,终于形成缗钱状红细胞串联,迅速沉淀,由此程序产生的浓集红细胞压积〈zetacrit〉分成真血细胞比容,从而得出 ZSR)

ration [ˈræʃən] *n* 定量,配给量;口粮,定粮(每日配给的饮食) | basal ~ 基本口粮(配给所需的能量,但缺少一种或多种维生素)

rational [ˈræʃənl] *a* 合理的;有理性的

rationale [ˌræʃəˈnɑːl] *n* 【拉】基本原理,理论基础

rationality [ˌræʃəˈnæləti] *n* 合理性

rationalize [ˈræʃənəlaiz] *vt* 使合理;文饰 | **rationalization** [ˌræʃənəlaiˈzeiʃən, -liˈz-] *n* 合理化;文饰[作用]

ratsbane [ˈrætsbein] *n* 杀鼠药(尤指白砷)

rat-tails [ˈræt teilz] *n* 鼠尾样肿(马腿)

rattle [ˈrætl] *n* 哮吼(临死前黏液阻塞气管时的气流声)

rattlesnake [ˈrætlsneik] *n* 响尾蛇

Rattus [ˈrætəs] *n* 【拉】鼠属 | ~ norvegicus 褐鼠,沟鼠 / ~ rattus 黑鼠 / ~ rattus alexandrinus 埃及鼠,屋顶鼠

Rauber's layer [ˈraubə] (August A. Rauber)劳贝尔层(胚胎早期构成胚盘的三层细胞中最外的一层,亦称胚盘外胚层或原始外胚层)

raucedo [rɔːˈsiːdəu] *n* 【拉】声嘶

Rauchfuss' sling [ˈrauhfus] (Karl A. Rauchfuss)劳黑富斯(脊柱)悬带(接于床铺,以供支撑脊柱,能使患部溢出物逸出) | ~ triangle 劳黑富斯三角(渗出性胸膜炎时,健侧脊柱旁有三角形的浊音区)

Rua's apophysis, process [rau] (Johann J. Rau 〈Ravius〉)锤骨前突,锤骨长突

rausch [rauʃ] *n* 【德】醚酩酊麻醉

rauschbrand [ˈrauʃbrʌnt] *n* 【德】气肿性炭疽,黑腿病

Rauwolfia [rɔːˈwulfiə] *n* 萝芙木属,萝芙藤属 | ~ serpentina 蛇根木,印度萝芙木

rauwolfia [rɔːˈwulfiə] *n* 蛇根木,印度萝芙木

RAV Rous associated virus 劳斯相关病毒

ray [rei] *n* 线,射线;幅肋(昆虫) | actinic ~, chemical ~ 光化射线 / antirachitic ~s 抗佝偻病射线(2 700 ~ 3 020 Å 单位紫外线) / astral ~, polar ~ 星射线,极射线 / bactericidal ~s 灭菌射线(1 850 ~ 2 600 Å 单位紫外线) / caloric ~ 致热射线 / canal ~ 极隧射线(真空管的阳极射线) / central ~ 中心光线,中心射线 / characteristic ~ 标识射线 / characteristic fluorescent ~s, fluorescent ~s 标识荧光射线,荧光射线(系由在原子内壳层的电子重排而发射的次级射线,与标识射线相同,不同之处:标识射线是由电子轰击 X 线管靶所致,而标识荧光射线是由原射线光子轰击吸收材料所致) / convergent ~ 会聚射线 / cosmic ~ 宇宙线 / digital ~ 指线,趾线 / direction ~ 目标射线 / erythema-producing ~s 致红斑射线 / grenz ~s, border ~s, borderline ~s, infra-roentgen ~s, transition ~s 跨界[射]线,境界[射]线(很软的 X 线,其波长约为 2 Å 单位,位于 X 线与紫外线之间) / H ~s 氢核束 / incident ~ 入射线 / infrared ~s 红外线(波长为 7 700 ~ 500 000 Å 单位) / intermediate ~s, W ~s 居间射线,W 射线(其波长介于紫外线与 X 线之间) / luminous ~s 光线(发光的射线) / n ~s n 射线(一种辐射线的衍生形式,尚未完全确定) / necrobiotic ~s 生物致死线(短波紫外线) / paracathodic ~s 旁阴极射线 / pigment-producing ~s 致色射线(可引起色素沉着,波长为 2 500 ~ 3 000 Å 单位) / positive ~s, anode ~s 阳极射线 / roentgen ~s X[射]线,伦琴[射]线 / ultraviolet ~s 紫外线 / vital ~s 疗效紫外线(2 900 ~ 3 200 Å 单位波长的紫外线) / X- ~s X

[射]线,伦琴[射]线

Raymond-Cestan syndrome [reiˈmɔŋ sesˈtæn] (F. Raymond; Etienne J. M. R. Cestan) 雷蒙-塞斯唐综合征(基底动脉小支栓塞后所致的脑桥病灶,表现为四肢麻痹、感觉缺失及眼球震颤)

Raymond's apoplexy [reiˈmɔŋ] (Fulgence Raymond) 雷蒙中风(一种渐重性卒中,表现为一侧手感觉异常,以后变为麻痹。亦称雷蒙型中风)

Raynaud's disease (gangrene) [reiˈnəu] (Maurice Raynaud) 雷诺病(坏疽)(①一种原发性或特发性血管疾病,特征为雷诺现象双侧发作,女性犯此病较男性多;②腮腺炎后咽肌麻痹,亦称局部窒息) | ~ phenomenon 雷诺现象(指、趾间歇性双侧缺血性发作,有时侵及耳鼻,特征为严重苍白,常伴有感觉异常和疼痛,由寒冷或情绪刺激所引起,保暖后即缓解,如病情为特发性或原发性的,则称为雷诺病) / ~ sign 雷诺征(肢端发绀)

razoxane [reiˈzɔksein] *n* 雷佐生(抗肿瘤药,可减少多柔比星〈doxorubicin〉和相关的抗肿瘤蒽环类药结合使用时对心脏的毒性)

Rb rubidium 铷

RBBB right bundle branch block 右束支传导阻滞

RBC red blood cell, red blood corpuscles 红细胞;red blood (cell) count 红细胞计数;relative bone conduction 相对骨导

RBC IT red blood cell iron turnover 红细胞铁转换

RBD REM sleep behavior disorder 快速眼动睡眠行为障碍

RBE relative biological effectiveness 相对生物效应

RBP retinol binding protein 维生素 A 结合蛋白

RCA regulator of complement activation 补体活化调节因子;right coronary artery 右冠状动脉

RCM Royal College of Midwives 皇家助产士学会

RCN Royal College of Nursing 皇家护理学会

RCOG Royal College of Obstetricians and Gynaecologists 皇家妇产科医师学会

RCP Royal College of Physicians 皇家内科医师学会

rcp reciprocal translocation 相互易位

RCS Royal College of Surgeons 皇家外科医师学会

RCSED Royal College of Surgeons of Edinburgh 爱丁堡皇家外科医师学会

RCSI Royal College of Surgeons in Ireland 爱尔兰皇家外科医师学会

RCU red cell utilization 红细胞利用率

RCVS Royal College of Veterinary Surgeons 皇家外科兽医学会

RD reaction of degeneration 变性反应

rd rutherford 卢[瑟福](放射性物质的蜕变单位,每秒钟 10^6 次衰变单位)

RDA recommended dietary allowance 推荐膳食供给量;right displacement of the abomasum 皱胃右移位

RDE receptor-destroying enzyme 受体破坏酶

RE radium emanation 镭射气;right eye 右眼;retinol equivalent 视黄醇当量

Re rhenium 铼

re- [前缀]再,复,反,回

reablement [ri(ː)ˈeiblmənt] *n* 复原,恢复

reabsorption [ˌriːəbˈsɔːpʃən] *n* 重吸收 | constant fraction ~ 恒定比率重吸收

react [ri(ː)ˈækt] *vi* 应答;反应;起化学作用,起反应

reactance [ri(ː)ˈæktəns] *n* 电抗,有感电阻

reactant [ri(ː)ˈæktənt] *n* 反应物 | acute phase ~ 急性期反应物(一种血浆蛋白,例如结合球蛋白,α_1-抗胰蛋白酶,血清类黏蛋白,C3,血浆铜蓝蛋白,纤维蛋白原和C-反应性蛋白,其浓度增加或减少与炎症的过程结合在一起)

reaction [ri(ː)ˈækʃən] *n* 反应 | accelerated ~ 加速反应 / acetic acid ~ 醋酸反应(见 Rivalta's reaction) / acetonitrile ~ 乙腈反应(见 Hunt's reaction) / acid ~ 酸性反应 / acrosome ~ 顶体反应(受精) / acute situational ~, acute stress ~ 急性境遇性反应状态,急性应激反应 / agglutinoid ~ 类凝集素反应(见 prozone) / alarm ~ 紧急反应(人体受到突然刺激而尚未适应时所引起的全部非特异性反应) / alkaline ~ 碱性反应 / allergic ~ 变应性反应 / allograft ~ 同种异体移植物反应 / alphanaphthol ~ α-萘酚反应(检尿葡萄糖、尿蛋白质) / anamnestic ~ 回忆反应,回忆应答(anamnestic response,见 response 项下相应术语) / anaphylactic ~ 过敏性反应 / anaphylactoid ~ 类过敏性反应,假过敏反应 / anatoxin ~ 类毒素反应(应用类毒素时的皮内反应) / anergastic ~ 脑活动力缺失性反应(状态)(器质性精神病) / antalgic ~ 防痛反应 / antigen ~ of Debré and Paraf 德布雷-帕拉夫抗原反应(诊断肾结核的补体结合试验,以患者尿作抗原,以已知结核抗血清作抗体进行试验) / antigen-antibody ~ 抗原-抗体反应(抗原与同种抗体的特异性结合形成可逆性的抗原抗体复合物,其溶解度随抗原抗体比率而有所不同,抗原抗体反应可出现沉淀反应、凝集反应、补体依赖性反应、中和反应或嗜细胞效应) / antiglobulin ~ 抗球蛋白反应 / antitryptic ~ 抗胰蛋白酶反应 / asphenamine ~ 胂凡纳明反应(见 Abelin's reaction) / associative ~ 联想反应 / axon ~, axonal ~ 轴索反应(轴突被截断后引起神经节细胞一连串变化,即中心核染质溶解和核移位) / bacteriolytic ~ 溶菌反应(引起特异溶菌作用的反应) / biphasic ~ 二相反应 / biuret ~ 双缩脲反应(见 test 项下相应术语) / blanching ~ 转白反应(见 Schultz-Charlton reaction) / cachexia ~ 恶病质反应(血清中抗胰蛋白酶力增大,见于

恶性疾病或其他以恶病质为特征的疾病)/ cadaveric ~ 尸反应(家族性周期性麻痹时,患肌电反应完全消失)/ cancer ~ 癌反应 / capsular ~ 荚膜反应(细菌荚膜物质与同种抗体的反应)/ carbamino ~ 氨基甲酰反应(用于研究蛋白质消化过程)/ chain ~ 连锁反应,链式反应(一种核〈中子〉反应)/ citochol ~ 快速胆固醇反应(见 Sachs-Witebsky test)/ chromaffin ~ 嗜铬反应 / coagulation ~, coagulo ~ 凝固反应(检梅毒的一种试验,根据的事实是,梅毒血清较正常血清更能妨碍凝血酶的产生,从而抑制血液的凝固)/ cockade ~ 花结状反应(见 Römer's test)/ colloidal gold ~ (脑脊液)胶体金反应/ complement fixation ~ 补体结合反应(见 test 项下相应术语)/ compluetic ~ 梅毒补体结合反应(见 Wassermann reaction)/ conglobation ~ 成团反应(检梅毒)/ conglutination ~ 胶固反应,团集反应,黏合反应(由胶固素、细胞〈例如细菌或红细胞〉、新鲜补体以及用吸收法除去凝集素的一种细胞特异性免疫血清混合而成的凝集反应)/ conjunctival ~ 结膜反应(见 ophthalmic ~)/ consensual ~ 交叉反应;同感反应 / conversion ~ 转换反应(指将内心冲突转换为运动或感觉症状)/ coupled ~ 连接反应 / cross ~ 交叉反应(抗体与并不特异性地促使其合成的抗原相互作用)/ cutaneous ~ 皮肤反应(见 cutireaction;取蛋白或花粉溶液注射于敏感者或擦在其磨损处后所引起的反应)/ cutituberculin ~ 皮上结核菌素反应(见 Moro's reaction)/ dark ~ 暗反应/ defense ~ 防御反应 / ~ of degeneration 变性反应 / delayed ~ 迟发型反应(接触诱发物后几小时至几天才出现的反应)/ delayed-blanch ~ 迟发型转白反应(皮内注射乙酰胆碱或乙酰甲胆碱引起的一种与异位性疾病相关的异常的相矛盾的反应,其特征不是通常的红斑疹块和潮红,而是在注射后 3 ~ 5 分钟于潮红处发生迟发型转白,并持续 15 ~ 30 分钟)/ delayed hypersensitivity ~, delayed-type hypersensitivity ~ 迟发型超敏反应 / depot ~ 储存反应(皮下结核菌素试验时,在针头进入点周围皮肤的红色反应)/ dermotuberculin ~ 皮肤结核菌素反应(见 Pirquet's reaction)/ desmoid ~ 硬纤维袋反应(检胃分泌及活动)/ desmoplastic ~ 纤维形成性反应 / diazo ~ 重氮反应(见 Ehrlich's diazo reaction)/ digitonin ~ 洋地黄皂苷反应(测甾醇)/ displacement ~ 置换反应(一种化学反应)/ downgrading ~ 下降反应(一种麻风反应,表面上类似逆转〈"上升"〉反应,对麻风分枝杆菌的免疫应答出现紊乱,麻风的临床症状恶化,组织内麻风分枝杆菌指数增加)/ dysergastic ~ 脑控制不良性反应 / E-E ~ 红斑水肿性反应(见 Foshay's reaction)/ egg yellow ~ 蛋黄反应(在埃利希〈Ehrlich〉重氮反应中未加入氨之前所出现的黄色泡沫,据认为表示患有急性肺炎)/ epiphanin ~ 血清显红反应(此反应曾用于梅毒血清学诊断)/ erythematous-edematous ~ 红斑水肿性反应(见 Foshay's reaction)/ erythrocyte sedimentation ~ 红细胞沉降反应 / erythrophore ~ 红色素细胞反应(雄鱼在注射性腺激素后变为红色)/ ~ of exhaustion 衰竭反应,虚脱反应 / false positive ~ 假阳性反应(梅毒试验时不是由于梅毒而是由于其他疾病引起的阳性反应)/ fatigue ~ 疲劳反应(肌肉运动过累引起的体温上升)/ fixation ~ 结合反应(补体结合 complement fixation,见 fixation 项下相应术语)/ flocculation ~ 絮状反应(见 Sachs-Georgi test)/ focal ~ 灶性反应(在感染或注射部位或其周围发生的反应,可能由于注射特异性物质,例如结核菌素、马疽菌素或菌苗所诱发,或由于使用非特异性物质而诱发)/ foreign body ~ 异物反应/ franklinic ~ of degeneration 静电变性反应 / gold ~ 金反应(见 Lange's test①解)/ graft-vs-host ~ 移植物抗宿主反应(含有大量免疫活性细胞的移植物,对基因型不同的受体组织发生的一种免疫反应。由于受体的免疫未成熟性,或由于受体的特殊遗传品种〈第一代杂种病〉或因受体全身曾受过射线照射或使用免疫抑制药,因而移植物并未受到排斥。含有大量能引起移植物对宿主反应的免疫活性细胞的组织,包括脾脏、淋巴结及胸导管淋巴结,其次是骨髓和外周血液。参阅 runt disease,见 disease 项下相应术语)/ group ~ 类属反应,类属凝集反应(group agglutination,见 agglutination 项下相应术语)/ hemagglutination-inhibition ~ 血凝抑制反应(利用抗体抑制病毒凝集红细胞)/ hemiopic pupillary ~ 偏盲性瞳孔反应(某些偏盲病例的反应,当光线投射到视网膜一边时,可引起虹膜收缩,但投射到另一边时则无反应)/ hemoclastic ~ 红细胞破坏反应 / heterophil antibody ~ 嗜异性抗体反应(抗体对嗜异性抗原所产生的反应,见 Paul-Bunnell test)/ homograft ~ 同种移植反应 / hunting ~ 摆动反应(手指或其他部分受 15 ℃以下温度刺激时交替发生血管收缩和血管扩张期)/ hyperkinetic ~ of childhood 儿童多动反应,注意缺陷障碍[伴多动](即 attention-deficit hyperactivity disorder,见 disorder 项下相应术语)/ hypersensitivity ~超敏反应,超敏感性反应 / ~ of identity 一致性反应,同一性反应(若两个溶液中的抗原完全相同,则它们与同原抗体溶液将形成一条连续的沉淀线,此时三个溶液分别置于在凝胶扩散平板上形成三角形的三个池内。若沉淀线连续,但具有骨刺样突出〈部分一致性反应〉,则抗原不相同,但有相同的抗原决定簇。若形成两个交叉线〈非一致性反应〉,则这两种抗原毫不相关)/ id ~ 附发疹反应(一种局部或全身无菌性继发性皮疹）/ immediate ~ 速发型反应，立即型反应（例如变应性反应，接触诱导物后几秒至几分钟内即出现的反应）/ immediate hypersensitivity ~ 速发型超敏反应 / immune ~ 免疫反应（接触抗原后动物体起特异变化的反应性，显示为抗体产生、细胞免疫或免疫耐受性；种痘后产生丘疹和红晕，而无水疱形成，表示有高度免疫力）/ indophenol ~ 靛酚反应（见 test 项下相应术语）/ intracutaneous ~ 皮内反应（注射皮肤试验抗原至皮内后所出现的反应，这样的反应可能有诊断价值，如锡克〈Schick〉试验，狄克〈Dick〉试验、结核菌素试验等）/ intracuti ~ 皮内反应（见 Frei test）/ intradermal ~ 皮内反应（见 intracutaneous ~）/ involutional psycotic ~ 衰老期忧郁症，更年期忧郁症 / johnin ~ 约尼反应，副结核菌素反应（副结核菌素引起的类似结核菌素反应的皮肤反应，用于诊断牛的约尼〈Johne〉病）/ K. H. ~ 补体结合血细胞凝集合并反应（检马鼻疽）/ lengthening ~ 伸长反应（伸肌延长以使肢体可以屈曲）/ lentochol ~ 缓慢胆固醇反应（见 Sachs-Georgi test）/ lepra ~ 麻风反应（在抗麻风治疗或在尚未治疗的各型麻风过程中出现的一种急性或亚急性超敏状态，其中包括两种类型的免疫反应，一是迟发型超敏反应〈见 reverse ~s〉，另一是免疫复合物反应）/ lepromin ~ 麻风菌素反应（见 test 项下相应术语）/ light ~ 光反应（光合作用时的光化学过程，在此过程中，光能参与的一系列反应导致产生 ATP 及还原型辅酶〈NADH 或 NADPH〉，然后这些物质参与暗反应）/ local ~ 局部反应（发生在注射部位类似灶性反应〈focal reaction〉的现象）/ manic-depressive ~ 躁狂-抑郁反应，躁郁症[反应] / miostagmin ~, miostagminic ~ 微滴反应（一种废弃的诊断肿瘤、梅毒、伤寒等的血清学试验，其根据是抗体与对应抗原结合时能降低混合物的表面张力）/ mixed cell agglutination ~ 混合细胞凝集反应（由于抗体与不同的抗原决定簇对细胞的反应，出现不同细胞型的混合凝集）/ mixed leukocyte ~ 混合白细胞反应（培养两个个体的白细胞，即出现母细胞；组织相容性与母细胞的数目成反比）/ myasthenic ~ 肌无力性反应 / myotonic ~ 肌强直反应 / neurotonic ~ 神经张力性肌反应 / neutral ~ 中性反应 / ninhydrin ~ [水合]茚三酮反应（triketohydrindene hydrate test，见 test 项下相应术语）/ nitritoid ~ 亚硝酸盐样反应（见 crisis 项下相应术语）/ ~ of nonidentity 非一致性反应，非同一性反应（见 ~ of identity）/ nucleal ~ 核反应（醛品红磺酸反应，即任何含醛溶液加品红磺酸反应，产生浅蓝与红色反应）/ ophthalmic ~ 眼反应（用伤寒和结核的毒素滴眼后眼结膜的局部反应，若患这些疾病其反应较健康者或患有其他疾病的人远为严重）/ orbicularis ~ 眼轮匝肌反应（见 Westphal-Piltz phenomenon）/ pain ~ 疼痛反应（因疼痛而有瞳孔放大）/ pancreatic ~ 胰反应（确定胰腺炎或胰脏恶性疾病的存在）/ paraserum ~ 副血清反应（伤寒和痢疾杆菌的菌株与副伤寒、大肠杆菌、突变性霍乱以及其他传染病的菌株的凝集反应）/ ~ of partial identity 部分一致性反应，部分同一性反应（在二维双向扩散中所见的一种反应型：抗原池和抗血清池之间的沉淀线之一在交叉点中止，而另一沉淀线则通过此交叉点，提示抗原样品具有几个〈但非全部〉共同的抗原决定簇，见 ~ of identity）/ passive cutaneous anaphylaxis（PCA）~ 被动皮肤过敏反应（参阅 passive cutaneous anaphylaxis，见 anaphylaxis）/ percutaneous ~ 皮上反应（见 Moro's reaction）/ periodic acid-Schiff ~, PAS ~ 过碘酸希夫反应（用于检测糖原、上皮黏蛋白、中性多糖和糖蛋白）/ P-K ~ 普-屈反应（即 Prausnitz-Küstner ~，检人体反应素的皮肤反应）/ precipitin ~ 沉淀素反应（检Ⅰ、Ⅱ和Ⅲ型肺炎球菌感染；可溶性抗原与对应抗体的特异性反应）/ prozone ~ 前带反应，前区反应（见 prozone）/ pseudoallergic ~ 假变态反应 / puncture ~ 穿刺反应（结核菌素皮下注射部位的红肿反应，用于结核病的诊断）/ quanti-Pirquet（QP）~ 定量皮尔盖反应，定量结核菌素划痕反应（用两种不同稀释度〈1/10 和 1/100〉的旧结核菌素作皮上划痕，以判断结核病感染程度和活动性的皮尔盖反应）/ quellung ~（肺炎球菌）荚膜肿胀反应（见 Neufeld's reaction）/ reversal ~ 逆转反应（通常在界线类麻风的化疗时发生的一种麻风反应，代表一种迟发型超敏反应，并伴麻风分枝杆菌的细胞介导免疫"上升"，促使此病趋向于结核样型麻风。主要特征为红斑、水肿、早先存在的静止病灶有触痛、出现新病灶、神经炎伴神经损坏、发热、腺病和白细胞计数上升，同样见 downgrading ~）/ reverse passive Arthus ~ 反向被动阿图斯反应（实验动物的皮肤部位注入沉淀抗体，然后 30 分钟到 2 小时后再静脉注入同种抗原而产生的反应，因而与阿图斯反应时沉淀抗体和抗原所在的常见解剖部位相反）/ second set ~ 二次反应（见 phenomenon 项下相应术语）/ sedimentation ~ 沉降反应，红细胞沉降反应 / seroanaphylactic ~ 血清过敏反应（应用血清防治时发生的过敏反应）/ seroenzyme ~ 血清酶反应（见 Abderhalden's ~）/ serological ~ 血清学反应 / serum sickness-like ~ 血清病样反应 / shortening ~ 缩短反应（肢体回至伸展位置时，在伸长反应后继之而起的缩短）/ sigma ~ 西格马反应，σ 反应（一种诊断梅毒的絮状反应，由萨克斯-格奥尔吉〈Sachs-Georgi〉反应改良而来，即作一系列试验以决定其中哪一个产生絮状反应）/ skin ~ 皮肤反应（见 cutaneous ~）/

small-drop ~ 小滴反应(见 miostagmin ~)/ sympathetic stress ~ 交感神经应激反应 / tendon ~ 腱反应(敲打肌腱产生肌肉的反射性收缩,亦称腱反射)/ thyroid function ~ 甲状腺功能反应 / toxin antitoxin ~ 毒素抗毒素反应(见 immunoreaction)/ trigger ~ 扳机反应,突发反应(见 action 项下相应术语)/ tryptophan ~ 色氨酸反应(见 test 项下相应术语)/ tuberculin ~ 结核菌素反应(见 test 项下相应术语)/ uniphasic ~ 单相反应(仅有屈曲的反应)/ upgrading ~ 上升反应(见 reversal ~)/ vaccination ~ 接种反应,种痘反应,牛痘接种反应(接种后的局部性与全身性反应)/ wheal and erythema ~, wheal-flare ~ 风团与红斑反应,风团潮红反应(特征性局部皮肤反应,系因肥大细胞中释放组胺所致,亦称刘易斯〈Lewis〉三联反应,参阅 triple response,见 response 项下相应术语)/ white-graft ~ 苍白移植物反应(对组织移植物例如皮肤移植物的一种免疫反应,由于这种反应的结果,移植的组织并没有得到血液供应,迅速被排斥)/ xanthoproteic ~ 黄色蛋白[质]反应(见 Mulder's test)/ xanthydrol ~ 黄嘌呤醇反应(取尿毒症患者的组织用黄醇的冰醋酸溶液固定时,在组织内即存积大量黄醇)/ zed ~ 饥饿终期反应(饥饿婴儿在饥饿缓解后出现的反应,包括体重微增、体温上升及出现含有大量细胞的水泻)

reaction-formation [ri(ː)ˈækʃən fɔːˈmeiʃən] *n* 心理反应形成,反相形成

reactivate [ri(ː)ˈæktiveit] *vt, vi* 复能,再活化

reactivation [ri(ː)ˌæktiˈveiʃən] *n* 复能[作用],再活化[作用] | ~ of serum 血清复能(加入新鲜补体使血清的免疫活性得以恢复)

reactivator [ri(ː)ˈæktiveitə] *n* 激活剂,激活因子 | cholinesterase ~ 胆碱酯酶激活剂

reactive [ri(ː)ˈæktiv] *a* 反应[性]的

reactivity [ˌri(ː)ækˈtivəti] *n* 反应性

reactogenic [riˌæktəuˈdʒenik] *a* 致反应性的(指疫苗)

reactor [ri(ː)ˈæktə] *n* 反应堆;反应器 | nuclear ~ [原子]核反应堆

reading [ˈriːdiŋ] *n* 阅读;读数 | lip ~, speech ~ 读唇,唇读

readjustment [ˌriːəˈdʒʌstmənt] *n* 再适应 | social ~ 社会再适应

Read's formula [riːd] (Jay M. Read)里德公式(0.75×脉搏率+0.75×脉压-72,近似基础代谢率)

reagent [ri(ː)ˈeidʒənt] *n* 试剂,试药;反应物 | acid molybdate ~ 酸性钼酸盐试剂 / arsenic-sulfuric acid ~ 砷硫酸试剂(检生物碱)/ benzidine ~ 联苯胺试剂(检隐血)/ dinitrosalicylic acid ~ 二硝基水杨酸试剂(见 Sumner's reagent)/ general ~ 类别试剂 / splenic ~ 脾试剂,脾收缩剂

reagin [ˈriːədʒin, riˈeidʒin] *n* 反应素(抗体) | atopic ~ 特应性反应素 | **~ic** [ˌriːəˈdʒinik] *a*

reattach [ˌriːəˈtætʃ] *vt* 再附着

reamer [ˈriːmə] *n* 扩孔钻(牙)

reamputation [ˌriːæmpjuˈteiʃən] *n* 再切断术

rearrange [ˌriːəˈreindʒ] *vt* 重排 | **~ment** *n*

reattach [ˌriːəˈtætʃ] *vt* 再附着 | **~ment** *n* 再附着;复置术

Réaumur's scale [reiəuˈmjuːr] (René A. F. Réaumur)列[奥米尔]氏温标(水的冰点在零度,但水的正常沸点为80度〈80°R〉) | ~ thermometer 列[奥米尔]氏温度计

rebase [riˈbeis] *vt* 垫底

rebound [riˈbaund] *vi, vt, n* 反跳,回跳 | REM ~ 快速眼动反跳(受试者长期被剥夺快速眼动〈rapid eye movement〉睡眠,一旦得以宁静地睡眠,就使快速眼动睡眠增加而得到补偿)

recalcification [riˌkælsifiˈkeiʃən] *n* 再钙化

recall [riˈkɔːl] *vt, n* 回忆

recanalization [riːˌkænəlaiˈzeiʃən, -liˈz-] *n* 再通(尤指血管阻塞物的疏通)

recapitulation [ˌriːkəˌpitjuˈleiʃən] *n* 再演,重演(见 theory 项下相应术语)

receiver [riˈsiːvə] *n* 收受者;收集器,接受器;接收机

receptaculum [ˌriːsepˈtækjuləm] ([复] **receptacula** [ˌriːsepˈtækjulə]) *n* 【拉】容器,[接]受器

receptive [riˈseptiv] *a* 接受的,感受的

receptor [riˈseptə] *n* 感受器;受体 | α-adrenergic ~s α 肾上腺素能受体 / β-adrenergic ~ β 肾上腺素能受体 / B cell antigen ~s B 细胞抗原受体(单体 IgM, IgD 及 IgG 附着在 B 淋巴细胞的细胞膜上,与 T 协助细胞连合,在与抗原接触时激发 B 细胞活化)/ cholinergic ~s 胆碱能受体 / complement ~s 补体受体(补体成分的细胞表面受体)/ contact ~ 触觉感受器 / contiguous ~ 接触感受器 / distance ~ 距离感受器 / dominant ~ 显性受体 / Fc ~s Fc 受体(抗原-抗体复合物或聚集免疫球蛋白的特异性细胞表面受体,在免疫球蛋白分子的 Fc 部分结合一个部位,并显示特定免疫球蛋白类的特异性)/ ~ of the first(second, third) order 第一类(第二类、第三类)受体(埃利希〈Ehrlich〉侧链学说中第一类受体只包括抗毒素,第二类包括凝集素、沉淀素和调理素,第三类包括溶素)/ gustatory ~ 味觉感受器 / H_1, H_2 ~s H_1, H_2 受体,组胺$_1$,组胺$_2$ 受体 / IgE ~s IgE 受体(免疫球蛋白 E〈IgE〉在肥大细胞和嗜碱细胞上的细胞表面受体)/ insulin ~s 胰岛素受体(靶细胞表面上的胰岛素特异性

受体) / low-density lipoprotein(LDL) ~s 低密度脂蛋白受体 / muscarinic ~s 毒蕈碱性受体 / N_1 - ~s N_1 受体(烟碱性受体,优先受到己双铵的阻断,此类受体在自主神经节细胞上发生) / N_2 - ~s N_2 受体(烟碱性受体,优先受到癸双铵的阻断,此类受体在横纹肌上发生) / nicotinic ~s 烟碱性受体(胆碱能受体,起先受到高剂量生物碱烟碱的刺激和阻断,然后受到筒箭毒碱的阻断,此类受体可在自主神经节细胞、横纹肌以及脊中枢神经元上找到) / pressure ~ 压觉感受器 / secondary ~s 第二级受体 / sessile ~ 固定受体(在埃利希〈Ehrlich〉侧链学说中指不能释出形成抗体的受体) / T cell antigen ~s T 细胞抗原受体(T 细胞上的受体,能识别①特异性外来抗原和②自身 MHC〈主要组织相容性复合体〉抗原,两者同时可见到激发 T 细胞活化) / visual ~ 视觉感受器 / volume ~s 容量感受器

recess [ri'ses, 'riːses] *n* 隐窝 | accessory ~ of elbow, sacciform ~ of articulation of elbow 肘关节囊状隐窝 / chiasmatic ~, optic ~ 视隐窝 / laryngopharyngeal ~, piriform ~ 喉咽隐窝,梨状隐窝 / ~ of pelvic mesocolon 乙状结肠间隐窝 / ~ of vestibule 前庭球囊隐窝

recession [ri'seʃən] *n* 退缩

recessive [ri'sesiv] *a* 退缩的;隐性的 *n* 隐性

recessus [ri'sesəs] ([复]**recessus**) *n*【拉】隐窝

recidivism [ri'sidivizəm], **recidivation** [riˌsidi'veiʃən] *n* (疾病)复发,再发;(罪行)累犯 | **recidivist** [ri'sidivist] *n* (疾病)复发者;累犯者,惯犯 / **recidivistic** [riˌsidi'vistik] *a*

recipe ['resipi] *n* 取(处方头语);处方

recipient [ri'sipiənt] *n* 受者(接受移植物的个体);受血者;接受者;接受器,容器 *a* 接受的,容纳的 | universal ~ 万能受血者,普适受血者 | **recipience** [ri'sipiəns], **recipiency** [ri'sipiənsi] *n* 接受,容纳

recipiomotor [riˌsipiəu'məutə] *a* 运动感受的

reciprocate [ri'siprəkeit] *vt*, *vi* 交互,往复,互换 | **reciprocation** [riˌsiprə'keiʃən] *n*

recirculation [riːˌsəːkju'leiʃən] *n* 再循环

Recklinghausen-Applebaum disease ['rekliˌhauzən 'æpəlbaum] (F. D. von Reckinghausen; L. Applebaum)雷-阿病,血色素沉着症

Recklinghausen's canals ['rekliŋhauzən] (Friedrich D. von Recklinghausen)雷克林豪森管(结缔组织内的毛细淋巴管) | ~ disease 神经纤维瘤病,多发性神经纤维瘤 / ~ disease of bone 囊状纤维性骨炎

Reclus' disease [rei'kljuː] (Paul Reclus) 雷克吕病(①无痛性乳腺囊性增大,特征为腺泡和腺管的多发性扩张;②硬结性蜂窝织炎)

recognin [riː'kɔgnin] *n* 细胞识别素

recognition [ˌrekəg'niʃən] *n* 识别 | maternal ~ of pregnancy 母体妊娠识别

recombinant [riː'kɔmbinənt] *n* 重组体(指遗传重组产生的新细胞或个体) | ~ DNA 重组 DNA / growth hormone ~ (hGHr)生长激素重组体

recombination [ˌriːkɔmbi'neiʃən] *n* 再组合,重组(遗传学上指基因重组) | bacterial ~ 细菌再组合(变异性的一种)

recompression [ˌriːkəm'preʃən] *n* 再压缩[作用]

recon ['riːkɔn] *n* 重组子,交换子(细菌遗传物质重组的最小单位,估计这单位可能包括一系列的三联体)

reconstitution [riːˌkɔnsti'tjuːʃən] *n* 再组成 | blood ~ 血液再组成

reconstruction [ˌriːkɔns'trʌkʃən] *n* 重建,改建 | image ~ from projections 投射影像重建(由一套数学投影法重建一个物体的二维或三维影像的 X 线摄影,如横断轴向体层摄影)

recontour [ri'kɔntuə] *vt* 修整外形(牙)

record ['rekɔːd] *n* 记录 [ri'kɔːd] *vt* 记录 | eccentric interocclusal ~ 非正中殆间记录 / facebow ~ 面弓记录 / functional chew-in ~ 功能性咀嚼记录 / interocclusal ~殆间记录 / jaw relation ~ 颌位记录 / maxillomandibular ~ 上下颌[关系]记录,上下颌间记录 / occluding centric relation ~ 中心性殆关系记录/ problem-oriented ~ (POR)面向问题记录(一种对病人护理记录的方法,重点指明病人哪些特有的保健问题需要特别注意,以及如何组织互助保健计划来处理那些业已鉴定的问题。其主要内容为数据库〈the data base〉,问题一览表〈the problem list〉,保健计划〈the plan〉和病程记录〈the progress notes〉。另见 SOAP) / profile ~ 侧面外形记录 / protrusive ~ 前突记录 / protrusive occlusal ~ 前突殆记录 / terminal jaw relation ~ 终颌关系记录

recovery [ri'kʌvəri] *n* 恢复,痊愈,复原;回收

recrement ['rekrimənt] *n* 回吸液,再吸收物质(分泌后再吸收的物质) | **~itious** [ˌrekrimen'tiʃəs] *a*

recrudesce [ˌriːkruː'des] *vi* (短期后)复发 | **~nce** *n* / **~nt** *a*

recruit [ri'kruːt] *vt* 充实,补充;使恢复

recruitment [ri'kruːtmənt] *n* 补充;恢复健康;征集,募集(反应或现象);复聪(耳科) | over ~ 超重振 / ~ of follicles 卵泡征集

Rect. rectificatus【拉】精馏的,精制的;矫正的;调整的

rectal ['rektəl] *a* 直肠的

rectalgia [rek'tældʒiə] *n* 直肠痛

rectectomy [rek'tektəmi] *n* 直肠切除术

rectification [ˌrektifiˈkeiʃən] *n* 精馏,精制;矫正,调整;整流 | spontaneous ~ 自发性矫正(分娩开始前自发矫正横位) / anomalous ~ 异常整流
rectified [ˈrektifaid] *a* 精馏的,精制的;矫正的,调整的;整流的
rectifier [ˈrektifaiə] *n* 整流器;精馏器;矫正者;矫正器 | thermionic ~ 热离子整流器
rectischiac [rekˈtiskiæk] *a* 直肠坐骨的
rectitis [rekˈtaitis] *n* 直肠炎
rect(o)- [构词成分]直;直肠
rectoabdominal [ˌrektəuæbˈdɔminl] *a* 直肠腹[部]的
rectocele [ˈrektəsiːl] *n* 直肠膨出
rectoclysis [rekˈtɔklisis] *n* 直肠滴注法
rectococcygeal [ˌrektəukɔkˈsidʒiə] *a* 直肠尾骨的
rectococcygeus [ˌrektəukɔkˈsidʒiəs] *a* 【拉】直肠尾骨的
rectococcypexy [ˌrektəuˈkɔksipeksi] *n* 直肠尾骨固定术
rectocolitis [ˌrektəukɔˈlaitis] *n* 直肠结肠炎
rectocutaneous [ˌrektəukju(ː)ˈteinjəs] *a* 直肠皮肤的
rectocystotomy [ˌrektəusisˈtɔtəmi] *n* 直肠膀胱切开术
rectolabial [ˌrektəuˈleibjəl] *n* 直肠阴唇的
rectoperineorrhaphy [ˌrektəuˌperiniˈɔrəfi] *n* 直肠会阴缝合术
rectopexy [ˈrektəˌpeksi] *n* 直肠固定术
rectoplasty [ˈrektəˌplæsti] *n* 直肠成形术
rectoromanoscope [ˌrektəurəuˈmænəskəup] *n* 直肠乙状结肠镜 | **rectoromanoscopy** [ˌrektəu-ˌrəuməˈnɔskəpi] *n* 直肠乙状结肠镜检查
rectorrhaphy [rekˈtɔrəfi] *n* 直肠缝合术
rectoscope [ˈrektəskəup] *n* 直肠镜 | **rectoscopy** [rekˈtɔskəpi] *n* 直肠镜检查
rectosigmoid [ˌrektəuˈsigmɔid] *a* 直肠乙状结肠的
rectosigmoidectomy [ˌrektəuˌsigmɔiˈdektəmi] *n* 直肠乙状结肠切除术
rectostenosis [ˌrektəustiˈnəusis] *n* 直肠狭窄
rectostomy [rekˈtɔstəmi] *n* 直肠造口术
rectotome [ˈrektətəum] *n* 直肠刀
rectotomy [rekˈtɔtəmi] *n* 直肠切开术
rectoureteral [ˌrektəujuəˈriːtərəl] *a* 直肠输尿管的,输尿管直肠的
rectourethral [ˌrektəujuəˈriːθrəl] *a* 直肠尿道的
rectouterine [ˌrektəuˈjuːtərain, -rin] *a* 直肠子宫的
rectovaginal [ˌrektəuˈvædʒinəl] *a* 直肠阴道的
rectovesical [ˌrektəuˈvesikəl] *a* 直肠膀胱的
rectovestibular [ˌrektəuvesˈtibjulə] *a* 直肠[阴道]前庭的(如瘘)
rectovulvar [ˌrektəuˈvʌlvə] *a* 直肠外阴的
rectum [ˈrektəm] ([复] **rectums** 或 **recta** [ˈrektə]) *n* 【拉】直肠
rectus [ˈrektəs] *a* 【拉】直的 *n* 直肌
recumbent [riˈkʌmbənt] *a* 斜卧的
recurrence [riˈkʌrəns] *n* 再发,复发
recurrent [riˈkʌrənt] *a* 再发的,复发的;回归的
recurvation [ˌriːkəːˈveiʃən] *n* 反屈,反弯
RED reference dose 参考剂量
red [red] *n* 红[色] *a* 红[色]的 | aniline ~ 苯胺红,碱性品红 / bordeaux ~ 波多尔红(枣红;酸性枣红) / carmine ~ 卡红,胭脂红/ Congo ~, cotton ~ 刚果红,茶红,棉红 / naphthol ~ 萘酚红,苋紫 / phenol ~ 酚红,酚磺酞 / scarlet ~, oil ~ Ⅳ 猩红,油红Ⅳ / trypan ~ 锥虫红,台盼红 / vital ~ 活染红 / wool ~ 羊毛红,苋紫
redecussate [ˌriːdiˈkʌseit] *n* 再交叉
redfoot [ˈredfut] *n* 红足症,红脚病(侵犯新生羔羊病因不明的致命性疾病)
redia [ˈriːdiə] ([复] **rediae** [ˈriːdiiː]) (F. Redi) *n* 雷蚴
redifferentiation [ˌriːdifəˌrenʃiˈeiʃən] *n* 再分化
Redig. in pulv. redigatur in pulverem 【拉】须成为粉末
Red. in pulv. reductus in pulverem 【拉】成为粉末
redintigrate [reˈdintigreit] *vt* 使恢复,使复原 | **redintegration** [reˌdintiˈgreiʃən] *n* 复原,恢复;重整[作用](指精神活动)
redislocation [ˌriːdisləuˈkeiʃən] *n* 再脱位
redox [ˈriːdɔks] *n* 氧化还原[作用]
redress [ˈriːˈdres] *vt* 重新敷裹(伤口),再包扎
redressement [ridresˈmɔŋ] *n* 【法】再包扎;矫正术 | ~ forcé 强制矫正术(尤指矫正膝外翻)
red tide [red taid] 红潮(水中有大量膝沟藻〈Gonyaulax〉时,能使水变色)
reduce [riˈdjuːs] *vt* 减少;使还原;使(骨折等)复位; *vi* 减少 | ~**d** *a* 复位的;还原的 / **reducible** *a* 可减少的;可复位的;可还原的
reducer [riˈdjuːsə] *n* 还原剂;减弱基因
reductant [riˈdʌktənt] *n* 还原剂
reductase [riˈdʌkteis] *n* 还原酶 | 5α-~ 5α-还原酶(此酶缺乏为一种常染色体隐性性状,可致男性假两性畸形)
reduction [riˈdʌkʃən] *n* 减少,减数;复位术;还原[作用] | ~ of chromosomes 染色体减数 / closed ~ 闭合复位术 / ~ en masse 连囊复位术(疝) / open ~ 切开复位术(骨折) / weight ~ 体重减轻
reductive [riˈdʌktiv] *a* 减少的;还原的
reductone [riˈdʌktəun] *n* 还原酮,二羟丙烯醛
reductor [riˈdʌktə] *n* 还原剂;还原器;复位器

reduplicate [riˈdjuːplikeit] *vt* 使加倍,重复 *vi* 重复,反复 [riˈdjuːplikit] *a* 重复的,加倍的 | **reduplication** [riˌdjuːpliˈkeiʃən] *n* 再重复,再复制 / **reduplicative** [riˈdjuːplikətiv] *a*

reduviid [riˈdjuːviid] *n* 猎蝽

Reduviidae [ˌriːdjuˈvaiidiː] *n* 猎蝽科

Reduvius [riˈdjuːviəs] *n* 猎蝽属 | ~ personatus 假装猎蝽

redwater [ˈredwɔːtə] *n* (牛、羊的)红尿病,血尿病(即得克萨斯〈Texas〉热;杆菌性血红蛋白尿)

Reed-Hodgkin disease [riːd ˈhɔdʒkin] (D. Reed; Thomas Hodgkin)里-霍病,霍奇金病(见 Hodgkin's disease)

Reed's cells, Reed-Sternberg cells [ˈriːd ˈstəːnbəːg] (Dorothy Reed; Carl Sternberg) 里德细胞,里-施细胞(见 Sternberg-Reed cells)

re-educate [ˈriː ˈedju(ː)keit] *vt* 再教育,再训练(使丧失能力的人或精神有病的人恢复其失去的能力) | **re-education** [ˈriː ˌedju(ː)ˈkeiʃən] *n*

reef [riːf] *n* 内折(组织)

reentry [riːˈentri] *n* 返回,折返(过早心搏时) | arterial blood ~ 动脉血返回

Rees's test [riːs] (George O. Rees) 里斯试验(检白蛋白)

reexamine [ˈriːigˈzæmin] *vt* 再检查 | **reexamination** [ˈriːigˌzæmiˈneiʃən] *n*

refect [riˈfekt] *n* 使恢复

refection [riˈfekʃən] *n* 恢复(特指鼠维生素 B 缺乏症状的恢复) | **refectious** [riˈfekʃəs] *a*

refeeding [riˈfiːdiŋ] *n* 再营养(禁食或饥饿后恢复正常营养)

refill [ˈriːˈfil] *vt*, *vi* 再充填;再配(处方)

refine [riˈfain] *vt*, *vi* 精制,精炼

refinement [riˈfainmənt] *n* 精制,精炼

reflect [riˈflekt] *vt* 反射;*vi* 反射 | **~ed** *a* 反射的

reflecting [riˈflektiŋ] *a* 反射的

reflection [riˈflekʃən] *n* 反射作用

reflective [riˈflektiv] *a* 反射的

reflector [riˈflektə] *n* 反光镜;反射器;反射层 | dental ~ 口腔镜

reflex [ˈriːfleks] *n* 反射[作用] | abdominal ~es 腹壁反射 / accommodation ~ 调节反射(视) / ankle ~ 踝反射,踝阵挛 / atriopressor ~ 心房加压反射 / attention ~ of pupil 注意性瞳孔反射 / attitudinal ~es 状态反射 / audito-oculogyric ~ 听音转眼反射 / biceps ~ 肱二头肌反射 / bladder ~, urinary ~ 膀胱反射,尿意反射 / bulbomimic ~, facial ~ 眼球颜面反射,颜面反射(中风昏迷时,压迫眼球引起损害对侧的面肌收缩,毒物引起的昏迷时,反射发生于两侧) / cat's eye ~ 猫眼反射(见于猫眼性黑矇,瞳孔遇光反射如猫的照膜) / clasp-knife ~ 折刀反射,伸长反应 / conditioned ~, conditional ~, acquired ~, behavior ~ 条件反射 / corneal ~, blink ~, eyelid closure ~, lid ~ 角膜反射,瞬目反射,睑闭反射 / crossed ~, indirect ~, consensual ~ 交叉反射,同感反射 / deep ~, deeper ~ 深层反射 / doll's eye ~ 玩偶眼反射(当早产儿的头部向一侧转动时,双眼即向对侧协同转动,然后回复到睑裂的中部) / gastropancreatic ~ 胃胰反射 / H- ~H 反射(刺激某一神经,尤其是用电休克刺激胫神经而激起的一种单突触反射) / heel-tap ~ 跟反射 / inverted radial ~ 桡骨倒错反射 / knee jerk ~ 膝反射 / let-down ~, milk ejection ~, milk let-down ~ 排乳反射 / mass ~ 总体反射 / nasolabial ~ 鼻唇反射 / obliquus ~ 腹外斜肌反射 / oculopupillary ~ 瞳孔反射 / oculovagal ~ 眼迷走神经反射 / orbicularis pupillary ~ 眼轮匝肌瞳孔反射 / palatal ~, swallowing ~ 腭反射 / pharyngeal ~, gag ~ 咽反射,呕反射 / plantar ~, sole ~ 跖反射,足底反射 / prepotential ~es 本能反射,本能 / pulmonocoronary ~ 肺冠状动脉反射 / pupillary ~, iris contraction ~ 瞳孔反射,虹膜收缩反射 / rectal ~, defecation ~ 直肠反射 / renointestinal ~ 肾肠反射 / reversed pupillary ~ 反向瞳孔反射 / righting ~ 翻正反射,正位反射 / rooting ~ 觅食反射(新生儿的一种反射,表现为刺激颊侧或上、下唇时新生儿的口和面转向刺激物) / shot-silk ~, water-silk ~ 闪缎反射,水彩样反射,闪缎样视网膜 / somatointestinal ~ 体肠反射 / stapedial ~ 镫骨肌[听]反射 / startle ~ 惊吓反射(见 Moro's reflex) / stretch ~, myotatic ~ 牵张反射,肌伸张反射 / tendon ~ 腱反射(一种深层反射) / triceps ~, elbow ~ 肱三头肌反射,肘反射 / unconditioned ~, inborn ~ 非条件反射,先天[性]反射 / vesicointestinal ~ 膀胱肠反射 / virile ~ ①球海绵体反射,阴茎反射;②男性反射(向上拉包皮或龟头而使软阴茎突然向下的反射,亦称休斯〈Hughes〉反射)

reflexogenic [riˌfleksəˈdʒenik], **reflexogenous** [ˌriːflekˈsɔdʒənəs] *a* 产生反射作用的,促反射作用的;反射作用引起的

reflexograph [riˈfleksəgrɑːf, -græf] *n* 反射描记器

reflexology [ˌriːflekˈsɔlədʒi] *n* 反射学

reflexometer [ˌriːflekˈsɔmitə] *n* 反射计(肌肉)

reflexophil [riˈfleksəfil] *a* 反射性的

reflexotherapy [riˌfleksəuˈθerəpi] *n* 反射疗法

refluent [ˈrefluənt] *a* 回流的,反流的 | **refluence** [ˈrefluəns] *n*

reflux [ˈriːflʌks] *n* 回流,反流 | gastroesophageal ~ 胃食管反流 / hepatojugular ~ 肝颈静脉反流[征] / intrarenal ~ 肾内反流 / urethrovesiculodifferential ~ 尿道精囊差别回流(指液体、精

子、注入物从后尿道进入生殖系统）/ vesicoureteral ~, vesicoureteric ~ 膀胱输尿管反流
refract [riˈfrækt] *vt* 使折射，对…验光 | **~ive** *a* 折射的，屈光的 / **~ivity** [ˌriːfrækˈtivəti] *n* 折射性；折射率差，折射系数
refracta dosi [riˈfræktə ˈdəusai]【拉】重复分剂量，分数[剂]量
refractile [riˈfræktail] *a* 折射的，可折射的
refraction [riˈfrækʃən] *n* 折射，屈光 | dynamic ~ 活动[眼]折射（正常视调节）
refractionist [riˈfrækʃənist] *n* 验光师
refractometer [ˌriːfrækˈtɔmitə] *n* 折射计，屈光计，折光仪 | **refractometry** *n* 屈光计检查
refractor [riˈfræktə] *n* 折射器
refractory [riˈfræktəri] *a* 不应[期]的；难治的，顽固性的 | **refractoriness** *n* 不应性；难治
refracture [riˈfræktʃə] *n* 再骨折
refrangible [riˈfrændʒibl] *a* 可折射的 | **refrangibility** [riˌfrændʒiˈbiləti] *n* 折射性，屈光性
refresh [riˈfreʃ] *vt* 使清新，使精力恢复；使复新（如使创口复新）*vi* 恢复精神
refreshment [riˈfreʃmənt] *n*（精神）恢复；使精力恢复的食物和饮料
refrigerant [riˈfridʒərənt] *a* 冷却的；退热的，清凉的 *n* 清凉剂，退热药
refrigerate [riˈfridʒəreit] *vt* 冷冻 | **refrigeration** [riˌfridʒəˈreiʃən] *n* 冷冻[作用] / **refrigerative**, **refrigeratory** [riˈfridʒərətəri] *a*
refrigerator [riˈfridʒəreitə] *n* 冰箱，冷藏器
refringent [riˈfrindʒənt] *a* 折射的，屈光的 | **refringency**, **refringence** *n*
Refsum's disease (syndrome) [ˈrefsum]（Sigvald Refsum）雷夫叙姆病（综合征），植烷酸贮积症（一种遗传性疾病，伴植烷酸代谢缺陷，主要表现为慢性多神经炎、色素性视网膜炎、共济失调等，可能有鳞癣、神经性聋和心电图异常，为常染色体隐性性状遗传。亦称多神经炎型遗传性共济失调）
refusion [riˈfjuːʒən] *n*（血）回输法
REG radioencephalography 放射脑电图学
regainer [riˈgeinə] *n*（牙间隙）恢复器
regainer-maintainer [riˈgeinə meinˈteinə] *n*（牙间隙）恢复保持器
Regaud residual body [rəˈgəu]（Claude Regaud）勒格残体（一种无核团块，由细小颗粒、脂质飞沫和变性细胞器组成，在精子发生时，其尾局部分化完成后脱落）
regel [ˈreigəl] *n*【德】月经，行经 | kleine ~ 排卵期月经
regenerate [riˈdʒenəreit] *vt*, *vi* 再生 [riˈdʒenərit] *a* 再生的
regeneration [riˌdʒenəˈreiʃən] *n* 再生 | epimorphic ~ 割处再生 / morphallactic ~ 变形再生
regenerative [riˈdʒenəreitiv] *a* 再生的
regime, régime [reiˈʒiːm] *n* 制度，生活制度
regimen [ˈredʒimen] *n*【拉】制度，生活制度；方案 | initial treatment ~ 初治方案 / chemotherapy ~ 化疗方案
regiment [ˈredʒimənt] *n* 团；一大群 | medical ~ 军医队
regio [ˈriːdʒiəu]（[复] **regiones** [riːdʒiˈəuniːz]）*n*【拉】区，部[位]
region [ˈriːdʒən] *n* 区，部[位] | abdominal ~s 腹部 / ~ of accommodation 调节区，调视范围 / basilar ~ 颅底区，颅底 / ciliary ~ 睫状体区 / deltoid ~ 三角肌区 / inguinal ~ 腹股沟区 / motor ~, rolandic ~ 运动区 / sensory ~, parietotemporal ~ 感觉区，顶颞区
regional [ˈriːdʒənəl] *a* 区的，部位的；局部的
register [ˈredʒistə] *n* 记录，登记，注册；登记簿，注册簿；声域，音域 *vt*, *vi* 登记，注册
registrant [ˈredʒistrənt] *n*（值班）登记护士
registrar [ˌredʒisˈtrɑː, ˈredʒis-] *n* 登记员，挂号员；专科住院医师
registration [ˌredʒisˈtreiʃən] *n* 注册，登记，挂号；记录（牙科中指颌关系记录）| maxillomandibular ~ 上下颌（关系）记录，上下颌间记录
registry [ˈredʒistri] *n* 挂号处，（值班护士）登记处；集中登记（收集病理资料以及有关的临床、化验、X线等方面的资料，以便集中研究）| central ~ 中心登记
regress [ˈriːgres] *n* 回归；退化，退行 [riˈgres] *vi* 回归；退化
regression [riˈgreʃən] *n* 退化，退行；（症状或病程的）消退；回归 | linear ~ 直线回归，线性回归（使直线回归适合于被观察数据的统计程序）
regressive [riˈgresiv] *a* 退化的，退行的；消退的；回归的
regular [ˈregjulə] *a* 规律的，有规律的；定时的；定期的；经常的 | **~ity** [ˌregjuˈlærəti] *n* 规律性；正规；定期 / **~ly** *ad*
regularize [ˈregjuləraiz] *vt* 使有规律，使系统化；调整 | **regularization** [ˌregjuləraiˈzeiʃən, -riˈz-] *n*
regulation [ˌregjuˈleiʃən] *n* 规则，条例；管理；调整；调节 | down ~ 减量调节 / up ~ 增量调节
regulator [ˈregjuleitə] *n* 调节剂；调节器；调节基因
Reg. umb. regio umbilici【拉】脐区
regurgitate [ri(ː)ˈgəːdʒiteit] *vi*, *vt* 反流；反胃 | **regurgitant** *a*
regurgitation [ri(ː)ˌgəːdʒiˈteiʃən] *n* 反流；反胃 | aortic ~ 主动脉瓣反流 / mitral ~ 二尖瓣反流 / pulmonic ~ 肺动脉瓣反流 / valvular ~ 瓣

膜性反流

rehabilitate [ˌriːhəˈbiliteit] *vt* 复原,恢复,康复 | **rehabilitation** [ˌriːhəbiliˈteiʃən] *n* 康复[学]

rehabilitee [ˌriːhəˈbiliˌtiː] *n* 复原者,康复者

rehalation [ˌriːhəˈleiʃən] *n* 再[呼]吸

Rehfuss' test(method) [ˈreifus] (Martin E. Rehfuss) 雷富斯试验(检胃分泌) | ~ tube 雷富斯管(取胃液管)

Rehmaniz [reiˈmæniə] *n* 地黄属

rehydration [ˌriːhaiˈdreiʃən] *n* 再水化[作用],再水合[作用]

Reichel's cloacal duct [ˈraiʃəl] (Friedrich P. Reichel) 赖歇尔一穴肛管(胎儿时期隔开道格拉斯〈Douglas〉隔与一穴肛的裂隙)

Reichert's canal [ˈraiʃət] (Karl B. Reichert) 连合管 | ~ cartilage 舌弓软骨(胚胎) / ~ recess (耳)蜗隐窝 / ~ substance 赖歇特质(前穿质后部)

Reichmann's disease (syndrome) [ˈraiʃmən] (Nikolas Reichmann) 持续性胃液分泌过多

Reid Hunt's reaction(test) [riːd hʌnt] 里德·亨特反应(试验)(见 Hunt's reaction)

Reid's base line [riːd] (Robert W. Reid) 里德基线(连接眶下嵴至外耳道及枕部中线之线,用于测颅)

Reifenstein's syndrome [ˈraifənstain] (Edward C. Reifenstein Jr.) 赖芬斯坦综合征(为男性促性腺激素过多性性腺功能减退症,系因对睾酮反应遗传性不能所致,伴有尿道下裂、男子女性型乳房、原发性性腺功能减退及青春期后睾丸萎缩和精子缺乏)

Reil's ansa [rail] (Johann C. Reil) 脑脚襻 | ~ insula 脑岛 / ~ ribbon 内侧丘系 / ~ sulcus 环状沟 / ~ trigone 丘系三角,蹄系三角

reimplantation [ˌriːimplɑːnˈteiʃən] *n* 移植

reinfection [ˌriːinˈfekʃən] *n* 再感染 | endogenous ~ 内源性感染再燃

reinforcement [ˌriːinˈfɔːsmənt] *n* 增强,加强,强化 | ~ of reflex 反射增强

reinforcer [ˌriːinˈfɔːsə] *n* 增强因子,增强剂

reinfusate [ˈriːinˌfjuːseit] *n* 再输注液,再输入液

reinfusion [ˌriːinˈfjuːʒən] *n* 再输注,再输入

Reinke's crystalloids (crystals) [ˈrainki] (Friedrich B. Reinke) 赖因克类晶体(晶体)(睾丸间质细胞〈Leydig cell〉内明显的形态多样的晶状结构) | ~ edema 赖因克水肿(称之为赖因克间隙的颈区经长期刺激后所致的炎症和水种,通常为长期滥用嗓子、吸烟或过多接触干燥空气或尘埃的结果) / ~ space 赖因克间隙(声韧带和覆盖其上的黏膜之间的一种潜在间隙,其炎症导致赖因克水肿)

reinnervation [ˌriːinəˈveiʃən] *n* 神经移植术,神经支配恢复术

reinoculation [ˌriːiˌnɔkjuˈleiʃən] *n* 再接种

reintegration [ˌriːintiˈgreiʃən] *n* 再整合[作用];重整[作用](指精神活动)

reintubation [ˌriːintjuˈbeiʃən] *n* 再插管[法]

reinversion [ˌriːinˈvəːʃən] *n* 复位术,翻回法(尤指内翻子宫复位术)

reinvocation [ˌriːinvəuˈkeiʃən] *n* 复能[作用],再活化[作用]

Reisseissen's muscles [ˈraisaisən] (Franz D. Reisseisen) 赖赛曾肌(最小支气管的平滑肌纤维)

Reissner's fiber [ˈraisnə] (Ernst Reissner) 赖斯纳纤维(脊髓中央管内的纵纤维) | ~ membrane 蜗管前庭壁,前庭膜

reiterature [riːˌitərəˈtjuəri] *vt* 【拉】重复,再配(处方)

Reiter's disease (syndrome) [ˈraitə] (Hans Reiter) 莱特尔病(综合征)(非淋病性尿道炎,继之为结膜炎和关节炎,其原因不明,主要发生于男子,常伴脓溢性皮肤角化病、口炎、龟头溃疡及龟头炎)

rejection [riˈdʒekʃən] *n* 排斥[反应] | acute ~, acute cellular ~ 急性排斥反应,急性细胞性排斥反应 / chronic ~ 慢性排斥反应 / hyperacute ~ 超急性排斥反应 / second-set ~ 二次排斥(见 phenomenon 项下相应术语)

rejuvenescence [ˌriːdʒuːviˈnesns] *n* 回春,复壮,返老还童 | **rejuvenescent** *a*

relapse [riˈlæps] *vi*, *n* 复发 | intercurrent ~ 间歇性复发 / mucocutaneous ~ 皮肤黏膜(梅毒)疹复发 / rebound ~ 反跳式复发(尤指类风湿关节炎患者停用可的松或 ACTH 后的疾病症状复发)

relation [riˈleiʃən] *n* 关系 | acquired eccentric jaw ~ 后天性非正中颌骨关系 / buccolingual ~ 颊舌关系 / centric ~, centric jaw ~ 正中颌骨关系 / dynamic ~s 动力关系 / eccentric ~, eccentric jaw ~, acentric ~ 非正中颌骨关系 / jaw ~ 颌骨关系 / lateral occlusal ~ 外侧闭合性颌关系 / median jaw ~ 正中颌关系 / median retruded jaw ~ 正中后退颌关系 / object ~ 对象关系(一个人与另一个人之间形成的感情连接) / posterior border jaw ~ 后缘颌关系 / protrusive jaw ~ 前凸颌关系 / rest jaw ~ 休止颌关系 / ridge ~ (上下)嵴关系 / static ~s 静止关系(指两个物体之间的关系) / unstrained jaw ~ 无紧张性颌关系

relaxant [riˈlæksənt] *a* 松弛的,弛缓的,舒张的 *n* 弛缓药 | muscle ~ 肌肉松弛药

relaxation [ˌriːlækˈseiʃən] *n* 松弛;弛缓,舒张 | isometric ~ 等长舒张(肌肉)

relaxin [riˈlæksin] *n* 松弛素,耻骨松弛激素,松弛肽

reliability [riˌlaiəˈbiləti] *n* 可靠性
relief [riˈliːf] *n* 缓解,减轻
relieve [riˈliːv] *vt* 缓解,减轻
reline [ˈriːˈlain] *vt* 重衬(义齿)
reluxation [ˌriːlʌkˈseiʃən] *n* 再脱位
REM rapid eye movements 快速眼动
rem [rem] (*r*oentgen-*e*quivalent-*m*an) *n* 雷姆,人体伦琴当量(1 rem〈雷姆〉= 1 rad〈拉德〉× RBE〈相对生物学效应〉)
Remak's band [ˈreimʌk] (Robert Remak)(神经)轴索 | ~ fibers 雷马克纤维,灰纤维(无髓神经纤维)/ ~ ganglion 窦房神经节/ ~ plexus 黏膜下丛
Remak's paralysis (type) [ˈreimʌk] (Ernst J. Remak)雷马克麻痹(型)(指与腕的伸肌麻痹) | ~ reflex 雷马克反射(刺激大腿前上部,引起一、二、三趾的跖屈)/ ~ symptom(sign) 雷马克症状(征)(多处感觉及延缓疼痛,均见于脊髓痨)
remedial [riˈmiːdjəl] *a* 治疗的;纠正的,修补的,补救的
remedy [ˈremidi] *n* 治疗[法];药[物] | concordant remedies 协调药 / inimic remedies 对抗药 / tissue ~s 组织药(根据顺势疗法生化学派的说法,有 12 种能构成身体矿物质基础的药物)
remifentanil hydrochloride [ˌremiˈfentənil] 盐酸瑞芬太尼(一种短效类阿片镇痛药,用作麻醉佐药)
Remijia [riˈmidʒiə] *n* 铜色树属
remineralization [riˌminərəlaiˈzeiʃən, -liˈz-] *n* 补充矿质(如对人体)
remission [riˈmiʃən] *n* 缓解,减轻,弛张 | **remissive** *a*
remittence [riˈmitəns] *n* 缓解,弛张
remittent [riˈmitənt] *a* 缓解的,弛张的,忽重忽轻的
remnant [ˈremnənt] *n* 遗留物,残余;[常用复]残存者 *a* 遗留的,残余的 | acroblastic ~ 原顶体残余 / gastric ~ 残胃
remodeling [riːˈmɔdəliŋ] *n* 重新塑造,改型 | bone ~ 骨质重建
remotivation [riːˌməutiˈveiʃən] *n* 重活跃(在精神病学中指一种由精神病院护理人员给予的团体治疗法,用以激发长期停药患者的交往技能和对环境的关心)
removal [riˈmuːvəl] *n* 摘除,切除 | manual ~ of placenta 手取胎盘术 / ~ of foreign body in brain 脑内异物摘除术
remyelination [riːˌmaiəliˈneiʃən] *n* 再髓鞘(因病或损伤发生脱髓鞘后,髓鞘恢复)
ren [ren] ([复] **renes** [ˈriːniːz]) *n*【拉】肾
renal [ˈriːnl] *a* 肾的
Renaut's bodies [reˈnəu] (Joseph L. Renaut) 雷诺体(肌营养不良时变性神经纤维中的灰色颗粒)
renculus [ˈrenkjuləs] ([复] **renculi** [ˈrenkjulai]) *n*【拉】肾小叶
Rendu-Osler-Weber disease, syndrome [rɔnˈdjuː ˈəuzlə ˈwiːbə] (H. J. L. M. Rendu; William Osler; Frederick P. Weber) 遗传性出血性毛细管扩张
Rendu's tremor [rɔnˈdjuː] (Henri J. L. M. Rendu) 郎杜震颤(癔症性的意向性震颤)
renes [ˈriːniːz] ren 的复数
renicapsule [ˈreniˌkæpsjuːl] *n* 肾上腺
reniculus [riˈnikjuləs] ([复] **reniculi** [riˈnikjulai]) *n*【拉】肾小叶
reniform [ˈrenifɔːm] *a* 肾形的
renin [ˈriːnin] *n* 肾素,高血压蛋白原酶,血管紧张肽原酶
reninism [ˈriːninizəm] *n* 肾素增多症 | primary ~ 原发性肾素增多症(高血压,低钾血症、醛固酮过多症以及血浆中肾素活性增强的一种综合征,系因肾小球细胞增生所致)
reninoma [ˌreniˈnəumə] *n* 近球细胞瘤
renipelvic [ˌreniˈpelvik] *a* 肾盂的
reniportal [ˌreniˈpɔːtl] *a* 肾门(静脉系统)的
renipuncture [ˌreniˈpʌŋktʃə] *n* 肾穿刺术
rennet [ˈrenit] *n* 粗制凝乳酶,干胃膜
rennin [ˈrenin] *n* 凝乳酶
renninogen [riˈninədʒən] *n* 凝乳酶原,前凝乳酶
ren(o)- [构词成分]肾
renocolic [ˌriːnəuˈkɔlik], **renocolonic** [ˌriːnəukəˈlɔnik] *a* 肾结肠的
renocortical [ˌriːnəuˈkɔːtikəl] *a* 肾皮质的
renocutaneous [ˌriːnəukjuˈteiniəs] *a* 肾[脏]皮[肤]的
renoduodenal [ˌriːnəuˌdju(ː)ˌəuˈdiːnəl)] *a* 肾十二指肠的
renogastric [ˌriːnəuˈgæstrik] *a* 肾胃的
renogram [ˈriːnəgræm], **renocystogram** [ˌriːnəuˈsistəgræm] *n* 肾图(用辐射探测器检肾功能的记录)
renography [riˈnɔgrəfi] *n* 肾造影[术]
renointestinal [ˌriːnəuinˈtestinl] *a* 肾肠的
renomedullary [ˌriːnəuˈmedjuˌlɛəri] *a* 肾髓质的
renopathy [riˈnɔpəθi] *n* 肾病
renoprival [ˌriːnəuˈpraivəl] *a* 肾功能缺乏的,肾无能的
renoscopy [riˈnɔskəpi] *n* 肾镜检查
renotrophic [ˌriːnəˈtrɔfik] *a* 促肾[营养]的,促肾增大的
renotropic [ˌriːnəˈtrɔpik] *a* 向肾的
renovascular [ˌriːnəuˈvæskjulə] *a* 肾血管的

Renshaw cells [ˈrenʃɔː] (Birdsey Renshaw) 闰绍细胞(脊髓腹侧正中区的中间神经元与运动神经元形成抑制性联系)

renule [ˈrenjuːl] *n* 肾段(由肾动脉分支供血的肾区)

renunculus [riˈnʌŋkjuləs] *n* 肾小叶

reorganize [ˈriːˈɔːɡənaiz] *vt*, *vi* 再机化,组织再生 | **reorganization** [ˈriːˌɔːɡənaiˈzeiʃən, -niˈz-] *n*

Reoviridae [ˌriːəuˈviridiː] *n* 呼肠孤病毒科

Reovirus [ˈriːəuˌvaiərəs] *n* 呼肠孤病毒属

reovirus [ˈriːəuˌvaiərəs] (*r*espiratory and *e*nteric *o*rphan + *virus*) *n* 呼吸道肠道孤儿病毒,呼肠孤病毒

reoxidation [riˌɔksiˈdeiʃən] *n* 再氧化

reoxygenation [riˌɔksidʒiˈneiʃən] *n* 再氧合

Rep. repetatur【拉】重复,再配

rep [rep] (*r*oentgen *e*quivalent *p*hysical) *n* 物理伦琴当量

repair [riˈpɛə] *vt n* 修补,修复 | perineal ~ 会阴修复术/ ~ of cervi 宫颈修补术

repatency [riˈpeitənsi] *n* 再开放,再通

repeat [riˈpiːt] *vt* 重复

repeatability [riˌpiːtəˈbiləti] *n* 可重复性

repellent [riˈpelənt] *a* 驱除的,驱散的,消肿的;排斥的;相斥的 *n* 驱除药,消肿药 | **repellency, repellence** *n* 抵抗性,排斥性

repeller [riˈpelə] *n* 退回器(兽医产科器械)

repercolation [ˌriːpəːkəˈleiʃən] *n* 再渗漉

repercussion [ˌriːpə(ː)ˈkʌʃən] *n* 消退法,消肿法;浮动诊胎法 | **repercussive** [ˌriːpə(ː)ˈkʌsiv] *a* 消肿的 *n* 消肿药

reperfusion [ˌriːpəːˈfjuːʒən] *n* 再灌注(对曾暂时局部缺血的某一区或部分的血流量恢复)

repetatur [ˌriːpiˈteitjuə] *vt* (被动语态)【拉】重复,再配

replacement [ri(ː)ˈpleismənt] *n* 置换术 | fluid ~ 补液 / total joint ~ 全关节置换(一种关节成形术)

replant [riːˈplɑːnt] *vt* 回植 | **~ation** [ˌriːplɑːnˈteiʃən] *n*

replenish [riˈpleniʃ] *vt*, *vi* 装满,充满 | **~er** *n* 显影液再生剂

replete [riˈpliːt] *a* 充实的,充满的 | **repletion** [riˈpliːʃən] *n*

replicase [ˈreplikeis] *n* 复制酶

replication [ˌrepliˈkeiʃən] *n* 复制(指复制相同的DNA 或 RNA 分子) | conservative ~ 保留复制(DNA 复制时,原来的分子保持完整,形成一个完全新的分子) / DNA ~ DNA 复制(通过解离双螺旋的双链以及形成新的互补链,而使 DNA 分子产生许多相同的复制品) / nonconservative ~, dispersive ~ 非保留复制,分散性复制(DNA 复制时,亲代核苷酸碱分布在每个子分子的双链上) / semiconservative ~ 半保留复制(DNA 复制时,DNA 双链纵分,以致每个子分子各有一个新合成链和一个亲代链)

replicon [ˈreplikɔn] *n* 复制子(指细菌内 DNA 一种自主复制凝聚物,如染色体、质体)

repolarization [riˌpəuləraiˈzeiʃən, -riˈz-] *n* 复极,复极化

repositioning [ˌriːpəˈziʃəniŋ] *n* 复位 | jaw ~ 颌复位术

repositor [riˈpɔzitə] *n* 复位器

repository [riˈpɔzitəri] *n* 贮藏处(一般指长效药物的肌内注射部位)

repression [riˈpreʃən] *n* 压制,抑制;压抑;阻遏 | coordinate ~ 并列性抑制(几种酶) / enzyme ~, endproduct ~ 酶抑制,终产物性抑制 / gene ~ 基因阻遏 / reactive ~ 压抑性精神病,压抑反应状态

repressor [riˈpresə] *n* 抑制子,阻抑物,阻遏物(遗传学上指调节基因所产生的物质)

reproducibility [ˌriːprəuˌdjuːsiˈbiləti] *n* 再现性,复验性

reproduction [ˌriːprəˈdʌkʃən] *n* 生殖,繁殖;复现(心理) | asexual ~ 无性生殖 / cytogenic ~ 细胞性生殖 / sexual ~ 有性生殖 / somatic ~分体生殖

reproductive [ˌriːprəˈdʌktiv] *a* 生殖的;复现的

repromicin [ˌreprəuˈmaisin] *n* 瑞普米星(抗生素)

reproterol hydrochloride [ˌriprəˈterəul] 盐酸瑞普特罗(支气管扩张药)

reptilase [ˈreptileis] *n* 蛇毒凝血酶(用于检测凝血时间)

reptile [ˈreptail] *n* 爬虫,爬行动物

Reptilia [repˈtiliə] *n* 爬行纲

repullulation [riˌpʌljuˈleiʃən] *n* 再发芽

repulse [riˈpʌls] *vt* 排斥,厌恶 | **repulsion** [riˈpʌlʃən] *n* 排斥,相斥;斥力

RES reticuloendothelial system 网状内皮系统

resazurin [riˈseizjurin] *n* 刃天青(一种醌亚胺化合物,用作 pH 指示剂,亦用作氧化还原电位的指示剂)

rescinnamine [riˈsinəmin] *n* 瑞西那明(用作镇静剂及抗高血压药)

rescue [ˈreskju] *vt*, *n* 援救,营救 | **~r** [ˈreskjuə] *n* 援救者,营救者

resect [ri(ː)ˈsekt] *vt* 切除 | **~able** *a* 可切除的

resection [ri(ː)ˈsekʃən] *n* 切除术 | gastric ~ 胃切除术 / root ~ (牙)根尖切除术 / submucous ~ 黏膜下(鼻中隔)切除术,开窗切除术 / transurethral ~ prostatic(TURP)经尿道前列腺切除术 / wedge ~ 楔形切除术 | **~al** *a*

resectoscope [ri(ː)ˈsektəskəup] *n* 电切镜
resectoscopy [ˌriːsekˈtɔskəpi] *n* 电切除术
resene [ˈresiːn] *n* 氧化树脂
reserpine [ˈresəpiːn, riˈsəːpin] *n* 利舍平(抗高血压药,亦用作镇静药)
reserpinized [ˈresəpinaizd] *a* 利舍平化的,利舍平治疗的
reserve [riˈzəːv] *vt* 储备;保留 *n* 储备[力],储量 | alkali ~, alkaline ~ 碱储量 / cardiac ~ 心力储备
reservoir [ˈrezəvwɑː] *n* 贮水池,贮器;储金池(牙);(寄生物或病菌的)贮主 | chromatin ~ 染色质核仁,核粒 / ~ of infection 传染贮主,传染贮源 / ~ of virus 病毒贮主 / venous ~ 静脉贮血器
reset [ˈriːˈset] *vt* 重调定;重接(断骨) [ˈriːset] *n*
reshaping [riˈʃeipiŋ] *n* 改形,矫形
resident [ˈrezidənt] *n* 住院医师
residual [riˈzidjuəl] *a* 剩余的,残余的,残留的 *n* 剩余;残渣
residue [ˈrezidjuː] *n* 残余,剩余;基,残基;渣,残余物 | day ~ 白昼残留印象(指梦中残留白天经验的痕迹)
residuum [riˈzidjuəm] ([复] **residua** [riˈzidjuə]) *n*【拉】残余,剩余;残渣 | gastric ~ 胃内残渣 / sporal ~ 孢子残渣(孢子形成后的残留胞质)
resilience [riˈziliəns], **resiliency** [riˈziliənsi] *n* 回弹,弹性;回弹能 | **resilient** *a*
resilin [riˈzilin] *n* 节枝弹性蛋白
resin [ˈrezin] *n* 树脂;松脂,松香 *vt* 涂树脂于;用树脂处理 | acrylic ~s 丙烯酸树脂 / activated ~ 自凝树脂 / anion-exchange ~ 阴离子交换树脂 / azure A carbacrylic ~ 天青 A 羧丙烯酸树脂 / carbacrylamine ~s 羧丙烯胺树脂 / cation-exchange ~ 阳离子交换树脂 / cholestyramine ~ 考来烯胺树脂,消胆胺,降脂一号树脂(降血脂药) / cold-curing ~ 冷凝树脂,自凝树脂 / composite ~ 复合树脂 / copolymer ~ 异分子聚合树脂 / direct filling ~ (牙用)直接填料树脂 / epoxy ~ 环氧树脂 / heat-curing ~ 热凝树脂 / ion exchange ~ 离子交换树脂 / podophyllum ~ 鬼臼[树]脂(局部腐蚀药,治疗乳头瘤,以前用作泻药) / quick-cure ~ 快凝树脂,自凝树脂 / polyaminemethylene ~ 聚胺甲烯树脂(抗胃酸药) / self-curing ~ 自凝树脂 / styrene ~ 苯乙烯树脂,聚苯乙烯/ synthetic ~ 合成树脂 / vinyl ~ 乙烯树脂
resina [riˈzainə] *n*【拉】树脂;松脂,松香
resinoid [ˈrezinɔid] *a* 树脂样的 *n* 类树脂;热固[性]树脂
resinotannol [ˌrezinəˈtænɔl] *n* 树脂鞣醇
resinous [ˈrezinəs] *a* 树脂性的,树脂的
resistance [riˈzistəns] *n* 抵抗力,抵抗性;耐药性;电阻,阻力 | airway ~ 呼吸道阻力,气道阻力 / drug ~ 抗药性 / electrical ~ 电阻 / environmental ~ 环境阻力 / total peripheral ~ 总外周阻力 / total pulmonary ~ 全肺阻力 / vascular ~ 血管阻力
resite [ˈresait] *n* 丙阶酚醛树脂,不熔酚醛树脂
resole [ˈresəul] *n* 甲阶酚醛树脂,可熔酚醛树脂
resolution [ˌrezəˈljuːʃən] *n* 消除;(炎症等的)消退,消散;分辨率 | longitudinal ~ 纵向分辨率
resolvent [riˈzɔlvənt] *a* 使溶解的;使分解的;消散的 *n* 消散药
resonance [ˈrezənəns] *n* 反响,叩响;共振;中介[现象] | amphoric ~ 空瓮音 / bandbox ~ 空匣音,空匣叩响(肺气肿时) / cough ~ 咳音,咳响 / cracked-pot ~ 破壶音,破壶响 / electron spin ~ 电子自旋共振 / nuclear magnetic ~ 核磁共振 / osteal ~ 骨性叩响 / paramagnetic ~ 顺磁共振 / shoulder-strap ~ 肩部叩响(锁骨上方肺尖处的肺部叩响) / tympanic ~ 鼓音,鼓响 / vesicular ~ 肺泡性叩响 / vesiculotympanic ~, wooden ~ 肺泡鼓性叩响,木性叩响 / vocal ~ 听觉语音 / whispering ~ 耳语响
resonant [ˈrezənənt] *a* 反响的,叩响的;共振的
resonator [ˈrezəneitə] *n* 共振器
resorb [riˈsɔːb] *vt, vi* 再吸收,重吸收;消溶
resorcinism [riˈzɔːsinizəm] *n* 雷琐辛中毒,间苯二酚中毒
resorcinol [riˈzɔːsinɔl] *n* 雷琐辛,间苯二酚(角质层分离剂) | ~ monoacetate 醋雷琐辛,间苯二酚单醋酸酯(抗皮脂溢药,角质层分离剂) | **resorcin** [riˈzɔːsin], **resorcinum** [riːzɔˈsainəm] *n*
resorcinolphthalein [riˌzɔːsinɔlˈθæliːn] *n* 间苯二酚酞,荧光素
resorption [riˈsɔːpʃən] *n* 吸收,吸回[作用],吸除[作用] | bone ~ 骨吸收 / idiopathic ~ 自发性吸收 / tubular ~ 肾小管吸收 | **resorptive** *a*
respirable [risˈpaiərəbl] *a* 可呼吸的,适于呼吸的
respiration [ˌrespəˈreiʃən] *n* 呼吸;呼吸音 | abdominal ~ 腹式呼吸 / absent ~ 呼吸音消失,无呼吸音呼吸 / accelerated ~ 呼吸加速(呼吸速度每分钟超过 25 次) / artificial ~ 人工呼吸 / bronchocavernous ~, metamorphosing ~ 支气管空洞呼吸音 / bronchovesicular ~, harsh ~, rude ~, transitional ~ 支气管肺泡呼吸音,粗糙呼吸音,粗杂呼吸音,过渡呼吸音 / cavernous ~ 空洞呼吸音 / cogwheel ~, interrupted ~, jerky ~, wavy ~ 齿轮状呼吸,间断性呼吸,急冲状呼吸,波浪状呼吸 / divided ~ 分割呼吸 / electrophrenic ~ 膈神经电刺激呼吸 / forced ~

强力呼吸 / internal ~, tissue ~ 内呼吸,组织呼吸 / paradoxical ~ 反常呼吸,逆呼吸 / periodic ~ 周期性呼吸,潮式呼吸 / puerile ~, supplementary ~ 小儿样呼吸音,代偿性呼吸音 / slow ~ 呼吸缓慢(呼吸速度每分钟少于 12 次) / tubular ~, bronchial ~ 管性呼吸音,支气管呼吸音 / vicarious ~ 代偿性呼吸

respirator [ˈrespəreitə] *n* 呼吸器,呼吸机;呼吸罩 | cabinet ~ 箱式呼吸器 / cuirass ~ 胸甲式呼吸器 / simple ~ 简易呼吸机

respiratory [risˈpaiərətəri] *a* 呼吸的

respire [risˈpaiə] *vi*, *vt* 呼吸

respirometer [ˌrespiˈrɔmitə] *n* 呼吸[运动]计

respond [risˈpɔnd] *vi*, *vt* 回答,响应 **responder** [risˈpɔndə] *n* 应答者,反应者 | first ~ 第一急救者

response [risˈpɔns] *n* 应答,反应 | anamnestic ~, memory ~, recall ~, booster ~, second set ~, secondary immune ~ 回忆应答,记忆应答,加强应答,二次应答,二次免疫应答(在免疫学中指注射过去已有过初次免疫应答的抗原之后血内抗体迅速重现) / autoimmune ~ 自身免疫应答(针对自身组织产生抗体或淋巴细胞的免疫应答) / delayed ~ 迟发型应答(见 reaction 项下相应术语) / galvanicskin ~ 皮肤电反应 / immediate ~ 速发型应答(见 reaction 项下相应术语) / immune ~ 免疫应答(机体对抗原产生的特异性应答,包括细胞免疫、体液免疫与免疫耐受性) / primary immune ~ 初次免疫应答(对抗原初次刺激的免疫应答,特征为特异性抗体合成开始前有一个潜伏期) / recall titer ~ 强化效价反应,回忆滴度应答(用加强注射使特异性凝集素增加的现象) / reticulocyte ~ 网状细胞增多反应 / triple ~ (of Lewis)(刘易斯)三重应答(用钝器划触皮肤后的一种生理应答:首先在划痕部位由于释放组胺或组胺样物质呈现红线,继而在红线周围形成潮红现象,最后由于局限性水肿而形成风团)

responsibility [risˌpɔnsəˈbiləti] *n* 责任,责任心;责任能力 | criminal ~ 刑事责任能力

rest [rest] *n* 剩余,胎性剩余;支托 | aberrant ~ 迷芽瘤 / adrenal ~, suprarenal ~ 肾上腺剩余(有时见于卵巢或睾丸内) / bed ~ 床支架;卧床休息 / carbon ~ [剩]余碳(指血滤液中) / embryonic ~, epithelial ~, fetal ~ 胎性剩余,上皮剩余 / incisal ~ 切端支托 / lingual ~ 舌侧支托/ occlusal ~ 殆支托 / precision ~ 精密支托 / recessed ~ 隐蔽支托 / semiprecision ~ 半精密支托 / surface ~ [牙]面支托

restbite [ˈrestbait] *n* 休止殆,休止咬合

restenosis [ˌriːstiˈnəusis] *n* 再狭窄(尤指心瓣的)

restenotic [ˌriːstəˈnɔtik] *a* 再狭窄的

restibrachium [ˌrestiˈbreikiəm] ([复] **restibrachia** [ˌrestiˈbreikiə]) *n* 绳状体,小脑下臂

restiform [ˈrestifɔːm] *a* 绳状的

restis [ˈrestis] ([复] **restes** [ˈrestiːz]) *n*【拉】绳状体

restitutio [ˌrestiˈtuːʃiəu] *n*【拉】整复,恢复;转回(胎头) | ~ ad integrum 完全恢复

restitution [ˌrestiˈtjuːʃən] *n* 整复,恢复;转回(胎头)

restoration [ˌrestəˈreiʃən] *n* 恢复,康复;复位,回复;修复 | buccal ~ 颊面窝洞修复 /prosthetic ~ 假体修复(口腔矫形修复)

restorative [risˈtɔrətiv] *a* 促恢复的 *n* 恢复药

restrainer [risˈtreinə] *n* 制动器;抑制剂

restraint [risˈtreint] *n* 抑制,制止;节制;约束,拘束 | chemical ~ 化学约束(用麻醉药品使精神病患者趋于平静)

restriction [risˈtrikʃən] *n* 限制,限定 | MHC ~ MHC 限制,主要组织相容性复合体限制

resublimed [riːsəˈblaimd] *a* 再升华的

resupination [ˌriːsjuːpiˈneiʃən] *n* 反转,颠倒;仰卧位

resupine [ˌriːsjuːˈpain] *a* 仰卧的

resuscitation [riˌsʌsiˈteiʃən] *n* 复苏 | ~ of heart 心脏复苏

resuscitator [riˈsʌsiteitə] *n* 复苏器

resuture [riˈsjuːtʃə] *n* 再缝术,二期缝术

resynchronization [riːˌsiŋkrəniˈzeiʃən] *n* 再同步

retainer [riˈteinə] *n* 固位体(牙);保留器,保持器 | direct ~直接固位体

retamine [ˈretəmin] *n* 鹰爪豆碱

retard [riˈtɑːd] *vt*, *n* 延迟,延缓 | expiratory flow ~ 呼气延缓

retardant [riˈtɑːdənt] *a* 使延迟的 *n* 抑制剂

retardate [riˈtɑːdeit] *n* 智力迟钝者

retardation [ˌriːtɑːˈdeiʃən] *n* 阻滞,迟缓,延滞发育;妨碍 | mental ~ 精神发育迟缓,智力低下 / psychomotor ~ 精神运动性阻滞 / ~ of thought 思想迟缓 | **retardative** [riˈtɑːdətiv], **retardatory** [riˈtɑːdətəri] *a*

retch [retʃ, riːtʃ] *vi* 干呕 | **~ing** *n*

rete [ˈriːtiː] ([复] **retia** [ˈriːʃiə]) *n*【拉】网 | acromial ~ 肩峰网 / articular cubital ~ 肘关节网 / calcaneal ~跟网 / dorsal carpal ~ 腕背网/ epidermal ~ 生发层 / plantar ~, plantar venous ~ 足底静脉网 | **retial** [ˈriːʃiəl] *a*

retentate [riˈtenteit] *a* 存留的

retention [riˈtenʃən] *n* 潴留,停滞;保留,保持;固位 | denture ~ 义齿固位 / direct ~ 直接固位 / indirect ~ 间接固位 / surgical ~ 外科手术固位 / ~ of urine 尿潴留

reteplase [ˈretəpleis] *n* 瑞替普酶(溶血栓药,治疗心肌梗死,静脉内给药)

retethelioma [ˌriːtiθiːliˈəumə] *n* 网状内皮肉瘤，恶性淋巴瘤
reticula [riˈtikjulə] reticulum 的复数
reticular [riˈtikjulə] *a* 网状的 | **~ly** *ad*
reticulate [riˈtikjulit] *a* 网状的 [riˈtikjuleit] *vt*, *vi*(使)成网状 | **~d** [riˈtikjuleitid] *a*
reticulation [riˌtikjuˈleiʃən] *n* 网状形成 | dust ~ 尘网形成(肺尘病的早期，尤见于煤矿工人，可能发展成炭末石末沉着病)
reticulin [riˈtikjulin] *n* 网霉素，羟基链霉素；网硬蛋白 | ~ M 网硬蛋白 M(网状内皮系统产生的一种内分泌物)
reticulitis [riˌtikjuˈlaitis] *n* 蜂窝胃炎(反刍动物第二胃的炎症)
reticul(o)- [构词成分]网，网状结构
reticulocyte [riˈtikjuləuˌsait] *n* 网状细胞，网织红细胞 | **reticulocytic** [riˌtikjuləuˈsitik] *a*
reticulocytogenic [riˌtikjuləuˌsaitəuˈdʒenik] *a* 网状细胞生成的
reticulocytopenia [riˌtikjuləuˌsaitəuˈpiːniə] *n* 网状细胞减少
reticulocytosis [riˌtikjuləusaiˈtəusis] *n* 网状细胞增多
reticuloendothelial [riˌtikjuləuˌendəuˈθiːliəl] *a* 网状内皮的
reticuloendothelioma [riˌtikjuləuˌendəuθiːliˈəumə] *n* 网状内皮瘤(恶性淋巴瘤)
reticuloendotheliosis [riˌtikjuləuˌendəuθiːliˈəusis] *n* 网状内皮组织增殖 | leukemic ~ 白细胞性网状内皮组织增殖，毛细胞白血病 / systemic aleukemic ~全身性非白血病性网状内皮组织增殖(见 Letterer-Siwe disease)
reticuloendothelium [riˌtikjuləuˌendəuˈθiːljəm] *n* 网状内皮组织
reticulohistiocytary [riˌtikjuləuˌhistiəˈsaitəri] *a* 网状组织细胞的
reticulohistiocytoma [riˌtikjuləu ˌhistiəsaiˈtəumə] *n* 网状组织细胞瘤
reticulohistiocytosis [riˌtikjuləuˌhistiəsaiˈtəusis] *n* 网状组织细胞瘤病 | multicentric ~ 多中心性网状(内皮系统)组织细胞瘤病，脂质皮肤关节炎
reticuloid [riˈtikjulɔid] *a* 网状细胞增多[症]样的 *n* 类网状细胞增多症 | actinic ~ 光线性类网状细胞增多症
reticuloma [riˌtikjuˈləumə] *n* 网状内皮细胞瘤(组织细胞恶性淋巴瘤)
reticulonodular [rəˌtikjuləuˈnɔdjulə] *a* 网结节的
reticulopenia [riˌtikjuləuˈpiːniə] *n* 网状细胞减少
reticulopericarditis [rəˌtikjuləuˌperikɑːˈdaitis] *n* 网心包炎
reticuloperithelium [riˌtikjuləuˌperiˈθiːljəm] *n* 网周上皮
reticuloperitonitis [rəˌtikjuləuˌperitəˈnaitis] *n* 网腹膜炎
reticulopituicyte [riˌtikjuləupiˈtju(ː)isait] *n* 垂体网状细胞
reticulopod [riˈtikjuləupɔd], **reticulopodium** [riˌtikjuləuˈpəudjəm] *n* 网状假足，网状伪足
reticulopodia [riˌtikjuləuˈpəudia] reticulopodium 的复数
reticulorumen [rəˌtikjuləuˈruːmən] *n* 网状瘤胃
reticuloruminal [rəˌtikjuləuˈruːminəl] *a* 网状瘤胃的(亦称瘤胃网状的)
reticulosarcoma [riˌtikjuləusɑːˈkəumə] *n* 网状细胞肉瘤(未分化的或组织细胞的恶性淋巴瘤)
reticulosis [riˌtikjuˈləusis] *n* 网状细胞增多[症] | histiocytic medullary ~, familial hemophagocytic ~, familial histiocytic ~ 组织细胞性髓性网状细胞增多，家族性嗜血细胞性网状细胞增多，家族性组织细胞性网状细胞增多 / lipomelanic ~ 脂肪黑变性网状细胞增多，皮肤病性淋巴结病/ pagetoid ~ 变形性骨炎样网状细胞增多
reticulothelium [riˌtikjuləuˈθiːljəm] *n* 网织上皮
reticulum [riˈtikjuləm] ([复] **reticula** [riˈtikjulə] *n* 【拉】网(尤指细胞原生质网)；网状组织；蜂窝胃(反刍动物第二胃) | endoplasmic ~ 内质网 / sarcoplasmic ~ 肌浆网，肌质网 / stellate ~ 星形网 / ~ trabeculare anguli iridocornealis 虹膜角膜角小梁网
retiform [ˈriːtifɔːm, ˈretifɔːm] *a* 网状的
retina [ˈretinə] ([复] **retinas** 或 **retinae** [ˈretiniː]) *n* 视网膜 | coarctate ~ 紧压性视网膜，漏斗状视网膜 / detached ~, detachment of ~ 视网膜脱离 / lower ~ 下半[部]视网膜 / nasal ~ 鼻半侧视网膜 / shot-silk ~, watered-silk ~ 闪缎样视网膜 / temporal ~ 颞半侧视网膜 / tigroid ~ 豹纹状视网膜 / upper ~ 上半[部]视网膜
retinaculum [ˌretiˈnækjuləm] ([复] **retinacula** [ˌretiˈnækjulə]) *n* 【拉】支持带，系带；持疝钩
retinal [ˈretinəl] *a* 视网膜的 *n* 视黄醛，维生素 A 醛
retinal$_1$ [ˈretinəl] *n* 视网醛，维生素 A 醛
retinal$_2$ [ˈretinəl] *n* 去氢视网醛，去氢维生素 A 醛
retinal isomerase [ˈretinəl aiˈsɔməreis] 视黄醛异构酶
retinal reductase [ˈretinəl riˈdʌkteis] 视黄醛还原酶(一种酶活性的旧称，现称醇脱氢酶〈NAD(P)$^+$〉)
retinascope [ˈretinəskəup] *n* 视网膜镜
retine [ˈretiːn] *n* 抑细胞素(抑制细胞的分裂和生长)

retinene [ˈretiniːn] *n* 视黄醛,维生素A醛

retinitis [ˌretiˈnaitis] *n* 视网膜炎 | apoplectic ~ 猝出血性视网膜炎 / azotemic ~ 氮血症性视网膜炎 / central angiospastic ~ 血管痉挛性中心视网膜炎 / gravidic ~ 妊娠性视网膜炎 / leukemic ~, splenic ~ 白血病性视网膜炎 / ~ pigmentosa sine pigmento 无色素性视网膜色素变性,无色素沉着的色素性视网膜炎 / punctate ~ 点状视网膜炎 / renal ~ 肾炎性视网膜炎 / ~ sclopetaria 射伤性视网膜炎/striate ~ 纹状视网膜炎

retinoblastoma [ˌretinəublæsˈtəumə] *n* 视网膜母细胞瘤,视网膜神经胶质瘤

retinochoroid [ˌretinəuˈkɔːrɔid] *a* 视网膜脉络膜的

retinochoroiditis [ˌretinəukɔːrɔiˈdaitis] *n* 视网膜脉络膜炎 | ~ juxtapapillaris 近视乳头性视网膜脉络膜炎 / toxoplasmic ~ 弓形体性视网膜脉络膜炎

retinocytoma [ˌretinəusaiˈtəumə] *n* 视网膜细胞瘤(亦称视网膜瘤)

retinodialysis [ˌretinəudaiˈælisis] *n* 视网膜断离

retinograph [ˈretinəgrɑːf, -græf] *n* 视网膜照片

retinography [ˌretiˈnɔgrəfi] *n* 视网膜照相术

retinoic acid [ˌretiˈnɔik] 维A酸,维生素A酸,视黄酸

retinoid [ˈretinɔid] *a* 视网膜样的;树脂样的 *n* 类维生素A

retinol [ˈretinɔl] *n* 视黄醇,维生素A;松香油

retinol$_1$ [ˈretinɔl] *n* 视黄醇,维生素A_1

retinol$_2$ [ˈretinɔl] *n* 去氢视黄醇,维生素A_2

retinol dehydrogenase [ˈretinɔl diːˈhaidrədʒəneis] 视黄醇脱氢酶

retinol *O*-fatty-acyltransferase [ˈretinɔl ˈfæti ˌæsilˈtrænsfəreis] 视黄醇*O*-脂[肪]酰基转移酶

retinoma [ˌretiˈnəumə] *n* 视网膜瘤,视网膜细胞瘤

retinomalacia [ˌretinəuməˈleiʃiə] *n* 视网膜软化

retinopapillitis [ˌretinəuˌpæpiˈlaitis] *n* 视网膜视乳头炎

retinopathy [ˌretiˈnɔpəθi] *n* 视网膜病变 | arteriosclerotic ~ 动脉硬化性视网膜病变 / central disk-shaped ~ 盘性中心性视网膜病变,盘性黄斑变性/ central serous ~, central angiospastic ~ 浆液性中心性视网膜病变,血管痉挛性中心性视网膜病变 / circinate ~ 环形视网膜病变(亦称环形视网膜炎) / diabetic ~ 糖尿病[性]视网膜病变 / exudative ~ 渗出性视网膜病变(亦称渗出性视网膜炎) / hemorrhagic ~ 出血性视网膜病变 / hypertensive ~ 高血压性视网膜病变 / ~ of prematurity 早产儿视网膜病变,晶状体后纤维组织形成 / pigmentary ~ 色素性视网膜病变 / proliferative ~ 增生性视网膜病变 / renal ~ 肾性视网膜病变 / stellate ~ 星状视网膜病变

retinoschisis [ˌretiˈnɔskisis] *n* 视网膜劈裂症

retinoscope [ˈretinəskəup] *n* 检影镜 | **retinoscopy** [ˌretiˈnɔskəpi] *n* 检影[法]

retinosis [ˌretiˈnəusis] *n* 视网膜变性

retinotopic [ˌretinəuˈtɔpik] *a* 视网膜区域定位的,视网膜定位的

retinotoxic [ˌretinəuˈtɔksik] *a* 毒害视网膜的

retinyl [ˈretinil] *n* 视黄基

retinyl-palmitate esterase [ˈretinil ˈpælmiteit ˈestəreis] 棕榈酸视黄酯酯酶

retisolution [ˌretisəˈljuːʃən] *n* 高尔基(Golgi)体溶解

retispersion [ˌretiˈspəːʃən] *n* 高尔基体移位(高尔基〈Golgi〉体从正常位置移到细胞周围)

retoperithelium [ˌriːtəuˌperiˈθiːljəm] *n* 网周上皮

Retortamonadida [riˌtɔːtəməuˈnædidə] *n* 曲滴虫目

Retortamonas [ˌriːtəˈtæmənəs] *n* 曲滴虫属

retothel [ˈriːtəθəl] *a* 网状内皮的

retothelium [ˌriːtəuˈθiːljəm] *n* 网织上皮 | **retothelial** *a*

retract [riˈtrækt] *vt, vi* 缩回,缩卷

retractile [riˈtræktail] *a* 可缩回的,可退缩的

retraction [riˈtrækʃən] *n* 退缩,缩回 | clot ~ 血块收缩 / gingival ~ 龈后缩 / mandibular ~ 下颌后缩

retractor [riˈtræktə] *n* 牵开器;缩肌

retrad [ˈriːtræd] *ad* 向后(向后方或背侧)

retrieval [riˈtriːvəl] *n* (记忆内容的)随意再现;检索

retr(o)- [前缀] 后,向后,在后

retroacetabular [ˌretrəuˌæsəˈtæbjulə] *a* 髋臼后的

retroact [ˌretrəuˈækt] *vi* 倒行,回动,起反作用

retroaction [ˌretrəuˈækʃən] *n* 反作用,逆作用

retroactive [ˌretrəuˈæktiv] *a* 倒行的,回动的,反作用的

retroauricular [ˌretrəuɔːˈrikjulə] *a* 耳后的

retrobronchial [ˌretrəuˈbrɔŋkiəl] *a* 支气管后的

retrobuccal [ˌretrəuˈbʌkəl] *a* 颊后的,口后的

retrobulbar [ˌretrəuˈbʌlbə] *a* 眼球后的;脑桥后的

retrocalcaneobursitis [ˌretrəukælˌkeiniəubəˈsaitis] *n* 跟腱(黏液)囊炎

retrocardiac [ˌretrəuˈkɑːdiæk] *a* 心后的

retrocatheterism [ˌretrəuˈkæθitərizəm] *n* 逆行插管法

retrocecal [ˌretrəuˈsiːkəl] *a* 盲肠后的

retrocervical [ˌretrəuˈsəːvikəl] *a* 子宫颈后的

retrocession [ˌretrəuˈseʃən] *n* 后退,后移(尤指子

宫后移);交还,归还

retrochiasmatic [ˌretrəukaiæsˈmætik] *a* 视交叉后的

retroclavicular [ˌretrəukləˈvikjulə] *a* 锁骨后的

retroclusion [ˌretrəuˈkluːʒən] *n* 逆压法,动脉后针压术

retrocochlear [ˌretrəuˈkɔkliə] *a* [耳]蜗后的

retrocolic [ˌretrəuˈkɔlik] *a* 结肠后的

retrocollic [ˌretrəuˈkɔlik] *a* 项的,颈后的

retrocollis [ˌretrəuˈkɔlis] *n* 颈后倾(头向后仰的痉挛性斜颈)

retrocrine [ˌretrauˈkrain] *n* 反分泌

retrocrural [ˌretrəuˈkruərəl] *a* 腿后的

retrodeviation [ˌretrəuˌdiːviˈeiʃən] *n* 后偏(后倾、后屈、后移的总称)

retrodisplacement [ˌretrəudisˈpleismənt] *n* 后移位

retroesophageal [ˌretrəui(ː)ˈsɔfədʒiəl] *a* 食管后的

retrofilling [ˌretrəuˈfiliŋ] *n* 倒充填[法](从根尖开始充填)

retroflex(ed) [ˈretrəufleks(t)] *a* 后屈的

retroflexion [ˌretrəuˈflekʃən] *n* 后屈(尤指子宫后屈)

retrogasserian [ˌretrəugæˈsiəriən] *a* 半月神经节后根的

retrognathia [ˌretrəuˈnæθiə], **retrognathism** [ˌretrəuˈnæθizəm] *n* 缩颌,颌后缩 | **retrognathic** *a*

retrograde [ˈretrəugreid] *a* 退行性的,逆行的;衰退的,退化的 *vi* 退行,逆行;退化 | **retrogradation** [ˌretrəugrəˈdeiʃən] *n*

retrography [riˈtrɔgrəfi] *n* 反写

retrogression [ˌretrəuˈgreʃən] *n* 退化,变性;退行(指退行至发育早期不太复杂的状态)

retroinfection [ˌriːtrəuinˈfekʃən] *n* 逆传染(由胎儿传染母体)

retroinsular [ˌretrəuˈinsjulə] *a* 岛后的

retroiridian [ˌretrəuaiˈridiən] *a* 虹膜后的

retrojection [ˌretrəuˈdʒekʃən] *n* 腔洞灌洗法

retrolabyrinthine [ˌretrəuˌlæbiˈrinθiːn] *a* 迷路后的

retrolental [ˌretrəuˈlentl], **retrolenticular** [ˌretrəulenˈtikjulə] *a* 晶状体后的

retrolingual [ˌretrəuˈliŋgwəl] *a* 舌后的

retrolisthesis [ˌretrəuˈlisθəsis] *n* 骶骨前移

retromammary [ˌretrəuˈmæməri] *a* 乳房后的

retromandibular [ˌretrəumænˈdibjulə] *a* 下颌后的

retromastoid [ˌretrəuˈmæstɔid] *a* 乳突后的

retromesenteric [ˌretrəuˌmesənˈterik] *a* 肠系膜后的

retromolar [ˌretrəuˈməulə] *a* 磨牙后的

retromorphosis [ˌretrəumɔːˈfəusis] *n* 退行性变态

retronasal [ˌretrəuˈneizəl] *a* 鼻后的

retro-ocular [ˌretrəuˈɔkjulə] *a* 眼后的

retroparotid [ˌretrəupəˈrɔtid] *a* 腮腺后的

retropatellar [ˌretrəupəˈtelə] *a* 髌后的

retroperitoneal [ˌretrəuˌperitəuˈniːəl] *a* 腹膜后的

retroperitoneum [ˌretrəuˌperitəuˈniːəm] *n* 腹膜后腔

retroperitonitis [ˌretrəuˌperitəuˈnaitis] *n* 腹膜后间隙炎

retropharyngeal [ˌretrəufəˈrindʒiəl] *n* 咽后的

retropharyngitis [ˌretrəuˌfærinˈdʒaitis] *n* 咽后炎

retropharynx [ˌretrəuˈfæriŋks] *n* 咽后部

retroplacental [ˌretrəupləˈsentl] *a* 胎盘后的

retroplasia [ˌretrəuˈpleisiə] *n* 退行性化生(组织或细胞变性为更原始型)

retropleural [ˌretrəuˈpluərəl] *a* 胸膜[腔]后的

retroposed [ˈretrəupəuzd] *a* 后移的

retroposition [ˌretrəupəˈziʃən] *n* 后位,后移;复位,回复

retropubic [ˌretrəuˈpjuːbik] *a* 耻骨弓后的

retropulsion [ˌretrəuˈpʌlʃən] *n* 推回,向后压(如分娩时的胎头);后退(如脊髓痨时),反步症;后退步态,后冲步态(一种异常步态)

retrorectal [ˌretrəuˈrektəl] *a* 直肠后的

retrorenal [ˌretrəuˈriːnəl] *a* 肾后的

retrorsine [ˈretrəsin] *n* 倒千里光碱(一种有毒的生物碱)

retrosigmoidal [ˌretrəusigˈmɔidəl] *a* 乙状窦后的

retrosinus [ˌretrəuˈsainəs] *n* 后窦(颞骨乳突)

retrospondylolisthesis [ˌretrəuˌspɔndiləulisˈθiːsis] *n* 骶骨前移

retrostalsis [ˌretrəuˈstælsis] *n* 逆蠕动

retrosternal [ˌretrəuˈstəːnəl] *a* 胸骨后的

retrosymphysial [ˌriːtrəusimˈfiziəl] *a* 耻骨联合后的

retrotarsal [ˌretrəuˈtɑːsəl] *a* 睑板后的

retrotorsion [ˌretrəuˈtɔːʃən] *n* 逆行性扭转

retrouterine [ˌretrəuˈjuːtərain] *a* 子宫后的

retrovaccination [ˌretrəuˌvæksiˈneiʃən] *n* 还原接种法(用从人获得的疫苗病毒接种至小母牛身上,同样亦指从曾接种疫苗病毒的母牛身上获取病毒再接种至小母牛身上)

retroversioflexion [ˌretrəuˌvəːsiəuˈflekʃən] *n* 后倾后屈

retroversion [ˌretrəuˈvəːʃən, -ʒən] *n* 后倾 | ~ of uterus 子宫后倾

retroverted [ˌretrəuˈvəːtid] *a* 后倾的

retrovesical [ˌretrəuˈvesikəl] *a* 膀胱后的

Retroviridae [ˌretrəuˈviridiː] *n* 反转录病毒科
retrovirus [ˈretrəuˌvaiərəs] *n* 反转录病毒
retrusion [riˈtruːʒən] *n* 后移(如牙齿在咬合线后的位置不良);下颌后移
Rett syndrome [ret] (Andreas Rett)雷特综合征(累及脑灰质的一种进行性病变,只见于女性,出生时即存在,特征为孤独行为、共济失调、痴呆、癫痫发作及失去有目的用手能力,伴大脑萎缩、血氨轻度升高及生物胺水平降低。亦称大脑萎缩性高氨血症)
return [riˈtəːn] *n* 回流;回归,复发 | cardiotomy blood ~ 心内血回收 / venous ~ 静脉回流
Retzius' fibers [ˈretsiəs] (Anders A. Retzius)雷济厄斯纤维(科尔蒂〈Corti〉器内戴特斯〈Deiters〉细胞的硬丝) / ~ space(cavity) 膀胱前隙,耻骨后隙 / ~ veins 雷济厄斯静脉(自小肠壁至下腔静脉的属支,即肠壁静脉)
Retzius' foramen [ˈretsiəs] (Magnus G. Retzius)第四脑室外侧孔 | ~ lines(striae)釉质生长线
reunient [riˈjuːniənt] *a* 再连合的
reunion [riːˈjuːnjən] *n* [断裂]重接
reuptake [riːˈʌpteik] *n* 重摄取,再摄取
Reuss's color charts(tables) [ˈrɔis] (August R. Von Reuss)罗伊斯比色图表(检色觉)
revaccination [ˌriːvæksiˈneiʃən] *n* 复种(第二次预防接种)
revascularization [riːˌvæskjuləraiˈzeiʃən, -riˈz-] *n* 血运重建
revehent [rəˈviːhənt] *a* 回流的(指静脉和动脉)
reverberate [riˈvəːbəreit] *vt*, *vi* 反响 | **reverberation** [riˌvəːbəˈreiʃən] *n* 反响;混响;回荡
Reverdin's graft [reivəˈdæn] (Jacques L. Reverdin)表皮移植片 | ~ method 雷维尔丹法(表皮移植) / ~ operation 雷维尔丹手术(一种表皮移植法)
Reverdin's needle [reivəˈdæn] (Albert Reverdin)雷维尔丹活眼针(外科用针)
reverie [ˈrevəri] *n* 出神,幻想
reversal [riˈvəːsəl] *n* 颠倒,逆转;反向,相反 | ~ of gradient (肠)梯度颠倒,粪便逆行 / sex ~ 性转换,性反转
reverse transcriptase [riˈvəːs trænsˈkripteiz] 逆转录酶,RNA 指导的 DNA 聚合酶
reversible [riˈvəːsəbl] *a* 可逆的 | **reversibility** [riˌvəːsəˈbiləti] *n* 可逆性
reversion [riˈvəːʃən] *n* 逆转,倒转,反向;回复变异;返祖遗传(某些远祖的遗传性状的重现) | antigenic ~ 抗原性逆转(成熟细胞的抗原结构转变为未成熟细胞的抗原结构,如某些肿瘤中所见)
Revilliod's sign [reiviˈjɔː] (Jean L. A. Revilliod)腊维约征,眼轮匝肌征(orbicularis sign, 见 sign 项下相应术语)
revivescent [ˌreviˈvesnt], **reviviscent** [ˌreviˈvisnt] *a* 复苏的,回生的;恢复的 | **revivescence** [ˌreviˈvesns], **reviviscence** [ˌreviˈvisns] *n* 复苏,回生,生命力复活;反应再现(指以前作过诊断性皮肤结核菌素试验的患者,在皮下注射结核菌素时,局部皮肤反应再现)
revivify [ri(ː)ˈvivifai] *vt*, *vi* 复苏,回生;恢复 | **revivification** [ri(ː)ˌvivifiˈkeiʃən] *n* 复新,复活(指创口等)
revolute [ˈrevəljuːt] *a* 后卷的,绕转的
revolution [ˌrevəˈljuːʃən] *n* 绕转,回转
révulseur [ˌreivjulˈsəː] *n* 【法】针刺器(用于邦夏特〈Baunscheidt〉针法)
Rexed's laminae [ˈreksed] (B. Rexed)雷克赛德板层(一种构造学方案,用以将脊髓的结构根据灰质不同区域的神经元细胞学特征加以分类。它包含 9 个板层〈Ⅰ-Ⅸ〉,延伸到整个脊髓,大体平行于灰质的背侧柱和腹侧柱,第 10 区〈板层Ⅹ〉围绕中央管,由背侧和腹侧连合以及中央胶质组成)
Reye-Johnson syndrome [rai ˈdʒɔnsn] (R. D. K. Reye; George M. Johnson)雷-约综合征(见 Reye's syndrome)
Reye's syndrome [rai] (Ralph D. K. Reye)雷亥综合征(一种罕见的儿童急性有时为致死性疾病,常作为水痘的后遗症或病毒性上呼吸道感染发生,特点为复发性呕吐及血清转氨酶水平升高,伴有肝脏及其他内脏的特殊改变,可继以一种脑病期,伴急性脑肿胀、意识障碍及癫痫发作)
Reynals 见 Duran-Reynals
Reynolds' number [ˈrenəldz] (Osborne Reynolds)雷诺数(液体的流速乘以管的直径,并除以循环液的运动黏度。此值对湍流来说是比较低的,对层流则较高)
Reynold's test [ˈrenəld] (James E. Reynold)雷诺尔德试验(检丙酮)
RF rheumatoid factor 类风湿因子
Rf rutherfordium 铲
RFA right frontoanterior 额右前(胎位)
RFLP restriction fragment length polymorphism 限制性[内切酶]片断长度多态性(见 polymorphism 项下相应术语)
RFP right frontoposterior 额右后(胎位)
RFPS(Glasgow) Royal Faculty of Physicians and Surgeons of Glasgow (格拉斯哥)皇家内外科医师协会
RFT right frontotransverse 额右横(胎位)
RGN Registered General Nurse(Scotland)注册普通护士(苏格兰)
Rh rhodium 铑
Rh_{null} Rh 因子缺乏,Rh 因子无(为一种罕见血型的符号,见 syndrome 项下相应术语)
Rhabdiasoidea [ˌræbdiəˈsɔidiə] *n* 棒线[虫]总科
rhabditic [ræbˈditik] *a* 小杆线虫的

Rhabditidae [ræb'ditidiː] *n* 小杆科
rhabditiform [ræb'ditifɔːm] *a* 杆状的
Rhabditis [ræb'daitis] *n* 小杆线虫属
rhabditoid ['ræbditɔid] *a* 杆状的
Rhabditoidea [ˌræbdi'tɔidiə] *n* 小杆总科
rhabdium ['ræbdiəm] *n* 横纹肌纤维
rhabd(o)- [构词成分] 杆;横纹
rhabdocyte ['ræbdəsait] *n* 杆状核细胞,晚幼粒细胞
rhabdoid ['ræbdɔid] *a* 杆状的
Rhabdomonadina [ˌræbdəuməunə'dainə] *n* 杆单胞虫亚目
Rhabdomonas [ˌræbdəu'məunəs] *n* 杆单胞菌属
rhabdomyoblast [ˌræbdəu'maiəuˌblæst] *n* 成横纹肌细胞 | **~ic** [ˌræbdəuˌmaiəu'blæstik] *a*
rhabdomyoblastoma [ˌræbdəuˌmaiəublæs'təumə] *n* 成横纹肌细胞瘤,横纹肌肉瘤
rhabdomyochondroma [ˌræbdəuˌmaiəukɔn'drəumə] *n* 横纹肌软骨瘤(良性间叶瘤)
rhabdomyolysis [ˌræbdəumai'ɔlisis] *n* 横纹肌溶解
rhabdomyoma [ˌræbdəumai'əumə] *n* 横纹肌瘤
rhabdomyomyxoma [ˌræbdəumaiəumik'səumə] *n* 横纹肌黏液瘤
rhabdomyosarcoma [ˌræbdəuˌmaiəusɑː'kəumə], **rhabdosarcoma** [ˌræbdəusɑː'kəumə] *n* 横纹肌肉瘤
Rhabdonema [ˌræbdəu'niːmə] *n* 小杆线虫属
rhabdos ['ræbdɔs] *n* 杆状体
rhabdosphincter [ˌræbdəu'sfiŋktə] *n* 横纹肌纤维括约肌
Rhabdoviridae [ˌræbdəu'viridiː] *n* 弹状病毒科
rhabdovirus ['ræbdəuˌvaiərəs] *n* 弹状病毒,棒状病毒
rhachi- 以 rhachi-起始的词,同样见以 rachi-起始的词
rhacoma [rei'kəumə] *n* 皮肤表皮脱落;阴囊下垂
rhaebocrania [ˌriːbə'kreinjə] *n* 斜颈
rhaeboscelia [ˌriːbə'siːliə] *n* 膝内翻(弓形腿);膝外翻
rhaebosis [riː'bəusis] *n* 弯曲(腿或任何直的部分的变弯)
rhagades ['rægədiːz] *n* 皲裂
rhagadiform [rei'gædifɔːm] *a* 皲裂状的
-rhage [构词成分]出血,流血;流出
rhagiocrine ['rædʒiəkrain] *a* 含胶体的(空泡)
rhagionid [ˌrædʒi'ɔnid] *n* 鹬虻
Rhagionidae [ˌrædʒi'ɔnidiː] *n* 鹬虻科
rhamninose ['ræmninəus] *n* 鼠李三糖
rhamnose ['ræmnəus] *n* 鼠李糖
rhamnoside ['ræmnəsaid] *n* 鼠李糖苷
rheotaxis [ˌriːə'tæksis] *n* 向流性 | negative ~ 负向流性(生物体的运动与液流的方向相同)/ positive ~ 正向流性(生物体的运动与液流的方向相反) | **rheotropism** [riː'ɔtrəpizəm] *n*
rheotome ['riːətəum] *n* 电流断续器,断流器
rheotrope ['riːətrəup] *n* 电流变向器
rhestocythemia [ˌrestəsai'θiːmiə] *n* 破裂红细胞血症
rhesus ['riːsəs] *n* 恒河猴,猕,罗猴
Rheum ['riːəm] *n* 大黄属
rheum [ruːm], **rheuma** ['ruːmə] *n* 稀黏液 | epidemic ~ 流行性感冒,流感
rheumapyra [ˌruːmə'paiərə] *n* 急性风湿病,风湿[性]热
rheumarthritis [ˌruːmɑː'θraitis] *n* 关节风湿病
rheumatic [ru(ː)'mætik] *a* (患)风湿病的,风湿性的 *n* 风湿病患者
rheumaticosis [ru(ː)ˌmæti'kəusis] *n* 小儿风湿状态
rheumatid ['ruːmətid] *n* 风湿疹
rheumatism ['ruːmətizəm] *n* 风湿病 | desert ~ 球孢子菌病 / gonorrheal ~ 淋病性风湿病(伴淋病性尿道炎,常产生关节强硬) / inflammatory ~ 炎性风湿病,风湿[性]热 / lumbar ~ 腰风湿病,腰痛 / muscular ~ 肌风湿病,纤维织炎 / nodose ~ 结节性风湿病,类风湿关节炎 / osseous ~ 骨风湿病,类风湿关节炎 / palindromic ~ 复发性风湿病(指关节炎及关节周炎一再发作) / tuberculous ~ 结核性风湿病(由于结核毒素所致) / visceral ~ 内脏风湿病(较常见的为心脏或心包)
rheumatismal [ˌruːmə'tizməl] *a* 风湿病的,风湿性的
rheumatocelis [ˌruːmətəu'kiːlis] *n* 风湿性紫癜
rheumatogenic [ˌruːmətəu'dʒenik] *a* 发生风湿的,致风湿病的
rheumatoid ['ruːmətɔid] *a* 风湿病样的,类风湿的
Rhamnus ['ræmnəs] *n* 鼠李属
Rh antiblody, blood group, factor (源于 Rhesus 恒河猴,1940 年在其血液中发现含有此因子)Rh 抗体,Rh 血型,Rh 因子(见 antibody, blood group 和 factor 项下相应术语)
rhaphania [rə'feiniə] *n* 野萝卜子中毒
rhaphe ['reifiː] *n* 缝[际]
-rhaphy [构词成分]缝合术
rheumatalgia [ˌruːmə'tældʒiə] *n* 风湿痛(慢性风湿性痛)
rhe [riː] *n* 流值(流度单位)
-rhea [构词成分] 溢出,流出
rhegma ['regmə] *n* 破裂,裂损;骨折
rhegmatogenous [ˌregmə'tɔdʒinəs] *a* 孔源性的

（如孔源性视网膜脱离）
rheic acid [ˈriːik] 大黄酸，大黄酚
Rhein's picks [rain]（M. L. Rhein）任氏牙签（在牙根管顶开孔及加宽用）
rhenium(Re) [ˈriːniəm] *n* 铼（化学元素）
rheo- [构词成分] 流，电流
rheobase [ˈriːəbeis] *n* 基强度（电流产生刺激作用所需的最小电位）| **rheobasic** [ˌriːəˈbeisik] *a*
rheocardiogram [ˌriːəˈkɑːdiəgræm] *n* 心电阻图
rheocardiography [ˌriːəuˌkɑːdiˈɔgrəfi] *n* 心电阻描记法
rheocord [ˈriːəkɔːd] *n* 变阻器
rheography [riːˈɔgrəfi] *n* 血流描记术
rheology [riːˈɔlədʒi] *n* 流变学，液流学（如研究血液在心脏和血管的流动）
rheometer [riːˈɔmitə] *n* 电流计；血流速度计
rheonome [ˈriːənəum] *n* 电流调节器；神经反应测定器
rheophore [ˈriːəfɔː] *n* 电极
rheoscope [ˈriːəskəup] *n* 检电器，验电器
rheostat [ˈriːəstæt] *n* 变阻器
rheostosis [ˌriːɔsˈtəusis] *n* 条纹状骨肥厚
rheotachygraphy [ˌriːətəˈkigrəfi] *n* 肌电波描记法
rheumatology [ˌruːməˈtɔlədʒi] *n* 风湿病学 | **rheumatologist** *n* 风湿病学家
rheumatopyra [ˌruːmətəuˈpaiərə] *n* 风湿[性]热
rheumatosis [ˌruːməˈtəusis] *n* 风湿病
rheumic [ˈruːmik] *a* 稀黏液的
rhexis [ˈreksis] *n* 破裂（器官或血管）
rhigosis [riˈgəusis] *n* 寒觉，冷觉 | **rhigotic** [riˈgɔtik] *a*
rhinal [ˈrainl] *a* 鼻的
rhinalgia [raiˈnældʒiə] *n* 鼻痛
rhinallergosis [ˌrainələˈgəusis] *n* 变应性鼻炎，过敏性鼻炎
rhinedema [ˌraini(ː)ˈdiːmə] *n* 鼻水肿
rhinencephalia [ˌrainensiˈfeiliə] *n* 喙状鼻[畸形]
rhinencephalon [ˌrainenˈsefəlɔn] *n* 嗅脑
rhinencephalus [ˌrainenˈsefələs] *n* 喙状鼻畸胎
rhinenchysis [raiˈnenkisis] *n* 鼻内注射
rhinesthesia [ˌrainisˈθiːzjə] *n* 嗅觉
rhineurynter [ˌrinjuˈrintə] *n* 鼻孔扩张器
Rhinocladiella [ˌrainəuˌklædiˈeilə] *n* 鼻毛癣菌属
rhinion [ˈrinjən] *n* 鼻缝点，下鼻点
rhinism [ˈrainizəm] *n* 鼻音
rhinitis [raiˈnaitis] *n* 鼻炎 | acute catarrhal ～ 急性卡他性鼻炎 / allergic ～, anaphylactic ～ 变应性鼻炎，过敏性鼻炎 / dyscrinic ～ 内分泌失调性鼻炎 / fibrinous ～, croupous ～ 纤维蛋白性鼻炎，格鲁布性鼻炎 / nonseasonal allergic ～, atopic ～, perennial ～ 非季节性变应性鼻炎，特应性鼻炎，常年性鼻炎 / ～ sicca 干燥性鼻炎 / tuberculous ～, scrofulous ～ 结核性鼻炎，腺病性鼻炎
rhin(o)- [构词成分] 鼻
rhinoanemometer [ˌrainəuˌæniˈmɔmitə] *n* 鼻气流计
rhinoantritis [ˌrainəuænˈtraitis] *n* 鼻上颌窦炎
rhinobyon [raiˈnəubiɔn] *n* 鼻塞[子]
rhinocanthectomy [ˌrainəukænˈθektəmi] *n* 内眦切除术
rhinocele [ˈrainəsiːl] *n* 嗅叶腔
rhinocephalus [ˌrainəuˈsefələs] *n* 喙状鼻畸胎
Rhinocephalus annulatus [ˌrainəuˈsefələs ˌænjuˈleitəs] 具环牛蜱（即 Boophilus annulatus）
rhinocephaly [ˌrainəuˈsefəli] *n* 喙状鼻[畸形]
rhinocheiloplasty [ˌrainəuˈkailəˌplæsti] *n* 鼻唇成形术
rhinocleisis [ˌrainəuˈklaisis] *n* 鼻塞，鼻堵
rhinocoele [ˈrainəsiːl] *n* 嗅叶腔
rhinodacryolith [ˌrainəuˈdækriəˌliθ] *n* 鼻泪管石
rhinodynia [ˌrainəuˈdiniə] *n* 鼻痛
rhinoentomophthoromycosis [ˌrainəuˈentəˌmɔfθərəumaiˈkəusis] *n* 鼻藻菌病
Rhinoestrus [raiˈnestrəs] *n* 鼻狂蝇属
rhinogenous [raiˈnɔdʒinəs] *a* 鼻原的，鼻性的
rhinokyphosis [ˌrainəukaiˈfəusis] *n* 鼻后凸
rhinolalia [ˌrainəuˈleiliə] *n* 鼻音 | ～ aperta, open ～ 开放性鼻音 / ～ clausa 闭合性鼻音
rhinolaryngitis [ˌrainəuˌlærinˈdʒaitis] *n* 鼻喉炎
rhinolaryngology [ˌrainəuˌlæriŋˈgɔlədʒi] *n* 鼻喉科学 | **rhinolaryngologist** *n* 鼻喉科学家，鼻喉科医生
rhinolith [ˈrainəliθ] *n* 鼻石
rhinolithiasis [ˌrainəuliˈθaiəsis] *n* 鼻石症
rhinology [raiˈnɔlədʒi] *n* 鼻科学 | **rhinologist** *n* 鼻科学家，鼻科医生
rhinomanometer [ˌrainəuməˈnɔmitə] *n* 鼻[塞测]压计
rhinomanometry [ˌrainəuməˈnɔmitri] *n* 鼻腔测压[法]
rhinometer [raiˈnɔmitə] *n* 鼻腔计，量鼻器
rhinommectomy [ˌrainɔˈmektəmi] *n* 内眦切除术
rhinomycosis [ˌrainəumaiˈkəusis] *n* 鼻真菌病
rhinonecrosis [ˌrainəuneˈkrəusis] *n* 鼻坏死
rhinonemmeter [ˌrainəuˈnemitə] *n* 鼻气流计
rhinoneurosis [ˌrainəunjuəˈrəusis] *n* 鼻神经官能病
rhinopathy [raiˈnɔpəθi], **rhinopathia** [ˌrainəuˈpæθiə] *n* 鼻病
rhinopharyngeal [ˌrainəufəˈrindʒiəl] *a* 鼻咽的
rhinopharyngitis [ˌrainəuˌfærinˈdʒaitis] *n* 鼻咽炎

| ~ mutilans 毁形性鼻咽炎

rhinopharyngocele [ˌrainəufəˌriŋgəsiːl] *n* 鼻咽[气]瘤,鼻咽[气]囊肿

rhinopharyngolith [ˌrainəufəˈriŋgəliθ] *n* 鼻咽石

rhinopharynx [ˌrainəuˈfæriŋks] *n* 鼻咽

rhinophonia [ˌrainəˈfəuniə] *n* 鼻音

rhinophore [ˈrainəfɔː] *n* 鼻通气管

rhinophycomycosis [ˌrainəuˌfaikəumaiˈkəusis] *n* 鼻藻菌病

rhinophyma [ˌrainəˈfaimə] *n* 肥大性酒渣鼻,鼻赘

rhinoplasty [ˈrainəˌplæsti] *n* 鼻成形术 | English ~ 英国式鼻成形术(颊部皮瓣鼻成形术) / Indian ~ 印度式鼻成形术(额部皮瓣鼻成形术) / Italian ~, tagliacotian ~ 意大利式鼻成形术(臂部皮瓣鼻成形术) | **rhinoplastic** [ˌrainəˈplæstik] *a*

rhinopneumonitis [ˌrainəuˌnjuːməuˈnaitis] *n* 鼻肺炎

rhinopolypus [ˌrainəuˈpɔlipəs] *n* 鼻息肉

rhinoptia [raiˈnɔpʃiə] *n* 内斜视

rhinoreaction [ˌrainəuri(ː)ˈækʃən] *n* 鼻反应(鼻内结核菌素反应,鼻黏膜在涂滴结核菌素后,结核患者鼻黏膜出现渗出液反应)

rhinorrhagia [ˌrainəˈreidʒiə] *n* 鼻出血

rhinorrhaphy [raiˈnɔrəfi] *n* 鼻缝合术

rhinorrhea [rainəˈriːə] *n* 鼻漏

rhinosalpingitis [ˌrainəusælpinˈdʒaitis] *n* 鼻咽鼓管炎

rhinoscleroma [ˌrainəuskliəˈrəumə] *n* 鼻硬结病

rhinoscope [ˈrainəskəup] *n* 鼻镜 | **rhinoscopic** [ˌrainəˈskɔpik] *a* 鼻镜检查的 / **rhinoscopy** [raiˈnɔskəpi] *n* 鼻镜检查[法]

rhinosinusitis [ˌrainəuˌsainəˈsaitis] *n* 鼻鼻窦炎,鼻窦炎

rhinosporidiosis [ˌrainəuspəˌridiˈəusis] *n* 鼻孢子菌病

Rhinosporidium [ˌrainəuspəˈridjəm] *n* 鼻孢子菌属 | ~ seeberi 西[伯]氏鼻孢子菌

rhinostegnosis [ˌrainəustegˈnəusis] *n* 鼻塞,鼻堵

rhinostenosis [ˌrainəustiˈnəusis] *n* 鼻道狭窄

rhinotomy [raiˈnɔtəmi] *n* 鼻切开术

rhinotracheitis [ˌrainəuˌtreikiˈaitis] *n* 鼻气管炎

rhinovaccination [ˌrainəuˌvæksiˈneiʃən] *n* 鼻接种(将疫苗或其他免疫制剂接种至鼻黏膜处)

Rhinovirus [ˈrainəuˌvaiərəs] *n* 鼻病毒属

rhinovirus [ˈrainəuˌvaiərəs] *n* 鼻病毒 | **rhinoviral** [ˌrainəuˈvaiərəl] *a*

rhiotin [ˈraiətin] *n* 根瘤菌生物素

Rhipicentor [ˌraipiˈsentə] *n* 扇革蜱属

Rhipicephalus [ˌraipiˈsefələs] *n* 扇头蜱属 | ~ appendicularis 具尾扇头蜱 / ~ bursa 囊状扇头蜱 / ~ capensis 好望角扇头蜱 / ~ decoloratus 脱色扇头蜱 / ~ sanguineus 血红扇头蜱 / ~ simus 拟态扇头蜱

rhitid(o)- 以 rhitid(o)-起始的词,同样见以 rhytid(o)-起始的词

rhizagra [raiˈzægrə] *n* 牙根钳(古代拔牙根用)

rhizanesthesia [raiˈzænisˈθiːzjə] *n* 神经根麻醉

rhiz(o)- [构词成分]根

Rhizobiaceae [raiˈzəubiˈeisiiː] *n* 根瘤菌科

Rhizobium [raiˈzəubiəm] *n* 根瘤菌属

rhizoblast [ˈraizəublæst] *n* 鞭毛根,生毛体

Rhizoctonia [raizɔkˈtəuniə] *n* 丝核菌属

rhizodontropy [ˌraizəuˈdɔntrəpi] *n* 牙根转动术;牙根冠固定术

rhizodontrypy [ˌraizəuˈdɔntripi] *n* 牙根钻孔术

Rhizoglyphus [raiˈzɔglifəs] *n* 根嗜螨属 | ~ parasiticus 寄生根嗜螨

rhizoid [ˈraizɔid] *a* 根样的 *n* 假根 | **~al** [raiˈzɔidl] *a* 根样的

rhizolysis [raiˈzɔlisis] *n* 经皮射频脊神经根切断术

Rhizomastigida [ˌraizəumæsˈtidʒidə] *n* 变形鞭毛目

rhizome [ˈraizəum] *n* 根茎

rhizomelic [raizəuˈmelik] *a* 肢根的(髋与肩的)

rhizomeningomyelitis [ˌraizəuməˌniŋgəumaiəˈlaitis] *n* 脊髓脊膜脊神经根炎

Rhizomucor [ˌraizəuˈmjuːkə] *n* 根毛霉菌属

rhizoneure [ˈraizənjuə] *n* 神经根细胞

rhizoplast [ˈraizəplæst] *n* 根丝体

Rhizopoda [raiˈzɔpədə] *n* 根足[虫]亚纲

rhizopodium [ˌraizəuˈpəudiəm] ([复] **rhizopodia** [ˌraizəuˈpəudiə]) *n* 根状假足

Rhizopus [raiˈzəupəs] *n* 根霉菌属,酒曲菌属

rhizotomist [raiˈzɔtəmist] *n* 采药者

rhizotomy [raiˈzɔtəmi] *n* 脊神经根切断术 | anterior ~ 脊神经前根切断术 / posterior ~ 脊神经后根切断术

rho [rəu] *n* 希腊语的第 17 个字母(Ρ, ρ)

rhodamine [ˈrəudəmiːn] *n* 若丹明,碱性蕊香红(一种红色荧光染料)

rhodanate [ˈrəudəneit] *n* 硫氰酸盐

rhodanic acid [rəuˈdænik] 硫氰酸

rhodanine [ˈrəudəniːn] *n* 硫氰酸

rhodium(Rh) [ˈrəudjəm] *n* 铑(化学元素)

Rhodnius prolixus [ˈrɔdniəs prəˈliksəs] 长红猎蝽

rhod(o)- [构词成分]蔷薇,玫瑰,红

Rhodobacteriineae [ˌrəudəuˌbæktəriˈainiiː] *n* 红色细菌亚目

Rhodococcus [ˌrəudəuˈkɔkəs] *n* 红球菌属

rhodocyte [ˈrəudəsait] *n* 红细胞

Rhododendron [ˌrəudəˈdendrən] *n* 杜鹃花属

rhodogenesis [ˌrəudəuˈdʒenisis] *n* 视紫质生成
Rhodomicrobium [ˌrəudəumaiˈkrəubjəm] *n* 蔷薇色丝状菌属
rhodophane [ˈrəudəfein] *n* 视红质(鸟类和鱼类的视网膜锥体的红色素)
rhodophylaxis [ˌrəudəu faiˈlæksis] *n* 视紫质保护性 | **rhodophylactic** *a* 保护视紫质的
rhodoporphyrin [ˌrəudəˈpɔːfirin] *n* 玫红卟啉
Rhodopseudomonas [ˌrəudəuˌpsjuːdəuˈməunəs] *n* 红假单胞菌属
rhodopsin [rəuˈdɔpsin] *n* 视紫质,视紫红质,视紫素
rhodopsin kinase [rəuˈdɔpsin ˈkaineis] 视紫红激酶
Rhodospirillaceae [ˌrəudəuˌspaiəriˈleisiiː] *n* 红螺菌科
Rhodospirillales [ˌrəudəuˌspaiəriˈleiliːz] *n* 红螺菌目
Rhodospirillum [ˌrəudəu spaiəˈriləm] *n* 红螺菌属
Rhodothece [ˌrəudəˈθiːsi] *n* 红鞘硫细菌属
Rhodotorula [ˌrəudəˈtɔrulə] *n* 红酵母菌属 | ~ glutinis 胶红酵母菌 / ~ rubra 深红酵母菌
rhodotoxin [ˌrəudəˈtɔksin] *n* 杜鹃毒素
rhomb [rɔm] *n* 菱形,斜方形
rhombencephalon [ˌrɔmbenˈsefələn] *n* 菱脑
rhombocoele [ˈrɔmbəsiːl] *n* 脊髓终室
rhomboid [ˈrɔmbɔid] *n* 菱形,菱形体 *a* 菱形的
rhombomere [ˈrɔmbəumiə] *n* 菱脑原节
Rhombomys [ˈrɔmbəumis] *n* 大沙鼠属
rhonchus [ˈrɔŋkəs] *n*【拉】干啰音 | **rhonchal**, **rhonchial** *a*
Rhopalopsyllus [ˌrəupələuˈsiləs] *n* 棒状蚤属
Rhopalopsyllus cavicola [ˌrəupələˈsiləs kəˈvikələ] 洞蚤
rhoptry [ˈrɔptri] *n* 棒状体
rhotacism [ˈrəutəsizəm] *n* r 音化(亦称 r 发音不正)
rhotanium [rəuˈteinjəm] *n* 金钯合金
rhubarb [ˈruːbɑːb] *n* 大黄(用于流浸膏剂或芳香酊,用作泻药)
r-HuEPO recombinant human erythropoietin 重组人红细胞生成素
Rhus [rʌs] *n* 漆树属
rhus [rʌs] *n* 漆树
Rhynchocoela [ˌrainkəˈsiːlə] *n* 纽形动物门
rhynchocoelan [ˌrainkəˈsiːlən] *n* 纽虫,纽形动物
Rhynchodea [rinˈkəudiə] *n* 吻毛总目
Rhynchodida [rinˈkəudidə] *n* 吻毛目
rhyostomaturia [ˌraiəuˌstəuməˈtjuəriə] *n* 尿性涎症
rhyparia [raiˈpeəriə] *n*【希】口垢,污物
rhythm [ˈriðəm] *n* 节律 | alpha ~ α 节律(脑电波) / beta ~ β 节律(脑电波) / biological ~ 生物节律 / circadian ~ 昼夜节律 / circus ~ 环转节律 / coupled ~ 二联律 / delta ~ δ 节律(脑电波) / ectopic ~ 异位节律 / escape ~ 逸搏心律 / fetal ~ 胎心节律,胎样心音 / gallop ~, cantering ~ 奔马律 / idioventricular ~ 心室自主心律 / infradian ~ 超昼夜节律 / isochronal ~ 等时节律 / metachronal ~ 异时节律 / nodal ~, atrioventricular ~ 结性心律,房室心律 / nyctohemeral ~ 昼夜性节律 / pendulum ~ 钟摆状节律 / reciprocal ~ 折返心律 / sinus ~ 窦性心律 / theta ~(脑电波)θ 节律 / triple ~ 三音律 / ultradian ~ 次昼夜节律 | **~ic(al)** [ˈriðmik(əl)] *a*
rhythmeur [riðˈməː] *n* 火花线圈(使 X 线机中的电流产生节律性中断)
rhythmicity [riðˈmisəti] *n* 节律性
rhythmotherapy [ˌriðməuˈθerəpi] *n* 节律疗法(如以节拍治口吃)
rhytid [ˈraitid]([复] **rhytides** [ˈraitidiːs]) *n* 皱纹
rhytidectomy [ˌritiˈdektəmi] *n* 除皱术(切除皮肤以消除皱纹)
rhytidoplasty [ˈritidəˌplæsti] *n* 皱纹切除术(消除皮肤皱纹)
rhytidosis [ˌritiˈdəusis] *n* 角膜皱缩(濒死现象)
rib [rib] *n* 肋[骨] | false ~s, abdominal ~s, asternal ~s, spurious ~s 假肋,腹肋,弓肋 / floating ~s, vertebral ~s 浮肋,浮动弓肋,椎肋 / true ~s, sternal ~s, vertebrosternal ~s 真肋,胸骨肋,椎胸肋 / vertebrocostal ~s 椎弓肋(两侧上三个假肋)
ribaminol [raiˈbæminəul] *n* 利巴米诺(记忆辅药)
ribavirin [ˌraibəˈvaiərin] *n* 利巴韦林(抗病毒药)
Ribbert's theory [ˈribət] (Moritz W. H. Ribbert) 里贝特学说(肿瘤系由残留细胞发育而成,因周围组织张力减少所致)
ribbon [ˈribən] *n* 带,系带,带状物,带状构造 | synaptic ~ 突触带
Ribes's ganglion [riːb] (François Ribes) 里伯神经节(大脑前交通动脉神经丛)
ribitol [ˈraibitɔl] *n* 核[糖]醇
ribodesose [raiˈbəudisəus] *n* 脱氧核糖
riboflavin [ˌraibəuˈfleivin] *n* 核黄素,维生素 B_2 | ~ -5′-phosphate 核黄素-5′-磷酸,黄素单核苷酸
riboflavin kinase [ˌraibəuˈfleivin ˈkaineis] 核黄素激酶
ribonic acid [raiˈbɔnik] 核糖酸
ribonuclease [ˌraibəuˈnjuːklieis] *n* 核糖核酸酶 | ~ Ⅰ 核糖核酸酶Ⅰ,胰核糖核酸酶(亦称 RNase, RNase I 和 RNase A)
ribonucleic acid (RNA) [ˌraibəunjuːˈkliːik] 核

糖核酸 | heterogenous nuclear RNA (hnRNA) 不均一核 RNA,核不均一 RNA / messenger RNA (mRNA) 信使 RNA / ribosomal RNA (rRNA) 核蛋白体 RNA,核糖体 RNA / transfer RNA (tRNA) 转移 RNA

ribonucleoprotein (RNP) [ˌraibəuˌnjuːkliəuˈprəutiːn] *n* 核糖核蛋白

ribonucleoside [ˌraibəuˈnjuːkliəsaid] *n* 核[糖核]苷

ribonucleoside diphosphate reductase [ˌraibəuˈnjuːkliəsaid daiˈfɔsfeit riˈdʌkteis] 核[糖核]苷二磷酸还原酶(亦称核糖核苷酸还原酶)

ribonucleotide [ˌraibəuˈnjuːkliətaid] *n* 核[糖核]苷酸

ribonucleotide reductase [ˌraibəuˈnjuːkliətaid riˈdʌkteis] 核[糖核]苷酸还原酶,核[糖核]苷二磷酸还原酶

riboprine [ˈraibəupriːn] *n* 利波腺苷(抗肿瘤药)

ribopyranose [ˌraibəuˈpaiərənəus, -ˈpirə-] *n* 吡喃核糖

ribose [ˈraibəus] *n* 核糖

ribose nucleic acid [ˈraibəus njuːˈkliːik] 核糖核酸

ribose-5-phosphate isomerase [ˈraibəus ˈfɔsfeit aiˈsɔməreis] 核糖-5-磷酸异构酶

ribose-phosphate pyrophosphokinase [ˈraibəus ˈfɔsfeit ˌpaiərəuˌfɔsfəˈkaineis] 核糖磷酸焦磷酸激酶(此酶活性增强为一种 X 连锁隐性性状,可导致嘌呤合成不断增加,并引起原发性痛风。亦称磷酸核糖焦磷酸合成酶)

ribosome [ˈraibəsəum] *n* 核[糖核]蛋白体,核糖体

ribosyl [ˈraibəsil] *n* 核糖基

5-ribosyluracil [ˌraibəsilˈjuərəsil] *n* 5′-尿苷,假尿[嘧啶核]苷

ribothymidine [ˌribəuˈθaimidiːn] *n* 胸腺嘧啶核糖核苷,胸苷

Ribot's law [riːˈbəu] (T. Ribot) 里博定律(此定律说明,一个能操多种语言的失语症患者首先恢复的是患者的母语,只有在本人以后学得的一种或多种语言不十分流利的情况下,才是正确的。同样见 Pitres' law)

ribovirus [ˈraibəuˌvaiərəs] *n* 核糖核酸病毒,RNA 病毒

ribulose [ˈraibjuləus] *n* 核酮糖

ribulose-phosphate 3-epimerase [ˈraibjuləus ˈfɔsfeit iˈpiməreis] 核酮糖-磷酸 3-差向异构酶

RIC Royal Institute of Chemistry 皇家化学学会

rice [rais] [单复同] *n* 米 | ~ polishings 米糠 / white ~ 精白米

Richardson's sign [ˈritʃədsn] (Benjamin W. Richardson) 理查森征(用止血带绑紧手臂,则其末梢部静脉渐次怒张,但死亡时则否)

Richards-Rundle syndrome [ˈritʃədz ˈrʌndəl] (B. W. Richards; A. T. Rundle) 里-伦综合征(一种先天性综合征,包括酮酸尿、智力迟钝、第二性征发育低下、耳聋、共济失调和外周性肌肉消瘦,此种消瘦在儿童期为进行性的,但最终会停止)

Richet's aneurysm [riˈʃei] (Didier D. A. Richet) 里歇动脉瘤(梭形动脉瘤)

Richner-Hanhart syndrome [ˈriknə ˈhænhɑːt] (Hermann Richner; Ernst Hanhart) 里-汉综合征,酪氨酸血症 Ⅱ 型

Richter-Monro line [ˈriʃtə mənˈrəu] 里希特-门罗线(见 Monro-Richter line)

Richter's hernia [ˈriʃtə, ˈriʃtə] (August G. Richter) 里希特疝(肠管仅一侧肠壁脱出,亦称肠壁疝)

Richter's syndrome [ˈriktə] (Maurice N. Richter) 里克特综合征(慢性淋巴细胞白血病伴弥漫性组织细胞性淋巴瘤)

ricin [ˈraisin] *n* 蓖麻毒蛋白

ricinism [ˈraisinizəm] *n* 蓖麻子中毒

ricinoleic acid [ˌraisinəuˈliːik] 蓖麻油酸,12-羟[基]油酸

Ricinus [ˈrisinəs] *n* 蓖麻属

rickets [ˈrikits] [复] *n* 佝偻病 | acute ~ 急性佝偻病,婴儿坏血病 / fat ~ 肥胖性佝偻病 / fetal ~ 胎性佝偻病,软骨发育不全 / hemorrhagic ~ 出血性佝偻病,婴儿坏血病 / hepatic ~ 肝病性佝偻病 / late ~, tardy ~ 迟发佝偻病 / renal ~ 肾性佝偻病 / vitamin D-resistant ~, pseudodeficiency ~, refractory ~, vitamin D-refractory ~ 抗维生素 D 佝偻病,假缺乏性佝偻病,难治性佝偻病,维生素 D 难治性佝偻病

rickettsemia [ˌrikeˈtsiːmiə] *n* 立克次体血症

Rickettsia [riˈketsiə] (Howard T. Ricketts) 立克次体属 | ~ akari 螨立克次体 / ~ australis 澳立克次体 / ~ burnetii, ~ diaporica 伯纳特立克次体(即 Coxiella burnetii) / ~ canis 犬立克次体 / ~ conorii 康诺尔立克次体 / ~ prowazekii 普氏立克次体 / ~ quintana, ~ pediculi, ~ wolhynica 五日热立克次体,体虱型立克次体,伏尔希尼地方立克次体 / ~ rickettsii 立氏立克次体 / ~ sennetsu 森纳苏立克次体 / ~ siberica, ~ sibericus 西伯利亚立克次体 / ~ tsutsugamushi, ~ akamushi, ~ nipponica, ~ orientalis 恙虫热立克次体,东方立克次体 / ~ typhi, ~ mooseri, ~ muricola 地方性斑疹伤寒立克次体,莫塞尔立克次体,鼠型立克次体

rickettsia [riˈketsiə] ([复] **rickettsias** 或 **rickettsiae** [riˈketsiiː]) *n* 立克次体 | **~l** *a*

Rickettsiaceae [riˌketsiˈeisiiː] *n* 立克次体科

Rickettsiae [riˈketsiiː] *n* 立克次体族

Rickettsiales [riˌketsiˈeiliːz] *n* 立克次体目

rickettsialpox [ri'ketsiəlˌpɔks] *n* 立克次体痘
rickettsicidal [riˌketsi'saidl] *a* 杀立克次体的
Rickettsieae [ˌriket'saiiː] *n* 立克次体族
Rickettsiella [riˌketsi'elə] *n* 小立克次体属
rickettsiosis [riˌketsi'əusis] *n* 立克次体病 | canine ~ 犬立克次体病 / chigger-borne ~ 沙螨(立克次体)热
rickettsiostatic [riˌketsiəu'stætik] *a* 抑制立克次体的
rickety ['rikiti] *a* 佝偻病的
Ricolesia [ˌraikəu'liːziə] (*Ri*ckettsia + J. D. W. A. *Coles*) *n* 立柯体属(衣原体科的一属)
rictus ['riktəs] *n*【拉】裂,裂口 | **rictal** *a* 裂的
RID radial immunodiffusion 辐射状免疫扩散
Riddoch's mass reflex ['ridɔk] (George Riddoch) 里多克总体反射(在脊髓剧烈外伤时,刺激伤处以下,引起下肢的屈曲反射、肠和膀胱排空和伤处以下的皮肤出汗)
Rideal-Walker coefficient ['ridiəl 'wɔːkə] (Samuel Rideal; J. F. A Walker) 石炭酸系数(用以表示某化合物杀菌力的方法)
ridge [ridʒ] *n* 嵴,脊;棱线 | basal ~ 舌面嵴(牙冠背面嵴) / bulbar ~s 心球嵴 / deltoid ~ 三角肌嵴,三角肌粗隆 / genital ~, germ ~ 生殖[腺]嵴 / mammary ~, milk ~ 乳腺嵴 / mylohyoid ~ 颌舌嵴,颌舌[骨]线 / superciliary ~, supraorbital ~ 眉嵴,眉弓 / taste ~s 味觉嵴,舌叶状乳头
ridging ['ridʒiŋ] *n* 脊皱(在整形外科中指手术平整区边缘可见的线或嵴)
ridgling ['ridʒliŋ], **ridgel** ['ridʒəl] *n* 单睾丸动物
ridgy ['ridʒi] *a* 有脊的,隆起的
Ridley's sinus ['ridli] (Humphrey Ridley) 环状窦
Riechert-Mundinger apparatus [ri'kəːt 'muːndiŋgə] (T. Riechert; F. Mundinger) 里-蒙器(用于里-蒙立体定位外科手术) | ~ technique 里-蒙技术(一种立体定位技术,使用一个半圆形弧导装置和一个环,以保持头部定位)
Riedel's lobe ['riːdəl] (Bernhard M. C. L. Riedel) 里德尔叶(肝附垂叶,即附于肝右叶肝的舌形部分) | ~ struma (disease, thyroiditis) 里德尔甲状腺肿(病、甲状腺炎)(一种慢性增生性纤维化炎症性过程,通常累及甲状腺一叶,有时为两叶,且波及邻近的气管及其肌肉、筋膜、神经、血管等。亦称板样甲状腺炎)
Rieder's cells ['riːdə] (Hermann Rieder) 里德尔细胞(一种原粒细胞,见于急性白血病患者) | ~ cell leukemia 里德尔细胞白血病(原粒细胞白血病的一型) / ~ lymphocyte 里德尔淋巴细胞(有核的淋巴细胞,其细胞核分叶而且扭转,见于慢性淋巴细胞白血病)
Riegel's pulse ['riːgəl] (Franz Riegel) 里格尔脉搏(呼气时脉搏变小)
Rieger's anomaly ['riːgə] (Herwigh Rieger) 里格异常(见里格综合征) | ~ syndrome 里格综合征(牙发育不全、肛门狭窄、器官距离过远、智力缺陷及面骨发育不全)
Riegler's test ['riːglə] (Emanuel Riegler) 里格勒试验(检尿白蛋白、胃液游离盐酸、尿葡萄糖)
Riehl's melanosis [riːl] (Gustav Riehl) 里尔黑变病(面部皮肤色素沉着,表现为皮肤痒、发红、脱屑及点状棕色沉着)
Riesman's pneumonia ['riːsmən] (David Riesman) 里斯曼肺炎(特殊型慢性支气管肺炎) | ~ sign 里斯曼征(①突眼性甲状腺肿时,用听诊器放在闭合的眼上可听到一种杂音;②糖尿病昏迷时眼球软化)
Rieux's hernia [ri'əː] (Léon Rieux) 盲肠后疝
RIF right iliac fossa 右髂窝
rifamide ['rifəmaid] *n* 利福米特(抗菌性抗生素)
rifampin ['rifəmpin], **rifampicin** ['rifəmpisin] *n* 利福平(抗生素类药)
rifamycin [ˌrifə'maisin] *n* 利福霉素(抗生素类药)
rifapentine [ˌrifə'pentiːn] *n* 利福喷汀(一种合成的利福霉素〈rifamycin〉抗生素,与其他抗结核药物结合使用,治疗肺结核,口服给药)
rifomycin [ˌrifə'maisin] *n* 利福霉素(rifamycin 的旧称)
Rift Valley fever [rift 'væli] 裂谷热(布雅病毒〈bunyavirus〉所致家畜〈如羊、牛〉和人的急性发热性感染,1915 年首次见于肯尼亚的裂谷,现遍及南非、东非至埃及)
Riga disease, Riga-Fede disease ['rigə 'feidei] (Antonio Riga; Francesco Fede) 里加病,里加-费代病(小儿舌系带肉芽肿,发生于下中央门牙擦伤后引起,亦称恶病质性口疮)
right-handed ['rait 'hændid] *a* 善用右手的,右利的 *ad* 用右手
rigidity [di'dʒidəti] *n* 强直 | anatomical ~ (分娩时子宫颈)非病理性强直 / cadaveric ~, postmortem ~ 死后强直,尸僵 / clasp-knife ~ 折刀样强直(伸肌抗力增加) / cogwheel ~ 齿轮样强直 / decerebrate ~ 去大脑强直,去大脑僵直 / lead-pipe ~ 铅管样强直 / muscle ~, muscular ~ 肌强直 / pathologic ~ (分娩时子宫颈)病理性强直 / spasmodic ~ (子宫颈)痉挛性强直
Riggs disease [rigz] (John M. Riggs) 边缘性牙周炎
rigor ['raigɔː, 'rigə] *n*【拉】寒战,发冷;强直,僵直 | acid ~ 酸僵,酸性肌强直 / heat ~ 热僵 / ~ mortis 尸僵,死后强直 / ~ nervorum 破伤风 / ~ tremens 震颤麻痹 / water ~ 水僵,水性肌强直

Riley-Day syndrome [ˈraili dei] (Conrad Milton Riley; Richard Lawrence Day) 赖利-戴综合征(即家族性自主神经功能异常 dysautonomia)

Riley-Smith syndrome [ˈraili smiθ] (H. D. Riley, Jr.; W. R. Smith) 赖利-史密斯综合征(巨头畸形但无脑积水,多发性血管瘤及假视神经乳头水肿,推测为常染色体显性遗传)

riluzole [ˈriljuzəul] *n* 利鲁唑(用于治疗肌萎缩侧索硬化的一种化合物,可延长存活时间,但不能增强肌力或改进神经功能)

rim [rim] *n* 边,缘 | bite ~, occlusion ~, record ~ 殆堤,殆缘

rima [ˈraimə] ([复] **rimae** [ˈraimiː]) *n*【拉】裂 | intercartilaginous ~ 软骨间裂,呼吸裂(声门裂软骨间部) / intermembranous ~ 膜间裂,声带裂(声门裂膜间部) | **~l** *a*

rimantadine hydrochloride [raiˈmæntədiːn] 盐酸金刚乙胺(抗病毒药,用于预防 A 型流感)

rimiterol hydrobromide [ˌrimiˈterəul] 氢溴酸利米特罗(拟肾上腺素药,用作支气管扩张药)

rimose [ˈraiməus], **rimous** [ˈraiməs] *a* 有皲裂的

rimula [ˈrimjulə] ([复] **rimulae** [ˈrimjuliː]) *n* 小裂(尤指脊髓或脑)

RIND reversible ischemic neurologic deficit 可逆性缺血性神经障碍

rinderpest [ˈrindəpest] *n* 牛疫,牛瘟

Rindfleisch's cells [ˌrintˈflaiʃi] (Georg E. Rindfleisch) 嗜酸细胞 | ~ folds 林德弗莱施褶(环绕主动脉开口,心包浆膜面的皱襞)

ring [riŋ] *n* 环,圈,环状物 | annular ~s, pleural ~s 环状阴影,胸膜环(X 线片所显环状影,表示肺结核空洞) / atrial ~ 心房环 / carbocyclic ~ 一碳环(环状化合物中只含一个碳原子) / cardiac lymphatic ~ 心淋巴管环 / constriction ~, contraction ~ 痉挛性狭窄环 / contact ~ 接触环(枪弹伤入口) / esophageal ~ 食管环 / homocyclic ~, isocyclic ~ 同素环;碳环 / periosteal bone ~ 骨周骨环 / polar ~ 极环 / signet ~ 环状体(疟原虫) / supermitral ~ 二尖瓣上环

ring-bone [ˈriŋ bəun] *n* 骹骨赘(马的外生骨疣) | low ~ 低位骹骨赘,锥突部骨炎(马)

Ringer's injection [ˈriŋə] (Sydney Ringer) 林格注射液(注射用的氯化钠、氯化钾和氯化钙无菌水溶液,用作电解质及水分的补充) | ~ lactated injection 乳酸盐林格注射液(注射用的氯化钙、氯化钾、氯化钠及乳酸钠无菌水溶液,用作电解质及水分的补充) / ~ solution (mixture) 林格[溶]液(合剂)(每 100 ml 含 820 ~ 900 mg 氯化钠、25 ~ 35 mg 氯化钾、30 ~ 36 mg 氯化钙及新沸纯净水,用作局部生理盐液)

Ringschwiele [ˈriŋʃviːlə] *n*【德】环状斑块

ringworm [ˈriŋwəːm] *n* 癣,癣菌病 | ~ of the beard 须癣 / ~ of the body 体癣 / ~ of feet 脚癣,皮真菌病 / ~ of groin 股癣 / ~ of the nails 甲癣,甲真菌病 / ~ of the scalp 发癣

Rinne's test [ˈrinə] (Heinrich A. Rinne) 林纳试验(气、骨导对比试验)

Riolan's anastomosis [ˌriəˈlɑːŋ] (Jean Riolan) 里奥郎吻合(肠系膜上动脉和肠系膜下动脉吻合) | ~ arch 里奥郎弓(横结肠肠系膜弓) / ~ bones 里奥郎骨(枕骨、颞骨岩部缝间小骨) / ~ muscle 里奥郎肌(①眼轮匝肌睫部;②睾提肌) / ~ nosegay 里奥郎束(起自颞骨茎突的肌肉束) / ~ ossicle 里奥郎小骨(枕骨颞骨乳突部缝间小骨)

riomitsin [ˌraiəˈmitsin] *n* 氧四环素,土霉素

rip [rip] *n* 裂口,裂缝

RIPA radioimmunoprecipitation assay 放射免疫沉淀测定

riparian [raiˈpɛəriən] *a* 缘的;丘脑带的

Ripault's sign [riˈpəu] (Louis H. A. Ripault) 里波征(活时压眼,瞳孔暂时改变,死后压眼,则永久改变)

ripazepam [riˈpæzəpæm] *n* 利帕西泮(弱安定药)

RIPHH Royal Institute of Public Health and Hygiene 皇家公共卫生和卫生学协会

risedronate sodium [riˈsedrəˌneit] 利塞膦酸钠(一种骨吸收的二磷酸盐抑制剂,用于预防和治疗骨质疏松,并治疗畸形性骨炎,口服给药)

risk [risk] *n* 危险,风险;危险率,危险度 | anesthesia ~ 麻醉危险性 / attributable ~ 属性危险度(接触某危险因子的群体中某病的发生率与未接触的群体中该病发生率之间的算术差) / empiric ~ 经验风险(仅根据经验而非其成因机制的有关知识决定某性状在某家族中发生或复发的概率) / genetic ~ 遗传危险率(根据遗传传递模式有关知识决定某性状在某家族中发生或复发的概率) / relative ~ 相对危险度(接触某特定危险因子的群体中某病的发生率与未接触的群体中该病发生率之比)

risperidone [risˈperidəun] *n* 利培酮(抗精神病药)

Risley's prism [ˈrizli] (Samuel D. Risley) 里斯利棱镜(用于测量眼肌不平衡现象)

risocaine [ˈraizəkein] *n* 利索卡因(局部麻醉药,止痒药)

Risser jacket [ˈrisə] (Joseph C. Risser) 里塞石膏背心(用于脊柱侧凸)

RIST radioimmunosorbent test 放射免疫吸附试验

Ristella melaninogenica [risˈtelə ˌmeleninəuˈdʒenikə] 黑色素拟杆菌

ristocetin [ˌristəˈsiːtin] *n* 利托菌素(抗生素类药)

risus [ˈraisəs] *n*【拉】笑,大笑 | ~ caninus, ~ sardonicus 痉笑,苦笑面容

Ritgen maneuver (method) [ˈritgən] (Ferdinand

A. M. F. von Ritgen）里特根（娩出）手法（宫缩间隔时，以手指在肛门后方将胎头向后压，并向上抬举，以利胎头仰伸而自阴户口娩出）

ritodrine hydrochloride [ˈritədriːn] 盐酸利托君（β_2 拟肾上腺素药，用作平滑肌〈子宫肌〉松弛药）

ritonavir [raiˈtəunəvir] *n* 利托那韦（一种 HIV 蛋白酶抑制剂，可致未成熟非感染的病毒颗粒形成，用于治疗人免疫缺陷病毒感染和获得性免疫缺陷综合征，口服给药）

Ritter-Rollet phenomenon (sign) [ˈritə rɔˈlei]（J. W. Ritter; Alexander Rollet）里特尔-罗勒特现象（征）（弱电刺激足屈，强电刺激足伸）

Ritter's disease [ˈritə]（Gottfried Ritter von Rittershain）葡萄球菌性烫伤样皮肤综合征，新生儿剥脱性皮炎

Ritter's law [ˈritə]（Johann W. Ritter）里特尔定律（通电与断电均对神经产生刺激作用）| ~ tetanus 里特尔强直（恒电流沿神经通电一段时间所发生的强直性收缩，见于手足搐搦）

Ritter-Valli law [ˈritə ˈvæli]（J. W. Ritter; Eusebio Valli）里特尔-瓦利定律（将神经由神经中枢切断时，所引起的向周边行走的兴奋性初期增强，继之消失）

ritual [ˈritjuəl] *n* 仪式动作（在精神病学中，指为缓解焦虑强迫进行一系列重复动作，如见于强迫性神经症）

rituximab [riˈtʌksimæb] *n* 利妥单抗（一种结合 CD 20 抗原的嵌合鼠-人单克隆抗体，用作抗肿瘤药，治疗 CD 20-阳性的 B 细胞非霍奇金〈Hodgkin〉淋巴瘤，静脉内给药）

rivalry [ˈraivəlri] *n* 竞争，敌对；拮抗 | binocular ~, retinal ~ 双眼拮抗，视网膜拮抗（注视同一物体时，双眼显像有明显的交互移位情况，无法融合成连续的影像）/ sibling ~ 同胞竞争（兄弟姐妹间为了争取双亲或双亲之一的抚爱、感情和注意，或为了得到其他承认或利益而开展的竞争）

Rivalta's reaction (test) [riˈvæltə]（Fabio Rivalta）里瓦尔塔反应（试验）（利用醋酸鉴别漏出液与渗出液）

Riva-Rocci sphygmomanometer [ˌrivəˈrəutʃi]（Scipione Riva-Rocci）里瓦·罗契血压计，水银血压计

rivastigmine tartrate [ˌrivəˈstigmiːn] 酒石酸利斯的明（一种胆碱酯酶抑制药，据认为可增加中枢神经系统内乙酰胆碱的水平，口服给药，用作佐药，治疗轻度到中度阿尔茨海默〈Alzheimer〉型痴呆）

Riverius' draft [riˈviəriəs] 里佛留斯顿服剂（见 Rivière's potion）

Rivière's potion [riviˈɛə]（Lázare Rivière）里维埃饮剂（一份柠檬酸与一份重碳酸钠或重碳酸钾混合制成）

Riviere's sign [riˈviə]（Clive Riviere）里维尔征（第 5、6、7 胸椎棘突平面叩音有一变化区，表明有一密度增高带通过背部，为肺结核之征）

rivinian [riˈviniən] *a* 里维纳斯（A. Q. Rivinus）的

Rivinus's ducts (canals) [riˈvinəs]（Augustus Q. Rivinus）舌下腺小管 | ~ gland 舌下腺 / ~ incisure (foramen, notch, segment) 鼓切迹

rivus [ˈraivəs]（[复] **rivi** [ˈraivai]）*n*【拉】河 | ~ lacrimalis 泪湖

riziform [ˈrizifɔːm] *a* 米粒形的

RKY roentgenkymography X 线记波摄影[术]，X 线记波法

RLF retrolental fibroplasia 晶体后纤维增生症

RLL right lower lobe 右下叶（肺）

RMA right mentoanterior 颏右前（胎位）

RML right middle lobe 右中叶（肺）

RMP right mentoposterior 颏右后（胎位）

RMT right mentotransverse 颏右横（胎位）

RN registered nurse 注册护士

Rn radon 氡

RNA ribonucleic acid 核糖核酸 | messenger RNA (mRNA) 信使核糖核酸，信使 RNA / ribosomal RNA (rRNA) 核糖体核糖核酸，核糖体 RNA，核蛋白体 RNA / soluble ~ 可溶性核糖核酸，可溶性 RNA / transfer RNA (tRNA) 转移核糖核酸，转移 RNA

RNA-directed DNA polymerase [pəˈliməreis] RNA 指导的 DNA 聚合酶（亦称反转录酶）

RNA directed RNA polymerase [pəˈliməreis] RNA 指导的 RNA 聚合酶

RNA nucleotidyltransferase [ˌnjuːkliəuˌtaidilˈtrænsfəreis] RNA 核苷酸[基]转移酶（RNA 聚合酶的旧称）

RNA polymerase [pəˈliməreis] RNA 聚合酶

RNA replicase [ˈreplikeis] RNA 复制酶，RNA 指导的 RNA 聚合酶

RNase ribonuclease 核糖核酸酶（有时专指胰核糖核酸酶）| ~ I pancreatic ribonuclease 胰核糖核酸酶 / ~ A pancreatic ribonuclease 胰核糖核酸酶

RNP ribonucleoprotein 核糖核蛋白

ROA right occipitoanterior 枕右前（胎位）

roach [rəutʃ] *n* 蜚蠊，油虫，蟑螂

roaring [ˈrɔːriŋ] *n* 喘鸣症（马）

robenidine hydrochloride [rəuˈbenidin] 盐酸罗贝胍（家禽抗球虫药）

Robert's ligament [rɔˈbɛə]（Cesar A. Robert）半月板股骨后韧带

Robertson's pupil [ˈrɔbətsn] 见 Argyll Robertson pupil

Robertson's sign [ˈrɔbətsn]（William E. Robertson）罗伯逊征（①心脏病患者垂危前心区胸肌

呈现纤维性收缩;②诈病时压迫诉痛部位仍不引起散瞳;③腹水时,令患者仰卧,检查者即可感知患者胁腹胀满及紧张)

Robert's pelvis [ˈrɔbɛət] (Heinrich L. F. Robert) 罗伯特骨盆(横斜径狭窄骨盆)

Roberts syndrome [ˈrɔbəts] (John B. Roberts) 罗伯茨综合征(一种遗传性综合征,为常染色体隐性性状遗传,包括肢体长骨发育不全,合并腭唇裂及其他异常)

Roberts' test [ˈrɔbəts] (William Roberts) 罗伯茨试验(检尿白蛋白、尿糖)

robin [ˈrəubin] *n* 刺槐毒素

Robinia [rəuˈbiniə] *n* 刺槐属

Robinow's syndrome (dwarfism) [ˈrɔbinəu] (Meinhard Robinow) 罗宾诺综合征(侏儒症)(侏儒症合并眶间距增宽,牙列不齐,前额膨出,凹陷性鼻梁及肢短)

Robin's anomalad, syndrome [rəuˈbæn] (Pierre Robin) 洛宾异常、综合征(即 Pierre Robin syndrome)

Robinson's circle [ˈrɔbinsn] (Frederick B. Robinson) 罗宾逊动脉环(由腹主动脉、髂总、髂内、子宫及卵巢动脉所形成的环)

Robison ester [ˈrɔbisn] (Robert Robison) 罗比森酯,葡糖-6-磷酸 | ~ ester dehydrogenase 罗比森酯脱氢酶,葡糖-6-磷酸脱氢酶

Robles' disease [ˈrəubleis] (Rudolfo V. Robles) 罗布莱病,盘尾丝虫病

roborant [ˈrɔbərənt] *a* 强壮的

Robson's line [ˈrɔbsn] (Arthur W. M. Robson) 罗布森线(从乳头至脐划出的一条假想线) | ~ point 罗布森点(胆囊炎最强压痛点,位于从右乳头至脐所设线的中1/3与下1/3交界点的相对处) | ~ position 罗布森卧位(病人仰卧,用沙袋垫在第11、12肋骨下,用于胆道手术)

robust [rəuˈbʌst] *a* 强健的

Rochalimaea [ˌrəukəlaiˈmiːə] (H. da Rocha-Lima) *n* 罗卡利马体属 | ~ quintana 五日热罗卡利马体(亦称五日热立克次体,伏尔希尼立克次体)

Rocher's sign [rəuˈʃɛə] (Henri G. L. Rocher) 罗歇征(睾丸扭转时不能分辨附睾与睾丸体,而在附睾炎时,附睾呈新月形扩大,方可摸到睾丸体)

Rochon-Duvigneaud's syndrome [rəuˈʃau duːviːˈnjəu] (André Rochon-Duvigneaud) 罗肖·杜维尼奥综合征,眶上裂综合征(即 superior orbital fissure syndrome,见 syndrome 项下相应术语)

rocking [ˈrɔkiŋ] *n* 摇摆 | body ~ 身体(前后)摇摆

rocuronium bromide [ˌrəukjuˈrəuniəm] 罗库溴铵(神经肌肉阻断药)

rod [rɔd] *n* 杆,柱(特指视网膜杆) | enamel ~s 釉柱 / germinal ~ 子孢子 / muscle ~ 肌原纤维 / olfactory ~ 嗅杆(嗅双极神经元的细顶部) / retinal ~s 视网膜杆

rodent [ˈrəudənt] *a* 咬的,嚼的;啮齿目的;侵蚀性的(溃疡) *n* 啮齿动物

Rodentia [rəuˈdenʃə] *n* 啮齿目

rodenticide [rəuˈdentisaid] *a* 杀啮齿类的 *n* 杀啮齿类剂,灭鼠剂

rodentine [rəuˈdentain] *a* 啮齿动物的

rodocaine [ˈrəudəkein] *n* 罗多卡因(局部麻醉药)

roentgen [ˈrentgən, ˈrɔnt-] (Wilhelm Conrad Röntgen) *n* 伦琴(X线或γ辐射的国际单位)

roentgen rays [ˈrentəgən] (W. K. Roentgen) 伦琴线,X[射]线

roentgenkymogram [ˌrentgənˈkaiməgræm] *n* X线记波照片

roentgenkymograph [ˌrentgənˈkaiməgrɑːf] *n* X线记波摄影机,X线记波摄影装置 | **~y** [ˌrentgənkaiˈmɔgrəfi] *n* X线记波摄影[术],X线记波法,X线描记法

roentgenocardiogram [ˌrentgənəuˈkɑːdiəgræm] *n* X线心搏描记图

roentgenocinematography [ˌrentgənəuˌsiniməˈtɔgrəfi] *n* X线电影摄影[术]

roentgenogram [ˌrentˈgenəgræm], **roentgenograph** [ˈrentgənəgrɑːf] *n* X线[照]片

roentgenography [ˌrentgəˈnɔgrəfi] *n* X线摄影[术] | body section ~ 体层X线摄影[术] / mass ~ 团体X线摄影[术](指居民普检) / miniature ~ 缩影X线摄影[术] / mucosal relief ~ 黏膜皱襞X线造影[术] / selective ~ 选择性X线摄影[术],居民抽检X线摄影[术] / spot film ~ 适时X线摄影[术],点片X线摄影[术] | **roentgenographic** [ˌrentgənəˈgræfik] *a* X线摄影的

roentgenokymograph [ˌrentgənəuˈkaiməgrɑːf, -græf] *n* X线记波摄影机,X线记波摄影装置

roentgenology [ˌrentgəˈnɔlədʒi] *n* X线学 | **roentgenologic** [ˌrentgənəˈlɔdʒik] *a* / **roentgenologist** *n* X线学家,X线科医师

roentgenolucent [ˌrentgənəuˈljuːsnt] *a* 可透X线的,X线可透的

roentgenometer [ˌrentgəˈnɔmitə] *n* X线量测定器,X线量计 | **roentgenometry** [ˌrəntgəˈnɔmitri] *n* X线量测定法;X线影像测量法

roentgenopaque [ˌrentgənəuˈpeik] *a* 不透X线的,X线不透的

roentgenoparent [ˌrentgənəuˈpɛərənt] *a* 可透X线的

roentgenoscope [rentˈgenəskəup] *n* X线荧光

屏,X线透视屏

roentgenoscopy [ˌrentgəˈnɔskəpi] *n* X线透视[法],X线检查,荧光屏检查

roentgenotherapy [ˌrentgənəuˈθerəpi] *n* X线治疗,X线疗法

roeteln [ˈretəln] *n* 【德】风疹

rofecoxib [ˌrəufəˈkɔksib] *n* 罗非考昔(非甾体消炎药,用于治疗骨关节炎、急性疼痛和痛经,口服给药)

Roger-Josué test [rɔˈʒei ʒɔzjuˈei] (H. L. Roger; Otto Josué) 水疱试验(检传染病)

Roger's disease [rɔˈʒei] (Henri L. Roger) 罗惹病(先天性心室间隔缺损) | ~ reaction 罗惹反应(痰内有白蛋白为结核病之征) / ~ symptom 罗惹症状(结核性脑膜炎第三期时体温低于正常)

Roger's reflex [rəuˈʒei] (Georges H. Roger) 罗惹反射,食管唾液反射

Rogers' sphygmomanometer [ˈrɔdʒəz] (Oscar H. Rogers) 罗杰斯血压计

Röhl's marginal corpuscles [reil] (Wilhelm Röhl) 勒尔边缘小体(投用化学药物后,动物红细胞边缘所见到的一种小体)

roka [ˈrəukə] *n* 罗卡栋(栋科植物)

Rokitansky-Cushing ulcers [ˌrɔːkiˈtʌnski ˈkuʃiŋ] (K. F. von Rokitansky; Harvey W. Cushing) 罗-库溃疡(中枢神经系统严重损害的一种偶发性溃疡性并发症,侵及食管下1/3、胃底或十二指肠)

Rokitansky-Küster-Hauser syndrome [ˌrɔːkiˈtʌnski ˈkiːstə ˈhauzə] (K. F. von Rokitansky; Hermann Küster; G. A. Hauser) 罗-屈-豪综合征(见 Mayer-Rokitansky-Küster-Hauser syndrome)

Rokitansky's disease [ˌrɔːkiˈtʌnski] (Karl F. von Rokitansky) 大块肝坏死 | ~ diverticulum 罗基坦斯基憩室(食管牵引性憩室) / ~ pelvis 脊柱滑出性骨盆

rolandic [rəuˈlændik] (Luigi Lorando) *a* 罗朗多的

rolandometer [ˌrəulənˈdɔmitə] *n* 脑裂计,脑裂测计器

Rolando's angle [rəuˈlændəu] (Luigi Rolando) 罗朗多角(中央沟角) | ~ area, zone 罗朗多区,皮质运动区 / ~ cells 罗朗多细胞(胶质神经细胞) / ~ column 罗朗多柱(延髓灰小结节) / ~ fasciculus 罗朗多束(延髓灰质后角扩大部) / ~ funiculus 外侧楔索 / ~ fissure 罗朗多裂,中央沟 / ~ line 中央沟线 / ~ gelatinous substance 罗朗多胶状质 / ~ tubercle 罗朗多结节,灰结节(延髓)

role [rəul] *n* 作用,功用 | gender ~ 性别作用(一个人藉以表明他或她是男或女而表现出来的形象,这是性别同一性〈gender identity〉的社会表达)

roletamide [rəuˈletəmaid] *n* 咯来米特(安眠药)

Rolfing [ˈrɔlfiŋ] (Ida Rolf) *n* 罗尔夫按摩治疗法

rolicyprine [ˌrəuliˈsaipriːn] *n* 罗利普令(抗抑郁药)

rolitetracycline [rəuliˌtetrəˈsaiklin] *n* 罗列环素(半合成广谱抗生素) | ~ nitrate 硝酸罗列环素

roll [rəul] *vi, vt* 滚动 *n* 卷 | cotton ~ 棉卷(牙科用) / iliac ~ 髂卷(腊肠样卷,位于左髂窝) / scleral ~ 巩膜回转缘,巩膜卷(睫状体依附之处)

roller [ˈrəulə] *n* 棉卷,纱布卷(外科用);滚轴 | massage ~ 电按摩滚轴

Roller's nucleus [ˈrɔlə] (Christian F. W. Roller) 罗勒核(①舌下神经核前部的一群小细胞;②橄榄核门附近的细胞)

Rolleston's rule [ˈrəulstən] (Humphrey D. Rolleston) 罗尔斯顿规律(成人的理想收缩压为年龄的1/2加100)

Rollet's chancre [rɔˈlei] (Joseph P. M. Rollet) 混合性下疳

Rollet's stroma [ˈrɔlət] (Alexander Rollet) 罗累特基质(血红蛋白除去后所遗留的红细胞部分)

Rollet's syndrome [rəuˈlei] (J. Rollet) 罗莱综合征,眶尖综合征(即 orbital apex syndrome,见 syndrome 项下相应术语)

Rollier's radiation [rɔˈljɛə] (Auguste Rollier) 罗利尔照射(结核病患者日光紫外线照射,逐渐增加其照射剂量) | ~ treatment 罗利尔疗法(日光治疗外科结核)

Romaña's sign [rəuˈmɑːnjə] (Cecilio Romaña) 罗曼尼亚征(偏侧性眼炎,伴睑水肿、结膜炎、局部淋巴结肿大,为南美洲锥虫病之征)

romanopexy [rəuˈmænəˌpeksi] *n* 乙状结肠固定术

romanoscope [rəuˈmænəskəup] *n* 乙状结肠镜

Romanovsky's (Romanowsky's) stain (method) [ˌrɔməˈnɔfski] (Dimitri L. Romanovsky) 罗曼诺夫斯染剂[法](染血液涂片显示疟原虫)

Romano-Ward syndrome [rəuˈmɑːnəu wɔːd] (C. Romano; O. C. Ward) 罗马诺-沃德综合征(一种常染色体显性遗传型Q-T间期延长综合征,特征为晕厥,有时伴心室颤动并猝死。参见 Jervell and Lange-Nielsen syndrome)

rombergism [ˈrɔmbəːgizəm] *n* 闭目难立征,龙贝格征(见 Romberg's sign)

Romberg's disease (trophoneurosis) [ˈrɔmbəːg] (Moritz H. Romberg) 进行性单侧面萎缩症 | ~ sign 龙贝格征,闭目难立征(闭目并足直立时身体摇摆,见于脊髓痨) / ~ spasm 龙贝格痉挛(第五脑神经支配肌肉的嚼肌痉挛) / ~ station 龙贝格姿势,闭目立正姿势 / ~ test 龙贝

格试验(鉴别周围性共济失调与小脑性共济失调)

Römer's test (reaction) [ˈriːmə] (Paul H. Römer) 勒梅尔试验(反应)(皮内注射结核菌素至患结核的豚鼠能引起产生中心出血坏死的丘疹。亦称花结状试验)

Rommelaere's sign [ˌrɔmeləˈɛə] (Guillaume Rommelaere) 罗梅拉尔征(癌性恶病质时尿中正磷酸盐及氯化钠含量异常减少)

Romney Marsh disease [ˈrɔmni mɑːʃ] (Romney Marsh 为英格兰地名,该地首次报道此病) 肠毒血病

rongeur [rɔŋˈʒəː] *n*【法】咬骨钳,修骨钳

ronidazole [rəuˈnidəzəul] *n* 罗硝唑(兽用抗原虫药)

ronnel [ˈrɔnel] *n* 皮蝇磷(即芬氯磷 fenclofos,杀虫药)

Rönne's nasal step [ˈrenə] 伦内鼻侧阶梯(视野鼻侧阶梯状缺损,见于青光眼)

röntgenography [ˌrentgəˈnɔgrəfi] *n* X 线摄影[术]

Rood method [ruːd] (Margaret Rood) 鲁德法(克服痉挛状态的一种技术,依据的理论是:刺激皮肤特定区会促使皮下的肌肉收缩,并导致相关的拮抗肌相互松弛;用一种特制的刷子或用冰块敲击造成刺激)

roof [ruːf] *n* 顶,盖 | ~ of orbit 眶顶 / ~ of skull 颅顶 / ~ of tympanum 鼓室顶

room [ruːm] *n* 房间,室 | delivery ~ 产房,分娩室 / intensive therapy ~ 加强治疗室 / operating ~ 手术室 / postdelivery ~ 产后室 / predelivery ~, labor ~ 待产室 / recovery ~ 恢复室(连接手术室或产房,对手术后或产后患者给予照顾至恢复,然后回病室护理) / utility ~ 杂用室

rooming-in [ˈruːmiŋin] *n* 新生儿母子同室

root [ruːt] *n* 根,解剖根(牙齿由牙骨质覆盖的部分) / bitter ~ 龙胆 / clinical ~ 临症根(牙) / ~ of clitoris 阴蒂脚 / deadly nightshade ~ 颠茄根 / facial ~ 面神经根 / ~ of hair 毛根 / insane ~ 莨菪根 / licorice ~, sweet ~ 甘草 / lingual ~ 舌侧根 / ~ of lung 肺根 / mandrake ~ 鬼臼根 / ~ of nail 甲根 / orizaba jalap ~ 药薯(根) / palatine ~ 腭侧根 / puccoon ~, red ~ 血根

rootlet [ˈruːtlit] *n* 小根,支根 | flagellar ~ 鞭毛小根(亦称鞭毛根,生毛体,根丝体)

ROP right occipitoposterior 枕右后(胎位)

ropinirole hydrochloride [rəuˈpiniˌrəul] 盐酸罗匹尼罗(多巴胺激动药,用作抗运动障碍药,治疗帕金森〈Parkinson〉病,口服给药)

ropivacaine hydrochloride [rəuˈpivəkein] 盐酸罗哌卡因(局部麻醉药)

ropizine [ˈrəupiziːn] *n* 罗匹嗪(抗惊厥药)

roridin [ˈrəuridin] *n* 杆孢菌素

Rorschach test [ˈrɔːʃʌh] (Hermann Rorschach) 罗尔沙赫试验,墨迹测验(测思想和情绪的病症,以 10 张印有黑色或彩色的墨迹卡片,让病人注视并讲出他所见的情形)

Rosa [ˈrəuzə] *n* 蔷薇属

rosacea [rəuˈzeiʃiə] *n* 酒渣鼻,红斑痤疮 | granulomatous ~, lupoid ~, papular ~ 肉芽肿性酒渣鼻,狼疮样酒渣鼻,丘疹性酒渣鼻

rosaceous [rəuˈzeiʃəs] *a* 蔷薇属的;蔷薇色的,玫瑰色的

rosacic acid [rəuˈzæsik] 尿赤素

Rosai-Dorfman disease [ˈrəuzai ˈdɔːfmən] (Juan Rosai; Ronald F. Dorfman) 罗-道病(一种罕见的综合征,通常见于儿童或青少年,颈淋巴结〈和有时为其他淋巴结〉巨大肿胀,并含有大量组织细胞;结节外疾病亦常见,有时伴发热、贫血、中性粒细胞增多症、红细胞沉降率增高以及高丙球蛋白血症。亦称窦组织细胞增生症伴巨大淋巴结病)

rosamicin [ˌrəuzəˈmaisin] *n* 罗沙米星(抗生素类药)

rosaniline [rəuˈzæniliːn] *n* 玫瑰苯胺,蔷薇苯胺,一甲基品红

rosaramicin [ˌrəusərəˈmaisin] *n* 罗沙米星(抗生素类药)

rosary [ˈrəuzəri] *n* 串珠形构造,串珠 | rachitic ~ 串珠肋

rose [rəuz] *n* 蔷薇,玫瑰;玫瑰红[色] *a* 玫瑰花的;玫瑰色的 | ~ bengal 孟加拉玫红,四碘四氯荧光素

rosein [ˈrəuziin] *n* 品红,复红;玫瑰菌素

rosemary [ˈrəuzməri, -ˌmeəri] *n* 迷迭香

Rosenbach's sign [ˈrɔːzənbʌh] (Ottomar Rosenbach) 罗森巴赫征(①肠炎性疾病时腹壁皮肤反射消失,②偏瘫时拧患侧腹部皮肤,腹壁皮肤反射缺失;③突眼性甲状腺肿时眼睑闭合时呈现急速细微震颤) | ~ syndrome 罗森巴赫综合征(阵发性心搏过速伴有胃及呼吸道并发症) / ~ test 罗森巴赫试验(检靛红、血中冷溶血素)

Rosenbach's tuberculin [ˈrɔːzənbʌh] (F. J. R. Rosenbach) 罗森巴赫结核菌素(从感染上一种发癣菌的结核杆菌培养物制备,此感染可减低结核杆菌的毒性)

Rosenberg-Bergstrom syndrome [ˈrəuzənbəːg ˈbəːstrəm] (Alan L. Rosenberg; Lavonne Bergstrom) 罗-伯综合征(一种常染色体隐性遗传综合征,特征为高尿酸血症、肾功能不全、共济失调及耳聋,或许由于核糖磷酸焦磷酸激酶缺乏所致)

Rosenberg-Chutorian syndrome [ˈrəuzənbəːg

tʃuː'tɔriən] (Roger N. Rosenberg; Abe M. Chutorian) 罗-丘综合征(一种罕见的 X 连锁遗传综合征,特征为视萎缩、进行性神经性聋和多神经病)

Rosen method ['rəuzən] (Marion Rosen) 罗森法(一种健身法)

Rosenmüller's body (organ) ['rɔːzənˌmilə] (Johann C. Rosenmüller) 罗森苗勒体(器),卵巢冠 | ~ gland (node) 泪腺睑部;[复]腹股沟深淋巴结 / ~ recess (cavity, fossa) 咽隐窝 / ~ valve 鼻泪管襞

Rosenthal's canal ['rɔːzəntʌl] (Isidor Rosenthal) 蜗轴螺旋管

Rosenthal's test ['rɔːzənθɔːl] (Sanford M. Rosenthal) 罗森索尔试验(检尿血、肝功能)

Rosenthal's vein ['rɔːzəntʌl] (Friedrich C. Rosenthal) 基底静脉

Rosenthal syndrome ['rəuzənθɔːl] (Robert L. Rosenthal) 罗森索尔综合征(一种遗传性出血性素质,临床上类似血友病,系缺乏凝血因子Ⅺ所致)

roseola [rəu'ziːələ, rəuzi'əulə] *n*【拉】玫瑰疹

Roseolovirus [ˌrəuzi'əuləuˌvaiərəs] *n* 玫瑰疹病毒属

Roser sign, Roser-Braun sign ['rəuzə braun] (Wilhelm Roser; Heirich Braun) 罗泽尔征,罗-布征(硬脑脊膜的搏动消失,为脑瘤或脑脓肿之征)

Rose's position ['rəuz] (Frank A. Rose) 罗斯卧位(垂头仰卧体位,以防止患者在口腔手术时吸入血,患者仰卧并垂头于手术台端外,尽量伸展,使患者之血可自上门牙缘溢出)

Rose's test ['rɔːzə] (Joseph C. Rose) 罗泽试验(检血)

Rose's tetanus ['rɔːzə] (Edmund Rose) 头部破伤风

roset [rəu'zet] *n* 玫瑰花结,玫瑰花形(见 rosette)

rosette [rəu'zet] *n*【法】玫瑰花结,玫瑰花形(任何类似玫瑰花的结构或形成物,例如播散性红斑狼疮试验时所见的溶化核质小球周围有多形核白细胞簇以及有丝分裂早期染色体形成的图形) | E ~ E 玫瑰花结,红细胞玫瑰花结 / EAC ~ EAC 玫瑰花结,红细胞-抗体-补体玫瑰花结

rosiglitazone maleate [rəusig'litəzəun] 马来酸罗西利宗(抗糖尿病药)

rosin ['rɔzin] *n* 松香

Rosin's test ['rɔːzin] (Heinrich Rosin) 罗辛试验(检靛红)

Rosmarinus [ˌrɔsmə'rainəs] *n*【拉】迷迭香属

rosolic acid [rəu'zɔlik] 蔷薇色酸,玫红酸

rosoxacin [rəu'sɔksəsin] *n* 罗索沙星,(抗菌药)

Rossbach's disease ['rɔsbʌh] (Michael J. Rossbach) 胃酸过多[症]

Ross' black spores [rɔs] (Ronald Ross) 罗斯黑孢子(在蚊胃壁内的色素性疟卵囊) | ~ cycle 罗斯周期(疟原虫在蚊体内的生活周期)

Ross' bodies ['rɔs] (Edward H. Ross) 罗斯体,梅毒白细胞虫(铜色球体,含深色颗粒,有时作阿米巴样运动,见于梅毒患者血液和组织液中)

Rossel's aloin test [rɔ'sel] (Otto Rossel) 罗塞尔芦荟素试验(检粪血)

Rossolimo's reflex (sign) [ˌrɔsə'liːməu] (Gregorij I. Rossolimo) 罗索利莫反射(征)(叩足趾跖面时,足趾屈曲,为锥体束病损)

Rostan's asthma [rɔs'tɑːŋ] (Louis L. Rostan) 心病性气喘

rostellum [rɔs'teləm] ([复] **rostella** [rɔs'telə]) *n*【拉】顶突(尤指绦虫头节的肉体隆凸,可能带钩或不带钩)

rostrad ['rɔstræd] *ad* 向嘴侧;向头侧

rostral ['rɔstrəl] *a* 嘴的,嘴侧的 *ad* 向嘴侧

rostralis [rɔs'treilis] *a*【拉】嘴的,嘴侧的

rostra ['rɔstrə] rostrum 的复数

rostrate ['rɔstreit] *a* 有嘴的,有喙的

rostriform ['rɔstrifɔːm] *a* 嘴状的,喙状的

rostrum ['rɔstrəm] ([复] **rostrums** 或 **rostra** ['rɔstrə]) *n*【拉】嘴,喙 | ~ of corpus callosum 胼胝体嘴 / sphenoidal ~ 蝶嘴

ROT right occipitotransverse 枕右横(胎位)

Rot 见 Roth

rot [rɔt] (-tt-) *vt, vi* 腐烂,腐败 *n* 腐烂,腐败;肝[双盘]吸虫病 | Barcoo ~ 沙漠疮 / black ~ 黑色腐败(有时见于贮蛋) / foot ~ 蹄坏疽病(亦称羊脚病) / pizzle ~, sheath ~ 地方性兽病龟头包皮炎

rotablation [ˌrəutæb'leiʃən] *n* 动脉粥样斑旋转切除

Rotaliina [ˌrəutə'laiinə] *n* 轮孔虫亚目

rotameter [rəu'tæmitə] *n* 转子流速计(测定麻醉气体的给予量)

rotary ['rəutəri] *a* 旋转的,轮转的,转动的

rotate [rəu'teit] *vt, vi* 旋转,转动

rotation [rəu'teiʃən] *n* 旋转;旋光度 | axial ~ of kidney 肾轴性旋转 / molar ~ 摩尔旋光度 / molecular ~ 分子旋光度;分子转动 / optical ~ 旋光性;旋光度 / specific ~ 旋光率

rotationplasty [rəuˌteiʃən'plæsti] *n* 旋转皮瓣成形术

rotator [rəu'teitə] *n* 转子,旋转器;回旋肌

rotatory ['rəutətəri, rəu'teitəri] *a* 旋转的,转动的

Rotavirus ['rəutəˌvaiərəs] *n* 轮状病毒属

rotavirus ['rəutəˌvaiərəs] *n* 轮状病毒

Roth-Bernhardt disease [rəut 'bəːnhɑːt] (V.

K. Roth; Martin Bernhardt) 感觉异常性股痛
Rotch's sign [rɔtʃ] (Thomas M. Rotch) 罗奇征(右第五肋间隙叩诊呈浊音,为心包积液之征)
röteln [ˈretəln] *n* 【德】风疹
rotenone [ˈrəutənəun] *n* 鱼藤酮(杀昆虫、杀疥螨药)
rotexed [ˈrəutekst] *a* 转屈的
rotexion [rəuˈtekʃən] *n* 转屈
Rothera's test [ˈrɔθərə] (Arthur C. H. Rothera) 罗瑟雷试验(检丙酮)
Rothia [ˈrɔθiə] (Genevieve D. Roth) *n* 罗氏菌属 | ~ dentocariosus 龋齿罗氏菌(亦称龋齿放线菌)
Rothman-Makai syndrome [ˈrəutmən ˈmɔːkɔi] (Max Rothman; Endre Makai) 罗-莫综合征(特发性局限性脂膜炎伴脂肪细胞坏死,噬脂性肉芽肿及囊肿形成,通常都能自动消失)
Rothmund-Thomson syndrome [ˈrəutmənd ˈtɔmsn] (August von Rothmund, Jr.; Mathew Sidney Thomson) 罗-汤综合征(主要发生在女性的一种常染色体隐性遗传性综合征,特征为皮肤出现网状萎缩性斑块,色素沉着过度,毛细血管扩张,常伴有幼年性白内障,鞍状鼻,先天性骨缺陷,发、甲与牙生长障碍及性腺功能减退。亦称先天性皮肤异色病)
Rothschild's sign [rəutˈʃiːld] (Henri J. N. C. de Rothschild) 罗特希尔德征(①胸骨角异常扁平并可移动,见于肺结核;②甲状腺功能不全时眉毛外 1/3 脱落)
Roth's (Rot's) disease (syndrome), Roth-Bernhardt disease (syndrome) [rɔːt ˈbɔːnhɑːt] (Vladimir K. Roth; Martin Bernhardt) 感觉异常性股痛
Roth's spots [rɔːt] (Moritz Roth) 罗特斑(圆形或卵圆形白斑,有时见于早期亚急性细菌性心内膜炎的视网膜内) | ~ vas aberrans 罗特迷管
rotifer [ˈrəutifə] *n* 轮虫
Rotifera [rəuˈtifərə] *n* 轮虫纲
rotlauf [ˈrɔtlauf] *n* 【德】猪丹毒
Rotor's syndrome [rəuˈtɔː] (Arthuro B. Rotor) 罗托综合征(慢性家族性非溶血性黄疸,与杜-约〈Dubin-Johnson〉综合征的区别在于无肝脏色素沉着)
rotoxamine [rəuˈtɔksəmiːn] *n* 罗托沙敏(抗组胺药) | ~ tartrate 酒石酸罗托沙敏(抗组胺药)
Rotter's test [ˈrɔtə] (H. Rotter) 罗特尔试验(检体内维生素 C)
rottlera [ˈrɔtlərə] *n* 粗糠柴,卡马拉(见 kamala)
rottlerin [ˈrɔtlərin] *n* 粗糠柴毒,卡马拉素
rotula [ˈrɔtjulə] *n* 【拉】髌;盘状骨突;糖丸,糖锭
rotulad [ˈrɔtjulæd] *ad* 向髌侧
rotular [ˈrɔtjulə] *a* 髌的
rotz [rəuts] *n* 【德】[马]鼻疽
rouge [ruːʒ] *n* 铁丹,红铁粉
rouget du porc [ruːˈʒei djuː ˈpɔːk] 【法】猪丹毒荨麻疹型
Rouget's bulb [ruˈʒei] (Antoine D. Rouget) 卵巢血管丛
Rouget's cells [ruˈʒei] (Charles M. B. Rouget) 鲁惹细胞(蛙毛细管壁的收缩细胞) | ~ muscle 鲁惹肌(睫状肌环行部)
rough [rʌf] *a* 粗糙的,不光滑的
roughage [ˈrʌfidʒ] *n* 粗糙食物(饮食中难消化的食物,如纤维、纤维素等)
Rougnon-Heberden disease [ruˈnjɔːŋ ˈhebədən] (Nicholas F. Rougnon de Magny; William Heberden) 心绞痛
rouleau [ruːˈləu] ([复] **rouleaus** 或 **rouleaux** [ruːˈləuz]) *n* 【法】红细胞钱串 | erythrocyte ~ 红细胞叠积
roundworm [ˈraundwəːm] *n* 线虫;蛔虫
Rous sarcoma [raus] (Francis P. Rous) 劳斯肉瘤(一种特异的肉瘤样新生物,见于某些禽类,从中可获得一种滤过性病毒〈首次获知可以致瘤〉,再接种于其他禽体内,可产生相同的新生物) | ~ sarcoma virus 劳斯肉瘤病毒(一种产生禽类纤维肉瘤的白血病毒,可使其他动物产生肿瘤) / ~ test 劳斯试验(检尿含铁血黄素)
Roussel's sign [ruˈsel] (Theophile Roussel) 罗塞尔征(轻叩锁骨及第四肋骨间锁骨下区产生锐痛,为初期肺结核之征)
Roussy-Dejerine syndrome [ruˈsi ˌdeʒəˈriːn] (Gustave Roussy; Joseph J. Dejerine) 丘脑综合征(thalamic syndrome, 见 syndrome 项下相应术语)
Roussy-Lévy syndrome (disease, hereditary areflexic dystasia) [ruˈsiː leiˈviː] (Gustave Roussy; Gabrielle Lévy) 罗-雷综合征(病,遗传性反射消失性起立不能)(一种慢性进行性遗传病,为常染色体显性遗传,特征为感觉性共济失调伴反射消失,远端肢体肌肉萎缩,尤其是腓骨肌萎缩,手静止时震颤,弓形足或爪形足,有时为脊柱后侧凸)
route [ruːt] *n* 径路 | intraracheal ~ 气管内径路 / operative ~ 手术入路
Rouvière's node [ruːviˈɛə] (Henri Rouvière) 罗维埃结(咽喉淋巴结外侧组的最上部,位于颅底)
Roux's anastomosis (operation) [ruː] (César Roux), **Roux-en-Y anastomosis** 鲁氏吻合术(手术)(包括小肠在内的任何Y形吻合术)
Roux's serum [ruː] (Pierre P. E. Roux) 抗白喉血清
Rovighi's sign [rɔˈvigi] (Alberto Rovighi) 罗维

季征(叩诊和触诊时可感知浅表肝棘球蚴囊震颤)

Rovsing's sign [ˈrɔvsiŋ] (Niels T. Rovsing) 罗符辛征(阑尾炎时,压迫麦氏〈McBurney〉点相当的左腹部,可引起麦氏点典型的疼痛) | ~ syndrome 罗符辛综合征(马蹄肾伴恶心、腹部不适及伸展过度时疼痛)

Rowntree-Geraghty test [ˈrauntri(ː) ˈgerəti] (Leonard G. Rowntree; John T. Geraghty) 酚磺酞试验(检肾功能)

roxarsone [rɔkˈsɑːsəun] *n* 罗沙胂(一种砷剂,兽医中用于治疗家禽球虫病和坏死性肠炎,并用于治疗猪痢疾)

RPF renal plasma flow 肾血浆流量

R Ph Registered Pharmacist 注册药师

RPLND retroperitoneal lymph node dissection 腹膜后淋巴结切除术

rpm revolutions per minute 每分钟绕转(现用 r/m)

RPS renal pressor substance 肾加压物质

RQ respiratory quotient 呼吸商

RRA Registered Record Administrator 注册病案管理员

-rrhage, -rrhagia [构词成分]出血,流血

-rrhaphy [构词成分]缝合术,修复术

-rrhea [构词成分]溢出,流出

-rrhexis [构词成分]破裂,折裂

-rrhoea 见-rrhea

rRNA ribosomal RNA 核糖体 RNA

RSA right sacroanterior 骶右前(胎位)

RScA right scapuloanterior 肩右前(胎位)

RSCN Registered Sick Children's Nurse 注册小儿科护士

RScP right scapuloposterior 肩右后(胎位)

RSM Royal Society of Medicine 皇家医学会

RSNA Radiological Society of North America 北美放射学会

RSP right sacroposterior 骶右后(胎位)

RST right sacrotransverse 骶右横(胎位)

RSTMH Royal Society of Tropical Medicine and Hygiene 皇家热带医学与卫生学会

RSV Rous sarcoma virus 劳斯肉瘤病毒;respiratory syncytial virus 呼吸道合孢病毒

RTA renal tubular acidosis 肾小管性酸中毒

RTF resistance transfer factor 抗性转移因子

RU rat unit 大鼠单位

RU-486 mifepristone 米非司酮(抗孕激素药)

Ru ruthenium 钌

rub [rʌb] (-bb-) *vt*, *vi* 摩擦 *n* 摩擦;摩擦音(一种听诊音) | friction ~ 摩擦音 / pericardial ~ 心包摩擦音 / pleuritic ~ 胸膜摩擦音

rubber [ˈrʌbə] *n* 橡胶;橡皮

rubefacient [ˌruːbiˈfeiʃjənt] *a* 使(皮肤等)发红的 *n* 发赤药(用以产生主动性或被动性充血使皮肤发红)

rubefaction [ˌruːbiˈfækʃən] *n* (皮肤)发红

rubella [ruˈbelə] *n* 风疹

Rubens flap [ˈruːbənz] (Peter P. Rubens,佛兰德斯画家)鲁本斯瓣

rubeola [ruːˈbiələ] *n* 麻疹

rubeosis [ˌruːbiˈəusis] *n* 发红,潮红

ruber [ˈruːbə] *a* 【拉】红的

ruberythric acid [ˌruːbəˈriθrik] 茜根酸

rubescent [ruːˈbesnt] *a* 变红的,发红的

rubidium (Rb) [ru(ː)ˈbidiəm] *n* 铷(化学元素)

rubidomycin [ru(ː)ˈbidəˌmaisin] *n* 柔红霉素(抗生素类药)

rubiginous [ru(ː)ˈbidʒinəs], **rubiginose** [ru(ː)ˈbidʒinəus] *a* 锈色的,赤褐色的(指痰)

rubin [ˈruːbin] *n* 品红,复红

Rubinstein's syndrome [ˈruːbinstain] (Jack H. Rubinstein) 鲁宾斯坦综合征(一种先天性病征,特征为智力和运动发育迟缓,拇指与大趾增宽,身材矮小,独特面容,包括硬腭高拱和直或钩形鼻,各种眼畸形,肺动脉狭窄,形成瘢痕疙瘩,枕骨大孔增大,并有肋骨与胸骨畸形)

Rubinstein-Taybi syndrome [ˈruːbinstain ˈteibi] (J. H. Rubinstein; Hooshang Taybi) 鲁宾斯坦-泰比综合征(即 Rubinstein's syndrome)

Rubin's test [ˈruːbin] (Isidor C. Rubin) 鲁宾试验(①输卵管通气术:用二氧化碳经子宫吹气,若输卵管通畅,气可进入腹膜腔内,可由荧光镜和 X 线照片测知;②检禽造白细胞组织增生病毒:如病毒存在,即对以后接种的劳斯〈Rous〉病毒产生一种细胞抵抗力〈抗性诱导因子〉,亦称 RIF test)

Rubivirus [ˈruːbiˌvaiərəs] *n* 风疹病毒属

Rubner's law [ˈruːbnə] (Max Rubner) 鲁布纳定律(①能量消耗不变律:生长速度与代谢过程的强度成正比;②生长商不变律:用于生长的能量占总能量的一定比数,此比数称为生长商) | ~ test 鲁布纳试验(检血一氧化碳及检尿乳糖、葡萄糖、麦芽糖)

rubor [ˈruːbə] *n* 【拉】红,发红(炎症主要征象之一)

rubriblast [ˈruːbriblæst] *n* 原正成红细胞,原[始]红细胞

rubric [ˈruːbrik] *a* 红的;红核的

rubricyte [ˈruːbrisait] *n* 多染性正成红细胞,中幼红细胞

rubrospinal [ˌruːbrəuˈspainl] *a* 红核脊髓的

rubrothalamic [ˌruːbrəuθəˈlæmik] *a* 红核丘脑的

rubrum [ˈruːbrəm] *n* 【拉】红(色) | ~ Congo 刚果红 / ~ scarlatinum 猩红

Rubus [ˈruːbəs] *n* 【拉】悬钩子属

Ruck's watery extract tuberculin [rʌk] (Karl

von Ruck）鲁克结核菌素水溶液（结核杆菌培养物在 55 ℃真空条件下浓缩至原量的 1/10，过滤。滤液用碘化铋钠酸性溶液沉淀，过滤，中和滤液后，再过滤。滤液加纯乙醇使成为 90% 乙醇，沉淀后再过滤，将干燥沉淀配成 1% 水溶液）

ructus [ˈrʌktəs] *n*【拉】嗳气

Rudbeckia [rʌdˈbekiə] *n* 金花菊属

rudiment [ˈruːdimənt] *n* 退化器官，残遗器官，痕迹器官，遗迹；原基，始基 | lens ~ 晶状体原基 / ~ of vaginal process 鞘突遗迹

rudimental [ˌruːdiˈmentl]，**rudimentary** [ˌruːdiˈmentəri] *a* 残遗的，已退化的；原基的

rudimentum [ˌruːdiˈmentəm] *n*【拉】原始，始基；残遗器官，痕迹器官，遗迹

Rudimicrosporea [ˌruːdiˌmaikrəuˈspɔːriə] *n* 二型孢子纲

Rud's syndrome [ruːd]（Einar Rud）鲁德综合征（为先天性综合征，包括单纯鱼鳞病、智力缺陷、癫痫及幼稚症）

rue [ruː] *n* 芸香

rufescine [ˈruːfəsin] *n* 蛤蛎色素

Ruffini's brushes (organ) [ruˈfini]（Angelo Ruffini）鲁菲尼终柱［器］（皮肤乳头内的一种神经末梢）| ~ corpuscles (cylinders) 鲁菲尼小体（圆柱体）（环层小体，尤指与压觉和温觉有关的神经末梢）

rufiopin [ˌruːfiˈəupin] *n* 绛阿片素

rufous [ˈruːfəs] *a* 暗红色的

ruga [ˈruːgə]（［复］**rugae** [ˈruːdʒiː]）*n*【拉】皱褶 | **rugate** [ˈruːgeit, ˈruːgit] *a*

Ruggeri's reflex (sign) [ruːˈdʒeiri]（Ruggero Ruggeri）鲁杰里反射（征），眼球脉搏反射（眼球强行会聚观察极近的某些物体后脉搏加速，表示交感神经兴奋）

rugine [ruˈʒiːn] *n* 骨锉，骨刮

rugitus [ˈruːdʒitəs] *n*【拉】肠鸣

rugose [ˈruːgəus]，**rugous** [ˈruːgəs] *a* 皱褶的，皱的 | **rugosity** [ruːˈgɔsəti] *n* 皱褶状态，皱褶

Rukavina type familial amyloid polyneuropathy (syndrome) [ruːkəˈvainə]（John G. Rukavina）鲁卡瓦纳型家族性淀粉样蛋白多神经病，印第安纳州型家族性淀粉样蛋白多神经病

RUL right upper lobe 右上叶（肺）

rule [ruːl] *n* 规则，条例；规律 | delivery date ~ 分娩日期规律（见 Nägele's rule）/ phase ~ 相律

rumbatron [ˈrʌmbətrɔn] *n* 电子加速器（一种高效能射频振荡器，用电子作为轰击粒子，使原子破碎）

rumen [ˈruːmen]（［复］**rumens** 或 **rumina** [ˈruːminə]）*n* 瘤胃（反刍动物的第一胃）

rumenitis [ˌruːməˈnaitis] *n* 瘤胃炎

rumenotomy [ˌruːməˈnɔtəmi] *n* 瘤胃切开术

ruminal [ˈruːminəl] *a* 瘤胃的

ruminant [ˈruːminənt] *n* 反刍动物 *a* 反刍动物的；反刍的；沉思的

Ruminantia [ˌruːmiˈnænʃiə] *n* 反刍亚目

ruminate [ˈruːmineit] *vi, vt* 反刍，反嚼；沉思，反复思考

rumination [ˌruːmiˈneiʃən] *n* 反刍，反嚼；沉思 | obsessive ~ 强迫性穷思竭虑

ruminative [ˈruːminətiv] *a* 沉思的，持续思考的

Ruminococcus [ˌruːminəuˈkɔkəs] *n* 瘤胃球菌属

ruminoreticular [ˌruːminəurəˈtikjulə] *a* 瘤胃网状的，网状瘤胃的

Rummo's disease [ˈruməu]（Gaetano Rummo）心脏下垂

rump [rʌmp] *n* 臀部，臀

Rumpel-Leede phenomenon (sign, test) [ˈrumpəl ˈleidə]（Theodor Rumpel; Stockbridge C. Leede）鲁姆普尔－雷德现象（征、试验）（用橡胶绷带将上臂轻缚 10 分钟后下方出现小的皮下出血点，为猩红热及出血性素质之征）

Rumpf's sign (symptom, reaction) [rumpf]（Heinrich T. M. Rumpf）鲁姆夫征（症状，反应）（①在强感应电疗法停止后，有交替的纤维性和强直性收缩，见于外伤性神经功能病，亦称鲁姆夫创伤性反应；②痛处受压时脉搏加快，见于神经衰弱）

Rundles-Falls syndrome [ˈrʌndlz fɔːlz]（Ralph W. Rundles; Harold F. Falls）遗传性铁粒幼红细胞性贫血

runt [rʌnt] *n* 侏儒（指矮小动植物，也贬指人）

Runyon classification, group [ˈrʌnjən]（Ernest H. Runyon）鲁尼恩分类法、类型（根据细菌的色素形成及生长情况的一种分枝杆菌分类法）

rupia [ˈruːpiə] *n* 蛎壳疮，蛎壳疹 | **~l** *a*

rupioid [ˈruːpiɔid] *a* 蛎壳疮样的

rupture [ˈrʌptʃə] *n* 破裂；疝 *vt, vi* 破裂，裂开 | defense ~ 防御［力］崩溃（如矿工吸入硅石粉太多而减低对结核病的抵抗力）/ ~ of membranes 胎膜破裂

Rusconi's anus [rusˈkəuni]（Mauro Rusconi）胚孔

Ruscus [ˈrʌskəs] *n* 假叶树属

rush [rʌʃ] *n* 冲，奔；蠕动波 | peristaltic ~s 蠕动冲

Russell effect [ˈrʌsl]（W. J. Russell）拉塞尔效应（靠光以外的物质作用而显影）

Russell's bodies [ˈrʌsl]（William Russell）拉塞尔小体（浆细胞内球形包涵体，为含有表面丙球蛋白的黏液蛋白，可能是由细胞内的免疫球蛋白聚集而成，亦称癌小体，品红小体）

Russell's dwarf, syndrome (dwarfism) [ˈrʌsl]

(Alexander Russell) 拉塞尔侏儒、综合征(侏儒症)(见 Silver-Russell syndrome)

Russell-Silver syndrome (dwarfism) [ˈrʌsl ˈsilvə] (A. Russell; Henry K. Silver) 拉塞尔-西尔弗综合征(侏儒症)(见 Silver-Russell syndrome)

Russell's viper [ˈrʌsl] (Patrick Russell) 鲁塞尔蝰(蛇) | ~ viper venom 鲁塞尔蝰蛇毒(在试管内,用作内在的凝血致活酶,并用于凝血因子 X 缺乏的确定)

Russell traction [ˈrʌsl] (R. H. Russell) 拉塞尔牵引(以一悬带紧依膝下连结顶置滑车所作的牵引)

Russo's reaction (test) [ˈrusəu] (Mario Russo) 鲁索反应(试验)(伤寒患者的一种尿反应,加 4 滴甲基蓝溶液于 15 ml 尿中,在伤寒第一期,尿呈淡绿色,病重时,呈翠绿色,病退时呈浅蓝色)

rust [rʌst] *n* 铁锈,铁锈色;锈病,锈菌(植物)

Rust's disease [rust] (Johann N. Rust) 鲁斯特病(颈椎骨的结核性脊椎炎) | ~ phenomenon (sign) 鲁斯特现象(征)(上部颈椎骨疽或癌症时,患者采取卧位或从卧位起坐时,须用双手扶持自己头部) / ~ syndrome 鲁斯特综合征(颈硬,头部硬,在卧位或从卧位起坐时,须用双手扶持头部,发生于结核病、癌症、脊椎骨折、风湿病或关节病、梅毒性骨膜炎)

rut [rʌt] *n* 雄性(动物)动情期;动情期

Ruta [ˈruːtə] *n* 芸香属

rutaecarpine [ˌruːtiːˈkɑːpin] *n* 吴[茱]萸次碱

rutamycin [ˌrutəˈmaisin] *n* 芦他霉素(抗生素类药)

ruthenium (Ru) [ru(ː)ˈθiːniəm] *n* 钌(化学元素)

rutherford (rd) [ˈrʌðəfəd] (Ernest Rutherford) *n* 卢[瑟福](放射性物质的蜕变单位,每秒蜕变一百万次)

rutherfordium (Rf) [ˌrʌðəˈfɔːdiəm] (Sir Ernest Rutherford) *n* 铲(化学元素)

rutidosis [ˌruːtiˈdəusis] *n* 角膜皱缩(濒死现象)

rutilism [ˈruːtilizəm] *n* 红发

rutin [ˈruːtin], **rutoside** [ˈruːtəsaid] *n* 芦丁,芸香苷(用以减少毛细血管的脆性)

rutinose [ˈruːtinəus] *n* 芸香[二]糖

Ruvalcaba's syndrome [ˌruːvælˈkeibə] (R. H. Ruvalcaba) 鲁瓦凯巴综合征(掌骨或跖骨过短,生殖器发育不全,病因不明的发育迟缓,但男子出生后就存在,特征为小头、骨骼畸形、生殖器发育不全及身心发育迟缓)

ruyschian [ˈrɔiʃiæn] *a* 鲁伊施(Frederic Ruysch)的

Ruysch's glomeruli [rɔiʃ] (Frederic Ruysch) 肾小球 | ~ membrane (tunic) 脉络膜毛细管层 / ~ muscle 鲁伊施肌(子宫底肌组织) / ~ tube 鲁伊施管(犁鼻器管遗迹) / ~ veins 涡静脉

RV residual volume 残气量

RVA rabies vaccine adsorbed 吸附狂犬病疫苗

RVAD right ventricular assist device 右心室辅助装置

RVH right ventricular hypertrophy 右心室肥大

rye [rai] *n* 黑麦 | spurred ~ 麦角

Rye classification [rai] (Rye 为纽约一地名,1965 年在此一次会议采用此分类法)拉伊分类法(霍奇金〈Hodgkin〉病分类法,根据组织学和病理学,分成以下类型:淋巴细胞为主型、混合细胞型、淋巴细胞耗竭型和结节硬化型)

Ryle tube [rail] (G. A. Ryle) 赖尔管(薄橡皮管,一端呈橄榄形,送入试餐用)

S

S spherical lens 球镜片；serine 丝氨酸；siemens 西门子；smooth（colony）光滑型菌落；substrate 底物；sulfur 硫；Svedberg unit 斯维特伯格单位；saeral vertebrae（S1 through S5）骶椎（1 到 5）
S. signa【拉】标记，用法签
S entropy 熵
S- sinister【拉】左的
S_1 first heart sound 第一心音
S_2 second heart sound 第二心音
S_3 third heart sound 第三心音
S_4 fourth heart sound 第四心音
S_f Sverdberg flotation unit 斯维德伯格漂浮单位
s second 秒
s. sinister【拉】左的；semis【拉】半，一半
$\bar{s}$ sine【拉】无
s 样本标准差（sample standard deviation）的符号
s^{-1} reciprocal second 秒的倒数（$ms^{-1} = m/s$）
Σ 希腊字母 sigma 的大写；数学中表示总和的符号
σ sigma 希腊语第 18 个字母；标准差（standard deviation）的符号
$σ^2$ variance 方差
SA sinoatrial 窦房的
S. A. secundum artem【拉】按技术，人工地
Saathoff's test [ˈsɑːtɔf]（Lübhard Saathoff）萨托夫试验（检粪内脂肪）
saber-legged [ˈseibə legd] *a* 军刀状腿的（指马）
Sabin-Feldman syndrome [ˈseibin ˈfeldmən]（Albert B. Sabin；Henry A. Feldman）萨-费综合征（脉络膜视网膜炎与脑钙化，类似弓形虫病的表现，但所有弓形虫病试验均为阴性）
sabinism [ˈsæbinizəm] *n* 沙比桧中毒
sabinol [ˈsæbinɔl] *n* 桧萜醇
Sabin's vaccine [ˈseibin]（Albert B. Sabin）萨宾疫苗，口服脊髓灰质炎活疫苗
Sabouraudia [ˌsæbuˈrəudiə] *n* 发癣菌属
Sabouraudites [ˌsæburəuˈdaitiːz] *n* 小孢子菌属
Sabouraud's dextrose agar [sɑːbuˈrəu]（Raymond J. A. Sabouraud）沙氏葡萄糖琼脂（培养真菌用）
sabulous [ˈsæbjuləs] *a* 沙样的，有沙的
saburra [səˈbəːrə] *n*【拉】口垢，口臭 | **~l** *a*
sac [sæk] *n* 囊 | air ~s 肺泡 / allantoic ~ 尿膜囊 / alveolar ~s 肺泡[小]囊 / amniotic ~ 羊膜囊，羊膜 / conjunctival ~ 结膜囊 / epiploic ~ 网膜囊 / laryngeal ~ 喉室 / heart ~ 心包 / serous ~ 浆膜囊（由胸膜、心包、腹膜组成）/ splenic ~ 脾囊，脾隐窝 / tear ~ 泪囊 / vitelline ~，yolk ~ 卵黄囊
sacbrood [ˈsækbruːd] *n* 幼蜂皱萎病
saccade [səˈkeid] *n* 扫视，眼急动 | **saccadic** [səˈkædik] *a*
saccate [ˈsækeit] *a* 囊状的；有囊的
saccharascope [ˈsækərəskəup] *n* 发酵糖定量器
saccharase [ˈsækəreis] *n* 蔗糖酶
saccharate [ˈsækəreit] *n* 蔗糖盐；糖二酸盐
saccharated [ˈsækəˌreitid] *a* 含糖的
saccharephidrosis [ˌsækərefiˈdrəusis] *n* 糖汗症；皮肤糖溢
saccharic acid [səˈkærik] 葡糖二酸；糖酸
saccharide [ˈsækəraid] *n* 糖类
sacchariferous [ˌsækəˈrifərəs] *a* 含糖的，生糖的
saccharify [səˈkærifai] *vt* 使糖化 | **saccharification** [ˌsækərifiˈkeiʃən] *n* 糖化[作用]
saccharimeter [ˌsækəˈrimitə] *n* 糖量计 | fermentation ~ 发酵糖量计
saccharin [ˈsækərin] *n* 糖精，邻磺酰苯甲酰亚胺 | ~ calcium 糖精钙（甜味药）/ ~ sodium 糖精钠（甜味药）| **saccharinol** [səˈkærinɔl]，**saccharinum** [ˌsækəˈrainəm] *n*
saccharine [ˈsækərain] *a* 似糖的，甜味的
sacchar(o)- [构词成分] 糖
saccharobiose [ˌsækərəuˈbaiəus] *n* 蔗[二]糖，二糖
saccharocoria [ˌsækərəuˈkɔːriə] *n* 厌糖[现象]
saccharogalactorrhea [ˌsækərəugəˌlæktəˈriːə] *n* 多糖乳，乳汁多糖
saccharolytic [ˌsækərəuˈlitik] *a* 糖分解的
saccharometabolism [ˌsækərəumeˈtæbəlizəm] *n* 糖[新陈]代谢 | **saccharometabolic** [ˌsækərəuˌmetəˈbɔlik] *a*
saccharometer [ˌsækəˈrɔmitə] *n* 糖量计
Saccharomyces [ˌsækərəuˈmaisiːz] *n* 酵母属 | ~ albicans [变] 白色酵母，白色念珠菌 / ~ anginae 咽峡炎酵母 / ~ apiculatus 尖端酵母 / ~ cantliei 坎氏酵母 / ~ capillitii 脱发酵母 / ~ cerevisiae 酿酒酵母 / ~ ellipsoideus 椭圆酵母 / ~ exiguus 少孢酵母 / ~ galacticolus 乳品酵母 / ~ glutinis 胶酵母 / ~ granulomatosus 肉芽肿酵母 / ~ guttulatus 点滴酵母 / ~ hansenii 汉森

酵母 / ~ hominis 人体酵母 / ~ lemonnieri 列氏酵母 / ~ lithogenes 石原酵母 / ~ rubrum 深红酵母
saccharomyces [ˌsækərəuˈmaisiːz] ([复] **saccharomycetes** [ˌsækərəumaiˈsiːtiːz]) *n* 酵母 | **saccharomycetic** [ˌsækərəumaiˈsetik] *a*
Saccharomycetaceae [ˌsækərəumaisiˈteisiiː] *n* 酵母科
saccharomycetolysis [ˌsækərəuˌmaisiˈtɔlisis] *n* 酵母溶解[现象]
Saccharomycopsis [ˌsækərəumaiˈkɔpsis] *n* 复膜孢酵母属 | ~ guttulatus 点滴复膜孢酵母
saccharonic acid [ˌsækəˈrɔnik] 糖酮酸,甲基糖二酸
saccharopine [ˈsækərəuˌpiːn] *n* 酵母氨酸
saccharopine dehydrogenase (NAD⁺, L-glutamate-forming) [ˈsækərəuˌpiːn diːˈhaidrədʒəneis ˈgluːtəmeit ˈfɔːmiŋ] 酵母氨酸脱氢酶(NAD⁺, L-谷氨酸形成的)(此酶活性在高赖氨酸血症及变异型酵母氨酸尿症中缺乏)
saccharopine dehydrogenase (NADP⁺, L-lysine-forming) [ˈsækərəuˌpiːn diːˈhaidrədʒəneis ˈlaisiːn ˈfɔːmiŋ] 酵母氨酸脱氢酶(NADP⁺, L-赖氨酸形成的)(此酶活性在高赖氨酸血症中缺乏,并在变异型酵母氨酸尿症中实质性减少,通常称赖氨酸酮戊二酸还原酶)
saccharopinemia [ˌsækərəupiˈniːmiə] *n* 酵母氨酸血[症](血内酵母氨酸过多,如高赖氨酸血症或酵母氨酸尿症时)
saccharopinuria [ˌsækərəupiˈnjuəriə] *n* 酵母氨酸尿症(①尿内排泄酵母氨酸;②一种变异型高赖氨酸血症,由于α-氨基己二酸半醛合酶活性部分缺乏所致)
saccharorrhea [ˌsækərəuˈriːə] *n* 糖尿
saccharosan [ˈsækərəsən] *n* 脱水蔗糖
saccharose [ˈsækərəus] *n* 蔗糖
saccharosuria [ˌsækərəuˈsjuəriə] *n* 蔗糖尿
Saccharum [ˈsækərəm] *n* 甘蔗属 | ~ officinarum 甘蔗
saccharum [ˈsækərəm] *n*【拉】糖(尤指蔗糖)
saccharuria [ˌsækəˈrjuəriə] *n* 糖尿
sacci [ˈsæksai] saccus 的所有格和复数
sacciform [ˈsæksifɔːm], **saccular** [ˈsækjulə] *a* 囊形的
sacculate [ˈsækjulit], **sacculated** [ˈsækjuˌleitid] *a* 囊状的,成囊的,有小囊的
sacculation [ˌsækjuˈleiʃən] *n* 成囊;小囊,袋 | ~s of colon 结肠袋
saccule [ˈsækjuːl] *n* 小囊;球囊 | air ~s, alveolar ~s 肺泡[小]囊 / laryngeal ~, ~ of larynx 喉小囊
sacculitis [ˌsækjuˈlaitis] *n* 小囊炎
sacculocochlear [ˌsækjuləuˈkɔkliə] *a* 球囊耳蜗的
sacculotomy [ˌsækjuˈlɔtəmi] *n* 球囊切开[术]
sacculus [ˈsækjuləs] ([复] **sacculi** [ˈsækjulai]) *n*【拉】小囊;球囊
saccus [ˈsækəs] ([复] **sacci** [ˈsæksai]) *n* 囊
SACH solid ankle cushion heel 软跟假脚
Sachs' disease [sæks] (Bernard 〈Barney〉 Sachs) 家族性黑矇性痴呆
Sachs-Georgi test (reaction) [zaːks geˈɔːgi] (Hans Sachs; Walter Georgi) 萨克斯-格奥尔吉试验(反应)(检梅毒:1 ml 人或牛心胆固醇化乙醇浸出液 1 份和 0.9% 氯化钠溶液 9 份的混合液,加至 0.3 ml 梅毒血清,能产生絮状沉淀。亦称缓慢胆固醇反应)
Sachsse's test [ˈzaːksə] (Georg R. Sachsse) 萨克塞试验(检尿糖)
Sachs-Witebsky test (reaction) [zaːks wiˈtebski] (Hans Sachs; Ernest Witebsky) 萨克斯-威特布斯基试验(反应)(检梅毒:一种快速梅毒血清反应,所用牛心胆固醇化浸出液比 Sachs-Georgi 试验所用的较浓。亦称快速胆固醇反应或加速胆固醇试验)
sacrad [ˈseikræd] *ad* 向骶骨,向骶侧
sacral [ˈseikrəl] *a* 骶骨的
sacralgia [seiˈkrældʒiə] *n* 骶骨痛
sacralization [ˌseikrəlaiˈzeiʃən, -liˈz-] *n* (第五腰椎)骶骨融合,骶化
sacrarthrogenic [ˌseikraːθrəuˈdʒenik] *a* 骶关节病的
sacrectomy [seiˈkrektəmi] *n* 骶骨切除术
sacrifice [ˈsækrifais] *n* 牺牲,牺牲品
sacr(o)- [构词成分]骶[骨]
sacroanterior [ˌseikrəuænˈtiəriə] *n* 骶前位(产位)
sacrococcygeal [ˌseikrəukɔkˈsidʒiəl] *a* 骶尾的
sacrococcyx [ˌseikrəuˈkɔksiks] *n* 骶尾骨
sacrocoxalgia [ˌseikrəukɔkˈsældʒiə] *n* 骶尾骨痛
sacrocoxitis [ˌseikrəukɔkˈsaitis] *n* 骶髋关节炎
sacrodynia [ˌseikrəuˈdiniə] *n* 骶[部]痛
sacroiliac [ˌseikrəuˈiliæk] *a* 骶髂的
sacroiliitis [ˌseikrəuˌiliˈaitis] *n* 骶髂关节炎
sacrolisthesis [ˌseikrəulisˈθiːsis] *n* 骶骨前移
sacrolumbar [ˌseikrəuˈlʌmbə] *a* 骶腰的
sacroperineal [ˌseikrəuˌperiˈniːəl] *a* 骶骨会阴的
sacroposterior [ˌseikrəupɔsˈtiəriə] *n* 骶后位(产位)
sacropromontory [ˌseikrəuˈprɔməntəri] *n* 骶骨岬
sacrosciatic [ˌseikrəusaiˈætik] *a* 骶骨坐骨的
sacrosidase [sæˈkrəusideis] *n* 蔗糖苷酶(一种从酵母衍生的酶,催化二糖包括蔗糖的末端果糖残余的水解,用作替代物,以取代蔗糖酶-异麦芽糖酶缺乏症时所缺乏的蔗糖酶活性,口服给药)

sacrospinal [ˌseikrəuˈspainl] *a* 骼棘的;骶脊的
sacrospinous [ˌseikrəuˈspainəs] *a* 骼棘的
sacrotomy [seiˈkrɔtəmi] *n* 骶骨[下部]切开术
sacrotransverse [ˌseikrəutrænsˈvəːs] *n* 骶横位(产位)
sacrouterine [ˌseikrəuˈjuːtərin] *a* 骶骨子宫的
sacrovertebral [ˌseikrəuˈvəːtibrəl] *a* 骶骨椎骨的
sacrum [ˈseikrəm] ([复] **sacrums** 或 **sacra** [ˈseikrə]) *n* 骶骨 | assimilation ~ 同化骶骨 / tilted ~ 骶骨倾斜
sactosalpinx [ˌsæktəuˈsælpiŋks] *n* 输卵管积液
SAD seasonal affective disorder 季节性情感障碍
saddle [ˈsædl] *n* 鞍;鞍状物;鞍基 | denture base ~ 假牙牙托
sadism [ˈsædizəm] *n* 施虐狂,施虐欲,施虐癖 | anal ~ 肛[欲]期施虐欲 / oral ~ 口期施虐欲 | **sadist** *n* 施虐者,施虐狂者,施虐癖者 / **sadistic** [sæˈdistik] *a*
sadomasochism [ˌsædəuˈmæsəkizəm] *n* 施虐受虐狂(一种既施虐又受虐的性变态) | **sadomasochist** *n* 施虐受虐狂者 / **sadomasochistic** [ˌsædəuˌmæ səuˈkistik] *a*
SADS Schedule for Affective Disorder and Schizophrenia 情感障碍和精神分裂症时间表
Saemisch's operation (section) [ˈseimiʃ] (Edwin T. Saemisch) 塞米施手术(切开术)(治眼前房积脓) | ~ ulcer 匐行性角膜溃疡
Saenger's macula [ˈzeŋgə] (Max Saenger) 淋病性斑
Saenger's sign (reflex) [ˈzeŋgə] (Alfred Saenger) 曾格尔征(反射)(消失的瞳孔对光反应,经过在黑暗中短暂停留后又告恢复,见于脑性梅毒,但不见于脊髓痨)
Saethre-Chotzen syndrome [ˈseitrə ˈkɔtzən] (Haakon Saethre; F. Chotzen) 塞-科综合征(见 Chotzen syndrome)
safflower [ˈsæflauə] *n* 红花,草红花
safranin O [ˈsæfrənin] 沙黄 O,番红 O(用作核染剂及用作革兰〈Gram〉染色法中的复染。亦可拼写成 safranine O)
safrene [ˈsæfriːn] *n* 黄樟烯
safrol [ˈsæfrɔl], **safrole** [ˈsæfrəul] *n* 黄樟脑,黄樟素(止痛药)
safrosin [ˈsæfrəsin] *n* 蓝曙红
sage [seidʒ] *n* 洋苏草
sagittal [ˈsædʒitl] *a* 矢状的,前后向的
sagittalis [ˌsædʒiˈteilis] *a* 【拉】矢状的,前后向的
sago [ˈseigəu] *n* 西[谷]米(西谷椰子淀粉)
Sahli's reaction [ˈsɑːli] (Herman Sahli) 萨利反应,硬纤维袋反应(检胃分泌及运动) | ~ method 萨利法(酸性高铁血红素测定法) / ~ test 萨利试验(检胃蠕动及消化能力)
Saint's triad [seint] (Charles F. M. Saint) 圣氏三联征(食管裂孔疝、结肠憩室和胆石症同时发生)
Sakati-Nyhan syndrome [ˈsækəti ˈnaihən] (Nadia Sakati; William L. Nyhan) 萨-纳综合征,尖头多指并指[畸形]Ⅲ型,尖头多趾并趾[畸形]Ⅲ型
Saksenaea [ˌsæksəˈniːə] *n* 瓶酶属
Saksenaeaceae [ˌsæksəniːˈeisiːiː] *n* 瓶酶科
S. A. L. secundum artis leges 【拉】按技术规定
sal [sæl] *n* 【拉】盐
salad [ˈsæləd] *n* 色拉 | word ~ 语词杂拌
salamander [ˈsæləˌmændə] *n* 蝾螈
salamanderin [ˌsæləˈmændərin] *n* 蝾螈毒碱
salantel [ˈsæləntəl] *n* 沙仑太尔(兽用抗蠕虫药)
Sala's cells [ˈsælə] (Luigi Sala) 萨拉细胞(形成心包感觉神经末梢纤维的结缔组织星形细胞)
salazosulfapyridine [ˌsæləzəuˌsʌlfəˈpiridiːn] *n* 柳氮磺吡啶(磺胺类药)
salbutamol [sælˈbjuːtəmɔl] *n* 沙丁胺醇(支气管扩张药)
salcolex [ˈsælkəleks] *n* 柳胆来司(抗炎、解热、镇痛药)
salethamide maleate [sæˈleθəmaid] 马来酸沙乙酰胺(镇痛药)
salicin [ˈsælisin] *n* 水杨苷(镇痛药)
salicyl [ˈsælisil] *n* 水杨基;邻羟苄基
salicylacetic acid [ˌsælisiləˈsiːtik] 水杨乙酸,水杨酰醋酸
salicylaldehyde [ˌsælisilˈældihaid] *n* 水杨醛;邻羟苯甲酸
salicylamide [ˌsælisilˈæmaid] *n* 水杨酰胺(口服解热镇痛药)
salicylanilide [ˌsælisilˈænilaid] *n* 水杨[酰]苯胺(局部抗真菌药,治疗头癣)
salicylase [səˈlisileis] *n* 水杨酶,水杨醛氧化酶
salicylate [sæˈlisileit] *n* 水杨酸盐(或酯) | ~ meglumine 水杨酸葡胺(抗风湿药和镇痛药)
salicylated [sæˈlisileitid, ˈsæli-] *a* 含水杨酸的,浸水杨酸的
salicylazosulfapyridine [ˌsæliˌsiləzəuˌsʌlfəˈpiridiːn] *n* 柳氮磺吡啶(磺胺类药)
salicylemia [ˌsælisiˈliːmiə] *n* 水杨酸盐血[症]
salicylic [ˌsæliˈsilik] *a* 水杨基的
salicylic acid [ˌsæliˈsilik] 水杨酸
salicylism [ˈsæliˌsilizəm] *n* 水杨酸中毒(常有耳鸣,恶心及呕吐)
salicyloacetic acid [ˌsælisiləuəˈsiːtik] 水杨酰醋酸
salicylsalicylic acid [sæˌlisilˌsæliˈsilik] 双水杨酯(见 salsalate)
salicylsulfonic acid [ˌsælisilsʌlˈfɔnik] 磺基水

杨酸
salicyltherapy [ˌsælisil'θerəpi] *n* 水杨酸疗法
salicyluric acid [ˌsælisi'ljuərik] 水杨尿酸,水杨酸甘氨酸
saliferous [sə'lifərəs] *a* 产盐的,含盐的
salifiable ['sæliˌfaiəbl] *a* (能变)成盐的
salification [ˌsælifi'keiʃən] *n* 成盐作用
salify ['sælifai] *vt* 使成盐
salimeter [sə'limitə] *n* 盐液浓度计,盐液比重计
saline ['seilain, -liːn] *a* 盐的,含盐的,咸的 [sə'lain; 'seilain, -liːn] *n* 盐水 | physiological ~, normal ~ 生理盐水
salinigrin [ˌsæli'naigrin] *n* 柳黑苷
salinometer [ˌsæli'nɔmitə] *n* 盐液密度计
saliva [sə'laivə] *n* 涎,唾液 | chorda ~ 鼓索性涎(刺激鼓索所分泌的颌下腺涎,较正常涎液清稀) / ganglionic ~ 神经节性涎(刺激颌下腺所分泌的涎液) / lingual ~ 舌腺涎 / parotid ~ 腮腺涎 / ropy ~ 黏性涎 / sublingual ~ 舌下腺涎 / submaxillary ~ 颌下腺涎 / sympathetic ~ 交感神经性涎
salivant ['sælivənt] *a* 催涎的 *n* 催涎药
salivaria [ˌsæli'vɛəriə] *n* 唾窦锥虫 | ~**n** *a*
salivary ['sælivəri] *a* 涎的,唾液的
salivate ['sæliveit] *vt* 使流涎,使过量分泌唾液 *vi* 流涎,分泌唾液 | **salivation** [ˌsæli'veiʃən] *n* 流涎,多涎
salivator ['sæliˌveitə] *n* 催涎剂
salivatory ['sælivətəri] *a* 催涎的
salivin ['sælivin] *n* 涎液素,涎淀粉酶
salivolithiasis [səˌlaivəuli'θaiəsis] *n* 涎石病
Salix ['sæliks] *n* 柳属
Salkowski's method [sæl'kɔfski] (Ernst L. Salkowski) 萨尔科夫斯基法(检嘌呤体及尿酸) | ~ test 萨尔科夫斯基试验(检血中一氧化碳、胆固醇、吲哚、葡萄糖及肌酸酐)
Salk vaccine [sɔːlk] (Jonas E. Salk) 索尔克疫苗(预防脊髓灰质炎的灭活疫苗)
salmeterol xinafoate [sæl'metərɔl] 辛那福酸沙美特罗(支气管扩张药)
salmiac ['sælmiæk] *n* 氯化铵
salmin(e) ['sælmin] *n* 鲑精蛋白
salmon ['sælmən] *n* 鲑;鲑肉色,橙红色
Salmonella [ˌsælmə'nelə] *n* 沙门菌属 | ~ abortus equi 马流产沙门菌 / ~ abortus ovis 绵羊流产沙门菌 / ~ agona 阿哥拉沙门菌 / ~ anatum 鸭沙门菌 / ~ arizonae 亚利桑那沙门菌 / ~ bongor 波哥沙门菌 / ~ chloleraesuis 猪霍乱沙门菌 / ~ enteritidis 肠炎沙门菌 / ~ gallinarum 鸡沙门菌 / ~ houtenae 豪顿沙门菌 / ~ morgani 摩根沙门菌,摩根变形杆菌 / ~ paratyphi, ~ paratyphi A 副伤寒沙门菌,甲型副伤寒沙门菌 / ~ paratyphi B, ~ schottmülleri 乙型副伤寒杆菌,肖特苗勒沙门菌 / ~ paratyphi C, ~ hirshfeldii 丙型副伤寒沙门菌,希施费尔德沙门菌 / ~ pullorum 鸡瘟沙门菌 / ~ salamae 塞拉姆沙门菌 / ~ sendai 仙台沙门菌 / ~ typhimurium, ~ aertrycke 鼠伤寒沙门菌 / ~ typhosa, ~ typhi 伤寒沙门菌,伤寒杆菌
salmonella [ˌsælmə'nelə] ([复] **salmonellae** [ˌsælmə'neliː]) *n* 沙门菌
salmonellal [ˌsælmə'nelәl] *a* 沙门菌引起的
Salmonelleae [ˌsælmə'neliiː] *n* 沙门菌族
salmonellosis [ˌsælməne'ləusis] *n* 沙门菌感染(食物中含有沙门菌引起,特征为急剧性腹泻,伴有急腹痛,里急后重和〈或〉副伤寒)
salocoll ['sæləkɔl] *n* 萨罗可(抗风湿药)
salol ['seilɔl] *n* 萨罗,水杨酸苯酯
Salomon's test ['zæləmən] (Hugo Salomon) 扎洛蒙试验(检胃溃疡性癌的白蛋白试验)
salpingectomy [ˌsælpin'dʒektəmi] *n* 输卵管切除术
salpingemphraxis [ˌsælpindʒem'fræksis] *n* 咽鼓管阻塞
salpingian [sæl'pindʒiən] *a* 输卵管的;咽鼓管的
salpingion [sæl'pindʒiɔn] *n* 咽鼓管点
salpingitis [ˌsælpin'dʒaitis] *n* 输卵管炎;咽鼓管炎 | chronic interstitial ~ 慢性间质性输卵管炎 / chronic vegetating ~ 慢性增殖性输卵管炎 / eustachian ~ 咽鼓管炎 / hemorrhagic ~ 出血性输卵管炎 / hypertrophic ~, mural ~, parenchymatous ~ 增殖性输卵管炎,肥厚性输卵管炎,实质性输卵管炎 / tuberculous ~ 结核性输卵管炎 | **salpingitic** [ˌsælpin'dʒitik] *a*
salping(o)- [构词成分] 管;输卵管;咽鼓管
salpingocatheterism [sælˌpiŋgəu'kæθitərizəm] *n* 咽鼓管插管法
salpingocele [sæl'piŋgəsiːl] *n* 输卵管疝
salpingocyesis [sælˌpiŋgəusai'iːsis] *n* 输卵管妊娠(异位妊娠的一种)
salpingography [ˌsælpiŋ'gɔgrəfi] *n* 输卵管造影[术]
salpingolithiasis [sælˌpiŋgəuli'θaiəsis] *n* 输卵管石病(输卵管壁钙质沉着)
salpingolysis [ˌsælpiŋ'gɔlisis] *n* 输卵管粘连分离术
salpingo-oophorectomy [sælˌpiŋgəu ˌəuɔfə'rektəmi], **salpingo-ovariectomy** [sælˌpiŋgəuəuˌvɛəri'ektəmi], **salpingo-ovariotomy** [sælˌpiŋgəu əuˌvɛəri'ɔtəmi] *n* 输卵管卵巢切除术
salpingo-oophoritis [sælˌpiŋgəu ˌəuɔfə'raitis], **salpingo-oothecitis** [sælˌpiŋgəu ˌəuəθi'saitis] *n* 输卵管卵巢炎
salpingo-oophorocele [sælˌpiŋgəu əu'ɔfərəsiːl],

salpingo-oothecocele [sælˌpiŋgəu ˌəuə'θiːkəsiːl] *n* 输卵管卵巢疝

salpingoperitonitis [sælˌpiŋgəuˌperitəu'naitis] *n* 输卵管腹膜炎

salpingopexy [sæl'piŋgəˌpeksi] *n* 输卵管固定术

salpingopharyngeal [sælˌpiŋgəufə'rindʒiːəl] *a* 咽鼓管咽的

salpingoplasty [sæl'piŋgəˌplæsti] *n* 输卵管成形术

salpingorrhaphy [ˌsælpiŋ'gɔrəfi] *n* 输卵管缝合术

salpingoscopy [ˌsælpiŋ'gɔskəpi] *n* 咽鼓管镜检查

salpingostaphyline [sælˌpiŋgəu'stæfilin] *a* 咽鼓管悬雍垂的

salpingostomatomy [sælˌpiŋgəustəu'mætəmi], **salpingostomatoplasty** [sælˌpiŋgəustəu'mætəˌplæsti] *n* 输卵管部分切除造口术

salpingostomy [ˌsælpiŋ'gɔstəmi] *n* 输卵管造口术

salpingotomy [ˌsælpiŋ'gɔtəmi] *n* 输卵管切开术

salpingoureteral [sælˌpiŋgəujuə'riːtərəl] *a* 输卵管输尿管的

salpinx ['sælpiŋks] *n*【希】管

salsalate ['sælsəleit] *n* 双水杨酯,水杨酰水杨酸,双水杨酸,水杨酸水杨酸酯(用于治骨关节炎和类风湿关节炎)

salt [sɔːlt] *n* 盐;食盐;[复]泻盐 *a* 含盐的 *vt* 加盐于,用盐处理 | acid ~ 酸性盐 / baker's ~ 碳酸铵 / basic ~ 碱性盐 / bile ~ 胆汁盐 / common ~ 食盐,氯化钠 / Epsom ~ 泻盐,硫酸镁 / pancreatic ~ 胰酶盐剂(用作消化药) / peptic ~ 胃蛋白酶盐剂(用作消化药) / smelling ~s 嗅盐 / table ~ (餐桌上用的)食盐

saltant ['sæltənt] *n* 突变型;菌落突变型

saltation [sæl'teiʃən] *n* 跳跃,舞蹈;突变,种群突变

saltatory ['sæltətəri], **saltatorial** [ˌsæltə'tɔːriəl], **saltatoric** [ˌsæltə'tɔːrik] *a* 跳跃的,舞蹈的;突变的

Salter's incremental lines ['sɔːltə] (James A. Salter)索尔特增长线(牙本质)

saltiness ['sɔːltinis] *n* 咸性

salting in ['sɔːltiŋ in] 盐溶(通过提高盐浓度溶解蛋白质,当少量中性盐加入时,不溶解于纯水的一定量蛋白质即可溶解)

salting-out ['sɔːltiŋ aut] *n* 盐析

saltpeter, saltpetre ['sɔːltˌpiːtə] *n* 硝石,硝酸钾 | Chile ~ 智利硝石,硝酸钠

salty ['sɔːlti] *a* 含盐的;咸的

salubrious [sə'ljuːbriəs] *a* 有益健康的,适于卫生的 | **salubrity** *n*

saluresis [ˌsælju'riːsis] *n* 尿食盐排泄(尿中钠和氯根离子的排泄) | **saluretic** [ˌsælju'retik] *a* [促]尿食盐排泄的 *n* 促尿食盐排泄药

salutarium [ˌsælju'tɛəriəm] *n* 疗养地

salutary ['sæljutəri] *a* 有益健康的,适于[恢复]健康的

salute [sə'ljuːt] *n* 致敬 | allergic "salute"变应性仪态

salvage ['sælvidʒ] *n* (疾病等的)抢救 | ~ at scene 现场抢救

salvarsan ['sælvəsən] *n* 胂凡钠明,六〇六(抗梅毒药)

salve [sɑːv, sælv] *n* 软膏,油膏 *vt* 敷软膏于 | fetron ~ 费特龙油膏(含硬脂酸苯胺及凡士林) / scarlet ~ 猩红油膏

Salvia ['sælviə] *n*【拉】鼠尾草属

Salzmann's nodular corneal dystrophy ['zælzmən] (Maximilian Salzmann) 扎尔茨曼结节性角膜营养不良(角膜上皮层、角膜前弹性层及角膜基质外部的进行性肥大性变性)

samaderin [sə'mædərin] *n* 黄楝树苦素

samandaridine [ˌsæmən'dæridin] *n* 蝾螈啶

samandarine [sə'mændəriːn] *n* 蝾螈碱

samarium (Sm) [sə'mɛəriəm] *n* 钐(化学元素)

Sambucus [sæm'bjuːkəs] *n* 接骨木属

SAMHSA Substance Abuse and Mental Health Services Agency 药物滥用和精神卫生服务处

sample ['sɑːmpl] *n* 样本,样品;标本 *vt* 取样 | random ~ 随机样本

sampling ['sɑːmpliŋ] *n* 取样,抽样 | chorionic villus ~ (CVS) 绒膜绒毛取样(用于 9~12 周妊娠时的产前诊断法。亦可拼写成 chorionic villous sampling,亦称绒膜绒毛活组织检查)

Sampson's cyst ['sæmpsn] (John A. Sampson) 桑普森囊肿,巧克力样囊肿(chocolate cyst,见 cyst 项下相应术语)

Sanarelli's serum [ˌsænə'reli] (Giuseppe Sanarelli) 萨内雷利血清(用于保护性接种以防黄热病)

sanative ['sænətiv] *a* 治愈的

sanatorium [ˌsænə'tɔːriəm] ([复] **sanatoriums** 或 **sanatoria** [ˌsænə'tɔːriə]) *n* 疗养院,疗养所(尤指对结核病患者或其他恢复期患者实施户外疗养的场所);疗养站(热带地区的疗养地)

sanatory ['sænətəri] *a* 有益健康的,促进健康的

sanctuary ['sæŋktʃuˌɛəri] *n* 药聚区

sancycline [sæn'saikliːn] *n* 山环素(抗生素类药)

sand [sænd] *n* 沙,沙土 | brain ~ 脑沙,松果体石 / intestinal ~ 肠沙

sandalwood ['sændlwud] *n* 檀香;檀香木

sandarac ['sændəræk] *n* 山达脂(牙科用作填齿泥) *vt* 用山达脂溶液处理

sand crack [sænd kræk] 蹄裂病(马)

Sander's disease [ˈsændə] (Wilhelm Sander) 赞德尔病(偏执狂的一种)
Sanders' disease [ˈsændəz] (Murray Sanders) 流行性角膜结膜炎
sandfly [ˈsændflai] *n* 白蛉
Sandhoff disease [ˈsɑːndhɔf] (K. Sandhoff) 桑德霍夫病(GM_2 神经节苷脂沉积症的一型〈变异型 O 或Ⅱ型〉,其临床特征类似泰-萨克斯〈Tay-Sachs〉病及 GM_2 神经节苷脂沉积症 B 变异型的其他型,但其特征为贮存或排泄含低聚糖的 *N*-乙酰氨基葡糖、有时为器官巨大症以及仅在非犹太人中发生。其基本缺陷为已糖胺酶 A 和 B 同工酶缺乏,系由该酶的 β 链内的一种缺损所致。本病发生有若干型〈婴儿型、少年型和成人型〉,随着起病年龄的增加,病情也随之减轻)
Sandifer's syndrome [ˈsændifə] (Paul Sandifer) 桑迪福综合征(间歇性斜颈,见于儿童,系作为回流性食管炎或食管裂孔疝的症状发生)
Sandström's bodies, glands [ˈzæntstreim] (Ivar V. Sandström) 甲状旁腺,副甲状腺
Sandwith's bald tongue [ˈsændwiθ] (Fleming M. Sandwith) 桑德韦思秃舌(见于糙皮病晚期)
sane [sein] *a* 神志正常的,精神健全的
Sanfilippo's syndrome [sænfiˈlipəu] (Sylvester J. Sanfilippo) 桑菲利波综合征(为四种不均一的在生化上各异而在临床上不能区别的黏多糖贮积症,其特征在生化上为尿中排泄硫酸乙酰肝素,在临床上为严重而迅速的精神衰退,躯体症状相对较轻。2～6 岁发病;头大,身高正常;轻度胡尔勒〈Hurler〉样特征〈多发性骨发育障碍,肝肿大〉;全身多毛;通常死于 20 岁之前。四种酶的类型为:A 型最严重,因乙酰肝素 *N*-硫酸酯酶缺乏所致;B 型为 α-*N*-乙酰氨基葡糖苷酶缺乏所致;C 型为乙酰肝素-α-氨基葡糖苷-*N*-乙酰基转移酶缺乏所致;D 型为 *N*-乙酰氨基葡糖-6-硫酸酯酶缺乏所致。亦称黏多糖贮积症Ⅲ型)
Sänger 见 Saenger
sangui- [构词成分]血
sanguicolous [sæŋˈgwikələs] *a* 住血的(生活在血中的)
sanguifacient [ˌsæŋgwiˈfeiʃənt] *a* 造血的,生血的
sanguiferous [sæŋˈgwifərəs] *a* 运血的,含血的
sanguification [ˌsæŋgwifiˈkeiʃən] *n* 血液生成;血液化
sanguimotor [ˌsæŋgwiˈməutə], **sanguimotory** [ˌsæŋgwiˈməutəri] *a* 血液循环的
sanguinaria [ˌsæŋgwiˈnɛəriə] *n* 血根(用作白松糖浆成分)
sanguinarine [ˌsæŋgwiˈneiriːn] *n* 血根碱
sanguine [ˈsæŋgwin] *a* 有血色的,多血质的
sanguineous [sæŋˈgwiniəs], **sanguinous** [ˈsæŋgwinəs] *a* 血的,含血的,多血质的
sanguinolent [sæŋˈgwinələnt] *a* 含血的,血色的
sanguinopoietic [ˌsæŋgwinəupɔiˈetik] *a* 生血的,造血的
sanguinopurulent [ˌsæŋgwinəuˈpjuərulənt] *a* 血液浓性的
sanguirenal [ˌsæŋgwiˈriːnl] *a* 血[与]肾的
sanguis [ˈsæŋgwis] *n*【拉】血,血液
sanguisuction [ˌsæŋgwiˈsʌkʃən] *n* 吸血法
sanguivorous [sæŋˈgwivərəs] *a* 食血的,吸血的(指雌蚊)
sanicult [ˈsænikʌlt] *n* 江湖医术
sanies [ˈseiniiːz] *n*【拉】腐液,败液 | sanious [ˈseiniəs] *a*
sanify [ˈsænifai] *vt* 使合卫生,改善…的环境卫生
saniopurulent [ˌseiniəuˈpjuərulənt] *a* 腐脓性的
sanioserous [ˌseiniəuˈsiərəs] *a* 腐浆液性的
sanitarian [ˌsæniˈtɛəriən] *a* 公共卫生[学]的,保健的 *n* 公共卫生学家,保健专家
sanitarium [ˌsæniˈtɛəriəm] *n* 疗养地;疗养院,疗养所
sanitary [ˈsænitəri] *a* 卫生的,保健的
sanitation [ˌsæniˈteiʃən] *n* 卫生,环境卫生[学];卫生设备;污水排放
sanitization [ˌsænitaiˈzeiʃən, -tiˈz-] *n* 卫生处理(尤指饮食用具)
sanitize [ˈsænitaiz] *vt* 使清洁,给…消毒,卫生处理;除去…中的有害成分
sanity [ˈsænəti] *n* 神志正常,精神健全
San Joaquin Valley fever (disease) [sæn wɑːˈkiːn ˈvæli] (San Joaquin Valley 在加利福尼亚州,此病在该地尤为明显)圣华金河谷热(病),原发性球孢子菌病
Sansom's sign [ˈsænsəm] (Arthur E. Sansom) 桑塞姆征(①心包积液时第二及第三肋间隙浊音明显增加;②患胸主动脉瘤时,置听诊器于口唇上可听到节律性杂音)
Sanson's images [ˈsænsɔn] (Louis J. Sanson) 桑松像(角膜前表面及晶状体前后面形成的投射像)
santalum [ˈsætələm] *n* 檀香;檀香木
Santavuori's disease (syndrome) [sɑntɑːˈvuəuri] (Pirkko Santavuori) 桑塔沃里病(综合征)(见 Haltia-Santavuori disease)
Santavuori-Haltia disease (syndrome) [sɑːntɑːˈvuəuri ˈhɑːltiɑː] (P. Santavuori; M. Haltia) 桑-霍病(综合征)(见 Haltia-Santavuori disease)
santenic acid [sænˈtenik] 檀烯酸
santonica [sænˈtɔnikə] *n*【拉】山道年花
santonic acid [sænˈtɔnik] 山道酸

santonin [ˈsæntənin] *n* 山道年(抗蠕虫药)
santoninic acid [ˌsæntəˈninik] 山道年酸
Santorini's cartilages [ˌsɑːntəuˈriːni] (Giovanni D. Santorini) 小角状软骨 | ~ circular muscle 尿道环行肌 / ~ duct 副胰管 / ~ fissures 外耳道软骨切迹 / ~ ligament 环咽韧带 / ~ muscle 笑肌 / ~ papilla 十二指肠壶腹 / ~ plexus 前列腺丛;前列腺静脉丛 / ~ tubercle 小角结节
SAP sphingolipid activator protein 鞘脂激活蛋白
sap [sæp] *n* 液,汁 | cell ~ 透明质 / nuclear ~ 核液,核淋巴 | ~**less** *a* 无液的
saphena [səˈfiːnə] *n*【拉】隐静脉 | **saphenous** *a*
saphenectomy [ˌsæfiˈnektəmi] *n* 隐静脉切除术
saphenography [ˌsæfəˈnɔgrəfi] *n* 隐静脉造影[术]
sapid [ˈsæpid] *a* 有香味的,美味的
sapin [ˈseipin] *n* 沙平(尸胺、脑胺的一种无毒异构体)
sapo [ˈseipəu] *n*【拉】肥皂,皂
sapogenin [səˈpɔdʒinin] *n* 皂苷元,皂角苷配基
saponaceous [ˌsæpəuˈneiʃəs] *a* 肥皂性的,肥皂般的
Saponaria [ˌseipəuˈnɛəriə] *n* 肥皂草属
saponarin [ˌseipəuˈneirin] *n* 肥皂草苷
saponatus [ˌseipəuˈneitəs] *a*【拉】含皂的
saponification [səˌpɔnifiˈkeiʃən] *n* 皂化[作用]
saponify [səˈpɔnifai] *vt, vi* 皂化 | **saponifiable** *a* 可皂化的 / **saponifier** *n* 皂化剂
saponin [ˈsæpənin] *n* 皂苷 | cholan ~s 胆烷皂苷 / triterpenoid ~s 三萜式皂苷
sapophore [ˈsæpəfɔː] *n* 生味基,生味团
sapotalene [ˈsæpəˌtæliːn] *n* 山榄烯
sapotoxin [ˌseipəuˈtɔksin] *n* 皂毒苷
Sappey's fibers [sɑːˈpei] (Marie P. C. Sappey) 萨佩纤维(眼翼状韧带内的平滑肌纤维) | ~ ligament 萨佩韧带(下颌关节囊的增厚后部) / ~ nucleus 红核 / ~ veins 附脐静脉
sapphism [ˈsæfizəm] *n* 女性同性恋
sapremia [sæˈpriːmiə] *n* 腐血症,脓毒中毒 | **sapremic** *a* 腐血症的,脓毒性的
saprin [ˈseiprin] *n* 腐尸碱(得自腐败的内脏物质的一种无毒尸碱)
sapr(o)- [构词成分]腐败
saprobe [ˈsæprəub] *n* 污水生物,腐生生物
saprobic [səˈprəubik] *a* 污水生物的,腐生生物的,污水生的,腐生的
saprogenic [ˌsæprəuˈdʒenik] *a* 生腐的,腐化的
Saprolegnia [ˌsæprəuˈlegniə] *n* 水霉属 | ~ ferax 水霉
Saprolegniales [ˌsæprəuˌlegniˈeiliːz] *n* 水霉目
sapronosis [ˌsæprəuˈnəusis] *n* 腐生病(由环境中微生物引起的一种疾病)
sapropel [ˈsæprəpel] *n* 腐泥(江、湖等的黑色腐殖质淤积,缺氧但富有硫化氢) | ~**ic** [ˌsæprəuˈpelik] *a*
saprophagous [səˈprɔfəgəs] *a* 食腐的,腐物寄生的
saprophyte [ˈsæprəfait] *n* 腐生菌,腐生生物
saprophytic [ˌsæprəuˈfitik], **saprophilous** [səˈprɔfiləs] *a* 腐物寄生的;食腐的,腐生的
saprophytism [ˈsæprəfaitizəm] *n* 腐物寄生;死物寄生
Saprospira [ˌsæprəuˈspaiərə] *n* 腐生螺旋体属
saprozoic [ˌsæprəuˈzəuik] *a* 腐生的,食腐的,腐物寄生的(尤指原生动物)
saprozoite [ˌsæprəuˈzəuait] *n* 食腐动物,腐[物寄]生动物
saquinavir [səˈkwinəvir] *n* 沙奎那韦(一种 HIV〈人免疫缺陷病毒〉蛋白酶抑制剂,可致未成熟非感染的病毒颗粒形成,用于治疗人免疫缺陷病毒感染和获得性人免疫缺陷综合征,口服给药)
saralasin acetate [səˈræləsin] 醋酸沙拉新(血管紧张素Ⅱ的拮抗剂,用作抗高血压药)
sarapus [ˈsærəpəs] *n* 扁平足者
Sarbó's sign [ˈsɑːbəu] (Arthur von Sarbó) 萨尔博征(脊髓痨时腓神经痛觉缺失)
Sarcina [ˈsɑːsinə] *n* 八叠球菌属
sarcina [ˈsɑːsinə] ([复] **sarcinae** [ˈsɑːsiniː]) *n* 八叠球菌
sarcitis [sɑːˈsaitis] *n* 肌炎
sarc(o)- [构词成分]肉,肌
sarcoblast [ˈsɑːkəblæst] *a* 成肌细胞
sarcocarcinoma [ˌsɑːkəuˌkɑːsiˈnəumə] *n* 癌肉瘤
sarcocele [ˈsɑːkəsiːl] *n* 睾丸肉样肿
sarcocol [ˈsɑːkəkɔl] *n* 甘草味胶
sarcocyst [ˈsɑːkəsist] *n* 肉孢子虫;肉孢子虫囊
sarcocystin [ˌsɑːkəuˈsistin] *n* 肉孢子虫毒素
Sarcocystis [ˌsɑːkəˈsistis] *n* 肉孢子虫属 | ~ bovihominis 牛-人肉孢子虫 | ~ suihominis 猪-人肉孢子虫
sarcocystosis [ˌsɑːkəsisˈtəusis] *n* 肉孢子虫病
sarcocyte [ˈsɑːkəsait] *n* 肉层(原虫外胞质的中层)
Sarcodina [ˌsɑːkəˈdainə] *n* 肉足亚门(原生动物门)
sarcodine [ˈsɑːkədiːn] *a* 肉足亚门的(Sarcodina) *n* 肉足[亚门]原虫
sarcodinian [ˌsɑːkəˈdiniən] *n* 肉足[亚门]原虫
sarcoenchondroma [ˌsɑːkəuˌenkɔnˈdrəumə] *n* 软骨肉瘤
sarcogenic [ˌsɑːkəuˈdʒenik] *a* 生肌的
sarcoglia [sɑːˈkɔgliə] *n* 肌胶质
sarcohydrocele [ˌsɑːkəuˈhaidrəsiːl] *n* 水囊肿性

睾丸肉样肿
sarcoid [ˈsɑːkɔid] *a* 肉样的 *n* 肉样瘤,类肉瘤;肉样瘤病,结节病
sarcoidosis [ˌsɑːkɔiˈdəusis] *n* 结节病 | ~ cordis 心脏结节病 / muscular ~ 肌肉结节病
sarcolactate [ˌsɑːkəuˈlækteit] *n* 肌乳酸盐
sarcolactic acid [ˌsɑːkəuˈlæktik] 肌乳酸
sarcolemma [ˌsɑːkəuˈlemə] *n* 肌膜 | **sarcolemmic**, **sarcolemmous** *a*
sarcoleukemia [ˌsɑːkəuljuːˈkiːmiə] *n* 淋巴肉瘤细胞白血病,白血病性肉瘤
sarcolysin [ˌsɑːkəuˈlaisin] *n* 溶肉瘤素 | L-sarcolysin *n* 左旋溶肉瘤素(抗肿瘤药)
sarcolysis [sɑˈkɔlisis] *n* 软组织溶解,肌肉分解 | **sarcolytic** [sɑːkəuˈlitik] *a* 溶软组织的,溶肌肉的
sarcolyte [ˈsɑːkəlait] *n* 溶软组织细胞,溶肉细胞
sarcoma [sɑːˈkəumə] ([复] **sarcomas** 或 **sarcomata** [sɑːˈkəumətə]) *n* 肉瘤 | adipose ~ 脂肉瘤 / alveolar soft part ~ 腺泡状软组织肉瘤 / ameloblastic ~ 成釉细胞肉瘤 / botryoid ~ 葡萄状肉瘤 / chloromatous ~ 绿色[肉]瘤 / ~ colli uteri hydropicum papillare 乳头状水泡状宫颈肉瘤,葡萄状肉瘤 / embryonal ~ 胚胎性肉瘤 / endometrial stromal ~ 宫内膜间质肉瘤 / granulocytic ~ 粒细胞性肉瘤,绿色瘤 / immunoblastic ~ of B cells 成免疫细胞性 B 细胞肉瘤 / immunoblastic ~ of T cells 成免疫细胞性 T 细胞肉瘤 / leukocytic ~ 白血病性肉瘤 / lymphatic ~ 淋巴肉瘤 / osteoblastic ~ 成骨细胞肉瘤 / osteogenic ~, osteoid ~, osteolytic ~ 骨原性肉瘤,骨样肉瘤,溶骨肉瘤 / reticulum cell ~, reticulocytic ~, reticuloendothelial ~, retothelial ~ 网状细胞肉瘤 / synovial ~ 滑膜肉瘤 / telangiectatic ~ 毛细管扩张性肉瘤 | **~tous** *a*
sarcomagenesis [ˌsɑːkəuməˈdʒenisis] *n* 肉瘤生成,肉瘤发生
sarcomagenic [ˌsɑːkəuməˈdʒenik] *a* 致肉瘤的
Sarcomastigophora [ˌsɑːkəuˌmæstiˈgɔfərə] *n* 肉鞭毛虫门
sarcomatoid [sɑːˈkəumətɔid] *a* 肉瘤样的
sarcomatosis [ˌsɑːkəuməˈtəusis] *n* 肉瘤病 | ~ cutis 皮肤肉瘤病 / general ~ 全身性肉瘤病
sarcomere [ˈsɑːkəmiə] *n* 肌(原纤维)节,肌小节
sarcomphalocele [ˌsɑːkɔmˈfæləsiːl] *n* 脐肉瘤
sarconeme [ˈsɑːkəniːm] *n* 微线体,短丝
sarcopenia [ˌsɑːkəuˈpiːniə] *n* 老年性肌肉萎缩
Sarcophaga [sɑːˈkɔfəgə] *n* 麻蝇属
Sarcophagidae [ˌsɑːkəuˈfædʒidiː] *n* 麻蝇科
sarcoplasm [ˈsɑːkəˌplæzəm] *n* 肌质 | **~ic** [ˌsɑːkəuˈplæzmik] *a*
sarcoplast [ˈsɑːkəplæst] *n* 肌间质细胞
sarcopoietic [ˌsɑːkəupɔiˈetik] *a* 生肌的
Sarcopsylla [ˌsɑːkɔpˈsilə] *n* 肉蚤属(即潜蚤属 Tunga) | ~ penetrans 穿皮肉蚤(即穿皮潜蚤 Tunga penetrans)
Sarcoptes [sɑːˈkɔptiːz] *n* 疥螨属 | ~ scabiei 疥螨
sarcoptic [sɑːˈkɔptik] *a* 疥螨的
Sarcoptidae [sɑːˈkɔptidiː] *n* 疥螨科
sarcoptidosis [sɑːˌkɔptiˈdəusis] *n* 疥,疥螨病
sarcosine [ˈsɑːkəsiːn] *n* 肌氨酸,*N*-甲基甘氨酸
sarcosine dehydrogenase [ˈsɑːkəsiːn diːˈhaidrədʒəneis] 肌氨酸脱氢酶(此酶缺乏为一种常染色体隐性性状,可致高肌氨酸血症)
sarcosinemia [ˌsɑːkəsiˈniːmiə] *n* 肌氨酸血症
sarcosinuria [ˌsɑːkəsiˈnjuəriə] *n* 肌氨酸尿[症]
sarcosis [sɑːˈkəusis] *n* 肉瘤病;肉过多
sarcosome [ˈsɑːkəsəum] *n* 肌粒,肉粒
Sarcosporidia [ˌsɑːkəuspəˈridiə] *n* 肉孢子虫目
sarcosporidiosis [ˌsɑːkəuspəˌridiˈəusis], **sarcosporidiasis** [ˌsɑːkəuˌspɔːriˈdaiəsis] *n* 肉孢子虫病
sarcosporidium [ˌsɑːkəuspəˈridiəm] ([复] **sarcosporidia** [ˌsɑːkəuspəˈridiə]) *n* 肉孢子虫
sarcostosis [ˌsɑːkɔsˈtəusis] *n* 肌骨化
sarcostyle [ˈsɑːkəstail] *n* 肌柱,肌原纤维束
sarcotherapeutics [ˌsɑːkəuˌθerəˈpjuːtiks], **sarcotherapy** [ˌsɑːkəuˈθerəpi] *n* 肉汁疗法,动物组织浸出物疗法
sarcotic [sɑːˈkɔtik] *a* 生肉的
sarcotubules [ˌsɑːkəuˈtjuːbjuːlz] *n* 肌[浆]小管
sarcous [ˈsɑːkəs] *a* 肉的,肌[肉组织]的
sardonic [sɑːˈdɔnik] *a* (不自主)痉笑的
sargramostim [sɑːˈgræməstim] *n* 沙格司亭(粒-巨噬细胞集落刺激因子,由重组技术形成,用作骨髓抑制性化疗治癌的佐剂,可加速造血系统的恢复)
sarin [sɑːˈriːn] *n* 沙林(一种有机磷化合物,为强效胆碱酯酶抑制剂,并用作神经毒气,中毒症状包括支气管缩窄、惊厥以及死亡)
sarmentocymarin [sɑːˌmentəuˈsaimərin] *n* 沙门苷
sarmentogenin [ˌsɑːmənˈtɔdʒənin] *n* 沙门苷元
sarmentose [ˈsɑːməntəus] *n* 沙门糖,箭毒羊角拗糖
Sarothamnus [ˌsærəˈθæmnəs] *n* 金雀花属
sarpicillin [ˌsɑːpiˈsilin] *n* 沙匹西林(抗菌药)
Sarracenia [ˌsærəˈsiːniə] *n* 瓶子草属
SARS severe acute respiratory syndrome 重症急性呼吸综合征
sarsaparilla [ˌsɑːsəpəˈrilə], **sarsa** [ˈsɑːsə] *n* 【拉;西】菝葜(治牛皮癣,也用作药物的调味剂)
sarsasapogenin [ˌsɑːsəˌsæpəˈdʒenin] *n* 菝葜皂苷

元,萨尔萨皂苷元

Sassafras [ˈsæsəfræs] *n*【拉】擦木属,黄樟属

satellite [ˈsætəlait] *n* 卫星;卫星病灶;卫星结节;伴行静脉,陪静脉(紧密伴随动脉的静脉,如肱静脉);随体(染色体的末端部分) | bacterial ~ 卫星菌,陪菌 / chromosomal ~ 染色体随体 / nucleolar ~ 核仁随体 / ~ DNA 卫星 DNA

satellitism [ˈsætəlitizəm] *n* 卫星现象(某些细菌菌种十分靠近其他无关细菌菌落时生长旺盛,例如流感嗜血杆菌即靠近链球菌菌落,这是由于后一菌种产生必需的代谢产物所致)

satellitosis [ˌsætəlaiˈtəusis] *n* 卫星现象,卫星状态(神经胶质细胞在神经元周围的堆积,见于神经元受损时)

satiety [səˈtaiəti] *n* 饱满感(食欲或渴感),厌腻

satratoxin [ˈseitrəˌtɔksin] *n* 黑葡萄穗霉毒素

Satterthwaite's method [ˈsætəθweit] (Thomas E. Satterthwaite) 萨特思韦特法(人工呼吸、轮流揿压和放松腹部)

Sattler's layer [ˈsætlə] (Hubert Sattler) 扎特勒层(脉络膜血管层中由中等大小血管所构成的部分)

satumomab [səˈtjuːməumæb] *n* 沙妥莫单抗(一种单克隆抗体,专用于结肠癌和卵巢腺癌的诊断用药)

saturable [ˈsætʃərəbl] *a* 可饱和的 | **saturability** [ˌsætʃərəˈbiləti] *n* 饱和额

saturant [ˈsætʃərənt] *a* 饱和的 *n* 饱和剂

saturate [ˈsætʃəreit] *vt* 使饱和 | **~d** *a* 饱和的

saturation [ˌsætʃəˈreiʃən] *n* 饱和,饱和度;饱和剂量(放射治疗时,在短时间内先给予组织能承受的最大剂量,然后在随后时间内给予较小分剂量以维持其生物效应);一次泡腾顿服量 | arterial oxygen ~ 动脉血氧饱和度 / oxygen ~ 氧饱和

saturnic [səˈtəːnik] *a* 中铅毒的

saturnine [ˈsætənain] *a* 铅的

saturnism [ˈsætənizəm] *n* 铅中毒

satyr [ˈsætə] *n* 色情狂者 | **~ic** [səˈtirik] *a* 色情狂的

satyriasis [ˌsætiˈraiəsis], **satyromania** [ˌsætirəuˈmeinjə] *n* 男子色情狂,求雌狂

sauce [sɔːs] *n* 调味汁,酱汁

saucer [ˈsɔːsə] *n* 托盘,碟 | auditory ~ 听窝(胚)

saucerization [ˌsɔːsəraiˈzeiʃən, -riˈz-] *n* 碟形手术;碟形凹陷(脊椎受压骨折形成)

Sauerbruch's prosthesis [ˈsauəbruh] (Ernst F. Sauerbruch) 绍尔布鲁赫假体(一种假体,使残肢的组织得以活动)

Sauer's vaccine [ˈsauə] (Louis W. Sauer) 索尔菌苗,百日咳菌苗(预防百日咳)

Saundby's test [ˈsɔːndbi] (Robert Saundby) 桑德比试验(检粪血)

Saunders' disease [ˈsɔːndəz] (Edward W. Saunders) 桑德斯病(一种危急的状态,见于给了高比例的碳水化合物而有消化性失调的婴儿,特征为呕吐、大脑症状及循环抑制) | ~ sign 桑德斯征(儿童在口张开时,产生手的联带运动,其中包括口张开、手指伸展和分开,亦称口手联带运动)

Saussure's hygrometer [sɔːˈsuə] (Horace B. de Saussure) 索苏尔湿度计,毛发湿度计

savin [ˈsævin] *n* 沙芬,新疆圆柏,沙比桧

saw [sɔː] *n* 锯 | amputating ~ 切断锯 / crown ~ 冠形锯 / hole ~ 钻锯,环钻 / separating ~ 分离锯(牙) / subcutaneous ~ 皮下骨锯

saxitoxin [ˌsæksiˈtɔksin] *n* 石房蛤毒素

Sayre's apparatus [ˈseiə] (Lewis A. Sayre) 塞尔吊架(上石膏背心时用)

SB sinus bradycardia 窦性心动过缓

Sb stibium 锑

SBE subacute bacterial endocarditis 亚急性细菌性心内膜炎

SC secretory component 分泌成分;closure of semilunar valves 半月瓣闭合

Sc scandium 钪

scab [skæb] *n* 痂 *vi* 结痂 | **~bed** [ˈskæbid] *a* 结痂的

scabby [ˈskæbi] *a* 痂的;疥疮的

scabicide [ˈskeibisaid] *a* 杀疥螨的 *n* 杀疥螨药

scabies [ˈskeibiiːz] *n* 疥疮;疥螨病 | Norwegian ~ 结痂性疥疮

scabietic [ˌskeibiˈetik], **scabetic** [skeˈbetik] *a* 疥疮的

scabious [ˈskeibjəs] *a* 痂的;疥疮的

SCAD deficiency short-chain acyl-CoA dehydrogenase deficiency 短链酰基辅酶 A 脱氢酶缺乏症

scala [ˈskeilə] ([复] **scalae** [ˈskeiliː]) *n*【拉】阶

scalar [ˈskeilə] *n*, *a* 纯量(的),标量(的),无向量(的)

scalariform [skəˈlærifɔːm] *a* 梯级形的,梯纹形的

scald [skɔːld] *vt* 烫伤;用沸水或蒸汽消毒 *n* 烫伤 | **~ing** *n* 烫伤;烧灼性痛

scale[1] [skeil] *n* 标,标度 | absolute ~ 绝对温标 / centigrade ~ 百分温标,摄氏温标 / Columbia Mental Maturity Scale 哥伦比亚智力成熟表(一种特殊形式的心理功能和普通能力的测验,适合于 3 ~ 12 岁不会说话或身体有缺陷的儿童,如患有大脑麻痹的儿童) / French ~ 法制标度(一种表示导尿管、尿道探子以及其他管状器械的型号标度,1 F 约等于 0.33 mm,即 18 F 表示直径为 6 mm) / hydrometer ~ 比重计标度(用以表示液体的比重) / intelligence ~ 智力量表 / ordinal ~ 顺序标度(标度中的样点用数字表示,如疾病症状的分级:轻度①,中度②或重度

③) / ratio ~ 比例尺度(用于对感觉的心理物理测量)

scale² [skeil] *n* 鳞片;(眼中的)翳障;(皮肤的)鳞屑;牙垢 *vt* 除垢 | adhesive ~ 黏着性鳞屑

scalene [ˈskeiliːn] *a* 不等边的(指三角形),偏三角的;斜角肌的

scalenectomy [ˌskeiliˈnektəmi] *n* 斜角肌切除术

scalenotomy [ˌskeiliˈnɔtəmi] *n* 斜角肌切开术

scalenus [skeiˈliːnəs] *n* 【拉】斜角肌

scaler¹ [ˈskeilə] *n* 洁治器(牙)

scaler² [ˈskeilə] *n* 定标器;换算装置;计数器

scaling [ˈskeiliŋ] *n* 刮治

scalp [skælp] *n* 头皮 | dissecting cellulitis of ~ 头皮切割性蜂窝织炎 / gyrate ~ 头皮松垂,回状头皮

scalpel [ˈskælpəl] *n* 解剖刀,手术刀

scalpriform [ˈskælprifɔːm] *a* 凿形的

scaly [ˈskeili] *a* 有鳞屑的;鳞状的

scammony [ˈskæməni] *n* 司格蒙旋花;药旋花(根)(驱虫药、泻药) | Mexican ~ 墨西哥司格蒙旋花,药薯(根) | **scammonia** [skəˈməu-niə] *n*

scan [skæn] *vt* 扫描,扫描检查 *vi* 扫描 *n* 扫描图;扫描 | CAT ~, CT ~ 计算体层摄影扫描,计算机轴向体层摄影(即 computerized axial tomography)

scandium (Sc) [ˈskændiəm] *n* 钪(化学元素)

scanner [ˈskænə] *n* 扫描仪,扫描器 | EMI ~ EMI 扫描器(在阴极射线管上显示出重建体层摄影影像的仪器) / scintillation ~ 闪烁扫描器

scanning [ˈskæniŋ] *n* 扫描[术];断续言语 | radioisotope ~ 放射性同位素扫描

scanography [skæˈnɔgrəfi] *n* 扫描检查

scansion [ˈskænʃən] *n* 断续言语

Scanzoni's maneuver (operation) [skænˈtsəuni] (Friedrich W. Scanzoni) 斯坎佐尼手法(产钳娩出手法,即使用产钳旋转胎头之法)

scapha [ˈskeifə] *n* 【拉】耳舟,舟状窝

scaphion [ˈskeifiən] *n* 颅底外面

scaph(o)- [构词成分]船,舟

scaphocephaly [ˌskæfəˈsefəli], **scaphocephalia** [ˌskæfəsiˈfeiliə], **scaphocephalism** [ˌskæfəˈsefəlizəm] *n* 舟状头[畸形] | **scaphocephalic** [ˌskæfəsəˈfælik], **scaphocephalous** [ˌskæfəˈsefələs] *a*

scaphohydrocephalus [ˌskæfəˌhaidrəuˈsefələs], **scaphohydrocephaly** [ˌskæfəˌhaidrəuˈsefəli] *n* 舟状头脑积水

scaphoid [ˈskæfɔid] *a* 舟状的 *n* 舟骨

scaphoiditis [ˌskæfɔiˈdaitis] *n* 舟骨炎

scapholunate [ˌskæfəuˈljuːneit] *a* 舟骨月骨的

scapula [ˈskæpjulə] ([复] **scapulas** 或 **scapulae** [ˈskæpjuliː]) *n* 肩胛[骨];肩板(昆虫) | elevated ~ 高位肩胛(先天性肩胛耸举症) / scaphoid ~ 舟状肩胛[骨] / winged ~, alar ~ 翼状肩胛[骨]

scapulalgia [ˌskæpjuˈlældʒiə] *n* 肩胛痛

scapular [ˈskæpjulə] *a* 肩胛[骨]的

scapulary [ˈskæpjuləri] *n* 肩悬带

scapulectomy [ˌskæpjuˈlektəmi] *n* 肩胛切除术

scapuloanterior [ˌskæpjuləuænˈtiəriə] *n* 肩前位(横产胎位之一)

scapuloclavicular [ˌskæpjuləukləˈvikjulə] *a* 肩胛锁骨的

scapulodynia [ˌskæpjuləuˈdiniə] *n* 肩[胛]痛

scapulohumeral [ˌskæpjuləuˈhjuːmərəl] *a* 肩胛肱骨的

scapuloperoneal [ˌskæpjuləuˌperəˈniəl] *a* 肩腓骨的

scapulopexy [ˈskæpjuləˌpeksi] *n* 肩胛固定术

scapuloposterior [ˌskæpjuləupɔsˈtiəriə] *n* 肩后位(横产胎位之一)

scapus [ˈskeipəs] ([复] **scapi** [ˈskeipai]) *n* 干,体,柄

scar [skɑː] *n* 瘢痕,疤痕 | hypertrophic ~ 肥厚性瘢痕 / white ~ of ovary 白体

scarification [ˌskεərifiˈkeiʃən] *n* 划破,划痕

scarifier [ˈskεərifaiə], **scarificator** [ˈskεərifiˌkeitə] *n* 划痕器

scarify [ˈskεərifai] *vt* 划破,划痕

scarlatina [ˌskɑːləˈtiːnə] *n* 【拉】猩红热 | puerperal ~ 产褥性猩红热 | **~l** [skɑːˈlætinl] *a*

scarlatinella [skɑːˌlætiˈnelə] *n* 轻型猩红热

scarlatiniform [ˌskɑːləˈtinifɔːm], **scarlatinoid** [skɑːˈlætinɔid] *a* 猩红热样的

scarlet [ˈskɑːlit] *n* 猩红色 *a* 猩红的 | ~ G 黄光油溶红,苏丹Ⅲ / ~ R 猩红 R,猩红

Scarpa's fascia [ˈskɑːpə] (Anthony Scarpa) 斯卡帕筋膜(腹壁浅筋膜深层) | ~ fluid 斯卡帕液(内淋巴液) / ~ foramen 鼻腭神经孔 / ~ ganglion 前庭神经节 / ~ ligament 镰缘上角 / ~ membrane 第二鼓膜,蜗窗膜 / ~ nerve 鼻腭神经 / ~ sheath 提睾筋膜 / ~ shoe 内翻足矫形靴 / ~ staphyloma (眼)后葡萄肿 / ~ triangle 股三角

scarring [ˈskɑːriŋ] *n* 瘢痕形成

SCAT sheep cell agglutination test 绵羊细胞凝集试验(测血清类风湿因子)

Scatchard plot [ˈskætʃəd] (George Scatchard) 斯卡查德图(用于分析配体和受体的可逆性结合的一种图,依据的是希尔〈Hill〉方程式,其中希尔系数为 1.0)

scatemia [skəˈtiːmiə] *n* 肠性毒血症

scat(o)- [构词成分]粪,粪质

scatol [ˈskeitɔl] *n* 粪臭素；甲基吲哚
scatologia [ˌskætəˈləudʒə] *n* 嗜粪癖
scatology [skəˈtɔlədʒi] *n* 粪便学 | **scatologic** [skætəˈlɔdʒik] *a*
scatoma [skəˈtəumə] *n* 粪结，粪瘤（肠内积粪）
scatophagy [skəˈtɔfədʒi] *n* 食粪癖
scatophilia [ˌskætəuˈfiliə] *n* 恋粪癖
scatoscopy [skəˈtɔskəpi] *n* 粪便检视法
scattergram [ˈskætəgræm] *n* 散点图（见 scatterplot）
scattering [ˈskætəriŋ] *a* 分散的 *n* 分散；散射，扩散；散布
scatterplot [ˈskætəplɔt] *n* 散点图（两个随机变量成对观察的直角坐标上的一种标绘图，每次观察在图上标上一个点，点的分散或集积表示两个变量之间的关系）
scatula [ˈskætjulə] *n* 盒，纸匣
scavenger [ˈskævindʒə] *n* 清除剂，净化剂；食腐动物
ScD Scientiae Doctor 理学博士
ScDA scapulodextra anterior【拉】肩右前（胎位）
ScDP scapulodextra posterior【拉】肩右后（胎位）
Scedosporium [siːdəˈspɔːriəm] *n* 足放线病菌属
scelalgia [skiˈlældʒiə səˈlæl-] *n* 小腿痛
scelotyrbe [ˌseləˈtəːbi] *n* 小腿痉瘫
Schacher's ganglion [ˈʃɑːhə] (Polycarp G. Schacher) 睫状神经节
Schachowa's spiral tubes [ˈʃɑːkəvə] (Seraphina Schachowa) 肾小管
Schafer's dumbbell, dumbbell of Schafer [ˈʃeifə] (Edward A. Sharpey-Schafer) 谢弗小体（在横纹肌组织内发现的小体）| ~ method 谢弗法（伏卧式人工呼吸法：令患者伏卧，前额置于一臂部，施术者两膝跨于患者两髋关节旁，两手紧压患者下方肋骨的上背部，然后慢慢抬身，同时两手放松，以每 5 秒做一次向前向后运动）
Schäfer's syndrome [ˈʃeifə] (Erich Schäfer) 谢弗综合征（先天性厚甲伴身心发育迟缓）
Schäffer's reflex [ˈʃefə] (Max Schäffer) 舍费尔反射（器质性偏瘫时，压迫跟腱的中 1/3，则足及趾屈曲）
Schamberg's disease (dermatosis, progressive pigmented purpuric dermatosis) [ˈʃæmbəːg] (Jay F. Schamberg) 山伯格病（皮肤病、进行性色素性紫癜性皮肤病，是青春期及青年男性的一种慢性无症状性皮肤病，局限于胫部、踝部及足背和趾骨，特征为长出橙色至浅黄褐色斑疹，边缘内或边缘上有红色小点〈红椒样斑点〉）
Schanz's disease [ˈʃʌnts] (Alfred Schanz) 尚茨病（外伤性跟腱炎）| ~ syndrome 尚茨综合征（脊椎病一系列症状，包括疲劳感、脊椎突压痛、伏卧时痛以及脊椎弯曲的病征）
Schardinger's enzyme [ˈʃɑːdiŋgə] (Franz Schardinger) 沙尔丁格酶，黄嘌呤氧化酶 | ~ reaction 沙尔丁格反应（用于区别鲜奶和加热过的牛奶：用醛和亚甲蓝或靛蓝处理牛奶，如为鲜奶，则染料还原为无色化合物）
scharlach R [ˈʃɑːlək] 猩红
Schatzki's ring [ˈʃɑːtski] (Richard Schatzki) 沙茨基环，食管环
Schaudinn's fluid [ʃɔːˈdin] (Fritz R. Schaudinn) 绍丁液（一种硬化液，含有氯化汞、醇及蒸馏水）
Schaumann's bodies [ˈʃɔːmən] (Jörgen Schaumann) 绍曼体（肉样瘤病时，患病处所见的红色或棕色结节性贝壳样病损）| ~ sarcoidosis (disease, syndrome) 肉样瘤病，结节病
Schauta's operation [ˈʃɔːtə] (Friedrich Schauta) 绍塔手术（经阴道广泛性子宫切除治疗宫颈癌）
Schauta-Wertheim operation [ˈʃɔːtə ˈvəːthaim] (Friedrich Schauta; Ernst Wertheim) 绍塔-韦特海姆手术（见 Wertheim-Schauta operation）
SChE serum cholinesterase 血清胆碱酯酶
Schede's clot [ˈʃeidə] (Max Schede) 谢德血块（谢德手术〈坏死骨取出术〉形成的血块）| ~ operation (method, resection, treatment) 谢德手术（法、切除术、疗法）（①脓胸胸壁切除术；②下肢静脉曲张手术；③坏死骨取出术）
schedule [ˈʃedjuːl, ˈskedʒu(ː)l] *n* 一览表，时间表，程序表 | Diagnostic Interview Schedule (DIS) 诊断性交谈时间表 / ~ of reinforcement 强化时间表
Scheibe's aplasia [ˈʃaibə] (A. Scheibe) 沙伊伯不发育（球囊和耳蜗管部分不发育）| ~ deafness 沙伊伯聋（一种先天性聋，因球囊和耳蜗管部分不发育〈沙伊伯不发育〉所致）
Scheie's syndrome [ʃei] (Harold G. Scheie) 沙伊综合征（为胡尔勒〈Hurler〉综合征比较轻的等位基因变异型，黏多糖贮积症 I 型中三种等位基因病中最轻的一种，特征为角膜混浊，鹰爪手，主动脉瓣受累，面容稍显粗糙，宽嘴，膝外翻及弓形足。身高、智力和寿命均正常，由于 L-艾杜糖苷酸酶缺乏所致。亦称黏多糖贮积症 IS 型，以前称黏多糖贮积症 V 型）
Scheiner's experiment [ˈʃainə] (Christoph Scheiner) 沙伊纳实验（通过卡片上相近两个针孔注视物体的实验，如物体在焦点上，只见到一个物像，如不在焦点上，则见到两个或两个以上的物像）
schema [ˈskiːmə] ([复] **schemata** [ˈskiːmətə]) *n* 计划，纲要；图解，格式，图式
schematic [skiˈmætik] *a* 纲要的；图解的，按照图式的
scheme [skiːm] *n* 计划，纲要，方案；图解，图式
Schepelmann's sign [ˈʃeipəlmæn] (Emil Schep-

elmann) 舍佩尔曼征(干性胸膜炎时,患者身体弯向健侧则疼痛增加;而肋间神经痛时,弯向患侧则疼痛增加)

Scherer's test [ˈʃeirə] (Johann J. von Scherer) 舍雷尔试验(检肌醇、纯白氨酸、酪氨酸)

scheroma [skiˈrəumə] *n* 干眼病,眼干燥(缺乏维生素 A)

Scheuermann's disease, kyphosis [ˈʃɔiəmən] (Holger W. Scheuermann) 舒尔曼病、脊柱后凸(椎骨骨软骨病)

Schick's sign [ʃik] (Béla Schick) 锡克征(患支气管淋巴结结核的婴儿呼气时可听到的喘鸣) | ~ test (reaction) 锡克试验(反应),白喉毒素皮内试验(检机体对白喉免疫性的试验)

Schiefferdecker's disk [ʃiːfəˈdekə] (Paul Schiefferdecker) 席费尔德克尔板(朗飞〈Ranvier〉节处施万〈Schwann〉鞘和轴索之间,用硝酸银染成黑色的物质) | ~ symbiosis theory 席费尔德克尔共生学说(认为人体各组织之间有某种共生现象,因而此组织的代谢产物能作为刺激使其他组织活动)

Schiff's biliary cycle [ʃif] (Moritz Schiff) 席夫胆汁循环(胆汁中的胆汁盐为肠绒毛所吸收,然后送回肝脏,在肝内再被利用的循环,亦称胆盐肠肝循环)

Schiff's reagent [ʃif] (Hugo Schiff) 希夫试剂(检醛) | ~ test 希夫试验(检尿碳水化合物、胆固醇、尿囊素及脲、尿酸、乳中甲醛)

Schilder's disease (encephalitis) [ˈʃildə] (Paul F. Schilder) 希尔德病(脑炎)(儿童和青少年亚急性或慢性型脑白质病,亦称弥漫性轴周性脑炎,进行性皮质下脑病)

Schiller's test [ˈʃilə] (Walter Schiller) 席勒试验,宫颈黏膜碘试验(检宫颈癌)

Schilling's leukemia [ˈʃiliŋ] (Victor T. A. G. Schilling) 希林白血病,急性单核细胞白血病

Schilling test [ˈʃiliŋ] (Robetr F. Schilling) 希林试验(检维生素 B_{12} 胃肠吸收,诊断原发性恶性贫血)

Schimmelbusch's disease [ˈʃiməlˌbuʃ] (Curt Schimmelbusch) 席梅尔布施病(增生性乳腺炎的一种,其特征为有许多小囊肿发生,亦称乳腺囊性病)

schindylesis [ˌskindiˈliːsis] *n* 夹合连接,沟缝

Schinus [ˈskainəs] *n* 秘鲁乳香属

Schinzel-Giedion syndrome [ˈʃintsel ˈgiːdiɔn] (Albert A. G. L. Schinzel; Andres Giedion) 幸-吉综合征(一种罕见的综合征,或许为常染色体隐性遗传,表现为肾盂积水、骨骼异常、面中部扁平、多毛症、癫痫发作以及重症生长发育迟缓)

Schiøtz's tonometer [ʃiˈets] (Hjalmar Schiøtz) 希厄茨眼压计(用于测定眼内压)

Schirmer's syndrome [ˈʃirmə] (Rudolf Schirmer) 席默综合征(一种斯-韦〈Sturge-Weber〉综合征,其中青光眼在疾病过程中很早发生)

-schisis [构词成分]裂

schistasis [ˈskistəsis] *n* 裂,分裂(尤指人体上的裂,一种先天性缺损,如躯裂畸形)

schist(o)- [构词成分]裂,分裂

schistocelia [ˌʃistəuˈsiːliə, -ˌskis-] *n* 腹裂[畸形]

schistocephalus [ˌʃistəˈsefələs, ˌski-] *n* 头裂畸胎

schistoc(o)elia [ˌʃistəˈsiːliə, ˌski-] *n* 先天性腹裂[畸形]

schistocormia [ˌʃistəˈkɔːmiə, ˌski-] *n* 躯裂[畸形]

schistocormus [ˌʃistəˈkɔːməs, ˌski-] *n* 躯裂畸胎

schistocystis [ˌʃistəˈsistis] *n* 膀胱裂

schistocyte [ˈʃistəsait, ˈski-] *n* 裂细胞,裂红细胞(常见于溶血性贫血患者的血液中)

schistocytosis [ˌʃistəsaiˈtəusis, ˌski-] *n* 裂细胞症

schistoglossia [ˌʃistəˈglɔsiə, ˌski-] *n* 舌裂[畸形]

Schistosomatidae [ˌʃistəsəuˈmætidiː, -ˌskis-] *n* 裂体科

schistomelia [ˌʃistəˈmiːliə, ski-] *n* 肢裂[畸形]

schistomelus [ʃisˈtɔmiləs, ski-] *n* 肢裂畸胎

schistometer [ʃisˈtɔmitə, ˌski-] *n* 声门裂测量计

schistoprosopia [ˌʃistəprəˈsəupiə, ˌski-] *n* 面裂[畸形]

schistoprosopus [ˌʃistəˈprɔsəpəs, ˌski-] *n* 面裂畸胎

schistorachis [ʃisˈtɔrəkis, ski-] *n* 脊柱裂[畸形]

schistosis [ʃisˈtəusis, ski-] *n* 肺石板屑沉着病

Schistosoma [ˌʃistəˈsəumə, ˌski-] *n* 裂体[吸虫]属,血吸虫属 | ~ bovis 牛裂体吸虫,牛血吸虫 / ~ haematobium 埃及裂体吸虫,埃及血吸虫 / ~ indicum 印度裂体吸虫,印度血吸虫 / ~ intercalatum 间插裂体吸虫,间插血吸虫 / ~ japonicum 日本裂体吸虫,日本血吸虫 / ~ mansoni 曼氏裂体吸虫,曼氏血吸虫 / ~ mattheei 羊裂体吸虫,羊血吸虫 / ~ spindale 梭形裂体吸虫 / ~ mekongi 湄公河裂体吸虫,湄公河血吸虫

schistosomacidal [ˌʃistəˌsəuməˈsaidl, ˌski-] *a* 杀血吸虫的

schistosomacide [ˌʃistəˈsəuməsaid, ˌski-] *n* 杀血吸虫药

schistosomal [ˌʃistəuˈsəuməl, ˌski-] *a* 血吸虫的

Schistosomatium [ˌʃistəsəuˈmeiʃiəm, ˌski-] *n* 小裂体吸虫属

schistosome [ˈʃistəsəum, ˌski-] *n* 裂体吸虫,血吸虫

schistosomia [ˌʃistəˈsəumiə, ˌski-] 体裂(下肢缺损)畸形(腹部有裂隙与下肢发育不全或缺损)

schistosomiasis [ˌʃistəsəuˈmaiəsis, ˌski-] *n* 血吸

虫病 | cutaneous ~ 皮肤血吸虫病,血吸虫皮炎,游泳癣 / ~ intercalatum 刚果血吸虫病,间插血吸虫病 / ~ japonica, eastern ~, oriental ~ 日本血吸虫病 / ~ mansoni 曼氏血吸虫病 / urinary ~, vesical ~, ~ haematobia 尿路血吸虫病,膀胱血吸虫病,埃及血吸虫病

schistosomicidal [ˌʃistəˌsəumiˈsaidl, ˌski-] *a* 杀血吸虫的

schistosomicide [ˌʃistəˈsəumisaid, ˌski-] *n* 杀血吸虫药

Schistosomum [ˌʃistəˈsəuməm, ˌski-] *n* 裂体[吸虫]属,血吸虫属(即 Schistosoma)

schistosomulum [ˌʃistəˈsɔmjuləm, ˌskis-] ([复] **schistosomula** [ˌʃistəˈsɔmjulə, ˌskis-]) *n* 血吸虫童虫

schistosomus [ˌʃistəuˈsəuməs, ˌski-] *n* 体裂(下肢缺损)畸胎

schistothorax [ˌʃistəˈθɔːræks, ˌski-], **schistosternia** [ˌʃistəˈstəːniə, ˌski-] *n* 胸裂[畸形]

schistotrachelus [ˌʃistətrəˈkiːləs, ˌski-] *n* 颈裂畸胎

schizamnion [ˌskizˈæmniən] *n* 裂隙羊膜

schizaxon [skiˈzæksɔn] *n* 轴索裂支

schizencephaly [ˌskizenˈsefəli] *n* 脑裂[畸形],脑裂性孔洞脑[畸形] | **schizencephalic** [ˌskizensiˈfælik] *a*

schiz(o)- [构词成分]裂,分裂

schizoaffective [ˌskizəuəˌfektiv, ˌskits-] *a* 分裂情感性的

Schizoblastosporion [ˌskizəuˌblæstəuˈspɔːriən] *n* 裂芽酵母孢子菌属

schizocephalia [ˌskizəusəˈfeiliə] *n* 头裂[畸形]

schizocyte [ˈskizəsait] *n* 裂细胞,裂红细胞

schizocytosis [ˌskizəusaiˈtəusis] *n* 裂细胞症

schizogenesis [ˌskizəuˈdʒenisis] *n* 裂殖[作用]

schizogenous [skiˈzɔdʒinəs] *a* 裂殖生殖的

schizogony [skiˈzɔgəni] *n* 裂体生殖(孢子中无性生殖器,尤指人体血细胞中的疟原虫生活周期)

schizogyria [ˌskizəuˈdʒaiəriə] *n* 脑回裂[畸形]

schizoid [ˈskizɔid, ˈskits-] *a* 精神分裂样的,类精神分裂症的 *n* 分裂性人格者

schizokinesis [ˌskizəukaiˈniːsis] *n* 反应分裂(指特异的条件反应已消退后,伴随的非特异的反应仍可由刺激引起)

schizomycete [ˌskizəumaiˈsiːt] *n* 裂殖菌

Schizomycetes [ˌskizəumaiˈsiːtiːz] *n* 裂殖菌纲

schizont [ˈskizɔnt] *n* 裂殖体

schizonticide [skiˈzɔntisaid] *n* 杀裂殖体药

schizonychia [ˌskizəuˈnikiə] *n* (指或趾)甲裂

schizophasia [ˌskizəuˈfeiziə] *n* 言语杂乱,分裂性言语(精神分裂症)

schizophrenia [ˌskizəuˈfriːniə, ˌskitsəu-] *n* 精神分裂症 | acute ~ 急性型精神分裂症 / ambulatory ~ 逍遥型精神分裂症(轻度精神分裂症,患者不需住院治疗) / borderline ~ 边缘型精神分裂症 / catatonic ~ 紧张型精神分裂症 / childhood ~ 儿童期精神分裂症(特征为孤独、退缩的行为,未能脱离母亲的个性,总发育不成熟) / disorganized ~ 错乱型精神分裂症 / hebephrenic ~ 青春型精神分裂症 / latent ~ 潜隐型精神分裂症(特征为具有明显的精神分裂症症状,但无精神分裂症发作史,其中包括边缘型、早期型、发病前驱型、先兆型、假神经症型和假病态人格型精神分裂症) / paranoid ~ 偏执型精神分裂症 / paraphrenic ~ 妄想痴呆型精神分裂症 / prepsychotic ~ 发病前驱型精神分裂症 / process ~, nuclear ~ 进行性精神分裂症,核心型精神分裂症 / pseudoneurotic ~ 假神经症型精神分裂症 / pseudopsychopathic ~ 假病态人格型精神分裂症 / reactive ~ 反应性精神分裂症 / residual ~ 残留型精神分裂症 / schizo-affective ~ 分裂情感型精神分裂症 / simple ~ 单纯型精神分裂症 | **schizophrenic** [ˌskizəuˈfrenik] *a* 精神分裂症的 *n* 精神分裂症患者

schizophreniform [ˌskizəuˈfrenifɔːm] *a* 精神分裂症样的

schizophrenosis [ˌskizəufriˈnəusis] *n* 精神分裂症(指早发性痴呆)

Schizophyceae [ˌskizəuˈfaisiiː] *n* 裂殖藻纲

schizoprosopia [ˌskizəuprəˈsəupiə] *n* 面裂[畸形](如兔唇、腭裂等)

Schizopyrenida [ˌskizəupiˈrenidə] *n* 裂黄目

Schizosaccharomyces hominis [ˌskizəuˌsækərəuˈmaisiːz ˈhɔminis] 人裂殖酵母菌,人体酵母菌

schizothorax [ˌskizəuˈθɔːræks] *n* 胸裂[畸胎]

schizotonia [ˌskizəuˈtəuniə] *n* 肌紧张分裂

schizotrichia [ˌskizəuˈtrikiə] *n* 毛发端分裂

schizotropic [ˌskizəuˈtrɔpik] *a* 向裂殖体的

schizotrypanosis [ˌskizəuˌtripəˈnəusis], **schizotrypanosomiasis** [ˌskizəuˌtripənəsəuˈmaiəsis] *n* 南美洲锥虫病

Schizotrypanum [ˌskizəuˈtripənəm] *n* 锥体虫属

schizotypal [ˌskizəuˈtaipəl, ˌskits-] *a* 精神分裂症型的

schizozoite [ˌskizəuˈzəuait] *n* 裂殖子,裂体性孢子

schlammfieber [ˈʃlɑːmfiːbə] *n* 【德】沼地热(类似钩端螺旋体性黄疸)

Schlatter-Osgood disease [ˈʃlætə ˈɔzgud] (Carl Schlatter; Robert B. Osgood) 见 Osgood-Schlatter disease

Schlatter's disease (sprain) [ˈʃlætə] (Carl Schlatter) 施莱特病(见 Osgood-Schlatter disease) | ~ operation 施莱特手术(全胃切除术,

治癌)
schlepper [ˈʃlepə] *n*【德】抗原载体
Schlemm's canal [ʃlem] (Friedrich S. Schlemm) 巩膜静脉窦 | ~ ligaments 盂肱韧带
Schlesinger's sign (phenomenon) [ˈʃleiziŋə] (Hermann Schlesinger) 施勒辛格尔征(现象)(手足搐搦时,患者之腿举至膝关节,并在髋关节处用力屈曲,则在短时间内即产生膝关节的伸肌痉挛,足极度旋后)
Schlichter test [ˈʃliktə] (Jakub G. Schlichter) 施立克特试验,血清杀菌活力试验
Schlösser's treatment (injection, method) [ˈʃlesə] (Carl Schlösser) 施勒塞尔疗法(注射法)(80%乙醇注入面神经孔,治疗面神经痛)
schlusskoagulum [ˌʃluskəuˈægjuləm] *n*【德】封锁凝块(胚细胞植入子宫内膜后,封闭裂口的凝块)
Schmidt-Lanterman incisures [ˈʃmit ˌlɑːntəˈmɑːn] (Henry D. Schmidt; A. J. Lanterman) 髓鞘切迹(有髓神经纤维鞘上的斜线或斜痕) | ~ segment 髓鞘节
Schmidt's diet [ʃmit] (Adolf Schmidt) 施密特饮食(每天饮食中含有 9 338 J 热量,以便于检查各种原因腹泻时的粪便) | ~ syndrome 施密特综合征(由于疑核及副神经核损害引起的一侧麻痹,影响声带、腭帆、斜方肌及胸锁乳突肌) / ~ test 施密特试验(检胆汁、糖、胰分解蛋白功能、肠消化不良、胃消化功能)
Schmidt's fibrinoplastin [ʃmit] (Eduard O. Schmidt) 副球蛋白
Schmidt's syndrome [ʃmit] (Martin Benno Schmidt) 施密特综合征(一种以上内分泌腺包括甲状腺、肾上腺、性腺、甲状旁腺及内分泌胰腺的功能减退,并以任何组合方式伴有可能由于自体免疫的非内分泌异常,如白斑、脱发及恶性贫血。本征主要发生于成年妇女,起初仅为肾上腺与甲状腺功能的原发性衰竭。亦称多内分泌腺自身免疫病Ⅱ型)
Schmincke tumor [ˈʃminkə] (Alexander Schmincke) 淋巴上皮瘤
Schmitz bacillus [ʃmits] (Karl E. F. Schmitz) 施米茨杆菌(志贺痢疾杆菌Ⅱ型)
Schmorl's body [ʃmɔːl] (Christian G. Schmorl) 施莫尔体(突入相邻脊椎的一部分髓核) | ~ disease 施莫尔病(①髓样核突出病;②家兔等坏死菌病) / ~ nodule 施莫尔结节(在脊椎X线摄片中所见的小结,由于髓核脱垂进入相邻椎骨所致)
schmutzdecke [ˈʃmutsdekə] *n*【德】去污层(细菌、藻类及其他微生物在慢速砂滤器表面上形成的地毯样层,有助于将水滤清)
Schnabel's caverns [ˈʃnæbəl] (Isidor Schnabel) 施纳贝尔腔(青光眼视神经中的病理性小腔)
schnauzkrampf [ˈʃnautskræmpt] *n*【德】噘嘴(见于某些紧张症患者)
schneiderian [ʃnaiˈdiːriːən] *a* 施耐德(Conrad Victor Schneider)的(如 schneiderian membrane 〈鼻黏膜〉)
schneiderian membrane [ʃnaiˈdiəriən] (Conrad V. Schneider) 鼻黏膜
Schneider's carmine [ˈʃnaidə] (Franz C. Schneider) 施奈德胭脂红(胭脂红在浓醋酸中的饱和溶液)
Schroeder van der Kolk's law [ˈʃrerdə vɑːn der kɔlk] (Jacob Ludwig Conrad Schroeder van der Kolk) 施罗德·范德科尔克定律(混合神经的感觉纤维其分布的部分即受同一神经的运动纤维刺激的肌肉所移动的部分)
Schoemaker's line [ˈʃimɑːkə] (Jan Scjoemaker) 舍马克线(大转子至髂前上棘的线)
Scholz's disease [ˈʃɔːlts] (Willibald O. Scholz) 朔尔茨病,异染性脑白质营养不良(幼年型)
Schönbein's reaction [ˈʃeinbain] (Christian F. Schönbein) 舍拜因反应(将碘化钾和硫酸铁加入过氧化氢溶液,则产生游离碘) | ~ test 舍拜因试验(检血、铜)
Schönlein-Henoch purpura (disease, syndrome) [ˈʃeinlain ˈhenɔh] (J. L. Schönlein; Edouard H. Henoch) 舍恩莱因-亨诺赫紫癜(病、综合征)(一种血小板不减少性紫癜,可能由于原因不明的脉管炎所致,儿童中最常见,伴有多种临床症状,如荨麻疹和红斑、关节病和关节炎、胃肠道症状及肾病。亦称变应性紫癜或过敏性紫癜)
Schönlein's purpura (disease) [ˈʃeinlain] (Johann L. Schönlein) 风湿性紫癜
Schön's theory [ʃein] (Wilhelm Schön) 舍恩学说(眼调节学说,即睫状肌对晶状体的作用与双手握橡皮球并用手指压缩所产生的作用相同)
Schottmüller's disease [ˈʃɔtmilə] (Hugo Schottmüller) 副伤寒
Schott's treatment (bath) [ʃɔt] (Theodor Schott) 朔特疗法(应用德国瑙海姆〈Nauheim〉的盐水温浴及系统性的医疗体育以治心脏病)
schradan [ˈʃrɑːdən] *n* 八甲磷胺(杀虫药)
Schreger's lines (band, striae, zones) [ˈʃreigə] (Bernhard G. Schreger) 施雷格线(带、纹)(釉质光暗带)
Schreiber's maneuver [ˈʃraibə] (Julius Schreiber) 施赖伯尔手法(检膝反射时摩擦大腿上部内侧)
Schridde's granules [ˈʃridə] (Hermann Schridde) 施里德粒(浆细胞和淋巴细胞内的微粒,类似线粒体,但较小)
Schroeder's disease [ˈʃreidə] (Robert Schroe-

der) 施勒德病(子宫内膜异位及大量出血,可能由于促性腺激素缺乏所致)

Schroeder's syndrome [ˈʃrəudə] (Henry A. Schroeder) 施勒德综合征(血压高,汗盐含量异常减少,由于肾上腺功能亢进所致,并且体重显著增加)

Schroeder's test [ˈʃreidə] (Woldemar von Schroeder) 施勒德试验(检脲)

Schroetter 见 Schrötter

Schrön-Much granules [ʃrein muh] (Otto von Schrön; Hans C. Much) 施-穆粒(即穆赫粒,见 Much's granules)

Schrön's granule [ˈʃrein] (Otto von Schrön) 施伦粒(卵胚斑中所见的一种小体,来源不明)

Schrötter's catheter [ˈʃretə] (Leopold Schrötter) 施勒特尔导管(扩张喉狭窄用) | ~ chorea 施勒特尔舞蹈病,膈痉挛(diaphragmatic chorea,见 chorea 项下相应术语)

Schuchardt's incision [ˈʃukɑːt] (Karl A. Schuchardt) 舒卡特切口,阴道旁切口(切开阴道和会阴以扩大外阴阴道出口,便于在癌手术时接近阴道,但极少用于分娩。亦称阴道会阴切开术)

Schüffner's dots (granules, punctuation, stippling) [ˈʃifnə] (Wilhelm A. P. Schüffner) 许夫纳小点(粒、斑点、点彩)(间日疟原虫在红细胞内的细小红点)

Schüle's sign [ˈʃiːlə] (Heinrich Schüle) 许勒征(忧郁面容)

Schüller-Christian disease (syndrome) [ˈʃilə ˈkristjən] (Artur Schüller; Henry A., Christian) 许勒尔-克里斯琴病(综合征)(见 Hand-Schüller-Christian disease 〈syndrome〉)

Schüller's disease (syndrome) [ˈʃilə] (Artur Schüller) 许勒尔病(综合征)(见 Hand-Schüller-Christian disease 〈syndrome〉) | ~ phenomenon 许勒尔现象(器质性偏瘫患者步行时易向患侧偏斜)

Schüller's ducts [ˈʃclə] (Karl Heinrich Anton Ludwig Max Schüller) 女尿道旁管 | ~ glands 尿道旁腺

Schüller's method [ˈʃilə] (Karl H. A. L. M. Schüller) 许勒尔法(一种人工呼吸法,用手指在肋骨下钩紧,有节奏地提高胸部)

Schultz-Charlton reaction (phenomenon, test) [ʃults ˈtʃɑːltən] (Werner Schultz; Willy Charlton) 舒尔茨-查尔顿反应(现象、试验),猩红热红疹消退反应,皮肤转白试验(当猩红热抗毒素或猩红热患者恢复期血清注入皮肤红斑处,注射部位的皮肤红斑消退转白,猩红热患者的血清并不产生此反应)

Schultz-Dale reaction [ˈʃults ˈdeil] (Werner Schultz; Henry H. Dale) 舒尔茨-戴尔反应(见 Dale's reaction)

Schultze-Chvostek sign [ˈʃultsə ˈvɔstek] (Friedrich Schultze; Franz Chvostek) 舒尔策-沃斯特克征(见 Chvostek's sign)

Schultze's bundle (tract) [ˈʃultsə] (Max J. S. Schultze) 束间束(脊髓) | ~ cells 嗅细胞

Schultze's cells [ˈʃuːltsə] (Max J. S. Schultze) 溴细胞 | ~ tract 束间束

Schultze's fold [ˈʃultsə] (Bernhard S. Schultz) 舒尔策褶(羊膜褶)

Schultze's sign [ˈʃultsə] (Friedrich Schultze) 舒尔策征(①见 Chvostek's sign; ②舌现象 tongue phenomenon,见 phenomenon 项下相应术语) | ~ type 舒尔策型,肢端感觉异常

Schultze's test [ˈʃultsə] (Ernst Schultze) 舒尔策试验(检纤维素、胆固醇、蛋白质)

Schultz's angina (disease, syndrome) [ˈʃults] (Werner Schultz) 粒细胞缺乏症

Schumm's test [ʃum] (Otto Schumm) 舒姆试验(检血及血浆正铁血红素)

Schürmann's test [ˈʃəːmən] (Walter Schürmann) 许尔曼试验(检梅毒)

Schutz's fasciculus (bundle, tract) [ʃits] (Hugo Schutz) 许茨束,背侧纵束

Schütz's micrococcus [ʃits] (Johann W. Schütz) 马链球菌

Schwabach's test [ˈʃvɑːbɑːh] (Dagobert Schwabach) 施瓦巴赫试验(检听力)

Schwalbe's corpuscles [ˈʃvɑːlbə] (Gustav A. Schwalbe) 施瓦尔布小体,味蕾 | ~ fissure 脉络膜裂 / ~ foramen 延髓盲孔 / ~ sheath 弹性纤维鞘 / ~ space 视神经鞘间隙

schwannoma [ʃwɔˈnəumə], **schwannoglioma** [ˌʃwɔnəglaiˈəumə] *n* 神经鞘瘤

schwannomin [ʃwɑːˈnəumin] *n* 神经膜蛋白(见 merlin)

schwannosis [ʃwɔˈnəusis], **schwannitis** [ʃwɔˈnaitis] *n* 神经鞘[肥厚]病,神经鞘炎

Schwann's cell [ʃvɔn] (Theodor Schwann) 施万细胞(神经膜细胞,神经鞘细胞) | ~ membrane (sheath) 神经膜(鞘) / ~ nucleus 施万细胞核 / ~ white substance 髓鞘质

Schwartze's sign [ʃwɑːtzə] (Hermann H. R. Schwartze) 施瓦策征(鼓膜后发红,有时见于耳硬化症患者,因岬周围的黏膜充血之故)

Schwartz-Jampel syndrome, Schwartz-Jampel-Aberfeld syndrome [ʃwɔːts ˈdʒæmpəl ˈeibəfeld] (Oscar Schwartz; Robert S. Jampel; D. C. Aberfeld) 施-詹综合征,施-詹-阿综合征(一种常染色体隐性疾病,特征为肌强直性肌病、侏儒症、睑裂狭小、关节挛缩和扁平面容。亦称软骨营养不良性肌强直)

Schwartz's test [ʃvɑːts] (Charles E. Schwartz)

施瓦茨试验(检静脉曲张)
Schwarz activator [ʃvɑːts] (A. Martin Schwarz) 施瓦茨活动矫正器,弓形活动矫正器 | ~ appliance 施瓦茨矫正器(一种可摘的正牙矫正器)
Schwarz's test [ʃvɑːts] (Karl L. H. Schwarz) 施瓦茨试验(检二乙眠砜);(Gottwald Schwarz)施瓦茨试验(检胃消化功能)
Schwediauer [ˈʃveidiˌauə] 见 Swediauer
Schweigger-Seidel sheath [ˈʃvaigə ˈsaidəl] (Franz Schweiger-Seidel) 施魏格尔·赛德尔鞘,脾椭圆体鞘(脾脏内动脉第二部分的壁梭形增厚,形成脾毛笔形动脉)
schweinerotlauf [ˌʃvainəˈrɔtlauf] *n* 【德】猪丹毒
schweineseuche [ˌʃvainəˈzɔiʃə] *n* 【德】猪出血性败血病
Schweitzer's reagent [ˈʃvaitsə] (Matthias E. Schweitzer) 施魏策尔试剂(以氢氧化铜溶于氨水中配成的溶液,用作溶剂检纤维素,亦称铜氨液)
schwelle [ˈʃvelə] *n* 【德】阈,界限
Schweninger-Buzzi anetoderma [ˈʃveningə ˈbuːtsi] (Ernst Schweninger; Fausto Buzzi) 施-布型皮肤松弛(进行性原发性皮肤松弛,无任何前驱性炎症,特征为突然出现许多淡蓝白色斑疹,有些斑疹隆起,常见于妇女)
Schweninger's method [ˈʃveningə] (Ernst Schweninger) 施文宁格法(限制饮食中的液体以减轻肥胖)
SCI spinal cord injury 脊髓损伤
scia- 以 scia-起始的词,同样见以 skia-起始的词
sciage [siˈɑːʒ] *n* 【法】锯木状按摩法
scialyscope [saiˈæliskəup] *n* 隔室传真装置(一种将手术现场投影于与手术室隔开的另一暗室中的装置)
Scianna blood group [siːˈɑːnɑː] (Scianna 为 20 世纪 60 年代首次报道的先证者的姓)赛安娜血型(一种含有红细胞抗原 Sc1〈以前为 Sm〉和 Sc2〈以前为 Bu[a]〉的血型)
sciatic [saiˈætik] *a* 坐骨的
sciatica [saiˈætikə] *n* 【拉】坐骨神经痛
SCID severe combined immunodeficiency 重度联合免疫缺陷病
science [ˈsaiəns] *n* 科学;学科 | applied ~ 应用科学 / behavioral ~ 行为科学 / natural ~, physical ~ 自然科学 / pure ~ 纯粹科学
scientist [ˈsaiəntist] *n* 科学家
scieropia [saiəˈrəupiə] *n* 雾视[症]
scilla [ˈsilə] *n* 【拉】海葱
scillabiose [ˌsiləˈbaiəus] *n* 海葱二糖,绵枣儿二糖,鼠李糖葡糖苷
scillaren [ˈsilərən] *n* 海葱苷(强心药)
scilliroside [ˈsilirəsaid] *n* 红海葱苷
scillism [ˈsilizəm] *n* 海葱中毒
scillitic [ˈsilitik] *a* 海葱的
scimitar [ˈsimitə] *a* 短弯刀形的
scintirenography [ˌsintiriːˈnɔgrəfi] *n* 肾闪烁摄影[术]
scintigram [ˈsintigræm] *n* 闪烁图
scintigraphy [sinˈtigrəfi] *n* 闪烁法,闪烁显像 | thyroidal lymph node ~ 甲状腺淋巴结闪烁显像,放射性同位素甲状腺淋巴显像[术] | **scintigraphic** [ˌsintiˈgræfik] *a*
scintilla [sinˈtilə] *n* 【拉】闪烁
scintillascope [sinˈtiləskəup] *n* 闪烁镜
scintillate [ˈsintileit] *vi* 闪烁
scintillation [ˌsintiˈleiʃən] *n* 闪烁[现象];光闪视;闪烁粒(放射性元素蜕变时放射的微粒)
scintillator [ˈsintileitə] *n* 闪烁器;闪烁体
scintillometer [ˌsintiˈlɔmitə] *n* 闪烁计数计
scintilloscope [sinˈtiləskəup] *n* 闪烁镜
scintiphotograph [ˌsintiˈfəutəgrɑːf, -græf], **scintiphoto** [ˌsintiˈfəutəu] *n* 闪烁[照]片
scintiphotography [ˌsintifəˈtɔgrəfi] *n* 闪烁摄影[术]
scintiscan [ˈsintiskæn] *n* 闪烁扫描
scintiscanner [ˌsintiˈskænə] *n* 闪烁扫描器
sciopody [skaiˈɔpədi] *n* 巨足,大足(尤指儿童)
scirrh(o)- [构词成分]硬
scirrhoid [ˈs(k)irɔid] *a* 硬癌样的
scirrhoma [s(k)iˈrəumə] *n* 硬癌 | ~ caminianorum 扫烟囱工人癌
scirrhophthalmia [ˌs(k)irɔfˈθælmiə] *n* 眼硬癌
scirrhous [ˈs(k)irəs] *a* 硬癌的
scirrhus [ˈs(k)irəs] ([复] **scirrhuses** 或 **scirrhi** [ˈs(k)irai]) *n* 硬癌
scissel [ˈsisəl, ˈsizəl] *n* 金属片(作牙托用)
scission [ˈsiʒən, ˈsiʃən] *n* 分裂;剪裂
scissors [ˈsizəz] [复] *n* 剪[刀] | canalicular ~ 泪管剪 / cannula ~ 开管剪 / craniotomy ~ 颅骨剪(胎儿穿颅剪)
scissors-bite [ˈsizəz ˈbait] *n* 剪式[反]殆
scissura [siˈsjuərə] ([复] **scissurae** [siˈsjuəriː]) *n* 【拉】分裂
Sciuridae [ˈsjuːridiː] *n* 松鼠科
ScLA scapulolaeva anterior 【拉】肩左前(胎位)
SCLC small cell lung carcinoma (or cancer) 小细胞肺癌
sclera [ˈskliərə] *n* 巩膜 | blue ~ 青色巩膜 | **~l** *a*
scleradenitis [ˌskliərædiˈnaitis] *n* 硬化性腺炎
scleratitis [ˌskliərəˈtaitis] *n* 巩膜炎
scleratogenous [ˌskliərəˈtɔdʒinəs] *a* 致硬化的
sclerectasia [ˌskliərekˈteiziə], **sclerectasis** [ˌskliəˈrektəsis] *n* 巩膜膨胀
sclerectoiridectomy [skliəˌrektəuˌiriˈdektəmi] *n*

巩膜虹膜切除术(治青光眼)

sclerectoiridodialysis [skliəˌrektəuˌiridəudaiˈælisis] *n* 巩膜切除虹膜分离术

sclerectome [skliəˈrektəum] *n* 巩膜刀

sclerectomy [skliəˈrektəmi] *n* 巩膜切除术;(中耳)硬化病变切除术

sclerema [skliəˈriːmə], **scleredema** [ˌskliəriˈdiːmə] *n* 硬肿病

sclerencephaly [ˌskliərenˈsefəli], **sclerencephalia** [ˌskliərensəˈfeiliə] *n* 脑硬化

sclerenchyma [ˌskliəˈreŋkimə] *n* 厚壁组织(植物)

sclererythrin [skliəˈreriθrin] *n* 麦角红质

scleriasis [skliəˈraiəsis] *n* 睑硬结

scleriritomy [ˌskliəriˈritəmi] *n* 巩膜虹膜切开术(治前葡萄肿)

scleritis [skliəˈraitis] *n* 巩膜炎 | annular ~ 环状巩膜炎 / brawny ~ 角膜缘性巩膜炎

scler(o)- [构词成分]巩膜;硬化

scleroadipose [ˌskliərəuˈædipəus] *a* 纤维组织[与]脂肪的

scleroblastema [ˌskliərəublæsˈtiːmə] *n* 成骨胚组织,生骨胚组织 | **scleroblastemic** [ˌskliərəublæsˈtemik] *a*

sclerocataracta [ˌskliərəuˌkætəˈræktə] *n* 硬性内障

sclerochoroiditis [ˌskliərəukɔːrɔiˈdaitis] *n* 巩膜脉络膜炎

scleroconjunctival [ˌskliərəukəndʒʌŋkˈtaivəl] *a* 巩膜结膜的

scleroconjunctivitis [ˌskliərəukənˌdʒʌŋktiˈvaitis] *n* 巩膜结膜炎

sclerocornea [ˌskliərəuˈkɔːniə] *n* 硬化性角膜 | **~l** *a*

sclerodactyly [ˌskliərəuˈdæktili], **sclerodactylia** [ˌskliərəudækˈtiliə] *n* 指端硬化

scleroderma [ˌskliərəuˈdəːmə] *n* 硬皮病 | circumscribed ~, localized ~ 局限性硬皮病,硬斑病 / systemic ~, diffuse ~, generalized ~ 全身性硬皮病 | **~tous** *a*

sclerodesmia [ˌskliərəuˈdezmiə] *n* 韧带硬化

sclerogenous [skliəˈrɔdʒinəs], **sclerogenic** [ˌskliərəuˈdʒenik] *a* 致硬化的

sclerogummatous [ˌskliərəuˈgʌmətəs] *a* 纤维组织[与]梅毒肿的

scleroid [ˈskliərɔid] *a* 硬质的,硬性的(指有硬组织的)

scleroiritis [ˌskliərəuaiəˈraitis] *n* 巩膜虹膜炎

sclerokeratitis [ˌskliərəuˌkerəˈtaitis], **sclerokeratosis** [ˌskliərəuˌkerəˈtəusis] *n* 巩膜角膜炎;硬化性角膜炎

sclerokeratoiritis [ˌskliərəuˌkerətəuaiəˈraitis] *n* 巩膜角膜虹膜炎

scleroma [skliəˈrəumə] ([复] **scleromata** [skliəˈrəumətə]) *n* 【希】硬结(尤指鼻或喉组织) | ~ respiratorium 呼吸道硬结[病],鼻硬结症

scleromalacia [ˌskliərəuməˈleiʃiə] *n* 巩膜软化(亦称穿通性巩膜软化)

scleromeninx [ˌskliərəuˈmiːniŋks] *n* 硬脑膜,硬脑脊膜

scleromere [ˈskliərəmiə] *n* 骨节;生骨板

sclerometer [skliəˈrɔmitə] *n* 硬度计

scleromucin [ˌskliərəuˈmjuːsin] *n* 麦角黏液质,麦角黏蛋白

scleromyxedema [ˌskliərəuˌmiksiˈdiːmə] *n* 硬化性黏液水肿

scleronychia [ˌskliərəuˈnikiə] *n* 指甲硬化,趾甲硬化

scleronyxis [ˌskliərəuˈniksis] *n* 巩膜穿刺术

sclero-oophoritis [ˌskliərəu əuˌɔfəˈraitis], **sclero-oothecitis** [ˌskliərəu ˌəuəθiˈsaitis] *n* 硬化性卵巢炎

sclerophthalmia [ˌskliərɔfˈθælmiə] *n* 巩膜化角膜,巩膜眼症(由于角膜和巩膜不完全分化,角膜周围不透明,只有中央部仍清晰)

scleroprotein [ˌskliərəuˈprəutiːn] *n* 硬蛋白

sclerosal [skliəˈrəusəl] *a* 硬的,硬化的

sclerosant [skliəˈrəusənt] *n* 组织硬化剂(一种化学刺激剂,先产生炎症,最后导致纤维化,用以治静脉曲张)

sclerosarcoma [ˌskliərəusɑːˈkəumə] *n* 纤维化肉瘤

scleroscope [ˌskliərəuˈskəup] *n* 硬度计

sclerose [skliəˈrəus] *vt, vi* 变硬,硬化 | **~d** *a* 硬化的 / **sclerosing** *a* 致硬化的,硬化的

sclérose en plaques [skleiˈrəuz ɔŋˈplæk] 【法】多发性硬化

sclerosis [skliəˈrəusis] ([复] **scleroses** [skliəˈrəusiːz]) *n* 【希】硬化 | amyotrophic lateral ~ 肌萎缩性(脊髓)侧索硬化 / anterolateral ~, ventrolateral ~ 脊髓前侧索硬化 / arterial ~, arteriocapillary ~, vascular ~ 动脉硬化 / arteriolar ~ 小动脉硬化 / bone ~ 骨硬化,骨质象牙化 / combined ~ 合并性硬化(脊髓亚急性合并性变性) / diffuse ~ (脑脊髓)弥漫性硬化 / endocardial ~ 心内膜硬化(纤维弹性组织增生) / gastric ~ 胃硬化,皮革状胃,皮囊胃 / lateral ~ (脊髓)侧索硬化 / lobar ~ 脑叶硬化 / multiple ~, disseminated ~, focal ~, insular ~ 多发性硬化 / posterior ~ (脊髓)后索硬化,脊髓痨 / posterolateral ~ (脊髓)后侧索硬化 / presenile ~ 老早性脑硬化,老早性痴呆 / systemic ~ 系统性硬化病 / unicellular ~ 细胞间硬化,细胞间纤维组织增生

scleroskeleton [ˌskliərəuˈskelitn] *n* 硬化骨骼
sclerostenosis [ˌskliərəustiˈnəusis] *n* 硬化性狭窄,硬缩
Sclerostoma [skliəˈrɔstəmə] *n* 硬口虫属(即圆线虫属 Strongylus) | ~ duodenale 十二指肠钩虫(即 Ancylostoma duodenale)/ ~ syngamus 气管比翼线虫(即 Syngamus trachea)
sclerostomy [skliəˈrɔstəmi] *n* 巩膜造口术
sclerotherapy [ˌskliərəuˈθerəpi] *n* 硬化治疗[术],硬化疗法(注射硬化性溶液,治疗痔或静脉曲张)
sclerotia [skliəˈrəuʃiə] sclerotium 的复数
sclerotic [skliəˈrɔtik] *a* 硬的,硬化的 *n* 巩膜
sclerotica [skliəˈrɔtikə] *n*【拉】巩膜
sclerotic acid [skliəˈrɔtik] 麦角硬酸
scleroticectomy [skliəˌrɔtiˈsektəmi] *n* 巩膜切除术
scleroticochoroiditis [skliəˌrɔtikəuˌkɔːrɔiˈdaitis] *n* 巩膜脉络膜炎
scleroticonyxis [skliəˌrɔtikəuˈniksis], **scleroticopuncture** [skliəˌrɔtikəuˈpʌŋktʃə] *n* 巩膜穿刺术
Sclerotinia [ˌskliərəuˈtiniə] *n* 核盘菌属
Sclerotiniaceae [ˌskliərəutiniˈeisiiː] *n* 核盘菌科
sclerotinic acid [ˌskiərəuˈtinik] 麦角硬酸
sclerotitis [ˌskliərəuˈtaitis] *n* 巩膜炎
sclerotium [skliəˈrəuʃiəm] *n* 菌核(由某些真菌如黑麦麦角所形成的黑色厚壁硬块) | **sclerotial** [skliəˈrəuʃiəl] *a*
sclerotome [ˈskliərətəum] *n* 巩膜刀;生骨节
sclerotomy [skliəˈrɔtəmi], **scleroticotomy** [skliəˌrɔtiˈkɔtəmi] *n* 巩膜切开术
sclerous [ˈskliərəs] *a* 硬的,硬化的
sclerozone [ˈskliərəzəun] *n* 附肌带,附着带
ScLP scapulo laeva posterior【拉】肩左后(胎位)
SCM State Certified Midwife 持有国家证书的助产士
scoleces [ˈskəulisiːz, skəuˈliːsiːz] scolex 的复数
scoleciasis [skəuliˈsaiəsis] *n* 蠋病
scoleciform [skəuˈlesifɔːm] *a* (绦虫)头节样的
scoleco- [构词成分]蠕虫;头节
scolecoid [ˈskəulikɔid] *a* 蠕虫样的;头节样的(包虫囊)
scolecology [ˌskəuliˈkɔlədʒi] *n* 蠕虫学
scolex [ˈskəuleks] ([复] **scoleces** [ˈskəulisiːz, skəuˈliːsiːz]) *n*【拉】头节(绦虫)
scolio- [构词成分]弯曲
scoliokyphosis [ˌskɔliəukaiˈfəusis] *n* 脊柱后凸侧弯
scoliorachitic [ˌskɔliəurəˈkitik] *a* 脊柱侧弯[与]佝偻病性的
scoliosiometry [ˌskɔliəusiˈɔmitri] *n* 脊柱凸度测量法
scoliosis [ˌskɔliˈəusis] *n* 脊柱侧弯 | coxitic ~ 髋关节炎性脊柱侧弯 / habit ~ 习惯性脊柱侧弯 / sciatic ~ 坐骨神经痛性脊柱侧弯 / static ~ 静止性脊柱侧弯 | **scoliotic** [ˌskɔliˈɔtik] *a*
scoliosometer [ˌskɔliəuˈsɔmitə] *n* 脊柱侧弯[测量]计
scoliotone [ˈskɔliətəun] *n* 脊柱侧弯矫正器
Scolopendra [ˌskɔləˈpendrə] *n* 蜈蚣属
scolopsia [skəˈlɔpsiə] *n* 可动骨缝
scombrine [ˈskɔmbrin] *n* 鲭精蛋白
scombroid [ˈskɔmbrɔid] *a* 鲭亚目的 *n* 鲭
Scombroidea [skrɔmˈbrɔidiə] *n* 鲭亚目
scombrone [ˈskɔmbrəun] *n* 鲭组蛋白
scombrotoxic [ˌskɔmbrəuˈtɔksik] *a* 鲭中毒的
scombrotoxin [ˌskɔmbrəuˈtɔksin] *n* 鲭毒素
scoop [skuːp] *n* 匙,杓 *vt* 用杓取出 | ear ~ 耳刮匙
scopafungin [ˌskəupəˈfʌndʒin] *n* 司可芬净(抗菌、抗真菌抗生素)
scoparin [skəˈpɛərin] *n* 金雀花素
scoparius [skəˈpɛəriəs] *n* 金雀花(有利尿、导泻、催吐作用)
-scope [构词成分]镜
scopin [ˈskəupin] *n* 东莨菪醇
scopola [skəˈpəulə] *n* 莨菪(抗胆碱药)
scopolagnia [ˌskəupəˈlægniə] *n* 窥视色情癖(窥淫癖;露阴癖)
scopolamine [skəˈpɔləmiːn] *n* 东莨菪碱(抗胆碱药) | ~ hydrobromide 氢溴酸东莨菪碱(大脑镇静、散瞳、睫状肌麻痹药) / ~ methylbromide 甲溴东莨菪碱(抗胆碱药)
scopoletin [skəˈpɔlitin] *n* 东莨菪亭,7-羟-6-甲氧香豆素
Scopolia [skəˈpəuliə] *n* 东莨菪属
scopometer [skəˈpɔmitə] *n* 浊度计,视测浊度计 | **scopometry** *n* 浊量法,视测浊度测定法
scopophilia [ˌskəupəuˈfiliə], **scoptolagnia** [ˌskɔptəuˈlægniə], **scoptophilia** [ˌskɔptəuˈfiliə] *n* 窥视色情癖(窥淫癖;露阴癖)
scopophobia [ˌskəupəuˈfəubiə], **scoptophobia** [ˌskɔptəuˈfəubiə] *n* 被窥视恐怖
scopula [ˈskɔpjulə] *n* 毛丛(围口纤毛虫的离口细胞器)
Scopulariopsis [ˌskɔpjuˌlɛəriˈɔpsis] *n* 帚霉属
scopulariopsosis [ˌskɔpjuˌlɛəriɔpˈsəusis] *n* 帚霉病
-scopy [构词成分]检查
scorbutic [skɔːˈbjuːtik] *a* 坏血病的
scorbutigenic [skɔːˌbjuːtiˈdʒenik] *a* 致坏血病的
scorbutus [skɔːˈbjuːtəs] *n*【拉】坏血病
scordinema [ˌskɔːdiˈniːmə] *n* 呵欠,欠伸(某些传染病的前驱症状)

score [skɔː] *n* 评分,分数 | recovery ~ 新生儿后期评分(评定新生儿在产后超过1分钟以上的不同时间的心率、呼吸力、肌张力、反射应激性和肤色所得出的总分) / injury severity ~ 创伤严重度评分

scorings ['skɔːriŋz] *n* (骨)生长残痕

scorpion ['skɔːpjən] *n* 蝎

scorpionism ['skɔːpjənizəm] *n* 蝎螫中毒

scot(o)- [构词成分]暗,盲

Scotobacteria [ˌskəutəbæk'tiəriə] *n* 暗细菌纲

scotobacterium [ˌskəutəbæk'tiəriəm] *n* 暗细菌

scotochromogen [ˌskɔtəu'krəumədʒən] *n* 暗产色菌株

scotochromogenicity [ˌskɔtəuˌkrəumədʒe'nisəti] *n* 暗产色性 | **scotochromogenic** [ˌskɔtəuˌkrəumə'dʒenik] *a*

scotodinia [ˌskɔtə'diniə] *n* 暗点性眩晕(伴有视力障碍及头痛)

scotogram ['skɔtəgræm], **scotograph** ['skɔtəgrɑːf, -græf] *n* X线[照]片;暗色显影片

scotographic [ˌskɔtə'græfik] *a* X线摄影的;暗室显影的

scotography [skə'tɔgrəfi] *n* X线摄影术;暗室显影术

scotoma [skə'təumə] ([复] **scotomata** [skə'təumətə]) *n* 暗点,盲点;精神"盲点" | arcuate ~ 弓形盲点 / aural ~ 音定向不能 / cecocentral ~ 哑铃形暗点 / color ~ 色盲暗点 / fluttering ~, scintillating ~ 闪光暗点 / hemianopic ~ 偏盲暗点 / mental ~ 精神"盲点",自省力缺乏 / mobile scotomata 能动暗点 / physiologic ~ 生理暗点 / ring ~, annular ~ 环状暗点 | **~tous** *a*

scotomagraph [skə'təuməgrɑːf, -græf] *n* 暗点描记器

scotometer [skə'tɔmitə] *n* 暗点计 | **scotometry** *n* 暗点定量[法]

scotomization [ˌskɔtəmai'zeiʃən, -mi'z-] *n* 暗点发生(尤指精神"盲点"形成,患者企图否认一切与其自我相冲突的事物的存在)

scotophilia [ˌskɔtəu'filiə] *n* 嗜黑暗癖

scotophobia [ˌskɔtəu'fəubiə] *n* 黑暗恐怖,恐暗症

scotophobin [ˌskəutəu'fəubin] *n* 黑暗恐怖肽(由15个氨基酸组成的肽,从黑暗恐怖情况下饲养的大鼠及小鼠脑组织中分离出来的,如将这种肽注射入正常啮齿动物体内,据称会引起对黑暗的恐怖)

scotopia [skə'təupiə] *n* 暗视,暗适应 | **scotopic** [skə'tɔpik] *a*

scotopsin [skə'tɔpsin] *n* 暗视蛋白(视网膜杆体色素中的蛋白质组成部分)

scotoscopy [skə'tɔskəpi] *n* 视网膜镜检查,检影法;X线透视检查

scototherapy [ˌskɔtəu'θerəpi] *n* 蔽光疗法

scours ['skauəz] [复] *n* 家畜腹泻病 | bloody ~ 血泻病(猪的黑泻病) / calf ~ 牛泻病(牛犊的白泻病) / winter ~ 冬季泻病(牛的黑泻病)

scr scruple 英分(药衡制重量单位,1英分=1.296 g)

scrapie ['skeipi] *n* 痒病(绵羊和山羊的一种脑病)

scratch [skrætʃ] *vt* 搔,抓;抓伤;擦;挖 *vi* 搔,抓 *n* 搔,抓,抓痕;抓伤,抓破;乱涂 | **~es** *n* 葡萄疮(马脚)

screatus [skri'eitəs] *n*【拉】阵发性响咳(或鼓鼻)(神经功能病所致)

screen [skriːn] *n* 屏,幕;保护剂,防护剂 *vt* 荧光屏检查(英国用语);筛选检查 | fluorescent ~ 荧光屏,荧光板 / intensifying ~ 增感屏 / tangent ~ 正切暗点计屏(正面视野计屏) / vestibular ~, oral ~ 口前庭屏,口腔保护剂

screening ['skriːniŋ] *n* 筛选;筛选检查,集体检诊;荧光屏检查(英国用语) | mass ~ 群体筛选检查 / multiphasic ~, multiple ~ 多种方法检诊,多相性集体检诊(同时使用多种实验室方法检查各种疾病或病理情况,如贫血、糖尿病、心脏病、高血压、梅毒、结核及其他肺病) / prescriptive ~ 指定性筛选(为健康状况表现良好的人进行早期检查疾病或疾病的前体,以便在发病时或疾病变得明显前及早提供医疗保健)

screw [skruː] *n* 螺旋,螺[丝]钉 | expansion ~ 扩弓螺旋器

screwworm ['skruːwəːm] *n* 旋蝇(蛆)

Scribner shunt ['skribnə] (Belding H. Scribner) 斯克里勃纳分流术(见 Quinton-Scribner shunt)

scribomania [ˌskribəu'meinjə] *n* 涂写癖,书写癖

scrobiculate [skrəu'bikjulit] *a* 小窝形的,有小凹的

scrobiculus [skrəu'bikjuləs] *n*【拉】小窝,小凹 | ~ cordis 心窝

scrofula ['skrɔfjulə] *n*【拉】淋巴结结核,瘰疬

scrofuloderma [ˌskrɔfjuləu'dəːmə] *n* 瘰疬性皮肤结核

scrofulous ['skrɔfjuləs] *a* 淋巴结结核的,瘰疬性的

scrotal ['skrəutl] *a* 阴囊的

scrotectomy [skrəu'tektəmi] *n* 阴囊切除术

scrotitis [skrəu'taitis] *n* 阴囊炎

scrotocele ['skrəutəsiːl] *n* 阴囊(腹股沟)疝

scrotoplasty ['skrəutəˌplæsti] *n* 阴囊成形术

scrotum ['skrəutəm] ([复] **scrota** ['skrəutə]) *n*【拉】阴囊 | lymph ~ 阴囊淋巴管扩张 / watering-can ~ 阴囊多发性尿瘘

scruple ['skruːpl] *n* 英分(药衡制重量单位,1英分=1.296 g)

scrupulosity [ˌskruːpju'lɔsəti] *n* 顾虑过多,过度

疑虑

scultetus [skəlˈtiːtəs] (Johann Schultes〈Scultetus〉) *n* 多头绷带

Scultetus bandage [skəlˈtiːtəs] (Johannes Scultes〈Scultetus〉) 舒尔蒂特斯绷带(一种多头绷带,其多头相互重叠包扎,用安全别针固定位置)

scu-PA single chain urokinase-type plasminogen activator 单链尿激酶型纤溶酶原激活物

scurvy [ˈskəːvi] *n* 坏血病 | infantile ~, hemorrhagic ~ 婴儿坏血病,出血性坏血病 / sea ~ 航海坏血病(真坏血病,因过去在海员中尤为常见而得名)

scutate [ˈskjuːteit] *a* 鳞的;鼓室盾板的

scute [skjuːt] *n* 鳞;鼓室盾板 | tympanic ~ 鼓室盾板

scutellum [skjuˈteləm] ([复] **scutella** [skjuˈtelə]) *n* 盾盖

Scuticociliatida [ˌskjuːtikəuˌsiliˈeitidə] *n* 膜纤目

scutiform [ˈskjuːtifɔːm] *a* 盾形的

scutulum [ˈskjuːtjuləm] ([复] **scutula** [ˈskjuːtjulə]) *n* 黄癣痂 | **scutular** *a*

scutum [ˈskjuːtəm] ([复] **scuta** [ˈskjuːtə]) *n* 【拉】鼓室盾板;甲状软骨;髌骨;盾片(指蜱科或硬体蜱) | ~ pectoris 胸骨

scybalum [ˈsibələm] ([复] **scybala** [ˈsibələ]) *n* 【希】硬粪块 | **scybalous** *a*

scyllite [ˈsilait] *n* 鲨肝已糖

scyllitol [ˈsilitɔl] *n* 鲨肌醇

scymnol [ˈsimnɔl] *n* 鲨胆固醇,鲨胆甾醇

scyphoid [ˈsaifɔid] *a* 杯状的

Scytalidium [ˌsaitəˈlidiəm] *n* 小柱孢菌属

scythropasmus [ˌsaiθrəˈpæzməs] *n* 面容憔悴

scytoblastema [ˌsaitəublæsˈtiːmə] *n* 皮基,皮胚

Scytonema [ˌsaitəuˈniːmə] *n* 双歧藻属

SD skin dose 皮肤量;standard deviation 标准差

SDA sacrodextra anterior【拉】骶右前(胎位);specific dynamic action 特殊动力作用

SDE specific dynamic effect (食物的)特殊动力效应

SDP sacrodextra posterior【拉】骶右后(胎位)

SDS sodium dodecyl sulfate 十二烷基硫酸钠

SDS-PAGE SDS-polyacrylamide gel electrophoresis 十二烷基硫酸钠-聚丙烯酰胺凝胶电泳

SDT sacrodextra transversa【拉】骶右横(胎位)

SE standard error 标准误;sphenoethmoidal suture 蝶筛[骨]缝

Se selenium 硒

Seabright bantam syndrome [ˈsiːbrait ˈbræntəm] (源自锡布赖特矮脚鸡,此品种中雄鸡患此病)假甲状旁腺功能减退症

seal [siːl] *n* 封蜡;熔封,封闭 | border ~ 周边封闭 / double ~ 双层封闭 / posterior palatal ~ 腭后封闭 / velopharyngeal ~ 咽帆封闭

sealant [ˈsiːlənt] *n* 封闭剂 | dental ~ 牙封闭剂(亦称牙科粘胶) / fissure ~ 沟封闭剂 / pit and fissure ~ 沟凹封闭剂

sealer [ˈsiːlə] *n* 封闭剂 | root canal ~, endodontic ~ 根管封闭剂,牙髓病封闭剂(亦称根管粘固粉)

seam [siːm] *n* 缝;接缝;骨缝 | pigment ~ 色素缝(在瞳孔边缘周围向前卷曲的虹膜色素上皮部分) | **~less** *a* 无缝的

sear [siə] *vt* 烙,烧灼

search [səːtʃ] *vi* 探究,调查 *n* 探索;调查 | **~er** *n* 膀胱石探杆

seasick [ˈsiːsik] *a* 晕船的 | **~ness** *n*

seat [siːt] *n* 座;座位 | basal ~ 基座 / rest ~ 支托座

seatworm [ˈsiːtwəːm] *n* 蛲虫

sea urchin [siː ˈəːtʃin] 海胆

seaweed [ˈsiːwiːd] *n* 海藻

sebaceous [siˈbeiʃəs] *a* 皮脂的,脂肪的;分泌皮脂的

sebacic acid [siˈbæsik] 癸二酸

Sebileau's hollow [ˈsebiləu] (Pierre Sebileau) 塞比洛凹(舌下凹,由口腔黏膜及舌下腺所形成)

sebiparous [siˈbipərəs], **sebiferous** [siˈbifərəs] *a* 生皮脂的

sebolith [ˈsebəliθ] *n* 皮脂石

seborrheid [ˌsebəˈriːid] *n* 皮脂溢疹,皮脂溢性皮炎

seborrhiasis [ˌsebəˈraiəsis] *n* 脂溢性银屑病,反向银屑病

seborrh(o)ea [ˌsebəˈriːə] *n* 皮脂溢出;皮脂溢性皮炎 | ~ adiposa, ~ oleosa 油性皮脂溢 / ~ congestiva 红斑狼疮 / ~ sicca 干性皮脂溢 | **~l**, **seborrheic** [ˌsebəˈriːik], **seborrhoic** [ˌsebəˈrəuik] *a*

sebotropic [ˌsebəˈtrɔpik] *a* 亲皮脂的

sebum [ˈsiːbəm] *n*【拉】羊脂,牛羊脂;脂肪;皮脂 | cutaneous ~ 皮脂

Secale [siːˈkeiliː] *n*【拉】黑麦属 | ~ cereale 黑麦

secale cornutum [siˈkeiliː kɔˈnjuːtəm] 麦角

secalin [ˈsekəlin] *n* 裸麦醇溶蛋白

secalintoxin [ˌsekəlinˈtɔksin] *n* 黑麦碱毒素

secalose [ˈsekələus] *n* 黑麦糖

Sechenoff's center [ˈsetʃenɔf] 见 Setschenow

Seckel's bird-headed dwarf (syndrome) [ˈsekəl] (Helmut P. G. Seckel) 塞克尔鸟头侏儒(综合征)(头小而匀称的侏儒,狭长鸟状脸,鼻鸟嘴状突出,大眼,睑裂先天愚型样倾斜及下颌后缩。亦称小头侏儒)

seclazone [ˈsekləzəun] *n* 司克拉宗(抗炎药,促尿酸排泄药)

secobarbital [ˌsikəˈbɑːbitæl] *n* 司可巴比妥(催眠药)
secodont [ˈsikədɔnt] *a* 切牙型
second(s) [ˈsekənd] *n* 秒
secondary [ˈsekəndəri] *a* 第二的,第二次的;继发性的,第二期的;次级的
second intention [ˈsekənd inˈtenʃən] 二期愈合
secreta [siˈkriːtə] [复] *n*【拉】分泌物
secretagogue [siˈkriːtəgɔg] *a* 促分泌的 *n* 促分泌素
secrete [siˈkriːt] *vt* 分泌
secretin [siˈkriːtin] *n* 促胰液素,肠促胰液肽,胰泌素(多肽激素类药) | gastric ~ 促胃液素
secretinase [siˈkriːtineis] *n* 促胰液素酶,肠促胰液肽酶
secretion [siˈkriːʃən] *n* 分泌[作用];分泌物 | antilytic ~ 非麻痹性分泌 / external ~ 外分泌 / internal ~ 内分泌 / paralytic ~ 麻痹性分泌(神经麻痹时)
secretive [siˈkriːtiv] *a* 分泌的,促进分泌的
secretogogue [siˈkriːtəgɔg] *a* 促分泌的 *n* 催分泌素
secretoinhibitory [siˌkriːtəuinˈhibitəri] *a* 抑制分泌的
secretomotor [siˌkriːtəuˈməutə], **secretomotory** [siˌkriːtəuˈməutəri] *a* 刺激分泌的(指神经)
secretor [siˈkriːtə] *n* 分泌管,分泌腺;分泌者(在遗传学中指在唾液和其他体液中含有 ABO 血型的 ABH 抗原的人);分泌[者]基因(决定分泌者遗传特性的基因)
secretory [siˈkriːtəri] *a* 分泌作用的,分泌性的
sect [sekt] *n* 部分,节,段
sectarian [sekˈtɛəriən] *n* 宗派医(拘于定见或教条的医师)
sectile [ˈsektail] *a* 可割的,可切的 *n* 分段,段
sectio [ˈsekʃiəu] ([复] **sectiones** [sekʃiˈəuniːz]) *n*【拉】切开[术];切[断]面,切片;节
section [ˈsekʃən] *n* 切开[术];切[断]面,截面;切片;节,部分 | abdominal ~ 剖腹术 / celloidin ~ 火棉胶切片 / cervical cesarean ~ 子宫下段剖腹产术 / cesarean ~ 剖宫产术 / corporeal cesarean ~ 子宫体切开剖腹产术 / cross ~ 横断面,横切面 / frontal ~, coronal ~ 额切面,冠状缝切面 / frozen ~ 冰冻切片 / paraffin ~ 石蜡切片 / perineal ~ 尿道外切开术 / sagittal ~ 矢状切面 / serial ~ 连续切片 / transverse ~ 横切面;横切片
sector [ˈsektə] *n* 弧三角形,扇形,扇面;部分,成分 *vt* 把…分成扇形;使分成部分 | **~al** *a*
sectorial [sekˈtɔːriəl] *a* 扇形的(在遗传学上,指一部分具有体细胞突变的组织,因而在表型上不同于身体其他组织;同样亦指具有这部分组织的个体〈镶嵌体〉);切割的,分段的
secundigravida [siˌkʌndiˈgrævidə] *n*【拉】第二次孕妇
secundina [ˌsikʌnˈdainə] ([复] **secundinae** [ˌsikʌnˈdainiː]) *n*【拉】产后物,胞衣(胎盘、胎膜);陪件
secundines [ˈsekʌndainz] *n* 产后物,胞衣(胎盘、胎膜);陪件
secundipara [ˌsikʌnˈdipərə] *n*【拉】二产妇 | **secundiparity** [siˌkʌndiˈpærəti] *n* 二产 / **secundiparous** [ˌsikʌnˈdipərəs] *a* 二产的
secundum artem【拉】按技术,人工地
securinine [siˈkjuəriniːn] *n* 一叶萩碱(中枢兴奋药)
SED skin erythema dose 皮肤红斑量
sedation [siˈdeiʃən] *n* 镇静作用,镇静状态
sedative [ˈsedətiv] *a* 镇静的 *n* 镇静药
sedentary [ˈsedntəri] *a* 静坐的;坐式的
Sédillot's operation [seidiˈjəu] (Charles E. Sédillot)塞迪约手术(①悬雍垂缝术;②上唇皮瓣修复手术)
sediment [ˈsedimənt] *n* 沉淀,沉积物 | urinary ~ 尿沉淀 | **~al** [ˌsediˈmentl] *a*
sedimentable [ˌsediˈmentəbl] *a* 能形成沉淀的
sedimentary [ˌsediˈmentəri] *a* 沉淀的,沉积的,沉降的
sedimentation [ˌsedimenˈteiʃən] *n* 沉淀作用,沉积,沉降 | erythrocyte ~ 红细胞沉降,血沉
sedimentator [ˌsedimenˈteitə] *n* [离心]沉淀器(分离尿沉淀物)
sedoheptulose [ˌsiːdəuˈheptjuləus] *n* 景天庚酮糖
sedopeptose [ˌsiːdəuˈpeptəus] *n* 景天糖,佛甲草庚酮糖
seed [siːd] *n* 种子,籽;精液;种子形小管(镭疗) *vt* 接种(用微生物接种在培养基上) *vi* 结实;播种 | larkspur ~ 飞燕草子 / plantago ~, psyllium ~ 车前子 / radiogold(^{198}Au) ~ 放射性^{198}金籽(一段金丝,约长 2.5 mm,厚 0.8 mm,治疗癌症用的永久性填隙式放射性植入管) / radon ~ 氡籽,氡小管(可插入组织内的密封型金属或玻璃制小管,用以治疗恶性病质) | **~less** *a* 无核的
Seeligmüller's sign [ˈzeiliʃˌmilə] (Otto L. G. A. Seeligmüller)泽利希苗勒征(面神经痛时,患侧瞳孔散大)
Seessel's pouch (pocket) [ˈseisəl] (Albert Seessel)西赛尔憩室(囊)(咽底憩室,胚咽的一种暂时性突出小囊,嘴向咽膜,尾向拉特克〈Rathke〉囊)
Séglas type [seiˈglɑː] (Jules E. Séglas)塞格拉型(偏执狂的精神运动型)
segment [ˈsegmənt] *n* 区段;节,段,节片 | cranial ~s 颅节 / medullary ~ 髓鞘节 / mesoblastic

~, mesodermal ~ 体节 / neural ~ 神经管节, 髓管节 / rod ~ 杆体节(视网膜) / sacral ~ 骶段(骨盆) / spinal ~ 脊髓(节)段 / uterine ~ 子宫分段 | **~ary** *a*

segmenta [segˈmentə] segmentum 的复数

segmental [segˈmentl] *a* 节的,段的,分节的,节片的

segmentation [ˌsegmənˈteiʃən] *n* 分割;分节,分节运动;分裂 | haustral ~ 结肠袋分节运动

segmentectomy [ˌsegmenˈtektəmi] *n* 段切除术(如肺或肝段切除)

segmenter [segˈmentə] *n* 裂殖体(疟原虫在血细胞内分成裂殖子)

Segmentina [ˌsegmənˈtainə] *n* 隔扁螺属(姜片虫的第一中间宿主)

segmentum [segˈmentəm] ([复] **segmenta** [segˈmentə]) *n* 【拉】节,段,节片

segregate [ˈsegrigeit] *vt* 使分离,使隔离 *vi* 分离,受隔离;分凝,分异 | **segregative** *a*

segregation [ˌsegriˈgeiʃən] *n* 分离(遗传学中指在生殖细胞成熟分裂过程中同源染色体的等位基因出现分离现象);分居,隔离(指居民);分离,分异(将合子中的效能逐渐限制于胚胎形成的不同区域) | adjacent ~ 相邻分离

segregator [ˈsegriˌgeitə] *n* (两肾)分隔采尿器

Séguin's signal symptom (sign) [seiˈgæn] (Edouard Séguin)塞甘先兆症状(征)(癫痫发作前肌肉不自主收缩)

Sehrt's clamp (compressor) [sεət] (Ernst Sehrt)泽尔特夹(压迫器)(一种夹子,压迫主动脉或一肢体以止血)

Seidelin bodies [ˈsaidəlin] (Harold Seidelin)赛德林小体(该名称一度被认为是黄热病患者红细胞内所见的结构,发现者认为此即为黄热病的病因)

Seidel's scotoma (sign) [ˈsaidəl] (Erich Seidel)赛德尔暗点(征)(青光眼早期征,弓形盲点的进一步发展,由生理盲点向上或〈与〉向下延伸的镰状暗点)

Seidlitz powder [ˈsaidlits] 塞得利兹粉(捷克波希米亚矿泉得名,是一种碳酸氢钠、酒石酸钾钠与酒石酸的混合,用作泻药,亦称复方泡腾散) | ~ powder test 塞得利兹粉试验(检腽肌疝)

Seignette's salt [saiˈnjet] (Pierre Seignette)酒石酸钾钠

seismesthesia [ˌsaismisˈθiːzjə], **seisesthesia** [ˌsaisisˈθiːzjə] *n* (液体或空气介质的)振动[感]觉

seismic [ˈsaizmik] *a* 地震的

seismocardiogram [ˌsaizməuˈkɑːdiəgræm] *n* 心震图

seismocardiography [ˌsaizməuˌkɑːdiˈɔgrəfi] *n* 心震描记法

seismotherapy [ˌsaizməuˈθerəpi] *n* [机械]振动疗法

Seitelberger's disease [ˈsaitəlˌbəːgə] (Franz Seitelberger)赛特贝格病,婴儿神经轴索营养不良

seizure [ˈsiːʒə] *n* (疾病的)发作;癫痫发作 | absence ~ 失神发作(亦称癫痫小发作) / audiogenic ~ 听原性癫痫发作(由于声音引起的癫痫发作) / cerebral ~ 脑病发作,癫痫发作 / febrile ~ 热性癫痫发作 / jackknife ~ 折刀状发作(一种严重的肌阵挛,出现于出生后头十八个月) / photogenic ~ 光原性癫痫发作 / psychic ~ 精神猝变,情绪猝变 / psychomotor ~ 精神运动性癫痫 / uncinate ~ 钩回发作(颞叶钩回区引起的癫痫发作)

sejunction [siˈdʒʌŋkʃən] *n* 联想阻隔

sekisanine [seˈkisənin] *n* 二氢石蒜碱

selachian [siˈleikiən] *n* 板鳃类鱼,软骨鱼

Seldinger technique [ˈseldiŋgə] (Sven I. Seldinger)塞尔丁格技术(将导管插入空心腔结构或体腔的一种方法,使用一根狭针进入结构,用导丝穿过此针,拔去此针,使导管在金属丝上向前推进。此法用于血管造影、心血管插管术及中心静脉系的套管插入术)

selection [siˈlekʃən] *n* 选择 | artificial ~ 人工选择 / directional ~ 定向选择 / disruptive ~, diversifying ~ 歧化选择,分裂选择,多样化选择 / natural ~ 自然选择 / progeny ~ 子代选择 / sexual ~ 性选择 / stabilizing ~ 稳定化选择,稳定性选择 / truncate ~ 分段选择(在医学遗传学中指为了遗传结构进行家系选择,即查证一个或一个以上的血缘关系,一般查证成员中未受遗传特性影响的血缘关系)

selectin [səˈlektin] *n* 选择蛋白

selective [siˈlektiv] *a* 选择的,有选择力的

selectivity [silekˈtivəti] *n* 选择性

selegiline hydrochloride [siˈledʒəliːn] 盐酸司来吉兰(单胺氧化酶 B 型抑制剂,与左旋多巴〈levodopa〉和卡巴多巴〈carbidopa〉合用,用作抗震颤麻痹药,口服给药)

selenate [ˈselineit] *n* 硒酸盐

selene [siˈliːni] *n* 【拉;希】月形 | ~ unguium 甲弧影

selenic acid [siˈlenik] 硒酸

selenide [ˈselinaid] *n* 硒化物

Selenidium [ˌseliˈnidiəm] *n* 月形簇虫属

seleniferous [ˌsiːləˈnifərəs] *a* 硒的

selenious acid [səˈliːniəs] 亚硒酸

selenium (Se) [siˈliːnjəm] *n* 硒(化学元素) | ~ sulfide 二硫化硒(局部抗真菌药,抗皮脂溢药)

selenodont [siˈliːnədɔnt] *a* 月牙型的

selenomethionine [ˌselənəume'θaiəniːn] *n* 硒蛋氨酸(硒取代硫原子的蛋氨酸;放射性型〈^{75}Se〉,用于检组织对蛋氨酸的摄入量)
selenomethylnorcholesterol (SMC) [səˌliːnəuˌmeθilˌnɔːkə'lestərəl] *n* 硒甲基降胆固醇(^{75}Se-6β-硒甲基降胆固醇,为以^{75}Se 标记的胆固醇类似物,用于肾上腺皮质放射核素成像)
Selenomonas [ˌsilinəu'məunəs] *n* 月形单胞菌属
selenoplegia [siˌliːnəu'pliːdʒiə], **selenoplexia** [siˌliːnəu'pleksiə] *n* 月光病(从前认为由于月光照射所致的病)
selenosis [ˌsili'nəusis] *n* 硒中毒
selenous acid [si'liːnəs] 亚硒酸
self [self] ([复]**selves** [selvz]) *n* 自我,自己;自身(表示动物自身的抗原成分,与表示外来抗原成分非自身"not self"相对应) *a* 同一性质的
self-antigen ['self ˌæntidʒən] *n* 自体抗原,自身抗原
self-assertion [ˌself ə'səːʃən] *n* 自我断言
self-differentiation ['self ˌdifərenʃi'eiʃən] *n* 非依赖性分化(某一部分自行发育过程,不受外界影响或环境改变的支配)
self-digestion [ˌself di'dʒestʃən] *n* 自体消化,自体溶解
self-fermentation [ˌself fəːmen'teiʃən] *n* 自体溶解,自体消化
self-fertilization [ˌself ˌfəːtilai'zeiʃən, -li'z-] *n* 自体受精
self-heal ['self ˌhiːl] *n* (有医疗作用的)自体愈合植物(尤指夏枯草)
self-hypnosis [ˌself hip'nəusis] *n* 自我催眠
self-inductance [ˌself in'dʌktəns] *n* 自感[电]
self-induction ['self in'dʌkʃən] *n* 自感应
self-infection [ˌself in'fekʃən] *n* 自体传染,自体感染,自身传染
selfing ['selfiŋ] *n* 自花受精;自体受精(如绦虫节片之间)
self-limited [ˌself 'limitid] *a* (病程)自限的,自身限制[性]的
self-observation [ˌself ɔbzə'veiʃən] *n* 自我观察
self-replication ['self ˌrepli'keiʃən] *n* (染色体)自我复制
self-suspension [ˌself səs'penʃən] *n* 自体悬吊法(头与腋悬吊或头悬吊以牵张脊柱)
self-tolerance ['self 'tɔlərəns] *n* 自体耐受性,自身耐受性(机体对自身抗原的免疫无反应性,亦称自身中毒禁忌)
selfwise ['selfwaiz] *a* 自向的(指胚细胞或胚组织,无论移植至任何新的部位,仍按照以前预定的型式发育)
Seliberia [ˌseli'biriə] (G. L. Seliber) *n* 塞里伯菌属 | ~ stellate 星状塞里伯菌
Selivanoff's (Seliwanow's) test (reaction) [seli'vɑːnɔf] (Feodor F. Selivanoff)塞利万诺夫试验(反应)(检尿果糖)
sella ['selə] ([复]**sellae** ['seliː]) *n*【拉】鞍 | **~r** *a* 蝶鞍的
sellanders ['seləndəz] [复] *n* 马膝湿疹
Sellards' test ['selɑːdz] (Andrew W. Sellards)塞拉兹试验(检酸中毒,亦称重碳酸盐耐量试验)
Sellick maneuver ['selik] (Brian A. Sellick)塞立克手法(气管内插管时,为了压迫食管并防止被动性反流而采用压迫环状软骨的手法)
Selter's disease ['seltə] (Paul Selter)肢痛症,红皮水肿性多神经病
Selye syndrome ['selii] (Hans Selye)塞莱综合征,全身适应综合征(即 general adaptation syndrome,见 syndrome 项下相应术语)
Semb's operation [seim] (Carl Semb)塞姆手术(筋膜外肺尖萎陷术,治肺结核)
semeiography [ˌsiːmai'ɔgrəfi] *n* 症状记录
semeiology [siːmai'ɔlədʒi], **semeiotics** [ˌsiːmai'ɔtiks] *n* 症状学
semeiotic(al) [ˌsiːmai'ɔtik(əl), -mi-] *a* 症状的;特殊病征的
semelincident [ˌseməl'insidənt] *a* 终身(罹病)一次的
semel in d. semel in die【拉】每日一次(亦可写成 s. i. d.)
semelparity [ˌseməl'pærəti] *n* 终身一胎[现象] | **semelparous** [se'melpərəs] *a*
semen ['siːmen] ([复]**semens** 或 **semina** ['seminə]) *n*【拉】种子;精液 | ~ contra 山道年花
semenology [ˌsiːmə'nɔlədʒi] *n* 精液学 | **semenologist** *n* 精液学家
semenuria [ˌsiːmə'njuəriə] *n* 精液尿
semi- [前缀]半
semialdehyde [ˌsemi'ældihaid] *n* 半醛 | glutamic-γ-~ 谷氨酸γ半醛
semiantigen [ˌsemi'æntidʒən] *n* 半抗原
semiapochromat [ˌsemiˌæpə'krəumət] *n* 半复消色差物镜 | **semiapochromatic** [ˌsemiˌæpəkrəu'mætik] *a* 半复消色差的
semiaxial [ˌsemi'æksiəl] *a* 半轴的
semicanal [ˌsemikə'næl] *n* 半管 | ~ of auditory tube 咽鼓管半管 / ~ of humerus 肱骨结节间沟 / ~ of tensor tympani muscle 鼓膜张肌半管
semicanalis [ˌsemikə'neilis] ([复]**semicanales** [ˌsemikə'neiliːz]) *n*【拉】半管
semicartilaginous [ˌsemiˌkɑːti'lædʒinəs] *a* 半软骨的
semicoma [ˌsemi'kəumə] *n* 轻昏迷,半昏迷 | **~tose** [ˌsemi'kəumətəus] *a*

semicrista [ˌsemiˈkristə] ([复] **semicristae** [ˌsemiˈkristiː]) *n*【拉】小嵴
semidecussation [ˌsemiˌdekʌˈseiʃən] *n* 半交叉(神经纤维);锥体交叉
semidiagrammatic [ˌsemiˌdaiəgrəˈmætik] *a* 半图式的
semidiameter [ˌsemidaiˈæmitə] *n* 半径
semidominance [ˌsemiˈdɔminəns] *n* 半显性,不完全显性
semiflexion [ˌsemiˈflekʃən] *n* 半屈;半屈位
semifluctuating [ˌsemiˈflʌktjuˌeitiŋ] *a* 半波动的
semifluid [ˌsemiˈflu(ː)id] *a* 半流质的 *n* 半流质
semiglutin [ˌsemiˈgluːtin] *n* 半明胶蛋白
Semih. semihora【拉】半小时
semilente [ˈsemilent] *a* 中效的
semilunar [ˌsemiˈljuːnə] *a* 半月形的,月牙形的
semilunare [ˌsemiljuˈnɛəri] *n*【拉】月骨(腕部)
semiluxation [ˌsemilʌkˈseiʃən] *n* 不全脱位,半脱位
semimembranous [ˌsemiˈmembrənəs] *a* 半膜的
semina [ˈseminə] semen 的复数
seminal [ˈsiːminl, ˈseminl] *a* 种子的;精液的
seminarcosis [ˌseminɑːˈkəusis] *n* 朦胧麻醉,半麻醉
semination [ˌsemiˈneiʃən] *n* 授精
seminiferous [ˌsemiˈnifərəs] *a* 生精子的,输精子的
seminology [ˌsiːmiˈnɔlədʒi] *n* 精液学 | **seminologic(al)** [ˌsiːminəˈlɔdʒik(əl)] *a* / **seminologist** *n* 精液学家
seminoma [ˌsemiˈnəumə, ˌsiː-] *n* 精原细胞瘤 | ovarian ~ 卵巢精原细胞瘤
seminormal [ˌsemiˈnɔːməl] *a* 半当量[浓度]的
seminose [ˈseminəus] *n* 甘露糖
seminuria [ˌsimiˈnjuəriə] *n* 精液尿
semiography [ˌsimiˈɔgrəfi] *n* 症状记录
semiology [ˌsiːmiˈɔlədʒi] *n* 症状学 | **semiologic(al)** [ˌsiːmiəˈlɔdʒik(əl)] *a* / **semiologist** *n* 症状学家
semiorbicular [ˌsemiɔːˈbikjulə] *a* 半圆形的,半环形的
semiotic(al) [ˌsiːmiˈɔtik(əl)] *a* 症状的;特殊病征的
semiotics [ˌsiːmiˈɔtiks] *n* 症状学(体征和症状的研究)
semiparametric [ˌsemiˌpærəˈmetrik] *a* 半参数的
semiparasite [ˌsemiˈpærəsait] *n* 半寄生物(既是腐生物,又是寄生物,具有致病性)
semipenniform [ˌsemiˈpenifɔːm] *a* 半羽状的
semipermeable [ˌsemiˈpəːmjəbl] *a* 半[渗]透性的
semiplacenta [ˌsemipləˈsentə] *n* 半胎盘(某些动物)
semiplegia [ˌsemiˈpliːdʒiə] *n* 偏瘫,半身不遂
semipronation [ˌsemiprəˈneiʃən] *n* 半俯卧位;半旋前
semiprone [ˌsemiˈprəun] *a* 半俯卧位的
semiquantitative [ˌsemiˈkwɔntitətiv] *a* 半定量的
semiquinone [ˌsemikwiˈnəun] *n* 半醌
semirecumbent [ˌsemiriˈkʌmbənt] *a* 半卧的
semis(ss.) [ˈsemis] *n*【拉】半,一半
semisideratio [ˌsemiˌsidəˈreiʃiəu] *n* 偏瘫,半身不遂
semisomnus [ˌsemiˈsɔmnəs], **semisopor** [ˌsemiˈsəupə] *n* 轻昏迷
semispeculum [ˌsemiˈspekjuləm] *n* 半窥镜(膀胱切石术用)
semistarvation [ˌsemistɑːˈveiʃən] *n* 半饥饿,饥饿疗法
semisulcus [ˌsemiˈsʌlkəs] *n* 半沟
semisupination [ˌsemiˌsjuːpiˈneiʃən] *n* 半仰卧位;半旋后
semisupine [ˌsemisjuːˈpain] *a* 半仰卧位的
semisynthetic [ˌsemisinˈθetik] *a* 半合成的
semitendinous [ˌsemiˈtendinəs] *a* 半腱的
semitransparent [ˌsemitrænsˈpɛərənt] *a* 半透明的
Semliki Forest encephalitis [semˈliːki] (Semliki Forest 在乌干达西部,在该地带蚊传播此病毒)塞姆利基森林脑炎 | ~ virus 塞姆利基森林病毒
Semon-Hering hypothesis, theory [ˈzeimən ˈheiriŋ] (Richard W. Semon; Ewald Hering)塞蒙-黑林假说、学说(亦称记忆学说,即细胞对所加之影响有遗传性"记忆",因此它倾向于经遗传而得到获得性特性)
Semon's law [ˈsiːmən] (Felix Semon)塞蒙定律(喉运动神经有进行性器质性疾病时,声带外展肌〈环杓后肌〉首先受到影响) | ~ sign 塞蒙征(恶性喉病时声带运动受损)
Semple's treatment [ˈsempl] (David Semple)森普尔疗法,狂犬病疗法(注射森普尔疫苗预防狂犬病) | ~ vaccine 森普尔疫苗,狂犬病疫苗
semustine [səˈmʌstiːn] *n* 司莫司汀(抗肿瘤药,主要用于治疗脑瘤、结肠直肠癌、胃癌、霍奇金〈Hodgkin〉病和恶性黑素瘤)
Senear-Usher syndrome [siˈniə ˈʌʃə] (Francis E. Senear; Barney Usher) 红斑性天疱疮
senecifolin [ˌseniˈsifəlin] *n* 千里光叶碱
senecine [ˈsenəsiːn] *n* 千里光因(一种生物碱)
Senecio [siˈniːʃiəu] *n*【拉】千里光属
seneciosis [səˌnəuʃiˈəusis] *n* 千里光中毒
senectitude [siˈnektitjuːd] *n* 老年时期,晚年
senega [ˈsenigə] *n*【拉】美远志(从前曾用于治肺

炎后期、气喘等)
senegenin [ˌseniˈdʒenin] *n* 美远志皂苷元
senegin [ˈsenidʒin] *n* 远志皂苷
senesce [siˈnes] *vi* 开始衰老
senescense [siˈnesns] *n* 衰老,老年化 | dental ~ 牙齿衰老
senescent [siˈnesnt] *a* 衰老的
Sengstaken-Blakemore tube [ˈseŋzteikən ˈbleikmɔː] (Robert W. Sengstaken; Arthur H. Blakemore)森-布管,三腔双囊管(一种多腔管,用以填塞出血的食管静脉曲张,一管通达气囊,使其在胃中充气,以保持此器具于原位并压迫贲门部周围血管,另一管通达一狭长气囊以此囊压迫食管壁,第三管附着于一抽吸器以吸出胃中的内容物)
senile [ˈsiːnail] *a* 老年的,衰老的 | **senility** [siˈniləti] *n*
senilism [ˈsiːnilizəm] *n* 早老,早衰
Senior-Loken syndrome [ˈsiːnjə ˈləukən] (Boris Senior; Aagot C. Loken)西-卢综合征(一种罕见的常染色体隐性遗传综合征,表现为毯层视网膜变性和家族性青年性肾消耗病,有些权威人士认为这是青年性肾消耗病-髓质囊性病综合征的一部分。亦称肾-视网膜综合征或发育不良)
senium [ˈsiːniəm] *n* 年老,衰老,老年
senna [ˈsenə] *n* 番泻叶
sennatin [ˈsenətin] *n* 番泻叶素(从番泻叶提出的有效成分,皮下注射用作泻药)
Senn's bone plates [sen] (Nicholas Senn)森氏骨板(用于对合及缝合肠段) | ~ operation 森氏手术(应用外侧密接及骨板作肠吻合术)
senograph [ˈsiːnəgrɑːf, -græf] *n* 低电压[X线]摄影器;低电压[X线]摄片 | **~y** [siˈnɔgrəfi] *n* 低电压[X线]摄影术(一种低电压恒电位X线摄影术,尤指乳房X线摄影术)
senopia [siˈnəupiə] *n* 老年期视力回春,老视减退现象(由于老年时期晶状体核心硬化而引起近视所造成,亦称第二视力)
sennoside [ˈsenəusaid] *n* 番泻苷
sennosides [ˈsenəusaidz] *n* 番泻苷合剂(用作泻药,口服给药)
sensation [senˈseiʃən] *n* 感觉 | cincture ~, girdle ~ 束勒感,束带状感觉 / general ~ 全身感觉 / gnostic ~s, new ~s 认识性感觉,新生感觉(指轻触觉、本体感觉等精细感觉) / objective ~, external ~ 客观感觉,外部感觉 / referred ~, reflex ~, transferred ~ 牵涉性感觉,反射性感觉,转移性感觉 / subjective ~, internal ~ 主观感觉,内部感觉
sense [sens] *n* 觉,感觉 | color ~ 色觉 / equilibrium ~, static ~ 平衡觉,静位觉 / form ~ 立体觉 / kinesthetic ~, muscle ~ 运动感觉,肌觉 / posture ~ 位置觉,姿势觉 / proprioceptive ~ 本体感觉 / seventh ~, visceral ~ 第七感觉,内脏感觉 / sixth ~ 第六感觉(一般机体觉,即 cenesthesia) / special ~ 特种感觉,五官觉
sensibiligen [ˌsensiˈbilidʒən], **sensibilisinogen** [ˌsensiˌbiliˈsinədʒən] *n* 过敏原,致敏原
sensibilin [ˌsensiˈbilin], **sensibilisin** [ˌsensiˈbilisin] *n* 过敏素,致敏素
sensibility [ˌsensiˈbiləti] *n* 感觉性,感受性,敏感性;感觉,感觉能力;灵敏度 | bone ~ 骨感觉,振动[感]觉 / deep ~, mesoblastic ~ 深部感觉 / epicritic ~ 精细感觉(区别皮肤触觉和温度的能力) / joint ~ 关节感觉 / proprioceptive ~, somesthetic ~ 本体感觉 / recurrent ~ 回反感觉 / splanchnesthetic ~ 内脏感觉
sensibilization [ˌsensibilaiˈzeiʃən, -liˈz-] *n* 增敏[作用];致敏[作用]
sensible [ˈsensəbl] *a* 感觉得到的
sensiferous [senˈsifərəs] *a* 传导感觉的
sensigenous [senˈsidʒinəs] *a* 产生感觉的
sensimeter [senˈsimitə] *n* 感觉计(测身体感觉缺失区和感觉过敏区的敏感度)
sensitin [ˈsensitin] *n* 迟发致敏素(从病原体如病毒、细菌或真菌制备的非抗原性物质,能引起迟发型敏感性)
sensitinogen [ˌsensiˈtinədʒən] *n* 致敏原,过敏原(统称)
sensitive [ˈsensitiv] *a* 敏感的,神经过敏的,(由于某种疾病而)过敏的 | **~ness** *n* 感受性,敏感性
sensitivity [ˌsensiˈtivəti] *n* 感受性,敏感性,过敏;灵敏度 | proportional ~ 相应敏感性(对刺激的强度具有某种定量代数关系的反应)
sensitization [ˌsensitaiˈzeiʃən, -tiˈz-] *n* 致敏作用;增敏 | active ~ 自动致敏 / autoerythrocyte ~ 自体红细胞致敏[作用],自身红细胞致敏(作用) / protein ~ 蛋白质致敏[作用] / passive ~ 被动致敏 / Rh ~ Rh 致敏(对 Rh 因子〈即 Rh 抗原,尤其是 D 抗原〉起致敏的过程或状态,如孕妇为 Rh〈 - 〉,胎儿为 Rh〈 + 〉,胎儿血进入母体循环使母体致敏)
sensitize [ˈsensitaiz] *vt* 使敏感;致敏(指对抗原) | **~d** *a* 致敏的 / **~r** *n* 致敏物质,敏化物
sensitizin [ˌsensiˈtaizin] *n* 致敏素,过敏原
sensitometer [ˌsensiˈtɔmitə] *n* 感光计
sensomobile [ˌsensəˈməubail] *a* 感觉移动的 | **sensomobility** [ˌsensəməuˈbiliti] *n* 感觉移动性
sensor [ˈsensə] *n* 传感器,感受器
sensorial [senˈsɔːriəl] *a* 感觉中枢的;皮质感觉中枢的;感觉的,知觉的
sensoriglandular [ˌsensəriˈglændjulə] *a* 感觉性分泌的

sensorimetabolism [ˌsensərimeˈtæbəlizəm] *n* 感觉性代谢
sensorimotor [ˌsensəriˈməutə], **sensomotor** [ˌsensəˈməutə] *a* 感觉运动的
sensorimuscular [ˌsensəriˈmʌskjulə] *a* 感觉性肌肉活动的
sensorineural [ˌsensəriˈnjuərəl] *a* 感觉神经的，感音神经性的
sensorium [senˈsɔːriəm] *n* 感觉中枢；（大脑）皮质感觉中枢；神志，感觉，知觉
sensorivascular [ˌsensəriˈvæskjulə], **sensorivasomotor** [ˌsensəriˌveizəuˈməutə] *a* 感觉性血管[运动]的
sensory [ˈsensəri] *a* 感觉的
sensual [ˈsensjuəl] *a* 耽于声色口腹之乐的；色情的；感觉的 | **~ity** [ˌsensjuˈæləti] *n* 耽于声色
sensualism [ˈsenʃuəlizəm] *n* 肉欲主义，感官享乐主义
sensuous [ˈsensjuəs] *a* 感官方面的，感觉上的
sentics [ˈsentiks] *n* 情感学（研究情感表达的学科） | **sentic** [ˈsentik] *a*
sentience [ˈsenʃəns], **sentiency** [ˈsenʃənsi] *n* 感觉能力
sentient [ˈsenʃənt] *a* 能感觉的，有感觉的
sentiment [ˈsentimənt] *n* 感情；情感，情操
sentimental [ˌsentiˈmentl] *a* 感伤的；多愁善感的；情感[上]的 | **~ity** [ˌsentimenˈtæləti] *n* 情感生活；多愁善感 / **~ist** *n* 感伤主义者
SEP somatosensory evoked potential 躯体感觉诱发电位
sepal [ˈsepəl, ˈsiː-] *n* 萼片
sepaloid [ˈsepəlɔid] *a* 萼片样的
separable [ˈsepərəbl] *a* 可分的 | **separability** [ˌsepərəˈbiləti] *n* 可分离性，可分性 *n*
separate [ˈsepərit] *a* 分离的；单独的；各别的 [ˈsepəreit] *vt* 使分离；把…分类；区分，使离析 *vi* 分离；离析；析出 | **~ly** *ad*
separation [ˌsepəˈreiʃən] *n* 分离，分开；离析 | placental ~ 胎盘剥离
separative [ˈsepərətiv] *a* 分离的
separator [ˈsepəreitə] *n* 分离器；分液器；分牙器
separatorium [ˌsepərəˈtɔːriəm] *n* 颅骨膜分离器
separatory [ˈsepərətəri] *a* 分离用的
sepazonium chloride [ˌsepəˈzəuniəm] 氯化三苯唑（局部抗感染药）
sepedon [ˌsepiˈdɔn] *n* 【希】腐败
sepedonogenesis [ˌsepəˌdəunəuˈdʒenisis], **sepedogenesis** [ˌsepədəuˈdʒenisis] *n* 败血病发生
seperidol hydrochloride [səˈperidəul] 盐酸氯氟哌醇（安定药）
sepia [ˈsiːpjə] *n* 【拉；希】乌贼墨汁 *a* 深棕色的
sepiapterin reductase [siːpiˈæptərin riˈdʌkteis] 墨蝶呤还原酶
sepium [ˈsiːpiəm] *n* 【拉】乌贼骨，海螵蛸
sepsin [ˈsepsin] *n* 腐败素，腐败蒜，腐败毒
sepsis [ˈsepsis] *n* 脓毒病，脓毒症 | ~ agranulocytica 粒细胞缺乏性脓毒病，粒细胞缺乏症 / incarcerated ~ 潜伏性脓毒病，箝闭性脓毒病 / ~ intestinalis 肠性脓毒病 / ~ lenta 慢性脓毒病 / mouse ~, murine ~ 鼠脓毒病 / puerperal ~ 产后脓毒病
Sepsis violacea [ˈsepsis ˌvaiəˈleisiə] 马粪蝇
sepsometer [sepˈsɔmitə] *n* 空气有机质测定计
Sept. septem 【拉】七
septa [ˈseptə] septum 的复数
septal [ˈseptl] *a* 中隔的，间隔的
septan [ˈseptən] *a* 每七日复发的
septanose [ˈseptənəus] *n* 环庚糖
septate [ˈsepteit] *a* 有隔的，分隔的
Septatina [ˌseptəˈtainə] *n* 有隔亚目
septation [sepˈteiʃən] *n* 分隔；中隔，隔[膜]
septatome [ˈseptətəum] *n* 鼻中隔刀
septavalent [ˌseptəˈveilənt] *a* 七价的
septectomy [sepˈtektəmi] *n* 鼻中隔切除术
septic [ˈseptik] *a* 腐败性的，脓毒性的；败血病的 *n* 腐败剂，腐烂物
septicemia [ˌseptiˈsiːmiə] *n* 败血病，败血症 | bronchopulmonary ~ 支气管肺性败血病 / cryptogenic ~ 隐原性败血病 / hemorrhagic ~ 出血性败血病（巴斯德菌病）/ melitensis ~ 波状热，布鲁[杆]菌病 / morphine injector's ~（人）类鼻疽 / plague ~ 鼠疫败血病，败血性鼠疫 / sputum ~ 痰菌性败血病 | **septemia** [sepˈtiːmiə] *n* / **septicemic** [ˌseptiˈsiːmik] *a*
septicine [ˈseptisiːn] *n* 腐鱼尸碱
septicophlebitis [ˌseptikəufliˈbaitis] *n* 脓毒性静脉炎
septicopyemia [ˌseptikəupaiˈiːmiə] *n* 脓毒败血病，脓毒败血症 | metastatic ~ 转移性脓毒败血病 / spontaneous ~, cryptogenic ~ 自发性脓毒败血病，隐原性脓毒败血病 | **septicopyemic** *a*
septicozymoid [ˌseptikəuˈzaimɔid] *n* 脓毒性类酶
septigravida [ˌseptiˈgrævidə] *n* 【拉】第七次孕妇
septile [ˈseptail] *a* 隔的
septimetritis [ˌseptimiˈtraitis] *n* 脓毒性子宫炎
septineuritis [ˌseptinjuəˈraitis] *n* 脓毒性神经炎
septipara [sepˈtipərə] *n* 【拉】七产妇
septivalent [ˌseptiˈveilənt] *a* 七价的
sept(o)- [构词成分] 隔
septomarginal [ˌseptəuˈmɑːdʒinəl] *a* 隔缘的
septometer [sepˈtɔmitə] *n* 鼻中隔厚度计；空气有机质测定计
septonasal [ˌseptəuˈneizəl] *a* 鼻中隔的
septoplasty [ˌseptəuˈplæsti] *n* 鼻中隔成形术

septorhinoplasty [ˌseptəuˈrainəuˌplæsti] *n* 鼻中隔成形术

septostomy [sepˈtɔstəmi] *n* 中隔造口术 | balloon atrial ~ 气囊房中隔造口术

septotome [ˈseptətəum] *n* 鼻中隔刀

septotomy [sepˈtɔtəmi] *n* 鼻中隔切开术

septulum [ˈseptjuləm] ([复] **septula** [ˈseptjulə]) *n*【拉】小隔

septum [ˈseptəm] ([复] **septums** 或 **septa** [ˈseptə]) *n*【拉】中隔,间隔,隔[膜] | atrioventricular ~ of heart 房室隔 / ~ of auditory tube, bony ~ of eustachian canal 肌咽鼓管隔 / bony ~ of nose 鼻中隔骨部 / bronchial ~ 气管隆凸 / enamel ~ 釉索 / femoral ~ 股环隔 / gingival ~, gum ~ 龈中隔 / ~ of glans penis 阴茎头隔 / interalveolar ~, interdental ~ 牙槽间隔,牙间隔 / interatrial ~ of heart, interauricular ~ 房间隔,房中隔 / mobile ~ of nose 鼻中隔活动部,鼻中隔膜部 / nasal ~ 鼻中隔 / neural ~ 髓管隔 / septa of testis 睾丸小隔 / transverse ~ of ampulla 壶腹嵴

septuplet [ˈseptʃuplit] *n* 七胎

seq. luce. sequenti luce【拉】第二日

sequel [ˈsiːkwəl] *n* 后遗症,后发病,遗患

sequela [siˈkwiːlə] ([复] **sequelae** [siˈkwiːliː]) *n*【拉】后遗症,后发病,遗患

sequence [ˈsiːkwəns] *n* 连续,顺序;后果,结果;序列征 *vt* 测序,定序 | flanking ~ 侧翼序列 / intervening ~ 内含子 / nearest neighbor ~ 最近邻序列

sequester [siˈkwestə] *vt* 隔绝,分离

sequestrant [siˈkwestrənt] *n* 多价螯合剂

sequestration [ˌsiːkwesˈtreiʃən] *n* 死骨形成;隔离(病人);分离;血管内血量净增值 | pulmonary ~ 肺隔离症

sequestrectomy [ˌsiːkwesˈtrektəmi], **sequestrotomy** [ˌsiːkwesˈtrɔtəmi] *n* 死骨切除术

sequestrum [siˈkwestrəm] ([复] **sequestrums** 或 **sequestra** [siˈkwestrə]) *n* 死骨片 | primary ~ 第一级死骨片 / secondary ~ 第二级死骨片 / tertiary ~ 第三级死骨片 | **sequestral** [siˈkwestrəl] *a*

sequoiosis [ˌsiːkwɔiˈəusis] *n* 红杉尘肺

Ser serine 丝氨酸

sera [ˈsiərə] serum 的复数

seractide acetate [səˈræktaid] 丝拉克肽醋酯,三十九肽促皮质素醋酯(合成促皮质素)

seral [ˈsiərəl] *a* 演替系列的(如演替系列期 seral stage)

seralbumin [ˌsiərælˈbjuːmin] *n* 血清白蛋白,血清清蛋白

serangitis [ˌsiərænˈdʒaitis] *n* (阴茎)海绵体炎

sere [siə] *n* (生态学中的)演替系列

serempion [siˈrempjəm] *n* 致命性麻疹(西印度群岛)

Serenoa [ˌseriˈnəuə] *n* 蓝棕属,锯叶棕属

seretin [ˈseritin] *n* 四氯化碳

Sergent's white adrenal line [sɛəˈʒɔŋ] (Emile Sergent)塞尔让肾上腺性白线(腹部指甲划痕后发生的白线,见于肾上腺功能不良)

serglobulin [səˈglɔbjulin] *n* 副球蛋白

serial [ˈsiəriəl] *a* 连续的,一系列的;序列的

serialograph [ˌsiəriˈæləgrɑːf, -græf] *n* 连续[X线]摄影器,系列[X线]摄影装置

seriatim [ˌsiəriˈeitim]【拉】*ad* 依次地,逐一地;连续地 *a* 依次的,逐一的;连续的

sericin [ˈserisin] *n* 丝胶蛋白

sericite [ˈsiərisait] *n* 绢云母(一种云母或白云母,能引起肺尘病)

Sericopelma [ˌserikəuˈpelmə] *n* 巨毛蜘蛛属

series [ˈsiəriːz] *n* 连续,系列;系,列,组,族,型 | aliphatic ~ 脂肪系,脂族 / aromatic ~ 芳香系 / basophil ~, basophilic ~ 嗜碱细胞族 / eosinophil ~, eosinophilic ~ 嗜酸性细胞族 / fatty ~ 脂芳系 / homologous ~ 同系,同源系,同系列 / leukocytic ~ 白细胞系 / lymphocyte ~, lymphocytic ~ 淋巴细胞系 / lyotropic ~ 离子促变序列 / monocyte ~, monocytic ~ 单核细胞系 / neutrophil ~, neutrophilic ~ 中性粒细胞系 / plasmacyte ~, plasmacytic ~ 浆细胞系

seriflux [ˈseriflʌks] *n* 浆水,浆液(水样排出物)

serifuge [ˈsiərifjuːdʒ] *n* 血清离心机

serine (Ser, S) [ˈseriːn, ˈsiə-] *n* 丝氨酸

L-serine dehydratase [ˈseriːn diːˈhaidrəteis] L-丝氨酸脱水酶

serine endopeptidase [ˈseriːn ˌendəuˈpeptideis] 丝氨酸内肽酶

serine hydroxymethyltransferase [ˈseriːn haiˌdrɔksiˌmeθilˈtrænsfəreis] 丝氨酸羟甲基转移酶,甘氨酸羟甲基转移酶

serine protease [ˈsiəriːn ˈprəutieis] 丝氨酸蛋白酶,丝氨酸内肽酶

serine proteinase [ˈseriːn ˈprəutiːneis] 丝氨酸蛋白酶,丝氨酸内肽酶

serine-type carboxypeptidase [ˈseriːnˌtaip kɑːˌbɔksiˈpeptideis] 丝氨酸型羧肽酶

serioscopy [ˌsiəriˈɔskəpi] *n* 连续(实体)照片投影检查

seriscission [ˌseriˈsiʒən] *n* 线切术

SERM selective estrogen receptor modulator 选择性雌激素受体调质

sermorelin acetate [ˌsermәuˈrelin] 醋酸舍莫瑞林(一种合成肽的醋酸盐,相当于一部分生长激素释放素,用于治疗青春期前儿童的特发性生

长激素缺乏症,皮下给药)
seroalbuminous [ˌsiərəuælˈbjuːminəs] *a* 血清白蛋白的
seroalbuminuria [ˌsiərəuælˌbjuːmiˈnjuəriə] *n* 血清白蛋白尿
seroanaphylaxis [ˌsiərəuˌænəfiˈlæksis] *n* 血清过敏反应,血清过敏症
serochrome [ˈsiərəkrəum] *n* 血清色素
serocolitis [ˌsiərəukɔˈlaitis] *n* 结肠浆膜炎
seroconversion [ˌsiərəukənˈvəːʃən] *n* 血清转化[现象](给予疫苗后的抗体产生)
seroconvert [ˌsiərəukənˈvəːt] *vt* 血清转化(对疫苗产生抗体)
seroculture [ˈsiərəkʌltʃə] *n* 血清培养物
serocystic [ˌsiərəuˈsistik] *a* 浆液性囊肿的
serodiagnosis [ˌsiərəuˌdaiəgˈnəusis] *n* 血清学诊断 | **serodiagnostic** [ˌsiərəuˌdaiəgˈnɔstik] *a*
seroenteritis [ˌsiərəuˌentəˈraitis] *n* 肠浆膜炎
seroenzyme [ˌsiərəuˈenzaim] *n* 血清酶
seroepidemiology [ˌsiərəuˌepiˌdiːmiˈɔlədʒi] *n* 血清流行病学 | **seroepidemiologic** [ˌsiərəuˌepiˌdiːmiəˈlɔdʒik] *a*
sero-fast [ˈsiərə ˈfɑːst] *a* 抗血清的(指细菌)
serofibrinous [ˌsiərəuˈfaibrinəs] *a* 浆液纤维蛋白性的
serofibrous [ˌsiərəuˈfaibrəs] *a* 浆液纤维性的
seroflocculation [ˌsiərəuˌflɔkjuˈleiʃən] *n* 血清絮凝[作用],血清絮状反应
serofluid [ˌsiərəuˈfluːid] *n* 浆液
serogastria [ˌsiərəuˈgæstriə] *n* 胃内积血清(蛋白质丧失性胃病)
serogenesis [ˌsiərəuˈdʒenisis] *n* 血清生成
seroglobulin [ˌsiərəuˈglɔbjulin] *n* 血清球蛋白
seroglycoid [ˌsiərəuˈglaikɔid] *n* 血清糖蛋白
serogroup [ˈsiərəugruːp] *n* 血清群(①含有共同抗原的一群细菌,可能包括一个以上的血清型、种或属。血清型为暂定非正式名称,用于某些细菌属的分类,例如 Leptospira, Salmonella, Shigella 和 Streptococcus;②在抗原上密切相关的一群病毒种)
serohemorrhagic [ˌsiərəuˌheməˈreidʒik] *a* 浆液出血性的
serohepatitis [ˌsiərəuˌhepəˈtaitis] *n* 肝[脏]浆膜炎
seroimmunity [ˌsiərəuiˈmjuːnəti] *n* 血清免疫(抗血清引起的免疫,即被动免疫)
serolactescent [ˌsiərəulækˈtesnt] *a* 血清乳状的
serolemma [ˌsiərəuˈlemə] *n* 胎浆膜
serolipase [ˌsiərəuˈlaipeis] *n* 血清脂酶
serology [siəˈrɔlədʒi] *n* 血清学(在体外研究抗原抗体反应的科学) | diagnostic ~ 诊断血清学,血清诊断 | **serologic(al)** [ˌsiərəˈlɔdʒik(əl)] *a* / **serologist** *n* 血清学家,血清学工作者
serolysin [siəˈrɔlisin] *n* 血清溶素
seroma [siəˈrəumə] *n* 血清肿(组织内有肿瘤样的血清血液性积液)
seromembranous [ˌsiərəuˈmembrənəs] *a* 浆液膜性的,浆膜的
seromucoid [ˌsiərəuˈmjuːkɔid] *a* 浆液黏液性的 *n* 血清[类]黏蛋白
seromucous [ˌsiərəuˈmjuːkəs] *a* 浆液黏液性的
seromucus [ˌsiərəuˈmjuːkəs] *n* 浆液黏液(混合分泌)
seromuscular [ˌsiərəuˈmʌskjulə] *a* (肠道)浆膜肌膜的
seromyotomy [ˌsiərəumaiˈɔtəmi] *n* 浆膜肌切开术
seronegative [ˌsiərəuˈnegətiv] *a* 血清阴性的 | **seronegativity** [ˌsiərəuˌnegəˈtivəti] *n*
seroperitoneum [ˌsiərəuˌperitəuˈniːəm] *n* 腹腔积液,腹水
serophilic [ˌsiərəuˈfilik] *a* 嗜血清的(指细菌)
serophysiology [ˌsiərəuˌfiziˈɔlədʒi] *n* 血清生理学
seroplastic [ˌsiərəuˈplæstik] *a* 浆液纤维蛋白性的
seropneumothorax [ˌsiərəuˌnjuːməuˈθɔːræks] *n* 浆液气胸
seropositive [ˌsiərəuˈpɔzətiv] *a* 血清阳性的 | **seropositivity** [ˌsiərəupɔziˈtivəti] *n*
seroprognosis [ˌsiərəuprəgˈnəusis] *n* 血清预后
seroprophylaxis [ˌsiərəuˌprɔfiˈlæksis] *n* 血清预防(注射免疫血清或恢复期血清预防疾病)
seropurulent [ˌsiərəuˈpjuərulənt] *a* 浆液脓性的
seropus [ˌsiərəuˈpʌs] *n* 浆液性脓
seroreaction [ˌsiərəuri(ː)ˈækʃən] *n* 血清反应
serorelapse [ˌsiərəuriˈlæps] *n* 血清复发(治疗后血清学效价明显上升)
seroresistance [ˌsiərəuriˈzistəns] *n* 血清不应性(治疗后血清学效价不能满意地下降)
seroresistant [ˌsiərəuriˈzistənt] *a* 血清不应性的(治疗后对病原体仍显示血清阳性反应的)
sero-reversal [ˌsiərəu riˈvəːsəl] *n* 血清逆转(治疗后血清学效价下降)
seroreversion [ˌsiərəuriːˈvəːʒən] *n* 血清反应逆转(从血清反应阳性状态自发或诱发转换到血清反应阴性状态)
serosa [siˈrəusə, siˈrəuzə] *n* 浆膜;绒[毛]膜 | **~l** *a*
serosamucin [siˌrəusəˈmjuːsin] *n* 浆膜黏蛋白(见于炎症性腹水渗出液)
serosanguineous [ˌsiərəusæŋˈgwiniəs] *a* 血清血液的
seroscopy [siəˈrɔskəpi] *n* 血清凝集镜检查
serose [ˈsiərəus] *n* 血清[蛋白]脲
seroserous [ˌsiərəuˈsiərəs] *a* 浆膜与浆膜的

serositis [ˌsiərəuˈsaitis] ([复]**serositides** [ˌsiərəuˈsaitidiːz]) *n* 浆膜炎 | multiple ~ 多浆膜炎
serosity [siəˈrɔsəti] *n* 浆液性
serosurvey [ˌsiərəuˈsəːvei] *n* 血清学调查(使用血清学试验对与某种传染病有过接触和具有免疫力的人群进行筛选性检查)
serosynovial [ˌsiərəusiˈnəuviəl] *a* 浆液滑液性的
serosynovitis [ˌsiərəuˌsinəˈvaitis] *n* 浆液性滑膜炎
serotherapist [ˌsiərəuˈθerəpist] *n* 血清疗法家,血清治疗工作者
serotherapy [ˌsiərəuˈθerəpi] *n* 血清[免疫]疗法 | **serotherapeutical** [ˌsiərəuˌθerəˈpjuːtikəl] *a*
serothorax [ˌsiərəuˈθɔːræks] *n* 浆液胸,胸膜[腔]积水,水胸
serotonergic [ˌsiərəutəuˈnəːdʒik] *a* 含血清素的;血清素激活的
serotonin [ˌserəˈtəunin] *n* 5-羟色胺,血清素
serotoninergic [ˌsiərəuˌtəuniˈnəːdʒik] *a* 含血清素的;血清素激活的
serotoxin [ˌsiərəuˈtɔksin] *n* 血清毒素
serotype [ˈsiərətaip] *n* 血清分型;血清型 | heterologous ~ 异[种]血清型 / homologous ~ 同[种]血清型
serous [ˈsiərəs] *a* 浆液的;血清的
serovaccination [ˌsiərəuˌvæksiˈneiʃən] *n* 血清疫苗接种(注射血清与疫苗接种同时进行,由前者产生被动免疫,由后者产生自动免疫)
serovar [ˈsiərəvɑː] *n* 血清型
serozyme [ˈsiərəzaim] *n* 凝血酶原(在血清中)
serpent [ˈsəːpənt] *n* 蛇,毒蛇
serpentarium [ˌsəːpənˈtɛəriəm] ([复]**serpentariums** 或 **serpentaria** [ˌsəːpənˈtɛəriə]) *n* 美蛇根,蛇根马兜铃(一种收敛苦味药)
Serpentes [ˈsəːpəntiːz] *n* 蛇类
serpentine [ˈsəːpəntain] *n* 蛇根碱
serpiginous [səːˈpidʒinəs] *a* 匐行的,匐行性的(如结节性溃疡性皮肤梅毒的损害)
serpin [ˈsəːpin] *n* 丝氨酸蛋白酶抑制剂
serrate [ˈserit, ˈsereit] *a* 有锯齿[边]的[ˈsereit] *vt* 使成锯齿状 | **~d** [seˈreitid] *a* 锯齿状的
Serratia [səˈreiʃiə] *n* 沙雷菌属 | ~ liquefaciens, ~ proteamaculans 解凝沙雷菌 / ~ marcescens 黏质沙雷菌,灵杆菌 / ~ odorifera 臭味沙雷菌 / ~ plymuthica 普利茅斯沙雷菌 / ~ rubidaea 深红沙雷菌
Serratieae [ˌserəˈtaiiiː] *n* 沙雷菌族
serration [səˈreiʃən] *n* 锯齿形,锯齿构造
serratus [səˈreitəs] *a*【拉】锯齿状的 *n* 锯肌
serrefine [sɛəˈfiːn] *n*【法】小弹簧镊(压迫出血性血管,用以止血)
Serres' angle [sɛəz] (Antoine E. R. A. Serres)面后角 | ~ glands 塞尔腺(在婴儿龈上形成的珠状上皮细胞小体)
serrulate [ˈserjuleit] *a* 细锯齿状的
Sertoli's cell [səˈtəuli] (Enrico Sertoli)塞托利细胞,[睾丸]支持细胞 | ~ cell junction complex 支持细胞连接复合体 / Sertoli-cell-only syndrome 塞托利细胞仅存综合征(单纯睾丸支持细胞综合征) / ~ cell tumor 塞托利细胞瘤(睾丸支持细胞瘤) / ~ column 塞托利柱(睾丸细精管体壁层中一种长形的塞托利细胞组成的细胞柱)
sertraline hydrochloride [ˈsəːtrəliːn] 盐酸舍曲林(5-羟色胺再摄取的选择性抑制剂,用作抗抑郁药,口服给药)
serum [ˈsiərəm] ([复]**serums** 或 **sera** [ˈsiərə]) *n* 血清;浆液 | active ~ 活性血清(含补体) / allergenic ~, allergic ~ 变应性血清,变态反应性血清 / anallergenic ~, anallergic ~ 抗变应性血清,抗变态反应性血清 / antibothropic ~ 抗响尾蛇血清 / anticholera ~ 抗霍乱血清 / anticomplementary ~ 抗补体血清 / anticrotalus ~ 抗响尾蛇血清 / antidiphtheric ~ 抗白喉血清,白喉抗毒素 / antihepatic ~ 抗肝血清 / antilymphocyte ~ (ALS) 抗淋巴细胞血清 / antimeningococcus ~ 抗脑膜炎球菌血清 / antiophidic ~ 抗眼镜蛇血清,抗毒蛇血清 / antipancreatic ~ 抗胰血清 / antipertussis ~ 抗百日咳血清 / antiphagocytic ~ 抗吞噬血清 / antiplague ~, antipest ~ 抗鼠疫血清 / antiplatelet ~ 抗血小板血清 / antipneumococcus ~ 抗肺炎球菌血清 / antirabies ~ 抗狂犬病血清 / antireticular cytotoxic ~ (ACS) 抗网状细胞毒性血清 / antisarcomatous ~ 抗肉瘤血清 / antiscarlatinal ~ 抗猩红热血清 / anti-snakebite ~ 抗蛇咬伤血清,抗毒蛇血清 / antispermotoxic ~ 抗精子毒素血清,抗精子毒素 / antistaphylococcus ~ 抗葡萄球菌血清 / antistreptococcus ~ 抗链球菌血清 / antitetanic ~ (ATS) 抗破伤风血清,破伤风抗毒素 / antitoxic ~ 抗毒血清 / antitubercle ~ 抗结核血清 / antitularense ~ 抗土拉血清,抗野兔热血清 / antityphoid ~ 抗伤寒血清 / antivenomous ~ 抗毒蛇血清 / articular ~ 滑液 / bacteriolytic ~ 溶菌血清 / blood ~ 血清 / blood grouping ~s 血液分型血清(用于测定血型) / chicken ~ 鸡免疫血清 / convalescence ~, convalescent ~, convalescents' ~ 恢复期血清 / cytotropic ~ 亲细胞性血清 / despeciated ~ 去种特异性血清 / endotheliolytic ~ 溶内皮细胞血清 / foreign ~ 异体血清 / gastrotoxic ~ 胃毒血清 / heterologous ~ 异种血清 / hog cholera ~ 猪霍乱血清 / homologous ~ 同种血清 / hyperimmune ~ 超免疫血清,高度免疫血清 / immune ~ 免疫血清 / inactivated ~ 灭活血清 / leukocytolytic ~ 溶白细胞血清 / leukotoxic ~ 白细胞毒血清 / lym-

phatolytic ~ 溶淋巴组织血清 / monovalent ~ 单价血清 / motile ~ 动力血清,动能型血清 / nephrolytic ~, nephrotoxic ~ 溶肾血清,肾毒血清 / normal ~ 正常血清 / pericardial ~ 心包液 / petit ~ 无毒血清沉淀 / plague ~ 鼠疫血清,抗鼠疫血清 / polyvalent ~, multipartial ~ 多价血清 / pooled ~ 混合血清 / pregnancy ~ 妊娠血清 / prophylactic ~ 预防用血清 / specific ~ 特异性血清 / streptococcus ~ 链球菌血清,抗链球菌血清 / thymotoxic ~ 胸腺毒血清 / thyrolytic ~, thyrotoxic ~ 溶甲状腺血清,甲状腺毒血清 / truth ~ "说真话"血清(这是一个使用不当的名称,指有时在麻醉心理分析时所使用的药物,尤指异戊巴比妥钠和硫喷妥钠,此药物并不是血清,使用这些药物并不保证说话的真实性) | **~al** [si'ruməl] *a*

serum-fast ['siərəm fɑːst] *a* 抗血清的(指细菌)

serumuria [ˌsiərə'mjuəriə] *n* 蛋白尿

Serv. serva【拉】保留,保存

service ['səːvis] *n* 服务;行政部门;公共设施 | free medical ~ 公费医疗 / health ~ 保健事业;卫生部门;卫生设施

servomechanism [ˌsəːvə'mekənizəm] *n* 伺服机构(一种控制系统,用反馈控制另一系统的误差;本词亦应用于生物系统,例如按入射光的量控制瞳孔直径的机制)

seryl ['siəril, 'seril] *n* 丝氨酰[基]

sesame ['sesəmi] *n* 芝麻,脂麻,胡麻

sesamoid ['sesəmɔid] *a* 籽样的,种子样的 *n* 籽骨

sesamoiditis [ˌsesəmɔi'daitis] *n* 籽骨炎(马足部)

Sesamum ['sesəməm] *n* 芝麻属,脂麻属

sesqui- [前缀]倍半,一个半

sesquih. sesquihora【拉】一小时半

sesquihora [seskwi'hɔrə] *n*【拉】一小时半

sesquioxide [ˌseskwi'ɔksaid] *n* 倍半氧化物,三氧化二某(化合物)

sesquisulfate [ˌseskwi'sʌlfeit] *n* 倍半硫酸盐,三硫酸化二某(化合物)

sesquisulfide [ˌseskwi'sʌlfaid] *n* 倍半硫化物,三硫化二某(化合物)

sessile ['sesil] *a* 无柄的,座生的,无蒂的;固着的,固定的

Sessilina [ˌsesi'lainə] *n* 固着亚目

Sessinia [sə'siniə] *n* 斑螯属

sestamibi [ˌsestə'mibi] *n* 司他米比(一种含有6个取代的异氢化物链的化合物,作为放射标记锝〈^{99m}Tc〉的络合物,用于研究心肌灌注成像以及甲状腺和甲状旁腺成像)

set [set] *vt* 使(骨等)复位 *vi* (骨)接合 *n* 定向 | phalangeal ~ 小趾娇形术

seta ['siːtə] ([复] **setae** ['siːtiː]) *n* 刚毛,刚毛样结构

setaceous [si'teiʃəs] *a* 有刚毛的,刚毛状的

Setaria [si'tɛəriə] *n* 鬃丝虫属 | ~ equina 马鬃丝虫 / ~ labiatopapillosa, ~ cervi, ~ cervina 唇突鬃丝虫

setback ['setbæk] *n* 挫折,障碍;(疾病的)复发

Setchenow's centers (nuclei) ['setʃinɔf] (Ivan M. Setchenow)谢切诺夫中枢(核)(脊髓和延髓内的反射抑制中枢)

set-fast ['setfæst] *n* 尿氮过多

setiferous [si'tifərəs], **setigerous** [si'tidʒərəs] *a* 有刚毛的,生刚毛的

set-in ['set-in] *a* 装入的,嵌入的; *n* 嵌入物

seton ['siːtn] *n*【法】泄液线

set-point ['setpɔint] *n* 调定点(由自动控制系统维持的控制变量的靶值,如由下丘脑恒温器控制体温的调定点)

Settegast's projection ['sætəgæst] (H. Settegast)塞特加斯特投照(一种头部斜位投照)

setter ['setə] *n* 安放者,镶嵌者 | bone ~ 接骨者

setup ['setʌp] *n* 机构;体制;体格;方案;(在试用基托上)装排(假牙)

Seutin's bandage [sju'tæn] (Louis J. Seutin)索丹绷带(淀粉石膏绷带)

sevelamer hydrochloride [sə'veləmə] 盐酸司凡拉美(一种磷酸盐黏合剂,口服,以减少血清磷浓度,治疗终末期肾病患者的高磷酸盐血症和异位性钙化)

sever ['sevə] *vt, vi* 切断

severe [si'viə] *a* 严重的,重度的

severity [si'verəti] *n* 严重程度 | ~ of illness scale 疾病严重程度量表

Sever's disease ['siːvə] (James W. Sever)塞佛病,跟骨骺炎

sevoflurane [ˌsiːvə'fluːrein] *n* 七氟烷,七氟醚(吸入性麻醉药)

sevum ['siːvəm] *n*【拉】羊脂

sewage ['sju(ː)idʒ] *n* (下水道的)污水,污物 | activated ~ 活性污水 / domestic ~ 生活污水 / septic ~ 腐败性污水

sewerage ['sjuəridʒ] *n* 污水工程,排水工程,下水道设备

sex [seks] *n* 性别,性 *vt* 区别(生物体的性别) | chromosomal ~, genetic ~ 染色体性别(体细胞内XX〈女〉遗传型或XY〈男〉遗传型所决定的性别) / nuclear ~ 核性别(根据性染色质的有无所决定的性别,在正常条件下若有则表明XX〈女〉遗传型,若无则为XY〈男〉遗传型) | **~less** *a* 无性[别]的

sex-[1] [构词成分]【拉】六

sex-[2] [构词成分]【拉】性,性别,性欲

sex-conditioned [ˌseks kən'diʃənd] *a* 从性的(指只出现在一个性别的基因,一个性别为显性,另

一个性别为隐性）

sexdigitate [seksˈdidʒiteit] *a* 六指的，六趾的

sexduction [seksˈdʌkʃən] *n* 性导（一个细菌的部分遗传物质由性因子 F 带到另一个细菌体内的过程，见 F-duction）

sex-influenced [ˌseksˈinfluənst] *a* 从性的（见 sex-conditioned）

sexivalent [sekˈsivələnt] *a* 六价的

sex-limited [seksˈlimitid] *a* 限性的，性限定的（指遗传性状）

sex-linked [seksˈliŋkt] *a* 伴性的，性连的，性连锁的（由性染色体的基因决定的，虽然一个遗传特性可以与 X 染色体伴连或与 Y 染色体伴连，但事实上临床上所有有意义的伴性遗传都是由 X 染色体上的基因所遗传，因此 sex-linked 与 X-linked用作同义词）

sexology [sekˈsɔlədʒi] *n* 性学

sexopathy [sekˈsɔpəθi] *n* 性欲异常

sextan [ˈsekstən] *a* 六日周期的，每六日复发的（指发热）*n* 六日热

sextigravida [ˌsekstiˈgrævidə] *n*【拉】第六次孕妇

sextipara [seksˈtipərə] *n*【拉】六产妇

sextuplet [ˈsekstjuplit, seksˈtʌplit] *n* 六胎

sexual [ˈseksjuəl] *a* 性的，性欲的 | contrary ~ 性欲反向者

sexuality [ˌseksjuˈæləti] *n* 性别；性欲 | infantile ~ 幼稚性欲（据弗洛伊德〈Freud〉学说，婴幼儿的性活动包括性心理发育的口欲期、肛欲期和阳具期）

Seyderhelm's solution [ˈsaidəhelm]（Richard Seyderhelm）赛德黑尔姆液（鉴别尿内沉淀细胞用）

Sézary cell [ˈseizəri]（Albert Sézary）赛塞利细胞（一种异常的单核细胞，核含染色质过多，有皱褶，筛状，周围为狭的胞质边缘，可含空泡，存在于皮肤 T 细胞淋巴瘤中）| ~ syndrome（erythroderma）赛塞利综合征（红皮病）（一种皮肤 T 细胞淋巴瘤，表现为泛发性剥脱性红皮病，剧烈瘙痒，外周淋巴结病以及皮肤、淋巴结和外周血中出现含染色质过多的异常单核细胞〈Sézary cells〉）

SFEMG single fiber electromyography 单纤维肌电描记法

SGOT serum glutamic-oxaloacetic transaminase 血清谷草转氨酶，血清谷氨酸草酰乙酸转氨酶

SGPT serum glutamic-pyruvic transaminase 血清谷丙转氨酶，血清谷氨酸丙酮酸转氨酶

SH serum hepatitis 血清肝炎

shadow [ˈʃædəu] *n* 阴影，影 | bat's wing ~ 蝙蝠翼样阴影（通过两肺由肺门向外周辐射的一种 X 线摄影影像，在肺尖、肺周和肺底留下一条清亮区）/ blood ~ 红细胞影 / heart ~ 心影，心脏影像（X 线片）| ~**less** *a* 无阴影的

shadow-casting [ˈʃædəu ˈkɑːstiŋ] *n* 阴影定型，定影[法]（标本表面涂金属物射影的方法）

shadowgram [ˈʃædəugræm], **shadowgraph** [ˈʃædəugrɑːf, -græf-] *n* X 线[照]片

shadowgraphy [ˈʃædəugrɑːfi] *n* X 线摄影[术]

Shaffer's method [ˈʃeifə]（Philip A. Shaffer）谢弗法（检肌酸酐）

shaft [ʃɑːft] *n* 干，柄，体，轴 | ~ of femur 股骨体 / ~ of fibula 腓骨体 / hair ~ 毛干 / ~ of humerus 肱骨体 / ~ of metacarpal bone 掌骨体 / ~ of penis 阴茎体 / ~ of phalanx of fingers（toes）指（趾）骨体 / ~ of radius 桡骨体 / ~ of rib 肋骨体（肋干）/ ~ of tibia 胫骨体 / ~ of ulna 尺骨体

shagreen [ʃæˈgriːn] *n* 鲨革；鲨革样皮；鲨革样皮损

shake [ʃeik] *n* 摇动；震动；[常用复]寒战 | hatter's ~s 毛皮帽工寒战（汞中毒）/ spelter ~s 黄铜铸工寒战（锌中毒）

shamanism [ˈʃɑːməˌnizəm, ˈʃei-] *n* 萨满教

sham-feeding [ʃæmˈfiːdiŋ] *n* 假饲

shank [ʃæŋk] *n* 胫，小腿

shaping [ˈʃeipiŋ] *n* 塑造（行为疗法使用的一种操作性条件反射技术，通过强化渐渐接近最后所要达到的行为从而产生新的行为。亦称逐步渐近 successive approximation）

Sharpey's fibers [ˈʃɑːpi]（William Sharpey）夏皮纤维（一种来自骨膜而包埋入骨膜板的纤维，亦称骨纤维、穿通性纤维）

shashitsu [ʃəˈʃitsu] *n* 沙螨（沙虱）

shear [ʃiə] *n* 切力，切应力

Shear's test [ʃiə]（Murray J. Shear）希尔试验（检维生素 D）

sheath [ʃiːθ] *n* 鞘 | bulbar ~ 眼球筋膜，眼球囊 / carotid ~ 颈动脉鞘 / crural ~ 小腿筋膜 / dentinal ~ 牙质小管鞘 / enamel rod ~s, enamel prism ~s 釉柱鞘 / female ~ 阴道 / lamellar ~ 神经束膜 / masculine ~ 前列腺囊 / mucous ~s 黏液鞘（黏液囊及滑液鞘）/ mucous ~ of tendon 腱黏液鞘 / myelin ~, medullary ~ 髓鞘 / nucleated ~, primitive ~ 神经鞘 / root ~ 根鞘（①齿根鞘：一种上皮细胞围模，在未生出牙的周围及牙囊的内侧；②毛根鞘：毛囊的上皮部分，分成内根鞘和产生皮脂腺的外根鞘）

Sheehan's syndrome [ˈʃiːən]（Harold L. Sheehan）希恩综合征，产后垂体坏死

sheep-pox [ˈʃiːp-pɔks] *n* 羊痘，羊天花

sheet [ʃiːt] *n* 被单；表 | draw ~ 抽单 / drip ~ 湿裹单

shelf [ʃelf]（[复] **shelves** [ʃelvz]）*n* 架，棚 | dental ~ 牙棚，釉棚 / mesocolic ~ 结肠系膜架（横结肠系膜与大网膜的合称）/ palatine ~ 腭突（胚）

shell [ʃel] *n* 壳(果壳,贝壳);外壳 | egg ~ 卵壳

shellac [ʃəˈlæk] *n* 虫胶,片胶(片状虫胶),虫胶制剂 *vt* 以虫胶清漆涂;以虫胶处理

shellfish [ˈʃelfiʃ] *n* 贝,贝壳类,牡蛎

shen【汉】神(按照中医指人体基本物质之一)

Shenton's line(arch) [ˈʃentən] (Thomas Shenton)申顿线(弓)(正常髋关节的X线曲线,为闭孔顶部所形成)

Shepherd's fracture [ˈʃəpəd] (Francis J. Shepherd)谢泼德骨折(距骨骨折,伴外保护缘分离)

Sherman-Bourquin unit [ˈʃəːmən ˈbuəkwin] (Henry C. Sherman; Ann Bourquin)谢尔曼-布奎因维生素 B_2 单位(核黄素的剂量单位,每天给标准的受试大鼠饲以该剂量8周,可使其体重每周增加3 g)

Sherman-Munsell unit [ˈʃəːmən ˈmʌnsəl] (Henry C. Sherman; Hazel E. Munsell)谢尔曼-芒塞尔维生素A单位(维生素A的剂量单位,每天给原先缺乏维生素A的标准大鼠在8周内饲以该剂量,足以维持其体重每周增加3 g)

Sherman plate [ˈʃəːmən] (Harry M. O'Neil Sherman)谢尔曼板(一种铬钴合金或不锈钢骨板,可用螺丝钉固定于骨折处,常用于下颌骨骨折的切开复位)

Sherman unit [ˈʃəːmən] (Henry C. Sherman)谢尔曼维生素A单位(见 Sherman-Munsell unit)

Sherrington's law [ˈʃeriŋtn] (Charles S. Sherrington)谢灵顿定律(①每一个脊神经后根支配皮肤一特定区域,而来自邻接脊髓节的纤维可能侵入该区;②当肌肉接受一神经冲动而收缩时,其拮抗肌也同时接受一神经冲动而松弛)

shiatsu [ʃiˈɔtsuː] *n*【日】指压法(日本式针刺疗法)

Shibley's sign [ˈʃibli] (Gerald S. Shibley)希伯利征(肺实变或胸腔积液时,通过听诊器听到患者所发出的全部元音都是"ah〈啊〉")

shield [ʃiːld] *n* 盾,罩,屏;防护物 | embryonic ~ 胚盾 / eye ~ 眼罩 / lead ~ 铅遮板,铅屏(放射学上用以保护工作人员) / nipple ~ 乳头罩 / oral ~ 口保护罩,口前庭屏 / phallic ~ 男阴防护物

shift [ʃift] *vt* 转移,移位 *vi* 转变;移动 *n* 转变,转移,移位 | chloride ~ 氯[离子]转移 / ~ to the left 核左移(血象中幼稚中性粒细胞占优势) / regenerative blood ~ 再生性血转移(由于骨髓受到急性刺激,幼稚型和髓细胞型白细胞迅速泻出) / ~ to the right 核右移(血象中成熟中性粒细胞占优势)

Shiga's bacillus [ˈʃigə] (Kiyoshe Shiga 志贺洁日)志贺杆菌(志贺痢疾杆菌Ⅰ型) | ~ toxin 志贺毒素(志贺痢疾杆菌Ⅰ型产生的外毒素)

Shigella [ʃiˈgelə] (Kiyoshe Shiga 志贺洁日)志贺[杆]菌属 | ~ alkalescens 碱性志贺菌 / ~ ambigua 不定志贺菌(志贺痢疾杆菌Ⅱ型) / ~ arabinotarda type A 甲型胶醇志贺菌 / ~ arabinotarda type B 乙型胶醇志贺菌 / ~ boydii 鲍氏志贺菌(丙群痢疾杆菌) / ~ ceylonesis 锡兰志贺菌 / ~ dispar 异型志贺菌 / ~ dysenteriae 志贺痢疾杆菌(甲群痢疾杆菌,分为若干血清型,第一型为志贺菌,第二型为施氏菌) / ~ etousae 伊杜沙志贺菌 / ~ flexneri 弗氏志贺菌(乙群痢疾杆菌) / ~ madampensis 马丹浦志贺菌 / ~ newcastle 新城志贺菌 / ~ paradysenteriae 副痢疾志贺菌 / ~ parashigae 副志贺菌 / ~ schmitzii 施氏志贺菌(志贺痢疾杆菌Ⅱ型) / ~ shigae 志贺志贺菌(志贺痢疾杆菌Ⅰ型) / ~ sonnei 宋内菌,宋内志贺菌,宋内痢疾杆菌(丁群痢疾杆菌)

shigella [ʃiˈgelə] ([复] **shigellae** [ʃiˈgeliː]) *n* 志贺菌

shigellosis [ˌʃigəˈləusis] *n* 细菌性痢疾

shikimene [ˈʃikimiːn] *n* 莽草素

shikimic acid [ʃiˈkimik] 莽草酸

shin [ʃin] *n* 胫,胫部 | cucumber ~ 黄瓜状胫(胫骨前凹) / saber ~ 军刀状胫(胫骨前凸,见于遗传性梅毒、雅司病及畸形性骨炎)

shinbone [ˈʃinbəun] *n* 胫骨

shingles [ˈʃiŋglz] *n* 带状疱疹

shiver [ˈʃivə] *n* 战栗,寒战

shivering [ˈʃivəriŋ] *n* 战栗(肌肉收缩所致的不随意颤抖);肌肉异常抽搐(一种马病)

SHML sinus histiocytosis with massive lymphoadenopathy 窦性组织细胞增生症伴巨大淋巴结病

shock [ʃɔk] *n* 休克 | anaphylactic ~, allergic ~ 过敏性休克,变[态反]应性休克 / anaphylactoid ~ 类过敏性休克,过敏样休克,胶体性猝衰 / bomb ~ 轰炸休克(由反复轰炸所造成的恐怖和精神病态) / break ~ 断电震 / burn ~ 烧伤性休克 / cardiogenic ~ 心源性休克(如心肌梗死时心排血量突然减少所致) / cerebral ~ 脑(外伤或病态)性休克 / colloid ~ 胶体性休克,假过敏反应 / colloidoclastic ~ 胶体平衡障碍性休克 / diastolic ~ (心)舒张期震荡 / electric ~ 电击,电震,电休克 / endotoxic ~, endotoxin ~ 内毒素性休克(伴有大量细菌感染,一般由革兰阴性细菌所致) / heart ~, cardiac ~ 心脏休克 / hemoclastic ~ 红细胞破坏性休克,血液崩解性危象 / hemorrhagic ~ 失血性休克 / histamine ~ 组胺休克 / hypovolemic ~, oligemic ~ 低血容量性休克 / insulin ~, hypoglycemic ~ 胰岛素休克,低血糖休克 / micro ~ 微[量]休克 / peptone ~ 胨休克 / septic ~ 感染性休克 / serum ~ 血清性休克 / shell ~ 炮弹休克,爆炸性精神异常 / surgical ~ 外科休克 / testicular ~ 睾丸性休克 / traumatic ~ 创伤性休克

Shope papilloma [ʃəup] (Richard E. Shope) 肖普乳头状瘤(兔乳头状瘤,兔的病毒性疾病,特征为角疣形成,这些乳头状瘤是第一种哺乳动物肿瘤,为一种病毒所引起,并为纯病毒 DNA 遗传的)

shortsighted [ˈʃɔːtˈsaitid] *a* 近视的 | **~ness** *n* 近视

shot [ʃɔt] *n* 注射

shoulder [ˈʃəuldə] *n* 肩;肩台 | drop ~ 肩下垂;肩垂病 / frozen ~ 冻肩(由于纤维织炎所致,肩关节不能自由转动) / knocked down ~ 敲落肩(肩峰锁骨关节处肩分离或脱位) / loose ~ 松弛肩(见于进行性肌萎缩) / stubbed ~ 肩扭伤

shoulder-blade [ˈʃəuldə bleid] *n* 肩胛[骨]

shoulder slip [ˈʃəuldə slip] 肩胛上麻痹(马)

Shouldice repair [ˈʃəuldis] (Edward E. Shouldice) 舒尔迪斯修复术(巴西尼〈Bassini〉手术的一种改良法,以便腹股沟疝修复,在此手术中使用连续缝合取代间断缝合)

show [ʃəu] *n* (分娩或行经前)现血,血先露,见红 | bloody ~ 见红

shower [ˈʃauə] *n* 淋浴;骤现,骤发 | uric acid ~ 尿酸骤增

Shprintzen syndrome [ˈʃprintsən] (Robert J. Shprintzen) 施普林曾综合征,腭帆心脏面部综合征(即 velocardiofacial syndrome,见 syndrome 项下相应术语)

Shrady's saw [ˈʃreidi] (George F. Shrady) 希雷迪锯,皮下骨锯

Shrapnell's membrane [ˈʃræpnəl] (Henry. J. Shrapnell) 施拉普内尔膜(鼓膜上方松弛部)

shrinkage [ˈʃriŋkidʒ] *n* 收缩,皱缩;减少;皱缩度

shroud [ʃraud] *n* 裹尸布

shudder [ˈʃʌdə] *vi*, *n* 震颤,战栗,发抖

Shulman's syndrome [ˈʃuːlmən] (Lawrence E. Shulman) 舒尔曼综合征,嗜酸性筋膜炎

shunt [ʃʌnt] *vt*, *vi* 分路;分流;吻合 *n* 支路,旁路,短路;分流;分流术 | arteriovenous (A-V) ~ 动静脉短路 / cardiovascular ~ 心肺分流 / hexose monophosphate ~, pentose ~ 磷酸己糖支路,戊糖磷酸途径 / left-to-right ~ 左向右分流 / peritoneovenous ~ 腹腔静脉分流 / portacaval ~, postcaval ~ 门腔静脉(吻合)分流术 / right to left ~ 右向左分流 / ventriculoatrial ~ 脑室心房分流术 / ventriculoperitoneal ~ 脑室腹腔分流术 / ventriculovenous ~ 脑室颈静脉分流术

shuttle [ˈʃʌtl] *n* 梭 *vt*, *vi* 往返机制,穿梭机制 | glycerol phosphate ~ 磷酸甘油穿梭作用 / malate-aspartate ~ 苹果酸-天冬氨酸穿梭作用 / space ~ 航天飞机

Shwachman-Diamond syndrome [ˈʃwɔkmən ˈdaiəmɔnd] (Harry Shwachman; Louis Klein Diamond) 舒-戴综合征(见 Shwachman syndrome)

Shwachman syndrome [ˈʃwɔkmən] (Harry Shwachman) 舒瓦克曼综合征(原发性胰腺功能不全与骨髓衰竭,特征为汗液氯化值正常、胰腺功能不全及中性粒细胞减少。本征可伴有侏儒及髋骨干骺端发育不全)

Shwartzman's phenomenon (reaction) [ˈʃwɑːtsmən] (Gregory Shwartzman) 施瓦茨曼现象(反应)(一种严重而有坏死的出血性反应,实验可用家兔先在腹皮内注射 0.25 ml 伤寒或其他培养物滤液,24 小时〈18～32 小时〉后,再由静脉注射 0.01 ml 同样滤液,注射部位中央变蓝,周围变红,皮肤光泽、平滑、水肿,表面下血管破裂及大量白细胞死亡)

Shy-Drager syndrome [ʃai ˈdreigə] (George M. Shy; Glenn A. Drager) 夏伊-德雷格综合征(一种原因不明的进行性病征,以自主神经功能不全的症状开始,包括男性阳萎、便秘、尿急或尿潴留及无汗,继之出现广泛性神经功能障碍的体征,如帕金森样紊乱、小脑性共济失调、肌消瘦与自发性收缩以及小腿粗大震颤。亦称慢性直立性低血压,慢性特发性直立性低血压,特发性直立性低血压)

Shy-Magee syndrome [ʃai məˈgiː] (G. M. Shy; Kenneth R. Magee) 夏-马综合征,中央轴空病(见 disease 项下 central core disease)

SI Système Internationale d'Unités 国际单位制; stimulation index 刺激指数(见 test 项下 lymphocyte proliferation test)

Si silicon 硅

SIADH syndrome of inappropriate antiuretic hormone 抗利尿激素分泌失调综合征

sialaden [saiˈælədən] *n* 涎腺,唾液腺

sialadenectomy [ˌsaiəˌlædiˈnektəmi] *n* 涎腺切除术

sialadenitis [ˌsaiəˌlædiˈnaitis] *n* 涎腺炎

sialadenography [ˌsaiəˌlædiˈnɔgrəfi] *n* 涎腺涎管X线造影[术]

sialadenoma [ˌsaiəˌlædiˈnəumə] *n* 涎腺瘤

sialadenopathy [ˌsaiəˌlædiˈnɔpəθi] *n* 涎腺病 | benign lymphoepithelial ~ 良性淋巴上皮性涎腺病,良性淋巴上皮性损害

sialadenosis [ˌsaiəlˌædiˈnəusis] *n* 涎腺病(亦称涎腺炎)

sialadenotomy [ˌsaiəˌlædiˈnɔtəmi] *n* 涎腺切开[引流]术

sialagogue [saiˈæləgɔg] *n* 催涎剂 | **sialagogic** [ˌsaiələˈgɔdʒik] *a* 催涎的

sialaporia [ˌsaiələˈpɔːriə] *n* 涎缺乏,唾液缺乏

sialate [ˈsaiəleit] *n* 唾液酸盐

sialectasia [ˌsaiəlekˈteiziə] *n* 涎管扩张
sialemesis [ˌsaiəˈlemisis] *n* 呕涎(癔症性吐涎)
sialic [saiˈælik] *a* 涎的,唾液的;唾液酸的
sialic acid [saiˈælik] 唾液酸
sialidase [saiˈælideis] *n* 唾液酸酶(①缺乏此酶为常染色体隐性性状,可致唾液酸沉积症,在 EC 命名法中,称外-α-唾液酸酶;②亦称神经氨酸酶)
sialidosis [saiˌæliˈdəusis] *n* 涎酸贮积症
sialine [ˈsaiəlain] *a* 涎的,唾液的
sialism [ˈsaiəlizəm], **sialismus** [ˌsaiəˈlizməs] *n* 流涎,多涎
sialitis [ˌsaiəˈlaitis] *n* 涎腺(或涎管)炎
sial(o)- [构词成分]涎,唾液
sialoadenectomy [ˌsaiələuˌædiˈnektəmi] *n* 涎腺切除术
sialoadenitis [ˌsaiələuˌædiˈnaitis] *n* 涎腺炎
sialoadenotomy [ˌsaiələuˌædiˈnɔtəmi] *n* 涎腺切开[引流]术
sialoaerophagia [ˌsaiələuˌεərəuˈfeidʒiə] *n* [吞]咽气涎癖
sialoaerophagy [ˌsaiələuεəˈrɔfədʒi] *n* 吞涎气症
sialoangiectasis [ˌsaiələuˌændʒiˈektəsis] *n* 涎管扩张
sialoangiitis [ˌsaiələuˌændʒiˈaitis], **sialoangitis** [ˌsaiələuænˈdʒaitis], **sialodochitis** [ˌsaiələudəˈkaitis], **sialoductitis** [ˌsaiələudʌkˈtaitis] *n* 涎管炎
sialoangiography [ˌsaiələuˌændʒiˈɔgrəfi] *n* 涎管 X 线造影[术]
sialocele [ˈsaiələuˌsiːl] *n* 涎囊肿
sialodacryoadenitis [ˌsaiələuˌdækriəuˌædəˈnaitis] *n* 涎腺泪腺炎
sialodochoplasty [ˌsaiələuˈdəukəˌplæsti] *n* 涎管成形术
sialogastrone [ˌsaiələuˈgæstrəun] *n* 涎[液]抑胃素
sialogenous [ˌsaiəˈlɔdʒinəs] *a* 生涎的
sialoglycoconjugate [saiˌæləuˌglaikəukɔnˈdʒugət] *n* 唾液酸糖结合物
sialogogue [saiˈæləgɔg] *n* 催涎剂 | **sialogogic** [ˌsaiələuˈgɔdʒik] *a* 催涎的
sialogram [saiˈæləgræm] *n* 涎管 X 线造影[照]片
sialograph [saiˈæləgrɑːf, -græf] *n* 涎管 X 线造影[照]片 | **~y** [ˌsaiəˈlɔgrəfi] *n* 涎管 X 线造影术
sialolith [saiˈæləliθ] *n* 涎石
sialolithiasis [ˌsaiələuliˈθaiəsis] *n* 涎石病
sialolithotomy [ˌsaiələuliˈθɔtəmi] *n* 涎石切除术(涎腺或涎管切开取石术)
sialology [ˌsaiəˈlɔlədʒi] *n* 涎学,唾液学
sialoma [ˌsaiəˈləumə] *n* 涎瘤
sialometaplasia [ˌsaiələuˌmetəˈpleizjə] *n* 涎腺化生 | necrotizing ~ 坏死性涎腺化生,坏死性涎管转化
sialomucin [ˌsaiələuˈmjuːsin] *n* 唾液黏蛋白
sialophagia [ˌsaiələuˈfeidʒiə] *n* 吞涎症
sialorrhea [ˌsaiələˈriə] *n* 流涎,多涎
sialoschesis [ˌsaiəˈlɔskisis] *n* 涎液分泌抑制
sialosemeiology [ˌsaiələuˌsiːmaiˈɔlədʒi] *n* 涎液诊断学(测定病人的生理状态,尤其测定代谢过程)
sialosis [ˌsaiəˈləusis] *n* 流涎,多涎
sialostenosis [ˌsaiələustiˈnəusis] *n* 涎管狭窄
sialosyrinx [ˌsaiələuˈsiriŋks] *n* 涎腺瘘;涎管注射器,涎管引流管
sialotic [ˌsaiəˈlɔtik] *a* 流涎的
sialyloligosaccharide [saiˌælilˌɔligəuˈsækəraid] *n* 唾液酸低聚糖
sialyltransferase [saiˌælilˈtrænsfəreis] *n* 唾液酸转移酶
Sia's test (Richard H. P.,中国内科学家谢和平)谢氏试验(检黑热病的一种血清试验,即 1 份血清加上 3 份蒸馏水,有絮状沉淀物即表明黑热病)
sib [sib] *n* 同胞(兄弟姊妹)
sibilant [ˈsibilənt] *a* 咝音的 *n* 咝音
sibilus [ˈsibiləs] *n*【拉】咝音,飞箭音
sibling [ˈsibliŋ] *n* 同胞(兄弟姊妹) | HLA identical ~ HLA 相同同胞
siboroxime [ˌsaibəuˈrɔksiːm] *n* 西布洛肟(一种化合物,与 ^{99m}Tc 络合,用于脑成像)
sibship [ˈsibʃip] *n* 血缘关系,同胞关系(出自共同父母的兄弟姊妹关系),同胞群(兄弟姊妹)
Sibson's aponeurosis (fascia) [ˈsibsn] (Francis Sibson)胸膜上膜 | ~ furrow, ~ groove 胸大肌下沟 / ~ notch 西布逊切迹(急性心包渗液时,心前区浊音左上界向内弯进) / ~ vestibule 主动脉前庭
sibutramine hydrochloride [siˈbjuːtrəmiːn] 盐酸西布曲明(去甲肾上腺素和 5-羟色胺重摄取的抑制剂,结构上与苯丙胺有关,用作食欲抑制剂,治疗肥胖症,口服给药)
Sicard's syndrome [siˈkɑː] (Jean A. Sicard)西卡尔综合征(见 Collet's syndrome)
siccant [ˈsikənt] *a* 干燥的
siccative [ˈsikətiv] *a* 干燥的,收湿的 *n* 干燥剂,除湿剂
sicchasia [siˈkeiziə] *n* 恶心
siccolabile [ˌsikəˈleibail] *a* 不耐干燥的
siccostabile [ˌsikəˈsteibail] *a* 耐干燥的
siccus [ˈsikəs] *a*【拉】干燥的
sick [sik] *a* 不舒服的,患病的;恶心的
sick bay [sik bei] 海上医院,海上诊疗所

sickle-cell [ˈsikl sel] *n* 镰状细胞(红细胞)
sicklemia [sikˈliːmiə] *n* 镰状细胞性贫血 / **sicklemic** *a*
sickling [ˈsikliŋ] *n* (红细胞)镰状化,(血内)镰状细胞形成
sickness [ˈsiknis] *n* 疾病 | African sleeping ~ 非洲昏睡病,非洲锥虫病 / air ~, aerial ~, aviation ~ 航空晕,航空病,晕飞机 / altitude ~ 高空病 / athletes' ~ 运动员病 / balloon ~ 气球病,高空病 / black ~ 黑热病 / car ~ 晕车[病] / decompression ~, caisson ~, compressed-air ~减压病,潜涵病,潜水员病,压缩空气病 / falling ~ 癫痫 / Gambian sleeping ~ 冈比亚昏睡病,冈比亚锥虫病 / green ~ 萎黄病,绿色贫血 / green tobacco ~ 烟草萎黄病 / Jamaican vomiting ~ 牙买加呕吐病(亦称阿吉中毒,西非荔枝果中毒) / laughing ~ 笑病,假性延髓麻痹 / milk ~ 乳[毒]病(因饮用震颤病牛羊的乳或乳制品所致);震颤病 / morning ~ 早孕反应 / motion ~ 运动病(如晕车、晕船、晕飞机) / mountain ~ 高山病 / radiation ~, X-ray ~ 放射病(X 线或镭疗后的急性反应) / Rhodesian sleeping ~ 罗得西亚昏睡病,罗得西亚锥虫病 / sea ~ 晕船[病] / serum ~ 血清病(亦称血清中毒) / sleeping ~ 非洲锥虫病 / sweating ~ 汗热病,流行性粟粒疹热 / talking ~ 多语症(流行性脑炎的一种) / vomiting ~ 呕吐病,牙买加呕吐病
Sid blood group [sid] (源自英国先证者名字的一部分,于 20 世纪 60 年代首次报道)锡德血型(含有大量公有红细胞抗原 Sd^a,称之为 Sd ⟨a^{++}⟩的血型)
s. i. d. semel in die【拉】每日一次(亦可写成 semel in d.)
side [said] *n* 边,面,侧 | balancing ~, nonfunctioning ~ 平衡侧,非功能侧(牙列) / working ~, functioning ~ 工作侧,功能侧(牙列)
side-bone [ˈsaidbəun] *n* 环骨肿(马)
side effect [ˈsaidiˌfekt] 副作用(药物)
sideration [ˌsidəˈreiʃən] *n* 闪电状发病;电击;电灼疗法
siderinuria [ˌsidəriˈnjuəriə] *n* 铁尿
siderism [ˈsidərizəm] *n* 金属疗法
sider(o)- [构词成分]铁
Siderobacter [ˌsidərəuˈbæktə] *n* 铁杆菌属
sideroblast [ˈsidərəˌblæst] *n* 成高铁红细胞,铁粒幼细胞 | **~ic** [ˌsidərəˈblæstik] *a*
Siderocapsa [ˌsidərəuˈkæpsə] *n* 铁囊菌属
Siderocapsaceae [ˌsidərəukæpˈseisiiː] *n* 铁囊菌科
Siderococcus [ˌsidərəuˈkɔkəs] *n* 铁球菌属
siderocyte [ˈsidərəsait] *n* 高铁红细胞
sideroderma [ˌsidərəˈdəːmə] *n* 铁色皮[症]
siderofibrosis [ˌsidərəufaiˈbrəusis] *n* (脾)铁末沉着性纤维变性
Sideromonas [ˌsidərəuˈməunəs] *n* 铁单胞菌属
sideromycin [ˌsidərəuˈmaisin] *n* 高铁霉素(任何一类结构上与氧肟酸相关的抗生素,通过干扰铁摄取而抑制细菌生长)
Sideronema [ˌsidərəuˈniːmə] *n* 铁线菌属
sideropenia [ˌsidərəuˈpiːniə] *n* 铁[质]缺乏 | **sideropenic** *a* 缺铁性的
Siderophacus [ˌsidəˈrəufəkəs] *n* 铁晶形菌属
siderophage [ˈsidərəˌfeidʒ] *n* 噬铁细胞
siderophil [ˈsidərəfil] *a* 嗜铁的 *n* 嗜铁体
siderophilin [ˌsidəˈrɔfilin] *n* 转铁蛋白,铁传递蛋白
siderophilous [ˌsidəˈrɔfiləs] *a* 嗜铁的
siderophone [ˈsidərəfəun] *n* (眼内)铁屑检查听音器
siderophore [ˈsidərəˌfɔː] *n* 含铁细胞;含铁血黄素巨噬细胞;载铁体
sideroscope [ˈsidərəskəup] *n* (眼内)铁屑测验器
siderosilicosis [ˌsidərəuˌsiliˈkəusis] *n* 铁[硅]末沉着,铁硅尘肺
siderosis [ˌsidəˈrəusis] *n* 铁沉着[病] | ~ bulbi 眼球铁质沉着 / ~ conjunctivae 结膜铁质沉着 / hematogenous ~ 血源性铁质沉着 / hepatic ~ 肝铁质沉着 / nutritional ~ 营养性血铁过多,营养性高铁血 / pulmonary ~ 肺铁质沉着病,铁尘肺 / urinary ~ 尿铁[色素]沉着,含铁血黄素尿 / xenogenous ~ 异物性铁质沉着 | **siderotic** [ˌsidəˈrɔtik] *a* 铁质沉着的
Siderosphaera [ˌsidərəuˈsfiərə] *n* 铁球形菌属
siderous [ˈsidərəs] *a* 含铁的
SIDS sudden infant death syndrome 婴儿猝死综合征(见 syndrome 项下相应术语)
Siegert's sign [ˈsiːgət] (Ferdinand Siegert)西格特征(指先天愚型或伸舌样白痴时,小指短而内向弯曲的特征)
Siegle's otoscope [ˈziːgl] (Emil Siegle)齐格尔耳镜(增减空气压力时,观察鼓膜变异)
siemens(S) [ˈsiːmənz] [单复同] *n* 西门子(电导的国际单位,亦称姆欧 mho)
Siemerling's nucleus [ˈsiːməliŋ] (Ernst Siemerling)西默林核(动眼神经核的前组)
Sieur's test (sign) [siˈəː] (Célestin Sieur)希厄尔试验征,钱币试验(coin test,见 test 项下相应术语)
sidewinder [ˈsaidwaində] *n* 角响尾蛇
sieve [siv] *n* 筛,滤网 | molecular ~ 分子筛(用于化学分离)
sievert(Sv) [ˈsiːvəːt] *n* 西[韦特](放射吸收剂量当量的国际单位,1 西 = 100 雷姆)
Sig. signetur【拉】标记,用法签

sigh [sai] *vi* 叹气 *n* 叹气

sight [sait] *n* 视力 | day ~ 夜盲[症](昼视) / far ~, long ~ 远视 / near ~, short ~ 近视 / night ~ 昼盲[症](夜视) / second ~ 视力再生,老年期视力回春

sigma [ˈsigmə] *n* 希腊语的第 18 字母(Σ, σ, s);用作千分之一秒、标准差及总和的符号

sigmatism [ˈsigmətizəm], **sigmasism** [ˈsigməsizəm] *n* s 发音困难;滥用 s 音

sigmoid [ˈsigmɔid] *a* S 形的;C 形的;乙状的(指乙状结肠曲) *n* 乙状结肠

sigmoidectomy [ˌsigmɔiˈdektəmi] *n* 乙状结肠切除术

sigmoiditis [ˌsigmɔiˈdaitis] *n* 乙状结肠炎

sigmoidocystoplasty [sigˌmɔidəuˈsistəuˌplæsti] *n* 乙状结肠膀胱扩大术

sigmoidopexy [sigˈmɔidəˌpeksi] *n* 乙状结肠固定术

sigmoidoproctostomy [sigˌmɔidəuprɔkˈtɔstəmi], **sigmoidorectostomy** [sigˌmɔidəurəkˈtɔstəmi] *n* 乙状结肠直肠吻合术

sigmoidoscope [sigˈmɔidəskəup] *n* 乙状结肠镜 | **sigmoidoscopy** [ˌsigmɔiˈdɔskəpi] *n* 乙状结肠镜检查[术]

sigmoidosigmoidostomy [sigˌmɔidəusigmɔiˈdɔstəmi] *n* 乙状结肠乙状结肠吻合术

sigmoidostomy [ˌsigmɔiˈdɔstəmi] *n* 乙状结肠造口术

sigmoidotomy [ˌsigmɔiˈdɔtəmi] *n* 乙状结肠切开术

sigmoidovesical [sigˌmɔidəuˈvesikəl] *a* 乙状结肠膀胱的

Sigmund's glands [ˈzigmund] (Karl L. Sigmund) 西格蒙德腺(滑车上淋巴结)

sign [sain] *n* 征兆,迹象;征,体征 | accessory ~, assistant ~ 副征 / air-cushion ~ 气垫征(见 Klemm's sign) / antecedent ~ 前驱征,先兆征 / anterior tibial ~ 胫前肌征(将痉挛性截瘫大腿强力屈向腹部时,胫前肌不随意收缩,见于痉挛性截瘫) / anticus ~ 胫前肌征,胫前肌反射(见 Piotrowski's sign) / cardinal ~s 主征(指炎征:痛、热、红、肿、功能障碍) / chin-retraction ~ 下颌回缩征(麻醉第三期的一种体征,在吸气时颏和喉向下移动) / clavicular ~ 锁骨征(右锁骨内 1/3 处的肿胀,见于先天性梅毒) / cogwheel ~ 齿轮征(齿轮现象 cogwheel phenomenon,见 phenomenon 项下相应术语) / coin ~ 钱币征(钱币试验 coin test,见 test 项下相应术语) / commemorative ~ 后遗体征 / contralateral ~ 对侧征(见 Brudzinski's sign②解) / DTP ~ (distal tingling on percussion)叩诊肢端麻刺感,蚁走感征(见 Tinel's sign) / duct ~ 腺管征(流行性腮腺炎时腮腺管口可见到红斑) / echo ~ 回声征(①在棘球蚴囊上可听到一种类似回声的叩诊音;②重复一个句子的最后一个字或分句,见于某些脑病;模仿言语) / ether ~ 乙醚征(为死征之一,皮下注射 1 或 2 ml 乙醚,若抽针时乙醚喷出,则人已死,若乙醚吸收,则生命尚存) / external malleolar ~ 足外踝征(见 Chaddock's reflex) / extinction ~ 皮肤红斑消退试验(见 Schultz-Charlton reaction) / fabere ~ 屈展旋伸征(见 Patrick's test) / facial ~ 面征(见 Chvostek's sign) / fan ~ 扇形征,开趾征(刺激足底,则足趾展开,为巴彬斯奇〈Babinski〉反射的一部分) / flush-tank ~ 水槽征(大量排尿同时腰部肿胀暂退,为肾盂积水之征) / forearm ~ 前臂征(见 Leri's sign) / formication ~ 蚁走感征(见 Tinel's sign) / hyperkinesis ~ 运动过度征(见 Claude's hyperkinesis sign) / interossei ~ 骨间肌征(见 Souques's phenomenon) / jugular ~ 颈静脉征(见 Queckenstedt's sign) / leg ~ 腿征(见 Schlesinger's sign) / ligature ~ 结扎征(血尿时,结扎一肢,则该肢末梢部出现瘀斑) / meniscus ~ 半月征(胃溃疡在 X 线像呈半月影,半月向外,则溃疡在小弯,半月向下,则溃疡在角切迹的远端) / neck ~ 颈征(见 Brudzinski's sign ①解) / niche ~ 龛影(见 Haudek's sign) / objective ~, physical ~ 他觉征,体征,物理征 / orange-peel ~ 橘皮状征(检脂瘤,以手紧压脂瘤基部,覆盖的皮肤可出现"桔皮"状) / orbicularis ~ 眼轮匝肌征(偏瘫时,开健侧眼则不能闭患侧眼) / palmoplantar ~ 掌跖征(见 Filipovitch's sign) / plumb-line ~ 垂直线征(在诊断胸腔积液时,用垂直线估计胸骨的移位) / pneumatic ~ 气压试验(见 Hennebert's sign) / pronation ~ 旋前征(见 Babinski's sign⑤解;Strümpell's sign③解) / pyramid ~, pyramidal ~ 锥体束征 / radialis ~ 桡神经征(见 Strümpell's sign②解) / setting-run ~ 斜下眼征(眼睛向下偏差,因此虹膜"落"在下睑之下,白色巩膜暴露在虹膜与上睑之间,为颅内压〈出血或脑膜室管膜炎〉或脑干受刺激〈如核黄疸〉之征) / spinal ~ 脊肌征(胸膜炎时,病侧脊肌强直性收缩) / spine ~ 脊柱征(脊髓灰质炎时,由于疼痛,患者不愿前屈脊柱) / stairs ~ 梯级征(脊髓痨患者下楼困难) / string ~ 线状征(见 Kantor's sign);索束征(在拉出完整睾丸或正在进行精子生成的睾丸组织时所见到的小管拉丝现象,此现象在睾丸萎缩时,小管会因纤维化和透明质化而中止) / swinging flashlight ~ 摆动电筒征(令患者双眼凝视远方,用强光照射健眼,即可见到瞳孔两侧收缩十分明显,电筒光移至患眼,两瞳孔即短时扩大,然后将电筒光回到健眼时,两瞳孔迅即收缩并保持收缩状态,提示视神经或视网膜有轻微损伤) / thermic ~ 温度征(见 Kashida's sign) / tibialis ~ 胫肌征(见 Strümpell's sign①解) / toe ~ 足趾征(见 Babinski's reflex) / trepidation ~ 震颤征,膝阵挛 / vein ~ 静脉征(沿腋中线由胸静脉和腹壁浅静脉肿胀的连合处所形成的一种蓝色素,见于支气管淋巴结结核及上腔静脉阻塞) / vital ~s 生命体征(指脉搏、呼吸及体温)

signa [ˈsignə] *n*【拉】标记,用法签

signalment [ˈsignəlmənt] *n* 特别标记(在兽医中,对动物的物种、品种、年龄和性别的记载)

signature [ˈsignitʃə] *n* 标记,用法签;药效形象(旧时认为表明与医药用途有关的植物外形特征,如苔类植物的肝形叶用于肝病,黄色的番红花表示对黄疸有用) | **signaturist** *n* 药效形象说者,象形药物说者

significance [sigˈnifikəns] *n* 显著性

signing [ˈsainiŋ] *n* 手势语

Signorelli's sign [siːnjɔˈreli] (Angelo Signorelli) 辛尼约雷利征(脑膜炎时,下颌骨后点有极度压痛)

Sig. n. pro. signa nomine proprio【拉】标记药名

siguatera [sigwəˈterə] *n*【西】鱼肉中毒

sikimi [ˈsikimi] *n*【日】莽草,毒八角

sikimin [ˈsikimin] *n* 莽草素

sikimitoxin [siˌkimiˈtɔksin] *n* 莽草毒素

silafilcon A [ˌsiləˈfilkɔn] 西拉费尔康 A(一种亲水性接触镜材料)

silafocon A [ˌsiləˈfəukɔn] 西拉福康 A(一种疏水性接触镜材料)

silandrone [siˈlændrəun] *n* 硅雄酮(雄激素类药)

sildenafil citrate [silˈdenəˌfil] 枸橼酸西登非尔(一种磷酸二酯酶抑制药,使阴茎平滑肌松弛,从而促使血液流向海绵体,在阳萎疗法中用于治疗勃起功能障碍)

silence [ˈsailəns] *n* 静止,无声 *vt* 消声 | electrocerebral ~ (ECS) 大脑电沉静 | **~r** *n* 消声器

silent [ˈsailənt] *a* 静止的;无症状的;无声的

silex [ˈsaileks] *n* 硅石,二氧化硅

Silex's sign [ˈsiːleks] (Paul Silex) 西勒克斯征(口周围放射状沟纹,见于先天梅毒患者)

Silfverskiöld's syndrome [ˈsilvəʃerid] (Nils G. Silfverskiöld) 西尔弗谢里德综合征(一种离心性骨软骨发育不良,骨骼改变主要在四肢,并作为显性性状遗传)

silhouette [ˌsiluːˈet] *n* 轮廓;廓影,侧影 | cardiac ~ 心影轮廓(X 线胸片上显现)

silica [ˈsilikə] *n* 硅石,二氧化硅

silicate [ˈsilikit, -keit] *n* 硅酸盐(或酯)

silicatosis [ˌsilikəˈtəusis] *n* 硅酸盐沉着病,硅酸盐肺

silicea [siˈlisiə] *n* 硅剂(顺势疗法的名称)

siliceous, silicious [siˈliʃəs] *a* 硅质的,含硅的

silicic [siˈlisik] *a* 硅的,硅石的 | ~ acid 硅酸

silicoanthracosis [ˌsilikəuˌænθrəˈkəusis] *n* 石末沉着病,硅肺

Silicoflagellida [ˌsilikəufləˈdʒelidə] *n* 硅鞭[毛虫]目

silicofluoride [ˌsilikəuˈfluːəraid] *n* 硅氟化物

silicol [ˈsilikɔl] *n* 偏磷酸酪蛋白氧化硅(治结核药剂)

silicon (Si) [ˈsilikən] *n* 硅(化学元素) | ~ carbide 碳化硅,金刚砂 / colloidal ~ dioxide 胶体二氧化硅 / ~ dioxide 二氧化硅

silicone [ˈsilikəun] *n* (聚)硅酮

silicoproteinosis [ˌsilikəuˌprəutiːˈnəusis] *n* 硅蛋白尘肺(一种迅速致命性尘肺,大量暴露于硅尘之中在数周到数月之后发生,特征为气腔内有蛋白液)

silicosiderosis [ˌsilikəuˌsidəˈrəusis] *n* 硅铁末沉着病,硅铁肺

silicosis [ˌsiliˈkəusis] *n* 硅沉着病,硅肺(亦称磨工病) | infective ~ 感染性硅肺,硅肺结核 | **silicotic** [ˌsiliˈkɔtik] *a* 硅肺的

silicotuberculosis [ˌsilikəutju(ː)ˌbəːkjuˈləusis] *n* 石末沉着性结核病,硅肺结核

silicotungstic acid [ˌsilikəuˈtʌŋstik] 硅钨酸

siliqua [ˈsilikwə] ([复] **siliquae** [ˈsilikwiː]) *n*【拉】长角果,长壳 | ~ olivae 橄榄体壳,橄榄体周纤维

siliquose [ˈsilikwəus] *a* 长角状的,长壳状的

silk [silk] *n* 丝

silkworm [ˈsilkwəːm] *n* 蚕

silkworm-gut [ˈsilkwəːmgʌt] *n* 蚕肠线

siloxane [saiˈlɔksein] *n* 硅氧烷

silver (Ag) [ˈsilvə] *n* 银 *vt* 镀银于 *vi* 变成银白色 | colloidal ~ iodide 胶体碘化银(一种抗菌剂,治黏膜炎症) / ~ iodide 碘化银(用于治梅毒、神经病及结膜炎) / mild ~ protein 弱蛋白银(局部抗感染药) / ~ nitrate 硝酸银(局部抗感染药,用于防止新生儿眼炎) / ~ orthophosphate 正磷酸银 / ~ picrate 苦味酸银(用于治前尿道炎、阴道毛滴虫及念珠菌感染) / strong ~ protein 强蛋白银(一种活性强的杀菌药) / ~ sulfadiazine 磺胺嘧啶银,烧伤宁,烫伤宁 / ~ sulfide 硫化银

Silverman's needle [ˈsilvəmən] (Irving Silverman) 西尔弗曼针(取组织标本用针)

Silverman's syndrome [ˈsilvəmən] (Frederis N. Silverman) 西尔弗曼综合征(见 Currarino-Silverman syndrome)

Silver-Russell syndrome (dwarfism) [ˈsilvə ˈrʌsəl] (H. K. Silver; Alexander Russell) 西尔弗-拉塞尔综合征(侏儒症)(此综合征包括出生时体重低〈尽管其妊娠足月〉,身材矮小,两侧不对

称,轻度至中度促性腺激素分泌增加,可伴有第5指〈小指〉内弯,咖啡牛奶斑,并指〈趾〉畸形,三角形脸,口角折向下及性早熟)

silverskin [ˈsilvəskin] *n* 银皮,谷皮,米皮

Silver's syndrome [ˈsilvə] (Henry K. Silver) 西尔弗综合征(见 Silver-Russell syndrome)

Silvester's method [silˈvestə] (Henry R. Silvester) 西尔维斯特法(一种人工呼吸法:置患者仰卧,用力拉其双臂过头以抬高肋骨,直至空气停止进入胸部为止,然后将其双臂拉至胸部以下,在胸部加压1秒左右,直至空气停止呼出,此法反复进行,每分钟16次)

silvestrene [silˈvestriːn] *n* 纵萜,松节油萜

Silvestrini-Corda syndrome [ˌsilvəsˈtriːni ˈkɔːdə] (R. Silvestrin; L. Corda) 西-科综合征(类无睾者体型,体毛缺失,性欲缺乏,睾丸萎缩,不育及男子女性型乳房,为一种雌激素活性异常增强的综合征,系肝脏不能灭活循环的雌激素所致)

Silvius [ˈsilviəs] *n* 斑虻属

Silybum [ˈsilibəm] *n* 水飞蓟属

Simaruba [ˌsiməˈruːbə] *n* 苦樗属

simarubidin [ˌsiməˈruːbidin] *n* 苦樗素

simazine [ˈsaiməziːn] *n* 西玛三嗪(除草剂)

simesthesia [ˌsimisˈθiːzjə] *n* 骨感觉

simethicone [siˈmeθikəun] *n* 二甲硅油(胃镜检查时用作消泡沫药,亦用作排气剂及制剂时用作释放剂,兽医用于治牛鼓胀病)

simian [ˈsimiən] *a* 猿的,猴的 *n* 猿,猴(尤指类人猿)

similia similibus curantur [siˈmiliə siˈmilibʌs kjuˈræntə]【拉】以毒攻毒(顺势疗法的一个原则,类似病用类似药治疗)

simillimum [siˈmiliməm] *n*【拉】类似药(顺势疗法药物)

Simmonds' disease (syndrome) [ˈsiməndz] (Morris Simmonds) 西蒙兹病(综合征),全垂体功能减退(垂体性恶病质)

Simonart's thread (band) [ˌsiːməˈnɑː] (Pierre J. C. Simonart) 西莫纳尔线(带)(当羊膜腔为羊水充胀时,羊膜与胎儿间粘连牵拉而形成羊膜线或带)

Simonea folliculorum [siˈməuniə fəˌlikjuˈlɔːrəm] 毛囊蠕螨(即 demodex folliculorum)

Simonelli's test [ˌsaiməˈneli] (F. Simonelli) 西莫内利试验(检肾功能不全)

Simons' disease [ˈsaimənz] (Arthur Simons) 西蒙斯病,部分脂肪营养不良

Simon's foci [ˈsaimən] 西蒙病灶(儿童肺尖的血源性区,据认为是成长后肺尖型结核病的前体)

Simonsiella [saiˌmɔnsiˈeilə] (Hellmuth Simons) *n* 西蒙斯菌属

Simonsiellaceae [ˌsaimənˌsieˈleisiiː] *n* 西蒙斯菌科

Simon's septic factor [ˈsaimən] (Charles E. Simon) 西蒙败血因子(脓性感染时血内嗜酸细胞减少,中性粒细胞增多) | ~ sign 西蒙征(吸气时脐回缩或不动)

Simon's sign [ˈsaimən] (John Simon) 西蒙征(脑膜炎初期,膈肌运动与胸廓运动的正常关系消失)

simple [ˈsimpl] *a* 简单的;单的,单一的;初级的;原始的 *n* 药草(古名) | **~r** *n* 草药医生

Simplexvirus [ˈsimpleksˌvaiərəs] *n* 单纯疱疹病毒属

Simpson light (lamp) [ˈsimpsn] (William S. Simpson) 辛普森灯(一种电弧光灯,从前用于治皮肤疾患)

Simpson's forceps [ˈsimpsn] (James Y. Simpson) 辛普森钳(一种产钳)

Simpson's splint [ˈsimpsn] (William K. Simpson) 辛普森夹(鼻内敷棉夹)

Sims's position [simz] (James M. Sims) 席姆斯卧位(病人以左侧胸部卧下,右膝及大腿上曲,左臂沿背放置,作阴道检查,亦称半伏卧位) | ~ speculum 席姆斯镜(双瓣鸭嘴形阴道窥器)

simul [ˈsiməl] *ad*【拉】同时

simulation [ˌsimjuˈleiʃən] *n* 诈病,装病;模仿,模拟(如以一种疾病模拟另一种疾病)

simulator [ˈsimjuleitə] *n* 模仿者;装病者,诈病者;模拟器,模拟装置 | electrocardiographic ~ 心电描记模拟装置

Simuliidae [ˌsaimjuˈliːidiː] *n* 蚋科

Simulium [saiˈmjuːljəm] *n* 蚋属

simultanagnosia [ˌsaimʌlˌteinægˈnəusiə] *n* 画片中动作失认 | **simultagnosia** [ˌsaimʌltægˈnəusiə] *n*

SIMV synchronized intermittent mandatory ventilation 同步间歇强制通气

simvastatin [ˌsimvəˈstætin] *n* 西伐他汀(抗高血脂药)

sinal [ˈsainl] *a* 窦的

sinalbin [siˈnælbin] *n* 白芥子硫苷,白芥子苷

sinapinic acid [ˌsinəˈpinik] 白芥子酸

Sinapis [ˈsinəpis] *n* 芥属

sinapism [ˈsinəpizəm] *n* 芥子泥,芥子硬膏

sincalide [ˈsinkəlaid] *n* 辛卡利特(利胆药)

sinciput [ˈsinsipʌt] ([复] **sinciputs** 或 **sincipita** [sinˈsipitə]) *n*【拉】前顶,前头(颅顶的前半部) | **sincipital** [sinˈsipitl] *a*

Sindbis fever [ˈsindbis] (Sindbis 为埃及一村名,20世纪50年代在该村首次观察到此热) 辛德毕斯热(库蚊传播的 α-病毒所致的流行性地方性热病) | ~ virus 辛德毕斯病毒(α-病毒属的一

种病毒,由库蚊传播,可致辛德毕斯热)

Sinding-Larsen disease [ˈsindiŋ ˈlɑːsən] (C. M. F. Sinding-Larsen)辛定-拉逊病(见 Larsen's disease)

Sinding-Larsen-Johansson disease [ˈsindiŋ ˈlɑːsən jəuˈhɑːnsən] (C. M. F. Sinding-Larsen; Sven C. Johansson)辛-约病(见 Larsen's disease)

sinefungin [ˌsinəˈfʌndʒin] *n* 西萘芬净(抗真菌抗生素)

sinew [ˈsinjuː] *n* 腱 | weeping ~ 腱鞘囊肿(手背)

sing. singulorum【拉】每一个,单一,各

single blind [ˈsiŋgl blaind] 单盲法的(指临床试验或其他实验,受试者不知道正在接受何种治疗)

singultation [ˌsiŋgʌlˈteiʃən] *n* 呃逆

singultus [siŋˈgʌltəs] *n*【拉】呃逆 | **singultous** [siŋˈgʌltəs] *a*

sinigrin [ˈsinigrin] *n* 黑芥子硫苷酸钾,芥子苷

sinister [ˈsinistə] *a* 左侧的

sinistrad [siˈnistræd] *ad* 左向,向左

sinistral [ˈsinistrəl] *a* 左侧的;左利的,善用左手的 *n* 善用左手的人,左利者

sinistrality [ˌsinisˈtræləti] *n* 左利,善用左侧器官(手、耳、眼、腿等)

sinistraural [ˌsinisˈtrɔːrəl] *a* 左利耳的,善用左耳的,左耳敏听的

sinistr(o)- [构词成分]左,左侧

sinistrocardia [ˌsinistrəuˈkɑːdiə] *n* 左位心,左移心

sinistrocerebral [ˌsinistrəuˈseribrəl] *a* 左大脑[半球]的

sinistrocular [ˌsinisˈtrɔkjulə] *a* 左利眼的,善用左眼的 | **~ity** [ˌsinisˌtrɔkjuˈlærəti] *n*

sinistrogyration [ˌsinistrəudʒaiəˈreiʃən] *n* 左旋(如眼或偏振面的移动)

sinistromanual [ˌsinistrəuˈmænjuəl] *a* 左利手的,善用左手的

sinistropedal [ˌsinisˈtrɔpədl] *a* 左利足的,善用左足的,左足多用的

sinistrorse [ˈsinistrɔːs] *a* 左旋的

sinistrose [ˈsinistrəus] *n* 左旋糖(有时在尿内见到)

sinistrotorsion [ˌsinistrəuˈtɔːʃən] *n* 左旋(主要指眼)

sinkaline [ˈsiŋkəlin] *n* 胆碱

Sinkler's phenomenon [ˈsiŋklə] (Wharton Sinkler)辛克勒现象(强力屈曲痉挛性瘫痪下肢的蹈趾时,髋及膝关节屈曲)

sin(o)- [构词成分]窦

sinoatrial [ˌsainəuˈeitriəl], **sinoauricular** [ˌsainəuɔːˈrikjulə] *a* 窦房的

sinobronchitis [ˌsainəubrɔŋˈkaitis] *n* 鼻窦支气管炎

sinography [saiˈnɔgrəfi] *n* 窦腔 X 线摄影[术]

sinomenine [saiˈnɔmiːniːn] *n* 汉防已碱,青藤碱

Sinomenium [ˌsainəuˈmiːniəm] *n* 防已属,青藤属

Si non val. si non valeat【拉】如不够,如无效

sinopulmonary [ˌsainəuˈpʌlməˌnəri] *a* 窦肺的

sinospiral [ˌsainəuˈspaiərəl] *a* 窦(螺)旋的(指心脏某些肌纤维)

sinoventricular [ˌsainəuvenˈtrikjulə] *a* 窦室的

sinter [ˈsintə] *n* 泉华(矿泉边缘沉积的钙或硅类物质)

sintoc [ˈsintɔk] *n* 辛脱克桂皮

sinuate [ˈsinjuit, -eit] *a* 波状的,具有波状边缘的;纡曲的

sinuatrial [ˌsinjuˈeitriəl], **sinuauricular** [ˌsinjuɔːˈrikjulə] *a* 窦房的

sinuitis [sinjuˈaitis] *n* 窦炎

sinuosity [ˌsinjuˈɔsəti] *n* 弯曲,纡曲[状态]

sinuotomy [ˌsainjuˈɔtəmi] *n* 窦切开术

sinuous [ˈsinjuəs] *a* 弯曲的,纡曲的

sinus [ˈsainəs] ([复] **sinus** 或 **sinuses**) *n*【拉】窦;窦道(脓液流出的管道);窦房结 | accessory ~es of the nose 鼻旁窦,鼻窦 / air ~ 含气窦(骨) / ~ of anterior chamber 眼前房窦 / aortic ~ 主动脉窦 / basilar ~ 基底窦,基底丛 / carotid ~ 颈动脉窦 / cerebral ~ 大脑窦 / coccygeal ~ 骶尾窦 / cranial ~es 硬[脑]膜窦 / dermal ~ 皮窦,皮洞 / laryngeal ~ 喉室 / mastoid ~ 乳突窦,乳突气房 / oral ~ 口道,口凹 / pilonidal ~ 藏毛窦(骶尾窦) / straight ~ 直窦 / traumatic ~ 创伤性窦道 / uterine ~es 子宫[静脉]窦(孕时) | **~al** *a*

sinusitis [ˌsainəˈsaitis] *n* 鼻窦炎

sinusoid [ˈsainəsɔid] *a* 窦状的 *n* 窦状隙(亦称窦状小管) | myocardial ~s 心肌窦状隙 | **~al** [ˌsainəˈsɔidl] *a* 窦状隙的;正弦[曲线]样的

sinusoidalization [ˌsainəˌsɔidəlaiˈzeiʃən] *n* 正弦电疗

sinusotomy [ˌsainəˈsɔtəmi] *n* 窦切开术

sinuspiral [ˌsainjuˈspaiərəl] *a* 窦螺旋的

sinuventricular [ˌsainjuvenˈtrikjulə] *a* 窦室的

Si op. sit si opus sit【拉】必要时

siphon [ˈsaifən] *n* 虹吸;虹吸管 *vt* 用虹吸管吸出;吮吸 *vi* 通过虹吸管 | **~age** [ˈsaifənidʒ] *n* 虹吸法;虹吸作用

Siphona irritans [saiˈfɔnə ˈiritəns] 扰血蝇(即 Haematobia irritans)

Siphonaptera [ˌsaifəˈnæptərə] *n* 蚤目

Siphunculata [saiˌfʌŋkjuˈleitə] *n* 虱目

Siphunculina [saiˌfʌnkjuˈlainə] *n* 小蝇属 | ~ funicola 眼蝇

Sipple's syndrome [ˈsipəl] (John H. Sipple)西普尔综合征,多发性内分泌腺瘤形成ⅡA型
Sippy diet [ˈsipi] (Bertram W. Sippy)西皮饮食(对消化性溃疡或对不能摄入大量食物的饮食法) | ~ treatment(method)西皮疗法(中和胃酸,治消化性溃疡)
siqua [ˈsaikwə] (从拉丁文 sidentis altitudinis quadratio〈坐高平方〉造成的新词) *n* 坐高平方(计算肠吸收表面面积的皮尔盖〈Pirquet〉单位,即坐高的平方,单位用公分)
sirenomelia [ˌsairənəuˈmiːliə] *n* (无足)并腿畸形
sirenomelus [ˌsaiəreˈnɔmiləs] *n* (无足)并腿畸胎
siriasis [siˈraiəsis] *n* 日射病,中暑
sirikaya [ˌsiriˈkeijə] *n* 番荔枝
sirolimus [siˈrəulimәs] *n* 西罗莫司(一种大环内酯抗生素,制自吸水链霉菌〈Streptomyces hygroscopicus〉,具有免疫抑制性质,用于预防肾移植排斥反应。口服给药)
sirup [ˈsirəp] *n* 糖浆[剂]
-sis [构词成分]状态,病态,病
SISI short increment sensitivity index 短增量敏感指数
sismotherapy [ˌsisməuˈθerəpi] *n* 振动疗法
sisomicin [ˌsisəuˈmaisin] *n* 西索米星,紫苏霉素(抗生素类药) | ~ sulfate 硫酸紫苏霉素
sissorexia [ˌsisəˈreksiə] *n* 脾内血细胞蓄积
sister [ˈsistə] *n* 护士长(英国用语);护士
Sister Mary Joseph's nodule [sistə ˈmɛəri ˈdʒəusəf] (Sister Mary Joseph Dempsey 为美国罗马天主教修女和医务工作者)修女玛丽·约瑟夫小结(深入脐区皮下组织的小结,伴发转移性腹内症,常为胃、卵巢、结肠、直肠或胰源性的)
Sisto's sign [ˈsistəu] (Genero Sisto)西斯托征(先天梅毒儿的经常哭叫)
Sistrunk operation [ˈsistrənk] (Walter Sistrunk) 西斯特伦克手术(一种切除骨状舌管囊肿和窦道的手术)
Sistrurus [sisˈtrurəs] *n* 小响尾蛇属
Sisyrinchium galaxioides [sisiˈriŋkiəm gəˌlæksiˈɔidiːz] 南美庭菖蒲(其球茎有通便利尿作用)
site [sait] *n* 位置,部位,位点 | active ~, catalytic ~ 活性部位,催化部位(酶分子的) / allosteric ~ 别构部位(酶分子的) / antigenic-binding ~, antigen-combining ~, combining ~ 抗原结合部位,结合部位 / binding ~s 结合部位(酶分子的) / immunologically privileged ~s 免疫特惠区 / operator ~ 操纵基因位点 / restriction ~ 限制[酶切]位点
sitfast [ˈsitfɑːst, -fæst] *n* 坐�散瘤(役畜)
sit(o)- [构词成分]食物
sitology [saiˈtɔlədʒi], **sitiology** [ˌsitiˈɔlədʒi] *n* 饮食学,营养学
sitomania [ˌsaitəuˈmeinjə], **sitiomania** [ˌsitiəuˈmeinjə] *n* 贪食狂;间发性善饥
sitophobia [ˌsaitəuˈfəubiə] *n* 畏食
sitosterol [saiˈtɔstərɔl] *n* 谷甾醇,谷固醇(降血脂药)
β-sitosterolemia [saiˌtɔstərəˈliːmiə] *n* β-谷固醇血症
sitotherapy [ˌsaitəuˈθerəpi] *n* 饮食疗法,营养疗法
sitotoxin [ˌsaitəuˈtɔksin] *n* 食物毒素
sitotoxism [ˌsaitəuˈtɔksizəm] *n* 食物中毒,食品中毒
sitotropism [ˌsaiˈtɔtrəpizəm], **sitotaxis** [ˌsaitəuˈtæksis] *n* 向食性,趋食性(细胞)
situation [ˌsitjuˈeiʃən] *n* 位置;情境(心理学上指作用于个体并影响其行为的身体、心理、社会与文化诸因素的总和)
situs [ˈsaitəs] *n*【拉】位置,部位,位点 | ~ inversus viscerum 内脏反位 / ~ perversus 内脏错位,内脏异位 / ~ solitus 内脏正位 / ~ transversus 内脏逆位
SIV simian immunodeficiency virus 猿猴免疫缺陷病毒
Si vir. perm. si vires permittant【拉】如体力能支持
Sjögren-Larsson syndrome [ˈʃəugren ˈlɑːsən] (Karl G. T. Sjögren; Tage K. L. Larsson) 舍-拉综合征(先天性智力发育不全,鱼鳞病及痉挛性锥体系统症状)
Sjögren's syndrome(disease) [ˈʃəugren] (Henrik S. C. Sjögren) 舍格伦综合征(病)(一种病因不明的综合征,常发生于中年或老年妇女,特点为干性角膜结膜炎、口腔干燥和结缔组织病〈通常为类风湿关节炎〉三联症。同样见 syndrome 项下 sicca syndrome)
Sjöqvist's method [ˈʃəukwist] (John A. Sjöqvist) 斯耶克维斯特法(用氧化钡合剂作尿中脲的定量测定)
skatole [ˈskætəul] *n* 粪臭素,3-甲基吲哚
skatology [skəˈtɔlədʒi] *n* 粪便学 | **skatologic** [ˌskætəˈlɔdʒik] *a*
skatophagy [skəˈtɔfədʒi] *n* 食粪癖
skatoxyl [skəˈtɔksil] *n* 羟甲基吲哚
skatoxylglycuronic acid [skəˌtɔksilglaikjuəˈrɔnik] 羟甲基吲哚葡萄糖醛酸
skatoxylsulfuric acid [skəˌtɔksilsʌlˈfjuərik] 羟甲基吲哚硫酸
skein [skein] *n* 染色质钮,丝球;线束,线胶 | test ~s 试验彩线(用于霍姆格伦〈Holmgren〉彩线试验,检彩色的辨别力)
skelalgia [skiˈlældʒiə] *n* 腿痛
skelasthenia [ˌskilæsˈθiːniə] *n* 腿无力

skeletal [ˈskelitl] *a* 骨骼的
skeletin [ˈskelitin] *n* 骨骼蛋白,骨骼胶(无脊椎动物的胶状物质,包括几丁质、丝胶、海绵硬蛋白等)
skeletization [ˌskelitaiˈzeiʃən, -tiˈz-] *n* 极度消瘦;骨骼剥制法(去除软组织)
skeletogenous [ˌskeliˈtɔdʒinəs] *a* 成骨骼的
skeletogeny [ˌskeliˈtɔdʒini] *n* 骨骼形成,骨骼发生
skeletography [ˌskeliˈtɔgrəfi] *n* 骨骼论
skeletology [ˌskeliˈtɔlədʒi] *n* 骨骼学
skeleton [ˈskelitn] *n* 骨骼 | appendicular ~ 附属骨骼(四肢骨骼) / axial ~ 中轴骨骼(颅骨、脊柱骨、肋骨和胸骨) / visceral ~ 脏腑骨骼(保护内脏的骨骼,如胸骨、肋骨、髋骨)
skeletopia [ˌskeliˈtəupiə], **skeletopy** [ˈskeliˌtəupi] *n* 骨骼关联
Skene's glands(ducts, tubules) [skiːn] (Alexander J. C. Skene)尿道旁腺
skenitis [skiˈnaitis] *n* 尿道旁腺炎
skenoscope [ˈskiːnəskəup] *n* 尿道旁腺镜
skeocytosis [ˌskiəusaiˈtəusis] *n* 幼稚白细胞症(亦称白细胞左移)
skepticism [ˈskeptisizəm] *n* 多疑癖
skeptophylaxis [ˌskeptəufiˈlæksis] *n* 辅助免疫,微量免疫;微量脱敏
skew [skjuː] *a* 斜的,偏的;偏斜的(概率分布不对称的) | **~ness** *n* 偏斜,偏斜度
skewfoot [ˈskjuːfut] *n* 内收内翻跖[畸形]
skia- [构词成分]影(尤指 X 线的)
skiagram [ˈskaiəgræm] *n* X 线摄影[照]片
skiagraph [ˈskaiəgrɑːf, -græf] *n* X 线摄影[照]片 | **~y** [skaiˈægrəfi] *n* X 线摄影[术]
skiameter [skaiˈæmitə] *n* X 线量测定器,X 线量计
skiametry [skaiˈæmitri] *n* 视网膜镜检查,检影法
skiascope [ˈskaiəskəup] *n* 视网膜镜,检影镜
skiascopy [skaiˈæskəpi] *n* 视网膜镜检查,检影[法];X 线透视检查
Skillern's fracture [ˈskilən] (Penn G. Skillern) 斯基勒伦骨折(桡尺骨合并骨折:桡骨下 1/3 的完全骨折,与尺骨下 1/3 的青枝骨折)
skimming [ˈskimiŋ] *n* 分液滑动 | plasma ~ 血浆分滑
skin [skin] *n* 皮,皮肤 | alligator ~, crocodile ~ 鳄皮状鳞癣,重鳞癣 / beaters' ~, goldbeaters' ~ 动物肠衣 / bronzed ~(肾上腺性)青铜色皮病 / colloidion ~ 火棉胶样皮(见于火棉胶样婴儿) / elastic ~, India rubber ~ 弹性皮肤,印度橡皮样皮 / lax ~ 皮肤松垂 / marble ~ 大理石样皮肤 / piebald ~ 花斑,斑驳病 / porcupine ~ 高起鱼鳞癣 / sailors' ~, farmer's ~ 光化性弹力纤维病 / shagreen ~ 鲨革样皮
skinfold [ˈskinfəuld] *n* 皮褶厚度
Skinner box [ˈskinə] (Burrhus Frederic Skinner) 斯金纳箱(测试动物条件反射用的一种实验围栏,实验动物做一动作〈如压杆〉即可获得奖赏)
Skinner classification [ˈskinə] (C. N. Skinner) 斯金纳分类法(一种以无牙间隙与剩余牙齿相互间位置关系为基础的部分无牙、部分义齿的分类法)
skler(o)- 以 skler(o)-起始的词,同样见以 scler(o)-起始的词
Sklowsky's symptom [ˈsklauski] (E. L. Sklowsky)斯克洛夫斯基症状(水痘时,用示指轻压附近健康皮肤,再压水痘的水疱,其壁易崩溃,内容物即溢出)
skodaic [skəˈdeiik] (Josef Skoda) *a* 斯科达的 | ~ resonance 斯科达叩响(胸上部叩响增强而胸下部呈实音)
Skoda's sign [ˈskɔːdə] (Josef Skoda)斯科达征(胸腔大量积液或肺炎实变区的上部,胸部叩诊可听到一种鼓音) | ~ tympany 斯科达鼓音,斯科达叩响(见 skodaic resonance)
skole- 以 skole-起始的词,同样见以 scole-起始的词
skopometer [skəˈpɔmitə] *n* 液体彩色浊度计
skot(o)- 以 skot(o)-起始的词,同样见以 scot(o)-起始的词
SKSD streptokinase-streptodornase 链激酶-链道酶
skull [skʌl] *n* 颅,头颅骨 | hot cross bun ~, natiform ~ 臀状头(先天梅毒特征) / lacuna ~ 颅顶骨内面凹陷 / maplike ~ 地图状头颅(见于慢性特发性黄瘤病颅骨 X 线摄片) / steeple ~, tower ~ 尖头[畸形]
sl slyke 斯莱克(缓冲值单位)
SLA sacro-laeva anterior 骶左前(胎位)
SLAC scapholunate advanced collapse 舟月骨进展型萎缩
slaframine [ˈslæfrəmiːn] *n* 根霉菌胺(一种催涎性真菌毒素,可致家畜流涎病)
SLE systemic lupus erythematosus 系统性红斑狼疮
sleep [sliːp] *n* 睡眠 | crescendo ~ 渐强性睡眠 / frozen ~ 冷冻睡眠法(治癌,局部组织温度为 4~10 ℃,全身体温下降到 21~32 ℃) / nonrapid eye movement ~, NREM ~, deep ~, orthodox ~, quiet ~, slow wave ~, synchronized ~ 非快速眼动睡眠,深睡眠,正相睡眠,平静睡眠,(脑电)慢波睡眠,同步睡眠 / paroxysmal ~ 发作性睡眠 / prolonged ~ 延续睡眠法(在药物麻醉下持续若干天治神经功能病) / rapid eye movement ~, REM ~, active ~, desynchronized ~, dreaming ~ (D ~), fast wave ~, paradoxical ~ 快速眼动睡眠,主动睡眠,非同步睡眠,作梦睡眠,(脑电)快波睡眠,异相睡

眠(睡眠倒错) / twilight ~ 朦胧麻醉,半麻醉
sleeptalking [ˈsliːptɔːkiŋ] *n* 梦呓
sleepwalking [ˈsliːpˌwɔːkiŋ] *n* 梦游,梦行[症] | **sleepwalk** *vt*/ **sleepwalker** *n* 梦游者
sleepygrass [ˈsliːpigræs] *n* 睡眠草,美洲醉马草
slice [slais] *n* 切片,片 | tissue ~ 组织切片
slide [slaid] *n* (显微镜用)载玻片,载物片
sling [sliŋ] *n* 悬带 | vascular ~ 血管悬吊
slit [slit] *n* 裂缝,裂隙 | gill ~ 鳃裂
slit-lamp [ˈslitˌlæmp] *n* 裂隙灯(检查眼睛用)
SLO scanning laser ophthalmoscope 扫描激光检眼镜
slobbers [ˈslɔbəz] *n* 垂肉皮炎(家兔);流涎病(家畜)
slope [sləup] *n* 倾斜,斜面;斜率,斜度 *vi*, *vt* 倾斜 | E-F ~ E-F 斜率
slough [slʌf] *n* 腐肉,腐痂 *vi* (痂等)脱落
sloughing [ˈslʌfiŋ] *n* 腐肉形成;腐肉分离
slows [sləuz] *n* (牛、羊)震颤病(人饮其乳可得乳毒病)
SLP sacrolaeva posterior【拉】骶左后(胎位)
SLT sacrolaeva transversa【拉】骶左横(胎位)
Sluder's neuralgia (syndrome) [ˈsluːdə] (Greenfield Sluder) 斯路德神经痛(综合征)(蝶腭节神经痛,引起上颌骨区灼痛和锥刺痛,此痛并辐射至颈和肩部) | ~ operation (method) 斯路德手术(法)(用扁桃体铡除刀切除扁桃体)
sludge [slʌdʒ] *n* 淤泥,污泥,泥浆 | activated ~ 活性污泥 | **sludgy** [slʌdʒi] *a* 有淤泥的,淤泥多的
sludging [ˈslʌdʒiŋ] *n* 淤沉,沉积 | ~ of blood (血管内)血液沉积
slug [slʌg] *n* 蛞蝓,蜒蚰
slurry [ˈsləːri] *n* 淤浆,泥浆
slush [slʌʃ] *n* 雪泥 | carbon dioxide ~ 二氧化碳雪泥(用于治疗各种皮肤病)
slyke (sl) [slaik] *n* 斯莱克(缓冲值的单位,自 D. D. Van Slyke 缓冲分析先驱者得名)
Sly syndrome [slai] (William S. Sly)斯赖综合征(β-葡糖苷酸酶缺乏引起的黏多糖贮积症,其生化特征为尿内排泄硫酸皮肤素和硫酸乙酰肝素,粒细胞中有颗粒状包涵体。1 ~ 2 岁之间发病,伴有轻度到中度胡尔勒〈Hurler〉样特点,其中包括多发性骨发育障碍、鸡胸、内脏巨大、心脏杂音、身材矮小和中度精神发育迟缓,也存在较轻的类型,亦称黏多糖贮积症Ⅶ型,β-葡糖苷酸酶缺乏症)
Sm samarium 钐
SMA 6/60 Sequential Multiple Analyzer 顺序多项分析仪 6/60(一种自动化学装置的商品名,60 分钟内可测定血清内 6 种物质的浓度,并以固定顺序报告检验结果,所测定的物质为肌酸酐或葡萄糖、尿素氮、氯化物、二氧化碳、钠和钾)
SMA 12/60 Sequential Multiple Analyzer 顺序多项分析仪 12/60(一种自动化学装置的商品名,60 分钟内可测定 12 种物质的浓度,并以固定顺序报告检验结果,所测定的物质为钙、无机磷、葡萄糖、尿素氮、尿酸、胆固醇、总蛋白、白蛋白、总胆红素、碱性磷酸酯酶、乳酸脱氢酶和天冬氨酸转氨酶)
SMAF specific macrophage arming factor 特异性巨噬细胞武装因子
small [smɔːl] *a* 小的 | ~ for gestational age infant 小于胎龄儿
smallpox [ˈsmɔːlpɔks] *n* 天花 | bovine ~ 牛痘 / coherent ~ 集合性天花 / confluent ~ 融合性天花 / discrete ~ 分离性天花 / equine ~ 马痘 / hemorrhagic ~, black ~ 出血性天花,黑痘 / inoculation ~ 接种痘,接种天花 / malignant ~ 恶性天花(出血性天花致死型) / mild ~ 轻型天花 / modified ~ 轻天花,变形天花/ ovine ~ 羊痘
SMC selenomethylnorcholesterol 硒甲基降胆固醇
smear [smiə] *n* 涂片 | cervical scraping ~ 宫颈刮片
smegma [ˈsmegmə] *n*【希】阴垢,包皮垢(皮脂腺分泌物,主要在包皮下) | ~ embryonum 胎垢,胎儿皮脂 | **~tic** [smegˈmætik] *a*
smegmolith [ˈsmegməliθ] *n* 包皮垢石
smell [smel] *n* 嗅觉,嗅;气味
smell-brain [ˈsmelbrein] *n* 嗅脑
Smellie's method [ˈsmeli] (William Smellie) 斯梅利法(后出胎头娩出法) | ~ scissors 斯梅利剪(外刃颅骨剪)
smilacin [ˈsmailəsin] *n* 菝葜皂苷
smilagenin [ˌsmailəˈdʒenin] *n* 异菝葜皂苷元
Smilax [ˈsmailæks] *n* 菝葜属 | ~ aristolochiaefolia 墨西哥菝葜
smile [smail] *n* 微笑 | high ~ 高位微笑
Smith-Lemli-Opitz syndrome [smiθ ˈlemli ˈəupits] (David W. Smith; Luc Lemli; John M. Opitz)史-莱-奥综合征(一种遗传性综合征,作为常染色体隐性性状遗传,特征为多种先天性异常,其中包括小头、智力迟钝、肌张力减退、男性生殖器发育不全、短鼻与鼻孔前倾、第 2 及第 3 趾并趾畸形等)
Smith-Petersen nail [ˈsmiθ ˈpiːtəsn] (Marius N. Smith-Petersen)史密斯-彼得森钉(股骨颈骨折时用以固定股骨头的三刃钉)
Smith's disease [smiθ] (Eustace Smith)黏液性结肠炎 | ~ sign 史密斯征(支气管淋巴结增大时,患者将头往后仰,在胸骨柄听诊可听到杂音)
Smith's dislocation [smiθ] (Robert W. Smith)史密斯脱位(跖骨和第一楔骨向上及向后的脱位) | ~ fracture 史密斯骨折(桡骨下端靠近关节面的骨折,下部碎片向前移位)

Smith's operation [smiθ] (Henry Smith) 史密斯手术(未成熟的白内障连同一个完整的囊一起摘除)

Smith's phenomenon [smiθ] (Theobald Smith) 史密斯现象(应用于标定白喉抗毒素的豚鼠,由于注射少量血清,对血清极为易感,在几周后如注射较大剂量的相同血清,可迅速导致死亡)

Smith's test [smiθ] (Walter G. Smith) 史密斯试验(检胆色素)

Smith-Strang disease [smiθ stræŋ] (Allan J. Smith; Leonard B. Strang) 史-斯病,蛋氨酸吸收障碍综合征(即 methionine malabsorption syndrome,见 syndrome 项下相应术语)

smog [smɔg] *n* 烟雾

SMON subacute myelo-opticoneuropathy 亚急性脊髓视神经病

SMR standardized mortality (or morbidity) ratio 标准化死亡率(或发病率)比; submucous resection (of nasal septum) (鼻中隔)黏膜下切除术

smut [smʌt] *n* 污斑;黑穗病 *vt* 使(农作物)患黑穗病 *vi* 患黑穗病 | corn ~ 玉蜀黍黑穗病 / rye ~ 麦角

Sn stannum 锡

S. N. secundum naturam【拉】按自然(规律),自然地,天然地

sn- (为 stereospecific numbering 的简写)立体特异编排(此为化学前缀,用以表示甘油衍生物的立体异构体)

snake [sneik] *n* 蛇 | brown ~ 褐蛇 / cabbage ~ 甘蓝蛇 / coral ~ 珊瑚蛇 / crotalid ~ 响尾蛇 / elapid ~ 眼镜蛇 / hair ~ 毛蛇 / harlequin ~ 花斑眼镜蛇 / poisonous ~ 毒蛇 / venomous ~ 毒蛇 / viperine ~ 蝰蛇

snakebite [ˈsneikbait] *n* 蛇咬伤

snakeroot [ˈsneikruːt] *n* 美蛇根,蛇根马兜铃(治蛇咬伤)

SNAP sensory nerve action potential 感觉神经动作电位

snap [snæp] *n* 弹响,锐声 | opening ~ 开瓣音(二尖瓣)

snapper [ˈsnæpə] *n* 笛鲷

snare [snɛə] *n* 圈套;圈套器,勒除器(勒除息肉和肿瘤用) | cold ~ 冷勒除器 / hot ~ 热勒除器,电烙勒除器

Sneddon's syndrome [ˈsnedən] (Ian B. Sneddon) 斯内顿综合征(一种罕见的疾病,在此病中脑动脉病和局部缺血常伴有弥散性非炎症性网状青斑)

Sneddon-Wilkinson disease [ˈsnednˈwilkinsn] (Lan Bruce Sneddon; Darrell Sheldon Wilkinson) 斯-威病,角层下脓疱性皮病

sneeze [sniːz] *vi* 打喷嚏 *n* 喷嚏

sneezweed [ˈsniːzwiːd] *n* 堆心菊

Snellen's chart [ˈsnelən] (Hermann Snellen) 斯内伦视力表(检视敏度) | ~ reform eye 斯内伦假眼(由两个凹凸板构成的人工空心假眼) / ~ test 斯内伦试验(检一侧诈盲及视敏度) / ~ test type 斯内伦测验标型(视力表)

Snell's law [snel] (Willebrord van Roijen Snell) 斯涅耳定律(对于两个已知的介质,其入射角的正弦对折射角的正弦呈恒定关系)

Snider match test [ˈsnaidə] (Thomas H. Snider) 斯奈特火柴试验(一种肺通气量筛选试验:将普通书夹式火柴点燃近半,置于距患者口腔 15 cm 处,嘱其深吸气后张嘴呼气熄灭火柴)

SNM Society of Nuclear Medicine 核医学学会

Snodgrass procedure [ˈsnɔdgræs] (Warren Snodgrass) 斯诺德格拉斯手术(手术矫正远端尿道的尿道下裂,即造一个肾小管新尿道,并配有一个去上皮化的肉膜和鞘膜的皮瓣)

snore [snɔː] *vi* 打鼾 *n* 打鼾,鼾声

snout [snaut] *n* (动物的)口鼻部

snow [snəu] *n* 雪 | carbon dioxide ~ 二氧化碳雪(干冰,固态二氧化碳,有时用于冷冻手术)

snowblind [ˈsnəublaind] *a* 雪盲的 | **~ness** *n* 雪盲[症]

SNP single nucleotide polymorphism 单核苷酸多态性

snRNA small nuclear RNA 核内小分子核糖核酸

snRNP small nuclear ribonucleoprotein 核内小分子核糖核蛋白

SNS sympathetic nervous system 交感神经系统

snuff [snʌf] *n* 嗅剂,鼻吸药

snuff-box [ˈsnʌfbɔks] *n* 鼻烟盒 | anatomical ~ 鼻烟窝(拇指背面的凹)

snuffles [ˈsnʌflz] *n* 婴儿鼻塞(婴儿鼻黏膜黏液溢,一般见于先天梅毒)

SO the spheno-occipital synchondrosis 蝶枕软骨结合(头颅测量学名词,蝶骨与枕骨结合处的最高点)

SOAP SOAP 护理计划(一种将面向问题记录〈problem-oriented record,见 record 项下相应术语〉中的病程记录〈progress notes〉记录下来的过程使之概念化的方案,S 表示取自患者等人的主观数据〈subjective data〉,O 为观察、体检、诊断等的客观数据〈objective data〉,A 为对患者的评价〈assessment〉,P 为患者护理计划〈plan〉)

soap [səup] *n* 肥皂 | animal ~, curd ~ 兽脂皂,家用皂 / castile ~ 橄榄油皂 / green ~, medicinal soft ~, potash ~, soft ~ 绿皂,药用软皂,钾皂,软皂 / guaiac ~ 愈创木酚钾皂 / liquid ~ 液体皂,肥皂溶液 / soda ~, hard ~ 钠皂,硬皂 / superfatted ~ 多脂皂 / zinc ~ 锌皂(作软膏或硬膏用)

soapstone [ˈsəupstəun] *n* 皂石(亦称滑石)

Soave operation [səuˈɑːvei] (F. Soave) 索阿韦手术(直肠内拖出术治疗先天性巨结肠,将正常

的结肠通过剥掉黏膜的直肠连接肛门)

SOB shortness of breath 呼吸短促,气促

socia [ˈsəuʃiə] *n* 副器官 | ~ parotides 副腮腺

socialize [ˈsəuʃəlaiz] *vt* 使社会化 | **socialization** [ˌsəuʃəlaiˈzeiʃən, -liˈz-] *n* 社会化

socioacusis [ˌsəusiəuəˈkjuːsis] *n* 社会性听力减退,社会性重听

sociobiology [ˌsəusiəubaiˈɔlədʒi] *n* 社会生物学 | **sociobiologic(al)** [ˌsəusiəubaiəˈlɔdʒik(əl)] *a* / **sociobiologist** *n* 社会生物学家

sociogenic [ˌsəusiəuˈdʒenik] *a* 社会原性的

sociology [ˌsəusiˈɔlədʒi] *n* 社会学 | **sociologist** *n* 社会学家

sociometry [ˌsəusiˈɔmitri] *n* 社会测量(社会学中关于测量人类社会行为的一门分支) | **sociometric** [ˌsəusiəˈmetrik] *a*

sociopath [ˈsəusiəpæθ] *n* 反社会者,对抗社会性病态人格者 | **~ic** [ˌsəusiəˈpæθik] *a* 反社会的

sociopathy [ˌsəusiˈɔpəθi] *n* 对抗社会性病态人格;社会病态

sociotherapy [ˌsəusiəuˈθerəpi] *n* 社会[适应]治疗

socket [ˈsɔkit] *n* 槽,臼,窝 | dry ~ 干槽症(牙槽窝骨髓炎) / tooth ~s 牙槽

soda [ˈsəudə] *n* 苏打,碳酸钠 | baking ~, bicarbonate of ~ 小苏打,碳酸氢钠,重碳酸钠 / caustic ~ 苛性钠,氢氧化钠 / chlorinated ~ 含氯苏打 / ~ lime 碱石灰 / washing ~ 洗衣碱,碳酸钠

sodiarsphenamine [ˌsəudaiɑːsˈfenəmin] *n* 胂凡钠明钠

sodii [ˈsəudiai] (sodium 的所有格) *n*【拉】钠

sodiocitrate [ˌsəudiəuˈsitrit] *n* 枸橼酸钠盐

sodiotartrate [ˌsəudiəuˈtɑːtrit] *n* 酒石酸钠盐

sodium(Na) [ˈsəudjəm] *n* 钠 | ~ acetate 醋酸钠(用于全身性与泌尿系的碱化剂,亦用于祛痰和利尿) / ~ acetrizoate 醋碘苯酸钠(X 线造影剂,用于尿路、胆道及心血管造影) / ~ alginate 藻酸钠,海藻酸钠 / ~ alizarinsulfonate 茜素磺酸钠,茜素红 / ~ aminosalicylate 对氨水杨酸钠(抗结核药) / ~ antimonyltartrate 酒石酸锑钠(治锥虫病) / ~ antimonyl-thioglycollate 巯基乙酸锑钠 / ~ arsenate 砷酸钠 / ~ ascorbate 维生素 C 钠(抗生素类药) / ~ aurothiomalate 金硫丁二钠(消炎镇痛药) / ~ aurothiosulfate 金硫代硫酸钠(消炎镇痛药) / ~ benzoate 苯甲酸钠(防腐药,亦用于肝功能试验) / ~ bicarbonate 碳酸氢钠(解胃酸药) / ~ biphosphate, ~ acid phosphate 磷酸二氢钠,酸性磷酸钠(抗高血钙药,尿酸化药) / ~ bisulfite 亚硫酸氢钠(用作各种药物制剂的抗氧化剂) / ~ borate 硼砂,四硼酸钠(用作药物制剂的碱化剂,亦用于洗剂、含漱液和漱口药) / ~ cacodylate 甲胂酸钠(从前用于治结核、贫血、疟疾等) / ~ calcium edetate, ~ calcium edetate 依地酸钙钠,依地酸二钙钠,乙二胺四乙酸钙钠,解铅乐(金属中毒解毒药) / ~ caprylate 辛酸钠(治皮肤真菌病) / ~ carbonate 碳酸钠(用于药物制剂的碱化剂) / ~ cellulose phosphate 磷酸纤维素钠(用于治疗复发性肾磷酸钙结石) / ~ chloride 氯化钠(电解质补充药) / ~ citrate 枸橼酸钠(抗凝药) / ~ folate 叶酸钠(用于治各种贫血及口炎性腹泻) / ~ glutamate 谷氨酸钠(治脑病等) / ~ gold thiosulfate 金硫代硫酸钠 / ~ hydroxide 氢氧化钠(用作药物制剂的碱化剂,亦称苛性钠、烧碱) / ~ hypochlorite 次氯酸钠(具有灭菌、除臭和漂白作用) / ~ hyposulfite 硫代硫酸钠 / ~ iodate 碘酸钠(用作黏膜性疾病的抗菌剂) / ~ iodide 碘化钠(造影剂) / ~ iopodate 碘泊酸钠(胆道造影剂) / ~ lactate 乳酸钠(治酸中毒) / ~ lauryl sulfate 月桂硫酸钠(用作润湿剂、去污剂等) / ~ metabisulfite 焦亚硫酸钠(用于药物制剂) / ~ monofluorophosphate 氟磷酸钠(龋齿预防药) / ~ nitrite 亚硝酸钠(解毒药,治氰化物中毒,亦用于缓解心绞痛、两侧间歇性小动脉痉挛症、气喘及铅绞痛、痉挛性结肠炎等) / ~ nitroprusside, ~ nitroferricyanide 硝普钠,亚硝基铁氰化钠(抗高血压药) / ~ oxybate 羟丁酸钠(安眠药,麻醉时用作辅药) / ~ paraaminosalicylate(PAS-Na)对氨水杨酸钠(抗结核药) / ~ phenolsulfonate 酚磺酸钠(肠抗菌药) / ~ phytate 肌醇六磷酸钠,植酸钠(钙螯合剂) / ~ polyphosphate 聚偏磷酸钠(制药助剂) / ~ polystyrene sulfonate 聚苯乙烯磺酸钠(钠型阳离子交换树脂,用于治疗高钾血症) / ~ salicylate 水杨酸钠(止痛、解热、抗风湿药) / ~ stibocaptate 锑卡酸钠(抗血吸虫药) / ~ thiamylal 硫戊巴比妥钠(全身麻醉药) / ~ thiosulfate 硫代硫酸钠(解氰中毒以及预防在游泳池和公共淋浴场所的脚癣感染) / ~ trimetaphosphate 三偏磷酸钠(制药助剂)

sodium-potassium adenosinetriphosphatase [əˌdenəsiːntraiˈfɔsfəteis] 钠钾腺苷三磷酸酶

sodokosis [ˌsəudəˈkəusis] *n* 鼠咬热

sodoku [ˈsəudəku] *n*【日】鼠咬热

sodomy [ˈsɔdəmi] *n* 鸡奸,兽奸 | **sodomist, sodomite** [ˈsɔdəmai] *n* 鸡奸者,兽奸者

sodophthalyl [ˌsəudəˈθælil] *n* 二钠醌酚酞(轻泻药)

Soemmering's ring [ˈsemərin] (Samuel T. von Soemmering) 泽默林环(亦称泽默林白内障) | ~ spot 视网膜黄斑 / ~ crystalline swelling 泽默林晶状体肿胀(白内障晶状体除去后,晶状体囊下部的环状肿胀)

SOFAS Social and Occupational Functioning Assess-

ment Scale 社会和职业功能评定表
softening [ˈsɔfniŋ] *n* 软化 | ~ of the brain 脑软化 / colliquative ~ 液化性软化 / mucoid ~ 黏液样软化,黏液性变性 / ~ of the stomach 胃软化 / yellow ~, pyriform ~ 黄色软化,梨状软化
Sohval-Soffer syndrome [ˈsəuvəlˈsɔfə] (Arthur R. Sohval; Louis J. Soffer) 苏-索综合征(一种先天性综合征,包括男性性腺功能减退,伴有颈椎与肋骨多处骨骼畸形和智力迟钝)
sokosha [səˈkəuʃə] *n* 鼠咬热
Sol. solution 溶液
sol [sɔl] *n* 溶胶;溶液
Solanaceae [ˌsəuləˈneisii:] *n* 茄科 | **solanaceous** [ˌsəuləˈneiʃəs] *a*
solandrine [səuˈlændrin] *n* 去甲莨菪碱,伪莨菪碱
solanine [ˈsəulənі:n] *n* 茄碱,龙葵碱
solanocyte [səˈlænəsait] *n* 焰状细胞
solanoid [ˈsəulənɔid] *a* 马铃薯状的(指某些恶性肿瘤)
Solanum [səuˈleinəm] *n*【拉】茄属 | ~ carolinense 美洲野茄 / ~ tuberosum 马铃薯
solapsone [səˈlæpsəun], **solasulfone** [ˌsəuləˈsʌlfəun] *n* 苯丙砜(抗麻风药)
solar [ˈsəulə] *a* 太阳[神经]丛的(尤指腹腔神经丛的)
solarium [səuˈlɛəriəm] ([复] **solariums** 或 **solaria**) *n*【拉】日光浴室
solation [sɔˈleiʃən] *n* 溶胶化[作用],胶溶[作用]
Soldaini's test (reagent) [ˌsɔldəˈi:ni] (Arturo Soldaini)索尔代尼试验(试剂)(检尿糖)
solder [ˈsɔldə, ˈsɔdə] *n* 焊料,焊锡 *vt, vi* 焊接
sole [səul] *n* 足底,跖 | convex ~, dropped ~ 凸状足底
solecism [ˈsɔlisizəm] *n* 文法不通,语法错误
solen(o)- [构词成分]管,沟
Solenoglypha [ˌsəuliˈnɔglifə] *n* 管牙(毒蛇)类
solenoid [ˈsəulinɔid] *n* 螺线管
solenonychia [ˌsəulinəuˈnikiə] *n* 管状甲,中裂甲,甲中部管状营养不良
Solenopotes [ˌsəulənəˈpəuti:z] *n* 盲虱属 | ~ capillatus 水牛盲虱
Solenopsis [ˌsəuliˈnɔpsis] *n* 水蚁属
sole plate, sole-plate [səul pleit] 终板
solferino [ˌsɔlfəˈri:nəu] *n* 品红,复红
solid [ˈsɔlid] *a* 固体的,实心的;立体的 *n* 固体;立体 | color ~ 色立体(用以表示色的深浅间的关系)
Solidago [ˌsɔliˈdeigəu] *n*【拉】一枝黄花属
solidism [ˈsɔlidizəm] *n* 固体病理学说
solipsism [ˈsəulipsizəm] *n* 唯我论 | **solipsistic** [ˌsəulipˈsistik] *a* / **solipsist** [ˈsəulipsist] *n* 唯我论者
sol-lunar [sɔl ˈlju:nə] *a* 日月的
solpugid [sɔlˈpju:dʒid] *n* 避日虫
Solpugida [ˌsɔlpjuˈdʒidə] *n* 避日虫目(一种毒蛛)
soluble [ˈsɔljubl] *a* 溶解的,可溶的 | **solubility** [ˌsɔljuˈbiləti] *n* 溶解度
solum [ˈsəuləm] ([复] **sola** [ˈsəulə]) *n*【拉】最下部;底
solute [ˈsɔlju:t] *n* 溶质
solutio [səˈlju:ʃiəu] *n*【拉】溶液
solution [səˌlju:ʃən] *n* 溶液;溶解[作用] | alcoholic ~ 醇溶液(溶剂) / alkaline aromatic ~ 碱性芳香溶液(漱口药) / aluminum acetate ~ 醋酸铝溶液(用于皮肤抗菌、止痒) / aluminum subacetate ~ 碱式醋酸铝溶液,次醋酸铝溶液(皮肤病抗菌用药) / anisotonic ~ 异渗溶液,不等渗溶液 / anticoagulant (acid) citrate dextrose ~ 枸橼酸盐葡萄糖抗凝溶液(保存全血的一种抗凝剂) / antiseptic ~ 抗菌溶液,防腐溶液 / aqueous ~ 水溶液(水用作溶剂) / arsenic chloride ~ 氯化砷溶液 / arsenical ~ 亚砷酸钾溶液(见 potassium arsenite ~) / arsenious acid ~ 亚砷酸溶液 / benzalkonium chloride ~ 苯扎氯铵溶液(表面抗感染药) / boric acid ~ 硼酸溶液(外用抗菌药) / buffer ~ 缓冲溶液 / carmine ~ 卡红溶液,胭脂红溶液 / centinormal ~ 百分之一当量溶液(见 hundredth-normal ~) / coal tar ~ 煤焦油溶液(稀释后用作表面抗湿疹药) / compound cresol ~ 复方甲酚溶液,复方皂溶液 / compound iodine ~ 复方碘溶液,浓碘溶液 / contrast ~ 造影溶液 / crystal violet ~ 结晶紫溶液(抗感染药) / decimolar ~ 十分之一摩尔溶液(0.1 mol/L 溶液) / decinormal ~ 十分之一当量溶液(见 tenthnormal ~) / diluted ammonia ~ 稀氨溶液,氨溶液 / disclosing ~ 显示液 / double-normal ~ 二当量溶液(2 N) / epinephrine ~ 肾上腺素溶液(用作血管收缩药) / epinephrine bitartrate ophthalmic ~ 重酒石酸肾上腺素眼溶液(用以散瞳及治青光眼) / ethereal ~ 醚性溶液(醚作溶剂) / ferric chloride ~ 氯化铁溶液 / fixative ~ 固定液 / formaldehyde ~ 甲醛溶液(消毒剂) / gentian violet ~ 甲紫溶液(抗感染药) / gram molecular ~ 摩尔溶液 / half-normal ~ 二分之一当量溶液(N/2) / hundredth-normal ~ 百分之一当量溶液(N/100 或 0.01 N) / hydrogen peroxide ~, hydrogen dioxide ~ 过氧化氢溶液(皮肤和黏膜表面抗感染药) / hyperbaric ~ 高比重溶液(如脊髓麻醉使用的一种) / iodine ~ 碘溶液(表面抗感染药) / isobaric ~ 等比重溶液(如脊髓麻醉使用的一种) / isofurophate ophthalmic ~ 异氟磷眼溶液

(治疗青光眼,局部用于结膜) / lead subacetate ~ 碱式醋酸铅溶液,次醋酸铅溶液(用作收敛剂及局部镇静剂) / liver ~ 肝溶液(能促使恶性贫血患者造血) / methylrosaniline chloride ~ 甲紫溶液,龙胆紫溶液(见 gentian violet ~) / molal ~ 重量摩尔溶液,重模溶液,摩尔溶液 / molar ~ 容积摩尔溶液,容模溶液,摩尔溶液 / normal ~ 当量溶液(N/1 或 1 N) / normal saline ~, normal salt ~ 当量盐溶液(见 physiological salt ~) / normobaric ~ 等比重溶液(见 isobaric ~) / parathyroid ~ 甲状旁腺溶液 / phenylephrine hydrochloride ophthalmic ~ 盐酸去氧肾上腺素眼溶液 / physiological salt ~, physiological sodium chloride ~ 生理盐溶液(一种氯化钠水溶液,其重量克分子〈摩尔〉渗透压浓度与血清相似) / pituitary ~, posterior pituitary ~ 垂体(后叶)溶液 / potassium arsenite ~ 亚砷酸钾溶液(治慢性髓细胞性白血病及慢性皮炎) / saline ~, salt ~ 盐溶液 / saponated cresol ~ 甲酚皂溶液(消毒剂) / saturated ~ 饱和溶液 / sclerosing ~ 硬化溶液 / seminormal ~ 半当量溶液(N/2) / sodium chloride ~ 氯化钠溶液(用作等渗压赋形剂) / standard ~ 标准溶液 / stock ~ 原液,母液(浓度较高的能长期保存的溶液) / strong ammonia ~ 浓氨溶液(溶剂) / strong iodine ~ 浓碘溶液 / stronger ammonium hydroxide ~ 浓氢氧化铵溶液,浓氨溶液 / sulfurated lime ~ 含硫石灰溶液(从前用作角质层分离剂治寻常粉刺和皮脂溢) / supersaturated ~ 过饱和溶液 / susa ~ 苏萨溶液(一种脱钙液) / tenth-normal ~ 十分之一当量溶液(N/10 或 0.1 N) / test ~s 试[溶]液 / thousandth-normal ~ 千分之一当量溶液(N/1000 或 0.001 N) / volumetric ~ 滴定[用]溶液,定量溶液

solv. solve【拉】溶解

solvable [ˈsɔlvəbl] *a* 可溶解的,可溶的 | **solvability** [ˌsɔlvəˈbiləti] *n* 溶解能力;溶剂化度

solvate [ˈsɔlveit] *n* 溶剂合物,溶[剂]化物 *vt* 使成溶剂化物 | **solvation** [səlˈveiʃən] *n* 溶合,溶[剂]化(溶质与溶剂的化学结合)

solvency [ˈsɔlvənsi] *n* 溶解能力

solvent [ˈsɔlvənt] *a* 溶解的,溶化的 *n* 溶剂,溶媒

solvolysis [səlˈvɔlisis] *n* 溶剂分解[作用],媒解[作用](水解、氨解、硫解的双分解反应的统称)

soma [ˈsəumə] *n* 体,躯体(有别于精神);体组织(有别于生殖细胞);体细胞

somacule [ˈsəuməkjuːl] *n* 原微粒(原生质)

somal [ˈsəuməl] *a* 体的,躯体的

somalin [ˈsɔməlin] *n* 索马林(强心苷)

soman [ˈsəumæn] *n* 索曼(一种有机磷化合物,为强效胆碱酯酶抑制剂,并用作神经毒气,中毒症状包括支气管缩窄、惊厥以及死亡)

somaplasm [ˈsəuməplæzəm] *n* 体浆,体质(见 somatoplasm)

somascope [ˈsəuməskəup] *n* 超声波检查仪

somasthenia [ˌsəumæsˈθiːniə], **somatasthenia** [ˌsəumətæsˈθiːniə] *n* 体无力,疲惫

somatalgia [ˌsəuməˈtældʒiə] *n* 躯体痛

somatesthesia [ˌsəumətisˈθiːzjə] *n* 躯体感觉,体觉 | **somatesthetic** [ˌsəumətisˈθetik] *a*

somatic [səuˈmætik] *a* 躯体的,体壁的;菌体的,体细胞的

somaticovisceral [səuˌmætikəuˈvisərəl], **somaticosplanchnic** [səuˌmætikəuˈsplæŋknik] *a* 躯体内脏的

somatist [ˈsəumətist] *n* 躯体论者(认为一切精神病及神经功能病均由躯体病变所致)

somatization [ˌsəumətaiˈzeiʃən, -tiˈz-] *n* 躯体症状化(指精神病学中,精神症状转化为躯体症状)

somat(o)- [构词成分]躯体,体

somatoceptor [səuˈmætəˌseptə] *n* 体[壁]感受器

somatochrome [səuˈmætəkrəum] *n* 体染色神经细胞

somatocrinin [ˌsumətəuˈkrainin] *n* 促生长素释放素

somatoderm [səuˈmætədəːm] *n* 体壁中胚层

somatodidymus [ˌsəumətəuˈdidiməs] *n* 单躯联胎

somatodymia [ˌsəumətəuˈdimiə] *n* 单躯联胎畸形,躯干联胎畸形

somatoform [səuˈmætəfɔːm] *a* 躯体形的(表示与躯体疾病相似的心因性症状)

somatogenesis [ˌsəumətəuˈdʒenisis] *n* 躯型发生,体质形成

somatogenetic [ˌsəumətəudʒiˈnetik] *a* 躯型发生的;体因性的

somatogenic [ˌsəumətəuˈdʒenik] *a* 体因性的

somatognosis [ˌsəumətɔgˈnəusis] *n* 躯体存在感觉(亦称存在感觉,躯体觉,或第 6 感觉)

somatogram [səuˈmætəgræm] *n* 躯体 X 线[照]片

somatoliberin [ˌsumətəuˈlibərin] *n* 促生长素释放素

somatology [ˌsəuməˈtɔlədʒi] *n* 躯体学,身体学 | **somatologic(al)** [ˌsəumətəˈlɔdʒik(ə)l] *a* | **somatologist** [ˌsəuməˈtɔlədʒist] *n* 躯体学家

somatomammotropin [ˌsəumətəuˌmæməuˈtrəupin] *n* 生长促乳素,生长催乳素 | chorionic ~ 绒毛膜生长催乳素,人胎盘催乳素

somatome [ˈsəumətəum] *n* 胎体刀;体节 | **somatomic** [ˌsəuməˈtɔmik] *a*

somatomedin [ˌsəumətəuˈmiːdin] *n* 生长素介质

somatomegaly [ˌsəumətəuˈmegəli] *n* 巨大发育,巨大畸形,巨人症

somatometry [səuməˈtɔmitri] *n* 活体测量[法]

somatopagus [ˌsəuməˈtɔpəgəs] *n* 单躯联胎,躯干联胎
somatopathy [ˌsəuməˈtɔpəθi] *n* 躯体病 | **somatopathic** [ˌsəumətəuˈpæθik] *a*
somatophrenia [ˌsəumətəuˈfriːniə] *n* 躯体病幻想
somatoplasm [ˈsəumətəˌplæzəm] *n* 体浆,体质(体细胞的原生质,有别于生殖质) | **somatoplastic** [ˌsəumətəuˈplæstik] *a*
somatopleure [ˈsəumətəpluə] *n* 胚体壁(外胚层和体壁中胚层) | **somatopleural** [ˌsəumətəuˈpluərəl] *a*
somatopsychic [ˌsəumətəuˈsaikik] *a* 躯体与精神的;身心的
somatopsychosis [ˌsəumətəusaiˈkəusis] *n* 躯体性精神病
somatoschisis [ˌsəuməˈtɔskisis] *n* 躯体裂
somatoscopy [ˌsəuməˈtɔskəpi] *n* 体格检查,身体检视法
somatosensory [ˌsəumətəuˈsensəri] *a* 躯体感觉的
somatosexual [ˌsəumətəuˈseksjuəl] *a* 体征与性征的,性发育体征的
somatosplanchnopleuric [ˌsəumətəuˌsplæŋknəuˈpluərik] *a* 体层[与]脏层的
somatostatin (SS) [ˌsəumətəuˈstætin] *n* 生长抑素,促生长素抑制素
somatostatinoma [ˌsəumətəuˌstætiˈnəumə] *n* 生长抑[制]素瘤
somatotherapy [ˌsəumətəuˈθerəpi] *n* 躯体治疗
somatotonia [ˌsəumətəuˈtəuniə] *n* 身体紧张型(一种人格特性,表现为肌肉活动和强有力的身体活动)
somatotopagnosia [ˌsəumətəuˌtɔpægˈnəuziə] *n* 自体部位觉缺失,自体部位失认
somatotopic [ˌsəumətəuˈtɔpik] *a* 躯体特定区的(指大脑运动区的组织机构,身体不同部位活动的控制,集中在皮质的特定区内)
somatotridymus [ˌsəumətəuˈtraidiməs] *n* 三躯联胎
somatotroph [səuˈmætətrəuf] *n* 生长激素细胞 | **somatotrope** [səuˈmætətrəup] *n*
somatotrophic [ˌsəumətəuˈtrɔfik] *a* 促生长的
somatotropic [ˌsəumətəuˈtrɔpik] *a* 亲躯体的,亲躯体细胞的;促生长的;生长激素性的
somatotropin [ˌsəumətəuˈtrəupin], **somatotrophin** [ˌsəumətəuˈtrəufin], **somatropin** [səuˈmætrəpin] *n* 生长激素,促生长素
somatotype [səuˈmætətaip] *n* 体型,体式
somatotyping [səuˈmætəˌtaipiŋ] *n* 体型决定法
somatotypy [səuˈmætəˌtaipi] *n* 体型决定
somatrem [ˈsəumətrem] *n* 人蛋氨生长素(一种生物合成的人生长激素制剂,由重组技术使用大肠埃希杆菌制得,与天然人激素的区别在于在末端含有一个附加的蛋氨酸残基。本品用于治疗生长停滞和艾滋病相关的恶病质或体重丧失,肌内或皮下给药)
-some [构词成分]体
somesthesia [ˌsəumisˈθiːzjə] *n* 躯体感觉,体觉 | **somesthetic** [ˌsəumisˈθetik] *a*
SOMI sternal-occipital-mandibular immobilizer (orthosis) 胸骨-枕骨-下颌骨制动装置(支具)
-somia [构词成分]体,躯体
somite [ˈsəumait] *n* 体节(亦称中胚叶节)
somnambulate [sɔmˈnæmbjuleit] *vi* 梦行 | **somnambulant** *a* / **somnambulation** [sɔmˌnæmbjuˈleiʃən] *n* / **somnambulator** *n* 梦行者
somnambulism [sɔmˈnæmbjulizəm], **somnambulance** [sɔmˈnæmbjuləns] *n* 梦行[症];催眠梦行症 | **somnambulist** *n* 梦行者 / **somnambulistic** [sɔmˌnæmbjuˈlistik] *a*
somni- [构词成分]睡眠
somnifacient [ˌsɔmniˈfeiʃənt] *a* 催眠的 *n* 催眠药,安眠药
somniferous [sɔmˈnifərəs], **somnific** [sɔmˈnifik] *a* 催眠的
somniloquism [sɔmˈniləkwizəm], **somniloquence** [sɔmˈniləkwəns], **somniloquy** [sɔmˈniləkwi] *n* 梦呓,梦语 | **somniloquist** *n* 梦呓者
somniloquous [sɔmˈniləkwəs] *a* 梦呓的
Somniosus [ˌsɔmniˈəusəs] *n* 睡鲨属
somnipathy [sɔmˈnipəθi] *n* 催眠性迷睡,催眠状态;睡眠障碍 | **somnipathist** *n* 催眠性迷睡者
somnocinematograph [ˌsɔmnəuˌsiniˈmætəgrɑːf] *n* 睡眠运动描记器
somnolent [ˈsɔmnələnt] *a* 瞌睡的,嗜眠的 | **somnolence, somnolency** *n*
somnolentia [ˌsɔmnəˈlenʃiə] *n* 【拉】瞌睡,嗜眠;睡眠性酩酊状态
somnolism [ˈsɔmnəlizəm] *n* 催眠状态
somnus [ˈsɔmnəs] *n* 【拉】睡眠
Somogyi effect (phenomenon) [ˈsəumədʒi] (Michael Somogyi)索莫吉效应(现象)(糖尿病时发生的一种反跳现象,即用胰岛素过多治疗会诱发低血糖,低血糖促使肾上腺素、ACTH、高血糖素和生长激素的释放,这些激素刺激脂肪分解、糖原异生和糖原分解,导致反跳性高血糖和酮病) | ~ unit 索莫吉单位(在规定条件下每 30 分钟可释放等于 1 mg 葡萄糖还原值的淀粉酶量)
somosphere [ˈsəuməsfiə] *n* 初质球,初浆球
sonant [ˈsəunənt] *n* 浊辅音
sonar [ˈsəunɑː] *n* 声呐,水声测位仪
sonarography [ˌsəunəˈrɔgrəfi] *n* 超声扫描术
sonde [sɔnd] *n* 【法】探子 | ~ coudé 弯探子

sone [səun] *n* 宋(响度单位,1 000 Hz 的纯音声压级在闻阈上 40 dB 时的响度)
sonic ['sɔnik] *a* 声波的;声速的
sonicate ['sɔnikeit] *vt* 声处理(借高频声波破坏细菌) ['sɔnikit] *n* 声处理标本(借高频声波破坏细菌所得到的产物)
sonication [ˌsɔni'keiʃən] *n* 声处理(借高频声波破坏细菌)
sonifer ['sɔnifə] *n* 助听器
sonitus ['sɔnitəs] *n*【拉】耳鸣
Sonne dysentery ['sɔni] (Carl O. Sonne)宋内菌痢(发生在温带地区,由丁群痢疾杆菌即宋内志贺菌所致)
sonogram ['səunəgræm] *n* 声像图
sonography [səu'nɔgrəfi] *n* 声像图检查,超声检查 | **sonographic** [ˌsəunəu'græfik] *a*
sonohysterography [ˌsɔnəuˌhistə'rɔgrəfi] *n* 子宫超声检查[术]
sonolucency [ˌsəunəu'ljuːsənsi] *n* 透声性
sonolucent [ˌsəunəu'ljuːsənt] *a* 透声性的
sonometer [səu'nɔmitə] *n* 听力计;弦音计,振动频率计
sonorant [sə'nɔːrənt] *n* 浊辅音
sonorous [səu'nɔːrəs] *a* 鼾声的
sonourethrography [ˌsəunəuˌjuərə'θrɔgrəfi] *n* 尿道超声检查[术]
soot [sut] *n* 煤烟,烟灰
sophisticate [sə'fistikeit] *vt* (食物或药品)掺假 | **sophistication** [səˌfisti'keiʃən] *n* (食物或药品)掺假
sophomania [ˌsɔfə'meinjə] *n* 大智妄想
Sophora [sə'fɔːrə] *n* 槐属
sophoretin [sɔfə'riːtin] *n* 槲皮素,槲皮黄素,栎精
sophorin ['sɔfərin] *n* 芸香苷,芦丁
sophorine ['sɔfəriːn] *n* 槐碱,金雀花碱,野靛碱
sopor ['səupə] *n*【拉】迷睡,酣睡
soporiferous [ˌsəupə'rifərəs] *a* 引起酣睡的,催眠的 | **~ly** *ad* | **~ness** *n*
soporific [ˌsəupə'rifik] *a* 催眠的 *n* 催眠药
soporous ['səupərəs], **soporose** ['səupərəus] *a* 迷睡的,酣睡的
S. op. s. si opus sit【拉】必要时
Sorangiaceae [səˌrændʒi'eisiiː] *n* 堆囊黏细菌科
Sorangium [sə'rændʒiəm] *n* 堆囊黏细菌属
sorb [sɔːb] *vt* 吸收,吸附
sorbefacient [ˌsɔːbi'feiʃənt] *a* 促吸收的 *n* 吸收剂
sorbent ['sɔːbənt] *n* 吸着剂
sorbic acid ['sɔːbik] 山梨酸,2, 4-己二烯酸(抗菌防腐药)
sorbin ['sɔːbin], **sorbinose** ['sɔːbinəus] *n* 山梨糖
sorbitan ['sɔːbi'tən] *n* 脱水山梨糖醇
sorbitol ['sɔːbitɔl], **sorbite** ['sɔːbait] 山梨糖醇(甜味剂,片剂赋形剂)
sorbitol dehydrogenase ['sɔːbitɔl diː'haidrədʒəneis] 山梨糖醇脱氢酶,L-艾杜糖醇脱氢酶
sorbose ['sɔːbəus] *n* 山梨糖
Sordariaciae [ˌsɔːdəri'eisiiː] *n* 粪壳科
Sordariales [sɔːˌdeiri'eilis] *n* 粪壳目
sordes ['sɔːdiːz] *n*【拉】口垢 | ~ gastricae 胃垢
sore [sɔː] *a* 痛的 *n* 疮,溃疡 | bed ~ 褥疮 / canker ~ 口溃疡,复发性滤泡性口炎 / chrome ~ 铬溃疡 / cold ~ 感冒疮,发热性疱疹 / Delhi ~ 皮肤利什曼病 / desert ~, veldt ~ 沙漠疮,热带溃疡 / fungating ~ 肉芽增生性软下疳 / hard ~ [硬]下疳 / Kandahar ~, Lahore ~, Madagascar ~, Moultan ~, Natal ~, oriental ~, Penjdeh ~, tropical ~ 皮肤利什曼病,东方疖,热带疮 / pressure ~ 褥疮 / soft ~ 软下疳 / venereal ~ 下疳(尤指软下疳) | **~ness** *n* 酸痛;溃疡
Sörensen's reagent ['sɔrənsn] (Sören P. L. Sörensen)索伦森试剂(醋酸缓冲液,检白蛋白)
Soret band [sɔ'rei] (C. Soret)索瑞[光谱]带(血红蛋白光谱的紫色外的吸收带) | ~ effect (phenomenon)索瑞效应(现象)(在温梯中溶液冷热两部分中间起浓度差)
sore throat [sɔː θrəut] 咽喉炎 | clergyman's ~ ~ 过用性发声困难,慢性咽喉炎发声困难 / diphtheria ~ ~ 白喉 / hospital ~ ~ 医院咽喉炎(咽和咽门脓毒性炎症,有时侵袭医院的护士和实习医师) / putrid ~ ~, ulcerated ~ ~ 坏疽性咽炎 / septic ~ ~, epidemic streptococcal ~ ~, streptococcal ~ ~ 脓毒性咽喉炎,链球菌性扁桃体炎(流行病时发生的一种严重型咽喉炎,一般由酿脓链球菌有时由类马链球菌所致) / spotted ~ ~ 滤泡性扁桃体炎
Sorghum ['sɔːgəm] *n* 蜀黍属
sori ['səurai] sorus 的复数
soroche, sorroche [sə'rəutʃiː] *n*【西】(南美洲安第斯山脉)高山病
sororiation [səˌrɔri'eiʃən] *n* 青春期乳房发大
Sorosphaera [ˌsɔːrə'sfiərə] *n* 球壶菌属
sorption ['sɔːpʃən] *n* (水在胶体内的)掺和,混合;吸收[作用](指物质经过胃肠道黏膜的双定向运动及其最后结果,其中包括吸收、肠吸收、外吸收和内吸收);吸着[作用](气体在金属或其他固体表面上的吸附或化学吸着)
Sorsby's syndrome [sɔːzbi] (Arnold Sorsby)索斯比综合征(一种先天性疾病,包括双侧黄斑缺损,伴手足末端营养不良及通常限于远端两指〈趾〉骨的短指〈趾〉畸形)
sorter ['sɔːtə] *n* 分类机,分类器 | fluorescence-

activated cell ~ (FACS)荧光激活细胞分类器

sorus [ˈsəurəs]([复]**sori** [ˈsəurai]) *n* 孢子团

S. O. S. si opus sit【拉】必要时

sotalol hydrochloride [ˈsəutələul] 盐酸索他洛尔(β受体阻滞药)

soterenol hydrochloride [səuˈterinəul] 盐酸索特瑞醇(拟肾上腺素药,具有扩张支气管作用)

soterocyte [ˈsəutərəusait] *n* 血小板

Soto-Hall sign [ˈsəutəuhɔːl](Ralph Soto-Hall)索托-霍尔征(患者仰卧躺平,开始从颈部屈曲脊柱,继续向下弯,即在背部病变损害部位出现疼痛)

Sotos' syndrome [ˈsəutəus](Juan F. Sotos)索托斯综合征,大脑性巨人症

Sottas disease [ˈsɔtəz](Jules Sottas)进行性肥大性间质性神经病

soudan [su(ː)ˈdæn] *n* 苏丹,苯偶氮间苯二酚(脂肪染色剂)

souffle [ˈsuːfl] *n* 杂音,吹气音 | cardiac ~ 心脏杂音 / fetal ~ 胎儿杂音 / funic ~, funicular ~, umbilical ~ 脐带杂音 / placental ~ 胎盘杂音 / splenic ~ 脾杂音 / uterine ~ 子宫杂音

sound¹ [saund] *n* 音,声 | bandbox ~ 纸箱样音(肺气肿时胸部叩响) / bell ~, coin ~ 金属音,钱币音 / bellows ~ 风箱音(心内膜杂音) / bottle ~ 空瓮性啰音;空瓮音 / cracked-pot ~ 破壶音 / entotic ~s 耳内杂音 / first ~ 第一心音 / flapping ~ 拍击音 / friction ~ 摩擦音 / heart ~s 心音 / hippocratic ~ 希波克拉底振荡音(脓气胸或浆液气胸形成) / pulmonic second ~ 肺动脉第二音(与肺动脉半月瓣有关,缩写 P_2) / second ~ 第二心音 / succussion ~s, shaking ~ 振荡音 / tick-tack ~s 滴嗒音(与第一心音和第二心音无大差别) / third ~ 第三心音 / to-and-fro ~ 来回摩擦音(心收缩和舒张时可听到) / water-wheel ~ 水车音 / xiphisternal crunching ~ 剑突摩擦音(一种奇特的声音,原因不明,20%健康人的胸骨下段和剑突处常可听到)

sound² [saund] *a* 健康的

sound³ [saund] *n* 探子,探条 | esophageal ~ 食管探子 / lacrimal ~ 泪管探子 / urethral ~ 尿道探子 / uterine ~ 子宫探子

sounding² [ˈsaundiŋ] *n* 测探,试探;调查;探通术 | ~ of uterine cavity 探宫腔术 / urethral ~ 尿道扩张

Souques's phenomenon [suˈke](Alexandre A. Souques)苏克现象(在不全偏瘫时,提高手臂出现手指不随意伸展和分开。亦称伸指现象) | ~ sign 苏克征(①坐在椅子上的患者突然受到往后拉时,下肢不能正常地伸展以达平衡,为晚期纹状体疾病;②苏克现象)

Southern blot technique (blot analysis, blot hybridization, blot test) [ˈsʌðən](E. M. Southern, 20 世纪英国生物学家)萨慎印迹技术(印迹分析,印迹杂交,印迹试验),DNA 印迹技术

Southwestern blot technique (blot analysis, blot hybridization, blot test) [sauθˈwestən] DNA-蛋白质印迹技术(印迹分析,印迹杂交,印迹试验)

Souttar's tube [ˈsautə](Henry S. Souttar)骚塔管(引入一根可屈性金属管,保持食管畅通,治疗不能手术的食管癌)

sowdah [ˈsaudə][阿拉伯语"black"] *n* 黑皮病(也门和沙特阿拉伯盘尾丝虫病的典型皮肤表现,通常局限在单侧或两侧下肢,特征为皮肤有黑色素沉着、增厚和粗糙、肿胀、剧烈瘙痒,有丘疹和近卫淋巴结肿大)

Soxhlet's apparatus [ˈsɔkslət](Franz R. von Soxhlet)索克斯雷特萃取器(以蒸馏溶剂连续从固体物质中萃取脂肪)

soybean [ˈsɔibiːn], **soya** [ˈsɔiə] *n* 大豆

Soymida febrifuga [ˈsɔimidə feˈbrifjugə] 印度红木

sp. spiritus【拉】乙醇;酊剂

SP-40, 40 clusterin 簇连蛋白

SPA sperm penetration assay 精子穿透测定

spa [spɑː] *n* 矿泉,矿泉疗养地

space [speis] *n* 空间,宇宙;隙,间隙;腔 | apical ~ 根尖隙(牙) / axillary ~ 腋窝 / bregmatic ~ 前囟 / cartilage ~s 软骨隙;软骨陷窝 / cell ~s 细胞空隙(结缔组织基质内) / dead ~ 无效腔;死隙(手术或创伤缝合后) / epidural ~ 硬膜外隙 / free way ~ 休止殆间隙 / interpleural ~ 胸膜间腔,纵隔 / popliteal ~ 腘窝 / subarachnoid ~ 蛛网膜下腔 | **~less** *a* 无限的;不占地位的

spacelab [ˈspeislæb] *n* 宇宙实验室,太空实验室

spacer [ˈspeisə] *n* 间隔区

spacing [ˈspeisiŋ] *n* 间距,间隔

spade [speid] *n* 铲;去睾者(阉人,阉兽)

spadic [ˈspeidik] *n* 古柯叶

spagyric [spəˈdʒirik] *a* 炼丹医术的,炼金医术的

spagyrist [ˈspædʒirist] *n* 炼丹医术家,化学医学家

Spalding's sign [ˈspɔːldiŋ](Alfred B. Spalding)斯波尔丁征(宫内胎儿X线片上颅顶骨重叠,表示胎儿已死亡)

Spallanzani's law [ˌspælənˈzæni](Lazaro Spallanzani)斯帕朗扎尼定律(年轻人细胞的再生能力较老年人强)

spallation [spɔːˈleiʃən] *n* 分裂,散裂

span [spæn] *n* 指距;全长;跨距;一段时间;广度 | life ~ 寿命

spanemia [spəˈniːmiə] *n* 贫血

spanemic [spəˈniːmik] *a* 贫血的 *n* 补血剂

Spaniopsis [ˌspæniˈɔpsis] *n* 鹬虻属
Spanish windlass [ˈspæniʃ ˈwindləs] 西班牙绞带(一种绞拉式止血带)
span(o)- [构词成分]缺乏,稀少
spanopnea [ˌspænɔpˈniːə] *n* 呼吸减少(一种神经性疾病,呼吸低而深,自觉呼吸困难)
spar [spɑː] *n* 晶石 | Iceland ~ 冰岛晶石(用于制造尼科尔〈Nicol〉棱镜)
sparfloxacin [spɑːˈflɔksəsin] *n* 司氟沙星(一种合成广谱抗菌药,口服给药)
sparganosis [ˌspɑːgəˈnəusis] *n* 裂头蚴病
sparganum [spɑːˈgeinəm] ([复] **spargana** [spɑːˈgeinə]) *n* 裂头蚴
sparsomycin [ˌspɑːsəuˈmaisin] *n* 司帕霉素(抗肿瘤抗菌素)
sparteine [ˈspɑːtiin] *n* 司巴丁,金雀花碱 | ~ sulfate 硫酸金雀花碱(催产药)
spartium [ˈspɑːʃiəm] *n* 金雀花
spasm [ˈspæzəm] *n* 痉挛 | ~ of accommodation 调节痉挛,调视痉挛(睫状肌痉挛,对近物产生过多调节) / bronchial ~ 支气管痉挛(气喘时) / cerebral ~ 大脑性痉挛 / clonic ~ 阵挛性痉挛 / cynic ~, canine ~ 痉笑 / facial ~ 面痉挛 / fixed ~ 持久性痉挛 / glottic ~ 声门痉挛,喉痉挛 / habit ~ 习惯性痉挛 / handicraft ~ 手艺工痉挛,职业性神经功能病 / intention ~ 意向性痉挛 / lock ~ 固定性痉挛,手指强直性痉挛 / mobile ~ 手足徐动症,指痉病 / nodding ~, salaam ~ 点头痉挛 / occupation ~, functional ~, professional ~ 职业性痉挛,职业性神经功能病 / rotatory ~ 旋头痉挛,转头痉挛 / saltatory ~, dancing ~ 痉跳病 / synclonic ~ 共同阵挛性痉挛 / tetanic ~ 破伤风痉挛;强直性痉挛,紧张性痉挛 / tonic ~ 强直性痉挛,紧张性痉挛 / winking ~, nictitating ~ 瞬目痉挛 / writers' ~ 书写痉挛
spasm(o)- [构词成分]痉挛
spasmodic [spæzˈmɔdik] *a* 痉挛的,抽搐的
spasmogen [ˈspæzmədʒən] *n* 致痉物
spasmogenic [ˌspæzməˈdʒenik] *n* 致痉的
spasmology [spæzˈmɔlədʒi] *n* 痉挛学
spasmolygmus [ˌspæzməˈligməs] *n* 痉挛性呃逆
spasmolysis [spæzˈmɔlisis] *n* 解痉[作用]
spasmolytic [ˌspæzməˈlitik], **spasmolysant** [spæzˈmɔlizənt] *a* 解痉的 *n* 解痉药
spasmophilia [ˌspæzməˈfiliə] *n* 痉挛素质 | **spasmophilic** [ˌspæzməˈfilik], **spasmophile** [ˈspæzməfail] *a*
spasmotin [ˈspæzmətin] *n* 麦角痉挛碱
spasmus [ˈspæzməs] *n* 【拉】痉挛 | ~ nutans 点头痉挛
spastic [ˈspæstik] *a* 痉挛[性]的;强直的,僵硬的 *n* 痉挛者
spasticity [spæsˈtisəti] *n* 痉挛状态;强直状态 | clasp-knife ~ 折刀式强直
spatia [ˈspeiʃiə] spatium 的复数
spatial [ˈspeiʃəl] *a* 空间的;隙的,间隙的,腔的 | **~ity** [speiʃiˈæləti] *n* 空间性
spatic [ˈspeitik] *a* 隙的,间隙的,腔的(尤指邻面间隙)
spatium [ˈspeiʃiəm] ([复] **spatia** [ˈspeiʃiə]) *n* 【拉】隙,间隙,腔
spatula [ˈspætjulə, -tʃə-] *n* 抹刀,刮铲;(调软膏用的)药刀,软膏刀;压舌板
spatular [ˈspætjulə, -tʃə-] *a* 抹刀状的,药刀状的
spatulate [ˈspætjulit, -tʃə-] *a* 抹刀状的,药刀状的 *vt* (用抹刀或软膏刀)调拌 | **spatulation** [ˌspætjuˈleiʃən, -tʃə-] *n* 调拌
spavin [ˈspævin] *n* 飞节内肿(马)
spavined [ˈspævind] *a* 患飞节内肿的
spawn [spɔːn] *n* 菌丝,菌柱,菌种体
spay [spei] *vt* 切除(动物的)卵巢,阉割
SPCA serum prothrombin conversion accelerator 血清凝血酶原转变加速因子(凝血因子Ⅶ)
Spearman's rank correlation coefficient(rho) [ˈspiəmən] (Charles Edward Spearman)斯皮尔曼秩相关系数(ρ)(指两个变量以秩代替实际值后计算出的积矩相关系数)
spearmint [ˈspiəmint] *n* 留兰香,绿薄荷
specialism [ˈspeʃəlizəm] *n* 专长,特长;专业,专门学科 | medical ~ 医学专业
specialist [ˈspeʃəlist] *n* 专家,专科医师 | clinical nurse ~, nurse ~ 护理专家,临床护理专业人员
speciality [ˌspeʃiˈæləti], **specialty** [ˈspeʃəlti] *n* 专业;特长;特性,特征
specialize [ˈspeʃəlaiz] *vt* 专门化;特化,专化 | **specialization** [ˌspeʃəlaiˈzeiʃən, -liˈz-] *n* 特殊化,专业化;特化,专化 / **~d** *a* 专门的;特化的,专化的
speciate [ˈspiːʃieit] *vi* 物种形成 | **speciation** [ˌspiːʃiˈeiʃən] *n*
species [ˈspiːʃiːz] [单复同] *n* 物种,种 | diovulatory ~ 二卵种 / fugitive ~ 易逝种(在某一地区短时期居住或生长的植物或动物种) / monovulatory ~ 单卵种 / polyovulatory ~ 多卵种 / type ~ 模式种
species-specific [ˈspiːʃiːz spiˈsifik] *a* 种特异性的(指抗原、药物或传染物)
specific [spiˈsifik] *a* 特有的,特异性的,专一性的;种的;有特效的;由一种病菌引起的 *n* 特效药
specificity [ˌspesiˈfisəti] *n* 特异性,特殊性;专一性;特性,特征 | organ ~ 器官特异性 / species ~ 种特异性

specimen [ˈspesimin] *n* 标本;样品,(检验用)抽样 | corrosion ~ 腐蚀标本

SPECT single photon emission computed tomography 单光子发射计算体层摄影[术]

spectacle [ˈspektəkl] *n* [复]眼镜 | compound ~s 复合眼镜 / decentered ~s 偏心眼镜 / divided ~s 双焦点眼镜 / pantoscopic ~s 双焦点眼镜 / periscopic ~s 周视眼镜 / prismatic ~s 三棱眼镜 / pulpit ~s 半片阅读镜 / stenopeic ~s 小孔镜 / tinted ~s 有色眼镜 / wire frame ~s 镍网眼镜

spectinomycin [ˌspektinəuˈmaisin] *n* 大观霉素(抗生素类药) | ~ hydrochloride 盐酸大观霉素

spectra [ˈspektrə] spectrum 的复数

spectral [ˈspektrəl] *a* 光谱的

spectrin [ˈspektrin] *n* 血影蛋白,红细胞膜内蛋白

spectr(o)- [构词成分]谱,光谱

spectrochrome [ˈspektrəukrəum] *a* 色光谱的

spectrocolorimeter [ˌspektrəuˌkʌləˈrimitə] *n* 单色盲分光镜

spectrofluorometer [ˌspektrəufluəˈrɔmitə] *n* 荧光分光计

spectrograph [ˈspektrəugrɑːf, -græf] *n* 光谱仪,摄谱仪 | mass ~ 质谱仪(即质谱计)

spectrometer [spekˈtrɔmitə] *n* 分光计;光谱计 | mass ~ 质谱计(亦称质谱仪)

spectrometry [spekˈtrɔmitri] *n* 分光术,光谱测定法

spectrophotofluorometer [ˌspektrəuˌfəutəuˌfluəˈrɔmitə] *n* 分光光度荧光计

spectrophotometer [ˌspektrəufəuˈtɔmitə] *n* 分光光度计 | **spectrophotometry** *n* 分光光度测定法

spectropolarimeter [ˌspektrəuˌpəuləˈrimitə] *n* 旋光分光计,分光偏振计

spectropyrheliometer [ˌspektrəupaiəˌhiːliˈɔmitə] *n* 日射光谱仪

spectroscope [ˈspektrəskəup] *n* 分光镜 | **spectroscopic** [ˌspektrəˈskɔpik] *a*

spectroscopy [spekˈtrɔskəpi] *n* 光谱学;分光术,分光镜检查

spectrum [ˈspektrəm] ([复] **spectrums** 或 **spectra** [ˈspektrə]) *n* 光谱,波谱,谱 | absorption ~ 吸收[光]谱 / broad- ~ 广谱(指抗生素) / action ~ 作用光谱 / continuous ~ 连续谱 / diffraction ~ 衍射光谱 / electromagnetic ~ 电磁波谱 / fortification ~ 闪光暗点 / ocular ~ 后像 / toxin ~ 毒素谱(抗毒素中和能力的图解说明) / x-ray X 线谱

specular [ˈspekjulə] *a* 用窥器[检查]的

speculum [ˈspekjuləm] ([复] **speculums** 或 **specula** [ˈspekjulə]) *n* 窥器,扩张器 | duck-billed ~ 鸭嘴式[阴道]窥器 / eye ~ 开睑器 / stop ~ 固定开睑器 / wire bivalve ~ 镍条双瓣窥器(检阴道)

speech [spiːtʃ] *n* 言语 | clipped ~, scamping ~, slurred ~ 缩简言语,言语不清(麻痹性痴呆特征之一) / echo ~ 模仿言语 / esophageal ~ 食管言语(喉切除术后) / incoherent ~ 语无伦次,言语散乱(连串思维障碍所致) / jumbled ~ 紊乱言语,言语讷吃 / mirror ~ 倒语,音节颠倒 / plateau ~ 单音调言语 / scanning ~ 断续言语 / staccato ~ 断音言语(见于多发性硬化症)

Spee's curve (curvature) [spei] (Ferdinand G. von Spee)施佩曲线(牙列殆面曲线)

spell [spel] *n* (病的)小发作

spelling [ˈspeliŋ] *n* 拼字;拼法,缀字法 | finger ~ 手指字母拼读,手指语

Spemann's induction [ˈʃpeimən] (Hans Spemann)施佩曼诱导(胎儿发育早期某些组织对相邻组织起刺激性与指引性作用)

Spencer-Parker vaccine [ˈspensə ˈpɑːkə] (Roscoe R. Spencer; Ralph R. Parker)斯宾塞-派克疫苗(落基山斑疹热疫苗,由感染的蜱研磨配制而成)

Spence's tail [spens] (James Spence)斯彭斯尾(乳腺组织突入腋区,有时形成一个可见的团块,此团块在月经前或哺乳期可能扩大)

Spengler's fragments [ˈspenglə] (Carl Spengler)斯彭格勒碎片(结核病患者痰中的圆形小片) | ~ immune bodies 斯彭格勒免疫体(从免疫动物〈经人和牛结核杆菌免疫者〉血细胞提取的制剂,这是基于结核病的免疫物质是在血细胞内,而不是在血清内的想法。此制剂曾一度用于治疗结核病) / ~ tuberculin 牛结核菌素

Spens' syndrome [spenz] (Thomas Spens)斯彭斯综合征(见 Adams-Stokes disease)

sperm [spəːm] *n* 精液;精子 | muzzled ~ 迟钝精子

sperma [ˈspəːmə] *n* 【拉】精液;精子

spermaceti [ˌspəːməˈseti] *n* 鲸蜡

spermacrasia [ˌspəːməˈkreiziə] *n* (精液中)精子缺乏

spermagglutination [ˌspəːməˌgluːtiˈneiʃən] *n* 精子凝集反应

spermalist [ˈspəːməlist] *n* 精源论者(见 spermist)

spermanucleic acid [ˌspəːmənjuːˈkliːik] 精子核酸

spermary [ˈspəːməri] *n* 睾丸;精巢

spermase [ˈspəːmeis] *n* 麦芽氧化酶

spermateliosis [ˌspəːməˌtiːliˈəusis] *n* 精子形成(由精细胞形成精子的过程)

spermatemphraxis [ˌspəːmətemˈfræksis] *n* 精液阻塞

spermatic [ˌspəːˈmætik] *a* 精子的;精液的
spermaticide [spəːˈmætisaid] *n* 杀精子药
spermatid [ˈspəːmətid] *n* 精细胞,精子细胞
spermatin [ˈspəːmətin] *n* 精液蛋白
spermatism [ˈspəːmətizəm] *n* 精子团;精液生成;射精
spermatitis [ˌspəːməˈtaitis] *n* 输精管炎;精索炎
spermat(o)-, sperm(o)- [构词成分] 种子;精子,精液
spermatoblast [ˈspəːmətəuˌblæst] *n* 精细胞,精子细胞
spermatocele [ˈspəːmətəuˌsiːl] *n* 精液囊肿(附睾或睾丸网囊肿)
spermatocelectomy [spəːˌmætəusiˈlektəmi] *n* 精液囊肿切除术
spermatocidal [ˌspəːmətəuˈsaidl] *a* 杀精子的
spermatocide [ˈspəːmətəuˌsaid] *n* 杀精子剂
spermatocyst [ˈspəːmətəuˌsist] *n* 精囊;精子囊肿
spermatocystectomy [ˌspəːmətəusisˈtektəmi] *n* 精囊切除术
spermatocystitis [ˌspəːmətəusisˈtaitis] *n* 精囊炎
spermatocystotomy [ˌspəːmətəusisˈtɔtəmi] *n* 精囊切开术
spermatocyte [ˈspəːmətəuˌsait] *n* 精母细胞 | primary ~ 初级精母细胞 / secondary ~ 次级精母细胞 | **spermatocytal** [ˌspəːmətəuˈsaitl] *a*
spermatocytogenesis [ˌspəːmətəuˌsaitəuˈdʒenisis] *n* 精母细胞发生
spermatocytoma [ˌspəːmətəusaiˈtəumə] *n* 精原细胞瘤
spermatogenesis [ˌspəːmətəuˈdʒenisis], **spermatogeny** [ˌspəːməˈtɔdʒini] *n* 精子发生,精子生成(精子形成的第一阶段,精原细胞生成精母细胞,然后生成精子)
spermatogenic [ˌspəːmətəuˈdʒenik], **spermatogenous** [ˌspəːməˈtɔdʒinəs] *a* 精子发生的,生精子的
spermatogenetic [ˌspəːmətəudʒəˈnetik] *a* 精子生成的,生精子的
spermatogonium [ˌspəːmətəuˈgəuniəm] ([复] **spermatogonia** [ˌspəːmətəuˈgəuniə]), **spermatogone** [ˈspəːmətəuˌgəun] *n* 精原细胞
spermatoid [ˈspəːmətɔid] *a* 精子样的
spermatology [ˌspəːməˈtɔlədʒi] *n* 精液学 | **spermatological** [ˌspəːmətəuˈlɔdʒikəl] *a* / **spermatologist** *n* 精液学家
spermatolysin [ˌspəːməˈtɔlisin] *n* 溶精子素
spermatolysis [ˌspəːməˈtɔlisis] *n* 精子溶解 | **spermatolytic** [ˌspəːmətəuˈlitik] *a* 溶解精子的
spermatomerite [ˌspəːmətəuˈmiərait], **spermatomere** [ˈspəːmətəuˌmiə] *n* 精核染色体
spermatomicron [ˌspəːmətəuˈmaikrɔn] *n* 精液微粒(用超显微镜可见其布朗〈brownian〉运动)
spermatopathia [ˌspəːmətəuˈpæθiə], **spermatopathy** [ˌspəːməˈtɔpəθi] *n* 精液病
spermatophore [ˈspəːmətəuˌfɔː] *n* 精原细胞;(一些低等动物所突出的)精子包囊,精包,精荚
spermatopoietic [ˌspəːmətəupɔiˈetik] *a* 生精子的;促精液分泌的
spermatorrhea [ˌspəːmətəˈriːə] *n* 遗精,溢精
spermatoschesis [ˌspəːməˈtɔskisis] *n* 精液分泌抑制
spermatosome [spəːˈmætəsəum] *n* 精子
spermatospore [spəːˈmætəspɔː] *n* 精原细胞
spermatotoxic [ˌspəːmətəuˈtɔksik] *a* 杀精子的,毒害精子的,精子毒的
spermatotoxin [ˌspəːmətəuˈtɔksin] *n* 精子毒素
spermatovum [ˌspəːməˈtəuvəm] *n* 受精卵
spermatoxin [ˌspəːməˈtɔksin] *n* 精子毒素
spermatozoicide [ˌspəːmətəuˈzəuisaid] *n* 杀精子剂
spermatozoid [ˈspəːmətəuzɔid] *n* 精子;游动精子(植物雄生殖细胞)
spermatozoon [ˌspəːmətəuˈzəuɔn] ([复] **spermatozoa** [ˌspəːmətəuˈzəuə]) *n* 精子 | **spermatozoal**, **spermatozoan**, **spermatozoic** *a*
spermaturia [ˌspəːməˈtjuəriə] *n* 精液尿
spermectomy [spəːˈmektəmi] *n* 精索切除术
spermia [ˈspəːmiə] spermium 的复数
spermiation [ˌspəːmiˈeiʃən] *n* 精子放出,放精(成熟精子从塞托利〈Sertoli〉细胞释放出来)
spermicidal [ˌspəːmiˈsaidl] *a* 杀精子的
spermicide [ˈspəːmisaid] *n* 杀精子剂
spermid [ˈspəːmid] *n* 精细胞,精子细胞
spermidine [ˈspəːmidiːn] *n* 精脒,亚精胺
spermiduct [ˈspəːmidʌkt] *n* 精管(射精管与输精管的合称)
spermine [ˈspəːmi(ː)n] *n* 精胺 | ~ phosphate 磷酸精胺
spermi(o)- 见 spermat(o)-
spermiocyte [ˈspəːmiəˌsait] *n* 初级精母细胞
spermiogenesis [ˌspəːmiəuˈdʒənisis] *n* 精子发生,精子形成(由精细胞转变成精子的过程)
spermiogonium [ˌspəːmiəuˈgəuniəm] *n* 精原细胞
spermiogram [ˈspəːmiəgræm] *n* 精子发生图
spermioteleosis [ˌspəːmiəuˌtiːliˈəusis] *n* 精子发育过程,精子成熟 | **spermioteleotic** [ˌspəːmiəuˌtiːliˈɔtik] *a*
spermist [ˈspəːmist] *n* 精源论者(胚中预成说的信仰者,认为精子是完整的微型人)
spermium [ˈspəːmiəm] ([复] **spermia** [ˈspəːmiə]) *n*【拉】[成熟]精子
sperm(o)- 见 spermat(o)-

spermoblast [ˈspəːməblæst] *n* 精细胞,精子细胞
spermocytoma [ˌspəːməusaiˈtəumə] *n* 精原细胞瘤
spermolith [ˈspəːməliθ] *n* 精管石
spermoloropexy [ˌspəːməuˈlɔrəˌpeksi], **spermoloropexis** [ˌspəːməuˌlɔrəˈpeksis] *n* 精索固定术
spermolysin [spəːˈmɔlisin] *n* 溶精子素,精子毒素
spermolysis [spəːˈmɔlisis] *n* 精子溶解 | **spermolytic** [ˌspəːməuˈlitik] *a* 溶解精子的
spermoneuralgia [ˌspəːməunjuəˈrældʒiə] *n* 精索神经痛
Spermophilus [spəˈmɔfiləs] *n* 掘地小栗鼠属
spermophlebectasia [ˌspəːməˌflibekˈteiziə] *n* 精索静脉曲张
spermoplasm [ˈspəːməplæzəm] *n* 精质(精细胞原生质)
spermosphere [ˈspəːməsfiə] *n* 精细胞球
spermospore [ˈspəːməspɔː] *n* 精原细胞
spermotoxin [ˌspəːməuˈtɔksin] *n* 精子毒素 | **spermotoxic** [ˌspəːməˈtɔksik] *a*
spes [spiːs] *n*【拉】希望 | ~ phthisica 结核病患者痊愈希望
SPF specific-pathogen free 无特殊病原体的(指用于实验饲养的定菌动物,并已知无特殊病原菌)
sp gr specific gravity 比重
sph spherical 球面的;spherical lens 球面透镜
sphacelate [ˈsfæsileit] *vt, vi* 生坏疽,坏疽化,形成腐肉 | **sphacelation** [ˌsfæsiˈleiʃən] *n* 坏疽形成,坏疽化,腐肉形成
sphacelinic acid [ˌsfæsiˈlinik] *n* 麦角毒酸
sphacelism [ˈsfæsilizəm] *n* 坏疽化,坏死,腐肉形成
sphaceloderma [ˌsfæsiləuˈdəːmə] *n* 皮坏疽(或由此产生的溃疡)
sphacelotoxin [ˌsfæsiləuˈtɔksin] *n* 痉挛毒素;麦角痉挛碱
sphacelous [ˈsfæsiləs] *a* 坏疽的,腐肉形成的
sphacelus [ˈsfæsiləs] *n*【拉】坏死物,腐肉
Sphaenacanthina [ˌsfenəkænˈθainə] *n* 楔棘虫亚目
Sphaeranthus [sfiˈrænθəs] *n* 戴星草属
Sphaerellarina [ˌsfiərelәˈrainə] *n* 球壳亚目
Sphaeria [ˈsfiəriə] *n* 球果菌属 | ~ sinensis 中华球果菌
Sphaeriales [ˌsfiəriˈeiliːz] *n* 球壳目
sphaer(o)- 以 sphaer(o)-起始的词,同样见以 spher(o)-起始的词
Sphaeroides maculatus [sfiəˈrɔidiːzmækjuˈleitəs] *n* 斑点圆鲀
Sphaeromyxa [ˌsfiərəuˈmiksə] *n* 球黏菌属
Sphaerophorus [sfiəˈrəufərəs] *n* 丝杆菌属 | ~ necrophorus 坏死厌氧丝杆菌
Sphaerotilus [sfiəˈrəutiləs] *n* 球衣细菌属
sphagiasmus [ˌsfeidʒiˈæzməs] *n* 颈肌痉挛(癫痫时);癫痫小发作
sphagitis [sfəˈdʒaitis] *n* 咽喉炎
Sphecidae [ˈsfiːsidiː] *n* 膜翅科
sphenethmoid [sfəˈneθmɔid] *a* 蝶筛[骨]的
sphenion [ˈsfiːniən] ([复] **sphenia** [ˈsfiːniə]) *n* 蝶点(测颅点,在顶骨蝶角部)
sphen(o)- [构词成分]楔形;蝶骨
sphenobasilar [ˌsfiːnəuˈbæsilə] *a* 蝶骨枕底部的
sphenoccipital [ˌsfiːnɔkˈsipitl] *a* 蝶枕[骨]的
sphenocephalus [ˌsfiːnəuˈsefələs] *n* 楔形头畸胎
sphenocephaly [ˌsfiːnəuˈsefəli] *n* 楔形头[畸形]
sphenoethmoid [ˌsfiːnəuˈeθmɔid] *a* 蝶筛[骨]的
sphenofrontal [ˌsfiːnəuˈfrʌntl] *a* 蝶额[骨]的
sphenoid [ˈsfiːnɔid] *a* 楔形的,楔状的;蝶骨的 *n* 蝶骨 | **~al** [sfiːˈnɔidl] *a* 蝶骨的
sphenoiditis [ˌsfiːnɔiˈdaitis] *n* 蝶窦炎
sphenoidostomy [ˌsfiːnɔiˈdɔstəmi] *n* 蝶窦开放术
sphenoidotomy [ˌsfiːnɔiˈdɔtəmi] *n* 蝶窦切开术
sphenomalar [ˌsfiːnəuˈmeilə] *a* 蝶颧[骨]的
sphenomaxillary [ˌsfiːnəuˈmæksiləri] *a* 蝶上颌的
sphenometer [sfiːˈnɔmitə] *n* (楔形)骨片测量器(测量手术中切除的楔形骨片,以纠正弯曲)
Sphenomonadina [ˌsfiːnəuˌməunəˈdainə] *n* 楔胞藻亚目
Sphenomonas [ˌsfiːnəuˈməunəs] *n* 楔胞藻属
spheno-occipital [ˌsfiːnəuɔkˈsipitl] *a* 蝶枕[骨]的
sphenopagus [sfiːˈnɔpəgəs] *n* 蝶骨互连双胎[畸形]
sphenopalatine [ˌsfiːnəuˈpælətin] *a* 蝶腭[骨]的
sphenoparietal [ˌsfiːnəupəˈraiitl] *a* 蝶顶[骨]的
sphenopetrosal [ˌsfiːnəupiˈtrəusəl] *a* 蝶骨岩部的
sphenorbital [sfiːˈnɔːbitl] *a* 蝶骨眶部的
sphenosquamosal [ˌsfiːnəuskweiˈməusəl] *a* 蝶骨鳞部的
sphenotemporal [ˌsfiːnəuˈtempərəl] *a* 蝶颞[骨]的
sphenotic [sfiːˈnɔtik] *a* 蝶骨的
sphenotresia [ˌsfiːnəuˈtriːziə] *n* 颅骨钻孔术
sphenotribe [ˈsfiːnətraib] *n* (胎儿)碎颅器
sphenotripsy [ˈsfiːnəˌtripsi] *n* (胎儿)碎颅术
sphenoturbinal [ˌsfiːnəuˈtəːbinl] *a* 蝶鼻甲的
sphenovomerine [ˌsfiːnəuˈvəumərin] *a* 蝶犁[骨]的
sphenozygomatic [ˌsfiːnəuzaigəˈmætik] *a* 蝶颧

[骨]的

sphere [sfiə] *n* 球,球形 | attraction ~ 吸引球,中心体 / embryotic ~ 桑葚胚 / segmentation ~ 桑葚胚;卵裂球 / vitelline ~, yolk ~ 卵黄球,桑葚胚

spheresthesia [ˌsfiəris'θiːzjə] *n* 球状感觉(喉部球状物阻塞感),癔球感

spheric(al) ['sferik(əl)] *a* 球的,球形的

spher(o)- [构词成分]球,球体

spherocylinder [ˌsfiərəu'silində] *n* 球柱[透]镜

spherocyte ['sfiərəsait] *n* 球形细胞(见于遗传性球形细胞增多症,亦见于获得性溶血性贫血) | **spherocytic** [ˌsfiərəu'sitik] *a*

spherocytosis [ˌsfiərəusai'təusis] *n* 球形细胞增多症 | hereditary ~ 遗传性球形细胞增多症(一种先天性家族型溶血性贫血)

spheroid ['sfiərɔid] *n* 球[形]体,球状体 *a* 球形的,球状的 | **~al** [sfiə'rɔidl] *a* 球形的,球状的

spheroidin [sfiə'rɔidin] *n* 河豚精蛋白,河豚毒素

spherolith ['sfiərəliθ] *n* 球状石(新生儿肾组织内沉积物)

spheroma [sfiə'rəumə] *n* 球状瘤

spherometer [sfiə'rɔmitə] *n* 球径计,测球仪

spherophakia [ˌsfiərəu'feikiə] *n* 球形晶状体

Spherophorus [sfiə'rəufərəs] *n* 丝杆菌属(即 Sphaerophorus)

spheroplast ['sferəplæst] *n* 球浆体,球形体

spherospermia [ˌsfiərəu'spəːmiə] *n* 球状精子,无尾精子,缺尾精子

spherule ['sferjuːl] *n* 小球[体] | **spherular** *a*

spherulin ['sfiərjulin] *n* 内孢囊素(一种皮肤试验抗原,由内孢囊-内孢子期的粗球孢子菌制成,可检测几乎全部球孢子菌素阳性者,也可检测以往接触过粗球孢子菌的球孢子菌素阴性者)

sphincter ['sfiŋktə] *n*【拉】括约肌 | cardiac ~, cardioesophageal ~ 贲门括约肌 / cornual ~, tubal ~ 子宫输卵管角括约肌,输卵管括约肌 / ~ of eye 眼括约肌,眼轮匝肌 / hepatic ~ 肝静脉括约肌 / inguinal ~ 腹股沟管括约肌 / pyloric ~ 幽门括约肌 / rectal ~ 直肠括约肌 | **~al** ['sfiŋktərəl], **~ic** [sfiŋk'terik] *a*

sphincteralgia [ˌsfiŋktə'rældʒiə] *n* (肛门)括约肌痛

sphincterectomy [ˌsfiŋktə'rektəmi] *n* 括约肌切除术

sphincterismus [ˌsfiŋktə'rizməs] *n* (肛门)括约肌痉挛

sphincteritis [ˌsfiŋktə'raitis] *n* 括约肌炎

sphincterolysis [ˌsfiŋktə'rɔlisis] *n* 虹膜前粘连分离术

sphincterometry [ˌsfiŋktə'rɔmətri] *n* 括约肌测压

sphincteroplasty ['sfiŋktərəuˌplæsti] *n* 括约肌成形术

sphincteroscope ['sfiŋktərəuˌskəup] *n* (肛门)括约肌镜 | **sphincteroscopy** [ˌsfiŋktə'rɔskəpi] *n* (肛门)括约肌镜检查

sphincterotome ['sfiŋktərəuˌtəum] *n* 括约肌切开器

sphincterotomy ['sfiŋktə'rɔtəmi] *n* 括约肌切开术 | internal ~ (肛门)内括约肌切开术

sphinganine ['sfiŋgəniːn] *n* 二氢鞘氨醇

sphingo- [构词成分][神经]鞘氨醇,[神经]鞘脂类

sphingogalactoside ['sfiŋgəugə'læktəsaid] *n* [神经]鞘半乳糖苷(戈谢〈Gaucher〉病时组成脾脏特有的部分物质)

sphingoglycolipid [ˌsfiŋgəuˌglaikəu'lipid] *n* [神经]鞘糖脂

sphingoin [ˌsfiŋgəuin] *n* [神经]鞘氨[基]脂

sphingol [ˌsfiŋgɔl] *n* [神经]鞘氨醇

sphingolipid [ˌsfiŋgəu'lipid] *n* [神经]鞘脂类

sphingolipidosis [ˌsfiŋgəuˌlipi'dəusis] ([复] **sphingolipidoses** [ˌsfiŋgəˌlipi'dəusiːz]) *n* 神经鞘脂贮积症(如家族性脾性贫血、类脂组织细胞增多病及黑矇性家族性白痴)

sphingolipodystrophy [ˌsfiŋgəuˌlipədistrəfi] *n* [神经]鞘脂代谢障碍(包括家族性脾性贫血、异染性白质营养障碍、类脂组织细胞增多病等)

sphingomyelin [ˌsfiŋgəu'maiəlin] *n* [神经]鞘磷脂

sphingomyelinase [ˌsfiŋgəu'maiəlineis] *n* [神经]鞘磷脂酶,[神经]鞘磷脂磷酸二酯酶

sphingomyelinase deficiency [神经]鞘磷脂酶缺乏症,尼曼-皮克〈Niemann-Pick〉病

sphingomyelinosis [ˌsfiŋgəu'maiəli'nəusis] *n* [神经]鞘髓磷脂沉积病

sphingomyelin phosphodiesterase [ˌsfiŋgəu'maiəlin ˌfɔsfədai'estəreis] [神经]鞘磷脂磷酸二酯酶(此酶缺乏为一种常染色体隐性性状,可致尼曼-皮克〈Nieman-Pick〉病,亦称[神经]鞘磷脂酶)

sphingophospholipid [ˌsfiŋgəuˌfɔsfə'lipid] *n* [神经]鞘磷脂(含鞘氨醇及磷酸胆碱)

sphingosine ['sfiŋgəsi(ː)n] *n* [神经]鞘氨醇

sphingosine *N*-acyltransferase ['sfiŋgəsi nˌæsil'trænsfəreis] [神经]鞘氨醇 *N*-酰基转移酶

sphygmic ['sfigmik] *a* 脉的

sphygm(o)- [构词成分]脉,脉搏

sphygmobologram [ˌsfigməu'bəuləgræm] *n* 脉能图,脉力图

sphygmobolometer [ˌsfigməubə'lɔmitə] *n* 脉能描记器(也同样间接描记心收缩力) | **sphyg-**

mobolometry [ˌsfigməubəˈlɔmitri] *n* 脉能描记法

sphygmocardiogram [ˌsfigməuˈkɑːdiəgræm] *n* 心动脉搏图

sphygmocardiograph [ˌsfigməuˈkɑːdiəgrɑːf, -græf] *n* 心动脉搏描记器

sphygmocardioscope [ˌsfigməuˈkɑːdiəskəup] *n* 心动心音脉搏描记器

sphygmochronograph [ˌsfigməuˈkrəunəgrɑːf, -græf] *n* 脉搏自动描记器

sphygmodynamometer [ˌsfigməuˌdainəˈmɔmitə] *n* 脉力计

sphygmogenin [sfigˈmɔdʒinin] *n* 肾上腺素

sphygmogram [ˈsfigməgræm] *n* 脉搏图

sphygmograph [ˈsfigməgrɑːf, -græf] *n* 脉搏描记器 | **~ic** [ˌsfigməˈgræfik] *a* 脉搏描记的 / **~y** [sfigˈmɔgrəfi] *n* 脉搏描记法

sphygmoid [ˈsfigmɔid] *a* 脉搏样的

sphygmology [sfigˈmɔlədʒi] *n* 脉学,脉搏学

sphygmomanometer [ˌsfigməuməˈnɔmitə] *n* 血压计

sphygmometer [sfigˈmɔmitə] *n* 脉搏计

sphygmometrograph [ˌsfigməuˈmetrəgrɑːf, -græf] *n* 血压描记器

sphygmometroscope [ˌsfigməuˈmetrəskəup] *n* 听脉血压计

sphygmo-oscillometer [ˌsfigməuˌɔsiˈlɔmitə] *n* 示波血压计

sphygmopalpation [ˌsfigməupælˈpeiʃən] *n* 切脉,按脉

sphygmophone [ˈsfigməfəum] *n* 脉音听诊器

sphygmoplethysmograph [ˌsfigməupliˈθizməgrɑːf] *n* 脉搏体积描记器,脉容[积]描记器

sphygmoscope [ˈsfigməskəup] *n* 脉搏检视器

sphygmoscopy [sfigˈmɔskəpi] *n* 脉搏检查

sphygmosystole [ˌsfigməuˈsistəli] *n* 收缩期脉搏曲线

sphygmotonometer [ˌsfigməutəˈnɔmitə] *n* 脉张力计;动脉管弹性计

sphygmoviscosimetry [ˌsfigməuˌviskəuˈsimitri] *n* 血压血液黏度测量法

sphyrectomy [sfaiˈrektəmi] *n* 锤骨切除术

sphyrotomy [sfaiˈrɔtəmi] *n* 锤骨切开术,锤骨切除术

spica [ˈspaikə] ([复] **spicas** 或 **spicae** [ˈspaisiː]) *n* 【拉】人字形绷带

spicular [ˈspikjulə] *a* 针的,刺的

spiculate [ˈspikjulit] *a* 针状的,刺状的

spicule [ˈspaikjuːl, ˈspikjuːl] *n* 针,刺;针状体;交合刺

spiculum [ˈspikjuləm] ([复] **spicula** [ˈspikjulə]) *n* 【拉】针,刺;交合刺

spider [ˈspaidə] *n* 蜘蛛;蛛状痣 | arterial ~, ~ burst, vascular ~ 蛛状痣 / banana ~ 疾行异足蛛 / black widow ~ 黑寡妇毒蛛,致命红斑毒蛛 / brown recluse ~ 棕色隐士蜘蛛 / cat-headed ~ 猫头蛛 / European wolf ~ 欧狼蛛 / funnel-web ~ 漏斗网蜘蛛 / lynx ~ 山猫蛛 / tree funnel-web ~ 树状漏斗网蜘蛛 / wandering ~ 游动蜘蛛

Spieghel's line [ˈʃpigəl] (Adrian van der Spieghel) 半月线(腹横肌)

Spiegler-Fendt pseudolymphoma (sarcoid) [ˈʃpiːglə fent] (Edward Spiegler; Heinrich Fendt) 施皮格勒-芬特假淋巴瘤(肉样瘤),皮肤淋巴细胞瘤

Spiegler's test (reagent) [ˈʃpiːglə] (Edouard Spiegler) 施皮格勒试验(试剂)(检白蛋白)

Spielmeyer-Vogt disease [ˈʃpiːlmiəfəukt] (Walter Spielmeyer; Heinrich Vogt) 施-福病,黑矇性白痴

Spigelia [spaiˈdʒiːliə] (Adriaan van der Spieghel) *n* 驱虫草属

spigelian [spaiˈdʒiːliən] (Adriaan van der Spieghel) *a* 斯皮格尔的(如 ~ line 半月线, ~ lobe 尾状叶)

spigeline [spaiˈdʒiːliːn] *n* 赤根驱虫草素

spignet [ˈspignet] *n* 美楤木

spike [spaik] *n* (曲线的)峰;(噬菌体)刺突;穗状花序,穗

spikenard [ˈspaiknɑːd] *n* 印度甘松香 | American ~ 美楤木 / false ~ 假甘松香

Spilanthes [spaiˈlænθiːz] *n* 千日菊属

spillway [ˈspilwei] *n* 溢出道,溢口(咀嚼时颊面间食物溢出口)

spin [spin] *n* 旋转,自旋

spina [ˈspainə] ([复] **spinae** [ˈspainiː]) *n* 【拉】棘,刺;脊柱 | ~ bifida 脊柱裂

spinach, spinage [ˈspinidʒ] *n* 波菜

spinacin [ˈspainəsin] *n* 菠菜蛋白,菠菜素

spinal [ˈspainl] *a* 棘的,刺的;脊柱的

spinalgia [spaiˈnældʒiə] *n* 脊痛

spinalis [spaiˈneilis] *n* 【拉】棘肌 *a* 棘的;脊柱的

spinant [ˈspainənt] *n* 脊髓兴奋药

spinate [ˈspaineit] *a* 有棘的,棘状的

spindle [ˈspindl] *n* 梭;纺锤体 | aortic ~ 主动脉梭 / central ~ 中心纺锤体 / cleavage ~ 卵裂纺锤体 / enamel ~s 釉梭 / muscle ~, neuromuscular ~ 肌梭,神经肌梭 / nuclear ~ 核纺锤体 / tendon ~ 腱梭 / tigroid ~s 虎斑小体

spine [spain] *n* 棘,刺;脊柱 | alar ~, angular ~ 角棘 / bamboo ~ 竹节样脊柱(见于类风湿脊柱炎的一种 X 线特征) / basilar ~ 咽结节 / cleft

~ 脊柱裂 / dorsal ~ 脊柱 / hemal ~ 血管棘 / hysterical ~ 癔症性脊柱病态 / ischial ~, ~ of ischium 坐骨棘 / kissing ~s 吻状棘突,接触棘突(椎骨) / pharyngeal ~ 咽棘 / poker ~, rigid ~ 脊柱强直 / railway ~ 铁路事故性脊柱(脊髓损伤后的外伤性神经功能病) / typhoid ~ 伤寒性脊柱(病)

Spinelli's operation [spiˈneli] (Pier G. Spinelli) 斯平内利手术(子宫翻出修复术)

spinifugal [spaiˈnifjugəl] *a* 离脊髓的,脊髓传出的

spinipetal [spaiˈnipitl] *a* 向脊髓的

Spinitectus gracilis [ˌspainiˈtektəsˈgræsilis] 薄脊四叠线虫

spinnbarkeit [ˌspinbɑːkait] *n* 【德】(子宫颈)黏液拉丝现象(用以观察卵巢排卵功能)

spinobulbar [ˌspainəuˈbʌlbə] *a* 脊髓延髓的

spinocellular [ˌspainəuˈseljulə] *a* 棘细胞的

spinocerebellar [ˌspainəuˌseriˈbelə] *a* 脊髓小脑的

spinocerebellum [ˌspainəuseriˈbeləm] *n* 脊髓小脑,旧小脑,原小脑

spinocortical [ˌspainəuˈkɔːtikəl] *a* 脊髓[大脑]皮质的

spinocostalis [ˌspainəukɔsˈteilis] *n* 棘肋肌(上后锯肌及下后锯肌的合称)

spinogalvanization [ˌspainəuˈgælvənaiˈzeiʃən, -niˈz-] *n* 脊髓[直]流电疗法

spinoglenoid [ˌspainəuˈgliːnɔid] *a* 肩胛冈关节盂的

spinogram [ˌspainəgræm] *n* 脊柱 X 线[照]片;脊髓造影[照]片

spinopetal [spaiˈnɔpitl] *a* 向脊髓的

spinose [ˈspainəus], **spinous** [ˈspainəs] *a* 棘状的;棘的,刺的;棘突的

spinotectal [ˌspainəuˈtektl] *a* 脊髓顶盖的,顶盖脊髓的

spinothalamic [ˌspainəuθəˈlæmik] *a* 脊髓丘脑的

spinthariscope [spinˈθæriskəup] *n* 闪烁镜(检察镭射气)

spintherism [ˈspinθərizəm], **spintheropia** [ˌspinθəˈrəupiə] *n* 闪光幻视(玻璃状体液内发生胆固醇结晶,是炎症或其他眼病后的蜕变)

spintherometer [ˌspinθəˈrɔmitə], **spintometer** [spinˈtɔmitə] *n* X 线透度计

spiperone [ˈspipərəun] *n* 螺哌隆(安定药,用于治疗精神分裂症)

spir. spiritus【拉】乙醇,酊剂

spiracle [ˈspirəkəl] *n* 喷水口;气门,气孔

spiradenoma [ˈspairædiˈnəumə] *n* 螺旋腺瘤(即汗腺腺瘤) | cylindromatous ~ 圆柱瘤状汗腺腺瘤,圆柱瘤 / eccrine ~ 小汗腺螺旋腺瘤

spiral [ˈspaiərəl] *a* 螺旋[形]的 *n* 螺旋[形];螺线;蜷线

spiramycin [ˌspaiərəˈmaisin] *n* 螺旋霉素(抗生素类药)

Spiranthes [spaiˈrænθiːz] *n* 绶草属

spireme [ˈspaiəriːm] *n* 染色质纽,丝球

spirilla [spaiəˈrilə] spirillum 的复数

Spirillaceae [ˌspaiəriˈleisiiː] *n* 螺菌科

spirillemia [ˌspaiəriˈliːmiə] *n* 螺菌血症

spirillicidal [spaiəˌriliˈsaidl] *a* 杀螺菌的

spirillicide [spaiəˈrilisaid] *a* 杀螺菌的 *n* 杀螺菌药

spirillicidin [spaiəˌriliˈsaidin] *n* 杀螺菌素

spirillolysis [ˌspaiəriˈlɔlisis] *n* 螺菌溶解

spirillosis [ˌspaiəriˈləusis] *n* 螺菌病

Spirillospora [ˌspaiərilәuˈspɔːrə] *n* 螺孢菌属 | ~ albida [带]白色螺孢菌

spirillotropic [ˌspaiərilәuˈtrɔpik] *a* 亲螺菌的

spirillotropism [ˌspaiəriˈlɔtrəpizəm] *n* 亲螺菌性

Spirillum [spaiəˈriləm] *n* 螺菌属 | ~ minus 小螺菌,鼠咬热螺旋体

spirillum [spaiəˈriləm] ([复] **spirilla** [spaiəˈrilə]) *n* 螺[旋]菌

spirit [ˈspirit] *n* 酒精;酊剂 | aromatic ammonia ~, ammonia ~ 芳香氨酊 / anise ~ 洋茴香酊 / benzaldehyde ~ 苯甲醛酊 / camphor ~ 樟脑酊 / compound orange ~ 复方橙皮酊 / ethylnitrite ~, ~ of nitrous ether, sweet ~ of nitre 亚硝酸乙酯酊 / methylated ~ 含甲醇酒精,变性酒精 / nitroglycerin ~, glyceryl trinitrate ~ 三硝酸甘油酊 / peppermint ~ 欧薄荷酊 / perfumed ~ 香料酒精 / proof ~ 规定酒精 / rectified ~ 精馏酒精 / spearmint ~ 绿薄荷酊 / ~ of wine 酒精,醇,乙醇

spir(o)- [构词成分]螺旋;呼吸

Spirocerca [ˌspaiərəuˈserkə] *n* 旋尾[线虫]属

spirocercosis [ˌspaiərəusəˈkəusis] *n* 旋尾线虫病

Spirochaeta [ˌspaiərəˈkiːtə] *n* 螺旋体属,波体属 | ~ pseudoicterogenes 假黄疸螺旋体(本名在德国用于表示双曲钩端螺旋体 Leptospira biflexa)

Spirochaetaceae [ˌspaiərəkiːˈteisiiː] *n* 螺旋体科

Spirochaetales [ˌspaiərəkiːˈteiliːz] *n* 螺旋体目

spirochete [ˈspaiərəkiːt] *n* 螺旋体 | **spirochetal** [ˌspaiərəˈkiːtl] *a*

spirochetemia [ˌspaiərəkiːˈtiːmiə] *n* 螺旋体血症

spirocheticidal [ˌspaiərəkiːtiˈsaidl] *a* 杀螺旋体的

spirocheticide [ˌspaiərəˈkiːtisaid] *n* 杀螺旋体药

spirochetogenous [ˌspaiərəkiːˈtɔdʒinəs] *a* 螺旋体原[性]的

spirochetolysin [ˌspaiərəkiːˈtɔlisin] *n* 溶螺旋体素

spirochetolysis [ˌspaiərəkiːˈtɔlisis] *n* 螺旋体溶解

[作用] | **spirochetolytic** [ˌspaiərəˌkiːtə'litik] *a*
spirochetosis [ˌspaiərəkiː'təusis] *n* 螺旋体病 | ~ arthritica 关节螺旋体病 / bronchopulmonary ~ 支气管(肺)螺旋体病 / fowl ~ 鸡螺旋体病 / icterogenic ~, ~ icterohaemorrhagica 黄疸性螺旋体病,出血性黄疸螺旋体病,钩端螺旋体性黄疸
spirocheturia [ˌspaiərəkiː'tjuəriə] *n* 螺旋体尿
spirofibrilla [ˌspaiərəufai'brilə] ([复] **spirofibrillae** [ˌspaiərəufai'briliː]) *n* 螺形纤丝
spirogram ['spaiərəgræm] *n* 肺量图,呼吸[描记]图
spirograph ['spaiərəgrɑːf, -græf] *n* 呼吸描记器 | **~y** [spaiə'rɔgrəfi] *n* 呼吸描记法
spirographin [spaiə'rɔgrəfin] *n* 血绿透明蛋白原
Spirogyra [ˌspaiərə'dʒaiərə] *n* 水绵属
spiroid ['spaiərɔid] *a* 螺旋样的
spiro-index [ˌspaiərə'indeks] *n* 呼吸指数(肺活量除以身高所得之值)
spirolactone [ˌspaiərəu'læktəun] *n* 螺甾内酯,螺旋内酯固醇
spiroma [spaiə'rəumə] *n* 汗腺瘤
spirometer [spaiə'rɔmitə] *n* 肺量计,呼吸量计 | **spirometric** [ˌspaiərə'metrik] *a* 肺量测定的;肺量计的 / **spirometry** *n* 肺量测定法,呼吸量测定法
Spirometra [ˌspaiərəu'metrə] *n* 迭宫[绦虫]属 | ~ erinaceieuropaei 刺猬迭宫绦虫
Spironema [ˌspaiərəu'niːmə] *n* 线螺旋体属
spironolactone [spaiəˌrəunə'læktəun] *n* 螺内酯(醛固酮拮抗药,利尿药)
spirophore ['spaiərəfɔː] *n* 柜式人工呼吸器
Spiroplasma [ˌspaiərəu'plæzmə] *n* 螺旋原体属
Spiroplasmataceae [ˌspaiərəuˌplæzmə'teisiiː] *n* 螺旋原体科
Spiroptera [spaiə'rɔptərə] *n* 螺线虫属
Spiroschaudinnia [ˌspaiərəuʃau'diniə] *n* 绍丁螺旋体属
spiroscope ['spaiərəskəup] *n* 呼吸量检视器 | **spiroscopy** [spaiə'rɔskəpi] *n* 呼吸量检视法
Spirosoma [ˌspaiərəu'səumə] *n* 螺状菌属
Spirosomaceae [ˌspaiərəusə'meisiiː] *n* 螺状菌科
spirosparta [ˌspaiərə'spɑːtə] ([复] **spirospartae** [ˌspairə'spɑːtiː]) *n* 螺形纤丝体(植物细胞)
Spiro's test ['spiːrəu] (Karl Spiro) 施皮罗试验(检氨和脲、检马尿酸)
Spirotrichia [ˌspairəu'trikiə] *n* 旋毛亚纲
Spirotrichonympha [ˌspaiərəuˌtrikə'nimfə] *n* 旋毛蛹虫属
Spiruroidea [ˌspaiəru'rɔidiə] *n* 旋尾超科
spissated ['spiseitid] *a* 蒸浓的;浓缩的;凝结了的
spissitude ['spisitjuːd] *n* 蒸浓;浓缩;稠度
Spitzka-Lissauer tract (column) ['spitskə 'lisauə] (E. C. Spitzka; Heinrich Lissauer) 背外侧束
Spitzka's nucleus ['spitskə] (Edward C. Spitzka) 斯皮茨卡核(见 Perlia's nucleus) | ~ tract 背外侧束
Spitz nevus [spits] (Sophie Spitz) 斯皮茨痣,梭形及上皮样细胞痣
Spivack's operation ['spivæk] (Julius L. Spivack) 斯皮瓦克手术(膀胱造口术的一种方法,其管由胃前壁所形成,其底部有一瓣膜)
splanchnapophysis [ˌsplæŋknə'pɔfisis] *n* 内脏骨突 | **splanchnapophyseal** [ˌsplæŋknæpə'fiziəl] *a*
splanchnectopia [ˌsplæŋknek'təupiə] *n* 内脏异位,内脏移位
splanchnesthesia [ˌsplæŋknis'θiːzjə] *n* 内脏感觉 | **splanchnesthetic** [ˌsplæŋknis'θetik] *a*
splanchnic ['splæŋknik] *a* 内脏的
splanchnicectomy [ˌsplæŋkni'sektəmi] *n* 内脏神经切除术(此术与交感神经切除术结合做,有利于原发性高血压的缓解)
splanchnicotomy [ˌsplæŋkni'kɔtəmi] *n* 内脏神经切断术
splanchn(o)- [构词成分]内脏;内脏神经
splanchnoblast ['splæŋknəblæst] *n* 内脏原基,内脏始基
splanchnocele ['splæŋknəsiːl] *n* 内脏突出,内脏疝
splanchnocoele ['splæŋknəsiːl] *n* 体腔,胸腹腔
splanchnocranium [ˌsplæŋknəu'kreinjəm] *n* 脏颅(自鳃弓发生的颅骨部分)
splanchnoderm ['splæŋknədəːm] *n* 胚脏壁,脏层
splanchnodiastasis [ˌsplæŋknəudai'æstəsis] *n* 内脏分离,内脏分裂;内脏异位,内脏移位
splanchnography [splæŋk'nɔgrəfi] *n* 内脏解剖论
splanchnolith ['splæŋknəliθ] *n* 内脏石(肠石)
splanchnology [splæŋk'nɔlədʒi], **splanchnologia** [ˌsplæŋknəu'ləudʒiə] *n* 内脏学
splanchnomegaly [ˌsplæŋknəu'megəli], **splanchnomegalia** [ˌsplæŋknəumi'geiliə] *n* 巨内脏,内脏巨大
splanchnomicria [ˌsplæŋknəu'mikriə] *n* 内脏过小
splanchnopathy [splæŋk'nɔpəθi] *n* 内脏病
splanchnopleure ['splæŋknəpluə] *n* 胚脏壁,脏层 | **splanchnopleural** [ˌsplæŋknəu'pluərəl] *a*
splanchnoptosis [ˌsplæŋknɔp'təusis] *n* 内脏下垂
splanchnosclerosis [ˌsplæŋknəuskliə'rəusis] *n* 内脏硬化
splanchnoscopy [splæŋk'nɔskəpi] *n* 内镜检查(用内镜对内脏检视)

splanchnoskeleton [ˌsplæŋknəuˈskelitn] *n* 内脏骨骼(尤指形成动物某些器官的骨骼结构,如鳃、舌、眼、阴茎等)
splanchnosomatic [ˌsplæŋknəusəuˈmætik] *a* 内脏[与]躯体的
splanchnotomy [splæŋkˈnɔtəmi] *n* 内脏解剖学,内脏解剖
splanchnotribe [ˈsplæŋknətraib] *n* 夹肠器
S-plasty [ˈesˈplæsti] *n* S 形成形术(成形外科学中使用 S 形切口的一种方法)
splayleg [ˈspleileg] *n* 外翻腿,肌原纤维发育不良
splayfoot [ˈspleifut] *n* 平跖外翻足 | **~ed** *a*
spleen [spliːn] *n* 脾 | accessory ~ 副脾 / bacon ~ 火腿脾,淀粉样脾 / cyanotic ~ 绀色脾 / diffuse waxy ~ 弥漫性蜡样脾 / enlarged ~ 脾肿大 / floating ~, movable ~, wandering ~ 游动脾 / hard baked ~ 烤硬状脾(霍奇金〈Hodgkin〉病时) / porphyry ~ 斑岩脾 / sago ~ 西米脾 / waxy ~, lardaceous ~ 蜡样脾,豚脂样脾
splen [splen] *n*【希】脾
splenadenoma [ˌspliːnædiˈnəumə] *n* 脾髓增殖性脾大,脾髓增生
splenalgia [spliˈnældʒiə] *n* 脾[神经]痛 | **splenalgic** [spliˈnældʒik] *a*
splenatrophy [spleˈnætrəfi] *n* 脾萎缩
splenauxe [spliˈnɔːksi], **splenectasis** [spliˈnektəsis] *n* 脾[肿]大
splenceratosis [ˌsplenserəˈtəusis] *n* 脾硬化
splenculus [ˈspleŋkjuləs] *n*【拉】副脾,小脾
Splendore-Hoeppli phenomenon [splenˈdɔːrei ˈhəːpliː] (Alphonso Splendore; Reinhard J. C. Hoeppli)斯-霍现象(致病生物周围有无定形的嗜伊红细胞的透明物质沉积,见于某些真菌性和寄生虫性疾病,为局部抗原-抗体反应的结果)
splenectomize [spliˈnektəmaiz] *vt* 脾切除
splenectomy [ˌspliˈnektəmi] *n* 脾切除术
splenectopia [splinekˈtəupiə], **splenectopy** [spliˈnektəpi] *n* 脾异位,脾移位,游动脾
splenelcosis [ˌspliːnelˈkəusis], *n* 脾溃疡[形成]
splenemia [spliˈniːmiə], **splenemphraxis** [ˌspliːnemˈfræksis] *n* 脾充血
spleneolus [spliˈniːələs] *n* 副脾,小脾
splenetic [spliˈnetik] *a* 脾病的
splenial [ˈspliːniəl] *a* 绷带的,压布的;夹肌的
splenic [ˈsplenik, ˈspliːnik] *a* 脾的
splenicterus [spleˈniktərəs] *n* 脾炎黄疸
splenification [ˌsplenifiˈkeiʃən] *n* 脾样变
spleniform [ˈsplenifɔːm] *a* 脾样的
spleniserrate [ˌspleniˈsereit] *a* 夹肌锯肌的
splenitis [spliˈnaitis] *n* 脾炎 | spodogenous ~ 废质原性脾炎(脾内异粒积聚所致)
splenium [ˈspliːniəm] *n*【拉】带状结构;绷带,压布;胼胝体压部 | ~ corporis callosi 胼胝体压部
splenius [ˈspliːniəs] *n* 夹肌
splenization [ˌspliːnaiˈzeiʃən, ˌsplen-, -niˈz-] *n* 脾样变 | hypostatic ~ 坠积性脾样变
splen(o)- [构词成分]脾
splenoblast [ˈspliːnəblæst] *n* 成脾细胞
splenocele [ˈspliːnəsiːl] *n* 脾疝
splenoceratosis [ˌspliːnəuˌserəˈtəusis] *n* 脾硬化
splenocleisis [ˌspliːnəuˈklaisis] *n* 脾[表面]刺激法(促进纤维组织增生)
splenocolic [ˌspliːnəuˈkɔlik] *a* 脾结肠的
splenocyte [ˈspliːnəsait] *n* 脾细胞
splenodynia [ˌspliːnəuˈdiniə] *n* 脾痛
splenogenous [spliˈnɔdʒinəs] *a* 脾源[性]的
splenogram [ˈspliːnəgræm] *n* 脾 X 线[照]片;脾细胞[分类]象
splenogranulomatosis [ˌsplenəuˌgrænjuˌləuməˈtəusis] *n* 脾肉芽肿病 | ~ siderotica 铁质沉着性脾肉芽肿病
splenography [spliˈnɔgrəfi] *n* 脾 X 线摄影[术];脾脏论
splenohepatomegaly [ˌspliːnəuhepətəuˈmegəli], **splenohepatomegalia** [ˌspliːnəuˌhepətəumiˈgeiliə] *n* 脾肝[肿]大
splenoid [ˈspliːnɔid] *a* 脾样的
splenokeratosis [ˌspliːnəukerəˈtəusis] *n* 脾硬化
splenolaparotomy [ˌspliːnəuˌlæpəˈrɔtəmi] *n* 剖腹脾切开术
splenology [spliˈnɔlədʒi] *n* 脾脏学
splenolymphatic [ˌspliːnəulimˈfætik] *a* 脾[与]淋巴结的
splenolysin [spliˈnɔlisin] *n* 溶脾素
splenolysis [spliˈnɔlisis] *n* 脾溶解,脾组织破坏
splenoma [spliˈnəumə] ([复] **splenomas** 或 **splenomata** [spliˈnəumətə]) *n* 脾瘤
splenomalacia [ˌspliːnəuməˈleiʃiə] *n* 脾软化
splenomedullary [ˌspliːnəuˈmedʌləri] *a* 脾[与]骨髓的
splenomegaly [ˌspliːnəuˈmegəli] *n* 脾[肿]大 | congestive ~ 充血性脾大(亦称脾性贫血) / Egyptian ~ 埃及脾大(曼氏血吸虫所致) / febrile tropical ~ 发热性热带脾大,黑热病 / hemolytic ~ 溶血性脾大(溶血性贫血) / infective ~, infectious ~ 感染性脾大 / myelophthisic ~ 骨髓痨性脾大 / siderotic ~ 铁质沉着性脾大(伴纤维化) / spodogenous ~ 废质原性脾大(脾内红细胞积聚所致) | **splenomegalia** [ˌspliːnəumiˈgeiliə]
splenometry [spliˈnɔmitri] *n* 脾[体积]测定法
splenomyelogenous [ˌspliːnəumaiəˈlɔdʒinəs] *a* 脾[与]骨髓[源]性的
splenomyelomalacia [ˌspliːnəuˌmaiələuməˈleiʃiə]

n 脾[与]骨髓软化
splenoncus [spliˈnɔŋkəs] *n* 脾瘤
splenonephric [ˌspliːnəuˈnefrik] *a* 脾肾的
splenonephroptosis [ˌspliːnəuˌnefrɔpˈtəusis] *n* 脾肾[同侧]下垂
splenopancreatic [ˌspliːnəuˌpæŋkriˈætik] *a* 脾胰的
splenoparectasis [ˌspliːnəupəˈrektəsis] *n* 脾过大
splenopathy [spliˈnɔpəθi] *n* 脾病
splenopexy [ˈspliːnəˌpeksi], splenopexia [ˌspliːnəuˈpeksiə], **splenopexis** [ˈspliːnəuˌpeksis] *n* 脾固定术
splenophrenic [spliːnəuˈfrenik] *a* 脾膈的
splenopneumonia [ˌspliːnəunju(ː)ˈməunjə] *n* 脾样变性肺炎
splenoportography [ˌspliːnəupəˈtɔgrəfi] *n* 脾门静脉造影术
splenoptosis [ˌspliːnɔpˈtəusis], **splenoptosia** [ˌspliːnɔpˈtəuziə] *n* 脾下垂
splenorenal [ˌspliːnəˈriːnl] *a* 脾肾的,脾肾静脉的
splenorenopexy [ˌspliːnəˈriːnəˌpeksi] *n* 脾肾固定术
splenorrhagia [ˌspliːnəˈreidʒiə] *n* 脾出血
splenorrhaphy [spliˈnɔrəfi] *n* 脾修补术
splenosis [spliˈnəusis] *n* 脾组织植入 | pericardial ~ 心包腔内脾组织植入(以增加心肌的血供)
splenotomy [spliˈnɔtəmi] *n* 脾切开术
splenotoxin [ˌspliːnəuˈtɔksin] *n* 脾毒素
splenulus [ˈsplenjuləs], **splenunculus** [spliˈnʌŋkjuləs] *n* 副脾,小脾
splice [splais] *vt*, *n* 剪接
splicing [ˈsplaisiŋ] *n* 剪接(遗传学中指在基因转录时内含子排除〈splicing out〉和外显子接合〈splicing together〉)
splint [splint] *n* 夹板,夹;[复](马的)掌骨疣 *vt* 用夹板夹 | Balkan ~ 巴尔干夹(用于骨折,作伸展用) / banjo traction ~ 球拍式牵引夹 / bracketed ~ 有架夹 / drop foot ~ 下垂足夹 / knee ~ 膝关节夹 / plaster ~ 石膏夹板 / poroplastic ~ 可塑性夹 / shin ~s 外胫夹(运动员在趾长屈肌劳损后,沿胫骨出现疼痛)
splinter [ˈsplintə] *n* 裂片
splintery [ˈsplintəri] *a* 裂片[状]的
splinting [ˈsplintiŋ] *n* 夹板用法,夹板疗法;夹板固定术(对松动牙)
splints [splints] *n* 掌骨赘(马)
split [split] (split; -tt-) *vt*, *vi* 分裂, 分离; *n* 分裂;裂缝,直裂口,隙 *a* 分裂的;分离的
splitting [ˈsplitiŋ] *n* 分解,分裂 | ~ of heart sounds 心音分裂
spodiomyelitis [ˌspəudiəuˌmaiəˈlaitis] *n* 脊髓灰质炎,急性脊髓前角灰质炎
spod(o)- [构词成分]灰;废质
spodogenous [spəˈdɔdʒinəs] *a* 废质[原]性的
spodogram [ˈspɔdəgræm] *n* 灰像(焚化少量组织或其他物质后造成的像)
spodography [spəˈdɔgrəfi] *n* 灰像检查,显微灰化法(焚化少量组织,并用超显微镜观察灰像,用以研究细胞的矿质成分)
spoke [spəuk] *n* 辐条,轮辐
spondee [ˈspɔndiː] *n* 扬扬格(两个音节的词〈例如 pancake〉在每个音节上具有相同的重音,用于测试言语接受阈)
spondylalgia [ˌspɔndiˈlældʒiə] *n* 脊椎痛
spondylarthritis [ˌspɔndilɑːˈθraitis] *n* [脊]椎关节炎
spondylarthrocace [ˌspɔndilɑːˈθrɔkəsi] *n* 脊椎结核
spondylarthropathy [ˌspɔndilɑːˈθrɔpəθi] *n* 脊椎关节病
spondylexarthrosis [ˌspɔndiˌleksɑːˈθrəusis] *n* 脊椎脱位
spondylitis [ˌspɔndiˈlaitis] *n* 脊椎炎 | hypertrophic ~ 肥大性脊椎炎 / reumatoid ~, ankylosing ~ 类风湿脊柱炎,强直性脊柱炎 | **spondylitic** [ˌspɔndiˈlitik] *a*
spondylizema [ˌspɔndilaiˈziːmə] *n* 脊椎下移
spondyl(o)- [构词成分] 脊椎,脊柱
spondyloarthropathy [ˌspɔndiləuɑːˈθrəpəθi] *n* 脊柱关节病
spondylocace [ˌspɔndiˈlɔkəsi] *n* 脊椎结核
spondylodesis [ˌspɔndiˈlɔdisis] *n* 脊椎融合术(结核性脊柱病时,用短骨移植使脊椎融合)
spondylodidymia [ˌspɔndiləudaiˈdimiə] *n* 脊柱联胎畸形
spondylodymus [ˌspɔndiˈlɔdiməs] *n* 脊柱联胎
spondylodynia [ˌspɔndiləuˈdiniə] *n* 脊椎痛
spondylolisthesis [ˌspɔndiləuˈlisθisis], **spondyloptosis** [ˌspɔndilɔpˈtəusis] *n* 脊椎前移 | **spondylolisthetic** [ˌspɔndiləulisˈθetik] *a*
spondylolysis [ˌspɔndiˈlɔlisis] *n* [脊]椎骨脱离
spondylomalacia [ˌspɔndiləuməˈleiʃiə] *n* 脊椎软化
spondylopathy [ˌspɔndiˈlɔpəθi] *n* 脊椎病,脊柱病
spondylopyosis [ˌspɔndiləupaiˈəusis] *n* 脊椎化脓
spondyloschisis [ˌspɔndiˈlɔskisis] *n* (先天性)椎弓裂
spondylosis [ˌspɔndiˈləusis] *n* 椎关节强硬,脊椎关节强硬 | cervical ~ 颈椎病 / lumbar ~ 腰椎关节强硬 | **spondylotic** [ˌspɔndiˈlɔtik] *a*
spondylosyndesis [ˌspɔndiləuˈsindisis] *n* 脊柱制动术,脊柱融合术
spondylotherapy [ˌspɔndiləuˈθerəpi] *n* 脊椎疗法
spondylotomy [ˌspɔndiˈlɔtəmi] *n* 脊椎切开术,椎

柱切开术

spondylous [ˈspɔndiləs] *a* 脊椎的,椎骨的

sponge [spʌnʤ] *n* 海绵;(外科用)纱布, *vt* 用海绵揩拭 | absorbable gelatin ~ 吸收性明胶海绵(局部止血用) / ear ~ 洗耳海绵 / fibrin ~ 纤维蛋白海绵(止血用) / gelatin ~ 明胶海绵(止血用,尤与凝血酶一起蘸用)

spongia [ˈspʌndʒiə] *n*【拉;希】海绵 | ~ gelatina absorbenda 吸收性明胶海绵

spongiform [ˈspʌndʒifɔːm] *a* 海绵状的

spongiitis, spongeitis [ˌspɔnʤiˈaitis] *n* 阴茎海绵体炎,尿道周炎

spongin [ˌspʌnʤin] *n* 海绵硬蛋白

spongi(o)- [构词成分] 海绵

spongioblast [ˈspɔnʤiəˌblæst] *n* 胶质母细胞;无轴索细胞

spongioblastoma [ˌspɔnʤiəublæsˈtəumə], **spongiocytoma** [ˌspɔnʤiəusaiˈtəumə] *n* 胶质母细胞瘤,恶性胶质瘤

spongiocyte [ˈspɔnʤiəsait] *n* (神经)胶质细胞;(肾上腺皮质)海绵状细胞

spongioid [ˈspʌnʤiɔid] *a* 海绵样的

spongioplasm [ˈspɔnʤiəplæzəm] *n* 海绵质;轴索浆粒(轴索粒状物质)

spongiosa [ˌspɔndʒiˈəusə] *a* 海绵状的(有时单独使用表示骨松质)

spongiosaplasty [ˌspɔndʒiəusəˈplæsti] *n* 骨松质成形术

spongiosis [spɔnʤiˈəusis] *n* (皮肤)海绵层水层 | **spongiotic** [spɔnʤiˈɔtik] *a*

spongiositis [ˌspɔnʤiəuˈsaitis] *n* 阴茎海绵体炎

spongosterol [spɔnˈgɔstərɔl] *n* 海绵甾醇,海绵固醇

spongy [ˈspʌnʤi] *a* 海绵状的

spontaneity [ˌspɔntəˈniːəti] *n* 自发性,自生;自发动作(或行为等)

spontaneous [spɔnˈteinjəs] *a* 自发的,特发的

spool [spuːl] *n* 线轴,卷轴(绕手术缝线等用)

spoon [spuːn] *n* 匙,调羹;一匙的量 | excavator ~ 匙形挖器(牙科) / marrow ~ 骨髓匙 / sharp ~ 锐匙(刮肉芽组织) | **~ful** *n* 一匙的量

spoon-fed [ˈspuːn fed] *a* 用匙喂的

sporadic [spəˈrædik] *a* 散发[性]的,散在的

sporadin [ˈspɔrədin] *n* 配子体;滋养体(原虫)

sporadoneure [spəˈrædənjuə] *n* 散在神经元

Sporadotrichina [ˌspəurədəutriˈkainə] *n* 散毛亚目

sporangiophore [spəˈrændʒiəfɔː] *n* 孢囊柄

sporangiospore [spəˈrændʒiəspɔː] *n* 孢囊孢子

sporangium [spəˈrændʒiəm] ([复] **sporangia** [spəˈrændʒiə]) *n* 孢子囊 | **sporangial** [spəˈrændʒiəl] *a*

sporation [spəˈreiʃən] *n* 孢子形成,芽胞形成

spore [spɔː] *n* 孢子,芽胞 *vi* 长孢子 | asexual ~ 无性孢子 / bacterial ~s 细菌芽胞 / swarm ~ 游动孢子 / washed ~s 洗净芽胞(已无毒素)

sporenrest [ˈspɔːrənrest] *n*【德】孢子残渣

sporetia [spəˈriːʃiə] *n* 生殖染色质

Sporichthya [spəˈrikθiə] *n* 鱼孢菌属

sporicidal [ˌspɔːriˈsaidl] *a* 杀芽孢的

sporicide [ˈspɔːrisaid] *n* 杀孢子剂

sporidesmin [ˌspɔːriˈdesmin] *n* 孢子素

Sporidiales [spəˌridiˈeiliːz] *n* 担孢子菌目

sporiferous [spɔːˈrifərəs] *a* 产孢子的,产芽胞的

sporiparous [spɔːˈripərəs] *a* 产孢子的

spor(o)- [构词成分]孢子,芽胞

sporoagglutination [ˌspɔːrəuəˌgluːtiˈneiʃən] *n* 孢子凝集反应(诊断孢子丝菌病的孢子凝集现象)

sporoblast [ˈspɔːrəblæst] *n* 成孢子细胞

Sporobolomyces [spəˌrɔbələuˈmaisiːz] *n* 掷孢酵母属

sporocyst [ˈspɔːrəsist] *n* 孢子囊;包蚴 | **~ic** [ˌspɔːrəˈsistik] *a*

Sporocytophaga [ˌspɔːrəusaiˈtɔfəgə] *n* 生孢噬纤维菌属

sporodochium [ˌspɔːrəuˈdəukiəm] *n* 分生孢子座

sporoduct [ˈspɔːrədʌkt] *n* 孢子管

sporogenesis [ˌspɔːrəuˈdʒenisis], **sporogeny** [spəˈrɔdʒini] *n* 孢子发生,孢子形成 | **sporogenic** [ˌspɔːrəˈdʒenik], **sporogenous** [spəˈrɔdʒinəs] *a* 产孢子的

sporogony [spəˈrɔgəni] *n* 孢子生殖;孢子发生

Sporolactobacillus [ˌspɔːrəuˌlæktəubəˈsiləs] *n* 芽胞乳杆菌属

sporont [ˈspɔːrɔnt] *n* 产孢体,孢子体(性周期的成熟原虫)

sporophore [ˈspɔːrəfɔː] *n* 孢子梗;孢囊柱(黏菌);子实体(真菌) | **sporophoric** [ˌspɔːrəˈfɔrik] *a*

sporophyte [ˈspɔːrəfait] *n* 孢子体(倍数世代交替时的二倍体或无性期) | **sporophytic** [ˌspɔːrəˈfitik] *a*

sporoplasm [ˈspɔːrəuplæzəm] *n* 孢原浆(生殖细胞原浆) | **~ic** [ˌspɔːrəuˈplæzmik] *a*

Sporosarcina [ˌspɔːrəusɑːˈsainə] *n* 芽胞八叠球菌属

Sporothrix [ˈspɔːrəθriks] *n* 孢子丝菌属

sporotrichin [spəˈrɔtrikin] *n* 孢子丝菌素(用于皮肤试验,以诊断孢子丝菌病)

sporotrichosis [ˌspɔːrəutraiˈkəusis] *n* 孢子丝菌病

sporotrichotic [ˌspɔːrəutraiˈkɔtik] *a* 孢子丝菌属的;孢子丝菌病的

Sporotrichum [spə'rɔtrikəm] *n* 孢子丝菌属
Sporozoa [ˌspɔːrəu'zəuə] *n* 孢子虫纲(即 Sporozoea);孢子虫亚门
sporozoa [ˌspɔːrəu'zəuə] sporozoon 的复数
sporozoan [ˌspɔːrə'rəuən] *a* 孢子虫的 *n* 孢子虫
Sporozoea [ˌspɔːrəu'zəuiə] *n* 孢子虫纲(亦称 Sporozoa)
sporozoite [ˌspɔːrəu'zəuait] *n* 子孢子,孢子体
sporozooid [ˌspɔːrəu'zəuɔid] *a* 孢子虫样的 *n* 类孢子虫
sporozoon [ˌspɔːrəu'zəuɔn] ([复] **sporozoa** [ˌspɔːrəu'zəuə]) *n* 孢子虫
sporozoosis [ˌspɔːrəuzəu'əusis] *n* 孢子虫病
sport [spɔːt] *n* 突变,芽变;先天畸形 *vt* 突变为;芽变出 *vi* 游戏;突变;芽变
sporular [ˌspɔːrjulə] *a* 孢子的,芽胞的
sporulation [ˌspɔːrju'leiʃən] *n* 孢子形成,芽胞形成
sporule ['spɔːrjuːl] *n* 小孢子
spot [spɔt] *n* 点,斑点 | acoustic ~s 听斑,位觉斑 / blind ~ 盲点(视网膜) / blue ~ 青斑;胎斑 / café au lait ~s【法】咖啡牛乳色[素]斑(如见于神经纤维瘤病和奥尔布赖特〈Albright〉综合征) / cherry-red ~ 樱桃红斑(通过幼稚型家族性黑矇性痴呆患者眼睛的视网膜中央凹可见到) / chromatin ~ 性染色质 / cold ~ 冷点(温度点的一种) / cotton-wool ~s 棉絮状渗出点,雪团状渗出点(见于高血压性视网膜病,红斑狼疮等病) / cribriform ~s 筛区,筛斑/ deaf ~ 聋点 / embryonic ~ 胚斑,胚区 / epigastric ~ 上腹[压痛]点 / eye ~ 眼点(胚胎期眼的原基;见 eyespot) / flame ~s 火焰状出血点 / focal ~ 焦点 / hot ~ 热点(温度点的一种;神经瘤点;阳性区,X 线胶片或热像图胶片上密度增高区) / hypnogenetic ~ 催眠点,引眠点 / light ~ 光点,光锥 / liver ~ 雀斑,褐黄斑(脸上褐色斑点的俗称) / mental blind ~ 精神盲点,心理盲点 / milk ~s 乳白斑;乳状斑 / milky ~s 乳色斑 / mongolian ~, sacral ~ 胎斑,骶斑 / pain ~s 痛点 / pelvic ~s 骨盆点(透视时在骼骨后下棘及耻骨水平支部位常见到的圆形或卵圆形阴影) / plague ~ 鼠疫斑(见于腺鼠疫) / rose ~s 玫瑰疹(伤寒开头七天出现于腹部和腰部上) / shin ~s 胫前斑,糖尿病性皮肤病 / soldier's ~s 军人斑,乳白斑 / spongy ~ 海绵斑,血管带 / temperature ~s 温度点(在皮肤上,包括热点和冷点) / tendinous ~s 腱样斑,乳白斑 / typhoid ~s 伤寒蔷薇疹(见 rose ~s) / vital ~ 生命点(指延髓呼吸中枢) / warm ~s 热点 / yellow ~ 黄斑(视网膜)
sprain [sprein] *vt* 扭伤 *n* 扭伤,捩伤
spray [sprei] *n* 飞沫;喷雾;喷雾器;喷雾剂 *vt, vi* 喷 | ether ~ 乙醚喷雾 / needle ~ 针孔喷雾 / tyrothricin ~ 短杆菌素喷雾
spreader ['spredə] *n* 摊开器,涂布器 | root canal filling ~ 根管充填涂布器
Sprengel's deformity ['ʃpreŋəl] (Otto G. K. Sprengel) 施普伦格畸形,高位肩胛(先天性翼状肩胛畸形,即先天性肩胛骨向上移位)
sprew [spruː] *n* 口炎性腹泻;铸道(牙)(见 sprue)
spring [spriŋ] *n* 弹簧 | auxiliary ~ 副簧,辅助簧
Sprinz-Dubin syndrome [ʃprints 'djuːbin] (Helmuth Sprinz; Isidore N. Dubin) 施-杜综合征(见 Dubin-Johnson syndrome)
Sprinz-Nelson syndrome [ʃprints 'nelsn] (H. Sprinz; R. S. Nelson) 施-纳综合征(见 Dubin-Johnson syndrome)
sprue [spruː] *n* 口炎性腹泻(热带和非热带慢性吸收不良综合征,亦称卡他性痢疾);铸道(牙) | nontropical ~ 非热带性口炎性腹泻(亦称成人乳糜泻、谷蛋白肠病) / tropical ~ 热带口炎性腹泻(亦称锡兰口疮,热带性口炎)
Spt. spiritus【拉】乙醇;酊剂
Spumavirinae [ˌspjuːmævi'rainiː] *n* 泡沫病毒亚科
Spumavirus ['spjuːməˌvaiərəs] *n* 泡沫病毒属
spumavirus ['spjuːməˌvaiərəs] *n* 泡沫病毒
Spumellarida [ˌspjuːme'lɛəridə] *n* 泡沫虫科
spur [spəː] *n* 骨刺,骨棘,骨距;金属突出片;刺(牙);支线 | calcaneal ~ 跟骨刺 / occipital ~ 枕骨刺 / olecranon ~ 鹰嘴刺 / ~ of nasal septum 鼻中隔骨棘
spurious ['spjuəriəs] *a* 假的,伪的
Spurway's syndrome ['spəːwei] (John Spurway) 斯帕尔韦综合征,成骨不全(Ⅰ型)
sputamentum [ˌspjuːtə'mentəm] *n*【拉】痰
sputum ['spjuːtəm] ([复] **sputa** ['spjuːtə]) *n* 痰,唾沫 | albuminoid ~ 蛋白样痰 / green ~ 绿痰 / rusty ~ 锈色痰
SQ subcutaneous 皮下的
squad ['skwɔd] *n* 队 | flying ~ 空中急救队
squalane ['skwɔlein] *n* 角鲨烷,异三十烷
squalene ['skweiliːn] *n* 角鲨烯,三十碳六烯
squama ['skweimə] ([复] **squamae** ['skweimiː]) *n*【拉】鳞 | external mental ~ 颏隆凸 / frontal ~, perpendicular ~ 额鳞 / occipital ~ 枕鳞 / temporal ~ 颞鳞
squamate ['skweimeit] *a* 有鳞(屑)的;鳞状的
squamatization [ˌskweimətai'zeiʃən, -ti'z-] *n* 鳞状[细胞]化
squame [skweim] *n* 鳞;鳞屑
squamocellular [ˌskweiməu'seljulə] *a* 鳞状细胞的
squamofrontal [ˌskweiməu'frʌntl] *a* 额鳞的
squamomastoid [ˌskweiməu'mæstɔid] *a* 颞鳞乳

突的

squamo-occipital [ˌskweiməu ɔk'sipitl] *a* 枕鳞的

squamoparietal [ˌskweiməupə'raiitl], **squamosoparietal** [skweiˌməusəupə'raiitl] *a* 鳞部顶骨的

squamopetrosal [ˌskweiməupi'trəusəl] *a* (颞骨)鳞岩的

squamosa [skwei'məusə] *a*【拉】鳞状的(如 pars ~ 鳞部) *n* 鳞部

squamosal [skwei'məusəl] *a* 鳞状的 *n* 鳞部(颞骨)

squamosphenoid [ˌskweiməu'sfiːnɔid] *a* 颞鳞蝶骨的

squamotemporal [ˌskweiməu'tempərəl] *a* 颞鳞的

squamous ['skweiməs] *a* 鳞状的

squamozygomatic [ˌskweiməuˌzaigə'mætik] *a* 颞鳞颧部的

square [skwɛə] *n* 正方形

squatting ['skwɔtiŋ] *n* 蹲位(产妇临产时及患有发绀性心脏缺损,尤其患法乐〈Fallot〉四联症的儿童常采用此式)

squeeze [skwiːz] *n* 压榨;压缩;挤压伤 | tussive ~ 咳嗽性肺压缩(肺在咳嗽时压缩,能迫使肺泡及细小的气道中的物质进入支气管)

squill [skwil] *n* 海葱 | **~itic** [skwi'litik] *a* 海葱的,含海葱的

squint [skwint] *vi* 斜视 *n* 斜视,斜眼 | accommodative ~ 调节性斜视 / comitant ~, concomitant ~ 共同性斜视 / convergent ~ 会聚性斜视,内斜视 / divergent ~ 散开性斜视,外斜视

Squire's catheter ['skwaiə] (Trumann H. Squire) 斯夸尔导管,分节导管(vertebrated catheter,见 catheter 项下相应术语) | ~ sign 斯夸尔征(瞳孔交替性收缩和扩大,提示基底性脑膜炎)

squirrel ['skwɔːrəl] *n* 松鼠

SR stimulation ratio 刺激率(见 test 项下 lymphocyte proliferation test)

Sr strontium 锶

sr steradian 立体弧度,球面度

SRBC sheep red blood cell 绵羊红细胞

SRF somatotropin releasing factor 生长激素释放因子;skin reactive factor 皮肤反应因子

SRH somatotropin releasing hormone 生长激素释放激素

SRN State Registered Nurse(England and Wales)国家注册护士(英格兰和威尔士)

sRNA soluble ribonucleic acid 可溶性核糖核酸

SRS-A slow reacting substance of anaphylaxis 过敏性慢反应物质

SS somatostatin 生长抑素,促生长素抑制素

ss. semis【拉】半,一半

Ssabanejew-Frank operation [sə'bɑːnejef 'fræŋk] (Ivan Ssabanejew; Rudolf Frank) 萨巴内耶夫-弗兰克手术(见 Frank's operation)

SSD source-skin distance (放射)源-皮[肤]距[离]

ssDNA single-stranded DNA 单链 DNA

SSPE subacute sclerosing panencephalitis 亚急性硬化性全脑炎

ssRNA single-stranded RNA 单链 RNA

SSS sick sinus syndrome 病态窦房结综合征;specific soluble substance 特异性可溶性物质

s. s. s stratum super stratum【拉】层上层,层叠

S. S. V. sub signo veneni【拉】毒药标记

ST sinus tachycardia 窦性心动过速

St stoke 池(动力黏度单位)

St. stet, stent【拉】放置

stab [stæb] *n* 穿刺(如穿刺培养 stab culture);杆(如杆状核细胞 stab cell);刺伤的伤口

stabilarsan [stei'bilɑːsən] *n* 斯塔比胂(胂凡纳明的双糖苷)

stabilate ['steibileit] *n* 稳定生物

stabile ['steibil, 'steibail] *a* 稳定[性]的 | heat ~ 耐热的

stability [stə'biləti] *n* 稳定;稳定性 | dimensional ~ 尺度稳定性

stabilize ['steibilaiz] *vt*, *vi* 稳定,安定 | **stabilization** [ˌsteibilai'zeiʃən, -li'z-] *n* 稳定[作用],安定[作用] | **~r** *n* 稳定器,安定器;安定剂,稳定剂

stabilograph [ˌsteibiləˌgrɑːf] *n* 稳定度测定器(戒酒时测运动不稳定的程度)

stable ['steibl] *a* 稳定的

staccato [stə'kɑːtəu] *a*, *ad* 断续的(地),不连贯的(地)

stachybotryotoxicosis [ˌstækiˌbɔtriəuˌtɔksi'kəusis] *n* 葡萄穗霉中毒症

Stachybotrys [ˌstæki'bɔtris] *n* 葡萄穗霉属

stachydrine [stə'kidrin] *n* 水苏碱,脯氨酸二甲内盐

stachyose ['stækiəus] *n* 水苏[四]糖

Stacke's operation ['stʌki] (Ludwig Stacke) 斯塔克手术(鼓室乳突根治术,即乳突及鼓室内容物切除,因此乳突窦、耳隐窝、鼓室及听道形成一个单一的腔)

stactometer [stæk'tɔmitə] *n* 测滴计,滴量计

Staderini's nucleus [ˌstædə'riːni] (Rutilio Staderini) 斯塔德里尼核,闰核(见 nucleus intercalatus)

Stader splint ['steidə] (Otto Stader) 斯塔德夹板(两头有洞的钢板,用螺丝钉固定骨折)

stadium ['steidjəm] ([复] **stadiums** 或 **stadia** ['steidjə]) *n* 期,病期 | ~ acmes(病)极期 / ~ caloris 发热期 / ~ decrementi (病势)减退期;退热期 / ~ fluorescentiae 出疹期 / ~ frigoris (间歇热的)发冷期 / ~ incrementi, ~ augmenti(病

势)加重期;(发热)进行期 / ~ invasionis 侵入期,侵袭期 / ~ sudoris 出汗期

Staehelin's test [ˈsteiəlin] (Rudolf Staehelin) 施特林试验(检心肌功能效率)

staff [stɑːf] ([复] **staffs** 或 **staves** [steivz]) *n* 棒,杆;探杆,导引探子;([复] **staffs**)(全体)工作人员 | attending ~ 负责医务人员 / consulting ~ 会诊医师 / house ~ 住院医师

stage [steidʒ] *n* 阶段,时期;(显微镜)镜台,载物台 | algid ~ 寒冷期,厥冷期 / anal ~ 肛[恋]期(精神分析,指婴儿性心理发展的第二期) / asphyxial ~ 绝厥期(霍乱) / cold ~ 发冷期(疟疾) / defervescent ~ 减退期,退热期 / expulsive ~ 排出期,第二产程(指胎儿) / first ~ 第一产程,/ fourth ~ 第四产程 / genital ~ 性器恋期,性器性欲期(精神分析) / hot ~ 发热期(疟疾) / incubative ~ 潜伏期(细菌进入人体) / ~ of latency 潜伏期(传染病);静息期(传染病) / mechanical ~ 机械台(显微镜) / oral ~ 口欲[性欲]期(精神分析,指婴儿性心理发展的最早期) / phallic ~ 阳具期(精神分析,指婴儿性心理发展的第三期) / rest ~ 静止期(子宫内膜) / resting ~, vegetative ~ 休眠期,静止期;滋养期(细胞及其核分裂时) / second ~ 第二产程 / sauroid ~ 正成红细胞期 / seral ~ 演替系列期(亦称演替系列群落) / sweating ~ 出汗期(疟疾) / third ~ 第三产程 / transitional pulp ~ [牙]髓转变期 / ugly duckling ~ 丑小鸭期(上切牙初萌于尖牙萌出之前的混合出牙期)

stagger [ˈstæɡə] *vi, vt, n* 摇晃,蹒跚;[复]蹒跚病(家畜晕倒病);眩晕(减压病时发生) | blind ~s 蹒跚病(家畜晕倒病);急性硒中毒(动物)

staging [ˈsteidʒiŋ] *n* 疾病分期:肿瘤分类 | TNM ~ TNM 分类,恶性肿瘤国际临床病期分类(根据三个基本组成部分:原发性肿瘤〈T〉、局部淋巴结〈N〉和转移〈M〉进行肿瘤分类。附加数字表示肿瘤侵袭的大小和程度,如 0 表示不能检出,1, 2, 3 和 4 表示大小或侵袭程度不断增加,这样一个肿瘤可描述为 T_1, M_2, M_0)

Stahl's ear [stɑːl] (Friedrich K. Stahl) 施塔尔耳(耳畸形,分二型:第一型为耳轮与对耳轮融合畸形;第二型为耳轮脚分裂畸形,对耳轮脚不是两个,而是分裂成三)

Stahl's gland [stɑːl] (Hermann Stahl) 施塔尔腺(位于面动脉上的淋巴结)

stain [stein] *vt* 染色 *vi* 被染色 *n* 染色剂;着色斑,色素斑 | after ~ 后染剂 / counter ~ 复染剂 / differential ~ 鉴别染剂 / electron ~s 电子染剂(显现超微结构) / heavymetal ~ 重金属染剂 / lipoid ~ 类脂染剂 / port-wine ~ 焰色痣 / tumor ~ 肿瘤染色(X 线摄影时由于造影剂集中在扭曲变形的和异常的血管内而出现的密度增高区,在动脉造影的毛细血管期和静脉期尤为明显,可以指示肿瘤) | **~able** *a* 可染色的

staining [ˈsteiniŋ] *n* 染色法,染色 | bipolar ~ 对极染色法 / differential ~ 鉴别染色法 / double ~ 复染色法 / fluorescent ~ 荧光染色法 / negative ~ 负染色法(背景染色法,细菌不染色) / polar ~ 端极染色法 /relief ~ 对比染色法(背景着色留下细胞不着色的一种染色法) / substantive ~ 直接染色法 / supravital ~ 离体活体染色 / telomeric ~, terminal ~ 端粒染色法,终极染色法(着色于染色体端粒区的染色体鉴别染色法) / vital ~, intravital ~ 活性染色,活体染色

stalagmometer [ˌstæləɡˈmɔmitə] *n* (表面张力)滴重计

stalagmon [stəˈlæɡmɔn] *n* (改变液体表面张力的)胶体质

stalk [stɔːk] *n* 茎,柄,蒂 | abdominal ~, belly ~ 腹蒂(脐带) / allantoic ~ 尿囊蒂 / body ~ 体蒂 / cerebellar ~ 小脑脚 / hypophyseal ~, neural ~ 垂体茎,垂体柄 / optic ~ 眼茎 / yolk ~ 卵黄蒂

stallimycin hydrochloride [ˌstæliˈmaisin] 盐酸司他霉素(抗菌药)

stamen [ˈsteimen, -mən] *n* 雄蕊

Stamey procedure (colposuspension) [ˈsteimi] (Thomas A. Stamey) 斯塔米手术(膀胱颈悬吊术)(一种膀胱颈悬吊术,类似 Borch 手术,藉助膀胱镜显形) | ~ procedure for stress urinary incontinence 斯塔米尿道悬吊术

stamina [ˈstæminə] *n* 精力,耐力

stammer [ˈstæmə] *vt, vi* 口吃地说 *n* 口吃,讷吃 | **~er** *n* 口吃者/ **~ing** *n* 口吃,讷吃 *a* [患]口吃的

Stamnosoma [ˌstæmnəˈsəumə] *n* 壶吸虫属

stance [stæns, stɑːns] *n* 姿态,态度

stanch [stɑːntʃ] *vt* 止血 | **~er** *n* 止血药

standard [ˈstændəd] *n* 标准,水准,规格,规范 | ~ of living 生活水平

standardize [ˈstændədaiz] *vt* 使标准化,用标准校验 | **standardization** [ˌstændədaiˈzeiʃən, -diˈz-] *n* 标准化,规格化;标定

standstill [ˈstænd*stil*] *n* 停止,停顿 | atrial ~, auricle ~ 心房停顿,心耳停顿 / cardiac ~ 心停顿 / respiratory ~ 呼吸停顿/ sinus ~ 窦性静止 / ventricular ~ 心室停顿

Stanford-Binet test [ˈstænfɔd biˈnei] (Stanford University,斯坦福大学对此测验经过修订后在美国使用;Alfred Binet,法国心理学家)斯坦福-比奈测验(一种比奈测验的修订,按美国儿童情况进行翻译、改编和规范化)

Stanley bacillus [ˈstænli] 斯坦利杆菌(沙门菌属的血清型,从英国斯坦利食物中毒患者分离而得)

Stanley Kent 见 Kent
stannate [ˈstæneit] *n* 锡酸盐
stannic [ˈstænik] *a* (正)锡的,四价锡的 | ~ acid 锡酸 / ~ chloride 氯化锡,四氯化锡
stanniferous [stæˈnifərəs] *a* 含锡的
Stannomida [stəˈnɔmidə] *n* 有线目
stannosis [stæˈnəusis] *n* 肺锡末沉着病,锡尘肺
stannous [ˈstænəs] *a* 亚锡的,二价锡的
stannum [ˈstænəm] *n*【拉】锡
stanolone [ˈstænələun] *n* 雄诺龙(雄激素,治疗不能手术的乳癌和手术后转移性乳癌)
stanozolol [stæˈnəuzələl] *n* 司坦唑(雄激素,同化激素类药)
stapedectomy [ˌsteipiˈdektəmi] *n* 镫骨足板切除术
stapedial [stəˈpiːdiəl] *a* 镫骨的
stapediolysis [stəˌpiːdiˈɔlisis] *n* 镫骨松动术(治耳硬化)
stapedioplasty [stəˌpiːdiəˈplæsti] *n* 镫骨成形术
stapediotenotomy [stəˌpiːdiəutiˈnɔtəmi] *n* 镫骨肌腱切断术
stapediovestibular [stəˌpiːdiəuvesˈtibjulə] *a* 镫骨前庭的
stapedotomy [ˌsteipiˈdɔtəmi] *n* 镫骨足板造孔术
stapes [ˈsteipiːz] *n*【拉】镫骨
staphisagria [ˌstæfiˈseigriə] *n* 虱草子
staphisagrine [ˌstæfiˈseigrin] *n* 虱草子碱
staphylagra [ˌstæfiˈleigrə] *n* 悬雍垂钳
staphylectomy [ˌstæfiˈlektəmi] *n* 悬雍垂切除术
staphyledema [ˌstæfiliˈdiːmə] *n* 悬雍垂水肿
staphylematoma [ˌstæfiˌleməˈtəumə] *n* 悬雍垂血肿
staphyline [ˈstæfilain] *a* 葡萄状的;悬雍垂的
staphylinid [stæfiˈlinid] *a* 隐翅虫的 *n* 隐翅虫
Staphylinidae [ˌstæfiˈlinidiː] *n* 隐翅虫属
staphylinus [ˌstæfiˈlainəs] *a*【拉】悬雍垂的
staphylion [stəˈfiliən] *n*【希】后鼻棘点(头颅测量名词,在硬腭正中面的后缘);悬雍垂;乳头
staphylitis [ˌstæfiˈlaitis] *n* 悬雍垂炎
staphyl(o)- [构词成分] 葡萄状;悬雍垂
staphyloangina [ˌstæfiləuænˈdʒɑinə] *n* 悬雍垂咽峡炎(喉内有假膜沉积,为葡萄球菌所致)
staphylobacterin [ˌstæfiləuˈbæktərin] *n* 葡萄球菌菌苗
staphylocoagulase [ˌstæfiləukəuˈægjuleis] *n* 葡萄球菌凝固酶
staphylococcal [ˌstæfiləuˈkɔkəl] *a* 葡萄球菌的
staphylococcemia [ˌstæfiləukɔkˈsiːmiə] *n* 葡萄球菌菌血症,葡萄球菌败血病
staphylococci [ˌstæfiləuˈkɔksai] staphylococcus 的复数
staphylococcic [ˌstæfiləuˈkɔksik] *a* 葡萄球菌的
staphylococcide [ˌstæfiləuˈkɔksaid], **staphylocide** [ˌstæfiləusaid] *n* 杀葡萄球菌剂
staphylococcin [ˌstæfiləuˈkɔksin] *n* 葡萄球菌素
staphylococcosis [ˌstæfiləukɔˈkəusis] *n* 葡萄球菌病
Staphylococcus [ˌstæfiləuˈkɔkəs] *n* 葡萄球菌属 | ~ albus 白色葡萄球菌 / ~ aureus 金黄色葡萄球菌 / ~ epidermidis 表皮葡萄球菌 / ~ pyogenes var. albus 白色化脓葡萄球菌 / ~ saprophyticus 腐生性葡萄球菌 / ~ simulans, ~ haemolyticus, ~ hominis 溶血性葡萄球菌
staphylococcus [ˌstæfiləuˈkɔkəs] ([复] **staphylococci** [ˌstæfiləuˈkɔksai]) *n* 葡萄球菌
staphyloderma [ˌstæfiləuˈdəːmə] *n* 葡萄球菌性皮肤化脓
staphylodialysis [ˌstæfiləudaiˈælisis] *n* 悬雍垂松弛
staphyloedema [ˌstæfiləuiˈdiːmə] *n* 悬雍垂水肿
staphylokinase [ˌstæfiləuˈkaineis] *n* 葡萄球菌激酶,链激酶
staphyloleukocidin [ˌstæfiləuˌljuːkəuˈsaidin] *n* 葡萄球菌杀白细胞素
staphylolysin [ˌstæfiˈlɔlisin] *n* 葡萄球菌溶血素 | α ~, alpha ~ α 葡萄球菌溶血素,甲型葡萄球菌溶血素 / β ~, beta ~ β 葡萄球菌溶血素,乙型葡萄球菌溶血素 / δ ~, delta ~ δ 葡萄球菌溶血素,丁型葡萄球菌溶血素 / ε ~, epsilon ~ ε 葡萄球菌溶血素,戊型葡萄球菌溶血素 / γ ~, gamma ~ γ 葡萄球菌溶血素,丙型葡萄球菌溶血素
staphyloma [ˌstæfiˈləumə] *n* 葡萄肿 | annular ~ 环行葡萄肿 / ciliary ~ 睫状体葡萄肿 / equatorial ~ 赤道部葡萄肿,中纬线葡萄肿 / intercalary ~ 箝嵌性葡萄肿 / projecting ~, ~ corneae 角膜葡萄肿 | **~tous** [ˌstæfiˈlɔmətəs] *a* 葡萄肿的,葡萄肿样的
staphyloncus [ˌstæfiˈlɔŋkəs] *n* 悬雍垂瘤,悬雍垂肿
staphylopharyngorrhaphy [ˌstæfiləuˌfæriŋˈgɔrəfi] *n* 腭咽缝合术
staphyloplasty [ˈstæfiləuˌplæsti] *n* 悬雍垂成形术
staphyloptosia [ˌstæfilɔpˈtəusiə], **staphyloptosis** [ˌstæfilɔpˈtəusis] *n* 悬雍垂下垂
staphylorrhaphy [ˌstæfiˈlɔrəfi] *n* 悬雍垂缝合术
staphyloschisis [ˌstæfiˈlɔskisis] *n* 悬雍垂裂
staphylotome [ˈstæfilətəum] *n* 悬雍垂刀
staphylotomy [ˌstæfiˈlɔtəmi] *n* 悬雍垂切除术;葡萄肿切除术
staphylotoxin [ˌstæfiləuˈtɔksin] *n* 葡萄球菌毒素
staphylotropic [ˌstæfiləuˈtrɔpik] *a* 亲葡萄球菌的
stapling [ˈsteipliŋ] *n* 纤维包扎 | gastric ~ 胃分隔

star [stɑː] *n* 星,星[形]体 | daughter ~ 子星体,双星体 / lens ~s 晶状体星线 / mother ~ 母星体,单星体 / polar ~s 双星星线;极星线

starch [stɑːtʃ] *n* 淀粉;[复]淀粉类食物 | animal ~ 糖原 / cassava ~ 卡沙瓦淀粉,木薯淀粉 / corn ~ 玉蜀黍淀粉 / ~ glycerite 亚甘油酸淀粉,淀粉甘油剂 / lichen ~, moss ~ 地衣聚糖,地衣多糖 | **~y** *a* 淀粉的,似淀粉的

starch phosphorylase [stɑːtʃ fɔs'fɔrileis] 淀粉磷酸化酶

stare [stɛə] *vi*, *vt*, *n* 凝视,注视 | postbasic ~ 后基底(脑膜炎)性凝视

Stargardt's disease (macular degeneration) ['ʃtɑːgɑːt] (Karl B. Stargardt) 施塔加特病(黄斑变性)(遗传性黄斑变性,一般见于6~20岁,特点为视力迅速消失,黄斑部外观异常,并有色素沉着)

Starling's curve ['stɑːliŋ] (Ernest H. Starling) 斯塔林曲线(图解表示心排血量或其他测定心室作功能力的曲线) | ~ hypothesis 斯塔林学说(毛细管血浆与组织间隙液之间的液体转移率和方向,与毛细管壁两侧的流体静压、血浆和组织液内蛋白渗透压以及作为滤膜的毛细管壁特性有关) / ~ law 斯塔林定律(①心收缩定律:心脏每搏排血量与舒张期回流量成正比;②心脏定律:心脏每次收缩所释放的能量是构成肌壁的纤维长度的简单函数)

Starr-Edwards heart valve prosthesis, valve [stɑː 'edwədz] (Albert Starr; M. L. Edwards) 斯塔尔-爱德华兹心脏瓣膜(一种笼罩球人工心脏瓣膜)

starter ['stɑːtə] *n* 引酵物,促酵物;起子

stasimorphy [ˌstæsi'mɔːfi], **stasimorphia** [ˌstæsi'mɔːfiə] *n* (器官)发育停滞畸形

stasis ['steisis] ([复] **stases** [steisiːz]) *n* 停滞,淤滞 | papillary ~ 视乳头淤血,视神经乳头水肿 / pressure ~ 压迫性(循环)停滞 / venous ~ 静脉淤滞

-stasis [构词成分]停滞,淤滞

Stas-Otto method [stɑːs 'ɔtəu] (Jean S. Stas) 斯塔斯-奥托法(分离生物碱与类似的氨基化合物)

Stat. statim【拉】立即

-stat [构词成分]生长抑制剂;稳定装置,稳定器

state [steit] *n* 状态,情况;(疾病发作等的)转折点 | acute confusional ~ 急性精神模糊状态,谵妄 / alpha ~ α脑波状态(松弛和宁静的觉醒状态) / anelectrotonic ~ 阳极电紧张状态 / anxiety tension ~ (ATS) 焦虑紧张状态,神经肌肉张力过强 / anxious ~ 焦虑状态 / borderline ~ 临界状态(诊断用语,当难以确定症状主要是神经症性还是精神病性时使用) / carrier ~ 带菌状态(带菌者) / catelectrotonic ~ 阴极电紧张状态 / central excitatory ~ 中枢兴奋状态 / correlated ~ 协调状态,动力平衡 / dreamy ~ 梦样状态(见于颞叶病变) / epileptic ~ 癫痫持续状态 / excited ~ 激发态(原子核、原子或分子所处的状态) / ground ~ 基态(原子核、原子或分子所处最低能量的状态) / hypnagogic ~ 入眠前状态 / hypnoidal ~ 催眠样状态 / hypnoidic ~ 类催眠状态 / hypnoleptic ~ 发作性睡眠状态 / hypnopompic ~ 半醒状态/ marble ~ 大理石状态(脑纹状体的一种病变) / metastable ~ 亚稳[状]态(原子核、原子或分子所处较低能量的状态)/ oxidation ~ 氧化态 / persistent vegetative ~ 持续性自主状态(由于脑损害而引起的在一种觉醒状态下的极度无反应状态) / refractory ~ 不应状态 / resting ~ 休眠状态 / steady ~ 稳态,动力平衡 / triplet ~ 三重态(原子或分子的电子激发态) / twilight ~ 朦胧状态

stathmokinesis [ˌstæθməkai'niːsis] *n* 细胞分裂完全抑制

static ['stætik] *a* 静止的,静态的,静位的;静力的

-static [后缀] 抑制的;抑制剂;停滞的

statics ['stætiks] *n* 静力学

statim ['steitim] *ad*【拉】立即(缩写为 stat.)

-statin [构词成分]抑制素

station ['steiʃən] *n* 站,所;站立姿势(运动失调疾病时此姿势有时显示为特殊病征);产位;救护站,救护所 | first aid ~ 急救站

stationary ['steiʃənəri] *a* 停滞的,静止的

statistic [stə'tistik] *n* 统计值,典型统计量

statistics [stə'tistiks] *n* 统计;统计学 | Baysian ~ 贝斯统计(一种有争议的统计方法学,它不像常规的统计学那样,把总体参数看作是固定的〈虽然是未知的〉值,而把参数看作是具有特殊概率分布的随机变量,称之为先验分布。争论点就在于先验分布,它代表着实验者的主观见解,作为各种参数值的先验可信度,譬如说,在估计已出现阳性试验结果的特定疾病存在的概率时,先验分布就代表着实验者对该疾病在研究的人群中流行情况的判断) / nonparametric ~ 非参数统计,无参数统计 / vital ~ 生命统计,人口统计

statoacoustic [ˌstætəuə'kuːstik] *a* 平衡听觉的

statoconium [ˌstætə'kəuniəm] ([复] **statoconia** [ˌstætə'kəuniə]) *n* 位觉砂

statocyst ['stætəsist] *n* 耳囊,平衡囊(耳迷路内)

statolith ['stætəuliθ] *n* 位觉砂,耳石;平衡石(动物耳囊内)

statolon ['stætəlɔn] *n* 维司托隆(抗病毒药)

statometer [stə'tɔmitə] *n* 眼球突出计

statosphere ['stætəsfiə] *n* 中心球,中心体

stature ['stætʃə] *n* 身材,身高 | short ~ 身材矮小症

status ['steitəs] *n*【拉】状态,情况;体质 | absence

~ 失神状态 / ~ anginosus 心绞痛状态(亦称心肌梗死前心绞痛) / ~ arthriticus 关节炎体质,痛风素质 / ~ asthmaticus 哮喘持续状态 / ~ calcifames 缺钙状态,钙饥饿 / ~ choreicus 舞蹈病持续状态 / ~ cribralis, ~ cribrosus 筛状脑 / ~ epilepticus, ~ convulsivus 癫痫持续状态,持续性抽搐状态 / ~ lymphaticus 淋巴体质 / ~ marmoratus 大理石状态 / petit mal ~ 小发作持续状态 / ~ quo 现状 / ~ praesens 现在状态,检查时情况 / ~ spongiosus 海绵状脑 / ~ thymicus 胸腺体质 / ~ verrucosus 疣状脑 / ~ vertiginosus 眩晕持续状态

statuvolence [stæ'tju:vələns], **statuvolism** [stæ'tju:vəlizəm] *n* 自我催眠[状态] | **statuvolent** [stæ'tju:vələnt], **statuvolic** [ˌstætju'vɔlik] *a* 自我催眠的

Staub-Traugott effect (test) [stɔ:b 'trɔ:gət] (Hans Staub; Carl Traugott) 斯-特效应(试验)(正常人口服首剂葡萄糖1小时后再服第二剂时,血糖水平并不升高) | ~ phenomenon 斯-特现象(给予一次葡萄糖负荷后相隔不长时间相继给予的葡萄糖负荷皆可加速处理。同样见 Stauber Traugott effect)

Stauffer syndrome ['stɔ:fə] (Maurice H. Stauffer) 斯道弗综合征(一种副癌综合征,见于肾细胞癌患者,特点为生化肝异常,无肝瘤转移)

staurion ['stɔ:riən] *n* 腭十字点(腭正中缝与腭横缝的交叉点)

stauroplegia [ˌstɔ:rə'pli:dʒiə] *n* 交叉性偏瘫

stavesacre ['steivzeikə] *n* 虱草子

stavudine ['stævjudi:n] *n* 司他优定(一种胸苷的核苷类似物,抑制人免疫缺陷病毒〈HIV〉复制,用于治疗 HIV 感染,口服给药)

staxis ['stæksis] *n*【希】滴流,渗血

stay [stei] *n* 支柱,支撑物 | ~ of white line 白线支座

STD sexually transmitted disease 性传播疾病

STE subperiosteal tissue expander 骨膜下组织扩展器

steal [sti:l] (动脉)盗血(血液从正常的流程改道) | subclavian ~ 锁骨下(动脉)盗血(锁骨下动脉闭塞性疾病时)

steapsin [sti'æpsin] *n* 胰脂酶

steapsinogen [ˌstiæp'sinədʒən] *n* 胰脂酶原

stearaldehyde [ˌstiə'rældihaid] *n* 硬脂醛

stearate ['stiəreit] *n* 硬脂酸盐

stearic [sti'ærik] *a* 硬脂的,似硬脂的 | ~ acid 硬脂酸

steariform [sti'ærifɔ:m] *a* 脂肪样的

stearin ['stiərin] *n* [三]硬脂酸甘油酯

Stearn's alcoholic amentia [stə:n] (Albert W. Stearn) 斯特恩酒中毒性意识模糊(暂时性酒中毒性精神病,维持时间较长,无明显兴奋躁动)

stear(o)-, [构词成分]脂,脂肪

stearolic acid [stiə'rɔlik] 十八碳炔酸

stearopten(e) [ˌstiə'rɔptən] *n* 硬脂萜,硬脂脑

stearoyl ['stiərɔil] *n* 硬脂酰基

stearoyl-CoA desaturase ['stiərɔil di:'sætʃjəreis] 硬脂酰基-辅酶A去饱和酶(亦称酰基-辅酶A去饱和酶)

stearrhea [ˌstiə'ri:ə] *n* 脂肪痢,皮脂溢

steatite ['stiətait] *n* 滑石

steatitis [ˌstiə'taitis] *n* 脂肪织炎

steat(o)- 见 stear(o)-

steatocele [sti'ætəsi:l] *n* 阴囊脂肿

steatocystoma [ˌstiətəusis'təumə] *n* 皮脂囊肿 | ~ multiplex 多发性皮脂囊肿

steatogenous [stiə'tɔdʒinəs] *a* 产生脂肪的

steatohepatitis [ˌstiətəuˌhepə'taitis] *n* 脂肪肝炎 | nonalcoholic ~ (NASH)非酒精性脂肪肝炎

steatolysis [ˌstiə'tɔlisis] *n* 脂肪分解(脂肪吸收前的乳化过程) | **steatolytic** [ˌstiətəu'litik] *a*

steatoma [ˌstiə'təumə] ([复] **steatomas** 或 **steatomata** [stiə'təumətə]) *n* 脂瘤;皮脂囊肿;粉瘤

steatomatosis [ˌstiətəumə'təusis] *n* 皮脂囊肿病

steatomery [ˌstiə'tɔməri] *n* 股臀部脂肪沉积,股臀过肥

steatonecrosis [ˌstiətəune'krəusis] *n* 脂肪[组织]坏死

steatopygia [ˌstiətəu'pidʒiə] *n* 臀脂过多,女臀过肥 | **steatopygous** [ˌstiə'tɔpigəs] *a*

steatorrhea [ˌstiətəu'ri:ə] *n* 脂肪泻 | idiopathic ~ 特发性脂肪泻(非热带性口炎性腹泻)

steatosis [ˌstiə'təusis] *n* 脂肪变性;皮脂腺病 | ~ cardiaca 心肌脂变

stechiology [ˌsteki'ɔlədʒi] *n* [组织]细胞生理学

stechiometry [ˌsteki'ɔmitri] *n* 化学计算[法],化学计量学

Steele-Richardson-Olszewski syndrome [sti:l 'ritʃədsən ɔl'ʃevski] (John C. Steele; John C. Richardson; Jerzy Olszewski) 斯-理-奥综合征(一种进行性神经障碍,60岁时发病,特征为核上性眼肌麻痹,尤其是向下凝视麻痹,假性延髓麻痹,构音障碍,颈与躯干肌张力障碍性强直及痴呆)

Steell's murmur [sti:l] (Graham Steell) 斯蒂尔杂音(见 Graham Steell murmur)

Steenbock unit ['sti:nbɔk] (Harry Steenbock) 斯廷博克单位(维生素D单位,能在10天内使标准的佝偻病大鼠桡骨和尺骨的远端患佝偻病干骺端产生一条钙沉积狭线的维生素D总量)

steffimycin [ˌstefi'maisin] *n* 司替霉素(抗菌药,

具有抗病毒作用)

stege [stiːdʒ] *n* 科尔蒂(Corti)杆内层(在内耳)

stegnosis [steg'nəusis] *n* 缩窄;狭窄 | **stegnotic** [steg'nɔtik] *a* 缩窄的;狭窄的;收敛的

Stegomyia [ˌstegə'maijə] *n* 覆蚊亚属

Steinach's operation (method) ['stainəh] (Eugen Steinach) 斯太纳赫手术(法)(结扎输精管,并切除其一部分,使睾丸的精子发生器萎缩而间质组织增生,从而助长患者性腺激素的输出量,而使之有返老还童之感)

Steinbrockers's syndrome ['steinbrɔkə] (Otto Steinbrocker) 施泰因布洛克综合征,肩-手综合征(即 shoulder-hand syndrome,见 syndrome 项下相应术语)

Steindler operation ['steindlə] (Arthur Steindler) 施泰因德勒手术(手术矫正弓形足,即从跖足跟表面剥去肌肉和筋膜)

Steiner's syndrome ['ʃtainə] (L. Steiner) 斯坦纳综合征(见 Curtius' syndrome)

Steiner's tumors ['stainə] (Gabriel Steiner) 斯坦纳瘤(三期梅毒或非性病性密旋螺体感染所致,亦称关节旁结节)

Steinert's disease ['ʃtainət] (Hans Steinert) 斯坦内特病,肌强直性营养不良

Stein-Leventhal syndrome ['stain 'levənθəl] (Irving F. Stein; Michael L. Leventhal) 斯坦因-利文撒尔综合征(一种临床综合征,特征为继发性经闭和排卵停止〈因此不孕〉,常伴双侧多囊性卵巢,促卵泡成熟激素及17-酮甾类的分泌基本正常)

Steinmann's extension ['ʃtainmən] (Fritz Steinmann) 施氏牵伸术,导钉牵伸术(nail extension,见 extension 项下相应术语) | ~ pin 施氏针(骨折内部固定用)

Stein's test [stain] (Stanislav A. F. von Stein) 斯坦因试验(闭双眼时一足不能站立,见于耳迷路病患者)

Steinstrasse ['ʃtainʃtrɑːsə] *n*【德】石街(体外冲击波碎石术后,存留于输尿管内的碎石片所致的尿道阻塞)

Stelangium [sti'lændʒiəm] *n* 柱囊黏细菌属

stele ['stiːli, stiːl] *n* 中柱(植物)

stella ['stelə] ([复] **stellae** ['steliː]) *n*【拉】星 | ~ lentis hyaloidea 晶状体后极 / ~ lentis iridica 晶状体前极

stellar ['stelə] *a* 星的,星形的;主要的

Stellaria [ste'lɛəriə] *n* 繁缕属

stellate ['steleit] *a* 星状的

Stellatosporea [ˌstelətəu'spɔːriə] *n* 星状孢子虫纲

stellectomy [stə'lektəmi] *n* 星状神经节切除术

stellreflexe [ˌstelri'fleksi] *n*【德】姿势反射

stellula ['steljulə] ([复] **stellulae** ['steljuliː]) *n*【拉】小星

Stellwag's sign (symptom) ['ʃtelvɑːk] (Carl Stellwag von Carion) 施特尔瓦格征(症状)(上睑退缩,睑裂明显增宽,瞬目运动稀少且不完全,见于突眼性甲状腺肿)

stem [stem] *n* 茎,干,梗 | brain ~ 脑干 / infundibular ~ 漏斗茎,漏斗柄;下丘脑漏斗

stem bromelain [stem 'brəuəlein] 茎菠萝蛋白酶(从凤梨植物的茎衍生)

Stemonitida [ˌstiːməu'naitidə] *n* 有钙目

Stemonitis [ˌstiːməu'naitis] *n* 有钙属

stench [stentʃ] *n* 恶臭

Stender dish ['stendə] (Wilhelm P Stender) 施坦德皿(组织标本制备及染色皿)

stenion ['steniən] ([复] **stenia** ['steniə]) *n* 横狭点(两颞凹最小横径)

Steno ['stiːnəu] 见 Stensen

steno- [构词成分]狭窄,狭小

stenobregmatic [ˌstenəubreg'mætik] *a* 前顶狭窄的,狭囟的

stenocardia [ˌstenəu'kɑːdiə] *n* 心绞痛,狭心症

stenocephaly [ˌstenəu'sefəli], **stenocephalia** [ˌstenəusi'feiliə] *n* 头狭窄 | **stenocephalous** [ˌstenəu'sefələs] *a*

stenochoria [ˌstenəu'kɔːriə] *n* 狭窄

stenocoriasis [ˌstenəukə'raiəsis] *n* 瞳孔狭小

stenocrotaphia [ˌstenəukrə'teifiə], **stenocrotaphy** [ˌstenə'krɔtəfi] *n* 颞部狭窄

stenopeic [ˌstenəu'piːik] *a* 狭隙的,裂隙的,小孔的

stenophotic [ˌstenəu'fəutik] *a* 弱光视力的

stenosed [sti'nəust, sti'nəuzd] *a* 狭窄的

stenosis [sti'nəusis] ([复] **stenoses** [sti'nəusiːz]) *n*【希】狭窄 | aortic ~ 主动脉瓣狭窄 / buttonhole mitral ~, fishmouth mitral ~ 钮孔状二尖瓣狭窄(二尖瓣尖粘连并缩短,形成一条膈裂,类似钮孔。亦称钮孔状畸形) / caroticovertebral ~ 椎动脉颈段狭窄 / cicatricial ~ 瘢痕性狭窄 / idiopathic hypertrophic subaortic ~, muscular subaortic ~ 特发性肥厚性主动脉瓣下狭窄,肌性主动脉瓣下狭窄 / mitral ~ 二尖瓣狭窄 / myocardial infundibular ~ 心肌性漏斗状狭窄 / postdiphtheritic ~ 白喉后狭窄 / pulmonary ~ 肺动脉瓣狭窄 / pyloric ~ 幽门狭窄 / subaortic ~, subvalvular aortic ~ 主动脉瓣下狭窄 / tricuspid ~ 三尖瓣狭窄 / valvular ~ 瓣膜狭窄 | **stenotic** [sti'nɔtik], **stenosal** [sti'nəusəl] *a*

stenostomia [ˌstenəu'stəumiə] *n* 口[嘴]狭窄

stenothermic [ˌstenə'θəːmik], **stenothermal** [ˌstenə'θəːməl] *a* 耐狭温的(指仅能耐小范围温度的细菌)

stenothorax [ˌstenəu'θɔːræks] *n* 胸狭窄

Stenotrophomonas [ˈstenəuˌtrəufəuˈməunəs] *n* 狭食单胞菌属 | ~ maltophilia 嗜麦芽狭食单胞菌

Stensen's canal, duct [ˈstensən] (Niels Stensen) 腮腺[导]管 | ~ experiment 斯滕森实验(压迫动物腹主动脉,以阻断脊髓腰段的血液供应,则引起两后肢麻痹) / ~ foramen 切牙孔 / ~ plexus 斯滕森丛(腮腺管静脉丛)

stent [stent] *n* 斯滕特印模(用塑性树脂质制成的口腔印);斯滕特固定模,支架(用塑性树脂质制的模型,以维持皮移植片,使不离位,或为施行吻合术的管形组织提供支持的一种装置或模型) | endovascular ~ 血管内支架

Stent graft [stent] (Charles R. Stent) 斯滕特移植物,嵌入移植物 | ~ mass 斯滕特印模膏

stephanion [stiˈfeiniən] *n* 冠状点(在颅侧,即冠状缝与上颞线的交叉点) | **stephanial** *a*

Stephanofilaria [ˌstefənəufiˈlɛəriə] *n* 冠丝虫属 | ~ stilesi 斯氏冠丝虫

stephanofilariasis [ˌstefənəuˌfiləˈraiəsis] *n* 冠丝虫病(见于牲口,亦称蠕虫皮炎)

stephanofilarosis [ˌtefənəuˌfiləˈrəusis] *n* 冠丝虫病

Stephanuridae [ˌstefəˈnjuəridiː] *n* 冠丝虫科

Stephanurus [ˌstefəˈnjuərəs] *n* 冠线虫属,肾线虫属 | ~ dentatus 有齿肾线虫(猪肾线虫)

steradian(sr) [stiˈreidiən] *n* 立体弧度,球面度(立体角单位,相当于半径平方的球面所对的立体角)

sterc(o)- [构词成分]粪

stercobilin [ˌstəːkəuˈbailin] *n* 粪胆[色]素,尿胆[色]素

stercobilinogen [ˌstəːkəubaiˈlinədʒən] *n* 粪胆[色]素原,尿胆[色]素原

stercolith [ˈstəːkəliθ] *n* 粪石

stercoporphyrin [ˌstəːkəuˈpɔːfirin] *n* 粪卟啉

stercoraceous [ˌstəːkəˈreiʃəs], **stercoral** [ˈstəːkərəl] *a* 粪的,含粪的

stercoraria [ˌstəːkəuˈrɛəriə] *n* 粪锥虫 | **stercorarian** [ˌstəːkəuˈrɛəriən] *a*

stercorin [ˈstəːkərin] *n* 粪甾醇

stercorolith [ˈstəːkərəliθ] *n* 粪石

stercoroma [ˌstəːkəˈrəumə] *n* 粪结,粪瘤(肠内积粪)

stercorous [ˈstəːkərəs] *a* 粪的,含粪的

Sterculia [stəˈkjuːliə] *n* 苹婆属,梧桐属

sterculia [stəˈkjuːliə] *n* 苹婆;卡拉牙胶,梧桐胶

stercus [ˈstəːkəs] ([复] **stercora** [ˈstəːkərə]) *n* 【拉】粪

stereo- [构词成分] 立体的,三维的;固体的,实体的

stereoagnosis [ˌstiəriəuægˈnəusis], **stereoanesthesia** [ˌstiəriəuˌænisˈθiːzjə] *n* 立体觉缺失

stereoarthrolysis [ˌstiəriəuɑːˈθrɔlisis] *n* 关节松解术

stereoauscultation [ˌstiəriəuˌɔːskəlˈteiʃən] *n* 实体听诊[法](用两架扩音听诊器听诊)

stereoblastula [ˌstiəriəuˈblæstjulə] *n* 实囊胚

stereocampimeter [ˌstiəriəukæmˈpimitə] *n* 立体平面视野计(研究一侧中心暗点及中心视网膜区内缺损)

stereochemistry [ˌstiəriəuˈkemistri] *n* 立体化学 | **stereochemical** *a*

stereocilium [ˌstiəriəuˈsiljəm] ([复] **stereocilia** [ˌstiəriəuˈsiliə]) *n* 【拉】静纤毛(在细胞游离面上不活动的细胞质丝)

stereocinefluorography [ˌstiəriəuˌsiniˌfluəˈrɔgrəfi] *n* 立体荧光电影摄影[术]

stereoencephalotome [ˌsteriəuenˈsefələtəum] *n* 脑定点切开器

stereoencephalotomy [ˌsteriəuenˌsefəˈlɔtəmi] *n* 脑定点切开术

stereofluoroscopy [ˌstiəriəuˌfluəˈrɔskəpi] *n* 立体荧光屏透视检查;立体 X 线透视法

stereognosis [ˌstiəriɔgˈnəusis], **stereocognosy** [ˌstiəriəuˈkɔgnəsi] *n* 实体觉,立体觉 | **stereognostic** [ˌstiəriɔgˈnɔstik] *a*

stereogram [ˈstiəriəgræm], **stereograph** [ˈstiəriəgrɑːf] *n* 立体 X 线(照)片;实体镜画

stereoisomer [ˌstiəriəuˈaisəmə] *n* 立体异构体,立体异构物

stereoisomerism [ˌsteriəuaiˈsɔmərizəm] *n* 立体异构[现象] | **stereoisomeric** [ˌstiəriəuˌaisəuˈmerik] *a*

stereology [ˌstiəriˈɔlədʒi] *n* 体视学(研究细胞或显微组织的三维性质)

stereometer [ˌstiəriˈɔmitə] *n* 体积计 | **stereometry** [ˌstiəriˈɔmitri] *n* 体积测定法

stereomicroscope [ˌstiəriəuˈmaikrəskəup] *n* 立体显微镜

Stereomyxida [ˌsteriəuˈmiksidə] *n* 坚胶丝目

stereo-ophthalmoscope [ˌstiəriəu ɔfˈθælməskəup] *n* 立体检眼镜,双目检眼镜

stereophorometer [ˌstiəriəufəˈrɔmitə] *n* 立体[隐]斜视矫正器

stereophoroscope [ˌstiəriəuˈfɔrəskəup] *n* 活动影片检视器

stereophotography [ˌstiəriəufəˈtɔgrəfi] *n* 立体摄影[术]

stereophotomicrograph [ˌstiəriəufəutəuˈmaikrəgrɑːf] *n* 立体显微照片

stereoplasm [ˈstiəriəˌplæzəm] *n* 固浆,固质(原生质固体部分)

stereopsis [ˌstiəriˈɔpsis] *n* 实体视觉

stereoradiometry [ˌstiəriəuˌreidiˈɔmitri] *n* 立体放射测量法

stereoroentgenography [ˌstiəriəuˌrentgəˈnɔgrəfi], **stereoradiography** [ˌstiəriəuˌreidiˈɔgrəfi] *n* 立体X线摄影[术]

stereoroentgenometry [ˌstiəriəuˌrentgəˈnɔmitri] *n* 立体X线测量法,立体X线影像测量法

stereosalpingography [ˌstiəriəuˌsælpiŋˈgɔgrəfi] *n* 立体输卵管X线摄影[术]

stereoscope [ˈstiəriəskəup] *n* 立体镜 | **stereoscopic** [ˌstiəriəˈskɔpik] *a*

stereoskiagraphy [ˌstiəriəuskiˈægrəfi] *n* 立体X线摄影[术]

stereospecific [ˌstiəriəuspiˈsifik] *a* 立体特异的(指酶或合成有机反应)

stereotaxic [ˌstiəriəuˈtæksik] **stereotactic** [ˌstiəriəuˈtæktik] *a* 趋实体的;立体定向的(尤指控制特定功能的大脑分立各区的定向);趋触性的

stereotaxis [ˌstiəriəuˈtæksis] *n* 趋实体性;趋触性;立体定向

stereotaxy [ˌstiəriəuˈtæksi] *n* 立体定向手术

stereotropism [ˌstiəriˈɔtrəpizəm] *n* 向实体性;亲实体性 | **stereotropic** [ˌstiəriəuˈtrɔpik] *a* 向异体的,向实体的

stereotypy [ˈstiəriəˌtaipi] *n* 刻板动作,刻板症(反复或坚持无意义的动作、体位或言语);刻板,定型 | ~ of speech 刻板言语

Stereum [ˈstiəriəm] *n* 韧革[真]菌属

steric [ˈsterik, ˈstiə-] *a* 空间[排列]的(指原子);立体化学的

sterid [ˈsterid] *n* 甾类化合物,类固醇

sterigma [stiˈrigmə] ([复] **sterigmata** [stiˈrigmətə]) *n*【希】担子柄;(种子植物)叶座;小梗

sterigmatocystin [stəˌrigmətəuˈsistin] *n* 柄曲霉素

Sterigmatocystis [stiˌrigmətəuˈsistis], **Sterigmocystis** [stiˌrigməuˈsistis] *n* 小梗囊孢菌属(即曲霉属 Aspergillus)

sterilant [ˈsterilənt] *n* 杀菌剂

sterile [ˈsterail, -rəl-] *a* 不生育的;不结果实的;无菌的,消毒的

sterility [steˈriləti] *n* 不育,不孕;无菌 | female ~ 女性不育,女性不孕 / male ~ 男性不育 / one-child ~ 一儿性不育症 / primary ~ 原发不孕症 / relative ~ 相对性不育 / secondary ~ 继发不孕症

sterilization [ˌsterilaiˈzeiʃən, -liˈz-] *n* 灭菌,消毒;绝育 | chemical ~ 化学灭菌法,药剂灭菌法 / eugenic ~ 优生学绝育 / fractional ~, intermittent ~ 分段灭菌法,间歇灭菌法 / mechanical ~ 器械灭菌法

sterilize [ˈsterilaiz] *vt* 消毒,灭菌;绝育 | **~r** *n* 灭菌器,消毒器

sternad [ˈstəːnæd] *ad* 向胸骨

sternal [ˈstəːnəl] *a* 胸骨的

sternalgia [stəːˈnældʒiə] *n* 胸骨痛;心绞痛

Sternberg-Reed cells [ˈstəːnbəːgˈriːd] (Carl Sternberg; Dorothy Reed)施-里细胞(多核分叶状巨大细胞,见于霍奇金〈Hodgkin〉病时的淋巴结内)

Sternberg's disease [ˈstəːnbəːg] (Carl Sternberg) 施特恩伯格病(见 Hodgkin's disease) | ~ giant cells 施特恩伯格巨大细胞(见 Sternberg-Reedcells)

sternebra [ˈstəːnibrə] ([复] **sternebrae** [ˈstəːnibriː]) *n* 胸骨节(指幼年期的胸骨节,以后才融合为胸骨体)

sternen [ˈstəːnən] *a* 胸骨的

stern(o)- [构词成分]胸骨

sternoclavicular [ˌstəːnəukləˈvikjulə], **sternocleidal** [ˌstəːnəuˈklaidl] *a* 胸锁[骨]的

sternoclavicularis [ˌstəːnəukləˌvikjuˈlɛəris] *a*【拉】胸锁[骨]的 *n* 胸锁肌

sternocleidomastoid [ˌstəːnəuˌklaidəˈmæstɔid] *a* 胸锁乳突的

sternocostal [ˌstəːnəuˈkɔstl] *a* 胸[骨]肋的

sternodymia [ˌstəːnəuˈdimiə] *n* 胸骨联胎畸形

sternodymus [stəːˈnɔdiməs] *n* 胸骨联胎

sternodynia [ˌstəːnəuˈdiniə] *n* 胸骨痛

sternogoniometer [ˌstəːnəuˌgəuniˈɔmitə] *n* 胸骨角度测量器

sternohyoid [ˌstəːnəuˈhaiɔid] *a* 胸骨舌骨的

sternoid [ˈstəːnɔid] *a* 胸骨样的

sternomastoid [ˌstəːnəuˈmæstɔid] *a* 胸骨乳突的

sternopagia [ˌstəːnəuˈpeidʒiə] *n* 胸骨联胎畸形

sternopagus [stəːˈnɔpəgəs] *n* 胸骨联胎

sternopericardial [ˌstəːnəuˌperiˈkɑːdiəl] *a* 胸骨心包的

sternoscapular [ˌstəːnəuˈskæpjulə] *a* 胸骨肩胛的

sternoschisis [stəːˈnɔskisis] *n* 胸骨裂[畸形]

Sternostoma [ˌstəːnəuˈstəumə] *n* 胸口螨属

sternothyreoideus [ˌstəːnəuˌθairiˈɔidiəs] *a* 胸骨甲状软骨的;胸骨甲状腺的 *n* 胸骨甲状肌

sternothyroid [ˌstəːnəuˈθairɔid] *a* 胸骨甲状软骨的;胸骨甲状腺的

sternotomy [stəːˈnɔtəmi] *a* 胸骨切开术

sternotracheal [ˌstəːnəutrəˈkiːəl] *a* 胸骨气管的

sternotrypesis [ˌstəːnəutraiˈpiːsis] *n* 胸骨穿孔术

sternovertebral [ˌstəːnəuˈvəːtibrəl] *a* 胸骨椎骨的

sternoxiphopagus [ˌstəːnəuzaiˈfɔpəgəs] *n* 胸骨剑突联胎

Stern's position [stəːn] (Heinrich Stern) 斯特恩卧位(患者仰卧,头下垂于检查台端,可使右房室瓣闭锁不全杂音听得更清楚)
sternum [ˈstəːnəm] *n* 胸骨 | cleft ~ 胸骨裂
sternutatio [ˌstəːnjuˈteiʃiəu] *n*【拉】喷嚏 | ~ convulsiva 痉挛性喷嚏
sternutation [ˌstəːnjuˈteiʃən] *n* 喷嚏
sternutator [ˈstəːnjuˌteitə] *n* 催嚏剂,催嚏物,催嚏气
sternutatory [stəːˈnjuːtəˌtəri] *a* 催嚏的 *n* 催嚏剂 | **sternutative** [stəːˈnjuːtətiv] *a*
sternzellen [ˈʃtəːntselən] *n*【德】星状细胞
steroid [ˈsterɔid, ˈstiə-] *n* 甾类化合物,类固醇 | anabolic ~ 促蛋白合成甾类,促蛋白合成类固醇
steroid 11*β*-monooxygenase [ˈsterɔid ˌmɔnəu-ˈɔksidʒineis] 类固醇11*β*-单加氧酶(此酶缺乏为一种常染色体隐性性状,称作11*β*-羟化酶缺乏症,并可致先天性肾上腺增生Ⅳ型。亦称11*β*-羟化酶)
steroid 17*α*-monooxygenase [ˈsterɔid ˌmɔnəuˈɔksidʒineis] *n* 类固醇17*α*-单加氧酶(此酶缺乏为一种常染色体隐性性状,称作17-*α*-羟化酶缺乏症,并可致先天性肾上腺增生Ⅴ型。亦称17*α*-羟化酶)
steroid 21-monooxygenase [ˈsterɔid ˌmɔnəuˈɔksidʒineis] 类固醇21-单加氧酶(此酶缺乏为一种常染色体隐性性状,称作21-羟化酶缺乏症,并可致先天性肾上腺增生Ⅲ型。亦称21-羟化酶)
steroidogenesis [stəˌrɔidəˈdʒenisis] *n* 类固醇生成
steroidogenic [stəˌrɔidəˈdʒenik] *a* 类固醇生成的
steroid sulfatase [ˈsterɔid ˈsʌlfəteis] 类固醇硫酸酯酶(即 steryl-sulfatase)
sterol [ˈsterɔl, ˈstiə-] *n* 甾醇,固醇
sterol *O*-acyltransferase [ˈsterɔl ˌæsilˈtrænsfəreis] 固醇*O*-酰基转移酶(亦称酰基辅酶A:胆固醇酰基转移酶,胆固醇酰基转移酶)
sterol esterase [ˈsterɔl ˈestəreis] 固醇酯酶(溶酶体酶缺乏,可致等位基因常染色体遗传病渥尔曼〈Wolman〉病和胆固醇酯贮积病。亦称酸性脂〈肪〉酶和胆固醇酯酶)
stertor [ˈstəːtə] *n*【拉】鼾息,鼾声 | hen-cluck ~ 鸡鸣状鼾息(见于咽后脓肿) | **~ous** [ˈstəːtərəs] *a*
steryl-sulfatase [ˈsteril ˈsʌlfəteis] 类固醇硫酸酯酶(此酶缺乏为一种X连锁性状,可致X连锁鱼鳞病。亦称 steroid sulfatase)
stethacoustic [ˌsteθəˈkuːstik] *a* 听诊器可听到的
stethalgia [steˈθældʒiə] *n* 胸痛,胸壁痛
stethemia [ˌsteˈθiːmiə] *n* 肺充血
stethendoscope [steˈθendəskəup] *n* 胸X线透视机
steth(o)- [构词成分]胸
stethocyrtograph [ˌsteθəuˈsəːtəgrɑːf] *n* 胸廓曲度描记器
stethogoniometer [ˌsteθəuˌgəuniˈɔmitə] *n* 胸廓曲度计
stethograph [ˈsteθəgrɑːf] *n* 胸动描记器
stethography [steˈθɔgrəfi] *n* 胸动描记法;心音描记法
stethokyrtograph [ˌsteθəuˈkəːtəgrɑːf] *n* 胸廓曲度描记器
stethometer [steˈθɔmitə] *n* 胸围计,胸廓张度计
Stethomyia [ˌsteθəuˈmaijə] *n* 胸蚊亚属(按蚊属)
stethomyositis [ˌsteθəuˌmaiəˈsaitis], **stethomyitis** [ˌsteθəumaiˈaitis] *n* 胸肌炎
stethoparalysis [ˌsteθəupəˈrælisis] *n* 胸肌麻痹
stethophone [ˈsteθəfəun] *n* 胸音传播器;听诊器
stethophonometer [ˌsteθəufəuˈnɔmitə] *n* 胸音计,听诊测音器
stethopolyscope [ˌsteθəuˈpɔliskəup] *n* 多管听诊器(几个人同时使用)
stethoscope [ˈsteθəskəup] *n* 听诊器 | **stethoscopic(al)** [ˌsteθəˈskɔpik(əl)] *a* 听诊器的 | **stethoscopy** [ˌsteˈθɔskəpi] *n* 听诊器检查
stethospasm [ˈsteθəspæzəm] *n* 胸肌痉挛
Stevens-Johnson syndrome [ˈstiːvnz ˈdʒɔnsn] (Albert M. Stevens; Frank C. Johnson)斯蒂文斯-约翰逊综合征(一种严重型多形性红斑,其损害可能累及口和肛门生殖器黏膜;并伴有全身症状,其中包括不适、衰竭、头痛、发热、关节痛和结膜炎。亦称多腔性糜烂性外胚层病,重症多形[性]红斑)
Stewart-Holmes sign [ˈstjuət həumz] (Purves Stewart; Gordon Holmes)斯图尔特-霍姆斯征,回缩现象(rebound phenomenon,见 phenomenon 项下相应术语)
Stewart's purple [stjuət] (Douglas H. Stewart)斯图尔特紫(1 喱〈grain〉碘溶于1英两凡士林中)
Stewart-Treves syndrome [ˈstjuət triːvz] (Fred W. Stewart; Norman Treves)斯-特综合征(淋巴管肉瘤是切除淋巴结后臂部严重淋巴水肿的晚期并发症,通常与根治性乳房切除术有关)
STH somatotropic(growth) hormone 生长激素
sthenia [ˈsθiːniə] *n* 强壮,壮健,有力 | **sthenic** [ˈsθenik] *a*
sthen(o)- [构词成分]力
sthenometer [sθeˈnɔmitə] *n* 肌力计
sthenometry [sθeˈnɔmitri] *n* 体力测量法
sthenophotic [ˌsθenəuˈfəutik] *a* 强光视力的
sthenoplastic [ˌsθenəuˈplæstik] *a* 强壮体型的(细长型)
STI systolic time intervals 收缩时间间期

stibamine [ˈstibəmiːn] *n* 脒胺(从前用于治利什曼病) | ~ glucoside 脒胺葡糖苷,锑巴葡胺(抗感染药) / urea ~ 脲脒胺(治利什曼病、血吸虫病及丝虫病)
stibanilic acid [ˌstibəˈnilik] *n* 对氨基苯胂酸
stibialism [ˈstibiəlizəm] *n* 锑中毒
stibiated [ˈstibiˌeitid] *a* 含锑的
stibiation [ˌstibiˈeiʃən] *n* (大量)锑疗法
stibium(Sb) [ˈstibiəm] *n*【拉】锑(化学元素)
stibocaptate [ˌstibəuˈkæpteit] *n* 二巯基琥珀酸锑钠(抗血吸虫药)
stibogluconate sodium [ˌstibəuˈgljuːkəneit] *n* 葡萄糖酸锑钠
stibonium [stiˈbəuniəm] *n* 四氢锑基,锑鎓
stibophen [ˈstibəfən] *n* 脒波芬(抗血吸虫药,尤治曼氏血吸虫、埃及血吸虫、日本血吸虫,也可治腹股沟肉芽肿)
stichochrome [ˈstikəkrəum] *n* 染色质纹(指有易染质的神经细胞)
Stichotrichina [ˌstikəutriˈkainə] *n* 鬃毛虫亚目
Sticker's disease [ˈstikə] (Georg Sticker)传染性红斑
Stickler's syndrome [ˈstiklə] (Gunnar B. Stickler)施蒂克勒综合征,遗传性进行性关节-眼病
sticky [ˈstiki] *a* 黏性的,胶黏的 | **stickiness** *n* 黏,黏稠
Sticta [ˈstiktə] *n* 牛皮叶属,镂苔属(地衣)
Stieda's disease [ˈstiːdə] (Alfred Stieda)施蒂达病(见 Pellegrini's disease) | ~ fracture 股骨内髁骨折
Stieda's process [ˈstiːdə] (L. Stieda)距骨后突
Stierlin's symptom(sign) [ˈstiəlin] (Eduard Stierlin)施蒂尔林症状(征)(硬化或溃疡的 X 线征,尤指盲肠及升结肠的结核)
stiffness [ˈstifnis] *n* 僵硬 | morning ~ 晨僵
stigma [ˈstigmə] ([复] **stigmas** 或 **stigmata** [ˈstigmətə]) *n*【希】特征(一种心理或身体的标记或特点,有助于鉴别或诊断病情);滤泡小斑;圣痕(手足紫癜性或出血性损害,类似基督殉难时的痕斑);柱头(植物);眼点 | costal ~ 肋骨特征(见 Stiller's sign) / ~ of degeneracy 变质特征 / follicular ~ 滤泡小斑(卵巢) / malpighian ~s 马尔皮基小孔(脾静脉上小静脉进入大静脉点) / psychic ~ 精神特征 / somatic ~ 躯体特征 | **~l, ~tic** [stigˈmætik] *a*
stigmasterol [stigˈmæstərɔl] *n* 豆甾醇,豆固醇(工业合成类固醇的重要原料)
Stigmatella [ˌstigməˈtelə] *n* 标桩菌属
stigmatism [ˈstigmətizəm] *n* 有小斑(状态);折光正常
stigmatization [ˌstigmətaiˈzeiʃən, -tiˈz-] *n* 斑痕形成,瘀斑形成;出血斑生成(用催眠暗示在皮肤上形成出血点或红线)
stigmatometer [ˌstigməˈtɔmitə] *n* 散光测定计(检查眼折光力及眼底镜直接检查)
stigmatophilia [ˌstigmətəuˈfiliə] *n* 文身癖(一种有赖于刺身或文身获得性兴奋的性变态)
stigmatoscope [stigˈmætəskəup] *n* 细孔屈光镜
stigmatoscopy [ˌstigməˈtɔskəpi] *n* 细孔屈光镜检查
stigmatose [ˈstigmətəus] *a* 有小斑的
stijfziekte [stiːfˈziːkti] *n*【荷】牛磷缺乏病
stilalgin [stiˈlældʒin] *n* 甲酚甘油醚(即美芬新 mephenesin,骨骼肌松弛药)
Stilbaceae [stilˈbeisiiː] *n* 束梗孢科
stilbazium iodide [stilˈbæziəm] 司替碘铵(抗蠕虫药)
Stilbellaceae [stilbəˈleisiiː] *n* 束梗孢科
stilbene [ˈstilbiːn] *n* 芪,1-2 二苯乙烯
stilbestrol [stilˈbestrɔl] *n* 己烯雌酚,乙芪酚
Stilesia [staiˈliːʒə] *n* 裸头绦虫属
stilet, stilette [stiˈlet] *n* 通管丝,管心针;细探子
stili [ˈstailai] stilus 的复数
stillbirth [ˈstilbəːθ] *n* 死产
stillborn [ˈstilbɔːn] *a* 死产的
Still-Chauffard syndrome [ˈstil ʃəuˈfɑː] (G. F. Still; Anatole M. E. Chauffard)斯蒂尔-肖法综合征(见 Chauffard's syndrome)
Stiller's rib [ˈstilə] (Berthold Stiller)斯蒂勒肋骨(第十肋骨异常移动) | ~ sign 斯蒂勒征(移动性第十肋骨,提示神经衰弱的倾向)
stillicidium [ˌstiliˈsidiəm] *n* 滴流,泪溢 | ~ lacrimarum 泪溢 / ~ narium [鼻]感冒,鼻卡他 / ~ urinae 尿意窘迫,痛性尿淋沥
Stillingia [stiˈlindʒiə] *n* 皇后根属
Stilling's canal [ˈstiliŋ] (Benedict Stilling)玻璃体管 | ~ column 胸核,背核(脊髓) / ~ fibers 施蒂林纤维(指小脑联合纤维是不正确的,正确的指延髓网状纤维) / ~ fleece 施蒂林毛丛(小脑齿状核周围白纤维) / ~ nucleus 施蒂林核(骶核;胸核,背核〈脊髓〉)
Stilling's syndrome [ˈʃtiliŋ] (Jakob Stilling)施蒂林综合征(见 Duane's syndrome)
Stilling-Türk-Duane syndrome [ˈʃtiliŋ tiək djuˈein] (J. Stilling; Siegmund Türk; Alexander Duane)施-蒂-杜综合征(见 Duane's syndrome)
Still's disease [stil] (George F. Still)斯蒂尔病(各种类型的儿童慢性多关节炎,特征为淋巴结肿大,尤其脾肿大,以及不规则热。亦称幼年类风湿关节炎)
stilus [ˈstailəs] ([复] **stili** [ˈstailai]) *n*【拉】通管丝,管心针;细探子;棒剂,药笔剂
Stimson's method [ˈstimsən] (Lewis A. Stimson)斯廷森法(肩前脱位的闭合复位术,即用小

砝码牵引悬于桌边的患臂,患者处于俯卧位)

stimulant [ˈstimjulənt] *a* 引起兴奋的,刺激的 *n* 兴奋药,兴奋剂,刺激剂,刺激物 | cardiac ~ 心兴奋药 / central ~ 中枢兴奋药 / general ~ 全身兴奋药 / genital ~ 性兴奋药,春药 / local ~, topical ~ 局部兴奋药 / nervous ~ 神经兴奋药

stimulate [ˈstimjuleit] *vt* 刺激,激发,促进,使兴奋 *vi* 起刺激作用

stimulation [ˌstimjuˈleiʃən] *n* 刺激[作用],兴奋[作用] | areal ~ 大面积刺激 / audiovisual-tactile ~ 听视触觉刺激 / paradoxical ~ 反常刺激 / punctual ~ 单点刺激

stimulative [ˈstimjulətiv] *a* 刺激的,促进的 *n* 刺激[物],促进因素

stimulator [ˈstimjuˌleitə, ˌstimjuˈleitə] *n* 刺激质,刺激素;刺激器 | human thyroid adenylate cyclase ~s(HTACS) 人甲状腺苷酸环化酶刺激因子,促甲状腺免疫球蛋白 / long-acting thyroid ~s (LATS) 长效甲状腺刺激物

stimulin [ˈstimjulin] *n* 刺激素

stimulon [ˈstimjulən] *n* 促病毒(繁殖)素

stimulus [ˈstimjuləs] ([复] **stimuli** [ˈstimjulai]) *n* 刺激,刺激物 | adequate ~ 适宜刺激 / aversive ~ 后抑刺激 / conditioned ~ 条件刺激 / discriminative ~ 辨别刺激 / eliciting ~ 诱发刺激,激发刺激 / heterologous ~ 异种刺激物 / liminal ~ 近阈刺激物 / nomotopic ~ 正位刺激物 / reinforcing ~ 增强刺激 / subliminal ~ 阈下刺激物 / supraliminal ~ 阈上刺激物 / thermal ~ 温刺激物 / threshold ~ 阈刺激物 / unconditioned ~ 无条件刺激,非制约刺激

sting [stiŋ] *vt* 刺,螫,叮;刺痛;刺激 *vi* 刺;刺痛;剧痛 *n* 刺,叮;刺痛,刺伤,螫伤

stinger [ˈstiŋə] *n* 刺痛,螫痛

stingray [ˈstiŋrei] *n* 魟

Stintzing's tables [ˈstintsiŋ] (Roderich Stintzing) 斯廷青表(肌肉及神经正常电兴奋的平均值表)

Stipa [ˈstaipə] *n* 针茅属

stipe [staip] *n* 菌柄,柄

stippling [ˈstipliŋ] *n* 点彩 | epiphyseal ~ 骺点彩(见于点状软骨发育不全) / gingival ~ 牙龈点彩 / malarial ~ 疟点彩(常见于含有间日疟原虫的染色红细胞内)

stirofos [ˈstairəfɔs] *n* 司替罗磷(兽用杀虫剂)

stirp [stəːp] *n* 世系,血统;种

stirpiculture [ˈstəːpiˌkʌltʃə] *n* 优种繁殖[法] | **stirpicultural** [ˌstəːpiˈkʌltʃərəl] *a*

stirps [stəːps] ([复] **stirpes** [ˈstəːpiːz]) *n* 族;族祖;群;种族;种;茎;(受精卵中的)遗传因子

stirrup [ˈstirəp] *n* 镫;镫骨

stitch [stitʃ] *n* 缝迹,缝线,线法;(肋骨边缘一侧)刺痛 *vt*, *vi* 缝,缝合

stithe [staiθ] *n* 砧骨

stizolobin [ˌstaizəˈləubin] *n* 龙爪黧豆球蛋白

St. John's wort [sein dʒəunz wɔːt] 金丝桃

stochastic [stəˈkæstik] *a* 随机的

stocking [ˈstɔkiŋ] *n* 长[统]袜 | elastic ~s 弹性袜(外科用橡皮袜子)

Stoerk's blennorrhea [stəːk] (Carl Stoerk) 施特尔克脓溢(伴慢性化脓,造成耳、咽、喉黏膜肥厚)

stoichiology [ˌstɔikiˈɔlədʒi], **stoechiology** [ˌstekiˈɔlədʒi] *n* 细胞生理学

stoichiometry [ˌstɔikiˈɔmitri] *n* 化学计算[法],化学计量学,化学数学 | **stoichiometric** [ˌstɔikiəˈmetrik] *a*

stoke(St) [stəuk] *n* 沲(旧动力黏度单位,液体的黏度为每立方厘米具有 1 泊的黏度和 1 克的密度)

Stokes-Adams disease (syndrome) [ˈstəuks ˈædəmz] (William Stokes; Robert Adams) 斯-亚病(综合征)(见 Adams-Stokes disease)

Stokes' amputation(operation) [stəuks] (William Stokes) 斯托克斯切断术(手术)(见 Gritti-Stokes amputation)

Stokes' disease [stəuks] (William Stokes) 斯托克斯病(见 Graves' disease) | ~ collar 斯托克斯颈圈(颈与胸部软组织水肿样肥厚,伴有自颈到膈部的静脉扩张,见于上腔静脉阻塞时) / ~ expectorant 祛痰合剂 / ~ law 斯托克斯定律(位于肌肉下面的黏膜发炎时则该肌经常发生麻痹) / ~ syndrome 斯托克斯综合征(见 Adams-Stokes syndrome)

Stokes' reagent (test) [stəuks] (William R. Stokes) 斯托克斯试剂(试验)(检氧合血红蛋白)

Stokvis' disease [ˈstɔkvis] (Barend J. E. Stokvis) 肠原性紫绀 | ~ test 斯托克维斯试验(检胆色素)

Stokvis-Talma syndrome [ˈstɔkvis ˈtælmə] (B. J. E. Stokvis; Sape Talma) 肠原性紫绀

stolon [ˈstəulən, -lɔn] *n* 匍匐菌丝

stoma [ˈstəumə] ([复] **stomas** 或 **stomata** [ˈstəumətə]) *n*【希】口,小孔;气孔(植物);人造口(指结肠造口术、回肠造口术时在腹壁造成之口)

stomacace [stəuˈmækəsi] *n* 溃疡性口炎

stomach [ˈstʌmək] *n* 胃 | aberrant umbilical ~ 脐部胃迷离(含有胃黏膜的脐结构) / aviator's ~ 飞行员胃病,飞行员神经功能病 / cardiac ~ 胃贲门部 / cascade ~ 瀑布形胃 / cup-and-spill ~ 杯溢胃(X 线摄影发现,在钡剂溢入胃主腔前在胃底滞留一段时间,这是由于结肠膨大压迫所

致）/ dumping ~ 胃倾倒症（在胃肠吻合术后）/ hourglass ~ , bilocular ~ 葫芦胃，沙漏胃 / leather bottle ~ , sclerotic ~ 皮革样胃，硬化胃 / thoracic ~ , upside-down ~ 胸位胃，高位胃 / trifid ~ 三腔胃 | **~al** *a*

stomachache [ˈstʌməkeik] *n* 胃痛

stomachalgia [ˌstʌməˈkældʒiə] *n* 胃痛

stomachic [stəˈmækik] *a* 胃的，健胃的 *n* 健胃药

stomachodynia [ˌstʌməkəuˈdiniə] *n* 胃痛

stomachoscopy [ˌstʌməˈkɔskəpi] *n* 胃镜检查

stomadeum [ˌstəuməˈdiːəm] *n* 口道，口凹（胚胎）

stomal [ˈstəuməl] *a* 口的，小孔的；人造口的（指经外科手术在腹壁造成之口）

stomata [ˈstəumətə] stoma 的复数

stomatal [ˈstəumətəl] *a* 小孔的

stomatalgia [ˌstəuməˈtældʒiə], **stomalgia** [stəˈmældʒiə] *n* 口[腔]痛

stomatic [stəuˈmætik] *a* 口的

stomatitis [ˌstəuməˈtaitis]（[复] **stomatitides** [ˌstəuməˈtaitidiːz]）*n* 口炎 | allergic ~ 变应性口炎 / angular ~ 口角炎 / aphthobullous ~ 口蹄疫 / aphthous ~ 口疮性口炎，疱疹性口炎 / contact ~ 接触性口炎 / denture ~ 义齿口炎（亦称义齿性口疮）/ epidemic ~ , epizootic ~ 流行性口炎，口蹄疫 / erythematopultaceous ~ 红斑软烂性口炎 / fusospirochetal ~ 梭状螺旋菌口炎 / gangrenous ~ 坏疽性口炎（亦称走马疳）/ herpetic ~ , vesicular ~ 疱疹性口炎，水泡性口炎 / lead ~ 铅毒性口炎 / mercurial ~ 汞毒性口炎 / mycotic ~ 霉菌性口炎，鹅口疮 / recurrent aphthous ~ 复发性阿弗他口炎 / ~ scarlatina 猩红热口炎 / ~ venenata 接触性毒性口炎

stomat(o)- [构词成分]口，口腔

stomatocace [ˌstəuməˈtɔkəsi] *n* 溃疡性口炎

stomatocyte [ˈstəumətəsait] *n* 裂口红细胞（偶见于溶血性贫血和肝病）

stomatocytosis [ˌstəumətəusaiˈtəusis] *n* 口形红细胞增多（一种先天性溶血性贫血）

stomatodynia [ˌstəumətəuˈdiniə] *n* 口[腔]痛

stomatodysodia [ˌstəumətəudiˈsəudiə] *n* 口臭

stomatogastric [ˌstəumətəuˈgæstrik] *a* 口胃的

stomatogenesis [ˌstəumətəuˈdʒenisis] *n* 口腔发生（见于纤毛原虫的一种形态学过程；所有口腔结构和有关的细胞器均在此过程中形成或被取代）

stomatoglossitis [ˌstəumətəugləˈsaitis] *n* 口舌炎

stomatognathic [ˌstəumətɔgˈnæθik] *a* 口颌的

stomatography [ˌstəuməˈtɔgrəfi] *n* 口腔论

stomatolalia [ˌstəumətəuˈleiliə] *n* 鼻塞语音

stomatology [ˌstəuməˈtɔlədʒi] *n* 口腔医学 | **stomatologic(al)** [ˌstəumətəuˈlɔdʒik(əl)] *a* / **stomatologist** *n* 口腔医学家

stomatomalacia [ˌstəumətəuməˈleiʃiə] *n* 口腔[结构]软化

stomatomenia [ˌstəumətəuˈmiːniə] *n* 月经期口[黏膜]出血

stomatomy [stəuˈmætəmi] *n* 子宫口切开术

stomatomycosis [ˌstəumətəumaiˈkəusis] *n* 口真菌病

stomatonecrosis [ˌstəumətəuneˈkrəusis] *n* 坏疽性口炎，走马疳

stomatopathy [ˌstəuməˈtɔpəθi] *n* 口[腔]病

stomatoplasty [ˈstəumətəˌplæsti] *n* 口[腔]成形术；子宫口成形术 | **stomatoplastic** [ˌstəumətəuˈplæstik] *a*

stomatorrhagia [ˌstəumətəˈreidʒiə] *n* 口出血 | ~ gingivarum 龈出血

stomatoschisis [ˌstəuməˈtɔskisis] *n* 口裂，唇裂

stomatoscope [stəuˈmætəskəup] *n* 口腔镜

stomatotomy [ˌstəuməˈtɔtəmi] *n* 子宫口切开术

stomatotyphus [ˌstəumətəuˈtaifəs] *n* 斑疹伤寒性口溃疡

stomencephalus [ˌstəumenˈsefələs] *n* 头颌不全长嘴畸胎

stomion [ˈstəumiən] *n*【希】口点（人体测量名词，唇闭时口裂的中心点）

stom(o)- 见 stomat(o)-

stomocephalus [ˌstəuməˈsefələs] *n* 头颌不全长嘴畸胎

stomodeum [ˌstəuməˈdiːəm] *n* 口道，口凹（胚胎外胚层内陷处以后即形成口）| **stomodeal** *a*

stomoschisis [stəuˈmɔskisis] *n* 口裂

Stomoxys [stəˈmɔksis] *n* 螫蝇属 | ~ bouffardi 鲍氏螫蝇 / ~ calcitrans 厩螫蝇

-stomy [构词成分]造口术，吻合术

stone [stəun] *n* 石；结石；磨石；英石（英制重量单位，用来表示体重时，等于 14 磅或约 6.34 kg）| artificial ~ 人造石（牙）/ bladder ~ 膀胱石 / blue ~ 胆矾（硫酸铜）/ chalk ~ 痛风石 / dental ~ 髓石（牙垢，牙积石）；人造石（牙）/ kidney ~ 肾石 / lung ~ 肺石 / metabolic ~ 代谢性结石，胆甾醇石 / rotten ~ 硅藻岩 / salivary ~ 涎石 / ~-searcher 结石探杆（探查膀胱石用）/ skin ~s 皮[下]石 / staghorn ~ 鹿角形石 / struvit ~ 鸟粪石（磷酸铵镁结石）/ tear ~ 泪[腺]石 / womb ~ 子宫石

stone-searcher [ˈstəun səːtʃə] *n* 膀胱石探杆

Stookey's reflex [ˈstuki]（Byron P. Stookey）斯图基反射（小腿半屈，曲于膝关节时，轻叩半膜肌及半腱肌的肌腱，小腿就更屈曲）

stool [stuːl] *n* 粪便 | bilious ~ 胆汁便 / caddy ~ 黑色泥状便（见于黄热病）/ fatty ~ 脂性便（见于胰病及吸收障碍综合征）/ lienteric ~ 不消化

便 / mucous ~ 黏液性便(见于肠炎或黏液性结肠炎) / rice-water ~ 米泔水样便(霍乱排出) / spinach ~ 菠菜绿便(婴儿使用甘汞所致) / watery ~ 水样便

stop [stɔp] *vt* 塞住;阻止;停止;充填(牙) *vi* 停止;阻塞 *n* 停止;阻碍;塞住,填塞 | centric ~ 牙接触面 / occlusal ~ 殆支托

storax [ˈstɔræks] *n*【拉】苏合香[脂](祛痰剂,杀寄生虫局部用药)

storiform [ˈstɔːrifɔːm] *a* 席纹状的

storm [stɔːm] *n* 暴发,发作,症状骤增 | thyroid ~, thyrotoxic ~ 甲状腺危象(甲状腺毒症〈突眼性甲状腺肿〉症状骤增,尤其出现在甲状腺切除术后)

Storm van Leeuwen's chamber [stɔːmvæn ˈljuːvən] (William Storm van Leeuwen) 斯托姆·范·勒文室(保持无空气传播抗原的防变应室)

stoss [stɔs] *n*【德】冲击(给药)(见 stosstherapy)

stosstherapy [ˈstɔsθerəpi] *n* 冲击疗法(一次给患者以大剂量疗法,或短期内给以过量药物疗法)

STP standard temperature and pressure 标准温度和压力(0 ℃和 101 kPa)

strabismology [ˌstræbizˈmɔlədʒi] *n* 斜视学

strabismometer [ˌstræbizˈmɔmitə] *n* 斜视计

strabismometry [ˌstræbizˈmɔmitri] *n* 斜视角测量[法]

strabismus [strəˈbizməs] *n* 斜视,斜眼 | comitant ~ 共同性斜视 / convergent ~ 内斜视 / divergent ~, external ~ 外斜视 / nonparalytic ~ 非麻痹性斜视 / suppressed ~ 隐斜视 | **strabismal, strabismic** *a*

strabometer [strəˈbɔmitə] *n* 斜视计

strabometry [strəˈbɔmitri] *n* 斜视[度]测量法

strabotome [ˈstræbətəum] *n* 斜视刀

strabotomy [strəˈbɔtəmi] *n* 斜视手术

Strachan-Scott syndrome [strɔn skɔt] (W. H. W. Strachan; Henry H. Scott) 斯-司综合征(见 Strachan's syndrome)

Strachan's syndrome [strɔn] (William H. W. Strachan) 斯特朗综合征(一种原因不明的营养性多神经病,见于牙买加和其他国家贫穷地区,可能由于饮食中缺乏维生素 B_1 或维生素 B_2 所致,特征为弱视、感觉异常、头晕、舌炎、口炎、感觉途径损害及其他不同症状)

straddle [ˈstrædl] *vi* 跨骑

strain[1] [strein] *vt* 扭伤;滤 *vi* 被过滤;渗出 *n* 过劳,劳损,扭伤 | high-jumper's ~ 跳高员劳损(跳高者股转肌扭伤) / ventricular ~ 心室劳损

strain[2] [strein] *n* 菌株,毒株,品系 | cell ~ 细胞株(通过选择或繁殖,从原始培养或细胞系得到的培养物) / heterologous ~ 异株 / homologous ~ 同株 / reference ~ 参照株 / resistant ~ 抗性株 / R ~, rough ~ 粗糙[型]菌株,R[型]菌株(细菌变异而形成的粗糙菌落的菌株。R 菌落粗糙、不整齐,在液体培养基中生长呈颗粒状,荚膜消失,致病力弱) / S ~, smooth ~ 光滑[型]菌株,S[型]菌株(细菌变异而形成的光滑菌落的菌株。S 菌落平滑、整齐,在液体培养基中生长呈弥散状,有荚膜者保持荚膜,致病力强) / Vi ~ Vi 菌株(伤寒杆菌中带有 Vi 抗原的菌株)

strainer [ˈstreinə] *n* 滤过器

strait [streit] *n* 窄道,狭口 | inferior pelvic ~ 骨盆出口 / superior pelvic ~ 骨盆入口

straitjacket [ˈstreitˌdʒækit] *n* 约束衣(尤指用以约束疯人的臂而言)

stramonium [strəˈməuniəm] *n* 曼陀罗[叶](治气喘病)

strand [strænd] *n* 线,丝条;(线等的)股,绞;串 | lateral enamal ~ 侧釉丝条,外侧牙板

strangalesthesia [ˌstræŋgəlisˈθiːzjə] *n* 束勒感;束带状感觉

strangles [ˈstræŋglz] [复] *n* (马等的)传染性卡他,腺疫

strangulate [ˈstræŋgjuleit] *vt* 勒死;使窒息,绞窄 *vi* 窒息;被抑住 | **strangulation** [ˌstræŋgjuˈleiʃən] *n* (呼吸)窒息;绞窄

strangulated [ˌstraŋgjuˈleitid] *a* 绞窄的

strangury [ˈstræŋgjuri], **stranguria** [stræŋˈgjuəriə] *n* 痛性尿淋沥

strap [stræp] *n* [条]带;橡皮膏 | crib ~ 马颈(喉吭)护带

strapping [ˈstræpiŋ] *n* 贴膏法;绑扎法

Strasburger's cell plate [ʃtrʌsˈbuəgəː] (Eduard A. Strasburger) 施特拉斯布格细胞板,中体

Strassburg's test [ˈʃtrʌsbuəg] (Gustav A. Strassburg) 施特拉斯布格试验(检无白蛋白尿中的胆汁酸)

strata [ˈstrɑːtə, ˈstreiːtə] stratum 的复数

stratiform [ˈstrætifɔːm] *a* 层状的

stratify [ˈstrætifai] *vt, vi* (使)分层 | **stratified** *a* / **stratification** [ˌstrætifiˈkeiʃən] *n*

stratigram [ˈstrætigræm] *n* 体层[照]片,断层[照]片

stratigraphy [strəˈtigrəfi] *n* 体层 X 线摄影[术],断层 X 线摄影[术]

stratum [ˈstrɑːtəm, ˈstreitəm] ([复] **strata**) *n* 层

Straus' reaction (phenomenon, test) [straus] (Isidore Straus) 施特劳斯反应(现象、试验)(含有毒性的马鼻疽菌的物质接种到雄豚鼠的腹腔内时,即产生阴囊损害)

Strauss' sign [ʃtraus] (Hermann Strauss) 施特劳

斯征(乳糜性腹水时,食用脂肪性食物后,则脂肪增加)

streak [striːk] *n* 条纹;划线 | medullary ~ 脊髓沟,神经沟 / meningeal ~ 脑膜[病]性划痕,脑(病)性划痕 / primitive ~, germinal ~ 原条,胚线

stream [striːm] *n* 流(水流或其他液体等) | axial ~ 轴流(如在血管腔内) / blood ~ 血流 / electron ~ 电子流

streaming [ˈstriːmiŋ] *n* 流,流动 | cytoplasmic ~, protoplasmic ~ 胞质环流

streblomicrodactyly [ˌstrebləuˌmaikrəuˈdæktili] *n* 小指弯曲

Streeter developmental horizons [ˈstriːtə] (George L. Streeter)斯特里特发育分期(人胚发育阶段分期方法,斯特里特将受精开始7周的时期,概括为23个人胚胎发育阶段,每个阶段跨度为2或3天)

stremma [ˈstremə] *n*【希】扭伤

strength [streŋθ] *n* 强度 | ionic ~ 离子强度

strep [strep] *n* 链球菌(streptococcus 的缩略式) *a* 链球菌的

strephenopodia [ˌstrefenəuˈpəudiə] *n* 足内翻

strephexopodia [ˌstrefeksəuˈpəudiə] *n* 足外翻

streph(o)- [构词成分]扭转,倒转

strephopodia [ˌstrefəuˈpəudiə] *n* 马蹄足

strephosymbolia [ˌstrefəusimˈbəuliə] *n* 视像倒反;读字倒反(如 b-d, q-p 辨识困难)

strepitus [ˈstrepitəs] *n*【拉】杂音,噪音(听诊音)

strepogenin [ˌstrepəˈdʒenin] *n* 促长肽(存在于酪蛋白和某些其他蛋白之中,且为动物最适生长所需要的一种因素)

strepsinema [ˌstrepsiˈniːmə] *n* 绞线(指绞线期的染色质线)

strepsitene [ˈstrepsitiːn] *n* 绞线期(减数分裂的一个阶段)

streptamine [ˈstreptəˌmiːn] *n* 链霉胺

streptavidin [strepˈtævidin] *n* 抗生蛋白链菌素(一种细菌蛋白,在免疫学及生物化学测定中用作探查物,因它对生物素有极大的亲和性和专一性)

strepticemia [ˌstreptiˈsiːmiə] *n* 链球菌菌血症

streptidine [ˈstreptidiːn] *n* 链霉胍

strept(o)- [构词成分]扭转;链球菌

streptoangina [ˌstreptəuænˈdʒainə] *n* 链球菌性咽峡炎

Streptobacillus [ˌstreptəubəˈsiləs] *n* 链[球]杆菌属

streptobacillus [ˌstreptəubəˈsiləs] ([复] **streptobacilli** [ˌstreptəubəˈsilai]) *n* 链[球]杆菌

streptobacteria [ˌstreptəubækˈtiəriə] *n* [复]链状菌

streptobacterin [ˌstreptəuˈbæktərin] *n* 链球菌菌苗

streptobiosamine [ˌstreptəubaiˈəusəmiːn] *n* 链霉二糖胺

streptocerciasis [ˌstreptəusəːkaiəsis] *n* 链尾线虫病

Streptococcaceae [ˌstreptəukɔkˈkeisiiː] *n* 链球菌科

streptococcal [ˌstreptəuˈkɔkəl] *a* 链球菌的

streptococcemia [ˌstreptəukɔkˈsiːmiə] *n* 链球菌菌血症

streptococci [ˌstreptəuˈkɔksai] streptococcus 的复数

streptococcic [ˌstreptəuˈkɔksik] *a* 链球菌的

streptococcicide [ˌstreptəuˈkɔksisaid] *n* 杀链球菌药

streptococcolysin [ˌstreptəukɔˈkɔlisin] *n* 链球菌溶血素,链溶素

streptococcosis [ˌstreptəukəuˈkəusis] *n* 链球菌病

Streptococcus [ˌstreptəuˈkɔkəs] *n* 链球菌属 | ~ acidominimus 少酸链球菌 / ~ agalactiae 无乳链球菌 / ~ anaerobius 厌氧性链球菌 / ~ anhemolyticus 不溶血性链球菌 / ~ avium 鸟链球菌 / ~ bovis 牛链球菌 / ~ cremoris 乳脂链球菌 / ~ durans 坚忍链球菌 / ~ equisimilis 类马链球菌 / ~ erysipelatis 丹毒链球菌 / ~ evolutus 展性链球菌 / ~ faecalis 粪链球菌 / ~ foetidus 恶臭链球菌 / ~ hemolyticus 溶血性链球菌 / ~ intermedius 中链球菌 / ~ lacticus, ~ lactis 乳链球菌 / ~ lanceolatus 矛形链球菌 / ~ liquefaciens 液化链球菌 / ~ mastitidis 无乳链球菌 / ~ micros 小链球菌 / ~ mitis 轻型链球菌 / ~ mutans 突变链球菌 / ~ pneumoniae 肺炎链球菌,肺炎双球菌 / ~ pyogenes 化脓链球菌 / ~ salivarius 唾液链球菌 / ~ sanguis 血链球菌 / ~ thermophilus 嗜热链球菌 / ~ uberis 乳房链球菌 / ~ zymogenes 产酶链球菌

streptococcus [ˌstreptəuˈkɔkəs] ([复] **streptococci** [ˌstreptəuˈkɔksai]) *n* 链球菌 | anhemolytic ~, gamma ~ 不溶血性链球菌,丙型链球菌 / group A, B, C(etc.) streptococci A、B、C(等)族链球菌 / hemolytic ~, α ~, β ~ 溶血性链球菌,甲型链球菌,乙型链球菌 / ~ MG MG 链球菌(非溶血性链球菌的一菌株,从原发性非典型肺炎患者的痰中分离出) / nonhemolytic ~, indifferent ~ 非溶血性链球菌 / viridans ~ 草绿色链球菌

streptodornase [ˌstreptəuˈdɔːneis] *n* 链道酶,链球菌 DNA 酶 | streptokinase-~ 链激酶-链道酶,双链酶(用作蛋白分解剂和纤维溶解剂)

streptoduocin [ˌstreptəuˈdjuəsin] *n* 双链霉素(含硫酸二氢链霉素和硫酸链霉素)

streptogenin [ˌstreptəuˈdʒenin] *n* 蛋白促生长肽(在牛奶和其他食物的蛋白中有一种假设的物质,为细菌和实验动物最适生长所需要的)
streptohemolysin [ˌstreptəuˌhiːməˈlaisin] *n* 链球菌溶血素
streptokinase [ˌstreptəuˈkaineis] *n* 链激酶 | ~-streptodornase 链激酶-链道酶,双链酶(用作蛋白分解剂和纤维溶解剂)
streptoleukocidin [ˌstreptəuˌljuːkəˈsaidin] *n* 链[球菌]杀白细胞素
streptolysin [strepˈtɔlisin] *n* 链球菌溶血素 | ~ O 链球菌溶血素 O,不耐氧链球菌溶血素 / ~ S 链球菌溶血素 S,耐氧链球菌溶血素
streptomicrodactyly [ˌstreptəuˌmaikrəuˈdæktili] *n* 小指弯曲
Streptomyces [ˌstreptəuˈmaisiːz] *n* 链霉菌属 | ~ paraguayensis 巴拉圭链霉菌 / ~ vinaceus 葡萄色链霉菌(产维生素 B_{12} 的菌种)
Streptomycetaceae [ˌstreptəuˌmaisiˈteisiiː] *n* 链霉菌科
streptomycin [ˌstreptəuˈmaisin] *n* 链霉素(抗菌抗生素) | ~ hydrochloride 盐酸链霉素 / ~ sulfate 硫酸链霉素
streptomycosis [ˌstreptəumaiˈkəusis] *n* 链霉菌病
Streptoneura [ˌstreptəuˈnjuərə] *n* 扭神经亚纲
streptonigrin [ˌstreptəuˈnaigrin] *n* 绛色霉素(抗肿瘤抗生素)
streptonivicin [ˌstreptəuˈnaivisin] *n* 新生霉素(抗生素类药)
streptose [ˈstreptəus] *n* 链霉糖
streptosepticemia [ˌstreptəuseptiˈsiːmiə] *n* 链球菌败血病
Streptosporangium [ˌstreptəuspəˈrændʒiəm] *n* 链孢子囊菌属
streptothricin [ˌstreptəuˈθraisin] *n* 链丝菌素
Streptothrix [ˈstreptəθriks] *n* 链丝菌属 | ~ bovis 牛链丝菌,刚果嗜皮菌 / ~ farcinica 皮疽链丝菌,鼻疽诺卡菌 / ~ nocardii 诺卡链丝菌,鼻疽诺卡菌
streptotrichal [strepˈtɔtrikəl] *a* 链丝菌的
streptotrichosis [ˌstreptəutraiˈkəusis], **streptothricosis** [ˌstreptəuθraiˈkəusis] *n* 链丝菌病
Streptoverticillium [ˌstreptəuvəːtiˈsiliəm] *n* 链轮枝孢属
streptozocin [ˌstreptəuˈzəusin], **streptozotocin** [ˌstreptəuzəˈtəusin] *n* 链佐星(抗肿瘤抗生素)
stress [stres] *n* 压力;应力;应激 | compressive ~ 压应力
stress-breaker [ˈstresbreikə] *n* 应力中断器(中断或减少作用于桥基牙的咬合力)
stretcher [ˈstretʃə] *n* 担架;伸张器
stretches [ˈstretʃəz] *n* 遗传性周期性痉挛
stria [ˈstraiə] ([复] **striae** [ˈstraiiː]) *n* 条纹,纹;线条 | purple ~e 紫纹
striascope [ˈstraiəskəup] *n* 屈光检查器
striatal [straiˈeitl] *a* 纹状体的
striate [ˈstraieit] *a* 纹状的 | **~d** [ˈstraieitid] *a* 纹状的
striation [straiˈeiʃən] *n* 纹理;条纹,抓痕
striatonigral [ˌstraiətəuˈnaigrəl] *a* 纹状体黑质的
striatum [straiˈeitəm] *n* 纹状体;新纹状体 *a* 有条纹的,有槽的
stricken [ˈstrikən] *a* 受(疾病、灾难、伤害)侵袭的
stricture [ˈstriktʃə] *n* 狭窄 | contractile ~, recurrent ~ 收缩性狭窄,再发性狭窄 / hysterical ~ 癔症性(食管)狭窄 / irritable ~ 敏感性狭窄 / organic ~ 器质性狭窄 | **~d** *a*
strictureplasty [ˈstriktʃəˌplæsti], **stricturoplasty** [ˈstriktʃərəuˌplæsti] *n* 狭窄缝合术(使用纵深切开并横向缝合狭窄,对变窄的肠段的管径施行手术扩大)
stricturization [ˌstriktʃəraiˈzeiʃən, -riˈz-] *n* 狭窄化
stricturotome [ˈstriktʃərəˌtəum] *n* 狭窄切开刀
stricturotomy [ˌstriktʃəˈrɔtəmi] *n* 狭窄切开术
strident [ˈstraidnt], **stridulous** [ˈstridjuləs] *a* 喘鸣的
stridor [ˈstraidə] *n*【拉】喘鸣
strike [straik] *n* 皮肤蝇蛆病
stringhalt [ˈstriŋhɔːlt] *n* 跛行症(马)
striocellular [ˌstraiəuˈseljulə] *a* 横纹肌纤维[与]细胞的
striocerebellar [ˌstraiəuˌseriˈbelə] *a* 纹状体[与]小脑的
striomotor [ˌstraiəuˈməutə] *a* 横纹肌运动的
striomuscular [ˌstraiəˈmʌskjulə] *a* 横纹肌的
strionigral [ˌstraiəuˈnaigrəl] *a* 纹状体黑质的
strip [strip] *vt* 剥,剥离,剥脱;挤出(如用手指沿血管压挤其内容物);磨光(缩小牙齿近中远中的宽度);除去(用电化学法除去牙冠内的金属,以增加内径) *n* 条,带,磨带 | abrasive ~ 研磨带(用以对牙或义齿的邻面进行磨光和外形修复) / linen ~ 亚麻带(一种研磨带)
stripe [straip] *n* 纹,条纹 | **~d** *a* 有条纹的
stripper [ˈstripə] *n* 剥除[静脉]器
strobila [strəˈbailə] ([复] **strobilae** [strəˈbailiː]), **strobilus** [ˈstrɔbələs] *n*【拉】链体(绦虫);孢子叶球(植物)
strobile [ˈstrɔbail] *n* 链体(绦虫);孢子叶球(植物)
strobiloid [ˈstrɔbəlɔid] *a* 链体样的(绦虫);球果状的(植物)
stroboscope [ˈstrəubəskəup] *n* 动态镜(观察快速

运动用),频闪观测器 | **stroboscopic** [ˌstrəubəˈskɔpik] *a*

stroke [strəuk] *n* 打,击;(病)突然发作,[脑]卒中;心搏动 | apoplectic ~ 卒中发作 / back ~ 反击,反冲 / effective ~ 有效摆动(指纤毛) / heat ~ 中暑,热射病 / light ~ 光射病 / lightning ~ 电击 / paralytic ~ 瘫痪发作 / recovery ~ 恢复摆动(指纤毛) / sun ~ 日射病,中暑

stroma [ˈstrəumə] ([复] **stromata** [ˈstrəumətə]) *n*【希】基质,间质;子座 | ~ of cornea 角膜基质,角膜固有质 / ~ of thyroid gland 甲状腺基质 / vitreous ~ 玻璃状体基质 | **~l, ~tic** [strəˈmætik] *a*

stromatin [ˈstrəumətin] *n* (红细胞)基质蛋白

stromatogenous [ˌstrəuməˈtɔdʒinəs] *a* 基质[原]性的

stromatolysis [ˌstrəuməˈtɔlisis] *n* 基质溶解

stromatosis [ˌstrəuməˈtəusis] *n* 基质性子宫内膜异位

stromelysin [strəuˈmelisin] *n* 溶基质素,基质溶素

Stromeyer's cephalhematocele [ˈʃtrəumaiə] (Georg F. L. Stromeyer)施特罗迈耶头血囊肿(与静脉通连的骨膜下头血囊肿,用力呼气时可引起其充血) | ~ splint 施特罗迈耶夹板(铰链腿夹板,可固定任何角度)

stromuhr [ˈstrɔːmuə] *n*【德】血流速度计

Strong's bacillus [strɔŋ] (Richard P. Strong)斯特朗杆菌,弗氏志贺菌(Shigella flexneri)

strongyli [ˈstrɔndʒilai] strongylus 的复数

strongyliasis [ˌstrɔndʒiˈlaiəsis] *n* 圆线虫病

strongylid [ˈstrɔndʒilid] *a* 圆线虫科的 *n* 圆线虫

Strongylidae [strɔnˈdʒilidiː] *n* 圆线虫科

Strongyloidea [ˌstrɔndʒiˈlɔidiə] *n* 类圆线虫总科

Strongyloides [ˌstrɔndʒiˈlɔidiːz] *n* 类圆线虫属 | ~ papillosus 乳头类圆线虫 / ~ ratti 鼠类圆线虫 / ~ stercoralis, ~ intestinalis 粪类圆线虫,肠类圆线虫

strongyloidiasis [ˌstrɔndʒilɔiˈdaiəsis], **strongyloidosis** [ˌstrɔndʒilɔiˈdəusis] *n* 类圆线虫病

strongylosis [ˌstrɔndʒiˈləusis] *n* 圆线虫病

Strongylus [ˈstrɔndʒiləs] *n* 圆线虫属 | ~ edentatus 无齿圆线虫 / ~ equinus 马圆线虫 / ~ filaria 丝圆线虫 / ~ gibsoni 吉[布逊]氏圆线虫(即指形长刺线虫 Mecistocirrhus digitatus) / ~ gigas 巨圆线虫(即肾膨结线虫 Dioctophyma renale) / ~ longevaginatus 长鞘圆线虫(即长后圆线虫 Metastrongylus elongatus) / ~ micrurus 小圆线虫 / ~ paradoxus 猪圆线虫(即长后圆线虫 Metastrongylus elongatus) / ~ renalis 肾圆线虫(即肾膨结线虫 Dioctophyma renale) / ~ subtilis 不定毛圆线虫(即蛇形毛圆线虫 Trichostrongylus colubriformis) / ~ vulgaris 寻常圆线虫

strongylus [ˈstrɔndʒiləs] ([复] **strongyli** [ˈstrɔndʒilai]) *n* 圆线虫

strontia [ˈstrɔnʃiə] *n* 氧化锶

strontium(Sr) [ˈstrɔnʃiəm] *n* 锶(化学元素)

strontiuresis [ˌstrɔnʃijuəˈriːsis] *n* 锶尿排泄 | **strontiuretic** [ˌstrɔnʃijuəˈretik] *a* 锶尿排泄的,促锶尿排泄的

strophanthidin [strəuˈfænθidin] *n* 毒毛旋花苷元,毒毛旋花子苷元

strophanthin [strəuˈfænθin] *n* 毒毛花苷 | G- ~, ~ -G 毒毛花苷 G(即哇巴因 ouabain,强心药)

Strophanthus [strəuˈfænθəs] *n* 毒毛旋花属

Strophariaceae [strəˌfeiriˈeisiiː] *n* 球盖菇科

strophocephalus [ˌstrɔfəuˈsefələs] *n* 扭头畸胎

strophocephaly [ˌstrɔfəuˈsefəli] *n* 扭头[畸形]

strophosomus [ˌstrɔfəuˈsəuməs] *n* 扭体露脏畸胎

strophulus [ˈstrɔfjuləs] *n*【拉】婴儿苔藓,丘疹性荨麻疹

struck [strʌk] *n* (传染性)羊肠毒血病

structural [ˈstrʌktʃərəl] *a* 结构[上]的

structure [ˈstrʌktʃə] *n* 结构 | denture-supporting ~ 义齿支持结构 / primary ~, covalent ~ 一级结构,共价结构(多肽链的氨基酸顺序或核酸链的碱基顺序) / quaternary ~ 四级结构(大分子亚单位的几何排列) / secondary ~ 二级结构(大分子的三维结构) / tertiary ~ 三级结构(单体大分子或多体大分子亚单位的三维结构) | **~-less** *a* 无结构的,无细胞结构的

struggle [ˈstrʌgl] *n*, *vi* 斗争;奋斗 | ~ for existence 生存竞争

struma [ˈstruːmə] ([复] **strumas** 或 **strumae** [ˈstruːmiː]) *n*【拉】甲状腺肿;腺病 | ~ lymphomatosa 淋巴瘤性甲状腺肿 / ~ maligna 恶性甲状腺肿,甲状腺体癌 | **strumous** *a*

strumectomy [struːˈmektəmi] *n* 甲状腺肿切除术 | median ~ 正中甲状腺肿切除术

strumiprivous [ˌstruːmiˈpraivəs], **strumiprival** [struːmiˈpraivəl], **strumiprivic** [ˌstruːmiˈpraivik] *a* 甲状腺缺乏的(甲状腺切除所致的)

strumitis [struːˈmaitis] *n* 甲状腺炎 | eberthian ~ 伤寒性甲状腺炎

Strümpell-Leichtenstern disease [ˈʃtrimpəl ˈlaiʃtənstəːn] (A. von Strümpell; Otto Leichtenstern)出血性脑炎

Strümpell-Marie disease [ˈʃtrimpəl məˈriː] (A. von Strümpell; Pierre Marie)类风湿脊柱炎

Strümpell's disease [ˈʃtrimpəl] (Adolf von Strümpell)施特吕姆佩尔病(①遗传型侧索硬化,主要是腿痉挛;②脑脊髓灰质炎) | ~ sign 施特吕姆佩尔征(①大腿向腹部屈曲时则足背屈,见于痉挛性下肢麻痹,亦称胫肌征;②如腕

不过度背屈则不能拳握,亦称桡神经征;③旋前征:前臂被动屈曲时则旋前,见于偏瘫)/ ~ type 施特吕姆佩尔型,遗传型侧索硬化

Strümpell-Westphal pseudosclerosis [ˈʃtrimpəl ˈvestfɑːl](A. von Strümpell; Carl F. O. Westphal)肝豆状核变性

Strunsky's sign [ˈstrunski](Max Strunsky)斯特伦斯基征(检足前弓疾患:检查者捏患者足趾,并突然屈曲,若前弓发炎,则引起疼痛)

Struther's ligament [ˈstrʌθəz](Sir John Struthers)斯特拉瑟斯韧带(一种纤维带,有时从肱骨髁上突延伸到正中上髁,围住正中神经和常为肱动脉以及为喙肱肌和部分旋前圆肌提供异常附着物)

Struve's test [ˈstruːvə](Heinrich Struve)斯特鲁甫试验(检尿血)

struvite [ˈstruːvait] *n* 鸟粪石

strychnine [ˈstrikniːn] *n* 士的宁(中枢兴奋药) | ~ hydrochloride 盐酸士的宁 / ~ nitrate 硝酸士的宁 / ~ phosphate 磷酸士的宁 / ~ sulfate 硫酸士的宁

strychninism [ˈstrikninizəm], **strychnism** [ˈstriknizəm] *n* 士的宁中毒

strychninization [ˌstrikninaiˈzeiʃən, -niˈz-] *n* 士的宁作用

strychninomania [ˌstrikninəuˈmeinjə] *n* 士的宁狂,士的宁中毒性精神病

strychnize [ˈstriknaiz] *vt* 使受士的宁作用

Strychnos [ˈstriknəs] *n*【希】马钱属

STS serologic test for syphilis 梅毒血清学试验;Society of Thoracic Surgeons 胸外科医师学会

Student's *t*-test [ˈstjuːdənt](“Student”为英国数学家 William Sealy Gossett 的笔名)“斯氏”*t* 检验(见 test 项下 *t*-test)

Studer neobladder [ˈstjuːdə](Urs E. Studer)斯图德新膀胱(一种低压型原位回肠新膀胱)

study [ˈstʌdi] *n* 检查,研究;研究项目 | electrophysiologic ~ 电生理检查 / prospective ~, cohort ~ 前瞻性研究,队列研究(一种流行病学研究)/ retrospective ~, case-control ~ 回顾性研究,病例对照研究(一种流行病学研究)

stump [ˈstʌmp] *n* 残肢;残株 | appendiceal ~ 阑尾残端 / conical ~ 圆锥形残肢,锥体状残肢(截肢后由于肌肉过分缩进所致)

stun [stʌn] *vt* 使晕眩,打昏,震晕 *n* 晕眩

stunning [ˈstʌniŋ] *n* 功能丧失(类似意识丧失) | myocardial ~ 心肌功能丧失(心肌功能暂时受损,由于短时期局部缺血所致,以后还会持续一段时间)

stunt [stʌnt] *vt* 阻碍发育(或成长) *n* 发育障碍

stupe [stjuːp] *n* 热敷布(用于热敷法) *vt* 热敷

stupefacient [ˌstjuːpiˈfeiʃənt] *a* 致木僵的,麻醉的 *n* 麻醉药 | **stupefactive** [ˌstjuːpiˈfæktiv] *a*

stupefaction [ˌstjuːpiˈfækʃən] *n* 麻木状态,昏迷

stupefy [ˈstjuːpifai] *vt* 使麻木,使失感觉

stupidity [stju(ː)ˈpidəti] *n* 愚蠢;迟钝

stupor [ˈstjuːpə] *n* 昏迷;木僵,昏呆 | anergic ~ 无力性木僵 / lethargic ~ 昏睡性木僵,迷睡 | **~ose** [ˈstjuːpərəus], **~ous** [ˈstjuːpərəs] *a*

stupp [stʌp] *n* 汞烟尘,粗汞华

sturdy [ˈstəːdi] *n* 羊蹒跚病

Sturge-Kalischer-Weber syndrome [stəːdʒ ˈkɑːliʃ ˈwebə](W. A. Sturge; Siegfried Kalischer; Frederick P. Weber)斯-卡-韦综合征(见 Sturge-Weber syndrome)

Sturge's disease, syndrome, Sturge-Weber syndrome [ˈstəːdʒ ˈwebə](William A. Sturge; Frederick P. Weber)斯特奇病、综合征,斯-韦综合征(一种先天性综合征,包括脸部焰色痣、软脑膜和脉络膜血管瘤、晚期青光眼,常伴有颅内钙化、智力迟缓、对侧偏瘫以及癫痫)

Sturm's conoid [stəːm](Johann C. Sturm)斯图姆类圆锥体(各种散光症对一点的漫射像的形状改变,其像可能为一椭圆体,一圆圈或一锐线) | ~ interval 散光间距

stutter [ˈstʌtə] *vt*, *vi* 结结巴巴地说 *n* 口吃 | **~er** *n* 口吃者

stuttering [ˈstʌtəriŋ] *n* 口吃 | labiochoreic ~ 唇痉挛性口吃,唇舞病 / urinary ~ 断续排尿

sty, stye [stai]([复] **sties** 或 **styes**) *n* 睑腺炎,麦粒肿

stycosis [staiˈkəusis] *n* 石膏沉着(硫酸钙沉着,主要在淋巴结)

style¹ [stail] *n* 风格,作风;式样,类型

style² [stail] *n* 通管丝,管心针;细探子

stylet [ˈstailit] *n* 通管丝,管心针;细探子 | intubating ~ 插管芯

styli [ˈstailai] stylus 的复数

styliform [ˈstailifɔːm] *a* 长而尖的,针状的,茎状的

styliscus [staiˈliskəs] *n*【拉】细柱形塞条

styl(o)- [构词成分]茎突,茎状

stylohyoid [ˌstailəuˈhaiɔid], **stylohyal** [ˌstailəuˈhaiəl] *a* 茎突舌骨的

styloid [ˈstailɔid] *a* 茎状的,柱样的 *n* 柱晶

styloiditis [ˌstailɔiˈdaitis] *n* 茎突炎

stylomandibular [ˌstailəumænˈdibjulə] *a* 茎突下颌的

stylomastoid [ˌstailəuˈmæstɔid] *a* 茎突乳突的

stylomaxillary [ˌstailəuˈmæksiləri] *a* 茎突上颌的

Stylommatophora [staiˌlɔməˈtɔfərə] *n* 柄眼亚目

stylomyloid [ˌstailəuˈmailɔid] *a* 茎突磨牙部的

stylopodium [ˌstailəuˈpəudjəm] *n* 柱骨(胚胎期的肱骨和股骨)

Stylosanthes [ˌstailəuˈsænθiːz] *n* 铅笔花属
stylostaphyline [ˌstailəuˈstæfilain] *a* 茎突腭帆的
stylosteophyte [staiˈlɔstiəfait] *n* 茎状骨赘
stylostixis [ˌstailəuˈstiksis] *n* 针[刺]术
stylus [ˈstailəs]（[复] **styluses** 或 **styli** [ˈstailai]）*n* 通管丝,管心针;细探子;棒剂,药笔剂
stymatosis [ˌstaiməˈtəusis] *n* 出血性阴茎异常勃起
stypage [ˈstaipidʒ, stiˈpɑːʒ] *n*【法】药栓使用(局部麻醉法)
stype [staip] *n* 药栓,药布
stypsis [ˈstipsis] *n*【希】收敛[作用];收敛疗法
styptic [ˈstiptik] *a* 收敛的,止血的 *n* 收敛剂,止血剂 | chemical ~ 化学止血剂 / mechanical ~ 机械性止血物 / vascular ~ 血管收缩性止血剂 | **~al** *a* / **~ity** [stipˈtisəti] *n* 收敛性,止血作用
styramate [ˈstirəmeit] *n* 司替氨酯(骨骼肌松弛药)
Styrax [ˈstaiəræks] *n* 安息香属
styrax [ˈstaiəræks] *n* 苏合香
styrol [ˈstaiərɔl], **styrene** [ˈstaiəriːn], **styrolene** [ˈstairəuliːn] *n* 苯乙烯
styron [ˈstaiərɔn], **styrone** [ˈstaiərəun] *n* 肉桂醇
su. sumat【拉】服用
sub- [前缀]在下,下;不足,不全;次,亚
subabdominal [ˌsʌbæbˈdɔminl] *a* 腹下的
subabdominoperitoneal [ˌsʌbæbˌdɔminəuˌperitəuˈniːəl] *a* 腹腔腹膜下的
subacetabular [ˌsʌbæsiˈtæbjulə] *a* 髋臼下的
subacetate [sʌbˈæsiteit] *n* 次醋酸盐,碱式醋酸盐
subacid [sʌbˈæsid] *a* 微酸[性]的 | **~ity** [ˌsʌbəˈsidəti] *n* 微酸性,酸不足,酸过少
subacromial [ˌsʌbəˈkrəumiəl] *a* 肩峰下的
subacute [ˌsʌbəˈkjuːt] *a* 亚急性的
subalimentation [ˌsʌbælimenˈteiʃən] *n* 营养不足
subanal [sʌbˈeinəl] *a* 肛门下的
subapical [sʌbˈæpikəl] *a* 根尖下的
subaponeurotic [ˌsʌbæpənjuəˈrɔtik] *a* 腱膜下的
subaquatic [ˌsʌbəˈkwætik] *a* 水下的;半水生性的,半水栖的
subaqueous [ˌsʌbˈeikwiəs] *a* 水下的
subarachnoid [ˌsʌbəˈræknɔid] *a* 蛛网膜下的
subarcuate [sʌbˈɑːkjuit] *a* 微弯的,稍呈弓状的
subareolar [ˌsʌbəˈriːələ] *a* 乳晕下的
subastragalar [ˌsʌbəˈstrægələ] *a* 距骨下的
subastringent [ˌsʌbəˈstrindʒənt] *a* 中度收敛的
subatloidean [ˌsʌbætˈlɔidiən] *a* 寰椎下的
subatomic [ˌsʌbəˈtɔmik] *a* 逊原子的,亚原子的
subaural [sʌbˈɔːrəl] *a* 耳下的
subaurale [ˌsʌbɔːˈreili] *a* 耳郭下点(人体测量名词,当受检者向前直视时,耳小叶下缘的最低点)
subauricular [ˌsʌbɔːˈrikjulə] *a* 耳郭下的
subaxial [sʌbˈæksiəl] *a* 轴下的
subaxillary [sʌbˈæksiləri] *a* 腋下的
subbasal [sʌbˈbeisl] *a* 基底下的
subbrachial [sʌbˈbreikiəl] *a* (脑)臂下的
subbrachycephalic [ˌsʌbbreikisəˈfælik] *a* 亚短头型的
subbranch [sʌbˈbrɑːntʃ] *n* 小分支
subbreed [ˈsʌbbriːd] *n* 亚品种
subcalcareous [ˌsʌbkælˈkεəriəs] *a* 微石灰性的
subcalcarine [sʌbˈkælkərain] *a* 距状裂下的
subcalorism [sʌbˈkælərizəm] *n* 受寒,感冒
subcapsular [sʌbˈkæpsjulə] *a* 囊下的,被膜下的
subcapsuloperiosteal [sʌbˌkæpsjuləuˌperiˈɔstiəl] *a* 关节囊[与]骨膜下的
subcarbonate [sʌbˈkɑːbənit] *n* 次碳酸盐,亚碳酸盐
subcarinal [ˌsʌbkəˈrainəl] *a* 气管隆嵴下的
subcartilaginous [ˌsʌbkɑːtiˈlædʒinəs] *a* 软骨下的;部分软骨的
subcentral [sʌbˈsentrəl] *a* 近中央的;中央裂下的
subception [sʌbˈsepʃən] *n* 下知觉,潜知觉
subchloride [sʌbˈklɔːraid] *n* 次氯化物,亚氯化物
subchondral [sʌbˈkɔndrəl] *a* 软骨下的
subchordal [sʌbˈkɔːdəl] *a* 脊索下的;声带下的
subchorionic [ˌsʌbkɔːriˈɔnik] *a* 绒毛膜下的
subchoroidal [ˌsʌbkɔːˈrɔidəl] *a* 脉络膜下的
subchronic [sʌbˈkrɔnik] *a* 亚慢性的(慢性与亚急性之间的)
subclass [ˈsʌbklɑːs] *n* 亚纲(生物分类)
subclavian [sʌbˈkleiviən], **subclavicular** [ˌsʌbkləˈvikjulə] *a* 锁骨下的
subclinical [sʌbˈklinikəl] *a* 亚临床的,临床症状不显的(指早期轻度疾病)
subclone [ˈsʌbkləun] *n* 亚克隆
subconjunctival [ˌsʌbkəndʒʌŋkˈtaivəl] *a* 结膜下的
subconscious [sʌbˈkɔnʃəs] *a* 下意识的 | **~ly** *ad* | **~ness** *n*
subcoracoid [sʌbˈkɔrəkɔid] *a* 喙突下的
subcortex [sʌbˈkɔːteks] *n* 下皮质,皮质下部
subcortical [sʌbˈkɔːtikəl] *a* 皮质下的,皮层下的
subcostal [sʌbˈkɔstl] *a* 肋骨下的
subcostalis [ˌsʌbkɔːsˈteilis]（[复] **subcostales** [ˌsʌbkɔːsˈteiliːz]）*a*【拉】肋骨下的
subcranial [sʌbˈkreinjəl] *a* 颅下的
subcrepitant [sʌbˈkrepitənt] *a* 亚捻发音的
subcrepitation [ˌsʌbkrepiˈteiʃən] *n* 亚捻发音
subcrystalline [ˌsʌbˈkristəlain] *a* 部分结晶的,结

晶不明显的
subculture [ˈsʌbkʌltʃə] *n* 传代培养物;传代培养法
subcutaneous (SC, SQ) [ˌsʌbkju(ː)ˈteinjəs] *a* 皮下的 | **~ly** *ad*
subcuticular [ˌsʌbkjuˈtikjulə] *a* 表皮下的
subcutis [sʌbˈkjuːtis] *n* 皮下组织
subdelirium [ˌsʌbdiˈliəriəm] *n* 轻度谵妄
subdeltoid [sʌbˈdeltɔid] *a* 三角肌下的
subdental [sʌbˈdentl] *a* 牙下的
subdiaphragmatic [ˌsʌbdaiəfrægˈmætik] *a* 膈下的
subdivision [ˈsʌbdiˌviʒən] *n* 再分,细分;亚门
subdominant [ˌsʌbˈdɔminənt] *a* 亚优势的 *n* 亚优势种
subdorsal [sʌbˈdɔːsəl] *a* 背部下的
subduct [sʌbˈdʌkt] *vt* 下转 | **~ion** [sʌbˈdʌkʃən] *n* 下转,眼球下转
subdural [sʌbˈdjuərəl] *a* 硬膜下的
subendocardial [ˌsʌbendəuˈkɑːdiəl] *a* 心内膜下的
subendocardium [ˌsʌbəndəuˈkɑːdiəm] *n* 心内膜下层
subendothelial [ˌsʌbendəuˈθiːljəl] *a* 内皮下的
subendothelium [ˌsʌbendəuˈθiːljəm] *n* 内皮下膜(见 Débove's membrane)
subendymal [sʌbˈendiməl], **subependymal** [ˌsʌbeˈpendiməl] *a* 室管膜下的
subependymoma [ˌsʌbeˌpendiˈməumə] *n* 亚室管膜瘤
subepicardial [ˌsʌbepiˈkɑːdiəl] *a* 心外膜下的
subepidermal [ˌsʌbepiˈdəːməl], **subepidermic** [ˌsʌbepiˈdəːmik] *a* 表皮下的
subepiglottic [ˌsʌbepiˈglɔtik] *a* 会厌下的
subepithelial [ˌsʌbepiˈθiːliəl] *a* 上皮下的
suberic acid [sjuːˈberik] 辛二酸
suberin [ˈsjuːbərin] *n* 软木脂
suberitin [sjuːˈberitin] *n* 皮海绵毒质
suberosis [ˌsjuːbəˈrəusis] *n* 软木尘肺
subextensibility [ˌsʌbeksˌtensiˈbiləti] *n* 伸延性不足,伸展性减少
subfamily [sʌbˈfæmili] *n* 亚科(生物分类)
subfascial [sʌbˈfæsʃəl] *a* 筋膜下的
subfertile [sʌbˈfəːtail] *a* 低生育力的
subfertility [ˌsʌbfə(ː)ˈtiləti] *n* 低生育力
Sub fin. coct. sub finem coctionis【拉】直到煮沸完毕
subflavous [sʌbˈfleivəs] *a* 淡黄[色]的
subfolium [sʌbˈfəuljəm] *n* 小脑小叶 | **subfoliar** *a*
subform [ˈsʌbfɔːm] *n* 从属形式,派生形式
subfrontal [sʌbˈfrʌntəl] *a* 额叶下的
subgaleal [sʌbˈgeiliəl] *a* 帽状腱膜下的
subgallate [sʌbˈgæleit] *n* 次没食子酸盐,次棓酸盐
subgemmal [sʌbˈdʒeməl] *a* 味蕾下的
subgenus [sʌbˈdʒiːnəs] *n* 亚属(生物分类)
subgerminal [sʌbˈdʒəːminl] *a* 胚下的
subgingival [sʌbˈdʒindʒivəl] *a* 龈下的
subglenoid [sʌbˈgliːnɔid] *a* 关节盂下的
subglossal [sʌbˈglɔsəl] *a* 舌下的
subglossitis [ˌsʌbglɔˈsaitis] *n* 舌下炎
subglottic [sʌbˈglɔtik] *a* 声门下的
subgranular [sʌbˈgrænjulə] *a* 亚粒状的
subgrondation [ˌsʌbgrɔnˈdeiʃən] *n*【法】骨嵌凹
subgroup [ˈsʌbgruːp] *n* 亚群,子群;族(周期表);副族(指周期表中的 B 族);亚[血]型
subgyrus [sʌbˈdʒaiərəs] *n* 隐[脑]回
subhepatic [ˌsʌbhiˈpætik] *a* 肝下的
subhumeral [sʌbˈhjuːmərəl] *a* 肱骨下的
subhyaloid [sʌbˈhaiəlɔid] *a* 透明膜下的
subhyoid [sʌbˈhaiɔid], **subhyoidean** [ˌsʌbhaiˈɔidiən] *a* 舌骨下的
subicteric [ˌsʌbikˈterik] *a* 轻黄疸的
subiculum [səˈbikjuləm] *n* (脑)下托 | **subicular** [səˈbikjulə] *a*
subiliac [sʌbˈiliæk] *a* 髂骨下的
subilium [sʌbˈiliəm] *n* 髂骨下部
subimbibitional [ˌsʌbimbiˈbiʃənl] *a* 液体吸取不足的
subinflammation [ˌsʌbinfləˈmeiʃən] *n* 轻[度]炎症 | **subinflammatory** [ˌsʌbinˈflæmətəri] *a*
subintimal [sʌbˈintiməl] *a* (血管)内膜下的
subintrance [sʌbˈintrəns] *n* 提前发作
subintrant [sʌbˈintrənt] *a* 提前发作的
subinvolution [ˌsʌbinvəˈljuːʃən] *n* 子宫复旧不全 | chronic ~ of uterus 慢性子宫复旧不全
subiodide [sʌbˈaiədaid] *n* 低碘化物
subjacent [sʌbˈdʒeisənt] *a* 在下的,下邻的,下面相连的
subject [ˈsʌbdʒikt] *a* 从属的;易受…的,常患…的 *n* 受治疗者,受实验者 [səbˈdʒekt] *vt* 使隶属,使服从;使受到,使遭遇
subjective [sʌbˈdʒektiv] *a* 主观的,自觉的,主觉性的 | **~ly** *ad* | **subjectivity** [ˌsʌbdʒekˈtivəti] *n* 主观,主观性
subjectoscope [sʌbˈdʒektəskəup] *n* 视觉检查器
subjugal [sʌbˈdʒuːgəl] *a* 颧骨下的
subkingdom [ˈsʌbˌkiŋdəm] *n* 亚界,门(生物分类)
sublate [ˈsʌbleit] *vt* 分离,脱离 | **sublation** [sʌbˈleiʃən] *n*
sublatio [sʌbˈleiʃiəu] *n*【拉】分离,脱离 | ~ reti-

nae 视网膜脱离
sublesional [sʌbˈliːʒənəl] *a* 损伤部下的
sublethal [sʌbˈliːθəl] *a* 亚致死的,次致死的
sublimate [ˈsʌblimeit] *vt*, *vi* 升华 [ˈsʌblimit] *a* 升华的 [ˈsʌblimit] *n* 升华物;升汞 | corrosive ~ 升汞,二氯化汞 | **sublimation** [ˌsʌbliˈmeiʃən] *n* 升华[作用]
sublime [səˈblaim] *vt*, *vi* 升华
subliminal [sʌbˈliminl] *a* 阈下的,限下的
sublimis [sʌbˈlaimis] *a* 【拉】浅的,表面的
sublingual [sʌbˈliŋgwəl] *a* 舌下的
sublinguitis [ˌsʌbliŋˈgwaitis] *n* 舌下腺炎
sublobe [ˈsʌbləub] *n* 分叶,小叶
sublobular [sʌbˈlɔbjulə] *a* 小叶下的
subluxate [sʌbˈlʌkseit] *vi* 不全脱位,半脱位,部分脱位
subluxation [ˌsʌblʌkˈseiʃən] *n* 不全脱位,半脱位 | ~ of lens 晶状体不全脱位 / radial head ~ 桡骨小头半脱位
sublymphemia [ˌsʌblimˈfiːmiə] *n* 血[内]淋巴细胞减少
submammary [sʌbˈmæməri] *a* 乳腺下的
submandibular [ˌsʌbmænˈdibjulə] *a* 下颌下的
submania [sʌbˈmeinjə] *n* 轻躁狂
submarginal [ˌsʌbˈmɑːdʒinəl] *a* 缘下的
submaxilla [ˌsʌbmækˈsilə] *n* 下颌,下颌骨
submaxillaritis [sʌbˌmæksiləˈraitis] *n* 颌下腺炎
submaxillary [sʌbˈmæksiləri] *a* 颌下的
submedial [sʌbˈmiːdjəl], **submedian** [sʌbˈmiːdjən] *a* 中线下的,近中线的
submembranous [sʌbˈmembrənəs] *a* 部分膜性的
submental [sʌbˈmentl] *a* 颏下的
submentovertex [sʌbˌmentəuˈvəːteks] *a* 颏下顶的
submetacentric [ˌsʌbmetəˈsentrik] *a* 亚中着丝粒的(染色体)
submicron [sʌbˈmaikrɔn] *n* 亚微[细]粒,次微子(一种胶体微粒,其大小从 5×10^{-7} cm ~ 1×10^{-5}cm 不等,只有用超显微镜才能看到)
submicroscopic(al) [sʌbˌmaikrəsˈkɔpik(əl)] *a* 亚微观的,亚显微的
subminiature [ˌsʌbˈminjətʃə] *a* 超小型的
subminiaturize [ˌsʌbˈminjətʃəraiz] *vt*, *vi* 超小型化 | **subminiaturization** [ˈsʌbˌminjətʃəraiˈzeiʃən, -riˈz-] *n*
submorphous [sʌbˈmɔːfəs] *a* 亚晶形的
submucosa [ˌsʌbmjuːˈkəusə] *n* 黏膜下层 | **~l** *a*
submucous [sʌbˈmjuːkəs] *a* 黏膜下的
subnarcotic [ˌsʌbnɑːˈkɔtik] *a* 中度麻醉的
subnasal [sʌbˈneizəl] *a* 鼻下的
subnasale [sʌbneiˈseili], **subnasion** [sʌbˈneiziən] *n* 鼻中隔下点(人体测量名词,鼻中隔以中矢状平面方向与上唇会合处所成之点)
subnatant [sʌbˈneitənt] *a* (位于)下层的 *n* 下层清液
subneural [sʌbˈnjuərəl] *a* 神经下的
subnitrate [sʌbˈnaitreit] *n* 次硝酸盐,碱式硝酸盐
subnormal [sʌbˈnɔːməl] *a* 低[于正]常的,正常下的
subnormality [ˌsʌbnɔːˈmæləti] *n* 低常状态 | mental ~ 精神低常状态,精神失常
subnotochordal [ˌsʌbnəutəˈkɔːdl] *a* 脊索下的
subnucleus [sʌbˈnjuːkliəs] *n* 亚核
subnutrition [ˌsʌbnju(ː)ˈtriʃən] *n* 营养不足
suboccipital [ˌsʌbɔkˈsipitl] *a* 枕骨下的
subocular [sʌbˈɔkjulə] *a* 眼下的
suboptimal [sʌbˈɔptiməl] *a* 最适度下的
suboptimum [sʌbˈɔptiməm] *n* 次最适度
suborbital [sʌbˈɔːbitl] *a* 眶下的
suborder [sʌbˈɔːdə] *n* 亚目(生物分类)
suboxide [sʌbˈɔksaid] *n* 低氧化物
subpapillary [sʌbˈpæpiləri] *a* 乳头层下的
subpapular [sʌbˈpæpjulə] *a* 亚丘疹性的
subparalytic [ˌsʌbpærəˈlitik] *a* 轻瘫的,不全麻痹的
subparietal [ˌsʌbpəˈraiitl] *a* 顶下的
subpatellar [ˌsʌbpəˈtelə] *a* 髌下的
subpectoral [sʌbˈpektərəl] *a* 胸肌下的
subpelviperitoneal [sʌbˌpelviˌperitəuˈniːəl] *a* 盆腔腹膜下的
subpericardial [ˌsʌbperiˈkɑːdiəl] *a* 心包下的
subperiosteal [ˌsʌbperiˈɔstiəl] *a* 骨膜下的
subperiosteocapsular [ˌsʌbperiˌɔstiəuˈkæpsjulə] *a* 关节囊[与]骨膜下的
subperitoneal [ˌsʌbperitəuˈniːəl], **subperitoneoabdominal** [ˌsʌbperitəuˌniəuæbˈdɔminl] *a* 腹膜下的,腹腔腹膜下的
subperitoneopelvic [ˌsʌbperitəuniəuˈpelvik] *a* 盆腔腹膜下的
subpharyngeal [ˌsʌbfəˈrindʒiəl] *a* 咽下的
subphrenic [sʌbˈfrenik] *a* 膈下的
subphylum [sʌbˈfailəm] ([复] **subphyla** [sʌbˈfailə]) *n* 亚门(生物分类)
subpial [sʌbˈpaiəl] *a* 软[脑脊]膜下的
subpituitarism [ˌsʌbpiˈtju(ː)itərizəm] *n* 垂体功能减退
subplacenta [ˌsʌbpləˈsentə] *n* 基蜕膜
subpleural [sʌbˈpluərəl] *a* 胸膜下的
subpreputial [ˌsʌbpriˈpjuːʃəl] *a* 包皮下的
subpubic [sʌbˈpjuːbik] *a* 耻骨[弓]下的
subpulmonary [sʌbˈpʌlmənəri] *a* 肺下的

subpulpal [sʌbˈpʌlpl] *a* 牙髓下的
subpyramidal [ˌsʌbpiˈræmidl] *a* 锥体下的
subrectal [sʌbˈrektəl] *a* 直肠下的
subregion [ˈsʌbriːdʒən] *n* 分区;亚区(生物分布) | **~al** [sʌbˈriːdʒənl] *a*
subretinal [sʌbˈretinl] *a* 视网膜下的
subscaphocephaly [ˌsʌbskæfəˈsefəli] *n* 中度舟状头[畸形]
subscapular [sʌbˈskæpjulə] *a* 肩胛下的
subscleral [sʌbˈskliərəl] *a* 巩膜下的
subsclerotic [sʌbskliəˈrɔtik] *a* 巩膜下的;部分硬化的
subscription [səbˈskripʃən] *n* 调配法,下标(处方)
subserosa [ˌsʌbsiəˈrəusə] *n* 浆膜下层
subserous [sʌbˈsiərəs] *a* 浆膜下的
subsibilant [sʌbˈsibilənt] *a* 轻咝音的
subside [səbˈsaid] *vi* 减退,消退 | **~nce** [səbˈsaidəns, ˈsʌbsidəns] *n*
subsonic [sʌbˈsɔnik] *a* 亚声速的;亚声频的;次声的
subspecialty [sʌbˈspeʃəlti] *n* 分科,亚专科(如内科中的胃肠科)
subspecies [ˈsʌbˌspiːʃi(ː)z] *n* 亚种(生物分类)
subspinale [ˌsʌbspaiˈneili] *n* 上颌牙槽座下点(亦称 A 点,见 point A)
subspinous [sʌbˈspainəs] *a* 棘突下的
subsplenial [sʌbˈspliːniəl] *a* 胼胝体压部下的
substage [ˈsʌbsteidʒ] *n* (显微镜的)镜台下部
substance [ˈsʌbstəns] *n* 质,物质 | accessory food ~ 辅助食物因素,维生素 / ad ~ 突触传递物质 / agglutinable ~ 可凝集物质 / agglutinating ~ 凝集物质(凝集素) / α-~, alpha ~, reticular ~ α 物质,网状物质(红细胞内) / anti-immune ~ 抗免疫物质,抗免疫体 / β-~, beta ~ β 物质,异染粒 / contact ~ 接触剂,催化剂 / H ~ H 物质(在具有 ABO 血型系 O 型的个体中的红细胞同族抗原;释放性物质,见 released ~) / molecular ~ 神经纤维网 / P-P ~, pellagra-preventing ~ 糙皮病预防物质 / preventive ~ 预防性物质(抗体) / red ~ of spleen 脾髓 / released ~ 释放性物质(炎症时释放的组胺样物质,能增加血管通透性) / ~ sensibilisatrice, sensibilizing ~, sensitizing ~ 致敏物质(抗体) / slow reacting ~ of anaphylaxis(SRS-A) 过敏性慢反应物质(过敏反应时释放的物质,能引起某些平滑肌长时间缓慢收缩,此物质由白细胞三烯〈leukotrienes〉 C_4, C_4,和 E_4 的混合物组成) / specific soluble ~ (SSS) 特异性可溶性物质
substantia [səbˈstænʃiə] ([复] **substantiae** [səbˈstænʃiiː]) *n* 【拉】质,物质
substernal [sʌbˈstəːnl] *a* 胸骨下的
substernomastoid [ˌsʌbstəːnəuˈmæstɔid] *a* 胸锁乳突肌下的
substituent [sʌbˈstitjuənt] *n* 取代基
substitute [ˈsʌbstitjuːt] *n* 替代药,代用品 | blood ~, plasma ~ 血液代用品,血浆代用品
substitution [ˌsʌbstiˈtjuːʃən] *n* 代替,替换;取代反应,置换反应 | creeping ~ of bone 匍匐性骨置换
substitutive [ˈsʌbstitjuːtiv] *a* 取代的,代用的,置换的
substrate [ˈsʌbstreit] *n* 底物
substratum [ˌsʌbˈstrɑːtəm, ˌsʌbˈstreitəm] ([复] **substrata** [ˌsʌbˈstrɑːtə, ˌsʌbˈstreitə]) *n* 【拉】底物,基质;下层,基层,低层
substructure [ˈsʌbˌstrʌktʃə] *n* 下部结构,基础 | implant ~ 植入结构(如骨膜下植入义齿)
subsulcus [sʌbˈsʌlkəs] *a* 隐沟
subsulfate [sʌbˈsʌlfeit] *a* 次硫酸盐,碱式硫酸盐
subsultus [sʌbˈsʌltəs] *n* (痉挛性)跳动 | ~ tendinum 腱跳动
subsurface [ˈsʌbˈsəːfis] *a* 表面下的
subsylvian [sʌbˈsilviən] *a* 大脑侧裂下的
subsystem [ˈsʌbˈsistim] *n* 分系统,支系统
subtalar [sʌbˈteilə] *a* 距骨下的(如 ~ joint 距跟关节)
subtarsal [sʌbˈtɑːsəl] *a* 跗骨下的
subtelocentric [ˌsʌbteləˈsentrik] *a* 亚端着丝粒的(染色体)
subtemperate [sʌbˈtempərit] *a* 副温带的,亚温带的
subtemporal [sʌbˈtempərəl] *a* 颞下的
subtenial [sʌbˈtiːniəl] *a* 带下的
subtentorial [sʌbˈtentəriəl] *a* (小脑)幕下的
subterhuman [ˌsʌbtəˈhjuːmən] *a* 低于人类的
subterminal [ˌsʌbˈtəːminl] *a* 近末端的,近端的
subtertian [ˌsʌbˈtəːʃən] *a* 亚间日的,近乎间日发作的
subtetanic [ˌsʌbtiˈtænik] *a* 轻度强直的,轻度抽搦的
subthalamic [ˌsʌbθəˈlæmik] *a* 丘脑下的
subthalamus [sʌbˈθæləməs] *n* 底丘脑
subthreshold [ˌsʌbˈθreʃhəuld] *a* (药物剂量)次于最低限度的,不足以起到作用的;阈下的,限值以下的
subthyroidism [sʌbˈθairɔidizəm] *n* 甲状腺功能减退
subtile [ˈsʌtl] *a* 锐敏的
subtilin [ˈsʌbtilin] *n* 枯草菌素
subtilisin [sʌbˈtilisin] *n* 枯草杆菌蛋白酶
subtle [ˈsʌtl] *a* 锐敏的;精细的
subtotal [ˈsʌbˌtəutl] *a* 次全的
subtransparent [ˌsʌbtrænsˈpeərənt] *a* 半透明的

subtrapezial [ˌsʌbtrəˈpiːziəl] *a* 斜方肌下的
subtribe [ˈsʌbtraib] *n* 亚族(生物分类)
subtrochanteric [ˌsʌbtrəukænˈterik] *a* 转子下的
subtrochlear [sʌbˈtrɔkliə] *a* 滑车下的
subtropic(al) [ˈsʌbˈtrɔpik(əl)] *a* 副热带的,亚热带的
subtuberal [sʌbˈtjuːbərəl] *a* 结节下的
subtympanic [ˌsʌbtimˈpænik] *a* 鼓室下的;轻鼓音的
subtypical [sʌbˈtipikəl] *a* 亚定型的
subulate [ˈsjuːbjulit] *a* 锥形的,钻形的
subumbilical [ˌsʌbʌmˈbilikəl] *a* 脐下的
subungual [sʌbˈʌŋgwəl] *a* 指甲下的,趾甲下的
suburethral [ˌsʌbjuəˈriːθrəl] *a* 尿道下的
subvaginal [sʌbˈvædʒinəl] *a* 鞘下的;阴道下的
subvertebral [sʌbˈvəːtibrəl] *a* 脊柱下的
subvirile [sʌbˈviril] *a* 男性征不足的
subvitaminosis [sʌbˌvaitəmiˈnəusis] *n* 维生素不足症,维生素缺乏症
subvitrinal [sʌbˈvitrinəl] *a* 玻璃[状]体下的
subvolution [ˌsʌbvəˈljuːʃən] *n* 翻转术(一种皮瓣反转术,尤指切除或反转翼状胬肉手术,使外表面或皮面与切除的肉面接触,以防再粘连)
subwaking [sʌbˈweikiŋ] *a* 半醒的
subzonal [sʌbˈzəunəl] *a* 带下的
subzygomatic [ˌsʌbzaigəˈmætik] *a* 颧下的
succagogue [ˈsʌkəgɔg] *a* 促分泌的 *n* 促分泌剂
succedaneum [ˌsʌksiˈdeiniəm] ([复] **succedanea** [ˌsʌksiˈdeiniə]) *n* 替代品,代用品 | **succedaneous** [ˌsʌksiˈdeiniəs] *a*
succenturiate [ˌsʌksenˈtjuəriit] *a* 副的;替代的
successor [səkˈsesə] *n* 继承牙
succi [ˈsʌkai, ˈsʌksai] succus 的复数
succimer(DMSA) [ˈsʌksimə] *n* 琥巯酸(一种螯合剂,二巯丙醇〈dimercaprol〉的类似物,口服治疗重金属中毒,一种与^{99m}Tc 的合剂用作肾功能试验的诊断用药)
succinate [ˈsʌksineit] *n* 丁二酸盐,琥珀酸盐(酯或阴离子型)
succinate-CoA ligase(GDP-forming) [ˈsʌksineit ˈlaigeis] 琥珀酸-CoA 连接酶(GDP 形成的)(亦称琥珀酰 CoA 合成酶)
succinate dehydrogenase [ˈsʌksineit diːˈhaidrədʒəneis] 琥珀酸脱氢酶
succinate dehydrogenase(ubiquinone) [ˈsʌksineit diːˈhaidrədʒəneis juːˈbikwiˌnəun] 琥珀酸脱氢酶(泛醌)
succinate-semialdehyde dehydrogenase [ˈsʌksineit ˌsemiˈældihaid diːˈhaidrədʒəneis] 琥珀酸半醛脱氢酶
succinic acid [səkˈsinik] 琥珀酸,丁二酸
succinic semialdehyde dehydrogenase dificiency 琥珀酸半醛脱氢酶缺乏症(一种常染色体隐性遗传氨基酸病,由于琥珀酸半醛脱氢酶缺乏所致,从而产生的 γ-氨基丁酸和 γ-羟丁酸的增加导致智力迟钝、张力减退和共济失调。亦称 γ-或 4-羟丁酸尿症)
succinimide [səkˈsinimaid] *n* 琥珀酰亚胺
Succinimonas [ˌsʌksiniˈməunəs] *n* 琥珀酸单胞菌属
Succinivibrio [ˌsʌksiniˈvibriəu] *n* 琥珀酸弧菌属
succinodehydrogenase [ˌsʌksinəudiːˈhaidrədʒəneis] *n* 琥珀酸脱氢酶
succinoresinol [ˌsʌksinəˈrezinɔl] *n* 琥珀树脂醇
succinous [ˈsʌksinəs] *a* 琥珀的
succinum [ˈsʌksinəm] *n*【拉】琥珀
succinyl [ˈsʌksinil] *n* 琥珀酰
succinylacetoacetate [ˌsʌksinilәˌsiːtəuˈæsiteit] *n* 琥珀酰乙酰乙酸
succinylacetone [ˌsʌksinilˈæsitəun] *n* 琥珀酰丙酮
succinylcholine chloride [ˌsʌksinilˈkəuliːn] 氯琥珀胆碱(神经肌肉阻断药)
succinyl CoA [ˈsʌksinil] 琥珀酰 CoA,琥珀酰辅酶 A
succinyl CoA synthetase [ˈsʌksinil ˈsinθiteis] 琥珀酰 CoA 合成酶,琥珀酸-CoA 连接酶(GDP 形成的)
succinylcoenzyme A [ˌsʌksinilˈkəuenzaim] 琥珀酰辅酶 A
succinyldihydrolipoamide [ˌsʌksinildaiˌhaidrəu-ˌlipəuˈæmaid] *n* 琥珀酰二氢硫辛酰胺
succinylsulfathiazole [ˌsʌksinilˌsʌlfəˈθaiəzəul] *n* 琥珀磺胺噻唑(磺胺类药)
succorrhea [ˌsʌkəˈriːə] *n* 分泌溢液;分泌过多
succulent [ˈsʌkjulənt] *a* 多汁的 | **succulence** *n*
succus [ˈsʌkəs] ([复] **succi** [ˈsʌkai, ˈsʌksai]) *n*【拉】汁,液
succuss [səˈkʌs] *vt* 振荡(摇动病人以确定体腔内有无积液) | **~ive** *a*
succussion [səˈkʌʃən] *n* 振荡[法];振荡音 | hippocratic ~ 希波克拉底振荡音(振荡身体时胸内有振水音,一般即诊断为水气胸)
sucholoalbumin [ˌsʌkəuləuˈælbjumin] *n* 猪胆汁白蛋白
sucker [ˈsʌkə] *n* 乳儿;吸管,吸盘
suckle [ˈsʌkl] *vt* 哺乳
suckling [ˈsʌkliŋ] *n* 乳儿;哺乳
Sucquet-Hoyer anastomosis(canal) [siˈkei ˈɔjɛə] (J. P. Sucquet; Henryk Hoyer) 苏盖-奥耶吻合(管)(球形动静脉吻合的动脉段)
sucralfate [sjuːˈkrælfeit] *n* 硫糖铝(抗胃溃疡药)
sucralose [ˈsjuːkrələus] *n* 三氯半乳蔗糖(用作甜

味剂)

sucrase [ˈsjuːkreis] *n* 蔗糖酶,转化酶

sucrase-isomaltase [ˈsjuːkreis ˌaisəuˈmɔːlteis] 蔗糖酶异麦芽糖酶

sucrase-isomaltase deficiency [ˈsjuːkreis ˌaisəuˈmɔːlteis] 蔗糖酶异麦芽糖酶缺乏症(为二糖酶缺乏症,肠黏膜蔗糖酶异麦芽糖酶复合物的活性缺乏可致蔗糖和淀粉糊精吸收不良。本症特征为水泻、渗透性发酵性腹泻,有时可导致脱水和营养不良,婴儿期尤为明显〈先天性蔗糖不耐症〉)

sucrate [ˈsjuːkreit] *n* [蔗]糖合物

sucre [ˈsjuːkrə] *n*【法】糖 | ~ actuelle 真糖(游离血糖)/ ~ virtuelle 假糖(胶态血糖)

sucroclastic [ˌsjuːkrəuˈklæstik] *a* 糖分解的,解糖的

sucrose [ˈsjuːkrəus] *n* 蔗糖 | ~ octaacetate 蔗糖八醋酸酯(酒精变性剂)

sucrose α-glucosidase [ˈsjuːkrəus ɡluːˈkəusideis] 蔗糖 α-葡糖苷酶(sucrase 的 EC 命名法)

sucrosemia [ˌsjuːkrəuˈsiːmiə] *n* 蔗糖血[症]

sucrosum [sjuˈkrəusəm] *n*【拉】蔗糖

sucrosuria [ˌsjuːkrəuˈsjuəriə] *n* 蔗糖尿[症]

suction [ˈsʌkʃən] *n* 吸引[术] | post-tussive ~ 咳后回吸声

Suctoria [sʌkˈtɔːriə] *n* 吸管亚纲

suctorial [sʌkˈtɔːriəl] *a* 吸吮的,适于吸吮的;有吸盘的

suctorian [sʌkˈtɔːriən] *n* 吸管虫 *a* 吸管亚纲的

Suctorida [ˌsʌkˈtɔridə] *n* 吸管虫目

sucuuba [ˈsʌsjubə] *n* 南美鸡蛋花

sudamen [suːˈdeimən] ([复] **sudamina** [suːˈdæminə]) *n*【拉】粟疹,痱子,汗疹 | **sudaminal** [suːˈdæminəl] *a*

sudanophil [suˈdænəfil] *a* 染苏丹的,嗜苏丹的 *n* 嗜苏丹体

sudanophilia [suˌdænəuˈfiliə] *n* 染苏丹性,嗜苏丹性

sudanophilic [suˌdænəuˈfilik], **sudanophilous** [ˌsuːdəˈnɔfiləs] *a* 染苏丹的,嗜苏丹的

sudarium [sjuːˈdeəriəm] *n*【拉】发汗浴

sudarshan shurna [suˈdɑːʃən ˈʃuənə] 印度解热合剂(含 50 种药)

sudation [sjuːˈdeiʃən] *n* 发汗,出汗;剧汗

sudatorium [ˌsjuːdəˈtɔːriəm] ([复] **sudatoria** [ˌsjuːdəˈtɔːriə]) *n*【拉】热气浴;热气浴室

sudatory [ˈsjuːdətəri] *a* 发汗的,利汗的 *n* 发汗剂;热气浴室

Sudeck-Leriche syndrome [ˈzudek ləˈriːʃ] (P. H. M. Sudeck; René Loriche) 祖德克-勒里什综合征(创伤后血管痉挛伴有骨质疏松)

Sudeck's atrophy (disease) [ˈzudek] (Paul H. M. Sudeck) 创伤后骨萎缩 | ~ critical point, point of Sudeck 祖德克临界点,祖德克点(位于最后乙状结肠动脉与直肠上动脉分支间的直肠点,过去认为在此点以下结扎直肠上动脉分支将引起直肠坏疽,但未经临床经验确证)

sudogram [ˈsjuːdəɡræm] *n* (全身)泌汗分布图

sudomotor [sjuːdəˈməutə] *a* 催汗的,促汗的

sudoresis [ˌsjuːdəˈriːsis] *n* 多汗

sudoriferous [ˌsjuːdəˈrifərəs] *a* 分泌汗的;生汗的,出汗的

sudorific [ˌsjuːdəˈrifik] *a* 发汗的 *n* 发汗药

sudoriparous [ˌsjuːdəˈripərəs] *a* 生汗的,出汗的

sudoxicam [sjuːˈdɔksikæm] *n* 舒多昔康(抗炎药)

SUDS sudden unexplained death syndrome 原因不明的猝死综合征(见 syndrome 项下相应术语)

suet [ˈsjuːlt] *n*【拉】兽脂,牛羊脂 | benzoinated ~ 安息香羊脂 / prepared ~ 精制羊脂

sufentanil [suːˈfentənil] *n* 舒芬太尼(镇痛药)

sufentanil citrate [suːˈfentənil] 枸橼酸舒芬太尼(全身麻醉时用作镇痛辅药)

suffocant [ˈsʌfəkənt] *n* 窒息剂

suffocate [ˈsʌfəkeit] *vt* 使窒息 *vi* 窒息 | **suffocation** [ˌsʌfəˈkeiʃən] *n* | **suffocative** [ˈsʌfəkeitiv] *a* 使人窒息的

suffuse [səˈfjuːz] *vt* (液体、光、色等)充满,弥漫于 | **suffusion** [səˈfjuːʒən] *n* 充满,弥漫;涨红;溢血

sugar [ˈʃuɡə] *n* 糖 | actual ~ 真糖(游离血糖) / blood ~ 血糖 / cane ~ 蔗糖 / compressible ~ 可压缩糖 / confectioner's ~ 糖粉(用作甜剂和片剂的赋形剂) / fruit ~ 果糖 / heart ~, muscle ~ 肌醇 / larch ~ 松三糖 / liver ~ 肝糖 / starch ~ 糊精 / threshold ~ 肾糖阈[值] / virtual ~ 假糖(胶态血糖)

sugarin [ˈʃuɡərin] *n* 甲糖精

suggest [səˈdʒest] *vt* 暗示,提示

suggestible [səˈdʒestəbl] *a* 可暗示的 | **suggestibility** [səˌdʒestiˈbiləti] *n* 暗示性

suggestion [səˈdʒestʃən] *n* 暗示 | hypnotic ~ 催眠暗示 / posthypnotic ~ 催眠后暗示

suggillation [ˌsədʒiˈleiʃən] *n* 紫斑,瘀斑

suicidal [sjuiˈsaidl] *a* 自杀的

suicide [ˈsjuisaid] *n* 自杀 | psychic ~ 精神性自杀(不用任何物理手段而结束自己生命)

suicidology [ˌsjuisaiˈdɔlədʒi] *n* 自杀学(研究自杀的原因及预防)

suid [ˈsjuid] *a* 猪的

suint [ˈsjuːint, swint] *n* 羊毛粗脂

suipestifer [ˌsjuːiˈpestifə] *n* 猪疫菌类(一组沙门菌,可引起人和猪的副伤寒性胃肠炎)

Suipoxvirus [ˈsjuiˌpɔksˌvaiərəs] *n* 猪痘病毒属

suit [sjuːt, suːt] *n* (一套)衣服 | antiblackout ~, anti-G ~, G ~ (飞行员)抗加速服,抗黑矇服 / antishock ~ 抗休克服(充气抗休克服)

Suker's sign [ˈsuːkə] (George F. Suker)苏克征(缺乏互补性凝视,见于突眼性甲状腺肿眼球外旋时)

sulazepam [sʌˈlæzəpæm] *n* 硫西泮(弱安定药)

sulbactam [səlˈbæktəm] *n* 舒巴坦(β-内酰胺酶抑制药) | ~ sodium 舒巴坦钠(舒巴坦的钠盐,增加青霉素和头孢菌素的抗菌活力)

sulbenox [sʌlˈbenɔks] *n* 舒贝诺司(兽用生长促进药)

sulcate [ˈsʌlkeit] *a* 有沟的 | **sulcation** [sʌlˈkeiʃən] *n* 沟形成,有沟[状态]

sulciform [ˈsʌlsifɔːm] *a* 沟状的

sulconazole nitrate [sʌlˈkɔnəzəul] 硝酸硫康唑(抗真菌药)

sulculus [ˈsʌlkjuləs] ([复] **sulculi** [ˈsʌlkjulai]) *n*【拉】小沟

sulcus [ˈsʌlkəs] ([复] **sulci** [ˈsʌlsai]) *n*【拉】沟 | angular ~ 角沟,角切迹 / aortic ~ 主动脉沟 / arterial sulci 动脉沟 / atrioventricular ~, coronary ~ of heart 房室沟,心冠状沟 / ~ of auditory tube 咽鼓管沟 / meningeal sulci 动脉沟 / precentral ~, vertical ~ 中央前沟,垂直沟 / venous sulci, sulci for veins 静脉沟

sulfa [ˈsʌlfə] *a* 磺胺的;[含]磺胺药物的

sulfabenzamide [ˌsʌlfəˈbenzəmaid] *n* 磺胺苯酰(抗菌药)

sulfacetamide [ˌsʌlfəˈsetəmaid] *n* 磺胺醋酰(磺胺类药,用于治疗尿路感染) | ~ sodium 磺胺醋酰钠(局部用于结膜,治疗对磺胺敏感的眼部感染)

sulfachlorpyridazine [ˌsʌlfəˌklɔːpiˈridəziːn] *n* 磺胺氯达嗪(兽用抗菌药)

sulfacid [sʌlˈfæsid] *n* 硫代酸;磺酸

sulfacytine [ˌsʌlfəˈsaitiːn] *n* 磺胺西汀(磺胺类药,用于治疗急性尿路感染)

sulfadiazine [ˌsʌlfəˈdaiəziːn] *n* 磺胺嘧啶(磺胺类药) | ~ silver 磺胺嘧啶银(外用抗菌药,在治疗二度和三度烧伤时用以预防创伤脓毒病) / ~ sodium 磺胺嘧啶钠

sulfadimethoxine [ˌsʌlfəˌdaimeˈθɔksiːn] *n* 磺胺地索辛(磺胺类药,用作抗菌药)

sulfadimetine [ˌsʌlfəˈdaimətiːn] *n* 磺胺异二甲嘧啶(即磺胺索嘧啶 sulfisomidine)

sulfadimidine [ˌsʌlfəˈdaimidiːn] *n* 磺胺二甲嘧啶(磺胺类药)

sulfadoxine [ˌsʌlfəˈdɔksiːn] *n* 磺胺多辛(磺胺类药,用于治疗麻风和恶性疟)

sulfaethidole [ˌsʌlfəˈeθidəul] *n* 磺胺乙二唑(磺胺类药,主要用作尿路防腐剂)

sulfafurazole [ˌsʌlfəˈfjuərəzəul] *n* 磺胺异噁唑(磺胺类药,用作抗菌药)

sulfaguanidine [ˌsʌlfəˈgwænidiːn] *n* 磺胺胍(磺胺类药,用作抗菌药,治疗胃肠道感染)

sulfaldehyde [sʌlˈfældihaid] *n* 硫醛

sulfalene [ˈsʌlfəliːn] *n* 磺胺林(磺胺类药,用作抗菌药,尤其用于治疗尿路感染)

sulfamerazine [ˌsʌlfəˈmerəziːn] *n* 磺胺甲嘧啶(抗菌药)

sulfameter [ˈsʌlfəmiːtə] *n* 磺胺对甲氧嘧啶(用作抗菌药,治疗急慢性尿路感染)

sulfamethazine [ˌsʌlfəˈmeθəziːn] *n* 磺胺二甲嘧啶(磺胺类药,用作抗菌药)

sulfamethizole [ˌsʌlfəˈmeθizəul] *n* 磺胺甲二唑(磺胺类药,用作抗菌药,主要用于治疗尿路感染)

sulfamethoxazole [ˌsʌlfəmeˈθɔksəzəul] *n* 磺胺甲噁唑(磺胺类药,用作抗菌药,尤其用于防治急性尿路感染、脓皮病及创伤与软组织的感染)

sulfamethoxypyridazine [ˌsʌlfəmeˌθɔksipiˈridəziːn] *n* 磺胺甲氧嗪(磺胺类药,用作抗菌药,治疗尿路感染及其他感染)

sulfamethyldiazine [ˌsʌlfəˌmeθilˈdaiəziːn] *n* 磺胺甲嘧啶(抗菌药)

sulfamethylthiadiazole [ˌsʌlfəˌmeθilˌθaiəˈdaiəzəul] *n* 磺胺甲二唑(即 sulfamethizole)

sulfamido [sʌlˈfæmidəu], **sulfamine** [sʌlˈfæmin] *n* 氨磺酰基,磺酰胺基

sulfamidochrysoidine [sʌlˌfæmidəukriˈsɔidiːn] *n* 磺胺米可定(磺胺类药)

sulfamonomethoxine [ˌsʌlfəˌmɔnəmeˈθɔksiːn] *n* 磺胺间甲氧嘧啶(抗菌性磺胺类药)

sulfamoxole [ˌsʌlfəˈmɔksəul] *n* 磺胺噁唑(抗菌性磺胺类药)

sulfanilamide [ˌsʌlfəˈniləmaid] *n* 磺胺(磺胺类药)

sulfanilate [sʌlˈfænileit] *n* 磺胺酸盐,对氨基苯磺酸盐

sulfanilic acid [ˌsʌlfəˈnilik] 对氨基苯磺酸

sulfanitran [ˌsʌlfəˈnaitræn] *n* 磺胺硝苯(家禽用抗菌性磺胺类药和抗球虫药)

sulfanuria [ˌsʌlfəˈnjuəriə] *n* 磺胺剂性无尿

sulfapyridine [ˌsʌlfəˈpiridiːn] *n* 磺胺吡啶(一种抗菌化合物,口服用作疱疹样皮炎抑制剂,曾用于治疗肺炎和链球菌性感染)

sulfaquinoxaline [ˌsʌlfəkwiˈnɔksəliːn] *n* 磺胺喹沙啉(兽用抗菌性磺胺类药)

sulfarsphenamine [ˌsʌlfɑːˈsfenəmiːn] *n* 硫胂凡纳明(曾用于治疗梅毒)

sulfasalazine [ˌsʌlfəˈsæləziːn] *n* 柳氮磺吡啶(磺胺类药)

sulfatase [ˈsʌlfəteis] *n* 硫酸酯酶 | multiple ~

deficiency 多硫酸酯酶缺乏症(一种溶酶体贮积症,为一种常染色体隐性性状,合并有异染性脑白质营养不良幼稚型和黏多糖贮积症,患儿既不会走路,也不会说话,并表现有鱼鳞病、粗糙面容、肝脾肿大、脊柱畸形和黏多糖尿。亦称黏硫脂病)

sulfate [ˈsʌlfeit] *n* 硫酸盐,硫酸酯 | acid ~ 酸性硫酸盐 / basic ~ 碱性硫酸盐 / chondroitin ~ 硫酸软骨素 / conjugated ~s, ethereal ~s 结合硫酸盐,硫酸乙酯 / cupric ~ 硫酸铜 / dermatan ~ 硫酸皮肤素,硫酸软骨素 B / mineral ~s, preformed ~s 无机硫酸盐 / neutral ~, normal ~ 中性硫酸盐,正硫酸盐

sulfatemia [ˌsʌlfeiˈtiːmiə] *n* 硫酸盐血症

sulfathiazole [ˌsʌlfəˈθaiəzəul] *n* 磺胺噻唑(曾广泛用作抗菌药,现已被低毒性磺胺类药及抗生素所取代)

sulfatidase [ˌsʌlfəˈtaideis] *n* 硫[脑]苷脂酶,芳香基硫酸酯酶

sulfatide [ˈsʌlfətaid] *n* 硫[脑]苷脂

sulfation [sʌlˈfeiʃən] *n* 硫酸盐化作用

sulfazamet [sʌlˈfæzəmit] *n* 磺胺吡唑(兽用抗菌性氨苯磺胺)

sulfhemoglobin [ˌsʌlfhiːməuˈgləubin] *n* 硫血红蛋白

sulfhemoglobinemia [ˌsʌlfhiːməuˌgləubiˈniːmiə] *n* 硫血红蛋白血症

sulfhydrate [sʌlfˈhaidreit] *n* 氢硫化物

sulfhydric acid [sʌlfˈhaidrik] 氢硫酸,硫化氢

sulfhydryl [sʌlfˈhaidril] *n* 硫氢[基],巯[基]

sulfide [ˈsʌlfaid] *n* 硫化物 | mercuric ~ 硫化汞(以前用于治疗梅毒)

sulfindigotate [sʌlˈfindigəteit] *n* 硫靛酸盐,靛蓝磺酸盐

sulfinic acid [ˌsʌlˈfinik] 亚磺酸

sulfinpyrazone [ˌsʌlfinˈpairəzəun] *n* 磺吡酮(促尿酸排泄药,用于治疗痛风)

sulfinyl [ˈsʌlfinil] *n* 亚硫酰基,亚磺酰基

sulfisomidine [sʌlfiˈsɔmidiːn] *n* 磺胺索嘧啶(磺胺类药)

sulfisoxazole [ˌsʌlfiˈsɔksəzəul] *n* 磺胺异噁唑(磺胺类药,用作抗菌药) | ~ acetyl 磺胺乙酰异噁唑 / ~ diolamine 磺胺异噁唑二乙醇胺盐

sulfite [ˈsʌlfait] *n* 亚硫酸盐

sulfite oxidase [ˈsʌlfait ˈɔksideis] 亚硫酸氧化酶(此酶先天性缺乏可致进行性神经系统异常、晶状体脱位和智力迟钝)

sulfmethemoglobin [ˌsʌlfmetˌhiːməuˈgləubin] *n* 硫血红蛋白

sulf(o)- [前缀]硫,磺基

sulfoacid [ˌsʌlfəuˈæsid] *n* 磺酸

sulfobromophthalein sodium [ˌsʌlfəuˌbrəum-əuˈθæliːn] *n* 磺溴酞钠(肝功能测定药)

sulfoconjugation [ˌsʌlfəuˌkɔndʒuˈgeiʃən] *n* 硫酸结合作用

sulfocyanate [ˌsʌlfəuˈsaiəneit] *n* 硫氰酸盐

sulfocyanic acid [ˌsʌlfəsaiˈænik] 硫氰酸

sulfogel [sʌlfədʒel] *n* 硫酸凝胶

***N*-sulfoglucosamine sulfohydrolase** [ˌsʌlfəug-luːˈkəusəmiːn ˌsʌlfəuˈhaidrəleis] *N*-磺基葡糖胺磺基水解酶(此酶缺乏可致桑菲利波〈Sanfilippo〉综合征 A 型,与乙酰肝素 *N*-硫酸酯酶可能完全相同)

sulfohydrate [ˌsʌlfəuˈhaidreit] *n* 氢硫化物

sulfoiduronate sulfatase [ˌsʌlfəuˌaidjuˈrɔneit ˈsʌlfəteis] 硫代艾杜糖醛酸硫酸酯酶,艾杜糖醛酸硫酸酯酶

sulfolipid [ˌsʌlfəuˈlipid] *n* 硫脂

sulfolithocholylglycine [ˌsʌlfəuˌliθəuˌkəulilˈglai-siːn] *n* 硫石胆酰苷氨酸

sulfolithocholyltaurine [ˌsʌlfəuˌliθəuˌkəulilˈtau-riːn] *n* 硫石胆酰牛磺酸

Sulfolobus [ˌsʌlfəuˈləubəs] *n* 硫叶菌属

sulfolysis [sʌlˈfɔlisis] *n* 硫酸[双分]解(硫酸进行的酸解)

sulfomucin [ˌsʌlfəuˈmjuːsin] *n* 硫黏蛋白

sulfonamide [sʌlˈfɔnəmaid] *n* 磺胺(磺胺类药,此类药已大部分被更有效而毒性低的抗生素所取代)

sulfonamidemia [ˌsʌlfəuˌnæmiˈdiːmiə] *n* 磺胺血

sulfonamidocholia [ˌsʌlfəuˌnæmidəuˈkəuliə] *n* 磺胺胆

sulfonamidotherapy [ˌsʌlfəuˌnæmidəuˈθerəpi] *n* 磺胺药物疗法,磺胺剂疗法

sulfonamiduria [ˌsʌlfəuˌnæmiˈdjuəriə] *n* 磺胺尿

sulfonate [ˈsʌlfəneit] *n* 磺酸盐(酯或阴离子)

sulfone [ˈsʌlfəun] *n* 砜;磺[基]

sulfonethylmethane [ˌsʌlfəuˌneθilˈmeθein] *n* 双乙磺丁烷(催眠药)

sulfonic [sʌlˈfɔnik] *a* 磺[基]的

sulfonic acid [sʌlˈfɔnik] 磺酸

sulfonmethane [ˌsʌlfəunˈmeθein] *n* 双乙磺丙烷(催眠药)

sulfonterol hydrochloride [sʌlˈfɔntərəul] 盐酸磺酰特罗(支气管扩张药)

sulfonyl [ˈsʌlfənil] *n* 磺酰,硫酰

sulfonylurea [ˌsʌlfəniljuəˈriə] *n* 磺酰脲(用于对不能单靠饮食与运动治疗的非胰岛素依赖性糖尿病患者控制高血糖)

sulfoprotein [ˌsʌlfəuˈprəutiːn] *n* 硫蛋白

sulfosalicylate [ˌsʌlfəusəˈlisileit] *n* 磺基水杨酸盐(或酯)

sulfosalicylic acid [ˌsʌlfəuˌsæliˈsilik] 磺基水杨酸

sulfosalt [ˈsʌlfəsɔːlt] *n* 磺酸盐
sulfosol [ˈsʌlfəsɔl] *n* 硫酸溶胶
sulfotransferase [ˌsʌlfəuˈtrænsfəreis] *n* 磺基转移酶
sulfoxidation [səlˌfɔksiˈdeiʃən] *n* 磺化氧化作用
sulfoxide [sʌlˈfɔksaid] *n* 硫氧化物;亚砜
sulfoxism [sʌlˈfɔksizəm] *n* 硫酸中毒
sulfoxone sodium [sʌlˈfɔksəun] 阿地砜钠(抗菌药,主要用作抑麻风杆菌药,治疗瘤型麻风和结核样型麻风,口服给药)
sulfur(S) [ˈsʌlfə] *n* 硫(化学元素) | colloidal ~ 胶态硫 / ~ dioxide 二氧化硫 / flower of ~, sublimed ~ 硫华,升华硫 / hepar- ~, liver of ~ 硫肝,含硫钾 / ~ hydride 硫化氢 / ~ iodide 碘化硫 / lac ~, precipitated ~ 硫黄乳,沉淀硫 / milk of ~ 硫乳,胶态硫 / radioactive ~ 放射性硫,射硫 / roll ~ 硫黄熔条 / ~ vasogen 硫凡士精(软膏) / vegetable ~ 石松子 washed ~, ~ lotum 洗制硫(精制硫)
sulfuraria [ˌsʌlfjuˈrɛəriə] *n* 温泉黄粉(用于皮肤病)
sulfurated [ˈsʌlfjuˌreitid], **sulfureted** [ˈsʌlfjuˌretid] *a* 含硫的,硫化的
sulfurator [ˈsʌlfjuˌreitə] *n* 硫黄烟熏器,硫黄熏蒸器
sulfureous [sʌlˈfjuəriəs] *a* 硫[黄]的
sulfuret [ˈsʌlfjurit] *n* 硫化物
sulfuric [sʌlˈfjuərik] *a* [正]硫的 | ~ acid 硫酸
sulfurize [ˈsʌlfjuəraiz] *vt* 硫化
sulfurous [ˈsʌlfərəs] *a* 亚硫的 | ~ acid 亚硫酸
sulfurtransferase [ˌsʌlfəˈtrænsfəreis] *n* 硫基转移酶
sulfuryl [ˈsʌlfəril] *n* 磺酰,硫酰
sulfydryl [sʌlˈfaidril] *n* 硫氢基,巯基
sulindac [sʌˈlindæk] *n* 舒林酸(消炎镇痛解热药)
sulisobenzone [ˌsʌlisəuˈbenzəun] *n* 舒利苯酮(紫外线遮光剂)
Sulkowitch's test [ˈsʌlkəuˌwitʃ] (Hirsh W. Sulkowitch)萨尔科维奇试验(检尿钙)
sullage [ˈsʌlidʒ] *n* 污水,污物
Sullivan's test [ˈsʌlivən] (Michael X. Sullivan) 沙利文试验(检尿半胱氨酸)
sulnidazole [sʌlˈnidəzəul] *n* 舒硝唑(抗滴虫药)
suloctidil [sʌlˈlɔktidil] *n* 舒洛地尔(周围血管扩张药)
suloxifen oxalate [sʌˈlɔksifən] 草酸舒洛昔芬(支气管扩张药)
sulph- 以 sulph-起始的词,同样见以 sulf-起始的词
sulpiride [ˈsʌlpiraid] *n* 舒必利(止吐药,抗抑郁药)
sulprostone [sʌlˈprɔstəun] *n* 硫前列酮(前列腺素)
sulthiame [sʌlˈθaieim] *n* 舒噻美(碳酸酐酶抑制剂,用作抗惊厥药)
Sulzberger-Garbe syndrome [sʌlzˈbəːgə ˈgɑːbi] (Marion B. Sulzberger; William Garbe)萨-加综合征,渗出性盘状苔藓样皮炎
sum. sumat【拉】令服用;sumendum【拉】服用
sumac [ˈsjuːmæk] *n* 漆树(属植物) | poison ~, swamp ~ 美国毒漆
sumatriptan succinate [ˌsjuːməˈtriptæn] 琥珀酸舒马普坦(一种选择性 5-羟色胺受体激动药,用于治疗急性偏头痛和丛集性头痛,口服、皮下或鼻内给药)
sumbul [sʌmˈbul] *n* 苏布,麝香草根(神经兴奋及镇痉药)
summation [sʌˈmeiʃən] *n* 总和 | central ~ 中枢[性]总和(连续发生的阈下刺激累积在反射中枢内,直到最后引起反射兴奋状态为止)
summit [ˈsʌmit] *n* 顶[点] | ~ of bladder 膀胱顶部 / ~ of nose 鼻根
Sumner's method [ˈsʌmnə] (James B. Sumner) 萨姆纳法(检尿糖) | ~ reagent 萨姆纳试剂(检测正常和糖尿病的尿糖)
Sumner's sign [ˈsʌmnə] (F. W. Sumner)萨姆纳征(轻触髂窝,腹肌紧张略为增加,即提示有阑尾炎、输尿管结石和肾结石或卵巢囊肿的蒂扭转)
sunbath [ˈsʌnbɑːθ] *n* 日光浴
sunbathe [ˈsʌnbeið] *vi* 沐日光浴
sunburn [ˈsʌnbəːn] *n* 晒斑,晒伤(长期接触太阳光或太阳灯所致)
suncillin sodium [sʌnˈsilin] 森西林钠(抗菌药)
sundowning [ˈsʌndauniŋ] *n* 日落精神错乱
sunscreen [ˈsʌnskriːn] *n* 遮光剂,防晒药
sunstroke [ˈsʌnstrəuk] *n* 日射病,中暑
super- [前缀]上,在上;过度,高度
superabduction [ˌsjuːpəræbˈdʌkʃən] *n* 外展过度
superacid [ˌsjuːpəˈræsid] *a* 酸过多的,过量酸的
superacidity [ˌsjuːpərəˈsidəti] *n* 酸过多,过度酸性
superacromial [ˌsjuːpərəˈkrəumiəl] *a* 肩峰上的
superactivity [ˌsjuːpərækˈtivəti] *n* 活动过强
superacute [ˌsjuːpərəˈkjuːt] *a* 超急性的
superalimentation [ˌsjuːpəˌrælimenˈteiʃən] *n* 超量营养疗法,强饲法,管饲法
superalkalinity [ˌsjuːpəˌrælkəˈlinəti] *n* 碱性过度
superantigen [ˌsjuːpəˈæntidʒən] *n* 超抗原
superaurale [ˌsjuːpərɔːˈreili] *n* 耳郭上点(人体测量名词,耳轮上缘的最高点)
supercarbonate [ˌsjuːpəˈkɑːbənit] *n* 重碳酸盐,碳酸氢盐
supercentral [ˌsjuːpəˈsentrəl] *a* 中心上的;中央沟上的

supercilium [ˌsjuːpəˈsiliəm] ([复] **supercilia** [ˌsjuːpəˈsiliə]) *n* 【拉】眉 | **superciliary** [ˌsjuːpəˈsiliəri] *a*
superclass [ˈsjuːpəklɑːs] *n* 超纲,总纲(生物分类)
supercoil [ˈsjuːpəkɔil] *n* 超螺旋(染色体)
supercool [sjuːpəˈkuːl] *vt* 使过冷 *vi* 过冷(指液体冷到凝固点以下而不凝结)
superdistention [ˌsjuːpədisˈtenʃən] *n* 膨胀过度
superduct [ˌsjuːpəˈdʌkt] *vt* 上转,上举
superduction [ˌsjuːpəˈdʌkʃən] *n* (眼)上转
superego [ˌsjuːpərˈiːgəu, -ˈe-] *n* 超我,超自我
superexcitation [ˌsjuːpəˌreksiˈteiʃən] *n* 兴奋过度
superextended [ˌsjuːpəriksˈtendid] *a* 伸展过度的
superextension [ˌsjuːpəriksˈtenʃən] *n* 伸展过度
superfamily [ˌsjuːpəˈfæmili] *n* 超科,总科(生物分类)
superfecundation [ˌsjuːpəˌfiːkənˈdeiʃən] *n* 同期复孕(指卵)
superfemale [ˌsjuːpəˈfiːmeil] *n* 超雌(雌性细胞内含有超常数的X染色体)
superfetation [ˌsjuːpəfiˈteiʃən] *n* 异期复孕(指卵)
superficial [ˌsjuːpəˈfiʃəl] *a* 浅[层]的,表面的
superficialis [ˌsjuːpəfiʃiˈeilis] *a* 【拉】浅的,表面的
superficies [ˌsjuːpəˈfiʃiiːz] *n* 【拉】表面
superflexion [ˌsjuːpəˈflekʃən] *n* 屈曲过度
superfunction [ˌsjuːpəˈfʌŋkʃən] *n* 功能亢进
superfusate [ˌsjuːpəˈfjuːzeit] *n* 灌注液
superfuse [ˌsjuːpəˈfjuːz] *vt* 用液体灌注(器官或组织)
superfusion [ˌsjuːpəˈfjuːʒən] *n* 液体灌注法
supergenual [ˌsjuːpəˈdʒenjuəl] *a* 膝上的
supergroup [ˈsjuːpəgruːp] *n* 超群(对抗原上相关的一群病毒性血清群的非正式名称)
superheat [ˈsjuːpəhiːt] *vt* 使过热 *n* 过热 | **~er** *n* 过热器
superhelix [ˌsjuːpˈheliks] *n* 超螺旋 | negative ~ 负超螺旋 / positive ~ 正超螺旋
superimpregnation [ˌsjuːpəˌrimpregˈneiʃən] *n* 复孕,重孕
superinduce [ˌsjuːpərinˈdjuːs] *vt* 重复诱导 | **superinduction** [ˌsjuːpərinˈdʌkʃən] *n* 超诱导
superinfection [ˌsjuːpərinˈfekʃən] *n* 重叠感染,二重感染(抗菌疗法过程中在原来感染部位或在较远部位发生的一种新的感染,由于抗药性的细菌或真菌入侵所致) | exogenous ~ 外源性重感染
superinvolution [ˌsjuːpəˌrinvəˈljuːʃən] *n* 复旧过度
superior [ˌsju(ː)ˈpiəriə] *a* 上的,在上的; *n* 上段支气管
superjacent [ˌsjuːpəˈdʒeisənt] *a* 盖在上面的,压在上面的
superlactation [ˌsjuːpəlækˈteiʃən] *n* 泌乳过多
superlattice [ˌsjuːpəˈlætis] *n* 超点阵(在固溶体中,原子或分子的一种排列,包括溶质的点阵与溶剂的点阵相互穿插)
superlethal [ˌsjuːpəˈliːθəl] *a* 超致死量的
supermaxilla [ˌsjuːpəmækˈsilə] *n* 上颌骨
supermedial [ˌsjuːpəˈmiːdjəl] *a* 中部上的
supermoron [ˌsjuːpəˈmɔːrən] *n* 高级愚蠢,临界愚蠢(指精神发育稍有缺陷的人)
supermotility [ˌsjuːpəməuˈtiləti] *n* 运动过度
supernatant [ˌsjuːpəˈneitənt] *a* 浮在上层的 *n* 上清液(离心沉淀后的上层液)
supernate [ˈsjuːpəneit] *n* 上清液
supernormal [ˌsjuːpəˈnɔːməl] *a* 超[正]常的,逾常的
supernumerary [ˌsjuːpəˈnjuːmərəri] *a* 多余的,额外的
supernutrition [ˌsjuːpənju(ː)ˈtriʃən] *n* 营养过度
superoccipital [ˌsjuːpərɔkˈsipitl] *a* 枕骨上部的,后头上的
superolateral [ˌsjuːpərəuˈlætərəl] *a* 上外侧的
superomedial [ˌsjuːpərəuˈmiːdiəl] *a* 中上的
superorder [ˈsjuːpərˌɔːdə] *n* 超目,总目(生物分类)
superovulation [ˌsjuːpəˌrəuvjuːˈleiʃən] *n* 超[数]排卵
superoxide [ˌsjuːpəˈrɔksaid] *n* 超氧化物
superoxide dismutase [ˌsjuːpəˈrɔksaid disˈmjuːteis] 超氧[化]物歧化酶
superparasite [ˌsjuːpəˈpærəsait] *n* 超寄生物,次级寄生物
superparasitism [ˌsjuːpəˈpærəˌsaitizəm] *n* 重复寄生[现象],过度寄生[现象],超寄生
superphosphate [ˌsjuːpəˈfɔsfeit] *n* 过磷酸盐(尤指过磷酸钙)
superpose [ˌsjuːpəˈpəuz] *vt* 叠加,重叠 | **superposition** [ˌsjuːpəpəˈziʃən] *n* 重叠
super-regeneration [ˌsjuːpəriˌdʒenəˈreiʃən] *n* 再生过度
supersalt [ˈsjuːpəsɔːlt] *n* 过酸盐,高(某酸)盐
supersaturate [ˌsjuːpəˈsætʃəreit] *vt* 使过饱和 | **supersaturation** [ˌsjuːpəˌsætʃəˈreiʃən] *n* 过饱和[现象]
superscription [ˌsjuːpəˈskripʃən] *n* 处方标记(处方上的符号℞)
supersecretion [ˌsjuːpəsiˈkriːʃən] *n* 分泌过多

supersede [ˌsjuːpəˈsiːd] *vt* 替代,取代
supersedent [ˌsjuːpəˈsiːdənt] *n* 减病药(部分治愈或防止疾病的药物)
supersensible [ˌsjuːpəˈsensəbl], **supersensory** [ˌsjuːpəˈsensəri] *a* 超越感觉的
supersensitive [ˌsjuːpəˈsensitiv] *a* 敏感过度的,过敏的 | **supersensitivity** [ˌsjuːpəˌsensiˈtivəti] *n* 超敏感性,过敏性
supersensitization [ˌsjuːpəˌsensitaiˈzeiʃən, -tiˈz-] *n* 促过敏作用,致超敏作用
supersensual [ˌsjuːpəˈsensjuəl] *a* 超[越]感觉的;精神上的
supersession [ˌsjuːpəˈseʃən] *n* 代替,取代
supersoft [ˌsjuːpəˈsɔft] *a* 超软的(指射线的波长长,吸收系数大,穿透力低)
supersonic [ˌsjuːpəˈsɔnik] *a* 超声[波]的;超声速的,超音速的
supersonics [ˌsjuːpəˈsɔniks] *n* 超声学
supersphenoid [ˌsjuːpəˈsfiːnɔid] *a* 蝶骨上的
superstructure [ˈsjuːpəˌstrʌktʃə] *n* 超结构
supertension [ˌsjuːpəˈtenʃən] *n* 张力过度,紧张过度
supervascularization [ˌsjuːpəˌvæskjuləraiˈzeiʃən, -riˈz-] *n* 超血管形成(在放射疗法中,指肿瘤细胞被破坏时血管供应相对增加,致使残留的肿瘤细胞得以经由未损伤的毛细血管基质提供较好的血流供应)
supervene [ˌsjuːpəˈviːn] *vi* 附加,并发 | **supervenient** [ˌsjuːpəˈviːniənt] *a* | **supervention** [ˌsjuːpəˈvenʃən] *n*
supervenosity [ˌsjuːpəviˈnɔsəti] *n* [血液]静脉性过度,静脉[血]氧过低
superversion [ˌsjuːpəˈvəːʒən] *n* (眼)上转
supervirulent [ˌsjuːpəˈvirjulənt] *a* 超毒力的,毒力过高的
supervisor [ˈsjuːpəvaizə] *n* 管理人员;护监(如管理医院特种病房或部门护理工作的护士)
supervitaminosis [ˌsjuːpəˌvaitəmiˈnəusis] *n* 维生素过多症
supervoltage [ˈsjuːpəˌvɔltidʒ] *n* 超电压,超高压(X 线治疗时,通常指电压范围在 500 kV 以内)
supinate [ˈsjuːpineit] *vt, vi* 仰卧;旋后(上下肢) | **supination** [ˌsjuːpiˈneiʃən] *n* / **supinator** *n* 旋后肌
supine [sjuːˈpain, sjuːpain] *a* 仰卧的;旋后的
suppedania [ˌsʌpəˈdeiniə] *n* 足底敷药[法]
support [səˈpɔːt] *vt* 支持;供养 *n* 支持;支柱,支持器,托 | advanced life ~ 加强生命支持 / basal life ~ 基础生命支持
suppositorium [səˌpɔziˈtɔːriəm] ([复]**suppositoria** [səˌpɔziˈtɔːriə]) *n*【拉】栓剂
suppository [səˈpɔzitəri] *n* 栓剂 | glycerin ~ 甘油栓
suppress [səˈpres] *vt* 压制,压抑,抑制 | **~ive** *a* | **~or** *n* 抑制器;抑制基因
suppressant [səˈpresnt] *a* 抑制的,遏抑的 *n* 抑制剂(对分泌排泄等的)
suppression [səˈpreʃən] *n* 抑制,制止;压抑(精神分析) | intergenic ~ 基因间抑制 / intragenic ~ 基因内抑制
suppurant [ˈsʌpjuərənt] *a* 化脓的 *n* 催脓剂
suppurantia [ˌsʌpjuəˈrænʃiə] *n* 催脓剂
suppurate [ˈsʌpjuəreit] *vi* 化脓 | **suppuration** [ˌsʌpjuəˈreiʃən] *n* | **suppurative** [ˈsʌpjuərətiv] *a*
supra- [前缀]在上,上
supra-acromial [ˌsjuːprəəˈkrəumiəl] *a* 肩峰上的
supra-anal [sjuːprəˈeinəl] *a* 肛门上的
supra-auricular [ˌsjuːprəɔːˈrikjulə] *a* 耳上的
supra-axillary [ˌsjuːprəˈæksiləri] *a* 腋上的
suprabuccal [ˌsjuːprəˈbʌkəl] *a* 颊上的
suprabulge [ˈsjuːprəbʌldʒ] *n* 凸上面(牙)
supracarinal [ˌsjuːprəkəˈrainəl] *a* 气管隆嵴上的
supracerebellar [ˌsjuːpreseriˈbelə] *a* 小脑上的
suprachoroid [ˌsjuːprəˈkɔːrɔid] *a* 脉络膜上的
suprachoroidea [ˌsjuːprəkɔːˈrɔidiə] *n* 脉络膜上层,脉络膜外层
supraciliary [ˌsjuːprəˈsiliəri] *a* 眉的,眉部的
supraclavicular [ˌsjuːprəkləˈvikjulə] *a* 锁骨上的
supraclavicularis [ˌsjuːprəkləˌvikjuˈleiris] *a*【拉】锁骨上的 *n* 锁骨上肌
supraclusion [ˌsjuːprəˈkluːʒən] *n* 超𬌗,超咬合
supracondylar [ˌsjuːprəˈkɔndilə], **supracondyloid** [ˌsjuːprəˈkɔndilɔid] *a* 髁上的
supracostal [ˌsjuːprəˈkɔstl] *a* 肋上的,肋外的
supracotyloid [ˌsjuːprəˈkɔtilɔid] *a* 髋臼上的
supracranial [ˌsjuːprəˈkreiniəl] *a* 颅上的
supradiaphragmatic [ˌsjuːprəˌdaiəfrægˈmætik] *a* 膈上的
supraduction [ˌsjuːprəˈdʌkʃən] *n* (眼)上转
supraepicondylar [ˌsjuːprəˌepiˈkɔndilə] *a* 上髁上的
supraepitrochlear [ˌsjuːprəˌepiˈtrɔkliə] *a* 肱骨内上髁上的
supraglenoid [ˌsjuːprəˈgliːnɔid] *a* 关节盂上的
supraglotitis [ˌsjuːprəgləˈtaitis] *n* 声门上炎
supraglottic [ˌsjuːprəˈglɔtik] *a* 声门上的
supraglottis [ˌsjuːprəˈglɔtis] *n* 声门上区
suprahepatic [ˌsjuːprəhiˈpætik] *a* 肝上的
suprahyoid [ˌsjuːprəˈhaiɔid] *a* 舌骨上的
suprainguinal [ˌsjuːprəˈiŋgwinl] *a* 腹股沟上的
supraintestinal [ˌsjuːprəinˈtestinl] *a* 肠上的
supraliminal [ˌsjuːprəˈliminl] *a* (感觉)阈上的

supralumbar [ˌsjuːprəˈlʌmbə] *a* 腰上的
supramalleolar [ˌsjuːprəməˈliːələ] *a* 踝上的
supramammary [ˌsjuːprəˈmæməri] *a* 乳腺上的,乳房上的
supramandibular [ˌsjuːprəmænˈdibjulə] *a* 下颌上的
supramarginal [ˌsjuːprəˈmɑːdʒinəl] *a* 缘上的
supramastoid [ˌsjuːprəˈmæstɔid] *a* [颞骨]乳突上的
supramaxilla [ˌsjuːprəmækˈsilə] *n* 上颌骨
supramaxillary [ˌsjuːprəˈmæksiləri] *a* 上颌的;上颌上的
supramaximal [ˌsjuːprəˈmæksiməl] *a* 超大的,最大度以上的
suprameatal [ˌsjuːprəmiˈeitl] *a* 口上的,道上的(尤指尿道口上的)
supramental [ˌsjuːprəˈmentl] *a* 颏上的
supramentale [ˌsjuːprəmenˈteili] *n* 下颌牙槽座点(即 B 点,见 point B)
supranasal [ˌsjuːprəˈneizəl] *a* 鼻上的
supranormal [ˌsjuːprəˈnɔːməl] *a* 超常的,正常以上的
supranuclear [ˌsjuːprəˈnjuːkliə] *a* 核上的
supraoccipital [ˌsjuːprəɔkˈsipitl] *a* 枕骨上的,后头上部的
supraocclusion [ˌsjuːprəɔˈkluːʒən] *n* 超𬌗,超咬合
supraocular [ˌsjuːprəˈɔkjulə] *a* 眼球上的
supraomohyoid [ˌsjuːprəˌəuməuˈhaiɔid] *a* 肩胛舌骨肌上的
supraoptimal [ˌsjuːprəˈɔptiməl] *a* 超最适的,最适度以上的
supraoptimum [ˌsjuːprəˈɔptiməm] *n* 超最适度
supraorbital [ˌsjuːprəˈɔːbitl] *a* 眶上的
suprapatellar [ˌsjuːprəpəˈtelə] *a* 髌上的
suprapelvic [ˌsjuːprəˈpelvik] *a* 骨盆上的
suprapharmacologic [ˌsjuːprəˌfɑːməkəˈlɔdʒik] *a* 超药理的(超出一般治疗剂量或药物的药理浓度)
supraphysiological [ˌsjuːprəˌfiziəuˈlɔdʒikəl] *a* 超生理学的
suprapontine [ˌsjuːprəˈpɔntain] *a* 脑桥上[部]的
suprapubic [ˌsjuːprəˈpjuːbik] *a* 耻骨弓上的
suprarenal [ˌsjuːprəˈriːnl] *a* 肾上的;肾上腺的
suprarenalectomy [ˌsjuːprəˌriːnəˈlektəmi] *n* 肾上腺切除术
suprarenalemia [ˌsjuːprəˌriːnəˈliːmiə] *n* 肾上腺素血
suprarenalism [ˌsjuːprəˈriːnəlizəm] *n* 肾上腺功能障碍
suprarenalopathy [ˌsjuːprəˌriːnəˈlɔpəθi], **suprarenopathy** [ˌsjuːprəriˈnɔpəθi] *n* 肾上腺(功能障碍)病
suprarene [ˌsjuːprəˈriːn] *n* 肾上腺
suprarenogenic [ˌsjuːprəˌriːnəuˈdʒenik] *a* 肾上腺源的
suprarenoma [ˌsjuːprəriˈnəumə] *n* 肾上腺瘤
suprarenotropic [ˌsjuːprəˌriːnəuˈtrɔpik] *a* 促肾上腺的
suprarenotropism [ˌsjuːprəriˈnɔtrəpizəm] *n* 促肾上腺性
suprascapular [ˌsjuːprəˈskæpjulə] *a* 肩胛上的
suprascleral [ˌsjuːprəˈskliərəl] *a* 巩膜外的
suprasellar [ˌsjuːprəˈselə] *a* 蝶鞍上的
supraseptal [ˌsjuːprəˈseptl] *a* 膈上的
suprasonics [ˌsjuːprəˈsɔniks] *n* 超声学
supraspinal [ˌsjuːprəˈspainl] *a* 棘上的;脊柱上的
supraspinous [ˌsjuːprəˈspainəs] *a* 棘上的,棘突上的
suprastapedial [ˌsjuːprəstəˈpiːdiəl] *a* 镫骨上的
suprasternal [ˌsjuːprəˈstəːnl] *a* 胸骨上的
suprasterol [ˌsjuːprəˈsterɔl] *n* 超甾醇,过照甾醇
suprasylvian [ˌsjuːprəˈsilviən] *a* 大脑侧裂上的
supratemporal [ˌsjuːprəˈtempərəl] *a* 颞上的
supratentorial [ˌsjuːprətenˈtɔːriəl] *a* (脑)幕上的
suprathoracic [ˌsjuːprəθɔːˈræsik] *a* 胸廓上的
suprathreshold [ˌsjuːprəˈθreʃəuld] *a* 阈上的
supratip [ˈsjuːprətip] *a* 鼻尖上的
supratonsillar [ˌsjuːprəˈtɔnsilə] *a* 扁桃体上的
supratrochlear [ˌsjuːprəˈtrɔkliə] *a* 滑车上的
supratympanic [ˌsjuːprətimˈpænik] *a* 鼓室上的
supraumbilical [ˌsjuːprəˌʌmbiˈlaikəl] *a* 脐上的
supravaginal [ˌsjuːprəˈvædʒinl] *a* 鞘上的;阴道上的
supravalvar [ˌsjuːprəˈvælvə] *a* 瓣膜上的(特指主动脉瓣上的或肺动脉瓣上的)
supraventricular [ˌsjuːprəvenˈtrikjulə] *a* 室上的
supraverge [ˈsjuːprəvəːdʒ] *n* 上转
supravergence [ˌsjuːprəˈvəːdʒəns] *n* 上转,眼上转
supraversion [ˌsjuːprəˈvəːʒən] *n* 高位牙;上转,眼上转
supravesical [ˌsjuːprəˈvesikəl] *a* 膀胱上的
supravital [ˌsjuːprəˈvaitl] *a* 体外活体的,超活体的(一种染色法,即将染料加在已脱离生物体的细胞培养基上)
supraxiphoid [ˌsjuːprəˈzaifɔid] *a* 剑突上的
suprazygomatic [ˌsjuːprəˌzaigəuˈmætik] *a* 颧骨上的
suprofen [sjuːˈprəufən] *n* 舒洛芬(前列腺素抑制剂,具有抗炎作用)
sura [ˈsjuərə] *n*【拉】腓肠(小腿肚) | **~l** *a*

Suragina [suːrəˈdʒainə] *n* 鹬虻属
suralimentation [ˌsəːrælimenˈteiʃən] *n* 超量营养法,强饲法
suramin hexasodium [ˈsuərəmin] 舒拉明六钠(抗锥虫和抗丝虫药,用于防治非洲锥虫病和盘尾丝虫病〈对此病的使用主要已被伊维菌素 ivermectin 所取代〉;本品亦抑制激素生长和由肾上腺皮质细胞造成的激素生成,用于治疗不宜手术的正在转移的肾上腺皮质癌。亦称舒拉明钠)
suramin sodium [ˈsjuərəmin] 舒拉明钠(抗锥虫药)
surd [səːd] *a* 清音的 *n* 清音
surdimute [ˈsəːdimjuːt] *a* 聋哑的 *n* 聋哑者
surdimutism [ˌsəːdiˈmjuːtizəm] *n* 聋哑症
surdimutitas [ˌsəːdiˈmjuːtitəs] *n*【拉】聋哑症
surditas [ˈsəːditəs] *n*【拉】聋
surdity [ˈsəːditi] *n* 聋
surexcitation [ˌsəːriksaiˈteiʃən] *n* 兴奋过度
surface [ˈsəːfis] *n* 面,表面 | distal ~ 远中面 / mesial ~, medial ~ 近中面
surface-active [ˈsəːfis ˌæktiv] *a* 表面活性的
surfactant [səːˈfæktənt] *n* 表面活性剂,表面活化剂
surge [səːdʒ] *vi* 汹涌 *n* 急剧上升,激增 | follicle-stimulating hormone ~ 促卵泡素激增 / luteinizing hormone ~ 黄体化激素激增
surgeon [ˈsəːdʒən] *n* 外科医师 | acting assistant ~, contract ~ 代理外科助理医师,订约军医 / ~ general (美国)军医处处长,(美国)卫生局局长;(英国)陆军军医 / house ~ 外科住院医师
surgery [ˈsəːdʒəri] *n* 外科,外科学;手术室;诊所(英国) | abdominal ~ 腹部外科 / antiseptic ~ 防腐外科 / arthrosteopedic ~ 骨科 / aseptic ~ 无菌外科 / cardiac ~ 心脏外科 / cerebral ~ 脑外科 / clinical ~ 临床外科 / cosmetic ~ 整容外科 / general ~ 普通外科学 / major ~ 大外科 / minor ~ 小外科 / open heart ~ 心脏直视手术 / operative ~ 外科手术学 / oral ~ 口腔外科 / oral and maxillofacial ~ 口腔及颌面外科 / orthopedic ~ 矫形外科 / pelvic ~ 盆腔外科 / plastic ~ 成形外科,整形外科,整复外科 / psychiatric ~ 精神病学外科(为治疗精神科疾患所实施的脑外科手术) / radical ~ 根治外科手术 / reconstructive ~ 整复外科 / sonic ~ 超声外科 / stereotactic ~, stereotaxic ~ 立体定向手术 / structural ~ 结构外科
surgibone [ˈsəːdʒibəun] *n* 外科用骨(矫形外科和整形外科时用作体内骨夹板,但由于异体反应,现很少使用)
surgical [ˈsəːdʒikəl] *a* 外科[术]的,外科[手术]用的
surinamine [sjuˈrinəmin] *n* 甲基酪氨酸,柯桠树碱
surma [suːmə] *n* 苏玛(一种硫化铅,在印度为了美容和医疗目的,传统上用于眼睑,可引起铅中毒)
surra [ˈsuərə] *n* 苏拉病,伊[凡斯]氏锥虫病(一种由伊氏锥虫引起马、骆驼、象、猪、山羊、狗等家畜的锥虫病)
surrogate [ˈsʌrəgit] *n* 替代物,代用品;替代者,替身 | father ~ 父亲替代者(精神分析)
sursanure [səːˈseinjuə] *n* 外愈内烂性顽疮,潜疮
sursumduction [ˌsəːsʌmˈdʌkʃən], **sursumvergence** [ˌsəːsʌmˈvəːdʒəns], **sursumversion** [ˌsəːsʌmˈvəːʒən] *n* (眼)上转
suruçucu [ˌsuːruːˈsuːkuː] *n* 丛林王
surveillance [səːˈveiləns] *n* 监视,监督(在免疫理论中,指免疫系统〈T 淋巴细胞〉经常监视体组织内异常细胞) | immune ~, immunological ~ 免疫监督(一种假说中的监督功能,免疫系统通过这种功能就能抗癌)
survival [səˈvaivəl] *n* 幸存,生存,存活;生存者 | ~ of the fittest 适者生存
survivin [səːˈvaivin] *n* 存活蛋白(能中和天冬氨酸特异性半胱氨酸蛋白酶活性,从而抑制细胞凋亡的一种蛋白)
susceptibility [səˌseptəˈbiləti] *n* 易感性,敏感性,感受性 | magnetic ~ 磁感受性,磁化率
susceptible [səˈseptəbl] *a* 易感的,敏感的 *n* 未经(天然或后天)免疫者
suspenopsia [ˌsʌspəˈnɔpsiə] *n* 视觉暂停
suspensiometer [səsˌpensiˈɔmitə] *n* 混悬度测定器
suspension [səsˈpenʃən] *n* 悬吊[术];固定术;混悬,悬浮[液] | cephalic ~ 头悬吊 / colloid ~ 悬[浮]胶体,胶体悬液 / ~ of uterus 子宫固定术
suspensoid [səsˈpensɔid] *n* 悬[浮]胶体,胶体悬液
suspensor [səsˈpensə] *n* 悬带,吊绷带
suspensorius [ˌsəspenˈsɔːriəs] *a*【拉】悬的 *n* 悬带
suspensory [səsˈpensəri] *a* 悬的 *n* 悬带
sustentaculum [ˌsʌstenˈtækjuləm] ([复] **sustentacula** [ˌsʌstenˈtækjulə]) *n*【拉】支柱;支持物 | **sustentacular** *a* 支柱的,支持的
susto [ˈsjuːstəu] *n* 急性惊恐症(见于拉丁美洲的文化特异综合征,包括对恶毒眼光〈evil eye〉、巫术和精神着魔的恐惧而引起的惊恐反应)
susurrus [sjuˈsʌrəs] *n*【拉】杂音
sutika [ˈsjuːtikə] *n* 孕妇贫血病(孕时消化不良、发热,产后有进行性恶性贫血)
sutilains [ˈsutileins] *n* 舒替兰酶,蛋白水解酶(得

自枯草杆菌)

Sutton's disease [ˈsʌtn] (Richard Lightburn Sutton Jr.)裂隙性肉芽肿

Sutton's disease [ˈsʌtn] (Richard Lightburn Sutton)复发性坏死性黏膜腺周围炎 | ~ nevus 晕痣

Suttonella [ˌsʌtəˈnelə] *n* 萨顿菌属

sutura [sjuːˈtjuərə] ([复]**suturae** [sjuːˈtjuəriː]) *n*【拉】缝

sutural [ˈsjuːtʃərəl] *a* 缝的,骨缝的

suturation [ˌsjuːtʃəˈreiʃən] *n* 缝(合)

suture [ˈsjuːtʃə] *n* 缝,缝合;缝线 *vt* 缝合 | absorbable ~ 可吸收缝线 / apposition ~, coaptation ~ 对位缝合 / basilar ~ 基底缝,蝶枕裂 / bolster ~ 枕垫缝合 / button ~ 纽扣缝合 / catgut ~ 肠线 / coronal ~, arcuate ~ 冠状缝 / false ~, bastard ~ 假缝 / figure-of-eight ~ 8字形缝合 / interrupted ~ 间断缝合 / lambdoid ~, occipitoparietal ~ 人字缝,枕顶缝 / primary ~ 一期缝合 / pursestring ~ 荷包缝合 / sagittal ~, biparietal ~, jugal ~ 矢状缝 / secondary ~ 二期缝合 / silk ~ 丝线

suxamethonium chloride [ˌsʌksəmeˈθəuniəm] 氯琥珀胆碱(神经肌肉阻断药)

suxemerid sulfate [sʌkˈsemərid] 硫酸琥甲哌酯(镇咳药)

Suzanne's gland [suˈzæn] (Jean G. Suzanne)苏赞腺(在牙槽舌沟下的口腔黏液腺)

SUZI subzonal insemination 带下受精

SV stroke volume 每搏量;sinus venosus 静脉窦;simian virus 猿猴病毒

SV40 simian virus 40 猿猴病毒 40

Sv sievert 西[韦特](放射吸收剂量当量的国际单位)

SVC superior vena cava 上腔静脉

Svedberg [ˈswedbəːg] *n* 斯维德伯格单位(即 Svedberg unit)

Svedberg unit [ˈswedbəːg] (Theodor Svedberg) 斯维德伯格单位(沉降系数单位,用以表示大分子沉降系数的单位,等于 10^{-13} s,符号为 S) | ~ flotation unit 斯维德伯格漂浮单位(用以表示在离心机中漂浮而不沉淀〈如脂蛋白〉的大分子负沉降系数的单位,等于 10^{-13} s,符号为 S_f)

SVT supraventricular tachycardia 室上性心动过速

swab [swɔb] *n* 拭子,药签;(用拭子取下的)化验标本 *vt* (用拭子等)拭抹

swaddler [ˈswɔdlə] *n* 婴儿服,新生儿保暖服 | silver ~ 银色婴儿服(由聚酯组成,用一层薄铝压成薄片衬在里面,防止新生儿身体处于低温状态)

swage [sweidʒ] *n* 型铁,型模 *vt* 用型铁以塑形

swager [ˈsweidʒə] *n* 压模器(牙)

Swainsona [ˈsweinsənə] *n* 苦马豆属

swallow [ˈswɔləu] *vt* 吞服 *n* 吞,咽

swallowing [ˈswɔləuiŋ] *n* 吞咽 | air ~ 吞气症

swarming [ˈswɔːmiŋ] *a* 丛集的(细菌) *n* 群游;现象

swayback [ˈsweibæk] *n* 马背凹陷,凹背;脊柱前凸;羊羔蹒跚病,羊缺铜病

sweat [swet] *vi* 出汗 *vt* 使出汗 *n* 汗;出汗 | bloody ~ 血汗[症] / blue ~ 青汗[症] / fetid ~ 臭汗 / green ~ 绿汗[症] / night ~ 盗汗 / phosphorescent ~ 磷光性汗

sweating [ˈswetiŋ] *n* 出汗 | gustatory ~ 味觉性出汗,耳颞综合征

Swediaur's (Schwediauer's) disease [ˌsweidiˈɔːə] (François X. Swediaur〈或 Schwediauer〉) 斯韦迪奥尔病(跟骨黏液囊炎)

sweeney, sweeny [ˈswiːni] *n* 肩胛上麻痹(马)

Sweet's syndrome [swiːt] (Robert Douglas Sweet)斯威特综合征,急性发热性嗜中性[细胞]皮肤病

swellhead [ˈswelhed] *n* 植物中毒热(羊);家禽白喉

swelling [ˈsweliŋ] *n* 肿胀;隆突 | arytenoid ~ 披裂突 / blennorrhagic ~ 淋病性膝肿 / Calabar ~s, Kamerun ~s 卡拉巴丝虫肿,罗阿丝虫性皮下肿 / capsular ~ 荚膜肿胀(具有荚膜的肺炎球菌接触型特异性抗体后,由于抗体与荚膜多糖结合而形成肿胀现象。亦称诺伊菲尔德〈Neufeld〉反应) / cloudy ~, albuminous ~ 混浊肿胀,蛋白性肿胀 / fugitive ~ 短时性肿胀 / genital ~, labioscrotal ~ 生殖突(胚胎),阴唇阴囊突 / giant ~ 血管神经性水肿 / glassy ~ 淀粉样变性 / hunger ~ 饥饿性水肿 / labial ~ 阴唇突(胚胎) / scrotal ~ 阴囊隆起 / tropical ~ 热带肿 / tympanic ~ 鼓室隆起 / white ~ 白色肿,结核性关节肿

Swenson's operation [ˈswensən] (Orvar Swenson)斯温森手术(一种先天性巨结肠手术,包括切除直肠和肠的无神经节段,以及回肠肛门拖出术并保留肛门括约肌)

Swift-Feer disease [swift fɛə] (H. Swift; Emil Feer)斯-费病,肢痛症

Swift's disease [swift] (H. Swift)斯维夫特病,肢痛症(见 acrodynia)

swim-up [ˈswimʌp] *n* 迁移 | sperm ~ 精子迁移

swine [swain] *n* 猪

swinepox [ˈswainpɔks] *n* 猪痘

switch [switʃ] *n* 转换,转移,改变;开关,电闸,电键 | class ~ 种类转换(B 细胞或浆细胞由产生 IgM 转换成产生 IgG, IgA,或 IgE 的过程)

Swyer-James syndrome [ˈswaiə dʒeimz] (Paul R. Swyer; G. C. W. James)苏-詹综合征(获得性单侧透明肺,伴有呼气时严重气道梗阻,血量过

少及肺门阴影缩小)

Swyer syndrome [ˈswaiə] (Gerald Isaac MacDonald Swyer) 46, XY 性腺发育不全

sycephalus [saiˈsefələs] *n* [四耳]并头联胎

sychnuria [sikˈnjuəriə] *n* 尿频

sycosiform [saiˈkəusifɔːm] *a* 须疮样的

sycosis [saiˈkəusis] *n* 须疮;睑疮 | coccogenic ~ 球菌性须疮 / lupoid ~ 狼疮样须疮 / parasitic ~ 寄生性须疮,须癣 / ~ tarsi 睑疮 / ~ vulgaris, ~ barbae, ~ staphylogenes 寻常须疮,须疮,葡萄球菌性须疮

Sydenham's chorea [ˈsidənhæm] (Thomas Sydenham) 小舞蹈病 | ~ cough 西登哈姆咳(呼吸肌的癔症性痉挛)

syllepsiology [siˌlepsiˈɔlədʒi] *n* 妊娠学

syllepsis [siˈlepsis] *n* 受孕,妊娠

sylvan [ˈsilvən] *n* 邻甲基呋喃 *a* 森林的

sylvatic [silˈvætik] *a* 森林的

Sylvest's disease [silˈvest] (Ejnar Sylvest) 流行性胸膜痛

sylvian [ˈsilviən] *a* 西尔维厄斯的 (Franciscus Sylvius de la Böe)(如 ~ artery 大脑中动脉, ~ fossa 大脑侧窝, ~ line 大脑侧裂后支线, ~ point 大脑外侧裂近点, ~ vein 大脑中静脉)

sylvian syndrome, sylvian aqueduct syndrome [ˈsilviən] 西尔维厄斯综合征,中脑水管综合征(垂直凝视障碍,退缩性眼球震颤,会聚性眼球震颤,会聚性痉挛,以及瞳孔对光或近距视觉反应减弱或缺失〈但瞳孔大小通常正常〉,因中脑水管周围的灰质发生肿瘤、炎症或血管损害所致)

Sylvius' angle [ˈsilviəs] (Franciscus Sylvius 〈François de la Böe〉) 西尔维厄斯角(大脑外侧沟接界与水平线垂直的半球顶点切线所形成之角) | ~ aqueduct 中脑水管 / ~ fissure 大脑外侧沟 / ~ fossa ①大脑外侧窝;②大脑外侧沟 / ~ sulcus 大脑外侧沟 / ~ valve 下腔静脉瓣 / ~ ventricle 透明隔腔

symballophone [simˈbæləfəun] *n* 定向听诊器

symbiology [ˌsimbaiˈɔlədʒi] *n* 共生学,共生生物学

symbiont [ˈsimbaiɔnt], **symbion** [ˈsimbaiɔn], **symbiote** [ˈsimbaiəut] *n* 共生体,共生生物

symbiosis [ˌsimbaiˈəusis] *n* 【希】共生(不同种类的两种生物共同生活在一起);依赖关系(在精神病学中,指互相加强两个相互依赖的人之间的关系) | antagonistic ~, antipathetic ~ 拮抗性共生 / conjunctive ~ 连接共生 / constructive ~ 积极共生 / disjunctive ~ 分离共生 | **symbionic** [ˌsimbaiˈɔnik], **symbiotic** [ˌsimbaiˈɔtik] *a* 共生的

symblepharon [simˈblefərɔn] *n* 睑球粘连 | anterior ~ 睑球前粘连 / posterior ~ 睑球后粘连 / total ~ 睑球全粘连

symblepharopterygium [simˌblefərəuteˈridʒiəm] *n* 睑球翼状粘连

symbol [ˈsimbəl] *n* 象征,符号 | phallic ~ 阳具象征(在精神分析中,任何尖形或直立的物体均可象征阴茎)

symbolia [simˈbɔliə] *n* 形体感觉(触觉识别形体能力)

symbolic(al) [simˈbɔlik(əl)] *a* 象征性的;符号的

symbolism [ˈsimbəlizəm] *n* 象征主义;象征癖(精神异常错乱时,每一件事情的发生都被想象为患者自己思想的象征);象征表示(在精神分析上,为一种潜意识思维机制,常与性有关)

symbolize [ˈsimbəlaiz] *vt* 象征,代表;用符号表示 *vi* 采用象征;使用符号 | **symbolization** [ˌsimbəlaiˈzeiʃən, -liˈz-] *n* 象征化,象征作用

symbrachydactyly [simˌbrækiˈdæktili], **symbrachydactylia** [simˌbrækidækˈtiliə], **symbrachydactylism** [simˌbrækiˈdæktilizəm] *n* 指短粘连畸形,趾短粘连畸形

symclosene [ˈsimkləsiːn] *n* 氯氧三嗪(局部抗感染药)

symdichloromethyl ether [ˌsimdaiˌklɔːrəuˈmeθil ˈiːθə] 对称二氯甲基醚

Syme's amputation [saim] (James Syme) 赛姆截肢术(踝关节下足切断术,两个踝一并切除) | ~ operation 赛姆手术(①赛姆截肢术;②尿道外切开术的一种方法)

Symington's body [ˈsaimiŋtən] (Johnson Symington) 肛尾韧带

symmelia [siˈmiːliə] *n* 并腿[畸形]

symmelus, symelus [ˈsiminləs] *n* 并腿畸胎

Symmers' disease [ˈsiməz] (Douglas Symmers) 结节性淋巴瘤

Symmer's fibrosis [ˈsiməz] (William St. Clair Symmers) 管干型纤维化

symmetric(al) [siˈmetrik(əl)] *a* 对称的

symmetry [ˈsimitri] *n* 对称[性] | bilateral ~ 两侧对称 / inverse ~ 反[面]对称 / radial ~ 辐射对称

sympathectomize [ˌsimpəˈθektəmaiz] *vt* 切除交感神经

sympathectomy [ˌsimpəˈθektəmi], **sympathetectomy** [ˌsimpəθiˈtektəmi] *n* 交感神经切除术

sympathetic [ˌsimpəˈθetik] *a* 同感的;交感的;交感神经的 *n* 交感神经,交感神经系统

sympatheticomimetic [ˌsimpəˌθetikəumiˈmetik, -maiˈme-] *a* 拟交感[神经]的,类交感[神经]的 *n* 拟交感神经药

sympatheticoparalytic [ˌsimpəˌθetikəupærəˈliti-

k] *a* 抗交感[神经]的,交感神经阻滞的
sympatheticotonia [ˌsimpəˌθetikəu'təuniə] *n* 交感神经过敏,交感神经紧张 | **sympatheticotonic** [ˌsimpəˌθetikəu'tɔnik] *a*
sympathetoblast [ˌsimpə'θetəblæst] *n* 成交感神经细胞
sympathic [sim'pæθik] *a* 同感的;交感的;交感神经的
sympathicectomy [simˌpæθi'sektəmi] *n* 交感神经切除术
sympathicoblast [sim'pæθikəuˌblæst] *n* 成交感神经细胞
sympathicoblastoma [simˌpæθikəublæs'təumə] *n* 成交感神经细胞瘤
sympathicodiaphtheresis [simˌpæθikəuˌdaiəfθi'riːsis] *n* (生殖腺)交感神经毁损术
sympathicogonioma [simˌpæθikəuˌgəni'əumə] *n* 交感神经原细胞瘤,成交感神经细胞瘤
sympathicolytic [simˌpæθikəu'litik] *a* 抗交感[神经]的,交感神经阻滞的 *n* 抗交感神经药,交感神经阻滞药
sympathicomimetic [simˌpæθikəumi'metik, -mai'me-] *a* 拟交感[神经]的,类交感[神经]的 *n* 拟交感神经药
sympathicopathy [simˌpæθi'kɔpəθi] *n* 交感神经系统病
sympathicotherapy [simˌpæθikəu'θerəpi] *n* 交感神经刺激疗法
sympathicotonia [simˌpæθikəu'təuniə] *n* 交感神经过敏,交感神经紧张 | **sympathicotonic** [simˌpæθikəu'tɔnik] *a*
sympathicotripsy [simˌpæθikəu'tripsi] *n* 交感神经压轧术
sympathicotrope [sim'pæθikətrəup] *a* 向交感神经的,趋交感神经的
sympathicotropic [simˌpæθikəu'trɔpik] *a* 向交感神经的,趋交感神经的 *n* 向交感神经药,趋交感神经药
sympathicus [sim'pæθikəs] *n* 交感神经系统
sympathin ['simpəθin] *n* 交感神经素,去甲肾上腺素
sympathism ['simpəθizəm] *n* 易受暗示性,同感性
sympathoadrenal [ˌsimpəθəuə'driːnl] *a* 交感肾上腺的
sympathoblast [sim'pæθəblæst] *n* 成交感神经细胞
sympathoblastoma [ˌsimpəθəublæs'təumə] *n* 成交感神经细胞瘤
sympathogone [ˌsimpəθəu'gəun] *n* 交感神经原细胞
sympathogonioma [ˌsimpəθəugəni'əumə] *n* 交感神经原细胞瘤,成交感神经细胞瘤
sympathogonium [ˌsimpəθəu'gəunjəm] ([复] **sympathogonia** [ˌsimpəθəu'gəuniə]) *n* 交感神经原细胞
sympatholytic [ˌsimpəθəu'litik] *a* 抗交感[神经]的,交感神经阻滞的 *n* 抗交感神经药,交感神经阻滞药
sympathomimetic [ˌsimpəθəumi'metik, -mai'm-] *a* 拟交感[神经]的,类交感[神经]的 *n* 拟交感神经药
sympathy ['simpəθi] *n* 同情;感应;交感[作用],同感[作用]
sympectothiene [simˌpektə'θaiiːn], **sympectothion** [simˌpektə'θaiən] *n* 巯组氨酸三甲[基]内盐,麦角硫因
sympexion [sim'peksiən] ([复] **sympexia** [sim'peksiə]) *n* 凝结物
sympexis [sim'peksis] *n* 红细胞集结(按表面张力原理)
symphalangia [ˌsimfə'lændʒiə], **symphalangism** [sim'fæləndʒizəm] *n* 指关节融合,趾关节融合
symphoricarpus [ˌsimfɔri'kɑːpəs] *n* 雪莓
Symphoromyia [ˌsimfərə'maijə] *n* 北美鹬虻属
Symphyacanthida [ˌsimfiə'kænθidə] *n* 黏合棘目
symphyocephalus [ˌsimfiəu'sefələs] *n* 并头联胎
symphyogenetic [ˌsimfiəudʒi'netik] *a* (先天与后天因素)联合作用的
symphyseal, symphysial [sim'fiziəl] *a* 联合的
symphyseorrhaphy [simˌfizi'ɔrəfi] *n* 耻骨联合缝合术
symphyses ['simfisiːz] symphysis 的复数
symphysic [sim'fizik] *a* [异常]联合的,融合的
symphysiectomy [simˌfizi'ektəmi] *n* 耻骨联合切除术
symphysiolysis [simˌfizi'ɔlisis] *n* 耻骨联合松解术
symphysion [sim'fiziən] *n* 下颌联合点(下颌骨齿槽突外缘中点)
symphysiorrhaphy [simˌfizi'ɔrəfi] *n* 耻骨联合缝合术
symphysiotome [sim'fiziətəum] *n* 耻骨联合[切开]刀
symphysiotomy [simˌfizi'ɔtəmi] *n* 耻骨联合切开术
symphysis ['simfisis] ([复] **symphyses** ['simfisiːz]) *n*【希】联合 | pubic ~ 耻骨联合 / sacrococcygeal ~ 骶尾联合 / sacroiliac ~ 骶髂关节
symphysodactyly [ˌsimfisəu'dæktili] *n* 并指畸形,并趾畸形
Symphytum ['simfitəm] *n* 西门肺草属
symphytum ['simfitəm] *n* 西门肺草

symplasm [ˈsimplæzəm], **symplast** [ˈsimplæst] *n* 共质体,共浆体
symplasmatic [ˌsimplæzˈmætik] *a* 共质的,共浆的
symplex [ˈsimpleks] *n* 松合物,疏合物(如血红蛋白与氧结合)
sympodia [simˈpəudiə] *n* [无足]无腿畸形
sympodial [simˈpəudiəl] *a* 合轴的
sympodula [simˈpɔdjulə] *n* 合轴产孢细胞
symport [ˈsimpɔːt] *n* 同向转运
symporter [simˈpɔːtə] *n* 膜转运蛋白
symptom [ˈsimptəm] *n* 症状 | abstinence ~s 脱瘾症状,戒断症状(见 withdrawal ~s) / cardinal ~ 主要症状(对医师确定疾病性质最有意义的症状);[复]基本症状(脉搏、体温及呼吸所显示的症状) / characteristic ~, guiding ~ 特征性症状,特殊症状 / concomitant ~ 伴发症状 / consecutive ~ 连续症状(出现在某一疾病恢复期的症状,但与此病无关) / constitutional ~, general ~ 全身症状 / deficiency ~ 缺乏症状(某些内分泌腺分泌缺乏所致的症状) / delayed ~ 迟发症状 / direct ~ 直接症状 / dissociation ~ (感觉)分离症状(对痛和冷、热的感觉丧失,但未失去触觉的感觉能力,见于脊髓空洞症) / endothelial ~ (血管)内皮症状(见 Rumpel-Leede phenomenon) / equivocal ~ 非特征性症状,不明确症状(几种不同疾病都能产生的症状) / esophagosalivary ~ 食管癌多涎症状 / halo ~, rainbow ~ 虹彩轮症状,晕轮症状(一个体光源周围所见的彩色环,为青光眼之征) / incarceration ~ 箝闭症状,游走肾危象(移位肾周期性复发症状,如肾痛、胃痛和严重虚脱) / indirect ~ 间接症状 / induced ~ 诱发症状 / labyrinthine ~s 迷路症状(提示内耳疾病的一组症状) / local ~ 局部症状 / localizing ~s 示位症状(提示损害位置的症状) / neighborhood ~ 周邻症状 / nostril ~ 鼻孔症状(呼气时鼻孔扩张,吸气时鼻孔下缩) / objective ~ 客观症状 / pathognomonic ~ 示病性症状,伴病性症状 / presenting ~ 主要症状,主诉 / reflex ~ 反射症状(远离受疾病影响的那一部分发生的症状) / signal ~ 先兆症状(能警告接近癫痫或其他发作的一种感觉、先兆或其他自觉经验) / static ~, passive ~ 静态症状 / subjective ~ 自觉症状,主观症状 / sympathetic ~ 交感症状,同感症状 / withdrawal ~s 戒断症状,脱瘾症状(已成瘾者于突然停药后的症状)
symptomatic [ˌsimptəˈmætik] *a* 症状的,根据症状的
symptomatize [ˈsimptəmətaiz], **symptomize** [ˈsimptəmaiz] *vt* 是…的症状;表明
symptomatology [ˌsimptəməˈtɔlədʒi] *n* 症状学
symptomatolytic [ˌsimptəmətəuˈlitik], **symptomolytic** [ˌsimptəməˈlitik] *a* 消除症状的
symptome [seŋˈtɔm] *n* 【法】症状 | ~s complice 综合征,征群,综合症状
symptosis [simpˈtəusis] *n* 消耗,消瘦(全身或某器官的)
sympus [ˈsimpəs] *n* 无足并腿畸胎
Syms's tractor [simz] (Parker Syms) 西姆斯牵引器(末端接一可充气的橡皮袋管子,用以把前列腺牵引到会阴切口中)
syn- [前缀]连,联,合,共
synadelphus [ˌsinəˈdelfəs] *n* 头躯联胎,单头单躯八肢畸胎
synaetion [siˈniːtiən] *n* 副[病]因
synalbumin [siˈnælbjumin] *n* 抗胰岛素(一种假设的胰岛素竞争抑制剂,结合在白蛋白上的胰岛素 B 链,对人糖尿病的意义尚未确定)
synalgia [siˈnældʒiə] *n* 连带痛,牵连痛 | **synalgic** [siˈnældʒik] *a*
synanamorph [sinˈænəˌmɔːf] *n* 共无性型(具有相同有性型〈teleomorph〉的两个或两个以上的无性型〈anamorph〉的任何一种)
synanche [siˈnænki] *n* 锁喉,咽峡炎
Synangium [siˈnændʒiəm] *n* 聚囊黏菌属
synanthrin [siˈnænθrin] *n* 菊糖,菊粉
synanthrose [siˈnænθrəus] *n* 块茎糖,多缩左旋糖
synaphymenitis [siˌnæfiməˈnaitis] *n* 结膜炎
synapse [ˈsinæps] *n* 突触 | axoaxonic ~ 轴轴突触 / axodendritic ~ 轴树突触 / axodendrosomatic ~ 轴树体突触 / axosomatic ~ 轴体突触 / dendrodendritic ~ 树树突触 / electrotonic ~ 电紧张性突触 / en passant 过往性突触 / loop ~ 环状突触
synapsis [siˈnæpsis] ([复] **synapses** [siˈnæpsiːz]) *n* 【希】联会(减数分裂的染色体配对);突触 | **synaptic** [siˈnæptik] *a*
synaptase [siˈnæpteis] *n* 苦杏仁酶
synaptene [siˈnæptiːn] *n* 偶线[期](见 amphitene)
synaptology [ˌsinæpˈtɔlədʒi] *n* 突触学(神经病学的一部分)
synaptosome [siˈnæptəˌsəum] *n* 突触体
synarthrophysis [ˌsinɑːθrəˈfaisis] *n* 关节粘连
synarthrosis [ˌsinɑːˈθrəusis] ([复] **synarthroses** [ˌsinɑːˈθrəusiːz]), **synarthrodia** [ˌsinɑːθrəudiə] *n* 【希】不动关节 | **synarthrodial** *a*
synathroisis [ˌsinəˈθrɔisis], **synathresis** [ˌsinəˈθriːsis] *n* [局部]充血
syncaine [siŋˈkein] *n* 盐酸普鲁卡因(局部麻醉药)
syncanthus [siŋˈkænθəs] *n* 眶球粘连
syncaryon [siŋˈkæriɔn] *n* 合核体(由两个原核融合而形成的核)

syncelom [sin'siːləm] *n* 体腔(包括胸膜腔、心包腔、腹膜腔以及鞘膜)

Syncephalastrum [sinˌsefə'læstrəm] *n* 并头状菌属

syncephalus [sin'sefələs] *n* [四耳]并头联胎

synchesis ['siŋkisis] *n* 玻璃体液化

synchilia [siŋ'kailiə] *n* 并唇[畸形]

synchiria [siŋ'kaiəriə] *n* 两侧错觉

syncholia [siŋ'kəuliə] *n* 胆汁内异质分泌

synchondrectomy [ˌsiŋkən'drektəmi] *n* 软骨结合切除术(尤指耻骨联合切除术)

synchondroseotomy [ˌsiŋkənˌdrəusi'ɔtəmi] *n* 软骨结合切开术(尤指骶髂联合切开术,治膀胱外翻)

synchondrosis [ˌsiŋkən'drəusis] ([复]**synchondroses** [ˌsiŋkən'drəusiːz]) *n*【希】[透明软骨]结合 | costoclavicular ~ 肋锁韧带 / synchondroses of cranium 颅软骨结合 / epiphyseal ~ 骺软骨结合 / intersphenoidal ~ 蝶间软骨结合 / pubic ~ 耻骨联合 / sternal ~ 胸骨软骨结合

synchondrotomy [ˌsiŋkən'drɔtəmi] *n* 软骨结合切开术(指耻骨联合切开术或任何其他软骨结合切开术)

synchorial [siŋ'kɔːriəl] *a* (多胎妊娠)同绒毛膜的

synchronia [siŋ'krəuniə] *n* 同时性,同步现象;准时发生

synchronism ['siŋkrənizəm], **synchrony** ['siŋkrəni] *n* 同时性,同步现象 | **synchronistic** [ˌsiŋkrə'nistik] *a* | **synchronistically** [ˌsiŋkrə'nistikəli] *ad*

synchronize ['siŋkrənaiz] *vi* 同时发生,同步 *vt* 同步化 | **synchronization** [siŋkrənai'zeiʃən, -ni'z-] *n* 同步化

synchronous ['siŋkrənəs] *a* 同时[发生]的,同步的 | **~ly** *ad* | **~ness** *n*

synchrotron ['siŋkrəutrɔn] *n* 同步加速器

synchysis ['siŋkisis] *n*【希】玻璃体液化 | ~ scintillans 闪光性玻璃体液化(玻璃状体液内发生胆固醇结晶,是炎症或其他眼病后的蜕变)

syncinesis [ˌsinsai'niːsis] *n* 联带运动

synciput ['sinsipʌt] *n* 前顶,前头

synclinal [siŋ'klainl] *a* 互倾的,向斜的

synclitism ['siŋklitizəm], **syncliticism** [siŋ'klitisizəm] *n* 胎头均倾,头盆倾势均匀;同时成熟(指血细胞核和胞质) | **synclitic** [siŋ'klitik] *a* (胎头)均倾的

synclonus ['sinklənəs] *n* 共同阵挛;共同阵挛病

syncope ['siŋkəpi] *n* 晕厥 | ~ anginosa 心绞痛晕厥 / carotid sinus ~ 颈动脉窦性晕厥,颈动脉窦综合征 / cough ~ 咳嗽晕厥 / digital ~ 指晕厥 / micturition ~ 排尿晕厥 / postural ~ 体位性晕厥 / stretching ~ 伸展性晕厥 / swallow ~ 吞咽晕厥 / tussive ~, laryngeal ~ 咳嗽晕厥,喉晕厥 / vasovagal ~, vasodepressor ~ 血管迷走神经性晕厥,血管降压性晕厥 | **syncopal** ['siŋkəpl], **syncopic** [siŋ'kɔpik] *a*

syncretio [siŋ'kriːʃiəu] *n*【拉】粘连(浆膜面)

syncytial [sin'siʃəl] *a* 多核的;合胞体的

syncytiolysin [ˌsinsiti'ɔlisin] *n* 合胞体溶素,融合细胞溶素(能破坏合胞体的溶素,将动物胎盘物质注射至另一动物所产生的溶素)

syncytioma [sinˌsiti'əumə] *n* 合胞体瘤 | ~ malignum 恶性合胞体瘤,绒毛膜上皮瘤

syncytiotoxin [sinˌsitiə'tɔksin] *n* 合胞体毒素,融合细胞毒素(对胎盘有特异性作用的毒素)

syncytiotrophoblast [sinˌsitiə'trɔfəblæst] *n* 合[胞]体滋养层

syncytiotrophoblastic [sinˌsitiəuˌtrɔfə'blæstik] *a* 合胞体滋养层的

syncytium [sin'siʃiəm] ([复] **syncytia** [sin'siʃiə]) *n* 多核体;合胞体

syncytoid ['sinsitɔid] *a* 合胞体样的

syncytotoxin [ˌsinsitə'tɔksin] *n* 融合细胞毒素(用胎盘细胞免疫动物后所产生的细胞溶解性毒素)

syndactylus [sin'dæktiləs] *n* 并指者,并趾者

syndactyly [sin'dæktili] *n* 并指畸形,并趾畸形 | complicated ~ 复杂并指,复杂并趾 / partial ~ 部分并指,部分并趾 / simple ~ 简单并指,简单并趾 / single ~ 两指并指,两趾并趾 | **syndactylia** [ˌsindæk'tiliə], **syndactylism** [sin'dæktilizəm] *n* | **syndactylous** *a*

syndectomy [sin'dektəmi] *n* 球结膜环切术

syndelphus [sin'delfəs] *n* 头躯联胎,单头单躯八肢畸胎

syndesis ['sindəsis] *n* 关节固定术;联会,接合

syndesmectomy [ˌsindez'mektəmi, -des-] *n* 韧带切除术

syndesmectopia [ˌsindezmek'təupiə, -des-] *n* 韧带异位

syndesmitis [ˌsindez'maitis, -des-] *n* 韧带炎;结膜炎 | ~ metatarsea 跖韧带炎,行军瘤

syndesm(o)- [构词成分]韧带;结缔组织

syndesmochorial [ˌsindəzməu'kɔːriəl] *a* 结膜绒膜的

syndesmography [ˌsindez'mɔgrəfi, -des-] *n* 韧带论

syndesmology [ˌsindez'mɔlədʒi, -des-], **syndesmologia** [ˌsindezmə'ləudʒiə, -des-] *n* 韧带学

syndesmo-odontoid [sinˌdezməu ɔ'dɔntɔid, -ˌdes-] *n* 齿突韧带联合(寰齿后关节)

syndesmopexy [sinˈdezməˌpeksi, -ˈdes-] *n* 韧带固定术

syndesmophyte [sinˈdezməfait, -ˈdes-] *n* 韧带骨赘

syndesmoplasty [sinˈdezməˌplæsti, -ˈdes-] *n* 韧带成形术

syndesmorrhaphy [ˌsindezˈmɔrəfi, -des-] *n* 韧带缝合术

syndesmosis [ˌsindezˈməusis, -des-] ([复] **syndesmoses** [ˌsindezˈməusiːz, -des-]) *n*【希】韧带连接 | **syndesmotic** [ˌsindezˈmɔtik, -des-] *a*

syndesmotomy [ˌsindezˈmɔtəmi, -des-] *n* 韧带切开术

syndrome [ˈsindrəum] *n* 综合征 | acquired immune deficiency ~, acquired immunodeficiency ~ (AIDS) 获得性免疫缺陷综合征(艾滋病)(由于感染人免疫缺陷病毒〈HIV〉而引起的一种流行性可传染的反转录病毒疾病,严重病例显示细胞免疫极度降低,并累及某些已知的高危人群,其中包括同性恋和异性恋男子、滥用静脉给药者、血友病患者和其他接受输血者、与HIV感染者有性接触以及感染此病毒的母亲刚生的婴儿。疾病控制与预防中心艾滋病诊断〈CDC/AIDS〉所确定的标准是:须确诊存在至少能中度提示细胞介导免疫基本缺陷的疾病〈例如60岁以下的人有卡波西〈Kaposi〉肉瘤或肺孢子虫病,或其他危及生命的机会性感染〉,同时须无已知基本免疫缺陷或报道过与此病有关的任何其他宿主防御缺陷的原因〈例如医源性免疫抑制或淋巴网状恶性肿瘤〉,或HIV感染者存在下列任何一种疾病:CD4⁺T淋巴细胞计数少于200/ml或CD4⁺T淋巴细胞百分比少于14%、肺结核、侵袭性宫颈癌或复发性肺炎) / acute brain ~, acute organic brain ~ 急性脑综合征,急性器质性脑综合征(见 organic brain ~) / addisonian ~ 艾迪生综合征(肾上腺功能不全引起的综合征,见 Addison's disease) / adiposogenital ~ 肥胖性生殖器退化综合征,肥胖性生殖器退化,脑性肥胖症 / adrenogenital ~ 肾上腺性征综合征(肾上腺皮质功能亢进,女性有假两性畸形和男性化,常在出生时证实,男性为早熟性性发育〈早熟性巨生殖器巨体〉,常于出生后3~4年才出现,临床检查所见为皮质醇〈cortisol〉产生不足及随之发生垂体ACTH分泌过多从而导致雄激素产生过多所致。亦称先天性肾上腺增生) / adult respiratory distress ~ (ARDS) 成人型呼吸窘迫综合征(暴发性肺间质性水肿和肺泡水肿,通常在创伤后数天内发生,推想为由于脑损伤或缺氧引起的大量交感神经物质排放以及由于毛细血管通透性增高所致。亦称休克肺) / AEC ~ AEC综合征(见 Hay-Wells syndrome) / "Alice in Wonderland" ~ "艾丽丝漫游奇境记"式综合征(一种妄想状态,表现为人格解体、体象紊乱、对时间流逝的感觉发生改变以及其他妄想或错觉,可能与精神分裂症、癫痫、偏头痛、顶叶疾患、催眠状态或使用致幻药有关) / amnestic ~ 遗忘综合征(见 Korsakoff's psychosis) / amyostatic ~ 肌震颤性综合征,肝豆状核变性 / anginal ~, anginose ~ 心绞痛综合征(冠状动脉功能不全的疼痛及其他症状) / ankyloblepharon-ectodermal dysplasia-clefting ~ 睑缘粘连-外胚层发育不良-唇腭裂综合征(见 Hay-Wells syndrome) / anorexia-cachexia ~ 厌食-恶病质综合征(一种对癌症的全身性反应,系由于厌食和恶病质之间某种目前不十分清楚的关系而产生,其表现为营养不良、体重减轻、肌肉软弱无力、酸中毒和毒血症) / anterior cornual ~ 脊髓前角综合征(由于脊髓前角的损害引起的肌肉萎缩) / anterior interosseous ~ 骨间前综合征(由骨间前神经损害引起的综合征,通常由于骨折或撕裂伤或有时由于受压所致,近侧前臂疼痛,神经支配的肌肉软弱无力) / anxiety ~ 焦虑综合征(伴以焦虑的体症,如心悸、呼吸快而浅、出汗、苍白及惊恐感) / aortic arch ~ 主动脉弓综合征(导致主动脉弓动脉闭塞的任何一组疾病,这样的闭塞可能由于动脉粥样硬化、动脉栓塞、梅毒性或结核性动脉炎等所致) / argentaffinoma ~ 嗜银细胞瘤综合征(见 carcinoid ~) / auriculotemporal ~ 耳颞综合征(颊部潮红及出汗,与进食有关,见于腮腺损害及由于耳颞神经所致) / autoerythrocyte sensitization ~ 自身红细胞致敏综合征(见 painful bruising ~) / autoimmune polyendocrine-candidiasis ~ 自身免疫性多内分泌腺-念珠菌病综合征,多内分泌腺自身免疫病Ⅰ型 / basal cell nevus ~ 基底细胞痣综合征(一种常染色体显性遗传综合征,特征为生命早期形成无数基底细胞癌,伴发皮肤异常〈尤其是手和足的一种红斑性凹陷水肿〉,以及骨、神经系统、眼和生殖道的异常,亦称戈林〈Gorlin〉综合征,戈林-戈尔茨〈Gorlin-Goltz〉综合征,痣样基底细胞癌综合征和痣样基底细胞瘤综合征) / battered-child ~ 受虐儿童综合征(儿童出现的无法解释或无适当解释的身体创伤及累遭〈通常受父母〉身体严重虐待所致的其他表现) / brachial ~ 臂丛综合征(臂丛的神经受压迫或刺激所致的一种病况) / brittle bone ~ 脆骨综合征,成骨不全 / brittle cornea ~ 脆性角膜综合征(一种X连锁隐性遗传综合征,特征为脆性角膜、蓝巩膜及红发) / bulbar ~ 延髓综合征(见 Dejerine's syndrome ②解) / capsular thrombosis ~ 内囊血栓形成综合征(内囊血管血栓形成所致的偏瘫) / capsulothalamic ~ 内囊丘脑综合征(由于丘脑和内囊损害所致的偏瘫、偏盲及痛觉反常) / carcinoid ~ 类癌综合征(伴有类癌瘤〈嗜银细胞瘤〉的一种综合征,其特征为皮肤青紫色发红,持续数分

钟到数天之久、腹泻水样粪、支气管收缩性发作、血压突然下降、水肿和腹水,这由于嗜银细胞瘤细胞所分泌的儿茶酚胺所致。亦称嗜银细胞瘤综合征)/ carotid sinus ~ 颈动脉窦综合征(晕厥有时伴有惊厥发作,由于一侧或两侧颈动脉窦受压时颈动脉窦反射兴奋过度所致)/ carpal tunnel ~ 腕管综合征(腕管内正中神经受压时,手指与手有疼痛及灼伤或麻刺样感觉异常,有时扩展至肘部)/ cat's cry ~ 猫叫综合征(见 cri du chat ~)/ cat-eye ~, cat's eye ~ 猫眼综合征(虹膜缺损伴肛门闭锁,还可能有许多其他异常,其中包括耳前皮赘或耳郭前瘘、器官距离过远、先天性心脏病、骨骼异常和肾脏畸形)/ cauda equina ~ 马尾综合征(会阴、膀胱、骶骨钝而酸痛,伴感觉异常和无反射性麻痹,由于脊髓神经根受压所致)/ cavernous sinus ~ 海绵窦综合征(结膜水肿、突眼、上睑及鼻根水肿,并有第三、第四及第六神经麻痹,由于海绵窦血栓形成所致)/ celiac ~ 乳糜泻综合征,乳糜泻 / centroposterior ~ 脊髓后中央灰质综合征(脊髓空洞症性感觉分离和血管运动障碍,由于脊髓灰质后中央部损害所致)/ cerebellar ~ 小脑综合征(遗传性小脑性共济失调)/ cerebrohepatorenal ~ 脑肝肾综合征(一种常染色体隐性遗传病,特征为颅面异常、肌张力减退、肝大、多囊肾、黄疸,并于婴儿早期死亡,伴肝与肾内过氧化物酶体缺乏)/ cervical ~ 颈神经(根)综合征(颈神经根受刺激或受压所引起的情况,特征为颈痛,辐射至肩、臂或前臂)/ cervical rib ~, cervicobrachial ~ 颈肋综合征(见 scalenus ~)/ chancriform ~ 下疳样综合征,原发性肺外球孢子菌病 / chiasma ~, chiasmatic ~ 视交叉综合征(表示视交叉损害的一种综合征,有视力损害、视野限制、中心暗点、头痛、眩晕和晕厥)/ Chinese restaurant ~ (CRS) 中国餐馆综合征(一种暂时性的动脉扩张综合征,由于摄食常用于有调味品的中国菜中的谷氨酸钠所致,特征为头搏动、头晕、背痛等)/ chorea ~ 舞蹈症样综合征(见 Hunt's striatal syndrome ②解)/ chronic brain ~, chronic organic brain ~ 慢性脑综合征,慢性器质性脑综合征(见 organic brain ~)/ closed head ~ 闭合性颅脑(损伤)综合征 / cold agglutinin ~ 冷凝集素综合征(循环抗体〈通常为 IgM〉的存在能使红细胞凝集,温度在 37 ℃以下这种作用更强)/ combined immunodeficiency ~ 联合免疫缺陷综合征 / ~ of corpus striatum 纹状体综合征(见 Vogt's syndrome)/ costoclavicular ~ 肋锁综合征(在颈臂出口的神经或血管受压迫、牵伸或摩擦所引起的臂及〈或〉手部疼痛或其他障碍)/ couvade ~ 拟娩综合征(妊娠妇女的配偶出现与妊娠有关的一些症状,如恶心、呕吐和腹痛)/ craniosynostosis-radial aplasia ~ 颅缝早闭-桡骨发育不良综合征(即巴-杰综合征 Baller-Gerald ~)/ CREST ~, CRST ~ CREST 综合征,CRST 综合征(一型全身性硬皮病,包括皮肤钙质沉着症〈*c*alcinosis cutis〉,雷诺现象〈*R*aynaud's phenomenon〉,食管功能不良〈*e*sophageal dysfunction〉,指〈趾〉硬皮病〈*s*clerodactyly〉及毛细血管扩张〈*t*elangiectasia〉,上述症状中食管功能不良不显著者则称为 CRST 综合征)/ cri du chat ~ 猫叫综合征(由于 B 组染色体〈4 或 5〉的短臂缺失所引起的遗传性先天性综合征,特征为眼距过宽、小头畸形、精神发育障碍,病孩哭声犹如猫叫)/ ~ of crocodile tears 鳄泪综合征(进食时流泪,见于面瘫患者)/ crush ~ 挤压综合征(身体某部受挤压后发生的水肿、尿少及其他肾衰竭的症状)/ cryptophthalmos ~ 隐眼(畸形)综合征(一种常染色体隐性遗传性异常,特征为睑孔缺失,一侧或双侧眼球结构破坏,耳畸形,腭裂,喉狭窄,并指〈趾〉,脑膜膨出,肛门闭锁,心脏缺陷和肾发育不良。亦称弗莱塞〈Fraser〉综合征)/ culture-specific ~ 文化特异综合征(有特定文化背景的一种紊乱行为,但不符合西医的疾病分类,例如 amok, koro, piblokto 和 windigo)/ diarrheogenic ~ 致腹泻综合征(见 Verner-Morrison syndrome)/ dumping ~ 倾倒综合征(已做过部分胃切除术和胃空肠吻合术的病人进食后发生的恶心、软弱、出汗、心悸、不同程度的晕厥,常有温暖感及有时腹泻,或许是由于胃内容物过分迅速排空所致的一种复杂反应)/ dyscontrol ~ 失控综合征(一型发作性、异常的并经常是激烈的和无法控制的社会行为,但并无挑衅行为,可能由于边缘系统或颞叶疾病所致,或可能伴有酗酒,或滥用某种精神作用物质所致。亦称发作性失控)/ dysmaturity ~ 成熟障碍综合征(由于胎盘功能不全所致的综合征,引起慢性应激反应和缺氧,见于过期妊娠的胎儿和婴儿,特征为皮下脂肪减少,皮肤脱屑和长指甲,常有黄色胎粪染上指〈趾〉甲、皮肤和胎脂。亦称过度成熟综合征,胎盘功能不全综合征)/ dysplastic nevus ~ 发育不良性痣综合征(有家族性的或有家族性危险的、或非家族性的恶性黑素瘤者出现的发育不良性痣)/ ectopic ACTH ~ 异位 ACTH 综合征(来自非内分泌组织的肿瘤产生 ACTH 而引起的病症,根据其持续时间,症状可能难以捉摸而类似真正的库欣〈Cushing〉病,但低钾血症性碱中毒和软弱无力常为突出表现)/ EEC ~, ectrodactyly-ectodermal dysplasia-clefting ~ EEC 综合征,缺指(趾)畸形-外胚层发育不良-唇腭裂综合征(一种常染色体显性遗传的综合征,涉及外胚层和中胚层各种组织,包括外胚层发育不良伴皮肤与毛发色素减退,毛发和眉毛稀疏,无睫毛,甲营养不良,牙少而小,缺指〈趾〉畸形及唇腭裂)/ effort ~ 奋力综合征(神经性循环衰竭)/ egg-white ~ 卵白综合征 / EMG ~, *e*xomphalos-*m*acroglossia-*g*igantism ~ 脐疝-巨舌-巨大发育综合征(即 Beckwith-Wiedemann ~) / empty-sella ~ 空蝶鞍综合征(由放射学诊断的一种综合征,表现为鞍膈退化,蝶鞍形成蛛网膜下腔的延伸部分并充满脑脊液,以及垂体窝出现空泡,脑垂体虽存在,但呈扁平状。垂体激素分泌可能正常、缺乏或过多) / epiphyseal ~ 松果体综合征(外生殖器和性功能早熟,长骨异常早熟性生长,出现脑内积水的体征,提示松果体受损的所有其他运动和感觉的症状缺失。亦称早熟性巨生殖器巨体) / erythrocyte autosensitization ~ 红细胞自身致敏综合征(见 painful bruising ~) / extrapyramidal ~ 锥体束外综合征(特征为不随意运动异常,其中包括震颤麻痹、手足徐动症及舞蹈症) / floppy infant ~ 婴儿松弛综合征(一种婴儿先天性肌病,临床特征为肌张力减退和肌软弱无力) / focal dermal hypoplasia ~ 局灶性皮肤发育不良综合征 / four-day ~ 四天综合征(新生儿呼吸窘迫综合征,因婴儿一般在四天之内康复或死亡,故名) / fragile X ~ 脆性 X[染色体]综合征(一种 X 连锁综合征,多数男性表现为精神发育迟缓、睾丸增大、前额高、颌大及耳长,多数杂合女性表现为轻度精神发育迟缓) / G ~ G 综合征(见 Opitz syndrome) / general adaptation ~ 全身适应综合征(指对紧张境遇的全身防御反应) / glucagonoma ~ 胰高血糖素瘤综合征(胰腺 α 细胞分泌高血糖素的肿瘤,伴有血清高血糖素水平升高、轻度糖尿病、体重减轻、贫血、舌炎、口炎、口角炎、睑炎和坏死松解性游走性红斑) / half base ~ 半底综合征(见 Garcin's syndrome) / happy puppet ~ 快乐木偶综合征(一种常染色体隐性遗传综合征,特征为忽动忽停木偶样运动,经常发笑,智力迟钝和运动性阻抑,独特的张嘴面容和癫痫发作。亦称安吉尔曼〈Angelman〉综合征) / HARD ~ HARD 综合征(见 Walker-Warburg syndrome) / haw ~ 瞬膜综合征(狗或猫瞬膜之一或两者均突出。亦称瞬膜) / heart-hand ~ 心-手综合征(见 Holt-Oram syndrome) / hemolytic-uremic ~ 溶血尿毒症综合征(一种罕见的综合征,病因不明,主要发生于 4 岁以下的儿童,特征为肾功能衰竭、微血管病性溶血性贫血、严重血小板减少和紫癜) / hereditary benign intraepithelial dyskeratosis ~ 遗传性良性上皮内角化不良综合征(特征为球结膜斑和口腔黏膜增厚,临床上类似白色皱褶性肥大〈Cannon 白色海绵状痣〉。本征为常染色体显性遗传,有高度的外显率) / 17-hydroxylase deficiency ~ 17-羟化酶缺乏综合征(17-α-羟化酶缺乏引起的先天性肾上腺增生导致雌激素和雄激素缺乏,从而导致性幼稚型,脱氧皮质酮和皮质酮的补偿性分泌增加引起低钾血症性碱中毒和高血压) / hyperactive child ~ 活动过强儿童综合征(见 disorder 项下 attention-deficit hyperactivity disorder) / hypercalcemia ~ 高钙血综合征(见 milk-alkali ~) / hypereosinophilic ~ 嗜酸细胞增多综合征(血中嗜酸细胞数大量增加,酷似白血病,特征为嗜酸细胞浸润心、脑、肝及肺,并表现为一种渐进性致死的病程) / hyperimmunoglobulinemia E ~ 高免疫球蛋白 E 血症综合征(一种原发性免疫缺陷病,特征为皮肤、肺、关节及其他部位复发性葡萄球菌性脓肿,瘙痒性皮炎,血清 IgE 水平很高,IgG, IgA 和 IgM 水平正常,血与痰中嗜酸细胞增多) / hyperkinetic ~ 多动综合征(见 disorder 项下 attention-deficit hyperactivity disorder) / hypertelorism-hypospadias ~ 器官距离过远-尿道下裂综合征(见 Opitz syndrome) / hypoplastic left heart ~ (HLHS) 左心发育不全综合征(任何一组先天性畸形,包括左心室发育不全或闭锁,主动脉瓣或二尖瓣或两者均发育不全或闭锁,以及升主动脉发育不全,特征为呼吸窘迫和极度紫绀,伴心脏衰竭,婴儿早期即死亡) / ~ of inappropriate antidiuretic hormone (SIADH) 抗利尿激素分泌失调综合征(持久性低钠血症,尿渗摩尔浓度不相适应地增高,无 ADH 释放的刺激物,可伴发于肿瘤〈尤其是肺的燕麦细胞癌或胰腺癌,由于肿瘤可产生异位性 ADH〉、肺及中枢神经系统疾病,包括头部创伤) / intrauterine parabiotic ~ 子宫内联体生活综合征(见 placental transfusion ~) / irritable bowel ~, irritable colon ~ 肠易激综合征,结肠易激综合征(一种慢性非炎性疾病,特征为腹痛、排便习惯改变,表现为腹泻或便秘,或两者均有,但无病理性变化。亦称过敏性结肠,痉挛性结肠) / jejunal ~ 倾倒综合征(见 dumping ~) / kinky-hair ~ 扭结发综合征(见 Menkes' syndrome) / kleeblattschädel (cloverleaf skull) ~ 三叶草形头颅综合征(一种先天性疾患,特征为多发性或全部颅缝骨性联接,伴有脑积水,某些病例有面骨发育不全及长骨异常) / lacrimo-auriculo-dento-digital ~, LADD ~ 泪-耳-牙-指(趾)综合征,LADD 综合征(一种常染色体显性遗传综合征,特征为鼻泪管、耳、四肢和牙畸形,常伴混合型听力丧失。可能发生唾液腺和泌尿生殖系统异常) / lazy leukocyte ~ 懒惰白细胞综合征(发生于儿童的一种综合征,特点为反复轻度感染,伴有中性粒细胞的趋化性不足及随机移动性缺陷) / LEOPARD ~ 豹斑综合征(常染色体显性遗传,表现为多发性雀斑样痣,无症状性心脏缺陷和典型粗糙面容,也可并发肺动脉瓣狭窄、感音神经性聋、骨骼改变、两眼间距过远及生殖系统畸形。亦称多发性雀斑样痣综合征) / locked-in ~ 闭锁综合征(四肢麻痹及缄默症,意识未损及,眼随意垂直运动仍保存并能眨眼,通常由于脑桥腹部血管损害所致。亦称睁眼昏迷,假性昏迷) / long Q-T ~ 长 Q-T 间期综合征(表现几种不同形式,可能是后天性的,通常由于代谢或心脏异常或服药所致,或可能是先天性的,发生时或伴耳聋〈Jervell and Lange-Nielsen syndrome〉或不伴耳聋〈Romano-Ward syndrome〉。本征可能导致严重心律失常和心源性猝死) / maternal deprivation ~ 失母爱综合征(由于失去母亲或缺乏适当的母爱而导致生长障碍、行为孤独及精神发育迟缓) / methionine malabsortion ~ 蛋氨酸吸收障碍综合征(为蛋氨酸吸收障碍的常染色体隐性遗传性疾病,其尿有类似烟叶烘房内的特殊气味,系细菌作用于未吸收的蛋氨酸形成 α-羟丁酸所致;其特征为白发,智力迟钝,惊厥及发作性呼吸深快。亦称烟叶烘房气味尿病,史-斯〈Smith-Strang〉病) / middle lobe ~ 中叶综合征(右肺中叶扩张不全伴慢性肺炎) / milk-alkali ~ 乳碱综合征(特征为血钙过多但无尿钙过多或血磷酸盐过少,仅有轻度碱中毒,血清磷酸酶正常,但有严重肾功能不全伴高氮血症及钙沉着,系长期摄入牛乳及可吸收的钙所致。亦称伯内特〈Burnett〉综合征和高钙血综合征) / mucocutaneous lymph node ~ (MLNS) 黏膜皮肤淋巴结综合征(一种最常累及婴幼儿的病因不明的综合征,特征为发热、结膜充血、唇及口腔变红、溃疡性龈炎、颈淋巴结肿大及呈手套-短袜状分布并逐渐融合成亮红色的红斑性皮疹。皮肤逐渐变硬及水肿、并有指趾脱皮。亦称川崎〈Kawasaki〉病) / multiple lentigines ~ 多发性雀斑样痣综合征(见 LEOPARD ~) / multiple pterygium ~ 多发性翼状赘蹼综合征(一种常染色体隐性遗传综合征,包括颈、腋、腘窝、肘前及股间区的翼状赘蹼,伴两眼间距过宽,腭裂,小颌,睑下垂及身材矮小,骨骼异常,包括指〈趾〉弯曲、并指〈趾〉畸形、马蹄内翻足和摇摆椅状足,此外还有脊椎融合和肋骨异常。男子有隐睾病,女子则无大阴唇) / myasthenic ~ 肌无力综合征(见 Eaton-Lambert syndrome) / nevoid basal cell carcinoma ~, nevoid basalioma ~ 痣样基底细胞癌综合征,痣样基底细胞瘤综合征(见 basal cell nevus ~) / neuroleptic malignant ~ 神经阻滞剂恶性综合征(一种罕见的有时是致死的反应,特征为高热、强直及昏迷) / OAV ~ 眼耳脊椎发育不良综合征(即眼耳脊椎发育不良 oculoauriculovertebral dysplasia) / oculocerebrorenal ~ 眼脑肾综合征(一种 X 连锁遗传病,特征为维生素 D 不应性佝偻病,眼积水、先天性青光眼与白内障、精神发育迟缓及肾小管重吸收功能障碍,还有低磷酸盐血症、酸中毒与氨基酸尿。亦称洛氏〈Lowe〉病) / oculomandibulofacial ~ 眼下颌面综合征(主要特征为颅面骨畸形〈通常为短头畸形〉,鹦鹉鼻,下颌发育不全,矮小但匀称,毛发稀少,先天性双侧白内障及眼小。亦称下颌眼面颅面骨畸形) / OFD ~, oral-facial-digital ~ 口-面-指综合征 / OMM ~ 眼下颌肢发育不良综合征,眼下颌肢发育不良 / one-and-a-half ~ 一个半综合征(一种眼运动障碍,由于一个展神经核和附近内侧纵束的脑干损害所致,同侧眼移动无法超出水平中线,对侧眼可外展并作双目注视的任何企图) / orbital apex ~ 眶尖综合征(眼肌麻痹伴视力减弱以致可能导致失明,眼睑肿胀,上睑下垂,上睑、半额和角膜感觉过敏或减退以及血管舒缩障碍,系由于外伤、炎症或肿瘤过程累及眶上裂和视神经管或它们所包含的结构所致) / orbital floor ~ 眶底综合征(眼球突出,复视以及在受三叉神经支配的区域内感觉缺失,与眶底内的损害一起发生) / organic brain ~ 器质性脑病综合征(见 organic mental ~) / organic mental ~ 器质性精神综合征(与一种或多种特异性器质性致病因素有关的一群精神性或行为性体征和症状。DSM Ⅲ-R〈美国精神病诊断统计手册〉包括 6 种特异性器质性脑病综合征:delirium and dementia〈谵妄与痴呆〉, amnestic syndrome or organic hallucinosis〈遗忘综合征或器质性幻觉症〉, organic delusional syndrome, organic mood syndrome, and organic anxiety syndrome〈器质性妄想综合征、器质性心境综合征和器质性焦虑综合征〉, organic personality syndrome〈器质性人格综合征〉, intoxication and withdrawal〈中毒与戒断〉, organic mental syndrome〈器质性精神综合征〉。当致病因素是对精神起显著作用的物质,则冠以该物质的名称,去掉"organic",并将"syndrome"改为"disorder",例如"alcohol amnestic disorder〈酒精性遗忘症〉"、"cannabis delusional disorder〈大麻妄想性精神障碍〉") / orofaciodigital (OFD) ~, type Ⅰ 口-面-指综合征Ⅰ型(即 oral-facial-digital ~, type Ⅰ) / orofaciodigital ~, type Ⅱ 口-面-指(综合征Ⅱ型,莫尔(Mohr)综合征) / outlet ~ 臂丛综合征(见 brachial ~) / painful bruising ~ 痛性淤紫综合征(主要在青年妇女发生的一种紫癜性反应,患者在无创伤情况下,任何部位可反复自发出现单个或多个痛性淤斑,多数情况下是由于对红细胞构架成分过敏,某些情况下是对白细胞成分过敏,情绪波动是诱因) / pancreatic cholera ~ 胰性霍乱综合征(见 Verner-Morrison syndrome) / paratrigeminal ~ 三叉神经旁综合征(见 Raeder's paratrigeminal syndrome) / PEP ~ [*p*lasma cell dyscrasia, *e*ndocrinopathy, *p*olyneuropathy] PEP 综合征(浆细胞病、内分泌病和多神经病综合征,见 POEMS ~) / PHC ~ PHC 综合征(一种常染色体显性遗传综合征,包括前磨牙发育不良〈premolar aplasia〉,多汗症〈hyperhidrosis〉和早年白发〈premature canities〉) / placental dysfunction ~ 胎盘功能不全综合征(由于胎盘内发生变性变化造成胎儿营养不良和缺氧。发育完全时,指〈趾〉

甲、皮肤和胎脂染成亮黄色,脐带呈黄绿色。亦称黄色胎脂综合征)/ placental transfusion ~ 胎盘输血综合征(孪生子出生时,一个贫血,另一个多血,系因一方血液经由两者间的连接血管驱入对方循环所致。亦称子宫内联体生活综合征)/ POEMS ~ POEMS 综合征(一种结合多神经病〈*p*olyneuropathy〉、器官肥大〈*o*rganomegaly〉、内分泌病〈*e*ndocrinopathy〉、M-蛋白〈*M*-protein〉和皮肤变化〈*s*kin changes〉的多系统综合征,可能与蛋白异常血症如存在异常单克隆蛋白和轻链有关。亦称克罗-深濑〈Crow-Fukase〉综合征,PEP 综合征)/ postmaturity ~ 过度成熟综合征(见 dysmaturity ~)/ postperfusion ~, post-transfusion ~ 灌注后综合征,输血后综合征(巨细胞病毒性单核细胞增多症,心脏直视手术或其他外科手术采用体外循环或多次输血后 3~6 周出现。亦称输血后单核细胞增多症)/ respiratory distress ~ of newborn 新生儿呼吸窘迫综合征(以呼吸困难伴发绀为特征的新生儿病状。本征包括两种类型:①透明膜病或综合征,②新生儿特发性呼吸窘迫。亦称先天性肺泡发育不全,先天性吸入性肺炎)/ restless leg ~ 下肢不宁综合征(坐或躺卧尤其在入睡前,深感小腿内部不适,而产生一种不可抗拒的冲动来活动小腿)/ retraction ~ 眼球后缩综合征(见 Duane's syndrome)/ Rh-null ~ Rh 因子缺乏综合征(慢性溶血性贫血,累及缺乏所有 Rh 因子〈Rh_{null}〉者。本征特点为球形红细胞症、裂口红细胞症以及渗透脆性增加)/ runting ~ 发育阻碍综合征(移植物抗宿主反应,特征为腹泻、皮炎、肝脾肿大、溶血性贫血及各类血细胞减少)/ salt-losing ~, salt-depletion 失盐综合征,缺盐综合征(由于体内大量缺钠所致的呕吐、脱水、高血压和突然死亡)/ scalenus ~, scalenus anticus ~ 斜角肌综合征,前斜角肌综合征(肩部疼痛,并常向下延伸至臂或向上放射到颈背部,因颈肋和前斜角肌之间的神经和血管受压所致。亦称纳夫济格〈Naffziger〉综合征,颈肋综合征)/ scimitar ~ 弯刀综合征(右肺静脉全部或部分引流入下腔静脉,常伴有右肺发育不全,因在胸部 X 线摄影时可见静脉畸形的阴影凸出于心脏下缘右侧而得名)/ ~ of sea-blue histocyte 海蓝色组织细胞综合征(一种罕见疾病,特征为存在着一种形态上很明显的海蓝色粒状组织细胞及脾肿大)/ severe acute respiratory ~ (SARS)重症急性呼吸综合征(一种传染性呼吸疾病,特征为发热、干咳和呼吸困难,常伴有头痛和全身疼痛,据认为是由一种冠状病毒所致)/ sicca ~ 干燥综合征(角膜结膜炎和口腔干燥,不伴有结缔组织病,参见 Sjögren's syndrome)/ shoulder-hand ~ 肩-手综合征(局限于上肢的交感反射性营养不良)/ sick sinus ~ 病态窦房结综合征(为一复杂的心律失常,表现为仅有严重的窦性心动过缓,或窦性心动过缓与心动过速交替发生,或窦性心动过缓伴有房室传导阻滞)/ sleep apnea ~ 睡眠呼吸暂停综合征(发作性呼吸停止,发生于由非快速眼动〈NREM〉向快速眼动〈REM〉过渡时,伴有反复觉醒与白天睡眠过多,最常发生于中年肥胖男性,据认为有若干原因,其中之一为气道萎陷或阻塞及肌张力抑制,而这正是 REM 睡眠的特征)/ space adaptation ~ 太空适应综合征(发生于宇宙飞行时失重环境下的一种运动病,伴有恶心、呕吐、厌食、头痛、不适、倦睡和嗜眠,可能由于位觉砂〈其功能有赖于重力的存在〉有关运动的信号与视觉系统〈可影响自主神经系统〉的信号相抵触所致。亦称宇宙病)/ spherophakia-brachymorphia ~ 球形晶状体-短身材综合征(见 Weill-Marchesani syndrome)/ steely hair ~ 钢发综合征(见 Menkes' syndrome)/ stiff-man ~ 僵人综合征(病因不明,特征为进行性波动性中轴和肢体肌肉僵硬而无大脑与脊髓病变的体征,但肌电图活动仍连续)/ stomatitis-pneumoenteritis ~ 口炎-肺肠炎综合征,小反刍动物疫(即 peste des petits ruminants,见 peste 项下相应术语)/ striatal ~ 纹状体综合征(见 Hunt's striatal syndrome)/ sudden infant death ~ (SIDS) 婴儿猝死综合征(cot death,见 death 项下相应术语)/ sudden unexplained death ~ (SUDS)原因不明的猝死综合征(2 岁或 2 岁以上东南亚裔的死亡,其内在原因尚未发现)/ superior orbital fissure ~ 眶上裂综合征(眶深部与单侧额头痛,伴有进行性第六、第三、第四脑神经麻痹,动眼神经麻痹,视野缩小以及其他眼病变,此征发生或由于蝶骨脑膜瘤压迫附近神经所致,或由于蝶窦炎感染扩展至眶上裂所致)/ tegmental ~ 大脑被盖综合征(偏瘫与眼球运动障碍交替出现,提示大脑被盖受损)/ temporomandibular dysfunction ~, temporomandibular joint ~ 颞颌关节功能障碍综合征,颞颌关节综合征(本征包括不全聋、耳内闭塞感、耳鸣、颞颌关节内咔嗒声或吧嗒声、头晕、头痛以及耳、喉、舌、鼻内灼痛)/ testicular feminization ~ 睾丸女性化综合征,雄激素不敏感综合征(男性假两性畸形的极端类型,特点为外观女性发育,包括第二性征,但睾丸存在而无子宫与输卵管,系因终末器对 5α-睾酮的抗拒作用所致)/ thalamic ~ 丘脑综合征(包括偏身麻木、轻度偏瘫、偏身共济失调、偏瘫一侧持续性剧痛。亦称丘脑感觉过敏性感觉缺失)/ thrombocytopenia-absent radius (TAR) 血小板减少-桡骨缺如综合征(一种常染色体隐性遗传综合征,包括血小板减少合并桡骨缺如或发育不全,有时伴先天性心脏病及肾脏异常)/ TINU ~ TINU 综合征(一种罕见肾小管间质性肾炎和葡萄膜炎〈tubulointerstitial nephritis and uveitis〉综合征,常伴发免疫变更)/

TORCH ~ (*t*oxoplasmosis, *o*ther agents, *r*ubella, *c*ytomegalovirus, *h*erpes simplex) TORCH 综合征(弓形虫病,其他病原体,风疹,巨细胞病毒,单纯疱疹)(一组感染的任何一种,见于新生儿,由于致病因子之一已经穿过胎盘屏障,这些致病因子在婴儿具有类似症状,在母亲可能在临床上并不明显) / toxic shock ~ 中毒性休克综合征(一种严重疾病,特征为突发高热、呕吐、腹泻和肌痛,继之血压降低,严重病例出现休克,急性期出现日晒样皮疹伴皮肤脱屑,尤其是手掌和足底部) / transfusion ~ 输血综合征(即胎盘输血综合征,见 placental transfusion ~) / translocation Down ~ 易位性唐氏综合征(多出的染色体物质〈21 号染色体长臂〉易位到另一近端着丝粒染色体上的唐氏综合征〈在标准的 21 三体中,是多出一个完整的 21 号染色体〉。易位染色体携带者共有 45 个染色体,其中包括易位染色体,其子女患唐氏综合征的概率将增加) / trisomy 8 ~, trisomy C ~ 8 三体综合征,C 三体综合征(伴有一个额外的 8 号染色体的综合征,特征为轻度到重度智力迟钝,前额隆凸,眼球深陷,唇厚,耳突起及指〈趾〉弯曲) / trisomy 11q ~ 11q 三体综合征(由于存在一个额外的 11 号染色体长臂所致的综合征;因可能累及不同片段,故伴发的异常也极其可变,包括耳郭前瘘,胆囊发育不全,小阴茎,双角子宫,小眼,心肺脑畸形,癫痫发作和反复感染) / trisomy 13 ~, trisomy D ~ 13 三体综合征,D 三体综合征(一种染色体畸变,系因一个额外的 13 号染色体引起中枢神经系统缺陷和智力迟钝,合并腭唇裂,多指〈趾〉,皮纹型异常以及心脏、内脏和生殖器异常。亦称帕陶〈Patau〉综合征) / trisomy 18 ~, trisomy E ~ 18 三体综合征,E 三体综合征(特征为智力迟钝,舟状头或其他头颅畸形,小颌,睑下垂,低位耳,角膜混浊,耳聋,蹼颈,短指〈趾〉,室间隔缺损,梅克尔〈Meckel〉憩室及其他畸形,系因一个额外的 18 号染色体存在所致。亦称爱德华兹〈Edwards〉综合征) / trisomy 21 ~ 21 三体综合征,唐氏综合征(见 Down syndrome) / trisomy 22 ~ 22 三体综合征(系因一个额外的 22 号染色体所致,典型特征为智力与生长发育迟缓,小头,低位或畸形耳,小额,长人中,耳前皮赘或瘘管及先天性心脏病。男性有阴茎小及〈或〉睾丸未降) / unilateral nevoid telangiectasia ~ 单侧痣样毛细血管扩张综合征(亦称单侧痣毛细血管扩张) / velocardiofacial ~ 腭帆心脏面部综合征(一种常染色体显性遗传综合征,包括心脏缺损和具有特征性的颅面异常,其中包括腭裂、颌异常和鼻突出。本征常伴有 22 号染色体异常,经常发生学习不能,身材矮小,手与指〈趾〉纤细且伸展过度,脊柱侧凸,智力迟钝,腹股沟疝,耳畸形,小头畸形不太常见。亦称施普林曾〈Shprintzen〉综合征,VCF 综合征) / WAGR ~ WAGR 综合征(维尔姆斯瘤〈*W*ilms' tumor〉、无虹膜〈*a*niridia〉、泌尿生殖器异常〈*g*enitourinary abnormalities〉或性腺母细胞瘤〈gonadoblastoma〉和智力迟钝〈mental *r*etardation〉综合征,由于 11 号染色体 p13 区小中间缺失所致) / WDHA ~ (*w*atery *d*iarrhea, *h*ypokalemia, *a*chlorhydria) WDHA 综合征(水泻、低血钾和胃酸缺乏综合征,见 Verner-Morrison syndrome) / WDHH ~ (*w*atery *d*iarrhea, *h*ypokalemia, *h*ypochlorhydria) WDHH 综合征(水泻、低血钾和胃酸过少综合征,见 Verner-Morrison ~) / whistling-face ~, whistling face-windmill vane hand ~ 吹口哨面容综合征,吹口哨面容-风车翼样手综合征,颅腕跗骨营养不良 / X-linked lymphoproliferative ~ X 连锁淋巴细胞增生综合征(一种免疫缺陷病,表现为对 Epstein-Barr 病毒〈EBV〉缺乏细胞或体液免疫反应。暴发性传染性单核细胞增多症、致死性 B 细胞恶性增生或低丙球蛋白血症可能由于 EBV 感染所致。亦称 X 连锁淋巴细胞增生症、邓肯〈Duncan〉病或综合征) XXY ~ XXY 染色体综合征,克莱恩费尔特(Klinefelter)综合征 / yellow nail ~ 黄甲综合征(与淋巴水肿特别是腿部淋巴水肿有关的综合征,包括指〈趾〉甲淡黄至淡绿变色) / yellow vernix ~ 黄色胎脂综合征(即胎盘功能不全综合征,见 placental dysfunction ~) | **syndromic** [sinˈdrəumik] *a*

syndromology [ˌsindrəˈmɔlədʒi] *n* 综合征学

synechia [siˈnekiə] ([复]**synechiae** [siˈnekiiː]) *n* 粘连;虹膜粘连 | annular ~, circular ~ 虹膜环形粘连 / anterior ~ 虹膜前粘连 / ~ pericardii 心包腔粘连 / posterior ~ 虹膜后粘连 / ~ vulvae 外阴闭锁

synechotome [siˈnekətəum] *n* 虹膜粘连[切开]刀

synechotomy [ˌsiniˈkɔtəmi] *n* 虹膜粘连切开术;粘连分离术

synechtenterotomy [ˌsinekˌtentəˈrɔtəmi] *n* 肠粘连切开术

synecology [ˌsiniˈkɔlədʒi] *n* 群落生态学

synencephalocele [ˌsinenˈsefələˌsiːl] *n* 粘连性脑突出

synencephalus [ˌsinenˈsefələs] *n* [四耳]并头联胎

synencephaly [ˌsinenˈsefəli] *n* 并头联胎畸形

syneresis [siˈnerəsis] *n* (胶体)凝缩[作用],(胶体)脱水收缩

synergenesis [ˌsinəˈdʒenisis] *n* 胞质传递说(每一个细胞将它的原生质传递至由原生质所衍生的每一代细胞)

synergetic [ˌsinəˈdʒetik] *a* 协同的,协作的

synergism [ˈsinədʒizəm] *n* 协同作用(两种作用物共同作用所引起的效果大于两者单独作用时

的总和,例如药物的协同作用) | **synergistic** [ˌsinəˈdʒistik] *a*

synergist [ˈsinədʒist] *n* 增效剂,协作剂;协同器[官] | pituitary ~ 垂体协作激素

synergy [ˈsinədʒi], **synergia** [siˈnəːdʒiə] *n* 协同作用(指药物) | **synergic** [siˈnəːdʒik] *a*

synesthesia [ˌsinisˈθiːzjə] *n* 联觉,牵连感觉(如闻声觉色) | ~ algica 疼痛联觉 | **synesthetic** [ˌsinisˈθetik] *a*

synesthesialgia [ˌsinisˌθiːziˈældʒiə] *n* 痛联觉,痛性牵连感觉(刺激患侧产生痛觉,但身体正常侧则无感觉甚至有快感)

synezesis [ˌsiniˈziːsis] *n* 闭合;凝线[期](见 synizesis)

Syngamidae [sinˈgæmidiː] *n* 比翼科

Syngamus [ˈsingəməs] *n* 比翼[线虫]属 | ~ trachea 气管比翼线虫

syngamy [ˈsiŋgəmi] *n* 有性生殖;[原]核融合 | **syngamic** [sinˈgæmik], **syngamous** [ˈsingəməs] *a*

syngeneic [ˌsindʒiˈneiik] *a* 同源的,同基因的,同系的(在移植生物学中指基因型相同的个体或组织)

syngenesioplastic [ˌsindʒiˌniziəuˈplæstik] *a* 同源移植的,同血统移植的(例如母儿、兄妹间)

syngenesiotransplantation [ˌsindʒiˌniziəuˌtrænsplɑːnˈteiʃən] *n* 同源移植术,同血统移植术

syngenesis [sinˈdʒenisis] *n* 有性生殖;群落发生,群落演替;共生,同生 | **syngenetic** [ˌsindʒiˈnetik] *a*

syngnathia [sinˈneiθiə] *n* 连颌畸形(上下颌间黏膜带先天性畸形)

syngonic [sinˈgɔnik] *a* 共生殖腺的(受精时决定性别的)

syngraft [ˈsingrɑːft, -græft] *n* 同种同基因移植(两个基因型相同个体之间的组织移植)

Synhymeniida [ˌsinhaimiˈniːidə] *n* 合膜目

synhymenium [ˌsinhaiˈmeniəm] *n* 合膜

synizesis [ˌsiniˈziːsis] *n*【希】闭合;凝线[期](有丝分裂的一个时期,此时核染色质浓缩成一团)

synkainogenesis [ˌsinkainəuˈdʒenisis] *n* 同时新生

synkaryon [sinˈkæriɔn] *n* 合核体(由两个原核融合而形成的核);受精核

synkinesis [ˌsinkaiˈniːsis] *n* 联带运动 | imitative ~ 模仿性联带运动 / mouth-and-hand ~ 口手联带运动(见 Saunders' sign) | **synkinetic** [ˌsinkaiˈnetik] *a* | **synkinesia** [ˌsinkaiˈniːziə] *n*

synnecrosis [ˌsineˈkrəusis] *n* 双损共亡(两种不同种类的生物共同生活在一起,双方都受到损害或死亡)

synnema [siˈniːmə] *n* 束丝

synneurosis [ˌsinjuəˈrəusis] *n* 韧带联合

synocha [ˈsinəkə] *n* 稽留热 | **synochus** [ˈsinəkəs] *n* / ~**l** *a*

synocytotoxin [ˌsinəˌsaitəuˈtɔksin] *n* 溶细胞毒素

synonychia [sinəˈnikiə] *n* 并甲

synophrys [siˈnɔfris], **synophridia** [ˌsinɔˈfridiə] *n* 连眉,一字眉

synophthalmia [ˌsinɔfˈθælmiə] *n* 并眼[畸形],独眼[畸形]

synophthalmus [ˌsinɔfˈθælməs] *n* 并眼畸胎,独眼畸胎

synopsy [ˈsinəpsi] *n* 视联觉,光联觉;并眼[畸形],独眼[畸形]

synoptophore [siˈnɔptəfɔː] *n* 同视机,斜视诊疗器

synoptoscope [siˈnɔptəskəup] *n* 同视镜,斜视检眼镜

synorchism [siˈnɔːkizəm], **synorchidism** [siˈnɔːkidizəm] *n* 睾丸融合[症]

synoscheos [siˈnɔskiəs] *n* 阴囊阴茎粘连

synosteology [ˌsinɔstiˈɔlədʒi] *n* 关节学,关节解剖学

synosteotomy [ˌsinɔstiˈɔtəmi] *n* 关节切开术

synostosis [ˌsinɔsˈtəusis] ([复] **synostoses** [ˌsinɔsˈtəusiːz]), **synosteosis** [ˌsinɔstiˈəusis] *n* 骨连接;骨结合 | **synostotic** [ˌsinɔsˈtɔtik], **synosteotic** [ˌsinɔstiˈɔtik] *a*

synotia [saiˈnəuʃiə] *n* 并耳[畸形]

synotus [saiˈnəutəs] *n* 并耳畸胎

synovectomy [ˌsinəˈvektəmi] *n* 滑膜切除术 | radioisotope ~ 滑膜照射法(见 synoviorthesis)

synovia [siˈnəuviə] *n*【拉】滑液 | ~**l** *a*

synovialis [siˌnəuviˈeilis] *a*【拉】滑液的 *n* 滑膜

synovialoma [siˌnəuviəˈləumə] *n* 滑膜瘤

synovianalysis [siˌnəuviəˈnælisis] *n* 滑液检验,滑液分析

synovin [ˈsinəvin] *n* 滑液蛋白

synovi(o)- [构词成分]滑液;滑膜

synovioblast [siˈnəuviəblæst] *n* 滑膜成纤维细胞,成滑膜细胞

synoviocyte [siˈnəuviəsait] *n* 滑膜细胞

synovioma [siˌnəuviˈəumə] *n* 滑膜瘤 | benign ~ 良性滑膜瘤(腱鞘的巨细胞瘤) / malignant ~ 恶性滑膜瘤,滑膜肉瘤

synoviorthese [siˌnəuviɔːˈθez] *n*【法】滑膜切除术(见 synoviorthesis)

synoviorthesis [siˌnəuviɔːˈθiːsis] *n* 滑膜切除术(关节内注射放射性胶体照射滑膜,以破坏发炎的滑膜组织)

synoviosarcoma [siˌnəuviəusɑːˈkəumə] *n* 滑膜肉瘤

synoviparous [ˌsinəˈvipərəs] *a* 产生滑液的

synovitis [ˌsinəˈvaitis] *n* 滑膜炎 | bursal ~ 黏液囊炎,滑囊炎 / dendritic ~ 绒毛状滑膜炎 / dry ~ 干性滑膜炎 / fungous ~ 真菌性关节炎,真菌性滑膜炎 / tendinous ~, vaginal ~ 腱鞘炎

synovium [siˈnəuviəm] *n* 滑膜

synphalangism [sinˈfæləndʒizəm] *n* 指关节融合,趾关节融合

synpneumonic [ˌsinju(ː)ˈmɔnik] *a* 伴同肺炎[发生]的

synprolan [ˈsinprələn] *n* 促性腺激素增强因子

synreflexia [ˌsinriˈfleksiə] *n* 联带反射,联合反射

syntax [ˈsintæks] *n* 句法 | **syntactic** [sinˈtæktik] *a*

syntaxis [sinˈtæksis] *n* 关节(联接)

syntectic [sinˈtektik] *a* 消瘦的

syntenosis [sintiˈnəusis] *n* 腱性联接

synteny [ˈsintini] *n* 同线性 | **syntenic** [sinˈtenik] *a* 同线的

synteresis [ˌsintəˈriːsis] *n* 预防疗法,预防 | **synteretic** [ˌsintəˈretik] *a*

syntexis [sinˈteksis] *n* 【希】消瘦

synthase [ˈsinθeis] *n* 合酶

synthermal [sinˈθəːməl] *a* 同温的,等温的

synthescope [ˈsinθəskəup] *n* 合成观测计(观测两个液体接触时可见作用的仪器)

synthesis [ˈsinθisis] ([复] **syntheses** [ˈsinθisiːz]) *n* 合成[法];综合;接合(创口) | ~ of continuity 连续性接合 / inducible enzyme ~ 诱导酶合成(在有代谢物存在时,细胞内一种酶的合成增加,此代谢物常为该酶的底物或底物的前体。此过程在原核生物内受基因转录的操纵子控制而发生〈表型适应〉,亦称酶的适应) / morphologic ~ 组织形态生成,组织发生

synthesize [ˈsinθisaiz] *vt* 合成;综合;接合

synthetase [ˈsinθiteis] *n* 合成酶 | glycogen ~ 糖原合成酶 / tryptophane ~ 色氨酸合成酶,色氨酸碳链酶

synthetic [sinˈθetik] *a* 合成的;综合[性]的;接合的 *n* 化学合成物,合成剂 | **~al** *a*

synthetism [ˈsinθitizəm] *n* 骨折接合术,接骨法

synthorax [sinˈθɔːræks] *n* 胸部联胎

syntomycin [ˌsintəˈmaisin], **synthomycin** [ˌsinθəˈmaisin] *n* 合霉素

syntone [ˈsintəun] *n* 精神和谐者,人格完整者

syntonic [sinˈtɔnik] *a* 精神和谐的,人格完整的(对环境反应正常的一种完整人格型,与类精神分裂症型相对照)

syntonin [ˈsintənin] *n* 辛托宁,酸白蛋白

syntopie, syntopy [ˈsintəpi] *n* 邻接关系,毗连关系(指器官)

syntripsis [sinˈtripsis] *n* 粉碎性骨折

syntrophism [ˈsintrəfizəm] *n* 共同生长,互养共栖(由于和另一个菌株相混合或接近促使微生物生长)

syntrophoblast [sinˈtrɔfəblæst] *n* 合胞体滋养层

syntrophus [ˈsintrəfəs] *n* 先天病,遗传病

syntropic [sinˈtrɔpik] *a* 同向的(如肋骨或脊椎);同调的,相互关联的(如一病对他病的发展或发生的关系)

syntropy [ˈsintrəpi] *n* 同向;同调,相关;健康整合状态

synulosis [ˌsinjuˈləusis] *n* 结瘢,瘢痕形成 | **synulotic** [ˌsinjuˈlɔtik] *a* 结瘢的,瘢痕形成的 *n* 结瘢药

Synura [sinˈjuərə] *n* 合尾滴虫属

synxenic [sinˈzenik] *a* 定菌[丛]的,既知菌[丛]的(实验动物)

Syphacia [saiˈfeiʃiə] *n* 管状线虫属 | ~ obvelata 鼠管状线虫

syphilid [ˈsifilid] *n* 梅毒疹 | macular ~ 梅毒蔷薇疹

syphilide [ˈsifilaid] ([复] **syphilides** [siˈfilidez]) *n* 【法】梅毒疹

syphilis [ˈsifilis] *n* 梅毒 | cardiovascular ~ 心血管梅毒 / cerebrospinal ~ 脑脊髓梅毒,埃尔布(Erb)痉挛性截瘫 / early ~ 早期梅毒 / endemic ~ 地方性梅毒 / late benign ~, gummatous ~ 晚期良性梅毒,梅毒瘤 / latent ~ 潜伏梅毒 / nonvenereal ~ 非性病梅毒 / parenchymatous ~ 主质性梅毒,主质性神经梅毒 / primary ~ 一期梅毒 / quaternary ~ 四期梅毒,终期梅毒 / secondary ~ 二期梅毒 / tertiary ~ 三期梅毒 | **syphilitic** [ˌsifiˈlitik] *a* 梅毒的 *n* 梅毒患者

syphiloma [ˌsifiˈləumə] *n* 梅毒瘤,树胶肿

syphilophobia [ˌsifiləuˈfəubjə], **syphiliphobia** [ˌsifiliˈfəubjə], **syphilomania** [ˌsifiləuˈmeinjə] *n* 梅毒恐怖 | **syphilophobic** [ˌsifiləuˈfəubik] *a*

syphilophyma [ˌsifiləuˈfaimə] *n* 梅毒性肿块

syphilopsychosis [ˌsifiləusaiˈkəusis] *n* 梅毒性精神病

syphilosis [ˌsifiˈləusis] *n* 全身梅毒病

syphilous [ˈsifiləs] *a* 梅毒的

syphitoxin [ˌsifiˈtɔksin] *n* 抗梅毒血清

Syr. syrupus 糖浆[剂]

syrigmophonia [ˌsirigməuˈfəuniə] *n* 笛音

syrigmus [siˈrigməs] *n* 耳鸣

syringadenoma [səˌriŋgædiˈnəumə] *n* 汗腺腺瘤 | ~ papilliferum 乳头状汗腺腺瘤

syringe [ˈsirindʒ, siˈrindʒ] *n* 注射器;冲洗器 *vt* (用注射器等)注射;冲洗 | chip ~, air ~ 吹干器,气枪 / dental ~ 牙科注射器 / fountain ~ 自流注射器 / hypodermic ~ 皮下注射器 / probe ~ 探查注射器

syringectomy [ˌsirinˈdʒektəmi] *n* 瘘管切除术

syringin [si'rindʒin] *n* [紫]丁香苷

syringitis [ˌsirin'dʒaitis] *n* 咽鼓管炎

syring(o)- [构词成分]管,瘘,洞

syringoacanthoma [səˌriŋgəuˌækæn'θəumə] *n* 汗管棘皮瘤

syringoadenoma [siˌriŋgəuædi'nəumə] *n* 汗腺腺瘤

syringobulbia [siˌriŋgəu'bʌlbiə] *n* 延髓空洞症

syringocarcinoma [siˌriŋgəuˌkɑːsi'nəumə] *n* 汗腺癌

syringocele [si'riŋgəsiːl] *n* 空洞性脊髓突出

syringocoele [si'riŋgəsiːl] *n* 脊髓中央管

syringocystadenoma [siˌriŋgəuˌsistædi'nəumə] *n* 汗腺腺瘤 | ~ papilliferum 乳头状汗腺腺瘤

syringocystoma [siˌriŋgəusis'təumə] *n* 汗腺囊瘤

syringoencephalia [siˌriŋgəuˌensi'feiliə] *n* 脑空洞症

syringoencephalomyelia [siˌriŋgəuenˌsefələum-ai'iːliə] *n* 脑脊髓空洞症

syringohydromyelia [səˌriŋgəuˌhaidrəumai'iːliə] *n* 脊髓积水空洞症

syringoid [si'riŋgɔid] *a* 管样的,瘘管样的

syringoma [ˌsiriŋ'gəumə] *n* 汗管瘤

syringomeningocele [siˌriŋgəumə'niŋgəsiːl] *n* 脊髓膜中央管突出

syringomyelia [siˌriŋgəumai'iːliə] *n* 脊髓空洞症 | traumatic ~ 外伤性脊髓空洞症

syringomyelitis [si'riŋgəuˌmaiə'laitis] *n* 空洞性脊髓炎

syringomyelocele [siˌriŋgəu'maiələˌsiːl] *n* 脊髓中央管突出

syringomyelus [siˌriŋgəu'maiələs] *n* 脊髓中央管扩张

syringopontia [siˌriŋgəu'pɔnʃiə] *n* 脑桥空洞症

Syringospora [ˌsairiŋ'gɔspərə] *n* 念珠菌属(现称 Candida)

syringotome [si'riŋgətəum] *n* 瘘管刀

syringotomy [ˌsiriŋ'gɔtəmi] *n* 瘘管切开术

syrinx ['siriŋks] ([复] **syrinxes** 或 **syringes** [si'riŋdʒiːz]) *n* 【希】瘘,瘘管;咽鼓管;鸣管(鸟类)

syrosingopine [ˌsaiərə'siŋgəpain] *n* 昔洛舍平(抗高血压药)

Syrphidae ['sifidiː] *n* 蚜蝇科

syrup ['sirəp] *n* 糖浆[剂] | acacia ~ 阿拉伯胶糖浆 / aromatic eriodictyon ~, aromatic Yerba santa ~ 芳香圣草糖浆 / cherry ~ 樱桃糖浆 / compound white pine ~ 复方白松糖浆 / compound white pine ~ with codeine 复方白松可待因糖浆 / glycyrrhiza ~, licorice ~ 甘草糖浆 / medicated ~ 含药糖浆 / orange ~ 橙皮糖浆 / simple ~ 单糖浆 | **~y** *a* 糖浆状的

syrupus ['sirəpəs] *n*【拉】糖浆[剂] | ~ aurantii 橙皮糖浆 / ~ cerasi 樱桃糖浆 / ~ corrigens 芳香圣草糖浆 / ~ pini albae compositus 复方白松糖浆 / ~ pini albae compositus cumcodeina 复方白松可待因糖浆 / ~ rubi idaei 覆盆子糖浆

syssarcosis [ˌsisɑː'kəusis] *n* 肌性骨联接 | **syssarcotic** [ˌsisɑː'kɔtik], **syssarcosic** [ˌsisɑː'kəusik] *a*

syssomus [ˌsi'səuməs] *n*【希】[两头单体]并躯联胎

systaltic [sis'tæltik] *a* 舒缩交替的;搏动的

systatic [sis'tætik] *a* 犯几种感觉的,(同时影响几种感觉功能的)

system ['sistim, 'sistəm] *n* 系统,系;制度,制;方式,方法;分类[法];学派 | absorbent ~ 吸收系统,淋巴系统 / adipose ~ 脂肪[组织]系统 / alimentary ~ 消化系统 / association ~ 联合系统(神经纤维) / autonomic nervous ~ 自主神经系统 / biologic amplification ~ 生物学扩大系统(增强免疫反应的各种成分组成的系统,其中包括补体成分和血管舒缓素系统) / biological ~ 生物系统 / blood group ~ 血型系,血型分类[法] / blood-vascular ~ 血管系统 / brain cooling ~ 脑降温装置 / buffer ~ 缓冲系统 / bulbospiral ~ 主动脉球螺旋系统(心脏) / cardiovascular ~ 心血管系统 / case ~ 病案教学制 / centimeter-gram-second ~ 厘米-克-秒制 / central nervous ~ (CNS)中枢神经系统 / centrencephalic ~ 中央脑系统 / cerebrospinal ~ 脑脊髓神经系统,中枢神经系统 / chromaffin ~ 嗜铬系统 / circulatory ~ 循环系统 / complement ~ 补体系统(一套复杂的、相互作用的蛋白质的体液免疫系统) / coordinate ~ 坐标系 / dentinal ~ 牙质管系统 / dermal ~, dermoid ~ 皮肤系统 / digestive ~ 消化系统 / dioptric ~ 屈光系 / disperse ~, dispersion ~ 分散系 / dosimetric ~ 剂量制 / ecological ~ 生态系 / endocrine ~ 内分泌系统 / endothelial ~ 内皮系统,网状内皮系统 / exteroceptive nervous ~ 外感受神经系统 / extrapyramidal ~, extracorticospinal ~ 锥体外系统,皮质脊髓外系统,锥体外束 / genitourinary ~ 生殖泌尿系统 / glandular ~ 腺系统 / hematopoietic ~ 造血系统 / heterogeneous ~ 非均匀系,多相系 / homogeneous ~ 均匀系 / hormonopoietic ~ 造激素系统,内分泌系统 / humoral amplification ~s 体液放大系统 / hypophyseoportal ~ 垂体门脉系统 / International System of Units 国际单位制(即 SI unit) / interrenal ~ 肾上腺皮质系统 / keratinizing ~, malpighian ~ 角[质]化系统 / kinety ~ 动体[列]系,动胞器列系统 / kinin ~, kallikrein ~ 激肽系统,血管舒缓素系统 / labyrinthine ~ 迷路系统 / limbic ~ 边缘系统(包括海马回、齿状回、扣带回等) /

lymphatic ~ 淋巴系统 / lymphoid ~ 淋巴样系统 / lymphoreticular ~ 淋巴网状系统 / macrophage ~ 巨噬细胞系统,网状内皮系统 / masticatory ~ 咀嚼系统 / mastigont ~ 鞭毛器系统 / meter-kilogram-second ~ 米-千克-秒制 / metric ~ 米制 / mononuclear phagocyte ~ (MPS)单核吞噬细胞系统 / nervous ~ 神经系统 / parasympathetic nervous ~ 副交感神经系统 / peripheral nervous ~ 外周神经系统,周围神经系统 / periventricular ~ (脑)室周系统 / pigmentary ~, melanocyte ~ 色素系统,黑素细胞系 / pituitary portal ~ 垂体门脉系统 / plenum ~ 流入式通风系统 / portal ~ 门静脉系统 / properdin ~ 备解素系统 / proprioceptive nervous ~ 本体感受神经系统 / resonating ~ 共振系统 / respiratory ~ 呼吸系统 / reticular activating ~ 网状激活系统 / reticuloendothelial ~ (RES)网状内皮系统 / sensory storage ~ 感觉贮存系统 / SI ~ 国际单位制(即 SI unit) / sinospiral ~ 静脉窦螺旋系统 / somatic nervous ~ 体干神经系统 / stomatognathic ~ 咀嚼系统 / sympathetic nervous ~ 交感神经系统 / T ~, triad ~ 横管系统,三联体系统 / urogenital ~ 泌尿生殖系统 / uropoietic ~ 泌尿系统 / vascular ~ 血管系统 / vasomotor ~ 血管舒缩系统 / vegetative nervous ~ 自主神经系统 / vestibular ~ 前庭系统 / visceral nervous ~ 内脏神经系统

systema [sisˈtiːmə] *n*【希】系统,系

systematic(al) [ˌsistiˈmætik(əl)] *a* 系统的,系的;分类的 | **~ally** *ad*

systematize [ˈsistimətaiz], **systemize** [ˈsistimaiz] *vt* 使系统化;把…分类 | **~d** *a* 系统化的,分类的 / **systematization** [ˌsistimətaiˈzei-ʃən, -tiˈz-] *n* 系统化;分类

systematology [ˌsistiməˈtɔlədʒi] *n* 体系论,组织系统学说

systemic [sisˈtemik] *a* 系统的;全身的 | **~ally** *ad*

systemoid [ˈsistimɔid] *a* 系统样的;多种组织的(指肿瘤)

système sécant [sisˈtem seiˈkɑːn]【法】交割系统(见于纤毛原虫缝线之一)

systogene [ˈsistədʒiːn] *n* 酥胺,酪胺(2-对羟苯基乙胺)

systole [ˈsistəli] *n* 心缩期 | aborted ~, frustrate ~ 顿挫性收缩 / atrial ~ 心房收缩 / extra ~ 期外收缩(过早收缩) / ventricular ~ 心室收缩 | **systolic** [sisˈtɔlik] *a*

systolometer [ˌsistəˈlɔmitə] *n* 心音鉴定器

systremma [sisˈtremə] *n*【希】腓肠痉挛,小腿肚痉挛

syzygiology [siˌzidʒiˈɔlədʒi] *n* 整体关系学

Syzygium [siˈzidʒiəm] *n* 蒲桃属

syzygy [ˈsizidʒi], **syzygium** [siˈzidʒiəm] *n* (器官)融合;融合虫,融合体 | **syzygial** [siˈzidʒiəl] *a*

Szabo's test [ˈsɑːbəu] (Dionys Szabo) 萨博试验(检胃盐酸)

Szent-Györgyi reaction [ˈsentˈ dʒəːrdʒi] (Albert Szent-Györgyi) 森特·哲尔吉维生素 C 反应(1% 的维生素 C 溶液混以硫酸亚铁时,则呈紫色,以硫代硫酸钠还原时,则紫色消失)

T

T tera- 垓;tesla 特斯拉;threonine 苏氨酸;thymine or thymidine 胸腺嘧啶或胸苷;tetanus toxoid 破伤风类毒素;thoracic vertebrae (T1 through T12) 胸椎(T1 到 T12);triangulation number 三角划分数;intraocular tension 眼内压

2, 4, 5-T 2, 4, 5-trichlorophenoxyacetic acid 2, 4, 5-三氯苯氧乙酸,245 涕(除莠剂)

T-1824 Evans blue 伊文思蓝,偶氮蓝

T absolute temperature 绝对温度;transmittance 透射比

$T_{1/2}$ half-life 半衰期,半存留期;half-time 半时值

$\mathbf{T_1}$ tricuspid valve closure 三尖瓣闭锁

$\mathbf{T_3}$ triiodothyronine 三碘甲腺原氨酸

$\mathbf{T_4}$ thyroxine 甲状腺素

$\mathbf{T_m}$ 熔解温度,解链温度(melting temperature)和肾小管最大排泄量(tubular maximum,用于报告肾功能检查结果,下标字母表明试验中所使用的物质,如 T_{mPAH}〈tubular maximum for paraaminohippuric acid〉,即肾小管排泄对氨马尿酸的最大量)的符号

t translocation 易位,移位作用

t time 时间;temperature 温度 *t*-test *t* 检测(见 test 项下相应术语)

$\mathbf{t_{1/2}}$ half-life 半衰期,半存留期;half-time 半时值的符号

θ theta 希腊语的第 8 个字母;角(angle)的符号

τ tau 希腊语的第 19 个字母;旋力(torque)和平均寿命(mean life)的符号

TA *Terminologia Anatomica*《解剖学术语》;toxin antitoxin 毒素-抗毒素

Ta tantalum 钽

tabacin [ˈtæbəsin] *n* 烟草苷,烟草素

tabacosis [ˌtæbəˈkəusis], **tabacism** [ˈtæbəsizəm] *n* 烟草中毒;烟末沉着病,烟尘肺

tabacum [ˈtæbəkəm] *n*【拉】烟,烟草

tabagism [ˈtæbədʒizəm] *n* 烟草中毒,烟碱中毒

taballa [təˈbelə] ([复] **tabellae** [təˈbeliː]) *n*【拉】片剂,锭剂,糖锭

tabanid [ˈtæbənid] *n* 虻

Tabanidae [təˈbæniədiː] *n* 虻科

Tabanus [təˈbeinəs] *n*【拉】虻属,原虻属 | ~ atratus 黑虻 / ~ bovinus 嗜牛原虻,牛虻 / ~ ditaeniatus, ~ fasciatus, ~ gratus 二带虻,二带原虻

tabardillo [ˈtæbɑːˈdiːljəu] *n*【西】鼠型斑疹伤寒

tabatière anatomique [təˌbætiˈɛəənətəˈmiːk]【法】鼻烟窝(手背拇指基部的凹)

tabella [təˈbelə] ([复] **tabellae** [təˈbeliː]) *n*【拉】片剂,锭剂,糖锭剂

tabernanthine [ˌtæbəˈnænθiːn] *n* 马山茶碱

tabes [ˈteibiːz] *n*【拉】消耗,消瘦;脊髓痨 | abortive ~, rudimentary ~ 顿挫性脊髓痨 / cervical ~, ~ superior 颈型脊髓痨,上肢型脊髓痨 / cerebral ~ 脊髓痨性全身麻痹症 / ~ dorsalis 脊髓痨,运动性共济失调 / peripheral ~ 假脊髓痨 | **tabetic** [təˈbetik], **tabic** [ˈtæbik] *a* 脊髓痨的

tabescent [təˈbesnt] *a* 消瘦的,干皱的 | **tabescence** *n*

tabetiform [təˈbetifɔːm] *a* 脊髓痨样的

tabid [ˈtæbid] *a* 脊髓痨的;消瘦的

tabification [ˌtæbifiˈkeiʃən] *n* 消瘦

tablature [ˈtæblətʃə] *n* 颅骨分层

table [ˈteibl] *n* 台,工作台;表,表格;骨板(颅骨的) | cohort life ~ 队列寿命表,群组寿命表(临床研究或试验中一组个体存活数据表) / demographic life ~, mortality ~ 人口寿命表,死亡表 / inner(outer) ~ of bones of skull 颅骨内(外)板 / inner ~ of frontal bone 额骨内面 / periodic ~ 周期表 / vitreous ~ 颅骨内板 / water ~ 地下水位

tablespoon [ˈteiblspuːn] *n* 汤匙,大匙(15 ml)

tablespoonful [ˈteiblˌspuːnful] *n* 一大汤匙容量

tablet [ˈtæblit] *n* 药片,片剂 | buccal ~ 口腔片 / dispensing ~ 调剂片,配方片 / enteric coated ~ 肠溶片剂 / hypodermic ~ 皮下注射用片剂 / throat ~s 润喉片 / triturate ~ 研制片剂,模印片

taboo [təˈbuː] *n* 禁忌,戒律

taboparesis [ˌteibəpəˈriːsis], **taboparalysis** [ˌteibəpəˈrælisis] *n* 脊髓痨性全身麻痹症

tabula [ˈtæbjulə] ([复] **tabulae** [ˈtæbjuliː]) *n*【拉】骨板

tabular [ˈtæbjulə] *a* 板状的

TAC tetracaine, epinephrine, and cocaine 丁卡因-肾上腺素-可卡因(溶液)

tacahout [ˌtækəˈhuːt] *n*【阿拉伯】印度柽柳瘿

tacamahac [ˈtækəmeiˌhæk] *n* 裂榄树胶

tache [tɑːʃ, tæʃ] *n*【法】斑点 | ~ blanche 白斑

(一种肝白斑,见于某些传染病) / ~s bleuâtres 青斑 / ~ cérébrale, ~ méningéale 脑[病]性划痕,脑膜[病]性划痕(用指甲在皮肤上划痕时所产生的充血性条纹,伴发于各种不同的神经病或脑病) / ~s laiteuses 乳状斑(网膜出现乳状小斑,由淋巴样细胞和巨噬细胞形成,尤以兔为明显) / ~ noire 黑斑(见于灌丛斑疹伤寒或地中海一带地方性立克次体病) / ~ spinale 脊髓病性斑

tachistoscope [tə'kistəskəup] *n* 速转实体镜,速示器 | **tachistoscopic** [təˌkistə'skɔpik] *a*

tach(o)- [构词成分]速,快速

tachogram ['tækəgræm] *n* 血液速度[描记]图

tachography [tə'kɔgrəfi] *n* 血流速度描记法

tachometer [tæ'kɔmitə] *n* 血流速度计

tachy- [构词成分]速,快速

tachyalimentation [ˌtækiˌælimen'teiʃən] *n* 食物进肠过速(见于胃切除术和胃肠吻合术后,为倾倒综合征的表现)

tachyarrhythmia [ˌtækiə'riðmiə] *n* 快速心律失常

tachyauxesis [ˌtækiɔːk'ziːsis] *n* 生长快速

tachycardia [ˌtæki'kɑːdiə] *n* 心动过速 | atrial ~ 房性心动过速 / paroxysmal ~ 阵发性心动过速 / ventricular ~ 室性心动过速

tachycardiac [ˌtæki'kɑːdiæk], **tachycardic** [ˌtæki'kɑːdik] *a* 心动过速的 *n* 心动加速药

tachydysrhythmia [ˌtækidis'riθmiə] *n* 快速[型]心律失常(本词使用时常被 tachyarrhythmia 所取代)

tachygastria [ˌtæki'gæstriə] *n* 胃窦电活动亢进

tachygenesis [ˌtæki'dʒenisis] *n* 快速发生(胚胎)

tachykinin [ˌtæki'kainin] *n* 速激肽(可引起平滑肌收缩和血管扩张)

tachylalia [ˌtæki'leiliə] *n* 言语快速,急语

tachylogia [ˌtæki'ləudʒə] *n* 言语快速,急语

tachymeter [tæ'kimitə] *n* 动速测量器

tachyphagia [ˌtæki'feidʒiə] *n* 速食癖

tachyphrasia [ˌtæki'freiziə], **tachyphasia** [ˌtæki'feiziə], **tachyphemia** [ˌtæki'fiːmiə] *n* 言语急速,急语

tachyphrenia [ˌtæki'friːniə] *n* 精神活动过速,精神活动亢进

tachyphylaxis [ˌtækifi'læksis], **tachysynthesis** [ˌtæki'sinθisis] *n* 快速免疫[法](由于过去的小剂量注射而对某种浸出物或血清的中毒剂量作用取得快速免疫);快速减敏[性](应用数剂后,机体对某种药物或生理活性药剂的反应性迅速减低)

tachypnea [ˌtæki'pniːə] *n* 呼吸急促

tachypragia [ˌtækip'rægiə] *n* 动作过速

tachyrhythmia [ˌtæki'riθmiə] *n* 心动过速(尤指机制不明时)

tachysterol [tæ'kistərɔl] *n* 速固醇

tachytrophism [ˌtæki'trəufizəm] *n* [新陈]代谢过速,代谢亢进

tachyzoite [ˌtæki'zəuait] *n* 速殖子,速殖体

taclamine hydrochloride ['tækləmiːn] 盐酸他克拉明(弱安定药)

tacrine hydrochloride ['tækriːn] 盐酸他克林(胆碱酯酶抑制药,用于改善轻度到中度阿尔茨海默〈Alzheimer〉型痴呆患者的认知行为表现,口服给药)

tacrolimus [ˌtaikrəu'laiməs] *n* 他克莫司(大环内酯免疫抑制药,作用类似环孢素,口服或静脉内给药,预防器官尤其是肝脏移植的排斥反应,局部用于治疗中度到重度特应性皮炎)

tactic ['tæktik] *a* 顺序的;有规立构的(指聚合物);(有)趋性的

tacticity [tæk'tisəti] *n* 顺序性,(顺序)排列性;立构规正度(指聚合物)

tactile ['tæktail] *a* 触觉的;能触知的 | **tactility** [tæk'tiləti] *n*

tactilogical [ˌtækti'lɔdʒikəl] *a* 触觉的

taction ['tækʃən] *n* 触;触觉

tactometer [tæk'tɔmitə] *n* 触觉测量器

tactor ['tæktə] *n* 触器(触觉末端器官)

tactual ['tæktjuəl] *a* 触觉的 | **~ly** *ad*

tactus ['tæktəs] *n*【拉】触,接触;触觉;触诊,指诊 | ~ eruditus, ~ expertus 熟练触诊

TAD 6-thioguanine, ara-C, and daunomycin 6-硫鸟嘌呤-阿糖胞苷-柔红霉素(联合化疗治癌方案)

tadpole ['tædpəul] *n* 蝌蚪

Taenia ['tiːniə] *n*【拉】绦虫属,带绦虫属 | ~ antarctica 南极绦虫 / ~ brachysoma 短体多头绦虫 / ~ cervi 獐绦虫 / ~ confusa, ~ bremneri 混杂绦虫 / ~ crassiceps 肥头绦虫 / ~ demarariensis 马达加斯加瑞列绦虫(即 Raillietina madagascariensis) / ~ echinococcus 细粒棘球绦虫(即 Echinococcus granulosus) / ~ elliptica 犬复殖绦虫,犬复孔绦虫(即 Dipylidium caninum) / ~ hydatigena, ~ marginata 水泡绦虫,有缘绦虫 / ~ krabbei 克拉绦虫 / ~ madagascariensis 马达加斯加瑞列绦虫(即 Raillietina madagascariensis) / ~ nana 短膜壳绦虫,微小膜壳绦虫(即 Hymenolepis nana) / ~ ovis 羊绦虫 / ~ pisiformis 豆状绦虫 / ~ saginata, ~ africana, ~ cucurbitina, ~ mediocanellata, ~ philippina 牛带绦虫,无钩绦虫 / ~ solium 猪带绦虫,有钩绦虫 / ~ taeniaeformis, ~ crassicollis 巨颈绦虫

taenia ['tiːniə] ([复]**taeniae** ['tiːniiː]) *n*【拉】带;绦虫

taenia- [构词成分]绦虫;带(同样见 tenia-,并以

此起始的词)

taeniacide [ˈtiːniəˌsaid] *a* 杀绦虫的 *n* 杀绦虫药 | **taeniacidal** [ˌtiːniəˈsaidl] *a*

taeniafugal [ˌtiːniəˈfjuːgəl] *a* 驱绦虫的

taeniafuge [ˈtiːniəˌfjuːdʒ] *n* 驱绦虫药

taenial [ˈtiːniəl] *a* 绦虫的;带的

Taeniarhynchus [ˌtiːniəˈriŋkəs] *n* 带吻[绦虫]属

taeniasis [tiːˈnaiəsis] *n* 绦虫病

taeniform [ˈtiːnifɔːm] *a* 绦虫状的;带状的

Taeniidae [tiːˈnaiidiː] *n* 带[绦虫]科

taenioid [ˈtiːniɔid] *a* 带状的;绦虫状的

taeniola [tiːˈnaiələ] *n* 【拉】小带

Taeniorhynchus [ˌtiːniəˈriŋkəs] *n* 曼蚊属

tag [tæg] *n* 附属物;签条,标签 | auricular ~s 耳赘,副耳 / cutaneous ~, skin ~ 皮赘,软垂疣 / radioactive ~ 放射性标记

tagatose [ˈtægətəus] *n* 塔格糖(一种己酮糖)

tagesrest [ˈtɑːgəzrest] *n* 【德】(导致夜梦的)白昼残留印象

tagliacotian rhinoplasty (operation) [ˌtɑːliəˈkəuʃiən] (Gasparo Tagliacozzi) 达利阿果齐鼻成形术(手术)(皮瓣取自臂部的意大利式人工鼻成形术)

tai chi 【汉】太极

taiga [ˈtaigə, -gɑː] *n* 泰加群落(森林)(即北方针叶林)

tail [teil] *n* 尾;尾状物 | ~ of caudate nucleus 尾状核尾 / occult ~ 隐尾 / polyadenylate (poly A) ~ 多(聚)腺苷酸尾 / ~ of spleen 脾尾,脾前端 / ~ of spermatozoon 精子尾部 | **~ed** *a* [用以构成复合词]有…(状)尾的 / **~less** *a* 无尾的

tailgut [ˈteilgʌt] *n* 尾肠

Taillefer's valve [ˌtɑːjiˈfei] (Louis A. H. S. T. Taillefer) 泰来福瓣(鼻泪管中部的黏膜襞)

taipan [taiˈpæn] *n* 眼镜蛇(澳大利亚北部和新几内亚产的一种毒蛇)

Takahara's disease [ˌtɑːkɑːˈhɑːrɑː] (Shigeo Takahara) 过氧化氢酶缺乏症

Takata-Ara test [təˈkɑːtə ˈɑːrə] (Maki Takata 高田蒔;Kiyoshi Ara 荒清) 高田-荒试验(检脑脊液蛋白质)

Takata's reagent [təˈkɑːtə] (Maki Takata 高田蒔) 高田试剂(氯化汞溶液和碱性品红溶液的混合物,用于高田-荒试验)

Takayasu's arteritis (disease, syndrome) [ˌtɑːkɑːˈjɑːsuː] (Mikito Takayasu) 高安动脉炎(病,综合征)(由于头臂干、锁骨下及颈总动脉在其主动脉弓起始上方的进行性闭塞,导致两臂及颈动脉脉搏丧失,然后可能伴有脑(如晕厥或短暂偏瘫)、眼(如短暂失明或视网膜萎缩)、面部(如肌肉萎缩)、两臂(如跛行)或肾等缺血症状。亦称主动脉弓动脉炎、臂头动脉炎或缺血和无脉病)

Tal. talis 【拉】这样的

talalgia [təˈlældʒiə] *n* 足跟痛,踝部痛

talampicillin hydrochloride [təˌlæmpiˈsilin] 盐酸酞氨西林(抗生素类药)

talantropia [ˌtælənˈtrəupiə] *n* 眼球震颤

talar [ˈteilə] *a* 距骨的

Talauma elegans [təˈlɔːmə ˈeligəns] 南洋玉兰

talbutal [ˈtælbjutəl] *n* 他布比妥(催眠镇静药)

talc [tælk] *n* 滑石,滑石粉 *vt* 用滑石处理

talcose [ˈtælkəus], **talcous** [ˈtælkəs] *a* 含滑石的,滑石的

talcosis [tælˈkəusis] *n* 滑石沉着病 | pulmonary ~ 肺滑石沉着病,滑石肺

talcum [ˈtælkəm] *n* 【拉】滑石,滑石粉

taleranol [təˈlerənəul] *n* 左环十四酮酚(一种抑制促性腺激素的酶)

tali [ˈteilai] talus 的复数

taliacotian [ˌtæliəˈkəuʃiən] *a* 见 tagliacotian

taliped [ˈtæliped] *a* 畸形足的 *n* 畸形足者

talipedic [ˌtæliˈpiːdik] *a* 畸形足的

talipes [ˈtælipiːz] *n* 【拉】畸形足 | ~ calcaneovalgus 仰趾外翻足 / ~ calcaneovarus 仰趾内翻足 / ~ calcaneus 仰趾足 / ~ cavus 弓形足,爪形足 / ~ equinovalgus 马蹄外翻足 / ~ equinovarus 马蹄内翻足 / ~ equinus 马蹄足 / ~ planovalgus 外翻平跖足,外翻扁平足 / ~ valgus 外翻足 / ~ varus 内翻足

talipomanus [ˌtæliˈpɔmənəs] *n* 畸形手

Tallqvist's scale [ˈtɑːlkvist] (Theodor W. Tallqvist) 塔尔克维斯特标度(为系列标度,以前用于测定血红蛋白含量)

Talma's disease [ˈtælmə] (Sape Talma) 后天性肌强直 | ~ operation 塔尔马手术(网膜固定术,治疗腹水)

talocalcaneal [ˌteiləukælˈkeiniəl], **talocalcanean** [ˌteiləukælˈkeiniən] *a* 距[骨]跟[骨]的

talocrural [ˌteiləuˈkkruːrəl] *a* 距骨小腿[骨]的

talofibular [ˌteiləuˈfibjulə] *a* 距[骨]腓[骨]的

talon [ˈtælɔn] *n* 【拉】牙座,磨牙低尖(上磨牙后部) | **~ed** *a*

talonavicular [ˌteiləunəˈvikjulə], **taloscaphoid** [ˌteiləuˈskæfɔid] *a* 距[骨]舟[骨]的

talonic acid [təˈlɔnik] 塔龙酸

talonid [ˈtælənid] *n* 下磨牙远中部,下牙座

talopram hydrochloride [ˈtæləpræm] 盐酸他洛普仑(儿茶酚胺强化剂)

talose [ˈteiləus] *n* 塔罗糖(一种己醛糖)

talotibial [ˌteiləuˈtibiəl] *a* 距[骨]胫[骨]的

talus [ˈteiləs] ([复] **tali** [ˈteilai]) *n* 【拉】距骨;踝

tama [ˈteimə] *n* 腿足肿胀

tambour [ˈtæmbuə] *n*【法】[记纹]气鼓

Tamm-Horsfall mucoprotein (protein) [tæm ˈhɔːsfæl] (Igor Tamm; Frank Lappin Horsfall, Jr.)塔-霍黏蛋白(蛋白),T-H 蛋白(由亨勒〈Henle〉襻升支的细胞所产生的一种物质,为尿的正常成分,也是尿中管型的主要蛋白成分)

tamoxifen citrate [təˈmɔksifən] 枸橼酸他莫昔芬(口服非甾体抗雌激素药,用于绝经期后妇女乳腺癌的姑息治疗,不孕症者用于促使排卵)

tampan [ˈtæmpæn] *n* 波斯锐缘蜱

tampicin [ˈtæmpisin] *n* 球根牵牛花苷

tampon [ˈtæmpən] *n*【法】塞子;(塞伤口等用的)棉塞,止血塞 *vt* 用棉塞塞(伤口) | tracheal ~ 气管套囊(口鼻手术时,用以防止血液流入气管)

tamponade [ˌtæmpəˈneid] *n* 填塞,压塞 | balloon ~ 气囊填塞(食管胃填塞) / cardiac ~, heart ~ 心脏压塞 / chronic ~ 慢性心脏压塞 / esophagogastric ~ 食管胃填塞 | **tamponage** [tæmpəˈnɑːʒ], **tamponing** [ˈtæmpəniŋ] *n*

tamponment [tæmˈpɔnmənt] *n* 填塞,压塞

tamsulosin hydrochloride [tæmˈsuːləusin] 盐酸坦洛新(α_1 受体阻滞药,专治前列腺受体,用以改进尿流速,减轻良性前列腺增生的症状,口服给药)

Tamus [ˈteiməs] *n* 浆果薯蓣属

tan [tæn] *n* 晒黑,晒成褐色 *a* 褐色的 *vt*, *vi* (受日光或紫外光)使成褐色

Tanacetum [ˌtænəˈsiːtəm] *n* 艾菊属 | ~ parthenium 银胶艾菊

tanapox [ˈtænəˌpɔks] (Tana River 为肯尼亚河流名) *n* 特纳河痘(一种由痘病毒引起的发生在肯尼亚和扎伊尔的病毒性疾病,特征为发热,四肢有一二处丘疹水疱性损害)

tandamine hydrochloride [ˈtændəmiːn] 盐酸坦达明(抗抑郁药)

tangentiality [tænˌdʒenʃiˈæləti] *n* 离题症(回答问题时说话不切题,与琐谈症〈circumstantiality〉不同,琐谈症者回答问题最终还能切题。本词大体上与 loosening of associations〈联想松弛〉同义)

tanghin [ˈtæŋgin] *n* 马达加斯加海杧果

Tangier disease [tænˈdʒiə] 丹吉尔病,高密度脂蛋白缺乏症(大西洋丹吉尔岛得名,一种家族性疾病,其特点为血清中缺乏高密度脂蛋白,在扁桃体及另一些组织内有胆固醇酯贮积)

tangle [ˈtæŋgl] *n* 缠结 | neurofibrillary ~s 神经纤维缠结(见于阿尔茨海默〈Alzheimer〉病时大脑皮质中)

tangoreceptor [ˌtæŋgəuriˈseptə] *n* 接触感受器

tank [tæŋk] *n* 槽,池 | activated sludge ~ 活化污泥池 / biological ~ 生物学处理池(一种改良的化粪池) / digestion ~ 隐化池 / oxygen ~ 氧气瓶 / septic ~, anaerobic ~, hydrolytic ~ 化粪池,水解槽

tannal [ˈtænæl] *n* 鞣酸铝 | insoluble ~ 不溶性鞣酸铝,碱性鞣酸铝(收敛剂)

tannalin [ˈtænəlin] *n* 坦纳林(一种甲醛溶液)

tannase [ˈtæneis] *n* 鞣酸酶

tannate [ˈtænit] *n* 鞣酸盐

tannic acid [ˈtænik] 鞣酸

tannin [ˈtænin] *n* 鞣质,鞣酸 | diacetyl ~, ~ diacetylate [二]乙酰鞣酸 / pathologic ~ 病害性鞣酸 / physiologic ~ 生理性鞣酸

tanning [ˈtæniŋ] *n* 鞣革[法];晒成褐色;鞣酸疗法(灼伤时用)

Tanret's reagent [tɑːnˈrei] (Charles Tanret)唐累试剂(检尿白蛋白) | ~ test (reaction) 唐累试验(反应)(检尿白蛋白)

Tansini's operation [tænˈsiːni] (Iginio Tansini) 汤西尼手术(乳房切除术的一种;肝囊肿切除法的一种;胃切除法的一种)

tantalum (Ta) [ˈtæntələm] *n* 钽(化学元素)

tantrum [ˈtæntrəm] *n* 暴怒

tanycyte [ˈtænisait] *n* 伸长细胞

tap¹ [tæp] *n* 轻叩 | front ~ 胫前轻叩(脊髓受刺激时,轻叩小腿前肌肉可引起小腿肌肉收缩) / heel ~ 足跟轻叩(轻叩足跟引起趾反射运动,见于锥体束受损)

tap² [tæp] *n* 抽液[术],穿刺术 *vt* 穿刺放液 | bloody ~ 血性腰椎穿刺 / spinal ~ 腰椎穿刺

tape [teip] *n* 带;磁带;胶带 | adhesive ~ 绊创膏

tapeinocephaly [ˌtæpinəuˈsefəli] *n* 矮型头,低型头 | **tapeinocephalic** [ˌtæpinəusəˈfælik] *a*

taper [ˈteipə] *n*, *vt*, *vi* 变细 | ~ing of mucosal fold 黏膜皱襞前端变细

tapetum [təˈpiːtəm] ([复] **tapeta** [təˈpiːtə]) *n*【拉】毯(表层膜或细胞层);脑毯 | **tapetal** *a* 毯的

tapeworm [ˈteipwəːm] *n* 绦虫 | African ~, beef ~, unarmed ~ 非洲绦虫,牛带绦虫,无钩绦虫(即 Taenia saginata) / armed ~, pork ~ 有钩绦虫,猪肉绦虫(即 Taenia solium) / broad ~, fish ~, Swiss ~ 阔节裂头绦虫(即 Diphyllobothrium latum) / dog ~ 犬绦虫(细粒棘球绦虫 Echinococcus granulosus;犬复孔绦虫 Dipylidium caninum) / double-pored dog ~ 犬复孔绦虫(即 Dipylidium caninum) / dwarf ~ 短小绦虫,短膜壳绦虫(即 Hymenolepis nana) / fringed ~ 放射状缕体绦虫(即 Thysanosoma actinioides) / heart-headed ~ 心形裂头绦虫(即 Diphyllobothrium cordatum) / hydatid ~ 细粒棘球绦虫(即 Echinococcus granulosus) / Madagascar ~ 马达加斯加瑞列绦虫(即 Reillietina madagascariensis) / Manson's larval ~ 曼[森]氏裂头绦虫(即 Diphyllobothrium mansonoides) / measly ~ 有钩绦虫,猪带绦虫(即 Taenia solium) / rat ~ 长膜壳绦虫,缩小膜壳绦虫(即 Hymenolepis diminuta) / Ward's Nebraskan ~ 混杂绦虫(即 Taenia confusa)

taphephobia [ˌtæfiˈfəubiə] *n* 活埋恐怖

taphophilia [ˌtæfəuˈfiliə] *n* 恋坟癖

Tapia's syndrome [ˈtæpiə] (Antonio G. Tapia)塔皮亚综合征(舌喉偏侧麻痹,腭帆不受侵)

tapinocephaly [ˌtæpinəuˈsefəli] *n* 矮型头,低型头 | **tapinocephalic** [ˌtæpinəusəˈfælik] *a*

tapioca [ˌtæpiˈəukə] *n* 木薯淀粉(食用)

tapiroid [ˈteipirɔid] *a* 貘嘴样的,突唇样的

tapotage [təpəuˈtɑːʒ] *n* 叩诊咳(叩诊锁骨上区时而引起的咳嗽吐痰,偶见于肺结核患者)

tapotement [təpɔtˈmɔŋ] *n*【法】叩抚法,轻叩式按摩法

tapping [ˈtæpiŋ] *n* 穿刺放液法;轻叩法,叩抚法

Taq polymerase [tæk] Taq 聚合酶(见于生活在温泉中的栖热水生菌的一种酶,此酶耐热,因而能耐受聚合酶链反应的高温)

tar [tɑː] *n* 焦油 | coal ~ 煤焦油(局部抗湿疹药,抗银屑病药) / gas ~ 煤[气]焦油 / juniper ~ 杜松焦油 / pine ~ 松焦油,木溜油

Taraktogenos kurzii [ˌtærəkˈtɔdʒinɔs ˈkəːzii] 缅甸大风子

tarantism [ˈtærəntizəm] *n* 毒蜘蛛舞蹈病(据说由狼蛛咬伤所致,可以跳舞治愈)

tarantula [təˈræntjulə] *n* 狼蛛(一种毒蛛,咬伤后引起局部炎症和疼痛,一般并不严重) | American ~ 美洲狼蛛 / black ~ 黑狼蛛 / European ~ 欧洲狼蛛

Taraxacum [təˈræksəkəm] *n*【拉】蒲公英属

taraxigen [təˈræksidʒən] *n* 过敏素原

taraxin [təˈræksin] *n* 过敏素

taraxy [təˈræksi] *n* 过敏性

tarbadillo [ˌtɑːbəˈdiːljəu] *n*【西】鼠型斑疹伤寒

tarbagan [ˈtɑːbəgən] *n* 土拨鼠

Tardieu's spots [tɑːˈdjuː] (Auguste A. Tardieu)塔迪厄点(窒息死后胸膜下的瘀斑) | ~ test 塔迪厄试验(检杀婴:胃黏膜中有空气泡说明胎儿曾有过呼吸)

tardive [ˈtɑːdiv] *a*【法】迟发的,延迟的(指典型病灶迟发的疾病)

tare [tɛə] *n* 皮重,称瓶重量;(平衡容器用的)配衡体 *vt* 确定容器的皮重(盛物后自总重量减去,可得物品净重量)

tarentism [ˈtærəntizəm] *n* 毒蜘蛛舞蹈病(见 tarantism)

tarentula [təˈtentjulə] *n* 狼蛛

target [ˈtɑːgit] *n* 靶,靶点

targeting [ˈtɑːgetiŋ] *n* 寻靶作用 | gene ~ 基因寻靶,基因导向

Taricha [təˈriːkə] *n* 蝾螈属

tarichatoxin [ˌtærikəˈtɔksin] *n* 蝾螈毒素,河豚毒素

Tarin fascia [tɑːˈrein] (Pierre Tarin ⟨Tarini, Tarinus⟩)齿状回 | ~ fossa 脚间窝 / ~ recess (space) 脚间窝前隐窝 / ~ valve(velum) 下髓帆

tariric acid [təˈririk] 十八碳炔酸

Tarlov's cyst [ˈtɑːlɔv] (Isadore M. Tarlov)塔洛夫囊肿,神经周囊肿

Tarnier's forceps [tɑːniˈɛə] (Etienne S. Tarnier)塔尼埃钳(一种轴牵引产钳)

tarsadenitis [ˌtɑːsædiˈnaitis] *n* 睑板腺炎

tarsal [ˈtɑːsəl] *a* 跗骨的;睑板的 *n* 跗骨;睑板

tarsalgia [tɑːˈsældʒiə] *n* 跗骨痛

tarsalia [tɑːˈseiliə] *n* 跗骨

tarsalis [tɑːˈseilis] *a*【拉】跗骨的;睑板的 *n* 睑板肌

tarsectomy [tɑːˈsektəmi] *n* 跗骨切除术;睑板切除术

tarsectopia [ˌtɑːsekˈtəupiə] *n* 跗骨脱位

tarsitis [tɑːˈsaitis] *n* 睑板炎,睑缘炎;跗骨炎

tars(o)- [构词成分]跗骨,跗;睑板

tarsocheiloplasty [ˌtɑːsəuˈkailəˌplæsti] *n* 睑缘成形术(如治疗倒睫)

tarsoclasis [tɑːˈsɔkləsis] *n* 跗骨折骨术

tarsomalacia [ˌtɑːsəuməˈleiʃiə] *n* 睑板软化

tarsomegaly [ˌtɑːsəuˈmegəli] *n* 巨跟骨,跟骨增大

tarsometatarsal [ˌtɑːsəuˌmetəˈtɑːsəl] *a* 跗[骨]跖[骨]的

tarso-orbital [ˌtɑːsəuˈɔːbitl] *a* 睑板眶壁的

tarsophalangeal [ˌtɑːsəufəˈlændʒiəl] *a* 跗[骨]趾[骨]的

tarsophyma [ˌtɑːsəuˈfaimə] *n* 睑板瘤

tarsoplasty [ˈtɑːsəuˌplæsti], **tarsoplasia** [ˌtɑːsəuˈpleiziə] *n* 睑成形术

tarsoptosis [ˌtɑːsɔpˈtəusis] *n* 扁平足,平足

tarsorrhaphy [tɑːˈsɔrəfi] *n* 睑缝合术

tarsotarsal [ˌtɑːsəuˈtɑːsəl] *a* 跗骨间的

tarsotibial [ˌtɑːsəuˈtibiəl] *a* 跗[骨]胫[骨]的

tarsotomy [tɑːˈsɔtəmi] *n* 跗骨切开术;睑板切开术

Tar's symptom [tɑː] (Aloys Tar)塔尔症状(肺浸润时,肺下界异常)

tarsus [ˈtɑːsəs] ([复] **tarsi** [ˈtɑːsai]) *n*【拉】跗,跗骨;睑板

tartar [ˈtɑːtə] *n* 酒石;牙垢,牙石 | borated ~ 硼酸酒石 / cream of ~ 酒石酸氢钾 / ~ emetic 吐酒石,酒石酸锑钾 / serumal ~ 牙根垢,龈下垢 / vitriolated ~ 硫酸酒石,硫酸钾

tartarated [ˈtɑːtəˌreitid], **tartarized** [ˈtɑːtəraizd] *a* 加酒石酸的

tartaric [tɑːˈtærik] *a* [含]酒石的,[含]酒石酸的 | ~ acid 酒石酸

tartarize [ˈtɑːtəraiz] *vt* 使酒石化,用酒石处理 | **tartarization** [ˌtɑːtəraiˈzeiʃən, -riˈz-] *n* 吐酒石疗法

tartarous [ˈtɑːtərəs] *a* 酒石[性]的,含酒石的;从酒石中提取的

tartrate [ˈtɑːtreit] *n* 酒石酸盐 | acid ~ 酸性酒石酸盐 / normal ~ 正酒石酸盐

tartrated [ˈtɑːtreitid] *a* 含酒石酸的

tartrobismuthate [ˌtɑːtrəuˈbizməθeit] *n* 酒石酸铋

tartronic acid [tɑːˈtrɔnik] 羟基丙二酸,丙醇二酸

Tarui disease [ˈtɑːruːi] (Seiichiro Tarui)糖原贮积症Ⅶ型

tasikinesia [ˌtæsikaiˈniːziə] *n* 起立行走癖,行动癖(静坐不能)

tastant [ˈteistənt] *n* 促味剂(如盐)

taste [teist] *n* 味觉,味 | color ~ 尝味觉色,色味联觉 / franklinic ~ 静电刺激性味觉

taste-blindness [teistˈblaindnis] *n* 味盲(缺乏辨别苯硫脲的苦味的现象)

tasteless [ˈteistlis] *a* 无味的,不能辨味的

taster [ˈteistə] *n* 尝味者(在遗传学研究中指对一种特别的试验物质如苯硫脲能辨别出苦味的人)

TAT thematic apperception test 主题统觉测验;toxin-antitoxin 毒素-抗毒素

Tatlockia micdadei [tætˈlɔkiə mikˈdeidiai] 匹茨堡肺炎病原体(Pittsburgh pneumonia agent)

tätte melk [ˈtetə melk] 特特奶(一种加捕虫堇叶的牛奶)

tattoo [təˈtuː] *n*, *vt* 文身

tattooing [təˈtuːiŋ] *n* 文身术 | ~ of the cornea 角膜墨针术,角膜染色术

Tatumella [ˌteitəˈmelə] (Harvey Tatum) *n* 塔特姆菌属

tau [tɔː] *n* 希腊语的第 19 个字母(Τ, τ); T 字形物

taurine [ˈtɔːri(ː)n] *n* 牛磺酸,氨基乙磺酸

taur(o)- [构词成分]牛磺酸

taurocarbamic acid [ˌtɔːrəukɑːˈbæmik] 牛磺脲酸,*N*-氨甲酰牛磺酸

taurochenodeoxycholate [ˌtɔːrəuˌkiːnəudiːˌɔksiˈkəuleit] *n* 牛磺鹅脱氧胆酸,鹅脱氧胆酰牛磺酸

taurochenodeoxycholic acid [ˌtɔːrəuˌkiːnəudiːˌɔksiˈkəulik] 牛磺鹅脱氧胆酸,鹅脱氧胆酰牛磺酸

taurocholaneresis [ˌtɔːrəˌkəuləˈnerisis] *n* 牛磺胆酸排出过多

taurocholanopoiesis [ˌtɔːrəukəuˌlænəupɔiˈiːsis] *n* 牛磺胆酸生成

taurocholate [ˌtɔːrəˈkəuleit] *n* 牛磺胆酸盐

taurocholemia [ˌtɔːrəkəˈliːmiə] *n* 牛磺酸血

taurocholic acid [ˌtɔːrəˈkəulik] *a* 牛磺胆酸

taurodontism [ˌtɔːrəˈdɔntizəm] *n* 长冠牙(一种异形牙,牙体长而牙根细)

taurylic acid [tɔːˈrilik] 牛磺酰酸

Taussig-Bing syndrome [ˈtɔːsig ˈbiŋ] (Helen B. Taussig; Richard J. Bing)陶-宾综合征(一种罕见的先天性心脏畸形,特征为大血管转位及为大的肺动脉所跨骑的心室间隔缺损,从血液动力学上来说,其特征为肺动脉高血压、肺动脉多血、发绀、肺动脉内血氧饱和度较主动脉为高)

taut(o)- [构词成分]相同

tautological [ˌtɔːtəˈlɔdʒikəl] *a* 重复的,赘述的 | **~ly** *ad*

tautomenial [ˌtɔːtəˈmiːniəl] *a* 同经期的

tautomer [ˌtɔːtəmə] *n* 互变异构体

tautomeral [tɔːˈtɔmərəl] *a* 同侧的(神经细胞)

tautomerase [tɔːˈtɔməreis] *n* 互变异构酶

tautomerism [tɔːˈtɔmərizəm] *a* 互变异构 | enol-keto ~ 烯醇-酮互变异构 / proton ~ 质子互变异构(亦称质子移变) / ring-chain ~ 环-链互变异构 | **tautomeric** [ˌtɔːtəˈmerik] *a*

Tawara's node [təˈwɑːrə] (Sunao Tawara 田原淳)田原结,房室结

tawny [ˈtɔːni] *n*, *a* 黄褐色(的),茶色(的)

taxa [ˈtæksə] taxon 的复数

taxane [ˈtæksein] *n* 紫杉烷

taxidermy [ˈtæksidəːmi] *n* 动物标本剥制术

taxine [ˈtæksiːn] *n* 紫杉碱

taxis [ˈtæksis] ([复]**taxes** [ˈtæksiːz]) *n*【希】向性,趋性(指能动的生物体对外界刺激应答的定向运动);整复[法](即用手法用力将异位或受损的器官或组织复回,如骨折和脱位的复位、疝的复位等)

-taxis [构词成分]趋…性

Taxodium distichum [tækˈsəudiəm ˈdistikəm] 落羽松

taxology [tækˈsɔlədʒi] *n* 分类学

taxon [ˈtæksɔn] ([复]**taxa** [ˈtæksə]) *n* 分类单位(指生物)

taxonomy [tækˈsɔnəmi] *n* 分类学 | numerical ~ 数值分类法(对数量较大的菌株分类法) | **taxonomic(al)** [ˌtæksəuˈnɔmik(əl)] *a* | **taxonomist** *n* 分类学家

Taxopodida [ˌtæksəuˈpəudidə] *n* 列足目

Taxus [ˈtæksəs] *n* 紫杉属 | ~ brevifolia 短叶紫杉(抗肿瘤药 taxol〈紫杉酚〉的来源)

Taylor brace (apparatus, splint) [ˈteilə] (Charles F. Taylor)泰勒支具(器、夹板)(一种胸

腰骶矫形器,用作脊柱支持架)
Tay-Sachs disease (TSD) [ˈtei ˈsæks] (Warren Tay; Bernard Sachs) 泰-萨克斯病(最常见的神经节苷脂贮积症,几乎只在东北欧犹太人中间发生,TSD 为一种 GM_2 神经节苷脂贮积症,其特征为婴儿期〈3~6 个月〉发病、洋娃娃样脸、樱桃红点、早期失明、听觉过敏、巨头、癫痫发作、张力减退,2~5 岁间死亡)
Tay's choroiditis (disease) [tei] (Warren Tay) 泰氏脉络膜炎(病)(脉络膜的变性,特征为黄斑周围显不规则黄色斑点,据认为是动脉粥样硬化所致,见于老年,亦称老年性点状脉络膜炎) | ~ sign (spot) 樱桃红点(在黄斑上)
tazarotene [tɑːˈzærəutiːn] *n* 他扎罗汀(一种前药,经受水解成为皮肤内的视黄醛衍生物,局部用于治疗寻常痤疮和银屑病)
tazettine [ˈteizətin] *n* 多花水仙碱
tazobactam [ˌtæzəuˈbæktæm] *n* 三唑巴坦(β-内酰胺酶抑制药) | ~ sodium 三唑巴坦钠
tazolol hydrochloride [ˈteizələul] 盐酸他佐洛尔(肾上腺素能药,强心药)
TB tuberculin 结核菌素
Tb terbium 铽
TBG thyroxine-binding globulin 甲状腺素结合球蛋白
TBI traumatic brain injury 创伤性脑损伤;total body irradiation 全身放射性照射
TBII TSH-binding inhibitory immunoglobulins 促甲状腺激素结合抑制性免疫球蛋白
TBP bithionol 硫氯酚
TBW total body water 全身含水量
TC transcobalamin 转钴胺素,钴胺素传递蛋白
Tc technetium 锝
TCD_{50} median tissue culture dose 半数组织培养量
TCDD 2, 3, 7, 8-tetrachlorodibenzo-*p*-dioxin 2, 3, 7, 8-四氯二苯并对二噁英
$TCID_{50}$ median tissue culture infective dose 半数组织培养感染量
TCM traditional Chinese medicine 中医
TCMI T cell-mediated immunity T 细胞[介导]免疫
TCR T cell antigen receptor T 细胞[抗原]受体
TCV total cell volume 细胞总容积
TD_{50} median toxic dose 半数中毒量
Td tetanus and diphtheria toxoids, adult type 成年型破伤风及白喉类毒素
TDA TSH-displacing antibody 促甲状腺激素置换抗体
TDE tetrachlorodiphenylethane 四氯二苯乙烷,滴滴滴(即 DDD〈dichlorodiphenyldichloroethane〉)
TDI toluene diisocyanate 二异氰酸甲苯酯
t. d. s. ter die sumendum【拉】一日服三次
TdT terminal deoxynucleotidyl transferase 末端脱氧核苷酸转移酶
Te tellurium 碲;tetanus 破伤风
TEA tetraethylammonium 四乙铵
tea [tiː] *n* 茶;茶剂,浸剂 | beef ~ 牛肉茶,牛肉汤 / black ~ 红茶 / green ~ 绿茶 / pectoral ~ 祛痰茶
Teale's amputation (operation) [tiːl] (Thomas P. Teale) 蒂尔切断术(手术)(肢的一侧保留长的长方形皮瓣和体被,另一侧保留短的长方形皮瓣)
team [tiːm] *n* 队,组 | first-aid ~ 救护队 / mobile medical ~ 巡回医疗队
tear¹ [tiə] *n* 眼泪;滴,珠(树脂或树胶) *vi* 流泪 | crocodile ~s 鳄泪(咀嚼及进食时流泪,见于面瘫患者)
tear² [tɛə] *vt* 撕[开] *vi* 撕,扯 *n* 撕,裂;裂伤 | cemental ~, cementum ~ 牙骨质撕裂
teart [təːt] *n* 高钼土壤,高钼植物;下泻疾病(以高钼土壤上生长的植物饲养牛羊所致的慢性钼中毒)
tease [tiːz] *vt* (用针)拨开,挑开(组织)
teaspoon [ˈtiːspuːn] *n* 茶匙(约合 5 ml)
teat [tiːt] *n* (乳房)乳头;橡皮奶头
TeBG testosterone-estradiol-binding globulin 睾酮-雌二醇结合球蛋白
teboroxime [ˌtebəˈrɔksiːm] *n* 锝硼酸肟(一种与 ^{99m}Tc 络合的化合物,构成 BATO,用作心血管成像时局部灌注的标记)
tebutate [ˈtebjuteit] *n* 叔丁乙酸盐,叔丁乙酸酯(tertiary butyl acetate 的 USAN 缩约词)
technetium (Tc) [tekˈniːʃiəm] *n* 锝(化学元素) | ~ 99m 锝-99m / ~ ^{99m}Tc albumin aggregated 锝 ^{99m}Tc 聚集白蛋白 / ~ ^{99m}Tc etidronate 锝 ^{99m}Tc 依替膦酸 / ~ 99m pertechnetate 锝-99m 高锝酸盐
technic [ˈteknik] *a* 技术的,工艺的 *n* 术,技术,操作[法](=technique) | ~s *n* 技术学,工艺学
technical [ˈteknikəl] *a* 技术的,工艺的
technician [tekˈniʃən] *n* 技术员,技师 | laboratory ~ 化验员
technique [tekˈniːk] *n*【法】术,技术,操作[法] | dilution-filtration ~ 稀释过滤技术(一种血培养技术) / Enzyme-Multiplied Immunoassay Technique (EMIT) 多元酶免疫测定法 / fluorescent antibody ~ 荧光抗体技术(一种免疫荧光技术) / hanging drop ~ 悬滴技术(显微镜检查生物体) / immunoperoxidase ~ 免疫过氧物酶技术(一种组织学染色法) / peroxidase-antiperoxidase (PAP) ~ 过氧化物酶-抗过氧化物酶技术(一种在组织切片中检测抗原或抗体技术) / push-back ~ 推后技术(使软腭向后复位重建腭咽功能的手术,亦称推后操作) / Rebuck skin window ~ 里巴克皮窗技术(一种研究炎症反应变化顺

序的技术）/ scintillation counting ~ 闪烁计数技术（测放射性量）/ squash ~ 挤压技术（为染色体研究的细胞制备法）/ time diffusion ~ 定时扩散术（一种脊髓麻醉法）

technocausis [ˌteknə*u*ˈkɔːsis] *n* 烙术

technologist [tekˈnɔlədʒist] *n* 技术人员

technology [tekˈnɔlədʒi] *n* 技术学，工艺学 | assisted reproductive ~ (ART) 辅助生殖技术（治不育）

teclozan [ˈtekləzæn] *n* 替克洛占（抗阿米巴药）

Tectibacter [ˌtektiˈbæktə] *n* 被菌属

tectocephaly [ˌtektəuˈsefəli] *n* 舟状头[畸形] | **tectocephalic** [ˌtektəusəˈfælik] *a*

tectology [tekˈtɔlədʒi] *n* 组织构造学

tectorial [tekˈtɔːriəl] *a* 盖膜的，覆膜的，顶盖的

tectorium [tekˈtɔːriəm] ([复] **tectoria** [tekˈtɔːriə]) *n* 【拉】（耳蜗）盖膜，覆膜

tectospinal [ˌtektəuˈspainl] *a* 顶盖脊髓的

tectum [ˈtektəm] *n* 顶盖

TED threshold erythema dose 红斑阈量

TEE transesophageal echocardiography 经食管超声心动描记术

teeth [tiːθ] tooth 的复数

teethe [tiːð] *vi* 出牙，生牙

teething [ˈtiːðiŋ] *n* 出牙，生牙

tegafur [ˈtegəfə] *n* 替加氟（抗肿瘤药）

tegmen [ˈtegmən] ([复] **tegmina** [ˈtegminə]) *n* 【拉】盖

tegmental [tegˈmentəl] *a* 盖的，被盖的

tegmentum [tegˈmentəm] ([复] **tegmenta** [tegˈmentə]) *n* 【拉】盖，被盖；大脑脚盖

tegument [ˈtegjumənt] *n* 体被，皮肤 | **~al** [ˌtegjuˈmentl]，**~ary** [ˌtegjuˈmentəri] *a*

Teichmann's crystals [ˈtaiʃmən] (Ludwig C. Teichmann) 泰希曼结晶（氯化血红素结晶）| ~ test 泰希曼试验（检血）

teichoic acids [taiˈkəuik] 磷壁酸，胞壁酸（革兰阳性细菌细胞壁和细胞膜内形形色色的聚合物）

teichopsia [taiˈkɔpsiə] *n* 闪光暗点

teicoplanin [ˌtaikəuˈplænin] *n* 替考拉宁（一种糖肽抗生素，用于治疗抗青霉素革兰阳性细菌引起的感染）

teinodynia [ˌtainəˈdiniə] *n* 腱痛

teknocyte [ˈteknəsait] *n* 幼稚[中性]白细胞

tektin [ˈtektin] *n* 筑丝蛋白

tela [ˈtiːlə] ([复] **telae** [ˈtiːliː]) *n* 【拉】组织

Teladorsagia [ˌtiːlədɔːˈseidʒə] *n* 毛圆线虫属

telalgia [teˈlældʒiə] *n* 牵涉性痛

telangiectasia [teˌlændʒiekˈteiziə]，**telangiectasis** [teˌlændʒiˈektəsis] ([复] **telangiectases** [teˌlændʒiˈektəsiːz]) *n* 毛细[血]管扩张 | spider ~ 蛛状痣 | **telangiectatic** [teˌlændʒiekˈtætik] *a*

telangiectodes [teˌlændʒiekˈtəudiːz] *a* 毛细管扩张的

telangiitis [teˌlændʒiˈaitis] *n* 毛细管炎

telangion [teˈlændʒiɔn] *n* 终动脉

telangiosis [ˌtelændʒiˈəusis] *n* 毛细管病

telar [ˈtiːlə] *a* 组织的，组织样的

telarche [tiːˈlɑːki] *n* 乳房初长，乳房开始发育

tele- [构词成分]终，末；远距

telebinocular [ˌtelibaiˈnɔkjulə] *n* 矫视三棱镜

telecanthus [ˌteliˈkænθəs] *n* 内眦距过宽

telecardiogram [ˌteliˈkɑːdiəgræm] *n* 遥测心电图

telecardiography [ˌteliˌkɑːdiˈɔgrəfi] *n* 远距心电描记法

telecardiophone [ˌteliˈkɑːdiəˌfəun] *n* 远距心音听诊器

teleceptor [ˈteliˌseptə] *n* 距离感受器 | **teleceptive** *a* 距离感受性的

telecinesia [ˌtelisaiˈniːziə]，**telecinesis** [ˌtelisaiˈniːsis] *n* 远距运动，心灵致动（见 telekinesis）

telecord [ˈtelikɔːd] *n* 心动周期 X 线摄影自动操纵装置

telecurietherapy [ˌteliˌkjuəriˈθerəpi] *n* 远距居里治疗，远距放射治疗（用放射源如镭进行远距治疗）

teledactyl [ˌteliˈdæktil] *n* 直腰拾物器（脊柱病患者用）

teledendrite [ˌteliˈdendrait]，**teledendron** [ˌteliˈdendrɔn] *n* 终树突

telediagnosis [ˌteliˌdaiəgˈnəusis] *n* 远距诊断（医生当与患者遥隔时通过传送的遥控监护资料或闭路电视进行会诊）

telefluoroscopy [ˌteliflu(ː)əˈrɔskəpi] *n* 远距荧光屏检查，遥测荧光屏检查

telegony [tiˈlegəni] *n* 前父影响，先父遗传（关于动物遗传的一种假想，认为先前公兽的特性能遗传给同一母兽与其他公兽交配所生的后代）| **telegonic** [ˌteliˈgɔnik] *a*

telekinesis [ˌtelikaiˈniːsis] *n* 远距运动，心灵致动（即不直接接触某物体，而能使其运动）| **telekinetic** [ˌtelikaiˈnetik] *a*

telelectrocardiogram [ˌteliˌlektrəuˈkɑːdiəgræm] *n* 远距心电图

telelectrocardiograph [ˌteliˌlektrəuˈkɑːdiəgrɑːf] *n* 远距心电描记器

telemedicine [ˌteliˈmedisin] *n* 遥控医学，远距医学（远离现场的医生通过闭路电视给在现场的医务人员提供咨询服务）

telemeter [ˈtelimiːtə] *n* 遥测计 | **telemetric** [ˈtelimiːtrik, ˌteliˈmetrik] *a* 遥测的 / **telemetry** [tiˈlemitri] *n* 远距测定法，遥测术

telemnemonike [ˌteliniˈmɔniki] *n* 隔体记忆（能

了解他人记忆中事物）

telencephalization [ˌtelenˌsefəlaiˈzeiʃən, -liˈz-] *n* 端脑分化（个体发育过程中较复杂的神经反应的方向转移到端脑）

telencephalon [ˌtelenˈsefəlɔn], **telencephal** [teˈlensifəl] *n* 端脑，终脑 | **telencephalic** [ˌtelensəˈfælik] *a*

teleneurite [ˌteliˈnjuərait] *n* 终轴突

teleneuron [ˌteliˈnjuərɔn] *n* 神经末端

telenzepine [təˈlenzəpiːn] *n* 替仑西平（用于胃酸过多和消化性溃疡时抑制胃液分泌）

tele(o)- [构词成分]末，终，端

teleology [ˌteliˈɔlədʒi] *n* 目的论（认为任何事物有其最终目标或适应于一定的目的） | **teleological** [ˌteliəˈlɔdʒikəl] *a* / **teleologist** *n* 目的论者

teleomitosis [ˌteliəumaiˈtəusis] *n* 终期分裂

teleomorph [ˈtiːliəumɔːf] *n* 有性型（真菌的有性〈完全〉状态）

teleonomy [ˌteliˈɔnəmi] *n* 存在价值说（一种未经证实的学说，认为有机体一种结构或功能的存在就表明它在进化过程中有其存在的价值） | **teleonomic** [ˌteliəuˈnɔmik] *a*

teleopsia [ˌteliˈɔpsiə] *n* 视物显远症

teleorganic [ˌteliɔːˈgænik] *a* 生命必需的

teleoroentgenogram [ˌteliəurentˈgenəgræm] *n* 远距 X 线[照]片

teleoroentgenography [ˌteliəuˌrentgəˈnɔgrəfi] *n* 远距 X 线摄影[术]（X 线管与片距为 $6\frac{1}{2}$ ~7 英尺〈2 ~2.13 m〉）

teleost [ˈteliɔst] *n* 硬骨鱼 | **teleostean** *a*

telepathize [tiˈlepəθaiz] *vt* 思想交通，思想感应

telepathology [ˌtelipəˈθɔlədʒi] *n* 远距病理学

telepathy [tiˈlepəθi] *n* 传心，通灵，心灵感通 | **telepathic** [ˌteliˈpæθik] *a* / **telepathist** *n* 传心术者，通灵术者

teleradiogram [ˌteliˈreidiəgræm] *n* 远距 X 线[照]片

teleradiography [ˌteliˌreidiˈɔgrəfi] *n* 远距 X 线摄影[术]

teleradium [ˌteliˈreidjəm] *n* 远距施镭，远距镭照射

telereceptor [ˌteliriˈseptə] *n* 距离感受器

telergic [teˈləːdʒik] *a* 远距作用的，心灵感应作用的

telergy [ˈtelədʒi] *n* 自动[症]；心灵感应作用

teleroentgenogram [ˌtelirentˈgenəgræm] *n* 远距 X 线[照]片

teleroentgenography [ˌteliˌrentgəˈnɔgrəfi] *n* 远距 X 线摄影[术]（X 线管与片距为 $6\frac{1}{2}$ ~7 英尺〈2 ~2.13 m〉）

teleroentgentherapy [ˌteliˌrentgənˈθerəpi] *n* 远距 X 线治疗

telestethoscope [ˌteliˈsteθəskəup] *n* 远距听诊器

telesthesia [ˌtelisˈθiːzjə] *n* 传心，通灵，心灵感通

telesthetoscope [ˌteliˈsθetəskəup] *n* 远距听诊器

telesyphilis [ˌteliˈsifilis] *n* 终期梅毒（指脊髓痨、全身麻痹症）

teletactor [ˌteliˈtæktə] *n* 触觉助听器

teletherapy [ˌteliˈθerəpi] *n* 远距[放射]疗法

telethermometer [ˌteliθəˈmɔmitə] *n* 遥测温度计

Teliomycetes [ˌtiːliəumaiˈsiːtiːz] *n* 冬孢菌纲

teliospore [ˈtiːliəuspɔː] *n* 冬孢子

tellurate [ˈteljureit] *n* 碲酸盐

telluric [tiˈljuərik] *a* 地球的，[正]碲的 | ~ acid 碲酸

telluride [ˈteljuraid] *n* 碲化物

tellurism [ˈteljurizəm] *n* 水土致病，地气致病

tellurite [ˈteljurait] *n* 亚碲酸盐

tellurium (Te) [teˈljuəriəm] *n* 碲（化学元素）

tellurous [ˈteljuərəs] *a* 亚碲的

Tellyesniczky's fluid (mixture) [ˌteljetsˈnitski] (Kálmár Tellyesniczky) 捷列斯尼茨基液（混合液）（由重铬酸钾、水、冰醋酸组成）

telmisartan [ˌtelmiˈsɑːtæn] *n* 替米沙坦（血管紧张素Ⅱ拮抗药）

tel(o)- [构词成分]末，终，端

telobiosis [ˌteləubaiˈəusis] *n* 对端并生（胚胎）

telobranchial [ˌteləuˈbræŋkiəl] *a* 端鳃的，终鳃的

telocentric [ˌteləuˈsentrik] *a* 端着丝粒的（指染色体）

telocinesia [ˌteləusaiˈniːziə], **telocinesis** [ˌteləusaiˈniːsis] *n* 末期（见 telophase）

telocoele [ˈteləsiːl] *n* 端脑腔

telodendrion [ˌteləuˈdendriɔn] ([复] **telodendria** [ˌteləuˈdendriə]), **telodendron** [ˌteləuˈdendrɔn] *n* 终树突

telogen [ˈtelədʒən] *n* 毛发生长终期

teloglia [teˈlɔgliə] *n* 终末胶质细胞，神经鞘细胞

telognosis [ˌteləgˈnəusis] *n* 远距诊断，电讯诊断

telokinesis [ˌteləukaiˈniːsis] *n* 末期（见 telophase）

telolecithal [ˌteləuˈlesiθəl] *a* 端黄[卵]的，偏黄[卵]的（卵黄偏于一端的）

telolemma [ˌteləuˈlemə] *n* 终膜（运动神经终板的两层被膜，由肉膜及亨勒〈Henle〉鞘的延伸部组成）

telomer [ˈteləmə] *n* 调聚物

telomerase [təˈləuməreis] *n* 端粒[末端转移]酶

telomere [ˈteləmiə] *n* 端粒（染色体两端的染色粒，端粒的存在使正常的染色体端间不发生融合）

telophase [ˈteləfeiz] *n* [分裂]末期（即丝裂末

期，指有丝分裂和减数分裂过程的最后一个阶段，这时染色体集中到两极，形成两个子细胞的核，整个细胞质缢分为二）

telophragma [ˌteləuˈfrægmə] *n* Z 膜（横纹肌间线）

teloreceptor [ˈtiːləriˌseptə] *n* 距离感受器

telorism [ˈteləriẓəm] *n* [器官]距离过远

telosynapsis [ˌteləusiˈnæpsis] *n* 衔接联会（染色体）

telotaxis [ˌteləuˈtæksis] *n* 趋端性（昆虫等）

telotism [ˈtelətizəm] *n* 功能完整；阴茎勃起

telson [ˈtelsn] *n* 尾节（昆虫）；毒刺（蝎类）

telstar [ˈtelstɑː] *n* 通信卫星

temazepam [təˈmæzəpæm] *n* 替马西泮（弱安定药）

temefos [ˈtemifɔs] *n* 替美福司（有机磷杀虫药，兽用杀外寄生虫药）

temodox [ˈteməd ɔks] *n* 替莫多司（兽用生长促进药）

temozolomide [ˌteməˈzəuləmaid] *n* 替莫唑胺（抗肿瘤药）

temp. dext. tempori dextro【拉】在右颞部

temperament [ˈtempərəmənt] *n* 气质 | bilious ~, choleric ~ 胆汁质 / lymphatic ~, phlegmatic ~ 淋巴质，黏液质 / melancholic ~, atrabilious ~ 忧郁质 / nervous ~ 神经质 / sanguine ~, sanguineous ~ 多血质

temperantia [ˌtempəˈrænʃiə] *n* 镇静药

temperature [ˈtempəritʃə] *n* 温度；体温 | basal body ~ 基础体温 / body ~ 体温 / critical ~ 临界温度 / mean ~ 平均温度 / normal ~ 正常体温 / optimum ~ 最适温度 / room ~ 室温 / subnormal ~ 正常下温度

template [ˈtemplit] *n* 模板（牙科中作装牙用；理论免疫学中指决定抗体分子结合部位构型的抗原；遗传学中指一条 DNA 单链是合成 RNA 互补链或 mRNA 的模板，又是合成核酸或蛋白质的模板）| surgical ~ 手术模板（作即时义齿修复用）

temple [ˈtempl] *n* 颞颥，颞部

tempolabile [ˌtempəuˈleibail] *a* 缓变的（随时间而变化的）

tempora [ˈtempərə] tempus 的复数

temporal [ˈtempərəl] *a* 颞的

temporalis [tempəˈreilis] *a*【拉】颞的 *n* 颞肌

temporoauricular [ˌtempərəuɔːˈrikjulə] *a* 颞耳[部]的

temporofacial [ˌtempərəuˈfeiʃəl] *a* 颞面的

temporofrontal [ˌtempərəuˈfrʌntl] *a* 颞额的；颞额束的

temporohyoid [ˌtempərəuˈhaiɔid] *a* 颞舌骨的

temporomalar [ˌtempərəuˈmeilə] *a* 颞颧的

temporomandibular [ˌtempərəumænˈdibjulə] *a* 颞下颌的

temporomaxillary [ˌtempərəuˈmæksiləri] *a* 颞上颌的

temporo-occipital [ˌtempərəuɔkˈsipitl] *a* 颞枕的

temporoparietal [ˌtempərəupəˈraiitl] *a* 颞顶的

temporoparietalis [ˌtempərəupəˌraiəˈteilis] *a*【拉】颞顶的

temporopontile [ˌtempərəuˈpɔntail] *a* 颞叶脑桥的

temporospatial [ˌtempərəuˈspeiʃəl] *a* 时间与空间的，时空的

temporosphenoid [ˌtempərəuˈsfiːnɔid] *a* 颞蝶的

temporozygomatic [ˌtempərəuˌzaigəˈmætik] *a* 颞颧的

tempostabile [ˌtempəusˈteibail] *a* 不缓变的（不随时间而变化的）

temp. sinist. tempori sinistro【拉】在左颞部

tempus [ˈtempəs]（[复] **tempora** [ˈtempərə]）*n*【拉】颞颥，颞部

temuline [ˈtemjuliːn] *n* 毒麦灵，毒麦碱

tenacious [tiˈneiʃəs] *a* 黏的；（记忆力等）强的

tenacity [tiˈnæsəti] *n* 黏性；韧性；强记 | cellular ~ 细胞韧性

tenaculum [tiˈnækjuləm]（[复] **tenaculums** 或 **tenacula** [tiˈnækjulə]）*n*【拉】持钩（外科手术用）；支持体

tenalgia [tiˈnældʒiə] *n* 腱痛

tenascin [ˈtenəsin] *n* 韧黏素

Tenckhoff catheter [ˈteŋkɔf]（H. Tenckhoff）坦科夫导管（腹膜透析用）

tenderness [ˈtendənis] *n* 触痛，压痛 | pencil ~ 铅笔头触痛 / rebound ~ 反跳痛

tendinitis [ˌtendiˈnaitis] *n* 腱炎 | stenosing ~ 狭窄性腱鞘炎

tendin(o)- [构词成分]腱

tendinoplasty [ˈtendinəuˌplæsti] *n* 腱成形术

tendinosuture [ˌtendinəuˈsjuːtʃə] *n* 腱缝合术

tendinous [ˈtendinəs] *a* 腱的，腱状的，腱性的

tendo [ˈtendəu]（[复] **tendines** [ˈtendiniːz]）*n*【拉】腱

tend(o)- [构词成分]腱

tendolysis [tenˈdɔlisis] *n* 腱粘连松解术

tendomucin [ˌtendəuˈmjuːsin] *n* 腱黏蛋白

tendon [ˈtendən] *n* 腱 | calcaneal ~ 跟腱 / common ~ 总腱 / conjoined ~ 联合腱，腹股沟镰 / pulled ~ 腱撕裂 / slipped ~ 滑动腱 / trefoil ~, cordiform ~ of diaphragm 膈中心腱

tendonitis [ˌtendəuˈnaitis] *n* 腱炎

tendoplasty [ˈtendəˌplæsti] *n* 腱成形术

tendosynovitis [ˌtendəuˌsinəˈvaitis] *n* 腱鞘炎

tendotome [ˈtendətəum] *n* 腱刀

tendotomy [tenˈdɔtəmi] *n* 腱切断术
tendovaginal [ˌtendəuˈvædʒinəl] *a* 腱鞘的
tendovaginitis [ˌtendəuˌvædʒiˈnaitis] *n* 腱鞘炎
tenebrimycin [tiˌnebriˈmaisin] *n* 暗霉素(即妥布霉素 tobramycin)
Tenebrio [təˈniːbriəu] *n* 拟步行虫属
tenecteplase [təˈnektəpleis] *n* 替尼普酶(一种改良型人组织纤维蛋白溶酶原激活药,由重组DNA技术产生,用作溶血栓药,治疗心肌梗死,静脉内给药)
tenectomy [tiˈnektəmi] *n* 腱切除术,腱鞘切除术
tenemycin [ˌteniˈmaisin] *n* 暗霉素(即妥布霉素 tobramycin)
Tenericutes [ˌtenəˈrikjutiːz, ˌtiːnəriˈkjuːtiːz] *n* 无壁[细]菌类
tenesmus [tiˈnezməs] *n*【拉】里急后重 | rectal ~ 里急后重 / vesical ~ 排尿里急后重 | **tenesmic** *a*
ten Horn 见 Horn
tenia [ˈtiːniə] ([复]**teniae** [ˈtiːniiː]) *n* 带;绦虫
teniacide [ˈtiːniəˌsaid] *a* 杀绦虫的 *n* 杀绦虫药
teniafugal [ˌtiːniəˈfjuːgəl] *a* 驱绦虫的
teniafuge [ˈtiːniəˌfjuːdʒ] *n* 驱绦虫药
tenial [ˈtiːniəl] *a* 绦虫的;带的
teniamyotomy [ˌtiːniəmaiˈɔtəmi] *n* 结肠带肌切开术
teniasis [tiˈnaiəsis] *n* 绦虫病
tenicide [ˈtenisaid] *a* 杀绦虫的 *n* 杀绦虫药
teniform [ˈtenifɔːm] *a* 绦虫状的;带状的
tenifugal [tiˈnifjugəl] *a* 驱绦虫的
tenifuge [ˈtenifjuːdʒ] *n* 驱绦虫药
tenioid [ˈtiːniɔid] *a* 绦虫状的;带状的
teniola [tiˈniːələ] *n* 小带,灰质小带
teniotoxin [ˌtiːniəuˈtɔksin] *n* 绦虫毒素
teniposide (VM-26) [ˌteniˈpəusaid] *n* 替尼泊苷(抗肿瘤药)
tennis [ˈtenis] *n* 网球
ten(o)-, tenont(o)- [构词成分]腱
tenodesis [tiˈnɔdisis] *n* 肌腱固定术
tenodynia [ˌtenəuˈdiniə] *n* 腱痛
tenofibril [ˈtenəuˈfaibril] *n* 张力原纤维
tenofovir [təˈnəufəuˌvir] *n* 替诺福韦(一种核苷酸类似物,用作抗反转录病毒药,以抑制反转录酶) | ~ disoproxil fumarate 替诺福韦地索普苷延胡索酸酯(替诺福韦的前药,用于治疗 HIV-1〈人免疫缺陷病毒-1〉感染)
tenolysis [teˈnɔlisis] *n* 肌腱松解术
tenomyoplasty [ˌtenəuˈmaiəˌplæsti] *n* 腱肌成形术
tenomyotomy [ˌtenəumaiˈɔtəmi] *n* 腱肌切除术
tenonectomy [ˌtenəuˈnektəmi] *n* 腱部分切除术,腱缩短术
tenonitis [ˌtenəˈnaitis] *n* 腱炎;眼球囊炎
tenonometer [ˌtenəˈnɔmitə] *n* 眼压计
tenonostosis [ˌtenənɔsˈtəusis] *n* 腱骨化
Tenon's capsule (fascia, membrane) [təˈnɔn] (Jacques R. Tenon)眼球筋膜,眼球囊 | ~ space 巩膜外层间隙
tenontagra [ˌtenənˈtægrə] *n* 腱痛风
tenontitis [ˌtenənˈtaitis] *n* 腱炎
tenont(o)- 见 teno-
tenontodynia [ˌtenəntəuˈdiniə] *n* 腱痛
tenontography [ˌtenənˈtɔgrəfi] *n* 腱论
tenontolemmitis [təˌnɔntəuleˈmaitis] *n* 腱鞘炎
tenontology [ˌtenənˈtɔlədʒi] *n* 腱学
tenontomyoplasty [təˌnɔntəuˈmaiəˌplæsti] *n* 腱肌成形术
tenontomyotomy [ˌtenɔntəumaiˈɔtəmi] *n* 腱肌切除术
tenontophyma [təˌnɔntəuˈfaimə] *n* 腱瘤
tenontoplasty [təˈnɔntəˌplæsti] *n* 腱成形术
tenontothecitis [təˈnɔntəuθiˈsaitis] *n* 腱鞘炎
tenontotomy [ˌtenənˈtɔtəmi] *n* 肌腱切断术
tenophyte [ˈtenəfait] *n* 腱赘
tenoplasty [ˈtenəˌplæsti] *n* 肌腱成形术 | **tenoplastic** [ˌtenəuˈplæstik] *a*
tenoreceptor [ˌtenəriˈseptə] *n* 腱感受器
tenorrhaphy [tiˈnɔrəfi] *n* 腱缝合术
tenositis [ˌtenəuˈsaitis] *n* 腱炎
tenostosis [ˌtenɔsˈtəusis] *n* 腱骨化
tenosuture [ˌtenəuˈsjuːtʃə] *n* 腱缝合术
tenosynitis [ˌtenəusaiˈnaitis] *n* 腱鞘炎
tenosynovectomy [ˌtenəuˌsinəˈvektəmi] *n* 腱鞘切除术
tenosynovitis [ˌtenəuˌsinəˈvaitis] *n* 腱鞘炎
tenotome [ˈtenətəum] *n* 腱刀
tenotomize [tiˈnɔtəmaiz] *vt* 肌腱切断
tenotomy [tiˈnɔtəmi] *n* 肌腱切断术 | curb ~ 眼肌后徙术(治斜视的一种手术) / graduated ~ 部分肌腱切断术
tenovaginitis [ˌtenəuˌvædʒiˈnaitis] *n* 腱鞘炎
TENS transcutaneous electrical nerve stimulation 经皮电刺激神经疗法
tense [tens] *a* 拉紧的,紧张的
tensible [ˈtensible] *a* 能拉长的,能伸展的
tensile [ˈtensail] *a* 张力的,可伸展的
tensio-active [ˌtensiəu ˈæktiv] *a* 表面张力活性的
tensiometer [ˌtensiˈɔmitə] *n* 表面张力计
tension [ˈtenʃən] *n* 压力,张力;紧张 | arterial ~ 动脉压 / electric ~ 电压 / intraocular ~ 眼球内压,眼压 / intravenous ~ 静脉压 / muscular ~ 肌紧张,肌张力 / premenstrual ~ 经前期紧张 / surface ~ 表面张力 / tissue ~ 组织张力
tensity [ˈtensəti] *n* 紧张,紧张度

tensive [ˈtensiv] *a* 张力的
tensometer [tenˈsɔmitə] *n* 张力计,张力测量仪
tensor [ˈtensə] *n*【拉】张肌
tent[1] [tent] *n* 帐篷;帐状物,帷幕 | oxygen ~ 氧幕,氧气帐 / steam ~ 蒸气帷(呼吸道疾病时用)
tent[2] [tent] *n* 塞条 *vt* 将塞条嵌进(伤口) | sponge ~ 海绵塞条(扩张宫颈管用)
tentacle [ˈtentəkl] *n* 触手;触须(动物) / **tentacular** [tenˈtækjulə] *a*
tentaculiform [tenˈtækjulifɔːm] *a* 触手状的
tenthmeter [tenθˈmiːtə] *n* 埃(波长单位, $=10^{-10}$ m)
tentorium [tenˈtɔːriəm] ([复] **tentoria** [tenˈtɔːriə]) *n*【拉】幕 | ~ of cerebellum 小脑幕 / ~ of hypophysis 鞍膈 | **tentorial** *a*
tentum [ˈtentəm] *n* 阴茎
tenulin [ˈtenjulin] *n* 细叶土木香苦素(嚏剂)
tenuous [ˈtenjuəs] *a* 稀薄的,纤细的,微弱的
TEOAE transient evoked otoacoustic emissions 短暂诱发性耳声发射
tephromalacia [ˌtefrəuməˈleiʃiə] *n* 灰质软化(脑或脊髓)
tephromyelitis [ˌtefrəumaiəˈlaitis] *n* 脊髓灰质炎
tephrosis [teˈfrəusis] *n* 焚化,灰化;火葬
tephrylometer [ˌtefriˈlɔmitə] *n* 脑灰质[厚度]测量计
tepor [ˈtiːpə] *n* 微热,微温
TEPP tetraethyl pyrophosphate 焦磷酸四乙酯,特普(杀虫剂)
teprotide [ˈteprətaid] *n* 替普罗肽(抗高血压药)
ter- [前缀]三,三倍
tera- [构词成分]垓,兆兆,万亿($=10^{12}$)
teracurie [ˌterəˈkjuəri] *n* 垓居里(旧放射单位, $=10^{12}$ Ci)
teras [ˈterəs] ([复] **terata** [ˈterətə]) *n*【拉;希】畸胎
teratic [teˈrætik] *a* 畸形的
teratism [ˈterətizəm] *n* [畸胎]畸形
terat(o)- [构词成分]畸胎,畸形
teratoblastoma [ˌterətəublæsˈtəumə] *n* 畸胎样瘤
teratocarcinogenesis [ˌterətəuˌkɑːsinəuˈdʒenisis] *n* 畸胎瘤发生
teratocarcinoma [ˌterətəuˌkɑːsiˈnəumə] *n* 畸胎癌
teratogen [ˈterətədʒən] *n* 致畸因子,致畸原,致畸剂
teratogenic [ˌterətəuˈdʒenik] *a* 畸形形成的,致畸形的
teratogenesis [ˌterətəuˈdʒenisis], **teratogeny** [ˌterəˈtɔdʒəni] *n* 畸形形成,畸形发生 | **teratogenetic** [ˌterətəudʒiˈnetik] *a*
teratogenous [ˌterəˈtɔdʒinəs] *a* 畸形性的
teratoid [ˈterətɔid] *a* 畸胎样的
teratology [ˌterəˈtɔlədʒi] *n* 畸形学,畸胎学 | **teratologic(al)** [terətəˈlɔdʒik(əl)] *a*
teratoma [ˌterəˈtəumə] ([复] **teratomas** 或 **teratomata** [ˌterəˈtəumətə]) *n* 畸胎瘤 | **~tous** *a*
teratosis [ˌterəˈtəusis] *n* [畸胎]畸形
teratospermia [ˌterətəuˈspəːmiə] *n* 畸形精子[症]
teratozoospermia [ˌterətəuˌzəuəuˈspəːmiə] *n* 畸形游动精子[症](亦称畸形精子[症])
terazosin hydrochloride [təˈreizəsin] 盐酸特拉唑嗪(抗高血压药)
terbinafine hydrochloride [ˈtəːbinəˌfiːn] 盐酸特比奈芬(一种合成抗真菌化合物,妨碍麦角固醇生物合成,破坏真菌细胞膜功能,表面用药以及口服治疗各种类型的癣和甲癣)
terbium(Tb) [ˈtəːbiəm] *n* 铽(化学元素)
terbutaline sulfate [təˈbjuːtəliːn] 硫酸特布他林(β 受体激动剂,用作支气管扩张药)
terchloride [təːˈklɔːraid] *n* 三氯化物
terconazole [teˈkəunəzəul] *n* 特康唑(抗真菌药)
tere [ˈtiəri] *vt*【拉】擦,研磨(调剂用词)
terebene [ˈterəbiːn] *n* 松节油萜,芸香烯
terebenthene [ˌterəˈbenθiːn] *n* 松节油
terebic acid [teˈrebik] 芸香酸
terebinth [ˈterəbinθ] *n* 笃耨香;松油脂
terebinthina [ˌterəˈbinθinə] *n*【拉】松油脂,松脂
terebinthinate [ˌterəˈbinθineit], **terebinthine** [terəˈbinθiːn] *a* 含松油脂的,似松油脂的
terebinthinism [ˌterəˈbinθinizəm] *n* 松节油中毒
terebrachesis [ˌterəbreiˈkiːsis] *n* (子宫)圆韧带减短术
terebrant [ˈterəbrənt], **terebrating** [ˈterəˌbreitiŋ] *a* 钻刺性的(如锥痛)
terebration [ˌteriˈbreiʃən] *n* 环钻术;锥痛
teres [ˈtiəriːz] *a*【拉】圆的 *n* 圆肌
terfenadine [təˈfenədiːn] *n* 特非那定(抗组胺药)
tergal [ˈtəːgəl] *a* 背的,背面的
ter in die [təː in diːei]【拉】一日三次
term [təːm] *n* 期;期限;足月,足孕;名词,术语 | ontogenetic ~ 胚胎学名词
terminad [ˈtəːminæd] *ad* 向末端
terminal [ˈtəːminl] *a* 端的;末端的 *n* 末端,终点 | C ~ C 末端,羧基末端(即 C-terminal) / N ~ N 末端,氨基末端(即 N-terminal)
terminal addition enzyme 末端加成酶,DNA 核苷酸基外转移酶
terminal deoxynucleotidyl transferase (**TdT**) [diːˌɔksiˌnjuːkliəuˈtaidil ˈtrænsfəreis] 末端脱氧核苷酸转移酶,DNA 核苷酸基外转移酶
terminate [ˈtəːmineit] *vt, vi* 终止,结束

terminatio [ˌtəːmiˈneiʃiəu] ([复] **terminationes** [ˌtəːmiˌneiʃiˈəuniːz]) *n*【拉】末端，端；终止

Terminologia Anatomica (**TA**) [ˌtəːminəuˈləudʒiə ˌænəˈtɔmikə]【拉】《解剖学术语》(即 *International Anatomical Terminology*《国际解剖学术语》，于1998年出版，取代 *Nomina Anatomica* [NA])

terminology [ˌtəːmiˈnɔlədʒi] *n* 术语；命名法 | *International Anatomical Terminology*《国际解剖学术语》(即 *Terminologia Anatomica*《解剖学术语》)

terminus [ˈtəːminəs] ([复] **terminuses** 或 **termini** [ˈtəːminai]) *n* 末端；名词，术语 | termini generales 通称 / termini ontogenetici 胚胎学名词

termolecular [ˌtəːməuˈlekjulə] *a* 三分子的

ternary [ˈtəːnəri] *a* 第三的；三元的 | ~acid 三元酸

Ternidens [ˈtəːnidənz] *n* 三齿[线虫]属 | ~ diminutus 缩小三齿线虫

ternitrate [təːˈnaitreit] *n* 三硝酸盐

terodiline hydrochloride [ˌtəːrəuˈdailiːn] 盐酸特罗地林(冠状动脉扩张药，用于治疗劳力性心绞痛)

teroxide [təːˈrɔksaid] *n* 三氧化物

terpene [ˈtəːpiːn] *n* 萜

terpenism [ˈtəːpənizəm] *n* 萜中毒

terpin [ˈtəːpin] *n* 萜品，萜二醇 | ~ hydrate 萜品醇，水合萜二醇(祛痰药)

terpineol [təˈpiniɔl] *n* 萜品醇，松油醇

terra [ˈterə] *n*【拉】土，土地 | ~ alba 白土，石膏粉 / ~ lemnia 赭土 / ~ merita 郁金，姜黄 / ~ ponderosa 重土，硫酸钡 / ~ sigillata 真赭土 / ~ silicea purificata 精制硅藻土

terrein [ˈteriin] *n* 土曲菌素，羟基环五烷酮

terrestric acid [teˈrestrik] 青地霉酸

Terridens [ˈteridəns] *n* 三齿[线虫]属 | diminutus 缩小三齿线虫

territoriality [ˌteriˌtɔːriˈæləti] *n* 地区性，地盘性(生物的一种行为型，指一个或一群动物划出地盘，有力地防御同种的其他成员的侵入)

territory [ˈteritəri] *n* 地盘(由一个或一群动物所占据的栖息区域，属于同种的其他成员进入这个地盘，它们就会被作为入侵者而受到攻击)

terror [ˈterə] *n* 惊吓，惊悸 | day ~s 昼惊 / night ~s 夜惊

Terry's syndrome [ˈteri] (Theodore L. Terry) 特里综合征，未熟儿视网膜病

Terson's syndrome [teˈsɔn] (Albert Terson) 德桑综合征，玻璃体出血

tersulfide [təːˈsʌlfaid] *n* 三硫化物

tertian [ˈtəːʃən] *a* 每三日[复发]的，间日的 *n* 间日热 | double ~ 复间日疟

tertiary [ˈtəːʃəri] *a* 第三的，第三位的，第三级的；(梅毒等)第三期的；(化学)叔的，特的，三代的，三发性的

tertigravida [ˌtəːʃiˈgrævidə] *n*【拉】第三次孕妇

tertipara [təːˈʃipərə] *n*【拉】三产妇

tervalent [təːˈveilənt] *a* 三价的

Teschen disease [ˈteʃən] (Teschen 为原捷克斯洛伐克一地区，1929年在该地区报道过此病)猪传染性脑脊髓炎

TESE testicular sperm extraction 睾丸精子提取

tesicam [ˈtesikæm] *n* 替昔康(抗炎药)

tesla (**T**) [ˈteslə] *n* 特斯拉(磁通量密度的国际单位制单位，以每平方米韦伯〈webers〉计算)

teslaization [ˌtesleiaiˈzeiʃən] (Nikola Tesla) *n* 特斯拉电疗法，高频电疗法

tessellated [ˈtesileitid] *a* 棋盘格状的，分成方格的

test¹ [test] *n* 壳，甲壳，介壳

test² [test] *n* 试验，测验；化验，化验结果；试剂 *vt* 试验，测试；化验，分析 | abortus Bang ring (ABR) ~ 流产班氏环状试验(检牛布鲁杆菌病的筛选试验，亦称乳汁环状试验) / acetic acid ~ 乙酸试验(检尿白蛋白) / acetic acid and potassium ferrocyanide ~ 乙酸[和]亚铁氰化钾试验(检蛋白质) / acid elution ~ 酸洗脱试验(检胎儿血红蛋白) / acidified serum ~ 酸化血清试验(检阵发性睡眠性血红蛋白尿) / acid-lability ~ 酸灭活试验(根据鼻病毒和肠病毒在不同的pH水平时的活力对两者进行鉴别的试验，鼻病毒在pH3~5的情况下孵育1~3小时即告灭活) / acoustic reflex ~ 听反射试验(测听反射阈，用以区分传导性聋和感音神经性聋以及诊断听神经瘤) / adrenalin ~ 肾上腺素试验(检甲状腺功能) / agglutination ~ 凝集试验(检细菌凝集，用于诊断细菌性疾病或病毒性及立克次体疾病以及类风湿关节炎) / air ~ 充气试验(检胎盘完整) / alizarin ~ 西素试验(检胃分泌) / alkali denaturation ~ 碱变性试验(一种中度敏感的分光光度测定法，以检测胎儿血红蛋白的浓度，此法系利用血红蛋白分子对其珠蛋白部分接触碱不致变性的特点进行的) / alternate binaural loudness balance (ABLB) ~ 双耳交替响度平衡试验，ABLB试验 / alternate cover ~ 交替遮盖试验(检测斜视和/或隐斜视的类型，即交替遮盖两眼并注意未遮盖眼的运动) / alternate loudness balance ~ 交替响度平衡试验 / antiglobulin ~ (AGT) 抗球蛋白试验 / antiglobulin consumption ~ 抗球蛋白消耗试验 / Army General Classification ~ 陆军通用分类测验(用于军队人员工作安排的一种智力测验) / arylsulfatase ~ 芳[香]基硫酸酯酶试验(鉴别快

速生长分枝杆菌的种属）/ augmented histamine ~ 组胺加重试验（检胃功能）/ autohemolysis ~ 自身溶血试验 / automated reagin ~（ART）自动反应素试验 / bar-reading ~ 障碍阅读试验 / bentonite flocculation ~ 皂土絮凝试验，皂土絮状试验 / benzidine ~ 联苯胺试验（检尿或粪便中潜血）/ bile solubility ~ 胆汁溶解度试验（鉴别肺炎双球菌与链球菌）/ binaural distorted speech ~s 对耳畸变言语试验 / biuret ~ 双缩脲试验（检蛋白质及脲）/ bracelet ~ 手镯试验（风湿样关节炎时，轻压桡尺骨下端侧面，引起疼痛）/ California mastitis ~（CMT）加利福尼亚乳腺炎试验（检牛的亚临床性乳腺炎）/ CAMP ~ *C*hristie, *A*tkins and *M*unch-*P*etersen CAMP 试验（对 B 族 β 溶血性链球菌的初步鉴定）/ carotid sinus ~ 颈动脉窦试验（检心绞痛）/ catalase ~ 过氧化氢酶试验，触酶试验（检细菌产生的过氧化氢酶）/ catoptric ~ 反光试验（观察角膜及晶体的反光情况以检内障）/ cephalin-cholesterol flocculation ~ 脑磷脂胆固醇絮状试验（从前用于肝功能试验）/ chemiluminescence ~ 化学发光试验（中性粒细胞杀灭微生物功能的敏感试验，包括检测由不稳定的和高度反应性的氧代谢物〈如噬菌作用后在突发性呼吸时所产生的单态氧〉所释放的化学发光能。本试验能检测慢性肉芽肿病的杂合携带者，亦能检测髓过氧物酶缺乏患者）/ chi-squared（χ^2）~ 卡方检验（一种统计检验，即期望值和观察值之差的平方，除以期望值〈在检验中的每一类〉各商数之和即为卡方〈符号为 χ^2〉，卡方值越小，则假设与实际频数之间的符合程度越接近）/ chromatin ~ 染色质试验（测定遗传型性别）/ cis-trans ~ 顺反测验，顺反位置效应测验（使两个拟等位突变基因分别处于顺式或反式构型而观察个体的表型，从而判断它们是否属于同一顺反子的测验）/ citrate ~ 枸橼酸试验（鉴别肠杆菌）/ cocaine ~ 可卡因试验（双眼滴入可卡因溶液，患霍纳〈Horner〉综合征那只眼的瞳孔要比正常眼小）/ coccidioidin ~ 球孢子菌素试验（一种检球孢子菌病的皮内试验）/ colloidal gold ~ 胶态金试验（检脑脊液蛋白-球蛋白，从而诊断某些中枢神经系统疾患，如神经梅毒、多发性硬化、脊髓灰质炎以及脑炎）/ complement fixation ~ 补体结合试验（检查血清中抗体与相应抗原结合后结合补体的一种血清学试验）/ concentration ~ 浓度试验（检肾功能）/ conglutinating complement absorption ~（CCAT）胶固补体吸收试验 / Congo red ~ 刚果红试验（检淀粉样变性）/ contact ~ 接触试验（见 patch ~）/ cover-uncover ~ 遮盖-不遮盖试验（检测隐斜视的类型，即遮盖一眼并注意不遮盖眼的运动）/ dark-adaptation ~ 暗适应试验（检维生素 A 缺乏症。此试验的依据为：维生素 A 摄入量缺乏则欲在暗室中见一微明物体的能力就减弱）/ Denver Development Screening ~ 丹佛发育筛选测验（鉴定婴儿和学龄前儿童发育迟缓的测验）/ deoxyribonuclease（DNase）~ 脱氧核糖核酸酶试验（检细菌的脱氧核糖核酸酶的存在）/ deoxyuridine suppression ~ 脱氧尿苷抑制试验（检测叶酸或钴胺缺乏）/ dexamethasone suppression ~ 地塞米松抑制试验（检测下丘脑-垂体-肾上腺皮质功能）/ differential ~ for infectious mononucleosis 传染性单核细胞增多症鉴别试验 / disk diffusion ~ 平板扩散试验（检细菌对抗生素的敏感性）/ double glucagon ~ 两次高血糖素试验（检淀粉 1, 6-葡萄苷酶缺乏）/ dye exclusion ~ 染料排斥试验（试管中测定细胞活力）/ early pregnancy ~ 早孕试验 / erythrocyte protoporphyrin（EP）~ 红细胞原卟啉试验（铅中毒筛选试验）/ esophageal acid infusion ~ 食管酸灌注试验（诊断胃食管回流）/ euglobulin lysis ~ 优球蛋白溶解试验（检测纤维蛋白溶酶原激活剂）/ FE_{Na} ~ 滤过钠排泄分数（excreted fraction of filtered sodium）试验（测定肾小管对钠的再吸收）/ femoral nerve stretch ~ 股神经牵张试验（检第三或第四腰椎间盘病损）/ fern ~ 羊齿状试验（检雌激素）/ ferric chloride ~ 氯化铁试验（检涎液中的硫氰酸；检水杨酸）/ finger-nose ~, finger-to-finger ~ 指鼻试验，指指试验（检肢体协调运动）/ flocculation ~ 絮凝试验，絮状试验 / fluorescent treponemal antibody absorption（FTA-ABS）~ 荧光[梅毒]密螺旋体抗体吸收试验（检梅毒）/ fundus reflex ~ 眼底反射试验（检影法，视网膜镜检查）/ glycerophosphate ~ 甘油磷酸盐试验（检肾功能）/ glycyltryptophan ~ 甘氨酰色氨酸试验（检胃癌）/ gold number ~, gold-sol ~ 金胶液试验，金值试验（检脑脊液球蛋白，从而诊断脑脊髓梅毒）/ guaiac ~ 愈创木脂试验（检潜血）/ hapten inhibition ~ 半抗原抑制试验（抗原决定簇血清学特性的鉴定）/ hatching ~ 孵化试验（检尿或粪中血吸虫卵）/ heel-knee ~ 跟膝试验（检两侧下肢协调运动）/ hemadsorption ~ 血[细胞]吸附试验（一种试管〈体外〉试验，血细胞凝集素存在时，红细胞吸附到受感染的组织的细胞上，以测定血细胞凝集的病毒）/ hemagglutination inhibition（HI, HAI）~ 血细胞凝集抑制试验，血凝抑制试验 / histamine ~ 组胺试验（检胃分泌、交感神经系统损害、嗜铬细胞瘤）/ histamine-flare ~ 组胺发红试验（检麻风和疱疹后神经痛）/ histidine loading ~ 组氨酸负荷试验（检叶酸缺乏）/ horse cell ~ 马细胞试验（保-邦-戴〈Paul-Bunnell-Davidsohn〉试验的一种改良，检伴有传染性单核细胞增多症的嗜异性抗体，即使用马红细胞而不用绵羊红细胞，不需要离心分离，整个试验几分钟即完成）/ hydrogen peroxide ~ 过氧化氢试验(检血) / hyperemia ~ 充血试验(检动脉硬化,见 Moschcowitz's test) / hypothesis ~ 假设检验(确定一系列观察是否符合思考中的假设的一种抽象方法,也是大多数统计检验的理论基础。假设检验是在两种假设间作出决定的,一种假设认为研究中的效应并不存在,即无效假设 null hypothesis, H_0,另一种则认为有某种特定效应存在,即备择假设 alternative hypothesis, H_1) / IMViC ~ IMViC 试验(为 *i*ndole〈吲哚〉、*m*ethyl red〈甲基红〉、*V*oges-Proskauer〈伏-普〉反应及 *c*itrate〈枸橼酸〉修改过的首字母缩写词,一系列代谢试验,用作鉴别肠杆菌科所属菌属的规范化操作) / indigo carmine ~ 靛卡红试验(检肾渗透性) / indophenol ~ 靛酚试验(检细胞内氧化酶及成髓细胞等) / inoculation ~ 接种试验(检急性脊髓前角灰质炎) / intracutaneous tuberculin ~ 结核菌素皮内试验(检结核病) / intradermal ~, intracutaneous ~ 皮内试验(皮内注射抗原的一种皮肤试验) / lactose ~ 乳糖试验(检肾功能) / latex agglutination ~, latex fixation ~ 胶乳凝集试验,胶乳结合试验(将可溶性抗原吸附在聚苯乙烯胶乳颗粒上,加上特异性抗体可使之凝集,此试验广泛用于检查类风湿因子,在妊娠试验中检尿人绒〈毛〉膜促性腺激素) / lepromin ~ 麻风菌素试验(检麻风) / levulose tolerance ~ 果糖耐量试验(检肝功能) / limulus ~ 鲎(溶解物)试验(马蹄蟹〈即鲎 Limulus polyphemus〉血细胞浸液接触患者血标本,如标本中含有革兰阴性菌内毒素,就会产生血细胞浸液的凝胶作用) / lipase ~ 脂酶试验(检肝功能) / litmus-milk ~ 石蕊牛乳试验(检胰脂酶) / lupus band ~ 狼疮带试验(一种免疫荧光试验,检测系统性红斑狼疮患者中真皮表皮交界部是否有免疫球蛋白和补体沉积及其程度) / lymphocyte proliferation ~ 淋巴细胞增生试验(检查淋巴细胞对致丝裂素、特定抗原或同种细胞反应能力的功能试验,淋巴细胞分别用刺激物或不用刺激物培养数日,然后用^{3}H 标记的胸苷培养数小时,刺激培养和对照培养中胸苷的摄取率则称为刺激指数〈SI〉或刺激率〈SR〉。亦称胚细胞样转变测定,淋巴细胞增生测定) / magnesionitric ~ 镁硝酸试验(检尿白蛋白) / mallein ~ 马鼻疽菌素试验(检鼻疽) / methylene blue ~ 亚甲蓝试验(检肾渗透性、检乳) / microprecipitation ~ 微量沉淀试验(使用微量血清做沉淀试验) / migration inhibitory factor (MIF) ~ 游走抑制因子试验(体外测试淋巴细胞在特异性抗原作用下产生 MIF 的试验) / milk ring ~ 乳汁环状试验(见 abortus Bang ring ~) / mirror ~ 镜面试验(检支气管分泌物) / monaural loudness balance (MLB) ~ 单耳响度平衡试验 / multiple-puncture ~ 多刺试验(一种皮内试验,以若干刺针或叉针蘸取试验材料〈例如结核菌素〉后刺压入皮内) / mumps-skin ~ 腮腺炎皮肤试验(检对腮腺炎的免疫力:此试验不可靠,很少使用,即皮内注射灭活腮腺炎病毒,结核菌素型迟发型超敏反应发生即为阳性反应) / neutralizaton ~ 中和试验(测定抗血清或其他物质对病毒或其他有关细菌致病性质的中和能力) / niacin ~ 烟酸试验(检结核分枝杆菌) / nitrate reduction ~ 硝酸盐还原试验(检硝酸盐经细菌培养还原为亚硝酸盐。此试验可用于肠杆菌科、分枝杆菌和某些需氧菌的可疑菌株的鉴定) / nitric acid ~ 硝酸试验(检白蛋白) / nitric acid-magnesium sulfate ~ 硝酸硫酸镁试验(检白蛋白) / nitroblue tetrazolium (NBT) ~ 四唑氮蓝试验(检中性粒细胞杀菌功能) / nitrogen partition ~ 氮分配试验(检肝功能) / nitroprusside ~ 硝基氢氰酸盐试验(检半胱氨酸、丙酮、肌酐) / one-tailed ~ 单尾检验,单侧检验(一种假设检验) / ONPG ~ ONPG 试验(检细菌中 β-D-半乳糖苷酶:细菌在含邻-硝基苯-β-D-半乳糖吡喃糖苷 *O*-nitrophenyl-β-D-galactopyranoside〈ONPG〉的缓冲胨培养基中生长,如出现黄色,即示有 β-半乳糖苷酶生成) / orcinol ~ 苔黑酚试验(检尿戊糖) / orthotoluidine ~ 邻甲基苯胺试验(检血) / osazone ~ 脎试验(检糖) / ovarian hyperemia ~ 卵巢充血试验(检孕) / palmin ~, palmitin ~ 软脂酸酯试验(检胰腺功能) / passive cutaneous anaphylaxis ~ 被动皮肤过敏反应试验(用于研究引起直接过敏性反应的抗体) / passive protection ~ 被动保护试验(在动物注射抗血清被动免疫后进行的保护试验) / passive transfer ~ 被动转移试验(一种皮肤反应,检测人的反应素 IgE) / patch ~ 斑贴试验(主要用于诊断变态反应:以小块纱布或滤纸浸透可疑变应原,贴于皮肤一段时候,出现红肿即为阳性反应) / PCA ~ 被动皮肤过敏反应试验(即 passive cutaneous anaphylaxis ~) / phenolphthalein ~ 酚酞试验(检粪中血及尿内血液) / phenolsulfonphthalein ~ 酚磺酞试验(检肾功能) / phenoltetrachlorophthalein ~ 四氯酚酞试验(检肝功能) / phlorhizin ~, phlorizin ~ 根皮苷试验(检肾功能不全) / phloroglucin ~, phloroglucinol ~ 间苯三酚试验(检尿中半乳糖、戊糖及糖醛酸) / phosphatase ~ 磷酸酶试验(鉴定消毒牛奶;检血清磷酸酶) / pineapple ~ 菠萝试验(检胃酪酸) / plantar ischemia ~ 跖缺血试验(检小腿和足部循环障碍) / pregnancy ~ 妊娠试验(一类以检出孕妇尿中绒毛膜促性腺激素来诊断妊娠的试验) / protection ~ 保护[力]试验,血清中和试验 / protein tyrosin ~ 蛋白酪氨酸试验(检疟疾) / quadriceps ~ 四头肌试验(检甲状腺功能亢进) / radioactive renogram ~ 放射肾 X 线摄片试验(静脉内注射放射性核素物质，并用外烁闪器检验肾对此物质的摄入和分泌）/ radioallergosorbent ~（RAST）放射变应原吸附试验（测定血清中特异性免疫球蛋白 E 抗体的试验）/ radioimmunosorbent ~（RIST）放射免疫吸附试验（一种高度敏感的放射免疫测定法，测定血清中免疫球蛋白 E 抗体的总浓度）/ radioisotope renal excretion ~ 放射性核素肾排泄试验（研究肾功能）/ rank sum ~ 秩和检验（一种无效假设对备择假设的非参数统计检验，无效假设的两种样本来自同一群体，备择假设的两种样本来自两个群体，其概率分布类型相同但位置不同，根据秩和的统计值，当双方样本以上升次序联合分级观察时，即可算出一种样本的秩和）/ rapid plasma reagin（RPR）~s 快速血浆反应素试验（一组诊断梅毒的絮凝试验，采用未加热的血清和一种改良的 VDRL〈美国性病研究所〉抗原〈含氯化胆碱和炭粒〉，就能目视絮凝现象，广泛用于筛选检查）/ rash-extinction ~ 红疹消退试验（见 Schultz-Charlton reaction）/ resorcinol ~ 间苯二酚试验（检盐酸）/ rheumatoid arthritis ~ 类风湿关节炎试验 / RIF（resistance-inducing factor）~ 抗性诱导因子试验（见 Rubin's test ②解）/ ring ~ 成环试验（检抗生素活性、鼻疽、蛋白质）/ rose bengal ~ 孟加拉玫红试验（检肝功能）/ salicylaldehyde ~ 水杨醛试验（检尿内丙酮）/ sand ~ 沙滤试验（检尿内胆汁及血红蛋白）/ santonin ~ 山道年试验（检肝抗毒效力）/ scarification ~ 划痕试验（一种皮肤试验，经划痕将抗原引入，如皮尔盖试验，见 Pirquet test）/ SCMC ~ SCMC 试验（精子-子宫颈精液接触〈*s*perm-*c*ervical *m*ucus *c*ontact〉，检子宫颈因子不育）/ scratch ~ 划痕试验（一种皮肤试验，将抗原用在表面划痕上）/ screen ~ 遮盖试验（交替遮盖试验，见 alternate cover ~；遮盖-不遮盖试验，见 coveruncover ~）/ screening ~ 筛选试验（用以排除那些肯定不患还在争议中的疾病的人，而对其余具有阳性反应的人则作较仔细的诊断试验）/ serologic ~ 血清学试验（任何用患者血清的实验室试验）/ serum ~ 血清试验（检血、肉、精液等，亦称生物试验）/ serologic ~ for syphilis（STS）梅毒血清学试验 / serum bactericidal activity ~ 血清杀菌活性试验 / serum neutralization ~ 血清中和试验（血清抗微生物活性试验，即将血清、病毒或其他受检微生物的混合物接种到易感的动物，亦称保护试验）/ shadow ~ 暗影试验（视网膜镜检查，检影法）/ sheep cell agglutination ~（SCAT）绵羊细胞凝集试验（任何使用绵羊红细胞的凝集试验）/ short increment sensitivity index（SISI）~ 短增量敏感指数试验 / sign ~ 符号检验（一种无效假说的非参数统计检验）/ signed rank ~ 符号秩检验（一种无效假设对备择假说的非参数统计检验）/ skin ~ 皮肤试验 / sniff ~ 鼻吸试验（病人作嗅闻动作时，X 线透视检查可见到膈膜麻痹侧上升，正常侧下降）/ sponge ~［热］海绵试验，热纱布试验（检脊柱病）/ Sterneedle tuberculin ~ 艉针结核菌素试验（使用自动六针头装置，即艉针 Sterneedle，浸有 1 ~ 2 滴结核菌素 P. P. D.，置于前臂，刺入皮下 1 mm 之深，从而使结核菌素沉积于皮肤外表面，3 ~ 7 日期间针刺部位有硬结，并大于 5 mm 者为阳性，此试验在英国称希夫〈Heaf〉试验）/ Student's *t*- ~ 斯氏 *t* 检验（见 *t*- ~）/ sucrose lysis ~ 蔗糖溶血试验（检阵发性夜间血红蛋白尿）/ sulfur ~ 硫试验（检蛋白质）/ susceptibility ~ 敏感试验（检病原菌对抗生素的敏感性）/ *t*-~ *t* 检验（根据 *t* 分布的一种统计假设检验，用于检验两组的均值差）/ tannic acid ~ 鞣酸试验（检核白蛋白）/ thematic apperception ~（TAT）主题统觉测验 / thermoagglutination ~ 热凝集试验（检细菌抗原性变种的一种试验，将细菌盐水悬液煮沸 2 小时后，略呈粗糙的菌株能发生凝集）/ thiochrome ~ 脱氢硫胺试验（检维生素 B_1）/ three-glass ~ 三杯试验（检尿道炎及膀胱炎）/ thymol turbidity ~ 麝香草酚浊度试验（从前用作检肝功能的一种絮凝试验）/ tolerance ~ 耐量试验（测循环效能；测机体对某一物质的代谢能力或对药物的耐受能力）/ thyroid suppression ~ 甲状腺抑制试验（检甲状腺功能亢进）/ tine ~，tine tuberculin ~（Rosenthal）结核菌素叉刺试验（2 mm 长尖叉 4 支接在塑料手柄上，尖叉浸蘸旧结核菌素，干后压入前臂掌侧皮内，以此方法在外层接种，48 ~ 72 小时后检查，是否有可触知的硬结，如在划刺处周围有 1 个以上直径超过 2 mm 的硬结，即为阳性）/ tone decay ~ 音衰变试验（一种听力计试验）/ tray agglutination ~ 托盘凝集试验（一型精子凝集试验，将精子和血清混合在显微镜托盘上以便检查）/ treponemal hemagglutination（TPHA）~ 梅毒螺旋体血凝试验（检梅毒）/ Treponema pallidum complement fixation（TPCF）~ 梅毒螺旋体补体结合试验（检梅毒）/ Treponema pallidum cryolysis complement fixation（TPCP）~ 梅毒螺旋体冻溶补体结合试验（检梅毒）/ Treponema pallidum immobilization（TPI）~ 梅毒螺旋体制动试验（检梅毒）/ trichophytin ~ 发癣菌素试验（检发癣菌感染）/ triketohydrindene hydrate ~ 水合茚三酮试验（检蛋白质及氨基酸）/ tryptophan ~ 色氨酸试验（检胃容物中有色氨酸即表明有胃癌）/ tuberculin ~ 结核菌素试验（检结核病）/ tuberculin titer ~ 结核菌素效价试验（用不同浓度的结核菌素进行注射以测定机体对结核菌素过敏性程度的试验）/ two-glass ~ 二杯试验（检尿道炎，早起时病人收集尿液，第一部分放于第一个玻璃杯中，第二部分放于第二个杯中，如患有前尿道炎,第一个玻璃杯中的尿混浊,第二个杯尿清澈,如前后尿道皆发炎,则二杯中的尿均混浊) / two-tailed ~ 双尾检验,双侧检验(一种假设检验) / unheated serum reagin (USR) ~ 未加热血清反应素试验(一种使用未加热血清 VDRL〈美国性病研究所〉试验的改良,主要用于筛选检查) / urea concentration ~ 脲浓度试验(检肾功能) / Urecholine supersensitivity ~ 乌拉胆碱超敏性反应(检神经源性膀胱) / VDRL [Venereal Disease Research Laboratory] VDRL (美国性病研究所)试验(检梅毒的规范化非梅毒螺旋体抗原的血清学试验,即使用热灭活血清和 VDRL 抗原的玻片絮凝试验) / ventilation ~ 换气试验(测运动时呼气量) / worsted ~ 彩线试验(检色彩视力) / χ^2 ~ 卡方检验(见 chi-squared ~) / D-xylose absorption ~, D-xylose tolerance ~ D-木糖吸收试验,D-木糖耐量试验(吸收不良综合征的鉴别诊断)

testa [ˈtestə] *n*【拉】壳,甲壳,介壳

Testacea [tesˈteiʃiə] *n* 有壳目

Testacealobosia [ˌtestəˌsiːələuˈbəusiə] *n* 壳叶亚纲

testacean [tesˈteiʃiən] *n*, *a* 壳叶[原]虫(的)

testaceous [tesˈteiʃiəs] *a* 有壳的,有介壳的,有甲壳的

Testacida [tesˈtæsidə] *n* 有壳目

testalgia [tesˈtældʒiə] *n* 睾丸痛

testate [ˈtesteit] *a* 有壳的(指壳叶亚纲阿米巴样原虫)

test card [test kɑːd] 视力卡 | stigmometric ~ ~ 文盲视力卡

testectomy [tesˈtektəmi] *n* 睾丸切除术

testee [tesˈtiː] *n* 受测验者,测验对象

tester [ˈtestə] *n* 试验者;检验器,测试器;(试验用的)对照物

testes [ˈtestiːz] testis 的复数

testicle [ˈtestikl] *n* 睾丸 | **testicular** [tesˈtikjulə] *a*

testicond [ˈtestikənd] *a* 隐睾的,睾丸未降的

testicular nucleic acid [tesˈtikjulə] 睾丸核酸

testiculate [tesˈtikjuleit] *a* 睾丸状的

testiculoma [tesˌtikjuˈləumə] *n* 男性细胞瘤,男胚瘤

testiculus [tesˈtikjuləs] ([复] **testiculi** [tesˈtikjulai]) *n*【拉】睾丸

testing [ˈtestiŋ] *n* 鉴定 | reality ~ 真实性鉴定

testis [ˈtestis] ([复] **testes** [ˈtestiːz]) *n*【拉】睾丸 | ectopic ~ 异位睾丸 / inverted ~ 睾丸反向 / ~ muliebris 卵巢 / obstructed ~ 睾丸受阻 / pulpy ~ 髓样睾丸 / retained ~, undescended ~ 隐睾,睾丸未降

testitis [tesˈtaitis] *n* 睾丸炎

testitoxicosis [ˌtestiˌtɔksiˈkəusis] *n* 睾丸中毒症

Testivin's sign [testiˈven] (G. Testivin) 特斯替文征(从尿中除去白蛋白,加酸处理,再加上 1/3 尿量的乙醚之后可形成一层火棉胶样表膜,据称可见于传染病的潜伏期)

test letter [test ˈletə] 视力标型,视力表

test meal [test ˈmiːl] 试验餐 | motor ~ ~ 胃肠运动试验餐

testoid [ˈtestɔid] *n* 睾丸激素[类]

testolactone [ˌtestəuˈlæktəun] *n* 睾内酯(抗赘生物类固醇)

testopathy [tesˈtɔpəθi] *n* 睾丸病

testosterone [tesˈtɔstərəun] *n* 睾酮,睾丸素 | ~ cyclopentylpropionate, ~ cypionate 环戊丙酸睾酮,睾酮环戊丙酸酯 / ~ enanthate, ~ heptanoate 庚酸睾酮 / ethinyl ~ 乙炔基睾酮 / ~ ketolaurate 睾酮十二酮酸酯,癸酰乙酸睾酮 / methyl ~ 甲睾酮,甲基睾酮,甲基睾丸素 / ~ phenylacetate 苯乙酸睾酮,苯乙酸睾丸素 / ~ propionate 丙酸睾酮,丙酸睾丸素

testosterone 17 β-dehydrogenase (NADP⁺) [tesˈtɔstərəun diːˈhaidrədʒəneis] 睾酮 17β-脱氢酶($NADP^+$)(此酶缺乏为一种常染色体隐性性状,可称为 17β-羟甾类脱氢酶缺乏症。亦称 17β-羟甾类脱氢酶,17β-酮甾类还原酶)

testotoxicosis [ˌtestəuˌtɔksiˈkəusis] *n* 睾酮中毒[症](一型男性性早熟,约 3 岁时发生,由于循环睾酮过量所致,为常染色体显性遗传,患者通常具有如成人一样的正常生育力)

test-tube [ˈtesttjuːb] *a* 试管的;在试管中发育(或生长)的;由人工授精而生长的

test type [test taip] 视力标型,视力表

TET treadmill exercise test 跑台运动试验; tubal embryo transfer 输卵管胚胎移植

tetanal [ˈtetənəl] *a* 破伤风的

tetania [tiˈteiniə] *n*【拉】手足搐搦;[肌]强直

tetanic [tiˈtænik] *a* 破伤风的;强直性的

tetaniform [tiˈtænifɔːm] *a* 破伤风样的;强直样的

tetanigenous [ˌtetəˈnidʒinəs] *a* 致破伤风的;致强直的

tetanilla [ˌtetəˈnilə] *n* 无强直手足搐搦;多发性肌阵挛

tetanism [ˈtetənizəm] *n* 破伤风样病,假破伤风

tetanization [ˌtetənaiˈzeiʃən, -niˈz-] *n* 促强直作用,致强直[作用]

tetanize [ˈtetənaiz] *vt* 使强直,致强直

tetanocannabin [ˌtetənəuˈkænəbin] *n* 大麻强直素

tetanode [ˈtetənəud] *n* 手足搐搦静止期

tetanoid [ˈtetənɔid] *a* 破伤风样的;强直样的

tetanolysin [ˌtetəˈnɔlisin] *n* 破伤风[菌]溶血素

tetanometer [ˌtetəˈnɔmitə] *n* 强直测验计

tetanospasmin [ˌtetənəuˈspæzmin] *n* 破伤风[菌]痉挛毒素

tetanus [ˈtetənəs] *n* 破伤风;[肌]强直 | acoustic ~ 听性强直(蛙肌) / anodal closure ~ 阳极通电强直 / anodal opening ~ 阳极断电强直 / apyretic ~ 手足搐搦 / cathodal closure ~ 阴极通电强直 / cathodal opening ~ 阴极断电强直 / cephalic ~ 头部破伤风 / cerebral ~ 脑破伤风 / cryptogenic ~ 隐原性破伤风 / drug ~ 药物性强直 / flexor ~ 屈肌强直 / intermittent ~ 手足搐搦,间歇性强直 / postserum ~ 血清注射后破伤风 / puerperal ~, uterine ~ 产后破伤风

tetany [ˈtetəni] *n* 手足搐搦;[肌]强直 | duration ~ 通电期间强直 / gastric ~ 胃病性手足搐搦 / hyperventilation ~ 过度呼吸性手足搐搦 / latent ~ 潜在性手足搐搦(在电或机械性刺激时出现的手足搐搦) / parathyroid ~, parathyroprival ~ 甲状旁腺缺乏性手足搐搦

tetartanope [teˈtɑːtənəup] *n* 象限盲者,四分之一盲者;蓝黄色盲者,第四型色盲者

tetartanopia [ˌtetɑːtəˈnəupiə], **tetartanopsia** [ˌtetɑːtəˈnɔpsiə] *n* 象限盲,四分之一盲;蓝黄色盲,第四型色盲 | **tetartanopic** [ˌtetɑːtəˈnɔpik] *a*

tetartocone [tiˈtɑːtəkəun], **tetarcone** [ˈtetɑːkəun] *n* 上后内尖,上颌双尖牙后内尖

tetartoconid [tiˌtɑːtəˈkəunid] *n* 下后内尖,下颌双尖牙后内尖

tetia [ˈtiːtiə] *n* 雅司病(即 yaws)

tetiothalein sodium [ˌtiːʃiəˈθæliːn] 四碘酚酞钠(造影剂)

tetmil [ˈtetmil] *n* 十毫米(度量单位)

tetra- [构词成分]四

tetra-amylose [ˌtetrəˈæmiləus] *n* 四戊基糖,四直链淀粉

tetrabasic [ˌtetrəˈbeisik] *a* 四碱价的,四元的

tetrablastic [ˌtetrəˈblæstik] *a* 四胚层的

tetraboric acid [ˌtetrəˈbɔːrik] 四硼酸,焦硼酸

tetrabrachius [ˌtetrəˈbreikiəs] *n* 四臂畸胎

tetrabromofluorescein [ˌtetrəˌbrəuməuˌfluəˈresiːn] *n* 四溴荧光素,曙红

tetrabromophenolphthalein [ˌtetrəˌbrəuməuˌfiːnɔlˈθæliːn] *n* 四溴酚酞(指示剂)

tetrabromophthalein sodium [ˌtetrəˌbrəuməu-ˈθæliːn] 四溴酚酞钠(胆囊造影剂)

tetracaine [ˈtetrəkein] *n* 丁卡因(局部麻醉药) | ~ hydrochloride 盐酸丁卡因(局部或表面麻醉药)

tetracetate [teˈtræsiteit] *n* 四乙酸盐

tetrachirus [ˌtetrəˈkaiərəs] *n* 四手畸胎

tetrachlorethane [ˌtetrəklɔːˈreθein] *n* 四氯乙烷(抗蠕虫药,亦用作溶剂和干洗时使用)

tetrachloride [ˌtetrəˈklɔːraid] *n* 四氯化物

tetrachlormethane [ˌtetrəklɔːˈmeθein] *n* 四氯甲烷,四氯化碳

2, 3, 7, 8-tetrachlorodibenzo-*p*-dioxin (TCDD) [ˌtetrəˌklɔːrəudaiˌbenzəu daiˈɔksin] 2, 3, 7, 8-四氯二苯并对二噁英(一种使除莠剂 2, 4, 5-T 污染的致畸和致癌的二噁英)

tetrachloroethane [ˌtetrəˌklɔːrəuˈeθein] *n* 四氯乙烷(一种毒害肝细胞的工业溶剂)

tetrachloroethylene [ˌtetrəˌklɔːrəˈeθiliːn] *n* 四氯乙烯(抗蠕虫药)

tetrachlorphenoxide [ˌtetrəˌklɔːfəˈnɔksaid] *n* 四氯苯酚(杀真菌剂)

tetrachromic [ˌtetrəˈkrəumik] *a* 四色的;四色视的

tetracid [ˈtetræsid] *a* 四[价]酸的 *n* 四[价]酸

tetracosanoic acid [ˌtetrəˌkəusəˈnəuik] 二十四[烷]酸

tetracrotic [ˌtetrəˈkrɔtik] *a* 四波[脉]的

tetracyclic [ˌtetrəˈsiklik] *a* 四环的

tetracycline [ˌtetrəˈsaiklin] *n* 四环素(抗生素类药) | ~ phosphate complex 四环素磷酸复盐(抗菌药)

tetrad [ˈtetræd] *n* 四价元素;四分体(染色体);四裂体(细菌);四联症

tetradactyly [ˌtetrəˈdæktili] *n* 四指[畸形],四趾[畸形] | **tetradactylous** *a*

tetradecanoate [ˌtetrəˌdekəˈnəueit] *n* 十四[烷]酸盐,肉豆蔻酸盐

tetradecanoyl phorbol acetate [ˌtetrəˈdekənɔil ˈfɔːbɔl ˈæsiteit] 十四[烷]酰佛波醇乙酸酯(一种佛波醇酯,为一种促癌物,用于促使实验动物生长皮肤癌)

tetradeconic acid [ˌtetrədiˈkɔnik] 十四[烷]酸,肉豆蔻酸

-tetraene [后缀]四烯

tetraerythrin [ˌtetrəˈeriθrin] *n* 四红素,甲壳红素

tetraethylammonium [ˌtetrəˌeθiləˈməuniəm] *n* 四乙铵

tetraethylpyrophosphate (TEPP) [ˌtetrəˌeθilˌpairəuˈfɔsfeik] *n* 焦磷酸四乙酯,特普(杀虫剂)

tetraethylthiuram disuifide [ˌtetrəˌeθilˈθaijuəˌræm] 二硫化四乙基秋兰姆(即双硫仑 disulfiram,抗乙醇中毒药)

tetragon [ˈtetrəgən], **tetragonum** [ˌtetrəˈgəunəm] *n* 方形,四边形

tetragonal [teˈtrægənl] *a* 四角形的,四边形的

tetragonus [ˌtetrəˈgəunəs] *n* 颈阔肌

tetrahedral [ˌtetrəˈhedrəl] *a* 有四面的,四面体的

tetrahedron [ˌtetrəˈhedrən] ([复] **tetrahedrons** 或 **tetrahedra** [ˌtetrəˈhedrə]) *n* 四面体

tetrahydric [ˌtetrəˈhaidrik] *a* 四氢的

tetrahydrobiopterin [ˌtetrəˌhaidrəubaiˈɔptərin] *n* 四氢生物蝶呤(可致恶性高苯丙氨血症)
tetrahydrocannabinol (**THC**) [ˌtetrəˌhaidrəu-kəˈnæbinɔl] *n* 四氢大麻酚(拟精神病药)
tetrahydrofolate (**THF**) [ˌtetrəˌhaidəˈfəuleit] *n* 四氢叶酸酯,四氢叶酸
tetrahydrofolic acid (**THF**) [ˌtetrəˌhaidrəˈfəu-lik] 四氢叶酸
tetrahydropalmatine [ˌtetrəˌhaidrəuˈpælmətin] *n* 四氢帕马丁(镇痛药)
tetrahydropteroylglutamate methyltransferase [ˌtetrəˌhaidrəˌterɔilˈgluːtəmeitˌmeθilˈtrænsfəreis] 四氢蝶酰[基]谷氨酸甲基转移酶,5-甲基四氢叶酸-高半胱氨酸甲基转移酶
tetrahydropteroylglutamic acid [ˌtetrəˌhaidr-əuˌterɔilgluːˈtæmik] 四氢蝶酰谷氨酸,四氢叶酸
tetrahydrozoline hydrochloride [ˌtetrəhaiˈdr-ɔzəliːn] 盐酸四氢唑啉(肾上腺素能药,局部用于鼻黏膜,并用于结膜,促使血管收缩)
Tetrahymena [ˌtetrəˈhaimenə] *n* 四膜虫属 | ~ pyriformis 梨形四膜虫
Tetrahymenina [ˌtetrəˌhaiməˈnainə] *n* 四膜虫亚目
tetraiodoethylene [ˌtetrəˌaiədəuˈeθiliːn] *n* 四碘乙烯,二碘仿
tetraiodophenolphthalein [ˌtetrəˌaiədəuˌfiːnɔl-ˈθæliːn] *n* 四碘酚酞(胆囊造影剂)
tetraiodophthalein sodium [ˌtetrəˌaiədəuˈθæ-liːn] 四碘酚酞钠
L-3, 5, 3′, 5′-tetraiodothyronine [ˌtetrəˌaiə-dəuˈθaiərəniːn] *n* 四碘甲腺原氨酸,甲状腺素
tetralogy [teˈtrælədʒi] *n* 四联症
tetramastigote [ˌtetrəˈmæstigəut] *a* 四鞭毛的 *n* 四鞭毛体
tetramazia [ˌtetrəˈmeiziə] *n* 四乳[畸形]
tetramer [ˈtetrəˌmə] *n* 四聚物,四聚体
Tetrameres [teˈtræməriːz] *n* 四棱线虫属 | ~ americana 美洲四棱线虫
tetrameric [ˌtetrəˈmerik], **tetramerous** [teˈtr-æmərəs] *a* 四部[分]的
tetramethyl [ˌtetrəˈmeθil] *n* 四甲基
tetramethylammonium hydroxide [ˌtetrəˌmeθ-iləˈməunjəm] *n* 羟化四甲铵
tetramethylbenzidine [ˌtetrəˌmeθilˈbenzidiːn] *n* 四甲联苯胺(联苯胺类似物,用作色原,在生化测定中检测辣根过氧化物酶活性)
tetramethylenediamine [ˌtetrəˌmeθiliːnˈdaiə-miːn] *n* 丁二胺,腐胺
tetramethylputrescine [tetrəˌmeθilpjuˈtresin] *n* 四甲基腐胺,四甲烯四甲基二胺
tetramethyluric acid [ˌtetrəˌmeθiˈljuərik] 四甲基尿酸
tetramine [ˈtetrəmiːn] *n* 羟化四甲铵
tetramisole hydrochloride [teˈtræmisəul] 盐酸四咪唑(抗蠕虫药)
Tetramitus mesnili [teˈtræmitəs mesˈnaili] 迈氏四鞭毛虫(即迈氏唇鞭毛虫 Chilomastix mesnili)
tetramylose [teˈtræmiləus] *n* 四戊基糖,四直链淀粉
tetranitrol [ˌtetrəˈnaitrɔl] *n* 丁四硝酯(即 erythrityl tetranitrate,抗心绞痛药,血管扩张药)
tetranophthalmos [ˌtetrənɔfˈθælmɔs] *n* 四眼畸胎
tetranopsia [ˌtetrəˈnɔpsiə] *n* 象限盲,四分之一盲
tetranucleotide [ˌtetrəˈnjuːkliətaid] *n* 四核苷酸,核酸
Tetranychus [teˈtrænikəs] *n* 叶螨属 | ~ autumnalis 秋恙螨(即 Trombicula autumnalis) / ~ molestissimus 剧扰叶螨 / ~ telarius 棉红叶螨
Tetraodon [ˌtetrəˈəudɔn] *n* 鲀属
Tetraodontoidea [ˌtetrəɔdɔnˈtɔidiə] *n* 河豚亚目,鲀亚目
tetraodontoxin [teˌtrelədɔnˈtɔksin] *n* 河豚毒素,河鲀毒素
tetraodontoxism [teˌtreiədɔnˈtɔksizəm] *n* 河豚中毒,河鲀中毒
tetraotus [ˌtetrəˈəutəs] *n* 四耳畸胎
tetraparesis [ˌtetrəˈpærisis] *n* 四肢轻瘫
tetrapeptide [ˌtetrəˈpeptid] *n* 四肽
Tetraphyllidea [ˌtetrəfiˈlidiə] *n* 四叶[绦虫]目
tetraplegia [ˌtetrəˈpliːdʒiə] *n* 四肢麻痹,四肢瘫
tetraploid [ˈtetrəplɔid] *a* 四倍的 *n* 四倍体(指一个个体或细胞具有四整套染色体) | **~y** *n* 四倍性
tetrapodisis [ˌtetrəpəuˈdaisis] *n* 四足行动
tetrapus [ˈtetrəpəs] *n* 四足畸胎
tetrapyrrole [ˈtetrəpiˌrəul] *n* 四吡咯
tetrasaccharide [ˌtetrəˈsækəraid] *n* 四糖
tetrascelus [teˈtræsiləs] *n* 四腿畸胎
tetrasomic [ˌtetrəˈsəumik] *a* 二倍加二的,四[染色]体的
tetrasomy [ˈtetrəˌsəumi] *n* 四[染色]体性
tetraspore [ˈtetrəspɔː] *n* 四分孢子
tetraster [teˈtræstə] *n* 四星体
tetrastichiasis [ˌtetrəstiˈkaiəsis] *n* 四列睫,四行睫
tetratomic [ˌtetrəˈtɔmik] *a* 四原子的;四羟[基]的
tetratrichomonas buccalis [ˌtetrətriˈkɔmənəs bəˈkeilis] 口腔[四]毛滴虫(即 Trichomonas tenax)
tetravaccine [ˌtetrəˈvæksiːn] *n* 四联疫苗,四联菌苗(含有伤寒杆菌、副伤寒杆菌甲和乙以及霍乱弧菌死菌液所制成的疫苗)

tetravalent [te'trævələnt] *a* 四价的
tetrodonic acid [ˌtetrə'dɔnik] 河鲀酸,河豚酸
tetrodotoxin [ˌtetrədə'tɔksin] *n* 河鲀毒素
tetrodotoxism [ˌtetrədə'tɔksizəm] *n* 河鲀中毒,河豚中毒
tetrofosmin [ˌtetrəu'fɔzmin] *n* 替曲膦(一种膦,与^{99m}Tc 标记时用于心肌灌注成像)
tetronal ['tetrənl] *n* 特妥那(催眠药)
tetronerythrin [ˌtetrə'neriθrin] *n* 羽毛红素
tetrophthalmos [ˌtetrɔf'θælmɔs] *n* 四眼畸胎
tetrose ['tetrəus] *n* 丁糖
tetrotus [te'trəutəs] *n* 四耳畸胎
tetroxide [te'trɔksaid] *n* 四氧化物
tetrulose ['tetruːləus] *n* 酮丁糖
tetrydamine [te'traidəmiːn] *n* 四氢甲吲胺(镇痛、抗炎药)
tetryl ['tetril] *n* 三硝基苯甲硝胺(可致工业性皮炎)
tetter ['tetə] *n* 皮肤病(俗名);动物痒症(传染人的畜类皮肤病) | milky ~ 乳痂,婴儿头皮脂溢
tetterwort ['tetəwət] *n* 血根[草]
teucrin ['tjuːkrin] *n* 石蚕苷
Teucrium ['tjuːkriəm] *n* 石蚕属
Teutleben's ligament ['tɔitləbən] (Friedrich Ernst Karl von Teutleben) 肺韧带
teutlose ['tjuːtləus] *n* 甜菜根糖
tewfikose ['tjuːfikəus] *n* 埃及牛乳糖
texis ['teksis] *n*【拉;希】分娩,生产
textiform ['tekstifɔːm] *a* 网状的;组织状的
textoblastic [ˌtekstəu'blæstik] *a* 生成新组织的,再生的
textometer [ˌtekstəu'miːtə] *n* 原生质,原浆
Textulariina [ˌtekstjulə'raiinə] *n* 织虫亚目
texture ['tekstʃə] *n* 结构,质地,组织;肌理 | **textural** *a*
textus ['tekstəs] *n*【拉】组织
TF transfer factor 转移因子;tuberculin filtrate 结核菌素滤液
6-TG 6-thioguanine 硫鸟嘌呤,6-硫鸟嘌呤(抗肿瘤药)
TGF transforming growth factor 转化生长因子
T-group training group 训练组
TGT thromboplastin generation test 凝血激酶生成试验
Th thorium 钍
THA total hip arthroplasty 全髋关节成形术
thalamectomy [ˌθælə'mektəmi] *n* 丘脑破坏法
thalamencephalon [ˌθæləmen'sefələn] *n* 丘脑 | **thalamencephalic** [ˌθæləˌmense'fælik] *a*
thalami ['θæləmai] thalamus 的复数
thalamic [θə'læmik] *a* 丘脑的
thalamocoele ['θæləməuˌsiːl] *n* 丘脑室,第三脑室
thalamocortical [ˌθæləməu'kɔːtikəl] *a* 丘脑皮质的
thalamolenticular [ˌθæləməulen'tikjulə] *a* 丘脑豆状核的
thalamomamillary [ˌθæləmə'mæmiləri] *a* 丘脑乳头体的
thalamotegmental [ˌθæləməuteg'mentl] *a* 丘脑被盖的
thalamotomy [ˌθælə'mɔtəmi] *n* 丘脑切开术 | anterior ~ 丘脑前核切开术 / dorsomedial ~ 丘脑背内侧核切开术
thalamus ['θæləməs] ([复] **thalami** ['θæləmai]) *n*【拉】丘脑
thalassanemia [θəˌlæsə'niːmiə] *n* 珠蛋白生成障碍性贫血,地中海贫血
thalassemia [ˌθælə'siːmiə] *n* 珠蛋白生成障碍性贫血,地中海贫血 | *α*- ~ *α*-珠蛋白生成障碍性贫血 / *β*- ~ *β*-珠蛋白生成障碍性贫血 / *δ*- ~ *δ*-地中海贫血 / hemoglobin C- ~ 血红蛋白 C 珠蛋白生成障碍性贫血 / hemoglobin E- ~ 血红蛋白 E 珠蛋白生成障碍性贫血 / hemoglobin S- ~ 血红蛋白 S 珠蛋白生成障碍性贫血 / ~ intermedia 中间型珠蛋白生成障碍性贫血 / sickle cell- ~ 镰状细胞珠蛋白生成障碍性贫血 / ~ major 重型珠蛋白生成障碍性贫血 / ~ minor 轻型珠蛋白生成障碍性贫血
thalassin [θə'læsin] *n* 海葵素
thalassoposia [θəˌlæsəu'pəuziə] *n* 饮[用]海水
thalassotherapy [θəˌlæsəu'θerəpi] *n* 海水浴疗法;海滨治疗
thalgrain ['θælgrein] *n* 铊谷(谷类中混入硫酸铊,杀鼠类药)
thalidomide [θə'lidəmaid] *n* 沙利度胺(催眠镇静药,20 世纪 50 年代和 60 年代初在欧洲广泛使用,但妊娠早期妇女服后引起胎儿畸形,故不再使用。本品对缓解急性麻风反应伴随而来的剧痛十分有效,但孕妇不宜)
thalleioquin [θə'laiəkwin] *n* 奎宁绿脂(奎宁试验时所产生的一种绿色树脂物质)
thallic ['θælik] *a* 铊的,三价铊的
thallitoxicosis [ˌθæliˌtɔksi'kəusis], **thallotoxicosis** [ˌθæləˌtɔksi'kəusis] *n* 铊中毒
thallium (Tl) ['θæliəm] *n* 铊(化学元素) | ~ 201 ^{201}Tl,铊 201(以氯化亚铊〈thallous chloride〉形式用作诊断辅助药)
thall(o)- [构词成分]枝,芽;叶状体;铊
Thallobacteria [ˌθailəubæk'tiəriə] *n* 叶状菌纲
Thallophyta [θə'lɔfitə] *n* 菌藻植物类,叶状植物类
thallophyte ['θæləfait] *n* 菌藻植物,叶状植物
thallospore ['θæləspɔː] *n* 原植体孢子,无梗孢

子,菌丝孢子

thallous [ˈθæləs] *a* 亚铊的,一价铊的

thallous chloride Tl 201 [ˈθæləs] 氯化亚^{201}Tl(静脉注射用于闪烁扫描,辅助诊断心脏病,亦称 thallium chloride 〈^{201}Tl Cl〉)

thallus [ˈθæləs] *n* 原植体;菌体

thalposis [θælˈpəusis] *n* 温觉 | **thalpotic** [θælˈpɔtik] *a*

Thal procedure [θæl] (Alan P. Thal) 萨尔手术(小于食管下段整个周缘的胃底折叠术,以纠正良性狭窄或胃食管反流)

THAM tromethamine, tris (hydroxymethyl) aminomethane 氨丁三醇,缓血酸胺,三羟甲基氨基甲烷(碱化剂,静脉注射矫治代谢性酸中毒)

Thamnidiaceae [θæmˌnidiˈeisiiː] *n* 枝霉科

Thamnidium [θæmˈnidiəm] *n* 枝霉属

thamuria [θæˈmjuəriə] *n* 频尿

thanat(o)- [构词成分]死

thanatobiologic [ˌθænətəuˌbaiəˈlɔdʒik] *a* 死[与]生的

thanatognomonic [ˌθænətəunəuˈmɔnik] *a* 死征的

thanatoid [ˈθænətɔid] *a* 似死的,假死的

thanatology [ˌθænəˈtɔlədʒi] *n* 死亡学

thanatometer [ˌθænəˈtɔmitə] *n* 检尸温度计

thanatophidia [ˌθænətəˈfidiə] *n* 毒蛇(总称) | **~l** *a*

thanatophoric [ˌθænətəuˈfɔrik] *a* 致命的,致死的

thanatopsia [ˌθænəˈtɔpsiə], **thanatopsy** [ˈθænəˌtɔpsi] *n* 尸体剖检

thanatosis [ˌθænəˈtəusis] *n* 坏死,坏疽

Thane's method [θein] (George D. Thane) 塞因法,(大脑)中央沟定位法

Thapsia [ˈθæpsiə] *n* 【拉;希】毒胡萝卜属

thapsic acid [ˈθæpsik] 十六碳二酸

thaumatropy [θɔːˈmætrəpi] *n* 器官转化,结构转化

Thaysen's disease [ˈθaisn] (Thornwald E. H. Thaysen) 非热带口炎性腹泻(肠道吸收不良综合征)

THC tetrahydrocannabinol 四氢大麻酚

thea [θiːə] *n* 【拉】茶

theaism [ˈθiːəizəm] *n* 茶中毒

theatre, theater [ˈθiətə] *n* (阶梯式的)教室,讲堂 | operating ~ 手术示教室,手术示范室

thebaic [θiˈbeiik] *a* 阿片的,鸦片的

thebaine [θiˈbeiin] *n* 蒂巴因,二甲基吗啡

thebesian [θiˈbiːziən] (Adam C. Thebesius) *a* 特贝西乌斯的 | ~ foramen 小静脉孔 / ~ valve 冠状窦瓣 / ~ veins 心最小静脉

thebolactic acid [θibəˈlæktik] 阿片乳酸

theca [ˈθiːkə] ([复] **thecae** [ˈθiːsiː]) *n* 【拉】膜,鞘 | **~l** *a*

thecitis [θiˈsaitis] *n* 腱鞘炎

thecodont [ˈθiːkədɔnt] *a* 牙槽包牙的

thecoma [θiˈkəumə] *n* 泡膜细胞瘤

thecomatosis [ˌθiːkəuməˈtəusis] *n* 泡膜细胞增生症(卵巢基质弥散性增生)

thecostegnosis [ˌθiːkəustegˈnəusis] *n* 腱鞘狭窄

Theden's bandage [ˈteidən] (Johann C. A. Theden) 特登绷带(一种止血绷带)

Theileria [θaiˈliəriə] (Arnold Theiler) *n* 泰累尔梨浆虫属 | ~ lawrencei 劳氏泰累尔梨浆虫 / ~ mutans 突变泰累尔梨浆虫 / ~ ovis 卵形泰累尔梨浆虫

theileriasis [ˌθailəˈraiəsis] *n* 泰累尔梨浆虫病 | tropical ~ 热带泰累尔梨浆虫病(牛的传染病。亦称地中海沿岸热,热带梨浆虫病) | **theileriosis** [θaiˌləriˈəusis] *n*

Theiler's disease [ˈtailə] (Max Theiler) 泰累尔病(鼠特发性脑脊髓炎) | ~ virus 泰累尔病毒(鼠特发性脑脊髓炎病毒)

Theile's canal [ˈtailə] (Friedrich W. Theile) 泰勒管(心包在主动脉和肺动脉起始部反转所形成的腔) | ~ glands 泰勒腺(胆囊盂及胆囊管壁内的腺样形成物) / ~ muscle 会阴浅横肌

Theimich's lip sign [ˈtaimik, -miʃ] (Martin Theimich) 泰米希唇征(轻叩口轮匝肌可引起唇部突出或撅起)

thein(e) [ˈθiːin] *n* 茶碱,咖啡因

theinism [ˈθiːinizəm], **theism** [ˈθiːizəm] *n* 茶中毒

thelalgia [θiːˈlældʒiə] *n* 乳头痛

thelarche [θiːˈlɑːki] *n* 乳房初发育

Thelazia [θiˈleiziə] *n* 吸吮线虫属

thelaziasis [ˌθeləˈzaiəsis] *n* 吸吮线虫病

Thelaziidae [ˌθiːləˈzaiidiː] *n* 吸吮科

thele-, thel(o)- [构词成分]乳头

theleplasty [ˈθiːliˌplæsti] *n* 乳头成形术

thelerethism [θiˈleriθizəm] *n* 乳头膨起

theliolymphocyte [ˌθiːliəuˈlimfəsait] *n* 上皮内淋巴细胞

thelitis [θiːˈlaitis] *n* 乳头炎

thelium [ˈθiːliəm] ([复] **thelia** [ˈθiːliə]) *n* 【拉】乳头

thel(o)- 见 thele-

Thelohania [ˌθiːləˈheiniə] *n* 单孢子虫属

thelorrhagia [ˌθiːləˈreidʒiə] *n* 乳头出血

thelothism [ˈθiːləθizəm], **thelotism** [ˈθiːlətizəm] *n* 乳头膨起

thelyblast [ˈθeliblæst] *n* 雌性原核 | **~ic** [ˌθeliˈblæstik] *a*

thelygenic [ˌθiːliˈdʒenik] *a* 产雌的(只产生雌性后代的)

thelykinin [ˌθiːliˈkainin] *n* 雌酮
thelytocia [ˌθeliˈtəuʃiə], **thelytoky** [θiˈlitəki] *n* 产雌单性生殖(只产生雌性后代的单性生殖) | **thelytocous** [θiˈlitəkəs] *a* 产雌的
thenad [ˈθiːnæd] *ad* 向鱼际,向掌
thenal [ˈθiːnəl] *a* 鱼际的,掌的
thenar [ˈθiːnɑː] *n*【希】鱼际 *a* 鱼际的,掌的
thenium closylate [ˈθeniəm ˈkləusileit] 氯苯磺酸西尼铵(兽用抗蠕虫药)
thenyldiamine hydrochloride [ˌθenilˈdaiəmiːn] 盐酸西尼二胺(抗组胺药)
thenylpyramine [ˌθenilˈpirəmiːn] *n* 噻吩甲吡胺(即美沙吡啉 methapyrilene,抗组胺药)
Theobaldia [ˌθiəˈbɔːldiə] (Frederic V. Theobald) *n* 赛保蚊属(即脉毛蚊属 Culiseta)
Theobroma [ˌθiəˈbrəumə] *n* 可可属
theobromine [ˌθiəˈbrəumiːn] *n* 可可碱(利尿药,平滑肌松弛药,心脏兴奋药,血管扩张药)
theolin [ˈθiəlin] *n* 庚烷
theophylline [ˌθiəˈfilin, θiˈɔfilin] *n* 茶碱(平滑肌松弛药,主要用作利尿药) | ~ aminoisobutanol 氨异丁醇茶碱(即安布茶碱 ambuphylline) / ~ cholinate 胆茶碱 / ~ olamine 茶碱乙醇胺 / ~ sodium glycinate 甘氨茶碱钠(主要用作平滑肌松弛药)
theorem [ˈθiərəm] *n* 定理,原理 | central limit ~ 中心极限定理(关于样本均数分布的定理)
theory [ˈθiəri] *n* 理论,学说 | aging ~ of atherosclerosis 动脉粥样硬化衰老说(认为动脉弱样硬化是衰老的不可避免的结果,因此是一种不可逆过程) / apposition ~ 外积[生长]学说(认为组织生长是由细胞外在存积所致) / avalanche ~ 雪崩学说(传出神经冲动逐渐加强学说) / cell ~ 细胞学说(认为一切生命物质是由细胞组成的,细胞的活动是生命的基本过程) / cell-chain ~ 细胞链学说(神经纤维含有特殊细胞链,而这些细胞与中枢细胞仅为续发性的关联) / clonal deletion ~ 克隆删除学说(对自身抗原具有免疫耐受性的学说,根据免疫细胞的"禁忌克隆",凡与自身抗原起反应的克隆,在胚胎期间一经与抗原接触即被删除。"clonal abortion〈克隆夭折〉","clonal anergy〈克隆反应缺失〉","clonal silencing〈克隆静止〉","clonal purging〈克隆清除〉"这些术语也可用来说明这种现象) / clonal-selection ~ of immunity 免疫克隆选择学说(由伯内特〈Burnet〉提出的一种抗体形成选择学说)。根据此学说,正常个体带有一整套能与一切可能的抗原决定簇起反应的淋巴细胞系。在胚胎时期,凡是能与自身抗原起反应的细胞系一与抗原相接触就被抑制,而在出生后,未被抑制的细胞系与相应抗原接触能改变应答性,表现为增生、形成抗体以及细胞免疫。免疫耐受性是细胞系被抑制的结果。原被抑制了的抗自身抗原的细胞系在以后再度获得活性时,则可导致自身免疫性疾病 / closed circulation ~ 封闭循环学说(解释脾内血液如何由动脉进入静脉窦的学说之一,认为毛细血管直接向静脉窦排空的。亦称快速循环学说) / closed-open circulation ~ 封闭-开放循环学说(认为脾内有开放循环也有封闭循环,例如当脾充血时,脾收缩时的封闭循环即变为开放循环) / contractile ring ~ 收缩环学说(解释分裂细胞中沟形成的学说,根据此学说,分裂细胞的外层中胶质环的收缩〈外层凝胶收缩〉像阿米巴的不动部分,故表面积减少,但实际上在分裂前,表面积却增加 26% 左右) / convergence-projection ~ 会聚投射学说(解释牵涉性痛) / core conductor ~ 核心导体学说(关于电紧张电位及其在神经纤维中伴随电流的形成学说,根据此学说,神经纤维可以看作核心导体,即含有导电液体材料的圆柱体和具有高度电阻的外鞘,周围有一层传导介质) / dualistic ~ 二元论,二元说(认为血细胞来源于两种不同的原始细胞:原始粒细胞与原始淋巴细胞) / ectopic focus ~ 异位病灶学说(心房纤维性颤动是由于从异位病灶迅速排出的结果而引起) / emergency ~ 应急学说(认为在情绪激动、疼痛和机体紧急需要时,肾上腺髓质即能分泌。亦称坎-巴〈Cannon-Bard〉学说) / emigration ~ 白细胞渗出学说(白细胞渗出是炎症的主要特征) / encrustation ~ 包壳学说(Rokitansky 提出的一种学说,认为血液中的纤维蛋白物质沉积在血管内膜的内表面,并认为脂肪变态即在此沉积物中继发形成的) / expanding surface ~ 表面扩张学说(一种细胞分裂学说,认为核质也许从染色体释出,引起两极的细胞扩张。随着极区扩张,赤道即收缩,从而导致细胞分裂) / fast circulation ~ 快速循环学说(即封闭循环学说 closed circulation ~) / gate ~, gate-control ~ 闸门学说,闸门控制学说(损害组织的疼痛刺激所产生的神经冲动,由直径小的 C 纤维和 A-δ 纤维传送到脊髓,在背角突触处由于大直径有髓鞘 A 纤维的同时刺激而被阻滞,因而疼痛冲动不能传至更高级的中枢神经系统,疼痛即受到抑制。亦称闸门假说)/ germ ~ 病菌学说(认为传染病是由微生物引起) / gestalt ~ 格式塔学说,完形心理学 / ground water ~ 地下水学说(病菌通过地下水传播疾病) / humoral ~ 体液学说(一种古代学说,认为身体含有四种体液:血液、黏液、黄胆汁及黑胆汁,此种体液适当调和则健康,不平衡或不规则分布则形成疾病) / information ~ 信息学说(主要通过统计方法对交流信息的特性进行分析的系统,以及对此进行编码、传递、变异、接收和破译的系统) / lateral-chain ~, side-chain ~ 侧链学说(见 Ehrlich's side-chain theory) / ~ of medicine 医学理论 / metabolic ~ of

atherosclerosis 动脉粥样硬化代谢学说(认为动脉粥样硬化是由于脂质代谢,特别是胆固醇代谢紊乱引起的) / mnemic ~ (细胞)记忆印迹学说(认为细胞对外界刺激的影响有遗传的记忆能力。因此经遗传而得到获得性性状) / monophyletic ~, unitarian ~ 一元论,一元说(各种形式的红、白细胞皆来源于一种形式或同一形式的原始血细胞,而各种类型的细胞是经过分化过程产生的) / ~ of mutations 突变说(根据遗传学说,遗传质的变异性有时可能不产生波动性变异,而产生明显的永久性变异,后者如对动物有利,则通过自然选择保存下来,这样永久性的变异称为突变) / open circulation ~ 开放循环学说(解释脾内血液如何由动脉进入静脉窦的学说之一,认为毛细血管直接沟通髓质网状结构,并认为血液是逐渐滤回进入静脉窦的。亦称徐缓循环学说) / open-closed circulation ~ 开放封闭循环学说(见 closed-open circulation ~) / place ~ (听觉)部位学说 / polarization-membrane ~ 极化膜学说(认为活细胞、休止细胞都有半透膜包围,膜上布有一系列电偶极子,负电荷在内表面,正电荷在外表面。当膜的电生理状态完整时,整个膜表面都由电偶极子包围,称为极化) / polyphyletic ~ 多元论,多系学说(认为各种血细胞皆来源于两个以上不同种类的原始〈母〉细胞) / P. O. U. ~ 胎盘卵巢子宫(placenta-ovary-uterus)产生内分泌学说 / quantum ~ 量子论(能量的辐射和吸收发生为一定量,称为量子〈E〉,量子大小不等,其关系式以 $E = h\nu$ 表示之,其中 h 是普朗克〈Planck〉常数,ν 为辐射频率) / recapitulation ~ 重演学说(个体发育重演种系发生,即认为生物在个体发育过程中经历如同其种系生命发展形式从低级到高级所经历的同样连续过程。亦称生物发生律) / recombinational germline ~ 重组种系学说(解释抗体多样性的缘起的学说,据此学说,一个免疫球蛋白链编码的 DNA 是由两个基因通过一次体细胞重组活动而组成的,一个是单一的恒定区基因,另一个则是几百万可变区基因之一。亦称德-贝〈Dreyer and Bennett〉假说) / resonance ~ (听觉)共振学说 / single hit ~ 单击学说(认为补体只须在红细胞表面诱导一个部位的损害,而不是几个部位的损害,即可导致溶血) / sliding filament ~ 肌丝滑行学说(①认为肌纤维的细丝和粗丝在肌收缩时互相滑行而长度不变。②认为纤毛收缩时的纤丝〈微管〉滑行与肌收缩时肌丝滑行的机制相似,见本条①) / slow circulation ~ 徐缓循环学说(即开放循环学说 open circulation ~) / spindle elongation ~ 纺锤体伸长学说(认为纺锤体和星体在细胞分裂中起决定性作用。此学说所依据的观察为细胞在后期的伸长,伴随着赤道皱缩,据信中心是被纺锤小管推开的,因为纺锤体和星体的结构似乎很坚硬) / target ~, hit ~ 靶子学说,击中学说(此学说在于说明电离辐射作用于细胞内某一很小的敏感部位引起的一些生物效应) / thermostat ~ 恒温器学说(认为脑中摄食中枢和饱觉中枢像体温调节中枢一样,也对体温敏感:体温降低使摄食中枢活化,饱觉中枢抑制,而体温升高则对两个中枢的作用相反) / trialistic ~ 三元论,三元说(认为血细胞来源于成原始粒细胞、原始淋巴细胞与单核细胞) / unitary ~ 疾病一元论 / wave ~, undulatory ~ 波动说(认为光、热、电都是以波的形式通过空间传播的)

theotherapy [ˌθiːəˈθerəpi] *n* 宗教疗法

theque [tek] *n*【法】痣细胞团(含黑色素的痣细胞,发生在皮肤的真皮与表皮结合处或完全在真皮处)

therapeusis [ˌθerəˈpjuːsis] *n* 治疗,疗法

therapeutic [ˌθerəˈpjuːtik] *a* 治疗[学]的,疗法的

therapeutics [ˌθerəˈpjuːtiks] *n* 治疗学;疗法,治疗

Theraphosidae [θerəˈfəusidiː] *n* 捕鸟蛛科

therapia [ˌθerəˈpiə] *n*【拉;希】疗法,治疗

therapist [ˈθerəpist], **therapeutist** [ˌθerəˈpjuːtist] *n* 治疗学家

therapy [ˈθerəpi] *n* 疗法,治疗 | anticoagulant ~ 抗凝[血]疗法 / autoserum ~ 自身血清疗法 / beam ~ 光束疗法(光谱疗法;远距镭疗法) / behavior ~ 行为疗法(亦称行为矫正,调整疗法) / biological ~ 生物(制剂)疗法(其中包括应用血清、抗毒素、疫苗及非特异性蛋白) / buffer ~ 缓冲疗法(静脉注射缓冲物质,如碳酸氢钠,其目的在于降低氢离子浓度) / carbon dioxide ~ 二氧化碳[吸入]疗法(一种罕用的休克疗法,治疗孤独的精神病患者) / carbonic ~ 二氧化碳疗法 / collapse ~ 萎陷疗法(治肺结核) / convulsive ~ 惊厥疗法(以诱发惊厥的方法治疗精神病,主要治疗抑郁症。现在几乎普遍使用电惊厥疗法〈ECT〉,即以电流诱发惊厥。惊厥疗法原先是以药物诱导惊厥的,最初用戊四氮 pentylenetrazol〈Metrazol〉,以后则用三氟乙醚 flurothyl〈Indoklon〉。以前称休克疗法) / diathermic ~ 透热疗法 / duplex ~ 二重电疗法,直流中波联合疗法 / electric convulsive ~, electroconvulsive ~ (ECT), electroshock ~ (EST) 电惊厥疗法,电休克治疗 / family ~ 家庭治疗(家庭成员的集体治疗,探索家庭关系以及探索一个以上的家庭成员中有精神病的潜在原因的过程) / gametocyte ~ 灭配子体疗法(消灭疟原虫配子体) / grid ~ (X 线)筛板疗法 / group ~ 集体治疗(一组病人或病人的亲属或病人与亲属间进行的心理治疗,其中包括在一个治疗师指导下利用集体成员间的相互作用以改变个别成员的适应不良行为。亦称集体心理治疗) /

heterovaccine ~ 异种菌苗疗法 / humidification ~ 湿化疗法(用水分过饱和的空气,治疗上、下呼吸道充血状态) / immunization ~ 免疫疗法(用抗血清以及用自动抗原物质如疫苗予以治疗) / immunosuppressive ~ 免疫抑制治疗(应用X线、皮质类甾醇及细胞毒性化学药物抑制对抗原的免疫反应,此法用于各种病情,其中包括自身免疫性疾病、变态反应、多发性骨髓瘤、慢性肾炎以及器官移植) / Indoklon convulsive ~ 三氟乙醚惊厥疗法(见 convulsive ~) / inhalation ~ 吸入疗法(旨在使心肺系统在气体交换方面的病理生理改变恢复正常的治疗,如应用呼吸机、气溶胶生成装置以及氧、氦氧和二氧化碳合剂所作的治疗) / Metrazol shock ~ 戊四氮休克疗法(见 convulsive ~) / narcosis ~ 麻醉疗法(一般用巴比妥盐类药物诱导长时间睡眠〈每日18~20小时,约2周〉以治疗某些剧烈焦虑反应、疲惫和高度激动。亦称睡眠疗法) / nonspecific ~ 非特异性疗法(注射非特异性物质如蛋白、脲、细菌菌苗等,对细胞活性产生全身性和非特异性效应以治传染病) / opsonic ~, bacterial ~ 调理素疗法,细菌疗法(注射菌苗增加血液调理指数的一种非特异性疗法) / organic ~ 器官疗法,内脏制剂疗法 / orthomolecular ~ 正分子治疗(对疾病,尤其是对精神科疾患的治疗,依据的理论为使体内正常存在的物质恢复最适浓度,即可治愈) / pharmacological ~ 药物性惊厥疗法(见 convulsive ~) / physical ~ 物理疗法,理疗 / primal ~ 基本疗法(鼓励病人重温早期创伤性经历的一种心理治疗) / play ~ 游戏疗法(一种心理治疗方法,用于治疗儿童的情绪障碍,病人与治疗师之间的言语交往在很大程度上以游戏来替代) / replacement ~ 补充疗法,补偿疗法(应用机体天然产物或合成代用品补充机体产物的形成不足或缺陷) / sleep ~ 睡眠疗法(即麻醉疗法 narcosis ~) / sparing ~, protective ~ 保护疗法(保护器官,尽可能让它休息,免受损害) / speech ~ 言语矫正法(以特殊方式矫正言语和语言障碍) / subcoma insulin ~ 亚昏迷性胰岛素疗法(应用胰岛素以引起轻度低血糖、镇静和体重增加,过去曾以此法治疗神经症性疾患和精神分裂症) / suggestion ~ 暗示疗法(以催眠暗示治病) / thread burial ~ 埋线疗法 / zone ~ 体区疗法(身体疾病区域作机械性刺激)

Theria [ˈθiəriə] *n* 兽亚纲

theriaca [θiˈraiəkə], **theriac** [ˈθeriæk] *n* 解毒糖剂

theriatrics [ˌθiriˈætriks] *n* 兽医学

Theridiidae [ˌθeriˈdaiidiː] *n* 球腹蛛科

theriogenology [ˌθiriˌəudʒəˈnɔlədʒi] *n* 动物生殖学(兽医学的一门学科) | **theriogenologic(al)** [ˌθiriəuˌdʒenəˈlɔdʒik(əl)] *a* | **theriogenologist** *n* 动物生殖学家

theriotherapy [ˌθiəriəuˈθerəpi] *n* 动物病疗法

therm [θəːm] *n* 克卡(旧热单位,即小卡);千卡(旧热单位,即大卡)

thermacogenesis [ˌθəːməkəuˈdʒenisis] *n* (药物)促体温上升作用

thermae [ˈθəːmi] *n*【拉】温泉;温泉疗养院

thermaerotherapy [θəːˌmɛərəuˈθerəpi] *n* 热汽疗法

thermal [ˈθəːməl] *a* 热的,热量的

thermalgesia [ˌθəːmælˈdʒiːzjə] *n* 热性痛觉

thermalgia [θəːˈmældʒiə] *n* 灼痛

thermanalgesia [ˌθəːmænælˈdʒiːzjə] *n* 热性痛觉缺失

thermanesthesia [ˌθəːmænesˈθiːzjə] *n* 温度觉缺失

thermatology [ˌθəːməˈtɔlədʒi] *n* 热疗学

thermel [ˈθəːmel] *n* 热电温度计

thermelometer [ˌθəːmeˈlɔmitə] *n* 电热温度计

thermesthesia [ˌθəːmesˈθiːzjə] *n* 温度觉

thermesthesiometer [ˌθəːmesˌθiːziˈɔmitə] *n* 温度觉测量器

thermhyperesthesia [ˌθəːmhaipəresˈθiːzjə] *n* 温度感过敏

thermhypesthesia [ˌθəːmhaipesˈθiːzjə] *n* 温度觉迟钝

thermic [ˈθəːmik] *a* 热的

thermion [ˈθəːmiən] *n* 热离子,热电子 | **~ic** [ˌθəːmiˈɔnik] *a*

thermionics [ˌθəːmiˈɔniks] *n* 热离子学

thermistor [θəːˈmistə] *n* 热敏电阻,热变电阻器

therm(o)- [构词成分]热,温

Thermoactinomyces [ˌθəːməuˌæktinəuˈmaisiːz] *n* 热放线菌属 | ~ vulgaris 普通热放线菌

thermoaesthesia [ˌθəːməuesˈθiːzjə] *n* 温度觉

thermoalgesia [ˌθəːməuælˈdʒiːzjə] *n* 热性痛觉

thermoanalgesia [ˌθəːməuænælˈdʒizjə] *n* 热性痛觉缺失

thermoanesthesia [ˌθəːməuˌænesˈθiːzjə] *n* 温度觉缺失

thermocauterectomy [ˌθəːməukɔːtəˈrektəmi] *n* 烙除法

thermocautery [ˌθəːməuˈkɔːtəri] *n* 热烙器

thermochemistry [ˌθəːməuˈkemistri] *n* 热化学 | **thermochemical** *a*

thermochroic [ˌθəːməuˈkrəuik] *a* 反射热线的,选吸热线的

thermochroism [θəːˈmɔkrəizəm], **thermochrosis** [θəːməuˈkrəusis] *n* 反射热线[作用],选吸热线[作用]

thermocoagulation [ˌθəːməukəuˌægjuˈleiʃən] *n* 热凝固术

thermocouple [ˈθəːməuˌkʌpl] *n* 温差电偶，热电偶
thermocurrent [ˌθəːməuˈkʌrənt] *n* 热电流
thermodiffusion [ˌθəːməudiˈfjuːʒən] *n* 热扩散
thermodilution [ˌθəːməudaiˈljuːʃən] *n* 热稀释法（测心室血容量和心排血量）
thermoduric [ˌθəːməuˈdjuərik] *a* 耐热的
thermodynamic [ˌθəːməudaiˈnæmik] *a* 热力[学]的
thermodynamics [ˌθəːməudaiˈnæmiks] *n* 热力学
thermoelectric [ˌθəːməuiˈlektrik] *a* 温差电的，热电的 ǀ **~ity** [ˌθəːməuilekˈtrisəti] *n*
thermoelectron [ˈθəːməuiˈlektrɔn] *n* 热电子
thermoelement [ˈθəːməuˈelimənt] *n* 温差电偶，热电偶
thermoesthesia [ˌθəːməuesˈθiːzjə] *n* 温度觉
thermoesthesiometer [ˌθəːməuesˌθiːziˈɔmitə] *n* 温度觉测量器
thermoexicitory [ˌθəːməuekˈsaitəri] *a* 刺激生热的
thermogenesis [ˌθəːməuˈdʒenisis] *n* 生热，生热作用 ǀ **thermogenetic** [ˌθəːməudʒiˈnetik]，**thermogenic** [ˌθəːməuˈdʒenik]，**thermogenous** [θəːˈmɔdʒinəs] *a*
thermogenics [ˌθəːməuˈdʒeniks] *n* 生热学
thermogenin [θəˈmɔdʒənin] *n* 生热蛋白，解偶联蛋白
thermogram [ˈθəːməgræm] *n* 温度记录图，温谱图；热像图
thermograph [ˈθəːməgrɑːf] *n* 温度图仪，温度记录器；热像图；温度描记器 ǀ continuous scan ~ 连续扫描温度记录器 ǀ **~y** [θəːˈmɔgrəfi] *n* 温度记录法，发热记录法，热像图检查法（如用于诊断乳腺肿瘤）/ **~ic** [ˌθəːməuˈgræfik] *a* 温度记录器的；热像图的；温度记录法的，热像图检查法的
thermogravimeter [ˌθəːməugrəˈvimitə] *n* 热解重量分析计
thermohyperalgesia [ˌθəːməuˌhaipərælˈdʒiːzjə] *n* 热性痛觉过敏
thermohyperesthesia [ˌθəːməuˌhaipəresˈθiːzjə] *n* 温度觉过敏
thermohypesthesia [ˌθəːməuˌhaipesˈθiːzjə]，**thermohypoesthesia** [ˌθəːməuˌhaipəuesˈθiːzjə] *n* 温度觉减退
thermoinactivation [ˌθəːməuinˌæktiˈveiʃən] *n* 热灭活法
thermoinhibitory [ˌθəːməuinˈhibitəri] *a* 抑制生热的
thermointegrator [ˌθəːməuˈintigreitə] *n* 体表温度测量器
thermolabile [ˌθəːməuˈleibail] *a* 不耐热的
thermolamp [ˈθəːməulæmp] *n* 热灯（用于热疗法）
thermolaryngoscope [ˌθəːməuləˈriŋgəskəup] *n* 电热喉镜
thermology [θəːˈmɔlədʒi] *n* 热学
thermoluminescence [ˌθəːməuljuːmiˈnesns] *n* 热致发光
thermolysis [θəˈmɔlisis] *n* 热解[作用]；散热[作用]（通过辐射、蒸发等）ǀ **thermolytic** [ˌθəːməuˈlitik] *a*
thermomagnetic [ˌθəːməumægˈnetik] *a* 热磁的
thermomassage [ˌθəːməuˈmæsɑːʒ] *n* 热按摩法
thermomastography [ˌθəːməumæsˈtɔgrəfi] *n* 乳房热图描记[术]（诊断乳房病变）
thermometer [θəˈmɔmitə] *n* 温度计，温度表 ǀ bimetal ~ 双金属温度计 / centigrade ~ 百分温度计，摄氏温度计 / clinical ~ 体温计 / differential ~ 差示温度计 / gas ~ 气体温度计 / kata ~ 干湿球温度计 / liquid-in-glass ~ 液测温度计 / metastatic ~ 易位温度计 / oral ~ 口腔温度计，口表 / recording ~，self-registering ~ 自记温度计 / rectal ~ 直肠温度计，肛表 / resistance ~ 电阻温度计 / thermocouple ~ 热电偶温度计
thermometric [ˌθəːməuˈmetrik] *a* 温度计的；温度测量的，测温的
thermometry [θəˈmɔmitri] *n* 温度测量法
Thermomicrobium [ˌθəːməumaiˈkrəubiəm] *n* 热菌属
Thermomonospora [ˌθəːməuməuˈnɔspɔrə] *n* 热单孢菌属
thermoneurosis [ˌθəːməunjuəˈrəusis] *n* 神经性发热
thermonuclear [ˌθəːməuˈnjuːkliə] *a* 热核的
thermopalpation [ˌθəːməupælˈpeiʃən] *n* 温度差别按诊法
thermopenetration [ˌθəːməuˌpeniˈtreiʃən] *n* 透热法，内科透热法
thermoperiodism [ˌθəːməuˈpiəriədizəm]，**thermoperiodicity** [ˌθəːməuˌpiəriəˈdisəti] *n* 温度周期现象
thermophile [ˈθəːməfail] *n* 嗜热生物，嗜热菌 ǀ **thermophilic** [ˌθəːməˈfilik] *a* 嗜热的
thermophore [ˈθəːməfɔː] *n* 保热器；温度觉检测器
thermopile [ˈθəːməpail] *n* 温差电堆，热电堆
thermoplacentography [ˌθəːməuˌplæsənˈtɔgrəfi] *n* 胎盘温度记录法（测胎盘附着位置）
Thermoplasma [ˌθəːməuˈplæzmə] *n* 热原体属
thermoplastic [ˌθəːməˈplæstik] *a* 热塑性的 *n* 热塑塑料
thermoplegia [ˌθəːməuˈpliːdʒiə] *n* 热射病，中暑

thermopolypnea [ˌθəːməuˌpɔli'pni(ː)ə] *n* 高热性气促 | **thermopolypneic** [ˌθəːməuˌpɔli'pniːik] *a*
thermoprecipitation [ˌθəːməupriˌsipi'teiʃən] *n* 热沉淀反应
thermoprecipitinogen [ˌθəːməupriˌsipi'tinədʒən] *n* 热沉淀原
thermoradiotherapy [ˌθəːməuˌreidiəu'θerəpi] *n* 透热 X 线疗法
thermoreceptor [ˌθəːməuri'septə] *n* 温度感受器
thermoregulation [ˌθəːməuˌregju'leiʃən] *n* 体温调节,温度调节 | **thermoregulator** [ˌθəːməu'regjuleitə] *n* 温度调节器
thermoresistance [ˌθəːməuri'zistəns] *n* 抗热性,耐热性
thermoresistant [ˌθəːməuri'zistənt] *a* 抗热的,耐热的
thermos [ˌθəːmɔs] *n* 保温瓶(热水瓶、冰瓶)
thermoscope ['θəːməskəup] *n* 验温器 | **thermoscopic** [ˌθəːməs'kɔpik] *a*
thermoset ['θəːməset] *a* 热固性的 *n* 热固性
thermosetting [ˌθəːməu'setiŋ] *a* 热固的
thermostabile [ˌθəːməu'steibail], **thermostable** [ˌθəːməu'steibl] *a* 耐热的 | **thermostability** [ˌθəːməustə'biləti] *n* 耐热性,热稳定性
thermostasis [ˌθəːməu'steisis] *n* 体温恒定,恒温[状态]
thermostat ['θəːməstæt] *n* 恒温器 | hypothalamic ~ 下丘脑恒温器
thermostatics [ˌθəːməs'tætiks] *n* 静热力学
thermosteresis [ˌθəːməusti'riːsis] *n* 热耗损,热损失
thermostromuhr [ˌθəːmə'strəumuə] *n* 电热血液流量计
thermosystaltism [ˌθəːməu'sistəltizəm] *n* 温度性收缩(温度变化引起的肌肉收缩) | **thermosystaltic** [ˌθəːməusis'tæltik] *a*
thermotaxis [ˌθəːmə'tæksis] *n* 体温调节;趋温性,向温性 | **thermotactic**, **thermotaxic** *a*
thermotherapy [ˌθəːməu'θerəpi] *n* 温热疗法
thermotics [θə'mɔtiks] *n* 热学
thermotolerant [ˌθəːməu'tɔlərənt] *a* 耐热的(指细菌的活性不因高温而终止)
thermotonometer [ˌθəːməutəu'nɔmitə] *n* 热性肌张力计(热引起的肌收缩测定)
thermotracheotomy [ˌθəːməutræki'ɔtəmi] *n* 热烙气管切开术
thermotropism [θə'mɔtrəpizəm] *n* 向温性(指细胞) | **thermotropic** [ˌθəːməu'trɔpik] *a*
Thermus ['θəːməs] *n* 栖热菌属
theroid ['θiərɔid] *a* 兽样的,兽性的
theromorph ['θiərəmɔːf], **theromorphism** [ˌθiərəu'mɔːfizəm] *n* 兽形部分,兽形结构(指生物体或人的形态部分有多余的、畸形的或残缺的部分,很像低等动物)
Theromyzon [θə'rɔmizɔn] *n* 兽蛭属
thesaurismosis [θiˌsɔːriz'məusis] *n* 贮积病,沉着病 | amyloid ~ 淀粉贮积病,淀粉样变性 / bilirubin ~ 胆红素贮积病,黄疸 / urate ~ 尿酸盐贮积症,痛风 / water ~ 水肿
thesaurosis [θiːsɔː'rəusis] *n* 贮积症,沉着病
theta ['θiːtə] *n* 希腊语的第 8 个字母(Θ, *θ*)
Thévenard's syndrome [teivə'nɑː] (André Thévenard) 泰文纳综合征,遗传性感觉根性神经病变
THF tetrahydrofolic acid 或 tetrahydrofolate 四氢叶酸
thiabendazole [ˌθaiə'bendəzəul] *n* 噻苯达唑(广谱抗蠕虫药)
thiacetarsamide sodium [θaiˌæsət'ɑːsəmaid] 硫胂胺钠(一种三价砷剂,兽医中用于治疗恶丝虫病)
thiacetazone [θaiə'setəzəun] *n* 氨硫脲(抗菌药,具有结核菌抑制和抗麻风作用)
thiadiazide [ˌθaiə'daiəzaid], **thiadiazine** [ˌθaiə'daiəziːn] *n* 噻嗪化物,噻嗪类(利尿药)
thiamazole [θai'æməzəul] *n* 甲巯咪唑(抗甲状腺药)
thiamin ['θaiəmin] *n* 硫胺,维生素 B_1
thiaminase [θai'æmineis] *n* 硫胺[素]酶
thiamine ['θaiəmiːn] *n* 硫胺,维生素 B_1 | ~ hydrochloride 盐酸硫胺(维生素 B_1) / ~ mononitrate 一硝酸硫胺 / phosphorylated ~, ~ pyrophosphate 硫胺焦磷酸,辅羧酶 / ~ propyldisulfide 丙硫硫胺,新维生素 B_1
thiamin pyridinylase ['θaiəmin piri'dinileis] 硫胺[素]吡啶基酶(亦称硫胺[素]酶 I)
thiamphenicol [θaiæm'fenikɔl] *n* 甲砜霉素(抗生素类药)
thiamytal [θai'æmitæl] *n* 硫戊比妥(麻醉药) | ~ sodium 硫戊比妥钠
Thiara [θai'ɑːrə] *n* 疾行螺属
thiasine ['θaiəsin] *n* 巯基组氨酸三甲基内盐
thiazide ['θaiəzaid] *n* 噻嗪化物,噻嗪类(利尿药)
-thiazide [后缀]噻嗪类利尿药
thiazole ['θaiəzəul] *n* 噻唑
thiazolidinedione [ˌθaiəˌzɔlidiːn'daiəun] *n* 硫阿二酮(口服抗高血糖药)
Thibierge-Weissenbach syndrome [tibi'əːʒ 'vaisənbɑːk] (Georges Thibierge; Raymond J. E. Weissenbach) 提-魏综合征,钙质沉着
thickening ['θikəniŋ] *n* 增厚(或粗、密、浓);增稠剂 | pleural ~ 胸膜增厚

thickness [ˈθiknəs] *n* 厚度 | half-value ~ 半值层 / triceps skinfold(TSF) ~ 三头肌皮褶厚度,皮下脂肪厚度

Thiele's syndrome [θiːl] (George H. Thiele) 锡尔综合征(骶骨和尾骨下部区的触痛和疼痛或邻近软组织和肌肉上的触痛和疼痛)

Thiemann's disease [ˈtiːmɑːn] (H. Thiemann) 提曼病(家族性指骨骺无血管性坏死,始于儿童期或青春期,造成指间关节畸形,亦称家族性指骨关节病。拇指及第一跗跖关节亦可见类似损害,此病情称为掌骨跖骨骨软骨炎)

thiemia [θaiˈiːmiə] *n* 硫血[症]

thienamycin [θaiˌenəˈmaisin] *n* 噻烯霉素,沙纳霉素(抗菌药)

Thiersch's graft [ˈtiːəʃ] (Karl Thiersch) 蒂尔施移植物(见 Ollier-Thiersch graft) | ~ operation 蒂尔施手术(①肛门环箍术;②用刀片或取皮机切取簿中厚皮片)

thiethylperazine [θaiˌeθilˈperəziːn] *n* 硫乙拉嗪(止吐药) | ~ malate 苹果酸硫乙拉嗪(止吐药) / ~ maleate 马来酸硫乙拉嗪(止吐药)

thigh [θai] *n* 股,大腿 | cricket ~ 板球股(进行板球或足球运动造成有些股直肌肌纤维破裂) / drivers' ~ 司机股(由于驾驶汽车时运用加速器受压引起坐骨神经痛)

thigmesthesia [ˌθigmisˈθiːzjə] *n* 触觉

thigm(o)- [构词成分]触

thigmotaxis [ˌθigməˈtæksis] *n* 趋触性 | **thigmotactic** [ˌθigməˈtæktik] *a*

Thigmotrichina [ˌθigməutriˈkainə] *n* 触毛亚目

thigmotropism [θigˈmɔtrəpizəm] *n* 向触性,趋触性 | **thigmotropic** [ˌθigməˈtrɔpik] *a*

thihexinol methylbromide [θai-ˈheksinəul] 甲溴噻昔诺(抗胆碱能药,止泻药)

thimble [ˈθimbəl] *n* 顶盖;蹄裂

thimbling [ˈθimbliŋ] *a* 套筒状的

thimerosal [θaiˈmerəsəl] *n* 硫柳汞(消毒防腐药)

thimethaphan camphorsulfonate [θaiˈmeθəfən ˌkæmfəˈsʌlfəneit] 樟磺咪芬(即 trimethaphan camsylate, 抗高血压药)

thinking [ˈθiŋkiŋ] *n* 思想,思维 | autistic ~ 内向性思维 / dereistic ~ 脱离现实思想,空想,幻想 / paralogic ~ 逻辑倒错性思维

thio [ˈθaiəu] *a* 硫的,含硫的

thi(o)- [前缀]硫

thio acid [ˌθaiəuˈæsid] *n* 硫代酸

thioalbumose [ˌθaiəuˈælbjuməus] *n* 硫脲

thioalcohol [ˌθaiəuˈælkəhɔl] *n* 硫醇

β-thio-α-aminopropionic acid [ˈbiːtəˈθaiəuˈælfəˌæminəuprəupiˈɔnik] 半胱氨酸

thioarsenite [ˌθaiəuˈɑːsinait] *n* 硫亚砷酸盐

Thiobacillus [ˌθaiəubəˈsiləs] *n* 硫杆菌属

Thiobacteriaceae [ˌθaiəubækˌtiəriˈeisiiː] *n* 硫细菌科

Thiobacterium [ˌθaiəubækˈtiəriəm] *n* 硫细菌属

thiobarbital [ˌθaiəuˈbɑːbitæl] *n* 硫巴比妥(甲状腺抑制药)

thiobarbiturate [ˌθaiəubɑːˈbitjuəreit] *n* 硫巴比土酸盐

thiobarbituric acid [ˌθaiəubɑːbiˈtjuərik] 硫巴比土酸

Thiocapsa [ˌθaiəuˈkæpsə] *n* 荚硫菌属

thiocarbamide [ˌθaiəuˈkɑːbəmaid] *n* 硫脲

thiochrome [ˈθaiəkrəum] *n* 硫色素,脱氢硫胺[素]

thioctic acid [θaiˈɔktik] 硫辛酸,维生素 B_{14}(治肝功能障碍药)

thiocyanate [ˌθaiəuˈsaiəneit] *n* 硫氰酸根,硫氰酸盐;硫氰酸酯

thiocyanic acid [ˌθaiəusaiˈænik] 硫氰酸

thiocyanide [ˌθaiəuˈsaiənaid] *n* 硫氰酸根,硫氰酸盐

Thiocystis [ˌθaiəuˈsistis] *n* 囊硫菌属

Thiodendron [ˌθaiəuˈdendrɔn] *n* 枝硫菌属

Thioderma [ˌθaiəuˈdəːmə] *n* 真皮硫菌属

Thiodictyon [ˌθaiəuˈdiktiɔn] *n* 网硫菌属

thiodiphenylamine [ˌθaiəudaiˌfeniˈlæmiːn] *n* 吩噻嗪(抗蠕虫药)

thiodotherapy [ˌθaiəudəuˈθerəpi] *n* 硫碘疗法

thioester [ˌθaiəuˈestə] *n* 硫酯

thioether [θaiəuˈiːθə] *n* 硫醚

thioethylamine [ˌθaiəuˌeθiˈlæmiːn] *n* 硫乙胺,氨基乙硫醇

thioflavine [ˌθaiəuˈfleiviːn] *n* 硫黄素,甲基脱硫氢对甲苯胺磺酸盐(黄色染料)

thiogenic [ˌθaiəuˈdʒenik] *a* 产硫的(指利用硫化氢合成高级硫化合物的细菌)

thioglucose [ˌθaiəuˈgluːkəus] *n* 硫葡糖

thioglucosidase [ˌθaiəugluˈkəusideis] *n* 硫葡糖苷酶,葡糖硫苷酶

thioguanine (6-TG) [ˌθaiəuˈgwæniːn] *n* 硫鸟嘌呤(抗肿瘤药)

thiokinase [ˌθaiəuˈkaineis] *n* 硫激酶

thiol [ˈθaiɔl] *n* 巯基,硫氢基;硫醇

thiolactic acid [ˌθaiəuˈlæktik] 硫乳酸

thiolase [ˈθaiəleis] *n* 硫解酶,硫醇酶,乙酰辅酶 A 转乙酰酶

thiol endopeptidase [ˈθaiɔl ˌendəuˈpeptideis] 硫醇内肽酶,半胱氨酸内肽酶

thiolhistidine [ˌθaiɔlˈhistidiːn] *n* 巯[基]组氨酸

thiomersalate [ˌθaiəuˈməːsəleit] *n* 硫柳汞(消毒防腐药)

thioneine [ˌθaiəuˈniiːn] *n* 巯基组氨酸三甲内盐,麦角硫因

thionic [θaiˈɔnik] *a* 硫的 | ~ acid 硫羰酸
thionin [ˈθaiənin] *n* 硫堇(异染〈色〉性染料)
thionyl [ˈθaiənil] *n* 亚硫酰(硫氧基)
thiopanic acid [ˌθaiəuˈpænik] 泛磺酸
thiopectic [ˌθaiəuˈpektik] *a* 固定硫的
Thiopedia [ˌθaiəuˈpiːdiə] *n* 板硫菌属
thiopental sodium [ˌθaiəuˈpentl], **thiopentone** [ˌθaiəuˈpentəun] *n* 硫喷妥钠(麻醉药)
thiopexic [ˌθaiəuˈpeksik] *a* 固定硫的
thiopexy [ˈθaiəpeksi] *n* 硫固定[作用]
Thioploca [ˌθaiəuˈpləukə] *n* 辫硫菌属
Thiopolycoccus [ˌθaiəuˌpɔliˈkɔkəs] *n* 多球硫菌属
thiopropazate hydrochloride [ˌθaiəuˈprəupəzeit] 盐酸奋乃静醋酸酯(吩噻嗪类安定药,用于治疗精神病)
Thiorhodaceae [ˌθaiəurəuˈdeisiiː] *n* 红硫菌科
thioridazine hydrochloride [ˌθaiəuˈridəziːn] 盐酸硫利达嗪(安定药)
thiosalicylic acid [ˌθaiəuˌsæliˈsilik] 硫柳酸,硫代水杨酸
Thiosarcina [ˌθaiəusɑːˈsainə] *n* 八叠球硫菌属
thiosinamine [ˌθaiəuˈsinəmiːn] *n* 烯丙硫脲(能促纤维织吸收)
Thiospira [ˌθaiəuˈspaiərə] *n* 硫螺菌属
Thiospirillopsis [ˌθaiəuˌspaiəriˈlɔpsis] *n* 拟硫螺菌属
Thiospirillum [ˌθaiəuˌspaiəˈriləm] *n* 紫硫螺菌属
thiostrepton [ˌθaiəuˈstreptɔn] *n* 硫链球菌(兽医用抗菌药)
thiosulfate [ˌθaiəuˈsʌlfeit] *n* 硫代硫酸盐
thiosulfate sulfurtransferase [ˌθaiəuˈsʌlfeit ˌsʌlfəˈtrænsfəreis] 硫代硫酸转硫酶
thiosulfuric acid [ˌθaiəusʌlˈfjuərik] 硫代硫酸
thiotepa [ˌθaiəuˈtiːpə] *n* 塞替派(抗肿瘤药)
Thiothece [ˌθaiəuˈtiːsi] *n* 鞘硫菌属
thiothixene [ˌθaiəuˈθiksiːn] *n* 替沃噻吨(抗精神病药) | ~ hydrochloride 盐酸替沃噻吨(抗精神病药)
Thiothrix [ˈθaiəθriks] *n* 丝硫菌属
thiouracil [ˌθaiəuˈjuərəsil] *n* 硫尿嘧啶(抗甲状腺药,治疗甲状腺功能亢进,并可治疗心绞痛及充血性心力衰竭)
thiourea [ˌθaiəuˈjuəriə] *n* 硫脲(对甲状腺功能起抑制作用,曾用作抗甲状腺药)
Thiovulum [θaiˈəuvjuːləm] *n* 卵硫菌属
thioxanthene [ˌθaiəuˈzænθiːn] *n* 噻吨(包括替沃噻吨〈thiothixene〉和氯普噻吨〈chlorprothixene〉任何一类结构上有关的抗精神病药)
thiozine [ˈθaiəziːn] *n* 巯基组氨酸三甲内盐,麦角硫因
thiphenamil hydrochloride [θaiˈfenəmil] 盐酸替芬那米(抗胆碱药,具有强解痉和平滑肌松弛作用)
thiram [ˈθairəm] *n* 塞仑(局部抗真菌药)
thirst [θəːst] *n* 渴感 | subliminal ~, insensible ~, twilight ~ 阈下渴感,不显性渴感,朦胧渴感 / true ~, real ~ 实际渴感
thirsty [ˈθəːsti] *a* 渴的
Thiry's fistula [ˈθairi] (Ludwig Thiry) 锡里瘘(在一段分离的肠管做一个人工开口,其近端缝合于腹壁,而远端则闭合,用于动物实验)
thistle [ˈθisl] *n* 蓟;蓟属植物
thixolabile [ˌθiksəˈleibail] *a* 易触变的,不耐触的
thixotropy [θikˈsɔtrəpi], **thixotropism** [θikˈsɔtrəpizəm] *n* 触变性,摇溶性 | **thixotropic** [ˌθiksəˈtrɔpik] *a* 触变的,摇溶的
thlipsencephalus [ˌθlipsenˈsefələs] *n* 颅不全畸胎
Thogoto virus [θəuˈgəutəu] (Thogoto 森林在肯尼亚,首次在此分离出该病毒)索哥托病毒(一种蜱传正黏病毒,传染非洲人、牛和羊。人感染有时导致重度脑炎和视神经炎)
Thoma's ampulla [ˈtɔmə] (Richard Thoma) 托马壶腹(脾髓内小叶间动脉终末膨大部) | ~ fluid 托马液(组织脱钙液,由酒精和纯硝酸组成)
Thomas shunt [ˈtɔməs] (G. I. Thomas) 托马斯分流(一种血液透析用的动静脉分流管,包含一个硅化橡胶插管和涤纶套囊,插入股动脉和股静脉之间)
Thomas sign [təuˈmɑːs] (Andre A. H. Thomas) 托马斯征(见 André Thomas sign)
Thomas' sign [ˈtɔməs] (Hugh O. Thomas) 托马斯征(托马斯试验时,可见髋部屈曲畸形) | ~ splint 托马斯夹板(一种腿用夹板) / ~ test 托马斯试验(患者仰卧,一腿屈曲,使膝触胸,腰椎变平,对侧髋部所取的角度,即屈曲畸形的程度)
Thoma-Zeiss counting chamber (cell) [ˈtɔmə tsais] (Richard Thoma; Carl Zeiss) 托马-蔡斯计数池(血细胞计数器)
Thompson arthroplasty [ˈtɔmpsn] (Frederick R. Thompson) 汤普森关节成形术(使用汤普森假体的髋关节功能重建手术) | ~ prosthesis 汤普森假体(髋关节成形术中使用的一种活合金〈Vitallium〉植入物)
Thompson's test [ˈtɔmpsn] (Henry Thompson) 汤普森试验,二杯试验(two glass test,见 test 项下相应术语)
Thomsen's disease [ˈtɔmsn] (Asmus J. T. Thomsen) 先天性肌强直
Thomson scattering [ˈtɔmsn] (Sir Joseph John Thomson) 汤姆森散射(未变散射,即光子与原子相互作用而产生的偏转,光子未丢失能量)

Thomson's disease [ˈtɔmsn] (Mathew S. Thomson)汤姆森病(一种常染色体隐性遗传性皮肤病,除鞍状鼻及白内障未表现外,其余均类似罗-汤〈Rothmund-Thomson〉综合征)

Thomson's sign [ˈθɔmsən] (Frederick H. Thomson)汤姆森征(见 Pastia's lines)

thonzonium bromide [θɔnˈzəuniəm] 通佐溴铵(阳离子去垢剂)

thonzylamine hydrochloride [θɔnˈziləmiːn] 盐酸宋齐拉敏(抗组胺药)

thoracalgia [ˌθɔːrəˈkældʒiə] *n* 胸痛

thoracectomy [ˌθɔːrəˈsektəmi] *n* 胸廓部分切除术

thoracentesis [ˌθɔːrəsenˈtiːsis] *n* 胸腔穿刺术

thoraces [ˈθəurəsiːz] thorax 的复数

thoracic [θɔːˈræsik], **thoracal** [ˈθɔːrəkəl] *a* 胸的,胸廓的

thoracicoabdominal [θɔːˌræsikəuæbˈdɔminl] *a* 胸腹的

thoracicohumeral [θɔːˌræsikəuˈhjuːmərəl] *a* 胸肱的

thoracispinal [θɔːˌræsiˈspainl] *a* 脊柱胸段的

thorac(o)- [构词成分]胸

thoracoabdominal [ˌθɔːrəkəuæbˈdɔminl] *a* 胸腹的

thoracoacromial [ˌθɔːrəkəuəˈkrəumiəl] *a* 胸肩峰的

thoracobronchotomy [ˌθɔːrəkəubrɔŋˈkɔtəmi] *n* 胸廓支气管切开术

thoracoceloschisis [ˌθɔːrəkəusiˈlɔskisis] *n* 胸腹裂[畸形]

thoracocentesis [ˌθɔːrəkəusenˈtiːsis] *n* 胸腔穿刺术

thoracocyllosis [ˌθɔːrəkəusaiˈləusis] *n* 胸畸形

thoracocyrtosis [ˌθɔːrəkəusəːˈtəusis] *n* 胸弯曲

thoracodelphus [ˌθɔːrəkəuˈdelfəs] *n* 脐上胸联胎

thoracodidymus [ˌθɔːrəkəuˈdidiməs] *n* 胸部联胎

thoracodynia [ˌθɔːrəkəuˈdiniə] *n* 胸痛

thoracogastrodidymus [ˌθɔːrəkəuˌgæstrəuˈdidiməs] *n* 胸腹联胎

thoracogastroschisis [ˌθɔːrəkəugæsˈtrɔskisis] *n* 胸腹裂

thoracograph [θɔːˈrækəgrɑːf, -græf] *n* 胸动描记器

thoracolaparotomy [ˌθɔːrəkəuˌlæpəˈrɔtəmi] *n* 胸腹切开术

thoracolumbar [ˌθɔːrəkəuˈlʌmbə] *a* 胸腰的,脊柱胸腰段的

thoracolysis [ˌθɔːrəˈkɔlisis] *n* 胸廓粘连松解术

thoracomelus [ˌθɔːrəˈkɔmiləs] *n* 胸部寄生肢畸胎,胸肢畸胎

thoracometer [ˌθɔːrəˈkɔmitə] *n* 胸围计,胸廓张度计

thoracometry [ˌθɔːrəˈkɔmitri] *n* 胸廓测量法

thoracomyodynia [ˌθɔːrəkəuˌmaiəuˈdiniə] *n* 胸肌痛

thoracoomphalopagus [ˌθɔːrəkəuˌɔmfəˈlɔpeigəs] *n* 胸脐部联胎

thoracopagus [ˌθɔːrəˈkɔpəgəs] *n* 胸联双胎

thoracoparacephalus [ˌθɔːrəkəuˌpærəˈsefələs] *n* 头不全胸部寄生胎

thoracopathy [ˌθɔːrəˈkɔpəθi] *n* 胸部疾病

thoracoplasty [ˌθɔːrəkəuˈplæsti] *n* 胸廓成形术

thoracopneumograph [ˌθɔːrəkəuˈnjuːməgrɑːf] *n* 胸肺描记器

thoracoschisis [ˌθɔːrəˈkɔskisis] *n* 胸裂[畸形]

thoracoscope [θɔːˈrækəskəup] *n* 胸腔镜 | **thoracoscopy** [ˌθɔːrəˈkɔskəpi] *n* 胸腔镜检查

thoracostenosis [ˌθɔːrəkəustiˈnəusis] *n* 胸廓狭窄

thoracostomy [ˌθɔːrəˈkɔstəmi] *n* 胸膜腔造口术

thoracotomy [ˌθɔːrəˈkɔtəmi] *n* 开胸术

thoradelphus [ˌθɔːrəˈdelfəs] *n* 脐上胸联胎

thorax [ˌθɔːræks] ([复] **thoraxes** 或 **thoraces** [ˈθɔːrəsiːz]) *n* 胸,胸廓 | amazon ~ 单孔胸 / barrel-shaped ~ 桶状胸 / cholesterol ~ 胆固醇性胸膜积液 / pyriform ~ 梨形胸

Thorel's bundle [ˈtɔːrəl] (Christen Thorel)托雷尔束(联接窦房结与房室结的心脏内一束肌纤维)

thoriagram [ˈθɔːriəgræm] *n* 钍照片

thorium(Th) [ˈθɔːriəm] *n* 钍(化学元素) | radioactive ~ 射钍 / ~ X 钍 X(由钍蜕变产生的一种放射性元素,镭的同位素,半衰期约 $3\frac{2}{3}$ 日,从前用于治疗浅表性皮肤病,现为软 X 线和跨界射线所取代)

Thormählen's test [ˈtɔːmeilən] (Johann Thormählen)托尔梅伦试验(检尿内黑素)

Thorn's syndrome [θɔːn] (George W. Thorn)索恩综合征,失盐性肾炎

Thornton's sign [ˈθɔːntən] (Knowsley Thornton)桑顿征(肾结石时胁腹部剧烈疼痛)

Thornwaldt [ˈtɔːnvɑːlt] 见Tornwaldt

thoron [ˈθɔːrɔn] *n* 钍射气

thoroughpin [ˈθʌrəpin] *n* 滑膜鞘[肌腱]肿胀(马)

thought [θɔːt] *n* 思想,思维 | audible ~ 思维化声

thought broadcasting [θɔːt ˈbrɔːdkɑːstiŋ] 思维播散(认为自己的思维被播散到外界)

thought insertion [θɔːt inˈsəːʃən] 思维插入(认为思维不是自己的,而被插入自己脑中的一种妄想)

thought withdrawal [θɔːt wiðˈdrɔːəl] 思维被夺

（认为某人或某物正从自己脑中思维被夺的一种妄想）
thozalinone [θɔ'zælinəun] *n* 托扎啉酮（抗抑郁药）
Thr threonine 苏氨酸
thread [θred] *n* 线 | celluloid ～ 赛璐珞线
threadworm ['θredwəːm] *n* 线虫；蛲虫
thremmatology [ˌθremə'tɔlədʒi] *n* 育种学（生物）
threonine（Thr，T） ['θriəniːn] *n* 苏氨酸
threonine dehydratase ['θriːəniːn diː'haidrəteis] 苏氨酸脱水酶
threonyl ['θriːənil] *n* 苏氨酰[基]
threose ['θriːəus] *n* 苏糖
threpsis ['θrepsis] *n*【希】营养
threpsology [θrep'sɔlədʒi] *n* 营养学
threptic ['θreptik] *a* 营养的
threshold ['θreʃhəuld] *n* 阈，阈值 | absolute ～，sensitivity ～，stimulus ～ 绝对阈，感受阈，刺激阈（能产生感觉的最低刺激限度）/ auditory ～ 听阈（最小感觉音）/ erythema ～ 红斑阈（引起皮肤红斑所需的放射剂量）/ galvanic ～ 基强度（产生刺激所需的最小电压）/ pyrogenic ～，parasite ～ 致热阈（血内致热所需的疟原虫数）/ renal ～ 肾阈（血浆内物质的浓度，到此浓度物质开始在尿内排出）/ ～ of visual sensation 视觉阈（产生视觉的最小刺激量）
thrill [θril] *n* 震颤 | aneurysmal ～ 动脉瘤震颤（动脉瘤触诊时）/ aortic ～ 主动脉震颤（主动脉瓣疾病时）/ diastolic ～ 舒张期震颤（主动脉瓣闭锁不全时）/ hydated ～ 棘球蚴震颤 / presystolic ～ 收缩期前震颤 / purring ～ 猫鸣状震颤 / systolic ～ 收缩期震颤（主动脉瓣狭窄、肺动脉瓣狭窄及室间隔缺损时）
thrix [θriks] *n*【希】毛，发
-thrix [构词成分]发，毛
throat [θrəut] *n* 咽，咽喉，喉；咽门；颈前部 | sore ～ 咽喉痛 / trench ～ 战壕咽炎，樊尚（Vincent）咽炎
throaty ['θrəuti] *a* 喉音的，沙哑的
throb [θrɔb]（-bb-）*vi*，*n* 跳动，悸动，搏动
throbbing ['θrɔbiŋ] *a* 跳动的，搏动的
Throckmorton's reflex ['θrɔkmɔːtn]（Thomas B. Throckmorton）思罗克莫顿反射（类似巴彬斯奇〈Babinski〉反射，叩击足背引起踇趾向背面翻屈，其他四趾分开）
thromballosis [ˌθrɔmbə'ləusis] *n* 静脉血凝固
thrombapheresis [ˌθrɔmbəfə'riːsis] *n* 血小板去除术
thrombase ['θrɔmbeis] *n* 凝血酶
thrombasthenia [ˌθrɔmbəs'θiːnjə] *n* 血小板功能不全
thrombectomy [θrɔm'bektəmi] *n* 血栓切除术
thrombembolia [ˌθrɔmbem'bəuliə] *n* 血栓栓塞
thrombi ['θrɔmbai] thrombus 的复数
thrombin ['θrɔmbin] *n* 凝血酶
thrombinogen [θrɔm'binədʒən] *n* 凝血酶原
thromb(o)- [构词成分]血栓
thromboagglutinin [ˌθrɔmbəuə'gluːtinin] *n* 血小板凝集素
thromboangiitis [ˌθrɔmbəuˌændʒi'aitis] *n* 血栓性脉管炎 | ～ obliterans 血栓闭塞性脉管炎
thromboarteritis [ˌθrɔmbəuˌɑːtə'raitis] *n* 血栓[性]动脉炎
thromboasthenia [ˌθrɔmbəuəs'θiːnjə] *n* 血小板功能不全
thrombocinase [ˌθrɔmbəu'kaineis] *n* 凝血酶原激酶
thromboclasis [θrɔm'bɔkləsis] *n* 血栓碎裂，血栓溶解
thromboclastic [ˌθrɔmbəu'klæstik] *a* 碎裂血栓的
thrombocyst ['θrɔmbəusist]，**thrombocystis** [ˌθrɔmbəu'sistis] *n* 血栓囊
thrombocytapheresis [ˌθrɔmbəuˌsaitəfə'riːsis] *n* 血小板去除术
thrombocyte ['θrɔmbəusait] *n* 血小板 | **thrombocytic** [ˌθrɔmbəu'sitik] *a*
thrombocythemia [ˌθrɔmbəusai'θiːmiə] *n* 血小板增多
thrombocytin [ˌθrɔmbəu'saitin] *n* 血小板素，5-羟色胺
thrombocytocrit [ˌθrɔmbəu'saitəkrit] *n* 血小板比容，血小板压积；血小板比容计
thrombocytolysis [ˌθrɔmbəusai'tɔlisis] *n* 血小板溶解
thrombocytopathia [ˌθrɔmbəuˌsaitəu'pæθiə] *n* 血小板病
thrombocytopathy [ˌθrɔmbəusai'tɔpəθi] *n* 血小板病 | **thrombocytopathic** [ˌθrɔmbəuˌsaitəu'pæθik] *a*
thrombocytopenia [ˌθrɔmbəuˌsaitəu'piːniə] *n* 血小板减少 | essential ～ 特发性血小板减少性紫癜 / immune ～ 免疫性血小板减少（与抗血小板抗体〈IgG〉的存在有关的血小板减少）
thrombocytopoiesis [ˌθrɔmbəuˌsaitəupɔi'iːsis] *n* 血小板发生 | **thrombocytopoietic** [ˌθrɔmbəuˌsaitəupɔi'etik] *a*
thrombocytosis [ˌθrɔmbəusai'təusis] *n* 血小板增多
thromboelastogram [ˌθrɔmbəui'læstəgræm] *n* 凝血弹性[描记]图
thromboelastograph [ˌθrɔmbəui'læstəgrɑːf] *n* 凝血弹性描记器 | **～y** [ˌθrɔmbəuˌiːlæs'tɔgrəfi] *n* 凝血弹性描记法
thromboembolic [ˌθrɔmbəuəm'bɔlik] *a* 血栓栓

塞的

thromboembolism [ˌθrɔmbəu'embəlizəm] **thromboembolia** [ˌθrɔmbəuem'bəuliə] *n* 血栓栓塞

thromboendarterectomy [ˌθrɔmbəuˌendɑːtə'rektəmi] *n* 血栓动脉内膜切除术

thromboendarteritis [ˌθrɔmbəuendˌɑːtə'raitis] *n* 血栓[性]动脉内膜炎,血栓[性]动脉炎

thromboendocarditis [ˌθrɔmbəuˌendəukɑː'daitis] *n* 血栓[性]心内膜炎

thrombogen ['θrɔmbədʒin] *n* 凝血酶原

thrombogenesis [ˌθrɔmbəu'dʒenisis] *n* 血栓形成

thrombogenic [ˌθrɔmbəu'dʒenik] *a* 形成血栓的

β-thromboglobulin [ˌθrɔmbəu'glɔbjulin] *n* β-血小板球蛋白

thromboid ['θrɔmbɔid] *a* 血栓样的

thrombokinase [ˌθrɔmbəu'kaineis] *n* 凝血酶原激酶

thrombokinesis [ˌθrɔmbəukai'niːsis] *n* 血栓形成,血液凝固

thrombokinetics [ˌθrɔmbəukai'netiks] *n* 血凝动力学

thrombolymphangitis [ˌθrɔmbəuˌlimfæn'dʒaitis] *n* 血栓[性]淋巴管炎

thrombolysis [θrɔm'bɔlisis] *n* 血栓溶解 | **thrombolytic** [ˌθrɔmbəu'litik] *a* 溶解血栓的 *n* 溶血栓药

thrombomodulin [ˌθrɔmbəu'mɔdjulin] *n* 血栓调节素,血栓调节蛋白

thrombon ['θrɔmbɔn] *n* 血小板系

thrombopathia [ˌθrɔmbəu'pæθiə], **thrombopathy** [θrɔm'bɔpəθi] *n* 血小板紊乱

thrombopenia [ˌθrɔmbəu'piːniə] *n* 血小板减少[症] | essential ~ 特发性血小板减少性紫癜 | **thrombopeny** ['θrɔmbəˌpiːni] *n*

thrombophilia [ˌθrɔmbəu'filiə] *n* 血栓形成倾向

thrombophlebitis [ˌθrɔmbəufli'baitis] *n* 血栓性静脉炎

thromboplastic [ˌθrɔmbəu'plæstik] *a* 形成血栓的,促凝血的

thromboplastid [ˌθrɔmbəu'plæstid] *n* 血小板

thromboplastin [ˌθrɔmbəu'plæstin] *n* 促凝血酶原激酶 | extrinsic ~ 外源性促凝血酶原激酶 / intrinsic ~ 内源性促凝血酶原激酶

thromboplastinogen [ˌθrɔmbəuplæs'tinədʒən] *n* 促凝血酶原激酶原(凝血因子Ⅷ或抗血友病因子 A 的旧名)

thrombopoiesis [ˌθrɔmbəupɔi'iːsis] *n* 血栓形成;血小板生成 | **thrombopoietic** [ˌθrɔmbəupɔi'etik] *a*

thrombopoietin [ˌθrɔmbəupɔi'iːtin] *n* 血小板生成素

thromboresistance [ˌθrɔmbəuri'sistəns] *n* 血栓阻力(血管对血栓形成的阻力,同样见 anticoagulation)

thrombosed ['θrɔmbəust] *a* 形成血栓的

thrombosinusitis [ˌθrɔmbəuˌsainə'saitis] *n* 血栓[性]硬膜窦炎

thrombosis [θrɔm'bəusis] *n* 血栓形成 | agonal ~ 濒死期血栓形成 / cardiac ~ 心内血栓形成 / cerebral ~ 脑血栓形成(可能导致脑梗死) / coronary ~ 冠状动脉血栓形成(常导致突然死亡或心肌梗死) / infective ~ 传染性血栓形成(与细菌感染有关) / marantic ~, marasmic ~, atrophic ~ 衰弱性血栓形成(主要指婴儿期和老年期消耗病时矢状窦血栓形成) / plate ~, platelet ~ 血小板性血栓形成 / sinus ~ 静脉窦血栓形成 / venous ~ 静脉血栓形成,血[栓]性静脉炎 | **thrombotic** [θrɔm'bɔtik] *a*

thrombospondin [ˌθrɔmbəu'spɔndin] *n* 血小板反应素,血小板凝血酶敏感蛋白

thrombostasis [θrɔm'bɔstəsis] *n* 血栓性淤血

thrombosthenin [ˌθrɔmbəu'sθiːnin] *n* 血栓收缩蛋白

thrombotest ['θrɔmbətest] *n* 凝血试验

thrombotonin [ˌθrɔmbəu'təunin] *n* 5-羟色胺

thromboxane [θrɔm'bɔksein] *n* 血栓烷,血栓素,凝血噁烷

thromboxane-A synthase [θrɔm'bɔksein 'sinθeis] 凝血噁烷-A 合酶(此酶活性缺乏为一种常染色体显性性状,可致血小板释放缺损)

thrombus ['θrɔmbəs] ([复] **thrombi** ['θrɔmbai]) *n* 血栓 | agonal ~, agony ~ 濒死期血栓 / antemortem ~ 死前血栓(死前在心脏或大血管内形成的血栓或血块) / calcified ~ 钙化血栓,静脉石 / marantic ~, marasmic ~ 衰弱性血栓(伴有严重消耗病) / mural ~ 附壁血栓 / phagocytic ~ 噬细胞栓(脑微细管的黑色素性白细胞积滞) / postmortem ~ 死后血栓(死后在心脏或大血管内形成的血栓或血块) / red ~ 红色血栓 / white ~ 白色血栓(一种不含有红细胞;一种主要由白细胞组成;还有一种主要由血小板和纤维蛋白组成,通常见于动脉血栓形成)

thrush [θrʌʃ] *n* 鹅口疮(亦称真菌性口炎);蹄叉腐烂(马)

thrust [θrʌst] *vt, vi, n* 猛推;挺伸,延伸 | paraspinal ~ 脊椎旁猛推法(治腰骶椎劳损) / spinal ~ 脊椎猛推法(治腰骶椎劳损) / tongue ~ 挺舌(幼稚型吮[吸]吞[咽]动作)

thrypsis ['θripsis] *n* 【希】粉碎性骨折

Thudichum's test ['tudiʃum] (John L. W. Thudichum) 土迪休姆试验(检肌酸酐)

Thuja ['θjuːdʒə] *n* 【拉】金钟柏属,岩柏属

thuja ['θjuːdʒə] *n* 侧柏,金钟柏(可利尿、解热、发汗、通经)

thujone [ˈθjuːdʒəun] *n* 侧柏酮
thulium(Tm) [ˈθjuːliəm] *n* 铥(化学元素)
thumb [θʌm] *n* 拇指,拇 | bifid ~ 分叉拇指 / tennis ~ 网球员拇病,拇长屈肌腱鞘炎
thumbnail [ˈθʌmneil] *n* 拇指甲
thumbprint [ˈθʌmprint] *n* 拇指纹
thumb-printing [ˈθʌmprintiŋ] *n* 指压征(一种 X 线摄影征,即结肠充钡时出现的匀称的压迹,好像是拇指压成的,见于各种结肠疾患,特别是缺血性结肠炎)
thumbstall [ˈθʌmstɔːl] *n* 拇指套
thumb-sucking [θʌmˈsʌkiŋ] *n* 吮拇癖
thump [θʌmp] *n* 重击,重击声 *vt*, *vi* 重击 | precordial ~ 心前区重击(见 thumpversion)
thumps [θʌmps] *n* 猪肺病(蛔虫幼虫所致);马噎病(膈痉挛所致)
thumpversion [θʌmpˈvəːʒən] *n* 击胸法(开始心肺复苏时击胸一二下以便起始搏动或使室性纤维性颤动转变成正常节律)
thylakoid [ˈθailəkɔid] *n* 类囊体(内含叶绿体光合色素及催化光依赖性反应的酶类)
thyme [taim] *n* 百里香,麝香草 | creeping ~, wild ~ 匐枝百里香,野麝香草
thymectomize [θaiˈmektəmaiz] *vt* 切除胸腺
thymectomy [θaiˈmektəmi] *n* 胸腺切除术
thymelcosis [ˌθaimelˈkəusis] *n* 胸腺溃疡
thymene [ˈθaimiːn] *n* 百里烯,麝香草萜,麝香草烯
thymergastic [ˈθaiməˈgæstik], **thymergasia** [ˌθaiməˈgeiziə] *n* 情感性精神病
-thymia [构词成分]情感,心境
thymian [ˈθimiən, ˈtimiən] *n*【德】百里香,麝香草
thymiasis [θaiˈmaiəsis] *n* 雅司病(即 yaws)
thymic [ˈθaimik] *a* 胸腺的;百里香的,麝香草的 | ~ acid 胸腺核苷酸
thymicolymphatic [ˌθaimikəulimˈfætik] *a* 胸腺淋巴结的
thymidine [ˈθaimidiːn] *n* 胸[腺嘧啶脱氧核]苷
thymidine kinase(TK) [ˈθaimidiːn ˈkaineis] 胸苷激酶
thymidylate [ˌθaimiˈdileit] *n* 胸苷酸
thymidylate synthase [ˌθaimiˈdileit ˈsinθeis] 胸苷酸合酶(在早先文献中不确切地称为 thymidylate synthetase〈胸苷酸合成酶〉)
thymidylic acid [ˌθaimiˈdilik] 胸[腺嘧啶脱氧核]苷酸
thymidylyl [ˌθaimiˈdilil] *n* 胸苷基
thymin [ˈθaimin] *n* 胸腺激素,胸腺素
thymine [ˈθaimiːn] *n* 胸腺嘧啶
thymine-uraciluria [ˌθaimiːn ˌjuərəsiˈljuəriə] *n* 胸腺嘧啶尿嘧啶尿(尿内嘧啶类胸腺嘧啶和尿嘧啶过多,如二氢嘧啶脱氢酶缺乏症时所发生的情况)
thyminic acid [θaiˈminik] 胸腺嘧啶原酸
thymion [ˈθimiɔn] *n*【希】皮肤疣
thymiosis [ˌθimiˈəusis] *n* 雅司病(即 yaws)
thymitis [θaiˈmaitis] *n* 胸腺炎
thym(o)- [构词成分]胸腺;精神,情感
thymocrescin [ˌθaiməuˈkresin] *n* 胸腺生长激素
thymocyte [ˈθaiməsait] *n* 胸腺细胞
thymoform [ˈθaiməfɔːm] *n* 麝莫仿,麝香草脑甲醛
thymogenic [ˌθaiməuˈdʒenik] *a* 情感性的
thymohydroquinone [ˌθaiməuˌhaidrəukwiˈnəun] *n* 麝香草氢醌
thymokesis [ˌθaiməuˈkiːsis] *n* 胸腺遗留(成人)
thymokinetic [ˌθaiməukaiˈnetik] *a* 刺激胸腺的
thymol [ˈθaimɔl] *n* 麝香草脑,麝香草酚,百里酚(制剂时用作稳定剂,并有防腐、抗菌及抗真菌作用,从前用作驱虫药) | ~ iodide 麝酚碘,麝香草酚碘(从前用作抗真菌、抗菌药) / ~ phthalein 麝香草酚酞
thymoleptic [ˌθaiməuˈleptik] *n* 抗抑郁药
thymolize [ˈθaiməlaiz] *vt* 用麝香草脑处理
thymolphthalein [ˌθaimɔlˈθæliːn] *n* 麝香草酚酞,百里酚酞(用作指示剂)
thymolysin [θaiˈmɔlisin] *n* 溶胸腺素(损害或杀死胸腺细胞的抗体)
thymolysis [θaiˈmɔlisis] *n* 胸腺溶解,胸腺破坏 | **thymolytic** [ˌθaiməuˈlitik] *a* 溶胸腺的,破坏胸腺的
thymoma [θaiˈməumə] *n* 胸腺瘤
thymometastasis [ˌθaiməumeˈtæstəsis] *n* 胸腺组织转移
thymonucleic acid [ˌθaiməuˈnjuːkliik] 胸腺核酸,脱氧核糖核酸
thymopathy [θaiˈmɔpəθi] *n* 胸腺病;情感性疾病 | **thymopathic** [ˌθaiməuˈpæθik] *a*
thymopentin [ˌθaiməuˈpentin] *n* 胸腺喷丁(一种五肽免疫刺激剂)
thymopoietin [ˌθaiməuˈpɔiətin] *n* 促胸腺生成素
thymoprivous [θaiˈmɔprivəs], **thymoprivic** [ˌθaiməuˈprivik] *a* 胸腺缺乏的
thymosin [ˈθaiməsin] *n* 胸腺素(一种体液因素,由胸腺分泌的一种激素,促使外周淋巴组织生长,尤其是促使胸腺依赖性区域的生长,亦称胸腺激素)
thymotoxic [ˌθaiməuˈtɔksik] *a* 胸腺毒性的
thymotoxin [ˌθaiməuˈtɔksin] *n* 胸腺毒素,溶胸腺素
thymotrophic [ˌθaiməuˈtrəufik] *a* 促胸腺的
thymovidin [θaiˈməuvidin] *n* (鸟)胸腺促卵激素
Thymus [ˈθaiməs] *n* 百里香属

thymus [ˈθaiməs] *n*【拉】胸腺 | accessory ~ 副胸腺 / persistent ~, ~ persistens hyperplastica 久存性胸腺 / ~ nucleic acid 胸腺核酸,脱氧核糖核酸

thymus-dependent [ˈθaiməs diˈpendənt] *a* 胸腺依赖的(指 T 淋巴细胞)

thymusectomy [ˌθaiməˈsektəmi] *n* 胸腺切除术

thymus-independent [θaiməsindiˈpendənt] *a* 非胸腺依赖的(指 B 淋巴细胞)

thynnin [ˈθinin] *n* 鲔精蛋白

thypar [ˈθaipə] *a* 甲状腺及甲状旁腺缺乏的

thyratron [ˈθairətrɔn] *n* 闸流管(用作矫正交流电的电瓣)

thyremphraxis [ˌθairemˈfræksis] *n* 甲状腺阻塞

thyre(o)- 以 thyre(o)-起始的词,同样见以 thyr(o)-起始的词

thyreoitis [ˌθairiəuˈaitis] *n* 甲状腺炎

thyr(o)- [构词成分]甲状腺,甲状

thyroactive [ˌθairəuˈæktiv] *a* 促甲状腺活性的

thyroadenitis [ˌθairəuædiˈnaitis] *n* 甲状腺炎

thyroaplasia [ˌθairəuəˈpleiziə] *n* 甲状腺发育不全

thyroarytenoid [ˌθairəuˌæriˈtiːnɔid] *a* 甲杓[软骨]的

thyrocalcitonin [ˌθairəuˌkælsiˈtəunin] *n* 甲状腺降钙素,降钙素

thyrocardiac [ˌθairəuˈkɑːdiæk] *a* 甲状腺[与]心脏的

thyrocarditis [ˌθairəukɑːˈdaitis] *n* 甲状腺性心炎

thyrocele [ˈθairəsiːl] *n* 甲状腺肿

thyrochondrotomy [ˌθairəukɔnˈdrɔtəmi] *n* 甲状软骨切开术

thyrocolloid [ˌθairəuˈkɔlɔid] *n* 甲状腺胶质

thyrocricotomy [ˌθairəukraiˈkɔtəmi] *n* 环甲膜切开术

thyrodesmic [ˌθairəuˈdezmik] *a* 促甲状腺的,亲甲状腺的

thyroepiglottic [ˌθairəuˌepiˈglɔtik] *a* 甲状会厌的

thyrofissure [ˌθairəuˈfiʃə] *n* 甲状软骨裂开术

thyrogenous [θaiˈrɔdʒinəs], **thyrogenic** [ˌθairəuˈdʒenik] *a* 甲状腺源的,甲状腺性的

thyroglobulin [ˌθairəuˈglɔbjulin] *n* 甲状腺球蛋白

thyroglossal [ˌθairəuˈglɔsəl] *a* 甲状舌[管]的

thyrohyal [ˌθairəuˈhaiəl] *a* 甲状舌骨的 *n* 舌骨大角

thyrohyoid [ˌθairəuˈhaiɔid] *a* 甲状舌骨的

thyroid [ˈθairɔid] *a* 甲状的 *n* 甲状腺;甲状腺[制]剂,甲状腺粉(获自人食用的驯养动物甲状腺,经洗净、干燥、变成粉末,含碘量 0.17% ~ 0.23%,为淡黄色无定形粉,从前用作甲状腺[激]素的来源,以治疗甲状腺功能减退) | aberrant ~ 异位甲状腺 / accessory ~ 副甲状腺 / intrathoracic ~ 胸内甲状腺 / retrosternal ~, substernal ~ 胸骨后甲状腺,胸骨下甲状腺

thyroidea [θaiˈrɔidiə] *n* 甲状腺

thyroidectomize [ˌθairɔiˈdektəmaiz] *vt* 切除甲状腺

thyroidectomy [ˌθairɔiˈdektəmi] *n* 甲状腺切除术

thyroidism [ˈθairɔidizəm] *n* 甲状腺功能亢进;甲状腺[制]剂中毒

thyroiditis [ˌθairɔiˈdaitis] *n* 甲状腺炎 | acute ~ 急性甲状腺炎 / autoimmune ~ 自身免疫性甲状腺炎 / chronic lymphadenoid ~, chronic lymphocytic ~ 慢性淋巴结样甲状腺炎,慢性淋巴细胞性甲状腺炎(即桥本〈Hashimoto〉甲状腺炎) / giant cell ~, giant follicular ~ 巨细胞性甲状腺炎,巨滤泡性甲状腺炎,亚急性肉芽肿性甲状腺炎 / granulomatous ~ 肉芽肿性甲状腺炎,亚急性肉芽肿性甲状腺炎 / invasive ~, ligneous ~ 侵袭性甲状腺炎,板样甲状腺炎 / pseudotuberculous ~ 假结核性甲状腺炎,亚急性肉芽肿性甲状腺炎 / subacutegranulomatous ~ 亚急性肉芽肿性甲状腺炎 / woody ~ 慢性纤维性甲状腺炎

thyroidization [ˌθairɔidaiˈzeiʃən, -diˈz-] *n* 甲状腺[制]剂疗法;(组织病理学中指组织的)甲状腺样出现

thyroidomania [ˌθairɔidəuˈmeinjə] *n* 甲状腺[功能亢进]性精神病

thyroidotherapy [ˌθairɔidəuˈθerəpi] *n* 甲状腺[制]剂疗法

thyroidotomy [ˌθairɔiˈdɔtəmi] *n* 甲状腺切开术

thyroidotoxin [ˌθairɔidəuˈtɔksin] *n* 甲状腺毒素

thyroid peroxidase [ˈθairɔid pəˈrɔksideis] 甲状腺过氧物酶,碘化物过氧物酶

thyroigenous [θaiˈrɔidʒinəs] *a* 甲状腺源的,甲状腺性的

thyrointoxication [ˌθairəuinˌtɔksiˈkeiʃən] *n* 甲状腺毒症,甲状腺中毒

thyroliberin [ˌθairəuˈlibərin] *n* 促甲状腺激素释放激素(即 thyroid stimulating hormone releasing hormone)

thyrolysin [θaiˈrɔlisin] *n* 溶甲状腺素

thyrolytic [ˌθairəuˈlitik] *a* 溶甲状腺的,破坏甲状腺的

thyromegaly [ˌθairəuˈmegəli] *n* 甲状腺肿大

thyromimetic [ˌθairəumaiˈmetik, -miˈm-] *a* 拟甲状腺素的,拟甲状腺的

thyroncus [θaiˈrɔŋkəs] *n* 甲状腺肿

thyronine [ˈθairəuniːn] *n* 甲状腺原氨酸

thyronucleoalbumin [ˌθairəuˌnjuːkliəˈælbjumin] *n* 甲状腺核白蛋白

thyro-oxyindole [ˌθairəu ˌɔksiˈindɔl] *n* 甲状腺素

thyroparathyroidectomy [ˌθairəuˌpærəˌθairɔiˈde-

ktəmi] *n* 甲状腺甲状旁腺切除术
thyroparathyroprivic [ˌθairəuˌpærəˌθairəu'privik] *a* 甲状腺甲状旁腺缺失的
thyropathy [θai'rɔpəθi] *n* 甲状腺病
thyropenia [ˌθairəu'piːniə] *n* 甲状腺分泌减少
thyroperoxidase [ˌθairəupə'rɔksideis] *n* 甲状腺过氧化物酶,碘化物过氧化物酶
thyrophyma [ˌθairəu'faimə] *n* 甲状腺瘤,甲状腺肿
thyroprival [ˌθairəu'praivəl], **thyroprivic** [ˌθairəu'privik], **thyroprivous** [θai'rɔprivəs] *a* 甲状腺缺乏的,甲状腺切除后的
thyroprivia [ˌθairəu'priviə] *n* 甲状腺缺乏症,甲状腺切除后状态
thyroptosis [ˌθairə'ptəusis] *n* 甲状腺下移,低位甲状腺
thyrosis [θai'rəusis] ([复] **thyroses** [θai'rəusiːz]) *n* 甲状腺功能病
thyrotherapy [ˌθairəu'θerəpi] *n* 甲状腺[制]剂疗法
thyrotome ['θairətəum] *n* 甲状软骨刀
thyrotomy [θai'rɔtəmi] *n* 甲状软骨切开术;甲状腺切开术
thyrotoxic [ˌθairəu'tɔksik] *a* 甲状腺毒性的
thyrotoxicosis [ˌθairəuˌtɔksi'kəusis], **thyrotoxemia** [ˌθairəutɔk'siːmiə], **thyrotoxia** [ˌθairəu 'tɔksiə] *n* 甲状腺毒症
thyrotoxin [ˌθairəu'tɔksin] *n* 甲状腺毒素
thyrotroph ['θairəutrəuf], **thyrotrope** ['θairətrəup] *n* 促甲状腺[激]素细胞(亦称 β-嗜碱细胞)
thyrotropic [ˌθairə'trɔpik], **thyrotrophic** [θairə'trɔfik] *a* 促甲状腺的
thyrotropin [θai'rɔtrəpin], **thyrotrophin** [θai'rɔtrəfin] *n* 促甲状腺[激]素(垂体激素类药)
thyroxine(T_4) [θai'rɔksi(ː)n] *n* 甲状腺素 | levo ~ 左甲状腺素,左旋甲状腺素(甲状腺激素) | **thyroxin** [θai'rɔksin] *n* / **thyroxinic** [ˌθairɔk'sinik] *a*
thyroxinemia [θaiˌrɔksi'niːmiə] *n* 甲状腺素血[症]
thyroxinsodium [θaiˌrɔksin'səudjəm] *n* 甲状腺素钠
thyrsus ['θəːsəs] *n* 聚伞圆锥花序
Thysanosoma [ˌθisənə'səumə] *n* 缝体绦虫属 | ~ actinioides 放射状缝体绦虫
Ti titanium 钛
TIA transient ischemic attack 短暂性脑缺血发作
tiacarana [ˌtiəkə'rænjə] *n* 溃烂型皮肤利什曼病
tiagabine hydrochloride [tai'ægəbiːn] 盐酸噻加宾(抗惊厥药,用作其他抗惊厥药的辅药,治疗部分发作,口服给药)
tiamenidine hydrochloride [ˌtaiə'menidiːn] 盐酸噻胺唑啉(抗高血压药)
tiaprofenic acid [ˌtaiəprəu'fenik] 噻洛芬酸(非甾体消炎药,用于治疗类风湿关节炎和骨关节炎,口服给药)
tiazuril [tai'æzjuəril] *n* 硫苯三嗪酮(家禽抗球虫药)
TIBC total iron-binding capacity 总铁结合力
tibia ['tibiə] ([复] **tibias** 或 **tibiae** ['tibiiː]) *n* 胫骨 | saber ~, sabershaped ~ 军刀状胫骨 | **~l** *a*
tibiad ['tibiæd] *ad* 向胫侧
tibiale [ˌtibi'eili] *n* 胫侧骨(胚)
tibialgia [ˌtibi'ældʒiə] *n* 胫骨痛(伴有淋巴细胞增多及嗜酸粒细胞增多)
tibialis [ˌtibi'eilis] *a* 胫骨的 *n* 胫骨肌
tibien ['tibiən] *a* 胫骨的
tibiocalcanean [ˌtibiəukæl'keiniən] *a* 胫[骨]跟[骨]的
tibiofemoral [ˌtibiəu'femərəl] *a* 胫[骨]股[骨]的
tibiofibular [ˌtibiəu'fibjulə], **tibioperoneal** [ˌtibiəuˌperə'niːəl] *a* 胫[骨]腓[骨]的
tibionavicular [ˌtibiəunə'vikjulə], **tibioscaphoid** [ˌtibiəu'skæfɔid] *a* 胫[骨]舟[骨]的
tibiotarsal [ˌtibiəu'tɑːsəl] *a* 胫[骨]跗[骨]的
tibolone ['tibələun] *n* 替勃龙(促蛋白合成类固醇)
tibric acid ['taibrik] 替贝酸(降血脂药)
tic [tik] *n*【法】抽搐 | bowing ~ 鞠躬状抽搐 / convulsive ~ 面肌抽搐 / ~ de pensée 思想暴露癖 / ~ douloureux 三叉神经痛,(面部)痛性痉挛 / facial ~, mimic ~ 面肌抽搐 / gesticulatory ~ 表演状抽搐 / local ~ 局部抽搐 / ~ nondouloureux 无痛性抽搐,肌阵挛 / rotatory ~ 旋转性抽搐,旋头痉挛
ticarbodine [tai'kɑːbədiːn] *n* 替卡波定(抗蠕虫药)
ticarcillin [ˌtaikə'silin] *n* 替卡西林(抗生素类药) | ~ cresyl sodium 替卡西林甲苯酯钠 / ~ disodium, ~ sodium 替卡西林钠
tick [tik] *n* 蜱,壁虱 | adobe ~ 波斯锐缘蜱(即 Argas persicus) / American dog ~ 美洲犬蜱(即变异革蜱 Dermacentor variabilis) / bandicoot ~ 袋鼠蜱(即硕鼠血蜱 Haemaphysalis humerosa) / beady-legged winter horse ~ 珠足冬季马蜱(即巨肢蜱 Margaropus winthemi) / black pitted ~ 黑凹蜱(即拟态扇头蜱 Rhipicephalus simus) / bont ~ 希伯来钝眼蜱(即 Amblyomma hebraeum) / British dog ~ 英国犬蜱(即犬硬蜱 Ixodes canisuga) / brown dog ~ 褐色犬蜱(即血红扇头蜱 Rhipicephalus sanguineus) / caster bean ~ 篦

子硬蜱(即 Ixodes ricinus) / cattle ~ 牛蜱(即具环牛蜱 Boophilus annulatus) / dog ~ 犬蜱(①犬血蜱 Haemaphysalis leachi; ②变异革蜱 Dermacentor variabilis; ③血红扇头蜱 Rhipicephalus sanguineus) /ear ~ 耳蜱(即耳残喙蜱 Otobius megnini) / Gulf Coast ~ 海湾蜱(即斑点钝眼蜱 Amblyomma maculatum) / hard ~, hardbodied ~ 硬蜱 / Kenya ~ 肯尼亚蜱(即具尾扇头蜱 Rhipicephalus appendiculatus) / Lone Star ~ 美洲钝眼蜱(即 Amblyommaamericanum) / miana ~ 波斯锐缘蜱(即 Argas persicus) / Pacific coast dog ~ 西海岸犬蜱(即西方革蜱 Dermacentoroccidentalis) / pajaroello ~ 皮革钝缘蜱(即 Ornithodoros coriaceus) / pigeon ~ 鸽锐缘蜱(即 Argasreflexus) / rabbit ~ 野兔血蜱(即 Haemaphysalis leporus-palustris) / Rocky Mountain wood ~ 落基山林蜱(即安氏革蜱 Dermacentor andersoni) / russet ~ 朽叶色蜱(即多毛硬蜱 Ixodes pilosus) / scrub ~ 灌木丛蜱(即全环硬蜱 Ixodes holocyclus) / seed ~ 幼虫期蜱 / sheep ~ 羊蜱蝇(即 Melophagus ovinus) / soft ~, soft-bodied ~ 软蜱 / spinous ear ~ 耳[刺]蜱(即耳残喙蜱 otobius megnini) / taiga ~ 全沟硬蜱(即 Ixodes persulcatus) / tampan ~ 毛白钝缘蜱(即 Ornithodoros moubata);波斯锐缘蜱(即 Argas persicus) / wood ~ 美国森林蜱(即安氏革蜱 Dermacentorandersoni)

tickicide [ˈtikisaid] *n* 杀蜱药

tickling [ˈtikliŋ] *n* 呵痒

tickover [ˈtikəuvə] *n* 空转,慢转(用以描述补体旁路的调节)

ticlatone [ˈtiklətəun] *n* 替克拉酮(抗菌药,抗真菌药)

ticlopidine hydrochloride [taiˈklɔpidiːn] 盐酸噻氯匹定(血小板抑制药)

ticpolonga [ˌtikpəˈlɔŋgə] *n* 锡兰大蒲蛇(亦称鲁塞尔蝰蛇〈Vipera russelli〉)

ticrynafen [taiˈkrinəfən] *n* 替尼酸(促尿酸排泄的利尿药,因对肝的毒性而停用)

tictology [tikˈtɔlədʒi] *n* 产科学

t. i. d. ter in die【拉】一天三次

tide [taid] *n* 潮,变异(指体液中某些成分的变异或增加) | acid ~ 酸潮(尿) / alkaline ~ 碱潮(尿) / fat ~ 脂肪潮(淋巴液及血液)

Tidy's test [ˈtaidi] (Charles M. Tidy)泰迪试验(检尿白蛋白)

Tiedemann's nerve [ˈtiːdəmən] (Friedrich Tiedemann)蒂德曼神经(围绕视网膜中央动脉的交感神经丛)

tienilic acid [taiəˈnilik] 替尼酸(利尿药,抗高血压药)

Tietze's syndrome(disease) [ˈtiːtsə] (Alexander Tietze)蒂策综合征(病)(①特发性痛性非化脓性肋软骨〈尤其是第二肋骨〉肿胀,前胸痛可能与冠状动脉病时的痛相似,亦称肋软骨炎;②白化病〈眼色素正常除外〉、聋哑及眉毛发育不全)

tigestol [taiˈdʒestɔl] *n* 替孕醇(孕激素类药)

tiglic acid [ˈtiglik] 顺芷酸,α-甲基巴豆酸

tiglium [ˈtigljəm] *n*【拉】巴豆

tigogenin [tiˈgɔdʒinin] *n* 提果皂苷元

tigonin [ˈtigənin] *n* 提果皂苷

tigroid [ˈtaigrɔid] *a* 虎斑状的

tigrolysis [taiˈgrɔlisis] *n* 虎斑溶解(神经细胞易染体溶解)

tiletamine hydrochloride [taiˈletəmiːn] 盐酸替来他明(麻醉药,抗惊厥药)

Tilia [ˈtiliə] *n* 椴属

tilidine hydrochloride [ˈtilidiːn] 盐酸替利定(麻醉性镇痛药)

Tillaux's disease [tiˈjəu] (Paul J. Tillaux)提奥病(乳腺炎并乳腺中形成多发性肿瘤)

Tilletia [tiˈliːʃiə] *n* 腥黑粉菌属

Tilletiaceae [tiˌliːʃiˈeisiiː] *n* 腥黑粉菌科

tilmicosin [ˌtilmiˈkɔsin] *n* 替米考星(兽医用抗菌药)

tilmus [ˈtilməs] *n* 摸空,捉空摸床[动作](见于高热或重病时)

tilorone [ˈtilərəun] *n* 替洛隆(抗病毒药) | ~ hydrochloride 盐酸替洛隆(抗病毒药)

tiltometer [tilˈtɔmitə] *n* 倾斜测定仪(脊髓麻醉时测量手术台倾斜度)

tiludronate disodium [tiˈljuːdrəneit] 替鲁膦酸二钠(骨吸收抑制药,用于治疗畸形性胃炎,口服给药)

timbre [ˈtimbə, ˈtæmbr] *n*【法】音色,音品 | ~ métallique 金属音

time(t) [taim] *n* 时间 | apex ~ 高峰时间(指肌肉的复合收缩) / bleeding ~ 出血时间 / chromoscopy ~ 胃液染色时间(测胃腺分泌) / clot retraction ~ 血块退缩时间,血块凝缩时间 / coagulation ~, clotting ~ 凝固时间 / decimal reduction ~ 拾-存活时间(存活微生物减少 10 倍所需的热力灭菌时间) / doubling ~ (对数期细胞)倍增时间 / generation ~ 增代时间,一代时间(两代相隔的时间,或细菌中的细胞由一次分裂到下一次分裂的时间) / prothrombin ~ 凝血酶原时间(脑组织浸出物和钙加到血浆后血块形成所需的时间) / recalcification ~ 再钙化时间(钙离子在经抗凝处理的血小板含量甚丰的血浆中被置换时血块形成所需的时间) / sedimentation ~ 沉降时间(红细胞沉降率) / thermal death ~ 热致死时间(指灭菌) / ventricular activation ~ 室壁激动时间

timer [ˈtaimə] *n* (自动)定时器,时计,限时器

Timme's syndrome [ˈtimə] (Walter Timme) 蒂姆综合征(卵巢及肾上腺功能不全,伴有代偿性垂体功能减退)

Timofeew's corpuscles [timəuˈfeief] (Dmitri A. Timofeew) 提莫费夫小体(尿道膜部和前列腺部黏膜下层所见的特异化型环层小体)

timolol maleate [ˈtaiməlɔl] 马来酸噻吗洛尔(β-肾上腺素能阻滞药)

timothy [ˈtiməθi] *n* 梯牧草

tin(Sn) [tin] *n* 锡

tina [ˈtinə] *n* 品他病(螺旋体性皮肤病)

tinct. tincture, tinctura 酊,酊剂

tinctable [ˈtiŋktəbl] *a* 可染的

tinction [ˈtiŋkʃən] *n* 染色;(药剂中)着色或调味

tinctorial [tiŋkˈtɔːriəl] *a* 染色的

tinctura [tiŋkˈtjuːrə] ([所有格、复] **tincturae** [tiŋkˈtjuːriː]) *n*【拉】酊,酊剂

tincturation [ˌtiŋktjuˈreiʃən] *n* 酊剂制备

tincture [ˈtiŋktʃə] *n* 酊,酊剂 | belladonna ~ 颠茄酊(抗胆碱能药) / camphorated opium ~ 樟脑阿片酊(镇痛酊) / capsicum ~ 辣椒酊(刺激剂及驱风剂) / compound benzoin ~ 复方安息香酊(表面保护剂) / compound cardamom ~ 复方豆蔻酊(调味剂) / compound gentian ~ 复方龙胆酊,苦味酊(苦味健胃药) / digitalis ~ 洋地黄酊(强心药) / ferric citrochloride ~ 氯化枸橼酸铁酊(止血药) / green soap ~ 绿肥皂酊,软肥皂搽剂 / iodine ~ 碘酊(俗名碘酒,皮肤消毒药) / lemon ~, lemon peel ~ 柠檬酊(调味剂) / nux vomica ~ 马钱子酊(苦味酊) / opium ~ 阿片酊 / strong iodine ~ 浓碘酊(刺激剂、抗菌剂及杀真菌剂)

tine [tain] *n* 叉,尖齿

tinea [ˈtiniə] *n*【拉】癣 | ~ amiantacea, asbestos-like ~ 石棉状癣 / ~ axillaris 腋癣,腋毛菌病 / ~ barbae 须癣,触染性须疮 / ~ capitis 头癣 / ~ ciliorum 睫癣 / ~ imbricata 叠瓦癣 / ~ kerion 脓癣 / ~ nigra 黑癣 / ~ nodosa 发结节病 / ~ pedis 脚癣 / ~ profunda 深癣,毛癣菌性肉芽肿 / ~ sycosis 触染性须疮,须癣 / ~ tonsurans 头癣 / ~ unguium 甲癣,甲真菌病 / ~ versicolor 花斑癣

Tinel's sign [tiˈnel] (Jules Tinel) 蒂内尔征(在已经切断神经的部位叩诊时肢远端有麻刺感,提示神经部分损害或开始再生。亦称蚁走感征)

tinfoil [ˈtinfɔil] *n* 锡箔

tingibility [ˌtindʒiˈbiləti] *n* 可染性

tingible [ˈtindʒibl] *a* 可染的

tingling [ˈtiŋgliŋ] *n* 麻刺感 | distal ~ on percussion 叩诊肢端麻刺感(见 Tinel's sign)

tinidazole [taiˈnidəzəul] *n* 替硝唑(抗滴虫药)

tinkle [ˈtiŋkl] *n* 叮叮声,叮当音(肺空洞或气胸时听到) | metallic ~ 金属叮当音(有时和其他呼吸音连在一起可听到)

tinnitus [tiˈnaitəs] *n*【拉】耳鸣 | ~ aurium 耳鸣 / clicking ~ 撞击性耳鸣 / nervous ~ 神经性耳鸣 / objective ~ 他觉性耳鸣

Tinospora [tiˈnɔspərə] *n* 青牛胆属

tinsel [ˈtinsəl] *n* 金属箔,金属丝

tint [tint] *n* 色调,色辉 | ~ B 色调 B 度(测定 X 线量的纸碟的色调,B 度指已达到使毛发脱落的辐射量)

Tintinnina [ˌtintiˈnainə] *n* 筒壳亚目

tintometer [tinˈtɔmitə] *n* 液体比色器,色调计,色辉计 | **tintometry** *n* 液体比色法 / **tintometric** [ˌtintəˈmetrik] *a* 液体比色的

tinzaparin sodium [tinˈzæpərin] 亭扎肝素钠(抗凝药和抗血栓药,并用作华法林钠的辅药,治疗深静脉血栓伴或不伴肺栓塞,皮下给药)

tioconazole [ˌtaiəuˈkəunəzəul] *n* 噻康唑(局部抗真菌药,阴道内应用治疗外阴阴道念珠菌病)

tioperidone hydrochloride [ˌtaiəuˈperidəun] 盐酸硫哌立酮(安定药)

tiopinac [taiˈəupinæk] *n* 硫平酸(抗炎、镇痛、解热药)

tiopronin [taiˈɔprənin] *n* 硫普罗宁(用于治疗胱氨酸尿症,口服给药)

tioxidazole [ˌtaiɔkˈsaidəzəul] *n* 噻昔达唑(抗蠕虫药)

tip [tip] *n* 梢尖,末端 | ~ of nose 鼻尖 / ~ of sacral bone 骶尖 / ~ of tongue 舌尖

tipping [ˈtipiŋ] *n* 翻动(牙齿改变其垂直位的运动);牙尖复位

tiprenolol hydrochloride [taiˈprenəlɔl] 盐酸替普洛尔(β 受体阻滞药)

TIPS transjugular intrahepatic portosystemic shunt 经颈静脉肝内门体静脉分流

tiqueur [tiˈkəː] *n* [患]抽搐者

tiquinamide hydrochloride [taiˈkwinəmaid] 盐酸替喹胺(胃抗胆碱药)

tirebal [tiəˈbɑːl] *n*【法】拔弹器

tirefond [tiəˈfɔŋ] *n*【法】起骨器;螺旋,提锥

tires [taiəz] *n* 震颤病(牛、羊);乳毒病(人)

tiring [ˈtaiəriŋ] *n* 轮箍术(治髌骨骨折)

tirofiban hydrochloride [ˌtairəuˈfaibæn] 盐酸替洛法班(血小板抑制药,用于预防急性冠心病综合征〈不稳定心绞痛或非 Q 波心肌梗死〉患者的血栓,静脉内给药)

Tiselius apparatus [tiˈseiliəs] (Arne W. K. Tiselius) 提塞留斯电泳仪(从血清、血浆和其他体液中分离出蛋白质)

tisic [ˈtizik] *a* [患]痨病的 *n* 痨病患者;气喘(旧名)

tisis [ˈtisis] *n* 痨病;肺痨

tissue [ˈtisjuː] *n* 组织;纱 | accidental ~ 偶发组织 / adenoid ~ 腺样组织,淋巴组织 / adrenogenic ~ 雄激素带 / areolar ~, cribriform ~ 蜂窝组织,蜂窝织 / cellular ~ 蜂窝组织,蜂窝织 / chromaffin ~ 嗜铬组织 / cicatrical ~ 瘢痕组织 / compact ~ 致密质(尤指骨密质) / connective ~ 结缔组织,结缔质 / erectile ~ 勃起组织 / extracellular ~ 细胞外组织 / extraperitoneal ~ 腹膜外组织,腹膜外筋膜 / fatty ~, adipose ~ 脂肪组织 / fibrous ~ 纤维组织,纤维织 / gut-associated lymphoid(GALT) ~ 肠相关淋巴组织 / heterotopic ~ 异位组织,迷芽瘤 / hyperplastic ~ 增生组织 / indifferent ~ 未分化组织 / interrenal ~ 肾上腺皮质组织 / interstitial ~ 间质组织 / loose connective ~ 疏松结缔组织 / lymphadenoid ~ 淋巴腺样组织 / lymphoid ~, lymphatic ~ 淋巴组织 / mesenchymal ~ 间叶组织,间充质 / muscular ~ 肌组织 / osteoid ~ 骨样组织(未钙化骨组织) / parenchymatous ~ 实质,主质 / reticular ~, reticulated ~ 网状组织 / rubber ~ 橡皮片(用于手术) / splenic ~ 脾组织,红髓 / target ~ 靶组织(指在体内或体外,体液免疫或细胞免疫所指向的组织或指对某一激素起应答的组织) / tuberculosis granulation ~ 结核性肉芽组织

tissular [ˈtisjuːlə] *a* 组织的

titanate [ˈtaitəneit] *n* 钛酸盐

titanic [taiˈtænik] *a* 钛的,四价钛的 | ~ acid 钛酸

titanium(Ti) [taiˈteinjəm] *n* 钛(化学元素) | ~ dioxide 二氧化钛

titer, titre [ˈtaitə] *n* 效价,滴度,值 | agglutination ~ 凝集反应效价(血清能引起细菌或其他颗粒性抗原发生凝集的最高稀释度)

titillate [ˈtitileit] *vt* 搔痒,撩痒 | **titillation** [ˌtitiˈleiʃən] *n*

titin [ˈtaitin] *n* 肌联蛋白,粗丝联接蛋白

titrant [ˈtaitrənt] *n* 滴定剂(滴定用标准液)

titrate [ˈtaitreit] *vt*, *vi* 滴定

titration [taiˈtreiʃən] *n* 滴定法 | colorimetric ~ 比色滴定法(测氢离子浓度) / complexometric ~ 络合滴定法 / coulometric ~ 库伦滴定 / formol ~ 甲醛滴定法(检尿氨基酸) / potentiometric ~ 电位滴定法(测氢离子浓度)

titrimetric [ˌtitriˈmetrik] *a* 滴定[测量]的

titrimetry [taiˈtrimitri] *n* 滴定测量

titubant [ˈtitjubənt] *n* 蹒跚者

titubation [ˌtitjuˈbeiʃən] *n* 蹒跚(步态) | lingual ~ 口吃,讷吃

Tityus [ˈtitiəs] *n* 钳蝎属 | ~ serrulatus 巴西钳蝎

tixanox [ˈtiksənɔks] *n* 替咕诺(抗变态反应药)

tixocortol pivalate [tikˈsəukɔːtɔl] 特戊酸替可的松(糖皮质激素,具有抗炎作用,直肠给药,治疗溃疡性结肠炎)

tizanidine hydrochloride [taiˈzænidiːn] 盐酸替扎尼定(解痉药)

Tizzoni's test [tiˈdzəuni] (Guido Tizzoni) 蒂佐尼试验(检组织中铁)

TJA total joint arlthroplasty 全关节成形术

TK thymidine kinase 胸苷激酶

TKA total knee arthroplasty 全膝关节成形术

TKD tokodynamometer 分娩力计

TKG tokodynagraph 分娩力[描记]图

Tl thallium 铊

TLC total lung capacity 肺总量; thin-layer chromatography 薄层色谱法,薄层层析

TLI total lymphoid irradiation 全淋巴照射

TLSO thoracolumbosacral orthosis 胸腰骶矫形器

TLV threshold limit value 阈限值

Tm thulium 铥

TMA trimellitic anhydrate 1, 2, 4-苯三酸酐

TMI transmandibular implant 经下颌植入物

TMST treadmill stress test 跑台应激试验

TMV tobacco mosaic virus 烟草花叶病毒

Tn normal intraocular tension 正常眼内压,正常眼压

TND transmissible neurodegenerative disease 传染性神经变性病

TNF tumor necrosis factor 肿瘤坏死因子

TNM tumor-nodes-metastasis 肿瘤-淋巴结-转移(见 staging)

TNS transcutaneous nerve stimulation 经皮神经刺激

TNT trinitrotoluene 三硝基甲苯

TO tinctura opii 阿片酊

toad [təud] *n* 蟾蜍

toadskin [ˈtəudskin] *n* 蟾皮病(缺乏维生素 A)

toadstool [ˈtəudstul] *n* 毒伞菌,蕈状毒菌

tobacco [təˈbækəu] *n* 烟草;烟叶 | mountain ~ 山金车(花) / poison ~ 莨菪

tobaccoism [təˈbækəizəm] *n* 烟草中毒

Töbey-Ayer test [ˈtoubi ˈeiə] (George L. Töbey, Jr.; James B. Ayer) 托比-艾尔试验(检静脉窦血栓形成)

Tobold's apparatus [ˈtɔːbɔlt] (Adelbert A. O. Tobold) 喉镜照明器

tobramycin [ˌtəubrəˈmaisin] *n* 妥布霉素,托布拉霉素(亦称暗霉素,抗生素类药)

tocainide hydrochloride [təuˈkeinaid] 盐酸托卡尼(口服抗心律失常药,结构和作用类似利多卡因〈lidocaine〉,用于治疗室性心律失常)

tocamphyl [təuˈkæmfil] *n* 托莰非(利胆药)

toc(o)- [构词成分] 分娩,产,生育

tocodynagraph [ˌtəukəuˈdainəgrɑːf] *n* 分娩力[描记]图

tocodynamometer [ˌtəukəuˌdainəˈmɔmitə] *n* 分娩力计

tocograph [ˈtɔkəgrɑːf, -græf] *n* 分娩力描记器 | **~y** [təuˈkɔgrəfi] *n* 分娩力描记法

tocokinin [ˌtɔkəˈkinin] *n* 激育素(获自酵母及数种植物,有雌激素的性质)

tocol [ˈtəukɔl] *n* 母育酚

tocology [təuˈkɔlədʒi] *n* 产科学 | **tocologist** *n* 产科学家

tocolysis [təuˈkɔlisis] *n* 安宫,保胎(早产时抑制子宫收缩)

tocolytic [ˌtəukəuˈlitik] *a* 子宫收缩抑制的 *n* 子宫收缩抑制药

tocometer [təuˈkɔmitə] *n* 分娩力计

tocopherol [təˈkɔfərɔl] *n* 生育酚,维生素 E | α-~, alpha-~ α-生育酚,维生素 E

tocopheryl [təuˈkɔfəril] *n* 生育酚酰基

tocophobia [ˌtəukəˈfəubjə] *n* 分娩恐怖

tocotrienol [ˌtəukəuˈtraiənɔl] *n* 生育三烯酚

tocus [ˈtəukəs] *n*【拉】生育,分娩

Todaro's tendon [təuˈdɑːrəu] (Francesco Todaro)托达罗腱(一个可触知的右心房壁内心内膜下胶原束,从纤维性中心体,经过主动脉圆枕,延伸至下腔静脉瓣的内侧端)

Toddalia [təuˈdæliə] *n* 簕钩属,飞龙掌血属

Todd bodies [tɔd] (John L. Todd)托德体(若干两栖动物的红细胞内)

Todd's cirrhosis [tɔd] (Robert B. Todd)原发性胆汁性肝硬化 | ~ paralysis(palsy)托德瘫痪(癫痫后偏瘫或单瘫,在癫痫发作后持续几分钟或若干小时,间或有数天之久) / ~ process 托德突,脚间纤维(连接腹股沟浅环内侧脚和外侧脚的纤维)

Todd-Wells apparatus [tɔd welz] (Edwin M. Todd; T. H. Wells, Jr.)托-韦器(用于托-韦立体定位性外科的技术) | ~ technique 托-韦技术(一种立体定位性技术)

toddy [ˈtɔdi] *n* 棕榈汁;棕榈酒(由杜松子酒或威士忌酒、糖和水制成的酒类饮料)

toe [təu] *n* 趾 | great ~ 踇趾,踇 / hammer ~, mallet ~ 锤状趾 / little ~ 小趾 / pigeon ~ 鸽趾,内收足 / webbed ~s 蹼趾

toeless [ˈtəulis] *a* 无趾的

toenail [ˈtəuneil] *n* 趾甲

Toepfer [ˈtepfə] *n* 见 Töpfer

tofenacin hydrochloride [təuˈfenəsin] 盐酸托芬那辛(抗胆碱药,具有抗抑郁作用)

tofu [ˈtəufuː] *n* 豆腐

tofukasu [tɔːfuˈkɑːsu] *n*【日】豆腐渣

Togaviridae [ˌtəugəˈviridiː] *n* 披膜病毒科

togavirus [ˈtəugəˌvaiərəs] *n* 披膜病毒,披盖病毒

toilet [tɔilit] *n* 盥洗室,厕所,卫生间;清洗创口

Toison's solution (fluid) [twəˈzɔŋ] (J. Toison)图瓦宗溶液(红细胞计数稀释液,含甲紫、氯化钠、硫酸钠、甘油和水)

tokelau [təukəˈlau] *n* 叠瓦癣(Tokelau 为南太平洋一个环状珊瑚岛)

tok(o)- 见 toco-

tokodynagraph (TKG) [ˌtəukəuˈdainəgrɑːf, -græf] *n* 分娩力[描记]图

tokodynamometer (TKD) [ˌtəukəuˌdainəˈmɔmitə] *n* 分娩力计

tolamolol [təuˈlæməlɔl] *n* 妥拉洛尔(β 受体阻滞药)

tolazamide [tɔˈlæzəmaid] *n* 妥拉磺脲(口服降血糖药)

tolazoline hydrochloride [tɔˈlæzəliːn] 盐酸妥拉唑啉(β 受体阻滞药及末梢血管扩张药)

tolbutamide [tɔlˈbjuːtəmaid] *n* 甲苯磺丁脲(口服降血糖药)

tolcapone [ˈtɔlkəˌpəun] *n* 托卡朋(抗震颤麻痹药)

tolciclate [təulˈsaikleit] *n* 托西拉酯(抗真菌药)

Toldt's membrane [təult] (Karl Toldt)托尔特膜(在肾之前的肾筋膜部分)

tolerance [ˈtɔlərəns] *n* 耐受;耐[药]量;耐受性,耐力 | acquired ~ 后天耐受[性](由于连续使用药物,对药物一般作用的抵抗力不断增加) / adoptive ~ 过继耐受[性](经过放射性照射的动物,接受了对某种抗原有耐受性的供者的淋巴细胞后,所获得的特异性免疫耐受性) / crossed ~ 交叉耐受性(对一种药物或毒物已获得耐受性的人此后对另一种药物的易感性则减少) / drug ~ 药物耐受性(由于连续使用药物,对药物作用的易感性逐渐减少) / glucose ~ 葡萄糖耐量(身体使葡萄糖产生代谢变化的能力) / high-dose ~, high-zone ~ 高剂量耐受[性],高区带耐受(经大量抗原刺激后形成的获得性免疫耐受性) / immunologic ~ 免疫耐受性(一种免疫应答,其特点为淋巴组织对正常情况下能引起免疫反应的抗原呈现特异性的无反应性。在胎儿或初生期接触抗原后,或在成年给予大量或很小量的某种抗原后均可发生。某一抗原所引起的免疫耐受性并不影响对一些不相关的抗原的免疫反应。亦称免疫麻痹) / impaired glucose ~ (IGT)糖耐量减低(空腹血糖水平或口服葡萄糖耐量试验结果异常,但尚未达诊断糖尿病的水平。以前称化学性糖尿病、隐性糖尿病、临床前糖尿病或亚临床糖尿病) / low-doze ~, low-zone ~ 低剂量耐受[性],低区带耐受性(经少量抗原持续刺激后形成的获得性免疫耐受性) / self ~ 自身耐受[性](对自身抗原的免疫无反应性是在胚胎期通过“自身识别”过程而获得的) / split ~ 分裂耐受[性](①对同种细胞诱发免疫耐受性后,对细胞表面一种或一组抗原发生耐受性,而对细胞表面的其他抗原仍具免疫应答;②指免疫耐受性要么

对体液免疫系统发生影响,要么对细胞免疫系统发生影响,但不会对两者都发生影响。亦称免疫偏移)

tolerant [ˈtɔlərənt] *a* 能忍受的

toleration [ˌtɔləˈreiʃən] *n* 忍受;耐量;耐受性,耐力

tolerogen [ˈtɔlərədʒən] *n* 耐受原(动物体内能诱导机体对以后注射攻击剂量时出现特异性免疫无反应性状态的抗原)

tolerogenesis [ˌtɔlərəuˈdʒenisis] *n* 致(免疫)耐受性,(免疫)耐受性形成

tolerogenic [ˌtɔlərəuˈdʒenik] *a* 致耐受性的(能诱发免疫耐受性);耐受原的

***o*-tolidine** [ˈtɔlidiːn] *n* *o*-联甲苯胺(以前用于检测隐血,因其致癌,现限止使用)

tolindate [təuˈlindeit] *n* 托林达酯(抗真菌药)

tolle causam [ˈtɔləˈkɔːzæm]【拉】根除病因(自然医术的医学原则,主张治疗的目的在于证实并根除病因)

Tollens' test [ˈtɔlənz] (Bernhard C. G. Tollens) 托伦斯试验(检醛、葡萄糖、戊糖、结合糖醛酸酯)

tolmetin sodium [ˈtɔlmetin] 托美丁钠(抗炎、镇痛、解热药)

tolnaftate [tɔlˈnæfteit] *n* 托萘酯(抗真菌药)

tolonium chloride [təˈləuniəm] 托洛氯铵(抗肝素药,亦称甲苯胺蓝O)

Tolosa-Hunt syndrome [təuˈləusɑː hʌnt] (Eduardo S. Tolosa; William E. Hunt) 托洛萨-亨特综合征(单侧眼肌麻痹合并眶后及三叉神经第1分支分布区疼痛,据认为系眶上裂或海绵窦内非特异性炎症与肉芽组织所致)

tolpyrramide [tɔlˈpiərəmaid] *n* 甲苯磺吡胺(口服降血糖药)

tolterodine tartrate [tɔlˈterədiːn] 酒石酸托特罗定(毒碱受体拮抗药,用于治疗活动过度性膀胱,伴有尿频、尿急或紧迫性尿失禁的症状,口服给药)

toluene [ˈtɔljuiːn], **toluol** [ˈtɔljuɔl] *n* 甲苯

toluic acid [təˈljuːik] 甲基苯甲酸

toluidine [təˈljuːidiːn] *n* 甲苯胺,氨基甲苯 | ~ blue O 甲苯胺蓝O(即托洛氯铵 tolonium chloride,抗肝素药)

tolusafranine [ˌtɔljuˈsæfrəniːn] *n* 番红T,亮藏红

toluyl [ˈtɔljuil] *n* 甲苯酰

toluylene [təˈljuːiliːn] *n* 二苯乙烯,芪

tolyl [ˈtɔlil] *n* 甲苯基 | ~ hydroxide 甲酚,煤酚

tomaculous [təuˈmækjuləs] *a* 腊肠样的(通常由于肿胀所致)

tomatin(e) [təˈmeitin] *n* 番茄素,番茄[碱糖]苷

-tome [构词成分]刀;片,节

tomentose [təuˈmentəus] *a* 被绒毛的

tomentum [təuˈmentəm] ([复] **tomenta** [təuˈmentə]) *n* 大脑绒被(大脑软膜和皮质的小血管网)

Tomes' fibers(fibrils) [təumz] (John Tomes) 成牙本质细胞突 | ~ granular layer 托姆斯颗粒层(靠近牙骨质的一层钙化不完全的牙本质) / ~ process①(Charles S. Tomes) 牙釉质细胞突;②(John Tomes) 成牙本质细胞突

tomite [ˈtəumait] *n* 藻煤

Tommaselli's disease (syndrome) [ˌtɔməˈseli] (Salvatore Tommaselli) 托马塞利病(综合征)(过量奎宁所致发热及血尿)

Tommasi's sign [tɔˈmæsi] (L. Tommasi) 托马西征(在下肢后外侧发生脱毛现象,几乎独见于患痛风的男子)

tom(o)- [构词成分]切割;层[面]

tomogram [ˈtəuməgræm] *n* X线体层[照]片,X线断层[照]片

tomograph [ˈtəuməgrɑːf, -græf] *n* X线体层摄影机,X线断层摄影机

tomography [təˈmɔgrəfi] *n* 体层摄影[术] | computed ~ (CT), computerized axial ~ (CAT) 计算机体层摄影[术],计算机轴向体层摄影[术](亦称 CAT scan) / hypocycloidal ~ 内摆线体层摄影[术],梅花状轨迹体层摄影[术] / positron emission ~ (PET) 正电子发射体层摄影[术] / ultrasonic ~ 体层声像图检查,超声体层扫描

tomont [ˈtəumɔnt] *n* 分裂前体

-tomy [构词成分]切开术,切断术

tonal [ˈtəunl] *a* 音调的,色调的

tonality [təuˈnæləti] *n* 音调,色调

tonaphasia [tɔnəˈfeiziə] *n* 音调性失语,乐歌不能

tone [təun] *n* 音,音调;色调;紧张性 *vt*, *vi* 具有某种音调(或色调) | feeling ~ 情调 / heart ~s 心音 / jecoral ~ 肝音,肝区叩音 / plastic ~ 成形性紧张

tonga [tɔŋgə] *n* 雅司病(即 yaws)

tongs [tɔŋz] *n* 钳,铗

tongue [tʌŋ] *n* 舌 | adherent ~ 粘连舌 / baked ~ 干烘舌(见于患伤寒症时) / bald ~ 光舌,秃舌 / bifid ~, cleft ~, double ~, split ~ 舌裂 / black ~, black hairy ~ 黑舌[病] / burning ~ 舌灼痛 / eardinal ~ 鲜红舌 / choreic ~ 舌舞蹈(舞蹈病时舌像蛇样伸缩) / coated ~, furred ~ 有苔舌,舌苔 / cobble-stone ~ 圆石子样舌 / earthy ~ 土样舌(钙苔舌) / encrusted ~ 厚苔舌 / filmy ~ 对称白斑舌 / fissured ~, crocodile ~, furrowed ~, grooved ~, plicated ~, scrotal ~, sulcated ~, wrinkled ~ 裂缝舌,沟舌 / geographic ~, mappy ~ 地图样舌,良性游走性舌炎 / hairy ~ 毛舌 / magenta ~

洋红舌 / parrot ~ 鹦鹉舌 / smoker's ~ 吸烟舌,舌白斑病 / stippled ~ , dotted ~ 点彩舌 / strawberry ~ 草莓舌 / wooden ~ , timber ~ 木样舌(牛的放线菌病)

tongue-tie [ˈtʌŋ tai] *n* 舌系带短缩

tongue-tied [ˈtʌŋ taid] *a* 舌系带短缩的

tonic [ˈtɔnik] *a* 紧张的;强直的 *n* 补药,强壮药 | bitter ~ 苦补药,苦味健胃药 / cardiac ~ 强心药 / digestive ~ 助消化药 / general ~ 全身强壮药 / intestinal ~ 健肠药 / stomachic ~ 健胃药 / vascular ~ 血管强壮药

tonic-clonic [ˌtɔnik ˈklɔnik] *a* 强直阵挛性的

tonicity [təˈnisəti] *n* 紧张性,张力

tonicize [ˈtɔnisaiz] *vt* 促进张力,促进紧张

tonicoclonic [ˌtɔnikəuˈklɔnik] *a* 强直阵挛性的

tonka bean [ˈtɔŋkə biːn] 香豆,香翅豆

ton(o)- [构词成分]紧张,张力,强直

tonoclonic [ˌtɔnəˈklɔnik] *a* 强直阵挛性的

tonofibril [ˈtɔnəˌfaibril] *n* 张力原纤维

tonofilament [ˌtəunəuˈfiləmənt] *n* 张力丝

tonogram [ˈtəunəgræm] *n* 张力[描记]图

tonograph [ˈtəunəgrɑːf, -græf] *n* 张力描记器

tonography [təuˈnɔgrəfi] *n* 张力描记法 | carotid compression ~ 颈动脉加压张力描记法(测颈动脉阻塞)

tonometer [təuˈnɔmitə] *n* 张力计,压力计(亦称眼压计) | air-puff ~ 气压眼压计 / applanation ~ 压平眼压计 / electronic ~ 电子眼压计 / impression ~ , indentation ~ 压陷眼压计

tonometric [tɔnəˈmetrik] *a* 张力计的,压力计的;张力测量的,压力测量的

tonometry [təuˈnɔmitri] *n* 张力测量法,压力测量法(尤指眼压测量法) | digital ~ 指诊眼压测量法

tonophant [ˈtɔnəfənt] *n* 音振动描记器

tonoplast [ˈtɔnəplæst] *n* 液泡膜;液泡形成体,成泡质

tonoscope [ˈtɔnəskəup] *n* 音波振动描记器;音振测脑器;张力计

tonotopic [ˌtɔnəuˈtɔpik] *a* 张力学说的(认为有一个空间排列结构,因此某些音频沿着此结构如在蜗神经核中那样的一个特殊部分传递的) | **~ity** [ˌtɔnəutəˈpisəti] *n*

tonsil [ˈtɔnsl] *n* 扁桃体(旧名扁桃腺) | ~ of cerebellum 小脑扁桃体 / eustachian ~ , tubal ~ 咽鼓管淋巴小结 / faucial ~ , palatine ~ 腭扁桃体 / lingual ~ 舌扁桃体 / resected ~ 切除后(遗留)扁桃体 / submerged ~ , buried ~ 埋入性扁桃体 / third ~ , pharyngeal ~ 咽扁桃体 | **~lar** *a*

tonsilla [tɔnˈsilə] ([复] **tonsillae** [tɔnˈsiliː]) *n* 【拉】扁桃体

tonsillectome [ˌtɔnsiˈlektəum] *n* 扁桃体切除器

tonsillectomy [ˌtɔnsiˈlektəmi] *n* 扁桃体切除术

tonsillith [ˈtɔnsiliθ] *n* 扁桃体石

tonsillitis [ˌtɔnsiˈlaitis] *n* 扁桃体炎 | diphtherial ~ 扁桃体白喉 / lacunar ~ , caseous ~ 陷窝性扁桃体炎 / ~ lenta 迁延性扁桃体炎 / preglottic ~ 舌扁桃体炎 / superficial ~ 表浅性扁桃体炎 | **tonsillitic** [ˌtɔnsiˈlitik] *a*

tonsill(o)- [构词成分]扁桃体

tonsilloadenoidectomy [ˌtɔnsiləuˌædinɔiˈdektəmi] *n* 扁桃体增殖腺切除术

tonsillohemisporosis [ˌtɔnsiləuˈhemispəˈrəusis] *n* 扁桃体半孢子菌病

tonsillolith [tɔnˈsiləliθ] *n* 扁桃体石

tonsillomoniliasis [ˌtɔnsiləuˌmɔniˈlaiəsis] *n* 扁桃体念珠菌病

tonsillomycosis [ˌtɔnsiləumaiˈkəusis] *n* 扁桃体真菌病

tonsillo-oidiosis [ˌtɔnsiləuəuˌidiˈəusis] *n* 扁桃体卵霉菌病,扁桃体念珠菌病

tonsillopathy [ˌtɔnsiˈlɔpəθi] *n* 扁桃体病

tonsilloprive [ˈtɔnsiləupraiv] *a* 已切除扁桃体的,扁桃体缺乏的

tonsilloscopy [tɔnsiˈlɔskəpi] *n* 扁桃体镜检查

tonsillotome [tɔnˈsilətəum] *n* 扁桃体刀

tonsillotomy [ˌtɔnsiˈlɔtəmi] *n* 扁桃体切开术,扁桃体部分切除术

tonsillotyphoid [ˌtɔnsiləuˈtaifɔid] *n* 咽型伤寒

tonsolith [ˈtɔnsəliθ] *n* 扁桃体结石

tonsure [ˈtɔnʃə] *n* 秃斑

tonus [ˈtəunəs] *n* 紧张 | acerebral ~ 去[大]脑紧张 / chemical ~ 化学紧张 / myogenic ~ 肌[源]性紧张 / neurogenic ~ 神经[源]性紧张

tooth [tuːθ] ([复] **teeth**) *n* 牙 | accessional teeth 恒磨牙 / anterior teeth, labial teeth 前牙 / artificial ~ 人工牙 / bicuspid teeth 前磨牙 / canine teeth, cuspid teeth 尖牙 / cheoplastic teeth 低熔铸牙 / crosspin teeth 横针牙 / deciduous teeth, milk teeth, primary teeth, temporary teeth 乳牙,暂牙 / diatoric teeth, pinless teeth 带孔假牙,无针假牙 / eye ~ 眼牙,上尖牙 / fused teeth 融合牙 / geminate ~ , connate ~ 双生牙,双连牙 / hag teeth 巨隙前牙 / hair teeth 毛牙,听牙 / impacted ~ 阻生牙 / incisor teeth 切牙 / lion's ~ 蒲公英 / malacotic teeth 软质牙 / malposed ~ 异位牙,错位牙 / molar teeth 磨牙 / permanent teeth 恒牙 / posterior teeth, buccal teeth, cheek teeth 后牙 / premolar teeth 前磨牙 / screwdriver teeth 凿状牙 / snaggle ~ 凸牙,歪牙 / wandering ~ 游走牙,移位牙 / wisdom ~ 智牙

toothache [ˈtuːθeik] *n* 牙痛

tooth-borne [ˈtuːθ bɔːn] *a* 牙支承的(假牙)

Tooth's atrophy, disease, type [tuːθ] (Howard H. Tooth)进行性神经病性腓骨肌萎缩症

topagnosia [ˌtɔpəɡˈnəuziə] *n* 位置觉缺失;环境认识不能

topagnosis [ˌtɔpəɡˈnəusis] *n* 位置觉缺失(触觉定位能力缺失)

topalgia [təˈpældʒiə] *n* 局部痛(见于神经衰弱)

-tope [构词成分]地方,位置

topectomy [təˈpektəmi] *n* 额叶皮质局部切除术(治疗精神病)

topesthesia [ˌtɔpesˈθiːzjə] *n* 位置觉

Töpfer's test [ˈtepfə] (Alfred E. Töpfer) 特普费尔试验(胃酸定量法)

tophaceous [təˈfeiʃəs] *a* 砂砾性的;痛风石的

topholipoma [ˌtɔfəliˈpəumə] *n* 松石脂[肪]瘤

tophus [ˈtəufəs] ([复] **tophi** [ˈtəufai]) *n*【拉】痛风石;松石(牙石或涎石) | auricular ~ 耳痛风石 / dental ~ 牙垢,牙石 / ~ syphiliticus 梅毒性结节

topical [ˈtɔpikəl] *a* 表面的,局部的(如皮肤表面抗感染药) | **~ly** *ad*

Topinard's angle [ˌtɔpiˈnɑː] (Paul Topinard) 眉棘角(耳穴及眉间至前鼻棘的两线所形成之角) | ~ line 托皮纳尔线(眉间与颏点之间的线)

topiramate [təuˈpairəmeit] *n* 托吡酯(抗惊厥药,治疗部分发作,口服给药)

top(o)- [构词成分]局部,部位

topoalgia [ˌtɔpəˈældʒiə] *n* 局部痛

topoanesthesia [ˌtɔpəuˌænesˈθiːzjə] *n* 位置觉缺失

topochemistry [ˌtɔpəuˈkemistri] *n* 局部化学(一个结构的特定部位〈如细胞表膜〉的化学组成)

topodysesthesia [ˌtɔpəuˌdisesˈθiːzjə] *n* 局部感觉迟钝

topognosis [ˌtɔpəɡˈnəusis] *n* 位置觉

topography [təˈpɔɡrəfi] *n* 局部解剖,局部记载 | **topographic(al)** [ˌtɔpəuˈɡræfik(əl)] *a*

topoisomer [ˌtəupəuˈaisəmə] *n* 拓扑异构体(一种DNA分子)

topoisomerase [ˌtəupəuaiˈsɔməreis] *n* 拓扑异构酶 | type Ⅰ ~ Ⅰ型拓扑异构酶,DNA 拓扑异构酶 / type Ⅱ ~ Ⅱ型拓扑异构酶,DNA 拓扑异构酶(ATP-水解的)

topology [təˈpɔlədʒi] *n* 局部解剖学;胎位产道关系 | **topologic(al)** [ˌtɔpəˈlɔdʒik(əl)] *a* 局部解剖学的 / **topologist** *n* 局部解剖学家

toponarcosis [ˌtɔpəunɑːˈkəusis] *n* 局部麻醉

toponym [ˈtɔpənim] *n* 部位名称(用以区别器官)

toponymy [təˈpɔnimi] *n* 部位命名法

topoparesthesia [ˌtɔpəuˌpæresˈθiːzjə] *n* 局部感觉异常

topophylaxis [ˌtɔpəufiˈlæksis] *n* 局部防卫法(使用松紧带加于注射胂凡纳明的肢体起防卫作用)

topotecan hydrochloride [ˌtəupəuˈtiːkæm] 盐酸拓扑替康(一种 DNA 拓扑异构酸〈Ⅰ型拓扑异构酶〉的细胞毒性抑制剂,防止 DNA 链在断裂之后通过 DNA 异构酶再接合,导致双链 DNA 断裂和细胞死亡,用作辅药,治疗转移性卵巢癌和难治性小细胞肺癌,静脉滴注给药)

topothermesthesiometer [ˌtɔpəuˌθəːmesθiːziˈɔmitə] *n* 局部温度觉测量器

topovaccinotherapy [ˌtɔpəuˌvæksinəuˈθerəpi] *n* 局部菌苗疗法(局部进行人工免疫的方法)

topterone [ˈtɔptərəun] *n* 托普雄酮(抗雌激素药)

TOPV poliovirus vaccine live oral trivalent 三价口服脊髓灰质炎病毒活疫苗

TORCH toxoplasmosis, other agents, rubella, cytomegalovirus, herpes simplex 弓形虫病,其他病原体,风疹,巨细胞病毒,单纯疱疹

torcular [ˈtɔːkjulə] *n* 中空膨胀区

Torek operation [ˈtɔrək] (Franz J. A. Torek) 托雷克手术(①睾丸下降固定术;②胸段食管切除术)

toremifene citrate [ˈtɔrəmiˌfiːn] 枸橼酸托瑞米芬(雌激素拮抗药,用于姑息性治疗转移性乳腺癌)

tori [ˈtɔːrai] torus 的复数

toric [ˈtɔːrik] *a* 隆凸的,圆枕状的

Torkildsen's shunt (operation) [ˈtɔːkildsn] (Arne Torkildsen) 托希尔森分流术(手术),脑室-脑池分流术

tormina [ˈtɔːminə] *n*【拉】绞痛 | **~l** *a*

tornwaldtitis [ˌtɔːnvɑːlˈtaitis] *n* 托恩瓦尔特黏液囊炎,咽囊炎(见 Tornwaldt's bursitis)

Tornwaldt's (Thornwaldt's) bursitis (disease) [ˈtɔːnvɑːlt] (Gustav L. Tornwaldt) 托恩瓦尔特黏液囊炎(咽囊慢性炎症,可形成含脓包囊及鼻咽狭窄。亦称咽部黏液囊炎,咽囊炎)

torose [ˈtɔːrəus], **torous** [ˈtɔːrəs] *a* 膨出的,隆凸的

Torovirus [ˌtɔːrəuˈvaiərəs] *n* 环曲病毒属

torovirus [ˈtɔːrəuˌvaiərəs] *n* 环曲病毒

torpent [ˈtɔːpənt] *a* 迟钝的 *n* 缓和[刺激]剂,保护剂

torpid [ˈtɔːpid] *a* 麻痹的,迟钝的 | **~ity** [tɔːˈpidəti] *n*

torpify [ˈtɔːpifai] *vt* 使麻木,使迟钝,使失去知觉

torpor [ˈtɔːpə] *n*【拉】迟钝(对正常刺激无反应) | ~ retinae 视网膜感光迟钝

torporific [ˌtɔːpəˈrifik] *a* 使麻木的,使迟钝的,使失去知觉的

torque [tɔːk] *n* 旋力;扭转力

torquing [ˈtɔːkiŋ] *n* 扭转(如扭转异位牙)

torr [tɔː] *n* 托(旧压力单位,相当于 1 mmHg〈= 133.322 Pa〉的压力)

torrefy [ˈtɔrifai] *vt* 烘烤,焙干 | **torrefaction** [ˌtɔriˈfækʃən] *n*

Torre's syndrome [ˈtɔri] (Douglas P. Torre) 托里综合征(多发性癌,主要是胃肠道癌,伴有大量皮脂腺瘤)

torricellian [ˌtɔːriˈtʃeliən] *a* 托里切利(Evangelista Torricelli)的(如 ~ vacuum 托里切利真空)

torrid [ˈtɔrid] *a* 热的 | **~ity** [tɔˈridəti] *n*

torsemide [ˈtɔːsəmaid] *n* 托塞米(利尿药,抗高血压药)

torsiometer [ˌtɔːsiˈɔmitə] *n* 眼旋计

torsion [ˈtɔːʃən] *n* 扭转,捩转 | negative ~ 反扭转 / positive ~ 顺扭转 | **~al** *a*

torsionometer [ˌtɔːʃəˈnɔmitə] *n* 脊柱扭转测量器

torsive [ˈtɔːsiv] *a* 扭转的

torsiversion [ˌtɔːsiˈvəːʃən] *n* 扭转位(牙)

torso [ˈtɔːsəu] *n* 躯干

torsoclusion [ˌtɔːsəuˈkluːʒən] *n* 扭转压法;扭转殆

torso-occlusion [ˌtɔːsəu ɔˈkluːʒən] *n* 扭转殆

torticollis [ˌtɔːtiˈkɔlis] *n* 斜颈 | **torticollar** [ˌtɔːtiˈkɔlə] *a*

tortile [ˈtɔːtail] *a* 扭转的

tortipelvis [ˌtɔːtiˈpelvis] *n* 骨盆扭转,变形性肌张力障碍

tortua [ˈtɔːtjuə] *n*【拉】剧痛

tortuosity [ˌtɔːtjuˈɔsəti] *n* 曲折,扭弯

tortuous [ˈtɔːtjuəs] *a* 弯曲的,扭弯的

Torula [ˈtɔrjulə] *n* 串酵母属,圆酿母属 | ~ capsulatus, ~ histolytica 荚膜串酵母,新型隐球菌

toruli [ˈtɔrjulai] torulus 的复数

toruliform [ˈtɔrjulifɔːm], **toruloid** [ˈtɔrjulɔid] *a* 串珠状的,念珠状的

torulin [ˈtɔrjulin] *n* 硫胺

toruloma [tɔrjuˈləumə] *n* 球拟酵母结节,隐球菌结节

Torulopsis [ˌtɔrjuˈlɔpsis] *n* 球拟酵母属 | ~ glabrata 光滑球拟酵母 / ~ histolytica 溶组织球拟酵母,新型隐球菌 / ~ pintolopesii 宾[吐罗比斯]氏球拟酵母

torulopsosis [ˌtɔrjuˈlɔpsəsis] *n* 球拟酵母病

torulosis [ˌtɔrjuˈləusis] *n* 球拟酵母病,隐球菌病

torulus [ˈtɔrjuləs] ([复] **toruli** [ˈtɔrjulai]) *n*【拉】隆凸,小圆凸

torus [ˈtɔːrəs] ([复] **tori** [ˈtɔːrai]) *n*【拉】圆枕

tosifen [ˈtəusifən] *n* 托西芬(抗心绞痛药)

tosyl [ˈtəusil] *n* 甲苯磺酰

tosylate [ˈtəusileit] *n* 甲苯磺酸盐(*p*-toluenesulfonate 的 USAN 缩约词)

totipotency [təuˈtipətənsi] *n* [分化]全能性

totipotential [ˌtəutipəuˈtenʃəl], **totipotent** [təuˈtipətənt] *a* 全能的(指细胞具有向各方向发展的能力)

totipotentiality [ˌtəutipəuˌtenʃiˈæləti] *n* 全能性

Toti's operation [ˈtəuti] (Addeo Toti) 泪囊鼻腔造口术

touch [tʌtʃ] *vt*, *vi* 触,接触;触诊,指诊;触痛 *n* 触,碰;触觉;触诊;微量,痕量 | abdominal ~ 腹部触诊 / double ~ 双指触诊(阴道与直肠同时指诊) / rectal ~ 直肠指诊 / vaginal ~ 阴道指诊 / vesical ~ 膀胱指诊

toucherism [ˈtʌtʃərizəm] *n* 触摸癖(一种性变态,通过触摸以达到性唤醒或性欲高潮)

Touraine-Solente-Golé syndrome [tuˈrein səuˈlɑːnt gəuˈlei] (Albert Touraine; G. Solente; L. Golé) 厚皮性骨膜病

Tourette 见 Gilles de la Tourette

tourmaline [ˈtuəməliːn] *n* 电气石(用于光学仪器)

Tournay's sign [tuːˈnei] (Auguste Tournay) 图尔内征(向极度外侧位凝视时,外展眼的瞳孔单侧扩大)

tournesol [ˈtuənisɔl] *n* 石蕊,石蕊素

tourniquet [ˈtuənikei] *n*【法】止血带,压脉器 | automatic rotating ~ 自动轮换止血带 / garrote ~, Spanish ~, torcular ~ 勒绞式止血带,西班牙绞带 / pneumatic ~ 充气止血带 / scalp ~ 头皮止血带

tousey [ˈtəuzi] (Sinclair Tousey) 陶西(X 线功率单位,其辐射性能相当于一烛光白炽灯对照相软片所产生的感光效应)

Touton giant cells [ˈtutɔn] (Karl Touton) 图顿巨细胞(含类脂质的多核巨细胞,见于黄瘤及组织细胞增多病 X)

towel [ˈtauəl] *n* 毛巾,手巾 | sanitary ~ 卫生带,月经带

Towne's projection [taun] (Edward B. Towne) 汤氏位投照(头部 X 线投照,投照时中心射线斜穿额骨,产生面部结构和枕骨的位观,这是前后半轴位投照)

Townes syndrome [taunz] (Philip L. Townes) 汤斯综合征(一种常染色体显性遗传综合征,包括心房异常和缺损,肢和指〈趾〉——尤其是拇指——异常,以及肾缺陷。本征常包括心脏病、耳聋或囊性卵巢)

Townsend ionization [ˈtaunsənd] (John Townsend) 汤森德电离(见 ionization 项下 avalanche ionization)

toxanemia [ˌtɔksəˈniːmiə] *n* 中毒性贫血

toxaphene [ˈtɔksəfiːn] *n* 毒杀芬(一种人工合成氯代烃类农业杀虫剂)

Toxascaris [tɔkˈsæskəris] *n* 弓蛔线虫属 | ~ leonina 狮弓蛔线虫

toxemia [tɔkˈsiːmiə] *n* 毒血症 | alimentary ~ 食物性毒血症 / preeclamptic ~ 子痫前毒血症 / ~ of pregnancy, eclamptic ~, eclamptogenic ~ 妊娠毒血症,子痫性毒血症 | **toxemic** *a*

toxenzyme [tɔksˈenzaim] *n* 毒[性]酶

toxi- 见 tox(o)-

toxic [ˈtɔksik] *a* 有毒的,毒物的;中毒的,毒性的

toxicant [ˈtɔksikənt] *a* 有毒性的 *n* 毒物

toxication [ˌtɔksiˈkeiʃən] *n* 中毒

toxicemia [tɔksiˈsiːmiə] *n* 毒血症

toxicide [ˈtɔksisaid] *n* 解毒药

toxicity [tɔkˈsisəti] *n* 毒性;毒力 | O_2 ~, oxygen ~ 氧中毒

toxic(o)- [构词成分]毒

toxicodendric acid [ˌtɔksikəuˈdendrik] 野葛酸

toxicodendrol [ˌtɔksikəuˈdendrɔl] *n* 野葛油,毒葛油

Toxicodendron [ˌtɔksikəuˈdendrən] *n* 漆树属

toxicogenic [ˌtɔksikəuˈdʒenik] *a* 产毒的,产生毒素的

toxicohemia [ˌtɔksikəuˈhiːmiə] *n* 毒血症

toxicoid [ˈtɔksikɔid] *a* 毒物样的

toxicology [ˌtɔksiˈkɔlədʒi] *n* 毒理学 | **toxicologic(al)** [ˌtɔksikəˈlɔdʒik(əl)] *a* / **toxicologist** *n* 毒理学家

toxicomania [ˌtɔksikəuˈmeinjə] *n* 毒物瘾,嗜毒癖,药物癖

toxicomaniac [ˌtɔksikəuˈmeiniæk] *n* 毒物瘾者,嗜毒癖者

toxicopathy [ˌtɔksiˈkɔpəθi] *n* 中毒[性]病 | **toxicopathic** [ˌtɔksikəuˈpæθik] *a*

toxicopexis [ˌtɔksikəuˈpeksis], **toxicopexy** [ˈtɔksikəuˌpeksi] *n* 毒物中和 | **toxicopectic** [ˌtɔksikəuˈpektik], **toxicopexic** [ˌtɔksikəuˈpeksik] *a* 中和毒物的

toxicophidia [ˌtɔksikəuˈfidiə] *n* 毒蛇

toxicophobia [ˌtɔksikəuˈfəubjə] *n* 毒物恐怖,中毒恐怖,恐毒症

toxicosis [ˌtɔksiˈkəusis] *n* 中毒 | alimentary ~ 食物中毒,食品中毒 / endogenic ~ 内因性中毒,自体中毒 / exogenic ~ 外因性中毒(如食物中毒) / gestational ~ 妊娠中毒 / hemorrhagic capillary ~ 出血性毛细管中毒,中毒性毛细管出血 / retention ~ 潴留性中毒,停滞性中毒

toxicosozin [ˌtɔksikəuˈsəuzin] *n* 抗毒防卫素拮抗蛋白

toxicyst [ˈtɔksisəst] *n* 毒胞,毒囊

toxidrome [ˈtɔksidrəum] *n* 毒物综合征

toxiferous [tɔkˈsifərəs] *a* 有毒的

toxigenic [ˌtɔksiˈdʒenik] *a* 产毒的,产生毒素的

toxigenicity [ˌtɔksidʒiˈnisəti] *n* 产毒性

toxignomic [ˌtɔksigˈnɔmik] *a* 示毒的(表示毒物的毒性作用)

toxin [ˈtɔksin] *n* 毒素 | amanita ~ 条蕈毒素 / anthrax ~ 炭疽毒素 / bacterial ~s 细菌毒素 / botulinus ~ 肉素杆菌毒素 / clostridial ~ 梭[状芽胞杆]菌毒素 / diphtheria ~ for Schick test 锡克试验用白喉毒素(用于锡克试验的白喉毒素标准化制剂,以前称诊断用白喉毒素 diagnostic diphtheria ~) / erythrogenic ~ 红斑毒素 / fusarial ~ 镰刀菌毒素 / gas gangrene ~ 气性坏疽毒素 / inactivated diagnostic diphtheria ~ 诊断用灭活白喉毒素(即锡克试验对照剂 Schick test control) / plague ~ 鼠疫毒素 / pseudomonal ~ 假单胞菌毒素 / tetanus ~ 破伤风毒素 / whooping cough ~ 百日咳毒素

toxin-antitoxin [ˌtɔksinˈæntiˌtɔksin] *n* 毒素-抗毒素(白喉毒素与白喉抗毒素的混合物,用于白喉免疫,混合物的比例应使白喉毒素 85% 的毒性为抗毒素中和)

toxinemia [ˌtɔksiˈniːmiə] *n* 毒血症

toxinology [ˌtɔksiˈnɔlədʒi] *n* 毒素学

toxinosis [ˌtɔksiˈnəusis] *n* 毒素病

toxinum [tɔkˈsainəm] *n* 【拉】毒素

toxipathy [tɔkˈsipəθi] *n* 中毒[性]病

toxiphobia [ˌtɔksiˈfəubiə] *n* 毒素恐怖,中毒恐怖,恐毒症

toxiphrenia [ˌtɔksiˈfriːniə] *n* 中毒型精神病;精神分裂症伴中毒谵妄状态

toxiresin [ˌtɔksiˈrezin] *n* 毒树脂

toxisterol [tɔkˈsistərɔl] *n* 毒甾醇

toxitabellae [ˌtɔksitəˈbeliː] *n* 毒[药]片剂

tox(o)- [构词成分]毒,毒素,毒物;弓

Toxocara [ˌtɔksəˈkærə] *n* 弓蛔虫属 | ~ canis 犬弓蛔虫 / ~ cati, ~ mystax 猫弓蛔虫

toxocaral [ˌtɔksəˈkærəl] *a* 弓蛔虫的

toxocariasis [ˌtɔksəkəˈraiəsis] *n* 弓蛔虫病 | human ~ 人弓蛔虫病,内脏幼虫移行症

toxogen [ˈtɔksədʒən] *n* 毒[素]原

toxogenin [tɔkˈsɔdʒinin] *n* 过敏毒原素,过敏毒反应质(注射抗原后血内形成一种物质,虽其本身不具活性,但若再度注射抗原,则产生过敏反应)

toxoglobulin [ˌtɔksəuˈglɔbjulin] *n* 毒球蛋白

toxoid [ˈtɔksɔid] *n* 类毒素 | adsorbed ~ 吸附类毒素 / adsorbed diphtheria ~s 吸附白喉类毒素 / adsorbed diphtheria and tetanus ~s 吸附白喉和破伤风类毒素 / adsorbed tetanus ~ 吸附破伤风类毒素 / alum ~, alum precicipitated ~ (A. P. T.) 明矾(沉淀)类毒素 / diphtheria ~ 白喉类毒素 / fluid ~ 液体类毒素 / formol ~ 甲醛类毒素 / precipitated ~ 沉淀类毒素 / tetanus ~ 破伤风类毒素

toxoid-antitoxoid [ˌtɔksɔid ˈæntiˌtɔksɔid] *n* 类毒素-抗类毒素
toxolecithin [ˌtɔksəuˈlesiθin], **toxolecithid** [ˌtɔksəuˈlesiθid] *n* 毒卵磷脂
toxolysin [tɔkˈsɔlisin] *n* 溶毒素,抗毒素
toxoneme [ˈtɔksəuniːm] *n* 棒状细胞器,棒状体
toxonosis [ˌtɔksəˈnəusis] *n* 中毒
toxopeptone [ˌtɔksəuˈpeptəun] *n* 毒[蛋白]胨
toxopexic [ˌtɔksəuˈpeksik] *a* 中和毒素的
toxophil [ˈtɔksəfil] *a* 亲毒的
toxophilic [ˌtɔksəuˈfilik], **toxophilous** [ˌtɔksəu ˈfiləs] *a* 亲毒的,易感毒素的
toxophore [ˈtɔksəfɔː] *n* 毒簇,毒性基团(指毒素分子中的原子团,当毒素分子与结合簇适当地结合后,即发挥其效能)
toxophorous [tɔkˈsɔfərəs] *a* 毒簇的,带毒素的
toxophylaxin [ˌtɔksəufiˈlæksin] *n* 抗毒防御素(能破坏和中和细菌毒性产物的防御物质)
Toxoplasma [ˌtɔksəuˈplæzmə] *n* 弓形虫属 | ~ gondii, ~ cuniculi 鼠弓形虫,兔弓形虫
toxoplasmin [ˌtɔksəuˈplæzmin] *n* 弓形虫素(从感染了弓形虫的小鼠腹腔液制备的抗原,皮内注射作为诊断弓形虫病的试验)
toxoplasmosis [ˌtɔksəuplæzˈməusis] *n* 弓形虫病 | ocular ~ 眼弓形虫病,弓形虫性脉络膜视网膜炎
toxoprotein [ˌtɔksəuˈprəutiːn] *n* 毒蛋白
Toxothrix [ˈtɔksəθriks] *n* 弓丝菌属
toxuria [tɔkˈsjuəriə] *n* 尿毒症
Toynbee's corpuscles [ˈtɔinbiː] (Joseph Toynbee) 角膜小体 | ~ experiment 托因比实验(紧闭口鼻后吞咽,使鼓室内压力降低) / ~ law 托因比定律(中耳炎引起脑脓肿时,由乳突引起者位于小脑及横窦,由鼓室顶引起者位于大脑) / ~ ligament 鼓膜张肌 / ~ otoscope 托因比耳镜(插入患者及检查者耳内之管,在中耳吹气法时借以对患者之耳作听诊)
TPA, t-PA tissue plasminogen activator 组织纤溶酶原激活物
TPHA *Treponema pallidum* hemagglutination assay 梅毒螺旋体血凝测定
t-plasminogen activator(t-PA, TPA) [plæzˈminəˌdʒən ˈætiveitə] 组织纤溶酶原激活物(亦称 tissue plasminogen activator)
TPN total parenteral nutrition 全胃肠外营养; triphosphopyridine nucleotide 三磷酸吡啶核苷酸
TPNH reduced triphosphopyridine nucleotide 还原型三磷酸吡啶核苷酸
TPP thiamine pyrophosphate 硫胺素焦磷酸
TR tricuspid regurgitation 三尖瓣反流
trabecula [trəˈbekjulə] ([复] **trabeculae** [trəˈbekjuliː]) *n* 【拉】小梁,柱 | **~r** [trəˈbekjulə] *a*
trabecularism [trəˈbekjulərizəm] *n* 小梁结构
trabeculate [trəˈbekjulit] *a* 有小梁的
trabeculation [trəˌbekjuˈleiʃən] *n* 小梁形成
trabeculectomy [trəˌbekjuˈlektəmi] *n* 小梁切除术(以利于引流青光眼时的水状液)
trabeculoplasty [trəˈbekjuləˌplæsti] *n* 小梁成形术 | laser ~ 激光小梁成形术(开角型青光眼手术)
trabs [træbs] ([复] **trabes** [ˈtreibiːz]) *n* 胼胝体(大脑)
trace [treis] *n* 痕量,微量;痕迹 | memory ~ 记忆痕迹
tracer [ˈtreisə] *n* 示踪器;示踪物;描记器 | needle-point ~, arrow-point ~ 针尖描记器(牙科) / radioactive ~ 放射性示踪物 / stylus ~ 细探子描记器(牙科)
trachea [ˈtreikiə, trəˈki(ː)ə] ([复] **tracheas** 或 **tracheae** [ˈtreikiiː, trəˈkiːiː]) *n*【拉】气管 | scabbard ~ 剑鞘形气管 | **~l** *a*
tracheaectasy [ˌtreikiəˈektəsi] *n* 气管扩张
trachealgia [ˌtreikiˈældʒiə] *n* 气管痛
tracheid [ˈtreikiid] *n* 管胞
tracheitis [ˌtreikiˈaitis] *n* 气管炎
trachelagra [ˌtrækiˈlægrə] *n* 颈痛风
trachelectomy [ˌtrækiˈlektəmi] *n* 宫颈切除术
trachelematoma [ˌtrækiˌleməˈtəumə] *n* 胸锁乳突肌血肿
trachelism [ˈtrækilizəm], **trachelismus** [ˌtrækiˈlizməs] *n* 颈肌痉挛
trachelitis [ˌtrækiˈlaitis] *n* 宫颈炎
trachel(o)- [构词成分]颈,项
trachelocele [ˈtrækiləsiːl] *n* 气管黏膜疝样突出
trachelocyllosis [ˌtrækiləusiˈləusis] *n* 斜颈
trachelocyrtosis [ˌtrækiləusəːˈtəusis] *n* 颈椎后凸
trachelocystitis [ˌtrækiləusisˈtaitis] *n* 膀胱颈炎
trachelodynia [ˌtrækiləuˈdiniə] *n* 颈痛
trachelokyphosis [ˌtrækiləukaiˈfəusis] *n* 颈椎后凸
trachelology [ˌtrækiˈlɔlədʒi] *n* 颈病学 | **trachelologist** *n* 颈病学家
trachelomyitis [ˌtrækiləumaiˈaitis] *n* 颈肌炎
trachelopexy [ˌtrækiləuˈpeksi], **trachelopexia** [ˌtrækiləuˈpeksiə] *n* 宫颈固定术
tracheloplasty [ˈtrækiləuˌplæsti] *n* 宫颈成形术
trachelorrhaphy [ˌtrækiˈlɔrəfi] *n* 宫颈修补术
tracheloschisis [ˌtrækiˈlɔskisis] *n* (先天性)颈裂[畸形]
trachelosyringorrhaphy [ˌtrækiləuˌsiriŋˈgɔrəfi] *n* 阴道瘘宫颈缝合术,阴道瘘宫颈修补术
trachelotomy [ˌtrækiˈlɔtəmi] *n* 宫颈切开术
trache(o)- [构词成分]气管

tracheoaerocele [ˌtreikiə*u*ˈεərə*u*siːl] *n* 气管气疝
tracheobronchial [ˌtreikiə*u*ˈbrɔŋkjəl] *a* 气管支气管的
tracheobronchitis [ˌtreikiə*u*brɔŋˈkaitis] *n* 气管支气管炎
tracheobronchomegaly [ˌtreikiə*u*ˌbrɔŋkə*u*ˈmegəli] *n* 气管支气管扩大
tracheobronchoscopy [ˌtreikiə*u*brɔŋˈkɔskəpi] *n* 气管支气管镜检查
tracheocele [ˈtreikiəˌsiːl] *n* 气管黏膜疝样突出
tracheoesophageal [ˌtreikiə*u*i(ː)ˈsɔfədʒiəl] *a* 气管食管的
tracheofissure [ˌtreikiə*u*ˈfiʃə] *n* 气管裂开术
tracheofistulization [ˌtreikiə*u*ˌfistjulaiˈzeiʃən, -liˈz-] *n* 气管穿刺投药法;气管瘘管形成
tracheogenic [ˌtreikiə*u*ˈdʒenik] *a* 气管原的
tracheolaryngeal [ˌtreikiə*u*ləˈrindʒiəl] *a* 气管喉的
tracheolaryngotomy [ˌtreikiə*u*ˌlæriŋˈgɔtəmi] *n* 气管喉切开术
tracheole [ˈtreikiəul] *n* 微气管
tracheomalacia [ˌtreikiə*u*məˈleiʃiə] *n* 气管软化
tracheopathia [ˌtreikiə*u*ˈpæθiə], **tracheopathy** [ˌtreikiˈɔpəθi] *n* 气管病
tracheopharyngeal [ˌtreikiə*u*fəˈrindʒiəl] *a* 气管咽的
Tracheophilus cymbius [ˌtreikiˈɔfiləsˈsimbiəs] 鸭气管吸虫
tracheophonesis [ˌtreikiə*u*fəuˈniːsis] *n* 气管部[心音]听诊
tracheophony [ˌtreikiˈɔfəni] *n* 气管音
tracheophyte [ˈtreikiəˌfait] *n* 微管植物
tracheoplasty [ˈtreikiəˌplæsti] *n* 气管成形术
tracheopyosis [ˌtreikiə*u*paiˈəusis] *n* 气管化脓,化脓性气管炎
tracheorrhagia [ˌtreikiə*u*ˈreidʒiə] *n* 气管出血
tracheorrhaphy [ˌtreikiˈɔrəfi] *n* 气管缝合术,气管修补术
tracheoschisis [ˌtreikiˈɔskisis] *n* 气管裂
tracheoscopy [ˌtreikiˈɔskəpi] *n* 气管镜检查 | percervical ~, low ~ 经(气管)切口气管镜检查,低位气管镜检查 / peroral ~, high ~ 经口气管镜检查,高位气管镜检查 | **tracheoscopic** [ˌtreikiə*u*ˈskɔpik] *a*
tracheostenosis [ˌtreikiə*u*stiˈnəusis] *n* 气管狭窄
tracheostoma [ˌtreikiˈɔstəmə] *n* 气管造口
tracheostomize [ˌtreikiˈɔstəmaiz] *vt* 作气管造口
tracheostomy [ˌtreikiˈɔstəmi] *n* 气管造口术
tracheotome [trəˈkiətəum] *n* 气管刀
tracheotomize [ˌtreikiˈɔtəmaiz] *vt* 切开气管
tracheotomy [ˌtreikiˈɔtəmi] *n* 气管切开术 | inferior ~ 气管下部切开术,低位气管切开术 / superior ~ 气管上部切开术,高位气管切开术
Trachinidae [trəˈkinidiː] *n* 龙臘科
trachitis [trəˈkaitis] *n* 气管炎
trachoma [trəˈkəumə]([复] **trachomata** [trəˈkəumətə]) *n* 【希】沙眼,粒性结膜炎 | ~ of vocal bands 结节性声带炎 | **~tous** [trəˈkɔmətəs] *a*
Trachybdella bistriata [ˌtreikiˈdelə ˌbistriˈɑːtə] 巴西水蛭
trachychromatic [ˌtreikikrə*u*ˈmætik] *a* 深染的
trachyonychia [ˌtrækiəˈnikiə] *n* 粗糙甲(甲粗糙并脆裂,常伴有银屑病、斑秃和扁平苔藓)
trachyphonia [ˌtreikiˈfəuniə] *n* 声嘶
tracing [ˈtreisiŋ] *n* 示踪,追踪;描记法 | arrow point ~, needle-point ~, stylus ~ 箭头描记法,尖形描记法 / extraoral ~ 口外描记法 / Gothic arch ~ 高腭弓描记法,尖形弓描记法 / intraoral ~ 口内描记法
track [træk] *n* 径迹 | fog ~ 雾迹(电子或其他粒子穿过过饱和的雾室时所留下的痕迹) / germ ~ 胚迹,生殖细胞连迹 / ionization ~ 电离径迹(见 path 项下相应术语)
tracking [ˈtrækiŋ] *n* 追踪,跟踪 | visual ~ 可视追踪
tract [trækt] *n* 束,道 | alimentary ~ 消化道 / ascending ~ 上行束 / biliary ~ 胆道 / bulbar ~ 延髓束 / bulbospinal ~ 橄榄脊髓束 / cerebellorubrospinal ~ 小脑红核脊髓束 / cerebellothalamic ~ 小脑丘脑束 / corticocerebellar ~s, corticopontile ~s, corticopontine ~s 皮质脑桥束 / corticothalamic ~ 皮质丘脑束 / descending ~ 下行束 / digestive ~ 消化道 / dorsal(或 posterior) spinocerebellar ~ 脊髓小脑后束 / extrapyramidal ~, extracorticospinal ~ 锥体外束 / fastigiobulbar ~ 顶核延髓束 / foraminous spiral ~ 螺旋孔束 / genitourinary ~ 生殖泌尿道 / habenulopeduncular ~ 缰核脚间束,后屈束 / iliotibial ~ 髂胫束 / lateral corticospinal ~ 皮质脊髓侧束 / mamillothalamic ~ 乳头丘脑束 / motor ~ 运动束 / olfactory ~ 嗅束 / olivocerebellar ~ 橄榄小脑束 / olivospinal ~ 橄榄脊髓束 / optic ~ 视束 / pyramidal ~ 锥体束 / respiratory ~ 呼吸道 / rubroreticular ~ 红核网状束 / rubrospinal ~ 红核脊髓束 / solitary ~ of medulla oblongata 延髓孤束 / spinal ~ of trigeminal nerve 三叉神经脊束 / spino-olivary ~ 脊髓橄榄束 / tectobulbar ~ 顶盖延髓束 / tectospinal ~ 顶盖脊髓束 / thalamocortical ~ 丘脑皮质束 / thalamooccipital ~ 视辐射线 / thalamoolivary ~ 丘脑橄榄束 / transverse peduncular ~ 脑脚横束 / ventral(或 anterior) spinocerebellar ~ 脊髓小脑腹束(或前束) / ves-

tibulospinal ~ 前庭脊[髓]束

tractellum [træk'teləm] ([复] **tractella** [træk'telə]) *n*【拉】前鞭毛

traction ['trækʃən] *n* 牵引[术] | axis ~ 轴牵引(如产科骨盆牵引) / skeletal ~ 骨骼牵引 | **~al** *a*

tractive ['træktiv] *a* 牵引的

tractor ['træktə] *n* 牵引器 | urethral ~ 尿道牵引器

tractoration [ˌtræktə'reiʃən] *n* 金属牵引器疗法

tractotomy [træk'tɔtəmi] *n* 神经束切断术

tractus [træktəs] [单复同] *n*【拉】束,道

tragacanth ['trægəkænθ] *n* 西黄蓍胶

tragal ['treigəl] *a* 耳屏的

Trager Approach ['treigə] (Nilton Trager) 特雷格入门(一种可缓解疼痛并促进身心放松的健身法使用要点)

tragi ['treidʒai] tragus 的复数

Tragia ['treidʒiə] *n* 刺痒藤属

tragion ['trædʒiɔn] *n* 耳屏点(人体测量名词,位于耳屏的上缘)

tragomaschalia [ˌtrægəumæs'keiliə] *n* 腋臭

tragophonia [ˌtrægəu'fəuniə], **tragophony** [trə'gɔfəni] *n* 羊音(支气管羊音)

tragopodia [ˌtrægəu'pəudiə] *n* 膝外翻

tragus ['treigəs] ([复] **tragi** ['treidʒai]) *n*【拉】耳屏;耳毛

train [trein] *vt* 培养,训练 *n* 成串;系列;顺序 | ~ of four stimulation 四个成串刺激

trainable ['treinəbl] *a* 可训练的(指中度精神发育迟缓者〈智商为35~50〉,学习能力不可能超过二年级水平,但能从职业培训中受益,并在监护下能生活自理)

training ['treiniŋ] *n* 训练,锻炼,培养 | assertiveness ~, expressive ~ 自信心确立训练法,表达训练法(行为疗法的一种,即对患者训练适宜的人际间反应,包括积极和消极情感的表达)

trait [trei, treit] *n* 特质;特性,性状 | secretor ~ 分泌者特性(ABO血型系中能在唾液中分泌ABH抗原的能力,这种特性是以单纯的孟德尔式遗传) / sickle cell ~ 镰状细胞特性(通常是无症状的,由血红蛋白S的杂合性所致)

trajector [trə'dʒektə] *n* 检弹探子(检创伤中子弹的位置)

TRALI transfusion-related acute lung injury 输血性急性肺损伤

tralonide ['treilənaid] *n* 曲萘德(糖皮质激素)

tramadol hydrochloride ['træmədəul] 盐酸曲马朵(镇痛药)

tramazoline hydrochloride [trə'mæzəliːn] 盐酸曲马唑啉(肾上腺素能药,具有减轻鼻充血作用)

Trambusti's reaction (test) [træm'busti] (Arnaldo Trambusti) 特拉姆布斯蒂反应(试验)(结核菌素注射至机体时,针头与皮肤表面平行插入,注射部位变红者为阳性反应,亦称皮内反应)

tramitis [trə'maitis] *n* 早期肺结核[X线]条痕(如胸膜粘连、纵隔偏移、硬化条索、淋巴结钙化、肺纹理增加等)

trance [trɑːns] *n* 迷睡,恍惚,迷睡性木僵 | alcoholic ~ 酒毒迷睡,酒毒性恍惚 / death ~ 死状迷睡,死状恍惚 / hypnotic ~ 催眠性迷睡

trandolapril [træn'dəuləˌpril] *n* 群多普利(血管紧张素转化酶抑制药,用于治疗高血压和心肌梗死后充血性心力衰竭或左心室功能紊乱,口服给药)

tranexamic acid [trænek'sæmik] 氨甲环酸(止血药)

tranquillizer ['træŋkwilaizə] *n* 安定药 | major ~ 强安定药,抗精神病药 / minor ~ 弱安定药,抗焦虑药

trans [trænz] *a* 反(在有机化学中指两种几何异构体中的一种,在遗传学中指反式结构)

trans- [前缀]经[由],越,横过,齐,透过,移;反[式]

transabdominal [ˌtrænsæb'dɔminl] *a* 经腹壁的

transacetylase [træns'æsitileis] *n* 转乙酰酶,乙酰基转移酶

transacetylation [trænsˌæsiti'leiʃən] *n* 转乙酰作用,乙酰基转移[作用]

transacylase [træns'æsileis] *n* 转酰酶,酰基转移酶

transacylation [trænsˌæsi'leiʃən] *n* 转酰基作用,酰基转移[作用]

transaldolase [træns'ældəleis] *n* 转醛醇酶,醛醇基转移酶

transamidinase [ˌtrænsə'midineis] *n* 转脒酶,脒基转移酶

transaminase [træn'sæmineis] *n* 转氨酶,氨基转移酶

transamination [ˌtrænsæmi'neiʃən] *n* 转氨作用,氨基转移[作用]

transanimation [trænˌsæni'meiʃən] *n* 口对口复苏法

transantral [træns'æntrəl] *a* 经窦的(如经窦施行的脑外科)

transaortic [ˌtrænsei'ɔːtik] *a* 经主动脉的

transatrial [træns'eitriəl] *a* 经[心]房的

transaudient [træns'ɔːdiənt] *a* 传声的

transaxial [træns'æksiəl] *a* 经轴的

transbasal [træns'beisl] *a* 经基底的(如经颅底的)

transbronchial [træns'brɔŋkiəl] *a* 经支气管的
transcalent [træns'keilənt] *a* 透[辐射]热的
transcallosal [trænskə'ləusəl] *a* 经胼胝体的
transcalvarial [ˌtrænskæl'vɛəriəl] *a* 经颅盖的
transcanal [trænskə'næl] *a* 经导管的,经耳道的
transcarbamoylase [trænsˌkɑːbə'mɔileis] *n* 转氨甲酰酶,氨甲酰基转移酶
transcarboxylase [ˌtrænskɑː'bɔksileis] *n* 转羧酶,羧基转移酶
transcatheter [træns'kæθitə] *a* 经导管的
transcellular [træns'seljulə] *a* 跨细胞的,穿过细胞的
transcervical [træn'səːvikəl] *a* 经宫颈的
transclomiphene [træns'kləumifiːn] *n* 反氯菧酚胺(即珠氯米芬 zuclomiphene)
transcobalamin(TC) [ˌtrænskəu'bæləmin] *n* 转钴胺素,运钴胺素蛋白,钴胺素传递蛋白 | ~ Ⅱ 转钴胺素Ⅱ,运钴胺素蛋白Ⅱ,钴胺素传递蛋白Ⅱ
transcochlear [træns'kɔkliə] *a* 经耳蜗的(如切除肿瘤)
transcondyloid [træns'kɔndilɔid] *a* 经髁的
transcortical [træns'kɔːtikəl] *a* 经皮质的;连接皮质的
transcortin [træns'kɔːtin] *n* 经皮质激素传递蛋白(亦称皮质类固醇结合球蛋白,皮质醇球蛋白)
transcranial [træns'kreiniəl] *a* 经颅的
transcricothyroid [trænsˌkraikəu'θairɔid] *a* 经环甲膜的
transcript ['trænskript] *n* 转录物 | primary ~ 前转录物(基因的第一 RNA 转录物,包含内含子和外显子)
transcriptase [træns'kripteis] *n* 转录酶(即 DNA 指导的 RNA 聚合酶 DNA-directed RNA polymerase) | reverse ~ 逆转录酶,RNA 指导的 DNA 聚合酶
transcription [ˌtræns'kripʃən] *n* 转录(蕴藏在 DNA 的遗传信息在 RNA 链上产生互补碱基顺序)
transcutaneous [ˌtrænskju(ː)'teinjəs] *n* 经皮的
transdermal [træns'dəːməl] *a* 经皮的
transducer [træns, trænz'djuːsə] *n* 换能器 | neuroendocrine ~ 神经内分泌换能器
transducin [træns'djuːsin] *n* 传导素,转导蛋白
transduction [træns'dʌkʃən] *n* 转导(细菌由于噬菌体的影响而引起遗传物质的重组,并将一个细菌体内的遗传物质通过噬菌体转移到另一个细菌体)
transdural [træns'djuərəl] *a* 经硬脑膜的,经硬脊膜的
transection [træn'sektʃən] *n* 横断 | ~ of aorta 主动脉横断
transepidermal [ˌtrænsepi'dəːməl] *a* 经表皮的
transethmoidal [trænseθ'mɔidəl] *a* 经筛骨的
transfaunation [ˌtrænsfɔː'neiʃən] *n* 转变宿主,转宿(寄生物转变其宿主)
transfection [træns'fekʃən] *n* 转染(通过病毒核酸的感染)
transfectoma [ˌtrænzfek'təumə] *n* 转染瘤(转染免疫球蛋白基因的淋巴样细胞,能产生从自己基因编码的特异性中分离的抗体分子)
transfemoral [træns'femərəl] *a* 经股骨的;经股动脉的
transfer [træns'fəː] *vt* 转移,传递,传输 *vi* 转移 ['trænsfə(ː)] *n* 转移,传递,传输;变换 | linear energy ~ (LET) 线性能量传递 / passive ~ 被动转移(即从免疫动物或呈致敏的动物采取抗体或淋巴细胞注射于正常同种机体,即可将免疫性输送给未免疫宿主)
transferase ['trænsfəreis] *n* 转移酶
transference ['trænsfərəns] *n* 转移(如症状的转移);移情(精神分析) | counter ~ 反移情
transferrin [træns'ferin] *n* 转铁蛋白,铁传递蛋白
transfinite [træns'fainait] *a* 超限的
transfixion [træns'fikʃən] *n* 缝扎
transforation [ˌtrænsfə'reiʃən] *n* 穿颅术(胎头)
transforator ['trænsfəˌreitə] *n* 穿颅器
transformation [ˌtrænsfə'meiʃən] *n* 变化,变形,转化 | asbestos ~ 石棉变形 / bacterial ~ 细菌性转形变异(细胞间遗传信息的转移过程) / G-F ~, globular-fibrous ~ 球状纤维状变形(肌肉收缩时的现象) / lymphocyte ~ 淋巴细胞转化(当有特异性抗原存在或有非特异性刺激物〈如植物血凝素、链球菌溶血毒素、抗淋巴细胞血清等〉时,培养的淋巴细胞发生形态学的改变)
transformer [træns'fɔːmə] *n* 性别转换基因
transformiminase [ˌtrænsfə'mimineis] *n* 转亚氨甲基酶,亚氨甲基转移酶
transformism [træns'fɔːmizəm] *n* 种变说,种族变化论
transfrontal [træns'frʌntəl] *a* 经额骨的
transfructosylase [trænsˌfrʌktə'sileis] *n* 转果糖酶,果糖基转移酶
transfuse [træns'fjuːz] *vt* 输血,输液
transfusion [træns'fjuːʒən] *n* 转输,输血,输液 | autologous ~ 自体输血 / exchange ~, exsanguination ~, replacement ~, substitution ~ 换血疗法,换血(用于患成红血细胞增多症的新生儿及严重尿毒症) / fetomaternal ~ 胎儿-母体输血(胎儿血液经胎盘输至母体血液循环) / immediate ~, direct ~ 直接输血法 / indirect ~, mediate ~ 间接输血法 / intrauter-

ine ~ 子宫内输血(治子宫内胎儿成红血细胞增多症)

transgenation [ˌtrænsdʒiˈneiʃən] *n* 突变

transgene [ˈtrænsdʒiːn] *n* 转基因

transgenic [trænsˈdʒenik] *a* 转基因的(指一段DNA从一个基因组实验性拼接到不同基因组的DNA上)

transglucosylase [ˌtrænsgluːkəuˈsileis] *n* 转葡糖基酶,葡糖基转移酶

transglutaminase [ˌtrænzgluːˈtæmineis] *n* 转谷氨酰胺酶

transglycosidation [trænsˌglaikəusiˈdeiʃən] *n* 转糖苷作用

transglycosylase [ˌtrænsglaiˈkəusileis] *n* 转糖酶,糖基转移酶

transhexosylase [trænsˌheksəˈsileis] *n* 转己糖酶,己糖基转移酶

transhiatal [ˌtrænshaiˈeitl] *a* 经裂孔的

transhumeral [trænsˈhjuːmərəl] *a* 经肱骨的

transient [ˈtrænziənt] *a* 短暂的,瞬时的 | **transience, transiency** *n*

transiliac [trænˈsiliæk] *a* 髂骨间的;经髂骨的

transilient [trænsˈiliənt] *a* 跳越的,跃过的

transilluminate [ˌtrænsiˈljuːmineit] *vt* 透照 | **transillumination** [ˌtrænsiˌljuːmiˈneiʃən] *n* 透照[法]

transinsular [trænsˈinsjulə] *a* 经[脑]岛的

transischiac [trænsˈiskiæk] *a* 坐骨间的

transisthmian [trænsˈismiən] *a* 经峡的(尤指穹窿回峡)

transistor [trænˈsistə] *n* 晶体管

transit [ˈtrænsit] *n* 通过,经过;运送,运输

transition [trænˈsiʒən] *n* 跃迁;转变,转换 | electron ~ 电子跃迁

transitory [ˈtrænsitəri] *a* 短暂的,暂时性的

transketolase [trænsˈkiːtəleis] *n* 转酮醇酶,酮醇基转移酶

translabyrinthine [trænsˌlæbəˈrinθiːn] *a* 经迷路的

translateral [trænsˈlætərəl] *a* 横侧的(X线摄影时,指病人卧位水平线投照的位观)

translation [trænsˈleiʃən] *n* 翻译;转化,转移;转译(在蛋白质生物合成中,以信使核糖核酸分子为模板合成蛋白质的过程)

translator [trænsˈleitə] *n* 翻译机,译码器(指细胞遗传信息)

translocase [trænsˈləukeis] *n* 移位酶

translocation [ˌtrænsləuˈkeiʃən] *n* 易位(遗传学上指一个染色体的片段移位到同源染色体另一部分或移位到一个非同源染色体) | balanced ~ 平衡易位(所产生的遗传物质比正常的二倍体或单倍体不多也不少) / reciprocal ~ 相互易位(在两个断裂的染色体之间相互交换片段,一个染色体的一部分与另一个染色体的一部分相联)

translucent [trænsˈljuːsnt] *a* 半透明的 | **translucence, translucency** *n* 半透明性,半透明度

transmeatal [ˌtrænsmiːˈætəl] *a* 经耳道的

transmembrane [trænsˈmembrein] *a* 跨膜的,越膜的

transmetatarsal [trænsˌmetəˈtɑːsəl] *a* 经跖骨的

transmethylase [trænsˈmeθileis] *n* 转甲基酶,甲基转移酶

transmethylation [ˌtrænsmeθiˈleiʃən] *n* 转甲基作用,甲基转移[作用]

transmigration [ˌtrænzmaiˈgreiʃən] *n* 移行,移动;血细胞渗出 | external ~ 外移行(卵由宫外移入对侧输卵管) / internal ~ 内移行(卵由宫内移入对侧输卵管)

transmissible [trænsˈmisəbl] *a* 可传播的,可传染的;可传递的;能透射的 | **transmissibility** [trænsˌmisəˈbiləti] *n* 传播性,传染性;传递性(遗传);可透性

transmission [trænsˈmiʃən] *n* 传播,传染;传递(遗传);传导,传递(神经);透射 | duplex ~ 两向传导(神经冲动) / horizontal ~ 水平传播(同一世代的传染散播,一般通过接触含有致病微生物的排泄物所致) / synaptic ~ 突触传导(神经冲动) / vertical ~ 垂直传播(不同世代的散播,如经初乳、胎盘传于子代)

transmit [trænsˈmit] *vt* 传播;传染;传导;传递(遗传)

transmitral [trænsˈmaitrəl] *a* 经二尖瓣的,经左房室瓣的

transmittance(T) [trænsˈmitəns] *n* 透光度;透射比

transmitter [trænsˈmitə] *n* 递质 | excitatory ~ 兴奋性递质

transmucosal [ˌtrænsmjuːˈkəusəl] *a* 经黏膜的

transmural [trænsˈmjuərəl] *a* 透壁的

transmutation [ˌtrænsmjuːˈteiʃən] *n* 演变,衍变(指物种演变);嬗变,蜕变(一种元素成为另一种元素的变化;核子学中,以核轰击使原子核成为不同原子数的原子核,引起质子和中子重新排列)

transmute [trænsˈmjuːt] *vt, vi* 演变,衍变;(使元素)嬗变,蜕变 | **transmutable** *a* 能变形的,能变质的;可嬗变的,可蜕变的

transocular [trænsˈɔkjulə] *a* 经眼的

transonance [ˈtrænsənəns] *n* (音)传响,(音)彻响

transonic [trænˈsɔnik] *a* 超声的,超声速的,跨声速的

transorbital [trænsˈɔːbitl] *a* 经[眼]眶的

transovarial [ˌtrænsəuˈvɛəriəl], **transovarian** [ˌtrænsəuˈvɛəriən] *a* 经卵巢的
transoximinase [ˌtrænsɔkˈsimineis] *n* 转肟酶,肟基转移酶
transpalatal [trænsˈpælətl] *a* 经腭的
transparency [trænsˈpɛərənsi], **transparence** [trænsˈpɛərəns] *n* 透明性,透明度
transparent [trænsˈpɛərənt] *a* 透明的,透光的
transparietal [ˌtrænspəˈraiitl] *a* 顶骨间的;穿过体壁的
transpentosylase [trænsˌpentəˈsileis] *n* 转戊糖酶,戊糖基转移酶
transpeptidase [trænsˈpeptideis] *n* 转肽酶,肽基转移酶
transperitoneal [ˌtrænsperitəuˈniːəl] *a* 经腹膜的
transphosphorylase [ˌtrænsfɔsˈfɔrileis] *n* 转磷酸酶,磷酸变位酶
transphosphorylation [trænsˌfɔsfəriˈleiʃən] *n* 转磷酸[作用]
transpiration [ˌtrænspiˈreiʃən] *n* 蒸散,蒸腾;不显[性出]汗 | pulmonary ~ 肺蒸散
transplacental [ˌtrænspləˈsentl] *a* 经胎盘的
transplant[1] [ˈtrænsplɑːnt, -plænt] *n* 移植物,移植片;移植
transplant[2] [trænsˈplɑːnt, -ˈplænt] *vt* 移植
transplantar [trænsˈplæntə] *a* 经跖的,经足底的
transplantation [ˌtrænsplɑːnˈteiʃən, -plænt-] *n* 移植[术] | allogeneic ~ 异基因移植 / heterotopic ~ 异位移植 / orthotopic ~, homotopic ~ 原位移植,同位移植 / syngeneic ~ 同系移植 / syngenesioplastic ~ 同血统移植(同种内近缘个体间,例如母子或兄妹间的组织移植) / tendon ~ 腱移植
transpleural [trænsˈpluərəl] *a* 经胸膜的
transport [ˈtrænspɔːt] *n* 运输,转运 | active ~ 主动转运(直接由于代谢能量消耗所产生的物质穿过细胞膜和上皮层的活动) / axoplasmic ~ 轴浆运输 / blood gas ~ 血液气体运输 / placental ~ 胎盘转运
transportation [ˌtrænspɔːˈteiʃən] *n* 输送,后送 | ~ of burn patient 烧伤病人转送
transporter [trænsˈpɔːtə] *n* 转运蛋白
transpose [trænsˈpəuz] *vt* 使互换位置,变换
transposition [ˌtrænspəˈziʃən] *n* 转位,反位(内脏);移位术(皮瓣);移位,换位(在一个分子内两个原子变换位置);转座 | corrected ~ of great vessels 矫正型大血管转位(亦称混合性左位心) / ~ of great vessels 大血管转位 / partial ~ of great vessels 大血管部分转位(见 Taussig-Bing syndrome)
transposon [trænzˈpəuzɔn] *n* 转座子,转位子
transpubic [trænsˈpjuːbik] *a* 经耻骨的
transradial [trænsˈreidiəl] *a* 经桡动脉的;经桡骨的
transsacral [trænsˈseikrəl] *a* 经骶骨的,横过骶骨的
transsection [trænˈsekʃən] *n* 横切,横断面
transsegmental [ˌtrænssegˈmentl] *a* 经肢节的
transseptal [trænsˈseptl] *a* 经中隔的,横过中隔的
transsexual [trænsˈseksjuəl] *n* 易性癖者 | **~ism** *n* 易性癖(一种变态心理)
trans-sonic [træns ˈsɔnik] *a* 超声的,超声速的,跨声速的
transsphenoidal [ˌtrænssfiːˈnɔidl] *a* 经蝶骨的
transsternal [trænsˈstəːnl] *a* 经胸骨的
transsuccinylase [ˌtrænssʌkˈsinileis] *n* 转琥珀酰基酶,二氢硫辛酰胺琥珀酰[基]转移酶
transtemporal [trænsˈtempərəl] *a* 经颞叶的,横过颞叶的
transthalamic [ˌtrænsθəˈlæmik] *a* 经丘脑的,横过丘脑的
transthermia [trænsˈθəːmiə] *n* 透热法
transthoracic [ˌtrænsθɔːˈræsik] *a* 经胸廓的,经胸腔的
transthyretin [ˌtrænsθaiˈretin] *n* 转甲状腺素,转甲状腺蛋白(由肝脏分泌的一种 α-球蛋白)
transtibial [trænsˈtibiəl] *a* 经胫骨的
transtracheal [trænsˈtreikiəl] *a* 经气管的,经气管壁的
transtrochanteric [trænstrəukənˈterik] *a* 经转子的(指手术)
transtympanic [ˌtrænstimˈpænik] *a* 经鼓室的
transubstantiate [ˌtrænsəbˈstænʃieit] *vt* 使变换 | **transubstantiation** [ˌtrænsəbˌstænʃiˈeiʃən] *n* 组织替换
transudate [ˈtrænsjudeit] *n* 漏出液,渗出液
transudation [trænsjuˈdeiʃən] *n* 漏出,渗出
transude [trænˈsjuːd] *vi, vt* 漏出,渗出
transuranic [ˌtrænsjuəˈrænik] *a* 超铀的 | **transuranium** [ˌtrænsjuəˈreinjəm] *n* 超铀元素 *a* 超铀的
transureteroureterostomy [ˌtrænsjuəˌriːtərəujuəˌriːtəˈrɔstəmi] *n* 经输尿管输尿管吻合术(断离的输尿管两端与对侧输尿管作端侧吻合)
transurethral [ˌtrænsjuəˈriːθrəl] *a* 经尿道的
transvaginal [trænsˈvædʒinl] *a* 经阴道的
transvaterian [ˌtrænsvəˈtiəriən] *a* 经十二指肠乳头的
transvector [trænsˈvektə] *n* 带毒体,传毒者(自己不产生毒物,而携带和传播外来毒物的生物,如蛤贝类)
transvenous [trænsˈviːnəs] *a* 经静脉的
transventricular [ˌtrænsvenˈtrikjulə] *a* 经[心]

室的
transversal [trænz'vəːsəl] *a* 横向的,横断的
transversalis [ˌtrænsvəː'seilis] *a* 横的(横贯体轴的)*n* 横肌
transverse ['trænzvəːs] *a* 横向的,横切的 | **~ly** *ad*
transversectomy [ˌtrænsvəː'sektəmi] *n* 椎骨横突切除术
transversion [træns'vəːʃən] *n* 易位牙;颠换(DNA 或 RNA 中的一个嘌呤被嘧啶替换或一个嘧啶被嘌呤替换所引起的突变)
transversocostal [trænsˌvəːsəu'kɔstl] *a* 肋[椎]横突的
transversotomy [ˌtrænsvəː'sɔtəmi] *n* 椎骨横突切开术
transversourethralis [trænsˌvəːsəuˌjuəri'θreilis] *n* 尿道横肌
transversus [træns'vəːsəs] *a* 横的 *n* 横肌
transvesical [træns'vesikəl] *a* 经膀胱的
transvestite [træns'vestait] *n* 易装癖者 | **transvestism** [træns'vestizəm], **transvestitism** [træns'vestitizəm] *n* 易装癖(如酷爱异性服装、发式、风度等)
Trantas' dots ['trænstəs] (Alexios Trantas) 特兰塔斯小点(春季结膜炎时,结膜缘部有石灰状小白斑点)
tranylcypromine sulfate [ˌtrænil'saiprəmiːn] 硫酸反苯环丙胺(抗抑郁药)
trap [træp] *n* 捕集器;防[臭]气阀;防臭曲管 *vt* 捕获 | air ~ping 空气滞留
trapeze [trə'piːz] *n* 斜方形
trapeziform [trə'pezifɔːm] *a* 斜方形的
trapeziometacarpal [trəˌpiːziəumetə'kɑːpl] *a* 大多角骨掌骨的
trapezium [trə'piːzjəm] *n* 斜方形;大多角骨 | **trapezial** [trə'piːziəl] *a*
trapezoid ['træpizɔid] *n* 斜方形;小多角骨 *a* 斜方形的 | **~al** [ˌtræpi'zɔidl] *a*
Trapp's formula (coefficient) [træp] (Julius Trapp) 特腊普公式(系数)(尿液比重最后两个数字,乘以 2〈特腊普系数〉所得之积,接近于 1 L 尿液所含固体的格令〈grain〉数)
TRAPS TNF-receptor-associated periodic syndrome 肿瘤坏死因子-受体相关的周期性综合征
trastuxumab [træs'tʌzjumæb] *n* 曲他单抗(一种重组 DNA 衍生的人源化单克隆抗体,与人生长因子受体 2〈HFR2〉结合,后者为某些乳腺癌患者过度表达出来的一种蛋白质,用作抗肿瘤药,治疗转移性乳腺癌及 HFR2 的过度表达,静脉内给药)
Traube-Hering waves ['traubi 'həːriŋ] (Ludwig Traube; Edwald Hering) 特-赫波(动脉压节律性升降,系血管收缩中枢的节律性活动所致)
Traube's sign ['traubə] (Ludwig Traube) 特劳伯征(主动脉反流时,在股动脉上听诊时可闻及一声响亮的枪击样声音。亦称枪击音) | ~ semilunar space 特劳伯半月状间隙(左前胸部的左下前方的一区域,胃内空气在此产生水鼓音)
trauma ['trɔːmə] ([复] **traumas** 或 **traumata** ['trɔːmətə]) *n*【拉;希】损伤,外伤,创伤 | birth ~ 产伤 / occlusal ~ 𬌗创伤 / potential ~ (牙)潜在伤 / psychic ~ 精神创伤
traumasthenia [ˌtrɔːmæs'θiːnjə] *n* 创伤性神经衰弱
traumatherapy [ˌtrɔːmə'θerəpi] *n* 创伤治疗学
traumatic [trɔː'mætik] *a* 创伤的,外伤的
traumatic acid [trɔː'mætik] 愈伤酸,2-十二烯二酸
traumatin ['trɔːmətin] *n* (植物)创伤激素
traumatism ['trɔːmətizəm] *n* 创伤病,外伤病;伤,伤口
traumatize ['trɔːmətaiz] *vt* 使受外伤;使受精神创伤
traumat(o)- [构词成分]创伤,外伤
traumatogenic [ˌtrɔːmətəu'dʒenik] *a* 创伤[原]性的;造成创伤的
traumatology [ˌtrɔːmə'tɔlədʒi] *n* 创伤学 | **traumatologist** *n* 创伤学家,伤科医生
traumatonesis [ˌtrɔːmətə'niːsis] *n* 创口缝术
traumatopathy [ˌtrɔːmə'tɔpəθi] *n* 创伤病,外伤病
traumatophilia [ˌtrɔːmətəu'filiə] *n* 嗜创伤癖
traumatopnea [ˌtrɔːmətɔp'niːə] *n* 创伤性气急(伴虚脱)
traumatopyra [ˌtrɔːmətə'paiərə] *n* 创伤性热
traumatosis [ˌtrɔːmə'təusis] *n* 创伤病,外伤病
traumatotherapy [ˌtrɔːmətəu'θerəpi] *n* 创伤治疗法
traumatropism [trɔː'mætrəpizəm] *n* 向[创]伤性(指生物体向创伤生长或活动)
Trautmann's triangle ['trəutmɑːn] (Moritz F. Trautmann) 特鲁特曼三角(为一间隙,其前角在含有迷路的突起处,后界为横窦,上界为下颞线。当此骨手术移去时,在此三角区的上后角将与岩上窦相遇)
travail ['træveil] *n* 分娩,生产
travoprost ['trævəuprɔst] *n* 曲拉前列(一种合成的前列腺素类似物,用于治疗开角型青光眼患者眼内压升高或高眼压症,局部用于结膜)
tray [trei] *n* [托]盘 | acrylic resin ~ 丙烯酸树脂盘(印模盘) / impression ~ 印模托盘(用以装印模物质以取颌或牙的模型)

trazodone hydrochloride [ˈtreizədəun] 盐酸曲唑酮(抗抑郁药,安定药,降压药)

Treacher Collins syndrome, Treacher Collins-Franceschetti syndrome [ˈtriːtʃə ˈkɔlinz frænsisˈketi] (Edward Treachen Collins; Adolphe Franceschetti) 下颌面骨发育不全

treacle [ˈtriːkl] *n* 糖浆,糖蜜

tread [ˈtred] *n* 践伤(马蹄)

treatment [ˈtriːtmənt] *n* 处理;治疗,疗法 | active ~ 直接疗法,积极疗法 / antigen ~ 抗原疗法(注射抗原使机体产生自动免疫的疗法,包括用细菌、疫苗、结核菌素等) / autoserosalvarsan ~ 自身血清胂凡纳明疗法(治麻痹性痴呆) / autoserous ~ 自身血清疗法(注射患者本人血清治疗传染病) / carbon dioxide ~ 二氧化碳疗法(见 therapy 项下相应术语) / causal ~ 病因疗法 / choline ~ 胆碱疗法(静脉注射硼酸胆碱和放射物质合并使用治癌) / conservative ~ 保守疗法 / curative ~ 祛病疗法 / dietetic ~ 饮食疗法 / eventration ~ (经腹部切口)露脏 X 线疗法 / gland ~ 性腺剂疗法,性激素疗法 / high-frequency ~ 高频电疗,透热法 / hypoglycemic shock ~ 低血糖休克疗法,胰岛素休克疗法 / malarial ~ 疟热疗法 / medicinal ~ 药物疗法 / oatmeal ~ 燕麦食疗法(饮食中限制蛋白质及碳水化合物,限于吃燕麦片,以治糖尿病) / organ ~ 脏器疗法,器官疗法,内脏制剂疗法 / palliative ~ 姑息疗法 / preventive ~, prophylactic ~ 预防法 / salicyl ~ 水杨酸盐疗法(治风湿病) / sand ~ 沙浴疗法 / sewage ~ 污水处理法 / slush ~ 雪泥疗法(以二氧化碳雪、丙酮和硫黄的混合剂治痤疮) / starvation ~ 禁食疗法 / string method ~ 线(扩张)疗法(治食管狭窄) / subcoma insulin ~ 亚昏迷性胰岛素疗法(见 therapy 项下相应术语) / surgical ~ 外科疗法 / terrain ~ 山地疗法(采取经常性体育锻炼、爬山、饮食调节,以治心脏衰竭及神经衰弱等) / thyroid ~ 甲状腺制剂疗法 / tonic ~ 补剂疗法;长期(小剂量)汞疗法(治梅毒) / underwater ~ 水下疗法(治脊髓灰质炎)

trebenzomine hydrochloride [triˈbenzəmiːn] 盐酸曲苯佐明(抗抑郁药)

tree [triː] *n* 树;世系图 | bronchial ~ 支气管树 / family ~ 家族世系图,家谱,系统树 / tracheobronchial ~ 气管支气管树

trefoil [ˈtriːfɔil] *n* 三叶草,三叶豆

trehala [triˈheilə] *n* 茧蜜

trehalase [triˈheileis] *n* 茧蜜糖酶,海藻糖酶

α, α-trehalase [triˈhɑːleis, -ˈhei-] *n* α, α-海藻糖酶(此酶缺乏为一种常染色体隐性遗传病,可致海藻糖吸收障碍,摄入大量食用蘑菇后可能出现呕吐和腹泻)

trehalose [triˈheiləus] *n* 海藻糖

Treitz's arch [ˈtraits] (Wenzel Treitz) 特赖茨弓(由左结肠上动脉和肠系膜下静脉形成的血管弓) | ~ fossa 十二指肠上隐窝,十二指肠空肠隐窝 / ~ hernia 特赖茨疝(经十二指肠上隐窝的腹膜后疝) / ~ muscle (ligament) 十二指肠提肌

treloxinate [triˈlɔksineit] *n* 曲洛酯(降胆固醇药)

Trematoda [ˌtreməˈtəudə] *n* 吸虫纲

trematode [ˈtremətəud] *n* 吸虫

trematodiasis [ˌtremətəuˈdaiəsis] *n* 吸虫病

tremble [ˈtrembl] *vi* 震颤;发抖 *n* 震颤;[复]震颤病(牛、羊),乳毒病(人)

tremelloid [ˈtreməlɔid], **tremellose** [ˈtreməl-əus] *a* 凝胶样的,胶冻样的

tremetol [ˈtremətɔl], **tremetone** [ˈtremətəun] *n* 佩兰毒素,白蛇根毒素

tremogram [ˈtriːməgræm] *n* 震颤描记图

tremograph [ˈtriːməgrɑːf, -græf] *n* 震颤描记器

tremolabile [ˌtriːməuˈleibail] *a* 不耐震的(指酵素易为震动而被抑制活力)

tremor [ˈtremə, ˈtriːmə] *n* 震颤 | action ~ 动作性震颤 / arsenic ~ 砷毒性震颤 / coarse ~ 粗大震颤 / continuous ~ 持续性震颤(持续发生的震颤,类似震颤麻痹) / ~ cordis 心震颤,心悸,心跳 / darkness ~ 暗光(眼球)震颤 / epidemic ~ 流行性震颤,鸟脑脊髓炎 / epileptoid ~ 癫痫样震颤 / essential ~, familial ~, hereditary essential ~ 特发性震颤,家族性震颤,遗传性特发性震颤 / fine ~ 频细震颤 / flapping ~ 扑翼样震颤 / forced ~ 强迫性震颤 / intention ~ 意向性震颤 / kinetic ~ 动作性震颤 / purring ~ 猫喘样震颤 / rest ~ 静止震颤(肢体放松并加支托时发生的震颤,如震颤麻痹时) / static ~ 静止性震颤 / striocerebellar ~ 纹状体小脑性震颤 / trombone ~ of tongue 舌拉管样震颤(即马尼安运动 Magnan's movement) / volitional ~ 意向性震颤 | **~ous** [ˈtremərəs] *a*

tremorgram [ˈtriːməgræm] *n* 震颤描记图

tremulor [ˈtremjulə] *n* 震颤机

tremulous [ˈtremjuləs] *a* 震颤的

trenching [ˈtrentʃiŋ] *n* 掘壕掩埋法(粪便处理)

Trendelenburg cannula [trenˈdelənbəːg] (Friedrich Trendelenburg) 特伦德伦堡套管(附橡皮袋的气管套管,用于气管切开术后闭合气管以防止血液流入) | ~ operation 特伦德伦堡手术(①曲张静脉切除术;②结扎大隐静脉以治静脉曲张;③骶髂联合切开术,治膀胱外翻;④经胸腔肺栓子切除术) / ~ position 特伦德伦堡卧位(头低脚高位) / ~ symptom 特伦德伦堡症状(臀肌麻痹引起的摇摆步态) / ~ test 特伦德伦堡试验(①检静脉瓣疾病;②检脊髓灰质炎、股骨颈骨折、髋内翻和先天脱位等)

trendscriber [ˈtrendskraibə] *n* 心电动向描记器
trendscription [trendˈskripʃən] *n* 心电动向描记术
trepan [triˈpæn] *n* 环钻,环锯 *vi* 用环锯在…上施行手术 | **~ation** [ˌtrepəˈneiʃən] *n* 环钻[术],环锯[术]
trepanner [triˈpænə] *n* 环钻者
trephine [triˈfiːn, triˈfain] *n* 环钻,环锯 *vt* 用环锯在…上施行手术 | **trephination** [ˌtrefiˈneiʃən] *n* 环钻[术],环锯[术]
trephinement [triˈfainmənt] *n* 环钻[术],环锯[术]
trephiner [triˈfainə] *n* 环钻者
trephocyte [ˈtrefəsait] *n* 滋养细胞
trepidant [ˈtrepidənt] *a* 震颤性的
trepidatio [ˌtrepiˈdeiʃiəu] *n*【拉】震颤,抖颤;悸惧 | ~ cordis 心悸
trepidation [ˌtrepiˈdeiʃən] *n* 震颤,抖颤;悸惧
trepo- [构词成分]旋转,转动
Trepomonas [ˌtrepəuˈməunəs] *n* 旋滴虫属
Treponema [ˌtrepəˈniːmə] *n* 密螺旋体属 | ~ buccale 颊密螺旋体(亦称颊包柔螺旋体 Borrelia buccalis) / ~ calligyrum 阴部密螺旋体,湿疣密螺旋体 / ~ carateum 品他病密螺旋体 / ~ cuniculi 家兔密螺旋体,家兔螺旋体 / ~ denticola 齿垢密螺旋体 / ~ genitalis 生殖器密螺旋体 / ~ herrejoni 赫雷云密螺旋体,品他病密螺旋体 / ~ macrodentium 大牙密螺旋体 / ~ microdentium 小牙密螺旋体,牙螺旋体 / ~ mucosum 黏膜密螺旋体 / ~ pallidum 苍白密螺旋体,梅毒螺旋体 / ~ pallidum subsp. pertenue 梅毒密螺旋体细弱密螺旋体亚种 / ~ paraluiscuniculi 脊髓痨兔密螺旋体(亦称家兔密螺旋体) / ~ pertenue 细弱密螺旋体,雅司螺旋体 / ~ recurrentis 回归热密螺旋体,回归热包柔螺旋体 / ~ refringens 屈折密螺旋体 / ~ reiteri 瑞氏密螺旋体 / ~ vincentii 奋森密螺旋体(亦称樊尚包柔密螺旋体 Borrelia vincentii,樊尚螺旋体 spirillum of Vincent)
treponema [ˌtrepəˈniːmə], **treponeme** [ˈtrepəniːm] *n* 密螺旋体 | **treponemal** [ˌtrepəˈniːməl], **treponematous** [ˌtrepəˈniːmətəs] *a*
Treponemataceae [ˌtrepəˌniːməˈteisiiː] *n* 密螺旋体科
treponematosis [ˌtrepəniːməˈtəusis] *n* 密螺旋体病
treponeme [ˌtrepəniːm] *n* 密螺旋体
treponemiasis [ˌtrepəniːˈmaiəsis] *n* 密螺旋体病,梅毒
treponemicidal [ˌtrepəˌniːmiˈsaidl] *a* 杀密螺旋体的
trepopnea [ˌtrepɔpˈniːə] *n* 转卧呼吸(取卧位时最舒适的呼吸状态)
treppe [ˈtrepə] *n*【德】阶梯现象(迅速反复刺激,使肌肉收缩程度逐渐增加的一种现象)
Tresilian's sign [triˈsiliən] (Frederick J. Tresilian) 特雷西里安征(流行性腮腺炎时腮腺管口发红)
tresis [ˈtriːsis] *n*【希】穿破,穿孔
trestolone acetate [ˈtrestələun] 醋酸曲托龙(抗肿瘤药,雄性类固醇)
tretinoin [ˈtretinɔin] *n* 维 A 酸(角质溶解药)
Treves' fold [triːvz] (Frederick Treves) 回盲襞 | ~ operation 特里维斯手术(波特〈Pott〉病的手术,经腰部将脓肿切开,洗涤及刮除脓囊,并将死骨刮除)
Trevor disease [ˈtrevə] (David Trevor) 特雷弗病,半肢畸形骨骺发育不良
TRH thyrotropin-releasing hormone 促甲状腺[激]素释放[激]素
tri- [前缀]三,三次
triable [ˈtraiəbl] *a* 可试[验]的
triacetate [traiˈæsiteit] *n* 三醋酸盐,三乙酸盐
triacetin [traiˈæsitin] *n* 三醋汀,乙酸甘油酯(局部抗真菌药)
triacetyloleandomycin [traiˌæsitiˌləuliˌændəˈmaisin] *n* 醋竹桃霉素(抗菌药)
triacid [traiˈæsid] *a* 三[酸]价的 *n* 三元酸
Triactinomyxon [ˌtraiækˌtinəuˈmiksɔn] *n* 三角孢子虫属
triacylglycerol [traiˌæsilˈglisərɔl] *n* 三酰[基]甘油
triacylglycerol lipase [traiˌæssilˈglisərɔl ˈlaipeis] 三酰甘油酯酶(亦称酯酶)
triad [ˈtraiəd] *n* 三联体;三价元素;三联;三征,三联征 | acute compression ~ 急性压塞三征(见 Beck's triad) / adrenomedullary ~ 肾上腺髓质三征(由肾上腺髓质活化作用产生的症状:心动过速、血管缩小、出汗) / hepatic ~s, portal ~s 肝三联(在肝小叶之角,肝动脉、肝静脉和胆管属支的汇集) | **~ic** [traiˈædik] *a*
triaditis [traiəˈdaitis] *n* 三体炎 | portal ~ 门三体炎(肝门管区的肝动脉、肝静脉和胆管周围的结缔组织炎症)
triafungin [ˌtraiəˈfʌndʒin] *n* 三嗪芬净(抗真菌药)
triage [triˈɑːʒ] *n*【法】伤员拣别分类(对战争或其他灾难造成的伤员,按轻重缓急分送适当地方治疗)
trial [ˈtraiəl] *n* 试,试用,试验 *a* 试验性的 | clinical ~ 临床试验 / crossover ~ 交叉试验 / ~ and error 尝试错误(反复试验以期获得最令人满意的结果)
trialism [ˈtraiælizəm] *n* 三元论(trialistic theory,

见 theory 项下相应术语)

triallylamine [ˌtraiæliˈlæmiːn] *n* 三丙烯胺,三烯丙基胺

triamcinolone [ˌtraiæmˈsinələun] *n* 曲安西龙(肾上腺皮质激素类药) | ~ acetonide 曲安奈德 / ~ acetonide sodium phosphate 曲安奈德磷酸钠 / ~ hexacetonide 己曲安奈德

triamine [traiˈæmiːn] *n* 三胺

triamterene [traiˈæmtəriːn] *n* 氨苯蝶啶(利尿降压药)

triamylose [traiˈæmiləus] *n* 葡萄三聚糖

triangle [ˈtraiæŋgl] *n* 三角[形] | auditory ~ 前庭区 / auricular ~ 耳郭三角 / ~ of auscultation 听诊三角(斜方肌下缘、背阔肌、肩胛骨内缘构成的三角) / crural ~ 下腹三角(由股内侧、下腹部、腹股沟部和外阴构成) / ~ of election 颈动脉上三角 / facial ~ 面三角(为一三角区,其尖端为颅底点、牙槽中点和鼻点) / inguinal ~ 腹股沟三角;股三角 / urogenital ~ 尿生殖膈 / vesical ~ 膀胱三角

triangular [traiˈæŋgjulə] *a* 三角[形]的

triangularis [ˌtraiæŋgjuˈlɛəris] *a* 【拉】三角的

triangulate [traiˈæŋgjuleit] *vt* 使成三角形 [traiˈæŋgjulit] *a* 三角形的

triantebrachia [ˌtraiæntiˈbreikiə] *n* 三前臂[畸形]

Triatoma [traiˈætəmə] *n* 锥蝽属 | ~ megista 大锥蝽 / ~ infestans 骚扰锥蝽 / ~ sanguisuga 吸血锥蝽

triatomic [ˌtraiəˈtɔmik] *a* 三原子的;三羟的

triazene [ˈtraiəziːn] *n* 三氮烯

triazolam [traiˈeizəlæm] *n* 三唑仑(安定药)

triazole [ˈtraiəzəul, traiˈeizəul] *n* 三唑;三唑类抗真菌化合物

tribadism [ˈtribədizəm], **tribady** [ˈtribədi] *n* 女性同性恋

tribasic [traiˈbeisik] *a* 三碱[价]的,三元的 | ~ acid 三元酸

tribe [traib] *n* 族(生物分类)

tribenoside [traiˈbenəsaid] *n* 三苄糖苷(毛细血管保护药)

Tribolium [traiˈbəuljəm] *n* 拟谷盗属(甲虫)

tribology [triˈbɔlədʒi] *n* 摩擦学(研究关节的润滑、摩擦和耗损)

triboluminescence [ˌtraibəuˌljuːmiˈnesns] *n* 摩擦[发]光

tribrachia [traiˈbreikiə] *n* 三臂[畸形]

tribrachius [traiˈbreikiəs] *n* 三臂畸胎;三臂联胎

tribromaloin [ˌtraibrəuˈmæləin] *n* 三溴芦荟苷

tribromide [traiˈbrəumaid] *n* 三溴化物

tribromoethanol [traiˌbrəuməuˈeθənɔl], **tribromethanol** [ˌtraibrəuˈmeθənɔl] *n* 三溴乙醇(麻醉药)

tribromsalan [traiˈbrɔmsəlæn] *n* 三溴沙仑(消毒药)

tribulosis [ˌtribjuˈləusis] *n* 蒺藜中毒

Tribulus [ˈtribjuləs] *n* 蒺藜属

tributyl citrate [traiˈbjuːtil] 枸橼酸三丁酯(药物制剂时用作增塑剂)

tributyrin [traiˈbjuːtirin] *n* 丁酸甘油酯

tributyrinase [ˌtraibjuˈtirineis] *n* [三]丁酸甘油酯酶

TRIC [trik] (*t*rachoma *i*nclusion *c*onjunctivitis) 沙眼包涵体结膜炎

tricalcic [traiˈkælsik] *a* 三钙的(含三个钙原子的)

tricellular [traiˈseljulə] *a* 三细胞的

tricephalus [traiˈsefələs] *n* 三头畸胎

triceps [ˈtraiseps] ([复] **triceps⟨es⟩**) *n* 【拉】三头肌 *a* 三头的

triceptor [traiˈseptə] *n* 三簇介体

tricheiria [traiˈkaiəriə] *n* 三手[畸形]

trichesthesia [ˌtrikesˈθiːzjə] *n* 毛发[感]觉

trichiasis [triˈkaiəsis] *n* 【希】倒睫;毛尿[症]

Trichiida [triˈkaiidə] *n* 有丝目

trichilemmoma [ˌtrikileˈməumə] *n* 毛根鞘瘤

trichina [triˈkainə] ([复] **trichinae** [triˈkainiː]) *n* 毛线虫

Trichinella [ˌtrikiˈnelə] *n* 毛线虫属 | ~ spiralis 旋毛线虫,旋毛虫 | **Trichina** [triˈkainə] *n*

Trichinellidae [ˌtrikiˈnelidiː] *n* 毛形科

trichiniferous [ˌtrikiˈnifərəs] *a* 含旋毛虫的

trichinization [ˌtrikinaiˈzeiʃən, -niˈz-] *n* 旋毛虫感染

trichinosis [ˌtrikiˈnəusis], **trichinelliasis** [ˌtrikinəˈlaiəsis], **trichinellosis** [ˌtrikinəˈləusis], **trichiniasis** [ˌtrikiˈnaiəsis] *n* 旋毛虫病

trichinous [ˈtrikinəs] *a* 有旋毛虫的

trichion [ˈtrikiɔn] ([复] **trichia** [ˈtrikiə]) *n* 【希】发际中点(人体测量名词,头正中矢状面与发型轮廓相交之点)

trichite [ˈtraikait] *n* 针形微晶(淀粉粒的);丝泡,线泡(原生动物的器官);丝带,线带(纤毛原生动物的器官);针形质体(稀毛纤毛虫的)

trichitis [traiˈkaitis] *n* 毛球炎(俗名发根炎)

trichlorethylene [traiklɔːˈreθiliːn] *n* 三氯乙烯

trichlorfon [traiˈklɔːfɔn] *n* 敌百虫(剧毒有机磷杀虫药,亦用作抗血吸虫药)

trichloride [traiˈklɔːraid] *n* 三氯化物

trichlormethane [ˌtraiklɔːˈmeθein] *n* 三氯甲烷,氯仿

trichlormethiazide [traiˌklɔːmiˈθaiəzaid] *n* 三氯噻嗪(利尿降压药)

trichloroacetaldehyde [traiˌklɔːrəuˌæsiˈtældihaid] *n* 三氯乙醛,氯醛

trichloroacetic acid [traiˌklɔːrəuəˈsiːtik] 三氯醋酸,三氯乙酸(腐蚀收敛药)
trichloroethylene [ˌtraiklɔːrəuˈeθiliːn] *n* 三氯乙烯(吸入性止痛和麻醉药,用于短时间的小手术)
trichloromethylchloroformate [ˌtraiklɔːrəuˌmeθilklɔːrəuˈfɔːmeit] *n* 氯甲酸三氯甲酯,三氯甲基氯甲酸酯(一种刺激肺的含氯毒气)
trichloromonofluoromethane [ˌtraiˌklɔːrəuˌmɔnəufluərəuˈmeθein] *n* 三氯氟甲烷(用作气溶胶抛射剂)
trichlorophenol [ˌtraiklɔːrəuˈfiːnɔl] *n* 三氯苯酚(消毒防腐药)
2, 4, 5-trichlorophenoxyacetic acid [traiˌklɔːrəufiˌnɔksiəˈsiːtik] 2, 4, 5-三氯苯氧乙酸,245 涕(即 2, 4, 5-T,除莠剂)
trichlorotrivinylarsine [traiˌklɔːrəutraiˌvainiˈlɑːsin] *n* 三氯三乙烯砷(一种致喷嚏性的军用毒气)
trichlorphon [traiˈklɔːfɔn] *n* 敌百虫(即 metrifonate)
trich(o)- [前缀]毛,发
trichoadenoma [ˌtrikəuˌædiˈnəumə] *n* 毛发腺瘤
trichoaesthesia [ˌtrikəesˈθiːzjə] *n* 毛发[感]觉
trichoanesthesia [ˌtrikəænisˈθiːzjə] *n* 毛发感觉缺失
trichobacteria [ˌtrikəbækˈtiəriə] *n* [有]毛菌;丝状菌
trichobasalioma hyalinicum [ˌtrikəbeiˌsæliˈəumə ˌhaiəˈlinikəm] 透明性毛基细胞瘤
trichobezoar [ˌtrikəˈbiːzəuə] 毛石
Trichobilharzia [ˌtrikəbilˈhɑːziə] *n* 毛毕吸虫属 | ~ ocellata 鸭毛毕吸虫
trichocardia [ˌtrikəˈkɑːdiə] *n* 绒毛心(由于渗出性心包炎)
trichocephaliasis [ˌtrikəˌsefəˈlaiəsis], **trichocephalosis** [ˌtrikəˌsefəˈləusis] *n* 鞭虫病
Trichocephalus [ˌtrikəˈsefələs] *n* 毛首鞭虫属,鞭虫属
trichoclasia [ˌtrikəˈkleisiə] *n* 结节性脆发病,发结节病
trichoclasis [triˈkɔkləsis] *n* 脆发[症]
Trichocomaceae [ˌtrikəukəuˈmeisiiː] *n* 毛发菌科
trichocyst [ˈtrikəsist] *n* 丝泡,线泡
Trichodectes [ˌtrikəˈdektiːz] *n* 啮毛虱属 | ~ canis 犬啮毛虱 / ~ climax 山羊啮毛虱(即山羊啮虱 Damalinia caprae) / ~ equi 马啮毛虱(即马啮虱 Damalinia equi) / ~ hermsi 赫姆斯啮毛虱(即赫姆斯啮虱 Damalinia hermsi) / ~ latus 犬啮毛虱 / ~ pilosus 马啮毛虱(即马啮虱 Damalinia pilosus) / ~ sphaerocephalus 红头啮毛虱
Trichoderma [trikəˈdəːmə] *n* 木霉属
Trichodina [triˈkɔdinə] *n* 车轮虫属
trichodiscoma [ˌtrikəudisˈkəumə] *n* 毛盘瘤
trichoepithelioma [ˌtrikəˌepiθiːliˈəumə] *n* 毛发上皮瘤
trichoesthesia [ˌtrikəesˈθiːzjə] *n* 毛发[感]觉
trichoesthesiometer [ˌtrikəesˌθiːziˈɔmitə] *n* 毛发感觉测量器
trichofolliculoma [ˌtrikəufəˌlikjuˈləumə] *n* 毛囊瘤
trichoglossia [ˌtrikəˈglɔsiə] *n* 毛舌
trichographism [triˈkɔgrəfizəm] *n* 立毛反射
trichohyalin [ˌtrikəˈhaiəlin] *n* 毛透明蛋白
trichoid [ˈtrikɔid] *a* 毛发状的
tricholemmoma [ˌtrikəuleˈməumə] *n* 毛根鞘瘤
tricholeukocyte [ˌtrikəuˈljuːkəusait] *n* 毛白细胞,多毛细胞
tricholith [ˈtrikəliθ] *n* 毛石;毛粪石(胃肠内)
trichologia [ˌtrikəˈləudʒiə] *n* 拔毛发癖,拔毛发狂
trichology [triˈkɔlədʒi] *n* 毛发学 | **trichologist** *n* 毛发学家
trichoma [traiˈkəumə] *n* 睑内翻;纠发病 | **~tous** [triˈkɔmətəs] *a*
trichomadesis [ˌtrikəməˈdiːsis] *n* (过速或过早)脱发,脱毛
trichomania [ˌtrikəˈmeinjə] *n* 拔毛发癖,拔毛发狂
trichome [ˈtraikəum] *n* [细菌]毛状体;藻丝 | **trichomic** [triˈkəumik] *a*
trichomegaly [ˌtrikəuˈmegəli] *n* 长睫毛(一种先天性综合征,包括睫毛和眉毛生长过多,伴侏儒、精神发育迟缓和视网膜色素变性)
trichomonacidal [ˌtrikəˌməunəˈsaidl], **trichomonadicidal** [ˌtrikəməuˌnædiˈsaidl] *n* 杀毛滴虫的
trichomonacide [ˌtrikəˈməunəsaid] *n* 杀毛滴虫药
trichomonad [ˌtrikəˈmɔnæd] *n* 毛滴虫 | **trichomonal** [ˌtrikəˈmɔnəl] *a*
Trichomonadida [ˌtrikəuməˈnædidə] *n* 毛滴虫目
Trichomonas [ˌtrikəuˈməunəs, ˌtrikəuˈmɔnəs, triˈkɔmənəs] *n* 毛滴虫属 | ~ foetus 胎毛滴虫 / ~ gallinae, ~ columbae, ~ columbarum 鸡毛滴虫 / ~ gallinarum 鹑鸡毛滴虫 / ~ hominis, ~ intestinalis 人毛滴虫,肠毛滴虫 / ~ muris 鼠毛滴虫 / ~ pulmonalis 肺毛滴虫 / ~ tenax, ~ buccalis, ~ elongata 口腔毛滴虫 / ~ vaginalis 阴道毛滴虫
trichomoniasis [ˌtrikəuməˈnaiəsis] *n* 毛滴虫病,滴虫病 | avian ~ 鸟毛滴虫病 / bovine ~ 牛毛滴虫病 / ~ vaginalis 阴道毛滴虫病
Trichomycetes [ˌtrikəmaiˈsiːtiːz] *n* 毛丝菌纲
trichomycosis [ˌtrikəmaiˈkəusis] *n* 毛发真菌病 |

~ axillaris, ~ chromatica 腋毛菌病 / ~ favosa 黄癣
trichon [ˈtrikɔn] *n* 发癣菌素,毛癣菌素
trichonodosis [ˌtrikəunəuˈdəusis] *n* 发结节病
Trichonympha [ˌtrikəuˈnimfə] *n* 披发虫属
Trichonymphina [ˌtrikəuˈnimfinə] *n* 披发亚目
trichopathy [triˈkɔpəθi] *n* 毛发病 | **trichopathic** [ˌtrikəˈpæθik] *a*
trichophagia [ˌtrikəˈfeidʒiə], **trichophagy** [traiˈkɔfədʒi] *n* 食毛癖
trichophytic [ˌtrikəˈfitik] *a* 毛癣菌的;促进毛发生长的
trichophytid [triˈkɔfitid] *n* 毛癣菌疹
trichophytin [triˈkɔfitin] *n* 毛癣菌素
trichophytobezoar [ˌtrikəˌfaitəˈbiːzɔː] *n* 毛植物石(由动物毛发和植物纤维组成)
Trichophyton [triˈkɔfitɔn] *n* 毛癣菌属 | ~ simii 猴毛癣菌
trichophytosis [ˌtrikəfaiˈtəusis] *n* 毛癣菌病
Trichoptera [traiˈkɔptərə] *n* 毛翅目
trichoptilosis [ˌtrikətiˈləusis] *n* 毛发纵裂病
trichorrhea [ˌtrikəˈriːə] *n* 骤脱发,骤脱毛
trichorrhexis [ˌtrikəˈreksis] *n* 脆发[症] | ~ nodosa 结节性脆发病,发结节病
trichoschisis [triˈkɔskisis] *n* 裂发[症]
trichoscopy [triˈkɔskəpi] *n* 毛发检查
Trichosida [triˈkəusidə] *n* 毛片目
trichosiderin [ˌtrikəˈsidərin] *n* 毛发铁色素
trichosis [triˈkəusis] *n* 毛发病;异处生毛症 | ~ carunculae 泪阜生毛症
Trichosoma [ˌtrikəˈsəumə] *n* 毛体线虫属(即毛细线虫属 Capillaria) | ~ contortum 扭转毛体线虫(即扭转毛细线虫 Capillaria contorta)
Trichosomoides [ˌtrikəsəuˈmɔidiːz] *n* 似毛体线虫属 | ~ crassicauda 粗尾似毛体线虫
Trichosporon [ˌtrikəuˈspɔːrɔn] *n* 毛孢子菌属 | ~ cutaneum, ~ giganteum 皮肤毛孢子菌,巨毛孢子菌
trichosporonosis [traiˌkɔspərəˈnəusis] *n* 毛孢子菌病(不包括白色毛结节菌病)
trichosporosis [ˌtrikəspəˈrəusis] *n* 毛孢子菌病
Trichosporum [ˌtrikəˈspɔːrəm] *n* 毛孢子菌属
trichostasis spinulosa [triˈkɔstəsis ˌspinjuˈləusə] 小棘状毛壅症
Trichostomatida [ˌtrikəustəˈmætidə] *n* 毛口目
Trichostomatina [ˌtrikəuˌstəuməˈtainə] *n* 毛口亚目
trichostrongyliasis [ˌtrikəˌstrɔndʒiˈlaiəsis], **trichostrongylosis** [ˌtrikəˌstrɔndʒiˈləusis] *n* 毛圆线虫病
Trichostrongylidae [ˌtrikəstrɔnˈdʒilidiː] *n* 毛圆线虫科
Trichostrongylus [ˌtrikəˈstrɔndʒiləs] *n* 毛圆线虫属 | ~ capricola 羊圆线虫 / ~ colubriformis, ~ instabilis 蛇形毛圆线虫,不定毛圆线虫 / ~ orientalis 东方毛圆线虫 / ~ probolurus 突尾毛圆线虫 / ~ vitrinus 透明毛圆线虫
trichothecene [traiˈkɔθəsiːn] *n* 单端孢毒素
Trichothecium [ˌtrikəˈθiːʃiəm] *n* 单端孢属 | ~ roseum 粉红单端孢
trichothiodystrophy [ˌtrikəuˌθaiəuˈdistrəfi] *n* 毛发硫营养不良
trichotillomania [ˌtrikəˌtiləˈmeinjə] *n* 拔毛狂
trichotomous [traiˈkɔtəməs] *a* 三分的,分三部的
trichotoxin [ˌtraikəˈtɔksin] *n* 毛发毒素(对上皮细胞有毒性作用的抗体)
trichroism [ˈtraikrəizəm], **trichromatism** [traiˈkrəumətizəm] *n* 三色[现象] | **trichroic** [traiˈkrəuik] *a*
trichromacy [traiˈkrəuməsi] *n* 三色视
trichromasy [traiˈkrəuməsi] *n* 三色视(能区分红、黄、蓝三原色及其混合色),正常色觉 | anomalous ~ 色弱(亦称异常三色型色觉)
trichromat [ˈtraikrəmæt] *n* 三色视者,正常色觉者
trichromatism [traiˈkrəumətizəm] *n* 三色[现象],三色视觉型(正常色觉) | anomalous ~ 异常三色型色觉,三色觉异常,色弱
trichromatopsia [ˌtraikrəuməˈtɔpsiə] *n* 三色视,正常色觉 | **trichromic** [traiˈkrəumik], **trichromatic** [ˌtraikrəuˈmætik] *a*
trichterbrust [ˈtriʃtəbrust] *n*【德】漏斗[状]胸
trichuriasis [ˌtrikjuˈraiəsis] *n* 鞭虫病
Trichuridae [ˌtrikjuˈridiː] *n* 鞭虫科,毛首科
Trichuris [triˈkjuəris] *n* 鞭虫属 | ~ trichiura 毛首鞭虫
Trichuroidea [ˌtrikjuəˈrɔidiː] *n* 鞭虫总科
tricipital [traiˈsipitl] *a* 三头肌的;三头的
tricitrates [traiˈsitreits] *n* 三枸橼酸盐(一种有枸橼酸钠、枸橼酸钾和枸橼酸的溶液,用作系统性或尿碱化剂、抗尿结石药和中和性缓冲液)
triclabendazole [ˌtraikləˈbendəzəul] *n* 三氯苯达唑(抗蠕虫药)
triclobisonium chloride [ˌtraikləubiˈsəunjəm] 曲比氯铵(消毒药)
triclocarban [ˌtraikləuˈkɑːbæn] *n* 三氯卡班(消毒药)
triclofenol piperazine [traiˈkləufənɔl] 三氯酚哌嗪(抗蠕虫药)
triclofos sodium [ˈtraikləfəus] 三氯福司钠(镇静、安眠药)
triclonide [traiˈkləunaid] *n* 三氯奈德(抗炎药)
triclosan [traiˈkləusæn] *n* 三氯生(抗菌药)
tricorn [ˈtraikɔːn] *n* 侧脑室

tricornute [traiˈkɔːnjuːt] *a* 有三个角的,三突的
tricresol [traiˈkriːsɔl] *n* 三甲酚,三煤酚
tricresyl phosphate [traiˈkresil] 磷酸三甲酚酯
tri-*o*-cresyl phosphate [traiˈkresil] 磷酸三邻甲酚酯
tricrotism [ˈtraikrətizəm] *n* 三波脉[现象] | **tricrotic** [traiˈkrɔtik] *a*
tricuspid [traiˈkʌspid] *a* 三尖的;三尖瓣的,右房室瓣的
tricyanic acid [ˌtraisaiˈænik] 三聚氰酸
tricyclamol chloride [traiˈsaikləmɔl] *n* 三环氯铵(抗胆碱药,解痉药)
tricyclic [traiˈsiklik] *a* 三环的
Trid. triduum【拉】三日
tridactyl [traiˈdæktil] *a* 三指的,三趾的
tridactylism [ˌtraiˈdæktilizəm] *n* 三指,三趾 | **tridactylous** [traiˈdæktiləs] *a* 三指的,三趾的
trident [ˈtraidənt], **tridentate** [traiˈdentit] *a* 三叉的,三尖的
tridermal [traiˈdəːməl] *a* 三胚层的
tridermic [traiˈdəːmik] *a* 三胚层(外、内、中胚层)的
tridermogenesis [ˌtraidəːməuˈdʒenisis] *n* 三胚层形成
tridermoma [ˌtraidəːˈməumə] *n* 三胚层瘤
tridihexethyl chloride [ˌtraidaihekˈseθil] 曲地氯铵(抗胆碱药,解痉药,抗消化性溃疡药)
tridymite [ˈtridimait] *n* 鳞石英
tried [traid] *a* 试验过的 | ~ and true 经考验证明是好的,实践证明可取的
trielcon [traiˈelkɔn] *n* 三爪钳
triencephalus [ˌtraienˈsefələs] *n* 无口鼻眼畸胎
-triene [后缀] 三烯
trientene hydrochloride [ˈtraientiːn] 盐酸曲恩汀(一种螯合剂,用于螯合和促进威尔逊〈Wilson〉病过多铜排泄)
triester [traiˈestə] *n* 三酯[化合]物
triethanolamine [ˌtraieθəˈnɔləmiːn] *n* 三乙醇胺
triethylamine [ˌtraieθiˈlæmiːn] *n* 三乙胺
triethyl citrate [traiˈeθil] 枸橼酸三乙酯(药物制剂时用作增塑剂)
triethylenemelamine [traiˌeθiliːnˈmeləmiːn] *n* 三亚胺嗪(即曲他胺 tretamine,抗肿瘤药)
triethylenethiophosphoramide [traiˌeθiliːnˌθaiəfɔsˈfɔrəmaid] *n* 塞替派(即 thiotepa,抗肿瘤药)
trifacial [traiˈfeiʃəl] *a* 三叉神经的
trifid [ˈtraifid] *a* 三裂的
triflocin [traiˈfləusin] *n* 三氟洛辛(利尿药)
triflumidate [traiˈfluːmideit] *n* 三氟米酯(抗炎药)
trifluoperazine hydrochloride [ˌtraifluəˈperəziːn] 盐酸三氟拉嗪(抗精神病药)
trifluperidol [traifluˈperidɔl] *n* 三氟哌多(安定药)
triflupromazine [ˌtraifluˈprəuməziːn] *n* 三氟丙嗪(抗精神病药) | ~ hydrochloride 盐酸三氟丙嗪
trifluridine [traiˈfluəridin] *n* 曲氟尿苷(眼科用抗病毒药)
trifluromethylthiazide [traiˌfluərəˌmeθilˈθaiəzaid] *n* 氟甲噻嗪(即 flumethiazide,利尿药)
triflutate [ˈtraifljuˌteit] *n* 三氟醋酸盐(trifluoroacetate 的 USAN 缩约词)
trifocal [traiˈfəukəl] *a* 三焦点的 *n* [复]三焦点眼镜
trifoliosis [ˌtraifəliˈəusis] *n* 香草木樨中毒,三叶草病(马)
Trifolium [traiˈfəuliəm] *n* 三叶草属
trifurcate [ˈtrifəːkeit] *vi* 分成三支 [traiˈfəːkit] *a* 有三叉的,分成三支的 | **trifurcation** [ˌtraifəˈkeiʃən] *n* 分成三支,三叉分支,三杈;三根分叉部
trigastric [traiˈgæstrik] *a* 三腹的(指肌肉)
trigeminal [traiˈdʒeminəl] *a* 三叉神经的;三联的
trigeminus [traiˈdʒeminəs] *n*【拉】三叉神经
trigeminy [traiˈdʒemini] *n* 三联律
trigenic [taiˈdʒenik] *a* 三基因的(在染色体任何位点上具有三种不同的等位基因)
trigger [ˈtrigə] *n* 扳机,发动中心;触发(指启动一系列连锁免疫反应的第一步)
Triglochin [traiˈləukin] *n* 水麦冬属
triglyceride [traiˈglisəraid] *n* 甘油三酯,三酸甘油酯
triglyceride lipase [traiˈglisəraid ˈlaipeis] 甘油三酯脂酶,三酰甘油脂酶
trigocephalus [ˌtraigəˈsefələs] *n* 三角头畸胎
trigona [traiˈgəunə] trigonum 的复数
trigone [ˈtraigəun] *n* 三角,三角区 | ~ of bladder, vesical ~ 膀胱三角[区] / carotid ~ 颈动脉三角 / cerebral ~ 大脑穹窿 / collateral ~ 侧副三角 / collateral ~ of fourth ventricle, ~ of vagus nerve 迷走神经三角(亦称灰翼) / iliopectineal ~ 髂耻窝 / interpeduncular ~ (脑)脚间窝 / urogenital ~ 尿生殖膈 | **trigonal** [ˈtraigənəl] *a*
trigonectomy [ˌtraigəuˈnektəmi] *n* 膀胱三角[区]切除术
Trigonella [traigəˈnelə] *n* 葫芦巴属
trigonelline [ˌtrigəˈnelin] *n* 葫芦巴碱,*N*-甲基烟酸内盐
trigonid [traiˈgɔnid] *n* 下三角座,下三尖(磨牙)
trigonitis [ˌtrigəˈnaitis] *n* 膀胱三角区炎
trigonocephalus [ˌtrigənəuˈsefələs] *n* 三角头畸胎

trigonocephaly [traiˌgəunəu'sefəli], **trigonocephalia** [ˌtrigənəusi'feiliə] *n* 三角头[畸形] | **trigonocephalic** [ˌtrigənəusə'fælik] *a*
trigonotome [trai'gəunətəum] *n* [切]膀胱三角[区]刀
trigonum [trai'gəunəm] ([复] **trigona** [trai'gəunə]) *n*【拉】三角,三角区
trihexosylceramide [traiˌheksəusil'serəmaid] *n* 三己糖基神经酰胺,神经酰胺三己糖苷
trihexyphenidyl hydrochloride [traiˌheksi'fenidil] 盐酸苯海索(抗震颤麻痹药)
trihybrid [trai'haibrid] *n* 三对基因杂种
trihydrate [trai'haidreit] *n* 三羟化物 | **~d** *a* / **trihydroxide** [ˌtraihai'drɔksaid] *n*
trihydric [trai'haidrik] *a* 三羟的,三元的,三羟基醇的
trihydrol [trai'haidrɔl] *n* 三分子水
trihydroxy [ˌtraihai'drɔksi] *n* 三羟基
trihydroxybenzoic acid [traihaiˌdrɔksiben'zəuik] 三羟基苯酸,没食子酸
trihydroxyestrin [ˌtraihaiˌdrɔksi'estrin] *n* 雌三醇
tri-iniodymus [ˌtraiini'ɔdiməs] *n* 枕部三头联胎
triiodide [trai'aiədaid] *n* 三碘化物
triiodoethionic acid [traiˌaiədəueθi'ɔnik] 碘酚酸(即碘芬酸 iophenoxic acid,胆囊造影剂)
triiodomethane [traiˌaiədəu'meθein] *n* 三碘甲烷(局部抗感染药)
triiodothyronine (T_3) [ˌtraiˌaiədəu'θairəniːn] *n* 三碘甲腺原氨酸(治甲状腺功能减退药)
trikates ['traikeits] *n* 三钾盐(一个溶于纯水中的醋酸钾、碳酸氢钾和枸橼酸钾溶液,用作钾补充剂,治疗和预防低钾血症,口服给药)
triketohydrindene hydrate [traiˌkiːtəuhai'drindiːn] *n* 水合茚三酮
triketopurine [ˌtraikiːtəu'pjuərin] *n* 三酮嘌呤,尿酸
trilabe ['traileib] *n* 三叉取[膀胱]石钳
trilaminar [trai'læminə] *a* 三层的
trilateral [tai'lætərəl] *a* 三边的
trilaurin [trai'lɔːrin] *n* 月桂酸甘油酯
trilinolein [ˌtraili'nəuliin] *n* 三亚油精,三亚麻油酸甘油酯
trill [tril] *n* 颤音;颤动
trilliin ['triliin] *n* 延龄草素,延龄草苷
Trillium ['triljəm] *n* 延龄草属 | ~ erectum 直立延龄草
trilobate [trai'ləubeit], **trilobed** [trai'ləubd] *a* 三叶的
trilobectomy [ˌtrailəu'bektəmi] *n* 三肺叶切除术
trilocular [trai'lɔkjulə] *a* 三室的
trilogy ['trilədʒi] *n* 三联,三联症
trilostane ['trailəstein] *n* 曲洛司坦(肾上腺皮质抑制药)
trimagnesium phosphate [ˌtraimæg'niːziəm] 三碱磷酸镁
trimastigamoeba [traiˌmæstigə'miːbə] *n* 三鞭毛阿米巴
trimastigote [trai'mæstigəut] *a* 三鞭毛的 *n* 三鞭毛细胞
trimazosin hydrochloride [trai'meizəsin] 盐酸曲马唑嗪(抗高血压药)
trimedoxime [ˌtraimi'dɔksiːm] *n* 双解磷(有机磷中毒解毒药)
trimenon [trai'miːnən] *n* 三个月,三月期
trimensual [trai'mensjuəl] *a* 每三个月[一发]的
trimeprazine tartrate [trai'meprəziːn] 酒石酸异丁嗪(镇定、止痒药)
trimer ['traimə] *n* 三[聚]体,三聚物;三壳粒(病毒壳体) | **~ic** [trai'merik] *a*
trimercuric [ˌtraiməː'kjuərik] *a* 三汞的,三高汞[原子]的
Trimeresurus [ˌtrimərə'surəs] *n* 竹叶青属(蛇)
trimester [trai'mestə] *n* 三个月,三月期 | ~ of pregnancy 妊娠期
trimetaphosphatase [ˌtraimetə'fɔsfəteis] *n* 三偏磷酸酶
trimethadione [ˌtraimeθə'daiəun] *n* 三甲双酮(抗惊厥药)
trimethaphan camsilate [trai'meθəfən] 樟磺咪芬(抗高血压药)
trimethidinium methosulfate [traiˌmeθi'diniəm] 甲硫酸曲美替定(神经节阻断药,抗高血压药)
trimethobenzamide hydrochloride [traiˌmeθə'benzəmaid] 盐酸曲美苄胺(止吐药)
trimethoprim [trai'meθəprim] *n* 甲氧苄啶(抗菌药)
trimethylamine [ˌtraimeθi'læmiːn] *n* 三甲胺
trimethylaminoacetic acid [ˌtraimeθiˌlæminəuə'siːtik] 三甲氨乙酸
trimethylene [trai'meθiliːn] *n* 三甲烯(麻醉药)
trimethylxanthine [traiˌmeθil'zænθin] *n* 三甲黄嘌呤,咖啡碱,咖啡因
trimetozine [trai'metəziːn] *n* 曲美托嗪(镇静药)
trimipramine [trai'miprəmiːn] *n* 曲米帕明(三环抗抑郁药) | ~ maleate 马来酸曲米帕明(三环抗抑郁药)
trimopam maleate ['traiməpæm] 马来酸曲匹泮(安定药)
trimorphous [trai'mɔːfəs] *a* (同质)三形的
trinal ['trainl], **trinary** ['trainəri] *a* 三倍的,三元的,三部分组成的
trine [train] *a* 三倍的,三部分组成的 *n* 三个一组
trinegative [trai'negətive] *a* 三价阴根的
trineural [trai'njuərəl] *a* 三神经的

trineuric [traiˈnjuərik] *a* 三神经元的
trinitrate [traiˈnaitreit] *n* 三硝酸酯(或盐)
trinitrin [traiˈnaitrin], **trinitroglycerin** [traiˌnaitrəuˈglisərin], **trinitroglycerol** [traiˌnaitrəuˈglisərɔl] *n* 硝酸甘油(抗心绞痛药)
trinitrocellulose [ˌtrainaitrəuˈseljuləuz] *n* 三硝基纤维素,火棉
trinitrocresol [ˌtrainaitrəuˈkriːsɔl] *n* 三硝基甲酚
trinitrophenol [ˌtrainaitrəuˈfiːnɔl] *n* 三硝基酚(防腐药,收敛药)
trinitrotoluene [ˌtrainaitrəuˈtɔljuiːn] *n* 三硝基甲苯(亦称 TNT)
trinucleate [traiˈnjuːkliit] *a* 有三核的
trinucleotide [traiˈnjuːkliətaid] *n* 三核苷酸
triocephalus [ˌtraiəuˈsefələs] *n* 无口鼻眼畸胎
Triodontophorus diminutus [ˌtraiɔdɔnˈtɔfərəs dimiˈnjuːtəs] 缩小三齿线虫
triokinase [ˌtraiəuˈkaineis] *n* 丙糖激酶
triolein [traiˈəuliin] *n* 油酸甘油酯
triolism [ˈtraiəlizəm] *n* 三人恋,三联淫
triophthalmos [ˌtraiɔfˈθælmɔs] *n* 三眼畸胎
triopodymus [ˌtraiəuˈpɔdiməs] *n* 三面畸胎
triorchid [traiˈɔːkid], **triorchis** [traiˈɔːkis] *n* 三睾[畸形]者
triorchidism [traiˈɔːkidizəm], **triorchism** [traiˈɔːkizəm] *n* 三睾[畸形]
triorthocresyl phosphate [traiˌɔːθəuˈkresil] 磷酸三邻甲酚酯
triorthotolyl phosphate [traiˌɔːθəuˈtɔlil] 磷酸三邻甲苯酯
triose [ˈtraiəuz] *n* 丙糖
triose kinase [ˈtraiəus ˈkaineis] 丙糖激酶
triosephosphate dehydrogenase [ˌtraiəusˈfɔsfeit diːˈhaidrədʒəneis] 磷酸丙糖脱氢酶,甘油醛-3-磷酸脱氢酶
triosephosphate isomerase [ˌtraiəusˈfɔsfeit aiˈsɔməreis] 磷酸丙糖异构酶(此酶缺乏为一种常染色体隐性性状,可致溶血性贫血、神经肌肉功能不良和易致感染)
triotus [traiˈəutəs] *n* 三耳畸胎
trioxide [traiˈɔksaid] *n* 三氧化物
trioxsalen [traiˈɔksələn] *n* 三甲沙林(治白癜风药)
trioxypurine [ˌtraiɔksiˈpjuərin] *n* 三氧嘌呤,尿酸
tripalmitin [traiˈpælmitin] *n* 棕榈酸甘油酯
tripara [ˈtripərə] *n* 三产妇
triparanol [traiˈpærənɔl] *n* 曲帕拉醇(降血脂药)
tripartite [traiˈpɑːtait] *a* 三部分的
tripelennamine [ˌtraipəˈlenəmiːn] *n* 曲吡那敏(抗组胺药)
tripeptide [traiˈpeptaid] *n* 三肽
tripeptidylpeptidase [traiˌpeptidilˈpeptideis] *n* 三肽基肽酶
triphalangeal [ˌtraifəˈlændʒiəl] *a* [拇指]三指节畸形的
triphalangism [traiˈfæləndʒizəm], **triphalangia** [traifəˈlændʒiə] *n* [拇指]三指节畸形
triphasic [traiˈfeizik] *n* 三相的(肌动电流)
triphenylethylene [traiˌfeniˈleθiliːn] *n* 三苯乙烯(合成雌激素)
triphenylmethane [traiˌfenilˈmeθein] *n* 三苯甲烷
triphosphate [traiˈfɔsfeit] *n* 三磷酸盐
triphosphopyridine nucleotide [traiˌfɔsfəuˈpiridiːn] 三磷酸吡啶核苷酸(现名烟酰胺腺嘌呤二核苷酸磷酸〈NADP〉。缩写为 TPN)
triphthemia [trifˈθiːmiə] *n* 血液废物潴留
Tripier's amputation [tripiˈɛə] (Léon Tripier)特里皮埃足切除术(此手术除切除跗骨一部分外,其余与肖帕尔〈Chopart〉切断术相似)
triple [ˈtripl] *a* 三倍的,三联的,三部分的
triple-angle [ˈtriplˈæŋgl] *n* 三角器(牙科)
triple blind [tripl blaind] 三盲法(临床试验或其他实验时,受试者、治疗者、评估治疗反应者都不知道任何一位受试者接受的是何种治疗)
triplegia [traiˈpliːdʒiə] *n* 三肢瘫(偏瘫兼对侧一肢麻痹)
triple mask [ˈtripəl mæsk] 三盲法(见 triple blind)
triplet [ˈtriplit] *n* 三个一组;三胞胎中的一个;[复]三胎;三合[透]镜;三联体(分子遗传学中指在 DNA 或 RNA 中三个连续核苷酸组成的一个单位,一个三联体为一种氨基酸的密码);三线态
triplex [ˈtripleks] *a* 三倍的,三联的,三部分的
triploblastic [ˌtripləuˈblæstik] *a* 三胚层的
triploid [ˈtriplɔid] *a* 三倍的 *n* 三倍体(个体或细胞含有三整套染色体) | **~y** *n* 三倍性(染色体)
triplokoria [ˌtripləuˈkɔːriə] *n* 三瞳[畸形]
triplopia [tripˈləupiə] *n* 三重复视(视一物为三)
tripod [ˈtraipɔd] *n* 三脚架,三脚台 | ~ of life, vital ~ 生命三柱(脑、心、肺)
tripodia [traiˈpəudiə] *n* 三足[畸形]
tripodial [traiˈpəudiəl] *a* 三足的
tripoding [ˈtraipɔdiŋ] *n* 三足支撑(如瘫痪病人由坐位或立位改变体位时所采取的三个支撑点)
tripoli [ˈtripəli] *n* 硅藻土(牙科用作磨光剂)
tripositive [traiˈpɔzətiv] *a* 三价阳根的
triprolidine hydrochloride [traiˈprəulidiːn] 盐酸曲普利啶(抗组胺药)
triprosopus [ˌtraiprəˈsəupəs] *n* 三面畸胎
tripsis [ˈtripsis] *n* 研磨,研碎;按摩
-tripsy [构词成分]压轧术
triptokoria [ˌtriptəuˈkɔːriə] *n* 三瞳[畸形]

triptophan hydroxylase [ˈtriptəfæn haiˈdrɔksileis] 色氨酸羟化酶,色氨酸5-单加氧酶
triptorelin [ˌtriptəˈrelin] *n* 曲普瑞林(一种合成戈那瑞林〈gonadorelin〉类似物,用作抗肿瘤药,用于姑息性治疗晚期卵巢癌和治疗前列腺癌)
triptorelin pamoate [ˌtriptəˈrelin] 帕姆酸曲普瑞林(合成戈那瑞林〈gonadorelin〉类似物,长期使用可抑制促性腺素;用作抗肿瘤药,姑息性治疗前列腺癌,亦用于治疗性早熟和子宫内膜异位症,肌内给药)
tripus [ˈtraipəs] *n* 三脚架;三足畸胎
triquetrous [traiˈkwiːtrəs] *n* 三角的,三角形的
triquetrum [traiˈkwiːtrəm] *n*【拉】三角骨 *a* 三角的
triradial [traiˈreidjəl], **triradiate** [traiˈreidieit] *a* 三向辐射的
triradiation [ˌtraireidiˈeiʃən] *n* 三向辐射
triradius [traiˈreidiəs] *n* 指纹三角,三叉点
TRIS tris (hydroxymethyl) aminomethane 氨丁三醇,缓血酸胺,三羟甲基氨基甲烷(碱化剂,静脉注射矫治代谢性酸中毒)
tris [tris] *n* 氨丁三醇;三(2, 3-二溴丙基)磷酸酯
trisaccharidase [traiˈsækərideis] *n* 三糖水解催化酶
trisaccharide [traiˈsækəraid] *n* 三糖
trisalicylate [ˌtraisæliˈsileit, traisəˈlisəleit] *n* 三水杨酸盐 | choline magnesium ~ 三水杨酸胆碱镁(水杨酸胆碱和水杨酸镁的结合,用作镇痛、解热、消炎和抗风湿药,口服给药)
tris (2, 3-dibromopropyl) phosphate [ˌtrisdaiˌbrəuməuˈprəupil ˈfɔsfeit] *n* 三(2, 3-二溴丙基)磷酸酯(一种黄色液体阻燃剂,从前用于制作儿童衣服,但因其致癌现已限止使用。亦称tris)
trisegmentectomy [traisegmenˈtektəmi] *n* 三段切除术(指肝三段切除)
Trisetum [traiˈsiːtəm] *n* 燕麦草属
tris (hydroxymethyl) aminomethane (TRIS, THAM) [ˌtris (haiˌdrɔksiˌmeθil) æminəuˈmeθein] 氨丁三醇,缓血酸胺,三羟甲基氨基甲烷(碱化剂,静脉注射矫治代谢性酸中毒)
trismoid [ˈtrizmɔid] *n* 类牙关紧闭(新生儿牙关紧闭的一种)
trismus [ˈtrizməs] *n* 牙关紧闭(破伤风早期症状) | ~ nascentium, ~ neonatorum 新生儿牙关紧闭,新生儿破伤风(婴儿由于脐感染破伤风所致,俗称"七日风") | **trismic** *a*
trisnitrate [trisˈnaitreit] *n* 三硝酸盐
trisodium phosphonoformate [traiˈsəudiəm ˌfɔsfɔnəuˈfɔːmeit] 膦甲酸三钠,膦甲酸钠
trisomic [traiˈsəumik] *a* 三[染色]体的 *n* 三体生物 | **trisomy** [ˈtraisəmi], **trisomia** [traiˈsəumiə] *n* 三(染色)体性(二倍体加另一染色体)
trisplanchnic [traiˈsplæŋknik] *a* 三大体腔的
tristearin [traiˈstiərin] *n* (三)硬脂酸甘油酯
tristichia [traiˈstikiə] *n* 三列睫,三行睫
tristimania [ˌtristiˈmeinjə] *n* 忧郁症
trisubstituted [traiˈsʌbstiˌtjuːtid] *a* 三代的,三元取代的
trisulcate [traiˈsʌlkeit] *a* 有三沟的
trisulfapyrimidines [traiˌsʌlfəpaiˈrimidiːnz] [复] *n* 三磺嘧啶复合剂(磺胺嘧啶〈sulfadiazine〉,磺胺甲基嘧啶〈sulfamerazine〉,磺胺二甲嘧啶〈sulfamethazine〉的混合制剂)
trisulfate [traiˈsʌlfeit] *n* 三硫酸盐
trisulfide [traiˈsʌlfaid] *n* 三硫化物
Trit. tritura【拉】研制,研磨
tritan [ˈtraitən] *a* 蓝色弱的,蓝色盲的 *n* 蓝色弱者,蓝色盲者
tritanomal [ˌtraitəˈnɔməl] *n* 蓝色弱者,第三色弱者
tritanomaly [ˌtraitəˈnɔməli] *n* 蓝色弱,第三色弱 | **tritanomalous** [ˌtraitəˈnɔmələs] *a*
tritanope [ˈtraitəˌnəup] *n* 黄蓝色盲者,第三型色盲者
tritanopia [ˌtraitəˈnəupiə], **tritanopsia** [ˌtraitəˈnɔpsiə] *n* 蓝色盲,第三色盲 | **tritanopic** [ˌtraitəˈnɔpik] *a*
triterpene [traiˈtəːpiːn] *n* 三萜
tritiate [ˈtritieit] *vt* 氚化,氚标记
triticeous [traiˈtiʃəs] *a* 麦粒样的
triticeum [traiˈtisiəm] *n*【拉】麦粒软骨
triticin [ˈtritisin] *n* 小麦糖
triticonucleic acid [ˌtritikəuˈnjuːkliik] 麦胚核酸
Triticum [ˈtritikəm] *n*【拉】小麦属
triticum [ˈtritikəm] *n* 小麦属植物(偃麦草根茎,有利尿作用)
Tritirachium [ˌtritiˈreikiəm] *n* 丝状菌属
tritium (^{3}H) [ˈtritiəm] *n* 氚(氢的放射性同位素)
tritocone [ˈtraitəkəun] *n* 上前第三尖(哺乳动物的上前磨牙远中颊尖)
tritoconid [ˌtraitəˈkəunid] *n* 下前第三尖(哺乳动物的下前磨牙远中颊尖)
tritolyl phosphate [traiˈtɔlil] 磷酸三甲苯酯
tri-*o*-tolyl phosphate [traiˈtɔlil] 磷酸三邻甲苯酯
triton [ˈtraitn] *n* 氚核
Tritrichomonas [traiˌtrikəˈməunəs] *n* 三毛滴虫属
triturate [ˈtritjureit] *vt* 研磨,研制 *n* 磨碎物,研制剂 | **triturable** [ˈtritjurəbl] *a* 可研制的,可研磨的 / **trituration** [ˌtritjuˈreiʃən] *n* 研制[法],研磨[法];研制剂;齐化 / **triturator** [ˌtritjuˈreitə] *n* 研磨器

trivalent [traiˈveilənt] *a* 三价的 *n* 三价体(在减数分裂中发生联会的三个同源染色体的总称) | **trivalence** *n* 三价

trivalve [ˈtraivælv] *a* 三瓣的(窥器)

trizonal [traiˈzəunəl] *a* 三带的,三个区域的

tRNA transfer-RNA 转移 RNA

trocar [ˈtrəukɑː] *n* 套针 | piloting ~ 导引套针(导引连接气管造口术的套针) / rectal ~ 经直肠膀胱套针

troch. trochiscus 锭剂,糖锭[剂]

trochanter [trəuˈkæntə] *n*【拉;希】转子 | ~ major, greater ~ 大转子 / ~ minor, lesser ~, small ~ 小转子 / ~ tertius, third ~, rudimentary ~ 第三转子 | **~ic** [ˌtrəukənˈterik], **~ian** [ˌtrəukənˈteriən] *a*

trochanterplasty [trəuˈkæntəˌplæsti] *n* 转子成形术

trochantin [trəuˈkæntin] *n* 小转子 | **~ian** [ˌtrəukənˈtiniən] *a*

troche [trəuʃ, trəuki] *n* 锭剂,糖锭[剂]

trochin [ˈtrəukin] *n* 肱骨小结节

trochiscus [trəˈkiskəs] ([复] **trochisci** [trəˈkis(k)ai]) *n*【拉】锭剂,糖锭[剂]

trochiter [ˈtrɔkitə] *n* 大转子;肱骨大结节 | **~ian** [ˌtrɔkiˈtiəriən] *a*

trochlea [ˈtrɔkliə] ([复] **trochleae** [ˈtrɔkliiː]) *n*【拉】滑车

trochlear [ˈtrɔkliə] *a* 滑车的;滑车神经的

trochleariform [ˌtrɔkliˈærifɔːm] *a* 滑车形的

trochlearis [ˌtrɔkliˈɛəris] *a* 滑车的 *n* 滑车神经;眼上斜肌

trochocephaly [ˌtrəukəuˈsefəli], **trochocephalia** [ˌtrəukəusəˈfeiliə] *n* 轮状头[畸形],圆头[畸形]

trochoid [ˈtrəukɔid], **trochoidal** [trəuˈkɔidl] *a* 车轴状的,滑车状的

trochoides [trəuˈkɔidiːz] *n*【希】车轴关节

trochophore [ˈtrəukəfɔː] *n* 担轮幼虫

troglitazone [ˌtrəugliˈteizəun] *n* 曲格列酮(抗高血糖药,降低胰岛素抗性,以前用于治疗非胰岛素依赖型糖尿病,由于肝细胞毒性,本品停止使用)

Troglostrongylus [ˌtrɔgləuˈstrɔndʒiləs] *n* 隐孔圆线虫属

Troglotrema [ˌtrɔgləˈtriːmə] *n* 隐孔[吸虫]属 | ~ salmincola 鲑隐孔吸虫

Troglotrematidae [ˌtrɔgləutriˈmætidiː] *n* 隐孔科

troilism [ˈtrɔilizəm] *n* 三人恋,三联淫

Troisier's ganglion [trwəziˈɛə] (Charles E. Troisier) 特鲁瓦西埃淋巴结(胸骨后肿瘤时锁骨上部有时见到肿大的淋巴结) | ~ node 信号结(signal node,见 node 项下相应术语) / ~ sign 特鲁瓦西埃征(锁骨上淋巴结肿大,为内腹部恶性病或胸骨后肿瘤之征) / ~ syndrome 特鲁瓦西埃综合征(糖尿病时青铜色恶病质)

trolamine [ˈtrəuləmiːn] *n* 三乙醇胺(药物制剂时用作碱化剂,亦称 triethanolamine;triethanolamine 的 USAN 缩约词)

troland [ˈtrəulənd] *n* 托兰(视网膜所受光刺激的单位)

Trolard's plexus (net) [trəˈlɑː] (Paulin Trolard) 舌下神经管静脉网 | ~ vein 下吻合静脉

troleandomycin [ˌtrəuliændəuˈmaisin] *n* 醋竹桃霉素(抗菌药)

trolnitrate phosphate [trɔlˈnaitreit] 磷酸三乙硝胺(血管扩张药)

Tröltsch's corpuscles [ˈtreltʃi] (Anton F. von Tröltsch) 特勒尔奇小体(鼓膜放射性纤维间小体) | ~ recesses (spaces) 特勒尔奇隐窝(鼓膜前及后隐窝)

Trombicula [trɔmˈbikjulə] *n* 恙螨属 | ~ akamushi 红恙螨 / ~ alfreddugèsi, ~ irritans, ~ tsalsahuatl 致痒恙螨,阿氏真恙螨(即 Eutrombicula alfreddugèsi) / ~ autaumnalis, ~ holosericeum 秋恙螨,日本恙虫 / ~ deliensis 地里恙螨 / ~ fletcheri 弗[莱彻]氏恙螨 / ~ intermedia 居中恙螨 / ~ pallida 苍白恙螨 / ~ scutellaris 小板恙螨

trombiculiasis [trɔmˌbikjuˈlaiəsis] *n* 恙螨病

trombiculid [trɔmˈbikjulid] *n* 恙螨

Trombiculidae [ˌtrɔmbikjuˈlaidiː] *n* 恙螨科

trombiculidiasis [trɔmˌbikjuliˈdaiəsis] *n* 恙螨病

trombidiiasis [trɔmˌbidiˈaiəsis], **trombidiosis** [trɔmˌbidiˈəusis] *n* 恙螨病

Trombidium [trɔmˈbidjəm] *n* 恙螨属(旧名)

tromethamine [trəˈmeθəmiːn] *n* 氨丁三醇(碱化剂,静脉注射矫治代谢性酸中毒)

Trommer's test [ˈtrɔmə] (Karl A. Trommer) 特罗默尔试验(检尿糖)

Trömner's sign [ˈtremnə] (Ernest L. O. Trömner) 特勒姆内征(指反射,见 Hoffmann's sign 2 解)

tromomania [ˌtrɔməˈmeinjə] *n* 震颤谵妄

tromophonia [ˌtrɔməˈfəuniə] *n* 颤音

trona [ˈtrəunə] *n* 天然碱,粗碳酸钠

tronchado [trɔnˈkɑːdəu] *n* 牛瘫痪病(中美洲和墨西哥)

tropate [ˈtrəupeit] *n* 托品酸盐,α-苯基-β-羟丙酸盐

tropesis [trəuˈpiːsis] *n* 倾向,动向

trophectoderm [trɔˈfektədəːm] *n* 滋养外胚层

trophedema [ˌtrɔfiˈdiːmə] *n* 营养性水肿(下肢永久性水肿) | congenital ~, hereditary ~ 先天性营养性水肿(见 Milroy's disease)

Tropheryma [trəu'ferimə] *n* 营养防御菌属 | ~ whippelii 惠氏营养防御菌

trophesy ['trɔfisi] *n* 神经性营养不良 | **trophesial** [trə'fiːziəl], **trophesic** [trə'fiːsik] *a*

trophic ['trɔfik] *a* 营养的

-trophic, -trophin [构词成分]营养

trophicity [trə'fisəti] *n* 营养功能

trophism ['trɔfizəm] *n* 营养作用,营养性

troph(o)- [构词成分]营养

trophoblast ['trɔfəblæst] *n* 滋养层 | **~ic** [ˌtrɔfəu'blæstik] *a*

trophoblastoma [ˌtrɔfəublæs'təumə] *n* 绒[毛]膜上皮癌

trophochromidia [ˌtrɔfəukrəu'midiə], **trophochromatin** [ˌtrɔfəu'krəumətin] *n* 核外滋养染色质,滋养染色质

trophocyte ['trɔfəsait] *n* 滋养细胞

trophoderm ['trɔfədəːm] *n* 滋养层

trophodermatoneurosis [ˌtrɔfəuˌdəːmətəunjuə'rəusis] *n* 营养性皮肤神经功能病

trophodynamics [ˌtrɔfəudai'næmiks] *n* 营养动力学

trophoedema [ˌtrɔfəui'diːmə] *n* 营养性水肿(见 trophedema)

tropholecithus [ˌtrɔfəu'lesiθəs] *n* 营养卵黄 | **tropholecithal** *a*

trophology [trə'fɔlədʒi] *n* 营养学

trophon ['trɔfən] *n* 神经元营养质

trophoneurosis [ˌtrɔfəunjuə'rəusis] *n* 营养神经[功能]病 | facial ~ 面部营养神经病,半面萎缩 / lingual ~ 舌营养神经病,进行性半侧舌萎缩 / muscular ~ 肌营养神经病,神经性肌营养不良症 | **trophoneurotic** [ˌtrɔfəunjuə'rɔtik] *a*

trophonosis [ˌtrɔfəu'nəusis] *n* 营养[性]病

trophont ['trəufɔnt] *n* 营养体(原虫)

trophonucleus [ˌtrɔfəu'njuːkliəs] *n* 滋养核,大核

trophopathy [trə'fɔpəθi], **trophopathia** [ˌtrɔfəu'pæθiə] *n* 营养[性]病

trophoplast ['trɔfəplæst] *n* 滋养质粒,原形体

trophospongium [ˌtrɔfəu'spʌndʒiəm] ([复] **trophospongia** [trɔfəu'spʌndʒiə]) *n* 【拉;希】胞管系;[复]滋养海绵层

trophotaxis [ˌtrɔfəu'tæksis] *n* 趋营养性

trophotherapy [ˌtrɔfəu'θerəpi] *n* 营养疗法

trophotropism [ˌtrɔfəu'trəupizəm] *n* 向营养性

trophozoite [ˌtrɔfəu'zəuait] *n* 滋养体(原虫)

-trophy [构词成分]食物,营养

tropia ['trəupiə] *n* 斜视,斜眼

-tropic [构词成分]向…的,亲…的

tropic acid ['trɔpik] 托品酸,α-苯(基)-*β*-羟(基)丙酸

tropical ['trɔpikəl] *a* 热带的

tropicamide [trəu'pikəmaid] *n* 托吡卡胺(抗胆碱能药,散瞳药)

tropidine ['trɔpidin] *n* 脱水托品(托品脱水产物)

tropin ['trəupin] *n* 亲[菌]素,调理素

-tropin [构词成分]亲…,促…

tropine ['trəupiːn] *n* 托品,莨菪醇

tropism ['trəupizəm] *n* 向性,嗜性 | **tropistic** [trəu'pistik] *a*

trop(o)- [构词成分]转变,反应,改变

tropochrome ['trəupəˌkrəum] *a* 拒染性的

tropocollagen [ˌtrəupəu'kɔlədʒən] *n* 原胶原

tropoelastin [ˌtrɔpəui'læstin] *n* 原弹性蛋白

tropometer [trə'pɔmitə] *n* 旋转计(检眼球;检长骨)

tropomyosin [ˌtrəupəu'maiəsin] *n* 原肌球蛋白 | ~ A 原肌球蛋白 A,副肌球蛋白

tropon ['trɔpən] *n* (动植物)白蛋白营养粉

troponin ['trɔpənin] *n* 肌钙蛋白

-tropy [构词成分]转变,改变

trotyl ['trəutil] *n* 三硝基甲苯

trough [trɔ(ː)f] *n* 沟,槽 | synaptic ~s 突触裂隙,初级突触裂隙

trousers ['trauzəs] *n* 裤子,长裤

Trousseau's phenomenon [tru'səu] (Armand Trousseau)特鲁索现象(压迫某肌肉的神经时,引起该肌痉挛性收缩现象,见于手足搐搦) | ~ sign 特鲁索征(低钙束臂征;脑[病]性划痕,见 tache cérébrale) / ~ spot 特鲁索点(脑[病]性划痕,见 tache cérébrale) / ~ twitching 面肌颤搐

trovafloxacin mesylate [ˌtrəuvə'flɔksəsin] 甲磺托氟沙星(抗菌药)

troxidone ['trɔksidəun] *n* 三甲双酮(抗惊厥药,抗癫痫药)

troy [trɔi] *n* 金衡[制]

Trp tryptophan 色氨酸

TRU turbidity reducing unit 浊度减低单位(透明质酸酶活性单位)

Trueta treatment (method, technique) [tru-'eitə] (José Trueta)图埃塔疗法(骨折处理,包括迅速外科疗法、清理创口、切除骨碎片及异物、骨折复位、裹创口及石膏固定、注射破伤风抗毒素)

truffles ['trʌflz] *n* 块菌

trumpet ['trʌmpit] *n* 呼吸管(蛹);助听筒(聋人用)

truncal ['trʌŋkəl] *a* 躯干的,干的

truncate ['trʌŋkeit] *vt* 截断,切断 *a* 截断的,截状的

truncus ['trʌŋkəs] *n* ([复] **trunci** ['trʌnsai])躯干,干

trunk [trʌŋk] *n* 躯干,干 | basilar ~ 基底动脉 / brachiocephalic ~ 头臂[动脉]干,无名动脉 / ~

of corpus callosum 胼胝体干 / intestinal lymphatic ~s 肠[淋巴]干

trusion [ˈtruʒən] *n* 错位,异位 | bimaxillary ~ 双颌牙错位 / bodily ~ 全牙错位 / coronal ~ 牙冠错位 / mandibular ~ 下牙错位 / maxillary ~ 上牙错位

truss [trʌs] *n* 疝带;桥筋,桥架 | nasal ~ 鼻夹(鼻骨折用) / yarn ~ 羊毛绒疝带(婴儿腹股疝用)

truxilline [ˈtrʌksilin] *n* 异托品基可卡因,组丝古柯碱

try-in [ˈtraiin] *n* 试戴(假牙)

trypaflavine [ˌtripəˈfleivin] *n* 吖啶黄,锥虫黄

trypanblau [ˈtraipənˌblau] *n*【德】台盼蓝,锥虫蓝

trypanid [ˈtripənid] *n* 锥虫病疹

trypanocidal [ˌtripənəuˈsaidl] *a* 杀锥虫的

trypanocide [triˈpænəsaid] *a* 杀锥虫的 *n* 杀锥虫药

trypanolysis [ˌtripəˈnɔlisis] *n* 溶锥虫[作用] | **trypanolytic** [ˌtripənəuˈlitic] *a*

Trypanoplasma [ˌtripənəuˈplæzmə] *n* 锥浆虫属

Trypanosoma [ˌtripənəuˈsəumə] *n* 锥虫属 | ~ americanum 美洲锥虫 / ~ avium 鸟锥虫 / ~ brucei, ~ pecaudi 布[鲁斯]氏锥虫,佩[克]氏锥虫 / ~ calmetii 卡[尔默特]氏锥虫 / ~ congolense, ~ nanum 刚果锥虫,短小锥虫 / ~ cruzi 克[鲁斯]氏锥虫 / ~ dimorpha 二形锥虫 / ~ equinum 马锥虫 / ~ equiperdum, ~ rougeti 马媾疫锥虫,马类性病锥虫 / ~ evansi, ~ hippicum 伊[凡斯]氏锥虫,马锥虫 / ~ gambiense, ~ hominis, ~ ugandense 冈比亚锥虫,人体锥虫,乌干达锥虫 / ~ lewisi 路[易士]氏锥虫 / ~ melophagium 蜱蝇锥虫 / ~ neotomae 林鼠锥虫 / ~ rhodesiense 罗德西亚锥虫 / ~ rotatorium 旋转锥虫/ ~ simiae 猿猴锥虫 / ~ theileri 泰[累尔]氏锥虫 / ~ triatomae 锥蝽锥虫 / ~ vivax, ~ uniforme 活动锥虫

trypanosomal [triˌpænəˈsəuməl] *a* 锥虫的

trypanosomatid [ˌtripənəuˈsəumətid] *n*, *a* 锥虫亚目原虫(的)

Trypanosomatina [ˌtripənəuˌsəuməˈtainə] *n* 锥虫亚目

trypanosomatosis [ˌtripənəuˌsəuməˈtəusis] *n* 锥虫病

trypanosomatotropic [triˌpænəˌsəumətəuˈtrɔpik] *a* 向锥虫的

trypanosome [triˈpænəsəum] *n* 锥虫

trypanosomiasis [ˌtripənəusəuˈmaiəsis] *n* 锥虫病 | African ~, Congo ~ 非洲锥虫病,刚果锥虫病 / American ~ , Brazilian ~, Cruz ~, South American ~ 美洲锥虫病,巴西锥虫病,克[鲁斯]氏锥虫病,南美洲锥虫病(即恰克斯病,见 Chagas' disease) / Rhodesian ~ 罗德西亚锥虫病

trypanosomicidal [ˌtripənəuˌsəumiˈsaidl] *a* 杀锥虫的

trypanosomicide [ˌtripənəuˈsəumisaid] *a* 杀锥虫的 *n* 杀锥虫药

trypanosomid [triˈpænəsəumid] *n* 锥虫病疹

Trypanozoon [ˌtripənəuˈzəuɔn] *n* 锥虫属

trypanroth [ˈtripənrɔθ] *n*【德】台盼红,锥虫红

tryparosan [traiˈpærəsæn] *n* 台盼罗散(副品红分子中引入卤根所得的制剂注射用于治锥虫病)

tryparsamide [triˈpɑːsəmaid] *n* 锥虫胂胺(抗锥虫药)

trypasafrol [ˌtraipəˈsæfrɔl] *n* 锥虫番红(番红色素类之一,治锥虫病)

trypesis [traiˈpiːsis] *n*【希】环钻术,环锯术

trypochete [ˈtraipəkiːt] *n* 德勒包涵体(见 Döhle's inclusion bodies)

trypomastigote [ˌtraipəˈmæstigəut] *n* 锥鞭体

tryponarsyl [ˌtraipəˈnɑːsil], **trypotan** [ˈtraipətən] *n* 锥虫胂胺(抗锥虫药)

trypsin [ˈtripsin] *n* 胰蛋白酶 | crystallized ~ 结晶胰蛋白酶 | **tryptic** *a*

trypsinize [ˈtripsinaiz] *vt* 受胰蛋白酶作用

trypsinogen [tripˈsinədʒən], **trypsogen** [ˈtripsədʒən] *n* 胰蛋白酶原

tryptamine [ˈtriptəmiːn] *n* 色胺

tryptase [ˈtripteis] *n* 类胰蛋白酶

tryptolysis [tripˈtɔlisis] *n* 胰胨分解 | **tryptolytic** [ˌtriptəuˈlitik] *a*

tryptone [ˈtriptəun] *n* 胰[蛋白]胨

tryptophan (**Trp**, **W**) [ˈtriptəfæn], **tryptophane** [ˈtriptəfein] *n* 色氨酸

tryptophanase [ˈtriptəfəneis] *n* 色氨酸酶

tryptophan 2, 3-dioxygenase [ˈtriptəfæn daiˈɔksidʒəneis] 色氨酸 2, 3-双加氧酶

trytophan hydroxylase [ˈtriptəfæn haiˈdrɔksileis] 色氨酸羟化酶,色氨酸 5-单加氧酶

tryptophan 5-monooxygenase [ˈtriptəfæn ˌmɔnəuˈɔksidʒəneis] 色氨酸 5-单加氧酶(此酶在中枢神经系统内发生,并在恶性高苯丙氨酸血症时失活)

tryptophan pyrrolase [ˈtriptəfæn piˈrəuleis] 色氨酸吡咯酶,色氨酸 2, 3-双加氧酶

tryptophanuria [ˌtriptəufəˈnjuəriə] *n* 色氨酸尿

tryptophyl [ˈtriptəfil] *n* 色氨酰

TS test solution 试[验溶]液;tricuspid stenosis 右房室瓣狭窄

TSA tumor-specific antigen 肿瘤特异性抗原

tsalsahuatl [ˌtsælseiˈwhɑːtl] *n* 阿氏真恙螨,致痒恙螨(即 Eutrombicula alfreddugèsi)

TSD Tay-Sachs disease 泰-萨克斯病,GM_2 神经节

苷脂贮积症变异型 B

TSE transmissible spongioform encephalopathy 传染性海绵状脑病

tsetse [ˈtsetsi] *n* 采采蝇(舌蝇属)

TSF triceps skinfold 三头肌皮褶(厚度)

TSH thyroid-stimulating hormone 促甲状腺[激]素

T-spine thoracic spine 胸脊柱

TSTA tumor-specific transplantation antigen 肿瘤特异性移植抗原

Tsuga [ˈtsuɡə] *n* 铁杉属

tsutsugamushi [tsuːtsuɡəˈmuːʃi] *n*【日】恙虫

TT therapeutic touch 治疗性触诊; thrombin time 凝血酶时间

TTV thrombotic threshold velocity 血栓形成阈速度

TU tuberculin unit 结核菌素单位

tuaminoheptane [tjuˌæminəuˈheptein] *n* 异庚胺(肾上腺素能药,吸入可使鼻黏膜血管收缩以减轻充血) | ~ sulfate 硫酸异庚胺(局部用于鼻黏膜)

tuba [ˈtjuːbə] ([复] **tubae** [ˈtjuːbiː]) *n*【拉】管

tubal [ˈtjuːbəl] *a* 管的(尤指输卵管的,如输卵管妊娠 tubal pregnancy)

tubatorsion [tjuːbəˈtɔːʃən] *n* 输卵管扭转

tubba [ˈtʌbə], **tubboe** [ˈtʌbəu] *n* 掌跖雅司病

tube [tjuːb] *n* 管 | air ~ 呼吸管,呼吸道 / auditory ~ 咽鼓管 / cathoderay ~ 阴极[射]线管 / collecting ~s 集合管(肾) / corneal ~s 角膜板层管 / digestive ~ 消化管,消化道 / discharge ~ 放电管 / drainage ~ 引流管 / dressed ~ 敷料引流管 / eustachian ~ 欧氏管,咽鼓管 / fallopian ~ 输卵管 / feeding ~ 饲管 / fusion ~s 融合[视]力测练管 / gas ~ 含气(X 线)管 / granulation ~ 喉肉芽压迫插管 / neural ~, medullary ~, cerebromedullary ~ 神经管(胚) / pus ~ 输卵管积脓 / roll ~ 旋转管 / salivary ~s 涎腺叶间管 / sputum ~ 容痰管(离心沉淀用) / tampon ~ 填塞管(填塞直肠止血,但可容气体排出) / tracheotomy ~ 气管切开插管 / uterine ~ 输卵管 / vacuum ~ 真空管 / valve ~ 真空整流管 / X-ray ~ X 线管

tubectomy [tjuːˈbektəmi] *n* 输卵管[部分]切除术

tuber [ˈtjuːbə] ([复] **tubers** 或 **tubera** [ˈtjuːbərə]) *n*【拉】结节 | eustachian ~ 欧氏结节,鼓室结节 / omental ~ of liver 肝网膜结节 / omental ~ of pancreas 胰网膜结节 / papillary ~ of liver 肝乳头突 / sciatic ~ 坐骨结节

tubercle [ˈtjuːbə(ː)kl] *n* 结节,结核[结]节;牙冠结节 | acoustic ~ 听结节 / anatomical ~, dissection ~ 剖尸疣,尸毒性疣 / anterior ~ of atlas 寰椎前结节 / anterior obturator ~ 闭孔前结节 / auricular ~, darwinian ~ 耳丘,达尔文结节 / calcaneal ~ 跟骨结节 / caseous ~s 干酪样结核[结]节 / caudal ~ of liver 肝尾状突 / crude ~ 粗隆,干酪样结核[结]节 / deltoid ~ 三角肌粗隆 / external(或 greater) ~ of humerus 肱骨大结节 / genital ~, cloacal ~ 生殖结节 / gray ~ 灰色结核[结]节;灰结节 / greater ~ of calcaneus 跟结节内侧突 / ~ of humerus 肱骨小头 / internal(或 lesser) ~ of humerus 肱骨小结节 / lesser ~ of calcaneus 跟结节外侧突 / mamillary ~ of hypothalamus 乳头体 / muscular ~ of atlas 寰椎前结节 / posterior ~ of atlas 寰椎后结节 / posterior obturator ~ 闭孔后结节 / transverse ~ of fourth tarsal bone 骰骨粗隆 / trochlear ~ 滑车棘 / ~ of ulna 尺骨粗隆 / yellow ~ 黄色结核[结]节,干酪样结核(结)节

tubercula [tju(ː)ˈbəːkjulə] tuberculum 的复数

tubercular [tju(ː)ˈbəːkjulə] *a* 结节的,结节状的

Tuberculariaceae [tju(ː)ˌbəːkjuˌlæriˈeisiiː] *n* 结节菌科

tuberculate [tju(ː)ˈbəːkjulit], **tuberculated** [tju(ː)ˈbəːkjuleitid] *a* 有结节的;患结核的

tuberculation [tju(ː)ˌbəːkjuˈleiʃən] *n* 结节形成;结核[结]节形成

tuberculid [tju(ː)ˈbəːkjulid] *n* 结核疹 | micronodular ~ 微结节性结核疹,肉芽肿性酒渣鼻 / papulonecrotic ~ 丘疹坏死性结核疹(亦称瘰疬性痤疮,丘疹坏死性结核病) / rosacea-like ~ 酒渣鼻样结核疹,肉芽肿性酒渣鼻

tuberculigenous [tju(ː)ˌbəːkjuˈlidʒinəs] *a* 引起结核[病]的

tuberculin [tju(ː)ˈbəːkjulin] *n* 结核菌素 | albumose-free(A. F.) ~, Tuberculin Albumose Frei (T. A. F.) 无胨结核菌素,脱胨结核菌素(用于皮下结核菌素试验) / alkaline ~ 碱性结核菌素(用 1/10N 碳酸钠溶液提取结核杆菌的制剂,相似于原始结核菌素) / autogenous ~ 自体结核菌素,自身结核菌素 / bacillary emulsion(B. E.) ~ (T. B. E.) 乳剂结核菌素,结核菌素乳剂 / bouillon filtrate(B. F.) 肉汤滤液结核菌素 / ~ contagious(T. C.) 接触传染性结核菌素(可被身体细胞所摄取,成为细胞的组分) / ~ filtrate(T. F.) 滤液结核菌素 / New ~, original ~ (T. O.), residual ~, ~ residue(T. R.)新结核菌素,原[始]结核菌素,沉渣结核菌素 / old ~ (O. T.) 旧结核菌素 / perlsucht ~, perlsucht tuberculin original (P. T. O.) 牛结核菌素,原(始)牛结核菌素 / perlsucht tuberculin rest(P. T. R.) 牛结核菌素沉淀 / ~ precipitation(T. P.) 沉淀结核菌素 / purified ~ 纯结核菌素 / purified protein derivative(PPD) ~ 纯蛋白衍生物结核菌素 / vacuum ~ (V. T.) 真空结核菌素 / vital ~ 减毒活结核菌素 / ~ zymoplastiche (TZ) 醇制结核菌素

tuberculinization [tjuˌbəːkjuˌlinaiˈzeiʃən, -niˈz-]

n 结核菌素应用法(应用结核菌素进行治疗或进行皮肤试验)

tuberculinose [tju(ː)ˈbəːkjuˌlinəus] *n* 变性结核菌素

tuberculinotherapy [tju(ː)ˌbəːkjuˌlinəuˈθerəpi] *n* 结核菌素疗法

tuberculinum [tju(ː)ˌbəːkjuˈlainəm] *n*【拉】结核菌素 | ~ pristinum 旧结核菌素

tuberculitis [ˌtjuːbə(ː)kjuˈlaitis] *n* 结核[结]节炎

tuberculization [tju(ː)ˌbəːkjulaiˈzeiʃən, -liˈz-] *n* 结核菌素疗法;结核化(形成或演变成结核)

tuberculoalbumin [tju(ː)ˌbəːkjuləuˈælbjumin] *n* 结核白蛋白

tuberculocele [tju(ː)ˈbəːkjuləuˌsiːl] *n* 睾丸结核

tuberculocidal [tju(ː)ˌbəːkjuləuˈsaidl] *a* 杀结核菌的

tuberculocide [tju(ː)ˈbəːkjuləuˌsaid] *n* 杀结核菌药

tuberculocidin [tju(ː)ˌbəːkjuləuˈsaidin] *n* 杀结核菌素(用氯化铂处理结核菌素而得的蛋白胨,应用如同结核菌素,据称无后者的副作用)

tuberculoderma [tju(ː)ˌbəːkjuləuˈdəːmə] *n* 皮[肤]结核

tuberculofibroid [tju(ː)ˌbəːkjuləuˈfaibrɔid] *a* 结核[结]节纤维样变性的

tuberculofibrosis [tju(ː)ˌbəːkjuləufaiˈbrəusis] *n* 纤维性结核

tuberculoid [tju(ː)ˈbəːkjulɔid] *a* 结核[结]节样的;结核[病]样的

tuberculoidin [tju(ː)ˌbəːkjuˈlɔidin] *n* 类结核菌素(一种改变的结核菌素,用酒精处理清除其杆菌)

tuberculoma [tju(ː)ˌbəːkjuˈləumə] *n* 结核球 | ~ en plaque 斑状结核球

tuberculomyces [tju(ː)ˌbəːkjuˈlɔmisiːz] *n* 结核菌类

tuberculo-opsonic [tju(ː)ˌbəːkjuləu ɔpˈsɔnik] *a* 结核菌调理素的

tuberculoprotein [tju(ː)ˌbəːkjuləuˈprəutiːn] *n* 结核菌蛋白

tuberculosarium [tju(ː)ˌbəːkjuləuˈsɛəriəm] *n* 结核病疗养院

tuberculosilicosis [tju(ː)ˌbəːkjuləuˌsiliˈkəusis] *n* 硅肺结核

tuberculosis [tju(ː)ˌbəːkjuˈləusis] *n* 结核病 | anthracotic ~ 肺尘埃沉着病,尘肺 / atypical ~ 非典型结核,分枝杆菌病 / basal ~ 肺底[部]结核,肺底痨 / ~ of bones and joints 骨与关节结核 / bovine ~ 牛结核 / cerebral ~ 结核性脑膜炎 / ~ cutis lichenoides 苔藓样皮肤结核,瘰疬性苔藓 / ~ cutis miliaris disseminata 播散性粟粒性皮肤结核,播散性粟粒性结核 / ~ cutis orificialis 腔口部皮肤结核 / exudative ~ 渗出性肺结核 / genital ~ 生殖器结核 / genito-urinary ~ 泌尿生殖系结核 / hematogenous ~ 血源性结核 / hilus ~ 肺门结核 / inhalation ~, aerogenic ~ 吸入性肺结核 / ~ of intestines 肠结核 / ~ of kidney 肾结核 / ~ lichenoides 瘰疬性苔藓 / ~ of lungs, pulmonary ~ 肺结核 / ~ miliaris disseminata 播散性粟粒性结核 / miliary ~ 粟粒性结核 / oral ~ 口腔结核 / postprimary ~, reinfection ~ 原发后结核,再感染性结核 / primary ~, childhood ~ 原发性结核 / primary inoculation ~ 原发性接种性结核(亦称原发性接种性复征,原发性结核性复征) / productive ~ 增生性结核 / ~ of skin 皮肤结核 / spinal ~, ~ of spine 脊柱结核 / tracheobronchial ~ 气管支气管结核 / warty ~ 疣状[皮]结核

tuberculostatic [tju(ː)ˌbəːkjuləuˈstætik] *n* 结核菌抑制药 *a* 抑制结核菌的

tuberculostearic acid [tju(ː)ˌbəːkjuləustiˈærik] 结核硬脂酸,10-甲基硬脂酸

tuberculotic [tju(ː)ˌbəːkjuˈlɔtik] *a* 结核病的,患结核病的

tuberculous [tju(ː)ˈbəːkjuləs] *a* 结核性的

tuberculum [tju(ː)ˈbəːkjuləm] ([复] **tubercula** [tju(ː)ˈbəːkjulə]) *n*【拉】结节

tuberin [ˈtjuːbərin] *n* 马铃薯球蛋白

tuberosis [ˌtjuːbəˈrəusis] *n* 结节形成[状态]

tuberositas [ˌtjuːbəˈrɔsitəs] ([复] **tuberositates** [ˌtjuːbəˌrɔsiˈtɑːtiːz]) *n*【拉】粗隆

tuberosity [ˌtjuːbəˈrɔsəti] *n* 粗隆 | ~ of cuboid bone 骰骨粗隆 / external(或 lateral) ~ of femur 股骨外上髁 / ~ of fifth metatarsal bone 第五跖骨粗隆 / ~ of first metatarsal bone 第一跖骨粗隆 / internal(或 medial) ~ of femur 股骨内上髁 / ischial ~, ~ of ischium 坐骨结节 / lesser ~ of humerus 肱骨小结节 / masseteric ~ 咬肌粗隆 / pyramidal ~ of palatine bone 腭骨锥突

tuberous [ˈtjuːbərəs] *a* 有结节的,结节状的,隆凸的;有块茎的,块茎状的

tubi [ˈtjuːbai] tubus 的复数

Tubifera [tjuˈbifərə] *n* 果蝇属

tubiferous [tjuˈbifərəs] *a* 有结节的;有块茎的

tub(o)- [构词成分]管

tuboabdominal [ˌtjuːbəuæbˈdɔminl] *a* 输卵管腹腔的

tuboadnexopexy [ˌtjuːbəuædˈneksəˌpeksi] *n* 子宫附件固定术

tubocurarine [ˌtjuːbəukjuˈrɑːrin] *n* 筒箭毒碱 | ~ chloride 氯筒箭毒碱(神经肌肉阻断药) / dimethyl ~ iodide 碘二甲筒箭毒碱(骨骼肌松

弛药）

tuboligamentous [ˌtjuːbəuˌligəˈmentəs] *a* 输卵管阔韧带的

tubo-ovarian [ˌtjuːbəuəuˈvεəriən] *a* 输卵管卵巢的

tubo-ovariotomy [ˌtjuːbəu əuˌvεəriˈɔtəmi] *n* 输卵管卵巢切除术

tubo-ovaritis [ˌtjuːbəuˌəuvəˈraitis] *n* 输卵管卵巢炎

tuboperitoneal [ˌtjuːbəuˌperitəuˈniːəl] *a* 输卵管腹膜的

tuboplasty [ˈtjuːbəuˌplæsti] *n* 管成形术（如输卵管成形术，咽鼓管成形术）| eustachian ~ 咽鼓管成形术

tuborrhea [ˌtjuːbəˈriːə] *n* 咽鼓管溢

tuboscopy [tjuːˈbɔskəpi] *n* 咽鼓管镜检查

tubotorsion [ˌtjuːbəuˈtɔːʃən] *n* 管扭转（尤指咽鼓管）

tubotympanal [ˌtjuːbəuˈtimpənl] *a* 咽鼓管鼓室的

tubotympanic [ˌtjuːbəutimˈpænik] *a* 咽鼓管鼓室的

tubotympanum [ˌtjuːbəuˈtimpənəm] *n* 咽鼓管鼓室

tubouterine [ˌtjuːbəuˈjuːtərain] *a* 输卵管子宫的

tubovaginal [ˌtjuːbəuˈvædʒinl] *a* 输卵管阴道的

tubular [ˈtjuːbjulə] *a* 小管的，管状的，管性的

tubulature [ˈtjuːbjulətʃə] *n*（容器）颈管，曲颈甑管

tubule [ˈtjuːbjuːl] *n* 小管，细管 | caroticotympanic ~s 颈鼓小管 / collecting ~s 集合小管（肾）/ convoluted ~s（肾）曲小管；曲细精管 / convoluted renal ~s 肾曲小管 / convoluted seminiferous ~s 曲细精管 / dental ~s, dentinal ~s 牙质小管 / discharging ~s 排泄小管，乳头管 / lactiferous ~ 输乳小管 / segmental ~s 中肾小管 / seminiferous ~s 细精管 / straight renal ~s 肾直小管；直细精管 / straight seminiferous ~s 直细精管 / uriniferous ~s, uriniparous ~s 肾小管 / vertical ~s 卵巢旁体小管

tubuli [ˈtjuːbjulai] tubulus 的复数

tubulin [ˈtjuːbjulin] *n* 微管蛋白

Tubulina [ˌtjuːbjuˈlainə] *n* 管足亚目

tubulitis [ˌtjuːbjuˈlaitis] *n* 肾小管炎

tubulization [ˌtjuːbjulaiˈzeiʃən] *n* 神经套管术（治疗神经损伤）

tubuloacinar [ˌtjuːbjuləuˈæsinə] *a* 管状腺泡的

tubulocyst [ˈtjuːbjuləusist] *n* 管囊肿

tubuloglomerular [ˌtjuːbjuləugləˈmərjulə] *a* 肾小球肾小管的，肾小管肾小球的

tubulointerstitial [ˌtjuːbjuləuˌintəˈstiʃəl] *a* 肾小管间质的

tubulopathy [ˌtjuːbjuˈlɔpəθi] *n* 肾小管病

tubuloracemose [ˌtjuːbjuləuˈræsiməus] *a* 管状葡萄状的

tubulorrhexis [ˌtjuːbjuləuˈreksis] *n* 肾小管破裂

tubulosaccular [ˌtjuːbjuləuˈsækjulə] *a* 管状囊状的

tubulose [ˈtjuːbjuləus], **tubulous** [ˈtjuːbjuləs] *a* 小管的，含小管的

tubulovesicle [ˌtjuːbjuləuˈvesikl] *n* 管状囊

tubulovesicular [ˌtjuːbjuləuvəˈsikjulə] *a* 管状囊状的

tubulus [ˈtjuːbjuləs]（[复] **tubuli** [ˈtjuːbjulai]）*n*【拉】小管，细管

tubus [ˈtjuːbəs]（[复] **tubi** [ˈtjuːbai]）*n*【拉】管

tuckahoe [ˈtʌkəhəu] *n* 茯苓

Tuerck 见 Türck

Tuffier's test [ˈtjuːfiεə]（Marin T. Tuffier）杜菲埃试验（在动脉瘤时，当肢体的主要动静脉被压住后，只有在侧支循环通畅时，手或足的静脉才会鼓胀）

tuft [tʌft] *n* 丛 | enamal ~s 釉丛 / hair ~s 毛丛 / malpighian ~s, renal ~s 肾小球 / synovial ~s（关节）滑膜绒毛

tufted [ˈtʌftid] *a* 丛生的，簇状的

tuftsin [ˈtʌftsin] *n* 促吞噬素，促吞噬肽

tug [tʌg] *vi*, *vt*, *n* 牵引

tugging [ˈtʌgiŋ] *n* 牵引感 | tracheal ~ 气管牵引感（见于主动脉弓动脉瘤）

tui na【汉】推拿

tularemia [ˌtjuləˈriːmiə] *n* 土拉菌病，兔热病 | gastrointestinal ~ 胃肠土拉菌病 / glandular ~ 腺型土拉菌病 / oculoglandular ~ 眼腺型土拉菌病 / oropharyngeal ~ 口咽型土拉菌病 / pulmonary ~, pulmonic ~ 肺土拉菌病 / ulceroglandular ~ 溃疡淋巴腺型土拉菌病

tularine [ˈtjuːləriːn] *n* 土拉菌素（土拉杆菌皮肤试验用的抗原，治土拉菌病）

tulase [ˈtjuːleiz] *n* 结核菌蜡（结核杆菌提取物，贝林〈von Behring〉曾用于治疗结核）

tulle gras [tuːlˈgrɑː]【法】润肤细布，敷伤巾

Tullio's phenomenon [ˈtuːliəu]（Pietro Tullio）图里奥现象（局限性迷路炎患者由于高强声而引起眩晕）

Tulpius valve [ˈtʌlpiəs]（Nikolaas Tulpius〈Nicolas Tulp〉）回盲瓣

tulsi [ˈtuːlsi] *n* 罗勒

tumefacient [ˌtjuːmiˈfeiʃənt] *a* 肿胀的，致肿胀的

tumefaction [ˌtjuːmiˈfækʃən] *n* 肿胀，肿大

tumefy [ˈtjuːmifai] *vt*, *vi*（使）肿起，（使）肿大

tumentia [tjuːˈmenʃiə] *n*【拉】肿胀 | vasomotor ~ 血管舒缩性肿胀

tumescence [tjuːˈmesns] *n* 肿胀,肿大 | **tumescent** *a*
tumeur [tuːˈmur] *n*【法】肿瘤 | ~ perlée [perˈlei]【法】胆脂瘤 / ~ pileuse [piˈluːz]【法】毛石
tumid [ˈtjuːmid] *a* 肿胀的 | **~ity** [tjuːˈmidəti] *n*
tumor [ˈtjuːmə] *n* [肿]瘤;肿胀,肿块 | acute splenic ~ 急性脾肿胀 / adenoid ~ 腺瘤 / adenomatoid ~ 类腺瘤样瘤(一种生殖系统内的良性肿瘤) / adipose ~, fatty ~ 脂[肪]瘤 / adrenal rest ~ 肾上腺剩余[组织]瘤 / ~ albus 白色肿,结核性关节肿 / aniline ~ 苯胺瘤 / benign ~, innocent ~ 良性瘤 / blood ~ 血肿;动脉瘤 / brown ~ 棕色瘤 / carcinoid ~ of bronchus 支气管类癌肿瘤 / carotid body ~ 颈动脉体瘤 / ~ colli 颈部肿瘤 / connective-tissue ~ 结缔组织肿瘤 / chromaffin-cell ~ 嗜铬细胞瘤 / colloid ~ 胶样瘤,黏液瘤 / embryonal ~ 胚(组织)瘤 / fibroid ~, fibrocellular ~ 纤维细胞瘤,纤维瘤 / germinal ~ 生发瘤,胚瘤 / glomus ~ 血管球瘤 / glomus jugulare ~ 颈静脉球瘤 / granulosa-theca cell ~ 粒层卵泡膜细胞瘤 / gummy ~ 梅毒瘤,树胶肿 / hilar cell ~ 卵巢门细胞瘤 / ivory-like ~ 象牙样瘤,密质骨瘤 / lacteal ~ 乳瘤,乳房脓肿;乳腺囊肿 / ~ lienis 脾肥,脾盈 / lipoid cell ~ of ovary 卵巢类脂质细胞瘤(亦称肾上腺剩余瘤,男化卵巢瘤) / malignant ~ 恶性[肿]瘤 / march ~ 行军瘤,跖韧带炎 / mast cell ~ 肥大细胞瘤 / melanotic neuroectodermal ~, retinal anlage ~ 黑素沉着性神经外胚层瘤,视网膜原基瘤 / organoid ~ 器官样瘤(一种畸胎瘤) / pearl ~, pearly ~ 珠光瘤,胆脂瘤 / plasma cell ~ 浆细胞瘤 / pregnancy ~ 孕期瘤(在孕期发生的牙龈脓性肉芽肿) / ranine ~ 舌下囊肿 / recurring digital fibrous ~s of childhood 儿童复发性指纤维瘤,儿童复发性趾纤维瘤 / vascular ~ 动脉瘤;血管瘤 / white ~ 白肿,白色肿胀,慢性结核性关节炎 / yolk sac ~ 卵黄囊瘤,中肾病(2型) | **~ous** [ˈtjuːmərəs] *a*
tumoraffin [ˌtjuːməˈræfin] *a* 亲瘤[细胞]的,嗜瘤[细胞]的
tumoricidal [ˌtjuːməriˈsaidl] *a* 破坏肿瘤细胞的,杀癌细胞的
tumorigenesis [ˌtjuːməriˈdʒenisis] *n* 肿瘤发生
tumorigenic [ˌtjuːməriˈdʒenik] *a* 致瘤的,肿瘤发生的
tumorlet [ˈtjuːməlit] *n* 小瘤
tumultus [tju(ː)ˈmʌltəs] *n*【拉】骚乱,骚动
Tunga [ˈtʌŋgə] *n* 潜蚤属 | ~ penetrans 穿皮潜蚤
tungiasis [tʌŋˈgaiəsis] *n* 潜蚤病
tungstate [ˈtʌŋsteit] *n* 钨酸盐
tungsten (W) [ˈtʌŋstən] *n* 钨(化学元素) | **~ic** [tʌŋsˈtenik] *a*
tungstic [ˈtʌŋstik] *a* 六价钨的,[正]钨的,五价钨的 | ~ acid 钨酸
tunic [ˈtjuːnik] *n* 膜,被膜 | fibrous ~ 纤维膜,纤维层 / mucous ~ 黏膜 / muscular ~ 肌层,肌织膜 / pharyngeal ~, pharyngobasilar ~ 咽颅底板 / proper ~ 固有膜,固有层
tunica [ˈtjuːnikə] ([复] **tunicae** [ˈtjuːnikiː]) *n*【拉】膜,被膜
tunicary [ˈtjuːnikəri] *a* 有膜的
Tunicata [ˌtjuːniˈkeitə] *n*【拉】被囊类(动物)
tunicate [ˈtjuːnikeit] *n* 被囊动物
tunicin [ˈtjuːnisin] *n* 动物纤维素,被囊(动物)纤维素
tunnel [ˈtʌnl] *n* 隧道,地道 | carpal ~, flexor ~ 腕管,屈肌管
turacin [ˈtjuərəsin] *n* 羽红素
turacoporphyrin [ˌtjuərəkəuˈpɔːfirin] *n* 羽红素卟啉
turanose [ˈtjuərənəus] *n* 松二糖
turban [ˈtəːbən] *n* 包头巾 | ice ~ 冰巾(化疗时用于防止脱发)
Turbatrix [təːˈbeitriks] *n* 线虫属 | ~ aceti 醋线虫
Turbellaria [ˌtəːbəˈlɛəriə] *n* 涡虫纲
turbid [ˈtəːbid] *a* 混浊的 | **~ity** [təːˈbidəti] *n* 浊度;混浊
turbidimeter [ˌtəːbiˈdimitə] *n* 比浊计,浊度计 | **turbidimetric** [ˌtəːbidiˈmetrik] *a* 比浊的,浊度计的 | **turbidimetry** *n* 比浊法,测浊法,浊度测定法
turbinate [ˈtəːbinit] *a* 甲介形的 *n* 鼻甲[骨] | sphenoid ~ 蝶骨甲 | **~d** [ˈtəːbineitid] *a* 甲介形的 / **turbinal** [ˈtəːbinl] *a*, *n*
turbinectomy [ˌtəːbiˈnektəmi] *n* 鼻甲切除术
turbinotome [təːˈbinətəum] *n* 鼻甲刀
turbinotomy [ˌtəːbiˈnɔtəmi] *n* 鼻甲切开术
TURBT transurethral resection of bladder tumor 经尿道膀胱肿瘤切除术
Türck's bundle [tiək] (Ludwig Türck) 颞桥束 | ~ column (fasciculus) 锥体前束,皮质脊髓前束 / ~ degeneration 继发性变性(脊髓神经) / ~ trachoma 慢性卡他性喉炎
Turck's zone [təːk] (Fenton B. Truck) 变性带(即肠壁结缔组织层,由肠穿入的细菌在此均被消灭)
Turcot's syndrome [təːˈkəu] (Jacques Turcot) 特科特综合征(家族性结肠息肉病,伴中枢神经系统恶性肿瘤〈神经胶质瘤〉)
turgescent [təːˈdʒesnt] *a* 肿大的,(开始)肿胀的 | **turgescence** *n* 肿胀,肿大
turgid [ˈtəːdʒid] *a* 肿胀的,浮肿的;充满的,胀

满的

turgidization [ˌtəːdʒidaiˈzeiʃən, -diˈz-] *n* 充满法,胀满法(注入液体使组织胀满的方法)

turgometer [təːˈgɔmitə] *n* 肿度测定器

turgor [ˈtəːgə] *n*【拉】充盈,充满,胀满 | ~ vitalis 血管(正常)充盈

turista [tuəˈristə] *n*【西】旅游者腹泻(墨西哥对 traveler's diarrhea 的称呼)

Türk's cell(irritation leukocyte) [tiək] (Wilhelm Türk) 蒂尔克细胞(刺激性白细胞)(一种单核无粒细胞,兼有非典型淋巴细胞和浆细胞两者形态特征,见于严重贫血、慢性感染和白血病样反应时的末梢血液)

turmeric [ˈtəːmərik] *n* 姜黄

turmschaedel [ˈtuːmʃɑːdel] *n*【德】颅骨高圆畸形

Turner's sign [ˈtəːnə] (George G. Turner) 特纳征(急性出血性胰腺炎时腰部皮肤变色)

Turner's sulcus [ˈtəːnə] (William A. Turner) 顶间沟(大脑)

Turner's syndrome [ˈtəːnə] (Henry H. Turner) 特纳综合征(躯体矮小,性腺发育不全,具有各种畸形,如蹼颈、低发际、肘外翻等,与第二个性染色体缺失有关,患者的表型是女性,通常不能生育。亦称性腺发育不全)

Turner tooth(hypoplasia) [ˈtəːnə] (Joseph G. Turner) 特纳牙(发育不全)(单个牙釉质发育不全,最常见的为上颌恒切牙或上、下颌前磨牙中的一颗,由于局部感染或外伤所致)

turnover [ˈtəːnˌəuvə] *n* 更新,周转,转换 | erythrocyte iron ~ (EIT), red blood cell iron ~ (RBCIT) 红细胞铁转换 / plasma iron ~ (PIT) 血浆铁转换

turnsick [ˈtəːnsik], **turnsickness** [ˈtəːnsiknis] *n* 蹒跚病(家畜晕倒病)

turnsol [ˈtəːnsɔl] *n* 石蕊,石蕊素

TURP transurethral resection of the prostate 经尿道前列腺切除[术]

turpentine [ˈtəːpəntain] *n* 松脂,松油脂,松节油

turricephaly [ˌtəːriˈsefəli] *n* 尖形头

turunda [tjuˈrʌndə] *n*【拉】(外科)塞条;栓剂,塞药

Turyn's sign [ˈtuːrin] (Felix Turyn) 图林征(坐骨神经痛时,如患者跗趾背曲,臀区即感到疼痛)

tus. tussis【拉】咳[嗽]

tussal [ˈtʌsəl] *a* 咳[嗽]的

tussicula [təˈsikjulə] *n*【拉】轻咳

tussicular [təˈsikjulə] *a* 咳的

tussiculation [təˌsikjuˈleiʃən] *n* 干咳,烦咳

tussigenic [ˌtʌsiˈdʒenik] *a* 致咳的

tussis [ˈtʌsis] *n*【拉】咳[嗽] | **tussive** *a*

tutamen [tjuˈteimən] ([复] **tutamina** [tjuˈtæminə]) *n*【拉】保护器,防御物

Tuttle's proctoscope [ˈtʌtl] (Edward G. Tuttle) 塔特尔直肠镜(顶端装有电灯光,并可对直肠壶腹充气)

tween-brain [ˈtwiːnbrein] *n* 间脑

tweezer(s) [ˈtwiːzə(z)] *n* 镊(俗称)

twig [twig] *n* 细支,小支(神经或血管)

twin [twin] *n* 双胎儿之一;[复]双胎儿,双胎,孪生 | acardiac ~ 无心双胎,无心畸胎 / allantoidoangiopagous ~s 脐血管联胎 / conjoined ~s, Siamese ~s 联体双胎,联体儿 / dizygotic ~s, binovular ~s, dissimilar ~s, dichorial ~s, dichorionic ~s, false ~s, fraternal ~s, heterologous ~s, two-egg ~s, unlike ~s 双卵双胎儿 / monozygotic ~s, identical ~s, monochorial ~s, monochorionic ~s, monoovular ~s, one-egg ~s, similar ~s, true ~s, uniovular ~s 单卵双胎儿,单卵孪生

twinge [twindʒ] *n* 刺痛

twinning [ˈtwiniŋ] *n* 双生,双胎生成

twinship [ˈtwinʃip] *n* 孪生,双生

twist [twist] *vt* 扭伤 *vi* 扭伤 *n* 扭转 | intestinal ~ 肠扭转

twitch [twitʃ] *vt*, *vi* 抽搐,颤搐 *n* 抽搐,颤搐;压板(兽医用具)

twitching [ˈtwitʃiŋ] *n* 颤搐 | fascicular ~ 肌束颤搐 / fibrillar ~ 原纤维性颤搐

Twort-d'Herelle phenomenon [twəːt dəˈrel] (Frederick W. Twort; Félix H. d'Herelle) 图尔特-代列尔现象(一种可传播的细菌溶解现象,即噬菌现象。当伤寒或痢疾细菌的肉汤培养物中加入一滴恢复期伤寒或痢疾病人过滤的粪便肉汤乳液时,细菌培养物将于数小时后完全溶解,若将一滴已溶解的培养物加于另一杆菌培养物时,将发生与第一次完全一样的溶解,然后加一滴这种培养物可溶解第三种培养物,且能如此转移达数百次)

TWZ triangular working zone 三角工作区(见 Kambin's triangular working zone)

TXA_2, TXB_2 thromboxanes A_2 and B_2 血栓烷 A_2,血栓烷 B_2

tybamate [ˈtaibəmeit] *n* 泰巴氨酯(弱安定药)

tying up [ˈtaiiŋ ʌp] 氮尿症(马)

tylectomy [taiˈlektəmi] *n* 肿块切除术

tylion [ˈtiliən] *n* 交叉沟中点(视交叉沟前缘的正中点)

tyloma [taiˈləumə] *n*【希】胼胝

Tylophora asthmatica [taiˈlɔfərə æsˈmætikə] 印度娃儿藤(催吐药并用于治痢疾及气喘)

tylophorine [taiˈlɔfərin] *n* 娃儿藤碱(催吐、镇喘药)

tylosin [ˈtailəusin] *n* 泰洛星(兽医用抗生素),泰乐菌素

tylosis [taiˈləusis] *n* 胼胝形成;胼胝 | ~ ciliaris 眼睑胼胝形成 / ~ linguae 颊黏膜白斑病 / ~ palmaris et plantaris 掌跖角化病 | **tylotic** [taiˈlɔtik] *a* 胼胝的

tyloxapol [taiˈlɔksəpɔl] *n* 泰洛沙泊(表面活性剂,祛痰药)

tympanal [ˈtimpənəl] *a* 鼓室的;鼓膜的

tympanectomy [ˌtimpəˈnektəmi] *n* 鼓膜切除术

tympania [timˈpæniə] *n* 气鼓,鼓胀 | ~ uteri 子宫气鼓

tympanic [timˈpænik] *a* 鼓室的;鼓响的

tympanicity [ˌtimpəˈnisəti] *n* 鼓响性

tympanion [timˈpæniən] *n* 鼓环点 | lower ~ 鼓环最低点 / upper ~ 鼓环最高点

tympanism [ˈtimpənizəm] *n* 气鼓,鼓胀

tympanites [ˌtimpəˈnaitiːz] *n* 气鼓,鼓胀 | false ~ 假性气鼓 / uterine ~ 子宫气肿,子宫积气 | **tympanitic** [ˌtimpəˈnitik] *a* 气鼓的;鼓响的

tympanitis [ˌtimpəˈnaitis] *n* 鼓室炎,中耳炎

tympan(o)- [构词成分]鼓室,鼓膜

tympanoacryloplasty [ˌtimpənəuəˈkriləˌplæsti] *n* 鼓室丙烯酸酯成形术

tympanocentesis [ˌtimpənəusenˈtiːsis] *n* 鼓膜穿刺

tympanoeustachian [ˌtimpənəujuːˈsteiʃjən] *a* 鼓室咽鼓管的

tympanogenic [ˌtimpənəuˈdʒenik] *a* 鼓室原的

tympanogram [timˈpænəˌgræm] *n* 鼓室导抗图

tympanohyal [ˌtimpənəuˈhaiəl] *a* 鼓室[与]舌骨弓的 *n* 鼓舌骨

tympanolabyrinthopexy [ˌtimpənəuˌlæbiˈrinθəpeksi] *n* 鼓室迷路连接术(治耳硬化症所致的进行性聋)

tympanomalleal [ˌtimpənəuˈmæliəl] *a* 鼓室锤骨的

tympanomandibular [ˌtimpənəumænˈdibjulə] *a* 鼓室下颌的

tympanomastoidectomy [ˌtimpənəuˌmæstɔiˈdektəmi] *n* 鼓室乳突切除术

tympanomastoiditis [ˌtimpənəuˌmæstɔiˈdaitis] *n* 鼓室乳突炎

tympanomeatal [ˌtimpənəumiːˈeitəl] *a* 鼓室耳道的

tympanometric [ˌtimpənəuˈmetrik] *a* 鼓室测压的

tympanometry [ˌtimpəˈnɔmitri] *n* 鼓室测压法,鼓室压测量法

tympanoplasty [ˌtimpənəuˈplæsti] *n* 鼓室成形术 | **tympanoplastic** [ˌtimpənəuˈplæstik] *a*

tympanosclerosis [ˌtimpənəuskliəˈrəusis] *n* 鼓膜硬化

tympanosclerotic [ˌtimpənəuskləˈrɔtik] *a* 鼓室硬化的

tympanosquamosal [ˌtimpənəuskweiˈməusəl] *a* 鼓室鳞部的

tympanostapedial [ˌtimpənəustəˈpiːdiːəl] *a* 鼓室镫骨的

tympanostomy [ˌtimpəˈnɔstəmi] *n* 鼓室造孔术

tympanosympathectomy [ˌtimpənəuˌsimpəˈθektəmi] *n* 鼓室丛切除术

tympanotemporal [ˌtimpənəuˈtempərəl] *a* 鼓室颞骨的

tympanotomy [ˌtimpəˈnɔtəmi] *n* 鼓室探查术

tympanous [ˈtimpənəs] *a* 鼓气的,鼓胀的

tympanum [ˈtimpənəm] *n*【拉】鼓室;中耳腔

tympany [ˈtimpəni] *n* 气鼓,鼓胀;鼓响,鼓音

Tyndall cone [ˈtindl] (John Tyndall) 延德尔锥(这种散射光锥可区分胶体与拟晶体) | ~ effect(phenomenon) 延德尔效应(现象)(强烈光束通过真性溶液为不可见,而通过胶体溶液轮廓分外明显,因为光受到移动的胶体颗粒的表面反射之故) / ~ light 延德尔光(气体或液体中分子反射光)

tyndallization [ˌtindəlaiˈzeiʃən, -liˈz-] (John Tyndall) *n* 间歇灭菌法

type [taip] *n* 型,式,类型;典型 | allotropic ~ 异我关怀型(一种非自我中心的人格) / amyostatic-kinetic ~ 肌震颤运动型(流行性脑炎的一型) / apoplectic ~ 中风型 / asthenic ~ 无力型,瘦长型 / athletic ~ 运动员型,健壮型 / bird's-head ~ 小头型(白痴) / blood ~s 血型 / body ~ 体型 / leg ~ 腿型(进行性遗传性肌萎缩) / leptosome ~ 瘦长型 / phthisic ~ 痨病型 / pyknic ~ 矮胖型 / seclusive ~ 隐士型,孤独隐退型 / test ~ 视力标型(视力表) / wild ~ 野生型(指遗传学中的表现型,亦指正常基因)

typembryo [taipˈembriəu] *n* 典型胚,类型胎

Typhaceae [taiˈfeisiiː] *n* 伤寒菌科(旧名)

typhemia [taiˈfiːmiə] *n* 伤寒菌血症

typhia [ˈtifiə] *n* 伤寒

typhic [ˈtaifik] *a* 伤寒的;斑疹伤寒的

typhlectasis [tifˈlektəsis] *n* 盲肠膨胀

typhlectomy [tifˈlektəmi] *n* 盲肠切除术

typhlenteritis [ˌtiflentəˈraitis] *n* 盲肠炎

typhlitis [tifˈlaitis] *n* 盲肠炎

typhl(o)- [构词成分]盲肠;盲

typhlocele [ˈtifləsiːl] *n* 盲肠突出

Typhlocoelum [ˌtifləˈsiːləm] *n* 盲腔[吸虫]属 | ~ cucumerinum 巴西鸡吸虫

typhlocolitis [ˌtifləukɔˈlaitis] *n* 盲肠结肠炎

typhlodicliditis [ˌtifləuˌdikliˈdaitis] *n* 回盲瓣炎

typhloempyema [ˌtifləuˌempaiˈiːmə] *n* 盲肠脓肿

typhloenteritis [ˌtifləuˌentəˈraitis] *n* 盲肠炎
typhlohepatitis [ˌtifləuˌhepəˈtaitis] *n* 传染性肠肝炎(火鸡)
typhlolexia [ˌtifləuˈleksiə] *n* 词盲,视性失读
typhlolithiasis [ˌtifləuliˈθaiəsis] *n* 盲肠石病
typhlology [tifˈlɔlədʒi] *n* 盲学
typhlomegaly [ˌtifləuˈmegəli] *n* 盲肠巨大,巨盲肠
typhlon [ˈtiflɔn] *n*【希】盲肠
typhlopexy [ˈtifləuˌpeksi], **typhlopexia** [ˌtifləuˈpeksiə] *n* 盲肠固定术
typhloptosis [ˌtifləuˈtəusis] *n* 盲肠下垂
typhlorrhaphy [tifˈlɔrəfi] *n* 盲肠缝合术
typhlosis [tifˈləusis] *n* 盲,视觉缺失
typhlostenosis [ˌtifləustiˈnəusis] *n* 盲肠狭窄
typhlostomy [tifˈlɔstəmi] *n* 盲肠造口术
typhloteritis [ˌtifləutəˈraitis] *n* 盲肠炎
typhlotomy [tifˈlɔtəmi] *n* 盲肠切开术
typhloureterostomy [ˌtifləujuˌriːtəˈrɔstəmi] *n* 盲肠输尿管吻合术
typhobacillosis [ˌtaifəuˌbæsiˈləusis] *n* 伤寒菌毒症 | ~ tuberculosa 伤寒型结核菌毒症
typhobacterin [ˌtaifəuˈbæktərin] *n* 伤寒菌苗
typhogenic [taifəuˈdʒenik] *a* 引起伤寒(或斑疹伤寒)的
typhohemia [ˌtaifəuˈhiːmiə] *n* 伤寒菌血症
typhoid [ˈtaifɔid] *a* 似斑疹伤寒的;伤寒的;伤寒样的 *n* 伤寒 | fowl ~ 鸡伤寒 / provocation ~ 激发性伤寒
typhoidal [taiˈfɔidl] *a* 伤寒的;伤寒样的
typhoidin [ˈtaifɔidin] *n* 伤寒菌素
typhomalarial [ˌtaifəuməˈlɛəriəl] *a* 伤寒型疟疾的
Typhonium trilobatum [taiˈfəunjəm ˌtrailəˈbætəm]【拉】裂叶犁头草
typhopaludism [ˌtaifəuˈpæljudizəm] *n* 伤寒型疟疾
typhopneumonia [ˌtaifəunju(ː)ˈməuniə] *n* 伤寒肺炎(伤寒并发肺炎)
typhus [ˈtaifəs] *n* 斑疹伤寒 | amarillic ~ 黄热病 / benign ~, recrudescent ~ 再燃性斑疹伤寒 / canine ~ 无黄疸型钩端螺旋体病 / collapsing ~ 虚脱性伤寒 / epidemic ~, classic ~, European ~, exanthematic ~, exanthematous ~, louse-borne ~ 流行性斑疹伤寒,欧洲斑疹伤寒,虱传斑疹伤寒 / Indian tick ~ 印度蜱传斑疹伤寒 / murine ~, endemic ~, fleaborne ~, Manchurian ~, Mexican ~, Moscow ~, Toulon ~ 鼠型斑疹伤寒,地方性斑疹伤寒,蚤传斑疹伤寒,满州斑疹伤寒,墨西哥斑疹伤寒,莫斯科斑疹伤寒,土伦斑疹伤寒 / North Queensland tick ~, Australian tick ~, Queensland tick ~ 北昆士兰蜱传斑疹伤寒,澳大利亚蜱传斑疹伤寒,昆士兰蜱传斑疹伤寒 / scrub ~, miteborne ~, tropical ~ 丛林斑疹伤寒,螨传斑疹伤寒,热带斑疹伤寒,恙虫病 / Siberian tick ~, North Asian tick ~ 西伯利亚蜱传斑疹伤寒,北亚蜱传斑疹伤寒 / tick ~, tick-borne ~, exanthematic ~ of São Paulo, São Paulo ~ 蜱传斑疹伤寒,落基山斑疹热 / urban ~, shop ~ 城市斑疹伤寒 | **typhous** *a*
typical [ˈtipikəl] *a* 典型的
typing [ˈtaipiŋ] *n* 分型,定型 | HLA ~, tissue ~ 人[类]白细胞抗原分型,组织分型 / ~ of blood 血型定型(用已知抗血清决定血细胞属于哪一型) / phage ~ 噬菌体分型 / primed lymphocyte ~ (PLT) 致敏淋巴细胞定型
typodont [ˈtaipədɔnt] *n* 模式牙(含有人工牙或天然牙供教学训练使用的人造模型),错𬌗模拟矫治𬌗架
typology [taiˈpɔlədʒi] *n* 类型学;血型学 | **typological** [ˌtaipəˈlɔdʒikəl] *a*
typonym [ˈtaipənim] *n* 同模式异名 | **~al** [taiˈpɔniməl] *a* / **~ic** [taipəˈnimik] *a*
typoscope [ˈtaipəskəup] *n* 弱视矫正器,助视器
Tyr tyrosine 酪氨酸
tyramine [ˈtaiərəmiːn] *n* 酪胺
tyrannism [ˈtirənizəm] *n* 暴虐狂,病态残暴
tyrein [ˈtaiəriːn] *n* 凝固[乳]酪蛋白
tyresin [taiˈriːsin] *n* 解蛇毒素
tyr(o)- [构词成分]干酪,酪
tyrocidin(e) [ˌtaiərəuˈsaidin] *n* 短杆菌酪肽
Tyrode's solution [ˈtairəud] (Maurice V. Tyrode) 蒂罗德[溶]液(一种含镁的洛克〈Locke〉溶液,尤用于灌注兔肠)
tyrogenous [taiəˈrɔdʒinəs] *a* 干酪原的
Tyroglyphus [taiəˈrɔglifəs] *n* 粉螨属(即食酪螨属 Tyrophagus) / ~ castellani 卡氏粉螨(即卡氏食酪螨 Tyrophagus castellani) / ~ farinae 粗脚粉螨(即粗脚食酪螨 Tyrophagus farinae) / ~ longior 长粉螨(即长食酪螨 Tyrophagus longior) / ~ siro 粗脚粉螨(即 Acarus siro)
tyroid [ˈtaiərɔid] *a* 干酪样的
tyroma [taiəˈrəumə] *n* 干酪样瘤;干酪样结块
tyromatosis [ˌtaiərəuməˈtəusis] *n* 干酪变性,干酪化
tyropanoate sodium [ˌtaiərəupəˈnəueit] 丁酰碘番酸钠(口服胆囊造影剂)
Tyrophagus [taiəˈrɔfəgəs] *n* 食酪螨属(亦称粉螨属) | ~ castellani 卡氏食酪螨 / ~ farinae 粗脚食酪螨 / ~ longior 长食酪螨 / ~ siro 粗脚食酪螨(即 Acarus siro)
tyrosamine [taiəˈrəusəmiːn] *n* 酪胺
tyrosinase [taiəˈrəusineis] *n* 酪氨酸酶

tyrosine (Tyr, Y) [ˈtaiərəsiːn] *n* 酪氨酸
tyrosine aminotransferase [ˈtaiərəsiːn əˌmiːnəuˈtrænsfəreis] 酪氨酸氨基转移酶,酪氨酸转氨酶(见 tyrosine transaminase)
tyrosine hydroxylase [ˈtairəsiːn haiˈdrɔksileis] 酪氨酸羟化酶,酪氨酸 3-单加氧酶
tyrosine kinase [ˈtairəsiːn ˈkaineis] 酪氨酸激酶,蛋白酪氨酸激酶
tyrosinemia [ˌtaiərəsiˈniːmiə] *n* 酪氨酸血[症]
tyrosine 3-monooxygenase [ˈtairəsiːn ˌmɔnəuˈɔksidʒəneis] 酪氨酸 3-单加氧酶(此酶在脑内发生,并在恶性高苯丙氨酸血症时失活)
tyrosine transaminase [ˈtairəsiːn trænsˈæmineis] 酪氨酸转氨酶(此酶缺乏为一种常染色体隐性性状,可致酪氨酸血症Ⅱ型)
tyrosinosis [ˌtaiərəsiˈnəusis] *n* 酪氨酸代谢病
tyrosinuria [ˌtaiərəsiˈnjuəriə] *n* 酪氨酸尿
tyrosis [taiəˈrəusis] *n* 干酪变性
tyrosyl [ˈtaiərəsil] *n* 酪氨酰[基]
tyrosyluria [ˌtaiərəsiˈljuəriə] *n* 酪氨酰基尿
tyrothricin [ˌtaiərəˈθraisin] *n* 短杆菌素(抗生素类药)
Tyrothrix [ˈtaiərəθriks] *n* 酪毛霉属
tyrotoxicon [ˌtaiərəˈtɔksikɔn] *n* 干酪毒碱,氢氧化重氮苯
tyrotoxicosis [ˌtaiərəˌtɔksiˈkəusis], **tyrotoxism** [ˌtaiərəˈtɔksizəm] *n* 干酪中毒
Tyrrell's fascia [ˈtirəl] (Frederick Tyrrell) 直肠前列腺筋膜 | ~ hook 蒂勒尔钩(用于眼手术)
tysonian [taiˈsəuniən] *a* 泰森(Edward Tyson)的
tysonitis [ˌtaisəˈnaitis] *n* 包皮腺炎
Tyson's crypts (glands) [ˈtaisn] (Edward Tyson) 泰森腺(包皮腺) | ~ cyst 泰森囊肿(尿道黏液囊肿)
tyvelose [ˈtaivələuz] *n* 泰威糖,伤寒菌糖,3,6-二脱氧-D 甘露糖
Tyzzeria [taiˈziəriə] *n* 泰泽球虫属
Tzanck cell [tsænk] (Arnault Tzanck) 棘层松解细胞(退化性上皮细胞,见于天疱疮) | ~ test 赞克试验(检疱疹性疾病的病灶基底部细胞)
Tzaneen disease [tsɑːˈniːn] (Tzaneen 为南非一地名,在该地首次报道此病)乍宁病(一种蜱传原虫病,见于南非,由于突变泰累尔梨浆虫〈Theileria mutans〉所致,发生于牛和水牛,表现为轻度发热,或可能是严重的,甚至是致死的)
tzetze [ˈtsetsi] *n* 采采蝇(舌蝇属)

U

U uranium 铀; uracil 尿嘧啶; uridine 尿苷; international unit of enzyme activity 酶活性国际单位; unit 单位

u atomic mass unit 原子质量单位

uarthritis [ˌjuːɑːˈθraitis] *n* 痛风,尿酸性关节炎

uberous [ˈjuːbərəs] *a* 多育的,繁殖的

uberty [ˈjuːbəti] *n* 生育力,繁殖力

ubiquinol [juːˈbikwinɔl] *n* 泛醌醇(泛醌〈ubiquinone〉的还原型)

ubiquinol-cytochrome-c reductase [juːˈbikwinɔlˈsaitəkrəumriˈdʌkteis] 泛醌醇-细胞色素 c 还原酶(亦称泛醌醇脱氢酶)

ubiquinol dehydrogenase [juːˈbikwinɔl diːˈhaidrədʒəneis] 泛醌醇脱氢酶,泛醌醇-细胞色素 c 还原酶

ubiquinone [juːˈbikwinəun] *n* 泛醌,辅酶 *Q*

ubiquitin [juːˈbikwitin] *n* 遍在蛋白质

Uchida technique [uːˈtʃiːdə] (Hajime Uchida) 内田技术(一种输卵管结扎法,在输卵管黏膜下注射盐溶液,使黏膜与下方的管分离,一部分黏膜予以切除,无黏膜的管回缩而形成残端,缝合封闭)

udder [ˈʌdə] *n* (牛,羊等的)乳房

UDP uridine diphosphate 尿苷二磷酸

UDP-*N*-acetylgalactosamine [ˌæsitilgəlækˈtəusəmiːn] 尿苷二磷酸-*N*-乙酰半乳糖胺

UDP-*N*-acetylglucosamine [ˌæsitilgluːˈkəusəmiːn] 尿苷二磷酸-*N*-乙酰葡糖胺

UDP-*N*-acetylglucosamine 4-epimerase [ˌæsitilgluːˈkəusəmiːn əˈpiməreis] 尿苷二磷酸-*N*-乙酰葡糖胺 4-差向异构酶

UDP-*N*-acetylglucosamine-lysosomal-enzyme *N*-acetylglucosaminephosphotransferase [ˌæsitilgluːˈkəusəmiːnˌlaisəsəumælˈenzaim ˌæsiˌtiːlgluːˌkəusəmiːnˌfɔsfəˈtrænsfəreis] 尿苷二磷酸-*N*-乙酰葡糖胺溶酶体酶 *N*-乙酰葡糖胺磷酸转移酶(此酶缺乏为一种常染色体隐性性状,可致黏脂贮积症Ⅱ型和Ⅲ型。亦称 *N*-乙酰氨基葡糖基磷酸转移酶)

UDP-*N*-acetylglucosamine pyrophosphorylase [ˌæsitilgluːˈkəusəmiːn ˌpairəufɔsˈfɔrileis] 尿苷二磷酸-*N*-乙酰葡糖胺焦磷酸化酶

UDPgalactose [gəˈlæktəus] 尿苷二磷酸半乳糖

UDP galactose 4-epimerase [gəˈlæktəus iˈpiməreis] 尿苷二磷酸半乳糖 4-差向异构酶,尿苷二磷酸葡萄糖 4-差向异构酶

UDPglucose [ˈgluːkəus] 尿苷二磷酸葡萄糖

UDPglucose 6-dehydrogenase [ˌgluːkəus diːˈhaidrədʒəneis] 尿苷二磷酸葡萄糖 6-脱氢酶

UDP glucose 4-epimerase [ˈgluːkəus iˈpiməreis] 尿苷二磷酸葡萄糖 4-差向异构酶(红细胞内此酶缺乏为一种常染色体隐性性状,可引起红细胞内半乳糖-1-磷酸的聚积。亦称尿苷二磷酸半乳糖 4-差向异构酶)

UDP glucose-hexose-1-phosphate uridylyltransferase [ˈgluːkəus ˈheksəus ˈfɔsfeit ˌjuəridililˈtrænsfəreis] 尿苷二磷酸葡萄糖-己糖-1-磷酸尿苷酰基转移酶(此酶活性缺乏为一种常染色体隐性性状,可致半乳糖血症。亦称半乳糖-1-磷酸尿苷酰转移酶,己糖-1-磷酸尿苷酰基转移酶和尿苷酰转移酶)

UDP glucose pyrophosphorylase [ˈgluːkəus ˌpæiərəufɔsˈfɔrileis] 尿苷二磷酸葡萄糖焦磷酸化酶,尿苷三磷酸葡萄糖-1-磷酸尿苷酰基转移酶

UDP glucuronate [gluːˈkjuərəneit] 尿苷二磷酸葡糖醛酸

UDP glucuronate-bilirubin-glucuronosyltransferase [gluːˈkjuərəneitˌbiliˈruːbingluːkjuərənəsilˈtrænsfəreis] 尿苷二磷酸葡糖醛酸-胆红素-葡糖醛酸基转移酶

UDPglucuronate decarboxylase [gluːˈkjuərəneit ˌdiːkɑːˈbɔksileis] 尿苷二磷酸葡糖醛酸脱羧酶

UDPhexose [ˈheksəus] 尿苷二磷酸己糖

UDPiduronate [ˌaidjuˈrɔneit] 尿苷二磷酸艾杜糖醛酸

UDPxylose [ˈzailəus] 尿苷二磷酸木糖

Udránszky's test [uˈdrænski] (László Udránszky) 乌德兰茨基试验(检胆汁酸或酪氨酸)

udruj [ˈʌdrʌdʒ] *n* 乌得鲁胶(一种药用树胶)

Uffelmann's test (reagent) [ˈuːfelmən] (Jules Uffelmann) 乌费尔曼试验(试剂)(检胃容纳物中盐酸和乳酸)

Uhlenhuth's test [ˈuːlənhut] (Paul T. Uhlenhuth) 乌冷呼特试验,血清试验(serum test,见 test 项下相应术语)

Uhl's anomaly [juːl] (Henry S. M. Uhl) 尤尔异

常(右心室心肌先天性发育不良,导致心脏右侧排血量减少)

Uhthoff's sign [ˈuːthɔf] (Wilhelm Uhthoff) 乌托夫征(多发性脑脊髓硬化时的眼球震颤)

UK urokinase 尿激酶

ulaganactesis [juːˌlæɡənækˈtiːsis] *n* 龈刺激,龈痒

ulalgia [juːˈlældʒiə] *n* 龈痛

ulatrophy [juːˈlætrəfi] *n* 龈萎缩 | afunctional ~ 功能缺失性龈萎缩 / calcic ~ 涎石性龈萎缩 / ischemic ~, atrophic ~ 缺血性龈萎缩 | **ulatrophia** [ˌjuːləˈtrəufiə] *n*

ulcer [ˈʌlsə] *n* 溃疡 | Aden ~ 东方疖,皮肤利什曼病 / amebic ~ 阿米巴性溃疡 / burrowing phagedenic ~ 洞穴崩蚀性溃疡(进行性协同性坏疽;米兰尼〈Meleney〉溃疡) / catarrhal corneal ~ 卡他性角膜溃疡 / chicle ~, chiclero ~ 糖胶树胶工人溃疡(一种地方性动物传染的森林病,皮肤利什曼病的一型,多侵犯耳郭) / corrosive ~ 腐蚀性溃疡,坏疽性口炎 / decubital ~, decubitus ~ 褥疮 / dendriform ~, dendritic ~ 树状(角膜)溃疡 / dental ~ 牙源性溃疡 / flask ~ 瓶状溃疡(阿米巴性痢疾患者的一种肠溃疡) / giant peptic ~s 巨大消化性溃疡 / girdle ~ 环状溃疡,肠壁结核性溃疡 / hypertensive ischemic ~ 高血压性局部缺血性溃疡 / kissing ~s 相对面溃疡(指胃) / marginal ~, stoma ~, stomal ~ 边缘性溃疡,吻合口溃疡 / perambulating ~, phagedentic ~, sloughing ~ 崩蚀性溃疡,腐[肉分]离性溃疡 / pneumococcus ~ 肺炎球菌性角膜溃疡,匐行性角膜溃疡 / pudendal ~ 阴部溃疡,腹股沟肉芽肿 / round ~ 圆形溃疡,胃消化性溃疡 / sea anemone ~ 海葵形溃疡(阿米巴肠溃疡) / serpiginous corneal ~ 匐行性角膜溃疡 / soft ~ 软下疳 / stress ~ 应激性溃疡 / submucous ~ 黏膜下溃疡 / tropical phagedenic ~ 热带崩蚀性溃疡 / undermining burrowing ~ 洞穴崩蚀性溃疡(进行性协同性坏疽;米兰尼〈Meleney〉溃疡)

ulcera [ˈʌlsərə] ulcus 的复数

ulcerate [ˈʌlsəreit] *vt, vi* 形成溃疡 | **ulceration** [ˌʌlsəˈreiʃən] *n* 溃疡形成;溃疡 / **ulcerative** [ˈʌlsərətiv] *a* 溃疡的,溃疡性的

ulcerocancer [ˌʌlsərəuˈkænsə] *n* 溃疡癌,癌性溃疡

ulcerogangrenous [ˌʌlsərəuˈɡæŋɡrinəs] *a* 溃疡坏疽的

ulcerogenic [ˌʌlsərəuˈdʒenik] *a* 致溃疡的,产生溃疡的

ulcerogranuloma [ˌʌlsərəuɡrænjuˈləumə] *n* 溃疡肉芽肿

ulceromembranous [ˌʌlsərəuˈmembrənəs] *a* 溃疡膜性的

ulcerous [ˈʌlsərəs] *a* 溃疡的,溃疡性的

ulcus [ˈʌlkəs] ([复] **ulcera** [ˈʌlsərə]) *n*【拉】溃疡

uldazepam [ʌlˈdeizəpæm] *n* 乌达西泮(安定药)

ule- 见 ul(o)-[1]

ulectomy[1] [juːˈlektəmi] *n* 瘢痕切除术

ulectomy[2] [juːˈlektəmi] *n* 龈切除术

ulegyria [ˌjuːliˈdʒaiəriə] *n* 瘢痕性脑回

ulemorrhagia [ˌjuːleməuˈreidʒiə] *n* 龈出血

ulerythema [ˌjuːleriˈθiːmə] *n* 瘢痕性红斑 | ~ ophryogenes 眉部瘢痕性红斑

Ulex europaeus L. (**Leguminosae**) [ˈjuːleks juəˈrəupiəs] 荆豆

ulexine [juːˈleksiːn] *n* 荆豆碱,金雀花碱,野靛碱

uliginous [juːˈlidʒinəs] *a* 多泥的,黏滑的

ulitis [juːˈlaitis] *n* 龈炎 | aphthous ~ 口疮性龈炎 / fungus ~ 真菌性龈炎 / mercurial ~ 汞毒性龈炎

ullem [ˈʌləm] *n* (北欧拉普兰地区的)消化不良症

Ullmann's line [ˈʌlmæn] (Emerich Ullmann) 乌尔曼线(脊椎前移时,从第一骶椎前缘垂直向上延伸至骶骨上表面的线,穿过最后一个腰椎)

Ullrich-Feichtiger syndrome [ˈuːlrik ˈfaiktiɡə] (Otto Ullrich; H. Feichtiger) 乌-法综合征(表现为小颌,六指〈趾〉畸形,生殖器异常,塌鼻梁,小眼,器官距离过远,耳郭凸起以及其他缺陷)

Ullrich-Turner syndrome [ˈuːlrik ˈtəːnə] (O. Ullrich; Henry H. Turner) 乌-特综合征(见 Noonan's syndrome)

Ulmus [ˈʌlməs] *n*【拉】榆属 | ~ fulva Michx 赤榆

ulna [ˈʌlnə] ([复] **ulnas** 或 **ulnae** [ˈʌlniː]) *n*【拉】尺骨 | **~d** [ˈʌlnæd] *ad* 向尺侧 / **~r** *a* 尺骨的,尺侧的

ulnare [ʌlˈnɛəri] *n*【拉】三角骨

ulnaris [ʌlˈnɛəris] *a*【拉】尺骨的,尺侧的

ulnen [ˈʌlnən] *a* 尺骨的

ulnocarpal [ˌʌlnəuˈkɑːpl] *a* 尺腕的

ulnoradial [ˌʌlnəuˈreidjəl] *a* 尺桡的

ul(o)-[1] [构词成分]瘢痕

ul(o)-[2] [构词成分]龈

ulocace [juːˈlɔkəsi] *n* 龈溃疡

ulocarcinoma [ˌjuːləukɑːsiˈnəumə] *n* 龈癌

uloglossitis [ˌjuːləuɡlɔˈsaitis] *n* 龈舌炎

uloncus [juːˈlɔŋkəs] *n* 龈瘤;龈肿

ulorrhagia [ˌjuːləuˈreidʒiə] *n* 龈出血

ulorrhea [ˌjuːləuˈriə] *n* 龈渗血

-ulose [后缀]酮糖

ulotomy[1] [juːˈlɔtəmi] *n* 瘢痕切开术

ulotomy[2] [juːˈlɔtəmi] *n* 龈切开术

ulotripsis [juːləuˈtripsis] *n* 龈按摩

ultimate [ˈʌltimit] *a* 最远的；最后的；极限的
ultimisternal [ˌʌltimiˈstəːnl] *a* 剑突的
ultimobranchial [ˌʌltiməuˈbræŋkiəl] *a* 后鳃的
ultimum moriens [ˈʌltiməm ˈmɔriənz]【拉】最后死者（指右心房，因其最后停止搏动；指斜方肌上部）
ult. praes. ultimum praescriptus【拉】最后处方
ultra- [前缀]超，过度，限外
ultrabrachycephalic [ˌʌltrəˌbrækisəˈfælik] *a* 超短头的
ultracentrifugation [ˌʌltrəsenˌtrifjuˈgeiʃən] *n* 超速离心法
ultracentrifuge [ˌʌltrəˈsentrifjuːdʒ] *n* 超速离心机 *vt* 用超速离心机使分离
ultradian [ʌlˈtreidiən] *a* 次昼夜的
ultradolichocephalic [ˌʌltrəˌdɔlikəusəˈfælik] *a* 超长头的
ultrafilter [ˌʌltrəˈfiltə] *n* 超滤器；超滤膜
ultrafiltrate [ˌʌltrəˈfiltreit] *n* 超滤液
ultrafiltration [ˌʌltrəfilˈtreiʃən] *n* 超滤法 | isolated ~ 单纯超滤
ultragaseous [ˌʌltrəˈgæsiəs] *a* 超气态的
ultralente [ˈʌltrəlent] *a* 超长效的
ultramicrochemistry [ˌʌltrəˌmaikrəuˈkemistri] *n* 超微量化学
ultramicron [ˌʌltrəˈmaikrɔn] *n* 超微粒
ultramicropipet [ˌʌltrəˌmaikrəupaiˈpet] *n* 超微量吸管，超微滴管（能吸极微量〈0.002～0.005 ml〉液体的吸管）
ultramicroscope [ˌʌltrəˈmaikrəskəup] *n* 超显微镜 | **ultramicroscopic** [ˌʌltrəˌmaikrəˈskɔpik] *a* 超显微镜的；超出普通显微镜可见度范围的 / **ultramicroscopy** [ˌʌltrəmaiˈkrɔskəpi] *n* 超显微术，超显微镜检查
ultramicrotome [ˌʌltrəˈmaikrətəum] *n* 超薄切片机
ultraphagocytosis [ˌʌltrəˌtægəsaiˈtəusis] *n* 超吞噬作用（摄取亚显微大小的颗粒）
ultraprophylaxis [ˌʌltrəprɔfiˈlæksis] *n* 超预防（限制身体有缺陷的人结婚以避免产生疾病或畸形儿童的预防措施）
ultraquinine [ˌʌltrəˈkwinin] *n* 超奎宁，高奎宁，后莫奎宁
ultra-red [ˌʌltrəˈred] *n* 红外线 *a* 红外[线]的
ultrashort [ˌʌltrəˈʃɔːt] *a* 极短的；超短[波]的
ultrasonic [ˌʌltrəˈsɔnik] *a* 超声[波]的 | **~s** *n* 超声[波]学
ultrasonogram [ˌʌltrəˈsɔnəgræm] *n* 超声图
ultrasonography [ˌʌltrəsəˈnɔgrəfi] *n* 超声检查[术] | endoscopic ~ 内镜超声检查[术] / gray-scale / ~ 灰阶超声检查 **ultrasonographic** [ˌʌltrəˌsɔnəˈgræfik] *a*
ultrasonometry [ˌʌltrəsəˈnɔmətri] *n* 超声测量法
ultrasound [ˈʌltrəsaund] *n* 超声
ultrastructure [ˌʌltrəˈstrʌktʃə] *n* 超微结构，亚显微结构 | **~al** [ˌʌltrəˈstrʌktʃərəl] *a*
ultratoxon [ˌʌltrəˈtɔksɔn] *n* 超减力毒素
ultraviolet [ˌʌltrəˈvaiəlit] *a* 紫外（线）的 *n* 紫外线 | far ~ 远紫外线（1 800～2 900Å）/ near ~ 近紫外线（2 900～3 900Å）
ultravisible [ˌʌltrəˈvizəbl] *a* 超视的，超显微镜的
ultromotivity [ˌʌltrəuməuˈtivəti] *n* 自动力，自动性
Ultzmann's test [ˈultsmən]（Robert Ultzmann）乌尔次曼试验（检胆色素）
ululation [ˌjuːljuˈleiʃən] *n*（癔症患者的）狂叫，嚎叫
umbauzonen [ˌʌmbauˈzɔnən] *n*【德】卢塞（Looser）变形区（骨 X 线照片所现黑线）
umbel [ˈʌmbel] *n* 伞形花序
umbellic acid [ʌmˈbelik] 伞形酸，2，4-二羟[基]肉桂酸
Umbelliferae [ˌʌmbəˈlifiriː] *n* 伞形科
umbelliferone [ˌʌmbeˈlifərəun] *n* 伞形酮，7-羟[基]香豆素
umbelliferous [ˌʌmbəˈlifərəs] *a* 伞形科的；伞形花序的
umber [ˈʌmbə] *n*，*a* 棕土（的），红棕色（的）
Umber's test [ˈumbə]（Friedrich Umber）乌姆贝尔试验（检猩红热）
umbilectomy [ˌʌmbiˈlektəmi] *n* 脐切除术
umbilical [ʌmˈbilikəl，ˌʌmbiˈlaikəl] *a* 脐的
umbilicate [ʌmˈbilikit]，**umbilicated** [ʌmˈbilikeitid] *a* 有脐的，脐形的，凹陷的 | **umbilication** [ʌmˌbiliˈkeiʃən] *n* 成脐形，凹陷
umbilicus [ʌmˈbilikəs]（[复] **umbilicuses** 或 **umbilici** [ʌmˈbilisai]）*n*【拉】脐 | amniotic ~ 羊膜脐 / decidual ~ 蜕膜脐 / posterior ~ 后脐，藏毛窦
umbo [ˈʌmbəu]（[复] **umbos** 或 **umbones** [ʌmˈbəuniːz]）*n*【拉】突，圆头 | ~ of tympanic membrane 鼓膜凸
umbonate [ˈʌmbəneit] *a* 凸形的，钮形的
umbra [ˈʌmbrə] *n* 全影区；锐区（放射学中指清晰对比区）
umbrascopy [ʌmˈbræskəpi] *n* X 线透视检查；视网膜镜检查
umbrella [ʌmˈbrelə] *n* 伞，伞形物
UMP uridine monophosphate 尿苷[一磷]酸
UMP synthase [ˈsinθeis] 尿苷[一磷]酸合酶
UMP synthase deficiency 尿苷[一磷]酸缺乏症，乳清酸尿症Ⅰ型
uña de gato [ˈuːnjaː dei ˈgɑːtəu]【西】钩藤；钩藤制剂

unazotized [ʌnˈæzətaizd] *a* 不含氮的
unbalance [ʌnˈbæləns] *vt* 使精神错乱,使紊乱 *n* 错乱,紊乱
uncal [ˈʌŋkəl] *a* 钩的
Uncaria [ʌnˈkɛəriə] *n*【拉】钩藤属
uncarthrosis [ˌʌŋkɑːˈθrəusis] *n* 钩骨病
unci [ˈʌnsai] uncus 的复数
uncia [ˈʌnsiə] ([复] **unciae** [ˈʌnsiiː]) *n*【拉】盎司;英寸
unciform [ˈʌnsifɔːm] *a* 钩状的,钩形的;钩骨的 *n* 钩骨
unciforme [ˌʌnsiˈfɔːmi] *n*【拉】钩骨
uncinal [ˈʌnsinəl] *a* 钩状的,有钩的;钩回的
Uncinaria [ˌʌnsiˈnɛəriə] *n* 钩虫属 | ~ americana 美洲钩虫(即美洲板口线虫 Necator americanus) / ~ duodenalis 十二指肠钩虫(即 Ancylostoma duodenale)
uncinariasis [ˌʌnsinəˈraiəsis] *n* 钩虫病 | **uncinariatic** [ˌʌnsiˌnɛəriˈætik] *a*
uncinate [ˈʌnsinit] *a* 钩状的,有钩的;钩回的
uncinatum [ˌʌnsiˈneitəm] *n*【拉】钩骨
uncipressure [ˈʌnsiˌpreʃə] *n* 钩压法(止血)
uncommitted [ˌʌnkəˈmitid] *a* 未遂的(指犯罪);不受(某些原则)约束的;未被监禁的;未送往精神病院的;未定型的(指免疫细胞尚未定型,即尚未接受抗原刺激,仍保持有多种免疫反应潜能的状况)
uncomplemented [ʌnˈkɔmpliˌmentid] *a* 未结合补体的(因此无活动性的)
uncomplicated [ʌnˈkɔmplikeitid] *a* 无并发症的
unconscious [ʌnˈkɔnʃəs] *a* 无意识的 *n* 潜意识 | collective ~ 集体潜意识 | **~ly** *ad* | **~ness** *n*
unco-ossified [ˌʌnkəuˈɔsifaid] *a* 未共同骨化的(未联合为一骨)
uncotomy [ʌŋˈkɔtəmi] *n* 海马回沟切开术
uncouple [ʌnˈkʌpl] *vt* 解开,松开 | **~r** *n* 解偶联剂
uncovertebral [ˌʌnkəuˈvəːtibrəl] *a* 椎骨钩突的
unction [ˈʌŋkʃən] *n* 油膏;涂油膏,涂药膏
unctuous [ˈʌŋktjuəs] *a* 油的,油膏的,含油脂的;油滑的,油样的
uncus [ˈʌŋkəs] ([复] **unci** [ˈʌnsai]) *n*【拉】钩
undecane [ˈʌndikein] *n* 十一[碳]烷
undecenoic acid [ˌʌndesiˈnəuik], **undecylenic acid** [ˌʌndesiˈlenik] 十一烯酸(抗真菌药)
underbite [ˈʌndəbait] *n* 下咬合(retrognathism 的俗称)
undercut [ˈʌndəˌkʌt] *n* 底切;底切部 [ˈʌndəˈkʌt] *vt* 从下部切开,底切 *vi* 切去下部,底切
under-developed [ˈʌndədiˈveləpt] *a* 发育不全的
undergrowth [ˈʌndəgrəuθ] *n* 发育不全
underhorn [ˈʌndəhɔːn] *n* 下角(侧脑室)
undersensing [ˈʌndəˌsensiŋ] *n* 检测不全(人工心脏起搏器的心脏电信号失检,导致传送刺激过于频繁和不规则,其原因包括磁头脱位,脉冲发生器功能不良,纤维变性,梗死和药物)
understain [ˈʌndəstein] *n* 浅染,染色不足
undertoe [ˈʌndətəu] *n* 践底趾(蹋趾移位于其他各趾下)
undertreat [ˌʌndəˈtriːt] *vt* 治疗不足
Underwood's disease [ˈʌndəwud] (Michael Underwood) 硬化病
undifferentiated [ˌʌndifəˈrenʃieitid] *a* 未分化的
undifferentiation [ˌʌndifəˌrenʃiˈeiʃən] *n* 未分化[作用];退行发育
undine [ʌnˈdiːn, ˈʌndain] *n* 洗眼壶
undinism [ˈʌndinizəm] *n* 弄水色情,水淫;排尿色情
Undritz anomaly [ˈuːndritz] (E. Undritz) 遗传性嗜中性粒细胞核分叶过多
undulant [ˈʌndjulənt] *a* 波动的,波状的
undulate [ˈʌndjuleit] *vt*, *vi* 波动
undulation [ˌʌndjuˈleiʃən] *n* 波动;颤动,振动 | jugular ~ 颈静脉波,静脉搏 / respiratory ~ 呼吸性血压波
ung. unguentum【拉】软膏
ungual [ˈʌŋgwəl] *a* 指甲的,趾甲的
unguent [ˈʌŋgwənt] *n* 药膏,软膏;润滑油
unguentum [ʌŋˈgwentəm] *n*【拉】软膏
unguiculate [ʌŋˈgwikjulit] *a* 有爪的,爪样的
unguiculus [ʌŋˈgwikjuləs] *n*【拉】小[指]甲
unguis [ˈʌŋgwis] ([复] **ungues** [ˈʌŋgwiːz]) *n*【拉】指甲,趾甲;眼前房积脓;爪 | ~ incarnatus 嵌甲
ungula [ˈʌŋgjulə] *n*【拉】蹄
ungulate [ˈʌŋgjuleit] *a* 有蹄的,蹄状的 *n* 有蹄动物
unguligrade [ˈʌŋgjuliˌgreid] *a* 蹄行的
uni- [前缀]一,单
uniarticular [ˌjuːniɑːˈtikjulə] *a* 单关节的
uniaural [ˌjuːniˈɔːrəl] *a* 单耳的
uniaxial [ˌjuːniˈæksiəl] *a* 单轴的
unibasal [ˌjuːniˈbeisl] *a* 单底的
unicaliceal [ˌjuːnikəˈlisiəl] *a* 单盏的(指异型肾,亦可拼写成 unicalyceal)
unicameral [ˌjuːniˈkæmərəl] *a* [有]单腔的
unicellular [ˌjuːniˈseljulə] *a* 单细胞的
unicentral [ˌjuːniˈsentrəl], **unicentric** [ˌjuːniˈsentrik] *a* 单中心的
uniceps [ˌjuːniˈseps] *a* 单头的(肌)
uniceptor [ˈjuːniˌseptə] *n* 单受体,单簇受体
unicollis [ˌjuːniˈkɔlis] *a*【拉】单颈的(如 uterus unicornis unicollis〈单颈单角子宫〉)
unicornous [ˌjuːniˈkɔːnəs] *a* 单角的

unicuspid [ˌjuːniˈkʌspid] *a* 单尖的 *n* 单尖牙

unicuspidate [ˌjuːniˈkʌspideit] *a* [有]单尖的

unidirectional [ˌjuːnidiˈrekʃənəl, -dai-] *a* 单向的

unifilar [ˌjuːniˈfailə] *a* 单丝的

uniflagellate [ˌjuːniˈflædʒeleit] *a* 单鞭毛的

unifocal [ˌjuːniˈfəukəl] *a* 单灶的,单病灶的

uniforate [ˌjuːniˈfɔːreit] *a* 单孔的

unigeminal [ˌjuːniˈdʒeminl] *a* 双胎之一的

unigerminal [ˌjuːniˈdʒəːminl] *a* 单胚的

uniglandular [ˌjuːniˈglændjulə] *a* 单腺的

unigravida [ˌjuːniˈgrævidə] *n* 初孕妇

unilaminar [ˌjuːniˈlæminə] *a* 单层的

unilateral [ˌjuːniˈlætərəl] *a* 单侧的,一侧的

unilobar [ˌjuːniˈləubə] *a* 单叶的

unilocular [ˌjuːniˈlɔkjulə] *a* 单房的

unimodal [ˌjuːniˈməudl] *a* 单式的;(曲线)单峰的

uninephrectomized [ˌjuːninəˈfrektəmaizd] *a* 单侧肾切除后的

uninephric [ˌjuːriˈnefrik] *a* 单肾的

uninjured [ʌnˈindʒəd] *a* 未受损伤的

uninuclear [ˌjuːniˈnjuːkliə], **uninucleated** [ˌjuːniˈnjuːklieitid] *a* 单核的

uniocular [ˌjuːniˈɔkjulə] *a* 单眼的

union [ˈjuːnjən] *n* 连接,结合;愈合 | faulty ~ 连接不良(指骨折) / primary ~ 第一期愈合 / vicious ~ 连接不正(指骨折骨)

uniovular [ˌjuːniˈɔvjulə] *a* 单卵的

unipapillary [ˌjuːniˈpæpiləri] *a* 单乳头的(指异型肾)

unipara [juːˈnipərə] *n* 初产妇

uniparental [ˌjuːnipəˈrentl] *a* 单亲的

uniparous [ju(ː)ˈnipərəs] *a* 一胎一仔的(每次产一卵〈或一仔〉的);初产的

unipolar [ˌjuːniˈpəulə] *a* 单极的(如神经细胞)

uniport [ˈjuːnipɔːt] *n* 单向转运,易化扩散

uniporter [ˈjuːnipɔːtə] *n* 单向转运蛋白

unipotential [ˌjuːnipəuˈtenʃəl], **unipotent** [ju(ː)ˈnipətənt] *a* 单能性的(指细胞) | **unipotency** [ˌjuːniˈpəutənsi] *n*

unirritable [ʌnˈiritəbl] *a* 无应激性的,不能刺激的

uniseptate [ˌjuːniˈsepteit] *a* 单[中]隔的

unisexual [ˌjuːniˈseksjuəl] *a* 单性的

unit [ˈjuːnit] *n* 单位;单元 | amboceptor ~ 介体单位(以过量补体能使一定量红细胞溶血的介体的最小量) / American Drug Manufacturers' Association ~ 美国制药商协会单位(斯廷博克〈Steenbock〉单位的十分之一) / Angström ~ 埃单位(波长单位,$Å = 10^{-7}$ mm) / antigen ~ 抗原单位(固定一单位补体以防止溶血所需的最小量抗原) / antitoxic ~ 抗毒素单位(表达抗毒素中和能力的单位) / atomic mass ~, atomic weight ~ 原子质量单位 / British thermal ~ 英国热量单位 / CGS ~ 厘米-克-秒制单位 / cat ~ 猫单位(猫的每千克〈kg〉体重计算的洋地黄剂量,以该剂量缓慢而持续地注入静脉时可使猫致死) / clinical ~ 临床单位(一种雌激素效能单位,相当于国际单位的六分之一) / colony-forming ~ 集落生成单位 / complement ~ 补体单位(在介体单位存在下,溶解一定量红细胞所需补体的最小量) / coronary care ~ 冠心病监护治疗病房 / ~ of current 电流单位 / dental ~ 牙单位(一种咀嚼单位,由一颗牙及其附件组成);牙科综合治疗台 / electromagnetic ~s 电磁系单位 / electrostatic ~s 静电系单位 / enzyme ~ 酶单位(见 international ~ of enzyme activity) / ~ of force 力单位 / ~ of heat 热量单位 / hemolytic ~ 溶血单位(见 complement ~) / intensive care ~ 重症监护治疗病房,重症监护室 / international ~ of enzyme activity 酶活性国际单位(在最适温度、最适 pH 和最适底物浓度的标准状况下,在 1 分钟的时间催化 1 μmol 的底物发生转化的酶的量,符号为 IU) / international ~ of penicillin 青霉素国际单位(在 0.6 μg 国际标准青霉素Ⅱ或 G 钠盐中含有的特定的青霉素活性) / international ~ of vitamin A 维生素 A 国际单位(相当于 0.6 μg 纯 β-胡萝卜素的活性) / international ~ of vitamin D 维生素 D 国际单位(1 mg 经过照射的麦角固醇的国际标准溶液〈1 mg 溶于 10 ml 橄榄油中〉的活性) / light ~ 光单位 / map ~ 图距单位(染色体上位点之间的相对距离,如由重组频度测定的距离) / morgan ~ 摩尔根单位(见 morgan) / mouse ~ 小鼠单位(雌激素的生物鉴定单位) / Oxford ~ 牛津单位(溶于 50 ml 肉羹培养中,恰好完全阻止金黄色葡萄球菌生长所需的青霉素量) / peripheral resistance ~ (PRU)外周阻力单位(血管阻力的常规单位,等于 1 ml/s 的血流可产生 1 mmHg〈=133.322 Pa〉的压力差) / physiologic ~ 胶粒,微胶粒 / quantum ~ 量子单位(见 Planck's constant) / rat ~ 大鼠单位(促动情激素〈雌激素〉的最大稀释度〈即最小量〉,即将该激素注入卵巢切除的成年大鼠,在第一天内每隔 4 小时注射一次,共注射三次,可引起阴道上皮角化和脱屑) / ~ of resistance 电阻单位 / SI ~ 国际单位制单位(指任何一种国际单位制〈Système International d'Unités 或 International System of Units〉的单位) / specific smell ~ 特殊嗅觉单位 / sudanophobic ~ 拒苏丹单位(垂体切除鼠〈至少有 2~3 只〉连续 8 日早晚注射而引起嫌苏丹区消失所需的促肾上腺皮质激素最小量) / toxic ~, toxin ~ 毒性单位,毒素单位(能使大约250 g重的豚鼠在 3~4 天内死亡的

最小的毒素量）/ tuberculin ～ 结核菌素单位（0.1 ml 结核菌素溶液中含有 0.000 02 mg 纯蛋白衍化物，相当于旧结核菌素 1∶10 000 稀释液的效能）/ turbidity reducing ～ 浊度减低单位（使 0.2 mg 透明质酸盐所产生的浊度加上酸化马血清后正好足以减低到 0.1 mg 产生的浊度的透明质酸酶量）/ urotoxic ～ 尿毒素单位（能杀死体重 1 g 动物的最小尿毒素量）/ USP ～ 美国药典单位 / vitamin A ～ 维生素 A 单位（见 international ～ of vitamin A）/ ～ of vitamin B_1 维生素 B_1 单位（3 μg国际标准制剂的抗神经炎活性）/ vitamin D ～ 维生素 D 单位（见 international ～ of vitamin D）/ vitamin G ～ 维生素 G 单位 / X-ray ～ X 线单位

unitage [ˈjuːnitidʒ] *n* 单位量

unitary [ˈjuːnitəri] *a* 单元的，一元的，单式的，酉的

United States Pharmacopeia《美国药典》

uniterminal [ˌjuːniˈtəːminl] *a* 单极的

unitless [ˈjuːnitləs] *a* 无单位的

Unitunicatae [ˌjuːniˌtjuːniˈkeitiː] *n* 单囊类

univalent [ˌjuːniˈveilənt] *a* 一价的，单价的 *n* 单价体（在减数分裂中期没有配对的单个染色体）| **univalence** *n* 一价，单价

univariate [ˌjuːniˈvɛəriət] *a* 单变量的

university [ˌjuːniˈvəːsəti] *n* 大学 | University of Wissconsin solution UW 液

univitelline [ˌjuːnivaiˈtelin] *a* 单卵的，单卵黄的

unmedullated [ʌnˈmedəˌleitid] *a* 无髓的（指神经纤维）

unmyelinated [ʌnˈmaiəliˌneitid] *a* 无髓［鞘］的（指神经纤维）

Unna-Pappenheim stain [ˈunə ˈpʌpənhaim]（Paul G. Unna; Artur Pappenheim）乌纳-帕彭海姆染剂（用甲基绿和派洛宁染浆细胞）

Unna's boot [ˈunə]（Paul G. Unna）乌纳糊靴（静脉曲张性溃疡敷料）| ～ alkaline methylene blue stain 乌纳碱性亚甲蓝染剂（染浆细胞）

Unna-Thost disease, syndrome [ˈunə tɔst]（Paul G. Unna; Arthur Thost）弥漫性掌跖角化病

unoprostone isopropyl [ˌjuːnəuˈprɔstəun] 异丙乌诺前列酮（抗青光眼药）

unorganized [ʌnˈɔːgənaizd] *a* 无结构的，无器官的

unorientation [ˌʌnɔːrienˈteiʃən] *n* 定向［力］障碍，定向力丧失

unphysiologic [ˌʌnfiziəˈlɔdʒik] *a* 非生理性的

unproductive [ˌʌnprəˈdʌktiv] *a* 不生痰的

unresectable [ˌʌnri(ː)ˈsektəbl] *a* 不可切除的

unrest [ʌnˈrest] *n* 不安 | peristaltic ～ 蠕动紊乱

unsaturated [ʌnˈsætʃəreitid] *a* 不饱和的，未饱和的 | **unsaturation** [ˌʌnsætʃəˈreiʃən] *n*

Unschuld's sign [ˈunʃuld]（Paul Unschuld）翁舒尔德征（糖尿病初期腓肠肌痉挛）

unsharpness [ʌnˈʃɑːpnis] *n* 模糊

unspecific monooxygenase [ˌʌnspəˈsifik mɔnəuˈɔksədʒəneis] 非特异性单加氧酶

unstriated [ˌʌnˈstraieitid] *a* 无横纹的

unthriftiness [ʌnˈθriftinis] *n* 不旺盛（指幼畜）

Unverricht-Lundborg disease [ˈunferikt ˈlundbɔːg]（H. Unverricht; Herman B. Lundborg）翁-隆病，波罗的海肌阵挛性癫痫

Unverricht's disease (syndrome) [ˈunferikt]（Heinrich Unverricht）肌阵挛性癫痫

unvoiced [ʌnˈvɔist] *a* 清音的

upas [ˈjuːpəs] *n* 见血封喉（桑科）

u-plasminogen activator [plæzˈminədʒən ˈæktiveitə] 尿纤溶酶原激活物（肾内产生并尿内排泄，诱发治疗血栓溶解。亦称尿激酶）

UPP urethral pressure profile 尿道压力图

UPPP uvulopalatopharyngoplasty 腭垂腭咽成形术，腭咽成形术

up-regulation [ʌp ˌregjuˈleiʃən] *n* 增量调节（狭义来说，表示某一基因的增加，亦即特异 mRNA 转录增加，而且更广泛地用于指某一特别基因由于任何原因其 mRNA 水平增加，如特异 mRNA的稳定性增加）

uprighting [ˈʌpraitiŋ] *n* 竖立（将倾斜牙翻动到更加垂直的牙轴斜度）

upsiloid [ˈjupsilɔid, ˈʌp-] *a* 倒人字形的，V 字形的（像希腊语字母 υ 或 Υ 的）

upsilon [juːpˈsailən, ˈjuːpsilən, ˈʌp-] *n* 希腊语的第 20 个字母（Υ, υ）

upstream [ˈʌpˌstriːm] *a* 上游的 *n* 上游区（在分子生物学中，本词表示位于基因的 5′位的核酸区或感兴趣区）

uptake [ˈʌpteik] *n* 摄取 | maximal oxygen ～ 最大摄氧量 / thyroid iodine ～ 甲状腺摄碘率

urachovesical [ˌjuərəkəuˈvesikəl] *a* 脐尿管膀胱的

urachus [ˈjuərəkəs] *n* 脐尿管 | **urachal** *a*

uracil [ˈjuərəsil] *n* 尿嘧啶 | 5-methyl ～ 5-甲基尿嘧啶，胸腺嘧啶

uracrasia [ˌjuərəˈkreisiə] *n* 尿性质不良

uracratia [ˌjuərəˈkreiʃiə] *n* 遗尿，尿失禁

uragogue [ˈjuərəgɔg] *a* 利尿的 *n* 利尿药

uramil [ˈjuərəmil] *n* 尿咪，氨基丙二酰脲，5-氨基巴比土酸

uramilic acid [juərəˈmilik] 缩-2-氨基丙二酰脲酸

uraminoacetic acid [ˌjuəˌræminəuəˈsiːtik] 脲乙酸

uraminobenzoic acid [ˌjuəˌræminəubenˈzəuik] 脲苯甲酸

uraminotauric acid [ˌjuəˌræminəuˈtɔːrik] 脲牛磺酸
uran-gallein [ˌjuərənˈgæliin] *n* 铀棓因(弹性组织染剂)
uranianism [juəˈreiniənizəm] *n* 同性恋
uranic [juəˈrænik] *a* [正]铀的,含有六价铀的
uranidin [juəˈrænidin] *n* 动物黄色素(海绵、珊瑚、水母及蠕虫中的某种黄色素)
uranin [ˈjuərənin] *n* 荧光素钠
uranisc(o)- [构词成分]腭
uraniscochasma [ˌjuərəˌniskəuˈkæzmə] *n* 腭裂
uraniscolalia [ˌjuərəˌniskəuˈleiliə] *n* 腭裂语声
uraniscoplasty [ˌjuərəˈniskəˌplæsti] *n* 腭成形术
uraniscorrhaphy [ˌjuərənisˈkɔrəfi] *n* 腭裂缝合术,腭修补术
uraniscus [ˌjuərəˈniskəs] *n* 腭
uranism [ˈjuərənizəm] *n* 同性恋
uranium(U) [juəˈreinjəm] *n* 铀(化学元素)
uran(o)- [构词成分]腭
uranoplasty [ˈjuərənəˌplæsti] *n* 腭成形术 | **uranoplastic** [ˌjuərənəuˈplæstik] *a*
uranoplegia [ˌjuərənəuˈpliːdʒiə] *n* 腭麻痹
uranorrhaphy [ˌjuərəˈnɔrəfi] *n* 腭裂缝合术
uranoschisis [ˌjuərəˈnɔskisis], **uranoschism** [juəˈrænəskizəm] *n* 腭裂
uranostaphyloplasty [ˌjuərənəuˈstæfiləuˌplæsti] *n* 软硬腭成形术
uranostaphylorrhaphy [ˌjuərənəuˌstæfiˈlɔrəfi] *n* 软硬腭缝合术
uranostaphyloschisis [ˌjuərənəuˌstæfiˈlɔskisis] *n* 软硬腭裂
uranosteoplasty [ˌjuərəˈnɔstiəˌplæsti] *n* 腭成形术
Uranotaenia [ˌjuərənəuˈtiːniə] *n* 蓝带蚊属 | ~ loashanensis 乐山蓝带蚊
uranous [ˈjuərənəs] *n* [亚]铀的,含有四价铀的
uranyl [ˈjuərənil] *n* 双氧铀,二氧化铀 | ~ acetate 乙酸双氧铀,醋酸双氧铀(用于鼻卡他)
urapostema [ˌjuərəpɔsˈtiːmə] *n* 含尿脓肿
urarthritis [ˌjuərɑːˈθraitis] *n* 痛风性关节炎
urase [ˈjuəreis] *n* 脲酶,尿素酶
urasin [juəˈræsin] *n* 细菌脲酶
urate [ˈjuəreit] *n* 尿酸盐
uratemia [ˌjuərəˈtiːmiə] *n* 尿酸盐血
urate oxidase [ˈjuəreit ˈɔksideis] 尿酸氧化酶(亦称尿酸酶)
uratic [juəˈrætik] *a* 尿酸盐的;痛风的
uratohistechia [ˌjuərətəuhisˈtekiə] *n* (组织)尿酸盐沉着
uratoma [ˌjuərəˈtəumə] *n* 痛风石,尿酸盐结石
uratosis [ˌjuərəˈtəusis] *n* (组织)尿酸盐沉着
uraturia [ˌjuərəˈtjuəriə] *n* 尿酸盐尿
urazin(e) [ˈjuərəzin] *n* 尿嗪,双尿,环二脲
urazole [ˈjuərəzəul] *n* 尿唑(双尿素缩合物)
Urbach-Oppenheim disease [ˈəːbək ˈɔpənhaim] (Erich Urbach; Maurice Oppenheim) 糖尿病脂性渐进性坏死
Urbach-Wiethe disease [ˈəːbək ˈwiːti] (Erich Urbach; Camillo Wiethe) 脂质蛋白沉积症
urceiform [əːˈsiːfɔːm], **urceolate** [ˈəːsiəlit] *a* 壶形的
ur-defense [ˌəːdiˈfens] *n* 原始信念,基本[心理]防御信念
urea [ˈjuəriə] *n* 脲,尿素(利尿药) | ~ nitrogen 尿素氮,脲氮 | **ureal** *a*
ureagenesis [juəˌriəˈdʒenəsis] *n* 脲生成,尿素生成
ureagenetic [juəriədʒiˈnetik] *a* 脲生成的,尿素生成的
ureametry [ˌjuəriˈæmitri] *n* 脲测定法,尿素测定法
Ureaplasma [juəˌriəˈplæzmə] *n* 脲原体属,尿素原体属 | ~ urealyticum 解脲脲原体,尿素分解尿素原体
ureaplasma [juəˌriəˈplæzmə] *n* 脲原体,尿素原体
ureapoiesis [juəˌriəpɔiˈiːsis] *n* 脲生成,尿素生成
urease [ˈjuərieis] *n* 脲酶,尿素酶
urecchysis [juəˈrekisis] *n* 尿浸润
Urechites suberecta [juəˈrekitiːz ˌsʌbəˈrektə] 黄龙葵(夹竹桃科植物)
urechitin [juəˈrekitin] *n* 黄龙葵苷
urechitoxin [juəˌrekiˈtɔksin] *n* 黄龙葵毒素
uredema [ˌjuəri(ː)ˈdiːmə] *n* 尿液性水肿
uredepa [əːriˈdiːpə] *n* 乌瑞替派(抗肿瘤药)
Uredinales [ˌjuərədiˈneiliːz] *n* 锈菌目
uredofos [juəˈriːdəfɔs] *n* 乌瑞磷(兽用抗蠕虫药)
ureic [juəˈriːik] *a* 脲的,尿素的
ureide [ˈjuəriid] *n* 酰脲
urein(e) [juəˈriːin] *n* 烷基脲
urelcosis [ˌjuərəlˈkəusis] *n* 尿路溃疡
uremia [juəˈriːmiə] *n* 尿毒症 | **uremic** *a*
uremigenic [juəˌriːmiˈdʒenik] *a* 尿毒症性的;致尿毒症的
ure(o)- 以 ure(o)-起始的词,同样见以 urea-起始的词
ureolysis [ˌjuəriˈɔlisis] *n* 尿素分解 | **ureolytic** [ˌjuəriəˈlitik] *a*
ureometer [ˌjuəriˈɔmitə] *n* 脲[量]测定器,脲素计 | **ureometry** *n* 脲测定法,尿素测定法
ureotelic [ˌjuəriəˈtelik] *a* 排尿素代谢的
uresiesthesis [juəˌriːsiesˈθiːsis] *n* 排尿感觉
uresis [juəˈriːsis] *n* 排尿

-uresis [构词成分]尿排出
uret [ˈjuəret] *n* 氮氧甲基
ureter [juəˈriːtə] *n* 输尿管 | ectopic ~ 异位输尿管 / postcaval ~, circumcaval ~, retrocaval ~ 腔静脉后输尿管 | ~**al** [juəˈriːtərəl], **uretal** [juəˈriːtəl] *a*
ureteralgia [juəˌriːtəˈrældʒiə] *n* 输尿管痛
ureterectasis [juəˌriːtəˈrektəsis], **ureterectasia** [juəˌriːtərekˈteiziə] *n* 输尿管扩张
ureterectomy [juəˌriːtəˈrektəmi] *n* 输尿管切除术
ureteric [ˌjuəriˈterik] *a* 输尿管的
ureteritis [juəˌriːtəˈraitis] *n* 输尿管炎
ureter(o)- [构词成分]输尿管
ureteroarterial [juəˌriːtərəuɑːˈtiəriəl] *a* 输尿管动脉的
ureterocele [juəˈriːtərəuˌsiːl] *n* 输尿管脱垂 | ectopic ~ 异位输尿管膨出
ureterocelectomy [juəˌriːtərəusiːˈlektəmi] *n* 输尿管膨出切除术
ureterocervical [juəˌriːtərəuˈsəːvikəl] *a* 输尿管子宫颈的
ureterocolostomy [juəˌriːtərəukəˈlɔstəmi] *n* 输尿管结肠吻合术
ureterocutaneostomy [juəˌriːtərəukjuˌteiniˈɔstəmi] *n* 输尿管皮肤造口术
ureterocystanastomosis [juəˌriːtərəuˌsistəˌnæstəˈməusis], **ureterocystoneostomy** [juəˌriːtərəuˌsistəniˈɔstəmi], **ureterocystostomy** [juəˌriːtərəusisˈtɔstəmi] *n* 输尿管膀胱吻合术
ureterocystoscope [juəˌriːtərəuˈsistəskəup] *n* 输尿管膀胱镜
ureterodialysis [juəˌriːtərəudaiˈælisis] *n* 输尿管破裂
ureteroduodenal [juəˌriːtərəuˌdju(ː)əuˈdiːnl] *a* 输尿管十二指肠的
ureteroenteric [juəˌriːtərəuenˈterik] *a* 输尿管肠的
ureteroenterostomy [juəˌriːtərəuentəˈrɔstəmi], **ureteroenteroanastomosis** [juəˌriːtərəuˌentərəuˌənæstəˈməusis] *n* 输尿管肠吻合术
ureterogram [juəˈriːtərəgræm] *n* 输尿管造影[照]片
ureterography [juəˌriːtəˈrɔgrəfi] *n* 输尿管造影[术]
ureteroheminephrectomy [juəˌriːtərəuˌhemineˈfrektəmi] *n* 输尿管肾部分切除术
ureterohydronephrosis [juəˌriːtərəuˌhaidrəunəˈfrəusis] *n* 输尿管肾盂积水
ureteroileal [juəˌriːtərəuˈiliəl] *a* 输尿管回肠的
ureteroileostomy [juəˌriːtərəuˌiliˈɔstəmi] *n* 输尿管回肠吻合术
ureterointestinal [juəˌriːtərəuinˈtestinl] *a* 输尿管肠的
ureterolith [juəˈriːtərəliθ] *n* 输尿管石
ureterolithiasis [juəˌriːtərəuliˈθaiəsis] *n* 输尿管石病
ureterolithotomy [juəˌriːtərəuliˈθɔtəmi] *n* 输尿管切开取石术
ureterolysis [juəˌriːtəˈrɔlisis] *n* 输尿管破裂;输尿管麻痹;输尿管松解术
ureteromeatotomy [juəˌriːtərəuˌmiːəˈtɔtəmi] *n* 输尿管口切开术
ureteroneocystostomy [juəˌriːtərəuˌni(ː)əusisˈtɔstəmi] *n* 输尿管膀胱吻合术
ureteroneopyelostomy [juəˌriːtərəuˌni(ː)əupaiiˈlɔstəmi] *n* 输尿管肾盂吻合术
ureteronephrectomy [juəˌriːtərəuneˈfrektəmi] *n* 输尿管肾切除术
ureteronephroscopy [juəˌriːtərəunəˈfrɔskəpi] *n* 输尿管肾镜检查[术]
ureteropathy [juəˌriːtəˈrɔpəθi] *n* 输尿管病
ureteropelvic [juəˌriːtərəuˈpelvik] *a* 输尿管肾盂的
ureteropelvioneostomy [juəˌriːtərəuˌpelviəuni(ː)ˈɔstəmi] *n* 输尿管肾盂吻合术
ureteropelvioplasty [juəˌriːtərəuˈpelviəˌplæsti] *n* 输尿管肾盂成形术
ureterophlegma [juəˌriːtərəuˈflegmə] *n* 输尿管黏液蓄积
ureteroplasty [juəˌriːtərəˌplæstiˈ] *n* 输尿管成形术
ureteroproctostomy [juəˌriːtərəuprɔkˈtɔstəmi] *n* 输尿管直肠吻合术
ureteropyelitis [juəˌriːtərəupaiiˈlaitis] *n* 输尿管肾盂炎
ureteropyelography [juəˌriːtərəupaiiˈlɔgrəfi] *n* 输尿管肾盂造影[术]
ureteropyeloneostomy [juəˌriːtərəuˌpaiiləuniˈɔstəmi] *n* 输尿管肾盂吻合术
ureteropyelonephritis [juəˌriːtərəuˌpaiiləuneˈfraitis] *n* 输尿管肾盂肾炎
ureteropyelonephrostomy [juəˌriːtərəuˌpaiiləu-neˈfrɔstəmi] *n* 输尿管肾盂吻合术
ureteropyeloplasty [juəˌriːtərəuˈpaiiləˌplæsti] *n* 输尿管肾盂成形术
ureteropyelostomy [juəˌriːtərəupaiiˈlɔstəmi] *n* 输尿管肾盂吻合术
ureteropyosis [juəˌriːtərəupaiˈəusis] *n* 输尿管化脓
ureterorectal [juəˌriːtərəuˈrektl] *a* 输尿管直肠的
ureterorectoneostomy [juəˌriːtərəurektəuniˈɔs-

təmi], **ureterorectostomy** [juəˌriːtərəurek'tɔstəmi] *n* 输尿管直肠吻合术

ureterorenoscope [juəˌriːterəu'riːnəskəup] *n* 输尿管肾镜 | **ureterorenoscopy** [juəˌriːtərəuri'nɔskəpi] *n* 输尿管肾镜检查

ureterorrhagia [juəˌriːtərəu'reidʒiə] *n* 输尿管出血

ureterorrhaphy [juəˌriːtə'rɔrəfi] *n* 输尿管缝合术

ureteroscope [juə'riːtərəuˌskəupi] *n* 输尿管镜

ureterosigmoidostomy [juəˌriːtərəuˌsigmɔi'dɔstəmi] *n* 输尿管乙状结肠吻合术

ureterostenosis [juəˌriːtərəusti'nəusis], **ureterostegnosis** [juəˌriːtərəusteg'nəusis], **ureterostenoma** [juəˌriːtərəusti'nəumə] *n* 输尿管狭窄

ureterostoma [juəˌriːtə'rɔstəumə] *n* 输尿管口，输尿管瘘

ureterostomy [juəˌriːtə'rɔstəmi], **ureterostomosis** [juəˌriːtərəustə'məusis] *n* 输尿管造瘘术

ureterotomy [juəˌriːtə'rɔtəmi] *n* 输尿管切开术

ureterotrigonoenterostomy [juəˌriːtərəutraiˌgənəuentə'rɔstəmi] *n* 输尿管膀胱三角肠吻合术

ureterotrigonosigmoidostomy [juəˌriːtərəutraiˌgənəuˌsigmɔi'dɔstəmi] *n* 输尿管膀胱三角乙状结肠吻合术

ureteroureteral [juəˌriːtərəujuə'riːtərəl] *a* 输尿管输尿管的

ureteroureterostomy [juəˌriːtərəujuəˌriːtə'rɔstəmi] *n* 输尿管输尿管吻合术

ureterouterine [juəˌriːtərəu'juːtərain] *a* 输尿管子宫的

ureterovaginal [juəˌriːtərəu'vædʒinl] *a* 输尿管阴道的

ureterovesical [juəˌriːtərəu'vesikəl] *a* 输尿管膀胱的

ureterovesicoplasty [ˌjuəˌriːtərəu'vesikəuˌplæsti] *n* 输尿管膀胱成形术

ureterovesicostomy [juəˌriːtərəuˌvesi'kɔstəmi] *n* 输尿管膀胱吻合术

urethan ['juərəθæn], **urethane** ['juərəθein] *n* 乌拉坦，尿烷，氨甲酸乙酯（抗肿瘤药）

urethra [juə'riːθrə] *n* 尿道 | double ~ 双尿道 | ~l *a*

urethralgia [ˌjuərə'θrældʒiə] *n* 尿道痛

urethrascope [juə'riːθrəskəup] *n* 尿道镜 | **urethrascopic** [juəˌriːθrə'skɔpik] *a*

urethratresia [juəˌriːθrə'triːziə] *n* 尿道闭锁

urethrectomy [ˌjuərə'θrektəmi] *n* 尿道切除术

urethremphraxis [juəˌriːθrem'fræksis] *n* 尿道梗阻

urethreurynter [juəˌriːθru'rintə] *n* 尿道扩张器

urethrism [juə'riːθrizəm] *n* 尿道痉挛

urethritis [ˌjuəri'θraitis] *n* 尿道炎 | ~ cystica 囊性尿道炎 / ~ glandularis 腺性尿道炎 / gonococcal ~ 淋病性尿道炎 / nongonococcal ~ 非淋病性尿道炎 / simple ~, nonspecific ~ 单纯性尿道炎，非特异性尿道炎 / specific ~ 特异性尿道炎，淋病性尿道炎 / ~ venerea 性病尿道炎，淋病

urethr(o)- [构词成分] 尿道

urethroanal [juəˌriːθrəu'einəl] *a* 尿道肛门的，肛门尿道的

urethroblennorrhea [juəˌriːθrəublenə'riːə] *n* 尿道脓溢

urethrobulbar [juəˌriːθrəu'bʌlbə] *a* 尿道球的

urethrocele [juə'riːθrəsiːl] *n* 尿道膨出；（女性）尿道憩室

urethrocystitis [juəˌriːθrəusis'taitis] *n* 尿道膀胱炎

urethrocystogram [juəˌriːθrəu'sistəgræm] *n* 尿道膀胱 X 线[照]片

urethrocystography [juəˌriːθrəusis'tɔgrəfi] *n* 尿道膀胱造影[术]

urethrocystometry [juəˌriːθrəusis'tɔmitri] *n* 尿道膀胱测量[法]

urethrocystopexy [juəˌriːθrəu'sistəˌpeksi] *n* 尿道膀胱固定术

urethrodynia [juəˌriːθrəu'diniə] *n* 尿道痛

urethrograph [juə'riːθrəgrɑːf, -græf] *n* 尿道内径描记器

urethrography [ˌjuərə'θrɔgrəfi] *n* 尿道造影[术]

urethroileal [juəˌriːθrəu'iliəl] *a* 尿道回肠的，回肠尿道的

urethrometer [ˌjuərə'θrɔmitə] *n* 尿道测量器

urethrometry [ˌjuərə'θrɔmitri] *n* 尿道阻力测定法；尿道测量法

urethropenile [juəˌriːθrəu'piːnail] *a* 尿道阴茎的

urethroperineal [juəˌriːθrəuperi'niːəl] *a* 尿道会阴的

urethroperineoscrotal [juəˌriːθrəupeˌriniːəu'skrəutl] *a* 尿道会阴阴囊的

urethropexy [juə'riːθrəˌpeksi] *n* 尿道固定术（矫正女性小便失禁）

urethrophraxis [juəˌriːθrəu'fræksis] *n* 尿道梗阻

urethrophyma [juəˌriːθrəu'faimə] *n* 尿道瘤

urethroplasty [juə'riːθrəˌplæsti] *n* 尿道成形术

urethroprostatic [juəˌriːθrəuprɔs'tætik] *a* 尿道前列腺的

urethrorectal [juəˌriːθrəu'rektl] *a* 尿道直肠的

urethrorrhagia [juəˌriːθrəu'reidʒiə] *n* 尿道出血

urethrorrhaphy [ˌjuərə'θrɔrəfi] *n* 尿道缝合术，尿道修补术

urethrorrhea [juəˌriːθrəu'riə] *n* 尿道溢液
urethroscope [juə'riːθrəskəup] *n* 尿道镜 | **urethroscopic** [juəˌriːθrə'skɔpik] *a* 尿道镜的;尿道镜检查的 | **urethroscopy** [ˌjuərə'θrɔskəpi] *n* 尿道镜检查术
urethroscrotal [juəˌriːθrəu'skrəutl] *a* 尿道阴囊的
urethrospasm [juə'riːθrəspæzəm] *n* 尿道痉挛
urethrostaxis [juəˌriːθrəu'stæksis] *n* 尿道渗血
urethrostenosis [juəˌriːθrəusti'nəusis] *n* 尿道狭窄
urethrostomy [ˌjuərə'θrɔstəmi] *n* 尿道造口术
urethrotome [juə'riːθrətəum] *n* 尿道刀
urethrotomy [ˌjuərə'θrɔtəmi] *n* 尿道切开术
urethrotrigonitis [juəˌriːθrəuˌtraigə'naitis] *n* 尿道膀胱三角炎
urethrovaginal [juəˌriːθrəu'vædʒinl] *a* 尿道阴道的
urethrovesical [juəˌriːθrəu'vesikəl] *a* 尿道膀胱的
uretic [juə'retik] *a* 利尿的 *n* 利尿药
urgency ['əːdʒənsi] *n* 尿急
Urginea [əː'dʒiniə] *n*【拉】海葱属
urhidrosis [ˌəːhi'drəusis] *n* 尿汗症 | ~ crystallina 结晶尿汗症
-uria [构词成分] 尿
urian ['juəriən] *n* 尿色素,尿色肽
uric ['juərik] *a* 尿的
uric acid ['juərik] 尿酸
uricacidemia [ˌjuərikˌæsi'diːmiə], **uricemia** [ˌjuəri'siːmiə] *n* 尿酸血症
uricaciduria [ˌjuərikˌæsi'djuəriə] *n* 尿酸尿
uricase ['juərikeis] *n* 尿酸酶
uric(o)- [构词成分] 尿;尿酸
uricocholia [ˌjuərikəu'kəuliə] *n* 尿酸胆汁[症]
uricolysis [ˌjuəri'kɔlisis] *n* 尿酸分解[作用] | **uricolytic** [ˌjuərikəu'litik] *a*
uricometer [ˌjuəri'kɔmitə] *n* 尿酸计,尿酸定量器
uricopoiesis [ˌjuərikəupɔi'iːsis] *n* 尿酸生成
uricosuria [ˌjuərikəu'sjuəriə] *n* 尿酸尿 | **uricosuric** *a* 促尿酸尿的 *n* 促尿酸尿药
uricotelic [ˌjuərikəu'telik] *a* 排尿酸代谢的
uricotelism [ˌjuərikəu'telizəm] *n* 排尿酸型代谢
uricoxidase [ˌjuəri'kɔksaideis] *n* 尿酸氧化酶
uridine ['juəridi(ː)n] *n* 尿苷 | ~ diphosphate (UDP)尿苷二磷酸 / ~ diphosphoglucuronate 尿苷二磷酸葡萄糖醛酸 / ~ monophosphate (UMP)尿苷[一磷]酸 / ~ triphosphate (UTP) 尿苷三磷酸
uridrosis [juəri'drəusis] *n* 尿汗症
uridylate [ˌjuəri'dileit] *n* 尿苷酸
uridylic acid [ˌjuəri'dilik] 尿苷酸
uridyl transferase ['juəridil 'trænsfəreis] 尿苷酰转移酶,尿苷二磷酸葡萄糖-己糖-1-磷酸尿苷酰基转移酶
uridylyl [ˌjuəri'dilil] *n* 尿苷酰基
uriesthesis [ˌjuəri'esθisis] *n* 排尿感觉
urina [juə'rainə] *n*【拉】尿
urinable ['juərinəbl] *a* 可尿出的(可由尿排泄的)
urinaccelerator [ˌjuərinæk'seləˌreitə] *n* 球海绵体肌
urinacidometer [ˌjuərinˌæsi'dɔmitə] *n* 尿 pH 计,尿氢离子[浓度]测定器
urinaemia [ˌjuəri'niːmiə] *n* 尿毒症
urinal ['juərinl] *n* 尿壶,贮尿器
urinalysis [ˌjuəri'næləsis] ([复] **urinalyses** [ˌjuəri'næləsiːz]) *n* 尿液分析 | mid-stream clean-catch ~ 中段净集尿液分析
urinary ['juərinəri] *a* 尿的,含尿的;泌尿的
urinate ['juərineit] *vi* 排尿
urination [ˌjuəri'neiʃən] *n* 排尿 | precipitant ~ 急迫排尿,尿意逼迫 / stuttering ~ 间歇性排尿
urinative ['juərinətiv] *a* 利尿的 *n* 利尿药
urine ['juərin] *n* 尿 | black ~ 黑尿(由黑素或尿黑酸所致) / chylous ~ 乳糜尿 / cloudy ~, nebulous ~ 混浊尿(一般由于磷酸盐尿或尿酸盐尿所致,但也可能由脓尿所致) / crude ~ 淡尿 / diabetic ~ 糖尿 / febrile ~ 热病性尿 / gouty ~ 痛风尿 / milky ~ 乳状尿(可能由乳糜尿或脓尿所致) / residual ~ 残余尿
urinemia [ˌjuəri'niːmiə] *n* 尿毒症
urine-mucoid [ˌjuərin'mjuːkɔid] *n* 尿黏液样物
urinidrosis [ˌjuərini'drəusis] *n* 尿汗症
uriniferous [ˌjuəri'nifərəs] *a* 输尿的
uriniparous [ˌjuəri'nipərəs], **urinific** [ˌjuəri'nifik] *a* 产尿的,泌尿的
urin(o)- [构词成分] 尿
urinocryoscopy [ˌjuərinəukrai'ɔskəpi] *n* 尿冰点测定法
urinogenital [ˌjuərinəu'dʒenitl] *a* 泌尿生殖的
urinogenous [ˌjuəri'nɔdʒinəs] *a* 尿原的;生尿的
urinoglucosometer [ˌjuərinəuˌgluːkəu'sɔmitə] *n* 尿糖定量器,尿糖计
urinology [ˌjuəri'nɔlədʒi] *n* 泌尿外科学 | **urinologist** *n* 泌尿外科医师,泌尿外科学家
urinoma [ˌjuəri'nəumə] *n* 尿性囊肿
urinometer [ˌjuəri'nɔmitə] *n* 尿比重计 | **urinometry** *n* 尿比重测量法
urinophilous [ˌjuəri'nɔfiləs] *a* 嗜尿的(如微生物)
urinoscopy [ˌjuəri'nɔskəpi] *n* 尿检查,检尿法
urinosexual [ˌjuərinəu'seksjuəl] *a* 泌尿生殖的

urinothorax [ˌjuərinəuˈθɔːræks] *n* 尿胸
urinous [ˈjuərinəs], **urinose** [ˈjuərinəus] *a* 尿的,尿质的
uriposia [ˌjuəriˈpəuziə] *n* 饮尿
urishiol [juːˈriʃiɔl] *n* 漆[儿茶]酚
urningism [ˈəːniŋizəm], **urnism** [ˈəːnizəm] *n* 同性恋
ur(o)- [构词成分]尿;尿道;排尿
uroacidimeter [ˌjuərəuˌæsiˈdimitə] *n* 尿酸度测定器
uroammoniac [ˌjuərəuəˈməuniæk] *a* [含]尿酸与氨的
uroanthelone [ˌjuərəuˈænθələun] *n* 尿抗溃疡素,尿抑胃素,尿抑肠素
uroazotometer [ˌjuərəuˌæzəˈtɔmitə] *n* 尿氮计,尿氮定量器
urobenzoic acid [ˌjuərəubenˈzəuik] 马尿酸
urobilin [ˌjuərəuˈbailin] *n* 尿胆素
urobilinemia [ˌjuərəuˌbiliˈniːmiə] *n* 尿胆素血
urobilinogen [ˌjuərəubiˈlinədʒən] *n* 尿胆素原
urobilinogenemia [ˌjuərəubiˌlinədʒiˈniːmiə] *n* 尿胆素原血
urobilinogenuria [ˌjuərəubiˌlinədʒiˈnjuəriə] *n* 尿胆素原尿
urobilinoid [ˌjuərəuˈbilinɔid] *a* 尿胆素样的
urobilinoiden [ˌjuərəuˌbiliˈnɔidən] *n* 类尿胆素
urobilinuria [ˌjuərəuˌbiliˈnjuəriə] *n* 尿胆素尿
urocanase [ˌjuərəuˈkæneis] *n* 尿刊酸酶,尿刊酸水合酶
urocanase deficiency 尿刊酸酶缺乏症(一种组氨酸分解代谢遗传性疾病,由于尿刊酸水合酶缺乏所致,特征为尿内大量排泄尿刊酸,发育迟缓,也可能伴有智力迟钝)
urocanate [ˌjuərəuˈkæneit] *n* 尿刊酸(阴离子型)
urocanate hydratase [ˌjuərəuˈkæneitˈhaidrəteis] 尿刊酸水合酶(此酶缺乏据认为是一种常染色体隐性性状,可致尿刊酸酶缺乏症。亦称尿刊酸酶)
urocanic acid [ˌjuərəuˈkænik] 尿刊酸,咪唑丙烯酸
urocele [ˈjuərəsiːl] *n* 阴囊积尿
urocheras [juəˈrɔkərəs] *n* 尿沙
urochezia [ˌjuərəuˈkiːziə] *n* 肛门排尿
urochloralic acid [ˌjuərəukləˈrælik], **urochloric acid** [ˌjuərəuˈklɔːrik] 尿氯酸
Urochordata [ˌjuərəuˈkɔːdeitə] *n* 尾索亚门
urochordate [ˌjuərəuˈkɔːdeit] *n* 尾索(动物)
urochrome [ˈjuərəkrəum] *n* 尿色素,尿色肽
urochromogen [ˌjuərəuˈkrəumədʒin] *n* 尿色素原,尿色肽原
urocinetic [ˌjuərəusaiˈnetik] *a* 泌尿器反射性的
uroclepsia [ˌjuərəuˈklepsiə] *n* 遗尿,尿失禁
urocoproporphyria [ˌjuərəuˌkɔprəpɔːˈfiriə] *n* 尿粪卟啉病,症状性迟发性皮肤卟啉病
urocrisia [ˌjuərəuˈkriziə] *n* 检尿诊病法
urocriterion [ˌjuərəukraiˈtiəriən] *n* 检尿判病[指征]
urocyanin [ˌjuərəuˈsaiənin] *n* 尿蓝质
urocyanogen [ˌjuərəusaiˈænədʒin] *n* 尿蓝质原
urocyanosis [ˌjuərəusaiəˈnəusis] *n* 尿蓝母尿
urocyst [ˈjuərəsist] *n* 膀胱 | **~ic** [ˌjuərəuˈsistik] *a*
Urocystis [ˌjuərəuˈsistis] *n* 条黑粉菌属 | ~ tritici 小麦秆条黑粉菌
urocystis [ˌjuərəuˈsistis] *n*【拉】膀胱
urocystitis [ˌjuərəusisˈtaitis] *n* 膀胱炎
urodeum [ˌjuərəuˈdiːəm] *n* 泄殖道
urodialysis [ˌjuərəudaiˈælisis] *n* 尿闭
urodilatin [ˌjuərəuˈdilətin] *n* 尿舒张肽
urodochium [ˌjuərəuˈdəukiəm] *n* 尿壶,贮尿器
urodynamics [ˌjuərəudaiˈnæmiks] *n* 尿动力学 | **urodynamic** *a*
urodynia [ˌjuərəuˈdiniə] *n* 排尿痛
uroedema [ˌjuərəui(ː)ˈdiːmə] *n* 尿液性水肿
uroenterone [ˌjuərəuˈentərəun] *n* 尿抑胃素(胃分泌抑制药)
uroerythrin [ˌjuərəuˈeriθrin] *n* 尿红质,尿赤素
uroferric acid [ˌjuərəuˈferik] 尿铁酸
uroflavin [ˌjuərəuˈfleivin] *n* 尿黄素
uroflometer, uroflowmeter [ˌjuərəuˈfləumitə] *n* 尿流计
uroflow [ˈjuərəufləu] *n* 尿流量
urofollitropin [ˌjuərəuˈfɔliˌtrəupin] *n* 尿促卵泡素(促性激素类药)
urofuscin [ˌjuərəuˈfʌsin] *n* 尿[紫]褐质
urofuscohematin [ˌjuərəuˌfʌskəuˈhemətin] *n* 尿紫褐血红质
urogaster [ˌjuərəuˈgæstə] *n* 尿肠(胚胎尿囊腔的一部分)
urogastrone [ˌjuərəuˈgæstrəun] *n* 尿抑胃素(胃分泌抑制药)
urogenesis [ˌjuərəuˈdʒenəsis] *n* 尿形成,尿生成
urogenital [ˌjuərəuˈdʒenitl] *a* 泌尿生殖[器]的
urogenous [juəˈrɔdʒinəs] *a* 尿源的;生尿的
uroglaucin [ˌjuərəuˈglɔːsin] *n* 尿蓝质
Uroglena [ˌjuərəˈgliːnə], **Uroglenopsis** [ˌjuərəgliˈnɔpsis] *n* 窝尾虫属
urogram [ˈjuərəgræm] *n* 尿路造影[照]片
urography [juəˈrɔgrəfi] *n* 尿路造影[术] | descending ~, excretion ~, excretory ~, intravenous ~ 下行性尿路造影[术],排泄性尿路造影[术],静脉尿路造影[术] / oral ~ 口服法尿路造影[术] /retrograde ~, ascending ~, cysto-

scopic ～ 逆行性尿路造影[术],上行性尿路造影[术],膀胱镜检查尿路造影[术]
urogravimeter [ˌjuərəugrəˈvimitə] *n* 尿比重计
urohematin [ˌjuərəuˈhemətin] *n* 尿血质,尿血红质
urohematonephrosis [ˌjuərəuˌhemətəuniˈfrəusis] *n* 肾积尿血
urohematoporphyrin [ˌjuərəuˌhemətəuˈpɔːfirin] *n* 尿血卟啉
urohypertensin [ˌjuərəuhaipə(ː)ˈtensin] *n* 尿血管紧张素
urokinase(UK) [ˌjuərəuˈkaineis] *n* 尿激酶(蛋白分解酶)
urokinetic [ˌjuərəukaiˈnetik] *a* 泌尿器反射性的(指一种消化不良)
urokymography [ˌjuərəukaiˈmɔgrəfi] *n* 泌尿(生殖)系统记波摄影[术]
urolagnia [ˌjuərəuˈlægniə] *n* 尿色情
uroleucic acid [ˌjuərəuˈljuːsik], **uroleucinic acid** [ˌjuərəuljuˈsinik] 尿亮酸
urolith [ˈjuərəliθ] *n* 尿石 | **~ic** [ˌjuərəˈliθik] *a*
urolithiasis [ˌjuərəuliˈθaiəsis] *n* 尿石形成,尿石病
urolithology [ˌjuərəuliˈθɔlədʒi] *n* 尿石学
urology [juəˈrɔlədʒi] *n* 泌尿外科学 | **urologic(al)** [ˌjuərəuˈlɔdʒik(əl)] *a* / **urologist** *n* 泌尿外科医生,泌尿外科学家
urolutein [ˌjuərəuˈljuːtiːn] *n* 尿黄色素
uromancy [ˈjuərəˌmænsi], **uromantia** [ˌjuərəuˈmænʃiə] *n* 检尿预后
uromelanin [ˌjuərəuˈmelənin] *n* 尿黑素
uromelus [juəˈrɔmiləs] *n* 单足并腿畸胎
urometer [juəˈrɔmitə] *n* 尿比重计
urometry [juəˈrɔmitri] *n* 尿压测定法 | **urometric** [ˌjuərəuˈmetrik] *a* 尿压测定的
uromodulin [ˌjuərəuˈmɔdjulin] *n* 尿调谐蛋白(即 Tamm-Horsfall mucoprotein)
uromucoid [ˌjuərəuˈmjuːkɔid] *n* 尿类黏蛋白(尿内一种不溶解的黏蛋白质)
uronate [ˈjuːrəneit] *n* 糖醛酸(盐、阴离子或酯)
uroncus [juəˈrɔŋkəs] *n* 尿肿
Uronema caudatum [ˌjuərəˈniːməkɔːˈdeitəm] 尾纤虫
uronephrosis [ˌjuərəuniˈfrəusis] *n* 肾盂积尿
uronic acid [juəˈrɔnik] 糖醛酸,糖羰酸
uron(o) -见 ur(o)-
uronology [ˌjuərəˈnɔlədʒi] *n* 泌尿外科学
urononcometry [ˌjuərəunɔŋˈkɔmitri] *n* 一日尿量测定法
uronophile [juəˈrɔnəfail] *a* 嗜尿的(指微生物)
uronoscopy [ˌjuərəˈnɔskəpi] *n* 尿检查
uropathogen [ˌjuərəˈpæθədʒən] *n* 尿路病原体
uropathy [juəˈrɔpəθi] *n* 尿路病变
uropenia [ˌjuərəuˈpiːniə] *n* 尿过少
uropepsin [ˌjuərəuˈpepsin] *n* 尿胃蛋白酶
uropepsinogen [ˌjuərəupepˈsinədʒən] *n* 尿胃蛋白酶原
urophanic [ˌjuərəuˈfænik] *a* 尿返物的
urophein [ˌjuərəˈfiːin] *n* 尿灰质
urophilia [ˌjuərəuˈfiliə] *n* 恋尿癖
urophobia [ˌjuərəˈfəubjə] *n* 排尿恐怖
urophosphometer [ˌjuərəufɔsˈfɔmitə] *n* 尿磷定量器
uropittin [ˌjuərəuˈpitin] *n* 尿焦质
uroplania [ˌjuərəuˈpleiniə] *n* 异地排尿(在泌尿道以外器官内存尿或排尿)
uropod [ˈjuərəupɔd] *n* 尾肢,尾足,腹足
uropoiesis [ˌjuərəupɔiˈiːsis] *n* 尿生成 | **uropoietic** [ˌjuərəupɔiˈetik] *a*
uroporphyria [ˌjuərəupɔːˈfiriə] *n* 尿卟啉病
uroporphyrin [ˌjuərəˈpɔːfirin] *n* 尿卟啉
uroporphyrinogen [ˌjuərəupɔːfiˈrinədʒən] *n* 尿卟啉原,六氢尿卟啉
uroporphyrinogen decarboxylase [ˌjuərəuˌpɔːfiˈrinədʒən diːkɑːˈbɔksileis] 尿卟啉原脱羧酶(此酶活性减少可伴有迟发性皮肤卟啉病和变异型肝性红细胞生成性卟啉病)
uroporphyrinogen Ⅲ cosynthase [ˌjuərəuˌpɔːfiˈrinədʒən kəuˈsinθeis] 尿卟啉Ⅲ同合酶,尿卟啉原-Ⅲ合酶
uroporphyrinogen-Ⅲ synthase [ˌjuərəuˌpɔːfiˌrinədʒən ˈsinθeis] 尿卟啉原-Ⅲ合酶(此酶缺乏为一种常染色体隐性性状,可致先天性红细胞生成性卟啉病。亦称尿卟啉原Ⅲ同合酶)
uroporphyrinogen Ⅰ synthase [ˌjuərəuˌpɔːfiˈrinədʒən ˈsinθeis] 尿卟啉原Ⅰ合酶,羟甲基[原]胆色烷合酶
uroprotection [ˌjuərəuprəuˈtekʃən] *n* 尿道保护
uroprotective [ˌjuərəuprəuˈtektiv] *a* 尿道保护的
uropsammus [ˌjuərəuˈsæməs] *n* 尿沙
uropterin [juəˈrɔptərin] *n* 尿硫蝶呤
uropyonephrosis [ˌjuərəupaiəniˈfrəusis] *n* 肾盂积脓尿
uropyoureter [ˌjuərəupaiəjuəˈriːtə] *n* 输尿管积脓尿
uroradiology [ˌjuərəuˌreidiˈɔlədʒi] *n* 泌尿放射学
uro-reaction [ˌjuərəuri(ː)ˈækʃən] *n* 尿变碱性反应(检结核病)
urorhythmography [ˌjuərəuriθˈmɔgrəfi] *n* 输尿管口喷尿描记法
urorosein [ˌjuərəuˈrəuziːn] *n* 尿绯质,尿蔷薇红素
uroroseinogen [ˌjuərəuˌrəusiˈinədʒən] *n* 尿绯

质原
urorrhagia [ˌjuərəuˈreidʒiə] *n* 多尿(如糖尿病)
urorrhea [ˌjuərəˈriə] *n* 遗尿
urorrhodin [ˌjuərəuˈrəudin] *n* 尿绯质,尿蔷薇红素(见于伤寒、肾炎、肺结核等病中)
urorrhodinogen [ˌjuərəurəuˈdinədʒən] *n* 尿绯质原
urorubin [ˌjuərəˈruːbin] *n* 尿红质
urorubinogen [ˌjuərəuruˈbinədʒən] *n* 尿红质原
urorubrohematin [ˌjuərəuˌruːbrəuˈhemətin] *n* 尿红高铁血红素(偶见于某些体质病如麻风的尿中)
urosaccharometry [ˌjuərəusækəˈrɔmitri] *n* 尿糖测定法
urosacin [juəˈrəusəsin] *n* 尿绯质,尿蔷薇红素
uroscheocele [juəˈrɔskiəˌsiːl] *n* 阴囊积尿
uroschesis [juəˈrɔskəsis] *n* 尿潴留
uroscopy [juəˈrɔskəpi] *n* 尿[诊断]检查 | **uroscopic** [ˌjuərəˈskɔpik] *a*
urosemiology [ˌjuərəuˌsiːmiˈɔlədʒi] *n* 尿诊断学
urosepsin [ˌjuərəuˈsepsin] *n* 尿脓毒素
urosepsis [ˌjuərəuˈsepsis] *n* 尿脓毒病,尿脓毒症 | **uroseptic** *a*
urosis [juəˈrəusis] *n* 尿路病
urospectrin [ˌjuərəuˈspektrin] *n* 尿分光色素
urostalagmometry [ˌjuərəuˌstæləgˈmɔmitri] *n* 尿表面张力检查;尿滴数检查
urostealith [ˌjuərəuˈstiəliθ] *n* 尿脂石
urothelium [ˌjuərəuˈθiːliəm] *n* 尿路上皮 | **urothelial** [ˌjuərəuˈθiːliəl] *a*
urotoxia [ˌjuərəˈtɔksiə] *n* 尿毒性;尿毒质;尿毒单位(足以杀死 1 kg 体重生物的量)
urotoxic [ˌjuərəˈtɔksik] *a* 尿毒素的
urotoxicity [ˌjuərəutɔkˈsisəti] *n* 尿毒性
urotoxin [ˌjuərəuˈtɔksin] *n* 尿毒素
urotoxy [ˈjuərəˌtɔksi] *n* 尿毒性;尿毒质;尿毒单位(见 urotoxia)
uroureter [ˌjuərəujuəˈriːtə] *n* 输尿管积尿
uroxanthin [ˌjuərəuˈzænθin] *n* 尿黄质,β-吲哚硫酸钾
uroxin [juəˈrɔksin] *n* 双四氧嘧啶
URR urea reduction ratio 尿素减少比
urrhodin [juəˈrəudin] *n* 尿绯质,尿蔷薇红素
ursodeoxycholate [ˌəːsəudiːˌɔksiˈkəuleit] *n* 熊去氧胆酸(石胆酸的解离型)
ursodeoxycholic acid [ˌəːsəudiːˌɔksiˈkəulik] 熊去氧胆酸(胆石溶解药)
ursodeoxycholylglycine [ˌəːsəudiːˌɔksiˌkəulilˈglaisiːn] *n* 熊去氧胆酰甘氨酸
ursodeoxycholyltaurine [ˌəːsəudiːˌɔksiˌkəulilˈtɔːri(ː)n] *n* 熊去氧胆酰牛磺酸
ursodiol [ˌəːsəuˈdaiɔl] *n* 熊去氧胆酸(胆石溶解药)
ursolic acid [əːˈsɔlik] 熊果酸
ursone [ˈəːsəun] *n* 熊果酸
Urtica [ˈəːtikə] *n* 荨麻属 | ~ dioica 大荨麻(具有兴奋、利尿、止血作用)
urticant [ˈəːtikənt] *a* 刺痒的
urticaria [ˌəːtiˈkεəriə] *n* 荨麻疹 | aquagenic ~ 水源性荨麻疹 / ~ bullosa 大疱性荨麻疹 / cholinergic ~ 胆碱能性荨麻疹 / cold ~ 寒冷性荨麻疹 / contact ~ 接触性荨麻疹 / giant ~ 巨大荨麻疹,血管神经性水肿 / heat ~ 热性荨麻疹 / ~ medicamentosa 药物性荨麻疹 / ~ multiformis endemica 地方性多形性荨麻疹(即白蛉皮炎) / papular ~ 丘疹性荨麻疹 / solar ~, light ~ 日光性荨麻疹 | **~l, urticarious** [ˌəːtiˈkεəriəs] *a*
urticariogenic [ˌəːtiˌkεəriəˈdʒenik] *a* 致荨麻疹的
urticate [ˈəːtikeit] *a* 有风块的 *vt* 用荨麻刺激 | **urtication** [ˌəːtiˈkeiʃən] *n* 荨麻疹形成;刺痒;荨麻刺激法
urushiol [juəˈruʃiɔl] *n* 漆[儿茶]酚
US ultrasound 超声
USAN [ˈjuːsən] 美国采用药名(United States Adopted Names 的首字母缩略词,为美国药物命名委员会采用的非专利药名)
Uschinsky's culture medium [usˈtʃinski] (Nikolaus Uschinsky)乌斯钦斯基培养基(天冬酰胺培养基,无蛋白质培养基)
USDA United States Department of Agriculture 美国农业部
Usher's syndrome [ˈʌʃə] (Charles H. Usher) 厄舍尔综合征(一种常染色体隐性遗传综合征,表现为先天性聋,伴色素性视网膜炎,常以失眠告终,有时也发生智力迟钝和步态障碍)
Usnea barbata [ˈʌsniə bɑːˈbeitə] 大松萝(有效成分包括地衣酸,具有抗菌能力)
usnein [ˈʌsniːn] *n* 地衣酸
usnic acid [ˈʌsnik] 地衣酸
USP *United States Pharmacopeia*《美国药典》
USPHS United States Public Health Service 美国公共卫生署
USRDS United States Renal Data System 美国肾数据系统
Ustilaginaceae [ˌʌstiˌlædʒiˈneisiiː] *n* 黑粉菌科
Ustilaginales [ˌʌstiˌlædʒiˈneiliːz] *n* 黑粉菌目
ustilaginism [ˌʌstiˈlædʒinizəm] *n* 黑粉菌中毒
Ustilago [ˌʌstiˈleigəu] *n*【拉】黑粉菌属,黑穗病菌属 | ~ maydis 玉蜀黍黑粉菌
ustion [ˈʌstʃən] *n* 烙
ustulation [ˌʌstjuˈleiʃən] *n* (将药)焙干,煅
ustus [ˈʌstəs] *a*【拉】煅制的

usustatus [juːˈsjuːsteitəs] *n* 站立姿势(指动物)
uta [ˈuːtə] *n* 黏膜皮肤利什曼病
Ut dict. ut dictum【拉】遵医嘱
Utend. utendus【拉】用,用于
uteralgia [ˌjuːtəˈrældʒiə] *n* 子宫痛
uteri [ˈjuːtərai] uterus 的复数
uterine [ˈjuːtərain, -rin] *a* 子宫的
uter(o)- [构词成分] 子宫;同样见以 hyster(o)-, metra-和 metr(o)-起始的词
uteroabdominal [ˌjuːtərəuæbˈdɔminl] *a* 子宫腹的
uterocervical [ˌjuːtərəuˈsəːvikəl] *a* 子宫宫颈的
uterodynia [ˌjuːtərəuˈdiniə] *n* 子宫痛
uterofixation [ˌjuːtərəufikˈseiʃən] *n* 子宫固定术
uterogenic [ˌjuːterəuˈdʒenik] *a* 子宫原的,子宫性的
uterogestation [ˌjuːtərəudʒesˈteiʃən] *n* 子宫妊娠;足月妊娠
uteroglobulin [ˌjuːtərəuˈglɔbjulin] *n* 子宫球蛋白,胚泡激肽
uterography [ˌjuːtəˈrɔgrəfi] *n* 子宫造影[术]
uterolith [ˈjuːtərəliθ] *n* 子宫石
uterometer [ˌjuːtəˈrɔmitə] *n* 子宫测量器 | **uterometry** *n* 子宫测量法
utero-ovarian [ˌjuːtərəuəuˈvɛəriən] *a* 子宫卵巢的
uteropexy [ˈjuːtərəˌpeksi] *n* 子宫固定术
uteroplacental [ˌjuːtərəupləˈsentl] *a* 子宫胎盘的
uteroplasty [ˈjuːtərəˌplæsti] *n* 子宫成形术
uterorectal [ˌjuːtərəuˈrektl] *a* 子宫直肠的
uterosacral [ˌjuːtərəuˈseikrəl] *a* 子宫骶骨的
uterosalpingography [ˌjuːtərəuˌsælpiŋˈgɔgrəfi] *n* 子宫输卵管造影[术],子宫输卵管 X 线摄影[术]
uterosclerosis [ˌjuːtərəuskliˈrəusis] *n* 子宫硬化
uteroscope [ˈjuːtərəskəup] *n* 子宫镜
uterothermometry [ˌjuːtərəuθəːˈmɔmitri] *n* 子宫温度测量法
uterotomy [ˌjuːtəˈrɔtəmi] *n* 子宫切开术
uterotonic [ˌjuːtərəuˈtɔnik] *a* 子宫收缩的 *n* 子宫收缩药
uterotropic [ˌjuːtərəuˈtrɔpik] *a* 向子宫的(如药物)
uterotubal [ˌjuːtərəuˈtjuːbəl] *a* 子宫输卵管的
uterotubography [ˌjuːtərəutjuːˈbɔgrəfi] *n* 子宫输卵管造影[术],子宫输卵管 X 线摄影[术]
uterovaginal [ˌjuːtərəuˈvædʒinl] *a* 子宫阴道的
uteroventral [ˌjuːtərəuˈventrəl] *a* 子宫腹腔的
uteroverdin [ˌjuːtərəuˈvəːdin] *n* 胆绿素
uterovesical [ˌjuːtərəuˈvesikəl] *a* 子宫膀胱的
uterus [ˈjuːtərəs] ([复] **uteri** [ˈjuːtərai]) *n*【拉】子宫
UTI urinary tract infection 尿道感染,尿路感染
utilization [ˌjuːtilaiˈzeiʃən, -liˈz-] *n* 利用 | red cell ~ (RCU)红细胞利用率
UTP uridine triphosphate 尿苷三磷酸
UTP-glucose-1-phosphate uridylyltransferase [ˈgluːkəusˈfɔsfeit ˌjuəridililˈtrænsfəreis] 尿苷三磷酸-葡萄糖-1-磷酸尿苷酰基转移酶(亦称尿苷二磷酸葡萄糖焦磷酸化酶)
UTP-hexose-1-phosphate uridylyltransferase [ˈheksəus ˈfɔsfeit ˌjuəriˌdililˈtrænsfəreis] 尿苷三磷酸-己糖-1-磷酸尿苷酰基转移酶(此酶存在于成人肝脏,但婴儿中缺如。亦称半乳糖-1-磷酸尿苷酰基转移酶)
utricle [ˈjuːtrikl] *n* 小囊;椭圆囊 | prostatic ~, urethral ~ 前列腺囊 | **utricular** [juːˈtrikjulə] *a* 椭圆囊的;囊状的
utriculitis [juːˌtrikjuˈlaitis] *n* 椭圆囊炎
utriculosaccular [juːˌtrikjuləuˈsækjulə] *a* 椭圆囊球囊的
utriculus [juːˈtrikjuləs] ([复] **utriculi** [juːˌtrikjulai]) *n*【拉】小囊;椭圆囊
utriform [ˈjuːtrifɔːm] *a* 囊状的;瓶状的
UV ultraviolet 紫外线
UVA ultraviolet A 紫外线 A
uva [ˈjuːvə] ([复] **uvae** [ˈjuːviː]) *n*【拉】葡萄干 | ~ **ursi** 熊果(叶)
UVB ultraviolet B 紫外线 B
UVC ultraviolet C 紫外线 C
uvea [ˈjuːviə] *n* 眼色素层,葡萄膜 | **~l** *a*
uveitis [ˌjuːviˈaitis] *n* 葡萄膜炎 | granulomatous ~ 肉芽肿性葡萄膜炎 / lens-induced ~ 晶状体性葡萄膜炎 / nongranulomatous ~ 非肉芽肿性葡萄膜炎 / phacoantigenic ~ 晶状体抗原性葡萄膜炎 / posterior ~ 后葡萄膜炎 / toxoplasmic ~ 弓形虫性葡萄膜炎 / tuberculous ~ 结核性葡萄膜炎 | **uveitic** [ˌjuːviˈitik] *a*
uveolabyrinthitis [ˌjuːviəulæbərinˈθaitis] *n* 葡萄膜迷路炎
uveomeningitis [ˌjuːviəuˌmeninˈdʒaitis] *n* 葡萄膜脑膜炎
uveoparotid [ˌjuːviəupəˈrɔtid] *a* 葡萄膜腮腺的
uveoparotitis [ˌjuːviəuˌpærəˈtaitis] *n* 葡萄膜腮腺炎
uveoscleritis [ˌjuːviəuskliəˈraitis] *n* 葡萄膜巩膜炎
uviform [ˈjuːvifɔːm] *a* 葡萄形的
uviofast [ˈjuːviəfɑːst] *a* 抗紫外线的
uviolize [ˈjuːviəlaiz] *vt* 紫外线照射
uviometer [ˌjuːviˈɔmitə] *n* 紫外线测量计
uvioresistant [ˌjuːviəuriˈzistənt] *a* 抗紫外线的
uviosensitive [ˌjuːviəˈsensitiv] *a* 紫外线敏感的
uvitic acid [juˈvitik] 5-甲基苯间二甲酸

uvula [ˈjuːvjulə] ([复] **uvulae** [ˈjuːvjuliː]) *n* 【拉】垂;腭垂 | bifid ~ 悬雍垂裂 / ~ of cerebellum 小脑垂,蚓垂 | **~r** *a*

uvularis [ˌjuːvjuˈlɛəris] *a* 【拉】腭垂的,悬雍垂的 *n* 悬雍垂肌

uvulectomy [ˌjuːvjuˈlektəmi] *n* 悬雍垂切除术

uvulitis [ˌjuːvjuˈlaitis] *n* 悬雍垂炎

uvulopalatopharyngoplasty (UPPP) [ˌjuːvjuləuˌpælətəufəˈriŋgəuˌplæsti] *n* 腭垂腭成形术,腭咽成形术

uvulopalatoplasty [ˌjuːvjuləuˈpælətəuˌplæsti] *n* 腭垂腭咽成形术,腭咽成形术

uvuloptosis [ˌjuːvjulɔpˈtəusis], **uvulaptosis** [ˌjuːvjulæpˈtəusis] *n* 悬雍垂下垂

uvulotome [ˈjuːvjuləutəum], **uvulatome** [ˈjuːvjulətəum] *n* 悬雍垂刀

uvulotomy [ˌjuːvjuˈlɔtəmi], **uvulatomy** [ˌjuːvjuˈlætəmi] *n* 悬雍垂切开术,悬雍垂(部分)切除术

uzara [juːˈzɑːrə] *n* 乌扎拉根(产于非洲,当地人用于治腹泻和痢疾)

uzarin [juːˈzærin] *n* 乌沙苷(止泻药)

V

V valine 缬氨酸;vanadium 钒;vision 视力;volf 伏［特］voltage 电压;volume 容量,容积,体积

$\mathbf{V_H}$ variable region of an immunoglobulin heavy chain 免疫球蛋白重链可变区

$\mathbf{V_L}$ variable region of an immunoglobulin light chain 免疫球蛋白轻链可变区

$\mathbf{V_{max}}$ maximum velocity of an enzyme-catalyzed reaction 酶催化反应的最大速度(见 Michaelis-Menten equation)

$\mathbf{v_T}$ tidal volume 潮气量(肺换气时)

v. vena【拉】静脉

v velocity 速度;voltage 电压

VA visual acuity 视力;Veterans Administration 退伍军人管理局(现称退伍军人事务部 Department of Veterans Affairs〈DVA〉)

VAC vincristine, dactinomycin, and cyclophosphamide 长春新碱-放线菌素 D-环磷酰胺(联合化疗治癌方案)

vaccenic acid ［væk'senik］ 11-十八［碳］烯酸

vaccigenous ［væk'sidʒinəs］ *a* 产生菌苗的

vaccina ［væk'sainə］ *n* 牛痘

vaccinable ［væk'sinəbl］ *a* 可接种的

vaccinal ［'væksinl］ *a* 菌苗的,疫苗的;牛痘的;接种的;有预防力的

vaccinate ［ˌvæksineit］ *vt* 接种疫苗

vaccination ［ˌvæksi'neiʃən］ *n* 疫苗接种,种痘 | BCG ~ 卡介苗接种

vaccinationist ［'væksi'neiʃənist］ *n* 主张种痘者,主张接种者

vaccinator ［'væksineitə］ *n* 接种员,种痘员;种痘刀

vaccine ［'væksiːn］ *n* 疫苗,菌苗;牛痘苗 | anaplasmosis ~ 微粒孢子虫病菌苗(用于预防牛微粒孢子虫病) / anthrax ~ 炭疽菌苗 / anthrax spore ~ 炭疽芽胞菌苗(用于接种家畜以预防炭疽病) / attenuated ~ 减毒疫苗 / autogenous ~ 自身疫苗,自身菌苗 / bacterial ~ 菌苗 / BCG ~, tuberculosis ~ 卡介苗,结核菌苗 / bluetongue ~ 蓝舌疫苗(用于预防绵羊的蓝舌病) / bovine virus diarrhea ~ 牛病毒性腹泻疫苗(用于免疫家畜、预防牛病毒性腹泻) / bronchitis ~ 支气管炎疫苗(用于预防鸡及其他禽类的传染性支气管炎) / Brucella abortus ~ 流产布鲁菌菌苗(用于免疫健康小牛,预防布鲁菌病) / bursal disease ~ 黏液囊病疫苗(用于免疫小鸡,预防传染性黏液囊病) / canine distemper ~ 犬瘟热病疫苗(用于免疫犬,以预防犬瘟热病) / cholera ~ 霍乱菌苗 / coccidiosis ~ 球虫病疫苗(用于诱发鸡的亚临床球虫感染,使之产生对临床感染的免疫力) / diptheria and tetanus toxoids and pertussis ~ 白喉、破伤风类毒素、百日咳菌苗混合制剂,百白破三联制剂 / duck embryo ~ 鸭胚疫苗(预防狂犬病) / duck virus hepatitis ~ 鸭病毒性肝炎疫苗(用于预防鸭病毒性肝炎) / encephalomyelitis ~ 脑脊髓炎疫苗(用于免疫马,预防东部和西部马脑脊髓炎) / equine influenza ~ 马流感疫苗(用于免疫马,预防由流感病毒 A 马株 1 和 2 引起的马流感) / equine rhinopneumonitis ~ 马鼻肺炎疫苗(用于免疫马,由于马疱疹病毒 1 型引起的马病毒性鼻肺炎) / Erysipelothrix rhusiopathiae ~ 猪红斑丹毒丝菌疫苗(用于预防猪的丹毒) / feline panleukopenia ~ 猫传染性粒细胞缺乏性疫苗(用于免疫猫,预防猫传染性粒细胞缺乏症) / feline rhinotracheitis ~ 猫鼻气管炎疫苗(用于免疫猫,预防猫鼻气管炎) / fowl laryngotracheitis ~ 鸡喉气管炎疫苗(用于预防鸡的喉气管炎) / fowlpox ~ 鸡痘疫苗(用于免疫小鸡和火鸡,预防鸡痘) / hepatitis B ~ 乙型肝炎疫苗(用于免疫高危人群,例如医务人员和牙科人员、免疫减弱的患者和需要透析或频繁输血的患者、医院附近的居民和职工、接触带病毒者的人以及男同性恋者) / heterologous ~, heterotypic ~ 异种疫苗,异型疫苗 / influenza virus ~ 流感病毒疫苗 / measles ~ 麻疹疫苗 / measles virus ~ live 麻疹病毒活疫苗(用于儿童的常规免疫以及未患过麻疹或已用活麻疹疫苗免疫过而无抗麻疹血清抗体的青少年和成人的免疫。儿童通常用麻疹-腮腺炎-风疹〈MMR〉三联疫苗免疫。美国药典［USP］正式名称为 mumps virus vaccine live〈腮腺炎病毒活疫苗〉, measles and mumps virus vaccine live〈麻疹和腮腺炎病毒活疫苗〉, measles, mumps and rubella virus vaccine live〈麻疹、腮腺炎和风疹病毒活疫苗〉rubella and mumps virus vaccine live〈风疹和腮腺炎病毒活疫苗〉) / meningococcal polysaccaride ~ 脑膜炎球菌多糖疫苗(在脑膜炎球菌病流行时,本疫苗可给 2 岁以上的儿童注射,常规仅用于军队征募新兵) / mink enteritis ~ 貂肠炎疫苗(用于免疫貂,预防貂病毒性肠炎) / mumps virus ~ live 腮腺炎病毒活疫苗(用于儿童的常规免疫和未患过腮腺炎或已用

活腮腺炎疫苗免疫过的青少年和成人的免疫。）/ Newcastle disease ～ 新城病疫苗（用于免疫鸡，预防新城病）/ ovine ecthyma ～ 羊臁疮疫苗（用于免疫绵羊和山羊，预防传染性臁疮）/ Pasteurella multocida ～ 出血败血性巴氏杆菌菌苗（用于预防由于出血败血性巴氏杆菌3型和4型引起的火鸡巴斯德菌病）/ pigeon pox ～ 鸽痘疫苗（用于预防小鸡和火鸡的鸡痘）/ pertussis ～ 百日咳菌苗 / plague ～ 鼠疫菌苗 / poliomyelitis ～ 脊髓灰质炎疫苗 / pneumococcal polysaccharide ～ 肺炎球菌多糖疫苗（用于免疫2岁以上患慢性心肺肝或肾病、糖尿病、镰状细胞贫血、解剖或功能性无脾症的人以及在肺炎球菌病高危的育婴室或其他在医院工作的人）/ poliovirus ～ inactivated（IPV）灭活脊髓灰质炎病毒疫苗（在美国只用于免疫那些有免疫缺陷的患者或初次免疫那些高危未免疫的成人。亦称索尔克〈Salk〉疫苗，以前称脊髓灰质炎疫苗）/ polyvalent ～ 多价疫苗 / rabies ～ 狂犬病疫苗 / poliovirus ～ live oral（OPV），poliovirus ～ live oral trivalent（TOPV）口服脊髓灰质炎病毒活疫苗，三价口服脊髓灰质炎病毒活疫苗（用于儿童常规免疫，预防脊髓灰质炎。亦称萨宾〈Sabin〉疫苗）/ reocorona viral calf diarrhea ～ 呼肠-冠状病毒性小牛腹泻疫苗（用于免疫新生小牛，预防呼肠病毒和冠状病毒引起的肠病）/ replicative ～ 复制性疫苗（任何一种含有能繁殖的生物体〈其中包括活的和减毒的病毒和细菌〉的疫苗）/ Rocky Mountain spotted fever ～ 落基山斑疹热疫苗 / rubella virus ～ live 风疹病毒活疫苗（用于儿童的常规免疫以及用于未进行过免疫并无风疹血清抗体的已届育龄的未孕妇女的免疫）/ smallpox ～ 牛痘苗，天花疫苗 / split-virus ～ 裂解病毒疫苗（即亚单位疫苗 subunit ～）/ streptococcus group E ～ 链球菌E族疫苗（用于预防猪的链球菌性淋巴结炎〈下颌或颈脓肿〉）/ subunit ～ 亚单位疫苗（由一种病毒的特异性蛋白质亚单位制成的疫苗，亦称裂解病毒疫苗，亚病毒粒子疫苗）/ subvirion ～ 亚病毒粒子疫苗（即亚单位疫苗 subunit ～）/ transmissible gastroenteritis ～ 传染性胃肠炎疫苗（用于预防猪的传染性胃肠炎）/ typhoid ～ 伤寒菌苗 / typhoid and paratyphoid ～ 伤寒和副伤寒菌苗 / typhus ～ 斑疹伤寒疫苗 / yellow fever ～ 黄热病疫苗

vaccinia [vækˈsiniə] *n*【拉】牛痘 | ～ gangrenosa, progressive ～ 坏疽性牛痘，进行性牛痘 / generalized ～ 全身性牛痘 | **~l** *a*

vacciniculturist [ˌvæksiniˈkʌltʃərist] *n* 牛痘苗制造者

vaccinid [ˈvæksinid], **vacciniola** [ˌvæksiniˈəulə] *n* 牛痘疹，全身性牛痘

vaccinifer [vækˈsinifə] *n* 供给痘苗者，可采痘苗者（作为牛痘苗来源的个体）

vacciniform [vækˈsinifɔːm] *a* 牛痘样的

vaccinin [ˈvæksinin] *n* 牛痘苗素

vaccinization [ˌvæksinaiˈzeiʃən, -niˈz-] *n* 连续接种

vaccinogen [vækˈsinədʒən] *n* 菌苗源，疫苗源

vaccinogenous [ˌvæksiˈnɔdʒinəs] *a* 产生菌苗的

vaccinostyle [vækˈsinəstail] *n* 接种刀（接种牛痘苗的双刃小刀）

vaccinotherapy [ˌvæksinəuˈθerəpi] *n* 疫苗疗法，菌苗疗法

Vaccinium [vækˈsːniəm] *n* 乌饭树属，越橘属

vaccinum [vækˈsainəm] *n*【拉】疫苗，菌苗 | ～ antityphicum 抗伤寒菌苗，伤寒菌苗 / ～ pertussis 百日咳菌苗 / ～ pestis 鼠疫菌苗 / ～ typhosum 伤寒菌苗 / ～ typhosum et paratyphosum 伤寒和副伤寒菌苗 / ～ vacciniae, ～ variolae 牛痘苗

VACTERL *v*ertebral, *a*nal, *c*ardiac, *t*racheal, *e*sophageal, *r*enal and *l*imb 脊椎的、肛门的、心脏的、气管的、食管的、肾的和肢体的（用以表示先天性畸形一型的首字母缩拼词，此畸形有时见于有些婴儿，其母亲曾服用过孕激素-雌激素节育丸）

vacua [ˈvækjuə] vacuum 的复数

vacuolate [ˈvækjuəleit] *vt* 形成空泡 [ˈvækjuəlit] *a* 有空泡的 | **~d** [ˈvækjuəˌleitid] *a* / **vacuolation** [ˌvækjuəˈleiʃən] *n* 空泡形成

vacuole [ˈvækjuəul] *a* 空泡，液泡 | autophagic ～ 自体吞噬泡，自噬液泡，自噬小体 / condensing ~s 浓缩泡 / contractile ～ 伸缩泡 / digestive ～ 消化泡，次级溶酶体 / food ～ 食物泡 / heterophagic ～ 异体吞噬泡，异噬体 / plasmocrine ～ 含晶体性空泡（在分泌细胞内）/ rhagiocrine ～ 含胶体性空泡（在分泌细胞内）/ water ～ 水泡（在细胞原生质内）| **vacuolar** [ˈvækjuələ] *a*

vacuolization [ˌvækjuəlaiˈzeiʃən, -liˈz-] *n* 空泡形成

vacuome [ˈvækjuəum] *n* 液泡系，中性红小泡系（细胞内）

vacuum [ˈvækjuəm]（[复] **vacuums** 或 **vacua** [ˈvækjuə]）*n* 真空 | high ～ 高度真空 / torricellian ～ 托里切利真空（气压计管内真空部分）/ ～ extraction 胎头吸引术

VAD ventricular assist device 心室辅助装置

vadum [ˈveidəm] *n*【拉】浅滩，沟滩（脑裂内的小隆）

vagal [ˈveigəl] *a* 迷走神经的

vagectomy [veiˈdʒektəmi] *n* 迷走神经切除术

vagi [ˈveidʒai] vagus 的复数

vagina [vəˈdʒainə]（[复] **vaginas** 或 **vaginae** [vəˈdʒainiː]）*n*【拉】鞘；阴道

vaginal [vəˈdʒainəl, ˈvædʒi-] *a* 鞘的；阴道的；睾

丸鞘膜的

vaginalitis [ˌvædʒinəˈlaitis] *n* 睾丸鞘膜炎 | plastic ~ 肥厚性睾丸鞘膜炎

vaginapexy [ˌvædʒinəˈpeksi] *n* 阴道固定术

vaginate [ˈvædʒinit] *a* 有鞘的

vaginectomy [ˌvædʒiˈnektəmi], **vaginalectomy** [ˌvædʒinəˈlektəmi] *n* 睾丸鞘膜切除术;阴道切除术

vaginiperineotomy [ˌvædʒiniˌperiniˈɔtəmi] *n* 阴道会阴切开术

vaginismus [ˈvædʒiˈnizməs] *n*【拉】阴道痉挛 | mental ~ 精神性阴道痉挛 / perineal ~ 会阴性阴道痉挛 / posterior ~ 后侧阴道痉挛 / vulvar ~ 外阴性阴道痉挛

vaginitis [ˌvædʒiˈnaitis] *n* 阴道炎;鞘炎 | atrophic ~, adhesive ~, senile ~ 萎缩性阴道炎,粘连性阴道炎,老年性阴道炎 / diphtheritic ~ 白喉性阴道炎 / emphysematous ~ 气肿性阴道炎 / granular ~ 粒状阴道炎 / ~ testis 睾丸鞘膜炎 / trichomonas ~ 滴虫阴道炎

vagin(o)- [构词成分]阴道

vaginoabdominal [ˌvædʒinəuæbˈdɔminl] *a* 阴道腹的

vaginocele [ˈvædʒinəˌsiːl] *n* 阴道疝;阴道脱垂

vaginocutaneous [ˌvædʒinəukju(ː)ˈteinjəs] *n* 阴道皮肤的

vaginodynia [ˌvædʒinəuˈdiniə] *n* 阴道痛

vaginofixation [ˌvædʒinəufikˈseiʃən] *n* 阴道[腹壁]固定术

vaginogram [ˈvædʒinəgræm] *n* 阴道 X 线[照]片

vaginography [ˌvædʒiˈnɔgrəfi] *n* 阴道 X 线造影[术]

vaginolabial [ˌvædʒinəuˈleibiəl] *a* 阴道阴唇的

vaginometer [ˌvædʒiˈnɔmitə] *n* 阴道测量器

vaginomycosis [ˌvædʒinəumaiˈkəusis] *n* 阴道霉菌病

vaginopathy [ˌvædʒiˈnɔpəθi] *n* 阴道病

vaginoperineal [ˌvædʒinəuperiˈniːəl] *a* 阴道会阴的

vaginoperineoplasty [ˌvædʒinəuˌperiˈniːəuˌplæsti] *n* 阴道会阴成形术

vaginoperineorrhaphy [ˌvædʒinəuˌperiniˈɔrəfi] *n* 阴道会阴缝合术(修补术)

vaginoperineotomy [ˌvædʒinəuˌperiniˈɔtəmi] *n* 阴道会阴切开术

vaginoperitoneal [ˌvædʒinəuˌperitəuˈniːəl] *a* 阴道腹膜的

vaginopexy [ˈvædʒinəˌpeksi] *n* 阴道固定术

vaginoplasty [ˈvædʒinəˌplæsti] *n* 阴道成形术

vaginoscope [ˈvædʒinəskəup] *n* 阴道镜,阴道窥器 | **vaginoscopy** [ˌvædʒiˈnɔskəpi] *n* 阴道镜检查,阴道窥器检查

vaginosis [ˌvædʒiˈnəusis] *n* 阴道病 | bacterial ~ 细菌性阴道病

vaginotomy [ˌvædʒiˈnɔtəmi] *n* 阴道切开术

vaginovesical [ˌvædʒinəuˈvesikəl] *a* 阴道膀胱的

vaginovulvar [ˌvædʒinəuˈvʌlvə] *a* 阴道外阴的

vagitus [vəˈdʒaitəs] *n*【拉】儿哭 | ~ uterinus 子宫内儿哭 / ~ vaginalis 阴道内儿哭

vagoaccessorius [ˌveigəuˌæksəˈsɔːriəs] *n*【拉】迷走副神经(指迷走神经与副神经脑部的联合)

vagoglossopharyngeal [ˌveigəuˌglɔsəufəˈrindʒiəl] *a* 迷走[与]舌咽神经的

vagogram [ˈveigəgræm] *n* 迷走神经电[流]图

vagolysis [veiˈgɔlisis] *n* 迷走神经(食管支)松解术(为缓解贲门痉挛) | **vagolytic** [ˌveigəuˈlitik] *a* 迷走神经松弛的

vagomimetic [ˌveigəumaiˈmetik, -mi-] *a* 类迷走[神经]的,拟迷走[神经]的

vagosplanchnic [ˌveigəuˈsplæŋknik] *a* 迷走内脏神经的,迷走交感神经的

vagosympathetic [ˌveigəusimpəˈθetik] *a* 迷走交感神经的

vagotomy [veiˈgɔtəmi] *n* 迷走神经切断术 | highly selective ~ 高选择性迷走神经切断术 / medical ~ 迷走神经药物切断术,迷走神经阻滞 / parietal cell ~ 胃壁细胞迷走神经切断术(治十二指肠溃疡) / surgical ~ 外科迷走神经切断术 / truncal ~ 迷走神经干切断术

vagotonia [ˌveigəuˈtəuniə], **vagotony** [veiˈgɔtəni] *n* 迷走神经过敏,迷走神经紧张 | **vagotonic** [ˌveigəuˈtɔnik] *a*

vagotonin [veiˈgɔtənin] *n* 迷走[神经]紧张素(获自胰腺的制剂,增加迷走[神经]紧张、缓慢心律及增加肝内糖原贮藏)

vagotropism [veiˈgɔtrəpizəm] *n* 向迷走[神经]性,亲迷走[神经]性 | **vagotropic** [ˌveigəˈtrɔpik], **vagotrope** [ˈveigətrəup] *a* 向迷走[神经]的

vagovagal [ˌveigəuˈveigəl] *a* 迷走迷走的

vagrant [ˈveigrənt] *a* 游动的

vagus [ˈveigəs] ([复] **vagi** [ˈveidʒai]) *n*【拉】迷走神经

vagusstoff [ˈveigəstɔf] *n* 迷走神经[激]素,迷走神经物质(迷走神经末梢释放的一种抑制心脏活动的物质,或许是乙酰胆碱,或是一种与此密切有关的物质)

Vahlkampfia [vɑːlˈkæmpfiə] *n* 瓦氏变形虫属

vaidya [ˈvaidiɑː] *n*【梵】医师,医生

Vail's neuralgia (syndrome), vidian neuralgia [veil] (Harris H. Vail) 威尔神经痛(综合征),维杜斯神经痛(影响翼管神经的神经痛,一般继发于蝶窦炎,伴发面、颈和肩疼痛)

Val valine 缬氨酸

valacyclovir hydrochloride [ˌvæləˈsaikləuvir] 盐酸伐昔洛韦(抗病毒药)

valamin [ˈvæləmin] *n* 瓦尔米,炔己蚁胺(曾用作催眠、镇静药)

valdecoxib [ˌvældəˈkɔksib] *n* 伐地考昔(非甾体消炎药)

valence [ˈveiləns] *n* 效价;价(化合价,原子价) | biologic ~ 生物学价(同种抗原与抗体分子的结合力) | **valency** *n* 效价;价(化合价,原子价)

Valentin's corpuscles [ˈvæləntiːn] (Gabriel G. Valentin)法伦廷小体(神经组织内的淀粉状蛋白小体) | ~ ganglion(pseudoganglion)法伦廷神经节(假神经节)(①鼓室隆起;②上牙槽神经上的神经节)

Valentine's position [ˈvæləntiːn] (Ferdinand C. Valentine)瓦伦丁卧位(仰卧,双髋屈曲,用于冲洗尿道)

***n*-valeraldehyde** [væləˈrældihaid] *n* 正戊醛,戊醛

valerate [ˈvæləreit] *n* 戊酸盐,戊酸酯

valerian [vəˈliəriən] *n* 缬草属植物(镇痉药和神经兴奋药) | Greek ~ 花葱(溃疡局部敷用)

Valeriana [vəliəˈriːeinə] *n* 缬草属

valerianic acid [vəˌliəriˈænik], **valeric acid** [vəˈliərik] 戊酸

valethamate bromide [vəˈleθəmeit]戊沙溴铵(季铵类抗胆碱能药,解痉药)

valetudinarian [væliˌtjuːdiˈnεəriən] *n* 虚弱者,久病虚弱者 | **~ism** *n* 虚弱,久病虚弱

valganciclovir hydrochloride [ˌvælgænˈsaikləuvir] 盐酸戊更昔洛韦(更昔洛韦〈ganciclovir〉的前药,用于治疗获得性免疫缺陷综合征患者的巨细胞病毒性视网膜炎)

valgus [ˈvælgəs] *a*【拉】外翻的(足),外偏的(手)

validation [ˌvæliˈdeiʃən] *n* 证实 | consensual ~ 同感效证

validity [vəˈlidəti] *n* 效度 | construct ~ 构想效度 / content ~ 内容效度 / criterion ~ 效标效度 / face ~ 表面效度

valine(Val, V) [ˈveiliːn, ˈvæliːn] *n* 缬氨酸

valinemia [ˌvæliˈniːmiə] *n* 缬氨酸血

valine transaminase [ˈveiliːn trænsˈæmineis] 缬氨酸转氨酶

vallate [ˈvæleit] *a* 轮廓形的,杯状的

vallecula [vəˈlekjulə] ([复] **valleculae** [vəˈlekjuliː]) *n*【拉】谷(也可表示会厌谷) | **~r**, **~te** [vəˈlekjulit] *a*

Valleix's points [vɑːˈlei] (Francois L. I. Valleix) 瓦雷点(神经痛时沿某些神经走行有压痛点)

valley [ˈvæli] *n* 谷 | ~ of cerebellum 小脑谷

vallicepobufagin [vəˌlisepəuˈbjuːfədʒin] *n* 垣头蟾蜍精,蟾酥(得自垣头蟾 Bufo valliceps 皮腺中的一种心脏毒)

Valli-Ritter law [ˈvæli ˈritə] (Eusebio Valli; Johann W. Ritter)瓦利-里特尔定律(见 Ritter-Valli law)

vallis [ˈvælis] *n*【拉】小脑谷

vallum [ˈvæləm] *n* ([复] **valla** [ˈvælə])【拉】冈,廓

valnoctamide [ˌvælˈnɔktəmaid] *n* 戊诺酰胺(安定药)

valone [ˈvæləun] *n* 异戊酰茚满二酮(杀虫药,灭鼠药)

valproate sodium [vælˈprəueit] 丙戊酸钠(抗癫痫药,尤其用于抑制癫痫小发作)

valproic acid [vælˈprəuik] 丙戊酸(抗癫痫药,用于治疗癫痫发作,尤其是癫痫小发作)

valrubicin [vælˈruːbisin] *n* 戊柔比星(抗肿瘤药)

Valsalva maneuver (experiment, method, test) [vɑːlˈsɑːlvə] (Antonio M. Valsalva) 瓦尔萨尔瓦动作(①用力呼气,抵住关闭的声门,由此产生的胸内压增加影响静脉回流心脏。亦称瓦尔萨尔瓦实验。②用力呼气,抵住闭合的鼻孔和嘴,引起咽鼓管和中耳内压力增加,以致鼓膜向外移动;从前用作咽鼓管未闭的试验。亦称瓦尔萨尔瓦法或试验)

valsartan [vælˈsɑːtæn] *n* 缬沙坦(血管紧张素Ⅱ拮抗药,促进血管扩张,减少醛固酮作用,用作抗高血压药,口服给药)

Valsuani's disease [ˌvælsjuˈæni] (Emilio Valsuani)瓦尔苏阿尼病(产后及哺乳期妇女的进行性恶性贫血)

value [ˈvæljuː] *n* 价值,值 | acetyl ~ 乙酰价,乙酰值 / acid ~ 酸值 / buffer ~ 缓冲值 / fuel ~ 燃料热值(指食物) / globular ~ 红细胞血红蛋白值,血色指数 / liminal ~, threshold ~ 阈值 / mean clinical ~ 平均临床价值,平均治疗效果

valva [ˈvælvə] ([复] **valvae** [ˈvælviː]) *n* 瓣,瓣膜

valval [ˈvælvəl], **valvar** [ˈvælvə] *a* 瓣的,瓣膜的

valvate [ˈvælveit] *a* [有]瓣的

valve [vælv] *n* 瓣,瓣膜 | artificial cardiac ~ 人造心脏瓣膜 / cage-ball ~ 球笼型瓣(一种人造心脏瓣膜) / porcine ~ 猪瓣膜(一种用戊二醛处理过的猪主动脉瓣制成的心脏瓣膜替代物) / tilting-disk prosthetic ~ 倾斜式碟瓣

valved [ˈvælvd] *a* 有瓣的

valviform [ˈvælvifɔːm] *a* 瓣状的

valvotome [ˈvælvətəum] *n* 瓣膜刀(切心瓣膜用)

valvotomy [vælˈvɔtəmi] *n* 瓣膜切开术

valvula [ˈvælvjulə] ([复] **valvulae** [ˈvælvjuliː]) *n*【拉】瓣,瓣膜

valvular [ˈvælvjulə] *a* 瓣的

valvulitis [ˌvælvjuˈlaitis] *n* 瓣炎;心瓣炎 | rheu-

matic ~ 风湿性心瓣炎(有时不确切地称为风湿性心内膜炎)
valvuloplasty [ˈvælvjuləˌplæsti] *n* 瓣膜成形术
valvulotome [ˈvælvjulətəum] *n* 瓣膜刀
valvulotomy [ˌvælvjuˈlɔtəmi] *n* 瓣膜切开术
valyl [ˈvælil, ˈveilil] *n* 缬氨酰
valylene [ˈvæliliːn] *n* 缬烯炔,异戊烯炔
VAMP vincristine, methotrexate, 6-mercaptopurine, and prednisone 长春新碱-甲氨蝶呤-6-巯基嘌呤-泼尼松(联合化疗治癌方案)
vampire [ˈvæmpaiə] *n* 吸血蝙蝠
Vampirovibrio [væmˌpaiərəuˈvibriəu] *n* 蝙蝠弧菌属
vanadate [ˈvænədeit] *n* 钒酸盐
vanadic acid [vəˈnædik] 钒酸
vanadium(V) [vəˈneidjəm] *n* 钒(化学元素)
vanadiumism [vəˈneidiəmizəm] *n* 钒中毒
Van Allen type familial amyloid polyneuropathy(syndrome) [vænˈælən] (Maurice W. Van Allen)范艾伦型家族性淀粉样蛋白多神经病,衣阿华州型家族性淀粉样蛋白多神经病
van Bogaert-Nyssen-Peiffer syndrome [vɑːnˌbəugεət ˈnaisen ˈpaifə] (L. van Bogaert; R. Nyssen; Jürgen Peiffer)范-奈-派综合征,异染性脑白质营养不良(成人型)
van Bogaert-Nyssen syndrome [vɑːn ˈbəugεət ˈnaisen] (L. van Bogaert; René Nyssen)范-奈综合征,异染性脑白质营养不良(成人型)
van Bogaert's encephalitis, sclerosing leukoencephalitis [vɑːnˈbəugεət] (Ludo van Bogaert)范布盖特脑炎、硬化性脑白质炎,亚急性硬化性全脑炎
van Buchem's syndrome [vɑːn ˈbuːkem] (Francis S. P. van Buchem)范布凯综合征,全身性骨皮质增生症
van Buren's disease [vænˈbjuərən] (William H. van Buren)范布伦病(见 Peyronie's disease)
vancomycin hydrochloride [ˈvæŋkəˌmaisin] 盐酸万古霉素(抗生素类药)
van Deen's test [væn ˈdiːn] (Izaak A. van Deen)范迪恩试验(见 Deen's test)
Van de Graaff machine [væn də ˈgrɑːf] (Robert J. Van de Graaff)范德格雷夫机(高电压静电发电机)
van den Bergh's disease [væn den ˈbəːg] (A. A. Hijmans〈Hymans〉van den Bergh)肠性发绀 | ~ test 范登伯格试验(检胆红素)
van der Hoeve's syndrome [vɑːn dəˈhuːvə] (Jan van der Hoeve)范德赫夫综合征,成骨不全(Ⅰ型)
van der Kolk's law 见 Schroeder van der Kolk's law
van der Velden's test [væn də ˈveldən] (Reinhardt van der Velden)范德韦尔登试验(检胃液内游离盐酸)
van der Waals forces [vɑːn də vɑːls] (Johannes D. van der Waals)范德瓦尔斯力(在原子和分子之间存在相对微弱的短程吸引力,致使非极性有机化合物互相吸引〈疏水结合〉)
Van der Woude's syndrome [vændə ˈwəudə] (Anne Van der Woude)范德伍德综合征(一种遗传性综合征,由常染色体显性遗传性状遗传,包括唇裂和(或)腭裂,伴有下唇囊肿)
van Gehuchten's cells [væn geiˈhuktən] (Arthur van Gehuchten)范格胡克滕细胞(高尔基〈Golgi〉Ⅱ型神经元,即具有分支性短突的神经元) | ~ method 范格胡克滕法(以冰醋酸 10 份、氯仿 30 份、乙醇 60 份的混合液作组织固定法)
Vanghetti's prosthesis [vənˈgeti] (Giuliano Vanghetti)旺盖蒂假体(类似索尔布鲁赫〈Sauerbruch〉的假体,可借残肢的肌肉活动)
van Gieson's stain [vænˈgiːsn] (Ira van Gieson)范吉逊染剂(含酸性品红及三硝基酚水溶液,染结缔组织)
van Helmont's mirror [væn ˈhelmɔnt] (Johannes B. van Helmont)膈中心腱
van Hook's operation [væn ˈhuk] (Weller van Hook)输尿管输尿管吻合术
van Hoorne's canal [væn ˈhɔːn] (Jean van Hoorne)胸导管
Vanilla [vəˈnilə] *n*【拉】香草属,香子兰属
vanilla [vəˈnilə] *n* 香草,香子兰
vanillal [vəˈniləl] *n* 乙基香草醛,乙基香子兰醛
vanillic acid [vəˈnilik] 香草酸
vanillin [ˈvænilin, vəˈnilin] *n* 香草醛,香子兰醛(制药时用作调味剂) | ethyl ~ 乙[基]香草醛(制药时用作调味剂)
vanillism [vəˈnilizəm] *n* 香草中毒,香子兰中毒
vanillylmandelic acid (VMA) [vəˌnililmænˈdelik] 香草扁桃酸,4-羟基-3-甲氧基扁桃酸(尿内 VMA 浓度可用于筛选嗜铬细胞瘤病人)
vanilmandelic acid [ˌvænəlmænˈdelik] 香草扁桃酸(见 vanillylmandelic acid)
Van Slyke-Cullen method (test) [væn ˈslaik ˈkʌlən] (Donald D. Van Slyke; Glenn E. Cullen)范斯莱克-卡伦法(试验)(检血中二氧化碳或血的碱储量及检脲)
Van Slyke-Fitz method [væn ˈslaikfits] (Donald D. Van Slyke; Reginald Fitz)范斯莱克-费茨法(检碱储量)
Van Slyke's formula [væn ˈslaik] (Donald D. Van Slyke)范斯莱公式(不同物质的尿系数 = $D/Bl \times \sqrt{Wt \times V}$,其中 D 表示每日排出尿内物质〈g〉,Bl 为每升血同一物质的克数,Wt 为病人的体重〈kg〉,V 表示 24 小时尿总容量) | ~

method 范斯莱法(检氨基氮) / ~ test 范斯莱试验(检氨基氮及脲)

van't Hoff's law [vænt ˈhɔf] (Jacobus H. van't Hoff)范托夫定律(①物体在溶液内的渗透压等于在同温同压情况下的气压,如果其分子为气体状态并占有与溶液相等的容积;②范托夫规律) | ~ rule 范托夫规律(温度每增高 10 ℃,化学反应的速度增加一倍或一倍以上)

Vanzetti's sign [vənˈtseti] (Tito Vanzetti)旺泽蒂征(坐骨神经痛时,尽管脊柱侧凸,骨盆总是在水平位,但其他伴有脊柱侧凸的损伤,则骨盆倾斜)

vapocauterization [ˌveipəuˌkɔːtəraiˈzeiʃən, -riˈz-] *n* 蒸气烙术

vapor [ˈveipə] *n* 蒸气;呼气

vaporific [ˌveipəˈrifik] *a* 形成蒸气的;蒸气状的,雾状的

vaporish [ˈveipəriʃ] *a* 蒸气状的,多蒸气的

vaporium [veiˈpɔːriəm], **vaporarium** [ˌveipəˈrɛəriəm] *n*【拉】蒸气疗器;蒸气疗室

vaporize [ˈveipəraiz] *vt*, *vi* 蒸发,汽化 | **vaparization** [ˌveipəraiˈzeiʃən, -riˈz-] *n*

vaporizer [ˌveipəˈraizə] *n* 蒸发器

vapors [ˈveipəz] *n* 癔症,疑病症,抑郁症

vapotherapy [ˌveipəuˈθerəpi] *n* 蒸汽治疗

Vaquez's disease [væˈkeiz] (Louis H. Vaquez)真性红细胞增多,红细胞增多症

var. variety 变种

variable [ˈvɛəriəbl] *a* 易变的,可变的,变异的 *n* 变量,变数 | random ~ 随机变量(有一个数值的随机过程的结果) | **variability** [ˌvɛəriəˈbiləti] *n* 变化性,变异性

variance [ˈvɛəriəns] *n* 变化,变异;方差(一个变数与平均数的偏差的平方的平均值)

variant [ˈvɛəriənt] *a* 变异的 *n* 变异体,变型,变种 | L-phase ~ L-相变种(某些细菌的变种相,由渗透压休克、温度休克或抗生素所诱发,由球形体或卵圆形体组成而无硬细胞壁。这些细胞能生长与繁殖,可能是稳定的,也可能回复到正常的菌细胞。亦称 L-型)

variate [ˈvɛəriit] *a* 易变的,可变的,可变异的

variation [ˌvɛəriˈeiʃən] *n* 变异 | allotypic ~ 同种异型变异 / antigenic ~ 抗原性变异 / continuous ~ 连续变异 / idiotypic ~ 个体基因型变异,个体遗传型变异 / impressed ~ 强制变异 / inborn ~ 先天变异 / isotypic ~ 同型变异 / meristic ~ 数量变异 / microbial ~ 微生物变异 / phenotypic ~ 表型变异 / quasicontinuous ~ 类似连续变异 / smooth-rough(S-R) ~ 光滑型-粗糙型(菌落)变异(指菌落型别的变异)

varication [ˌværiˈkeiʃən] *n* 静脉曲张形成;静脉曲张

variceal [ˌværiˈsiːəl] *a* 静脉曲张的,脉管曲张的

varicella [ˌværiˈselə] *n*【拉】水痘 | ~ gangrenosa 坏疽性水痘 / ~ inoculata, vaccination ~ 接种性水痘

varicellation [ˌværiseˈleiʃən], **varicellization** [ˌværiselaiˈzeiʃən, -liˈz-] *n* 水痘接种

Varicellavirus [ˌværiˈseləˌvaiərəs] *n* 水痘病毒属

varicelliform [ˌværiˈselifɔːm] *a* 水痘样的

varicelloid [ˌværiˈselɔid] *a* 水痘样的

varices [ˈværisiːz] varix 的复数

variciform [væˈrisifɔːm] *a* [静脉]曲张样的,[静脉]曲张的

varic(o)- [构词成分]静脉曲张

varicoblepharon [ˌværikəuˈblefərɔn] *n* 睑静脉曲张

varicocele [ˈværikəusiːl] *n* 精索静脉曲张 | ovarian ~, pelvic ~ 卵巢静脉曲张,骨盆静脉曲张 / utero-ovarian ~ 子宫卵巢静脉曲张 | **varicole** [ˈværikəul] *n*

varicocelectomy [ˌværikəusiˈlektəmi] *n* 精索静脉曲张切除术

varicography [ˌværiˈkɔgrəfi] *n* 曲张静脉 X 线摄影[术],曲张静脉造影[术]

varicoid [ˈværikɔid] *a* 静脉曲张样的

varicomphalus [ˌværiˈkɔmfələs] *n* 脐静脉曲张

varicophlebitis [ˌværikəufliˈbaitis] *n* 曲张静脉炎

varicose [ˈværikəus] *a* 曲张的(静脉)

varicosis [ˌværiˈkəusis] *n*【拉】静脉曲张

varicosity [ˌværiˈkɔsəti] *n* 静脉曲张;静脉曲张状态

varicotomy [ˌværiˈkɔtəmi] *n* 曲张静脉切除术

varicula [vəˈrikjulə] *n*【拉】结膜静脉曲张

variety [vəˈraiəti] *n* 变种;品种

variola [vəˈraiələ] *n*【拉】天花 | ~ caprina 山羊痘疮,山羊天花 / ~ crystallina 水痘 / ~ hemorrhagica 出血性天花,黑痘 / ~ inserta 接种后天花 / ~ major 重型天花 / ~ miliaris 粟粒性天花,小疱性天花 / ~ minor, ~ mitigata 类天花 / ~ pemphigosa 天疱疮样天花 / ~ siliquosa 空疱天花 / ~ vera [真性]天花 / ~ verrucosa 疣状天花 | **~r** *a* 天花的,痘的

Variolaria amara [ˌvɛəriəˈlɛəriə əˈmeirə] 苦地衣(石蕊来源)

variolate [ˈvɛəriəleit] *a* 天花样的 *vt* 接种人痘,引痘

variolation [ˌvɛəriəˈleiʃən] *n* 天花接种,人痘接种,引痘法 | bovine ~ 牛天花接种 | **variolization** [ˌvɛəriəlaiˈzeiʃən, -liˈz-] *n*

variolic [ˌværiˈɔlik] *a* 天花的,痘的

varioliform [ˌvɛəriˈəulifɔːm] *a* 天花样的

varioloid [ˈvɛəriəlɔid] *n* 变形天花,轻天花 *a* 天花样的

variolous [vəˈraiələs] *a* 天花的,痘的
variolovaccine [vəˌraiələuˈvæksiːn] *a* 牛痘的 *n* 牛痘苗
variolovaccinia [vəˌraiələuvækˈsiniə] *n* 引种后牛痘(牛接种人痘后所得的痘)
varistor [vəˈristə] *n* 变阻器
varix [ˈvɛəriks] ([复] **varices** [ˌvɛəriˈsiːz]) *n* 【拉】静脉曲张 | anastomotic ~ 吻合性静脉曲张 / aneurysmal ~, aneurysmoid ~ 动静脉瘤性静脉曲张 / arterial ~ 动脉曲张,曲张状动脉瘤 / cirsoid ~ 曲张状动脉瘤,蜿蜒状动脉瘤 / lymph ~, ~ lymphaticus 淋巴管曲张,淋巴管扩张 / papillary varices 辣椒斑,玉红斑
varnish [ˈvɑːniʃ] *n* 涂剂
varolian [vəˈrəuliən] *a* 瓦罗里(Costanzo Varolius)的;脑桥的
Varolius' bridge [vəˈrəuliəs] (Costanzo Varolius 〈Varoli, Varolio〉)脑桥 | ~ valve 回盲瓣
varus [ˈvɛərəs] *a*【拉】内翻的(只与名词连用,如 talipes ~〈内翻足〉)
vas [væs] ([复] **vasa** [ˈveisə])【拉】管,脉管 | **~al** [ˈveisəl, ˈveizəl] *a*
vasalgia [vəˈsældʒiə] *n* 脉管痛
vasalium [vəˈseiljəm] *n* 脉管组织
vascular [ˈvæskjulə] *a* 血管的,脉管的 | **~ity** [ˌvæskjuˈlærəti] *n* 多血管[状态],血管供应,血管分布
vascularize [ˈvæskjuləraiz] *vt, vi* 形成血管,血管化 | **vascularization** [ˌvæskjuləraiˈzeiʃən, -riˈz-] *n*
vasculature [ˈvæskjulətʃə] *n* 脉管系统,血管系统
vasculitis [ˌvæskjuˈlaitis] *n* 血管炎 | hypersensitivity ~, allergic ~, leukocytoclastic ~ 过敏性血管炎,变应性血管炎,白细胞破碎性血管炎 / nodular ~ 结节性血管炎 / segmented hyalinizing ~, livedo ~ 节段性透明性血管炎,青斑血管炎(指下肢慢性复发性血管炎) | **vasculitic** [ˌvæskjuˈlitik] *a*
vasculogenesis [ˌvæskjuləuˈdʒenisis] *n* 血管发生
vasculogenic [ˌvæskjuləuˈdʒenik] *a* 形成血管的,血管化的
vasculolymphatic [ˌvæskjuləulimˈfætik] *a* 血管淋巴管的
vasculomotor [ˌvæskjuləuˈməutə] *a* 血管舒缩的,血管运动的
vasculopathy [ˌvæskjuˈlɔpəθi] *n* 血管病变
vasculotoxic [ˌvæskjuləuˈtɔksik] *a* 血管毒性的
vasculum [ˈvæskjuləm] ([复] **vascula** [ˈvæskjulə]) *n*【拉】小管
vasectomized [væˈsektəmaizd] *a* 切除输精管的
vasectomy [væˈsektəmi] *n* 输精管切除术
vaseline [ˈvæsiliːn] *n* 凡士林,黄石蜡,软石脂
vasifactive [ˌvæsiˈfæktiv] *a* 血管形成的
vasiform [ˈvæsifɔːm] *a* 脉管状的
vasitis [vəˈsaitis] *n* 输精管炎
vas(o)- [构词成分]血管;管
vasoactive [ˌveizəuˈæktiv, ˌvæs-] *a* 血管作用的,作用于血管的
vasoconstriction [ˌveizəukənˈstrikʃən, ˌvæs-] *n* 血管收缩 | **vasoconstrictive** *a*
vasoconstrictor [ˌveizəukənˈstriktə, ˌvæs-] *a* 血管收缩的 *n* 血管收缩药
vasocorona [ˌveizəukəˈrəunə, ˌvæs-] *n* 动脉冠
vasodentin [ˌveizəuˈdentin, ˌvæs-] *n* 血管性牙本质
vasodepression [ˌveizəudiˈpreʃən, ˌvæs-] *n* 血管减压
vasodepressor [ˌveizəudiˈpresə, væs-] *a* 血管减压的 *n* 血管减压药
vasodilatation [ˌveizəuˌdaileiˈteiʃən, ˌvæs-] *n* 血管舒张,血管扩张 | **vasodilative** [ˌveizəuˈdaileitiv, ˌvæs-] *a*
vasodilation [ˌveizəudaiˈleiʃən, ˌvæs-] *n* 血管舒张,血管扩张 | reflex ~ 反射性血管舒张
vasodilator [ˌveizəudaiˈleitə, ˌvæs-] *a* 血管舒张的 *n* 血管舒张药,血管扩张药
vasoepididymography [ˌveizəuˌepiˌdidiˈmɔgrəfi, ˌvæs-] *n* 输精管附睾造影[术]
vasoepididymostomy [ˌveizəuˌepididiˈmɔstəmi, ˌvæs-] *n* 输精管附睾吻合术
vasoformative [ˌveizəuˈfɔːmətiv, ˌvæs-], **vasofactive** [ˌveizəuˈfæktiv, ˌvæs-] *a* 血管形成的
vasoganglion [ˌveizəuˈgæŋgliən, ˌvæs-] *n* 血管网
vasography [vəˈsɔgrəfi] *n* 血管造影[术];输精管造影[术]
vasohypertonic [ˌveizəuˌhaipə(ː)ˈtɔnik, ˌvæs-] *a* 血管增压的
vasohypotonic [ˌveizəuˌhaipəuˈtɔnik, ˌvæs-] *a* 血管减压的
vasoinert [ˌveizəuiˈnəːt, ˌvæs-] *a* 不影响血管舒缩的,无血管舒缩作用的
vasoinhibitor [ˌveizəuinˈhibitə, ˌvæs-] *n* 血管抑制药 | vasoinhibitory *a* 血管抑制的
vasoligation [ˌveizəulaiˈgeiʃən, ˌvæs-], **vasoligature** [ˌveizəuˈligətʃə, ˌvæs-] *n* 输精管结扎术
vasomotion [ˌveizəuˈməuʃən, ˌvæs-] *n* 血管舒缩
vasomotor [ˌveizəuˈməutə, ˌvæs-] *a* 血管舒缩的,血管运动性的 *n* 血管舒缩药
vasomotorial [ˌveizəuməuˈtɔːriəl, ˌvæs-] *a* 血管舒缩的,血管运动性的
vasomotoricity [ˌveizəuˌməutəˈrisəti, ˌvæs-] *n* 血管舒缩能力
vasomotorium [ˌveizəuməuˈtɔːriəm, ˌvæs-] *n* 血

管舒缩系统

vasomotory [ˌveizəuˈməutəri, ˌvæs-] *a* 血管舒缩的,血管运动性的

vasoneuropathy [ˌveizəunjuəˈrɔpəθi, ˌvæs-] *n* 血管神经病

vasoneurosis [ˌveizəuˈnjuəˈrəusis, ˌvæs-] *n* 血管神经病

vaso-orchidostomy [ˌveizəuˌɔːkiˈdɔstəmi, ˌvæs-] *n* 输精管睾丸吻合术

vasoparesis [ˌveizəupəˈriːsis, ˌvæs-] *n* 血管轻瘫

vasopermeability [ˌveizəuˌpəːmiəˈbiləti, ˌvæs-] *n* 血管通透性

vasopressin [ˌveizəuˈpresin, ˌvæs-] *n* 血管升压素,加压素

vasopressor [ˌveizəuˈpresə, ˌvæs-] *a* 血管加压的 *n* 血管加压药

vasopuncture [ˌveizəuˈpʌŋktʃə, ˌvæs-] *n* 输精管穿刺术

vasoreflex [ˌveizəuˈriːfleks, ˌvæs-] *n* 血管反射

vasorelaxation [ˌveizəuriːlækˈseiʃən, ˌvæs-] *n* 血管舒张

vasoresection [ˌveizəuri(ː)ˈsekʃən, ˌvæs-] *n* 输精管切除术

vasorrhaphy [væˈsɔrəfi] *n* 输精管缝合术

vasosection [ˌveizəuˈsekʃən, ˌvæs-] *n* 输精管切断术

vasosensory [ˌveizəuˈsensəri, ˌvæs-] *a* 血管感觉的

vasospasm [ˈveizəuˌspæzəm, ˌvæs-] *n* 血管痉挛

vasospasmolytic [ˌveizəuˌspæzməˈlitik, ˌvæs-] *a* 解[除]血管痉挛的

vasospastic [ˌveizəuˈspæstik, ˌvæs-] *a* 血管痉挛的

vasostimulant [ˌveizəuˈstimjulənt, ˌvæs-] *a* 刺激血管的,促血管舒缩的

vasostomy [vəˈsɔstəmi] *n* 输精管造口术

vasotocin [ˌveizəuˈtəusin, ˌvæs-] *n* 加压催产素,8-精催产素

vasotomy [vəˈsɔtəmi] *n* 输精管切断术

vasotonia [ˌveizəuˈtəuniə, ˌvæs-] *n* 血管紧张 | **vasotonic** [ˌveizəuˈtɔnik, ˌvæs-] *a*

vasotribe [ˈveizəutraib, ˌvæs-] *n* 血管压轧钳,血管压轧器

vasotripsy [ˈveizəuˌtripsi, ˈvæs-] *n* 血管压轧术

vasotrophic [ˌveizəuˈtrɔfik, ˌvæs-] *a* 血管营养的

vasotropic [ˌveizəuˈtrɔpik, ˌvæs-] *a* 促血管的,向血管的

vasovagal [ˌveizəuˈveigəl, ˌvæs-] *a* 血管迷走神经的

vasovasostomy [ˌveizəuvəˈsɔstəmi, ˌvæs-] *n* 输精管输精管吻合术

vasovesiculectomy [ˌveizəuviˌsikjuˈlektəmi, ˌvæs-] *n* 输精管精囊切除术

vasovesiculitis [ˌveizəuviˌsikjuˈlaitis, ˌvæs-] *n* 输精管精囊炎

vastus [ˈvæstəs] *a*【拉】巨大的 *n* 股肌(如股外侧肌 musculus vastus lateralis)

VATER *v*ertebral defects, imperforate *a*nus, *t*racheo *e*sophageal fistula, and *r*adial and *r*enal dysplasia 脊椎缺损,肛门闭锁,气管食管瘘,桡骨及肾脏发育异常(表示一种非随机结合的先天性缺陷的首字母缩拼词)

Vateria indica [vəˈtiəriə ˈindikə] 白达麻香(龙脑香料)

Vater-Pacini corpucles [ˈfɑːtə peiˈsiːni] (Abraham Vater; Filippo Pacini) 环层小体

Vater's ampulla [ˈfɑːtə] (Abraham Vater) 法特壶腹,肝胰管壶腹 | ~ corpuscles 环层小体 / ~ papilla 十二指肠乳头

VATS video-assisted thoracic (or thoracoscopic) surgery 电视胸腔(或胸腔镜)外科

Vaughan-Novy's test [vɔːn ˈnɔvi] (Victor C. Vaughan; Frederick G. Novy) 沃恩-诺维试验(检干酪毒碱)

vault [vɔːlt] *n* 穹窿 | ~ of pharynx 咽穹窿

VC vital capacity 肺活量

VCG vectorcardiogram 心向量图

VCU voiding cystourethrography 排尿期膀胱尿道造影

VCUG voiding cystourethrogram 排尿期膀胱尿道造影片; voiding cystourethrography 排尿期膀胱尿道造影

VD venereal disease 性病

VDEL Venereal Disease Experimental Laboratory 性病实验研究室

VDH valvular disease of the heart 心瓣膜病

VDRL Venereal Disease Research Laboratories 性病研究所

vecordia [viˈkɔːdiə] *n* 轻度精神障碍

vection [ˈvekʃən] *n* 媒介过程

vectis [ˈvektis] *n* 助产杠杆

vector [ˈvektə] *n* 媒介物(尤指动物〈常为节肢动物〉传病媒介);[运]载体;矢量,向量 | biological ~ 生物性媒介物(病原体在媒介动物中能生长繁殖) / mechanical ~ 机械(带虫或带菌)媒介物(仅能携带病原体,而病原体不能在动物体中生长繁殖) / spatial ~ 空间向量 | **~ial** [vekˈtɔːriəl] *a*

vector-borne [ˈvektə ˌbɔːn] *a* 媒介传播的,传病媒介传染的

vectorcardiogram (VCG) [ˌvektəˈkɑːdiəgræm] *n* 心向量图

vectorcardiograph [ˌvektəˈkɑːdiəgrɑːf] *n* 心向量描记器

vectorcardiography [ˌvektəkɑːdiˈɔgrəfi] *n* 心向

量描记术 | spatial ~ 空间心向量描记术
vectoscope [ˈvektəskəup] *n* 矢量显示器
vecuronium bromide [ˌvekjuˈrəuniəm] 维库溴铵(神经肌肉阻断药)
Vedder's culture medium (agar) [ˈvedə] (E. B. Vedder)维德培养基(淀粉琼脂) | ~ signs 维德征(轻压腓肠肌即引起疼痛,以针刺腿前面,可测知其麻木存在,注意膝盖反射的任何改变,当病人蹲踞于脚跟上时,注意病人不使用手则不能起立,为脚气病的体征)
VEE Venezuelan equine encephalomyelitis 委内瑞拉马脑脊髓炎
vegan [ˈvedʒən, ˈviːgən] *n* 绝对素食者 | **~ism** *n* 绝对素食主义
vegetable [ˈvedʒitəbl] *a* 植物的 *n* 植物;蔬菜
vegetal [ˈvedʒitl] *a* 植物的,植物性的;生长的,营养的
vegetality [ˌvedʒiˈtæləti] *n* 植物性
vegetarian [ˌvedʒiˈtɛəriən] *n* 素食者 *a* 素食主义的,素食者的,素食的 | **~ism** *n* 素食主义
vegetate [ˈvedʒiteit] *vi* (赘疣等)生长;长大
vegetation [ˌvedʒiˈteiʃən] *n* 赘生物,赘疣,增殖体;生长,增殖 | adenoid ~ 腺样增殖体(在鼻咽) / bacterial ~s 细菌性赘生物(心瓣膜或心内膜上) / dendritic ~ 树枝状赘疣(一种绒毛状癌) / verrucous ~s 疣状赘生物(在心内膜) | **~al** *a*
vegetative [ˈvedʒitətiv] *a* 生长的,营养的;植物性的,自主[性]的(如自主神经系统)
vegetoanimal [ˌvedʒitəuˈænimәl] *a* 动植物的
VEGF vascular endothelial growth factor 血管内皮细胞生长因子
vehicle [ˈviːikl] *n* [运]载体;赋形剂;媒介物;载色剂
veil [veil] *n* 帆,帘,幕,盖;面纱;羊膜;胎膜
Veillonella [veijɔˈnelə] (Adrien Veillon) *n* 韦荣球菌属
Veillonellaceae [ˌveijɔneˈleisiiː] *n* 韦荣球菌科
Veillon tube [veiˈjɔː] (Adrien Veillon) 韦荣管(一段玻管,一端塞以橡皮塞,一端塞以棉花,培养细菌用)
vein [vein] *n* 静脉(详见附录) | aqueous ~s 房水静脉 / emulgent ~ 泄出静脉(左精索静脉合于左肾静脉处) / hypophysioportal ~s 垂体门静脉(输送垂体的血液至丘脑下部) / primary head ~s 原头静脉(胚胎头内循脑旁连接前主静脉的静脉) / varicose ~s 静脉曲张
veinlet [ˈveinlit] *n* 小静脉
vela [ˈviːlə] velum 的复数
velamen [viˈleimən] ([复] **velamina** [viˈlæminə])【拉】帆,膜 | ~ vulvae 阴门帘
velamentous [veləˈmentəs] *a* 帆状的,膜状的
velamentum [ˌveləˈmentəm] ([复] **velamenta** [ˌveləˈmentə]) *n* 帆,膜
velar [ˈviːlə] *a* 帆的(尤指腭帆)
veliform [ˈvelifɔːm] *a* 帆状的,膜状的
Vella's fistula [ˈviːlə] (Luigi Vella)维拉瘘(一种肠瘘,即在一段分离的肠管,做一个人工开口,其各端均缝于腹壁)
vellosine [veˈləusin] *n* 中美毒葛藤碱
vellus [ˈveləs] *n*【拉】毫毛
velocimeter [ˌveləˈsimitə] *n* 速度计
velocimetry [ˌviːləˈsimitri] *n* 速度测量法 | laser-Doppler ~ 激光-多普勒测速法(利用激光测量红细胞在微循环床的流速)
velocity (*v*) [viˈlɔsəti] *n* 速度,速率 | nerve conduction ~ 神经传导速度
velonoskiascopy [ˌviːlənəskaiˈæskəpi] *n* 针动检影器
velopharyngeal [ˌviːləufəˈrindʒiəl] *a* 腭咽的
velosynthesis [ˌviːləuˈsinθisis] *n* 腭帆缝合术
Velpeau's bandage [velˈpəu] (Alfred A. L. M. Velpeau)维尔波绷带(肩部骨折时用) | ~ deformity 银叉样变形 / ~ hernia 维尔波疝(股血管前股疝)
velum [ˈviːləm] ([复] **vela** [ˈviːlə]) *n* 帆 | artificial ~ 人造腭帆 / nursing ~ (腭裂)哺乳帆
velutinous [vəˈljuːtinəs] *a* 天鹅绒状的,有短绒毛的
vena [ˈviːnə] ([复] **vanae** [ˈviːniː]) *n*【拉】静脉(详见附录)
vena-caval [ˈviːnəˈkeivəl] *a* 腔静脉的
vena caval 腔静脉的
venacavogram [ˌviːnəˈkeivəgræm] *n* 腔静脉造影[照]片
venacavography [ˌviːnəkeiˈvɔgrəfi] *n* 腔静脉造影[术](一般指下腔静脉)
Vena medinensis [ˈviːnə ˌmediˈnensis] 麦地那龙线虫(即 Dracunculus medinensis)
venation [viːˈneiʃən] *n* 静脉分布;脉序
venectasia [ˌviːnekˈteiziə] *n* 静脉扩张
venectomy [viːˈnektəmi] *n* 静脉切除术
veneer [viˈniə] *n* 贴面
venenate [ˈvenineit] *vt* 使中毒 | **venenation** [ˌveniˈneiʃən] *n* 中毒
veneniferous [ˌveniˈnifərəs] *a* 带毒的
venenific [ˌveniˈnifik] *a* 生毒物的
Venenosa [ˌveniˈnəusə] [复] *n* 毒蛇类
venenosalivary [ˌveninəuˈsælivəri] *a* 毒涎的,毒唾液的
venenosity [ˌveniˈnɔsəti] *n* 毒性
venenous [ˈveninəs] *a* 有毒的,毒性的
venenum [viˈniːnəm] ([复] **venena** [viˈniːnə]) *n*【拉】毒物
venepuncture [ˈveniˌpʌŋktʃə] *n* 静脉穿刺术

venereal [vi'niəriəl] *a* 性交的,性病的
venereology [viˌniəri'ɔlədʒi], **venerology** [ˌvenə'rɔlədʒi] *n* 性病学 | **venereologist** [viˌniəri'ɔlədʒist] *n* 性病学家
venerupin [ˌvenə'rupin] *n* 蛤仔毒素
venery ['venəri] *n* 交媾,性交
venesection [ˌveni'sekʃən] *n* 静脉切开术
venesuture [ˌveni'sjuːtʃə] *n* 静脉缝合术
venin ['venin] *n* 蛇毒
veniplex ['venipleks] *n* 静脉丛
venipuncture ['veniˌpʌŋktʃə] *n* 静脉穿刺[术]
venisection [ˌveni'sekʃən] *n* 静脉切开术
venisuture ['veniˌsjuːtʃə] *n* 静脉缝合术
venlafaxine hydrochloride [ˌvenlə'fæksiːn] 盐酸文拉法辛(抗抑郁药,抗焦虑药)
ven(o)- [构词成分]静脉
venoatrial [ˌviːnəu'eitriəl], **venoauricular** [ˌviːnəuɔː'rikjulə] *a* 腔静脉心房的
venoclysis [viː'nɔklisis] *n* 静脉输注
venoconstriction [ˌviːnəukən'strikʃən] *n* 静脉收缩
venofibrosis [ˌviːnəufai'brəusis] *n* 静脉纤维化,静脉[中层]纤维变性
venogram ['viːnəgræm] *n* 静脉造影[照]片;静脉脉搏描记
venography [viː'nɔgrəfi] *n* 静脉造影[术];静脉脉搏描记法 | portal ~ 门静脉造影[术]/ splenic ~ 脾门静脉造影[术]
venom ['venəm] *n* 毒[物],毒液,动物毒素 | snake ~ 蛇毒 / spider ~ 蜘蛛毒
venomization [ˌvenəmai'zeiʃən, -mi'z-] *n* 蛇毒疗法
venomosalivary [ˌvenəməu'sælivəri] *a* 毒涎的,毒唾液的
venomotor [ˌviːnəu'məutə] *a* 静脉舒缩的,静脉运动的
venomous ['venəməs] *a* 毒的,有毒的,分泌毒液的
venoocclusion [ˌviːnəuə'kluːʒən] *n* 静脉闭塞
veno-occlusive [ˌviːnəu ə'kluːsiv] *a* 静脉闭塞的
venoperitoneostomy [ˌviːnəuperiˌtəuni'ɔstəmi] *n* 隐静脉腹膜造口[引流]术
venopressor [viːnə'presə] *a* 静脉血压的 *n* 静脉收缩药
venorrhaphy [viː'nɔːrəfi] *n* 静脉缝合术
venosclerosis [ˌviːnəuskliə'rəusis] *n* 静脉硬化
venose ['viːnəus] *a* 静脉的
venosinal [ˌviːnəu'sainəl] *a* 腔静脉心房窦的
venosity [viː'nɔsəti] *n* 静脉血过多;静脉血供应充裕
venostasis [viː'nɔstəsis] *n* 静脉淤滞
venotomy [viː'nɔtəmi] *n* 静脉切开
venous ['viːnəs] *a* 静脉的
venovenostomy [ˌviːnəuviː'nɔstəmi] *n* 静脉静脉吻合术
venovenous [ˌviːnəu'viːnəs] *a* 静脉静脉的
vent [vent] *n* [气]孔,口(尤指肛孔,肛门);排脓口 | pulmonic alveolar ~s 肺泡间孔
ventage ['ventidʒ] *n* 小孔,小口;气孔
venter ['ventə] ([复] **ventres** ['ventriːz]) *n* 【拉】腹;胃;子宫;窝,凹
ventilate ['ventileit] *vt* 通风;通气 | **ventilative** *a*
ventilation [ˌventi'leiʃən] *n* 通风;通气;言语表达(自己的问题、情绪等,用于精神病学) | assist / control mode ~ 辅助 / 控制式通气 / control-mode ~ 控制式通气 / exhausting ~ 抽气通风 / intermittent mandatory ~ (IMV) 间歇强制通气 / minute ~ 每分钟通气量(亦称总通气量) / plenum ~ 扇入供气 / synchronized intermittent mandatory ~ (SIMV) 同步间歇强制通气
ventilator ['ventileitə] *n* 通风器;通气机 | cuirass ~ 胸甲式通气机 / negative pressure ~ 负压通气机
ventilatory ['ventiləˌtɔːri] *a* 通气的
ventouse [vɔŋ'tuːz] *n* 【法】吸(疗)杯,吸罐,拔罐,火罐
ventrad ['ventræd] *ad* 向腹侧,向前
ventral ['ventrəl] *a* 腹的;腹侧的,前侧的
ventralis [ven'treilis] *a* 【拉】腹的;腹侧的,前侧的
ventralward ['ventrəlwəd] *ad* 向腹侧,向前
ventri- 见 ventro-
ventricle ['ventrikl] *n* 室(如脑室、心室等) | aortic ~ of heart 左心室 / ~s of the brain 脑室 / ~ of cord 脊髓室(中央管) / left ~ of heart 左心室 / pineal ~ 松果体隐窝 / right ~ of heart 右心室 | **ventricular** [ven'trikjulə] *a*
ventricornu [ˌventri'kɔːnju] *n* 脊髓前角 | **~al** *a*
ventricose ['ventrikəus] *a* 一侧膨出的
ventriculi [ven'trikjulai] ventriculus 的复数
ventriculitis [venˌtrikju'laitis] *n* 脑室炎
ventricul(o)- [构词成分]室(脑室,心室)
ventriculoatriostomy [venˌtrikjuləuˌeitri'ɔstəmi] *n* 脑室心房造口[引流]术
ventriculocisternostomy [venˌtrikjuləuˌsistə'nɔstəmi] *n* 脑室脑池造口[引流]术
ventriculocordectomy [venˌtrikjuləukɔː'dektəmi] *n* 喉室声带切除术
ventriculoencephalitis [venˌtrikjuləuenˌsefə'laitis] *n* 脑室性脑炎
ventriculogram [ven'trikjuləˌgræm] *n* 脑室造影[照]片;心室造影[照]片,心室图
ventriculography [venˌtrikju'lɔgrəfi] *n* 脑室造影[术];心室造影[术]

ventriculomegaly [venˌtrikjuləuˈmegəli] *n* 脑室异常扩大
ventriculometry [venˌtrikjuˈlɔmitri] *n* 脑室压测量法
ventriculomyotomy [venˌtrikjuləumaiˈɔtəmi] *n* 室肌切开术(切开闭塞肌带以治疗主动脉下狭窄)
ventriculonector [venˌtrikjuləuˈnektə] *n* 房室束
ventriculopuncture [venˈtrikjuləˌpʌŋktʃə] *n* 脑室穿刺术
ventriculoscope [venˈtrikjuləskəup] *n* 脑室镜 | **ventriculoscopy** [venˌtrikjuˈlɔskəpi] *n* 脑室镜检查
ventriculostium [venˌtrikjuˈlɔstiəm] *n* 脑室瘘
ventriculostomy [venˌtrikjuˈlɔstəmi] *n* 脑室造瘘术
ventriculosubarachnoid [venˌtrikjuləuˌsʌbəˈræknɔid] *a* 脑室[与]蛛网膜下腔的
ventriculotomy [venˌtrikjuˈlɔtəmi] *n* 心室切开术
ventriculovenostomy [venˌtrikjuləuviˈnɔstəmi] *n* 脑室颈静脉造口[引流]术
ventriculus [venˈtrikjuləs] ([复] **ventriculi** [venˈtrikjulai]) *n*【拉】室;胃
ventricumbent [ˌventriˈkʌmbənt] *a* 伏卧的
ventriduct [ˈventridʌkt] *vt* 引向腹侧 | **ventriduction** [ˌventriˈdʌkʃən] *n* 腹侧牵引
ventriflexion [ˌventriˈflekʃən] *n* 前屈
ventrimeson [venˈtrimisn] *n* 腹中线 | **ventrimesal** [ˌventriˈmiːsəl] *a*
ventr(o)-, ventri- [构词成分]腹,腹侧,前
ventrocystorrhaphy [ˌventrəusisˈtɔrəfi] *n* 膀胱腹壁缝合术
ventrodorsad [ˌventrəuˈdɔːsæd] *ad* 向腹背
ventrodorsal [ˌventrəuˈdɔːsəl] *a* 腹背[侧]的
ventrofixation [ˌventrəufikˈseiʃən] *n* 子宫悬吊术
ventrohysteropexy [ˌventrəuˈhistərəˌpeksi] *n* 腹壁子宫固定术
ventroinguinal [ˌventrəuˈiŋgwin] *a* 腹腹股沟的
ventrolateral [ˌventrəuˈlætərəl] *a* 腹外侧的
ventromedian [ˌventrəuˈmiːdjən] *a* 腹侧正中的
ventroposterior [ˌventrəupɔsˈtiəriə] *a* 腹侧[与]后部的
ventroptosia [ˌventrɔpˈtəusiə], **ventroptosis** [ˌventrɔpˈtəusis] *n* 胃下垂
ventroscopy [venˈtrɔskəpi] *n* 腹腔镜检查
ventrose [ˈventrəus] *a* 腹状膨凸的
ventrosuspension [ˌventrəusəsˈpenʃən] *n* 子宫悬吊术
ventrotomy [venˈtrɔtəmi] *n* 剖腹术
venturimeter [ˌventjuəˈrimitə] (G. B. Venturi) *n* 文丘里流量计(如测血液流量)
venula [ˈvenjulə] ([复] **venulae** [ˈvenjuliː]) *n*【拉】小静脉,微静脉
venule [ˈvenjuːl] *n* 小静脉,微静脉 | **venular** [ˈvenjulə] *a*
venulitis [ˌvenjuˈlaitis] *n* 小静脉炎 | cutaneous necrotizing ~ 皮肤坏死性小静脉炎
VEP visual evoked potential 视觉诱发电位
verapamil hydrochloride [vəˈræpəmil] 盐酸维拉帕米(冠状动脉扩张药)
veratric acid [vəˈrætrik] 藜芦酸,3,4-二甲氧[基]苯甲酸
veratroidine [ˌverəˈtrɔidin] *n* 藜芦次碱(神经兴奋药,心脏抑制药)
Veratrum [vəˈreitrɔm] *n*【拉】藜芦属 | ~ album 白藜芦,蒜藜芦(用于治高血压) / ~ viride 绿藜芦(用于治高血压)
verbal [ˈvəːbəl] *a* 言语的,词句的;口头的,口述的
Verbena [vəːˈbiːnə] *n* 马鞭草属
verbenol [və(ː)ˈbiːnɔl] *n* 马鞭草烯醇
verbenone [və(ː)ˈbiːnəun] *n* 马鞭草烯酮
verbigeration [vəˌbidʒəˈreiʃən] *n* 重复言语
verbomania [ˌvəːbəˈmeinjə] *n* 多言狂,饶舌癖
verdigris [ˈvəːdigris] *n* 铜绿(一种碱性醋酸铜,收敛药)
verdohemin [ˌvəːdəˈhiːmin] *n* 氯铁胆绿素
verdohemochromogen [ˌvəːdəuˌhiːməuˈkrəumədʒən] *n* 血绿原,胆绿血色原
verdohemoglobin [ˌvəːdəuˌhiːməuˈgləubin] *n* 胆绿蛋白,胆珠蛋白
verdoperoxidase [ˌvəːdəupəˈrɔksideis] *n* 绿过氧化物酶
Veress needle [vəˈres] (J. Veress)维里斯穿刺针(用于体腔吹气法,如微创外科时用于气腹)
Verga'a lacrimal groove [ˈvəːgə] (Andrea Verga)韦尔加泪沟(从鼻泪管的下口往下通的沟) | ~ ventricle 韦尔加室(穹窿与胼胝体间的裂隙,亦称第六脑室)
verge [vəːdʒ] *n* 边缘;环 | anal ~ 痔环
vergence [ˈvəːdʒəns], **vergency** [ˈvəːdʒənsi] *n* (眼)倾向,(眼)转向
Verheyen's stars [vəˈhaiən] (Philippe Verheyen) 韦海恩星(肾表面星状静脉丛,亦称肾星形小静脉)
Verhoeff's operation [ˈvəːhef] (Frederick H. Verhoeff) 维尔赫夫手术(巩膜后切开术及电离穿刺术,用于视网膜剥离手术) | ~ stain 维尔赫夫染剂(染弹性组织)
Vermale's operation [vəˈmæl] (Raymond de Vermale)韦马尔手术(双瓣贯穿切断术)
vermes [ˈvəːmiːz] vermis 的复数
vermetoid [ˈvəːmitɔid] *a* 蠕虫样的
vermian [ˌvəːmiən] *a* 小脑蚓部的

Vermicella [ˌvəːmiˈselə] *n* 线蛇属
vermicidal [ˌvəːmiˈsaidl] *a* 杀蠕虫的
vermicide [ˈvəːmisaid] *n* 杀蠕虫药
vermicular [vəːˈmikjulə] *a* 蠕虫样的
vermiculate [vəːˈmikjulit] *a* 蠕虫形的
vermiculation [vəːˌmikjuˈleiʃən] *n* 蠕动
vermicule [ˈvəːmikjuːl] *n* 小蠕虫;虫样体 | traveling ~ 动合子
vermiculous [vəˈmikjuləs], **vermiculose** [vəˈmikjuləus] *a* 蠕虫样的;患蠕虫病的
vermiform [ˈvəːmifɔːm] *a* 蠕虫样的
vermifugal [vəˈmifjugəl] *a* 驱[蠕]虫的
vermifuge [ˈvəːmifjuːdʒ] *a* 驱[蠕]虫的 *n* 驱[蠕]虫药
vermilion [vəˈmiljən] *n* 红唇
vermilionectomy [vəˌmiljəˈnektəmi] *n* 红唇缘切除术
vermin [ˈvəːmin] *n* 虫,体外寄生虫(如虱、臭虫、蚤等) | **~al** *a* 蠕虫的,虫的
vermination [ˌvəːmiˈneiʃən], **verminosis** [ˌvəːmiˈnəusis] *n* 蠕虫病,虫病
verminotic [ˌvəːmiˈnɔtik] *a* 蠕虫病的,虫病的
verminous [ˈvəːminəs] *a* 蠕虫的,害虫孳生的
vermis [ˈvəːmis] *n*【拉】蠕虫;蚓部 | inferior ~ 下蚓部(小脑) / superior ~ 上蚓部(小脑)
vermix [ˈvəːmiks] *n* 阑尾
vermography [vəːˈmɔgrəfi] *n* 阑尾造影[术]
vernal [ˈvəːnl] *a* 春天的,春天发生的;青春的
Verner-Morrison syndrome [ˈvəːnə ˈmɔrisn] (John V. Verner; Ashton B. Morrison) 弗纳-莫里森综合征(一种罕见的大量水泻、低血钾和胃酸缺乏综合征,通常伴有血管活性肠多肽含量过多,系因胰内血管活性肠[多]肽瘤〈vipoma〉所致。亦称致腹泻综合征,胰性霍乱或胰性霍乱综合征和 WDHA 综合征)
Vernes' test [ˈvɛənz] (Arthur Vernes) 韦尔恩试验(检梅毒、结核病)
Vernet's syndrome [vəˈnei] (Maurice Vernet) 韦内综合征(第九,十,十一脑神经麻痹,由于颈静脉孔区损害所致,亦称颈静脉孔综合征)
Verneuil's canals [vəˈneiiː] (Aristide A. S. Verneuil) 韦尔讷伊管(静脉侧支) | ~ disease 韦尔讷伊病(梅毒性黏液囊病) / ~ neuroma 韦尔讷伊神经瘤(丛状神经瘤)
vernier [ˈvəːnjə] *n* 游尺,游标尺
vernin [ˈvəːnin] *n* 蚕豆嘌呤核苷,蚕豆腺嘌呤戊糖苷
vernix [ˈvəːniks] *n*【拉】涂剂
Vernonia anthelmintica [vəˈnəuniə ˌænθəlˈmintikə] 驱虫斑鸠菊
Verocay bodies [ˈverəkei] (José Verocay) 维罗凯体(神经纤维瘤中的螺旋状细胞群)
verocytotoxin [ˌverəuˌsaitəuˈtɔksin] *n* 绿猴肾细胞毒素(亦称志贺〈Shiga〉杆菌样毒素)
vérole [veiˈrəul] *n*【法】梅毒 | ~ nerveuse 神经梅素
verotoxin [ˌverəuˈtɔksin] *n* 绿猴肾细胞毒素(Vero cell 为非洲绿猴肾细胞株系)
verruca [vəˈruːkə] ([复] **verrucae** [veˈruːsiː]) *n*【拉】疣,瘊 | ~ acuminata 尖锐湿疣 / ~ digitata 指状疣 / ~ filiformis 丝状疣, ~ peruana, ~ peruviana 秘鲁疣 / ~ plana, ~ plana juvenilis 扁平疣,青年扁平疣 / ~ plantaris 跖疣,足底疣 / ~ seborrheica, ~ senilis 老年疣,皮脂溢性角化病 / ~ vulgaris 寻常疣
verrucarin [vəˈruːkərin] *n* 疣孢菌素
verruciform [veˈruːsifɔːm] *a* 疣状的
verrucosis [ˌveruːˈkəusis] *n* 疣病
verrucous [ˈverukəs], **verrucose** [veˈruːkəus] *a* 有疣的,疣的
verruga [veˈruːgə] *n*【西】疣,瘊 | ~ peruana 秘鲁疣
versicolor [ˈvəːsikʌlə] *a* 杂色的,多色的,花斑的
version [ˈvəːʃən, -ʒən] *n* 转向,转位;子宫倾侧;(胎位)倒转术,转胎位术;(两眼)共轭旋转 | bimanual ~, combined ~ 内外倒转术,联合转胎位术 / bipolar ~ 两极倒转术 / cephalic ~ 胎头倒转术 / external ~, abdominal ~ 外转胎位术 / internal ~ 内转胎位术 / pelvic ~ 胎臀倒转术 / podalic ~ 胎足倒转术 / spontaneous ~ 自然倒转
vertebra [ˈvəːtibrə] ([复] **vertebras** 或 **vertebrae** [ˈvəːtibriː]) *n*【拉】椎骨,脊椎 | abdominal ~e 腰椎 / basilar ~ 基椎,末腰椎 / false ~e 假椎(骶尾椎) / prominent ~ 隆椎(第七颈椎) / sternal ~ 胸骨节,胸杠 | **~l** *a*
vertebrarium [ˌvəːtiˈbrɛəriəm] *n*【拉】脊柱
vertebrate collagenase [ˈvəːtibreit ˈkɔlədʒeneis] 脊椎动物胶原酶
vertebrarterial [ˌvəːtibrɑːˈtiəriəl] *a* 椎动脉的
Vertebrata [ˌvəːtiˈbreitə] *n* 脊椎动物亚门
vertebrate [ˈvəːtibrit] *a* 有脊椎的,脊椎动物的 *n* 脊椎动物 | **~d** [ˈvəːtibreitid] *a* 脊椎状的;有脊椎的
vertebrectomy [ˌvəːtiˈbrektəmi] *n* 椎骨切除术
vertebr(o)- [构词成分]椎骨,脊椎
vertebroarterial [ˌvəːtibrəuɑːˈtiəriəl] *a* 椎动脉的
vertebrobasilar [ˌvəːtibrəuˈbæsilə] *a* 脊椎基底动脉的
vertebrocarotid [ˌvəːtibrəukəˈrɔtid] *a* 椎动脉颈动脉的,颈动脉椎动脉的
vertebrochondral [ˌvəːtibrəuˈkɔndrəl] *a* 椎骨肋软骨的

vertebrocostal [ˌvəːtibrəuˈkɔstl] *a* 椎肋的
vertebrodidymus [ˌvəːtibrəuˈdidiməs], **vertebrodymus** [ˌvəːtiˈbrɔdiməs] *n* 脊柱联胎
vertebrofemoral [ˌvəːtibrəuˈfemərəl] *a* 椎股的
vertebrogenic [ˌvəːtibrəuˈdʒenik] *a* 脊椎源性的,脊柱源性的
vertebroiliac [ˌvəːtibrəuˈiliæk] *a* 椎髂的
vertebromammary [ˌvəːtibrəuˈmæməri] *a* 椎骨乳房的
vertebroplasty [ˈvəːtibrəuˌplæsti] *n* 椎骨成形术
vertebrosacral [ˌvəːtibrəuˈseikrəl] *a* 椎骶的
vertebrosternal [ˌvəːtibrəuˈstəːnəl] *a* 椎骨胸骨的
verteporfin [ˌvəːtəˈpɔːfin] *n* 维替卟吩(光致敏药)
vertex [ˈvəːteks] ([复] **vertexes** 或 **vertices** [ˈvəːtisiːz]) *n*【拉】顶点;顶,头顶 | ~ of bony cranium 颅骨顶 / ~ cordis 心尖 / ~ of cornea 角膜顶 / ~ of urinary bladder 膀胱顶,膀胱尖
vertical [ˈvəːtikəl] *a* 垂直的;顶点的,头顶的
verticalis [ˌvəːtiˈkeilis] *a*【拉】垂直的
verticillate [vəːˈtisilit] *a* 轮生的,环生的
Verticillium [ˌvəːtiˈsiljəm] *n* 轮枝孢菌属 | ~ graphii 耳炎轮枝孢菌,圆轮霉菌(有时见于外耳炎和真菌性角膜炎)
verticine [ˈvəːtisin] *n* 浙贝母碱甲
verticomental [ˌvəːtikəuˈmentl] *a* 顶颏的
vertiginous [vəːˈtidʒinəs] *a* 眩晕的
vertigo [ˈvəːtigəu, vəːˈtaigəu] *n* 眩晕 | ~ ab aure laeso 耳性眩晕 / alterobaric ~, pressure ~ 变压性眩晕 / auditory ~, aural ~ 耳性眩晕 / benign paroxysmal positional (or postural) ~ 良性阵发性体位性眩晕 / central ~ 中枢性眩晕 / disabling positional ~ 体位性失能眩晕 / encephalic ~ 脑性眩晕 / essential ~ 特发性眩晕 / gastric ~ 胃性眩晕 / height ~ 高处俯视性眩晕 / horizontal ~ 水平位眩晕 / laryngeal ~ 喉性眩晕,剧咳后晕厥 / objective ~ 客观眩晕,物景(转动)性眩晕 / primary ~ 原发性眩晕 / residual ~ 残余性眩晕 / riders' ~ 乘车性眩晕,晕车 / subjective ~ 自体性眩晕,主观眩晕 / vertical ~ 垂直视性眩晕 / vestibular ~ 前庭性眩晕 / villous ~ 肝病性眩晕
vertigraphy [vəːˈtigrəfi] *n* 体层 X 线摄影[术]
verumontanitis [ˌviːrjuˌmɔntəˈnaitis] *n* 精阜炎
verumontanum [ˌviːrjumɔnˈteinəm] *n* 精阜
vesalian [viˈseiliən] (Andreas Vesalius) *a* 韦萨留斯的(如 ~ bone 第五跖骨粗隆)
vesalianum [viˌseiliˈeinəm] (Andreas Vesalius) *n* 韦萨留斯骨(由第五跖骨粗隆分离而成的籽骨)
Vesalius' foramen [viˈseiliəs] (Andreas Vesalius) 韦萨留斯孔(蝶骨卵圆孔内侧的小孔) | ~ ligament 腹股沟韧带
vesania [viˈseiniə] *n*【拉】精神错乱,精神病(指严重的精神障碍,分四期:躁狂症、忧郁症、偏执狂与痴呆) | **vesanic** [viˈsænik] *a* 精神病的,躁狂的,疯癫的
Vesic. vesicula, vesicatorium【拉】囊,泡;[小]水疱
vesica [ˈvesikə, viˈsai-] ([复] **vesicae** [ˈvesisiː, viˈsai-]) *n*【拉】膀胱;囊,泡
vesical [ˈvesikəl] *a* 囊的,泡的;膀胱的
vesicant [ˈvesikənt], **vesicatory** [ˌvesiˈkeitəri] *a* 发疱的,起疱的 *n* 起疱剂
vesicate [ˈvesikeit] *vt, vi* 发疱,起疱 | **vesication** [ˌvesiˈkeiʃən] *n* 发疱,起疱;疱
vesicle [ˈvesikl] *n* 囊,泡;小水泡 | acrosomal ~ 顶体泡 / auditory, otic ~ 听泡,听囊 / brain ~s 脑泡 / chorionic ~ 绒毛膜 / concentrating ~s 浓缩泡 / false spermatic ~ 前列腺囊 / germinal ~ 胚泡(未熟卵核) / intermediate ~s 中间泡,运输小泡 / matrix ~ 基质小泡 / multilocular ~, compound ~, kerionic ~ 多房水泡(皮肤) / ocular ~, ophthalmic ~, optic ~ 眼泡 / phagocytotic ~ 吞噬体,吞噬泡 / pinocytotic ~ 胞饮小体,胞饮泡,饮液泡 / seminal ~ 精囊 / synaptic ~s 突触小泡 / transfer ~s, transitional ~, transport ~ 运输小泡(亦称中间泡) / water expulsion ~ 排水泡,收缩泡
vesic(o)- [构词成分]膀胱;囊,泡,水疱
vesicoabdominal [ˌvesikəuæbˈdɔminəl] *a* 膀胱腹的
vesicocavernous [ˌvesikəuˈkævənəs] *a* 肺泡空洞性的
vesicocele [ˈvesikəˌsiːl] *n* 膀胱膨出
vesicocervical [ˌvesikəuˈsəːvikəl] *a* 膀胱宫颈的
vesicoclysis [ˌvesiˈkɔklisis] *n* 膀胱灌洗术
vesicocolic [ˌvesikəuˈkɔlik] *a* 膀胱结肠的
vesicocolonic [ˌvesikəukəˈlɔnik] *a* 膀胱结肠的
vesicofixation [ˌvesikəufikˈseiʃən] *n* 膀胱固定术
vesicoileal [ˌvesikəuˈiliəl] *a* 膀胱回肠的,回肠膀胱的
vesicointestinal [ˌvesikəuinˈtestinl], **vesicoenteric** [ˌvesikəuenˈterik] *a* 膀胱肠的
vesicolithotomy [ˌvesikəuliˈθɔtəmi] *n* 膀胱切开取石术
vesicoperineal [ˌvesikəuˌperiˈniːəl] *a* 膀胱会阴的
vesicopexy [ˈvesikəuˌpeksi] *n* 膀胱固定术
vesicoprostatic [ˌvesikəuprɔsˈtætik] *a* 膀胱前列腺的
vesicopubic [ˌvesikəuˈpjubik] *a* 膀胱耻骨的
vesicopustule [ˌvesikəuˈpʌstjuːl] *n* 水脓疱,脓性水泡
vesicorectal [ˌvesikəuˈrektəl] *a* 膀胱直肠的

vesicorenal [ˌvesikəuˈriːnl] *a* 膀胱肾的
vesicosigmoid [ˌvesikəuˈsigmɔid] *a* 膀胱乙状结肠的
vesicosigmoidostomy [ˌvesikəuˌsigmɔiˈdɔstəmi] *n* 膀胱乙状结肠吻合术
vesicospinal [ˌvesikəuˈspainl] *a* 膀胱脊椎的
vesicostomy [ˌvesiˈkɔstəmi] *n* 膀胱造口术
vesicotomy [ˌvesiˈkɔtəmi] *n* 膀胱切开术
vesicoumbilical [ˌvesikəuʌmˈbilikəl] *a* 膀胱脐的
vesicourachal [ˌvesikəuˈjuərəkəl] *a* 膀胱脐尿管的
vesicoureteral [ˌvesikəujuəˈriːtərəl], **vesicoureteric** [ˌvesikəuˌjuəriˈterik] *a* 膀胱输尿管的
vesicourethral [ˌvesikəujuəˈriːθrəl] *a* 膀胱尿道的
vesicouterine [ˌvesikəuˈjuːtərin] *a* 膀胱子宫的
vesicouterovaginal [ˌvesikəuˌjuːtərəuˈvædʒinəl] *a* 膀胱子宫阴道的
vesicovaginal [ˌvesikəuˈvædʒinəl] *a* 膀胱阴道的
vesicovaginorectal [ˌvesikəuˌvædʒinəuˈrektəl] *a* 膀胱阴道直肠的
vesicula [viˈsikjulə] ([复] **vesiculae** [viˈsikjuliː]) *n*【拉】囊,泡;[小]水疱
vesicular [viˈsikjulə] *a* 囊状的,泡状的;水疱的
vesiculase [viˈsikjuleis] *n* 精液凝固酶
vesiculate [viˈsikjulit] *a* 有小泡的;小囊状的 [viˈsikjuleit] *vt*, *vi* 起疱,成疱 | **~d** [viˈsikjuˌleitid] *a* 起疱的,成疱的 | **vesiculation** [viˌsikjuˈleiʃən] *n* 起泡,水疱形成
vesiculectomy [viˌsikjuˈlektəmi] *n* 囊切除术(尤指精囊切除术)
vesiculiform [viˈsikjuliˌfɔːm] *a* 囊状的,泡状的
vesiculitis [viˌsikjuˈlaitis] *n* 囊炎(尤指精囊炎) | seminal ~ 精囊炎
vesiculobronchial [viˌsikjuləuˈbrɔŋkiəl] *a* 肺泡支气管性的
vesiculocavernous [viˌsikjuləuˈkævənəs] *a* 肺泡空洞性的
vesiculogram [viˈsikjuləgræm] *n* 精囊造影[照]片
vesiculography [viˌsikjuˈlɔgrəfi] *n* 精囊造影[术]
vesiculopapular [viˌsikjuləuˈpæpjulə] *a* 水疱丘疹的
vesiculopustular [viˌsikjuləuˈpʌstjulə] *a* 水疱脓疱的
vesiculotomy [viˌsikjuˈlɔtəmi] *n* 囊切开术
vesiculotubular [viˌsikjuləuˈtjuːbjulə] *a* 肺泡支气管性的
vesiculotympanic [viˌsikjuləutimˈpænik] *a* 肺泡鼓性的
vesiculotympanitic [viˌsikjuləutimpɔˈnitik] *a* 肺泡鼓性的
Vesiculovirus [vəˈsikjuləuˌvaiərəs] *n* 水疱性病毒属
Vespa [ˈvespə] *n* 黄蜂属
vesperal [ˈvespərəl] *a* 黄昏的,夜晚的
Vespidae [ˈvespidiː] *n* 黄蜂科
Vespula [ˈvespjulə] *n* 黄蜂属
vessel [ˈvesl] *n* 管,脉管 | arterioluminal ~s 小动脉心腔小管 / arteriosinusoidal ~s 小动脉血窦小管 / bile ~ 胆管 / blood ~ 血管 / chyliferous ~s, lacteal ~s 乳糜管 / collateral ~ 并行管;侧副管 / hemorrhoidal ~s 痔血管(直肠曲张静脉) / lymphatic ~s, absorbent ~s 淋巴管 / nutrient ~s 营养血管
vessicnon [ˈvesiknɔn], **vessignon** [ˌvesiˈnjɔn] *n*【法】后胭滑膜瘤(马)
vestibula [vesˈtibjulə] vestibulum 的复数
vestibule [ˈvestibjuːl] *n* 前庭 | ~ of ear 耳前庭 / ~ of mouth 口腔前庭 / ~ of pharynx 咽门;口咽 / ~ of vagina, ~ of vulva 阴道前庭 | **vestibular** [vesˈtibjulə] *a*
Vestibuliferia [vesˌtibjuliˈfiəriə] *n* 前庭亚纲
vestibulitis [vesˌtibjuˈlaitis] *n* 前庭炎
vestibulocerebellum [vesˌtibjuləuˌseriˈbeləm] *n* 前庭小脑,古小脑
vestibulocochlear [vesˌtibjuləuˈkɔkliə] *a* 前庭蜗的
vestibulogenic [vesˌtibjuləuˈdʒenik] *a* 前庭源性的
vestibulo-ocular [vesˌtibjuləuˈɔkjulə] *a* 前庭眼的
vestibuloplasty [vesˈtibjuləˌplæsti] *n* 前庭成形术
vestibulotomy [vesˌtibjuˈlɔtəmi] *n* (耳)前庭切开术
vestibulourethral [vesˌtibjuləujuəˈriːθrəl] *a* (阴道)前庭[与]尿道的
vestibulum [vesˈtibjuləm] ([复] **vestibula** [vesˈtibjulə]) *n*【拉】前庭
vestige [ˈvestidʒ] *n* 遗迹,剩件,剩余 | coccygeal ~ 神经管尾端遗迹 / ~ of vaginal process 鞘突遗迹 | **vestigial** [vesˈtidʒiəl] *a*
vestigium [vesˈtidʒiəm] ([复] **vestigia** [vesˈtidʒiə]) *n*【拉】遗迹,剩件,剩余
vesuvine [viˈsjuːviːn] *n* 苯胺棕,俾斯麦棕 R(即 Bismark brown R)
veta [ˈveitə] *n*【西】高山病
vetch [vetʃ] *n* 豌豆,巢菜;山黧豆
veterinarian [ˌvetəriˈnɛəriən] *n* 兽医
veterinary [ˈvetərinəri] *a* 兽医的 *n* 兽医
VF vocal fremitus 语音震颤

vf field of vision 视野
VFib ventricular fibrillation 心室纤颤,心室颤动
VFl ventricular flutter 心室扑动
VHDL very-high-density lipoprotein 极高密度脂蛋白
viable [ˈvaiəbl] *a* 能生存的,能活的(尤指胎儿已发育到在子宫外能活的阶段) | **viability** [ˌvaiəˈbiləti] *n* 生活能力,生存能力
vial [ˈvaiəl] *n* 小瓶 *vt* 放…于小瓶中
vibesate [ˈvaibəseit] *n* 维必塞(一种聚乙烯制剂,用以封闭伤口)
vibex [ˈvaibeks] ([复] **vibices** [viˈbaisiːz]) *n* 淤线(一种线形皮下血性渗出物)
vibratile [ˈvaibrətail] *a* 振动的,震动的
vibration [vaiˈbreiʃən] *n* 振动,震动;震颤法,振动按摩法 | photoelectric ~ 光电振动(在圆锥,圆柱细胞内)
vibrative [ˈvaibrətiv] *a* 振动的,震动的 [ˈvibrətiv] *n* 振动音,震颤音
vibratode [ˈvaibrətəud] *n* 振动器极
vibrator [vaiˈbreitə] *n* 振动器
vibratory [ˈvaibrətəri] *a* 振动的,震动的
Vibrio [ˈvibriəu] *n* 弧菌属 | ~ alginolyticus 溶藻弧菌 / ~ anguillarum 鳗弧菌 / ~ cholerae 霍乱弧菌 / ~ cholerae biotype albensis 霍乱弧菌易北河型 / ~ cholerae biotype cholerae 霍乱弧菌霍乱型 / ~ cholerae biotype eltor 霍乱弧菌埃尔托型 / ~ cholerae biotype proteus 霍乱弧菌变形型(即麦奇尼科夫弧菌 ~ metschnikovii) / ~ coli 大肠弧菌,空肠弯曲菌 / ~ comma 逗点状弧菌,霍乱弧菌 / ~ danubicus 多瑙河弧菌 / ~ eltor 埃尔托弧菌 / ~ fetus 胎弧菌 / ~ fluvialis 河流弧菌 / ~ ghinda 京达弧菌 / ~ group EF-6, ~ group F EF-6 群弧菌,F 群弧菌 / ~ harveyi 哈氏弧菌 / ~ hollisae 霍氏弧菌 / ~ jejuni 空肠弧菌 / ~ massauah 马萨奥弧菌(假弧菌) / ~ metchnikovii 麦奇尼科夫弧菌 / ~ mimicus 拟态弧菌 / noncholera ~s (NCVs) 非霍乱弧菌 / ~ parahaemolyticus 副溶血性弧菌 / ~ phosphorescens 磷光弧菌,霍乱弧菌易北河型 / ~ proteus 变形弧菌 / ~ piscium 鱼弧菌 / ~ septicus 败血型弧菌 / ~ succinogenes 产琥珀弧菌 / ~ tyrogenus 干酪弧菌
vibrio [ˈvibriəu] ([复] **vibrios** 或 **vibriones** [vibriˈəuniːz]) *n* 弧菌 | Celebes ~ 西里伯斯弧菌 / El Tor ~ 埃尔托弧菌 / NAG ~s, nonagglutinating ~s 非凝集弧菌 / paracholera ~s 副霍乱弧菌
vibriocidal [ˌvibriəuˈsaidl] *a* 杀弧菌的(尤杀霍乱弧菌)
vibrion [ˌvibriˈɔn] *n*【法】弧菌 | ~ septique 败血型弧菌,败血梭状芽胞杆菌
Vibrionaceae [ˌvibriəuˈneisiiː] *n* 弧菌科
vibriones [vibriˈəuniːz] vibrio 的复数
vibriosis [ˌvibriˈəusis] *n* 弧菌病
vibrissa [vaiˈbrisə] ([复] **vibrissae** [vaiˈbrisiː]) *n*【拉】鼻毛(人的);触须(犬、猫等动物的)
vibroacoustic [ˌvaibrəuəˈkuːstik] *a* 振动声学的
vibrocardiogram [ˌvaibrəuˈkɑːdiəgræm] *n* 心振动[描记]图
vibrocardiography [ˌvaibrəuˌkɑːdiˈɔgrəfi] *n* 心振动描记术
vibrolode [ˈvaibrələud] *n* 振动器极
vibromasseur [ˌvibrəuməˈsəː] *n*【法】振动按摩器
vibrometer [vaiˈbrɔmitə] *n* 振动治聋器
vibrophone [ˈvibrəfəun] *n* 鼓膜振动器
vibrophonocardiograph [ˌvaibrəuˌfəunəuˈkɑːdiəgrɑːf] *n* 心振动心音描记器
vibrotherapeutics [ˌvaibrəuθerəˈpjuːtiks] *n* 振动疗法
viburnic acid [vaiˈbəːnik] 荚蒾酸
Viburnum [vaiˈbəːnəm] *n*【拉】荚蒾属 | ~ opulus 雪球荚蒾(其干树皮曾用作镇痉剂和子宫镇静药) / ~ prunifolium 樱叶荚蒾(其干根或茎皮曾用作子宫镇静药)
vicarious [vaiˈkεəriəs] *a* 替代的,错位的(如 ~ menstruation 代偿性月经,异位月经,倒经)
vicho [ˈviːtʃəu] *n* 痢疾(秘鲁俗语)
Vicia [ˈviʃiə] *n* 蚕豆属,巢菜属 | ~ faba(fava) 蚕豆
vicianose [ˈvaisiənəus] *n* 蚕豆糖,荚豆二糖
vicilin [ˈvaisilin] *n* 豌豆球蛋白
vicine [ˈvaisin] *n* 蚕豆嘧啶葡糖苷
Vicq d'Azyr's band [viːk dəˈziə] (Félix Vicq d'Azyr) 维克达济尔带(大脑皮质锥体细胞层内的白色带) | ~ fasciculus 乳头丘脑束 / ~ foramen 延髓盲孔
Vidal's disease [viˈdɑːl] (Jean B. É. Vidal) 单纯慢性苔藓
Vidal's operation [viˈdɑːl] (Auguste T. Vidal) 维达尔手术(精索静脉曲张皮下静脉结扎术)
vidarabine [vaiˈdεərəbiːn] *n* 阿糖腺苷(表面抗病毒药,治疗单纯性疱疹性角膜炎,静脉注射治疗单纯性疱疹性脑炎)
video- [构词成分]电视,视频
videodensitometry [ˌvidiəuˌdensiˈtɔmitri] *n* 视频测密术,视频密度测量法
videoendoscope [ˌviːdiəuˈendəuskəup] *n* 电视内镜
videoendoscopy [ˌviːdiəuenˈdɔskəpi] *n* 电视内镜检查术
videofluoroscopy [ˌvidiəufluəˈrɔskəpi] *n* 电视透视检查

videognosis [ˌvidiəɡˈnəusis] *n* X 线[照]片电视诊断
videokymography [ˌviːdiəukaiˈmɔɡrəfi] *n* 电视记纹法
videolaparoscope [ˌviːdiəuˈlæpərəuˌskəup] *n* 电视剖腹镜
videolaparoscopy [ˌviːdiəuˌlæpəˈrɔskəpi] *n* 电视剖腹镜检查[术]
videolaseroscopy [ˌvidiəuleizəˈrɔskəpi] *n* 视频激光腹腔镜检查
videomicroscopy [ˌvidiəumaiˈkrɔskəpi] *n* 电视显微镜检查,电视显微术
vidian artery [ˈvidiən] (Guido Guidi〈拉 Vidjus〉) 翼管动脉 | ~ canal 翼管 / ~ nerve 翼管神经 / deep ~ nerve 岩深神经
Vieussens' ansa [viəˈsæn] (Raymond de Vieussens) 锁骨下襻 | ~ foramina 小静脉孔 / ~ limbus 卵圆窝缘 / ~ valve 前髓帆 / ~ veins 心前静脉 / ~ ventricle 透明隔腔
view [vjuː] *n* 观,观察位观(投照) | apical four-chamber ~ 心尖四腔观 / long-axis ~ 长轴观 / short-axis ~ 短轴观 / two-chamber ~ 二腔观
VIG vaccinia immune globulin 牛痘免疫球蛋白
vigabatrin [vaiˈɡeibətrin] *n* 氨己烯酸(抗癫痫药)
vigilambulism [ˌvidʒiˈlæmbjulizəm] *n* 醒性梦行症
vigilance [ˈvidʒiləns] *n* 不眠症,警醒症
vigintinormal [vaiˌdʒintiˈnɔːməl] *a* 二十分之一当量的(溶液)
Vignal's cells [viːˈnjɑːl] (Guillaume Vignal) 维尼阿尔细胞(胚胎结缔组织细胞)
vignin [ˈvignin] *n* 豇豆球蛋白
vigor [ˈviɡə] *n* 活力,精力;壮健 | hybrid ~ 杂种优势 | **vigorous** [ˈviɡərəs] *a* 精力充沛的,壮健的;强有力的
Vigouroux's sign [ˌviːɡuˈruː] (Auguste Vigouroux) 维古鲁征(突眼性甲状腺肿时,皮肤对电流刺激的抵抗减少)
Villard's button [viˈlɑː] (Eugêne Villard) 维拉德钮(一种改良的墨菲〈Murphy〉钮)
Villaret's syndrome [viləˈrei] (Maurice Villaret) 维拉雷综合征(第 9, 10, 11, 12 对,有时为第 7 对脑神经一侧麻痹,由于腮腺后隙损害所致,特征为咽上缩肌麻痹吞咽困难、软腭和咽门麻痹及这些部位与咽感觉丧失、舌后 1/3 的味觉丧失、声带麻痹和喉感觉丧失、胸锁乳突肌和斜方肌麻痹以及颈交感神经麻痹。亦称腮腺后间隙综合征)
Villarsia nymphaeoides [viˈlɑːziə ˌnimfiˈɔidiːz] 荇菜(有抗坏血病作用)
villi [ˈvilai] villus 的复数
villiferous [viˈlifərəs] *a* 有绒毛的
villikinin [ˌviliˈkainin] *n* 缩肠绒毛素
villin [ˈvilin] *n* 绒毛蛋白
villitis [viˈlaitis] *n* 胎盘绒毛炎;绒毛炎(马蹄)
villoma [viˈləumə], **villioma** [ˌviliˈəumə] *n* 绒毛瘤
villonodular [ˌviləˈnɔdjulə] *a* 绒毛(与)结节性的(指滑膜组织增生病)
villose [ˈviləus], **villous** [ˈviləs] *a* 绒毛的,有绒毛的,绒毛状的
villositis [ˌviləˈsaitis] *n* 胎盘绒毛炎
villosity [viˈlɔsəti] *n* 绒毛状态;绒毛
villus [ˈviləs] ([复] **villi** [ˈvilai]) *n*【拉】绒毛 | amniotic ~ 羊膜绒毛 / anchoring ~ 固定绒毛 / arachnoid villi 蛛网膜粒 / chorionic ~ 绒毛膜绒毛 / intestinal villi 肠绒毛 / lingual villi 丝状乳头 / pericardial ~ 心包绒毛 / pleural villi 胸膜绒毛 / synovial villi 滑膜绒毛
villusectomy [ˌviləˈsektəmi] *n* 滑膜[绒毛]切除术
viloxazine hydrochloride [viˈlɔksəziːn] 盐酸维洛沙秦(抗抑郁药)
vimentin [viˈmentin] *n* 波形蛋白
vinbarbital [vinˈbɑːbitæl] *n* 戊烯比妥(催眠镇静药)
vinblastine sulfate [vinˈblæstiːn] 硫酸长春碱(抗肿瘤药,尤用于治疗霍奇金〈Hodgkin〉病)
Vinca [ˈviŋkə] *n* 长春花属
vinca [ˈviŋkə] *n* 长春花
vincamine [ˈvinkəmiːn] *n* 长春胺(用于帮助脑血管障碍患者改善智能)
Vincent's angina [ˈvinsənt] (Henri Vincent) 樊尚咽峡炎(痛性膜性溃疡,伴水肿,口咽及喉部有充血性斑点,由于急性坏死溃疡性龈炎扩散所致) | ~ gingivitis 樊尚龈炎,急性坏死溃疡性龈炎/ ~ infection 樊尚感染,急性坏死溃疡性龈炎 / ~ spirillum 樊尚螺菌,樊尚密螺旋体 / ~ stomatitis 樊尚口炎,急性坏死溃疡性龈炎 / ~ tonsillitis 樊尚扁桃体炎(急性坏死性龈炎,只累及扁桃体)
vincofos [ˈvinkəfɔs] *n* 乙烯磷(抗蠕虫药)
vincristine sulfate [vinˈkristiːn] 硫酸长春新碱(抗肿瘤药,主要用于联合化疗,治疗霍奇金〈Hodgkin〉病、急性淋巴细胞白血病、非霍奇金淋巴瘤,也可治疗维尔姆斯〈Wilms〉瘤、成神经细胞瘤、乳癌、横纹肌肉瘤和其他肉瘤,以及某些脑瘤。其主要副作用为混合性运动感觉神经病变和自主性末梢神经病变)
vinculin [ˈvinkjulin] *n* 纽带蛋白
vinculum [ˈviŋkjuləm] ([复] **vinculums** 或 **vincula** [ˈviŋkjulə]) *n* 纽,系带 | vincula of tendons of fingers 指腱纽 / vincula of tendons of toes

趾腱纽

vindesine sulfate [ˈvindəsiːn] 硫酸长春地辛(抗肿瘤药,治疗急性淋巴细胞白血病)

Vineberg operation [ˈvainbəːg] (Arthur M. Vineberg)范堡手术(把胸廓内动脉移植于心肌内,以增强侧支循环的血供)

vinegar [ˈvinigə] *n* 醋,醋剂

vinegaroon [ˌvinigəˈruːn] *n* 醋蝎(因其分泌物有臭气似醋,故名)

vinometer [viˈnɔmitə] *n* 酒精比重计,酒类醇量计

vinorelbine tartrate [viˈnɔːrelbiːn] 酒石酸长春瑞滨(抗肿瘤药)

Vinson's syndrome [ˈvinsn] (Porter P. Vinson) 文森综合征(见 Plummer-Vinson syndrome)

vinum [ˈvainəm] *n*【拉】酒[剂]

vinyl [ˈvainil] *n* 乙烯基 | ~ ether 乙烯醚(吸入麻醉药,因其可燃性现已少用)

viocid [ˈvaiəsid] *n* 龙胆紫

Viola [ˈvaiələ] *n*【拉】堇菜属 | ~ odorata 香堇菜 / ~ tricolor 三色堇,蝴蝶花

violacein [ˌvaiəˈleisiːn] *n* 紫色杆菌素,青紫色素杆菌素

violaceous [ˌvaiəuˈleisiəs] *a* 紫色的,青紫色的(通常指皮肤变色)

violaquercitrin [vaiˌəuləˈkwəːsitrin] *n* 紫槲皮苷,芸香苷,芦丁

violate [ˈvaiəleit] *vt* 违反,侵犯;强奸;妨碍 | **violation** [ˌvaiəˈleiʃən] *n*

violence [ˈvaiələns] *n* 暴力 | direct ~ 直接暴力

violescent [ˌvaiəˈlesnt] *a* 淡紫色的

violet [ˈvaiəlit] *n* 紫色 | amethyst ~, iris ~ 水晶紫(四乙基酚藏红) / chrome ~ 色紫(玫红酸的衍生物) / cresyl ~, cresylecht ~ 甲酚紫(用于病理染色) / gentian ~, ~ G, ~ 7B or C, crystal ~, methyl ~, Paris ~, pentamethyl ~, hexamethyl ~ 龙胆紫,甲紫 / visual ~ 视紫蓝质

violuric acid [vaiəˈljuərik] 紫尿酸

viomycin sulfate [ˈvaiəˌmaisin] 硫酸紫霉素(抗结核药)

viosterol [vaiˈɔstərɔl] *n* 麦角骨化醇,钙化[甾]醇,维生素 D_2

VIP vasoactive intestinal polypeptide 血管活性肠[多]肽

viper [ˈvaipə] *n* 蝰蛇 | European ~ 欧洲蝰 / Gaboon ~ 加蓬蝰 / palm ~ 掌蝰 / rhinocerous ~ 犀角蝰 / sand ~, nose-horned ~沙蝰,鼻角蝰

Vipera [ˈvaipərə] *n* 蝰蛇属

Viperidae [vaiˈperidiː] *n* 蝰蛇科

viperine [ˈvaipərin], **viperid** [ˈvaipərid] *n* 蝰蛇 *a* 蝰蛇的,毒蛇的

vipoma, VIPoma [viˈpəumə] [*v*asoactive*i*ntestinal *p*olypeptide + *-oma*] *n* 血管活性肠[多]肽瘤(一种内分泌瘤,常发生于胰腺,分泌过多的血管活性肠多肽,可致弗纳-莫里森〈Verner-Morrison〉综合征。亦称致泻瘤)

viraginity [ˌvaiərəˈdʒinəti] *n* 女子男征

viral [ˈvaiərəl] *a* 病毒的

Virales [vaiəˈreiliːz] *n* 病毒目

Virchow-Robin spaces [ˈfirkəu rɔˈbæn] (Rudolf L. K. Virchow; Charles P. Robin) 魏尔啸-罗宾隙(血管在进入脑时其周围的间隙,形成内壁的是蛛网膜样的膜的延长,外壁是软脑膜的连续,插入的管道与蛛网膜下隙沟通)

Virchow's angle [ˈfirkəu, -ʃəu] (Rudolf L. K. Virchow) 魏尔啸角(介于鼻基线与鼻鼻下线之间) | ~ cells 麻风细胞 / ~ corpuscles 角膜小体 / ~ crystal 魏尔啸结晶(胆红素黄色结晶) / ~ degeneration 淀粉样变性 / ~ line 魏尔啸线(鼻根至人字缝尖的连线) / ~ node 信号结(signal node,见 node 项下相应术语)

Virchow-Seckel syndrome [ˈfirkəu ˈsekəl] (R. L. K. Virchou; H. P. G. Seckel) 魏尔啸-塞克尔综合征(见 Seckel syndrome)

viremia [vaiəˈriːmiə] *n* 病毒血[症]

virgin [ˈvəːdʒin] *n* 处女 *a* 纯洁的;未接触的

virginal [ˈvəːdʒinl] *a* 处女的,童贞的

virginiamycin [vəːˌdʒiniəˈmaisin] *n* 维吉霉素(抗生素类药)

virginity [vəːˈdʒinəti] *n* 童贞,纯洁

virginium [vəːˈdʒiniəm] *n* 锫(元素钫〈francium〉的旧名)

viricide [ˈvirisaid] *n* 杀病毒药 | viricidal [viriˈsaidl] *a* 杀病毒的

viridin [vaiˈridin] *n* 绿啶;绿胶霉素(抗真菌抗生素)

viridobufagin [ˌviridəuˈbjuːfədʒin] *n* 绿蟾蜍精

virile [ˈvirail, ˈvaiərail] *a* 男性的;有男性征的(尤指有性交能力的)

virilescence [ˌviriˈlesns] *n* 男性化(指女子)

virilia [vaiəˈriliə] *n*【拉】男性生殖器

viriligenic [ˌvirilaiˈdʒenik] *a* 促男性化的

virilism [ˈvirilizəm] *n* 男性化(指女子) | adrenal ~ 肾上腺性男性化 / prosopopilary ~ 须眉性男性化

virility [viˈriləti] *n* 有男性征;男性

virilization [ˌvirilaiˈzeiʃən, -liˈz-] *n* 男性化(指女子)

virilizing [ˈviriˌlaiziŋ] *a* 致男性化的

virion [ˈvaiəriɔn] *n* 病毒粒体

viripotent [vaiˈripətənt] *a* 性成熟的(指男子);可婚嫁的(指女子)

virogene [ˈvaiərədʒiːn] *n* 病毒基因

virogenetic [ˌvaiərəudʒiˈnetik] *a* 病毒所致的,病毒源的
viroid [ˈvaiərɔid] *n* 类病毒
virolactia [ˌvaiərəuˈlækʃiə] *n* 乳汁病毒
virology [ˌvaiəˈrɔlədʒi] *n* 病毒学 | **virologic(al)** [ˌvaiərəˈlɔdʒik(əl)] *a* / **virologist** *n* 病毒学家
viromicrosome [ˌvaiərəuˈmaikrəsəum] *n* 病毒微粒(不全病毒颗粒)
viropexis [ˌvaiərəuˈpeksis] *n* 病毒入胞现象(病毒固定在动物细胞膜上,进而被细胞吞没)
viroplasm [ˈvaiərəplæzəm] *n* 病毒粒质
virose [ˈvaiərəus], **virous** [ˈvaiərəs] *a* 有毒[性]的
virosis [ˌvaiəˈrəusis] ([复] **viroses** [ˌvaiəˈrəusiːz]) *n* 病毒病(病毒所致)
virostatic [ˌvaiərəuˈstætik] *a* 抑制病毒的 *n* 病毒抑制药
virucide [ˈvaiərəsaid] *n* 杀病毒剂 | **virucidal** [ˌvaiərəˈsaidl] *a* 杀病毒的
virulence [ˈvirjuləns] *n* 毒力,毒性,致病力
virulent [ˈvirjulənt] *a* 有毒力的,毒性的,致病力强的,毒害的
virulicidal [ˌvirəˈlisidl] *a* 灭毒性的
viruliferous [ˌvirəˈlifərəs] *a* 带病毒的,产毒的
viruria [vaiəˈrjuəriə] *n* 病毒尿症
virus [ˈvaiərəs] *n* 【拉】病毒 | acute laryngotracheobronchitis ~ 急性喉气管炎支气管炎病毒,副流感病毒 2 型 / adeno-associated ~ 腺病毒相关病毒 / Amapari ~ 阿马帕里病毒(从巴西啮齿动物分离出的一种沙粒病毒) / animal ~ 动物病毒 / ~ animatum 活病毒 / Argentine hemorrhagic fever ~ 阿根廷出血热病毒(即呼宁病毒 Junin ~) / attenuated ~ 减毒病毒 / Australian X disease ~ 澳大利亚 X 病病毒 / avian leukosis ~ 禽白血病病毒 / B ~ B 病毒,猴疱疹病毒 / bacterial ~ 细菌病毒,噬菌体 / Bittner ~ 比特纳病毒,小鼠乳腺瘤病毒 / Bolivian hemorrhagic fever ~ 玻利维亚出血热病毒(即马丘波病毒 Machupo ~) / Brunhilde ~ 布伦希尔得病毒(脊髓灰质炎病毒第一型) / Bunyamwera ~ 布尼安维拉病毒(一种虫媒病毒,见于乌干达西部森林地区) / bushy stunt ~ 丛缩病毒(一种小球形植物病毒,引起番茄丛缩病) / Bwamba fever ~ 布汪巴热病毒(一种虫媒病毒,布汪巴为乌干达一地名) / C ~, Coxsackie ~ 柯萨奇病毒(一种肠道病毒,柯萨奇为美国一地名) / CA ~, croup-associated ~ 格鲁布相关病毒,哮吼相关病毒,致哮吼病毒,副流感乙型病毒 / Cache Valley ~ 卡奇谷病毒(一种虫媒病毒,首次见于美国犹他州的卡奇谷) / cancer inducing ~ 致癌病毒(使感染细胞进行不受控制的增殖的病毒,包括 RNA 病毒和 DNA 病毒) / Catu ~ 卡图病毒(与瓜马〈Guama〉病毒密切相关的一种虫媒病毒) / CCA ~ (chimpanzee coryza agent)黑猩猩鼻炎因子,呼吸道合胞体病毒 / CELO(chicken-embryo-lethal orphan) ~ 鸡胚致死性孤儿病毒(一种肠道孤病毒) / Chagres ~ 恰格尔斯病毒(一种引起发热的虫媒病毒,伴有不适、头痛、局部和全身疼痛,见于巴拿马) / Chenuda ~ 秦纽达病毒(一种与夸兰菲尔〈Quaranfil〉病毒密切有关的虫媒病毒) / Chikungunya ~ 奇昆古尼亚病毒(一种虫传病毒,见于坦桑尼亚) / Columbia SK ~ 哥伦比亚 SK 病毒,哥伦比亚脑-心肌炎病毒 / Congo-Crimean hemorrhagic fever ~, Crimean hemorrhagic fever ~ 刚果-克里米亚出血热病毒,克里米亚出血热病毒 / coryza ~ 鼻病毒 / cytomegalic inclusion disease ~ 巨细胞性包涵体病病毒 / defective ~ 缺陷病毒,缺损病毒(见 helper ~) / EB ~, Epstein Barr ~ EB 病毒,非洲淋巴细胞瘤病毒(一种疱疹病毒) / Ebola ~ 埃博拉病毒(一种未分类的 RNA 病毒,形态上类似马尔堡〈Marburg〉病毒,但抗原性有区别,可引起急性、高度致死性出血热,见于苏丹和刚果西北部邻近地区) / ECBO ~ 牛肠道细胞病变孤儿病毒 / ECDO ~ 犬肠道细胞病变孤儿病毒 / ECHO ~ 人肠道细胞病变孤儿病毒,艾柯病毒 / ECMO ~ 猴肠道细胞病变孤儿病毒 / ECSO ~ 猪肠道细胞病变孤儿病毒 / EEE(eastern equine encephalomyelitis) ~ 东方马脑脊髓炎病毒(一组虫媒病毒引起马、骡以及人的脑脊髓炎,见于美国、加拿大、墨西哥以及中南美洲) / exanthematous disease ~ 疹病病毒 / FA ~ FA 病毒(可引起小鼠脊髓炎的一株病毒) / ~ fixé, fixed ~ 固定病毒(狂犬病病毒,经过接种失去感染性,但仍保持抗原性) / Friend ~ 弗里德病毒(可引起小鼠恶性网状组织病变的鼠白血病病毒) / Germistan ~ 杰米斯顿病毒(可引起南非轻度热病的布尼安维拉〈Bunyamwera〉群的一种虫媒病毒) / granulosis ~ 杆状病毒 / Guama ~ 瓜马病毒(从巴西贝伦地区患有高热、头痛、肌和关节痛,有时有恶心和眩晕的林业人员中分离出的一种虫媒病毒) / Hantaan(Hataan) ~ 汉滩病毒(流行性出血热的病原体,亦称朝鲜出血热病毒) / helper ~ 辅助病毒(一种病毒,如劳斯相关〈Rous-associated〉病毒,它能使缺损病毒〈如劳斯病毒〉形成蛋白外壳) / hemagglutinating ~ of Japan 日本血凝病毒(即仙台病毒 Sendai ~) / hepatitis A ~ (HAV)甲型肝炎病毒 / hepatitis B ~ (HBV)乙型肝炎病毒 / hepatitis C ~ 丙型肝炎病毒 / hepatitis delta ~ δ 型肝炎病毒 / herpes ~ 疱疹病毒 / human immunodeficiency ~ (HIV)人免疫缺陷病毒(一种人 T 细胞白血病 / 淋巴瘤病毒,是获得性免疫缺陷综合征即艾滋病的病原体) / human T-cell leuke-

mia / lymphoma ~, human T-cell lymphotrophic ~(HTLV)人T细胞白血病 / 淋巴瘤病毒,人嗜T淋巴细胞病毒(其中一型,即人免疫缺陷病毒为获得性免疫缺陷综合征〈艾滋病〉的病原体) / Ilheus ~ 伊刘斯病毒(巴西的一种虫传脑炎病毒) / infectious porcine encephalomyelitis ~ 传染性猪脑脊髓炎病毒 / infectious wart ~ 传染性疣病毒 / influenza ~ 流感病毒 / iridescent ~ 虹彩病毒 / Japanese B encephalitis ~ 流行性乙型脑炎病毒 / JH ~ 人肠道病变孤儿病毒 28 / Kemerovo ~ 克麦罗沃病毒(一种蜱传虫媒病毒,与西伯利亚西部良性热病有关) / Korean hemorrhagic fever ~ 朝鲜出血热病毒(即汉滩病毒 Hantaan ~) / Kumba ~ 昆巴病毒(西非喀麦隆昆巴地区的一种虫媒病毒,抗原性与塞姆利基〈Semliki〉森林病毒相同) / Langat ~ 兰加特病毒(一种蜱传虫媒病毒,可引起人与小鼠的脑炎) / Lansing ~ 蓝辛病毒(脊髓灰质炎病毒Ⅱ型的原型株) / Lassa ~ 拉沙病毒(原于1969年在尼日利亚拉沙分离出的一种毒力极强的沙拉病毒,可引起急性热病,死亡率高) / Latino ~ 拉丁美洲病毒(从玻利维亚噬鼠动物中分离出的一种沙粒病毒) / LCM ~, lymphocytic choriomeningitis ~ 淋巴细胞性脉络丛脑膜炎病毒 / louping ill ~ 羊跳跃病病毒 / lymphadenopathy-associated ~(LAV)淋巴结病相关病毒,人免疫缺陷病毒 / M-25 ~ M-25 病毒(从人上呼吸道疾病中分离出的一种具有黏病毒性质的病毒) / Machupo ~ 马丘波病毒(最初于1959年在玻利维亚出血热流行期分离出的一种沙粒病毒,为玻利维亚出血热的病原体,亦称玻利维亚出血热病毒) / Makonde ~ 马康德病毒(在坦桑尼亚马康德高原地区与奇昆古尼亚〈chikungunya〉病毒一起分离出的一种虫媒病毒) / mammary tumor ~ 乳腺瘤病毒,小鼠乳腺瘤病毒 / Marburg ~ 马尔堡病毒(一种未分离的 RNA 病毒,可引起一种急性高致死型出血热,即为马尔堡病。马尔堡为德国中部一城市) / masked ~, latent ~ 隐性病毒,潜伏性病毒 / Mayaro ~ 马雅罗病毒(一种虫媒病毒,见于特立尼达的马雅罗以及巴西地区) / Mengo ~ 门戈病毒(一种脑心肌炎病毒,见于乌干达) / milker's node ~ 挤奶者结节病毒,副痘苗病毒 / MM ~ MM 病毒,脑心肌炎病毒 / monkey-pox ~ 猴痘病毒 / Mossuril ~ 莫苏里病毒(一种蚊传虫媒病毒) / mouse mammary tumor ~ 小鼠乳腺瘤病毒 / murine leukemia ~ 鼠白血病病毒 / newborn pneumonitis ~ 新生儿肺炎病毒(即仙台病毒 Sendai ~) / non-A, non-B hepatitis ~ 非甲非乙肝炎病毒,丙型肝炎病毒 / non-oncogenic ~ 非致癌病毒 / Norwalk ~ 诺沃克病毒(急性胃肠炎流行病的常见病原体,腹泻与呕吐持续 24 ~ 48 小时。诺沃克为美国俄亥俄州一城市) / Ntaya ~ 恩塔亚病毒(原于1943年从乌干达西部恩塔亚沼泽各种蚊子〈包括库蚊和伊蚊〉中分离出的一种病毒,注射小鼠脑内,可感染致死) / oncogenic ~ 致癌病毒 / O'nyong-nyong ~ 奥尼翁-尼翁病毒(一种虫媒病毒,见于乌干达和肯尼亚) / orphan ~es 孤儿病毒(指一些未证明与疾病有关的病毒,如肠道孤儿病毒) / papilloma ~ 乳头瘤病毒 / pappataci fever ~ 白蛉热病毒 / parainfluenza ~ 副流感病毒(从不同程度的上呼吸道疾病患者分离出的病毒。副流感病毒分为副流感病毒1型,含有两种免疫性相关但不相同的病毒,即仙台病毒和血〈细胞〉吸附病毒Ⅱ型;副流感病毒Ⅱ型为从急性喉气管支气管炎患者分离出的一种病毒,亦称致哮吼病毒 CA ~ 或 croup-associated ~;副流感病毒Ⅲ型为一种可引起尤其是儿童的支气管炎和肺炎的病毒,亦称血〈细胞〉吸附病毒1型;副流感病毒4型为一种与儿童呼吸道疾病有关的病毒) / Parana ~ 巴拉那病毒(从巴拉圭啮齿动物中分离出的一种沙粒病毒) / paravaccinia ~ 副痘苗病毒(亦称挤奶者结节病毒,假牛痘病毒) / pharyngoconjunctival fever ~ 咽结膜热病毒,腺病毒Ⅲ型 / Pichinde ~ 皮秦德病毒(一种感染哥伦比亚啮齿动物的沙粒病毒,并可从人亚临床感染中分离出) / Piry ~ 皮里病毒(从东非急性发热性综合征患者中分离的一种沙粒病毒) / polyoma ~ 多瘤病毒 / poliomyelitis ~ 脊髓灰质炎病毒 / Pongola ~ 庞哥拉病毒(在非洲可引起热病的一种虫媒病毒) / pseudocowpox ~ 假牛痘病毒,副痘苗病毒 / Quaranfil ~ 夸兰菲尔病毒(在埃及发现的一种虫媒病毒) / rabbit fibroma ~ 兔纤维瘤病毒 / Rauscher leukemia ~ 劳舍尔白血病病毒(一种鼠白血病病毒,可引起小鼠淋巴样白血病) / Rous-associated ~ (RAV)劳斯相关病毒(一种辅助病毒,能使有缺损的劳斯肉瘤病毒形成蛋白外壳) / RS ~, respiratory syncytial ~ 呼吸道合胞体病毒(亦称黑猩猩鼻炎因子) / SA ~ SA 病毒(从仓鼠脑中分离出的一种病毒) / St. Louis encephalitis ~ 圣路易斯脑炎病毒 / satellite ~ 卫星病毒(需有辅助病毒存在方能复制的病毒株,据认为是由于衣壳编码区缺陷所致) / Semliki Forest ~ 塞姆利基森林病毒(一种虫媒病毒,见于乌干达) / Sendai ~ 仙台病毒(副流感1型病毒的一株,仙台是日本地名) / sigma ~ σ 病毒(使果蝇成为对二氧化碳呈敏感状态的病毒) / Sindbis ~ 辛德比斯病毒(埃及的一种虫媒病毒) / Spondweni ~ 斯庞德温尼病毒(原于1955年从非洲蚊子中分离出的一种虫媒病毒,可引起人的短期热病) / street ~ 通常毒,街病毒(普通狂犬病病毒) / Tacaribe ~ 塔卡里伯病毒(从特立尼达的蝙蝠中分离出的一种沙粒病毒,免疫性与呼宁〈Junin〉病毒和马丘波〈Machupo〉病毒有关) / Tahyna ~ 塔希纳病毒(一种与加利福尼亚病毒血清学相关的病毒,在欧洲各国可分离出,可能使人和动物致病) / Tamiami ~ 太米阿米病毒(从佛罗里达州啮齿动物中分离出的一种沙粒病毒) / temperate ~ 温和噬菌体 / tickborne ~ 蜱传病毒 / tobacco mosaic ~ 烟草花叶病毒 / tumor ~ 肿瘤病毒 / U ~ U 病毒(类似副流感病毒 2 型,但分类未定,发现于患声门下喉炎的儿童。亦称乌普塞拉病毒 Uppsala ~) / Uganda S ~ 乌干达 S 病毒(一种虫媒病毒) / Uppsala ~ 乌普塞拉病毒(即 U 病毒) / vacuolating ~, simian ~ 40 (SV 40)空泡形成病毒,猿猴病毒 / VEE ~, Venezuelan equine encephalomyelitis ~ 委内瑞拉马脑脊髓炎病毒 / WEE ~, western equine encephalomyelitis ~ 西方马脑脊髓炎病毒 / Wesselsbron ~ 韦塞尔斯布朗病毒(南非的一种虫媒病毒) / West Nile ~ 西尼罗河病毒,西尼罗河脑炎病毒 / Wyeomyia ~ 怀俄米亚病毒(布尼安维拉〈Bunyamwera〉病毒群中的一种病毒) / Yaba ~ 亚巴病毒(一种能产生猴浅表性良性肿瘤的病毒) / Yale SK ~ 耶鲁大学 SK 病毒(一株脊髓灰质炎病毒) / Zika ~ 齐卡病毒(原先于 1947 年在乌干达齐卡森林的猴中分离出的一种虫媒病毒,以后发现可能传染非洲伊蚊,人也感染)

virusemia [ˌvaiərəˈsiːmiə] *n* 病毒血[症]

virustatic [ˌvaiərəˈstætik] *a* 抑制病毒的

vis [vis]([复] **vires** [ˈvaiəriːz]) *n*【拉】力 | ~ in situ 固有力,本力 / ~ medicatrix naturae 自愈力 / ~ vitae, ~ vitalis 活力

viscera [ˈvisərə] viscus 的复数

viscerad [ˈvisəræd] *ad* 向内脏

visceral [ˈvisərəl] *a* 内脏的

visceralgia [ˌvisəˈrældʒiə] *n* 内脏痛

visceralism [ˈvisərəlizəm] *n* 内脏病原说

viscerimotor [ˌvisəriˈməutə] *a* 内脏运动的

viscer(o)-[构词成分] 内脏

viscerocranium [ˌvisərəuˈkreinjəm] *n* 脏颅

viscerography [ˌvisəˈrɔgrəfi] *n* 脏器 X 线造影[术]

visceroinhibitory [ˌvisərəuinˈhibitəri] *a* 抑制内脏[运动]的

visceromegaly [ˌvisərəuˈmegəli] *n* 内脏肥大

visceromotor [ˌvisərəuˈməutə] *a* 内脏运动的

visceroperietal [ˌvisərəupəˈraiitl] *a* 内脏腹壁的

visceroperitoneal [ˌvisərəuˌperitəuˈniːəl] *a* 内脏腹膜的

visceropleural [ˌvisərəuˈpluərəl] *a* 内脏胸膜的

visceroptosis [ˌvisərɔpˈtəusis] *n* 内脏下垂

viscerosensory [ˌvisərəuˈsensəri] *a* 内脏感觉的

visceroskeletal [ˌvisərəuˈskelitl] *a* 内脏骨骼的

viscerosomatic [ˌvisərəusəuˈmætik] *a* 内脏躯体的

viscerotome [ˈvisərətəum] *n* 肝组织刺取器(尸体);脏节,脏区(腹部内脏上受单一脊神经后根支配的、分布输入神经纤维的一区)

viscerotomy [visəˈrɔtəmi] *n* 肝组织刺取术(尸体)

viscerotonia [ˌvisərəuˈtəuniə] *n* 内脏强健型性格

viscerotrophic [ˌvisərəuˈtrɔfik] *a* 内脏营养的

viscerotropic [ˌvisərəuˈtrɔpik] *a* 亲内脏的

viscid [ˈvisid] *a* 黏的 | **~ity** [viˈsidəti] *n* 黏质,黏性

viscin [ˈvisin] *n* 槲寄生素

viscoelastic [ˌviskəuiˈlæstik] *a* 黏弹性的(指黏性物质,用于白内障手术时或对前房施行其他手术时恢复或维持眼尤其是前房的形状)

viscogel [ˈviskədʒel] *n* 黏凝胶

viscosaccharase [ˌviskəuˈsækəreis] *n* 黏蔗糖酶,产胶蔗糖酶

viscose [ˈviskəus] *n* 黏胶;黏胶丝 *a* 黏的,黏性的

viscosimeter [ˌviskəuˈsimitə], **viscometer** [visˈkɔmitə] *n* 黏度计 | **viscosimetry** [ˌviskəuˈsimitri], **viscometry** [visˈkɔmitri] *n* 黏度测量法

viscosity [visˈkɔsəti] *n* 黏[滞]性;黏[滞]度 | ~ of thinking 思维黏滞

Viscum [ˈviskəm] *n* 槲寄生

viscous [ˈviskəs] *a* 黏的,黏性的

viscus [ˈviskəs]([复] **viscera** [ˈvisərə]) *n*【拉】内脏

visile [ˈvizil] *a* 视觉的

vision [ˈviʒən] *n* 视,视觉;视力(符号为 V) | achromatic ~ 全色盲 / chromatic ~ 色觉;色视症 / day ~, photopic ~ 白昼视觉,明视觉 / dichromatic ~ 二色视 / double ~ 复视 / facial ~ 面部[感觉]测距能力 / half ~ 偏盲 / halo ~, iridescent ~, rainbow ~ 虹[彩]视 / multiple ~ 视物显多症 / night ~, scotopic ~, twilight ~ 夜间视觉,暗视觉 / ~ nul 阴性盲点(不自觉盲点) / ~ obscure 阳性盲点(自觉盲点) / pseudoscopic ~ 虚性视觉,非实体视觉 / scoterythrous ~ 红色盲(弱视) / stereoscopic ~, haploscopic ~, solid ~ 实体视觉,立体视觉 / triple ~ 三重复视(视一物为三) / tunnel ~, shaft ~ 视野狭窄,管状视野 / violet ~ 紫幻视 / word ~ 文字视觉 / yellow ~ 黄视症,视物显黄症

visna [ˈvisnə] *n* 绵羊脱髓鞘性脑白质炎

visual [ˈvizjuəl] *a* 视觉的,视力的 *n* 视觉性记忆优势者

visualization [ˌvizjuəlaiˈzeiʃən, -liˈz-] *n* 显影,造影术 | double contrast ~ 对衬造影术,双对比造影术

visualize [ˈvizjuəlaiz] *vt* 使显影

visuoauditory [ˌvizjuəuˈɔːditəri] *a* 视听的,声光感觉的
visuognosis [ˌvizjuəgˈnəusis] *n* 视觉辨认,辨视力
visuometer [ˌvizjuˈɔmitə] *n* 视力计
visuomotor [ˌvizjuəuˈməutə] *a* 视觉眼肌运动的
visuopsychic [ˌvizjuəˈsaikik] *a* 精神视觉的
visuosensory [ˌvizjuəˈsensəri] *a* 视觉的
visuospatial [ˌvizjuəuˈspeiʃəl], **visual-spatial** [ˈvizjuəl ˈspeiʃəl] *a* 视觉空间的
vitagonist [vaiˈtægənist] *n* 维生素拮抗物
vital [ˈvaitl] *a* 生命的,生活的;维持生命所必需的;重要的,紧要的 *n* [复]活命器官,紧要器官 ǀ **~ly** *ad*
vitalism [ˈvaitəlizəm] *n* 生机论,生活力说 ǀ **vitalist** *n* 生机论者,生活力说者 / **vitalistic** [ˌvaitəˈlistik] *a*
Vitali's test [viˈtæli] (Dioscoride Vitali) 维塔利试验(检生物碱、胆色素、麝香草脑、尿脓)
vitality [vaiˈtæləti] *n* 生命力;生机,活力;生活力
vitalize [ˈvaitəlaiz] *vt* 使有生机,活力化,激发 ǀ **vitalization** [ˌvaitəlaiˈzeiʃən, -liˈz-] *n*
vitamer [ˈvaitəmə] *n* 同效维生素
vitameter [vaiˈtæmitə] *n* 维生素分析器
vitamin [ˈvitəmin, ˈvaitəmin] *n* 维生素 ǀ ~ A 维生素 A,视黄醇 / ~ A_1 维生素 A_1,视黄醇 / ~ A_2 维生素 A_2,去氢视黄醇 / ~ B complex 复合维生素 B / ~ B_1 维生素 B_1,硫胺[素] / ~ B_2 维生素 B_2,核黄素 / ~ B_6 维生素 B_6,吡多辛 / ~ B_{12} 维生素 B_{12},氰钴胺 / ~ B_{12a} 维生素 B_{12a},羟钴胺 / ~ B_c 维生素 B_c,叶酸 / ~ B_c conjugate 维生素 B_c 轭合物,叶酸 / ~ C 维生素 C,抗坏血酸 / ~ D 维生素 D,骨化醇(抗佝偻病维生素) / ~ D_2 维生素 D_2,麦角骨化醇,[麦角]钙化醇 / ~ D_3 维生素 D_3,胆骨化醇,胆钙化醇 / ~ E 维生素 E(抗不育维生素的总称,如 α-生育酚) / ~ G 维生素 G,核黄素 / ~ H 维生素 H,生物素 / ~ K 维生素 K(抗出血维生素的总称) / ~ K_1 维生素 K_1,植物甲萘醌 / ~ K_2 维生素 K_2,四烯甲萘醌 / ~ K_3 维生素 K_3,甲萘醌 / ~ L 维生素 L,鼠乳汁分泌因子 / ~ M 维生素 M,叶酸 / anticantic ~ 抗白发维生素,对氨基苯甲酸 / antihemorrhagic ~ 抗出血维生素,维生素 K / anti-infection ~ 抗感染维生素,维生素 A / antineuritic ~ 抗神经炎维生素,硫胺 / antipellagra ~ 抗糙皮病维生素,烟酸 / antiscorbutic ~ 抗坏血病维生素,抗坏血酸 / antisterility ~ 抗不育维生素,维生素 E / antixerophthalmic ~ 抗干眼病维生素,维生素 A / fat-soluble ~s 脂溶性维生素(维生素 A, D, E 和 K) / water-soluble ~s 水溶性维生素(即除维生素 A, D, E 和 K 以外的所有维生素)
vitamin A acid 维 A 酸,维生素 A 酸
vitaminization [ˌvitəminaiˈzeiʃən, -niˈz-] *n* 维生素治疗
vitaminogenic [vaiˌtæminəuˈdʒenik] *a* 维生素源的
vitaminoid [ˈvaitəminɔid] *a* 维生素样的
vitaminology [ˌvaitəmiˈnɔlədʒi] *n* 维生素学
vitaminoscope [ˌvaitəˈminəskəup] *n* 维生素 A 缺乏检眼器
vitanition [ˌvaitəˈniʃən] *n* 维生素缺乏性营养障碍
vitellarium [ˌvitəˈlɛəriəm] *n* 卵黄腺
vitellary [ˈvitələri] *a* 卵黄的
vitellicle [viˈtelikl, vai-] *n* 卵黄囊
vitellin [viˈtelin, vai-] *n* 卵黄磷蛋白
vitelline [ˌviˈtelin, vai-] *a* 卵黄的
vitellogenesis [ˌvaitələuˈdʒenisis] *n* 卵黄生成[作用]
vitellolutein [ˌvaitələuˈljuːtiːn] *n* 卵黄黄质,卵黄黄素
vitellorubin [ˌvaitələuˈruːbin] *n* 卵黄红素,卵黄红质;甲壳红素
vitellose [vaiˈteləus] *n* 卵磷[蛋白]脲,卵黄[蛋白]脲
vitellus [vaiˈteləs] *n* 【拉】卵黄
Vitex [ˈvaiteks] *n* 黄荆属
vitiate [ˈviʃieit] *vt* 使(作用等)有缺陷,使失效 ǀ **vitiation** [ˌviʃiˈeiʃən] *n* 缺陷,失效
vitiatin [vaiˈtaiətin] *n* 维提阿丁(胆碱的同系物,有时出现于尿中)
vitiliginous [ˌvitiˈlidʒinəs] *a* 白斑的
vitiligo [ˌvitiˈlaigəu] ([复] **vitiligines** [ˌvitiˈlidʒiniːz]) *n* 【拉】白斑(皮肤脱色斑,如白癜风或白纹) ǀ circumscribed ~, perinevic ~ 痣周白斑 / ~ iridis 虹膜退色
Vitis [ˈvaitis] *n* 【拉】葡萄属 ǀ ~ vinifera 葡萄
vitium [ˈviʃiəm] ([复] **vitia** [ˈviʃiə]) *n* 【拉】缺陷,缺损,错误,病 ǀ ~ conformationis 畸形 / ~ cordis 器质性心脏病 / ~ primae formationis 先天(性)畸形
vitochemical [ˌvaitəˈkemikəl] *a* 生命化学的,有机化学的
vitodynamics [ˌvaitəudaiˈnæmiks] *n* 生物动态学,生物力学
vit. ov. sol. vitello ovi solutus 【拉】溶于卵黄的
vitrectomy [viˈtrektəmi] *n* 玻璃体切割术
vitreitis [ˌvitriˈaitis] *n* 玻璃体炎
vitreocapsulitis [ˌvitriəuˌkæpsjuˈlaitis] *n* 玻璃体炎;玻璃体囊炎
vitreodentin [ˌvitriəuˈdentin] *n* 透明牙质,硬牙质
vitreoretinal [ˌvitriəuˈretinəl] *a* 玻璃体视网膜的
Vitreoscilla [ˌvitriɔˈsilə] *n* 透明颤菌属

Vitreoscillaceae [ˌvitriˌɔsiˈleisiiː] *n* 透明颤菌科

vitreous [ˈvitriəs] *a* 玻璃体的,透明的 *n* 玻璃体 | detached ~ 玻璃体脱离 / primary ~ 原玻璃体 / primary persistent hyperplastic ~ 原发性玻璃体持续增生 / secondary ~ 第二玻璃体,后成玻璃体 / tertiary ~ 第三玻璃体

vitrescence [viˈtresns] *n* 玻[璃]态;玻[璃]状

vitreum [ˈvitriəm] *n* (眼)玻璃体

vitrify [ˈvitrifai] *vt*, *vi* 玻璃化 | **vitrification** [ˌvitrifiˈkeiʃən] *n*

vitrina [viˈtrainə] *n* 玻璃体(一种透明或玻璃样物质) | ~ auditoria, ~ auris 内淋巴 / ~ ocularis, ~ oculi 玻璃体

vitriol [ˈvitriəl] *n* 矾,硫酸盐晶体 *vt* 浸于稀硫酸中,用硫酸处理 | blue ~ 胆矾,蓝矾,硫酸铜 / elixir of ~ 芳香族硫酸 / green ~绿矾,硫酸亚铁 / oil of ~ 硫酸 / white ~, zinc ~ 皓矾,锌矾,硫酸锌

vitriolated [ˈvitriəˌleitid] *a* 含矾的;含硫酸的

vitriolic [ˌvitriˈɔlik] *a* 硫酸的

vitronectin [ˌvitrəuˈnektin] *n* 玻连蛋白

vitrum [ˈvitrəm] *n*【拉】玻璃

vivi- [构词成分]活,生命

vividialysis [ˌvividaiˈælisis] *n* 活[体]膜透析

vividiffusion [ˌvividiˈfjuːʒən] *n* 活[体]扩散法,人工扩散法

vivification [ˌvivifiˈkeiʃən] *n* 活质化(同化为活质)

viviparous [viˈvipərəs, vai-] *a* 胎生的 | **viviparity** [viviˈpærəti, vai-] *n*

Viviparus [vaiˈvipərəs] *n* 田螺属

vivipation [ˌviviˈpeiʃən] *n* 胎生[作用]

viviperception [ˌvivipəˈsepʃən] *n* 活体研究,活体观察

vivisect [ˌviviˈsekt] *vt*, *vi* 活体解剖(动物) | ~**ion** *n*

vivisectionist [ˌviviˈsekʃənist] *n* 活体解剖者(指动物实验)

vivosphere [ˈvaivəsfiə] *n* 生存空间;生物圈,生命层

VLA very late activation (antigen) 极晚活化(抗原)

Vladimiroff-Mikulicz amputation [ˌvlædiˈmiərɔf ˈmikjulitʃ] (Alexander A. Vladimiroff; Johann von Mikulicz-Radecki) 弗-米切断术(切除跟骨和距骨的足骨成形切断术)

Vladimiroff's operation [ˌvlædiˈmiərɔf] (Alexander A. Vladimiroff) 弗拉季米洛夫手术(跗骨切除术)

VLBW very low birth weight (infant) 极低出生体重(儿)

VLCD very low calorie diet 极低热量膳食

VLDL very low-density lipoproteins 极低密度脂蛋白

Vleminckx solution [ˈvleminks] (Jean F. Vleminckx) 含硫石灰溶液

VM-26 teniposide 替尼泊苷

VMA vanillylmandelic acid 香草扁桃酸,3-甲氧-4 羟扁桃酸

VMD Doctor of Veterinary Medicine (【拉】Veterinariae Medicinae Doctor) 兽医博士

vocal [ˈvəukəl] *a* 嗓音的;言语的;发声的,发音的;声带的(如 ~ nodule 声带小结)

Voegtlin's unit [ˈvegtlin] (Carl Voegtlin) 弗格特林单位(用 0.5 mg 垂体后叶标准粉末制剂能导致离体的豚鼠子宫收缩的量)

Voges-Proskauer test (reaction) [ˈfɔːgəs ˈprɔskauə] (O. Voges; Bernhard Proskauer) 福格斯-普罗斯考尔试验(反应)(检测乙酰甲基原醇的存在,从而鉴别大肠杆菌与产气杆菌)

Vogt-Koyanagi-Harada syndrome [fəukt kəujɑːˈnɑːgi hɑːˈrɑːdɑː] (Alfred Vogt; Y. Koyanagi; Einosuke Harada) 福格特-小柳-原田综合征(双侧色素层炎伴渗出性虹膜睫状体炎、脉络膜炎、假性脑〈脊〉膜炎和暂时性或永久性视网膜剥离,发生时伴有脱发、白癜疯、白发症、视敏度丧失、头痛、呕吐、耳聋及有时眩晕或青光眼。本综合征可能是一种炎性自体免疫疾病)

Vogt-Koyanagi syndrome [fəukt kəujɑːˈnɑːgi] (Alfred Vogt; Yoshizo Koyanagi) 福格特-小柳综合征(以渗出性虹膜睫体炎与脉络膜炎为特征的眼色素层脑膜炎,合并皮肤与毛发片块状色素减退,睫毛与眉毛也变白,可能还有视网膜剥离并伴有耳聋及耳鸣)

Vogt's angle [fəukt] (Karl Vogt) 福格特角(介于鼻颅底线与牙槽鼻线间的角)

Vogt Spiclmcycr discase [fəukt ˈʃpiːlmaiə] (Heinrich Vogt; Walter Spielmeyer) 福-施病,黑矇性白痴

Vogt's point, Vogt-Hueter point [fəukt ˈhiːtə] (Paul F. E. Vogt; Karl Hueter) 福格特点,福格特-许特点(环钻颅骨点)

Vogt's syndrome (disease) [fəukt] (Oskar Vogt) 福格特综合征(常伴有产伤的一种综合征,特征为两侧手足徐动症、行走困难、痉挛性哭笑、言语障碍、纹状体神经纤维髓鞘形成过多,呈现大理石纹样,有时为智能缺陷,亦称纹状体综合征)

Vohwinkel's syndrome [fəuˈvinkel] (Karl Hermann Vohwinkel) 沃温凯尔综合征,遗传性残毁性角化瘤

voice [vɔis] *n* 语音,语声 | cavernous ~, amphoric ~ 空洞语音 / double ~ 复音,双音 / eunuchoid ~ 类无睾者语音 / whispered ~ 耳语声

voiced [vɔist] *a* 浊音的

voiceless [ˈvɔisləs] *a* 清音的
void [vɔid] *vt* 排泄
Voigt's boundary lines [fɔit] (Christian A. Voigt) 伏伊特界线(周围神经分布界限)
Voillemier's point [vwɑːlmiˈɛə] (Léon C. Voillemier) 瓦尔米埃点(两髂前上嵴连接一条线,此线向下6.5 cm处,即肥胖者或水肿患者的膀胱穿刺点)
Voit's nucleus [fɔit] (Carl von Voit) 福伊特核(小脑内副齿状核)
voix [vwɑː] *n*【法】语音,语声 | ~ depolichinelle 笨拙音,傀儡音(羊音的一种)
vola [ˈvəulə] *n*【拉】掌,跖 | **~r** *a*
volardorsal [ˌvəuləˈdɔːsəl] *a* 掌背的,跖背的
volaris [vəuˈlɛəris] *a* 手掌的,掌侧的
volatile [ˈvɔlətail] *a* 挥发性的 | **volatility** [ˌvɔləˈtiləti] *n* 挥发性,挥发度
volatilize [vɔˈlætilaiz], *vt*, *vi* 挥发 | **volatilizable** [vɔˈlætilaizəbl] *a* 可挥发的,可发散的 / **volatilization** [vɔˌlætilaiˈzeiʃən, -liˈz-] *n* 挥发作用,发散 / **~r** 挥发器
vole [vəul] *n* 野鼠,田鼠
Volhard's test [ˈfɔːlhɑːd] (Franz Volhard) 福尔哈德试验(①测氯化物;②尿比重试验,检肾功能)
volition [vəuˈliʃən] *n* 意志;意志力;决断 | **~al** *a*
Volkmann's canals [ˈfɔlkmən] (Alfred W. Volkmann)福尔克曼管,穿通管(骨膜下层容纳血管的小管) | ~ membrane 福尔克曼膜(结核性脓肿纤维包囊壁)
Volkmann's contracture [ˈfɔlkmən] (Richard von Volkmann) 福尔克曼挛缩(肘部由于严重外伤或止血带应用不当,以致肌力丧失,迅速发生手指或腕部缺血性挛缩。亦称肌缺血性萎缩) | ~ disease 福尔克曼病(由于胫跗关节脱位所致的足先天性畸形) / ~ ischemic paralysis 局部缺血性麻痹 / ~ spoon 福尔克曼匙,锐匙(用以刮除肉芽组织)
volley [ˈvɔli] *n* 冲动排,一列冲动(由人工诱发的一种节律性连续肌颤搐或由单一刺激所致神经冲动的集合) | antidromic ~ 逆行冲动排(指在反射弧中通过前根向中心运行的逆向兴奋)
volsella [vɔlˈselə] *n*【拉】双爪钳
volt(V) [ˈvəult] *n* 伏[特] | electron ~ (eV) 电子伏[特]
voltage [ˈvəultidʒ] *n* 电压
voltaic [vɔlˈteiik] *a* 伏打电的,[直]流电的
voltaism [ˈvɔltəizəm] *n* 伏打电,[直]流电
voltameter [vɔlˈtæmitə] *n* 电量计
voltammeter [ˌvəultˈæmitə] *n* 伏安计,电压电量计
voltampere [vəultˈæmpɛə] *n* 伏(特)安[培]
voltmeter [ˈvəultmiːtə] *n* 伏特计,电压计
Voltolini's disease [vɔltəˈliːni] (Frederic E. R. Voltolini) 伏尔托利尼病(急性化脓性内耳炎) | ~ tube 伏尔托利尼管(切开鼓膜时,用以保持其切口开放)
volume [ˈvɔlju(ː)m] *n* 容积,容量,体积 | atomic ~ 原子体积 / blood ~ 血量 / circulation ~, ~ of circulation 循环血量 / ~ of distribution 分布容量 / end-diastolic ~ 舒张期末容积 / expiratory reserve ~ 补呼气量 / inspiratory reserve ~ 补吸气量 / mean corpuscular ~ 红细胞平均容量 / minute ~ 分钟量(每分钟肺呼出气体量) / packed-cell ~ (PCV), ~ of packed red cells (VPRC) 血细胞比容,红细胞压积 / plasma ~ 血浆容量 / red cell ~ 红细胞容积 / residual ~ 残气量 / stroke ~ 每搏量 / tidal ~ 潮气量
volumeter [vɔˈljuːmitə] *n* 容量计,容积计 | **volumetric(al)** [ˌvɔljuˈmetrik(əl)] *a* 容量的,容积的;测容量的,测容积的 / **volumetry** *n* 容量测定,容量分析
volumette [ˌvɔljuˈmet] *n* 重复定量滴管
volumination [ˌvɔlju(ː)miˈneiʃən] *n* 菌体肿胀
volumometer [ˌvɔljuˈmɔmitə], **volumenometer** [ˌvɔljumiˈnɔmitə] *n* 容积计
voluntary [ˈvɔləntəri] *a* 随意的
voluntomotory [ˌvɔləntəuˈməutəri] *a* 随意运动的
volute [vəˈljuːt] *n* 涡旋形;涡囊;涡螺 *a* 涡旋的,涡卷的
volutin [vəˈljutin] *n* 异染质
volutrauma [ˌvɔljuˈtraumə] *n* 过度通气性肺损伤
Volvocida [vɔlˈvɔsidə] *n* 团藻虫目
Volvox [ˈvɔlvɔks] *n* 团藻虫属
volvulate [ˈvɔlvjuleit] *vt*, *vi* 扭转,扭结
volvulosis [ˌvɔlvjuˈləusis] *n* 盘尾丝虫病
volvulus [ˈvɔlvjuləs] *n* 肠扭转 | ~ neonatorum 新生儿肠扭转
vomer [ˈvəumə] *n*【拉】犁骨 | **~ine** [ˈvəumərin] *a*
vomerobasilar [ˌvəumərəuˈbæsilə] *a* 犁骨颅底的
vomeronasal [ˌvəumərəuˈneizəl] *a* 犁[骨]鼻骨的
vomica [ˈvɔmikə] ([复] **vomicae** [ˈvɔmisiː]) *n*【拉】咳脓痰;脓腔(肺)
vomicose [ˈvɔmikəus] *a* 多脓的,多溃疡的
vomit [ˈvɔmit] *n* 呕吐;呕吐物;催吐药 *vt*, *vi* 呕吐 | bilious ~ 胆性呕吐物 / black ~ 黑色呕吐物 / coffee-ground ~ 咖啡渣呕吐物
vomiting [ˈvɔmitiŋ] *n* 呕吐 | cerebral ~ 脑性呕吐 / cyclic ~, periodic ~, recurrent ~ 周期性呕吐,阵发性呕吐 / dry ~ 干呕 / nervous ~ 神经性呕吐 / pernicious ~ 恶性孕吐 / ~ of preg-

nancy 妊娠呕吐 / projectile ~ 喷射性呕吐 / stercoraceous ~, fecal ~ 呕粪,吐粪
vomitive [ˈvɔmitiv] *a* 呕吐的,催吐的 *n* 催吐药
vomito [ˈvɔmitəu] *n*【西】呕吐;呕吐物 | ~ negro 黑色呕吐物
vomitory [ˈvɔmitəri] *n* 吐剂
vomiturition [ˌvɔmitjuəˈriʃən] *n* 干呕
vomitus [ˈvɔmitəs] *n*【拉】呕吐;呕吐物 | ~ cruentus 血性呕吐物,呕血 / ~ matutinus (慢性胃卡他性)晨吐
von Arlt 见 Arlt
von Behring 见 Behring
von Bezold 见 Bezold
v-*onc* viral *onc*ogene 病毒肿瘤基因
von Economo 见 Economo
von Frisch 见 Frisch
von Gierke 见 Gierke
von Graefe 见 Graefe
von Haller 见 Haller
von Hansemann cells [fəunˈhɑːnsəmɑːn] (David Paul von Hansemann) 冯·汉则曼细胞(含有米-古〈Michaelis-Gutmann〉小体的巨噬细胞,见于泌尿道和肾脏软斑病时的细胞内)
von Hippel 见 Hippel
von Langenbeck 见 Langenbeck
von Leyden 见 Leyden
von Mikulicz 见 Mikulicz
von Monakow 见 Monakow
von Pirquet 见 Pirquet
von Recklinghausen 见 Recklinghausen
von Tröltsch 见 Tröltsch
von Willebrand 见 Willebrand disease
von Zenker 见 Zenker
von Zumbusch 见 Zumbusch
Voorhees' bag [vuəˈriːz] (James D. Voorhees) 伏希斯袋(宫颈注水扩张袋)
vorbeireden [ˈfɔːbireidən] *n* 答非所问症(见于甘塞〈Ganser〉综合征和其他心理障碍)
Voronoff's operation [ˈvəurənɔf] (Serge Voronoff) 伏龙诺夫手术(将类人猿的睾丸移植至人,以期使受试者返老还童)
vortex [ˈvɔːteks] ([复] **vortexes** 或 **vortices** [ˈvɔːtisiːz]) *n*【拉】涡 | coccygeal ~ 尾毛涡 / ~ of heart 心涡
Vorticella [ˌvɔːtiˈselə] *n* 钟虫属
v. o. s vitello ovi solutus【拉】溶于卵黄的
Vossius lenticular ring [ˈvɔsiəs] (Adolf Vossius) 沃祖斯晶体环(虹膜震荡环)
vox [vɔks] ([复] **voces** [ˈvəusiz]) *n*【拉】嗓音,语音,语声 | ~ cholerica 霍乱嘶哑声
voxel [ˈvɔksel] *n* 体素(计算机轴向体层摄影时经扫描的每一像素的体积单位)
voyeur [vwɑːˈjəː] *n* 窥阴癖者 | **~ism** *n* 窥阴癖
VP variegate porphyria 杂斑卟啉病
VP-16 etoposide 依托泊苷
VPB ventricular premature beat 室性期前搏动
VPC ventricular premature complex 室性期前复合波
VPD ventricular premature depolarization 室性期前除极
VPF vascular permeability factor 血管通透性因子
VPRC volume of packed red cells 血细胞比容
VR vocal resonance 语响
VRE vancomycin-resistant enterococci 抗万古霉素肠球菌
Vrolik's disease [ˈvrəulik] (Willem Vrolik) 伏洛利克病,隐性遗传型成骨不全(Ⅱ型)
VS volumetric solution 滴定溶液,定量溶液
VSG variable surface glycoprotein 可变表面糖蛋白
VSV Vesiculovirus 水泡性病毒属
VT ventricular tachycardia 室性心动过速
vuerometer [ˌvjuəˈrɔmitə] *n* 眼距测量器
vulcanite [ˈvʌlkənait] *n* 硬橡皮,硫化橡皮
vulgaris [vʌlˈgɛəris] *a*【拉】寻常的,普通的
vulnerable [ˈvʌlnərəbl] *a* 易损的;易患病的 | **vulnerability** [ˌvʌlnərəˈbiləti] *n* 易损性;易患病性
vulnerant [ˈvʌlnərənt] *a* 致创伤的 *n* 致伤物
vulnerary [ˈvʌlnərəri] *a* 治创伤的 *n* 创伤药
vulnerate [ˈvʌlnəreit] *vt* 致伤,造成创伤
vulnus [ˈvʌlnəs] *n*【拉】创伤,伤口
Vulpian's atrophy [ˈvulpiæn] (Edme F. A. Vulpian) 伍尔皮安萎缩(肩肱型脊髓肌萎缩) | ~ law 伍尔皮安定律(脑部分损坏时,该处功能即由其余部分执行) / ~ test 伍尔皮安试验(检肾上腺素)
vulpic acid [ˈvʌlpik], **vulpinic acid** [ˌvʌlˈpinik] 枕酸甲酯
vulsella [vʌlˈselə], **vulsellum** [vʌlˈseləm] *n*【拉】双爪钳
vulva [ˈvʌlvə] ([复] **vulvae** [ˈvʌlviː]) *n*【拉】外阴,女阴 | fused ~ 外阴闭锁 | **~l**, **~r**, **~te** [ˈvʌlveit] *a*
vulvectomy [vʌlˈvektəmi] *n* 外阴切除术
vulvismus [vʌlˈvizməs] *n* 阴道痉挛
vulvitis [vʌlˈvaitis] *n* 外阴炎 | diabetic ~ 糖尿病性外阴炎 / erosive ~, phlegmonous ~ 腐蚀性外阴炎,蜂窝织炎性外阴炎 / leukoplakic ~ 白斑病外阴炎,外阴干皱 / plasma cell ~, ~ plasmocellularis 浆细胞性外阴炎 / pseudoleukoplakic ~ 假白斑病外阴炎
vulvocrural [vʌlvəˈkruərəl] *a* 外阴股的
vulvopathy [vʌlˈvɔpəθi] *n* 外阴病
vulvorectal [ˌvʌlvəˈrektl] *a* 外阴直肠的
vulvouterine [ˌvʌlvəˈjuːtərin] *a* 外阴子宫的

vulvovaginal [ˌvʌlvəˈvædʒinəl] *a* 外阴阴道的

vulvovaginitis [ˌvʌlvəˌvædʒiˈnaitis] *n* 外阴阴道炎 | infectious pustular ~ 感染性脓疱性外阴阴道炎 / senile ~ 老年性外阴阴道炎

vv. venae【拉】静脉

v / v volume (of solute) per volume (of solvent) (溶质)容量 / (溶剂)容量

VW vessel wall 血管壁,管壁

vWF von Willebrand's factor 冯 · 维勒布兰德因子

VX VX 神经毒气

V-Y plasty V-Y 成形术(即 V-Y 法, V-Y procedure)

VZIG varicella-zoster immune globulin 水痘-带状疱疹免疫球蛋白

W

W tryptophan 色氨酸；tungsten 钨；watt 瓦特

W work 功

Waardenburg's syndrome [ˈvɑːʌdənbəːg] (Petrus J. Waardenburg) 瓦登伯格综合征(①为一种常染色体显性遗传病,特征为内眦和泪点横向移位所致的鼻梁增宽,色素紊乱,其中包括白色额发、虹膜异色、白睫毛、白斑病以及有时伴耳蜗性聋;②为一种常染色体显性遗传病,特征为尖头畸形、眶和面部畸形以及短指〈趾〉畸形,伴轻度软组织并指〈趾〉畸形、腭裂、眼积水、心脏畸形以及可能还有肘与膝的挛缩。亦称尖头并指〈趾〉畸形Ⅳ型和克-瓦〈Klein-Waardenberg〉综合征)

Wachendorf's membrane [ˈvɑːhəndɔːf] (Eberhard J. Wachendorf) 瓦肯多夫膜(①瞳孔膜;②质膜)

Wada's test [ˈwɑːdə] (Juhn A. Wada) 和田试验(检语言功能的优势半球)

wagaga [wəˈgægə] *n* 丝虫病(斐济群岛的土名)

Wagner-Jauregg treatment [ˈvɑːgnəˈjaureg] (Julius Wagner von Jauregg) 瓦格纳·约雷格疗法(麻痹性痴呆的疟原虫接种疗法)

Wagner's corpuscles [ˈvɑːgnə] (Rudolf Wagner) 触觉小体 | ~ spot 瓦格纳点(人卵的核仁)

Wagner's disease [ˈvɑːgnə] (Ernst L. Wagner) 胶状粟粒疹

Wagner's hammer [ˈvɑːgnə] (Johann P. Wagner) 瓦格纳锤(见 Neef's hammer)

Wagner's operation [ˈvɑːgnə] (Wilhelm Wagner) 瓦格纳手术(颅骨成形性切除术)

Wagstaffe's fracture [ˈwægstɑːf] (William W. Wagstaffe) 瓦格斯塔夫骨折(内踝离解)

WAIS Wechsler Adult Intelligence Scale 韦克斯勒成人智力量表

waist [weist] *n* 腰,腰部

Waldenburg's apparatus [ˈvɑːldənbəːg] (Louis Waldenburg) 瓦尔登伯格器(助呼吸器,即压缩患者吸入的空气或让呼气排出)

Waldenström's disease [ˈvɑːldənstrem] (Johan H. Waldenström) 瓦尔登斯特伦病(股骨小头的骨软骨病)

Waldenström's macroglobulinemia [ˈvɑːldnstrem] (Jan Waldenström) 瓦尔登斯特伦巨球蛋白血症(一种类似白血病的浆细胞病,淋巴细胞、浆细胞及中间型形态的细胞分泌 IgM M 成分,骨髓呈弥散性浸润,虚弱、倦怠和视力障碍)

Waldeyer's fluid [ˈvɑːldaiə] (Heinrich W. G. von Waldeyer) 氯化钯脱钙液 | ~ fossa 十二指肠结肠系膜隐窝 / ~ glands 瓦尔代尔腺(睑缘内管泡腺) / ~ layer 卵巢血管层 / ~ tonsillar ring 瓦尔代尔扁桃体环(由舌、咽、腭扁桃体所形成的环状淋巴组织) / ~ sulcus 瓦尔代尔沟(螺旋沟)

walk [wɔːk] *vi* 走,步行 *n* 步态

walker [ˈwɔːkə] *n* 助行器

Walker's lissencephaly [ˈwɔːkə] (Arthur E. Walker) 沃克无脑回(见 Walker-Warburg syndrome)

Walker-Warburg syndrome [ˈwɔːkə ˈvɑːrbəːg] (A. E. Walker; Mette Warburg) 沃-瓦综合征(一种先天性综合征,通常在1岁前即死亡,包括脑积水,无脑回,各种眼异常,诸如视网膜发育不全、角膜混浊或小眼,有时为脑突出。亦称 HARD 综合征)

walking [ˈwɔːkiŋ] *n* 行走,步行,步度;步态 *a* 能行走的;不需卧床休息的 | chromosome ~ 染色体步查,染色体步移(在分子遗传学中,按顺序分离基因文库中携带重叠 DNA 序列的亚克隆,因此过程很像是沿部分染色体"步行",最终寻找到并分离出目标基因,故而得名) / heel ~ 足跟步态(见于周围神经炎) / sleep ~ 睡行[症]

wall [wɔːl] *n* 壁 | axial ~ 轴壁(牙) / cavity ~ 洞壁(牙) / cell ~ 细胞壁 / germ ~ 胚壁 / nail ~ 甲廓 / parietal ~ 壁层,胚体壁 / periotic ~ 听泡壁 / splanchnic ~ 脏层,胚脏壁 / subpulpal ~ 髓底壁

Wallenberg's syndrome [ˈvɑːlənbəːg] (Adolf Wallenberg) 瓦伦贝格综合征(由后下小脑动脉栓塞所致的综合征,特征为同侧面部温度觉和痛觉丧失、对侧四肢和躯干温觉和痛觉丧失、同侧共济失调、吞咽困难、构音障碍以及眼球震颤)

wallerian degeneration [wɔˈliəriən] (Augustus V. Waller) 沃勒变性(指已与营养中枢断离的神经纤维的脂肪变性,亦称继发变性) | ~ law, Waller's law 沃勒定律(在神经节中枢侧切断脊神经根感觉纤维,则切断纤维的周边部分未变性,而与脊髓相连的纤维则变性)

walleye [ˈwɔːlai] *n* 角膜白斑;散开性斜视,外

斜视

Wallhauser-Whitehead's method [ˈwɔlhausə ˈwaithed] (A. Wallhauser; J. M. Whitehead) 沃尔豪泽-怀特黑德法(用自身腺滤出液治疗霍奇金〈Hodgkin〉病)

wall-plate [ˈwɔl pleit] *n* 低压电流机

Walter's bromide test [ˈvɑːltə] (Friedrich K. Walter) 华尔特溴化物试验(正常人血内溴化物含量与脑脊液内的含量的比率是不变的,但在精神病患者的比率则有改变)

Walthard's islets (cell rests, inclusions) [ˈvɑːltɑːd] (Max Walthard) 瓦尔塔德小岛(细胞残余、包涵物)(卵巢生殖上皮的微小包涵物,由此可发生卵巢纤维上皮瘤)

Walther's ducts [ˈvɑːltə] (August F. Walther) 舌下腺小管 | ~ ganglion 尾骨球 / ~ oblique ligament 距腓后韧带

wambles [ˈwɑːmblz] *n* 乳毒病

wanderer [ˈwɑːdərə] *n* 患失调综合征的幼驹

wandering [ˈwɔndəriŋ] *a* 游动的,游走的 *n* 游动;神志恍惚,精神错乱 | mind ~ 冥思,出神,心不在焉 / pathologic tooth ~ 病理性牙游动

wanganga [wænˈgæŋgə] *n* 象皮病样热(斐济土语)

Wangensteen drainage [ˈwæŋgənstiːn] (Owen H. Wangensteen) 旺根斯滕引流(用胃管或十二指肠管持续吸引引流,以治肠梗阻等) | ~ tube (apparatus, suction) 旺根斯滕管(器、抽吸)(胃肠吸引器,用以保持胃、十二指肠的减压)

Wangiella [wæŋiːˈelə] *n* 瓶霉属

Wang's test (Wang Chung Tik, 中国病理学家王宠益)王氏试验(尿蓝母定量试验)

Wanscher's mask [ˈvɑːnʃə] (Oscar Wanscher) 万舍面罩(乙醚麻醉时用)

warbles [ˈwɔːblz] *n* (牛)皮瘤(由皮下蝇蛆所致囊肿) | ox ~ 牛皮蝇蛆

Warburg's coenzyme [ˈwɑːrburk] (Otto H. Warburg) 烟酰胺腺嘌呤二核苷酸磷酸,三磷酸吡啶核苷酸

Warburg's syndrome [ˈwɑːrbərg] (Mette Warburg) 瓦氏综合征(见 Walker-Warburg syndrome)

ward [wɔːd] *n* 病房,病室 | isolation ~ 隔离病室 / psychopathic ~ 精神病室

Ward-Romano syndrome [wɔːd rəuˈmɑːnəu] (O. C. Ward; C. Romano) 沃德-罗马诺综合征(见 Romano-Ward syndrome)

warfarin [ˈwɑːfərin] *n* 华法林(抗凝药)

Waring's method (system) [ˈwɛəriŋ] (George E. Waring) 华林法(系统)(污水地下灌溉处置法)

Warren's fat columns [ˈwɔrən] (John C. Warren) 华伦皮下脂肪柱(自皮肤结缔组织至毛囊和汗腺的脂肪组织柱) | ~ incision 华伦切口(乳房手术的切口,即沿胸乳皱襞切开,可达到乳房任何部分)

Warren shunt [ˈwɔːrən] (W. Dean Warren) 沃伦分流,远端脾肾分流

wart [wɔːt] *n* 疣,肉赘 | acuminate ~, pointed ~, venereal ~ 尖锐湿疣,性病湿疣 / anatomical ~, necrogenic ~ 解剖疣,剖尸疣,尸毒性疣,疣状皮结核 / common ~ 寻常疣 / flat ~, juvenile ~, plane ~ 扁平疣,青年疣 / moist ~ 扁头湿疣,梅毒湿疣 / mosaic ~ 镶嵌疣 / mother ~ 母疣 / peruvian ~ 秘鲁疣 / postmortem ~, prosector's ~, tuberculous ~ 剖尸疣,尸毒性疣,解剖者疣,疣状皮结核 / seborrheic ~, senile ~ 脂溢性疣,脂溢性角化病,老年疣 / seed ~ 子疣 / soot ~ 煤烟疣,煤灰癌 / telangiectatic ~ 血管扩张性疣,血管角质瘤 | **~y** *a* 有疣的,疣状的

Wartenberg's disease [ˈwɔːtənbəːg] (Robert Wartenberg) 华滕伯格病(感觉异常性手痛) | ~ sign 华滕伯格征(①小指外展为尺神经麻痹体征;②小脑病患者步行时两臂摆动减少或无摆动) / ~ symptom 华滕伯格症状(①鼻孔、鼻尖发痒显示脑瘤;②锥体病时,其他手指因阻力屈曲,拇指也屈曲)

Warthin-Finkeldey cell [ˈwɔːθin ˈfiŋkəldei] (A. S. Warthin; Wilhelm Finkeldey) 沃-芬细胞(多核巨细胞并有核内包涵体,为淋巴网状源性,见于各种器官,其中包括淋巴结、扁桃体、阑尾及胸腺,恰好在麻疹之前或麻疹前驱期的时期)

Warthin's tumor [ˈwɔːθin] (Alfred S. Warthin) 沃辛瘤,淋巴瘤性乳头状囊腺瘤

wash [wɔʃ] *vt*, *vi* 洗 *n* 洗,洗涤;洗剂,洗液 | eye ~ 洗眼剂 / mouth ~ 漱[口]药,含漱剂

washer [ˈwɔʃə] *n* 洗涤器 | centrifugal cell ~ 离心式细胞清洗器

washing [ˈwɔːʃiŋ] *n* 洗[涤],漂[洗] | sperm ~ 精子清洗(试管内受精时用)

washout [ˈwɔːʃaut] *n* 洗去,冲去 | nitrogen ~ 氮洗脱

Wasielewskia [ˌwæsieˈljuːskiə] 瓦西列夫斯基变形虫属,双鞭变形虫属

Waskia [ˈwæskiə] *n* 华斯克内滴虫属,内滴虫属

wasp [wɔsp] *n* 胡蜂,黄蜂

wasserhelle [ˈvʌːsəˌheli] *a*【德】明的,水样透明的(细胞)

Wassermann-fast [ˈwʌsəmən ˌfɑːst] *a* 华氏反应固定的,梅毒补体结合反应固定的(虽经抗梅毒药物治疗,而始终显示华氏反应阳性的)

Wassermann reaction (test) [ˈwʌsəmən] (August P. von Wassermann) 华[色曼]氏反应(试验),梅毒补体结合反应(试验)(根据补体结合诊断梅毒的一种试验) | provocative ~ reaction

激发性华氏反应(先使用砷剂的华氏反应,此法可使原为阴性反应者转为阳性反应)

Wassilieff's disease [wə'silief] (Nikolai P. Wassilieff) 钩端螺旋体性黄疸

waste [weist] *vt*, *vi* 消耗;消瘦 *a* 排泄的 *n* 排泄物;消耗 | phonetic ~ of the breath 环杓侧肌麻痹性呼气过速 / sodium ~ 钠消耗

wasting [weistiŋ] *n* 消耗;消瘦 *a* 消耗[性]的;使消瘦的

water ['wɔːtə] *n* 水,水剂;芳香水;净化水 | ammonia ~ 氨水,稀氨溶液 / bound ~ 结合水 / capillary ~ 毛细管水(在土壤中) / carbon dioxide-free ~ 无二氧化碳水 / distilled ~ 蒸馏水 / free ~ 游离水 / ground ~ 地下水 / hamamelis ~, witch-hazel ~ 北美金缕梅水 / hard ~ 硬水 / heavy ~ 重水,氧化氘 / ~ for injection 注射用水 / lead ~ 铅水(稀次醋酸铅溶液) / metabolic ~, ~ of combustion 代谢水,燃烧水 / mineral ~ 矿水,泉水 / ~ on the brain 脑积水 / ~ on the knee 膝关节水肿 / orange flower ~ 橙花水 / potable ~ 饮用水 / purified ~ 净化水 / raw ~ 未经纯化的水 / saline ~ 盐水 / serum ~ 血清水(制备细菌培养基用) / soft ~ 软水 / stronger ammonia ~ 浓氨水,浓氨溶液 / tap ~ 自来水

water-bite ['wɔːt bait] *n* 战壕足

water-borne ['wɔːtə bɔːn] *a* 水传播的

water brash ['wɔːtə bræʃ] 胃灼热,反酸

Waterhouse-Friderichsen syndrome ['wɔːtəhaus ˌfridə'riksən] (Rupert Waterhouse; Carl Friderichsen), 沃-弗综合征,暴发性脑膜炎球菌败血症(恶性或暴发型流行性脑脊膜炎,特征为突然发作及病程短、发热、昏迷、虚脱、发绀、皮肤与黏膜出血及两侧肾上腺出血)

waters ['wɔːtəz] *n* 羊水(俗称)

watershed ['wɔːtəʃed] *n* 分水岭,分水界 | abdominal ~s 腹腔分水岭

Waters' position ['wɔːtəz] (Charles A. Waters) 沃特斯位(沃特斯投照时头的位置) | ~ projection 沃特斯投照(前头的放射投照,用以位观上颌窦和蝶骨,中心射线以通过颏的角度进入)

Waterston operation (anastomosis, shunt) ['wɔːtəstən] (David J. Waterston) 沃特斯顿手术(吻合术、分流术)(升主动脉和右肺动脉之间的吻合术,作为先天性肺动脉瓣狭窄的姑息性疗法)

Watkins' operation ['wɔtkinz] (Thomas J. Watkins) 沃特金斯手术(用于子宫脱垂的一种手术,其膀胱由子宫的前壁剥离,使子宫位于支持全部膀胱的位置)

Watson-Crick helix ['wɔtsn krik] (James D. Watson; Francis H. C. Crick) 沃森-克里克螺旋结构形(指 DNA 分子的一种双螺旋结构形)

Watsonius watsoni [wɔt'səuniəs wɔt'səunai] (Malcolm Watson) 瓦[生]氏瓦生吸虫

Watson-Schwartz test ['wɔtsn ʃwɑːts] (Cecil J. Watson; Samuel Schwartz) 沃森-施瓦茨试验(诊断急性卟啉病)

watt (W) [wɔt] *n* 瓦[特](电功率单位)

wattage ['wɔtidʒ] *n* 瓦[特]数

watt-hour ['wɔt auə] *n* 瓦[特小]时

wattmeter ['wɔtmitə] *n* 瓦特计

wave [weiv] *n* 波 | alpha ~s α 波(频率为每秒 8~13 次的脑电波) / anacrotic ~ 升线一波 / anadicrotic ~ 升线二波 / beta ~s β 波(频率为每秒 18~30 次的脑电波) / catacrotic ~ 降线一波 / catadicrotic ~ 降线二波 / contraction ~ 收缩波 / delta ~s δ 波(频率为每秒 $3\frac{1}{2}$ 次以下的脑电波;心电图早期 QRS 波) / dicrotic ~ 降中波 / excitation ~ 兴奋波 / F ~s F 波(心电图) / fibrillary ~s 纤维性颤动波(心电图)/ P ~ P 波(心电图) / papillary ~, percussion ~ 脉首波(静脉波曲线的主要升支) / phrenic ~ 膈运动波 / pulse ~ 脉波 / Q ~ Q 波(心电图) / R ~ R 波(心电图) / random ~ 任意波(睡眠初期发生于脑电波中的一种不规则的电波) / recoil ~ 反冲波 / S ~ S 波(心电图) / short ~ 短波 / sonic ~ 声波 / T ~ T 波(心电图) / theta ~s θ 波(频率为每秒 4~7 次的脑电波) / tricrotic ~ 三波脉波 / ultrashort ~ 超短波,微波 / ultrasonic ~ 超声波

waveform ['weivfɔːm] *n* 波形(常用作 wave 的同义词) | sinusoidal ~ 正弦波

wavelength (λ) ['weivleŋθ] *n* 波长 | effective ~, equivalent ~ 有效波长 / minimum ~ 最短波长

wax [wæks] *n* 蜡 | blockout ~ 平整蜡 / bone ~ 骨蜡 / boxing ~ 围模蜡 / candelilla ~ 小烛树蜡 / carnauba ~, palm ~ 巴西棕榈蜡 / casting ~ 铸造蜡 / cetyl esters ~ 十六烷基酯蜡(药物制剂时用作硬化剂,亦称合成鲸蜡) / Chinese ~ 虫白蜡 / dental ~ 牙蜡 / dental inlay casting ~, inlay casting ~, inlay pattern ~ 牙嵌体铸模蜡 / ear ~ 耵聍,耳垢 / grave ~ 尸蜡 / inlay ~ 嵌体蜡 / set-up ~ 校准蜡 / try-in ~ 基板蜡 / tubercle bacillus ~ 结核杆菌蜡质 / vegetable ~ 植物蜡 / white ~ 白[蜂]蜡 / yellow ~ 黄[蜂]蜡

waxing ['wæksiŋ] *n* 蜡型制作

waxing up ['wæksiŋ ʌp] 上蜡,蜡模形成

Wb weber 韦伯(磁通量单位)

WBC white blood cell 白细胞; white blood (cell) count 白细胞计数

wean [wiːn] *vt* 断奶

weanling ['wiːnliŋ] *n* 刚断奶婴儿(或幼畜) *a* 刚

断奶的

web [web] *n* 网,丝;网状物;蛛网状组织;蹼 | esophageal ~ 食管蹼(此术语常与 esophageal ring〈食管环〉换用) / subsynaptic ~ 突触下网 / terminal ~ 闭锁网,终网 / laryngeal ~ 喉蹼[畸形]

webbed [webd] *a* 有蹼的

weber(Wb) [ˈveibə] *n* 韦伯(磁通量单位)

Weber-Christian disease, panniculitis, syndrome [ˈwebə ˈkristjən] (F. P. Weber; Henry A. Christian) 复发性结节性非化脓性脂膜炎

Weber-Cockayne syndrome [ˈwebə ˈkɔkein] (F. P. Weber; Edward A Cockyne) 局限性大疱性表皮松解

Weber-Fechner law [ˈveibə ˈfeknə] (Ernest H. Weber; Gustav T. Fechner) 韦-费定律(感觉等量增加〈算术级数〉,刺激必须以几何级数增加。亦称精神物理定律)

Weber-Gubler syndrome [ˈwebə ˈguːblə] (H. D. Weber; Adolphe M. Gubler) 韦-古综合征(见 Weber's syndrome)

Weber-Leyden syndrome [ˈwebə ˈlaidən] (H. D. Weber; Ernst Victor von Leyden) 韦-莱综合征(见 Weber's syndrome)

Weber's corpuscle(organ) [ˈveibə] (Moritz I. Weber) 前列腺囊 | ~ glands 舌黏液腺 / ~ zone 髋关节轮匝带

Weber's disease [ˈwebə] (Frederick P. Weber) 韦伯病(①局部性大疱性表皮松解;②斯特奇-韦伯综合征,见 Sturge-Weber syndrome)

Weber's douche [ˈveibə] (Theodor Weber) 韦伯灌洗(一种鼻灌洗)

Weber's law [ˈveibə] (Ernest H. Weber) 韦伯定律(当刺激强度改变时,可感觉的最小刺激差异,与全部刺激之间,维持一定的比例) | ~ paradox 韦伯奇异现象(肌肉伸长不能收缩) / ~ test 韦伯试验(检尿蓝母、血)

Weber's sign(symptom) [ˈwebə] (Hermann D. Weber) 韦伯征(症状)(一侧动眼神经麻痹,对侧偏瘫) | ~ syndrome(paralysis) 韦伯综合征(麻痹)(同侧动眼神经麻痹,对侧痉挛性偏瘫,亦称动眼神经交叉性偏瘫)

Weber's test [ˈveibə] (Friedrich E. Weber) 韦伯试验(检耳聋、尿蓝母、血)

Webster's operation [ˈwebstə] (John C. Webster) 韦伯斯特手术(治子宫后移位,圆韧带穿过阔韧带,固定于子宫的背面)

Webster's test [ˈwebstə] (John Webster) 韦伯斯特试验(检尿中三硝基甲苯)

Wechsler Adult Intelligence Scale, Intelligence Scale for Children [ˈwekslə] (David Wechsler) 韦克斯勒成人智力量表,韦克斯勒儿童智力量表

weddellite [ˈwedəlait] *n* (首次在南极洲 Weddell Sea 发现)二水草酸钙(见于尿石内)

Wedensky facilitation [vəˈdenski] (Nikolai Yevgenyevich Wedensky) 韦金斯基易化作用(穿越阻滞的易化作用,当神经传导完全阻滞时,阻滞部以下神经对电刺激的阈值下降) | ~ inhibition 韦金斯基抑制(神经的部分传导阻滞可仍有低频率的传导冲动,但不会出现高频率的传导冲动) / ~ phenomenon 韦金斯基现象(对一神经使用一系列快速反复刺激,肌肉对首次刺激迅速收缩,然后再也不起反应,但如果对神经的刺激速度较慢,则肌肉对所有刺激均有反应)

wedge [wedʒ] *n* 楔;楔形物 *vt, vi* 楔入 | step ~ 楔形梯级(楔形梯级式〈X 线〉透度计,用以测量 X 线的透度)

WEE western equine encephalomyelitis 西方马脑脊髓炎

Weeks' bacillus [wiːks] (John E. Weeks) 结膜炎嗜血杆菌

weep [wiːp] *vi* 流泪 *n* 流泪;渗出;滴下

weever fish [ˈwiːvə fiʃ] 鲈鱼

weevil [ˈwiːvəl] *n* 象鼻虫 | wheal ~ 麦粒象鼻虫

Wegener's granulomatosis [ˈvegənə] (F. Wegener) 韦格纳肉芽肿病(一种多系统疾病,主要侵袭男子,特征为累及上、下呼吸道的坏死性肉芽肿性血管炎、肾小球性肾炎和程度不同的系统性小血管血管炎,一般认为代表一种对不明抗原的异常过敏性反应)

Wegner's disease [ˈvegnə] (Friedrich R. G. Wegner) 韦格纳病(遗传性梅毒骨软骨炎所致骨骺分离) | ~ sign 韦格纳征(遗传梅毒致死婴儿的骺线增宽变色)

wehnelt [ˈveinəlt] *n* 韦内(X 线硬度单位,X 线穿透力单位)

Weichbrodt's reaction [ˈvaiʃbrɔt] (Raphael Weichbrodt) 魏希布罗特反应(检梅毒) | ~ test 魏希布罗特试验(检球蛋白)

Weichselbaum's diplococcus [ˈvaikselˌbaum] (Anton Weichselbaum) 魏克塞尔包姆双球菌,脑膜炎奈瑟菌(Neisseria meningitides)

Weidel's test [ˈvaidəl] (Hugo Weidel) 魏德尔试验(检尿酸、黄嘌呤、黄嘌呤体)

Weigert's law [ˈvaigət] (Karl Weigert) 魏格尔特定律(损耗过补律:在有机界中失去或破坏一元素时,则有一补偿作用随之而来,使该元素过量生产)

weight [weit] *n* 重,重量 | apothecaries' ~ 药用衡量 / atomic ~ 原子量 / avoirdupois ~ 常衡制(英制) / combining ~ 化合量,结合量 / equivalent ~ 当量 / molecular ~ 分子量 / troy ~ 金衡制(英制)

weightless [ˈweitlis] *a* 失重的 | **~ness** *n* 失重

weights and measures 度量衡的,有影响的

Weil-Felix reaction (test) [vail ˈfeiliks] (Edmund Weil; Arthur Felix) 外-斐反应(试验)(斑疹伤寒病人血清能使变形杆菌 X 菌产生有诊断价值的凝集反应,这显然由于有共同抗原存在所致)

Weill-Marchesani syndrome [vail mɑːkəˈsɑːni] (Georges Weill; Oswald Marchesani) 韦-马综合征(一种先天性结缔组织的疾病,作为常染色体显性或隐性性状遗传,特征为短头,短指〈趾〉,身材矮小,胸廓宽大及肌肉系统过于发达,关节活动度减少,球形晶状体,晶状体异位,近视及青光眼。亦称先天性中胚叶增生性营养不良,球形晶状体-短身材综合征)

Weill's sign [vail] (Edmond Weill) 韦尔征(婴儿肺炎的病侧锁骨下部无膨胀)

Weil's basal layer (zone) [vail] (L. A. Weil) 魏尔基底层(区)(在牙髓的成牙质细胞层内)

Weil's stain [wail] (Arthur Weil) 韦尔染剂(染髓鞘)

Weil's syndrome (disease) [vail] (Adolf Weil) 魏尔综合征(病)(一种重型钩端螺旋体病,特征为黄疸,通常伴有氮血症、出血、贫血、意识障碍和持续发热。亦称钩端螺旋体性黄疸,传染性黄疸,出血性黄疸钩端螺旋体病)

Weil's test [wail] (Richard Weil) 韦尔试验,眼镜蛇毒试验(检梅毒)

Weinberg's test (reaction) [ˈvainbəːg] (Michel Weinberg) 温伯格试验(反应)(诊断包虫病的一种补体结合试验)

Weingarten's syndrome [ˈwaingɑːtən] (R. J. Weingarten) 热带嗜酸粒细胞增多症

Weinmannia [wainˈmæniə] *n* 万灵木属(树皮具有收敛作用)

Weir Mitchel [wir ˈmitʃəl] 见 Mitchel

Weir's operation [wiə] (Robert F. Weir) 阑尾造口术

Weisbach's angle [ˈvaisbɑːh] (Albin Weisbach) 魏斯巴赫角(在牙槽中点处)

Weismann's theory [ˈwaismən] (August Weismann), **weismannism** [ˈwaismənizəm] *n* 魏斯曼学说(后天特性不遗传)

Weiss' reflex [vais] (Leopold Weiss) 魏斯反射(近视反射)

Weiss' sign [vais] (Nathan Weiss) 魏斯征(轻叩面神经时面肌痉挛)

Weiss' test [vais] (Moriz Weiss) 魏斯试验(检尿色素原)

Weitbrecht's cartilage [ˈvirbrekt] (Josias Weitbrecht) 肩锁关节关节盘 | ~ cord(ligament) 前臂骨间膜斜索 / ~ foramen 魏特布雷希特孔(肩关节囊孔,滑膜经由此孔至肩胛下肌下面的滑囊) / ~ retinaculum 魏特布雷希特支持带(附着于股骨颈的支持带纤维)

Welander's distal myopathy (myopathy, syndrome) [ˈveilɑːndə] (Lisa Welander) 范伦德远端肌病(肌病、综合征),晚期远端遗传性肌病

Welch's bacillus [ˈwelʃ] (William H. Welch) 产气荚膜(梭状芽胞)杆菌

Welcker's angle [ˈvelkə] (Hermann Welcker) 顶骨蝶角 | ~ method 威尔克法(先放血,然后冲洗血管以测定全血量)

Wells syndrome [welz] (G. C. Wells) 威尔斯综合征(蜂窝织炎,表现为红斑、水肿及皮肤经常水疱形成,伴有嗜酸粒细胞增多、火焰形皮肤损伤和轻度发热;一次发作持续 2 ~ 6 周,经常复发和病情加剧)

welt [welt] *n* 风团,风疹块

wen [wen] *n* 皮脂腺囊肿

Wenckebach block [ˈvenkəbɑːh] (Karel F. Wenckebach) 温克巴赫传导阻滞(一型第 I 度房室传导阻滞,在 P-R 间期一系列稳定增长后,周期性发生一次或多次心搏脱漏,这通常由于房室结内传导阻滞之故) / ~ period 温克巴赫期(发生于温克巴赫传导阻滞连续心动周期时的 P-R 间期稳定延长) / ~ phenomenon 温克巴赫现象(见 ~ block)

Wender's test [ˈvendə] (Neumann Wender) 文德尔试验(检葡萄糖)

Wenzell's test [ˈwenzəl] (William T. Wenzell) 温策尔试验(检士的宁)

Werdnig-Hoffmann spinal muscular atrophy (disease) [ˈvəːdnig ˈhɔfmɑːn] (Guido Werdnig; Ernst Hoffmann) 韦德尼希-霍夫曼脊髓性肌萎缩(病)(一种遗传性进行性幼稚型肌萎缩。亦称家族脊髓性肌萎缩、婴儿进行性脊髓性肌萎缩)

Werlhof's disease [ˈvəːlhɔf] (Paul G. Werlhof) 特发性血小板减少性紫癜

Wermer's syndrome [ˌwəːmə] (Paul Wermer) 多发性内分泌腺瘤形成 I 型

Werner-His disease [ˈvəːnə ˈhis] (Heinrich Werner; William His) 战壕热

Werner Schultz disease [ˈvernə ʃults] (Werner Schultz) 韦尔纳·舒尔茨病,粒细胞缺乏症

Werner's syndrome [ˈvəːnə] (C. W. Otto Werner) 维尔纳综合征,成人早老症(为常染色体隐性遗传的成人过早衰老,主要特征为硬皮病样皮肤改变〈尤其累及肢体〉、白内障、皮下钙化、肌肉萎缩、糖尿病倾向、面部呈现衰老外观、白发秃头以及肿瘤发生率高。常见身材矮小都是从儿童期开始,其他特征通常是在成人期形成。)

Wernicke-Korsakoff syndrome [ˈvəːnikə kɔːˈsækɔːf] (Karl Wernicke; Sergei S. Korsakoff) 韦尼克-科尔萨科夫综合征(硫胺〈维生素 B_1〉

缺乏所致的神经精神疾患,最常见的为长期滥用酒精所致,并伴发其他营养性多神经病)

Wernicke-Mann hemiplegia (type) [ˈvəːnikə mɑːn] (Karl Wernicke; Ludwig Mann) 韦尼克曼偏瘫(型)(四肢的不全性偏瘫)

Wernicke's aphasia [ˈvəːnikə] (Karl Wernicke) 感觉性失语[症],记言不能 | ~ area, ~ center, ~ field, ~ zone 韦尼克区(言语中枢) / ~ encephalopathy (disease, syndrome) 韦尼克脑病(病、综合征)(一种神经性疾病,特征为精神错乱、情感淡漠、瞌睡、共济失调步态、眼球震颤和眼肌麻痹。现知本病为硫胺〈维生素 B_1〉缺乏所致,最常见的为长期滥用酒精所致,几乎都伴发 Korsakoff 综合征〈器质性遗忘症〉,并常伴有其他营养性多神经病) / ~ reaction 韦尼克反应,偏盲性瞳孔反应(hemiopic pupillary reaction,见 reaction 项下相应术语) / ~ triangle 韦尼克三角(内囊后脚内之区,在此区内视辐射线刚离开外侧膝状体,接近听辐射线和躯体感觉辐射线)

Wertheim-Schauta operation [ˈvəːtaim ˈʃautə] (Ernst Wertheim; Friedrich Schauta) 韦特海姆-绍特手术(膀胱突出修补术,将子宫放在膀胱底和阴道前壁之间)

Wertheim's operation [ˈvəːthaim] (Ernst Wertheim) 韦特海姆手术(根治性子宫切除术,治宫颈癌手术)

Westberg's space [ˈvestbɛəg] (Friedrich Westberg) 韦斯特贝格隙(心包主动脉隙)

Westergren method [ˈvestergren] (Alf Westergren) 韦斯特格伦法(检红细胞沉降率) | ~ tube 韦斯特格伦管(在韦斯特格伦法中用于测定红细胞沉降率)

Westermark's sign [ˈvestəmɑːk] (N. Westermark) 韦斯特马克征(肺栓塞远端的肺组织,正常放射阴影暂时消失〈无血管〉)

Western blot technique (blot analysis, blot hybridization, blot test) [ˈwestən] (仿 Southern blot technique 诙谐式造词) 蛋白质印迹技术(印迹分析,印迹杂交,印迹试验)

West Nile encephalitis (fever) [west nail] (乌干达北部西尼罗河谷和地区于 1937 年首次观察到此病)西尼罗河脑炎(热)(一种由黄病毒西尼罗河病毒所致的轻度发热性散发性疾病,由库蚊传播) | ~ virus 西尼罗河病毒(黄病毒属的一种病毒,可致西尼罗河脑炎)

Weston Hurst disease [ˈwestən həːst] (Edward Weston Hurst) 韦斯顿·赫斯特病,急性坏死性出血性脑脊髓炎

Westphal-Piltz phenomenon [ˈvestfɑːl ˈpilts] (A. K. O. Westphal; Jan Piltz) 韦斯特法尔-皮尔茨现象(用力闭上眼睑,瞳孔即收缩,并随之散大,由于轮匝肌紧张所致) | ~ reflex 韦斯特法尔-皮尔茨反射(瞳孔收缩伴闭眼或试图闭眼)

Westphal's nucleus [ˈvestfɑːl] (Carl F. O. Westphal) 副核 | ~ sign (phenomenon, symptom) 韦斯特法尔征(现象、症状)(脊髓痨时膝反射消失)

Westphal's phenomenon [ˈvestfɑːl] (Alexander K. O. Westphal) 韦斯特法尔现象(①见 Westphal-Piltz phenomenon; ②见 Westphal sign) | ~ pupillary reflex 韦斯特法尔瞳孔反射(见 Westphal-Piltz reflex)

Westphal-Strümpell disease, pseudosclerosis [ˈvestfɑːl ˈstrimpəl] (C. F. O. Westphal; Ernst A. G. G. von Strümpell) 肝豆状核变性

West's syndrome [west] (Charles West) 韦斯特综合征,婴儿痉挛

wet-nurse [ˈwetnəːs] *n* 奶妈,乳母

wet-pack [ˈwetpæk] *n* 湿裹法

wetpox [ˈwetpɔks] *n* 湿痘(类似禽痘,生于口腔内,常因窒息而引起死亡)

wet-scald [ˈwetskɔːld] *n* 羊湿疹

Wetzel's grid [ˈwetsel] (Norman C. Wetzel) 韦策尔网格(可由小框格直读儿童生长、发育及基础代谢数值)

Wetzel's test [ˈvetsel] (Georg Wetzel) 韦策尔试验(检血内一氧化碳)

Wever-Bray phenomenon [ˈwiːvə brei] (Ernest G. Wever; Charles W. Bray) 耳蜗微音

Weyers' oligodactyly syndrome [ˈvaiəz] (Helmut Weyers) 维耶斯少指(趾)畸形综合征(一种先天性综合征,包括尺骨及尺侧掌骨与指骨缺失,肘前翼状胬肉,胸骨节段减少,肾脾畸形及唇裂与腭裂)

Weyl's test [vail] (Theodor Weyl) 魏尔试验(检肌酸酐、尿硝酸)

Wharton's duct [ˈhwɔːtn] (Thomas Wharton) 下颌下腺管 | ~ jelly (gelatin) 脐带胶质

wheal [hwiːl] *n* 风团

wheel [hwiːl] *n* 轮,磨盘 | rag ~ 布[质]磨盘

wheelchair [ˈhwiːlˌtʃɛə] *n* (病人等用的)轮椅

Wheelhouse's operation [ˈhwiːlhaus] (Claudius G. Wheelhouse) 惠尔豪斯手术(会阴部尿道切开术)

wheeze [hwiːz] *vi* 喘气,喘息 *n* 哮鸣 | asthmatoid ~ 哮喘样哮鸣

whelk [welk] *n* 酒刺,面部丘疹

whelp [hwelp] *vt* 下崽,产仔(指母狗) *n* 小狗

whewellite [ˈhjuːwəlait] (William Whewell) *n* 一水草酸钙(见于尿石内)

whey [hwei] *n* 乳清 | wine ~ 甜乳清酒 | **~ey** [ˈhweiiː] *a* 似乳清的

WHHL Watanabe heritable hyperlipidemic (rabbit) 渡边可遗传的高脂血(家兔)

whip [hwip] *vt*, *n* 鞭打 | catheter ~ 导管伪压

whiplash [ˈhwiplæʃ] *n* 鞭打;鞭子式损伤(whiplash injury, 见 injury 项下相应术语)

Whipple's disease [ˈhwipl] (George H. Whipple) 惠普尔病(一种养料吸收障碍综合征,亦称肠源性脂肪代谢障碍) | ~ test 惠普尔试验(检肝功能)

Whipple's operation [ˈhwipl] (Allen O. Whipple) 惠普尔手术(根治性胰头十二指肠切除术) | ~ triad 惠普尔三联征(分泌胰岛素肿瘤的主要临床征象:①自发性低血糖〈血糖低于 50 mg/100 ml〉,②伴有中枢神经或血管舒缩症状,③口服或静脉注射葡萄糖使症状缓解)

whipworm [ˈhwipwəːm] *n* [毛首]鞭虫

whisper [ˈhwispə] *vi* 低语,耳语 *n* 低语,耳语

Whitaker test [ˈhwitəkə] (Robert H. Whitaker) 怀特克试验(一种压力-流速研究,通过肾盂的顺行肾盂造影[术]和膀胱内导管测定输尿管对尿一定流速的阻力)

white [hwait] *a* 白的 *n* 白色;[复]白带 | Spanish ~ 次硝酸铋 / visual ~ 视白质

whitecomb [ˈhwaitkəum] *n* 白冠病,鸡冠癣病

whitehead [ˈhwaithed] *n* 粟粒疹

Whitehead's operation [ˈhwaithed] (Walter Whitehead) 怀特黑德手术(以切除法治疗痔疮)

Whitehorn's method [ˈhwaithɔːn] (John C. Whitehorn) 怀特霍恩法(检血中氯化物)

whiteleg [ˈhwaitleg] *n* 股白肿

whitepox [ˈhwaitpɔks] *n* 轻型天花,乳白痘,类天花

White's operation [ˈhwait] (J. W. White) 怀特手术(睾丸切除术,治前列腺肥大)

Whitfield's ointment [ˈhwitfiːld] (Arthur Whitfield) 怀特菲尔德软膏(苯甲酸及水杨酸软膏)

whitlockite [ˈhwitləkait] (Herbert P. Whitlock) *n* 三元磷酸钙(见于尿石内)

whitlow [ˈhwitləu] *n* 瘭疽,化脓性指头炎 | herpetic ~ 疱疹性瘭疽 / melanotic ~ 黑变性瘭疽 / thecal ~ 腱鞘瘭疽(手指末节化脓性腱鞘炎)

Whitman's operation [ˈhwitmən] (Royal Whitman) 惠特曼手术(①髋关节成形术;②距骨切除术)

Whitmore's bacillus [ˈhwitmɔː] (Major A. Whitmore) 假鼻疽杆菌 | ~ disease(fever) 类鼻疽

Whitnall's tubercle [ˈhwitnæl] (Samuel E. Whitnall) 怀特纳尔结节(颧骨眶面中内侧部分的小隆起,亦称眶外侧结节或睑结节)

WHO World Health Organization 世界卫生组织

whooping cough [ˈhuːpiŋkɔf] 百日咳

whorl [hwəːl] *n* 螺环;斗形纹 | bone ~ 内生骨疣 / lens ~ 晶体环 | **~ed** *a* 有螺环的;有斗形纹的

Whytt's disease [hwit] (Robert Whytt) 惠特病(结核性脑膜炎引起的急性脑积水)

Wichmann's asthma [ˈviʃmən] (Johann E. Wichmann) 喘鸣性喉痉挛

Wickersheimer's fluid(medium) [ˈvikəˌʃaimə] (J. Wickersheimer) 维克沙伊默尔液(保存解剖标本用)

Wickham's striae [ˈwikəm] (Louis-Frédéric Wickham) 威克姆纹(丘疹上的灰白色网纹,为扁平苔藓的特征)

Widal-Abrami disease [viˈdɑːl əˈbrɑːmi] (G. F. I. Widal; Pierre Abrami) 肥-阿病,后天溶血性黄疸

Widal's syndrome [viˈdɑːl] (Georges F. I. Widal) 溶血性黄疸贫血病 | ~ test(reaction, serum test) 肥达试验(反应,血清试验),伤寒凝集反应(试验)(检伤寒)

Widowitz' sign [ˈvidəuvits] (Jannak Widowitz) 维多维茨征(眼球突出,眼球及眼睑运动迟缓,见于白喉性麻痹)

width [widθ] *n* 宽度 | pulse ~ 脉冲宽度 / window ~ 窗宽(γ 射线的能量范围)

Wigand's version(maneuver) [ˈviːgənt] (Justus H. Wigand) 维甘德手法(横位胎儿外倒转术)

Wiggers diagram [ˈwigəz] (Carl J. Wiggers) 威格斯图(以图表示心搏周期的变化)

Wilbur-Addis test [ˈwilbə ˈædis] (Ray Lyman Wilbur; Thomas Addis) 韦-艾试验(检尿胆素原及尿胆素)

Wilcoxon's rank sum test, signed rank test [wilˈkɔksn] (Frank Wilcoxon) 威尔科克森秩和检验、符号秩检验(见 test 项下 rank sum test 和 signed rank test)

wild [waild] *a* 野生的;野生型的

Wildbolz test (reaction) [ˈviltbəults] (Hans Wildbolz) 威尔特博尔茨试验(反应),自尿试验(反应)(检结核病)

Wildermuth's ear [ˈvildəmut] (Hermann A. Wildermuth) 维尔达穆特耳(对耳轮较显,耳轮发育不全)

Wilder's diet [ˈwaildə] (Russell M. Wilder, Sr.) 魏尔德饮食(低钾饮食,从前用于治疗艾迪生〈Addison〉病)

Wilder's law of initial value [ˈwaildə] (Joseph Wilder) 怀尔德初期值定律(自主性器官的功能越强,其对刺激引起的兴奋能力越弱,而对抑制因子的反应则越强,由于初期值过高或过低,常有明显的反常反应的趋势,即和正常反应方向相反)

Wilder's sign [ˈwaildə] (William H. Wilder) 怀尔德征(突眼性甲状腺肿时的早期体征,即眼球由内向外或由外向内转动时出现轻度震颤)

Wilde's cords [waild] (William R. W. Wilde) 胼胝体横纹 | ~ incision 怀尔德切开(耳后乳突切开,治乳突脓肿)

Willan's lepra [ˈwilən] (Robert Willan) 牛皮癣,银屑病

Willebrand disease [ˈvilibrɑːnt] (Erik A. von Willebrand) 维勒布兰特病,血管性血友病(即 von Willebrand's disease〈冯·维勒布兰特病〉,先天性出血素质,作为常染色体显性性状遗传,特征为出血时间延长,凝血因子Ⅷ缺乏,血小板贴附于玻璃小珠经常受损,伴鼻出血和外伤或手术后出血增多,子宫出血和产后出血) | ~ factor 维勒布兰特因子(即 von Willebrand's factor〈冯·维勒布兰特因子〉,因子Ⅷ的属性,为血小板黏附于血管成分所必需,此因子缺乏,可导致出血时间延长,见于冯·维勒布兰特病。亦称 factor $Ⅷ_{VWF}$)

Willett forceps (clamp) [ˈwilit] (J. A. Willett) 威利特钳(头皮钳)

Willia [ˈwiliə] *n* 威立酵母属(现名汉逊酵母属 Hansenula)

Williams-Beuren syndrome [ˈwiliəmz ˈbɔirən] (J. C. P. Williams; Alois J. Beuren) 威-布综合征(见 Williams syndrome)

Williams-Campbell syndrome [ˈwiljəmz ˈkæmbl] (Howard Williams; Peter E. Campbell) 威-坎综合征(先天性支气管软化,系因末梢支气管第一分枝远端的环状软骨缺失所致,特点为支气管扩张)

Williamson's blood test [ˈwiljəmsn] (Richard T. Williamson) 威廉森血液试验(检糖尿病)

Williamson's sign [ˈwiljəmsn] (Oliver K. Williamson) 威廉森征(气胸及胸膜积液时下肢血压与同侧臂血压相比显著降低)

Williams' sign (tracheal tone) [ˈwiljəmz] (Charles J. B. Williams) 威廉斯征(气管音)(胸膜大量积液时第二肋间呈浊鼓音)

Williams syndrome [ˈwiljəmz] (J. C. P. Williams) 威廉斯综合征(主动脉瓣上方狭窄、精神发育迟缓、小精灵面容及婴儿暂时性高钙血症。亦称小精灵面容综合征)

Willis' antrum [ˈwilis] (Thomas Willis) 幽门窦 | ~ circle 大脑动脉环 / ~ cords 威利斯索(上矢状窦横索) / ~ nerve 副神经(第十一对脑神经) / ~ paracusis 威利斯误听(在嘈杂环境下听力增强)

willow [ˈwiləu] *n* 柳;柳皮制剂(用作消炎解热药)

Wilms' tumor [ˈvilmz] (Marx Wilms) 肾母细胞瘤(一种迅速形成的恶性混合型肾瘤,由胚胎性瘤组成,一般是 5 岁前儿童患此病,可能见之于胎儿。亦称胚性腺肌肉瘤,胚性癌肉瘤)

Wilson-Mikity syndrome [ˈwilsn ˈmikəti] (Miriam G. Wilson; Victor G. Mikity) 威-米综合征(一种罕见的低出生体重儿肺功能不全,特点为起病隐匿,生后一月发生呼吸过度与发绀,常致死亡。X 线摄影见全肺有多发性囊状充气过度病灶与间质性支持结构粗糙增厚。本症被认为系肺实质成熟度不同,特别是肺泡增生方面的差异,因此被称为肺成熟障碍)

Wilson's degeneration, disease, syndrome [ˈwilsn] (Samuel A. K. Wilson) 肝豆状核变性

Wilson's muscle [ˈwilsn] (James Wilson) 尿道膜部括约肌

Wimberger's sign [ˈvimbəːg] (Heinrich Wimberger) 温博格征(近端胫骨对称性糜烂,患先天性梅毒婴儿 X 线摄影时所见)

Wimshurst machine [ˈwimzhəːst] (James Wimshurst) 温姆斯赫斯特起电机

Winchester syndrome [ˈwintʃestə] (Patricia Winchester) 温彻斯特综合征(一种常染色体隐性遗传综合征,包括身材矮小、关节挛缩、骨质疏松、角膜混浊以及类似类风湿关节炎的关节病变)

Winckel's disease [ˈviŋkəl] (Franz K. L. W. von Winckel) 温克尔病(新生儿的一种致死性疾病,其特点为黄疸、出血、血红蛋白尿等)

windage [ˈwindidʒ] *n* 气压伤

windburn [ˈwindbəːn] *n* 吹风性皮肤伤(过度吹风引起的皮肤皲裂)

windchill [ˈwindtʃil] *n* 风力降温,吹风冷却

windgall [ˈwindgɔːl] *n* 后腘滑膜瘤(马)

windigo [ˈwindigəu] *n* 巨神温第高(因纽特人和美国某些印第安人神话中的食人肉巨神,同样也是一种特定文化的综合征,表现为被巨神温第高着魔的妄想,惧怕成为食人肉者,有时确有食人肉行为和激越性忧郁症。亦称 witigo)

windlass [ˈwindləs] *n* 起锚机,卷扬机 | Spanish ~ 西班牙纹带(一种急救用的肢体止血带)

window [ˈwindəu] *n* 窗,窗口 | aortic ~ 主动脉窗 / aorticopulmonary ~ 主-肺动脉窗,主动脉中隔缺损 / oval ~ 卵圆窗,前庭窗 / round ~ 圆窗,蜗窗

windowing [ˈwindəuiŋ] *n* 开窗术(在骨皮质上的外科开口)

windpipe [ˈwindpaip] *n* 气管

windpuff [ˈwindpʌf] *n* 球节下肿(马)

windsucking [ˈwindsʌkiŋ] *n* 咬槽咽气癖(马)

wing [wiŋ] *n* 翼 | ash-like ~ 灰翼,迷走神经三角 / ~ of nose 鼻翼 / ~ of vomer 犁骨翼

Winiwarter-Buerger disease [ˈviniˌvɑːtə ˈbiəgə] (Felix von Winiwarter; Leo Buerger) 维-伯病,血栓闭塞性脉管炎

Winiwarter's operation [ˈviniˌvɑːtə] (Alexander von Winiwarter) 胆囊小肠吻合术

winking [ˈwiŋkiŋ] *n* 眨眼,瞬目 | jaw ~ 颌动瞬目(反射)

Winkler's disease [ˈvinklə] (Max Winkler) 慢性

结节性耳轮软骨皮炎

Winslow's foramen [ˈwinzləu] (Jacob B. Winslow) 网膜孔 | ~ ligament 腘斜韧带 / ~ pancreas 钩突(胰) / ~ stars 温斯娄毛细血管涡(眼)

Winterbottom's sign (symptom) [ˈwintəˌbɔtəm] (Thomas M. Winterbottom) 温特博特姆征(症状)(患非洲锥虫病时后颈淋巴结肿大)

wintergreen [ˈwintəgriːn] *n* 冬绿树;冬青油

Winternitz's sound [ˈvintəˌnits] (Wilhelm Winternitz) 温特尼茨探子(双腔导管)

Winter's syndrome [ˈwintə] (Jeremy S. D. Winter) 温特综合征(一种先天性综合征,包括肾性发育不良、内生殖器异常,尤其是阴道闭锁以及中耳小骨异常)

winterberry [ˈwintəˌberi] *n* 美洲冬青

Wintrich's sign [ˈvintriʃ] (Anton Wintrich) 温特里希征(肺空洞时,胸部叩音的音调随开口和闭口而变化)

Wintrobe hematocrit tube [ˈwintrəub] (Maxwell M. Wintrobe) 温特罗布血细胞比容管(一种厚壁玻璃管,以毫米从 0 到 105 刻度) | ~ method 温特罗布法(测血红细胞沉降率)

wire [ˈwaiə] *n* 丝,金属丝 | arch ~ 弓丝(牙科用) / ligature ~ 结扎丝 / separating ~ 分离丝(正牙学用)

wireworm [ˈwaiəwəːm] *n* 捻转血矛线虫

wiring [ˈwaiəriŋ] *n* 结扎术,栓结术,线缝法,接线法;架线缝法(骨折) | circumferential ~ 环绕结扎术 / continuous loop ~ 连续小环结扎术 / craniofacial suspension ~ 颅面悬吊栓结术 / perialveolar ~ 牙槽周栓结术 / piriform aperture ~ 犁状口栓结术

Wirsung's canal (duct) [ˈviəsuːŋ] (Johann G. Wirsung) 胰管

wiry [ˈwaiəri] *a* 弦样的(指脉搏细而紧,如腹膜炎时)

WISC Wechsler Intelligence Scale for Children 韦克斯勒儿童智力量表

Wishart test [ˈwiʃɑːt] (Mary B. Wishart) 威夏尔特试验(检丙酮血)

Wiskott-Aldrich syndrome [ˈviskɔt ˈɔːldritʃ] (Alfred Wiscott; Robert Anderson Aldrich) 威-奥综合征(一种 X 连锁免疫缺陷综合征,特征为湿疹、血小板减少及复发性化脓性感染。对多糖抗原不能产生抗体,从而增加了对荚膜杆菌〈流感嗜杆菌,脑膜炎球菌,肺炎球菌〉的易感性。通常 IgM 降低,IgA 和 IgE 升高,皮肤通常无变应性,淋巴网状内皮细胞恶性病的发生率亦高。亦称奥尔德里奇〈Aldrich〉综合征,伴有血小板减少和湿疹的免疫缺陷症)

witch hazel [witʃ ˈheizəl] 北美金缕梅;金缕梅酊剂(局部用作轻度收敛药,亦称北美金缕梅水)

Withania [wiˈθeiniə] *n* 茄属

withdrawal [wiðˈdrɔːəl] *n* (病理性)退隐;药物戒断病 | substance ~ 药物戒断病

withers [ˈwiðəz] *n* 鬐甲(马肩胛间隆起部分) | fistulous ~ (马的)鬐甲瘘

witigo [wiˈtaigəu] *n* 巨神温第高(见 windigo)

witkop [ˈwitkɔp] *n* 头皮白痂病,黄癣(见于南非班图人)

Witzel's gastrostomy (operation) [ˈvitsel] (Friedrich O. Witzel) 威策尔胃造口术

witzelsucht [ˈvitselzuːht] *n* 【德】诙谐癖

Wladimiroff's operation [ˌvlædiˈmiːrɔf] 弗拉季米罗夫手术(跗骨切除术)

WMA World Medical Association 世界医学协会

wobble [ˈwɔbl] *vi, vt* 摇摆,摆动 *n* 摇摆,摆动

wobbles [ˈwɔblz] [复] *n* 马摇摆病

Wohlfahrtia [vɔːlˈfɑːtiə] *n* 污蝇属 | ~ magnifica 壮丽污蝇 / ~ vigil 迈[根]氏污蝇

Wohlfart-Kugelberg-Welander syndrome [ˈvəulfɑːt ˈkuːgəlbəːg ˈveləndə] (Karl G. V. Wohlfart; Eric K. H. Kugelberg; Lisa Welander) 沃-库-韦综合征(见 Kugelberg-Welander syndrome)

Wohlgemuth's test [ˈvɔːlgiːmut] (Julius Wohlgemuth) 沃尔格穆特试验(检肾功能不全)

Wolbachia [wɔlˈbækiə] (Simeon Burt Wolbach) *n* 沃尔巴克体属

Wolbachieae [ˌwɔlbəˈkaiiː] (S. B. Wolbach) *n* 沃尔巴克体族

Woldman's test [ˈwɔldmən] (Edward E. Woldman) 沃尔德曼试验(检胃肠病变)

Wolfe-Krause free skin graft [vulf krauz] (J. R. Wolfe; Fedor Krause) 全厚皮片

Wolfenden's position [ˈwɔlfəndən] (Richard N. Wolfenden) 沃尔芬登卧位(头部悬垂床边)

Wolfe's graft [wulf] (John R. Wolfe) 沃尔夫移植片(全厚皮片)

Wolff-Eisner reaction (test) [vɔlfˈaiznə] (Alfred Wolff-Eisner) 午非・埃斯纳反应(试验)(用伤寒和结核的毒素滴眼后,眼结膜的局部反应)

wolffian [ˈwulfiən] (Kaspar F. Wolff) *a* 午非的(如 ~ body 午非体〈中肾〉, ~ cyst 午非管囊肿〈一种子宫阔韧带囊肿〉, ~ duct 午非管〈中肾管〉, ~ ridge 中肾嵴)

Wolff-Parkinson-White syndrome [ˈwulf ˈpɑːkinsn ˈhwait] (Louis Wolff; John Parkinson; Paul D. White) 沃-帕-怀综合征(阵发性心动过速〈或心房纤颤〉和预激相联系,心电图显示短 P-R 间期及宽 QRS 波群。有时使用时与预激综合征同义,亦称 WPW 综合征)

Wolff's duct [vuːlf] (Kaspar F. Wolff) 中肾管

Wolff's law [vɔlf] (Julius Wolff) 沃尔夫定律(正

常的或异常的骨,其形成的结构最适于抵抗在其上作用之力)

Wolf-Hirschhorn syndrome [vɔlf ˈhəːʃhɔːn] (Ulrich Wolf; Kurt Hirschhorn) 沃-赫综合征(一种与4号染色体短臂部分缺失有关的综合征,特征为小头,眼距过宽,内眦赘皮,腭裂,小颌,简化型低位耳,隐睾及尿道下裂)

Wölfler's glands [ˈvelflə] (Anton Wölfler) 副甲状腺 | ~ operation 韦尔夫勒手术(前胃空肠吻合术,治幽门梗阻)

wolfram(W) [ˈwulfrəm] *n* 钨(化学元素)

Wolfram syndrome [ˈwulfrəm] (D. J. Wolfram) 沃尔弗拉姆综合征(一种常染色体隐性遗传综合征,包括糖尿病、尿崩症、视神经萎缩及神经性聋)

Wolfring's glands [ˈvɔːlfriŋ] (Emilij F. von Wolfring) 沃尔弗林腺(结膜下管泡腺)

wolfsbane [ˈwulfsbein] *n* 欧乌头;山金车花

Wolinella [ˌwəuliˈnelə] (M. J. Wolin) *n* 沃林菌属 | ~ recta 直肠沃林菌,直肠弯曲杆菌 / ~ succinogenes 产琥珀沃林菌(亦称产琥珀弧菌)

Wollaston's doublet [ˈwuləstən] (William H. Wollaston) 沃拉斯顿双合透镜(纠正色象差)

Wolman disease [ˈwɔlmən] (Moshe Wolman) 渥尔曼病,酸性脂酶缺乏症(溶酶体固醇酯酶缺乏所致的溶酶体贮积症,婴儿早期开始发病,1岁前即死亡。临床特征包括肝脾肿大、脂泻、腹胀、贫血、营养不良和肾上腺钙化)

Womach procedure [ˈwuːmæk] 沃麦克手术(脾切除术并切除胃大弯上半部,血行阻断,穿胃缝合静脉曲张;施行此手术是为了治疗门静脉高压导致的静脉曲张出血)

womb [wuːm] *n* 子宫

Wong's method (San Yin Wong 中国生化学家黄新彦)黄氏法(检血红蛋白中铁)

Woodbridge treatment [ˈwudbridʒ] (John E. Woodbridge) 伍德布里奇疗法(用小剂量甘汞、鬼臼脂及肠消毒剂治伤寒)

woodchuch [ˈwudtʃʌk] *n* 旱獭

Wood's light (filter, glass) [wud] (Robert W. Wood) 伍德光(滤器、玻璃)(汞蒸气灯的紫外线照射,通过氧化镍滤器〈即伍德滤器或玻璃〉透射,可见光谱中只有一部分紫外线可透过,诊断头癣等用)

Wood's sign [wud] (Horatio C. Wood) 伍德征(轮匝肌松弛、眼球凝视和散在性斜视,为深度麻醉的指征)

wool [wul] *n* 羊毛;绒毛;棉[花] | collodion ~ 火棉,二硝化纤维素 / cotton ~ 原棉,脱脂棉,药棉 / gut ~ 肠线绒 / styptic ~ 止血棉(浸过氯化铁的棉花)

Woolner's tip [ˈwulnə] (Thomas Woolner) 耳郭结节

word-blind [ˈwəːd blaind] *a* 无读字能力的,患失读症的

word salad [wəːd ˈsæləd] 言语杂乱,言语芜杂

Woringer-Kolopp disease (syndrome) [ˌvəurinˈʒεə kəˈlɔp] (Frédéric Woringer; P. Kolopp) 伏-科病(综合征),佩吉特病样网状细胞增生病(即 pagetoid reticulosis)

work(*W*) [wəːk] *n* 功 | ~ of breathing 呼吸功 / cardiac ~ 心脏作功 / stroke ~ 每搏作功

work-up [ˈwəːkʌp] *n* 检查(指化验、X线等)

World Health Organization (WHO) 世界卫生组织

worm [wəːm] *n* 虫,蠕虫;蚓部 | bilharzia ~ 裂体吸虫,血吸虫(即 Schistosoma) / bladder ~ 囊虫 / blinding ~ 旋盘尾丝虫(即 Onchocerca volvulus) / case ~ 棘球绦虫(即 Echinococcus) / cayor ~ 病蝇蛆 / ~ of cerebellum 小脑蚓部 / dragon ~, guinea ~, Medina ~, serpent ~ 麦地那龙线虫(即 Dracunculus medinensis) / eel ~, maw ~ 蛔虫(即 Ascaris) / eye ~ 眼丝虫,罗阿丝虫(即 Loa loa) / flat ~ 扁形动物,扁虫 / fluke ~ 吸虫 / heart ~ 犬恶丝虫(即 Dirofilaria immitis) / horsehair ~ 铁线虫(即 Gordius) / kidney ~ 肾膨结线虫(即 Dioctophyma renale) / lung ~ 肺蠕虫(如肺吸虫) / meal ~ 拟谷盗甲虫 / palisade ~ 马圆线虫(即 Strongylus equinus) / pork ~ 旋毛线虫,旋毛虫(即 Trichinella spiralis) / screw ~ 旋蝇 / spinyheaded ~, thorny-headed ~ 棘头虫(即 Acanthocephala) / stomach ~ 捻转血矛线虫(即 Haemonchus contortus) / tongue ~ 舌形虫(即 Pentastomida) / trichina ~ 旋毛虫(即 Trichinella)

wormian bones [ˈwəːmiən] (Olaus Worm) 缝间骨

Wormley's test [ˈwəːmli] (Theodore G. Wormley) 沃姆利试验(检生物碱)

Worm-Müller's test [vəːm ˈmilə] (Jacob Worm-Müller) 沃姆·苗勒试验(检尿葡萄糖)

wormseed [ˈwəːmsiːd] *n* 山道年草;土荆芥

wormwood [ˈwəːmwud] *n* 苦艾

Woulfe's bottle [wulf] (Peter Woulfe) 沃尔夫瓶(三颈洗气瓶)

wound [wuːnd] *n* 伤,创伤,伤口 | aseptic ~ 无菌伤口 / blowing ~ 开放性气胸 / contused ~ 挫伤 / incised ~ 切伤 / lacerated ~ 撕裂伤 / non-penetrating ~ 非贯通伤 / open ~ 开放性创伤 / penetrating ~ 贯通伤 / perforating ~ 穿透伤 / poisoned ~ 染毒创伤,感染性创伤 / puncture ~ 戳伤 / septic ~ 脓毒性伤口 / seton ~ 串线伤(指伤口的入口与出口均在受伤部位的同侧) / sucking ~, traumatopneic ~ 吸气性创伤 / tangential ~ 切线伤 | ~**ed** *a* 受伤的 *n* [the ~ed] 伤员(尤指战争中的伤员、伤兵)

W-plasty [ˈplæsti] W 形成形术

wrapping [ˈræpiŋ] *n* 包装 | fundic ~ 胃底折叠术

wreath [riːθ] ([复] **wreaths** [riːðz]) *n* 花冠,花冠体(细胞核分裂的一时期) | daughter ~ 双星体 / hippocratic ~ 希波克拉底花冠,花冠秃

Wreden's sign [ˈvreidən] (Robert R. Wreden) 伏雷登征(出生时死亡的婴儿,其外耳道内有一种胶状物质)

Wright's blood group [rait] (Wright 为英国先证者的姓,1953 年首次报道)赖特血型(含有红细胞抗原 Wr^a 和 Wr^b 的一种血型)

Wright's stain [rait] (James H. Wright) 瑞特染剂(曙红和亚甲蓝的混合物,用于显示血细胞和疟原虫)

Wright's syndrome [rait] (Irving S. Wright) 赖特综合征(①臂过度外展所致的一种神经血管综合征,这样过度外展可引起锁骨下动脉闭塞,导致坏死或臂丛牵张引起感觉症状;②一种疾病,其特征为多病灶性纤维性骨炎,皮肤色素沉着及性早熟)

Wrisberg's cartilage [ˈrisbəːg] (Heinrich A. Wrisberg) 楔状软骨 | ~ ganglion, ganglion Wrisbergi 心神经节,半月神经节 / ~ ligament 半月板股骨后韧带 / ~ lines 里斯贝格线(连接三叉神经的运动根和感觉根的丝束) / ~ nerve 中间神经;臂内侧皮神经 / ~ tubercle 楔状结节

wrist [rist] *n* 腕 | tennis ~ 网球员腕病(腕部腱鞘炎)

wristdrop [ˈristdrɔp] *n* 腕下垂

writing [ˈraitiŋ] *n* 书写 | mirror ~, specular ~ 镜像书写,反向书写

wryneck [ˈrainek] *n* 斜颈

wt weight 重,重量

wucheratrophie [ˌvuːkeˈrætrəfi] (【德】"proliferation atrophy〈增生性萎缩〉") *n* 脂肪替代性萎缩(即 wucher atrophy)

Wuchereria [ˌvukəˈriːriə] *n* 吴策线虫属 | ~ bancrofti 班[克罗夫特]氏吴策线虫,班[克罗夫特]氏线虫 / ~ malayi 马来吴策线虫,马来丝虫(即 Brugia malayi)

wuchereriasis [ˌvukəriˈraiəsis] *n* 吴策线虫病

Wunderlich's curve [ˈvundəliʃ] (Carl R. A. Wunderlich) 温德利希曲线(伤寒病人体温的典型变化曲线)

Wundt's tetanus [vunt] (Wilhelm Wundt) 冯特强直(因电流或损伤引起的蛙肌肉持续强直收缩)

Wurster's test [ˈvuəstə] (Casimir Wurster) 武斯特试验(检过氧化氢、酪氨酸)

w/v weight (of solute) per volume (of solvent) 重/容(溶质重量与溶剂重量比)

Wyburn-Mason's syndrome [ˈwaibəːn ˈmeisən] (Roger Wyburn-Mason) 怀伯恩·梅森综合征(脑一侧或两侧动静脉瘤,眼异常〈尤其在视网膜内〉,面痣,有时为精神发育迟缓)

Wyeomyia [ˌwiːəuˈmaijə] *n* 维欧米亚蚊属

Wyeth's operation [ˈwaiəθ] (John A. Wyeth) 韦思手术(髋关节离断术)

Wylie's drain [ˈwaili] (Walker G. Wylie) 怀利引流管(一种有柄的硬橡皮子宫托,沿柄有沟)

Wynn method [win] (Sidney Keth Wynn) 温氏法(用狭长三角形皮瓣修复双侧唇裂)

X

X Kienbock's unit 金伯克单位; xanthine 黄嘌呤; xanthosine 黄苷

$\underline{X}$ reactance 电抗

$\overline{X}$ sample mean 样本平均值

x abscissa 横坐标

ξ xi,希腊语的第 14 个字母

xanchromatic [ˌzænkrəuˈmætik] *a* 黄色的

xanoxate sodium [zəˈnɔkseit] 异丙氧蒽酸钠(支气管扩张药)

xanthate [ˈzænθeit] *n* 黄原酸盐

xanthelasma [ˌzænθəˈlæzmə] *n* 黄斑瘤(亦称睑黄瘤);黄瘤

xanthelasmatosis [ˌzænθəlæzməˈtəusis] *n* 黄瘤病

xanthematin [zænˈθemətin] *n* 血黄素,黄色高铁血红素(血红素黄色衍生物)

xanthemia [zænˈθiːmiə] *n* 胡萝卜素血

xanthene [ˈzænθiːn] *n* 呫吨,[夹]氧杂蒽

xanthic [ˈzænθik] *a* 黄色的;黄嘌呤的

xanthin [ˈzænθin] *n* 植物黄质

xanthine(X) [ˈzænθiːn] *n* 黄嘌呤

xanthine dehydrogenase [ˈzænθiːn diːˈhaidrədʒəneis] 黄嘌呤脱氢酶(此酶活性缺乏可致黄嘌呤尿和黄嘌呤石沉积)

xanthine oxidase [ˈzænθiːn ˈɔksideis] 黄嘌呤氧化酶(此酶缺乏为一种常染色体隐性性状,可致黄嘌呤尿症)

xanthinin [ˈzænθinin] *n* 黄质宁(硫脲酸胺加热分解产生的结晶性物质);苍耳素

xanthinuria [ˌzænθiˈnjuəriə], **xanthiuria** [ˌzænθiˈjuəriə] *n* 黄嘌呤尿 | **xanthinuric** *a*

xanthism [ˈzænθizəm] *n* 黄化,黄素沉着病,暗红色白化病

xanth(o)- [构词成分] 黄色

Xanthobacter [ˌzænθəuˈbæktə] *n* 黄色[无芽胞]杆菌属

xanthochromia [ˌzænθəˈkrəumiə] *n* 黄变(脑脊液或皮肤) | ~ striata palmaris 掌条纹状黄变

xanthochromic [ˌzænθəˈkrəumik], **xanthochromatic** [ˌzæθəukrəuˈmætik] *a* 黄变的;黄色的(专指脑脊液)

xanthocyanopsia [ˌzænθəusaiəˈnɔpsiə] *n* 红绿色盲(黄蓝色视)

xanthocystine [ˌzænθəuˈsistin] *n* 黄胱氨酸(从死体结节中发现的一种物质)

xanthocyte [ˈzænθəsait] *n* 黄色细胞

xanthoderma [ˌzænθəˈdəːmə] *n* 黄肤,皮肤变黄

xanthodontous [ˌzænθəuˈdɔntəs] *a* 黄牙的

xanthoerythrodermia [ˌzænθəuiˌriθrəuˈdəːmiə] *n* 黄红皮肤(皮肤变黄红色) | ~ perstans 持久性黄红皮病,小斑块状银屑病

xanthofibroma thecocellulare [ˌzænθəufaiˈbrəumə ˌθiːkəuˌseljuˈlɛəri] 黄体瘤,皮肤纤维瘤

xanthogranuloma [ˌzænθəugrænjuˈləumə] *n* 黄肉芽肿 | juvenile ~ 幼年黄色肉芽肿

xanthokyanopy [ˌzænθəukaiˈænəpi] *n* 红绿色盲(黄蓝色视)

xanthoma [zænˈθəumə] ([复] **xanthomas** 或 **xanthomata** [zænˈθəumətə]) *n* 黄[色]瘤 | craniohypophyseal ~ 颅垂体部黄瘤 / diabetic ~ 糖尿病性黄瘤 / ~ disseminatum, ~ multiplex 播散性黄瘤,多数性黄瘤 / eruptive ~, ~ eruptivum 丘疹性黄瘤 / planar ~, plane ~, ~ planum, generalized plane ~ 扁平黄瘤,泛发性扁平黄瘤 / ~ striatum palmare 掌纹黄瘤 / tendinous ~, ~ tendinosum 腱黄瘤 / tuberoeruptive ~ 结节丘疹性黄瘤 / tuberosum, ~ tuberosum multiplex, tuberous ~ 结节性黄瘤,多发性结节性黄瘤 | **~tous** *a*

xanthomatosis [ˌzænθəuməˈtəusis] *n* 黄[色]瘤病 | biliary hypercholesterolemic ~ 胆汁性高胆固醇血症性黄瘤病 / ~ bulbi 眼球黄瘤病(角膜脂变) / cerebrotendinous ~ 脑腱黄瘤病 / chronic idiopathic ~ 慢性特发性黄瘤病 / ~ corneae 角膜黄瘤病,角膜脂肪性营养不良 / ~ iridis 虹膜黄瘤病 / primary familial ~ 原发性家族性黄瘤病

Xanthomonas [ˌzænθəuˈməunəs] *n* 黄[单胞]杆菌属

xanthone [ˈzænθəun] *n* 呫吨酮,氧杂蒽酮

xanthophane [ˈzænθəfein] *n* 视网膜黄素,视黄素

xanthophore [ˈzænθəfɔː] *n* 黄色素细胞(冷血动物)

xanthophose [ˈzænθəfəuz] *n* 黄[光]幻视

xanthophyll [ˈzænθəufil] *n* 叶黄素,胡萝卜醇 | **~ous** [ˌzænθəuˈfiləs] *a*

xanthoproteic [ˌzænθəuprəuˈtiːik] *a* 黄色蛋白的 | ~ acid 黄色蛋白酸

xanthoprotein [ˌzænθəuˈprəutiːn] *n* 黄色蛋白

xanthopsia [ˌzænˈθɔpsiə], **xanthopia** [zænˈθəu-piə] *n* 黄视症,视物显黄症

xanthopsin [zænˈθɔpsin] *n* 视黄质

xanthopsis [zænˈθɔpsis] *n* [癌]黄色素沉着

xanthopterin [zænˈθɔptərin] *n* 黄蝶呤,2-氨基-4,6-二羟基蝶呤

xanthorhamnin [ˌzænθəuˈræmnin] *n* 黄鼠李苷,鼠李精

xanthorubin [ˌzænθəˈruːbin] *n* 血清黄色素

xanthosarcoma [ˌzænθəusɑːˈkəumə] *n* 黄肉瘤,黄髓瘤

xanthosine(X) [ˈzænθəsiːn] *n* 黄苷 | ~ monophosphate (XMP) 黄苷酸

xanthosis [zænˈθəusis] *n* 黄皮症,黄变症

xanthotoxin [ˌzænθəˈtɔksin] *n* 氧化补骨脂素,黄原毒

xanthous [ˈzænθəs] *a* 黄的,黄色的

xanthurenic acid [ˌzænθjuəˈrenik] 黄尿酸,4, 8-二羟基喹啉甲酸

xanthuria [zænˈθjuəriə] *n* 黄嘌呤尿

xanthyl [ˈzænθil] *n* 呫吨基,氧[杂]蒽基

xanthylic [zænˈθilik] *a* 黄嘌呤的 | ~ acid 黄苷酸

X-bite crossbite 反殆,反咬合

Xe xenon 氙

xenembole [zeˈnembəli], **xenenthesis** [ˌzenen-ˈθiːsis] *n* 异物导入,异物侵入

xenia [ˈziːniə] *n*【希】种子直感(花粉对于胚以外的组织的影响);异粉性(指胚乳)

xen(o)- [构词成分] 外;异物

xenoantigen [ˌzenəuˈæntidʒən] *n* 异种抗原(有机体中出现一种以上的抗原,如 ABO 血型的 A 和 B 抗原)

xenobiotic [ˌzenəubaiˈɔtik] *n*, *a* 异生物(的),异生物素(的)(生物系统中外来的化合物)

xenocytophilic [ˌzenəuˌsaitəuˈfilik] *a* 嗜异种细胞的

xenodiagnosis [ˌzenəudaiəgˈnəusis] *n* 异体接种诊断法(用在实验室培育的臭虫粪便中找出传染型致病菌的方法,以诊断早期恰加斯〈Chagas〉病);宿主诊断法(用可疑感染了毛线虫的食用肉饲养实验室培育的大鼠或小鼠,使毛线虫在宿主中繁殖,然后检查实验动物有无该种寄生虫寄生) | **xenodiagnostic** [ˌzenəuˌdaiəg-ˈnɔstik] *a* 异体接种诊断的,宿主诊断的

xenogeneic [ˌzenəudʒeˈneiik] *a* 异种的,异种基因的

xenogenesis [ˌzenəuˈdʒenisis] *n* 世代交替,异配生殖;亲子异型 | **xenogenetic** [ˌzenəudʒiˈne-tik], **xenogenic** [ˌzenəuˈdʒenik] *a* 世代交替的;异种的,异种基因的

xenogenous [zeˈnɔdʒinəs] *a* 异体的,体外性的;异种的,异种基因的

xenograft [ˈzenəgrɑːft, -græft] *n* 异种移植;异种移植物

xenology [ziˈnɔlədʒi] *n* (寄生物)宿主学

xenomenia [ˌzenəuˈmiːniə] *n* 代偿性月经,异位月经,倒经

xenon(Xe) [ˈzenɔn] *n* 氙(化学元素)

xenoparasite [ˌzenəuˈpærəsait] *n* 异常寄生物(在宿主体弱时寄生)

xenophobia [ˌzenəˈfəubjə] *n* 生客恐怖,陌生恐怖

xenophonia [ˌzenəˈfəuniə] *n* 音调变异

xenophthalmia [ˌzenɔfˈθælmiə] *n* 异物性眼炎

Xenophyophorea [ˌziːnəuˌfaiəuˈfəuriə] *n* 丸壳纲

Xenopsylla [ˌzenɔpˈsilə] *n* 客蚤属 | ~ astia 亚洲客蚤,亚洲鼠蚤 / ~ brasiliensis 巴西客蚤 / ~ cheopis 印鼠客蚤,开皇客蚤,印度鼠蚤,鼠疫蚤 / ~ vexabilis, ~ hawaiiensis 夏威夷客蚤

Xenopus [ˈzenɔpəs] *n* 非洲蟾蜍属 | ~ laevis 有爪蟾蜍(供妊娠试验用)

xenorexia [ˌzenəˈreksiə] *n* 异食癖

xenotropic [ˌzenəuˈtrɔpik] *a* 异嗜的(指异嗜性病毒)

xenyl [ˈzenil] *n* 联苯基

xenylamine [zəˈniləmiːn] *n* 联苯基胺

xeransis [ziəˈrænsis] *n* 干燥,除湿

xerantic [ziəˈræntik] *a* 致干燥的,除湿的

xeraphium [ziəˈræfiəm] *n* 干燥粉,除湿粉

xer(o)- [构词成分] 干燥

xerocheilia [ˌziərəuˈkailiə] *n* 唇干燥

xerocollyrium [ˌziərəukəˈliriəm] *n* 干眼膏

xerocyte [ˈziːrəusait] *n* 干燥细胞

xerocytosis [ˌziːrəusaiˈtəusis] *n* 干燥细胞病

xeroderma [ˌziərəuˈdəːmə] *n* 干皮病,皮肤干燥病 | ~ pigmentosum 着色性干皮病 | **xerodermia** [ˌziərəuˈdəːmiə] *n* | **~tic** [ˌziərəudəˈmæ-tik] *a* 干皮病的,皮肤干燥的

xerodermoid [ˌziərəuˈdəːmɔid] *n* 类干皮病 | pigmented ~ 着色性类干皮病

xeroform [ˈziərəfɔːm] *n* 干仿,塞罗仿,三溴酚铋

xerogel [ˈziərədʒel] *n* 干凝胶

xerography [ziəˈrɔgrəfi] *n* 干板 X 线摄影[术] | **xerographic** [ˌziərəˈgræfik] *a*

xeroma [ziəˈrəumə] *n* 结膜干燥,干眼病

xeromammography [ˌziərəumæˈmɔgrəfi] *n* 干板乳房 X 线摄影[术]

xeromenia [ˌziərəuˈmiːniə] *n* 干经,干性月经

xeromycteria [ˌziərəumikˈtiəriə] *n* 鼻[黏膜]干燥

xerophagia [ˌziərəuˈfeidʒiə], **xerophagy** [ziə-ˈrɔfədʒi] *n* 干食[法]

xerophobia [ˌziərəuˈfəubjə] *n* 恐惧(愤怒或情绪

激动)性唾液分泌抑制;干燥恐怖

xerophthalmia [ˌziərɔf'θælmiə], **xerophthalmus** [ziərɔf'θælməs] *n* 眼干燥症 | **xerophthalmic** *a*

xeroradiography [ˌziərəureidi'ɔgrəfi] *n* 干板 X 线摄影[术]

xerosialography [ˌziərəuˌsaiə'lɔgrəfi] *n* 干板涎管 X 线造影[术]

xerosis [ziə'rəusis] *n*【希】干燥[病]

xerostomia [ziərə'stəumiə] *n* 口腔干燥,口干燥[症]

xerotes [ziə'rəutiːz, 'zerətiːz] *n*【希】干燥

xerothermic [ziərə'θəːmik] *a* 干热的;适应干热环境的

xerotic [ziə'rɔtik] *a* 干燥的

xerotomography [ˌziərəutə'mɔgrəfi] *n* 干板体层摄影[术]

xerotripsis [ˌziərəu'tripsis] *n* 干擦

X-His dipeptidase [dai'peptideis] 氨酰基组氨酸二肽酶(此血清同工酶缺乏可致血清肌肽酶缺乏症。亦称肌肽酶和 aminoacyl-histidine dipeptidase)

xi [gzai, ksai, zai] *n* 希腊语的第 14 个字母(Ξ, ξ)

xilobam ['zailəbæm] *n* 希洛班(肌肉松弛药)

Ximenia [zai'miːniə] *n* 西门木属

xipamide ['zipəmaid] *n* 希帕胺(利尿、降压药)

xiphi- 见 xiph(o)-

xiphin ['zifin] *n* 剑鱼精蛋白

xiphisternum [ˌzifi'stəːnəm] ([复] **xiphisterna** [ˌzifi'stəːnə]) *n* 剑突 | **xiphisternal** *a*

xiph(o)-, xiphi- [构词成分] 剑,剑突

xiphocostal [ˌzifəu'kɔstl] *a* 剑突肋骨的

xiphodynia [ˌzifəu'diniə] *n* 剑突痛

xiphoid ['zifɔid, 'zai-] *a* 剑状的 *n* 剑突

xiphoiditis [ˌzifɔi'daitis] *n* 剑突炎

xiphoomphaloischiopagus [ˌzaifəuˌɔmfələuˌiski'ɔpəgəs] *n* 剑突脐坐骨联胎

xiphopagotomy [zaiˌfɔpə'gɔtəmi] *n* 剑突联胎切分术

xiphopagus [zai'fɔpəgəs], **xiphodidymus** [ˌzifəu'didiməs], **xiphodymus** [zai'fɔdiməs] *n* 剑突联体

X-linked ['eks liŋkt] *a* 伴性的,X 连锁的(由 X 染色体上的基因遗传的)

XMP xanthosine monophosphate 黄苷酸

XO XO 型(只有一个性染色体,而缺乏另一个 X 或 Y 染色体)

XOAN X-linked (Nettleship) ocular albinism X 连锁(内氏型)眼白化病

X-Pro dipeptidase [dai'peptideis] 氨酰基脯氨酸二肽酶(此酶活性减少为一种常染色体隐性性状,可致氨酰基脯氨酸〈二肽〉酶缺乏症。亦称氨酰基脯氨酸酶和脯氨酸二肽酶)

X-ray ['eks'rei] *n* X 线,X 射线,伦琴线 *a* X 射线的,X 光的 *vt* 用 X 光检查(治疗或摄影) | spark ~s 刷形放电,电刷疗法

xylanthrax [zai'lænθræks] *n* 木炭,炭

xylazine hydrochloride ['zailəziːn] 盐酸赛拉嗪(兽用止痛、镇静和肌肉松弛药)

xylem ['zailem] *n* 木质部(植物纤维束的)

xylene ['zailiːn] *n* 二甲苯(显微镜检查时用作溶剂和清洁剂)

xylenol ['zailinɔl] *n* 二甲酚,二甲苯酚

xylic acid ['zailik] 二甲苯酸,二甲苯甲酸

xylidic acid ['zailidik] 甲苯二酸

xylidine ['zailidi(ː)n] *n* 二甲苯胺

xylitol ['zailitɔl] *n* 木糖醇

xylitol dehydrogenase ['zailitɔl diː'haidrədʒəneis] 木糖醇脱氢酶,L-木酮糖还原酶

xylitone ['zailitəun] *n* 丙酮油

xyl(o)- [构词成分] 木

xylogen ['zailədʒən] *n* 木素,木质素

Xylohypha [ˌzailəu'haifə] *n* 丝状菌属

xyloketose [ˌzailəu'kiːtəus] *n* 木酮糖

xyloketosuria [ˌzailəukiːtəu'sjuəriə] *n* 木酮糖尿

xylol ['zailɔl] *n* 二甲苯

xyloma [zai'ləumə] *n* 木质瘤(植物)

xylometazoline hydrochloride [ˌzailəumetə'zəuliːn] 盐酸赛洛唑啉(肾上腺素能药,局部用作血管收缩药,以减轻鼻黏膜肿胀和充血)

xylonic acid [zai'lɔnik] 木糖酸

xylopyranose [ˌzailəu'pairənəus] *n* 吡喃木糖,木糖

Xylorrhiza [ˌzailə'raizə] *n* 菊属

xylosazone [zai'ləusəzəun] *n* 木糖脎

xylose ['zailəus] *n* 木糖

xyloside ['zailəsaid] *n* 木糖苷

xylosidoglucose [ˌzailəuˌsaidəu'gluːkəus] *n* 木糖葡萄糖苷,樱草糖,报春花糖

xylosuria [ˌzailə'sjuəriə] *n* 木糖尿

xylotherapy [ˌzailəu'θerəpi] *n* 木[质]疗法

xylulose ['zailjuləus] *n* 木酮糖

L-xylulose reductase ['zailjuləus ri'dʌkteis] L-木酮糖还原酶(此酶缺乏为一种常染色体隐性性状,可致戊糖尿症)

L-xylulosuria [ˌzailjulə'sjuəriə] *n* 左旋木酮糖尿

xylyl ['zailil] *n* 二甲苯基

xylylenediamine [ˌzaililiːn'daiəmiːn] *n* 二甲苯二胺

xyphoid ['zaifɔid, 'zi-] *a* 剑状的 *n* 剑突

xysma ['zismə] *n*【希】絮片,假膜片(见于腹泻粪便中)

xyster ['zistə] *n*【希】刮骨刀,刮器,骨刮

Y

Y tryosine 酪氨酸; yttrium 钇
y ordinate 纵坐标
Υ 希腊语大写字母 upsilon
υ upsilon, 希腊语的第 20 个字母
yabapox [ˈjæbəˌpɔks] *n* 亚巴痘(由痘病毒引起的一种病毒性疾病,亚巴〈Yaba〉为尼日利亚一地名)
yahourth [ˈjɑːəːt] *n* 酸乳
yam [jæm] *n* 薯蓣,薯蓣属植物 | Chinese ~ 山药,薯蓣,家山药
yang【汉】阳
yarrow [ˈjærəu] *n* 洋蓍草;洋蓍草制剂
Yatapoxvirus [ˈjætəˌpɔksˌvaiərəs] [*ya*bapox + *ta*-napox + *virus*] *n* 亚特痘病毒属(由亚巴痘病毒和特纳河痘病毒组成)
yatobyo [ˌjɑːtəˈbaijəu] *n*【日】土拉菌病,兔热病
yaw [jɔː] *n* 雅司疹 | guinea corn ~ 玉米粒状雅司疹 / mother ~ 初发雅司疹 / ringworm ~ 环状雅司疹
yawey [ˈjɔːi] *a* 雅司病的
yawning [ˈjɔːniŋ] *n* 呵欠
yaws [jɔːz] [复] *n* 雅司病(一种由雅司螺旋体引起的皮肤病,多见于热带地区的儿童中,与梅毒相似,脸、手、足的皮肤出现红霉样损害) | carb ~ 角化过度性雅司病 / forest ~ 皮肤利什曼病
Ya Yan Tzu 鸦胆子(中药,亦可译为 Ya Tan Tzu,即 Brucea,其籽用于治阿米巴痢疾)
Yb ytterbium 镱
yeast [jiːst] *n* 酵母(菌),酿母(菌) | bakers' ~, brewers' ~ 啤酒酵母,药用酵母 / dried ~ 干酵母 / imperfect ~ 半知酵母 / perfect ~ 完全酵母
yeast nucleic acid [jiːst njuːˈkliːik] 酵母核酸,核糖核酸
yellow [ˈjeləu] *a* 黄[色]的;(因病等)发黄的 *n* 黄[色];黄色染料 | alizarin ~ 茜素黄(指示剂) / brilliant ~ 煌黄(指示剂) / butter ~ 甲基黄,对二甲氨基偶氮苯 / chrome ~ 铬黄,贡黄,铬酸铅 / corallin ~ 玫红酸黄,玫红酸钠 / fast ~, acid ~ 坚牢黄,酸性黄,氨基偶氮苯磺酸钠 / imperial ~ 金橙黄(染料) / visual ~ 视黄质
yellowjacket [ˈjeləuˌdʒækət] *n* 黄蜂
yellows [ˈjeləuz] *n* 钩端螺旋体性黄疸;羊霍乱
Yeo's treatment [ˈjiəu] (Isaac B. Yeo) 伊奥疗法(禁食糖类应用大量热饮料以治肥胖病)
yerba [ˈjəːbə] *n*【西】草,草本,草药
yerba santa [ˈjerbə ˈsɑːntə]【西】散塔草,北美圣草
yerbine [ˈjəːbin] *n* 巴拉圭茶碱
Yerkes-Bridges test [ˈjəːkiːz ˈbridʒiz] (Robert M. Yerkes; James W. Bridges) 耶基斯-布里奇测验(检智力)
Yerkes discrimination box [ˈjəːkiːz] (Robert M. Yerkes) 耶尔克斯辨别箱(一种门很多的迷津,用于实验室,以研究动物的视觉辨别能力,开正确的门得到奖赏,开错误的门则受到电击)
Yersinia [jəːˈsiniə] (A. J. E. Yersin) *n* 耶尔森菌属 | ~ enterocolitica 小肠结肠炎耶尔森菌 / ~ frederiksenii 费氏耶尔森菌 / ~ intermedia 中间耶尔森菌 / ~ kristensenii 克氏耶尔森菌 / ~ pestis 鼠疫耶尔森菌(以前称鼠疫杆菌,鼠疫巴斯德菌) / ~ pseudotuberculosis 假结核耶尔森菌(以前称假结核巴斯德菌) / ~ ruckeri 红色耶尔森菌
yersinia [jəːˈsiniə] *n* 耶尔森菌
Yersinieae [jəːˈsiniiː] *n* 耶尔森菌科
yersiniosis [jəːˌsiniˈəusis] *n* 耶尔森菌病;小肠结肠炎耶尔森菌病
Yersin's serum [ˈjəːsin] (Alexandre E. J. Yersin) 耶尔森血清,抗鼠疫血清
yew [jəu] *n* 紫杉 | Pacific ~ 短叶紫杉
yin【汉】阴
-yl [化学后缀] 基(尤指一价烃基)
ylang-ylang [ˌiːlɑːŋˈiːlɑːŋ] *n* 夷兰(产于马来亚的一种乔木)
-ylene [后缀] 撑(在化学中表示二价烃基)
yochubio [jəuˈtʃuːbiəu] *n* 恙虫病
yoga [jəugə] *n*【梵】瑜伽 | hatha ~ 瑜伽气功
yogurt [ˈjəugəːt] *n* 酸乳
yohimbine hydrochloride [jəuˈhimbiːn] 盐酸育亨宾(化学上类似利舍平〈reserpine〉的一种生物碱,具有 α 受体阻滞作用,用作交感神经阻滞药和扩瞳药,以及用于治疗阳萎,口服给药)
yoke [jəuk] *n* 连接结构;轭 | alveolar ~s of mandible 下颌骨牙槽轭 / aleveolar ~s of maxilla 上颌骨牙槽轭 / sphenoidal ~ 蝶轭
yolk [jəuk] *n* 蛋黄,卵黄;羊毛脂 | accessory ~, nutritive ~ 副卵黄,营养卵黄 / egg ~ 蛋黄 /

formative ~ 成胚卵黄

Young-Helmholtz theory [jʌŋ ˈhelmhɔːlts] (Thomas Young; H. L. F, von Helmholtz) 杨-黑尔姆霍尔茨学说(色觉依三组视网膜纤维而定,与红、绿、紫色相符)

Young's operation [jʌŋ] (Hugh H. Young) 杨氏手术(①前列腺穿孔切除术;②精囊及部分射精管切除术)

Young's rule [jʌŋ] (Thomas Young) 杨氏规则(小儿药量计算规则,即将小儿岁数加 12 乘成人剂量除岁数即得)

yperite [ˈiːpərait] *n* 芥子气,二氯二乙硫醚

ypsiliform [ipˈsilifɔːm], **ypsiloid** [ˈipsilɔid] *a* 倒人字形的,V 字形的

ytterbium(Yb) [iˈtəːbjəm] *n* 镱(化学元素)

yttric [ˈitrik] *a* 钇的,含钇的

yttrium(Y) [ˈitriəm] *n* 钇(化学元素)

yukon [ˈjuːkɔn] *n* 重电子(为纪念日本物理学家汤川而定的名称)

Yvon's coefficient [ˈiːvɔn] (Paul Yvon) 伊冯系数(尿中脲与磷酸盐含量的比率) | ~ test 伊冯试验(①检尿中乙酰苯胺;②检生物碱)

Z

Z atomic number 原子序数; **impedence** 阻抗

Z-[德 zusammen (together)] Z 型(用于表明具有双键化合物的绝对构型的立体标码)

ζ zeta, 希腊语第 6 个字母

zafirlukast [zəˈfirluːkæst] *n* 扎非鲁卡(白细胞三烯受体拮抗药,用作抗哮喘药,口服给药)

Zahn's infarct [tsɑːn] (Friedrich W. Zahn) 蔡恩梗死(肝内红蓝脱色区,伴有淤滞和肝细胞萎缩,见于门静脉肝内分支阻塞后,并非真的梗死,因为未见坏死) | ~ lines (ribs) 蔡恩线(死前血块中可见的层状结构,由灰白色纤维蛋白与明显的红蓝色血块狭带交织而成)

Zahorsky's disease [zəˈhɔski] (John Zahorsky) 柴霍斯基病,幼儿急疹,猝发疹

zaire [ˈzairei] *n* 流行性霍乱(发生于葡萄牙)

zalcitabine [zælˈsaitəbiːn] *n* 扎西他滨(抗反转录病毒药,用于治疗人免疫缺陷病毒〈HIV〉感染,口服给药)

zaleplon [ˈzæləplɔn] *n* 扎来普隆(镇静催眠药,用于短期治疗失眠症,口服给药)

Zamia [ˈzeimiə] *n* 泽米属(泽米棕榈的一属)

zamia [ˈzeimiə] *n* 泽米(美洲苏铁科泽米属植物);苏铁科植物(cycad 的误用名)

zanamivir [zəˈnæmivir] *n* 扎纳米韦(病毒性神经氨酸酶抑制药,用于防治 A 型流感和 B 型流感,吸入用药)

Zander apparatus [ˈzændə] (Jonas G. W. Zander) 赞德理疗器(为锻炼身体各部分而设计的一套器械,目前很少采用)

Zangemeister's test [ˌzæŋgəˈmaistə] (Wilhelm Zangemeister) 粲格迈斯特试验(父儿关系鉴定,即将小儿的血清和父亲的血清混合,利用光度计即可测定其透光度减弱,如将父亲以外的男人血清加入小儿血清中,则透光度不减弱)

Zang's space [zæŋ] (Christoph B. Zang) 锁骨上小窝

Zappert's chamber [ˈtsæpət] (Julius Zappert) 扎佩特计数池

zaranthan [zəˈrænθən] *n*【希伯来文】乳房硬化

Zaufal's sign [ˈtsaufɑːl] (Emanuel Zaufal) 鞍状鼻,塌鼻

Z-DNA Z 型 DNA

Zea [ˈziːə] *n* 玉米属,玉蜀黍属 | ~ mays L. 玉米,玉蜀黍

zearalenol [zəˈrælənɔl] *n* 折伦诺(见 zeranol)

zearalenone [zəˈrælənəun] *n* 玉米赤霉烯酮

zeatin [ˈziətin] *n* 玉米素,N^6-异戊烯腺嘌呤

zeaxanthin [ziəˈzænθin] *n* 玉米黄质

zedoary [ˈzedəuəri] *n* 蓬莪术(块茎)

Zeeman effect [ˈtsiːmən] (Pieter Zeeman) 济曼效应(光谱中的单线受适当的磁场作用而分离)

zein [ˈziːin] *n* 玉米醇溶蛋白

zeinolysis [ˌziːiˈnɔlisis] *n* 玉米蛋白分解[作用] | **zeinolytic** [ˌziːinəˈlitik] *a* 分解玉米蛋白的

zeiosis [zaiˈəusis] *n* 沸腾运动(见于人工培养基上所培养的细胞周围)

Zeis' glands [tsais] (Eduard Zeis) 蔡斯腺,睑板皮脂腺

zeisian [ˈzaisiən] *a* 蔡斯(Eduard Zeis) 的(如 ~ stye 外睑腺炎)

zeism [ˈziːizəm], **zeismus** [ziˈismәs] *n* 玉米中毒,玉米红斑

zeistic [ziːˈistik] *a* 玉米的

zeitgeber [ˈzaitgeibə] *n*【德】授时因子

Zeller's test [ˈzelə] (O. Zeller) 策勒试验(①检尿内黑素;②莫洛尼试验,见 Moloney's test)

Zellweger syndrome [ˈzelwegə] (Hans Ulrich Zellweger) 泽尔韦格综合征(即脑肝肾综合征 cerebrohepatorenal syndrome,见 syndrome 项下相应术语)

zenkerism [ˈzeŋkərizəm] (F. A. Zenker) *n* 岑克尔变性(见 Zenker's degeneration)

zenkerize [ˈzeŋkəraiz] (K. Zenker) *vt* 用岑克尔溶液固定

Zenker's crystals [ˈzeŋkə] (Friedrich A. von Zenker) 岑克尔晶体(气喘晶体,白细胞晶体) | ~ degeneration (necrosis) 岑克尔变性(坏死),蜡样坏死(横纹肌坏死和透明变性) / ~ diverticulum 咽下部憩室

Zenker's fixative (fluid, solution) [ˈzeŋkə] (Konrad Zenker) 岑克尔固定液(液、溶液)(含腐蚀性的氯化汞、重铬酸、硫酸钠、冰醋酸和水)

zeolite [ˈziːəlait] *n* 沸石

zeoscope [ˈziːəskəup] *n* 沸点检醇器

zeranol [ˈzerənɔl] *n* 折仑诺(同化激素类药,主要用于兽医)

zero [ˈziərəu] ([复] **zeros** 或 **zeroes**) 零,零点,零度 *a* 零的 *vt* 调节(仪器等)到零点 | absolute ~ 绝对零度(= −273.15 ℃或 −459.67 ℉) /

limes ~ 无毒界量,不致死界 / physiologic ~ 生理零度(不引起感觉的)

Zero Balancing [ˈziərəuˈbælənsiŋ] 零平衡(根据西方解剖学原理与东方关于身体能量的概念相结合的一种健身法,即在骨骼的关键区施行轻揉)

zero-zero [ˈziərəuˈziərəu] *a* 视程零的

zerumbet [ziˈrʌmbet] *n* 球姜(其根茎为一种香料或药物,现在少用)

zestocausis [ˌzestəˈkɔːsis] *n* 蒸汽灼法

zestocautery [ˌzestəˈkɔːtəri] *n* 蒸汽烙管,蒸汽烙器

zeta [ˈziːtə] *n* 希腊语第6个字母(Z, ζ)

zetacrit [ˈzeitəkrit] *n* 浓集红细胞压积(见 ratio 项下 zeta sedimentation ratio)

zeugopodium [ˌzjuːgəˈpəudiəm] *n* 接合骨(胚胎期的桡尺骨和胫腓骨)

zidometacin [ˌzaidəˈmetəsin] *n* 齐多美辛(抗炎药)

zidovudine [zaiˈdəuvjudiːn] *n* 齐多夫定(即 azidothymidine,抗病毒药)

ziega [ziˈeigə] *n* 凝乳

Ziegler's operation [ˈziːglə] (Samuel L. Ziegler) 齐格勒手术(V 形虹膜切除术,以形成人工瞳孔)

Ziehen-Oppenheim disease [ˈziːhənˈɔpənhaim] (Georg T. Ziehen; Herman Oppenheim) 变形性肌张力障碍

Ziehen's test [ˈziːhən] (Georg T. Ziehen) 齐恩测验(检精神疾病,令患者指出客体的区别,如水与冰,猫与犬等)

Ziehl-Neelsen's stain (method) [ˈziːlˈniːlsən] (Franz Ziehl; Friederich K. A. Neelsen) 齐-尼染色法(一种检查抗酸细菌染色法) | ~ carbolfuchsin 齐-尼石炭酸品红

Zielke instrumentation [ˈtsilkə] (K. Zielke) 齐尔格器械用法(矫正脊柱侧凸的一种方法,现主要被杜韦尔〈Dwyer〉器械用法所取代)

Ziemssen's motor points [ˈziːmsən] (Hugo W. von Ziemssem) 齐姆森运动点(运动神经进入肌肉处,选为肌肉电疗之点)

Zieve syndrome [ziːv] (Leslie Zieve) 齐夫综合征(摄入大量乙醇后引起的高胆固醇血症,肝脾肿大,肝脏脂肪浸润,溶血性贫血及高甘油三酯血症)

ZIFT zygote intrafallopian transfer 合子输卵管内移植

zigzagplasty [ˈzigzægˌplæsti] *n* Z 字形整形术

zilantel [ziˈlæntəl] *n* 齐仑太尔(抗蠕虫药)

zileuton [zaiˈljuːtən] *n* 齐留通(脂氧化酶抑制药,用于防治慢性哮喘的症状,口服给药)

zimb [zim] *n* 刷蛇

zimelidine hydrochloride [ziˈmelidiːn] 盐酸齐美利定(抗抑郁药)

Zimmerlin's atrophy (type) [ˈziməlin] (Franz Zimmerlin) 济默林萎缩(型)(从身体上部开始的遗传进行性肌萎缩)

Zimmermann's arch [ˈziməmən] (Karl W. Zimmermann) 济默曼弓(胚胎时偶尔出现的动脉弓,在第四动脉弓与肺动脉弓之间)

Zimmermann's pericyte [ˈziməmən] (Karl Wilhem Bruno Zimmermann) 济默曼外膜细胞(即 pericyte)

zinc (Zn) [ziŋk] *n* 锌(化学元素) | ~ oxide, white ~ 氧化锌,锌白(收敛药、保护剂) / ~ phenolsulfonate, ~ sulfocarbolate 酚磺酸锌(曾用作抗菌药和收敛药,并用于制造杀虫药) / ~ pyrithione 巯氧吡啶锌,吡硫锌(抗菌药,局部抗真菌药,抗皮脂溢药) / ~ stearate 硬脂酸锌(用作扑粉) / ~ sulfanilate 氨苯磺酸锌(抗菌药) / ~ sulfate, ~ vitriol 硫酸锌,锌矾(用作黏膜的收敛药,用于各种皮肤科制剂,内服用作止吐药,尤其在治疗中毒时,亦称皓矾) / ~ undecylenate 十一烯酸锌(以20%配成软膏,用于皮肤真菌病) | **~ic** [ˈziŋkik], **~ky**, **~y**, **zinky** [ˈziŋki], **~ous** *a* 锌的;含锌的

zincalism [ˈziŋkəlizəm] *n* 慢性锌中毒

zincative [ˈziŋkətiv] *a* 负电的

zinciferous [ziŋˈkifərəs] *a* 含锌的

zincoid [ˈziŋkɔid] *a* 似锌的,锌的

zincum [ˈziŋkəm] *n*【拉】锌

Zinn's artery [zin] (Johann G. Zinn) 视网膜中央动脉 | ~ aponeurosis 小带纤维 / ~ circle 视神经血管环 / ~ ligament 总腱环 / ~ zone 睫状小带

Zinsser-Cole-Engman syndrome [ˈzinsə kəul ˈiŋgmən] (Ferdinand Zinsser; Harold Newton Cole; Martin Feeney Engman) 津-科-英综合征,先天性角化不良

Zinsser inconsistency [ˈzinsə] (Hans Zinsser) 津泽不协调现象(局部和全身性过敏症状缺乏平行)

zinterol hydrochloride [ˈzintərəul] 盐酸净特罗(支气管扩张药)

zipp [zip] *n* 锡普糊,氧化锌碘仿糊(由氧化锌、碘仿和液体石蜡研磨而成的一种糊剂,兽医外科用以涂布伤口)

zipper [ˈzipə] *n* 拉链 | leucine ~ 亮氨酸拉链

ziprasidone hydrochloride [ziˈpreisidəun] 盐酸齐培西酮(抗精神病药,用于治疗精神分裂症,口服给药)

zirconium (Zr) [zəːˈkəunjəm] *n* 锆(化学元素) | ~ dioxide, ~ oxide 二氧化锆,氧化锆(曾用作消化道 X 线造影剂,并可制成软膏曾用于治毒

葛性皮炎)

zisp [zisp] *n* 锡斯普糊(一种改良型锡普糊〈zipp〉,用过氧化锌代替氧化锌)

Zn zinc 锌

zoacanthosis [ˌzəuækənˈθəusis] *n* 动物残体性皮炎

zoanthropy [zəuˈænθrəpi] *n* 变兽妄想 | **zoanthropic** [ˌzəuænˈθrɔpik] *a*

zoescope [ˈzəuiskəup] *n* 动态镜

zoetic [zəuˈetik] *a* 生命的

zoetrope [ˈzəuitrəup] *n* 活动幻镜

zoic [ˈzəuik] *a* 动物的,动物生活的

zolamine hydrochloride [ˈzəuləmin] 盐酸佐拉敏(抗组胺药,局部麻醉药)

zolazepam hydrochloride [ˈzəuleisəpæm] 盐酸唑拉西泮(一种镇静催眠化合物,用于兽医,与盐酸替来他明〈tiletamine〉结合使用)

zoledronic acid [ˌzəuləˈdrɔnik] 佐来膦酸(破骨细胞骨吸收的二膦酸盐抑制药,用于治疗恶性高钙血症,静脉内给药)

Zollinger-Ellison syndrome [ˈzɔlindʒə ˈelisn] (Robert M. Zollinger; Edwin H. Ellison) 佐林格-埃利森综合征(消化性溃疡、极度胃酸过多、胰岛细胞瘤三联征)

Zöllner's lines (figures) [ˈzelnə] (Johann C. F. Zöllner) 策尔纳线(图形)(一组特别排列的线,用于眼检查)

zolmitriptan [ˌzəulmiˈtriptæn] *n* 佐米曲坦(选择性5-羟色胺受体激动药,用于缓解急性偏头痛,伴有或不伴有先兆,口服给药)

zolpidem tartrate [zəulˈpidem] 酒石酸唑吡坦(镇静催眠药,短期治疗失眠症,口服给药)

zomepirac sodium [ˌzəumiˈpiəræk] 佐美酸钠(消炎镇痛药)

zometapine [zəuˈmetəpiːn] *n* 氯苯吡草(抗抑郁药)

zomidin [ˈzəumidin] *n* 肉浸质

zomotherapy [ˌzəuməuˈθerəpi] *n* 肉汁疗法,肉食疗法

zona [ˈzəunə] ([复] **zonae** [ˈzəuniː]) *n*【拉】区,带;带状疱疹

zonal [ˈzəunəl] *a* 带的,区的,区带的;分区的;地区性的

zonary [ˈzəunəri] *a* 带的,区的

Zondek-Aschheim test [ˈtsɔndek ˈʌʃhaim] (Bernhardt Zondek; Selmar Aschheim) 仓德克-阿希海姆试验,小白鼠妊娠试验(检孕)

zone [zəun] *n* 带,区 | androgenic ~, X ~ 雄激素带,X带(胚) / ~ of antibody excess 抗体过剩带(在沉淀素反应中抗体浓度相对高的区带,形成可溶性复合物,反应受到抑制,亦称前带,前区) / ~ of antigen excess 抗原过剩带(在沉淀素反应中抗原浓度相对高的区带,形成可溶性复合物,反应受到抑制,亦称后带,后区) / arcuate ~ 弓状带,螺旋管 / biokinetic ~ 生物活动带(活细胞进行生命活动的温度范围,在10°~45°之间) / ciliary ~ 睫状区 / contact area ~ 接触区(邻近牙齿的接触区) / dolorogenic ~, trigger ~ 发痛区,扳机区 / ~ of equivalence 等价带,最适比例带(见 ~ of optimal proportions) / erogenous ~, erotogenic ~ 性欲发生区 / ~ of exclusion 排斥区(胞质中除高尔基〈Golgi〉复合体外无任何细胞器存在的区域) / glomerular ~ 丝球带,小球带 / hemorrhoidal ~ 痔带,肛静脉丛 / inhibition ~ 抑制带(见 prozone) / keratogenous ~ 角质增生区 / Looser's transformation ~s 卢塞变形区,假骨折线(骨X线片所见的暗线,据认为是某些骨病时发生疲劳骨折后的病理性愈合期) / motor ~ 运动区(脑皮质区) / nuclear ~ 晶状体涡 / ~ of optimal proportions 最适比例带(在沉淀素反应中的最高沉淀区带,抗原和抗体结合形成一交联网格。亦称等价带) / proagglutinoid ~ 前凝集带(见 prozone) / tendinous ~s of heart 心纤维环 / thymus-dependent ~ 胸腺依赖区 / thymus-independent ~ 胸腺非依赖区 / umbau ~s【德】卢塞变形区(即 Looser's transformation ~s) / visual ~ 视区

zonesthesia [ˌzəunesˈθiːzjə] *n* 束勒感,束带状感觉

zonifugal [zəuˈnifjugəl] *a* 离区的,远区的

zoning [ˈzəuniŋ] *n* 带现象(使用较少量可疑血清而出现较强的补体结合)

zonipetal [zəuˈnipitl] *a* 向区的

zonisamide [zəuˈnisəˌmaid] *n* 唑尼沙胺(抗惊厥药)

zonoskeleton [ˌzounəˈskelitn] *n* 肢带骨(胚胎期的肩胛锁骨和髋骨)

zonula [ˈzəunjulə] ([复] **zonulae** [ˈzəunjuliː]) *n*【拉】小带

zonule [ˈzəunjuːl] *n* 小带 | ciliary ~, lens ~ 睫状小带,晶状体悬器 | **zonular** [ˈzəunjulə] *a* 小带[状]的

zonulitis [ˌzəunjuˈlaitis] *n* 睫状小带炎

zonulolysis [ˌzɔnjuˈlɔlisis], **zonulysis** [ˌzɔujuˈlaisis] *n* 晶状体悬勒带松解术

zonulotomy [ˌzɔnjuˈlɔtəmi] *n* 晶状体悬勒带切断术

zo(o)- [构词成分]动物

zoo-agglutinin [ˌzəuəuəˈgluːtinin] *n* 动物凝集素(动物毒中能凝集红细胞的物质)

zoo-anaphylactogen [ˌzəuəuˌænəfiˈlæktədʒən] *n* 动物过敏原(能引起过敏反应的动物蛋白质)

zoobiology [ˌzəuəubaiˈɔlədʒi] *n* 动物生物学

zoobiotism [ˌzəuəuˈbaiətizəm] *n* 生命学

zooblast [ˈzəuəblæst] *n* 动物细胞
zoochemistry [ˌzəuəuˈkemistri] *n* 动物化学 | **zoochemical** *a*
zoodermic [ˌzəuəuˈdəːmik] *a* 动物皮肤的(供移植用)
zoodetritus [ˌzəuəudiˈtraitəs] *n* 动物碎屑
zoodynamics [ˌzəuəudaiˈnæmiks] *n* 动物[动]力学,动物生理学 | **zoodynamic** *a*
zooerastia [ˌzəuəuiːˈræstiə] *n* 兽奸
zooflagellate [ˌzəuəuˈflædʒileit] *n* 鞭毛动物
zoofulvin [ˌzəuəuˈfʌlvin] *n* 鸟羽黄色素
zoogenic [zəuəuˈdʒenik] *a* 动物的
zoogenous [zəuˈɔdʒinəs] *a* 动物源的;胎生的
zoogeny [zəuˈɔdʒini], **zoogenesis** [ˌzəuəuˈdʒenisis] *n* 动物发生,动物进化
zoogeography [ˌzəuəudʒiˈɔgrəfi] *n* 动物地理学
zooglea, zoogloea [ˌzəuəˈgliːə] *n* 菌胶团 | **zoogleic, zoogloeic** [ˌzəuəˈgliːik] *a*
zoogleal [ˌzəuəˈgliːəl] *a* 菌胶团的
Zoogloea [ˌzəuəˈgliːə] *n* 菌胶团属
zoogonous [zəuˈɔgənəs] *a* 胎生的
zoogony [zəuˈɔgəni] *n* 胎生
zoografting [ˈzəuəˌgrɑːftiŋ] *n* 动物组织移植术
zoography [zəuˈɔgrəfi] *n* 动物志 | **zoographic (al)** [ˌzəuəˈgræfik(əl)] *a*
zoohormone [ˌzəuəuˈhɔːməun] *n* 动物激素
zooid [ˈzəuɔid] *a* 动物样的 *n* 动物样体;个体(动物群体的一个);游动孢子
zookinase [ˌzəuəuˈkineis] *n* 动物激酶
zoolagnia [ˌzəuəuˈlægniə] *n* 恋兽欲,戏兽色情
zoology [zəuˈɔlədʒi] *n* 动物学 | experimental ~ 实验动物学 | **zoologist** *n* 动物学家 / **zoologic (al)** [ˌzəuəˈlɔdʒik(əl)] *a*
zoomania [ˌzəuəuˈmeinjə] *n* 嗜兽癖
Zoomastigophora [ˌzəuəuˌmæstiˈgɔfərə] *n* 动鞭毛亚纲
Zoomastigophorea [ˌzəuəuˌmæstiˌgɔfəˈriːə] *n* 动鞭纲,动物鞭毛虫纲
zoomastigophorean [ˌzəuəuˌmæstiˌgɔfəˈriːən] *n* 动鞭毛虫
Zoon balanitis (erythroplasia) [zəun] (Johannes J. Zoon) 佐氏龟头炎(增殖性红斑),浆细胞性局限性龟头炎
zoonerythrin [ˌzəuɔnˈeriθrin] *n* 动物红素,甲壳红素
zoonite [ˈzəuənait] *n* 脑脊髓节
zoonomy [zəuˈɔnəmi] *n* 动物生物学
zoonosis [zəuˈɔnəsis] ([复] **zoonoses** [zəuˈɔnəsiːz]) *n* 动物源性寄生虫病,人畜共患病(如炭疽、鹦鹉热等均可传染于人) | **zoonotic** [ˌzəuəˈnɔtik] *a* 人畜互传的
zoonosology [ˌzəuəunəuˈsɔlədʒi] *n* 动物疾病分类学
Zoopagales [ˌzəuəpəˈgeiliːs] *n* 接合菌目
zooparasite [ˌzəuəuˈpærəsait] *n* 寄生动物 | **zooparasitic** [ˌzəuəuˌpærəˈsitik] *a*
zoopathology [ˌzəuəupəˈθɔlədʒi] *n* 动物病理学
zoopery [zəuˈɔpəri] *n* 动物实验 | **zooperal** *a*
zoophagous [zəuˈɔfəgəs] *a* 食动物的,食肉的
zoopharmacology [ˌzəuəuˌfɑːməˈkɔlədʒi] *n* 动物药理学,兽医药理学
zoopharmacy [zəuəˈfɑːməsi] *n* 动物药剂学,兽医药剂学
zoophile [ˈzəuəfail] *a* 嗜动物[血]的(指蚊) *n* 嗜动物癖者,反对[动物]活体解剖者
zoophilia [ˌzəuəˈfiliə] *n* 嗜动物癖,动物爱好;恋兽欲,戏兽色情
zoophilic [ˌzəuəˈfilik], **zoophilous** [zəuˈɔfiləs] *a* 爱好动物的;嗜动物[血]的(指蚊)
zoophilism [zəuˈɔfilizəm] *n* 嗜动物癖,动物爱好;反对[动物]活体解剖主义 | erotic ~ 动物色情狂
zoophobia [ˌzəuəuˈfəubjə] *n* 动物恐怖,恐兽症
zoophysiology [ˌzəuəuˌfiziˈɔlədʒi] *n* 动物生理学
zoophyte [ˈzəuəfait] *n* 植虫,植物性动物(如海绵) | **zoophytic (al)** [ˌzəuəˈfitik(əl)] *a*
zooplankton [ˌzəuəuˈplæŋktən] *n* 浮游动物 | **~ic** [ˌzəuəplæŋkˈtɔnik] *a*
zooplasty [ˌzəuəuˈplæsti] *n* 动物组织成形术,动物组织移植术
zooprecipitin [ˌzəuəupriˈsipitin] *n* 动物沉淀素
zooprophylaxis [ˌzəuəuprɔfiˈlæksis] *n* 动物病预防法;家畜诱蚊预防法
zoopsia [zəuˈɔpsiə] *n* 动物幻视
zoopsychology [ˌzəuəusaiˈkɔlədʒi] *n* 动物心理学
zoosadism [ˌzəuəuˈsædizəm] *n* 动物虐待[色情]狂,动物施虐癖
zooscopy [zəuˈɔskəpi] *n* 动物幻视;动物研究
zoosensitinogen [ˌzəuəuˌsensiˈtinədʒən] *n* 动物致敏原,动物过敏原
zoosis [zəuˈəusis] *n* 动物性病,动物源病
zoosperm [ˈzəuəspəːm] *n* 游动精子
zoospermia [ˌzəuəˈspəːmiə] *n* (所射精液内)活精子存在
zoosporangium [ˌzəuəuspəˈrændʒiəm] ([复] **zoosporangia** [ˌzəuəuspəˈrændʒiə]) *n* 游动孢子囊
zoospore [ˈzəuəspɔː] *n* 游动孢子 | **zoosporic** [ˌzəuəˈspɔrik], **zoosporous** [zəuˈɔspərəs] *a*
zoosteroid [ˌzəuəuˈsterɔid] *n* 动物甾类
zoosterol [zəuˈɔstərɔl] *n* 动物甾醇
zootechnics [ˌzəuəuˈtekniks] *n* 动物驯养术

zootechny [ˌzəuəuˈtekni] *n* 动物驯养术
zootic [zəuˈɔtik] *a* 低等动物的
zootomy [zəuˈɔtəmi] *n* 动物解剖;动物解剖学,比较解剖学 | **zootomic(al)** [ˌzəuəuˈtɔmik(əl)] *a* | **zootomist** *n* 比较解剖学家
zootoxin [ˌzəuəˈtɔksin] *n* 动物毒素
zootrophic [ˌzəuəuˈtrɔfik] *a* 动物式营养的
zootrophotoxism [ˌzəuəuˌtrɔfəuˈtɔksizəm] *n* 动物性食物中毒,兽肉中毒
zooxanthella [ˌzəuəuzænˈθelə] ([复] **zooxanthellae** [ˌzəuəuzænˈθeliː]) *n* 虫黄藻,动物黄藻
Zopfius [ˈzɔpfiəs] *n* 佐普夫杆菌属(旧名,现称库尔特杆菌属 Kurthia)
zopiclone [ˈzəupiˌkləun] *n* 佐匹克隆(镇静催眠药,用于短期治疗失眠症,口服给药)
zorbamycin [zɔːbəˈmaisin] *n* 佐尔博霉素
zorubicin hydrochloride [zəuˈruːbisin] 盐酸佐柔比星(抗肿瘤药)
zoster [ˈzɔstə] *n*【希】带状疱疹
Zostera marina [ˈzɔstərə məˈrainə] 大叶藻
zosteriform [zɔsˈterifɔːm], **zosteroid** [ˈzɔstərɔid] *a* 带状疱疹样的
zoxazolamine [ˌzɔksəˈzɔləmiːn] *n* 氯苯唑胺(骨骼肌松弛药,促尿酸排泄药治疗痛风)
Z-plasty [zed ˈplæsti] *n* Z 成形术(一种解除瘢痕挛缩手术)
Zr (zirconium) 锆
Zsigmondy's gold number method, test [sigˈmɔndi] (Richard A. Zsigmondy) 希格蒙迪金值法、试验,胶态金试验(见 test 项下 colloidal gold test)
ZSR zeta sedimentation rate Z 血沉比率
Zuberella [ˌzubəˈrelə] *n* 佐勃杆菌属(革兰阴性厌氧菌的一属)
zuckergussdarm [ˈtsukəˌgusdɑːm] *n*【德】糖衣肠,慢性纤维包围性腹膜炎
zuckergussleber [ˈtsukəˌgusleibə] *n*【德】糖衣肝,慢性增生性肝周炎
Zuckerkandl's bodies (organs) [ˈtsuːkerˌkɑːndl] (Emil Zuckerkandl) 主动脉旁体 | ~ convolution 终板旁回 / ~ dehiscences 祖克坎德尔裂(偶见于筛骨层内的小裂隙) / ~ fascia 祖克坎德尔筋膜(肾筋膜的后部)
zuclomiphene [zuːˈkləumifiːn] *n* 珠氯米芬(抗不育症药)
Zumbusch's psoriasis [ˈtsumbuʃ] (Leo von Zumbusch) 楚姆布什银屑病,泛发性脓疱性银屑病
Zuntz's theory [ˈzuːnts] (Nathan Zuntz) 宗兹学说(一种肌肉收缩学说)
zwischenferment [ˈtsviʃənˌfəːmənt] *n*【德】间酶,6-磷酸葡糖脱氢酶
zwischenkörper [ˈtsviʃənˌkəːpə] *n*【德】介体
zwischenscheibe [ˈtsviʃənˌʃaibə] *n*【德】Z 盘(即克劳斯〈Krause〉膜,横纹肌间线)
zwitterion [ˈtsvitəˌraiən] *n* 两性离子 | **~ic** [ˌtsvitəraiˈɔnik] *a*
zwölffingerdarm [tsvelfˈfiŋgədɑːm] *n*【德】十二指肠
zygadenine [zaiˈgædinin] *n* 棋盘花碱
zygal [ˈzaigəl] *a* 轭状的
zygapophysis [ˌzaigəˈpɔfisis] *n* 椎骨关节突 | **zygapophyseal** [ˌzaigəpəˈfiziəl] *a*
zygion [ˈzidʒiən] ([复] **zygia** [ˈzidʒiə]) *n*【希】轭点(测颅点)
zyg(o)- [构词成分]轭,接合
Zygocotyle lunatum [ˌzaigəuˈkəutili ljuːˈneitəm] 镰形轭吸虫
zygocyte [ˈzaigəsait], **zygoite** [ˈzaigəait] *n* 合子
zygodactyly [ˌzaigəˈdæktili] *n* 并指[畸形],并趾[畸形]
zygoma [zaiˈgəumə] *n*【希】颞[骨]颧突;颧弓;颧骨 | **~tic** [ˌzaigəˈmætik] *a*
zygomaticofacial [ˌzaigəuˌmætikəuˈfeiʃəl] *a* 颧面的
zygomaticofrontal [ˌzaigəuˌmætikəuˈfrʌntl] *a* 颧额的
zygomaticomaxillary [ˌzaigəuˌmætikəuˈmækˈsiləri] *a* 颧上颌的
zygomatico-orbital [ˌzaigəuˌmætikəuˈɔːbitl] *a* 颧眶的
zygomaticosphenoid [ˌzaigəuˌmætikəuˈsfiːnɔid] *a* 颧蝶的
zygomaticotemporal [ˌzaigəuˌmætikəuˈtempərəl] *a* 颧颞的
zygomaxillare [ˌzaiqəuˈmæksiˌlɛəri] *n*【拉】颧颌点
zygomaxillary [ˌzaigəuˈmæksiləri] *a* 颧上颌的
Zygomycetes [ˈzaigəumaiˈsiːtiːz] *n* 接合菌亚纲
zygomycosis [ˌzaigəumaiˈkəusis] *n* 接合菌病 | rhinofacial ~ 鼻藻菌病(即 rhinoentomophthoromycosis) / subcutaneous ~ 蛙粪虫霉病(即 entomophthoromycosis basidiobolae)
Zygomycota [ˌzaigəumaiˈkəutə] *n* 接合菌门
Zygomycotina [ˌzaigəuˌmaikəuˈtainə] *n* 接合菌亚门
zygon [ˈzaigɔn] *n*【希】接合嵴
zygoneure [ˈzaigənjuə] *n* 接合[神经]细胞
zygophore [ˈzaigəufɔː] *n* 接合枝
zygoplast [ˈzaigəplæst] *n* 根丝体(原虫体内与核联接的小体)
zygopodium [ˌzaigəuˈpəudiəm] *n* 肢干,接合骨(胚胎期的桡尺骨和胫腓骨)
zygosis [zaiˈgəusis] *n* 接合(单细胞生物)

zygosity [zaiˈgɔsəti] *n* 接合性
zygosphere [ˈzaigəsfiə] *n* 接合配子
zygospore [ˈzaigəspɔː], **zygosperm** [ˈzaigəspəːm] *n* 接合孢子 | **zygosporic** [ˌzaigəˈspɔrik] *a*
zygostyle [ˈzaigəstail] *n* [终]末尾椎
zygote [ˈzaigəut] *n* [接]合子 | duplex ~ 复式合子,双显性组合合子 / multiplex ~ 多式合子,无显性组合合子 / simplex ~ 单式合子,单显性组合合子 | **zygotic** [zaiˈgɔtik] *a*
zygotene [ˈzaigətiːn] *n* 偶线期(减数分裂的接合期)
zygotoblast [zaiˈgəutəblæst] *n* 子孢子
zygotomere [zaiˈgəutəmiə] *n* 成孢子细胞
zylonite [ˈzailənait] *n* 赛璐珞,假象牙
zymase [ˈzaimeis] *n* 酶;微胶粒;酿酶,酒化酶
zymasis [ˈzaiməsis] *n* 酵母成分压出[法]
zyme [zaim] *n*【希】酶;病菌(致病酶)
zymetology [ˌzaimiˈtɔlədʒi] *n* 酶学
zymic [ˈzaimik] *a* 酶的
zymin [ˈzaimin] *n* 胰酶制剂(治疗用);酶
zymo- [构词成分]酶,发酵
Zymobacterium [ˌzaiməubækˈtiəriəm] *n* 发酵菌属
zymochemistry [ˌzaiməuˈkemistri] *n* 酶化学
zymoexcitator [ˌzaiməuˈeksaiˌteitə], **zymoexciter** [ˌzaiməuekˈsaitə] *n* 酶原激活剂,酶激活剂
zymogen [ˈzaimədʒən] *n* 酶原 | lab ~ 凝乳酶原
zymogenesis [ˌzaiməuˈdʒenisis] *n* 酶生成[作用]
zymogenic [ˌzaiməuˈdʒenik], **zymogenous** [zaiˈmɔdʒinəs], **zymogic** [zaiˈmɔdʒik] *a* 发酵的;引起发酵的
zymogram [ˈzaiməgræm] *n* 酶谱
zymohexase [ˌzaiməuˈhekseis] *n* 醛缩酶,醛醇缩合酶
zymoid [ˈzaimɔid] *a* 类酶的 *n* 腐组织毒
zymolysis [zaiˈmɔlisis], **zymohydrolysis** [ˌzaiməuhaiˈdrɔlisis] *n* 酶解作用 | **zymolytic** [ˌzaiməˈlitik] *a*
zymome [ˈzaiməum] *n* 微胶粒
Zymomonas [ˌzaiməˈməunəs] *n* 酵单胞菌属
Zymonema [ˌzaiməuˈniːmə] *n* 酵丝菌属 | ~ albicans 白色酵丝菌(即白念珠菌 Candida albicans) / ~ capsulatum, ~ dermatitidis, ~ gilchristi 荚膜酵丝菌,皮炎酵丝菌,吉氏酵丝菌(即皮炎芽生菌 Blastomyces dermatitidis) / ~ farciminosum 马淋巴腺炎酵丝菌(即马淋巴腺炎组织胞浆菌 Histoplasma farciminosus)
zymophore [ˈzaiməfɔː] *n* 酶支持体,酶活性簇,催凝簇(酶分子上显示其特异作用的原子团,是酶的活性部位) | **zymophorous** [zaiˈmɔfərəs] *a*
zymophosphate [ˌzaiməuˈfɔsfeit] *n* 酵母己糖磷酸
zymoprotein [ˌzaiməuˈprəutiːn] *n* 酶蛋白
zymosan [ˈzaiməsən] *n* 酵母多糖,酵母聚糖(抗补体因子的一种)
zymoscope [ˈzaiməskəup] *n* 发酵测定器
zymose [ˈzaiməus] *n* 转化酶
zymosis [zaiˈməusis] *n*【希】发酵;发酵病;传染病 | **zymotic** [zaiˈmɔtik] *a* 发酵的;发酵病的;传染病的 *n* 传染病
zymosterol [zaiˈmɔstərɔl] *n* 霉菌甾醇,酵母甾醇
zymosthenic [ˌzaiməsˈθenik] *a* 增强酶活性的
zytase [ˈzaiteis] *n* 木聚糖酶,木糖胶酶
Zz. zingiber【拉】姜

附　　录

一　动脉名对照表

arteria

~ alveolaris inferior [TA], inferior alveolar artery 下牙槽动脉

~e alveolares superiores anteriores [TA], anterior superior alveolar arteries 上牙槽前动脉

~ alveolaris superior posterior [TA], posterior superior alveolar artery 上牙槽后动脉

~ angularis [TA], angular artery 内眥动脉

~ appendicularis [TA], appendicular artery 阑尾动脉

~ arcuata pedis [TA], arcuate artery of foot 足弓状动脉

~e arcuatae renis [TA], arcuate arteries of kidney 肾弓状动脉

~ auricularis posteria [TA], posterior auricular artery 耳后动脉

~ auricularis profunda [TA], deep auricular artery 耳深动脉

~ axillaris [TA], axillary artery 腋动脉

~ basilaris [TA], basilar artery 基底动脉

~ brachialis [TA], brachial artery 肱动脉

~ brachialis superficialis [TA], superficial brachial artery 浅肱动脉

~ buccalis [TA], buccal artery 颊动脉

~ bulbi penis [TA], artery of bulb of penis 尿道球动脉

~ bulbi vestibuli [TA], artery of bulb of vestibule 前庭球动脉

~ canalis pterygoidei [TA], artery of pterygoid canal 翼管动脉

~ carotis communis [TA], common carotid artery 颈总动脉

~ carotis externa [TA], external carotid artery 颈外动脉

~ carotis interna [TA], internal carotid artery 颈内动脉

~ centralis retinae [TA], central artery of retina 视网膜中央动脉

~ cerebelli inferior anterior, anterior inferior cerebellar artery 小脑下前动脉

~ cerebelli inferior posterior, posterior inferior cerebellar artery 小脑下后动脉

~ cerebelli superior, superior cerebellar artery 小脑上动脉

~ cerebri anterior [TA], anterior cerebral artery 大脑前动脉

~ cerebri media [TA], middle cerebral artery 大脑中动脉

~ cerebri posterior [TA], posterior cerebral artery 大脑后动脉

~ cervicalis ascendens [TA], ascending cervical artery 颈升动脉

~ cervicalis profunda [TA], deep cervical artery 颈深动脉

~ choroidea anterior [TA], anterior choroidal artery 脉络丛前动脉

~e ciliares anteriores [TA], anterior ciliary arteries 睫前动脉

~e ciliares posteriores breves [TA], short posterior ciliary arteries 睫后短动脉

~e ciliares posteriores longea [TA], long posterior ciliary arteries 睫后长动脉

~ circumflexa femoris lateralis [TA], lateral circumflex femoral artery 旋股外侧动脉

~ circumflexa femoris medialis [TA], medial circumflex femoral artery 旋股内侧动脉

~ circumflexa humeri anterior [TA], anterior circumflex humeral artery 旋肱前动脉

~ circumflexa humeri posterior [TA], posterior circumflex humeral artery 旋肱后动脉

~ circumflexa ilium profunda [TA], deep circumflex iliac artery 旋髂深动脉

~ circumflexa ilium superficialis [TA], superficial circumflex iliac artery 旋髂浅动脉

~ circumflexa scapulae [TA], circumflex artery of scapula 旋肩胛动脉

~ colica dextra [TA], right colic artery 右结肠动脉

~ colica media [TA], middle colic artery 中结肠动脉

~ colica sinistra [TA], left colic artery 左结肠动脉

~ collateralis media [TA], middle collateral artery 中副动脉

~ collateralis radialis [TA], radial collateral artery 桡侧副动脉

~ collateralis ulnaris inferior [TA], inferior ulnar

collateral artery 尺侧下副动脉
~ collateralis ulnaris superior [TA], superior ulnar collateral artery 尺侧上副动脉
~ comitans nervi ischiadici [TA], accompanying artery of ischiadic nerve 坐骨神经伴行动脉
~ communicans anterior [TA], anterior communicating artery 前交通动脉
~ communicans posterior [TA], posterior communicating artery 后交通动脉
~e conjunctivales anteriores [TA], anterior conjunctival arteries 结膜前动脉
~e conjunctivales posteriores [TA], posterior conjunctival arteries 结膜后动脉
~ coronaria dextra [TA], right coronary artery 右冠状动脉
~ coronaria sinistra [TA], left coronary artery 左冠状动脉
~ cremasterica [TA], cremasteric artery 提睾肌动脉
~ cystica [TA], cystic artery 胆囊动脉
~e digitales dorsales manus [TA], dorsal digital arteries of hand 指背动脉
~e digitales dorsales pedis [TA], dorsal digital arteries of foot 趾背动脉
~e digitales palmares communes [TA], common palmar digital arteries 指掌侧总动脉
~e digitales palmares propriae [TA], proper palmar digital arteries 指掌侧固有动脉
~e digitales plantares communes [TA], common plantar digital arteries 趾底总动脉
~e digitales plantares propriae [TA], proper plantar digital arteries 趾足底固有动脉
~ dorsalis clitoridis [TA], dorsal artery of clitoris 阴蒂背动脉
~ dorsalis nasi [TA], dorsal artery of nose 鼻背动脉
~ dorsalis pedis [TA], dorsal artery of foot 足背动脉
~ dorsalis penis [TA], dorsal artery of penis 阴茎背动脉
~ ductus deferentis [TA], artery of ductus deferens 输精管动脉
~ epigastrica inferior [TA], inferior epigastric artery 腹壁下动脉
~ epigastrica superficialis [TA], superficial epigastric artery 腹壁浅动脉
~ epigastrica superior [TA], superior epigastric artery 腹壁上动脉
~e episclerales [TA], episcleral arteries 巩膜外动脉
~ ethmoidalis anterior [TA], arterior ethmoidal artery 筛前动脉
~ ethmoidalis posterior [TA], posterior ethmoidal artery 筛后动脉
~ facialis [TA], facial artery 面动脉
~ femoralis [TA], femoral artery 股动脉
~e gastricar breves [TA], short gastric arteries 胃短动脉
~ gastrica dextra [TA], right gastric artery 胃右动脉
~ gastrica sinistra [TA], left gastric artery 胃左动脉
~ gastroduodenalis [TA], gastroduodenal artery 胃十二指肠动脉
~ gastroepiploica dextra, right gastroepiploic artery 胃网膜右动脉
~ gastroepiploica sinistra, left gastroepiploic artery 胃网膜左动脉
~ genus inferior lateralis, lateral inferior genicular artery 膝下外侧动脉
~ genus inferior medialis, medial inferior genicular artery 膝下内侧动脉
~ genus media, middle genicular artery 膝中动脉
~ genus superior medialis, medial superior genicular artery 膝上内动脉
~ glutea inferior, inferior gluteal artery 臀下动脉
~ glutea superior, superior gluteal artery 臀上动脉
~e helicinae penis [TA], helicine arteries of penis 阴茎螺旋动脉
~ hepatica communis [TA], common hepatic artery 肝总动脉
~ hepatica propria [TA], proper hepatic artery 肝固有动脉
~ hyaloidea [TA], hyaloid artery 玻璃体动脉
~ hypogastrica, hypogastric artery 髂内动脉
~e ilei [TA], ileal arteries 回肠动脉
~ ileocolica [TA], ileocolic artery 回结肠动脉
~ iliaca communis [TA], common iliac artery 髂总动脉
~ iliaca externa [TA], external iliac artery 髂外动脉
~ iliaca interna [TA], internal iliac artery 髂内动脉
~ iliolumbalis [TA], iliolumbar artery 髂腰动脉
~ infraorbitalis [TA], infraorbital artery 眶下动脉
~e intercostales posteriores [TA], posterior intercostal arteries 肋间后动脉
~ intercostalis suprema [TA], highest intercostal artery 肋间最上动脉
~e interlobares renis [TA], interlobar arteries of kidney 肾叶间动脉
~e interlobulares hepatis [TA], interlobular arteries of liver 肝小叶间动脉
~e interlobulares renis, interlobular arteries of kidney 肾小叶间动脉
~ interossea anterior [TA], anterior interosseous

artery 骨间前动脉
~ interossea communis [TA], common interosseous artery 骨间总动脉
~ interossea posterior [TA], posterior interosseous artery 骨间后动脉
~ interossea recurrens [TA], recurrent interosseous artery 骨间返动脉
~e jejunales [TA], jejunal arteries 空肠动脉
~ labialis inferior [TA], inferior labial artery 下唇动脉
~ labialis superior [TA], superior labial artery 上唇动脉
~ labyrinthi [TA], artery of labyrinth 迷路动脉
~ lacrimalis [TA], lacrimal artery 泪腺动脉
~ laryngea inferior [TA], inferior laryngeal artery 喉下动脉
~ laryngea superior [TA], superior laryngeal artery 喉上动脉
~ lienalis splenic artery 脾动脉
~ ligamenti teretis uteri [TA], artery of round ligament of uterus 子宫圆韧带动脉
~e lumbales [TA], lumbar arteries 腰动脉
~ malleolaris anterior lateralis [TA], lateral anterior malleolar artery 外踝前动脉
~ malleolaris anterior medialis [TA], medial anterior malleolar artery 内踝前动脉
~ masseterica [TA], masseteric artery 咬肌动脉
~ maxillaris [TA], maxillary artery 上颌动脉
~ mediana, median artery 正中动脉
~ meningea anterior, anterior meningeal artery 脑膜前动脉
~ meningea media [TA], middle meningeal artery 脑膜中动脉
~ meningea posterior [TA], posterior meningeal artery 脑膜后动脉
~ mentalis [TA], mental artery 颏动脉
~ mesenterica inferior [TA], inferior mesenteric artery 肠系膜下动脉
~ mesenterica superior [TA], superior mesenteric artery 肠系膜上动脉
~e metacarpeae dorsales [TA], dorsal metacarpal arteries 掌背动脉
~e metacarpeae palmares [TA], palmar metacarpal arteries 掌心动脉
~e metatarsales dorsales [TA], dorsal metatarsal arteries 跖背动脉
~e metatarsales plantares [TA], plantar metatarsal arteries 足心动脉
~ musculophrenica [TA], musculophrenic artery 肌膈动脉
~e nasales posteriores laterales [TA], posterior lateral nasal arteries 鼻后外侧动脉
~e nutriciae humeri [TA], nutrient arteries of humerus 肱骨滋养动脉
~ obturatoria [TA], obturator artery 闭孔动脉
~ obturatoria accessoria [TA], accessory obturator artery 副闭孔动脉
~ occipitalis [TA], occipital artery 枕动脉
~ ophthalmica [TA], ophthalmic artery 眼动脉
~ ovarica [TA], ovarian artery 卵巢动脉
~ palatina ascendens [TA], ascending palatine artery 腭升动脉
~ palatina descendens [TA], descending palatine artery 腭降动脉
~ palatina major [TA], greater palatine artery 腭大动脉
~e palatinae minores [TA], lesser palatine arteries 腭小动脉
~e palpebrales laterales [TA], lateral palpebral arteries 睑外侧动脉
~e palpebrales mediales [TA], medial palpebral arteries 睑内侧动脉
~e pancreaticoduodenales inferiores [TA], inferior pancreaticoduodenal arteries 胰十二指肠下动脉
~e perforantes [TA], perforating arteries 穿动脉
~ pericardiacophrenica [TA], pericardiacophrenic artery 心包膈动脉
~ perinealis [TA], perineal artery 会阴动脉
~ peronea, peroneal artery 腓动脉
~ pharyngea ascendens [TA], ascending pharyngeal artery 咽升动脉
~e phrenicae inferiores [TA], inferior phrenic arteries 膈下动脉
~e phrenicae superiores [TA], superior phrenic arteries 膈上动脉
~ plantaris lateralis [TA], lateral plantar artery 足底外侧动脉
~ plantaris medialis [TA], medial plantar artery 足底内侧动脉
~ poplitea [TA], popliteal artery 腘动脉
~ princeps pollicis [TA], principal artery of thumb 拇主要动脉
~ profunda brachii [TA], deepbrachial artery 肱深动脉
~ profunda clitoridis [TA], deep artery of clitoris 阴蒂深动脉
~ profunda femoris [TA], deep femoral artery 股深动脉
~ profunda linguae [TA], deep lingual artery 舌深动脉
~ profunda penis [TA], deep artery of penis 阴茎深动脉
~ pudenda interna [TA], internal pudental artery 阴部内动脉
~ pulmonalis dextra [TA], right pulmonary artery 右肺动脉

~ pulmonalis sinistra［TA］, left pulmonary artery 左肺动脉
~ radialis［TA］, radial artery 桡动脉
~ radialis indicis［TA］, radial artery of index finger 示指桡侧动脉
~ rectalis inferior［TA］, inferior rectal artery 直肠下动脉
~ rectalis media［TA］, middle rectal artery 直肠中动脉
~ rectalis superior［TA］, superior rectal artery 直肠上动脉
~ recurrens radialis［TA］, radial recurrent artery 桡侧返动脉
~ recurrens tibialis anterior［TA］, anterior tibial recurrent artery 胫前返动脉
~ recurrens tibialis posterior［TA］, posterior tibial recurrent artery 胫后返动脉
~ recurrens ulnaris［TA］, ulnar recurrent artery 尺侧返动脉
~ renalis［TA］, renal artery 肾动脉
~e sacrales laterales［TA］, lateral sacral arteries 骶外侧动脉
~ sacralis mediana［TA］, median sacral artery 骶正中动脉
~e sigmoideae［TA］, sigmoid arteries 乙状结肠动脉
~ sphenopalatina［TA］, sphinopalatine artery 蝶腭动脉
~ spinalis anterior［TA］, anterior spinal artery 脊髓前动脉
~ spinalis posterior［TA］, posterior spinal artery 脊髓后动脉
~ stylomastoidea［TA］, stylomastoid artery 茎乳动脉
~ subclavia［TA］, subclavian artery 锁骨下动脉
~ subcostalis［TA］, subcostal artery 肋下动脉
~ sublingualis［TA］, sublingual artery 舌下动脉
~ submentalis［TA］, submental artery 颏下动脉
~ subscapularis［TA］, subscapular artery 肩胛下动脉
~ supraorbitalis［TA］, supraorbital artery 眶上动脉
~ suprarenalis inferior［TA］, inferior suprarenal artery 肾上腺下动脉
~ suprarenalis media［TA］, middle suprarenal artery 肾上腺中动脉
~e suprarenales superiores［TA］, superior suprarenal arteries 肾上腺上动脉
~ suprascapularis［TA］, suprascapular artery 肩胛上动脉
~ supratrochlearis［TA］, supratrochlear artery 滑车上动脉
~e surales［TA］, sural arteries 腓肠动脉
~ tarsea lateralis［TA］, lateral tarsal artery 跗外侧动脉
~e tarseae mediales, medial tarsal arteries 跗内侧动脉
~ temporalis media［TA］, middle temporal artery 颞中动脉
~ temporalis superficialis［TA］, superficial temporal artery 颞浅动脉
~ testicularis［TA］, testicular artery 睾丸动脉
~ thoracica interna［TA］, internal thoracic artery 胸廓内动脉
~ thoracica lateralis［TA］, lateral thoracic artery 胸外侧动脉
~ thoracoacromialis［TA］, thoracoacromial artery 胸肩峰动脉
~ thoracodorsalis［TA］, thoracodorsal artery 胸背动脉
~ thyroidea inferior［TA］, inferior thyroid artery 甲状腺下动脉
~ thyroidea superior［TA］, superior thyroid artery 甲状腺上动脉
~ tibialis anterior［TA］, anterior tibial artery 胫前动脉
~ tibialis posterior［TA］, posterior tibial artery 胫后动脉
~ transversa colli, transverse cervical artery 颈横动脉
~ transversa faciei［TA］, transverse facial artery 面横动脉
~ tympanica anterior［TA］, anterior tympanic artery 鼓室前动脉
~ tympanica inferior［TA］, inferior tympanic artery 鼓室下动脉
~ tympanica posterior［TA］, posterior tympanic artery 鼓室后动脉
~ tympanica superior［TA］, superior tympanic artery 鼓室上动脉
~ umbilicalis［TA］, umbilical artery 脐动脉
~ urethralis［TA］, urethral artery 尿道动脉
~ uterina［TA］, uterine artery 子宫动脉
~ vaginalis［TA］, vaginal artery 阴道动脉
~ vertebralis［TA］, vertebral artery 椎动脉
~ vesicalis inferior［TA］, inferior vesical artery 膀胱下动脉
~e vesicales superiores［TA］, superior vesical arteries 膀胱上动脉
~ zygomaticoorbitalis［TA］, zygomaticoorbital artery 颧眶动脉

二 肌名对照表

musculus

~ abductor digiti minimi manus［TA］, abductor muscle of little finger 小指展肌

~ abductor digiti minimi pedis [TA], abductor muscle of little toe 小趾展肌
~ abductor hallucis [TA], abductor muscle of great toe 踇展肌
~ abductor pollicis brevis [TA], short abductor muscle of thumb 拇短展肌
~ abductor pollicis longus [TA], long abductor muscle of thumb 拇长展肌
~ adductor brevis [TA], short adductor muscle 短收肌
~ adductor hallucis [TA], adductor muscle of great toe 踇收肌
~ adductor longus [TA], long adductor muscle 长收肌
~ adductor magnus [TA], great adductor muscle 大收肌
~ adductor pollicis [TA], adductor muscle of thumb 拇收肌
~ anconeus [TA], anconeus muscle 肘肌
~ antitragicus [TA], antitragus muscle 对耳屏肌
~ arrector pili [TA], arrector muscle of hair 立毛肌
~ articularis cubiti [TA], articular muscle of elbow 肘关节肌
~ articularis genus [TA], articular muscle of knee 膝关节肌
~ aryepiglotticus [TA], aryepiglottic muscle 杓会厌肌
~ arytenoideus obliquus [TA], oblique arytenoid muscle 杓斜肌
~ arytenoideus transversus [TA], transverse arytenoid muscle 杓横肌
~ auricularis anterior [TA], anterior auricular muscle 耳前肌
~ auricularis posterior [TA], posterior auricular muscle 耳后肌
~ auricularis superior [TA], superior auricular muscle 耳上肌
~ biceps brachii [TA], biceps muscle of arm 肱二头肌
~ biceps femoris [TA], biceps muscle of thigh 股二头肌
~ brachialis [TA], brachial muscle 肱肌
~ brachioradialis [TA], brachioradial muscle 肱桡肌
~ bronchoesophageus [TA], bronchoesophageal muscle 支气管食管肌
~ buccinator [TA], buccinator muscle 颊肌
~ bulbospongiosus [TA], ~ bulbocavernosus, bulbocavernous muscle 球海绵体肌
~ ceratocricoideus [TA], ceratocricoid muscle 角环肌
~ chondroglossus [TA], chondroglossus muscle 小角舌肌
~ ciliaris [TA], ciliary muscle 睫状肌
~ coccygeus [TA], coccygeus muscle 尾骨肌
~ constrictor pharyngis inferior [TA], inferior constrictor muscle of pharynx 咽下缩肌
~ constrictor pharyngis medius [TA], middle constrictor muscle of pharynx 咽中缩肌
~ constrictor pharyngis superior [TA], superior constrictor muscle of pharynx 咽上缩肌
~ coracobrachialis [TA], coracobrachial muscle 喙肱肌
~ corrugator supercilii [TA], superciliary corrugator muscle 皱眉肌
~ cremaster [TA], cremaster muscle 提睾肌
~ cricoarytenoideus lateralis [TA], lateral cricoarytenoid muscle 环杓侧肌
~ cricoarytenoideus posterior [TA], posterior cricoarytenoid muscle 环杓后肌
~ cricothyroideus [TA], cricothyroid muscle 环甲肌
~ deltoideus [TA], deltoid muscle 三角肌
~ depressor anguli oris [TA], depressor muscle of angle of mouth 降口角肌
~ depressor labii inferioris [TA], depressor muscle of lower lip 降下唇肌
~ depressor septi nasi [TA], depressor muscle of nasal septum 降鼻中隔肌
~ depressor supercilii [TA], super ciliary depressor muscle 降眉肌
~ digastricus [TA], digastric muscle 二腹肌
~ dilator pupillae [TA], dilator papillae muscle 瞳孔开大肌
~ epicranius [TA], epicranial muscle 颅顶肌
~ erector spinae [TA], erector muscle of spine 竖脊肌
~ extensor carpi radialis brevis [TA], short radial extensor muscle of wrist 桡侧腕短伸肌
~ extensor carpi radialis longus [TA], long radial extensor muscle of wrist 桡侧腕长伸肌
~ extensor carpi ulnaris [TA], ulnar extensor muscle of wrist 尺侧腕伸肌
~ extensor digiti minimi [TA], extensor muscle of little finger 小指伸肌
~ extensor digitorum [TA], extensor muscle of fingers 指伸肌
~ extensor digitorum brevis [TA], short extensor muscle of toes 趾短伸肌
~ extensor digitorum longus [TA], long extensor muscle of toes 趾长伸肌
~ extensor hallucis brevis [TA], short extensor muscle of great toe 踇短伸肌
~ extensor hallucis longus [TA], long extensor muscle of great toe 踇长伸肌

~ extensor indicis [TA], extensor muscle of index finger 示指伸肌
~ extensor pollicis brevis [TA], short extensor muscle of thumb 拇短伸肌
~ extensor pollicis longus [TA], long extensor muscle of thumb 拇长伸肌
~ flexor carpi radialis [TA], radial flexor muscle of wrist 桡侧腕屈肌
~ flexor carpi ulnaris [TA], ulnar flexor muscle of wrist 尺侧腕屈肌
~ flexor digiti minimi brevis manus [TA], short flexor muscle of little finger 小指短屈肌
~ flexor digiti minimi brevis pedis [TA], short flexor muscle of little toe 小趾短屈肌
~ flexor digitorum brevis [TA], short flexor muscle of toes 趾短屈肌
~ flexor digitorum longus [TA], long flexor muscle of toes 趾长屈肌
~ flexor digitorum profundus [TA], deep flexor muscle of fingers 指深屈肌
~ flexor digitorum superficialis [TA], superficial flexor muscle of fingers 指浅屈肌
~ flexor hallucis brevis [TA], short flexor muscle of great toe 跗短屈肌
~ flexor hallucis longus [TA], long flexor muscle of great toe 跗长屈肌
~ flexor pollicis brevis [TA], short flexor muscle of thumb 拇短屈肌
~ flexor pollicis longus [TA], long flexor muscle of thumb 拇长屈肌
~ gastrocnemius [TA], gastrocnemius muscle 腓肠肌
~ gemellus inferior [TA], inferior gemellus muscle 下孖肌
~ gemellus superior [TA], superior gemellus muscle 上孖肌
~ genioglossus [TA], genioglossus muscle 颏舌肌
~ geniohyoideus [TA], geniohyoid muscle 颏舌骨肌
~ gluteus maximus [TA], greatest gluteal muscle 臀大肌
~ gluteus medius [TA], middle gluteal muscle 臀中肌
~ gluteus minimus [TA], least gluteal muscle 臀小肌
~ gracilis [TA], gracilis muscle 股薄肌
~ helicis major [TA], helicis major muscle 耳轮大肌
~ helicis minor [TA], helicis minor muscle 耳轮小肌
~ hyoglossus [TA], hyoglossal muscle 舌骨舌肌
~ iliacus [TA],iliac muscle 髂肌
~ iliococcygeus [TA], iliococcygeal muscle 髂尾肌
~ iliocostalis [TA], iliocostal muscle 髂肋肌
~ iliocostalis cervicis [TA], iliocostal muscle of neck 颈髂肋肌
~ iliocostalis lumborum [TA], iliocostal muscle of loins 腰髂肋肌
~ iliocostalis thoracis, iliocostal muscle of thorax 胸髂肋肌
~ iliopsoas [TA], iliopsoas muscle 髂腰肌
musculi incisivi labii inferioris, incisive muscles of inferior lip 下唇切牙肌
musculi incisivi labii superioris, incisive muscles of superior lip 上唇切牙肌
~ infraspinatus [TA], infraspinous muscle 冈下肌
musculi intercostales externi [TA], external intercostal muscles 肋间外肌
musculi intercostales interni [TA], internal intercostal muscles 肋间内肌
musculi interossei dorsales manus [TA], dorsal interosseous muscles of hand 手骨间背侧肌
musculi interossei dorsales pedis [TA], dorsal interosseous muscles of foot 足骨间背侧肌
musculi interossei palmares [TA], palmar interosseous muscles 骨间掌侧肌
musculi interossei plantares [TA], plantar interosseous muscles 骨间足底肌
musculi interspinales [TA], interspinal muscles 棘间肌
musculi intertransversarii [TA], intertransverse muscles 横突间肌
~ ischiocavernosus [TA], ichiocavernosus muscle 坐骨海绵体肌
~ latissimus dorsi [TA], latissimus dorsi muscle 背阔肌
~ levator anguli oris [TA], levator muscle of angle of mouth 提口角肌
~ levator ani [TA], levator ani muscle 肛提肌
musculi levatores costarum [TA], levator muscles of ribs 肋提肌
~ levator glandulae thyroideae [TA], levator muscle of thyroid gland 甲状腺提肌
~ levator labii superioris [TA], levator muscle of upper lip 提上唇肌
~ levator labii superioris alaeque nasi [TA], levator muscle of upper lip and ala of nose 提上唇鼻翼肌
~ levator palpebrae superioris [TA], levator muscle of upper eyelid 上睑提肌
~ levator prostatae [TA], levator muscle of prostate 前列腺提肌
~ levator scapulae [TA], levator muscle of scapula 肩胛提肌
~ levator veli palatini [TA], levator muscle of palatine velum 腭帆提肌

~ longissimus capitis [TA], longissimus muscle of head 头最长肌
~ longissimus cervicis [TA], longissimus muscle of neck 颈最长肌
~ longissimus thoracis [TA], longissimus muscle of thorax 胸最长肌
~ longitudinalis inferior linguae [TA], inferior longitudinal muscle of tongue 舌下纵肌
~ longitudinalis superior linguae [TA], superior longitudinal muscle of tongue 舌上纵肌
~ longus capitis [TA], long muscle of head 头长肌
~ longus colli [TA], long muscle of neck 颈长肌
musculi lumbricales manus [TA], lumbrical muscles of hand 手蚓状肌
musculi lumbricales pedis [TA], lumbrical muscles of foot 足蚓状肌
~ masseter [TA], masseter muscle 咬肌
~ mentalis [TA], chin muscle 颏肌
musculi multifidi, multifidus muscles 多裂肌
~ mylohyoideus [TA], mylohyoid muscle 下颌舌骨肌
~ nasalis [TA], nasal muscle 鼻肌
~ obliquus auriculae [TA], oblique muscle of auricle 耳郭斜肌
~ obliquus capitis inferior [TA], inferior oblique muscle of head 头下斜肌
~ obliquus capitis superior [TA], superior oblique muscle of head 头上斜肌
~ obliquus externus abdominis [TA], external oblique muscle of abdomen 腹外斜肌
~ obliquus inferior bulbi [TA], inferior oblique muscle of eyeball 眼下斜肌
~ obliquus internus abdominis [TA], internal oblique muscle of abdomen 腹内斜肌
~ obliquus superior bulbi [TA], superior oblique muscle of eyeball 眼上斜肌
~ obturatorius externus [TA], external obturator muscle 闭孔外肌
~ obturatorius internus [TA], internal oburator muscle 闭孔内肌
~ occipitofrontalis [TA], occipitofrontal muscle 枕额肌
~ omohyoideus [TA], omohyoid muscle 肩胛舌骨肌
~ opponens digiti minimi [TA], opposing muscle of little finger 小指对掌肌
~ opponens pollicis [TA], opposing muscle of thumb 拇对掌肌
~ orbicularis oculi [TA], orbicular muscle of eye 眼轮匝肌
~ orbicularis oris [TA], orbicular muscle of mouth 口轮匝肌
~ orbitalis [TA], orbital muscle 眶肌
~ palatoglossus [TA], palatoglossus muscle 腭舌肌
~ palatopharyngeus [TA], palatopharyngeal muscle 腭咽肌
~ palmaris brevis [TA], short palmar muscle 掌短肌
~ palmaris longus [TA], long palmar muscle 掌长肌
musculi papillares [TA], papillary muscles 乳头肌
musculi pectinati, pectinate muscles 梳状肌
~ pectineus [TA], pectineal muscle 耻骨肌
~ pectoralis major [TA], greater pectoral muscle 胸大肌
~ pectoralis minor [TA], smaller pectoral muscle 胸小肌
~ peroneus brevis [TA], short peroneal muscle 腓骨短肌
~ peroneus longus [TA], long peroneal muscle 腓骨长肌
~ peroneus tertius [TA], third peroneal muscle 第三腓骨肌
~ piriformis [TA], periform muscle 梨状肌
~ plantaris [TA], plantar muscle 跖肌
~ pleuroesophageus [TA], pleuroesophageal muscle 胸膜食管肌
~ popliteus [TA], popliteal muscle 腘肌
~ procerus [TA], procerus muscle 降眉间肌
~ pronator quadratus [TA], quadrate pronator muscle 旋前方肌
~ pronator teres [TA], round pronator muscle 旋前圆肌
~ psoas major [TA], greater psoas muscle 腰大肌
~ psoas minor [TA], smaller psoas muscle 腰小肌
~ pterygoideus lateralis [TA], lateral pterygoid muscle 翼外肌
~ pterygoideus medialis [TA], medial pterygoid muscle 翼内肌
~ pubococcygeus [TA], pubococcygeal muscle 耻尾肌
~ puboprostaticus [TA], puboprostatic muscle 耻骨前列腺肌
~ puborectalis [TA], puborectal muscle 耻骨直肠肌
~ pubovaginalis [TA], pubovaginal muscle 耻骨阴道肌
~ pubovesicalis [TA], pubovesical muscle 耻骨膀胱肌
~ pyramidalis [TA], pyramidal muscle 锥状肌
~ pyramidalis auriculae [TA], pyramidal muscle of auricle 耳郭锥状肌
~ quadratus femoris [TA], quadrate muscle of thigh 股方肌

~ quadratus lumborum [TA], quadrate muscle of loins 腰方肌
~ quadratus plantae [TA], quadrate muscle of sole 足底方肌
~ quadriceps femoris [TA], quadriceps muscle of thigh 股四头肌
~ rectococcygeus [TA], rectococcygeal muscle 直肠尾骨肌
~ rectourethralis [TA], rectourethral muscle 直肠尿道肌
~ rectouterinus [TA], rectouterine muscle 直肠子宫肌
~ rectovesicalis [TA], rectovesical muscle 直肠膀胱肌
~ rectus abdominis [TA], rectus muscle of abdomen 腹直肌
~ rectus capitis anterior [TA], anterior rectus muscle of head 头前直肌
~ rectus capitis lateralis [TA], lateral rectus muscle of head 头外侧直肌
~ rectus capitis posterior major [TA], greater posterior rectus muscle of head 头后大直肌
~ rectus capitis posterior minor [TA], smaller posterior rectus muscle of head 头后小直肌
~ rectus femoris [TA], rectus muscle of thigh 股直肌
~ rectus inferior bulbi [TA], inferior rectus muscle of eyeball 眼下直肌
~ rectus lateralis bulbi [TA], lateral rectus muscle of eyeball 眼外直肌
~ rectus medialis bulbi [TA], medial rectus muscle of eyeball 眼内直肌
~ rectus superior bulbi [TA], superior rectus muscle of eyeball 眼上直肌
~ rhomboideus major [TA], greater rhomboid muscle 大菱形肌
~ rhomboideus minor [TA], smaller rhomboid muscle 小菱形肌
~ risorius [TA], risorius muscle 笑肌
musculi rotatores [TA], rotator muscles 回旋肌
~ sacrococcygeus dorsalis, dorsal sacrococcygeal muscle 骶尾后肌
~ sacrococcygeus ventralis, ventral sacrococcygeal muscle 骶尾前肌
~ salpingopharyngeus [TA], salpingopharyngeal muscle 咽鼓管咽肌
~ sartorius [TA], sartorius muscle 缝匠肌
~ scalenus anterior [TA], anterior scalene muscle 前斜角肌
~ scalenus medius [TA], middle scalene muscle 中斜角肌
~ scalenus minimus [TA], smallest scalene muscle 小斜角肌
~ scalenus posterior [TA], posterior scalene muscle 后斜角肌
~ semimembranosus [TA], semimembranous muscle 半膜肌
~ semispinalis capitis [TA], semispinal muscle of head 头半棘肌
~ semispinalis cervicis [TA], semispinal muscle of neck 颈半棘肌
~ semispinalis thoracis [TA], semispinal muscle of thorax 胸半棘肌
~ semitendinosus [TA], semitendinous muscle 半腱肌
~ serratus anterior [TA], anterior serratus muscle 前锯肌
~ serratus posterior inferior [TA], inferior posterior serratus muscle 下后锯肌
~ serratus posterior superior [TA], superior posterior serratus muscle 上后锯肌
~ soleus [TA], soleus muscle 比目鱼肌
~ sphincter ampullae hepatopancreaticae [TA], sphincter muscle of hepatopancreatic ampulla 肝胰壶腹括约肌
~ sphincter ani externus [TA], external sphincter muscle of anus 肛门外括约肌
~ sphincter ani internus [TA], internal sphincter muscle of anus 肛门内括约肌
~ sphincter ductus choledochi [TA], sphincter muscle of bile duct 胆总管括约肌
~ sphincter pupillae [TA], sphincter muscle of pupil 瞳孔括约肌
~ sphincter pylori [TA], sphincter muscle of pylorus 幽门括约肌
~ sphincter urethrae [TA], sphincter muscle of urethra 尿道括约肌
~ sphincter vesicae urinariae, sphincter muscle of urinary bladder 膀胱括约肌
~ spinalis capitis [TA], spinal muscle of head 头棘肌
~ spinalis cervicis [TA], spinal muscle of neck 颈棘肌
~ spinalis thoracis [TA], spinal muscle of thorax 胸棘肌
~ splenius capitis [TA], splenius muscle of head 头夹肌
~ splenius cervicis [TA], splenius muscle of neck 颈夹肌
~ stapedius [TA], stapedius muscle 镫骨肌
~ sternalis [TA], sternal muscle 胸骨肌
~ sternocleidomastoideus [TA], sternocleidomastoid muscle 胸锁乳突肌
~ sternohyoideus [TA], sternohyoid muscle 胸骨舌骨肌
~ sternothyroideus [TA], sternothyroid muscle 胸

骨甲状肌
~ styloglossus［TA］, styloglossus muscle 茎突舌肌
~ stylohyoideus［TA］, stylohyhoid muscle 茎突舌骨肌
~ stylopharyngeus［TA］, stylopharyngeal muscle 茎突咽肌
~ subclavius［TA］, subclavius muscle 锁骨下肌
musculi subcostales［TA］, subcostal muscles 肋下肌
~ subscapularis［TA］, subscapular muscle 肩胛下肌
~ supinator［TA］, supinator muscle 旋后肌
~ supraspinatus［TA］, supraspinous muscle 冈上肌
~ suspensorius duodeni［TA］, suspensory muscle of duodenum 十二指肠悬肌
~ tarsalis inferior［TA］, inferior tarsal muscle 下睑板肌
~ tarsalis superior［TA］, superior tarsal muscle 上睑板肌
~ temporalis［TA］, temporal muscle 颞肌
~ temporoparietalis［TA］, temporoparietal muscle 颞顶肌
~ tensor fasciae latae［TA］, tensor muscle of fascia lata 阔筋膜张肌
~ tensor tympani［TA］, tensor muscle of tympanum 鼓膜张肌
~ tensor veli palatini［TA］, tensor muscle of palatine velum 腭帆张肌
~ teres major［TA］, teres major muscle 大圆肌
~ teres minor［TA］, teres minor muscle 小圆肌
~ thyroarytenoideus［TA］, thyroarytenoid muscle 甲杓肌
~ thyroepiglotticus［TA］, thyroepiglottic muscle 甲状会厌肌
~ thyrohyoideus［TA］, thyrohyoid muscle 甲状舌骨肌
~ tibialis anterior［TA］, anterior tibial muscle 胫骨前肌
~ tibialis posterior［TA］, posterior tibial muscle 胫骨后肌
~ trachealis［TA］, tracheal muscle 气管肌
~ tragicus［TA］, muscle of tragus 耳屏肌
~ transversospinalis［TA］, transversospinal muscle 横突棘肌
~ transversus abdominis［TA］, transverse muscle of abdomen 腹横肌
~ transversus auriculae［TA］, transverse muscle of auricle 耳郭横肌
~ transversus linguae［TA］, transverse muscle of tongue 舌横肌
~ transversus menti［TA］, transverse muscle of chin 颏横肌
~ transversus nuchae［TA］, transverse muscle of neck 项横肌
~ transversus perinei profundus［TA］, deep transverse muscle of perineum 会阴深横肌
~ transversus perinei superficialis［TA］, superficial transverse muscle of perineum 会阴浅横肌
~ transversus thoracis［TA］, transverse muscle of thorax 胸横肌
~ trapezius［TA］, trapezius muscle 斜方肌
~ triceps brachii［TA］, triceps muscle of arm 肱三头肌
~ triceps surae［TA］, triceps muscle of calf 小腿三头肌
~ uvulae［TA］, muscle of uvula 腭垂肌
~ vastus intermedius［TA］, intermediate vastus muscle 股中间肌
~ vastus lateralis［TA］, lateral vastus muscle 股外侧肌
~ vastus medialis［TA］, medial vastus muscle 股内侧肌
~ verticalis linguae［TA］, vertical muscle of tongue 舌垂直肌
~ vocalis［TA］, vocal muscle 声带肌
~ zygomaticus major［TA］, greater zygomatic muscle 颧大肌
~ zygomaticus minor［TA］, smaller zygomatic muscle 颧小肌

三　神经名对照表

nervus
~ abducens［TA］, abducent nerve 展神经
~ accessorius［TA］, accessory nerve 副神经
~ alveolaris inferior［TA］, inferior alveolar nerve 下牙槽神经
nervi alveolares superiores［TA］, superior alveolar nerves 上牙槽神经
~ ampullaris anterior［TA］, anterior ampullary nerve 前壶腹神经
~ ampullaris lateralis［TA］, lateral ampullary nerve 外壶腹神经
~ ampullaris posterior［TA］, posterior ampullary nerve 后壶腹神经
nervi anococcygei［TA］, anococcygeal nerves 肛尾神经
nervi auriculares anteriores［TA］, anterior auricular nerves 耳前神经
~ auricularis magnus［TA］, great auricular nerve 耳大神经
~ auricularis posterior［TA］, posterior auricular nerve 耳后神经
~ auriculotemporalis［TA］, auriculotemporal nerve 耳颞神经

~ axillaris [TA], axillary nerve 腋神经
~ buccalis [TA], buccal nerve 颊神经
~ canalis pterygoidei [TA], nerve of pterygoid canal 翼管神经
~ cardiacus cervicalis inferior [TA], inferior cervical cardiac nerve 颈下心神经
~ cardiacus cervicalis medius [TA], middle cervical cardiac nerve 颈中心神经
~ cardiacus cervicalis superior [TA], superior cervical cardiac nerve 颈上心神经
nervi cardiaci thoracici, thoracic cardiac nerves 胸心神经
nervi caroticotympanici [TA], caroticotympanic nerves 颈鼓神经
nervi carotici externi [TA], external carotid nerves 颈外动脉神经
~ caroticus internus [TA], internal carotid nerve 颈内动脉神经
nervi cavernosi clitoridis [TA], cavernous nerves of clitoris 阴蒂海绵体神经
nervi cavernosi penis [TA], cavernous nerves of penis 阴茎海绵体神经
nervi cervicales [TA], cervical nerves 颈神经
nervi ciliares breves [TA], short ciliary nerves 睫状短神经
nervi ciliares longi [TA], long ciliary nerves 睫状长神经
nervi clunium inferiores [TA], inferior clunial nerves 臀下皮神经
nervi clunium medii [TA], middle clunial nerves 臀中皮神经
nervi clunium superiores [TA], superior clunial nerves 臀上皮神经
~ coccygeus [TA], coccygeal nerve 尾神经
nervi craniales [TA], cranial nerves 脑神经
~ cutaneus antebrachii lateralis [TA], lateral cutaneous nerve of forearm 前臂外侧皮神经
~ cutaneus antebrachii medialis [TA], medial cutaneous nerve of forearm 前臂内侧皮神经
~ cutaneus antebrachii posterior [TA], posterior cutaneous nerve of forearm 前臂后皮神经
~ cutaneus brachii lateralis inferior [TA], inferior lateral cutaneous nerve of arm 臂外侧下皮神经
~ cutaneus brachii lateralis superior [TA], superior lateral cutaneous nerve of arm 臂外侧上皮神经
~ cutaneus brachii medialis [TA], medial cutaneous nerve of arm 臂内侧皮神经
~ cutaneus brachii posterior [TA], posterior cutaneous nerve of arm 臂后皮神经
~ cutaneus dorsalis intermedius [TA], intermediate dorsal cutaneous nerve 背中间皮神经
~ cutaneus dorsalis lateralis [TA], lateral dorsal cutaneous nerve 背外侧皮神经
~ cutaneus dorsalis medialis [TA], medial dorsal cutaneous nerve 背内侧皮神经
~ cutaneus femoris lateralis [TA], lateral cutaneous nerve of thigh 股外侧皮神经
~ cutaneus femoris posterior [TA], posterior cutaneous nerve of thigh 股后皮神经
~ cutaneus surae lateralis [TA], lateral sural cutaneous nerve 腓肠外侧皮神经
~ cutaneus surae medialis [TA], medial sural cutaneous nerve 腓肠内侧皮神经
nervi digitales dorsales hallucis lateralis et digiti secundi medialis [TA], dorsal digital nerves of lateral surface of great toe and of medial surface of second toe 踇背外侧及第二趾背内侧神经
nervi digitales dorsales nervi radialis [TA], dorsal digital nerves of radial nerve 桡神经的指背神经
nervi digitales dorsales nervi ulnaris [TA], dorsal digital nerves of ulnar nerve 尺神经的指背神经
nervi digitales dorsales pedis, dorsal digital nerves of foot 趾背神经
nervi digitales palmares communes nervi mediani [TA], common palmar digital nerves of median nerve 正中神经的指掌侧总神经
nervi digitales palmares communes nervi ulnaris [TA], common palmar digital nerves of ulnar nerve 尺神经的指掌侧总神经
nervi digitales palmares proprii nervi mediani [TA], proper palmar digital nerves of median nerve 正中神经的指掌侧固有神经
nervi digitales palmares proprii nervi ulnaris [TA], proper palmar digital nerves of ulnar nerve 尺神经的指掌侧固有神经
nervi digitales plantares communes nervi plantaris lateralis [TA], common plantar digital nerves of lateral plantar nerve 足底外侧神经的趾足底总神经
nervi digitales plantares communes nervi plantaris medialis [TA], common plantar digital nerves of medial plantar nerve 足底内侧神经的趾足底总神经
nervi digitales plantares proprii nervi plantaris lateralis [TA], proper plantar digital nerves of lateral plantar nerve 足底外侧神经的趾足底固有神经
nervi digitales plantares proprii nervi plantaris medialis [TA], proper plantar digital nerves of medial plantar nerve 足底内侧神经的趾足底固有神经
~ dorsalis clitoridis [TA], dorsal nerve of clitoris 阴蒂背神经
~ dorsalis penis [TA], dorsal nerve of penis 阴茎背神经
~ dorsal scapulae [TA], dorsal scapular nerve 肩胛背神经
~ ethmoidalis anterior [TA], anterior ethmoidal

nerve 筛前神经
~ ethmoidalis posterior [TA], posterior ethmoidal nerve 筛后神经
~ facialis [TA], facial nerve 面神经
~ femoralis [TA], femoral nerve 股神经
~ frontalis [TA], frontal nerve 额神经
~ genitofemoralis [TA], genitofemoral nerve 生殖股神经
~ glossopharyngeus [TA], glossopharyngeal nerve 舌咽神经
~ gluteus inferior [TA], inferior gluteal nerve 臀下神经
~ gluteus superior [TA], superior gluteal nerve 臀上神经
~ hypogastricus [TA], hypogastric nerve 腹下神经
~ hypoglossus [TA], hypoglossal nerve 舌下神经
~ iliohypogastricus [TA], iliohypogastric nerve 髂腹下神经
~ ilioinguinalis [TA], ilioinguinal nerve 髂腹股沟神经
~ infraorbitalis [TA], infraorbital nerve 眶下神经
~ infratrochlearis [TA], infratrochlear nerve 滑车下神经
nervi intercostobrachiales [TA], intercostobrachial nerves 肋间臂神经
~ intermedius [TA], intermediate nerve 中间神经
~ interosseus antebrachii anterior [TA], anterior interosseous nerve of forearm 前臂骨间前神经
~ interosseus antebrachii posterior [TA], posterior interosseous nerve of forearm 前臂骨间后神经
~ interosseus cruris [TA], interosseous nerve of leg 小腿骨间神经
~ ischiadicus [TA], sciatic nerve 坐骨神经
~ jugularis [TA], jugular nerve 颈静脉神经
nervi labiales anteriores [TA], anterior labial nerves 阴唇前神经
nervi labiales posteriores [TA], posterior labial nerves 阴唇后神经
~ lacrimalis [TA], lacrimal nerve 泪腺神经
~ laryngeus inferior, inferior laryngeal nerve 喉下神经
~ laryngeus recurrens [TA], recurrent laryngeal nerve 喉返神经
~ laryngeus superior [TA], superior laryngeal nerve 喉上神经
~ lingualis [TA], lingual nerve 舌神经
nervi lumbales [TA], lumbar nerves 腰神经
~ mandibularis [TA], mandibular nerve 下颌神经
~ massetericus [TA], masseteric nerve 咬肌神经
~ maxillaris [TA], maxillary nerve 上颌神经
~ meatus acustici externi [TA], nerve of external acoustic meatus 外耳道神经
~ medianus [TA], median nerve 正中神经
~ mentalis [TA], mental nerve 颏神经
~ musculocutaneus [TA], musculocutaneous nerve 肌皮神经
~ mylohyoideus [TA], mylohyoid nerve 下颌舌骨肌神经
~ nasociliaris [TA], nasociliary nerve 鼻睫神经
~ nasopalatinus [TA], nasopalatine nerve 鼻腭神经
~ obturatorius [TA], obturator nerve 闭孔神经
~ occipitalis major [TA], greater occipital nerve 枕大神经
~ occipitalis minor [TA], lesser occipital nerve 枕小神经
~ occipitalis tertius [TA], third occipital nerve 第三枕神经
~ oculomotorius [TA], oculomotor nerve 动眼神经
nervi olfactorii, olfactory nerves 嗅神经
~ ophthalmicus [TA], ophthalmic nerve 眼神经
~ opticus [TA], optic nerve 视神经
~ palatinus major [TA], greater palatine nerve 腭大神经
nervi palatini minores [TA], lesser palatine nerves 腭小神经
nervi perineales [TA], perineal nerves 会阴神经
~ peroneus communis, common peroneal nerve 腓总神经
~ peroneus profundus, deep peroneal nerve 腓深神经
~ peroneus superficialis, superficial peroneal nerve 腓浅神经
~ petrosus major [TA], greater petrosal nerve 岩大神经
~ petrosus minor [TA], lesser petrosal nerve 岩小神经
~ petrosus profundus [TA], deep petrosal nerve 岩深神经
~ phrenicus [TA], phrenic nerve 膈神经
nervi phrenici accessorii [TA], accessory phrenic nerves 副膈神经
~ plantaris lateralis [TA], lateral plantar nerve 足底外侧神经
~ plantaris medialis [TA], medial plantar nerve 足底内侧神经
~ pterygoideus lateralis [TA], lateral pterygoid nerve 翼外肌神经
~ pterygoideus medialis [TA], medial pterygoid nerve 翼内肌神经
nervi pterygopalatini, pterygopalatine nerves 翼腭神经
~ pudendus [TA], pudendal nerve 阴部神经
~ radialis [TA], radial nerve 桡神经
nervi rectales inferiores, inferior rectal nerves 直肠

下神经
~ saccularis [TA], saccular nerve 球囊神经
nervi sacrales [TA], sacral nerves 骶神经
~ saphenus [TA], saphenous nerve 隐神经
nervi scrotales anteriores [TA], anterior scrotal nerves 阴囊前神经
nervi scrotales posteriores [TA], posterior scrotal nerves 阴囊后神经
nervi spinales [TA], spinal nerves 脊神经
~ splanchnicus imus [TA], lowest splanchnic nerve 内脏最下神经
nervi splanchnici lumbales [TA], lumbar splanchnic nerves 腰内脏神经
~ splanchnicus major [TA], greater splanchnic nerve 内脏大神经
~ splanchnicus minor [TA], lesser splanchnic nerve 内脏小神经
nervi splanchnici pelvici, pelvic splanchnic nerves 盆内脏神经
nervi splanchnici sacrales [TA], sacral splanchnic nerves 骶内脏神经
~ stapedius [TA], stapedius nerve 镫骨肌神经
~ subclavius [TA], subclavian nerve 锁骨下肌神经
~ subcostalis [TA], subcostal nerve 肋下神经
~ sublingualis [TA], sublingual nerve 舌底神经
~ suboccipitalis [TA], suboccipital nerve 枕下神经
~ subscapularis [TA], subscapular nerve 肩胛下神经
nervi supraclaviculares intermedii [TA], intermediate supraclavicular nerves 锁骨上中间神经
nervi supraclaviculares laterales [TA], lateral supraclavicular nerves 锁骨上外侧神经
nervi supraclaviculares mediales [TA], medial supraclavicular nerves 锁骨上内侧神经
~ supraorbitalis [TA], supraorbital nerve 眶上神经
~ suprascapularis [TA], suprascapular nerve 肩胛上神经
~ supratrochlearis [TA], supratrochlear nerve 滑车上神经
~ suralis [TA], sural nerve 腓肠神经
nervi temporales profundi [TA], deep temporal nerves 颞深神经
~ tensoris tympani [TA], nerve of tensor tympani 鼓膜张肌神经
~ tensoris veli palatini, nerve of tensor veli palatini 腭帆张肌神经
nervi thoracici [TA], thoracic nerves 胸神经
~ thoracicus longus [TA], long thoracic nerve 胸长神经
~ thoracodorsalis [TA], thoracodorsal nerve 胸背神经
~ tibialis [TA], tibial nerve 胫神经
~ transversus colli [TA], transverse cervical nerve 颈横神经
~ trigeminus [TA], trigeminal nerve 三叉神经
~ trochlearis [TA], trochlear nerve 滑车神经
~ tympanicus [TA], tympanic nerve 鼓室神经
~ ulnaris [TA], ulnar nerve 尺神经
~ utricularis [TA], utricular nerve 椭圆囊神经
~ utriculoampullaris [TA], utriculoampullary nerve 椭圆囊壶腹神经
nervi vaginales [TA], vaginal nerves 阴道神经
~ vagus [TA], vagus nerve 迷走神经
~ vertebralis [TA], vertebral nerve 椎动脉神经
~ vestibulocochlearis [TA], vestibulocochlear nerve 前庭蜗神经
~ zygomaticus [TA], zygomatic nerve 颧神经

四 骨名对照表

os
~ capitatum [TA], capitate bone 头状骨
~sa carpi [TA], carpal bones 腕骨
~ coccygis [TA], coccyx 尾骨
~ coxae [TA], hip bone 髋骨
~ cuboideum [TA], cuboid bone 骰骨
~ cuneiforme intermedium [TA], intermediate cuneiform bone 中间楔骨
~ cuneiforme laterale [TA], lateral cuneiform bone 外侧楔骨
~ cuneiforme mediale [TA], medial cuneiform bone 内侧楔骨
~ ethmoidale [TA], ethmoid bone 筛骨
~ frontale [TA], frontal bone 额骨
~ hamatum [TA], hamate bone 钩骨
~ hyoideum [TA], hyoid bone 舌骨
~ ilium [TA], ilium 髂骨
~ ischii [TA], ischium 坐骨
~ lacrimale [TA], lacrimal bone 泪骨
~ lunatum [TA], lunate bone 月骨
~sa metacarpalia, metacarpal bones 掌骨
~sa metatarsalis, metatarsal bones 跖骨
~ nasale [TA], nasal bone 鼻骨
~ naviculare [TA], navicular bone 足舟骨
~ occipitale [TA], occipital bone 枕骨
~ palatinum [TA], palatine bone 腭骨
~ parietale [TA], parietal bone 顶骨
~ pisiforme [TA], pisiform bone 豌豆骨

~ pubis [TA], pubic bone 耻骨
~ sacrum [TA], sacrum 骶骨
~ scaphoideum [TA], scaphoid bone 手舟骨
~sa sesamoidea, sesamoid bones 籽骨
~ sphenoidale [TA], sphenoid bone 蝶骨
~sa tarsi [TA], tarsal bones 跗骨
~ temporale [TA], temporal bone 颞骨
~ trapezium [TA], trapezium bone 大多角骨
~ trapexoideum [TA], trapezoid bone 小多角骨
~ triquetrum [TA], triquetral bone 三角骨
~ zygomaticum [TA], zygomatic bone 颧骨

五 静脉名对照表

vena

~ anastomotica inferior [TA], inferior anastomotic vein 下吻合静脉
~ anastomotica superior [TA], superior anastomotic vein 上吻合静脉
~ angularis [TA], angular vein 内眥静脉
~ appendicularis [TA], appendicular vein 阑尾静脉
~ aqueductus vestibuli [TA], vein of aqueduct of vestibule 前庭水管静脉
~e auriculares anteriores [TA], anterior auricular veins 耳前静脉
~ auricularis posterior [TA], posterior auricular vein 耳后静脉
~ axillaris [TA], axillary vein 腋静脉
~ azygos [TA], azygos vein 奇静脉
~ basalis [TA], basal vein 基底静脉
~ basilica [TA], basilic vein 贵要静脉
~e basivertebrales [TA], basivertebral veins 椎体静脉
~e brachiales [TA], brachial veins 肱静脉
~ brachiocephalica [TA], brachiocephalic vein 头臂静脉
~e bronchiales [TA], bronchial veins 支气管静脉
~ bulbi penis [TA], vein of bulb of penis 尿道球静脉
~ bulbi vestibuli [TA], vein of bulb of vestibule 前庭球静脉
~ canaliculi cochleae, vein of cochlear canal 蜗小管静脉
~ canalis pterygoidei [TA], vein of pterygoid canal 翼管静脉
~ cava inferior [TA], inferior vena cava 下腔静脉
~ cava superior [TA], superior vena cava 上腔静脉
~e cavernosae penis [TA], cavernous veins of penis 阴茎海绵体静脉
~ centralis glandulae suprarenalis [TA], central vein of suprarenal gland 肾上腺中央静脉
~e centrales hepatis [TA], central veins of liver 肝中央静脉
~ centralis retinae [TA], central vein of retina 视网膜中央静脉
~ cephalica [TA], caphalic vein 头静脉
~ cephalica accessoria [TA], accessory cephalic vein 副头静脉
~e cerebelli inferiores, inferior cerebellar veins 小脑下静脉
~e cerebelli superiores, superior cerebellar veins 小脑上静脉
~ cerebri anterior, anterior cerebral vein 大脑前静脉
~e cerebri inferiores, inferior cerebral veins 大脑下静脉
~e cerebri internae, internal cerebral veins 大脑内静脉
~ cerebri magna, great cerebral vein 大脑大静脉
~ cerebri media profunda, deep middle cerebral vein 大脑中深静脉
~ cerebri media superficialis, superficial middle cerebral vein 大脑中浅静脉
~e cerebri superiores, superior cerebral veins 大脑上静脉
~ cervicalis profunda [TA], deep cervical vein 颈深静脉
~ choroidea, choroid vein 脉络丛静脉
~e ciliares [TA], ciliary veins 睫状静脉
~e circumflexae femoris laterales [TA], lateral circumflex femoral veins 旋股外侧静脉
~e circumflexae femoris mediales, medial circumflex femoral veins 旋股内侧静脉
~ circumflexa ilium profunda [TA], deep circumflex iliac vein 旋髂深静脉
~ circumflexa ilium superficialis, superficial circumflex iliac vein 旋髂浅静脉
~ colica dextra [TA], right colic vein 右结肠静脉
~ colica media [TA], middle colic vein 中结肠静脉
~ colica sinistra [TA], left colic vein 左结肠静脉
~ comitans nervi hypoglossi [TA], accompanying vein of hypoglossal nerve 舌下神经伴行静脉
~e conjunctivales [TA], conjunctival veins 结膜静脉
~e cordis anteriores, anterior cardiac vein 心前静脉
~ cordis magna, great cardiac vein 心大静脉
~ cordis media, middle cardiac vein 心中静脉

~e cordis minimae, smallest cardiac veins 心最小静脉
~ cutanea [TA], cutaneous vein 皮静脉
~ cystica [TA], cystic vein 胆囊静脉
~e digitales dorsales pedis [TA], dorsal digital veins of foot 趾背静脉
~e digitales palmares [TA], palmar digital veins 指掌侧静脉
~e digitales plantares [TA], plantar digital veins 趾足底静脉
~ diploica frontalis [TA], frontal diploic vein 额板障静脉
~ diploica occipitalis [TA], occipital diploic vein 枕板障静脉
~ diploica temporalis anterior [TA], anterior temporal diploic vein 颞前板障静脉
~ diploica temporalis posterior [TA], posterior temporal diploic vein 颞后板障静脉
~ dorsalis clitoridis profunda [TA], deep dorsal vein of clitoris 阴蒂背深静脉
~e dorsales clitoridis superficiales, superficial dorsal veins of clitoris 阴蒂背浅静脉
~e dorsales linguae [TA], dorsal lingual veins, dorsal veins of tongue 舌背静脉
~ dorsalis penis profunda [TA], deep dorsal vein of penis 阴茎背深静脉
~e dorsales penis superficiales [TA], superficial dorsal veins of penis 阴茎背浅静脉
~ emissaria condylaris [TA], condylar emissary vein 髁导静脉
~ emissaria mastoidea [TA], mastoid emissary vein 乳突导静脉
~ emissaria occipitalis [TA], occipital emissary vein 枕导静脉
~ emissaria parietalis [TA], parietal emissary vein 顶导静脉
~ epigastrica inferior [TA], inferior epigastric vein 腹壁下静脉
~ epigastrica superficialis [TA], superficial epigastric vein 腹壁浅静脉
~e epigastricae superiores [TA], superior epigastric veins 腹壁上静脉
~e episclerales [TA], episcleral veins 巩膜外静脉
~e esophageae, esophageal veins 食管静脉
~e ethmoidales [TA], ethmoidal veins 筛静脉
~ facialis [TA], facial vein 面静脉
~ faciei profunda, deep facial vein 面深静脉
~ femoralis [TA], femoral vein 股静脉
~e fibulares [TA], fibular veins 腓静脉
~e gastricae breves [TA], short gastric veins 胃短静脉
~ gastrica dextra [TA], right gastric vein 胃右静脉
~ gastrica sinistra [TA], left gastric vein 胃左静脉
~ gastroepiploica dextra, right gastroepiploic vein 胃网膜右静脉
~ gastroepiploica sinistra, left gastroepiploic vein 胃网膜左静脉
~e gluteae inferiores [TA], inferior gluteal veins 臀下静脉
~e gluteae superiores [TA], superior gluteal veins 臀上静脉
~ hemiazygos [TA], hemiazygos vein 半奇静脉
~ hemiazygos accessoria [TA], accessory hemiazygos vein 副半奇静脉
~e hepaticae [TA], hepatic veins 肝静脉
~ ileocolica [TA], ileocolic vein 回结肠静脉
~ iliaca communis [TA], common iliac vein 髂总静脉
~ iliaca externa [TA], external iliac vein 髂外静脉
~ iliaca interna [TA], internal iliac vein 髂内静脉
~ iliolumbalis [TA], iliolumbar vein 髂腰静脉
~e intercapitales [TA], intercapital veins 掌骨头间静脉,跖骨头间静脉
~e intercostales anteriores [TA], anterior intercostal veins 肋间前静脉
~e intercostales posteriores [TA], posterior intercostal veins 肋间后静脉
~ intercostalis superior dextra [TA], right superior intercostal vein 右肋间上静脉
~ intercostalis superior sinistra [TA], left superior intercostal vein 左肋间上静脉
~ intercostalis suprema [TA], highest intercostal vein 肋间最上静脉
~e interlobares renis [TA], interlobar veins of kidney 肾叶间静脉
~e interlobulares hepatis [TA], interlobular veins of liver 肝小叶间静脉
~e interlobulares renis [TA], interlobular veins of kidney 肾小叶间静脉
~ intervertebralis [TA], intervertebral vein 椎间静脉
~ jugularis anterior [TA], anterior jugular vein 颈前静脉
~ jugularis externa [TA], external jugular vein 颈外静脉
~ jugularis interna [TA], internal jugular vein 颈内静脉
~e labiales anteriores [TA], anterior labial veins 阴唇前静脉

~e labiales inferiores [TA], inferior labial veins 下唇静脉
~e labiales posteriores [TA], posterior labial veins 阴唇后静脉
~ labialis superior[TA], superior labial vein 上唇静脉
~e labyrinthi [TA], labyrinthine veins 迷路静脉
~ lacrimalis [TA], lacrimal vein 泪腺静脉
~ laryngea inferior [TA], inferior laryngeal vein 喉下静脉
~ laryngea superior [TA], superior laryngeal vein 喉上静脉
~ lienalis, splenic vein 脾静脉
~ lingualis [TA], lingual vein 舌静脉
~e lumbales, lumbar veins 腰静脉
~ lumbalis ascendens [TA], ascending lumbar vein 腰升静脉
~e maxillares [TA], maxillary veins 上颌静脉
~ mediana antebrachii [TA], median antebrachial vein 前臂正中静脉
~ mediana basilica [TA], median basilic vein 贵要正中静脉
~ mediana cephalica [TA], median cephalic vein 头正中静脉
~ mediana cubiti [TA], median cubital vein 肘正中静脉
~e mediastinales [TA], mediastinal veins 纵隔静脉
~e meningeae [TA], meningeal veins 脑膜静脉
~e meningeae mediae [TA], middle meningeal veins 脑膜中静脉
mesenterica inferior [TA], inferior mesenteric vein 肠系膜下静脉
~ mesenterica superior [TA], superior mesenteric vein 肠系膜上静脉
~e metacarpales dorsales [TA], dorsal metacarpal veins 掌背静脉
~e metacarpales palmares [TA], palmar metacarpal veins 掌心静脉
~e metatarsales dorsales [TA], dorsal metatarsal veins 跖背静脉
~e metatarsales plantares [TA], plantar metatarsal veins 足心静脉
~e musculophrenicae [TA], musculophrenic veins 肌膈静脉
~e nasales externae [TA], external nasal veins 鼻外静脉
~ nasofrontalis [TA], nasofrontal vein 鼻额静脉
~ obliqua atrii sinistri [TA], oblique vein of left atrium 左房斜静脉
~e obturatoriae [TA], obturator vein 闭孔静脉
~ occipitalis [TA], occipital vein 枕静脉
~ ophthalmica inferior [TA], inferior ophthalmic vein 眼下静脉
~ ophthalmica superior [TA], superior ophthalmic vein 眼上静脉
~ ovarica dextra [TA], right ovarian vein 右卵巢静脉
~ ovarica sinistra [TA], left ovarian vein 左卵巢静脉
~ palatina externa [TA], external palatine vein 腭外静脉
~e palpebrales [TA], palpebral veins 睑静脉
~e palpebrales inferiores [TA], inferior palpebral veins 下睑静脉
~e palpebrales superiores [TA], superior palpebral veins 上睑静脉
~e pancreaticae [TA], pancreatic veins 胰静脉
~e pancreaticoduodenales [TA], pancreaticoduodenal veins 胰十二指肠静脉
~e paraumbilicales [TA], paraumbilical veins 附脐静脉
~e parotideae [TA], parotid veins 腮腺静脉
~e perforantes [TA], perforating veins 穿静脉
~e pericardiacae [TA], pericardiac veins 心包静脉
~e pericardiacophrenicae [TA], pericardiacophrenic veins 心包膈静脉
~e peroneae [TA], peroneal veins 腓静脉
~e pharyngeae [TA], pharyngeal veins 咽静脉
~e phrenicae inferiores [TA], inferior phrenic veins 膈下静脉
~ poplitea [TA], popliteal vein 腘静脉
~ posterior ventriculi sinistri cordis, posterior vein of left ventricle 左室后静脉
~ prepylorica [TA], prepyloric vein 幽门前静脉
~e profundae clitoridis [TA], deep veins of clitoris 阴蒂深静脉
~ profunda femoris [TA], deep femoral vein 股深静脉
~ profunda linguae [TA], deep lingual vein 舌深静脉
~e profundae penis [TA], deep veins of penis 阴茎深静脉
~e pudendae externae [TA], external pudendal veins 阴部外静脉
~ pudenda interna [TA], internal pudendal vein 阴部内静脉
~ pulmonalis dextra inferior [TA], right inferior pulmonary vein 右下肺静脉
~ pulmonalis dextra superior [TA], right superior pulmonary vein 右上肺静脉

~ pulmonalis sinistra inferior [TA], left inferior pulmonary vein 左下肺静脉
~ pulmonalis sinistra superior [TA], left superior pulmonary vein 左上肺静脉
~e radiales [TA], radial veins 桡静脉
~e rectales inferiores [TA], inferior rectal veins 直肠下静脉
~e rectales mediae [TA], middle rectal veins 直肠中静脉
~ rectalis superior [TA], superior rectal vein 直肠上静脉
~e renales [TA], renal veins 肾静脉
~ retromandibularis [TA], retromandibular vein 下颌后静脉
~e sacrales laterales [TA], lateral sacral veins 骶外侧静脉
~ sacralis mediana [TA], median sacral vein 骶正中静脉
~ saphena accessoria [TA], accessory saphenous vein 副隐静脉
~ saphena magna [TA], great saphenous vein 大隐静脉
~ saphena parva [TA], small saphenous vein 小隐静脉
~e scrotales anteriores [TA], anterior scrotal veins 阴囊前静脉
~e scrotales posteriores [TA], posterior scrotal veins 阴囊后静脉
~ septi pellucidi [TA], vein of septum pellucidum 透明隔静脉
~e sigmoideae [TA], sigmoid veins 乙状结肠静脉
~ spiralis modioli, spiral vein of modiolus 蜗轴螺旋静脉
~e stellatae renis [TA], stellate veins of kidney 肾星状小静脉
~ sternocleidomastoidea [TA], sternocleidomastoid vein 胸锁乳突肌静脉
~e striatae [TA], striate veins 纹状体静脉
~ stylomastoidea [TA], stylomastoid vein 茎乳静脉
~ subclavia [TA], subclavian vein 锁骨下静脉
~ subcostalis [TA], subcostal vein 肋下静脉
~e subcutaneae abdominis [TA], subcutaneous veins of abdomen 腹皮下静脉
~ sublingualis [TA], sublingual vein 舌下静脉
~ submentalis [TA], submental vein 颏下静脉
~ supraorbitalis [TA], supraorbital vein 眶上静脉
~ suprarenalis dextra [TA], right suprarenal vein 右肾上腺静脉
~ suprarenalis sinistra [TA], left suprarenal vein 左肾上腺静脉
~ suprascapularis [TA], suprascapular vein 肩胛上静脉
~e supratrochleares [TA], supratrochlear veins 滑车上静脉
~ temporalis media [TA], middle temporal vein 颞中静脉
~e temporales profundae [TA], deep temporal veins 颞深静脉
~e temporales superficiales [TA], superficial temporal veins 颞浅静脉
~ testicularis dextra [TA], right testicular vein 右睾丸静脉
~ testicularis sinistra [TA], left testicular vein 左睾丸静脉
~e thoracicae internae [TA], internal thoracic veins 胸廓内静脉
~ thoracica lateralis [TA], lateral thoracic vein 胸外侧静脉
~ thoracoacromialis [TA], thoracoacromial vein 胸肩峰静脉
~e thoracoepigastricae [TA], thoracoepigastric veins 胸腹壁静脉
~e thymicae [TA], thymic veins 胸腺静脉
~ thyroidea inferior [TA], inferior thyroid vein 甲状腺下静脉
~e thyroideae mediae [TA], middle thyroid vein 甲状腺中静脉
~ thyroidea superior [TA], superior thyroid vein 甲状腺上静脉
~e tibiales anteriores [TA], anterior tibial veins 胫前静脉
~e tibiales posteriores [TA], posterior tibial veins 胫后静脉
~e tracheales [TA], tracheal veins 气管静脉
~e transversae colli, transverse cervical veins 颈横静脉
~ transversa faciei, transverse facial vein 面横静脉
~e tympanicae [TA], tympanic veins 鼓室静脉
~e ulnares [TA], ulnar veins 尺静脉
~ umbilicalis, umbilical vein 脐静脉
~ umbilicalis sinistra [TA], left umbilical vein of fetus 左脐静脉
~e uterinae [TA], uterine veins 子宫静脉
~ vertebralis [TA], vertebral vein 椎静脉
~ vertebralis accessoria [TA], accessory vertebral vein 副椎静脉
~ vertebralis anterior [TA], anterior vertebral vein 椎前静脉
~e vesicales [TA], vesical veins 膀胱静脉
~e vestibulares [TA], vestibular veins 前庭静脉
~e vorticosae [TA], vorticose veins 涡静脉

六　摄氏华氏温标对照表

FAHRENHEIT : CELSIUS

℃ = (℉ −32) ×5/9

℉	℃	℉	℃	℉	℃
−50	−46.7	87	30.5	131	55.0
−40	−40.0	88	31.0	132	55.5
−35	−37.2	89	31.6	133	56.1
−30	−34.4	90	32.2	134	56.6
−25	−31.7	91	32.7	135	57.2
−20	−28.9	92	33.3	136	57.7
−15	−26.6	93	33.8	137	58.3
−10	−23.3	94	34.4	138	58.8
−5	−20.6	95	35.0	139	59.4
0	−17.7	96	35.5	140	60.0
+1	−17.2	97	36.1	141	60.5
5	−15.0	98	36.6	142	61.1
10	−12.2	98.6	37.0	143	61.6
15	−9.4	99	37.2	144	62.2
20	−6.6	100	37.7	145	62.7
25	−3.8	101	38.3	146	63.3
30	−1.1	102	38.8	147	63.8
31	−0.5	103	39.4	148	64.4
32	0	104	40.0	149	65.0
33	+0.5	105	40.5	150	65.5
34	1.1	106	41.1	151	66.1
35	1.6	107	41.6	152	66.6
36	2.2	108	42.2	153	67.2
37	2.7	109	42.7	154	67.7
38	3.3	110	43.3	155	68.3
39	3.8	111	43.8	156	68.8
40	4.4	112	44.4	157	69.4
41	5.0	113	45.0	158	70.0
42	5.5	114	45.5	159	70.5
43	6.1	115	46.1	160	71.1
44	6.6	116	46.6	161	71.6
45	7.2	117	47.2	162	72.2
46	7.7	118	47.7	163	72.7
47	8.3	119	48.3	164	73.3
48	8.8	120	48.8	165	73.8
49	9.4	121	49.4	166	74.4
50	10.0	122	50.0	167	75.0
55	12.7	123	50.5	168	75.5
60	15.5	124	51.1	169	76.1
65	18.3	125	51.6	170	76.6
70	21.1	126	52.2	171	77.2
75	23.8	127	52.7	172	77.7
80	26.6	128	53.3	173	78.3
85	29.4	129	53.8	174	78.8
86	30.0	130	54.4	175	79.4

（续表）

FAHRENHEIT : CELSIUS

℃ = (℉ −32) ×5/9

℉	℃	℉	℃	℉	℃
176	80.0	189	87.2	202	94.4
177	80.5	190	87.7	203	95.0
178	81.1	191	88.3	204	95.5
179	81.6	192	88.8	205	96.1
180	82.2	193	89.4	206	96.6
181	82.7	194	90.0	207	97.2
182	83.3	195	90.5	208	97.7
183	83.8	196	91.1	209	98.3
184	84.4	197	91.6	210	98.8
185	85.0	198	92.2	211	99.4
186	85.5	199	92.7	212	100.0
187	86.1	200	93.3	213	100.5
188	86.6	201	93.8	214	101.1